LANGE

2010

CURRENT
Medical Diagnosis & Treatment

FORTY-NINTH EDITION

Edited by

Stephen J. McPhee, MD
Professor of Medicine
Division of General Internal Medicine
Department of Medicine
University of California, San Francisco

Maxine A. Papadakis, MD
Professor of Clinical Medicine
Associate Dean for Student Affairs
School of Medicine
University of California, San Francisco

With Associate Authors

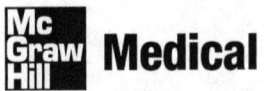
Medical

New York   Chicago   San Francisco   Lisbon   London   Madrid   Mexico City
Milan   New Delhi   San Juan   Seoul   Singapore   Sydney   Toronto

Current Medical Diagnosis & Treatment 2010, Forty-Ninth Edition

1 2 3 4 5 6 7 8 9 0   DOW/DOW   12 11 10 9

ISBN 978-0-07-162444-2
MHID 0-07-162444-9
ISSN 0092-8682

NOTICE

Medicine is an ever-changing science. As new research and clinical experience broaden our knowledge, changes in treatment and drug therapy are required. The authors and the publisher of this work have checked with sources believed to be reliable in their efforts to provide information that is complete and generally in accord with the standards accepted at the time of publication. However, in view of the possibility of human error or changes in medical sciences, neither the authors nor the publisher nor any other party who has been involved in the preparation or publication of this work warrants that the information contained herein is in every respect accurate or complete, and they disclaim all responsibility for any errors or omissions or for the results obtained from use of the information contained in this work. Readers are encouraged to confirm the information contained herein with other sources. For example and in particular, readers are advised to check the product information sheet included in the package of each drug they plan to administer to be certain that the information contained in this work is accurate and that changes have not been made in the recommended dose or in the contraindications for administration. This recommendation is of particular importance in connection with new or infrequently used drugs.

This book was set by Silverchair Science + Communications, Inc.
The editors were James Shanahan, Harriet Lebowitz, and Barbara Holton.
The production supervisor was Phil Galea.
The designer was Alan Barnett Design.
Cover art direction by Margaret Webster-Shapiro; series design by Mary McKeon.
The index was prepared by Katherine Pitcoff.
RR Donnelley was printer and binder.

This book is printed on acid-free paper.

Cover photos: Top left: Ischemic stroke shown on MRI image of the brain. Credit, Medical Body Scans/Photo Researchers, Inc. Right: Phlebitis shown on a phlebogram. Credit, VEM/Photo Researchers, Inc. Bottom left: Credit, CORBIS.

McGraw-Hill books are available at special quantity discounts to use as premiums and sales promotions, or for use in corporate training programs. To contact a representative please e-mail us at bulksales@mcgraw-hill.com.

Contents

Authors   xi
Preface   xvii

1. Disease Prevention & Health Promotion   1

Michael Pignone, MD, MPH, & René Salazar, MD

Prevention of Infectious Diseases   3
Prevention of Cardiovascular Disease   6
Prevention of Osteoporosis   12
Prevention of Physical Inactivity   12
Prevention of Overweight & Obesity   14
Cancer Prevention   16
Prevention of Injuries & Violence   18
Substance Abuse: Alcohol & Illicit Drugs   19

2. Common Symptoms   22

Ralph Gonzales, MD, MSPH, & Paul L. Nadler, MD

Cough   22
Dyspnea   24
Hemoptysis   27
Chest Pain   28
Palpitations   30
Acute Knee Pain   33
Lower Extremity Edema   36
Fever & Hyperthermia   38
Involuntary Weight Loss   40
Fatigue & Chronic Fatigue Syndrome   41
Acute Headache   44
Dysuria   46

3. Preoperative Evaluation & Perioperative Management   49

Hugo Q. Cheng, MD

Evaluation of the Asymptomatic Patient   49
Cardiac Risk Assessment & Reduction   49
Pulmonary Evaluation in Non–Lung
    Resection Surgery   53
Evaluation of the Patient with Liver Disease   54
Preoperative Hematologic Evaluation   55
Neurologic Evaluation   56
Management of Endocrine Diseases   57
Kidney Disease   58
Antibiotic Prophylaxis of Surgical Site Infections   59

4. Geriatric Disorders   61

C. Bree Johnston, MD, MPH, G. Michael Harper, MD, & C. Seth Landefeld, MD

General Principles of Geriatric Care   61
Assessment of the Older Adult   61
Management of Common Geriatric Problems   63
   Dementia   63
   Depression   66
   Delirium   67
   Immobility   68

Falls & Gait Disorders   68
Urinary Incontinence   70
Undernutrition & Frailty   72
Pressure Ulcers   72
Pharmacotherapy & Polypharmacy   74
Vision Impairment   74
Hearing Impairment   75
Elder Abuse   75

5. Palliative Care & Pain Management   76

Michael W. Rabow, MD, FAAHPM, & Steven Z. Pantilat, MD

Definition & Scope of Palliative Care   76
Pain Management   76
   Principles of Pain Management   76
   Pain at the End of Life   77
   Pharmacologic Pain Management Strategies   78
   Nonpharmacologic Treatments   86
Palliation of Other Common Symptoms   86
   Dyspnea   86
   Nausea & Vomiting   86
   Constipation   87
   Delirium & Agitation   87
End-of-Life Care   87
   Tasks after Death   93

6. Dermatologic Disorders   94

Timothy G. Berger, MD

Principles of Dermatologic Therapy   94
Common Dermatoses   99
   Pigmented Lesions   99
   Scaling Disorders   101
   Vesicular Dermatoses   113
   Weeping or Crusted Lesions   118
   Pustular Disorders   120
   Erythemas   125
   Blistering Diseases   130
   Papules   131
   Violaceous to Purple Papules & Nodules   134
   Pruritus (Itching)   136
   Inflammatory Nodules   140
   Epidermal Inclusion Cyst   141
   Photodermatitis   142
   Ulcers   143
Miscellaneous Dermatologic Disorders   144
   Pigmentary Disorders   144
   Baldness (Alopecia)   145
   Nail Disorders   146
   Dermatitis Medicamentosa
     (Drug Eruption)   147

7. Disorders of the Eyes & Lids   151

Paul Riordan-Eva, FRCS, FRCOphth

Refractive Errors   151

Disorders of the Lids & Lacrimal Apparatus	152
Conjunctivitis	153
Pinguecula & Pterygium	155
Corneal Ulcer	156
Acute Angle-Closure Glaucoma	157
Chronic Glaucoma	158
Uveitis	159
Cataract	161
Retinal Detachment	161
Vitreous Hemorrhage	162
Age-Related Macular Degeneration	162
Central & Branch Retinal Vein Occlusions	163
Central & Branch Retinal Artery Occlusions	164
Transient Monocular Blindness	165
Retinal Disorders Associated with Systemic Diseases	166
Ischemic Optic Neuropathy	168
Optic Neuritis	168
Optic Disk Swelling	169
Ocular Motor Palsies	169
Dysthyroid Eye Disease	170
Orbital Cellulitis	170
Ocular Trauma	171
Ultraviolet Keratitis (Actinic Keratitis)	172
Chemical Conjunctivitis & Keratitis	172
Treatment of Ocular Disorders	172
Precautions in Management of Ocular Disorders	172
Adverse Ocular Effects of Systemic Drugs	176

8. Ear, Nose, & Throat Disorders 179

Lawrence R. Lustig, MD, & Joshua S. Schindler, MD

Diseases of the Ear	179
Diseases of the Nose & Paranasal Sinuses	192
Diseases of the Oral Cavity & Pharynx	201
Diseases of the Salivary Glands	206
Diseases of the Larynx	207
Tracheostomy & Cricothyrotomy	211
Foreign Bodies in the Upper Aerodigestive Tract	212
Diseases Presenting as Neck Masses	212

9. Pulmonary Disorders 215

Mark S. Chesnutt, MD, Alex H. Gifford, MD, & Thomas J. Prendergast, MD

Disorders of the Airways	215
Pulmonary Infections	243
Pulmonary Neoplasms	259
Interstitial Lung Disease (Diffuse Parenchymal Lung Disease)	262
Disorders of the Pulmonary Circulation	266
Environmental & Occupational Lung Disorders	277
Pleural Diseases	282
Disorders of Control of Ventilation	287
Acute Respiratory Failure	289
Acute Respiratory Distress Syndrome	291

10. Heart Disease 294

Thomas M. Bashore, MD, Christopher B. Granger, MD, Patrick Hranitzky, MD, & Manesh R. Patel, MD

Congenital Heart Disease	294
Valvular Heart Disease	302
Coronary Heart Disease (Atherosclerotic CAD, Ischemic Heart Disease)	316
Disturbances of Rate & Rhythm	340
Bradycardias & Conduction Disturbances	354
Congestive Heart Failure	358
Myocarditis & the Cardiomyopathies	368
Acute Rheumatic Fever & Rheumatic Heart Disease	374
Diseases of the Pericardium	376
Pulmonary Hypertension & Pulmonary Heart Disease	380
Neoplastic Diseases of the Heart	382
Cardiac Involvement in Miscellaneous Systemic Diseases	383
Traumatic Heart Disease	384
The Cardiac Patient & Surgery	384
The Cardiac Patient & Pregnancy	384
Cardiovascular Screening of Athletes	385

11. Systemic Hypertension 387

Michael Sutters, MD, MRCP (UK)

How Is Blood Pressure Measured and Hypertension Diagnosed?	387
Prehypertension	387
Approach to Hypertension	388
Drug Therapy: Current Antihypertensive Agents	398
Resistant Hypertension	411
Hypertensive Urgencies & Emergencies	411

12. Blood Vessel & Lymphatic Disorders 415

Joseph H. Rapp, MD, Rajabrata Sarkar, MD, PhD, & Christopher D. Owens, MD, MSc

Atherosclerotic Peripheral Vascular Disease	415
Nonatherosclerotic Vascular Disease	422
Arterial Aneurysms	423
Venous Diseases	427
Diseases of the Lymphatic Channels	432
Shock	434

13. Blood Disorders 439

Charles A. Linker, MD

Anemias	439
Neutropenia	456
Leukemias & Other Myeloproliferative Disorders	457
Lymphomas	469
Stem Cell Transplantation	474
Blood Transfusions	476

14. Disorders of Hemostasis, Thrombosis, & Antithrombotic Therapy   480

Patrick F. Fogarty, MD, & Tracy Minichiello, MD

Platelet Disorders   480
Disorders of Coagulation   490
Antithrombotic Therapy   495

15. Gastrointestinal Disorders   502

Kenneth R. McQuaid, MD

Symptoms & Signs of Gastrointestinal
  Disease   502
Diseases of the Peritoneum   524
Diseases of the Esophagus   529
Diseases of the Stomach & Duodenum   544
Diseases of the Small Intestine   557
Diseases of the Colon & Rectum   569
Anorectal Diseases   593

16. Liver, Biliary Tract, & Pancreas Disorders   598

Lawrence S. Friedman, MD

Jaundice   598
Diseases of the Liver   601
Diseases of the Biliary Tract   634
Diseases of the Pancreas   641

17. Breast Disorders   649

Armando E. Giuliano, MD, & Sara A. Hurvitz, MD

Benign Breast Disorders   649
  Fibrocystic Condition   649
  Fibroadenoma of the Breast   650
  Nipple Discharge   651
  Fat Necrosis   651
  Breast Abscess   651
  Disorders of the Augmented Breast   652
Carcinoma of the Female Breast   652
Carcinoma of the Male Breast   673

18. Gynecologic Disorders   674

H. Trent MacKay, MD, MPH

Abnormal Premenopausal Bleeding   674
Postmenopausal Vaginal Bleeding   676
Premenstrual Syndrome
  (Premenstrual Tension)   676
Dysmenorrhea   677
Vaginitis   677
Cervical Polyps   679
Cyst & Abscess of Bartholin Duct   679
Effects of Exposure to Diethylstilbestrol
  In Utero   679
Cervical Intraepithelial Neoplasia (Dysplasia
  of the Cervix)   680
Carcinoma of the Cervix   682
Leiomyoma of the Uterus (Fibroid Tumor)   683
Carcinoma of the Endometrium   684
Carcinoma of the Vulva   685

Endometriosis   686
Pelvic Organ Prolapse   687
Pelvic Inflammatory Disease (Salpingitis,
  Endometritis)   687
Ovarian Cancer & Ovarian Tumors   689
Polycystic Ovary Syndrome   690
Female Sexual Dysfunction   691
Infertility   692
Contraception   694
Rape   701
Menopausal Syndrome   703

19. Obstetrics & Obstetric Disorders   705

Vanessa L. Rogers, MD, Susan Cox, MD, & William R. Crombleholme, MD, FACOG

Diagnosis of Pregnancy   705
Essentials of Prenatal Care   705
Nutrition in Pregnancy   708
Prevention of Hemolytic Disease of the
  Newborn (Erythroblastosis Fetalis)   709
Lactation   709
Travel & Immunizations during Pregnancy   710
Obstetric Complications of the First &
  Second Trimester   710
  Vomiting of Pregnancy (Morning Sickness)
    & Hyperemesis Gravidarum
    (Pernicious Vomiting of Pregnancy)   710
  Spontaneous Abortion   711
  Recurrent (Habitual) Abortion   712
  Ectopic Pregnancy   713
  Gestational Trophoblastic Disease
    (Hydatidiform Mole &
    Choriocarcinoma)   714
Obstetric Complications of the Second &
  Third Trimester   715
  Preeclampsia-Eclampsia   715
  Acute Fatty Liver of Pregnancy   718
  Preterm (Premature) Labor   719
  Third-Trimester Bleeding   720
Obstetric Complications of the
  Peripartum Period   720
  Puerperal Mastitis   720
  Chorioamnionitis & Endometritis   720
Medical Conditions Complicating
  Pregnancy   721
  Anemia   721
  Lupus Anticoagulant Anticardiolipin-
    Antiphospholipid Antibody   721
  Thyroid Disease   722
  Diabetes Mellitus   722
  Hypertensive Disease   723
  Heart Disease   724
  Asthma   724
  Seizure Disorders   724
Infectious Conditions Complicating
  Pregnancy   724
  Urinary Tract Infection   724
  Group B Streptococcal Infection   725
  Varicella   725

Tuberculosis   726
HIV/AIDS during Pregnancy   726
Maternal Hepatitis B & C Carrier State   726
Herpes Genitalis   727
Syphilis, Gonorrhea, & *Chlamydia
    trachomatis* Infection   727
Surgical Complications during Pregnancy   727
Choledocholithiasis, Cholecystitis, &
    Idiopathic Cholestasis of Pregnancy   727
Appendicitis   728
Carcinoma of the Breast   728
Ovarian Tumors   728

20. Musculoskeletal &
Immunologic Disorders   729

*David B. Hellmann, MD, MACP,
& John B. Imboden, Jr., MD*

Diagnosis & Evaluation   729
Degenerative & Crystal-Induced Arthritis   729
Pain Syndromes   736
Autoimmune Diseases   747
Vasculitis Syndromes   764
Seronegative Spondyloarthropathies   773
Infectious Arthritis   777
Infections of Bones   780
Other Rheumatic Disorders   783
Allergic Diseases   784
Atopic Disease   784
Primary Immunodeficiency Disorders   786

21. Fluid & Electrolyte Disorders   788

Kerry C. Cho, MD

Disorders of Sodium Concentration   789
Hyperosmolar Disorders & Osmolar Gaps   795
Disorders of Potassium Concentration   795
Disorders of Calcium Concentration   798
Disorders of Phosphorus Concentration   802
Disorders of Magnesium Concentration   805
Acid–Base Disorders   806
Fluid Management   815

22. Kidney Disease   816

Suzanne Watnick, MD, & Gail Morrison, MD

Assessment of Kidney Disease   816
Acute Kidney Injury (Acute Renal Failure)   819
Chronic Kidney Disease   825
Glomerulonephropathies   833
Nephrotic Disease in Primary Renal
    Disorders   840
Nephrotic Disease from Systemic
    Disorders   841
Diseases Demonstrating Nephritic
    & Nephrotic Components   843
Tubulointerstitial Diseases   844
Cystic Diseases of the Kidney   846
Multisystem Diseases with Variable
    Kidney Involvement   848

23. Urologic Disorders   850

*Maxwell V. Meng, MD, FACS, Marshall L. Stoller,
MD, & Thomas Walsh, MD*

Hematuria   850
Genitourinary Tract Infections   851
    Acute Cystitis   851
    Acute Pyelonephritis   852
    Acute Bacterial Prostatitis   853
    Chronic Bacterial Prostatitis   854
    Nonbacterial Prostatitis   855
    Prostatodynia   855
    Acute Epididymitis   856
Urinary Stone Disease   857
Interstitial Cystitis   861
Male Erectile Dysfunction & Sexual
    Dysfunction   862
Male Infertility   864
Benign Prostatic Hyperplasia   866

24. Nervous System Disorders   872

Michael J. Aminoff, MD, DSc, FRCP

Headache   872
Facial Pain   876
Epilepsy   878
Dysautonomia   884
Sensory Disturbances   885
Weakness & Paralysis   886
Transient Ischemic Attacks   886
Stroke   888
Intracranial & Spinal Tumors   897
Nonmetastatic Neurologic Complications
    of Malignant Disease   902
Pseudotumor Cerebri (Benign Intracranial
    Hypertension)   903
Selected Neurocutaneous Diseases   903
Movement Disorders   904
Dementia   912
Multiple Sclerosis   912
Neuromyelitis Optica   914
Vitamin E Deficiency   914
Spasticity   914
Myelopathies in AIDS   915
Myelopathy of Human T Cell Leukemia
    Virus Infection   915
Subacute Combined Degeneration of the
    Spinal Cord   915
Wernicke Encephalopathy   915
Stupor & Coma   915
Head Injury   918
Spinal Trauma   919
Syringomyelia   920
Degenerative Motor Neuron Diseases   920
Peripheral Neuropathies   921
Discogenic Neck Pain   929
Brachial & Lumbar Plexus Lesions   929
Disorders of Neuromuscular Transmission   932
Myopathic Disorders   934
Periodic Paralysis Syndrome   936

25. Psychiatric Disorders 937

*Stuart J. Eisendrath, MD, &
Jonathan E. Lichtmacher, MD*

Common Psychiatric Disorders 937
Substance Use Disorders (Drug Dependency,
 Drug Abuse) 977
Delirium, Dementia, & Other Cognitive
 Disorders (Formerly: Organic
 Brain Syndrome) 985
Psychiatric Problems Associated with
 Hospitalization & Illness 988

26. Endocrine Disorders 991

Paul A. Fitzgerald, MD

Diseases of the Hypothalamus &
 Pituitary Gland 991
Diseases of the Thyroid Gland 1002
The Parathyroids 1030
Metabolic Bone Disease 1038
Diseases of the Adrenal Cortex 1046
Pheochromocytoma & Paraganglioma 1058
Pancreatic & Duodenal
 Neuroendocrine Tumors 1062
Diseases of the Testes & Male Breast 1063
Amenorrhea & Menopause 1067
Multiple Endocrine Neoplasia 1075
Clinical Use of Corticosteroids 1077

27. Diabetes Mellitus & Hypoglycemia 1079

Umesh Masharani, MB, BS, MRCP(UK)

Diabetes Mellitus 1079
Diabetic Coma 1111
The Hypoglycemic States 1117

28. Lipid Disorders 1123

Robert B. Baron, MD, MS

Lipoproteins & Atherogenesis 1123
Lipid Fractions & the Risk of Coronary
 Heart Disease 1124
Therapeutic Effects of Lowering Cholesterol 1124
Secondary Conditions That Affect
 Lipid Metabolism 1125
Clinical Presentations 1125
Screening for High Blood Cholesterol 1126
Treatment of High Low-Density
 Lipoprotein Cholesterol 1130
High Blood Triglycerides 1133

29. Nutritional Disorders 1134

Robert B. Baron, MD, MS

Protein-Energy Malnutrition 1134
Obesity 1135
Eating Disorders 1138
Disorders of Vitamin Metabolism 1140
Diet Therapy 1145
Nutritional Support 1147

**30. Common Problems in Infectious
 Diseases & Antimicrobial Therapy** 1153

*Peter V. Chin-Hong, MD, MAS, B. Joseph Guglielmo,
PharmD, & Richard A. Jacobs, MD, PhD*

Common Problems in Infectious Diseases 1153
Fever of Unknown Origin 1153
Infections in the Immunocompromised
 Patient 1155
Hospital-Associated Infections 1159
Infections of the Central Nervous System 1162
Animal & Human Bite Wounds 1165
Sexually Transmitted Diseases 1166
Infections in Drug Users 1168
Acute Infectious Diarrhea 1169
Infectious Diseases in the
 Returning Traveler 1172
Traveler's Diarrhea 1173
Antimicrobial Therapy 1175
Selected Principles of Antimicrobial
 Therapy 1175
Hypersensitivity Tests & Desensitization 1180
Immunization Against Infectious Diseases 1186
Recommended Immunization of Infants,
 Children, & Adolescents 1186
Recommended Immunization of Adults 1186
Recommended Immunization for
 Travelers 1200
Vaccine Safety 1204

31. HIV Infection & AIDS 1205

Andrew R. Zolopa, MD, & Mitchell H. Katz, MD

Epidemiology 1205
Etiology 1208
Pathogenesis 1208
Pathophysiology 1208
Clinical Findings 1208
Differential Diagnosis 1218
Prevention 1218
Treatment 1221
Course & Prognosis 1233
When to Refer 1233
When to Admit 1234

32. Viral & Rickettsial Infections 1235

*Vicente F. Corrales-Medina, MD, &
Wayne X. Shandera, MD*

Viral Diseases 1235
Human Herpesviruses 1235
Major Vaccine-Preventable Viral
 Infections 1247
Other Neurotrophic Viruses 1255
Other Systemic Viral Diseases 1262
Common Viral Respiratory Infections 1268
Adenovirus Infections 1275
Other Exanthematous Viral Infections 1276
Viruses & Gastroenteritis 1278
Enteroviruses That Produce
 Several Syndromes 1278

Rickettsial Diseases 1280
  Typhus Group 1280
  Spotted Fevers 1283
  Other Rickettsial & Rickettsial-Like
    Diseases 1285
  Kawasaki Disease 1287

33. Bacterial & Chlamydial Infections 1289

Brian S. Schwartz, MD, & Henry F. Chambers, MD

Infections Caused by Gram-Positive Bacteria 1289
Infective Endocarditis 1303
Infections Caused by Gram-Negative
  Bacteria 1307
Actinomycosis 1323
Nocardiosis 1324
Infections Caused by Mycobacteria 1324
Infections Caused by Chlamydiae 1327

34. Spirochetal Infections 1330

Susan S. Philip, MD, MPH

Syphilis 1330
Non-Sexually Transmitted Treponematoses 1338
Selected Spirochetal Diseases 1339
  Relapsing Fever 1339
  Rat-Bite Fever 1340
  Leptospirosis 1341
  Lyme Disease (Lyme Borreliosis) 1342

35. Protozoal & Helminthic Infections 1348

Philip J. Rosenthal, MD

Protozoal Infections 1348
  African Trypanosomiasis
    (Sleeping Sickness) 1348
  American Trypanosomiasis
    (Chagas Disease) 1349
  Leishmaniasis 1351
  Malaria 1353
  Babesiosis 1362
  Toxoplasmosis 1363
  Amebiasis 1365
  Infections with Pathogenic
    Free-Living Amebas 1368
  Coccidiosis (Cryptosporidiosis, Isosporiasis,
    Cyclosporiasis, Sarcocystosis)
    & Microsporidiosis 1369
  Giardiasis 1371
  Other Intestinal Flagellate Infections 1372
  Trichomoniasis 1372
Helminthic Infections 1373
  Trematode (Fluke) Infections 1373
  Liver, Lung, & Intestinal Flukes 1375
  Cestode Infections 1376
  Intestinal Nematode (Roundworm)
    Infections 1379
  Invasive Nematode (Roundworm)
    Infections 1382
  Filariasis 1386

36. Mycotic Infections 1390

Samuel A. Shelburne, MD, & Richard J. Hamill, MD

Candidiasis 1390
Histoplasmosis 1391
Coccidioidomycosis 1392
Pneumocystosis (*Pneumocystis jiroveci*
  Pneumonia) 1394
Cryptococcosis 1396
Aspergillosis 1397
Mucormycosis 1398
Blastomycosis 1399
Paracoccidioidomycosis (South American
  Blastomycosis) 1399
Sporotrichosis 1399
Penicillium marneffei Infections 1400
Chromoblastomycosis (Chromomycosis) 1400
Mycetoma (Maduromycosis
  & Actinomycetoma) 1400
Other Opportunistic Mold Infections 1402
Antifungal Therapy 1402

37. Disorders Due to Physical Agents 1403

*Jacqueline A. Nemer, MD, FACEP, &
Brent R. W. Moelleken, MD, FACS*

Cold & Heat 1403
Burns 1408
Electrical Injury 1412
Radiation Exposure 1413
Near Drowning 1415
Disorders Due to Environmental Factors 1416

38. Poisoning 1420

Kent R. Olson, MD

Initial Evaluation: Poisoning or Overdose 1420
The Symptomatic Patient 1420
Antidotes & Other Treatment 1423
Diagnosis of Poisoning 1426
Selected Poisonings 1428

39. Cancer 1450

Patricia A. Cornett, MD, & Tiffany O. Dea, PharmD

Etiology 1450
Modifiable Risk Factors 1450
Staging 1451
  The Paraneoplastic Syndromes 1451
Types of Cancer 1452
  Lung Cancer 1452
  Hepatobiliary Cancers 1459
  Alimentary Tract Cancers 1465
  Cancers of the Genitourinary Tract 1484
Cancer Complications & Emergencies 1494
Primary Cancer Treatment 1498
  Systemic Cancer Therapy 1498
  Toxicity & Dose Modification of
    Chemotherapeutic Agents 1499
Prognosis 1511

40. Clinical Genetic Disorders 1512

Reed E. Pyeritz, MD, PhD

Acute Intermittent Porphyria	1512
Alkaptonuria	1513
Down Syndrome	1514
Fragile X Mental Retardation	1515
Gaucher Disease	1515
Disorders of Homocysteine Metabolism	1516
Klinefelter Syndrome	1517
Marfan Syndrome	1518
Hereditary Hemorrhagic Telangiectasia	1519

41. Complementary & Alternative Medicine 1520

Ellen F. Hughes, MD, PhD, & Kevin Barrows, MD

Herbal Medicines	1521
Dietary Supplements	1527
Acupuncture	1532
Mind-Body Medicine	1534

Appendix: Therapeutic Drug Monitoring & Laboratory Reference Intervals 1544

C. Diana Nicoll, MD, PhD, MPA, & Chuanyi Mark Lu, MD

Index 1557

ONLINE-ONLY CHAPTERS

www.AccessMedicine.com/CMDT

Anti-infective Chemotherapeutic & Antibiotic Agents

B. Joseph Guglielmo, PharmD

Penicillins
Cephalosporins
Other β-Lactam Drugs
Erythromycin Group (Macrolides)
Ketolides
Tetracycline Group
Glycylcyclines
Chloramphenicol
Aminoglycosides
Polymyxins

Antituberculous Drugs
Alternative Drugs in Tuberculosis Treatment
Rifamycins
Sulfonamides & Antifolate Drugs
Sulfones Used in the Treatment of Leprosy
Specialized Drugs Used Against Bacteria
Streptogramins
Oxazolidinediones
Daptomycin
Quinolones
Pentamidine & Atovaquone
Urinary Antiseptics
Antifungal Drugs
Antiviral Chemotherapy

Diagnostic Testing & Medical Decision Making

C. Diana Nicoll, MD, PhD, MPA, Michael Pignone, MD, MPH, & Chuanyi Mark Lu, MD

Benefits, Costs, & Risks
Performance of Diagnostic Tests
Test Characteristics
Use of Tests in Diagnosis & Management
Odds-Likelihood Ratios

Basic Genetics

Reed E. Pyeritz, MD, PhD

Introduction to Medical Genetics
   Genes & Chromosomes
   Mutation
   Genes in Individuals
   Genes in Families
   Disorders of Multifactorial Causation
   Chromosomal Aberrations
The Techniques of Medical Genetics
   Family History & Pedigree Analysis
   Cytogenetics
   Biochemical Genetics
   DNA Analysis
   Prenatal Diagnosis
   Neoplasia: Chromosomal & DNA Analysis

Information Technology in Patient Care

Russ Cucina, MD, MS

Clinical Uses of E-mail
Electronic Medical Records
Computerized Provider Order Entry
Clinical Decision Support Systems
Websites & Online Health-Related Forums
Mobile Computing for Clinicians
Telemedicine

Authors

Michael J. Aminoff, MD, DSc, FRCP
Professor of Neurology, University of California, San Francisco; Attending Physician, University of California Medical Center, San Francisco
aminoffm@neurology.ucsf.edu
Nervous System Disorders

David M. Barbour, PharmD, BCPS
Regional Scientific Associate Director, Novartis Pharmaceuticals Corporation, Denver, Colorado
dave.barbour@comcast.net
Drug References

Robert B. Baron, MD, MS
Professor of Medicine; Associate Dean for Graduate and Continuing Medical Education; Vice Chief, Division of General Internal Medicine, University of California, San Francisco
baron@medicine.ucsf.edu
Lipid Disorders; Nutritional Disorders

Kevin Barrows, MD
Associate Physician, Osher Center for Integrative Medicine; Department of Family and Community Medicine, University of California, San Francisco
barrowsk@ocim.ucsf.edu
Complementary & Alternative Medicine

Thomas M. Bashore, MD
Professor of Medicine; Vice Chief for Clinical Affairs and Education, Division of Cardiology, Duke University Medical Center, Durham, North Carolina
thomas.bashore@duke.edu
Heart Disease

Timothy G. Berger, MD
Professor of Clinical Dermatology, Department of Dermatology, University of California, San Francisco
bergert@derm.ucsf.edu
Dermatologic Disorders

Henry F. Chambers, MD
Professor of Medicine, University of California, San Francisco; Chief, Division of Infectious Diseases, San Francisco General Hospital
hchambers@medsfgh.ucsf.edu
Bacterial & Chlamydial Infections

Hugo Q. Cheng, MD
Clinical Professor of Medicine, Division of Hospital Medicine, University of California, San Francisco; Director, Medical Consultation Service, University of California Medical Center, San Francisco
quinny@medicine.ucsf.edu
Preoperative Evaluation & Perioperative Management

Mark S. Chesnutt, MD
Associate Professor of Medicine, Pulmonary & Critical Care Medicine, Oregon Health & Science University, Portland, Oregon; Chief, Critical Care, Portland Veterans Affairs Medical Center
chesnutm@ohsu.edu
Pulmonary Disorders; Lung Cancer (in Chapter 39)

Peter V. Chin-Hong, MD, MAS
Associate Professor of Medicine; Director, Transplant & Immunocompromised Host Infectious Diseases Program; Associate Director, Pathways to Careers in Clinical and Translational Research, University of California, San Francisco
phong@php.ucsf.edu
Common Problems in Infectious Diseases & Antimicrobial Therapy

Kerry C. Cho, MD
Assistant Clinical Professor of Medicine, Division of Nephrology, University of California San Francisco
kerry.cho@ucsf.edu
Fluid & Electrolyte Disorders

Patricia A. Cornett, MD
Professor of Medicine, University of California, San Francisco; Chief, Hematology/Oncology, San Francisco Veterans Affairs Medical Center, San Francisco, California
Cancer

Vicente F. Corrales-Medina, MD
Infectious Diseases Fellow, Department of Internal Medicine, Baylor College of Medicine, Houston, Texas
vfmedina@bcm.tmc.edu
Viral & Rickettsial Infections

Susan M. Cox, MD
Associate Dean for Medical Education, Gillette Professor of Obstetrics and Gynecology, University of Texas Southwestern Medical Center, Dallas, Texas
Obstetrics & Obstetric Disorders

William R. Crombleholme, MD, FACOG
Professor of Obstetrics and Gynecology, University of Connecticut, Farmington, Connecticut; Director of Labor and Delivery, Department of Women's Health, Hartford Hospital, Hartford, Connecticut
wcrombleholme@harthosp.org
Obstetrics & Obstetric Disorders

Russ Cucina, MD, MS

Assistant Professor of Medicine, Division of Hospital Medicine; Associate Medical Director, Information Technology, UCSF Medical Center; University of California, San Francisco
rcucina@medicine.ucsf.edu
CMDT Online—Information Technology in Patient Care

Elizabeth S. Davis, MD

Clinical Instructor, Division of Hospital Medicine, Department of Medicine, University of California, San Francisco
davise@medsfgh.ucsf.edu
References

Lukejohn Day, MD

Fellow, Gastroenterology, Department of Medicine, University of California, San Francisco
lukejohn.day@ucsf.edu
References

Tiffany O. Dea, PharmD

Oncology Pharmacist, Veterans Affairs Medical Center, San Francisco, California; Adjunct Professor, Thomas J. Long School of Pharmacy and Health Sciences, Stockton, California
Cancer

Stuart J. Eisendrath, MD

Professor of Psychiatry; Director of Clinical Services and The UCSF Depression Center, Langley Porter Psychiatric Hospital and Clinics, University of California, San Francisco
stuart.eisendrath@ucsf.edu
Psychiatric Disorders

Tania F. Esakoff, MD

Fellow, Maternal Fetal Medicine, Obstetrics, Gynecology and Reproductive Sciences, University of California, San Francisco
esakofft@obgyn.ucsf.edu
References

Charles K. Everett, MD

Chief Resident, Moffitt-Long Hospital, Department of Medicine, University of California, San Francisco; Fellow, Division of Pulmonary and Critical Care Medicine, University of California, San Francisco
charles.everett@ucsf.edu
References

Paul A. Fitzgerald, MD

Clinical Professor of Medicine, Department of Medicine, Division of Endocrinology, University of California, San Francisco
paul.fitzgerald@ucsf.edu
Endocrine Disorders

Patrick F. Fogarty, MD

Associate Clinical Professor of Medicine, Department of Medicine; Director, Adult Hemophilia Program, University of California, San Francisco
pfogarty@medicine.ucsf.edu
Disorders of Hemostasis, Thrombosis, & Antithrombotic Therapy

Lawrence S. Friedman, MD

Professor of Medicine, Harvard Medical School; Professor of Medicine, Tufts University School of Medicine, Boston, Massachusetts; Chair, Department of Medicine, Newton-Wellesley Hospital, Newton, Massachusetts; Assistant Chief of Medicine, Massachusetts General Hospital, Boston, Massachusetts
lfriedman@partners.org
Liver, Biliary Tract, & Pancreas Disorders; Hepatobiliary Cancers (in Chapter 39)

Alex H. Gifford, MD

Fellow in Pulmonary and Critical Care Medicine, Section of Pulmonary and Critical Care Medicine, Dartmouth-Hitchcock Medical Center, Lebanon, New Hampshire
Pulmonary Disorders

Armando E. Giuliano, MD

Chief of Science and Medicine, John Wayne Cancer Institute; Director, John Wayne Cancer Institute Breast Center, Saint John's Health Center, Santa Monica, California
giulianoa@jwci.org
Breast Disorders

Ralph Gonzales, MD, MSPH

Professor of Medicine; Professor of Epidemiology & Biostatistics, Division of General Internal Medicine, Department of Medicine, University of California, San Francisco
ralphg@medicine.ucsf.edu
Common Symptoms

Christopher B. Granger, MD

Associate Professor of Medicine; Director, Cardiac Care Unit, Duke University Medical Center, Durham, North Carolina
grang001@mc.duke.edu
Heart Disease

B. Joseph Guglielmo, PharmD

Professor and Chair, Department of Clinical Pharmacy, School of Pharmacy, University of California, San Francisco
guglielmoj@pharmacy.ucsf.edu
Common Problems in Infectious Diseases & Antimicrobial Therapy; CMDT Online—Anti-infective Chemotherapeutic & Antibiotic Agents

Richard J. Hamill, MD

Professor, Division of Infectious Diseases, Departments of Medicine and Molecular Virology & Microbiology, Baylor College of Medicine, Houston, Texas
richard.hamill@med.va.gov
Mycotic Infections

G. Michael Harper, MD

Associate Professor of Medicine, Geriatric Medicine, University of California, San Francisco; Director of Geriatrics Fellowship Training Program, San Francisco Veterans Affairs Medical Center, San Francisco, California
michael.harper3@med.va.gov
Geriatric Disorders

David B. Hellmann, MD, MACP

Aliki Perroti Professor of Medicine; Vice Dean for Johns Hopkins Bayview; Chairman, Department of Medicine, Johns Hopkins Bayview Medical Center, Johns Hopkins University School of Medicine, Baltimore, Maryland
hellmann@jhmi.edu
Musculoskeletal & Immunologic Disorders

Patrick Hranitzky, MD

Assistant Professor of Medicine; Director, Clinical Cardiac Electrophysiology; Director, Clinical Cardiac Electrophysiology Fellowship Program, Duke University Medical Center, Durham, North Carolina
patrick.hranitzky@duke.edu
Heart Disease

William Huen MD, MS, MPH

Assistant Clinical Professor, Department of Medicine, Division of Hospital Medicine, San Francisco General Hospital, University of California, San Francisco
huenw@medsfgh.ucsf.edu
References

Ellen F. Hughes, MD, PhD

Clinical Professor of Medicine, Division of General Internal Medicine, Department of Medicine, University of California, San Francisco
ehughes@medicine.ucsf.edu
Complementary & Alternative Medicine

Erick K. Hung, MD

Assistant Clinical Professor, Department of Psychiatry, University of California, San Francisco; Director of Mental Health, San Francisco Veterans Affairs Downtown Clinic
ehung@1ppi.ucsf.edu
References

Sara A. Hurvitz, MD

Assistant Professor; Director, Breast Oncology Program, Division of Hematology/Oncology, Department of Internal Medicine, University of California, Los Angeles
Breast Disorders

John B. Imboden, Jr., MD

Alice Betts Endowed Chair for Arthritis Research; Professor of Medicine, University of California, San Francisco; Chief, Division of Rheumatology, San Francisco General Hospital
jimboden@medsfgh.ucsf.edu
Musculoskeletal & Immunologic Disorders

Richard A. Jacobs, MD, PhD

Emeritus Clinical Professor of Medicine, Division of Infectious Diseases, Department of Medicine, University of California, San Francisco
jacobsd@medicine.ucsf.edu
Common Problems in Infectious Diseases & Antimicrobial Therapy

Prasanna Jagannathan, MD

Fellow, Infectious Diseases, Department of Medicine, University of California, San Francisco
jagannathanp@medsfgh.ucsf.edu
References

C. Bree Johnston, MD, MPH

Professor of Medicine, Division of Geriatrics, Department of Medicine, Veterans Affairs Medical Center, University of California, San Francisco
bree.johnston@ucsf.edu
Geriatric Disorders

Mitchell H. Katz, MD

Clinical Professor of Medicine, Epidemiology & Biostatistics, University of California, San Francisco; Director of Health, San Francisco Department of Public Health
mitch.katz@sfdph.org
HIV Infection & AIDS

Geoffrey A. Kerchner, MD, PhD

Clinical Instructor, Department of Neurology, Memory and Aging Center, University of California, San Francisco
kerchnerg@neurology.ucsf.edu
References

C. Seth Landefeld, MD

Professor; Chief, Division of Geriatrics; Director, UCSF-Mt. Zion Center on Aging, University of California, San Francisco; Director, Quality Scholars Fellowship Program, San Francisco Veterans Affairs Medical Center
sethl@medicine.ucsf.edu
Geriatric Disorders

Jonathan E. Lichtmacher, MD

Health Sciences Associate Clinical Professor of Psychiatry; Director, Adult Psychiatry Clinic, Langley Porter Hospitals and Clinics, University of California, San Francisco
jonathanl@lppi.ucsf.edu
Psychiatric Disorders

Charles A. Linker, MD

Clinical Professor of Medicine; Director, Bone Marrow Transplant Program, Division of Hematology/Oncology, University of California, San Francisco
linkerc@medicine.ucsf.edu
Blood Disorders

Chuanyi Mark Lu, MD

Associate Professor, Department of Laboratory Medicine, University of California, San Francisco; Chief, Hematology and Hematopathology, Laboratory Medicine Service, Veterans Affairs Medical Center, San Francisco, California
Appendix: Therapeutic Drug Monitoring & Laboratory Reference Intervals; CMDT Online—Diagnostic Testing & Medical Decision Making

Lawrence R. Lustig, MD

Francis A. Sooy, MD Professor of Otolaryngology – Head & Neck Surgery; Division Chief of Otology & Neurotology, Department of Otolaryngology – Head & Neck Surgery, University of California, San Francisco
llustig@ohns.ucsf.edu
Ear, Nose, & Throat Disorders

H. Trent MacKay, MD, MPH

Professor of Obstetrics and Gynecology, Uniformed Services University of the Health Sciences, Bethesda, Maryland; Staff Physician, Department of Obstetrics and Gynecology, National Naval Medical Center, Bethesda, Maryland
Gynecologic Disorders

Umesh Masharani, MB, BS, MRCP(UK)

Professor of Medicine, Division of Endocrinology and Metabolism, Department of Medicine, University of California, San Francisco
umesh.masharani@ucsf.edu
Diabetes Mellitus & Hypoglycemia

Kenneth R. McQuaid, MD

Professor of Clinical Medicine, University of California, San Francisco; Chief, Gastroenterology Section, San Francisco Veterans Affairs Medical Center
kenneth.mcquaid@med.va.gov
Gastrointestinal Disorders; Alimentary Tract Cancers (in Chapter 39)

Maxwell V. Meng, MD, FACS

Associate Professor, Department of Urology, University of California, San Francisco
mmeng@urology.ucsf.edu
Urologic Disorders; Cancers of the Genitourinary Tract (in Chapter 39)

Tracy Minichiello, MD

Associate Professor of Medicine, University of California, San Francisco; Chief, Anticoagulation and Thrombosis Services, San Francisco Veterans Affairs Medical Center
Disorders of Hemostasis, Thrombosis, & Antithrombotic Therapy

Brent R. W. Moelleken, MD, FACS

Associate Clinical Professor, Division of Plastic Surgery; Attending Physician, University of California, Los Angeles Medical Center; Private Practice in Plastic and Reconstructive Surgery, Beverly Hills, California
drbrent@drbrent.com
Disorders Due to Physical Agents

Gail Morrison, MD

Vice Dean for Education; Director of Academic Programs; Professor of Medicine, School of Medicine, Renal-Electrolyte and Hypertension Division, University of Pennsylvania Health System, Philadelphia, Pennsylvania
morrisog@mail.med.upenn.edu
Kidney Disease

James A. Murray, DO

Fellow, Section of Pulmonary and Critical Care Medicine, Dartmouth-Hitchcock Medical Center, Lebanon, New Hampshire
james.a.murray@hitchock.org
Lung Cancer (in Chapter 39)

Paul L. Nadler, MD

Associate Clinical Professor of Medicine; Director, Screening and Acute Care Clinic, Division of General Internal Medicine, University of California, San Francisco
nadler@medicine.ucsf.edu
Common Symptoms

Jacqueline A. Nemer, MD, FACEP

Associate Professor of Emergency Medicine, Department of Emergency Medicine, University of California, San Francisco
jacquelinea.nemer@ucsfmedctr.org
Disorders Due to Physical Agents

C. Diana Nicoll, MD, PhD, MPA

Clinical Professor and Vice Chair, Department of Laboratory Medicine; Associate Dean, University of California, San Francisco; Chief of Staff and Chief, Laboratory Medicine Service, San Francisco Veterans Affairs Medical Center
diana.nicoll@va.gov
Appendix: Therapeutic Drug Monitoring & Laboratory Reference Intervals; CMDT Online—Diagnostic Testing & Medical Decision Making

Kent R. Olson, MD

Clinical Professor of Medicine, Pediatrics, and Pharmacy, University of California, San Francisco; Medical Director, San Francisco Division, California Poison Control System
kent.olson@ucsf.edu
Poisoning

Christopher D. Owens, MD, MSc

Assistant Professor of Surgery, Division of Vascular and Endovascular Surgery, University of California, San Francisco
Blood Vessel & Lymphatic Disorders

Steven Z. Pantilat, MD

Professor of Clinical Medicine, Department of Medicine; Alan M. Kates and John M. Burnard Endowed Chair in Palliative Care; Director, Palliative Care Program, University of California, San Francisco
stevep@medicine.ucsf.edu
Palliative Care & Pain Management

Manesh R. Patel, MD

Assistant Professor of Medicine, Division of Cardiology, Duke University Medical Center, Durham, North Carolina
patel017@notes.duke.edu
Heart Disease

Susan S. Philip, MD, MPH

Assistant Clinical Professor of Medicine, Division of Infectious Diseases, Department of Medicine, University of California, San Francisco; Medical Director, San Francisco City Clinic, San Francisco Department of Public Health
susan.philip@sfdph.org
Spirochetal Infections

Michael Pignone, MD, MPH

Associate Professor of Medicine; Chief, Division of General Internal Medicine, Department of Medicine, University of North Carolina, Chapel Hill
pignone@med.unc.edu
Disease Prevention & Health Promotion; CMDT Online— Diagnostic Testing & Medical Decision Making

Thomas J. Prendergast, MD

Associate Professor of Medicine, Pulmonary and Critical Care Medicine, Oregon Health and Science University, Portland, Oregon; Staff Physician, Portland Veterans Affairs Medical Center
thomas.prendergast@va.gov
Pulmonary Disorders; Lung Cancer (in Chapter 39)

Reed E. Pyeritz, MD, PhD

Professor of Medicine and Genetics; Vice-Chair, Department of Medicine, University of Pennsylvania School of Medicine, Philadelphia
reed.pyeritz@uphs.upenn.edu
Clinical Genetic Disorders; CMDT Online—Basic Genetics

Michael W. Rabow, MD, FAAHPM

Professor of Medicine, Division of General Internal Medicine; Director, Symptom Management Service, Helen Diller Family Comprehensive Cancer Center, University of California, San Francisco
mrabow@medicine.ucsf.edu
Palliative Care & Pain Management

Joseph H. Rapp, MD

Professor of Surgery in Residence, University of California, San Francisco; Chief, Vascular Surgery Service, Veterans Affairs Medical Center, San Francisco, California
rappj@surgery.ucsf.edu
Blood Vessel & Lymphatic Disorders

Paul Riordan-Eva, FRCS, FRCOphth

Consultant Ophthalmologist, King's College Hospital, Honorary Senior Lecturer (Teaching), King's College London School of Medicine at Guy's, King's College, and St. Thomas' Hospitals, London, United Kingdom
paul.riordan-eva@kingsch.nhs.uk
Disorders of the Eyes & Lids

Vanessa L. Rogers, MD

Assistant Professor, Obstetrics and Gynecology, University of Texas Southwestern Medical Center, Dallas, Texas
vanessa.rogers@utsouthwestern.edu
Obstetrics & Obstetric Disorders

Philip J. Rosenthal, MD

Professor, Division of Infectious Diseases, Department of Medicine, University of California, San Francisco; San Francisco General Hospital
prosenthal@medsfgh.ucsf.edu
Protozoal & Helminthic Infections

René Salazar, MD

Assistant Clinical Professor, Division of General Internal Medicine, Department of Medicine, University of California, San Francisco
salazarr@medicine.ucsf.edu
Disease Prevention & Health Promotion

Rajabrata Sarkar, MD, PhD

Associate Professor of Surgery, Division of Vascular Surgery, University of California, San Francisco
sarkarr@surgery.ucsf.edu
Blood Vessel & Lymphatic Disorders

Joshua S. Schindler, MD

Assistant Professor, Department of Otolaryngology, Oregon Health & Science University, Portland, Oregon; Medical Director, OHSU-Northwest Clinic for Voice and Swallowing
schindlj@ohsu.edu
Ear, Nose, & Throat Disorders

Brian S. Schwartz, MD

Assistant Clinical Professor, Division of Infectious Diseases, Department of Medicine, University of California, San Francisco
brian.schwartz@ucsf.edu
Bacterial & Chlamydial Infections

Wayne X. Shandera, MD

Assistant Professor, Department of Internal Medicine, Baylor College of Medicine, Houston, Texas
shandera@bcm.tmc.edu
Viral & Rickettsial Infections

Samuel A. Shelburne, MD

Assistant Professor, Department of Internal Medicine, Baylor College of Medicine, Houston, Texas
samuels@bcm.tmc.edu
Mycotic Infections

Marshall L. Stoller, MD

Professor and Vice Chairman, Department of Urology, University of California, San Francisco
mstoller@urology.ucsf.edu
Urologic Disorders

Michael Sutters, MD, MRCP(UK)

Affiliate Assistant Professor of Medicine, Division of Nephrology, University of Washington School of Medicine, Seattle, Washington
michael.sutters@vmmc.org
Systemic Hypertension

Laura Tarter, MD

Rheumatology Fellow, University of California, San Francisco
laura.tarter@ucsf.edu
References

Brindusa Truta, MD

Fellow, Gastroenterology, Department of Medicine, University of California, San Francisco
brindusa.truta@ucsf.edu
References

Thomas Walsh, MD

Assistant Professor, Department of Urology, University of Washington School of Medicine, Seattle, Washington
walsht@u.washington.edu
Urologic Disorders

Sunny Wang, MD

Fellow, Division of Hematology and Oncology, University of California, San Francisco
Lung Cancer (in Chapter 39)

Suzanne Watnick, MD

Associate Professor of Medicine, Division of Nephrology and Hypertension, Oregon Health & Science University, Portland; Director, Dialysis Unit, Portland Veterans Affairs Medical Center, Portland, Oregon
watnicks@ohsu.edu
Kidney Disease

Katherine C. Yung, MD

Assistant Professor, Division of Laryngology, Department of Otolaryngology, Head and Neck Surgery, University of California, San Francisco
kyung@ohns.ucsf.edu
References

Andrew R. Zolopa, MD

Associate Professor of Medicine, Division of Infectious Diseases and Geographic Medicine, Stanford University, Stanford, California
azolopa@stanford.edu
HIV Infection & AIDS

Preface

Current Medical Diagnosis & Treatment 2010 is the 49th annual volume of this single-source reference for practitioners in both hospital and ambulatory settings. Annually updated, this book emphasizes the practical features of clinical diagnosis and patient management in all fields of internal medicine and in specialties of interest to primary care practitioners and to subspecialists who provide general care.

INTENDED AUDIENCE

House officers, medical students, and all other health professions students will find the descriptions of diagnostic and therapeutic modalities, with citations to the current literature, of everyday usefulness in patient care.

Internists, family physicians, hospitalists, nurse practitioners, physicians' assistants, and all primary care providers will appreciate *CMDT* as a ready reference and refresher text. Physicians in other specialties, pharmacists, and dentists will find the book a useful basic medical reference text. Nurses, nurse-practitioners, and physicians' assistants will welcome the format and scope of the book as a means of referencing medical diagnosis and treatment.

Patients and their family members who seek information about the nature of specific diseases and their diagnoses and treatment may also find this book to be a valuable resource.

NEW IN THIS EDITION

- Newly introduced topics include H1N1 influenza A (swine flu), Chikungunya fever, acute knee pain, neuromyelitis optica, and vaccine safety
- Cancer chapter totally rewritten by new authors
- Substantially updated Treatment sections for HIV infection & AIDS, female breast cancer, Kawasaki disease, and pneumocystosis
- New recommendations for use of nonsteroidal anti-inflammatory agents, coxib agents, and antiplatelet agents in patients with peptic ulcer disease
- Significant revision of antithrombotic therapy
- New recommendations for intervention in patients with patent ductus arteriosus
- New ACC/AHA Task Force Guidelines for management of congenital heart disease in pregnant women
- Reorganization of obstetric complications by trimester
- Extensive revision of hypokalemia, hyperkalemia, hypophosphatemia, and mixed acid-base disorders; sexually transmitted diseases; penicillin-resistant pneumococcus; ionizing radiation exposure
- Drug information, bibliographies, and Web sites updated through June 2009
- Expanded 24-page color insert

OUTSTANDING FEATURES

- Medical advances up to time of annual publication
- Detailed presentation of all primary care topics, including gynecology, obstetrics, dermatology, ophthalmology, otolaryngology, psychiatry, neurology, toxicology, urology, geriatrics, preventive medicine, and palliative care
- Concise format, facilitating efficient use in any practice setting
- More than 1000 diseases and disorders
- Only text with annual update on HIV infection
- Specific disease prevention information
- Easy access to drug dosages, with trade names indexed and costs updated in each edition
- Recent references, with unique identifiers (PubMed, PMID numbers) for rapid downloading of article abstracts and, in some instances, full-text reference articles
- ICD-9 codes listed on the inside covers

CMDT Online (www.AccessMedicine.com) provides full electronic access to CMDT 2010 plus expanded basic science information. CMDT Online is updated quarterly and includes a dedicated Media Gallery as well as links to related Web sites. Subscribers also receive access to Diagnosaurus with 1000+ differential diagnoses and *CURRENT Practice Guidelines in Primary Care, 2008.*

The four online-only chapters (Anti-infective Chemotherapeutic & Antibiotic Agents, Diagnostic Testing & Medical Decision Making, Basic Genetics, and Information Technology in Patient Care) are available at www.AccessMedicine.com/CMDT.

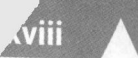
ACKNOWLEDGMENTS

We wish to thank our associate authors for participating once again in the annual updating of this important book. We are especially grateful to seven authors who are leaving *CMDT* this year: Joshua S. Adler, MD; Catherine K. Chang, MD; Masafumi Fukagawa, MD, PhD; Christopher J. Kane, MD, FACS; Kiyoshi Kurokawa, MD, MACP; James A. Murray, DO; and Hope S. Rugo, MD. These authors have contributed hours upon hours of work in culling and distilling the literature in their specialty areas and we have all benefited from their clinical wisdom and commitment.

Many students and physicians also have contributed useful suggestions to this and previous editions, and we are grateful. We continue to welcome comments and recommendations for future editions in writing or via electronic mail. The editors' and authors' institutional and e-mail addresses are given in the Authors section.

Stephen J. McPhee, MD
Maxine A. Papadakis, MD
San Francisco, California
September 2009

From inability to let alone; from too much zeal for the new and contempt for what is old; from putting knowledge before wisdom, and science before art and cleverness before common sense; from treating patients as cases; and from making the cure of the disease more grievous than the endurance of the same, Good Lord, deliver us.

—Sir Robert Hutchison

Table 1–2. Expert recommendations for preventive care for asymptomatic, low-risk adults.

Preventive Service	USPSTF[1]	CTF[2]	Other Organizations
Screening tests			
Blood pressure	Recommended for all adults; interval not stated	Fair evidence for inclusion in routine care	Joint National Committee VII: Recommended for all adults at each clinical encounter
Serum lipids	Recommended for all middle-aged and older adults and for young adults with multiple risk factors	Insufficient evidence for or against inclusion	National Cholesterol Education Panel Adult Treatment Panel III: Recommended for all adults age 21 and older
Depression screening	Recommended when support systems in place (B recommendation)	Recommended when support systems in place	
Counseling			
Healthy diet	Recommended for patients with increased risk; insufficient evidence for or against in average-risk patients	Fair evidence for inclusion	
Physical activity	Recommended	Fair evidence for inclusion	
Immunizations and chemoprevention			
Aspirin chemoprevention	Recommended for adults at increased risk for coronary heart disease (CHD)	Insufficient evidence for or against use	American Heart Association: Recommended for adults at increased risk for CHD
Influenza vaccination	Recommended for all adults 65 and older and for selected high-risk groups	Not addressed	
Pneumococcal vaccination	Recommended for immunocompetent adults older than age 65 or for adults younger than age 65 at increased risk	Recommended for healthy adults	

[1]United States Preventive Services Task Force; recommendations available at http://www.ahrq.gov.
[2]Canadian Task Force on Preventive Health Care; recommendations available at http://www.ctfhe.org/.

Shenson D et al. Delivery of preventive services to adults aged 50-64: monitoring performance using a composite measure, 1997–2004. J Gen Intern Med. 2008 Jun;23(6):733–40. [PMID: 18317846]

PREVENTION OF INFECTIOUS DISEASES

Much of the decline in the incidence and fatality rates of infectious diseases is attributable to public health measures—especially immunization, improved sanitation, and better nutrition.

Immunization remains the best means of preventing many infectious diseases. In the United States, childhood immunization has resulted in near elimination of measles, mumps, rubella, poliomyelitis, diphtheria, pertussis, and tetanus. *Haemophilus influenzae* type b invasive disease has been reduced by more than 95% since the introduction of the first conjugate vaccines.

However, substantial vaccine-preventable morbidity and mortality continue to occur among adults from vaccine-preventable diseases, such as hepatitis A, hepatitis B, influenza, and pneumococcal infections. For example, in adults in the United States, there are an estimated 50,000–70,000 deaths annually from influenza, hepatitis B, and invasive pneumococcal disease. Influenza vaccination is recommended for adults age 50 and older, and it has been documented that annual influenza immunization with inactivated vaccine (administered intramuscularly) prevents cardiovascular morbidity and all-cause mortality in persons with coronary and other atherosclerotic vascular disease. Rates of influenza vaccination have increased. Self-reported rates of influenza vaccine coverage in adults older than 65 years increased from 30% in 1989 to 70% in 2004. However, vaccination rates were higher for non-Hispanic whites compared with other ethnic minority groups.

The American College of Physicians recommends that clinicians should review each adult's immunization status at age 50; assess risk factors that would indicate a need for pneumococcal vaccination and annual influenza immunizations; reimmunize at age 65 those who received an immunization against pneumococcus more than 6 years before; ensure that all adults have completed a primary diphtheria-tetanus immunization series, and administer a single booster at age 50; and assess the postvaccination serologic response to hepatitis B vaccination in all recipients who have ongoing risks of exposure to blood or body fluids (eg, sharp injuries, blood splashes).

Strategies have also been proposed to improve influenza, pneumococcal polysaccharide, and hepatitis B vaccination. Strategies to enhance vaccinations in general include increasing community demand for vaccinations; enhancing access to vaccination services; and provider- or system-based interventions, such as reminder systems. Increasing reports of pertussis among US adolescents, adults, and their infant contacts have stimulated vaccine development for older age groups. A safe and effective tetanus-diphtheria 5-component acellular pertussis vaccine (Tdap) is available for use in adolescents and in adults younger than age 65. The

Advisory Committee on Immunization Practices (ACIP) recommends routine use of a single dose of Tdap for adults aged 19–64 years to replace the next booster dose of tetanus and diphtheria toxoids vaccine (Td). Further research is needed to elucidate the role of vaccination in persons older than 65 years and to determine whether future booster doses of Tdap are needed.

A new recombinant protein hepatitis E vaccine has been developed that has proven safe and efficacious in preventing hepatitis E among high-risk populations (such as those in Nepal). Both hepatitis A vaccine and immune globulin provide protection against hepatitis A; however, administration of immune globulin may provide a modest benefit over vaccination in some settings.

Recommended immunization schedules for children and adolescents and adults are set forth in Tables 30–12 and 30–13. Thimerosal-free hepatitis B vaccination is available for newborns and infants, and despite the disproved relationship between vaccines and autism, thimerosal-free vaccines are available for pregnant women.

Human papillomavirus (HPV) virus-like particle (VLP) vaccines have demonstrated effectiveness in preventing persistent HPV infections, and thus may impact the rate of cervical intraepithelial neoplasia (CIN) II–III. The American Cancer Society and the American Academy of Pediatrics (AAP) recommends routine HPV vaccination for girls aged 11–12 years. The AAP also recommends that all unvaccinated girls and women ages 13–26 years receive the HPV vaccine. Trials demonstrate efficacy of bivalent HPV (16/18) or quadrivalent HPV (6/11/16/18)L1 virus-like particle vaccines in preventing new HPV infection and cervical lesions but not in women with preexisting infection. It is estimated that routine use of HPV vaccination of females at 11 to 12 years of age and catch-up vaccination of females at age 13–16 (with vaccination of girls age 9 and 10 at the discretion of the physician) could prevent 95% to 100% of CIN and adenocarcinoma in situ, 99% of genital warts and approximately 70% of cervical cancer cases worldwide; thus, the role of HPV testing will need redefinition. Despite the effectiveness of the vaccine, rates of immunization are low. Interventions addressing personal beliefs and system barriers to vaccinations may help address the slow adoption of this vaccine.

Persons traveling to countries where infections are endemic should take precautions described in Chapter 30. Immunization registries—confidential, population-based, computerized information systems that collect vaccination data about all residents of a geographic area—can be used to increase and sustain high vaccination coverage.

Skin testing for tuberculosis and treating selected patients reduce the risk of reactivation tuberculosis (see Table 9–11). Two blood tests, which are not confounded by prior BCG (bacille Calmette-Guérin) vaccination, have been developed to detect tuberculosis infection by measuring in vitro T-cell interferon-gamma release in response to two antigens (the enzyme-linked immunospot [ELISpot], [T-SPOT.TB] and the other, a quantitative ELISA [QuantiFERON-TBGold] test). These T-cell–based assays have an excellent specificity that is higher than tuberculin skin testing in BCG-vaccinated populations. The rate of tuber-

culosis in the United States has been declining since 1992, although this decline has slowed in recent years. In 2007, the tuberculosis rate was the lowest recorded since national reporting began in 1953. The Advisory Council for the Elimination of Tuberculosis has called for a renewed commitment to eliminating tuberculosis in the United States, and the Institute of Medicine has published a detailed plan for achieving that goal. Patients with HIV infection are at an especially high risk for tuberculosis, and tuberculosis preventive therapy in the era of HIV will require further work to overcome implementation barriers and to identify optimal duration of preventive therapy and treatment approach for individuals receiving highly active antiretroviral therapy (HAART).

Treatment of tuberculosis poses a risk of hepatotoxicity and thus requires close monitoring of liver transaminases. Alanine aminotransferase (ALT) monitoring during the treatment of latent tuberculosis infection is recommended for certain individuals (preexisting liver disease, pregnancy, chronic alcohol consumption). ALT should be monitored in HIV-infected patients during treatment of tuberculosis disease and should be considered in patients over the age of 35. Symptomatic patients with an ALT elevation three times the upper limit of normal (ULN) or asymptomatic patients with an elevation five times the ULN should be treated with a modified or alternative regimen.

HIV infection is now the major infectious disease problem in the world, and it affects 850,000–950,000 persons in the United States. Since sexual contact is a common mode of transmission, primary prevention relies on eliminating unsafe sexual behavior by promoting abstinence, later onset of first sexual activity, decreased number of partners, and use of latex condoms. Appropriately used, condoms can reduce the rate of HIV transmission by nearly 70%. In one study, couples with one infected partner who used condoms inconsistently had a considerable risk of infection: the rate of seroconversion was estimated to be 13% after 24 months. No seroconversions were noted with consistent condom use. Unfortunately, as many as one-third of HIV-positive persons continue unprotected sexual practices after learning that they are HIV-infected. Tailored group educational intervention focused on practicing "safer sex" can reduce their transmission-risk behaviors with partners who are not HIV-positive. Other approaches to prevent HIV infection include treatment of sexually transmitted diseases, development of vaginal microbicides, and vaccine development. Increasingly, cases of HIV infection are transmitted by injection drug use. HIV prevention activities should include provision of sterile injection equipment for these individuals.

With regard to secondary prevention, many HIV-infected persons in the United States receive the diagnosis at advanced stages of immunosuppression, and almost all will progress to AIDS if untreated. On the other hand, HAART substantially reduces the risk of clinical progression or death in patients with advanced immunosuppression. Screening tests for HIV are extremely (> 99%) accurate. While the benefits of HIV screening appear to outweigh its harms, current screening is generally based on individual patient risk factors. Such screening can identify persons at risk for AIDS but misses a substantial proportion of those infected.

Nonetheless, the yield from screening higher prevalence populations is substantially greater than that from screening the general population, and more widespread screening of the population remains controversial.

In immunocompromised patients, live vaccines are contraindicated but many killed or component vaccines are safe and recommended. *Asymptomatic* HIV-infected patients have not shown adverse consequences when given live MMR and influenza vaccinations as well as tetanus, hepatitis B, *H influenzae* type b, and pneumococcal vaccinations—all should be given. However, if poliomyelitis immunization is required, the inactivated poliomyelitis vaccine is indicated. In *symptomatic* HIV-infected patients, live virus vaccines such as MMR should generally be avoided, but annual influenza vaccination is safe.

Whenever possible, immunizations should be completed before procedures that require or induce immunosuppression (organ transplantation or chemotherapy), or that reduce immunogenic responses (splenectomy). However, if this is not possible, the patient may mount only a partial immune response, yet even this partial response can be beneficial. Patients who undergo allogeneic bone marrow transplantation lose preexisting immunities and should be revaccinated. In many situations, family members should also be vaccinated to protect the immunocompromised patient, although oral live polio vaccine should be avoided because of the risk of infecting the patient.

New cases of poliomyelitis have been reported in the United States, Haiti, and the Dominican Republic recently, slowing its eradication in the Western Hemisphere. Worldwide eradication of poliovirus, including endemic areas such as India, remains challenging.

The current epidemic of highly pathogenic H5N1 avian influenza within duck and poultry populations in Southeast Asia raises serious concerns that genetic reassortment will result in a human influenza pandemic. In 2003 through 2005, there were 138 confirmed cases of human infection with H5N1 avian influenza in Vietnam, Thailand, Indonesia, China, and Cambodia, with a mortality rate of > 50%. To prevent and prepare for an increase in human cases, public health officials are working to improve detection methods and to stockpile effective antivirals, such as oseltamivir. The development of an H5N1 vaccine is underway. Two trials have demonstrated development of neutralizing antibodies using a vaccine with varying doses of hemagglutinin antigen.

Herpes zoster, caused by reactivation from previous varicella zoster virus (VZV) infection, affects many older adults and people with immune system dysfunction. Whites are at higher risk than other ethnic groups and the incidence in adults age 65 and older may be higher than previously described. It can cause postherpetic neuralgia, a potentially debilitating chronic pain syndrome. A varicella vaccine is available for the prevention of herpes zoster. Several clinical trials have shown that this vaccine (Zostavax) is safe, elevates VZV-specific cell-mediated immunity, and significantly reduces the incidence of herpes zoster and postherpetic neuralgia in persons older than 60 years. In one randomized, double-blind, placebo-controlled trial among more than 38,000 older adults, the vaccine reduced the incidence of postherpetic neuralgia by 66% and the incidence of herpes zoster by 51%. The vaccine is administered as a one-time subcutaneous dose (0.65 mL) and is approved for adults 60 years of age and older. However, durability of vaccine response and whether any booster vaccination is needed are still uncertain. The cost effectiveness of the vaccine varies substantially, and the patient's age should be considered in vaccine recommendations. One study reported a cost-effectiveness exceeding $100,000 per quality-adjusted life year saved.

In 2008, the United States Preventive Services Task Force (USPSTF) reviewed evidence to reaffirm its recommendation on screening for asymptomatic bacteriuria in adults. New evidence was reviewed, which continues to support routine screening in pregnant women but not in other groups of adults.

American Academy of Pediatrics Committee on Infectious Diseases. Prevention of human papillomavirus infection: provisional recommendations for immunization of girls and women with quadrivalent human papillomavirus vaccine. Pediatrics. 2007 Sep;120(3):666–8. [PMID: 17766541]

Centers for Disease Control and Prevention (CDC). Trends in tuberculosis–United States, 2007. MMWR Morb Mortal Wkly Rep. 2008 Mar 21;57(11):281–5. [PMID: 18354371]

Chaves SS et al. Chickenpox exposure and herpes zoster disease incidence in older adults in the U.S. Public Health Rep. 2007 Mar-Apr;122(2):155–9. [PMID: 17357357]

Churchyard GJ et al. Tuberculosis preventative therapy in the era of HIV infection: overview and research priorities. J Infect Dis. 2007 Aug 15;196 (Suppl 1):S52–62. [PMID: 17624827]

Committee on Adolescent Health Care; ACOG Working Group on Immunization. ACOG Committee Opinion No. 344: Human papillomavirus vaccination. Obstet Gynecol. 2006 Sep;108(3 Pt 1):699–705. [PMID: 16946235]

Davis MM et al; American Heart Association; American College of Cardiology; American Association of Cardiovascular and Pulmonary Rehabilitation; American Association of Critical Care Nurses; American Association of Heart Failure Nurses; American Diabetes Association; Association of Black Cardiologists, Inc; Heart Failure Society of America; Preventive Cardiovascular Nurses Association; American Academy of Nurse Practitioners; Centers for Disease Control and Prevention and the Advisory Committee on Immunization. Influenza vaccination as secondary prevention for cardiovascular disease: a science advisory from the American Heart Association/American College of Cardiology. J Am Coll Cardiol. 2006 Oct 3;48(7):1498–502. [PMID: 17010820]

Ehrlich HJ et al; Baxter H5N1 Pandemic Influenza Vaccine Clinical Study Team. A clinical trial of a whole-virus H5N1 vaccine derived from cell culture. N Engl J Med. 2008 Jun 12;358(24):2573–84. [PMID: 18550874]

FUTURE II Study Group. Quadrivalent vaccine against human papillomavirus to prevent high-grade cervical lesions. N Engl J Med. 2007 May 10;356(19):1915–27. [PMID: 17494925]

Garland SM et al. Quadrivalent vaccine against human papillomavirus to prevent anogenital diseases. N Engl J Med. 2007 May 10;356(19):1928–43. [PMID: 17494926]

Gershon AA et al. Varicella vaccine in the United States: a decade of prevention and the way forward. J Infect Dis. 2008 Mar 1;197(Suppl 2):S39–40. [PMID: 18419405]

Gidengil CA et al. Tetanus-diphtheria-acellular pertussis vaccination of adults in the USA. Expert Rev Vaccines. 2008 Jul;7(5):621–34. [PMID: 18564017]

Kahn JA et al. Rates of human papillomavirus vaccination, attitudes about vaccination, and human papillomavirus prevalence in young women. Obstet Gynecol. 2008 May;111(5):1103–10. [PMID: 18448742]

Lalvani A. Diagnosing tuberculosis infection in the 21st century: new tools to tackle an old enemy. Chest. 2007 Jun 131(6):1898–906. [PMID: 17565023]

Levie K et al. An adjuvanted, low-dose, pandemic influenza A (H5N1) vaccine candidate is safe, immunogenic, and induces cross-reactive immune responses in healthy adults. J Infect Dis. 2008 Sep 1;198(5):642–9. [PMID: 18576945]

Lu P et al. Influenza vaccination of recommended adult populations, U.S., 1989–2005. Vaccine. 2008 Mar 25;26(14):1786–93. [PMID: 18336965]

Lin K et al; U.S. Preventive Services Task Force. Screening for asymptomatic bacteriuria in adults: evidence for the U.S. Preventive Services Task Force reaffirmation recommendation statement. Ann Intern Med. 2008 Jul 1;149(1):W20–4. [PMID: 18591632]

Paavonen J et al. Efficacy of a prophylactic adjuvanted bivalent L1 virus-like-particle vaccine against infection with human papillomavirus types 16 and 18 in young women: an interim analysis of a phase III double-blind, randomized controlled trial. Lancet. 2007 Jun 30;369(9580):2161–70. [PMID: 17602732]

Pai M et al. Systematic review: T-cell-based assays for the diagnosis of latent tuberculosis infection: an update. Ann Intern Med. 2008 Aug 5;149(3):177–84. [PMID: 18593687]

Rambout L. Prophylactic vaccination against human papillomavirus infection and disease in women: a systemic review of randomized controlled trials. CMAJ. 2007 Aug 28;177(5):469–79. [PMID: 17671238]

Rothberg MB et al. Cost-effectiveness of a vaccine to prevent herpes zoster and postherpetic neuralgia in older adults. Clin Infect Dis. 2007 May 15;44(10):1280–8. [PMID: 17443464]

Saslow D et al. American Cancer Society Guideline for human papillomavirus (HPV) vaccine use to prevent cervical cancer and its precursors. CA Cancer J Clin. 2007 Jan–Feb;57(1):7–28. [PMID: 17237032]

Saukkonen JJ et al. An official ATS statement: hepatotoxicity of antituberculosis therapy. Am J Respir Crit Care Med. 2006 Oct 15;174(8):935–52. [PMID: 17021358]

Schiffman M. Integration of human papillomavirus vaccination, cytology and human papillomavirus testing. Cancer. 2007 Jun 25;111(3):145–53. [PMID: 17448822]

Shrestha MP et al. Safety and efficacy of a recombinant hepatitis E vaccine. N Engl J Med. 2007 Mar 1;356(9)895–903. [PMID: 17329696]

Thompson KM et al. Eradication versus control for poliomyelitis: an economic analysis. Lancet. 2007 Apr 21;369(9570):1363–71. [PMID: 17448822]

Treanor JJ et al. Safety and immunogenicity of an inactivated subvirion influenza A (H5N1) vaccine. N Engl J Med. 2006 Mar 30;354(13):1343–51. [PMID: 16571878]

Victor JC et al. Hepatitis A vaccine versus immune globulin for postexposure prophylaxis. N Engl J Med. 2007 Oct 25;357(17):1685–94. [PMID: 17947390]

Willis BC et al; Task Force on Community Preventive Services: Improving influenza, pneumococcal polysaccharide, and hepatitis B vaccination coverage among adults aged < 65 years at high risk: a report on recommendations of the Task Force on Community Preventive Services. MMWR Recomm Rep 2005;54(RR-5):1. [PMID: 15800472]

Zimmerman RK. HPV vaccine and its recommendations, 2007. J Fam Pract. 2007 Feb;56 (2 Suppl Vaccines):S1–5, C1. [PMID: 17270106]

PREVENTION OF CARDIOVASCULAR DISEASE

Cardiovascular diseases, including coronary heart disease (CHD) and stroke, represent two of the most important causes of morbidity and mortality in developed countries.

Several risk factors increase the risk for coronary disease and stroke. They can be divided into those that are modifiable (eg, lipid disorders, hypertension, cigarette smoking) and those that are not (eg, gender, age, family history of early coronary disease). This section considers the role of screening for and treating modifiable risk factors.

Impressive declines in age-specific mortality rates from heart disease and stroke have been achieved in all age groups in North America during the past 2 decades. The chief reasons for this favorable trend appear to be modification of risk factors, especially cigarette smoking and hypercholesterolemia, plus more aggressive detection and treatment of hypertension and better care for patients with heart disease. African-Americans appear to have a greater proportion of risk attributable to these key risk factors, suggesting that focusing on better control could help reduce disparities in health outcomes.

Hozawa A. Absolute and attributable risks of cardiovascular disease incidence in relation to optimal and borderline risk factors: comparison of African American with white subjects–Atherosclerosis Risk in Communities Study. Arch Intern Med. 2007 Mar 26;167(6):573–9. [PMID: 17389288]

Kahn R et al. The impact of prevention on reducing the burden of cardiovascular disease. Circulation. 2008 Jul 29;118(5):576–85. [PMID: 18606915]

▶ Abdominal Aortic Aneurysm

Screening for abdominal aortic aneurysm in men aged 65–75 years is associated with a significant reduction in condition-specific mortality (odds ratio, 0.57 [95% CI, 0.45 to 0.74]). This benefit is sustained through 7 years of follow-up. Women do not appear to benefit, and most of the benefit in men appears to accrue among current or former smokers.

Fleming C et al. Screening for abdominal aortic aneurysm: a best-evidence systematic review for the U.S. Preventive Services Task Force. Ann Intern Med. 2005 Feb 1;142(3):203–11. [PMID: 15684209]

Kim LG et al; Multicentre Aneurysm Screening Study Group. A sustained mortality benefit from screening for abdominal aortic aneurysm. Ann Intern Med. 2007 May 15;146(10):699–706. [PMID: 17502630]

▶ Cigarette Smoking

Cigarette smoking remains the most important cause of preventable morbidity and early mortality. In 2000, there were an estimated 4.8 million premature deaths in the world attributable to smoking, 2.4 million in developing countries and 2 million in industrialized countries. More than three-quarters (3.8 million) of these deaths were in men. The leading causes of death from smoking were cardiovascular diseases (1.7 million deaths), chronic obstructive pulmonary disease (COPD) (1 million deaths), and lung cancer (0.9 million deaths). Nicotine is highly addictive, raises brain levels of dopamine, and produces withdrawal symptoms on discontinuation. Cigar smoking has also increased; there is also continued use of smokeless tobacco (chewing tobacco and snuff), particularly among young people. Tobacco dependence may have a genetic component.

Cigarettes are responsible for one in every five deaths in the United States, yet smoking prevalence rates have been increasing among high school and college students. Currently, 23% of US adults and 26% of US young adults are smokers.

Smokers have twice the risk of fatal heart disease, 10 times the risk of lung cancer, and several times the risk of cancers of the mouth, throat, esophagus, pancreas, kidney, bladder, and cervix; a twofold to threefold higher incidence of stroke and peptic ulcers (which heal less well than in nonsmokers); a twofold to fourfold greater risk of fractures of the hip, wrist, and vertebrae; four times the risk of invasive pneumococcal disease; and a twofold increase in cataracts. In the United States, over 90% of cases of COPD occur among current or former smokers. Both active smoking and passive smoking are associated with deterioration of the elastic properties of the aorta (increasing the risk of aortic aneurysm) and with progression of carotid artery atherosclerosis. Smoking has also been associated with increased risks of leukemia, of colon and prostate cancers, of breast cancer among postmenopausal women who are slow acetylators of N-acetyl-transferase-2 enzymes, osteoporosis, and Alzheimer's disease. In cancers of the head and neck, lung, esophagus, and bladder, smoking is linked to mutations of the P53 gene, the most common genetic change in human cancer. Patients with head and neck cancer who continue to smoke during radiation therapy have lower rates of response than those who do not smoke. Olfaction and taste are impaired in smokers, and facial wrinkles are increased. Heavy smokers have a 2.5 greater risk of age-related macular degeneration. Smokers die 5–8 years earlier than never-smokers.

The children of smokers have lower birth weights, are more likely to be mentally retarded, have more frequent respiratory infections and less efficient pulmonary function, have a higher incidence of chronic ear infections than children of nonsmokers, and are more likely to become smokers themselves.

In addition, exposure to environmental tobacco smoke has been shown to increase the risk of cervical cancer, lung cancer, invasive pneumococcal disease, and heart disease; to promote endothelial damage and platelet aggregation; and to increase urinary excretion of tobacco-specific lung carcinogens. The incidence of breast cancer may be increased as well. Of approximately 450,000 smoking-related deaths in the United States annually, as many as 53,000 are attributable to environmental tobacco smoke.

Smoking cessation reduces the risks of death and of myocardial infarction in people with coronary artery disease; reduces the rate of death and acute myocardial infarction in patients who have undergone percutaneous coronary revascularization; lessens the risk of stroke; slows the rate of progression of carotid atherosclerosis; and is associated with improvement of COPD symptoms. On average, women smokers who quit smoking by age 35 add about 3 years to their life expectancy, and men add more than 2 years to theirs. Smoking cessation can increase life expectancy even for those who stop after the age of 65.

Although tobacco use constitutes the most serious common medical problem, it is undertreated. Almost 40% of smokers attempt to quit each year, but only 4% are success-

ful. Factors associated with successful cessation include having a rule against smoking in the home, being older, and having greater education. Persons whose physicians advise them to quit are 1.6 times as likely to attempt quitting. Over 70% of smokers see a physician each year, but only 20% of them receive any medical quitting advice or assistance.

Several effective interventions are available to promote smoking cessation, including counseling, pharmacotherapy, and combinations of the two. The five steps for helping smokers quit are summarized in Table 1–3.

Common elements of supportive smoking cessation treatments are reviewed in Table 1–4. A system should be implemented to identify smokers, and advice to quit should be tailored to the patient's level of readiness to change. Pharmacotherapy to reduce cigarette consumption is ineffective in smokers who are unwilling or not ready to quit. Conversely, all patients trying to quit should be offered pharmacotherapy except those with medical contraindications, women who are pregnant or breast-feeding, and adolescents.

Several pharmacologic therapies have been shown to be effective in promoting cessation. Nicotine replacement therapy doubles the chance of successful quitting. Guidelines for its use are presented in Table 1–5. Suggestions for the nicotine patch are listed in Table 1–6 and for nicotine gum in Table 1–7. The nicotine patch, gum, and lozenges are available over-the-counter, and nicotine nasal spray and inhalers by prescription. When the spray is combined with the patch, cessation rates are substantially higher. The sustained-release antidepressant drug bupropion (150–300 mg/d orally) is an effective smoking cessation agent and is associated with minimal weight gain, although seizures are a contraindication. It acts by boosting brain levels of dopamine and norepinephrine, mimicking the effect of nicotine. Weight gain was less in the combined program (Table 1–8). More recently, varenicline, a partial nicotinic acetylcholine-receptor agonist, has shown promise as an effective agent, although its adverse effects are incompletely understood. No single pharmacotherapy is clearly more effective than others, so patient preferences should be taken into account in selecting a treatment.

Weight gain occurs in most patients (80%) following smoking cessation. For many it averages 2 kg, but for others (10–15%) major weight gain—over 13 kg—may occur.

Clinicians should not show disapproval of patients who have not stopped smoking or who are not ready to make a quit attempt. Thoughtful advice that emphasizes the benefits of cessation and recognizes common barriers to success can increase motivation to quit and quit rates. An intercurrent illness such as acute bronchitis or acute myocardial infarction may motivate even the most addicted smoker to quit. Individualized or group counseling is very cost-effective, even more so than treating hypertension. Smoking cessation counseling by telephone ("quitlines") has proved effective. An additional strategy is to recommend that any smoking take place out of doors to limit the effects of passive smoke on housemates and coworkers. This can lead to smoking reduction and quitting. The clinician's role in smoking cessation is summarized in Table 1–3. Public policies, including higher cigarette taxes and more restrictive public smoking laws, have also been shown to encourage cessation.

Table 1–3. Actions and strategies for the primary care clinician to help patients quit smoking.

Action	Strategies for Implementation
Step 1. Ask—Systematically Identify All Tobacco Users at Every Visit	
Implement an officewide system that ensures that for *every* patient at *every* clinic visit, tobacco-use status is queried and documented[1]	Expand the vital signs to include tobacco use. Data should be collected by the health care team. The action should be implemented using preprinted progress note paper that includes the expanded vital signs, a vital signs stamp or, for computerized records, an item assessing tobacco-use status. Alternatives to the vital signs stamp are to place tobacco-use status stickers on all patients' charts or to indicate smoking status using computerized reminder systems.
Step 2. Advise—Strongly Urge All Smokers to Quit	
In a *clear, strong,* and *personalized* manner, urge every smoker to quit	Advice should be Clear: "I think it is important for you to quit smoking now, and I will help you. Cutting down while you are ill is not enough." Strong: "As your clinician, I need you to know that quitting smoking is the most important thing you can do to protect your current and future health." Personalized: Tie smoking to current health or illness and/or the social and economic costs of tobacco use, motivational level/readiness to quit, and the impact of smoking on children and others in the household. Encourage clinic staff to reinforce the cessation message and support the patient's quit attempt.
Step 3. Attempt—Identify Smokers Willing to Make a Quit Attempt	
Ask every smoker if he or she is willing to make a quit attempt at this time	If the patient is willing to make a quit attempt at this time, provide assistance (see step 4). If the patient prefers a more intensive treatment or the clinician believes more intensive treatment is appropriate, refer the patient to interventions administered by a smoking cessation specialist and follow up with him or her regarding quitting (see step 5). If the patient clearly states he or she is not willing to make a quit attempt at this time, provide a motivational intervention.
Step 4. Assist—Aid the Patient in Quitting	

A. Help the patient with a quit plan	*Set a quit date.* Ideally, the quit date should be within 2 weeks, taking patient preference into account.
	Help the patient prepare for quitting. The patient must:
	  Inform family, friends, and coworkers of quitting and request understanding and support.
	  Prepare the environment by removing cigarettes from it. Prior to quitting, the patient should avoid smoking in places where he or she spends a lot of time (eg, home, car).
	  Review previous quit attempts. What helped? What led to relapse?
	  Anticipate challenges to the planned quit attempt, particularly during the critical first few weeks.

B. Encourage nicotine replacement therapy except in special circumstances	Encourage the use of the nicotine patch or nicotine gum therapy for smoking cessation (see Table 1–5, Table 1–6, and Table 1–7 for specific instructions and precautions).
C. Give key advice on successful quitting	Abstinence: Total abstinence is essential. Not even a single puff after the quit date. Alcohol: Drinking alcohol is highly associated with relapse. Those who stop smoking should review their alcohol use and consider limiting or abstaining from alcohol use during the quit process. Other smokers in the household: The presence of other smokers in the household, particularly a spouse, is associated with lower success rates. Patients should consider quitting with their significant others and/or developing specific plans to maintain abstinence in a household where others still smoke.
D. Provide supplementary materials	Source: Federal agencies, including the National Cancer Institute and the Agency for Health Care Policy and Research; nonprofit agencies (American Cancer Society, American Lung Association, American Heart Association); or local or state health departments. Selection concerns: The material must be culturally, racially, educationally, and age appropriate for the patient. Location: Readily available in every clinic office.
Step 5. Arrange—Schedule Follow-Up Contact	
Schedule follow-up contact, either in person or via telephone[1]	Timing: Follow-up contact should occur soon after the quit date, preferably during the first week. A second follow-up contact is recommended within the first month. Schedule further follow-up contacts as indicated. Actions during follow-up: Congratulate success. If smoking occurred, review the circumstances and elicit recommitment to total abstinence. Remind the patient that a lapse can be used as a learning experience and is not a sign of failure. Identify the problems already encountered and anticipate challenges in the immediate future. Assess nicotine replacement therapy use and problems. Consider referral to a more intense or specialized program.

[1]Repeated assessment is not necessary in the case of the adult who has never smoked or not smoked for many years and for whom the information is clearly documented in the medical record.

Adapted and reproduced, with permission, from: The Agency for Health Care Policy and Research. Smoking Cessation Clinical Practice Guideline. JAMA. 1996 Apr 24;275(16):1270–80.

Table 1–4. Common elements of supportive smoking treatments.

Component	Examples
Encouragement of the patient in the quit attempt	Note that effective cessation treatments are now available. Note that half the people who have *ever* smoked have now quit. Communicate belief in the patient's ability to quit.
Communication of caring and concern	Ask how the patient feels about quitting. Directly express concern and a willingness to help. Be open to the patient's expression of fears of quitting, difficulties experienced, and ambivalent feelings.
Encouragement of the patient to talk about the quitting process	Ask about Reasons that the patient wants to quit. Difficulties encountered while quitting. Success the patient has achieved. Concerns or worries about quitting.
Provision of basic information about smoking and successful quitting	Inform the patient about The nature and time course of withdrawal. The addictive nature of smoking. The fact that any smoking (even a single puff) increases the likelihood of full relapse.

Adapted, with permission, from: The Agency for Health Care Policy and Research. Smoking Cessation Clinical Practice Guideline. JAMA. 1996 Apr 24;275(16):1270–80.

Brender E et al. JAMA patient page. Smoking cessation. JAMA. 2006 Jul 5;296(1):130. [PMID: 16820554]

Eisenberg MJ et al. Pharmacotherapies for smoking cessation: a meta-analysis of randomized controlled trials. CMAJ. 2008 Jul 15;179(2):135–44. [PMID: 18625984]

Lee CW et al. Factors associated with successful smoking cessation in the United States, 2000. Am J Public Health. 2007 Aug;97(8):1503–9. [PMID: 17600268]

Ranney L. Systematic review: smoking cessation intervention strategies for adults and adults in special populations. Ann Intern Med. 2006 Dec 5;145(11):845–56. [PMID: 16954352]

Stead LF et al. Physician advice for smoking cessation. Cochrane Database Syst Rev. 2008 Apr 16;(2):CD000165. [PMID: 18253970]

Yanbaeva DG et al. Systemic effects of smoking. Chest. 2007 May;131(5):1557–66. [PMID: 17494805]

▶ Lipid Disorders

Higher low-density lipoprotein (LDL) cholesterol concentrations and lower high-density lipoprotein (HDL) levels are associated with an increased risk of CHD. Elevated triglyceride levels and elevated plasma lipoprotein(a) are also independent risk factors for CHD. The absolute benefits of screening for—and treating—abnormal lipid levels depend on the presence and number of other cardiovascular risk factors. If other risk factors are present, cardiovascular risk is higher and the benefits of therapy are greater. Patients with diabetes mellitus or known cardiovascular disease are at still higher risk and benefit from treatment even when lipid levels are normal.

Table 1–5. Clinical guidelines for prescribing nicotine replacement products.

1. Who should receive nicotine replacement therapy?
Available research shows that nicotine replacement therapy generally increases rates of smoking cessation. Therefore, except in special circumstances, the clinician should encourage the use of nicotine replacement with patients who smoke. Little research is available on the use of nicotine replacement with light smokers (ie, those smoking ≤ 10–15 cigarettes/d). If nicotine replacement is to be used with light smokers, a lower starting dose of the nicotine patch or nicotine gum should be considered.

2. Should nicotine replacement therapy be tailored to the individual smoker?
Research does not support the tailoring of nicotine patch therapy (except with light smokers as noted above). Patients should be prescribed the patch dosages outlined in Table 1–6.
Research supports tailoring nicotine gum treatment. Specifically, research suggests that 4-mg gum rather than 2-mg gum be used with patients who are highly dependent on nicotine (eg, those smoking > 20 cigarettes/d, those who smoke immediately upon awakening, and those who report histories of severe nicotine withdrawal symptoms). Clinicians may also recommend the higher gum dose if patients request it or have failed to quit using the 2-mg gum.

Adapted, with permission, from: The Agency for Health Care Policy and Research. Smoking Cessation Clinical Practice Guideline. JAMA. 1996 Apr 24;275(16):1270–80.

Evidence for the effectiveness of statin-type drugs is better than for the other classes of lipid-lowering agents or dietary changes specifically for improving lipid levels. Multiple large randomized, placebo-controlled trials have demonstrated important reductions in total mortality, major coronary events, and strokes with lowering levels of LDL cholesterol by statin therapy for patients with known cardiovascular disease. Statins also reduce cardiovascular events for patients with diabetes mellitus. For patients with no previous history of cardiovascular events or diabetes, statins reduce coronary events for men, but less data are available for women. The recent JUPITER trial, however, showed relatively similar benefit for both men and women.

Guidelines for therapy are discussed in Chapter 28.

Cholesterol Treatment Trialists' (CTT) Collaborators, Kearney PM et al. Efficacy of cholesterol-lowering therapy in 18,686 people with diabetes in 14 randomised trials of statins: a meta-analysis. Lancet. 2008 Jan 12;371(9607):117–25. [PMID: 18191683]

Ridker PM et al; JUPITER Study Group. Rosuvastatin to prevent vascular events in men and women with elevated C-reactive protein. N Engl J Med. 2008 Nov 20;359(21):2195–207. [PMID: 18997196]

Thavendiranathan P. Primary prevention of cardiovascular diseases with statin therapy: a meta-analysis of randomized controlled trials. Arch Intern Med. 2006 Nov 27;166(21):2307–13. [PMID: 17130382]

▶ Hypertension

Over 43 million adults in the United States have hypertension, but 31% are unaware of their elevated blood pressure; 17% are aware but untreated; 29% are being treated but

Table 1–6. Suggestions for the clinical use of the nicotine patch.

Parameter of Clinical Use	Suggestions
Patient selection	Appropriate as a primary pharmacotherapy for smoking cessation.
Precautions	*Pregnancy:* Pregnant smokers should first be encouraged to attempt cessation without pharmacologic treatment. The nicotine patch should be used during pregnancy only if the increased likelihood of smoking cessation, with its potential benefits, outweighs the risk of nicotine replacement and potential concomitant smoking. Similar factors should be considered in lactating women.
	Cardiovascular diseases: While not an independent risk factor for acute myocardial events, the nicotine patch should be used only after consideration of risks and benefits among particular cardiovascular patient groups: those in the immediate (within 2 weeks) post-myocardial infarction period, those with serious arrhythmias, and those with severe or worsening angina pectoris.
	Skin reactions: Up to 50% of patients using the nicotine patch will have a local skin reaction. Skin reactions are usually mild and self-limiting but may worsen over the course of therapy. Local treatment with hydrocortisone cream (2.5%) or triamcinolone cream (0.5%) and rotating patch sites may ameliorate such local reactions. In fewer than 5% of patients do such reactions require the discontinuation of nicotine patch treatment.
Dosage[1]	Treatment of 8 weeks or less has been shown to be as efficacious as longer treatment periods. Based on this finding, we suggest the following treatment schedules as reasonable for most smokers. Clinicians should consult the package insert for other treatment suggestions. Finally, clinicians should consider individualizing treatment based on specific patient characteristics such as previous experience with the patch, number of cigarettes smoked, and degree of addiction.

Brand	Duration (weeks)	Dosage (mg/h)
Nicoderm and Habitrol	4	21/24
	then 2	14/24
	then 2	7/24
Prostep	4	22/24
	then 4	11/24
Nicotrol	4	15/16
	then 2	10/16
	then 2	5/16

Parameter of Clinical Use	Suggestions
Prescribing instructions	*Abstinence from smoking:* The patient should refrain from smoking while using the patch.
	Location: At the start of each day, the patient should place a new patch on a relatively hairless location between the neck and the waist.
	Activities: There are no restrictions while using the patch.
	Time: Patches should be applied as soon as patients awaken on their quit day.

[1]These dosage recommendations are based on a review of the published research literature and do not necessarily conform to package insert information.
Reproduced, with permission, from: The Agency for Health Care Policy and Research. Smoking Cessation Clinical Practice Guideline. JAMA. 1996 Apr 24;275(16):1270–80. Updated and revised from Treating Tobacco Use and Dependence. U.S. Public Health Service. www.surgeongeneral.gov/tobacco/default.htm.

have not controlled their blood pressure (still greater than 140/90 mm Hg); and only 23% are well controlled. In every adult age group, higher values of systolic and diastolic blood pressure carry greater risks of stroke and congestive heart failure. Systolic blood pressure is a better predictor of morbid events than diastolic blood pressure. Home monitoring is better correlated with target organ damage than clinic-based values. Clinicians can apply specific blood pressure criteria, such as those of the Joint National Committee, along with consideration of the patient's cardiovascular risk, to decide at what levels treatment should be considered in individual cases. Table 11–1 presents a classification of hypertension based on blood pressures.

Primary prevention of hypertension can be accomplished by strategies aimed at both the general population and special high-risk populations. The latter include persons with high-normal blood pressure or a family history of hypertension, blacks, and individuals with various behavioral risk factors such as physical inactivity; excessive consumption of salt, alcohol, or calories; and deficient intake of potassium. Effective interventions for primary prevention of hypertension include reduced sodium and alcohol consumption, weight loss, and regular exercise. Potassium supplementation lowers blood pressure modestly, and a diet high in fresh fruits and vegetables and low in fat, red meats, and sugar-containing beverages also reduces blood pressure.

Table 1–7. Suggestions for the clinical use of nicotine gum.

Parameter of Clinical Use	Suggestions
Patient selection	Appropriate as a primary pharmacotherapy for smoking cessation.
Precautions	*Pregnancy:* Pregnant smokers should first be encouraged to attempt cessation without pharmacologic treatment. Nicotine gum should be used during pregnancy only if the increased likelihood of smoking cessation, with its potential benefits, outweighs the risk of nicotine replacement and potential concomitant smoking. *Cardiovascular diseases:* Although not an independent risk factor for acute myocardial events, nicotine gum should be used only after consideration of risks and benefits among particular cardiovascular patient groups: those in the immediate (within 2 weeks) post-myocardial infarction period, those with serious arrhythmias, and those with serious or worsening angina pectoris. *Adverse effects:* Common adverse effects of nicotine chewing gum include mouth soreness, hiccups, dyspepsia, and jaw ache. These effects are generally mild and transient and can often be alleviated by correcting the patient's chewing technique (see "Prescribing instructions" below).
Dosage	Nicotine gum is available in doses of 2 mg and 4 mg per piece. Patients who smoke less than 25 cigarettes per day should be prescribed the 2-mg gum initially. The 4-mg gum should be prescribed to patients who express a preference for it, have failed with the 2-mg gum but remain motivated to quit, and/or smoke more than 25 cigarettes per day. The gum is most commonly prescribed for the first few months of a quit attempt. Clinicians should tailor the duration of therapy to fit the needs of each patient. Patients using the 2-mg strength should use not more than 30 pieces per day, whereas those using the 4-mg strength should not exceed 20 pieces per day.
Prescribing instructions	*Abstinence from smoking:* The patient should refrain from smoking while using the gum. *Chewing technique:* The gum should be chewed slowly until a "peppery" taste emerges, then "parked" between cheek and gum to facilitate nicotine absorption through the oral mucosa. Gum should be slowly and intermittently chewed and parked for about 30 minutes. *Absorption:* Acidic beverages (eg, coffee, juices, soft drinks) interfere with the buccal absorption of nicotine, so eating and drinking anything except water should be avoided for 15 minutes before and during chewing. *Scheduling of dose:* A common problem is that patients do not use enough gum to get the maximum benefit: they chew too few pieces per day and do not use the gum for a sufficient number of weeks. Instructions to chew the gum on a fixed schedule (at least 1 piece every 1 to 2 hours) for at least 1 to 3 months may be more beneficial than ad lib use.

Reproduced, with permission, from: The Agency for Health Care Policy and Research. Smoking Cessation Clinical Practice Guideline. JAMA. 1996 Apr 24;275(16):1270–80. Updated and revised from Treating Tobacco Use and Dependence. U.S. Public Health Service. www.surgeongeneral.gov/tobacco/default.htm.

Table 1–8. Suggestions for the clinical use of bupropion SR.

Parameter of Clinical Use	Suggestions
Patient selection	Appropriate as a first-line pharmacotherapy for smoking cessation.
Precautions	*Pregnancy:* Pregnant smokers should be encouraged to quit first without pharmacologic treatment. Bupropion SR should be used during pregnancy only if the increased likelihood of smoking abstinence, with its potential benefits, outweighs the risk of bupropion SR treatment and potential concomitant smoking. Similar factors should be considered in lactating women (FDA Class B). *Cardiovascular diseases:* Generally well tolerated; infrequent reports of hypertension. *Side effects:* The most common side effects reported by bupropion SR users were insomnia (35–40%) and dry mouth (10%). *Contraindications:* Bupropion SR is contraindicated in individuals with a history of seizure disorder, a history of an eating disorder, who are using another form of bupropion (Wellbutrin or Wellbutrin SR), or who have used an MAO inhibitor in the past 14 days.
Dosage	Patients should begin with a dose of 150 mg every morning for 3 days, then increase to 150 mg twice daily. Dosing at 150 mg twice daily should continue for 7–12 weeks following the quit date. Unlike nicotine replacement products, patients should begin bupropion SR treatment 1–2 weeks before they quit smoking. For maintenance therapy, consider bupropion SR 150 mg twice daily for up to 6 months.
Prescribing instructions	*Cessation prior to quit date:* Recognize that some patients will lose their desire to smoke prior to their quit date, or will spontaneously reduce the amount they smoke. *Scheduling of dose:* If insomnia is marked, taking the evening dose earlier (in the afternoon, at least 8 hours after the first dose) may provide some relief. *Alcohol:* Use alcohol only in moderation.

MAO, monoamine oxidase.
Adapted from Treating Tobacco Use and Dependence. U.S. Public Health Service. www.surgeongeneral.gov/tobacco/default.htm.

Interventions of unproven efficacy include pill supplementation of potassium, calcium, magnesium, fish oil, or fiber; macronutrient alteration; and stress management.

Improved identification and treatment of hypertension is a major cause of the recent decline in stroke deaths. Because hypertension is usually asymptomatic, screening is strongly recommended to identify patients for treatment. Despite strong recommendations in favor of screening and treatment, hypertension control remains suboptimal. An intervention that included patient education and provider education was more effective than provider education alone in achieving control of hypertension, suggesting the benefits of patient participation. Pharmacologic management of hypertension is discussed in Chapter 11.

Chobanian AV et al. The Seventh Report of the Joint National Committee on Prevention, Detection, Evaluation, and Treatment of High Blood Pressure: the JNC 7 report. JAMA. 2003 May 21;289(19):2560–72. [PMID: 12748199]

Messerli FH et al. Essential hypertension. Lancet. 2007 Aug 18;370(9587):591–603. [PMID: 17707755]

Roumie CL et al. Improving blood pressure control through provider education, provider alerts, and patient education: a cluster randomized trial. Ann Intern Med. 2006 Aug 1;145 (3):165–75. [PMID: 16880458]

Taylor JR et al. Home monitoring of glucose and blood pressure. Am Fam Physician. 2007 Jul 15;76(2):255–60. [PMID: 17695570]

Wolff T et al. Evidence for the reaffirmation of the U.S. Preventive Services Task Force recommendation on screening for high blood pressure. Ann Intern Med. 2007 Dec 4;147(11):787–91. [PMID: 18056663]

▶ Chemoprevention

As discussed in Chapters 10 and 24, regular use of low-dose aspirin (81–325 mg) can reduce the incidence of myocardial infarction in men. Low-dose aspirin reduces stroke but not myocardial infarction in middle-aged women. Based on its ability to prevent cardiovascular events, aspirin use is cost-effective for men and women who are at increased risk. Nonsteroidal anti-inflammatory drugs may reduce the incidence of colorectal adenomas and polyps but may also increase heart disease and gastrointestinal bleeding, and thus are not recommended for colon cancer prevention in average risk patients. Antioxidant vitamin (vitamin E, vitamin C, and beta-carotene) supplementation produced no significant reductions in the 5-year incidence of—or mortality from—vascular disease, cancer, or other major outcomes in high-risk individuals with coronary artery disease, other occlusive arterial disease, or diabetes mellitus.

Berger JS. Aspirin for the primary prevention of cardiovascular events in women and men: a sex-specific meta-analysis of randomized controlled trials. JAMA. 2006 Jan 18;295(3):306–13. [PMID: 16418466]

Greving JP et al. Cost-effectiveness of aspirin treatment in the primary prevention of cardiovascular disease events in subgroups based on age, gender, and varying cardiovascular risk. Circulation. 2008 Jun 3;117(22):2875–83. [PMID: 18506010]

Rostom A. Nonsteroidal anti-inflammatory drugs and cyclooxygenase-2 inhibitors for primary prevention of colorectal cancer: a systematic review prepared for the U.S. Preventive Services Task Force. Ann Intern Med. 2007 Mar 6;146(5):376–89. [PMID: 17339623]

Vivekananthan DP et al. Use of antioxidant vitamins for the prevention of cardiovascular disease: meta-analysis of randomised trials. Lancet. 2003 Jun 14;361(9374):2017–23. [PMID: 12814711]

PREVENTION OF OSTEOPOROSIS

Osteoporosis, characterized by low bone mineral density, is common and associated with an increased risk of fracture. The lifetime risk of an osteoporotic fracture is approximately 50% for women and 30% for men. Osteoporotic fractures can cause significant pain and disability. As such, research has focused on means of preventing osteoporosis and related fractures. Primary prevention strategies include calcium supplementation, vitamin D supplementation, and exercise programs. A recent systematic review and meta-analysis found that calcium supplementation of 1200 mg per day or more (with or without vitamin D) could decrease fracture risk for adults (mainly women were studied) over age 50. Screening for osteoporosis on the basis of low bone mineral density is also recommended for women over age 60, based on indirect evidence that screening can identify women with low bone mineral density and that treatment of women with low bone density with bisphosphonates is effective in reducing fractures. The effectiveness of screening for osteoporosis in younger women and in men has not been established. In addition, real-world adherence to pharmacologic therapy for osteoporosis is low: one-third to one-half of patients do not take their medication as directed. Vitamin D deficiency is common and can increase the risk of fracture. Screening to detect vitamin D deficiency in older adults has been proposed, but has not yet been rigorously evaluated.

Cherniack EP et al. Hypovitaminosis D: a widespread epidemic. Geriatrics. 2008 Apr;63(4):24–30. [PMID: 18376898]

Kanis JA et al; European Society for Clinical and Economic Aspects of Osteoporosis and Osteoarthritis (ESCEO). European guidance for the diagnosis and management of osteoporosis in postmenopausal women. Osteoporos Int. 2008 Apr;19(4):399–428. [PMID: 18266020]

Kothawala P et al. Systematic review and meta-analysis of real-world adherence to drug therapy for osteoporosis. Mayo Clin Proc. 2007 Dec;82(12):1493–501. [PMID: 18053457]

Nelson HD. Screening for postmenopausal osteoporosis: a review of the evidence for the U.S. Preventive Services Task Force. Ann Intern Med. 2002 Sep 17;137(6):529–41. [PMID: 12230356]

Schousboe JT. Cost-effectiveness of bone densitometry followed by treatment of osteoporosis in older men. JAMA. 2007 Aug 8;298(6):629–37. [PMID: 17684185]

Tang BM. Use of calcium or calcium in combination with vitamin D supplementation to prevent fractures and bone loss in people aged 50 years and older: a meta-analysis. Lancet. 2007 Aug 25;370(9588):657–66. [PMID: 17720017]

PREVENTION OF PHYSICAL INACTIVITY

Lack of sufficient physical activity is the second most important contributor to preventable deaths, trailing only tobacco use. A sedentary lifestyle has been linked to 28% of deaths from leading chronic diseases. The Centers for Disease Control and Prevention (CDC) has recommended that every adult in the United States should engage in 30 minutes or more of moderate-intensity physical activity on most days of the week. This guideline complements previous advice urging at least 20–30 minutes of more vigorous aerobic exercise three to five times a week.

Patients who engage in regular moderate to vigorous exercise have a lower risk of myocardial infarction, stroke, hypertension, hyperlipidemia, type 2 diabetes mellitus, diverticular disease, and osteoporosis. Current evidence supports the recommended guidelines of 30 minutes of moderate physical activity on most days of the week in both the primary and secondary prevention of CHD. Between 1980 and 2000, an estimated 5% of the decrease in US deaths from CHD among adults aged 25–84 years resulted from increases in physical activity.

In older nonsmoking men, walking 2 miles or more per day is associated with an almost 50% lower age-related mortality. The relative risk of stroke was found to be less than one-sixth in men who exercised vigorously compared with those who were inactive; the risk of type 2 diabetes mellitus was about half among men who exercised five or more times weekly compared with those who exercised once a week. Glucose control is improved in diabetics who exercise regularly, even at a modest level. In sedentary individuals with dyslipidemia, high amounts of high-intensity exercise produce significant beneficial effects on serum lipoprotein profiles. Physical activity is associated with a lower risk of colon cancer (although not rectal cancer) in men and women and of breast and reproductive organ cancer in women. Finally, weight-bearing exercise (especially resistance and high-impact activities) increases bone mineral content and retards development of osteoporosis in women and contributes to a reduced risk of falls in older persons. Resistance training has been shown to enhance muscular strength, functional capacity, and quality of life in men and women with and without CHD and is endorsed by the American Heart Association.

Exercise may also confer benefits on those with chronic illness. Men and women with chronic symptomatic osteoarthritis of one or both knees benefited from a supervised walking program, with improved self-reported functional status and decreased pain and use of pain medication. Exercise produces sustained lowering of both systolic and diastolic blood pressure in patients with mild hypertension. In addition, physical activity can help patients maintain ideal body weight. Individuals who maintain ideal body weight have a 35–55% lower risk for myocardial infarction than with those who are obese. Physical activity reduces depression and anxiety; improves adaptation to stress; improves sleep quality; and enhances mood, self-esteem, and overall performance.

In longitudinal cohort studies, individuals who report higher levels of leisure time physical activity are less likely to gain weight. Conversely, individuals who are overweight are less likely to stay active. However, at least 60 minutes of daily moderate-intensity physical activity may be necessary to maximize weight loss and prevent significant weight regain. Moreover, adequate levels of physical activity appear to be important for the prevention of weight gain and the development of obesity. Physical activity also appears to have an independent effect on health-related outcomes such as development of type 2 diabetes mellitus in patients with impaired glucose tolerance when compared with body weight, suggesting that adequate levels of activity may counteract the negative influence of body weight on health outcomes.

However, physical exertion can rarely trigger the onset of acute myocardial infarction, particularly in persons who are habitually sedentary. Increased activity increases the risk of musculoskeletal injuries, which can be minimized by proper warm-up and stretching, and by gradual rather than sudden increase in activity. Other potential complications of exercise include angina pectoris, arrhythmias, sudden death, and asthma. In insulin-requiring diabetics who undertake vigorous exercise, the need for insulin is reduced; hypoglycemia may be a consequence.

Only about 20% of adults in the United States are active at the moderate level—and only 8% currently exercise at the more vigorous level—recommended for health benefits. Instead, 60% report irregular or no leisure time physical activity.

The value of routine electrocardiography stress testing prior to initiation of an exercise program in middle-aged or older adults remains controversial. Patients with ischemic heart disease or other cardiovascular disease require medically supervised, graded exercise programs. Medically supervised exercise prolongs life in patients with congestive heart failure. Exercise should not be prescribed for patients with decompensated congestive heart failure, complex ventricular arrhythmias, unstable angina pectoris, hemodynamically significant aortic stenosis, or significant aortic aneurysm. Five- to 10-minute warm-up and cool-down periods, stretching exercises, and gradual increases in exercise intensity help prevent musculoskeletal and cardiovascular complications.

Physical activity can be incorporated into any person's daily routine. For example, the clinician can advise a patient to take the stairs instead of the elevator, to walk or bike instead of driving, to do housework or yard work, to get off the bus one or two stops earlier and walk the rest of the way, to park at the far end of the parking lot, or to walk during the lunch hour. The basic message should be the more the better and anything is better than nothing.

To be more effective in counseling about exercise, clinicians can also incorporate motivational interviewing techniques, adopt a whole practice approach (eg, use practice nurses to assist), and establish linkages with community agencies. Clinicians can incorporate the "5 As" approach:

1. Ask (identify those who can benefit).
2. Assess (current activity level).
3. Advise (individualize plan).
4. Assist (provide a written exercise prescription and support material).
5. Arrange (appropriate referral and follow-up).

Such interventions have a moderate effect on self-reported physical activity and cardiorespiratory fitness, even if they do not always help patients achieve a predetermined level of physical activity. In their counseling, clinicians should advise patients about both the benefits and risks of exercise, prescribe an exercise program appropriate for each patient, and provide advice to help prevent injuries or cardiovascular complications.

Although primary care providers regularly ask patients about physical activity and advise them with verbal counseling, few providers provide written prescriptions or perform fitness assessments. Tailored interventions may potentially help increase physical activity in individuals. Exercise counseling with a prescription, eg, for walking at either a hard intensity or a moderate intensity-high frequency, can produce significant long-term improvements in cardiorespiratory fitness. To be effective, exercise prescriptions must include recommendations on type, frequency, intensity, time, and progression of exercise and must follow disease-specific guidelines. In addition, published research suggests that getting patients to change physical activity levels requires motivational strategies beyond simple exercise instruction including patient education about goal-setting, self-monitoring, and problem-solving. For example, helping patients identify emotionally rewarding and physically appropriate activities, meet contingencies, and find social support will increase rates of exercise continuation.

Some physical activity is always preferable to a sedentary lifestyle. For home-bound elderly who have limited mobility and strength, such physical activity could focus on "functional fitness," such as mobility, transfers, and performing activities of daily living. Exercise-based rehabilitation can protect against falls and fall-related injuries and improve functional performance.

Duncan GE et al. Prescribing exercise at varied levels of intensity and frequency: a randomized trial. Arch Intern Med. 2005 Nov 14;165(20):2362–9. [PMID: 16287765]

Ford ES et al. Explaining the decrease in U.S. deaths from coronary disease, 1980–2000. N Engl J Med. 2007 Jun 7;356(23):2388–98. [PMID: 17554120]

Laaksonen DE et al; Finnish diabetes prevention study. Physical activity in the prevention of type 2 diabetes: the Finnish diabetes prevention study. Diabetes. 2005 Jan;54(1):158–65. [PMID: 15616024]

McDermott AY et al. Exercise and older patients: prescribing guidelines. Am Fam Physician. 2006 Aug 1;74(3):437–44. [PMID: 16913163]

Means KM et al. Balance, mobility, and falls among community-dwelling elderly persons: effects of a rehabilitation exercise program. Am J Phys Med Rehabil. 2005 Apr;84(4):238–50. [PMID: 1578256]

Ogilvie D et al. Interventions to promote walking: systematic review. BMJ. 2007 Jun 9;334(7605):1204. [PMID: 17540909]

Struck BD et al. Health promotion in older adults. Prescribing exercise for the frail and home bound. Geriatrics. 2006 May;61(5):22–7. [PMID: 16649815]

Petrella RJ et al. Physical activity counseling and prescription among Canadian primary care physicians. Arch Intern Med. 2007 Sep 10;167(16):1774–81. [PMID: 17846397]

Williams MA et al. Resistance exercise in individuals with and without cardiovascular disease: 2007 update: a scientific statement from the American Heart Association Council on Clinical Cardiology and Council on Nutrition, Physical Activity, and Metabolism. Circulation. 2007 Jul 31;116(5):572–84. [PMID: 17638929]

PREVENTION OF OVERWEIGHT & OBESITY

Obesity is now a true epidemic and public health crisis that both clinicians and patients must face. Normal body weight is defined as a body mass index (BMI), calculated as the weight in kilograms divided by the height in meters squared, of < 25 kg/m^2; overweight is defined as a BMI = 25.0–29.9 kg/m^2, and obesity as a BMI > 30 kg/m^2. The prevalence of obesity in US children, adolescents, and adults has grown dramatically since 1990. In 2003–2004, 17% of US children and adolescents were overweight and 32% of adults were obese. Among men, the prevalence of obesity increased significantly between 1999 and 2000 (28%) and between 2003 and 2004 (31%). Among women, no significant increase in the prevalence of obesity was observed between 1999 and 2000 (33%) or between 2003 and 2004 (33%). The prevalence of extreme obesity (BMI ≥ 40) in 2003–2004 was 3% in men and 7% in women. Prevalence varies by race and age, with older African American and Latina women having the greatest prevalence of obesity. This trend has been linked both to declines in physical activity and to increased caloric intake in diets rich in fats and carbohydrates.

Adequate levels of physical activity appear to be important for the prevention of weight gain and the development of obesity. However, as noted above, only about 20% of Americans are physically active at a moderate level, and only 8% at a more vigorous level, and 60% report irregular or no leisure time physical activity. In addition, only 3% of Americans meet four of the five recommendations for the intake of grains, fruits, vegetables, dairy products, and meat of the Food Guide Pyramid. Only one of four Americans eats the recommended five or more fruits and vegetables per day.

Risk assessment of the overweight and obese patient begins with determination of BMI, waist circumference for those with a BMI of 35 or less, presence of comorbid conditions, and a fasting blood glucose and lipid panel. Obesity is clearly associated with type 2 diabetes mellitus, hypertension, hyperlipidemia, cancer, osteoarthritis, cardiovascular disease, obstructive sleep apnea, and asthma. One of the most important sequelae of the rapid surge in prevalence of overweight and obesity between 1990 and 2000 has been a dramatic 30–40% increase in the prevalence of type 2 diabetes mellitus. In addition, almost one-quarter of the US population currently has the metabolic syndrome, putting them at high risk for the development of CHD. The relationship between overweight and obesity and diabetes, hypertension, and coronary artery disease is thought to be due to insulin resistance and compensatory hyperinsulinemia. Persons with a BMI ≥ 40 have death rates from cancers that are 52% higher for men and 62% higher for women than the rates in men and women of normal weight. Significant trends of increasing risk of death with higher BMIs are observed for cancers of the stomach and prostate in men and for cancers of the breast, uterus, cervix, and ovary in women, and for cancers of the esophagus, colon and rectum, liver, gallbladder, pancreas, and kidney, non-Hodgkin lymphoma, and multiple myeloma in both men and women.

In the Framingham Heart Study, overweight and obesity were associated with large decreases in life expectancy. For example, 40-year-old female nonsmokers lost 3.3 years and 40-year-old male nonsmokers lost 3.1 years of life expectancy because of overweight, and 7.1 years and 5.8 years of life expectancy, respectively, because of obesity. Obese female smokers lost 7.2 years and obese male smokers lost 6.7 years of life expectancy compared with normal-weight smokers, and 13.3 years and 13.7 years, respectively, compared with normal-weight nonsmokers. Clinicians must work to identify and provide the best prevention and treatment strategies for patients who are overweight and obese. Patients with abdominal obesity (high waist to hip size ratio) are at particularly increased risk. Control of visceral obesity in addition to other cardiovascular risk factors (hypertension, insulin resistance, and dyslipidemia) is essential to reducing cardiovascular risk.

Prevention of overweight and obesity involves both increasing physical activity and dietary modification to reduce caloric intake. Clinicians can help guide patients to develop personalized eating plans to reduce energy intake, particularly by recognizing the contributions of fat, concentrated carbohydrates, and large portion sizes (see Chapter 29). Patients typically underestimate caloric content, especially when consuming food away from home. Providing patients with caloric and nutritional information may help address the current obesity epidemic. To prevent the long-term chronic disease sequelae of overweight or obesity, clinicians must work with patients to modify other risk factors, eg, by smoking cessation (see above) and strict glycemic and blood pressure control (see Chapters 27 and 11).

Lifestyle modification, including diet, physical activity, and behavior therapy has been shown to induce clinically significant weight loss. Other treatment options for obesity include pharmacotherapy and surgery. One potentially effective diet strategy is the replacement of caloric beverages with low-calorie or noncaloric beverages. As noted above, in overweight and obese persons, at least 60 minutes of moderate-high intensity physical activity may be necessary to maximize weight loss and prevent significant weight regain. Counseling interventions or pharmacotherapy can produce modest (3–5 kg) sustained weight loss over 6–12 months. Pharmacotherapy appears safe in the short term; long-term safety is still not established. As an example, in a multicenter trial, treatment with 20 mg/d of rimonabant, a selective cannabinoid-1 receptor blocker, plus diet for 2 years produced modest but sustained reductions in weight and waist circumference and favorable changes in metabolic risk factors. Counseling appears to be most effective when intensive and combined with behavioral therapy. Maintenance strategies can help preserve weight loss.

In dietary therapy, results from the Women's Health Initiative Dietary Modification Trial showed that a low-fat diet high in vegetables, fruits, and grains produced a modest (2.2 kg, $P < .001$) weight loss that was sustained over prolonged follow-up (1.9 kg, $P < .001$ at 1 year, 0.4 kg, $P = .01$ at 7.5 years). A recent study comparing various diets revealed that Mediterranean (moderate fat, restricted calorie) and low-carbohydrate (non-restricted calorie) diets are effective alternatives to low-fat diets.

Weight loss strategies using dietary, physical activity, or behavioral interventions can produce significant improvements in weight among persons with prediabetes and a significant decrease in diabetes incidence. Multicomponent interventions including very-low-calorie or low-calorie diets hold promise for achieving weight loss in adults with type 2 diabetes mellitus.

Bariatric surgical procedures, eg, vertical banded gastroplasty and Roux-en-Y gastric bypass, are reserved for patients with morbid obesity whose BMI exceeds 40, or for less severely obese patients (with BMIs between 35 and 40) with high-risk comorbid conditions such as life-threatening cardiopulmonary problems (eg, severe sleep apnea, Pickwickian syndrome, and obesity-related cardiomyopathy) or severe diabetes mellitus. In selected patients, surgery can produce substantial weight loss (10 to 159 kg) over 1 to 5 years, with rare but sometimes severe complications. Nutritional deficiencies are one complication of bariatric surgical procedures and close monitoring of a patient's metabolic and nutritional status is essential.

Clinicians seem to share a general perception that almost no one succeeds in long-term maintenance of weight loss. However, research demonstrates that approximately 20% of overweight individuals are successful at long-term weight loss (defined as losing ≥ 10% of initial body weight and maintaining the loss for ≥ 1 year). National Weight Control Registry members who lost an average of 33 kg and maintained the loss for more than 5 years have provided useful information about how to maintain weight loss. Members report engaging in high levels of physical activity (approximately 60 min/d), eating a low-calorie, low-fat diet, eating breakfast regularly, self-monitoring weight, and maintaining a consistent eating pattern from weekdays to weekends. The development and implementation of innovative public health strategies is essential in the fight against obesity. Lessons learned from smoking cessation campaigns may be helpful in the battle against this significant public health concern.

Berman M et al. Obesity prevention in the information age: caloric information at the point of purchase. JAMA. 2008 Jul 23;300(4):433–5. [PMID: 18647987]

Flood JE et al. The effect of increased beverage portion size on energy intake at a meal. J Am Diet Assoc. 2006 Dec;10(12):1984–90. [PMID: 17126628]

Garson A Jr et al. Attacking obesity: lessons learned from smoking. J Am Coll Cardiol. 2007 Apr 24;49(16):1673–5. [PMID: 17448367]

Howard BV et al. Low-fat dietary pattern and weight change over 7 years: the Women's Health Initiative Dietary Modification Trial. JAMA. 2006 Jan 4;295(1):39–49. [PMID: 16391215]

Ogden CL et al. Prevalence of overweight and obesity in the United States, 1999–2004. JAMA. 2006 Apr 5;295(13):1549–55. [PMID: 16595758]

Pi-Sunyer FX et al; RIO-North America Study Group. Effect of rimonabant, a cannabinoid-1 receptor blocker, on weight and cardiometabolic risk factors in overweight or obese patients: RIO-North America: a randomized controlled trial. JAMA. 2006 Feb 15;295(7):761–75. [PMID: 16478899]

Ritz E. Total cardiovascular risk management. Am J Cardiol. 2007 Aug 6;100(3A):53J–60J. [PMID: 17666199]

Shai I et al; Dietary Intervention Randomized Controlled Trial (DIRECT) Group. Weight loss with a low-carbohydrate, Mediterranean, or low-fat diet. N Engl J Med. 2008 Jul 17;359(3):229–41. [PMID: 18635428]

Tucker ON et al. Nutritional consequences of weight-loss surgery. Med Clin North Am. 2007 May;91(3):499–514. [PMID: 17509392]

Wadden et al. Lifestyle modification for the management of obesity. Gastroenterology. 2007 May;132(6):2226–38. [PMID: 17498514]

CANCER PREVENTION

▶ Primary Prevention

Mortality rates of cancer have begun to decrease in the past 2 years; part of this decrease results from reductions in tobacco use, since cigarette smoking is the most important preventable cause of cancer. Preventive health examinations and preventive gynecologic examinations are among the most common reasons for ambulatory care visits, although the use and content of these types of visits remains controversial. Primary prevention of skin cancer consists of restricting exposure to ultraviolet light by wearing appropriate clothing and use of sunscreens. In the past 2 decades, there has been a threefold increase in the incidence of squamous cell carcinoma and a fourfold increase in melanoma in the United States. Persons who engage in regular physical exercise and avoid obesity have lower rates of breast and colon cancer. Prevention of occupationally induced cancers involves minimizing exposure to carcinogenic substances such as asbestos, ionizing radiation, and benzene compounds. Chemoprevention has been widely studied for primary cancer prevention (see above Chemoprevention section and Chapter 39). Use of tamoxifen, raloxifene, and aromatase inhibitors for breast cancer prevention is discussed in Chapters 17 and 39. Hepatitis B vaccination can prevent hepatocellular carcinoma (HCC), and screening and vaccination programs may be cost-effective and useful in preventing HCC in high-risk groups such as Asians and Pacific Islanders. The use of HPV vaccine to prevent cervical cancer is discussed above in the Prevention of Infectious Disease section.

Hutton DW et al. Cost-effectiveness of screening and vaccinating Asian and Pacific Islander adults for hepatitis B. Ann Intern Med. 2007 Oct 2;147(7):460–9. [PMID: 17909207]

Mehrotra A et al. Preventive health examinations and preventive gynecological examinations in the United States. Arch Intern Med. 2007 Sep 24;167(17):1876–83. [PMID: 17893309]

▶ Screening & Early Detection

Screening has been shown to prevent death from cancers of the breast, colon, and cervix. Current cancer screening recommendations from the American Cancer Society, the Canadian Task Force on Preventive Health Care, and the United States Preventive Services Task Force are shown in Table 1–9.

The appropriate form and frequency of screening for breast cancer is controversial. A large randomized trial of breast self-examination conducted among factory workers in Shanghai found no benefit. A systematic review performed for the United States Preventive Services Task Force found that mammography was moderately effective in reducing breast cancer mortality for women 40–74 years of age. The absolute benefit was greater for older women, and the risk of false-positive results was high for all women. Digital mammography is more sensitive in women with dense breasts and younger women; however, studies exploring outcomes are lacking. Several organizations, including the American Cancer Society and the National Cancer Institute, recommend routine mammography screening, and changes in screening guidelines appear to impact women's beliefs about how frequently they should obtain screening. Although delays to following up an abnormal mammogram exist, the use of patient navigation programs to reduce such delays appears beneficial, especially among poor and minority populations. The use of MRI is not currently recommended for general screening, although the American Cancer Society does recommend screening MRI for women at high risk ($\geq$ 20–25%), including those with a strong family history of breast or ovarian cancer. A recent systematic review reported that screening with both MRI and mammography might be superior to mammography alone in ruling out cancerous lesions in women with an inherited predisposition to breast cancer.

All current recommendations call for cervical and colorectal cancer screening. Prostate cancer screening, however, is controversial, as no completed studies have answered the question whether early detection and treatment after screen detection produce sufficient benefits to outweigh harms of treatment. A 2008 USPSTF review of current evidence on benefits and harm of screening asymptomatic men for prostate cancer with prostate-specific antigen (PSA) testing revealed that PSA screening is associated with increased psychological harm with uncertain potential benefits. Providers and patients are advised to discuss how to proceed in light of this uncertainty. Whether early detection through screening and subsequent treatment alters the natural course of the disease remains to be seen. There are still no data on the morbidity and mortality benefits of screening. Unlike the American College of Physicians, the American Cancer Society recommends that providers offer annual PSA testing for men over age 50. Screening is not recommended by any group for men who have estimated life expectancies of less than 10 years. Decision aids have been developed to help men weigh the arguments for and against PSA screening.

Annual or biennial fecal occult blood testing reduces mortality from colorectal cancer by 16–33%. The risk of death from colon cancer among patients undergoing at least one sigmoidoscopic examination is reduced by 60–80% compared with that among those not having sigmoidoscopy. Colonoscopy has also been advocated as a screening examination. It is more accurate than flexible sigmoidoscopy for detecting cancer and polyps, but its value in reducing colon cancer mortality has not been studied directly. Recent studies have shown that CT colography (virtual colonoscopy) is also able to detect cancers and polyps with reasonable accuracy.

Screening for cervical cancer with a Papanicolaou smear is indicated in sexually active adolescents and in adult women every 1–3 years. Screening for vaginal cancer

Table 1–9. Cancer screening recommendations for average-risk adults.

Test	ACS[1]	CTF[2]	USPSTF[3]
Breast self-examination (BSE)	An option for women over age 20.	Fair evidence that BSE *should not* be used.	Insufficient evidence to recommend for or against.
Clinical breast examination	Every 3 years age 20–40 and annually thereafter.	Good evidence for annual screening women aged 50–69 by clinical examination and mammography.	Insufficient evidence to recommend for or against.
Mammography	Annually age 40 and older.	Current evidence does not support the recommendation that screening mammography be included in or excluded from the periodic health examination of women aged 40–49.	Recommended every 1–2 years for women aged 40 and over (B).
Papanicolaou test	Annually beginning within 3 years after first vaginal intercourse or no later than age 21. Screening may be done every 2 years with the liquid-based Pap test. After age 30, women with three normal tests may be screened every 2–3 years or every 3 years by Pap test plus the HPV DNA test. Women may choose to stop screening after age 70 if they have had three normal (and no abnormal) results within the last 10 years.	Annually at age of first intercourse or by age 18; can move to every-2-year screening after two normal results to age 69.	Every 3 years beginning at onset of sexual activity or age 21 (A). Recommends against routinely screening women older than age 65 if they have had adequate recent screening with normal Pap tests and are not otherwise at high risk for cervical cancer (D).
Annual stool test for occult blood[4] or fecal immunochemical test (FIT) Sigmoidoscopy (every 5 years) Double-contrast barium enema (every 5 years) Colonoscopy (every 10 years)	Screening recommended, with the combination of fecal occult blood test or fecal immunochemical test (FIT) and sigmoidoscopy preferred over stool test or sigmoidoscopy alone. Double-contrast barium enema and colonoscopy also considered reasonable alternatives.	Good evidence for screening every 1–2 years over age 50. Fair evidence for screening over age 50 (insufficient evidence about combining stool test and sigmoidoscopy). Not addressed. Insufficient evidence for or against use in screening.	Screening strongly recommended (A), but insufficient evidence to determine best test.
Prostate-specific antigen (PSA) blood test Digital rectal examination (DRE)	PSA and DRE should be offered annually to men age 50 and older who have at least a 10-year life expectancy. Men at high risk (African-American men and men with a strong family history) should begin at age 45. Information should be provided to men about the benefits and risks, and they should be allowed to participate in the decision. Men without a clear preference should be screened.	Fair evidence *against* including in routine care. Insufficient evidence for or against including in routine care.	Insufficient evidence to recommend for or against. Insufficient evidence to recommend for or against.
Cancer-related checkup	For people aged 20 or older having periodic health exams, a cancer-related checkup should include counseling and perhaps oral cavity, thyroid, lymph node, or testicular examinations.	Not assessed.	Not assessed.

[1]American Cancer Society recommendations, available at http://www.cancer.org.
[2]Canadian Task Force on Preventive Health Care recommendations available at http://www.ctfphc.org.
[3]United States Preventive Services Task Force recommendations available at http://www.ahrq.gov/clinic/prevention.htm.
[4]Home test with three samples.
Recommendation A: The USPSTF strongly recommends that clinicians routinely provide the service to eligible patients. (The USPSTF found good evidence that the service improves important health outcomes and concludes that benefits substantially outweigh harms.)
Recommendation B: The USPSTF recommends that clinicians routinely provide the service to eligible patients. (The USPSTF found at least fair evidence that the service improves important health outcomes and concludes that benefits substantially outweigh harms.)
Recommendation D: The USPSTF recommends against routinely providing the service to asymptomatic patients. (The USPSTF found at least fair evidence that the service is ineffective or that harms outweigh benefits.)

with a Papanicolaou smear is not indicated in women who have undergone hysterectomies for benign disease with removal of the cervix—except in diethylstilbestrol (DES)-exposed women (see Chapter 18). Women over age 70 who have had normal results on three or more previous Papanicolaou smears may elect to stop screening.

Screening for lung cancer with spiral CT can detect early stage disease; however, its efficacy in reducing lung cancer mortality has not been evaluated in a randomized trial, although a recent study of survival in asymptomatic patients at risk for lung cancer who were screened annually with spiral CT revealed that such screening detected lung cancer at a curable stage.

Andriole GL et al; PLCO Project Team. Prostate cancer screening in the Prostate, Lung, Colorectal and Ovarian (PLCO) Cancer Screening Trial: findings from the initial screening round of a randomized trial. J Natl Cancer Inst. 2005 Mar 16;97(6):433–8. [PMID: 15770007]

Aus G et al. Individualized screening interval for prostate cancer based on prostate-specific antigen level: results of a prospective, randomized, population-based study. Arch Intern Med. 2005 Sep 12;165(16):1857–61. [PMID: 16157829]

Battaglia TA. Improving follow-up to abnormal breast cancer screening in an urban population. A patient navigation intervention. Cancer. 2007 Jan 15;109(2 Suppl):359–67. [PMID: 17123275]

Calvocoressi L et al. Mammography screening of women in their 40s: impact of changes in screening guidelines. Cancer. 2008 Feb 1;112(3):473–80. [PMID: 18072258]

Denny L et al. Screen-and-treat approaches for cervical cancer prevention in low-resource settings: a randomized controlled trial. JAMA. 2005 Nov 2;294(17):2173–81. [PMID: 16264158]

International Early Lung Cancer Action Program Investigators, Henschke CI et al. Survival of patients with stage I lung cancer detected on CT screening. N Engl J Med. 2006 Oct 26;355(17):1763–71. [PMID: 17065637]

Knutson D et al. Screening for breast cancer: current recommendations and future directions. Am Fam Physician. 2007 Jun 1;75(11):1660–6. [PMID: 17575656]

Lin K et al; U.S. Preventive Services Task Force. Benefits and harms of prostate-specific antigen screening for prostate cancer: an evidence update for the U.S. Preventive Services Task Force. Ann Intern Med. 2008 Aug 5;149(3):192–9. [PMID: 18678846]

New York Early Lung Cancer Action Project Investigators. CT screening for lung cancer: diagnoses resulting from the New York Early Lung Cancer Action Project. Radiology. 2007 Apr;243(1):239–49. [PMID: 17392256]

Prochaska JO et al. Stage-based expert systems to guide a population of primary care patients to quit smoking, eat healthier, prevent skin cancer, and receive regular mammograms. Prev Med. 2005 Aug;41(2):406–16. [PMID: 15896835]

Saslow D et al. American Cancer Society guidelines for breast screening with MRI as an adjunct to mammography. CA Cancer J Clin. 2007 Mar–Apr;57(2):75–89. [PMID: 17392385]

Torpy JM et al. JAMA patient page. Colon cancer screening. JAMA. 2006 Mar 8;295(10):1208. [PMID: 16522847]

Warner E et al. Systematic review: using magnetic resonance imaging to screen women at high risk for breast cancer. Ann Intern Med. 2008 May 6;148(9):671–9. [PMID: 18458280]

Weissfeld JL et al; PLCO Project Team. Flexible sigmoidoscopy in the PLCO cancer screening trial: results from the baseline screening examination of a randomized trial. J Natl Cancer Inst. 2005 Jul 6;97(13):989–97. [PMID: 15998952]

PREVENTION OF INJURIES & VIOLENCE

Injuries remain the most important cause of loss of potential years of life before age 65. Homicide and motor vehicle accidents are a major cause of injury-related deaths among young adults, and accidental falls are the most common cause of injury-related death in the elderly. Other causes of injury-related deaths include suicide and accidental exposure to smoke, fire, and flames.

Although there has been a steady decline in motor vehicle accident deaths per miles driven, road traffic injuries remain the tenth leading cause of death and the ninth leading cause of the burden of disease. Although seat belt use protects against serious injury and death in motor vehicle accidents, at least one-fourth of adults and one-third of teenagers do not use seat belts routinely. Air bags are protective for adults but not for small children.

Each year in the United States, more than 500,000 people are nonfatally injured while riding bicycles. The rate of helmet use by bicyclists and motorcyclists is significantly increased in states with helmet laws. Young men appear most likely to resist wearing helmets. Clinicians should try to educate their patients about seat belts, safety helmets, the risks of using cellular telephones while driving, drinking and driving—or using other intoxicants or long-acting benzodiazepines and then driving—and the risks of having guns in the home.

Long-term alcohol abuse adversely affects outcome from trauma and increases the risk of readmission for new trauma. Alcohol and illicit drug use are associated with an increased risk of violent death. There is a causal link between alcohol intoxication and injury due to assault. Harm reduction can be achieved through practical measures, such as using plastic glasses and bottles in licensed premises; controlling prices of drinks; and targeted policing based on police, accident, and emergency data.

Males aged 16–35 are at especially high risk for serious injury and death from accidents and violence, with blacks and Latinos at greatest risk. For 16- and 17-year-old drivers, the risk of fatal crashes increases with the number of passengers. Deaths from firearms have reached epidemic levels in the United States and will soon surpass the number of deaths from motor vehicle accidents. Having a gun in the home increases the likelihood of homicide nearly threefold and of suicide fivefold. In 2002, an estimated 877,000 individuals successfully committed suicide. Educating physicians to recognize and treat depression as well as restricting access to lethal methods have been found to reduce suicide rates.

In elderly patients, the risk of hip fracture when falling can be reduced by as much as 80% by wearing hip protectors, but only about half of patients use them regularly. Oral vitamin D supplementation with 700–800 international units/d appears to reduce the risk of hip and other nonvertebral fractures in both ambulatory and institutionalized elderly persons, but 400 international units/d is not sufficient for fracture prevention.

Finally, clinicians have a critical role in detection, prevention, and management of physical or sexual abuse—in particular, routine assessment of women for risk of domestic violence. In a trial, the 12-month prevalence of intimate partner violence ranged from 4% to 18% depending on the screening method, instrument, and health care setting. Rates of current domestic violence on exit questionnaire were 21% in suburban emergency department and 26% in urban emergency department settings. Inclusion of a single question about domestic violence in the medical history—"At any time, has a partner ever hit you, kicked you, or otherwise physically hurt you?"—can increase identification of this common problem. Another screen consists of three questions: (1) "Have you ever been hit, kicked, punched, or otherwise hurt by someone within the past year? If so, by whom?" (2) "Do you feel safe in your current relationship?" (3) "Is there a partner from a previous relationship who is making you feel unsafe now?" Women seem to prefer written, self-completed screening questionnaires to face-to-face questioning. Alternatively, computer prompts to clinicians may serve as useful reminders to inquiry. Assessment for abuse and offering of referrals to community resources creates potential to interrupt and prevent recurrence of domestic violence and associated trauma. Screening patients in emergency departments for intimate partner violence appears to have no adverse effects related to screening and may lead to increased patient contact with community resources.

Physical and psychological abuse, exploitation, and neglect of older adults are serious underrecognized problems. Clues to elder mistreatment include the patient's appearance, recurrent urgent-care visits, missed appointments, suspicious physical findings, and implausible explanations for injuries.

Bischoff-Ferrari HA et al. Fracture prevention with vitamin D supplementation: a meta-analysis of randomized controlled trials. JAMA. 2005 May 11;293(18):2257–64. [PMID: 15886381]

Collins KA. Elder maltreatment: a review. Arch Pathol Lab Med. 2006 Sep;130(9):1290–6. [PMID: 16948513]

Cusens B et al. Prevention of alcohol-related assault and injury. Hosp Med. 2005 Jun;66(6):346–8. [PMID: 15974163]

Houry D et al. Does screening in the emergency department hurt or help victims of intimate partner violence? Ann Emerg Med. 2008 Apr;51(4):433–42. [PMID: 18313800]

Jackson RD et al; Women's Health Initiative Investigators. Calcium plus vitamin D supplementation and the risk of fractures. N Engl J Med. 2006 Feb 16;354(7):669–83. [PMID: 16481635]

Koroukian SM et al. Analysis of injury- and violence-related fatalities in the Ohio Medicaid population: identifying opportunities for prevention. J Trauma. 2007 Apr;62(4):989–95. [PMID: 17426588]

MacMillan HL et al; McMaster Violence Against Women Research Group. Approaches to screening for intimate partner violence in health care settings: a randomized trial. JAMA. 2006 Aug 2;296(5):530–6. [PMID: 16882959]

Mann JJ et al. Suicide prevention strategies: a systematic review. JAMA. 2005 Oct 26;294(16):2064–74. [PMID: 16249421]

McClure R et al. Population-based interventions for the prevention of fall-related injuries in older people. Cochrane Database Syst Rev 2005;(1):CD004441. [PMID: 15674948]

McFarlane JM et al. Secondary prevention of intimate partner violence: a randomized controlled trial. Nurs Res. 2006 Jan–Feb;55(1):52–61. [PMID: 16439929]

Rhodes KV et al. Lowering the threshold for discussions of domestic violence: a randomized controlled trial of computer screening. Arch Intern Med. 2006 May 22;166(10):1107–14. [PMID: 16717173]

PREVENTION OF SUBSTANCE ABUSE: ALCOHOL & ILLICIT DRUGS

Substance abuse is a major public health problem in the United States. The lifetime prevalence of alcohol abuse is approximately 18%, whereas the lifetime prevalence of alcohol dependence is near 13%. Rates appear to be higher in men, whites, and younger and unmarried individuals. Approximately two-thirds of high school seniors are regular users of alcohol. Alcohol dependence often coexists with other substance disorders as well as with mood, anxiety, and personality disorders. Underdiagnosis and treatment of alcohol abuse is substantial, both because of patient denial and lack of detection of clinical clues. Treatment rates for alcohol dependence have slightly declined over the last several years. Only a quarter of alcohol-dependent patients have ever been treated.

As with cigarette use, clinician identification and counseling about alcoholism may improve the chances of recovery. About 10% of all adults seen in medical practices are problem drinkers. An estimated 15–30% of hospitalized patients have problems with alcohol abuse or dependence, but the connection between patients' presenting complaints and their alcohol abuse is often missed. The CAGE test (see Table 1–10) is both sensitive and specific for chronic alcoholism. However, it is less sensitive in detecting heavy or binge drinking in elderly patients and has been criticized for being less applicable to minority groups or to women. Others recommend asking three questions: (1) How many days per week do you drink (frequency)? (2) On a day when you drink alcohol, how many drinks do you have in one day (quantity)? (3) On how many occasions in the last month did you drink more than five drinks (binge drinking)? The Alcohol Use Disorder Identification Test (AUDIT) consists of questions on the quantity and frequency of alcohol consumption, on alcohol dependence symptoms, and on alcohol-related problems (Table 1–10). The AUDIT questionnaire is a cost-effective and efficient diagnostic tool for routine screening of alcohol use disorders in primary care settings. Choice of therapy remains controversial. However, use of screening procedures and brief intervention methods (Table 1–11; see Chapter 25) can produce a 10–30% reduction in long-term alcohol use and alcohol-related problems. However, brief advice and counseling without regular follow-up and reinforcement cannot sustain significant long-term reductions in unhealthy drinking behaviors.

Several pharmacologic agents are effective in reducing alcohol consumption. In acute alcohol detoxification, standard treatment regimens use long-acting benzodiazepines, the preferred medications for alcohol detoxification, because they can be given on a fixed schedule or through "front-loading" or "symptom-triggered" regimens. Adjuvant sympatholytic medications can be used to treat hyperadrenergic symptoms that persist despite adequate sedation. Three drugs are FDA approved for treatment of alcohol dependence—disulfiram, naltrexone, and acamprosate. Disulfiram, an aversive agent, has significant adverse effects and consequently, compliance difficulties have resulted in no clear evidence that it increases absti-

Table 1-10. Screening for alcohol abuse.

A. CAGE screening test[1]	
Have you ever felt the need to	Cut down on drinking?
Have you ever felt	Annoyed by criticism of your drinking?
Have you ever felt	Guilty about your drinking?
Have you ever taken a morning	Eye opener?

INTERPRETATION: Two "yes" answers are considered a positive screen. One "yes" answer should arouse a suspicion of alcohol abuse.

B. The Alcohol Use Disorder Identification Test (AUDIT).[2] (Scores for response categories are given in parentheses. Scores range from 0 to 40, with a cutoff score of $\geq$ 5 indicating hazardous drinking, harmful drinking, or alcohol dependence.)

1. How often do you have a drink containing alcohol?

(0) Never	(1) Monthly or less	(2) Two to four times a month	(3) Two or three times a week	(4) Four or more times a week

2. How many drinks containing alcohol do you have on a typical day when you are drinking?

(0) 1 or 2	(1) 3 or 4	(2) 5 or 6	(3) 7 to 9	(4) 10 or more

3. How often do you have six or more drinks on one occasion?

(0) Never	(1) Less than monthly	(2) Monthly	(3) Weekly	(4) Daily or almost daily

4. How often during the past year have you found that you were not able to stop drinking once you had started?

(0) Never	(1) Less than monthly	(2) Monthly	(3) Weekly	(4) Daily or almost daily

5. How often during the past year have you failed to do what was normally expected of you because of drinking?

(0) Never	(1) Less than monthly	(2) Monthly	(3) Weekly	(4) Daily or almost daily

6. How often during the past year have you needed a first drink in the morning to get yourself going after a heavy drinking session?

(0) Never	(1) Less than monthly	(2) Monthly	(3) Weekly	(4) Daily or almost daily

7. How often during the past year have you had a feeling of guilt or remorse after drinking?

(0) Never	(1) Less than monthly	(2) Monthly	(3) Weekly	(4) Daily or almost daily

8. How often during the past year have you been unable to remember what happened the night before because you had been drinking?

(0) Never	(1) Less than monthly	(2) Monthly	(3) Weekly	(4) Daily or almost daily

9. Have you or has someone else been injured as a result of your drinking?

(0) No	(2) Yes, but not in the past year	(4) Yes, during the past year

10. Has a relative or friend or a doctor or other health worker been concerned about your drinking or suggested you cut down?

(0) No	(2) Yes, but not in the past year	(4) Yes, during the past year

[1]Source: Mayfield D et al. The CAGE questionnaire: validation of a new alcoholism screening instrument. Am J Psychiatry. 1974;131:1121.
[2]Adapted, with permission, from Piccinelli M et al. Efficacy of the alcohol use disorders identification test as a screening tool for hazardous alcohol intake and related disorders in primary care: a validity study. BMJ. 1997 Feb 8;314(7078):420–4.

nence rates, decreases relapse rates, or reduces cravings. Persons who receive short-term treatment with naltrexone have a lower chance of alcoholism relapse. Compared with placebo, naltrexone can lower the risk of treatment withdrawal in alcohol-dependent patients. Compared with placebo, long-acting intramuscular formulation of naltrexone has been found to be well-tolerated and to reduce drinking significantly among treatment-seeking alcoholics over a 6-month period. In a randomized, controlled trial, patients receiving medical management with naltrexone, a combined behavioral intervention, or both fared better on drinking outcomes, whereas acamprosate showed no evidence of efficacy with or without combined behavioral intervention. Topiramate, although not yet FDA approved for this indication, is a promising treatment for alcohol dependence. In a recent randomized control trial, topiramate was more effective than placebo at reducing the percentage of heavy drinking days from baseline to week 14.

Use of illegal drugs—including cocaine, methamphetamine, and so-called "designer drugs"—either sporadically or episodically remains an important problem. Lifetime prevalence of drug abuse is approximately 8% and is generally greater among men, young and unmarried individuals, Native Americans, and those of lower socioeconomic status. As with alcohol, drug abuse disorders often coexist with personality, anxiety, and other substance abuse disorders.

Abuse of anabolic-androgenic steroids has been associated with use of other illicit drugs, alcohol, and cigarettes and with violence and criminal behavior. As with alcohol abuse, the lifetime treatment rate for drug abuse is low (8%). The recognition of drug abuse presents special

Table 1–11. Basic counseling steps for patients who abuse alcohol.

Establish a therapeutic relationship
Make the medical office or clinic off-limits for substance abuse
Present information about negative health consequences
Emphasize personal responsibility and self-efficacy
Convey a clear message and set goals
Involve family and other supports
Establish a working relationship with community treatment resources
Provide follow-up

Reproduced, with permission, from the United States Department of Health Human Services, U.S. Public Health Service, Office of Disease Prevention Health Promotion. Clinician's Handbook of Preventive Services: Put Prevention Into Practice. U.S. Government Printing Office, 1994.

problems and requires that the clinician actively consider the diagnosis. Clinical aspects of substance abuse are discussed in Chapter 25.

Currently, evidence does not support the use of carbamazepine, disulfiram, mazindol, phenytoin, nimodipine, lithium, antidepressants, or dopamine agonists in the treatment of cocaine dependence. In a methadone maintenance population, the combination of contingency management with bupropion is more effective than bupropion alone for the treatment of cocaine addiction.

Buprenorphine has potential as a medication to ameliorate the symptoms and signs of withdrawal from opioids and has been shown to be effective in reducing concomitant cocaine and opiate abuse. A stepped treatment program for heroin dependence using buprenorphine/naloxone, escalated to methadone if needed, has been shown to be equally effective as methadone maintenance therapy. Cessation of methadone maintenance is possible using buprenorphine by transfer from methadone to buprenorphine and subsequent buprenorphine reductions. Evidence does not support the use of naltrexone in maintenance treatment of opioid addiction. Rapid opioid detoxification with opioid antagonist induction using general anesthesia has emerged as an approach to treat opioid dependence. However, a randomized comparison of buprenorphine-assisted rapid opioid detoxification with naltrexone induction and clonidine-assisted opioid detoxification with delayed naltrexone induction found no significant differences in rates of completion of inpatient detoxification, treatment retention, or proportions of opioid-positive urine specimens, and the anesthesia procedure was associated with more potentially life-threatening adverse events. Finally, cognitive behavior therapy, contingency management, couples and family therapy, and other types of behavioral treatment have been shown to be effective interventions for drug addiction.

Anton RF. Naltrexone for the management of alcohol dependence. N Engl J Med. 2008 Aug 14;359(7):715–21. [PMID: 18703474]

Anton RF et al; COMBINE Study Research Group. Combined pharmacotherapies and behavioral interventions for alcohol dependence: the COMBINE study: a randomized controlled trial. JAMA. 2006 May 3;295(17):2003–17. [PMID: 16670409]

Blondell RD. Ambulatory detoxification of patients with alcohol dependence. Am Fam Physician. 2005 Feb 1;71(3):495–502. [PMID: 15712624]

Compton WM et al. Prevalence, correlates, disability, and comorbidity of DSM-IV drug abuse and dependence in the United States: results from the national epidemiologic survey on alcohol and related conditions. Arch Gen Psychiatry. 2007 May;64(5):566–76. [PMID: 17485608]

Coulton S et al; Stepwice Research Team. Opportunistic screening for alcohol use disorders in primary care: comparative study. BMJ. 2006 Mar 4;332(7540):511–7. [PMID: 16488896]

Garbutt JC et al; Vivitrex Study Group. Efficacy and tolerability of long-acting injectable naltrexone for alcohol dependence: a randomized controlled trial. JAMA. 2005 Apr 6;293(13):1617–25. [PMID: 15811981]

Hasin DS et al. Prevalence, correlates, disability, and comorbidity of DSM-IV alcohol abuse and dependence in the United States: results from the National Epidemiologic Survey on Alcohol and Related Conditions. Arch Gen Psychiatry. 2007 Jul;64(7):830–42. [PMID: 17606817]

Isaacson JH et al. Prescription drug use and abuse. Risk factors, red flags, and prevention strategies. Postgrad Med. 2005 Jul;118(1):19–26. [PMID: 16106916]

Johnson BA et al; Topiramate for Alcoholism Advisory Board; Topiramate for Alcoholism Study Group. Topiramate for treating alcohol dependence: a randomized controlled trial. JAMA. 2007 Oct 10;298(14):1641–51. [PMID: 17925516]

Kakko J et al. A stepped care strategy using buprenorphine and methadone versus conventional methadone maintenance in heroin dependence: a randomized controlled trial. Am J Psychiatry. 2007 May;164(5):797–803. [PMID: 17475739]

Poling J et al. Six-month trial of bupropion with contingency management for cocaine dependence in a methadone-maintained population. Arch Gen Psychiatry. 2006 Feb;63(2):219–28. [PMID: 16461866]

Saitz R. Clinical practice. Unhealthy alcohol use. N Engl J Med. 2005 Feb 10;352(6):596–607. [PMID: 15703424]

Srisurapanont M et al. Opioid antagonists for alcohol dependence. Cochrane Database Syst Rev. 2005;(1):CD001867. [PMID: 15674887]

Williams SH. Medications for treating alcohol dependence. Am Fam Physician. 2005 Nov 1;72(9):1775–80. [PMID: 16300039]

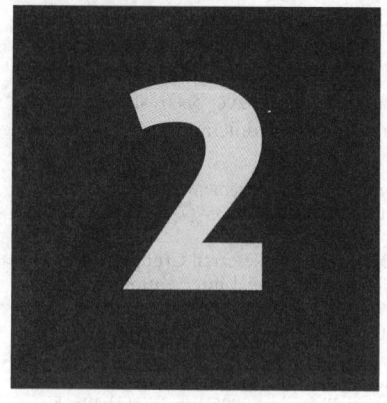

Common Symptoms

Ralph Gonzales, MD, MSPH,
& Paul L. Nadler, MD

COUGH

ESSENTIAL INQUIRIES

- ► Age.
- ► Duration of cough.
- ► Dyspnea (at rest or with exertion).
- ► Tobacco use history.
- ► Vital signs (heart rate, respiratory rate, body temperature).
- ► Chest examination.
- ► Chest radiography when unexplained cough lasts more than 3–6 weeks.

General Considerations

Cough adversely affects personal and work-related interactions, disrupts sleep, and often causes discomfort of the throat and chest wall. Most people seeking medical attention for acute cough desire symptom relief; few are worried about serious illness. Cough results from stimulation of mechanical or chemical afferent nerve receptors in the bronchial tree. Effective cough depends on an intact afferent–efferent reflex arc, adequate expiratory and chest wall muscle strength, and normal mucociliary production and clearance.

Clinical Findings

A. Symptoms

Distinguishing acute (< 3 weeks), persistent (> 3 weeks), and chronic (> 8 weeks) cough illness syndromes is a useful first step in evaluation. In healthy adults, most acute cough syndromes are due to viral respiratory tract infections. Postinfectious cough lasting 3–8 weeks has also been referred to as subacute cough to distinguish this common, distinct clinical entity from acute and chronic cough. Additional features of infection such as fever, nasal congestion, and sore throat help confirm the diagnosis. Dyspnea (at rest or with exertion) may reflect a more serious condition, and further

evaluation should include assessment of oxygenation (pulse oximetry or arterial blood gas measurement), airflow (peak flow or spirometry), and pulmonary parenchymal disease (chest radiography). The timing and character of the cough have not been found to be very useful in establishing the cause of acute cough syndromes, although cough-variant asthma should be considered in adults with prominent nocturnal cough, and persistent cough with phlegm increases the patient's likelihood of chronic obstructive pulmonary disease (COPD). Uncommon causes of acute cough illness should be suspected in those with heart disease (congestive heart failure [CHF]) or hay fever (allergic rhinitis) and those with environmental risk factors (such as farm workers).

Cough due to acute respiratory tract infection resolves within 3 weeks in the vast majority of patients (over 90%). Pertussis infection should be considered in previously immunized adults with persistent or severe cough lasting more than 2–3 weeks and approaches a prevalence of 20% when cough has persisted beyond 3 weeks.

When angiotensin-converting enzyme (ACE) inhibitor therapy, acute respiratory tract infection, and chest radiograph abnormalities are absent, up to 90% of cases of persistent cough are due to or exacerbated by postnasal drip, asthma, or gastroesophageal reflux disease (GERD). A history of nasal or sinus congestion, wheezing, or heartburn should direct subsequent evaluation and treatment, though these conditions frequently cause persistent cough in the absence of typical symptoms. Bronchogenic carcinoma is suspected when cough is accompanied by unexplained weight loss and fevers with night sweats, particularly in persons with significant tobacco or occupational exposures. Persistent cough accompanied by excessive mucus secretions increases the likelihood of COPD, particularly among smokers, or bronchiectasis in a patient with a history of recurrent or complicated pneumonia; chest radiographs are helpful in diagnosis. Dyspnea at rest or with exertion is not commonly reported among patients with persistent cough. The report of dyspnea requires assessment for other evidence of chronic lung disease, CHF, or anemia.

B. Physical Examination

Examination can direct subsequent diagnostic testing for acute and persistent cough. Pneumonia is suspected when

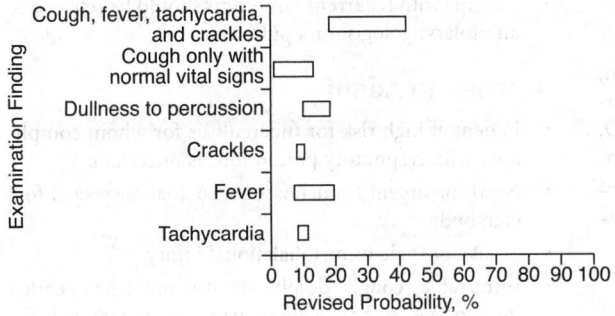

▲ **Figure 2–1.** Revised pneumonia probabilities based on history and physical examination findings. (Reproduced, with permission, from Metlay JP et al. Testing strategies in the initial management of patients with community-acquired pneumonia. Ann Intern Med. 2003 Jan 21;138(2):109–18.)

acute cough is accompanied by vital sign abnormalities (tachycardia, tachypnea, fever). Findings suggestive of airspace consolidation (rales, decreased breath sounds, fremitus, egophony) are significant predictors of community-acquired pneumonia but are present in a small number of cases. Purulent sputum is associated with bacterial infections in patients with structural lung disease (eg, COPD, cystic fibrosis), but it is a poor predictor of pneumonia in the otherwise healthy adult. Wheezing and rhonchi are frequent findings in adults with acute bronchitis and do not represent adult-onset asthma in most cases.

Physical examination of adults with persistent cough should look for evidence of chronic sinusitis, contributing to postnasal drip syndrome or asthma. Chest and cardiac signs may help distinguish COPD from CHF. In patients with cough and dyspnea, a normal match test (ability to blow out a match from 25 cm away) and maximum laryngeal height > 4 cm (measured from the sternal notch to the cricoid cartilage at end expiration) substantially decrease the likelihood of COPD. Similarly, normal jugular venous pressure and negative hepatojugular reflux decrease the likelihood of biventricular CHF.

C. Diagnostic Studies

1. Acute cough—Chest radiography should be considered for any adult with acute cough who shows abnormal vital signs or in whom the chest examination is suggestive of pneumonia. The relationship between specific clinical findings and the probability of pneumonia is shown in Figure 2–1. In patients with dyspnea, pulse oximetry and peak flow help exclude hypoxemia or obstructive airway disease. However, a normal pulse oximetry value (eg, > 93%) does not rule out a significant alveolar–arterial (A–a) gradient when patients have effective respiratory compensation. During documented influenza outbreaks, the positive predictive value of clinical diagnosis of influenza approaches 70% and usually obviates the usefulness of rapid diagnostic tests.

2. Persistent and chronic cough—Chest radiography is indicated when ACE inhibitor therapy–related and postinfectious cough are excluded by history or further diagnostic testing. If pertussis infection is suspected, testing should be performed using polymerase chain reaction on a nasopharyngeal swab or nasal wash specimen—keeping in mind that the ability to detect pertussis decreases as the duration of cough increases. When the chest film is normal, postnasal drip, asthma, and GERD are the most likely causes. The presence of typical symptoms of these conditions directs further evaluation or empiric therapy, though typical symptoms are often absent. Definitive procedures for determining the presence of each are available (Table 2–1). However, empiric treatment with a maximum-strength regimen for postnasal drip, asthma, or GERD for 2–4 weeks is one recommended approach since documenting the presence of postnasal drip, asthma, and GERD does not mean they are the cause of the cough illness. Other alternative approaches include the following: first, identify patients who have corticosteroid-responsive cough by examining induced sputum for increased eosinophil counts (> 3%); second, measure increased exhaled nitric oxide levels; or third, start an empiric trial of prednisolone, 30 mg daily for 2 weeks. Spirometry may help identify large airway obstruction in patients who have persistent cough and wheezing and who are not responding to asthma treatment. When empiric treatment trials are not helpful, additional evaluation with pH manometry, endoscopy, barium swallow, sinus CT or high-resolution chest CT may identify the cause.

▶ Differential Diagnosis

A. Acute Cough

Acute cough may be a symptom of acute respiratory tract infection, asthma, allergic rhinitis, and CHF, as well as a myriad of other less common causes.

Table 2–1. Empiric treatments or tests for persistent cough.

Suspected Condition	Step 1 (Empiric Therapy)	Step 2 (Diagnostic Testing)
Postnasal drip	Therapy for allergy or chronic sinusitis	ENT referral; sinus CT scan
Asthma	β_2-Agonist	Spirometry; consider methacholine challenge if normal
GERD	Proton pump inhibitors	Esophageal pH monitoring

ENT, ear, nose, and throat; GERD, gastroesophageal reflux disease.

B. Persistent and Chronic Cough

Causes of persistent cough include environmental exposures (cigarette smoke, air pollution), pertussis infection, postnasal drip syndrome (or upper airway cough syndrome), asthma (including cough-variant asthma), GERD, COPD, bronchiectasis, eosinophilic bronchitis, tuberculosis or other chronic infection, interstitial lung disease, and bronchogenic carcinoma. Persistent cough may also be psychogenic.

▶ Treatment

A. Acute Cough

Treatment of acute cough should target the underlying etiology of the illness, the cough reflex itself, and any additional factors that exacerbate the cough. When influenza is diagnosed, treatment with amantadine, rimantadine, oseltamivir, or zanamivir is equally effective (1 less day of illness) when initiated within 30–48 hours of illness onset. In the setting of *Chlamydia* or *Mycoplasma*-documented infection or outbreaks, first-line antibiotics include erythromycin, 250 mg orally four times daily for 7 days, or doxycycline, 100 mg orally twice daily for 7 days. In patients diagnosed with acute bronchitis, inhaled β_2-agonist therapy reduces severity and duration of cough in some patients. Evidence supports a modest benefit of dextromethorphan, but not codeine, on cough severity in adults with cough due to acute respiratory tract infections. Treatment of postnasal drip (with antihistamines, decongestants, or nasal corticosteroids) or GERD (with H_2-blockers or proton-pump inhibitors), when accompanying acute cough illness, can also be helpful. There is good evidence that vitamin C and echinacea are not effective in reducing the severity of acute cough illness after it develops; however, evidence does support vitamin C (at least 1 g daily) for prevention of colds among persons with major physical stressors (eg, post-marathon) or malnutrition.

B. Persistent and Chronic Cough

Evaluation and management of persistent cough often requires multiple visits and therapeutic trials, which frequently lead to frustration, anger, and anxiety. When pertussis infection is suspected or confirmed, treatment with macrolide antibiotics is appropriate to reduce shedding and transmission of the organism. When pertussis infection has lasted more than 7–10 days, antibiotic treatment does not affect the duration of cough, which can last up to 6 months. There is no evidence to guide how long treatment for persistent cough due to postnasal drip, asthma, or GERD should be continued.

▶ When to Refer

- Failure to control persistent or chronic cough following empiric treatment trials. The small percentage of patients with idiopathic persistent cough should be managed in consultation with an otolaryngologist or a pulmonologist; treatment options include nebulized lidocaine therapy and morphine sulfate, 5–10 mg orally twice daily.

- Patients with recurrent symptoms should be referred to an otolaryngologist or a pulmonologist.

▶ When to Admit

- Patient at high risk for tuberculosis for whom compliance with respiratory precautions is uncertain.

- Need for urgent bronchoscopy, such as suspected foreign body.

- Smoke or toxic fume inhalational injury.

- Intractable cough despite treatment, when cough impairs gas exchange or in patients at high risk for barotraumas (eg, recent pneumothorax).

Call SA et al. Does this patient have influenza? JAMA. 2005 Feb 23;293(8):987–97. [PMID: 15728170]

Chung KF et al. Prevalence, pathogenesis and causes of chronic cough. Lancet. 2008 Apr 19;371(9621):1364–74. [PMID: 18424325]

Hewlett EL et al. Clinical practice. Pertussis—not just for kids. N Engl J Med. 2005 Mar 24;352(12):1215–22. [PMID: 15788498]

Metlay JP et al. Testing strategies in the initial management of patients with community-acquired pneumonia. Ann Intern Med. 2003 Jan 21;138(2):109–18. [PMID: 12529093]

Morice AH et al. Opiate therapy in chronic cough. Am J Respir Crit Care Med. 2007 Feb 15;175(4):312–5. [PMID: 17122382]

Pavord ID et al. Management of chronic cough. Lancet. 2008 Apr 19;371(9621):1375–84. [PMID: 18424326]

Pratter MR et al. An empiric integrative approach to the management of cough: ACCP evidence-based clinical practice guidelines. Chest. 2006 Jan;129(1 Suppl):222S–231S. [PMID: 16428715]

Wenzel RP et al. Acute bronchitis. N Engl J Med. 2006 Nov 16;355(20):2125–30. [PMID: 17108344]

Yu L et al. Clinical benefit of sequential three-step empirical therapy in the management of chronic cough. Respirology. 2008 May;13(3):353–8. [PMID: 18399856]

DYSPNEA

 ESSENTIAL INQUIRIES

- ▶ Fever.
- ▶ Cough.
- ▶ Chest pain.
- ▶ Vital sign measurements; pulse oximetry.
- ▶ Cardiac and chest examination.
- ▶ Chest radiography.
- ▶ Arterial blood gas measurement.

▶ General Considerations

Dyspnea is a subjective experience or *perception* of uncomfortable breathing. However, the relationship between level of dyspnea and the severity of underlying disease varies widely across individuals. Dyspnea can result from conditions that increase the mechanical effort of breathing (eg, COPD, restrictive lung disease, respiratory muscle weakness), from conditions that produce compensatory tachypnea (eg, hypoxemia or acidosis), or from psychogenic origins. Rate of onset, previous dyspnea, medications, comorbidities, psychological profile, and severity of underlying disorder play a role in how and when persons present with dyspnea. In patients with established COPD, the patient-reported severity of dyspnea is superior to forced expiratory volume in 1 second (FEV_1) in predicting quality of life and 5-year mortality.

▶ Clinical Findings

A. Symptoms

The duration, severity, and periodicity of dyspnea influence the tempo of the clinical evaluation. Rapid onset, severe dyspnea in the absence of other clinical features should raise concern for pneumothorax, pulmonary embolism, or increased left ventricular end-diastolic pressure (LVEDP). Spontaneous pneumothorax is usually accompanied by chest pain and occurs most often in thin, young males, or in those with underlying lung disease. Pulmonary embolism should always be suspected when a patient reports a recent history (previous 4 weeks) of prolonged immobilization, estrogen therapy, or other risk factors for deep venous thrombosis (DVT) (eg, previous history of thromboembolism, cancer, obesity) and when the cause of dyspnea is not apparent. Silent myocardial infarction, which occurs more frequently in diabetic persons and women, can result in acute heart failure and dyspnea.

Accompanying symptoms provide important clues to various etiologies of dyspnea. When cough and fever are present, pulmonary disease (particularly infections) is the primary concern, although myocarditis, pericarditis, and septic emboli can also present in this manner. Chest pain should be further characterized as acute or chronic, pleuritic or exertional. Although acute pleuritic chest pain is the rule in acute pericarditis and pneumothorax, most patients with pleuritic chest pain in the outpatient clinic have pleurisy due to acute viral respiratory tract infection. Periodic chest pain that precedes the onset of dyspnea is suspicious for myocardial ischemia as well as pulmonary embolism. When associated with wheezing, most cases of dyspnea are due to acute bronchitis; however, when acute bronchitis seems unlikely, the clinician should also consider new-onset asthma, foreign body, and vocal cord dysfunction.

When a patient reports prominent dyspnea with mild or no accompanying features, consider noncardiopulmonary causes of impaired oxygen delivery (anemia, methemoglobinemia, cyanide ingestion, carbon monoxide), metabolic acidosis due to a variety of conditions, panic disorder, and chronic pulmonary embolism.

B. Physical Examination

A focused physical examination should include evaluation of the head and neck, chest, heart, and lower extremities. Visual inspection of the patient's respiratory pattern can suggest obstructive airway disease (pursed-lip breathing, use of extra respiratory muscles, barrel-shaped chest),

Table 2–2. Clinical findings suggesting obstructive airway disease.

	Adjusted Likelihood Ratios	
	Factor Present	Factor Absent
> 40 pack-years smoking	11.6	0.9
Age ≥ 45 years	1.4	0.5
Maximum laryngeal height ≤ 4 cm	3.6	0.7
All three factors	58.5	0.3

Reproduced, with permission, from Straus SE et al. The accuracy of patient history, wheezing, and laryngeal measurements in diagnosing obstructive airway disease. CARE-COAD1 Group. Clinical Assessment of the Reliability of the Examination—Chronic Obstructive Airways Disease. JAMA. 2000 Apr 12;283(14):1853–7.

pneumothorax (asymmetric excursion), or metabolic acidosis (Kussmaul respirations). Patients with impending upper airway obstruction (eg, epiglottitis, foreign body), or severe asthma exacerbation, sometimes assume a tripod position. Focal wheezing raises the suspicion for a foreign body or other bronchial obstruction. Maximum laryngeal height (the distance between the top of the thyroid cartilage and the suprasternal notch at end expiration) is a measure of hyperinflation. Obstructive airway disease is virtually nonexistent when a nonsmoking patient younger than 45 years has a maximum laryngeal height ≤ 4 cm (Table 2–2).

A systematic review has identified several clinical predictors of increased LVEDP useful in the evaluation of dyspneic patients with no prior history of CHF (Table 2–3). When none is present, there is a very low probability (< 10%) of increased LVEDP, and when two or more are present, there is a very high probability (> 90%) of increased LVEDP.

Table 2–3. Clinical findings suggesting increased left ventricular end-diastolic pressure.

Tachycardia
Systolic hypotension
Jugular venous distention (> 5-7 cm H_2O)[1]
Hepatojugular reflux (> 1 cm)[2]
Crackles, especially bibasilar
Third heart sound[3]
Lower extremity edema
Radiographic pulmonary vascular redistribution or cardiomegaly[1]

[1]These findings are particularly helpful.
[2]Proper abdominal compression for evaluating hepatojugular reflux requires > 30 seconds of sustained right upper quadrant abdominal compression.
[3]Cardiac auscultation of the patient at 45-degree angle in left lateral decubitus position doubles the detection rate of third heart sounds.
Source: Badgett RG et al. Can the clinical examination diagnose left-sided heart failure in adults? JAMA. 1997 Jun 4;277(21):1712–9.

C. Diagnostic Studies

Causes of dyspnea that can be managed without chest radiography are few: ingestions causing lactic acidosis, methemoglobinemia, and carbon monoxide poisoning. The diagnosis of pneumonia should be confirmed by chest radiography in most patients. When COPD exacerbation is severe enough to require hospitalization, results of chest radiography can influence management decisions in up to 20% of patients. Chest radiography is fairly sensitive and specific for new-onset CHF (represented by redistribution of pulmonary venous circulation) and can help guide treatment decisions in patients with dyspnea secondary to cardiac disease. End-expiratory chest radiography enhances detection of a small pneumothorax.

A normal chest radiograph has substantial diagnostic value. When there is no physical examination evidence of COPD or CHF and the chest radiograph is normal, the major remaining causes of dyspnea include pulmonary embolism, upper airway obstruction, foreign body, anemia, and metabolic acidosis. If a patient has tachycardia and hypoxemia but a normal chest radiograph and electrocardiogram (ECG), then further tests to exclude pulmonary emboli are warranted (see Chapter 9), provided blood tests exclude significant anemia or metabolic acidosis. High-resolution chest CT is particularly useful in the evaluation of pulmonary embolism and has the added benefit of providing information about interstitial and alveolar lung disease.

Serum or whole blood brain natriuretic peptide (BNP) testing can be useful in distinguishing cardiac from noncardiac causes of dyspnea in the emergency department, since elevated BNP levels are both sensitive and specific for increased LVEDP in symptomatic persons.

Persistent uncertainty following clinical examination and routine diagnostic testing warrants arterial blood gas measurement. With two notable exceptions (carbon monoxide poisoning and cyanide toxicity), arterial blood gas measurement distinguishes increased mechanical effort causes of dyspnea (respiratory acidosis with or without hypoxemia) from compensatory tachypnea (respiratory alkalosis with or without hypoxemia or metabolic acidosis) from psychogenic dyspnea (respiratory alkalosis). Carbon monoxide and cyanide impair oxygen delivery with minimal alterations in PO_2; percent carboxyhemoglobin identifies carbon monoxide toxicity. Cyanide poisoning should be considered in a patient with profound lactic acidosis following a theater fire. Suspected carbon monoxide poisoning or methemoglobinemia can also be confirmed with venous carboxyhemoglobin or methemoglobin levels.

Because arterial blood gas testing is impractical in most outpatient settings, **pulse oximetry** has assumed a central role in the office evaluation of dyspnea. Oxygen saturation values above 96% almost always correspond with a $PO_2 > 70$ mm Hg, and values less than 94% almost always represent clinically significant hypoxemia. Important exceptions to this rule include carbon monoxide toxicity, which leads to a normal oxygen saturation (due to the similar wavelengths of oxyhemoglobin and carboxyhemoglobin), and methemoglobinemia, which results in an oxygen saturation of about 85% that fails to increase with supplemental oxygen. A normal or mildly abnormal oxygen saturation (< 90%) in a delirious or obtunded patient with obstructive lung disease warrants immediate measurement of arterial blood gases to exclude hypercapnia and the need for intubation. When pulse oximetry yields equivocal results, assessment of desaturation with ambulation (eg, a brisk walk around the clinic) can be a useful finding (eg, when *Pneumocystis jiroveci* pneumonia is suspected).

Episodic dyspnea can be challenging if an evaluation cannot be performed during symptoms. Life-threatening causes include recurrent pulmonary embolism, myocardial ischemia, and reactive airway disease. When associated with audible wheezing, vocal cord dysfunction should be considered, particularly in a young woman who does not respond to asthma therapy. Spirometry is very helpful in further classifying patients with obstructive airway disease but is rarely needed in the initial or emergent evaluation of patients with acute dyspnea.

▶ Differential Diagnosis

Acute dyspnea, particularly as the chief complaint, demands urgent evaluation. Urgent and emergent conditions causing acute dyspnea include pneumonia, COPD, asthma, pneumothorax, pulmonary embolism, cardiac disease (eg, CHF, acute myocardial infarction, valvular dysfunction, arrhythmia, cardiac shunt), metabolic acidosis, cyanide toxicity, methemoglobinemia, and carbon monoxide poisoning.

▶ Treatment

The treatment of urgent or emergent causes of dyspnea should aim to relieve the underlying cause. Pending diagnosis, patients with hypoxemia should be immediately provided supplemental oxygen unless significant hypercapnia is present or strongly suspected pending arterial blood gas measurement. Dyspnea frequently occurs in patients nearing the end of life; whereas opioid therapy can provide substantial relief independent of the severity of hypoxemia, oxygen therapy appears to be most beneficial to patients with significant hypoxemia (see Chapter 5). In patients with severe COPD, oxygen therapy improves mortality and exercise performance. Pulmonary rehabilitation programs are another therapeutic option for patients with moderate to severe COPD or interstitial pulmonary fibrosis.

▶ When to Refer

- Patients with advanced COPD should be referred to a pulmonologist, and patients with CHF or valvular heart disease should be referred to a cardiologist following acute stabilization.
- Cyanide toxicity should be managed in conjunction with a toxicologist.

▶ When to Admit

- Impaired gas exchange from any cause or high risk of pulmonary embolism pending definitive diagnosis.
- Suspected cyanide poisoning.

Collins SP et al. Diagnostic and prognostic usefulness of natriuretic peptides in emergency department patients with dyspnea. Ann Emerg Med. 2003 Apr;41(4):532–45. [PMID: 12658254]

Cranston JM et al. Oxygen therapy for dyspnoea in adults. Cochrane Database Syst Rev. 2008 Jul 16;(3):CD004769. [PMID: 18646110]

Kapoor JR et al. Diagnostic and therapeutic approach to acute decompensated heart failure. Am J Med. 2007 Feb;120(2):121–7. [PMID: 17275448]

Karnani NG et al. Evaluation of chronic dyspnea. Am Fam Physician. 2005 Apr 15;71(8):1529–37. [PMID: 15864893]

Nonoyama ML et al. Effect of oxygen on health quality of life in patients with chronic obstructive pulmonary disease with transient exertional hypoxemia. Am J Respir Crit Care Med. 2007 Aug 15;176(4):343–9. [PMID: 17446339]

Voll-Aanerud M et al. Changes in respiratory symptoms and health-related quality of life. Chest. 2007 Jun;131(6):1890–7. [PMID: 17505046]

HEMOPTYSIS

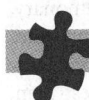

ESSENTIAL INQUIRIES

▸ Smoking history.

▸ Fever, cough, and other symptoms of lower respiratory tract infection.

▸ Nasopharyngeal or gastrointestinal bleeding.

▸ Chest radiography and complete blood count.

General Considerations

Hemoptysis is the expectoration of blood that originates below the vocal cords. It is commonly classified as trivial, mild, or massive—the latter defined as more than 200–600 mL (about 1–2 cups) in 24 hours. The dividing lines are arbitrary, since the amount of blood is rarely quantified with precision. Massive hemoptysis can be usefully defined as any amount that is hemodynamically significant or threatens ventilation, in which case the initial management goal is not diagnostic but therapeutic.

The lungs are supplied with a dual circulation. The pulmonary arteries arise from the right ventricle to supply the pulmonary parenchyma in a low-pressure circuit. The bronchial arteries arise from the aorta or intercostal arteries and carry blood under systemic pressure to the airways, blood vessels, hila, and visceral pleura. Although the bronchial circulation represents only 1–2% of total pulmonary blood flow, it can increase dramatically under conditions of chronic inflammation—eg, chronic bronchiectasis—and is frequently the source of hemoptysis.

The causes of hemoptysis can be classified anatomically. Blood may arise from the airways in COPD, bronchiectasis, and bronchogenic carcinoma; from the pulmonary vasculature in left ventricular failure, mitral stenosis, pulmonary embolism, and arteriovenous malformations; or from the pulmonary parenchyma in pneumonia, inhalation of crack cocaine, or autoimmune diseases (such as Goodpasture disease or Wegener granulomatosis). Diffuse alveolar hemorrhage is due to small vessel bleeding usually caused by autoimmune or hematologic disorders and results in alveolar infiltrates on chest radiography. Most cases of hemoptysis presenting in the outpatient setting are due to infection (eg, acute or chronic bronchitis, pneumonia, tuberculosis). Hemoptysis due to lung cancer increases with age, accounting for up to 20% of cases among the elderly. Less commonly (< 10% of cases), pulmonary venous hypertension (eg, mitral stenosis, pulmonary embolism) causes hemoptysis. Most cases of hemoptysis that have no visible cause on CT scan or bronchoscopy will resolve within 6 months without treatment, with the notable exception of patients at high risk for lung cancer (smokers older than 40 years). Iatrogenic hemorrhage may follow transbronchial lung biopsies, anticoagulation, or pulmonary artery rupture due to distal placement of a balloon-tipped catheter. No cause is identified in up to 15–30% of cases.

Clinical Findings

A. Symptoms

Blood-tinged sputum in the setting of an upper respiratory tract infection in an otherwise healthy, young (age < 40 years) nonsmoker does not warrant an extensive diagnostic evaluation if the hemoptysis subsides with resolution of the infection. However, hemoptysis is frequently a sign of serious disease, especially in patients with a high prior probability of underlying pulmonary pathology. One should not distinguish between blood-streaked sputum and cough productive of blood alone with regard to the evaluation plan. The goal of the history is to identify patients at risk for one of the disorders listed above. Pertinent features include past or current tobacco use, duration of symptoms, and the presence of respiratory infection. Nonpulmonary sources of hemorrhage—from the nose or the gastrointestinal tract—should also be excluded.

B. Physical Examination

Elevated pulse, hypotension, and decreased oxygen saturation suggest large volume hemorrhage that warrants emergent evaluation and stabilization. The nares and oropharynx should be carefully inspected to identify a potential upper airway source of bleeding. Chest and cardiac examination may reveal evidence of CHF or mitral stenosis.

C. Diagnostic Studies

Diagnostic evaluation should include a chest radiograph and complete blood count. Kidney function tests, urinalysis, and coagulation studies are appropriate in specific circumstances. Hematuria that accompanies hemoptysis may be a clue to Goodpasture syndrome or vasculitis. Flexible bronchoscopy reveals endobronchial cancer in 3–6% of patients with hemoptysis who have a normal (nonlateralizing) chest radiograph. Nearly all of these patients are smokers over the age of 40, and most will have had symptoms for more than 1 week. Bronchoscopy is indicated in such patients. High-resolution chest CT scan complements bronchoscopy and should be strongly considered in patients with normal chest radiograph and low risk for malignancy. It can visualize unsuspected bronchiectasis and arteriovenous malformations and will show central endobronchial lesions in many cases. High-resolution chest CT scanning is the test of choice for suspected small peripheral malignancies. CT angiography has become the initial test of choice for evaluating patients with suspected pulmonary embolism, although caution should be taken to avoid large contrast loads in patients with even mild chronic kidney disease (serum creatinine > 2.0 g/dL or rapidly rising creatinine in normal range).

Treatment

The management of mild hemoptysis consists of identifying and treating the specific cause. Massive hemoptysis is life-threatening. The airway must be protected, ventilation ensured, and effective circulation maintained. If the location of the bleeding site is known, the patient should be placed in the decubitus position with the involved lung dependent. Uncontrollable hemorrhage warrants rigid bronchoscopy and surgical consultation. In stable patients, flexible bronchoscopy may localize the site of bleeding, and angiography can embolize the involved bronchial arteries. Embolization is effective initially in 85% of cases, although rebleeding may occur in up to 20% of patients over the following year. The anterior spinal artery arises from the bronchial artery in up to 5% of people, and paraplegia may result if it is inadvertently cannulated.

When to Refer

- When bronchoscopic evaluation of lower respiratory tract is required, refer patients to a pulmonologist.
- Patients should be referred to an otolaryngologist for evaluation of upper respiratory tract bleeding source.
- Patients with severe coagulopathy complicating management should be referred to a hematologist.

When to Admit

- To stabilize bleeding process in patients at risk for or experiencing massive hemoptysis.
- To correct disordered coagulation (clotting factors or platelets, or both).
- To stabilize gas exchange.

Bidwell JL et al. Hemoptysis: diagnosis and management. Am Fam Physician. 2005 Oct 1;72(7):1253–60. [PMID: 16225028]

Corder R. Hemoptysis. Emerg Med Clin North Am. 2003 May;21(2):421–35. [PMID: 12793622]

Flume PA et al. Massive hemoptysis in cystic fibrosis. Chest. 2005 Aug;128(2):729–38. [PMID: 16100161]

Jones R et al. Alarm symptoms in early diagnosis of cancer in primary care: cohort study using General Practice Research Database. BMJ. 2007 May 19;334(7602):1040. [PMID: 17493982]

Tsoumakidou M et al. A prospective analysis of 184 hemoptysis cases: diagnostic impact of chest X-ray, computed tomography, bronchoscopy. Respiration. 2006;73(6):808–14. [PMID: 16446530]

CHEST PAIN

▶ Chest pain onset, character, location/size, duration, periodicity, and exacerbators.

▶ Shortness of breath.

▶ Vital signs.

▶ Chest and cardiac examination.

▶ Electrocardiography.

▶ Biomarkers of myocardial necrosis.

General Considerations

Chest pain (or chest discomfort) is a common symptom that can occur as a result of cardiovascular, pulmonary, pleural, or musculoskeletal disease, esophageal or other gastrointestinal disorders, or anxiety states. The frequency and distribution of life-threatening causes of chest pain, such as acute coronary syndrome (ACS), pericarditis, aortic dissection, pulmonary embolism, pneumonia, and esophageal perforation, vary substantially between clinical settings. Systemic lupus erythematosus, rheumatoid arthritis, and HIV are conditions that until only recently have been recognized as conferring a strong risk for coronary artery disease. Because pulmonary embolism can present with a wide variety of symptoms, consideration of the diagnosis and rigorous risk factor assessment for venous thromboembolism (VTE) is critical. Classic VTE risk factors include cancer, trauma, recent surgery, prolonged immobilization, pregnancy, oral contraceptives, and family history and prior history of VTE. Other conditions associated with increased risk of pulmonary embolism include CHF and COPD. Although uncommon in the office setting, delays in diagnosing life-threatening causes of chest pain can result in serious morbidity and mortality.

Clinical Findings

A. Symptoms

Myocardial ischemia is usually described as dull, aching sensation of "pressure," "tightness," "squeezing," or "gas," rather than as sharp or spasmodic. Ischemic symptoms usually subside within 5–20 minutes but may last longer. Progressive symptoms or symptoms at rest may represent unstable angina due to coronary plaque rupture and thrombosis. Prolonged chest pain episodes might represent myocardial infarction, although up to one-third of patients with acute myocardial infarction do not report chest pain. When present, pain due to myocardial ischemia is commonly accompanied by a sense of anxiety or uneasiness. The location is usually retrosternal or left precordial. Because the heart lacks somatic innervation, precise localization of pain due to cardiac ischemia is difficult; the pain is commonly referred to the throat, lower jaw, shoulders, inner arms, upper abdomen, or back. Ischemic pain may

Table 2–4. Likelihood ratios (LRs) for clinical features associated with acute myocardial infarction.

Clinical Feature	LR+ (95% CI)
History	
Chest pain that radiates to the left arm	2.3 (1.7–3.1)
Chest pain that radiates to the right shoulder	2.9 (1.4–3.0)
Chest pain that radiates to both arms	7.1 (3.6–14.2)
Pleuritic chest pain	0.2 (0.2–0.3)
Sharp or stabbing chest pain	0.3 (0.2–0.5)
Positional chest pain	0.3 (0.2–0.4)
Chest pain reproduced by palpation	0.2–0.4[1]
Nausea or vomiting	1.9 (1.7–2.3)
Diaphoresis	2.0 (1.9–2.2)
Physical examination	
Systolic blood pressure ≤ 80 mm Hg	3.1 (1.8–5.2)
Pulmonary crackles	2.1 (1.4–3.1)
Third heart sound	3.2 (1.6–6.5)
Electrocardiogram	
Any ST segment elevation (≥ 1 mm)	11.2 (7.1–17.8)
Any ST segment depression	3.2 (2.5–4.1)
Any Q wave	3.9 (2.7–7.7)
Any conduction defect	2.7 (1.4–5.4)
New ST segment elevation (≥ 1 mm)	5.7–53.9[1]
New ST segment depression	3.0–5.2[1]
New Q wave	5.3–24.8[1]
New conduction defect	6.3 (2.5–15.7)

[1]Heteregenous studies do not allow for calculation of a point estimate.
Adapted, with permission, from Panju AA et al. The rational clinical examination. Is this patient having a myocardial infarction? JAMA. 1998 Oct 14;280(14):1256–63.

be precipitated or exacerbated by exertion, cold temperature, meals, stress, or combinations of these factors and is usually relieved by rest. However, many episodes do not conform to these patterns; and atypical presentations of ACS are more common in the elderly, women, and persons with diabetes. Other symptoms that are associated with ACS include shortness of breath; dizziness; a feeling of impending doom; and vagal symptoms, such as nausea and diaphoresis. In the elderly, fatigue is a common presenting complaint of ACS. Likelihood ratios for cardinal symptoms considered in the evaluation of acute myocardial infarction are summarized in Table 2–4.

Hypertrophy of either ventricle or aortic stenosis may also give rise to chest pain with less typical features. Pericarditis may produce pain that is greater when supine than upright and may increase with respiration, coughing, or swallowing. Pleuritic chest pain is usually not ischemic, and pain on palpation should signal a musculoskeletal cause. Aortic dissection classically produces an abrupt onset of tearing pain of great intensity that often radiates to the back; however, this classic presentation occurs in a small proportion of cases. Anterior aortic dissection can also lead to myocardial or cerebrovascular ischemia.

Pulmonary embolism has a wide range of clinical presentations, with chest pain present in only 75% of cases. The chief objective in evaluating patients with suspected pulmonary embolism is to assess the patient's clinical risk for VTE based on medical history and associated signs and symptoms (see above and Chapter 9). Esophageal perforation of the thoracic region is another cause of chest pain, with most cases resulting from medical procedures of the esophagus.

B. Physical Examination

Findings on physical examination can occasionally yield important clues to the underlying cause of chest pain; however, a normal physical examination should never be used as the sole basis for ruling-out most diagnoses, particularly ACS and aortic dissection. Vital sign measurement, including pulse oximetry, is always the first step for assessing the urgency and tempo of the subsequent examination and diagnostic work-up.

Findings that increase the likelihood of ACS include diaphoresis, hypotension, S3 or S4 gallop, pulmonary crackles, or elevated jugular venous pressure (see Table 2–4). Although chest pain that is reproducible or worsened with palpation strongly suggests a musculoskeletal cause, up to 15% of patients with ACS will have reproducible chest wall tenderness. Pointing to the location of the pain with one finger has been shown to be highly correlated with nonischemic chest pain. Aortic dissection can result in differential blood pressures (> 20 mm Hg), pulse amplitude deficits, and new diastolic murmurs. Although hypertension is considered the rule in patients with aortic dissection, systolic blood pressure < 100 mm Hg is present in up to 25% of patients.

A cardiac friction rub represents pericarditis until proven otherwise. It can best be heard with the patient sitting forward at end-expiration. Tamponade should be excluded in all patients with a clinical diagnosis of pericarditis by assessing pulsus paradoxus (a decrease in systolic blood pressure during inspiration > 10 mm Hg) and inspection of jugular venous pulsations. Subcutaneous emphysema is common following cervical esophageal perforation but present in only about one-third of thoracic perforations (ie, those most commonly presenting with chest pain).

The absence of physical examination findings in patients with suspected pulmonary embolism usually serves to *increase* the likelihood of pulmonary embolism, although a normal physical examination is also compatible with the much more common conditions of panic/anxiety disorder and musculoskeletal disease.

C. Diagnostic Studies

Unless a competing diagnosis can be confirmed, an ECG is warranted in the initial evaluation of most patients with acute chest pain to help exclude ACS. ST segment elevation is the ECG finding that is the strongest predictor of acute myocardial infarction (see Table 2–4); however, up to 20%

of patients with ACS can have a normal ECG. A recent study concluded that patients with suspected ACS can be safely removed from cardiac monitoring in the emergency department if they are pain-free at initial physician assessment and have a normal or nonspecific ECG. This decision rule had 100% sensitivity for serious arrhythmia (95% confidence interval, 80–100%), but deserves further validation. Clinically stable patients with cardiovascular disease risk factors, normal ECG, normal cardiac biomarkers and no alternative diagnosis should be followed-up with a timely exercise stress test that includes perfusion imaging. The ECG can also provide evidence for alternative diagnoses, such as pericarditis and pulmonary embolism. Chest radiography is often useful in the evaluation of chest pain, and is always indicated when cough or shortness of breath accompanies chest pain. Findings of pneumomediastinum or new pleural effusion are consistent with esophageal perforation. CT is the study of choice at most centers for the diagnosis of esophageal perforation as well as for aortic dissection (helical CT).

In the evaluation of pulmonary embolism, diagnostic test decisions and results must be interpreted in the context of the clinical likelihood of VTE. A negative D-dimer test is helpful for excluding pulmonary embolism in patients with low clinical probability of VTE (3 month incidence = 0.5%); however, the 3-month risk of VTE among patients with intermediate and high risk of VTE is sufficiently high in the setting of a negative D-dimer test (3.5% and 21.4%, respectively) to warrant further imaging given the life-threatening nature of this condition if left untreated. CT angiography (with helical or multidetector CT imaging) has replaced ventilation-perfusion scanning as the preferred diagnostic test for pulmonary embolism, having approximately 90–95% sensitivity and 95% specificity for detecting pulmonary embolism (compared with pulmonary angiography). However, according to guidelines published by the American Academy of Family Physicians and the American College of Physicians (AAFP/ACP), the sensitivity of helical CT is probably not sufficiently high to exclude pulmonary embolism among patients with high clinical probability of VTE, in whom lower extremity ultrasound or pulmonary angiogram may be appropriate. When ventilation-perfusion scanning is performed, only results that are normal or high probability are useful for improving one's clinical assessment of pulmonary embolism.

Panic disorder is a common cause of chest pain, accounting for up to 25% of cases that present to emergency departments and a higher proportion of cases presenting in primary care office practices. Features that correlate with an increased likelihood of panic disorder include absence of coronary artery disease, atypical quality of chest pain, female sex, younger age, and a high level of self-reported anxiety.

► Treatment

Treatment of chest pain should be guided by the underlying etiology. The term "noncardiac chest pain" is used to describe patients who evade diagnosis after receiving extensive work-up. Although under-studied, one small trial of patients with noncardiac chest pain found that about half fulfilled criteria for anxiety or depression and almost half reported symptom improvement with high-dose proton-pump inhibitor therapy.

► When to Refer

- Refer patients with poorly controlled, noncardiac chest pain to a pain specialist.
- Refer with sickle cell anemia to a hematologist.

► When to Admit

- Failure to adequately exclude (to a sufficient degree) life-threatening causes of chest pain, particularly myocardial infarction, dissecting aortic aneurysm, pulmonary embolism, and esophageal rupture.
- Pain control for rib fracture that impairs gas exchange.

Candell-Riera J et al. Yield of early rest and stress myocardial perfusion single-photon emission computed tomography and electrocardiographic exercise test in patients with atypical chest pain, nondiagnostic electrocardiogram, and negative biochemical markers in the emergency department. Am J Cardiol. 2007 Jun 15;99(12):1662–6. [PMID: 17560871]

Fletcher GF et al. Update on exercise stress testing. Am Fam Physician. 2006 Nov 15;74(10):1749–54. [PMID: 17137006]

Gatien M et al. A clinical decision rule to identify which chest pain patients can safely be removed from cardiac monitoring in the emergency department. Ann Emerg Med. 2007 Aug;50(2):136–43. [PMID: 17498844]

Kass SM et al. Pleurisy. Am Fam Physician. 2007 May 1;75(9):1357–64. [PMID: 17508531]

Marcus GM et al. The utility of gestures in patients with chest discomfort. Am J Med. 2007 Jan;120(1):83–9. [PMID: 17208083]

Qaseem A et al. Current diagnosis of venous thromboembolism in primary care: a clinical practice guideline from the American Academy of Family Physicians and the American College of Physicians. Ann Fam Med. 2007 Jan–Feb;5(1):57–62. [PMID: 17261865]

Winters ME et al. Identifying chest pain emergencies in the primary care setting. Prim Care. 2006 Sep;33(3):625–42. [PMID: 17088152]

PALPITATIONS

ESSENTIAL INQUIRIES

- ► Forceful, rapid, or irregular beating of the heart.
- ► Rate, duration, and degree of regularity of heart beat.
- ► Age at first episode.
- ► Factors that precipitate or terminate episodes.
- ► Light-headedness or syncope.
- ► Chest pain.

► General Considerations

Palpitations are defined as an unpleasant awareness of the forceful, rapid, or irregular beating of the heart. They are a common presenting complaint and are usually benign; however, they are occasionally the symptom of a life-threatening arrhythmia. To avoid missing a dangerous cause of the patient's symptom, clinicians sometimes pursue expensive and invasive testing when a conservative diagnostic evaluation is sufficient. The converse is also true; in one study, 54% of patients with supraventricular tachycardia were initially wrongly diagnosed with panic, stress, or anxiety disorder. A disproportionate number of these misdiagnosed patients are women.

▶ Clinical Findings

A. Symptoms

Although described by patients in a myriad of ways, guiding the patient through a careful description of their palpitations may indicate a mechanism and narrow the differential diagnosis. Pertinent questions include the age at first episode; precipitants; and the rate, duration, and degree of regularity of the heart beat during the subjective palpitations. The examiner can ask the patient to "tap out" the rhythm with their fingers. The circumstances associated with onset and termination can also be helpful in determining the cause. Palpitations that start and stop abruptly suggest supraventricular or ventricular tachycardias. Patient-terminated palpitations using vagal maneuvers (such as the Valsalva maneuver) suggests supraventricular tachycardia.

Three common descriptions of palpitations are (1) "flip-flopping" (or "stop and start"), often caused by premature contraction of the atrium or ventricle, with the perceived "stop" from the pause following the contraction, and the "start" from the subsequent forceful contraction; (2) rapid "fluttering in the chest," with regular "fluttering" suggesting supraventricular or ventricular arrhythmias (including sinus tachycardia) and irregular "fluttering" suggesting atrial fibrillation, atrial flutter, or tachycardia with variable block; and (3) "pounding in the neck" or neck pulsations, often due to "cannon" A waves in the jugular venous pulsations that occur when the right atrium contracts against a closed tricuspid valve.

Palpitations associated with chest pain suggests ischemic heart disease, or if the chest pain is relieved by leaning forward, pericardial disease is suspected. Palpitations associated with light-headedness, presyncope, or syncope suggests hypotension and may signify a life-threatening cardiac arrhythmia. Palpitations that occur regularly with exertion suggests a rate-dependent bypass tract or hypertrophic cardiomyopathy. If a benign etiology for these concerning symptoms cannot be ascertained at the index visit, then ambulatory monitoring or prolonged cardiac monitoring in the hospital might be warranted.

Noncardiac symptoms should also be elicited since the palpitations may be caused by a normal heart responding to a metabolic or inflammatory condition. Weight loss may suggest hyperthyroidism. Palpitations can be precipitated by vomiting or diarrhea that leads to electrolyte disorders and hypovolemia. Palpitations associated with hyperventilation, hand tingling, and nervousness are common when anxiety or panic disorder is the root cause.

B. Physical Examination

It is uncommon for the clinician to have the opportunity to examine a patient during an episode of palpitations. However, careful cardiovascular examination can find abnormalities that can increase the likelihood of specific cardiac arrhythmias. The midsystolic click of mitral valve prolapse can suggest the diagnosis of a supraventricular arrhythmia as the cause for the palpitations. The harsh holosystolic murmur of hypertrophic cardiomyopathy, which occurs along the left sternal border and increases with the Valsalva maneuver, suggests atrial fibrillation or ventricular tachycardia. The presence of dilated cardiomyopathy, suggested on examination by a displaced and enlarged cardiac point-of-maximal impulse, increases the likelihood of ventricular tachycardia and atrial fibrillation. In patients with chronic atrial fibrillation, in-office exercise (eg, a brisk walk in the hallway) may reveal an intermittent accelerated ventricular response as the cause of the palpitations. The clinician should also look for signs of hyperthyroidism, such as tremulousness, brisk deep tendon reflexes, fine hand tremor, or signs of stimulant drug use (such as dilated pupils or skin or nasal septal lesions).

C. Diagnostic Studies

The two cardiac studies that are commonly used in the initial evaluation of a patient with palpitations are the 12-lead ECG and ambulatory monitoring devices, such as the Holter monitor or the event recorder.

A 12-lead ECG should be performed on all patients reporting palpitations because it can provide evidence for a wide variety of causes. Although in most instances a specific arrhythmia will not be detected on the tracing, a careful evaluation of the ECG can help the clinician deduce a likely etiology in certain circumstances.

For instance, bradyarrhythmias and heart block can be associated with ventricular ectopy or escape beats that may be experienced as palpitations by the patient. Evidence of prior myocardial infarction by history or on ECG (eg, Q waves) increases the patient's risk for nonsustained or sustained ventricular tachycardia. Ventricular preexcitation (Wolff-Parkinson-White syndrome) is suggested by a short PR interval (< 0.20 ms) and delta waves (upsloping PR segments). Left ventricular hypertrophy with deep septal Q waves in I, AVL, and V4 through V6 is seen in patients with hypertrophic obstructive cardiomyopathy. The presence of left atrial enlargement as suggested by a terminal P-wave force in V1 more negative than 0.04 msec and notched in lead II reflects a patient at increased risk for atrial fibrillation. A prolonged QT interval and abnormal T-wave morphology suggests the long-QT syndrome, which puts patients at increased risk for ventricular tachycardia.

For high-risk patients (Table 2–5), further diagnostic studies are warranted. A step-wise approach has been suggested—starting with ambulatory monitoring devices (Holter monitoring if the palpitations are expected to occur within the subsequent 72-hour period, event monitoring if less frequent), followed by invasive electrophysiologic testing if the ambulatory monitor records a worrisome arrhythmia or if serious arrhythmias are strongly

Table 2–5. Palpitations: Patients at high risk for a cardiovascular cause.

Historical risk factors
Family history of significant arrhythmias
Personal or family history of syncope or resuscitated sudden death
History of myocardial infarction (and likely scarred myocardium)
Physical examination findings
Structural heart disease such as dilated or hypertrophic cardio-myopathies
Valvular disease (stenotic or regurgitant)
ECG findings
Long QT syndrome
Bradycardia
Second- or third-degree heart block
Sustained ventricular arrhythmias

suspected despite normal findings on an appropriate ambulatory monitor.

In patients with a prior myocardial infarction, ambulatory cardiac monitoring or signal-averaged-ECG are appropriate next steps to assess ventricular tachycardia. ECG exercise testing is appropriate in patients who have palpitations with physical exertion and patients with suspected coronary artery disease. Echocardiography is useful when physical examination or ECG suggests structural abnormalities or decreased ventricular function.

Differential Diagnosis

When assessing a patient with palpitations in an urgent care setting, the clinician must ascertain whether the symptoms represent (1) an arrhythmia that is minor and transient, (2) significant cardiovascular disease, (3) a cardiac manifestation of a systemic disease such as thyrotoxicosis, or (4) a benign somatic symptom that is amplified by underlying psychosocial characteristics of the patient.

Patients who seek medical attention in the emergency department instead of a medical clinic are more likely to have a cardiac etiology (47% versus 21%), while psychiatric causes are more common among patients with palpitations who seek medical attention in office practices (45% versus 27%). In a study of patients who went to a university medical clinic with the chief complaint of palpitations, etiologies were cardiac in 43%, psychiatric in 31%, and miscellaneous in 10% (including illicit drugs, medications, anemia, thyrotoxicosis, and mastocytosis).

Cardiac arrhythmias that can result in symptoms of palpitations include sinus bradycardia; sinus, supraventricular, and ventricular tachycardia; premature ventricular and atrial contractions; sick sinus syndrome; and advanced atrioventricular block.

Nonarrhythmic cardiac causes of palpitations include valvular heart diseases, such as aortic insufficiency or stenosis, atrial or ventricular septal defect, cardiomyopathy, congenital heart disease, and pericarditis.

Noncardiac causes of palpitations include fever, dehydration, hypoglycemia, anemia, thyrotoxicosis, and pheochromocytoma. Drugs such as cocaine, alcohol, caffeine, and pseudoephedrine can precipitate palpitations, as can prescription medications, including digoxin, phenothiazines, theophylline, and β-agonists as well as ephedra-containing herbal remedies or supplements (now banned by the US Food and Drug Administration).

The most common psychiatric causes of palpitations are anxiety and panic disorder. The release of catecholamines during a panic attack or significant stress can trigger an arrhythmia. Asking a single question, "Have you experienced brief periods, for seconds or minutes, of an overwhelming panic or terror that was accompanied by racing heartbeats, shortness of breath, or dizziness?" can help identify patients with panic disorder.

▶ Treatment

After ambulatory monitoring, most patients with palpitations are found to have benign atrial or ventricular ectopy and nonsustained ventricular tachycardia. In patients with structurally normal hearts, these arrhythmias are not associated with adverse outcomes. Abstention from caffeine and tobacco may help. Often, reassurance suffices. If not, or in very symptomatic patients, a trial of a β-blocker may be prescribed. For treatment of specific atrial or ventricular arrhythmias, see Chapter 10.

▶ When to Refer

- For electrophysiologic studies.
- For advice regarding treatment of atrial or ventricular arrhythmias.

▶ When to Admit

- Palpitations associated with syncope or near-syncope, particularly when the patient is aged 75 years or older and has an abnormal ECG, hematocrit < 30%, shortness of breath, respiratory rate > 24/min, or a history of CHF.
- Patients with risk factors for a serious arrhythmia.

Abbott AV. Diagnostic approach to palpitations. Am Fam Physician. 2005;71(4):743–50. [PMID: 15742913]

Barsky AJ. Palpitations, arrhythmias, and awareness of cardiac activity. Ann Intern Med. 2001;134(9 Pt 2):832–7. [PMID: 11346318]

Delacrétaz E. Clinical practice. Supraventricular tachycardia. N Engl J Med. 2006 Mar 9;354(10):1039–51. [PMID: 16525141]

Ehlers A et al. Psychological and perceptual factors associated with arrhythmias and benign palpitations. Psychosomat Med. 2000;62(5):693–702. [PMID: 11020100]

Giada F et al. Recurrent unexplained palpitations (RUP) study comparison of implantable loop recorder versus conventional diagnostic strategy. J Am Coll Cardiol. 2007 May 15;49(19):1951–6. [PMID: 17498580]

Pittler MH et al. Adverse events of herbal food supplements for body weight reduction: systematic review. Obes Rev. 2005;6:93–111. [PMID: 15836459]

Rao A et al. Ambulatory cardiac rhythm monitoring. Br J Hosp Med (Lond). 2007;68:132–8. [PMID: 17419460]

Taggart NW et al. Diagnostic miscues in congenital long-QT syndrome. Circulation. 2007 May 22;115(20):2613–20. [PMID: 17502575]

ACUTE KNEE PAIN

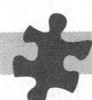

ESSENTIAL INQUIRIES

▶ Trauma.

▶ Swelling.

▶ Fever.

▶ Symptoms of "locking" or "catching."

General Considerations

The knee is the largest joint in the body and is susceptible to injury from trauma, inflammation from infection and arthritis, and degenerative changes.

The knee is a hinge joint. The joint line exists between the femoral condyles and tibial plateaus. Separating and cushioning these bony surfaces is the lateral and medial **meniscal cartilage**, which functions as a shock absorber during weight bearing. The patella is a large sesamoid bone anterior to the joint line. It is embedded in the quadriceps tendon, and it articulates with the trochlear groove of the femur. The knee is stabilized by the collateral ligaments from varus (lateral collateral ligament) and valgus (medial collateral ligament) stresses. The tibia is limited in its anterior movement by the anterior cruciate ligament and in its posterior movement by the posterior cruciate ligament. The bursae of the knee are located between the skin and bony prominences. They are sac-like structures with a synovial lining. They act to decrease friction of tendons and muscles as they move over adjacent bony structures. Excessive external pressure, overuse (friction), or inflammation can lead to swelling and pain of the bursae. The most common bursa to cause "knee pain" when inflamed are the prepatellar bursae (located between the skin and patella), and the pes anserine bursa (which is medial and inferior to the patella, just below the tibial plateau).

When there is a knee joint effusion caused by increased fluid in the interarticular space, physical examination will demonstrate swelling in the hollow around the patella and distention into the suprapatellar space (superior to the patella). Joint fluid, when excessive due to synovitis or trauma, can track posteriorly through a potential space, resulting in a popliteal cyst (also called Baker cyst). Other structures that are susceptible to injury and that may cause a patient to report knee pain (but that are not formally part of the knee joint) are the iliotibial band and the fibular head. The iliotibial band is a fascial structure that crosses the prominence of the lateral femoral condyle to attach to the fibular head. The fibular head is susceptible to fracture from trauma.

Clinical Findings

A careful history, coupled with a physical examination that specifically tests anatomic structures is frequently sufficient to establish a diagnosis. Radiologic studies and laboratory testing of aspirated joint fluid, when indicated, can

Table 2–6. Differential diagnosis of knee pain.

Mechanical dysfunction or disruption
"Internal derangement of the knee"—injury to the menisci or ligaments
Degenerative changes caused by osteoarthritis
Dynamic dysfunction or misalignment of the patella
Fracture as a result of trauma
Increased intra-articular pressure or inflammation
"Internal derangement of the knee"—injury to the menisci or ligaments
Inflammation or infection of the knee joint
Ruptured popliteal ("Baker") cyst
Peri-articular inflammation
"Internal derangement of the knee"—injury to the menisci or ligaments
Prepatellar or anserine bursitis
Ligamentous sprain

lead to a definitive diagnosis in most patients. The differential diagnosis of knee pain is found in Table 2–6.

A. History

Evaluation of knee pain should begin with general questions regarding duration and rapidity of symptom onset; a history of trauma; stress or compression from sports, hobbies, or occupation; symptoms of infection (fever, recent bacterial infections, risk factors for sexually transmitted infections [such as gonorrhea] or other bacterial infections [such as staphylococcal infection]). Previous orthopedic problems with, or surgery to, the affected knee should also be specifically queried.

B. Symptoms

1. Presence of clicking or popping, although nonspecific, may be indicative of osteoarthritis or the patellofemoral syndrome.

2. "Locking" or "catching" when walking suggests meniscal injury.

3. Difficulty bending or swelling of the knee (due to effusion) may indicate synovitis, bursitis, or popliteal (Baker) cyst; however, it may also be associated with meniscal injury if it follows a rotational injury. If acute swelling occurs following a trauma, it may indicate a fracture. If swelling occurs rapidly after a sudden twisting or hyperextension stress, an anterior cruciate ligament injury should be suspected.

4. Lateral "snapping" with flexion and extension of the knee may indicate inflammation of the iliotibial band.

5. Pain that is worsened when walking downstairs suggests the patellofemoral syndrome, or chondromalacia of the patella, degeneration of the subpatellar cartilage.

6. Pain that occurs when rising after prolonged sitting suggests a problem with tracking of the patella.

C. Physical Examination

To arrive at an accurate diagnosis, the physical examination should specifically test each anatomic structure.

Table 2–7. Location of common causes of knee pain.

Medial knee pain
Medial compartment osteoarthritis
Anserine bursitis (pain over the medial tibial plateau)
Medial collateral ligament strain
Medial meniscal injury
Anterior knee pain
Patellofemoral syndrome (often bilateral)
Osteoarthritis
Prepatellar bursitis (associated with swelling anterior to the patella)
"Jumper's knee" (pain at the inferior pole of the patella)
Septic arthritis
Gout or other inflammatory disorder
Lateral knee pain
Lateral collateral ligament sprain
Lateral meniscal injury
Lateral knee pain at the femoral condyle–inflammation of the iliotibial band (the iliotibial band syndrome)
Posterior (popliteal) pain
Effusion
Popliteal ("Baker") cyst

1. Localization—Prior to palpation of the knee by the clinician, it is useful for the patient to specifically identify the location of the pain if possible. Specific localization of the painful area can help identify the likely affected structures. Table 2–7 outlines the location of common causes of knee pain.

2. Inspection and palpation—To elicit joint line tenderness, flex the patient's knee while he or she is supine and feel for the soft area between the femur and tibia laterally and medially (this is the joint line). Pain and tenderness along the joint line supports the diagnosis of a meniscal injury or osteoarthritis. Pain over the tibial plateau following impact trauma suggests a tibial-plateau fracture (positive likelihood ratio [LR] = 1.1; negative LR = 0.8). Tenderness or swelling, or both, over the medial tibial plateau suggests anserine bursitis. Swelling and erythema over the patella is suggestive of prepatellar bursitis. A knee effusion is suggested by limitation of range of motion, patellar ballotment, fluid wave, concavity or fullness in the suprapatellar space, or loss of peripatellar dimples. Popliteal fullness or pain is indicative of an effusion or popliteal (Baker) cyst. If a popliteal cyst ruptures, there may be calf swelling accompanying the knee effusion. Finally, localized pain or palpable snapping over the lateral femoral condyle is characteristic of iliotibial band syndrome.

D. Specific Orthopedic Examination Maneuvers

1. Tests of ligamentous laxity—Ligamentous laxity is best ascertained if the physical examination is performed with relaxed knee muscles. This is most easily accomplished with the patient supine, leg/knee extended, popliteal space supported with a rolled up towel if needed, and the quadriceps femoris muscle relaxed. Otherwise, when significant pain and inflammation exist, maneuvers that test ligamentous laxity can be unreliable since voli-tional muscle contractions in response to or in anticipation of pain can obscure a positive result.

A. COLLATERAL LIGAMENTS—These ligaments can be examined by two tests.

(1) The valgus stress test—This test assesses stability of the medial collateral ligament. It should be done with the knee in extension, and repeated with the knee flexed at 25 degrees. With the thigh supported by the examination table, buttress the lateral side of the knee with one hand, and pull against the medial distal tibia with the other. This test is considered positive when valgus laxity is noted compared with the other knee. Laxity during this test with a fully extended knee indicates a more severe injury.

(2) The varus stress test—This test assesses stability of the lateral collateral ligament. It should also be done with the knee in extension, and repeated with the knee flexed at 25 degrees. Support the medial side of the knee with one hand, hold and pull the lateral distal tibia with the other (adducting the knee). This test is considered positive when varus laxity is noted compared with the other knee. Lateral collateral ligament laxity during a test of the fully extended knee indicates a more severe injury.

B. ANTERIOR CRUCIATE LIGAMENTS—The anterior cruciate ligaments can be examined by three tests: the anterior drawer test, the Lachman test, and the pivot shift test. Of the commonly used maneuvers to test for the integrity of the anterior cruciate ligaments, the Lachman and pivot shift tests have the best performance characteristics, whereas the anterior drawer sign is considered the easiest to perform. Small amounts of ligamentous laxity are common and can vary between individuals. Thus, interpretation of results of these maneuvers requires comparison with the contralateral side. A difference of > 1 cm in translation generally indicates a tear of the anterior cruciate ligament.

(1) The anterior drawer test—Have the patient lie supine and flex the knee to 90 degrees. Stabilize the patient's foot by leaning against it (or asking an assistant to do so), and grasp the proximal tibia with both hands around the calf and pull anteriorly. A positive test finds anterior cruciate ligament laxity compared with the unaffected side. (Sensitivity, 48%; specificity, 87%; positive LR = 3.7, negative LR = 0.6.)

(2) The Lachman test—Have the patient lie supine, and flex the knee to 25 degrees. Grasp the distal femur (lateral side), and the proximal tibia with the other hand on the medial side. With the knee in neutral position, stabilize the femur, and pull the tibia anteriorly. Excessive anterior translation of the tibia (compared with the other side) indicates injury to the anterior cruciate ligament. (Sensitivity, 84–87%; specificity, 93%; positive LR = 12.4, negative LR = 0.14.)

(3) The pivot shift test—Place the patient's knee in full extension, and then slowly flex it while applying internal rotation and a valgus stress. Feel for a subluxation at 20–40 degrees of knee flexion. (Positive LR = 20.4, negative LR = 0.4.)

C. POSTERIOR CRUCIATE LIGAMENT—This ligament can be examined by the posterior drawer (or "sag") test. With the patient supine, flex the knee to 90 degrees. Observe the anterior tibial plateau. It should be 10 mm anterior to the femoral condyles. Grasp the proximal tibia with both hands and push the tibia posteriorly. Compare movement, indicating laxity and possible tear of the posterior cruciate ligament, to the uninjured knee.

2. Tests of meniscal injury—There are two commonly used tests to assess meniscal injury.

A. The McMurray test— Flex the knee until the patient reports pain. (For this test to be valid, it must be flexed pain-free beyond 90 degrees.) Externally rotate the foot and then extend the knee. Palpating the medial knee for pain or "click" in the medial compartment of the knee is indicative of medial meniscus injury. To test the lateral meniscus, repeat the test, while rotating the foot internally. (Sensitivity, 53%; specificity, 59–97% depending on examiners studied; positive LR = 17.3, negative LR = 0.5.)

B. The Apley "grind" test—With patient lying prone on the examination table, flex the knee to 90 degrees. Grasp the foot in the palm of the hand. While applying downward pressure on the sole of the foot to axial load the lower leg (thereby compressing the menisci between the femoral condyles and the tibial plateau), carefully rotate the lower leg in a "grinding" motion, assessing for pain.

3. Testing for patella-femoral syndrome—There are three commonly used tests for the patella-femoral syndrome.

A. Patellar compression test—If compression of the patella against the femur reproduces the patient's pain (or causes "clicking" perceived by the patient), it is diagnostic of the patella-femoral syndrome.

B. Patellar grind test—With the patient supine and the knee extended, push the patella inferiorly by grasping the knee superior to the patella and pushing it downward. Ask the patient to contract the quadriceps muscle to oppose this downward translation. Pain or grinding is positive for chondromalacia of the patella.

C. Patellar apprehension test—Have the patient sit on the end of the examination table. Lift the lower leg into extension (asking the patient to relax the quadriceps muscle). Push the patella laterally, and then flex the knee to 30 degrees. Patellar instability is diagnosed if the patient experiences pain or apprehension.

E. Radiologic Studies

Under selected circumstances, radiologic studies can be useful in the diagnosis of acute knee pain. Plain radiographs can confirm osteoarthritic changes and identify fractures. MRI can assess soft-tissue injuries that may need urgent surgery (eg, ruptured anterior cruciate ligament). However, most causes of acute knee pain can be diagnosed in the absence of radiographic studies (see Ottawa Knee Rules below).

1. Plain knee radiographs

A. Osteoarthritis—Obtain bilateral weight-bearing knee films. Changes due to osteoarthritis include diminished width of articular cartilage, presence of osteophytes, and subchondral sclerosis.

Table 2–8. "Ottawa Knee Rules": Indications for radiographs in acute knee injury.

Consider knee radiography if <u>any one</u> of the following features is present:
Age ≥ 55 years
Fibular head tenderness
Isolated patella tenderness
Impaired knee flexion to 90 degrees
Inability to bear weight for four steps after the injury and in the emergency department

Reproduced, with permission, from Stiell IG et al. Prospective validation of a decision rule for the use of radiography in acute knee injuries. JAMA. 1996;275:611–5.

B. Acute fracture—In patients with acute knee trauma, the decision to obtain radiographs to exclude fracture should be guided by the "Ottawa Knee Rules" (Table 2–8) (sensitivity, ~100%; specificity 49%).

C. Patella-femoral syndrome—Although usually unnecessary for establishing the diagnosis of the patella-femoral syndrome, bilateral "sunrise" radiographs of the patellofemoral joint suggest chondromalacia of the patella when any of the following are present: subluxation, subchondral bony changes, osteophytes, or loose bodies. These findings are especially evident in advanced cases.

2. MRI of the knee—MRI of the knee is the most sensitive test for diagnosis and evaluation of soft tissue pathology, including injuries to the ligaments and menisci. MRI is useful to confirm an anterior cruciate ligament tear suspected from the history and Lachman test. MRI is helpful in determining the need for arthroscopy and surgery. It may also detect fracture after trauma when it is clinically suspected but plain radiographs are negative.

F. Arthrocentesis (see Chapter 20)

If a knee joint effusion is present, arthrocentesis and analysis of joint fluid is useful diagnostically, particularly for distinguishing infection from sterile inflammation (see Table 20–2). In addition, when knee pain is due to an effusion, joint fluid aspiration has therapeutic value by improving flexion and reducing pain. To avoid infecting the joint, arthrocentesis should not be performed when the aspirating needle will penetrate an active infection of the skin, such as cellulitis or abscess. It is also contraindicated if there is a significant coagulopathy, such as excessive anticoagulation with warfarin.

Arthrocentesis must be performed promptly to rule out an infection when acute knee pain with effusion is present as well as when inflammation is present and the patient is unable to actively flex the joint. An anterior cruciate ligament tear often leads to hemarthrosis. Thus, a physical examination that shows anterior cruciate ligament laxity combined with a joint aspiration that demonstrates bloody fluid is diagnostic of an anterior cruciate ligament tear.

Arthrocentesis and joint fluid analysis demonstrating crystals will lead to the diagnosis of gout (negatively birefringent, needle-shaped crystals) or pseudogout (positively birefringent, rectangular-shaped crystals). In bland knee joint effusions, removal of excessive joint fluid improves joint range of motion (flexion) and patient comfort.

Treatment

If infection, fracture, and ligamentous or meniscal tear are excluded, many acute knee conditions improve with conservative treatment consisting of low-impact activities and exercises (such as swimming, biking, walking, or cross-country skiing) to improve muscular strength and flexibility. For example, the patella-femoral syndrome is effectively treated with exercises to strengthen the vastus medialis muscle and with stretching of the hamstring and quadriceps muscles. A formal physical therapy program is usually not required.

The initial drugs of choice for the treatment of pain in knee osteoarthritis are acetaminophen and topical capsaicin. If a traditional nonsteroidal anti-inflammatory drug (NSAID) is indicated, the choice should be based on cost. The cyclooxygenase (COX)-2 inhibitor, celecoxib, is no more effective than traditional NSAIDs; it may offer short-term, but probably not long-term, advantage in preventing gastrointestinal complications. Due to its cost and potential risk of heart attack, this COX-2 inhibitor should be reserved for carefully selected patients.

When to Refer

Refer patients with fracture or internal derangement of the knee to an orthopedist.

When to Admit

- Admit patients with septic joints (in consultation with rheumatologist or orthopedist).
- Admit patients who are unable to ambulate and who lack home support for performing activities of daily living.

Bachmann LM et al. The accuracy of the Ottawa knee rule to rule out knee fractures: a systematic review. Ann Intern Med. 2004 Jan 20;140(2):121–4. [PMID: 14734335]

Blackham et al. Does regular exercise reduce the pain and stiffness of osteoarthritis? J Fam Pract. 2008 Jul;57(7):476–7. [PMID: 18625172]

Ebell MH. Evaluating the patient with a knee injury. Am Fam Physician. 2005 Mar 15;71(6):1169–72. [PMID: 15791893]

Englund M et al. Incidental meniscal findings on knee MRI in middle-aged and elderly persons. N Engl J Med. 2008 Sep 11;359(11):1108–15. [PMID: 18784100]

Jackson JL et al. Evaluation of acute knee pain in primary care. Ann Intern Med. 2003 Oct 7;139(7):575–88. [PMID: 14530229]

May TJ. Persistent anterior knee pain. Am Fam Physician. 2007 Jul 15;76(2):277–8. [PMID: 17695576]

Pavlov H et al. Acute trauma to the knee. American College of Radiology. ACR Appropriateness Criteria. Radiology. 2000 Jun;215(Suppl):365–73. [PMID: 11037449]

Porcheret M et al; Primary Care Rheumatology Society. Treatment of knee pain in older adults in primary care: development of an evidence-based model of care. Rheumatology (Oxford). 2007 Apr;46(4):638–48. [PMID: 17062646]

Silvis ML et al. Clinical inquiries. What is the best way to evaluate an acute traumatic knee injury? J Fam Pract. 2008 Feb;57(2):116–8. [PMID: 18248732]

Solomon DH et al. The rational clinical examination. Does this patient have a torn meniscus or ligament of the knee? Value of the physical examination. JAMA. 2001 Oct 3;286(13):1610–20. [PMID: 11585485]

Vincken PW et al. Effectiveness of MR imaging in selection of patients for arthroscopy of the knee. Radiology. 2002 Jun;223(3):739–46. [PMID: 12034943]

LOWER EXTREMITY EDEMA

ESSENTIAL INQUIRIES

- ▶ History of venous thromboembolism.
- ▶ Symmetry.
- ▶ Pain.
- ▶ Dependence.
- ▶ Skin findings.

General Considerations

Acute and chronic lower extremity edema present important diagnostic and treatment challenges. Lower extremities can swell in response to increased venous or lymphatic pressures, decreased intravascular oncotic pressure, increased capillary leak, and local injury or infection. **Chronic venous insufficiency** is by far the most common cause, affecting up to 2% of the population, and the incidence of venous insufficiency has not changed during the past 25 years. Venous insufficiency is a common complication of DVT; however, only a small number of patients with chronic venous insufficiency report a history of this disorder. Venous ulcer formation commonly affects patients with chronic venous insufficiency, and management of venous ulceration is labor-intensive and expensive.

Clinical Findings

A. Symptoms and Signs

Normal lower extremity venous pressure (in the erect position: 80 mm Hg in deep veins, 20–30 mm Hg in superficial veins) and cephalad venous blood flow require competent bicuspid venous valves, effective muscle contractions, and normal respirations. When one or more of these components fail, venous hypertension may result. Chronic exposure to elevated venous pressure by the postcapillary venules in the legs leads to leakage of fibrinogen and growth factors into the interstitial space, leukocyte aggregation and activation, and obliteration of the cutaneous lymphatic network. These changes account for the brawny, fibrotic skin changes observed in patients with chronic venous insufficiency, and the predisposition toward skin ulceration, particularly in the medial malleolar area.

Among common causes of lower extremity swelling, DVT is the most life-threatening. Clues suggesting DVT include a history of cancer, recent limb immobilization, or confinement to bed for at least 3 days following major surgery within the past month (Table 2–9). A search for

Table 2–9. Risk stratification of adults referred for ultrasound to rule out DVT.

Step 1: Calculate risk factor score
Score 1 point for each
Untreated malignancy
Paralysis, paresis, or recent plaster immobilization
Recently bedridden for > 3 days due to major surgery within 4 weeks
Localized tenderness along distribution of deep venous system
Entire leg swelling
Swelling of one calf > 3 cm more than the other (measured 10 cm below tibial tuberosity)
Pitting edema
Collateral superficial (nonvaricose) veins
Alternative diagnosis as likely as or more likely than DVT: subtract 2 points

Step 2: Obtain ultrasound		
Score	Ultrasound Positive	Ultrasound Negative
≤ 0	Confirm with venogram	DVT ruled out
1–2	Treat for DVT	Repeat ultrasound in 3–7 days
≥ 3	Treat for DVT	Confirm with venogram

DVT, deep venous thrombosis.

alternative explanations is equally important in excluding DVT. Bilateral involvement and significant improvement upon awakening favor systemic causes (eg, venous insufficiency, CHF, and cirrhosis). "Heavy legs" are the most frequent symptom among patients with chronic venous insufficiency, followed by itching. Pain, particularly if severe, is uncommon in uncomplicated venous insufficiency. Lower extremity swelling and inflammation in a limb recently affected by DVT could represent anticoagulation failure and thrombus recurrence but more often are caused by **postphlebitic syndrome** with valvular incompetence. Other causes of a painful, swollen calf include ruptured popliteal cyst, calf strain or trauma, and cellulitis.

Lower extremity swelling is a familiar complication of therapy with calcium channel blockers (particularly felodipine and amlodipine), thioglitazones, and minoxidil. Bilateral lower extremity edema can be a presenting symptom of nephrotic syndrome or volume overload caused by renal failure. Prolonged airline flights (> 10 hours) are associated with increased risk of edema. In those with low to medium risk of thromboembolism (eg, women taking oral contraceptives), long flights are associated with a 2% incidence of asymptomatic popliteal DVT.

B. Physical Examination

Physical examination should include assessment of the heart, lungs, and abdomen for evidence of pulmonary hypertension (primary, or secondary to chronic lung disease), CHF, or cirrhosis. Some patients with the latter have pulmonary hypertension without lung disease. There is a

spectrum of skin findings related to chronic venous insufficiency that depends on the severity and chronicity of the disease, ranging from hyperpigmentation and stasis dermatitis to abnormalities highly specific for chronic venous insufficiency: lipodermatosclerosis (thick brawny skin; in advanced cases, the lower leg resembles an inverted champagne bottle) and atrophie blanche (small depigmented macules within areas of heavy pigmentation). The size of both calves should be measured 10 cm below the tibial tuberosity and elicitation of pitting and tenderness performed. Swelling of the entire leg or swelling of one leg 3 cm more than the other suggests deep venous obstruction. In normal persons, the left calf is slightly larger than the right as a result of the left common iliac vein coursing under the aorta.

An ulcer located over the medial malleolus is a hallmark of chronic venous insufficiency but can be due to other causes. Shallow, large, modestly painful ulcers are characteristic of venous insufficiency, whereas small, deep, and more painful ulcers are more apt to be due to arterial insufficiency, vasculitis, or infection (including cutaneous diphtheria). Diabetic vascular ulcers, however, may be painless. When an ulcer is on the foot or above the mid calf, causes other than venous insufficiency should be considered.

C. Diagnostic Studies

Most causes of lower extremity swelling can be demonstrated with color duplex ultrasonography. Patients without an obvious cause of acute lower extremity swelling (eg, calf strain) should have an ultrasound performed, since DVT is difficult to exclude on clinical grounds. Recently, a predictive rule has been developed that allows a clinician to exclude a lower extremity DVT in patients without an ultrasound if the patient has low pretest probability for DVT and has a negative sensitive D-dimer test (the "Wells rule"). Assessment of the ankle-brachial pressure index (ABPI) is important in the management of chronic venous insufficiency, since peripheral arterial disease may be exacerbated by compression therapy. This can be performed at the same time as ultrasound. Caution is required in interpreting the results of ABPI in older patients and diabetics due to decreased compressibility of their arteries. A dipstick urine test that is strongly positive for protein can suggest nephrotic syndrome, and a serum creatinine can help estimate kidney function.

Differential Diagnosis

Possible causes include chronic venous insufficiency, DVT, cellulitis, musculoskeletal disorders (Baker cyst rupture, gastrocnemius tear or rupture), lymphedema, CHF, cirrhosis, and nephrotic syndrome as well as side effects from calcium channel blockers, minoxidil, or thioglitazones.

Treatment

Treatment of lower extremity edema should be guided by the underlying etiology. See relevant chapters for treatment of edema in patients with congestive heart failure (Chapter 10), nephrosis (Chapter 22), cirrhosis (Chapter 16), and lymphedema (Chapter 12). Edema resulting from calcium channel blocker therapy responds to concomitant therapy with ACE inhibitors or angiotensin receptor blockers.

In patients with chronic venous insufficiency without a comorbid volume overload state (eg, CHF), it is best to avoid diuretic therapy. These patients have relatively decreased intravascular volume, and administration of diuretics may result in acute renal insufficiency and oliguria. The most effective treatment involves (1) leg elevation, above the level of the heart, for 30 minutes three to four times daily, and during sleep; and (2) compression therapy. A wide variety of stockings and devices are effective in decreasing swelling and preventing ulcer formation. They should be put on with awakening, before hydration forces result in edema. Horse chestnut seed extract has been shown in several randomized trials to be equivalent to compression stockings and can be quite useful in nonambulatory patients. Patients with decreased ABPI should be managed in concert with a vascular surgeon. Compression stockings (12–18 mm Hg at the ankle) are effective in preventing edema and asymptomatic thrombosis associated with long airline flights in low- to medium-risk persons.

When to Refer

- Chronic lower extremity ulcerations requiring specialist wound care.
- Nephrotic syndrome should be managed with nephrology consultation.
- When there is coexisting severe arterial insufficiency (claudication) complicating treatment with compression stockings.

When to Admit

- Pending definitive diagnosis in patients at high risk for DVT with normal lower extremity ultrasound.
- Concern for impending compartment syndrome.
- Severe edema that impairs ability to ambulate or perform activities of daily living.

Amsler F et al. Compression therapy for occupational leg symptoms and chronic venous disorders—a meta-analysis of randomised controlled trials. Eur J Vasc Endovasc Surg. 2008 Mar;35(3):366–72. [PMID: 18063393]

Bamigboye AA et al. Interventions for varicose veins and leg oedema in pregnancy. Cochrane Database Syst Rev. 2007 Jan 24;(1):CD001066. [PMID: 17253454]

Bergan JJ et al. Chronic venous disease. N Engl J Med. 2006 Aug 3;355(5):488–98. [PMID: 16885552]

Jull A et al. Pentoxifylline for treating venous leg ulcers. Cochrane Database Syst Rev. 2007 Jul 18;(3):CD001733. [PMID: 17636683]

Mockler J et al. Clinical inquiries. What is the differential diagnosis of chronic leg edema in primary care? J Fam Pract. 2008 Mar;57(3):188–9. [PMID: 18321457]

O'Brien JG et al. Treatment of edema. Am Fam Physician. 2005 Jun 1;71(11):2111–7. [PMID: 15952439]

Palfreyman SJ et al. Dressings for healing venous leg ulcers. Cochrane Database Syst Rev. 2006 Jul 19;3:CD001103. [PMID: 16855958]

Wells PS et al. Does this patient have deep vein thrombosis? JAMA. 2006 Jan 11;295(2):199–207. [PMID: 16403932]

FEVER & HYPERTHERMIA

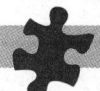

ESSENTIAL INQUIRIES

- Age.
- Localizing symptoms.
- Weight loss.
- Joint pain.
- Injection substance use.
- Immunosuppression or neutropenia.
- History of cancer.
- Medications.
- Travel.

General Considerations

The average normal oral body temperature taken in midmorning is 36.7 °C (range 36–37.4 °C). This spectrum includes a mean and 2 standard deviations, thus encompassing 95% of a normal population, measured in midmorning (normal diurnal temperature variation is 0.5–1 °C). The normal rectal or vaginal temperature is 0.5 °C higher than the oral temperature, and the axillary temperature is correspondingly lower. Rectal temperature is more reliable than oral temperature, particularly in mouth breathers or in tachypneic states.

Fever is a regulated rise to a new "set point" of body temperature. When proper stimuli act on appropriate monocyte-macrophages, these cells elaborate pyrogenic cytokines, causing elevation of the set point through effects in the hypothalamus. These cytokines include interleukin-1 (IL-1), tumor necrosis factor (TNF), interferon-γ, and interleukin-6 (IL-6). The elevation in temperature results from either increased heat production (eg, shivering) or decreased loss (eg, peripheral vasoconstriction). Body temperature in cytokine-induced fever seldom exceeds 41.1 °C unless there is structural damage to hypothalamic regulatory centers.

1. Fever

Fever as a symptom provides important information about the presence of illness—particularly infections—and about changes in the clinical status of the patient. The fever pattern, however, is of marginal value for most specific diagnoses except for the relapsing fever of malaria, borreliosis, and occasional cases of lymphoma, especially Hodgkin disease. Furthermore, the degree of temperature elevation does not necessarily correspond to the severity of the illness. In general, the febrile response tends to be greater in children than in adults. In older persons, neonates, and in persons receiving certain medications (eg, NSAIDs or corticosteroids), a normal temperature or even hypothermia may be observed. Markedly elevated body temperature may result in profound metabolic disturbances. High temperature during the first trimester of pregnancy may cause birth defects, such as anencephaly. Fever increases insulin requirements and alters the metabolism and disposition of drugs used for the treatment of the diverse diseases associated with fever.

2. Hyperthermia

Hyperthermia—not mediated by cytokines—occurs when body metabolic heat production or environmental heat load exceeds normal heat loss capacity or when there is impaired heat loss; heat stroke is an example. Body temperature may rise to levels (> 41.1 °C) capable of producing irreversible protein denaturation and resultant brain damage; no diurnal variation is observed.

Neuroleptic malignant syndrome is a rare and potentially lethal idiosyncratic reaction to major tranquilizers, particularly haloperidol and fluphenazine; however, it has also been reported with the atypical neuroleptics (such as olanzapine or risperidone). Serotonin syndrome resembles neuroleptic malignant syndrome but occurs within hours of ingestion of agents that increase levels of serotonin in the central nervous system, including serotonin reuptake inhibitors, monoamine oxidase inhibitors, tricyclic antidepressants, meperidine, dextromethorphan, bromocriptine, tramadol, lithium, and psychostimulants (such as cocaine, methamphetamine, and MDMA). Clonus and hyperreflexia are more common in serotonin syndrome whereas "lead pipe" rigidity is more common in neuroleptic malignant syndrome. Neuroleptic malignant and serotonin syndromes share common clinical and pathophysiologic features to malignant hyperthermia of anesthesia (see Chapters 25 and 38).

▶ Treatment

Discontinuation of the offending agent is mandatory. Treatment of neuroleptic malignant syndrome includes dantrolene in combination with bromocriptine or levodopa. Treatment of serotonin syndrome includes administration of a central serotonin receptor antagonist—cyproheptadine or chlorpromazine—alone or in combination with a benzodiazepine. In patients for whom it is difficult to distinguish which syndrome is present, treatment with a benzodiazepine may be the safest therapeutic option. Regardless of cause, alcohol sponges, cold sponges, ice bags, ice-water enemas, and ice baths can also help lower body temperature.

3. Fever of Undetermined Origin

(See Fever of Unknown Origin, Chapter 30)

Most febrile illnesses are due to common infections, are short-lived, and are relatively easy to diagnose. In certain instances, however, the origin of the fever may remain obscure ("fever of undetermined origin," FUO) even after protracted diagnostic examination. In upper respiratory tract infections, fever typically lasts no more than 3–5 days, beyond which additional evaluation should be considered. The term "FUO" has traditionally been reserved for unexplained cases of fever exceeding 38.3 °C on several occasions for at least 3 weeks in patients without neutropenia or immunosuppression (see Chapter 30). Some authors have advocated for changing the definition of FUO in frail elderly

Table 2–10. Differential diagnosis of fever and hyperthermia.

Fever—common causes
Infections: bacterial, viral, rickettsial, fungal, parasitic
Autoimmune diseases
Central nervous system disease, including head trauma and mass lesions
Malignant disease, especially renal cell carcinoma, primary or metastatic liver cancer, leukemia, and lymphoma
Fever—less common causes
Cardiovascular diseases, including myocardial infarction, thrombophlebitis, and pulmonary embolism
Gastrointestinal diseases, including inflammatory bowel disease, alcoholic hepatitis, and granulomatous hepatitis
Miscellaneous diseases, including drug fever, sarcoidosis, familial Mediterranean fever, tissue injury, hematoma, and factitious fever
Hyperthermia
Peripheral thermoregulatory disorders, including heat stroke, malignant hyperthermia of anesthesia, and malignant neuroleptic syndrome

nursing home patients to a persistent oral or tympanic membrane temperature of 37.2 °C (99 °F) or greater, or persistent rectal temperature of 37.5 °C (99.5 °F) or greater.

▶ Differential Diagnosis

See Table 2–10. The causes of FUO among elderly patients differ from those in younger patients, and a definitive diagnosis can be achieved in a larger proportion of elderly patients (up to 70%). Although the general diagnostic approach and distribution of infectious and noninfectious causes are roughly similar between age groups, tuberculosis and temporal arteritis are particularly more common causes of FUO in the elderly.

▶ Treatment

Most fever is well tolerated. When the temperature is greater than 40 °C, symptomatic treatment may be required. A reading over 41 °C is likely to be hyperthermia and thus not cytokine mediated, and emergent management is indicated. (See Heat Stroke, Chapter 37.)

A. Measures for Removal of Heat

Alcohol sponges, cold sponges, ice bags, ice-water enemas, and ice baths will lower body temperature. They are more useful in hyperthermia, since patients with cytokine-related fever will attempt to override these therapies.

B. Antipyretic Drugs

Antipyretic therapy is not needed except for patients with marginal hemodynamic status. Aspirin or acetaminophen, 325–650 mg every 4 hours, is effective in reducing fever. These drugs are best administered continuously rather than as needed, since "prn" dosing results in periodic chills and sweats due to fluctuations in temperature caused by varying levels of drug.

C. Antimicrobial Therapy

In most febrile patients, empiric antibiotic therapy should be deferred pending further evaluation. However, empiric antibiotic therapy is sometimes warranted. Prompt broad-spectrum antimicrobials are indicated for febrile patients who are clinically unstable, even before infection can be documented. These include patients with hemodynamic instability, those with neutropenia (neutrophils < 500/mcL), others who are asplenic (surgically or secondary to sickle cell disease) or immunosuppressed (including individuals taking systemic corticosteroids, azathioprine, cyclosporine, or other immunosuppressive medications), and those who are HIV infected (see Chapter 31). For treatment of fever during neutropenia following chemotherapy, outpatient parenteral antimicrobial therapy with an agent such as ceftriaxone can be provided effectively and safely. If a fungal infection is suspected in patients with prolonged fever and neutropenia, fluconazole is an equally effective but less toxic alternative to amphotericin B.

▶ When to Refer

Once the diagnosis of FUO is made, referral to infectious disease specialist or rheumatologist may be appropriate to guide specific additional tests.

▶ When to Admit

- Malignant hyperthermia.
- Heat stroke.
- For measures to control temperature when it is > 41 °C or when associated with seizure or other mental status changes.

Bleeker-Rovers CP et al. A prospective multicenter study on fever of unknown origin: the yield of a structured diagnostic protocol. Medicine (Baltimore). 2007 Jan;86(1):26–38. [PMID: 17220753]
Bottieau E et al. Fever after a stay in the tropics: diagnostic predictors of the leading tropical conditions. Medicine (Baltimore). 2007 Jan;86(1):18–25. [PMID: 17220752]
Norman DC et al. Fever of unknown origin in older persons. Infect Dis Clin North Am. 2007 Dec;21(4):937–45. [PMID: 18061083]
Rusyniak DE et al. Toxin-induced hyperthermic syndromes. Med Clin North Am. 2005 Nov;89(6):1277–96. [PMID: 16227063]
Watson JT et al. Clinical characteristics and functional outcomes of West Nile Fever. Ann Intern Med. 2004 Sep 7;141(5):360–5. [PMID: 15353427]
Woolery WA et al. Fever of unknown origin: keys to determining the etiology in older patients. Geriatrics. 2004 Oct;59 (10):41–5. [PMID: 15508555]

INVOLUNTARY WEIGHT LOSS

ESSENTIAL INQUIRIES

- ▶ Age.
- ▶ Caloric intake.
- ▶ Fever.
- ▶ Change in bowel habits.
- ▶ Secondary confirmation (eg, changes in clothing size).
- ▶ Substance use.
- ▶ Age-appropriate cancer screening history.

▶ General Considerations

Body weight is determined by a person's caloric intake, absorptive capacity, metabolic rate, and energy losses. The metabolic rate can be affected by a multitude of medical conditions through the release of various cytokines such as cachectin and interleukins. Body weight normally peaks by the fifth or sixth decade and then gradually declines at a rate of 1–2 kg per decade. In NHANES II, a national survey of community-dwelling elders (age 50–80 years), recent involuntary weight loss (> 5% usual body weight) was reported by 7% of respondents, and this was associated with a 24% higher mortality.

▶ Etiology

Involuntary weight loss is regarded as clinically significant when it exceeds 5% or more of usual body weight over a 6- to 12-month period and often indicates serious physical or psychological illness. Physical causes are usually evident during the initial evaluation. Cancer (about 30%), gastrointestinal disorders (about 15%), and dementia or depression (about 15%) are the most common causes. When an adequately nourished-appearing patient complains of weight loss, inquiry should be made about exact weight changes (with approximate dates) and about changes in clothing size. Family members can provide confirmation of weight loss, as can old documents such as driver's licenses. A mild, gradual weight loss occurs in some older individuals. It is due to changes in body composition, including loss of height and lean body mass and lower basal metabolic rate, leading to decreased energy requirements. However, rapid involuntary weight loss is predictive of morbidity and mortality in any population. In addition to various disease states, causes in older individuals include loss of teeth and consequent difficulty with chewing, alcoholism, and social isolation.

▶ Clinical Findings

Once the weight loss is established, the history, medication profile, physical examination, and conventional laboratory and radiologic investigations (such as complete blood count, serologic tests including HIV, thyroid-stimulating hormone (TSH) level, urinalysis, fecal occult blood test, chest radiography, and upper gastrointestinal series) usually reveal the cause. When these tests are normal, the second phase of evaluation should focus on more definitive gastrointestinal investigation (eg, tests for malabsorption; endoscopy) and cancer screening (eg, Papanicolaou smear, mammography, prostate specific antigen [PSA]).

If the initial evaluation is unrevealing, follow-up is preferable to further diagnostic testing. Death at 2-year follow-up was not nearly as high in patients with unexplained involuntary weight loss (8%) as in those with weight loss due to malignant (79%) and established non-malignant diseases (19%). Psychiatric consultation should be considered when there is evidence of depression, dementia, anorexia nervosa, or other emotional problems. Ultimately, in approximately 15–25% of cases, no cause for the weight loss can be found.

Differential Diagnosis

Malignancy, gastrointestinal disorders (eg, malabsorption, pancreatic insufficiency), dementia, depression, anorexia nervosa, hyperthyroidism, alcoholism, and social isolation are all established causes. "Meals on Wheels" is a useful mnemonic for remembering the common treatable causes of involuntary weight loss in the elderly (see box below).

Treatment

Weight stabilization occurs in most surviving patients with both established and unknown causes of weight loss through treatment of the underlying disorder and caloric supplementation. Nutrient intake goals are established in relation to the severity of weight loss, in general ranging from 30 to 40 kcal/kg/d. In order of preference, route of administration options include oral, temporary nasojejunal tube, or percutaneous gastric or jejunal tube. Parenteral nutrition is reserved for patients with serious associated problems. A variety of pharmacologic agents have been proposed for the treatment of weight loss. These can be categorized into appetite stimulants (corticosteroids, progestational agents, dronabinol, and serotonin antagonists); anabolic agents (growth hormone and testosterone derivatives); and anticatabolic agents (omega-3 fatty acids, pentoxifylline, hydrazine sulfate, and thalidomide).

When to Refer

- Weight loss caused by malabsorption.
- Persistent nutritional deficiencies despite adequate supplementation.
- Weight loss as a result of anorexia or bulimia.

When to Admit

- Severe protein-energy malnutrition, including the syndromes of kwashiorkor and marasmus.
- Vitamin deficiency syndromes.
- Cachexia with anticipated progressive weight loss secondary to unmanageable psychiatric disease.
- To carefully manage electrolyte and fluid replacement in protein-energy malnutrition and avoid "re-feeding syndrome."

Alibhai SM et al. An approach to the management of unintentional weight loss in elderly people. CMAJ. 2005 Mar 15;172(6):773–80. [PMID: 15767612]

Chapman IM. Nutritional disorders in the elderly. Med Clin North Am. 2006 Sep;90(5):887–907. [PMID: 16962848]

Johnson DK et al. Accelerated weight loss may precede diagnosis in Alzheimer disease. Arch Neurol. 2006 Sep;63(9):1312–7. [PMID: 16966511]

Mattox TW. Treatment of unintentional weight loss in patients with cancer. Nutr Clin Pract. 2005 Aug;20(4):400–10. [PMID: 16207680]

Morley JE et al. Cachexia: pathophysiology and clinical relevance. Am J Clin Nutr. 2006 Apr;83(4):735–43. [PMID: 16600922]

FATIGUE & CHRONIC FATIGUE SYNDROME

ESSENTIAL INQUIRIES

▶ Weight loss.
▶ Fever.
▶ Sleep-disordered breathing.
▶ Medications.
▶ Substance use.

General Considerations

Fatigue, as an isolated symptom, accounts for 1–3% of visits to generalists. The symptom of fatigue is often poorly described and less well defined by patients than symptoms associated with specific dysfunction of organ systems. Fatigue or lassitude and the closely related complaints of weakness, tiredness, and lethargy are often attributed to overexertion, poor physical conditioning, sleep disturbance,

---

MEALS ON WHEELS: A Mnemonic
for Common Treatable
Causes of Unintentional
Weight Loss in the Elderly.

Medication effects

Emotional problems, especially depression

Anorexia tardive (nervosa), alcoholism

Late-life paranoia

Swallowing disorders

Oral factors (eg, poorly fitting dentures, cavities)

No money

Wandering and other dementia-related behaviors

Hyperthyroidism, hypothyroidism, hyperparathyroidism, hypoadrenalism

Enteric problems (eg, malabsorption)

Eating problems (eg, inability to feed self)

Low-salt, low-cholesterol diets

Social problems (eg, isolation, inability to obtain preferred foods), gallstones

Adapted, with permission, from Morley JE et al. Nutritional issues in nursing home care. Ann Intern Med. 1995 Dec 1;123(11):850–9.

obesity, undernutrition, and emotional problems. A history of the patient's daily living and working habits may obviate the need for extensive and unproductive diagnostic studies.

▶ Clinical Findings

A. Fatigue

Clinically relevant fatigue is composed of three major components: generalized weakness (difficulty in initiating activities); easy fatigability (difficulty in completing activities); and mental fatigue (difficulty with concentration and memory). Important diseases that can cause fatigue include hyperthyroidism and hypothyroidism, CHF, infections (endocarditis, hepatitis), COPD, sleep apnea, anemia, autoimmune disorders, irritable bowel syndrome, and cancer. Alcoholism, side effects from such drugs as sedatives and β-blockers may be the cause. Psychological conditions, such as insomnia, depression, anxiety, panic attacks, dysth-

mia, and somatization disorder, may cause fatigue. Common outpatient infectious causes include mononucleosis and sinusitis. These conditions are usually associated with other characteristic signs, but patients may emphasize fatigue and not reveal their other symptoms unless directly asked. The lifetime prevalence of significant fatigue (present for at least 2 weeks) is about 25%. Fatigue of unknown cause or related to psychiatric illness exceeds that due to physical illness, injury, medications, drugs, or alcohol.

B. Chronic Fatigue Syndrome

A working case definition of chronic fatigue syndrome indicates that it is not a homogeneous abnormality, and there is no single pathogenic mechanism (Figure 2–2). No physical finding or laboratory test can be used to confirm the diagnosis of this disorder.

With regard to its pathophysiology, early theories postulated an infectious or immune dysregulation mecha-

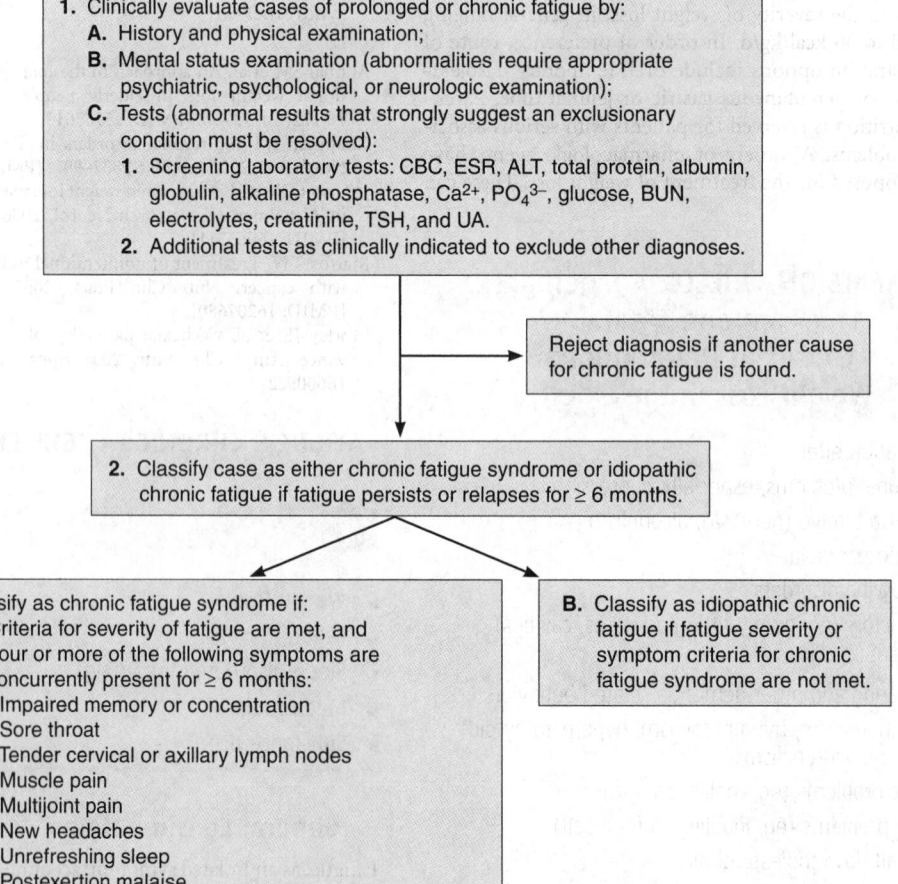

1. Clinically evaluate cases of prolonged or chronic fatigue by:
   A. History and physical examination;
   B. Mental status examination (abnormalities require appropriate psychiatric, psychological, or neurologic examination);
   C. Tests (abnormal results that strongly suggest an exclusionary condition must be resolved):
      1. Screening laboratory tests: CBC, ESR, ALT, total protein, albumin, globulin, alkaline phosphatase, Ca^{2+}, PO_4^{3-}, glucose, BUN, electrolytes, creatinine, TSH, and UA.
      2. Additional tests as clinically indicated to exclude other diagnoses.

Reject diagnosis if another cause for chronic fatigue is found.

2. Classify case as either chronic fatigue syndrome or idiopathic chronic fatigue if fatigue persists or relapses for ≥ 6 months.

A. Classify as chronic fatigue syndrome if:
   1. Criteria for severity of fatigue are met, and
   2. Four or more of the following symptoms are concurrently present for ≥ 6 months:
      • Impaired memory or concentration
      • Sore throat
      • Tender cervical or axillary lymph nodes
      • Muscle pain
      • Multijoint pain
      • New headaches
      • Unrefreshing sleep
      • Postexertion malaise

B. Classify as idiopathic chronic fatigue if fatigue severity or symptom criteria for chronic fatigue syndrome are not met.

▲ **Figure 2–2.** Evaluation and classification of unexplained chronic fatigue. (CBC, complete blood count; ESR, erythrocyte sedimentation rate; ALT, alanine aminotransferase; Ca^{2+}, calcium; PO_4^{3-}, phosphate; BUN, blood urea nitrogen; TSH, thyroid-stimulating hormone; UA, urinalysis.) (Modified and reproduced, with permission, from Fukuda K et al. The chronic fatigue syndrome: a comprehensive approach to its definition and study. Ann Intern Med. 1994 Dec 15;121(12):953–9.)

nism. Persons with confirmed chronic fatigue syndrome report a much greater frequency of childhood trauma and psychopathology and demonstrate higher levels of emotional instability and self-reported stress than non-fatigued controls. Neuropsychological, neuroendocrine, and brain imaging studies have confirmed the occurrence of neurobiologic abnormalities in most patients. Sleep disorders have been reported in 40–80% of patients with chronic fatigue syndrome, but their treatment has provided only modest benefit, suggesting that it is an effect rather than a cause of the fatigue. MRI scans may show brain abnormalities on T_2-weighted images—chiefly small, punctate, subcortical white matter hyperintensities, predominantly in the frontal lobes. Veterans of the Gulf War show a tenfold greater incidence of chronic fatigue syndrome compared with nondeployed military personnel.

In evaluating chronic fatigue, after the history and physical examination process is completed, standard investigation includes complete blood count, erythrocyte sedimentation rate, serum chemistries—blood urea nitrogen (BUN), electrolytes, glucose, creatinine, and calcium; liver and thyroid function tests—antinuclear antibody, urinalysis, and tuberculin skin test; and screening questionnaires for psychiatric disorders. Other tests to be performed as clinically indicated are serum cortisol, rheumatoid factor, immunoglobulin levels, Lyme serology in endemic areas, and tests for HIV antibody. More extensive testing is usually unhelpful, including antibody to Epstein-Barr virus. There may be an abnormally high rate of postural hypotension; some of these patients report response to increases in dietary sodium as well as antihypotensive agents such as fludrocortisone, 0.1 mg/d.

▶ Treatment

A. Fatigue

Management of fatigue involves identification and treatment of conditions that contribute to fatigue, such as cancer, pain, depression, disordered sleep, weight loss, and anemia. Resistance training and aerobic exercise lessens fatigue and improves performance for a number of chronic conditions associated with a high prevalence of fatigue, including CHF, COPD, arthritis, and cancer. Continuous positive airway pressure is an effective treatment for obstructive sleep apnea. Psychostimulants such as methylphenidate have shown inconsistent results in randomized trials of treatment of cancer-related fatigue.

B. Chronic Fatigue Syndrome

A variety of agents and modalities have been tried for the treatment of chronic fatigue syndrome. Acyclovir, intravenous immunoglobulin, nystatin, and low-dose hydrocortisone/fludrocortisone do not improve symptoms. There is a greater prevalence of past and current psychiatric diagnoses in patients with this syndrome. Affective disorders are especially common, but fluoxetine alone, 20 mg daily, is not beneficial. Patients with chronic fatigue syndrome have benefited from a comprehensive multidisciplinary intervention, including optimal medical management, treating any ongoing affective or anxiety disorder pharmacologically, and implementing a comprehensive cognitive-behavioral treatment program. **Cognitive-behavioral therapy,** a form of nonpharmacologic treatment emphasizing self-help and aiming to change perceptions and behaviors that may perpetuate symptoms and disability, is helpful. Although few patients are cured, the treatment effect is substantial. Response to cognitive-behavioral therapy is not predictable on the basis of severity or duration of chronic fatigue syndrome, although patients with low interest in psychotherapy rarely benefit. Graded exercise has also been shown to improve functional work capacity and physical function. At present, intensive individual cognitive-behavioral therapy administered by a skilled therapist and graded exercise are the treatments of choice for patients with chronic fatigue syndrome.

In addition, the clinician's sympathetic listening and explanatory responses can help overcome the patient's frustrations and debilitation by this still mysterious illness. All patients should be encouraged to engage in normal activities to the extent possible and should be reassured that full recovery is eventually possible in most cases.

▶ When to Refer

- Infections not responsive to standard treatment.
- Difficult to control hyperthyroidism or hypothyroidism.
- Severe psychological disease.
- Malignancy.

▶ When to Admit

- Failure to thrive.
- Fatigue severe enough to impair activities of daily living.
- Fatigue combined with poor social support making it unlikely for patient to comply with medical therapy or reliably return for follow-up appointments.

de Lange FP et al. Increase in prefrontal cortical volume following cognitive behavioural therapy in patients with chronic fatigue syndrome. Brain. 2008 Aug;131(Pt 8):2172–80. [PMID: 18587150]

Evans WJ et al. Physiological basis of fatigue. Am J Phys Med Rehabil. 2007 Jan;86(1 Suppl):S29–46. [PMID: 17370370]

Heim C et al. Early adverse experience and risk for chronic fatigue syndrome: results from a population-based study. Arch Gen Psychiatry. 2006 Nov;63(11):1258–66. [PMID: 17088506]

Kato K et al. Premorbid predictors of chronic fatigue. Arch Gen Psychiatry. 2006 Nov;63(11):1267–72. [PMID: 17088507]

Prins JB et al. Chronic fatigue syndrome. Lancet. 2006 Jan 28;367(9507):346–55. [PMID: 16443043]

Viner R et al. Fatigue and somatic symptoms. BMJ. 2005 Apr 30;330(7498):1012–5. [PMID: 15860829]

Whiting P et al. Interventions for the treatment and management of chronic fatigue syndrome: a systematic review. JAMA. 2001 Sep 19;286(11):1360–8. [PMID: 11560542]

Wolkove N et al. Sleep and aging: 2. Management of sleep disorders in older people. CMAJ. 2007 May 8;176(10):1449–54. [PMID: 17485699]

ACUTE HEADACHE

ESSENTIAL INQUIRIES

▶ Age > 50 years.

▶ Rapid onset and severe intensity (ie, "thunderclap" headache).

▶ Fever.

▶ Trauma.

▶ Vision changes.

▶ HIV infection.

▶ Current or past history of hypertension.

▶ Neurologic findings (mental status changes, motor or sensory deficits).

General Considerations

Headache is a common reason that adults seek medical care, accounting for approximately 13 million visits each year in the United States to physicians' offices, urgent care clinics, and emergency departments. A broad range of disorders can cause headache. This chapter will deal only with the approach to a new acute headache—not due to trauma—in adolescents and adults. The challenge in the initial evaluation of acute headache is to identify which patients are presenting with an uncommon but life-threatening condition. In the emergency department setting, approximately 1% of patients seeking medical attention for acute headache will have a life-threatening condition, whereas the prevalence of life-threatening conditions in the office practice setting is considerably lower.

Regardless of the underlying cause, headache is currently believed to occur as a result of the release of neuropeptides from trigeminal nerve endings that encapsulate the blood vessels of the pia mater and dura mater, resulting in neurogenic inflammation. Because this represents a final common pathway for many etiologies, diminution of headache in response to typical migraine therapies (such as serotonin receptor antagonists or ketorolac) does not rule out critical conditions such as subarachnoid hemorrhage or meningitis as the underlying cause.

Clinical Findings

A. Symptoms

A careful history and physical examination should aim to identify causes of acute headache that require immediate treatment. These causes can be broadly classified as imminent or completed **vascular events** (intracranial hemorrhage, thrombosis, vasculitis, malignant hypertension, arterial dissection, or aneurysm), **infections** (abscess, encephalitis, meningitis), **intracranial masses** causing intracranial hypertension, **preeclampsia,** and **carbon monoxide poisoning.** Having the patient carefully describe the onset of headache can be helpful in diagnosing a serious cause. Report of a sudden-onset headache that reaches maximal and severe

Table 2–11. Clinical features associated with acute headache that warrant urgent or emergent neuroimaging.

Prior to lumbar puncture
Abnormal neurologic examination
Abnormal mental status
Abnormal funduscopic examination (papilledema; loss of venous pulsations)
Meningeal signs
Emergent (conduct prior to leaving office or emergency department)
Abnormal neurologic examination
Abnormal mental status
Thunderclap headache
Urgent (scheduled prior to leaving office or emergency department)
HIV-positive patient[1]
Age > 50 years (normal neurologic examination)

[1]Use CT with or without contrast or MRI if HIV positive.
Source: American College of Emergency Physicians. Clinical Policy: critical issues in the evaluation and management of patients presenting to the emergency department with acute headache. Ann Emerg Med. 2002 Jan;39(1):108–22.

intensity within seconds or a few minutes is the classic description of a "thunderclap headache" and should precipitate workup for subarachnoid hemorrhage, since the estimated prevalence of subarachnoid hemorrhage in the setting of a thunderclap headache is 43%.

The general medical history can also guide the need for additional work-up. A new headache in a patient of advanced age or with a history of HIV disease under most circumstances (including a normal neurologic examination) warrants neuroimaging immediately (Table 2–11). When the patient has a medical history of hypertension—particularly uncontrolled hypertension—a complete search for criteria satisfying a diagnosis of "malignant hypertension" is appropriate to determine the correct urgency level of hypertension management (see Chapter 11). Headache and hypertension associated with pregnancy may be due to preeclampsia. Episodic headache associated with the triad of hypertension, heart palpitations, and sweats is suggestive of pheochromocytoma. In the absence of thunderclap headache, advanced age, and HIV disease, a careful physical examination and detailed neurologic examination will usually determine acuity of the work-up and need for further diagnostic testing.

Patient symptoms can also be useful for diagnosing migraine headache in the absence of the "classic" migraine pattern involving scintillating scotoma followed by unilateral headache, photophobia, and nausea and vomiting (Table 2–12). It is evident that the presence of three or more of these features can establish the diagnosis of migraine (in the absence of other clinical features that warrant neuroimaging studies), and the presence of none or one of these features (provided it is not nausea) can help to rule out migraine.

B. Physical Examination

Critical components of the physical examination of the patient with acute headache include vital sign measure-

Table 2–12. Summary likelihood ratios (LRs) for individual clinical features associated with migraine diagnosis.

Clinical Feature	LR+ (95% CI)	LR− (95% CI)
Nausea	19 (15–25)	0.19 (0.18–0.20)
Photophobia	5.8 (5.1–6.6)	0.24 (0.23–0.26)
Phonophobia	5.2 (4.5–5.9)	0.38 (0.36–0.40)
Exacerbation by physical activity	3.7 (3.4–4.0)	0.24 (0.23–0.26)

ments, neurologic examination, and vision testing with funduscopic examination. The finding of fever with acute headache warrants additional maneuvers to elicit evidence of meningeal inflammation, such as Kernig and Brudzinski signs. Besides malignant hypertension, significant hypertension can also be a sign of intracranial hemorrhage, preeclampsia, and pheochromocytoma. Patients over 60 years of age should be examined for scalp or temporal artery tenderness.

Careful assessment of visual acuity, ocular gaze, visual fields, pupillary defects, the optic disk, and retinal vein pulsations is crucial. Diminished visual acuity is suggestive of glaucoma, temporal arteritis, or optic neuritis. Ophthalmoplegia or visual field defects may be signs of venous sinus thrombosis, tumor, or aneurysm. Afferent pupillary defects can be due to intracranial masses or optic neuritis. Ipsilateral ptosis and miosis suggest Horner syndrome and in conjunction with acute headache may signify carotid artery dissection. Finally, papilledema or absent retinal venous pulsations are signs of elevated intracranial pressure—findings that should be followed by neuroimaging prior to performing lumbar puncture (Table 2–11).

Mental status and complete neurologic evaluations are also critical and should include assessment of motor and sensory systems, reflexes, gait, cerebellar function, and pronator drift. Any abnormality on mental status or neurologic evaluation warrants emergent neuroimaging (Table 2–11).

C. Diagnostic Studies

Guidance on when to perform neuroimaging is summarized in Table 2–11. Under most circumstances, a noncontrast head CT is sufficient to exclude intracranial hypertension with impending herniation, intracranial hemorrhage, and many types of intracranial masses (notable exceptions include lymphoma and toxoplasmosis in HIV-positive patients, herpes simplex encephalitis, and brain abscess). When appropriate, a contrast study can often be ordered to follow a normal noncontrast study. A normal neuroimaging study does not sufficiently exclude subarachnoid hemorrhage and should be followed by lumbar puncture. In patients for whom there is a high level of suspicion for subarachnoid hemorrhage or aneurysm, a normal CT and lumbar puncture should be followed by angiography within the next few days (provided the patient is medically stable). Lumbar puncture is also indi-cated to exclude infectious causes of acute headache, particularly in patients with fever or meningeal signs. Cerebrospinal fluid tests should routinely include Gram stain, white blood cell count with differential, red blood cell count, glucose, total protein, and bacterial culture. In appropriate patients, also consider testing cerebrospinal fluid for VDRL (syphilis), cryptococcal antigen (HIV-positive patients), acid-fast bacillus stain and culture, and complement fixation and culture for coccidioidomycosis. Storage of an extra tube with 5 mL of cerebrospinal fluid is also prudent for conducting unanticipated tests in the immediate future. Consultation with infectious disease experts regarding local availability of newer polymerase chain reaction tests for specific infectious pathogens (eg, herpes simplex 2) should also be considered in patients with evidence of central nervous system infection but no identifiable pathogen.

In addition to neuroimaging and lumbar puncture, additional diagnostic tests for exclusion of life-threatening causes of acute headache include erythrocyte sedimentation rate (temporal arteritis; endocarditis), urinalysis (malignant hypertension; preeclampsia), and sinus CT or radiograph (bacterial sinusitis, independently or as a cause of venous sinus thrombosis).

► Treatment

Treatment should be directed at the cause of acute headache. In patients in whom migraine or migraine-like headache has been diagnosed, early treatment with NSAIDs or triptans can often abort or provide significant relief of symptoms. The effectiveness of NSAIDs and triptans appears to be equivalent, although combination sumatriptan-naproxen appears to provide a greater sustained response (2–24 hours) compared with monotherapy with either agent alone. Nonoral medication administration is often necessary for patients with significant nausea and vomiting, in which case nasal and subcutaneous triptans and intramuscular ketorolac are therapeutic options. Other causes of acute headache, such as subarachnoid hemorrhage, intracranial mass, or meningitis, usually require emergent treatment in the hospital.

► When to Refer

- Frequent migraines not responsive to standard therapy.
- Migraines with atypical features.
- Chronic daily headaches due to medication overuse.

► When to Admit

- Need for repeated doses of parenteral pain medication.
- To facilitate an expedited work-up requiring a sequence of procedures and neuroimaging.
- Monitoring for progression of symptoms and neurologic consultation when the initial emergency department work-up is inconclusive.
- Pain severe enough to impair activities of daily living or limit participation in follow-up appointments or consultation.

Beck E et al. Management of cluster headache. Am Fam Physician. 2005 Feb 15;71(4):717–24. [PMID: 15742909]

Brandes JL et al. Sumatriptan-naproxen for acute treatment of migraine: a randomized trial. JAMA 2007 Apr 4;297(13):1443–54. [PMID: 17405970]

Detsky ME et al. Does this patient have migraine? JAMA. 2006 Sep 13;296(10):1274–83. [PMID: 16968852]

Dodik DW. Chronic daily headache. N Engl J Med. 2006 Jan 12;354(2):158–65. [PMID: 16407511]

Gladstein J. Headache. Med Clin North Am. 2006 Mar;90(2):275–90. [PMID: 16448875]

Locker TE et al. The utility of clinical features in patients presenting with nontraumatic headache: an investigation of adult patients attending an emergency department. Headache. 2006 Jun;46(6):954–61. [PMID: 16732841]

van Gijn J et al. Subarachnoid hemorrhage. Lancet. 2007 Jan 27;369(9558):306–18. [PMID: 17258671]

DYSURIA

ESSENTIAL INQUIRIES

▸ Fever.

▸ Nausea or vomiting.

▸ New back or flank pain.

▸ Vaginal discharge.

▸ Pregnancy risk.

▸ Structural abnormalities.

▸ Instrumentation of urethra or bladder.

▸ General Considerations

Dysuria (painful urination) is a common reason for adolescents and adults to seek urgent medical attention. An inflammatory process (eg, infection; autoimmune disorder) underlies most causes of dysuria. In women, cystitis will be diagnosed in up to 50–60% of cases and has an incidence of 0.5–0.7% per year in sexually active young women. The key objective in evaluating women with dysuria is to exclude serious upper urinary tract disease, such as acute pyelonephritis, and sexually transmitted diseases. In contrast, in men, urethritis accounts for the vast majority of cases of dysuria.

▸ Clinical Findings

A. Symptoms

Well-designed cohort studies have shown that some women can be reliably diagnosed with uncomplicated cystitis without a physical examination or urinalysis, and randomized controlled trials show that telephone management of uncomplicated cystitis is safe and effective. An increased likelihood of cystitis is present when women report multiple irritative voiding symptoms (dysuria, urgency, frequency), fever, or back pain (likelihood ratios = 1.6–2.0). Inquiring about symptoms of vulvovaginitis is imperative, since the presence of vaginal discharge or itching substantially decreases the likelihood of cystitis (likelihood ratios = 0.2–0.3). When women report dysuria and urinary frequency, and deny vaginal discharge and irritation, the likelihood ratio for culture-confirmed cystitis is 24.5. In contrast, when vaginal discharge or irritation is present, as well as dysuria or urinary frequency, the likelihood ratio is 0.7. Gross hematuria in women with voiding symptoms usually represents hemorrhagic cystitis, but can also be a sign of bladder cancer (particularly in older patients) or upper tract disease. Failure of hematuria to resolve with antibiotic treatment should prompt further evaluation of the bladder and kidneys. Chlamydial infection should be strongly considered among women age 25 years or younger who are sexually active and seeking medical attention for a suspected urinary tract infection for the first time or have a new partner.

Because fever and back pain, as well as nausea and vomiting, are considered harbingers of (or clinical criteria for) acute pyelonephritis, women with these symptoms should usually be examined by a clinician prior to treatment in order to exclude coexistent urosepsis, hydronephrosis, or nephrolithiasis. Other major risk factors for acute pyelonephritis (among women 18–49 years of age) relate to sexual behaviors (frequency of sexual intercourse three or more times per week, new sexual partner in previous year, recent spermicide use), as well as diabetes mellitus and recent urinary tract infection or incontinence. Finally, pregnancy risk, underlying structural factors (polycystic kidney disease, nephrolithiasis, neurogenic bladder), immunosuppression, diabetes, and a history of recent bladder or urethral instrumentation usually alter the treatment regimen (antibiotic choice or duration of treatment, or both) of uncomplicated cystitis.

B. Physical Examination

The presence of fever, tachycardia, or hypotension should alert the clinician to the possibility of urosepsis and the potential need for hospitalization. A focused examination in women, in uncomplicated circumstances, could be limited to ascertainment of costovertebral angle tenderness and to a lower abdominal and pelvic examination, if the history suggests vulvovaginitis or cervicitis.

C. Diagnostic Studies

1. Urinalysis—Urinalysis is probably overutilized in the evaluation of dysuria. The probability of culture-confirmed urinary tract infection among women with a history and physical examination compatible with uncomplicated cystitis is about 70–90%. Urinalysis is most helpful when the woman with dysuria does not have other typical features of cystitis. Dipstick detection (> trace) of leukocytes, nitrites, or blood supports a diagnosis of cystitis. When both leukocyte and nitrite tests are positive, the likelihood ratio is 4.2, and when both are negative, the likelihood ratio is 0.3. The negative predictive value of urinalysis is not sufficient to exclude culture-confirmed urinary tract infection in women with multiple and typical symptoms; and randomized trial evidence shows that antibiotic treatment is beneficial to women with typical symptoms and negative urinalysis dipstick tests.

2. Urine culture—Urine culture should be considered for all women with upper tract symptoms (prior to initiating antibi-

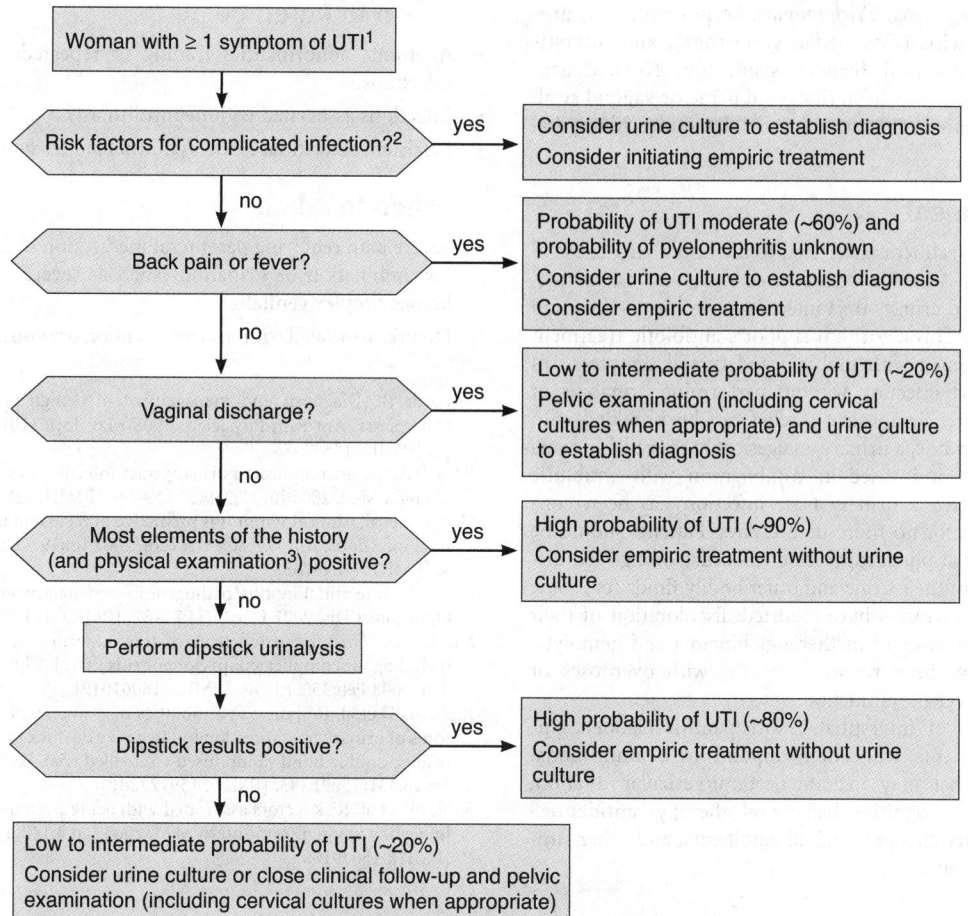

Woman with ≥ 1 symptom of UTI[1]

Risk factors for complicated infection?[2] — yes →
Consider urine culture to establish diagnosis
Consider initiating empiric treatment

no

Back pain or fever? — yes →
Probability of UTI moderate (~60%) and probability of pyelonephritis unknown
Consider urine culture to establish diagnosis
Consider empiric treatment

no

Vaginal discharge? — yes →
Low to intermediate probability of UTI (~20%)
Pelvic examination (including cervical cultures when appropriate) and urine culture to establish diagnosis

no

Most elements of the history (and physical examination[3]) positive? — yes →
High probability of UTI (~90%)
Consider empiric treatment without urine culture

no

Perform dipstick urinalysis

Dipstick results positive? — yes →
High probability of UTI (~80%)
Consider empiric treatment without urine culture

no

Low to intermediate probability of UTI (~20%)
Consider urine culture or close clinical follow-up and pelvic examination (including cervical cultures when appropriate)

[1] In women who have risk factors for sexually transmitted diseases, consider testing for chlamydia. The US Preventive Services Task Force recommends screening for *Chlamydia* for all women 25 years or younger and women of any age with more than one sexual partner, a history of sexually transmitted disease, or inconsistent use of condoms.

[2] A complicated UTI is one in an individual with a functional or anatomic abnormality of the urinary tract, including a history of polycystic renal disease, nephrolithiasis, neurogenic bladder, diabetes mellitus, immunosuppression, pregnancy, indwelling urinary catheter, or recent urinary tract instrumentation.

[3] The only physical examination finding that increases the likelihood of UTI is costovertebral angle tenderness, and clinicians may consider not performing this test in patients with typical symptoms of acute uncomplicated UTI (as in telephone management).

▲ **Figure 2–3.** Proposed algorithm for evaluating women with symptoms of acute urinary tract infection (UTI). (Modified and reproduced, with permission, from Bent S et al. Does this woman have an acute uncomplicated urinary tract infection? JAMA. 2002 May 22–29;287(20):2701–10.)

otic therapy), as well as those with dysuria and a negative urine dipstick test. In symptomatic women, a clean-catch urine culture is considered positive when 10^2–10^3 colony-forming units/mL of a uropathogenic organism is detected.

3. Renal imaging—When severe flank or back pain is present, the possibility of complicated kidney infection (perinephric abscess, nephrolithiasis) or of hydronephrosis should be considered. Depending on local availability, acceptable imaging options to assess for hydronephrosis include abdominal radiographs, renal ultrasound, or CT

scanning. To exclude nephrolithiasis, noncontrast helical CT scanning is more accurate than intravenous urography and is rapidly becoming the diagnostic test of choice for this purpose. In a meta-analysis, the positive and negative likelihood ratios of helical CT scanning for diagnosis of nephrolithiasis were 23.2 and 0.05, respectively.

▶ **Differential Diagnosis**

The differential diagnosis of dysuria in women includes acute cystitis, acute pyelonephritis, vaginitis (*Candida*, bacterial vaginosis, *Trichomonas*, herpes simplex), urethritis/cervicitis (*Chlamydia*, gonorrhea), and interstitial cystitis/painful bladder syndrome. Nucleic acid amplification tests from first-void urine or vaginal swab specimens are highly sensitive for detecting chlamydial infection.

Treatment

Definitive treatment is directed to the underlying cause of the dysuria. An evidence-informed algorithm for managing suspected urinary tract infection in women is shown in Figure 2–3. This algorithm supports antibiotic treatment of most women with multiple and typical symptoms of urinary tract infection without performing urinalysis or urine culture. Symptomatic relief can be provided with phenazopyridine, a urinary analgesic that is available over-the-counter; it is used in combination with antibiotic therapy (when a urinary tract infection has been confirmed) but for no more than 2 days. Patients should be informed that phenazopyridine will cause orange/red discoloration of their urine and other bodily fluids (eg, some contact lens wearers have reported discoloration of their lenses). Rare cases of methemoglobinemia and hemolytic anemia have been reported, usually with overdoses or underlying renal dysfunction.

In cases of interstitial cystitis/painful bladder syndrome, patients will often respond to a multimodal approach that may include urethral/vesicular dilation, biofeedback, cognitive behavioral therapy, antidepressants, dietary changes, vaginal emollients, and other supportive measures.

When to Refer

- Anatomic abnormalities leading to repeated urinary infections.
- Infections associated with nephrolithiasis.
- Persistent interstitial cystitis/painful bladder syndrome.

When to Admit

- Severe pain requiring parenteral medication or impairing ambulation or urination (such as severe primary herpes simplex genitalis).
- Dysuria associated with urinary retention or obstruction.

Edwards JL. Diagnosis and management of benign prostatic hyperplasia. Am Fam Physician. 2008 May 15;77(10):1403–10. [PMID: 18533373]

Fihn S. Acute uncomplicated urinary tract infection in women. N Engl J Med. 2003 Jul 17;349(3):259–66. [PMID: 12867610]

Gopal M et al. Clinical symptoms predictive of recurrent urinary tract infections. Am J Obstet Gynecol. 2007 Jul;197(1):74.e1–4. [PMID: 17618765]

Mayer R. Interstitial cystitis pathogenesis and treatment. Curr Opin Infect Dis. 2007 Feb;20(1):77–82. [PMID: 17197886]

Nicolle LE. Uncomplicated urinary tract infection in adults including uncomplicated pyelonephritis. Urol Clin North Am. 2008 Feb;35(1):1–12. [PMID: 18061019]

Richards D et al. Response to antibiotics of women with symptoms of urinary tract infection but negative dipstick urine test results: double blind randomised controlled trial. BMJ. 2005 Jul 16;331(7509):143. [PMID: 15972728]

Sholes D et al. Risk factors associated with acute pyelonephritis in healthy women. Ann Intern Med. 2005 Jan 4;142(1):20–7. [PMID: 15630106]

Preoperative Evaluation & Perioperative Management

Hugo Q. Cheng, MD

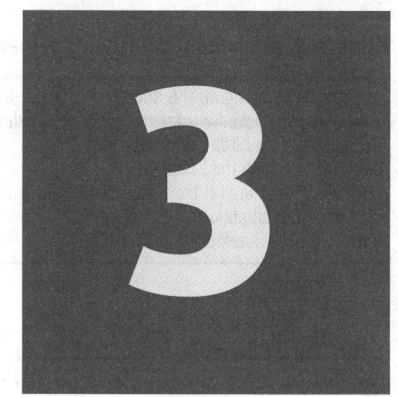

EVALUATION OF THE ASYMPTOMATIC PATIENT

Patients without significant medical problems—especially those under age 50—are at very low risk for perioperative complications. Their preoperative evaluation should include a complete history and physical examination. Special emphasis is placed on the assessment of functional status, exercise tolerance, and cardiopulmonary symptoms and signs in an effort to reveal previously unrecognized disease (especially cardiopulmonary disease) that may require further evaluation prior to surgery. In addition, a directed bleeding history (Table 3–1) should be taken to uncover coagulopathies that could contribute to excessive surgical blood loss. Routine preoperative testing of asymptomatic healthy patients under age 50 has not been found to help predict or prevent complications.

Patients who are older than 50 years and those with risk factors for coronary artery disease should have a 12-lead ECG because evidence of clinically silent coronary artery disease should prompt further cardiac evaluation. Minor ECG abnormalities such as bundle branch block, T wave changes, and premature ventricular contractions do not predict adverse postoperative outcomes. Of note, patients undergoing minor or minimally invasive procedures (such as cataract surgery) may not require any routine preoperative tests.

Minchota FA Jr. The preoperative evaluation and use of laboratory testing. Cleve Clin J Med. 2006 Mar;73(Suppl 1):S4–7. [PMID: 16570540]

van Klei WA et al. Role of history and physical examination in preoperative evaluation. Eur J Anaesthesiol. 2003 Aug;20(8):612–8. [PMID: 12932061]

CARDIAC RISK ASSESSMENT & REDUCTION

Cardiac complications of noncardiac surgery are a major cause of perioperative morbidity and mortality. The most important perioperative cardiac complications are myocardial infarction (MI) and cardiac death. Other complications include congestive heart failure (CHF), arrhythmias, and unstable angina. The principal patient-specific risk factor is the presence of end-organ cardiovascular disease. This includes not only coronary artery disease and CHF, but also cerebrovascular disease and chronic renal insufficiency. Diabetes mellitus is treated as a cardiovascular disease equivalent and has also been shown to increase the risk of cardiac complications. Major abdominal, thoracic, and vascular surgical procedures (especially abdominal aortic aneurysm repair) carry a higher risk of postoperative cardiac complications, likely due to their associated major fluid shifts, hemorrhage, and hypoxemia. These risk factors were identified in a validated multifactorial risk prediction index: the Revised Cardiac Risk Index (Table 3–2). The Revised Cardiac Risk Index has become a widely used tool for assessing and communicating cardiac risk and has been incorporated into routine perioperative care guidelines. Severely limited exercise capacity and greater severity of cardiac symptoms also predict higher cardiac risk. Emergency operations are also associated with greater cardiac risk. However, emergency operations should not be delayed by extensive cardiac evaluation. Instead, patients facing emergency surgery should be medically optimized for surgery as quickly as possible and closely monitored for cardiac complications during the perioperative period.

Role of Preoperative Noninvasive Ischemia Testing

Candidates for noninvasive ischemia testing independent of the planned noncardiac surgery should generally have such testing prior to elective surgery. Conversely, stress testing should be omitted if the results will not alter management.

Most patients can be accurately risk-stratified by history, physical examination, and electrocardiogram (ECG). Patients without clinical predictors for cardiac complications (Table 3–2) or who have at least fair functional capacity are at low risk for cardiac complications. Noninvasive testing in these patients is generally not helpful. Patients with more severe cardiac symptoms, such as New York Heart Association class III or IV angina (see Chapter 10), poor functional capacity, or a high Revised Cardiac Risk Index score are much more likely to suffer cardiac complications. Stress testing of these patients may be able to

Table 3–1. Findings suggestive of a bleeding disorder.

Unprovoked bruising on the trunk of > 5 cm in diameter
Frequent unprovoked epistaxis or gingival bleeding
Menorrhagia with iron deficiency
Hemarthrosis with mild trauma
Prior excessive surgical blood loss or reoperation for bleeding
Family history of abnormal bleeding
Presence of severe kidney or liver disease

Table 3–2. Revised Cardiac Risk Index.

Independent Predictors of Postoperative Cardiac Complications	
1. Intrathoracic, intraperitoneal, or infrainguinal vascular surgery	
2. History of ischemic heart disease	
3. History of congestive heart failure	
4. Insulin treatment for diabetes mellitus	
5. Serum creatinine level > 2 mg/dL	
6. History of cerebrovascular disease	

Scoring (Number of Predictors Present)	Risk of Major Cardiac Complications[1]
None	0.4%
One	0.9%
Two	7.0%
More than two	11%

[1]Myocardial infarction, pulmonary edema, ventricular fibrillation, cardiac arrest, and complete heart block.
Adapted, with permission, from Lee TH et al. Derivation and prospective validation of a simple index for prediction of cardiac risk of major noncardiac surgery. Circulation. 1999 Sept 7; 100(10):1043–9.

stratify them into low-risk and high-risk subgroups, particularly when major vascular surgery is planned. For patients who will undergo vascular surgery and who have multiple Revised Cardiac Risk Index predictors, the absence of inducible ischemia or the presence of only mild, limited ischemia on dipyridamole scintigraphy or dobutamine stress echocardiography predicts a generally acceptable risk of perioperative cardiac death or MI. In contrast, extensive inducible ischemia in this population predicts a very high risk of cardiac complications, which may not be modifiable by either medical management or coronary revascularization. An approach to perioperative cardiac risk assessment and management in patients with known or suspected stable coronary artery disease is shown in Figure 3–1.

► Perioperative Management of Patients with Coronary Artery Disease

Patients with acute coronary syndromes are at extremely high risk for complications and require immediate management of their cardiac disease prior to any preoperative evaluation (see Chapter 10). Patients with stable coronary artery disease have a 1–5% risk of MI and about a 1% mortality rate. In some patients, preoperative cardioprotective strategies can minimize these risks. Postoperative myocardial ischemia or infarction often presents atypically or may be asymptomatic. Symptoms and signs that should prompt consideration of postoperative MI include unexplained hypotension, hypoxemia, or delirium. However, current evidence is insufficient to formulate specific recommendations for screening asymptomatic patients for ischemia through the use of ECG or cardiac enzyme monitoring.

A. Medications

Preoperative antianginal medications, including β-blockers, calcium channel blockers, and nitrates, should be continued preoperatively and during the postoperative period. Early, small clinical trials demonstrated a reduction in perioperative cardiac morbidity and mortality with prophylactic β-blocking agents. A randomized trial in vascular surgery patients with ischemia on dobutamine stress echocardiography found that bisoprolol reduced the 30-day risk of cardiac mortality or nonfatal MI from 34% to 3% in these high-risk patients. In contrast, subsequent trials found a much smaller cardioprotective effect of β-blockers in lower risk patients. In the largest of these studies, extended-released metoprolol reduced the

absolute risk of cardiac complications by only 1.1% in patients with at least one Revised Cardiac Risk Index predictor who were undergoing major surgery. This was offset, however, by a 0.8% absolute increase in total mortality. Hypotension and bradycardia were more common when patients received β-blockers; in addition, the risk of stroke was higher in these patients. Because of the uncertain benefit-to-risk ratio of perioperative β-blockade, it should be reserved for patients with a relatively high risk of cardiac complications. Suggested indications for prophylactic β-blockade are presented in Table 3–3. Comparative trials between different β-blockers are lacking, although all cardioselective agents (eg, metoprolol or atenolol) are believed to be equivalent. The dose should be adjusted to maintain a heart rate under 65 beats per minute. Ideally, β-blockers should be started well in advance of surgery, to allow time to gradually titrate up the dose without causing excessive bradycardia or hypotension. β-Blockers should be continued for at least 3–7 days after surgery.

Observational studies show an association between the use of HMG-CoA reductase inhibitors (statins) during the perioperative period and lower rates of mortality and postoperative MI. A randomized trial in statin-naïve patients undergoing vascular surgery found that extended-release fluvastatin reduced the 30-day risk of cardiac death or nonfatal MI from 10.1% to 4.8%. Although there are insufficient data to make a strong recommendation regarding the perioperative use of prophylactic statins, they should be considered in patients undergoing vascular surgery and other patients deemed to be at high risk for cardiac complications. Patients already taking statins should continue these agents during the perioperative period.

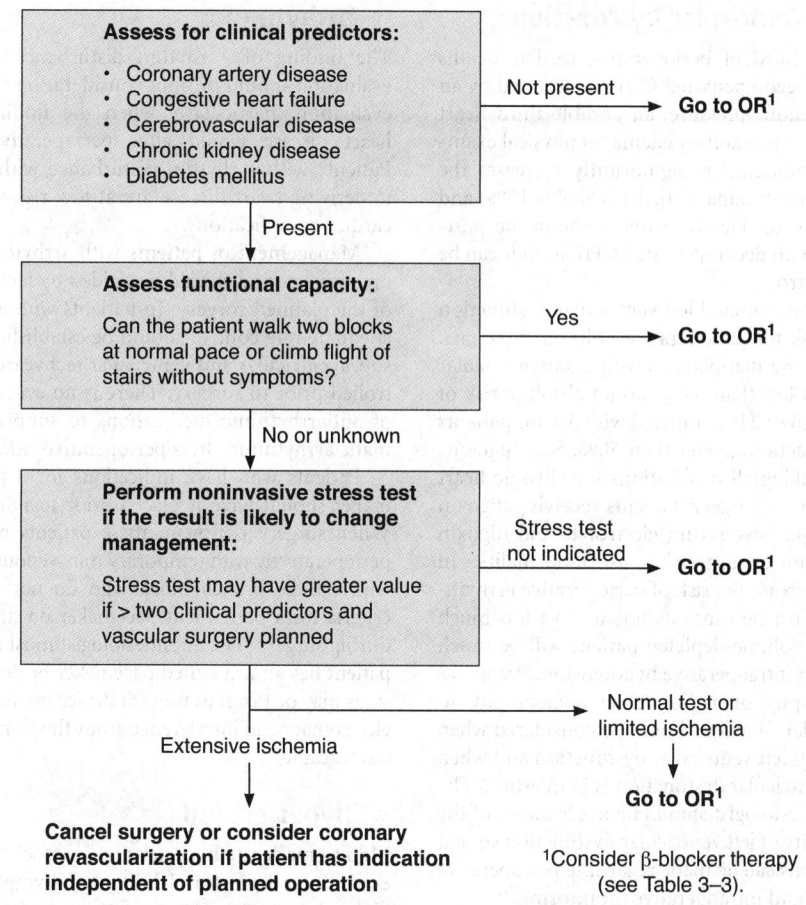

▲ Figure 3–1. Assessment and management of patients with known or suspected stable coronary artery disease (CAD) undergoing elective major noncardiac surgery. (OR, operating room.)

B. Coronary Revascularization

Retrospective studies suggest that patients who had previously undergone coronary artery bypass grafting (CABG) surgery or percutaneous coronary interventions (PCI) have

Table 3–3. Indications for prophylactic perioperative β-blockade.

Strong indications	Patient already taking β-blocker to treat ischemia, arrhythmia, or hypertension Patient with potential for myocardial ischemia (eg, reversibility on stress test) undergoing major vascular surgery
Possible indications	Patients with potential for myocardial ischemia undergoing major nonvascular surgery Patient with coronary disease or multiple other clinical predictors (heart failure, chronic kidney disease, diabetes mellitus) undergoing any major surgery

a relatively low risk of cardiac complications when undergoing subsequent noncardiac surgery. However, one trial randomized over 500 patients with angiographically proven coronary artery disease to either coronary revascularization (with either CABG or PCI) or medical management alone before vascular surgery. Postoperative nonfatal MI, 30-day mortality, and long-term mortality did not differ, suggesting that prophylactic revascularization before noncardiac surgery does not prevent cardiac complications. Thus, current data argue that preoperative CABG or PCI should only be performed on patients who have indications for the procedure independent of the planned noncardiac operation. In patients who have undergone recent intracoronary stenting, observational studies suggest that perioperative cardiac mortality rate may be very high if antiplatelet therapy is stopped due to concern for surgical site bleeding. The presumed mechanism of this increased mortality is acute stent thrombosis that results from premature discontinuation of antiplatelet therapy. Therefore, elective surgery should be deferred for at least 1 month after placement of a bare-metal stent and for a year after placement of a drug-eluting stent if antiplatelet therapy must be stopped perioperatively.

CHF & Left Ventricular Dysfunction

An estimated one-third of perioperative cardiac deaths result from CHF. Decompensated CHF, manifested by an elevated jugular venous pressure, an audible third heart sound, or evidence of pulmonary edema on physical examination or chest radiography, significantly increases the risk of perioperative pulmonary edema (roughly 15%) and cardiac death (2–10%). Elective surgery should be postponed in patients with decompensated CHF until it can be brought under control.

Patients with compensated left ventricular dysfunction are at increased risk for perioperative pulmonary edema. One large study found that patients with a left ventricular ejection fraction of less than 50% had an absolute risk of 12% for postoperative CHF compared with 3% for patients with an ejection fraction greater than 50%. Such patients should continue taking all medications for chronic heart failure up to the day of surgery. Patients receiving digoxin and diuretics should have serum electrolyte and digoxin levels measured prior to surgery because abnormalities in these levels may increase the risk of perioperative arrhythmias. Clinicians must be cautious not to give too much diuretic, since the volume-depleted patient will be much more susceptible to intraoperative hypotension. Preoperative echocardiography or radionuclide angiography to assess left ventricular function should be considered when there is suspicion of left ventricular dysfunction and when the cause of left ventricular dysfunction is in question. The surgeon and anesthesiologist should be made aware of the presence and severity of left ventricular dysfunction so that appropriate decisions can be made regarding perioperative fluid management and intraoperative monitoring.

Valvular Heart Disease

There are few data available regarding the perioperative risks of valvular heart disease for noncardiac surgery independent of associated coronary artery disease or CHF. The severity of valvular lesions should be evaluated by echocardiography or cardiac catheterization before noncardiac surgery to allow for appropriate fluid management and consideration of invasive intraoperative monitoring. Patients with severe symptomatic aortic stenosis are clearly at increased risk for cardiac complications and should not undergo elective surgery. In a series of patients with aortic stenosis who underwent noncardiac surgery, death or nonfatal MI occurred in 31% in patients with severe aortic stenosis (aortic valve area < 0.7 cm²), in 11% in those with moderate aortic stenosis (aortic valve area 0.7–1.0 cm²), and in 2% in those without aortic stenosis. Other studies have found that patients with asymptomatic aortic stenosis appeared to be at lower risk than patients with symptomatic aortic stenosis. Patients with mitral stenosis require heart rate control to maintain diastolic filling time. Patients with aortic or mitral regurgitation likely benefit from afterload reduction and careful attention to volume status. Candidates for valve replacement surgery or balloon valvuloplasty (if only short-term relief is needed) independent of the planned noncardiac surgery should have the valve correction procedure performed first.

Arrhythmias

The finding of a rhythm disturbance on preoperative evaluation should prompt consideration of further cardiac evaluation, particularly when the finding of structural heart disease would alter perioperative management. Patients with a rhythm disturbance without evidence of underlying heart disease are at low risk for perioperative cardiac complications.

Management of patients with arrhythmias in the preoperative period should be guided by factors independent of the planned surgery. In patients with atrial fibrillation, adequate rate control should be established. Symptomatic supraventricular and ventricular tachycardia must be controlled prior to surgery. There is no evidence that the use of antiarrhythmic medications to suppress an asymptomatic arrhythmia alters perioperative risk.

Patients who have indications for a permanent pacemaker should have it placed prior to noncardiac surgery. When surgery is urgent, these patients may be managed perioperatively with temporary transvenous pacing. Patients with bundle branch block who do not meet recognized criteria for a permanent pacemaker do not require pacing during surgery. The anesthesiologist must be notified that a patient has an implanted pacemaker or defibrillator so that steps may be taken to prevent device malfunction caused by electromagnetic interference from the intraoperative use of electrocautery.

Hypertension

Mild to moderate hypertension is associated with intraoperative blood pressure lability and asymptomatic myocardial ischemia but does not appear to be an independent risk factor for cardiac complications. No evidence supports delaying surgery in order to better control mild to moderate hypertension. Medications for chronic hypertension should generally be continued up to and including the day of surgery. Consideration should be given to holding angiotensin-converting enzyme inhibitors and angiotensin receptor blockers on the day of surgery, as these agents may increase the risk of intraoperative hypotension.

Severe hypertension, defined as a systolic pressure greater than 180 mm Hg or diastolic pressure greater than 110 mm Hg, appears to be an independent predictor of perioperative cardiac complications, including MI and CHF. It seems wise to delay surgery in patients with severe hypertension until blood pressure can be controlled, although it is not known whether the risk of cardiac complications is reduced with this approach.

Auerbach A et al. Assessing and reducing the cardiac risk of noncardiac surgery. Circulation. 2006 Mar 14;113(10):1361–76. [PMID: 16534031]

Fleisher LA et al. ACC/AHA 2007 guidelines on perioperative cardiovascular evaluation and care for noncardiac surgery: a report of the American College of Cardiology/American Heart Association Task Force on Practice Guidelines. J Am Coll Cardiol. 2007 Oct 23;50(17):1707–32. [PMID: 17950159]

Kapoor AS et al. Strength of evidence for perioperative use of statins to reduce cardiovascular risk: systematic review of controlled studies. BMJ. 2006 Dec 2;333(7579):1149. [PMID: 17088313]

Kertai MD et al. Aortic stenosis: an underestimated risk factor for perioperative complications in patients undergoing noncardiac surgery. Am J Med. 2004 Jan 1;116(1):8–13. [PMID: 14706659]

Makaryus AN et al. Nuclear stress testing in elderly patients: a review of its use in the assessment of cardiac risk, particularly in patients undergoing preoperative risk assessment. Drugs Aging. 2007;24(6):467–79. [PMID: 17571912]

POISE Study Group; Devereaux PJ et al. Effects of extended-release metoprolol succinate in patients undergoing non-cardiac surgery (POISE trial): a randomised controlled trial. Lancet. 2008 May 31;371(9627):1839–47. [PMID: 18479744]

Rabitts JA et al. Cardiac risk of noncardiac surgery after percutaneous coronary intervention with drug-eluting stents. Anesthesiology. 2008 Oct;109(4):596–604. [PMID: 18813037]

Winkler MH et al. Therapy insight: prophylaxis, monitoring and treatment of perioperative myocardial ischemia with emphasis on urological surgery. Nat Clin Pract Urol. 2007 Jun;4(6):333–40. [PMID: 17551537]

PULMONARY EVALUATION IN NON–LUNG RESECTION SURGERY

Pneumonia and respiratory failure requiring prolonged mechanical ventilation are the most important postoperative pulmonary complications and occur in 2–19% of surgical procedures. The occurrence of a postoperative pulmonary complication has been associated with a significant increase in hospital length of stay.

Risk Factors for the Development of Postoperative Pulmonary Complications

The risk of developing a pulmonary complication is highest in patients undergoing cardiac, thoracic, and upper abdominal surgery, with reported complication rates ranging from 9% to 19%. The risk in patients undergoing lower abdominal or pelvic procedures ranges from 2% to 5%, and for extremity procedures the range is less than 1–3%. The pulmonary complication rate for laparoscopic procedures appears to be much lower than that for open procedures. In one series of over 1500 patients who underwent laparoscopic cholecystectomy, the pulmonary complication rate was less than 1%. Other procedure-related risk factors include prolonged anesthesia time, need for general anesthesia, and emergency operations.

Among the many patient-specific risk factors for postoperative pulmonary complications, the strongest predictor appears to be advanced age. A meta-analysis found that surgical patients in their seventh decade had a fourfold higher risk of pulmonary complications compared with patients under age 50. Patients with chronic obstructive pulmonary disease (COPD) or CHF have at least twice the risk compared with patients without these conditions. In a single large prospective cohort of US military veterans, additional clinical risk factors for the development of postoperative pneumonia included dependent functional status, impaired sensorium, and prior stroke, long-term corticosteroid use, heavy alcohol consumption, and current cigarette smoking. In another study, cigarette smoking was also found to double the risk of postoperative pneumonia, even when controlling for underlying lung disease.

Patients with asthma are at increased risk for bronchospasm during tracheal intubation and extubation and during the postoperative period. However, if patients are at their optimal pulmonary function (as determined by symptoms, physical examination, or peak flow rate) at the time of surgery, they are not at increased risk for other pulmonary complications. Mild or moderate obesity also does not appear to increase the risk of clinically important pulmonary complications, but postoperative pneumonia was found to be twice as likely to develop in morbidly obese patients—those weighing over 113 kg (250 lb)—than in patients weighing less. Obese patients are prone to obstructive sleep apnea. This condition has been associated with a variety of postoperative complications, particularly in patients undergoing bariatric surgery. A summary of risk factors for pulmonary complications is presented in Table 3–4.

Pulmonary Function Testing & Laboratory Studies

Most studies have shown that preoperative pulmonary function testing (PFT) in unselected patients is not helpful in predicting postoperative pulmonary complications. The data are conflicting regarding the usefulness of preoperative PFT in certain selected groups of patients, such as the morbidly obese or those with COPD, especially when undergoing upper abdominal or cardiothoracic surgery. Assessment of the severity of COPD using PFT has not been shown to improve upon the clinical risk assessment with the exception that patients with a forced expiratory volume in 1 second (FEV_1) under 500 mL or an FEV_1 below 50% of the predicted value appear to be at particularly high risk. However, there is no clear degree of PFT abnormality that can be used as an absolute contraindication to non–lung resection surgery. Definitive recommendations regarding the indications for preoperative PFT cannot be made. In general terms, such testing may be helpful to confirm the diagnosis of COPD or asthma, to assess the severity of known pulmonary disease, and perhaps as part of the risk assessment for patients undergoing upper abdominal, cardiac, or thoracic surgery. Some experts have also advocated polysomnography to diagnose obstructive sleep apnea prior to bariatric surgery, but the benefits of this approach are unproven. Abnormally low or high blood urea nitrogen levels (indicating malnutrition and renal insufficiency, respectively) have been found to predict postoperative pulmonary complica-

Table 3–4. Clinical risk factors for postoperative pulmonary complications.

Upper abdominal or cardiothoracic surgery
Prolonged anesthesia time (> 4 hours)
Age > 60 years
Chronic obstructive pulmonary disease
Congestive heart failure
Tobacco use (> 20 pack-years)
Impaired cognition or sensorium
Functional dependency or prior stroke
Morbid obesity
Low serum albumin level
Obstructive sleep apnea

tions. In addition, several studies have found that a low serum albumin level is associated with a higher risk of pulmonary complications and a higher overall mortality.

Arterial blood gas measurement is not routinely recommended except in patients with known lung disease and suspected hypoxemia or hypercapnia.

▶ Perioperative Management

Retrospective studies have shown that smoking cessation reduced the incidence of pulmonary complications, but only if it was initiated at least 1–2 months before surgery. The incidence of postoperative pulmonary complications in patients with COPD or asthma may be reduced by preoperative optimization of pulmonary function. Patients who are wheezing will probably benefit from preoperative therapy with bronchodilators and, in certain cases, corticosteroids. Antibiotics may be beneficial for patients who cough with purulent sputum if the sputum can be cleared before surgery. On the other hand, the use of antibiotics in unselected patients undergoing head and neck cancer surgery did not reduce the occurrence of pulmonary complications. Patients receiving oral theophylline should continue taking the drug perioperatively. A serum theophylline level should be measured to rule out toxicity. Most patients with COPD can be treated with cardioselective β-blockers if indicated to prevent perioperative cardiac complications without suffering respiratory compromise.

Postoperative risk reduction strategies have centered on promoting lung expansion through the use of incentive spirometry, continuous positive airway pressure (CPAP), intermittent positive-pressure breathing (IPPB), and deep breathing exercises. Although trial results have been mixed, all these techniques have been shown to reduce the incidence of postoperative atelectasis and, in a few studies, to reduce the incidence of postoperative pulmonary complications. In most comparative trials, these methods were equally effective. Given the higher cost of CPAP and IPPB, incentive spirometry and deep breathing exercises are the preferred methods for most patients. However, in a randomized trial of patients undergoing esophageal or gastric resection, CPAP was more effective at preventing respiratory failure than incentive spirometry or deep breathing exercises and thus may be preferable after these operations. Incentive spirometry must be performed for 15 minutes every 2 hours. Deep breathing exercises must be performed hourly and consist of 3-second breath-holding, pursed lip breathing, and coughing. These measures should be started preoperatively and be continued for 1–2 days postoperatively.

Bapoje SR et al. Preoperative evaluation of the patient with pulmonary disease. Chest. 2007 Nov;132(5):1637–1645. [PMID: 17998364]

Catheline JM et al. Preoperative cardiac and pulmonary assessment in bariatric surgery. Obes Surg. 2008 Mar;18(3):271–7. [PMID: 18204992]

Dronkers J et al. Prevention of pulmonary complications after upper abdominal surgery by preoperative intensive inspiratory muscle training: a randomized controlled pilot study. Clin Rehabil. 2008 Feb;22(2):134–142. [PMID: 18057088]

Hulzebos EH et al. Preoperative intensive inspiratory muscle training to prevent postoperative pulmonary complications in high-risk patients undergoing CABG surgery. JAMA. 2006 Oct 18;296(15):1851–7. [PMID: 17047215]

Qaseem A et al; Clinical Efficacy Assessment Subcommittee of the American College of Physicians. Risk assessment for and strategies to reduce perioperative pulmonary complications for patients undergoing noncardiothoracic surgery: a guideline from the American College of Physicians. Ann Intern Med. 2006 Apr 18;144(8):575–80. [PMID: 16618955]

EVALUATION OF THE PATIENT WITH LIVER DISEASE

Patients with serious liver disease are at increased risk for perioperative morbidity and demise. Appropriate preoperative evaluation requires consideration of the effects of anesthesia and surgery on postoperative liver function and of the complications associated with anesthesia and surgery in patients with preexisting liver disease.

▶ The Effects of Anesthesia & Surgery on Liver Function

Postoperative elevation of serum aminotransferase levels is a relatively common finding after major surgery. Most of these elevations are transient and not associated with hepatic dysfunction. Studies in the 1960s and early 1970s showed that patients with liver disease are at increased relative risk for postoperative deterioration in hepatic function, although the absolute risk is not known. General anesthetic agents may cause deterioration of hepatic function via intraoperative reduction in hepatic blood flow leading to ischemic injury. Medications used for regional anesthesia produce similar reductions in hepatic blood flow and thus may be equally likely to lead to ischemic liver injury. Intraoperative hypotension, hemorrhage, and hypoxemia may also contribute to liver injury.

▶ Risk Factors for Surgical Complications

Observational studies have found that surgery in patients with serious liver disease is associated with a variety of complications, including hemorrhage, infection, renal failure, and encephalopathy, and with a substantial mortality rate. A key limitation in interpreting these data is our inability to determine the contribution of the liver disease to the observed complications independent of the surgical procedure.

Acute hepatitis appears to increase surgical risk. In three small series of patients with acute viral hepatitis who underwent abdominal surgery, the mortality rate was roughly 10%. Cirrhotic patients undergoing portosystemic shunt surgery who have evidence of alcoholic hepatitis on the preoperative liver biopsy also have a significantly increased surgical mortality rate compared with patients without alcoholic hepatitis. It seems reasonable to delay elective surgery in patients with acute viral or alcoholic hepatitis until the acute episode has resolved. These data are not sufficient to warrant substantial delays in urgent or emergent surgery.

There are few data regarding the risks of surgery in patients with chronic hepatitis. In a series of 272 patients with chronic hepatitis undergoing a variety of surgical procedures for variceal hemorrhage, the in-hospital mortality rate was less than 2%. Patients with serum aminotransferase levels greater than 150 units/L were excluded from this analysis. In a study of patients undergoing hepatectomy for hepatocellular carcinoma, patients with both cirrhosis and active hepatitis on the preoperative liver biopsy had a fourfold increase in mortality (8.7%) compared with patients with cirrhosis alone or active hepatitis alone.

In patients with cirrhosis, postoperative complication rates correlate with the severity of liver dysfunction. Traditionally, severity of dysfunction has been assessed with the Child-Turcotte-Pugh score (see Chapter 16). Patients with Child-Turcotte-Pugh class C cirrhosis who underwent portosystemic shunt surgery, biliary surgery, or trauma surgery during the 1970s and 1980s had a 50–85% mortality rate. Patients with Child-Turcotte-Pugh class A or B cirrhosis who underwent abdominal surgery during the 1990s, however, had relatively low mortality rates (hepatectomy 0–8%, open cholecystectomy 0–1%, laparoscopic cholecystectomy 0–1%). A recent multivariate analysis found that the Model for End-stage Liver Disease (MELD) score (which incorporates bilirubin and creatinine levels, and the prothrombin time expressed as the International Normalized Ratio) was the strongest predictor of postoperative mortality and outperformed the Child-Turcotte-Pugh classification. Patients with a MELD score above the median score of 8 had a 30-day mortality risk exceeding 10%. A conservative approach would be to avoid elective surgery in patients with Child-Turcotte-Pugh class C cirrhosis or in patients with a MELD score greater than 8. In addition, when surgery is elective, it is prudent to attempt to reduce the severity of ascites, encephalopathy, and coagulopathy preoperatively.

Bell CL et al. Management of the cirrhotic patient that needs surgery. Curr Treat Options Gastroenterol. 2005 Dec;8(6):473–80. [PMID: 16313865]
Filsoufi F et al. Early and late outcome of cardiac surgery in patients with liver cirrhosis. Liver Transpl. 2007 Jul;13(7):990–5. [PMID: 17427174]
Teh SH et al. Risk factors for mortality after surgery in patients with cirrhosis. Gastroenterology. 2007 Apr;132(4):1261–9. [PMID: 17408652]

PREOPERATIVE HEMATOLOGIC EVALUATION

Three of the more common clinical situations faced by the medical consultant are the patient with preexisting anemia, the assessment of bleeding risk, and the perioperative management of oral anticoagulation.

The key issue in the anemic patient is to determine the need for preoperative diagnostic evaluation and the need for transfusion. When feasible, the diagnostic evaluation of the patient with previously unrecognized anemia should be done prior to surgery because certain types of anemia (particularly sickle cell disease and immune hemolytic anemias) may have implications for perioperative management. Preoperative anemia is common, with a prevalence of 43% in a large cohort of elderly veterans undergoing surgery. In this cohort, morbidity and mortality increased as the preoperative hemoglobin level decreased, even after

adjusting for comorbidities. No data exist to identify a specific preoperative hemoglobin level that should prompt transfusion prior to surgery. It is also not known whether such transfusions will improve postoperative outcomes. Determination of the need for preoperative transfusion in an individual patient must consider factors other than the absolute hemoglobin level, including the presence of cardiopulmonary disease, the type of surgery, and the likely severity of surgical blood loss. The few studies that have compared different postoperative transfusion thresholds failed to demonstrate improved outcomes with a more aggressive transfusion strategy. The traditional recommendation had been to maintain a hemoglobin concentration greater than 10 g/dL. This may be too cautious in otherwise young and healthy patients. In fact, several observational studies and one randomized trial (which included 305 postoperative patients) have not found a benefit to transfusion above a threshold of 7 g/dL.

The most important component of the bleeding risk assessment is a directed bleeding history (see Table 3–1). Patients who are reliable historians and who reveal no suggestion of abnormal bleeding on directed bleeding history and physical examination are at very low risk for having an occult bleeding disorder. Laboratory tests of hemostatic parameters in these patients are generally not needed. When the directed bleeding history is unreliable or incomplete or when abnormal bleeding is suggested, a formal evaluation of hemostasis should be done prior to surgery and should include measurement of the prothrombin time, activated partial thromboplastin time, and platelet count (see Chapter 13).

Patients receiving long-term oral anticoagulation are at risk for thromboembolic complications when an operation requires interruption of their therapy. In a cohort study of 1293 interruptions of warfarin therapy for invasive procedures, the 30-day thromboembolic risk was 0.7%. There are insufficient data to determine the excess risk incurred by holding warfarin therapy or whether this risk may be mitigated through the practice of "bridging" anticoagulation, where unfractionated or low-molecular-weight heparin is administered parenterally while oral anticoagulants are held until just prior to surgery. The bleeding risk associated with bridging anticoagulation can be substantial. Patients in this cohort who received bridging anticoagulation had a 13% incidence of clinically significant bleeding, compared with 0.8% for patients who did not receive bridging anticoagulation. Although firm evidence-based guidelines for perioperative bridging are lacking, most experts recommend bridging therapy only in patients at high risk for thromboembolism. It is important to consider the patient's preferences when weighing the risks and consequences of a thromboembolic event versus major bleeding. A practical approach to perioperative anticoagulation management is shown in Table 3–5.

Dunn A. Perioperative management of oral anticoagulation: when and how to bridge. J Thromb Thrombolysis. 2006 Feb;21(1):85–9. [PMID: 16475048]
Garcia DA et al. Risk of thromboembolism with short-term interruption of warfarin therapy. Arch Intern Med. 2008 Jan 14;168(1):63–9. [PMID: 18195197]

Table 3–5. Recommendations for perioperative anticoagulation management.

Thromboembolic Risk without Anticoagulation	Recommendation
Low (< 8% annual risk) (eg, atrial fibrillation or mechanical bileaflet aortic valve prosthesis with fewer than two other stroke risk factors)	1. Stop oral anticoagulation 4–5 days before surgery 2. Measure INR the day before surgery to confirm that it is < 1.6 3. Resume oral anticoagulation the night of surgery, if possible 4. No bridging
High (> 8% annual risk) (eg, atrial fibrillation or mechanical heart valve with prior stroke, mechanical mitral valve prosthesis, arterial thromboembolism < 1 month ago, or venous thrombosis < 3 months ago)	1. Stop oral anticoagulation 4–5 days before surgery 2. Measure INR the day before surgery to confirm that it is < 1.6 3. Begin therapeutic dose UH or LMWH 2–3 days after stopping oral anticoagulation, and discontinue it 12–24 hours before surgery 4. Resume oral anticoagulation the night of surgery, if possible 5. If procedure has a low risk of bleeding, consider therapeutic dose UH or LMWH beginning 24 hours after surgery and continuing until the INR is therapeutic

LMWH, low-molecular-weight heparin; UH, unfractionated heparin.

Karkouti K et al. Risk associated with preoperative anemia in cardiac surgery: a multicenter cohort study. Circulation. 2008 Jan 29;117(4):478–84. [PMID: 18172032]

Wu WC et al. Preoperative hematocrit levels and postoperative outcomes in older patients undergoing noncardiac surgery. JAMA. 2007 June 13;297(22):2481–8. [PMID: 17565082]

NEUROLOGIC EVALUATION

Delirium occurs after major surgery in 5–50% of patients over the age of 50 years and is particularly common after hip fracture repair and aortic surgery, occurring in 30–60% of such patients. Postoperative delirium has been associated with higher rates of major postoperative cardiac and pulmonary complications, poor functional recovery, an increased length of hospital stay, an increased risk of subsequent dementia and functional decline, and increased mortality at 1 and 5 years. Several preoperative and postoperative factors, most notably age, preoperative cognitive impairment, preoperative psychotropic drug use, postoperative use of meperidine, and postoperative hyperglycemia have been associated with the development of postoperative delirium. Patients with multiple risk factors are at especially high risk. Delirium occurred in half of the patients with at least three of the risk factors listed in Table 3–6.

Two types of delirium reducing interventions have been evaluated: focused geriatric care and psychotropic medications. In a randomized, controlled trial of hip fracture surgery patients, those who received daily visits and targeted recommendations from a geriatrician had a lower risk of postoperative delirium (32%) than the control patients (50%). The most frequent interventions to prevent delirium were maintenance of the hematocrit greater than 30%; minimizing the use of benzodiazepines and anticholinergic and antihistamine medications; maintenance of regular bowel function; and early discontinuation of urinary catheters. Other studies comparing postoperative care in specialized geriatrics units with standard orthopedics wards have shown similar reductions in the incidence of delirium. Limited data support the use of neuroleptic medications to prevent postoperative delirium. A randomized trial in cardiac surgery patients demonstrated that risperidone (1 mg sublingual after regaining consciousness) reduced the incidence of postoperative delirium compared with placebo (11.1% vs. 31.7%). Another trial found that prophylactic oral haloperidol in orthopedic surgery patients failed to prevent delirium but did reduce its severity and duration. Postoperative cognitive dysfunction is defined as a reduction in memory, language comprehension, visuospatial comprehension, attention, or concentration. Postoperative cognitive dysfunction may occur in up to 25% patients after cardiopulmonary bypass and in 15% of patients after major noncardiac surgery. The symptoms are generally transient, lasting less than 3 months. It is more common in older patients and occurs with equal frequency after general or regional anesthesia.

Stroke may occur in 1–6% of patients undergoing cardiac or carotid artery surgery, but it occurs in less than 1% of all other surgical procedures. Most of the available data on postoperative stroke are in cardiac surgery patients. Most postoperative strokes are embolic in origin, and about half occur within the first postoperative day. Stroke after cardiac surgery is associated with significantly increased mortality, up to 22% in some studies. The risk factors for stroke after cardiac surgery include age > 60 years, a calcified aorta,

Table 3–6. Risk factors for the development of postoperative delirium.

Preoperative factors
Age > 70 years
Alcohol abuse
Cognitive impairment
Poor physical function status
Markedly abnormal serum sodium, potassium, or glucose level
Aortic, thoracic, hip fracture surgery, or emergency surgery
Postoperative factors
Use of meperidine or benzodiazepines, anticholinergics, antihistamines
Postoperative hematocrit < 30%
Use of urinary catheters

prior stroke, symptomatic carotid stenosis > 50%, peripheral vascular disease, cigarette smoking, diabetes mellitus, and renal failure. Most studies suggest that asymptomatic carotid bruits are associated with little or no increased risk of stroke in noncardiac, noncarotid surgery. The importance of asymptomatic carotid artery stenoses > 50% is not known. Postoperative heart failure, hypovolemia, and hyperglycemia may also increase the risk of stroke.

Prophylactic carotid endarterectomy in most patients with asymptomatic carotid artery disease is unlikely to be beneficial. On the other hand, patients with carotid disease who are candidates for carotid endarterectomy anyway (see Chapter 12) should probably have the carotid surgery prior to the elective surgery. In a recent observational study of 1566 patients who underwent carotid endarterectomy, the use of a statin medication was associated with a significant reduction in the rate of perioperative stroke and overall mortality. Given the broad indications for statin therapy in patients with vascular disease, it is prudent to begin statin treatment in patients with appropriate indications prior to their undergoing carotid surgery.

Bryson GL et al. Evidence-based clinical update: general anesthesia and the risk of delirium and postoperative cognitive dysfunction. Can J Anesth. 2006 Jul;53(7):669–77. [PMID: 16803914]

Dasgupta M et al. Preoperative risk assessment for delirium after noncardiac surgery: a systematic review. J Am Geriatr Soc. 2006 Oct;54(10):1578–89. [PMID: 17038078]

McGirt MJ et al. 3-Hydroxy-3-methylglutaryl coenzyme A reductase inhibitors reduce the risk of perioperative stroke and mortality after carotid endarterectomy. J Vasc Surg. 2005 Nov;42(5):829–36. [PMID: 16275430]

Prakanrattana U et al. Efficacy of risperidone for prevention of postoperative delirium in cardiac surgery. Anaesth Intensive Care. 2007 Oct;35(5):714–9. [PMID: 17933157]

Schrader SL et al. Adjunctive haloperidol prophylaxis reduces postoperative delirium severity and duration in at-risk elderly patients. Neurologist. 2008 Mar;14(2):134–7. [PMID: 18332845]

Selim M. Perioperative stroke. N Engl J Med. 2007 Feb 15;356(7):706–13. [PMID: 17301301]

MANAGEMENT OF ENDOCRINE DISEASES

▶ Diabetes Mellitus

Patients with diabetes are at increased risk for postoperative infections, particularly those involving the surgical site. Patients with a preoperative hemoglobin A_{1c} < 7% have roughly half the risk for developing a postoperative infection compared with those with a hemoglobin A_{1c} > 7%. Furthermore, diabetic patients are more likely to have cardiovascular disease and thus are at increased risk for postoperative cardiac complications. The most challenging issue in diabetics, however, is the maintenance of glucose control during the perioperative period. The increased secretion of cortisol, epinephrine, glucagon, and growth hormone during surgery is associated with insulin resistance and hyperglycemia in diabetic patients. The goal of management is the prevention of severe hyperglycemia or hypoglycemia in the perioperative period.

The ideal blood glucose level is not known, but studies suggest that tighter perioperative glycemic control leads to better clinical outcomes. Existing data pertain primarily to cardiac surgery patients. In observational studies, cardiac surgery patients with mean postoperative glucose levels < 180 mg/dL had fewer serious surgical site infections, a lower risk of acute kidney failure, and a shorter hospital stay than patients with higher mean levels. In a study of 1200 patients in a critical care unit, most of whom had undergone cardiac surgery, those randomized to strict normalization of serum glucose (80–110 mg/dL) had significantly less morbidity and a shorter length of stay in the critical care unit than patients who were treated only for serum glucose > 215 mg/dL. Based on these data, current guidelines recommend maintaining perioperative glucose levels as close to 110 mg/dL as possible in critically ill patients and between 90–130 mg/dL before meals in other patients. These goals must be adjusted based on a patient's individual circumstances, including their risk of hypoglycemia.

The specific pharmacologic management of diabetes during the perioperative period depends on the type of diabetes (insulin-dependent or not), the level of glycemic control, and the type and length of surgery. In general, patients who require insulin to control the diabetes (whether type 1 or type 2) will need intraoperative insulin with any surgical procedure. Patients with type 2 diabetes who take oral agents may require insulin during major or prolonged surgery. Perioperative management of all diabetic patients requires frequent blood glucose monitoring to prevent hypoglycemia and to ensure prompt treatment of hyperglycemia. Recommendations for glycemic control in patients who generally do not need intraoperative insulin are shown in Table 3–7. For patients who do require intraoperative insulin, no single regimen has been found to be superior in comparative trials. Three commonly used

Table 3–7. Perioperative management of diabetic patients who do not need insulin.

Patient	Recommended Management
Diabetes well controlled on diet alone	Measure glucose every 4 hours while fasting or NPO and give subcutaneous regular insulin as needed to maintain blood glucose < 130 mg/dL
	Avoid glucose-containing solutions during surgery
Diabetes well controlled on an oral sulfonylurea, metformin, or a thiazolidinedione	The last dose of medication should be taken on the evening before surgery
	Measure glucose every 4 hours while fasting or NPO and give subcutaneous regular insulin as needed to maintain blood glucose < 130 mg/dL
	Measure blood glucose level every 4 hours (or more frequently as indicated) during surgery
	Resume oral hypoglycemic therapy when the patient returns to baseline diet

NPO, nothing by mouth.

Table 3–8. Intraoperative insulin administration methods.

Method	Intravenous Insulin Administration	Glucose Administration	Blood Glucose Monitoring
Subcutaneous insulin	One-half to two-thirds of the usual dose of insulin is administered on the morning of surgery	Infuse 5% glucose-containing solution at a rate of at least 100 mL/h beginning on the morning of surgery and continuing until the patient begins eating	Every 2–4 hours beginning the morning of surgery
Continuous intravenous insulin infusion in glucose-containing solution	On the morning of surgery, infuse 5–10% glucose solution containing 5–15 units regular insulin per liter of solution at a rate of 100 mL/h. This provides 0.5–1.5 units of insulin per hour. Additional insulin may be added as needed to keep blood sugar 100–200 mg/dL.	Every 2–4 hours during intravenous insulin infusion
Separate intravenous insulin and glucose infusions	Infuse intravenous regular insulin at a rate of 0.5–1.5 units/h, adjusting as needed to keep blood sugar 100–200 mg/dL	Infuse 5–10% glucose-containing solution at a rate of 100 mL/h	Every 2–4 hours during intravenous insulin infusion

insulin administration methods are shown in Table 3–8. The subcutaneous route is used most often because it is easier to access and is less expensive. Intravenous insulin, which offers more rapid onset, shorter duration of action, and ease of dose titration, may be preferable for patients who are in the intensive care unit, patients who have poorly controlled diabetes, and patients who are undergoing cardiac surgery. Perioperative use of corticosteroids, common in neurosurgical and organ transplant procedures, increases glucose intolerance. Patients receiving corticosteroids often require additional regular insulin with meals, while their fasting glucose levels may remain relatively unchanged.

Corticosteroid Replacement

Perioperative complications (predominantly hypotension) resulting from primary or secondary adrenocortical insufficiency are rare. The common practice of administering high-dose corticosteroids during the perioperative period in patients at risk for adrenocortical has not been rigorously studied. While definitive recommendations regarding perioperative corticosteroid therapy cannot be made, a conservative approach would be to consider any patient to be at risk for having adrenocortical insufficiency who has received either the equivalent of 20 mg of prednisone daily for 3 weeks or the equivalent of 7.5 mg of prednisone daily for 1 month within the past year. A commonly used regimen is 50–100 mg of hydrocortisone given intravenously every 8 hours beginning before induction of anesthesia and continuing for 24–48 hours. Tapering the dose is not necessary. Patients being maintained on long-term corticosteroids should also continue their usual dose throughout the perioperative period.

Thyroid Disease

Severe symptomatic hypothyroidism has been associated with several perioperative complications, including intraoperative hypotension, CHF, cardiac arrest, and death. Elective surgery should be delayed in patients with severe hypothyroidism until adequate thyroid hormone replacement can be achieved. Similarly, patients with symptomatic hyperthyroidism are at risk for perioperative thyroid storm and should not undergo elective surgery until their thyrotoxicosis is controlled. An endocrinologist should be consulted if emergency surgery is needed in such patients. Conversely, patients with asymptomatic or mild hypothyroidism generally tolerate surgery well, with only a slight increase in the incidence of intraoperative hypotension; surgery need not be delayed for the month or more required to ensure adequate thyroid hormone replacement.

American Diabetes Association. Standards of medical care in diabetes–2006. Diabetes Care. 2006 Jan;29 (Suppl 1):S4–42. [PMID: 16373931]

Ascione R et al. Inadequate blood glucose control is associated with in-hospital mortality and morbidity in diabetic and nondiabetic patients undergoing cardiac surgery. Circulation. 2008 Jul 8;118(2):113–23. [PMID: 18591441]

Dronge AS et al. Long-term glycemic control and postoperative infectious complications. Arch Surg. 2006 Apr;141(4):375–80. [PMID: 16618895]

Hoogwerf BJ. Perioperative management of diabetes mellitus: how should we act on the limited evidence? Cleve Clin J Med. 2006 Mar;73 (Suppl 1):S95–9. [PMID: 16570557]

KIDNEY DISEASE

The risk for development of a significant reduction in kidney function, including dialysis requiring acute kidney failure, after major surgery has been estimated to be between 0.5% and 10%. The mortality associated with the development of postoperative acute kidney failure that requires dialysis exceeds 50%. Risk factors that have been associated with postoperative deterioration in kidney function are shown in Table 3–9. The most important of these are the presence of preoperative kidney dysfunction and cardiac or vascular surgery. In patients with normal preoperative kidney function (calculated creatinine clear-

Table 3–9. Risk factors for the development of postoperative acute renal failure.

Preoperative chronic renal insufficiency
Aortic surgery
Cardiac surgery
Peripheral vascular disease
Severe heart failure
Preoperative jaundice
Age > 70 years
Diabetes mellitus
COPD requiring daily bronchodilator therapy

COPD, chronic obstructive pulmonary disease.

ance > 80 mL/min) undergoing major noncardiac surgery, 0.8% developed significant acute kidney injury and 0.1% required renal replacement therapy. Several medications, including "renal dose" dopamine, mannitol, N-acetylcysteine, and furosemide, have been evaluated in an attempt to preserve kidney function during the perioperative period. None of these, however, have proved effective in clinical trials. Maintenance of adequate intravascular volume is likely to be the most effective method to reduce the risk of perioperative deterioration in kidney function.

Although the mortality rate for elective major surgery is low (1–4%) in patients with dialysis-dependent chronic kidney disease, the risk for perioperative complications, including postoperative hyperkalemia, pneumonia, fluid overload, and bleeding, is substantially increased. Postoperative hyperkalemia requiring emergent hemodialysis has been reported to occur in 20–30% of patients. Patients should undergo dialysis preoperatively within 24 hours before surgery, and their serum electrolyte levels should be measured just prior to surgery and monitored closely during the postoperative period.

Aronson S et al. Risk index for perioperative renal dysfunction/failure: critical dependence on pulse pressure hypertension. Circulation. 2007 Feb;116(6):733–742. [PMID: 17283267]

Craig RG et al. Recent developments in the perioperative management of adult patients with chronic kidney disease. Br J Anaesth. 2008 Sep;101(3):296–310. [PMID: 18617576]

Kheterpal S et al. Predictors of postoperative acute renal failure after noncardiac surgery in patients with previously normal renal function. Anesthesiology. 2007 Dec;107(6):892–902. [PMID: 18043057]

ANTIBIOTIC PROPHYLAXIS OF SURGICAL SITE INFECTIONS

Surgical site infection is a common and important cause of morbidity and prolonged hospital stays. There are an estimated 0.5–1 million surgical site infections annually in the United States. Surgical site infection is estimated to occur in roughly 4% of general or vascular operations. For most major procedures, the use of prophylactic antibiotics has been demonstrated to reduce the incidence of surgical site infections significantly. For example, antibiotic prophylaxis in colorectal surgery reduces the incidence of surgical site infection from 25–50% to below 20%. In addition, in a case control study of Medicare beneficiaries, the use of preoperative antibiotics within 2 hours of surgery was associated with a twofold reduction in 60-day mortality. Prophylactic antibiotics are considered standard care for all but "clean" surgical procedures. Clean procedures are those that are elective, nontraumatic, not associated with acute inflammation, and that do not enter the respiratory, gastrointestinal, biliary, or genitourinary tract. The surgical site infection rate for clean procedures is thought to be roughly 2%. However, in certain clean procedures, such as those that involve the insertion of a foreign body or breast cancer surgery, antibiotic prophylaxis is still recommended because the consequences of infection are serious. Antibiotic prophylaxis recommendations for a variety of procedures are shown in Table 3–10.

Multiple studies have evaluated the effectiveness of different antibiotic regimens for various surgical procedures. In most cases, no single antibiotic regimen has been shown to be superior. Several general conclusions can be drawn from these data. First, substantial evidence suggests that a single dose of an appropriate intravenous antibiotic—or combination of antibiotics—is as effective as multiple-dose regimens that extend into the postoperative period. For longer procedures, the dose should be repeated every 3–4 hours to ensure maintenance of a therapeutic serum level. Second, for most procedures, a first-generation cephalosporin is as effective as later-generation agents. Third, prophylactic antibiotics should be given intravenously at induction of anesthesia or roughly 30–60 minutes prior to the skin incision. Although the type of procedure is the main factor determining the risk of developing a surgical site infection, certain patient factors have been associated with increased risk, including diabetes, older age, obesity, heavy alcohol consumption, admission from a long-term care facility, and multiple medical comorbidities.

Other strategies to prevent surgical site infections have proven to be controversial. Evidence suggests that nasal carriage with *Staphylococcus aureus* is associated with a twofold to ninefold increased risk of surgical site and catheter-related infections in surgical patients. Treatment of nasal carriers of *S aureus* with 2% mupirocin ointment (twice daily intranasally for 3 days) prior to cardiac surgery decreases the risk of surgical site infections. However, in a recent large prospective cohort study, universal screening for methicillin-resistant *S aureus* in surgical patients failed to reduce infection rates from this pathogen. Data on the use of supplemental oxygen to prevent surgical site infections are also mixed. An early trial found that high concentration oxygen delivered in the immediate postoperative period reduced surgical site infections. The most recent study found an increased risk of surgical site infections with the use of 80% oxygen compared with 35% postoperatively. Thus, high-flow supplemental oxygen specifically to prevent these infections is presently not recommended. Preoperative bathing with antiseptic agents and preoperative

Table 3–10. Recommended antibiotic prophylaxis for selected surgical procedures.

Procedure	Recommended Antibiotic	Adult Dose
Superficial cutaneous	None	
Head and neck	Cefazolin	1–2 g intravenously
Neurologic	Cefazolin	1–2 g intravenously
Thoracic	Cefazolin	1–2 g intravenously
Noncardiac vascular	Cefazolin	1–2 g intravenously
Orthopedic, clean, without implantation of foreign material	None	
Orthopedic, all other	Cefazolin	1–2 g intravenously
Cesarean delivery	Cefazolin	2 g intravenously
Hysterectomy	Cefazolin or cefotetan	1–2 g intravenously
Breast cancer surgery	Cefazolin	1–2 g intravenously
Gastroduodenal	Cefazolin (high risk only)[1]	1–2 g intravenously
Biliary	Cefazolin (high risk only)[1]	1–2 g intravenously
Urologic	Cefazolin (high risk only)[2]	1–2 g intravenously
Appendectomy for uncomplicated appendicitis	Cefotetan or cefoxitin	1–2 g intravenously
Colorectal[3]	Ertapenem or	1 g intravenously
	Cefotetan or cefoxitin	1–2 g intravenously every 8 hours for 3 total doses
	–or–	
	Neomycin sulfate plus erythromycin base	1 g of each agent given orally at 19, 18, and 9 hours before surgery
	Cefazolin (high risk only)[1]	1–2 g intravenously
Breast and hernia	Cefazolin (high risk only)[1]	1–2 g intravenously

[1]High risk defined as patients with risk factors for surgical site infection such as older age, diabetes, or multiple medical comorbidities.
[2]High risk defined as prolonged postoperative catheterization or positive urine cultures.
[3]All patients should have mechanical bowel preparation with polyethylene glycol, mannitol, or magnesium citrate.

hair removal are common practices but have not demonstrated a reduction in surgical site infections in randomized trials. The use of razors for hair removal actually seems to increase the risk of surgical site infections and is therefore specifically not recommended. If preoperative hair removal is indicated, the use of clippers is preferred.

Fonseca SNS et al. Implementing 1-dose antibiotic prophylaxis for prevention of surgical site infection. Arch Surg. 2006 Nov;141(11):1109–13. [PMID: 17116804]

Forbess SS et al. Implementation of evidence-based practices for surgical site infection prophylaxis: results of a pre- and post-intervention study. J Am Coll Surg. 2008 Sep;207(3):336–41. [PMID: 18722937]

Harbarth S et al. Universal screening for methicillin-resistant *Staphylococcus aureus* at hospital admission and nosocomial infection in surgical patients. JAMA. 2008 Mar 12;299(10):1149–57. [PMID: 18334690]

Tanner J et al. Preoperative hair removal to reduce surgical site infection. Cochrane Database Syst Rev. 2006 Jul 19;3:CD004122. [PMID: 16856029]

Weber WP et al. The timing of surgical antimicrobial prophylaxis. Ann Surg. 2008 Jun;247(6):918–26. [PMID: 18520217]

Geriatric Disorders

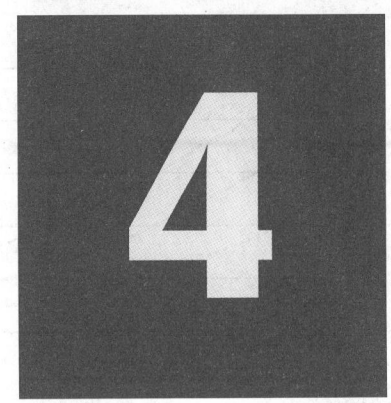

C. Bree Johnston, MD, MPH,
G. Michael Harper, MD,
& C. Seth Landefeld, MD

GENERAL PRINCIPLES OF GERIATRIC CARE

The following principles are helpful to keep in mind while caring for older adults:

1. Many disorders are multifactorial in origin and are best managed by multifactorial interventions.
2. Diseases often present atypically.
3. Not all abnormalities require evaluation and treatment.
4. Complex medication regimens, adherence problems, and polypharmacy are common challenges.

ASSESSMENT OF THE OLDER ADULT

Comprehensive assessment addresses three topics in addition to conventional assessment of symptoms and diseases: prognosis, values and preferences, and ability to function independently. Comprehensive assessment is warranted before major clinical decisions (eg, whether major surgery should be performed, or whether a patient should be treated for pneumonia at home or in the hospital), and each topic merits at least brief consideration in each clinical decision.

▶ Assessment of Prognosis

When an older person's life expectancy is greater than 10 years (ie, 50% of similar persons live longer than 10 years), it is reasonable to consider effective tests and treatments much as they are considered in younger persons. When life expectancy is less than 10 years (and especially when it is much less), choices of tests and treatments should be made on the basis of their ability to improve that particular patient's prognosis and quality of life in the shorter term of that patient's life expectancy. The relative benefits and harms of tests and treatments often change as prognosis worsens.

When an older patient's clinical situation is dominated by a single disease process (eg, lung cancer metastatic to brain), prognosis can be estimated well with a disease-specific instrument. Even in this situation, however, prognosis generally worsens with age (especially age greater than 90 years) and with the presence of serious age-related conditions, such as dementia, malnutrition, or impaired ability to walk.

When an older patient's clinical situation is not dominated by a single disease process, prognosis can be estimated initially by considering the patient's age, gender, and general health (Figure 4–1). For example, less than 25% of men age 95 years will live 5 years, whereas nearly 75% of women age 70 years will live 10 years.

The prognosis of older persons living at home can be estimated by considering age, gender, comorbid conditions, and function (Table 4–1). The prognosis of older persons discharged from the hospital is worse than that of those living at home and can be estimated by considering gender, comorbid conditions, and function at discharge (Table 4–2). The sum of risk points indicates the mortality rate for similar patients.

▶ Assessment of Values & Preferences

Values and preferences are determined by speaking directly with a patient or, when the patient cannot express preferences reliably, with the patient's surrogate. Values and preferences can be assessed most readily in the context of a specific medical decision. For example, the clinician might ask a patient considering a hip replacement, "How would you like your hip pain and function to be different? Tell me about the risk and discomfort you are willing to go through to achieve that improvement."

In assessing values and preferences, it is important to keep in mind the following:

1. Patients are experts about their preferences for outcomes and experiences; however, they often do not have adequate information to express informed preferences for specific tests or treatments.
2. Patients' preferences often change over time. For example, some patients find living with a certain degree of disability more acceptable than they thought before experiencing the disability.

▶ Assessment of Function

People often lose function in multiple domains as they age, with the results that they may not be able to do some activities as quickly or capably and may need assistance with other activities. Assessment of function improves prognos-

Women

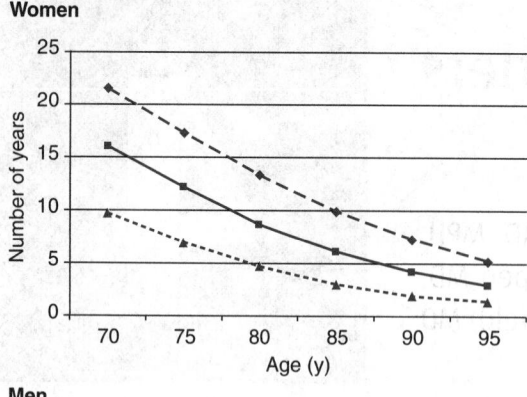

Men

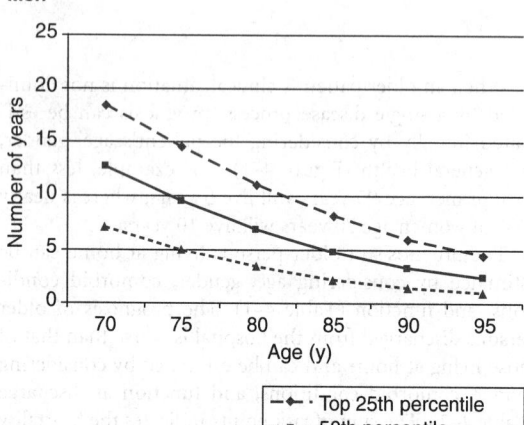

▲ **Figure 4–1.** Median life expectancy of older women and men. (Adapted, with permission, from Walter LC et al. Screening for colorectal, breast, and cervical cancer in the elderly: a review of the evidence. Am J Med. 2005 Oct;118(10):1078–86.)

Table 4–1. Prognostic factors, "risk points," and 4-year mortality rates for older persons living at home.

Prognostic Factor	Risk Points
Age	
60–64 years	1
64–69 years	2
70–74 years	3
74–79 years	4
80–84 years	5
85 years and older	7
Male sex	2
Comorbid conditions reported by patients	
Diabetes mellitus	1
Cancer	2
Lung disease	2
Heart failure	2
Body mass index < 25	1
Current smoker	2
Function	
Bathing difficulty	2
Difficulty handling finances	2
Difficulty walking several blocks	2
Sum of Risk Points	**4-year Mortality Rate**
1–2	2%
3–6	7%
7–10	19%
> 10	53%

Reprinted, with permission, from Lee SJ et al. Development and validation of a prognostic index for 4-year mortality in older adults. JAMA. 2006 Feb 15;295(7):801–8.

tic estimates (see above). Assessment of function is essential to determining an individual's needs in the context of their values and preferences, and the possible effects of prescribed treatment.

About one-fourth of patients over 65 have impairments in their IADLs (instrumental activities of daily living: transportation, shopping, cooking, using the telephone, managing money, taking medications, housecleaning, laundry) or ADLs (basic activities of daily living: bathing, dressing, eating, transferring from bed to chair, continence, toileting). Half of those persons older than 85 years have these latter impairments.

In general, persons who need help only with IADLs can usually live independently with minimal supports, such as financial services (eg, a representative payee) or a chore worker. If institutional care is needed, residential care, board-and-care, or assisted living is usually sufficient. While many persons who need help with ADLs may require a nursing home level of care, most live at home with caregivers and other community services (eg, day care).

► **Caregiver Issues**

Most elders with functional impairment live in the community with the help of an "informal" caregiver, most commonly a spouse or daughter. The health and well-being of the patient and caregiver are closely linked. High levels of functional dependency place an enormous burden on a caregiver, and may result in caregiver "burnout," depression, morbidity, and even increased mortality.

An older patient's need for nursing home placement is often better predicted from assessment of the caregiver characteristics and stress than the severity of the patient's illness. Therefore, part of caring for a frail elder involves paying attention to the well-being of the caregiver. The older patient who is also a caregiver is at risk for depression and should be screened for it. For the stressed caregiver, a social worker may help identify programs such as caregiver

The legend for Figure 4–1:
- Top 25th percentile
- 50th percentile
- Lowest 25th percentile

Table 4–2. Prognostic factors, "risk points," and 1-year mortality rates for patients discharged from the hospital after an acute medical illness.

Prognostic Factor	Risk Points
Male sex	1
Comorbid conditions reported by patients	
Cancer, metastatic	8
Cancer, not metastatic	3
Serum creatinine > 3 mg/dL	2
Albumin < 3 mg/dL	2
Albumin 3.0–3.4 mg/dL	1
Function	
Dependent in 1–4 ADL[1]	2
Dependent in 5 ADL	5

Sum of Risk Points	1-year Mortality Rate
0–1	4%
2–3	19%
4–6	34%
> 6	64%

[1]ADL refers to five activities of daily living: bathing, dressing, transferring, using the toilet, and eating.
Reprinted, with permission, from Walter LC et al. Development and validation of a prognostic index for 1-year mortality in older adults after hospitalization. JAMA. 2001 Jun 20;285(23):2987–94.

support groups, respite programs, adult day care, or hired home health aides.

Functional Screening Instrument

Functional screening should include assessment of ADL and IADL and questions to detect weight loss, falls, incontinence, depressed mood, self neglect, fear for personal safety, and common serious impairments (eg, hearing, vision, cognition, and mobility). Standard functional screening measures may not be useful in capturing subtle impairments in highly functional independent elders. One technique for these patients is to identify and regularly ask about a target activity, such as bowling or gardening. If the patient begins to have trouble with or discontinues such an "advanced activity of daily living," it may indicate early impairment, such as dementia, incontinence, or worsening hearing loss, which additional gentle questioning or assessment may uncover.

Busy primary care providers may find it more manageable to perform the elements of functional geriatric assessment over three or four visits or to train office personnel to perform some elements of the assessment.

Ensberg M et al. Incremental geriatric assessment. Prim Care. 2005 Sep;32(3):619–43. [PMID: 16140119]

Fried TR et al. Inconsistency over time in the preferences of older persons with advanced illness for life-sustaining treatment. J Am Geriatr Soc. 2007 Jul;55(7):1007–14. [PMID: 17608872]

Lee SJ et al. Development and validation of a prognostic index for 4-year mortality in older adults. JAMA. 2006 Feb 15;295(7):801–8. [PMID: 16478903]

MANAGEMENT OF COMMON GERIATRIC PROBLEMS

1. Dementia

 ESSENTIALS OF DIAGNOSIS

► Progressive decline of intellectual function.
► Loss of short-term memory and at least one other cognitive deficit.
► Deficit severe enough to cause impairment of function.
► Not delirious.

General Considerations

Dementia is an acquired persistent and progressive impairment in intellectual function, with compromise of memory and at least one other cognitive domain, most commonly language impairment, apraxia (inability to perform motor tasks, such as cutting a loaf of bread, despite intact motor function), agnosia (inability to recognize objects), and impaired executive function (poor abstraction, mental flexibility, planning, and judgment). The diagnosis of dementia requires a significant decline in function that is severe enough to interfere with work or social life.

Dementia has a prevalence that doubles every 5 years in the older population, reaching 30–50% at age 85. Women suffer disproportionately, both as patients (even after age adjustment) and as caregivers. Alzheimer disease (AD) accounts for roughly two-thirds of dementia cases in the United States, with vascular dementia (either alone or combined with AD) and dementia with Lewy bodies accounting for much of the rest. Some of the risk factors for AD are older age, family history, lower education level, and female gender. Education, cognitive "exercises," and social support may be protective. Risk factors for vascular dementia are those for stroke, ie, older age, hypertension, cigarette use, atrial fibrillation, diabetes mellitus, and hyperlipidemia.

Depression and delirium are also common in elders, may coexist with dementia, and may also present with cognitive impairment. Depression is a common concomitant of early dementia. A patient with depression and cognitive impairment whose intellectual function improves with treatment of the mood disorder has an almost fivefold greater risk of suffering irreversible dementia later in life. Delirium, characterized by acute confusion, occurs much more commonly in patients with underlying dementia.

Clinical Findings

A. Screening

1. Cognitive impairment—Although there is no consensus at present on whether older patients should be screened for dementia, the benefits of early detection include identification of potentially reversible causes, planning for the future (including discussing values and completing advance care directives), and providing support and counseling for the caregiver.

The combination of a clock drawing task with a three-item word recall (also known as the "mini-cog") is a simple screening test that is fairly quick to administer. Although a number of different methods for administering and scoring the clock draw test have been described, the authors of this chapter favor the approach of pre-drawing a four inch circle on a sheet of paper and instructing the patient to "draw a clock" with the time set at 10 minutes after 11. Scores are classified as normal, almost normal, or abnormal. When a patient is able to draw a clock normally and can remember all 3 objects, dementia is unlikely. When a patient fails this simple screen, further cognitive evaluation with the Folstein Mini Mental State Exam (MMSE) or other instruments is warranted.

2. Decision-making capacity—It is common for a cognitively impaired elder to face a serious medical decision and for the clinicians involved in his care to ascertain whether the capacity exists to make the choice. There are five components of a thorough assessment: (1) ability to express a choice; (2) understanding relevant information about the risks and benefits of planned therapy and the alternatives, in the context of one's values, including no treatment; (3) comprehension of the problem and its consequences; (4) ability to reason; and (5) consistency. A patient's choice should follow rationally from an understanding of the consequences.

Cultural sensitivity must be used in applying these five components to people of various cultural backgrounds. Decision-making capacity varies over time: A delirious patient may regain his capacity after an infection is treated, and so reassessments are often appropriate. Furthermore, the capacity to make a decision is a function of the decision in question. A woman with mild dementia may lack the capacity to consent to coronary artery bypass grafting yet retain the capacity to designate a surrogate decision maker.

B. Symptoms and Signs

The clinician can gather important information about the type of dementia that may be present by asking about: (1) the rate of progression of the deficits as well as their nature (including any personality or behavioral change); (2) the presence of other neurologic symptoms, particularly motor problems; (3) risk factors for HIV; (4) family history of dementia; and (5) medications, with particular attention to recent changes.

Work-up is directed at identifying any potentially reversible causes of dementia. However, such cases are indeed rare.

AD typically presents with early problems in memory and visuospatial abilities (eg, becoming lost in familiar surroundings, inability to copy a geometric design on paper), yet social graces may be retained despite advanced cognitive decline. Personality changes and behavioral difficulties (wandering, inappropriate sexual behavior, agitation) may develop as the disease progresses. Hallucinations may occur in moderate to severe dementia. End-stage disease is characterized by near-mutism; inability to sit up, hold up the head, or track objects with the eyes; difficulty with eating and swallowing; weight loss; bowel or bladder incontinence; and recurrent respiratory or urinary infections.

"Subcortical" dementias (eg, the dementia of Parkinson disease, and some cases of vascular dementia) are characterized by psychomotor slowing, reduced attention, early loss of executive function, and personality changes.

Dementia with Lewy bodies may be confused with delirium, as fluctuating cognitive impairment is frequently observed. Rigidity and bradykinesia are the primary signs, and tremor is rare. Response to dopaminergic agonist therapy is poor. Complex visual hallucinations—typically of people or animals—may be an early feature that can help distinguish dementia with Lewy bodies from AD. These patients demonstrate a hypersensitivity to neuroleptic therapy, and attempts to treat the hallucinations may lead to marked worsening of extrapyramidal symptoms.

Frontotemporal dementias are a group of diseases that include Pick disease, dementia associated with amyotrophic lateral sclerosis, and others. Patients manifest personality change (euphoria, disinhibition, apathy) and compulsive behaviors (often peculiar eating habits or hyperorality). In contrast to AD, visuospatial function is relatively preserved.

Dementia in association with motor findings, such as extrapyramidal features or ataxia, may represent a less common disorder (eg, progressive supranuclear palsy, corticobasal ganglionic degeneration, olivopontocerebellar atrophy).

C. Physical Examination

The neurologic examination emphasizes assessment of mental status but should also include evaluation for sensory deficits, possible previous strokes, parkinsonism, or peripheral neuropathy. The remainder of the physical examination should focus on identifying comorbid conditions that may aggravate the individual's disability.

D. Laboratory Findings

Laboratory studies should include a complete blood count, electrolytes, calcium, creatinine, glucose, thyroid-stimulating hormone (TSH), and vitamin B_{12} levels. HIV testing, RPR (rapid plasma reagin) test, heavy metal screen, and liver biochemical tests may be informative in selected patients but should not be considered part of routine testing.

E. Imaging

Most patients should receive neuroimaging as part of the diagnostic work-up to rule out subdural hematoma, tumor, previous stroke, and hydrocephalus (usually normal pressure). Those who are younger and those who have focal neurologic symptoms or signs, seizures, gait abnormalities, and an acute or subacute onset are most likely to yield positive findings and most likely to benefit from MRI scanning. In older patients with a more classic picture of AD in whom neuroimaging is desired, a noncontrast CT scan is sufficient.

Differential Diagnosis

Older individuals experience occasional difficulty retrieving items from memory (usually manifested as word-finding complaints) and experience a slowing in their rate of information processing. **Mild cognitive impairment** is an increasingly recognized condition in which a patient complains of memory problems, demonstrates mild deficits (most commonly in short-term memory) on formal testing, but does not meet criteria for dementia. Dementia will develop in more than half of people with mild cognitive impairment within 5 years. Acetylcholinesterase inhibitors have not consistently demonstrated a delay in the progression of mild cognitive impairment to AD. An elderly patient with intact cognition but with severe impairments in vision or hearing commonly becomes confused in an unfamiliar medical setting and consequently may be falsely labeled as demented. Cognitive testing is best performed after optimal correction of the sensory deficits.

Delirium can be distinguished from dementia by its acute onset, fluctuating course, and deficits in attention rather than memory. Because delirium and dementia often coexist, it may not be possible to determine how much impairment is attributable to each condition until the patient is fully recovered and back in their usual setting. Many medications have been associated with delirium and other types of cognitive impairment in older patients. Anticholinergic agents, hypnotics, neuroleptics, opioids, nonsteroidal anti-inflammatory drugs (NSAIDs), antihistamines (including H_2-antagonists), and corticosteroids are just some of the medications that have been associated with cognitive impairment in elders.

Treatment

Soon after diagnosis, patients and families should be made aware of the Alzheimer's Association (http://www.alz.org) as well as the wealth of helpful community and online resources and publications available. Caregiver support, education, and counseling can prevent or delay nursing home placement. Education should include the manifestations and natural history of dementia as well as the availability of local support services such as respite care. Even under the best of circumstances, caregiver stress can be substantial. Collaborative care models and disease management programs appear to improve the quality of care for patients with dementia.

A. Cognitive Impairment

Because demented patients have greatly diminished cognitive reserve, they are at high risk for experiencing acute cognitive or functional decline in the setting of new medical illness. Consequently, fragile cognitive status may be best main-

tained by ensuring that comorbid diseases such as congestive heart failure and infections are detected and treated.

1. Acetylcholinesterase inhibitors—The majority of experts recommend considering a trial of acetylcholinesterase inhibitors (eg, donepezil, galantamine, rivastigmine) in most patients with mild to moderate AD. These medications produce a modest improvement in cognitive function that is not likely to be detected in routine clinical encounters. Acetylcholinesterase inhibitors may also have similarly modest cognitive benefits in patients with vascular dementia or dementia with Lewy bodies. However, acetylcholinesterase inhibitors have not been shown to delay institutionalization or functional decline.

Starting doses, respectively, of donepezil, galantamine, and rivastigmine, are 5 mg orally once daily (maximum 10 mg once daily), 4 mg orally twice daily (maximum 12 mg twice daily), and 1.5 mg orally twice daily (maximum 6 mg twice daily). The doses are increased gradually as tolerated. The most bothersome side effects include diarrhea, nausea, anorexia, and weight loss. In those patients who have had no apparent benefit, experience side effects, or for whom the financial outlay is a burden, the authors of this chapter recommend a trial of discontinuation.

2. Memantine—In clinical trials, patients with more advanced disease have been shown to have statistical benefit from the use of memantine, an *N*-methyl-D-aspartate (NMDA) antagonist, with or without concomitant use of an acetylcholinesterase inhibitor. Long-term and meaningful functional outcomes have yet to be demonstrated.

B. Behavioral Problems

1. Nonpharmacologic approaches—Behavioral problems in demented patients are often best managed with a nonpharmacologic approach. Initially, it should be established that the problem is not unrecognized delirium, pain, urinary obstruction, or fecal impaction. It also helps to inquire whether the caregiver or institutional staff can tolerate the behavior, as it is often easier to find ways to accommodate to the behavior than to modify it. If not, the caregiver is asked to keep a brief log in which the behavior is described along with antecedent events and consequences. Recurring precipitants of the behavior are often found to be present or it may be that the behavior is rewarded—for example, by increased attention. Caregivers are taught to use simple language when communicating with the patient, to break down activities into simple component tasks, and to use a "distract, not confront" approach when the patient seems disturbed by a troublesome issue. Additional steps to address behavioral problems include the discontinuation of all medications except those considered absolutely necessary and correction, if possible, of sensory deficits.

2. Pharmacologic approaches—There is no clear consensus about pharmacologic approaches to treatment of behavioral problems in patients who have not benefited from nonpharmacologic therapies. The target symptoms—depression, anxiety, psychosis, mood lability, or pain—may suggest which class of medications might be most helpful in a given patient. Patients with depressive symptoms may show improvement with antidepressant therapy. Patients with dementia with Lewy bodies have shown clinically significant improvement in behavioral symptoms when treated with rivastigmine (3–6 mg orally twice daily).

For those with AD and agitation, no agents, including acetylcholinesterase inhibitors and antipsychotics, have demonstrated consistent efficacy. Despite the lack of strong evidence, antipsychotic medications have remained a mainstay for the treatment of behavioral disturbances, largely because of the lack of alternative agents. The newer atypical antipsychotic agents (risperidone, olanzapine, quetiapine, aripiprazole, clozapine, ziprasidone) are reported to be better tolerated than older agents but should be avoided in patients with vascular risk factors due to an increased risk of stroke and weight gain; they are also considerably more expensive. The US Food and Drug Administration has issued a public health advisory warning that atypical agents, when used to treat elderly demented patients with behavioral disturbances, increase mortality rates when compared with placebo. Studies have also linked haloperidol and other typical antipsychotics with increased mortality rates when used in patients with dementia. When the choice is made to use these agents, patients and caregivers should be carefully warned of the risks. Starting and target dosages should be much lower than those used in schizophrenia (eg, haloperidol, 0.5–2 mg orally; risperidone, 0.25–2 mg orally). Federal regulations require that if antipsychotic agents are used in treatment of a nursing home patient, drug reduction efforts must be made at least every 6 months.

▶ Prognosis

Life expectancy after a diagnosis of AD is typically 3–15 years; it may be shorter than previously reported. Other neurodegenerative dementias, such as dementia with Lewy bodies, show more rapid decline. Hospice is often appropriate for patients with end-stage dementia.

▶ When to Refer

Referral for neuropsychological testing may be helpful in the following circumstances: to distinguish dementia from depression, to diagnose dementia in persons of very poor education or very high premorbid intellect, and to aid diagnosis when impairment is mild.

Ballard C et al; DART-AD Investigators. The dementia antipsychotic withdrawal trial (DART-AD): long-term follow-up of a randomised placebo-controlled trial. Lancet Neurol. 2009 Feb;8(2):151–7. [PMID: 19138567]

Callahan CM et al. Effectiveness of collaborative care for older adults with Alzheimer disease in primary care: a randomized controlled trial. JAMA. 2006 May 10;295:2148–57. [PMID: 16684985]

Howard RJ et al. Donepezil for the treatment of agitation in Alzheimer's disease. N Engl J Med. 2007 Oct 4;357(14):1382–92. [PMID: 17914039]

Qaseem A et al; American College of Physicians/American Academy of Family Physicians Panel on Dementia. Current pharmacologic treatment of dementia: a clinical practice guideline from the American College of Physicians and the American Academy of Family Physicians. Ann Intern Med. 2008 Mar 4;148(5):370–8. [PMID: 18316755]

Schneider LS et al; CATIE-AD Study Group. Effectiveness of atypical antipsychotic drugs in patients with Alzheimer's disease. N Engl J Med. 2006 Oct 12;355(15):1525–38. [PMID: 17035647]

Vickrey BG et al. The effectiveness of a disease management intervention on quality and outcomes in dementia care. A randomized controlled trial. Ann Intern Med. 2006 Nov 21;145(10):713–26. [PMID: 17116916]

2. Depression

ESSENTIALS OF DIAGNOSIS

▶ Depressed elders may not admit to depressed mood.

▶ Depression screening in elders should include a question about anhedonia.

▶ General Considerations

Although the prevalence of major depression is similar in younger and older populations, depressive symptoms— often related to loss, disease, and life changes—may be present in more than 25% of elders. Depression is particularly common in hospitalized and institutionalized elders. Older single men have the highest suicide rate of any demographic group. Geriatric patients with depression are more likely to have somatic complaints, less likely to report depressed mood, and more likely to experience delusions than younger patients. In addition, depression may be an early symptom of a neurodegenerative condition such as dementia.

▶ Clinical Findings

A simple two-question screen—which consists of asking "During the past 2 weeks, have you felt down, depressed, or hopeless?" and "During the past 2 weeks, have you felt little interest or pleasure in doing things?"—is highly sensitive for detecting major depression in persons over age 65. Positive responses can be followed up with more comprehensive, structured interviews, such as the Geriatric Depression Scale (http://www.stanford.edu/~yesavage/) or the PHQ-9 (http://www.depression-primarycare.org).

Elderly patients with depressive symptoms should be questioned about medication use, since many drugs (eg, benzodiazepines, corticosteroids) may contribute to the clinical picture. Similarly, several medical problems can cause fatigue, lethargy, or hypoactive delirium, all of which may be mistaken for depression. Laboratory examination should include a complete blood count; liver, thyroid, and kidney function tests; and serum calcium. If delirium is in the differential diagnosis, the work-up should include a urinalysis and an electrocardiogram.

▶ Treatment

Choice of antidepressant agent in elders is usually based on side effect profile and cost. In general, fluoxetine is avoided because of its long duration of action and tricyclic antidepressants are avoided because of their high anticholinergic side effects. Regardless of the drug chosen, many experts recommend starting elders at a relatively low dose, titrating to full dose slowly, and continuing for a longer trial (at least 9 weeks) before trying a different medication. Cognitive behavioral therapy can improve outcomes alone or in combination with medication therapy. Depressed elders may do better with a collaborative care model that includes socialization and other support elements than with usual care. Recurrence of major depression is common in elders; any elder with a history of depression should be closely monitored for recurrence and considered for longer-term maintenance medication therapy.

When to Refer

Referral should be considered for patients who have not responded to an initial antidepressant drug trial and for patients with have symptoms of mania, suicidality, or psychosis.

When to Admit

Patients who are suicidal, homicidal, psychotic, or a danger to self or others should be considered for acute psychiatric hospitalization.

Hunkeler EM et al. Long term outcomes from the IMPACT randomized trial for depressed elderly patients in primary care. BMJ. 2006 Feb 4;332(7536):259–63. [PMID: 16428253]
Reynolds CF 3rd et al. Maintenance treatment of major depression in old age. N Engl J Med. 2006 Mar 16;354(11):1130–8. [PMID: 16540613]

3. Delirium

ESSENTIALS OF DIAGNOSIS

▶ Rapid onset and fluctuating course.
▶ Primary deficit in attention rather than memory.
▶ May be hypoactive or hyperactive.
▶ Dementia frequently coexists.

General Considerations

Delirium is an acute, fluctuating disturbance of consciousness, associated with a change in cognition or the development of perceptual disturbances (see also Chapter 25). It is the pathophysiologic consequence of an underlying general medical condition such as infection, coronary ischemia, hypoxemia, or metabolic derangement. Delirium persists in up to 25% of patients and is associated with worse clinical outcomes (higher in-hospital and postdischarge mortality, longer lengths of stay, greater probability of placement in a nursing facility).

Although the acutely agitated elderly patient often comes to mind when considering delirium, many episodes are more subtle. Such quiet, or hypoactive, delirium may only be suspected if one notices new cognitive slowing or inattention.

Cognitive impairment is an important risk factor for delirium. Approximately 25% of delirious patients are demented, and 40% of demented hospitalized patients are delirious. Other risk factors are male sex, severe illness, hip fracture, fever or hypothermia, hypotension, malnutrition, polypharmacy and use of psychoactive medications, sensory impairment, use of restraints, use of intravenous lines or urinary catheters, metabolic disorders, depression, and alcoholism.

Clinical Findings

A key component of a delirium work-up is review of medications because a large number of drugs, the addition of a new drug, or the discontinuation of a medication known to cause withdrawal symptoms are all associated with the development of delirium.

Laboratory evaluation of most patients should include a complete blood count, electrolytes, blood urea nitrogen (BUN) and serum creatinine, glucose, calcium, albumin, liver function studies, urinalysis, and electrocardiography. In selected cases, serum magnesium, serum drug levels, arterial blood gas measurements, blood cultures, chest radiography, urinary toxin screen, head CT scan, and lumbar puncture may be helpful.

Prevention

Prevention is the best approach in the management of delirium. Measures include improving cognition (frequent reorientation, activities, socialization with family and friends, when possible), sleep (massage, noise reduction, minimizing interruptions at night), mobility, vision (visual aids and adaptive equipment), hearing (portable amplifiers, cerumen disimpaction), and hydration status (volume repletion).

Treatment

Management of established episodes of delirium is largely supportive and includes treatment of any underlying causes, eliminating unnecessary medications, and avoidance of indwelling catheters and restraints. Antipsychotic agents (such as haloperidol, 0.5–1 mg, or quetiapine, 25 mg, at bedtime or twice daily) are considered the medication of choice when drug treatment of delirium is necessary. In emergency situations, starting haloperidol at 0.5 mg orally or intramuscularly and repeating every 30 minutes until the agitation is controlled may be necessary, but such treatment is often followed by prolonged sedation or other complications. Other medications (eg, trazodone, donepezil, mood stabilizers) have also been used, but evidence in support of these approaches is weak.

Most episodes of delirium clear in a matter of days after correction of the precipitant, but some patients suffer episodes of longer duration, and a few never return to their former baseline level of functioning. These individuals merit closer follow-up for the development of dementia if not already diagnosed.

When to Refer

If an initial evaluation does not reveal the cause of delirium or if entities other than delirium are in the differential diagnosis, referral to a neuropsychologist, neurologist, or geropsychiatrist should be considered.

When to Admit

Patients with delirium of unknown cause should be admitted for an expedited work-up if consistent with the patient's goals of care.

Young J et al. Delirium in older people. BMJ. 2007 Apr 21;334(7598):842–6. [PMID: 17446616]

4. Immobility

Although common in older people, reduced mobility is never normal and is often treatable if its causes are identified. Bedrest is an important cause of hospital-induced functional decline. Among hospitalized medical patients over 70, about 10% experience a decline in function, much of which results from preventable reductions in mobility.

The hazards of bed rest in older adults are multiple, serious, quick to develop, and slow to reverse. Deconditioning of the cardiovascular system occurs within days and involves fluid shifts, decreased cardiac output, decreased peak oxygen uptake, and increased resting heart rate. More striking changes occur in skeletal muscle, with loss of contractile velocity and strength. Pressure sores, deep venous thrombosis, and pulmonary embolism are additional serious risks. Within days after being confined to bed, the risk of postural hypotension, falls, and skin breakdown rises rapidly in the older patient. Moreover, recovery from these changes usually takes weeks to months.

Prevention & Treatment

When immobilization cannot be avoided, several measures can be used to minimize its consequences. Skin, particularly areas over pressure points, should be inspected at least daily. If the patient is unable to shift position, staff should do so every 2 hours. To minimize cardiovascular deconditioning, patients should be positioned as close to the upright position as possible, several times daily. To reduce the risks of contracture and weakness, range of motion and strengthening exercises should be started immediately and continued as long as the patient is in bed. Whenever possible, patients should assist with their own positioning, transferring, and self-care. As long as the patient remains immobilized, antithrombotic measures should be used if that is consistent with the patient's goals of care.

Avoiding restraints and discontinuing invasive devices (intravenous lines, urinary catheters) may increase an elderly patient's prospects for early mobility. Graduated ambulation should begin as soon as it is feasible. Advice from a physical therapist is often helpful both before and after discharge. Prior to discharge, physical therapists can recommend appropriate exercises and assistive devices; after discharge, they can recommend safety modifications and maintenance exercises.

5. Falls & Gait Disorders

Falls are the leading cause of nonfatal injuries in older persons, and their complications are the leading cause of death from injury in persons over age 65. Hip fractures are common precursors to functional impairment, nursing home placement, and death. Furthermore, fear of falling may lead some elders to restrict their activities. About one-third of people over 65 fall each year, and the frequency increases markedly with advancing age.

Every older person should be asked about falls; many will not volunteer such information. A thorough gait assessment should be performed in all older people. Gait and balance can be readily assessed by the "Up and Go Test," in which the patient is asked to stand up from a sitting position without use of hands, walk 10 feet, turn around, walk back, and sit down. Patients who take less than 10 seconds are usually normal, patients who take longer than 30 seconds tend to need assistance with many mobility tasks, and those in between tend to vary widely with respect to gait, balance, and function. The ability to recognize common patterns of gait disorders is an extremely useful clinical skill to develop. Examples of gait abnormalities and their causes are listed in Table 4–3.

Causes of Falls

Balance and ambulation require a complex interplay of cognitive, neuromuscular, and cardiovascular function. With age, balance mechanisms can become compromised and postural sway increases. These changes predispose the older person to a fall when challenged by an additional insult to any of these systems.

A fall may be the clinical manifestation of an occult problem, such as pneumonia or myocardial infarction, but much more commonly falls are due to the interaction between an impaired patient and an environmental risk factor. Falls in older people are rarely due to a single cause, and effective intervention entails a comprehensive assessment of the patient's intrinsic deficits (usually diseases and medications), the activity engaged in at the time of the fall, and environmental obstacles.

Intrinsic deficits are those that impair sensory input, judgment, blood pressure regulation, reaction time, and balance and gait. Dizziness may be closely related to the deficits associated with falls and gait abnormalities. While it may be impossible to isolate a sole "cause" or a "cure" for falls, gait abnormalities, or dizziness, it is often possible to identify and ameliorate some of the underlying contributory conditions and improve the patient's overall function.

As for most geriatric conditions, medication use is one of the most common, significant, and reversible causes of falling. Benzodiazepines, sedative-hypnotics, cardiac medications, antidepressants, neuroleptics, and the use of multiple medications simultaneously have been associated with an increased fall risk. Other often overlooked but treatable contributors include postural hypotension, (particularly postprandial, which peaks 30–60 minutes after a meal), insomnia, and urinary urgency.

Since most falls occur in or around the home, a visit by a visiting nurse, physical therapist, or health care provider reaps substantial benefits in identifying environmental obstacles and is generally reimbursed by third-party payers, including Medicare.

Table 4–3. Evaluation of gait abnormalities.

Gait Abnormality	Possible Cause
Inability to stand without use of hands	Deconditioning Myopathy (hyperthyroidism, alcohol, statin-induced) Hip or knee pain
Unsteadiness upon standing	Orthostatic hypotension Balance problem (peripheral neuropathy, vision problem, vestibular, other central nervous system causes) Generalized weakness
Stagger with eyes closed	Often indicates that vision is compensating for another deficit
Short steps	Weakness Parkinson disease or related condition
Asymmetry	Cerebrovascular accident Focal pain or arthritis
Wide-based gait	Fear, balance problems
Flexed knees	Contractures, quadriceps weakness
Slow gait	Fear of falling, weakness, deconditioning, peripheral vascular disease, chronic obstructive pulmonary disease, congestive heart failure, angina

Complications of Falls

The most common fractures resulting from falls are of the wrist, hip, and vertebrae. There is a high mortality rate (approximately 20% in 1 year) in elderly women with hip fractures, particularly if they were debilitated prior to the time of the fracture.

Fear of falling again is a common, serious, but treatable factor in the elderly person's loss of confidence and independence. Referral to a physical therapist for gait training with special devices is often all that is required.

Chronic subdural hematoma is an easily overlooked complication of falls that must be considered in any elderly patient presenting with new neurologic symptoms or signs. Headache or known history of trauma may both be absent.

Patients who are unable to get up from a fall are at risk for dehydration, electrolyte imbalance, pressure sores, rhabdomyolysis, and hypothermia.

Prevention & Management

The risk of falling and consequent injury, disability, and potential institutionalization can be reduced by modifying those factors outlined in Table 4–4. Emphasis is placed on treating all contributory medical conditions (eg, peripheral edema, delirium), minimizing environmental hazards, and reducing the number of medications—particularly those that induce orthostasis and parkinsonism (eg, α-blockers, nitrates, antipsychotics). Also important are strength, balance, and gait training as well as screening and treatment for osteoporosis, if present. There is evidence that vitamin D at doses of 800 international units daily or higher may help prevent falls and fractures. The recommended dose for vitamin D is 800–1000 international units daily for most elders who have no contraindications.

Assistive devices, such as canes and walkers, are useful for many older adults but are often used incorrectly.

Table 4–4. Fall risk factors and targeted interventions.

Risk Factor	Targeted Intervention
Postural hypotension (> 20 mm Hg drop in systolic blood pressure, or systolic blood pressure < 90 mm Hg)	Behavioral recommendations, such as hand clenching, elevation of head of bed; discontinuation or substitution of high-risk medications
Use of benzodiazepine or sedative-hypnotic agent	Education about sleep hygiene; discontinuation or substitution of medications
Use of multiple prescription medications	Review of medications
Environmental hazards	Appropriate changes; installation of safety equipment (eg, grab bars)
Gait impairment	Gait training, assistive devices, balance or strengthening exercises
Impairment in transfer or balance	Balance exercises, training in transfers, environmental alterations (eg, grab bars)
Impairment in leg or arm muscle strength or limb range of motion	Exercise with resistance bands or putty, with graduated increases in resistance

Canes should be used on the "good" side. The height of walkers and canes should generally be about the level of the wrist. Physical therapists are invaluable in assessing the need for an assistive device, selecting the best device, and training a patient in its correct use.

Patients with repeated falls are often reassured by the availability of phones at floor level, a portable phone, or a lightweight radio call system. Their therapy should also include training in techniques for arising after a fall. The clinical utility of anatomically designed external hip protectors in reducing fractures is currently uncertain.

▶ When to Refer

Patients with a recent history of falls should be referred for physical therapy, eye examination, and home safety evaluation.

▶ When to Admit

If the patient has new falls that are unexplained, particularly in combination with a change in the physical examination, hospitalization should be considered.

Bischoff-Ferrari HA et al. Effect of vitamin D on falls: a meta-analysis. JAMA. 2004 Apr 28;291(16):1999–2006. [PMID: 15113819]
Ganz DA et al. Will my patient fall? JAMA. 2007 Jan 3;297(1):77–86. [PMID: 17200478]
Järvinen TL et al. Shifting the focus in fracture prevention from osteoporosis to falls. BMJ. 2008 Jan 19;336(7636):124–6. [PMID: 18202065]

6. Urinary Incontinence

 ESSENTIALS OF DIAGNOSIS

- ▶ Involuntary loss of urine.
- ▶ *Stress* incontinence: leakage of urine upon coughing, sneezing, or standing.
- ▶ *Urge* incontinence: urgency and inability to delay urination.
- ▶ Overflow incontinence may have variable presentation.

▶ General Considerations

Incontinence in older adults is common, and interventions can improve most patients. Many patients fail to tell their providers about it. A simple question about involuntary leakage of urine is a reasonable screen: "Do you have a problem with urine leaks or accidents?"

▶ Classification

Because continence requires adequate mobility, mentation, motivation, and manual dexterity, problems outside the bladder often result in geriatric incontinence. In general, the authors of this chapter find it useful to differentiate between "transient" or "potentially reversible" causes of incontinence and more "established" causes.

A. Transient Causes

Use of the mnemonic "DIAPPERS" may be helpful in remembering the categories of transient incontinence.

1. Delirium—A clouded sensorium impedes recognition of both the need to void and the location of the nearest toilet. Delirium is the most common cause of incontinence in hospitalized patients; once it clears, incontinence usually resolves.

2. Infection—Symptomatic urinary tract infection commonly causes or contributes to urgency and incontinence. Asymptomatic bacteriuria does not.

3. Atrophic urethritis or vaginitis—Atrophic urethritis can usually be diagnosed presumptively by the presence of vaginal mucosal telangiectasia, petechiae, erosions, erythema, or friability. Urethral inflammation, if symptomatic, may contribute to incontinence in some women. Some experts suggest a trial of topical estrogen in these cases.

4. Pharmaceuticals—Drugs are one of the most common causes of transient incontinence. Typical offending agents include potent diuretics, anticholinergics, psychotropics, opioid analgesics, α-blockers (in women), α-agonists (in men), and calcium channel blockers.

5. Psychological factors—Severe depression with psychomotor retardation may impede the ability or motivation to reach a toilet.

6. Excess urinary output—Excess urinary output may overwhelm the ability of an older person to reach a toilet in time. In addition to diuretics, common causes include excess fluid intake; metabolic abnormalities (eg, hyperglycemia, hypercalcemia, diabetes insipidus); and disorders associated with peripheral edema, with its associated heavy nocturia when previously dependent legs assume a horizontal position in bed.

7. Restricted mobility—(See Immobility section, above.) If mobility cannot be improved, access to a urinal or commode (eg, at the bedside) may improve continence.

8. Stool impaction—This is a common cause of urinary incontinence in hospitalized or immobile patients. Although the mechanism is still unknown, a clinical clue to its presence is the onset of both urinary and fecal incontinence. Disimpaction usually restores urinary continence.

B. Established Causes

Causes of established incontinence should be addressed after the transient causes have been uncovered and managed appropriately. Risk factors for incontinence include older age, female gender, increased body mass index, and limited physical activity.

1. Detrusor overactivity (urge incontinence)—Detrusor overactivity refers to uninhibited bladder contractions that cause leakage. It is the most common cause of established geriatric incontinence, accounting for two-thirds of cases, and is usually idiopathic. Women will complain of urinary leakage after the onset of an intense urge to urinate that cannot be forestalled. In men the symptoms are similar, but detrusor overactivity commonly coexists with urethral obstruction from benign prostatic hyperplasia. Because detrusor overactivity also may be due to bladder stones or tumor, the abrupt onset of otherwise unexplained urge incontinence—especially if accompanied by perineal or suprapubic discomfort or sterile hematuria—should be investigated by cystoscopy and cytologic examination of a urine specimen.

2. Urethral incompetence (stress incontinence)— Urethral incompetence is the second most common cause of established urinary incontinence in older women. Stress incontinence is most commonly seen in men after radical prostatectomy. Stress incontinence is characterized by instantaneous leakage of urine in response to a stress maneuver. It commonly coexists with detrusor overactivity. Typically, urinary loss occurs with laughing, coughing, or lifting heavy objects. Leakage is worse or occurs only during the day, unless another abnormality (eg, detrusor overactivity) is also present. To test for stress incontinence, have the patient relax her perineum and cough vigorously (a single cough) while standing with a full bladder. Instantaneous leakage indicates stress incontinence if urinary retention has been excluded by postvoiding residual determination using ultrasound. A delay of several seconds or persistent leakage suggests that the problem is instead caused by an uninhibited bladder contraction induced by coughing.

3. Urethral obstruction— Urethral obstruction (due to prostatic enlargement, urethral stricture, bladder neck contracture, or prostatic cancer) is a common cause of established incontinence in older men but is rare in older women. It can present as dribbling incontinence after voiding, urge incontinence due to detrusor overactivity (which coexists in two-thirds of cases), or overflow incontinence due to urinary retention. Renal ultrasound is required to exclude hydronephrosis in men whose postvoiding residual urine exceeds 150 mL.

4. Detrusor underactivity (overflow incontinence)— Detrusor underactivity is the least common cause of incontinence. It may be idiopathic or due to sacral lower motor nerve dysfunction. When it causes incontinence, detrusor underactivity is associated with urinary frequency, nocturia, and frequent leakage of small amounts. The elevated postvoiding residual urine (generally over 450 mL) distinguishes it from detrusor overactivity and stress incontinence, but only urodynamic testing differentiates it from urethral obstruction in men. Such testing usually is not required in women, in whom obstruction is rarely present.

▶ **Treatment**

A. Transient Causes

Each identified transient cause should be treated regardless of whether an established cause coexists. For patients with urinary retention induced by an anticholinergic agent, discontinuation of the drug should first be considered. If this is not feasible, substituting a less anticholinergic agent

(eg, sertraline instead of desipramine for depression) may be useful.

B. Established Causes

1. Detrusor overactivity— The cornerstone of treatment is bladder training. Patients start by voiding on a schedule based on the shortest interval recorded on a bladder record. They then gradually lengthen the interval between voids by 30 minutes each week using relaxation techniques to postpone the urge to void. For cognitively impaired patients who are unable to manage on their own, timed voiding initiated by caregivers is an alternative.

Pelvic floor muscle ("Kegel") exercises, with or without biofeedback, can reduce the frequency of incontinence episodes when performed correctly and sustained. If behavioral approaches prove insufficient, drug therapy with antimuscarinic agents may provide additional benefit. The two oral drugs for which there is the most experience are tolterodine and oxybutynin. Available regimens of these drugs follow: short-acting tolterodine, 1–2 mg twice a day; long-acting tolterodine, 2–4 mg daily; short-acting oxybutynin, 2.5–5 mg twice or three times a day; long-acting oxybutynin, 5–15 mg daily; and oxybutynin transdermal patch, 3.9 mg per day applied twice weekly. All of these agents can produce delirium, dry mouth, or urinary retention; long-acting preparations may be better tolerated. Newer agents such as trospium chloride (20 mg orally once or twice daily), darifenacin (7.5–15 mg orally daily), and solifenacin (5–10 mg orally daily) appear to have similar efficacy and are reported to be better tolerated than oxybutynin and tolterodine, but limited data exist in older patients.

The combination of behavioral therapy and antimuscarinics appears to be more effective than either alone.

In men with both benign prostatic hyperplasia and detrusor overactivity, an antimuscarinic agent may provide relief over an α-agonist alone but should not be prescribed to men with an elevated postvoid residual urine volume (ie, > 200 mL) because of the risk of causing acute urinary retention.

2. Urethral incompetence (stress incontinence)— Lifestyle modifications, including limiting caffeine intake and timed voiding, may be helpful for some women, particularly women with mixed stress/urge incontinence. Pelvic floor muscle exercises are effective for women with mild to moderate stress incontinence who wish to avoid surgery and who can use them indefinitely; the exercises can be combined, if necessary, with biofeedback, electrical stimulation, or vaginal cones. Pelvic floor muscle exercises can be taught during bimanual vaginal examination or by asking the patient to try to contract the muscle that they use to stop the flow of urine. It is often necessary to perform 30–60 exercises daily for 6 weeks before significant improvement will be noticed. Pessaries or vaginal cones may be helpful in some women but should be prescribed by providers who are experienced with using these modalities.

Although a last resort, surgery is the most effective treatment for stress incontinence, resulting in a cure rate of 75–85% even in older women. Drug therapy is limited. Several trials have shown that duloxetine, a serotonin and norepinephrine reuptake inhibitor, reduces stress incontinence episodes in women. It is approved for use for this indication in some countries but not the United States. Side effects, including nausea, are common.

3. Urethral obstruction—Surgical decompression is the most effective treatment for obstruction, especially in the setting of urinary retention due to benign prostatic hyperplasia. A variety of newer, less invasive techniques make decompression feasible even for frail men. For the nonoperative candidate with urinary retention, intermittent or indwelling catheterization is used. For a man with prostatic obstruction who does not require or desire immediate surgery, treatment with α-blocking agents (eg, terazosin, 1–10 mg daily; prazosin, 1–5 mg orally twice daily; tamsulosin, 0.4–0.8 mg daily) can improve symptoms and delay obstruction. Finasteride, 5 mg daily, can provide additional benefit to an α-blocking agent in men with an enlarged prostate. The potential for finasteride to reduce the risk of prostate cancer is under investigation.

4. Detrusor underactivity—For the patient with a poorly contractile bladder, augmented voiding techniques (eg, double voiding, suprapubic pressure) often prove effective. If further emptying is needed, intermittent or indwelling catheterization is the only option. Antibiotics should be used only for symptomatic upper urinary tract infection or as prophylaxis against recurrent symptomatic infections in a patient using intermittent catheterization; they should not be used as prophylaxis with an indwelling catheter.

When to Refer

- Men with urinary obstruction who do not respond to medical therapy should be referred to a urologist.
- Women who do not respond to medical and behavioral therapy should be referred to a urogynecologist or urologist.

Burgio KL et al; Urinary Incontinence Treatment Network. Behavioral therapy to enable women with urge incontinence to discontinue drug treatment: a randomized trial. Ann Intern Med. 2008 Aug 5;149(3):161–69. [PMID: 18678843]

Kaplan SA et al. Tolterodine and tamsulosin for treatment of men with lower urinary tract symptoms and overactive bladder: a randomized controlled trial. JAMA. 2006 Nov 15;296(19):2319–28. [PMID: 17105794]

Norton P et al. Urinary incontinence in women. Lancet. 2006 Jan 7;367(9504):57–67. [PMID: 16399154]

7. Undernutrition & Frailty

General Considerations

Undernutrition affects substantial numbers of elderly persons and may be the clinical trigger that prompts the label of "failure to thrive." The degree of unintended weight loss that deserves evaluation is not agreed upon, although a reasonable threshold is loss of 5% of body weight in 1 month or 10% of body weight in 6 months.

"Frailty" is a term that may be clinically useful for describing a subgroup of patients—almost always elders—who have decreased functional reserve. Common clinical features of frailty include weakness, slowness, weight loss, low activity, and fatigue. Frailty may be accompanied by physiologic changes in inflammatory and neuroendocrine systems. The label of "failure to thrive" is typically applied when some triggering event—loss of social support, a bout of depression or pneumonia, the addition of a new medication—pulls a struggling elderly person below the threshold of successful independent living.

Clinical Findings

Useful laboratory and radiologic studies for the patient with weight loss or "failure to thrive" include complete blood count, serum chemistries (including glucose, TSH, creatinine, calcium), urinalysis, and chest radiograph. Exploring the patient's social situation, cognition, mood, and dental health are at least as important as looking for a purely medical cause of weight loss. These studies are intended to uncover an occult metabolic or neoplastic cause but are not exhaustive.

Treatment

Oral nutritional supplements of 200–1000 kcal/d can increase weight and improve outcomes in malnourished hospitalized elders. Megestrol acetate as an appetite stimulant has not been shown to increase body mass or lengthen life in the elderly population. For those who have lost the ability to feed themselves, assiduous hand feeding may allow maintenance of weight. Although artificial nutrition and hydration ("tube feeding") may seem a more convenient alternative, it deprives the patient of the taste and texture of food as well as the social milieu typically associated with mealtime; before this option is chosen, the patient or his or her surrogate will wish to review the benefits and burdens of the treatment in light of overall goals of care. If the patient makes repeated attempts to pull out the tube during a trial of artificial nutrition, the treatment burden becomes substantial, and the utility of tube feeding should be reconsidered. Although commonly used, there is no evidence that tube feeding prolongs life in patients with end-stage dementia.

The ideal strategies for diagnosing and managing "frailty" or "failure to thrive" are uncertain but are usually supportive, multifactorial, and individualized based on patient goals, life expectancy, and comorbidities. Sometimes, transitioning a patient to a palliative approach or a hospice program is the most appropriate clinical intervention.

Milne AC et al. Meta-analysis: Protein and energy supplementation in older people. Ann Intern Med. 2006 Jan 3;144(1):37–48. [PMID: 16389253]

8. Pressure Ulcers

ESSENTIALS OF DIAGNOSIS

- ► Examine at-risk patients on admission to hospital and daily thereafter.
- ► Pressure ulcers should be described by one of six stages:
  - Blanchable hyperemia (stage I).

- Extension through epidermis (stage II).
- Full thickness skin loss (stage III).
- Full thickness wounds with extension into muscle, bone, or supporting structures (stage IV).
- If eschar or slough overlies the wound, the wound is unstageable.
- Suspected deep tissue injury is an area of discolored or blistered skin.

General Considerations

The majority of pressure ulcers develop during a hospital stay for an acute illness. Incident rates range from 3% to 30% and vary according to patient characteristics. The primary risk factor for pressure ulcers is immobility. Other contributing risk factors include reduced sensory perception, moisture (urinary and fecal incontinence), poor nutritional status, and friction and shear forces.

In 2007, the National Pressure Ulcer Advisory Panel added two stages to the original four pressure ulcer stages: suspected deep tissue injury and unstageable. Ulcers in which the base is covered by slough (yellow, tan, gray, green or brown) and/or eschar (tan, brown or black) are considered unstageable. Suspected deep tissue injury is an area of purple or maroon discolored intact skin or blood-filled blister. The area may be preceded by tissue that is painful, firm, mushy, boggy, warmer or cooler compared with adjacent tissue.

A number of risk assessment instruments including the Braden Scale and the Norton score can be used to assess the risk of developing pressure ulcers; both have reasonable performance characteristics. These instruments can be used to identify the highest risk patients who might benefit most from scarce resources such as mattresses that reduce or relieve pressure.

As of October 2008, Medicare will no longer reimburse for hospital-acquired pressure ulcers. Pressure ulcers present on admission will qualify for a higher reimbursement. The medical record must contain documentation of pressure ulcers present on admission, and coders are required to use physician documentation as the basis for coding and reporting; therefore, physicians should include a full skin assessment on every admission history and physical.

Prevention

Using specialized support surfaces (including mattresses, beds, and cushions), patient repositioning, optimizing nutritional status, and moisturing sacral skin are strategies that have been shown to reduce pressure ulcers. For moderate- to high-risk patients, mattresses or overlays that reduce tissue pressure below a standard mattress appear to be superior to standard mattresses. The literature comparing specific products is sparse and inconclusive.

Evaluation

Evaluation of pressure ulcers should include patient's risk factors and goals of care, wound stage, size, depth, presence or absence of exudate, type of exudate present, appearance of the wound bed, and whether there appears to be surrounding infection, sinus tracking, or cellulitis. In poorly healing or atypical pressure ulcers, biopsy should be performed to rule out malignancy or other less common lesions such as pyoderma gangrenosum.

Treatment

Treatment is aimed toward removing necrotic debris and maintaining a moist wound bed that will promote healing and formation of granulation tissue. The type of dressing that is recommended depends on the location and depth of the wound, whether necrotic tissue or dead space is present, and the amount of exudate (Table 4–5). Pressure-reducing devices (eg, air-fluid beds and low air loss beds) are associated with improved healing rates. Although poor nutritional status is a risk factor for the development of pressure ulcers, the results of trials of nutritional supplementation in the treatment of pressure ulcers have been disappointing.

Providers can become easily overwhelmed by the array of products available for treatment of established pressure ulcers. Most institutions should designate a wound care expert or wound care team to select a streamlined wound care product line that has simple guidelines. In a patient with end-stage disease who is receiving palliative care, appropriate treatment might be directed toward comfort (including minimizing dressing changes and odors) rather than efforts directed at healing.

Complications

Pressure ulcers are associated with increased mortality rates, although a causal link has not been proven. Compli-

Table 4–5. Treatment of pressure ulcers.

Ulcer Type	Dressing Type and Considerations
Stage I and suspected deep tissue injury	Polyurethane film Hydrocolloid wafer Semipermeable foam dressing
Stage II	Hydrocolloid wafers Semipermeable foam dressing Polyurethane film
Stage III/IV	**For highly exudative wounds**, use highly absorptive dressing or packing, such as calcium alginate Wounds with necrotic debris must be debrided Debridement can be autolytic, mechanical (wet to moist), or surgical **Shallow, clean wounds** can be dressed with hydrocolloid wafers, semipermeable foam, or polyurethane **Deep wounds** can be packed with gauze; if the wound is deep and highly exudative, an absorptive packing should be used
Heel ulcer	Do not remove eschar on heel ulcers because it can help promote healing (eschar in other locations should be debrided)
Unstageable	Debride before deciding on further therapy

cations include pain, cellulitis, osteomyelitis, systemic sepsis, and prolongation of lengths of stay in the inpatient or nursing home setting.

► When to Refer

Ulcers that are large or nonhealing should be referred to a plastic or general surgeon or dermatologist for biopsy, debridement, and possible skin grafting.

► When to Admit

Patients with pressure ulcers should be admitted if the primary residence is unable to provide adequate wound care or pressure reduction, if the wound is infected, or for complex or surgical wound care.

National Pressure Ulcer Advisory Panel Website: http://www.npuap.org/pr2.htm
Reddy M et al. Preventing pressure ulcers: a systematic review. JAMA. 2006 Aug 23;296(8):974–84. [PMID: 16926357]
Reddy M et al. Treatment of pressure ulcers: a systematic review. JAMA. 2008 Dec 10;300(22):2647–62. [PMID: 19066385]
Zeller JL et al. JAMA patient page. Pressure ulcers. JAMA. 2006 Aug 23;296(8):1020. [PMID: 16926361]

9. Pharmacotherapy & Polypharmacy

There are several reasons for the greater incidence of iatrogenic drug reactions in the elderly population, the most important of which is the high number of medications that are taken by elders, especially those with multiple comorbidities. Drug metabolism is often impaired in this group due to a decrease in glomerular filtration rate as well as reduced hepatic clearance. The latter is due to decreased activity of microsomal enzymes and reduced hepatic perfusion with aging. The volume of distribution of drugs is also affected. Since older adults have a decrease in total body water and a relative increase in body fat, water-soluble drugs become more concentrated and fat-soluble drugs have longer half-lives. Older individuals often have varying responses to a given serum drug level. Thus, they are more sensitive to some drugs (eg, opioids) and less sensitive to others (eg, β-blocking agents).

► Precautions in Administering Drugs

Nonpharmacologic interventions can often be a first-line alternative to drugs (eg, diet for mild hypertension or type 2 diabetes mellitus). Therapy is begun with less than the usual adult dosage and the dosage increased slowly, consistent with its pharmacokinetics in older patients. However, age-related changes in drug distribution and clearance are variable among individuals, and some require full doses. After determining acceptable measures of success and toxicity, the dose is increased until one or the other is reached.

Despite the importance of beginning new drugs in a slow, measured fashion, all too often an inadequate trial is attempted (in terms of duration or dose) before discontinuation. Antidepressants, in particular, are frequently stopped before therapeutic dosages are reached.

A number of simple interventions can help improve adherence to the prescribed medical regimen. When possible, the provider should keep the dosing schedule simple, the number of pills low, the medication changes as infrequent as possible, and encourage the patient to use a single pharmacy. Pillboxes or "medi-sets" help some patients with adherence.

Having the patient or caregiver bring in all medications at each visit can help the provider perform medication reconciliation and reinforce reasons for drug use, dosage, frequency of administration, and possible adverse effects. Medication reconciliation is particularly important if the patient sees multiple providers.

Although serum drug levels may be useful for monitoring certain drugs with narrow therapeutic windows (eg, digoxin), toxicity can still occur even with "normal" therapeutic levels of many drugs. The risk of toxicity goes up with the number of medications prescribed. Certain combinations of medications (eg, warfarin and many types of antibiotics, digoxin and clarithromycin, angiotensin-converting enzyme inhibitors and NSAIDs) are particularly likely to cause drug-drug interactions, and should be watched carefully.

Trials of individual drug discontinuation should be considered (including sedative-hypnotics, antipsychotic medications, digoxin, proton pump inhibitors, NSAIDs) when the original indication is unclear, the goals of care have changed, or the patient might be experiencing side effects.

The Medicare prescription drug benefit in the United States certainly helps many elders with burdensome prescription drug costs. However, its benefits are complex and difficult to understand, particularly for those elders with limited cognition, literacy, and Internet access. Reforms are being debated in Congress that could alter the benefits. Information is available at www.medicare.gov.

► When to Refer

Patients with poor or uncertain adherence may benefit from referral to a pharmacist or a home health nurse.

Pham CB et al. Minimizing adverse drug events in older patients. Am Fam Physician. 2007 Dec 15;76(12):1837–44. [PMID: 18217523]

10. Vision Impairment

Although visual loss is not severe in many elders, visual impairment is an independent risk factor for falls; it also has a significant impact on quality of life. The prevalence of serious and correctable visual disorders in elders is sufficient to warrant a complete eye examination by an ophthalmologist or optometrist annually or biannually for most elders. Many patients with visual loss benefit from a referral to a low vision program, and primary care providers should not assume that an ophthalmologist or optometrist will automatically make this referral.

Rosenberg EA et al. The visually impaired patient. Am Fam Physician. 2008 May 15;77(10):1431–6. [PMID: 18533377]

11. Hearing Impairment

Over one-third of persons over age 65 and half of those over age 85 have some hearing loss. This deficit is correlated with social isolation and depression. A reasonable screen is to ask patients if they have hearing impairment. Those who answer "yes" should be referred for audiometry. Those who answer "no" may still have hearing impairment and can be screened by a handheld audioscope or the whispered voice test. The whispered voice test is administered by standing 2 feet behind the subject, whispering three random numbers, and simultaneously rubbing the external auditory canal of the non-tested ear to mask the sound. If the patient is unable to identify all three numbers, the test should be repeated with different numbers, and if still abnormal, a referral should be made to audiometry. To determine the degree to which hearing impairment interferes with functioning, the provider may ask if the patient becomes frustrated when conversing with family members, is embarrassed when meeting new people, has difficulty watching TV, or has problems understanding conversations. Caregivers or family members often have important information on the impact of hearing loss on the patient's social interactions.

Compliance with hearing amplification can be a challenge because of the stigma associated with hearing aid use as well as the cost of such devices, which are not paid for under most Medicare plans. Special telephones, amplifiers for the television, and many other devices are available to aid the person with hearing loss. Portable amplifiers are pager-sized units with earphones attached; they can be purchased inexpensively at many electronics stores and can be useful in health care settings for improving communication with hearing impaired patients. In general, facing the patient and speaking slowly in a low tone is a more effective communication strategy than yelling.

Folate supplementation was found to slow age-associated hearing loss in a country without widespread dietary folate fortification; it is unknown whether this practice is beneficial in countries that practice folate fortification.

Begai A et al. Does this patient have hearing impairment? JAMA. 2006 Jan 25;295(4):416–28. [PMID: 16434632]

Table 4–6. Questions that may elicit a history of elder abuse.

1. Has anyone ever hurt you?
2. Has anyone ever touched you without your consent?
3. Has anyone ever made you do things you didn't want to do?
4. Has anyone taken anything of yours without asking?
5. Has anyone ever scolded or threatened you?
6. Have you signed any papers that you didn't understand?
7. Is there anyone at home you are fearful of?
8. Are you alone much?
9. Has anyone ever refused to help you take care of yourself when you needed help?

Durga J et al. Effects of folic acid supplementation on hearing in older adults: a randomized, controlled trial. Ann Intern Med. 2007 Jan 2;146(1):1–9. [PMID: 17200216]

12. Elder Abuse

According to the best available estimates, between 1 and 2 million Americans age 65 or older have been injured, exploited, or otherwise mistreated by someone on whom they depended for care or protection. Neglect, both by self and caregiver, are the most common forms of abuse, followed by financial and emotional abuse.

Clues to the possibility of elder abuse include behavioral changes in the presence of the caregiver, delays between occurrence of injuries and sought treatment, inconsistencies between an observed injury and associated explanation, lack of appropriate clothing or hygiene, and not filling prescriptions. Many elders with cognitive impairment become targets of financial abuse.

It is helpful to observe and talk with every older person alone for at least part of a visit in order to question directly about possible abuse and neglect (Table 4–6). The laws in most states require health care providers to report suspected abuse or neglect. Adult protective services (APS) agencies are available in all 50 states to assist in cases of suspected elder abuse. The Web site for the National Center for Elder Abuse is http://www.ncea.aoa.gov.

Palliative Care & Pain Management

Michael W. Rabow, MD

Steven Z. Pantilat, MD

DEFINITION & SCOPE OF PALLIATIVE CARE

The focus of palliative care is to improve symptoms and quality of life at any stage of illness, utilizing the expertise of an interdisciplinary team. At the end of life, palliative care often becomes the only focus of care, but a palliative care approach is beneficial throughout the course of serious chronic and terminal illnesses, regardless of prognosis, whether the goal is to cure disease or manage chronic illness.

The World Health Organization defines palliative care as "an approach that improves the quality of life of patients and their families facing the problem associated with life-threatening illness, through the prevention and relief of suffering by means of early identification and impeccable assessment and treatment of pain and other problems, physical, psychosocial and spiritual." Palliative care commonly involves management of pain and other symptoms, including dyspnea, nausea and vomiting, constipation, and agitation; emotional distress, such as depression, anxiety, and interpersonal strain; and existential distress, such as spiritual crisis. While palliative care has been recognized formally as a medical subspecialty by the American Board of Medical Specialties and palliative care experts are increasingly available in hospital and outpatient settings, all clinicians should possess the basic skills to be able to manage pain; treat dyspnea; identify possible depression; communicate about important issues, such as prognosis and patient preferences for care; and help address spiritual distress.

Symptoms that cause significant suffering are a medical emergency that should be managed aggressively with frequent elicitation, continuous reassessment, and individualized treatment. While patients at the end of life may experience a host of distressing symptoms, pain, dyspnea, and delirium are among the most feared and burdensome. The palliation of these common symptoms is described later in this chapter. The principles of palliative care dictate that properly informed patients or their surrogates may decide to pursue aggressive symptom relief at the end of life even if, as a known but unintended consequence, the treatments preclude further unwanted curative interventions or even hasten death. There is a growing awareness that scrupulous symptom control for patients with end-stage illness may even prolong life.

PAIN MANAGEMENT

PRINCIPLES OF PAIN MANAGEMENT

The experience of pain includes the patient's emotional reaction to it and is influenced by many factors, including the patient's prior experiences with pain, meaning given to the pain, emotional stresses, and family and cultural influences. Pain is a subjective phenomenon, and clinicians cannot reliably detect its existence or quantify its severity without asking the patient directly. A useful means of assessing pain and evaluating the effectiveness of analgesia is to ask the patient to rate the degree of pain along a numeric or visual pain scale (Table 5–1).

General guidelines for management of pain are recommended for the treatment of all patients with pain (Table 5–2). Clinicians should ask about the nature, severity, timing, location, quality, and aggravating and relieving factors of the pain. Distinguishing between somatic, visceral, and neuropathic pain is essential to proper tailoring of pain treatments. The goal of pain management is properly decided by the patient. Some patients may wish to be completely free of pain even at the cost of significant sedation, while others will wish to control pain to a level that still allows maximal functioning.

Chronic severe pain should be treated continuously. For ongoing pain, a long-acting analgesic can be given around the clock with a short-acting medication as needed for "breakthrough" pain. For patients near the end of life, the oral route of administration is preferred because it is easier to administer at home, is not painful, and imposes no risk from needle exposure. Rectal, transdermal, and subcutaneous administration are also frequently used, as is intravenous or, rarely, intrathecal administration when necessary. Patient-controlled analgesia (PCA) of intravenous medications can provide better analgesia with less medication use and its principles have been adapted for use with oral administration.

Table 5–1. Pain assessment scales.

A. Numeric Rating Scale

No pain   Worst pain

0   1   2   3   4   5   6   7   8   9   10

B. Numeric Rating Scale Translated into Word and Behavior Scales

Pain intensity	Word scale	Nonverbal behaviors
0	No pain	Relaxed, calm expression
1–2	Least pain	Stressed, tense expression
3–4	Mild pain	Guarded movement, grimacing
5–6	Moderate pain	Moaning, restless
7–8	Severe pain	Crying out
9–10	Excruciating pain	Increased intensity of above

C. Wong Baker FACES Pain Rating Scale[1]

 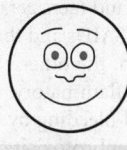 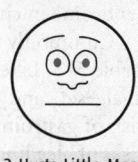 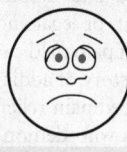 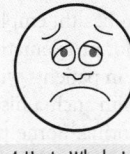 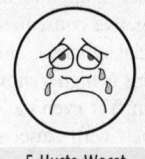

| 0 No hurt | 1 Hurts Little Bit | 2 Hurts Little More | 3 Hurts Even More | 4 Hurts Whole Lot | 5 Hurts Worst |

[1]Especially useful for patients who cannot read English and for pediatric patients.
Reprinted, with permission, from Hockenberry M, Wilson D, Winkelstein ML. *Wong's Essentials of Pediatric Nursing,* ed. 7. Copyright, Mosby.

When possible, the underlying cause of pain should be diagnosed and treated, balancing the burden of diagnostic tests with the patient's suffering. Treating the underlying cause of pain, such as radiation therapy for painful bone metastases, can obviate the need for ongoing treatment with analgesics along with their side effects. Regardless of

Table 5–2. Recommended clinical approach to pain management.

Ask about pain regularly. Assess pain systematically (quality, description, location, intensity or severity, aggravating and ame-liorating factors, cognitive responses). Ask about goals for pain control, management preferences.
Believe the patient and family in their reports of pain and what relieves it.
Choose pain control options appropriate for the patient, family, and setting. Consider drug type, dosage, route, contraindications, side effects. Consider nonpharmacologic adjunctive measures.
Deliver interventions in a timely, logical, coordinated manner.
Empower patients and their families. Enable patients to control their course to the greatest extent possible.
Follow up to reassess persistence of pain, changes in pain pattern, development of new pain.

Adapted from Jacox AK et al. *Management of Cancer Pain: Quick Reference Guide No. 9.* AHCPR Publication No. 94-0593. Rockville, MD: Agency for Health Care Policy and Research, Public Health Service, U.S. Department of Health and Human Services. March 1994.

decisions about seeking and treating its underlying cause, every patient should be offered prompt relief of pain.

PAIN AT THE END OF LIFE

► Definition & Prevalence

Pain is a common problem for patients at the end of life—up to 75% of patients dying of cancer experience pain—and it is what many people say they fear most about dying. Pain is also a common complaint among patients with noncancer diagnoses and is routinely undertreated. Up to 50% of severely ill hospitalized patients spent half of their time during the last 3 days of life in moderate to severe pain. The Joint Commission now includes pain management standards for all patient care organizations that it accredits.

► Barriers to Good Care

Deficiencies in pain management at the end of life have been documented in many settings. Some clinicians refer pain management to others when they believe that a patient's pain is not due to the disease for which they are treating the patient. Even oncologists often misperceive the origin of their patients' pain and inappropriately ignore complaints of pain.

Many clinicians have limited training and clinical experience with pain management and thus are understandably reluctant to attempt to manage severe pain. Lack of knowledge about the proper selection and dosing of analgesic medications carries with it attendant and typically exaggerated fears about the side effects of pain medications, including the possibility of respiratory depression from opioids. Most clinicians, however, can develop good pain management skills, and nearly all pain, even at the end of life, can be managed without hastening death through respiratory depression. In rare instances, palliative sedation may be necessary to control intractable agony as an intervention of last resort.

A misunderstanding of the physiologic effects of opioids can lead to unfounded concerns on the part of clinicians, patients, or family members that patients will become addicted to opioids. While physiologic **tolerance** (requiring increasing dosage to achieve the same analgesic effect) and **dependence** (requiring continued dosing to prevent symptoms of medication withdrawal) are expected with regular opioid use, the use of opioids at the end of life for relief of pain and dyspnea is not generally associated with a risk of psychological **addiction** (misuse of a substance for purposes other than one for which it was prescribed and despite negative consequences in health, employment, or legal and social spheres). The risk for problematic use of pain medications is higher, however, in patients with a history of addiction. Yet even patients with such a history need pain relief, albeit with closer monitoring. Some patients who demonstrate behaviors associated with addiction (demand for specific medications and doses, anger and irritability, poor cooperation or disturbed interpersonal reactions) may have **pseudo-addiction,** defined as exhibiting behaviors associated with addiction but only because their pain is inadequately treated. Once pain is relieved, these behaviors cease. In all cases, clinicians must be prepared to use appropriate doses of opioids in order to relieve distressing symptoms for patients at the end of life.

Some clinicians fear legal repercussions from prescribing the high doses of opioids sometimes necessary to control pain at the end of life. Some states have enacted special licensing and documentation requirements for opioid prescribing. However, governmental and professional medical groups, regulators, and the US Supreme Court have made it clear that appropriate treatment of pain is the right of the patient and a fundamental responsibility of the clinician. In fact, clinicians have been successfully sued for undertreatment of pain. Although clinicians may feel trapped between consequences of over- or under-prescribing opioids, there remains a wide range of practice in which clinicians can appropriately treat pain. Referral to pain or palliative care experts is appropriate whenever pain cannot be controlled expeditiously by the primary clinician.

PHARMACOLOGIC PAIN MANAGEMENT STRATEGIES

In general, pain can be well controlled with analgesic medications—both opioid and nonopioid—at any stage of illness. Evidence-based summaries and guidelines are available from the Agency for Healthcare Research and Quality (http://www.ncbi.nlm.nih.gov/books/bv.fcgi?rid=hstat1. chapter. 86205) and other organizations (http://www.nccn. org/professionals/physician_gls/PDF/pain.pdf). For mild to moderate pain, acetaminophen, aspirin, and nonsteroidal anti-inflammatory drugs (NSAIDs) may be sufficient. For moderate to severe pain, these agents combined with opioids may be helpful. Severe pain typically requires opioids.

▶ Acetaminophen & NSAIDs

Appropriate doses of acetaminophen may be just as effective an analgesic and antipyretic as NSAIDs but without the risk of gastrointestinal bleeding or ulceration. Acetaminophen can be given at a dosage of 500–1000 mg orally every 6 hours, although it can be taken every 4 hours as long as the risk of hepatotoxicity is kept in mind. Hepatotoxicity is a concern at doses greater than 4 g/d long-term, and doses for older patients and those with liver disease should not exceed 2 g/d.

Aspirin (325–650 mg orally every 4 hours) is an effective analgesic, antipyretic, and anti-inflammatory medication. Gastrointestinal irritation and bleeding, bleeding from other sources, allergy, and an association with Reye syndrome in children and teenagers limit its use.

Commonly used NSAIDs and their dosages are listed in Table 5–3. Like aspirin, the other NSAIDs are antipyretic, analgesic, and anti-inflammatory. NSAIDs increase the risk of gastrointestinal bleeding by 1.5 times normal. The risks of bleeding and nephrotoxicity from NSAIDs are both increased in elders. Gastrointestinal bleeding and ulceration may be prevented with the concurrent use of proton pump inhibitors (eg, omeprazole, 20–40 mg orally daily) or with the class of NSAIDs that inhibit only cyclooxygenase (COX)-2. Because of concerns about an association of COX-2 inhibitors with an increased risk of myocardial infarction, only celecoxib is still available. Celecoxib (100 mg/d to 200 mg orally twice daily) should be used with caution in patients with cardiac disease. The NSAIDs, including COX-2 inhibitors, can lead to exacerbations of congestive heart failure and should be used with caution in patients with that condition.

▶ Opioid Medications

For many patients, opioids are the mainstay of pain management. Opioids are appropriate for severe pain due to any cause, including neuropathic pain. Opioid medications are listed in Table 5–4. Full opioid agonists such as morphine, hydromorphone, oxycodone, methadone, fentanyl, hydrocodone, and codeine are used most commonly. Hydrocodone and codeine are typically combined with acetaminophen or an NSAID. Short-acting formulations of oral morphine sulfate (starting dosage 4–12 mg orally every 3–4 hours), hydromorphone (1–4 mg orally every 3–4 hours), or oxycodone (5–10 mg orally every 3–4 hours) are useful for acute pain not controlled with other analgesics. These same oral medications, or oral transmucosal fentanyl (200 mcg dissolved in mouth) or buccal fentanyl (100 mcg dissolved in the mouth), can be used for "rescue" treatment for patients experiencing pain that breaks through long-acting medications. For chronic stable pain, long-acting medications are preferred, such as oral sustained-release morphine (one to three times a day) or oxycodone (two or three times a day) or methadone (three or four times a day).

Table 5–3. Acetaminophen, COX-2 inhibitors, and useful nonsteroidal anti-inflammatory drugs.

Drug	Usual Dose for Adults ≥ 50 kg	Usual Dose for Adults < 50 kg[1]	Cost per Unit	Cost for 30 Days[2]	Comments[3]
Acetaminophen[4] (Tylenol, Datril, etc)	650 mg q4h or 975 mg q6h	10–15 mg/kg q4h (oral); 15–20 mg/kg q4h (rectal)	$0.02/325 mg (oral) OTC; $0.52/650 mg (rectal) OTC	$7.20 (oral); $93.60 (rectal)	Not an NSAID because it lacks peripheral anti-inflammatory effects. Equivalent to aspirin as analgesic and antipyretic agent.
Aspirin[5]	650 mg q4h or 975 mg q6h	10–15 mg/kg q4h (oral); 15–20 mg/kg q4h (rectal)	$0.02/325 mg OTC; $0.31/600 mg (rectal) OTC	$7.20 (oral); $55.80 (rectal)	Available also in enteric-coated form that is more slowly absorbed but better tolerated.
Celecoxib[4] (Celebrex)	200 mg once daily (osteoarthritis); 100–200 mg twice daily (rheumatoid arthritis)	100 mg once or twice daily	$2.45/100 mg; $4.02/200 mg	$120.60 OA; $241.20 RA	Cyclooxygenase-2 inhibitor. No antiplatelet effects. Lower doses for elderly who weigh < 50 kg. Lower incidence of endoscopic gastrointestinal ulceration. Not known if true lower incidence of gastrointestinal bleeding. Possible link to cardiovascular toxicity. Celecoxib is contraindicated in sulfonamide allergy.
Choline magnesium salicylate[6] (Trilasate, others)	1000–1500 mg three times daily	25 mg/kg three times daily	$0.46/500 mg	$124.20	Salicylates cause less gastrointestinal distress and kidney impairment than NSAIDs but are probably less effective in pain management than NSAIDs.
Diclofenac (Voltaren, Cataflam, others)	50–75 mg two or three times daily		$0.86/50 mg; $1.04/75 mg	$77.40; $93.60	May impose higher risk of hepatotoxicity. Low incidence of gastrointestinal side effects. Enteric-coated product; slow onset.
Diclofenac sustained release (Voltaren-XR, others)	100–200 mg once daily		$2.81/100 mg	$168.60	
Diflunisal[7] (Dolobid, others)	500 mg q12h		$1.29/500 mg	$77.40	Fluorinated acetylsalicylic acid derivative.
Etodolac (Lodine, others)	200–400 mg q6–8h		$1.47/400 mg	$176.40	Perhaps less gastrointestinal toxicity.
Fenoprofen calcium (Nalfon, others)	300–600 mg q6h		$0.51/600 mg	$61.20	Perhaps more side effects than others, including tubulointerstitial nephritis.
Flurbiprofen (Ansaid)	50–100 mg three or four times daily		$0.79/50 mg; $1.19/100 mg	$94.80; $142.80	Adverse gastrointestinal effects may be more common among elderly.
Ibuprofen (Motrin, Advil, Rufen, others)	400–800 mg q6h	10 mg/kg q6–8h[1]	$0.28/600 mg Rx; $0.05/200 mg OTC	$33.60; $9.00	Relatively well tolerated. Less gastrointestinal toxicity.
Indomethacin (Indocin, Indometh, others)	25–50 mg two to four times daily		$0.38/25 mg; $0.64/50 mg	$45.60; $76.80	Higher incidence of dose-related toxic effects, especially gastrointestinal and bone marrow effects.
Ketoprofen (Orudis, Oruvail, others)	25–75 mg q6–8h (max 300 mg/d)		$0.96/50 mg Rx; $1.07/75 mg Rx; $0.09/12.5 mg OTC	$172.80; $128.40; $16.20	Lower doses for elderly.
Ketorolac tromethamine (Toradol)	10 mg q4–6h to a maximum of 40 mg/d orally		$1.02/10 mg	Not recommended	Short-term use (< 5 days) only; otherwise, increased risk of gastrointestinal side effects.

(continued)

Table 5–3. Acetaminophen, COX-2 inhibitors, and useful nonsteroidal anti-inflammatory drugs. (continued)

Drug	Usual Dose for Adults ≥ 50 kg	Usual Dose for Adults < 50 kg[1]	Cost per Unit	Cost for 30 Days[2]	Comments[3]
Ketorolac tromethamine[8] (Toradol)	60 mg IM or 30 mg IV initially, then 30 mg q6h IM or IV		$1.44/30 mg	Not recommended	Intramuscular or intravenous NSAID as alternative to opioid. Lower doses for elderly. Short-term use (< 5 days) only.
Magnesium salicylate (various)	467 mg q4h		$0.08/467 mg OTC	$9.60	
Meclofenamate sodium[9] (Meclomen)	50–100 mg q6h		$3.40/100 mg	$408.00	Diarrhea more common.
Mefenamic acid (Ponstel)	250 mg q6h		$5.85/250 mg	$702.00	
Nabumetone (Relafen)	500–1000 mg once daily (max dose 2000 mg/d)		$1.30/500 mg; $1.53/750 mg	$91.80	May be less ulcerogenic than ibuprofen, but overall side effects may not be less.
Naproxen (Naprosyn, Anaprox, Aleve [OTC], others)	250–500 mg q6–8h	5 mg/kg q8h	$1.30/500 mg Rx; $0.08/220 mg OTC	$156.00; $7.20 OTC	Generally well tolerated. Lower doses for elderly.
Oxaprozin (Daypro, others)	600–1200 mg once daily		$1.51/600 mg	$90.60	Similar to ibuprofen. May cause rash, pruritus, photosensitivity.
Piroxicam (Feldene, others)	20 mg daily		$2.64/20 mg	$79.20	Not recommended in the elderly due to high adverse drug reaction rate. Single daily dose convenient. Long half-life. May cause higher rate of gastrointestinal bleeding and dermatologic side effects.
Sodium salicylate	325–650 mg q3–4h		$0.08/650 mg OTC	$19.20	
Sulindac (Clinoril, others)	150–200 mg twice daily		$0.98/150 mg; $1.21/200 mg	$58.80; $72.60	May cause higher rate of gastrointestinal bleeding. May have less nephrotoxic potential.
Tolmetin (Tolectin)	200–600 mg four times daily		$0.75/200 mg; $1.80/600 mg	$90.00; $216.00	Perhaps more side effects than others, including anaphylactic reactions.

[1]Acetaminophen and NSAID dosages for adults weighing less than 50 kg should be adjusted for weight.
[2]Average wholesale price (AWP, for AB-rated generic when available) for quantity listed. Source: *Red Book Update*, Vol. 28, No. 3, March 2009. AWP may not accurately represent the actual pharmacy cost because wide contractual variations exist among institutions.
[3]The adverse effects of headache, tinnitus, dizziness, confusion, rashes, anorexia, nausea, vomiting, gastrointestinal bleeding, diarrhea, nephrotoxicity, visual disturbances, etc, can occur with any of these drugs. Tolerance and efficacy are subject to great individual variations among patients. Note: All NSAIDs can increase serum lithium levels.
[4]Acetaminophen and celecoxib lack antiplatelet effects.
[5]May inhibit platelet aggregation for 1 week or more and may cause bleeding.
[6]May have minimal antiplatelet activity.
[7]Administration with antacids may decrease absorption.
[8]Has the same gastrointestinal toxicities as oral NSAIDs.
[9]Coombs-positive autoimmune hemolytic anemia has been associated with prolonged use.
OTC, over-the-counter; Rx, prescription; OA, osteoarthritis; RA, rheumatoid arthritis.
Adapted from Jacox AK et al: *Management of Cancer Pain: Quick Reference Guide for Clinicians No. 9.* AHCPR Publication No. 94-0593. Rockville, MD: Agency for Health Care Policy and Research, Public Health Service, U.S. Department of Health and Human Services. March 1994.

Table 5-4. Useful opioid agonist analgesics.

Drug	Approximate Equianalgesic Dose[1]		Usual Starting Dose					Potential Advantages	Potential Disadvantages
			Adults ≥ 50 kg Body Weight		Adults < 50 kg Body Weight				
	Oral	Parenteral	Oral	Parenteral	Oral	Parenteral			
Opioid agonists[2]									
Fentanyl	Not available	0.1 (100 mcg) q1h	Not available	50-100 mcg IV/IM q1h or 0.5-1.5 mcg/kg/h IV infusion $0.98/100 mcg	Not available	0.5-1 mcg/kg IV q1-4h or 1-2 mcg/kg IV × 1, then 0.5-1 mcg/kg/h infusion		Possibly less neuroexcitatory effects, including in kidney failure.	
Fentanyl oral transmucosal (Actiq); buccal (Fentora)		Not available	200 mcg transmucosal; 100 mcg buccal; $33.80/200 mcg transmucosal; $17.27/200 mcg buccal	Not available		Not available		For pain breaking through long-acting opioid medication.	Transmucosal and buccal formulations are not bioequivalent; there is higher bioavailability of buccal formulation.
Fentanyl transdermal	Conversion to fentanyl patch is based on total daily dose of oral morphine[2]: morphine 60-134 mg/d orally = fentanyl 25 mcg/h patch; morphine 135-224 mg/d orally = fentanyl 50 mcg/h patch; morphine 225-314 mg/day orally = fentanyl 75 mcg/h patch; and morphine 315-404 mg/d orally = fentanyl 100 mcg/h patch	Not available	Not available orally 12.5-25 mcg/h patch q72h; $14.42/25 mcg/h	Not available	12.5-25 mcg/h patch q72h	Not available		Stable medication blood levels.	Not for use in opioid-naïve patients.
Hydromorphone[3] (Dilaudid)	7.5 mg q3-4h	1.5 mg q3-4h	1-4 mg q3-4h; $0.37/2 mg	1.5 mg q3-4h; $1.02/2 mg	0.06 mg/q3-4h	0.015 mg/kg q3-4h		Similar to morphine. Available in injectable high-potency preparation, rectal suppository.	Short duration.

(continued)

Table 5–4. Useful opioid agonist analgesics. (continued)

Drug	Approximate Equianalgesic Dose[1]		Usual Starting Dose				Potential Advantages	Potential Disadvantages
			Adults ≥ 50 kg Body Weight		Adults < 50 kg Body Weight			
	Oral	Parenteral	Oral	Parenteral	Oral	Parenteral		
Levorphanol (Levo-Dromoran)	4 mg q6-8h	2 mg q6-8h	4 mg q6-8h; $1.07/2 mg	2 mg q6-8h; $3.96/2 mg	0.04 mg/kg q6-8h	0.02 mg q6-8h	Longer-acting than morphine sulfate.	
Meperidine[4] (Demerol)	300 mg q2-3h; normal dose 50-150 mg q3-4h	100 mg q3h; $0.69/50 mg	Not recommended; $0.69/50 mg	100 mg q3h; $0.86/100 mg	Not recommended	0.75 mg/kg q2-3h	Use only when single dose, short duration analgesia is needed as for outpatient procedures like colonoscopy. Not recommended for chronic pain or for repeated dosing.	Short duration. Normeperidine metabolite accumulates in kidney failure and other situations, and in high concentrations may cause irritability and seizures.
Methadone (Dolophine, others)	10-20 mg q6-8h (when converting from < 100 mg long-term daily oral morphine)	5-10 mg q6-8h	5-20 mg q6-8h; $0.15/10 mg	2.5-10 mg q6-8h; $4.10/10 mg	0.2 mg/kg q6-8h	0.1 mg/kg q6-8h	Somewhat longer-acting than morphine. Useful in cases of intolerance to morphine. May be particularly useful for neuropathic pain. Available in liquid formulation.	Analgesic duration shorter than plasma duration. May accumulate, requiring close monitoring during first weeks of treatment. Equianalgesic ratios vary with opioid dose.
Morphine[3] immediate release (Morphine sulfate tablets, Roxanol liquid)	30 mg q3-4h (repeat around-the-clock dosing); 60 mg q3-4h (single or intermittent dosing)	10 mg q3-4h	4-12 mg q3-4h; $0.18/15 mg	10 mg q3-4h; $1.22/10 mg	0.3 mg/kg q3-4h	0.1 mg/kg q3-4h	Standard of comparison; multiple dosage forms available.	No unique problems when compared with other opioids.
Morphine controlled-release[3] (MS Contin, Oramorph)	90-120 mg q12h	Not available	15-60 mg q12h; $1.69/30 mg	Not available	Not available	Not available		
Morphine extended release (Kadian, Avinza)	180-240 mg q24h	Not available	20-30 mg q24h; $3.71/30 mg	Not available	Not available	Not available	Once-daily dosing.	
Oxycodone (Roxicodone, OxyIR)	20-30 mg q3-4h	Not available	5-10 mg q3-4h; $0.33/5 mg	Not available	0.2 mg/kg q3-4h	Not available	Similar to morphine.	

Drug	Approximate equianalgesic oral dose	Approximate equianalgesic parenteral dose	Usual starting dose (oral, adults ≥50 kg)	Usual starting dose (parenteral, adults ≥50 kg)	Usual starting dose (oral, children & adults <50 kg)	Usual starting dose (parenteral, children & adults <50 kg)	Comments
Oxycodone controlled release (Oxycontin)	40 mg q12h	Not available	20–40 mg q12h; $3.69/20 mg				
Oxymorphone[5] injectable (Numorphan)	Not available	1 mg q3–4h	Not available	1 mg q3–4h; $3.13/1 mg			Active metabolite of oxycodone.
Oxymorphone[5] oral, immediate release (Opana)	10 mg q3–4h	Not available	5–10 mg q3–4h; $2.37/5 mg	Not available			New formulation with less known about equianalgesic dosing.
Oxymorphone[5] extended release (Opana ER)	30–40 mg q12h	Not available	15–30 mg q12h; $3.31/10 mg	Not available			New formulation with less known about equianalgesic dosing.
Combination Opioid-NSAID Preparations							
Codeine[6,7] (with aspirin or acetaminophen)[8]	180–200 mg q3–4h; normal dose, 15–60 mg q4–6h	130 mg q3–4h	60 mg q4–6h; $0.64/60 mg	60 mg q2h (IM/SC); $2.48/60 mg	0.5–1 mg/kg q3–4h	Not recommended	Similar to morphine. Closely monitor for efficacy as patients vary in their ability to convert the prodrug codeine to morphine.
Hydrocodone[5] (in Lorcet, Lortab, Vicodin, others)[8]	30 mg q3–4h	Not available	10 mg q3–4h; $0.32/5 mg	Not available	0.2 mg/kg q3–4h	Not available	Combination with acetaminophen limits dosage titration.
Oxycodone[6] (in Percocet, Percodan, Tylox, others)[8]	30 mg q3–4h	Not available	10 mg q3–4h; $0.31/5 mg	Not available	0.2 mg/kg q3–4h	Not available	Similar to morphine. Combination with acetaminophen and aspirin limits dosage titration.

[1] Published tables vary in the suggested doses that are equianalgesic to morphine. Clinical response is the criterion that must be applied for each patient; titration to clinical efficacy is necessary. Because there is not complete cross-tolerance among these drugs, it is usually necessary to use a lower than equianalgesic dose initially when changing drugs and to retitrate to response.

[2] Conversion is conservative; therefore, do not use these equianalgesic doses for converting back from fentanyl patch to other opioids because they may lead to inadvertent overdose. Patients may require breakthrough doses of short-acting opioids during conversion to transdermal fentanyl.

[3] **Caution:** For morphine, hydromorphone, and oxymorphone, rectal administration is an alternative route for patients unable to take oral medications. Equianalgesic doses may differ from oral and parenteral doses. A short-acting opioid should normally be used for initial therapy.

[4] Not recommended for chronic pain. Doses listed are for brief therapy of acute pain only. Switch to another opioid for long-term therapy.

[5] **Caution:** Recommended doses do not apply for adult patients with kidney or hepatic insufficiency or other conditions affecting drug metabolism.

[6] **Caution:** Doses of aspirin and acetaminophen in combination products must also be adjusted to the patient's body weight.

[7] **Caution:** Doses of codeine above 60 mg often are not appropriate because of diminishing incremental analgesia with increasing doses but continually increasing nausea, constipation, and other side effects.

[8] **Caution:** Monitor total acetaminophen dose carefully, including any OTC use. Total acetaminophen dose maximum 4 g/d. If liver impairment or heavy alcohol use, maximum is 2 g/d.

Note: Average wholesale price (AWP, generic when available) for quantity listed. Source: *Red Book Update*, Vol. 28, No. 3, March 2009. AWP may not accurately represent the actual pharmacy cost because wide contractual variations exist among institutions.

Adapted from Jacox AK et al. *Management of Cancer Pain: Quick Reference Guide for Clinicians No. 9.* AHCPR Publication No. 94-0593. Rockville, MD. Agency for Health Care Policy and Research, Public Health Service, U.S. Department of Health and Human Services. March 1994. (Erstad BL. A rational approach to the management of acute pain states.) Advanstar Communications, Inc. Reproduced in part, with permission, from Hosp Formul 1994;29(8 Part 2):586.

Transdermal fentanyl is appropriate for patients already tolerant to other opioids at a dose equivalent to at least 60 mg/d of oral morphine (equivalent to transdermal fentanyl 25 mcg/h every 72 hours) but should not be the first opioid used. Medications that inhibit cytochrome P450 3A4, such as ritonavir, ketoconazole, itraconazole, troleandomycin, clarithromycin, nelfinavir, nefazodone, amiodarone, amprenavir, aprepitant, diltiazem, erythromycin, fluconazole, fosamprenavir, and verapamil, and grapefruit juice can cause increased levels and duration of transdermal fentanyl. Since the fentanyl patch can require 24–48 hours to achieve pharmacologic "steady state," patients should be given short-acting opioids while awaiting the full analgesic effect of transdermal fentanyl.

Meperidine is not useful for chronic pain because it has a short half-life and a toxic metabolite, normeperidine, which can cause irritability and seizures. Partial agonists such as buprenorphine are limited by a dose-related ceiling effect. Mixed agonist-antagonists such as pentazocine and butorphanol tartrate also have a ceiling effect and are contraindicated in patients already receiving full agonist opioids since they may reverse the pain control achieved by the full agonist and cause a withdrawal effect.

A useful technique for opioid management of chronic pain is equianalgesic dosing (Table 5–4). The dosages of any full opioid agonists used to control pain can be converted into an equivalent dose of any other opioid. In this way, 24-hour opioid requirements and dosing regimens established using shorter-acting opioid medications can be converted into equivalent dosages of long-acting medications or formulations. Cross-tolerance is often incomplete, however, so less than the full calculated equianalgesic dosage is generally administered initially when switching between opioid formulations. Equianalgesic dosing for methadone is more complex and varies by dose and duration of use.

While some clinicians and patients inexperienced with the management of severe chronic pain may feel more comfortable with combined nonopioid-opioid agents, full agonist opioids are typically a better choice in patients with severe pain because the dose of opioid is not limited by the toxicities of the acetaminophen, aspirin, or NSAID component of combination preparations. There is no maximal allowable or effective dose for full opioid agonists. The dose should be increased to whatever is necessary to relieve pain, remembering that certain types of pain, such as neuropathic pain, may respond better to agents other than opioids, or to combinations of opioids with these other agents (see below).

While physiologic tolerance is possible with opioids, failure of a previously effective opioid dose to adequately relieve pain is usually due to worsening of the underlying condition causing pain, such as growth of a tumor or a new metastasis in a patient with cancer. In this case, for moderate unrelieved pain, the dose of opioid can be increased by 25–50%. For severe unrelieved pain, a dose increase of 50–100% may be appropriate. The frequency of dosing should be adjusted so that pain control is continuous. Long-term dosing may then be adjusted by adding the amount of short-acting opioid necessary for breakthrough pain over the preceding 24–48 hours to the long-acting medication dose. In establishing or reestablishing adequate dosing,

frequent reassessment of the patient's pain and medication side effects is necessary.

As opioids are titrated upwards, increasing difficulty with the side effects can be expected. Constipation is common at any dose of opioid and should be anticipated and prevented in all patients. The prophylaxis and management of opioid-induced constipation are outlined below.

Sedation can be expected with opioids, although tolerance to this effect typically develops within 24–72 hours at a stable dose. Sedation typically appears well before significant respiratory depression. If treatment for sedation is desired, dextroamphetamine (2.5–7.5 mg orally at 8 AM and noon) or methylphenidate (2.5–10 mg orally at 8 AM and noon) may be helpful. Caffeinated beverages can also help manage minor opioid sedation.

Although sedation is more common, patients may experience euphoria when first taking opioids or when the dose is increased. However, tolerance to this effect typically develops after a few days at a stable dose. At very high doses of opioids, multifocal myoclonus may develop. This symptom may resolve after lowering the dose or switching opioids. While waiting for the level of the offending medication to fall, low doses of lorazepam or dantrolene may be helpful for treating myoclonus.

Nausea due to opioids may occur with initiation of therapy and resolve after a few days. If it is severe or persistent, it can be treated with prochlorperazine, 10 mg orally or intravenously every 8 hours or 25 mg rectally every 6 hours. The most common cause of nausea in patients taking opioids, however, is unrelieved constipation.

Although clinicians may worry about respiratory depression with opioids, that side effect is uncommon when a low dose is given initially and titrated upward slowly. Patients at particular risk for respiratory depression include those with chronic obstructive pulmonary disease and baseline CO_2 retention, those with liver or kidney or combined liver-kidney failure, and those with adrenal insufficiency or frank myxedema. Yet, even patients with severe pulmonary disease can tolerate low-dose opioids, but they should be monitored carefully. Clinicians should not allow concerns about respiratory depression to prevent them from treating pain adequately.

True allergy (with urticaria) to opioids is rare. More commonly, patients will describe intolerance due to side effects such as nausea, pruritus, or urinary retention in response to a particular opioid. If such symptoms develop, they can usually be relieved by lowering the dose or switching to another opioid.

▶ Medications for Neuropathic Pain

It is essential when taking a patient's history to listen for descriptions such as burning, shooting, pins and needles, or electricity, and for pain associated with numbness. Such a history suggests neuropathic pain, which is treated with some medications not typically used for other types of pain. While opioids are effective for neuropathic pain, a number of nonopioid medications have been found to be effective in randomized trials (Table 5–5). The tricyclic antidepressants (TCAs) may provide the greatest relative efficacy and are a

Table 5–5. Pharmacologic management of neuropathic pain.

Drug[1]	Starting Dose	Typical Dose
Antidepressants[2]		
Amitriptyline[3]	10 mg orally at bedtime	10–150 mg orally at bedtime
Nortriptyline	10 mg orally at bedtime	10–150 mg orally at bedtime
Desipramine	10 mg orally at bedtime	10–200 mg orally at bedtime
Calcium-channel $\alpha2$-δ ligands		
Gabapentin[4]	100–300 mg orally once to three times daily	300–1200 mg orally three times daily
Pregabalin[5]	50 mg orally three times daily	100 mg orally three times daily
Selective serotonin norepinephrine reuptake inhibitors		
Duloxetine	60 mg orally daily or 20 mg orally twice daily in elders	60 mg orally daily
Venlafaxine[6]	75 mg orally daily divided into two or three doses	150–225 mg orally daily divided into two or three doses
Opioids	(see Table 5–4)	(see Table 5–4)
Other medications		
Lidocaine transdermal	5% patch applied daily, for a maximum of 12 hours	1–3 patches applied daily for a maximum of 12 hours
Tramadol hydrochloride	50 mg orally four times daily	100 mg orally two to four times daily

[1]Begin at the starting dose and titrate up every 4 or 5 days.
[2]Begin with a low dose. Pain relief may be achieved at doses below antidepressant doses, thereby minimizing adverse side effects.
[3]Avoid in elders because it has more severe anticholinergic effects.
[4]Common side effects include nausea, somnolence, and dizziness. Take medication on a full stomach. Do not combine with serotonin or norepinephrine uptake inhibitors, or with tricyclic antidepressants.
[5]Common side effects include dizziness, somnolence, peripheral edema, and weight gain. Must adjust dose for kidney impairment.
[6]Caution: Can cause hypertension and ECG changes. Obtain baseline ECG and monitor.

good first-line therapy. They usually have an effect within days at lower doses than are needed for an antidepressant effect. Desipramine, 10–200 mg/d orally, and nortriptyline, 10–150 mg/d orally, are good first choices because they cause less orthostatic hypotension and have fewer anticholinergic effects than amitriptyline. Start with a low dosage (10 mg orally daily) and titrate upward every 4 or 5 days.

The calcium channel $\alpha2$-δ ligands gabapentin and pregabalin are also considered first-line therapy for neuropathic pain. Both medications can cause sedation, dizziness, ataxia, and gastrointestinal side effects but have no significant drug interactions. Both drugs require dose adjustments in patients with kidney dysfunction. Gabapentin should be started at low dosages of 100–300 mg orally three times a day and titrated upward by 300 mg/d every 4 or 5 days with a typical effective dose of 1800–3600 mg/d. Pregabalin should be started at 150 mg/d in two or three divided doses. If necessary, the dose of pregabalin can be titrated upward to 300–600 mg/d in two or three divided doses. Both drugs are relatively safe in accidental overdosage and may be preferred over TCAs for a patient with a history of congestive heart failure or arrhythmia or if there is a risk of suicide. Gabapentin plus morphine in combination is more effective at lower doses of each drug than when each is used as a single agent.

The selective serotonin norepinephrine reuptake inhibitors (SSNRIs), duloxetine (60 mg/d or 20 mg twice daily in elders), and venlafaxine (150–225 mg/d) are also considered first-line treatments for neuropathic pain. Patients should be advised to take duloxetine on a full stomach because nausea is a common side effect. Duloxetine should not be combined with other serotonin or norepinephrine uptake inhibitors, but it can be combined with gabapentin or pregabalin. Because venlafaxine can cause hypertension and induce ECG changes, patients with cardiovascular risk factors should be carefully monitored when starting this drug.

Opioids and tramadol are also effective for neuropathic pain. Tramadol should be started at 50 mg orally daily and can be titrated up to 100 mg orally four times daily.

The 5% lidocaine patch (1–4 patches at a time) is effective in postherpetic neuralgia and may be effective in other types of localized neuropathic pain. A new patch is applied to the painful region daily for up to 12 hours.

Successful management of neuropathic pain often requires the use of more than one effective medication.

▶ Adjuvant Pain Medications & Treatments

If pain cannot be controlled without uncomfortable medication side effects, clinicians should consider using lower doses of multiple medications, as is done commonly for neuropathic pain, rather than larger doses of one or two medications. For bone pain, the anti-inflammatory effect of NSAIDs can be particularly helpful. Radiation therapy and bisphosphonates may also relieve bone pain. For some patients, a nerve block can provide substantial relief, such as a celiac plexus block for pain from pancreatic cancer. Intrathecal pumps may be useful for patients with severe pain responsive to opioids but who require such large doses that systemic side effects (eg, sedation and constipation) become limiting. There is some evidence for the use of cannabinoids as analgesics. Chemotherapeutic agents can be used for symptom management with palliative intent.

Corticosteroids such as dexamethasone or prednisone can be helpful for patients with headache due to increased intracranial pressure, pain from spinal cord compression, metastatic bone pain, and neuropathic pain due to invasion or infiltration of nerves by tumor. Because of the side effects of long-term corticosteroid administration, they are most appropriate in patients with end-stage disease. Low-dose intravenous or oral ketamine has been used successfully for neuropathic and other pain syndromes poorly responsive to opioids. Haloperidol and benzodiazepines may be used prophylactically to minimize ketamine's psychotomimetic side effects.

NONPHARMACOLOGIC TREATMENTS

Nonpharmacologic therapies are also valuable in treating pain. Hot or cold packs, massage, and physical therapy can be helpful for musculoskeletal pain. Similarly, biofeedback, acupuncture, chiropractic, meditation, music therapy, cognitive behavioral therapy, guided imagery, cognitive distraction, and framing may be of help in treating pain. Because mood and psychological issues play an important role in the patient's perception of and response to pain, psychotherapy, support groups, prayer, and pastoral counseling can also help in the management of pain. Major depression, which may be instigated by chronic pain or may alter the response to pain, should be treated aggressively.

► When to Refer

- Pain not responding to opioids at typical doses.
- Neuropathic pain not responding to first-line treatments.
- Complex methadone management issues.
- Intolerable side effects from oral opioids.
- Severe pain from bone metastases.
- For a surgical or anesthesia-based procedure, intrathecal pump, or nerve block.

► When to Admit

- Patients should be hospitalized for severe exacerbation of pain that is not responsive to previous stable oral opioid around-the-clock plus breakthrough doses.
- Patients whose pain is so severe that they cannot be cared for at home should be hospitalized.
- Uncontrollable side effects from opioids, including nausea, vomiting, and altered mental status, should prompt hospitalization.

Abrams DI et al. Cannabis in painful HIV-associated sensory neuropathy: a randomized placebo-controlled trial. Neurology. 2007 Feb 13;68(7):515–21. [PMID: 17296917]

Dworkin RH et al. Pharmacologic management of neuropathic pain: evidence-based recommendations. Pain. 2007 Dec 5;132(3):237–51. [PMID: 17920770]

Morrison RS et al. Cost savings associated with US hospital palliative care consultation programs. Arch Intern Med. 2008 Sep 8;168(16):1783–90. [PMID: 18779466]

Moryl N et al. Managing an acute pain crisis in a patient with advanced cancer: "This is as much of a crisis as a Code." JAMA. 2008 Mar 26;299(12):1457–67. [PMID: 18364488]

▼ PALLIATION OF OTHER COMMON SYMPTOMS

DYSPNEA

Dyspnea is the subjective experience of difficulty breathing and may be characterized by patients as tightness in the chest, shortness of breath, or a feeling of suffocation. Up to 50% of terminally ill patients may experience severe dyspnea.

Treatment of dyspnea is usually first directed at the cause (see Chapter 9). At the end of life, dyspnea is often treated nonspecifically with opioids. Immediate-release morphine orally or intravenously treats dyspnea effectively and typically at doses lower than would be necessary for the relief of moderate pain. Supplemental oxygen may be useful for the dyspneic patient who is hypoxic and may provide subjective benefit to other dyspneic patients as well. However, a nasal cannula and face mask are sometimes not well tolerated, and fresh air from a window or fan may provide relief. Judicious use of nonpharmacologic relaxation techniques such as meditation and guided imagery may be beneficial for some patients. Benzodiazepines may be useful for the anxiety associated with dyspnea but do not appear to act directly to relieve dyspnea.

NAUSEA & VOMITING

Nausea and vomiting are common and distressing symptoms. As with pain, the management of nausea may be maximized by regular dosing. An understanding of the four major inputs to the vomiting center may help direct treatment (see Chapter 15).

Vomiting associated with a particular opioid may be relieved by dose reduction or substitution with an equianalgesic dose of another opioid or a sustained-release formulation. In addition to the other dopamine receptor antagonist antiemetics listed in Table 15–2 that block the trigger zone, haloperidol (0.5–2 mg orally every 4–6 hours) is commonly used.

Vomiting may be due to stimulation of peripheral afferent nerves from the gut. Offering patients small amounts of food only when they are hungry may prevent nausea and vomiting. Nasogastric suction may provide rapid, short-term relief for vomiting associated with constipation, gastroparesis, or gastric outlet obstruction, with the addition of laxatives, prokinetic agents (only in the setting of partial not complete obstruction) such as metoclopramide (10–20 mg orally or intravenously four times a day), scopolamine (1.5-mg patch every 3 days), and high-dose corticosteroids as more definitive treatment. Nausea often requires treatment with more than one agent; when it is refractory to other treatments or due to increased intracranial pressure, it may respond to high-dose corticosteroids (eg, dexamethasone, 20 mg orally or intravenously daily in divided doses).

Vomiting due to disturbance of the vestibular apparatus may be treated with anticholinergic and antihistaminic agents (including diphenhydramine, 25 mg orally or intravenously every 8 hours, or scopolamine, 1.5-mg patch every 3 days).

Benzodiazepines can be effective in preventing the anticipatory nausea associated with chemotherapy but are otherwise not indicated for nausea and vomiting. Finally, many patients find medical marijuana or dronabinol (2.5–20 mg orally every 4–6 hours) helpful in the management of nausea and vomiting.

CONSTIPATION

Given the frequent use of opioids, poor dietary intake, and physical inactivity, constipation is a common problem among the dying. Clinicians must inquire about any difficulty with hard or infrequent stools. Constipation is an easily preventable and treatable cause of discomfort, distress, and nausea and vomiting (see Chapter 15).

Constipation may be prevented or relieved if patients can increase their activity and their intake of dietary fiber and fluids. Simple considerations such as privacy, undisturbed toilet time, and a bedside commode rather than a bedpan may be important for some patients.

For patients taking opioids, anticipating and preventing constipation is important. A prophylactic bowel regimen of stool softeners (docusate) and stimulants (bisacodyl or senna) should be started when opioid treatment is begun. Table 15–4 lists other agents that can be added as needed. Methylnaltrexone, a new subcutaneous medication, is a peripherally acting mu-receptor antagonist and holds promise for severe, unrelieved, opioid-induced constipation.

DELIRIUM & AGITATION

Many terminally ill patients die in a state of delirium—a disturbance of consciousness and a change in cognition that develops over a short time and is manifested by misinterpretations, illusions, hallucinations, disturbances in the sleep-wake cycle, psychomotor disturbances (eg, lethargy, restlessness), and mood disturbance (eg, fear, anxiety). Delirium complicated by myoclonus or convulsions at the end of life has been called **terminal restlessness.**

Careful attention to patient safety and nonpharmacologic strategies to help the patient remain oriented (clocks, calendars, a familiar environment, reassurance and redirection from caregivers) may be sufficient to prevent or manage minor delirium. Some delirious patients may be "pleasantly confused," and a decision by the patient's family and the clinician not to treat delirium may be justified.

More commonly, however, delirium at the end of life is distressing to patients and family and requires treatment. Delirium may interfere with the family's ability to feel comforting to the patient and may prevent a patient from being able to recognize and report important symptoms.

While there are many reversible causes of delirium (see Chapter 25), identifying and correcting the underlying cause at the end of life is often simply a question of attention to the choice and dosing of psychoactive medications.

When the cause of delirium cannot be identified, treated, or corrected rapidly enough, delirium may be treated symptomatically with neuroleptics, such as haloperidol (1–10 mg orally, subcutaneously, intramuscularly, or intravenously twice or three times a day) or risperidone (1–3 mg orally twice a day). The benefits of neuroleptics in the treatment of agitation must be weighed carefully against potential harms, based on mounting data showing an association between antipsychotic medications and increased mortality for older adults with dementia. When delirium is refractory to treatment and remains intolerable, sedation may be required to provide relief and may be achieved rapidly with midazolam (0.5–5 mg/h subcutaneously or intravenously) or barbiturates.

Clemens KE et al. Is there a higher risk of respiratory depression in opioid-naïve palliative care patients during symptomatic therapy of dyspnea with strong opioids? J Palliat Med. 2008 Mar;11(2):204–16. [PMID: 18333735]

Gill SS et al. Antipsychotic drug use and mortality in older adults with dementia. Ann Intern Med. 2007 Jun 5;146(11):775–86. [PMID: 17548409]

Thomas J et al. Methylnaltrexone for opioid-induced constipation in advanced illness. N Engl J Med. 2008 May 29;358(22):2332–43. [PMID: 18509120]

Wood GJ et al. Management of intractable nausea and vomiting in patients at the end of life: "I was feeling nauseous all of the time . . . nothing was working." JAMA. 2007 Sep 12;298(10):1196–207. [PMID: 17848654]

Yennurajalingam S et al. Palliative management of fatigue at the close of life: "It feels like my body is just worn out." JAMA. 2007 Jan 17;297(3):295–304. [PMID: 17227981]

► END-OF-LIFE CARE

In the United States, approximately 2.5 million people die each year. Caring for patients at the end of life is an important responsibility and a rewarding opportunity for clinicians. Clinicians battling to prolong life must recognize when life is ending in order to continue caring properly for their patients. Unfortunately, most clinical practice guidelines do not include significant attention to end-of-life care. End-of-life care refers to focusing care for those approaching death on the goals of relieving distressing symptoms and promoting quality of life rather than attempting to cure underlying disease. From the medical perspective, the end of life may be defined as that time when death—whether due to terminal illness or acute or chronic illness—is expected within weeks to months and can no longer be reasonably forestalled by medical intervention.

► Prognosis at the End of Life

Clinicians must help patients understand when they are approaching the end of life. This information influences patients' treatment decisions and may change how they spend their remaining time. While certain diseases such as

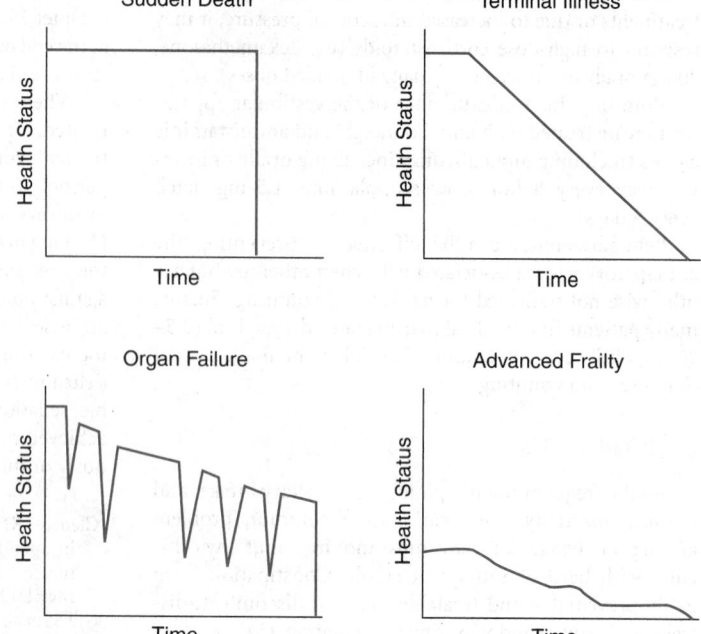

▲ Figure 5–1. Theoretical trajectories of dying. (Adapted, with permission, from Lunney JR et al. Profiles of older Medicare decedents. J Am Geriatr Soc 2002 Jun;50(6): 1108–12.)

cancer are more amenable to prognostic estimates regarding the time course to death, the other common causes of mortality in the United States—including heart disease, stroke, chronic lung disease, and dementia—have more variable trajectories and difficult to predict prognoses (Figure 5–1). Even for patients with cancer, clinician estimates of prognosis are often inaccurate and generally overly optimistic. Nonetheless, clinical experience, epidemiologic data, guidelines from professional organizations (eg, the National Hospice Organization), and computer modeling and prediction tools (eg, the Acute Physiology and Chronic Health Evaluation [APACHE] system, the Study to Understand Prognoses and Preferences for Outcomes and Risks of Treatment [SUPPORT] model, or the Palliative Performance Scale) may be used to help patients identify the end period of their lives. Clinicians can also ask themselves "Would I be surprised if this patient died in the next year?" to determine whether a discussion of prognosis and focus on end-of-life care would be appropriate. If the answer is "no," then the clinician should initiate a discussion. Recognizing that patients may have different levels of comfort with prognostic information, clinicians can introduce the topic by simply saying, "I have information about the likely time course of your illness. Would you like to talk about it?"

▶ Expectations About the End of Life

Patients' experiences at the end of life are influenced by their expectations about how they will die and the meaning of death. Many people fear how they will die more than death itself. Patients report fears of dying in pain or of suffocation, of loss of control, indignity, isolation, and of being a burden to their families. All of these anxieties may be ameliorated with good supportive care provided by an attentive group of caretakers.

Death is often regarded by clinicians, patients, and families as a failure of medical science. This attitude can create or heighten a sense of guilt about the failure to prevent dying. Both the general public and clinicians often are complicit in denying death, treating dying persons merely as patients and death as an enemy to be battled furiously in hospitals rather than as an inevitable outcome to be experienced as a part of life at home. As a result, approximately 75–80% of people in the United States die in hospitals or long-term care facilities.

Even when the clinician continues to pursue cure of potentially reversible disease, offering comfort and helping the patient prepare for death are foremost considerations. Patients at the end of life and their families identify a number of elements as important to quality end-of-life care: managing pain and other symptoms adequately, avoiding inappropriate prolongation of dying, preserving dignity, preparing for death, achieving a sense of control, relieving the burden on others, and strengthening relationships with loved ones.

▶ Communication & Care of the Patient

Caring for patients at the end of life requires the same skills clinicians use in other tasks of medical care: diagnosing treatable conditions, providing patient education, facilitating decision-making, and expressing understanding and caring. Communication skills are vitally important. Higher-quality communication is associated with greater satisfaction and awareness of patient wishes. When needed, the use of a professional interpreter can facilitate clear

Table 5–6. Suggestions for the delivery of bad news.

Prepare an appropriate place and time.
Address basic information needs.
Be direct; avoid jargon and euphemisms.
Allow for silence and emotional ventilation.
Assess and validate patient reactions.
Respond to immediate discomforts and risks.
Listen actively and express empathy.
Achieve a common perception of the problem.
Reassure about pain relief.
Ensure basic follow-up and make specific plans for the future.

Table 5–7. Clinician interventions helpful to families of dying patients.

Excellent communication, including physician willingness to talk about death, timely and clear information, proactive guidance, listening, and empathic responses
Advance care planning and clear decision-making, including culturally sensitive communication, achieving consensus among family members and an understanding that surrogate decision-makers are trying to determine what the *patient* would have wanted, not what the surrogate would want
Support for home care, including orienting family members to the scope and details of family caregiving, providing clear direction about how to contact professional caregivers, and informing patients and families of the benefits of hospice care
Empathy for family emotions and relationships, including recognizing and validating common positive and negative feelings
Attention to grief and bereavement, including support for anticipatory grief and follow-up with the family after the patient's death

Adapted, with permission, from Rabow MW et al. Supporting family caregivers at the end of life: "they don't know what they don't know." JAMA. 2004 Jan 28;291(4):483–91.

communication and help broker cultural issues. In particular, clinicians must become proficient at delivering bad news and then dealing with its consequences (Table 5–6).

Three further obligations are central to the clinician's role at this time. First, he or she must work to identify, understand, and relieve suffering, which may include physical, psychological, social, or spiritual distress. In assisting with redirection and growth, providing support, assessing meaning, and fostering transcendence, clinicians can help ameliorate their patients' suffering and help the patient live fully during this stage of life.

Second, clinicians can serve as facilitators or catalysts for hope. While a particular outcome may be extremely unlikely (such as cure of advanced cancer following exhaustive conventional and experimental treatments), hope may be defined as the patient's belief in what is *still* possible. Although expecting a "miraculous cure" may be simplistic and even harmful, hope for relief of pain, for reconciliation with loved ones, for discovery of meaning, and for spiritual transformation is realistic at the end of life. With such questions as "What is still possible now for you?" "When you look to the future, what do you hope for?" "What good might come of this?" clinicians can help patients uncover hope, explore meaningful and realistic goals, and develop strategies to realize them.

Third, dying patients' feelings of isolation and fear demand that clinicians assert that care will continue to be provided throughout the final stage of life. The promise of nonabandonment is perhaps the central principle of end-of-life care and is a clinician's pledge to an individual patient to serve as a caring partner, a resource for creative problem-solving and relief of suffering, a guide during uncertain times, and a witness to the patient's experiences—no matter what happens. Clinicians can say to a patient, "I will care for you whatever happens." Dying patients need their clinicians to offer their presence—not necessarily the ability to solve all problems but rather a commitment to recognize and receive the patients' difficulties and experiences with respect and empathy. At its best, the patient-clinician relationship can be a covenant of compassion and a recognition of common humanity.

Caring for the Family

In caring for patients at the end of life, clinicians must appreciate the central role played by family, friends, and romantic partners and often must deal with strong emotions of fear, anger, shame, sadness, and guilt experienced by those individuals. While significant others may support and comfort a patient at the end of life, the threatened loss of a loved one may also create or reveal dysfunctional or painful family dynamics. Furthermore, clinicians must be attuned to the potential impact of illness on the patient's family: substantial physical caregiving responsibilities and financial burdens as well as increased rates of anxiety, depression, chronic illness, and even mortality. Family caregivers, typically women, commonly provide the bulk of care for patients at the end of life, yet their work is often not acknowledged or compensated.

Clinicians can help families confront the imminent loss of a loved one (Table 5–7) and often must negotiate amid complex and changing family needs. Identifying a spokesperson for the family, conducting family meetings, allowing all to be heard, and providing time for consensus may help the clinician work effectively with the family.

Clinician Self-Care

Many clinicians find caring for patients at the end of life to be one of the most rewarding aspects of practice. However, working with the dying requires tolerance of uncertainty, ambiguity, and existential challenges. Clinicians must recognize and respect their own limitations and attend to their own needs in order to avoid being overburdened, overly distressed, or emotionally depleted.

Apatira L et al. Hope, truth, and preparing for death: perspectives of surrogate decision makers. Ann Intern Med. 2008 Dec 16;149(12):861–8. [PMID: 19075205]

Hallenbeck J. Palliative care in the final days of life: "They were expecting it at any time." JAMA. 2005 May 11;293(18):2265–71. [PMID: 15886382]

Lau F et al. Use of Palliative Performance Scale in end-of-life prognostication. J Palliat Med. 2006 Oct;9(5):1066–75. [PMID: 17040144]

McMillan SC. Interventions to facilitate family caregiving at the end of life. J Palliat Med. 2005;8(Suppl 1):S132–9. [PMID: 16499461]

Mitsumoto H et al. Palliative care for patients with amyotrophic lateral sclerosis: "Prepare for the worst and hope for the best." JAMA. 2007 Jul 11;298(2):207–16. [PMID: 17622602]

Wright AA et al. Associations between end-of-life discussions, patient mental health, medical care near death, and caregiver bereavement adjustment. JAMA. 2008 Oct 8;300(14):1665–73. [PMID: 18840840]

Decision-Making, Advance Care Planning, & Advance Directives

Well-informed, competent adults have a right to refuse medical intervention even if this is likely to result in death. Many are willing to sacrifice some quantity of life to protect a certain quality of life. In order to promote patient autonomy, clinicians are obligated to inform patients about the risks, benefits, alternatives, and expected outcomes of end-of-life medical interventions such as cardiopulmonary resuscitation (CPR), mechanical ventilation, vasopressor medication, hospitalization and ICU care, and nutrition and hydration. Advance directives are oral or written statements made by patients when they are competent that are intended to guide care should they become incompetent. Advance directives allow patients to project their autonomy into the future and are an important part of advance care planning—a process whereby patients consider various paths their illness may take and contingencies for responding to these possible developments based on their care goals and values. Advance directives take effect when the patient can no longer communicate his or her preferences directly. While oral statements about these matters are ethically binding, they are not legally binding in all states. State-specific advance directive forms are available from a number of sources, including http://www.caringinfo.org.

In addition to documenting patient preferences for care, the Durable Power of Attorney for Health Care (DPOA-HC) allows the patient to designate a surrogate decision-maker. The DPOA-HC is important since it is often difficult to anticipate what decisions will need to be made. The responsibility of the surrogate is to provide "substituted judgment"—to decide as the *patient* would, not as the *surrogate* wants. Clinicians should encourage patients to talk with their surrogates about their preferences generally and about scenarios that are likely to arise, such as the need for mechanical ventilation in a patient with end-stage emphysema. In the absence of a designated surrogate, clinicians usually turn to family members or next of kin. Clinicians should educate all patients—ideally, well before the end of life—about the opportunity to formulate an advance directive. Most patients with serious illness have already thought about end-of-life issues, want to discuss them with their clinician, want the clinician to bring up the subject, and feel better for having had the discussion. Despite regulations requiring health care institutions to inform patients of their rights to formulate an advance directive, only about 10% of people in the United States (including clinicians themselves) actually have completed them.

Do Not Attempt Resuscitation Orders

As part of advance care planning, clinicians can encourage patients to express their preferences about the use of CPR. Most patients and many clinicians are uninformed or misinformed about the nature and success of CPR. Only about 15% of all patients who undergo CPR in the hospital survive to hospital discharge. Moreover, among certain populations—especially those with serious systemic noncardiac disease, metastatic cancer, and sepsis—the likelihood of survival to hospital discharge following CPR is virtually nil.

Patients may ask their clinician to write an order that CPR not be attempted on them. Although this order initially was referred to as a DNR (do not resuscitate) order, many clinicians prefer the term "DNAR" (do not attempt resuscitation) to emphasize the low likelihood of success.

Patients deciding about CPR preferences should also be informed about the sequelae of surviving CPR. These may include fractured ribs, lacerated internal organs, and neurologic disability, and the frequent need for other aggressive interventions, such as ICU care, if CPR is successful.

For some patients at the end of life, decisions about CPR may not be about whether they will live but about how they will die. Clinicians should correct the misconception that withholding CPR in appropriate circumstances is tantamount to "not doing everything" or "just letting someone die." While respecting the patient's right ultimately to make the decision—and keeping in mind their own biases and prejudices—clinicians should offer explicit recommendations about DNAR orders and protect dying patients and their families from feelings of guilt and from the sorrow associated with vain hopes. Clinicians should encourage patients and their families to make proactive decisions about what is wanted in end-of-life care rather than focusing only on what is not to be done. For patients with pacemakers and internal cardiac defibrillators, clinicians must also address issues of turning off these devices as death approaches to prevent them from discharging during the dying process.

Hospice & Other Palliative Care Institutions

Hospice is an approach to end-of-life care where the most urgent objective is to address the physical and emotional needs of the dying. In the United States, 39% of people who die use hospice. While some hospice care is provided in hospitals and institutional residences, about 80% of patients receiving hospice care remain at home where they can be cared for by their family and visiting hospice staff. Hospice care focuses on the patient and family rather than the disease and on providing comfort and pain relief rather than on treating illness or prolonging life. Hospices provide intensive caring with the goal of helping people live well until they die.

Hospice embodies the palliative care philosophy that emphasizes individualized attention, human contact, and an interdisciplinary team approach. Hospice care can include arranging for respite for family caregivers and providing legal, financial, and other services. Primary care clinicians are strongly encouraged to continue caring for their patients during the time they are receiving hospice care.

Hospice care is highly rated by families and has been shown to increase patient satisfaction, to reduce costs (depending on when patients are referred to hospice care), and even to decrease family caregiver mortality. Hospice care tends to be used late in the course of the end of life. The average length of stay in hospices in the United States is 67 days, with 31% of patients dying within 7 days after beginning hospice care.

Most hospice organizations require clinicians to estimate the patient's probability of survival to be less than 6 months, since this is a criterion for eligibility to receive Medicare or other insurance coverage. Regrettably, the hospice benefit can be difficult to provide to people who are homeless or isolated or who have terminal prognoses that are difficult to quantify.

Cultural Issues

The individual patient's experience of dying occurs in the context of a complex interaction of personal, philosophic, and cultural influences. Various religious, ethnic, gender, class, and cultural traditions help determine patients' styles of communication, comfort in discussing particular topics, expectations about dying and medical interventions, and attitudes about the appropriate disposition of dead bodies. There are differences in knowledge and beliefs regarding advance directives, autopsy, organ donation, hospice care, and withdrawal of life-sustaining interventions among patients of different ethnic groups. Clinicians must appreciate recent evidence suggesting that palliative care is susceptible to some of the same racial biases previously documented in other medical disciplines. While each patient is an individual, being sensitive to a person's cultural beliefs and respecting ethnic traditions are important responsibilities of the clinician caring for a patient at the end of life, especially when the cultures of origin of the clinician and patient differ. A clinician may ask a patient, "What do I need to know about you and your beliefs that will help me take care of you?"

Demme RA et al. Ethical issues in palliative care. Anesthesiol Clin. 2006 Mar;24(1):129–44. [PMID: 16487899]

Gomes B et al. Where people die (1974–2030): past trends, future projections and implications for care. Palliat Med. 2008 Jan;22(1):33–41. [PMID: 18216075]

Hanson LC et al. Meeting palliative care needs in post-acute care settings: "to help them live until they die." JAMA. 2006 Feb 8;295(6):681–6. [PMID: 16467237]

Kushel MB et al. End-of-life care for homeless patients: "She says she is there to help me in any situation." JAMA. 2006 Dec 27;296(24):2959–66. [PMID: 17190897]

Shalowitz DI et al. The accuracy of surrogate decision makers: a systematic review. Arch Intern Med. 2006 Mar 13;166(5):493–7. [PMID: 16534034]

Tulsky JA. Beyond advance directives: importance of communication skills at the end of life. JAMA. 2005 Jul 20;294(3):359–65. [PMID: 16030281]

Nutrition & Hydration

Individuals at the end of life have a right to refuse nutrition and hydration. However, providing or withholding oral food and water is not simply a medical decision because feeding may have profound social and cultural significance for patients, families, and clinicians themselves. Withholding supplemental enteral or parenteral nutrition and hydration challenges the assumption that offering food is an expression of compassion and love and invokes distressing images of starvation. In fact, individuals at the end of life who choose to forgo nutrition and hydration are unlikely to suffer from hunger or thirst. Family and friends can be encouraged to express their love and caring in ways other than intrusive attempts at force feeding or hydration.

Tube feedings do not prevent aspiration pneumonia, and there is debate about whether artificial nutrition prolongs life in the terminally ill. In fact, there has been a growing awareness of the potential medical benefits of forgoing unwanted or artificial nutrition and hydration (including tube feedings, parenteral nutrition, and intravenous hydration) at the end of life.

Eating when not hungry and artificial nutrition are associated with a number of potential complications. Force feeding may cause nausea and vomiting in ill patients, and eating will lead to diarrhea in the setting of malabsorption. Nutrition may increase oral and airway secretions and the risk of choking, aspiration, and dyspnea. Nasogastric and gastrostomy tube feeding and parenteral nutrition impose risks of infection, epistaxis, pneumothorax, electrolyte imbalance, and aspiration—as well as the need to physically restrain the delirious patient to prevent dislodgment of catheters and tubes.

Withholding nutrition at the end of life causes remarkably little hunger or distress. Ill people often have no hunger with total caloric deprivation, and the associated ketonemia produces a sense of well-being, analgesia, and mild euphoria. However, carbohydrate intake even in small amounts (such as that provided by 5% intravenous dextrose solution) blocks ketone production and may blunt the positive effects of total caloric deprivation.

Withholding hydration may lead to death in a few days to a month. The quality of life for those at the end of life may be adversely affected by supplemental hydration because of its contribution to oral and airway secretions (leading to aspiration or the "death rattle"), polyuria, and the development or worsening of ascites, pleural or other effusions, and peripheral and pulmonary edema.

Although it is unclear to what extent withholding hydration at the end of life creates an uncomfortable sensation of thirst, any such sensation is usually relieved by simply moistening the dry mouth. Ice chips, hard candy, swabs, and minted mouthwash or a solution of equal parts nystatin solution, viscous lidocaine, and diphenhydramine for pain or discomfort associated with dry mouth are effective.

Withdrawal of Curative Efforts

Requests from appropriately informed and competent patients or their surrogates for withdrawal of life-sustaining interventions must be respected. In addition, clinicians may determine unilaterally that particular interventions are medically inappropriate—eg, continuing kidney dialysis in a patient dying of multiorgan failure. In such cases, the clinician's intention to withdraw a specific intervention should be communicated to the patient and family. If differences of opinion exist about the appropriateness of what is being done, the assistance of an institutional ethics committee should be sought.

Limitation of life support prior to death is an increasingly common practice in intensive care units. The withdrawal of life-sustaining interventions such as mechanical ventilation must be approached carefully to avoid needless patient suffering and distress for those in attendance. Clinicians should educate the patient and family about the expected course of events and the difficulty of determining the precise timing of death after withdrawal of interventions. Sedative and analgesic agents should be administered to ensure patient comfort even at the risk of respiratory depression or hypotension. Scopolamine (10 mcg/h subcutaneously or intravenously, or a 1.5-mg patch every 3 days), glycopyrrolate (1 mg orally every 4 hours), or atropine (1% ophthalmic solution, 1 or 2 drops sublingually as often as every hour) can be used for controlling airway secretions and the resultant "death rattle." A guideline for withdrawal of mechanical ventilation is provided in Table 5–8.

Psychological, Social, & Spiritual Issues

Dying is not exclusively or even primarily a biomedical event. It is an intimate personal experience with profound psychological, interpersonal, and existential meanings. For many people at the end of life, the prospect of impending death stimulates a deep and urgent assessment of their identity, the quality of their relationships, and the meaning and purpose of their existence.

A. Psychological Challenges

In 1969, Elisabeth Kübler-Ross identified five psychological stages or patterns of emotions that patients at the end of life may experience: denial and isolation, anger, bargaining, depression, and acceptance. Not every patient will experience all these emotions, and typically not in an orderly progression. In addition to these five stages are the perpetual challenges of anxiety and fear of the unknown. Simple information, listening, assurance, and support may help patients with these psychological challenges. In fact, patients and families rank emotional support as one of the most important aspects of good end-of-life care. Psychotherapy and group support may be beneficial as well.

Despite the significant emotional stress of facing death, clinical depression is not normal at the end of life and should be treated. Cognitive and affective signs of depression (such as hopelessness) may help distinguish depression from the low energy and other vegetative signs common with end-stage illness. Although traditional antidepressant treatments such as selective serotonin reuptake inhibitors are effective, more rapidly acting medications such as dextroamphetamine or methylphenidate (in doses used for sedation described earlier in this chapter) may be particularly useful when the end of life is near or while waiting for other antidepressant medication to take effect.

B. Social Challenges

At the end of life, patients should be encouraged to discharge personal, professional, and business obligations. This might include completing important work or personal projects, distributing possessions, writing a will, and making funeral and burial arrangements. The prospect of death often prompts patients to examine the quality of their interpersonal relationships and to begin the process of saying goodbye (Table 5–9). Dying may intensify a patient's need to feel cared for by the doctor and the need for clinician empathy and compassion. Concern about estranged relationships or "unfinished business" with significant others and interest in reconciliation may become paramount at this time.

C. Spiritual Challenges

Spirituality is the attempt to understand or accept the underlying meaning of life, one's relationships to oneself

---

Table 5–8. Guidelines for withdrawal of mechanical ventilation.

1. Stop neuromuscular blocking agents.
2. Administer opioids or sedatives to eliminate distress.
   If not already sedated, begin with fentanyl 100 mcg (or morphine sulfate 10 mg) by intravenous bolus and infusion of fentanyl 100 mcg/h intravenously (or morphine sulfate 10 mg/h intravenously).
   Distress is indicated by RR > 24, nasal flaring, use of accessory muscles of respiration, HR increase > 20%, MAP increase > 20%, grimacing, clutching.
3. Discontinue vasoactive agents and other agents unrelated to patient comfort, such as antibiotics, intravenous fluids, and diagnostic procedures.
4. Decrease Fio_2 to room air and PEEP to 0 cm H_2O.
5. Observe patient for distress.
   If patient is distressed, increase opioids by repeating bolus dose and increasing hourly infusion rate by 50 mcg fentanyl (or 5 mg morphine sulfate),[1] then return to observation.
   If patient is not distressed, place on T piece and observe.
   If patient continues without distress, extubate patient and continue to observe for distress.

[1]Ventilatory support may be increased until additional opioids have effect.
RR, respiratory rate; HR, heart rate; MAP, mean airway pressure; Fio_2, fraction of inspired oxygen; PEEP, positive end-expiratory pressure.
Adapted, with permission, from San Francisco General Hospital Guidelines for Withdrawal of Mechanical Ventilation/Life Support.

Table 5–9. Five statements often necessary for the completion of important interpersonal relationships.

(1) "Forgive me."	(An expression of regret)
(2) "I forgive you."	(An expression of acceptance)
(3) "Thank you."	(An expression of gratitude)
(4) "I love you."	(An expression of affection)
(5) "Goodbye."	(Leave-taking)

Reprinted, with permission, from Byock I. *Dying Well: Peace and Possibilities at the End of Life.* New York: Riverhead Books, 1997.

nd other people, one's place in the universe, and the possibility of a "higher power" in the universe. Spirituality is distinguished from particular religious practices or beliefs and is generally considered a universal human concern.

Perhaps because of an inappropriately exclusive attention to the biologic challenge of forestalling death or perhaps from feelings of discomfort or incompetence, clinicians frequently ignore their patients' spiritual concerns or reflexively refer these important issues to chaplains, psychiatrists or other caretakers (nurses, social workers, clergy). However, the existential challenges of dying are central to the well-being of people at the end of life and are the proper concern of clinicians. Clinicians can help dying patients by providing care to the whole person—by providing physical comfort and social support and by helping patients discover their own unique meaning in the world and an acceptance of death as a part of life.

Unlike physical ailments such as infections and fractures, which usually require a clinician's intervention to be treated, the patient's spiritual concerns often require only a clinician's attention, listening, and witness. Clinicians might choose to inquire about the patient's spiritual concerns and ask whether the patient wishes to discuss them. For example, asking, "How are you within yourself?" communicates that the clinician is interested in the patient's whole experience and provides an opportunity for the patient to share perceptions about his or her inner life. Questions that might constitute an existential "review of systems" are presented in Table 5–10.

While dying may be a period of inevitable loss of physical functioning, the end of life also offers an opportunity for psychological, interpersonal, and spiritual development. Individuals may grow—even achieve a heightened sense of well-being or transcendence—in the process of dying. Through listening, support, and presence, clinicians may help foster this learning and be a catalyst for this transformation. Rather than thinking of dying simply as the termination of life, clinicians and patients may be guided by a developmental model of dying that recognizes a series of lifelong developmental tasks and landmarks and allows for growth at the end of life.

Table 5–10. An existential review of systems.

Intrapersonal
What does your illness/dying mean to you?
What do you think caused your illness?
How have you been healed in the past?
What do you think is needed for you to be healed now?
What is right with you now?
What do you hope for?
Interpersonal
Who is important to you?
To whom does your illness/dying matter?
Do you have any unfinished business with significant others?
Transpersonal
What is your source of strength, help, or hope?
Do you have spiritual concerns or a spiritual practice?
If so, how does your spirituality relate to your illness/dying, and how can I help integrate your spirituality into your health care?
What do you think happens after we die?
What purpose might your illness/dying serve?
What do you think is trying to happen here?

Block SD. Psychological issues in end-of-life care. J Palliat Med. 2006 Jun;9(3):751–72. [PMID: 16752981]

Harrington SE et al. The role of chemotherapy at the end of life: "When is enough, enough?" JAMA. 2008 Jun 11;299(22):2667–78. [PMID: 18544726]

Koretz RL et al. Does enteral nutrition affect clinical outcome? A systematic review of the randomized trials. Am J Gastroenterol. 2007 Feb;102(2):412–29. [PMID: 17311654]

Sulmasy DP. Spiritual issues in the care of dying patients: ". . . It's okay between me and God." JAMA. 2006 Sep 20;296(11):1385–1392. [PMID: 16985231]

TASKS AFTER DEATH

After the death of a patient, the clinician is called upon to perform a number of tasks, both required and recommended. The clinician must plainly and directly inform the family of the death, complete a death certificate, contact an organ procurement organization, and request an autopsy.

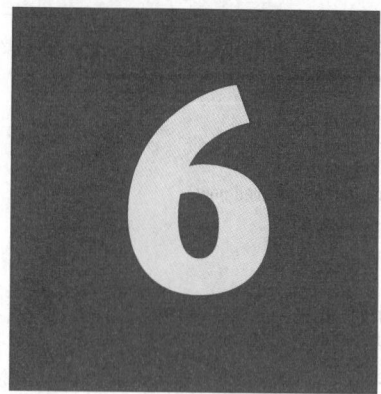

Dermatologic Disorders

Timothy G. Berger, MD

Dermatologic diseases are diagnosed by the types of lesions they cause. To make a diagnosis: (1) identify the type of lesion(s) the patient exhibits by morphology establishing a differential diagnosis (Table 6–1); and (2) obtain the elements of the history, physical examination, and appropriate laboratory tests to confirm the diagnosis. Unique clinical situations, such as the ill ICU patient, lead to different diagnostic considerations.

PRINCIPLES OF DERMATOLOGIC THERAPY

▶ Frequently Used Treatment Measures

A. Bathing

Soap should be used only in the axillae and groin and on the feet by persons with dry or inflamed skin. Soaking in water for 10–15 minutes before applying topical corticosteroids enhances their efficacy. Bath oils can be used, but add little above the use of moisturizers and may make the tub slippery, increasing the risk of falling.

B. Topical Therapy

Nondermatologists should become familiar with a representative agent in each category for each indication (eg, topical corticosteroid, topical retinoid, etc).

1. Corticosteroids—Topical corticosteroid creams, lotions, ointments, gels, foams, and sprays are presented in Table 6–2. Topical corticosteroids are divided into classes based on potency. There is little (except price) to recommend one agent over another within the same class. For a given agent, an ointment is more potent than a cream. The potency of a topical corticosteroid may be dramatically increased by applying an occlusive dressing over the corticosteroid. At least 4 hours of occlusion is required to enhance penetration. Such dressings may include gloves, plastic wrap, or plastic occlusive suits for patients with generalized erythroderma or atopy. Caution should be used in applying topical corticosteroids to areas of thin skin (face, scrotum, vulva, skin folds). Topical corticosteroid use on the eyelids may result in glaucoma or cataracts. One may estimate the amount of topical corticosteroid needed by using the "rule of nines" (as in burn evaluation; see Figure 37–2). In general, it takes an average of 20–30 g to cover the body surface of an adult once. Systemic absorption does occur, but adrenal suppression, diabetes, hypertension, osteoporosis, and other complications of systemic corticosteroids are very rare with topical corticosteroid therapy.

2. Emollients for dry skin ("moisturizers")—Dry skin is not related to water intake but to abnormal function of the epidermis. Many types of emollients are available. Petrolatum, mineral oil, Aquaphor, Vanicream, and Eucerin cream are the heaviest and best. Emollients are most effective when applied to wet skin. If the skin is too greasy after application, pat dry with a damp towel. Vanicream is relatively allergen-free and can be used if allergic contact dermatitis to topical products is suspected.

The scaly appearance of dry skin may be improved by urea, lactic acid, or glycolic acid-containing products provided no inflammation (erythema or pruritus) is present.

3. Drying agents for weepy dermatoses—If the skin is weepy from infection or inflammation, drying agents may be beneficial. The best drying agent is water, applied as repeated compresses for 15–30 minutes, alone or with aluminum salts (Burow solution, Domeboro tablets) or colloidal oatmeal (Aveeno).

4. Topical antipruritics—Lotions that contain 0.5% each of camphor and menthol (Sarna) or pramoxine hydrochloride 1%, are effective antipruritic agents (with or without 0.5% menthol, eg, Prax, PrameGel, Aveeno Anti-Itch lotion). Hydrocortisone, 1% or 2.5%, may be incorporated for its anti-inflammatory effect (Pramosone cream, lotion, or ointment). Doxepin cream 5% may reduce pruritus but may cause drowsiness. Pramoxine and doxepin are most effective when applied with topical corticosteroids. Monoamine oxidase inhibitors should be discontinued at least 2 weeks before treatment with doxepin.

5. Systemic antipruritic drugs

A. ANTIHISTAMINES—H_1-blockers are the agents of choice for pruritus when due to histamine, such as in urticaria. Otherwise, they appear to relieve pruritus only by their sedating effects. Except in the case of urticaria, nonsedating antihistamines are of limited value in inflammatory skin diseases.

Hydroxyzine 25–50 mg nightly is typically used for its sedative effect in pruritic diseases. Sedation can limit daytime

Table 6–1. Morphologic categorization of skin lesions and diseases.

Pigmented	Freckle, lentigo, seborrheic keratosis, nevus, blue nevus, halo nevus, atypical nevus, melanoma
Scaly	Psoriasis, dermatitis (atopic, stasis, seborrheic, chronic allergic contact or irritant contact), xerosis (dry skin), lichen simplex chronicus, tinea, tinea versicolor, secondary syphilis, pityriasis rosea, discoid lupus erythematosus, exfoliative dermatitis, actinic keratoses, Bowen disease, Paget disease, intertrigo
Vesicular	Herpes simplex, varicella, herpes zoster, dyshidrosis (vesicular dermatitis of palms and soles), vesicular tinea, dermatophytid, dermatitis herpetiformis, miliaria, scabies, photosensitivity
Weepy or encrusted	Impetigo, acute contact allergic dermatitis, any vesicular dermatitis
Pustular	Acne vulgaris, acne rosacea, folliculitis, candidiasis, miliaria, any vesicular dermatitis
Figurate ("shaped") erythema	Urticaria, erythema multiforme, erythema migrans, cellulitis, erysipelas, erysipeloid, arthropod bites
Bullous	Impetigo, blistering dactylitis, pemphigus, pemphigoid, porphyria cutanea tarda, drug eruptions, erythema multiforme, toxic epidermal necrolysis
Papular	Hyperkeratotic: warts, corns, seborrheic keratoses Purple-violet: lichen planus, drug eruptions, Kaposi sarcoma Flesh-colored, umbilicated: molluscum contagiosum Pearly: basal cell carcinoma, intradermal nevi Small, red, inflammatory: acne, miliaria, candidiasis, scabies, folliculitis
Pruritus[1]	Xerosis, scabies, pediculosis, bites, systemic causes, anogenital pruritus
Nodular, cystic	Erythema nodosum, furuncle, cystic acne, follicular (epidermal) inclusion cyst
Photodermatitis (photodistributed rashes)	Drug, polymorphic light eruption, lupus erythematosus
Morbilliform	Drug, viral infection, secondary syphilis
Erosive	Any vesicular dermatitis, impetigo, aphthae, lichen planus, erythema multiforme
Ulcerated	Decubiti, herpes simplex, skin cancers, parasitic infections, syphilis (chancre), chancroid, vasculitis, stasis, arterial disease

[1]Not a morphologic class but included because it is one of the most common dermatologic presentations.

use. The least sedating antihistamines are loratadine and fexofenadine. Cetirizine causes drowsiness in about 15% of patients. Some antidepressants, such as doxepin, mirtazapine, sertraline, and paroxetine can be effective antipruritics.

B. SYSTEMIC CORTICOSTEROIDS—(See Chapter 26.)

Carstens E. Scratching the brain to understand neuropathic itch. J Pain. 2008 Nov;9(11):973–4. [PMID: 18984500]

Hercogova J. Topical anti-itch therapy. Dermatol Ther. 2005 Jul–Aug;18(4):341–3. [PMID: 16297007]

Lovell P et al. Management and treatment of pruritus. Skin Therapy Lett. 2007 Feb;12(1):1–6. [PMID: 17361313]

Weisshaar E. Intractable chronic pruritus in a 67-year-old man. Acta Derm Venereol. 2008;88(5):488–90. [PMID: 18779888]

Weldon D. What lies beneath the surface of the itch in adults? Allergy Asthma Proc. 2007 Mar–Apr;28(2):153–62. [PMID: 17479598]

Sunscreens

Protection from ultraviolet light should begin at birth and will reduce the incidence of actinic keratoses and some nonmelanoma skin cancers when initiated at any age. The best protection is shade, but protective clothing, avoidance of direct sun exposure during the peak hours of the day, and daily use of chemical sunscreens are important.

Fair-complexioned persons should use a sunscreen with an SPF (sun protective factor) of at least 15 and preferably 30–40 every day. Sunscreens with high SPF values (> 30) afford some protection against UVA as well as UVB and may be helpful in managing photosensitivity disorders. Physical blockers (titanium dioxide and zinc oxide) are available in vanishing formulations. Aggressive sunscreen use should be accompanied by vitamin D supplementation in persons at risk for osteopenia (eg, organ transplant recipients).

American Academy of Family Physicians. Information from your family doctor. Saving your skin from sun damage. Am Fam Physician. 2006 Sep 1;74(5):815–6. [PMID: 16970028]

Lautenschlager S et al. Photoprotection. Lancet. 2007 Aug 11;370(9586):528–37. [PMID: 17693182]

Complications of Topical Dermatologic Therapy

Complications of topical therapy can be largely avoided. They fall into several categories:

A. Allergy

Of the topical antibiotics, neomycin and bacitracin have the greatest potential for sensitization. Diphenhydramine, benzocaine, vitamin E, aromatic essential oils, and bee pollen are potential sensitizers in topical medications. Preservatives and even the topical corticosteroids themselves can cause allergic contact dermatitis.

Table 6–2. Useful topical dermatologic therapeutic agents.

Agent	Formulations, Strengths, and Prices[1]	Apply	Potency Class	Common Indications	Comments
Corticosteroids					
Hydrocortisone acetate	Cream 1%: $3.00/30 g Ointment 1%: $3.00/30 g Lotion 1%: $7.19/120 mL	Twice daily	Low	Seborrheic dermatitis Pruritus ani Intertrigo	Not the same as hydrocortisone butyrate or valerate! Not for poison oak! OTC lotion (Aquinil HC) OTC solution (Scalpicin, T Scalp)
	Cream 2.5%: $12.81/30 g	Twice daily	Low	As for 1% hydrocortisone	Perhaps better for pruritus ani Not clearly better than 1% More expensive Not OTC
Alclometasone dipropionate (Aclovate)	Cream 0.05%: $20.29/15 g Ointment 0.05%: $39.70/45 g	Twice daily	Low	As for hydrocortisone	More efficacious than hydrocortisone Perhaps causes less atrophy
Clocortolone (Cloderm)	Cream 0.1%: $75.00/30 g	Three times daily	Medium	Contact dermatitis Atopic dermatitis	Does not cross react with other corticosteroids chemically and can be used in patients allergic to other corticosteroids
Desonide	Cream 0.05%: $15.47/15 g Ointment 0.05%: $39.88/60 g Lotion 0.05%: $32.83/60 mL	Twice daily	Low	As for hydrocortisone For lesions on face or body folds resistant to hydrocortisone	More efficacious than hydrocortisone Can cause rosacea or atrophy Not fluorinated
Prednicarbate (Dermatop)	Emollient cream 0.1%: $24.59/15 g Ointment 0.1%: $25.13/15 g	Twice daily	Medium	As for triamcinolone	May cause less atrophy No generic formulations Preservative-free
Triamcinolone acetonide	Cream 0.1%: $3.60/15 g Ointment 0.1%: $3.60/15 g Lotion 0.1%: $42.44/60 mL	Twice daily	Medium	Eczema on extensor areas Used for psoriasis with tar Seborrheic dermatitis and psoriasis on scalp	Caution in body folds, face Economical in 0.5-lb and 1-lb sizes for treatment of large body surfaces Economical as solution for scalp
	Cream 0.025%: $3.00/15 g Ointment 0.025%: $6.25/80 g	Twice daily	Medium	As for 0.1% strength	Possibly less efficacy and few advantages over 0.1% formulation
Fluocinolone acetonide	Cream 0.025%: $3.05/15 g Ointment 0.025%: $4.20/15 g	Twice daily	Medium	As for triamcinolone	
	Solution 0.01%: $11.00/60 mL	Twice daily	Medium	As for triamcinolone solution	
Mometasone furoate (Elocon)	Cream 0.1%: $26.90/15 g Ointment 0.1%: $23.90/15 g Lotion 0.1%: $55.71/60 mL	Once daily	Medium	As for triamcinolone	Often used inappropriately on the face or in children Not fluorinated
Diflorasone diacetate	Cream 0.05%: $36.78/15 g Ointment 0.05%: $51.86/30 g	Twice daily	High	Nummular dermatitis Allergic contact dermatitis Lichen simplex chronicus	
Amcinonide (Cyclocort)	Cream 0.1%: $18.42/15 g Ointment 0.1%: $46.12/60 g	Twice daily	High	As for betamethasone	
Fluocinonide (Lidex)	Cream 0.05%: $9.00/15 g Gel 0.05%: $20.87/15 g Ointment 0.05%: $21.04/15 g Solution 0.05%: $27.00/60 mL	Twice daily	High	As for betamethasone Gel useful for poison oak	Economical generics Lidex cream can cause stinging on eczema Lidex emollient cream preferred

(continued)

Table 6–2. Useful topical dermatologic therapeutic agents. (continued)

Agent	Formulations, Strengths, and Prices[1]	Apply	Potency Class	Common Indications	Comments
Betamethasone dipropionate (Diprolene)	Cream 0.05%: $7.80/15 g Ointment 0.05%: $9.40/15 g Lotion 0.05%: $38.85/60 mL	Twice daily	Ultra-high	For lesions resistant to high-potency corticosteroids Lichen planus Insect bites	Economical generics available
Clobetasol propionate (Temovate)	Cream 0.05%: $24.71/15 g Ointment 0.05%: $24.71/15 g Lotion 0.05%: $51.26/50 mL	Twice daily	Ultra-high	As for betamethasone dipropionate	Somewhat more potent than diflorasone Limited to 2 continuous weeks of use Limited to 50 g or less per week Cream may cause stinging; use "emollient cream" formulation Generic available
Halobetasol propionate (Ultravate)	Cream 0.05%: $31.49/15 g Ointment 0.05%: $31.49/15 g	Twice daily	Ultra-high	As for clobetasol	Same restrictions as clobetasol Cream does not cause stinging Compatible with calcipotriene (Dovonex)
Flurandrenolide (Cordran)	Tape: $34.93/80" × 3" roll Lotion 0.05%: $132.00/60 mL	q12h	Ultra-high	Lichen simplex chronicus	Protects the skin and prevents scratching
Nonsteroidal anti-inflammatory agents					
Tacrolimus[2] (Protopic)	Ointment 0.1%: $103.32/30 g Ointment 0.03%: $103.32/30 g	Twice daily	N/A	Atopic dermatitis	Steroid substitute not causing atrophy or striae Burns in ≥ 40% of patients with eczema
Pimecrolimus[2] (Elidel)	Cream 1%: $87.52/30 g	Twice daily	N/A	Atopic dermatitis	Steroid substitute not causing atrophy or striae
Antibiotics (for acne)					
Clindamycin phosphate	Solution 1%: $12.09/30 mL Gel 1%: $38.13/30 mL Lotion 1%: $53.06/60 mL Pledget 1%: $46.40/60	Twice daily	N/A	Mild papular acne	Lotion is less drying for patients with sensitive skin
Erythromycin	Solution 2%: $4.80/60 mL Gel 2%: $25.19/30 g Pledget 2%: $27.73/60	Twice daily	N/A	As for clindamycin	Many different manufacturers Economical
Erythromycin/ Benzoyl peroxide (Benzamycin)	Gel: $58.35/23.3 g Gel: $111.64/46.6 g	Twice daily	N/A	As for clindamycin Can help treat comedonal acne	No generics More expensive More effective than other topical antibiotic Main jar requires refrigeration
Clindamycin/ Benzoyl peroxide (BenzaClin)	Gel: $93.53/25 g Gel: $159.67/50 g	Twice daily	N/A	As for benzamycin	No generic More effective than either agent alone
Antibiotics (for impetigo)					
Mupirocin (Bactroban)	Ointment 2%: $44.65/22 g Cream 2%: $29.10/15 g	Three times daily	N/A	Impetigo, folliculitis	Because of cost, use limited to tiny areas of impetigo Used in the nose twice daily for 5 days to reduce staphylococcal carriage

(continued)

Table 6–2. Useful topical dermatologic therapeutic agents. (continued)

Agent	Formulations, Strengths, and Prices[1]	Apply	Potency Class	Common Indications	Comments
Antifungals: *Imidazoles*					
Clotrimazole	Cream 1%: $4.25/15 g OTC Solution 1%: $6.00/10 mL	Twice daily	N/A	Dermatophyte and *Candida* infections	Available OTC Inexpensive generic cream available
Econazole (Spectazole)	Cream 1%: $17.50/15 g	Once daily	N/A	As for clotrimazole	No generic Somewhat more effective than clotrimazole and miconazole
Ketoconazole	Cream 2%: $16.46/15 g	Once daily	N/A	As for clotrimazole	No generic Somewhat more effective than clotrimazole and miconazole
Miconazole	Cream 2%: $3.20/30 g OTC	Twice daily	N/A	As for clotrimazole	As for clotrimazole
Oxiconazole (Oxistat)	Cream 1%: $45.20/15 g Lotion 1%: $82.89/30 mL	Twice daily	N/A		
Sertaconazole (Ertaczo)	Cream 2%: $71.52/30 g	Twice daily	N/A	Refractory tinea pedis	By prescription More expensive
Sulconazole (Exelderm)	Cream 1%: $14.50/15 g Solution 1%: $31.20/30 mL	Twice daily	N/A	As for clotrimazole	No generic Somewhat more effective than clotrimazole and miconazole
Other antifungals					
Butenafine (Mentax)	Cream 1%: $49.53/15 g	Once daily	N/A	Dermatophytes	Fast response; high cure rate; expensive Available OTC
Ciclopirox (Loprox) (Penlac)	Cream 0.77%: $51.10/30 g Lotion 0.77%: $96.15/60 mL Solution 8%: $216.01/6.6 mL	Twice daily	N/A	As for clotrimazole	No generic Somewhat more effective than clotrimazole and miconazole
Naftifine (Naftin)	Cream 1%: $77.86/30 g Gel 1%: $156.60/60 mL	Once daily	N/A	Dermatophytes	No generic Somewhat more effective than clotrimazole and miconazole
Terbinafine (Lamisil)	Cream 1%: $8.15/12 g OTC	Once daily	N/A	Dermatophytes	Fast clinical response OTC
Antipruritics					
Camphor/menthol	Compounded lotion (0.5% of each)	Two to three times daily	N/A	Mild eczema, xerosis, mild contact dermatitis	
Pramoxine hydrochloride (Prax)	Lotion 1%: $15.89/120 mL OTC	Four times daily	N/A	Dry skin, varicella, mild eczema, pruritus ani	OTC formulations (Prax, Aveeno Anti-Itch Cream or Lotion; Itch-X Gel) By prescription mixed with 1% or 2% hydrocortisone
Doxepin (Zonalon)	Cream 5%: $103.14/30 g	Four times daily	N/A	Topical antipruritic, best used in combination with appropriate topical corticosteroid to enhance efficacy	Can cause sedation
Emollients					
Aveeno	Cream, lotion, others	Once to three times daily	N/A	Xerosis, eczema	Choice is most often based on personal preference by patient
Aqua glycolic	Cream, lotion, shampoo, others	Once to three times daily	N/A	Xerosis, ichthyosis, keratosis pilaris Mild facial wrinkles Mild acne or seborrheic dermatitis	Contains 8% glycolic acid Available from other makers, eg, Alpha Hydrox, or generic 8% glycolic acid lotion May cause stinging on eczematous skin

(continued)

Table 6–2. Useful topical dermatologic therapeutic agents. (continued)

Agent	Formulations, Strengths, and Prices[1]	Apply	Potency Class	Common Indications	Comments
Aquaphor	Ointment: $4.99/50 g	Once to three times daily	N/A	Xerosis, eczema For protection of area in pruritus ani	Not as greasy as petrolatum
Carmol	Lotion 10%: $12.05/180 mL Cream 20%: $14.63/90 g	Twice daily	N/A	Xerosis	Contains urea as humectant Nongreasy hydrating agent (10%); debrides keratin (20%)
Complex 15	Lotion: $6.48/240 mL Cream: $4.82/75 g	Once to three times daily	N/A	Xerosis Lotion or cream recommended for split or dry nails	Active ingredient is a phospho-lipid
DML	Cream, lotion, facial moisturizer: $5.95/240 mL	Once to three times daily	N/A	As for Complex 15	Face cream has sunscreen
Eucerin	Cream: $5.10/120 g Lotion: $5.10/240 mL	Once to three times daily	N/A	Xerosis, eczema	Many formulations made Eucerin Plus contains alphahydroxy acid and may cause stinging on eczematous skin Facial moisturizer has SPF 25 sunscreen
Lac-Hydrin-Five	Lotion: $10.54/240 mL OTC	Twice daily	N/A	Xerosis, ichthyosis, keratosis pilaris	Rx product is 12%
Lubriderm	Lotion: $7.36/480 mL	Once to three times daily	N/A	Xerosis, eczema	Unscented usually preferred
Neutrogena	Cream, lotion, facial moisturizer: $7.39/240 mL	Once to three times daily	N/A	Xerosis, eczema	Face cream has titanium-based sunscreen
Ceratopic Cream	Cream: $39.50/4 oz	Twice daily	N/A	Xerosis, eczema	Contains ceramide; anti-inflammatory and non-greasy moisturizer
U-Lactin	Lotion: $7.13/240 mL OTC	Once daily	N/A	Hyperkeratotic heels	Moisturizes and removes keratin

[1]Average wholesale price (AWP, for AB-rated generic when available) for quantity listed. AWP may not accurately represent the actual pharmacy cost because wide contractual variations exist among institutions. Source: *Red Book Update*, Vol. 28, No. 3, March 2009.
[2]Topical tacrolimus and pimecrolimus should only be used when other topical treatments are ineffective. Treatment should be limited to an area and duration to be as brief as possible. Treatment with these agents should be avoided in persons with known immunosuppression, HIV infection, bone marrow and organ transplantation, lymphoma, at high risk for lymphoma, and those with a prior history of lymphoma. N/A, not applicable; OTC, over-the-counter.

B. Irritation

Preparations of tretinoin, benzoyl peroxide, and other acne medications should be applied sparingly to the skin.

C. Overuse

Topical corticosteroids may induce acne-like lesions on the face (steroid rosacea) and atrophic striae in body folds.

▼ **COMMON DERMATOSES**

PIGMENTED LESIONS

MELANOCYTIC NEVI (Normal Moles)

In general, a **benign mole** is a small (< 6 mm) lesion with a well-defined border and a single shade of pigment from beige or pink to dark brown. The physical examination must take precedence over the history.

Moles have a normal natural history. In the patient's first decade of life, moles often appear as flat, small, brown lesions. They are called **junctional nevi** because the nevus cells are at the junction of the epidermis and dermis. Over the next 2 decades, these moles grow in size and often become raised, reflecting the appearance of a dermal component, giving rise to **compound nevi** (Plate 1). Moles may darken and grow during pregnancy. As white patients enter their seventh and eighth decades, most moles have lost their junctional component and dark pigmentation. At every stage of life, normal moles should be well-demarcated, symmetric, and uniform in contour and color.

Bishop JN et al. The prevention, diagnosis, referral and management of melanoma of the skin: concise guidelines. Clin Med. 2007 Jun;7(3):283–90. [PMID: 17633952]

ATYPICAL NEVI

The term "atypical nevus" or "atypical mole" has supplanted "dysplastic nevus." The diagnosis of atypical moles is made clinically and not histologically, and moles should be removed only if they are suspected to be melanomas. Clinically, these moles are large (≥ 6 mm in diameter), with an ill-defined, irregular border and irregularly distributed pigmentation (Plate 2). It is estimated that 5–10% of the white population in the United States has one or more atypical nevi. Studies have defined an increased risk of melanoma in the following populations: patients with 50 or more nevi with one or more atypical moles and one mole at least 8 mm or larger, and patients with a few to many definitely atypical moles. These patients deserve education and regular (usually every 6–12 months) follow-up. Kindreds with familial melanoma (numerous atypical nevi and a strong family history) deserve even closer attention, as the risk of developing single or even multiple melanomas in these individuals approaches 50% by age 50.

Cyr PR. Atypical moles. Am Fam Physician. 2008 Sep 15;78(6):735–40. [PMID: 18819240]
de Snoo FA et al. From sporadic atypical nevi to familial melanoma: risk analysis for melanoma in sporadic atypical nevus patients. J Am Acad Dermatol. 2007 May;56(5):748–52. [PMID: 17276542]

BLUE NEVI

Blue nevi are small, slightly elevated, blue-black lesions that favor the dorsal hands (Plate 3). They are common in persons of Asian descent, and an individual patient may have several of them. If present without change for many years, they may be considered benign, since malignant blue nevi are rare. However, blue-black papules and nodules that are new or growing must be evaluated to rule out nodular melanoma.

Bogart MM et al. Blue nevi: a case report and review of the literature. Cutis. 2007 Jul;80(1):42–4. [PMID: 17725063]

FRECKLES & LENTIGINES

Freckles (ephelides) and lentigines are flat brown spots. Freckles first appear in young children, darken with ultraviolet exposure, and fade with cessation of sun exposure. In adults, flat brown spots (lentigines) gradually appear in sun-exposed areas, particularly the dorsa of the hands. They do not fade with cessation of sun exposure. They should be evaluated like all pigmented lesions: If the pigmentation is homogeneous and they are symmetric and flat, they are most likely benign. They can be treated with topical 0.1% tretinoin, tazarotene 0.1%, 2% 4-hydroxyanisole with tretinoin 0.01% (Solage), laser therapy, and cryotherapy.

Ortonne JP et al. Treatment of solar lentigines. J Am Acad Dermatol. 2006 May;54(5 Suppl 2):S262–71. [PMID: 16631967]

SEBORRHEIC KERATOSES

Seborrheic keratoses are benign plaques, beige to brown or even black, 3–20 mm in diameter, with a velvety or warty surface (Plate 4). They appear to be stuck or pasted onto the skin. They are extremely common—especially in the elderly—and may be mistaken for melanomas or other types of cutaneous neoplasms. Although they may be frozen with liquid nitrogen or curetted if they itch or are inflamed, no treatment is needed.

Askari SK et al. Evaluation of prospectively collected presenting signs/symptoms of biopsy-proven melanoma, basal cell carcinoma, squamous cell carcinoma, and seborrheic keratosis in an elderly male population. J Am Acad Dermatol. 2007 May;56(5):739–47. [PMID: 17258839]

MALIGNANT MELANOMA

 ESSENTIALS OF DIAGNOSIS

▶ May be flat or raised.
▶ Should be suspected in any pigmented skin lesion with recent change in appearance.
▶ Examination with good light may show varying colors, including red, white, black, and bluish.
▶ Borders typically irregular.

▶ General Considerations

Malignant melanoma is the leading cause of death due to skin disease. There were an estimated 59,940 new cases of melanoma in the United States in 2007, with 8110 deaths. One in four cases of melanoma occurs before the age of 40. Overall survival for melanomas in whites has risen from 60% in 1960–1963 to more than 85% currently, primarily due to earlier detection of lesions.

Tumor thickness is the single most important prognostic factor. Ten-year survival rates—related to thickness in millimeters—are as follows: < 1 mm, 95%; 1–2 mm, 80%; 2–4 mm, 55%; and > 4 mm, 30%. With lymph node involvement, the 5-year survival rate is 30%; with distant metastases, it is less than 10%.

▶ Clinical Findings

Primary malignant melanomas may be classified into various clinicohistologic types, including lentigo maligna melanoma (arising on chronically sun-exposed skin of older individuals); superficial spreading malignant melanoma (two-thirds of all melanomas arising on intermittently sun-exposed skin); nodular malignant melanoma; acral-lentiginous melanomas (arising on palms, soles, and nail beds); and malignant melanomas on mucous membranes. Clinical features of pigmented lesions suspicious for melanoma are an irregular notched border where the pigment appears to be leaking into the normal surrounding skin; a topography that may be irregular, ie, partly raised and partly flat (Plates 5 and 6). Color variegation is present, and colors such as pink, blue, gray, white, and black are indications for referral. A useful mnemonic is the ABCD rule: "ABCD = Asymmetry, Border irregularity, Color variegation, and Diameter greater than 6 mm." "E" for Evolution can be added. The history of a changing mole (evolution) is the single most important historical reason for close evaluation and possible referral. Bleeding and ulceration are ominous signs. A mole that stands out from the patient's other moles deserves special scrutiny—the "ugly duckling sign." A patient with a large number of moles is statistically at increased risk for melanoma and deserves careful and periodic examination, particularly if the lesions are atypical. Referral of suspicious pigmented lesions is always appropriate.

While superficial spreading melanoma is largely a disease of whites, persons of other races are at risk for other types of melanoma, particularly acral lentiginous melanoma. These occur as dark, sometimes irregularly shaped lesions on the palms and soles and as new, often broad and solitary, darkly pigmented longitudinal streaks in the nails. Acral lentiginous melanoma may be a difficult diagnosis because benign pigmented lesions of the hands, feet, and nails occur commonly in more darkly pigmented persons and clinicians may hesitate to biopsy the palms, soles, and nail beds. As a result, the diagnosis is often delayed until the tumor has become clinically obvious and histologically thick. Clinicians should give special attention to new or changing lesions in these areas.

Dermoscopy—use of a special magnifying device to evaluate pigmented lesions—helps select suspicious lesions that require biopsy. In experienced hands, the specificity is 85% and the sensitivity 95%.

▶ **Treatment**

Treatment of melanoma consists of excision. After histologic diagnosis, the area is usually reexcised with margins dictated by the thickness of the tumor. Thin low-risk and intermediate-risk tumors require only conservative margins of 1–3 cm. More specifically, surgical margins of 0.5 cm for melanoma in situ and 1 cm for lesions less than 1 mm in thickness are recommended.

Sentinel lymph node biopsy (selective lymphadenectomy) using preoperative lymphoscintigraphy and intraoperative lymphatic mapping is effective for staging melanoma patients with intermediate risk without clinical adenopathy and is recommended for all patients with lesions over 1 mm in thickness or with high-risk histologic features. Referral of intermediate-risk and high-risk patients to centers with expertise in melanoma is strongly recommended.

Bataille V et al. Melanoma—Part 1: epidemiology, risk factors, and prevention. BMJ. 2008 Nov 20;337:a2249. [PMID: 19022841]

Bishop JN et al. The prevention, diagnosis, referral and management of melanoma of the skin: concise guidelines. Clin Med. 2007 Jun;7(3):283–90. [PMID: 17633952]

Markovic SN et al; Melanoma Study Group of the Mayo Clinic Cancer Center. Malignant melanoma in the 21st century, part 1: epidemiology, risk factors, screening, prevention, and diagnosis. Mayo Clin Proc. 2007 Mar;82(3):364–80. [PMID: 17352373]

Markovic SN et al; Melanoma Study Group of Mayo Clinic Cancer Center. Malignant melanoma in the 21st century, part 2: staging, prognosis, and treatment. Mayo Clin Proc. 2007 Apr;82(4):490–513. [PMID: 17418079]

Miller AJ et al. Melanoma. N Engl J Med. 2006 Jul 6;355(1):51–65. [PMID: 16822996]

Thompson JF et al. Case records of the Massachusetts General Hospital. Case 2-200 pigmented lesion on the arm. N Engl J Med. 2007 Jan 18:356(3):285–92. [PMID: 17229956]

Swetter SM. Malignant melanoma. Medscape. 2008 Jan 23; http://emedicine.medscape.com/article/1100753-overview.

Thirlwell C et al. Melanoma—Part 2: management. BMJ. 2008 Dec 1;337:a2488. [PMID: 19047194]

SCALING DISORDERS

ATOPIC DERMATITIS (Eczema)

 ESSENTIALS OF DIAGNOSIS

▶ Pruritic, exudative, or lichenified eruption on face, neck, upper trunk, wrists, and hands and in the antecubital and popliteal folds.

▶ Personal or family history of allergic manifestations (eg, asthma, allergic rhinitis, atopic dermatitis).

▶ Tendency to recur.

▶ Onset in childhood in most patients. Onset after age 30 is very uncommon.

▶ **General Considerations**

Atopic dermatitis looks different at different ages and in people of different races. Diagnostic criteria for atopic dermatitis must include pruritus, typical morphology and distribution (flexural lichenification, hand eczema, nipple eczema, and eyelid eczema in adults), onset in childhood, and chronicity. Also helpful are: (1) a personal or family history of atopic disease (asthma, allergic rhinitis, atopic dermatitis), (2) xerosis-ichthyosis, (3) facial pallor with infraorbital darkening, (4) elevated serum IgE, and (5) repeated skin infections.

▶ **Clinical Findings**

A. Symptoms and Signs

Itching may be severe and prolonged. Rough, red plaques usually without the thick scale and discrete demarcation of psoriasis affect the face, neck, and upper trunk. The flexural surfaces of elbows and knees are often involved. In chronic cases, the skin is dry, leathery, and lichenified. Pigmented persons may have poorly demarcated hypopigmented patches (pityriasis alba) on the cheeks and extremities. In black patients with severe disease, pigmentation may be lost in lichenified areas. During acute flares, widespread redness with weeping, either diffusely or in discrete plaques, is common.

B. Laboratory Findings

Food allergy is an uncommon cause of flares of atopic dermatitis in adults. Radioallergosorbent tests (RASTs) or skin tests may suggest dust mite allergy. Eosinophilia and increased serum IgE levels may be present.

▶ Differential Diagnosis

Atopic dermatitis must be distinguished from seborrheic dermatitis (less pruritic, frequent scalp and face involvement, greasy and scaly lesions, and quick response to therapy). Secondary staphylococcal infections may exacerbate atopic dermatitis, and should be considered during hyperacute, weepy flares of atopic dermatitis. Since virtually all patients with atopic dermatitis have skin disease before age 5, a new diagnosis of atopic dermatitis in an adult over age 30 should be made cautiously and only after consultation. Atopic-like dermatitis associated with marked elevation of IgE; recurrent, sometimes cold, staphylococcal abscesses; recurrent pneumonia with pneumatocele formation; and retained primary dentition may indicate hyper-IgE syndrome.

▶ Treatment

Patient education regarding gentle skin care and exactly how to use medications is critical in the successful management of atopic dermatitis.

A. General Measures

Atopic patients have hyperirritable skin. Anything that dries or irritates the skin will potentially trigger dermatitis. Atopic individuals are sensitive to low humidity and often get worse in the winter. Adults with atopic disorders should not bathe more than once daily. Soap should be confined to the armpits, groin, scalp and feet. Washcloths and brushes should not be used. After rinsing, the skin should be patted dry (not rubbed) and then immediately—within three minutes—covered with a thin film of an emollient such as Aquaphor, Eucerin, petrolatum, Vanicream, or a corticosteroid as needed. Vanicream can be used if contact dermatitis resulting from additives in medication is suspected. Atopic patients may be irritated by scratchy fabrics, including wools and acrylics. Cottons are preferable, but synthetic blends also are tolerated. Other triggers of eczema in some patients include sweating, ointments, hot baths, and animal danders. In adults, food allergy is a very uncommon cause of atopic dermatitis or its flares.

B. Local Treatment

Corticosteroids should be applied sparingly to the dermatitis once or twice daily and rubbed in well. Their potency should be appropriate to the severity of the dermatitis. In general, one should begin with triamcinolone 0.1% or a stronger corticosteroid then taper to hydrocortisone or another slightly stronger mild corticosteroid (alclometasone, desonide). It is vital that patients taper off corticosteroids and substitute emollients as the dermatitis clears to avoid the side effects of corticosteroids. Tapering is also important to avoid rebound flares of the dermatitis that may follow their abrupt cessation. Tacrolimus ointment (Protopic 0.03% or 0.1%) and pimecrolimus cream (Elidel 1%) can be effective in managing atopic dermatitis when applied twice daily. Burning on application occurs in about 50% of patients using Protopic and in 10–25% of Elidel users, but it may resolve with continued treatment. These medications do not appear to cause skin atrophy or striae, and are safe for application on the face and even the eyelids.

The US Food and Drug Administration (FDA) has issued a black box warning for both topical tacrolimus and pimecrolimus due to concerns about the development of T-cell lymphoma. The agents should be used sparingly and only in locations where less expensive corticosteroids cannot be used. Tacrolimus and pimecrolimus should be avoided in patients at high risk for lymphoma (ie, those with HIV, iatrogenic immunosuppression, prior lymphoma). The treatment of atopic dermatitis is dictated by the stage of the dermatitis.

1. Acute weeping lesions—Use water or aluminum subacetate solution (Domeboro tablets, one in a pint of cool water) or colloidal oatmeal (Aveeno; dispense one box, and use as directed on box) as soothing or astringent soaks, baths, or wet dressings for 10–30 minutes two to four times daily. Lesions on extremities particularly may be bandaged for protection at night. Use high-potency corticosteroids after soaking but spare the face and body folds. Tacrolimus is usually not tolerated at this stage. Systemic corticosteroids may be required (see below).

2. Subacute or scaly lesions—At this stage, the lesions are dry but still red and pruritic. Mid- to high-potency corticosteroids in ointment form should be continued until scaling and elevated skin lesions are cleared and itching is decreased substantially. At that point, patients should begin a 2- to 4-week taper from twice-daily to daily to alternate-day dosing with topical corticosteroids to reliance on emollients, with occasional use of corticosteroids on specific itchy areas. Instead of tapering the frequency of usage of a more potent corticosteroid, it may be preferable to switch to a low-potency corticosteroid. Tacrolimus and pimecrolimus are more expensive alternatives and may be added if corticosteroids cannot be stopped. They avoid the complications of long-term topical corticosteroid use.

3. Chronic, dry, lichenified lesions—Thickened and usually well-demarcated, they are best treated with high-potency to ultra-high-potency corticosteroid ointments. Nightly occlusion for 2–6 weeks may enhance the initial response. Occasionally, adding tar preparations such as LCD (liquor carbonis detergens) 10% in Aquaphor or 2% crude coal tar may be beneficial.

4. Maintenance treatment—Once symptoms have improved, constant application of effective moisturizers is recommended to prevent flares. In patients with moderate disease, weekend only use of topical corticosteroids can prevent flares.

C. Systemic and Adjuvant Therapy

Systemic corticosteroids are indicated only for severe acute exacerbations. Oral prednisone dosages should be high enough to suppress the dermatitis quickly, usually starting with 40–60 mg daily for adults. The dosage is then tapered to nil over a period of 2–4 weeks. Owing to the chronic nature of atopic dermatitis and the side effects of chronic systemic corticosteroids, long-term use of these agents is not recommended for maintenance therapy. Classic antihistamines may relieve severe pruritus. Hydroxyzine, diphenhydramine, or doxepin may be useful—the dosage increased gradually to avoid drowsiness. Fissures, crusts, erosions, or pustules indicate staphylococcal infection clinically. Antistaphylococcal antibiotics given systemically—such as a first-generation cephalosporin—may be helpful in management. Cultures to exclude methicillin-resistant *Staphylococcus aureus* are recommended. Phototherapy can be an important adjunct for severely affected patients, and the properly selected patient with recalcitrant disease may benefit greatly from therapy with UVB with or without coal tar or PUVA (psoralen plus ultraviolet A). Oral cyclosporine, mycophenolate mofetil, or azathioprine may be used for the most severe and recalcitrant cases.

Complications of Treatment

The clinician should monitor for skin atrophy. **Eczema herpeticum,** a generalized herpes simplex infection manifested by monomorphic vesicles, crusts, or scalloped erosions superimposed on atopic dermatitis or other extensive eczematous processes, is treated successfully with oral acyclovir, 200 mg five times daily, or intravenous acyclovir in a dose of 10 mg/kg intravenously every 8 hours (500 mg/ m² every 8 hours). Tacrolimus and pimecrolimus may increase the risk of eczema herpeticum.

Smallpox vaccination is absolutely contraindicated in patients with atopic dermatitis or a history thereof because of the risk of eczema vaccinatum. Generalized vaccinia may develop in patients with atopic dermatitis who have contact with recent vaccine recipients who still have pustular or crusted vaccination sites. Eczema vaccinatum and generalized vaccinia are indications for vaccinia immune globulin.

Prognosis

Atopic dermatitis runs a chronic or intermittent course. Affected adults may have only hand dermatitis. Poor prognostic factors for persistence into adulthood in atopic dermatitis include onset early in childhood, early generalized disease, and asthma. Only 40–60% of these patients have lasting remissions.

Akdis CA et al; European Academy of Allergology and Clinical Immunology/American Academy of Allergy, Asthma and Immunology. Diagnosis and treatment of atopic dermatitis in children and adults: European Academy of Allergology and Clinical Immunology/American Academy of Allergy, Asthma and Immunology/PRACTALL Consensus Report. J Allergy Clin Immunol. 2006 Jul;118(1):152–69. [PMID: 16815151]

Bieber T. Atopic dermatitis. N Engl J Med. 2008 Apr 3;358(14):1483–94. [PMID: 18385500]

Buys LM. Treatment options for atopic dermatitis. Am Fam Physician. 2007 Feb 15;75(4):523–8. [PMID: 17323714]

Yosipovitch G et al. What causes itch in atopic dermatitis? Curr Allergy Asthma Rep. 2008 Jul;8(4):306-11. [PMID: 18606082]

LICHEN SIMPLEX CHRONICUS (Circumscribed Neurodermatitis)

ESSENTIALS OF DIAGNOSIS

► Chronic itching and scratching.
► Lichenified lesions with exaggerated skin lines overlying a thickened, well-circumscribed scaly plaque.
► Predilection for nape of neck, wrists, external surfaces of forearms, lower legs, scrotum, and vulva.

General Considerations

Lichen simplex chronicus represents a self-perpetuating scratch-itch cycle—a learned behavior that is hard to disrupt.

Clinical Findings

Intermittent itching incites the patient to scratch the lesions. Itching may be so intense as to interfere with sleep. Dry, leathery, hypertrophic, lichenified plaques appear on the neck, ankles, or perineum (Plate 7). The patches are rectangular, thickened, and hyperpigmented. The skin lines are exaggerated.

Differential Diagnosis

This disorder can be differentiated from plaque-like lesions such as psoriasis (redder lesions having whiter scales on the elbows, knees, and scalp and nail findings), lichen planus (violaceous, usually smaller polygonal papules), and nummular (coin-shaped) dermatitis. Lichen simplex chronicus may complicate chronic atopic dermatitis.

Treatment

For lesions in extra-genital regions, superpotent topical corticosteroids are effective, with or without occlusion, when used twice daily for several weeks. In some patients, flurandrenolide (Cordran) tape may be effective, since it prevents scratching and rubbing of the lesion. The injection of triamcinolone acetonide suspension (5–10 mg/mL) into the lesions may occasionally be curative. Continuous occlusion with a flexible hydrocolloid dressing for 7 days at a time for 1–2 months may also be helpful. The area should be protected and the patient encouraged to become aware of when he or she is scratching. For genital lesions, see the section Pruritus Ani.

Prognosis

The disease tends to remit during treatment but may recur or develop at another site.

PSORIASIS

ESSENTIALS OF DIAGNOSIS

► Silvery scales on bright red, well-demarcated plaques, usually on the knees, elbows, and scalp.

- Nail findings including pitting and onycholysis (separation of the nail plate from the bed).
- Mild itching (usually).
- May be associated with psoriatic arthritis.
- Histopathology is not often useful and can be confusing.

General Considerations

Psoriasis is a common benign, chronic inflammatory skin disease with a genetic basis. Injury or irritation of normal skin tends to induce lesions of psoriasis at the site (Koebner phenomenon). Psoriasis has several variants—the most common is the plaque type. Eruptive (guttate) psoriasis consisting of myriad lesions 3–10 mm in diameter occurs occasionally after streptococcal pharyngitis. Rarely, grave, occasionally life-threatening forms (generalized pustular and erythrodermic psoriasis) may occur. Plaque type or extensive erythrodermic psoriasis with abrupt onset may accompany HIV infection.

Clinical Findings

There are often no symptoms, but itching may occur and be severe. Favored sites include the scalp, elbows, knees, palms and soles, and nails (Plate 8). The lesions are red, sharply defined plaques covered with silvery scales (Plate 9). The glans penis and vulva may be affected. Occasionally, only the flexures (axillae, inguinal areas) are involved. Fine stippling ("pitting") in the nails is highly suggestive of psoriasis. Patients with psoriasis often have a pink or red intergluteal fold. Not all patients have findings in all locations, but the occurrence of a few may help make the diagnosis when other lesions are not typical. Some patients have mainly hand or foot dermatitis and only minimal findings elsewhere. There may be associated arthritis that is most commonly distal and oligoarticular, although the rheumatoid variety with a negative rheumatoid factor may occur. The psychosocial impact of psoriasis is a major factor in determining the treatment of the patient.

Differential Diagnosis

The combination of red plaques with silvery scales on elbows and knees, with scaliness in the scalp or nail findings, is diagnostic (Plate 8). Psoriasis lesions are well demarcated and affect extensor surfaces—in contrast to atopic dermatitis, with poorly demarcated plaques in flexural distribution. In body folds, scraping and culture for *Candida* and examination of scalp and nails will distinguish psoriasis from intertrigo and candidiasis. Dystrophic changes in nails may simulate onychomycosis, but again, the general examination combined with a potassium hydroxide (KOH) or fungal culture will be valuable in diagnosis. The cutaneous features of reactive arthritis (Reiter syndrome) mimic psoriasis.

Treatment

There are many therapeutic options in psoriasis to be chosen according to the extent (BSA affected) and the presence of other findings (for example, arthritis). Certain drugs, such as β-blockers, antimalarials, statins, and lithium, may flare or worsen psoriasis. Even tiny doses of systemic corticosteroids given to patients with psoriasis may lead to severe rebound flares of their disease. Never use systemic corticosteroids to treat flares of psoriasis. In general, patients with moderate to severe psoriasis should be managed by or in conjunction with a dermatologist.

A. Limited Disease

For patients with limited disease (less than 10% of the patient's BSA), in whom lesions are composed of small plaques, phototherapy is the best therapy (see below). For patients with large plaques, the easiest regimen is to use a high-potency to ultra-high-potency topical corticosteroid cream or ointment. It is best to restrict the ultra-high-potency corticosteroids to 2–3 weeks of twice-daily use and then use them in a pulse fashion three or four times on weekends or switch to a midpotency corticosteroid. Topical corticosteroids rarely induce a lasting remission. They may cause psoriasis to become unstable. Additional measures are therefore commonly added to topical corticosteroid therapy. Calcipotriene ointment 0.005%, a vitamin D analog, is used twice daily for plaque psoriasis. Initially, patients are treated with twice-daily corticosteroids plus calcipotriene twice daily. This rapidly clears the lesions. Calcipotriene is then used alone once daily and with the corticosteroid once daily for several weeks. Eventually, the topical corticosteroids are stopped, and once- or twice-daily calcipotriene is continued long-term. Calcipotriene usually cannot be applied to the groin or on the face because of irritation. Treatment of extensive psoriasis with calcipotriene may result in hypercalcemia. Calcipotriene is incompatible with many topical corticosteroids (but not halobetasol), so if used concurrently it must be applied at a different time. Tar preparations such as Fototar cream, LCD (liquor carbonis detergens) 10% in Nutraderm lotion, alone or mixed directly with triamcinolone 0.1%, are useful adjuncts when applied twice daily. Occlusion alone has been shown to clear isolated plaques in 30–40% of patients. Occlusive hydrocolloid dressings such as thin DuoDerm are placed on the lesions and left undisturbed for as long as possible (a minimum of 5 days, up to 7 days) and then replaced. Responses may be seen within several weeks.

For the scalp, start with a tar shampoo, used daily if possible. For thick scales, use 6% salicylic acid gel (eg, Keralyt), P & S solution (phenol, mineral oil, and glycerin), or fluocinolone acetonide 0.01% in oil (Derma-Smoothe/FS) under a shower cap at night, and shampoo in the morning. In order of increasing potency, triamcinolone 0.1%, or fluocinolone, betamethasone dipropionate, fluocinonide or amcinonide, and clobetasol are available in solution form for use on the scalp twice daily. For psoriasis in the body folds, treatment is difficult, since potent corticosteroids cannot be used and other agents are poorly tolerated. Tacrolimus ointment 0.1% or 0.03% or pimecrolimus cream 1% may be effective in penile, groin, and facial psoriasis.

B. Moderate Disease

Psoriasis affecting 10–30% of the patient's BSA is frequently treated with UV phototherapy, either in a medical office or via a home light unit. Systemic agents listed below may also be used.

C. Generalized Disease

If psoriasis involves more than 30% of the body surface, it is difficult to treat with topical agents. The treatment of choice is outpatient narrowband UVB (NB-UVB) three times weekly. Clearing occurs in an average of 7 weeks, but maintenance may be required. Severe psoriasis unresponsive to outpatient ultraviolet light may be treated in a psoriasis day care center with the Goeckerman regimen, which involves use of crude coal tar for many hours and exposure to UVB light. Such treatment may offer the best chance for prolonged remissions.

PUVA may be effective even in patients who have not responded to standard NB-UVB treatment. Long-term use of PUVA is associated with an increased risk of skin cancer (especially squamous cell carcinoma and perhaps melanoma), particularly in persons with fair complexions. Thus, periodic examination of the skin is imperative. Atypical lentigines are a common complication. There can be rapid aging of the skin in fair individuals. Cataracts have not been reported with proper use of protective glasses. PUVA may be used in combination with other therapy, such as acitretin or methotrexate.

Methotrexate is very effective for severe psoriasis in doses up to 25 mg once weekly. It should be used according to published protocols. Liver biopsy is performed initially after methotrexate has been used long enough by the patient to demonstrate that it is effective and well tolerated, and then at intervals depending on the cumulative dose, usually every 1.5–2 g. Administration of folic acid, 1–2 mg daily, will eliminate nausea caused by methotrexate without compromising efficacy.

Acitretin, a synthetic retinoid, is most effective for pustular psoriasis in dosages of 0.5–0.75 mg/kg/d, but it also improves erythrodermic and plaque types and psoriatic arthritis. Liver enzymes and serum lipids must be checked periodically. Because acitretin is a teratogen and persists for long periods in fat, women of childbearing age must wait at least 3 years after completing acitretin treatment before considering pregnancy. When used as single agents, retinoids will flatten psoriatic plaques, but will rarely result in complete clearing. Retinoids find their greatest use when combined with phototherapy—either UVB or PUVA, with which they are synergistic.

Cyclosporine dramatically improves psoriasis and may be used to control severe cases. Rapid relapse (rebound) is the rule after cessation of therapy, so another agent must be added if cyclosporine is stopped. The tumor necrosis factor (TNF) inhibitors etanercept (Enbrel), 50 mg twice weekly; infliximab (Remicade); and adalimumab (Humira) have shown antipsoriatic activity. Infliximab provides the most rapid response and can be used for severe pustular or erythrodermic flares. Etanercept is used more frequently for long-term treatment at a dose of 50 mg twice weekly for 3

months, then 25 mg twice weekly. All three TNF inhibitors can also induce psoriasis. Alefacept (Amevive) and efalizumab (Raptiva) have moderate efficacy. The role of the latter two immunomodulators is unclear. IL-12/23 monoclonal antibodies can be dramatically effective in psoriasis.

Prognosis

The course tends to be chronic and unpredictable, and the disease may be refractory to treatment.

Friedewald VE et al. AJC editor's consensus: psoriasis and coronary artery disease. Am J Cardiol. 2008 Dec 15;102(12):1631–43. [PMID: 19064017]

Griffiths CE et al. Pathogenesis and clinical features of psoriasis. Lancet. 2007 Jul 21;370(9583):263–71. [PMID: 17658397]

Krueger GG et al; CNTO 1275 Psoriasis Study Group. A human interleukin-12/23 monoclonal antibody for the treatment of psoriasis. N Engl J Med. 2007 Feb 8;356(6):580–92. [PMID: 17287478]

Menter A et al. Current and future management of psoriasis. Lancet. 2007 Jul 21;370(9583):272–84. [PMID: 17658398]

Schmitt J et al. Efficacy and tolerability of biologic and nonbiologic systemic treatments for moderate-to-severe psoriasis: meta-analysis of randomized controlled trials. Br J Dermatol. 2008 Sep;159(3):513–26. [PMID: 18627372]

Thaci D. Long-term data in the treatment of psoriasis. Br J Dermatol. 2008 Aug;159(Suppl 2):18–24. [PMID: 18700911]

PITYRIASIS ROSEA

 ESSENTIALS OF DIAGNOSIS

▶ Oval, fawn-colored, scaly eruption following cleavage lines of trunk.

▶ Herald patch precedes eruption by 1–2 weeks.

▶ Occasional pruritus.

General Considerations

This is a common mild, acute inflammatory disease that is 50% more common in females. Young adults are principally affected, mostly in the spring or fall. Concurrent household cases have been reported.

Clinical Findings

Itching is common but is usually mild. The diagnosis is made by finding one or more classic lesions. The lesions consist of oval, fawn-colored plaques up to 2 cm in diameter (Plate 10). The centers of the lesions have a crinkled or "cigarette paper" appearance and a collarette scale, ie, a thin bit of scale that is bound at the periphery and free in the center. Only a few lesions in the eruption may have this characteristic appearance, however. Lesions follow cleavage lines on the trunk (so-called Christmas tree pattern, Plate 11), and the proximal portions of the extremities are often involved. A variant that affects the flexures (axillae and groin), so called inverse pityriasis rosea, and a papular variant, especially in black patients, also occur. An initial lesion ("herald patch") that is often larger than the later lesions often precedes the general eruption by 1–2 weeks. The eruption usually lasts 6–8 weeks and heals without scarring.

Differential Diagnosis

A serologic test for syphilis should be performed if at least a few perfectly typical lesions are not present and especially if there are palmar and plantar or mucous membrane lesions or adenopathy, features that are suggestive of secondary syphilis. For the nonexpert, an RPR (rapid plasma reagin) test in all cases is not unreasonable. Tinea corporis may present with red, slightly scaly plaques, but rarely are there more than a few lesions of tinea corporis compared to the many lesions of pityriasis rosea. Seborrheic dermatitis on occasion presents on the body with poorly demarcated patches over the sternum, in the pubic area, and in the axillae. Tinea versicolor, viral exanthems, and drug eruptions may simulate pityriasis rosea.

Treatment

Pityriasis rosea often requires no treatment. In Asians, Hispanics, or blacks, in whom lesions may remain hyperpigmented for some time, more aggressive management may be indicated. Treatment is, otherwise, only indicated if the patient is symptomatic. No treatment has been demonstrated efficacious in pityriasis rosea in adequately controlled and reproduced trials. Most dermatologists recommend UVB treatments, or prednisone as used for contact dermatitis for severe or severely symptomatic cases. For mild to moderate cases, topical corticosteroids of medium strength (triamcinolone 0.1%) and oral antihistamines may also be used if pruritus is bothersome. Oral erythromycin for 14 days was reported to clear 73% of patients within 2 weeks (compared with none of the patients receiving placebo).

Prognosis

Pityriasis rosea is usually an acute self-limiting illness that disappears in about 6 weeks.

Chuh AA et al. Interventions for pityriasis rosea. Cochrane Database Syst Rev. 2007 Apr 18;(2):CD005068. [PMID: 17443568]

SEBORRHEIC DERMATITIS & DANDRUFF

 ESSENTIALS OF DIAGNOSIS

- ► Dry scales and underlying erythema.
- ► Scalp, central face, presternal, interscapular areas, umbilicus, and body folds.

General Considerations

Seborrheic dermatitis is an acute or chronic papulosquamous dermatitis that often coexists with psoriasis.

Clinical Findings

Pruritus is an inconstant finding. The scalp, face, chest, back, umbilicus, eyelid margins, and body folds have dry scales or oily yellowish scurf (Plate 12). Patients with Parkinson disease, HIV infection, and patients who become acutely ill and are hospitalized often have seborrheic dermatitis.

Differential Diagnosis

There is a spectrum from seborrheic dermatitis to scalp psoriasis. Extensive seborrheic dermatitis may simulate intertrigo in flexural areas, but scalp, face, and sternal involvement suggests seborrheic dermatitis.

Treatment

A. Seborrhea of the Scalp

Shampoos that contain zinc pyrithione or selenium are used daily if possible. These may be alternated with ketoconazole shampoo (1% or 2%) used twice weekly. A combination of shampoos is used in refractory cases. Tar shampoos are also effective for milder cases and for scalp psoriasis. Topical corticosteroid solutions or lotions are then added if necessary and are used twice daily. (See treatment for scalp psoriasis, above.)

B. Facial Seborrheic Dermatitis

The mainstay of therapy is a mild corticosteroid (hydrocortisone 1%, alclometasone, desonide) used intermittently and not near the eyes. If the disorder cannot be controlled with intermittent use of a mild topical corticosteroid alone, ketoconazole (Nizoral) 2% cream is added twice daily. Topical tacrolimus (Protopic) and pimecrolimus (Elidel) are steroid-sparing alternatives.

C. Seborrheic Dermatitis of Nonhairy Areas

Low-potency corticosteroid creams—ie, 1% or 2.5% hydrocortisone, desonide, or alclometasone dipropionate—are highly effective.

D. Seborrhea of Intertriginous Areas

Apply low-potency corticosteroid lotions or creams twice daily for 5–7 days and then once or twice weekly for maintenance as necessary. Ketoconazole or clotrimazole cream may be a useful adjunct. Tacrolimus or pimecrolimus topically may avoid corticosteroid atrophy in chronic cases.

E. Involvement of Eyelid Margins

"Marginal blepharitis" usually responds to gentle cleaning of the lid margins nightly as needed, with undiluted Johnson and Johnson Baby Shampoo using a cotton swab.

Prognosis

The tendency is for lifelong recurrences. Individual outbreaks may last weeks, months, or years.

Schwartz RA et al. Seborrheic dermatitis: an overview. Am Fam Physician. 2006 Jul 1;74(1):125–30. [PMID: 16848386]

FUNGAL INFECTIONS OF THE SKIN

Mycotic infections are traditionally divided into two principal groups—superficial and deep. In this chapter, we will discuss only the superficial infections: tinea corporis and tinea cruris; dermatophytosis of the feet and dermatophytid of the hands; tinea unguium (onychomycosis); and tinea versicolor. See Chapter 36 for discussion of deep mycoses.

The diagnosis of fungal infections of the skin is usually based on the location and characteristics of the lesions and on the following laboratory examinations: (1) Direct demonstration of fungi in 10% KOH of scrapings from suspected lesions. "If it's scaly, scrape it" is a time-honored maxim. (2) Cultures of organisms from skin scrapings. (3) Histologic sections of biopsies stained with periodic acid-Schiff (Hotchkiss-McManus) technique may be diagnostic if scrapings and cultures are negative.

Principles of Treatment

A diagnosis should always be confirmed by KOH preparation, culture, or biopsy. Many other diseases cause scaling, and use of an antifungal agent without a firm diagnosis makes subsequent diagnosis more difficult. In general, fungal infections are treated topically except for those involving the nails, those that are very extensive, or those that involve the hair follicles.

Griseofulvin is safe and effective for treating dermatophyte infections of the skin (except for the scalp and nails). Itraconazole, an azole antifungal, and terbinafine, an allylamine oral antifungal, have excellent activity against dermatophytes and can be used in shorter courses than griseofulvin.

Fluconazole has excellent activity against yeasts and may be the treatment of choice for many forms of mucocutaneous candidiasis. Itraconazole, fluconazole, and terbinafine can all cause elevation of liver function tests and—though rarely in the dosing regimens used for the treatment of dermatophytosis—clinical hepatitis. Ketoconazole is no longer recommended for the treatment of dermatophytosis (except for tinea versicolor) because of the higher rate of hepatitis when it is used for more than a month.

General Measures & Prevention

Since moist skin favors the growth of fungi, dry the skin carefully after bathing or after perspiring heavily. Talc or other drying powders may be useful. The use of topical corticosteroids for other diseases may be complicated by intercurrent tinea or candidal infection, and topical antifungals are often used in intertriginous areas with corticosteroids to prevent this.

1. Tinea Corporis or Tinea Circinata (Body Ringworm)

ESSENTIALS OF DIAGNOSIS

► Ring-shaped lesions with an advancing scaly border and central clearing or scaly patches with a distinct border.

► On exposed skin surfaces or the trunk.

► Microscopic examination of scrapings or culture confirms the diagnosis.

General Considerations

The lesions are often on exposed areas of the body such as the face and arms. A history of exposure to an infected cat may occasionally be obtained, usually indicating *Microsporum* infection. *Trichophyton rubrum* is the most common pathogen, usually representing extension onto the trunk or extremities of tinea cruris, pedis, or manuum.

Clinical Findings

A. Symptoms and Signs

Itching may be present. In classic lesions, rings of erythema have an advancing scaly border and central clearing (Plates 13 and 14).

B. Laboratory Findings

The diagnosis may be confirmed by KOH preparation or culture.

Differential Diagnosis

Positive fungal studies distinguish tinea corporis from other skin lesions with annular configuration, such as the annular lesions of psoriasis, lupus erythematosus, syphilis, granuloma annulare, and pityriasis rosea. Psoriasis has typical lesions on elbows, knees, scalp, and nails. Secondary syphilis is often manifested by characteristic palmar, plantar, and mucous membrane lesions. Tinea corporis rarely has the large number of lesions seen in pityriasis rosea. Granuloma annulare lacks scales.

Complications

Complications include extension of the disease down the hair follicles (in which case it becomes much more difficult to cure) and pyoderma.

Prevention

Treat infected household pets (*Microsporum* infections).

Treatment

A. Local Measures

Tinea corporis responds to most topical antifungals, including miconazole, clotrimazole, butenafine, and terbinafine, which are available over the counter (Table 6–2). Terbinafine and butenafine require shorter courses and lead to the most rapid response. Treatment should be continued for 1–2 weeks after clinical clearing. Betamethasone dipropionate with clotrimazole (Lotrisone) is not recommended. Long-term improper use may result in side effects from the high-potency corticosteroid component, especially in body folds. Cases of tinea that are clinically resistant to this combination but respond to topical antifungals without the topical corticosteroid can occur.

B. Systemic Measures

Griseofulvin (ultramicrosize), 250–500 mg twice daily, is used. Typically, only 4–6 weeks of therapy are required. Itraconazole as a single week-long pulse of 200 mg daily is also effective in tinea corporis. Terbinafine, 250 mg daily for 1 month, is an alternative.

▶ Prognosis

Body ringworm usually responds promptly to conservative topical therapy or to an oral agent within 4 weeks.

2. Tinea Cruris (Jock Itch)

ESSENTIALS OF DIAGNOSIS

- ▶ Marked itching in intertriginous areas, usually sparing the scrotum.
- ▶ Peripherally spreading, sharply demarcated, centrally clearing erythematous lesions.
- ▶ May have associated tinea infection of feet or toenails.
- ▶ Laboratory examination with microscope or culture confirms diagnosis.

▶ General Considerations

Tinea cruris lesions are confined to the groin and gluteal cleft. Intractable pruritus ani may occasionally be caused by a tinea infection.

▶ Clinical Findings

A. Symptoms and Signs

Itching may be severe, or the rash may be asymptomatic. The lesions have sharp margins, cleared centers, and active, spreading scaly peripheries (Plate 15). Follicular pustules are sometimes encountered. The area may be hyperpigmented on resolution.

B. Laboratory Findings

Hyphae can be demonstrated microscopically in KOH preparations. The organism may be cultured.

▶ Differential Diagnosis

Tinea cruris must be distinguished from other lesions involving the intertriginous areas, such as candidiasis, seborrheic dermatitis, intertrigo, psoriasis of body folds ("inverse psoriasis"), and erythrasma. Candidiasis is generally bright red and marked by satellite papules and pustules outside of the main border of the lesion. *Candida* typically involves the scrotum. Seborrheic dermatitis also often involves the face, sternum, and axillae.

Intertrigo tends to be more red, less scaly, and present in obese individuals in moist body folds with less extension onto the thigh. Inverse psoriasis is characterized by distinct plaques. Other areas of typical psoriatic involvement should be checked, and the KOH examination will be negative. Erythrasma is best diagnosed with Wood's (ultraviolet) light—a brilliant coral-red fluorescence is seen.

▶ Treatment

A. General Measures

Drying powder (eg, miconazole nitrate [Zeasorb-AF]) can be dusted into the involved area in patients with excessive perspiration or occlusion of skin due to obesity. Underwear should be loose-fitting.

B. Local Measures

Any of the preparations listed in Table 6–2 may be used. Terbinafine cream is curative in over 80% of cases after once-daily use for 7 days.

C. Systemic Measures

Griseofulvin ultramicrosize is reserved for severe cases. Give 250–500 mg orally twice daily for 1–2 weeks. One week of either itraconazole, 200 mg daily, or terbinafine, 250 mg daily, can be effective.

▶ Prognosis

Tinea cruris usually responds promptly to topical or systemic treatment but often recurs.

3. Tinea Manuum & Tinea Pedis (Dermatophytosis, Tinea of Palms & Soles, "Athlete's Foot")

ESSENTIALS OF DIAGNOSIS

- ▶ Most often presenting with asymptomatic scaling.
- ▶ May progress to fissuring or maceration in toe web spaces.
- ▶ Common cofactor in lower leg cellulitis.
- ▶ Itching, burning, and stinging of interdigital web; scaling palms, and soles; vesicles of soles in inflammatory cases.
- ▶ The fungus is shown in skin scrapings examined microscopically or by culture of scrapings.

▶ General Considerations

Tinea of the feet is an extremely common acute or chronic dermatosis. Certain individuals appear to be more susceptible than others. Most infections are caused by *Trichophyton* species.

Clinical Findings

A. Symptoms and Signs

The presenting symptom may be itching, burning, or stinging. Pain may indicate secondary infection with complicating cellulitis. Interdigital tinea pedis is the most common predisposing cause of lower leg cellulitis in healthy individuals. Tinea pedis has several presentations that vary with the location. On the sole and heel, tinea may appear as chronic noninflammatory scaling, occasionally with thickening and fissuring. This may extend over the sides of the feet in a "moccasin" distribution. The KOH preparation is usually positive. Tinea pedis often appears as a scaling or fissuring of the toe webs, perhaps with sodden maceration (Plate 16). As the web spaces become more macerated, the KOH preparation and fungal culture are less often positive because bacterial species begin to dominate. Finally, there may also be grouped vesicles distributed anywhere on the soles, generalized exfoliation of the skin of the soles, or nail involvement in the form of discoloration and thickening and crumbling of the nail plate.

B. Laboratory Findings

KOH and culture does not always demonstrate pathogenic fungi from macerated areas.

Differential Diagnosis

Differentiate from other skin conditions involving the same areas, such as interdigital erythrasma (use Wood's light). Psoriasis may be a cause of chronic scaling on the palms or soles and may cause nail changes. Repeated fungal cultures should be negative, and the condition will not respond to antifungal therapy. Contact dermatitis (from shoes) will often involve the dorsal surfaces and will respond to topical or systemic corticosteroids. Vesicular lesions should be differentiated from pompholyx (dyshidrosis) and scabies by proper scraping of the roofs of individual vesicles. Rarely, gram-negative organisms may cause toe web infections, manifested as an acute erosive flare of interdigital disease. This entity is treated with aluminum salts (see below) and imidazole antifungal agents or ciclopirox.

Prevention

The essential factor in prevention is personal hygiene. Wear open-toed sandals if possible. Use of sandals in community showers and bathing places is often recommended, though the effectiveness of this practice has not been studied. Careful drying between the toes after showering is essential. A hair dryer used on low setting may be used. Socks should be changed frequently, and absorbent nonsynthetic socks are preferred. Apply dusting and drying powders as necessary. The use of powders containing antifungal agents (eg, Zeasorb-AF) or chronic use of antifungal creams may prevent recurrences of tinea pedis.

Treatment

A. Local Measures

1. Macerated stage—Treat with aluminum subacetate solution soaks for 20 minutes twice daily. Broad-spectrum antifungal creams and solutions (containing imidazoles or ciclopirox instead of tolnaftate and haloprogin) will help combat diphtheroids and other gram-positive organisms present at this stage and alone may be adequate therapy. If topical imidazoles fail, 1 week of once-daily topical allylamine treatment (terbinafine or butenafine) will often result in clearing.

2. Dry and scaly stage—Use any of the agents listed in Table 6–2. The addition of urea 10–20% lotion or cream may increase the efficacy of topical treatments in thick ("moccasin") tinea of the soles.

B. Systemic Measures

Griseofulvin may be used for severe cases or those recalcitrant to topical therapy. If the infection is cleared by systemic therapy, the patient should be encouraged to begin maintenance with topical therapy, since recurrence is common. Itraconazole, 200 mg daily for 2 weeks or 400 mg daily for 1 week, or terbinafine, 250 mg daily for 2–4 weeks, may be used in refractory cases.

Prognosis

For many individuals, tinea pedis is a chronic affliction, temporarily cleared by therapy only to recur.

Crawford F et al. Topical treatments for fungal infections of the skin and nails of the foot. Cochrane Database Syst Rev. 2007 Jul 18;(3):CD001434. [PMID: 17636672]
Nadalo D et al. What is the best way to treat tinea cruris? J Fam Pract. 2006 Mar;55(3):256–8. [PMID: 16428155]

4. Tinea Versicolor (Pityriasis Versicolor)

 ESSENTIALS OF DIAGNOSIS

► Velvety, tan, or pink macules or white macules that do not tan.

► Fine scales that are not visible but are seen by scraping the lesion.

► Central upper trunk the most frequent site.

► Yeast and short hyphae observed on microscopic examination of scales.

General Considerations

Tinea versicolor is a mild, superficial *Malassezia* infection of the skin (usually of the upper trunk). This yeast is a colonizer of all humans, which accounts for the high recurrence rate after treatment. The eruption is often called to patients' attention by the fact that the involved areas will not tan, and the resulting hypopigmentation may be mistaken for vitiligo. A hyperpigmented form is not uncommon.

Clinical Findings

A. Symptoms and Signs

Lesions are asymptomatic, but a few patients note itching. The lesions are velvety, tan, pink, or white macules that vary from 4–5 mm in diameter to large confluent areas. The lesions initially do not look scaly, but scales may be readily obtained by scraping the area. Lesions may appear on the trunk, upper arms, neck, and groin.

B. Laboratory Findings

Large, blunt hyphae and thick-walled budding spores ("spaghetti and meatballs") are seen on KOH. Fungal culture is not useful.

Differential Diagnosis

Vitiligo usually presents with larger periorificial lesions. Vitiligo (and not tinea versicolor) is characterized by total depigmentation, not just a lessening of pigmentation. Vitiligo does not scale. Pink and red-brown lesions on the chest are differentiated from seborrheic dermatitis of the same areas by the KOH preparation.

Treatment & Prognosis

Topical treatments include selenium sulfide lotion, which may be applied from neck to waist daily and left on for 5–15 minutes for 7 days; this treatment is repeated weekly for a month and then monthly for maintenance. Ketoconazole shampoo, 1% or 2%, lathered on the chest and back and left on for 5 minutes may also be used weekly for treatment and to prevent recurrence. Clinicians must stress to the patient that the raised and scaly aspects of the rash are being treated; the alterations in pigmentation may take months to fade or fill in.

Ketoconazole, 200 mg daily orally for 1 week or 400 mg as a single oral dose, with exercise to the point of sweating after ingestion, results in short-term cure of 90% of cases. Patients should be instructed not to shower for 8–12 hours after taking ketoconazole, because it is delivered in sweat to the skin. The single dose may not work in more hot and humid areas, and more protracted therapy carries a small risk of drug-induced hepatitis. Two doses of oral fluconazole, 300 mg, 14 days apart has similar efficacy. Without maintenance therapy, recurrences will occur in over 80% of "cured" cases over the subsequent 2 years. Imidazole creams, solutions, and lotions are quite effective for localized areas but are too expensive for use over large areas such as the chest and back.

Khachemoune A. Tinea versicolor. Dermatol Nurs. 2006 Apr; 18(2):167. [PMID: 16708681]

Yazdanpanah MJ et al. Comparison between fluconazole and ketoconazole effectivity in the treatment of pityriasis versicolor. Mycoses. 2007 Jul;50(4):311–3. [PMID: 17576325]

DISCOID LUPUS ERYTHEMATOSUS (Chronic Cutaneous Lupus Erythematosus)

▶ Localized red plaques, usually on the face.

▶ Scaling, follicular plugging, atrophy, dyspigmentation, and telangiectasia of involved areas.

▶ Histology distinctive.

▶ Photosensitive.

General Considerations

The two most common forms of chronic cutaneous lupus erythematosus (CCLE) are chronic scarring (discoid) lesions (DLE) and erythematous non-scarring red plaques (subacute cutaneous LE) (SCLE). Both occur most frequently in areas exposed to solar irradiation. Permanent hair loss and loss of pigmentation are common sequelae of discoid lesions. Systemic lupus erythematosus (SLE) is discussed in Chapter 20. Patients with SLE may have DLE or SCLE lesions.

Clinical Findings

A. Symptoms and Signs

Symptoms are usually mild. The lesions consist of dusky red, well-localized, single or multiple plaques, 5–20 mm in diameter, usually on the head in DLE and the trunk in SCLE. In DLE, the scalp, face, and external ears may be involved. In discoid lesions there is atrophy, telangiectasia, depigmentation, and follicular plugging. On the scalp, significant permanent hair loss may occur in lesions of DLE.

B. Laboratory Findings

If antinuclear antibody (ANA) is positive in high titer, or when lesions are widespread (not localized to the head), the findings of antibody to double-stranded DNA and hypocomplementemia suggest the diagnosis of SLE. Rare patients with marked photosensitivity and a picture otherwise suggestive of lupus have negative ANA tests but are positive for antibodies against Ro/SSA (SCLE).

Differential Diagnosis

The diagnosis is based on the clinical appearance confirmed by skin biopsy in all cases. In DLE, the scales are dry and "thumbtack-like" and can thus be distinguished from those of seborrheic dermatitis and psoriasis. Older lesions that have left depigmented scarring (classically in the concha of the ear) or areas of hair loss will also differentiate lupus from these diseases. Ten percent of patients with SLE have discoid skin lesions, and 5% of patients with discoid lesions have SLE. Medications (hydrochlorothiazide, calcium channel blockers, terbinafine) may induce SCLE with a positive Ro/SSA.

Treatment

A. General Measures

Protect from sunlight. Use high-SPF (> 50) sunblock with UVB and UVA coverage daily. **Caution:** Do not use any form of radiation therapy. Avoid using drugs that are potentially photosensitizing when possible.

B. Local Treatment

For limited lesions, the following should be tried before systemic therapy: high-potency corticosteroid creams applied each night and covered with airtight, thin, pliable plastic film (eg, Saran Wrap); or Cordran tape; or ultra-high-potency corticosteroid cream or ointment applied twice daily without occlusion.

C. Local Infiltration

Triamcinolone acetonide suspension, 2.5–10 mg/mL, may be injected into the lesions once a month.

D. Systemic Treatment

1. Antimalarials—Caution: These drugs should be used only when the diagnosis is secure because they have been associated with flares of psoriasis, which may be in the differential diagnosis. They may also cause ocular changes, and ophthalmologic evaluation is required at the onset of therapy and at regular intervals during treatment.

A. HYDROXYCHLOROQUINE SULFATE—0.2–0.4 g orally daily for several months may be effective and is often used prior to chloroquine. A minimum 3-month trial is recommended.

B. CHLOROQUINE SULFATE—250 mg daily may be effective in some cases where hydroxychloroquine is not.

C. QUINACRINE (ATABRINE)—100 mg daily may be the safest of the antimalarials, since eye damage has not been reported. It colors the skin yellow and is therefore not acceptable to some patients. It may be added to the other antimalarials for incomplete responses.

2. Isotretinoin—Isotretinoin, 1 mg/kg/d, is effective in CCLE or SCLE. Recurrences are prompt and predictable on discontinuation of therapy.

3. Thalidomide—Thalidomide is effective in refractory cases in doses of up to 300 mg daily. Monitor for neuropathy.

   Both isotretinoin and thalidomide are teratogens and should be used with appropriate contraception and monitoring in women of childbearing age.

Prognosis

The disease is persistent but not life-endangering unless systemic lupus is present. Treatment with antimalarials is effective in perhaps 60% of cases. Although the only morbidity may be cosmetic, this can be of overwhelming significance in more darkly pigmented patients with widespread disease. Scarring alopecia can be prevented or lessened with close attention and aggressive therapy.

Callen JP. Cutaneous lupus erythematosus: a personal approach to management. Australas J Dermatol. 2006 Feb;47(1)13–27. [PMID: 16405478]

Lee HJ et al. Cutaneous lupus erythematosus: understanding of clinical features, genetic basis, and pathobiology of disease guides therapeutic strategies. Autoimmunity. 2006 Sep;39(6):433–44. [PMID: 17060022]

CUTANEOUS T CELL LYMPHOMA (Mycosis Fungoides)

 ESSENTIALS OF DIAGNOSIS

▸ Localized or generalized erythematous scaling patches and plaques.

▸ Pruritus.

▸ Lymphadenopathy.

▸ Distinctive histology.

General Considerations

Mycosis fungoides is a cutaneous T cell lymphoma that begins on the skin and may involve only the skin for years or decades. Certain medications (including selective serotonin reuptake inhibitors) may produce eruptions clinically and histologically identical to those of mycosis fungoides.

Clinical Findings

A. Symptoms and Signs

Localized or generalized erythematous patches or plaques are present usually on the trunk. Plaques are almost always over 5 cm in diameter. Pruritus is a frequent complaint. The lesions often begin as nondescript or nondiagnostic patches, and it is not unusual for the patient to have skin lesions for more than a decade before the diagnosis can be confirmed. In more advanced cases, tumors appear. Lymphadenopathy may occur locally or widely. Lymph node enlargement may be due to benign expansion of the node (dermatopathic lymphadenopathy) or by specific involvement with mycosis fungoides.

B. Laboratory Findings

The skin biopsy remains the basis of diagnosis, though at times numerous biopsies are required before the diagnosis can be confirmed. In more advanced disease, circulating atypical cells (Sézary cells) can be detected in the blood by sensitive methods. Eosinophilia may be present.

Differential Diagnosis

Mycosis fungoides may be confused with psoriasis, a drug eruption, an eczematous dermatitis, Hansen disease (leprosy), or tinea corporis. Histologic examination can distinguish these conditions.

Treatment

The treatment of mycosis fungoides is complex. Early and aggressive treatment has not proved to cure or prevent progression of the disease. Skin-directed therapies including topical corticosteroids, topical mechlorethamine, bexarotene gel, and UV phototherapy, are used initially. If the disease progresses, PUVA plus retinoids, PUVA plus interferon, extracorporeal photophoresis, bexarotene, alpha-interferon with or without retinoids, interleukin 12, denileukin, and total skin electron beam are used if the condition progresses. If these low toxicity systemic and biologic agents fail, standard chemotherapies, starting with single agents, are used.

Prognosis

Mycosis fungoides is usually slowly progressive (over decades). Prognosis is better in patients with patch or plaque stage disease and worse in patients with erythroderma, tumors, and lymphadenopathy. Survival is not reduced in patients with limited patch disease. Elderly patients with patch and plaque stage disease commonly die of other causes. Overly aggressive treatment may lead to complications and premature demise.

Hymes KB. Choices in the treatment of cutaneous T-cell lymphoma. Oncology (Williston Park). 2007 Feb;21(2 Suppl 1):18–23. [PMID: 17474355]

Olsen E et al. Revisions to the staging and classification of mycosis fungoides and Sézary syndrome: a proposal of the International Society for Cutaneous Lymphomas (ISCL) and the cutaneous lymphoma task force of the European Organization of Research and Treatment of Cancer (EORTC). Blood. 2007 Sep 15;110(6):1713–22. [PMID: 17540844]

EXFOLIATIVE DERMATITIS
(Exfoliative Erythroderma)

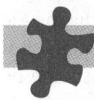 ESSENTIALS OF DIAGNOSIS

▶ Scaling and erythema over most of the body.
▶ Itching, malaise, fever, chills, weight loss.

General Considerations

Erythroderma describes generalized redness and scaling of the skin of more than 30% BSA. A preexisting dermatosis is the cause of exfoliative dermatitis in two-thirds of cases, including psoriasis, atopic dermatitis, contact dermatitis, pityriasis rubra pilaris, and seborrheic dermatitis. Reactions to topical or systemic drugs account for perhaps 20–40% of cases and cancer (cutaneous T cell lymphoma, Sézary syndrome) for 10–20%. Causation of the remainder is indeterminable. At the time of acute presentation, without a clear-cut prior history of skin disease or drug exposure, it may be impossible to make a specific diagnosis of the underlying condition, and diagnosis may require observation.

Clinical Findings

A. Symptoms and Signs

Symptoms may include itching, weakness, malaise, fever, and weight loss. Chills are prominent. Redness and scaling is widespread. Loss of hair and nails can occur. Generalized lymphadenopathy may be due to lymphoma or leukemia or may be reactive. The mucosae are spared.

B. Laboratory Findings

A skin biopsy is required and may show changes of a specific inflammatory dermatitis or cutaneous T cell lymphoma or leukemia. Peripheral leukocytes may show clonal rearrangements of the T cell receptor in Sézary syndrome.

Differential Diagnosis

It may be impossible to identify the cause of exfoliative erythroderma early in the course of the disease, so careful follow-up is necessary.

Complications

Debility (protein loss) and dehydration may develop in patients with generalized inflammatory exfoliative erythroderma; or sepsis may occur.

Treatment

A. Topical Therapy

Home treatment is with cool to tepid baths and application of mid-potency corticosteroids under wet dressings or with the use of an occlusive plastic suit. If the exfoliative erythroderma becomes chronic and is not manageable in an outpatient setting, hospitalize the patient. Keep the room at a constant warm temperature and provide the same topical treatment as for an outpatient.

B. Specific Measures

Stop all drugs, if possible. Systemic corticosteroids may provide spectacular improvement in severe or fulminant exfoliative dermatitis, but long-term therapy should be avoided (see Chapter 26). In addition, systemic corticosteroids must be used with caution because some patients with erythroderma have psoriasis and could develop pustular psoriasis. For cases of psoriatic erythroderma and pityriasis rubra pilaris, either acitretin or methotrexate may be indicated. Erythroderma secondary to lymphoma or leukemia requires specific topical or systemic chemotherapy. Suitable antibiotic drugs with coverage for *Staphylococcus* should be given when there is evidence of bacterial infection.

Prognosis

Most patients recover completely or improve greatly over time but may require long-term therapy. Deaths are rare in the absence of cutaneous T cell lymphoma. A minority of patients will suffer from undiminished erythroderma for indefinite periods.

Jaffer AN et al. Exfoliative dermatitis. Erythroderma can be a sign of a significant underlying disorder. Postgrad Med. 2005 Jan;117(1):49–51. [PMID: 15672891]

MISCELLANEOUS SCALING DERMATOSES

Isolated scaly patches may represent actinic (solar) keratoses, nonpigmented seborrheic keratoses, or Bowen or Paget disease.

1. Actinic Keratoses

Actinic keratoses are small (0.2–0.6 cm) macules or papules—flesh-colored, pink, or slightly hyperpigmented—that feel like sandpaper and are tender when the finger is drawn over them. They occur on sun-exposed parts of the body in persons of fair complexion. Actinic keratoses are considered premalignant, but only 1:1000 lesions per year progress to become squamous cell carcinomas.

Application of liquid nitrogen is a rapid and effective method of eradication. The lesions crust and disappear in 10–14 days. An alternative treatment is the use of fluorouracil cream. This agent may be rubbed into the lesions morning and night until they become first red and sore and then crusted and eroded (usually 2–3 weeks). Carac (0.5% fluorouracil) may be used once daily for a longer period (4 weeks to several months). Keratoses may clear with less irritation. Imiquimod 5% cream applied two to three times weekly for 3–6 weeks is the more costly alternative to topical fluorouracil (5FU). Any lesions that persist should be evaluated for possible biopsy.

McIntyre WJ et al. Treatment options for actinic keratoses. Am Fam Physician. 2007 Sep 1;76(5):667–71. [PMID: 17894135]

2. Bowen Disease & Paget Disease

Bowen disease (intraepidermal squamous cell carcinoma) occurs either on sun-exposed or sun-protected skin. The lesion is usually a small (0.5–3 cm), well-demarcated, slightly raised, pink to red, scaly plaque and may resemble psoriasis or a large actinic keratosis. These lesions may progress to invasive squamous cell carcinoma. Excision or other definitive treatment is indicated.

Extramammary Paget disease, a manifestation of intraepidermal carcinoma or underlying genitourinary or gastrointestinal cancer, resembles chronic eczema and usually involves apocrine areas such as the genitalia. Mammary Paget disease of the nipple, a unilateral or rarely bilateral red scaling plaque that may ooze, is associated with an underlying intraductal mammary carcinoma (Plate 17).

Cox NH et al; Therapy Guidelines and Audit Subcommittee, British Association of Dermatologists. Guidelines for management of Bowen's disease: 2006 update. Br J Dermatol. 2007 Jan;156(1):11–21. [PMID: 17199561]
Kanitakis J. Mammary and extramammary Paget's disease. J Eur Acad Dermatol Venereol. 2007 May;21(5):581–90. [PMID: 17447970]

INTERTRIGO

Intertrigo is caused by the macerating effect of heat, moisture, and friction. It is especially likely to occur in obese persons and in humid climates. The symptoms are itching, stinging, and burning. The body folds develop fissures, erythema, and sodden epidermis, with superficial denudation. Candidiasis may complicate intertrigo. "Inverse psoriasis," seborrheic dermatitis, tinea cruris, erythrasma, and candidiasis must be ruled out.

Maintain hygiene in the area, and keep it dry. Compresses may be useful acutely. Hydrocortisone 1% cream plus an imidazole or nystatin cream is effective. Recurrences are common.

VESICULAR DERMATOSES

HERPES SIMPLEX (Cold or Fever Sore; Genital Herpes)

ESSENTIALS OF DIAGNOSIS

▸ Recurrent small grouped vesicles on an erythematous base, especially in the orolabial and genital areas.

▸ May follow minor infections, trauma, stress, or sun exposure; regional lymph nodes may be swollen and tender.

▸ Viral cultures and direct fluorescent antibody tests are positive.

▸ General Considerations

Over 85% of adults have serologic evidence of herpes simplex type 1 (HSV-1) infections, most often acquired asymptomatically in childhood. Occasionally, primary infections may be manifested as severe gingivostomatitis. Thereafter, the patient may have recurrent self-limited attacks, provoked by sun exposure, orofacial surgery, fever, or a viral infection.

About 25% of the United States population has serologic evidence of infection with herpes simplex type 2 (HSV-2). HSV-2 causes lesions whose morphology and natural history are similar to those caused by HSV-1 on the genitalia of both sexes. The infection is acquired by sexual contact. In monogamous heterosexual couples where one partner has HSV-2 infection, seroconversion of the noninfected partner occurs in 10% over a 1-year period. Up to 70% of such infections appeared to be transmitted during periods of asymptomatic shedding. Genital herpes may also be due to HSV-1.

▸ Clinical Findings

A. Symptoms and Signs

The principal symptoms are burning and stinging. Neuralgia may precede or accompany attacks. The lesions consist of small, grouped vesicles that can occur anywhere but which most often occur on the vermilion border of the lips, the penile shaft, the labia, the perianal skin, and the buttocks (Plates 18 and 19). Any erosion in the genital region can be due to HSV-2 (or HSV-1). Regional lymph nodes may be swollen and tender. The lesions usually crust and heal in 1 week. Herpes simplex is the most common cause of painful genital ulcerations in patients with HIV infection.

B. Laboratory Findings

Lesions of herpes simplex must be distinguished from chancroid, syphilis, pyoderma, or trauma. Direct immunofluorescent antibody slide tests offer rapid, sensitive diagnosis. Viral culture may also be helpful. Herpes serology is not used in the diagnosis of an acute genital ulcer. However, specific HSV-2 serology by Western blot assay or enzyme-linked immunosorbent assay (ELISA) can determine who is HSV-infected and potentially infectious. Such testing is very useful in couples in which only one partner reports a history of genital herpes.

▶ Complications

Complications include pyoderma, eczema herpeticum, herpetic whitlow, herpes gladiatorum (epidemic herpes in wrestlers transmitted by contact), proctitis, esophagitis, neonatal infection, keratitis, and encephalitis.

▶ Prevention

Sunscreens are useful adjuncts in preventing sun-induced recurrences. Prophylactic use of oral acyclovir may prevent recurrences. Acyclovir should be started at a dosage of 200 mg four times daily beginning 24 hours prior to ultraviolet light exposure, dental surgery, or orolabial cosmetic surgery. Comparable doses are 500 mg twice daily for valacyclovir and 250 mg twice daily for famciclovir.

▶ Treatment

A. Systemic Therapy

Three systemic agents are available for the treatment of herpes infections: acyclovir, its valine analog valacyclovir, and famciclovir. All three agents are very effective and, when used properly, virtually nontoxic. Only acyclovir is available for intravenous administration. In the immunocompetent, with the exception of severe orolabial herpes, only genital disease is treated. For first clinical episodes of herpes simplex, the dosage of acyclovir is 200 mg orally five times daily (or 800 mg three times daily); of valacyclovir, 1000 mg twice daily; and of famciclovir, 250 mg three times daily. The duration of treatment is from 7 to 10 days depending on the severity of the outbreak. Most cases of recurrent herpes are mild and do not require therapy. In addition, pharmacotherapy of recurrent HSV is of limited benefit, with studies finding a reduction in the average outbreak by only 12–24 hours. To be effective, the treatment must be initiated by the patient at the first sign of recurrence. If treatment is desired, recurrent genital herpes outbreaks may be treated with 3 days of valacyclovir, 500 mg twice daily; or with 5 days of acyclovir, 200 mg five times a day, or famciclovir, 125 mg twice daily. Valacyclovir, 2 g twice daily for 1 day, or famciclovir, 1 g once or twice in 1 day, are equally effective short-course alternatives, and can abort impending recurrences of both orolabial or genital herpes. The addition of a potent topical corticosteroid three times daily reduces the duration, size, and pain of orolabial herpes treated with an oral antiviral agent.

In patients with frequent or severe recurrences, suppressive therapy is most effective in controlling disease. Suppressive treatment will reduce outbreaks by 85% and reduces viral shedding by more than 90%. This results in about a 50% reduced risk of transmission. The recommended suppressive doses, taken continuously, are acyclovir, 400 mg twice daily; valacyclovir, 500 mg once daily; or famciclovir, 125–250 mg twice daily. Long-term suppression appears very safe, and after 5–7 years a substantial proportion of patients can discontinue treatment. The use of condoms and patient education have proved effective in reducing genital herpes transmission in some studies and in others have not been beneficial. No single or combination intervention absolutely prevents transmission.

B. Local Measures

In general, topical therapy is not effective. It is strongly urged that 5% acyclovir ointment, if used at all, be limited to the restricted indications for which it has been approved, ie, initial herpes genitalis and mucocutaneous herpes simplex infections in immunocompromised patients. Penciclovir cream, to be applied at the first symptom every 2 hours while awake for 4 days for recurrent orolabial herpes, reduces the average attack duration from 5 days to 4.5 days.

▶ Prognosis

Aside from the complications described above, recurrent attacks last several days, and patients recover without sequelae.

Cernik C et al. The treatment of herpes simplex infections: an evidence-based review. Arch Intern Med. 2008 Jun 9;168 (11):1137–44. [PMID: 18541820]

Gupta R et al. Genital herpes. Lancet. 2007 Dec 22;370(9605):2127–37. [PMID: 18156035]

Spruance S et al. Short-course therapy for recurrent genital herpes and herpes labialis. J Fam Pract. 2007 Jan;56(1):30–6. [PMID: 17217895]

HERPES ZOSTER (Shingles)

 ESSENTIALS OF DIAGNOSIS

▶ Pain along the course of a nerve followed by grouped vesicular lesions.

▶ Involvement is unilateral; some lesions (< 20) may occur outside the affected dermatome.

▶ Lesions are usually on face or trunk.

▶ Direct fluorescent antibody positive, especially in vesicular lesions.

▶ General Considerations

Herpes zoster is an acute vesicular eruption due to the varicella-zoster virus. It usually occurs in adults. With rare exceptions, patients suffer only one attack. Dermatomal herpes zoster does not imply the presence of a visceral malignancy. Generalized disease, however, raises the suspicion of an associated immunosuppressive disorder such as Hodgkin disease or HIV infection. HIV-infected patients are 20 times more likely to develop zoster, often before other clinical findings of HIV disease are present. A history of HIV risk factors and HIV testing when appropriate should be considered, especially in patients with zoster who are younger than 55 years.

Clinical Findings

Pain usually precedes the eruption by 48 hours or more and may persist and actually increase in intensity after the lesions have disappeared. The lesions consist of grouped, tense, deep-seated vesicles distributed unilaterally along a dermatome (Plate 20). The most common distributions are on the trunk or face. Up to 20 lesions may be found outside the affected dermatomes. Regional lymph glands may be tender and swollen.

Differential Diagnosis

Since poison oak and poison ivy dermatitis can occur unilaterally, they must be differentiated at times from herpes zoster. Allergic contact dermatitis is pruritic; zoster is painful. One must differentiate herpes zoster from lesions of herpes simplex, which occasionally occurs in a dermatomal distribution. Doses of antivirals appropriate for zoster should be used in the absence of a clear diagnosis. Facial zoster may simulate erysipelas initially, but zoster is unilateral and shows vesicles after 24–48 hours. The pain of preeruptive herpes zoster may lead the clinician to diagnose migraine, myocardial infarction, acute abdomen, herniated disc, etc, depending on the dermatome involved.

Complications

Sacral zoster may be associated with bladder and bowel dysfunction. Persistent neuralgia, anesthesia or scarring of the affected area, facial or other nerve paralysis, and encephalitis may occur. Postherpetic neuralgia is most common after involvement of the trigeminal region, and in patients over the age of 55. Early (within 72 hours after onset) and aggressive antiviral treatment of herpes zoster reduces the severity and duration of postherpetic neuralgia. Zoster ophthalmicus (V_1) can result in visual impairment.

Prevention

An effective live herpes zoster vaccine (Zostavax) is available to prevent both herpes zoster and postherpetic neuralgia. It should be considered in persons aged 60 and older.

Treatment

A. General Measures

1. Immunocompetent host—Since early treatment of zoster reduces postherpetic neuralgia, those with a risk of developing this complication should be treated, ie, those over age 50 and those with nontruncal eruption. In addition, younger patients with acute moderate to severe pain or rash may benefit from effective antiviral therapy. Treatment can be given with oral acyclovir, 800 mg five times daily; famciclovir, 500 mg three times daily; or valacyclovir, 1 g three times daily—all for 7 days (see Chapter 32). For reasons of increased bioavailability and ease of dosing schedule, the preferred agents are those given three times daily. Patients should maintain good hydration. The dose of antiviral should be adjusted for kidney function as recommended. Nerve blocks may be used in the management of initial severe pain. Ophthalmologic consultation is vital for involvement of the first branch of the trigeminal nerve. Systemic corticosteroids are effective in reducing acute pain, improving quality of life, and returning patients to normal activities much more quickly. They do not increase the risk of dissemination in immunocompetent hosts. If not contraindicated, a tapering 3-week course of prednisone, starting at 60 mg/d, should be considered for its adjunctive benefit in immunocompetent patients. Oral corticosteroids do not reduce the prevalence, severity, or duration of postherpetic neuralgia beyond that achieved by effective antiviral therapy.

2. Immunocompromised host—Given the safety and efficacy of currently available antivirals, most immunocompromised patients with herpes zoster are candidates for antiviral therapy. The dosage schedule is as listed above, but treatment should be continued until the lesions have completely crusted and are healed or almost healed (up to 2 weeks). Because corticosteroids increase the risk of dissemination in immunosuppressed patients, they should not be used in these patients. Progression of disease may necessitate intravenous therapy with acyclovir, 10 mg/kg intravenously, three times daily. After 3–4 days, oral therapy may be substituted if there has been a good response to intravenous therapy. Adverse effects include decreased kidney function from crystallization, nausea and vomiting, and abdominal pain.

Foscarnet, administered in a dosage of 40 mg/kg two or three times daily intravenously, is indicated for treatment of acyclovir-resistant varicella-zoster virus infections.

B. Local Measures

Calamine or starch shake lotions may be of some help.

C. Postherpetic Neuralgia Therapy

The most effective treatment is prevention with vaccination of those at risk for developing zoster and early and aggressive antiviral therapy once zoster has occurred. Once established, postherpetic neuralgia may be treated with capsaicin ointment, 0.025–0.075%, or lidocaine (Lidoderm) topical patches. Chronic postherpetic neuralgia may be relieved by regional blocks (stellate ganglion, epidural, local infiltration, or peripheral nerve), with or without corticosteroids added to the injections. Amitriptyline, 25–75 mg as a single nightly dose, is the first-line oral therapy beyond simple analgesics. Gabapentin, up to 3600 mg daily (starting at 300 mg three times daily), may be added for additional pain relief. Referral to a pain management clinic should be considered in moderate to severe cases and in those failing the above treatments.

Prognosis

The eruption persists 2–3 weeks and usually does not recur. Motor involvement in 2–3% of patients may lead to temporary palsy.

Dworkin RH et al. Recommendations for the management of herpes zoster. Clin Infect Dis. 2007 Jan 1;44(Suppl 1):S1–S26. [PMID: 17143845]

Opstelten W et al. Treatment of herpes zoster. Can Fam Physician. 2008 Mar;54(3):373–7. [PMID: 18337531]

Oxman MN et al; Shingles Prevention Study Group. A vaccine to prevent herpes zoster and postherpetic neuralgia in older adults. N Engl J Med. 2005 Jun 2;352(22):2271–84. [PMID: 15930418]

Schmader K. Herpes zoster and postherpetic neuralgia in older adults. Clin Geriatr Med. 2007 Aug;23(3):615–32. [PMID: 17631237]

Woolery WA. Herpes zoster virus vaccine. Geriatrics. 2008 Oct;63(10):6–9. [PMID: 18828650]

VARIOLA (Smallpox) & VACCINIA

 ESSENTIALS OF DIAGNOSIS

▶ Prodromal high fever.

▶ Eruption progressing from papules to vesicles to pustules, then crusts.

▶ All lesions in the same stage.

▶ Face and distal extremities (including palms and soles) favored.

General Considerations

Concern for the use of smallpox virus as a bioterrorist weapon has led to the reintroduction of vaccination in some segments of the population (first responders and the military).

Clinical Findings

The incubation period for variola averages 12 days (7–17 days). The prodrome begins with abrupt onset of high fever, severe headaches, and backaches. At this stage, the infected person appears quite ill. The infectious phase begins with the appearance of an enanthem, followed in 1–2 days by a skin eruption. The lesions begin as macules, progressing to papules, then pustules, and finally crusts over 14–18 days. The face and distal extremities are favored. The face is affected first, followed by the upper extremities, then the lower extremities and trunk, completely evolving over 1 week. Lesions are relatively monomorphous, especially in each anatomic region.

Inoculation with vaccinia produces a papular lesion on day 2–3 that progresses to an umbilicated papule by day 4 and a pustular lesion by the end of the first week. The lesion then collapses centrally, and crusts. The crust eventually detaches up to a month after the inoculation. Persons with eczema should not be immunized as they may suffer widespread vaccinia (eczema vaccinatum) whose lesions might resemble those of smallpox. Vaccinia is moderately contagious, and patients with atopic dermatitis and Darier disease may acquire severe generalized disease by exposure to a recently vaccinated person. Generalized vaccinia may be fatal. Prior vaccination does not prevent generalized vaccinia, but previously vaccinated individuals have milder disease. Progressive vaccinia (vaccinia gangrenosum)—progression of the primary inoculation site to a large ulceration—occurs in persons with systemic immune deficiency. It can have a fatal outcome.

Differential Diagnosis

Smallpox and vaccinia are to be distinguished from generalized varicella zoster virus infection or generalized herpes simplex. The latter two viral infections are not associated with a severe febrile prodrome. Lesions are at various stages at each anatomic site. Varicella usually appears in waves or crops. Multiple palm and sole lesions are common in variola and uncommon in generalized varicella-zoster and herpes simplex infection.

Direct fluorescent antibody testing for HSV and varicella zoster virus are the first-line diagnostic tests to differentiate varicella zoster virus, HSV, vaccinia, and variola. Until the diagnosis is confirmed, strict isolation of the patient is indicated. Similar fluorescent testing for variola can be performed in special laboratories.

Treatment

There is no specific and proven antiviral therapy for vaccinia or variola. Vaccinia immune globulin is used to treat eczema vaccinatum and progressive vaccinia. Cidofovir may have some activity against these poxviruses.

Moore ZS et al. Smallpox. Lancet. 2006 Feb 4;367(9508):425–35. [PMID: 16458769]

POMPHOLYX; VESICULOBULLOUS HAND ECZEMA (Formerly Known as Dyshidrosis, Dyshidrotic Eczema)

 ESSENTIALS OF DIAGNOSIS

▶ "Tapioca" vesicles of 1–2 mm on the palms, soles, and sides of fingers, associated with pruritus.

▶ Vesicles may coalesce to form multiloculated blisters.

▶ Scaling and fissuring may follow drying of the blisters.

▶ Appearance in the third decade, with lifelong recurrences.

General Considerations

This is an extremely common form of hand dermatitis, preferably called pompholyx (Gr "bubble") or vesiculobullous dermatitis of the palms and soles. Patients often have an atopic background and report flares with stress. Patients with widespread dermatitis due to any cause may develop pompholyx-like eruptions as a part of an autoeczematization response.

Clinical Findings

Small clear vesicles stud the skin at the sides of the fingers and on the palms or soles (Plate 21). They look like the grains in tapioca. They may be associated with intense itching. Later, the vesicles dry and the area becomes scaly and fissured.

Differential Diagnosis

Unroofing the vesicles and examining the blister roof with a KOH preparation will reveal hyphae in cases of bullous tinea. Patients with inflammatory tinea pedis may have a vesicular dermatophytid of the palms. Always examine the feet of a patient with a hand eruption. Nonsteroidal anti-inflammatory drugs (NSAIDs) may produce an eruption very similar to that of dyshidrosis on the hands.

Prevention

There is no known way to prevent attacks.

Treatment

Topical and systemic corticosteroids help some patients dramatically. Since this is a chronic problem, systemic corticosteroids are generally not appropriate therapy. A high-potency topical corticosteroid used early in the attack may help abort the flare and ameliorate pruritus. Topical corticosteroids are also important in treating the scaling and fissuring that are seen after the vesicular phase. It is essential that patients avoid anything that irritates the skin; they should wear cotton gloves inside vinyl gloves when doing dishes or other wet chores, use long-handled brushes instead of sponges, and use a hand cream after washing the hands. Patients respond to PUVA therapy and injection of botulinum toxin into the palms as for hyperhidrosis.

Prognosis

For most patients, the disease is an inconvenience. For some, vesiculobullous hand eczema can be incapacitating.

Lofgren SM et al. Dyshidrosis: epidemiology, clinical characteristics, and therapy. Dermatitis. 2006 Dec;17(4):165–81. [PMID: 17150166]

PORPHYRIA CUTANEA TARDA

    ESSENTIALS OF DIAGNOSIS

► Noninflammatory blisters on sun-exposed sites, especially the dorsal surfaces of the hands.

► Hypertrichosis, skin fragility.

► Associated liver disease.

► Elevated urine porphyrins.

General Considerations

Porphyria cutanea tarda is the most common type of porphyria. Cases are sporadic or hereditary. The disease is associated with ingestion of certain medications (eg, estrogens), and liver disease from alcoholism or hepatitis C. In patients with liver disease, hemosiderosis is often present.

Clinical Findings

A. Symptoms and Signs

Patients complain of painless blistering and fragility of the skin of the dorsal surfaces of the hands (Plate 22). Facial hypertrichosis and hyperpigmentation are common.

B. Laboratory Findings

Urinary uroporphyrins are elevated twofold to fivefold above coproporphyrins. Patients may also have abnormal liver function tests, evidence of hepatitis C infection, increased liver iron stores, and hemochromatosis gene mutations. Multiple triggering factors are often discovered.

Differential Diagnosis

Skin lesions identical to those of porphyria cutanea tarda may be seen in patients who receive maintenance dialysis and in those who take certain medications (tetracyclines and NSAIDs, especially naproxen, and voriconazole). In this so-called pseudoporphyria, the biopsy results are identical to those associated with porphyria cutanea tarda, but urine porphyrins are normal.

Prevention

Although the lesions are triggered by sun exposure, the wavelength of light triggering the lesions is beyond that absorbed by sunscreens, which for that reason are ineffective. Barrier sun protection with clothing is required.

Treatment

Stopping all triggering medications and substantially reducing or stopping alcohol consumption may alone lead to improvement. Phlebotomy without oral iron supplementation at a rate of 1 unit every 2–4 weeks will gradually lead to improvement. Very low dose antimalarials (as low as 200 mg of hydroxychloroquine twice weekly), alone or in combination with phlebotomy, will increase the excretion of porphyrins, improving the skin disease. Treatment is continued until the patient is asymptomatic. Urine porphyrins may be monitored.

Prognosis

Most patients improve with treatment. Sclerodermoid skin lesions may develop on the trunk, scalp, and face.

Sassa S. Modern diagnosis and management of the porphyrias. Br J Haematol. 2006 Nov;135(3):281–92. [PMID: 16956347]

DERMATITIS HERPETIFORMIS

Dermatitis herpetiformis is an uncommon disease manifested by pruritic papules, vesicles, and papulovesicles mainly on the elbows, knees, buttocks, posterior neck, and scalp. It appears to have its highest prevalence in Scandinavia and is associated with HLA antigens -B8, -DR3, and -DQ2. The diagnosis is made by light microscopy, which demonstrates neutrophils at the dermal papillary tips. Direct immunofluorescence studies show granular deposits of IgA in the dermal papillae. Circulating antibodies to tissue transglutaminase are present in 90% of cases. NSAIDs may cause a flare. Patients have gluten-sensitive enteropathy, but for the great majority it is subclinical. However, ingestion of gluten is the cause of the disease, and strict long-term avoidance of dietary gluten has been shown to decrease the dose of dapsone (usually 100–200 mg/d) required to control the disease and may even eliminate the need for treatment. Patients with dermatitis herpetiformis are at increased risk for development of gastrointestinal lymphoma, and this risk is reduced by a gluten-free diet.

Zone JJ. Skin manifestations of celiac disease. Gastroenterology. 2005 Apr;128(4 Suppl 1):S87–91. [PMID: 15825132]

WEEPING OR CRUSTED LESIONS

IMPETIGO

ESSENTIALS OF DIAGNOSIS

▶ Superficial blisters filled with purulent material that rupture easily.

▶ Crusted superficial erosions.

▶ Positive Gram stain and bacterial culture.

General Considerations

Impetigo is a contagious and autoinoculable infection of the skin caused by staphylococci or streptococci.

Clinical Findings

A. Symptoms and Signs

The lesions consist of macules, vesicles, bullae, pustules, and honey-colored gummy crusts that when removed leave denuded red areas (Plate 23). The face and other exposed parts are most often involved. **Ecthyma** is a deeper form of impetigo caused by staphylococci or streptococci, with ulceration and scarring. It occurs frequently on the extremities.

B. Laboratory Findings

Gram stain and culture confirm the diagnosis. In temperate climates, most cases are associated with *S aureus* infec-

tion. *Streptococcus* species are more common in tropical infections. Community-associated methicillin-resistant *S aureus* (CA-MRSA) can be isolated from lesions of impetigo and ecthyma.

Differential Diagnosis

The main differential diagnoses are acute allergic contact dermatitis and herpes simplex. Contact dermatitis may be suggested by the history or by linear distribution of the lesions, and culture should be negative for staphylococci and streptococci. Herpes simplex infection usually presents with grouped vesicles or discrete erosions and may be associated with a history of recurrences. Viral cultures are positive.

Treatment

Soaks and scrubbing can be beneficial, especially in unroofing lakes of pus under thick crusts. Topical agents such as bacitracin, mupirocin, or retapamulin can be attempted for infections limited to small areas. Mupirocin and retapamulin are more expensive than systemic treatments. In most cases, systemic antibiotics are indicated. Cephalexin, 250 mg four times daily, is usually effective. Doxycycline, 100 mg twice daily, is a reasonable alternative. CA-MRSA may cause impetigo, and initial coverage for MRSA could include doxycycline, clindamycin, or trimethoprim-sulfamethoxazole (TMP-SMZ). About 50% of CA-MRSA cases are quinolone resistant. Recurrent impetigo is associated with nasal carriage of *S aureus*, treated with rifampin, 600 mg daily. Intranasal mupirocin ointment twice daily for 5 days clears the carriage of 40% of MRSA strains. Bleach baths ($^1/_2$ to 1 cup per 20 liters of bathwater for 15 minutes 3–5 times weekly) for all family members, and the use of dilute household bleach to clean showers and other bath surfaces may help reduce the spread. Individuals should not share towels if there is a case of impetigo in the household.

Cole C et al. Diagnosis and treatment of impetigo. Am Fam Physician. 2007 Mar 15;75(6):859–64. [PMID: 17390597]

ALLERGIC CONTACT DERMATITIS

ESSENTIALS OF DIAGNOSIS

▶ Erythema and edema, with pruritus, often followed by vesicles and bullae in an area of contact with a suspected agent.

▶ Later, weeping, crusting, or secondary infection.

▶ A history of previous reaction to suspected contactant.

▶ Patch test with agent positive.

General Considerations

Contact dermatitis is an acute or chronic dermatitis that results from direct skin contact with chemicals or allergens. Eighty percent of cases are due to excessive exposure to or additive effects of primary or universal irritants (eg, soaps, detergents, organic solvents) and are called irritant contact dermatitis. This appears red and scaly but not vesicular. The most common causes of allergic contact dermatitis are poison ivy or poison oak; topically applied antimicrobials (especially bacitracin and neomycin), anesthetics (benzocaine); hair-care products; preservatives; jewelry (nickel); rubber; vitamin E; essential oils; propolis (from bees); and adhesive tape. Occupational exposure is an important cause of allergic contact dermatitis. Weeping and crusting are typically due to allergic and not irritant dermatitis.

► Clinical Findings

A. Symptoms and Signs

In allergic contact dermatitis, the acute phase is characterized by tiny vesicles and weepy and crusted lesions, whereas resolving or chronic contact dermatitis presents with scaling, erythema, and possibly thickened skin (Plate 24). Itching, burning, and stinging may be severe. The lesions, distributed on exposed parts or in bizarre asymmetric patterns, consist of erythematous macules, papules, and vesicles. The affected area is often hot and swollen, with exudation and crusting, simulating—and at times complicated by—infection. The pattern of the eruption may be diagnostic (eg, typical linear streaked vesicles on the extremities in poison oak or ivy dermatitis). The location will often suggest the cause: Scalp involvement suggests hair dyes or shampoos; face involvement, creams, cosmetics, soaps, shaving materials, nail polish; and neck involvement, jewelry, hair dyes.

B. Laboratory Findings

Gram stain and culture will rule out impetigo or secondary infection (impetiginization). If itching is generalized, then scabies should be considered. After the episode has cleared, patch testing may be useful if the triggering allergen is not known.

► Differential Diagnosis

Asymmetric distribution, blotchy erythema around the face, linear lesions, and a history of exposure help distinguish acute contact dermatitis from other skin lesions. The most commonly mistaken diagnosis is impetigo. Chronic allergic contact dermatitis must be differentiated from scabies, atopic dermatitis, pompholyx, and other eczemas.

► Prevention

Prompt and thorough removal of the causative oil by washing with liquid dishwashing soap (eg, Dial Ultra) may be effective if done within 30 minutes after exposure to poison oak or ivy. The three most effective over-the-counter barrier creams which are applied prior to exposure and prevent/reduce the severity of the dermatitis are Stokogard, Hollister Moisture Barrier, and Hydropel.

    The mainstay of prevention is identification of the agent causing the dermatitis and avoidance of exposure or use of protective clothing and gloves. In industry-related cases, prevention may be accomplished by moving or retraining the worker.

► Treatment

A. Overview

While local measures are important, severe or widespread involvement is difficult to manage without systemic corticosteroids because even the highest-potency topical corticosteroids seem not to work well on vesicular and weepy lesions. Localized involvement (except on the face) can often be managed solely with topical agents. Irritant contact dermatitis is treated by protection from the irritant and use of topical corticosteroids as for atopic dermatitis (described above). The treatment of allergic contact dermatitis is detailed below.

B. Local Measures

1. Acute weeping dermatitis—Compresses are most often used. It is unwise to scrub lesions with soap and water. Calamine lotion may be used between wet dressings, especially for involvement of intertriginous areas or when oozing is not marked. Lesions on the extremities may be bandaged with wet dressings for 30–60 minutes several times a day. High potency topical corticosteroids in gel or cream form (eg, fluocinonide, clobetasol, or halobetasol) may help suppress acute contact dermatitis and relieve itching. This treatment should be followed by tapering of the number of applications per day or use of a mid-potency corticosteroid such as triamcinolone 0.1% cream to prevent rebound of the dermatitis. A soothing formulation is 2 oz of 0.1% triamcinolone acetonide cream in 7.5 oz Sarna lotion (0.5% camphor, 0.5% menthol, 0.5% phenol) mixed by the patient.

2. Subacute dermatitis (subsiding)—Mid-potency (triamcinolone 0.1%) to high-potency corticosteroids (clobetasol, amcinonide, fluocinonide, desoximetasone) are the mainstays of therapy.

3. Chronic dermatitis (dry and lichenified)—High-potency to superpotency corticosteroids are used in ointment form.

C. Systemic Therapy

For acute severe cases, prednisone may be given orally for 12–21 days. Prednisone, 60 mg for 4–7 days, 40 mg for 4–7 days, and 20 mg for 4–7 days without a further taper is one useful regimen. Another is to dispense seventy-eight 5-mg pills to be taken 12 the first day, 11 the second day, and so on. The key is to use enough corticosteroid (and as early as possible) to achieve a clinical effect and to taper slowly enough to avoid rebound. A Medrol Dosepak (methylprednisolone) with 5 days of medication is inappropriate on both counts. (See Chapter 26.)

► Prognosis

Allergic contact dermatitis is self-limited if reexposure is prevented but often takes 2–3 weeks for full resolution.

Craig K et al. What is the best duration of steroid therapy for contact dermatitis (rhus)? J Fam Pract. 2006 Feb;55(2):166–7. [PMID: 16451787]

Mark BJ et al. Allergic contact dermatitis. Med Clin North Am. 2006 Jan;90(1):169–85. [PMID: 16310529]

PUSTULAR DISORDERS

ACNE VULGARIS

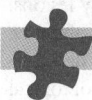 ESSENTIALS OF DIAGNOSIS

▶ Occurs at puberty, though onset may be delayed into the third or fourth decade.

▶ Open and closed comedones are the hallmark of acne vulgaris.

▶ The most common of all skin conditions.

▶ Severity varies from purely comedonal to papular or pustular inflammatory acne to cysts or nodules.

▶ Face and upper trunk may be affected.

▶ Scarring may be a sequela of the disease or picking and manipulating by the patient.

▶ General Considerations

Acne vulgaris is polymorphic. Open and closed comedones, papules, pustules, and cysts are found. The disease is activated by androgens in those who are genetically predisposed.

Acne vulgaris is more common and more severe in males. It does not always clear spontaneously when maturity is reached. Twelve percent of women and 3% of men over age 25 have acne vulgaris. This rate does not decrease until after age 44. The skin lesions parallel sebaceous activity. Pathogenic events include plugging of the infundibulum of the follicles, retention of sebum, overgrowth of the acne bacillus (*Propionibacterium acnes*) with resultant release of and irritation by accumulated fatty acids, and foreign body reaction to extrafollicular sebum. The mechanism of antibiotics in controlling acne is not clearly understood, but they may work because of their antibacterial or anti-inflammatory properties.

When a resistant case of acne is encountered in a woman, hyperandrogenism may be suspected. This may or may not be accompanied by hirsutism, irregular menses, or other signs of virilism. Polycystic ovary syndrome (PCOS) is the most common identifiable cause.

▶ Clinical Findings

There may be mild soreness, pain, or itching. The lesions occur mainly over the face, neck, upper chest, back, and shoulders. Comedones are the hallmark of acne vulgaris (Plate 25). Closed comedones are tiny, flesh-colored, non-inflamed bumps that give the skin a rough texture or appearance. Open comedones typically are a bit larger and have black material in them. Inflammatory papules, pustules, ectatic pores, acne cysts, and scarring are also seen.

Acne may have different presentations at different ages. Preteens often present with comedones as their first lesions. Inflammatory lesions in young teenagers are often found in the middle of the face, extending outward as the patient becomes older. Women in their third and fourth decades (often with no prior history of acne) commonly present with papular lesions on the chin and around the mouth.

▶ Differential Diagnosis

In adults, acne rosacea presents with papules and pustules in the middle third of the face, but telangiectasia, flushing, and the absence of comedones distinguish this disease from acne vulgaris. A pustular eruption on the face in patients receiving antibiotics or with otitis externa should be investigated with culture to rule out an uncommon gram-negative folliculitis. Acne may develop in patients who use systemic corticosteroids or topical fluorinated corticosteroids on the face. Acne may be exacerbated or caused by irritating creams or oils. Pustules on the face can also be caused by tinea infections. Lesions on the back are more problematic. When they occur alone, staphylococcal folliculitis, miliaria ("heat rash") or, uncommonly, *Malassezia* folliculitis should be suspected. Bacterial culture, trial of an antistaphylococcal antibiotic, and observing the response to therapy will help in the differential diagnosis. In patients with HIV infection, folliculitis is common and may be either staphylococcal folliculitis or eosinophilic folliculitis.

▶ Complications

Cyst formation, pigmentary changes in pigmented patients, severe scarring, and psychological problems may result.

▶ Treatment

A. General Measures

1. Education of the patient—When scarring seems out of proportion to the severity of the lesions, clinicians must suspect that the patient is manipulating the lesions. It is essential that the patient be educated in a supportive way about this complication. Anxiety and depression are often the underlying cause of young women excoriating minor acne. It is wise to let the patient know that at least 4–6 weeks will be required to see improvement and that old lesions may take months to fade. Therefore, improvement will be judged according to the number of new lesions forming after 6–8 weeks of therapy. Additional time will be required to see improvement on the back and chest, as these areas are slowest to respond. If hair pomades are used, they should contain glycerin and not oil. Avoid topical exposure to oils, cocoa butter (theobroma oil), and greases.

2. Diet—A low glycemic diet that results in weight loss has been reported to improve acne in males aged 15–25. This improvement was associated with a reduction in insulin resistance. Hyperinsulinemia has also been associated with acne in eumenorrheic women. The metabolic syndrome with insulin resistance can also be a feature of PCOS in women. This finding suggests a possible common pathogenic mechanism for acne in both adult women and men.

B. Comedonal Acne

Treatment of acne is based on the type and severity of lesions. Comedones require treatment different from that of pustules and cystic lesions. In assessing severity, take the sequelae of the lesions into account. An individual who gets only a few new lesions per month that scar or leave postinflammatory hyperpigmentation must be treated much more aggressively than a comparable patient whose lesions clear without sequelae. Soaps play little role in acne treatment, and unless the patient's skin is exceptionally oily, a mild soap should be used to avoid irritation that will limit the usefulness of other topicals, all of which are themselves somewhat irritating.

1. Topical retinoids—Tretinoin is very effective for comedonal acne or for treatment of the comedonal component of more severe acne, but its usefulness is limited by irritation. Start with 0.025% cream (not gel) and have the patient use it at first twice weekly at night, then build up to as often as nightly. A few patients cannot use even this low-strength preparation more than three times weekly but even that may cause improvement. A lentil-sized amount is sufficient to cover the entire face. To avoid irritation, have the patient wait 20 minutes after washing to apply. Adapalene gel 0.1% and reformulated tretinoin (Renova, Retin A Micro, Avita) are other options for patients irritated by standard tretinoin preparations. Some patients—especially teenagers—do best on 0.01% gel. Although the absorption of tretinoin is minimal, its use during pregnancy is contraindicated. Some patients report photosensitivity with tretinoin. Patients should be warned that they may flare in the first 4 weeks of treatment. Tazarotene gel (0.05% or 0.1%) (Tazorac) is another topical retinoid approved for treatment of psoriasis and acne, and may be used in patients intolerant of the other retinoids.

2. Benzoyl peroxide—Benzoyl peroxide products are available in concentrations of 2.5%, 4%, 5%, 8%, and 10%, but it appears that 2.5% is as effective as 10% and less irritating. In general, water-based and not alcohol-based gels should be used to decrease irritation.

3. Antibiotics—Use of topical antibiotics (see below) has been demonstrated to decrease pustular and comedonal lesions.

4. Comedo extraction—Open and closed comedones may be removed with a comedo.

C. Papular Inflammatory Acne

Antibiotics are the mainstay for treatment of inflammatory acne. They may be used topically or orally. The oral antibiotics of choice are tetracycline and doxycycline. Minocycline is often effective in acne unresponsive or resistant to treatment with these antibiotics but it is more expensive. Rarely, other antibiotics such as TMP-SMZ (one double-strength tablet twice daily), clindamycin (150 mg twice daily), or a cephalosporin (cefadroxil or cephalexin) may be used. Topical clindamycin phosphate and erythromycin are also used (see below). Topicals are probably the equivalent of about 500 mg/d of tetracycline given orally, which is half the usual starting dose. Topical antibiotics are used in three situations: for mild papular acne that can be controlled by topicals alone, for patients who refuse or cannot tolerate oral antibiotics, or to wean patients under good control from oral to topical preparations. To decrease resistance, benzoyl peroxide should be used in combination with the topical antibiotic.

1. Mild acne—The first choice of topical antibiotics in terms of efficacy and relative lack of induction of resistant *P acnes* is the combination of erythromycin or clindamycin with benzoyl peroxide topical gel. Clindamycin (Cleocin T) lotion (least irritating), gel, or solution, or one of the many brands of topical erythromycin gel or solution, may be used twice daily and the benzoyl peroxide in the morning. (A combination of erythromycin or clindamycin with benzoyl peroxide is available as a prescription item.) The addition of tretinoin 0.025% cream or 0.01% gel at night may increase improvement, since it works via a different mechanism.

2. Moderate acne—Tetracycline, 500 mg twice daily, doxycycline, 100 mg twice daily, and minocycline, 50–100 mg twice daily, are all effective though minocycline is more expensive. When initiating minocycline therapy, start at 100 mg in the evening for 4–7 days, then 100 mg twice daily, to decrease the incidence of vertigo. Plan a return visit in 6 weeks and at 3–4 months after that. If the patient's skin is quite clear, instructions should be given for tapering the dose by 250 mg for tetracycline, by 100 mg for doxycycline, or by 50 mg for minocycline every 6–8 weeks—while treating with topicals—to arrive at the lowest systemic dose needed to maintain clearing. In general, lowering the dose to zero without other therapy results in prompt recurrence of acne. Tetracycline, minocycline, and doxycycline are contraindicated in pregnancy, but oral erythromycin may be used.

It is important to discuss the issue of contraceptive failure when prescribing antibiotics for women taking oral contraceptives. Women may need to consider using barrier methods as well, and should report breakthrough bleeding. Oral contraceptives or spironolactone (50–200 mg daily) may be added as an antiandrogen in women with antibiotic-resistant acne or in women in whom relapse occurs after isotretinoin therapy.

3. Severe acne

A. ISOTRETINOIN—A vitamin A analog, isotretinoin is used for the treatment of severe cystic acne that has not responded to conventional therapy. A dosage of 0.5–1 mg/kg/d for 20 weeks for a cumulative dose of at least 120 mg/kg is usually adequate for severe cystic acne. Patients should be offered isotretinoin therapy before they experience significant scarring if they are not promptly and adequately controlled by antibiotics. The drug is *absolutely contraindicated during pregnancy* because of its teratogenicity; two serum pregnancy tests should be obtained before starting the drug in a female and every month thereafter. Sufficient medication for only 1 month should be dispensed. Two forms of effective contraception must be used. Informed consent must be obtained before its use and patients must be enrolled in a monitoring program (iPledge). Side effects occur in most patients, usually related to dry skin and mucous membranes (dry lips, nosebleed, and dry eyes). If headache occurs, pseudotumor cerebri must be considered. Depression has been reported. Hypertriglyceridemia will develop in about 25% of patients, hypercholesterolemia in 15%, and a lowering of high-density lipoproteins in 5%. Minor elevations in liver function tests may develop in some patients. Fasting blood sugar may be elevated. Miscellaneous adverse reactions include decreased night vision, musculoskeletal or bowel symptoms, dry skin, thinning of hair, exuberant granulation tissue in lesions, and bony hyperostoses (seen only with very high doses or with long duration of therapy). Moderate to severe myalgias rarely necessitate decreasing the dosage or stopping the drug. Laboratory tests to be performed in all patients before treatment and after 4 weeks on therapy include cholesterol, triglycerides, and liver function studies.

Elevations of liver enzymes and triglycerides return to normal upon conclusion of therapy. The drug may induce long-term remissions in 40–60%, or acne may recur that is more easily controlled with conventional therapy. Occasionally, acne does not respond or promptly recurs after therapy, but it may clear after a second course.

B. INTRALESIONAL INJECTION—In otherwise moderate acne, intralesional injection of dilute suspensions of triamcinolone acetonide (2.5 mg/mL, 0.05 mL per lesion) will often hasten the resolution of deeper papules and occasional cysts.

C. LASER, DERMABRASION—Cosmetic improvement may be achieved by excision and punch-grafting of deep scars and by abrasion of inactive acne lesions, particularly flat, superficial scars. The technique is not without untoward effects, since hyperpigmentation, hypopigmentation, grooving, and scarring have been known to occur. Dark-skinned individuals do poorly. Corrective surgery within 12 months after isotretinoin therapy may not be advisable. Active acne of all types can be treated with certain laser and photodynamic therapies. This can be considered when standard treatments are contraindicated or fail.

Prognosis

Acne vulgaris eventually remits spontaneously, but when this will occur cannot be predicted. The condition may persist throughout adulthood and may lead to severe scarring if left untreated. Patients treated with antibiotics continue to improve for the first 3–6 months of therapy. Relapse during treatment may suggest the emergence of resistant *P acnes*. The disease is chronic and tends to flare intermittently in spite of treatment. Remissions following systemic treatment with isotretinoin may be lasting in up to 60% of cases. Relapses after isotretinoin usually occur within 3 years and require a second course in up to 20% of patients.

Goodman G. Managing acne vulgaris effectively. Aust Fam Physician. 2006 Sep;35(9):705–9. [PMID: 16969442]

James WD. Clinical practice. Acne. N Engl J Med. 2005 Apr 7;352(14):1463–72. [PMID: 15814882]

Smith RN et al. The effect of a high-protein, low glycemic-load diet versus a conventional, high glycemic-load diet on biochemical parameters associated with acne vulgaris: a randomized, investigator-masked, controlled trial. J Am Acad Dermatol. 2007 Aug;57(2):247–56. [PMID: 17448569]

ROSACEA

 ESSENTIALS OF DIAGNOSIS

▶ A chronic facial disorder.

▶ A neurovascular component (erythema and telangiectasis and a tendency to flush easily).

▶ An acneiform component (papules and pustules) may also be present.

▶ A glandular component accompanied by hyperplasia of the soft tissue of the nose (rhinophyma).

General Considerations

The pathogenesis of this disorder is not known. Topical corticosteroids applied to the lower face can induce rosacea-like conditions.

Clinical Findings

Patients frequently report flushing or exacerbation of their rosacea by heat or cold, hot drinks, spicy food, sunlight, exercise, alcohol, emotions, and menopausal flushing. The cheeks, nose, and chin—at times the entire face—may have a rosy hue. No comedones are seen. In its mildest form, erythema and dilated vessels are seen on the cheeks. Inflammatory papules may be superimposed on this background and may evolve to pustules (Plate 26). Associated seborrhea may be found. The patient often complains of burning or stinging with episodes of flushing. Patients may have associated ophthalmic disease, including blepharitis and keratitis, that often requires systemic antibiotic therapy.

Differential Diagnosis

Rosacea is distinguished from acne by the presence of the neurovascular component and the absence of comedones. The rosy hue of rosacea and telangiectasis will pinpoint the diagnosis. Lupus is often misdiagnosed, but the presence of pustules excludes that diagnosis.

Treatment

Educating patients to avoid the factors they know to produce exacerbations is important. Patients should wear a broad-spectrum sunscreen with UVA coverage; however, exquisite sensitivity to topical preparations may limit patient options. Zinc- or titanium-based sunscreens are better tolerated, and barrier protective silicones in the sunblock may enhance tolerance. Medical management is effective only for the inflammatory papules and pustules and the erythema that surrounds them. Rosacea is usually a lifelong condition, so maintenance therapy is required.

A. Local Therapy

Metronidazole (available as creams, gels, or lotions), 0.75% applied twice daily or 1% applied once daily, is the topical treatment of choice. If metronidazole is not tolerated, topical clindamycin (solution, gel, or lotion) 1% applied twice daily is effective. Response is noted in 4–8 weeks. Sulfur-sodium sulfacetamide-containing topicals are helpful in patients only partially responsive to topical antibiotics. Benzoyl peroxide, as in acne vulgaris, may be helpful in reducing the pustular component. Topical retinoids can be carefully added for maintenance.

B. Systemic Therapy

Tetracycline, 250 or 500 mg orally twice daily on an empty stomach, should be used when topical therapy is inadequate. Minocycline or doxycycline, 50–100 mg daily to twice daily, is also effective. Metronidazole or amoxicillin, 250–500 mg twice daily, may be used in refractory cases. Side effects are few, although metronidazole may produce a disulfiram-like effect when the patient ingests alcohol and it may cause neuropathy with long-term use. Isotretinoin may succeed where other measures fail. A dosage of 0.5 mg/kg/d orally for 12–28 weeks is recommended. See precautions above. Telangiectasias are benefitted by laser therapy, and phymatous overgrowth of the nose can be treated by surgical reduction.

Prognosis

Rosacea tends to be a persistent process. With the regimens described above, it can usually be controlled adequately.

van Zuuren EJ et al. Interventions for rosacea. Cochrane Database Syst Rev. 2005 Jul 20;(3):CD003262. [PMID: 16034895]
van Zuuren EJ et al. Systematic review of rosacea treatments. J Am Acad Dermatol. 2007 Jan;56(1):107–15. [PMID: 17190628]

FOLLICULITIS (Including Sycosis)

ESSENTIALS OF DIAGNOSIS

▶ Itching and burning in hairy areas.
▶ Pustules in the hair follicles.

General Considerations

Folliculitis has multiple causes. It is frequently caused by staphylococcal infection and may be more common in the diabetic patient. When the lesion is deep-seated, chronic, and recalcitrant on the head and neck, it is called sycosis.

Gram-negative folliculitis, which may develop during antibiotic treatment of acne, may present as a flare of acne pustules or nodules. *Klebsiella, Enterobacter, Escherichia coli,* and *Proteus* have been isolated from these lesions.

"Hot tub folliculitis," caused by *Pseudomonas aeruginosa,* is characterized by pruritic or tender follicular, pustular lesions occurring within 1–4 days after bathing in a contaminated hot tub, whirlpool, or public swimming pool. Rarely, systemic infections may result. Neutropenic patients should avoid these exposures.

Nonbacterial folliculitis may also be caused by friction and oils. Occlusion, perspiration, and rubbing, such as that resulting from tight jeans and other heavy fabrics on the upper legs can worsen this type of folliculitis.

Steroid acne may be seen during topical or systemic corticosteroid therapy.

A form of sterile folliculitis called eosinophilic folliculitis consisting of urticarial papules with prominent eosinophilic infiltration is common in patients with AIDS. It may appear first with institution of highly active antiretroviral therapy (HAART) and be mistaken for a drug eruption.

Pseudofolliculitis is caused by ingrowing hairs in the beard area. It occurs in men and women with tightly curled beard hair. In this entity, the papules and pustules are located at the side of and not in follicles. It may be treated by growing a beard, by using chemical depilatories, or by shaving with a foil-guard razor. Laser hair removal is dramatically beneficial in patients with pseudofolliculitis, requires limited maintenance, and can be done on patients of any skin color. Pseudofolliculitis is a true medical indication for such a procedure and should not be considered cosmetic.

Clinical Findings

The symptoms range from slight burning and tenderness to intense itching. The lesions consist of pustules of hair follicles (Plate 27).

Differential Diagnosis

It is important to differentiate bacterial from nonbacterial folliculitis. The history is important for pinpointing the causes of nonbacterial folliculitis, and a Gram stain and culture are indispensable. One must differentiate folliculitis from acne vulgaris or pustular miliaria (heat rash) and from infections of the skin such as impetigo or fungal infections. Pseudomonas folliculitis is often suggested by the history of hot tub use. Eosinophilic folliculitis in AIDS often requires biopsy for diagnosis.

Complications

Abscess formation is the major complication of bacterial folliculitis.

Prevention

Correct any predisposing local causes such as oils or friction. Be sure that the water in hot tubs and spas is treated properly. If staphylococcal folliculitis is persistent, treatment of nasal or perineal carriage with rifampin, 600 mg daily for 5 days, or with topical mupirocin ointment 2% twice daily for 5 days, may help. Prolonged oral clindamycin, 150–300 mg/d for 4–6 weeks, or oral TMP-SMZ given 1 week per month for 6 months can be effective in preventing recurrent staphylococcal folliculitis and furunculosis. Bleach baths ($^1/_2$ to 1 cup per 20 liters of bathwater for 15 minutes 3–5 times weekly) may reduce cutaneous staphylococcal carriage and not contribute to antibiotic resistance. Control of blood glucose in diabetes may reduce the number of these infections.

► Treatment

A. Local Measures

Anhydrous ethyl alcohol containing 6.25% aluminum chloride (Xerac AC), applied to lesions and environs, may be helpful, especially for chronic frictional folliculitis of the buttocks. Topical antibiotics are generally ineffective if bacteria have invaded the hair follicle.

B. Specific Measures

Pseudomonas folliculitis will clear spontaneously in non-neutropenic patients if the lesions are superficial. It may be treated with ciprofloxacin, 500 mg twice daily for 5 days.

Systemic antibiotics are recommended for bacterial folliculitis due to other organisms. Extended periods of treatment (4–8 weeks or more) with antistaphylococcal antibiotics are required if infection has involved the scalp or densely hairy areas such as the axilla, beard, or groin.

Gram-negative folliculitis in acne patients may be treated with isotretinoin in compliance with all precautions discussed above (see Acne Vulgaris).

Eosinophilic folliculitis may be treated initially by the combination of potent topical corticosteroids and oral antihistamines. In more severe cases, treatment is with one of the following: topical permethrin (application for 12 hours every other night for 6 weeks); itraconazole, 200–400 mg daily; UVB or PUVA phototherapy; or isotretinoin, 0.5 mg/kg/d for up to 5 months. A remission may be induced by some of these therapies, but long-term treatment may be required.

► Prognosis

Bacterial folliculitis is occasionally stubborn and persistent, requiring prolonged or intermittent courses of antibiotics.

Nervi SJ et al. Eosinophilic pustular folliculitis: a 40 year retrospect. J Am Acad Dermatol. 2006 Aug;55(2):285–9. [PMID: 16844513]

MILIARIA (Heat Rash)

ESSENTIALS OF DIAGNOSIS

► Burning, itching, superficial aggregated small vesicles, papules, or pustules on covered areas of the skin, usually the trunk.

► More common in hot, moist climates.

► Rare forms associated with fever and even heat prostration.

► General Considerations

Miliaria occurs most commonly on the trunk and intertriginous areas. A hot, moist environment is the most frequent cause. Bedridden febrile patients are susceptible. Plugging of the ostia of sweat ducts occurs, with ultimate rupture of the sweat duct, producing an irritating, stinging reaction. Increase in numbers of resident aerobes, notably cocci, plays a role. Drugs that enhance sweat gland function (eg, clonidine, β-blockers, opiates), may contribute.

► Clinical Findings

The usual symptoms are burning and itching. The lesions consist of small, superficial, red, thin-walled, discrete vesicles (miliaria crystallina), papules (miliaria rubra), or vesicopustules or pustules (miliaria pustulosa). The reaction virtually always affects the back in a hospitalized patient.

► Differential Diagnosis

Miliaria is to be distinguished from drug eruption and folliculitis.

► Prevention

Use of an antibacterial preparation such as chlorhexidine prior to exposure to heat and humidity may help prevent the condition. Frequent turning or sitting of the hospitalized patient may reduce miliaria on the back.

► Treatment

The patient should keep cool and wear light clothing. Triamcinolone acetonide, 0.1% in Sarna lotion, or a mid-potency corticosteroid in a lotion or cream should be applied two to four times daily. Secondary infections (superficial pyoderma) are treated with appropriate antistaphylococcal antibiotics. Anticholinergic drugs given by mouth may be helpful in severe cases, eg, glycopyrrolate, 1 mg twice daily.

► Prognosis

Miliaria is usually a mild disorder, but severe forms (tropical anhidrosis and asthenia) result from interference with the heat-regulating mechanism.

Howe AS et al. Heat-related illness in athletes. Am J Sports Med. 2007 Aug;35(8):1384–95. [PMID: 17609528]

MUCOCUTANEOUS CANDIDIASIS

ESSENTIALS OF DIAGNOSIS

► Severe pruritus of vulva, anus, or body folds.

► Superficial denuded, beefy-red areas with or without satellite vesicopustules.

► Whitish curd-like concretions on the oral and vaginal mucous membranes.

► Yeast and pseudohyphae on microscopic examination of scales or curd.

General Considerations

Mucocutaneous candidiasis is a superficial fungal infection that may involve almost any cutaneous or mucous surface of the body. It is particularly likely to occur in diabetics, during pregnancy, and in obese persons who perspire freely. Systemic antibiotics, oral corticosteroids, and oral contraceptive agents may be contributory. Oral candidiasis may be the first sign of HIV infection (see Chapter 31).

Clinical Findings

A. Symptoms and Signs

Itching may be intense. Burning is reported, particularly around the vulva and anus. The lesions consist of superficially denuded, beefy-red areas in the depths of the body folds such as in the groin and the intergluteal cleft, beneath the breasts, at the angles of the mouth, and in the umbilicus (Plate 28). The peripheries of these denuded lesions are superficially undermined, and there may be satellite vesicopustules. Whitish, curd-like concretions may be present on mucosal lesions. Paronychia may occur (Plate 29).

B. Laboratory Findings

Clusters of budding cells and pseudohyphae can be seen under high power when skin scales or curd-like lesions have been cleared in 10% KOH. Culture can confirm the diagnosis.

Differential Diagnosis

Intertrigo, seborrheic dermatitis, tinea cruris, "inverse psoriasis," and erythrasma involving the same areas may mimic mucocutaneous candidiasis.

Complications

Systemic invasive candidiasis with candidemia may be seen with immunosuppression and in patients receiving broad-spectrum antibiotic and hypertonic glucose solutions, as in hyperalimentation. There may or may not be clinically evident mucocutaneous candidiasis.

Treatment

A. General Measures

Affected parts should be kept dry and exposed to air as much as possible. If possible, discontinue systemic antibiotics. For treatment of systemic invasive candidiasis, see Chapter 36.

B. Local Measures

1. Nails and paronychia—Apply clotrimazole solution 1% twice daily. Thymol 4% in ethanol applied once daily is an alternative.

2. Skin—Apply nystatin ointment or clotrimazole cream 1%, either with hydrocortisone cream 1%, twice daily.

3. Vulvar and anal mucous membranes—For vaginal candidiasis, single-dose fluconazole (150 mg) is effective.

Intravaginal clotrimazole, miconazole, terconazole, or nystatin may also be used. Long-term suppressive therapy may be required for recurrent or "intractable" cases. Non-*albicans* candidal species may be identified by culture in some refractory cases and may respond to oral itraconazole, 200 mg twice daily for 2–4 weeks.

4. Balanitis—This is most frequent in uncircumcised men, and *Candida* usually plays a role. Topical nystatin ointment is the initial treatment if the lesions are mildly erythematous or superficially erosive. Soaking with dilute aluminum acetate for 15 minutes twice daily may quickly relieve burning or itching. Chronicity and relapses, especially after sexual contact, suggest reinfection from a sexual partner who should be treated. Severe purulent balanitis is usually due to bacteria. If it is so severe that phimosis occurs, oral antibiotics—some with activity against anaerobes—are required; if rapid improvement does not occur, urologic consultation is indicated.

5. Mastitis—Lancinating breast pain and nipple dermatitis in breastfeeding women may be a manifestation of *Candida* colonization/infection of the breast ducts. Treatment with oral fluconazole, 200 mg/d can be dramatically effective.

Prognosis

Cases of cutaneous candidiasis range from the easily cured to the intractable and prolonged.

Academy of Breastfeeding Medicine Protocol Committee. ABM clinical protocol #4: mastitis. Revision, May 2008. Breastfeed Med. 2008 Sep;3(3):177–80. [PMID: 18778213]

Sobel JD. Vulvovaginal candidosis. Lancet. 2007 Jun 9;369 (9577):1961–71. [PMID: 17560449]

ERYTHEMAS

REACTIVE ERYTHEMAS

1. Urticaria & Angioedema

 ESSENTIALS OF DIAGNOSIS

- ▶ Eruptions of evanescent wheals or hives.
- ▶ Itching is usually intense but may on rare occasions be absent.
- ▶ Special forms of urticaria have special features (dermatographism, cholinergic urticaria, solar urticaria, or cold urticaria).
- ▶ Most incidents are acute and self-limited over a period of 1–2 weeks.
- ▶ Chronic urticaria (episodes lasting > 6 weeks) may have an autoimmune basis.

General Considerations

Urticaria can result from many different stimuli on an immunologic or nonimmunologic basis. The most common immunologic mechanism is mediated by IgE, as seen in the majority of patients with acute urticaria; another involves activation of the complement cascade. Some patients with chronic urticaria demonstrate autoantibodies directed against mast cell IgE receptors. Angiotensin-converting enzyme inhibitor and angiotensin II receptor antagonist therapy may be complicated by urticaria or angioedema. In general, extensive costly workups are not indicated in patients who have urticaria. A careful history and physical examination are more helpful.

Clinical Findings

A. Symptoms and Signs

Lesions are itchy red swellings of a few millimeters to many centimeters (Plate 30). The morphology of the lesions may vary over a period of minutes to hours, resulting in geographic or bizarre patterns. Individual lesions in true urticaria last less than 24 hours, and often only 2–4 hours. Angioedema is involvement of deeper subcutaneous tissue with swelling of the lips, eyelids, palms, soles, and genitalia. Angioedema is no more likely than urticaria to be associated with systemic complications such as laryngeal edema or hypotension. In cholinergic urticaria, triggered by a rise in core body temperature (hot showers, exercise), wheals are 2–3 mm in diameter with a large surrounding red flare. Cold urticaria is acquired or inherited and triggered by exposure to cold and wind (see Chapter 37).

B. Laboratory Findings

Laboratory studies are not likely to be helpful in the evaluation of acute or chronic urticaria. The most common causes of acute urticaria are foods, infections, and medications. The cause of chronic urticaria is often not found. In patients with individual slightly purpuric lesions that persist past 24 hours, skin biopsy may confirm neutrophilic urticaria or urticarial vasculitis. A functional ELISA test can detect patients with an autoimmune basis for their chronic urticaria.

Differential Diagnosis

Papular urticaria resulting from insect bites persists for days. A central punctum can usually be seen. Streaked urticarial lesions may be seen in the 24–48 hours before blisters appear in acute allergic plant dermatitis, eg, poison ivy, oak, or sumac. Urticarial response to heat, sun, water, and pressure are quite rare. Urticarial vasculitis may be seen as part of serum sickness, associated with fever and arthralgia. In this setting, a low serum complement level may be associated with severe systemic disease.

In hereditary angioedema, there is generally a positive family history and gastrointestinal or respiratory symptoms. Urticaria is not part of the syndrome, and lesions are not pruritic.

Treatment

A. General Measures

A detailed search by history for a cause of acute urticaria should be undertaken, and treatment may then be tailored to include the provocative condition. The chief causes are drugs—eg, aspirin, NSAIDs, morphine, and codeine; arthropod bites—eg, insect bites and bee stings (though the latter may cause anaphylaxis as well as angioedema); physical factors such as heat, cold, sunlight, and pressure; and, presumably, neurogenic factors, as in cholinergic urticaria induced by exercise, excitement, hot showers, etc. Other causes may include penicillins and other medications; inhalants such as feathers and animal danders; ingestion of shellfish, tomatoes, or strawberries; vaccines; external contactants, including various chemicals and cosmetics; and infections such as viral hepatitis (causing urticarial vasculitis).

B. Systemic Treatment

The mainstay of treatment initially includes H_1-antihistamines (see above). Initial therapy is hydroxyzine, 10 mg twice daily to 25 mg three times daily, or as one dose of 50–75 mg at night to reduce sedation. Cyproheptadine, 4 mg four times daily, may be especially useful for cold urticaria. "Nonsedating" or less sedating antihistamines are added if the generic sedating antihistamines are not effective. Options include fexofenadine, 60 mg twice daily (or 180 mg once daily); or loratadine, 10 mg/d. Higher doses of these second-generation antihistamines may be required to suppress urticaria (up to four times the standard recommended dose) than are required for allergic rhinitis. These high doses are safe and can be used in refractory cases. Cetirizine, a metabolite of hydroxyzine, is less sedating (13% of patients) and is given in a dosage of 10 mg/d.

Doxepin (a tricyclic antidepressant), 10–75 mg at bedtime, can be very effective in chronic urticaria. It has anticholinergic side effects.

H_2-antihistamines in combination with H_1-blockers may be helpful in patients with symptomatic dermatographism and to a lesser degree in chronic urticaria. UVB phototherapy can suppress some cases of chronic urticaria.

A few patients with chronic urticaria may respond to elimination of salicylates and tartrazine (coloring agent). Asymptomatic foci of infection—sinusitis, vaginal candidiasis, cholecystitis, and intestinal parasites—may rarely cause chronic urticaria. Systemic corticosteroids in a dose of about 40 mg daily will usually suppress acute and chronic urticaria. However, the use of corticosteroids is rarely indicated, since properly selected combinations of antihistamines with less toxicity are usually effective. Once corticosteroids are withdrawn, the urticaria virtually always returns if it had been chronic. Instead of instituting systemic corticosteroids, consultation should be sought from a dermatologist or allergist with experience in managing severe urticaria. Cyclosporine (3–5 mg/kg/d) may be effective in severe cases of autoimmune chronic urticaria.

C. Local Treatment

Local treatment is rarely rewarding.

Prognosis

Acute urticaria usually lasts only a few days to weeks. Half of patients whose urticaria persists for more than 6 weeks will have it for years.

Grob JJ et al. Non-sedating antihistamines in the treatment of chronic idiopathic urticaria using patient-reported outcomes. Curr Med Res Opin. 2008 Aug;24(8):2423–8. [PMID: 18651988]

Wakefield YS et al. Angiotensin converting enzyme inhibitors and delayed onset, recurrent angioedema of the head and neck. Br Dent J. 2008 Nov 22;205(10):553–6. [PMID: 19023310]

Zuberbier T et al. Urticaria: current opinions about etiology, diagnosis and therapy. Acta Derm Venereol. 2007;87(3):196–205. [PMID: 17533484]

2. Erythema Multiforme

ESSENTIALS OF DIAGNOSIS

▶ Sudden onset of symmetric erythematous skin lesions with history of recurrence.

▶ May be macular, papular, urticarial, bullous, or purpuric.

▶ "Target" lesions with clear centers and concentric erythematous rings or "iris" lesions may be noted in erythema multiforme minor. These are rare in drug-associated erythema multiforme major (Stevens-Johnson syndrome).

▶ Erythema multiforme minor on extensor surfaces, palms, soles, or mucous membranes. Erythema multiforme major favors the trunk.

▶ Herpes simplex is the most common cause of erythema multiforme minor.

▶ Drugs are the most common cause of erythema multiforme major in adults.

General Considerations

Erythema multiforme is an acute inflammatory skin disease. Erythema multiforme is divided clinically into minor and major types based on the clinical findings. Approximately 90% of cases of erythema multiforme minor follow outbreaks of herpes simplex, and so is now preferably termed "herpes-associated erythema multiforme" (HAEM). The term "erythema multiforme major" has been replaced by three terms: Stevens-Johnson syndrome, with less than 10% BSA skin loss; toxic epidermal necrolysis when there is greater than 30% BSA skin loss; and Stevens-Johnson syndrome/toxic epidermal necrolysis overlap for cases with between 10% and 30% BSA denudation. All these clinical scenarios are characterized by toxicity and involvement of two or more mucosal surfaces (often oral and conjunctival). They are most often caused by drugs, especially sulfonamides, NSAIDs, allopurinol, and anticonvulsants. *Mycoplasma pneumoniae* may trigger a skin eruption closely resembling Stevens-Johnson syndrome and may be the cause of Stevens-Johnson syndrome in up to 50% of children in some series. Erythema multiforme may also present as chronic or recurring ulceration localized to the oral mucosa, with skin lesions present in only half of the cases. The exposure to drugs associated with erythema multiforme may be systemic or topical (eg, eyedrops).

Clinical Findings

A. Symptoms and Signs

A classic target lesion, found most commonly in herpes-associated erythema multiforme, consists of three concentric zones of color change, most often found acrally on the hands and feet (Plate 31). Not all lesions will have this appearance. Drug-associated bullous eruptions in the Stevens-Johnson syndrome/toxic epidermal necrolysis spectrum present with raised purpuric target-like lesions, with only two zones of color change and a central blister, or nondescript reddish or purpuric macules. Pain on eating, swallowing, and urination can occur if the appropriate mucosae are involved. Inability to eat is common if the oral mucosa is extensively involved.

B. Laboratory Findings

Blood tests are not useful for diagnosis. Skin biopsy is diagnostic. Direct immunofluorescence studies are negative.

Differential Diagnosis

Urticaria and drug eruptions are the chief entities that must be differentiated from erythema multiforme minor. Individual lesions of true urticaria should come and go within 24 hours and are usually responsive to antihistamines. In erythema multiforme major, the differential diagnosis includes autoimmune bullous diseases (including pemphigus and pemphigoid) and acute generalized exanthematous pustulosis. The presence of a blistering eruption requires biopsy and consultation for appropriate diagnosis and treatment.

Complications

The tracheobronchial mucosa and conjunctiva may be involved in severe cases with resultant scarring. Ophthalmologic consultation is required if ocular involvement is present.

Treatment

A. General Measures

Toxic epidermal necrolysis is best treated in a burn unit. Otherwise, patients need not be admitted unless mucosal involvement interferes with hydration and nutrition. Patients who begin to blister should be seen daily. Open lesions should be managed like second-degree burns. Immediate discontinuation of the inciting medication (before blistering occurs) is a significant predictor of outcome. Delay in establishing the diagnosis and inadvertently continuing the offending medication results in higher morbidity and mortality.

B. Specific Measures

The most important aspect of treatment is to stop the offending medication and to move patients with more than 25–30% BSA involvement to a burn unit. Nutritional and fluid support and high vigilance for infection are the most important aspects of care. Recent reviews of systemic treatments for Stevens-Johnson syndrome and toxic epidermal necrolysis have been conflicting, but the largest series have failed to show statistically significant benefit with treatment. Some data support the use of high-dose corticosteroids. If corticosteroids are to be tried in more severe cases, they should be used early, before blistering occurs, and in moderate to high doses (prednisone, 100–250 mg) and stopped within days if there is no dramatic response. Intravenous immunoglobulin (IVIG) (0.75 g/kg/d for 4 days) has become standard of care at some centers for toxic epidermal necrolysis cases and can be considered in cases with greater than 30% BSA involvement. It has not been proven to reduce mortality. Oral and topical corticosteroids are useful in the oral variant of erythema multiforme. Oral acyclovir prophylaxis of herpes simplex infections may be effective in preventing recurrent herpes-associated erythema multiforme minor.

C. Local Measures

Topical therapy is not very effective in this disease. For oral lesions, 1% diphenhydramine elixir mixed with Kaopectate or with 1% dyclonine may be used as a mouth rinse several times daily.

▶ Prognosis

Erythema multiforme minor usually lasts 2–6 weeks and may recur. Erythema multiforme major may be serious with a mortality of about 30% in cases with greater than 30% BSA involvement.

Mittmann N et al. IVIG for the treatment of toxic epidermal necrolysis. Skin Therapy Lett. 2007 Feb;12(1):7–9. [PMID: 17361314]
Schneck J et al. Effects of treatments on the mortality of Stevens-Johnson syndrome and toxic epidermal necrolysis: A retrospective study on patients included in the prospective EuroSCAR Study. J Am Acad Dermatol. 2008 Jan;58(1):33–40. [PMID: 17919775]

3. Erythema Migrans (See also Chapter 34)

Erythema migrans is a unique cutaneous eruption that characterizes the localized or generalized early stage of Lyme disease (borreliosis). Three to 32 days (median: 7 days) after a tick bite, there is gradual expansion of redness around the papule representing the bite site (Plate 32). The advancing border is usually slightly raised, warm, red to bluish-red, and free of any scale. Centrally, the site of the bite may clear, leaving only a rim of peripheral erythema, or it may become indurated, vesicular, or necrotic. The annular erythema usually grows to a median diameter of 15 cm (range: 3–68 cm, but virtually always > 5 cm). It is accompanied by a burning sensation in half of patients; rarely, it is pruritic or painful. Multiple secondary annular lesions similar in appearance to the primary lesion but without indurated centers and generally of smaller size will develop in 20% of patients. In the southeastern United States, similar lesions are seen in patients who are not as ill and who tend to have classic central clearing of their lesions. These patients have negative Lyme serology tests.

This condition has been called Southern tick-associated rash illness (STARI). This illness is transmitted by the lonestar tick; some cases are caused by *Borrelia lonestari*, for which the white tail deer is the animal reservoir. Systemic symptoms are uncommon in STARI and the skin lesions respond to the same antibiotic agents used for Lyme disease, suggesting that a spirochete (probably as yet unidentified *Borrelia* species) is causative in all these cases.

Without treatment, erythema migrans and the secondary lesions fade in a median of 28 days, though some may persist for months. Ten percent of untreated patients experience recurrences over the ensuing months. Treatment with systemic antibiotics (see Table 34–4) is necessary to prevent systemic involvement. However, only 60–70% of those with systemic involvement have experienced erythema migrans.

Bratton RL et al. Diagnosis and treatment of Lyme disease. Mayo Clin Proc. 2008 May;83(5):566–71. [PMID: 18452688]
Centers for Disease Control and Prevention (CDC). Lyme disease—United States, 2003-2005. MMWR Morb Mortal Wkly Rep. 2007 Jun 15;56(23):573–6. [PMID: 17568368]
Dandache P et al. Erythema migrans. Infect Dis Clin North Am. 2008 Jun;22(2):235–60. [PMID: 18452799]
Fritch P. European Dermatology Forum: skin diseases in Europe. Skin diseases with high public health impact: toxic epidermal necrolysis and Stevens-Johnson syndrome. Eur J Dermatol. 2008 Mar–Apr;18(2):216–7. [PMID: 18424404]
Hazin R et al. Stevens-Johnson syndrome: pathogenesis, diagnosis, and management. Ann Med. 2008;40(2):129–38. [PMID: 18293143]
Masters EJ et al. STARI, or Masters disease: Lone star tick-vectored Lyme-like illness. Infect Dis Clin North Am. 2008 Jun;22(2):361–76. [PMID: 18452807]
Tibbles CD et al. Does this patient have erythema migrans? JAMA. 2007 Jun 20;297(23):2617–27. [PMID: 17579230]

INFECTIOUS ERYTHEMAS

1. Erysipelas

 ESSENTIALS OF DIAGNOSIS

▶ Edematous, spreading, circumscribed, hot, erythematous area, with or without vesicles or bullae.

▶ Central face frequently involved.

▶ Pain, chills, fever, and systemic toxicity may be striking.

▶ General Considerations

Erysipelas is a superficial form of cellulitis that occurs classically on the cheek, caused by β-hemolytic streptococci.

▶ Clinical Findings

A. Symptoms and Signs

The symptoms are pain, malaise, chills, and moderate fever. A bright red spot appears first, very often near a fissure at the angle of the nose. This spreads to form a tense, sharply demarcated, glistening, smooth, hot plaque (Plate 33). The margin characteristically makes noticeable advances in days or even hours. The lesion is somewhat edematous and can be pitted slightly with the finger. Vesicles or bullae occasionally develop on the surface. The lesion does not usually become pustular or gangrenous and heals without scar formation. The disease may complicate any break in the skin that provides a portal of entry for the organism.

B. Laboratory Findings

Leukocytosis is almost invariably present; blood cultures may be positive.

Differential Diagnosis

Erysipeloid is a benign bacillary infection producing cellulitis of the skin of the fingers or the backs of the hands in fishermen and meat handlers.

Complications

Unless erysipelas is promptly treated, death may result from extension of the process and systemic toxicity, particularly in the elderly.

Treatment

Place the patient at bed rest with the head of the bed elevated. Intravenous antibiotics effective against group A β-hemolytic streptococci and staphylococci are indicated for the first 48 hours in all but the mildest cases. A 7-day course is completed with penicillin VK, 250 mg, dicloxacillin, 250 mg, or a first-generation cephalosporin, 250 mg, orally four times a day. Alternatives in penicillin-allergic patients are clindamycin or erythromycin, the latter only if the infection is known to be due to streptococci.

Prognosis

Erysipelas was at one time a life-threatening infection. It can now usually be quickly controlled with systemic penicillin or erythromycin therapy.

Bartholomeeusen S et al. Epidemiology and comorbidity of erysipelas in primary care. Dermatology. 2007;215(2):118–22. [PMID: 17684373]
Leclerc S et al. Recurrent erysipelas: 47 cases. Dermatology. 2007;214(1):52–7. [PMID: 17191048]
See references in the next section.

2. Cellulitis

ESSENTIALS OF DIAGNOSIS

▶ Edematous, expanding, erythematous, warm plaque with or without vesicles or bullae.

▶ Lower leg is frequently involved.

▶ Pain, chills, and fever are commonly present.

▶ Septicemia may develop.

General Considerations

Cellulitis, a diffuse spreading infection of the dermis and subcutaneous tissue, is usually on the lower leg and most commonly due to gram-positive cocci, especially group A β-hemolytic streptococci and *S aureus*. Rarely, gram-negative rods or even fungi can produce a similar picture. In otherwise healthy persons, the most common portal of entry for lower leg cellulitis is toe web intertrigo with fissuring. Venous insufficiency can also predispose to lower leg cellulitis. Injection drug use and open ulcerations may also be complicated by cellulitis. Cellulitis in the diabetic foot may be a major problem and is often associated with neuropathy and hyperkeratotic nodules from ill-fitting shoes and abnormal weight bearing.

Clinical Findings

A. Symptoms and Signs

Cellulitis begins as a small patch, which from its onset is tender. Swelling, erythema, and pain are often present. The lesion expands over hours, so that from onset to presentation is usually 6 to 36 hours. As the lesion grows, the patient becomes more ill with progressive chills, fever, and malaise. If septicemia develops, hypotension may develop, followed by shock.

B. Laboratory Findings

Leukocytosis or at least a neutrophilia (left shift) is present from early in the course. Blood cultures may be positive. If a central ulceration, pustule, or abscess is present, culture may be of value. Aspiration of the advancing edge has a low yield (20%) and is usually not performed. Instead, if an unusual organism is suspected and there is no loculated site to culture, a full thickness skin biopsy taken before antibiotics are given can be useful. Part is cultured and part processed for histologic evaluation with Gram stain. This technique is particularly useful in the immunocompromised patient. If a primary source for the infection is identified (wound, leg ulcer, toe web intertrigo), cultures from these sites isolate the causative pathogen in half of cases and can be used to guide antibiotic therapy.

Differential Diagnosis

Two potentially life threatening entities that can mimic cellulitis (ie, present with a painful, red, swollen lower extremity) include deep venous thrombosis and necrotizing fasciitis. The diagnosis of necrotizing fasciitis should be suspected in a patient who has a very toxic appearance, bullae, crepitus or anesthesia of the involved skin, overlying skin necrosis, and laboratory evidence of rhabdomyolysis (elevated creatine kinase [CK]) or disseminated intravascular coagulation. While these findings may be present with severe cellulitis and bacteremia, it is essential to rule out necrotizing fasciitis because rapid surgical debridement is essential. Other skin lesions that may resemble cellulitis include sclerosing panniculitis, an acute, exquisitely tender red plaque on the medial lower legs above the malleolus in patients with venous stasis or varicosities, and acute severe contact dermatitis on a limb, which produces erythema, vesiculation, and edema as seen in cellulitis, but with itching instead of pain.

▶ Treatment

Intravenous or parenteral antibiotics may be required for the first 2–5 days, with adequate coverage for *Streptococcus* and *Staphylococcus*. Hospitalization is required in cases with severe local symptoms and signs, hypotension, elevated serum creatinine, low serum bicarbonate, elevated creatine kinase, elevated white blood cell count with marked left shift, or elevated C-reactive protein. If CA-MRSA is suspected, therapy is vancomycin, clindamycin, or TMP-SMZ plus a β-lactam. In mild cases or following the initial parenteral therapy, dicloxacillin or cephalexin, 250–500 mg four times daily for 5–10 days, is usually adequate. If MRSA is suspected, use of TMP-SMZ, clindamycin, or the combination of doxycycline plus rifampin should be considered. In patients in whom intravenous treatment is not instituted, the first dose of oral antibiotic can be doubled to achieve rapid high blood levels.

Anaya DA et al. Necrotizing soft-tissue infection: diagnosis and management. Clin Infect Dis. 2007 Mar 1;44(5):705–10. [PMID: 17278065]
Corwin P et al. Randomized controlled trial of intravenous antibiotic treatment for cellulitis at home compared with hospital. BMJ. 2005 Jan 15;330(7483):129. [PMID: 15604157]
Gabillot-Carre M et al. Acute bacterial skin infections and cellulitis. Curr Opin Infect Dis. 2007 Apr;20(2):118–23. [PMID: 17496568]

BLISTERING DISEASES

PEMPHIGUS

ESSENTIALS OF DIAGNOSIS

▶ Relapsing crops of bullae.

▶ Often preceded by mucous membrane bullae, erosions, and ulcerations.

▶ Superficial detachment of the skin after pressure or trauma variably present (Nikolsky sign).

▶ Acantholysis on biopsy.

▶ Immunofluorescence studies are confirmatory.

▶ General Considerations

Pemphigus is an uncommon intraepidermal blistering disease occurring on skin and mucous membranes. It is caused by autoantibodies to adhesion molecules expressed in the skin and mucous membranes. The cause is unknown, and in the preantibiotic, presteroid era, the condition was usually fatal within 5 years. The bullae appear spontaneously and are tender and painful when they rupture. Drug-induced pemphigus from penicillamine, captopril, and others has been reported. There are several forms of pemphigus: **pemphigus vulgaris** and its variant, **pemphigus vegetans;** and the more superficially blistering **pemphigus foliaceus** and its variant, **pemphigus erythematosus.** All forms may occur at any age but most commonly in middle age. The vulgaris form begins in the mouth in over 50% of cases. The foliaceus form is especially apt to be associated with other autoimmune diseases, or it may be drug-induced. Paraneoplastic pemphigus, a unique form of the disorder, is associated with numerous types of benign and malignant neoplasms but most frequently non-Hodgkin lymphoma.

▶ Clinical Findings

A. Symptoms and Signs

Pemphigus is characterized by an insidious onset of flaccid bullae, crusts, and erosions in crops or waves (Plate 34). In pemphigus vulgaris, lesions often appear first on the oral mucous membranes. These rapidly become erosive. The scalp is another site of early involvement. Rubbing a cotton swab or finger laterally on the surface of uninvolved skin may cause easy separation of the epidermis (**Nikolsky sign**).

B. Laboratory Findings

The diagnosis is made by light microscopy and by direct and indirect immunofluorescence (IIF) microscopy. Autoantibodies to intercellular adhesion molecules can be detected with ELISA assays and have replaced the use of IIF in some centers.

▶ Differential Diagnosis

Blistering diseases include erythema multiforme, drug eruptions, bullous impetigo, contact dermatitis, dermatitis herpetiformis, and bullous pemphigoid, but flaccid blisters are not typical of these diseases, and acantholysis is not seen on biopsy. All of these diseases have clinical characteristics and different immunofluorescence test results that distinguish them from pemphigus.

Paraneoplastic pemphigus is clinically, histologically, and immunologically distinct from other forms of the disease. Oral erosions and erythematous plaques resembling erythema multiforme are seen. Survival rates are low because of the underlying malignancy.

▶ Complications

Secondary infection commonly occurs; this is a major cause of morbidity and mortality. Disturbances of fluid, electrolyte, and nutritional intake can occur as a result of painful oral ulcers.

▶ Treatment

A. General Measures

When the disease is severe, hospitalize the patient at bed rest and provide antibiotics and intravenous feedings as indicated. Anesthetic troches used before eating ease painful oral lesions.

B. Systemic Measures

Pemphigus very often requires systemic therapy as early in its course as possible. However, the main morbidity in this disease is due to the side effects of such therapy. Initial therapy is with systemic corticosteroids: prednisone, 60–80 mg daily. In all but the most mild cases, a steroid-sparing agent is added from the beginning, since the course of the disease is long and the steroid-sparing agents take several weeks to exert their activity. Azathioprine (100–200 mg daily) or mycophenolate mofetil (1–1.5 g twice daily) is used most frequently, the latter seeming to be the most reliable and recommended for most cases. Rituximab may be given in refractory cases to diminish the amount of autoantibody production. If this fails, monthly IVIG at 2 g/kg intravenously over 3 days with rituximab is dramatically beneficial and has replaced high-dose corticosteroids plus cyclophosphamide and pulse intravenous corticosteroids as rescue therapy. Increased risk of thromboembolism is associated with IVIG therapy in these doses.

C. Local Measures

In patients with limited disease, skin and mucous membrane lesions should be treated with topical corticosteroids. Complicating infection requires appropriate systemic and local antibiotic therapy.

▶ Prognosis

The course tends to be chronic in most patients, though about one-third appear to experience remission. Infection is the most frequent cause of death, usually from *S aureus* septicemia.

Ahmed AR et al. Treatment of pemphigus vulgaris with rituximab and intravenous immune globulin. N Engl J Med. 2006 Oct 26;355(17):1772–9. [PMID: 17065638]
Dick SE. Pemphigus: a treatment update. Autoimmunity. 2006 Nov;39(7):591–9. [PMID: 17101503]

BULLOUS PEMPHIGOID

Many other autoimmune skin disorders are characterized by formation of bullae, or blisters. These include bullous pemphigoid, cicatricial pemphigoid, dermatitis herpetiformis, and pemphigoid gestationis.

Bullous pemphigoid is a relatively benign pruritic disease characterized by tense blisters in flexural areas, usually remitting in 5 or 6 years, with a course characterized by exacerbations and remissions. Most affected persons are over the age of 60 (often in their 70s or 80s), and men are affected twice as frequently as women. The appearance of blisters may be preceded by urticarial or edematous lesions for months. Oral lesions are present in about one-third of affected persons. The disease may occur in various forms, including localized, vesicular, vegetating, erythematous, erythrodermic, and nodular.

The diagnosis is made by biopsy and direct immunofluorescence examination. Light microscopy shows a subepidermal blister. With direct immunofluorescence, IgG and C3 are found at the dermal-epidermal junction. If the

patient has mild disease, ultrapotent corticosteroids may be adequate. Prednisone at a dosage of 0.75 mg/kg/d is often used to achieve rapid control of more widespread disease. Although slower in onset of action, tetracycline or erythromycin, 500 mg three times daily, alone or combined with nicotinamide—*not nicotinic acid or niacin!*—(up to 1.5 g/d), if tolerated, may control the disease in patients who cannot use corticosteroids or may allow decreasing or eliminating corticosteroids after control is achieved. Dapsone is particularly effective in mucous membrane pemphigoid. If these drugs are not effective, methotrexate, 5–25 mg weekly, or azathioprine, 50 mg one to three times daily, may be used as steroid-sparing agents. Mycophenolate mofetil (1 g twice daily) may be used in refractory cases.

Khumalo N et al. Interventions for bullous pemphigoid. Cochrane Database Syst Rev. 2005 Jul 20;(3):CD002292. [PMID: 16034874]

PAPULES

WARTS

 ESSENTIALS OF DIAGNOSIS

- ▶ Verrucous papules anywhere on the skin or mucous membranes, usually no larger than 1 cm in diameter.
- ▶ Prolonged incubation period (average 2–18 months). Spontaneous "cures" are frequent (50% at 2 years for common warts).
- ▶ "Recurrences" (new lesions) are frequent.

▶ General Considerations

Warts are caused by human papillomaviruses (HPVs). Typing of HPV lesions is NOT a part of standard medical evaluation except in the case of genital dysplasia. Genital HPV types are divided into low-risk and high-risk depending on the likelihood of their association with cervical and anal cancer.

▶ Clinical Findings

There are usually no symptoms. Tenderness on pressure occurs with plantar warts; itching occurs with anogenital warts (Plate 35). Flat warts are most evident under oblique illumination. Periungual warts may be dry, fissured, and hyperkeratotic and may resemble hangnails or other nonspecific changes. Plantar warts resemble plantar corns or calluses.

▶ Differential Diagnosis

Some warty-looking lesions are actually hypertrophic actinic keratoses or squamous cell carcinomas. Some genital warty lesions may be due to secondary syphilis (condylomata lata). The lesions of molluscum contagiosum are pearly with a central dell. In AIDS, wart-like lesions may be caused by varicella zoster virus.

▶ Prevention

Administration of a vaccine against certain genital HPV types can prevent infection with these wart types and reduce cervical dysplasia. It is recommended for teenage and young adult women (see Chapter 1).

▶ Treatment

Treatment is aimed at inducing "wart-free" intervals for as long as possible without scarring, since no treatment can guarantee a remission or prevent recurrences. In immunocompromised patients, the goal is even more modest, ie, to control the size and number of lesions present.

A. Removal

For common warts of the hands, patients are usually offered liquid nitrogen or keratolytic agents. The former may work in fewer treatments but requires office visits and is painful.

1. Liquid nitrogen—Liquid nitrogen is applied to achieve a thaw time of 20–45 seconds. Two freeze-thaw cycles are given every 2–4 weeks for several visits. Scarring will occur if it is used incorrectly. Liquid nitrogen may cause permanent depigmentation in pigmented individuals. Cryotherapy is first-line physician applied surgical treatment for condyloma acuminata.

2. Keratolytic agents and occlusion—Salicylic acid products may be used against common warts or plantar warts. They are applied then occluded. Plantar warts may be treated by applying a 40% salicylic acid plaster (Mediplast) after paring. The plaster may be left on for 5–6 days, then removed, the lesion pared down, and another plaster applied. Although it may take weeks or months to eradicate the wart, the method is safe and effective with almost no side effects. Chronic occlusion alone with water-impermeable tape (duct tape, adhesive tape) for months may be effective.

3. Podophyllum resin—For genital warts, the purified active component of the podophyllum resin, podofilox, is applied by the patient twice daily 3 consecutive days a week for cycles of 4–6 weeks. It is less irritating and more effective than "physician-applied" podophyllum resin. After a single 4-week cycle, 45% of patients were wart-free; but of these, 60% relapsed at 6 weeks. Thus, multiple cycles of treatment are often necessary. Patients unable to obtain the take home podofilox may be treated by in the clinician's office by painting each wart carefully (protecting normal skin) every 2–3 weeks with 25% podophyllum resin (podophyllin) in compound tincture of benzoin. Pregnant patients should not be so treated. Podophyllin is ineffective for common warts and plantar warts.

4. Imiquimod—A 5% cream of this local interferon inducer has moderate activity in clearing external genital warts (EGWs). Treatment is once daily on 3 alternate days per week. Response may be slow, with patients who eventually cleared having responses at 8 weeks (44%) or 12 weeks (69%). There is a marked gender difference with respect to response, with 77% of women and 40% of men

having complete clearing of their lesions. Once cleared, about 13% have recurrences in the short term.

In accidental exposure during pregnancy, there is less risk with imiquimod than with podophyllum resin (category B versus category X). Imiquimod is considerably more expensive than podophyllotoxin, but given the high rate of response in women and its safety, it appears to be the "patient-administered" treatment of choice for EGWs in women. In men, the more rapid response, lower cost, and similar efficacy make podophyllotoxin the initial treatment of choice, with imiquimod used for recurrences or refractory cases. Imiquimod has no demonstrated efficacy for—and should not be used to treat—plantar or common warts.

5. Operative removal—Plantar warts may be removed by blunt dissection. For hemostasis, trichloroacetic acid or Monsel solution on a tightly wound cotton-tipped applicator may be painted on the wound, or light electrocautery may be used. For genital warts, snip biopsy (scissors) removal followed by light electrocautery is more effective than cryotherapy, especially for patients with pedunculated or large lesions.

6. Laser therapy—The CO_2 laser can be effective for treating recurrent warts, periungual warts, plantar warts, and condylomata acuminata. It leaves open wounds that must fill in with granulation tissue over 4–6 weeks and is best reserved for warts resistant to all other modalities. Lasers with emissions of 585, 595, or 532 nm may also be used every 3–4 weeks to gradually ablate common or plantar warts. This is no more effective than cryotherapy in controlled trials. For genital warts, it has not been shown that laser therapy is more effective than electrosurgical removal.

7. Other agents—Bleomycin diluted to 1 unit/mL may be injected into common and plantar warts. It has been shown to have a high cure rate. It should be used with caution on digital warts because of the potential complications of Raynaud phenomenon, nail loss, and terminal digital necrosis.

B. Immunotherapy

Squaric acid dibutylester may be effective. It is applied in a concentration of 0.2–2% directly to the warts from once weekly to five times weekly to induce a mild contact dermatitis. Between 60% and 80% of warts clear over 10–20 weeks. Injection of *Candida* antigen starting at 1:50 dilution and repeated every 3–4 weeks may be similarly effective in stimulating immunologic regression of common and plantar warts.

C. Physical Modalities

Soaking warts in hot (42.2 °C) water for 10–30 minutes daily for 6 weeks has resulted in involution in some cases.

▶ Prognosis

There is a striking tendency to the development of new lesions. Warts may disappear spontaneously or may be unresponsive to treatment.

Gibbs S et al. Topical treatments for cutaneous warts. Cochrane Database Syst Rev. 2006 Jul 19;3:CD001781. [PMID: 16855978]

Mayeaux EJ Jr et al. Modern management of external genital warts. J Low Genit Tract Dis. 2008 Jul;12(3):185–92. [PMID: 18596459]

Partridge JM et al. Genital human papillomavirus infection in men. Lancet Infect Dis. 2006 Jan;6(1):21–31. [PMID: 16377531]

Scheinfeld N et al. An evidence-based review of medical and surgical treatments of genital warts. Dermatol Online J. 2006 Mar 30;12(3):5. [PMID: 16638419]

Zimet GD et al. Appropriate use of cervical cancer vaccine. Annu Rev Med. 2008 Feb 18;59:223–36. [PMID: 18186704]

CALLOSITIES & CORNS OF FEET OR TOES

Callosities and corns are caused by pressure and friction due to faulty weight-bearing, orthopedic deformities, improperly fitting shoes, or neuropathies.

Tenderness on pressure and "after-pain" are the only symptoms. The hyperkeratotic well-localized overgrowths always occur at pressure points. Dermatoglyphics (fingerprint lines) are preserved over the surface (not so in warts). When the surface is shaved with a 15 blade, a glassy core is found (which differentiates them from plantar warts, which have multiple capillary bleeding points or black dots when pared).

Treatment consists of correcting mechanical abnormalities that cause friction and pressure. Callosities may be removed by careful paring of the callus after a warm water soak or with keratolytic agents as found in various brands of corn pads.

Plantar hyperkeratosis of the heels can be treated successfully by using 20% urea (Ureacin 20) or 12% lactic acid (Lac-Hydrin) or combinations nightly and a pumice stone after soaking in water.

Callosities on diabetic feet, especially in the setting of hyposensate neuropathy, can be a major problem and the value of early podiatric management to prevent complications is very important.

Menz HB. Footwear characteristics and foot problems in older people. Gerontology. 2005 Sep–Oct;51(5):346–51. [PMID: 16110238]

Rathur HM et al. The diabetic foot. Clin Dermatol. 2007 Jan–Feb;25(1):109–20. [PMID: 17276208]

MOLLUSCUM CONTAGIOSUM

Molluscum contagiosum, caused by a poxvirus, presents as single or multiple dome-shaped, waxy papules 2–5 mm in diameter that are umbilicated (Plate 36). Lesions at first are firm, solid, and flesh-colored but upon reaching maturity become soft, whitish, or pearly gray and may suppurate. The principal sites of involvement are the face, lower abdomen, and genitals.

The lesions are autoinoculable and spread by wet skin-to-skin contact. In sexually active individuals, they may be confined to the penis, pubis, and inner thighs and are considered a sexually transmitted infection.

Molluscum contagiosum is common in patients with AIDS, usually with a helper T cell count < 100/mcL. Extensive lesions tend to develop over the face and neck as well as in the genital area.

The diagnosis is easily established in most instances because of the distinctive central umbilication of the dome-shaped lesion. The best treatment is by curettage or applications of liquid nitrogen as for warts—but more briefly. When lesions are frozen, the central umbilication often becomes more apparent. Light electrosurgery with a fine needle is also effective. It has been estimated that individual lesions persist for about 2 months. They are difficult to eradicate in patients with AIDS unless immunity improves. However, in AIDS, with highly effective anti-retroviral treatment molluscum does not need to be treated because they usually spontaneously clear.

van der Wouden JC et al. Interventions for cutaneous molluscum contagiosum. Cochrane Database Syst Rev. 2006 Apr 19;(2):CD004767. [PMID: 16625612]

BASAL CELL CARCINOMA

 ESSENTIALS OF DIAGNOSIS

▶ Pearly papule, erythematous patch > 6 mm, or nonhealing ulcer, in sun exposed areas (face, trunk, lower legs).

▶ History of bleeding.

▶ Fair-skinned person with a history of sun exposure (often intense, intermittent).

General Considerations

Basal cell carcinomas are the most common form of cancer. They occur on sun-exposed skin in otherwise normal fair-skinned individuals; ultraviolet light is the cause. The most common presentation is a papule or nodule that may have a central scab or erosion (Plate 37). Occasionally the nodules have stippled pigment (pigmented basal cell carcinoma). Intradermal nevi without pigment on the face of older white individuals may resemble basal cell carcinomas. Basal cell carcinomas grow slowly, attaining a size of 1–2 cm or more in diameter, usually only after years of growth. There is a waxy, "pearly" appearance, with telangiectatic vessels easily visible (Plate 38). It is the pearly or translucent quality of these lesions that is most diagnostic, a feature best appreciated if the skin is stretched. On the back and chest, basal cell carcinomas appear as reddish, somewhat shiny, scaly patches.

Clinicians should examine the whole skin routinely, looking for bumps, patches, and scabbed lesions. When examining the face, look at the eyelid margins and medial canthi, the nose and alar folds, the lips, and then around and behind the ears. While metastases almost never occur, therapy of basal cell carcinomas may cause significant cosmetic deformity in these areas, particularly for inadequately treated or recurrent lesions.

Treatment

Lesions suspected to be basal cell carcinomas should be biopsied, by shave or punch biopsy. Therapy is then aimed at eradication with minimal cosmetic deformity, often by excision and suturing with recurrence rates of 5% or less. The technique of three cycles of curettage and electrodesiccation depends on the skill of the operator and is not recommended for head and neck lesions. After 4–6 weeks of healing, it leaves a broad, hypopigmented, at times hypertrophic scar. Radiotherapy is effective and sometimes appropriate for older individuals (over 65), but recurrent tumors after radiation therapy are more difficult to treat and may be more aggressive. Radiation therapy is the most expensive method to treat basal cell carcinoma and should only be used if other treatment options are not appropriate. Mohs surgery—removal of the tumor followed by immediate frozen section histopathologic examination of margins with subsequent reexcision of tumor-positive areas and final closure of the defect—gives the highest cure rates (98%) and results in least tissue loss. It is appropriate therapy for tumors of the eyelids, nasolabial folds, canthi, external ear, and temple; for recurrent lesions; or where tissue sparing is needed for cosmesis. Since up to half of patients with a basal cell carcinoma will develop a second lesion, patients with basal cell carcinomas must be monitored to detect new or recurrent lesions.

Bath-Hextall FJ et al. Interventions for basal cell carcinoma of the skin. Cochrane Database Syst Rev. 2007 Jan 24;(1):CD003412. [PMID: 17253489]
Madan V et al. Genetics and risk factors for basal cell carcinoma. Br J Dermatol. 2006 May;154 Suppl 1:5–7. [PMID: 16712709]
Neville JA et al. Management of nonmelanoma skin cancer in 2007. Nat Clin Pract Oncol. 2007 Aug;4(8):462–9. [PMID: 17657251]

SQUAMOUS CELL CARCINOMA

ESSENTIALS OF DIAGNOSIS

▶ Nonhealing ulcer or warty nodule.

▶ Skin damage due to long-term sun exposure.

▶ Common in fair-skinned organ transplant recipients.

Squamous cell carcinoma usually occurs subsequent to prolonged sun exposure on exposed parts in fair-skinned individuals who sunburn easily and tan poorly. It may arise from an actinic keratosis. The lesions appear as small red, conical, hard nodules that occasionally ulcerate (Plate 39). The frequency of metastasis is not precisely known, though metastatic spread is said to be less likely with squamous cell carcinoma arising out of actinic keratoses than with those that arise de novo. In actinically induced squamous cell cancers, rates of metastasis are estimated from retrospective studies to be 3–7%. Squamous cell carcinomas of the lip, oral cavity, tongue, and genitalia have much higher rates of metastasis and require special management.

Examination of the skin and therapy are essentially the same as for basal cell carcinoma. The preferred treatment of squamous cell carcinoma is excision. Electrodesiccation and curettage and x-ray radiation may be used for some lesions, and fresh tissue microscopically controlled excision (Mohs) is recommended for high-risk lesions (lips,

temples, ears, nose) and for recurrent tumors. Follow-up for squamous cell carcinoma must be more frequent and thorough than for basal cell carcinoma, starting at every 3 months, with careful examination of lymph nodes. In addition, palpation of the lips is essential to detect hard or indurated areas that represent early squamous cell carcinoma. All such cases must be biopsied. Multiple squamous cell carcinomas are very common on the sun-exposed skin of organ transplant patients. The intensity of immunosuppression, not the use of any particular immunosuppressive agent, is the primary risk factor in determining the development of skin cancer after transplant. The tumors begin to appear after 5 years of immunosuppression. Regular dermatologic evaluation in at-risk organ transplant recipients is recommended. Biologic behavior of skin cancer in organ transplant recipients may be aggressive, and careful management is required. Other forms of immunosuppression such as chronic lymphocytic leukemia, HIV/AIDS, and chronic iatrogenic immunosuppression may also increase skin cancer risk and be associated with more aggressive skin cancer behavior.

Zafar SY et al. Malignancy after solid organ transplantation: an overview. Oncologist. 2008 Jul;13(7):769–78. [PMID: 18614590]

VIOLACEOUS TO PURPLE PAPULES & NODULES

LICHEN PLANUS

ESSENTIALS OF DIAGNOSIS

▶ Pruritic, violaceous, flat-topped papules with fine white streaks and symmetric distribution.

▶ Lacy lesions of the buccal mucosa.

▶ Commonly seen along linear scratch marks (Koebner phenomenon) on anterior wrists, penis, legs.

▶ Histopathologic examination is diagnostic.

▶ General Considerations

Lichen planus is an inflammatory pruritic disease of the skin and mucous membranes characterized by distinctive papules with a predilection for the flexor surfaces and trunk. The three cardinal findings are typical skin lesions, mucosal lesions, and histopathologic features of band-like infiltration of lymphocytes in the upper dermis. The most common drugs causing lichen planus-like reactions include sulfonamides, tetracycline, quinidine, NSAIDs, and hydrochlorothiazide. Hepatitis C infection is found with greater frequency in lichen planus patients than in controls. Allergy to mercury amalgams can trigger oral lesions identical to lichen planus.

▶ Clinical Findings

Itching is mild to severe. The lesions are violaceous, flat-topped, angulated papules, up to 1 cm in diameter, discrete or in clusters, with very fine white streaks (Wickham striae) on the flexor surfaces of the wrists and on the penis, lips, tongue as well as buccal, vaginal, and anorectal mucous membranes (Plate 40). The papules may become bullous or eroded. The disease may be generalized. Mucous membrane lesions have a lacy white network overlying them that may be confused with leukoplakia. The Koebner phenomenon (appearance of lesions in areas of trauma) may be seen.

A special form of lichen planus is the erosive or ulcerative variety, a major problem in the mouth or genitalia. Squamous cell carcinoma develops in 5% of patients with erosive oral or genital lichen planus.

▶ Differential Diagnosis

Lichen planus must be distinguished from similar lesions produced by medications (see above) and other papular lesions such as psoriasis, lichen simplex chronicus, graft-versus-host disease, and syphilis. Lichen planus on the mucous membranes must be differentiated from leukoplakia. Erosive oral lesions require biopsy and often direct immunofluorescence for diagnosis since lichen planus may simulate other erosive diseases.

▶ Treatment

A. Topical Therapy

Superpotent topical corticosteroids applied twice daily are most helpful for localized disease in nonflexural areas. Alternatively, high-potency corticosteroid cream or ointment may be used nightly under thin pliable plastic film.

Topical tacrolimus appears effective in oral and vaginal erosive lichen planus, but long-term therapy is required to prevent relapse. If tacrolimus is used, lesions must be observed carefully for development of cancer. Since absorption can occur through mucous membranes, serum tacrolimus levels should be checked at least once if widespread mucosal application ($> 5–10 \ cm^2$) is used. If the erosive oral lichen planus lesions are adjacent to a mercury containing amalgam, removal of the amalgam may result in clearing of the erosions.

B. Systemic Therapy

Corticosteroids (see Chapter 26) may be required in severe cases or in circumstances where the most rapid response to treatment is desired. Unfortunately, relapse almost always occurs as the corticosteroids are tapered, making systemic corticosteroid therapy an impractical option for the management of chronic lichen planus. NB-UVB, bath PUVA, oral PUVA, and the combination of an oral retinoid plus PUVA (re-PUVA) are all forms of phototherapy that can improve lichen planus. Hydroxychloroquine, 200 mg orally twice daily, can also be effective in mucosal lichen planus.

▶ Prognosis

Lichen planus is a benign disease, but it may persist for months or years and may be recurrent. Hypertrophic lichen planus and oral lesions tend to be especially persistent, and neoplastic degeneration has been described in chronically eroded lesions.

Carrozzo M et al. Lichen planus and hepatitis C virus infection: an updated critical review. Minerva Gastroenterol Dietol. 2008 Mar;54(1):65–74. [PMID: 18299669]
Torti DC et al. Oral lichen planus: a case series with emphasis on therapy. Arch Dermatol. 2007 Apr;143(4):511–5. [PMID: 17438185]

KAPOSI SARCOMA

▶ General Considerations

Before 1980 in the United States, this rare malignant skin lesion was seen mostly in elderly men, had a chronic clinical course, and was rarely fatal. Kaposi sarcoma occurs endemically in an often aggressive form in young black men of equatorial Africa, but it is rare in American blacks. Kaposi sarcoma continues to occur largely in homosexual men with HIV infection as an AIDS-defining illness. Kaposi sarcoma may complicate immunosuppressive therapy, and stopping the immunosuppression may result in improvement. Human herpes virus 8 (HHV-8), or Kaposi sarcoma-associated herpes virus (KSHV), is universally present in all forms of Kaposi sarcoma.

Red or purple plaques or nodules on cutaneous or mucosal surfaces are characteristic (Plate 41). Marked edema may occur with few or no skin lesions. Kaposi sarcoma commonly involves the gastrointestinal tract and can be screened for by fecal occult blood testing. In asymptomatic patients, these lesions are not sought or treated. Pulmonary Kaposi sarcoma can present with shortness of breath, cough, hemoptysis, or chest pain; it may be asymptomatic, appearing only on chest radiograph. Bronchoscopy may be indicated. The incidence of AIDS-associated Kaposi sarcoma is diminishing.

▶ Treatment

For Kaposi sarcoma in the elderly, palliative local therapy with intralesional chemotherapy or radiation is usually all that is required. In the setting of iatrogenic immunosuppression, the treatment of Kaposi sarcoma is primarily reduction of doses of immunosuppressive medications. In AIDS-associated Kaposi sarcoma, the patient should first be given effective anti-HIV antiretrovirals because in most cases this treatment alone is associated with improvement. Other therapeutic options include cryotherapy or intralesional vinblastine (0.1–0.5 mg/mL) for cosmetically objectionable lesions; radiation therapy for accessible and space-occupying lesions; and laser surgery for certain intraoral and pharyngeal lesions. Systemic therapy is indicated in patients with rapidly progressive skin disease (more than ten new lesions per month), with edema or pain, and with symptomatic visceral disease or pulmonary disease. Liposomal doxorubicin is highly effective in controlling these cases and has considerably less toxicity—and greater efficacy—than anthracycline monotherapy or combination chemotherapeutic regimens. α-Interferon may also be used. Paclitaxel and other taxanes can be effective even in patients who do not respond to anthracycline treatment. Col-3, a tetracycline derivative, has produced responses in refractory cases.

Di Lorenzo G et al. Management of AIDS-related Kaposi's sarcoma. Lancet Oncol. 2007 Feb;8(2):167–76. [PMID: 17267331]

Sullivan RJ et al. HIV/AIDS: epidemiology, pathophysiology, and treatment of Kaposi sarcoma associated herpesvirus disease: Kaposi sarcoma, primary effusion lymphoma and multicentric Castleman disease. Clin Infect Dis. 2008 Nov 1:47(9):1209–15. [PMID: 18808357]

PRURITUS (ITCHING)

Pruritus is a disagreeable sensation that provokes a desire to scratch. It is modulated by central factors, including anxiety, depression, and amphetamine and cocaine use. Many cases of pruritus are not mediated by histamine.

Dry skin is the first cause of itch that should be sought, since it is common and easily treated. Other causes include scabies, atopic dermatitis, insect bites, pediculosis, contact dermatitis, drug reactions, urticaria, psoriasis, lichen planus, lichen simplex chronicus, and fiberglass dermatitis.

Persistent pruritus not explained by cutaneous disease or association with a primary skin eruption should prompt a staged workup for systemic causes. Perhaps the most common cause of pruritus associated with systemic disease is uremia in conjunction with hemodialysis. Both this condition and the pruritus of liver disease may be helped by phototherapy with ultraviolet B or PUVA. Naltrexone and nalmefene have been shown to relieve the pruritus of liver disease. Naltrexone is not effective in pruritus associated with advanced chronic kidney disease, but gabapentin may be effective. Endocrine disorders such as hypothyroidism or hyperthyroidism, psychiatric disturbances, lymphoma, leukemia, and other internal malignant disorders, iron deficiency anemia, and certain neurologic disorders may also cause pruritus. Antihistamines reduce pruritus only by their sedating effect (except in urticaria). Nonsedating, second-generation antihistamines are of limited value in nonurticarial pruritus.

▶ Prognosis

Elimination of external factors and irritating agents may give complete relief. Pruritus accompanying a specific skin disease will subside when the skin disease is controlled. Pruritus accompanying serious internal disease may not respond to any type of therapy.

Greaves MW. Itch in systemic disease: therapeutic options. Dermatol Ther. 2005 Jul–Aug;18(4):323–7. [PMID: 16297004]

Heymann WR. Itch. J Am Acad Dermatol. 2006 Apr;54(4):705–6. [PMID: 16546594]

Lovell P et al. Management and treatment of pruritus. Skin Therapy Lett. 2007 Feb;12(1):1–6. [PMID: 17361313]

Yelverton CB et al. Exogenous factors in itch response. Curr Probl Dermatol. 2007;35:146–53. [PMID: 17641496]

ANOGENITAL PRURITUS

ESSENTIALS OF DIAGNOSIS

▸ Itching, chiefly nocturnal, of the anogenital area.

▸ Examination is highly variable, ranging from no skin findings to excoriations and inflammation of any degree, including lichenification.

▶ General Considerations

Anogenital pruritus may be due to intertrigo, psoriasis, lichen simplex chronicus, or seborrheic or contact dermatitis (from soaps, colognes, douches, contraceptives, and perhaps scented toilet tissue), or it may be due to irritating secretions, as in diarrhea, leukorrhea, or trichomoniasis, or to local disease (candidiasis, dermatophytosis, erythrasma), and at times oxyuriasis (pinworms). Lichen sclerosus may at times be the cause. Erythrasma is easily diagnosed by demonstration of coral-red fluorescence with Wood's light; it is easily cured with erythromycin orally or topically (Plate 42).

In pruritus ani, hemorrhoids are often found, and leakage of mucus and bacteria from the distal rectum onto the perianal skin may be important in cases in which no other skin abnormality is found.

Many women experience pruritus vulvae. Pruritus vulvae does not usually involve the anal area, though anal itching may spread to the vulva. In men, pruritus of the scrotum is most commonly seen in the absence of pruritus ani. Up to one-third of causes of anogenital pruritus may be due to nerve impingements of the lumbosacral spine, so referral for evaluation of lumbosacral spine disease is appropriate if no skin disorder is identified, and topical therapy is ineffective.

Squamous cell carcinoma of the anus and extramammary Paget disease are rare causes of genital pruritus.

▶ Clinical Findings

A. Symptoms and Signs

The only symptom is itching. Physical findings are usually not present, but there may be erythema, fissuring, maceration, lichenification, excoriations, or changes suggestive of candidiasis or tinea.

B. Laboratory Findings

Urinalysis and blood glucose testing may lead to a diagnosis of diabetes mellitus. Microscopic examination or culture of tissue scrapings may reveal yeasts or fungi. Stool examination may show pinworms. Radiologic studies may demonstrate spinal cord disease.

▶ Differential Diagnosis

The etiologic differential diagnosis consists of *Candida* infection, parasitosis, local irritation from contactants or irritants, nerve impingement and other primary skin disorders of the genital area such as psoriasis, seborrhea, intertrigo, or lichen sclerosus et atrophicus.

▶ Prevention

Instruct the patient in proper anogenital hygiene after treating systemic or local conditions. If appropriate, physical therapy and exercises to support the lower spine are recommended.

Treatment

A. General Measures

Treating constipation, preferably with high-fiber management (psyllium), may help. Instruct the patient to use very soft or moistened tissue or cotton after bowel movements and to clean the perianal area thoroughly with cool water if possible. Women should use similar precautions after urinating.

B. Local Measures

Pramoxine cream or lotion or hydrocortisone-pramoxine (Pramosone), 1% or 2.5% cream, lotion, or ointment, is helpful in managing pruritus in the anogenital area. The ointment or cream should be applied after a bowel movement. Topical doxepin cream 5% is similarly effective, but it may be sedating. The use of strong corticosteroids on the scrotum may lead to persistent severe burning upon withdrawal of the drug. Underclothing should be changed daily. Balneol Perianal Cleansing Lotion or Tucks premoistened pads, ointment, or cream may be very useful for pruritus ani. About one-third of patients with scrotal or anal pruritus will respond to capsaicin 0.006%. Treatment for underlying spinal neurologic disease may be required.

Prognosis

Although benign, anogenital pruritus is often persistent and recurrent.

Boardman LA et al. Recurrent vulvar itching. Obstet Gynecol. 2005 Jun;105(6):1451–5. [PMID: 15932843]

Cohen AD et al. Neuropathic scrotal pruritus: anogenital pruritus is a symptom of lumbosacral radiculopathy. J Am Acad Dermatol. 2005 Jan;52(1):61–6. [PMID: 15627082]

Siddiqi S et al. Pruritus ani. Ann R Coll Surg Engl. 2008 Sep;90(6):457–63. [PMID: 18765023]

SCABIES

ESSENTIALS OF DIAGNOSIS

▶ Generalized very severe itching.

▶ Pruritic burrows, vesicles and pustules, especially on finger webs and in wrist creases.

▶ Mites, ova, and brown dots of feces visible microscopically.

▶ Red papules or nodules on the scrotum and on the penile glans and shaft are pathognomonic.

General Considerations

Scabies is caused by infestation with *Sarcoptes scabiei*. The infestation usually spares the head and neck (though even these areas may be involved in infants, in the elderly, and in patients with AIDS). Scabies is usually acquired by sleeping with or in the bedding of an infested individual or by other close contact. The entire household may be affected. Hospital-associated scabies is increasingly common, primarily in long-term care facilities. Index patients are usually elderly and immunosuppressed. When these patients are hospitalized, hospital-based epidemics can occur. These epidemics are difficult to eradicate since many health care workers become infected and spread the infestation to other patients.

Clinical Findings

A. Symptoms and Signs

Itching is almost always present and can be quite severe. The lesions consist of more or less generalized excoriations with small pruritic vesicles, pustules, and "burrows" in the web spaces and on the heels of the palms, wrists, elbows, around the axillae, and on the breasts of women (Plate 43). The feet are a good place to identify burrows, since they may have been scratched off in other locations. The burrow appears as a short irregular mark, 2–3 mm long and the width of a hair. Characteristic nodular lesions may occur on the scrotum or penis and along the posterior axillary line.

B. Laboratory Findings

The diagnosis should be confirmed by microscopic demonstration of the organism, ova, or feces in a mounted specimen, examined with tap water. Best results are obtained when multiple lesions are scraped, choosing the best unexcoriated lesions from interdigital webs, wrists, elbows, or feet. A No. 15 blade is used to scrape each lesion until it is flat. Pinpoint bleeding may result from the scraping. Patients with crusted/hyperkeratotic scabies must be evaluated for immunosuppression (especially HIV and HTLV-1 infections) if no iatrogenic cause of immunosuppression is present.

Differential Diagnosis

Scabies must be distinguished from the various forms of pediculosis, from bedbug and flea bites, and from other causes of pruritus.

Treatment & Prognosis

Treatment is aimed at killing scabies mites and controlling the dermatitis, which can persist for months after effective eradication of the mites. Bedding and clothing should be laundered or cleaned or set aside for 14 days in plastic bags. High heat (60 °C) is required to kill the mites and ova. Unless treatment is aimed at all infected persons in a family or institutionalized group, reinfestations will probably occur.

Permethrin 5% cream is highly effective and safe in the management of scabies. Treatment consists of a single application for 8–12 hours, repeated in 1 week.

Pregnant patients should be treated only if they have documented scabies themselves. Permethrin 5% cream once for 12 hours—or 5% or 6% sulfur in petrolatum applied nightly for 3 nights from the collarbones down—may be used.

Patients will continue to itch for several weeks after treatment. Use of triamcinolone 0.1% cream will help resolve the dermatitis. Scabies in nursing home patients, institutionalized or mentally impaired (especially Down syndrome) patients, and AIDS patients may be much more difficult to treat.

Most failures in normal persons are related to incorrect use or incomplete treatment of the housing unit. In these cases, repeat treatment with permethrin once weekly for 2 weeks, with reeducation regarding the method and extent of application, is suggested. In immunocompetent individuals, ivermectin in a dose of 200 mcg/kg is effective in about 75% of cases with a single dose and 95% of cases with two doses 2 weeks apart. In immunosuppressed hosts and those with crusted (hyperkeratotic) scabies, multiple doses of ivermectin (every 2 weeks for two or three doses) plus topical therapy with permethrin once weekly may be effective when topical treatment and oral therapy alone fail. Oral ivermectin can be very beneficial in mass treatment to eradicate infections in institutions or villages.

If secondary pyoderma is present, it is treated with systemic antibiotics. In areas where nephritogenic streptococcal strains are prevalent, infestation with scabies or exposure to scabies-infested dogs may be followed by acute post-streptococcal glomerulonephritis.

Persistent pruritic postscabietic papules may be treated with mid- to high-potency corticosteroids or with intralesional triamcinolone acetonide (2.5–5 mg/mL).

Chosidow O. Clinical practices. Scabies. N Engl J Med. 2006 Apr 20;354(16):1718–27. [PMID: 16625010]

Heukelbach J et al. Scabies. Lancet. 2006 May 27;367(9524):1767–74. [PMID: 16731272]

Page TL et al. Clinical inquiries. When should you treat scabies empirically? J Fam Pract. 2007 Jul;56(7):570–2. [PMID: 17605950]

Mumcuoglu KY et al. Treatment of scabies infestations. Parasite. 2008 Sep;15(3):248–51. [PMID: 18814689]

Vorou R et al. Nosocomial scabies. J Hosp Infect. 2007 Jan;65(1):9–14. [PMID: 17141368]

PEDICULOSIS

ESSENTIALS OF DIAGNOSIS

► Pruritus with excoriation.
▸ Nits on hair shafts; lice on skin or clothes.
► Occasionally, sky-blue macules (maculae ceruleae) on the inner thighs or lower abdomen in pubic louse infestation.

General Considerations

Pediculosis is a parasitic infestation of the skin of the scalp, trunk, or pubic areas. Body lice usually occur among people who live in overcrowded dwellings with inadequate hygiene facilities. Pubic lice may be sexually transmitted. Head lice may be transmitted by shared use of hats or combs. Adults contacting children with head lice frequently acquire the infestation.

There are three different varieties: (1) pediculosis pubis, caused by *Phthirus pubis* (pubic louse, "crabs"); (2) pediculosis corporis, caused by *Pediculus humanus* var *corporis* (body louse); and (3) pediculosis capitis, caused by *Pediculus humanus* var *capitis* (head louse).

Head and body lice are similar in appearance and are 3–4 mm long. The body louse can seldom be found on the body, because the insect comes onto the skin only to feed and must be looked for in the seams of the clothing. Trench fever, relapsing fever, and typhus are transmitted by the body louse in countries where those diseases are endemic.

Clinical Findings

Itching may be very intense in body louse infestations, and scratching may result in deep excoriations, especially over the upper shoulders, posterior flanks, and neck. In some cases, only itching is present, with few excoriations seen. Pyoderma may be the presenting sign. Head lice can be found on the scalp or may be manifested as small nits resembling pussy willow buds on the scalp hairs close to the skin. They are easiest to see above the ears and at the nape of the neck. Pubic louse infestations are occasionally generalized, particularly in hairy individuals; the lice may even be found on the eyelashes and in the scalp.

Differential Diagnosis

Head louse infestation must be distinguished from seborrheic dermatitis, body louse infestation from scabies and bedbug bites, and pubic louse infestation from anogenital pruritus and eczema.

Treatment

Body lice are treated by disposing of the infested clothing and addressing the patient's social situation. For pubic lice, permethrin rinse 1% for 10 minutes and permethrin cream 5% applied for 8 hours are effective. Sexual contacts should be treated. Clothes and bedclothes should be washed and dried at high temperature if possible.

Permethrin 1% cream rinse (Nix) is a topical over-the-counter pediculicide and ovicide and is the treatment of choice for head lice. It is applied to the scalp and hair and left on for 8 hours before being rinsed off. Permethrin resistance of head lice is common. Malathion lotion 1% (Ovide) is very effective, but it is highly volatile and flammable, so application must be done in a well-ventilated room or out of doors. For involvement of eyelashes, petrolatum is applied thickly twice daily for 8 days, and remaining nits are then plucked off.

Leone PA. Scabies and pediculosis pubis: an update of treatment regimens and general review. Clin Infect Dis. 2007 Apr 1;44(Suppl 3):S153–9. [PMID: 17342668]

SKIN LESIONS DUE TO OTHER ARTHROPODS

ESSENTIALS OF DIAGNOSIS

► Localized rash with pruritus.
► Furuncle-like lesions containing live arthropods.

- Tender erythematous patches that migrate ("larva migrans").
- Generalized urticaria or erythema multiforme in some patients.

General Considerations

Some arthropods (eg, mosquitoes and biting flies) are readily detected as they bite. Many others are not, eg, because they are too small, because there is no immediate reaction, or because they bite during sleep. Reactions are allergic and may be delayed for hours to days. Patients are most apt to consult a clinician when the lesions are multiple and pruritus is intense.

Many persons will react severely only to their earliest contacts with an arthropod, thus presenting pruritic lesions when traveling, moving into new quarters, etc. Body lice, fleas, bedbugs, and mosquitoes should be considered. Spiders are often incorrectly believed to be the source of bites; they rarely attack humans, though the brown spider (Loxosceles laeta, Loxosceles reclusa) may cause severe necrotic reactions and death due to intravascular hemolysis, and the black widow spider (Latrodectus mactans) may cause severe systemic symptoms and death. (See also Chapter 38.) The majority of patient-diagnosed, physician-diagnosed, and even published cases of brown recluse spider bites (or loxoscelism) are incorrect, especially if made in areas where these spiders are not endemic. Many of these lesions are actually due to CA-MRSA.

In addition to arthropod bites, the most common lesions are venomous stings (wasps, hornets, bees, ants, scorpions) or bites (centipedes), furuncle-like lesions due to fly maggots or sand fleas in the skin, and a linear creeping eruption due to a migrating larva.

Clinical Findings

The diagnosis may be difficult when the patient has not noticed the initial attack but suffers a delayed reaction. Individual bites are often in clusters and tend to occur either on exposed parts (eg, midges and gnats) or under clothing, especially around the waist or at flexures (eg, small mites or insects in bedding or clothing). The reaction is often delayed for 1–24 hours or more. Pruritus is almost always present and may be all but intolerable once the patient starts to scratch. Secondary infection may follow scratching. Urticarial wheals are common. Papules may become vesicular. The diagnosis is aided by searching for exposure to arthropods and by considering the patient's occupation and recent activities.

The principal arthropods are as follows:

1. **Fleas:** Fleas are bloodsucking ectoparasites that feed on dogs, cats, humans, and other species. Flea saliva produces papular urticaria in sensitized individuals. To break the life cycle of the flea, one must treat the home and pets, using quick-kill insecticides, residual insecticides, and a growth regulator.
2. **Bedbugs:** In crevices of beds or furniture; bites tend to occur in lines or clusters. Papular urticaria is a characteristic lesion of bedbug (Cimex lectularius) bites. Bedbugs are not restricted to any socioeconomic group and are a major health problem in some major metropolitan areas, especially in commercial and residential hotels.
3. **Ticks:** Usually picked up by brushing against low vegetation.
4. **Chiggers or red bugs:** These are larvae of trombiculid mites. A few species confined to particular regions and locally recognized habitats (eg, berry patches, woodland edges, lawns, brush turkey mounds in Australia, poultry farms) attack humans, often around the waist, on the ankles, or in flexures, raising intensely itching erythematous papules after a delay of many hours. The red chiggers may sometimes be seen in the center of papules that have not yet been scratched.
5. **Bird and rodent mites:** Larger than chiggers, bird mites infest birds and their nests. Bites are multiple anywhere on the body. Room air conditioning units may suck in bird mites and infest the inhabitants of the room. Rodent mites from mice or rats may cause similar effects. If the domicile has evidence of rodent activity, then rodent mite dermatitis should be suspected, as the mites are rarely found. Pet rodents or birds may be infested with mites, maintaining the infestation.
6. **Mites in stored products:** These are white and almost invisible and infest products such as copra, vanilla pods, sugar, straw, cottonseeds, and cereals. Persons who handle these products may be attacked, especially on the hands and forearms and sometimes on the feet.
7. **Caterpillars of moths with urticating hairs:** The hairs are blown from cocoons or carried by emergent moths, causing severe and often seasonally recurrent outbreaks after mass emergence. The gypsy moth is a cause in the eastern United States.
8. **Tungiasis:** Tungiasis is due to the burrowing flea known as Tunga penetrans and is found in Africa, the West Indies, and South and Central America. The female burrows under the skin, sucks blood, swells to 0.5 cm, and then ejects her eggs onto the ground. Ulceration, lymphangitis, gangrene, and septicemia may result, in some cases with lethal effect. Simple surgical removal is usually performed.

Differential Diagnosis

Arthropods should be considered in the differential diagnosis of skin lesions showing any of the above symptoms.

Prevention

Arthropod infestations are best prevented by avoidance of contaminated areas, personal cleanliness, and disinfection of clothing, bedclothes, and furniture as indicated. Chiggers and mites can be repelled by permethrin applied to the head and clothing. (It is not necessary to remove clothing.) Bedbugs are no longer repelled by permethrin. Aggressive hygiene and removal of the infested occupant from the domicile may be required to eradicate bedbug infestation in a residence.

Treatment

Living arthropods should be removed carefully with tweezers after application of alcohol and preserved in alcohol for identification. In endemic Rocky Mountain spotted fever areas, ticks should not be removed with the bare fingers.

Corticosteroid lotions or creams are helpful. Topical antibiotics may be applied if secondary infection is suspected. Localized persistent lesions may be treated with intralesional corticosteroids.

Stings produced by many arthropods may be alleviated by applying papain powder (Adolph's Meat Tenderizer) mixed with water, or aluminum chloride hexahydrate (Xerac AC).

Extracts from venom sacs of bees, wasps, yellow jackets, and hornets are available for immunotherapy of patients at risk for anaphylaxis.

Scarupa MD et al. Bedbug bites masquerading as urticaria. J Allergy Clin Immunol. 2006 Jun;117(6):1508–9. [PMID: 16751024]
Swanson DL et al. Bites of brown recluse spiders and suspected necrotic arachnidism. N Engl J Med. 2005 Feb 17;352(7):700–7. [PMID: 15716564]
Vetter RS et al. Of spiders and zebras: publication of inadequately documented loxoscelism case reports. J Am Acad Dermatol. 2007 Jun;56(6):1063–4. [PMID: 17504721]

INFLAMMATORY NODULES

ERYTHEMA NODOSUM

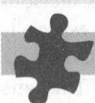 ESSENTIALS OF DIAGNOSIS

▶ Painful red nodules without ulceration on anterior aspects of legs.

▶ Slow regression over several weeks to resemble contusions.

▶ Women are predominantly affected by a ratio of 10:1 over men.

▶ Some cases associated with infection or drug exposure.

General Considerations

Erythema nodosum is a symptom complex characterized by tender, erythematous nodules that appear most commonly on the extensor surfaces of the lower legs. It usually lasts about 6 weeks and may recur. The disease may be associated with various infections—streptococcosis, primary coccidioidomycosis, other deep fungal infections, tuberculosis, *Yersinia pseudotuberculosis* and *Yersinia enterocolitica* infection, or syphilis. It may accompany sarcoidosis, Behçet disease, and inflammatory bowel disease. Erythema nodosum may be associated with pregnancy or with use of oral contraceptives or other medication.

Clinical Findings

A. Symptoms and Signs

The subcutaneous swellings are exquisitely tender and may be preceded by fever, malaise, and arthralgia. They are most often

located on the anterior surfaces of the legs below the knees but may occur on the arms, trunk, and face. The lesions, 1–10 cm in diameter, are at first pink to red; with regression, all the various hues seen in a contusion can be observed (Plate 44).

B. Laboratory Findings

Evaluation of patients presenting with acute erythema nodosum should include a careful history (including drug exposures) and physical examination for prior upper respiratory infection or diarrheal illness, symptoms of any deep fungal infection endemic to the area, a chest radiograph, a PPD, and two consecutive ASO/DNAseB titers at 2- to 4-week intervals. If no underlying cause is found, only a small percentage of patients will go on to develop a significant underlying illness (usually sarcoidosis) over the next year.

Differential Diagnosis

Erythema induratum from tuberculosis is seen on the posterior surfaces of the legs and may ulcerate. Lupus panniculitis presents as tender nodules on the buttocks and posterior arms that heal with depressed scars. In polyarteritis nodosa, the subcutaneous nodules are often associated with a fixed livedo. In the late stages, erythema nodosum must be distinguished from simple bruises and contusions.

Treatment

First, the underlying cause should be identified and treated. Primary therapy is with NSAIDs in usual doses. Saturated solution of potassium iodide, 5–15 drops three times daily, results in prompt involution in many cases. Complete bed rest may be advisable if the lesions are painful. Systemic therapy directed against the lesions themselves may include corticosteroid therapy (see Chapter 26) unless contraindicated by associated infection.

Prognosis

The lesions usually disappear after about 6 weeks, but they may recur.

Campen RB et al. Case records of the Massachusetts General Hospital. Case 25-2006. A 41-year-old woman with painful subcutaneous nodules. N Engl J Med. 2006 Aug 17;355(7):714–22. [PMID: 16914708]
Schwartz RA et al. Erythema nodosum: a sign of systemic disease. Am Fam Physician. 2007 Mar 1;75(5):695–700. [PMID: 17375516]

FURUNCULOSIS (Boils) & CARBUNCLES

 ESSENTIALS OF DIAGNOSIS

▶ Extremely painful inflammatory swelling based on a hair follicle that forms an abscess.

▶ Predisposing condition (diabetes mellitus, HIV disease, injection drug use) sometimes present.

▶ Coagulase-positive *Staphylococcus aureus* is the causative organism.

General Considerations

A furuncle (boil) is a deep-seated infection (abscess) caused by *S aureus* and involving the entire hair follicle and adjacent subcutaneous tissue. The most common sites of occurrence are the hairy parts exposed to irritation and friction, pressure, or moisture. Because the lesions are autoinoculable, they are often multiple. Diabetes mellitus (especially if using insulin injections), injection drug use, allergy injections, and HIV disease all increase the risk of staphylococcal infections by increasing the rate of carriage. Certain other exposures including hospitalization, athletic teams, prisons, military service, and homelessness may also increase the risk of infection.

A carbuncle consists of several furuncles developing in adjoining hair follicles and coalescing to form a conglomerate, deeply situated mass with multiple drainage points.

Clinical Findings

A. Symptoms and Signs

Pain and tenderness may be prominent. The abscess is either rounded or conical. It gradually enlarges, becomes fluctuant, and then softens and opens spontaneously after a few days to 1–2 weeks to discharge a core of necrotic tissue and pus. The inflammation occasionally subsides before necrosis occurs. Infection of the soft tissue around the nails (paronychia) may be due to staphylococci when it is acute or *Candida* when chronic.

B. Laboratory Findings

There may be slight leukocytosis, but a white blood cell count is rarely required. Pus should be cultured to rule out MRSA or other bacteria. Culture of the anterior nares may identify chronic staphylococcal carriage in cases of recurrent cutaneous infection.

Differential Diagnosis

The most common entity in the differential is an inflamed epidermal inclusion cyst that suddenly becomes red, tender, and expands greatly in size over one to a few days. The history of a prior cyst in the same location, the presence of a clearly visible cyst orifice, and the extrusion of malodorous cheesy rather than purulent material helps in the diagnosis. Tinea profunda (deep dermatophyte infection of the hair follicle) may simulate recurrent furunculosis. Furuncle is also to be distinguished from deep mycotic infections, such as sporotrichosis; from other bacterial infections, such as anthrax and tularemia (rare); from atypical mycobacterial infections; and from acne cysts. Hidradenitis suppurativa presents with recurrent tender sterile abscesses in the axillae and groin, on the buttocks, or below the breasts. The presence of old scars or sinus tracts plus negative cultures suggests this diagnosis.

Complications

Serious and sometimes fatal complications of staphylococcal infection such as septicemia can occur.

Prevention

Identifying and eliminating the source of infection is critical to prevent recurrences after treatment. The source individual may have chronic dermatitis or be an asymptomatic carrier. Local measures such as meticulous handwashing; no sharing of towels and clothing; aggressive scrubbing of showers, bathrooms and surfaces with bleach; bleach baths ($^1/_2$ to 1 cup per 20 liters of bathwater for 15 minutes 3–5 times weekly) and isolation of infected patients who reside in institutions to prevent spread are all effective measures.

Treatment

A. Specific Measures

Incision and drainage is recommended for all loculated suppurations and is the mainstay of therapy. Systemic antibiotics are usually given, although they offer little beyond adequate incision and drainage. Sodium dicloxacillin or cephalexin, 1 g daily in divided doses by mouth for 10 days, is usually effective. Doxycycline 100 mg twice daily, trimethoprim-sulfamethoxazole DS one tablet twice daily, and clindamycin 150–300 mg twice daily are effective in treating MRSA. Recurrent furunculosis may be effectively treated with a combination of cephalexin, 250–500 mg four times daily for 2–4 weeks, and rifampin, 300 mg twice daily for 5 days during this period. Chronic clindamycin, 150–300 mg daily for 1–2 months, may also cure recurrent furunculosis. Family members and intimate contacts may need evaluation for staphylococcal carrier state and perhaps concomitant treatment. Applications of topical 2% mupirocin to the nares, axillae, and anogenital areas twice daily for 5 days may eliminate the staphylococcal carrier state, although resistance is increasing.

B. Local Measures

Immobilize the part and avoid overmanipulation of inflamed areas. Use moist heat to help larger lesions "localize." Use surgical incision and drainage *after* the lesions are "mature." To incise and drain an acute staphylococcal paronychia, insert a flat metal spatula or sharpened hardwood stick into the nail fold where it adjoins the nail. This will release pus from a mature lesion.

Prognosis

Recurrent crops may harass the patient for months or years.

Elston DM. Community-acquired methicillin-resistant *Staphylococcus aureus*. J Am Acad Dermatol. 2007 Jan;56(1):1–16. [PMID: 17190619]

Embil JM et al. A man with recurrent furunculosis. CMAJ. 2006 Jul 18;175(2):143. [PMID: 16804121]

EPIDERMAL INCLUSION CYST

ESSENTIALS OF DIAGNOSIS

► Firm dermal papule or nodule.

- Overlying black comedone or "punctum."
- Expressible foul-smelling cheesy material.
- May become red and drain, mimicking an abscess.

General Considerations

Epidermal inclusion cysts (EICs) are common, benign growths of the upper portion of the hair follicle. They are common in Gardner syndrome and may be the first stigmata of the condition.

Epidermal inclusion cysts favor the face and trunk and may complicate nodulocystic acne vulgaris. Individual lesions range in size from 0.3 cm to several centimeters. An overlying pore or punctum is characteristic. Lateral pressure may lead to extrusion of a foul-smelling, cheesy material.

Differential Diagnosis

EICs are distinguished from lipomas by being more superficial (in the dermis not the subcutaneous fat) and by their overlying punctum. Many other benign and malignant tumors may superficially resemble EICs, but all lack the punctum.

Complications

EICs may rupture, creating an acute inflammatory nodule very similar to an abscess. Cultures of the expressed material will be sterile.

Treatment

Treatment is not required if asymptomatic. Inflamed lesions may be treated with incision and drainage or intralesional triamcinolone acetomide 5–10 mg/mL. For large or symptomatic cysts, surgical excision is curative.

Lee HE et al. Comparison of the surgical outcomes of punch incision and elliptical excision in treating epidermal inclusion cysts: a prospective, randomized study. Dermatol Surg. 2006 Apr;32(4):520–5. [PMID: 16681659]

Sukal SA et al. Safer and less unpleasant incision and drainage of epidermal inclusion cysts. Dermatol Surg. 2006 Sep;32(9):1214–5. [PMID: 16970709]

PHOTODERMATITIS

 ESSENTIALS OF DIAGNOSIS

- Painful or pruritic erythema, edema, or vesiculation on sun-exposed surfaces: the face, neck, hands, and "V" of the chest.
- Inner upper eyelids spared, as is the area under the chin.

General Considerations

In most cases, photosensitivity is an acute or chronic skin reaction due to hypersensitivity to ultraviolet radiation. It is caused by certain drugs, by lupus erythematosus, and some inherited disorders including the porphyrias. Contact photosensitivity may occur with plants, perfumes, and sunscreens.

Photodermatitis is manifested as phototoxicity—a tendency for the individual to sunburn more easily than expected—or, as photoallergy, a true immunologic reaction that often presents with dermatitis.

Clinical Findings

A. Symptoms and Signs

The acute inflammatory skin reaction, if severe enough, is accompanied by pain, fever, gastrointestinal symptoms, malaise, and even prostration, but this is very rare. Signs include erythema, edema, and possibly vesiculation and oozing on exposed surfaces. Peeling of the epidermis and pigmentary changes often result. The key to diagnosis is localization of the rash to photoexposed areas, though these eruptions may become generalized with time to involve even photoprotected areas. The lower lip may be affected.

B. Laboratory Findings

Blood and urine tests are generally not helpful unless porphyria cutanea tarda is suggested by the presence of blistering, scarring, milia (white cysts 1–2 mm in diameter) and skin fragility of the dorsal hands, and facial hypertrichosis. Eosinophilia may be present in chronic photoallergic responses.

Differential Diagnosis

The differential diagnosis is long. If a clear history of the use of a topical or systemic photosensitizer is not available and if the eruption is persistent, then a workup including biopsy and light testing may be required. Photodermatitis must be differentiated from contact dermatitis that may develop from one of the many substances in suntan lotions and oils, as these may often have a similar distribution. Sensitivity to actinic rays may also be part of a more serious condition such as porphyria cutanea tarda or lupus erythematosus. These disorders are diagnosed by appropriate blood or urine tests. Phenothiazines, quinine or quinidine, griseofulvin, sulfonylureas (especially hydrochlorothiazide), NSAIDs, and antibiotics (eg, some tetracyclines, quinolone, trimethoprim-sulfamethoxazole) may photosensitize the skin. PMLE is a very common idiopathic photodermatitis and often has its onset in the third to fourth decades except in Native Americans and Latinos, in whom it may present in childhood. PMLE is chronic in nature. Transitory periods of spontaneous remission do occur. The action spectrum of PMLE may also extend into the long ultraviolet wavelengths (UVA; 320–400 nm). Drug-induced photosensitivity is triggered by UVA.

Complications

Some individuals continue to be chronic light reactors even when they apparently are no longer exposed to photosensitizing drugs.

Prevention

While sunscreens are useful agents in general and should be used by persons with photosensitivity, patients may react to such low amounts of energy that sunscreens alone may not be sufficient. Sunscreens with an SPF of 30–60 and broad UVA coverage, containing dicamphor sulfonic acid (Mexoryl SX), avobenzone (Parasol 1789), titanium dioxide, and micronized zinc oxide, are especially useful in patients with photoallergic dermatitis. Photosensitivity due to porphyria is not prevented by sunscreens and requires barrier protection (clothing) to prevent outbreaks.

Treatment

A. Specific Measures

Drugs should be suspected in cases of photosensitivity even if the particular medication (such as hydrochlorothiazide) has been used for months.

B. Local Measures

When the eruption is vesicular or weepy, treatment is similar to that of any acute dermatitis, using cooling and soothing wet dressing.

Sunscreens should be used as described above. Mid-potency to high-potency topical corticosteroids are of limited benefit in sunburn reactions but may help in PMLE and photoallergic reactions. Since the face is often involved, close monitoring for corticosteroid side effects is recommended.

C. Systemic Measures

Aspirin may have some value for fever and pain of acute sunburn. Systemic corticosteroids in doses as described for acute contact dermatitis may be required for severe photosensitivity reactions. Otherwise, different photodermatoses are treated in specific ways.

Patients with severe photoallergy may require immunosuppressives, such as azathioprine, in the range of 50–150 mg/d, or cyclosporine, 3–5 mg/kg/d.

Prognosis

The most common phototoxic sunburn reactions are usually benign and self-limited. PMLE and some cases of photoallergy can persist for years.

Lautenschlager S et al. Photoprotection. Lancet. 2007 Aug 11;370(9586):528–37. [PMID: 17693182]
Morison WL. Clinical practice. Photosensitivity. N Engl J Med. 2004 Mar 11;350(11):1111–7. [PMID: 15014184]

ULCERS

LEG ULCERS SECONDARY TO VENOUS INSUFFICIENCY

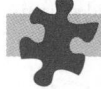

ESSENTIALS OF DIAGNOSIS

▸ Past history of varicosities, thrombophlebitis, or post-phlebitic syndrome.

▸ Irregular ulceration, often on the medial aspect of the lower legs above the malleolus.

▸ Edema of the legs, varicosities, hyperpigmentation, and red and scaly areas (stasis dermatitis) and scars from old ulcers support the diagnosis.

General Considerations

Patients at risk may have a history of venous insufficiency, either with obvious varicosities or with a past history of thrombophlebitis, or with immobility of the calf muscle group (paraplegics, etc). Red, pruritic patches of stasis dermatitis often precede ulceration. Because venous insufficiency plays a role in between 75% and 90% of lower leg ulcerations, testing of venous competence is a required part of a leg ulcer evaluation even when no changes of venous insufficiency are present.

Clinical Findings

A. Symptoms and Signs

Classically, chronic edema is followed by a dermatitis, which is often pruritic. These changes are followed by hyperpigmentation, skin breakdown, and eventually sclerosis of the skin of the lower leg (Plate 45). The ulcer base may be clean, but it often has a yellow fibrin eschar that may require surgical removal. Ulcers that appear on the feet, toes, or above the knees should be approached with other diagnoses in mind.

B. Laboratory Findings

Thorough evaluation of the patient's vascular system (including measurement of the ankle/brachial index [ABI]) is essential. If the ABI is less than 0.7, the patient should be referred to a vascular surgeon for surgical evaluation. Doppler and light rheography examinations as office procedures are usually sufficient (except in the diabetic) to elucidate the cause of most vascular cases of lower leg ulceration.

Differential Diagnosis

The differential includes vasculitis, pyoderma gangrenosum, arterial ulcerations, infection, trauma, skin cancer, arachnid bites, and sickle cell anemia. When the diagnosis is in doubt, a punch biopsy from the border (not base) of the lesion may be helpful.

Prevention

Compression stockings to reduce edema are the most important means of prevention. Compression should achieve a pressure of 30 mm Hg below the knee and 40 mm Hg at the ankle. The stockings should not be used in patients with arterial insufficiency with an ABI less than 0.7. Pneumatic sequential compression devices may be of great benefit when edema is refractory to standard compression dressings.

Treatment

A. Local Measures

Clean the base of the ulcer with saline or cleansers such as Saf-Clens. A curette or small scissors can be used to remove the yellow fibrin eschar; local anesthesia may be used if the areas are very tender.

The ulcer is treated with metronidazole gel to reduce bacterial growth and odor. Any red dermatitic skin is treated with a medium- to high-potency corticosteroid ointment. The ulcer is then covered with an occlusive hydroactive dressing (DuoDerm, Hydrasorb or Cutinova) or a polyurethane foam (Allevyn) followed by an Unna zinc paste boot. This is changed weekly. The ulcer should begin to heal within weeks, and healing should be complete within 4–6 months. If the patient is diabetic, becaplermin (Regranex) may be applied to those ulcers that are not becoming smaller or developing a granulating base. Some ulcerations require grafting. Full- or split-thickness grafts often do not take, and pinch grafts (small shaves of skin laid onto the bed) may be effective. Cultured epidermal cell grafts may accelerate wound healing, but they are very expensive. They should be considered in refractory ulcers, especially those that have not healed after a year or more of conservative therapy.

No topical intervention has evidence to suggest that it will improve healing of arterial leg ulcers.

B. Systemic Therapy

Pentoxifylline, 400 mg three times daily administered with compression dressings, is beneficial in accelerating healing of venous insufficiency leg ulcers. Zinc supplementation is occasionally beneficial in patients with low serum zinc levels. If cellulitis accompanies the ulcer, systemic antibiotics are recommended: dicloxacillin, 250 mg orally four times a day, or levofloxacin, 500 mg once daily for 1–2 weeks is usually adequate. Routine use of antibiotics and treating bacteria isolated from a chronic ulcer without clinical evidence of infection is discouraged. If the ulcer fails to heal or there is a persistent draining tract in the ulcer, an underlying osteomyelitis should be sought.

Prognosis

The combination of compression stockings and newer dressings enables venous stasis ulcers to heal within months. Topical growth factors, antibiotics, debriding agents, and xenografts and autografts can be considered in recalcitrant cases. If the ABI is less than 0.5, the prognosis for healing is poor. Ongoing control of edema is essential to prevent recurrent ulceration.

Lopez P et al. Effectiveness of dressings for healing venous leg ulcers. Am Fam Physician. 2007 Mar 1;75(5):649–50. [PMID: 17375509]

Nelson EA et al. Dressings and topical agents for arterial leg ulcers. Cochrane Database Syst Rev. 2007 Jan 24;(1):CD001836. [PMID: 17253465]

Palfreyman S et al. Dressings for venous leg ulcers: systematic review and meta-analysis. BMJ. 2007 Aug 4;335(7613):244. [PMID: 17631512]

▼ MISCELLANEOUS DERMATOLOGIC DISORDERS*

PIGMENTARY DISORDERS

Although the color of skin may be altered by many diseases and agents, the vast majority of patients have either an increase or decrease in pigment secondary to some inflammatory disease such as acne or atopic dermatitis.

Other pigmentary disorders include those resulting from exposure to exogenous pigments such as carotenemia, argyria, and tattooing. Other endogenous pigmentary disorders are attributable to metabolic substances—including hemosiderin (iron)—in purpuric processes; or to homogentisic acid in ochronosis; and bile pigments.

Classification

First, determine whether the disorder is hyperpigmentation or hypopigmentation, ie, an increase or decrease in normal skin colors. Each may be considered to be primary or to be secondary to other disorders.

A. Primary Pigmentary Disorders

1. Hyperpigmentation—The disorders in this category are nevoid, congenital or acquired, and include pigmented nevi, ephelides (juvenile freckles), and lentigines (senile freckles). Hyperpigmentation occurs also in arsenical melanosis or in association with Addison disease. **Melasma (chloasma)** occurs as patterned hyperpigmentation of the face, usually as a direct effect of estrogens. It occurs not only during pregnancy but also in 30–50% of women taking oral contraceptives, and rarely in men. One report suggests that such men have low testosterone and elevated luteinizing hormone levels.

2. Hypopigmentation and depigmentation—The disorders in this category are vitiligo, albinism, and piebaldism. In vitiligo, pigment cells (melanocytes) are destroyed (Plate 46). Vitiligo, present in approximately 1% of the population, may be associated with other autoimmune disorders such as autoimmune thyroid disease, pernicious anemia, diabetes mellitus, and Addison disease.

B. Secondary Pigmentary Disorders

Any damage to the skin (irritation, allergy, infection, excoriation, burns, or dermatologic therapy such as chemical peels and freezing with liquid nitrogen) may result in hyperpigmentation or hypopigmentation. Several disorders of clinical importance are described below.

1. Hyperpigmentation—The most common type of secondary hyperpigmentation occurs after another dermatologic condition, such as acne, and is most commonly seen in moderately complexioned persons (Asians, Hispanics, and light-skinned African Americans). It is called postinflammatory hyperpigmentation.

---

*Hirsutism is discussed in Chapter 26.

Pigmentation may be produced by certain drugs, eg, chloroquine, chlorpromazine, minocycline, and amiodarone. Fixed drug eruptions to phenolphthalein in laxatives, to trimethoprim-sulfamethoxazole, to NSAIDs, and to tetracyclines, for example, are further causes.

2. Hypopigmentation—Leukoderma is a disorder that may complicate atopic dermatitis, lichen planus, psoriasis, DLE, and lichen simplex chronicus. Practitioners must exercise special care in using liquid nitrogen on any patient with olive or darker complexions, since doing so may result in hypopigmentation or depigmentation, at times permanent. Intralesional or intra-articular injections of high concentrations of corticosteroids may also cause localized temporary hypopigmentation.

Differential Diagnosis

The evaluation of pigmentary disorders is helped by Wood's light, which accentuates epidermal pigmentation and highlights hypopigmentation. Depigmentation, as seen in vitiligo, enhances with Wood's light examination, whereas postinflammatory hypopigmentation does not.

Complications

Actinic keratoses and skin cancers are more likely to develop in persons with vitiligo. Severe emotional trauma may occur in extensive vitiligo and other types of hypopigmentation and hyperpigmentation, particularly in naturally dark-skinned persons.

Treatment & Prognosis

A. Hyperpigmentation

Therapeutic bleaching preparations generally contain hydroquinone. Hydroquinone has occasionally caused unexpected hypopigmentation, hyperpigmentation, or even secondary ochronosis and pigmented milia, particularly with prolonged use.

The role of exposure to ultraviolet light cannot be overstressed as a factor promoting or contributing to most disorders of hyperpigmentation, and such exposure should be minimized. Melasma, ephelides, and postinflammatory hyperpigmentation may be treated with varying success with 3–4% hydroquinone cream, gel, or solution and a sunscreen containing UVA photoprotectants (Avobenzone, Mexoryl, zinc oxide, titanium dioxide). Tretinoin cream, 0.025–0.05%, may be added. Superficial melasma responds well, but if there is predominantly dermal deposition of pigment (does *not* enhance with Wood's light), the prognosis is poor. Response to therapy takes months and requires avoidance of sunlight. Hyperpigmentation often recurs after treatment if the skin is exposed to ultraviolet light. Solar lentigines respond to liquid nitrogen application. Tretinoin, 0.1% cream and tazarotene 0.1% used over 10 months, will fade solar lentigines (liver spots), hyperpigmented facial macules in Asians, and postinflammatory hyperpigmentation in blacks. New laser systems for the removal of epidermal and dermal pigments are available, and referral should be considered for patients whose responses to medical treatment are inadequate.

B. Hypopigmentation

In secondary hypopigmentation, repigmentation may occur spontaneously. Cosmetics such as Covermark and Dermablend are highly effective for concealing disfiguring patches. Therapy of vitiligo is long and tedious, and the patient must be strongly motivated. If less than 20% of the skin is involved (most cases), topical tacrolimus 0.1% twice daily is the first-line therapy. A superpotent corticosteroid may also be used, but local skin atrophy from prolonged use may ensue. With 20–25% involvement, narrowband UVB or oral PUVA is best. Severe phototoxic response (sunburn) may occur with PUVA. The face and upper chest respond best, and the fingertips and the genital areas do not respond as well to treatment. Years of treatment may be required. Newer techniques of using epidermal autografts and cultured epidermis combined with PUVA therapy give hope for surgical correction of vitiligo.

Taïeb A et al. Clinical practice. Vitiligo. N Engl J Med. 2009 Jan 8;360(2):160–9. [PMID: 19129529]
Whitton ME et al. Interventions for vitiligo. Cochrane Database Syst Rev. 2006 Jan 25;(1):CD003263. [PMID: 16437451]

BALDNESS (Alopecia)

Baldness Due to Scarring (Cicatricial Alopecia)

Cicatricial baldness may occur following chemical or physical trauma, lichen planopilaris, bacterial or fungal infections, severe herpes zoster, chronic DLE, scleroderma, and excessive ionizing radiation. The specific cause is often suggested by the history, the distribution of hair loss, and the appearance of the skin, as in lupus erythematosus. Biopsy is useful in the diagnosis of scarring alopecia, but specimens must be taken from the active border and not from the scarred central zone.

Scarring alopecias are irreversible and permanent. It is important to diagnose and treat the scarring process as early in its course as possible.

Baldness Not Associated with Scarring

Nonscarring alopecia may occur in association with various systemic diseases such as SLE, secondary syphilis, hyperthyroidism or hypothyroidism, iron deficiency anemia, and pituitary insufficiency. The only treatment necessary is prompt and adequate control of the underlying disorder and usually leads to regrowth of the hair.

Androgenetic (pattern) baldness, the most common form of alopecia, is of genetic predetermination. The earliest changes occur at the anterior portions of the calvarium on either side of the "widow's peak" and on the crown (vertex). The extent of hair loss is variable and unpredictable. Minoxidil 5% is available over the counter and can be specifically recommended for persons with recent onset (< 5 years) and smaller areas of alopecia. Approximately 40% of patients treated twice daily for a year will have moderate to dense growth. Finasteride (Propecia), 1 mg orally daily, has similar efficacy and may be additive to minoxidil. As opposed to minoxidil, finasteride is used only in males.

Hair loss or thinning of the hair in women results from the same cause as common baldness in men (androgenetic alopecia) and may be treated with topical minoxidil. A workup consisting of determination of serum testosterone, DHEAS, iron, total iron binding capacity, thyroid function tests, and a complete blood count will identify most other causes of hair thinning in premenopausal women. Women who complain of thin hair but show little evidence of alopecia need follow-up, because more than 50% of the scalp hair can be lost before the clinician can perceive it.

Telogen effluvium is transitory increase in the number of hairs in the telogen (resting) phase of the hair growth cycle. This may occur spontaneously, may appear at the termination of pregnancy, may be precipitated by "crash dieting," high fever, stress from surgery or shock, malnutrition, or may be provoked by hormonal contraceptives. Whatever the cause, telogen effluvium usually has a latent period of 2–4 months. The prognosis is generally good. The condition is diagnosed by the presence of large numbers of hairs with white bulbs coming out upon gentle tugging of the hair. Counts of hairs lost by the patient on combing or shampooing often exceed 150 per day, compared to an average of 70–100. In one study, a major cause of telogen effluvium was found to be iron deficiency, and the hair counts bore a clear relationship to serum iron levels.

Alopecia areata is of unknown cause but is believed to be an immunologic process. Typically, there are patches that are perfectly smooth and without scarring. Tiny hairs 2–3 mm in length, called "exclamation hairs," may be seen. Telogen hairs are easily dislodged from the periphery of active lesions. The beard, brows, and lashes may be involved. Involvement may extend to all of the scalp hair (alopecia totalis) or to all scalp and body hair (alopecia universalis). Severe forms may be treated by systemic corticosteroid therapy, although recurrences follow discontinuation of therapy. Alopecia areata is occasionally associated with Hashimoto thyroiditis, pernicious anemia, Addison disease, and vitiligo.

Intralesional corticosteroids are frequently effective for alopecia areata. Triamcinolone acetonide in a concentration of 2.5–10 mg/mL is injected in aliquots of 0.1 mL at approximately 1- to 2-cm intervals, not exceeding a total dose of 30 mg per month for adults. Alternatively, anthralin 0.5% ointment, used daily, may help some patients. Alopecia areata is usually self-limiting, with complete regrowth of hair in 80% of patients with focal disease. Some mild cases are resistant to treatment, as are the extensive totalis and universalis types. Both topical diphencyprone and squaric acid dibutylester, have been used to treat persistent alopecia areata. The principle is to sensitize the skin, then intermittently apply weaker concentrations to produce and maintain a slight dermatitis. Hair regrowth in 3–6 months in some patients has been reported to be remarkable. Long-term safety and efficacy have not been established. Support groups for patients with extensive alopecia areata are very beneficial.

In **trichotillomania** (the pulling out of one's own hair), the patches of hair loss are irregular and short growing hairs are always present, since they cannot be pulled out until they are long enough. The patches are often unilateral, occurring on the same side as the patient's dominant hand. The patient may be unaware of the habit.

Han A et al. Clinical approach to the patient with alopecia. Semin Cutan Med Surg. 2006 Mar;25(1):11–23. [PMID: 16616299]
Rogers NE et al. Medical treatments for male and female pattern hair loss. J Am Acad Dermatol. 2008 Oct;59(4):547–66. [PMID: 18793935]

NAIL DISORDERS

1. Morphologic Abnormalities of the Nails

▶ Classification

Acquired nail disorders may be classified as local or those associated with systemic or generalized skin diseases.

A. Local Nail Disorders

Onycholysis (distal separation of the nail plate from the nail bed, usually of the fingers) is caused by excessive exposure to water, soaps, detergents, alkalies, and industrial cleaning agents. Candidal infection of the nail folds and subungual area, nail hardeners, and drug-induced photosensitivity may cause onycholysis, as may hyperthyroidism, hypothyroidism, and psoriasis.

1. Distortion of the nail occurs as a result of chronic inflammation of the nail matrix underlying the eponychial fold. Such changes may also be caused by warts, tumors, or cysts, impinging on the nail matrix.

2. Discoloration and crumbly thickened nails are noted in dermatophyte infection and psoriasis.

3. Allergic reactions (to resins in undercoats and polishes or to nail glues) are characterized by onycholysis or by grossly distorted, hypertrophic, and misshapen nails.

B. Nail Changes Associated with Systemic or Generalized Skin Diseases

Beau lines (transverse furrows) may follow any serious systemic illness.

1. Atrophy of the nails may be related to trauma or to vascular or neurologic disease.

2. Clubbed fingers may be due to the prolonged hypoxemia associated with cardiopulmonary disorders (Plate 47). (See Chapter 9.)

3. Spoon nails may be seen in anemic patients.

4. Stippling or pitting of the nails is seen in psoriasis, alopecia areata, and hand eczema.

5. Nail hyperpigmentation may be caused by many chemotherapeutic agents, but especially the taxanes.

▶ Differential Diagnosis

Onychomycosis may cause nail changes identical to those seen in psoriasis. Careful examination for more characteristic lesions elsewhere on the body is essential to the diagnosis of the nail disorders. Cancer should be suspected (eg, Bowen disease or squamous cell carcinoma) as the cause of any persistent solitary subungual or periungual lesion.

Complications

Toenail changes may lead to an ingrown nail—in turn often complicated by bacterial infection and occasionally by exuberant granulation tissue. Poor manicuring and poorly fitting shoes may contribute to this complication. Cellulitis may result.

Treatment & Prognosis

Treatment consists usually of careful debridement and manicuring and, above all, reduction of exposure to irritants (soaps, detergents, alkali, bleaches, solvents, etc). Longitudinal grooving due to temporary lesions of the matrix, such as warts, synovial cysts, and other impingements, may be cured by removal of the offending lesion.

2. Tinea Unguium (Onychomycosis)

Tinea unguium is a trichophyton infection of one or more (but rarely all) fingernails or toenails. The species most commonly found is *T rubrum*. "Saprophytic" fungi may rarely (< 5%) cause onychomycosis.

The nails are lusterless, brittle, and hypertrophic, and the substance of the nail is friable. Laboratory diagnosis is mandatory since only 50% of dystrophic nails are due to dermatophytosis. Portions of the nail should be cleared with 10% KOH and examined under the microscope for hyphae. Fungi may also be cultured. Periodic acid-Schiff stain of a histologic section of the nail plate will also demonstrate the fungus readily. Each technique is positive in only 50% of cases so several different tests may need to be performed.

Onychomycosis is difficult to treat because of the long duration of therapy required and the frequency of recurrences. Fingernails respond more readily than toenails. For toenails, treatment is limited to patients with discomfort, inability to exercise, and immune compromise.

In general, systemic therapy is required to effectively treat nail onychomycosis. Topical therapy has limited value and the adjunctive value of surgical procedures is unproven. Fingernails can virtually always be cured and toenails are cured 35–50% of the time and are clinically improved about 75% of the time. In all cases, before treatment, the diagnosis should be confirmed. The costs of the various treatment options should be known and the most cost-effective treatment chosen. Drug interactions must be avoided. Ketoconazole, due to its higher risk for hepatotoxicity, is not recommended to treat any form of onychomycosis. For fingernails, ultramicronized griseofulvin 250 mg orally three times daily for 6 months can be effective. Alternative treatments are (in order of preference) oral terbinafine 250 mg/d for 6 weeks, oral itraconazole 400 mg/d for 7 days each month for 2 months, and oral itraconazole 200 mg/d for 2 months. Off-label use of fluconazole, 400 mg once weekly for 6 months, can also be effective, but there is limited evidence for this option. Once clear, fingernails usually remain free of disease for some years.

Onychomycosis of the toenails does not respond to griseofulvin therapy or topical treatments. The best treatment, which is also FDA approved, is oral terbinafine 250 mg daily for 12 weeks. Liver function tests and a complete blood count with platelets are performed monthly during treatment. Pulse oral itraconazole 200 mg twice daily for 1 week per month for 3 months is inferior to standard terbinafine treatments, but it is an acceptable alternative for those unable to take terbinafine. The courses of terbinafine or itraconazole may need to be repeated 6 months after the first treatment cycle if fungal cultures of the nail are still positive.

Crawford F et al. Topical treatments for fungal infections of the skin and nails of the foot. Cochrane Database Syst Rev. 2007 Jul 18;(3):CD001434. [PMID: 17636672]

Scher RK et al. Onychomycosis: diagnosis and definition of cure. J Am Acad Dermatol. 2007 Jun;56(6):939–44. [PMID: 17307276]

Wilcock M et al. Inappropriate use of oral terbinafine in family practice. Pharm World Sci. 2003 Feb;25(1):25–6. [PMID: 12661473]

DERMATITIS MEDICAMENTOSA (Drug Eruption)

ESSENTIALS OF DIAGNOSIS

▶ Usually, abrupt onset of widespread, symmetric erythematous eruption.

▶ May mimic any inflammatory skin condition.

▶ Constitutional symptoms (malaise, arthralgia, headache, and fever) may be present.

General Considerations

As is well recognized, only a minority of cutaneous drug reactions result from allergy. True allergic drug reactions involve prior exposure, an "incubation" period, reactions to doses far below the therapeutic range, manifestations different from the usual pharmacologic effects of the drug, involvement of only a small portion of the population at risk, restriction to a limited number of syndromes (anaphylactic and anaphylactoid, urticarial, vasculitic, etc), and reproducibility.

Rashes are among the most common adverse reactions to drugs and occur in 2–3% of hospitalized patients. Amoxicillin, trimethoprim-sulfamethoxazole, and ampicillin or penicillin are the most common causes of urticarial and maculopapular reactions. Toxic epidermal necrolysis and Stevens-Johnson syndrome are most commonly produced by sulfonamides and anticonvulsants. Phenolphthalein, pyrazolone derivatives, tetracyclines, NSAIDs, trimethoprim-sulfamethoxazole, and barbiturates are the major causes of fixed drug eruptions.

Clinical Findings

A. Symptoms and Signs

Drug eruptions are generally classified as "simple" or "complex." Simple drug eruptions involve an exanthem, usually appear in the second week of drug therapy, and have no associated constitutional or laboratory findings. Antibiotics, including the penicillins and quinolones are the most common causes. Complex drug eruptions occur during the third week of treatment on average and have constitutional and laboratory findings. These may include fevers, chills, hematologic abnormalities (especially eosinophilia), and abnormal liver or kidney function. A mnemonic for complex eruptions is "DRESS" (DRug Eruption with Eosinophilia and Systemic Symptoms). The most common causes are the long-acting sulfonamides, allopurinol, and anticonvulsants. The use of anticonvulsants to treat bipolar disorder and chronic pain has led to an apparent increase in these reactions. Coexistent reactivation of Epstein-Barr virus, HHV-6, or cytomegalovirus is often present and may be important in the pathogenesis of these complex drug eruptions. Table 6–3 summarizes the types of skin reactions, their appearance and distribution, and the common offenders in each case.

B. Laboratory Findings

Routinely ordered blood work is of no value in the diagnosis of simple drug eruptions. In complex drug eruptions, the CBC, liver biochemical tests, and renal function tests should be monitored. Skin biopsies may be helpful in making the diagnosis.

Table 6–3. Skin reactions due to systemic drugs.

Reaction	Appearance	Distribution and Comments	Common Offenders
Toxic erythema	Morbilliform, maculopapular, exanthematous reactions.	The most common skin reaction to drugs. Often more pronounced on the trunk than on the extremities. In previously exposed patients, the rash may start in 2–3 days. In the first course of treatment, the eruption often appears about the seventh to ninth days. Fever may be present.	Antibiotics (especially ampicillin and tri-methoprim-sulfamethoxazole), sulfonamides and related compounds (including thiazide diuretics, furosemide, and sulfonylurea hypoglycemic agents), and barbiturates.
Erythema multiforme major	Target-like lesions. Bullae may occur. Mucosal involvement.	Usually trunk and proximal extremities.	Sulfonamides, anticonvulsants, and NSAIDs.
Erythema nodosum	Inflammatory cutaneous nodules.	Usually limited to the extensor aspects of the legs. May be accompanied by fever, arthralgias, and pain.	Oral contraceptives.
Allergic vasculitis	Inflammatory changes may present as urticaria that lasts over 24 hours, hemorrhagic papules ("palpable purpura"), vesicles, bullae, or necrotic ulcers.	Most severe on the legs.	Sulfonamides, phenytoin, propylthiouracil.
Exfoliative dermatitis and erythroderma	Red and scaly.	Entire skin surface.	Allopurinol, sulfonamides, isoniazid, anticonvulsants, gold, or carbamazepine.
Photosensitivity: increased sensitivity to light, often of ultraviolet A wavelengths, but may be due to UVB or visible light as well	Sunburn, vesicles, papules in photodistributed pattern.	Exposed skin of the face, the neck, and the backs of the hands and, in women, the lower legs. Exaggerated response to ultraviolet light.	Sulfonamides and sulfonamide-related compounds (thiazide diuretics, furosemide, sulfonylureas), tetracyclines, phenothiazines, sulindac, amiodarone, voriconazole, and NSAIDs.
Drug-related lupus erythematosus	May present with a photo-sensitive rash, annular lesions or psoriasis on upper trunk.	Less severe than systemic lupus erythematosus, sparing the kidneys and central nervous system. Recovery often follows drug withdrawal.	Diltiazem, etanercept, hydrochlorothiazide, infliximab, lisinopril.
Lichenoid and lichen planus-like eruptions	Pruritic, erythematous to violaceous polygonal papules that coalesce or expand to form plaques.	May be in photo- or nonphotodistributed pattern.	Carbamazepine, furosemide, gold salts, hydroxychloroquine, methyldopa, phenothiazines, propranolol, quinidine, quinine, sulfonylureas, tetracyclines, thiazides, and triprolidine.

(continued)

Table 6–3. Skin reactions due to systemic drugs. (continued)

Reaction	Appearance	Distribution and Comments	Common Offenders
Fixed drug eruptions	Single or multiple demarcated, round, erythematous plaques that often become hyperpigmented.	Recur at the same site when the drug is repeated. Hyperpigmentation, if present, remains after healing.	Numerous drugs, including antimicrobials, analgesics, barbiturates, cardiovascular drugs, heavy metals, antiparasitic agents, antihistamines, phenolphthalein, ibuprofen, and naproxen.
Toxic epidermal necrolysis	Large sheets of erythema, followed by separation, which looks like scalded skin.	Rare.	In adults, the eruption has occurred after administration of many classes of drugs, particularly anticonvulsants (lamotrigine and others), antibiotics, sulfonamides, and NSAIDs.
Urticaria	Red, itchy wheals that vary in size from < 1 cm to many centimeters. May be accompanied by angioedema.	Chronic urticaria is rarely caused by drugs.	Acute urticaria: penicillins, NSAIDs, sulfonamides, opiates, and salicylates. Angioedema is common in patients receiving ACE inhibitors.
Pigmentary changes	Flat hyperpigmented areas.	Forehead and cheeks (chloasma, melasma). The most common pigmentary disorder associated with drug ingestion. Improvement is slow despite stopping the drug.	Oral contraceptives are the usual cause.
	Blue-gray discoloration.	Light-exposed areas.	Chlorpromazine and related phenothiazines.
	Brown or blue-gray pigmentation.	Generalized.	Heavy metals (silver, gold, bismuth, and arsenic).
	Yellow color.	Generalized.	Usually quinacrine.
	Blue-black patches on the shins.		Minocycline, chloroquine.
	Blue-black pigmentation of the nails and palate and depigmentation of the hair.		Chloroquine.
	Slate-gray color.	Primarily in photoexposed areas.	Amiodarone.
	Brown discoloration of the nails.	Especially in more darkly pigmented patients.	Hydroxyurea.
Psoriasiform eruptions	Scaly red plaques.	May be located on trunk and extremities. Palms and soles may be hyperkeratotic. May cause psoriasiform eruption or worsen psoriasis.	Antimalarials, lithium, β-blockers, and tumor necrosis factor (TNF)-inhibitors.
Pityriasis rosea–like eruptions	Oval, red, slightly raised patches with central scale.	Mainly on the trunk.	Barbiturates, bismuth, captopril, clonidine, gold salts, methopromazine, metoprolol, metronidazole, and tripelennamine.

ACE, angiotensin-converting enzyme; NSAIDs, nonsteroidal anti-inflammatory drugs.

Differential Diagnosis

Observation after discontinuation, which may be a slow process, helps establish the diagnosis. Rechallenge, though of theoretical value, may pose a danger to the patient and is best avoided.

Complications

Some cutaneous drug reactions may be associated with visceral involvement. The organ systems involved depend on the individual medication or drug class. Most common is an infectious mononucleosis-like illness and hepatitis associated with administration of anticonvulsants.

Treatment

A. General Measures

Systemic manifestations are treated as they arise (eg, anemia, icterus, purpura). Antihistamines may be of value in urticarial and angioneurotic reactions. Epinephrine 1:1000, 0.5–1 mL intravenously or subcutaneously, should be used as an emergency measure. In complex eruptions, systemic corticosteroids may be required, starting at about 1 mg/kg/d and tapering very slowly.

B. Local Measures

Extensive blistering eruptions resulting in erosions and superficial ulcerations demand hospitalization and nursing care as for burn patients.

▶ Prognosis

Drug rash usually disappears upon withdrawal of the drug and proper treatment.

Bahna SL et al. New concepts in the management of adverse drug reactions. Allergy Asthma Proc. 2007 Sep–Oct;28(5):517–24. [PMID: 18034968]

Chia FL et al. Severe cutaneous adverse reactions to drugs. Curr Opin Allergy Clin Immunol. 2007 Aug;7(4):304–9. [PMID: 17620821]

Ganeva M et al. Carbamazepine-induced drug reaction with eosinophilia and systemic symptoms (DRESS) syndrome: report of four cases and brief review. Int J Dermatol. 2008 Aug;47(8):853–60. [PMID: 18717872]

Greenberger PA. 8. Drug allergy. J Allergy Clin Immunol. 2006 Feb;117(2 Suppl Mini-Primer):S464–70. [PMID: 16455348]

Disorders of the Eyes & Lids

Paul Riordan-Eva, FRCS, FRCOphth

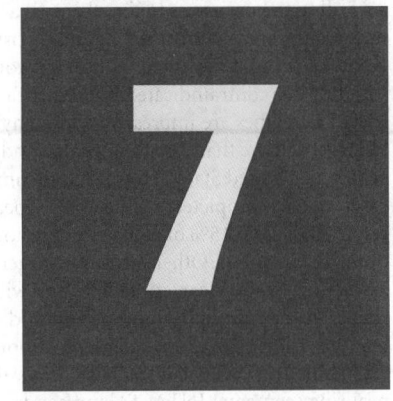

REFRACTIVE ERRORS

Refractive errors are the most common cause of reduced clarity of vision (visual acuity) and may be a readily treatable component of poor vision in patients with other diagnoses. In **emmetropia** (the normal state), objects at infinity are seen clearly with the unaccommodated eye. Objects nearer than infinity are seen with the aid of accommodation, which increases the refractive power of the lens. In **hyperopia**, objects at infinity are not seen clearly unless accommodation is used, and near objects may not be seen because accommodative capacity is finite. Hyperopia is corrected with plus (convex) lenses. In **myopia**, the unaccommodated eye focuses on objects closer than infinity; the distance of such objects from the patient becomes progressively shorter with increasing myopia. Thus, the high myope is able to focus on very near objects without glasses. Objects beyond this distance cannot be seen without the aid of corrective (minus, concave) lenses. In **astigmatism**, the refractive errors in the horizontal and vertical axes differ. **Presbyopia** is the natural loss of accommodative capacity with age. Persons with emmetropia usually notice inability to focus on objects at a normal reading distance at about age 45. Persons with hyperopia experience symptoms at an earlier age. Presbyopia is corrected with plus lenses for near work.

Use of a pinhole will overcome most refractive errors and thus allows their identification as a cause of reduced visual acuity.

1. Contact Lenses

Contact lenses are used mostly for correction of refractive errors, for which they provide better optical correction than glasses, as well as for management of diseases of the cornea, conjunctiva, or lids. The major types of lenses are rigid (gas-permeable) and soft. Rigid lenses are more durable and easier to care for than soft lenses but are more difficult to tolerate.

Contact lens care includes cleaning and sterilization whenever the lenses are removed and removal of protein deposits as required. Sterilization is usually by chemical methods. For individuals developing reactions to preserva-

tives in contact lens solutions, preservative-free systems are available. All contact lenses can be inserted in the morning and removed at night. Soft lenses are also available for extended wear. Disposable soft lenses to avoid the necessity for lens cleaning and sterilization are available for daily or extended wear.

The major risk from contact lens wear is bacterial, amebic, or fungal corneal infection, potentially a blinding condition. Such infections occur more commonly with soft lenses, particularly extended wear, for which there is at least a fivefold increase in risk of corneal ulceration compared with daily wear. Contact lens wearers should be made aware of the risks they face and ways to minimize them, such as avoiding extended-wear soft lenses and maintaining meticulous lens hygiene, including not using tap water or saliva for lens cleaning. Whenever there is ocular discomfort or redness, contact lenses should be removed. Ophthalmologic care should be sought if symptoms persist.

► When to Refer

Any contact lens wearer with an acute painful red eye must be referred emergently to an ophthalmologist.

Dart JK et al. Risk factors for microbial keratitis with contemporary contact lenses: a case-control study. Ophthalmology. 2008 Oct;115(10):1647–54. [PMID: 18597850]

Patel A et al. Contact lens-related microbial keratitis: recent outbreaks. Curr Opin Ophthalmol. 2008 Jul;19(4):302–6. [PMID: 18545011]

Stapleton F et al. The incidence of contact lens-related microbial keratitis in Australia. Ophthalmology. 2008 Oct;115(10):1655–62. [PMID: 18538404]

2. Surgical Correction

Various surgical techniques are available for the correction of refractive errors, particularly myopia. Laser corneal refractive surgery reshapes the mid-portion (stroma) of the cornea with an excimer laser. Laser assisted in situ keratomileusis (LASIK), including femtosecond laser assisted LASIK (IntraLASIK), and the surface ablation techniques epithelial LASIK (Epi-LASIK), laser epithelial keratomileusis (LASEK), and photorefractive keratectomy (PRK) differ according to how access to the stroma is achieved. LASIK is most commonly performed because postoperative visual recovery is rapid and there is little postoperative discomfort, but it is contraindicated if the cornea is relatively thin. Visual outcomes are impressive and many individuals seek treatment; more than 1 million people undergo LASIK each year in the United States. However, outcomes for individual cases are not completely predictable. Repeated treatment is required in up to 15% of patients and serious complications occur in up to 5%. Other refractive surgery techniques are extraction of the clear crystalline lens with insertion of a single vision, multifocal or accommodative intraocular lens, insertion of an intraocular lens without removal of the crystalline lens (phakic intraocular lens), intrastromal corneal ring segments (INTACS), and conductive keratoplasty (CK). Topical atropine and pirenzepine, a selective muscarinic antagonist, and rigid contact lens wear during sleep (orthokeratology) are also being investigated for myopia.

Fong CS. Refractive surgery: the future of perfect vision? Singapore Med J. 2007 Aug;48(8):709–18. [PMID: 17657376]

Sakimoto T et al. Laser eye surgery for refractive errors. Lancet. 2006 Apr 29;367(9520):1432–47. [PMID: 16650653]

Van Meter WS et al. Safety of overnight orthokeratology for myopia: a report by the American Academy of Ophthalmology. 2008 Dec;115(12):2301–13. [PMID: 18804868]

DISORDERS OF THE LIDS & LACRIMAL APPARATUS

1. Hordeolum

Hordeolum is a common staphylococcal abscess that is characterized by a localized red, swollen, acutely tender area on the upper or lower lid (Plate 48). Internal hordeolum is a meibomian gland abscess that points onto the conjunctival surface of the lid; external hordeolum or sty is smaller and on the margin.

Warm compresses are helpful. Incision may be indicated if resolution does not begin within 48 hours. An antibiotic ointment (bacitracin or erythromycin) applied to the eyelid every 3 hours may be beneficial during the acute stage. Internal hordeolum may lead to generalized cellulitis of the lid.

2. Chalazion

Chalazion is a common granulomatous inflammation of a meibomian gland that may follow an internal hordeolum. It is characterized by a hard, nontender swelling on the upper or lower lid with redness and swelling of the adjacent conjunctiva. If the chalazion is large enough to impress the cornea, vision will be distorted. Treatment is usually by incision and curettage but corticosteroid injection may also be effective.

3. Blepharitis

Blepharitis is a common chronic bilateral inflammatory condition of the lid margins. **Anterior blepharitis** involves the eyelid skin, eyelashes, and associated glands.

It may be ulcerative, because of infection by staphylococci, or seborrheic in association with seborrhea of the scalp, brows, and ears. **Posterior blepharitis** results from inflammation of the meibomian glands. There may be bacterial infection, particularly with staphylococci, or primary glandular dysfunction, in which there is a strong association with acne rosacea.

▶ Clinical Findings

Symptoms are irritation, burning, and itching. In **anterior blepharitis**, the eyes are "red-rimmed," and scales or granulations can be seen clinging to the lashes. In **posterior blepharitis**, the lid margins are hyperemic with telangiectasias; the meibomian glands and their orifices are inflamed, with dilation of the glands, plugging of the orifices, and abnormal secretions. The lid margin is frequently rolled inward to produce a mild entropion, and the tears may be frothy or abnormally greasy.

Blepharitis is a common cause of recurrent conjunctivitis. Both anterior and, more particularly, posterior blepharitis may be complicated by hordeola or chalazions; abnormal lid or lash positions, producing trichiasis; epithelial keratitis of the lower third of the cornea; marginal corneal infiltrates; and inferior corneal vascularization and thinning.

▶ Treatment

Anterior blepharitis is usually controlled by cleanliness of the lid margins, eyebrows, and scalp. Scales should be removed from the lids daily with a hot wash cloth or a damp cotton applicator and baby shampoo. In acute exacerbations, an antistaphylococcal antibiotic eye ointment such as bacitracin or erythromycin is applied daily to the lid margins. Antibiotic sensitivity studies may be helpful in severe cases.

In **mild posterior blepharitis,** regular meibomian gland expression may be sufficient to control symptoms. Inflammation of the conjunctiva and cornea indicates a need for more active treatment, including long-term low-dose oral antibiotic therapy, usually with tetracycline (250 mg twice daily), doxycycline (100 mg daily), minocycline (50–100 mg daily) or erythromycin (250 mg three times daily), and possibly short-term topical corticosteroids, eg, prednisolone, 0.125% twice daily. Topical therapy with antibiotics such as ciprofloxacin 0.3% ophthalmic solution twice daily may be helpful but should be restricted to short courses.

4. Entropion & Ectropion

Entropion (inward turning of usually the lower lid) occurs occasionally in older people as a result of degeneration of the lid fascia, or may follow extensive scarring of the conjunctiva and tarsus. Surgery is indicated if the lashes rub on the cornea. Botulinum toxin injections may also be used for temporary correction of the involutional lower eyelid entropion of older people.

Ectropion (outward turning of the lower lid) is common with advanced age. Surgery is indicated if there is excessive tearing, exposure keratitis, or a cosmetic problem.

Hintschich C. Correction of entropion and ectropion. Dev Ophthalmol. 2008;41:85–102. [PMID: 18453763]

5. Tumors

Basal cell carcinoma, squamous cell carcinoma, meibomian gland carcinoma, and malignant melanoma are the common cancers of the skin of the eyelids. Surgery for any lesion involving the lid margin should be performed by an ophthalmologist or suitably trained plastic surgeon to avoid deformity of the lid. Otherwise, small lesions can often be excised by the nonophthalmologist. Histopathologic examination of eyelid tumors should be routine, since 2% of lesions thought to be benign clinically are found to be malignant. The Mohs technique of intraoperative examination of excised tissue is particularly valuable in ensuring complete excision so that the risk of recurrence is reduced.

Bernardini FP. Management of malignant and benign eyelid lesions. Curr Opin Ophthalmol. 2006 Oct;17(5):480–4. [PMID: 16932064]

6. Dacryocystitis

Dacryocystitis is infection of the lacrimal sac due to obstruction of the nasolacrimal system. It may be acute or chronic and occurs most often in infants and in persons over 40 years. It is usually unilateral.

The usual infectious organisms are *Staphylococcus aureus* and β-hemolytic streptococci in acute dacryocystitis and *Staphylococcus epidermidis*, anaerobic streptococci, or *Candida albicans* in chronic dacryocystitis.

Acute dacryocystitis is characterized by pain, swelling, tenderness, and redness in the tear sac area; purulent material may be expressed. In chronic dacryocystitis, tearing and discharge are the principal signs, and mucus or pus may also be expressed.

Acute dacryocystitis responds well to systemic antibiotic therapy. Surgical relief of the underlying obstruction is usually done electively but may be performed urgently in acute cases. The chronic form may be kept latent with antibiotics, but relief of the obstruction is the only cure. In adults, the standard procedure for obstruction of the lacrimal drainage system is dacryocystorhinostomy, which involves surgical exploration of the lacrimal sac and formation of a fistula into the nasal cavity. Laser-assisted endoscopic dacryocystorhinostomy and balloon dilation or probing of the nasolacrimal system are alternatives. Congenital nasolacrimal duct obstruction is common and often resolves spontaneously but, if necessary, can be treated by probing of the nasolacrimal system, for example.

Kapadia MK et al. Evaluation and management of congenital nasolacrimal duct obstruction. Otolaryngol Clin North Am. 2006 Oct;39(5):959–77. [PMID: 16982257]

Mills DM et al. Acquired nasolacrimal duct obstruction. Otolaryngol Clin North Am. 2006 Oct;39(5):979–99. [PMID: 16982258]

CONJUNCTIVITIS

Conjunctivitis is the most common eye disease. It may be acute or chronic. Most cases are due to viral or bacterial (including gonococcal and chlamydial) infection. Other causes include keratoconjunctivitis sicca, allergy, chemical irritants, and deliberate self-harm. The mode of transmission of infectious conjunctivitis is usually direct contact via fingers, towels, handkerchiefs, etc, to the fellow eye or to other persons. It may be through contaminated eye drops.

Conjunctivitis must be differentiated from acute uveitis, acute glaucoma, and corneal disorders (Table 7–1).

Table 7–1. The inflamed eye: Differential diagnosis of common causes.

	Acute Conjunctivitis	Acute Anterior Uveitis (Iritis)	Acute Angle-Closure Glaucoma	Corneal Trauma or Infection
Incidence	Extremely common	Common	Uncommon	Common
Discharge	Moderate to copious	None	None	Watery or purulent
Vision	No effect on vision	Often blurred	Markedly blurred	Usually blurred
Pain	Mild	Moderate	Severe	Moderate to severe
Conjunctival injection	Diffuse; more toward fornices	Mainly circumcorneal	Mainly circumcorneal	Mainly circumcorneal
Cornea	Clear	Usually clear	Steamy	Clarity change related to cause
Pupil size	Normal	Small	Moderately dilated and fixed	Normal or small
Pupillary light response	Normal	Poor	None	Normal
Intraocular pressure	Normal	Usually normal but may be low or elevated	Markedly elevated	Normal
Smear	Causative organisms	No organisms	No organisms	Organisms found only in corneal infection

1. Viral Conjunctivitis

One of the most common causes of viral conjunctivitis is adenovirus type 3. Conjunctivitis due to this agent is usually associated with pharyngitis, fever, malaise, and preauricular adenopathy (pharyngoconjunctival fever). Locally, the palpebral conjunctiva is red, and there is a copious watery discharge and scanty exudate. Children are more often affected than adults, and contaminated swimming pools are sometimes the source of infection. The disease usually lasts 10 days. Epidemic keratoconjunctivitis is caused by adenovirus types 8, 19, 29, and 37. It is more likely to be complicated by visual loss due to corneal subepithelial infiltrates. The disease lasts at least 2 weeks.

Topical sulfonamides prevent secondary bacterial infection and cold compresses reduce the discomfort of the associated lid edema.

2. Bacterial Conjunctivitis

The organisms isolated most commonly in bacterial conjunctivitis are staphylococci, streptococci (particularly *S pneumoniae*), *Haemophilus* species, *Pseudomonas*, and *Moraxella*. All may produce a copious purulent discharge. There is no blurring of vision and only mild discomfort. In severe cases, examination of stained conjunctival scrapings and cultures is recommended.

The disease is usually self-limited, lasting about 10–14 days if untreated. Topical sulfonamide (eg, sulfacetamide, 10% ophthalmic solution or ointment three times a day) will usually clear the infection in 2–3 days but the need for antibacterial therapy is disputed. Povidone-iodine may also be effective. The use of topical fluoroquinolones is rarely justified for treatment of a generally self-limiting, benign infection.

Høvding G. Acute bacterial conjunctivitis. Acta Ophthalmol Scan. 2008 Feb;86(1):5–17. [PMID: 17970823]

A. Gonococcal Conjunctivitis

Gonococcal conjunctivitis, usually acquired through contact with infected genital secretions, typically causes copious purulent discharge. It is an ophthalmologic emergency because corneal involvement may rapidly lead to perforation. The diagnosis should be confirmed by stained smear and culture of the discharge. A single 1-g dose of intramuscular ceftriaxone is usually adequate. Topical antibiotics such as erythromycin and bacitracin may be added. Other sexually transmitted diseases, including chlamydiosis, syphilis, and HIV infection, should be considered.

B. Chlamydial Keratoconjunctivitis

1. Trachoma—Trachoma is a major cause of blindness worldwide. Recurrent episodes of infection in childhood manifest as bilateral follicular conjunctivitis, epithelial keratitis, and corneal vascularization (pannus). Cicatrization of the tarsal conjunctiva leads to entropion and trichiasis in adulthood, with secondary central corneal scarring.

Immunologic tests or polymerase chain reaction on conjunctival samples will confirm the diagnosis but treatment should be started on the basis of clinical findings. Single-dose therapy with oral azithromycin, 20 mg/kg, is effective. Alternatively, oral tetracycline or erythromycin, 250 mg four times a day, or doxycycline, 100 mg twice a day, is given for 3–4 weeks. Local treatment is not necessary. Surgical treatment includes correction of eyelid deformities and corneal transplantation.

Wright HR et al. Trachoma. Lancet. 2008 Jun 7;371(9628):1945–54. [PMID: 18539226]

2. Inclusion conjunctivitis—The agent of inclusion conjunctivitis is a common cause of genital tract disease in adults. The eye is usually involved following contact with genital secretions. The disease starts with acute redness, discharge, and irritation. The eye findings consist of follicular conjunctivitis with mild keratitis. A nontender preauricular lymph node can often be palpated. Healing usually leaves no sequelae. Diagnosis can be rapidly confirmed by immunologic tests or polymerase chain reaction on conjunctival samples. Treatment is with oral tetracycline or erythromycin, 500 mg four times a day, or doxycycline, 100 mg twice a day, for 1–2 weeks. Single-dose therapy with azithromycin, 1 g, may also be effective. Before treatment, all cases should be assessed for genital tract infection so that management can be adjusted accordingly, and other venereal diseases sought.

3. Dry Eyes (Keratoconjunctivitis Sicca)

This is a common disorder, particularly in older women. Hypofunction of the lacrimal glands, causing loss of the aqueous component of tears, may be due to aging, hereditary disorders, systemic disease (eg, Sjögren syndrome), or systemic and topical drugs. Excessive evaporation of tears may be due to environmental factors (eg, a hot, dry, or windy climate) or abnormalities of the lipid component of the tear film, as in blepharitis. Mucin deficiency may be due to malnutrition, infection, burns, or drugs.

▶ **Clinical Findings**

The patient complains of dryness, redness, or a scratchy feeling of the eyes. In severe cases, there is persistent marked discomfort, with photophobia, difficulty in moving the eyelids, and often excessive mucus secretion. In many cases, inspection reveals no abnormality, but on slit-lamp examination there are subtle abnormalities of tear film stability and reduced volume of the tear film meniscus along the lower lid. In more severe cases, damaged corneal and conjunctival cells stain with 1% rose bengal, which is to be avoided in severe cases because of the intense pain. In the most severe cases, there is marked conjunctival injection, loss of the normal conjunctival and corneal luster, epithelial keratitis that may progress to frank ulceration, and mucous strands. Schirmer test, which measures the rate of production of the aqueous component of tears, may be helpful.

▶ **Treatment**

Aqueous deficiency can be treated by replacement of the aqueous component of tears with various types of artificial tears. The simplest preparations are physiologic (0.9%) or hypo-osmotic (0.45%) solutions of sodium chloride. Balanced salt solution is more physiologic but also more expensive. All of these drop preparations can be used as frequently as every half-hour, but in most cases are needed only three or four times a day. More prolonged duration of action can be achieved with drop preparations containing methylcellulose (eg, Isopto Plain), polyvinyl alcohol (eg, Liquifilm Tears or HypoTears), or polyacrylic acid (carbomers) (eg, Gel-Tears or Viscotears) or by using petrolatum ointment (Lacri-Lube). Such mucomimetics are particularly indicated when there is mucin deficiency. If there is tenacious mucus, mucolytic agents (eg, acetylcysteine, 20% six times daily) may be helpful. Autologous serum eye drops are used in severe dry eye. The presence of ocular surface and lacrimal gland inflammation in dry eyes has prompted the use of anti-inflammatory agents, such as topical cyclosporine.

Lacrimal punctal occlusion by canalicular plugs or surgery is useful in severe cases. Blepharitis is treated as described above. Associated blepharospasm may benefit from botulinum toxin injections.

Artificial tear preparations are generally very safe and without side effects. However, the preservatives necessary to maintain their sterility are potentially toxic and allergenic and may cause keratitis and cicatrizing conjunctivitis in frequent users. Furthermore, the development of such reactions may be misinterpreted by both the patient and the doctor as a worsening of the dry eye state requiring more frequent use of the artificial tears and leading in turn to further deterioration, rather than being recognized as a need to change to a preservative-free preparation.

Latkany R. Dry eyes: etiology and management. Curr Opin Ophthalmol. 2008 Jul;19(4):287–91. [PMID: 18545008]
Tost FH et al. Plugs for occlusion of the lacrimal drainage system. Dev Ophthalmol. 2008;41:193–212. [PMID: 18453770]

4. Allergic Eye Disease

Allergic eye disease takes a number of different forms but all are expressions of atopy, which may also manifest as atopic asthma, atopic dermatitis, or allergic rhinitis.

▶ Clinical Findings

Symptoms include itching, tearing, redness, stringy discharge and, occasionally, photophobia and visual loss. **Allergic conjunctivitis** is a benign disease, occurring usually in late childhood and early adulthood. It may be seasonal (hay fever), developing usually during the spring or summer, or perennial. Clinical signs are limited to conjunctival hyperemia and edema (chemosis), the latter at times being marked and sudden in onset. **Vernal keratoconjunctivitis** also tends to occur in late childhood and early adulthood. It is usually seasonal, with a predilection for the spring. Large "cobblestone" papillae are noted on the upper tarsal conjunctiva. There may be lymphoid follicles at the limbus. **Atopic keratoconjunctivitis** is a more chronic disorder of adulthood. Both the upper and the lower tarsal conjunctivas exhibit a fine papillary conjunctivitis with fibrosis, resulting in forniceal shortening

and entropion with trichiasis. Staphylococcal blepharitis is a complicating factor. Corneal involvement, including refractory ulceration, is frequent during exacerbations of both vernal and atopic keratoconjunctivitis. The latter may be complicated by herpes simplex keratitis.

▶ Treatment

A. Mild and Moderately Severe Allergic Eye Disease

Apply a topical histamine H_1-receptor antagonist, such as levocabastine hydrochloride 0.05% or emedastine difumarate 0.05%, or ketorolac tromethamine 0.5%, a nonsteroidal anti-inflammatory agent, four times daily. Ketotifen 0.025%, which has histamine H_1-receptor antagonist, mast cell stabilizer, and eosinophil inhibitor activity, is applied two to four times daily; olopatadine, 0.2% once daily or 0.1% twice daily, azelastine 0.05% twice daily, and epinastine 0.05% twice daily reduce symptoms by a similar mechanism. Topical mast cell stabilizers, such as cromolyn sodium 4% or lodoxamide tromethamine 0.1%, applied four times daily, or nedocromil sodium 2%, applied twice daily, produce longer-term prophylaxis but the therapeutic response may be delayed. Topical vasoconstrictors and antihistamines are of limited efficacy in allergic eye disease and may produce rebound hyperemia and follicular conjunctivitis. Systemic antihistamines may be useful in prolonged atopic keratoconjunctivitis. In allergic conjunctivitis, specific allergens may be identifiable and thus avoidable. In vernal keratoconjunctivitis, a cooler climate often provides significant benefit.

B. Acute Exacerbations and Severe Allergic Eye Disease

Topical corticosteroids are essential to the control of acute exacerbations of both vernal and atopic keratoconjunctivitis. Corticosteroid-induced side effects, including cataracts, glaucoma, and exacerbation of herpes simplex keratitis, are major problems but may be attenuated by the ester corticosteroid, loteprednol 0.5%. Topical cyclosporine is also effective. Systemic corticosteroid therapy and even plasmapheresis may be required in severe atopic keratoconjunctivitis.

Bielory L et al. Allergic conjunctivitis. Immunol Allergy Clin North Am. 2008 Feb;28(1):43–58. [PMID: 18282545]

PINGUECULA & PTERYGIUM

Pinguecula is a yellow elevated conjunctival nodule, more commonly on the nasal side, in the area of the palpebral fissure. It is common in persons over age 35 years. Pterygium is a fleshy, triangular encroachment of the conjunctiva onto the nasal side of the cornea and is usually associated with constant exposure to wind, sun, sand, and dust (Plate 49). Pinguecula and pterygium are often bilateral.

Pingueculae rarely grow but may become inflamed (pingueculitis). Pterygia become inflamed and may grow. No treatment is usually required for inflammation of pinguecula or pterygium, but artificial tears are often beneficial, and short courses of topical nonsteroidal anti-inflammatory agents or weak corticosteroids (predniso-lone, 0.125% three times a day) may be necessary.

The indications for excision of pterygium are growth that threatens vision by approaching the visual axis, marked induced astigmatism, or severe ocular irritation. Recurrence is common and often more aggressive than the primary lesion.

Ang LP et al. Current concepts and techniques in pterygium treatment. Curr Opin Ophthalmol. 2007 Jul;18(4):308–13. [PMID: 17568207]

CORNEAL ULCER

Corneal ulcers are most commonly due to infection by bacteria, viruses, fungi, or amebas. Noninfectious causes—all of which may be complicated by infection—include neurotrophic keratitis (resulting from loss of corneal sensation), exposure keratitis (due to inadequate eyelid closure), severe dry eyes, severe allergic eye disease, and various inflammatory disorders that may be purely ocular or part of a systemic vasculitis. Delayed or ineffective treatment of corneal infection may lead to devastating consequences with corneal scarring or intraocular infection. Prompt referral is essential.

Patients complain of pain, photophobia, tearing, and reduced vision. The eye is red, with predominantly circum-corneal injection, and there may be purulent or watery discharge. The corneal appearance varies according to the organisms involved.

▶ When to Refer

Any patient with an acute painful red eye and corneal abnormality should be referred emergently to an ophthalmologist.

Thomas PA et al. Infectious keratitis. Curr Opin Infect Dis. 2007 Apr;20(20):129–41. [PMID: 17496570]

1. Bacterial Keratitis

Bacterial keratitis usually pursues an aggressive course. Precipitating factors include contact lens wear—especially overnight wear—and corneal trauma, including refractive surgery. The pathogens most commonly isolated are *Pseudomonas aeruginosa, Pneumococcus, Moraxella* species, and staphylococci. The cornea is hazy, with a central ulcer and adjacent stromal abscess. Hypopyon is often present. The ulcer is scraped to recover material for Gram stain and culture prior to starting treatment with high-concentration topical antibiotics applied hourly day and night for at least the first 48 hours. Fluoroquinolones such as levofloxacin 0.5%, ofloxacin 0.3%, norfloxacin 0.3%, or ciprofloxacin 0.3% are commonly used as first-line agents as long as local prevalence of resistant organisms is low. The fourth-generation fluoroquinolones (moxifloxacin 0.5% and gatifloxacin 0.3% [not available in the United States]), are also active against mycobacteria but otherwise may not be preferable. Gram-positive cocci can also be treated with a cephalosporin such as cefazolin, 100 mg/mL; and gram-negative bacilli can be treated with an aminoglycoside such as tobramycin, 15 mg/mL. If no organisms are seen on Gram stain, these two agents can be used together in areas where resistance to fluoroquinolones is common. Adjunctive topical corticosteroid therapy should only be prescribed by an ophthalmologist.

▶ When to Refer

Any patient with suspected bacterial keratitis must be referred emergently to an ophthalmologist.

2. Herpes Simplex Keratitis

Herpes simplex keratitis is an important cause of ocular morbidity. The ability of the virus to colonize the trigeminal ganglion leads to recurrences precipitated by fever, excessive exposure to sunlight, or immunodeficiency.

The dendritic (branching) ulcer is the most characteristic manifestation. More extensive ("geographic") ulcers also occur, particularly if topical corticosteroids have been used. These ulcers are most easily seen after instillation of fluorescein and examination with a blue light. Such epithelial disease in itself does not lead to corneal scarring. It responds well to simple debridement and patching. More rapid healing can be achieved by the addition of topical antivirals such as trifluridine drops or acyclovir ointment. Long-term oral acyclovir reduces the rate of recurrent epithelial disease, for which topical corticosteroids must not be used.

Stromal herpes simplex keratitis produces increasingly severe corneal opacity with each recurrence. Topical antivirals alone are insufficient to control stromal disease. Thus, topical corticosteroids are used in combination, but steroid dependence is a common consequence. Corticosteroids may also enhance viral replication, exacerbating epithelial disease. Oral acyclovir, 200–400 mg five times a day, is often helpful in the treatment of severe herpetic keratitis and for prophylaxis against recurrences, particularly in atopic or HIV-infected individuals. Severe stromal scarring may require corneal grafting, but the overall outcome is relatively poor. **Caution:** For patients with known or possible herpetic disease, topical corticosteroids should be prescribed only with ophthalmologic supervision.

▶ When to Refer

Any patient with a history of herpes simplex keratitis and an acute red eye should be referred urgently to an ophthalmologist.

Guess S et al. Evidence-based treatment of herpes simplex virus keratitis: a systematic review. Ocul Surf. 2007 Jul;5(3):240–50. [PMID: 17660897]

Wilhelmus KR. Therapeutic interventions for herpes simplex virus epithelial keratitis. Cochrane Database Syst Rev. 2008 Jan 23;(1):CD002898. [PMID: 18254009]

3. Herpes Zoster Ophthalmicus

Herpes zoster frequently involves the ophthalmic division of the trigeminal nerve. It presents with malaise, fever, headache, and periorbital burning and itching. These symptoms may precede the eruption by a day or more. The rash is initially vesicular, quickly becoming pustular and then crusting. Involvement of the tip of the nose or the lid margins predicts involvement of the eye. Ocular signs include conjunctivitis, keratitis, episcleritis, and anterior uveitis, often with elevated intraocular pressure. Recurrent anterior segment inflammation, neurotrophic keratitis, and posterior subcapsular cataract are long-term complications. Optic neuropathy, cranial nerve palsies, acute retinal necrosis, and cerebral angiitis are infrequent problems in the acute stage. HIV infection is an important risk factor for herpes zoster ophthalmicus and increases the likelihood of complications.

High-dose oral acyclovir (800 mg five times a day), valacyclovir (1 g three times a day), or famciclovir (250–500 mg three times a day) started within 72 hours after the appearance of the rash reduces the incidence of ocular complications but not necessarily of postherpetic neuralgia. Anterior uveitis requires treatment with topical corticosteroids and cycloplegics. Neurotrophic keratitis is an important cause of long-term morbidity.

When to Refer

Any patient with herpes zoster ophthalmicus and ocular symptoms or signs should be referred urgently to an ophthalmologist.

Opstelten W et al. Treatment of herpes zoster. Can Fam Physician. 2008 Mar;54(3):373–7. [PMID: 18337531]
Tyring SK. Management of herpes zoster and postherpetic neuralgia. J Am Acad Dermatol. 2007 Dec;57(6 Suppl):S136–142. [PMID: 18021865]

4. Fungal Keratitis

Fungal keratitis tends to occur after corneal injury involving plant material or in an agricultural setting, in eyes with chronic ocular surface disease, and increasingly in contact lens wearers. It is usually an indolent process, with the cornea characteristically having multiple stromal abscesses and relatively little epithelial loss. Intraocular infection is common. Corneal scrapings are cultured on media suitable for fungi whenever the history or corneal appearance is suggestive of fungal disease. Diagnosis is often delayed and treatment is difficult. Natamycin and amphotericin are the most commonly used topical agents. Systemic imidazoles may be helpful. Corneal grafting is often required.

5. Acanthamoeba Keratitis

Acanthamoeba infection is an important cause of keratitis in contact lens wearers. Although severe pain with perineural and ring infiltrates in the corneal stroma is characteristic, earlier forms with changes confined to the corneal epithelium are identifiable. Diagnosis is often delayed but is facilitated by confocal microscopy. Culture requires specialized media. Treatment is hampered by the organism's ability to encyst within the corneal stroma. Various agents have been used, principally biguanides and diamidines. Epithelial debridement may be useful in early infections. Corneal grafting may be required in the acute stage

to arrest the progression of infection or after resolution to restore vision. Systemic immunosuppression may be needed if there is scleral involvement.

Hammersmith KM. Diagnosis and management of Acanthamoeba keratitis. Curr Opin Ophthalmol. 2006 Aug;17(4):327–31. [PMID: 16900022]

ACUTE ANGLE-CLOSURE GLAUCOMA

ESSENTIALS OF DIAGNOSIS

▶ Older age group, particularly hyperopes, Inuits, and Asians.

▶ Rapid onset of severe pain and profound visual loss with "halos around lights."

▶ Red eye, steamy cornea, dilated pupil.

▶ Hard eye to palpation.

General Considerations

Primary acute angle-closure glaucoma occurs only with closure of a preexisting narrow anterior chamber angle, found in older age groups (owing to enlargement of the lens), hyperopes, Inuits, and Asians. The value of prophylactic laser therapy in high-risk populations is being assessed. In the United States, about 1% of people over age 35 years have narrow anterior chamber angles, but acute glaucoma rarely develops and prophylactic therapy is not generally indicated. Angle closure may be precipitated by pupillary dilation and thus can occur from sitting in a darkened theater, at times of stress or, rarely, from pharmacologic mydriasis (see Precautions in Management of Ocular Disorders, below). Anticholinergic or sympathomimetic agents (eg, nebulized bronchodilators, atropine for preoperative medication, antidepressants, nasal decongestants, or tocolytics) are also causes. Secondary acute angle-closure glaucoma may be observed with anterior uveitis, dislocation of the lens, or topiramate therapy. Symptoms are the same as in primary acute angle-closure glaucoma, but differentiation is important because of differences in management. Chronic angle-closure glaucoma is particularly common in eastern Asia. It presents in the same way as open-angle glaucoma (see below).

Clinical Findings

Patients with acute glaucoma usually seek treatment immediately because of extreme pain and blurred vision, though there are subacute cases. The blurred vision is associated with halos around lights. Nausea and abdominal pain may occur. The eye is red, the cornea steamy, and the pupil moderately dilated and nonreactive to light. Intraocular pressure is usually over 50 mm Hg, producing a hard eye on palpation.

Differential Diagnosis

Acute glaucoma must be differentiated from conjunctivitis, acute uveitis, and corneal disorders (Table 7–1).

Treatment

A. Primary

Initial treatment in primary angle-closure glaucoma is control of intraocular pressure. A single 500-mg intravenous dose of acetazolamide, followed by 250 mg orally four times a day, is usually sufficient. Osmotic diuretics such as oral glycerol and intravenous urea or mannitol—the dosage of all three being 1–2 g/kg—may be necessary if there is no response to acetazolamide. Laser therapy to the peripheral iris (iridoplasty) or anterior chamber paracentesis is also effective. Once the intraocular pressure has started to fall, topical 4% pilocarpine, 1 drop every 15 minutes for 1 hour and then four times a day, is used to reverse the underlying angle closure. The definitive treatment is laser peripheral iridotomy or surgical peripheral iridectomy, which should also be performed prophylactically on the fellow eye. Cataract extraction is a possible alternative. If it is not possible to control the intraocular pressure medically, glaucoma drainage surgery as for uncontrolled open-angle glaucoma (see below) may be required.

B. Secondary

In secondary acute angle-closure glaucoma, systemic acetazolamide is also used, with or without osmotic agents. Further treatment is determined by the cause.

Prognosis

Untreated acute angle-closure glaucoma results in severe and permanent visual loss within 2–5 days after onset of symptoms. Affected patients need to be observed for development of chronic glaucoma.

When to Refer

Any patient with suspected acute angle-closure glaucoma must be referred emergently to an ophthalmologist.

Gandhewar RR et al. Acute glaucoma presentations in the elderly. Emerg Med J. 2005 Apr;22(4):306–7. [PMID: 15788849]

Lachkar Y et al. Drug-induced acute angle closure glaucoma. Curr Opin Ophthalmol. 2007 Mar;18(2):129–33. [PMID: 17301614]

CHRONIC GLAUCOMA

ESSENTIALS OF DIAGNOSIS

- No symptoms in early stages.
- Insidious progressive bilateral loss of peripheral vision, resulting in tunnel vision but preserved visual acuities.
- Pathologic cupping of the optic disks.
- Usually associated with persistent elevation of intraocular pressure.

General Considerations

Chronic glaucoma is characterized by gradually progressive excavation ("cupping") and pallor of the optic disk with loss of vision progressing from slight constriction of the peripheral fields to complete blindness. In chronic open-angle glaucoma, primary or secondary, the intraocular pressure is elevated due to reduced drainage of aqueous fluid through the trabecular meshwork. In chronic angle-closure glaucoma, flow of aqueous fluid into the anterior chamber angle is obstructed. In normal-tension glaucoma, intraocular pressure is not elevated but the same pattern of optic nerve damage occurs, probably due to vascular insufficiency.

Primary open-angle glaucoma is bilateral. There is an increased prevalence in first-degree relatives of affected individuals and in diabetic patients. In blacks, it is more frequent, occurs at an earlier age, and results in more severe optic nerve damage. Secondary open-angle glaucoma may result from uveitis; ocular trauma; or corticosteroid therapy, whether it be topical, systemic, inhaled, or administered by nasal spray.

In the United States, it is estimated that 2% of people over 40 years of age have glaucoma, affecting more than 2 million individuals and being three times more prevalent in blacks. At least 25% of cases are undetected. Over 90% of cases are of the open-angle type, either primary open-angle or normal-tension glaucoma. Worldwide, about 50% of all cases of glaucoma are due to acute (see above) or chronic angle closure due to the very high prevalence of angle closure in Asians.

Clinical Findings

Because initially there are no symptoms, chronic glaucoma is often suspected at a routine eye test. Diagnosis requires consistent and reproducible abnormalities in at least two of three parameters—optic disk, visual field, and intraocular pressure. Optic disk cupping is identified as an absolute increase or an asymmetry between the two eyes of the ratio of the diameter of the optic cup to the diameter of the whole optic disk (cup-disk ratio, Plates 50 and 51). (Cup-disk ratio of greater than 0.5 or asymmetry of cup-disk ratio of 0.2 or more is suggestive.) Visual field abnormalities initially develop in the paracentral region, followed by constriction of the peripheral visual field. Central vision remains good until late in the disease. The normal range of intraocular pressure is 10–21 mm Hg.

In many individuals, elevated intraocular pressure is not associated with optic disk or visual field abnormalities. These persons with **ocular hypertension** are at increased risk for glaucoma. Treatment to reduce intraocular pressure is justified if there is a moderate to high risk, determined by several factors, including age, optic disk appearance, level of intraocular pressure, and corneal thickness. A significant proportion of eyes with primary open-angle glaucoma have normal intraocular pressure when it is first measured, and only repeated measurements identify the abnormally high pressure. In normal-tension glaucoma, intraocular pressure is always within the normal range despite repeated measurement.

There are many other causes of optic disk abnormalities or visual field changes that mimic glaucoma, and visual field testing may prove unreliable in some patients, particularly in the older age group. Taken together, these factors mean that the diagnosis of glaucoma is not always straightforward, hampering the effectiveness of screening programs.

Prevention

All persons over age 40 years should have intraocular pressure measurement and optic disk examination every 2–5 years. In persons with diabetes and in individuals with a family history of glaucoma, annual examination is indicated. Regular ophthalmic screening should be considered in patients taking long-term oral or combined intranasal and inhaled corticosteroid therapy.

Treatment

A. Medications

The prostaglandin analogs (latanoprost 0.005%, bimatoprost 0.03%, and travoprost 0.004% once daily at night, and unoprostone 0.15% twice daily) are commonly used as first-line therapy because of their efficacy, their lack of systemic side effects, as well as the convenience of once-daily dosing of latanoprost, bimatoprost, and travoprost. All may produce conjunctival hyperemia, permanent darkening of the iris and eyebrow color, and increased eyelash growth. Latanoprost has been associated with reactivation of uveitis and macular edema. Topical β-adrenergic blocking agents such as timolol 0.25% or 0.5%, carteolol 1%, levobunolol 0.5%, and metipranolol 0.3% solutions twice daily or timolol 0.5% gel once daily may be used alone or in combination with a prostaglandin analog. They are contraindicated in patients with reactive airway disease or heart failure. Betaxolol, 0.25% or 0.5%, a β-receptor selective blocking agent, is theoretically safer in reactive airway disease but less effective at reducing intraocular pressure. Brimonidine 0.2%, a selective α_2-agonist, and dorzolamide 2% or brinzolamide 1%, topical carbonic anhydrase inhibitors, also can be used in addition to a prostaglandin analog or a β-blocker (twice daily) or as initial therapy when prostaglandin analogs and β-blockers are contraindicated (brimonidine twice daily, dorzolamide and brinzolamide three times daily). Both are associated with allergic reactions. Combination drops Xalacom (latanoprost 0.005% and timolol 0.5%), Ganfort (bimatoprost 0.03% and timolol 0.5%), and DuoTrav (travoprost 0.004% and timolol 0.5%), each used once daily, and Cosopt (dorzolamide 2% and timolol 0.5%) and Combigan (brimonidine 0.2% and timolol 0.5%), each used twice daily improve compliance when multiple medications are required.

Apraclonidine, 0.5–1%, another α_2-agonist, can be used three times a day to postpone the need for surgery in patients receiving maximal medical therapy, but long-term use is limited by drug reactions. It is more commonly used to control acute rises in intraocular pressure such as after laser therapy. Pilocarpine 1–4%, epinephrine, 0.5–1%, and the prodrug dipivefrin, 0.1%, are rarely used because of adverse effects. Oral carbonic anhydrase inhibitors (eg, acetazolamide) may still be used on a long-term basis if topical therapy is inadequate and surgical or laser therapy is inappropriate.

B. Laser Therapy and Surgery

Laser trabeculoplasty is used as an adjunct to topical therapy to defer surgery and is also advocated as primary treatment. Surgery is generally undertaken when intraocular pressure is inadequately controlled by medical and laser therapy, but it may also be used as primary treatment. Trabeculectomy remains the standard procedure. Adjunctive treatment with subconjunctival mitomycin or fluorouracil is used perioperatively or postoperatively in difficult cases. Viscocanalostomy and deep sclerectomy with collagen implant—two alternative procedures that avoid a full-thickness incision into the eye—may be as effective as trabeculectomy but are more difficult to perform.

In chronic angle-closure glaucoma, laser peripheral iridotomy or surgical peripheral iridectomy may be helpful.

Prognosis

Untreated chronic glaucoma that begins at age 40–45 years will probably cause complete blindness by age 60–65. Early diagnosis and treatment can preserve useful vision throughout life. In primary open-angle glaucoma—and if treatment is required in ocular hypertension—the aim is to reduce intraocular pressure to a level that will adequately reduce progression of visual field loss. In eyes with marked visual field or optic disk changes, intraocular pressure must be reduced to less than 16 mm Hg. In normal-tension glaucoma with progressive visual field loss, it is necessary to achieve even lower intraocular pressure such that surgery is often required.

When to Refer

All patients with suspected chronic glaucoma should be referred to an ophthalmologist.

Chadha V et al. Advanced glaucomatous visual loss and oral steroids. BMJ. 2008 Aug 1;337:a670. [PMID: 18676441]

Hennis A et al. Awareness of incident open-angle glaucoma in a population study: the Barbados Eye Studies. Ophthalmology. 2007 Oct;114(10):1816–21. [PMID: 17698198]

Trikudanathan S et al. Optimum management of glucocorticoid-treated patients. Nat Clin Pract Endocrinol Metab. 2008 May;4(5):262–71. [PMID: 18349823]

Vistamehr S et al. Glaucoma screening in a high-risk population. J Glaucoma. 2006 Dec;15(6):534–40. [PMID: 17106368]

UVEITIS

ESSENTIALS OF DIAGNOSIS

► Usually immunologic but possibly infective or neoplastic.

▶ Acute nongranulomatous anterior uveitis: pain, redness, photophobia, and visual loss.

▶ Granulomatous anterior uveitis: blurred vision in a mildly inflamed eye.

▶ Posterior uveitis: gradual loss of vision in a quiet eye.

General Considerations

Intraocular inflammation (uveitis) is classified into acute or chronic, and nongranulomatous or granulomatous according to the clinical signs, or by its distribution—anterior or posterior uveitis, predominantly affecting the anterior or posterior segments of the eye, or panuveitis, in which both segments are affected equally. The common types are acute nongranulomatous anterior uveitis, granulomatous anterior uveitis, and posterior uveitis.

In most cases, the pathogenesis of uveitis is primarily immunologic, but infection may be the cause, particularly in immunodeficiency states. The systemic disorders associated with acute nongranulomatous anterior uveitis are the HLA-B27-related conditions ankylosing spondylitis, reactive arthritis, psoriasis, ulcerative colitis, and Crohn disease. Behçet syndrome produces both anterior uveitis, with recurrent hypopyon but little discomfort, and posterior uveitis, characteristically with branch retinal vein occlusions. Both herpes simplex and herpes zoster infections may cause nongranulomatous anterior uveitis as well as retinitis (acute retinal necrosis), which has a very poor prognosis.

Diseases producing granulomatous anterior uveitis also tend to be causes of posterior uveitis. These include sarcoidosis, toxoplasmosis, tuberculosis, syphilis, Vogt-Koyanagi-Harada syndrome (bilateral uveitis associated with alopecia, poliosis [depigmented eyelashes, eyebrows, or hair], vitiligo, and hearing loss), and sympathetic ophthalmia following penetrating ocular trauma. In toxoplasmosis, there may be evidence of previous episodes of retinochoroiditis. Syphilis characteristically produces a "salt and pepper" fundus but may present with a wide variety of clinical manifestations. The other principal pathogens responsible for ocular inflammation in HIV infection (see below) are cytomegalovirus (CMV), herpes simplex and herpes zoster viruses, mycobacteria, *Cryptococcus*, *Toxoplasma*, and *Candida*.

Autoimmune retinal vasculitis and pars planitis (intermediate uveitis) are idiopathic conditions that produce posterior uveitis.

Retinal detachment, intraocular tumors, and central nervous system lymphoma may all masquerade as uveitis.

Clinical Findings

Anterior uveitis is characterized by inflammatory cells and flare within the aqueous. In severe cases, there may be hypopyon (layered collection of white cells) and fibrin within the anterior chamber. Cells may also be seen on the corneal endothelium as keratic precipitates (KPs). In granulomatous uveitis, these are large "mutton-fat" KPs, and iris nodules may be seen. In nongranulomatous uveitis, the KPs are smaller and iris nodules are not seen. The pupil is usually small, and with the development of posterior

synechiae (adhesions between the iris and anterior lens capsule), it also becomes irregular.

Nongranulomatous anterior uveitis tends to present acutely with unilateral pain, redness, photophobia, and visual loss. Granulomatous anterior uveitis is more indolent, causing blurred vision in a mildly inflamed eye.

In **posterior uveitis,** there are cells in the vitreous. Inflammatory lesions may be present in the retina or choroid. Fresh lesions are yellow, with indistinct margins, and there may be retinal hemorrhages, whereas older lesions have more definite margins and are commonly pigmented. Retinal vessel sheathing may occur adjacent to such lesions or more diffusely. In severe cases, vitreous opacity precludes visualization of retinal details.

Posterior uveitis tends to present with gradual visual loss in a relatively quiet eye. Bilateral involvement is common. Visual loss may be due to vitreous haze and opacities, inflammatory lesions involving the macula, macular edema, retinal vein occlusion or, rarely, associated optic neuropathy.

Treatment

Anterior uveitis usually responds to topical corticosteroids. Occasionally, periocular corticosteroid injections or even systemic corticosteroids may be required. Dilation of the pupil is important to relieve discomfort and prevent posterior synechiae. **Posterior uveitis** more commonly requires systemic or intravitreal corticosteroid therapy and occasionally systemic immunosuppression with agents such as azathioprine, tacrolimus, cyclosporine, or mycophenolate. Pupillary dilation is not usually necessary. Biologic therapies are being investigated for recalcitrant anterior or posterior uveitis.

If an infectious cause is identified, specific antimicrobial therapy may be indicated. In general, the prognosis for anterior uveitis, particularly the nongranulomatous type, is better than that for posterior uveitis.

When to Refer

- Any patient with suspected acute uveitis should be referred urgently to an ophthalmologist or emergently if visual loss or pain is severe.

- Any patient with suspected chronic uveitis should be referred to an ophthalmologist urgently if there is more than mild visual loss.

When to Admit

Patients with severe uveitis, particularly those requiring intravenous therapy, may require hospital admission.

Ali A et al. Seronegative spondyloarthropathies and the eye. Curr Opin Ophthalmol. 2007 Nov;18(6):476–80. [PMID: 18162999]

Khanna A et al. Pattern of ocular manifestations in patients with sarcoidosis in developing countries. Acta Ophthalmol Scand. 2007 Sep;85(6):609–12. [PMID: 17651463]

Zeboulon N et al. Prevalence and characteristics of uveitis in spondylarthropathies: a systematic literature review. Ann Rheum Dis. 2008 Jul;67(7):955–9. [PMID: 17962239]

CATARACT

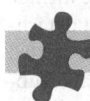

▶ Gradually progressive blurred vision.

▶ No pain or redness.

▶ Lens opacities (may be grossly visible).

General Considerations

Cataract is a lens opacity. It is the leading cause of blindness worldwide, but access to treatment is still limited in many areas. Cataracts are usually bilateral. They may be congenital (owing to intrauterine infections such as rubella and CMV, or inborn errors of metabolism such as galactosemia); traumatic; or secondary to systemic disease (diabetes, myotonic dystrophy, atopic dermatitis), systemic or inhaled corticosteroid treatment, or uveitis. Senile cataract is by far the most common type; most persons over age 60 have some degree of lens opacity. Cigarette smoking increases the risk of cataract formation.

Clinical Findings

Even in its early stages, a cataract can be seen through a dilated pupil with an ophthalmoscope or slit lamp. As the cataract matures, the retina will become increasingly more difficult to visualize, until finally the fundus reflection is absent and the pupil is white.

Treatment

In adults, functional visual impairment is the prime criterion for surgery. The cataract is usually removed by one of the techniques in which the posterior lens capsule remains (extracapsular), thus providing support for a prosthetic intraocular lens that dispenses with the need for heavy cataract glasses or contact lenses. Laser treatment may be required subsequently if the posterior capsule opacifies. Ultrasonic fragmentation (phacoemulsification) of the lens nucleus and foldable intraocular lenses allow cataract surgery to be performed through a small incision without the need for sutures, thus reducing the postoperative complication rate and accelerating visual rehabilitation. Multifocal and accommodative intraocular lenses reduce the need for both distance and reading glasses.

Management of congenital cataract is complicated by additional technical difficulties during surgery, changes in the optics of the eye with growth influencing choice of intraocular lens power, and treatment of associated amblyopia.

Prognosis

Cataract surgery in adults improves visual acuity in 95% of cases and can have a profound impact on quality of life, although expectations must be realistic. In the other 5%, there is preexisting retinal damage or operative or postoperative complications.

When to Refer

Patients with cataract should be referred to an ophthalmologist when their visual impairment adversely affects their everyday activities.

Bollinger KE et al. What can patients expect from cataract surgery? Cleve Clin J Med. 2008 Mar;75(3):193–6, 199–200. [PMID: 18383928]

Rosenberg EA et al. The visually impaired patient. Am Fam Physician. 2008 May 15;77(10):1431–6. [PMID: 18533377]

RETINAL DETACHMENT

▶ Curtain spreading across field of vision or sudden onset of visual loss in one eye.

▶ No pain or redness.

▶ Detachment seen by ophthalmoscopy.

General Considerations

Most cases of retinal detachment are due to development of a retinal tear (rhegmatogenous retinal detachment). This is usually spontaneous, is related to changes in the vitreous, and generally occurs in persons over 50 years of age. Myopia and cataract extraction are the two most common predisposing causes. Retinal tear may also be caused by penetrating or blunt ocular trauma. Once there is a tear in the retina, fluid vitreous is able to pass through the tear and lodge behind the sensory retina. This, combined with vitreous traction and the pull of gravity, results in progressive detachment. The superior temporal area is the most common site of detachment. The area involved rapidly increases, causing corresponding visual loss usually spreading upward across the field of vision. Central vision remains intact until the macula becomes detached.

Tractional retinal detachment occurs when there is preretinal fibrosis, such as in association with proliferative retinopathy secondary to diabetic retinopathy or retinal vein occlusion. Serous retinal detachment results from accumulation of subretinal fluid, such as in neovascular age-related macular degeneration or secondary to choroidal tumors.

Clinical Findings

On ophthalmoscopic examination in rhegmatogenous retinal detachment, the retina is seen hanging in the vitreous like a gray cloud. One or more retinal tears will usually be found on further examination. In traction retinal detachment, there is irregular retinal elevation with fibrosis. With serous retinal detachment, the retina is dome-shaped and the subretinal fluid may shift position with changes in posture.

Treatment

Treatment of rhegmatogenous retinal detachments is directed at closing the retinal tears. A permanent adhesion between the neurosensory retina, the retinal pigment epithelium, and the choroid is produced in the region of the tears by applying cryotherapy to the sclera or laser photocoagulation to the retina. To achieve apposition of the neurosensory retina to the retinal pigment epithelium while this adhesion is developing, indentation of the sclera with a silicone sponge or buckle; subretinal fluid drainage via an incision in the sclera; and injection of an expansile gas into the vitreous cavity, possibly following intraocular surgery to remove the vitreous (pars plana vitrectomy), may be required. Certain types of uncomplicated retinal detachment may be treated by pneumatic retinopexy, in which an expansile gas is initially injected into the vitreous cavity followed by positioning of the patient's head to facilitate reattachment of the retina. Once the retina is repositioned, the tear is sealed by laser photocoagulation or cryotherapy; these two methods are also used to seal retinal tears without associated detachment.

In complicated retinal detachments—particularly those in which fibroproliferative tissue has developed on the surface of the retina or within the vitreous cavity, ie, traction retinal detachments—retinal reattachment can be accomplished only by pars plana vitrectomy, direct manipulation of the retina, and internal tamponade of the retina with air, expansile gases, or even silicone oil. (The presence of an expansile gas within the eye is a contraindication to air travel, mountaineering at high altitude, and nitrous oxide anesthesia. Such gases persist in the globe for weeks after surgery.) (See Chapter 37.) Treatment of serous retinal detachments is determined by the underlying cause.

▶ Prognosis

About 80% of uncomplicated rhegmatogenous retinal detachments can be cured with one operation; an additional 15% will need repeated operations; and the remainder never reattach. The visual prognosis is worse if the macula is detached or if the detachment is of long duration. Without treatment, retinal detachment often becomes total within 6 months. Spontaneous detachments are ultimately bilateral in up to 25% of cases.

▶ When to Refer

All cases of retinal detachment must be referred urgently to an ophthalmologist, emergently if central vision is good. During transportation, the patient's head is positioned so that the detached portion of the retina will fall back with the aid of gravity.

Kang HK et al. Management of retinal detachment: a guide for non-ophthalmologists. BMJ. 2008 May 31;336(7655):1235–40. [PMID: 18511798]

VITREOUS HEMORRHAGE

Patients with vitreous hemorrhage complain of sudden visual loss, abrupt onset of floaters that may progressively increase in severity or, occasionally, "bleeding within the eye." Visual acuity ranges from 20/20 to light perception only. The eye is not inflamed, and the clue to diagnosis is the inability to see fundal details clearly despite the presence of a clear lens. Causes of vitreous hemorrhage include diabetic retinopathy, retinal tears (with or without detachment), retinal vein occlusions, neovascular age-related macular degeneration, blood dyscrasias, trauma, and subarachnoid hemorrhage. In all cases, examination by an ophthalmologist is essential. Retinal tears and detachments necessitate urgent treatment (see above).

▶ When to Refer

All patients with suspected vitreous hemorrhage must be referred urgently to an ophthalmologist.

Goff MJ et al. Causes and treatment of vitreous hemorrhage. Compr Ophthalmol Update. 2006 May–Jun;7(3):97–111. [PMID: 16882398]

AGE-RELATED MACULAR DEGENERATION

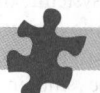

ESSENTIALS OF DIAGNOSIS

▶ Older age group.

▶ Acute or chronic deterioration of central vision in one or both eyes.

▶ Distortion or abnormal size of images.

▶ No pain or redness.

▶ Macular abnormalities seen by ophthalmoscopy.

▶ General Considerations

Age-related macular degeneration is the leading cause of permanent visual loss in the older population. The exact cause is unknown, but the prevalence increases with each decade over age 50 years (to almost 30% by age 75), and there is an association with genetically determined variations in the complement pathway. Other associated factors are race (usually white), sex (slight female predominance), family history, and a history of cigarette smoking.

Age-related macular degeneration is classified into atrophic ("dry," "geographic") and neovascular ("wet," "exudative"). Although both are progressive and usually bilateral, they differ in manifestations, prognosis, and management.

▶ Clinical Findings

The precursor to age-related macular degeneration is age-related maculopathy, characterized by retinal drusen. Hard drusen appear ophthalmoscopically as discrete yellow deposits. Soft drusen are larger, paler, and less distinct. Large, confluent soft drusen are particularly associated with neovascular age-related macular degeneration.

Atrophic degeneration is characterized by gradually progressive bilateral visual loss of moderate severity due to atrophy and degeneration of the outer retina and retinal pigment epithelium. In **neovascular degeneration,** choroidal new vessels grow between the retinal pigment epithelium and Bruch membrane, leading to accumulation of serous fluid, hemorrhage, and fibrosis. The onset of visual loss is more rapid and more severe in neovascular degeneration than in atrophic degeneration. The two eyes are frequently affected sequentially over a period of a few years. Neovascular disease accounts for about 90% of all cases of legal blindness due to age-related macular degeneration. Macular degeneration results in loss of central vision only. Peripheral fields and hence navigational vision are maintained, though these may become impaired by cataract formation for which surgery may be helpful.

Treatment

Treatment with oral vitamins and antioxidants reduces the risk of disease progression in patients with moderate age-related maculopathy or severe disease in one eye. Inhibitors of vascular endothelial growth factors (VEGF), including ranibizumab, pegaptanib, and bevacizumab, which reverse the choroidal neovascularization, result in stabilization and less frequently improvement in vision in neovascular degeneration. They have to be administered by intravitreal injection every 4–6 weeks. However, treatment is well tolerated with minimal adverse effects, although there is a small risk of intraocular infection and inflammation, retinal detachment, or traumatic cataract. Photodynamic laser therapy (PDT), involving intravenous injection of verteporfin activated by subsequent retinal laser irradiation to produce selective vascular damage, possibly supplemented by intravitreal or periocular triamcinolone, is beneficial for well-defined ("classic") and predominantly classic, as well as some small poorly-defined ("occult") choroidal neovascular membranes. Treatment may need to be repeated every 3 months. PDT may allow reduced frequency of intravitreal injections of VEGF inhibitors. Conventional laser retinal photocoagulation is only suitable for well-defined ("classic") choroidal neovascular membranes away from the fovea (extrafoveal), but these are uncommon.

Various surgical techniques to excise subfoveal neovascular membranes—or to reposition the macula away from them—have produced limited benefit.

There is no specific treatment for atrophic degeneration, but—as with the neovascular form—patients may benefit from low vision aids.

When to Refer

Older patients developing sudden visual loss due to macular disease—particularly paracentral distortion or scotoma with preservation of central acuity—should be referred urgently to an ophthalmologist.

Coleman HR et al. Age-related macular degeneration. Lancet. 2008 Nov 22;372(9652):1835–45. [PMID: 19027484]
Cook HL et al. Age-related macular degeneration: diagnosis and management. Br Med Bull. 2008;85:127–49. [PMID: 18334518]
Jager RD et al. Age-related macular degeneration. N Engl J Med. 2008 Jun 12;358(24):2606–12. [PMID: 18550876]
Parmet S et al. JAMA patient page. Age-related macular degeneration. JAMA. 2006 May 24;295(20):2438. [PMID: 16720828]
Rosenberg EA et al. The visually impaired patient. Am Fam Physician. 2008 May 15;77(10):1431–6. [PMID: 18533377]

CENTRAL & BRANCH RETINAL VEIN OCCLUSIONS

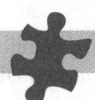

ESSENTIALS OF DIAGNOSIS

▶ Sudden monocular loss of vision.

▶ No pain or redness.

▶ Widespread or sectoral retinal hemorrhages seen by ophthalmoscopy.

General Considerations

All patients with retinal vein occlusion should be screened for diabetes, systemic hypertension, hyperlipidemia, and glaucoma. In younger patients, antiphospholipid antibodies, inherited thrombophilia, and hyperhomocysteinemia should be considered. Rarely, hyperviscosity syndromes, including myeloproliferative disorders, are associated with retinal vein occlusions and particularly should be considered in bilateral disease.

Clinical Findings

A. Symptoms and Signs

The visual impairment in central retinal vein occlusion is commonly first noticed upon waking. Ophthalmoscopic signs include widespread retinal hemorrhages, retinal venous dilation and tortuosity, retinal cotton-wool spots, and optic disk swelling.

Branch retinal vein occlusions may present in a variety of ways. Sudden loss of vision may occur at the time of occlusion if the fovea is involved or some time afterward from vitreous hemorrhage due to retinal new vessels. More gradual visual loss may occur with development of macular edema. In acute branch retinal vein occlusion, the retinal abnormalities (hemorrhages, venous dilation and tortuosity, and cotton-wool spots) are confined to the area drained by the obstructed vein.

B. Laboratory Findings

Obtain screening studies for diabetes and hyperlipidemia. In younger patients, consider obtaining antiphospholipid antibodies, platelet counts to check for thrombophilia, and plasma homocysteine levels. Very high paraproteins, found on serum protein electrophoresis (particularly IgM), can cause hyperviscosity.

Complications

If central retinal vein occlusion is associated with widespread retinal ischemia, manifesting as poor visual acuity (20/200 or worse), florid retinal abnormalities, and extensive areas of capillary closure on fluorescein angiography, there is a high risk of development of neovascular (rubeotic) glaucoma, typically within first 3 months.

Branch retinal vein occlusion may be complicated by peripheral retinal neovascularization or chronic macular edema.

Treatment

Eyes at risk of neovascular glaucoma following ischemic central retinal vein occlusion can be treated by panretinal laser photocoagulation either prophylactically or as soon as there is evidence of neovascularization, the latter approach necessitating frequent monitoring. Regression of iris neovascularization has been achieved with intravitreal injections of bevacizumab, an inhibitor of VEGF. In branch retinal vein occlusion complicated by retinal neovascularization, the ischemic retina should be laser photocoagulated.

Chronic macular edema responds to laser photocoagulation in branch but not central retinal vein occlusion. Intravitreal triamcinolone or inhibitors of VEGF, such as bevacizumab, may improve chronic macular edema in both branch and nonischemic central retinal vein occlusion.

Improvement in vision has been reported after vitrectomy with direct injection of tissue plasminogen activator into the retinal venous system or incision of the sclera at the edge of the optic disk (radial optic neurotomy). Improvement has also been reported after isovolemic hemodilution in central retinal vein occlusion and after vitrectomy alone or combined with surgical incision of the retinal vascular adventitia (arteriovenous sheathotomy) and injection of tissue plasminogen activator in branch retinal vein occlusion. However, the overall value of each technique remains uncertain.

Prognosis

In central retinal vein occlusion, severity of visual loss initially is a good guide to visual outcome. Good initial visual acuity (20/60 or better) indicates a good prognosis. Visual prognosis is poor for eyes with neovascular glaucoma.

Visual outcome in branch retinal vein occlusion is determined by the severity of macular damage from hemorrhage, ischemia, or edema.

When to Refer

All patients with retinal vein occlusion should be referred urgently to an ophthalmologist.

Margolis R et al. Branch retinal vein occlusion: clinical findings, natural history, and management. Compr Ophthalmol Update. 2006 Nov–Dec;7(6):265–76. [PMID: 17244442]

Suvajac G et al. Ocular manifestations in antiphospholipid syndrome. Autoimmun Rev. 2007 Jun;6(6):409–14. [PMID: 17537387]

Vortmann M et al. Acute monocular visual loss. Emerg Med Clin North Am. 2008 Feb;26(1):73–96. [PMID: 18249258]

CENTRAL & BRANCH RETINAL ARTERY OCCLUSIONS

ESSENTIALS OF DIAGNOSIS

▶ Sudden monocular loss of vision.

▶ No pain or redness.

▶ Widespread or sectoral retinal pallid swelling seen by ophthalmoscopy.

General Considerations

In patients 55 years of age or older with central retinal artery occlusion, giant cell arteritis must be considered. Carotid and cardiac sources of emboli must be sought in central and in branch retinal artery occlusion in particular, even if no retinal emboli are identified, so that appropriate treatment can be given to reduce the risk of stroke (see Chapter 12). Migraine, oral contraceptives, systemic vasculitis, congenital or acquired thrombophilia, and hyperhomocysteinemia should be considered in young patients. Internal carotid artery dissection should be considered when there is neck pain or a recent history of neck trauma. Diabetes, hyperlipidemia, and systemic hypertension should be considered in all patients.

Clinical Findings

A. Symptoms and Signs

Central retinal artery occlusion presents as sudden profound monocular visual loss. Visual acuity is usually reduced to counting fingers or worse, and visual field is restricted to an island of vision in the temporal field. Ophthalmoscopy reveals pallid swelling of the retina, most obvious in the posterior segment, with a cherry-red spot at the fovea. The retinal arteries are attenuated, and "box-car" segmentation of blood in the veins may be seen. Occasionally, emboli are seen in the central retinal artery or its branches. The retinal swelling subsides over a period of 4–6 weeks, leaving a relatively normal retinal appearance but a pale optic disk and attenuated arterioles.

Branch retinal artery occlusion may also present with sudden loss of vision if the fovea is involved, but more commonly sudden loss of visual field is the presenting complaint. Fundal signs of retinal swelling and adjacent cotton-wool spots are limited to the area of retina supplied by the occluded artery.

Clinical features of giant cell arteritis, which generally occurs in patients 55 years or older, include jaw claudication (in particular) but also may include headache, scalp tenderness, general malaise, weight loss, symptoms of polymyalgia rheumatica, and tenderness, thickening, or absence of pulse of the superficial temporal arteries. Table 20–14 lists the clinical manifestations of vasculitis.

B. Laboratory Findings

Screen for diabetes and hyperlipidemia in all patients. Erythrocyte sedimentation rate and C-reactive protein are usually markedly elevated in giant cell arteritis but one or both may be normal. Consider screening for other types of vasculitis (see Table 20–13). In younger patients, consider obtaining a platelet count to check for congenital or acquired thrombophilia and a plasma homocysteine level.

C. Imaging

Obtain duplex ultrasonography of the carotid arteries and echocardiography to seek out carotid and cardiac sources of emboli as well as internal carotid artery dissection.

▶ Treatment

If the patient is seen within a few hours after onset, emergency treatment—including laying the patient flat, ocular massage, high concentrations of inhaled oxygen, intravenous acetazolamide, and anterior chamber paracentesis—may influence the visual outcome. Studies of early thrombolysis, particularly by local intra-arterial injection but also intravenously, have shown good results in central retinal artery occlusion not due to giant cell arteritis.

In giant cell arteritis, there is risk—highest in the first few days—of involvement of the other eye. When the diagnosis is suspected, high-dose corticosteroids (oral prednisolone 1–1.5 mg/kg/d, if necessary preceded by intravenous hydrocortisone 250–500 mg stat, or methylprednisolone 0.5–1 g/d for 1–3 days followed by oral prednisolone, especially in patients with bilateral visual loss) must be instituted immediately, possibly together with low-dose aspirin. The patient must be monitored closely to ensure that treatment is adequate. A temporal artery biopsy should be performed promptly, and if necessary, assistance should be sought from a rheumatologist.

▶ When to Refer

• Patients with central retinal artery occlusion should be referred emergently to an ophthalmologist.

• Patients with branch retinal artery occlusion should be referred urgently.

▶ When to Admit

Patients with visual loss due to giant cell arteritis may require emergency admission for high-dose corticosteroid therapy and close monitoring to ensure that treatment is adequate.

Fraser JA et al. The treatment of giant cell arteritis. Rev Neurol Dis. 2008 Summer;5(3):140–52. [PMID: 18838954]

Mason JO 3rd et al. Branch retinal artery occlusion: visual prognosis. Am J Ophthalmol. 2008 Sep;146(3):455–7. [PMID: 18599018]

Noble J et al. Intra-arterial thrombolysis for central retinal artery occlusion: a systematic review. Br J Ophthalmol. 2008 May;92(5):588–93. [PMID: 18441166]

Vortmann M et al. Acute monocular visual loss. Emerg Med Clin North Am. 2008 Feb;26(1):73–96. [PMID: 18249258]

TRANSIENT MONOCULAR BLINDNESS

ESSENTIALS OF DIAGNOSIS

▶ Monocular loss of vision lasting a few minutes with complete recovery.

▶ No retinal abnormality on ophthalmoscopy.

Transient monocular blindness results from temporary reduction in ocular perfusion. It is usually caused by retinal emboli from ipsilateral carotid disease, in which case the visual loss is characteristically described as a curtain passing vertically across the visual field with complete monocular visual loss lasting a few minutes and a similar curtain effect as the episode passes (amaurosis fugax; also called "fleeting blindness"). Other causes include cardiac emboli and severe occlusive carotid disease; giant cell arteritis and antiphospholipid syndrome may cause episodes that characteristically occur on exposure to bright light. More transient episodes occur in patients with raised intracranial pressure; these episodes last only a few seconds to 1 minute, affect one or both eyes, and are due to optic nerve head ischemia. In young patients, there is a benign entity that has been ascribed to choroidal or retinal vascular spasm.

▶ Diagnostic Studies

The most reliable method of evaluating carotid stenosis is intra-arterial angiography. The noninvasive techniques of duplex ultrasonography, CT angiography, and magnetic resonance angiography are suitable screening methods. Electrocardiography should be performed in all cases, particularly to identify atrial fibrillation. Echocardiography, with transesophageal studies (if necessary), should be performed in young patients and in any patient with clinical evidence of a potential cardiac source of emboli.

▶ Treatment

To reduce the risk of stroke, all patients with transient monocular blindness due to retinal emboli from ipsilateral carotid disease should be treated with low-dose aspirin or another antiplatelet drug, and their vascular risk factors should be controlled. Those patients with high-grade stenosis (70–99%), and possibly those with medium-grade (30–69%) stenosis, should be considered for carotid endarterectomy or possibly angioplasty with stenting, but surgery is less likely to be necessary than in patients with cerebral hemispheric events (see Chapter 12).

In younger patients with the benign variant of transient monocular blindness, calcium channel blockers, such as slow-release nifedipine, 60 mg/d, may be effective.

▶ When to Refer

In all cases of episodic visual loss, early ophthalmologic consultation is advisable.

Sadek M et al. Carotid angioplasty and stenting, success relies on appropriate patient selection. J Vasc Surg. 2008 May;47(5):946–51. [PMID: 18455640]

Suvajac G et al. Ocular manifestations in antiphospholipid syndrome. Autoimmun Rev. 2007 Jun;6(6):409–14. [PMID: 17537387]

RETINAL DISORDERS ASSOCIATED WITH SYSTEMIC DISEASES

1. Diabetic Retinopathy

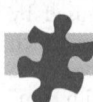 ESSENTIALS OF DIAGNOSIS

▸ Present in about 40% of diagnosed diabetic patients.

▸ Present in up to 20% of type 2 diabetic patients at diagnosis.

▸ Mild retinal abnormalities without visual loss in background retinopathy.

▸ Macular edema, exudates, or ischemia in maculopathy.

▸ Retinal new vessels in proliferative retinopathy.

General Considerations

In the United States, diabetic retinopathy is present in about 40% of diagnosed diabetic patients. It is the leading cause of new blindness among adults aged 20–65 years; the number of affected individuals aged 65 years or older is particularly increasing. Retinopathy increases in prevalence and severity with increasing duration and poorer control of diabetes. In type 1 diabetes, retinopathy is not detectable for at least 3 years after diagnosis. In type 2 diabetes, retinopathy is present in up to 20% of patients at diagnosis and may be the presenting feature. It is broadly classified as **nonproliferative**, comprising **background retinopathy** and **maculopathy, or proliferative**. Maculopathy and proliferative retinopathy may coexist, particularly in severe disease.

Clinical Findings

Nonproliferative retinopathy manifests as dilation of veins, microaneurysms, retinal hemorrhages, retinal edema, and hard exudates. In **background retinopathy,** the abnormalities are mild and do not cause any impairment of visual acuity. Pre-proliferative retinopathy is characterized by marked vascular abnormalities and retinal hemorrhages.

Maculopathy manifests as edema, exudates, or ischemia involving the macula (Plate 52). Assessment requires stereoscopic examination of the retina, retinal imaging with optical coherence tomography (OCT), and sometimes fluorescein angiography. Visual acuity is a poor guide to the presence of treatable maculopathy—hence the need for regular ophthalmologic follow-up. Maculopathy is the most common cause of legal blindness in type 2 diabetes.

Proliferative retinopathy is characterized by neovascularization, arising from either the optic disk or the major vascular arcades. Vitreous hemorrhage is a common sequela. Proliferation into the vitreous of blood vessels, with their associated fibrous component, may lead to tractional retinal detachment. Without treatment, the visual prognosis with proliferative retinopathy is generally much worse than that with nonproliferative retinopathy.

▸ Screening

Adult and adolescent patients with diabetes should undergo at least yearly screening, by fundal photography, preferably after pupil dilation (mydriasis), or by slit-lamp examination after pupil dilation. (Failure to identify diabetic retinopathy by direct ophthalmoscopy is common, particularly if the pupils are not dilated. Non-mydriatic fundal photography, possibly with centralized screening by telemedicine, may increase rates of participation.) More frequent monitoring is required in women during pregnancy, and who plan to become pregnant.

▸ Treatment

Treatment includes optimizing blood glucose, blood pressure, renal function, and serum lipids, although such measures are probably more important in preventing the development of retinopathy than in influencing its subsequent course.

Macular edema and exudates, but not ischemia, may respond to laser photocoagulation, intravitreal injection of corticosteroid or a VEGF inhibitor, or vitrectomy.

Proliferative retinopathy is usually treated by panretinal laser photocoagulation, preferably before vitreous hemorrhage or tractional detachment has occurred. Regression of neovascularization can also be achieved by intravitreal injection of a VEGF inhibitor. Determining whether panretinal laser photocoagulation should be undertaken for pre-proliferative retinopathy may be helped by assessing the degree of retinal ischemia on fluorescein angiography. Vitrectomy is necessary for removal of persistent vitreous hemorrhage, to improve vision and allow panretinal laser photocoagulation for the underlying retinal neovascularization, for treatment of tractional retinal detachment involving the macula, and for management of rapidly progressive proliferative disease.

Proliferative diabetic retinopathy, especially after successful laser treatment, is not a contraindication to treatment with thrombolytic agents, aspirin, or warfarin unless there has been recent vitreous or pre-retinal hemorrhage.

▸ When to Refer

- All diabetic patients with sudden loss of vision or retinal detachment should be referred emergently to an ophthalmologist.

- Proliferative retinopathy or maculopathy requires urgent referral to an ophthalmologist.

- Pre-proliferative retinopathy or unexplained reduction of visual acuity requires early referral to an ophthalmologist.

Chew EY. Screening options for diabetic retinopathy. Curr Opin Ophthalmol. 2006 Dec;17(6):519–22. [PMID: 17065919]

Kohner EM. Microvascular disease: what does the UKPDS tell us about diabetic retinopathy? Diabet Med. 2008 Aug;25 (Suppl) 2:20–4. [PMID: 18717974]

Massin P et al. The elderly diabetic's eyes. Diabetes Med. 2007 Apr;33 (Suppl) 1:S4–9. [PMID: 17702094]

Mohamed Q et al. Management of diabetic retinopathy: a systematic review. JAMA. 2007 Aug 22;298(8):902–16. [PMID: 17712074]

Saaddine JB et al. Projection of diabetic retinopathy and other major eye diseases among people with diabetes mellitus: United States, 2005–2050. Arch Ophthalmol. 2008 Dec;126(12):1740–7. [PMID: 19064858]

Scanlon PH et al. Visual acuity measurement and ocular co-morbidity in diabetic retinopathy screening. Br J Ophthalmol. 2008 Jun;92(6):775–8. [PMID: 18356262]

2. Hypertensive Retinochoroidopathy

Systemic hypertension affects both the retinal and choroidal circulations. The clinical manifestations vary according to the degree and rapidity of rise in blood pressure and the underlying state of the ocular circulation. The most florid disease occurs in young patients with abrupt elevations of blood pressure, such as may occur in pheochromocytoma, malignant hypertension, or pre-eclampsia-eclampsia.

Chronic hypertension accelerates the development of atherosclerosis. The retinal arterioles become more tortuous and narrow and develop abnormal light reflexes ("silver-wiring" and "copper-wiring"). There is increased venous compression at the retinal arteriovenous crossings ("arteriovenous nicking"), an important factor predisposing to branch retinal vein occlusions. Flame-shaped hemorrhages occur in the nerve fiber layer of the retina.

Acute elevations of blood pressure result in loss of autoregulation in the retinal circulation, leading to the breakdown of endothelial integrity and occlusion of precapillary arterioles and capillaries. These pathologic changes are manifested as cotton-wool spots, retinal hemorrhages, retinal edema, and retinal exudates, often in a stellate appearance at the macula. In the choroid, vasoconstriction and ischemia result in serous retinal detachments and retinal pigment epithelial infarcts. These infarcts later develop into pigmented lesions that may be focal, linear, or wedge-shaped. The abnormalities in the choroidal circulation may also affect the optic nerve head, producing ischemic optic neuropathy with optic disk swelling. Malignant hypertensive retinopathy was the term previously used to describe the constellation of clinical signs resulting from the combination of abnormalities in the retinal, choroidal, and optic disk circulation. When there is such severe disease, there is likely to be permanent retinal, choroidal, or optic nerve damage. Precipitous reduction of blood pressure may exacerbate such damage.

Wong TY et al. The eye in hypertension. Lancet. 2007 Feb 3;369(9559):425–35. [PMID: 17276782]

3. Blood Dyscrasias

In conditions characterized by thrombocytopenia or severe anemia, various types of hemorrhages occur in both the retina and choroid and may lead to visual loss. If macular hemorrhages have not occurred, it is possible to regain normal vision with treatment.

Sickle cell retinopathy is particularly common in hemoglobin SC disease but may also occur with other hemoglobin S variants. Manifestations include "salmon-patch" preretinal/intraretinal hemorrhages, "black sunbursts" resulting from intraretinal hemorrhage, and new vessels. Severe visual loss is rare. Retinal laser photocoagulation reduces the frequency of vitreous hemorrhage from new vessels. Surgery is occasionally needed for persistent vitreous hemorrhage or tractional retinal detachment.

4. AIDS

Cotton-wool spots, retinal hemorrhages, and microaneurysms are the most common ophthalmic abnormalities in AIDS patients.

CMV retinitis occurs when CD4 counts are below 50/mcL. It is characterized by progressively enlarging yellowish-white patches of retinal opacification, which are accompanied by retinal hemorrhages; they usually begin adjacent to the major retinal vascular arcades (Plate 53). Patients are often asymptomatic until there is involvement of the fovea or optic nerve or until retinal detachment develops.

Choices for initial therapy are (1) intravenous—ganciclovir 5 mg/kg twice a day, foscarnet 60 mg/kg three times a day, or cidofovir 5 mg/kg once weekly, usually for 2 weeks; (2) oral—valganciclovir 900 mg twice daily; or (3) local administration, using either intravitreal injection of ganciclovir, foscarnet, or fomivirsen or the sustained-release ganciclovir intravitreal implant. Intravitreal cidofovir is effective, but there is a high incidence of uveitis, low intraocular pressure, and ciliary body necrosis. Other major side effects are neutropenia and thrombocytopenia with systemic ganciclovir and nephrotoxicity with foscarnet and cidofovir. Doses of both ganciclovir and foscarnet are adjusted in patients with renal failure. Oral probenecid and intravenous hydration are used to minimize nephrotoxicity from cidofovir. All available agents are virostatic. Maintenance therapy can be conducted with lower-dose intravenous therapy (ganciclovir 3.75 mg/kg/d or foscarnet 60 mg/kg/d for 5 days each week, or cidofovir 5 mg/kg once every 2 weeks), with oral ganciclovir (3 g/d) or oral valganciclovir 900 mg once daily, or with intravitreal therapy. Local therapy tends to be more effective than systemic therapy and avoids systemic side effects, but there is a risk of intraocular complications, and the incidence of retinitis in the fellow eye and of extraocular CMV infection is higher. Unresponsive disease or reactivation during maintenance therapy can be managed by changing to a different agent or by use of combination therapy. Retinal detachment, either due to retinitis or as a complication of intravitreal therapy, requires vitrectomy and intravitreal silicone oil. Oral ganciclovir as prophylaxis against CMV retinitis in patients with low CD4 counts or high CMV burdens has not been found to be worthwhile.

Antiretroviral therapy may result in reduction of HIV virus load and increase in CD4 counts, and even regression of CMV retinitis without the use of anti-CMV therapy. If the CD4 count is maintained above 100/mcL, it may be possible to discontinue maintenance anti-CMV therapy. In patients with regressed CMV retinitis and restored CD4 counts, highly active antiretroviral therapy (HAART) commonly leads to "immune recovery" uveitis, which may lead to visual loss from cataract or retinal complications.

Other ophthalmic manifestations of opportunistic infections occurring in AIDS patients include herpes simplex retinitis, toxoplasmic and candidal chorioretinitis, herpes zoster ophthalmicus, and various entities due to syphilis or tuberculosis. Kaposi sarcoma of the conjunctiva and orbital lymphoma may also be seen on rare occasions (see Chapter 31).

Holland GN. AIDS and ophthalmology: the first quarter century. Am J Ophthalmol. 2008 Mar;145(3):397–408. [PMID: 18282490]

Jabs DA et al. Longitudinal study of the ocular complications of AIDS: 1. Ocular diagnoses at enrollment. Ophthalmology. 2007 Apr;114(4):780–6. [PMID: 17258320]

Jabs DA et al. Longitudinal study of the ocular complications of AIDS: 2. Ocular examination results at enrollment. Ophthalmology. 2007 Apr;114(4):787–93. [PMID: 17210182]

ISCHEMIC OPTIC NEUROPATHY

ESSENTIALS OF DIAGNOSIS

▸ Sudden painless visual loss with signs of optic nerve dysfunction.

▸ Optic disc swelling in anterior ischemic optic neuropathy.

Anterior ischemic optic neuropathy—due to inadequate perfusion of the posterior ciliary arteries that supply the anterior portion of the optic nerve—produces sudden visual loss, usually with an altitudinal field defect, and optic disk swelling. In older patients, it is often caused by giant cell arteritis, which necessitates emergency high-dose systemic corticosteroid treatment to prevent visual loss in the other eye. (See Central & Branch Retinal Artery Occlusions, above and Polymyalgia Rheumatica & Giant Cell Arteritis, Chapter 20.) The predominant factor predisposing to nonarteritic anterior ischemic optic neuropathy is congenitally crowded optic disks. Other causative factors include systemic hypertension, diabetes, hyperlipidemia, systemic vasculitis, inherited or acquired thrombophilia, and possibly ingestion of sildenafil and sleep apnea.

Ischemic optic neuropathy, usually involving the retrobulbar optic nerve and thus not causing any optic disk swelling (**posterior ischemic optic neuropathy**), may occur after severe blood loss or nonocular surgery, particularly prolonged lumbar spine surgery. Early correction of anemia and systemic hypotension may be beneficial.

▸ When to Refer

Patients with ischemic optic neuropathy should be referred urgently to an ophthalmologist.

▸ When to Admit

Patients with ischemic optic neuropathy due to giant cell arteritis may require emergency admission for high-dose corticosteroid therapy and close monitoring to ensure that treatment is adequate.

Danesh-Meyer HV et al. Erectile dysfunction drugs and risk of anterior ischaemic optic neuropathy: casual or causal association? Br J Ophthalmol. 2007 Nov;91(11):1551–5. [PMID: 17947271]

Luneau K et al. Ischemic optic neuropathies. Neurologist. 2008 Nov;14(6):341–54. [PMID: 19008740]

Newman NJ. Perioperative visual loss after nonocular surgeries. Am J Ophthalmol. 2008 Apr;145(4):604–10. [PMID: 18358851]

Preechawat P et al. Anterior ischemic optic neuropathy in patients younger than 50 years. Am J Ophthalmol. 2007 Dec;144(6):953–60. [PMID: 17854756]

OPTIC NEURITIS

ESSENTIALS OF DIAGNOSIS

▸ Subacute unilateral visual loss with signs of optic nerve dysfunction.

▸ Pain exacerbated by eye movements.

▸ Optic disc usually normal in acute stage but subsequently developing pallor.

▸ General Considerations

Inflammatory optic neuropathy (optic neuritis) is strongly associated with demyelinating disease, particularly multiple sclerosis but also acute disseminated encephalomyelitis. It also occurs in sarcoidosis; as a component of neuromyelitis optica (Devic syndrome); with viral infections (including measles, mumps, influenza and those caused by the varicella zoster virus); with various autoimmune disorders, particularly systemic lupus erythematosus; and by spread of inflammation from meninges, orbital tissues, or paranasal sinuses.

▸ Clinical Findings

Optic neuritis in demyelinating disease is characterized by unilateral loss of vision, which usually develops over a few days. Vision ranges from 20/30 to no perception of light. Commonly there is pain in the region of the eye, particularly on eye movements. Field loss is usually a central scotoma, but a wide range of monocular field defects is possible. There is marked loss of color vision and a relative afferent pupillary defect. In about two-thirds of cases, the optic nerve is normal during the acute stage (retrobulbar optic neuritis). In the remainder, the optic disk is swollen (papillitis) with occasional flame-shaped peripapillary hemorrhages. Visual acuity usually improves within 2–3 weeks and returns to 20/40 or better in 95% of previously unaffected eyes. Optic atrophy subsequently develops if there has been destruction of sufficient optic nerve fibers. Any patient with presumed demyelinating optic neuritis in which visual recovery does not occur or there are other atypical features should undergo further investigation, including imaging studies to exclude a compressive lesion.

Treatment

In acute demyelinating optic neuritis, intravenous methylprednisolone therapy for 3 days followed by a tapering course of oral prednisolone accelerates visual recovery, although in clinical practice the oral taper is rarely prescribed. Use in an individual patient is determined by the degree of visual loss, the state of the fellow eye, and the patient's visual requirements.

Optic neuritis due to sarcoidosis, neuromyelitis optica, herpes zoster, or systemic lupus erythematosus generally has a poorer prognosis and requires more prolonged corticosteroid therapy.

Prognosis

Among patients with a first episode of clinically isolated optic neuritis, multiple sclerosis will develop in 50% within 15 years but the visual and neurologic prognosis is good. The major risk factors are female gender, multiple white matter lesions on brain MRI scan, and cerebrospinal fluid oligoclonal bands. In patients with multiple cerebral white matter lesions, long-term interferon therapy reduces the risk of subsequent development of multiple sclerosis by 25% at 5 years, although the effect on long-term disability remains uncertain and some patients do not respond.

When to Refer

All patients with optic neuritis should be referred urgently for ophthalmologic or neurologic assessment.

Balcer LJ. Clinical practice. Optic neuritis. N Engl J Med. 2006 Mar 23;354(12):1273–80. [PMID: 16554529]

Germann CA et al. Ophthalmic diagnoses in the ED: optic neuritis. Am J Emerg Med. 2007 Sep;25(7):834–7. [PMID: 17870491]

Optic Neuritis Study Group. Multiple sclerosis risk after optic neuritis: final optic neuritis treatment trial follow-up. Arch Neurol. 2008 Jun;65(6):727–32. [PMID: 18541792]

Optic Neuritis Study Group. Visual function 15 years after optic neuritis: a final follow-up report from the Optic Neuritis Treatment Trial. Ophthalmology 2008 Jun;115(6):1079–82. [PMID: 17976727]

Volpe NJ. The optic neuritis treatment trial: a definitive answer and profound impact with unexpected results. Arch Ophthalmol. 2008 Jul;126(7):996–9. [PMID: 18625952]

OPTIC DISK SWELLING

Optic disk swelling may result from intraocular disease, orbital and optic nerve lesions, severe hypertensive retinochoroidopathy, or raised intracranial pressure, the last necessitating urgent imaging to exclude an intracranial mass or cerebral venous sinus occlusion. Intraocular causes include central retinal vein occlusion, posterior uveitis, and posterior scleritis. Optic nerve lesions causing disk swelling include optic neuritis; anterior ischemic optic neuropathy; optic disk drusen; optic nerve sheath meningioma; and nerve infiltra-

tion by sarcoidosis, leukemia, or lymphoma. Any orbital lesion causing nerve compression may produce disk swelling.

Papilledema (optic disk swelling due to raised intracranial pressure) is usually bilateral and most commonly produces enlargement of the blind spot without loss of acuity (Plate 54). Chronic papilledema, as in idiopathic intracranial hypertension and dural venous sinus occlusion, or severe acute papilledema may be associated with visual field loss and occasionally with profound loss of acuity. All patients with chronic papilledema must be monitored carefully—especially their visual fields—and cerebrospinal fluid shunt or optic nerve sheath fenestration should be considered in those with progressive visual failure not controlled by medical therapy (weight loss where appropriate and acetazolamide).

Optic disk drusen and congenitally crowded optic disks, which are associated with hyperopia, cause optic disk elevation that may be mistaken for swelling (pseudopapilledema). Exposed optic disk drusen may be obvious clinically or can be demonstrated by their autofluorescence. Buried drusen are best detected by orbital ultrasound or CT scanning. Other family members may be similarly affected.

OCULAR MOTOR PALSIES

In complete **third nerve paralysis**, there is ptosis with a divergent and slightly depressed eye. Extraocular movements are restricted in all directions except laterally (preserved lateral rectus function). Intact fourth nerve (superior oblique) function is detected by the presence of inward rotation on attempted depression of the eye.

Pupillary involvement (dilated pupil that does not react to light shone in either eye) is an important sign differentiating "surgical," including traumatic, from "medical" causes of isolated third nerve palsy. Compressive lesions of the third nerve—eg, aneurysm of the posterior communicating artery and uncal herniation due to a supratentorial mass lesion—characteristically have pupillary involvement. Patients with painful acute isolated third nerve palsy and pupillary involvement are assumed to have a posterior communicating artery aneurysm until this has been excluded. Pituitary apoplexy is a rarer cause. Medical causes of isolated third nerve palsy include diabetes, hypertension, and giant cell arteritis.

Fourth nerve paralysis causes upward deviation of the eye with failure of depression on adduction. There is vertical and torsional diplopia that becomes most apparent on attempted reading and descending stairs. Many cases with similar clinical features are due to congenital orbital musculo-facial anomaly, although labeled as congenital fourth nerve palsy. Trauma is a major cause of acquired—particularly bilateral—fourth nerve palsy, but posterior fossa tumor and medical causes such as in third nerve palsies should also be considered.

Sixth nerve paralysis causes convergent squint in the primary position with failure of abduction of the affected eye, producing horizontal diplopia that increases on gaze to the affected side and on looking into the distance. It is an important sign of raised intracranial pressure. Sixth nerve palsy may also be due to trauma, neoplasms, brainstem lesions, or medical causes.

An intracranial or intraorbital mass lesion should be considered in any patient with an isolated ocular motor palsy. In patients with isolated ocular motor nerve palsies presumed to be due to medical causes, brain MRI is generally only necessary if recovery has not begun within 3 months, although some authors suggest that it should be undertaken in all cases.

Ocular motor nerve palsies occurring in association with other neurologic signs may be due to lesions in the brainstem, the cavernous sinus, or in the orbit. Lesions around the cavernous sinus involve the upper divisions of the trigeminal nerve, the ocular motor nerves, and occasionally the optic chiasm. Orbital apex lesions involve the optic nerve and the ocular motor nerves.

Myasthenia and dysthyroid eye disease should also be considered in the differential diagnosis of disordered extraocular movements.

When to Refer

- Any patient with recent onset isolated third nerve palsy, particularly if there is pupillary involvement or pain, must be referred emergently for neurologic assessment and possible investigation for intracranial aneurysm.

- All patients with recent onset double vision should be referred urgently to an ophthalmologist or neurologist, particularly if there is multiple cranial nerve dysfunction or other neurologic abnormalities.

When to Admit

Patients with double vision due to giant cell arteritis may require emergency admission for high-dose corticosteroid therapy and close monitoring to ensure that treatment is adequate.

Reich SG. Teaching video is it III alone, or III and IV? Neurology. 2007 May 22;68(21):E34. [PMID: 17515533]
Woodruff MM et al. Evaluation of third nerve palsy in the Emergency Department, J Emerg Med. 2008 Oct;35(3):239–46. [PMID: 17976817]

DYSTHYROID EYE DISEASE

Dysthyroid eye disease is a syndrome of clinical and orbital imaging abnormalities caused by deposition of mucopolysaccharides and infiltration with chronic inflammatory cells of the orbital tissues, particularly the extraocular muscles. It usually occurs in association with autoimmune hyperthyroidism, when it is known as Graves disease. However clinical or laboratory evidence of thyroid dysfunction and thyroid autoantibodies may not be detectable at presentation or even on long-term follow-up. Radioiodine therapy and cigarette smoking increase its severity.

The primary clinical features are proptosis, lid retraction and lid lag, conjunctival chemosis and episcleral inflammation, and extraocular muscle dysfunction. Resulting symptoms are cosmetic abnormalities, surface irritation, which usually responds to artificial tears, and diplopia, which should be treated conservatively (eg, with prisms) in the active stages of the disease and only by surgery when the disease has been static for at least 6 months. The important complications are corneal exposure and optic nerve compression, both of which may lead to marked visual loss. The primary imaging features are enlargement of the extraocular muscles, usually affecting both orbits.

Treatment

Treatment options for optic nerve compression or severe corneal exposure are intravenous pulse methylprednisolone therapy (eg, 1 g daily for 3 days, repeated weekly for 3 weeks), oral prednisolone 80–100 mg/d, radiotherapy, or surgery (usually consisting of extensive removal of bone from the medial, inferior, and lateral walls of the orbit), either singly or in combination.

The optimal management of moderately severe dysthyroid eye disease without visual loss is controversial. Systemic corticosteroids and radiotherapy have not been shown to provide definite long-term benefit. Peribulbar corticosteroid injections have been advocated. Surgical decompression may be justified in patients with marked proptosis. Lateral tarsorrhaphy may be used for moderately severe corneal exposure. Other procedures are particularly useful for correcting lid retraction but should not be undertaken until the orbital disease is quiescent and orbital decompression or extraocular muscle surgery has been undertaken. Establishing and maintaining euthyroidism are important in all cases.

When to Refer

All patients with dysthyroid eye disease should be referred to an ophthalmologist, urgently if there is reduced vision.

Kuriyan AE et al. The eye and thyroid disease. Curr Opin Ophthalmol. 2008 Nov;19(6):499–506. [PMID: 18854695]
Wiersinga WM. Management of Graves' ophthalmopathy. Nat Clin Pract Endocrinol Metab. 2007 May;3(5):396–404. [PMID: 17452966]
Zoumalan CI et al. Efficacy of corticosteroids and external beam radiation in the management of moderate to severe thyroid eye disease. J Neuroophthalmol. 2007 Sep;27(3):205–14. [PMID: 17895822]

ORBITAL CELLULITIS

Orbital cellulitis is characterized by fever, proptosis, restriction of extraocular movements, and swelling with redness of the lids. Infection of the paranasal sinuses is the usual underlying cause. Immediate treatment with intravenous antibiotics is necessary to prevent optic nerve damage and spread of infection to the cavernous sinuses, meninges, and brain. The response to antibiotics is usually excellent, but abscess formation may necessitate surgical drainage. In immunocompromised patients, zygomycosis must be considered.

When to Refer

All patients with suspected orbital cellulitis must be referred emergently to an ophthalmologist.

Armstrong PA et al. An eye for trouble: orbital cellulitis. Emerg Med J. 2006 Dec;23(12):e66. [PMID: 17130587]

OCULAR TRAUMA

1. Conjunctival & Corneal Foreign Bodies

If a patient complains of "something in my eye" and gives a consistent history, a foreign body is usually present on the cornea or under the upper lid even though it may not be visible. Visual acuity should be tested before treatment is instituted, as a basis for comparison in the event of complications.

After a local anesthetic (eg, proparacaine, 0.5%) is instilled, the eye is examined with a hand flashlight, using oblique illumination, and loupe. Corneal foreign bodies may be made more apparent by the instillation of sterile fluorescein. They are then removed with a sterile wet cotton-tipped applicator or hypodermic needle. Polymyxin-bacitracin ophthalmic ointment should be instilled. It is not necessary to patch the eye.

Steel foreign bodies usually leave a diffuse rust ring. This requires excision of the affected tissue and is best done under local anesthesia using a slit lamp. **Caution:** Anesthetic drops should not be given to the patient for self-administration.

If there is no infection, a layer of corneal epithelial cells will line the crater within 24 hours. The intact corneal epithelium forms an effective barrier to infection, but once it is disturbed the cornea becomes extremely susceptible to infection. Early infection is manifested by a white necrotic area around the crater and a small amount of gray exudate.

In the case of a foreign body under the upper lid, a local anesthetic is instilled and the lid is everted by grasping the lashes gently and exerting pressure on the mid portion of the outer surface of the upper lid with an applicator. If a foreign body is present, it can easily be removed by passing a wet sterile cotton-tipped applicator across the conjunctival surface.

▶ When to Refer

Urgent referral to an ophthalmologist should be arranged if a corneal foreign body cannot be removed or if there is suspicion of corneal infection.

2. Intraocular Foreign Body

Intraocular foreign body requires emergency treatment by an ophthalmologist. Patients giving a history of "something hitting the eye"—particularly while hammering on metal or using grinding equipment—must be assessed for this possibility, especially when no corneal foreign body is seen, a corneal or scleral wound is apparent, or there is marked visual loss or media opacity. Such patients must be treated as for corneal laceration (see below) and referred without delay. Intraocular foreign bodies significantly increase the risk of intraocular infection.

▶ When to Refer

Patients with suspected intraocular foreign body must be referred emergently to an ophthalmologist.

Peate WF. Work-related eye injuries and illnesses. Am Fam Physician. 2007 Apr 1;75(7):1017–22. [PMID: 17427615]

3. Corneal Abrasions

A patient with a corneal abrasion complains of severe pain and photophobia. There is often a history of trauma to the eye, commonly involving a fingernail, piece of paper, or contact lens. Visual acuity is recorded, and the cornea and conjunctiva are examined with a light and loupe to rule out a foreign body. If an abrasion is suspected but cannot be seen, sterile fluorescein is instilled into the conjunctival sac: the area of corneal abrasion will stain a deeper green than the surrounding cornea.

Treatment includes polymyxin-bacitracin ophthalmic ointment, mydriatic (cyclopentolate 1%), and analgesics either topical or oral nonsteroidal anti-inflammatory agents. Padding the eye is probably not helpful for small abrasions. Recurrent corneal erosion may follow corneal abrasions.

4. Contusions

Contusion injuries of the eye and surrounding structures may cause ecchymosis ("black eye"), subconjunctival hemorrhage, edema or rupture of the cornea, hemorrhage into the anterior chamber (hyphema), rupture of the root of the iris (iridodialysis), paralysis of the pupillary sphincter, paralysis of the muscles of accommodation, cataract, dislocation of the lens, vitreous hemorrhage, retinal hemorrhage and edema (most common in the macular area), detachment of the retina, rupture of the choroid, fracture of the orbital floor ("blowout fracture"), or optic nerve injury. Many of these injuries are immediately obvious; others may not become apparent for days or weeks. The possibility of globe injury must always be considered in patients with facial injury, particularly if there is an orbital fracture. Patients with moderate to severe contusions should be seen by an ophthalmologist.

Any injury causing hyphema involves the danger of secondary hemorrhage, which may cause intractable glaucoma with permanent visual loss (Plate 55). The patient should be advised to rest until complete resolution has occurred. Daily ophthalmologic assessment is essential. Aspirin and any drugs inhibiting coagulation increase the risk of secondary hemorrhage and are to be avoided. Sickle cell anemia or trait adversely affects outcome.

▶ When to Refer

Patients with moderate or severe ocular contusion should be referred to an ophthalmologist, emergently if there is hyphema.

Ashaye AO. Traumatic hyphaema: a report of 472 consecutive cases. BMC Ophthalmol. 2008 Nov 26;8(1):24. [PMID: 19036128]

5. Lacerations

A. Lids

If the lid margin is lacerated, the patient should be referred for specialized care, since permanent notching may result. Lacerations of the lower eyelid near the inner canthus often sever the lower canaliculus. Lid lacerations not involving the margin may be sutured like any skin laceration.

B. Conjunctiva

In lacerations of the conjunctiva, sutures are not necessary. To prevent infection, sulfonamides or other antibiotics are instilled into the eye until the laceration is healed.

C. Cornea or Sclera

Patients with suspected corneal or scleral lacerations must be seen promptly by an ophthalmologist (Plate 56). Manipulation is kept to a minimum, since pressure may result in extrusion of the intraocular contents. The eye is bandaged lightly and covered with a metal shield that rests on the orbital bones above and below. The patient should be instructed not to squeeze the eye shut and to remain still. The eye is routinely imaged by radiography, and CT scanning if necessary, to identify and localize any metallic intraocular foreign body. MRI is contraindicated because of the risk of movement of the foreign body in the magnetic field. Endophthalmitis occurs in over 5% of open globe injuries.

▶ When to Refer

Patients with suspected globe laceration must be referred emergently to an ophthalmologist.

ULTRAVIOLET KERATITIS (Actinic Keratitis)

Ultraviolet burns of the cornea are usually caused by use of a sunlamp without eye protection, exposure to a welding arc, or exposure to the sun when skiing ("snow blindness"). There are no immediate symptoms, but about 6–12 hours later the patient complains of agonizing pain and severe photophobia. Slit-lamp examination after instillation of sterile fluorescein shows diffuse punctate staining of both corneas.

Treatment consists of binocular patching and instillation of 1–2 drops of 1% cyclopentolate (to relieve the discomfort of ciliary spasm). All patients recover within 24–48 hours without complications. Local anesthetics should not be prescribed because they delay corneal epithelial healing.

CHEMICAL CONJUNCTIVITIS & KERATITIS

Chemical burns are treated by copious irrigation of the eyes with saline solution, plain water, or buffering solution if available as soon as possible after exposure. Neutralization of an acid with an alkali or vice versa generates heat and may cause further damage. Alkali injuries are more serious and require prolonged irrigation, since alkalies are not precipitated by the proteins of the eye as are acids. It is important to remove any retained particulate matter such as is typically present in injuries involving cement and building plaster. This may require double eversion of the upper lid. The pupil should be dilated with 1% cyclopentolate, 1 drop twice a day, to relieve discomfort and prophylactic topical antibiotics should be started. In moderate to severe injuries, intensive topical corticosteroids and topical and systemic vitamin C are

also necessary. Complications include mucus deficiency, scarring of the cornea and conjunctiva, symblepharon (adhesions between the tarsal and bulbar conjunctiva), tear duct obstruction, and secondary infection. It can be difficult to assess severity of chemical burns without slit-lamp examination.

Peate WF. Work-related eye injuries and illnesses. Am Fam Physician. 2007 Apr 1;75(7):1017–22. [PMID: 17427615]

TREATMENT OF OCULAR DISORDERS

Table 7–2 lists commonly used ophthalmic drugs and their indications and costs.

PRECAUTIONS IN MANAGEMENT OF OCULAR DISORDERS

1. Use of Local Anesthetics

Unsupervised self-administration of local anesthetics is dangerous because the patient may further injure an anesthetized eye without knowing it. The drug may also interfere with the normal healing process.

2. Pupillary Dilation

Dilating the pupil can very occasionally precipitate acute glaucoma if the patient has a narrow anterior chamber angle and should be undertaken with caution if the anterior chamber is obviously shallow (readily determined by oblique illumination of the anterior segment of the eye). A short-acting mydriatic such as tropicamide should be used and the patient warned to report immediately if ocular discomfort or redness develops. Angle closure is more likely to occur if pilocarpine is used to overcome pupillary dilation than if the pupil is allowed to constrict naturally.

3. Corticosteroid Therapy

Repeated use of local corticosteroids presents several hazards: herpes simplex (dendritic) keratitis, fungal infection, open-angle glaucoma, and cataract formation. Furthermore, perforation of the cornea may occur when the corticosteroids are used for herpes simplex keratitis. Topical nonsteroidal anti-inflammatory agents are being used increasingly. The potential for causing or exacerbating systemic hypertension, diabetes mellitus, gastritis, osteoporosis, or glaucoma must always be borne in mind when systemic corticosteroids are prescribed, such as for uveitis or giant cell arteritis.

4. Contaminated Eye Medications

Ophthalmic solutions are prepared with the same degree of care as fluids intended for intravenous administration, but once bottles are opened there is always a risk of contamination, particularly with solutions of tetracaine, proparacaine, fluorescein, and any preservative-free preparations. The most dangerous is fluorescein, as this solution is frequently contaminated with *P aeruginosa*,

Table 7-2. Topical ophthalmic agents.

Agent	Cost/Size[1]	Recommended Regimen	Indications
Antibacterial Agents[2]			
Bacitracin 500 units/g ointment (various)[3]	$4.75/3.5 g	Refer to package insert (instructions vary)	Ocular surface infection involving lid, conjunctiva, or cornea.
Chloramphenicol 1% (10 mg/g) ointment (compounding pharmacy)[4]	No U.S. price		
Ciprofloxacin HCl (Ciloxan)	0.3% solution: $45.89/5 mL		
	0.3% ointment: $79.38/3.5 g		
Erythromycin 0.5% ointment (various)[5]	$5.73/3.5 g		
Fusidic acid 1% in gel (Fucithalmic)	Not available in United States		
Gatifloxacin 0.3% solution (Zymar)	$74.54/5 mL		
Gentamicin sulfate 0.3% solution (various)	$9.50/5 mL		
Gentamicin sulfate 0.3% ointment (various)	$17.70/3.5 g		
Levofloxacin 0.5% solution (Iquix 1.5%)	$67.20/5 mL		
Moxifloxacin sulfate 0.5% solution (Vigamox)	$70.68/3 mL		
Norfloxacin 0.3% solution (Chibroxin)	Not available in United States		
Ofloxacin 0.3% solution (Ocuflox)	$40.46.17/5 mL		
Polymyxin B/Trimethoprim sulfate 10,000 U/mL/1 mg/mL[6]	$17.42/10 mL		
Tobramycin 0.3% solution (various)	$15.00/5 mL		
Tobramycin 0.3% ointment (Tobrex)	$67.62/3.5 g		
Sulfacetamide sodium 10% solution (various)	$5.08/15 mL	1 or 2 drops every 1–3 hours	
Sulfacetamide sodium 10% ointment (various)	$15.25/3.5 g	Apply small amount (0.5 inch) into lower conjunctival sac once to four times daily and at bedtime	
Antifungal Agents			
Natamycin 5% suspension (Natacyn)	$189.00/15 mL	1 drop every 1–2 hours	Fungal ocular infections.
Antiviral Agents			
Acyclovir 3% ointment (Zovirax)	Not available in United States	5 times daily	Herpes simplex virus keratitis.
Trifluridine 1% solution (Viroptic)	$95.64/7.5 mL	1 drop onto cornea every 2 hours while awake for a maximum daily dose of 9 drops until resolution occurs; then an additional 7 days of 1 drop every 4 hours while awake (minimum five times daily)	
Anti-Inflammatory Agents			
Antihistamines[7]			
Azelastine HCl 0.05% ophthalmic solution (Optivar)	$97.93/6 mL	1 drop two to four times daily (up to 6 weeks)	Allergic eye disease.
Levocabastine HCl 0.05% ophthalmic solution (Livostin)	$96.40/10 mL	1 drop four times daily (up to 2 weeks)	
Emedastine difumarate 0.05% solution (Emadine)	$70.62/5 mL	1 drop four times daily	
Epinastine HCl 0.05% ophthalmic solution (Elestat)	$99.29/ 5 mL	1 drop twice daily (up to 8 weeks)	

(continued)

Table 7–2. Topical ophthalmic agents. (continued)

Agent	Cost/Size[1]	Recommended Regimen	Indications
Mast cell stabilizers			
Cromolyn sodium 4% solution (Crolom)	$37.20/10 mL	1 drop four to six times daily	Allergic eye disease.
Ketotifen fumarate 0.025% solution (Zaditor)	$12.19/5 mL	1 drop two to four times daily	
Lodoxamide tromethamine 0.1% solution (Alomide)	$91.20/10 mL	1 or 2 drops four times daily (up to 3 months)	
Nedocromil sodium 2% solution (Alocril)	$89.40/5 mL	1 drop twice daily	
Olopatadine hydrochloride 0.1% solution (Patanol)	$98.10/5 mL	1 drop twice daily	
Nonsteroidal anti-inflammatory agents[8]			
Bromfenac 0.09% solution (Xibrom)	$113.38/2.5 mL	1 drop to operated eye twice daily beginning 24 hours after cataract surgery and continuing through first 2 postoperative weeks	Treatment of postoperative inflammation following cataract extraction.
Diclofenac sodium 0.1% solution (Voltaren)	$55.15/5 mL	1 drop to operated eye four times daily beginning 24 hours after cataract surgery and continuing through first 2 postoperative weeks	Treatment of postoperative inflammation following cataract extraction and laser corneal surgery.
Flurbiprofen sodium 0.03% solution (various)	$8.73/2.5 mL	1 drop every half hour beginning 2 hours before surgery; 1 drop to operated eye four times daily beginning 24 hours after cataract surgery	Inhibition of intraoperative miosis. Treatment of cystoid macular edema and inflammation after cataract surgery.
Ketorolac tromethamine 0.5% solution (Acular)	$100.87/5 mL	1 drop four times daily	Treatment of allergic eye disease, postoperative inflammation following cataract extraction and laser corneal surgery.
Nepafenac 0.1% suspension (Nevanac)	$92.88/3 mL	1 drop to operated eye three times daily beginning 24 hours after cataract surgery and continuing through first 2 postoperative weeks	Treatment of postoperative inflammation following cataract extraction.
Corticosteroids[9]			
Dexamethasone sodium phosphate 0.1% solution (various)	$17.31/5 mL	1 or 2 drops as often as indicated by severity; use every hour during the day and every 2 hours during the night in severe inflammation; taper off as inflammation decreases	Treatment of steroid-responsive inflammatory conditions of anterior segment.
Dexamethasone sodium phosphate 0.05% ointment (various)	$6.34/3.5 g	Apply thin coating on lower conjunctival sac three or four times daily	
Fluorometholone 0.1% suspension (various)[10]	$16.01/10 mL	1 or 2 drops as often as indicated by severity; use every hour during the day and every 2 hours during the night in severe inflammation; taper off as inflammation decreases	
Fluorometholone 0.25% suspension (FML Forte)[10]	$38.63/10 mL		
Fluorometholone 0.1% ointment (FML S.O.P.)	$34.92/3.5 g	Apply thin coating on lower conjunctival sac three or four times daily	
Loteprednol etabopate 0.5% (Lotemax)	$117.04/10 mL	1 or 2 drops four times daily	

(continued)

Table 7–2. Topical ophthalmic agents. (continued)

Agent	Cost/Size[1]	Recommended Regimen	Indications
Prednisolone acetate 0.12% suspension (Pred Mild)	$36.14/10 mL	1 or 2 drops as often as indicated by severity of inflammation; use every hour during the day and every 2 hours during the night in severe inflammation; taper off as inflammation decreases	
Prednisolone sodium phosphate 0.125% solution (compounding pharmacy)	No U.S. price		
Prednisolone acetate 1% suspension (various)	$23.10/10 mL		
Prednisolone sodium phosphate 1% solution (various)	$24.06/10 mL		
Rimexolone 1% suspension (Vexol)	$64.74/10 mL		
Immunomodulator			
Cyclosporine 0.05% emulsion (Restasis) 0.4 mL/container	$123.32/30 containers	1 drop twice daily	Dry eyes and severe allergic eye disease.
Agents for Glaucoma and Ocular Hypertension			
Sympathomimetics			
Apraclonidine HCl 0.5% solution (Iopidine)	$86.22/5 mL	1 drop three times daily	Reduction of intraocular pressure. Expensive. Reserve for treatment of resistant cases.
Apraclonidine HCl 1% solution (Iopidine)	$14.33/unit dose	1 drop 1 hour before and immediately after anterior segment laser surgery	To control or prevent elevations of intraocular pressure after laser trabeculoplasty or iridotomy.
Brimonidine tartrate 0.2% solution (Alphagan)	$32.65/5 mL	1 drop two or three times daily	Reduction of intraocular pressure.
Dipivefrin HCl 0.1% solution (Propine)[11]	$14.06/5 mL	1 drop every 12 hours	Open-angle glaucoma.
β-Adrenergic blocking agents			
Betaxolol HCl 0.5% solution and 0.25% suspension (Betoptic S)[12]	0.5%: $46.68/10 mL 0.25%: $109.50/10 mL	1 drop twice daily	Reduction of intraocular pressure.
Carteolol HCl 1% and 2% solution (Various, Teoptic[13])	1%: $37.07/10 mL 2%: TEOPTIC not available in the U.S.	1 drop twice daily	
Levobunolol HCl 0.25% and 0.5% solution (Betagan)[13]	0.5%: $32.25/10 mL	1 drop once or twice daily	
Metipranolol HCl 0.3% solution (OptiPranolol)[13]	$26.85/10 mL	1 drop twice daily	
Timolol 0.25% and 0.5% solution (Betimol)[13]	0.5%: $64.80/10 mL	1 drop once or twice daily	
Timolol maleate 0.25% and 0.5% solution (Timoptic) and 0.25% and 0.5% gel (Timoptic-XE)[13]	0.5% solution: $32.35/10 mL 0.5% gel: $27.00/5 mL	1 drop once or twice daily	
Miotics			
Pilocarpine HCl (various)[14] 1–4%, 6%, 8%, and 10%	2%: $11.80/15 mL	1 drop three or four times daily	Reduction of intraocular pressure, treatment of acute or chronic angle-closure glaucoma, and pupillary constriction.
Pilocarpine HCl 4% gel (Pilopine HS)	$54.24/4 g	Apply 0.5-inch ribbon in lower conjunctival sac at bedtime	
Carbonic anhydrase inhibitors			
Dorzolamide HCl 2% solution (Trusopt)	$71.28/10 mL	1 drop three times daily	Reduction of intraocular pressure.
Brinzolamide 1% suspension (Azopt)	$91.38/10 mL	1 drop three times daily	
Prostaglandin analogs			
Bimatoprost 0.03% solution (Lumigan)	$80.53/2.5 mL	1 drop once daily at night	Reduction of intraocular pressure.

(continued)

Table 7–2. Topical ophthalmic agents. (continued)

Agent	Cost/Size[1]	Recommended Regimen	Indications
Latanoprost 0.005% solution (Xalatan)	$77.26/2.5 mL	1 drop once or twice daily at night	Reduction of intraocular pressure.
Travoprost 0.004% solution (Travatan)	$80.88/2.5 mL	1 drop once daily at night	
Unoprostone isopropyl 0.15% solution (Rescula)	Not available in United States	1 drop twice daily	
Combined preparations			
Xalacom (latanoprost 0.005% and timolol 0.5%)	Not available in United States	1 drop daily in the morning	Reduction of intraocular pressure.
Ganfort (bimatoprost 0.03% and timolol 0.5%)	Not available in United States	1 drop daily in the morning	
DuoTrav (travoprost 0.004% and timolol 0.5%)	Not available in United States	1 drop daily	
Cosopt (dorzolamide 2% and timolol 0.5%)	$130.80/10 mL	1 drop twice daily	
Combigan (brimonidine 0.2% and timolol 0.5%)	Not available in United States	1 drop twice daily	

[1]Average wholesale price (AWP, for AB-rated generic when available) for quantity listed. Source: *Red Book Update*, Vol. 28, No. 3, March 2009. AWP may not accurately represent the actual pharmacy cost because wide contractual variations exist among institutions.
[2]Many combination products containing antibacterials or antibacterials and corticosteroids are available.
[3]Little efficacy against gram-negative organisms (except *Neisseria*).
[4]Aplastic anemia has been reported with prolonged ophthalmic use.
[5]Also indicated for prophylaxis of neonatal conjunctivitis due to *Neisseria gonorrhoeae* or *Chlamydia trachomatis*.
[6]No gram-positive coverage.
[7]May produce rebound hyperemia and local reactions.
[8]Cross-sensitivity to aspirin and other nonsteroidal anti-inflammatory drugs.
[9]Long-term use increases intraocular pressure, causes cataracts and predisposes to bacterial, herpes simplex virus, and fungal keratitis.
[10]Less likely to elevate intraocular pressure.
[11]Macular edema occurs in 30% of patients.
[12]Cardioselective (β_1) β-blocker.
[13]Teoptic is not available in the United States.
[14]Nonselective (β_1 and β_2) β-blocker. Monitor all patients for systemic side effects, particularly exacerbation of asthma.
[15]Decreased night vision, headaches possible.

which can rapidly destroy the eye. Sterile fluorescein filter paper strips are recommended for use in place of fluorescein solutions.

Whether in plastic or glass containers, eye solutions should not remain in use for long periods after the bottle is opened. Four weeks after opening is an absolute maximal time to use a solution containing preservatives before discarding. Preservative-free preparations should be kept refrigerated and discarded within 1 week after opening.

If the eye has been injured accidentally or by surgical trauma, it is of the greatest importance to use freshly opened bottles of sterile medications or single-use eye-dropper units.

5. Toxic & Hypersensitivity Reactions to Topical Therapy

In patients receiving long-term topical therapy, local toxic or hypersensitivity reactions to the active agent or preservatives may develop, especially if there is inadequate tear secretion. Preservatives in contact lens cleaning solutions may produce similar problems. Burning and soreness are exacerbated by drop instillation or contact lens insertion; occasionally, fibrosis and scarring of the conjunctiva and cornea may occur.

An antibiotic instilled into the eye can sensitize the patient to that drug and cause an allergic reaction upon subsequent systemic administration.

6. Systemic Effects of Ocular Drugs

The systemic absorption of certain topical drugs (through the conjunctival vessels and lacrimal drainage system) must be considered when there is a systemic medical contraindication to the use of the drug. Ophthalmic solutions of the nonselective β-blockers, eg, timolol, may worsen congestive heart failure or asthma. Phenylephrine eye drops may precipitate hypertensive crises and angina. Also to be considered are adverse interactions between systemically administered and ocular drugs. Using only 1 or 2 drops at a time and a few minutes of nasolacrimal occlusion or eyelid closure ensure maximum efficacy and decrease systemic side effects of topical agents.

ADVERSE OCULAR EFFECTS OF SYSTEMIC DRUGS

Systemically administered drugs produce a wide variety of adverse effects on the visual system. Table 7–3 lists the major examples.

Table 7–3. Adverse ophthalmic effects of systemic drugs.

Drug	Possible Side Effects
Respiratory drugs	
Oxygen	Retinopathy of prematurity.
Anticholinergic bronchodilators	Angle-closure glaucoma due to mydriasis, blurring of vision due to cycloplegia, dry eyes.
Sympathomimetic bronchodilators and decongestants	Angle-closure glaucoma due to mydriasis.
Cardiovascular system drugs	
Digitalis	Disturbance of color vision, photopsia.
Thiazides	Xanthopsia (yellow vision), myopia.
Carbonic anhydrase inhibitors (acetazolamide)	Stevens-Johnson syndrome, myopia.
Amiodarone	Corneal deposits (vortex keratopathy), optic neuropathy, thyroid ophthalmopathy.
Sildenafil	Ischemic optic neuropathy.
Statins	Myasthenic syndrome.
Gastrointestinal drugs	
Anticholinergic agents	Angle-closure glaucoma due to mydriasis, blurring of vision due to cycloplegia, dry eyes.
Central nervous system drugs	
Anticholinergic agents including preoperative medications	Angle-closure glaucoma due to mydriasis, blurring of vision due to cycloplegia, dry eyes.
Phenothiazines	Deposits of pigment in conjunctiva, cornea, lens, and retina, oculogyric crises.
Haloperidol	Capsular cataract.
Lithium carbonate	Proptosis, oculogyric crisis, nystagmus.
Amphetamines	Widening of palpebral fissure, blurring of vision due to mydriasis.
Monoamine oxidase inhibitors	Nystagmus.
Tricyclic agents	Angle-closure glaucoma due to mydriasis, blurring of vision due to cycloplegia.
Phenytoin	Nystagmus.
Neostigmine	Nystagmus, miosis.
Morphine	Miosis.
Diazepam	Nystagmus.
Topiramate	Angle-closure glaucoma, myopia.
Paroxetine	Angle-closure glaucoma.
Vigabatrin	Visual field constriction.
Obstetric drugs	
Sympathomimetic tocolytics	Angle-closure glaucoma due to mydriasis.
Hormonal agents	
Corticosteroids	Cataract (posterior subcapsular); susceptibility to viral (herpes simplex), bacterial, and fungal infections; steroid-induced glaucoma.
Female sex hormones	Retinal artery occlusion, retinal vein occlusion, papilledema, extraocular muscle palsies, ischemic optic neuropathy.
Tamoxifen	Crystalline retinal and corneal deposits, optic neuropathy.
Immunomodulators	
Cyclosporine	Posterior reversible leukoencephalopathy.
Tacrolimus	Optic neuropathy, posterior reversible leukoencephalopathy.
Antibacterials	
Chloramphenicol	Optic neuropathy.
Streptomycin	Optic neuropathy, Stevens-Johnson syndrome.
Tetracycline, doxycycline, minocycline	Papilledema.

(continued)

Table 7–3. Adverse ophthalmic effects of systemic drugs. (continued)

Drug	Possible Side Effects
Sulfonamides	Stevens-Johnson syndrome, myopia.
Ethambutol	Optic neuropathy.
Isoniazid	Optic neuropathy.
Antimalarial agents	
Chloroquine, hydroxychloroquine	Retinal degeneration principally involving the macula, keratopathy.
Amebicides	
Iodochlorhydroxyquin	Optic neuropathy.
Chemotherapeutic agents	
Chlorambucil	Optic neuropathy.
Fluorouracil	Lacrimal obstruction.
Vincristine	Optic neuropathy.
Heavy metals	
Gold salts	Deposits in the cornea, conjunctiva, and lens.
Lead compounds	Optic neuropathy, papilledema, ocular palsies.
Chelating agents	
Penicillamine	Ocular pemphigoid, optic neuropathy, myasthenic syndrome.
Desferrioxamine	Retinopathy, optic neuropathy, lens opacity.
Oral hypoglycemic agents	
Chlorpropamide	Refractive error, Stevens-Johnson syndrome, optic neuropathy.
Vitamins	
Vitamin A	Papilledema.
Vitamin D	Band-shaped keratopathy.
Antirheumatic agents	
Salicylates	Subconjunctival or retinal hemorrhages, nystagmus.
Indomethacin	Corneal deposits.
Phenylbutazone	Retinal hemorrhages.
Dermatologic agents	
Retinoids (isotretinoin, tretinoin, acitretin, and etretinate)	Papilledema, blepharoconjunctivitis, corneal opacities, decreased contact lens tolerance, decreased dark adaptation, teratogenic ocular abnormalities.
Bisphosphonates	
Pamidronate	Scleritis, episcleritis, uveitis.
Alendronate	Scleritis, episcleritis, uveitis.

Fraunfelder FW. Ocular & systemic side effects of drugs. In: *Vaughan & Asbury's General Ophthalmology*, 17th ed. Riordan-Eva P, Whitcher JP (editors). McGraw-Hill, 2008.

Santaella RM et al. Ocular adverse effects associated with systemic medications: recognition and management. Drugs. 2007;67(1):75–93. [PMID: 17209665]

Ear, Nose, & Throat Disorders

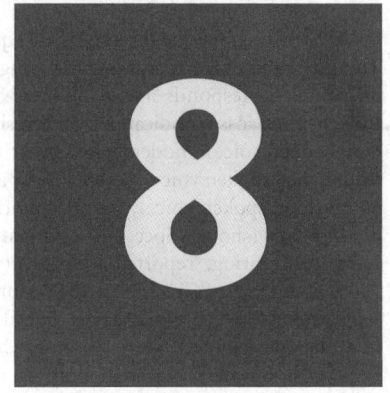

Lawrence R. Lustig, MD, & Joshua Schindler, MD

▼ DISEASES OF THE EAR

HEARING LOSS

 ESSENTIALS OF DIAGNOSIS

▶ Three main types of hearing loss: conductive, sensory, and neural.

▶ Most commonly due to cerumen impaction, transient eustachian tube dysfunction associated with upper respiratory tract infection, or age-related hearing loss.

Classification & Epidemiology

A. Conductive Hearing Loss

Conductive hearing loss results from dysfunction of the external or middle ear. There are four mechanisms, each resulting in impairment of the passage of sound vibrations to the inner ear: (1) obstruction (eg, cerumen impaction), (2) mass loading (eg, middle ear effusion), (3) stiffness effect (eg, otosclerosis), and (4) discontinuity (eg, ossicular disruption). Conductive losses in adults are most commonly due to cerumen impaction or transient eustachian tube dysfunction associated with upper respiratory tract infection. Persistent conductive losses usually result from chronic ear infection, trauma, or otosclerosis. Conductive hearing loss is usually correctable with medical or surgical therapy—or in some cases both.

B. Sensory Hearing Loss

Sensory hearing loss results from deterioration of the cochlea, usually due to loss of hair cells from the organ of Corti. Sensorineural losses in adults are common. The most common form is a gradually progressive, predominantly high-frequency loss with advancing age (presbyacusis). Additional common causes include excessive noise exposure, head trauma, and systemic diseases. An individual's genetic make-up influences all of these causes of sensory hearing loss. Sensory hearing loss is usually not

correctable with medical or surgical therapy but often may be prevented or stabilized. An exception is a sudden sensory hearing loss, which may respond to corticosteroids if delivered within several weeks of onset.

Marchese MR et al. Role of stapes surgery in improving hearing loss caused by otosclerosis. J Laryngol Otol. 2007 May;121(5):438–43. [PMID: 17112393]
O'Malley MR et al. Sudden hearing loss. Otolaryngol Clin North Am. 2008 Jun;41(3):633–49. [PMID: 18436003]
Van Eyken E et al. The complexity of age-related hearing impairment: contributing environmental and genetic factors. Audiol Neurootol. 2007;12(6):345–58. [PMID: 17664866]

C. Neural Hearing Loss

Neural hearing loss occurs with lesions involving the eighth nerve, auditory nuclei, ascending tracts, or auditory cortex. It is the least common clinically recognized cause of hearing loss. Causes include acoustic neuroma, multiple sclerosis, and auditory neuropathy.

Vlastarakos PV et al. Auditory neuropathy: endocochlear lesion or temporal processing impairment? Implications for diagnosis and management. Int J Pediatr Otorhinolaryngol. 2008 Aug;72(8):1135–50. [PMID: 18502518]

Evaluation of Hearing (Audiology)

In a quiet room, the hearing level may be estimated by having the patient repeat aloud words presented in a soft whisper, a normal spoken voice, or a shout. A 512-Hz tuning fork is useful in differentiating conductive from sensorineural losses. In the **Weber test**, the tuning fork is placed on the forehead or front teeth. In conductive losses, the sound appears louder in the poorer-hearing ear, whereas in sensorineural losses it radiates to the better side. In the **Rinne test**, the tuning fork is placed alternately on the mastoid bone and in front of the ear canal. In conductive losses, bone conduction exceeds air conduction; in sensorineural losses, the opposite is true.

Formal audiometric studies are performed in a soundproofed room. Pure-tone thresholds in decibels (dB) are obtained over the range of 250–8000 Hz for both air and bone conduction. Conductive losses create a gap between the air and bone thresholds, whereas in sensorineural losses both air and bone thresholds are equally diminished. The threshold of normal hearing is roughly from 0 to 20 dB, which corresponds to the loudness of a soft whisper. Mild hearing loss is indicated by a threshold of 20–40 dB (soft spoken voice), moderate loss by a threshold of 40–60 dB (normal spoken voice), severe loss by a threshold of 60–80 dB (loud spoken voice), and profound loss by a threshold of 80 dB (shout). Speech discrimination measures the clarity of hearing, reported as percentage correct (90–100% is normal). The site of the lesion responsible for sensorineural loss (cochlea versus central auditory system) may be determined with auditory brainstem-evoked responses; however, an MRI scan is usually preferred method because it has both better sensitivity and specificity for evaluating central lesions.

Every patient who complains of a hearing loss should be referred for audiologic evaluation unless the cause is easily remediable (eg, cerumen impaction, otitis media). Since some forms of sudden hearing loss do not respond to treatment (corticosteroids) after several weeks, any new-onset hearing loss without obvious ear pathology needs an immediate audiometric referral. Routine audiologic screening is recommended for adults who have been exposed to potentially injurious levels of noise or in those who have reached the age of 65, after which screening evaluations may be done every few years.

Bagai A et al. Does this patient have hearing impairment? JAMA. 2006 Jan 25;295(4):416–28. [PMID: 16434632]

▶ Hearing Rehabilitation

Patients with hearing loss not correctable by medical therapy may benefit from hearing amplification. Contemporary hearing aids are comparatively free of distortion and have been miniaturized to the point where they often may be contained entirely within the ear canal. To optimize the benefit, a hearing aid must be carefully selected to conform to the nature of the hearing loss. Digitally programmable hearing aids are now widely available and allow optimization of speech intelligibility and improved performance in difficult listening circumstances. Aside from hearing aids, many assistive devices are available to improve comprehension in individual and group settings, to help with hearing television and radio programs, and for telephone communication.

For patients with conductive loss or unilateral profound sensorineural loss, the bone-anchored hearing aid uses an oscillating post drilled into the mastoid, directly stimulating the ipsilateral cochlea (for conductive losses) or contralateral ear (profound unilateral hearing loss).

For patients with severe to profound sensory hearing loss, the cochlear implant—an electronic device that is surgically implanted into the cochlea to stimulate the auditory nerve—offers socially beneficial auditory rehabilitation to most adults with acquired deafness. New trends in cochlear implantation include its use for patients with only partial deafness, preserving residual hearing and allowing both acoustic and electrical hearing in the same ear, as well as bilateral cochlear implantation.

Brown KD et al. Benefits of bilateral cochlear implantation: a review. Curr Opin Otolaryngol Head Neck Surg. 2007 Oct;15(5):315–8. [PMID: 17823546]

Dorman MF et al. The benefits of combining acoustic and electric stimulation for the recognition of speech, voice and melodies. Audiol Neurootol. 2007 Nov 29;13(2):105–112. [PMID: 18057874]

Lloyd S et al. Updated surgical experience with bone-anchored hearing aids in children. J Laryngol Otol. 2007 Sep;121(9):826–31. [PMID: 17210090]

Palmer CV et al. Hearing loss and hearing aids. Neurol Clin. 2005 Aug;23(3):901–18. [PMID: 16026682]

Papsin BC et al. Cochlear implants for children with severe-to-profound hearing loss. N Engl J Med. 2007 Dec 6;357(23):2380–7. [PMID: 18057340]

DISEASES OF THE AURICLE

Disorders of the auricle are for the most part dermatologic. Skin cancers due to sun exposure are common and may be treated with standard techniques. Traumatic auricular hematoma must be recognized and drained to prevent significant cosmetic deformity (cauliflower ear) or canal blockage resulting from dissolution of supporting cartilage. Similarly, cellulitis of the auricle must be treated promptly to prevent development of perichondritis and its resultant deformity. Relapsing polychondritis is a rheumatologic disorder often associated with recurrent, frequently bilateral, painful episodes of auricular erythema and edema. Treatment with corticosteroids may help forestall cartilage dissolution. Respiratory compromise may occur as a result of progressive involvement of the tracheobronchial tree. Chondritis and perichondritis may be differentiated from auricular cellulitis by sparing of involvement of the lobule, which does not contain cartilage.

Rapini RP et al. Relapsing polychondritis. Clin Dermatol. 2006 Nov–Dec;24(6):482–5. [PMID: 17113965]

DISEASES OF THE EAR CANAL

1. Cerumen Impaction

Cerumen is a protective secretion produced by the outer portion of the ear canal. In most persons, the ear canal is self-cleansing. Recommended hygiene consists of cleaning the external opening with a washcloth over the index finger without entering the canal itself. In most cases, cerumen impaction is self-induced through ill-advised attempts at cleaning the ear. It may be relieved with detergent ear drops (eg, 3% hydrogen peroxide; 6.5% carbamide peroxide), mechanical removal, suction, or irrigation. Irrigation is performed with water at body temperature to avoid a vestibular caloric response. The stream should be directed at the ear canal wall adjacent to the cerumen plug. Irrigation should be performed only when the tympanic membrane is known to be intact.

Use of jet irrigators designed for cleaning teeth (eg, WaterPik) for wax removal should be avoided since they may result in tympanic membrane perforations. Following professional irrigation, the ear canal should be thoroughly dried (eg, by instilling isopropyl alcohol or using a hair blow-dryer on low-power setting) to reduce the likelihood of inducing external otitis. Specialty referral for cleaning under microscopic guidance is indicated when the impaction is frequently recurrent, has not responded to routine measures, or if the patient has a history of chronic otitis media or tympanic membrane perforation.

McCarter DF et al. Cerumen impaction. Am Fam Physician. 2007 May 15;75(10):1523–8. [PMID: 17555144]

2. Foreign Bodies

Foreign bodies in the ear canal are more frequent in children than in adults. Firm materials may be removed with a loop or a hook, taking care not to displace the object medially toward the tympanic membrane; microscopic guidance is helpful. Aqueous irrigation should not be performed for organic foreign bodies (eg, beans, insects), because water may cause them to swell. Living insects are best immobilized before removal by filling the ear canal with lidocaine.

Heim SW et al. Foreign bodies in the ear, nose, and throat. Am Fam Physician. 2007 Oct 15;76(8):1185–9. [PMID: 17990843]

3. External Otitis

 ESSENTIALS OF DIAGNOSIS

▶ Painful erythema and edema of the ear canal skin.

▶ Often with purulent exudate.

▶ Persistent external otitis in the diabetic or immuno-compromised patient may evolve into osteomyelitis of the skull base, often called malignant external otitis.

External otitis presents with otalgia, frequently accompanied by pruritus and purulent discharge. There is often a history of recent water exposure or mechanical trauma (eg, scratching, cotton applicators). External otitis is usually caused by gram-negative rods (eg, *Pseudomonas, Proteus*) or fungi (eg, *Aspergillus*), which grow in the presence of excessive moisture.

Examination reveals erythema and edema of the ear canal skin, often with a purulent exudate. Manipulation of the auricle often elicits pain. Because the lateral surface of the tympanic membrane is ear canal skin, it is often erythematous. However, in contrast to acute otitis media, it moves normally with pneumatic otoscopy. When the canal skin is very edematous, it may be impossible to visualize the tympanic membrane.

Fundamental to the treatment of external otitis is protection of the ear from additional moisture and avoidance of further mechanical injury by scratching. Acidic otic antibiotic drops that contain either an aminoglycoside or fluoroquinolone antibiotic, with or without corticosteroids, are usually effective (eg, neomycin sulfate, polymyxin B sulfate, and hydrocortisone). Purulent debris filling the ear canal should be gently removed to permit entry of the topical medication. Drops should be used abundantly (five or more

drops three or four times a day) to penetrate the depths of the canal. When substantial edema of the canal wall prevents entry of drops into the ear canal, a wick is placed to facilitate entry of the medication. In recalcitrant cases—particularly when cellulitis of the periauricular tissue has developed—oral fluoroquinolones (eg, ciprofloxacin, 500 mg twice daily for 1 week) are the drugs of choice because of their effectiveness against *Pseudomonas* species. Any case of persistent otitis externa in an immunocompromised or diabetic individual must be referred for specialty evaluation.

Rahman A et al. Pooled analysis of two clinical trials comparing the clinical outcomes of topical ciprofloxacin/dexamethasone otic suspension and polymyxin B/neomycin/hydrocortisone otic suspension for the treatment of acute otitis externa in adults and children. Clin Ther. 2007 Sep;29(9):1950–6. [PMID: 18035194]
Stone KE. Otitis externa. Pediatr Rev. 2007 Feb;28(2):77–8. [PMID: 17272526]

4. Pruritus

Pruritus of the external auditory canal, particularly at the meatus, is a common problem. While it may be associated with external otitis or with dermatologic conditions such as seborrheic dermatitis and psoriasis, most cases are self-induced either from excoriation or by overly zealous ear cleaning. To permit regeneration of the protective cerumen blanket, patients should be instructed to avoid use of soap and water or cotton swabs in the ear canal and avoid any scratching. Patients with excessively dry canal skin may benefit from application of mineral oil, which helps counteract dryness and repel moisture. When an inflammatory component is present, topical application of a corticosteroid (eg, 0.1% triamcinolone) may be beneficial. Symptomatic reduction of pruritus may also be obtained by use of oral antihistamines (eg, diphenhydramine, 25 mg orally at bedtime). Topical application of isopropyl alcohol promptly relieves ear canal pruritus in many patients.

Harth W et al. Topical tacrolimus treatment for chronic dermatitis of the ear. Eur J Dermatol. 2007 Sep–Oct;17(5):405–11. [PMID: 17673384]

5. Malignant External Otitis

Persistent external otitis in the diabetic or immunocompromised patient may evolve into osteomyelitis of the skull base, often called malignant external otitis. Usually caused by *Pseudomonas aeruginosa*, osteomyelitis begins in the floor of the ear canal and may extend into the middle fossa floor, the clivus, and even the contralateral skull base. The patient usually presents with persistent foul aural discharge, granulations in the ear canal, deep otalgia, and in advanced cases, progressive cranial nerve palsies involving nerves VI, VII, IX, X, XI, or XII. Diagnosis is confirmed by the demonstration of osseous erosion on CT and radionuclide scanning.

Treatment is medical, requiring prolonged antipseudomonal antibiotic administration, often for several months. Although intravenous therapy is often required, selected patients may be managed with ciprofloxacin (500–1000 mg orally twice daily), which has proved effective against many of the causative *Pseudomonas* strains. To avoid relapse, antibiotic therapy should be continued, even in the asymptomatic patient, until gallium scanning indicates a marked reduction in the inflammatory process. Surgical debridement of infected bone is reserved for cases of deterioration despite medical therapy.

Mani N et al. Cranial nerve involvement in malignant external otitis: implications for clinical outcome. Laryngoscope. 2007 May;117(5):907–10. [PMID: 17473694]

Narozny W et al. Infectious skull base osteomyelitis–still a life-threatening disease. Otol Neurotol. 2006 Oct;27(7):1047–8. [PMID: 17006357]

6. Exostoses & Osteomas

Bony overgrowths of the ear canal are a frequent incidental finding and occasionally have clinical significance. Clinically, they present as skin-covered bony mounds in the medial ear canal obscuring the tympanic membrane to a variable degree. Solitary osteomas are of no significance as long as they do not cause obstruction or infection. Multiple exostoses, which are generally acquired from repeated exposure to cold water (eg, "surfer's ear") often progress and require surgical removal.

Hetzler DG. Osteotome technique for removal of symptomatic ear canal exostoses. Laryngoscope. 2007 Jan;117(1 Part 2 Suppl 113):1–E4. [PMID: 17220810]

7. Neoplasia

The most common neoplasm of the ear canal is squamous cell carcinoma (SCC). When an apparent otitis externa does not resolve on therapy, SCC should be suspected and biopsy performed. This disease carries a very high 5-year mortality rate because the tumor tends to invade the lymphatics of the cranial base and must be treated with wide surgical resection and radiation therapy. Adenomatous tumors, originating from the ceruminous glands, generally follow a more indolent course.

Ogawa K et al. Treatment and prognosis of squamous cell carcinoma of the external auditory canal and middle ear: a multi-institutional retrospective review of 87 patients. Int J Radiat Oncol Biol Phys. 2007 Aug 1;68(5):1326–34. [PMID: 17446002]

DISEASES OF THE EUSTACHIAN TUBE

1. Eustachian Tube Dysfunction

ESSENTIALS OF DIAGNOSIS

▸ Aural fullness.

▸ Fluctuating hearing.

▸ Discomfort with barometric pressure change.

▸ At risk for serous otitis media.

The tube that connects the middle ear to the nasopharynx—the eustachian tube—provides ventilation and drainage for the middle ear cleft. It is normally closed,

opening only during swallowing or yawning. When eustachian tube function is compromised, air trapped within the middle ear becomes absorbed and negative pressure results. The most common causes of eustachian tube dysfunction are diseases associated with edema of the tubal lining, such as viral upper respiratory tract infections and allergy. The patient usually reports a sense of fullness in the ear and mild to moderate impairment of hearing. When the tube is only partially blocked, swallowing or yawning may elicit a popping or crackling sound. Examination may reveal retraction of the tympanic membrane and decreased mobility on pneumatic otoscopy. Following a viral illness, this disorder is usually transient, lasting days to weeks. Treatment with systemic and intranasal decongestants (eg, pseudoephedrine, 60 mg orally every 4 hours; oxymetazoline, 0.05% spray every 8–12 hours) combined with auto-inflation by forced exhalation against closed nostrils may hasten relief. Autoinflation should not be recommended to patients with active intranasal infection, since this maneuver may precipitate middle ear infection. Allergic patients may also benefit from desensitization or intranasal corticosteroids (eg, beclomethasone dipropionate, two sprays in each nostril twice daily for 2–6 weeks). Air travel, rapid altitudinal change, and underwater diving should be avoided during an active phase of the disease.

Conversely, an overly patent eustachian tube, termed "patulous eustachian tube," is a relatively uncommon problem, though may be quite distressing. Typical complaints include fullness in the ear and autophony, an exaggerated ability to hear oneself breathe and speak. A patulous eustachian tube may develop during rapid weight loss, or it may be idiopathic. In contrast to a hypofunctioning eustachian tube, the aural pressure is often made worse by exertion and may diminish during an upper respiratory tract infection. Although physical examination is usually normal, respiratory excursions of the tympanic membrane may occasionally be detected during vigorous breathing. Treatment includes avoidance of decongestant products, insertion of a ventilating tube to reduce the outward stretch of the eardrum during phonation, and, rarely, surgical narrowing of the eustachian tube.

Poe DS. Diagnosis and management of the patulous eustachian tube. Otol Neurotol. 2007 Aug;28(5):668–77. [PMID: 17534202]

Poe DS et al. Laser eustachian tuboplasty: two-year results. Laryngoscope. 2007 Feb;117(2):231–7. [PMID: 17277615]

2. Serous Otitis Media

ESSENTIALS OF DIAGNOSIS

▸ Blocked eustachian tube remains for a prolonged period.

▸ Resultant negative pressure will result in transudation of fluid.

Prolonged eustachian tube dysfunction with resultant negative middle ear pressure may cause a transudation of fluid.

This condition, known as serous otitis media, is especially common in children because their eustachian tubes are narrower and more horizontal in orientation than those in adults. Serous otitis media is less common in adults, in whom it usually occurs after an upper respiratory tract infection, with barotraumas, or with chronic allergic rhinitis. In any adult with persistent unilateral serous otitis media, nasopharyngeal carcinoma must be excluded. The tympanic membrane in serous otitis media is dull and hypomobile, occasionally accompanied by air bubbles in the middle ear and conductive hearing loss. The treatment of serous otitis media is similar to that for eustachian tube dysfunction. A short course of oral corticosteroids (eg, prednisone, 40 mg/d for 7 days) has been advocated by some clinicians, as have oral antibiotics (eg, amoxicillin, 250 mg orally three times daily for 7 days)—or even a combination of the two. The role of these regimens remains controversial, but they are probably of little lasting benefit.

When medication fails to bring relief after several months, a ventilating tube placed through the tympanic membrane may restore hearing and alleviate the sense of aural fullness. Endoscopically guided laser expansion of the nasopharyngeal orifice of the eustachian tube may improve function in recalcitrant cases.

Corbeel L. What is new in otitis media? Eur J Pediatr. 2007 Jun;166(6):511–9. [PMID: 17364173]
Seibert JW et al. Eustachian tube function and the middle ear. Otolaryngol Clin North Am. 2006 Dec;39(6):1221–35. [PMID: 17097443]

3. Barotrauma

Persons with poor eustachian tube function (eg, congenital narrowness or acquired mucosal edema) may be unable to equalize the barometric stress exerted on the middle ear by air travel, rapid altitudinal change, or underwater diving. The problem is generally most acute during airplane descent, since the negative middle ear pressure tends to collapse and block the eustachian tube. Several measures are useful to enhance eustachian tube function and avoid otic barotrauma. The patient should be advised to swallow, yawn, and autoinflate frequently during descent, which may be painful if the eustachian tube collapses. Systemic decongestants (eg, pseudoephedrine, 60–120 mg) should be taken several hours before anticipated arrival time so that they will be maximally effective during descent. Topical decongestants such as 1% phenylephrine nasal spray should be administered 1 hour before arrival.

For acute negative middle ear pressure that persists on the ground, treatment includes decongestants and attempts at autoinflation. Myringotomy (creation of a small eardrum perforation) provides immediate relief and is appropriate in the setting of severe otalgia and hearing loss. Repeated episodes of barotrauma in persons who must fly frequently may be alleviated by insertion of ventilating tubes.

Underwater diving may represent an even a greater barometric stress to the ear than flying. The problem occurs most commonly during the descent phase, when pain develops within the first 15 feet if inflation of the middle ear via the eustachian tube has not occurred. Divers must descend slowly and equilibrate in stages to avoid the development of severely negative pressures in the tympanum that may result in hemorrhage (hemotympanum) or perilymphatic fistula. In the latter, the oval or round window ruptures, resulting in sensory hearing loss and acute vertigo. Emesis due to acute labyrinthine dysfunction can be very dangerous during an underwater dive. Sensory hearing loss or vertigo, which develops during the ascent phase of a saturation dive, may be the first (or only) symptom of decompression sickness. Immediate recompression will return intravascular gas bubbles to solution and restore the inner ear microcirculation. Patients should be warned to avoid diving when they have upper respiratory infections or episodes of nasal allergy. Tympanic membrane perforation is an absolute contraindication to diving, as the patient will experience an unbalanced thermal stimulus to the semicircular canals and may experience vertigo, disorientation, and even emesis. Finally, persons with only one hearing ear should be advised of the dangers of diving because of the potential risk of otologic injury.

Klingmann C et al. Barotrauma and decompression illness of the inner ear: 46 cases during treatment and follow-up. Otol Neurotol. 2007 Jun;28(4):447–54. [PMID: 17417111]

DISEASES OF THE MIDDLE EAR

1. Acute Otitis Media

ESSENTIALS OF DIAGNOSIS

▶ Otalgia, often with an upper respiratory tract infection.
▶ Erythema and hypomobility of tympanic membrane.

General Considerations

Acute otitis media is a bacterial infection of the mucosally lined air-containing spaces of the temporal bone. Purulent material forms not only within the middle ear cleft but also within the pneumatized mastoid air cells and petrous apex. Acute otitis media is usually precipitated by a viral upper respiratory tract infection that causes eustachian tube obstruction. This results in accumulation of fluid and mucus, which becomes secondarily infected by bacteria. The most common pathogens both in adults and in children are *Streptococcus pneumoniae*, *Haemophilus influenzae*, and *Streptococcus pyogenes*.

Clinical Findings

Acute otitis media is most common in infants and children, although it may occur at any age. Presenting symptoms and signs include otalgia, aural pressure, decreased hearing, and often fever. The typical physical findings are erythema and decreased mobility of the tympanic membrane. Occasionally, bullae will be seen on the tympanic membrane.

Rarely, when middle ear empyema is severe, the tympanic membrane can bulge outward. In such cases, tympanic membrane rupture is imminent. Rupture is accompanied by a sudden decrease in pain, followed by the onset of otorrhea. With appropriate therapy, spontaneous healing of the tympanic membrane occurs in most cases. When perforation persists, chronic otitis media may evolve. Mastoid tenderness often accompanies acute otitis media and is due to the presence of pus within the mastoid air cells. This alone does not indicate suppurative (surgical) mastoiditis. Frank swelling over the mastoid bone or the association of cranial neuropathies or central findings indicates severe disease requiring urgent care.

▶ Treatment

The treatment of acute otitis media is specific antibiotic therapy, often combined with nasal decongestants. The first-choice oral antibiotic treatment is amoxicillin (20–40 mg/kg/d) or erythromycin (50 mg/kg/d) plus sulfonamide (150 mg/kg/d) for 10 days. Alternatives useful in resistant cases are cefaclor (20–40 mg/kg/d) or amoxicillin-clavulanate (20–40 mg/kg/d) combinations.

Tympanocentesis for bacterial (aerobic and anaerobic) and fungal culture may be performed by any experienced physician. A 20-gauge spinal needle bent 90 degrees to the hub attached to a 3-mL syringe is inserted through the inferior portion of the tympanic membrane. Interposition of a pliable connecting tube between the needle and syringe permits an assistant to aspirate without inducing movement of the needle. Tympanocentesis is useful for otitis media in immunocompromised patients and when infection persists or recurs despite multiple courses of antibiotics.

Surgical drainage of the middle ear (myringotomy) is reserved for patients with severe otalgia or when complications of otitis (eg, mastoiditis, meningitis) have occurred.

Recurrent acute otitis media may be managed with long-term antibiotic prophylaxis. Single daily oral doses of sulfamethoxazole (500 mg) or amoxicillin (250 or 500 mg) are given over a period of 1–3 months. Failure of this regimen to control infection is an indication for insertion of ventilating tubes.

Ramakrishnan K et al. Diagnosis and treatment of otitis media. Am Fam Physician. 2007 Dec 1;76(11):1650–8. [PMID: 18092706]

2. Chronic Otitis Media & Cholesteatoma

Chronic infection of the middle ear and mastoid generally develops as a consequence of recurrent acute otitis media, although it may follow other diseases and trauma. Perforation of the tympanic membrane is usually present. This may be accompanied by mucosal changes such as polypoid degeneration and granulation tissue and osseous changes such as osteitis and sclerosis. The bacteriology of chronic otitis media differs from that of acute otitis media. Common organisms include *P aeruginosa, Proteus* species, *Staphylococcus aureus,* and mixed anaerobic infections. The clinical hallmark of chronic otitis media is purulent aural discharge. Drainage may be continuous or intermittent, with increased severity during upper respiratory tract infection or following water exposure. Pain is uncommon

except during acute exacerbations. Conductive hearing loss results from destruction of the tympanic membrane or ossicular chain, or both. The medical treatment of chronic otitis media includes regular removal of infected debris, use of earplugs to protect against water exposure, and topical antibiotic drops for exacerbations. The activity of ciprofloxacin against *Pseudomonas* may help dry a chronically discharging ear when given in a dosage of 500 mg orally twice a day for 1–6 weeks.

Definitive management is surgical in most cases. Tympanic membrane repair may be accomplished with temporalis muscle fascia. Successful reconstruction of the tympanic membrane may be achieved in about 90% of cases, often with elimination of infection and significant improvement in hearing. When the mastoid air cells are involved by irreversible infection, they should be exenterated at the same time through a mastoidectomy.

Cholesteatoma is a special variety of chronic otitis media (Plate 57). The most common cause is prolonged eustachian tube dysfunction, with resultant chronic negative middle ear pressure that draws inward the upper flaccid portion of the tympanic membrane. This creates a squamous epithelium-lined sac, which—when its neck becomes obstructed—may fill with desquamated keratin and become chronically infected. Cholesteatomas typically erode bone, with early penetration of the mastoid and destruction of the ossicular chain. Over time they may erode into the inner ear, involve the facial nerve, and on rare occasions spread intracranially. Otoscopic examination may reveal an epitympanic retraction pocket, marginal tympanic membrane perforation that exudes keratin debris, or granulation tissue. The treatment of cholesteatoma is surgical marsupialization of the sac or its complete removal. This may require the creation of a "mastoid bowl" in which the ear canal and mastoid are joined into a large common cavity that must be periodically cleaned.

Isaacson G. Diagnosis of pediatric cholesteatoma. Pediatrics. 2007 Sep;120(3):603–8. [PMID: 17766534]

Ramakrishnan Y et al. A review of retraction pockets: past, present and future management. J Laryngol Otol. 2007 Jun;121(6):521–5. [PMID: 17201990]

▶ Complications of Otitis Media

A. Mastoiditis

Acute suppurative mastoiditis usually evolves following several weeks of inadequately treated acute otitis media. It is characterized by postauricular pain and erythema accompanied by a spiking fever. Radiography reveals coalescence of the mastoid air cells due to destruction of their bony septa. Initial treatment consists of intravenous antibiotics and myringotomy for culture and drainage. Failure of medical therapy indicates the need for surgical drainage (mastoidectomy).

Stähelin-Massik J et al. Mastoiditis in children: a prospective, observational study comparing clinical presentation, microbiology, computed tomography, surgical findings and histology. Eur J Pediatr. 2008 May;167(5):541–8. [PMID: 17668240]

B. Petrous Apicitis

The medial portion of the petrous bone between the inner ear and clivus may become a site of persistent infection when the drainage of its pneumatic cell tracts becomes blocked. This may cause foul discharge, deep ear and retro-orbital pain, and sixth nerve palsy (Gradenigo syndrome); meningitis may be a complication. Treatment is with prolonged antibiotic therapy (based on culture results) and surgical drainage via petrous apicectomy.

Hafidh MA et al. Otogenic intracranial complications. A 7-year retrospective review. Am J Otolaryngol. 2006 Nov–Dec; 27(6):390–5. [PMID: 17084222]

C. Facial Paralysis

Facial palsy may be associated with either acute or chronic otitis media. In the acute setting, it results from inflammation of the seventh nerve in its middle ear segment, perhaps mediated through bacterially secreted neurotoxins. Treatment consists of myringotomy for drainage and culture, followed by intravenous antibiotics (based on culture results). The use of corticosteroids is controversial. The prognosis is excellent, with complete recovery in most cases.

Facial palsy associated with chronic otitis media usually evolves slowly due to chronic pressure on the seventh nerve in the middle ear or mastoid by cholesteatoma. Treatment requires surgical correction of the underlying disease. The prognosis is less favorable than for facial palsy associated with acute otitis media.

Kitsko DJ et al. Inner ear and facial nerve complications of acute otitis media, including vertigo. Curr Allergy Asthma Rep. 2007 Nov;7(6):444–50. [PMID: 17986375]

D. Sigmoid Sinus Thrombosis

Trapped infection within the mastoid air cells adjacent to the sigmoid sinus may cause septic thrombophlebitis. This is heralded by signs of systemic sepsis (spiking fevers, chills), at times accompanied by signs of increased intracranial pressure (headache, lethargy, nausea and vomiting, papilledema). Diagnosis can be made noninvasively by magnetic resonance venography. Primary treatment is with intravenous antibiotics (based on culture results). Surgical drainage with ligation of the internal jugular vein may be indicated when embolization is suspected.

Kuczkowski J et al. Lateral sinus thrombosis in chronic otitis media. Otol Neurotol. 2007 Oct;28(7):992–3. [PMID: 17909438]

E. Central Nervous System Infection

Otogenic meningitis is by far the most common intracranial complication of ear infection. In the setting of acute suppurative otitis media, it arises from hematogenous spread of bacteria, most commonly H influenzae and S pneumoniae. In chronic otitis media, it results either from passage of infections along preformed pathways such as the petrosquamous suture line or from direct extension of disease through the dural plates of the petrous pyramid.

Epidural abscesses arise from direct extension of disease in the setting of chronic infection. They are usually asymptomatic but may present with deep local pain, headache, and low-grade fever. They are often discovered as an incidental finding at surgery. Brain abscess may arise in the temporal lobe or cerebellum as a result of septic thrombophlebitis adjacent to an epidural abscess. The predominant causative organisms are S aureus, S pyogenes, and S pneumoniae. Rupture into the subarachnoid space results in meningitis and often death. (See Chapter 30.)

Hafidh MA et al. Otogenic intracranial complications. A 7-year retrospective review. Am J Otolaryngol. 2006 Nov–Dec; 27(6):390–5. [PMID: 17084222]

3. Otosclerosis

Otosclerosis is a progressive disease with a marked familial tendency that affects the bony otic capsule. Lesions involving the footplate of the stapes result in increased impedance to the passage of sound through the ossicular chain, producing conductive hearing loss. This may be treated either through the use of a hearing aid or surgical replacement of the stapes with a prosthesis (stapedectomy). When otosclerotic lesions impinge on the cochlea ('cochlear otosclerosis'), permanent sensory hearing loss occurs. Some evidence suggests that hearing loss associated with cochlear otosclerosis may be stabilized by treatment with oral sodium fluoride over prolonged periods of time (Florical—8.3 mg sodium fluoride and 364 mg calcium carbonate—two tablets orally each morning).

Siddiq MA. Otosclerosis: a review of aetiology, management and outcomes. Br J Hosp Med (Lond). 2006 Sep;67(9):470–6. [PMID: 17017609]

4. Trauma to the Middle Ear

Tympanic membrane perforation may result from impact injury or explosive acoustic trauma (Plate 58). Spontaneous healing occurs in most cases. Persistent perforation may result from secondary infection brought on by exposure to water. Patients should be advised to wear earplugs while swimming or bathing during the healing period. Hemorrhage behind an intact tympanic membrane (hemotympanum) may follow blunt trauma or extreme barotrauma. Spontaneous resolution over several weeks is the usual course. When a conductive hearing loss greater than 30 dB persists for more than 3 months following trauma, disruption of the ossicular chain should be suspected. Middle ear exploration with reconstruction of the ossicular chain, combined with repair of the tympanic membrane when required, will usually restore hearing.

Conoyer JM et al. Otologic surgery following ear trauma. Otolaryngol Head Neck Surg. 2007 Nov;137(5):757–61. [PMID: 17967641]

5. Middle Ear Neoplasia

Primary middle ear tumors are rare. Glomus tumors arise either in the middle ear (glomus tympanicum) or in the jugular bulb with upward erosion into the hypotympanum (glomus jugulare). They present clinically with pulsatile tinnitus and hearing loss. A vascular mass may be visible behind an intact tympanic membrane. Large glomus jugulare tumors are often associated with multiple cranial neuropathies, especially involving nerves VII, IX, X, XI, and XII. Treatment usually requires surgery, radiotherapy, or both. Pulsatile tinnitus thus warrants magnetic resonance angiography and venography to rule out a vascular mass.

Kaylie DM et al. Neurotologic surgery for glomus tumors. Otolaryngol Clin North Am. 2007 Jun;40(3):625–49. [PMID: 17544699]

EARACHE

Earache can be caused by a variety of otologic problems, but most commonly external otitis and acute otitis media. Differentiation of the two should be apparent by pneumatic otoscopy (see above relevant sections on otitis externa and otitis media). Pain out of proportion to the physical findings may be due to herpes zoster oticus, especially when vesicles appear in the ear canal or concha. Persistent pain and discharge from the ear suggest osteomyelitis of the skull base or cancer, and patients with these complaints should be referred for specialty evaluation.

Nonotologic causes of otalgia are numerous. The sensory innervation of the ear is derived from the trigeminal, facial, glossopharyngeal, vagal, and upper cervical nerves. Because of this rich innervation, referred otalgia is quite frequent. Temporomandibular joint dysfunction is a common cause of referred ear pain. Pain is exacerbated by chewing or psychogenic grinding of the teeth (bruxism) and may be associated with dental malocclusion. Management includes soft diet, local heat to the masticatory muscles, massage, nonsteroidal anti-inflammatory medications, and dental referral. Repeated episodes of severe lancinating otalgia may occur in glossopharyngeal neuralgia. Treatment with carbamazepine (100–300 mg orally every 8 hours) often confers substantial symptomatic relief. Severe glossopharyngeal neuralgia, which is refractory to medical management, may respond to microvascular decompression of the ninth cranial nerve. Infections and neoplasia that involve the oropharynx, hypopharynx, and larynx frequently cause otalgia. Persistent earache demands specialty referral to exclude cancer of the upper aerodigestive tract.

Charlett SD et al. Referred otalgia: a structured approach to diagnosis and treatment. Int J Clin Pract. 2007 Jun;61(6):1015–21. [PMID: 17504363]

DISEASES OF THE INNER EAR

1. Sensory Hearing Loss

Diseases of the cochlea result in sensory hearing loss, a condition that is usually irreversible. Most cochlear diseases result in bilateral symmetric hearing loss. The presence of unilateral or asymmetric sensorineural hearing loss suggests a lesion proximal to the cochlea. Lesions affecting the eighth cranial nerve and central auditory system are discussed in the section on neural hearing loss. The primary goals in the management of sensory hearing loss are prevention of further losses and functional improvement with amplification and auditory rehabilitation.

A. Presbyacusis

Presbyacusis, or age-related hearing loss, is the most frequent cause of sensory hearing loss and is progressive, predominantly high-frequency, and symmetrical. It is difficult to separate the various etiologic factors (eg, noise trauma, drug exposure) that may contribute to presbyacusis, but genetic predisposition and prior noise exposure appear to play an important role. Most patients notice a loss of speech discrimination that is especially pronounced in noisy environments. About 25% of people between the ages of 65 and 75 years and almost 50% of those over 75 experience hearing difficulties.

Van Eyken E et al. The complexity of age-related hearing impairment: contributing environmental and genetic factors. Audiol Neurootol. 2007;12(6):345–58. [PMID: 17664866]

B. Noise Trauma

Noise trauma is the second most common cause of sensory hearing loss. Sounds exceeding 85 dB are potentially injurious to the cochlea, especially with prolonged exposures. The loss typically begins in the high frequencies (especially 4000 Hz) and progresses to involve the speech frequencies with continuing exposure. Among the more common sources of injurious noise are industrial machinery, weapons, and excessively loud music. Personal music devices (eg, MP3 and CD players) used at excessive loudness levels may also be potentially injurious. In recent years, monitoring of noise levels in the workplace by regulatory agencies has led to preventive programs that have reduced the frequency of occupational losses. Individuals of all ages, especially those with existing hearing losses, should wear earplugs when exposed to moderately loud noises and specially designed earmuffs when exposed to explosive noises.

Daniel E. Noise and hearing loss: a review. J Sch Health. 2007 May;77(5):225–31. [PMID: 17430434]

C. Physical Trauma

Head trauma has effects on the inner ear similar to those of severe acoustic trauma. Some degree of sensory hearing loss may occur following simple concussion and is frequent after skull fracture. Deployment of air bags during an automobile accident has also been associated with hearing loss.

Ulug T et al. Contralateral labyrinthine concussion in temporal bone fractures. J Otolaryngol. 2006 Dec;35(6):380–3. [PMID: 17380831]

D. Ototoxicity

Ototoxic substances may affect both the auditory and vestibular systems. The most commonly used ototoxic medications are aminoglycosides; loop diuretics; and several antineoplastic agents, notably cisplatin. These medications may cause irreversible hearing loss even when administered in therapeutic doses. When using these medications, it is important to identify high-risk patients such as those with preexisting hearing losses or renal insufficiency. Patients simultaneously receiving multiple ototoxic agents are at particular risk owing to ototoxic synergy. Useful measures to reduce the risk of ototoxic injury include serial audiometry and monitoring of serum peak and trough levels and substitution of equivalent nonototoxic drugs whenever possible. Efforts are underway to develop strategies, known as ototoxic chemoprotection, using drugs that shield the inner ear from damage during ototoxic exposure.

It is possible for topical agents that enter the middle ear to be absorbed into the inner ear via the round window. When the tympanic membrane is perforated, use of potentially ototoxic ear drops (eg, neomycin, gentamicin) is best avoided.

Rizzi MD et al. Aminoglycoside ototoxicity. Curr Opin Otolaryngol Head Neck Surg. 2007 Oct;15(5):352–7. [PMID: 17823553]
Rybak LP. Mechanisms of cisplatin ototoxicity and progress in otoprotection. Curr Opin Otolaryngol Head Neck Surg. 2007 Oct;15(5):364–9. [PMID: 17823555]

E. Sudden Sensory Hearing Loss

Idiopathic sudden loss of hearing in one ear may occur at any age, but typically, it occurs in persons over age 20 years. The cause is unknown; however, one hypothesis is that it results from a viral infection or a sudden vascular occlusion of the internal auditory artery. Prognosis is mixed, with many patients suffering permanent deafness in the involved ear while others have complete recovery. Prompt treatment with corticosteroids has been shown to improve the odds of recovery. A common regimen is oral prednisone, 80 mg/d, followed by a tapering dose over a 10-day period. Intratympanic administration of corticosteroids alone or in association with oral corticosteroids is increasingly being used for this problem and has been associated with more favorable prognosis in some reports. Because treatment appears to be most effective as close to the onset of the loss as possible, and appears not to be effective after 6 weeks, a prompt audiogram should be obtained in all patients who present with sudden hearing loss without obvious middle ear pathology.

Haynes DS et al. Intratympanic dexamethasone for sudden sensorineural hearing loss after failure of systemic therapy. Laryngoscope. 2007 Jan;117(1):3–15. [PMID: 17202923]
Wei B et al. Steroids for idiopathic sudden sensorineural hearing loss. Cochrane Database Syst Rev. 2006;(1):CD003998. [PMID: 16437471]

F. Hereditary Hearing Loss

Sensory hearing loss with onset during adult life often runs in families. The mode of inheritance may be either autosomal dominant or recessive. The age at onset, the rate of progression of hearing loss, and the audiometric pattern (high-frequency, low-frequency, or flat) can often be predicted by studying family members. In recent years, great strides have been made in identifying the molecular genetic errors associated with hereditary hearing loss. The con-

nexin-26 mutation, the most common cause of genetic deafness, may be tested clinically. Hearing loss is also frequently found in hereditary mitochondrial disorders. Progress is being made toward the development of methods to restore lost hair cells in genetic and other forms of deafness via gene therapy or stem cell–mediated techniques.

Eisen MD et al. Hearing molecules: contributions from genetic deafness. Cell Mol Life Sci. 2007 Mar;64(5):566–80. [PMID: 17260086]
Kochhar A et al. Clinical aspects of hereditary hearing loss. Genet Med. 2007 Jul;9(7):393–408. [PMID: 17666886]
Richardson RT et al. Inner ear therapy for neural preservation. Audiol Neurootol. 2006;11(6):343–56. [PMID: 16988498]

G. Autoimmune Hearing Loss

Sensory hearing loss may be associated with a wide array of systemic autoimmune disorders such as systemic lupus erythematosus, Wegener granulomatosis, and Cogan syndrome (hearing loss, keratitis, aortitis). The loss is most often bilateral and progressive. The hearing level often fluctuates, with periods of deterioration alternating with partial or even complete remission. The tendency is for the gradual evolution of permanent hearing loss, which usually stabilizes with some remaining auditory function but occasionally proceeds to complete deafness. Vestibular dysfunction, particularly dysequilibrium and postural instability, may accompany the auditory symptoms. A syndrome resembling Ménière disease may also occur with intermittent attacks of severe vertigo.

In many cases, the autoimmune pattern of audiovestibular dysfunction presents in the absence of recognized systemic autoimmune disease. Use of laboratory tests to screen for autoimmune disease (eg, antinuclear antibody, rheumatoid factor, erythrocyte sedimentation rate) may be informative. Specific tests of immune reactivity against inner ear antigens (anticochlear antibodies, lymphocyte transformation tests) are available but are currently of interest for research purposes only, demonstrating limited clinical value to date. Responsiveness to oral corticosteroid treatment is helpful in making the diagnosis and constitutes first-line therapy. If stabilization of hearing becomes dependent on long-term corticosteroid use, steroid-sparing immunosuppressive regimens may become necessary.

Agrup C et al. Immune-mediated inner-ear disorders in neurotology. Curr Opin Neurol. 2006 Feb;19(1):26–32. [PMID: 16415674]
Bovo R et al. Immune-mediated inner ear disease. Acta Otolaryngol. 2006 Oct;126(10):1012–21. [PMID: 16923703]

2. Tinnitus

Tinnitus is the perception of abnormal ear or head noises. Persistent tinnitus often, though not always indicates the presence of sensory hearing loss. Intermittent periods of mild, high-pitched tinnitus lasting seconds to minutes are common in normal-hearing persons. When severe and persistent, tinnitus may interfere with sleep and the ability to concentrate, resulting in considerable psychological distress.

The most important treatment of tinnitus is avoidance of exposure to excessive noise, ototoxic agents, and other factors that may cause cochlear damage. Masking the tinnitus with music or through amplification of normal sounds with a hearing aid may also bring some relief. Among the numerous drugs that have been tried, oral antidepressants (eg, nortriptyline at an initial dosage of 50 mg orally at bedtime) have proved to be the most effective. Habituation techniques, such as tinnitus retraining therapy, and masking techniques may prove beneficial in those with refractory symptoms. Transcranial magnetic stimulation of the central auditory system has recently been shown to improve symptoms in some patients.

Pulsatile tinnitus—often described by the patient as listening to one's own heartbeat—should be distinguished from tonal tinnitus. Although often ascribed to conductive hearing loss, this symptom may be far more serious and may indicate a vascular abnormality such as glomus tumor, venous sinus stenosis, carotid vaso-occlusive disease, arteriovenous malformation, or aneurysm. Magnetic resonance angiography and venography should be considered to establish the diagnosis.

In contrast, a staccato "clicking" tinnitus may result from middle ear muscle spasm, sometimes associated with palatal myoclonus. The patient typically perceives a rapid series of popping noises, lasting seconds to a few minutes, accompanied by a fluttering feeling in the ear.

Jastreboff MM. Sound therapies for tinnitus management. Prog Brain Res. 2007;166:435–40. [PMID: 17956808]
Kleinjung T et al. Transcranial magnetic stimulation (TMS) for treatment of chronic tinnitus: clinical effects. Prog Brain Res. 2007;166:359–67. [PMID: 17956800]
Liyanage SH et al. Pulsatile tinnitus. J Laryngol Otol. 2006 Feb;120(2):93–7. [PMID: 16359136]

3. Hyperacusis

Excessive sensitivity to sound may occur in normal-hearing individuals either for psychological reasons, in association with ear disease, or following noise trauma. Patients with cochlear dysfunction commonly experience "recruitment," an abnormal sensitivity to loud sounds despite a reduced sensitivity to softer ones. Fitting hearing aids and other amplification devices to patients with recruitment requires use of compression circuitry to avoid uncomfortable overamplification. For normal-hearing individuals with hyperacusis, use of an earplug in noisy environments may be beneficial, though attempts should be made at habituation.

Hiller W et al. Factors influencing tinnitus loudness and annoyance. Arch Otolaryngol Head Neck Surg. 2006 Dec;132(12): 1323–30. [PMID: 17178943]

4. Vertigo

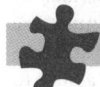
ESSENTIALS OF DIAGNOSIS

▶ Either a sensation of motion when there is no motion or an exaggerated sense of motion in response to a given bodily movement.

▶ Duration of discrete vertiginous events is key to diagnosis.

▶ Must differentiate peripheral from central etiologies of vestibular dysfunction.

▶ Peripheral: Onset is sudden; often associated with tinnitus and hearing loss; horizontal nystagmus may be present.

▶ Central: Onset is gradual; no associated auditory symptoms.

▶ Evaluation includes audiogram and electronystagmography (ENG) or videonystagmography (VNG).

▶ Clinical Findings

A. Symptoms and Signs

Vertigo is the cardinal symptom of vestibular disease. It is either a sensation of motion when there is no motion or an exaggerated sense of motion in response to a given bodily movement. While vertigo is typically experienced as a distinct "spinning" sensation, it may also present as a sense of tumbling or of falling forward or backward. It should be distinguished from imbalance, light-headedness, and syncope, all of which are nonvestibular in origin. The vertigo that results from peripheral vestibulopathy is usually of sudden onset, may be so severe that the patient is unable to walk or stand, and is frequently accompanied by nausea and vomiting. Tinnitus and hearing loss may be associated and provide strong support for a peripheral (ie, otologic) origin.

A thorough history will often narrow down, if not confirm the diagnosis. Critical elements of the history include the duration of the discrete vertiginous episodes (seconds, minutes to hours, or days), and associated symptoms. Triggers should also be sought, including diet (eg, high salt in the case of Ménière disease), stress, fatigue, and bright lights (eg, migraine-associated dizziness).

The physical examination of the patient with vertigo includes evaluation of the ears, eye motion in response to head turning and observation for nystagmus, cranial nerve examination, and Romberg testing. In acute peripheral lesions, nystagmus is usually horizontal with a rotatory component; the fast phase usually beats away from the diseased side. Visual fixation tends to inhibit nystagmus except in very acute peripheral lesions or with central nervous system disease. Dix-Hallpike testing (quickly lowering the patient to the supine position with the head extending over the edge and placed 30 degrees lower than the body, turned either to the left or right) will elicit a delayed onset (~10 sec) fatiguable nystagmus in cases of benign positional vertigo. Nonfatigable nystagmus in this position indicates a central etiology for the dizziness.

Since visual fixation often suppresses observed nystagmus, many of these maneuvers are performed with Frenzel goggles, which prevent visual fixation, and often bring out subtle forms of nystagmus. The Fukuda test, in which the patient consistently rotates when walking in place with eyes closed, can also demonstrate vestibular asymmetry.

In contrast to peripheral forms of vertigo, dizziness arising from central etiologies tends to develop gradually and then become progressively more severe and debilitating. Nystagmus is not always present but can occur in any direction and may be dissociated in the two eyes. The associated nystagmus is often nonfatigable, vertical rather than horizontal in orientation, without latency, and unsuppressed by visual fixation. ENG is useful in documenting these characteristics. The evaluation of central audiovestibular dysfunction requires imaging of the brain with MRI.

Episodic vertigo can occur in patients with diplopia from external ophthalmoplegia and is maximal when the patient looks in the direction where the separation of images is greatest. Cerebral lesions involving the temporal cortex may also produce vertigo, which is sometimes the initial symptom of a seizure. Finally, vertigo may be a feature of a number of systemic disorders and can occur as a side effect of certain anticonvulsant, antibiotic, hypnotic, analgesic, and tranquilizing drugs or of alcohol.

B. Laboratory Findings

Laboratory investigations such as audiologic evaluation, caloric stimulation, ENG, or VNG, and MRI are indicated in patients with persistent vertigo or when central nervous system disease is suspected. Vestibular-evoked myogenic potentials (VEMPs) are increasingly becoming part of the diagnostic evaluation. These studies will help distinguish between central and peripheral lesions and to identify causes requiring specific therapy. ENG consists of objective recording of the nystagmus induced by head and body movements, gaze, and caloric stimulation. It is helpful in quantifying the degree of vestibular hypofunction and may help with the differentiation between peripheral and central lesions. Computer-driven rotatory chairs and posturography platforms offer additional diagnostic modalities from specialized centers.

Honaker JA et al. Vestibular-evoked myogenic potentials. Curr Opin Otolaryngol Head Neck Surg. 2007 Oct;15(5):330–4. [PMID: 17823549]
Wuyts FL et al. Vestibular function testing. Curr Opin Neurol. 2007 Feb;20(1):19–24. [PMID: 17215684]

▶ Vertigo Syndromes Due to Peripheral Lesions

A. Endolymphatic Hydrops (Ménière Syndrome)

The cause of Ménière syndrome is unknown. Distention of the endolymphatic compartment of the inner ear is a pathologic finding and thought to be part of the pathogenesis of the disorder. Although a precise cause of hydrops cannot be established in most cases, two known causes are syphilis and head trauma. The classic syndrome consists of episodic vertigo, with discrete vertigo spells lasting 20 minutes to several hours in association with fluctuating low-frequency sensorineural hearing loss, tinnitus (usually low-tone and "blowing" in quality), and a sensation of aural pressure. These symptoms in the absence of hearing fluctuations suggests migraine-associated dizziness. Symptoms wax and wane as the endolymphatic pressure rises and falls.

Caloric testing commonly reveals loss or impairment of thermally induced nystagmus on the involved side. Primary treatment involves a low salt diet and diuretics (eg, acetazolamide). In refractory cases, patients may undergo intratympanic corticosteroid injections, endolymphatic sac decompression or vestibular ablation either through transtympanic gentamicin, vestibular nerve section, or surgical labyrinthectomy.

Ghossaini SN et al. An update on the surgical treatment of Ménière's diseases. J Am Acad Audiol. 2006 Jan;17(1):38–44. [PMID: 16640059]
Wittner S. Diagnosis and treatment Meniere's disease. JAAPA. 2006 May;19(5):34–9. [PMID: 16722043]

B. Labyrinthitis

Patients with labyrinthitis suffer from acute onset of continuous, usually severe vertigo lasting several days to a week, accompanied by hearing loss and tinnitus. During a recovery period that lasts for several weeks, the vertigo gradually improves. Hearing may return to normal or remain permanently impaired in the involved ear. The cause of labyrinthitis is unknown. Treatment consists of antibiotics if the patient is febrile or has symptoms of a bacterial infection, and supportive care. Vestibular suppressants are useful during the acute phase of the attack (eg, diazepam or meclizine) but should be discontinued as soon as feasible to avoid long-term dysequilibrium from inadequate compensation.

Pullen RL Jr. Spin control: caring for a patient with inner ear disease. Nursing. 2006 May;36(5):48–51. [PMID: 16670600]

C. Benign Paroxysmal Positioning Vertigo

Patients suffering from recurrent spells of vertigo, lasting under several minutes per spell, associated with changes in head position (often provoked by rolling over in bed), usually have benign paroxysmal positioning vertigo. The term "positioning vertigo" is more accurate than "positional vertigo" because it is provoked by changes in head position rather than by the maintenance of a particular posture.

The typical symptoms of positioning vertigo occur in clusters that persist for several days. There is a brief (10–15 sec) latency period following a head movement before symptoms develop, and the acute vertigo subsides within 10–60 seconds, though the patient may remain imbalanced for several hours. Constant repetition of the positional change leads to habituation. Since some central nervous system disorders can mimic BPPV (eg, vertebrobasilar insufficiency), recurrent cases warrant MRI scanning of the head. In central lesions, there is no latent period, fatigability, or habituation of the symptoms and signs. Treatment of BPPV involves physical therapy protocols (eg, the Epley maneuver or Brandt-Daroff exercises), based on the theory that peripheral positioning vertigo results from free-floating otoconia within a semicircular canal.

Kovar M et al. Diagnosing and treating benign paroxysmal positional vertigo. J Gerontol Nurs. 2006 Dec;32(12):22–9. [PMID: 17190403]

D. Vestibular Neuronitis

In vestibular neuronitis, a paroxysmal, usually single attack of vertigo occurs without accompanying impairment of auditory function and will persist for several days to a week before gradually clearing. During the acute phase, examination reveals nystagmus and absent responses to caloric stimulation on one or both sides. The cause of the disorder is unclear though presumed to be viral. Treatment consists of supportive care, including diazepam or meclizine during the acute phases of the vertigo only, followed by vestibular therapy if the patient does not completely compensate.

Huppert D et al. Low recurrence rate of vestibular neuritis: a long-term follow-up. Neurology. 2006 Nov 28;67(10):1870–1. [PMID: 17130428]

E. Traumatic Vertigo

The most common cause of vertigo following head injury is labyrinthine concussion. Symptoms generally diminish within several days but may linger for a month or more. Basilar skull fractures that traverse the inner ear usually result in severe vertigo lasting several days to a week and deafness in the involved ear. Chronic posttraumatic vertigo may result from cupulolithiasis. This occurs when traumatically detached statoconia (otoconia) settle on the ampulla of the posterior semicircular canal and cause an excessive degree of cupular deflection in response to head motion. Clinically, this presents as episodic positioning vertigo. Treatment consists of supportive care and vestibular suppressant medication (diazepam or meclizine) during the acute phase of the attack, and vestibular therapy.

Hoffer ME et al. Posttraumatic balance disorders. Int Tinnitus J. 2007;13(1):69–72. [PMID: 17691667]

F. Perilymphatic Fistula

Leakage of perilymphatic fluid from the inner ear into the tympanic cavity via the round or oval window is often discussed as a cause of vertigo and sensory hearing loss but is actually very rare. Most cases result from either physical injury (eg, blunt head trauma, hand slap to ear); extreme barotrauma during airflight, scuba diving, etc; or vigorous Valsalva maneuvers (eg, during weight lifting). Treatment may require middle ear exploration and window sealing with a tissue graft; however, this is seldom indicated without a clear-cut history of a precipitating traumatic event.

Alharethy SE. Oval window perilymph fistula caused by accidental stapedectomy during ear toilet. Saudi Med J. 2008 Jun;29(6):910–2. [PMID: 18521478]

G. Cervical Vertigo

Position receptors located in the facets of the cervical spine are important physiologically in the coordination of head and eye movements. Cervical proprioceptive dysfunction is a common cause of vertigo triggered by neck movements. This disturbance often commences after neck injury, particularly hyperextension. An association also exists with degenerative cervical spine disease. Although symptoms vary, vertigo may be triggered by assuming a particular head position as opposed to moving to a new head position (the latter typical of labyrinthine dysfunction). Management consists of neck movement exercises to the extent permitted by orthopedic considerations.

Endo K et al. Cervical vertigo and dizziness after whiplash injury. Eur Spine J. 2006 Jun;15(6):886–90. [PMID: 16432749]

H. Migrainous Vertigo

Episodic vertigo is frequently associated with a migraine type of headache. Most commonly, the vertigo is temporally related to the headache and lasts up to several hours. Some patients experience a positioning vertigo pattern. Occasionally, vertigo occurs independently of the head pain. It may appear identical to Ménière disease but without associated hearing loss or tinnitus. The importance of recognizing this association is that antimigraine pharmacotherapy often relieves the vestibular symptoms; other treatments include dietary changes and migraine prophylaxis.

Eggers SD. Migraine-related vertigo: diagnosis and treatment. Curr Pain Headache Rep. 2007 Jun;11(3):217–26. [PMID: 17504649]
Vitkovic J et al. Neuro-otological findings in patients with migraine- and nonmigraine-related dizziness. Audiol Neurootol. 2007 Nov 29;13(2):113–122. [PMID: 18057875]

I. Superior Semicircular Canal Dehiscence

Deficiency in the bony covering of the superior semicircular canal may be associated with vertigo triggered by loud noise exposure and an apparent conductive hearing loss. Diagnosis is with coronal high-resolution CT scan and VEMPs. Surgically sealing the dehiscent canal can improve symptoms.

Zhou G et al. Clinical and diagnostic characterization of canal dehiscence syndrome: a great otologic mimicker. Otol Neurotol. 2007 Oct;28(7):920–6. [PMID: 17955609]

▶ Vertigo Syndromes Due to Central Lesions

Central nervous system causes of vertigo include brainstem vascular disease, arteriovenous malformations, tumor of the brainstem and cerebellum, multiple sclerosis, and vertebrobasilar migraine. Vertigo of central origin often becomes unremitting and disabling. The associated nystagmus is often nonfatigable, vertical rather than horizontal in orientation, without latency, and unsuppressed by visual fixation. ENG is useful in documenting these characteristics. There are commonly other signs of brainstem dysfunction (eg, cranial nerve palsies; motor, sensory, or cerebellar deficits in the limbs) or of increased intracranial pressure. Auditory function is generally spared. The underlying cause should be treated.

Dieterich M. Central vestibular disorders. J Neurol. 2007 May;254(5):559–68. [PMID: 17417688]
Seemungal BM. Neuro-otological emergencies. Curr Opin Neurol. 2007 Feb;20(1):32–9. [PMID: 17215686]

Table 8-1. Common vestibular disorders: Differential diagnosis based on classic presentations.

Duration of Typical Vertiginous Episodes	Auditory Symptoms Present	Auditory Symptoms Absent
Seconds	Perilymphatic fistula	Positioning vertigo (cupulolithiasis), vertebrobasilar insufficiency, cervical vertigo
Hours	Endolymphatic hydrops (Ménière syndrome, syphilis)	Recurrent vestibulopathy, vestibular migraine
Days	Labyrinthitis, labyrinthine concussion	Vestibular neuronitis
Months	Acoustic neuroma, ototoxicity	Multiple sclerosis, cerebellar degeneration

DISEASES OF THE CENTRAL AUDITORY & VESTIBULAR SYSTEMS (Table 8-1)

Lesions of the eighth cranial nerve and central audiovestibular pathways produce neural hearing loss and vertigo. One characteristic of neural hearing loss is deterioration of speech discrimination out of proportion to the decrease in pure tone thresholds. Another is auditory adaptation, wherein a steady tone appears to the listener to decay and eventually disappear. Auditory evoked responses are useful in distinguishing cochlear from neural losses and may give insight into the site of lesion within the central pathways.

The evaluation of central audiovestibular disorders usually requires imaging of the internal auditory canal, cerebellopontine angle, and brain with enhanced MRI.

1. Vestibular Schwannoma (Acoustic Neuroma)

Eighth cranial nerve schwannomas are among the most common intracranial tumors. Most are unilateral, but about 5% are associated with the hereditary syndrome, neurofibromatosis type 2, in which bilateral eighth nerve tumors may be accompanied by meningiomas and other intracranial and spinal tumors. These benign lesions arise within the internal auditory canal and gradually grow to involve the cerebellopontine angle, eventually compressing the pons and resulting in hydrocephalus. Their typical auditory symptoms are unilateral hearing loss with a deterioration of speech discrimination exceeding that predicted by the degree of pure tone loss. Nonclassic presentations, such as sudden unilateral hearing loss, are fairly common. Any individual with a unilateral or asymmetric sensorineural hearing loss should be evaluated for an intracranial mass lesion. Vestibular dysfunction more often takes the form of continuous dysequilibrium than episodic vertigo. Other lesions of the cerebellopontine angle such as meningioma and epidermoids may have similar audiovestibular manifestations. Diagnosis is made by enhanced MRI. Treatment consists of observation, microsurgical excision, or stereotactic radiotherapy, depending on such factors as patient age, underlying health, and size of the tumor at presentation.

Abram S et al. Stereotactic radiation techniques in the treatment of acoustic schwannomas. Otolaryngol Clin North Am. 2007 Jun;40(3):571–88. [PMID: 17544696]

Bennett M et al. Surgical approaches and complications in the removal of vestibular schwannomas. Otolaryngol Clin North Am. 2007 Jun;40(3):589–609. [PMID: 1754469]

Myrseth E et al. Treatment of vestibular schwannomas. Why, when and how? Acta Neurochir (Wien). 2007;149(7):647–60. [PMID: 17558460]

Roehm PC et al. Management of acoustic neuromas in patients 65 years or older. Otol Neurotol. 2007 Aug;28(5):708–14. [PMID: 17667776]

2. Vascular Compromise

Vertebrobasilar insufficiency is a common cause of vertigo in the elderly. It is often triggered by changes in posture or extension of the neck. Reduced flow in the vertebrobasilar system may be demonstrated noninvasively through magnetic resonance angiography. Empiric treatment is with vasodilators and aspirin.

Vascular loops that impinge upon the brainstem root entry zone of cranial nerves have been shown to cause dysfunction. Widely recognized examples are hemifacial spasm and tic douloureux. It has been suggested that hearing loss, tinnitus, and disabling positioning vertigo may result from a vascular loop abutting the eighth cranial nerve, although this is controversial.

de Castro Junior NP et al. Sudden sensorineural hearing loss and vertigo associated with arterial occlusive disease: three case reports and literature review. Sao Paulo Med J. 2007 May 3;125(3):191–5. [PMID: 17923946]

Kim HA et al. Acute peripheral vestibular syndrome of a vascular cause. J Neurol Sci. 2007 Mar 15;254(1-2):99–101. [PMID: 17257625]

3. Multiple Sclerosis

Patients with multiple sclerosis may suffer from episodic vertigo and chronic imbalance. Hearing loss in this disease is most commonly unilateral and of rapid onset. Spontaneous recovery may occur.

Zeigelboim BS et al. High-frequency hearing threshold in adult women with multiple sclerosis. Int Tinnitus J. 2007;13(1):11–4. [PMID: 17691657]

OTOLOGIC MANIFESTATIONS OF AIDS

The otologic manifestations of AIDS are protean. The pinna and external auditory canal may be affected by Kaposi sarcoma as well as persistent and potentially invasive fungal infections, particularly due to *Aspergillus fumigatus*. The most common middle ear manifestation of AIDS is serous otitis media due to eustachian tube dysfunction arising from adenoidal hypertrophy (HIV lymphadenopathy), recurrent mucosal viral infections, or an obstructing nasopharyngeal tumor (eg, lymphoma). For middle ear effusions, ventilating tubes are seldom helpful and may trigger profuse watery otorrhea. Acute otitis media is usually caused by the typical bacterial organisms that occur in nonimmunocompromised patients, although *Pneumocystis jiroveci* (formerly *Pneumocystis carinii*) otitis has been reported. Sensorineural hearing loss is common and in some cases appears to result from viral central nervous system infection. In cases of progressive hearing loss, it is important to evaluate for cryptococcal meningitis and syphilis. Acute facial paralysis due to herpes zoster infection (Ramsay Hunt syndrome) is quite common and follows a clinical course similar to that in nonimmunocompromised patients. Treatment is primarily with high-dose acyclovir (see Chapters 6 and 32). Corticosteroids may also be effective.

Prasad HK et al. HIV manifestations in otolaryngology. Am J Otolaryngol. 2006 May–Jun;27(3):179–85. [PMID: 16647982]

DISEASES OF THE NOSE & PARANASAL SINUSES

INFECTIONS OF THE NOSE & PARANASAL SINUSES

1. Viral Rhinitis (Common Cold)

> ESSENTIALS OF DIAGNOSIS

▶ Clear rhinorrhea, hyposmia and nasal congestion.

▶ Associated symptoms, including malaise, headache, and cough.

▶ Erythematous, engorged nasal mucosa on exam.

▶ Absence of intranasal purulence.

▶ Clinical Findings

The nonspecific symptoms of the ubiquitous common cold are present in the early phases of many diseases that affect the upper aerodigestive tract. Because there are numerous serologic types of rhinoviruses, adenoviruses, and other viruses, patients remain susceptible throughout life. These infections, while generally quite benign and self-limited, have been implicated in the development of more serious conditions, such as acute bacterial sinusitis, acute otitis media, asthma and cystic fibrosis exacerbation and bronchitis. Nasal congestion, decreased sense of smell, watery rhinorrhea, and sneezing accompanied by general malaise, throat discomfort and, occasionally, headache are typical in viral infections. Nasal examination usually shows erythematous, edematous mucosa and a watery discharge. The presence of purulent nasal discharge suggests bacterial rhinosinusitis.

▶ Treatment

Despite ongoing research into viral chemotherapy, at this time, there are no effective antiviral therapies for either the prevention or treatment of viral rhinitis. There is a common misperception among patients that antibiotics are helpful. Supportive measures such as decongestants (pseudoephedrine, 30–60 mg every 4–6 hours or 120 mg twice daily) may provide some relief of rhinorrhea and nasal obstruction. Nasal sprays such as oxymetazoline or phenylephrine are rapidly effective. They should not be used for more than a few days at a time, since prolonged use leads to an almost addictive need to prevent rebound congestion from withdrawal of the drug called **rhinitis medicamentosa**. Treatment requires mandatory cessation of the sprays, and this is often extremely frustrating for patients. Topical intranasal corticosteroids (eg, flunisolide, 2 sprays in each nostril twice daily), intranasal anticholinergic (ipratropium 0.06% nasal spray, 2–3 sprays every 8 hours as needed) or a short tapering course of oral prednisone may help during the process of withdrawal.

▶ Complications

Other than eustachian tube dysfunction or transient middle ear effusion, complications of viral rhinitis are unusual. Secondary bacterial rhinosinusitis may occur and is suggested by persistence of symptoms beyond a week accompanied both by purulent green or yellow nasal secretions and unilateral facial or tooth pain. (See Acute Bacterial Rhinosinusitis below.)

Doyle WJ et al. Use of diagnostic algorithms and new technologies to study the incidence and prevalence of viral upper respiratory tract infections and their complications in high risk populations. Curr Opin All Clin Immunol. 2007 Feb;7(1):11–16. [PMID: 17218805]

Patick AK. Rhinovirus chemotherapy. Antiviral Res. 2006 Sep;71(2–3):391–6. [PMID: 16675037]

2. Acute Bacterial Rhinosinusitis (Sinusitis)

> ESSENTIALS OF DIAGNOSIS

▶ Purulent yellow-green nasal discharge or expectoration.

▶ Facial pain or pressure over the affected sinus or sinuses.

▶ Nasal obstruction.

▶ Acute onset of symptoms (between 1 and 4 week duration).

▶ Associated symptoms, including cough, malaise, fever, and headache.

▶ General Considerations

Acute sinus infections are uncommon compared with viral rhinitis, but they still affect nearly 20 million Americans annually, accounting for over 2 billion dollars in health care expenditures for sinusitis annually. When chronic sinus infection is included, the cost rises to at least 5.8 billion dollars annually. Such infections are often associated with inflammation of the mucosal of the nasal cavity near the drainage pores of the sinuses. To acknowledge this inflammation as a major component of the disease and to differentiate it from such processes as allergic or acute viral rhinitis, otolaryngologists prefer the term "bacterial rhinosinusitis."

Acute bacterial rhinosinusitis usually is a result of impaired mucociliary clearance and obstruction of the osteomeatal complex, or sinus "pore." Edematous mucosa causes obstruction of the complex, resulting in the accumulation of mucous secretion in the sinus cavity that becomes secondarily infected by bacteria. The largest of these osteomeatal complexes is deep to the middle turbinate in the middle meatus. This complex is actually a confluence of complexes draining the maxillary, ethmoid, and frontal sinuses. The sphenoid drains from a separate complex between the septum and superior turbinate.

The typical pathogens of bacterial sinusitis are the same as those that cause acute otitis media: *S pneumoniae*, other streptococci, *H influenzae* and, less commonly, *S aureus* and *Moraxella catarrhalis*. Pathogens vary regionally in both prevalence and drug resistance. It should be kept in mind that about 25% of healthy asymptomatic individuals may, if sinus aspirates are cultured, harbor such bacteria as well. Understanding of the anatomy, pathogenesis and microbiology of acute bacterial rhinosinusitis can help the clinician afford the most expeditious and cost-effective diagnosis and treatment while avoiding serious complications.

► Clinical Findings

A. Symptoms and Signs

The maxillary sinus, the largest of the paranasal sinuses, is the most commonly affected sinus. Unilateral facial fullness, pressure and tenderness over the cheek are common symptoms, but may not be present in many cases. Pain may refer to the upper incisor and canine teeth via branches of the trigeminal nerve, which traverse the floor of the sinus. Purulent nasal drainage should be noted with nasal obstruction or facial pain (pressure), or both. Maxillary sinusitis may result from dental infection, and teeth that are tender should be carefully examined for signs of abscess. Removal of the diseased tooth or drainage of the periapical abscess typically resolves the sinus infection. Nonspecific symptoms include fever, malaise, halitosis, headache, hyposmia, and cough. Bacterial rhinosinusitis can be distinguished from viral rhinitis by persistence of symptoms more than 10 days after onset or worsening of symptoms within 10 days after initial improvement.

Acute ethmoiditis in adults is often accompanied by maxillary sinusitis and symptoms are similar to those described above. Localized ethmoid sinusitis may present with pain and pressure over the high lateral wall of the nose between the eyes that may radiate to the orbit.

Sphenoid sinusitis is usually seen in the setting of pansinusitis, or infection of all the paranasal sinuses on at least one side. The patient may complain of a headache "in the middle of the head" and often points to the vertex.

Acute frontal sinusitis usually causes pain and tenderness of the forehead. This is most easily elicited by palpation of the orbital roof just below the medial end of the eyebrow.

Hospital-associated sinusitis is a form of acute bacterial rhinosinusitis that may present without any symptoms in the head and neck. It is a common source of fever in critically ill patients and is often associated with prolonged presence of a nasogastric tube causing inflammation of the nasal mucosa and osteomeatal complex obstruction. Pansinusitis on the side of the tube is common on imaging studies.

B. Imaging

It is usually possible to make the diagnosis of acute bacterial rhinosinusitis on clinical grounds alone. Although more sensitive than clinical examination, routine radiographs are not cost-effective and are not recommended by the Agency for Health Care Policy and Research or American Association of Otolaryngology Guidelines in the routine diagnosis of acute bacterial rhinosinusitis. They may, however, be helpful when clinically based criteria are difficult to evaluate or when symptoms of more serious infection are noted.

When necessary, noncontrast, screening coronal CT scans are more cost-effective and provide more information than conventional sinus films. CT provides a rapid and effective means to assess all of the paranasal sinuses, identify areas of greater concern (such as bony dehiscence, periosteal elevation or maxillary tooth root exposure within the sinus), and speed appropriate therapy.

Occasionally, a CT scan may be indicated to exclude acute bacterial rhinosinusitis. While reasonably sensitive, CT scans are not specific. Swollen soft tissue and fluid may be difficult to distinguish when opacification of the sinus is present from other conditions, such as chronic rhinosinusitis, nasal polyposis, or mucus retention cysts. Sinus abnormalities can be seen in most patients with an upper respiratory infection, while bacterial rhinosinusitis develops in only 2%.

If malignancy, intracranial extension or opportunistic infection is suspected, MRI with gadolinium should be ordered instead of, or in addition to, CT. MRI will distinguish tumor from fluid, inflammation, and inspissated mucus far better than CT, as well as better delineating tumor extent with respect to adjacent structures such as the orbit, skull base, and palate. Bone destruction can be demonstrated as well by MRI as by CT.

► Treatment

All patients with acute bacterial rhinosinusitis should have careful evaluation of pain. Nonsteroidal anti-inflammatories are generally recommended. Sinus symptoms may be improved with oral or nasal decongestants (or both)—eg, oral pseudoephedrine, 30–120 mg per dose, up to 240 mg/d; nasal oxymetazoline, 0.05%, or xylometazoline, 0.05–0.1%, one or two sprays in each nostril every 6–8 hours for up to 3 days.

Two-thirds patients with acute bacterial rhinosinusitis will improve symptomatically within 2 weeks without the use of antibiotics. However, antibiotics may be considered

Table 8–2. Oral antibiotic regimens for acute sinusitis.

Drug	Dose	Duration	Notes
First-line therapy			
Amoxicillin	1000 mg three times daily	7–10 days	
Trimethoprim-sulfamethoxazole	160/800 twice daily	7–10 days	Suitable in penicillin allergy
Doxycycline	200 mg once daily × 1 day, 100 mg twice daily thereafter	7–10 days	Suitable in penicillin allergy
First-line therapy after recent antibiotic use[1]			
Levofloxacin	500 mg once daily	10 days	
Amoxicillin-clavulanate	875 mg-125 mg twice daily	10 days	
Second-line therapy			
Amoxicillin-clavulanate	1000 mg-62.5 mg ER 2 tablets twice daily	10 days	If no improvement after 3 days on first-line therapy
Moxifloxacin	400 mg once daily	10 days	If no improvement after 3 days on first-line therapy
Telithromycin[2]	800 mg once daily	10 days	If no improvement after 10–14 days of first-line therapy

[1]Within last 4–6 weeks.
[2]Contraindicated in myasthenia gravis; recent reports of hepatic failure.
Adapted, with permission, from Marple BF et al. Acute bacterial rhinosinusitis: a review of U.S. treatment guidelines. Otolaryngol Head Neck Surg. 2006 Sep;135(3):341–8.

when symptoms last more than 10–14 days or when symptoms (including fever; facial pain; and periorbital, facial, or forehead swelling) are severe. Administration of antibiotics does, however, reduce by 50% the incidence of clinical failure and, coupled with clinical criteria-based diagnosis, represents the most cost-effective treatment strategy. Double-blinded studies exist to support numerous antibiotic choices. A summary of recent national guidelines for the treatment of acute sinusitis can be found in Table 8–2.

Selection of antibiotics is usually empiric and based on a number of factors including regional patterns of antibiotic resistance, antibiotic allergy, cost, and patient tolerance. Unless the patient is allergic to penicillin, amoxicillin should be used as the first-line agent. Treatment is usually for 10 days (or as stated above), although longer courses are sometimes required to prevent relapses. Macrolide therapy has been recommended as first-line therapy in patients with penicillin allergy.

Multidrug resistant *S pneumoniae* prevalence is growing in many urban areas of the United States as are β-lactamase/β-lactam inhibitor producing strains of *H influenza* and *M catarrhalis*. In such regions, guidelines call for empiric use of amoxicillin-clavulanate or second- or third-generation cephalosporins. Fluoroquinolones are reserved for treatment failures or for patients with a recent history of antibiotic therapy for another infection. Recurrent sinusitis or sinusitis that does not appear to respond clinically warrants CT imaging and evaluation by a specialist.

Hospital-associated infections in critically ill patients are treated differently from community-acquired infections. Broad-spectrum antibiotic coverage for bacteria including *P aeruginosa*, *S aureus* (including methicillin-resistant strains) and anaerobes must be considered. Removal of the nasogastric tube and improved nasal hygiene (nasal saline sprays, humidification of supplemental nasal oxygen, and nasal decongestants) are critical interventions and often curative in mild cases without aggressive antibiotic use. Endoscopic or transantral cultures may help direct medical therapy in complicated cases.

▶ **Complications**

Local complications of acute bacterial rhinosinusitis include orbital cellulitis and abscess, osteomyelitis, intracranial extension and cavernous sinus thrombosis.

Any change in the ocular examination in a patient with acute bacterial rhinosinusitis necessitates immediate CT imaging. Orbital complications typically occur by extension of ethmoid sinusitis through the lamina papyracea, a thin layer of bone that comprises the medial orbital wall. Extension in this area may cause orbital cellulitis leading to proptosis, gaze restriction, and orbital pain. Select cases are responsive to intravenous antibiotics with or without corticosteroids and should be managed in close conjunction with an ophthalmologist or otolaryngologist, or both. Extension through the lamina papyracea can also lead to subperiosteal abscess formation (orbital abscess). Such abscesses cause marked proptosis, ophthalmoplegia and pain with medial gaze. While some of these abscesses will respond to antibiotics, such findings should prompt an immediate referral to a specialist for consideration of decompression and evacuation. Failure to intervene quickly may lead to permanent visual impairment and "frozen globe."

Osteomyelitis requires prolonged antibiotics as well as removal of necrotic bone. The frontal sinus is most commonly affected, with bone involvement suggested by a tender puffy swelling of the forehead (Pott puffy tumor).

Following treatment, secondary cosmetic reconstructive procedures may be necessary.

Intracranial complications of sinusitis can occur either through hematogenous spread, as in cavernous sinus thrombosis and meningitis, or by direct extension, as in epidural and intraparenchymal brain abscesses. Fortunately, they are rare today. Cavernous sinus thrombosis is heralded by ophthalmoplegia, chemosis, and visual loss. The diagnosis is most commonly confirmed by MRI and, when identified early, it typically responds to intravenous antibiotics. Frontal epidural and intracranial abscesses are often clinically silent, but may present with altered metal status, persistent fever, or severe headache.

▶ When to Refer

Failure of acute bacterial rhinosinusitis to resolve after an adequate course of oral antibiotics may necessitate referral to an otolaryngologist for evaluation. Endoscopic cultures may direct further treatment choices. Nasal endoscopy and CT scan are indicated when symptoms persist longer than 4–12 weeks.

▶ When to Admit

- Facial swelling and erythema indicative of facial cellulitis.
- Proptosis.
- Vision change or gaze abnormality indicative of orbital cellulitis.
- Abscess or cavernous sinus involvement.
- Mental status changes suggestive of intracranial extension.
- Immunocompromised status.

Mafee MF et al. Imaging of rhinosinusitis and its complications: plain film, CT and MRI. Clin Rev Allergy Immunol. 2006 Jun; 30(3):165–86. [PMID: 16949962]

Pearlman AN et al. Review of current guidelines related to the diagnosis and treatment of rhinosinusitis. Curr Opin Otolaryngol Head Neck Surg. 2008 Jun;16(3):226–30. [PMID: 18475076]

Rosenfeld RM. Clinical practice guideline on adult sinusitis. Otolaryngol Head Neck Surg. 2007 Sep;137(3):365–77. [PMID: 17765760]

Rosenfeld RM et al. Systematic review of antimicrobial therapy in patients with acute rhinosinusitis. Otolaryngol Head Neck Surg. 2007 Sep;137(3 Suppl):S32–45. [PMID: 17761282]

3. Nasal Vestibulitis

Inflammation of the nasal vestibule may result from folliculitis of the hairs that line this orifice and is usually the result of nasal manipulation or hair trimming. Systemic antibiotics effective against S aureus (such as dicloxacillin, 250 mg orally four times daily for 7–10 days) are indicated. Topical mupirocin or bacitracin (applied two or three times daily) may be a helpful addition and may prevent future occurrences. If recurrent, the addition of rifampin (10 mg/kg orally twice daily for the last 4 days of treatment) may eliminate the S aureus carrier state. If a furuncle exists, it should be incised and drained, preferably intranasally. Adequate treatment of these infections is important to prevent retrograde spread of infection through valveless veins into the cavernous sinus and intracranial structures.

4. Invasive Fungal Sinusitis

Invasive fungal sinusitis is rare and includes both rhinocerebral mucormycosis (*Mucor, Absidia,* and *Rhizopus sp.*) and other invasive fungal infections, such as *Aspergillus.* The fungus spreads rapidly through vascular channels and may be lethal if not detected early. Patients with mucormycosis almost invariably have a contributing factor that results in some degree of immunocompromise, such as diabetes mellitus, long-term corticosteroid therapy, or end-stage renal disease. Mucormycosis is more common, however, in patients who are profoundly immunocompromised for the treatment of hematologic malignancies. Occasional cases have been reported in patients with AIDS though *Aspergillus sp.* is more common in this setting. The initial symptoms may be similar to those of acute bacterial rhinosinusitis, although facial pain is often more severe. Nasal drainage is typically clear or straw-colored, rather than purulent, and visual symptoms may be noted at presentation in the absence of significant nasal findings. On examination, the pathognomic finding of mucormycosis is a black eschar on the middle turbinate. This finding is not universal and may be inapparent if the infection is deep or high within the nasal bones. Often the mucosa appears normal or simply pale and dry. Early diagnosis requires suspicion of the disease and nasal biopsy with silver stains, revealing broad nonseptate hyphae within tissues and necrosis with vascular occlusion. Because CT or MRI may initially show only soft tissue changes, biopsy and ultimate debridement should be based on the clinical setting rather than radiographic demonstration of bony destruction or intracranial changes.

Invasive fungal sinusitis represents a medical and surgical emergency. Once recognized, prompt wide surgical debridement and amphotericin B by intravenous infusion are indicated for patients with reversible immune deficiency. Lipid-based amphotericin B (Ambisome) may be used in patients who have renal insufficiency or in those in whom it develops secondary to nephrotoxic doses of non-lipid amphotericin. Other antifungals, including voriconazole and caspofungin, may be appropriate therapy depending on the speciation of the organism. There is evidence that suggests that iron chelator therapy may also be a useful adjunct. While necessary for any possibility of cure, surgical management often results in tremendous disfigurement and functional deficits. Even with early diagnosis and immediate appropriate intervention, the prognosis is guarded and often results in the loss of at least one eye. In persons with diabetes, the mortality rate is about 20%; in patients with renal failure, it is over 50%; in AIDS and hematologic malignancy, it is close to 100%.

Anselmo-Lima WT et al. Invasive fungal rhinosinusitis in immunocompromised patients. Rhinology. 2004 Sep;42(3):141–4. [PMID: 15521667]

Aribandi M et al. Imaging features of invasive and noninvasive fungal sinusitis: a review. Radiographics. 2007 Sep–Oct;27(5):1283–96. [PMID: 17848691]

Epstein VA et al. Invasive fungal sinusitis and complications of rhinosinusitis. Otolaryngol Clin North Am. 2008 Jun;41(3):497–524. [PMID: 18435995]

ALLERGIC RHINITIS

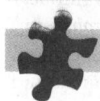

ESSENTIALS OF DIAGNOSIS

▶ Clear rhinorrhea, sneezing, tearing, eye irritation, and pruritus.

▶ Associated symptoms, including cough, bronchospasm, eczematous dermatitis.

▶ Environmental allergen exposure with presence of allergen specific IgE.

► General Considerations

Allergic rhinitis is very common in the United States. Population studies have reported the prevalence as between 14% and 40% among Americans, with most consensus panels agreeing on 20%. The total costs to society is estimated as up to 6 billion dollars annually. Seasonal allergic rhinitis is most commonly caused by pollens and spores. Flowering shrub and tree pollens are most common in the spring, flowering plants and grasses in the summer, and ragweed and molds in the fall. Dust, household mites, air pollution, and pet dander may produce year-round symptoms, termed "perennial rhinitis."

Allergic rhinitis is caused by exposure to an airborne allergen in a predisposed individual. Activation of both humoral (B-cell) and cytotoxic (T-cell) immune responses with subsequent allergen-specific IgE responses causes release of inflammatory mediators. The response is increased as antigen is passed to regional lymph nodes for greater T-cell activation. Interleukin and cytokine release causes specific activation of mast cells, eosinophils, plasma cells, basophils and other T-cells. Many of these circulating cells then migrate into the nasal and ocular epithelium where they contribute directly to symptoms through proinflammatory mediators, including histamine, prostaglandins, and kinins.

► Clinical Findings

The symptoms of "hay fever" are similar to those of viral rhinitis but are usually persistent and may show seasonal variation. Nasal symptoms are often accompanied by eye irritation, pruritus, conjunctival erythema, and excessive tearing. Many patients will note a strong family history of atopy or allergy.

The clinician should be careful to distinguish allergic rhinitis from nonallergic or vasomotor rhinitis. Vasomotor rhinitis is caused by increased sensitivity of the vidian nerve and is a common cause of clear rhinorrhea in the elderly. Often patients will report that they have troubling rhinorrhea in response to numerous nasal stimuli, including warm or cold air, odors or scents, light, or particulate matter.

On physical examination, the mucosa of the turbinates is usually pale or violaceous because of venous engorgement. This is in contrast to the erythema of viral rhinitis. Nasal polyps, which are yellowish boggy masses of hypertrophic mucosa, are associated with long-standing allergic rhinitis.

► Treatment

A. Antihistamines

Treatment of allergic and perennial rhinitis has improved in recent years. Antihistamines offer temporary, but immediate, control of many of the most troubling symptoms of allergic rhinitis. Numerous over-the-counter antihistamines, such as brompheniramine or chlorpheniramine (4 mg orally every 6–8 hours, or 8–12 mg orally every 8–12 hours as a sustained-release tablet) and clemastine (1.34–2.68 mg orally twice daily) offer the benefit of reduced cost though usually associated with higher rates of drowsiness compared with the newer prescription antihistamines. Exceptions may be loratadine (10 mg orally once daily) and the minimally sedating cetirizine (10 mg orally once daily), which are now available over the counter. Other prescription oral H_1-receptor antagonists include fexofenadine (60 mg orally twice daily or 120 mg once daily) and desloratadine (5 mg orally once daily). Fexofenadine appears to be nonsedating; desloratadine is minimally sedating. Also shown to be effective in randomized trials are ebastine (10–20 mg orally once daily) and misolastine (10 mg once daily). Two H_1-receptor antagonist antihistamine nasal sprays have also been shown to be effective in randomized trials: levocabastine (0.2 mg twice daily) and azelastine (two sprays per nostril, 1.1 mg/d). Topical nasal sprays are particularly useful in patients who complain of side effects, mostly xerostomia and sedation, of oral antihistamines. Many patients who find initial benefit from an antihistamine complain that allergy symptoms eventually return after several months of use. In such patients, typically with perennial allergy problems, antihistamine tolerance seems to develop and alternating effective antihistamines periodically can control symptoms over the long term.

B. Intranasal Corticosteroids

Intranasal corticosteroid sprays have revolutionized the treatment of allergic rhinitis. Evidence-based literature reviews show that these are more effective—and frequently less expensive—than nonsedating antihistamines. Patients should be reminded that there may be a delay in onset of relief of 2 or more weeks. Corticosteroid sprays may also shrink hypertrophic nasal mucosa and nasal polyps, thereby providing an improved nasal airway and osteomeatal complex drainage. Because of this effect, intranasal corticosteroids are critical in treating allergy in patients prone to recurrent acute bacterial rhinosinusitis or chronic rhinosinusitis. There are many available preparations, including beclomethasone (42 mcg/spray twice daily per nostril), flunisolide (25 mcg/spray twice daily per nostril), mometasone furoate (200 mcg once daily per nostril), budesonide (100 mcg twice daily per nostril) and fluticasone propionate (200 mcg once daily per nostril). The latter two synthetic corticosteroids appear to have higher topical potencies and lipid solubility and reduced systemic bioavailability, suggesting possible practical advantages; however, in practice, all intranasal corticosteroids are considered equally effective. Probably the most critical factor is compliance with regular use and proper introduction into the nasal cavity. In order to deliver medication to the region of the middle meatus, proper application involves holding the bottle straight up with the head tilted forward and pointing the bottle toward the ipsilateral ear when spraying. Side effects are limited and the most annoying is epistaxis. Some experts believe that this is related to incorrect delivery to the nasal septum, rather than correct delivery to the region of the middle meatus.

C. Adjunctive Treatment Measures

In addition to intranasal corticosteroid sprays and antihistamines, including H_1-receptor antagonists, the literature supports the use of antileukotriene medications such as montelukast (10 mg/d orally) alone or with cetirizine (10 mg/d orally) or loratadine (10 mg/d orally). There are proinflammatory effects of cysteinyl leukotrienes in upper airway disease, including allergic rhinitis, and hyperplastic polyposis, and sinusitis. Improved nasal rhinorrhea, sneezing, and congestion are seen with the use of leukotriene receptor antagonists, often in conjunction with antihistamines. Cromolyn sodium and sodium nedocromil are also useful adjunct agents for allergic rhinitis. They work by stabilizing mast cells and preventing proinflammatory mediator release. They are not absorbed by the gastrointestinal tract but do function topically and have very few side effects. The most useful form of cromolyn is probably the ophthalmologic preparation; the nasal preparation is not nearly as effective as inhaled corticosteroids. Intranasal cromolyn is cleared rapidly and must be administered four times daily for continued relief of symptoms.

Intranasal anticholinergic agents, such as ipratropium bromide 0.03% or 0.06% sprays (42–84 mcg per nostril three times daily), may be helpful adjuncts when rhinorrhea is a major symptom. Ipratropium nasal sprays are not as effective as intranasal corticosteroids for treating allergic rhinitis but are useful for treating vasomotor rhinitis.

Avoiding or reducing exposure to airborne allergens is the most effective means of alleviating symptoms of allergic rhinitis. Depending on the allergen, this can be extremely difficult, however. Maintaining an allergen-free environment by covering pillows and mattresses with plastic covers, substituting synthetic materials (foam mattress, acrylics) for animal products (wool, horsehair), and removing dust-collecting household fixtures (carpets, drapes, bedspreads, wicker) is worth the attempt to help more troubled patients. Air purifiers and dust filters (such as Bionaire models) may also aid in maintaining an allergen-free environment. Nasal saline irrigations are a very useful adjunct in the treatment of allergic rhinitis to mechanically flush the allergens from the nasal cavity. Though debated, there is no clear benefit to hypertonic saline over commercially available normal saline preparations (eg, Ayr or Ocean Spray). When symptoms are extremely bothersome, a search for offending allergens may prove helpful. This can either be done by skin testing or by serum RAST testing by an allergist.

In some cases, allergic rhinitis symptoms are inadequately relieved by medication and avoidance measures. Often, such patients have a strong family history of atopy and may also have lower respiratory manifestations such as allergic asthma. Referral to an allergist may be appropriate in such cases for consideration of immunotherapy. This treatment course is quite involved, with proper identification of offending allergens, progressively increasing doses of allergen(s) and eventual maintenance dose administration over a period of 3–5 years. Immunotherapy has been proven to reduce circulating IgE levels in patients with allergic rhinitis and reduce the need for allergy medications. While oral allergen exposure is actively being investigated, currently the primary mode of allergen exposure is by subcutaneous injection. Treatments are given at a suitable medical facility with monitoring following treatment because of the risk of anaphylaxis during dose escalation. Local reactions are common and usually self-limited.

Brunton SA et al. Treatment options for the management of perennial allergic rhinitis, with a focus on intranasal corticosteroids. South Med J. 2007 Jul;100(7):701–8. [PMID: 17639750]

Calderon MA et al. Allergen injection immunotherapy for seasonal allergic rhinitis. Cochrane Database Syst Rev. 2007 Jan 24;(1):CD001936. [PMID: 17253469]

Greiner AN. Allergic rhinitis: impact of the disease and considerations for management. Med Clin North Am. 2006 Jan;90(1):17–38. [PMID: 16310522]

Portnoy JM et al. Evidence-based strategies for treatment of allergic rhinitis. Curr Allergy Asthma Rep. 2004 Nov;4(6):439–46. [PMID: 15462709]

Prenner ME et al. Allergic rhinitis: treatment based on patient profiles. Am J Med. 2006 Mar;119(3):230–7. [PMID: 16490466]

Quillen DM et al. Diagnosing rhinitis: allergic vs. nonallergic. Am Fam Physician. 2006 May 1;73(9):1583–90. [PMID: 16719251]

Sheikh A et al. House dust mite avoidance measures for perennial allergic rhinitis. Cochrane Database Syst Rev. 2007 Jan 24;(1):CD001563. [PMID: 17253461]

OLFACTORY DYSFUNCTION

The physiology of olfaction is less well understood than that of the other special senses. The taste of foods is strongly affected by our sense of smell, and studies have shown a moderate correlation between taste discrimination ability and odor discrimination ability. In the past few years, discovery of the family of odorant receptor genes as well as inositol phosphate and cyclic nucleotide signaling pathways has led to a molecular basis of olfactory reception. Clinically, odorant molecules traverse the nasal vault to reach the cribriform area and become soluble in the mucus overlying the exposed dendrites of receptor cells. Anatomic blockage of the nasal cavity with subsequent airflow disruption is the most common cause of olfactory dysfunction (hyposmia or anosmia). Polyps, septal deformities, and nasal tumors may be the cause. Transient olfactory dysfunction often accompanies the common cold, nasal allergies, and perennial rhinitis through changes in the nasal and olfactory epithelium. About 20% of olfactory dysfunction is idiopathic, although it often follows a viral illness. Some have suggested administering large doses of vitamin A and zinc to such patients, although little evidence supports their use. Central nervous system neoplasms, especially those that involve the olfactory groove or temporal lobe, may affect olfaction and must be considered in patients with no other explanation for their hyposmia or other neurologic signs. Head trauma accounts for less than 5% of cases of hyposmia but is more commonly associated with anosmia. Absent, diminished, or distorted smell or taste has been reported in a wide variety of endocrine, nutritional, and nervous disorders. In particular, olfactory dysfunction in Parkinson disease and Alzheimer disease has been the subject of recent research. A great many medications have also been implicated in altering olfaction.

Evaluation of olfactory dysfunction should include a thorough history of systemic illnesses and medication use as well as a physical examination focusing on the nose and nervous system. Most clinical offices are not set up to test olfaction, but such tests may at times be worthwhile if only to assess whether a patient possesses any sense of smell at all. The University of Pennsylvania Smell Identification Test (UPSIT) is available commercially and is a simple, self-administered "scratch-and-sniff" test that is useful in differentiating hyposmia, anosmia, and malingering. Odor threshold can be tested at regional specialty centers using increasing concentrations of various odorants. In permanent hyposmia, counseling should be offered about seasoning foods with spices (eg, pepper) that stimulate the trigeminal as well as olfactory chemoreceptors, abuse of table salt as a seasoning, and safety issues such as the use of smoke alarms and electric rather than gas home appliances.

McNeill E et al. Diagnosis and management of olfactory disorders: survey of UK-based consultants and literature review. J Laryngol Otol. 2007 Aug;121(8):713–20. [PMID: 17359559]

Nordin S et al. Complaints of olfactory disorders: epidemiology, assessment and clinical implications. Curr Opin Allergy Clin Immunol. 2008 Feb;8(1):10–15. [PMID: 18188011]

EPISTAXIS

ESSENTIALS OF DIAGNOSIS

▶ Bleeding from the unilateral anterior nasal cavity most commonly.

▶ Most cases may be successfully treated by direct pressure on the bleeding site for 15 minutes. When this is inadequate, topical sympathomimetics and various nasal tamponade methods are usually effective.

▶ Posterior, bilateral, or large volume epistaxis should be triaged immediately to a specialist in a critical care setting.

General Considerations

Epistaxis is an extremely common problem in the primary care setting. Predisposing factors include nasal trauma (nose picking, foreign bodies, forceful nose blowing), rhinitis, drying of the nasal mucosa from low humidity or supplemental nasal oxygen, deviation of the nasal septum, hypertension, atherosclerotic disease, hereditary hemorrhagic telangiectasia (Osler-Weber-Rendu syndrome), inhaled nasal cocaine or other drug use, and alcohol use. Anticoagulation or antiplatelet medications may be associated with a higher incidence of epistaxis, more frequent recurrence of epistaxis, and greater difficulty controlling bleeding, but they do not cause epistaxis. Bleeding is most common in the anterior septum where a confluence of veins creates a superficial venous plexus (Kisselbach plexus).

Clinical Findings

It is important in all patients with epistaxis to consider underlying causes of the bleeding. Laboratory assessment of bleeding parameters may be indicated, especially in recurrent cases. Once the acute episode has passed, careful examination of the nose and paranasal sinuses to rule out neoplasia and hereditary hemorrhagic telangiectasia is wise.

Patients presenting with epistaxis often have higher blood pressures than control patients, but in many cases, blood pressure returns to normal following treatment of acute bleeding. Repeat evaluation for clinically significant hypertension and treatment should be performed following control of epistaxis and removal of any packing.

Treatment

Most cases of anterior epistaxis may be successfully treated by direct pressure on the site by compression of the nares continuously for 15 min. Venous pressure is reduced in the sitting position, and slight leaning forward lessens the swallowing of blood. Short-acting topical nasal decongestants (eg, phenylephrine, 0.125–1% solution, one or two sprays), which act as vasoconstrictors, may also be helpful. When the bleeding does not readily subside, the nose should be examined, using good illumination and suction, in an attempt to locate the bleeding site. Topical 4% cocaine applied either as a spray or on a cotton strip serves both as an anesthetic and as a vasoconstricting agent. If cocaine is unavailable, a topical decongestant (eg, oxymetazoline) and a topical anesthetic (eg, tetracaine or lidocaine) provide equivalent results. When visible, the bleeding site may be cauterized with silver nitrate, diathermy, or electrocautery. A supplemental patch of Surgicel or Gelfoam may be helpful with a moisture barrier, such as petroleum-based ointment, to prevent drying and crusting.

Occasionally, a site of bleeding may be inaccessible to direct control, or attempts at direct control may be unsuccessful. In such cases there are a number of alternatives. When the site of bleeding is anterior, a hemostatic sealant, pneumatic nasal tamponade, or anterior packing may suffice. There are a number of ways to do this, such as with several feet of lubricated iodoform packing systematically placed in the floor of the nose and then the vault of the nose, or with various manufactured products designed for nasal tamponade.

About 5% of nasal bleeding originates in the **posterior nasal cavity.** Such bleeds are more commonly associated with atherosclerotic disease and hypertension. If an anteriorly placed pneumatic nasal tamponade is unsuccessful, it may be necessary to consult an otolaryngologist for a pack to occlude the choana before placing a pack anteriorly. In emergency settings, new double balloon packs (Epistat) may facilitate rapid control of bleeding with little or no mucosal trauma. Because such packing is uncomfortable, bleeding may persist, and vasovagal syncope is quite possible, hospitalization for monitoring and stabilization is indicated. Opioid analgesics are needed to reduce the considerable discomfort and elevated blood pressure caused by a posterior pack.

Surgical management of epistaxis, through ligation of the nasal arterial supply (internal maxillary artery and ethmoid arteries) is an alternative to posterior nasal packing. Endovascular embolization of the internal maxillary artery or facial artery is also quite effective and can allow very specific control of hemorrhage. Such alternatives are necessary when packing fails to control life-threatening hemorrhage. On very rare occasions, ligation of the external carotid artery may be necessary.

After control of epistaxis, the patient is advised to avoid straining and vigorous exercise for several days. Nasal saline should be applied to the packing frequently to keep the packing moist. Avoidance of hot or spicy foods and tobacco is also advisable, since these may cause nasal vasodilation. Avoiding nasal trauma, including nose picking, is an obvious necessity. Lubrication with petroleum jelly or bacitracin ointment and increased home humidity may also be useful ancillary measures. Finally, antistaphylococcal antibiotics are indicated to reduce the risk of toxic shock syndrome developing while the packing remains in place (at least 5 days).

> ### When to Refer

Patients with recurrent epistaxis, large volume epistaxis, epistaxis that persists beyond 15 minutes of direct pressure, and episodic epistaxis with associated nasal obstruction should be referred to an otolaryngologist for endoscopic evaluation and possible imaging.

Douglas R et al. Update on epistaxis. Curr Opin Otolaryngol Head Neck Surg. 2007 Jun;15(3):180–3. [PMID: 17483687]
Randall DA. Epistaxis packing. Practical pointers for nosebleed control. Postgrad Med. 2006 Jun–Jul;119(1):77–82. [PMID: 16913650]

NASAL TRAUMA

The nasal pyramid is the most frequently fractured bone in the body. Fracture is suggested by crepitance or palpably mobile bony segments. Epistaxis and pain are common, as are soft tissue hematomas ("black eye"). It is important to make certain that there is no palpable step-off of the infraorbital rim, which would indicate the presence of a zygomatic complex fracture. Radiologic confirmation may at times be helpful but is not necessary in uncomplicated nasal fractures. It is also important to assess for possible concomitant additional facial, pulmonary, or intracranial injuries when the circumstances of injury are suggestive, as in the case of automobile and motorcycle accidents.

Treatment is aimed at maintaining long-term nasal airway patency and nasal aesthetics. Closed reduction, using topical 4% cocaine and locally injected 1% lidocaine,

should be attempted within 1 week of injury. In the presence of marked nasal swelling, it is best to wait several days for the edema to subside before undertaking reduction. Persistent functional or cosmetic defects may be repaired by delayed reconstructive nasal surgery.

Intranasal examination should be performed in all cases to rule out septal hematoma, which appears as a widening of the anterior septum, visible just posterior to the columella. The septal cartilage receives its only nutrition from its closely adherent mucoperichondrium. An untreated subperichondrial hematoma will result in loss of the nasal cartilage with resultant saddle nose deformity. Septal hematomas may become infected, with *S aureus* the predominant organism, and should be drained with an incision in the inferior mucoperichondrium on both sides. Antibiotics should be given and the drained fluid sent for culture.

Alvi A et al. Facial fractures and concomitant injuries in trauma patients. Laryngoscope. 2003 Jan;113(1):102–6. [PMID: 12514391]
Green KM. Reduction of nasal fractures under local anaesthetic. Rhinology. 2001 Mar;39(1):43–6. [PMID: 11340695]

TUMORS & GRANULOMATOUS DISEASE

1. Benign Nasal Tumors

A. Nasal Polyps

Nasal polyps are pale, edematous, mucosally covered masses commonly seen in patients with allergic rhinitis, but compelling evidence argues against a purely allergic pathogenesis. They may result in chronic nasal obstruction and a diminished sense of smell. In patients with nasal polyps and a history of asthma, aspirin should be avoided as it may precipitate a severe episode of bronchospasm, known as triad asthma (Samter triad). Such patients may have an immunologic salicylate sensitivity. The presence of polyps in children should suggest the possibility of cystic fibrosis.

Initial treatment with topical nasal corticosteroids (see Allergic Rhinitis section for specific drugs) for 1–3 months is usually successful for small polyps and may reduce the need for operation. A short course of oral corticosteroids (eg, prednisone, 6-day course using 21 5-mg tablets: 30 mg on day 1 and tapering by 5 mg each day) may also be of benefit. When polyps are massive or medical management is unsuccessful, polyps may be removed surgically. In healthy persons, this is a minor outpatient procedure. In recurrent cases or when surgery itself is associated with increased risk (such as in patients with asthma), a more complete procedure, such as ethmoidectomy, may be advisable. In recurrent polyposis, it may be necessary to remove polyps from the ethmoid, sphenoid, and maxillary sinuses to provide longer-lasting relief. Intranasal corticosteroid should be continued following polyp removal to prevent recurrence, and the clinician should consider allergen testing to determine the offending allergen and avoidance measures.

Alobid I et al. Nasal polyposis and its impact on quality of life: comparison between the effects of medical and surgical treatments. Allergy. 2005 Apr;60(4):452–8. [PMID: 15727575]

Bhattacharyya N. Progress in surgical management of chronic rhinosinusitis and nasal polyposis. Curr Allergy Asthma Rep. 2007 Jun;7(3):216–20. [PMID: 17448334]

Patiar S et al. Oral steroids for nasal polyps. Cochrane Database Syst Rev. 2007 Jan 24;(1):CD005232. [PMID: 17253548]

Williams AN et al. The clinical effectiveness of aspirin desensitization in chronic rhinosinusitis. Curr Allergy Asthma Rep. 2008 May;8(3):245–52. [PMID: 18589844]

B. Inverted Papilloma

Inverted papillomas are benign tumors caused by human papillomavirus (HPV) that usually arise on the lateral nasal wall. They present with unilateral nasal obstruction and occasionally hemorrhage. They are often easily seen on anterior rhinoscopy as cauliflower-like growths in or around the middle meatus. Because SCC is seen in about 10% of inverted or schneiderian papillomas, complete excision is strongly recommended. This usually requires a medial maxillectomy, but in selected cases an endoscopic approach may be possible. Because recurrence rates for inverted papilloma are reported to be as high as 20%, subsequent clinical and radiologic follow-up is imperative. All excised tissue (not just a portion) should be carefully reviewed by the pathologist to be sure no carcinoma is present.

Melroy CT et al. Benign sinonasal neoplasms: a focus on inverting papilloma. Otolaryngol Clin North Am. 2006 Jun;39(3):601–17. [PMID: 16757234]

C. Juvenile Angiofibroma

These highly vascular tumors arise in the nasopharynx, typically in adolescent males. Initially, they cause nasal obstruction and hemorrhage. Any adolescent male with recurrent epistaxis should be evaluated for an angiofibroma. The clinician should take great care when considering a biopsy because these masses can bleed profusely. Although benign, these tumors expand locally from the sphenopalatine foramen to the pterygopalatine fossa at the pterygoid canal and extend to the pterygoid base, the greater wing of the sphenoid, the nasal cavity, and the paranasal sinuses. They may involve the skull base, usually extradurally, and extend into the superior clivus. Treatment consists of preoperative embolization followed by surgical excision via an approach appropriate for the tumor extent. Small angiofibromas that do not involve the infratemporal fossa may be resected endoscopically. Extensive ones may require skull base approaches. Recurrences are not uncommon and should be resected if possible. Unresectable recurrences that do not appear to grow significantly may be followed radiologically with serial MR scans in expectation of possible eventual involution stabilization or involution of tumor. Low-dose (30 Gy) irradiation may be helpful in nonresectable, continually growing tumors.

Carrillo JF et al. Juvenile nasopharyngeal angiofibroma: clinical factors associated with recurrence, and proposal of a staging system. J Surg Oncol. 2008 Aug 1;98(2):75–80. [PMID: 18623038]

Glad H et al. Juvenile nasopharyngeal angiofibromas in Denmark 1981–2003: diagnosis, incidence, and treatment. Acta Otolaryngol. 2007 Mar;127(3):292–9. [PMID: 17364367]

2. Malignant Nasopharyngeal & Paranasal Sinus Tumors

Though rare, malignant tumors of the nose, nasopharynx, and paranasal sinuses are quite problematic as they tend to remain asymptomatic until late in their course. Although the prognosis is poor for advanced tumors, the results of treating resectable tumors of paranasal sinus origin have improved with the wider use of skull base resections and intensity-modulated radiation therapy. Cure rates are often 45–60%. Early symptoms are nonspecific, mimicking those of rhinitis or sinusitis. Unilateral nasal obstruction, otitis media, and discharge are common, with pain and recurrent hemorrhage often clues to the diagnosis of cancer. Any adult with persistent unilateral nasal symptoms or new otitis media should be thoroughly evaluated by a specialist. A high index of suspicion remains a key to the earlier diagnosis of these tumors. Patients often present with advanced symptoms such as proptosis, expansion of a cheek, or ill-fitting maxillary dentures. Malar hypesthesia, due to involvement of the infraorbital nerve, is common in maxillary sinus tumors. Biopsy is necessary for definitive diagnosis, and MRI is the best imaging study to delineate the extent of disease and plan appropriate surgery and radiation.

SCC is the most common cancer found. It is especially common in the nasopharynx, where it obstructs the eustachian tube and results in serous otitis media. Nasopharyngeal carcinoma (poorly differentiated SCC, nonkeratinizing SCC, or lymphoepithelioma) is usually associated with elevated IgA antibody to the viral capsid antigen of the Epstein-Barr virus (EBV). It is particularly common in patients of southern Chinese descent. Adenocarcinomas, mucosal melanomas, sarcomas, and non-Hodgkin lymphomas are less commonly encountered neoplasms of this area.

Treatment depends on the tumor type and the extent of disease. Nasopharyngeal carcinoma at this time is best treated by concomitant radiation and cisplatin followed by adjuvant chemotherapy with cisplatin and fluorouracil—this protocol significantly decreases local, nodal, and distant failures and increased progression-free and overall survival. Locally recurrent nasopharyngeal carcinoma may in selected cases be treated with repeat irradiation protocols or surgery with moderate success and a high degree of concern about local wound healing. Other SCCs are best treated—when resectable—with a combination of surgery and irradiation. Numerous protocols investigating the role of chemotherapy are under evaluation. Cranial base surgery appears to be an effective modality in improving the overall prognosis in paranasal sinus malignancies eroding the ethmoid roof.

Bourhis J et al; Meta-Analysis of Chemotherapy in Head, Neck Cancer Collaborative Group; Meta-Analysis of Radiotherapy in Carcinoma of Head, Neck Collaborative Group; Meta-Analysis of Chemotherapy in Nasopharynx Carcinoma Collaborative Group. Individual patients' data meta-analyses in head and neck cancer. Curr Opin Oncol. 2007 May;19(3):188–94. [PMID: 17414635]

Maghami E et al. Cancer of the nasal cavity and paranasal sinuses. Expert Rev Anticancer Ther. 2004 Jun;4(3):411–24. [PMID: 15161440]

Myers LL et al. Differential diagnosis and treatment options in paranasal sinus cancers. Surg Oncol Clin N Am. 2004 Jan;13(1):167–86. [PMID: 15062368]

3. Sinonasal Inflammatory Disease (Wegener Granulomatosis & Sarcoidosis)

The nose and paranasal sinuses are involved in over 90% of cases of Wegener granulomatosis. It is often not realized that involvement at these sites is more common than involvement of lungs or kidneys. Examination shows bloodstained crusts and friable mucosa. Biopsy, when positive, shows necrotizing granulomas and vasculitis. Other recognized sites of Wegener granulomatosis in the head and neck include the subglottis and the middle ear.

Sarcoidosis also commonly involves the paranasal sinuses and is clinically similar to other chronic sinonasal inflammatory processes. Sinonasal symptoms, including rhinorrhea, nasal obstruction, and hyposmia or anosmia may precede diagnosis of sarcoidosis in other organ systems. Clinically, the turbinates appear engorged with small white granulomas. Biopsy shows classic noncaseating granulomas. Notably, patients with sinonasal involvement generally have more trouble managing sarcoidosis in other organ systems.

Polymorphic reticulosis (midline malignant reticulosis, idiopathic midline destructive disease, lethal midline granuloma), as the multitude of apt descriptive terms suggest, is not well understood but appears to be a nasal T-cell or NK cell lymphoma. In contrast to Wegener granulomatosis, involvement is limited to the mid face, and there may be extensive bone destruction. Many destructive lesions of the mucosa and nasal structures labeled as polymorphic reticulosis are in fact non-Hodgkin lymphoma of either NK cell or T cell origin. Immunophenotyping, especially for CD56 expression, is essential in the histologic evaluation. Even when apparently localized, these lymphomas have a poor prognosis, with progression and death within a year the rule.

For treatment of Wegener granulomatosis, see Chapter 20.

Aubart FC et al. Sinonasal involvement in sarcoidosis: a case-control study of 20 patients. Medicine (Baltimore). 2006 Nov;85(6):365–71. [PMID: 17108780]

Erickson VR et al. Wegener's granulomatosis: current trends in diagnosis and management. Curr Opin Otolaryngol Head Neck Surg. 2007 Jun;15(3):170–6. [PMID: 17483685]

Mendenhall WM et al. Lethal midline granuloma-nasal natural killer/T-cell lymphoma. Am J Clin Oncol. 2006 Apr;29(2):202–6. [PMID: 16601443]

DISEASES OF THE ORAL CAVITY & PHARYNX

LEUKOPLAKIA, ERYTHROPLAKIA, ORAL LICHEN PLANUS, & ORAL CANCER

 ESSENTIALS OF DIAGNOSIS

▸ **Leukoplakia**—A white lesion that, unlike oral candidiasis, cannot be removed by rubbing the mucosal surface.

▸ **Erythroplakia**—Similar to leukoplakia except that it has a definite erythematous component.

▸ **Oral Lichen Planus**—Most commonly presents as lacy leukoplakia but may be erosive; definitive diagnosis requires biopsy.

▸ **Oral Cancer**—Early lesions appear as leukoplakia or erythroplakia; more advanced lesions will be larger, with invasion into tongue such that a mass lesion is palpable.

▸ Ulceration may be present.

Leukoplakic regions range from small to several centimeters in diameter (Plate 59). Histologically, they are often hyperkeratoses occurring in response to chronic irritation (eg, from dentures, tobacco, lichen planus); about 2–6%, however, represent either dysplasia or early invasive SCC. Distinguishing between **erythroplakia** and **leukoplakia** is important because about 90% of cases of erythroplakia are either dysplasia or carcinoma. **SCC** accounts for 90% of oral cancer. Alcohol and tobacco use are the major epidemiologic risk factors.

The differential diagnosis may include oral candidiasis, necrotizing sialometaplasia, pseudoepitheliomatous hyperplasia, median rhomboid glossitis, and vesiculoerosive inflammatory disease such as erosive lichen planus. This should not be confused with the brown-black gingival melanin pigmentation—diffuse or speckled—common in nonwhites, blue-black embedded fragments of dental amalgam, or other systemic disorders associated with general pigmentation (neurofibromatosis, familial polyposis, Addison disease). Intraoral melanoma is extremely rare.

Any area of **erythroplakia**, enlarging area of **leukoplakia**, or a lesion that has submucosal depth on palpation should have an incisional biopsy or an exfoliative cytologic examination. Ulcerative lesions are particularly suspicious and worrisome. Specialty referral should be sought early both for diagnosis and treatment. A systematic intraoral examination—including the lateral tongue, floor of the mouth, gingiva, buccal area, palate, and tonsillar fossae—and palpation of the neck for enlarged lymph nodes should be part of any general physical examination, especially in patients over the age of 45 who smoke tobacco or drink immoderately. Indirect or fiberoptic examination of the nasopharynx, oropharynx, hypopharynx, and larynx by an otolaryngologist, head and neck surgeon, or radiation oncologist should also be considered for such patients when there is unexplained or persistent throat or ear pain, oral or nasal bleeding, or oral erythroplakia. Fine-needle aspiration (FNA) biopsy may expedite the diagnosis if an enlarged lymph node is found. To date, there are no approved therapies for reversing or stabilizing leukoplakia or erythroplakia.

Oral lichen planus is a relatively common (0.5–2% of the population) chronic inflammatory autoimmune disease that may be difficult to diagnose clinically because of its numerous distinct phenotypic subtypes. For example, the reticular pattern may mimic candidiasis or hyperkeratosis, while the erosive pattern may mimic SCC. Management begins with distinguishing it from other oral lesions. Exfoliative cytology or a small incisional or excisional biopsy is indicated, especially if SCC is suspected. Therapy is aimed at managing pain and discomfort. Corticosteroids have been used widely both locally and systemically. Cyclosporines and retinoids have also been used. Many think there is a low rate (1%) of SCC arising within lichen planus (in addition to the possibility of clinical misdiagnosis).

Hairy leukoplakia occurs on the lateral border of the tongue and is a common early finding in HIV infection (see Chapter 31). It often develops quickly and appears as slightly raised leukoplakic areas with a corrugated or "hairy" surface (Plate 60). Clinical response following administration of zidovudine or acyclovir has been reported, and treatment is under active investigation.

Early detection of **SCC** is the key to successful management (Plate 61). Lesions less than 4 mm in depth have a low propensity to metastasize. Most patients in whom the tumor is detected before it is 2 cm in diameter are cured by local resection. Radiation is an alternative but not generally used as first-line therapy for small lesions. Large tumors are usually treated with a combination of resection, neck dissection, and external beam radiation. Reconstruction, if required, is done at the time of resection and can involve the use of myocutaneous flaps or vascularized free flaps with or without bone.

A number of clinical trials have suggested a role for beta-carotene, cyclooxygenase (COX)-2 inhibitors, vitamin E, and retinoids in producing regression of leukoplakia and reducing the incidence of recurrent SCCs. Retinoids suppress head and neck and lung carcinogenesis in animal models and inhibit carcinogenesis in individuals with premalignant lesions. They also seem to reduce the incidence of second primary cancers in head and neck and lung cancer patients previously treated for a primary.

Brennan M et al. Management of oral epithelial dysplasia: a review. Oral Surg Oral Med Oral Pathol Oral Radiol Endod. 2007 Mar;103 (Suppl):S19.e1–12. [PMID: 17257863]
Eisen D et al. Number V. Oral lichen planus: clinical features and management. Oral Dis. 2005 Nov;11(6):338–49. [PMID: 16269024]
Konkimalla VB et al. Diagnosis and therapy of oral squamous cell carcinoma. Expert Rev Anticancer Ther. 2007 Mar;7(3):317–29. [PMID: 17338652]

CANDIDIASIS

▶ Clinical Findings

A. Symptoms and Signs

Oral candidiasis (thrush) is usually painful and looks like creamy-white curd-like patches overlying erythematous mucosa (see Plate 28). Because these white areas are easily rubbed off (eg, by a tongue depressor)—unlike leukoplakia or lichen planus—only the underlying irregular erythema may be seen. Oral candidiasis is commonly encountered among the following patients: (1) those who wear dentures, (2) those who are debilitated, (3) those with diabetes, (4) those with anemia, (5) those undergoing chemotherapy or local irradiation, and (6) those receiving corticosteroids or broad-spectrum antibiotics. Angular cheilitis is another manifestation of candidiasis, although it is also seen in nutritional deficiencies (Plate 62).

B. Diagnostic Studies

The diagnosis is made clinically. A wet preparation using potassium hydroxide will reveal spores and may show nonseptate mycelia. Biopsy will show intraepithelial pseudomycelia of *Candida albicans*.

Candidiasis is often the first manifestation of HIV infection, and HIV testing should be considered in patients with no known predisposing cause for *Candida* overgrowth (see also Chapter 31). The US Department of Health Services Clinical Practice Guideline for Evaluation and Management of Early HIV Infection recommends examination of the oral mucosa with each clinician visit as well as at a dental examination every 6 months.

▶ Treatment

Effective antifungal therapy may be achieved with any of the following: fluconazole (100 mg/d for 7–14 days), ketoconazole (200–400 mg with breakfast [requires acidic gastric environment for absorption] for 7–14 days), clotrimazole troches (10 mg dissolved orally five times daily), or nystatin vaginal troches (100,000 units dissolved orally five times daily) or mouth rinses (500,000 units [5 mL of 100,000 units/mL] held in the mouth before swallowing three times daily). Shorter-duration therapy using fluconazole has proved effective. In patients with HIV infection, however, longer courses may be needed, and oral itraconazole (200 mg/d) may be indicated in fluconazole-refractory cases. Many of the *Candida* species in these patients are resistant to first-line azoles and may require newer drugs, such as voriconazole. In addition, 0.12% chlorhexidine or half-strength hydrogen peroxide mouth rinses may provide local relief. Nystatin powder (100,000 units/g) applied to dentures three or four times daily for several weeks may help denture wearers.

Pankhurst C. Candidiasis (oropharyngeal). Clin Evid. 2005 Jun;(13):1701–16. [PMID: 16135307]
Pienaar ED et al. Interventions for the prevention and management of oropharyngeal candidiasis associated with HIV infection in adults and children. Cochrane Database Syst Rev. 2006 Jul 19;3:CD003940. [PMID: 16856025]
Worthington HV et al. Interventions for treating oral candidiasis for patients with cancer receiving treatment. Cochrane Database Syst Rev. 2007 Apr 18;(2):CD001972. [PMID: 17443513]

GLOSSITIS, GLOSSODYNIA, DYSGEUSIA, & BURNING MOUTH SYNDROME

Inflammation of the tongue with loss of filiform papillae leads to a red, smooth-surfaced tongue (glossitis). Rarely painful, it may be secondary to nutritional deficiencies (eg, niacin, riboflavin, iron, or vitamin E), drug reactions, dehydration, irritants, foods and liquids, and possibly autoimmune reactions or psoriasis. If the primary cause cannot be identified and corrected, empiric nutritional replacement therapy may be of value.

Glossodynia is burning and pain of the tongue, which may occur with or without glossitis. In the absence of any clinical findings, it has been termed "the burning mouth syndrome." Glossodynia with glossitis has been associated with diabetes mellitus, drugs (eg, diuretics), tobacco, xerostomia, and candidiasis as well as the listed causes of glossitis. Periodontal disease is not apt to be a factor. The burning mouth syndrome typically has no identifiable associated risk factors and seems to be most common in postmenopausal women. Treating possible underlying causes, changing long-term medications to alternative ones, and smoking cessation may resolve symptoms of glossitis. Both glossodynia and the burning mouth syndrome are benign, and reassurance that there is no infection or tumor is likely to be appreciated. Effective treatments for the burning mouth syndrome include alpha-lipoic acid and clonazepam. Clonazepam is most effective as a rapid dissolving tablet placed on the tongue in doses from 0.25 mg to 0.5 mg every 8–12 hours. Behavioral therapy has also been shown to be effective. Unilateral symptoms, symptoms that cannot be related to a specific medication, and symptoms and signs involving regions supplied by other cranial nerves all may suggest neuropathology, and imaging of the brain, brainstem, and skull base with MRI should be considered.

Byrd JA et al. Glossitis and other tongue disorders. Dermatol Clin. 2003 Jan;21(1):123–34. [PMID: 12622275]

Patton LL et al. Management of burning mouth syndrome: systematic review and management recommendations. Oral Surg Oral Med Oral Pathol Oral Radiol Endod. 2007 Mar;103 (Suppl):S39:e1–13. [PMID: 17379153]

Speciali JG et al. Burning mouth syndrome. Curr Pain Headache Rep. 2008 Aug;12(4):279–84. [PMID: 18625105]

INTRAORAL ULCERATIVE LESIONS

1. Necrotizing Ulcerative Gingivitis (Trench Mouth, Vincent Infection)

Necrotizing ulcerative gingivitis, often caused by an infection of both spirochetes and fusiform bacilli, is common in young adults under stress (classically at examination time). Underlying systemic diseases may also predispose to this disorder. Clinically, there is painful acute gingival inflammation and necrosis, often with bleeding, halitosis, fever, and cervical lymphadenopathy. Warm half-strength peroxide rinses and oral penicillin (250 mg three times daily for 10 days) may help. Dental gingival curettage may prove necessary.

Necrotizing ulcerative periodontitis is discussed later in this chapter in the section on AIDS.

2. Aphthous Ulcer (Canker Sore, Ulcerative Stomatitis)

Aphthous ulcers are very common and easy to recognize. Their cause remains uncertain, although an association with human herpesvirus 6 has been suggested. Found on nonkeratinized mucosa (eg, buccal and labial mucosa and not attached gingiva or palate), they may be single or multiple, are usually recurrent, and appear as painful small (usually 1–2 mm, but sometimes 1–2 cm) round ulcerations with yellow-gray fibrinoid centers surrounded by red halos (Plate 63). The painful stage lasts 7–10 days; healing is completed in 1–3 weeks.

Treatment is nonspecific. Topical corticosteroids (triamcinolone acetonide, 0.1%, or fluocinonide ointment, 0.05%) in an adhesive base (Orabase Plain) do appear to provide symptomatic relief. Other topical therapies shown to be effective in controlled studies include diclofenac 3% in hyaluronan 2.5%, doxymycine-cyanoacrylate, mouthwashes containing the enzymes amyloglucosidase and glucose oxidase, and amlexanox 5% oral paste. A 1-week tapering course of prednisone (40–60 mg/d) has also been used successfully. Cimetidine maintenance therapy may be useful in patients with recurrent aphthous ulcers. Thalidomide has been used selectively in recurrent aphthous ulcerations in HIV-positive patients.

Large or persistent areas of ulcerative stomatitis may be secondary to erythema multiforme or drug allergies, acute herpes simplex, pemphigus, pemphigoid, epidermolysis bullosa acquisita, bullous lichen planus, Behçet disease, or inflammatory bowel disease. SCC may occasionally present in this fashion. When the diagnosis is not clear, incisional biopsy is indicated.

Femiano F et al. Guidelines for diagnosis and management of aphthous stomatitis. Pediatr Infect Dis J. 2007 Aug;26(8):728–32. [PMID: 17848886]

Scully C et al. Oral mucosal disease: recurrent aphthous stomatitis. Br J Oral Maxillofac Surg. 2008 Apr;46(3):198–206. [PMID: 17850936]

3. Herpetic Stomatitis

Herpetic gingivostomatitis is common, mild, and short-lived and requires no intervention in most adults. In immunocompromised persons, however, reactivation of herpes simplex virus infection is frequent and may be severe. Clinically, there is initial burning, followed by typical small vesicles that rupture and form scabs. Acyclovir (200–800 mg five times daily for 7–14 days) may shorten the course and reduce postherpetic pain. Differential diagnosis includes aphthous stomatitis (see above), erythema multiforme, syphilitic chancre, and carcinoma. Coxsackievirus-caused lesions (grayish white tonsillar and palatal ulcers of herpangina or buccal and lip ulcers in hand-foot-and-mouth disease) are seen more commonly in children under age 6.

Arduino PG et al. Oral and perioral herpes simplex virus type 1 (HSV-1) infection: review of its management. Oral Dis. 2006 May;12(3):254–70. [PMID: 16700734]

Sciubba JJ. Oral mucosal diseases in the office setting–part I: Aphthous stomatitis and herpes simplex infections. Gen Dent. 2007 Jul–Aug;55(4):347–56. [PMID: 17682646]

PHARYNGITIS & TONSILLITIS

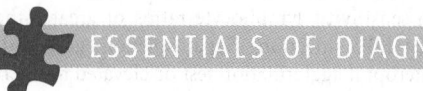

ESSENTIALS OF DIAGNOSIS

► Sore throat.

► Fever.

► Anterior cervical adenopathy.

- Tonsillar exudate.
- Focus is to treat group A β-hemolytic streptococcus infection to prevent rheumatic sequelae.

General Considerations

Pharyngitis and tonsillitis account for over 10% of all office visits to primary care clinicians and 50% of outpatient antibiotic use. The most appropriate management continues to be debated because some of the issues are deceptively complex, but consensus has increased in recent years. The main concern is determining who is likely to have a group A β-hemolytic streptococcal infection (GABHS), as this can lead to subsequent complications such as rheumatic fever and glomerular nephritis. A second public health policy concern is reducing the extraordinary cost (both in dollars and in the development of antibiotic-resistant *S pneumoniae*) in the United States associated with unnecessary antibiotic use. Questions now being asked: Is there still a role for culturing a sore throat, or have the rapid antigen tests supplanted this procedure under most circumstances? Are clinical criteria alone a sufficient basis for decisions about which patients should be given antibiotics? Should any patient receive any antibiotic other than penicillin (or erythromycin if penicillin-allergic)? For how long should treatment be continued? Numerous well-done studies in the past few years as well as increasing experience with rapid laboratory tests for detection of streptococci (eliminating the delay caused by culturing) appear to make a consensus approach more possible.

Clinical Findings

The clinical features most suggestive of group A β-hemolytic streptococcal pharyngitis include fever over 38 °C, tender anterior cervical adenopathy, lack of a cough, and a pharyngotonsillar exudate (Plates 64 and 65). These four features (the Centor criteria), when present, strongly suggest GABHS, and some would treat regardless of laboratory results. When three of the four are present, laboratory sensitivity of rapid antigen testing exceeds 90%. When only one criterion is present, GABHS is unlikely. Sore throat may be severe, with odynophagia, tender adenopathy, and a scarlatiniform rash. An elevated white count and left shift are also possible. Hoarseness, cough, and coryza are not suggestive of this disease.

Marked lymphadenopathy and a shaggy white-purple tonsillar exudate, often extending into the nasopharynx, suggest mononucleosis, especially if present in a young adult. Recently, the lymphocyte-white blood cell count ratio has been reported to efficiently and specifically differentiate tonsillitis from infectious mononucleosis. With about 90% sensitivity, lymphocyte ratios of greater than 35% suggest EBV infection. Hepatosplenomegaly and a positive heterophil agglutination test or elevated anti-EBV titer are corroborative. However, about one-third of patients with infectious mononucleosis have secondary streptococcal tonsillitis, requiring treatment. Ampicillin should routinely be avoided if mononucleosis is suspected

because it induces a rash that might be misinterpreted by the patient as a penicillin allergy. Diphtheria (extremely rare but described in the alcoholic population) presents with low-grade fever and an ill patient with a gray tonsillar pseudomembrane.

The most common pathogens other than group A β-hemolytic streptococci in the differential diagnosis of "sore throat" are viruses, *Neisseria gonorrhoeae*, *Mycoplasma*, and *Chlamydia trachomatis*. Rhinorrhea and lack of exudate would suggest a virus, but in practice it is not possible to confidently distinguish viral upper respiratory infection from GABHS on clinical grounds alone. Infections with *Corynebacterium diphtheriae*, anaerobic streptococci, and *Corynebacterium haemolyticum* (which responds better to erythromycin than penicillin) may also mimic pharyngitis due to group A β-hemolytic streptococci.

Treatment

Given the availability of many well-documented studies in recent years, one would think that a consensus might develop as to the most appropriate way to treat a sore throat. The Infectious Diseases Society of America recommends laboratory confirmation of the clinical diagnosis by means of either throat culture or a rapid antigen detection test. The American College of Physicians–American Society of Internal Medicine (ACP-ASIM), in collaboration with the Centers for Disease Control and Prevention, advocates use of a clinical algorithm alone—in lieu of microbiologic testing—for confirmation of the diagnosis in adults for whom the suspicion of streptococcal infection is high. Others examine the assumptions of the ACP-ASIM guideline for using a clinical algorithm alone and question whether those recommendations will achieve the stated objective of dramatically decreasing excess antibiotic use. Convincing clinical trials as well as clinician reminders and patient-based interventions may be needed before clinicians are likely to abandon long-held teachings (even though different clinicians appear to have been taught different strategies) regarding diagnosis and management of group A streptococcal pharyngitis. A Cochrane review concluded that multifaceted interventions where educational interventions occur on many levels were the only interventions whose effects were of sufficient magnitude to potentially reduce the incidence of antibiotic-resistant bacteria.

Thirty years ago, a single injection of benzathine penicillin or procaine penicillin was standard antibiotic treatment. This remains effective, but the injections are painful. If compliance is an issue, it may be the best choice. Oral treatment is also effective. Antibiotic choice aims to reduce the already low (10–20%) incidence of treatment failures (positive culture after treatment despite symptomatic resolution) and recurrences. A review of recent controlled studies suggests that penicillin V potassium (250 mg orally three times daily or 500 mg twice daily for 10 days) or cefuroxime axetil (250 mg orally twice daily for 5–10 days) are both effective. The efficacy of a 5-day regimen of penicillin V appears to be similar to that of a 10-day course, with a 94% clinical response rate and an 84% streptococcal eradication rate. Erythromycin (active against *Mycoplasma* and *Chlamydia*) is a reasonable alternative to penicillin in allergic patients. Cephalosporins are somewhat more effective than penicillin in producing bacteriologic cures; 5-day administration has been successful for cefpodoxime and cefuroxime. The macrolide antibiotics have also been reported to be successful in shorter-duration regimens. Azithromycin (500 mg once daily), because of its long half-life, need be taken for only 3 days.

Adequate antibiotic treatment usually avoids the streptococcal complications of scarlet fever, glomerulonephritis, rheumatic myocarditis, and local abscess formation.

Antibiotics for treatment failures are also somewhat controversial. Surprisingly, penicillin-tolerant strains are not isolated more frequently in those who fail treatment than in those treated successfully with penicillin. The reasons for failure appear to be complex, and a second course of treatment with the same drug is not unreasonable. Alternatives to penicillin include cefuroxime and other cephalosporins, dicloxacillin (which is β-lactamase–resistant), and amoxicillin with clavulanate. When there is a history of penicillin allergy, alternatives should be used, such as erythromycin. Erythromycin resistance—with failure rates of about 25%—is an increasing problem in many areas. In cases of severe penicillin allergy, cephalosporins should be avoided as the cross-reaction is common (8% or more).

Ancillary treatment of pharyngitis includes analgesics and anti-inflammatory agents, such as aspirin or acetaminophen. Some patients find that salt water gargling is soothing. In severe cases, anesthetic gargles and lozenges (eg, benzocaine) may provide additional symptomatic relief. Occasionally, odynophagia is so intense that hospitalization for intravenous hydration and antibiotics is necessary. (See Chapter 33.)

Arnold SR et al. Interventions to improve antibiotic prescribing practices in ambulatory care. Cochrane Database Syst Rev 2005 Oct 19;(4):CD003539. [PMID: 16235325]
Colletti T et al. Strep throat: guidelines for diagnosis and treatment. JAAPA. 2005 Sep;18(9):38–44. [PMID: 16184870]
Tewfik TL et al. Tonsillopharyngitis: clinical highlights. J Otolaryngol. 2005 Jun;34(Suppl 1):S45–9. [PMID: 16089240]

PERITONSILLAR ABSCESS & CELLULITIS

When infection penetrates the tonsillar capsule and involves the surrounding tissues, peritonsillar cellulitis results. Peritonsillar abscess and cellulitis present with severe sore throat, odynophagia, trismus, medial deviation of the soft palate and peritonsillar fold, and an abnormal muffled ("hot potato") voice. Following therapy, peritonsillar cellulitis usually either resolves over several days or evolves into peritonsillar abscess, also known as quinsy. The existence of an abscess may be confirmed by aspirating pus from the peritonsillar fold just superior and medial to the upper pole of the tonsil. A No. 19 or No. 21 needle should be passed medial to the molar and no deeper than 1 cm, because the internal carotid artery may lie more medially than its usual location and pass posterior and deep to the tonsillar fossa. There is controversy regarding the three ways to treat a peritonsillar abscess: needle aspiration, incision and drainage, or tonsillectomy. Some clinicians incise and drain the

area and continue with parenteral antibiotics, whereas others aspirate only and monitor as an outpatient. To drain the abscess and avoid recurrence, it may be appropriate to consider immediate tonsillectomy (quinsy tonsillectomy). About 10% of patients with peritonsillar abscess exhibit relative indications for tonsillectomy. All three approaches are effective and have support in the literature. Regardless of the method used, one must be sure the abscess is adequately treated, since complications such as extension to the retropharyngeal, deep neck, and posterior mediastinal spaces are possible. Bacteria may also be aspirated into the lungs, resulting in pneumonia. While there is controversy about whether a single abscess is sufficient indication for tonsillectomy, most would agree that patients with recurrent abscesses should have a tonsillectomy.

Johnson RF et al. The contemporary approach to diagnosis and management of peritonsillar abscess. Curr Opin Otolaryngol Head Neck Surg. 2005 Jun;13(3):157–60. [PMID: 15908813]
Khayr W et al. Management of peritonsillar abscess: needle aspiration versus incision and drainage versus tonsillectomy. Am J Ther. 2005 Jul–Aug;12(4):344–50. [PMID: 16041198]

TONSILLECTOMY

Despite the frequency with which tonsillectomy is performed, the indications for the procedure remain controversial. Most clinicians would agree that airway obstruction causing sleep apnea or cor pulmonale is an absolute indication for tonsillectomy. Similarly, persistent marked tonsillar asymmetry should prompt an excisional biopsy to rule out lymphoma. Relative indications include recurrent streptococcal tonsillitis, causing considerable loss of time from school or work, recurrent peritonsillar abscess, and chronic tonsillitis.

Tonsillectomy is not an entirely benign procedure. The pros and cons of tonsillectomy need to be discussed with each prospective patient. Postoperative bleeding occurs in 2–4% of cases and on rare occasions can lead to laryngospasm and airway obstruction. Pain may be considerable, especially in the adult. Protracted emesis or fever may also occasionally occur. Secondary bleeding 5–8 days postoperatively is far more common than bleeding in the first 24 hours. There is increasing economic pressure for these procedures to be done as outpatient surgery. At present, it seems clear that outpatient tonsillectomy is usually safe when followed by a 6-hour period of uneventful observation, but individual circumstances may mandate hospitalization.

Although reports in the 1970s suggested an association of tonsillectomy with Hodgkin disease, careful review of this literature reveals no conclusively causative association.

Alho OP et al. Tonsillectomy versus watchful waiting in recurrent streptococcal pharyngitis in adults: randomised controlled trial. BMJ. 2007 May 5;334(7600):939. [PMID: 17347187]
Bhattacharyya N et al. Economic benefit of tonsillectomy in adults with chronic tonsillitis. Ann Otol Rhinol Laryngol. 2002 Nov;111(11):983–8. [PMID: 12450171]
Darrow DH et al. Indications for tonsillectomy and adenoidectomy. Laryngoscope. 2002 Aug;112(8 Pt 2 Suppl 100):6–10. [PMID: 12172229]

DEEP NECK INFECTIONS

Deep neck abscesses usually present with marked neck pain and swelling in a toxic febrile patient. They are emergencies because they may rapidly compromise the airway. They may also spread to the mediastinum or cause septicemia. Most commonly, they originate from odontogenic infections. Other causes include suppurative lymphadenitis, direct spread of pharyngeal infection, penetrating trauma, pharyngoesophageal foreign bodies, cervical osteomyelitis, and intravenous injection of the internal jugular vein, especially in drug abusers. Recurrent deep neck infection may suggest an underlying congenital lesion such as a branchial cleft cyst. Suppurative lymphadenopathy in middle-age persons who smoke and drink alcohol regularly should be considered a manifestation of malignancy (typically metastatic SCC) until proven otherwise.

Fundamentals of treatment include securing the airway, intravenous antibiotics, and incision and drainage. In highly selected patients without airway compromise, needle aspiration and catheter drainage or even conservative management without antibiotics alone has been reported to be successful in uniloculated abscesses. The airway may be secured, when indicated, either by intubation or tracheotomy. Tracheotomy is preferable in the patients with substantial pharyngeal edema, since attempts at intubation may precipitate acute airway obstruction. Bleeding in association with a deep neck abscess suggests the possibility of carotid artery or internal jugular vein involvement and requires prompt neck exploration both for drainage of pus and for vascular control.

Contrast-enhanced CT usually augments the clinical examination in defining the extent of the infection. It often will distinguish inflammation (requiring antibiotics) from abscess (requiring drainage) and define for the surgeon the extent of an abscess. CT with MRI may also identify thrombophlebitis of the internal jugular vein secondary to oropharyngeal inflammation. This condition, known as Lemierre syndrome, may be associated with septic emboli and requires prompt institution of antibiotics appropriate for *Fusobacterium necrophorum* as well as the more usual upper airway pathogens. The presence of pulmonary infiltrates (or septic arthritis) in the setting of a neck abscess should lead one to suspect Lemierre syndrome.

Ludwig angina is the most commonly encountered neck space infection. It is a cellulitis of the sublingual and submaxillary spaces, often arising from infection of the mandible. Clinically, there is edema and erythema of the upper neck under the chin and often of the floor of the mouth. The tongue may be displaced upward and backward by the posterior spread of cellulitis. This may lead to occlusion of the airway and necessitate tracheotomy. Microbiologic isolates include streptococci, staphylococci, *Bacteroides*, and *Fusobacterium*. Usual doses of penicillin plus metronidazole, ampicillin-sulbactam, clindamycin, or selective cephalosporins are good initial choices. Culture and sensitivity data will then refine the choice. Dental consultation is advisable. External drainage via bilateral submental incisions is required if the airway is threatened or when medical therapy has not reversed the process.

Reynolds SC et al. Life-threatening infections of the peripharyngeal and deep fascial spaces of the head and neck. Infect Dis Clin North Am. 2007 Jun;21(2):557–76. [PMID: 17561083]

Vieira F et al. Deep neck infection. Otolaryngol Clin North Am. 2008 Jun;41(3):459–83. [PMID: 18435993]

▼ DISEASES OF THE SALIVARY GLANDS

ACUTE INFLAMMATORY SALIVARY GLAND DISORDERS

1. Sialadenitis

Acute bacterial sialadenitis in the adult most commonly affects either the parotid or submandibular gland. It typically presents with acute swelling of the gland, increased pain and swelling with meals, and tenderness and erythema of the duct opening. Pus often can be massaged from the duct. Sialadenitis often occurs in the setting of dehydration or in association with chronic illness. Underlying Sjögren syndrome may contribute. Ductal obstruction, often by an inspissated mucous plug, is followed by salivary stasis and secondary infection. The most common organism recovered from purulent draining saliva is *S aureus*. Treatment consists of intravenous antibiotics such as nafcillin (1 g intravenously every 4–6 hours) and measures to increase salivary flow, including hydration, warm compresses, sialagogues (eg, lemon drops), and massage of the gland. Usually one can switch to an oral agent based on clinical and microbiologic improvement to complete a 10-day course. Failure of the process to resolve on this regimen suggests abscess formation, ductal stricture, stone, or tumor causing obstruction. Ultrasound or CT scan may be helpful in establishing the diagnosis. In the setting of acute illness, a severe and potentially life-threatening form of sialadenitis, sometimes called "suppurative sialadenitis" may develop. The causative organism is usually *S aureus*, but often no pus will drain from Stensen papilla. These patients often do not respond to rehydration and intravenous antibiotics and thus may require operative incision and drainage to resolve the infection.

2. Sialolithiasis

Calculus formation is more common in Wharton duct (draining the submandibular glands) than in Stensen duct (draining the parotid glands). Clinically, a patient may note postprandial pain and local swelling, often with a history of recurrent acute sialadenitis. Stones in Wharton duct are usually large and radiopaque, whereas those in Stensen duct are usually radiolucent and smaller. Those very close to the orifice of Wharton duct may be palpated manually in the anterior floor of the mouth and removed intraorally by dilating or incising the distal duct. The duct proximal to the stone must be temporarily clamped (using, for instance, a single throw of a suture) to keep manipulation of the stone from pushing it back toward the submandibular gland. Those more than 1.5–2 cm from the duct are too close to the lingual nerve to be removed safely in this manner. Similarly, dilation of Stensen duct, located on the buccal surface opposite the second maxillary molar, may relieve distal stricture or allow a small stone to pass. Extracorporeal shock-wave lithotripsy and fluoroscopically guided basket retrieval have been used successfully, but are being replaced by sialoendoscopy for the management of chronic sialolithiasis. Repeated episodes of sialadenitis are usually associated with stricture and chronic infection. If the obstruction cannot be safely removed or dilated, excision of the gland may be necessary to relieve recurrent symptoms.

Brook I. Aerobic and anaerobic microbiology of suppurative sialadenitis. J Med Microbiol. 2002 Jun;51(6):526–9. [PMID: 12018662]
Papadaki ME et al. Interventional sialoendoscopy: early clinical results. J Oral Maxillofac Surg. 2008 May;66(5):954–62. [PMID: 18423286]

CHRONIC INFLAMMATORY & INFILTRATIVE DISORDERS OF THE SALIVARY GLANDS

Numerous infiltrative disorders may cause unilateral or bilateral parotid gland enlargement. Sjögren disease and sarcoidosis are examples of lymphoepithelial and granulomatous diseases that may affect the salivary glands. Metabolic disorders, including alcoholism, diabetes mellitus, and vitamin deficiencies, may also cause diffuse enlargement. Several drugs have been associated with parotid enlargement, including thioureas, iodine, and drugs with cholinergic effects (eg, phenothiazines), which stimulate salivary flow and cause more viscous saliva.

Salomonsson S et al. Minor salivary gland immunohistology in the diagnosis of primary Sjögren's syndrome. J Oral Pathol Med. 2009 Mar;38(2):282–8. [PMID: 18793250]

SALIVARY GLAND TUMORS

Approximately 80% of salivary gland tumors occur in the parotid gland. In adults, about 80% of these are benign. In the submandibular triangle, it is sometimes difficult to distinguish a primary submandibular gland tumor from a metastatic submandibular space node. Only 50–60% of primary submandibular tumors are benign. Tumors of the minor salivary glands are most likely to be malignant, with adenoid cystic carcinoma predominating.

Most parotid tumors present as an asymptomatic mass in the superficial part of the gland. Their presence may have been noted by the patient for months or years. Facial nerve involvement correlates strongly with malignancy. Tumors may extend deep to the plane of the facial nerve or may originate in the parapharyngeal space. In such cases, medial deviation of the soft palate is visible on intraoral examination. MRI and CT scans have largely replaced sialography in defining the extent of tumor.

When the clinician encounters a patient with an otherwise asymptomatic salivary gland mass where tumor is the most likely diagnosis, the choice is whether to simply excise the mass via a parotidectomy with facial nerve dissection or submandibular gland excision or to obtain an FNA biopsy first. Although the accuracy of

FNA biopsy for malignancy has been reported to be quite high, results vary among institutions. If a negative FNA biopsy would lead to a decision not to proceed to surgery, then it should be considered. Poor overall health of the patient and the possibility of inflammatory disease as the cause of the mass are situations where FNA biopsy might be helpful. In otherwise straightforward nonrecurrent cases, excision is indicated. In benign and small low-grade malignant tumors, no additional treatment is needed. Postoperative irradiation is indicated for larger and high-grade cancers.

Bhattacharyya N et al. Determinants of survival in parotid gland carcinoma: a population-based study. Am J Otolaryngol. 2005 Jan–Feb;26(1):39–44. [PMID: 15635580]
Mendenhall WM et al. Salivary gland pleomorphic adenoma. Am J Clin Oncol. 2008 Feb;31(1):95–9. [PMID: 18376235]
Scianna JM et al. Contemporary management of tumors of the salivary glands. Curr Oncol Rep. 2007 Mar;9(2):134–8. [PMID: 17288880]

DISEASES OF THE LARYNX

DYSPHONIA, HOARSENESS, & STRIDOR

The primary symptoms of laryngeal disease are hoarseness and stridor. Hoarseness is caused by an abnormal vibration of the vocal folds. The voice is breathy when too much air passes incompletely apposed vocal folds, as in unilateral vocal fold paralysis or vocal fold mass. The voice is harsh when the vocal folds are stiff and vibrate irregularly, as is the case in laryngitis or malignancy. Heavy, edematous vocal folds produce a rough vocal quality. Stridor (a high-pitched, typically inspiratory, sound) is the result of turbulent airflow from a narrowed glottis. Airway narrowing at or above the vocal folds produces inspiratory stridor. Airway narrowing below the vocal fold level produces either expiratory or biphasic stridor. The timing and rapidity of onset of stridor are critically important in determining the seriousness of the airway problem. All cases of stridor should be evaluated by a specialist and rapid-onset stridor should be evaluated emergently.

Evaluation of an abnormal voice begins with obtaining a history of the circumstances preceding its onset and an examination of the airway.

Any patient with hoarseness that has persisted beyond 2 weeks should be evaluated by an otolaryngologist with laryngoscopy. Especially when the patient has a history of tobacco use, laryngeal cancer or lung cancer (leading to paralysis of a recurrent laryngeal nerve) must be strongly considered. In addition to structural causes of dysphonia, laryngoscopy can help identify functional problems with the voice including vocal fold paralysis, muscle tension dysphonia, and spasmodic dysphonia.

Klein AM et al. Vocal emergencies. Otolaryngol Clin North Am. 2007 Oct;40(5):1063–80. [PMID: 17765695]
Richardson BE et al. Clinical evaluation of vocal fold paralysis. Otolaryngol Clin North Am. 2004 Feb;37(1):45–58. [PMID: 15062686]

COMMON LARYNGEAL DISORDERS

1. Epiglottitis

Epiglottitis (or, more correctly, supraglottitis) in adults should be suspected when a patient presents with a rapidly developing sore throat or when odynophagia (pain on swallowing) is out of proportion to apparently minimal oropharyngeal findings on examination. It is more common in diabetics and may be viral or bacterial in origin. Rarely in the era of *H influenzae* type b vaccine is this bacterium isolated in adults. Unlike in children, indirect laryngoscopy is generally safe and may demonstrate a swollen, erythematous epiglottis. Lateral plain radiographs may demonstrate an enlarged epiglottis (the epiglottis "thumb sign"). Initial treatment is hospitalization for intravenous antibiotics—eg, ceftizoxime, 1–2 g intravenously every 8–12 hours; or cefuroxime, 750–1500 mg intravenously every 8 hours; and dexamethasone, usually 4–10 mg as initial bolus, then 4 mg intravenously every 6 hours—and observation of the airway. Corticosteroids may be tapered as symptoms and signs resolve. Similarly, substitution of oral antibiotics may be appropriate to complete a 10-day course. Less than 10% of adults require intubation. Indications for intubation are dyspnea, rapid pace of sore throat (where progression to airway compromise may occur before the effects of corticosteroids and antibiotics), and endolaryngeal abscess noted on CT imaging. If the patient is not intubated, prudence suggests monitoring oxygen saturation with continuous pulse oximetry and initial admission to a monitored unit.

Glynn F et al. Diagnosis and management of supraglottitis (epiglottitis). Curr Infect Dis Rep. 2008 May;10(3):200–4. [PMID: 18510881]

Sobol SE et al. Epiglottitis and croup. Otolaryngol Clin North Am. 2008 Jun;41(3):551–66. [PMID: 18435998]

2. Recurrent Respiratory Papillomatosis

Papillomas are common lesions of the larynx and other sites where ciliated and squamous epithelia meet. Unlike oral papillomas, recurrent respiratory papillomatosis is likely to be symptomatic, with hoarseness that occasionally progresses to stridor over weeks to months. These papillomas are almost always HPV types 6 and 11. The disease is more common in children. Repeated laser vaporizations or cold knife resections via operative laryngoscopy are usually the mainstay of treatment. Severe cases can require treatment as often as every 6 weeks to maintain airway patency. Extension can occur into the trachea and lungs. Tracheotomy should be avoided, if possible, since it introduces an additional squamociliary junction for which papillomas appear to have a tropism. Interferon treatment has been under investigation for over two decades but is only indicated in severe cases with pulmonary involvement. Rarely, cases of malignant transformation have been reported (often in smokers), but recurrent respiratory papillomatosis should generally be thought of as a benign condition. Cidofovir (a cytosine nucleotide analog in use to treat cytomegalovirus retinitis) is also being investigated as intralesional therapy for recurrent respiratory papillo-matosis and has had reported success in both adults and children. Because cidofovir causes adenocarcinomas in laboratory animals, its potential for carcinogenesis is being monitored. A quadrivalent recombinant human HPV vaccine (Gardasil) has been approved by the FDA, with HPV type 6 and 11 epitopes conferring immunity in the patient. While not useful as a treatment option for patients with recurrent respiratory papillomatosis, this vaccine offers hope for the eventual eradication of this benign, but terribly morbid, disease.

Chadha NK. Antiviral agents for the treatment of recurrent respiratory papillomatosis: a systematic review of the English-language literature. Otolaryngol Head Neck Surg. 2007 Jun;136(6):863–9. [PMID: 17547971]

Derkay CS et al. Recurrent respiratory papillomatosis. Ann Otol Rhinol Laryngol. 2006 Jan;115(1):1–11. [PMID: 16466093]

3. Acute Laryngitis

Acute laryngitis is probably the most common cause of hoarseness, which may persist for a week or so after other symptoms of an upper respiratory infection have cleared. The patient should be warned to avoid vigorous use of the voice (singing, shouting) until their voice returns to normal, since persistent use may lead to the formation of traumatic vocal polyps, nodules and cysts. Although thought to be usually viral in origin, both *M catarrhalis* and *H influenzae* may be isolated from the nasopharynx at higher than expected frequencies. Erythromycin may reduce the severity of hoarseness and cough.

Reveiz L et al. Antibiotics for acute laryngitis in adults. Cochrane Database Syst Rev. 2005 Jan 25;(1):CD004783. [PMID: 15674965]

4. Laryngopharyngeal Reflux

Gastroesophageal reflux into the larynx (laryngopharyngeal reflux) is considered a possible cause of chronic hoarseness when other causes of abnormal vocal fold vibration (such as tumor or nodules) have been excluded by laryngoscopy. Gastroesophageal reflux disease (GERD) has also been suggested as a contributing factor to other symptoms such as throat clearing, throat discomfort, chronic cough, a sensation of postnasal drip, and esophageal spasm; as well as in many cases of posterior laryngitis and some cases of asthma. Since less than half of patients with laryngeal acid exposure have typical symptoms of heartburn and regurgitation, the lack of such symptoms should not be construed as eliminating this cause. Indeed, most patients with symptomatic laryngopharyngeal reflux, as it is now called, do not meet criteria for GERD by pH probe testing and these entities must be considered separately.

Management should initially exclude other causes of dysphonia through laryngoscopy and consultation with an otolaryngologist is advisable. Many clinicians opt for an empiric trial of a proton pump inhibitor as a practical alternative to an initial pH study. If used, the American Academy of Otolaryngology Head and Neck Surgery recommends twice daily therapy with full strength proton pump inhibitor (eg, omeprazole 40 mg orally twice daily, or equivalent) for a minimum of 3 months. Patients may note improvement in symptoms after 3 months, but the changes in the larynx often take 6 months to resolve. If symptoms improve and cessation of therapy leads to symptoms again, then a proton pump inhibitor is resumed at the lowest dose effective for remission, usually daily but at times on a demand basis. Although H_2-receptor antagonists are an alternative to proton pump inhibitors, they are generally both less clinically effective and less cost-effective. Nonresponders should undergo pH testing and manometry. Twenty-four-hour pH monitoring of the pharynx should best document laryngopharyngeal reflux and is advocated by some as the initial management step but it is costly, more difficult, and less available than lower esophageal monitoring alone. Lower esophageal pH monitoring does not correlate well with laryngopharyngeal reflux symptoms and double pH probe (proximal and distal) testing is accepted as the standard of care for evaluation of laryngopharyngeal reflux.

Ford CN. Evaluation and management of laryngopharyngeal reflux. JAMA. 2005 Sep 28;294(12):1534–40. [PMID: 16189367]

Hopkins C et al. Acid reflux treatment for hoarseness. Cochrane Database Syst Rev. 2006 Jan 25;(1):CD005054. [PMID: 16437513]

Koufman JA et al. Laryngopharyngeal reflux: Position statement of the Committee on Speech, Voice, and Swallowing Disorders of the American Academy of Otolaryngology-Head and Neck Surgery. Otolaryngol Head Neck Surg. 2002 Jul;127(1):32–5. [PMID: 12161727]

TUMORS OF THE LARYNX

1. Traumatic Lesions of the Vocal Folds

Vocal fold nodules are smooth, paired lesions that form at the junction of the anterior one-third and posterior two-thirds of the vocal folds. They are a common cause of hoarseness resulting from vocal abuse. In adults, they are referred to as "singer's nodules"; in children, "screamer's nodules." Treatment requires modification of voice habits, and referral to a speech therapist is indicated. While nearly all true nodules will resolve with behavior modification, recalcitrant nodules may require surgical excision. Often, additional pathology, such as a polyp or cyst, may be encountered.

Vocal fold polyps are unilateral masses that form within the superficial lamina propria of the vocal fold. They are related to vocal trauma and seem to follow resolution of vocal fold hemorrhage. Small, sessile polyps may resolve with conservative measures, such as voice rest and corticosteroids, but larger polyps are often irreversible and require operative resection.

Vocal fold cysts are also considered traumatic lesions of the vocal folds and are either true cysts with an epithelial lining or pseudocysts. They typically form from mucus-secreting glands on the inferior aspect of the vocal folds. Cysts may fluctuate in size from week to week and cause a variable degree of hoarseness. They rarely, if ever, resolve completely and may leave behind a sulcus, or vocal fold scar, if they decompress or are marsupialized. Such scarring can be a frustrating cause of permanent dysphonia.

Polypoid corditis is different from vocal fold polyps and may form from loss of elastin fibers and loosening of the intracellular junctions within the lamina propria. This loss allows swelling of the gelatinous matrix of the superficial lamina propria (called Reinke edema). These changes in the vocal folds are strongly associated with smoking, but also with vocal abuse, chemical industrial irritants, and hypothyroidism. While this problem is common in both male and female smokers, women seem more troubled by the characteristic decline in modal pitch caused by the increased mass of the vocal folds. If the habits change or the lesions cause stridor and airway obstruction, surgical resection of the hyperplastic vocal fold mucosa may be indicated to improve the airway and voice.

A common but often unrecognized cause of hoarseness is contact ulcers or granulomas on the vocal processes of the arytenoid cartilages. The cause of these ulcers is disputed, but they are clearly related to trauma and may be related to exposure of the underlying perichondrium. They are common following intubation and generally resolve quite quickly. Chronic ulceration or granuloma formation has been associated with esophageal reflux but is also common in patients with muscle tension dysphonia. Treatment is often multimodal with proton pump inhibitor therapy (omeprazole 40 mg orally twice daily, or equivalent) and voice therapy with special attention to vocal hygiene. Rare cases can be quite stubborn and persistent without adequate therapy.

Altman KW. Vocal fold masses. Otolaryngol Clin North Am. 2007 Oct;40(5):1091–108. [PMID: 17765697]

Gökcan KM et al. Vascular lesions of the vocal fold. Eur Arch Otorhinolaryngol. 2008 Aug 13 [Epub ahead of print]. [PMID: 18704472]

2. Laryngeal Leukoplakia

Leukoplakia of the vocal folds is commonly found in association with hoarseness in smokers. Direct laryngoscopy with biopsy is advised in almost all cases. Histologic examination usually demonstrates mild, moderate, or severe dysplasia. In some cases, invasive SCC is present in the initial biopsy specimen. Cessation of smoking may reverse or stabilize mild or moderate dysplasia. A certain percentage of patients—estimated to be less than 5% of those with mild dysplasia and about 35–60% of those with severe dysplasia—will subsequently develop SCC. Treatment options include close follow-up with laryngovideostroboscopy, serial resection, and external beam radiation therapy. Despite their cost and the lack of any evidence for their use in the treatment of leukoplakia, proton pump inhibitors have become the mainstay of treatment for these lesions.

Isenberg JS et al. Institutional and comprehensive review of laryngeal leukoplakia. Ann Otol Rhinol Laryngol. 2008 Jan;117(1):74–9. [PMID: 18254375]

3. Squamous Cell Carcinoma of the Larynx

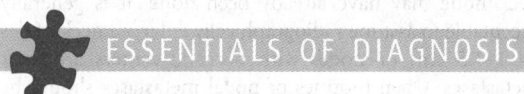

ESSENTIALS OF DIAGNOSIS

▸ New and persistent (more than 2 weeks duration) hoarseness in a smoker.

▸ Persistent throat or ear pain, especially with swallowing.

▸ Neck mass.

▸ Hemoptysis.

▸ Stridor or other symptoms of a compromised airway.

▸ Clinical Findings

A. Symptoms and Signs

SCC of the larynx, the most common malignancy of the larynx, occurs almost exclusively in patients with a history of significant tobacco use, and often with alcohol. SCC is usually seen in men age 50–70 years; about 13,000 new cases are seen in United States each year. A change in voice quality is most often the presenting complaint, although throat or ear pain, hemoptysis, dysphagia, weight loss, and airway compromise may occur. Neck metastases are not common in early glottic (true vocal fold) cancer in which the vocal folds are mobile, but a third of patients in whom there is impaired fold mobility will also have involved lymph nodes at neck dissection. Supraglottic carcinoma (false vocal folds, aryepiglottic folds, epiglottis), on the other hand, often metastasizes to both sides of the neck early in the disease. Complete head and neck examination, including laryngoscopy, by an experienced clinician is mandated for any person with the concerning symptoms listed under Essentials of Diagnosis.

B. Imaging and Laboratory Studies

Radiologic evaluation by CT or MRI is helpful in assessing tumor extent. Imaging evaluates neck nodes, tumor volume, and cartilage sclerosis or destruction. A chest CT scan is indicated if there are level VI enlarged nodes (around the trachea and the thyroid gland) or IV enlarged nodes (inferior to the cricoid cartilage along the internal jugular vein) or if a chest film is concerning for a second primary lesion or metastases. Laboratory evaluation includes complete blood count and liver function tests. Formal cardiopulmonary evaluation may be indicated, especially if partial laryngeal surgery is being considered. A positron emission tomography (PET) scan or CT-PET scan may be indicated to assess for distant metastases when there appears to be advanced local or regional disease.

C. Biopsy

Diagnosis is made by biopsy at the time of laryngoscopy. At that time, true fold mobility and arytenoid fixation, as well as surface tumor extent, can be evaluated. Most otolaryngologists recommend flexible esophagoscopy and flexible bronchoscopy at the same time to exclude synchronous primary tumor. Although an FNA biopsy of an enlarged neck node may have already been done, it is generally acceptable to assume radiographically enlarged neck nodes (> 1–1.5 cm) or nodes with necrotic centers are neck metastases. Open biopsies of nodal metastases should be discouraged because they may lead to higher rates of tumor treatment failure.

D. Tumor Staging

Staging is helpful in discussing laryngeal cancer, but a number of factors that are not included in the TNM staging are also important in deciding treatment recommendations.

▸ Treatment

Treatment of laryngeal carcinoma has four goals: cure, preservation of safe effective swallowing, preservation of useful voice, and avoidance of a permanent tracheostoma. For early glottic and supraglottic cancers, radiation therapy is the standard of care since cure rates are greater than 95% and 80%, respectively. That said, radiation therapy carries substantial morbidity and many early tumors (T1 and T2 lesions, without involved nodes) and selected advanced tumors (T3 and T4) may be treated with partial laryngectomy if at least one cricoarytenoid unit can be preserved. Five-year locoregional cure rates exceed 80–90% with surgery, and patient-reported satisfaction is excellent. In supraglottic tumors, even when clinically N0, elective limited neck dissection is indicated following surgical resection because of the high risk of neck node involvement.

For very advanced tumors, cisplatin-based chemoradiation protocols are used. Twenty-five years ago, total laryngectomy was often recommended for such patients. However, the 1994 VA study (with induction cisplatin and 5-fluorouracil followed by irradiation alone in responders) demonstrated that two-thirds of patients could preserve their larynx. Since that study, cisplatin-based chemotherapy concomitant with radiation therapy has been shown to be superior to either irradiation alone or induction chemotherapy followed by radiation. However, chemoradiation is associated with prolonged gastrostomy-dependent dysphagia. This high rate of chemoradiation-associated dysphagia has prompted a reevaluation of the role of extended, but less-than-total, laryngeal surgery for selected advanced laryngeal carcinoma in which at least one cricoarytenoid unit is intact. In addition, overall success in the treatment of larynx cancer has declined in parallel with the increase in organ preservation chemoradiation therapy. Some experts have proposed that this decline is the direct result of the shift in management of advanced laryngeal cancer away from surgery. Organ preservation surgery should be considered and discussed as an alternative to chemoradiation. Patient comorbidities and patient choice, after thorough discussion, play an important role in the choice between surgery and chemoradiation. The patient and treating clinicians must carefully consider *different* side effects and complications associated with different treatment modalities.

The presence of malignant adenopathy in the neck affects the prognosis greatly. Supraglottic tumors metastasize early and bilaterally to the neck, and this must be included in the treatment plans even when the neck is apparently uninvolved. Glottic tumors in which the true vocal folds are mobile (T1 or T2) have less than a 5% rate of nodal involvement; when a fold is immobile, the rate of ipsilateral nodal involvement climbs to about 30%. An involved neck is treated by surgery or chemoradiation, or both. This decision will depend on the treatment chosen for the larynx and the extent of neck involvement.

Total laryngectomy is largely reserved for patients with far-advanced resectable tumors with extralaryngeal spread or cartilage involvement, for those with persistent tumor following chemoradiation, and for patients with recurrent or second primary tumor following previous radiation therapy. Voice rehabilitation via a primary (or at times secondary) tracheoesophageal puncture produces intelligible and serviceable speech in about 75–85% of patients. Indwelling prostheses that are changed every 3–6 months are a common alternative to patient-inserted prostheses, which need changing more frequently.

Long-term follow-up is critical in head and neck cancer patients. In addition to the 3–4% annual rate of second tumors and monitoring for recurrence, psychosocial aspects of treatment are common. Dysphagia, impaired communication, and altered appearance, may result in patient difficulties adapting to the workplace and to social interactions. In addition, smoking cessation and alcohol abatement are common challenges. Nevertheless, about 65% of patients with larynx cancer are cured, most have useful speech, and many resume their prior livelihoods with adaptations.

Agrawal A et al. Transoral carbon dioxide laser supraglottic laryngectomy and irradiation in stage I, II, and III squamous cell carcinoma of the supraglottic larynx: report of Southwest Oncology Group Phase 2 Trial S9709. Arch Otolaryngol Head Neck Surg. 2007 Oct;133(10):1044–50. [PMID: 17938330]

Bernier J et al; European Organization for Research and Treatment of Cancer Trial 22931. Postoperative irradiation with or without concomitant chemotherapy for locally advanced head and neck cancer. N Engl J Med. 2004 May 6;350(19):1945–52. [PMID: 15128894]

Ganly I et al. Results of surgical salvage after failure of definitive radiation therapy for early-stage squamous cell carcinoma of the glottic larynx. Arch Otolaryngol Head Neck Surg. 2006 Jan;132(1):59–66. [PMID: 16415431]

Hashibe M et al. Alcohol drinking in never users of tobacco, cigarette smoking in never drinkers, and the risk of head and neck cancer: pooled analysis in the International Head and Neck Cancer Epidemiology Consortium. J Natl Cancer Inst. 2007 May 16;99(10):777–89. [PMID: 17505073]

Hoffman HT et al. Laryngeal cancer in the United States: changes in demographics, patterns of care, and survival. Laryngoscope. 2006 Sep;116(9 Pt 2 Suppl 111):1–13. [PMID: 16946667]

VOCAL FOLD PARALYSIS

Vocal fold paralysis can result from a lesion or damage to either the vagus or recurrent laryngeal nerve and usually results in breathy dysphonia and effortful voicing. Common causes of unilateral recurrent laryngeal nerve involvement include thyroid surgery (and occasionally thyroid cancer), other neck surgery (anterior discectomy and carotid endarterectomy), and mediastinal or apical involvement by lung cancer. Skull base tumors often involve or abut upon lower cranial nerves and may affect the vagus nerve directly, or the vagus nerve may be damaged during surgical management of the lesion. While iatrogenic injury is the most common cause of unilateral vocal fold paralysis, the second most common cause is idiopathic. However, before deciding whether the paralysis is due to iatrogenic injury or is idiopathic, the clinician must exclude other causes, such as malignancy. In the absence of other cranial neuropathies, a CT scan with contrast from the skull base to the aorto-pulmonary window (the span of the recurrent laryngeal nerve) should be performed. If other cranial nerve deficits are noted, a MRI scan of the brain and brainstem is warranted.

Unlike unilateral fold paralysis, bilateral fold paralysis usually causes inspiratory stridor with deep inspiration. If the onset of bilateral fold paralysis is insidious, it may be asymptomatic at rest and the patient may have a normal voice. However, the acute onset of bilateral vocal fold paralysis with inspiratory stridor at rest should be managed by a specialist immediately in a critical care environment. Causes of bilateral fold paralysis include thyroid surgery, esophageal cancer, and ventricular shunt malfunction. Unilateral or bilateral fold immobility may also be seen in cricoarytenoid arthritis secondary to advanced rheumatoid arthritis, intubation injuries, glottic and subglottic stenosis and, of course, laryngeal cancer. The goal of intervention is the creation of a safe airway with minimal reduction in voice quality and airway protection from aspiration. A number of fold lateralization procedures for bilateral paralysis have been advocated as a means of removing the tracheotomy tube.

Unilateral vocal fold paralysis is occasionally temporary and may take over a year to resolve spontaneously. Surgical management of persistent or irrecoverable symptomatic unilateral vocal fold paralysis has evolved over the last several decades. The primary goal is medialization of the paralyzed fold in order to create a stable platform for vocal fold vibration. Additional goals include improving pulmonary toilet by facilitating of cough and advancing diet. Success has been reported for years with injection laryngoplasty using Teflon, Gelfoam, fat and collagen. Teflon is the only permanent injectable material, but its use is discouraged because of granuloma formation within the vocal folds of some patients. Temporary injectable materials, such as collagen or fat, provide excellent temporary restoration of voice and can be placed under local or general anesthesia. Once the paralysis is determined to be permanent, formal medialization thyroplasty may be performed by creating a small window in the thyroid cartilage and placing an implant between the thyroarytenoid muscle and inner table of the thyroid cartilage. This procedure moves the vocal fold medially and creates a stable platform for bilateral, symmetric mucosal vibration.

Ollivere B et al. Swallowing dysfunction in patients with unilateral vocal fold paralysis: aetiology and outcomes. J Laryngol Otol. 2006 Jan;120(1):38–41. [PMID: 16359143]

Sulica L et al. Vocal fold paralysis. Otolaryngol Clin North Am. 2004 Feb;37(1):xi–xiv. [PMID: 15062695]

TRACHEOSTOMY & CRICOTHYROTOMY

There are two primary indications for tracheostomy: airway obstruction at or above the level of the larynx and respiratory failure requiring prolonged mechanical ventilation. In an acute emergency, cricothyrotomy secures an airway more rapidly than tracheostomy, with fewer potential immediate complications such as pneumothorax and hemorrhage. Percutaneous dilatational tracheostomy as an elective bedside (or intensive care unit) procedure has undergone scrutiny in recent years as an alternative to tracheostomy. In experienced hands, the various methods of percutaneous tracheostomy have been documented to be safe in carefully selected patients. Simultaneous video-bronchoscopy can reduce the incidence of major complications. The major cost reduction comes from avoiding the operating room. Bedside tracheostomy (in the intensive care unit) achieves similar cost reduction and is advocated by some experts as slightly less costly than the percutaneous procedures.

The most common indication for elective tracheostomy is the need for prolonged mechanical ventilation. There is no firm rule about how many days a patient must be intubated before conversion to tracheostomy should be advised. The incidence of serious complications such as subglottic stenosis increases with extended endotracheal intubation. As soon as it is apparent that the patient will require protracted ventilatory support, tracheostomy should replace the endotracheal tube. Less frequent indications for tracheostomy are life-threatening aspiration pneumonia, the need to improve pulmonary toilet to correct problems related to insufficient clearing of tracheobronchial secretions, and sleep apnea.

Posttracheostomy care requires humidified air to prevent secretions from crusting and occluding the inner cannula of the tracheostomy tube. The tracheostomy tube should be cleaned several times daily. The most frequent early complication of tracheostomy is dislodgment of the tracheostomy tube. Surgical creation of an inferiorly based tracheal flap sutured to the inferior neck skin may make reinsertion of a dislodged tube easier. It should be recalled that the act of swallowing requires elevation of the larynx, which is limited by tracheostomy. Therefore, frequent tracheal and bronchial suctioning is often required to clear the aspirated saliva as well as the increased tracheobronchial secretions. Care of the skin around the stoma is important to prevent maceration and secondary infection.

Epstein SK. Late complications of tracheostomy. Respir Care. 2005 Apr;50(4):542–9. [PMID: 15807919]

Groves DS et al. Tracheostomy in the critically ill: indications, timing and techniques. Curr Opin Crit Care. 2007 Feb; 13(1):90–7. [PMID: 17198055]

Homewood J et al. Tracheostomy care. Br J Hosp Med (Lond). 2005 Nov;66(11):M72–3. [PMID: 16308953]

FOREIGN BODIES IN THE UPPER AERODIGESTIVE TRACT

FOREIGN BODIES OF THE TRACHEA & BRONCHI

Aspiration of foreign bodies occurs less frequently in adults than in children. The elderly and denture wearers appear to be at greatest risk. Wider familiarity with the Heimlich maneuver has reduced deaths. If the maneuver is unsuccess-ful, cricothyrotomy may be necessary. Plain chest radiographs may reveal a radiopaque foreign body. Detection of radiolucent foreign bodies may be aided by inspiration-expiration films that demonstrate air trapping distal to the obstructed segment. Atelectasis and pneumonia may occur later.

Tracheal and bronchial foreign bodies should be removed under general anesthesia by a skilled endoscopist working with an experienced anesthesiologist.

Digoy GP. Diagnosis and management of upper aerodigestive tract foreign bodies. Otolaryngol Clin North Am. 2008 Jun;41(3):485–96. [PMID: 18435994]

ESOPHAGEAL FOREIGN BODIES

Foreign bodies in the esophagus create urgent but not life-threatening situations as long as the airway is not compromised. There is probably time to consult an experienced clinician for management. Patients are likely to have difficulty handling secretions and may be spitting out their saliva. It is a useful diagnostic sign of complete obstruction if the patient is drooling or cannot handle secretions. They may often point to the exact level of the obstruction. Indirect laryngoscopy often shows pooling of saliva at the esophageal inlet. Plain films may detect radiopaque foreign bodies such as chicken bones. Coins tend to align in the coronal plane in the esophagus and sagittally in the trachea. If a foreign body is suspected, a barium swallow may help make the diagnosis.

The treatment of an esophageal foreign body depends very much on identification of its nature. In children, swallowed nonfood objects are common. In adults, however, food foreign bodies are more common, and there is the greater possibility of underlying esophageal pathology. Endoscopic removal and examination is usually best, via flexible esophagoscopy or rigid laryngoscopy and esophagoscopy. If there is nothing sharp such as a bone, some clinicians advocate a hospitalized 24-hour observation period prior to esophagoscopy, noting that spontaneous passage of the foreign body will occur in 50% of adult patients. In the management of meat obstruction, the use of papain (meat tenderizer) should be discouraged because it can damage the esophageal mucosa. Obstruction may sometimes occur from a metal stent placed in the treatment of esophageal cancer.

Weissberg D et al. Foreign bodies in the esophagus. Ann Thorac Surg. 2007 Dec;84(6):1854–7. [PMID: 18036898]

DISEASES PRESENTING AS NECK MASSES

The differential diagnosis of neck masses is heavily dependent on the location in the neck, the age of the patient, and the presence of associated disease processes. Rapid growth and tenderness suggest an inflammatory process, while firm, painless, and slowly enlarging masses are often neoplastic. In young adults, most neck masses are benign (branchial cleft cyst, thyroglossal duct cyst, reactive lymphadenitis), although malignancy should always be considered (lymphoma, metastatic thyroid carcinoma). Lymphadenopathy is common in HIV-positive persons, but a growing or dominant mass may well represent lymphoma. In adults over age 40, cancer is the most common cause of persistent neck mass. A metastasis from SCC arising within the mouth, pharynx, larynx, or upper esophagus should be suspected, especially if there is a history of tobacco or significant alcohol use. Especially among patients younger than 30 or older than 70, lymphoma should be considered. In any case, a comprehensive otolaryngologic examination is needed. Cytologic evaluation of the neck mass via FNA biopsy is likely to be the next step if an obvious primary tumor is not obvious on physical examination.

CONGENITAL LESIONS PRESENTING AS NECK MASSES IN ADULTS

1. Branchial Cleft Cysts

Branchial cleft cysts usually present as a soft cystic mass along the anterior border of the sternocleidomastoid muscle. These lesions are usually recognized in the second or third decades of life, often when they suddenly swell or become infected. To prevent recurrent infection and possible carcinoma, they should be completely excised, along with their fistulous tracts.

First branchial cleft cysts present high in the neck, sometimes just below the ear. A fistulous connection with the floor of the external auditory canal may be present. Second branchial cleft cysts, which are far more common, may communicate with the tonsillar fossa. Third branchial cleft cysts, which may communicate with the piriform sinus, are rare.

Acierno SP et al. Congenital cervical cysts, sinuses and fistulae. Otolaryngol Clin North Am. 2007 Feb;40(1):161–76. [PMID: 17346566]

2. Thyroglossal Duct Cysts

Thyroglossal duct cysts occur along the embryologic course of the thyroid's descent from the tuberculum impar of the tongue base to its usual position in the low neck. Although they may occur at any age, they are most common before age 20. They present as a midline neck mass, often just below the hyoid bone, which moves with swallowing. Surgical excision is recommended to prevent recurrent infection. This requires removal of the entire fistulous tract along with the middle portion of the hyoid bone through which many of the fistulas pass. Preoperative evaluation should include a thyroid ultrasound to confirm anatomic position of the thyroid.

Lin ST et al. Thyroglossal duct cyst: a comparison between children and adults. Am J Otolaryngol. 2008 Mar–Apr;29(2):83–7. [PMID: 18314017]

INFECTIOUS & INFLAMMATORY NECK MASSES

1. Reactive Cervical Lymphadenopathy

Normal lymph nodes in the neck are usually less than 1 cm in length. Infections involving the pharynx, salivary glands, and scalp often cause tender enlargement of neck nodes. Enlarged nodes are common in HIV-infected persons. Except for the occasional node that suppurates and requires incision and drainage, treatment is directed against the underlying infection. An enlarged node (> 1.5 cm) or node with a necrotic center that is not associated with an obvious infection should be further evaluated, especially if the patient has a history of smoking, alcohol use, or prior cancer. Other common indications for FNA biopsy of a node include its persistence or continued enlargement. Common causes of cervical adenopathy include tumor (SCC, lymphoma, occasional metastases from non-head and neck sites) and infection (eg, reactive nodes, mycobacteria [discussed below], and cat scratch disease). Rare causes of adenopathy include Kikuchi disease (histiocytic necrotizing lymphadenitis) and autoimmune adenopathy.

Ridder GJ et al. Role of cat-scratch disease in lymphadenopathy in the head and neck. Clin Infect Dis. 2002 Sep 15;35(6):643–9. [PMID: 12203159]

2. Tuberculous & Nontuberculous Mycobacterial Lymphadenitis

Granulomatous neck masses are not uncommon. The differential diagnosis includes mycobacterial adenitis, sarcoidosis, and cat-scratch disease due to *Bartonella henselae*. Although mycobacterial adenitis can extend to the skin and drain externally (as described for atypical mycobacteria and referred to as scrofula), this late presentation is no longer common. The usual presentation of granulomatous disease in the neck is simply single or matted nodes. FNA biopsy is usually the best initial diagnostic approach: cytology, smear for acid-fast bacilli, culture, and sensitivity test; and polymerase chain reaction (PCR) can all be done.

Mycobacterial lymphadenitis is on the rise both in immunocompromised and immunocompetent individuals. Identification of *Mycobacterium tuberculosis* can usually be confirmed by a combination of FNA smear and culture, but excisional biopsy of a node may be needed. PCR from FNA (or from excised tissue) is the single most sensitive test and is particularly useful when conventional methods have not been diagnostic but clinical impression remains consistent for tuberculous infection.

Short-course therapy (6 months) consisting of an initial 4 months of streptomycin, isoniazid, rifampin, and pyrazinamide followed by 2 months of rifampin is the current recommended treatment for tuberculous lymphadenopathy (see Table 9–11). For atypical (nontuberculous) lymphadenopathy, treatment depends on sensitivity results of culture, but antibiotics likely to be useful include 6 months of isoniazid and rifampin and, for at least the first 2 months, ethambutol—all in standard dosages. Some would totally excise the involved nodes prior to chemotherapy, depending on location and other factors, but this can lead to chronic draining fistulas.

Koo V et al. Fine needle aspiration cytology (FNAC) in the diagnosis of granulomatous lymphadenitis. Ulster Med J. 2006 Jan;75(1):59–64. [PMID: 16457406]

Polesky A et al. Peripheral tuberculous lymphadenitis: epidemiology, diagnosis, treatment, and outcome. Medicine (Baltimore). 2005 Nov;84(6):350–62. [PMID: 16267410]

3. Lyme Disease

Lyme disease, caused by the spirochete *Borrelia burgdorferi* and transmitted by ticks of the *Ixodes* genus, may have protean manifestation, but over 75% of patients have symptoms involving the head and neck. Facial paralysis, dysesthesias, dysgeusia, or other cranial neuropathies are most common. Headache, pain, and cervical lymphadenopathy may occur. See Chapter 34 for a more detailed discussion.

DePietropaolo DL et al. Diagnosis of Lyme disease. Am Fam Physician. 2005 Jul 15;72(2):297–304. [PMID: 16050454]

Ljostad U et al. Acute peripheral facial palsy in adults. J Neurol. 2005 Jun;252(6):672–6. [PMID: 15778908]

TUMOR METASTASES

In older adults, 80% of firm, persistent, and enlarging neck masses are metastatic in origin. The great majority of these arise from SCC of the upper aerodigestive tract. A complete head and neck examination may reveal the tumor of origin, but examination under anesthesia with direct laryngoscopy, esophagoscopy, and bronchoscopy is usually required to fully evaluate the tumor and exclude second primaries.

It is often helpful to obtain a cytologic diagnosis if initial head and neck examination fails to reveal the primary tumor. An open biopsy should be done only when neither physical examination by an experienced clinician specializing in head and neck cancer nor FNA biopsy performed by an experienced cytopathologist yields a diagnosis. In such a setting, one should strongly consider obtaining an MRI or PET scan prior to open biopsy, as these methods may yield valuable information about a possible presumed primary site or another site for FNA.

With the exception of papillary thyroid carcinoma, non–squamous cell metastases to the neck are infrequent. While tumors that are not primary in the head or neck seldom metastasize to the cervical lymph nodes, the supraclavicular lymph nodes are quite often involved by lung, gastroesophageal, and breast tumors. Infradiaphragmatic tumors, with the exception of renal cell carcinoma and testicular cancer, rarely metastasize to the neck.

Barzilai G et al. Pattern of regional metastases from cutaneous squamous cell carcinoma of the head and neck. Otolaryngol Head Neck Surg. 2005 Jun;132(6):852–6. [PMID: 15944554]

Landry CS et al. The evolution of the management of regional lymph nodes in melanoma. J Surg Oncol. 2007 Sep 15;96(4):316–21. [PMID: 17879333]

LYMPHOMA

About 10% of lymphomas present in the head and neck. Lymphoma arising in AIDS patients is an increasing concern. Multiple rubbery nodes, especially in the young adult, are suggestive of this disease. A thorough physical examination may demonstrate other sites of nodal or organ involvement. FNA biopsy may be diagnostic, but open biopsy is often required to determine architecture and an appropriate treatment course.

Howlett DC et al. Diagnostic adequacy and accuracy of fine needle aspiration cytology in neck lump assessment: results from a regional cancer network over a one year period. J Laryngol Otol. 2007 Jun;121(6):571–9. [PMID: 17134537]

Pulmonary Disorders

Mark S. Chesnutt, MD
Alex H. Gifford, MD
Thomas J. Prendergast, MD

DISORDERS OF THE AIRWAYS

Airway disorders have diverse causes but share certain common pathophysiologic and clinical features. Airflow limitation is characteristic and frequently causes dyspnea and cough. Other symptoms are common and typically disease-specific. Disorders of the airways can be classified as those that involve the upper airways—loosely defined as those above and including the vocal folds—and those that involve the lower airways.

DISORDERS OF THE UPPER AIRWAYS

Upper airway obstruction may occur acutely or present as a chronic condition. **Acute upper airway obstruction** can be immediately life-threatening and must be relieved promptly to avoid asphyxia. Causes of acute upper airway obstruction include trauma to the larynx or pharynx, foreign body aspiration, laryngospasm, laryngeal edema from thermal injury or angioedema, infections (acute epiglottitis, Ludwig angina, pharyngeal or retropharyngeal abscess), and acute allergic laryngitis.

Chronic obstruction of the upper airway may be caused by carcinoma of the pharynx or larynx, laryngeal or subglottic stenosis, laryngeal granulomas or webs, or bilateral vocal fold paralysis. Laryngeal or subglottic stenosis may become evident weeks or months following a period of translaryngeal endotracheal intubation. Inspiratory stridor, intercostal retractions on inspiration, a palpable inspiratory thrill over the larynx, and wheezing localized to the neck or trachea on auscultation are characteristic findings. Flow-volume loops may show flow limitations characteristic of obstruction. Soft tissue radiographs of the neck may show supraglottic or infraglottic narrowing. CT and MRI scans can reveal exact sites of obstruction. Flexible endoscopy may be diagnostic, but caution is necessary to avoid exacerbating upper airway edema and precipitating critical airway narrowing.

Vocal fold dysfunction syndrome is a condition characterized by paradoxical vocal fold adduction, resulting in both acute and chronic upper airway obstruction. It can cause dyspnea and wheezing that may present as asthma or exercise-induced asthma but may be distinguished from asthma by the lack of response to bronchodilator therapy, normal spirometry immediately after an attack, spirometric evidence of upper airway obstruction, a negative bronchial provocation test, or direct visualization of adduction of the vocal folds on both inspiration and expiration. The condition appears to be psychogenic in nature. Bronchodilators are of no therapeutic benefit. Treatment consists of speech therapy, which uses breathing, voice, and neck relaxation exercises to abort the symptoms.

Mikita JA et al. Vocal cord dysfunction. Allergy Asthma Proc. 2006 Jul–Aug;27(4):411–4. [PMID: 16948360]
Sohrab S et al. Management of central airway obstruction. Clin Lung Cancer. 2007 Mar;8(5):305–12. [PMID: 17562229]

DISORDERS OF THE LOWER AIRWAYS

Tracheal obstruction may be intrathoracic (below the suprasternal notch) or extrathoracic. Fixed tracheal obstruction may be caused by acquired or congenital tracheal stenosis, primary or secondary tracheal neoplasms, extrinsic compression (tumors of the lung, thymus, or thyroid; lymphadenopathy; congenital vascular rings; aneurysms, etc), foreign body aspiration, tracheal granulomas and papillomas, and tracheal trauma.

Acquired **tracheal stenosis** is usually secondary to previous tracheotomy or endotracheal intubation. Dyspnea, cough, and inability to clear pulmonary secretions occur weeks to months after tracheal decannulation or extubation. Physical findings may be absent until tracheal diameter is reduced 50% or more, when wheezing, a palpable tracheal thrill, and harsh breath sounds may be detected. The diagnosis is usually confirmed by plain films or CT of the trachea. Complications include recurring pulmonary infection and life-threatening respiratory failure. Management is directed toward ensuring adequate ventilation and oxygenation and avoiding manipulative procedures that may increase edema of the tracheal mucosa. Surgical reconstruction, endotracheal stent placement, or laser photoresection may be required.

Bronchial obstruction may be caused by retained pulmonary secretions, aspiration, foreign bodies, bronchogenic carcinoma, compression by extrinsic masses, and tumors metastatic to the airway. Clinical and radiographic findings vary depending on the location of the obstruction and the degree of airway narrowing. Symptoms include dyspnea, cough, wheezing, and, if infection is present, fever and chills. A history of recurrent pneumonia in the same lobe or segment or slow resolution (> 3 months) of pneumonia on successive radiographs suggests the possibility of bronchial obstruction and the need for bronchoscopy.

Roentgenographic findings include **atelectasis** (local parenchymal collapse), postobstructive infiltrates, and air trapping caused by unidirectional expiratory obstruction. CT scanning may demonstrate the nature and the exact location of obstruction of the central bronchi. MRI may be superior to CT for delineating the extent of underlying disease in the hilum, but it is usually reserved for cases in which CT findings are equivocal. Bronchoscopy is the definitive diagnostic study, particularly if tumor or foreign body aspiration is suspected. The finding of bronchial breath sounds on physical examination or an air bronchogram on chest radiograph in an area of atelectasis rules out complete airway obstruction. Bronchoscopy is unlikely to be of therapeutic benefit in this situation.

Right middle lobe syndrome is recurrent or persistent atelectasis of the right middle lobe. This collapse is related to the relatively long length and narrow diameter of the right middle lobe bronchus and the oval ("fish mouth") opening to the lobe, in the setting of impaired collateral ventilation. Fiberoptic bronchoscopy or CT scan is often necessary to rule out obstructing tumor. Foreign body or other benign causes are common.

Duggan M et al. Pulmonary atelectasis: a pathogenic perioperative entity. Anesthesiology. 2005 Apr;102(4):838–54. [PMID: 15791115]
Kwon KY et al. Middle lobe syndrome: a clinicopathological study of 21 patients. Hum Pathol. 1995 Mar;26(3):302–7. [PMID: 7890282]

ASTHMA

ESSENTIALS OF DIAGNOSIS

▶ Episodic or chronic symptoms of airflow obstruction: breathlessness, chest tightness, wheezing, and cough.

▶ Complete or partial reversibility of airflow obstruction, either spontaneously or following bronchodilator therapy.

▶ Symptoms frequently worse at night or in the early morning.

▶ Prolonged expiration and diffuse wheezes on physical examination.

▶ Limitation of airflow on pulmonary function testing or positive bronchoprovocation challenge.

▶ General Considerations

Asthma is a common disease, affecting approximately 5% of the population. It is slightly more common in male

children (< 14 years old) and in female adults. A genetic predisposition to asthma is recognized. Prevalence, hospitalizations, and fatal asthma have all increased in the United States over the past 20 years. Each year, approximately 470,000 hospital admissions and 5000 deaths in the United States are attributed to asthma. Hospitalization rates have been highest among blacks and children, and death rates for asthma are consistently highest among blacks aged 15–24 years.

▶ Definition & Pathogenesis

Asthma is a chronic inflammatory disorder of the airways. No single histopathologic feature is pathognomonic but common findings include inflammatory cell infiltration with eosinophils, neutrophils, and lymphocytes (especially T lymphocytes); goblet cell hyperplasia, sometimes with plugging of small airways with thick mucus; collagen deposition beneath the basement membrane; hypertrophy of bronchial smooth muscle; airway edema; mast cell activation; and denudation of airway epithelium. This airway inflammation underlies disease chronicity and contributes to airway hyper-responsiveness, airflow limitation, and respiratory symptoms, including recurrent episodes of wheezing, breathlessness, chest tightness, and cough.

The strongest identifiable predisposing factor for the development of asthma is atopy, but obesity is increasingly recognized as a risk factor. Exposure of sensitive patients to inhaled allergens increases airway inflammation, airway hyper-responsiveness, and symptoms. Symptoms may develop immediately (immediate asthmatic response) or 4–6 hours after allergen exposure (late asthmatic response). Common allergens include house dust mites (often found in pillows, mattresses, upholstered furniture, carpets, and drapes), cockroaches, cat dander, and seasonal pollens. Substantially reducing exposure reduces pathologic findings and clinical symptoms.

Nonspecific precipitants of asthma include exercise, upper respiratory tract infections, rhinitis, sinusitis, postnasal drip, aspiration, gastroesophageal reflux, changes in the weather, and stress. Exposure to environmental tobacco smoke increases asthma symptoms and the need for medications and reduces lung function. Increased air levels of respirable particles, ozone, SO_2, and NO_2 precipitate asthma symptoms and increase emergency department visits and hospitalizations. Selected individuals may experience asthma symptoms after exposure to aspirin, nonsteroidal anti-inflammatory drugs, or tartrazine dyes. Certain other medications may also precipitate asthma symptoms (see Table 9–21). Occupational asthma is triggered by various agents in the workplace and may occur weeks to years after initial exposure and sensitization. Women may experience catamenial asthma at predictable times during the menstrual cycle. Exercise-induced bronchoconstriction begins during exercise or within 3 minutes after its end, peaks within 10–15 minutes, and then resolves by 60 minutes. This phenomenon is thought to be a consequence of the airways' attempt to warm and humidify an increased volume of expired air during exer-

Components of Severity		Classification of Asthma Severity $\geq$ 12 years of age			
			Persistent		
		Intermittent	Mild	Moderate	Severe
Impairment Normal FEV$_1$/FVC: 8–19 yr 85% 20–39 yr 80% 40–59 yr 75% 60–80 yr 70%	Symptoms	$\leq$ 2 days/week	> 2 days/week but not daily	Daily	Throughout the day
	Nighttime awakenings	$\leq$ 2x/month	3–4x/month	> 1x/week but not nightly	Often 7x/week
	Short-acting β_2-agonist use for symptom control (not prevention of EIB)	$\leq$ 2 days/week	> 2 days/week but not daily, and not more than 1x on any day	Daily	Several times per day
	Interference with normal activity	None	Minor limitation	Some limitation	Extremely limited
	Lung function	• Normal FEV$_1$ between exacerbations • FEV$_1$ > 80% predicted • FEV$_1$/FVC normal	• FEV$_1$ > 80% predicted • FEV$_1$/FVC normal	• FEV$_1$ > 60% but < 80% predicted • FEV$_1$/FVC reduced 5%	• FEV$_1$ < 60% predicted • FEV$_1$/FVC reduced > 5%
Risk	Exacerbations requiring oral systemic corticosteroids	0–1/year (see note)	$\geq$ 2/year (see note) ———————————————————→		
			←——————— Consider severity and interval since last exacerbation. ———————————→ Frequency and severity may fluctuate over time for patients in any severity category. Relative annual risk of exacerbations may be related to FEV$_1$.		
Recommended Step for Initiating Treatment (See Figure 9–2 for treatment steps.)		Step 1	Step 2	Step 3 and consider short course of oral systemic corticosteroids	Step 4 or 5
		In 2–6 weeks, evaluate level of asthma control that is achieved and adjust therapy accordingly.			

EIB, exercise-induced bronchospasm; FEV$_1$, forced expiratory volume in 1 second; FVC, forced vital capacity; ICU, intensive care unit.

Notes:
- The stepwise approach is meant to assist, not replace, the clinical decision-making required to meet individual patient needs.

- Level of severity is determined by assessment of both impairment and risk. Assess impairment domain by patient's/caregiver's recall of previous 2–4 weeks and spirometry. Assign severity to the most severe category in which any feature occurs.

- At present, there are inadequate data to correspond frequencies of exacerbations with different levels of asthma severity. In general, more frequent and intense exacerbations (eg, requiring urgent, unscheduled care, hospitalization, or ICU admission) indicate greater underlying disease severity. For treatment purposes, patients who had $\geq$ 2 exacerbations requiring oral systemic corticosteroids in the past year may be considered the same as patients who have persistent asthma, even in the absence of impairment levels consistent with persistent asthma.

▲ **Figure 9–1.** Classifying asthma severity and initiating treatment. (Adapted from National Asthma Education and Prevention Program. Expert Panel Report 3: Guidelines for the Diagnosis and Management of Asthma. National Institutes of Health Pub. No. 08-4051. Bethesda, MD, 2007. http://www.nhlbi.nih.gov/guidelines/asthma/asthgdln.htm.)

cise. "Cardiac asthma" is wheezing precipitated by uncompensated congestive heart failure.

Clinical Findings

Symptoms and signs vary widely from patient to patient as well as individually over time. General clinical findings in stable asthma patients are listed in Figure 9–1 and Table 9–1;

findings seen during asthma exacerbations are listed in Tables 9–2 and 9–3.

A. Symptoms and Signs

Asthma is characterized by episodic wheezing, difficulty in breathing, chest tightness, and cough. Excess sputum production is common. The frequency of asthma symptoms is

Table 9–1. Assessing asthma control.

Components of Control		Classification of Asthma Control (≥ 12 years of age)		
		Well Controlled	Not Well Controlled	Very Poorly Controlled
Impairment	Symptoms	≤ 2 days/week	> 2 days/week	Throughout the day
	Nighttime awakenings	≤ 2×/month	1–3×/week	≥ 4×/week
	Interference with normal activity	None	Some limitation	Extremely limited
	Short-acting β_2-agonist use for symptom control (not prevention of EIB)	≤ 2 days/week	>2 days/week	Several times/day
	FEV_1 or peak flow	> 80% predicted/personal best	60–80% predicted/personal best	< 60% predicted/personal best
	Validated questionnaires			
	ATAQ	0	1–2	3–4
	ACQ	≤ 0.75[1]	≥ 1.5	N/A
	ACT	≥ 20	16–19	≤ 15
Risk	Exacerbations requiring oral system corticosteroids	0–1/year	≥ 2/year (see note)	
		Consider severity and interval since last exacerbation		
	Progressive loss of lung function	Evaluation requires long-term follow-up care		
	Treatment-related adverse effects	Medication side effects can vary in intensity from none to very troublesome and worrisome. The level of intensity does not correlate to specific levels of control but should be considered in the overall assessment of risk.		
Recommended Action for Treatment (see Figure 9–2 for steps)		• Maintain current step • Regular follow-ups every 1–6 months to maintain control. • Consider step down if well controlled for at least 3 months.	• Step up 1 step and • Reevaluate in 2–6 weeks. • For side effects, consider alternative treatment options.	• Consider short course of oral systemic corticosteroids, • Step up 1–2 steps, and • Reevaluate in 2 weeks. • For side effects, consider alternative treatment options.

[1]ACQ values of 0.76–1.4 are indeterminate regarding well-controlled asthma.

EIB, exercise-induced bronchospasm; ICU, intensive care unit.

Notes:

· The stepwise approach is meant to assist, not replace, the clinical decision-making required to meet individual patient needs.

· The level of control is based on the most severe impairment or risk category. Assess impairment domain by patient's recall of previous 2–4 weeks and by spirometry or peak flow measures. Symptom assessment for longer periods should reflect a global assessment, such as inquiring whether the patient's asthma is better or worse since the last visit.

· At present, there are inadequate data to correspond frequencies of exacerbations with different levels of asthma control. In general, more frequent and intense exacerbations (eg, requiring urgent, unscheduled care, hospitalization, or ICU admission) indicate poorer disease control. For treatment purposes, patients who had ≥ 2 exacerbations requiring oral systemic corticosteroids in the past year may be considered the same as patients who have not-well-controlled asthma, even in the absence of impairment levels consistent with not-well-controlled asthma.

· Validated Questionnaires for the impairment domain (the questionnaire did not assess lung function or the risk domain).

  ATAQ = Asthma Therapy Assessment Questionnaire©

  ACQ = Asthma Control Questionnaire© (user package may be obtained at www.qoltech.co.uk or juniper@qoltech.co.uk)

  ACT = Asthma Control Test™

  Minimal Importance Difference: 1.0 for the ATAQ; 0.5 for the ACQ; not determined for the ACT.

· Before step up in therapy:

  —Review adherence to medication, inhaler.

  —If an alternative treatment option was used in a step, discontinue and use the preferred treatment for that step.

Adapted from National Asthma Education and Prevention Program. Expert Panel Report 3: Guidelines for the Diagnosis and Management of Asthma. National Institutes of Health Pub. No. 08-4051. Bethesda, MD, 2007. www.nhlbi/nih.gov/guidelines/asthma/asthgdln.htm.

highly variable. Some patients have infrequent, brief attacks of asthma while others may suffer nearly continuous symptoms. Asthma symptoms may occur spontaneously or may be precipitated or exacerbated by many different triggers as discussed above. Asthma symptoms are frequently worse at night; circadian variations in bronchomotor tone and bronchial reactivity reach their nadir between 3 AM and 4 AM, increasing symptoms of bronchoconstriction.

Table 9–2. Classifying severity of asthma exacerbations.

Note: Patients are instructed to use quick-relief medications if symptoms occur or if PEF drops below 80% predicted or personal best. If PEF is 50–79%, the patient should monitor response to quick relief medications carefully and consider contacting a clinician. If PEF is below 50%, immediate medical care is usually required. In the urgent or emergency care setting, the following parameters describe the severity and likely clinical course of an exacerbation.

	Symptoms and Signs	Initial PEF (or FEV_1)	Clinical Course
Mild	Dyspnea only with activity (assess tachypnea in young children)	PEV ≥ 70% predicted or personal best	• Usually cared for at home • Prompt relief with inhaled SABA • Possible short course of oral systemic corticosteroids
Moderate	Dyspnea interferes with limits of usual activity	PEF 40–69% predicted or personal best	• Usually requires office or ED visit • Relief from frequent inhaled SABA • Oral systemic corticosteroids; some symptoms last for 1–2 days after treatment is begun
Severe	Dyspnea at rest; interferes with conversation	PEF < 40% predicted or personal best	• Usually requires ED visit and likely hospitalization • Partial relief from frequent inhaled SABA • Oral systemic corticosteroids; some symptoms last for > 3 days after treatment is begun • Adjunctive therapies are helpful
Subset: Life-threatening	Too dyspneic to speak; perspiring	PEF < 25% predicted or personal best	• Requires ED/hospitalization; possible ICU • Minimal or no relief from frequent inhaled SABA • Intravenous corticosteroids • Adjunctive therapies are helpful

ED, emergency department; FEV_1, forced expiratory volume in 1 second; ICU, intensive care unit; PEF, peak expiratory flow; SABA, short-acting β_2-agonist.
Adapted from National Asthma Education and Prevention Program. Expert Panel Report 3: Guidelines for Diagnosis and Management of Asthma. National Institutes of Health Pub. No. 08-4051. Bethesda, MD, 2007. www.nhibi.nih.gov/guidelines/asthma/asthgdln.htm.

Some physical examination findings increase the probability of asthma. Nasal mucosal swelling, increased nasal secretions, and nasal polyps are often seen in patients with allergic asthma. Eczema, atopic dermatitis, or other manifestations of allergic skin disorders may also be present. Wheezing during normal breathing or a prolonged forced expiratory phase correlates well with the presence of airflow obstruction. Wheezing during forced expiration does not. Chest examination may be normal between exacerbations in patients with mild asthma. During severe asthma exacerbations, airflow may be too limited to produce wheezing, and the only diagnostic clue on auscultation may be globally reduced breath sounds with prolonged expiration. Hunched shoulders and use of accessory muscles of respiration suggest an increased work of breathing.

B. Pulmonary Function Testing

Clinicians are able to identify airflow obstruction on examination, but they have limited ability to assess it or to predict whether it is reversible. The evaluation for asthma should therefore include spirometry (FEV_1, FVC, FEV_1/FVC) before and after the administration of a short-acting bronchodilator. These measurements help determine the presence and extent of airflow obstruction and whether it is immediately reversible. Airflow obstruction is indicated by a reduced FEV_1/FVC ratio. Significant reversibility of airflow obstruction is defined by an increase of ≥ 12% and 200 mL in FEV_1 or ≥ 15% and 200 mL in FVC after inhaling a short-acting bronchodilator. A positive bronchodilator

response strongly confirms the diagnosis of asthma but a lack of responsiveness in the pulmonary function laboratory does not preclude success in a clinical trial of bronchodilator therapy. Severe airflow obstruction results in significant air trapping, with an increase in residual volume and consequent reduction in FVC, resulting in a pattern that suggests a restrictive ventilatory defect.

Bronchial provocation testing with inhaled histamine or methacholine may be useful when asthma is suspected but spirometry is nondiagnostic. Bronchial provocation is not recommended if the FEV_1 is less than 65% of predicted. A positive methacholine test is defined as a ≥ 20% fall in the FEV_1 at exposure to a concentration of 8 mg/mL or less. A negative test has a negative predictive value for asthma of 95%. Exercise challenge testing may be useful in patients with symptoms of exercise-induced bronchospasm.

Arterial blood gas measurements may be normal during a mild asthma exacerbation, but respiratory alkalosis and an increase in the alveolar-arterial oxygen difference ($A–a–DO_2$) are common. During severe exacerbations, hypoxemia develops and the $PaCO_2$ returns to normal. The combination of an increased $PaCO_2$ and respiratory acidosis may indicate impending respiratory failure and the need for mechanical ventilation.

Peak expiratory flow (PEF) meters are handheld devices designed as personal monitoring tools. PEF monitoring can establish peak flow variability, quantify asthma severity, and provide both the patient and the clinician with objective measurements on which to base treatment deci-

Table 9–3. Evaluation of asthma exacerbation severity.

	Mild	Moderate	Severe	Subset: Respiratory Arrest Imminent
Symptoms				
Breathlessness	While walking	While at rest (infant—softer, shorter cry, difficulty feeding)	While at rest (infant—stops feeding)	
	Can lie down	Prefers sitting	Sits upright	
Talks in	Sentences	Phrases	Words	
Alertness	May be agitated	Usually agitated	Usually agitated	Drowsy or confused
Signs				
Respiratory rate	Increased	Increased	Often > 30/minute	
		Guide to rates of breathing in awake children: Age — Normal Rate < 2 months — < 60/minute 2–12 months — < 50/minute 1–5 years — < 40/minute 6–8 years — < 30/minute		
Use of accessory muscles; suprasternal retractions	Usually not	Commonly	Usually	Paradoxical thoracoabdominal movement
Wheeze	Moderate, often only and expiratory	Loud; throughout exhalation	Usually loud; throughout inhalation and exhalation	Absence of wheeze
Pulse/minute	< 100	100–120	> 120	Bradycardia
		Guide to normal pulse rates in children: Age — Normal Rate 2–12 months — < 160/minute 1–2 years — < 120/minute 2–8 years — < 110/minute		
Pulsus paradoxus	Absent < 10 mm Hg	May be present 10–25 mm Hg	Often present > 25 mm Hg (adult) 20–40 mm Hg (child)	Absence suggests respiratory muscle fatigue
Functional Assessment				
PEF Percent predicted or percent personal best	≥ 70%	Approx. 40–69% or response lasts < 2 hours	< 40%	< 25% Note: PEF testing may not be needed in very severe attacks
Pao₂ (on air)	Normal (test not usually necessary)	≥ 60 mm Hg (test not usually necessary)	< 60 mm Hg: possible cyanosis	
and/or Pco₂	< 42 mm Hg (test not usually necessary)	< 42 mm Hg (test not usually necessary)	≥ 42 mm Hg: possible respiratory failure	
Sao₂ percent (on air) at sea level	> 95% (test not usually necessary)	90–95% (test not usually necessary)	< 90%	
	Hypercapnia (hypoventilation) develops more readily in young children than in adults and adolescents.			

PEF, peak expiratory low; Sao₂, oxygen saturation.
Notes:
· The presence of several parameters, but not necessarily all, indicates the general classification of the exacerbation.
· Many of these parameters have not been systematically studied, especially as they correlate with each other. Thus, they serve only as general guides.
· The emotional impact of asthma symptoms on the patient and family is variable but must be recognized and addressed and can affect approaches to treatment and follow-up.
Adapted from National Asthma Education and Prevention Program. Expert Panel Report 3: Guidelines for the Diagnosis and Management of Asthma. National Institutes of Health Pub. No. 08-4051. Bethesda, MD, 2007. http://www.nhlbi.nih.gov/guidelines/asthma/asthgdln.htm.

sions. There are conflicting data about whether measuring PEF improves asthma outcomes, but doing so is recommended to help confirm the diagnosis of asthma, to improve asthma control in patients with poor perception of airflow obstruction, and to identify environmental and occupational causes of symptoms. Predicted values for PEF vary with age, height, and gender but are poorly standardized. Comparison with reference values is less helpful than comparison with the patient's own baseline. PEF shows diurnal variation. It is generally lowest on first awakening and highest several hours before the midpoint of the waking day. PEF should be measured in the morning before the administration of a bronchodilator and in the afternoon after taking a bronchodilator. A 20% change in PEF values from morning to afternoon or from day to day suggests inadequately controlled asthma. PEF values less than 200 L/min indicate severe airflow obstruction.

C. Additional Testing

Routine chest radiographs in patients with asthma are usually normal or show only hyperinflation. Other findings may include bronchial wall thickening and diminished peripheral lung vascular shadows. Chest imaging is indicated when pneumonia, another disorder mimicking asthma, or a complication of asthma such as pneumothorax is suspected.

Skin testing or in vitro testing to assess sensitivity to environmental allergens can identify atopy in patients with persistent asthma who may benefit from therapies directed at their allergic diathesis. Evaluations for paranasal sinus disease or gastroesophageal reflux should be considered in patients with pertinent symptoms and in asthmatics with severe or refractory symptoms.

Noninvasive assessment of underlying airway inflammation through measurement of eosinophilia in induced sputum, or fractional nitric oxide concentration in exhaled breath condensates (FeNO), offers the promise of improved diagnosis and treatment strategies. Adjusting corticosteroid dose to minimize sputum eosinophilia appears to reduce the frequency of exacerbations compared with conventional clinical management, but the data are conflicting regarding the impact of FeNO on asthma outcomes. This is an exciting and rapidly changing area of asthma care.

▶ Complications

Complications of asthma include exhaustion, dehydration, airway infection, and tussive syncope. Pneumothorax occurs but is rare. Acute hypercapnic and hypoxic respiratory failure occurs in severe disease.

▶ Differential Diagnosis

It is prudent to consider conditions that mimic asthma in patients who have atypical symptoms or poor response to therapy. These disorders typically fall into one of four categories: upper airway disorders, lower airway disorders, systemic vasculitides, and psychiatric disorders. Upper airway disorders that mimic asthma include vocal fold paralysis, vocal fold dysfunction syndrome, foreign body aspiration, laryngotracheal masses, tracheal narrowing, tracheomalacia, and airway edema as in the setting of angioedema or inhalation injury. Lower airway disorders include nonasthmatic COPD (chronic bronchitis or emphysema), bronchiectasis, allergic bronchopulmonary mycosis, cystic fibrosis, eosinophilic pneumonia, and bronchiolitis obliterans. Systemic vasculitides with pulmonary involvement may have an asthmatic component, such as Churg-Strauss syndrome. Psychiatric causes include conversion disorders, which have been variably referred to as functional asthma, emotional laryngeal wheezing, vocal fold dysfunction, or episodic laryngeal dyskinesia. Münchausen syndrome or malingering may rarely explain a patient's complaints.

▶ NAEPP 3 Diagnosis & Management Guidelines

The National Asthma Education and Prevention Program (NAEPP), in conjunction with the Global Initiative for Asthma (GINA), a collaboration between the National Institutes of Health (NIH)/National Heart, Lung, and Blood Institute (NHLBI) and the World Health Organization (WHO), recently released its third Expert Panel Report providing guidelines for diagnosis and management of asthma (NAEPP 3). This report identifies four components of chronic asthma diagnosis and management: (1) assessing and monitoring asthma severity and asthma control, (2) patient education designed to foster a partnership for care, (3) control of environmental factors and comorbid conditions that affect asthma, and (4) pharmacologic agents for asthma.

1. Assessing and monitoring asthma severity and asthma control—Severity is the intrinsic intensity of the disease process. Control is the degree to which symptoms and limitations on activity are minimized by therapy. Responsiveness is the ease with which control is achieved with therapy. NAEPP 3 guidelines now emphasize control over classifications of severity, since the latter is variable over time and in response to therapy. A measure of severity on initial presentation (see Figure 9–1) is helpful, however, in guiding the initiation of therapy. Control of asthma is assessed in terms of **impairment** (frequency and intensity of symptoms and functional limitations) and **risk** (the likelihood of acute exacerbations or chronic decline in lung function). A key insight is that these two domains of control may respond differently to treatment: some patients may have minimal impairment yet remain at risk for severe exacerbations, for example, in the setting of an upper respiratory tract infection. Table 9–1 is used to assess the adequacy of asthma control and is used in conjunction with Figure 9–2 to guide adjustments in therapy based on the level of control.

2. Patient education designed to foster a partnership for care—Active self-management reduces urgent care visits and hospitalizations and improves perceived control of asthma. Therefore, an outpatient preventive approach that includes self-management education is an integral part of effective asthma care. All patients, but particularly

Intermittent Asthma	**Persistent Asthma: Daily Medication** Consult with asthma specialist if step 4 care or higher is required. Consider consultation at step 3.

Step 1

Preferred:

SABA PRN

Step 2

Preferred:

Low-dose ICS

Alternative:

Cromolyn, LTRA, nedocromil, or theophylline

Step 3

Preferred:

Low-dose ICS + LABA OR Medium-dose ICS

Alternative:

Low-dose ICS + either LTRA, theophylline, or zileuton

Step 4

Preferred:

Medium-dose ICS + LABA

Alternative:

Low-dose ICS + either LTRA, theophylline, or zileuton

Step 5

Preferred:

High-dose ICS + LABA

AND

Consider omalizumab for patients who have allergies

Step 6

Preferred:

High-dose ICS + LABA + oral corticosteroid

AND

Consider omalizumab for patients who have allergies

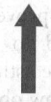

Step up if needed

(first, check adherence, environmental control, and comorbid conditions)

Assess control

Step down if possible

(and asthma is well controlled at least 3 months)

Each step: Patient education, environmental control, and management of comorbidities.

Steps 2–4: Consider subcutaneous allergen immunotherapy for patients who have allergic asthma (see notes).

Quick-Relief Medication for All Patients

- SABA as needed for symptoms. Intensity of treatment depends on severity of symptoms: up to three treatments at 20-minute intervals as needed. Short course of oral systemic corticosteroids may be needed.
- Use of SABA > 2 days a week for symptom relief (not prevention of EIB) generally indicates inadequate control and the need to step up treatment.

Key: *Alphabetical order is used when more than one treatment option is listed within either preferred or alternative therapy.* EIB, exercise-induced bronchospasm; ICS, inhaled corticosteroid; LABA, inhaled long-acting β₂-agonist; LTRA, leukotriene receptor antagonist; SABA, inhaled short-acting β₂-agonist

Notes:

- The stepwise approach is meant to assist, not replace, the clinical decision-making required to meet individual patient needs.
- If alternative treatment is used and response is inadequate, discontinue it and use the preferred treatment before stepping up.
- Zileuton is a less desirable alternative as adjunctive therapy due to limited studies and the need to monitor liver function. Theophylline requires monitoring of serum concentration levels.
- In step 6, before oral systemic corticosteroids are introduced, a trial of high-dose ICS + LABA + either LTRA, theophylline, or zileuton may be considered, although this approach has not been studied in clinical trials.
- Step 1, 2, and 3 preferred therapies are based on Evidence A; step 3 alternative therapy is based on Evidence A for LTRA, Evidence B for theophylline, and Evidence D for zileuton. Step 4 preferred therapy is based on Evidence B, and alternative therapy is based on Evidence B for LTRA and theophylline and Evidence D for zileuton. Step 5 preferred therapy is based on Evidence B. Step 6 preferred therapy is based on (EPR 2 1997) and Evidence B for omalizumab.
- Immunotherapy for steps 2–4 is based on Evidence B for house-dust mites, animal danders, and pollens; evidence is weak or lacking for molds and cockroaches. Evidence is strongest for immunotherapy with single allergens. The role of allergy in asthma is greater in children than in adults.
- Clinicians who administer immunotherapy or omalizumab should be prepared and equipped to identify and treat anaphylaxis that may occur.

▲ **Figure 9–2.** Stepwise approach to managing asthma. (Adapted from National Asthma Education and Prevention Program. Expert Panel Report 3: Guidelines for the Diagnosis and Management of Asthma. National Institutes of Health Pub. No. 08-4051. Bethesda, MD, 2007. http://www.nhlbi.nih.gov/guidelines/asthma/asthgdln.htm.)

those with poorly controlled symptoms or a history of severe exacerbations, should have a written asthma action plan that includes instructions for daily management and measures to take in response to specific changes in status. Patients should be taught to recognize symptoms—especially patterns indicating inadequate asthma control or predicting the need for additional therapy.

3. Control of environmental factors and comorbid conditions that affect asthma—Significant reduction in exposure to nonspecific airway irritants or to inhaled allergens in atopic patients may reduce symptoms as well as medication needs. Comorbid conditions that impair asthma management, such as rhinosinusitis, gastroesophageal reflux, obesity, and obstructive sleep apnea, should be identified and treated. This search for complicating conditions is particularly crucial in the initial evaluation of a new diagnosis, and in patients whose asthma is difficult to control or subject to frequent exacerbations.

4. Pharmacologic agents for asthma—Asthma medications can be divided into two categories: quick-relief (**reliever**) medications that act principally by direct relaxation of bronchial smooth muscle, thereby promoting prompt reversal of acute airflow obstruction to relieve accompanying symptoms, and long-term control (**controller**) medications that act primarily to attenuate airway inflammation and are taken daily independent of symptoms to achieve and maintain control of persistent asthma. NAEPP 3 recommendations emphasize daily anti-inflammatory therapy with inhaled corticosteroids as the cornerstone of treatment of persistent asthma.

Most asthma medications are administered orally or by inhalation. Inhalation of an appropriate agent results in a more rapid onset of pulmonary effects as well as fewer systemic effects compared with oral administration of the same dose. Metered-dose inhalers (MDIs) propelled by chlorofluorocarbons (CFCs) have been the most widely used delivery system, but non-CFC propellant systems such as hydrofluoroalkane (HFA), and dry powder inhalers (DPIs) are increasingly available. Proper MDI technique and the use of an inhalation chamber improve drug delivery to the lung and decrease oropharyngeal deposition. Nebulizer therapy is reserved for acutely ill patients and those who cannot use MDIs because of difficulties with coordination or cooperation.

► Treatment

The goals of asthma therapy are to minimize chronic symptoms that interfere with normal activity (including exercise), to prevent recurrent exacerbations, to reduce or eliminate the need for emergency department visits or hospitalizations, and to maintain normal or near-normal pulmonary function. These goals should be met while providing pharmacotherapy with the fewest adverse effects and while meeting patients' and families' expectations of satisfaction with asthma care.

A. Long-Term Control Medications

Anti-inflammatory agents, long-acting bronchodilators, and leukotriene modifiers comprise the important long-term control medications (Tables 9–4 and 9–5). Other classes of agents are mentioned briefly below.

1. Anti-inflammatory agents—Corticosteroids are the most potent and consistently effective anti-inflammatory agents currently available. They reduce both acute and chronic inflammation, resulting in fewer asthma symptoms, improvement in airflow, decreased airway hyperresponsiveness, and fewer asthma exacerbations. These agents may also potentiate the action of β-adrenergic agonists.

Inhaled corticosteroids are preferred, first-line agents for all patients with persistent asthma. Patients with persistent symptoms or asthma exacerbations who are not taking inhaled corticosteroids should be started on an inhaled corticosteroid. The most important determinants of agent selection and appropriate dosing are the patient's status and response to treatment. Dosages for inhaled corticosteroids vary depending on the specific agent and delivery device. For most patients, twice-daily dosing provides adequate control of asthma. Once-daily dosing may be sufficient in selected patients. Maximum responses from inhaled corticosteroids may not be observed for months. The use of an inhalation chamber coupled with mouth washing after MDI use decreases local side effects (cough, dysphonia, oropharyngeal candidiasis) and systemic absorption. DPIs are not used with an inhalation chamber. Systemic effects (adrenal suppression, osteoporosis, skin thinning, easy bruising, and cataracts) may occur with high-dose inhaled corticosteroid therapy.

Systemic corticosteroids (oral or parenteral) are most effective in achieving prompt control of asthma during exacerbations or when initiating long-term asthma therapy in patients with severe symptoms. In patients with refractory, poorly controlled asthma, systemic corticosteroids may be required for the long-term suppression of symptoms. Repeated efforts should be made to reduce the dose to the minimum needed to control symptoms. Alternate-day treatment is preferred to daily treatment. Rapid discontinuation of systemic corticosteroids after chronic use may precipitate adrenal insufficiency. Concurrent treatment with calcium supplements and vitamin D should be initiated to prevent corticosteroid-induced bone mineral loss in long-term administration. Bisphosphonates may offer additional protection to these patients.

2. Long-acting bronchodilators

A. MEDIATOR INHIBITORS—Cromolyn sodium and nedocromil are long-term control medications that prevent asthma symptoms and improve airway function in patients with mild persistent asthma or exercise-induced symptoms. These agents modulate mast cell mediator release and eosinophil recruitment and inhibit both early and late asthmatic responses to allergen challenge and exercise-induced bronchospasm. They can be effective when taken before an exposure or exercise but do not relieve asthmatic symptoms once present. The clinical response to these agents is less predictable than the response to inhaled corticosteroids. Nedocromil may help reduce the dose requirements for inhaled corticosteroids. Both agents have excellent safety profiles.

Table 9–4. Long-term control medications for asthma.

Medication	Dosage Form	Adult Dose	Comments
Inhaled Corticosteroids			(See Table 9–5)
Systemic Corticosteroids			(Applies to all three corticosteroids)
Methylpred-nisolone	2, 4, 6, 8, 16, 32 mg tablets	7.5–60 mg daily in a single dose in AM or every other day as needed for control	• For long-term treatment of severe persistent asthma, administer single dose in AM either daily or on alternate days (alternate-day therapy may produce less adrenal suppression). Short courses or "bursts" are effective for establishing control when initiating therapy or during a period of gradual deterioration.
Prednisolone	5 mg tablets, 5 mg/5 mL, 15 mg/5 mL	Short-course "burst": to achieve control, 40–60 mg per day as single or 2 divided doses for 3–10 days	
Prednisone	1, 2.5, 5, 10, 20, 50 mg tablets; 5 mg/mL, 5 mg/mL		• There is no evidence that tapering the dose following improvement in symptom control and pulmonary function prevents relapse.
Inhaled Long-Acting β₂-Agonists			Should not be used for symptom relief or exacerbations. Use with inhaled corticosteroids.
Salmeterol	DPI 50 mcg/blister	1 blister every 12 hours	• Decreased duration of protection against EIB may occur with regular use.
Formoterol	DPI 12 mcg/single-use capsule	1 capsule every 12 hours	• Decreased duration of protection against EIB may occur with regular use.
			• Each capsule is for single use only; additional doses should not be administered for at least 12 hours.
			• Capsules should be used only with the Aerolizor™ inhaler and should not be taken orally.
Combined Medication			
Fluticasone/ Salmeterol	DPI 100 mcg/50 mcg, 250 mcg/50 mcg, or 500 mcg/50 mcg HFA 45 mcg/21 mcg 115 mcg/21 mcg 230 mcg/21 mcg	1 inhalation twice daily; dose depends on severity of asthma	• 100/50 DPI or 45/21 HFA for patient not controlled on low- to medium-dose inhaled corticosteroids • 250/50 DPI or 115/21 HFA for patients not controlled on medium- to high-dose inhaled corticosteroids
Budesonide/ Formoterol	HFA MDI 80 mcg/4.5 mcg 160 mcg/4.5 mcg	2 inhalations twice daily; dose depends on severity of asthma	• 80/4.5 for patients who have asthma not controlled on low- to medium-dose inhaled corticosteroids • 160/4.5 for patients who have asthma not controlled on medium- to high-dose inhaled corticosteroids
Cromolyn and Nedocromil			
Cromolyn	MDI 0.8 mg/puff	2 puffs four times daily	• 4–6 week trial may be needed to determine maximum benefit.
	Nebulizer 20 mg/ampule	1 ampule four times daily	• Dose by MDI may be inadequate to affect hyperrespon-siveness.
Nedocromil	MDI 1.75 mg/puff	2 puffs four times daily	• One dose before exercise or allergen exposure provides effective prophylaxis for 1–2 hours. Not as effective for EIB as SABA.
			• Once control is achieved, the frequency of dosing may be reduced.
Leukotriene Modifiers			
Leukotriene Receptor Antagonists			
Montelukast	4 mg or 5 mg chewable tablet 10 mg tablet	10 mg each night at bedtime	• Montelukast exhibits a flat dose-response curve. Doses > 10 mg will not produce a greater response in adults.

(continued)

Table 9–4. Long-term control medications for asthma. (continued)

Medication	Dosage Form	Adult Dose	Comments
Zafirlukast	10 or 20 mg tablet	40 mg daily (20 mg tablet twice daily)	• For zafirlukast, administration with meals decreases bioavailability; take at least one hour before or 2 hours after meals. • Monitor for symptoms and signs of hepatic dysfunction.
5-Lipoxygenase Inhibitor			
Zileuton	600 mg tablet	2400 mg daily (600 mg four times daily)	• For zileuton, monitor hepatic enzymes (ALT).
Methylxanthines			
Theophylline	Liquids, sustained-release tablets, and capsules	Starting dose 10 mg/kg/d up to 300 mg maximum; usual maximum dose 800 mg/d	• Adjust dosage to achieve serum concentration of 5–15 mcg/mL at steady-state (at least 48 hours on same dosage). • Due to wide interpatient variability in theophylline metabolic clearance, routine serum theophylline level monitoring is important. • See below for factors that can affect theophylline levels.
Immunomodulators			
Omalizumab	Subcutaneous injection, 150 mg/1.2 mL following reconstitution with 1.4 mL sterile water for injection	150–375 mg SC every 2–4 weeks, depending on body weight and pretreatment serum IgE level	• Do not administer more than 150 mg per injection site. • Monitor for anaphylaxis for 2 hours following at least the first 3 injections.

Factor[1,2]	Decreases Theophylline Concentrations	Increases Theophylline Concentrations	Recommended Action
Food	↓ or delays absorption of some sustained-release theophylline (SRT) products	↑ rate of absorption (fatty foods)	Select theophylline preparation that is not affected by food.
Diet	↑ metabolism (high protein)	↓ metabolism (high carbohydrate)	Inform patients that major changes in diet are not recommended while taking theophylline.
Systemic, febrile viral illness (eg, influenza)		↓ metabolism	Decrease theophylline dose according to serum concentration. Decrease dose by 50% if serum concentration measurement is not available.
Hypoxia, cor pulmonale, and decompensated congestive heart failure, cirrhosis		↓ metabolism	Decrease dose according to serum concentration.
Age	↑ metabolism (1–9 years)	↓ metabolism (< 6 months, elderly)	Adjust dose according to serum concentration.
Phenobarbital, phenytoin, carbamazepine	↑ metabolism		Increase dose according to serum concentration.
Cimetidine		↓ metabolism	Use alternative H_2 blocker (eg, famotidine or ranitidine).
Macrolides: erythromycin, clarithromycin		↓ metabolism	Use alternative macrolide antibiotic, azithromycin, or alternative antibiotic or adjust theophylline dose.
Quinolones: ciprofloxacin, enoxacin, pefloxacin		↓ metabolism	Use alternative antibiotic or adjust theophylline dose. Circumvent with ofloxacin if quinolone therapy is required.
Rifampin	↑ metabolism		Increase dose according to serum concentration.
Ticlopidine		↓ metabolism	Decrease dose according to serum concentration.
Smoking	↑ metabolism		Advise patient to stop smoking; increase dose according to serum concentration.

[1]Factors affecting serum theophylline concentration.
[2]This list is not all inclusive; for discussion of other factors, see package inserts.
DPI, dry powder inhaler; EIB, exercise-induced bronchospasm; HFA, hydrofluoroalkane; IgE, immunoglobulin E; MDI, metered-dose inhaler; SABA, short-acting β_2-agonist.
Adapted from National Asthma Education and Prevention Program. Expert Panel Report 3: Guidelines for the Diagnosis and Management of Asthma. National Institutes of Health Pub. No. 08-4051. Bethesda, MD, 2007. http://www.nhlbi.nih.gov/guidelines/asthma/asthgdln.htm.

Table 9–5. Estimated comparative daily dosages for inhaled corticosteroids for asthma.

Drug	Low Daily Dose Adult	Medium Daily Dose Adult	High Daily Dose Adult
Beclomethasone HFA 40 or 80 mcg/puff	80–240 mcg	> 240–480 mcg	> 480 mcg
Budesonide DPI 90, 180, or 200 mcg/inhalation	180–600 mcg	> 600–1200 mcg	> 1200 mcg
Flunisolide 250 mcg/puff	500–1000 mcg	> 1000–2000 mcg	> 2000 mcg
Flunisolide HFA 80 mcg/puff	320 mcg	> 320–640 mcg	> 640 mcg

Fluticasone
  HFA/MDI: 44, 110, or 220
  mcg/puff
	88–264 mcg	> 264–440 mcg	> 440 mcg

DPI: 50, 100, or 250 mcg/ inhalation	100–300 mcg	> 300–500 mcg	> 500 mcg
Mometasone DPI 200 mcg/puff	200 mcg	400 mcg	> 400 mcg
Triamcinolone acetonide 75 mcg/puff	300–750 mcg	> 750–1500 mcg	> 1500 mcg

DPI, dry power inhaler; HFA, hydrofluoroalkaline; MDI, metered-dose inhaler.
Notes:
· **The most important determinant of appropriate dosing is the clinician's judgment of the patient's response to therapy.**
The clinician must monitor the patient's response on several clinical parameters and adjust the dose accordingly. The stepwise approach to therapy emphasizes that once control of asthma is achieved, the dose of medication should be carefully titrated to the minimum dose required to maintain control, thus reducing the potential for adverse effect.
· Some doses may be outside packaging labeling, especially in the high-dose range.
· MDI dosages are expressed as the actuator dose (the amount of drug leaving the actuator and delivered to the patient), which is the labeling required in the United States. This is different from the dosage expressed as the valve dose (the amount of drug leaving the valve, not all of which is available to the patient), which is used in many European countries and in some scientific literature. DPI doses are expressed as the amount of drug in the inhaler following activation.
· Comparative dosages are based on published comparative clinical trials. The rationale for some key comparisons is summarized as follows:
  —The high dose is the dose that appears likely to be the threshold beyond which significant hypothalamic-pituitary-adrenal (HPA) axis suppression is produced, and, by extrapolation, the risk is increased for other clinically significant systemic effects if used for prolonged periods of time.
  —The low- and medium-doses reflect findings from dose-ranging studies in which incremental efficacy within the low- to medium-dose ranges was established without increased systemic effect as measured by overnight cortisol excretion. The studies demonstrated a relatively flat-dose response curve for efficacy at the medium-dose range; that is, increasing the dose of high-dose range did not significantly increase efficacy but did increase systemic effect.
  —The dose for budesonide DPI is based on recently available comparative data with other medications. These new data, including meta-analyses, show that budesonide DPI is comparable to approximately twice the microgram dose of fluticasone MDI or DPI.
  —The dose for beclomethasone in HFA inhaler should be approximately one-half the dose for beclomethasone in chlorofluorocarbon (CFC) inhaler for adults and children, based on studies demonstrating that the different pharmaceutical properties of the medications result in enhanced lung delivery for the HFA (a less forceful spray from the HFA propellant and a reengineered nozzle that allows a smaller particle size) and clinical trials demonstrating similar potency to fluticasone at 1:1 dose ratio.
  —The dose for mometasone DPI is based on product information and current literature. Mometasone is approved for once daily administration. Mometasone furoate by dry powder achieved effects similar to twice the dose of budesonide by dry powder and comparable to a slightly higher dose of fluticasone propionate by dry powder.
  —The dose for flunisolide HFA is based on product information and current literature.

(continued)

Table 9–5. Estimated comparative daily dosages for inhaled corticosteroids for asthma. (continued)

- **Bioavailability**
  Both the relative potency and the relative bioavailability (systemic availability) determine the potential for systemic activity of an inhaled corticosteroid preparation. As illustrated here, the bioavailability of an inhaled corticosteroid is dependent on the absorption of the dose delivered to the lungs and the oral bioavailability of the swallowed portion of the dose received.
  —Absorption of the dose delivered to the lungs:
    · Approximately 10–50% of the dose from the MDI is delivered to the lungs. This amount varies among preparations and delivery devices.
    · Nearly all of the amount delivered to the lungs is bioavailable.
  —Oral bioavailability of the swallowed portion of the dose received:
    · Approximately 50–80% of the dose from the MDI without a spacer/holding chamber is swallowed.
    · The oral bioavailability of this amount varies:

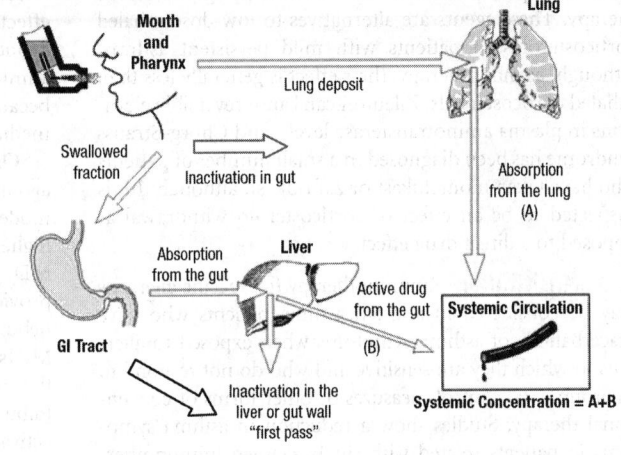

  Either a high first-pass metabolism or the use of a spacer/holding chamber with an MDI can decrease oral bioavailability, thus enhancing safety.

  The approximate oral bioavailability of inhaled corticosteroids has been reported as: beclomethasone dipropionate, 20%; flunisolide, 21%; triamcinolone acetonide, 10.6%; budesonide, 11%; fluticasone propionate, 1%; mometasone, < 1%.

- **Potential drug interactions**
  A number of the inhaled corticosteroids, including fluticasone, budesonide, and mometasone, are metabolized in the gastrointestinal tract and liver by CYP 3A4 isoenzymes. Potent inhibitors of CYP 3A4, such as ritonavir and ketoconazole, have the potential for increasing systemic concentrations of these inhaled corticosteroids by increasing oral availability and decreasing systemic clearance. Some cases of clinically significant Cushing syndrome and secondary adrenal insufficiency have been reported.

Adapted from National Asthma Education and Prevention Program. Expert Panel Report 3: Guidelines for the Diagnosis and Management of Asthma. National Institutes of Health Pub. No. 08-4051. Bethesda, MD, 2007. http://www.nhlbi.nih.gov/guidelines/asthma/asthgdln.htm.

B. β-ADRENERGIC AGONISTS—Long-acting β_2-agonists provide bronchodilation for up to 12 hours after a single dose. Salmeterol and formoterol are the two long-acting β_2-agonists available in the United States. They are administered via dry powder delivery devices. They are indicated for long-term prevention of asthma symptoms, nocturnal symptoms, and for prevention of exercise-induced bronchospasm. When added to standard doses of inhaled corticosteroids, long-acting β_2-agonists provide control equivalent to what is achieved by doubling the inhaled corticosteroid dose. Side effects are minimal at standard doses. Long-acting β_2-agonists should not be used as monotherapy since they have no anti-inflammatory effect and since monotherapy with long-acting β_2-agonists has been associated in two large studies with a small but statistically significant increased risk of severe or fatal asthma attacks. This increased risk may relate to genetic variation in the β-adrenergic receptor, but it has not been fully explained and remains an area of controversy. The efficacy of combined inhaled corticosteroid and long-acting β_2-agonist therapy has led to marketing of combination medications that deliver both agents simultaneously (see Table 9–4). Combination inhalers containing formoterol and budesonide have shown efficacy in both maintenance and rescue, given formoterol's short time to onset.

C. PHOSPHODIESTERASE INHIBITORS—Theophylline provides mild bronchodilation in asthmatic patients. This drug has modest anti-inflammatory properties, enhances mucociliary clearance, and strengthens diaphragmatic contractility. Sustained-release theophylline preparations are effective in controlling nocturnal asthma and are usually reserved for use as adjuvant therapy in patients with moderate or severe persistent asthma. Theophylline serum concentrations need to be monitored closely owing to the drug's narrow toxic-therapeutic range, individual differences in metabolism, and the effects of many factors on drug absorption and metabolism. Decreases in theophylline clearance accompany the use of cimetidine, macrolide and quinolone antibiotics, and oral contraceptives. Increases in theophylline clearance are caused by rifampin, phenytoin, barbiturates, and tobacco.

Adverse effects at therapeutic doses include insomnia, upset stomach, aggravation of dyspepsia and gastroesophageal reflux symptoms, and urination difficulties in elderly men with prostatism. Dose-related toxicities are common and include nausea, vomiting, tachyarrhythmias, headache, seizures, hyperglycemia, and hypokalemia.

3. Leukotriene modifiers—Leukotrienes are potent biochemical mediators that contribute to airway obstruction and asthma symptoms by contracting airway smooth muscle, increasing vascular permeability and mucus secretion, and attracting and activating airway inflammatory cells. Zileuton is a 5-lipoxygenase inhibitor that decreases leukotriene production, and zafirlukast and montelukast are cysteinyl leukotriene receptor antagonists. They cause modest improvements in lung function and reductions in asthma symptoms and lessen the need for β_2-agonist rescue therapy. These agents are alternatives to low-dose inhaled corticosteroids in patients with mild persistent asthma, although, as monotherapy, their effect is generally less than inhaled corticosteroids. Zileuton can cause reversible elevations in plasma aminotransferase levels, and Churg-Strauss syndrome has been diagnosed in a small number of patients who have taken montelukast or zafirlukast, although this is suspected to be an effect of corticosteroid withdrawal as opposed to a direct drug effect.

4. Desensitization—Immunotherapy for specific allergens may be considered in selected asthma patients who have exacerbations of asthma symptoms when exposed to allergens to which they are sensitive and who do not respond to environmental control measures or other forms of conventional therapy. Studies show a reduction in asthma symptoms in patients treated with single-allergen immunotherapy. Because of the risk of immunotherapy-induced bronchoconstriction, it should be administered only in a setting where such complications can be immediately treated.

5. Vaccination—Patients with asthma should receive pneumococcal vaccination (Pneumovax) and annual influenza vaccinations. Inactive vaccines (Pneumovax) are associated with few side effects but use of the live attenuated influenza vaccine intranasally may be associated with an increase in asthma exacerbations in young children.

6. Miscellaneous agents—Oral sustained-release β_2-agonists are reserved for patients with bothersome nocturnal asthma symptoms or moderate to severe persistent asthma who do not respond to other therapies. Omalizumab is a recombinant antibody that binds IgE without activating mast cells. In clinical trials in moderate to severe asthmatic patients with elevated IgE levels, it reduces the need for corticosteroids. Etanercept, a soluble TNF-α receptor antagonist, has shown modest efficacy in one small study of severe asthma.

B. Quick-Relief Medications

Short-acting bronchodilators and systemic corticosteroids comprise the important medications in this group of agents (Table 9–6).

1. β-Adrenergic agonists—Short-acting inhaled β_2-agonists, including albuterol, levalbuterol, bitolterol, pirbuterol, and terbutaline, are the most effective bronchodilators during exacerbations. All patients with acute symptoms should take one of these agents. There is no convincing evidence to support the use of one agent over another. β_2-Agonists relax airway smooth muscle and cause a prompt increase in airflow and reduction of symptoms. Administration before exercise effectively prevents exercise-induced bronchoconstriction. β_2-Selective agents may produce less cardiac stimulation than those with mixed β_1 and β_2 activities, although clinical trials have not consistently demonstrated this finding.

Inhaled β-adrenergic therapy is as effective as oral or parenteral therapy in relaxing airway smooth muscle and improving acute asthma and offers the advantages of rapid onset of action (< 5 minutes) with fewer systemic side effects. Repetitive administration produces incremental bronchodilation. Intravenous and subcutaneous routes of administration should be reserved for patients who because of age or mechanical factors are unable to inhale medications.

One or two inhalations of a short-acting inhaled β_2-agonist from an MDI are usually sufficient for mild to moderate symptoms. Severe exacerbations frequently require higher doses: 6–12 puffs every 30–60 minutes of albuterol by MDI with an inhalation chamber or 2.5 mg by nebulizer provide equivalent bronchodilation. Administration by wet nebulization does not offer more effective delivery than MDIs but does provide higher doses. With most β_2-agonists, the recommended dose by nebulizer for acute asthma (albuterol, 2.5 mg) is 25–30 times that delivered by a single activation of the MDI (albuterol, 0.09 mg). This difference suggests that standard dosing of inhalations from an MDI will often be insufficient in the setting of an acute exacerbation. Independent of dose, nebulizer therapy may be more effective in patients who are unable to coordinate inhalation of medication from an MDI because of age, agitation, or severity of the exacerbation.

Scheduled daily use of short-acting β_2-agonists is not recommended. Increased use (more than one canister a month) or lack of expected effect indicates diminished asthma control and dictates the need for additional long-term control therapy.

2. Anticholinergics—Anticholinergic agents reverse vagally mediated bronchospasm but not allergen- or exercise-induced bronchospasm. They may decrease mucus gland hypersecretion seen in asthma. Ipratropium bromide, a quaternary derivative of atropine free of atropine's side effects, is less effective than β_2-agonists for relief of acute bronchospasm, but it is the inhaled drug of choice for patients with intolerance to β_2-agonists and with bronchospasm due to β-blocker medications. Ipratropium bromide reduces the rate of hospital admissions when added to inhaled short-acting β_2-agonists in patients with moderate to severe asthma exacerbations. The role of anticholinergic agents in long-term management of asthma has not been clarified.

3. Phosphodiesterase inhibitors—Methylxanthines are not recommended for therapy of asthma exacerbations. Aminophylline has clearly been shown to be less effective than β_2-agonists when used as single-drug therapy for acute asthma and adds little except toxicity to the acute bronchodilator effects achieved by nebulized metaproterenol alone. Patients with exacerbations who are currently taking a theophylline-containing preparation should have their serum theophylline concentration measured to exclude theophylline toxicity.

4. Corticosteroids—Systemic corticosteroids are effective primary treatment for patients with moderate to severe asthma exacerbations and for patients with exacerbations who do not respond promptly and completely to inhaled

Table 9–6. Quick-relief medications for asthma.

Medication	Dosage Form	Adult Dose	Comments
Inhaled Short-Acting β₂-Agonists			
	MDI		
Albuterol CFC	90 mcg/puff, 200 puffs/canister	2 puffs 5 minutes before exercise	• An increasing use or lack of expected effect indicates diminished control of asthma.
Albuterol HFA	90 mcg/puff, 200 puffs/canister	2 puffs every 4–6 hours as needed	• Not recommended for long-term daily treatment. Regular use exceeding 2 days/week for symptom control (not prevention of EIB) indicates the need to step up therapy.
Pirbuterol CFC	200 mcg/puff, 400 puffs/canister		• Differences in potency exist, but all products are essentially comparable on a per puff basis.
Levalbuterol HFA	45 mcg/puff, 200 puffs/canister		• May double usual dose for mild exacerbations.
			• Should prime the inhaler by releasing four actuations prior to use.
			• Periodically clean HFA activator, as drug may block/plug orifice.
			• Nonselective agents (ie, epinephrine, isoproterenol, metaproterenol) are not recommended due to their potential for excessive cardiac stimulation, especially in high doses.
	Nebulizer solution		
Albuterol	0.63 mg/3 mL 1.25 mg/3 mL 2.5 mg/3 mL 5 mg/mL (0.5%)	1.25–5 mg in 3 mL of saline every 4–8 hours as needed	• May mix with budesonide inhalant suspension, cromolyn or ipratropium nebulizer solutions. May double dose for severe exacerbations.
Levalbuterol (R-albuterol)	0.31 mg/3 mL 0.63 mg/3 mL 1.25 mg/0.5 mL 1.25 mg/3 mL	0.63 mg–1.25 mg every 8 hours as needed	• Compatible with budesonide inhalant suspension. The product is a sterile-filled, preservative-free, unit dose vial.
Anticholinergics			
	MDI		
Ipratropium HFA	17 mcg/puff, 200 puffs/canister	2–3 puffs every 6 hours	• Evidence is lacking for anticholinergics producing added benefit to β₂-agonists in long-term control asthma therapy.
	Nebulizer solution		
	0.25 mg/mL (0.025%)	0.25 mg every 6 hours	
	MDI		
Ipratropium with albuterol	18 mcg/puff of ipratropium bromide and 90 mcg/puff of albuterol 200 puffs/canister	2–3 puffs every 6 hours	
	Nebulizer solution		
	0.5 mg/3 mL ipratropium bromide and 2.5 mg/3 mL albuterol	3 mL every 4–6 hours	• Contains EDTA to prevent discolorations of the solution. This additive does not induce bronchospasm.
Systemic Corticosteroids			
Methylprednisolone	2, 4, 6, 8, 16, 32 mg tablets	Short course "burst": 40–60 mg/d as single or 2 divided doses for 3–10 days	• Short courses or "bursts" are effective for establishing control when initiating therapy or during a period of gradual deterioration.
Prednisolone	5 mg tablets, 5 mg/5 mL, 15 mg/5 mL		• The burst should be continued until symptoms resolve and the PEF is at least 80% of personal best. This usually requires 3–10 days but may require longer. There is no evidence that tapering the dose following improvements prevents relapse.
Prednisone	1, 2.5, 5, 10, 20, 50 mg tablets; 5 mg/mL, 5 mg/5mL		• May be used in place of a short burst of oral corticosteroids in patients who are vomiting or if adherence is a problem.

(continued)

Table 9–6. Quick-relief medications for asthma. (continued)

Medication	Dosage Form	Adult Dose	Comments
	Repository injection		
(Methylprednisolone acetate)	40 mg/mL 80 mg/mL	240 mg IM once	

CFC, chlorofluorocarbon; EIB, exercise-induced bronchospasm; HFA, hydrofluoroalkane; IM, intramuscular; MDI, metered-dose inhaler; PEF, peak expiratory flow.
Adapted from National Asthma Education and Prevention Program. Expert Panel Report 3: Guidelines for the Diagnosis and Management of Asthma. National Institutes of Health Pub. No. 08-4051. Bethesda, MD, 2007. http://www.nhlbi.gov/guidelines/asthma/asthgdln.htm.

β_2-agonist therapy. These medications speed the resolution of airflow obstruction and reduce the rate of relapse. Delays in administering corticosteroids may result in delayed benefits from these important agents. Therefore, oral corticosteroids should be available for early administration at home in many patients with moderate to severe asthma. The minimal effective dose of systemic corticosteroids for asthma patients has not been identified. Outpatient prednisone "burst" therapy is 0.5–1 mg/kg/d (typically 40–60 mg) as a single or in two divided doses for 3–10 days. Severe exacerbations requiring hospitalization typically require 1 mg/kg of prednisone equivalent every 6–12 hours for 48 hours or until the FEV_1 (or PEF rate) returns to 50% of predicted (or 50% of baseline). The dose is then decreased to 60–80 mg/d until the PEF reaches 70% of predicted or personal best. No clear advantage has been found for higher doses of corticosteroids in severe exacerbations. It may be prudent to administer corticosteroids to critically ill patients via the intravenous route in order to avoid concerns about altered gastrointestinal absorption.

5. Antimicrobials—Empiric antibiotics are not recommended in routine asthma exacerbations, although antibiotics that cover atypical organisms (eg, telithromycin) are an area of ongoing research. Antibiotics may be useful if bacterial respiratory tract infections are thought to contribute. Thus, patients with fever or purulent sputum and evidence of pneumonia or bacterial sinusitis are reasonable candidates for such therapy.

▶ Treatment of Asthma Exacerbations

NAEPP 3 asthma treatment algorithms begin with an assessment of the severity of a patient's baseline asthma. Adjustments to that algorithm follow a stepwise approach based on a careful assessment of asthma control. Most instances of uncontrolled asthma are mild and can be managed successfully by patients at home with the telephone assistance of a clinician (Figure 9–3).

More severe exacerbations require evaluation and management in an urgent care or emergency department setting (Figure 9–4).

A. Mild Exacerbations

Mild asthma exacerbations are characterized by only minor changes in airway function (PEF > 80%) and minimal symptoms and signs of airway dysfunction (see Tables 9–2 and 9–3). The majority of such exacerbations can be managed at home with the telephone assistance of a clinician. Many patients respond quickly and fully to an inhaled short-acting β_2-agonist alone. However, an inhaled short-acting β_2-agonist may need to be continued at increased doses, eg, every 3–4 hours for 24–48 hours. In patients not taking an inhaled corticosteroid, initiation of this agent should be considered.

In patients already taking an inhaled corticosteroid, a 7-day course of oral corticosteroids (0.5–1.0 mg/kg/d) may be necessary. Doubling the dose of inhaled corticosteroid is not effective and is not recommended in the NAEPP 3 guidelines.

B. Moderate Exacerbations

The principal goals of treatment of moderate asthma exacerbations are correction of hypoxemia, reversal of airflow obstruction, and reduction of the likelihood of recurrence of obstruction. Early intervention may lessen the severity and shorten the duration of an exacerbation. Of paramount importance is correction of hypoxemia through the use of supplemental oxygen. Airflow obstruction is treated with continuous administration of an inhaled short-acting β_2-agonist and the early administration of systemic corticosteroids. Serial measurements of lung function to quantify the severity of airflow obstruction and its response to treatment are useful. The improvement in FEV_1 after 30 minutes of treatment correlates significantly with a broad range of indices of the severity of asthma exacerbations. Serial measurement of airflow in the emergency department is an important factor in disposition and may reduce the rate of hospital admissions for asthma exacerbations. The post-exacerbation care plan is an important aspect of management. Regardless of the severity, all patients should be provided with necessary medications and education in how to use them, instruction in self-assessment, a follow-up appointment, and instruction in an action plan for managing recurrence.

C. Severe Exacerbations

Owing to the life-threatening nature of severe exacerbations of asthma, treatment should be started immediately once the exacerbation is recognized. All patients with a severe exacerbation should immediately receive oxygen,

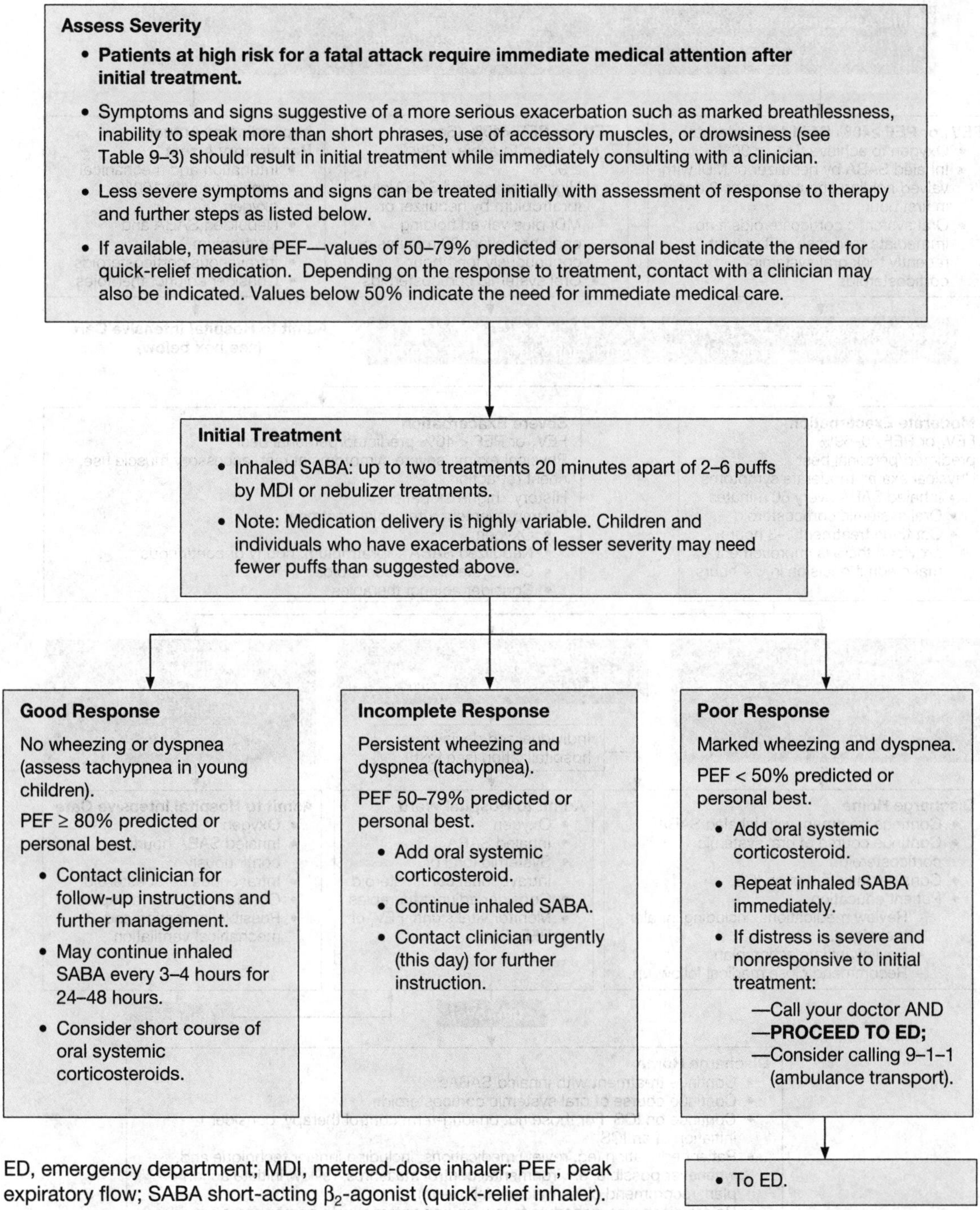

Assess Severity

- **Patients at high risk for a fatal attack require immediate medical attention after initial treatment.**

- Symptoms and signs suggestive of a more serious exacerbation such as marked breathlessness, inability to speak more than short phrases, use of accessory muscles, or drowsiness (see Table 9–3) should result in initial treatment while immediately consulting with a clinician.

- Less severe symptoms and signs can be treated initially with assessment of response to therapy and further steps as listed below.

- If available, measure PEF—values of 50–79% predicted or personal best indicate the need for quick-relief medication. Depending on the response to treatment, contact with a clinician may also be indicated. Values below 50% indicate the need for immediate medical care.

Initial Treatment

- Inhaled SABA: up to two treatments 20 minutes apart of 2–6 puffs by MDI or nebulizer treatments.

- Note: Medication delivery is highly variable. Children and individuals who have exacerbations of lesser severity may need fewer puffs than suggested above.

Good Response

No wheezing or dyspnea (assess tachypnea in young children).

PEF ≥ 80% predicted or personal best.

- Contact clinician for follow-up instructions and further management.

- May continue inhaled SABA every 3–4 hours for 24–48 hours.

- Consider short course of oral systemic corticosteroids.

Incomplete Response

Persistent wheezing and dyspnea (tachypnea).

PEF 50–79% predicted or personal best.

- Add oral systemic corticosteroid.

- Continue inhaled SABA.

- Contact clinician urgently (this day) for further instruction.

Poor Response

Marked wheezing and dyspnea.

PEF < 50% predicted or personal best.

- Add oral systemic corticosteroid.

- Repeat inhaled SABA immediately.

- If distress is severe and nonresponsive to initial treatment:

  —Call your doctor AND
  —**PROCEED TO ED;**
  —Consider calling 9–1–1 (ambulance transport).

ED, emergency department; MDI, metered-dose inhaler; PEF, peak expiratory flow; SABA short-acting β₂-agonist (quick-relief inhaler).

- To ED.

▲ **Figure 9–3.** Management of asthma exacerbations: home treatment. (Adapted from National Asthma Education and Prevention Program. Expert Panel Report 3: Guidelines for the Diagnosis and Management of Asthma. National Institutes of Health Pub. No. 08-4051. Bethesda, MD, 2007. http://www.nhlbi.nih.gov/guidelines/asthma/asthgdln.htm.)

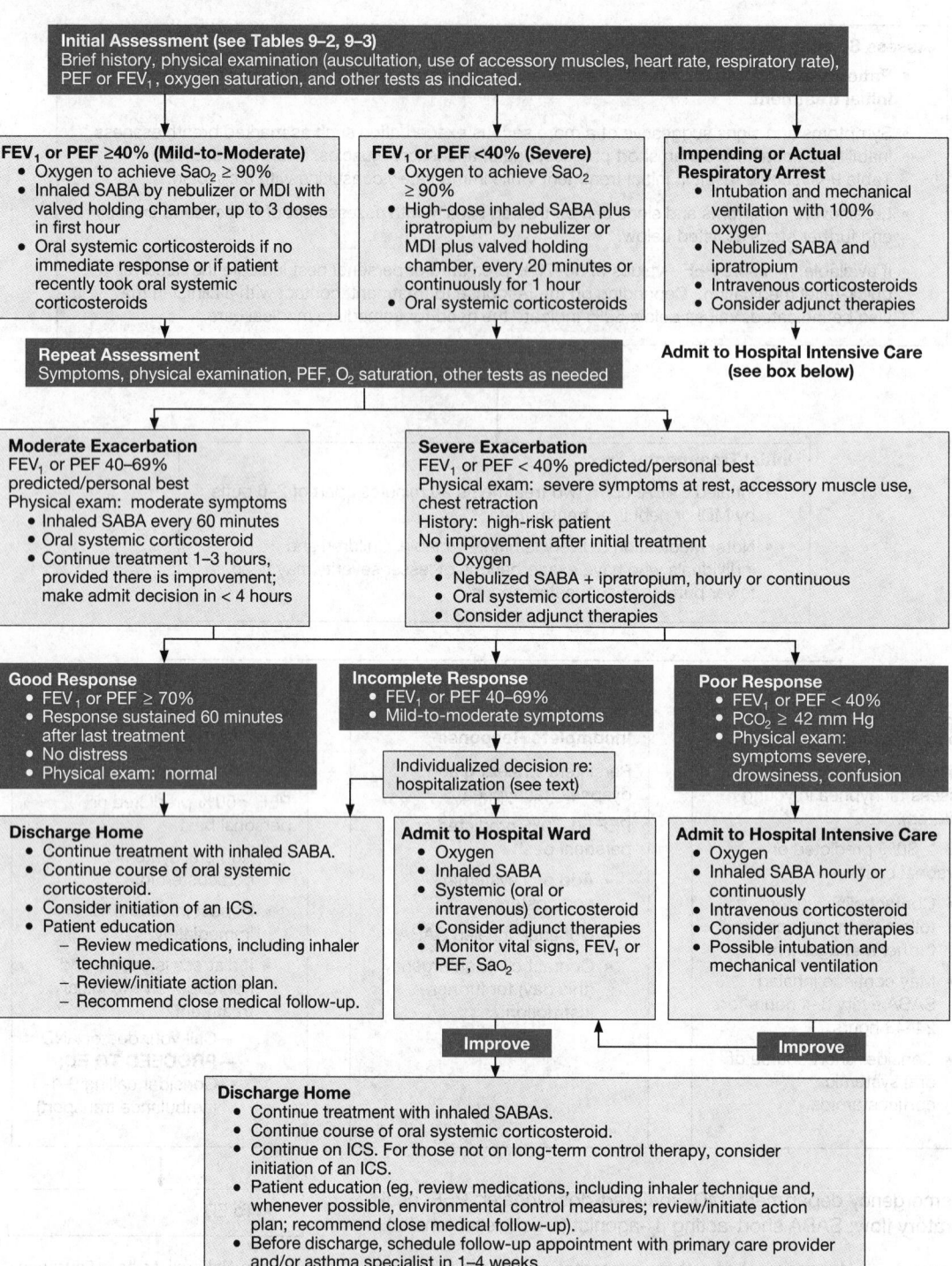

FEV$_1$, forced expiratory volume in 1 second; ICS, inhaled corticosteroid; MDI, metered-dose inhaler; PEF, peak expiratory flow; SABA, short-acting β$_2$-agonist; SaO$_2$, oxygen saturation.

▲ **Figure 9–4.** Management of asthma exacerbations: emergency department and hospital-based treatment. (Adapted from National Asthma Education and Prevention Program. Expert Panel Report 3: Guidelines for the Diagnosis and Management of Asthma. National Institutes of Health Pub. No. 08-4051. Bethesda, MD, 2007. http://www.nhlbi.nih.gov/guidelines/asthma/asthgdln.htm.)

high doses of an inhaled short-acting β_2-agonist, and systemic corticosteroids. A brief history pertinent to the exacerbation can be completed while treatment is being initiated. More detailed assessments, including laboratory studies, usually add little in the early phase of evaluation and management and should be postponed until after therapy is instituted.

Asphyxia is a common cause of fatal asthma, and oxygen therapy is therefore very important. Supplemental oxygen should be given to maintain an $SaO_2 > 90\%$ or a $PaO_2 > 60$ mm Hg. Oxygen-induced hypoventilation is extremely rare, and concern for hypercapnia should never delay correction of hypoxemia.

Frequent high-dose delivery of an inhaled short-acting β_2-agonist is indicated and is usually well tolerated in the setting of severe airway obstruction. Some studies suggest that continuous therapy is more efficacious than intermittent administration of these agents, but there is no clear consensus as long as similar doses are administered. At least three MDI or nebulizer treatments should be given in the first hour of therapy. Thereafter, the frequency of administration varies according to the improvement in airflow and associated symptoms and the occurrence of side effects. Ipratropium bromide reduces the rate of hospital admissions when added to inhaled short-acting β_2-agonists in patients with moderate to severe asthma exacerbations.

Systemic corticosteroids are administered as detailed above. Mucolytic agents (eg, acetylcysteine, potassium iodide) may worsen cough or airflow obstruction. Anxiolytic and hypnotic drugs are generally contraindicated in severe asthma exacerbations because of their respiratory depressant effects. In acute severe asthma ($FEV_1 < 25\%$ of predicted on presentation, or failure to respond to initial treatment), intravenous magnesium sulfate (2 g intravenously over 20 minutes) produces a detectable improvement in airflow and may reduce hospitalization rates.

Repeat assessment of patients with severe exacerbations should be made after the initial dose of inhaled bronchodilator and after three doses of inhaled bronchodilators (60–90 minutes after initiating treatment). The response to initial treatment is a better predictor of the need for hospitalization than is the severity of an exacerbation on presentation. The decision to hospitalize a patient should be based on the duration and severity of symptoms, severity of airflow obstruction, course and severity of prior exacerbations, medication use at the time of the exacerbation, access to medical care and medications, adequacy of social support and home conditions, and presence of psychiatric illness. In general, discharge to home is appropriate if the PEF or FEV_1 has returned to $\geq 60\%$ of predicted or personal best and symptoms are minimal or absent. Patients with a rapid response to treatment should be observed for 30 minutes after the most recent dose of bronchodilator to ensure stability of response before discharge to home.

A small subset of patients will not respond well to treatment and will show signs of impending respiratory failure due to a combination of worsening airflow obstruction and respiratory muscle fatigue (see Table 9–3). Such patients can deteriorate rapidly and thus should be monitored in a critical care setting. Intubation of an acutely ill asthma patient is technically difficult and is best done semi-electively, before the crisis of a respiratory arrest. At the time of intubation, close attention should be given to maintaining intravascular volume because hypotension commonly accompanies the administration of sedation and the initiation of positive-pressure ventilation in patients dehydrated due to poor recent oral intake and high insensible losses.

The main goals of mechanical ventilation are to ensure adequate oxygen and to avoid barotrauma. Controlled hypoventilation with permissive hypercapnia is often required to limit airway pressures. Frequent high-dose delivery of inhaled short-acting β_2-agonists should be continued along with anti-inflammatory agents as discussed above. Many questions remain regarding the optimal delivery of inhaled β_2-agonists to intubated, mechanically ventilated patients. Further studies are needed to determine the comparative efficacy of MDIs and nebulizers, optimal ventilator settings to use during drug delivery, ideal site along the ventilator circuit for introduction of the delivery system, and maximal acceptable drug doses. Unconventional therapies such as helium-oxygen mixtures and inhalational anesthetic agents are of unclear benefit but may be appropriate in selected patients.

▶ When to Refer

- Atypical presentation or uncertain diagnosis, particularly if additional diagnostic testing is required (bronchoprovocation challenge, skin testing for allergies, rhinoscopy, consideration of occupational exposure).
- Complicating comorbid problems, such as rhinosinusitis, tobacco use, multiple environmental allergies, suspected allergic bronchopulmonary aspergillosis.
- Suboptimal response to therapy.
- Patient is not meeting goals of asthma therapy after 3–6 months of treatment.
- Adult patient requires high-dose inhaled corticosteroids for control.
- Patient has required more than two courses of oral prednisone therapy in the past 12 months.
- Patient has an exacerbation requiring hospitalization in the past 12 months.
- Patient has had a life-threatening asthma exacerbation.
- Presence of social or psychological issues interfering with asthma management.

Aldington S et al. Asthma exacerbations. 5: Assessment and management of severe asthma in adults in hospital. Thorax. 2007 May;62(5):447–58. [PMID: 17468458]

Global Initiative for Asthma. Full text available online: http://www.ginasthma.com

Ibrahim WH et al. Paradoxical vocal cord motion disorder: past, present and future. Postgrad Med J. 2007 Mar;83(977):164–72. [PMID: 17344570]

National Asthma Education and Prevention Program: Expert panel report III: Guidelines for the diagnosis and management of asthma. Bethesda, MD: National Heart, Lung, and Blood Institute, 2007. (NIH publication no. 08-4051). Full text available online: http://www.nhlbi.nih.gov/guidelines/asthma/asthgdln.htm

Panettieri RA Jr. In the clinic. Asthma. Ann Intern Med. 2007 Jun 5;146(11):ITC6-1–ITC6-16. [PMID: 17548407]

Pinnock H et al. Asthma. BMJ. 2007 Apr 21;334(7598):847–50. [PMID: 17446617]

Rey E et al. Asthma in pregnancy. BMJ. 2007 Mar 17;334(7593):582–5. [PMID: 17363831]

Tilles SA. Differential diagnosis of adult asthma. Med Clin North Am. 2006 Jan;90(1):61–76. [PMID: 16310524]

CHRONIC OBSTRUCTIVE PULMONARY DISEASE

 ESSENTIALS OF DIAGNOSIS

▸ History of cigarette smoking.

▸ Chronic cough, dyspnea (in emphysema), and sputum production (in chronic bronchitis).

▸ Rhonchi, decreased intensity of breath sounds, and prolonged expiration on physical examination.

▸ Airflow limitation on pulmonary function testing that is not fully reversible and most often progressive.

General Considerations

COPD is a disease state characterized by the presence of airflow obstruction due to chronic bronchitis or emphysema; the airflow obstruction is generally progressive, may be accompanied by airway hyperreactivity, and may be partially reversible (American Thoracic Society). The NHLBI estimates that 14 million Americans have been diagnosed with COPD; an equal number are thought to be afflicted but remain undiagnosed. Grouped together, COPD and asthma now represent the fourth leading cause of death in the United States, with over 120,000 deaths reported annually. The death rate from COPD is increasing rapidly, especially among elderly men.

Most patients with COPD have features of both emphysema and chronic bronchitis. **Chronic bronchitis** is a clinical diagnosis defined by excessive secretion of bronchial mucus and is manifested by daily productive cough for 3 months or more in at least 2 consecutive years. **Emphysema** is a pathologic diagnosis that denotes abnormal permanent enlargement of air spaces distal to the terminal bronchiole, with destruction of their walls and without obvious fibrosis.

Cigarette smoking is clearly the most important cause of COPD in North America and Western Europe. Nearly all smokers suffer an accelerated decline in lung function that is dose- and duration-dependent. Fifteen percent develop progressively disabling symptoms in their 40s and 50s. It is estimated that 80% of patients seen for COPD have significant exposure to tobacco smoke. The remaining 20% frequently have a combination of exposures to environmental tobacco smoke, occupational dusts and chemicals, and indoor air pollution from biomass fuel used for cooking and heating in poorly ventilated buildings. Outdoor air pollution, airway infection, familial factors, and allergy have also been implicated in chronic bronchitis, and hereditary factors (deficiency of α_1-antiprotease [α_1-antitrypsin])

have been implicated in COPD. The pathogenesis of emphysema may involve excessive lysis of elastin and other structural proteins in the lung matrix by elastase and other proteases derived from lung neutrophils, macrophages, and mononuclear cells. Atopy and the tendency for bronchoconstriction to develop in response to nonspecific airway stimuli may be important risks for COPD.

▸ Clinical Findings

A. Symptoms and Signs

Patients with COPD characteristically present in the fifth or sixth decade of life complaining of excessive cough, sputum production, and shortness of breath. Symptoms have often been present for 10 years or more. Dyspnea is noted initially only on heavy exertion, but as the condition progresses it occurs with mild activity. In severe disease, dyspnea occurs at rest. As the disease progresses, two symptom patterns tend to emerge, historically referred to as "pink puffers" and "blue bloaters" (Table 9–7). These patterns were once thought to represent pure forms of emphysema and bronchitis, respectively, but this is a simplification of the anatomy and pathophysiology. Most COPD patients have pathologic evidence of both disorders, and their clinical course may reflect other factors such as central control of ventilation and concomitant sleep-disordered breathing.

Pneumonia, pulmonary hypertension, cor pulmonale, and chronic respiratory failure characterize the late stage of COPD. A hallmark of COPD is the exacerbation of symptoms beyond normal day-to-day variation, often including increased dyspnea, an increased frequency or severity of cough, increased sputum volume or change in sputum character. These exacerbations are commonly precipitated by infection (more often viral than bacterial) or environmental factors. Exacerbations of COPD vary widely in severity but typically require a change in regular therapy.

B. Laboratory Findings

Spirometry provides objective information about pulmonary function and assesses the results of therapy. Pulmonary function tests early in the course of COPD reveal only evidence of abnormal closing volume and reduced midexpiratory flow rate. Reductions in FEV_1 and in the ratio of forced expiratory volume to vital capacity (FEV_1% or FEV_1/FVC ratio) occur later. In severe disease, the FVC is markedly reduced. Lung volume measurements reveal a marked increase in residual volume (RV), an increase in total lung capacity (TLC), and an elevation of the RV/TLC ratio, indicative of air trapping, particularly in emphysema.

Arterial blood gas measurements characteristically show no abnormalities early in COPD other than an increased $A–a–DO_2$. Indeed, they are unnecessary unless (1) hypoxemia or hypercapnia is suspected, (2) the FEV_1 is < 40% of predicted, or (3) there are clinical signs of right heart failure. Hypoxemia occurs in advanced disease, particularly when chronic bronchitis predominates. Compensated respiratory acidosis occurs in patients with chronic respiratory failure, particularly in chronic bronchitis, with worsening of acidemia during acute exacerbations.

Table 9–7. Patterns of disease in advanced COPD.

	Type A: Pink Puffer (Emphysema Predominant)	Type B: Blue Bloater (Bronchitis Predominant)
History and physical examination	Major complaint is dyspnea, often severe, usually presenting after age 50. Cough is rare, with scant clear, mucoid sputum. Patients are thin, with recent weight loss common. They appear uncomfortable, with evident use of accessory muscles of respiration. Chest is very quiet without adventitious sounds. No peripheral edema.	Major complaint is chronic cough, productive of mucopurulent sputum, with frequent exacerbations due to chest infections. Often presents in late 30s and 40s. Dyspnea usually mild, though patients may note limitations to exercise. Patients frequently overweight and cyanotic but seem comfortable at rest. Peripheral edema is common. Chest is noisy, with rhonchi invariably present; wheezes are common.
Laboratory studies	Hemoglobin usually normal (12–15 g/dL). Pa_{O_2} normal to slightly reduced (65–75 mm Hg) but Sa_{O_2} normal at rest. Pa_{CO_2} normal to slightly reduced (35–40 mm Hg). Chest radiograph shows hyperinflation with flattened diaphragms. Vascular markings are diminished, particularly at the apices.	Hemoglobin usually elevated (15–18 g/dL). Pa_{O_2} reduced (45–60 mm Hg) and Pa_{CO_2} slightly to markedly elevated (50–60 mm Hg). Chest radiograph shows increased interstitial markings ("dirty lungs"), especially at bases. Diaphragms are not flattened.
Pulmonary function tests	Airflow obstruction ubiquitous. Total lung capacity increased, sometimes markedly so. $D_{L_{CO}}$ reduced. Static lung compliance increased.	Airflow obstruction ubiquitous. Total lung capacity generally normal but may be slightly increased. $D_{L_{CO}}$ normal. Static lung compliance normal.
Special evaluations		
$\dot{V}/\dot{Q}$ matching	Increased ventilation to high $\dot{V}/\dot{Q}$ areas, ie, high dead space ventilation.	Increased perfusion to low $\dot{V}/\dot{Q}$ areas.
Hemodynamics	Cardiac output normal to slightly low. Pulmonary artery pressures mildly elevated and increase with exercise.	Cardiac output normal. Pulmonary artery pressures elevated, sometimes markedly so, and worsen with exercise.
Nocturnal ventilation	Mild to moderate degree of oxygen desaturation not usually associated with obstructive sleep apnea.	Severe oxygen desaturation, frequently associated with obstructive sleep apnea.
Exercise ventilation	Increased minute ventilation for level of oxygen consumption. Pa_{O_2} tends to fall, Pa_{CO_2} rises slightly.	Decreased minute ventilation for level of oxygen consumption. Pa_{O_2} may rise; Pa_{CO_2} may rise significantly.

$D_{L_{CO}}$, single-breath diffusing capacity for carbon monoxide; $\dot{V}/\dot{Q}$, ventilation-perfusion.

Examination of the sputum may reveal *Streptococcus pneumoniae*, *H influenzae*, or *Moraxella catarrhalis*. Positive sputum cultures are poorly correlated with acute exacerbations, and research techniques demonstrate evidence of preceding viral infection in a majority of patients with exacerbations. The ECG may show sinus tachycardia and, in advanced disease, chronic pulmonary hypertension may produce electrocardiographic abnormalities typical of cor pulmonale. Supraventricular arrhythmias (multifocal atrial tachycardia, atrial flutter, and atrial fibrillation) and ventricular irritability also occur.

C. Imaging

Radiographs of patients with chronic bronchitis typically show only nonspecific peribronchial and perivascular markings. Plain radiographs are insensitive for the diagnosis of emphysema; they show hyperinflation with flattening of the diaphragm or peripheral arterial deficiency in about half of cases. CT of the chest, particularly using a high-resolution reconstruction algorithm, is more sensitive and specific than plain radiographs for the diagnosis of emphysema. Pulmonary hypertension may be suggested by enlargement of central pulmonary arteries in advanced disease. Doppler echocardiography is an effective noninvasive way to estimate pulmonary artery pressure if pulmonary hypertension is suspected.

Differential Diagnosis

Clinical, imaging, and laboratory findings should enable the clinician to distinguish COPD from other obstructive pulmonary disorders such as bronchial asthma, bronchiectasis, cystic fibrosis, bronchopulmonary mycosis, and central airflow obstruction. Simple asthma is characterized by complete or near-complete reversibility of airflow obstruction. Bronchiectasis is distinguished from COPD by features such as recurrent pneumonia and hemoptysis, digital clubbing, and characteristic imaging abnormalities. Patients with severe α_1-antiprotease (α_1-antitrypsin) deficiency are recognized by family history and the appearance of panacinar bibasilar emphysema early in life, usually in the third or fourth decade; hepatic cirrhosis and hepatocellular carcinoma may occur. Cystic fibrosis occurs in children and younger adults. Rarely, mechanical obstruction of the central airways simulates COPD. Flow-volume loops may help separate patients with central airway obstruction from those with diffuse intrathoracic airway obstruction characteristic of COPD.

► Complications

Acute bronchitis, pneumonia, pulmonary thromboembolism, and concomitant left ventricular failure may worsen otherwise stable COPD. Pulmonary hypertension, cor pulmonale, and chronic respiratory failure are common in advanced COPD. Spontaneous pneumothorax occurs in a small fraction of patients with emphysema. Hemoptysis may result from chronic bronchitis or may signal bronchogenic carcinoma.

► Prevention

COPD is largely preventable through elimination of long-term exposure to tobacco smoke. Smokers with early evidence of airflow limitation can significantly alter their disease by smoking cessation. Smoking cessation slows the decline in FEV_1 in middle-aged smokers with mild airways obstruction. Vaccination against influenza and pneumococcal infection may also be of benefit.

► Treatment

The treatment of COPD is guided by the severity of symptoms or the presence of an exacerbation or stable symptoms. Standards for the management of patients with stable COPD and COPD exacerbations have been published by the American Thoracic Society and the Global Initiative for Obstructive Lung Disease (GOLD), a joint expert committee of the NHLBI and the WHO. See Chapter 37 for a discussion of air travel in patients with lung disease.

A. Ambulatory Patients

1. Smoking cessation—The single most important intervention in smokers with COPD is to encourage smoking cessation. Simply telling a patient to quit succeeds 5% of the time. Behavioral approaches, ranging from clinician advice to intensive group programs, may improve cessation rates. Pharmacologic therapy includes nicotine replacement (transdermal patch, gum, lozenge, inhaler, or nasal spray), bupropion, and varenicline (a partial agonist of nicotine acetylcholine receptors) (see Chapter 1). Combined pharmacotherapies (two forms of nicotine replacement, or nicotine replacement and bupropion), with or without behavioral approaches have also been recommended. The Lung Health Study reported 22% sustained abstinence at 5 years in their intervention group (behavior modification plus nicotine gum). Varenicline has proved effective but wider use has revealed significant CNS side effects, including some reports of an increase in suicide.

2. Oxygen therapy—The only drug therapy that is documented to improve the natural history of COPD is supplemental oxygen in those patients with resting hypoxemia. Proved benefits of home oxygen therapy in hypoxemic patients include longer survival, reduced hospitalization needs, and better quality of life. Survival in hypoxemic patients with COPD treated with supplemental oxygen therapy is directly proportionate to the number of hours per day oxygen is administered: in patients treated with continuous oxygen, the survival after 36 months is about 65%—significantly better than the survival rate of about 45% in those who are treated with only nocturnal oxygen. Oxygen by nasal prongs must be given at least 15 hours a day unless therapy is intended only for exercise or sleep.

Requirements for Medicare coverage for a patient's home use of oxygen and oxygen equipment are listed in Table 9–8. Arterial blood gas analysis is preferred over oximetry to guide initial oxygen therapy. Hypoxemic patients with pulmonary hypertension, chronic cor pulmonale, erythrocytosis, impaired cognitive function, exercise intolerance, nocturnal restlessness, or morning headache are particularly likely to benefit from home oxygen therapy.

Home oxygen may be supplied by liquid oxygen systems (LOX), compressed gas cylinders, or oxygen concentrators. Most patients benefit from having both stationary and portable systems. For most patients, a flow rate of 1–3 L/min achieves a PaO_2 greater than 55 mm Hg. The monthly cost of home oxygen therapy ranges from $300.00 to $500.00 or more, higher for liquid oxygen systems. Medicare covers approximately 80% of home oxygen expenses. **Transtracheal oxygen** is an alternative method of delivery and may be useful for patients who require higher flows of oxygen than can be delivered via the nose or who are experiencing troublesome side effects from nasal delivery such as nasal drying or epistaxis. Reservoir

Table 9–8. Home oxygen therapy: Requirements for Medicare coverage.[1]

Group I (any of the following):
1. $PaO_2 \leq 55$ mm Hg or $SaO_2 \leq 88\%$ taken at rest breathing room air, while awake.
2. During sleep (prescription for nocturnal oxygen use only):
   a. $PaO_2 \leq 55$ mm Hg or $SaO_2 \leq 88\%$ for a patient whose awake, resting, room air PaO_2 is ≥ 56 mm Hg or $SaO_2 \geq 89\%$,
   or
   b. Decrease in $PaO_2 > 10$ mm Hg or decrease in $SaO_2 > 5\%$ associated with symptoms or signs reasonably attributed to hypoxemia (eg, impaired cognitive processes, nocturnal restlessness, insomnia).
3. During exercise (prescription for oxygen use only during exercise):
   a. $PaO_2 \leq 55$ mg Hg or $SaO_2 \leq 88\%$ taken during exercise for a patient whose awake, resting, room air PaO_2 is ≥ 56 mm Hg or $SaO_2 \geq 89\%$,
   and
   b. There is evidence that the use of supplemental oxygen during exercise improves the hypoxemia that was demonstrated during exercise while breathing room air.

Group II[2]:
$PaO_2 = 56$–59 mm Hg or $SaO_2 = 89\%$ if there is evidence of any of the following:
1. Dependent edema suggesting congestive heart failure.
2. P pulmonale on ECG (P wave > 3 mm in standard leads II, III, or aVF).
3. Hematocrit > 56%.

[1]Health Care Financing Administration, 1989.
[2]Patients in this group must have a second oxygen test 3 months after the initial oxygen set-up.

nasal cannulas or "pendants" and demand (pulse) oxygen delivery systems are also available to conserve oxygen.

3. Inhaled bronchodilators—Bronchodilators are agents in the pharmacologic management of patients with COPD. Bronchodilators do not alter the inexorable decline in lung function that is a hallmark of the disease, but they offer some patients improvement in symptoms, exercise tolerance, and overall health status. Aggressiveness of bronchodilator therapy should be matched to the severity of the patient's disease. In patients who experience no symptomatic improvement, bronchodilators should be discontinued.

The most commonly prescribed short-acting bronchodilators are the anticholinergic ipratropium bromide and β_2-agonists (eg, albuterol, metaproterenol), delivered by MDI or as an inhalation solution by nebulizer. Ipratropium bromide is generally preferred to the short-acting β_2-agonists as a first-line agent because of its longer duration of action and absence of sympathomimetic side effects. Some studies have suggested that ipratropium achieves superior bronchodilation in COPD patients. Typical doses are two to four puffs (36–72 mcg) every 6 hours. Short-acting β_2-agonists are less expensive and have a more rapid onset of action, commonly leading to greater patient satisfaction. At maximal doses, β_2-agonists have bronchodilator action equivalent to that of ipratropium but may cause tachycardia, tremor, or hypokalemia. There does not appear to be any advantage of scheduled use of short-acting β_2-agonists compared with as-needed administration. Use of both short-acting β_2-agonists and anticholinergics at submaximal doses leads to improved bronchodilation compared with either agent alone but does not improve dyspnea.

Long-acting β_2-agonists (eg, formoterol, salmeterol) and anticholinergics (tiotropium) appear to achieve bronchodilation that is equivalent or superior to what is experienced with ipratropium, in addition to similar improvements on health status. Although they are more expensive than short-acting agents, long-acting bronchodilators may have superior clinical efficacy in persons with advanced disease. A recent large randomized controlled trial (RCT) of long-term administration of tiotropium added to standard therapy reported fewer exacerbations or hospitalizations, and improved dyspnea scores, in the tiotropium group. Tiotropium had no effect on long-term decline in lung function, however. Another RCT comparing the effects of tiotropium with those of salmeterol-fluticasone in COPD over 2 years reported no difference in the risk of exacerbation. However, the incidence of pneumonia was higher in the salmeterol-fluticasone group, yet the dyspnea scores were lower, and there was a mortality benefit compared with tiotropium. This last finding awaits confirmation in further studies.

Whether there is a mortality benefit associated with salmeterol-fluticasone therapy remains controversial since serious concerns have been raised about the safety of both long-acting β_2-agonists and anticholinergics. Two large RCTs in asthmatic patients reported an increase in exacerbations and mortality in patients treated with salmeterol. These findings have not been observed in COPD patients, however, and several studies report a trend toward lower mortality in patients treated with salmeterol alone, compared with placebo. Several small studies and a recent meta-analysis have reported an increase in cardiovascular events among patients treated with long- and short-acting anticholinergics. In contrast, the 4-year tiotropium trial reported fewer cardiovascular events in the intervention group. Most practitioners believe that the documented benefits of anticholinergic therapy outweigh the potential risks, but this is an area of uncertainty and ongoing study.

4. Corticosteroids—Multiple large clinical trials have reported a reduction in the frequency of COPD exacerbations and an increase in self-reported functional status in COPD patients treated with inhaled corticosteroids. These same trials demonstrate no effect of inhaled corticosteroids on mortality or the characteristic decline in lung function experienced by COPD patients. At this time, inhaled corticosteroids alone should not be considered first-line therapy in stable COPD patients, who benefit more from bronchodilators, smoking cessation, and pulmonary rehabilitation.

Combination therapy with an inhaled corticosteroid and a long-acting β_2-agonist reduces the frequency of COPD exacerbations and improves self-reported functional status in COPD patients, compared with placebo or sole use of inhaled corticosteroids, long-acting β_2-agonists, or anticholinergics. Addition of an inhaled corticosteroid/long-acting β_2-agonist to tiotropium therapy in COPD patients does not reduce the frequency of COPD exacerbations but did improve hospitalization rates as well as self-reported functional status in one RCT.

Apart from acute exacerbations, COPD is not generally responsive to oral corticosteroid therapy. Only 10–20% of stable outpatients with COPD given oral corticosteroids will have a greater than 20% increase in FEV_1 compared with patients receiving placebo. There may be a subset of steroid-responsive COPD patients more likely to benefit from long-term oral or inhaled corticosteroids. Since there are no clinical predictors to identify such responders, empiric trials of oral corticosteroids are common. Current research provides little guidance to interpret clinically relevant benefit and clinically significant changes in spirometry, however. If empiric trials of oral corticosteroids are conducted, rigorous outcome assessment as advocated by the McMaster group is appropriate. The use of oral or systemic corticosteroids has well-recognized adverse effects, and it seems prudent management to seek to minimize cumulative oral corticosteroid exposure. Some patients may be truly "corticosteroid-dependent," but clinical experience suggests that this is rare when all other available therapies are optimized.

5. Theophylline—Oral **theophylline** is a fourth-line agent for treating patients with COPD who do not achieve adequate symptom control with anticholinergics, β_2-agonists, and inhaled corticosteroid therapy. Sustained-release theophylline improves hemoglobin saturation during sleep in COPD patients and is a first-line agent for those with sleep-related breathing disorders. Theophylline has fallen out of favor because of its narrow therapeutic window and the availability of potent inhaled bronchodilators. Nonetheless, theophylline does improve dyspnea, exercise performance, and pulmonary function in many patients with stable COPD. Its benefits may result from anti-inflammatory properties and extrapulmonary effects on diaphragm strength, myocardial contractility, and kidney function.

6. Antibiotics—Antibiotics are commonly prescribed to outpatients with COPD for the following indications: (1) to treat an acute exacerbation, (2) to treat acute bronchitis, and (3) to prevent acute exacerbations of chronic bronchitis (prophylactic antibiotics). Antibiotics appear to improve outcomes slightly in the first two situations, but there is no convincing evidence to support the use of prophylactic antibiotics in patients with COPD. Patients with a COPD exacerbation associated with dyspnea and a change in the quantity or character of sputum benefit the most from antibiotic therapy. In the past, common agents included trimethoprim-sulfamethoxazole (160/800 mg every 12 hours), amoxicillin (500 mg every 8 hours), or doxycycline (100 mg every 12 hours) given for 7–10 days. Prescribing patterns have changed, and a recent meta-analysis of antibiotic therapy in acute bronchitis complicating COPD found macrolides (azithromycin 500 mg followed by 250 mg daily for 5 days), fluoroquinolones (ciprofloxacin 500 mg every 12 hours), and amoxicillin-clavulanate (875/125 mg every 12 hours) to be more effective than older therapies. There are few controlled trials of antibiotics in severe COPD exacerbations but prompt administration of antibiotics is appropriate, particularly in those with risk factors for poor outcomes.

7. Pulmonary rehabilitation—Graded aerobic physical exercise programs (eg, walking 20 minutes three times weekly or bicycling) are helpful to prevent deterioration of physical condition and to improve patients' ability to carry out daily activities. Training of inspiratory muscles by inspiring against progressively larger resistive loads reduces dyspnea and improves exercise tolerance, health status, and respiratory muscle strength in some but not all patients. Pursed-lip breathing to slow the rate of breathing and abdominal breathing exercises to relieve fatigue of accessory muscles of respiration may reduce dyspnea in some patients. Many patients undergo these exercise and educational interventions in a structured rehabilitation program. In a number of studies, pulmonary rehabilitation has been shown to improve exercise capacity, decrease hospitalizations, and enhance quality of life. Referral to a comprehensive rehabilitation program is recommended in patients who have severe dyspnea, reduced quality of life, or frequent hospitalizations despite optimal medical therapy.

8. Other measures—In patients with chronic bronchitis, increased mobilization of secretions may be accomplished through the use of adequate systemic hydration, effective cough training methods, or use of a hand-held flutter device and postural drainage, sometimes with chest percussion or vibration. Postural drainage and chest percussion should be used only in selected patients with excessive amounts of retained secretions that cannot be cleared by coughing and other methods; these measures are of no benefit in pure emphysema. Expectorant-mucolytic therapy has generally been regarded as unhelpful in patients with chronic bronchitis. Cough suppressants and sedatives should be avoided as routine measures.

Human α_1-antitrypsin is available for replacement therapy in emphysema due to congenital deficiency (PiZZ or null genotype) of α_1-antiprotease (α_1-antitrypsin). Patients over 18 years of age with airflow obstruction by spirometry and serum levels less than 11 mcmol/L (~50 mg/dL) are potential candidates for replacement therapy. There is no evidence that replacement therapy is beneficial to heterozygotes (eg, PiMZ) with low-normal serum levels, although such patients may be at slightly increased risk for emphysema, especially in the setting of tobacco smoke exposure. α_1-Antitrypsin is administered intravenously in a dose of 60 mg/kg body weight once weekly.

Severe dyspnea in spite of optimal medical management may warrant a clinical trial of an opioid. Sedative-hypnotic drugs (eg, diazepam, 5 mg three times daily) are controversial in intractable dyspnea but may benefit very anxious patients. Intermittent negative-pressure (cuirass) ventilation and transnasal positive-pressure ventilation at home to rest the respiratory muscles are promising approaches to improve respiratory muscle function and reduce dyspnea in patients with severe COPD. A bilevel transnasal ventilation system has been reported to reduce dyspnea in ambulatory patients with severe COPD, but the long-term benefits of this approach and compliance with it have not been defined.

B. Hospitalized Patients

Management of the hospitalized patient with an acute exacerbation of COPD includes supplemental oxygen, inhaled ipratropium bromide plus β_2-agonists, and broad-spectrum antibiotics, corticosteroids and, in selected cases, chest physiotherapy. Theophylline should not be initiated in the acute setting, but patients taking theophylline prior to acute hospitalization should have their theophylline serum levels measured and maintained in the therapeutic range. Oxygen therapy should not be withheld for fear of worsening respiratory acidemia; hypoxemia is more detrimental than hypercapnia. Cor pulmonale usually responds to measures that reduce pulmonary artery pressure, such as supplemental oxygen and correction of acidemia; bed rest, salt restriction, and diuretics may add some benefit. Cardiac arrhythmias, particularly multifocal atrial tachycardia, usually respond to aggressive treatment of COPD itself. Atrial flutter may require DC cardioversion after initiation of the above therapy. If progressive respiratory failure ensues, tracheal intubation and mechanical ventilation are necessary. In clinical trials of COPD patients with hypercapnic acute respiratory failure, noninvasive positive-pressure ventilation (NPPV) delivered via face mask reduced the need for intubation and shortened lengths of stay in the intensive care unit (ICU). Other studies have suggested a lower risk of health care-associated infections and less use of antibiotics in COPD patients treated with NPPV. These benefits do not appear to extend to hypoxemic respiratory failure or to patients with acute lung injury or ARDS.

C. Surgery for COPD

1. Lung transplantation—Experience with both single and bilateral sequential lung transplantation for severe COPD is extensive. Requirements for lung transplantation are severe lung disease, limited activities of daily living, exhaustion of medical therapy, ambulatory status, potential for pulmonary rehabilitation, limited life expectancy without transplantation, adequate function of other organ systems, and a good social support system. Average total charges for lung transplantation through the end of the first postoperative year exceed $250,000. The 2-year survival rate after lung transplantation for COPD is 75%. Complications include acute rejection, opportunistic infection, and obliterative bronchiolitis. Substantial improvements in pulmonary function and exercise performance have been noted after transplantation.

2. Lung volume reduction surgery—Lung volume reduction surgery (LVRS), or reduction pneumoplasty, is a surgical approach to relieve dyspnea and improve exercise tolerance in patients with advanced diffuse emphysema and lung hyperinflation. Bilateral resection of 20–30% of lung volume in selected patients results in modest improvements in pulmonary function, exercise performance, and dyspnea. The duration of any improvement as well as any mortality benefit remains uncertain. Prolonged air leaks occur in up to 50% of patients postoperatively. Mortality rates in centers with the largest experience with LVRS range from 4% to 10%.

The National Emphysema Treatment Trial compared LVRS with medical treatment in a randomized, multicenter clinical trial of 1218 patients with severe emphysema. Overall, surgery improved exercise capacity but not mortality when compared with medical therapy. The persistence of this benefit remains to be defined. Subgroup analysis suggested that patients with upper lobe predominant emphysema and low exercise capacity might have improved survival, while other groups suffered excess mortality when randomized to surgery.

3. Bullectomy—Bullectomy is an older surgical procedure for palliation of dyspnea in patients with severe bullous emphysema. Bullectomy is most commonly pursued when a single bulla occupies at least 30–50% of the hemithorax. In this procedure, the surgeon removes a large emphysematous bulla that demonstrates no ventilation or perfusion on lung scanning and compresses adjacent lung with preserved function. Bullectomy can be performed with a CO_2 laser via thoracoscopy.

Prognosis

The outlook for patients with clinically significant COPD is poor. The degree of pulmonary dysfunction at the time the patient is first seen is an important predictor of survival: median survival of patients with severe $FEV_1 \leq 1$ L is about 4 years. A multidimensional index (the BODE index), which includes body mass index (BMI), airway obstruction (FEV_1), dyspnea (Medical Research Council dyspnea score), and exercise capacity is a tool that predicts death and hospitalization better than FEV_1 alone. Comprehensive care programs, cessation of smoking, and supplemental oxygen may reduce the rate of decline of pulmonary function, but therapy with bronchodilators and other approaches probably has little, if any, impact on the natural course of COPD.

Dyspnea at the end of life can be extremely uncomfortable and distressing to the patient and family. Dyspnea can be effectively managed with a combination of medications and mechanical interventions. As patients near the end of life, meticulous attention to palliative care is essential (see Chapter 5).

When to Refer

- COPD onset occurs before the age of 40.
- Frequent exacerbations (two or more a year) despite optimal treatment.
- Severe or rapidly progressive COPD.
- Symptoms disproportionate to the severity of airflow obstruction.
- Need for long-term oxygen therapy.
- Onset of comorbid illnesses (such as bronchiectasis, heart failure, or lung cancer).

When to Admit

- Severe symptoms or acute worsening that fails to respond to outpatient management.
- Acute or worsening hypoxemia, hypercapnia, peripheral edema, or change in mental status.
- Inadequate home care, or inability to sleep or maintain nutrition/hydration due to symptoms.
- The presence of high-risk comorbid conditions.

Ambrosino N et al. The clinical management in extremely severe COPD. Respir Med. 2007 Aug;101(8):1613–24. [PMID: 17383170]

Cote CG et al. Predictors of mortality in chronic obstructive pulmonary disease. Clin Chest Med. 2007 Sep;28(3):515–24. [PMID: 17720040]

Nannini L et al. Combined corticosteroid and long-acting beta-agonist in one inhaler versus placebo for chronic obstructive pulmonary disease. Cochrane Database of Syst Rev. 2007 Oct 17;(4):CD003794. [PMID: 17943798]

Qaseem A et al. Diagnosis and management of stable chronic obstructive pulmonary disease: a clinical practice guideline from the American College of Physicians. Ann Intern Med. 2007 Nov 6;147(9):633–8. [PMID: 17975186]

Rabe KF et al; Global Initiative for Chronic Obstructive Lung Disease. Global strategy for the diagnosis, management, and prevention of chronic obstructive pulmonary disease: GOLD executive summary. Am J Respir Crit Care Med. 2007 Sep 15;176(6):532–55. [PMID: 17507545]

Singh S et al. Inhaled anticholinergics and risk of major adverse cardiovascular events in patients with chronic obstructive pulmonary disease: a systematic review and meta-analysis. JAMA. 2008 Sep 24;300(12):1439–50. [PMID: 18812535]

Tashkin DP et al. A 4-year trial of tiotropium in chronic obstructive pulmonary disease. N Engl J Med. 2008 Oct 9;359(15):1543–54. [PMID: 18836213]

Viegi G et al. Definition, epidemiology and natural history of COPD. Eur Respir J. 2007 Nov 30;(5):993–1013. [PMID: 17978157]

Wedzicha JA et al; INSPIRE Investigators. The prevention of chronic obstructive pulmonary disease exacerbations by salmeterol/fluticasone propionate or tiotropium bromide. Am J Respir Crit Care Med. 2008 Jan 1;177(1):19–26. [PMID: 17916806]

Wilson JF. In the clinic. Smoking cessation. Ann Intern Med. 2007 Feb 6;146(3):ITC2-1–ITC2-16. [PMID: 17283345]

Wilt TJ et al. Management of stable chronic obstructive pulmonary disease: a systemic review for a clinical practice guideline. Ann Intern Med. 2007 Nov 6;147(9):639–653. [PMID: 17975187]

Yang IA et al. Inhaled corticosteroids for stable chronic obstructive pulmonary disease. Cochrane Database of Syst Rev. 2007 Apr 18;(2):CD002991. [PMID: 17443520]

Zuwallack R. The nonpharmacologic treatment of chronic obstructive pulmonary disease: advances in our understanding of pulmonary rehabilitation. Proc Am Thorac Soc. 2007 Oct 1;4(7):549–53. [PMID: 17878468]

BRONCHIECTASIS

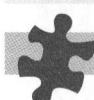 **ESSENTIALS OF DIAGNOSIS**

▶ Chronic productive cough with dyspnea and wheezing.

▶ Recurrent pulmonary infections requiring antibiotics.

▶ A preceding history of recurrent pulmonary infections or inflammation, or a predisposing condition.

▶ Radiographic findings of dilated, thickened airways and scattered, irregular opacities.

General Considerations

Bronchiectasis is a congenital or acquired disorder of the large bronchi characterized by permanent, abnormal dilation and destruction of bronchial walls. It may be caused by recurrent inflammation or infection of the airways and may be localized or diffuse. Cystic fibrosis causes about half of all cases of bronchiectasis. Other causes include lung infection (tuberculosis, fungal infections, lung abscess, pneumonia), abnormal lung defense mechanisms (humoral immunodeficiency, α_1-antiprotease [α_1-antitrypsin] deficiency with cigarette smoking, mucociliary clearance disorders, rheumatic diseases), and localized airway obstruction (foreign body, tumor, mucoid impaction). Immunodeficiency states that may lead to bronchiectasis include congenital or acquired panhypogammaglobulinemia; common variable immunodeficiency; selective IgA, IgM, and IgG subclass deficiencies; and acquired immunodeficiency from cytotoxic therapy, AIDS, lymphoma, multiple myeloma, leukemia, and chronic kidney and liver diseases. However, most patients with bronchiectasis have panhypergammaglobulinemia, presumably reflecting an immune system response to chronic airway infection. Acquired primary bronchiectasis is now uncommon in the United States because of improved control of bronchopulmonary infections.

Clinical Findings

A. Symptoms and Signs

Symptoms of bronchiectasis include chronic cough with production of copious amounts of purulent sputum, hemoptysis, and pleuritic chest pain. Dyspnea and wheezing occur in 75% of patients. Weight loss, anemia, and other systemic manifestations are common. Physical findings are nonspecific, but persistent crackles at the lung bases are common. Clubbing is infrequent in mild cases

but is common in severe disease (see Plate 47). Copious, foul-smelling, purulent sputum is characteristic. Obstructive pulmonary dysfunction with hypoxemia is seen in moderate or severe disease.

B. Imaging

Radiographic abnormalities include dilated and thickened bronchi that may appear as "tram-tracks" or as ring-like markings. Scattered irregular opacities, atelectasis, and focal consolidation may be present. High-resolution CT is the diagnostic study of choice.

▶ Treatment

Treatment of acute exacerbations consists of antibiotics (selected on the basis of sputum smears and cultures), daily chest physiotherapy with postural drainage and chest percussion, and inhaled bronchodilators. Hand-held flutter valve devices may be as effective as chest physiotherapy in clearing secretions. Empiric oral antibiotic therapy for 10–14 days with amoxicillin or amoxicillin-clavulanate (500 mg every 8 hours), ampicillin or tetracycline (250–500 mg four times daily), or trimethoprim-sulfamethoxazole (160/800 mg every 12 hours) is reasonable therapy in an acute exacerbation if a specific bacterial pathogen cannot be isolated. It is important to screen patients for infection with nontuberculous mycobacteria because these organisms may underlie a lack of treatment response. Preventive or suppressive treatment is sometimes given to stable outpatients with bronchiectasis who have copious purulent sputum. Clinical trial data to guide this practice are scant. Common regimens include macrolides (azithromycin, 500 mg three times a week; erythromycin, 500 mg twice daily), high-dose (3 g/d) amoxicillin or alternating cycles of the antibiotics listed above given orally for 2–4 weeks. In patients with underlying cystic fibrosis, inhaled aerosolized aminoglycosides reduce colonization by *Pseudomonas* species, improve FEV_1 and reduce hospitalizations; in non–cystic fibrosis bronchiectasis, adding inhaled tobramycin to oral ciprofloxacin for acute exacerbations due to *Pseudomonas* decreases microbial sputum burden but without apparent clinical benefit. Complications of bronchiectasis include hemoptysis, cor pulmonale, amyloidosis, and secondary visceral abscesses at distant sites (eg, brain). Bronchoscopy is sometimes necessary to evaluate hemoptysis, remove retained secretions, and rule out obstructing airway lesions. Massive hemoptysis may require embolization of bronchial arteries or surgical resection. Surgical resection is otherwise reserved for the few patients with localized bronchiectasis and adequate pulmonary function in whom conservative management fails.

Barker AF. Bronchiectasis. N Engl J Med. 2002 May 2;346(18):1383–93. [PMID: 11986413]

Ilowite J et al. Bronchiectasis: new findings in the pathogenesis and treatment of this disease. Curr Opin Infect Dis. 2008 Apr;21(2):163–7. [PMID: 18317040]

Morrissey BM. Pathogenesis of bronchiectasis. Clin Chest Med. 2007 Jun;28(2):289–96. [PMID: 17467548]

Noone PG et al. Primary ciliary dyskinesia: diagnostic and phenotypic features. Am J Respir Crit Care Med. 2004 Feb 15;169(4):459–67. [PMID: 14656747]

ALLERGIC BRONCHOPULMONARY MYCOSIS

Allergic bronchopulmonary mycosis is a pulmonary hypersensitivity disorder caused by allergy to fungal antigens that colonize the tracheobronchial tree. It usually occurs in atopic asthmatic individuals who are 20–40 years of age, in response to antigens of *Aspergillus* species. For this reason, the disorder is commonly referred to as allergic bronchopulmonary aspergillosis (ABPA). Primary criteria for the diagnosis of ABPA include (1) a clinical history of asthma, (2) peripheral eosinophilia, (3) immediate skin reactivity to *Aspergillus* antigen, (4) precipitating antibodies to *Aspergillus* antigen, (5) elevated serum IgE levels, (6) pulmonary infiltrates (transient or fixed), and (7) central bronchiectasis. If the first six of these seven primary criteria are present, the diagnosis is almost certain. Secondary diagnostic criteria include identification of *Aspergillus* in sputum, a history of brown-flecked sputum, and late skin reactivity to *Aspergillus* antigen. High-dose prednisone (0.5–1 mg/kg orally per day) for at least 2 months is the treatment of choice, and the response in early disease is usually excellent. Depending on the overall clinical situation, prednisone can then be cautiously tapered. Relapses are frequent, and protracted or repeated treatment with corticosteroids is not uncommon. Patients with corticosteroid-dependent disease may benefit from itraconazole (200 mg orally once or twice daily) without added toxicity. Bronchodilators (Table 9–6) are also helpful. Complications include hemoptysis, severe bronchiectasis, and pulmonary fibrosis.

Gibson PG. Allergic bronchopulmonary aspergillosis. Semin Respir Crit Care Med. 2006 Apr;27(2):185–91. [PMID: 16612769]

Virnig C et al. Allergic bronchopulmonary aspergillosis: a US perspective. Curr Opin Pulm Med. 2007 Jan;13(1):67–71. [PMID: 17133128]

CYSTIC FIBROSIS

ESSENTIALS OF DIAGNOSIS

▶ Chronic or recurrent cough, sputum production, dyspnea, and wheezing.

▶ Recurrent infections or chronic colonization of the airways with nontypeable *H influenzae,* mucoid and nonmucoid *Pseudomonas aeruginosa, Staphylococcus aureus,* or *Burkholderia cepacia.*

▶ Pancreatic insufficiency, recurrent pancreatitis, distal intestinal obstruction syndrome, chronic hepatic disease, nutritional deficiencies, or male urogenital abnormalities.

▶ Bronchiectasis and scarring on chest radiographs.

▶ Airflow obstruction on spirometry.

▶ Sweat chloride concentration above 60 mEq/L on two occasions or gene mutation known to cause cystic fibrosis.

General Considerations

Cystic fibrosis is the most common cause of severe chronic lung disease in young adults and the most common fatal hereditary disorder of whites in the United States. It is an autosomal recessive disorder affecting about 1 in 3200 whites; 1 in 25 is a carrier. Cystic fibrosis is caused by abnormalities in a membrane chloride channel (the cystic fibrosis transmembrane conductance regulator [CFTR] protein) that results in altered chloride transport and water flux across the apical surface of epithelial cells. Almost all exocrine glands produce an abnormal mucus that obstructs glands and ducts. Obstruction results in glandular dilation and damage to tissue. In the respiratory tract, inadequate hydration of the tracheobronchial epithelium impairs mucociliary function. High concentration of DNA in airway secretions (due to chronic airway inflammation and autolysis of neutrophils) increases sputum viscosity. Over 1000 mutations in the gene that encodes CFTR have been described, and at least 230 mutations are known to be associated with clinical abnormalities. The mutation referred to as ΔF508 accounts for about 60% of cases of cystic fibrosis.

Over one-third of the nearly 30,000 cystic fibrosis patients in the United States are adults. Because of the wide range of alterations seen in the CFTR protein structure and function, cystic fibrosis in adults may present with a variety of pulmonary and nonpulmonary manifestations. Pulmonary manifestations in adults include acute and chronic bronchitis, bronchiectasis, pneumonia, atelectasis, and peribronchial and parenchymal scarring. Pneumothorax and hemoptysis are common. Hypoxemia, hypercapnia, and cor pulmonale occur in advanced cases. Biliary cirrhosis and gallstones may occur. Nearly all men with cystic fibrosis have congenital bilateral absence of the vas deferens with azoospermia. Patients with cystic fibrosis have an increased risk of malignancies of the gastrointestinal tract, osteopenia, and arthropathies.

Clinical Findings

A. Symptoms and Signs

Cystic fibrosis should be suspected in a young adult with a history of chronic lung disease (especially bronchiectasis), pancreatitis, or infertility. Cough, sputum production, decreased exercise tolerance, and recurrent hemoptysis are typical complaints. Patients also often complain of facial (sinus) pain or pressure and purulent nasal discharge. Steatorrhea, diarrhea, and abdominal pain are also common. Digital clubbing, increased anteroposterior chest diameter, hyperresonance to percussion, and apical crackles are noted on physical examination. Sinus tenderness, purulent nasal secretions, and nasal polyps may also be seen.

B. Laboratory Findings

Arterial blood gas studies often reveal hypoxemia and, in advanced disease, a chronic, compensated respiratory acidosis. Pulmonary function studies show a mixed obstructive and restrictive pattern. There is a reduction in FVC, airflow rates, and TLC. Air trapping (high ratio of RV to

TLC) and reduction in pulmonary diffusing capacity are common.

C. Imaging

Hyperinflation is seen early in the disease process. Peribronchial cuffing, mucus plugging, bronchiectasis (ring shadows and cysts), increased interstitial markings, small rounded peripheral opacities, and focal atelectasis may be seen separately or in various combinations. Pneumothorax can also be seen. Thin-section CT scanning may confirm the presence of bronchiectasis.

D. Diagnosis

The quantitative pilocarpine iontophoresis sweat test reveals elevated sodium and chloride levels (> 60 mEq/L) in the sweat of patients with cystic fibrosis. Two tests on different days are required for accurate diagnosis. Facilities must perform enough tests to maintain laboratory proficiency and quality. A normal sweat chloride test does not exclude the diagnosis. Genotyping or other alternative diagnostic studies (such as measurement of nasal membrane potential difference, semen analysis, or assessment of pancreatic function) should be pursued if the test is repeatedly negative but there is a high clinical suspicion of cystic fibrosis. Standard genotyping is a limited diagnostic tool because it screens for only a fraction of the known cystic fibrosis mutations, although complete genetic testing is available.

▶ Treatment

Early recognition and comprehensive multidisciplinary therapy improve symptom control and the chances of survival. Referral to a regional cystic fibrosis center is strongly recommended. Conventional treatment programs focus on the following areas: clearance and reduction of lower airway secretions, reversal of bronchoconstriction, treatment of respiratory tract infections and airway bacterial burden, pancreatic enzyme replacement, and nutritional and psychosocial support (including genetic and occupational counseling). The Pulmonary Therapies Committee, established by the Cystic Fibrosis Foundation, has issued evidenced-based recommendations regarding long-term use of medications for maintenance of lung function and reduction of exacerbations in patients with cystic fibrosis.

Clearance of lower airway secretions can be promoted by postural drainage, chest percussion or vibration techniques, positive expiratory pressure (PEP) or flutter valve breathing devices, directed cough, and other breathing techniques; these approaches require detailed patient instruction by experienced personnel. Sputum viscosity in cystic fibrosis is increased by the large quantities of extracellular DNA that result from chronic airway inflammation and autolysis of neutrophils. Inhaled recombinant human deoxyribonuclease (rhDNase, dornase alpha) cleaves extracellular DNA in sputum; when administered long-term at a daily nebulized dose of 2.5 mg, this therapy leads to improved FEV_1 and reduces the risk of cystic fibrosis–related respiratory exacerbations and the need for intravenous antibiotics. Pharyngitis, laryngitis, and voice alterations are common

adverse effects. Inhalation of hypertonic saline has been associated with small improvements in pulmonary function and fewer pulmonary exacerbations. The beneficial effects of hypertonic saline in cystic fibrosis may derive from improved airway mucous clearance. Short-term antibiotics are used to treat active airway infections based on results of culture and susceptibility testing of sputum. S aureus (including methicillin-resistant strains) and a mucoid variant of P aeruginosa are commonly present. H influenzae, Stenotrophomonas maltophilia, and B cepacia (a highly drug-resistant organism) are occasionally isolated. Long-term antibiotics (azithromycin, 500 mg orally three times a week, and inhalation of an aerosolized tobramycin solution) are helpful in slowing disease progression and reducing exacerbations in patients with cultures of airway secretions persistently positive for P aeruginosa.

Inhaled bronchodilators (eg, albuterol, two puffs every 4 hours as needed) should be considered in patients who demonstrate an increase of at least 12% in FEV_1 after an inhaled bronchodilator. Vaccination against pneumococcal infection and annual influenza vaccination are advised. Screening of family members and genetic counseling are suggested.

Lung transplantation is currently the only definitive treatment for advanced cystic fibrosis. Double-lung or heart-lung transplantation is required. A few transplant centers offer living lobar lung transplantation to selected patients. The 3-year survival rate following transplantation for cystic fibrosis is about 55%.

▶ Prognosis

The longevity of patients with cystic fibrosis is increasing, and the median survival age is over 35 years. Death occurs from pulmonary complications (eg, pneumonia, pneumothorax, or hemoptysis) or as a result of terminal chronic respiratory failure and cor pulmonale.

Davis PB. Cystic fibrosis since 1938. Am J Respir Crit Care Med. 2006 Mar 1;173(5):475–82. [PMID: 16126935]

Flume PA et al. Cystic fibrosis pulmonary guidelines: chronic medications for maintenance of lung health. Am J Respir Crit Care Med. 2007 Nov 15;176(10):957–69. [PMID: 17761616]

Vender RL. Cystic fibrosis lung disease in adult patients. Postgrad Med. 2008 Apr;120(1):64–74. [PMID: 18467811]

BRONCHIOLITIS

Bronchiolitis is a generic term applied to varied inflammatory processes that affect the bronchioles, which are small conducting and respiratory airways < 2 mm in diameter. In infants and children, bronchiolitis is common and usually caused by respiratory syncytial virus or adenovirus infection. In adults, bronchiolitis is encountered in a variety of clinical settings, including infections, connective tissue diseases, inhalational injuries, drug reactions, and allograft transplantation. No single classification scheme has been widely accepted and, as a result, there is a confusing and overlapping array of terms to describe these disorders from the viewpoints of the clinician, the radiologist, and the pathologist.

The pathologic classification has two variants. **Constrictive bronchiolitis** (also referred to as obliterative bronchiolitis, or bronchiolitis obliterans) is characterized by chronic inflammation, concentric scarring, and smooth muscle hypertrophy causing luminal obstruction. These patients have airflow obstruction on spirometry, minimal radiographic abnormalities, and a progressive, deteriorating clinical course. **Proliferative bronchiolitis** occurs when there is an organizing intraluminal exudate, consisting of fibroblasts, foamy macrophages, and other cells that obstruct the lumen. When this exudate extends to the alveolar space, the pattern is referred to as bronchiolitis obliterans with organizing pneumonia (BOOP; now more commonly referred to as **cryptogenic organizing pneumonitis** [COP]) (see Table 9–14).

The clinical classification approach divides patients into groups based primarily upon etiology. Inhalational injuries, postinfectious, and drug-induced causes are identified by association with a known exposure or illness prior to the onset of symptoms. Disorders associated with bronchiolitis include organ transplantation, connective tissue diseases, and hypersensitivity pneumonitis. Idiopathic cases are characterized by the insidious onset of dyspnea or cough, and include **COP.** This disorder affects men and women between the ages of 50 and 70 years, typically with a dry cough, dyspnea, and constitutional symptoms present for weeks to months prior to presentation. Pulmonary function testing typically shows a restrictive ventilatory defect. The chest radiograph frequently shows bilateral patchy, ground-glass or alveolar infiltrates, although other patterns have been described (see Table 9–14). Corticosteroids are effective in two-thirds of patients, and improvement can be prompt. Therapy is initiated with prednisone at 1 mg/kg/d for 1–3 months. The dose is then tapered slowly to 20–40 mg/d, depending on the response, and weaned over the subsequent 3–6 months as tolerated. Relapses are common if corticosteroids are stopped prematurely or tapered too quickly.

Other idiopathic disorders associated with bronchiolitis include **respiratory bronchiolitis,** which is a disorder of small airways in cigarette smokers. It usually occurs without symptoms or physiologic evidence of lung disease. In some patients, however, it can cause diffuse parenchymal infiltrates, a syndrome referred to as respiratory bronchiolitis–associated interstitial lung disease (RB-ILD) and is often considered with desquamative interstitial pneumonia (DIP) to represent the spectrum of the smoking-related interstitial lung diseases. **Diffuse panbronchiolitis** is an idiopathic disorder of respiratory bronchioles, more frequently diagnosed in Japan. Men are affected about twice as often as women, two-thirds are nonsmokers, and most patients have a history of chronic pansinusitis. Marked dyspnea, cough, and sputum production are frequent, and chest examination shows crackles and rhonchi. Pulmonary function tests reveal obstructive abnormalities, and the chest radiograph shows a distinct pattern of diffuse, small, nodular shadows with hyperinflation.

It is important to consider both the clinical and pathologic classification schemes when evaluating bronchiolitis. Both "constrictive" and "proliferative" pathology can be seen in postinfectious and connective tissue diseases, and integration with the clinical history is important. Compared with constrictive bronchiolitis, proliferative bronchiolitis is overall more common, more likely to show a restrictive or mixed ventilatory defect, more likely to have an abnormal chest radiograph, and more likely to be responsive to corticosteroids. Constrictive bronchiolitis is relatively infrequent but can be seen in a variety of inhalation disorders; hypersensitivity pneumonitis; and chronic rejection in heart-lung, lung, and bone marrow transplant recipients. There is often an obstructive defect with hyperinflation, and chest radiographs may be normal or show hyperinflation. Constrictive bronchiolitis is relatively unresponsive to corticosteroids and is frequently progressive. For both constrictive and proliferative bronchiolitis, open or thoracoscopic lung biopsy is required to make the definitive diagnosis in the majority of cases.

Cordier JF. Cryptogenic organising pneumonia. Eur Respir J. 2006 Aug;28(2):422–46. [PMID: 16880372]

Ryu JH. Classification and approach to bronchiolar diseases. Curr Opin Pulm Med. 2006 Mar;12(2):145–51. [PMID: 16456385]

Smyth RL et al. Bronchiolitis. Lancet. 2006 Jul 22;368(9532):312–22. [PMID: 16860701]

▼ PULMONARY INFECTIONS

PNEUMONIA

Lower respiratory tract infections continue to be a major health problem despite advances in the identification of etiologic organisms and the availability of potent antimicrobial drugs. In addition, there is still much controversy regarding optimal diagnostic approaches and treatment choices for pneumonia.

Characteristics of pneumonia caused by specific agents and appropriate antimicrobial therapy are presented in Table 9–9. Pneumonias are typically classified as being either community-acquired or health care–associated. Anaerobic pneumonias and lung abscess can occur in both settings and warrant separate consideration.

This section sets forth the evaluation and management of pulmonary infiltrates in immunocompetent hosts separately from the approach to immunocompromised hosts—defined as patients with HIV disease, absolute neutrophil counts < 1000/mcL, current or recent exposure to myelosuppressive or immunosuppressive drugs, or those currently taking prednisone in a dosage of over 5 mg/d.

1. Community-Acquired Pneumonia

 ESSENTIALS OF DIAGNOSIS

► Symptoms and signs of an acute lung infection: fever or hypothermia, cough with or without sputum, dyspnea, chest discomfort, sweats, or rigors.

► Bronchial breath sounds or rales are frequent auscultatory findings.

Table 9–9. Characteristics and treatment of selected pneumonias.

Organism; Appearance on Smear of Sputum	Clinical Setting	Complications	Laboratory Studies	Antimicrobial Therapy[1,2]
Streptococcus pneumoniae (pneumococcus). Gram-positive diplococci.	Chronic cardiopulmonary disease; follows upper respiratory tract infection	Bacteremia, meningitis, endocarditis, pericarditis, empyema	Gram stain and culture of sputum, blood, pleural fluid	Preferred[3]: Penicillin G, amoxicillin. Alternative: Macrolides, cephalosporins, doxycycline, fluoroquinolones, clindamycin, vancomycin, TMP-SMZ, linezolid.
Haemophilus influenzae. Pleomorphic gram-negative coccobacilli.	Chronic cardiopulmonary disease; follows upper respiratory tract infection	Empyema, endocarditis	Gram stain and culture of sputum, blood, pleural fluid	Preferred[3]: Cefotaxime, ceftriaxone, cefuroxime, doxycycline, azithromycin, TMP-SMZ. Alternative: Fluoroquinolones, clarithromycin.
Staphylococcus aureus. Plump gram-positive cocci in clumps.	Residence in chronic care facility, health care–associated, influenza epidemics; cystic fibrosis, bronchiectasis, injection drug use	Empyema, cavitation	Gram stain and culture of sputum, blood, pleural fluid	For methicillin-susceptible strains: Preferred: A penicillinase-resistant penicillin with or without rifampin, or gentamicin. Alternative: A cephalosporin; clindamycin, TMP-SMZ, vancomycin, a fluoroquinolone. For methicillin-resistant strains: Vancomycin with or without gentamicin or rifampin, linezolid.
Klebsiella pneumoniae. Plump gram-negative encapsulated rods.	Alcohol abuse, diabetes mellitus; health care–associated	Cavitation, empyema	Gram stain and culture of sputum, blood, pleural fluid	Preferred: Third-generation cephalosporin. For severe infections, add an aminoglycoside. Alternative: Aztreonam, imipenem, meropenem, β-lactam/β-lactamase inhibitor, an aminoglycoside, or a fluoroquinolone.
Escherichia coli. Gram-negative rods.	Health care–associated; rarely, community-acquired	Empyema	Gram stain and culture of sputum, blood, pleural fluid	Same as for *Klebsiella pneumoniae.*
Pseudomonas aeruginosa. Gram-negative rods.	Health care–associated; cystic fibrosis, bronchiectasis	Cavitation	Gram stain and culture of sputum, blood	Preferred: An antipseudomonal β-lactam plus an aminoglycoside. Alternative: Ciprofloxacin plus an aminoglycoside or an antipseudomonal β-lactam.
Anaerobes. Mixed flora.	Aspiration, poor dental hygiene	Necrotizing pneumonia, abscess, empyema	Culture of pleural fluid or of material obtained by transtracheal or transthoracic aspiration	Preferred: Clindamycin, β-lactam/β-lactamase inhibitor, imipenem.
Mycoplasma pneumoniae. PMNs and monocytes; no bacteria.	Young adults; summer and fall	Skin rashes, bullous myringitis; hemolytic anemia	PCR. Culture.[4] Complement fixation titer.[5] Cold agglutinin serum titers are not helpful as they lack sensitivity and specificity.	Preferred: Doxycycline or erythromycin. Alternative: Clarithromycin; azithromycin, or a fluoroquinolone.
Legionella species. Few PMNs; no bacteria.	Summer and fall; exposure to contaminated construction site, water source, air conditioner; community-acquired or health care–associated	Empyema, cavitation, endocarditis, pericarditis	Direct immunofluorescent examination or PCR of sputum or tissue; culture of sputum or tissue.[4] Urinary antigen assay for *L pneumophila* serogroup 1.	Preferred: A macrolide with or without rifampin; a fluoroquinolone. Alternative: Doxycycline with or without rifampin, TMP-SMZ.
Chlamydophila pneumoniae. Nonspecific.	Clinically similar to *M pneumoniae,* but prodromal symptoms last longer (up to 2 weeks). Sore throat with hoarseness common. Mild pneumonia in teenagers and young adults.	Reinfection in older adults with underlying COPD or heart failure may be severe or even fatal	Isolation of the organism is very difficult. Serologic studies include microimmunofluorescence with TWAR antigen. PCR at selected laboratories.	Preferred: Doxycycline. Alternative: Erythromycin, clarithromycin, azithromycin, or a fluoroquinolone.

(continued)

Table 9–9. Characteristics and treatment of selected pneumonias. (continued)

Organism; Appearance on Smear of Sputum	Clinical Setting	Complications	Laboratory Studies	Antimicrobial Therapy[1,2]
Moraxella catarrhalis. Gram-negative diplococci.	Preexisting lung disease; elderly; corticosteroid or immunosuppressive therapy	Rarely, pleural effusions and bacteremia	Gram stain and culture of sputum, blood, pleural fluid	Preferred: A second- or third-generation cephalosporin; a fluoroquinolone. Alternative: TMP-SMZ, amoxicillin-clavulanic acid, or a macrolide.
Pneumocystis jiroveci. Nonspecific.	AIDS, immunosuppressive or cytotoxic drug therapy, cancer	Pneumothorax, respiratory failure, ARDS, death	Methenamine silver, Giemsa, or DFA stains of sputum or bronchoalveolar lavage fluid	Preferred: TMP-SMZ or pentamidine isethionate plus prednisone. Alternative: Dapsone plus trimethoprim; clindamycin plus primaquine; trimetrexate plus folinic acid.

[1]Antimicrobial sensitivities should guide therapy when available. (Modified from: The choice of antibacterial drugs. Med Lett Drugs Ther. 2001 Aug 20;43(1111–1112):69–78. [PMID: 11518876], and from Bartlett JG et al: Practice guidelines for the management of community-acquired pneumonia in adults. Clin Infect Dis. 2000 Aug;31(2):347–82. [PMID 10987697].)

[2]For additional antimicrobial therapy information, see Chapter 30, Infectious Disease: Antimicrobial Therapy: Tables 30–4 (drugs of choice), 30–6, and 30–7, 30–8, and 30–11 (pharmacology and dosage adjustment for kidney dysfunction).

[3]Consider penicillin resistance when choosing therapy. See text.

[4]Selective media are required.

[5]Fourfold rise in titer is diagnostic.

ARDS, acute respiratory distress syndrome; COPD, chronic obstructive pulmonary disease; PCR, polymerase chain reaction; TMP-SMZ, trimethoprim-sulfamethoxazole.

▶ Parenchymal infiltrate on chest radiograph.

▶ Occurs outside of the hospital or less than 48 hours after admission in a patient who is not hospitalized or residing in a long-term care facility.

General Considerations

Community-acquired pneumonia is a common disorder, with approximately 2–3 million cases diagnosed each year in the United States. It is the most deadly infectious disease in the United States and the sixth leading cause of death. Mortality is estimated to be approximately 14% among hospitalized patients and less than 1% for patients who do not require hospitalization. Important risk factors for increased morbidity and mortality from community-acquired pneumonia include advanced age, alcoholism, comorbid medical conditions, altered mental status, respiratory rate ≥ 30 breaths/min, hypotension (defined by systolic blood pressure < 90 mm Hg or diastolic blood pressure < 60 mm Hg), and increased blood urea nitrogen (BUN).

In immunocompetent patients, the history, physical examination, radiographs, and sputum examination are neither sensitive nor specific for identifying the microbiologic cause of community-acquired pneumonia. While helpful in selected patients, these modalities do not consistently differentiate bacterial from viral causes or distinguish "typical" from "atypical" causes. As a result, the American Thoracic Society and Infectious Disease Society of America recommend empiric treatment based on epidemiologic data.

▶ Definition & Pathogenesis

Community-acquired pneumonia is most often diagnosed outside of the hospital in ambulatory patients who are not residents of nursing homes and other long-term care facilities. It may also be diagnosed in a previously ambulatory patient within 48 hours after admission to the hospital.

Pulmonary defense mechanisms (cough reflex, mucociliary clearance system, immune responses) normally prevent the development of lower respiratory tract infections following aspiration of oropharyngeal secretions containing bacteria or inhalation of infected aerosols. Community-acquired pneumonia occurs when there is a defect in one or more of the normal host defense mechanisms or when a very large infectious inoculum or a highly virulent pathogen overwhelms the host.

Prospective studies have failed to identify the cause of community-acquired pneumonia in 40–60% of cases; two or more causes are identified in up to 5% of cases. Bacteria are more commonly identified than viruses. The most common bacterial pathogen identified in most studies of community-acquired pneumonia is *S pneumoniae*, accounting for approximately two-thirds of bacterial isolates. Other common bacterial pathogens include *H influenzae*, *M pneumoniae*, *C pneumoniae*, *S aureus*, *Neisseria meningitidis*, *M catarrhalis*, *Klebsiella pneumoniae*, other gram-negative rods, and *Legionella* species. Common viral causes of community-acquired pneumonia include influenza virus, respiratory syncytial virus, adenovirus, and parainfluenza virus. A detailed assessment of epidemiologic risk factors may aid in diagnosing pneumonias due to the following causes: *Chlamydia psittaci* (psittacosis), *Coxiella burnetii* (Q fever), *Francisella tularensis* (tularemia), endemic fungi (*Blastomyces, Coccidioides, Histoplasma*), and sin nombre virus (hantavirus pulmonary syndrome).

Clinical Findings

A. Symptoms and Signs

Most patients with community-acquired pneumonia experience an acute or subacute onset of fever, cough with or without sputum production, and dyspnea. Other common symptoms include rigors, sweats, chills, chest discomfort, pleurisy, hemoptysis, fatigue, myalgias, anorexia, headache, and abdominal pain.

Common physical findings include fever or hypothermia, tachypnea, tachycardia, and mild arterial oxygen desaturation. Many patients will appear acutely ill. Chest examination is often remarkable for altered breath sounds and rales. Dullness to percussion may be present if a parapneumonic pleural effusion is present.

The differential diagnosis of lower respiratory tract symptoms and signs is extensive and includes upper respiratory tract infections, reactive airway diseases, congestive heart failure, COP, lung cancer, pulmonary vasculitis, pulmonary thromboembolic disease, and atelectasis.

B. Laboratory Findings

Controversy surrounds the role of Gram stain and culture analysis of expectorated sputum in patients with community-acquired pneumonia. Most reports suggest that these tests have poor positive and negative predictive value in most patients. Some argue, however, that the tests should still be performed to try to identify etiologic organisms in the hope of reducing microbial resistance to drugs, unnecessary drug costs, and avoidable side effects of empiric antibiotic therapy. Expert panel guidelines suggest that sputum Gram stain should be attempted in all patients with community-acquired pneumonia and that sputum culture should be obtained for all patients who require hospitalization. Sputum should be obtained before antibiotics are initiated except in a case of suspected antibiotic failure. The specimen is obtained by deep cough and should be grossly purulent. Culture should be performed only if the specimen meets strict cytologic criteria, eg, more than 25 neutrophils and fewer than 10 squamous epithelial cells per low power field. These criteria do not apply to cultures of legionella or mycobacteria.

Additional testing is generally recommended for patients who require hospitalization: preantibiotic blood cultures (at least two sets with needle sticks at separate sites), arterial blood gases, complete blood count with differential, and a chemistry panel (including serum glucose, electrolytes, urea nitrogen, creatinine, bilirubin, and liver enzymes). The results of these tests help assess the severity of the disease and guide evaluation and therapy. HIV testing should be considered in all adult patients, and performed in those with risk factors.

C. Imaging

Chest radiography may confirm the diagnosis and detect associated lung diseases. It can also be used to help assess severity and response to therapy over time. Radiographic findings can range from patchy airspace infiltrates to lobar consolidation with air bronchograms to diffuse alveolar or interstitial infiltrates. Additional findings can include pleural effusions and cavitation. No pattern of radiographic abnormalities is pathognomonic of a specific cause of pneumonia.

Progression of pulmonary infiltrates during antibiotic therapy or lack of radiographic improvement over time are poor prognostic signs and also raise concerns about secondary or alternative pulmonary processes. Clearing of pulmonary infiltrates in patients with community-acquired pneumonia can take 6 weeks or longer and is usually fastest in young patients, nonsmokers, and those with only single lobe involvement.

D. Special Examinations

Sputum induction is reserved for patients who cannot provide expectorated sputum samples or who may have *P jiroveci* or *Mycobacterium tuberculosis* pneumonia. Transtracheal aspiration, fiberoptic bronchoscopy, and transthoracic needle aspiration techniques to obtain samples of lower respiratory secretions or tissues are reserved for selected patients.

Thoracentesis with pleural fluid analysis (Gram stain and cultures; glucose, lactate dehydrogenase (LD), and total protein levels; leukocyte count with differential; pH determination) should be performed on most patients with pleural effusions to assist in diagnosis of the etiologic agent and assess for empyema or complicated parapneumonic process. Serologic assays, polymerase chain reaction tests, specialized culture tests, and other new diagnostic tests for organisms such as *Legionella, M pneumoniae*, and *C pneumoniae* are performed when these diagnoses are suspected. Limitations of many of these tests include delay in obtaining test results and poor sensitivity and specificity.

Treatment

Antimicrobial therapy should be initiated promptly after the diagnosis of pneumonia is established and appropriate specimens are obtained, especially in patients who require hospitalization. Delays in obtaining diagnostic specimens or the results of testing should not preclude the early administration of antibiotics to acutely ill patients. Decisions regarding hospitalization should be based on prognostic criteria as outlined above in the section on general considerations. Treatment recommendations can be divided into those for patients who can be treated as outpatients and those for patients who require hospitalization.

Special consideration must be given to penicillin-resistant strains of S pneumoniae. Intermediate resistance to penicillin is defined as a minimum inhibitory concentration (MIC) of 0.1–1 mcg/mL. Strains with high-level resistance usually require an MIC ≥ 2 mcg/mL for penicillin. Resistance to other antibiotics (β-lactams, trimethoprim-sulfamethoxazole, macrolides, others) often accompanies resistance to penicillin. The prevalence of resistance varies by patient group, geographic region, and over time. Local resistance pattern data should therefore guide empiric therapy of suspected or documented *S pneumoniae* infections until specific susceptibility test results are available.

A. Treatment of Outpatients

Empiric antibiotic options for patients with community-acquired pneumonia who do not require hospitalization include the following: (1) Macrolides (clarithromycin, 500 mg orally twice a day, or azithromycin, 500 mg orally as a first dose and then 250 mg once a day for 4 days, or 500 mg daily for 3 days). (2) Doxycycline (100 mg orally twice a day). (3) Fluoroquinolones (with enhanced activity against *S pneumoniae*, such as levofloxacin 500 mg orally once a day, or moxifloxacin 400 mg orally once a day). Some experts prefer doxycycline or macrolides for patients under 50 years of age without comorbidities and a fluoroquinolone for patients with comorbidities or who are older than 50 years of age. Alternatives include erythromycin (250–500 mg orally four times daily), amoxicillin-potassium clavulanate—especially for suspected aspiration pneumonia—500 mg orally three times a day or 875 mg orally twice a day, and some second- and third-generation cephalosporins such as cefuroxime axetil (250–500 mg orally twice a day), cefpodoxime proxetil (100–200 mg orally twice a day), or cefprozil (250–500 mg orally twice a day).

There are limited data to guide recommendations for duration of treatment. The decision is influenced by the severity of illness, the etiologic agent, response to therapy, other medical problems, and complications. Therapy until the patient is afebrile for at least 72 hours is usually sufficient for pneumonia due to *S pneumoniae*. A minimum of 2 weeks of therapy is appropriate for pneumonia due to *S aureus*, *P aeruginosa*, *Klebsiella*, anaerobes, *M pneumoniae*, *C pneumoniae*, or *Legionella* species.

B. Treatment of Hospitalized Patients

Empiric antibiotic options for patients with community-acquired pneumonia who require hospitalization can be divided into those for patients who can be cared for on a general medical ward and those for patients who require care in an ICU. Patients who only require general medical ward care usually respond to an extended-spectrum β-lactam (such as ceftriaxone or cefotaxime) with a macrolide (clarithromycin or azithromycin is preferred if *H influenzae* infection is suspected) or a fluoroquinolone (with enhanced activity against *S pneumoniae*) such as levofloxacin or moxifloxacin. Alternatives include a β-lactam/β-lactamase inhibitor (ampicillin-sulbactam or piperacillin-tazobactam) with a macrolide.

Patients requiring admission to the ICU require a macrolide or a fluoroquinolone (with enhanced activity against *S pneumoniae*) plus an extended-spectrum cephalosporin (ceftriaxone, cefotaxime) or a β-lactam/β-lactamase inhibitor (ampicillin-sulbactam or piperacillin-tazobactam). Patients with penicillin allergies can be treated with a fluoroquinolone (with enhanced activity against *S pneumoniae*) with or without clindamycin. Patients with suspected aspiration pneumonia should receive a fluoroquinolone (with enhanced activity against *S pneumoniae*) with or without clindamycin, metronidazole, or a β-lac-

tam/β-lactamase inhibitor. Patients with structural lung diseases such as bronchiectasis or cystic fibrosis benefit from empiric therapy with an antipseudomonal penicillin, carbapenem, or cefepime plus a fluoroquinolone (including high-dose ciprofloxacin) until sputum culture and sensitivity results are available. For expanded discussions of specific antibiotics, see Chapter 30.

Almost all patients who are admitted to a hospital for therapy of community-acquired pneumonia receive intravenous antibiotics. Despite this preference, no studies demonstrate superior outcomes when hospitalized patients are treated intravenously instead of orally if patients can tolerate oral therapy and the drug is well absorbed. Duration of antibiotic treatment is the same as for outpatients with community-acquired pneumonia.

▶ Prevention

Polyvalent pneumococcal vaccine (containing capsular polysaccharide antigens of 23 common strains of *S pneumoniae*) has the potential to prevent or lessen the severity of the majority of pneumococcal infections in immunocompetent patients. Indications for pneumococcal vaccination include the following: age ≥ 65 years or any chronic illness that increases the risk of community-acquired pneumonia (see Chapter 30). Immunocompromised patients and those at highest risk of fatal pneumococcal infections should receive a single revaccination 6 years after the first vaccination. Immunocompetent persons 65 years of age or older should receive a second dose of vaccine if the patient first received the vaccine 6 or more years previously and was under 65 years old at the time of vaccination.

The influenza vaccine is effective in preventing severe disease due to influenza virus with a resulting positive impact on both primary influenza pneumonia and secondary bacterial pneumonias. The influenza vaccine is administered annually to persons at risk for complications of influenza infection (age ≥ 65 years, residents of long-term care facilities, patients with pulmonary or cardiovascular disorders, patients recently hospitalized with chronic metabolic disorders) as well as health care workers and others who are able to transmit influenza to high-risk patients.

Hospitalized patients who would benefit from pneumococcal and influenza vaccines should be vaccinated during hospitalization. The vaccines can be given simultaneously, and there are no contraindications to use immediately after an episode of pneumonia.

▶ When to Admit

- Failure of outpatient therapy, including inability to maintain oral intake and medications.
- Exacerbations of underlying disease that would benefit from hospitalization.
- Complications of pneumonia (such as hypoxemia, pleural effusion, sepsis, encephalopathy).
- Other medical or psychosocial needs (such as cognitive dysfunction, psychiatric disease, homelessness, drug abuse, lack of outpatient resources, or poor overall functional status).

Armitage K et al. New guidelines for the management of adult community-acquired pneumonia. Curr Opin Infect Dis. 2007 Apr;20(2):170–6. [PMID: 17496576]

Mandell LA et al. Infectious Diseases Society of America/American Thoracic Society consensus guidelines on the management of community-acquired pneumonia in adults. Clin Infect Dis. 2007 Mar 1;44(Suppl 2):S27–72. [PMID: 17278083]

Mizgerd JP. Acute lower respiratory tract infection. N Engl J Med. 2008 Feb 14;358(7):716–27. [PMID: 18272895]

Niederman MS. Recent advances in community-acquired pneumonia: inpatient and outpatient. Chest. 2007 Apr;131(4):1205–15. [PMID: 17426229]

2. Health Care–Associated Pneumonia

 ESSENTIALS OF DIAGNOSIS

► Occurs more than 48 hours after admission to the hospital or other health care facility and excludes any infection present at the time of admission.

► At least two of the following: fever, cough, leukocytosis, purulent sputum.

► New or progressive parenchymal infiltrate on chest radiograph.

► Especially common in patients requiring intensive care or mechanical ventilation.

General Considerations

Health care–associated pneumonia is an important cause of morbidity and mortality despite widespread use of preventive measures, advances in diagnostic testing, and potent new antimicrobial agents. Health care–associated pneumonia is the second most common cause of infection among hospital inpatients and is the leading cause of death due to infection with mortality rates ranging from 20% to 50%. While the majority of cases occur in patients who are not in an ICU, the highest-risk patients are those in such units or who are being mechanically ventilated; these patients also experience higher morbidity and mortality from health care-associated pneumonias.

Definition & Pathogenesis

Health care–associated pneumonia is defined as pneumonia developing more than 48 hours after admission to the hospital or other health care facility. Ventilator-associated pneumonia develops in a mechanically ventilated patient more than 48 hours after intubation.

Colonization of the pharynx and possibly the stomach with bacteria is the most important step in the pathogenesis of health care–associated pneumonia. Pharyngeal colonization is promoted by exogenous factors (instrumentation of the upper airway with nasogastric and endotracheal tubes, contamination by dirty hands and equipment, and treatment with broad-spectrum antibiotics that promote the emergence of drug-resistant organisms) and patient factors (malnutrition, advanced age, altered consciousness, swallowing disorders, and underlying pulmonary and systemic diseases). Aspiration of infected pharyngeal or gastric secretions delivers bacteria directly to the lower airway. Impaired cellular and mechanical defense mechanisms in the lungs of hospitalized patients raise the risk of infection after aspiration has occurred. Tracheal intubation increases the risk of lower respiratory infection by mechanical obstruction of the trachea, impairment of mucociliary clearance, trauma to the mucociliary escalator system, and interference with coughing. Tight adherence of bacteria such as *Pseudomonas* to the tracheal epithelium and the biofilm that lines the endotracheal tube makes clearance of these organisms from the lower airway difficult. Less important pathogenetic mechanisms of health care–associated pneumonia include inhalation of contaminated aerosols and hematogenous dissemination of microorganisms.

The role of the stomach in the pathogenesis of health care–associated pneumonia remains controversial. Observational studies have suggested that elevation of gastric pH due to antacids, H_2-receptor antagonists, or enteral feeding is associated with gastric microbial overgrowth, tracheobronchial colonization, and health care–associated pneumonia. Sucralfate, a cytoprotective agent that does not alter gastric pH, is associated with a trend toward a lower incidence of ventilator-associated pneumonia.

The most common organisms responsible for health care–associated pneumonia are *P aeruginosa*, *S aureus*, *Enterobacter*, *K pneumoniae*, and *Escherichia coli*. *Proteus*, *Serratia marcescens*, *H influenzae*, and streptococci account for most of the remaining cases. Infection by *P aeruginosa* and *Acinetobacter* tend to cause pneumonia in the most debilitated patients, those with previous antibiotic therapy, and those requiring mechanical ventilation. Anaerobic organisms (bacteroides, anaerobic streptococci, fusobacterium) may also cause pneumonia in the hospitalized patient; when isolated, they are commonly part of a polymicrobial flora. Mycobacteria, fungi, chlamydiae, viruses, rickettsiae, and protozoal organisms are uncommon causes of health care–associated pneumonia.

Clinical Findings

A. Symptoms and Signs

The symptoms and signs associated with health care–associated pneumonia are nonspecific; however, one or more clinical findings (fever, leukocytosis, purulent sputum, and a new or progressive pulmonary infiltrate on chest radiograph) are present in most patients. Other findings associated with health care–associated pneumonia include those listed above for community-acquired pneumonia.

The differential diagnosis of new lower respiratory tract symptoms and signs in hospitalized patients includes congestive heart failure, atelectasis, aspiration, ARDS, pulmonary thromboembolism, pulmonary hemorrhage, and drug reactions.

B. Laboratory Findings

The minimum evaluation for suspected health care–associated pneumonia includes blood cultures from two different sites and an arterial blood gas or pulse oximetry determination. Blood cultures can identify the pathogen in up to 20% of all patients with health care–associated pneumonia; positivity is associated with increased risk for complications and other sites of infection. The assessment of oxygenation helps define the severity of illness and determines the need for supplemental oxygen. Blood counts and clinical chemistry tests are not helpful in establishing a specific diagnosis of health care–associated pneumonia; however, they can help define the severity of illness and identify complications. Thoracentesis for pleural fluid analysis (stains, cultures; glucose, LD, and total protein levels; leukocyte count with differential; pH determination) should be performed in patients with pleural effusions.

Examination of sputum is attended by the same disadvantages as in community-acquired pneumonia. Gram stains and cultures of sputum are neither sensitive nor specific in the diagnosis of health care–associated pneumonia. The identification of a bacterial organism by culture of sputum does not prove that the organism is a lower respiratory tract pathogen. However, it can be used to help identify antibiotic sensitivity patterns of bacteria and as a guide to therapy. If health care–associated pneumonia from *Legionella pneumophila* is suspected, direct fluorescent antibody staining can be performed. Sputum stains and cultures for mycobacteria and certain fungi may be diagnostic.

C. Imaging

Radiographic findings are nonspecific and can range from patchy airspace infiltrates to lobar consolidation with air bronchograms to diffuse alveolar or interstitial infiltrates. Additional findings can include pleural effusions and cavitation. Progression of pulmonary infiltrates during antibiotic therapy and lack of radiographic improvement over time are poor prognostic signs and also raise concerns about secondary or alternative pulmonary processes. Clearing of pulmonary infiltrates can take 6 weeks or longer.

D. Special Examinations

Endotracheal aspiration using a sterile suction catheter and fiberoptic bronchoscopy with bronchoalveolar lavage or a protected specimen brush can be used to obtain lower respiratory tract secretions for analysis, most commonly in patients with ventilator-associated pneumonias. Endotracheal aspiration cultures have significant negative predictive value but limited positive predictive value in the diagnosis of specific etiologic agents in patients with health care–associated pneumonia. An invasive diagnostic approach using quantitative culture of bronchoalveolar lavage samples or protected specimen brush samples in patients suspected of having ventilator-associated pneumonia leads to significantly less antibiotic use, earlier attenuation of organ dysfunction, and fewer deaths at 14 days.

▶ Treatment

Treatment of health care–associated pneumonia, like treatment of community-acquired pneumonia, is usually empiric. Because of the high mortality rate, therapy should be started as soon as pneumonia is suspected. Initial regi-

mens must be broad in spectrum and tailored to the specific clinical setting. There is no uniform consensus on the best regimens.

Recommendations for the treatment of health care–associated pneumonia have been proposed by many organizations, including the American Thoracic Society. Initial empiric therapy with antibiotics is determined by the severity of illness, risk factors, and the length of hospitalization. Empiric therapy for mild to moderate health care–associated pneumonia in a patient without unusual risk factors or a patient with severe early-onset (within 5 days after admission) health care–associated pneumonia may consist of a second-generation cephalosporin, a non-antipseudomonal third-generation cephalosporin, or a combination of a β-lactam and β-lactamase inhibitor.

Empiric therapy for patients with severe, late-onset (≥ 5 days after admission) health care–associated pneumonia or with ICU- or ventilator-associated pneumonia should include a combination of antibiotics directed against the most virulent organisms, particularly *P aeruginosa*, *Acinetobacter* species, and *Enterobacter* species. The antibiotic regimen should include an aminoglycoside or fluoroquinolone plus one of the following: an antipseudomonal penicillin, an antipseudomonal cephalosporin, a carbapenem, or aztreonam—aztreonam alone with an aminoglycoside will be inadequate if coverage for gram-positive organisms or *H influenzae* is required. Vancomycin is added if infection with methicillin-resistant *S aureus* is of concern (especially in patients with coma, head trauma, diabetes mellitus, or advanced chronic kidney disease, or who are in the ICU). Anaerobic coverage with clindamycin or a β-lactam/β-lactamase inhibitor combination may be added for patients who have risk factors for anaerobic pneumonia, including aspiration, recent thoracoabdominal surgery, or an obstructing airway lesion. A macrolide is added when patients are at risk for *Legionella* infection, such as those receiving high-dose corticosteroids. After results of sputum, blood, and pleural fluid cultures have been obtained, it may be possible to switch to a regimen with a narrower spectrum. Duration of antibiotic therapy should be individualized based on the pathogen, severity of illness, response to therapy, and comorbid conditions. Therapy for gram-negative bacterial pneumonia is typically continued for at least 14 days. Data from a large trial assessing treatment outcomes in ventilator-associated pneumonia suggest that 8 days of antibiotics is as good as 15 days, except in cases caused by *P aeruginosa*.

Craven DE. What is healthcare-associated pneumonia, and how should it be treated? Curr Opin Infect Dis. 2006 Apr;19(2):153–60. [PMID: 16514340]

Klompas M. Does this patient have ventilator-associated pneumonia? JAMA. 2007 Apr 11;297(14):1583–93. [PMID: 17426278]

Masterton R. The place of guidelines in hospital-acquired pneumonia. J Hosp Infect. 2007 Jun;66(2):116–22. [PMID: 17482718]

Sinuff T et al; Canadian Critical Care Trials Group. Ventilator-associated pneumonia: improving outcomes through guideline implementation. J Crit Care. 2008 Mar;23(1):118–25. [PMID: 18359429]

3. Anaerobic Pneumonia & Lung Abscess

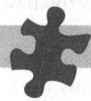

ESSENTIALS OF DIAGNOSIS

▸ History of or predisposition to aspiration.

▸ Indolent symptoms, including fever, weight loss, malaise.

▸ Poor dentition.

▸ Foul-smelling purulent sputum (in many patients).

▸ Infiltrate in dependent lung zone, with single or multiple areas of cavitation or pleural effusion.

General Considerations

Aspiration of small amounts of oropharyngeal secretions occurs during sleep in normal individuals but rarely causes disease. Sequelae of aspiration of larger amounts of material include nocturnal asthma, chemical pneumonitis, mechanical obstruction of airways by particulate matter, bronchiectasis, and pleuropulmonary infection. Individuals predisposed to disease induced by aspiration include those with depressed levels of consciousness due to drug or alcohol use, seizures, general anesthesia, or central nervous system disease; those with impaired deglutition due to esophageal disease or neurologic disorders; and those with tracheal or nasogastric tubes, which disrupt the mechanical defenses of the airways.

Periodontal disease and poor dental hygiene, which increase the number of anaerobic bacteria in aspirated material, are associated with a greater likelihood of anaerobic pleuropulmonary infection. Aspiration of infected oropharyngeal contents initially leads to pneumonia in dependent lung zones, such as the posterior segments of the upper lobes and superior and basilar segments of the lower lobes. Body position at the time of aspiration determines which lung zones are dependent. The onset of symptoms is insidious. By the time the patient seeks medical attention, necrotizing pneumonia, lung abscess, or empyema may be apparent.

Most aspiration patients with necrotizing pneumonia, lung abscess, and empyema are found to be infected with multiple species of anaerobic bacteria. Most of the remainder are infected with both anaerobic and aerobic bacteria. *Prevotella melaninogenica*, *Peptostreptococcus*, *Fusobacterium nucleatum*, and *Bacteroides* species are commonly isolated anaerobic bacteria.

Clinical Findings

A. Symptoms and Signs

Patients with anaerobic pleuropulmonary infection usually present with constitutional symptoms such as fever, weight loss, and malaise. Cough with expectoration of foul-smelling purulent sputum suggests anaerobic infection, though the absence of productive cough does not rule out such an infection. Dentition is often poor. Patients are rarely eden-

tulous; if so, an obstructing bronchial lesion is usually present.

B. Laboratory Findings

Expectorated sputum is inappropriate for culture of anaerobic organisms because of contaminating mouth flora. Representative material for culture can be obtained only by transthoracic aspiration, thoracentesis, or bronchoscopy with a protected brush. Transthoracic aspiration is rarely indicated, because drainage occurs via the bronchus and anaerobic pleuropulmonary infections usually respond well to empiric therapy.

C. Imaging

The different types of anaerobic pleuropulmonary infection are distinguished on the basis of their radiographic appearance. **Lung abscess** appears as a thick-walled solitary cavity surrounded by consolidation. An air-fluid level is usually present. Other causes of cavitary lung disease (tuberculosis, mycosis, cancer, infarction, Wegener granulomatosis) should be excluded. **Necrotizing pneumonia** is distinguished by multiple areas of cavitation within an area of consolidation. **Empyema** is characterized by the presence of purulent pleural fluid and may accompany either of the other two radiographic findings. Ultrasonography is of value in locating fluid and may also reveal pleural loculations.

Treatment

Penicillins have been the standard treatment for anaerobic pleuropulmonary infections. However, an increasing number of anaerobic organisms produce β-lactamases, and up to 20% of patients do not respond to penicillins. Improved responses have been documented with clindamycin (600 mg intravenously every 8 hours until improvement, then 300 mg orally every 6 hours) or amoxicillin-clavulanate (875 mg orally every 12 hours). Penicillin (amoxicillin, 500 mg every 8 hours, or penicillin G, 1–2 million units intravenously every 4–6 hours) plus metronidazole (500 mg orally or intravenously every 8–12 hours) is another option. Antibiotic therapy should be continued until the chest radiograph improves, a process that may take a month or more; patients with lung abscesses should be treated until radiographic resolution of the abscess cavity is demonstrated. Anaerobic pleuropulmonary disease requires adequate drainage with tube thoracostomy for the treatment of empyema. Open pleural drainage is sometimes necessary because of the propensity of these infections to produce loculations in the pleural space.

Paintal HS et al. Aspiration syndromes: 10 clinical pearls every physician should know. Int J Clin Pract. 2007 May;61(5):846–52. [PMID: 17493092]

Schiza S et al. Clinical presentation and management of empyema, lung abscess and pleural effusion. Curr Opin Pulm Med. 2006 May;12(3):205–11. [PMID: 16582676]

Shigemitsu H et al. Aspiration pneumonias: under-diagnosed and under-treated. Curr Opin Pulm Med. 2007 May;13(3):192–8. [PMID: 17414126]

PULMONARY INFILTRATES IN THE IMMUNOCOMPROMISED HOST

Pulmonary infiltrates in immunocompromised patients may arise from infectious or noninfectious causes. Infection may be due to bacterial, mycobacterial, fungal, protozoal, helminthic, or viral pathogens. Noninfectious processes such as pulmonary edema, alveolar hemorrhage, drug reactions, pulmonary thromboembolic disease, malignancy, and radiation pneumonitis may mimic infection.

Although almost any pathogen can cause pneumonia in a compromised host, two clinical tools help the clinician narrow the differential diagnosis. The first is knowledge of the underlying immunologic defect. Specific immunologic defects are associated with particular infections. Defects in humoral immunity predispose to bacterial infections; defects in cellular immunity lead to infections with viruses, fungi, mycobacteria, and protozoa. Neutropenia and impaired granulocyte function predispose to infections from *S aureus*, *Aspergillus*, gram-negative bacilli, and *Candida*. Second, the time course of infection also provides clues to the etiology of pneumonia in immunocompromised patients. A fulminant pneumonia is often caused by bacterial infection, whereas an insidious pneumonia is more apt to be caused by viral, fungal, protozoal, or mycobacterial infection. Pneumonia occurring within 2–4 weeks after organ transplantation is usually bacterial, whereas several months or more after transplantation *P jiroveci*, viruses (eg, cytomegalovirus), and fungi (eg, *Aspergillus*) are encountered more often.

Chest radiography is rarely helpful in narrowing the differential diagnosis. Examination of expectorated sputum for bacteria, fungi, mycobacteria, *Legionella*, and *P jiroveci* is important and may preclude the need for expensive, invasive diagnostic procedures. Sputum induction is often necessary for diagnosis. The sensitivity of induced sputum for detection of *P jiroveci* depends on institutional expertise, number of specimens analyzed, and detection methods.

Routine evaluation frequently fails to identify a causative organism. The clinician may begin empiric antimicrobial therapy and proceed to invasive procedures such as bronchoscopy, transthoracic needle aspiration, or open lung biopsy. The approach to management must be based on the severity of the pulmonary infection, the underlying disease, the risks of empiric therapy, and local expertise and experience with diagnostic procedures. Bronchoalveolar lavage using the flexible bronchoscope is a safe and effective method for obtaining representative pulmonary secretions for microbiologic studies. It involves less risk of bleeding and other complications than bronchial brushing and transbronchial biopsy. Bronchoalveolar lavage is especially suitable for the diagnosis of *P jiroveci* pneumonia in patients with AIDS when induced sputum analysis is negative. Surgical lung biopsy, now often performed by video-assisted thoracoscopy, provides the best opportunity for diagnosis of pulmonary infiltrates in the immunocompromised host. However, a specific diagnosis is obtained in only about two-thirds of cases, and the information obtained rarely affects the outcome. Therefore, empiric treatment is often preferred.

Rano A et al. Pulmonary infections in non-HIV-immunocompromised patients. Curr Opin Pulm Med. 2005 May;11(3): 213–7. [PMID: 15818182]

Rosen MJ. Pulmonary complications of HIV infection. Respirology. 2008 Mar;13(2):181–90. [PMID: 18339015]

Scaglione S et al. Evaluation of pulmonary infiltrates in patients after stem cell transplantation. Hematology. 2005 Dec;10(6):469–81. [PMID: 16321812]

PULMONARY TUBERCULOSIS

 ESSENTIALS OF DIAGNOSIS

▸ Fatigue, weight loss, fever, night sweats, and cough.

▸ Pulmonary infiltrates on chest radiograph, most often apical.

▸ Positive tuberculin skin test reaction (most cases).

▸ Acid-fast bacilli on smear of sputum or sputum culture positive for *M tuberculosis*.

▸ General Considerations

Tuberculosis is one of the world's most widespread and deadly illnesses. *M tuberculosis*, the organism that causes tuberculosis infection and disease, infects an estimated 20–43% of the world's population. Each year, 3 million people worldwide die of the disease. In the United States, it is estimated that 15 million people are infected with *M tuberculosis*. Tuberculosis occurs disproportionately among disadvantaged populations such as the malnourished, homeless, and those living in overcrowded and substandard housing. There is an increased occurrence of tuberculosis among HIV-positive individuals.

Infection with *M tuberculosis* begins when a susceptible person inhales airborne droplet nuclei containing viable organisms. Tubercle bacilli that reach the alveoli are ingested by alveolar macrophages. Infection follows if the inoculum escapes alveolar macrophage microbicidal activity. Once infection is established, lymphatic and hematogenous dissemination of tuberculosis typically occurs before the development of an effective immune response. This stage of infection, **primary tuberculosis**, is usually clinically and radiographically silent. In most persons with intact cell-mediated immunity, T cells and macrophages surround the organisms in granulomas that limit their multiplication and spread. The infection is contained but not eradicated, since viable organisms may lie dormant within granulomas for years to decades.

Individuals with this **latent tuberculosis infection** do not have active disease and cannot transmit the organism to others. However, reactivation of disease may occur if the host's immune defenses are impaired. Active tuberculosis will develop in approximately 10% of individuals with latent tuberculosis infection who are not given preventive therapy; half of these cases occur in the 2 years following primary infection. Up to 50% of HIV-infected patients will develop active tuberculosis within 2 years after infection with tuberculosis. Diverse conditions such as gastrectomy, silicosis, diabetes mellitus, and disorders associated with immunosuppression (eg, HIV infection or therapy with corticosteroids or other immunosuppressive drugs) are associated with an increased risk of reactivation.

In approximately 5% of cases, the immune response is inadequate and the host develops **progressive primary tuberculosis**, accompanied by both pulmonary and constitutional symptoms that are described below. Standard teaching has held that 90% of tuberculosis in adults represents activation of latent disease. New diagnostic technologies such as DNA fingerprinting suggest that as many as one-third of new cases of tuberculosis in urban populations are primary infections resulting from person-to-person transmission.

The percentage of patients with atypical presentations—particularly elderly patients, patients with HIV infection, and those in nursing homes—has increased. Extrapulmonary tuberculosis is especially common in patients with HIV infection, who often display lymphadenitis or miliary disease.

Strains of M tuberculosis resistant to one or more first-line antituberculous drugs are being encountered with increasing frequency. Risk factors for drug resistance include immigration from parts of the world with a high prevalence of drug-resistant tuberculosis, close and prolonged contact with individuals with drug-resistant tuberculosis, unsuccessful previous therapy, and patient noncompliance. Resistance to one or more antituberculous drugs has been found in 15% of tuberculosis patients in the United States. Outbreaks of multidrug-resistant tuberculosis in hospitals and correctional facilities in Florida and New York have been associated with mortality rates of 70–90% and median survival rates of 4–16 weeks.

► Clinical Findings

A. Symptoms and Signs

The patient with pulmonary tuberculosis typically presents with slowly progressive constitutional symptoms of malaise, anorexia, weight loss, fever, and night sweats. Chronic cough is the most common pulmonary symptom. It may be dry at first but typically becomes productive of purulent sputum as the disease progresses. Blood-streaked sputum is common, but significant hemoptysis is rarely a presenting symptom; life-threatening hemoptysis may occur in advanced disease. Dyspnea is unusual unless there is extensive disease. Rarely, the patient is asymptomatic. On physical examination, the patient appears chronically ill and malnourished. On chest examination, there are no physical findings specific for tuberculosis infection. The examination may be normal or may reveal classic findings such as posttussive apical rales.

B. Laboratory Findings

Definitive diagnosis depends on recovery of M tuberculosis from cultures or identification of the organism by DNA or RNA amplification techniques. Three consecutive morning sputum specimens are advised. Sputum induction may be helpful in patients who cannot voluntarily produce satisfactory specimens. Fluorochrome staining with rhodamine-auramine of concentrated, digested sputum specimens is performed initially as a screening method, with confirmation by the Kinyoun or Ziehl-Neelsen stains. Demonstration of acid-fast bacilli on sputum smear does not confirm a diagnosis of tuberculosis, since saprophytic nontuberculous mycobacteria may colonize the airways and rarely may cause pulmonary disease.

In patients thought to have tuberculosis despite negative sputum smears, fiberoptic bronchoscopy can be considered. Bronchial washings are helpful; however, transbronchial lung biopsies increase the diagnostic yield. Postbronchoscopy expectorated sputum specimens may also be useful. Early morning aspiration of gastric contents after an overnight fast is an alternative to bronchoscopy but is suitable only for culture and not for stained smear, because nontuberculous mycobacteria may be present in the stomach in the absence of tuberculous infection. M tuberculosis may be cultured from blood in up to 15% of patients with tuberculosis.

Cultures on solid media to identify M tuberculosis may require 12 weeks. Liquid medium culture systems allow detection of mycobacterial growth in several days, although this depends on the number of organisms in the inoculum. The slow rate of mycobacterial growth has fostered interest in rapid diagnostic techniques. Nucleic acid amplification or high-performance liquid chromatography can be used to identify the type of mycobacterium within hours of sputum processing. Rapid confirmation of M tuberculosis is valuable in the mobilization of public health resources.

Nucleic acid amplification (DNA and RNA) tests for M tuberculosis should be interpreted in the clinical context and on the basis of local laboratory performance. A patient whose sputum culture is positive for acid-fast bacilli but whose nucleic acid amplification test result is negative for M tuberculosis may have a false-negative amplification test, a false-positive smear, or a nontuberculous mycobacterial infection. Clinical suspicion remains a critical factor in interpreting these studies. Drug susceptibility testing of culture isolates is considered routine for the first isolate of M tuberculosis, when a treatment regimen is failing, and when sputum cultures remain positive after 2 months of therapy.

Needle biopsy of the pleura reveals granulomatous inflammation in approximately 60% of patients with pleural effusions caused by M tuberculosis. Pleural fluid cultures for M tuberculosis are positive in less than 25% of cases of pleural tuberculosis. Culture of three pleural biopsy specimens combined with microscopic examination of a pleural biopsy yields a diagnosis in up to 90% of patients with pleural tuberculosis.

C. Imaging

Radiographic abnormalities in primary tuberculosis include small homogeneous infiltrates, hilar and paratracheal lymph node enlargement, and segmental atelectasis. Pleural effusion may be present, especially in adults, sometimes as the sole radiographic abnormality. Cavitation may be seen with progressive primary tuberculosis (Plate 66). Ghon (calcified primary focus) and Ranke (calcified primary focus and calcified hilar lymph node) complexes are seen in a minority of patients and represent residual evidence of healed primary tuberculosis.

Reactivation tuberculosis is associated with various radiographic manifestations, including fibrocavitary apical disease, nodules, and pneumonic infiltrates. The usual location is in the apical or posterior segments of the upper lobes or in the superior segments of the lower lobes; up to 30% of patients may present with radiographic evidence of disease in other locations. This is especially true in elderly patients, in whom lower lobe infiltrates with or without pleural effusion are encountered with increasing frequency. Lower lung tuberculosis may masquerade as pneumonia or lung cancer. A "miliary" pattern (diffuse small nodular densities) can be seen with hematologic or lymphatic dissemination of the organism. Resolution of reactivation tuberculosis leaves characteristic radiographic findings. Dense nodules in the pulmonary hila, with or without obvious calcification, upper lobe fibronodular scarring, and bronchiectasis with volume loss are common findings.

In patients with early HIV infection, the radiographic features of tuberculosis resemble those in patients without HIV infection. In contrast, atypical radiographic features predominate in patients with late stage HIV infection. These patients often display lower lung zone, diffuse, or miliary infiltrates, pleural effusions, and involvement of hilar and, in particular, mediastinal lymph nodes.

D. Special Examinations

The tuberculin **skin test** identifies individuals who have been infected with M tuberculosis but does not distinguish between active and latent infection. The test is used to evaluate a person who has symptoms of tuberculosis, an asymptomatic person who may be infected with M tuberculosis (eg, after contact exposure), or to establish the prevalence of tuberculous infection in a population. Routine testing of individuals at low risk for tuberculosis is not recommended. The Mantoux test is the preferred method: 0.1 mL of purified protein derivative (PPD) containing 5 tuberculin units is injected intradermally on the volar surface of the forearm using a 27-gauge needle on a tuberculin syringe. The transverse width in millimeters of induration at the skin test site should be measured after 48–72 hours. Table 9–10 summarizes the criteria established by the Centers for Disease Control and Prevention (CDC) for interpretation of the Mantoux tuberculin skin test. Different criteria for determination of a positive reaction are used, based on the prior likelihood of infection, to maximize the performance of the test. In patients who have serial testing, a **tuberculin skin test conversion** is defined as an increase of ≥ 10 mm of induration within a 2-year period regardless of patient age.

In general, it takes 2–10 weeks after tuberculosis infection for an immune response to PPD to develop. Both false-positive and false-negative results occur. False-positive tuberculin skin test reactions occur in persons previously vaccinated against M tuberculosis with bacillus Calmette-Guérin (BCG) (extract of Mycobacterium bovis) and in those infected with nontuberculous mycobacteria. False-negative tuberculin skin test reactions may result from improper testing technique, concurrent infections, malnutrition, advanced age, immunologic disorders, lymphoreticular malignancies, corticosteroid therapy, chronic kidney

Table 9–10. Classification of positive tuberculin skin test reactions.[1]

Reaction Size	Group
≥ 5 mm	1. HIV-positive persons. 2. Recent contacts of individuals with active tuberculosis. 3. Persons with fibrotic changes on chest x-rays suggestive of prior tuberculosis. 4. Patients with organ transplants and other immunosuppressed patients (receiving the equivalent of > 15 mg/d of prednisone for 1 month or more).
≥ 10 mm	1. Recent immigrants (< 5 years) from countries with a high prevalence of tuberculosis (eg, Asia, Africa, Latin America). 2. HIV-negative injection drug users. 3. Mycobacteriology laboratory personnel. 4. Residents of and employees[2] in the following high-risk congregate settings: correctional institutions; nursing homes and other long-term facilities for the elderly; hospitals and other health care facilities; residential facilities for AIDS patients; and homeless shelters. 5. Persons with the following medical conditions that increase the risk of tuberculosis: gastrectomy, ≥ 10% below ideal body weight, jejunoileal bypass, diabetes mellitus, silicosis, advanced chronic kidney disease, some hematologic disorders, (eg, leukemias, lymphomas), and other specific malignancies (eg, carcinoma of the head or neck and lung). 6. Children < 4 years of age or infants, children, and adolescents exposed to adults at high risk.
≥ 15 mm	1. Persons with no risk factors for tuberculosis.

[1]A tuberculin skin test reaction is considered positive if the transverse diameter of the *indurated* area reaches the size required for the specific group. All other reactions are considered negative.

[2]For persons who are otherwise at low risk and are tested at entry into employment, a reaction of > 15 mm induration is considered positive.

Source: Screening for tuberculosis and tuberculosis infection in high-risk populations: recommendations of the Advisory Council for the Elimination of Tuberculosis. MMWR Morb Mortal Wkly Rep 1995 Sep 8;44(RR-11):19–34. [PMID: 7565540]

disease, HIV infection, and fulminant tuberculosis. Some individuals with latent tuberculosis infection may have a negative skin test reaction when tested many years after exposure.

Serial testing may create a false impression of skin test conversion. Dormant mycobacterial sensitivity is sometimes restored by the antigenic challenge of the initial skin test. This phenomenon is called "boosting." A two-step testing procedure is used to reduce the likelihood that a boosted tuberculin reaction will be misinterpreted as a recent infection. Following a negative tuberculin skin test, the person is retested in 1–3 weeks. If the second test is negative, the person is uninfected or anergic; if positive, a boosted reaction is likely. Two-step testing should be used for the initial tuberculin skin testing of individuals who will be tested repeatedly, such as health care workers. Anergy testing is not recommended for routine use to distinguish a true-negative result from anergy. Poor anergy test standardization and lack of outcome data limit the evaluation of its effectiveness. Interpretation of the tuberculin skin test in persons who have previously received BCG vaccination is the same as in those who have not had BCG.

Novel in vitro T-cell based assays promise significant change in the identification of persons with latent M tuberculosis infection. Potential advantages of in vitro testing include reduced variability and subjectivity associated with placing and reading the PPD, fewer false-positive results from prior BCG vaccination, and better discrimination of positive responses due to nontuberculous mycobacteria.

Persons with concomitant HIV and tuberculosis infection usually respond best when the HIV infection is treated concurrently. In some cases, prolonged antituberculous therapy may be warranted. Therefore, all patients with tuberculosis infection should be tested for HIV within 2 months after diagnosis.

▶ Treatment

A. General Measures

The goals of therapy are to eliminate all tubercle bacilli from an infected individual while avoiding the emergence of clinically significant drug resistance. The basic principles of antituberculous treatment are (1) to administer multiple drugs to which the organisms are susceptible; (2) to add at least two new antituberculous agents to a regimen when treatment failure is suspected; (3) to provide the safest, most effective therapy in the shortest period of time; and (4) to ensure adherence to therapy.

All suspected and confirmed cases of tuberculosis should be reported promptly to local and state public health authorities. Public health departments will perform case investigations on sources and patient contacts to determine if other individuals with untreated, infectious tuberculosis are present in the community. They can identify infected contacts eligible for treatment of latent tuberculous infection, and ensure that a plan for monitoring adherence to therapy is established for each patient with tuberculosis. Patients with tuberculosis should be treated by physicians who are skilled in the management of this infection. Clinical expertise is especially important in cases of drug-resistant tuberculosis.

Nonadherence to antituberculous treatment is a major cause of treatment failure, continued transmission of tuberculosis, and the development of drug resistance. Adherence to treatment can be improved by providing detailed patient education about tuberculosis and its treatment in addition to a case manager who oversees all aspects of an individual patient's care. **Directly observed therapy (DOT)**, which requires that a health care worker physically observe the patient ingest antituberculous medications in the home, clinic, hospital, or elsewhere, also improves adherence to treatment. The importance of direct observation of therapy cannot be overemphasized. The CDC recommends DOT for all patients with drug-resistant tuberculosis and for those receiving intermittent (twice- or thrice-weekly) therapy.

Hospitalization for initial therapy of tuberculosis is not necessary for most patients. It should be considered if a patient is incapable of self-care or is likely to expose new, susceptible individuals to tuberculosis. Hospitalized patients with active disease require a private room with negative-pressure ventilation until tubercle bacilli are no longer found in their sputum ("smear-negative") on three consecutive smears taken on separate days.

Additional treatment considerations can be found in Chapter 33. Characteristics of antituberculous drugs are provided in Table 9–11. More complete information can be obtained from the CDC's Division of Tuberculosis Elimination Web site at http://www.cdc.gov/tb/.

B. Treatment of Tuberculosis in HIV-Negative Persons

Most patients with previously untreated pulmonary tuberculosis can be effectively treated with either a 6-month or a 9-month regimen, though the 6-month regimen is preferred. The initial phase of a 6-month regimen consists of 2 months of daily isoniazid, rifampin, pyrazinamide, and ethambutol. Once the isolate is determined to be isoniazid-sensitive, ethambutol may be discontinued. If the M tuberculosis isolate is susceptible to isoniazid and rifampin, the second phase of therapy consists of isoniazid and rifampin for a minimum of 4 additional months, with treatment to extend at least 3 months beyond documentation of conversion of sputum cultures to negative for M tuberculosis. If DOT is used, medications may be given intermittently using one of three regimens: (1) Daily isoniazid, rifampin, pyrazinamide, and ethambutol for 2 months, followed by isoniazid and rifampin two or three times each week for 4 months if susceptibility to isoniazid and rifampin is demonstrated. (2) Daily isoniazid, rifampin, pyrazinamide, and ethambutol for 2 weeks, then administration of the same agents twice weekly for 6 weeks followed by administration of isoniazid and rifampin twice each week for 4 months if susceptibility to isoniazid and rifampin is demonstrated. (3) Thrice-weekly administration of isoniazid, rifampin, pyrazinamide, and ethambutol for 6 months.

Patients who cannot or should not (eg, pregnant women) take pyrazinamide should receive daily isoniazid

Table 9–11. Characteristics of antituberculous drugs.

Drug	Most Common Side Effects	Tests for Side Effects	Drug Interactions	Remarks
Isoniazid	Peripheral neuropathy, hepatitis, rash, mild CNS effects.	AST and ALT; neurologic examination.	Phenytoin (synergistic); disulfiram.	Bactericidal to both extracellular and intracellular organisms. Pyridoxine, 10 mg orally daily as prophylaxis for neuritis; 50–100 mg orally daily as treatment.
Rifampin	Hepatitis, fever, rash, flu-like illness, gastrointestinal upset, bleeding problems, kidney failure.	CBC, platelets, AST and ALT.	Rifampin inhibits the effect of oral contraceptives, quinidine, corticosteroids, warfarin, methadone, digoxin, oral hypoglycemics; aminosalicylic acid may interfere with absorption of rifampin. Significant interactions with protease inhibitors and nonnucleoside reverse transcriptase inhibitors.	Bactericidal to all populations of organisms. Colors urine and other body secretions orange. Discoloring of contact lenses.
Pyrazinamide	Hyperuricemia, hepatotoxicity, rash, gastrointestinal upset, joint aches.	Uric acid, AST, ALT.	Rare.	Bactericidal to intracellular organisms.
Ethambutol	Optic neuritis (reversible with discontinuance of drug; rare at 15 mg/kg); rash.	Red-green color discrimination and visual acuity (difficult to test in children under 3 years of age).	Rare.	Bacteriostatic to both intracellular and extracellular organisms. Mainly used to inhibit development of resistant mutants. Use with caution in kidney disease or when ophthalmologic testing is not feasible.
Streptomycin	Eighth nerve damage, nephrotoxicity.	Vestibular function (audiograms); BUN and creatinine.	Neuromuscular blocking agents may be potentiated and cause prolonged paralysis.	Bactericidal to extracellular organisms. Use with caution in older patients or those with kidney disease.

ALT, alanine aminotransferase; AST, aspartate aminotransferase; BUN, blood urea nitrogen; CBC, complete blood count.

and rifampin along with ethambutol for 4–8 weeks. If susceptibility to isoniazid and rifampin is demonstrated or drug resistance is unlikely, ethambutol can be discontinued and isoniazid and rifampin may be given twice a week for a total of 9 months of therapy. If drug resistance is a concern, patients should receive isoniazid, rifampin, and ethambutol for 9 months. Patients with smear- and culture-negative disease (eg, pulmonary tuberculosis diagnosed on clinical grounds) and patients for whom drug susceptibility testing is not available can be treated with 6 months of isoniazid and rifampin combined with pyrazinamide for the first 2 months. This regimen assumes low prevalence of drug resistance. Previous guidelines have used streptomycin interchangeably with ethambutol. Increasing worldwide streptomycin resistance has made this drug less useful as empiric therapy.

When a twice-weekly or thrice-weekly regimen is used instead of a daily regimen, the dosages of isoniazid, pyrazinamide, and ethambutol or streptomycin must be increased. Recommended dosages for the initial treatment of tuberculosis are listed in Table 9–12. Fixed-dose combinations of isoniazid and rifampin (Rifamate) and of isoniazid, rifampin, and pyrazinamide (Rifater) are available

to simplify treatment. Single tablets improve compliance but are more expensive than the individual drugs purchased separately.

C. Treatment of Tuberculosis in HIV-Positive Persons

Management of tuberculosis is rendered even more complex in patients with concomitant HIV disease. Experts in the management of both tuberculosis and HIV disease should be involved in the care of such patients. The CDC has published detailed recommendations for the treatment of tuberculosis in HIV-positive patients. These documents can be obtained by accessing the CDC Division of Tuberculosis Elimination Web site at http://www.cdc.gov/tb/.

The basic approach to HIV-positive patients with tuberculosis is similar to that detailed above for patients without HIV disease. Additional considerations in HIV-positive patients include: (1) longer duration of therapy and (2) drug interactions between rifamycin derivatives such as rifampin and rifabutin, used to treat tuberculosis, and some of the protease inhibitors and nonnucleoside reverse transcriptase inhibitors (NNRTIs), used to treat

Table 9–12. Recommended dosages for the initial treatment of tuberculosis.

Drugs	Daily	Cost[1]	Twice a Week[2]	Cost[1]/wk	Three Times a Week[2]	Cost[1]/wk
Isoniazid	5 mg/kg Max: 300 mg/dose	$0.21/300 mg	15 mg/kg Max: 900 mg/dose	$1.26	15 mg/kg Max: 900 mg/dose	$1.89
Rifampin	10 mg/kg Max: 600 mg/dose	$5.15/600 mg	10 mg/kg Max: 600 mg/dose	$10.30	10 mg/kg Max: 600 mg/dose	$15.45
Pyrazinamide	15–30 mg/kg Max: 2 g/dose	$4.84/2 g	50–70 mg/kg Max: 4 g/dose	$19.36	50–70 mg/kg Max: 3 g/dose	$21.78
Ethambutol	5–25 mg/kg Max: 2.5 g/dose	$11.33/2.5 g	50 mg/kg Max: 2.5 g/dose	$22.66	25–30 mg/kg Max: 2.5 g/dose	$33.99
Streptomycin	15 mg/kg Max: 1 g/dose	$9.10/1 g	25–30 mg/kg Max: 1.5 g/dose	$36.40	25–30 mg/kg Max: 1.5 g/dose	$54.60

[1]Average wholesale price (AWP, for AB-rated generic when available) for quantity listed. Source: *Red Book Update,* Vol. 28, No. 3, March 2009. AWP may not accurately represent the actual pharmacy cost because wide contractual variations exist among institutions.
[2]All intermittent dosing regimens should be used with directly observed therapy.

HIV (see above Web site). DOT should be used for all HIV-positive tuberculosis patients. Pyridoxine (vitamin B_6), 25–50 mg orally each day, should be administered to all HIV-positive patients being treated with isoniazid to reduce central and peripheral nervous system side effects.

D. Treatment of Drug-Resistant Tuberculosis

Patients with drug-resistant *M tuberculosis* infection require careful supervision and management. Clinicians who are unfamiliar with the treatment of drug-resistant tuberculosis should seek expert advice. Tuberculosis resistant only to isoniazid can be successfully treated with a 6-month regimen of rifampin, pyrazinamide, and ethambutol or streptomycin or a 12-month regimen of rifampin and ethambutol. When isoniazid resistance is documented during a 9-month regimen without pyrazinamide, isoniazid should be discontinued. If ethambutol was part of the initial regimen, rifampin and ethambutol should be continued for a minimum of 12 months. If ethambutol was not part of the initial regimen, susceptibility tests should be repeated and two other drugs to which the organism is susceptible should be added. Treatment of *M tuberculosis* isolates resistant to agents other than isoniazid and treatment of drug resistance in HIV-infected patients require expert consultation.

Multidrug-resistant tuberculosis (MDRTB) calls for an individualized daily directly observed treatment plan under the supervision of a clinician experienced in the management of this entity. Treatment regimens are based on the patient's overall status and the results of susceptibility studies. Most MDRTB isolates are resistant to at least isoniazid and rifampin and require a minimum of three drugs to which the organism is susceptible. These regimens are continued until culture conversion is documented, and then a two-drug regimen is continued for at least another 12 months. Some experts recommend at least 18–24 months of a three-drug regimen.

E. Treatment of Extrapulmonary Tuberculosis

In most cases, regimens that are effective for treating pulmonary tuberculosis are also effective for treating extrapulmonary disease. However, many experts recommend 9 months of therapy when miliary, meningeal, or bone and joint disease is present. Treatment of skeletal tuberculosis is enhanced by early surgical drainage and debridement of necrotic bone. Corticosteroid therapy has been shown to help prevent cardiac constriction from tuberculous pericarditis and to reduce neurologic complications from tuberculous meningitis (see Chapter 33).

F. Treatment of Pregnant or Lactating Women

Tuberculosis in pregnancy is usually treated with isoniazid, rifampin, and ethambutol. Ethambutol can be excluded if isoniazid resistance is unlikely. Therapy is continued for 9 months. Since the risk of teratogenicity with pyrazinamide has not been clearly defined, pyrazinamide should be used only if resistance to other drugs is documented and susceptibility to pyrazinamide is likely. Streptomycin is contraindicated in pregnancy because it may cause congenital deafness. Pregnant women taking isoniazid should receive pyridoxine (vitamin B_6), 10–25 mg orally once a day, to prevent peripheral neuropathy.

Small concentrations of antituberculous drugs are present in breast milk and are not known to be harmful to nursing newborns. Therefore, breastfeeding is not contraindicated while receiving antituberculous therapy.

G. Treatment Monitoring

Adults should have measurements of serum bilirubin, hepatic enzymes, urea nitrogen, creatinine, and a complete blood count (including platelets) before starting chemotherapy for tuberculosis. Visual acuity and red-green color vision tests are recommended before initiation of ethambutol and serum uric acid before starting pyrazinamide.

Audiometry should be performed if streptomycin therapy is initiated.

Routine monitoring of laboratory tests for evidence of drug toxicity during therapy is not recommended, unless baseline results are abnormal or liver disease is suspected. Monthly questioning for symptoms of drug toxicity is advised. Patients should be educated about common side effects of antituberculous medications and instructed to seek medical attention should these symptoms occur. Monthly follow-up of outpatients is recommended, including sputum smear and culture for *M tuberculosis* until cultures convert to negative. Patients with negative sputum cultures after 2 months of treatment should have at least one additional sputum smear and culture performed at the end of therapy. Patients with MDRTB should have sputum cultures performed monthly during the entire course of treatment. A chest radiograph at the end of therapy provides a useful baseline for any future films.

Patients whose cultures do not become negative or whose symptoms do not resolve despite 3 months of therapy should be evaluated for drug-resistant organisms and for nonadherence to the treatment regimen. DOT is required for the remainder of the treatment regimen, and the addition of at least two drugs not previously given should be considered pending repeat drug susceptibility testing. The clinician should seek expert assistance if drug resistance is newly found, if the patient remains symptomatic, or if smears or cultures remain positive.

Patients with only a clinical diagnosis of pulmonary tuberculosis (smears and cultures negative for *M tuberculosis*) whose symptoms and radiographic abnormalities are unchanged after 3 months of treatment usually either have another process or have had tuberculosis in the past.

H. Treatment of Latent Tuberculosis

Treatment of latent tuberculous infection is essential to controlling and eliminating tuberculosis in the United States. Treatment of latent tuberculous infection substantially reduces the risk that infection will progress to active disease. Targeted testing is used to identify persons who are at high risk for tuberculosis and who stand to benefit from treatment of latent infection. Table 9–10 defines high-risk groups and gives the tuberculin skin test criteria for treatment of latent tuberculous infection. In general, patients with a positive tuberculin skin test who are at increased risk for exposure or disease are treated. It is essential that each person who meets the criteria for treatment of latent tuberculous infection undergo a careful assessment to exclude active disease. A history of past treatment for tuberculosis and contraindications to treatment should be sought. All patients at risk for HIV infection should be tested for HIV. Patients suspected of having tuberculosis should receive one of the recommended multidrug regimens for active disease until the diagnosis is confirmed or excluded.

Some close contacts of persons with active tuberculosis should be evaluated for treatment of latent tuberculous infection despite a negative tuberculin skin test reaction (< 5 mm induration). These include immunosuppressed persons and those who may develop disease quickly after tuberculous infection. Close contacts who have a negative tuberculin skin test reaction on initial testing should be retested 10–12 weeks later.

Several treatment regimens for both HIV-negative and HIV-positive persons are available for the treatment of latent tuberculous infection: (1) **Isoniazid:** A 9-month regimen (minimum of 270 doses administered within 12 months) is considered optimal. Dosing options include a daily dose of 300 mg or twice-weekly doses of 15 mg/kg. Persons at risk for developing isoniazid-associated peripheral neuropathy (diabetes mellitus, uremia, malnutrition, alcoholism, HIV infection, pregnancy, seizure disorder) may be given supplemental pyridoxine (vitamin B_6), 10–50 mg/d. (2) **Rifampin and pyrazinamide:** A 2-month regimen (60 doses administered within 3 months) of daily rifampin (10 mg/kg up to a maximum dose of 600 mg) and pyrazinamide (15–20 mg/kg up to a maximum dose of 2 g) is recommended. (3) **Rifampin:** Patients who cannot tolerate isoniazid or pyrazinamide can be considered for a 4-month regimen (minimum of 120 doses administered within 6 months) of rifampin. HIV-positive patients receiving protease inhibitors or NNRTIs who are given rifampin require management by experts in both tuberculosis and HIV disease (see Treatment of Tuberculosis in HIV-Positive Persons, above).

Contacts of persons with isoniazid-resistant, rifampin-sensitive tuberculosis should receive a 2-month regimen of rifampin and pyrazinamide or a 4-month regimen of daily rifampin alone. Contacts of persons with MDRTB should receive two drugs to which the infecting organism has demonstrated susceptibility. Tuberculin skin test-negative and HIV-negative contacts may be observed without treatment or treated for 6 months. HIV-positive contacts should be treated for 12 months. All contacts of persons with MDRTB should have 2 years of follow-up regardless of treatment.

Persons with a positive tuberculin skin test (≥ 5 mm of induration) and fibrotic lesions suggestive of old tuberculosis on chest radiographs who have no evidence of active disease and no history of treatment for tuberculosis should receive 9 months of isoniazid, or 2 months of rifampin and pyrazinamide, or 4 months of rifampin (with or without isoniazid). Pregnant or breastfeeding women with latent tuberculosis should receive either daily or twice-weekly isoniazid with pyridoxine (vitamin B_6).

Baseline laboratory testing is indicated for patients at risk for liver disease, patients with HIV infection, women who are pregnant or within 3 months of delivery, and persons who use alcohol regularly. Patients receiving treatment for latent tuberculous infection should be evaluated once a month to assess for symptoms and signs of active tuberculosis and hepatitis and for adherence to their treatment regimen. Routine laboratory testing during treatment is indicated for those with abnormal baseline laboratory tests and for those at risk for developing liver disease.

Vaccine BCG is an antimycobacterial vaccine developed from an attenuated strain of *M bovis*. Millions of individuals worldwide have been vaccinated with BCG. However, it is not generally recommended in the United States because of the low prevalence of tuberculous infection, the vaccine's interference with the ability to determine latent tuberculous infection using tuberculin skin test reactivity, and its variable effectiveness against pulmonary tuberculosis. BCG vaccination in the United States should only be undertaken after consultation with local health officials and experts in the management of tuberculosis. Vaccination of health care workers should be considered on an individual basis in settings in which a high percentage of tuberculosis patients are infected with strains resistant to both isoniazid and rifampin, in which transmission of such drug-resistant *M tuberculosis* and subsequent infection are likely, and in which comprehensive tuberculous infection-control precautions have been implemented but have not been successful. The BCG vaccine is contraindicated in persons with impaired immune responses due to disease or medications.

Prognosis

Almost all properly treated patients with tuberculosis can be cured. Relapse rates are less than 5% with current regimens. The main cause of treatment failure is nonadherence to therapy.

American Thoracic Society; Centers for Disease Control and Prevention; Infectious Diseases Society of America. Controlling tuberculosis in the United States. Am J Respir Crit Care Med. 2005 Nov 1;172(9):1169–227. [PMID: 16249321]

Blumberg HM et al; American Thoracic Society/Centers for Disease Control and Prevention/Infectious Diseases Society of America: Treatment of tuberculosis. Am J Respir Crit Care Med. 2003 Feb 15;167(4):603–62. [PMID: 12588714]

Diagnostic Standards and Classification of Tuberculosis in Adults and Children. American Thoracic Society and Centers for Disease Control and Prevention. Am J Respir Crit Care Med 2000 Apr;161(4 Part 1):1376–95. [PMID: 10764337]

Grant A et al. Managing drug resistant tuberculosis. BMJ. 2008 Aug 28;337:a1110. [PMID: 18755763]

PULMONARY DISEASE CAUSED BY NONTUBERCULOUS MYCOBACTERIA

 ESSENTIALS OF DIAGNOSIS

▸ Chronic cough, sputum production, and fatigue; less commonly: malaise, dyspnea, fever, hemoptysis, and weight loss.

▸ Parenchymal infiltrates on chest radiograph, often with thin-walled cavities, that spread contiguously and often involve overlying pleura.

▸ Isolation of nontuberculous mycobacteria in a sputum culture.

General Considerations

Mycobacteria other than *M tuberculosis*—nontuberculous mycobacteria (NTM), sometimes referred to as "atypical" mycobacteria—are ubiquitous in water and soil and have been isolated from tap water. There appears to be a continuing increase in the number and prevalence of NTM species. Marked geographic variability exists, both in the NTM species responsible for disease and in the prevalence of disease. These organisms are not considered communicable from person to person, have distinct laboratory characteristics, and are often resistant to most antituberculous drugs. See Chapter 33 for further information.

Definition & Pathogenesis

The diagnosis of lung disease caused by NTM is based on a combination of clinical, radiographic, and bacteriologic criteria and the exclusion of other diseases that can resemble the condition. Specific diagnostic criteria are discussed below. Complementary data are important for diagnosis because NTM organisms can reside in or colonize the airways without causing clinical disease, especially in patients with AIDS, and many patients have preexisting lung disease that may make their chest radiographs abnormal.

Mycobacterium avium complex (MAC) is the most frequent cause of NTM pulmonary disease in humans in the United States. *Mycobacterium kansasii* is the next most frequent pulmonary pathogen. Other NTM causes of pulmonary disease include *Mycobacterium abscessus*, *Mycobacterium xenopi*, and *Mycobacterium malmoense*; the list of more unusual etiologic NTM species is long. Most NTM cause a chronic pulmonary infection that resembles tuberculosis but tends to progress more slowly. Disseminated disease is rare in immunocompetent hosts; however, disseminated MAC disease is common in patients with AIDS.

Clinical Findings

A. Symptoms and Signs

NTM infection among immunocompetent hosts frequently presents in one of three prototypical patterns: cavitary, upper lobe lesions in older male smokers that may mimic *M tuberculosis*; nodular bronchiectasis affecting the mid lung zones in middle-aged women with chronic cough; and hypersensitivity pneumonitis following environmental exposure. Most patients with NTM infection experience a chronic cough, sputum production, and fatigue. Less common symptoms include malaise, dyspnea, fever, hemoptysis, and weight loss. Symptoms from coexisting lung disease (COPD, bronchiectasis, previous mycobacterial disease, cystic fibrosis, and pneumoconiosis) may confound the evaluation. In patients with bronchiectasis, coinfection with NTM and *Aspergillus* is a negative prognostic factor. New or worsening infiltrates as well as adenopathy or pleural effusion (or both) are described in HIV-positive patients with NTM infection as part of the immune reconstitution inflammatory syndrome following institution of highly active antiretroviral therapy.

B. Laboratory Findings

The diagnosis of NTM infection rests on recovery of the pathogen from cultures. Sputum cultures positive for atypical mycobacteria do not prove infection because NTM may exist as saprophytes colonizing the airways or may be environmental contaminants. Bronchial washings are considered to be more sensitive than expectorated sputum samples; however, their specificity for clinical disease is not known.

Bacteriologic criteria have been proposed based on studies of patients with cavitary disease with MAC or *M kansasii*. Diagnostic criteria in immunocompetent persons include the following: positive culture results from at least two separate expectorated sputum samples; or positive culture from at least one bronchial wash; or a positive culture from pleural fluid or any other normally sterile site. The diagnosis can also be established by demonstrating NTM cultured from a lung biopsy, bronchial wash, or sputum plus histopathologic changes such as granulomatous inflammation in a lung biopsy. Rapid species identification of some NTM is possible using DNA probes or high-pressure liquid chromatography.

Diagnostic criteria are less stringent for patients with severe immune suppression. HIV-infected patients may show significant MAC growth on culture of bronchial washings without clinical infection; therefore, HIV patients being evaluated for MAC infection must be considered individually.

In general, drug susceptibility testing on cultures of NTM is not recommended except for the following NTM: (1) *M kansasii* to rifampin; and (2) rapid growers (such as *Mycobacterium fortuitum*, *Mycobacterium chelonae*, *M abscessus*) to amikacin, doxycycline, imipenem, fluoroquinolones, clarithromycin, cefoxitin, and sulfonamides.

C. Imaging

Chest radiographic findings include infiltrates that are progressive or persist for at least 2 months, cavitary lesions, and multiple nodular densities. The cavities are often thin-walled and have less surrounding parenchymal infiltrate than is commonly seen with MTB infections. Evidence of contiguous spread and pleural involvement is often present. High-resolution CT of the chest may show multiple small nodules with or without multifocal bronchiectasis. Progression of pulmonary infiltrates during therapy or lack of radiographic improvement over time are poor prognostic signs and also raise concerns about secondary or alternative pulmonary processes. Clearing of pulmonary infiltrates due to NTM is slow.

▶ Treatment

Establishing NTM infection does not mandate treatment in all cases, for two reasons. First, clinical disease may never develop in some patients, particularly asymptomatic patients with few organisms isolated from single specimens. Second, the spectrum of clinical disease severity is very wide; in patients with mild or slowly progressive symptoms, traditional chemotherapeutic regimens using a combination of agents may lead to drug-induced side effects worse than the disease itself.

Specific treatment regimens and responses to therapy vary with the species of NTM. Non-HIV-infected patients with MAC pulmonary disease usually receive a combination of daily clarithromycin or azithromycin, rifampin or rifabutin, and ethambutol. Streptomycin is considered for the first 2 months as tolerated. The optimal duration of treatment is unknown, but therapy should be continued for 12 months after sputum conversion. Medical treatment is initially successful in about two-thirds of cases, but relapses after treatment are common; long-term benefit is demonstrated in about half of all patients. Those who do not respond favorably generally have active but stable disease. Surgical resection is an alternative for the patient with progressive disease that responds poorly to chemotherapy; the success rate with surgical therapy is good. Disease caused by *M kansasii* responds well to drug therapy. A daily regimen of rifampin, isoniazid, and ethambutol for at least 18 months with a minimum of 12 months of negative cultures is usually successful. Rapidly growing mycobacteria (*M abscessus*, *M fortuitum*, *M chelonae*) are generally resistant to standard antituberculous therapy.

▶ When to Refer

Patients with rapidly growing mycobacteria infection should be referred for expert management.

Glassroth J. Pulmonary disease due to non-tuberculous mycobacteria. Chest. 2008 Jan;133(1):243–51. [PMID: 18187749]

Griffith DE et al. An official ATS/IDSA statement: diagnosis, treatment, and prevention of nontuberculous mycobacterial diseases. Am J Respir Crit Care Med. 2007 Feb 15;175(4):367–416. [PMID: 17277290]

▼ PULMONARY NEOPLASMS

See Chapter 39 for discussions of Lung Cancer, Secondary Lung Cancer, and Mesothelioma.

SCREENING FOR LUNG CANCER

Periodic evaluation of asymptomatic people at high risk for lung cancer is an attractive strategy without demonstrated benefit. Available evidence from the Mayo Lung Project suggests that serial chest radiographs can identify a significant number of early stage malignancies but that neither disease-specific mortality from lung cancer nor all-cause mortality is affected by screening. The illusory benefits of screening have been attributed to lead time, length time, and overdiagnosis biases. To date, no major advisory organization recommends screening for lung cancer.

The availability of rapid-acquisition, low-dose helical computed tomography (LDCT) has rekindled enthusiasm for lung cancer screening. LDCT is a very sensitive test. Compared with chest radiography, LDCT identifies between four and ten times the number of asymptomatic lung malignancies. LDCT may also increase the number of false-positive tests, unnecessary diagnostic procedures, and overdiagnosis. A mortality benefit remains to be proved. The National Lung Cancer Screening Trial is an ongoing NCI-funded multicenter trial to determine whether using LDCT to screen current or former heavy smokers for lung cancer will improve mortality in this population. Information is available at http://www.cancer.gov/NLST/.

Screening for lung cancer with biomolecular markers remains an area of study. A variety of strategies that evaluate patterns of volatile organic compounds in exhaled breath, or DNA alterations in exhaled breath condensate have been described, although lack clinical validation.

Bach PB et al. Screening for lung cancer: ACCP evidence-based clinical practice guidelines (2nd edition). Chest. 2007 Sep;132(3 Suppl):69S–77S. [PMID: 17873161]

SOLITARY PULMONARY NODULE

A solitary pulmonary nodule, sometimes referred to as a "coin lesion," is a < 3 cm isolated, rounded opacity on the chest imaging outlined by normal lung and not associated with infiltrate, atelectasis, or adenopathy. Most are asymptomatic and represent an unexpected finding on chest radiography or CT scanning. The finding is important because it carries a significant risk of malignancy. The frequency of malignancy in surgical series ranges from 10% to 68% depending on patient population. Most benign nodules are infectious granulomas. **Benign neoplasms** such as hamartomas account for less than 5% of solitary nodules.

The goals of evaluation are to identify and resect malignant tumors in patients who stand to benefit from resection while avoiding invasive procedures in benign disease. The task is to identify nodules with a sufficiently high probability of malignancy to warrant biopsy or resection or a sufficiently low probability of malignancy to justify observation.

Symptoms alone rarely establish the cause, but clinical and radiographic data can be used to assess the probability of malignancy. The patient's age is important. Malignant nodules are rare in persons under age 30. Above age 30, the likelihood of malignancy increases with age. Smokers are at increased risk, and the likelihood of malignancy increases with the number of cigarettes smoked daily. Patients with a prior malignancy have a higher likelihood of having a malignant solitary nodule.

The first and most important step in the radiographic evaluation is to review old radiographs. Comparison with prior studies allows estimation of doubling time, which is an important marker for malignancy. Rapid progression (doubling time less than 30 days) suggests infection; long-term stability (doubling time greater than 465 days) suggests benignity. Certain radiographic features help in estimating the probability of malignancy. Size is correlated with malignancy. A recent study of solitary nodules identified by CT scan showed a 1% malignancy rate in those measuring 2–5 mm, 24% in 6–10 mm, 33% in 11–20 mm, and 80% in 21–45 mm. The appearance of a smooth, well-defined edge is characteristic of a benign process. Ill-defined margins or a lobular appearance suggest malignancy. A high-resolution CT finding of spiculated margins and a peripheral halo are both highly associated with malignancy. Calcification and its pattern are also helpful clues. Benign lesions tend to have dense calcification in a central or laminated pattern. Malignant lesions are associated with sparser calcification that is typically stippled or eccentric. Cavitary lesions with thick (> 16 mm) walls are much more likely to be malignant. High-resolution CT offers better resolution of these characteristics than chest radiography and is more likely to detect lymphadenopathy or the presence of multiple lesions. Chest CT is indicated in any suspicious solitary pulmonary nodule.

► Treatment

Based on clinical and radiologic data, the clinician should assign a specific probability of malignancy to the lesion. The decision whether and how to obtain a diagnostic biopsy depends on the interpretation of this probability in light of the patient's unique clinical situation. The probabilities in parentheses below represent guidelines only and should not be interpreted as prescriptive.

In the case of solitary pulmonary nodules, a continuous probability function may be grouped into three categories. In patients with a low probability (< 5%) of malignancy (eg, age under 30, lesions stable for more than 2 years, characteristic pattern of benign calcification), watchful waiting is appropriate. Management consists of serial imaging studies (CT scans or chest radiographs) at intervals that would identify growth that would suggest malignancy. Three-dimensional reconstruction of high-resolution CT images provides a more sensitive test for growth.

Patients with a high probability (> 60%) of malignancy should proceed directly to resection following staging, provided the surgical risk is acceptable. Biopsies rarely yield a specific benign diagnosis and are not indicated.

Optimal management of patients with an intermediate probability of malignancy (5–60%) remains controversial. The traditional approach is to obtain a diagnostic biopsy either through transthoracic needle aspiration (TTNA) or bronchoscopy. Bronchoscopy yields a diagnosis in 10–80% of procedures depending on the size of the nodule and its location. In general, the bronchoscopic yield for nodules that are < 2 cm and peripheral is low, although complications are generally rare. Newer bronchoscopic modalities such as electromagnetic navigation and ultrathin bronchoscopy are being studied, although their impact upon diagnostic yield remains uncertain. TTNA has a higher diagnostic yield, reported to be between 50% and 97%. The yield is strongly operator-dependent, however, and is affected by the location and size of the lesion. Complications are higher than bronchoscopy, with pneumothorax occurring in up to 30% of patients, with up to one-third of these patients requiring placement of a chest tube.

Disappointing diagnostic yields and a high false-negative rate (up to 20–30% in TTNA) have prompted alternative approaches. Positron emission tomography (PET) detects increased glucose metabolism within malignant lesions with high sensitivity (85–97%) and specificity (70–85%). Many diagnostic algorithms have incorporated PET into the assessment of patients with inconclusive high-resolution CT findings. A positive PET increases the likelihood of malignancy, and a negative PET correctly excludes cancer in most cases. False-negative PET scans can occur with tumors with low metabolic activity (well-differentiated adenocarcinomas, carcinoids, and bronchioloalveolar tumors), and follow-up imaging is typically performed at discrete intervals to ensure absence of growth. PET has several drawbacks, however: resolution below 1 cm is poor, the test is expensive, and availability remains limited.

Sputum cytology is highly specific but lacks sensitivity. It is used in central lesions and in patients who are poor candidates for invasive diagnostic procedures. Researchers have attempted to improve the sensitivity of sputum cytology through the use of monoclonal antibodies to proteins that are up-regulated in pulmonary malignancies. Such tests offer promise but remain research tools at this time.

Video-assisted thoracoscopic surgery (VATS) offers a more aggressive approach to diagnosis. VATS is more invasive than bronchoscopy or TTNA but is associated with less postoperative pain, shorter hospital stays, and more rapid return to function than traditional thoracotomy. These advantages have led some centers to recommend VATS resection of all solitary pulmonary nodules with intermediate probability of malignancy. In some cases, surgeons will remove the nodule and evaluate it in the operating room with frozen section. If the nodule is malignant, they will proceed to lobectomy and lymph node sampling, either thoracoscopically or through conversion to standard thoracotomy.

All patients should be provided with an estimate of the likelihood of malignancy, and their preferences should be used to help guide diagnostic and therapeutic decisions. A strategy that recommends observation may not be preferred by a patient who desires a definitive diagnosis. Similarly, a surgical approach may not be agreeable to all patients unless the presence of cancer is definitive. Patient preferences should be elicited, and patients should be well informed regarding the specific risks and benefits associated with the recommended approach as well as the alternative strategies.

Gould MK et al. Evaluation of patients with pulmonary nodules: when is it lung cancer? ACCP evidence-based clinical practice guidelines (2nd edition). Chest. 2007 Sep;132(3 Suppl):108S–130S. [PMID: 17873164]

MacMahon H et al. Guidelines for management of small pulmonary nodules detected on CT scans: a statement from the Fleischner Society. Radiology. 2005 Nov;237(2):395–400. [PMID: 16244247]

Mott TF et al. Clinical inquiries. What is the best approach to a solitary pulmonary nodule identified by chest x-ray? J Fam Pract. 2007 Oct;56(10):845–7. [PMID: 17908518]

Winer-Muram HT. The solitary pulmonary nodule. Radiology. 2006 Apr;239(1):34–49. [PMID: 16567482]

BRONCHIAL CARCINOID TUMORS

Carcinoid and bronchial gland tumors are sometimes termed "bronchial adenomas." This term should be avoided because it implies that the lesions are benign when, in fact, carcinoid tumors and bronchial gland carcinomas are low-grade malignant neoplasms.

Carcinoid tumors are about six times more common than bronchial gland carcinomas, and most of them occur as pedunculated or sessile growths in central bronchi. Men and women are equally affected. Most patients are under 60 years of age. Common symptoms of bronchial carcinoid tumors are hemoptysis, cough, focal wheezing, and recurrent pneumonia. Peripherally located bronchial carcinoid tumors are rare and present as asymptomatic solitary pulmonary nodules. Carcinoid syndrome (flushing, diarrhea, wheezing, hypotension) is rare. Fiberoptic bronchoscopy may reveal a pink or purple tumor in a central airway. These lesions have a well-vascularized stroma, and biopsy may be complicated by significant bleeding. CT scanning is helpful to localize the lesion and to follow its growth over time. Octreotide scintigraphy is also available for localization of these tumors.

Bronchial carcinoid tumors grow slowly and rarely metastasize. Complications involve bleeding and airway obstruction rather than invasion by tumor and metastases. Surgical excision of clinically symptomatic lesions is often necessary, and the prognosis is generally favorable. Most bronchial carcinoid tumors are resistant to radiation and chemotherapy.

Chong S et al. Neuroendocrine tumors of the lung: clinical, pathologic, and imaging findings. Radiographics. 2006 Jan–Feb;26(1):41–57. [PMID: 16418242]

Oberg K et al; ESMO Guidelines Working Group. Neuroendocrine bronchial and thymic tumors: ESMO clinical recommendation for diagnosis, treatment and follow-up. Ann Oncol. 2008 May;19(Suppl 2):ii102–3. [PMID: 18456740]

MEDIASTINAL MASSES

Various developmental, neoplastic, infectious, traumatic, and cardiovascular disorders may cause masses that appear in the mediastinum on chest radiograph. A useful convention arbitrarily divides the mediastinum into three compartments—anterior, middle, and posterior—in order to classify mediastinal masses and assist in differential diagnosis. Specific mediastinal masses have a predilection for one or more of these compartments; most are located in the anterior or middle compartment. The differential diagnosis of an anterior mediastinal mass includes thymoma, teratoma, thyroid lesions, lymphoma, and mesenchymal tumors (lipoma, fibroma). The differential diagnosis of a middle mediastinal mass includes lymphadenopathy, pulmonary artery enlargement, aneurysm of the aorta or innominate artery, developmental cyst (bronchogenic, enteric, pleuropericardial), dilated azygous or hemiazygous vein, and foramen of Morgagni hernia. The differential diagnosis of a posterior mediastinal mass includes hiatus hernia, neurogenic tumor, meningocele, esophageal tumor, foramen of Bochdalek hernia, thoracic spine disease, and extramedullary hematopoiesis. The neurogenic tumor group includes neurilemmoma, neurofibroma, neurosarcoma, ganglioneuroma, and pheochromocytoma.

Symptoms and signs of mediastinal masses are nonspecific and are usually caused by the effects of the mass on surrounding structures. Insidious onset of retrosternal chest pain, dysphagia, or dyspnea is often an important clue to the presence of a mediastinal mass. In about half of cases, symptoms are absent, and the mass is detected on routine chest radiograph. Physical findings vary depending on the nature and location of the mass.

CT scanning is helpful in management; additional radiographic studies of benefit include barium swallow if esophageal disease is suspected, Doppler sonography or venography of brachiocephalic veins and the superior vena cava, and angiography. MRI is useful; its advantages include better delineation of hilar structures and distinction between vessels and masses. MRI also allows imaging in multiple planes, whereas CT permits only axial imaging. Tissue diagnosis is necessary if a neoplastic disorder is suspected. Treatment and prognosis depend on the underlying cause of the mediastinal mass.

Duwe BV et al. Tumors of the mediastinum. Chest. 2005 Oct;128(4):2893–909. [PMID: 16236967]

Whitten CR et al. A diagnostic approach to mediastinal abnormalities. Radiographics. 2007 May–Jun;27(3):657–71. [PMID: 17495284]

INTERSTITIAL LUNG DISEASE (DIFFUSE PARENCHYMAL LUNG DISEASE)

Interstitial lung disease, or diffuse parenchymal lung disease, comprises a heterogeneous group of disorders that share common presentations (dyspnea), physical findings (late inspiratory crackles), and chest radiographs (septal thickening and reticulonodular changes).

The term "interstitial" is misleading since the pathologic process usually begins with injury to the alveolar epithelial or capillary endothelial cells. Persistent alveolitis may lead to obliteration of alveolar capillaries and reorganization of the lung parenchyma, accompanied by irreversible fibrosis. The process does not affect the airways proximal to the respiratory bronchioles. At least 180 disease entities may present as interstitial lung disease. Table 9–13 outlines a selected list of differential diagnoses of interstitial lung disease. In most patients, no specific cause can be identified. In the remainder, drugs and a variety of organic and inorganic dusts are the principal causes. The history—particularly the occupational and medication history—may provide evidence of a specific cause.

The connective tissue diseases are a group of immunologically mediated inflammatory disorders including rheumatoid arthritis, systemic lupus erythematosus, scleroderma, polymyositis-dermatomyositis, Sjögren syndrome, and other overlap conditions. The presence of diffuse parenchymal lung disease in the setting of an established connective tissue disease is suggestive of the etiology. In some cases, lung disease precedes the more typical manifestations of the underlying connective tissue disease by months or years.

▶ Clinical Findings

A. Symptoms and Signs

The clinical consequence of widespread lung fibrosis is diminished lung compliance, which presents as restrictive lung disease. Patients usually describe an insidious onset of exertional dyspnea and cough. Sputum production is minimal. Chest examination reveals fine, late inspiratory crackles at the lung bases in 60–90% of patients. Digital clubbing is seen in 25–50% of patients at diagnosis (see Plate 47).

B. Laboratory Findings

Serologic tests for antinuclear antibodies and rheumatoid factor are positive in 20–40% of patients but are rarely

Table 9–13. Differential diagnosis of interstitial lung disease.

Drug-related
  Antiarrhythmic agents (amiodarone)
  Antibacterial agents (nitrofurantoin, sulfonamides)
  Antineoplastic agents (bleomycin, cyclophosphamide, methotrexate, nitrosoureas)
  Antirheumatic agents (gold salts, penicillamine)
  Phenytoin
Environmental and occupational (inhalation exposures)
  Dust, inorganic (asbestos, silica, hard metals, beryllium)
  Dust, organic (thermophilic actinomycetes, avian antigens, *Aspergillus* species)
  Gases, fumes, and vapors (chlorine, isocyanates, paraquat, sulfur dioxide)
  Ionizing radiation
  Talc (injection drug users)
Infections
  Fungus, disseminated (*Coccidioides immitis, Blastomyces dermatitidis, Histoplasma capsulatum*)
  Mycobacteria, disseminated
    Pneumocystis jiroveci
  Viruses
Primary pulmonary disorders
  Cryptogenic organizing pneumonitis (COP)
  Idiopathic fibrosing interstitial pneumonia: Acute interstitial pneumonitis, desquamative interstitial pneumonitis, nonspecific interstitial pneumonitis, usual interstitial pneumonitis, respiratory bronchiolitis-associated interstitial lung disease
  Pulmonary alveolar proteinosis
Systemic disorders
  Acute respiratory distress syndrome
  Amyloidosis
  Ankylosing spondylitis
  Autoimmune disease: Dermatomyositis, polymyositis, rheumatoid arthritis, systemic sclerosis (scleroderma), systemic lupus erythematosus
  Chronic eosinophilic pneumonia
  Goodpasture syndrome
  Idiopathic pulmonary hemosiderosis
  Inflammatory bowel disease
  Langerhans cell histiocytosis (eosinophilic granuloma)
  Lymphangitic spread of cancer (lymphangitic carcinomatosis)
  Lymphangioleiomyomatosis
  Pulmonary edema
  Pulmonary venous hypertension, chronic
  Sarcoidosis
  Wegener granulomatosis

diagnostic. Antineutrophil cytoplasmic antibodies (ANCAs) may be diagnostic in some clinical settings. Pulmonary function testing shows a loss of lung volume with normal to increased airflow rates. The $D_{L_{CO}}$ is decreased, and hypoxemia with exercise is common. In advanced cases, pulmonary hypertension and resting hypoxemia may be present.

C. Imaging

The chest radiograph is normal on presentation in up to 10% of patients. More typically, it shows patchy distribution of ground-glass, reticular, or reticulonodular infiltrates. In advanced disease, there are multiple small, thick-walled cystic spaces in the lung periphery ("honeycomb" lung). Honeycombing indicates the presence of locally advanced fibrosis with destruction of normal lung architecture. Conventional CT and high-resolution CT imaging reveal in greater detail the findings described on chest radiograph. In some cases, high-resolution CT may be strongly suggestive of a specific pathologic process.

D. Other Studies

Three diagnostic techniques are in common use: bronchoalveolar lavage, transbronchial biopsy, and surgical lung biopsy, either through an open procedure or using VATS.

Bronchoalveolar lavage may provide a specific diagnosis in cases of infection, particularly with *P jiroveci* or mycobacteria, or when cytologic examination reveals the presence of malignant cells. The findings may be suggestive and sometimes diagnostic of eosinophilic pneumonia, Langerhans cell histiocytosis, and alveolar proteinosis. Analysis of the cellular constituents of lavage fluid may suggest a specific disease, but these findings are not diagnostic.

Transbronchial biopsy through the flexible bronchoscope is easily performed in most patients. The risks of pneumothorax (5%) and hemorrhage (1–10%) are low. However, the tissue specimens recovered are small, sampling error is common, and crush artifact may complicate diagnosis. Transbronchial biopsy can make a definitive diagnosis of sarcoidosis, lymphangitic spread of carcinoma, pulmonary alveolar proteinosis, miliary tuberculosis, and Langerhans cell histiocytosis. Transbronchial biopsy cannot establish a specific diagnosis of idiopathic interstitial pneumonia. These patients generally require surgical lung biopsy.

Surgical lung biopsy is the standard for diagnosis of interstitial lung disease. Two or three biopsies taken from multiple sites in the same lung, including apparently normal tissue, may yield a specific diagnosis as well as prognostic information regarding the extent of fibrosis versus active inflammation. Patients under age 60 without a specific diagnosis generally should undergo surgical lung biopsy. In older and sicker patients, the risks and benefits must be weighed carefully for three reasons: (1) the morbidity of the procedure can be significant; (2) a definitive diagnosis may not be possible even with surgical lung biopsy; and (3) when a specific diagnosis is made, there may be no effective treatment. Empiric therapy or no treatment may be preferable to surgical lung biopsy in some patients.

Known causes of interstitial lung disease are dealt with in their specific sections. The important idiopathic forms are discussed below.

IDIOPATHIC FIBROSING INTERSTITIAL PNEUMONIA (Formerly Idiopathic Pulmonary Fibrosis)

The most common diagnosis among patients with interstitial lung disease is idiopathic fibrosing interstitial pneumonia, formerly known in the United States as "idiopathic pulmonary fibrosis" (known in the United Kingdom as "cryptogenic fibrosing alveolitis"). Historically, this diagnosis was based on clinical and radiographic criteria with only a small number of patients undergoing surgical lung biopsy. When biopsies were obtained, the common element of fibrosis led to the grouping together of several histologic patterns under the category of "idiopathic pulmonary fibrosis." These distinct histopathologic features are now recognized as being associated with different natural histories and responses to therapy (see Table 9–14). Therefore, in the evaluation of patients with idiopathic interstitial lung disease, clinicians should attempt to identify specific disorders and reserve the terms "idiopathic fibrosing interstitial pneumonia," or "cryptogenic fibrosing alveolitis" to denote only the histologic pattern of usual interstitial pneumonitis (UIP).

Patients with idiopathic fibrosing interstitial pneumonia may have any of the histologic patterns described in Table 9–14. The first step in evaluation is to identify patients whose disease is truly idiopathic. As indicated in Table 9–13, most identifiable causes of interstitial lung disease are infectious, drug-related, or environmental or occupational agents. Interstitial lung diseases associated with other medical conditions (pulmonary-renal syndromes, collagen-vascular disease) may be identified through a careful medical history. Apart from acute interstitial pneumonia, the clinical presentations of the idiopathic interstitial pneumonias are sufficiently similar to preclude a specific diagnosis. Chest radiographs and high-resolution CT scans are occasionally diagnostic. Ultimately, many patients with apparently idiopathic disease require surgical lung biopsy to make a definitive diagnosis. The importance of accurate diagnosis is twofold. First, it allows the clinician to provide accurate information about the cause and natural history of the illness. Second, accurate diagnosis helps distinguish patients most likely to benefit from therapy. Surgical lung biopsy may spare patients with UIP treatment with potentially morbid therapies.

The diagnosis of UIP can be made on clinical grounds alone in selected patients. A diagnosis of UIP can be made with 90% confidence in patients over 65 years of age who have (1) idiopathic disease by history and who demonstrate inspiratory crackles on physical examination; (2) restrictive physiology on pulmonary function testing; (3) characteristic radiographic evidence of progressive fibrosis over several years; and (4) diffuse, patchy fibrosis with pleural-based honeycombing on high-resolution CT scan. Such patients do not need surgical lung biopsy. Note that the diagnosis of UIP cannot be confirmed on transbronchial lung biopsy since the histologic diagnosis requires a pattern of changes rather than a single pathognomonic finding. Transbronchial biopsy may exclude UIP by confirming a specific alternative diagnosis.

Treatment of idiopathic fibrosing interstitial pneumonia is controversial. No randomized study has demonstrated that any treatment improves survival or quality of life compared with no treatment. Clinical experience suggests that patients with DIP or RB-ILD, nonspecific interstitial pneumonia (NSIP), or COP (see Table 9–14) frequently respond to corticosteroids and should be given a trial of therapy—typically prednisone, 1–2 mg/kg/d for a minimum of 2 months. The same therapy is almost uni-

Table 9–14. Idiopathic fibrosing interstitial pneumonias.

Name and Clinical Presentation	Histopathology	Radiographic Pattern	Response to Therapy and Prognosis
Usual interstitial pneumonia (UIP) Age 55–60, slight male predominance. Insidious dry cough and dyspnea lasting months to years. Clubbing present at diagnosis in 25–50%. Diffuse fine late inspiratory crackles on lung auscultation. Restrictive ventilatory defect and reduced diffusing capacity on pulmonary function tests. ANA and RF positive in ~25% in the absence of documented collagen-vascular disease.	Patchy, temporally and geographically nonuniform distribution of fibrosis, honeycomb change, and normal lung. Type I pneumocytes are lost, and there is proliferation of alveolar type II cells. "Fibroblast foci" of actively proliferating fibroblasts and myofibroblasts. Inflammation is generally mild and consists of small lymphocytes. Intra-alveolar macrophage accumulation is present but is not a prominent feature.	Diminished lung volume. Increased linear or reticular bibasilar and subpleural opacities. Unilateral disease is rare. High-resolution CT scanning shows minimal ground-glass and variable honeycomb change. Areas of normal lung may be adjacent to areas of advanced fibrosis. Between 2% and 10% have normal chest radiographs and high-resolution CT scans on diagnosis.	No randomized study has demonstrated improved survival compared with untreated patients. Inexorably progressive. Response to corticosteroids and cytotoxic agents at best 15%, and these probably represent misclassification of histopathology. Median survival approximately 3 years, depending on stage at presentation. Current interest in antifibrotic agents.
Respiratory bronchiolitis-associated interstitial lung disease (RB-ILD)[1] Age 40–45. Presentation similar to that of UIP though in younger patients. Similar results on pulmonary function tests, but less severe abnormalities. Patients with respiratory bronchiolitis are invariably heavy smokers.	Increased numbers of macrophages evenly dispersed within the alveolar spaces. Rare fibroblast foci, little fibrosis, minimal honeycomb change. In RB-ILD the accumulation of macrophages is localized within the peribronchiolar air spaces; in DIP[1], it is diffuse. Alveolar architecture is preserved.	May be indistinguishable from UIP. More often presents with a nodular or reticulonodular pattern. Honeycombing rare. High-resolution CT more likely to reveal diffuse ground-glass opacities and upper lobe emphysema.	Spontaneous remission occurs in up to 20% of patients, so natural history unclear. Smoking cessation is essential. Prognosis clearly better than that of UIP: median survival greater than 10 years. Corticosteroids thought to be effective, but there are no randomized clinical trials to support this view.
Acute interstitial pneumonitis (AIP) Clinically known as Hamman-Rich syndrome. Wide age range, many young patients. Acute onset of dyspnea followed by rapid development of respiratory failure. Half of patients report a viral syndrome preceding lung disease. Clinical course indistinguishable from that of idiopathic ARDS.	Pathologic changes reflect acute response to injury within days to weeks. Resembles organizing phase of diffuse alveolar damage. Fibrosis and minimal collagen deposition. May appear similar to UIP but more homogeneous and there is no honeycomb change—though this may appear if the process persists for more than a month in a patient on mechanical ventilation.	Diffuse bilateral airspace consolidation with areas of ground-glass attenuation on high-resolution CT scan.	Supportive care (mechanical ventilation) critical but effect of specific therapies unclear. High initial mortality: Fifty to 90 percent die within 2 months after diagnosis. Not progressive if patient survives. Lung function may return to normal or may be permanently impaired.
Nonspecific interstitial pneumonitis (NSIP) Age 45–55. Slight female predominance. Similar to UIP but onset of cough and dyspnea over months, not years.	Nonspecific in that histopathology does not fit into better-established categories. Varying degrees of inflammation and fibrosis, patchy in distribution but uniform in time, suggesting response to single injury. Most have lymphocytic and plasma cell inflammation without fibrosis. Honeycombing present but scant. Some have advocated division into cellular and fibrotic subtypes.	May be indistinguishable from UIP. Most typical picture is bilateral areas of ground-glass attenuation and fibrosis on high-resolution CT. Honeycombing is rare.	Treatment thought to be effective, but no prospective clinical studies have been published. Prognosis overall good but depends on the extent of fibrosis at diagnosis. Median survival greater than 10 years.
Cryptogenic organizing pneumonia (COP, formerly bronchiolitis obliterans organizing pneumonia [BOOP]) Typically age 50–60 but wide variation. Abrupt onset, frequently weeks to a few months following a flu-like illness. Dyspnea and dry cough prominent, but constitutional symptoms are common: fatigue, fever, and weight loss. Pulmonary function tests usually show restriction, but up to 25% show concomitant obstruction.	Included in the idiopathic interstitial pneumonias on clinical grounds. Buds of loose connective tissue (Masson bodies) and inflammatory cells fill alveoli and distal bronchioles.	Lung volumes normal. Chest radiograph typically shows interstitial and parenchymal disease with discrete, peripheral alveolar and ground-glass infiltrates. Nodular opacities common. High-resolution CT shows subpleural consolidation and bronchial wall thickening and dilation.	Rapid response to corticosteroids in two-thirds of patients. Long-term prognosis generally good for those who respond. Relapses are common.

[1]Includes desquamative interstitial pneumonia (DIP).

ANA, antinuclear antibody; ARDS, acute respiratory distress syndrome; RF, rheumatoid factor; UIP, usual interstitial pneumonia.

formly ineffective in patients with UIP. Since this therapy carries significant morbidity, experts do not recommend routine use of corticosteroids in patients with UIP. There are a number of ongoing clinical trials of antifibrotic therapies, such as pirfenidone and interferon gamma-1b, as well as smaller investigations of sildenafil, thalidomide, and biologic modifiers.

Collard HR et al. Acute exacerbations of idiopathic pulmonary fibrosis. Am J Respir Crit Care Med. 2007 Oct 1;176(7):636–43. [PMID: 17585107]

Noth I et al. Recent advances in idiopathic pulmonary fibrosis. Chest. 2007 Aug;132(2):637–50. [PMID: 17699135]

Ryu JH et al. Diagnosis of interstitial lung diseases. Mayo Clin Proc. 2007 Aug;82(8):976–86. [PMID: 17673067]

SARCOIDOSIS

 ESSENTIALS OF DIAGNOSIS

▶ Symptoms related to the lung, skin, eyes, peripheral nerves, liver, kidney, heart, and other tissues.

▶ Demonstration of noncaseating granulomas in a biopsy specimen.

▶ Exclusion of other granulomatous disorders.

General Considerations

Sarcoidosis is a systemic disease of unknown etiology characterized in about 90% of patients by granulomatous inflammation of the lung. The incidence is highest in North American blacks and northern European whites; among blacks, women are more frequently affected than men. Onset of disease is usually in the third or fourth decade.

Clinical Findings

A. Symptoms and Signs

Patients may present with malaise, fever, and dyspnea of insidious onset. Symptoms referable to the skin, eyes, peripheral nerves, liver, kidney, or heart may also cause the patient to seek care (Plate 67). Some individuals are asymptomatic and come to medical attention after abnormal findings (typically bilateral hilar and right paratracheal lymphadenopathy) on chest radiographs. Physical findings are atypical of interstitial lung disease in that crackles are uncommon on chest examination. Other findings may include erythema nodosum, parotid gland enlargement, hepatosplenomegaly, and lymphadenopathy.

B. Laboratory Findings

Laboratory tests may show leukopenia, an elevated erythrocyte sedimentation rate, and hypercalcemia (about 5% of patients) or hypercalciuria (20%). Angiotensin-converting enzyme (ACE) levels are elevated in 40–80% of patients with active disease. This finding is neither sensitive nor specific enough to have diagnostic significance. Physiologic testing may reveal evidence of airflow obstruction, but restrictive changes with decreased lung volumes and diffusing capacity are more common. Skin test anergy is present in 70%. ECG may show conduction disturbances and dysrhythmias.

C. Imaging

Radiographic findings are variable and include bilateral hilar adenopathy alone (radiographic stage I), hilar adenopathy and parenchymal involvement (radiographic stage II), or parenchymal involvement alone (radiographic stage III). Parenchymal involvement is usually manifested radiographically by diffuse reticular infiltrates, but focal infiltrates, acinar shadows, nodules and, rarely, cavitation may be seen. Pleural effusion is noted in fewer than 10% of patients.

D. Special Examinations

The diagnosis of sarcoidosis generally requires histologic demonstration of noncaseating granulomas in biopsies from a patient with other typical associated manifestations. Other granulomatous diseases (eg, berylliosis, tuberculosis, fungal infections) and lymphoma must be excluded. Biopsy of easily accessible sites (eg, palpable lymph nodes, skin lesions, or salivary glands) is likely to be positive. Transbronchial lung biopsy has a high yield (75–90%) as well, especially in patients with radiographic evidence of parenchymal involvement. Some clinicians believe that tissue biopsy is not necessary when stage I radiographic findings are detected in a clinical situation that strongly favors the diagnosis of sarcoidosis (eg, a young black woman with erythema nodosum). Biopsy is essential whenever clinical and radiographic findings suggest the possibility of an alternative diagnosis such as lymphoma. Bronchoalveolar lavage fluid in sarcoidosis is usually characterized by an increase in lymphocytes and a high CD4/CD8 cell ratio. Bronchoalveolar lavage does not establish a diagnosis but may be useful in following the activity of sarcoidosis in selected patients. All patients require a complete ophthalmologic evaluation.

Treatment

Indications for treatment with oral corticosteroids (prednisone, 0.5–1.0 mg/kg/d) include disabling constitutional symptoms, hypercalcemia, iritis, uveitis, arthritis, central nervous system involvement, cardiac involvement, granulomatous hepatitis, cutaneous lesions other than erythema nodosum, and progressive pulmonary lesions. Long-term therapy is usually required over months to years. Serum ACE levels usually fall with clinical improvement. Immunosuppressive drugs and cyclosporine have been tried, primarily when corticosteroid therapy has been exhausted, but experience with these drugs is limited. Anti-tumor necrosis factor (TNF) therapy with infliximab has shown some promise in extra-pulmonary sarcoidosis.

Prognosis

The outlook is best for patients with hilar adenopathy alone; radiographic involvement of the lung parenchyma is associated with a worse prognosis. Erythema nodosum portends a good outcome. About 20% of patients with lung involvement suffer irreversible lung impairment, characterized by progressive fibrosis, bronchiectasis, and cavitation. Pneumothorax, hemoptysis, mycetoma formation in lung cavities, and respiratory failure often complicate this advanced stage. Myocardial sarcoidosis occurs in about 5% of patients, sometimes leading to restrictive cardiomyopathy, cardiac dysrhythmias, and conduction disturbances. Death from pulmonary insufficiency occurs in about 5% of patients.

Patients require long-term follow-up; at a minimum, yearly physical examination, pulmonary function tests, chemistry panel, ophthalmologic evaluation, chest radiograph, and ECG.

Iannuzzi MC et al. Sarcoidosis. N Engl J Med. 2007 Nov 22;357(21):2153–65. [PMID: 18032765]

Judson MA. Sarcoidosis: clinical presentation, diagnosis, and approach to treatment. Am J Med Sci. 2008 Jan;335(1):26–33. [PMID: 18195580]

Mihailovic-Vucinic V et al. Pulmonary sarcoidosis. Clin Chest Med. 2008 Sep;29(3):459–73. [PMID: 18539238]

PULMONARY ALVEOLAR PROTEINOSIS

Pulmonary alveolar proteinosis is a rare disease in which phospholipids accumulate within alveolar spaces. The condition may be primary (idiopathic) or secondary (occurring in immune deficiency; hematologic malignancies; inhalation of mineral dusts; or following lung infections, including tuberculosis and viral infections). Progressive dyspnea is the usual presenting symptom, and chest radiograph shows bilateral alveolar infiltrates suggestive of pulmonary edema. The diagnosis is based on demonstration of characteristic findings on bronchoalveolar lavage (milky appearance and PAS-positive lipoproteinaceous material) in association with typical clinical and radiographic features. In some cases, transbronchial or surgical lung biopsy (revealing amorphous intra-alveolar phospholipid) is necessary.

The course of the disease varies. Some patients experience spontaneous remission; others develop progressive respiratory insufficiency. Pulmonary infection with nocardia or fungi may occur. Therapy for alveolar proteinosis consists of periodic whole lung lavage.

Ioachimescu OC et al. Pulmonary alveolar proteinosis. Chron Respir Dis. 2006;3(3):149–59. [PMID: 16916009]

EOSINOPHILIC PULMONARY SYNDROMES

Eosinophilic pulmonary syndromes are a diverse group of disorders typically characterized by eosinophilic pulmonary infiltrates, dyspnea, and cough. Many patients have constitutional symptoms, including fever. Common causes include exposure to medications (nitrofurantoin, phenytoin, ampicillin, acetaminophen, ranitidine) or infection with helminths (eg, *Ascaris*, hookworms, *Strongyloides*) or filariae (eg, *Wuchereria bancrofti*, *Brugia malayi*, tropical pulmonary eosinophilia). **Löffler syndrome** refers to acute eosinophilic pulmonary infiltrates in response to transpulmonary passage of helminth larvae. Pulmonary eosino-

philia can also be a feature of other illnesses, including ABPA, Churg-Strauss syndrome, systemic hypereosinophilic syndromes, eosinophilic granuloma of the lung (properly referred to as pulmonary Langerhans cell histiocytosis), neoplasms, and numerous interstitial lung diseases. If an extrinsic cause is identified, therapy consists of removal of the offending drug or treatment of the underlying parasitic infection.

One-third of cases are idiopathic, and there are two common syndromes. **Chronic eosinophilic pneumonia** is seen predominantly in women and is characterized by fever, night sweats, weight loss, and dyspnea. Asthma is present in half of cases. Chest radiographs often show peripheral infiltrates, the "photographic negative" of pulmonary edema. Bronchoalveolar lavage typically has a marked eosinophilia; peripheral blood eosinophilia is present in greater than 80%. Therapy with oral prednisone (1 mg/kg/d for 1–2 weeks followed by a gradual taper over many months) usually results in dramatic improvement; however, most patients require at least 10–15 mg of prednisone every other day for a year or more (sometimes indefinitely) to prevent relapses. **Acute eosinophilic pneumonia** is an acute, febrile illness characterized by cough and dyspnea, sometimes rapidly progressing to respiratory failure. The chest radiograph is abnormal but nonspecific. Bronchoalveolar lavage frequently shows eosinophilia but peripheral blood eosinophilia is rare at the onset of symptoms. The response to corticosteroids is usually dramatic.

Alam M et al. Chronic eosinophilic pneumonia: a review. South Med J. 2007 Jan;100(1):49–53. [PMID: 17269525]

Wechsler ME. Pulmonary eosinophilic syndromes. Immunol Allergy Clin North Am. 2007 Aug;27(3):477–92. [PMID: 17868860]

DISORDERS OF THE PULMONARY CIRCULATION

PULMONARY VENOUS THROMBOEMBOLISM

ESSENTIALS OF DIAGNOSIS

▶ Predisposition to venous thrombosis, usually of the lower extremities.

▶ One or more of the following: dyspnea, chest pain, hemoptysis, syncope.

▶ Tachypnea and a widened alveolar-arterial P_{O_2} difference.

▶ Characteristic defects on ventilation-perfusion lung scan, helical CT scan of the chest, or pulmonary angiogram.

▶ General Considerations

Pulmonary venous thromboembolism, often referred to as pulmonary embolism (PE), is a common, serious, and potentially fatal complication of thrombus formation within the deep venous circulation. PE is estimated to cause 200,000 deaths each year in the United States and is the third leading cause of death among hospitalized patients. Despite this prevalence, most cases are not recognized antemortem, and less than 10% of patients with fatal emboli have received specific treatment for the condition. Management demands a vigilant systematic approach to diagnosis and an understanding of risk factors so that appropriate preventive therapy can be given.

Many substances can embolize to the pulmonary circulation, including air (during neurosurgery, from central venous catheters), amniotic fluid (during active labor), fat (long bone fractures), foreign bodies (talc in injection drug users), parasite eggs (schistosomiasis), septic emboli (acute infectious endocarditis), and tumor cells (renal cell carcinoma). The most common embolus is thrombus, which may arise anywhere in the venous circulation or heart but most often originates in the deep veins of the lower extremities. Thrombi confined to the calf rarely embolize to the pulmonary circulation. However, about 20% of calf vein thrombi propagate proximally to the popliteal and ileofemoral veins, at which point they may break off and embolize to the pulmonary circulation. Pulmonary emboli will develop in 50–60% of patients with proximal deep venous thrombosis (DVT); half of these embolic events will be asymptomatic. Approximately 50–70% of patients who have symptomatic pulmonary emboli will have lower extremity DVT when evaluated.

PE and DVT are two manifestations of the same disease. The risk factors for PE are the risk factors for thrombus formation within the venous circulation: venous stasis, injury to the vessel wall, and hypercoagulability (Virchow triad). Venous stasis increases with immobility (bed rest—especially postoperative—obesity, stroke), hyperviscosity (polycythemia), and increased central venous pressures (low cardiac output states, pregnancy). Vessels may be damaged by prior episodes of thrombosis, orthopedic surgery, or trauma. Hypercoagulability can be caused by medications (oral contraceptives, hormonal replacement therapy) or disease (malignancy, surgery) or may be the result of inherited gene defects. The most common inherited cause in white populations is resistance to activated protein C, also known as factor V Leiden. The trait is present in approximately 3% of healthy American men and in 20–40% of patients with idiopathic venous thrombosis. Other major risks for hypercoagulability include the following: deficiencies or dysfunction of protein C, protein S, and antithrombin III; prothrombin gene mutation; and the presence of antiphospholipid antibodies (lupus anticoagulant and anticardiolipin antibody).

PE has multiple physiologic effects. Physical obstruction of the vascular bed and vasoconstriction from neurohumoral reflexes both increase pulmonary vascular resistance. Massive thrombus may cause right ventricular failure. Vascular obstruction increases physiologic dead space (wasted ventilation) and leads to hypoxemia through right-to-left shunting, decreased cardiac output, and surfactant depletion causing atelectasis. Reflex bronchoconstriction promotes wheezing and increased work of breathing.

▶ Clinical Findings

A. Symptoms and Signs

The clinical diagnosis of PE is notoriously difficult for two reasons. First, the clinical findings depend on both the size of the embolus and the patient's preexisting cardiopulmonary status. Second, common symptoms and signs of pulmonary emboli are not specific to this disorder (Table 9–15).

Indeed, no single symptom or sign or combination of clinical findings is specific to PE. Some findings are fairly sensitive: dyspnea and pain on inspiration occur in 75–85% and 65–75% of patients, respectively. Tachypnea is the only sign reliably found in more than half of patients. A common clinical strategy is to use combinations of clinical findings to identify patients' risk for PE. For example, 97% of patients in the original Prospective Investigation of Pulmonary Embolism Diagnosis (PIOPED I) study with angiographically proved pulmonary emboli had one or more of three findings: dyspnea, chest pain with breathing, or tachypnea. Wells and colleagues have published and validated a simple clinical decision rule that quantifies and dichotomizes this clinical risk assessment, allowing diversion of patients deemed unlikely to have PE to a simpler diagnostic algorithm (see Integrated Approach to Diagnosis of Pulmonary Embolism).

B. Laboratory Findings

The **ECG** is abnormal in 70% of patients with PE. However, the most common abnormalities are sinus tachycardia and nonspecific ST and T wave changes, each seen in approximately 40% of patients. Five percent or less of patients in the PIOPED I study had P pulmonale, right ventricular hypertrophy, right axis deviation, and right bundle branch block.

Arterial blood gases usually reveal acute respiratory alkalosis due to hyperventilation. The arterial PO_2 and the alveolar-arterial oxygen difference (A–a–DO_2) are usually abnormal in patients with PE compared with healthy, age-matched controls. However, arterial blood gases are not diagnostic: among patients who were evaluated in the PIOPED I study, neither the PO_2 nor the A–a–DO_2 differentiated between those with and those without pulmonary emboli. Profound hypoxia with a normal chest radiograph in the absence of preexisting lung disease is highly suspicious for PE.

Plasma levels of **D-dimer**, a degradation product of cross-linked fibrin, are elevated in the presence of thrombus. Using a D-dimer threshold between 300 and 500 ng/mL, a rapid quantitative enzyme-linked immunosorbent assay (ELISA) has shown a sensitivity for venous thromboembolism of 95–97% and a specificity of 45%. Therefore, a D-dimer < 500 ng/mL using the rapid ELISA provides strong evidence against venous thromboembolism, with a likelihood ratio of 0.11–0.13. Appropriate diagnostic thresholds have not been established for patients in whom D-dimer is elevated.

Serum troponin I, troponin T, and plasma beta-natriuretic peptide (BNP) levels are typically higher in patients with PE compared with those without embolism; the pres-

Table 9–15. Frequency of specific symptoms and signs in patients at risk for pulmonary thromboembolism.

	UPET[1] PE+ (n = 327)	PIOPED[2] PE+ (n = 117)	PIOPED[2] PE− (n = 248)
Symptoms			
Dyspnea	84%	73%	72%
Respirophasic chest pain	74%	66%	59%
Cough	53%	37%	36%
Leg pain	nr	26%	24%
Hemoptysis	30%	13%	8%
Palpitations	nr	10%	18%
Wheezing	nr	9%	11%
Anginal pain	14%	4%	6%
Signs			
Respiratory rate ≥ 16 UPET, ≥ 20 PIOPED I	92%	70%	68%
Crackles (rales)	58%	51%	40%[3]
Heart rate ≥ 100/min	44%	30%	24%
Fourth heart sound (S_4)	nr	24%	13%[3]
Accentuated pulmonary component of second heart sound (S_2P)	53%	23%	13%[3]
T ≥ 37.5 °C UPET, ≥ 38.5 °C PIOPED	43%	7%	12%
Homans sign	nr	4%	2%
Pleural friction rub	nr	3%	2%
Third heart sound (S_3)	nr	3%	4%
Cyanosis	19%	1%	2%

[1]Data from the Urokinase-Streptokinase Pulmonary Embolism Trial, as reported in Bell WR, et al. The clinical features of submassive and massive pulmonary emboli. Am J Med. 1977 Mar;62(3):355–60. [PMID: 842555]
[2]Data from patients enrolled in the PIOPED I study, as reported in Stein PD et al. Clinical, laboratory, roentgenographic, and electrocardiographic findings in patients with acute pulmonary embolism and no preexisting cardiac or pulmonary disease. Chest. 1991 Sep;100(3):598–603. [PMID: 1909617]
[3]$P < .05$ comparing patients in the PIOPED I study.
PE+, confirmed diagnosis of pulmonary embolism; PE−, diagnosis of pulmonary embolism ruled out; nr, not reported.

ence and magnitude of the elevation are not useful in diagnosis, but correlate with adverse outcomes, including death, mechanical ventilation and prolonged hospitalization.

C. Imaging and Special Examinations

1. Chest radiography—The chest radiograph is necessary to exclude other common lung diseases and to permit interpretation of the ventilation-perfusion ($\dot{V}/\dot{Q}$) scan, but it does not establish the diagnosis by itself. The chest radiograph was normal in only 12% of patients with confirmed PE in the PIOPED I study. The most frequent findings were atelectasis, parenchymal infiltrates, and pleural effusions. However, the prevalence of these findings was the same in hospitalized patients without PE. A prominent central pulmonary artery with local oligemia (Westermark sign) or pleural-based areas of increased opacity that represent intraparenchymal hemorrhage (Hampton hump) are uncommon. Paradoxically, the chest radiograph may be most helpful when normal in the setting of hypoxemia.

2. Lung scanning—A perfusion scan is performed by injecting radiolabeled microaggregated albumin into the venous system, allowing the particles to embolize to the pulmonary capillary bed. To perform a ventilation scan, the patient breathes a radioactive gas or aerosol while the distribution of radioactivity in the lungs is recorded.

A defect on perfusion scanning represents diminished blood flow to that region of the lung. This finding is not specific for PE. Defects in the perfusion scan are interpreted in conjunction with the ventilation scan to give a high, low, or intermediate (indeterminate) probability that PE is the cause of the abnormalities. Criteria for the combined interpretation of ventilation and perfusion scans (commonly referred to as a single test, the $\dot{V}/\dot{Q}$ scan) are complex, confusing, and not completely standardized. A normal perfusion scan excludes the diagnosis of clinically significant PE (negative predictive value of 91% in the PIOPED I study). A high-probability $\dot{V}/\dot{Q}$ scan is most often defined as having two or more segmental perfusion defects in the presence of normal ventilation and is sufficient to make the diagnosis of

PE in most instances (positive predictive value of 88% among PIOPED I patients). $\dot{V}/\dot{Q}$ scans are most helpful when they are either normal or indicate a high probability of PE. Such readings are reliable—interobserver agreement is best for normal and high-probability scans—and they carry predictive power: The likelihood ratios associated with normal and high-probability scans are 0.10 and 18, respectively, indicating significant and frequently conclusive changes from pretest to posttest probability.

However, 75% of PIOPED I $\dot{V}/\dot{Q}$ scans were nondiagnostic, ie, of low or intermediate probability. At angiography, these patients had an overall incidence of PE of 14% and 30%, respectively.

One of the most important findings of PIOPED I was that the clinical assessment of pretest probability could be used to aid the interpretation of the $\dot{V}/\dot{Q}$ scan. For patients with low-probability $\dot{V}/\dot{Q}$ scans and a low (20% or less) clinical pretest probability of PE, the diagnosis was confirmed in only 4%. Such patients may reasonably be observed off therapy without angiography. All other patients with nondiagnostic $\dot{V}/\dot{Q}$ scans require further testing to determine the presence of venous thromboembolism.

3. CT—Helical CT pulmonary angiography has essentially supplanted $\dot{V}/\dot{Q}$ scanning as the initial diagnostic study in North America for suspected PE. Helical CT pulmonary angiography requires administration of intravenous radiocontrast dye but is otherwise noninvasive. A high quality study is very sensitive for the detection of thrombus in the proximal pulmonary arteries but less so in more distal arteries where it may miss as many as 75% of subsegmental defects, compared with pulmonary angiography. Comparing helical CT pulmonary angiography to the $\dot{V}/\dot{Q}$ scan as the initial test for PE, detection of thrombi is roughly comparable, although more alternative pulmonary diagnoses are made with CT scanning.

Test characteristics of helical CT pulmonary angiography vary widely by study and facility. Factors influencing results include patient size and cooperation, the type and quality of the scanner, the imaging protocol, and the experience of the interpreting radiologist. Early studies comparing single-detector helical CT with standard angiography reported sensitivity of 53–60% and specificity of 81–97% for the diagnosis of PE. The 2006 PIOPED II study, using multidetector (four-row) helical CT and excluding the 6% of patients whose studies were "inconclusive," reported sensitivity of 83% and specificity of 96%.

A 15–20% false-negative rate is high for a screening test, and raises the practical question whether it is safe to withhold anticoagulation in patients with a negative helical CT. Research data provide two complementary answers. The insight of PIOPED I, that the clinical assessment of pretest probability improves the performance of the $\dot{V}/\dot{Q}$ scan, was confirmed with helical CT pulmonary angiography in PIOPED II, where positive and negative predictive values were highest in patients with concordant clinical assessments but poor with conflicting assessments: The negative predictive value of a normal helical CT in patients with a high pretest probability was only 60%. Therefore, a normal helical CT alone does not exclude PE in high-risk

patients, and either empiric therapy or further testing is indicated.

A large, prospective trial called the Christopher Study incorporated objective, validated pretest clinical assessment into diagnostic algorithms using D-dimer measurement. In this study, patients with a high pretest probability and a negative helical CT pulmonary angiogram who were not receiving anticoagulation had a low (< 2%) 3-month incidence of subsequent PE. This low rate of complications supports the contention that many false-negative studies represent clinically insignificant, small distal thrombi and provides support for monitoring most patients with a high-quality negative helical CT pulmonary angiogram off therapy (see Integrated Approach to Diagnosis of Pulmonary Embolism below). The rate of false-positive helical CT pulmonary angiograms and overtreatment of PE has not been as well studied to date.

4. Venous thrombosis studies—Seventy percent of patients with PE will have DVT on evaluation, and approximately half of patients with DVT will have PE on angiography. Since the history and physical examination are neither sensitive nor specific for PE and since the results of $\dot{V}/\dot{Q}$ scanning are frequently equivocal, documentation of DVT in a patient with suspected PE establishes the need for treatment and may preclude further testing.

Commonly available diagnostic techniques include venous ultrasonography, impedance plethysmography, and contrast venography. In most centers, venous ultrasonography is the test of choice to detect proximal DVT. Inability to compress the common femoral or popliteal veins in symptomatic patients is diagnostic of first-episode DVT (positive predictive value of 97%); full compressibility of both sites excludes proximal DVT (negative predictive value of 98%). The test is less accurate in distal thrombi, recurrent thrombi, or in asymptomatic patients. Impedance plethysmography relies on changes in electrical impedance between patent and obstructed veins to determine the presence of thrombus. Accuracy is comparable though not quite as high as ultrasonography. Both ultrasonography and impedance plethysmography are useful in the serial examination of patients with high clinical suspicion of venous thromboembolism but negative leg studies. In patients with suspected first-episode DVT and a negative ultrasound or impedance plethysmography examination, multiple studies have confirmed the safety of withholding anticoagulation while conducting two sequential studies on days 1–3 and 7–10. Similarly, patients with nondiagnostic $\dot{V}/\dot{Q}$ scans and an initial negative venous ultrasound or impedance plethysmography examination may be monitored off therapy with serial leg studies over 2 weeks. When serial examinations are negative for proximal DVT, the risk of subsequent venous thromboembolism over the following 6 months is less than 2%.

Contrast venography remains the reference standard for the diagnosis of DVT. An intraluminal filling defect is diagnostic of venous thrombosis. However, venography has significant shortcomings and has been replaced by venous ultrasound as the diagnostic procedure of choice. Venography may be useful in complex situations where there is discrepancy between clinical suspicion and noninvasive testing.

5. Pulmonary angiography—Pulmonary angiography remains the reference standard for the diagnosis of PE. An intraluminal filling defect in more than one projection establishes a definitive diagnosis. Secondary findings highly suggestive of PE include abrupt arterial cutoff, asymmetry of blood flow—especially segmental oligemia—or a prolonged arterial phase with slow filling. Pulmonary angiography was performed in 755 patients in the PIOPED I study. A definitive diagnosis was established in 97%; in 3% the studies were nondiagnostic. Four patients (0.8%) with negative angiograms subsequently had pulmonary thromboemboli at autopsy. Serial angiography has demonstrated minimal resolution of thrombus prior to day 7 following presentation. Thus, negative angiography within 7 days of presentation excludes the diagnosis.

Pulmonary angiography is a safe but invasive procedure with well-defined morbidity and mortality data. Minor complications occur in approximately 5% of patients. Most are allergic contrast reactions, transient kidney dysfunction, or related to percutaneous catheter insertion; cardiac perforation and arrhythmias are reported but rare. Among the PIOPED I patients who underwent angiography, there were five deaths (0.7%) directly related to the procedure.

The appropriate role of pulmonary angiography in the diagnosis of PE remains a subject of ongoing debate. There is wide agreement that angiography is indicated in any patient in whom the diagnosis is in doubt when there is a high clinical pretest probability of PE or when the diagnosis of PE must be established with certainty, as when anticoagulation is contraindicated or placement of an inferior vena cava filter is contemplated.

6. MRI—MRI has sensitivity and specificity equivalent to contrast venography in the diagnosis of DVT. It has improved sensitivity when compared with venous ultrasound in the diagnosis of DVT, without loss of specificity. The test is noninvasive and avoids the use of potentially nephrotoxic radiocontrast dye. However, it remains expensive and not widely available. Artifacts introduced by respiratory and cardiac motion have limited the use of MRI in the diagnosis of PE. New techniques have improved sensitivity and specificity to levels comparable with helical CT, but MRI remains primarily a research tool for PE.

▶ Integrated Approach to Diagnosis of Pulmonary Embolism

An integrated approach to diagnosis of PE uses the clinical likelihood of venous thromboembolism derived from a clinical prediction rule (Table 9–16) along with the results of diagnostic tests to come to one of three decision points: to establish venous thromboembolism (PE or DVT) as the diagnosis, to exclude venous thromboembolism with sufficient confidence to follow the patient off anticoagulation, or to refer the patient for additional testing. An ideal diagnostic algorithm would proceed in a cost-effective, stepwise fashion to come to these decision points at minimal risk to the patient. The standard $\dot{V}/\dot{Q}$ scan based

Table 9–16. Clinical prediction rule for pulmonary embolism (PE).

Variable	Points
Clinical symptoms and signs of deep venous thrombosis (DVT) (leg swelling and pain with palpation of deep veins)	3.0
Alternative diagnosis less likely than PE	3.0
Heart rate > 100 beats/min	1.5
Immobilization for more than 3 days or surgery in previous 4 weeks	1.5
Previous PE or DVT	1.5
Hemoptysis	1.0
Cancer (with treatment within past 6 months or palliative care)	1.0
Three-tiered clinical probability assessment	**Score**
High	> 6.0
Moderate	2.0 to 6.0
Low	< 2.0
Dichotomous clinical probability assessment	**Score**
PE likely	> 4.0
PE unlikely	< or = 4.0

Data from Wells PS et al. Derivation of a simple clinical model to categorize patients probability of pulmonary embolism: increasing the models utility with the SimpliRED D-dimer. Thromb Haemost. 2000 Mar;83(3):416–20. [PMID: 10744147]

algorithm (Table 9–17) has been replaced in most North American centers by a rapid D-dimer and helical CT pulmonary angiography based diagnostic algorithm (Figure 9–5). The $\dot{V}/\dot{Q}$ scan remains useful in many patients, especially those who are not able to undergo CT pulmonary angiography (eg, those with advanced chronic kidney disease), but there is a growing evidence to support the CT-based approach. In the rigorously conducted Christopher Study, the incidence of venous thromboembolism was only 1.3% and fatal PE occurred in just 0.5% of persons monitored for 3 months off anticoagulation therapy after objective, validated tools for clinical assessment, quantitative rapid D-dimer assays and a negative helical CT pulmonary angiography. The incidence of PE following a negative evaluation by these three means is comparable to that seen following negative pulmonary angiography.

▶ Prevention

Venous thromboembolism is often clinically silent until it presents with significant morbidity or mortality. It is a prevalent disease, clearly associated with identifiable risk factors. For example, the incidence of proximal DVT, PE, and fatal PE in untreated patients undergoing hip fracture surgery is reported to be 10–20%, 4–10%, and 0.2–5%, respectively. There is unambiguous evidence of the efficacy of prophylactic therapy in this and other clinical situations,

Table 9–17. Pulmonary ventilation-perfusion scan based diagnostic algorithm for PE.

Clinical concern for PE:

1. Analyze by three-tiered clinical probability assessment
2. Obtain V̇/Q̇ scan
3. Match results in the following table

		Clinical suspicion for PE by clinical probability assessment		
		HIGH	**MODERATE**	**LOW**
V̇/Q̇ Scan Results	**High probability**	STOP. Diagnosis established. Treat for PE.	STOP. Diagnosis established. Treat for PE.	Diagnosis likely (56% in PIOPED I, but small number of patients). Treat for PE or evaluate further with LE US or CT-PA.
	Indeterminate	Diagnosis highly likely (66% in PIOPED I). Treat for PE or evaluate further with LE US or CT-PA.	Uncertain diagnosis. Evaluate further with LE US or CT-PA.	Uncertain diagnosis. Evaluate further with LE US or CT-PA.
	Low probability	Uncertain diagnosis. Evaluate further with LE US or CT-PA.	Uncertain diagnosis. Evaluate further with LE US or CT-PA.	STOP. Diagnosis excluded; monitor off anticoagulation. Consider alternative diagnoses.
	Normal	STOP. Diagnosis excluded; monitor off anticoagulation. Consider alternative diagnoses.	STOP. Diagnosis excluded; monitor off anticoagulation. Consider alternative diagnoses.	STOP. Diagnosis excluded; monitor off anticoagulation. Consider alternative diagnoses.

Source: The PIOPED Investigators. Value of the ventilation/perfusion scan in acute pulmonary embolism: results of the Prospective Investigation of Pulmonary Embolism Diagnosis (PIOPED). JAMA. 1990 May 23–30;263(20):2753–9. [PMID: 2332918]
CT-PA, helical CT pulmonary angiography; LE US, lower extremity venous ultrasound for DVT; PE, pulmonary embolism.

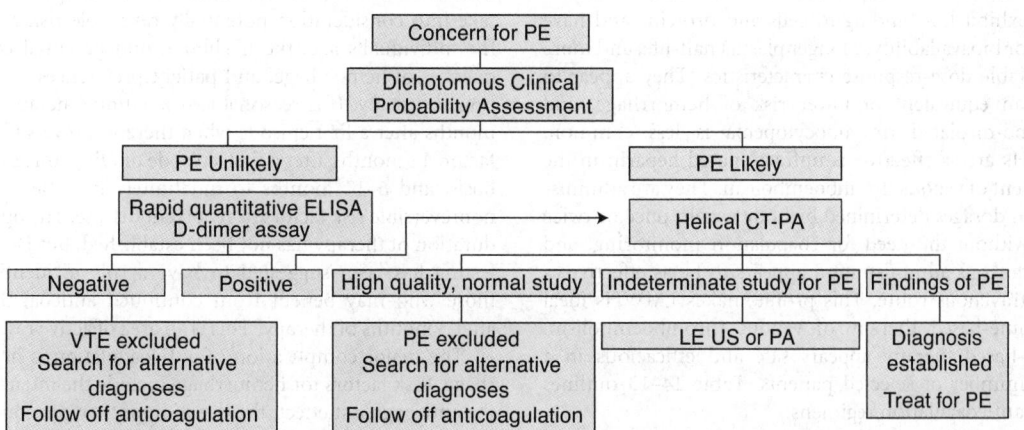

▲ **Figure 9–5.** D-dimer and helical CT-PA based diagnostic algorithm for PE. CT-PA, CT pulmonary angiogram; PE, pulmonary embolism; ELISA, enzyme-linked immunosorbent assay; VTE, venous thromboembolic disease; LE US, lower extremity venous ultrasound for deep venous thrombosis; PA, pulmonary angiogram. (Reproduced, with permission, from van Belle A et al. Effectiveness of managing suspected pulmonary embolism using an algorithm combining clinical probability, D-dimer testing, and computed tomography. JAMA 2006 Jan 11;295(2):172–9.)

yet it remains underused. Only about 50% of surgical deaths from PE had received any form of preventive therapy. A discussion of strategies for the prevention of venous thromboembolism can be found in Chapter 14.

▶ Treatment

A. Anticoagulation

Anticoagulation is not definitive therapy but a form of secondary prevention. Heparin binds to and accelerates the ability of antithrombin to inactivate thrombin, factor Xa, and factor IXa. It thus retards additional thrombus formation, allowing endogenous fibrinolytic mechanisms to lyse existing clot. The standard regimen of heparin followed by 6 months of oral warfarin results in an 80–90% reduction in the risk of both recurrent venous thrombosis and death from PE.

Heparin has troublesome pharmacokinetics. Its clearance is dose-dependent, it is highly protein-bound, and a minimum or threshold level is necessary to achieve an antithrombotic effect. It is necessary to monitor the activated partial thromboplastin time (aPTT) and adjust dosing to maintain the aPTT 1.5–2.5 times control. In patients with a moderate to high clinical likelihood of PE and no contraindications, full anticoagulation with heparin should begin with the diagnostic evaluation. Once the diagnosis of proximal DVT or PE is established, it is critical to ensure adequate therapy. Failure to achieve therapeutic heparin levels within 24 hours is associated with a fivefold increased risk of clot propagation. Heparin causes immune-mediated thrombocytopenia in 3% of patients; therefore, the platelet count should be determined frequently for the first 14 days of therapy. A subcutaneous, weight-adjusted regimen of unfractionated heparin has been proposed as a therapeutic alternative to intravenous or subcutaneous low-molecular-weight heparin (LMWH), when lack of intravenous access or resources prevent the favored approach.

LMWHs are depolymerized preparations of heparin with multiple advantages over unfractionated heparin. They exhibit less binding to cells and proteins and have superior bioavailability, a longer plasma half-life, and more predictable dose-response characteristics. They appear to carry an equivalent or lower risk of hemorrhage, and immune-mediated thrombocytopenia is less common. LMWHs are as effective as unfractionated heparin in the treatment of venous thromboembolism. They are administered in dosages determined by body weight once or twice daily without the need for coagulation monitoring, and subcutaneous administration appears to be as effective as the intravenous route. This profile makes LMWHs ideal for home-based therapy of venous thromboembolism. Home-based therapy appears safe and efficacious in a small number of selected patients. Table 14–13 outlines initial anticoagulation regimens.

Anticoagulation therapy for venous thromboembolism is continued for a minimum of 3 months, so oral anticoagulant therapy with warfarin is usually initiated concurrently with heparin. Warfarin affects hepatic synthesis of vitamin K–dependent coagulant proteins. It usually requires 5–7 days to become therapeutic; therefore, heparin is generally continued for 5 days. Warfarin is safe if begun concurrently with heparin, initially at a dose of 2.5–10 mg/d. The lower dose is preferred in elderly patients. Maintenance therapy usually requires 2–15 mg/d. Adequacy of therapy must be monitored by following the prothrombin time, most often adjusted for differences in reagents and reported as the international normalized ratio (INR). The target INR is 2.5, with the acceptable range from 2.0 to 3.0; below 2.0, there is an increased risk of thrombosis; above 4.0, there is an increased risk of hemorrhage. Warfarin has interactions with many drugs. Meticulous attention to medications is part of the routine management of every patient receiving warfarin. Warfarin is a pregnancy category X medication, indicating known fetopathic and teratogenic effects. When oral anticoagulation with warfarin is contraindicated, LMWH is a convenient alternative.

The optimal duration of anticoagulation therapy for venous thromboembolism is unknown. There appears to be a protective benefit to continued anticoagulation in first-episode venous thromboembolism (twice the rate of recurrence in 6 weeks compared with 6 months of therapy) and recurrent disease (eightfold risk of recurrence in 6 months compared with 4 years of therapy). These studies do not distinguish patients with reversible risk factors, such as surgery or transient immobility, from patients who have a nonreversible hypercoagulable state such as factor V Leiden, inhibitor deficiency, antiphospholipid syndrome, or malignancy. A RCT of low-dose warfarin (INR 1.5–2.0) versus no therapy following 6 months of standard therapy in patients with idiopathic DVT was stopped early. The protective benefits of continued anticoagulation include fewer DVTs in addition to a trend toward lower mortality despite more hemorrhage in the warfarin group. Risk reductions were consistent across groups with and without inherited thrombophilia.

For many patients, venous thrombosis is a recurrent disease, and continued therapy results in a lower rate of recurrence at the cost of an increased risk of hemorrhage. Therefore, the appropriate duration of therapy needs to take into consideration potentially reversible risk factors, the individual's age, the likelihood and potential consequences of hemorrhage, and patient preferences for continued therapy. It is reasonable to continue therapy for 6 months after a first episode when there is a reversible risk factor, 12 months after a first-episode of idiopathic thrombosis, and 6–12 months to indefinitely in patients with nonreversible risk factors or recurrent disease. The optimal duration of therapy has not been established, but D-dimer testing has been suggested to have a role in identifying those who may benefit from continued anticoagulation after 3 months of therapy. This is an area of active research.

The major complication of anticoagulation is hemorrhage. Risk factors for hemorrhage include the intensity of the anticoagulant effect; the duration of therapy; concomitant administration of drugs such as aspirin that interfere with platelet function; and patient characteristics, particularly increased age, previous gastrointestinal hemorrhage, and coexistent chronic kidney disease.

The reported incidence of major hemorrhage following intravenous administration of unfractionated heparin is nil to

7%; that of fatal hemorrhage is nil to 2%. The incidence with LMWHs is not statistically different. There is no information comparing hemorrhage rates at different doses of heparin. The risk of subtherapeutic heparin administration in the first 24–48 hours after diagnosis is significant; it appears to outweigh the risk of short-term supratherapeutic heparin levels. The incidence of hemorrhage during therapy with warfarin is reported to be between 3% and 4% per patient year. The frequency varies with the target INR and is consistently higher when the INR exceeds 4.0. There is no apparent additional antithrombotic benefit in venous thromboembolism with a target INR above 2.0–3.0 (see Chapter 14).

B. Thrombolytic Therapy

Streptokinase, urokinase, and recombinant tissue plasminogen activator (rt-PA; alteplase) increase plasmin levels and thereby directly lyse intravascular thrombi. In patients with established PE, thrombolytic therapy accelerates resolution of emboli within the first 24 hours compared with standard heparin therapy. This is a consistent finding using angiography, $\dot{V}/\dot{Q}$ scanning, echocardiography, and direct measurement of pulmonary artery pressures. However, at 1 week and 1 month after diagnosis, these agents show no difference in outcome compared with heparin and warfarin. There is no evidence that thrombolytic therapy improves mortality. Subtle improvements in pulmonary function, including improved single-breath diffusing capacity and a lower incidence of exercise-induced pulmonary hypertension, have been observed. The reliability and clinical importance of these findings is unclear. The major disadvantages of thrombolytic therapy compared with heparin are its greater cost and a significant increase in major hemorrhagic complications. The incidence of intracranial hemorrhage in patients with PE treated with alteplase is 2.1% compared with 0.2% in patients treated with heparin.

Current evidence supports thrombolytic therapy for PE in patients at high risk for death in whom the more rapid resolution of thrombus may be lifesaving. Such patients are usually hemodynamically unstable despite heparin therapy. Absolute contraindications to thrombolytic therapy include active internal bleeding and stroke within the past 2 months. Major contraindications include uncontrolled hypertension and surgery or trauma within the past 6 weeks. The role of thrombolysis in patients who are hemodynamically stable but with echocardiographic evidence of right heart strain is unclear and is subject to considerable practice variation.

C. Additional Measures

Interruption of the inferior vena cava may be indicated in patients with a major contraindication to anticoagulation who have or are at high risk for development of proximal DVT or PE. Placement of an inferior vena cava filter is also recommended for recurrent thromboembolism despite adequate anticoagulation, for chronic recurrent embolism with a compromised pulmonary vascular bed (eg, in pulmonary hypertension), and with the concurrent performance of surgical pulmonary embolectomy or pulmonary thromboendarterectomy. Percutaneous transjugular placement of a mechanical filter is the preferred mode of inferior vena cava

interruption. These devices reduce the short-term incidence of PE in patients presenting with proximal lower extremity DVT. However, they are associated with a twofold increased risk of recurrent DVT in the first 2 years following placement.

In rare critically ill patients for whom thrombolytic therapy is contraindicated or unsuccessful, mechanical or surgical extraction of thrombus may be indicated. Pulmonary embolectomy is an emergency procedure of last resort with a very high mortality rate. It is now performed only in a few specialized centers. Several catheter devices to fragment and extract thrombus through a transvenous approach have been reported in small numbers of patients. Comparative outcomes with surgery, thrombolytic therapy, or heparin have not been studied.

▶ Prognosis

PE is estimated to cause more than 50,000 deaths annually. In the majority of deaths, PE is not recognized antemortem or death occurs before specific treatment can be initiated. These statistics highlight the importance of preventive therapy in high-risk patients (Chapter 14). The outlook for patients with diagnosed and appropriately treated PE is generally good. Overall prognosis depends on the underlying disease rather than the PE itself. Death from recurrent thromboemboli is uncommon, occurring in less than 3% of cases. Perfusion defects resolve in most survivors. Chronic thromboembolic pulmonary hypertension develops in approximately 1% of patients. Selected patients may benefit from pulmonary endarterectomy.

Kearon C et al. Antithrombotic therapy for venous thromboembolic disease: American College of Chest Physicians Evidence-Based Clinical Practice Guidelines (8th Edition). Chest. 2008 Jun;133(6 Suppl):454S–545S. [PMID: 18574272]

Quiroz R et al. Clinical validity of a negative computed tomography scan in patients with suspected pulmonary embolism: a systematic review. JAMA. 2005 Apr 27;293(16):2012–7. [PMID: 15855435]

Roy PM et al. Systematic review and meta-analysis of strategies for the diagnosis of suspected pulmonary embolism. BMJ. 2005 Jul 30;331(7511):259. [PMID: 16052017]

Stein PD et al. Challenges in the diagnosis of acute pulmonary embolism. Am J Med. 2008 Jul;121(7):565–71. [PMID: 18589050]

Tapson VF. Acute pulmonary embolism. N Engl J Med. 2008 Mar 6;358(10):1037–52. [PMID: 18322285]

van Belle A et al; Christopher Study Investigators. Effectiveness of managing suspected pulmonary embolism using an algorithm combining clinical probability, D-dimer testing, and computed tomography. JAMA. 2006 Jan 11;295(2):172–9. [PMID: 16403929]

PULMONARY HYPERTENSION

ESSENTIALS OF DIAGNOSIS

▶ Dyspnea, fatigue, chest pain, and syncope on exertion.

▶ Narrow splitting of second heart sound with loud pulmonary component; findings of right ventricular hypertrophy and cardiac failure in advanced disease.

▶ Hypoxemia and increased wasted ventilation on pulmonary function tests.

▶ Electrocardiographic evidence of right ventricular strain or hypertrophy and right atrial enlargement.

▶ Enlarged central pulmonary arteries on chest radiograph.

▶ General Considerations

The pulmonary circulation is unique because of its high blood flow, low pressure (normally 25/8 mm Hg, mean 12), and low resistance (normally 200–250 dynes/sec/cm^{-5}). It can accommodate large increases in blood flow during exercise with only modest increases in pressure because of its ability to recruit and distend lung blood vessels. Contraction of smooth muscle in the walls of pulmonary arteriolar resistance vessels becomes an important factor in numerous pathologic states. Pulmonary hypertension is present when pulmonary artery pressure rises to a level inappropriate for a given cardiac output. Once present, pulmonary hypertension is self-perpetuating. It introduces secondary structural abnormalities in pulmonary vessels, including smooth muscle hypertrophy and intimal proliferation, and these may eventually stimulate atheromatous changes and in situ thrombosis, leading to further narrowing of the arterial bed.

Selected mechanisms responsible for **secondary pulmonary hypertension** and examples of corresponding clinical conditions are set forth in Table 9–18.

Pulmonary arteriolar vasoconstriction due to chronic hypoxemia may complicate any chronic lung disease and compound the effects of loss of pulmonary blood vessels (as seen with disorders such as emphysema and pulmonary fibrosis) and obstruction of the pulmonary vascular bed (as seen with disorders such as chronic pulmonary thromboembolic disease). Sustained increases in pulmonary venous pressure from left ventricular failure (systolic, diastolic, or both), mitral stenosis, and pulmonary veno-occlusive disease may cause "postcapillary" pulmonary hypertension. Increased pulmonary blood flow due to intracardiac shunts and increased blood viscosity due to polycythemia can also cause pulmonary hypertension. Pulmonary hypertension has also been associated with hepatic cirrhosis and portal hypertension.

Idiopathic (formerly **primary**) **pulmonary hypertension** (see Chapter 10) is pulmonary arterial hypertension that occurs in the absence of the identified cardiopulmonary disorders above or significant connective tissue disease. It occurs with hepatic cirrhosis and portal hypertension, HIV infection, use of anorectic drugs and sporadically in young and middle-aged women, some of whom have a familial form. Untreated, it is characterized by progressive dyspnea, a rapid downhill course, and an invariably fatal outcome. This condition is also called **plexogenic pulmonary arteriopathy,** in reference to the characteristic histopathologic plexiform lesion found in muscular pulmonary arteries.

Pulmonary veno-occlusive disease is a rare cause of postcapillary pulmonary hypertension occurring in chil-

Table 9–18. Mechanisms of pulmonary hypertension and examples of corresponding clinical conditions.

Reduction in cross-sectional area of pulmonary arterial bed
Vasoconstriction
Hypoxemia from any cause (chronic lung disease, sleep-disordered breathing, etc)
Acidosis
Loss of vessels
Lung resection
Emphysema
Vasculitis
Interstitial lung disease
Collagen-vascular disease
Obstruction of vessels
Pulmonary embolism (thromboemboli, tumor emboli, etc)
In situ thrombosis
Schistosomiasis
Sickle cell disease
Narrowing of vessels
Secondary structural changes due to pulmonary hypertension
Increased pulmonary venous pressure
Constrictive pericarditis
Left ventricular failure or reduced compliance
Mitral stenosis
Left atrial myxoma
Pulmonary veno-occlusive disease
Mediastinal diseases compressing pulmonary veins
Increased pulmonary blood flow
Congenital left-to-right intracardiac shunts
Increased blood viscosity
Polycythemia
Miscellaneous
Pulmonary hypertension occurring in association with hepatic cirrhosis and portal hypertension
HIV infection

dren and young adults. The cause is unknown, but associations with various conditions such as viral infection, bone marrow transplantation, chemotherapy, and malignancy have been described. The disease is characterized by progressive fibrotic occlusion of pulmonary veins and venules, along with secondary hypertensive changes in the pulmonary arterioles and muscular pulmonary arteries. Nodular areas of pulmonary congestion, edema, hemorrhage, and hemosiderosis are found. Chest radiography reveals prominent, symmetric interstitial markings, Kerley B lines, pulmonary artery dilation, and normally sized left atrium and left ventricle. Antemortem diagnosis is often difficult but is occasionally established by open lung biopsy. There is no effective therapy, and most patients die within 2 years as a result of progressive pulmonary hypertension.

▶ Clinical Findings

A. Symptoms and Signs

Secondary pulmonary hypertension is difficult to recognize clinically in the early stages, when symptoms and signs are primarily those of the underlying disease. Pulmonary hypertension may cause or contribute to dyspnea, present initially on exertion and later at rest. Dull, retrosternal chest pain resembling angina pectoris may be present.

Fatigue and syncope on exertion also occur, presumably a result of reduced cardiac output related to elevated pulmonary artery pressures or bradycardia.

The signs of pulmonary hypertension include narrow splitting of the second heart sound, accentuation of the pulmonary component of the second heart sound, and a systolic ejection click. In advanced cases, tricuspid and pulmonary valve insufficiency and signs of right ventricular failure and cor pulmonale are found.

B. Laboratory Findings

Polycythemia is found in many cases of pulmonary hypertension that are associated with chronic hypoxemia. Electrocardiographic changes are those of right axis deviation, right ventricular hypertrophy, right ventricular strain, or right atrial enlargement.

C. Imaging and Special Examinations

Radiographs and high-resolution CT scans of the chest can assist in the diagnosis of pulmonary hypertension and determination of the cause. In chronic disease, dilation of the right and left main and lobar pulmonary arteries and enlargement of the pulmonary outflow tract are seen; in advanced disease, right ventricular and right atrial enlargement are seen. Peripheral "pruning" of large pulmonary arteries is characteristic of pulmonary hypertension in severe emphysema.

Echocardiography is helpful in evaluating patients thought to have mitral stenosis, left atrial myxoma, and pulmonary valvular disease and may also reveal right ventricular enlargement and paradoxical motion of the interventricular septum. Doppler ultrasonography is a reliable noninvasive means of estimating pulmonary artery systolic pressure. However, precise hemodynamic measurements can only be obtained with right heart catheterization, which is helpful when postcapillary pulmonary hypertension, intracardiac shunting, or thromboembolic disease is considered as part of the differential diagnosis.

The diagnosis of pulmonary hypertension cannot be made on routine pulmonary function tests. Some results may help identify the cause; eg, diminution of the pulmonary capillary bed may cause reduction in the single breath diffusing capacity.

The following studies may be useful to exclude causes of secondary pulmonary hypertension: liver function tests, HIV test, collagen-vascular serologic studies, polysomnography, $\dot{V}/\dot{Q}$ lung scanning, pulmonary angiography, and surgical lung biopsy. $\dot{V}/\dot{Q}$ lung scanning is very helpful in identifying patients with pulmonary hypertension caused by recurrent pulmonary thromboemboli, a condition that is often difficult to recognize clinically.

▶ Treatment

Treatment of idiopathic (primary) pulmonary hypertension is discussed in Chapter 10. Treatment of secondary pulmonary hypertension consists mainly of treating the underlying disorder. Early recognition of pulmonary hypertension is crucial to interrupt the self-perpetuating

cycle responsible for rapid clinical progression. Most patients who present with symptoms and signs of pulmonary hypertension, however, already have advanced disease. If hypoxemia or acidosis is detected, corrective measures should be started immediately. Supplemental oxygen administered for at least 15 hours per day has been demonstrated to slow the progression of pulmonary hypertension in patients with hypoxemic COPD.

Permanent anticoagulation is indicated in idiopathic pulmonary hypertension but should be given only to those patients with secondary pulmonary hypertension at high risk for thromboembolism. Vasodilator therapy using various pharmacologic agents (eg, calcium antagonists, hydralazine, isoproterenol, diazoxide, nitroglycerin) has shown disappointing results in secondary pulmonary hypertension. Patients most likely to benefit from long-term pulmonary vasodilator therapy are those who respond favorably to a vasodilator challenge at right heart catheterization. It is clear that long-term oral vasodilator therapy should be used only if hemodynamic benefit is documented. Complications of pulmonary vasodilator therapy include systemic hypotension, hypoxemia, and even death.

Continuous long-term intravenous infusion (using a portable pump) of prostacyclin (PGI_2; epoprostenol), a potent pulmonary vasodilator, has been shown to confer hemodynamic and symptomatic benefits in selected patients with idiopathic pulmonary hypertension. This is the first therapy to demonstrate improved survival of patients with idiopathic pulmonary hypertension. Limitations of continuous infusion prostacyclin are difficulties in titration, technical problems with portable delivery systems, and the high cost of the drug. Newer agents in research trials include subcutaneous (treprostinil), inhaled (iloprost), and oral (beraprost) prostacyclin analogues, endothelin receptor antagonists (bosentan), and phosphodiesterase inhibitors (sildenafil). Some of these agents have shown improvement in functional status but, so far, there is no evidence for improved outcomes. Combination therapy is an area of active research.

Patients with marked polycythemia (hematocrit > 60%) should undergo repeated phlebotomy in an attempt to reduce blood viscosity. Cor pulmonale complicating pulmonary hypertension is treated by managing the underlying pulmonary disease and by using diuretics, salt restriction and, in appropriate patients, supplemental oxygen. The use of digitalis in cor pulmonale remains controversial. Pulmonary thromboendarterectomy may benefit selected patients with pulmonary hypertension secondary to chronic thrombotic obstruction of major pulmonary arteries.

Single or double lung transplantation may be performed on patients with end-stage idiopathic (primary) pulmonary hypertension. The 2-year survival rate is 50%.

▶ Prognosis

The prognosis in secondary pulmonary hypertension depends on the course of the underlying disease. The prognosis is favorable when pulmonary hypertension is detected early and the conditions leading to it are readily reversed. Patients with pulmonary hypertension due to fixed obliteration of the pulmonary vascular bed generally respond poorly to therapy; development of cor pulmonale in these cases implies a poor prognosis.

Ghofrani HA et al. Uncertainties in the diagnosis and treatment of pulmonary arterial hypertension. Circulation. 2008 Sep 9;118(11):1195–201. [PMID: 18779455]

Humbert M. Update in pulmonary arterial hypertension 2007. Am J Respir Crit Care Med. 2008 Mar 15;177(6):574–9. [PMID: 18316769]

Michelakis ED et al. Emerging concepts and translational priorities in pulmonary arterial hypertension. Circulation. 2008 Sep 30;118(14):1486–95. [PMID: 18824655]

PULMONARY VASCULITIS

Wegener granulomatosis is an idiopathic disease manifested by a combination of glomerulonephritis, necrotizing granulomatous vasculitis of the upper and lower respiratory tracts, and varying degrees of small vessel vasculitis. Chronic sinusitis, arthralgias, fever, skin rash, and weight loss are frequent presenting symptoms. Specific pulmonary complaints occur less often. The most common sign of lung disease is nodular pulmonary infiltrates, often with cavitation, seen on chest radiography. Tracheal stenosis and endobronchial disease are sometimes seen. The diagnosis is most often based on serologic testing and biopsy of lung, sinus tissue, or kidney with demonstration of necrotizing granulomatous vasculitis. See Chapter 20.

Allergic angiitis and granulomatosis (Churg-Strauss syndrome) is an idiopathic multisystem vasculitis of small and medium-sized arteries that occurs in patients with asthma. Histologic features include fibrinoid necrotizing epithelioid and eosinophilic granulomas. The skin and lungs are most often involved, but other organs, including the paranasal sinuses, the heart, gastrointestinal tract, liver, and peripheral nerves, may also be affected. Peripheral eosinophilia > 1500 cells/mcL or > 10% of peripheral WBCs is the rule. Abnormalities on chest radiographs range from transient infiltrates to multiple nodules. This illness may be part of a spectrum that includes polyarteritis nodosa.

Treatment of pulmonary vasculitis usually requires corticosteroids and cyclophosphamide. Oral prednisone (1 mg/kg ideal body weight per day initially, tapering slowly to alternate-day therapy over 3–6 months) is the corticosteroid of choice; in Wegener granulomatosis, some clinicians may use cyclophosphamide alone. For fulminant vasculitis, therapy may be initiated with intravenous methylprednisolone (up to 1 g intravenously per day) for several days. Cyclophosphamide (1–2 mg/kg ideal body weight per day initially, with dosage adjustments to avoid neutropenia) is given daily by mouth until complete remission is obtained and then is slowly tapered, and often replaced with methotrexate or azathioprine for maintenance therapy.

Five-year survival rates in patients with these vasculitis syndromes have been improved by the combination therapy. Complete remissions can be achieved in over 90% of patients with Wegener granulomatosis. The addition of trimethoprim-sulfamethoxazole (one double-strength tablet by mouth twice daily) to standard therapy may help prevent relapses.

Alberts WM. Pulmonary manifestations of the Churg-Strauss syndrome and related idiopathic small vessel vasculitis syndromes. Curr Opin Pulm Med. 2007 Sep;13(5):445–50. [PMID: 17940492]

Brown KK. Pulmonary vasculitis. Proc Am Thorac Soc. 2006;3(1):48–57. [PMID: 16493151]

Langford CA. Update on Wegener granulomatosis. Cleve Clin J Med. 2005 Aug;72(8):689–90. [PMID: 16122054]

ALVEOLAR HEMORRHAGE SYNDROMES

Diffuse alveolar hemorrhage may occur in a variety of immune and nonimmune disorders. Hemoptysis, alveolar infiltrates on chest radiograph, anemia, dyspnea, and occasionally fever are characteristic. Rapid clearing of diffuse lung infiltrates within 2 days is a clue to the diagnosis of diffuse alveolar hemorrhage. Pulmonary hemorrhage can be associated with an increased $D_{L_{CO}}$.

Causes of **immune alveolar hemorrhage** have been classified as anti-basement membrane antibody disease (Goodpasture syndrome), vasculitis and collagen vascular disease (systemic lupus erythematosus, Wegener granulomatosis, systemic necrotizing vasculitis, and others), and pulmonary capillaritis associated with idiopathic rapidly progressive glomerulonephritis. **Nonimmune causes** of diffuse hemorrhage include coagulopathy, mitral stenosis, necrotizing pulmonary infection, drugs (penicillamine), toxins (trimellitic anhydride), and idiopathic pulmonary hemosiderosis.

Goodpasture syndrome is idiopathic recurrent alveolar hemorrhage and rapidly progressive glomerulonephritis. The disease is mediated by anti-glomerular basement membrane antibodies. Goodpasture syndrome occurs mainly in men who are in their 30s and 40s. Hemoptysis is the usual presenting symptom, but pulmonary hemorrhage may be occult. Dyspnea, cough, hypoxemia, and diffuse bilateral alveolar infiltrates are typical features. Iron deficiency anemia and microscopic hematuria are usually present. The diagnosis is based on characteristic linear IgG deposits in glomeruli or alveoli by immunofluorescence and on the presence of anti-glomerular basement membrane antibody in serum. Combinations of immunosuppressive drugs (initially methylprednisolone, 30 mg/kg intravenously over 20 minutes every other day for three doses, followed by daily oral prednisone, 1 mg/kg/d; with cyclophosphamide, 2 mg/kg by mouth per day) and plasmapheresis have yielded excellent results.

Idiopathic pulmonary hemosiderosis is a disease of children or young adults characterized by recurrent pulmonary hemorrhage; in contrast to Goodpasture syndrome, renal involvement and anti-glomerular basement membrane antibodies are absent, but iron deficiency is typical. Treatment of acute episodes of hemorrhage with corticosteroids may be useful. Recurrent episodes of pulmonary hemorrhage may result in interstitial fibrosis and pulmonary failure.

Gómez-Román JJ. Diffuse alveolar hemorrhage. Arch Bronconeumol. 2008 Aug;44(8):428–36. Spanish. [PMID: 18775255]

ENVIRONMENTAL & OCCUPATIONAL LUNG DISORDERS

SMOKE INHALATION

The inhalation of products of combustion may cause serious respiratory complications. As many as one-third of patients admitted to burn treatment units have pulmonary injury from smoke inhalation. Morbidity and mortality due to smoke inhalation exceed those attributed to the burns themselves. The death rate of patients with both severe burns and smoke inhalation exceeds 50%.

All patients suspected of having significant smoke inhalation must be assessed for three consequences of smoke inhalation: impaired tissue oxygenation, thermal injury to the upper airway, and chemical injury to the lung. Impaired tissue oxygenation results from inhalation of carbon monoxide or cyanide and is an immediate threat to life. The management of patients with carbon monoxide and cyanide poisoning is discussed in Chapter 38. The clinician must recognize that patients with carbon monoxide poisoning display a normal partial pressure of oxygen in arterial blood (PaO_2) but have a low *measured* (ie, not oximetric) hemoglobin saturation (SaO_2). Immediate treatment with 100% oxygen is essential and should be continued until the measured carboxyhemoglobin level falls to less than 10% and concomitant metabolic acidosis has resolved.

Thermal injury to the mucosal surfaces of the upper airway occurs from inhalation of hot gases. Complications become evident by 18–24 hours. These include edema, impaired ability to clear oral secretions, and upper airway obstruction, producing inspiratory stridor. Respiratory failure occurs in severe cases. Early management (see also Chapter 37) includes the use of a high-humidity face mask with supplemental oxygen, gentle suctioning to evacuate oral secretions, elevation of the head 30 degrees to promote clearing of secretions, and topical epinephrine to reduce edema of the oropharyngeal mucous membrane. Helium-oxygen gas mixtures (Heliox) may reduce labored breathing due to upper airway narrowing. Close monitoring with arterial blood gases and later with oximetry is important. Examination of the upper airway with a fiberoptic laryngoscope or bronchoscope is superior to routine physical examination. Endotracheal intubation is often necessary to establish airway patency and is likely to be necessary in patients with deep facial burns or oropharyngeal or laryngeal edema. Tracheotomy should be avoided if possible because of an increased risk of pneumonia and death from sepsis.

Chemical injury to the lung results from inhalation of toxic gases and products of combustion, including aldehydes and organic acids. The site of lung injury depends on the solubility of the gases inhaled, the duration of exposure, and the size of inhaled particles that transport noxious gases to distal lung units. Bronchorrhea and bronchospasm are seen early after exposure along with dyspnea, tachypnea, and tachycardia. Labored breathing and cyanosis may follow. Physical examination at this stage reveals diffuse wheezing and rhonchi. Bronchiolar and alveolar edema (eg, ARDS) may develop within 1–2 days after exposure. Sloughing of the bronchiolar mucosa may occur within 2–3 days, leading to airway obstruction, atelectasis, and worsening hypoxemia. Bacterial colonization and pneumonia are common by 5–7 days after the exposure.

Treatment of smoke inhalation consists of supplemental oxygen, bronchodilators, suctioning of mucosal debris and mucopurulent secretions via an indwelling endotracheal tube, chest physical therapy to aid clearance of secretions, and adequate humidification of inspired gases. Positive end-expiratory pressure (PEEP) has been advocated to treat bronchiolar edema. Judicious fluid management and close monitoring for secondary bacterial infection with daily sputum Gram stains round out the management protocol.

The routine use of corticosteroids for chemical lung injury from smoke inhalation has been shown to be ineffective and may even be harmful. Routine or prophylactic use of antibiotics is not recommended.

Patients who survive should be watched for the late development of bronchiolitis obliterans.

Mlcak RP et al. Respiratory management of inhalation injury. Burns. 2007 Feb;33(1):2–13. [PMID: 17223484]

PULMONARY ASPIRATION SYNDROMES

Aspiration of foreign material into the tracheobronchial tree results from various disorders that impair normal deglutition, especially disturbances of consciousness and esophageal dysfunction.

1. Aspiration of Inert Material

Aspiration of inert material may cause asphyxia if the amount aspirated is massive and if cough is impaired, in which case immediate tracheobronchial suctioning is necessary. Most patients suffer no serious sequelae from aspiration of inert material.

2. Aspiration of Toxic Material

Aspiration of toxic material into the lung usually results in clinically evident pneumonia. **Hydrocarbon pneumonitis** is caused by aspiration of ingested petroleum distillates, eg, gasoline, kerosene, furniture polish, and other household petroleum products. Lung injury results mainly from vomiting and secondary aspiration. Therapy is supportive. The lung should be protected from repeated aspiration with a cuffed endotracheal tube if necessary. **Lipoid pneumonia** is a chronic syndrome related to the repeated aspiration of oily materials, eg, mineral oil, cod liver oil, and oily nose drops; it often occurs in elderly patients with impaired swallowing. Patchy infiltrates in dependent lung zones and lipid-laden macrophages in expectorated sputum are characteristic findings.

3. "Café Coronary"

Acute obstruction of the upper airway by food is associated with difficulty swallowing, old age, dental problems that impair chewing, and use of alcohol and sedative drugs. The Heimlich procedure is lifesaving in many cases.

4. Retention of an Aspirated Foreign Body

Retention of an aspirated foreign body in the tracheobronchial tree may produce both acute and chronic conditions, including recurrent pneumonia, bronchiectasis, lung abscess, atelectasis, and postobstructive hyperinflation. Occasionally, a misdiagnosis of asthma, COPD, or lung cancer is made in adult patients who have aspirated a foreign body. The plain chest radiograph usually suggests the site of the foreign body. In some cases, an expiratory film, demonstrating regional hyperinflation due to a check-valve effect, is helpful. Bronchoscopy is usually necessary to establish the diagnosis and attempt removal of the foreign body.

5. Chronic Aspiration of Gastric Contents

Chronic aspiration of gastric contents may result from primary disorders of the larynx or the esophagus, such as achalasia, esophageal stricture, systemic sclerosis (scleroderma), esophageal carcinoma, esophagitis, and gastroesophageal reflux. In the last condition, relaxation of the tone of the lower esophageal sphincter allows reflux of gastric contents into the esophagus and predisposes to chronic pulmonary aspiration, especially at night. Cigarette smoking, consumption of alcohol, and use of theophylline are known to relax the lower esophageal sphincter. Pulmonary disorders linked to gastroesophageal reflux and chronic aspiration include bronchial asthma, pulmonary fibrosis, and bronchiectasis. Even in the absence of aspiration, acid in the esophagus may trigger bronchospasm through reflex mechanisms.

The diagnosis of chronic aspiration is difficult. Ambulatory monitoring of esophageal pH for 24 hours detects esophageal reflux. Esophagogastroscopy and barium swallow are sometimes necessary to rule out esophageal disease. Management consists of elevation of the head of the bed, cessation of smoking, weight reduction, and antacids, H_2-receptor antagonists (eg, cimetidine, 300–400 mg), or proton pump inhibitors (eg, omeprazole, 20 mg) at night. Metoclopramide (10–15 mg orally four times daily or 20 mg at bedtime) or bethanechol (10–25 mg at bedtime) may also be helpful in some patients with gastroesophageal reflux.

6. Acute Aspiration of Gastric Contents (Mendelson Syndrome)

Acute aspiration of gastric contents is often catastrophic. The pulmonary response depends on the characteristics and amount of the gastric contents aspirated. The more acidic the material, the greater the degree of chemical pneumonitis. Aspiration of pure gastric acid (pH < 2.5) causes extensive desquamation of the bronchial epithelium, bronchiolitis, hemorrhage, and pulmonary edema. Acute gastric aspiration is one of the most common causes of ARDS. The clinical picture is one of abrupt onset of respiratory distress, with cough, wheezing, fever, and tachypnea. Crackles are audible at the bases of the lungs. Hypoxemia may be noted immediately after aspiration occurs. Radiographic abnormalities, consisting of patchy alveolar infiltrates in dependent lung zones, appear within a few hours. If particulate food matter has been aspirated

along with gastric acid, radiographic features of bronchial obstruction may be observed. Fever and leukocytosis are common even in the absence of superinfection.

Treatment of acute aspiration of gastric contents consists of supplemental oxygen, measures to maintain the airway, and the usual measures for treatment of acute respiratory failure. There is no evidence to support the routine use of corticosteroids or prophylactic antibiotics after gastric aspiration has occurred. Secondary pulmonary infection, which occurs in about one-fourth of patients, typically appears 2–3 days after aspiration. Management of this complication depends on the observed flora of the tracheobronchial tree. Hypotension secondary to alveolocapillary membrane injury and intravascular volume depletion is common and is managed with the judicious administration of intravenous fluids.

Paintal HS et al. Aspiration syndromes: 10 clinical pearls every physician should know. Int J Clin Pract. 2007 May;61(5):846–52. [PMID: 17493092]

OCCUPATIONAL PULMONARY DISEASES

Many acute and chronic pulmonary diseases are directly related to inhalation of noxious substances encountered in the workplace. Disorders that are due to chemical agents may be classified as follows: (1) pneumoconioses, (2) hypersensitivity pneumonitis, (3) obstructive airway disorders, (4) toxic lung injury, (5) lung cancer, (6) pleural diseases, and (7) miscellaneous disorders.

1. Pneumoconioses

Pneumoconioses are chronic fibrotic lung diseases caused by the inhalation of coal dust and various other inert, inorganic, or silicate dusts (Table 9–19). Pneumoconioses due to inhalation of inert dusts may be asymptomatic disorders with diffuse nodular infiltrates on chest radiograph. Clinically important pneumoconioses include coal workers' pneumoconiosis, silicosis, and asbestosis. Treatment for each is supportive.

A. Coal Worker's Pneumoconiosis

In coal worker's pneumoconiosis, ingestion of inhaled coal dust by alveolar macrophages leads to the formation of coal macules, usually 2–5 mm in diameter, that appear on chest radiograph as diffuse small opacities that are especially prominent in the upper lung. Simple coal worker's pneumoconiosis is usually asymptomatic; pulmonary function abnormalities are unimpressive. Cigarette smoking does not increase the prevalence of coal worker's pneumoconiosis but may have an additive detrimental effect on ventilatory function. In complicated coal worker's pneumoconiosis ("**progressive massive fibrosis**"), conglomeration and contraction in the upper lung zones occur, with radiographic features resembling complicated silicosis. **Caplan syndrome** is a rare condition characterized by the presence of necrobiotic rheumatoid nodules (1–5 cm in diameter) in the periphery of the lung in coal workers with rheumatoid arthritis.

Table 9–19. Selected pneumoconioses.

Disease	Agent	Occupations
Metal dusts		
Siderosis	Metallic iron or iron oxide	Mining, welding, foundry work
Stannosis	Tin, tin oxide	Mining, tin-working, smelting
Baritosis	Barium salts	Glass and insecticide manufacturing
Coal dust		
Coal worker's pneumoconiosis	Coal dust	Coal mining
Inorganic dusts		
Silicosis	Free silica (silicon dioxide)	Rock mining, quarrying, stone cutting, tunneling, sandblasting, pottery, diatomaceous earth
Silicate dusts		
Asbestosis	Asbestos	Mining, insulation, construction, shipbuilding
Talcosis	Magnesium silicate	Mining, insulation, construction, shipbuilding
Kaolin pneumoconiosis	Sand, mica, aluminum silicate	Mining of china clay; pottery and cement work
Shaver disease	Aluminum powder	Manufacture of corundum

B. Silicosis

In silicosis, extensive or prolonged inhalation of free silica (silicon dioxide) particles in the respirable range (0.3–5 mcm) causes the formation of small rounded opacities (silicotic nodules) throughout the lung. Calcification of the periphery of hilar lymph nodes ("eggshell" calcification) is an unusual radiographic finding that strongly suggests silicosis. Simple silicosis is usually asymptomatic and has no effect on routine pulmonary function tests; in complicated silicosis, large conglomerate densities appear in the upper lung and are accompanied by dyspnea and obstructive and restrictive pulmonary dysfunction. The incidence of pulmonary tuberculosis is increased in patients with silicosis. All patients with silicosis should have a tuberculin skin test and a current chest radiograph. If old, healed pulmonary tuberculosis is suspected, multidrug treatment for tuberculosis (not single-agent preventive therapy) should be instituted.

C. Asbestosis

Asbestosis is a nodular interstitial fibrosis occurring in workers exposed to asbestos fibers (shipyard and construction workers, pipe fitters, insulators) over many years (typically 10–20 years). Patients with asbestosis usually

seek medical attention at least 15 years after exposure with the following symptoms and signs: progressive dyspnea, inspiratory crackles, and in some cases, clubbing and cyanosis. The radiographic features of asbestosis include linear streaking at the lung bases, opacities of various shapes and sizes, and honeycomb changes in advanced cases. The presence of pleural calcifications may be a clue to diagnosis. High-resolution CT scanning is the best imaging method for asbestosis because of its ability to detect parenchymal fibrosis and define the presence of coexisting pleural plaques. Cigarette smoking in asbestos workers increases the prevalence of radiographic pleural and parenchymal changes and markedly increases the incidence of lung carcinoma. It may also interfere with the clearance of short asbestos fibers from the lung. Pulmonary function studies show restrictive dysfunction and reduced diffusing capacity. The presence of a ferruginous body in tissue suggests significant asbestos exposure; however, other histologic features must be present for diagnosis. There is no specific treatment.

O'Reilly KM et al. Asbestos-related lung disease. Am Fam Physician. 2007 Mar 1;75(5):683–8. [PMID: 17375514]

Scarisbrick D. Silicosis and coal workers' pneumoconiosis. Practitioner. 2002 Feb;246(1631):114, 117–9. [PMID: 11852619]

2. Hypersensitivity Pneumonitis

Hypersensitivity pneumonitis (also called extrinsic allergic alveolitis) is a nonatopic, nonasthmatic allergic pulmonary disease. It is manifested mainly as an occupational disease (Table 9–20), in which exposure to inhaled organic antigens leads to an acute illness characterized by sudden onset of malaise, chills, fever, cough, dyspnea, and nausea 4–8 hours after exposure to the offending antigen. This may occur after the patient has left work or even at night and thus may mimic paroxysmal nocturnal dyspnea. Bibasilar crackles, tachypnea, tachycardia, and (occasionally) cyanosis are noted. Small nodular densities sparing the apices and bases of the lungs are noted on chest radiograph. Pulmonary function studies reveal restrictive dysfunction and reduced diffusing capacity. Laboratory studies reveal an increase in the white blood cell count with a shift to the left, hypoxemia, and the presence of precipitating antibodies to the offending agent in serum. Hypersensitivity pneumonitis antibody panels against common offending antigens are available; positive results, while supportive, do not establish a definitive diagnosis. The histopathology of acute hypersensitivity pneumonitis is characterized by interstitial infiltrates of lymphocytes and plasma cells, with noncaseating granulomas in the interstitium and air spaces.

Prompt diagnosis is essential since symptoms are usually reversible if the offending antigen is removed from the patient's environment early in the course of illness. Continued exposure may lead to progressive disease. A subacute hypersensitivity pneumonitis syndrome (15% of cases) is characterized by the insidious onset of chronic cough and slowly progressive dyspnea, anorexia, and weight loss. Chronic exposure leads to progressive respiratory insufficiency and the appearance of pulmonary fibrosis on chest imaging. Surgical lung biopsy may be necessary

Table 9–20. Selected causes of hypersensitivity pneumonitis.

Disease	Antigen	Source
Farmer's lung	*Micropolyspora faeni, Thermoactinomyces vulgaris*	Moldy hay
"Humidifier" lung	Thermophilic actino-mycetes	Contaminated humidifiers, heating systems, or air conditioners
Bird fancier's lung ("pigeon-breeder's disease")	Avian proteins	Bird serum and excreta
Bagassosis	*Thermoactinomyces sacchari* and *T vulgaris*	Moldy sugar cane fiber (bagasse)
Sequoiosis	Graphium, Aureoba-sidium, and other fungi	Moldy redwood sawdust
Maple bark strip-per's disease	*Cryptostroma (Coniosporium) corticale*	Rotting maple tree logs or bark
Mushroom picker's disease	Same as farmer's lung	Moldy compost
Suberosis	*Penicillium frequentans*	Moldy cork dust
Detergent worker's lung	*Bacillus subtilis* enzyme	Enzyme additives

for the diagnosis of subacute and chronic hypersensitivity pneumonitis. Even with surgical lung biopsy, however, chronic hypersensitivity pneumonitis may be difficult to diagnose because histopathologic patterns overlap with several idiopathic interstitial pneumonias.

Treatment of acute hypersensitivity pneumonitis consists of identification of the offending agent and avoidance of further exposure. In severe acute or protracted cases, oral corticosteroids (prednisone, 0.5 mg/kg daily as a single morning dose for 2 weeks, tapered to nil over 4–6 weeks) may be given. Change in occupation is often unavoidable.

Ismail T et al. Extrinsic allergic alveolitis. Respirology. 2006 May;11(3):262–8. [PMID: 16635083]

3. Obstructive Airway Disorders

Occupational pulmonary diseases manifested as obstructive airway disorders include occupational asthma, industrial bronchitis, and byssinosis.

A. Occupational Asthma

It has been estimated that from 2% to 5% of all cases of asthma are related to occupation. Offending agents in the workplace are numerous; they include grain dust, wood dust, tobacco, pollens, enzymes, gum arabic, synthetic dyes, isocyanates (particularly toluene diisocyanate), rosin (soldering flux), inorganic chemicals (salts of nickel, platinum, and chromium), trimellitic anhydride, phthalic anhydride, formaldehyde, and various pharmaceutical agents. Diagnosis of occupational asthma depends on a high index of suspicion, an appropriate history, spirometric studies before and after exposure to the offending substance, and peak flow rate measurements in the workplace. Bronchial provocation testing may be helpful in some cases. Treatment consists of avoidance of further exposure to the offending agent and bronchodilators, but symptoms may persist for years after workplace exposure has been terminated.

B. Industrial Bronchitis

Industrial bronchitis is chronic bronchitis found in coal miners and others exposed to cotton, flax, or hemp dust. Chronic disability from industrial bronchitis is infrequent.

C. Byssinosis

Byssinosis is an asthma-like disorder in textile workers caused by inhalation of cotton dust. The pathogenesis is obscure. Chest tightness, cough, and dyspnea are characteristically worse on Mondays or the first day back at work, with symptoms subsiding later in the week. Repeated exposure leads to chronic bronchitis.

4. Toxic Lung Injury

Toxic lung injury from inhalation of irritant gases is discussed in the section on smoke inhalation. **Silo-filler's disease** is acute toxic high-permeability pulmonary edema caused by inhalation of nitrogen dioxide encountered in recently filled silos. Bronchiolitis obliterans is a common late complication, which may be prevented by early treatment of the acute reaction with corticosteroids. Extensive exposure to silage gas may be fatal. Inhalation of the compound diacetyl, a constituent of butter-flavoring, has been linked to the development of bronchiolitis obliterans among microwave popcorn production workers.

5. Lung Cancer

Many industrial pulmonary carcinogens have been identified, including asbestos, radon gas, arsenic, iron, chromium, nickel, coal tar fumes, petroleum oil mists, isopropyl oil, mustard gas, and printing ink. Cigarette smoking acts as a cocarcinogen with asbestos and radon gas to cause bronchogenic carcinoma. Asbestos alone causes malignant mesothelioma. Almost all histologic types of lung cancer have been associated with these carcinogens. Chloromethyl methyl ether specifically causes small cell carcinoma of the lung.

6. Pleural Diseases

Occupational diseases of the pleura may result from exposure to asbestos (see above) or talc. Inhalation of talc causes pleural plaques that are similar to those caused by asbestos. Benign asbestos pleural effusion occurs in some asbestos workers and may cause chronic blunting of the costophrenic angle on chest radiograph.

7. Other Occupational Pulmonary Diseases

Occupational agents are also responsible for other pulmonary disorders. These include **berylliosis**, an acute or chronic pulmonary disorder related to exposure to beryllium, which is absorbed through the lungs or skin and widely disseminated throughout the body. Acute berylliosis is a toxic, ulcerative tracheobronchitis and chemical pneumonitis following intense and severe exposure to beryllium. Chronic berylliosis, a systemic disease closely resembling sarcoidosis, is more common. Chronic pulmonary beryllium disease is thought to be an alveolitis mediated by the proliferation of beryllium-specific helper-inducer T cells in the lung. Exposure to beryllium now occurs in machining and handling of beryllium products and alloys. Beryllium miners are not at risk for berylliosis. Beryllium is no longer used in fluorescent lamp production, which was a source of exposure before 1950.

Beach J et al. A systematic review of the diagnosis of occupational asthma. Chest. 2007 Feb;131(2):569–78. [PMID: 17296663]
Mapp CE et al. Occupational asthma. Am J Respir Crit Care Med. 2005 Aug 1;172(3):280–305. [PMID: 15860754]

DRUG-INDUCED LUNG DISEASE

Typical patterns of pulmonary response to drugs implicated in drug-induced respiratory disease are summarized in Table 9–21. Pulmonary injury due to drugs occurs as a result of allergic reactions, idiosyncratic reactions, overdose, or undesirable side effects. In most patients, the mechanism of pulmonary injury is unknown.

Precise diagnosis of drug-induced pulmonary disease is often difficult, because results of routine laboratory studies are not helpful and radiographic findings are not specific. A high index of suspicion and a thorough medical history of drug usage are critical to establishing the diagnosis of drug-induced lung disease. The clinical response to cessation of the suspected offending agent is also helpful. Acute episodes of drug-induced pulmonary disease usually disappear 24–48 hours after the drug has been discontinued, but chronic syndromes may take longer to resolve. Challenge tests to confirm the diagnosis are risky and rarely performed.

Treatment of drug-induced lung disease consists of discontinuing the offending agent immediately and managing the pulmonary symptoms appropriately.

Inhalation of crack cocaine may cause a spectrum of acute pulmonary syndromes, including pulmonary infiltration with eosinophilia, pneumothorax and pneumomediastinum, bronchiolitis obliterans, and acute respiratory failure associated with diffuse alveolar damage and alveolar hemorrhage. Corticosteroids have been used with variable success to treat alveolar hemorrhage.

Babu KS et al. Drug-induced airway diseases. Clin Chest Med. 2004 Mar;25(1):113–22. [PMID: 15062603]

Table 9–21. Pulmonary manifestations of selected drug toxicities.

Asthma	**Pulmonary edema**
β-Blockers	Noncardiogenic
Aspirin	Aspirin
Nonsteroidal anti-inflamma-	Chlordiazepoxide
tory drugs	Cocaine
Histamine	Ethchlorvynol
Methacholine	Heroin
Acetylcysteine	Cardiogenic
Aerosolized pentamidine	β-Blockers
Any nebulized medication	**Pleural effusion**
Chronic cough	Bromocriptine
Angiotensin-converting	Nitrofurantoin
enzyme inhibitors	Any drug inducing systemic
Pulmonary infiltration	lupus erythematosus
Without eosinophilia	Methysergide
Amitriptyline	Chemotherapeutic agents
Azathioprine	**Mediastinal widening**
Amiodarone	Phenytoin
With eosinophilia	Corticosteroids
Sulfonamides	Methotrexate
L-Tryptophan	**Respiratory failure**
Nitrofurantoin	Neuromuscular blockade
Penicillin	Aminoglycosides
Methotrexate	Succinylcholine
Crack cocaine	Gallamine
Drug-induced systemic lupus	Dimethyltubocurarine
erythematosus	(metocurine)
Hydralazine	Central nervous system
Procainamide	depression
Isoniazid	Sedatives
Chlorpromazine	Hypnotics
Phenytoin	Opioids
Interstitial pneumonitis/	Alcohol
fibrosis	Tricyclic antidepressants
Nitrofurantoin	Oxygen
Bleomycin	
Busulfan	
Cyclophosphamide	
Methysergide	
Phenytoin	

Huggins JT et al. Drug-induced pleural disease. Clin Chest Med. 2004 Mar;25(1):141–53. [PMID: 15062606]

RADIATION LUNG INJURY

The lung is an exquisitely radiosensitive organ that can be damaged by external beam radiation therapy. The degree of pulmonary injury is determined by the volume of lung irradiated, the dose and rate of exposure, and potentiating factors (eg, concurrent chemotherapy, previous radiation therapy in the same area, and simultaneous withdrawal of corticosteroid therapy). Symptomatic radiation lung injury occurs in about 10% of patients treated for carcinoma of the breast, 5–15% of patients treated for carcinoma of the lung, and 5–35% of patients treated for lymphoma. Two phases of the pulmonary response to radiation are apparent: an acute phase (radiation pneumonitis) and a chronic phase (radiation fibrosis).

1. Radiation Pneumonitis

Radiation pneumonitis usually occurs 2–3 months (range 1–6 months) after completion of radiotherapy and is characterized by insidious onset of dyspnea, intractable dry cough, chest fullness or pain, weakness, and fever. The pathogenesis of acute radiation pneumonitis is unknown, but there is speculation that hypersensitivity mechanisms are involved. The dominant histopathologic findings are a lymphocytic interstitial pneumonitis progressing to an exudative alveolitis. Inspiratory crackles may be heard in the involved area. In severe disease, respiratory distress and cyanosis occur that are characteristic of ARDS. An increased white blood cell count and elevated sedimentation rate are common. Pulmonary function studies reveal reduced lung volumes, reduced lung compliance, hypoxemia, reduced diffusing capacity, and reduced maximum voluntary ventilation. Chest radiography, which correlates poorly with the presence of symptoms, usually demonstrates an alveolar or nodular infiltrate limited to the irradiated area. Air bronchograms are often observed. Sharp borders of the infiltrate may help distinguish radiation pneumonitis from other conditions such as infectious pneumonia, lymphangitic spread of carcinoma, and recurrent tumor. No specific therapy is proved to be effective in radiation pneumonitis, but prednisone (1 mg/kg/d orally) is commonly given immediately for about 1 week. The dose is then reduced and maintained at 20–40 mg/d for several weeks, then slowly tapered. Radiation pneumonitis may improve in 2–3 weeks following onset of symptoms as the exudative phase resolves. Acute respiratory failure, if present, is treated supportively. Death from ARDS is unusual in radiation pneumonitis.

2. Pulmonary Radiation Fibrosis

Pulmonary radiation fibrosis occurs in nearly all patients who receive a full course of radiation therapy for cancer of the lung or breast. Patients who experience radiation pneumonitis develop pulmonary fibrosis after an intervening period (6–12 months) of well-being. Most patients are asymptomatic, though slowly progressive dyspnea may occur. Radiation fibrosis may occur with or without antecedent radiation pneumonitis. Cor pulmonale and chronic respiratory failure are rare. Radiographic findings include obliteration of normal lung markings, dense interstitial and pleural fibrosis, reduced lung volumes, tenting of the diaphragm, and sharp delineation of the irradiated area. No specific therapy is proven effective, and corticosteroids have no value.

3. Other Complications of Radiation Therapy

Other complications of radiation therapy directed to the thorax include pericardial effusion, constrictive pericarditis, tracheoesophageal fistula, esophageal candidiasis, radiation dermatitis, and rib fractures. Small pleural effusions, radiation pneumonitis outside the irradiated area, spontaneous pneumothorax, and complete obstruction of central airways are unusual occurrences.

Abratt RP et al. Pulmonary complications of radiation therapy. Clin Chest Med. 2004 Mar;25(1):167–77. [PMID: 15062608]

Camus P et al. Interstitial lung disease induced by drugs and radiation. Respiration. 2004 Jul–Aug;71(4):301–26. [PMID: 15316202]

▼ PLEURAL DISEASES

PLEURITIS

Pain due to acute pleural inflammation is caused by irritation of the parietal pleura. Such pain is localized, sharp, and fleeting; it is made worse by coughing, sneezing, deep breathing, or movement. When the central portion of the diaphragmatic parietal pleura is irritated, pain may be referred to the ipsilateral shoulder. There are numerous causes of pleuritis. The setting in which pleuritic pain develops helps narrow the differential diagnosis. In young, otherwise healthy individuals, pleuritis is usually caused by viral respiratory infections or pneumonia. The presence of pleural effusion, pleural thickening, or air in the pleural space requires further diagnostic and therapeutic measures. Simple rib fracture may cause severe pleurisy.

Treatment of pleuritis consists of treating the underlying disease. Analgesics and anti-inflammatory drugs (eg, indomethacin, 25 mg orally two or three times daily) are often helpful for pain relief. Codeine (30–60 mg orally every 8 hours) may be used to control cough associated with pleuritic chest pain if retention of airway secretions is not a likely complication. Intercostal nerve blocks are sometimes helpful but the benefit is usually transient.

PLEURAL EFFUSION

ESSENTIALS OF DIAGNOSIS

▶ May be asymptomatic; chest pain frequently seen in the setting of pleuritis, trauma, or infection; dyspnea is common with large effusions.

▶ Dullness to percussion and decreased breath sounds over the effusion.

▶ Radiographic evidence of pleural effusion.

▶ Diagnostic findings on thoracentesis.

▶ General Considerations

There is constant movement of fluid from parietal pleural capillaries into the pleural space at a rate of 0.01 mL/kg body weight/h. Absorption of pleural fluid occurs through parietal pleural lymphatics. The resultant homeostasis leaves 5–15 mL of fluid in the normal pleural space. A pleural effusion is an abnormal accumulation of fluid in the pleural space. Pleural effusions may be classified by differential diagnosis (Table 9–22) or by underlying pathophysiology. Five pathophysiologic processes account for most pleural effusions: increased production of fluid in the setting of

Table 9–22. Causes of pleural fluid transudates and exudates.

Transudates	Exudates
Congestive heart failure (> 90% of cases)	Pneumonia (parapneumonic effusion)
Cirrhosis with ascites	Cancer
Nephrotic syndrome	Pulmonary embolism
Peritoneal dialysis	Bacterial infection
Myxedema	Tuberculosis
Acute atelectasis	Connective tissue disease
Constrictive pericarditis	Viral infection
Superior vena cava obstruction	Fungal infection
Pulmonary embolism	Rickettsial infection
	Parasitic infection
	Asbestos
	Meigs syndrome
	Pancreatic disease
	Uremia
	Chronic atelectasis
	Trapped lung
	Chylothorax
	Sarcoidosis
	Drug reaction
	Post-myocardial infarction syndrome

normal capillaries due to increased hydrostatic or decreased oncotic pressures (transudates); increased production of fluid due to abnormal capillary permeability (exudates); decreased lymphatic clearance of fluid from the pleural space (exudates); infection in the pleural space (empyema); and bleeding into the pleural space (hemothorax).

Diagnostic thoracentesis should be performed whenever there is a new pleural effusion and no clinically apparent cause. Observation is appropriate in some situations (eg, symmetric bilateral pleural effusions in the setting of congestive heart failure), but an atypical presentation or failure of an effusion to resolve as expected warrants thoracentesis. Sampling allows visualization of the fluid in addition to chemical and microbiologic analyses to identify the pathophysiologic processes listed above. A definitive diagnosis is made through positive cytology or identification of a specific causative organism in approximately 25% of cases. In another 50–60% of patients, identification of relevant pathophysiology in the appropriate clinical setting greatly narrows the differential diagnosis and leads to a presumptive diagnosis.

► **Clinical Findings**

A. Symptoms and Signs

Patients with pleural effusions most often report dyspnea, cough, or respirophasic chest pain. Symptoms are more common in patients with existing cardiopulmonary disease. Small pleural effusions are less likely to be symptomatic than larger effusions. Physical findings are usually absent in small effusions. Larger effusions may present with dullness to percussion and diminished or absent breath sounds over the effusion. Compressive atelectasis may cause bronchial breath sounds and egophony just above the effusion. A massive effusion with increased intrapleural pressure may cause contralateral shift of the trachea and bulging of the intercostal spaces. A pleural friction rub indicates infarction or pleuritis.

B. Laboratory Findings

The gross appearance of pleural fluid helps identify several types of pleural effusion. Grossly purulent fluid signifies empyema, an infection of the pleural space. Milky white pleural fluid should be centrifuged. A clear supernatant above a pellet of white cells indicates empyema, whereas a persistently turbid supernatant suggests a chylous effusion. Analysis of this supernatant reveals chylomicrons and a high triglyceride level (> 100 mg/dL), often from traumatic disruption of the thoracic duct. Hemorrhagic pleural effusion is a mixture of blood and pleural fluid. Ten thousand red cells per milliliter create blood-tinged pleural fluid; 100,000/mL create grossly bloody pleural fluid. Hemothorax is the presence of gross blood in the pleural space, usually following chest trauma or instrumentation. It is defined as a ratio of pleural fluid hematocrit to peripheral blood hematocrit > 0.5.

Pleural fluid samples should be sent for measurement of protein, glucose, and LD in addition to total and differential white blood cell counts. Chemistry determinations are used to classify effusions as transudates or exudates. This classification is important because the differential diagnosis for each entity is vastly different (Table 9–22). A pleural exudate is an effusion that has one or more of the following laboratory features: (1) ratio of pleural fluid protein to serum protein > 0.5; (2) ratio of pleural fluid LD to serum LD > 0.6; (3) pleural fluid LD greater than two-thirds the upper limit of normal serum LD.

Transudates have none of these features. Transudates occur in the setting of normal capillary integrity and suggest the absence of local pleural disease. Distinguishing laboratory findings include a glucose equal to serum glucose, pH between 7.40 and 7.55, and fewer than 1000 white blood cells/mcL with a predominance of mononuclear cells. Causes include increased hydrostatic pressure (congestive heart failure accounts for 90% of transudates), decreased oncotic pressure (hypoalbuminemia, cirrhosis), and greater negative pleural pressure (acute atelectasis). Exudates form as a result of pleural disease associated with increased capillary permeability or reduced lymphatic drainage. Bacterial pneumonia and cancer are the most common causes of exudative effusion, but there are many other causes with characteristic laboratory findings. These findings are summarized in Table 9–23.

Pleural fluid pH is useful in the assessment of parapneumonic effusions. A pH below 7.30 suggests the need for drainage of the pleural space. An elevated amylase level in pleural fluid suggests pancreatitis, pancreatic pseudocyst, adenocarcinoma of the lung or pancreas, or esophageal rupture.

Thoracentesis with culture and pleural biopsy is indicated in suspected tuberculous pleural effusion. Pleural fluid culture

Table 9–23. Characteristics of important exudative pleural effusions.

Etiology or Type of Effusion	Gross Appearance	White Blood Cell Count (cells/mcL)	Red Blood Cell Count (cells/mcL)	Glucose	Comments
Malignant effusion	Turbid to bloody; occasionally serous	1000 to < 100,000 M	100 to several hundred thousand	Equal to serum levels; < 60 mg/dL in 15% of cases	Eosinophilia uncommon; positive results on cytologic examination
Uncomplicated parapneumonic effusion	Clear to turbid	5000–25,000 P	< 5000	Equal to serum levels	Tube thoracostomy unnecessary
Empyema	Turbid to purulent	25,000–100,000 P	< 5000	Less than serum levels; often very low	Drainage necessary; putrid odor suggests anaerobic infection
Tuberculosis	Serous to serosanguineous	5000–10,000 M	< 10,000	Equal to serum levels; occasionally < 60 mg/dL	Protein > 4.0 g/dL and may exceed 5 g/dL; eosinophils (> 10%) or mesothelial cells (> 5%) make diagnosis unlikely
Rheumatoid effusion	Turbid; greenish yellow	1000–20,000 M or P	< 1000	< 40 mg/dL	Secondary empyema common; high LD, low complement, high rheumatoid factor, cholesterol crystals are characteristic
Pulmonary infarction	Serous to grossly bloody	1000–50,000 M or P	100 to > 100,000	Equal to serum levels	Variable findings; no pathognomonic features
Esophageal rupture	Turbid to purulent; red-brown	< 5000 to > 50,000 P	1000–10,000	Usually low	High amylase level (salivary origin); pneumothorax in 25% of cases; effusion usually on left side; pH < 6.0 strongly suggests diagnosis
Pancreatitis	Turbid to serosanguineous	1000–50,000 P	1000–10,000	Equal to serum levels	Usually left-sided; high amylase level

LD, lactate dehydrogenase; M, mononuclear cell predominance; P, polymorphonuclear leukocyte predominance.

is 44% sensitive, and the combination of closed pleural biopsy with culture and histologic examination for granulomas is 70–90% sensitive for the diagnosis of pleural tuberculosis.

Pleural fluid specimens should be sent for cytologic examination in all cases of exudative effusions in patients suspected of harboring an underlying malignancy. The diagnostic yield depends on the nature and extent of the underlying malignancy. Sensitivity is between 50% and 65%. A negative cytologic examination in a patient with a high prior probability of malignancy should be followed by one repeat thoracentesis. If that examination is negative, thoracoscopy (by a pulmonologist or by VATS) is preferred to closed pleural biopsy. The sensitivity of thoracoscopy is 92–96%.

C. Imaging

The lung is less dense than water and floats on pleural fluid that accumulates in dependent regions. Subpulmonary fluid may appear as lateral displacement of the apex of the diaphragm with an abrupt slope to the costophrenic sulcus or a greater than 2-cm separation between the gastric air bubble and the lung. On a standard upright chest radiograph, approximately 75–100 mL of pleural fluid must accumulate in the posterior costophrenic sulcus to be visible on the lateral view, and 175–200 mL must be present in the lateral costophrenic sulcus to be visible on the frontal view. Chest CT scans may identify as little as 10 mL of fluid. At least 1 cm of fluid on the decubitus view is necessary to permit blind thoracentesis. Ultrasonography is useful to guide thoracentesis in the setting of smaller effusions.

Pleural fluid may become trapped (loculated) by pleural adhesions, thereby forming unusual collections along the lateral chest wall or within lung fissures. Round or oval fluid collections in fissures that resemble intraparenchymal masses are called pseudotumors. Massive pleural effusion causing opacification of an entire hemithorax is most commonly caused by cancer but may be seen in tuberculosis and other diseases.

▶ Treatment

A. Transudative Pleural Effusion

Transudative pleural effusions characteristically occur in the absence of pleural disease. Treatment is directed at the underlying condition. Therapeutic thoracentesis for severe dyspnea typically offers only transient benefit. Pleurodesis and tube thoracostomy are rarely indicated.

B. Malignant Pleural Effusion

Approximately 15% of patients dying of cancer are reported to have malignant pleural effusions. Almost any form of cancer may cause effusions, but the most common causes are lung cancer (one-third of cases) and breast cancer. In 5–10% of malignant pleural effusions, no primary tumor is identified.

Between 40% and 80% of exudative pleural effusions are malignant, while over 90% of malignant pleural effusions are exudative. The most common mechanisms contributing to the formation of malignant effusions include direct tumor involvement of the pleura, local inflammation in response to tumor spread, and impairment or disruption of lymphatics. The term "paramalignant pleural effusion" refers to an effusion in a patient with cancer when repeated attempts to identify tumor cells in the pleura or pleural fluid are nondiagnostic but when there is a presumptive relation to the underlying malignancy. For example, superior vena cava syndrome with elevated systemic venous pressures causing a transudative effusion would be "paramalignant."

Most patients with malignant effusions have advanced disease and multiple symptoms. Dyspnea occurs in over half of patients with malignant pleural effusions. The cause of dyspnea is probably related to mechanical distortion of the lung and chest wall. Hypoxemia from intrapulmonary shunting and $\dot{V}/\dot{Q}$ mismatching is common and may be severe. Treatment may be systemic, with therapy for the underlying malignancy; or local, to address specific symptoms related to the effusion itself. Local treatment usually involves drainage through repeated thoracentesis or placement of a chest tube. Pleurodesis is a procedure by which an irritant is placed into the pleural space following chest tube drainage and lung reexpansion. The goal is to form fibrous adhesions between the visceral and parietal pleura, resulting in obliteration of the pleural space to prevent or significantly reduce reaccumulation of pleural fluid. Multiple agents have been used for pleurodesis, but the two in most common use are doxycycline (500 mg in 50–100 mL saline) and sterile, asbestos-free talc (by poudrage at thoracoscopy using 5 g or instillation of talc slurry through a chest tube using 4–5 g in 50 mL saline). Doxycycline and talc are associated with a 70–75% and a 90% success rate, respectively. Major side effects are pain and fever, which appear to be less common with talc. Pain associated with pleurodesis can be extreme. Patients should be premedicated with an anxiolytic-amnestic agent in addition to opioid analgesics.

Alternative strategies include an indwelling pleural catheter (eg, Pleurex) to facilitate home drainage. These catheters provide suitable ambulatory patients symptom relief while avoiding hospitalization, with approximately a 40% rate of spontaneous pleurodesis.

C. Parapneumonic Pleural Effusion

Parapneumonic pleural effusions are exudates that accompany approximately 40% of bacterial pneumonias. They are divided into three categories: simple or uncomplicated, complicated, and empyema. Uncomplicated parapneumonic effusions are free-flowing sterile exudates of modest size that resolve quickly with antibiotic treatment of pneumonia. They do not need drainage. Empyema is gross infection of the pleural space indicated by positive Gram stain or culture. Empyema should always be drained by tube thoracostomy to facilitate clearance of infection and to reduce the probability of fibrous encasement of the lung, causing permanent pulmonary impairment.

Complicated parapneumonic effusions present the most difficult management decisions. They tend to be larger than simple parapneumonic effusions and to show more evidence of inflammatory stimuli such as low glucose level, low pH, or evidence of loculation. Inflammation probably reflects ongoing bacterial invasion of the pleural space despite rare positive bacterial cultures. The morbidity associated with complicated effusions is due to their tendency to form a fibropurulent pleural "peel," trapping otherwise functional lung and leading to permanent impairment. Tube thoracostomy is indicated when pleural fluid glucose is < 60 mg/dL or the pH is < 7.2. These thresholds have not been prospectively validated and should not be interpreted strictly. The clinician should consider drainage of a complicated effusion if the pleural fluid pH is between 7.2 and 7.3 or the LD is > 1000 units/mL. Pleural fluid cell count and protein have little diagnostic value in this setting.

Tube thoracostomy drainage of empyema or parapneumonic effusions is frequently complicated by loculation that prevents adequate drainage. Intrapleural injection of fibrinolytic agents (streptokinase, 250,000 units, or urokinase, 100,000 units, in 50–100 mL of normal saline once or twice daily) is often used to improve drainage, although data are mixed as to whether this intervention improves outcomes.

D. Hemothorax

A small-volume hemothorax that is stable or improving on chest radiographs may be managed by close observation. In all other cases, hemothorax is treated by immediate insertion of a large-bore thoracostomy tube to: (1) drain existing blood and clot, (2) quantify the amount of bleeding, (3) reduce the risk of fibrothorax, and (4) permit apposition of the pleural surfaces in an attempt to reduce hemorrhage. Thoracotomy may be indicated to control hemorrhage, remove clot, and treat complications such as bronchopleural fistula formation.

Froudarakis ME. Diagnostic work-up of pleural effusions. Respiration. 2008;75(1):4–13. [PMID: 18185024]

Heffner JE et al. Recent advances in the diagnosis and management of malignant pleural effusions. Mayo Clin Proc. 2008 Feb;83(2):235–50. [PMID: 18241636]

Sahn SA. The value of pleural fluid analysis. Am J Med Sci. 2008 Jan;335(1):7–15. [PMID: 18195577]

SPONTANEOUS PNEUMOTHORAX

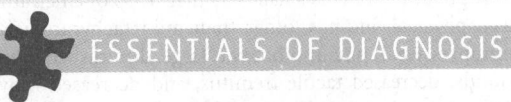
ESSENTIALS OF DIAGNOSIS

► Acute onset of unilateral chest pain and dyspnea.

▶ Minimal physical findings in mild cases; unilateral chest expansion, decreased tactile fremitus, hyperresonance, diminished breath sounds, mediastinal shift, cyanosis and hypotension in tension pneumothorax.

▶ Presence of pleural air on chest radiograph.

General Considerations

Pneumothorax, or accumulation of air in the pleural space, is classified as spontaneous (primary or secondary) or traumatic. Primary spontaneous pneumothorax occurs in the absence of an underlying lung disease, whereas secondary spontaneous pneumothorax is a complication of preexisting pulmonary disease. Traumatic pneumothorax results from penetrating or blunt trauma. Iatrogenic pneumothorax may follow procedures such as thoracentesis, pleural biopsy, subclavian or internal jugular vein catheter placement, percutaneous lung biopsy, bronchoscopy with transbronchial biopsy, and positive-pressure mechanical ventilation. Tension pneumothorax usually occurs in the setting of penetrating trauma, lung infection, cardiopulmonary resuscitation, or positive-pressure mechanical ventilation. In tension pneumothorax, the pressure of air in the pleural space exceeds ambient pressure throughout the respiratory cycle. A check-valve mechanism allows air to enter the pleural space on inspiration and prevents egress of air on expiration.

Primary pneumothorax affects mainly tall, thin boys and men between the ages of 10 and 30 years. It is thought to occur from rupture of subpleural apical blebs in response to high negative intrapleural pressures. Family history and cigarette smoking may also be important factors.

Secondary pneumothorax occurs as a complication of COPD, asthma, cystic fibrosis, tuberculosis, *Pneumocystis* pneumonia, menstruation (catamenial pneumothorax), and a wide variety of interstitial lung diseases including sarcoidosis, lymphangioleiomyomatosis, Langerhans cell histiocytosis, and tuberous sclerosis. Aerosolized pentamidine and a prior history of *Pneumocystis* pneumonia are considered risk factors for the development of pneumothorax. One-half of patients with pneumothorax in the setting of recurrent *Pneumocystis* pneumonia will develop pneumothorax on the contralateral side. The mortality rate of pneumothorax in *Pneumocystis* pneumonia is high.

Clinical Findings

A. Symptoms and Signs

Chest pain ranging from minimal to severe on the affected side and dyspnea occur in nearly all patients. Symptoms usually begin during rest and usually resolve within 24 hours even if the pneumothorax persists. Alternatively, pneumothorax may present with life-threatening respiratory failure if underlying COPD or asthma is present.

If pneumothorax is small (less than 15% of a hemithorax), physical findings, other than mild tachycardia, are unimpressive. If pneumothorax is large, diminished breath sounds, decreased tactile fremitus, and decreased movement of the chest are often noted. Tension pneumothorax should be suspected in the presence of marked tachycardia, hypotension, and mediastinal or tracheal shift.

B. Laboratory Findings

Arterial blood gas analysis is often unnecessary but reveals hypoxemia and acute respiratory alkalosis in most patients. Left-sided primary pneumothorax may produce QRS axis and precordial T wave changes on the ECG that may be misinterpreted as acute myocardial infarction.

C. Imaging

Demonstration of a visceral pleural line on chest radiograph is diagnostic and may only be seen on an expiratory film. A few patients have secondary pleural effusion that demonstrates a characteristic air-fluid level on chest radiography. In supine patients, pneumothorax on a conventional chest radiograph may appear as an abnormally radiolucent costophrenic sulcus (the "deep sulcus" sign). In patients with tension pneumothorax, chest radiographs show a large amount of air in the affected hemithorax and contralateral shift of the mediastinum.

Differential Diagnosis

If the patient is a young, tall, thin, cigarette-smoking man, the diagnosis of primary spontaneous pneumothorax is usually obvious and can be confirmed by chest radiograph. In secondary pneumothorax, it is sometimes difficult to distinguish loculated pneumothorax from an emphysematous bleb. Occasionally, pneumothorax may mimic myocardial infarction, pulmonary embolization, or pneumonia.

Complications

Tension pneumothorax may be life-threatening. Pneumomediastinum and subcutaneous emphysema may occur as complications of spontaneous pneumothorax. If pneumomediastinum is detected, rupture of the esophagus or a bronchus should be considered.

Treatment

Treatment depends on the severity of pneumothorax and the nature of the underlying disease. In a reliable patient with a small (< 15% of a hemithorax), stable spontaneous primary pneumothorax, observation alone may be appropriate. Many small pneumothoraces resolve spontaneously as air is absorbed from the pleural space; supplemental oxygen therapy may increase the rate of reabsorption. Simple aspiration drainage of pleural air with a small-bore catheter (eg, 16 gauge angiocatheter or larger drainage catheter) can be performed for spontaneous primary pneumothoraces that are large or progressive. Placement of a small-bore chest tube (7F to 14F) attached to a one-way Heimlich valve provides protection against development of tension pneumothorax and may permit observation from home. The patient should be treated symptomatically for cough and chest pain, and followed with serial chest radiographs every 24 hours.

Patients with secondary pneumothorax, large pneumothorax, tension pneumothorax, or severe symptoms or those who have a pneumothorax on mechanical ventilation should undergo chest tube placement (tube thoracostomy). The chest tube is placed under water-seal drainage, and suction is applied until the lung expands. The chest tube can be removed after the air leak subsides.

All patients who smoke should be advised to discontinue smoking and warned that the risk of recurrence is 50%. Future exposure to high altitudes, flying in unpressurized aircraft, and scuba diving should be avoided.

Indications for thoracoscopy or open thoracotomy include recurrences of spontaneous pneumothorax, any occurrence of bilateral pneumothorax, and failure of tube thoracostomy for the first episode (failure of lung to reexpand or persistent air leak). Surgery permits resection of blebs responsible for the pneumothorax and pleurodesis by mechanical abrasion and insufflation of talc.

Management of pneumothorax in patients with *Pneumocystis* pneumonia is challenging because of a tendency toward recurrence, and there is no consensus on the best approach. Use of a small chest tube attached to a Heimlich valve has been proposed to allow the patient to leave the hospital. Some clinicians favor its insertion early in the course.

▶ **Prognosis**

An average of 30% of patients with spontaneous pneumothorax experience recurrence of the disorder after either observation or tube thoracostomy for the first episode. Recurrence after surgical therapy is less frequent. Following successful therapy, there are no long-term complications.

Baumann MH. Management of spontaneous pneumothorax. Clin Chest Med. 2006 Jun;27(2):369–81. [PMID: 16716824]

Tschopp JM et al. Management of spontaneous pneumothorax: state of the art. Eur Respir J. 2006 Sep;28(3):637–50. [PMID: 16946095]

DISORDERS OF CONTROL OF VENTILATION

The principal influences on ventilatory control are arterial P_{CO_2}, pH, P_{O_2}, and brainstem tissue pH. These variables are monitored by peripheral and central chemoreceptors. Under normal conditions, the ventilatory control system maintains arterial pH and P_{CO_2} within narrow limits; arterial P_{O_2} is more loosely controlled.

Abnormal control of ventilation can be seen with a variety of conditions ranging from rare disorders such as Ondine curse, neuromuscular disorders, myxedema, starvation, and carotid body resection to more common disorders such as asthma, COPD, obesity, congestive heart failure, and sleep-related breathing disorders. A few of these disorders will be discussed in this section.

Annane D et al. Nocturnal mechanical ventilation for chronic hypoventilation in patients with neuromuscular and chest wall disorders. Cochrane Database Syst Rev. 2007 Oct 17;(4):CD001941. [PMID: 17943762]

PRIMARY ALVEOLAR HYPOVENTILATION

Primary alveolar hypoventilation ("Ondine curse") is a rare syndrome of unknown cause characterized by inadequate alveolar ventilation despite normal neurologic function and normal airways, lungs, chest wall, and ventilatory muscles. Hypoventilation is even more marked during sleep. Individuals with this disorder are usually nonobese males in their third or fourth decades who have lethargy, headache, and somnolence. Dyspnea is absent. Physical examination may reveal cyanosis and evidence of pulmonary hypertension and cor pulmonale. Hypoxemia and hypercapnia are present and improve with voluntary hyperventilation. Erythrocytosis is common. Treatment with ventilatory stimulants is usually unrewarding. Augmentation of ventilation by mechanical methods (phrenic nerve stimulation, rocking bed, mechanical ventilators) has been helpful to some patients. Adequate oxygenation should be maintained with supplemental oxygen, but nocturnal oxygen therapy should be prescribed only if diagnostic nocturnal polysomnography has demonstrated its efficacy and safety. Primary alveolar hypoventilation resembles—but should be distinguished from—**central alveolar hypoventilation**, in which impaired ventilatory drive with chronic respiratory acidemia and hypoxemia follows an insult to the brainstem (eg, bulbar poliomyelitis, infarction, meningitis, encephalitis, trauma).

OBESITY-HYPOVENTILATION SYNDROME (Pickwickian Syndrome)

In obesity-hypoventilation syndrome, alveolar hypoventilation appears to result from a combination of blunted ventilatory drive and increased mechanical load imposed upon the chest by obesity. Voluntary hyperventilation returns the P_{CO_2} and the P_{O_2} toward normal values, a correction not seen in lung diseases causing chronic respiratory failure such as COPD. Most patients with obesity-hypoventilation syndrome also suffer from obstructive sleep apnea (see below), which must be treated aggressively if identified as a comorbid disorder. Therapy of obesity-hypoventilation syndrome consists mainly of weight loss, which improves hypercapnia and hypoxemia as well as the ventilatory responses to hypoxia and hypercapnia. NPPV is helpful in some patients. Respiratory stimulants may be helpful and include theophylline, acetazolamide, and medroxyprogesterone acetate, 10–20 mg every 8 hours orally. Improvement in hypoxemia, hypercapnia, erythrocytosis, and cor pulmonale are goals of therapy.

Crummy F et al. Obesity and the lung: 2. Obesity and sleep-disordered breathing. Thorax. 2008 Aug;63(8):738–46. [PMID: 18663071]

Mokhlesi B et al. Assessment and management of patients with obesity hypoventilation syndrome. Proc Am Thorac Soc. 2008 Feb 15;5(2):218–25. [PMID: 18250215]

HYPERVENTILATION SYNDROMES

Hyperventilation is an increase in alveolar ventilation that leads to hypocapnia. It may be caused by a variety of conditions, such as pregnancy, hypoxemia, obstructive and infiltrative lung diseases, sepsis, hepatic dysfunction, fever, and pain. The term "central neurogenic hyperventilation" denotes a monotonous, sustained pattern of rapid and deep breathing seen in comatose patients with brainstem injury of multiple causes. Functional hyperventilation may be acute or chronic. **Acute hyperventilation** presents with hyperpnea, paresthesias, carpopedal spasm, tetany, and anxiety. **Chronic hyperventilation** may present with various nonspecific symptoms, including fatigue, dyspnea, anxiety, palpitations, and dizziness. The diagnosis of chronic hyperventilation syndrome is established if symptoms are reproduced during voluntary hyperventilation. Once organic causes of hyperventilation have been excluded, treatment of acute hyperventilation consists of rebreathing expired gas from a paper bag held over the face in order to decrease respiratory alkalemia and its associated symptoms. Anxiolytic drugs may also be useful.

Foster GT et al. Respiratory alkalosis. Respir Care. 2001 Apr;46(4):384–91. [PMID: 11262557]

Laffey JG et al. Hypocapnia. N Engl J Med. 2002 Jul 4;347(1):43–53. [PMID: 12097540]

SLEEP-RELATED BREATHING DISORDERS

Abnormal ventilation during sleep is manifested by apnea (breath cessation for at least 10 seconds) or hypopnea (decrement in airflow with drop in hemoglobin saturation of at least 4%). Episodes of apnea are **central** if ventilatory effort is absent for the duration of the apneic episode, **obstructive** if ventilatory effort persists throughout the apneic episode but no airflow occurs because of transient obstruction of the upper airway, and **mixed** if absent ventilatory effort precedes upper airway obstruction during the apneic episode. Pure central sleep apnea is uncommon; it may be an isolated finding or may occur in patients with primary alveolar hypoventilation or with lesions of the brainstem. Obstructive and mixed sleep apneas are more common and may be associated with life-threatening cardiac arrhythmias, severe hypoxemia during sleep, daytime somnolence, pulmonary hypertension, cor pulmonale, systemic hypertension, and secondary erythrocytosis.

Definitive diagnostic evaluation for suspected sleep apnea should include otorhinolaryngologic examination and overnight polysomnography (the monitoring of multiple physiologic factors during sleep). Electroencephalography, electro-oculography, electromyography, electrocardiography, pulse oximetry, and measurement of respiratory effort and airflow are performed in a complete evaluation. Screening may be performed using home nocturnal pulse oximetry, which when normal has a high negative predictive value in ruling out significant sleep apnea.

OBSTRUCTIVE SLEEP APNEA

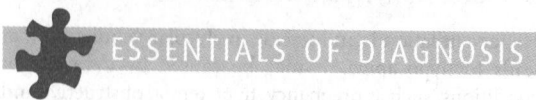

ESSENTIALS OF DIAGNOSIS

▶ Daytime somnolence or fatigue.

▶ A history of loud snoring with witnessed apneic events.

▶ Overnight polysomnography demonstrating apneic episodes with hypoxemia.

General Considerations

Upper airway obstruction during sleep occurs when loss of normal pharyngeal muscle tone allows the pharynx to collapse passively during inspiration. Patients with anatomically narrowed upper airways (eg, micrognathia, macroglossia, obesity, tonsillar hypertrophy) are predisposed to the development of obstructive sleep apnea. Ingestion of alcohol or sedatives before sleeping or nasal obstruction of any type, including the common cold, may precipitate or worsen the condition. Hypothyroidism and cigarette smoking are additional risk factors for obstructive sleep apnea. Before making the diagnosis of obstructive sleep apnea, a drug history should be obtained and a seizure disorder, narcolepsy, and depression should be excluded.

Clinical Findings

A. Symptoms and Signs

Most patients with obstructive or mixed sleep apnea are obese, middle-aged men. Systemic hypertension is common. Patients may complain of excessive daytime somnolence, morning sluggishness and headaches, daytime fatigue, cognitive impairment, recent weight gain, and impotence. Bed partners usually report loud cyclical snoring, breath cessation, witnessed apneas, restlessness, and thrashing movements of the extremities during sleep. Personality changes, poor judgment, work-related problems, depression, and intellectual deterioration (memory impairment, inability to concentrate) may also be observed.

Physical examination may be normal or may reveal systemic and pulmonary hypertension with cor pulmonale. The patient may appear sleepy or even fall asleep during the evaluation. The oropharynx is frequently found to be narrowed by excessive soft tissue folds, large tonsils, pendulous uvula, or prominent tongue. Nasal obstruction by a deviated nasal septum, poor nasal airflow, and a nasal twang to the speech may be observed. A "bull neck" appearance is common.

B. Laboratory Findings

Erythrocytosis is common. A hemoglobin level and thyroid function tests should be obtained. Observation of the sleeping patient reveals loud snoring interrupted by episodes of increasingly strong ventilatory effort that fail to produce airflow. A loud snort often accompanies the first breath following an apneic episode. **Polysomnography** reveals apneic episodes lasting as long as 60 seconds. Oxygen saturation falls, often to very low levels. Bradydysrhythmias such as sinus bradycardia, sinus arrest, or atrioventricular block may occur. Tachydysrhythmias, including paroxysmal supraventricular tachycardia, atrial fibrillation, and ventricular tachycardia, may be seen once airflow is reestablished.

Treatment

Weight loss and strict avoidance of alcohol and hypnotic medications are the first steps in management. Weight loss may be curative, but most patients are unable to lose the 10–20% of body weight required. **Nasal continuous positive airway pressure (nasal CPAP)** at night is curative in many patients. Polysomnography is frequently necessary to determine the level of CPAP (usually 5–15 cm H_2O) necessary to abolish obstructive apneas. Unfortunately, only about 75% of patients continue to use nasal CPAP after 1 year. Pharmacologic therapy for obstructive sleep apnea is disappointing. Supplemental oxygen may lessen the severity of nocturnal desaturation but may also lengthen apneas; it should not be routinely prescribed. Polysomnography is necessary to assess the effects of oxygen therapy. Mechanical devices inserted into the mouth at bedtime to hold the jaw forward and prevent pharyngeal occlusion have modest effectiveness in relieving apnea; however, patient compliance is not optimal.

Uvulopalatopharyngoplasty (UPPP), a procedure consisting of resection of pharyngeal soft tissue and amputation of approximately 15 mm of the free edge of the soft palate and uvula, is helpful in approximately 50% of selected patients. It is more effective in eliminating snoring than apneic episodes. UPPP may now be performed on an outpatient basis with a laser. **Nasal septoplasty** is performed if gross anatomic nasal septal deformity is present. **Tracheotomy** relieves upper airway obstruction and its physiologic consequences and represents the definitive treatment for obstructive sleep apnea. However, it has numerous adverse effects, including granuloma formation, difficulty with speech, and stoma and airway infection. Furthermore, the long-term care of the tracheotomy, especially in obese patients, can be difficult. Tracheotomy and other maxillofacial surgery approaches are reserved for patients with life-threatening arrhythmias or severe disability who have not responded to conservative therapy.

Some patients with sleep apnea have nocturnal bradycardia. A pilot study in 15 patients with either central or obstructive sleep apnea showed some improvement in oxygen saturation with atrial pacing. This single study must be considered preliminary.

Eckert DJ et al. Central sleep apnea: Pathophysiology and treatment. Chest. 2007 Feb;131(2):595–607. [PMID: 17296668]

Kakkar RK et al. Positive airway pressure treatment for obstructive sleep apnea. Chest. 2007 Sep;132(3):1057–72. [PMID: 17873201]

Patil SP et al. Adult obstructive sleep apnea: pathophysiology and diagnosis. Chest. 2007 Jul;132(1):325–37. [PMID: 17625094]

ACUTE RESPIRATORY FAILURE

Respiratory failure is defined as respiratory dysfunction resulting in abnormalities of oxygenation or ventilation (CO_2 elimination) severe enough to threaten the function of vital organs. Arterial blood gas criteria for respiratory failure are not absolute but may be arbitrarily established as a Po_2 under 60 mm Hg or a Pco_2 over 50 mm Hg. Acute respiratory failure may occur in a variety of pulmonary and

Table 9–24. Selected causes of acute respiratory failure in adults.

Airway disorders	Neuromuscular and related disorders
Asthma	Primary neuromuscular diseases
Acute exacerbation of chronic bronchitis or emphysema	Guillain-Barré syndrome
Obstruction of pharynx, larynx, trachea, main stem bronchus, or lobar bronchus by edema, mucus, mass, or foreign body	Myasthenia gravis
	Poliomyelitis
	Polymyositis
	Drug- or toxin-induced
Pulmonary edema	Botulism
Increased hydrostatic pressure	Organophosphates
Left ventricular dysfunction (eg, myocardial ischemia, heart failure)	Neuromuscular blocking agents
Mitral regurgitation	Aminoglycosides
Left atrial outflow obstruction (eg, mitral stenosis)	Spinal cord injury
	Phrenic nerve injury or dysfunction
Volume overload states	Electrolyte disturbances: hypokalemia, hypophosphatemia
Increased pulmonary capillary permeability	Myxedema
Acute respiratory distress syndrome	**Central nervous system disorders**
Acute lung injury	Drugs: sedative, hypnotic, opioid, anesthetics
Unclear etiology	Brainstem respiratory center disorders: trauma, tumor, vascular disorders, hypothyroidism
Neurogenic	
Negative pressure (inspiratory airway obstruction)	
Reexpansion	Intracranial hypertension
Tocolytic-associated	Central nervous system infections
Parenchymal lung disorders	**Increased CO_2 production**
Pneumonia	Fever
Interstitial lung diseases	Infection
Diffuse alveolar hemorrhage syndromes	Hyperalimentation with excess caloric and carbohydrate intake
Aspiration	Hyperthyroidism
Lung contusion	Seizures
Pulmonary vascular disorders	Rigors
Thromboembolism	Drugs
Air embolism	
Amniotic fluid embolism	
Chest wall, diaphragm, and pleural disorders	
Rib fracture	
Flail chest	
Pneumothorax	
Pleural effusion	
Massive ascites	
Abdominal distention and abdominal compartment syndrome	

nonpulmonary disorders (Table 9–24). A complete discussion of treatment of acute respiratory failure is beyond the scope of this chapter. Only a few selected general principles of management will be reviewed here.

► Clinical Findings

Symptoms and signs of acute respiratory failure are those of the underlying disease combined with those of hypoxemia or hypercapnia. The chief symptom of hypoxemia is dyspnea, though profound hypoxemia may exist in the absence of complaints. Signs of hypoxemia include cyanosis, restlessness, confusion, anxiety, delirium, tachypnea, bradycardia or tachycardia, hypertension, cardiac dysrhythmias, and tremor. Dyspnea and headache are the cardinal symptoms of hypercapnia. Signs of hypercapnia include peripheral and conjunctival hyperemia, hypertension, tachycardia, tachypnea, impaired consciousness, papilledema, and asterixis. The symptoms and signs of acute respiratory failure are both insensitive and nonspecific; therefore, the physician must maintain a high index of suspicion and obtain arterial blood gas analysis if respiratory failure is suspected.

► Treatment

Treatment of the patient with acute respiratory failure consists of: (1) specific therapy directed toward the underlying disease; (2) respiratory supportive care directed toward the maintenance of adequate gas exchange; and (3) general supportive care. Only the last two aspects are discussed below.

A. Respiratory Support

Respiratory support has both nonventilatory and ventilatory aspects.

1. Nonventilatory aspects—The main therapeutic goal in acute hypoxemic respiratory failure is to ensure adequate oxygenation of vital organs. Inspired oxygen concentration should be the lowest value that results in an arterial hemoglobin saturation of $\geq$ 90% ($P_{O_2} \geq$ 60 mm Hg). Higher arterial oxygen tensions are of no proven benefit. Restoration of normoxia may rarely cause hypoventilation in patients with chronic hypercapnia; however, *oxygen therapy should not be withheld for fear of causing progressive respiratory acidemia*. Hypoxemia in patients with obstructive airway disease is usually easily corrected by administering low-flow oxygen by nasal cannula (1–3 L/min) or Venturi mask (24–40%). Higher concentrations of oxygen are necessary to correct hypoxemia in patients with ARDS, pneumonia, and other parenchymal lung diseases.

2. Ventilatory aspects—Ventilatory support consists of maintaining patency of the airway and ensuring adequate alveolar ventilation. Mechanical ventilation may be provided via face mask (noninvasive) or through tracheal intubation.

A. NONINVASIVE POSITIVE-PRESSURE VENTILATION—NPPV delivered via a full face mask or nasal mask has become first-line therapy in COPD patients with hypercapnic respiratory failure who can protect and maintain the patency of their airway, handle their own secretions, and tolerate the mask apparatus. Several studies have demonstrated the effectiveness of this therapy in reducing intubation rates and ICU stays in patients with ventilatory

failure. Patients with acute lung injury or ARDS or those who suffer from severely impaired oxygenation do not benefit and should be intubated if they require mechanical ventilation. A bilevel positive pressure ventilation mode is preferred for most patients.

B. TRACHEAL INTUBATION—Indications for tracheal intubation include: (1) hypoxemia despite supplemental oxygen, (2) upper airway obstruction, (3) impaired airway protection, (4) inability to clear secretions, (5) respiratory acidosis, (6) progressive general fatigue, tachypnea, use of accessory respiratory muscles, or mental status deterioration, and (7) apnea. In general, orotracheal intubation is preferred to nasotracheal intubation in urgent or emergency situations because it is easier, faster, and less traumatic. The position of the tip of the endotracheal tube at the level of the aortic arch should be verified by chest radiograph immediately following intubation, and auscultation should be performed to verify that both lungs are being inflated. Only tracheal tubes with high-volume, low-pressure air-filled cuffs should be used. Cuff inflation pressure should be kept below 20 mm Hg if possible to minimize tracheal mucosal injury.

C. MECHANICAL VENTILATION—Indications for mechanical ventilation include: (1) apnea, (2) acute hypercapnia that is not quickly reversed by appropriate specific therapy, (3) severe hypoxemia, and (4) progressive patient fatigue despite appropriate treatment.

Several modes of positive-pressure ventilation are available. Controlled mechanical ventilation (CMV; also known as assist-control or A-C) and synchronized intermittent mandatory ventilation (SIMV) are ventilatory modes in which the ventilator delivers a minimum number of breaths of a specified tidal volume each minute. In both CMV and SIMV, the patient may trigger the ventilator to deliver additional breaths. In CMV, the ventilator responds to breaths initiated by the patient above the set rate by delivering additional full tidal volume breaths. In SIMV, additional breaths are not supported by the ventilator unless the pressure support mode is added. Numerous alternative modes of mechanical ventilation now exist, the most popular being pressure support ventilation (PSV), pressure control ventilation (PCV), and CPAP.

PEEP is useful in improving oxygenation in patients with diffuse parenchymal lung disease such as ARDS. It should be used cautiously in patients with localized parenchymal disease, hyperinflation, or very high airway pressure requirements during mechanical ventilation.

D. COMPLICATIONS OF MECHANICAL VENTILATION—Potential complications of mechanical ventilation are numerous. Migration of the tip of the endotracheal tube into a main bronchus can cause atelectasis of the contralateral lung and overdistention of the intubated lung. **Barotrauma** (alternatively referred to as "volutrauma"), manifested by subcutaneous emphysema, pneumomediastinum, subpleural air cysts, pneumothorax, or systemic gas embolism, may occur in patients whose lungs are overdistended by excessive tidal volumes, especially those with hyperinflation caused by airflow obstruction. Subtle parenchymal lung injury due to overdistention of alveoli is another potential hazard. Strategies to avoid barotrauma include deliberate hypoventilation through the use of low mechanical tidal volumes and respiratory rates, resulting in "permissive hypercapnia."

Acute respiratory alkalosis caused by overventilation is common. Hypotension induced by elevated intrathoracic pressure that results in decreased return of systemic venous blood to the heart may occur in patients treated with PEEP, those with severe airflow obstruction, and those with intravascular volume depletion. Ventilator-associated pneumonia is another serious complication of mechanical ventilation.

B. General Supportive Care

Maintenance of adequate nutrition is vital; parenteral nutrition should be used only when conventional enteral feeding methods are not possible. Overfeeding, especially with carbohydrate-rich formulas, should be avoided, because it can increase CO_2 production and may potentially worsen or induce hypercapnia in patients with limited ventilatory reserve. However, failure to provide adequate nutrition is more common. Hypokalemia and hypophosphatemia may worsen hypoventilation due to respiratory muscle weakness. Sedative-hypnotics and opioid analgesics are frequently used. They should be titrated carefully to avoid oversedation, leading to prolongation of intubation. Temporary paralysis with a nondepolarizing neuromuscular blocking agent is occasionally used to facilitate mechanical ventilation and to lower oxygen consumption. Prolonged muscle weakness due to an acute myopathy is a potential complication of these agents. Myopathy is more common in patients with kidney dysfunction and in those given concomitant corticosteroids.

Psychological and emotional support of the patient and family, skin care to avoid decubitus ulcers, and meticulous avoidance of health care–associated infection and complications of tracheal tubes are vital aspects of comprehensive care for patients with acute respiratory failure.

Attention must also be paid to preventing complications associated with serious illness. Stress gastritis and ulcers may be avoided by administering sucralfate, histamine H_2-receptor antagonists, or proton pump inhibitors. There is some concern that the latter two agents, which raise the gastric pH, may permit increased growth of gram-negative bacteria in the stomach, predisposing to pharyngeal colonization and ultimately health care–associated pneumonia; many clinicians therefore prefer sucralfate. The risk of DVT and PE may be reduced by subcutaneous administration of heparin (5000 units every 12 hours), the use of LMWH, or placement of a sequential compression device on an extremity.

Course & Prognosis

The course and prognosis of acute respiratory failure vary and depend on the underlying disease. The prognosis of acute respiratory failure caused by uncomplicated sedative or narcotic drug overdose is excellent. Acute respiratory failure in patients with COPD who do not require intubation and mechanical ventilation has a good immediate

prognosis. On the other hand, ARDS associated with sepsis has an extremely poor prognosis, with mortality rates of about 90%. Overall, adults requiring mechanical ventilation for all causes of acute respiratory failure have survival rates of 62% to weaning, 43% to hospital discharge, and 30% to 1 year after hospital discharge.

Crummy F et al. Non-invasive positive pressure ventilation for acute respiratory failure: justified or just hot air? Intern Med J. 2007 Feb;37(2):112–8. [PMID: 17229254]
Garpestad E et al. Noninvasive ventilation for critical care. Chest. 2007 Aug;132(2):711–20. [PMID: 17699147]
MacIntyre NR et al; National Association for Medical Direction of Respiratory Care. Management of patients requiring prolonged mechanical ventilation: report of a NAMDRC consensus conference. Chest. 2005 Dec;128(6):3937–54. [PMID: 16354866]

ACUTE RESPIRATORY DISTRESS SYNDROME

ESSENTIALS OF DIAGNOSIS

▶ Acute onset of respiratory failure.

▶ Bilateral radiographic pulmonary infiltrates.

▶ Absence of elevated left atrial pressure (if measured, pulmonary capillary wedge pressure ≤ 18 mm Hg).

▶ Ratio of partial pressure of oxygen in arterial blood (Pao_2) to fractional concentration of inspired oxygen (Fio_2) < 200, regardless of the level of PEEP.

General Considerations

ARDS denotes acute hypoxemic respiratory failure following a systemic or pulmonary insult without evidence of heart failure. ARDS is the most severe form of acute lung injury and is characterized by bilateral, widespread radiographic pulmonary infiltrates, normal pulmonary capillary wedge pressure (≤ 18 mm Hg) and a Pao_2/Fio_2 ratio < 200. ARDS may follow a wide variety of clinical events (Table 9–25). Common risk factors for ARDS include sepsis, aspiration of gastric contents, shock, infection, lung contusion, nonthoracic trauma, toxic inhalation, near-drowning, and multiple blood transfusions. About one-third of ARDS patients initially have sepsis syndrome. Pro-inflammatory cytokines released from stimulated inflammatory cells appear to be pivotal in lung injury. Although the mechanism of lung injury varies with the cause, damage to capillary endothelial cells and alveolar epithelial cells is common to ARDS regardless of cause. Damage to these cells causes increased vascular permeability and decreased production and activity of surfactant; these abnormalities lead to interstitial and alveolar pulmonary edema, alveolar collapse, and hypoxemia.

Clinical Findings

ARDS is marked by the rapid onset of profound dyspnea that usually occurs 12–48 hours after the initiating event.

Table 9–25. Selected disorders associated with ARDS.

Systemic Insults	Pulmonary Insults
Trauma	Aspiration of gastric contents
Sepsis	Embolism of thrombus, fat, air, or
Pancreatitis	amniotic fluid
Shock	Miliary tuberculosis
Multiple transfusions	Diffuse pneumonia (eg, SARS)
Disseminated intravascular	Acute eosinophilic pneumonia
coagulation	Cryptogenic organizing pneumonitis
Burns	Upper airway obstruction
Drugs and drug overdose	Free-base cocaine smoking
Opioids	Near-drowning
Aspirin	Toxic gas inhalation
Phenothiazines	Nitrogen dioxide
Tricyclic antidepressants	Chlorine
Amiodarone	Sulfur dioxide
Chemotherapeutic agents	Ammonia
Nitrofurantoin	Smoke
Protamine	Oxygen toxicity
Thrombotic thrombocytopenic	Lung contusion
purpura	Radiation exposure
Cardiopulmonary bypass	High-altitude exposure
Head injury	Lung reexpansion or reperfusion
Paraquat	

ARDS, acute respiratory distress syndrome; SARS, severe acute respiratory syndrome.

Labored breathing, tachypnea, intercostal retractions, and crackles are noted on physical examination. Chest radiography shows diffuse or patchy bilateral infiltrates that rapidly become confluent; these characteristically spare the costophrenic angles. Air bronchograms occur in about 80% of cases. Upper lung zone venous engorgement is distinctly uncommon. Heart size is normal, and pleural effusions are small or nonexistent. Marked hypoxemia occurs that is refractory to treatment with supplemental oxygen. Many patients with ARDS demonstrate multiple organ failure, particularly involving the kidneys, liver, gut, central nervous system, and cardiovascular system.

Differential Diagnosis

Since ARDS is a physiologic and radiographic syndrome rather than a specific disease, the concept of differential diagnosis does not strictly apply. Normal-permeability ("cardiogenic" or hydrostatic) pulmonary edema must be excluded, however, because specific therapy is available for that disorder. Measurement of pulmonary capillary wedge pressure by means of a flow-directed pulmonary artery catheter may be required in selected patients with suspected cardiac dysfunction. Routine use of the Swan-Ganz catheter in ARDS is discouraged.

Prevention

No measures that effectively prevent ARDS have been identified; specifically, prophylactic use of PEEP in patients at risk for ARDS has not been shown to be effective. Intrave-

nous methylprednisolone does not prevent ARDS when given early to patients with sepsis syndrome or septic shock.

Treatment

Treatment of ARDS must include identification and specific treatment of the underlying precipitating and secondary conditions (eg, sepsis). Meticulous supportive care must then be provided to compensate for the severe dysfunction of the respiratory system associated with ARDS and to prevent complications (see above).

Treatment of the hypoxemia seen in ARDS usually requires tracheal intubation and positive-pressure mechanical ventilation. The lowest levels of PEEP (used to recruit atelectatic alveoli) and supplemental oxygen required to maintain the PaO_2 above 60 mm Hg or the SaO_2 above 90% should be used. Efforts should be made to decrease FIO_2 to less than 60% as soon as possible in order to avoid oxygen toxicity. PEEP can be increased as needed as long as cardiac output and oxygen delivery do not decrease and airway pressures do not increase excessively. Prone positioning may transiently improve oxygenation in selected patients by helping recruit atelectatic alveoli; however, great care must be taken during the maneuver to avoid dislodging catheters and tubes.

A variety of mechanical ventilation strategies are available. A multicenter study of 800 patients demonstrated that a protocol using volume-cycled ventilation with low tidal volumes (6 mL/kg of ideal body weight) resulted in a 10% absolute mortality reduction over therapy with standard tidal volumes (defined as 12 mL/kg of ideal body weight); this trial reported the lowest mortality (31%) of any intervention to date for ARDS.

Cardiac output that falls when PEEP is used may be improved by reducing the level of PEEP or by the judicious use of inotropic drugs (eg, norepinephrine); administering fluids to increase intravascular volume should be done only with great caution because increases in pulmonary capillary pressure worsen pulmonary edema in the presence of increased capillary permeability. Therefore, the goal of fluid management is to maintain pulmonary capillary wedge pressure at the lowest level compatible with adequate cardiac output. Crystalloid solutions should be used when intravascular volume expansion is necessary. Diuretics should be used to reduce intravascular volume if pulmonary capillary wedge pressure is elevated.

Oxygen delivery can be increased in anemic patients by ensuring that hemoglobin concentrations are at least 7 g/dL; patients are not likely to benefit from higher levels. Increasing oxygen delivery to supranormal levels through the use of inotropes and high hemoglobin concentrations is not clinically useful and may be harmful. Strategies to decrease oxygen consumption include the appropriate use of sedatives, analgesics, and antipyretics.

A large number of innovative therapeutic interventions to improve outcomes in ARDS patients have been or are being investigated. Unfortunately, to date, none have consistently shown benefit in clinical trials. Systemic corticosteroids have been studied extensively with variable and inconsistent results. While recent studies suggest some specific improved outcomes when given within the first 2 weeks after the onset of ARDS, the routine use of cortico-steroids is not recommended.

▶ Course & Prognosis

The mortality rate associated with ARDS is 30–40%. If ARDS is accompanied by sepsis, the mortality rate may reach 90%. The major causes of death are the primary illness and secondary complications such as multiple organ system failure or sepsis. Median survival is about 2 weeks. Many patients who succumb to ARDS and its complications die after withdrawal of support (see Withdrawal of Support in Chapter 5). Most survivors of ARDS are left with some pulmonary symptoms (cough, dyspnea, sputum production), which tend to improve over time. Mild abnormalities of oxygenation, diffusing capacity, and lung mechanics persist in some individuals.

Deja M et al. Evidence-based therapy of severe acute respiratory distress syndrome: an algorithm-guided approach. J Int Med Res. 2008 Mar–Apr;36(2):211–21. [PMID: 18380929]

Menitove JE. Transfusion related acute lung injury (TRALI): a review. Mo Med. 2007 May–Jun;104(3):270–5. [PMID: 17619505]

Petrucci N et al. Lung protective ventilation strategy for the acute respiratory distress syndrome. Cochrane Database Syst Rev. 2007 Jul 18;(3):CD003844. [PMID: 17636739]

Wheeler AP et al. Acute lung injury and the acute respiratory distress syndrome: a clinical review. Lancet. 2007 May 5;369(9572):1553–64. [PMID: 17482987]

Wheeler AP et al; National Heart, Lung, and Blood Institute. Acute Respiratory Distress Syndrome (ARDS) Clinical Trials Network. Pulmonary-artery versus central venous catheter to guide treatment of acute lung injury. N Engl J Med. 2006 May 25;354(21):2213–24. [PMID: 16714768]

Wiedemann HP. A perspective on the Fluids and Catheters Treatment Trial (FACTT). Fluid restriction is superior in acute lung injury and ARDS. Cleve Clin J Med. 2008 Jan;75(1):42–8. [PMID: 18236729]

Wiedemann HP et al; National Heart, Lung, and Blood Institute Acute Respiratory Distress Syndrome (ARDS) Clinical Trials Network. Comparison of two fluid-management strategies in acute lung injury. N Engl J Med. 2006 Jun 15;354(24):2564–75. [PMID: 16714767]

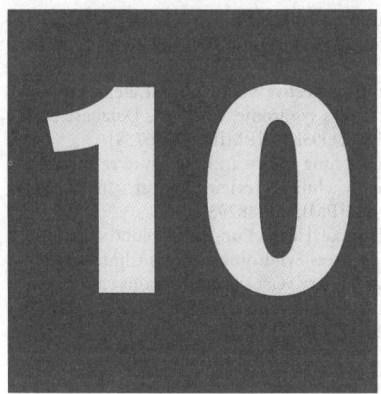

10

Heart Disease

Thomas M. Bashore, MD
Christopher B. Granger, MD
Patrick Hranitzky, MD
Manesh R. Patel, MD

FUNCTIONAL CLASSIFICATION OF HEART DISEASE

In the management of patients with heart disease, it is important to quantify and monitor the severity of symptoms. A commonly used classification system is that of the New York Heart Association (NYHA), shown below. However, in monitoring individual patients, it is better to document specific activities that produce symptoms, such as walking a distance; climbing stairs; or performing activities of daily living, such as using a vacuum sweeper or going grocery shopping.

Class I: No limitation of physical activity. Ordinary physical activity does not cause undue fatigue, dyspnea, or anginal pain.

Class II: Slight limitation of physical activity. Ordinary physical activity results in symptoms.

Class III: Marked limitation of physical activity. Comfortable at rest, but less than ordinary activity causes symptoms.

Class IV: Unable to engage in any physical activity without discomfort. Symptoms may be present even at rest.

Other classifications have been proposed, but these are universally accepted, and clinically can be applied to both heart failure and anginal symptoms. Some experts use the category of **Class V** to describe symptoms that are atypical and can occur either at rest or with exertion.

A task force from the American College of Cardiology/American Heart Association (ACC/AHA) proposed that patients with heart failure be classified into four stages:

Stage A: Those at high risk for congestive heart failure (CHF) but no structural heart disease (ie, hypertension, coronary artery disease [CAD]) and no symptoms.

Stage B: Those with structural heart disease associated with CHF and no symptoms.

Stage C: Those with structural heart disease who have current or prior symptoms.

Stage D: Those with refractory CHF requiring some device or special intervention.

Bonow RO et al. ACC/AHA clinical performance measures for adults with chronic heart failure: a report of the American College of Cardiology/American Heart Association Task Force on Performance Measures (Writing Committee to Develop Heart Failure Clinical Performance Measures) endorsed by the Heart Failure Society of America. J Am Coll Cardiol. 2005 Sep 20;46(6):1144–78. [PMID: 16168305]

CONGENITAL HEART DISEASE

Congenital lesions account for only about 2% of heart disease that presents in adulthood. As surgical and medical techniques have improved, more and more children are now reaching adulthood, and it is estimated that there are well over 1 million adults in the United States surviving with congenital heart disease. In fact, there are more adults with congenital heart disease than children. The ACC/AHA has published guidelines for the management of adults with congenital heart disease.

Bédard E et al. Adult congenital heart disease: a 2008 overview. Br Med Bull. 2008;85:151–80. [PMID: 18334519]
Khairy P et al. Adult congenital heart disease: toward prospective risk assessment of a multisystemic condition. Circulation. 2008 May 6;117(18):2311–2. [PMID: 18458179]
Warnes CA et al. ACC/AHA 2008 Guidelines for the Management of Adults With Congenital Heart Disease. A Report of the American College of Cardiology/American Heart Association Task Force on Practice Guidelines. Circulation. 2008 Dec 2;118(23):e714–833. [PMID: 18997169]

PULMONARY STENOSIS

 ESSENTIALS OF DIAGNOSIS

► Asymptomatic unless patient has at least moderately severe lesions.

► Severe cases may present with right-sided heart failure.

► Echocardiography/Doppler is diagnostic.

► Patients with peak pulmonic valve gradients > 60 mm Hg or mean of 40 mm Hg by echocardiography/Doppler should undergo intervention regardless of symptoms.

► A dysplastic pulmonary valve usually requires surgical treatment, while a domed pulmonary valve stenosis usually can be treated with balloon valvuloplasty.

General Considerations

Stenosis of the pulmonary valve or RV infundibulum increases the resistance to RV outflow, raises the RV pressure, and limits pulmonary blood flow. Pulmonic stenosis is often associated with other cardiac lesions. Pulmonary blood flow preferentially goes to the left lung in valvular pulmonic stenosis. Most patients with valvular pulmonic stenosis have a domed valve, though some patients have a dysplastic valve, especially those with Noonan syndrome. The phenotype of Noonan syndrome includes short stature, web neck, dental malocclusion, antimongoloid slanting of the eyes, mental retardation, and hypogonadism. Unlike those with a domed valve, patients with a dysplastic valve do not have a dilated main pulmonary artery (PA) or commissural fusion. In the absence of associated shunts, arterial saturation is normal. Infundibular stenosis may be so severe that the right ventricle (RV) is divided into a low-pressure and high-pressure chamber (double-chambered RV). Peripheral pulmonic stenosis can accompany valvular pulmonic stenosis and may be part of a variety of clinical syndromes, including the congenital rubella syndrome. Patients who have had the Ross procedure (transfer of the pulmonary valve to the aortic position with a homograft pulmonary valve placed in the pulmonary position) may experience postoperative pulmonic stenosis due to an immune response in the homograft.

Clinical Findings

A. Symptoms and Signs

While most of the older data rely on gradients obtained at cardiac catheterization, now the gradients by echo/Doppler are used clinically. Mild PS is present if the peak gradient by echo/Doppler is < 30 mm Hg, moderate PS is present if the peak gradient is between 30 mm Hg and 60 mm Hg, and severe PS is present if the peak gradient is > 60 mm Hg or the mean gradient is > 40 mm Hg. Mild cases of pulmonic stenosis are asymptomatic; moderate to severe pulmonic stenosis may cause symptoms of dyspnea on exertion, syncope, chest pain, and eventually RV failure.

On examination, there is often a palpable parasternal lift due to right ventricular hypertrophy (RVH) and the pulmonary outflow tract may be palpable if it is enlarged. A loud, harsh systolic murmur and occasionally a prominent thrill are present in the left second and third interspaces parasternally. The murmur radiates toward the left shoulder and increases with inspiration. In mild to moderate pulmonic stenosis, a loud ejection click can be heard to precede the murmur; this sound decreases with inspiration

as the increased RV filling from inspiration prematurely opens the valve during atrial systole. This is the only right-sided auscultatory event that decreases with inspiration. The valve excursion in systole, therefore, is less with inspiration, and the click diminishes in intensity. The second sound is obscured by the murmur in severe cases; the pulmonary component may be diminished, delayed, or absent. A right-sided S_4 and a prominent *a* wave in the venous pulse are present when there is RV diastolic dysfunction or a *c-v* wave if there is tricuspid regurgitation present. Right-sided S_4 gallops may be best heard in the right subclavicular area (where left-sided gallops would be distinctly uncommon). Pulmonic valve regurgitation is relatively uncommon in pulmonary stenosis and may be very difficult to hear, as the gradient between the reduced PA diastolic pressure and the elevated RV diastolic pressure may be quite small (low-pressure pulmonic regurgitation).

B. ECG and Chest Radiography

Right axis deviation or RVH is noted; peaked P waves provide evidence of right atrial (RA) overload. Heart size may be normal on radiographs, or there may be a prominent RV and RA or gross cardiac enlargement, depending on the severity. There is often poststenotic dilation of the main and left pulmonary arteries. The dilatation is primarily due to intrinsic abnormalities of the vessel wall. Pulmonary vascularity is usually normal. A careful look at the chest radiograph may reveal greater vascular perfusion of the left than the right base (Chen sign). Calcium may also be present in the main PA or pulmonic valve.

C. Diagnostic Studies

Echocardiography/Doppler is the diagnostic tool of choice, can provide evidence for a doming valve versus a dysplastic valve, can determine the gradient across the valve, and can provide information regarding subvalvular obstruction and the presence or absence of tricuspid or pulmonic valvular regurgitation. Catheterization is usually unnecessary for the diagnosis; it should be used only if the data are unclear or in preparation for either a percutaneous intervention or surgery. MRI and CT do not add additional information unless there is concern regarding associated cardiac lesions or peripheral pulmonary arterial lesions.

Prognosis & Treatment

Patients with mild pulmonic stenosis have a normal life span with no intervention. Moderate stenosis may be asymptomatic in childhood and adolescence, but symptoms often appear as patients grow older. The degree of stenosis does worsen with time in many patients, so serial follow-up is important. Severe stenosis is rarely associated with sudden death but can cause right heart failure in patients as early as in their 20s and 30s. Pregnancy and exercise tends to be well tolerated except in severe stenosis.

Class I indications for intervention include all symptomatic patients and all those with a resting peak gradient over 60 mm Hg or mean > 40 mm Hg, regardless of symptoms. Percutaneous balloon valvuloplasty is highly successful in domed valve patients and is the treatment of choice. Surgical commissurotomy can also be done, or pulmonary valve replacement (with either a bioprosthetic valve or homograft) when pulmonic regurgitation is too severe or the valve is dysplastic. In accordance with the newest guideline recommendations, endocarditis prophylaxis is unnecessary unless there has been prior pulmonary valve endocarditis (a very rare entity).

When to Refer

All symptomatic patients and all asymptomatic patients whose peak gradient is > 60 mm Hg or mean gradient > 40 mm Hg should be referred to a cardiologist with an interest and expertise in adult congenital heart disease.

Bashore TM. Adult congenital heart disease: right ventricular outflow tract lesions. Circulation. 2007 Apr 10;115(14):1933–47. [PMID: 17420363]

Khambadkone S et al. Percutaneous pulmonary valve implantation in humans: results in 59 consecutive patients. Circulation. 2005 Aug 23;112(8):1189–97. [PMID: 16103239]

Warnes CA et al. ACC/AHA 2008 Guidelines for the Management of Adults With Congenital Heart Disease. A Report of the American College of Cardiology/American Heart Association Task Force on Practice Guidelines. Circulation. 2008 Dec 2;118(23):e714–833. [PMID: 18997169]

Wilson W et al. Prevention of infective endocarditis: guidelines from the American Heart Association: a guideline from the American Heart Association Rheumatic Fever, Endocarditis, and Kawasaki Disease Committee, Council on Cardiovascular Disease in the Young, and the Council on Clinical Cardiology, Council on Cardiovascular Surgery and Anesthesia, and the Quality of Care and Outcomes Research Interdisciplinary Working Group. Circulation. 2007 Oct 9;116(15):1736–54. [PMID: 17446442]

COARCTATION OF THE AORTA

ESSENTIALS OF DIAGNOSIS

► Usual presentation is systemic hypertension.

► A gradient of > 20 mm Hg by echo/Doppler may be significant.

► Associated bicuspid aortic valve (in 50% of patients).

► Some patients have a webbed neck (XO karyotype, Turner syndrome).

► Absent or weak femoral pulses. Delay of the palpable pulse between the femoral and brachial artery.

► Systolic pressure is higher in upper extremities than in lower extremities; diastolic pressures are similar.

► ECG shows left ventricular hypertrophy; chest radiograph shows rib notching; echocardiography/Doppler is diagnostic.

General Considerations

Coarctation of the aorta consists of localized narrowing of the aortic arch just distal to the origin of the left subclavian artery. Its development is thought to be related to accessory ductal material that contracts soon after birth. Therefore, it is not usually present in the fetus. Collateral circulation develops around the coarctation through the intercostal arteries and the branches of the subclavian arteries and can lower the transcoarctation gradient. Coarctation is a cause of secondary hypertension and should be considered in young patients with elevated blood pressure (BP). The renin–angiotensin system is reset and this contributes to the hypertension. Elevated BP may not return to normal after coarctation repair. A bicuspid valve is seen in over 50% of the cases, and there is an increased incidence of cerebral berry aneurysms.

Clinical Findings

A. Symptoms and Signs

If cardiac failure does not occur in infancy, there are usually no symptoms until the hypertension produces left ventricular (LV) failure or cerebral hemorrhage occurs. Strong arterial pulsations are seen in the neck and suprasternal notch. Hypertension is present in the arms, but the pressure is normal or low in the legs. This difference is exaggerated by exercise. Femoral pulsations are weak and are delayed in comparison with the brachial or radial pulse. Patients may have severe coarctation, but with large collaterals may have relatively small gradients because of high flow through the collaterals to the aorta distal to the coarctation. A significant gradient is, therefore, > 20 mm Hg. Late systolic ejection murmurs at the base are often heard better posteriorly, especially over the spinous processes. There may be an associated aortic insufficiency or stenosis murmur due to the bicuspid aortic valve.

B. ECG and Chest Radiography

The ECG usually shows LV hypertrophy (LVH). Radiography shows scalloping of the ribs due to enlarged collateral intercostal arteries, dilation of the left subclavian artery and poststenotic aortic dilation, and LV enlargement. The coarctation region and the poststenotic dilation of the descending aorta may result in a "3" sign along aortic shadow on the PA chest radiograph (the notch in the "3" representing the area of coarctation).

C. Diagnostic Studies

Echocardiography/Doppler is usually diagnostic and may provide additional evidence for a bicuspid aortic valve. Both MRI and CT can also provide excellent images of the coarctation local anatomy. MRI and echocardiography/Doppler can also provide estimates of the gradient across the lesion. Cardiac catheterization provides definitive gradient information and is necessary if percutaneous stenting is to be considered.

Prognosis & Treatment

Cardiac failure is common in infancy and in older untreated patients; it is uncommon in late childhood and young adulthood. Patients with a demonstrated gradient of

> 20 mm Hg should be considered for intervention. Most untreated patients with the adult form of coarctation die before age 50 years from the complications of hypertension, rupture of the aorta, infective endarteritis, or cerebral hemorrhage. Aortic dissection also occurs with increased frequency. Coarctation of any significance may be poorly tolerated in pregnancy because of the inability to support the placental flow.

Resection of the coarctation site has a surgical mortality rate of 1–4% and includes risk of spinal cord injury. The percutaneous interventional procedure of choice is stenting when anatomically feasible. Otherwise, surgical resection (usually with end-to-end anastomosis) should be performed. About 25% of surgically corrected patients continue to be hypertensive years after surgery because of the changes in the renin–angiotensin system.

When to Refer

All patients should be referred to a cardiologist with an interest in adult congenital heart disease.

Golden AB et al. Coarctation of the aorta: stenting in children and adults. Catheter Cardiovasc Interv. 2007 Feb 1;69(2):289–99. [PMID: 17191237]
Warnes CA et al. ACC/AHA 2008 Guidelines for the Management of Adults With Congenital Heart Disease. A Report of the American College of Cardiology/American Heart Association Task Force on Practice Guidelines. Circulation. 2008 Dec 2;118(23):e714–833. [PMID: 18997169]

ATRIAL SEPTAL DEFECT & PATENT FORAMEN OVALE

 ESSENTIALS OF DIAGNOSIS

▸ Often asymptomatic and discovered on routine physical examination.

▸ All atrial septal defects should be closed either by a percutaneous device or by surgery if there is any evidence of an RV volume overload regardless of symptoms.

▸ Echocardiography/Doppler is diagnostic.

▸ A patent foramen ovale is present in 25% of the population but can lead to paradoxic emboli and cerebrovascular events. Suspicion should be highest in patients who have cryptogenic stroke before age 55 years.

General Considerations

The most common form of atrial septal defect (ASD) (80% of cases) is persistence of the ostium secundum in the mid septum; less common is the persistence of the ostium primum (low in the septum). In many patients with an ostium primum defect, there are mitral or tricuspid valve clefts as well as a ventricular septal defect (VSD) as part of the atrioventricular (AV) canal defect. A third form of ASD is the **sinus venosus defect,** a hole usually at of the upper

part of the atrial septum due to failure of the embryonic superior vena cava (SVC) or the inferior vena cava (IVC) to merge with the atria properly. The IVC sinus venosus defect is very rare. The SVC sinus venosus is often associated with anomalous drainage of the right upper pulmonary vein into the SVC. A very uncommon form of ASD is the **coronary sinus ASD** that is basically an unroofed coronary sinus. In all cases, normally oxygenated blood from the higher-pressure LA passes into the RA, increasing RV output and pulmonary blood flow. In children, the degree of shunting across these defects may be quite large (3:1 or so). As the RV diastolic pressure rises from the chronic volume overload, the RA pressure may rise and the degree of left-to-right shunting may decrease. Eventually, if the RA pressure exceeds the LA, the shunt may be right-to-left and cyanosis appears.

The pulmonary pressures are modestly elevated in most patients with an ASD due to the high pulmonary blood flow, but severe pulmonary hypertension with cyanosis (Eisenmenger physiology) is actually unusual, occurring in only about 15% of the patients with an ASD alone. Eventual RV failure may occur though, and most shunts should be corrected unless they are quite small (< 1.5:1 right-to-left shunt). In adults, a large right-to-left shunt may have begun to reverse, so the absolute left-to-right shunt measurement (Qp/Qs, where Qp=pulmonary flow and Qs=systemic flow) at the time the patient is studied may underestimate what it was some years ago. In addition, in most patients the LV compliance normally declines more over time than the RV, and the natural history of small atrial septal shunts is to increase as the patient ages (unless RV failure ensues) as the LA compliance worsens more than the RA.

ASDs predispose to atrial fibrillation due to RA enlargement, and paradoxic right-to-left emboli do occur. Interestingly, paradoxic emboli may be more common in patients with a patent foramen ovale (PFO) than a true ASD, as the eustachian valve in the RA directs flow from the IVC toward the septum, and the usual significant left-to-right flow from an ASD is often not present with a simple PFO. An **aneurysm of the atrial septum** is when there is redundancy of the septum primum through the foramen ovale, although it may include redundancy of the septum secundum as well. When present with a PFO, there is more shunting right to left as the atrial septum swings back and forth. This latter anatomic issue may explain why more right to left shunting occurs in patients with an atrial septal aneurysm and PFO than in those with a PFO alone.

Clinical Findings

A. Symptoms and Signs

Patients with small or moderate ASDs or with a PFO are asymptomatic unless a complication occurs. With large shunts, exertional dyspnea or cardiac failure may develop, most commonly in the fourth decade of life or later. Prominent RV and PA pulsations are readily visible and palpable. A moderately loud systolic ejection murmur can be heard in the second and third interspaces parasternally as a result of increased PA flow. S_2 is widely split and does not vary with breathing due to the fact that the left-to-right shunt decreases as the RA pressure increases with inspiration. In very large left-to-right shunts, a tricuspid rumble may be heard due to the high flow.

B. ECG and Chest Radiography

Right axis deviation or RVH may be present depending on the size of the RV volume overload. Incomplete or complete right bundle branch block is present in nearly all cases of ASD, and superior axis deviation is noted in the AV canal defect, where complete heart block is often seen as well. With sinus venosus defects, the P axis is leftward of +15° due to abnormal atrial activation with loss of the upper RA tissue from around the sinus node. The chest radiograph shows large pulmonary arteries, increased pulmonary vascularity, an enlarged RA and RV, and a small aortic knob with all pre-tricuspid valve cardiac left-to-right shunts.

C. Diagnostic Studies

Echocardiography demonstrates evidence of RA and RV volume overload. The atrial defect is usually observed, though sinus venosus defects may be elusive. Many patients with a PFO also have an atrial septal aneurysm. Echocardiography with agitated saline bubble contrast can demonstrate a right-to-left shunt and both pulsed and color flow Doppler flow studies can demonstrate shunting in either direction. A transesophageal echocardiogram (TEE) is helpful when transthoracic echocardiography quality is not optimal, and it improves the sensitivity for small shunts and provides a better assessment of PFO anatomy. Radionuclide flow studies quantify left-to-right shunting by observing the bolus of contrast within the lung fields and demonstrating early recirculation. Both CT and MRI can elucidate the atrial septal anatomy and demonstrate associated lesions. Cardiac catheterization is often helpful, especially if there are associated anomalous pulmonary veins. The size and location of the shunt can be determined and the pulmonary pressure and pulmonary vascular resistance (PVR) measured. Cardiac catheterization is required if percutaneous closure is to be contemplated.

▶ Prognosis & Treatment

Patients with small atrial shunts may live a normal life span. Large shunts usually cause disability by age 40 years. Because left-to-right shunts tend to increase with age-related changes in LV compliance, most clinicians believe that closure of all left-to-right shunts over 1.5:1 should be accomplished. This situation always results in RV volume overload. Current guidelines suggest that all ASDs should be closed if there is evidence of RV volume overload on echocardiogram. Increased PVR and hypertension secondary to pulmonary vascular disease rarely occur in childhood or young adult life in secundum defects but are more common in primum defects. After age 40 years, cardiac arrhythmias (especially atrial fibrillation) and heart failure may occur due to the chronic right heart volume overload. Paradoxical systemic arterial embolization becomes more of a concern as RV compliance is lost and the left-to-right shunt begins to reverse.

PFOs are not associated with significant shunting, and therefore the patients are asymptomatic and the heart size is normal. However, PFOs are responsible for most paradoxical emboli and are one of the most frequent causes of cryptogenic strokes in patients under age 55 years.

Small ASDs do not require intervention if echocardiography shows that the shunt is not creating an RV volume overload. Surgery involves anything from simple stitching of the foramen closed to patching of the hole with Dacron or a pericardial patch. Anomalous pulmonary venous connections are baffled to the LA through the sinus venosus defect when such anomalous veins are present. For ostium secundum ASDs, percutaneous closure by use of a variety of devices is now preferred over surgery. The percutaneous closure devices often resemble double umbrellas that lock the septum between the Dacron umbrellas when opened, though many designs are becoming available.

Patients with a PFO who have symptoms related to stroke or transient ischemic attack (especially if the age is under 55) or who have hypoxemia (especially upon standing—so called platypnea orthodeoxia) should probably have the PFO closed if no other cause for symptoms is evident. Migraine headaches may be more common in patients with a PFO, suggesting some unknown substance normally metabolized in the lung is entering the systemic circulation through the PFO, but current data remain unclear in this regard. For patients with cryptogenic stroke or transient ischemic attack, it is uncertain whether closure of the PFO, either by open surgical or percutaneous techniques, has any advantage over anticoagulation with either warfarin or aspirin. Although there are no data yet suggesting that PFO closure is better than medical therapy, ongoing randomized trials will help settle this issue.

▶ When to Refer

- All patients with an ASD initially discovered at echo/Doppler should be evaluated by a cardiologist with expertise in adult congenital disease to ensure no other structural disease is present.
- If the RA and RV sizes remain normal, serial echocardiography (yearly) should be performed.
- If the RA and RV volumes increase, then referral to a cardiologist who performs percutaneous closure is warranted.

Kim MS et al. Transcatheter closure of intracardiac defects in adults. J Interv Cardiol. 2007 Dec;20(6):524–45. [PMID: 18042058]

Kizer JR. Patent foramen ovale and cryptogenic stroke. Am J Med. 2007 Dec;120(12):e13. [PMID: 18060903]

Warnes CA et al. ACC/AHA 2008 Guidelines for the Management of Adults With Congenital Heart Disease. A Report of the American College of Cardiology/American Heart Association Task Force on Practice Guidelines. Circulation. 2008 Dec 2;118(23):e714–833. [PMID: 18997169]

VENTRICULAR SEPTAL DEFECT

ESSENTIALS OF DIAGNOSIS

▶ A restrictive VSD is small and makes a louder murmur than an unrestricted one.

▶ Small defects may be asymptomatic.

▶ Larger defects may result in pulmonary hypertension (Eisenmenger physiology) if not repaired.

▶ Echocardiography/Doppler is diagnostic.

► General Considerations

De novo VSDs are uncommon in adults. Congenital VSDs occur in various parts of the ventricular septum. Four types are often described: in **type A,** the VSD lies underneath the semilunar valves; in **type B,** the VSD is membranous with three variations; in **type C,** the inlet VSD is present below the tricuspid valve and often part of the AV canal defect; and **type D** is the muscular VSD. Membranous and muscular septal defects may spontaneously close in childhood as the septum grows and hypertrophies. A left-to-right shunt is present unless there is associated RV hypertension. The smaller the defect, the greater the gradient from the LV to the RV and the louder the murmur. The presentation in adults is dependent on the size of the shunt and whether there is associated pulmonic or subpulmonic stenosis that has protected the lung from the systemic pressure and volume. Unprotected lungs with large shunts invariably lead to pulmonary vascular disease and severe pulmonary hypertension (Eisenmenger physiology).

► Clinical Findings

A. Symptoms and Signs

The clinical features depend on the size of the defect and the presence or absence of RV outflow obstruction or an increased PVR. Small shunts are associated with loud, harsh holosystolic murmurs in the left third and fourth interspaces along the sternum. Larger shunts may create RV volume and pressure overload. If pulmonary hypertension occurs, high-pressure pulmonic regurgitation may result. A systolic thrill is common. Right heart failure may gradually become evident late in the course, and the shunt will begin to reverse as RV and LV systolic pressures equalize with the advent of pulmonary hypertension. Cyanosis from right-to-left shunting may then occur.

B. ECG and Chest Radiography

The ECG may be normal or may show right, left, or biventricular hypertrophy, depending on the size of the defect and the PVR. With large shunts, the RV, the LV the LA, and the pulmonary arteries are enlarged, and pulmonary vascularity is increased on chest radiographs. If PVR (pulmonary hypertension) evolves, an enlarged PA with pruning of the distal pulmonary vascular bed is seen. In rare cases of a VSD high in the ventricular septum, an

aortic cusp may prolapse into the VSD and reduce the VSD shunt but result in acute aortic regurgitation.

C. Diagnostic Studies

Echocardiography can demonstrate the size of the overloaded chambers and can usually define the defect anatomy. Doppler can qualitatively assess the magnitude of shunting by noting the gradient from LV to RV and, if some tricuspid regurgitation is present, the RV systolic pressure can be estimated. Color flow Doppler helps delineate the shunt defect and the presence of valvular regurgitation. MRI and cardiac CT can often visualize the defect and describe any other anatomic abnormalities. MRI can provide quantitative shunt data as well. Radionuclide flow studies are sometimes used to quantify the relative size of the left-to-right shunt. Cardiac catheterization is usually reserved for those with at least moderate shunting to determine the PVR and the degree of pulmonary hypertension. A PVR of > 7.0 absolute units or a PVR/systemic vascular resistance (SVR) ratio of greater than 0.67 (two-thirds systemic) usually implies inoperability.

► Prognosis & Treatment

Patients with the typical murmur as the only abnormality have a normal life expectancy except for the threat of infective endocarditis. Endocarditis is more typical of smaller shunts due to the high velocity of the jet lesion damaging the tricuspid septal leaflet or RV free wall. Antibiotic prophylaxis is still recommended. With large shunts, CHF may develop early in life, and survival beyond age 40 years is unusual without intervention.

The newest guidelines for the management of patients with VSD include the following:

1. Medical management (class 2b recommendation): Pulmonary vasodilatory therapy is appropriate for adults with a VSD and severe pulmonary hypertension.

2. Surgical management (class 1 recommendation): Closure is indicated when the left-to-right shunt ratio is > 2.0 or there is clinical LV volume overload. In addition, closure is recommended if there has been a history of infective endocarditis.

3. Surgical management (class 2b recommendation): Closure is reasonable if the left-to-right shunt is > 1.5 and pulmonary pressure and PVR are less than two-thirds systemic pressure and SVR. Closure is also reasonable if the shunt ratio is > 1.5 and there is evidence for heart failure.

Small shunts (pulmonary-to-systemic flow ratio < 1.5) in asymptomatic patients do not require surgery or other intervention. Defects causing large shunts should be repaired to prevent pulmonary hypertension or late heart failure. The presence of RV infundibular stenosis distal or pulmonary valve stenosis may protect the pulmonary circuit such that some patients even with a large VSD may still be operable as adults.

Surgical repair of a VSD is generally a low risk procedure unless there is significant Eisenmenger physiology. Currently, several new percutaneous closure devices are under investigation for nonsurgical closure of VSDs. Devices for muscular VSDs are approved and those for membranous VSDs are being implanted with promising results. The device is also approved for closure of a VSD related to acute myocardial infarction, although the results in this very high-risk patient population have not been great to date.

When to Refer

All patients with a VSD should be referred to a cardiologist with expertise in adult congenital disease initially to decide if long-term follow-up is warranted.

Fu YC et al. Transcatheter closure of perimembranous ventricular septal defects using the new Amplatzer membranous VSD occluder: results of the U.S. phase I trial. J Am Coll Cardiol. 2006 Jan 17;47(2):319–25. [PMID: 16412854]
Warnes CA et al. ACC/AHA 2008 Guidelines for the Management of Adults With Congenital Heart Disease. A Report of the American College of Cardiology/American Heart Association Task Force on Practice Guidelines. Circulation. 2008 Dec 2;118(23):e714–833. [PMID: 18997169]

TETRALOGY OF FALLOT

ESSENTIALS OF DIAGNOSIS

▶ Four features are characteristic:
- VSD.
- RVH.
- RV outflow obstruction from infundibular stenosis.
- Overriding aorta (< 50%); a right-sided aortic arch is seen in 25%.

▶ Echocardiography/Doppler may underestimate significant pulmonic regurgitation. Be wary if the RV is enlarged.

▶ Arrhythmias are common and periodic Holter monitoring is recommended.

▶ If the QRS width is > 180 msec, then the patient is subject to serious arrhythmias and sudden death.

General Considerations

Patients with tetralogy of Fallot have a VSD, RV infundibular stenosis, RVH, and a dilated aorta (in about 50% of patients it overrides the septum). There may or may not be pulmonary valve stenosis as well, usually due to a bicuspid pulmonary valve. The aorta can be quite enlarged and aortic regurgitation may occur. If more than 50% of the aorta overrides into the RV outflow tract, the situation is not unlike a double outlet RV. Two vascular abnormalities are common: a right-sided aortic arch (in 25%) and anomalous left anterior descending coronary artery from the right cusp. The latter is important in that surgical correction must avoid cutting this vessel when repairing the RV outflow obstruction and producing an anterior myocardial infarction.

Most adult patients have undergone prior surgery. If significant RV outflow obstruction is present in infancy, a Blalock-Taussig (or similar) shunt is often the initial surgical procedure to improve pulmonary blood flow. This procedure enables blood to reach the underperfused lung either by directly attaching one of the subclavian arteries to the PA (**classic Blalock shunt**) or by creating a conduit between the two (**modified Blalock shunt**). Other types of systemic to pulmonary shunts no longer in use include a window between the right PA and the aorta (**Waterston-Cooley shunt**) or a window between the left PA and the descending aorta (**Potts shunt**). In the adult, there may be a reduced upper extremity pulse on the side used for the Blalock procedure. **Total repair** of the tetralogy of Fallot generally includes a VSD patch and usually an enlarging RV outflow tract patch, as well as a take-down of the Blalock shunt. Often the RV outflow tract patch extends through the pulmonary valve into the PA (transannular patch), and the patient is left with wide-open pulmonic regurgitation. Over the years, the volume overload from the severe pulmonary regurgitation becomes the major hemodynamic problem. Ventricular arrhythmias can also originate from the edge of the patch, and tend to correlate with the size of the RV.

Clinical Findings

Most patients are relatively asymptomatic unless right heart failure occurs or arrhythmias become an issue. Patients can be active and generally require no specific therapy except endocarditis prophylaxis.

A. Symptoms and Signs

Physical examination should include checking both arms for any loss of pulse from a prior shunt procedure in infancy. The jugular venous pulsations (JVP) may reveal an increased a wave from poor RV compliance or rarely a c-v wave due to tricuspid regurgitation. The right-sided arch has no consequence. The precordium may be active, often with a persistent pulmonary outflow murmur. P_2 may or may not be present. A right-sided gallop may be heard. A residual VSD or aortic regurgitation may also be present. At times, the insertion site of a prior Blalock or other shunt may create a stenotic area in the PA and a continuous murmur occurs as a result.

B. ECG and Chest Radiography

The ECG reveals RVH and right axis deviation; in repaired tetralogy, there is often a right bundle branch block pattern. The chest radiograph shows a classic boot-shaped heart with prominence of the RV and a concavity in the RV outflow tract. This may be less impressive following repair. The aorta may be enlarged and right-sided. Importantly, the width of the QRS should be examined yearly. There are data that persons at greatest risk for sudden death are those with a QRS width of greater than 180 msec. The width of the QRS corresponds to the RV size, and in many patients, the QRS width actually decreases following repair of the pulmonary insufficiency.

C. Diagnostic Studies

Echocardiography/Doppler usually establishes the diagnosis by noting the unrestricted (large) VSD, the RV infundibular stenosis, and the enlarged aorta. In patients who have had tetralogy of Fallot repaired, echocardiography/Doppler also provides data regarding the amount of pulmonic regurgitation, RV and LV function, and the presence of aortic regurgitation.

Cardiac MRI and CT can quantitate both the pulmonary insufficiency and the RV volumes. In addition, cardiac MRI and CT can identify whether there is either a native pulmonary arterial branch stenosis or a stenosis at the distal site of a prior Blalock or other shunt. Cardiac catheterization is sometimes required to document the degree of pulmonic regurgitation because noninvasive studies depend on velocity gradients. Pulmonary angiography demonstrates the degree of pulmonic regurgitation, and RV angiography helps assess any postoperative outflow tract aneurysm.

Prognosis & Treatment

A few patients with "just the right amount" of pulmonic stenosis enter adulthood without having had surgery. However, most patients have had surgical repair of tetralogy of Fallot, including VSD closure, resection of infundibular muscle, and insertion of an outflow tract patch. Many have a transannular patch resulting in pulmonic regurgitation. Patients should be monitored to ensure the RV volume does not increase. Low-pressure pulmonic regurgitation is difficult to diagnose except during cardiac catheterization due to the fact that the RV diastolic pressures tend to be high and the pulmonary arterial diastolic pressure is low. This means there is little gradient between the PA and the RV in diastole, so that there may be little murmur or evidence for turbulence on color flow Doppler. If the RV begins to enlarge, it must be assumed that this is due to pulmonic regurgitation until proven otherwise.

If an anomalous coronary is present, then an extracardiac conduit around it from the RV to the PA may be necessary. By 20-year follow-up, reoperation is needed in about 10–15%, not only for severe pulmonic regurgitation but also for residual infundibular stenosis. Usually the pulmonic valve is replaced with a pulmonary homograft, though a porcine bioprosthetic valve is also suitable. Cryoablation of tissue giving rise to arrhythmias is sometimes performed at the time of reoperation. Branch pulmonary stenosis may be percutaneously opened by stenting. All patients require endocarditis prophylaxis. Most adults with stable hemodynamics can be quite active, and most women can carry a pregnancy adequately.

When to Refer

All patients with tetralogy of Fallot should be referred to a cardiologist with expertise in adult congenital heart disease.

Bashore TM. Adult congenital heart disease: Right ventricular outflow tract lesions. Circulation. 2007 Apr 10;115(14):1933–47. [PMID: 17420363]

PATENT DUCTUS ARTERIOSUS

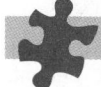 ESSENTIALS OF DIAGNOSIS

▶ Rare in adults.

▶ Adults with small or moderate size patent ductus arteriosus are usually asymptomatic, at least until middle age.

▶ Widened pulse pressure; loud S_2.

▶ Continuous murmur over left pulmonary area; thrill common.

▶ Echocardiography/Doppler is helpful, but the lesion is best visualized by MRI, CT, or contrast angiography.

General Considerations

The embryonic ductus arteriosus allows shunting of blood from the PA to the aorta in utero. The ductus arteriosus normally closes immediately after birth so that pulmonary blood flows to the pulmonary arteries. Failure to close normally results in a persistent shunt connecting the left PA and aorta, usually near the origin of the left subclavian artery. Prior to birth, the ductus is kept patent by the effect of circulating prostaglandins; in the neonate, a patent ductus can often be closed by administration of a prostaglandin inhibitor such as indomethacin. The effect of the persistent left-to-right shunt on the pulmonary circuit is dependent on the size of the ductus. If large enough, pulmonary hypertension (Eisenmenger physiology) may occur. A small ductus may be well tolerated until adulthood.

Clinical Findings

A. Symptoms and Signs

There are no symptoms unless LV failure or pulmonary hypertension develops. The heart is of normal size or slightly enlarged, with a hyperdynamic apical impulse. The pulse pressure is wide, and diastolic pressure is low. A continuous rough "machinery" murmur, accentuated in late systole at the time of S_2, is heard best in the left first and second interspaces at the left sternal border. Thrills are common. If pulmonary hypertension is present (Eisenmenger physiology), the shunt may reverse and the lower body receives desaturated blood, while the upper body receives saturated blood. Thus, the hands appear normal while the toes are cyanotic and clubbed.

B. ECG and Chest Radiography

A normal tracing or LVH is found, depending on the magnitude of shunting. On chest radiographs, the heart is normal in size and contour, or there may be LV and LA enlargement. The PA, aorta, and LA are prominent because they all are in the shunt pathway.

C. Diagnostic Studies

Echocardiography/Doppler can determine LV, RV, and atrial dimensions. Color flow Doppler allows visualization of the high velocity shunt jet into the proximal left PA. Cardiac MRI and CT can demonstrate the abnormality and assess the size of the pulmonary arteries. Cardiac catheterization can establish the shunt size and direction, and define the size and anatomic features of the ductus. It can also help determine whether pulmonary hypertension has occurred. If percutaneous closure is feasible, catheterization can be therapeutic.

Table 10-1. Recommendations for interventions in patients with patent ductus arteriosus.[1]

Class I
A. Closure of a patent ductus arteriosus either percutaneously or surgically is indicated for the following:
  1. Presence of left atrial or left ventricular enlargement, pulmonary artery hypertension, or net left-to-right shunting (level of evidence: C)
  2. Prior endarteritis (level of evidence: C)
B. Consultation with adult congenital heart disease interventional cardiologists is recommended before surgical closure is selected as the method of repair for patients with a calcified patent ductus arteriosus (level of evidence: C).
C. Surgical repair by a surgeon experienced in coronary heart disease surgery is recommended when:
  1. The patent ductus arteriosus is too large for device closure (level of evidence: C).
  2. Distorted ductal anatomy precludes device closure (eg, aneurysm or endarteritis) (level of evidence: B).
Class IIa
A. It is reasonable to close an asymptomatic small patent ductus arteriosus by catheter device (level of evidence: C).
B. Patent ductus arteriosus closure is reasonable for patients with pulmonary artery hypertension with a net left-to-right shunt (level of evidence: C).
Class III
Patent ductus arteriosus closure is not indicated for patients with pulmonary artery hypertension and net right-to-left shunt (level of evidence: C).

[1]Class 1 indicates treatment is useful and effective, IIa indicates weight of evidence is in favor of usefulness/efficacy, class IIb indicates weight of evidence is less well established, and class III indicates intervention is not useful/effective and may be harmful. Type A recommendations are derived from large-scale randomized trials, and B recommendations are derived from smaller randomized trials or carefully conducted observational analyses. ACC/AHA, American College of Cardiology/American Heart Association.

▶ Prognosis & Treatment

Large shunts cause a high mortality rate from cardiac failure early in life. Smaller shunts are compatible with long survival, CHF being the most common complication. Infective endocarditis or endarteritis may also occur, and antibiotic prophylaxis is recommended.

Surgical ligation of the patent ductus can be accomplished with excellent results. If the ductus has a "neck" and is of small enough size, percutaneous approaches using either coils or occluder devices are the preferred therapy. Newer duct occluder devices have a high success rate at a very low risk.

Table 10–1 outlines the new recommendations for intervention in patients with a patent ductus arteriosus.

▶ When to Refer

All patients with PDA should be referred to a cardiologist with expertise in adult congenital disease.

Warnes CA et al. ACC/AHA 2008 Guidelines for the Management of Adults With Congenital Heart Disease. A Report of the American College of Cardiology/American Heart Association Task Force on Practice Guidelines. Circulation. 2008 Dec 2;118(23):e714–833. [PMID: 18997169]

▼ VALVULAR HEART DISEASE

At one time, most cases of valvular disease in the United States were due to rheumatic heart disease (still true in developing countries), other causes are now much more common. In the elderly, "degenerative" calcific aortic valvular disease is now believed due to the same process that produces atherosclerosis, and studies have suggested that about 25% of adults over age 65 have some thickening of their aortic valve (aortic sclerosis) while 2–3% have frank aortic stenosis. Aortic sclerosis alone is a marker for future cardiovascular events and death. Calcium deposition may also occur in the mitral annulus creating enough dysfunction of the valve that either stenosis or regurgitation (or both) results. There is also increasing information that genetic markers associated with aortic stenosis may play a role in the expression of the disease. Mitral valve prolapse is still frequently seen and may be associated with the hyperadrenergic syndrome in younger patients. Valvular regurgitation may be due to LV dysfunction (mitral regurgitation) or RV dysfunction (tricuspid regurgitation).

The typical findings of each native lesion are described in Table 10–2. Table 10–3 shows how to use bedside maneuvers to distinguish the various murmurs.

Bonow RO et al. 2008 focused update incorporated into the ACC/AHA 2006 guidelines for the management of patients with valvular heart disease: a report of the American College of Cardiology/American Heart Association Task Force on Practice Guidelines. Endorsed by the Society of Cardiovascular Anesthesiologists, Society for Cardiovascular Angiography and Interventions, and Society of Thoracic Surgeons. J Am Coll Cardiol. 2008 Sep 23;52(13):e1–142. [PMID: 18848134]
Nishimura RA et al. ACC/AHA 2008 guideline update on valvular heart disease: focused update on infective endocarditis: a report of the American College of Cardiology/American Heart Association Task Force on Practice Guidelines: endorsed by the Society of Cardiovascular Anesthesiologists, Society for Cardiovascular Angiography and Interventions, and Society of Thoracic Surgeons. Circulation. 2008 Aug 19;118(8):887–96. [PMID: 18663090]

MITRAL STENOSIS

ESSENTIALS OF DIAGNOSIS

▶ Exertional dyspnea, orthopnea, and paroxysmal nocturnal dyspnea when the stenosis becomes severe.

▶ Symptoms often precipitated by onset of atrial fibrillation or pregnancy.

▶ Two syndromes occur; one with moderate mitral stenosis and pulmonary edema, and one with severe mitral stenosis, pulmonary hypertension, and low cardiac output.

▶ Echocardiography/Doppler is diagnostic.

▶ Surgery indicated for symptoms or evidence of pulmonary hypertension. Most symptomatic patients have a valve area less than 1.5 cm^2.

Table 10–2. Differential diagnosis of valvular heart disease.

	Mitral Stenosis	Mitral Regurgitation	Aortic Stenosis	Aortic Regurgitation	Tricuspid Stenosis	Tricuspid Regurgitation
Inspection	Malar flush, precordial bulge, and diffuse pulsation in young patients.	Usually prominent and hyperdynamic apical impulse to left of MCL.	Sustained PMI, prominent atrial filling wave.	Hyperdynamic PMI to left of MCL and downward. Visible carotid pulsations. Pulsating nailbeds (Quincke), head bob (deMusset).	Giant a wave in jugular pulse with sinus rhythm. Peripheral edema or ascites, or both.	Large v wave in jugular pulse; time with carotid pulsation. Peripheral edema or ascites, or both.
Palpation	"Tapping" sensation over area of expected PMI. Right ventricular pulsation left third to fifth ICS parasternally when pulmonary hypertension is present. P_2 may be palpable.	Forceful, brisk PMI; systolic thrill over PMI. Pulse normal, small, or slightly collapsing.	Powerful, heaving PMI to left and slightly below MCL. Systolic thrill over aortic area, sternal notch, or carotid arteries in severe disease. Small and slowly rising carotid pulse. If bicuspid AS check for delay at femoral artery to exclude coarctation.	Apical impulse forceful and displaced significantly to left and downward. Prominent carotid pulses. Rapidly rising and collapsing pulses (Corrigan pulse).	Pulsating, enlarged liver in ventricular systole.	Right ventricular pulsation. Systolic pulsation of liver.
Heart sounds, rhythm, and blood pressure	S_1 loud if valve mobile. Opening snap following S_2. The worse the disease, the closer the S_2-opening snap interval.	S_1 normal or buried in early part of murmur (exception is mitral prolapse where murmur may be late). Prominent third heart sound when severe MR. Atrial fibrillation common. Blood pressure normal. Midsystolic clicks may be present and may be multiple.	A_2 normal, soft, or absent. Prominent S_4. Blood pressure normal, or systolic pressure normal with high diastolic pressure.	S_1 normal or reduced, A_2 loud. Wide pulse pressure with diastolic pressure < 60 mm Hg. When severe, gentle compression of femoral artery with diaphragm of stethoscope may reveal diastolic flow (Duroziez) and pressure in leg on palpation > 40 mm Hg than arm (Hill).	S_1 often loud.	Atrial fibrillation may be present.
Murmurs						
Location and transmission	Localized at or near apex. Diastolic rumble best heard in left lateral position; may be accentuated by having patient do sit-ups. Rarely, short diastolic murmur along lower left sternal border (Graham Steell) in severe pulmonary hypertension.	Loudest over PMI; posteriorly directed jets (ie, anterior mitral prolapse) transmitted to left axilla, left infrascapular area; anteriorly directed jets (ie, posterior mitral prolapse) heard over anterior precordium. Murmur unchanged after premature beat.	Right second ICS parasternally or at apex, heard in carotid arteries and occasionally in upper interscapular area. May sound like MR at apex (Gallaverdin phenomenon), but murmur occurs after S_1 and stops before S_2. The later the peak in the murmur, the more severe the AS.	Diastolic: louder along left sternal border in third to fourth interspace. Heard over aortic area and apex. May be associated with low-pitched middiastolic murmur at apex (Austin Flint) due to functional mitral stenosis. If due to an enlarged aorta, murmur may radiate to right sternal border.	Third to fifth ICS along left sternal border out to apex. Murmur increases with inspiration.	Third to fifth ICS along left sternal border. Murmur hard to hear but increases with inspiration. Sit-ups can increase cardiac output and accentuate.

(continued)

Table 10–2. Differential diagnosis of valvular heart disease. (continued)

	Mitral Stenosis	Mitral Regurgitation	Aortic Stenosis	Aortic Regurgitation	Tricuspid Stenosis	Tricuspid Regurgitation
Timing	Relation of opening snap to A_2 important. The higher the LA pressure the earlier the opening snap. Presystolic accentuation before S_1 if in sinus rhythm. Graham Steell begins with P_2 (early diastole) if associated pulmonary hypertension.	Pansystolic: begins with S_1 and ends at or after A_2. May be late systolic in mitral valve prolapse.	Begins after S_1, ends before A_2. The more severe the stenosis, the later the murmur peaks.	Begins immediately after aortic second sound and ends before first sound (blurring both); helps distinguish from MR.	Rumble often follows audible opening snap.	At times, hard to hear. Begins with S_1, and fills systole. Increases with inspiration.
Character	Low-pitched, rumbling; presystolic murmur merges with loud S_1.	Blowing, high-pitched; occasionally harsh or musical.	Harsh, rough.	Blowing, often faint.	As for mitral stenosis.	Blowing, coarse, or musical.
Optimum auscultatory conditions	After exercise, left lateral recumbency. Bell chest piece lightly applied.	After exercise; use diaphragm chest piece. In prolapse, findings may be more evident while standing.	Use stethoscope diaphragm. Patient resting, leaning forward, breath held in full expiration.	Use stethoscope diaphragm. Patient leaning forward, breath held in expiration.	Use stethoscope bell. Murmur usually louder and at peak during inspiration. Patient recumbent.	Use stethoscope diaphragm. Murmur usually becomes louder during inspiration.
Radiography	Straight left heart border from enlarged LA appendage. Elevation of left mainstem bronchus. Large right ventricle and pulmonary artery if pulmonary hypertension is present. Calcification in mitral valve in rheumatic mitral stenosis or in annulus in calcific mitral stenosis.	Enlarged left ventricle and LA.	Concentric left ventricular hypertrophy. Prominent ascending aorta. Calcified aortic valve common.	Moderate to severe left ventricular enlargement. Aortic root often dilated.	Enlarged right atrium with prominent SVC and azygous shadow.	Enlarged right atrium and right ventricle.
ECG	Broad P waves in standard leads; broad negative phase of diphasic P in V_1. If pulmonary hypertension is present, tall peaked P waves, right axis deviation, or right ventricular hypertrophy appears.	Left axis deviation or frank left ventricular hypertrophy. P waves broad, tall, or notched in standard leads. Broad negative phase of diphasic P in V_1.	Left ventricular hypertrophy.	Left ventricular hypertrophy.	Tall, peaked P waves. Possible right ventricular hypertrophy.	Right axis usual.

Echocardiography

Two-dimensional echocardiography	Thickened, immobile mitral valve with anterior and posterior leaflets moving together. "Hockey stick" shape to opened anterior leaflet in rheumatic mitral stenosis. Annular calcium with thin leaflets in calcific mitral stenosis. LA enlargement, normal to small left ventricle. Orifice can be traced to approximate mitral valve orifice area.	Thickened mitral valve in rheumatic disease; mitral valve prolapse; flail leaflet or vegetations may be seen. Dilated left ventricle in volume overload. Operate for left ventricular end-systolic dimension > 4.5 cm.	Dense persistent echoes from the aortic valve with poor leaflet excursion. Left ventricular hypertrophy late in the disease. Bicuspid valve in younger patients.	Abnormal aortic valve or dilated aortic root. Diastolic vibrations of the anterior leaflet of the mitral valve and septum. In acute aortic insufficiency, premature closure of the mitral valve before the QRS. When severe, dilated left ventricle with normal or decreased contractility. Operate when left ventricular end-systolic dimension > 5.0 cm.	In rheumatic disease, tricuspid valve thickening, decreased early diastolic filling slope of the tricuspid valve. In carcinoid, leaflets fixed, but no significant thickening.	Enlarged right ventricle with paradoxical septal motion. Tricuspid valve often pulled open by displaced chordae.
Continuous and color flow Doppler and TEE	Prolonged pressure half-time across mitral valve allows estimation of gradient. MVA estimated from pressure half-time. Indirect evidence of pulmonary hypertension by noting elevated right ventricular systolic pressure measured from the tricuspid regurgitation jet.	Regurgitant flow mapped into LA. Use of PISA helps assess MR severity. TEE important in prosthetic mitral valve regurgitation.	Increased transvalvular flow velocity; severe AS when peak jet > 4 m/sec (64 mm Hg). Valve area estimate using continuity equation is poorly reproducible.	Demonstrates regurgitation and qualitatively estimates severity based on percentage of left ventricular outflow filled with jet and distance jet penetrates into left ventricle. TEE important in aortic valve endocarditis to exclude abscess. Mitral inflow pattern describes diastolic dysfunction.	Prolonged pressure half-time across tricuspid valve can be used to estimate mean gradient. Severe tricuspid stenosis present when mean gradient > 5 mm Hg.	Regurgitant flow mapped into right atrium and venae cavae. Right ventricular systolic pressure estimated by tricuspid regurgitation jet velocity.

A_2, aortic second sound; AS, aortic stenosis; ICS, intercostal space; LA, left atrial; MCL, midclavicular line; MR, mitral regurgitation; MVA, measured valve area; P_2, pulmonary second sound; PISA, proximal isovelocity surface area; PMI, point of maximal impulse; S_1, first heart sound; S_2, second heart sound; S_4, fourth heart sound; SVC, superior vena cava; TEE, transesophageal echocardiography; V_1, chest ECG lead 1.

Table 10–3. Effect of various interventions on systolic murmurs.

Intervention	Hypertrophic Obstructive Cardiomyopathy	Aortic Stenosis	Mitral Regurgitation	Mitral Prolapse
Valsalva	↑	↓	↓ or ×	↑ or ↓
Standing	↑	↑ or ×	↓ or ×	↑
Handgrip or squatting	↓	↓ or ×	↑	↓
Supine position with legs elevated	↓	↑ or ×	×	↓
Exercise	↑	↑ or ×	↓	↑

↑, increased; ↓, decreased; ×, unchanged.
Modified, with permission, from Paraskos JA. Combined valvular disease. In: *Valvular Heart Disease.* Dalen JE, Alpert JS (editors). Little, Brown, LWW, 2000.

General Considerations

Patients with mitral stenosis are usually presumed to have underlying rheumatic heart disease, though a history of rheumatic fever is usually noted in only about one-third. Rheumatic mitral stenosis results in thickening of the leaflets, fusion of the mitral commissures, retraction, thickening and fusion of the chordae, and calcium deposition in the valve. Mitral stenosis can also occur due to congenital disease with chordal fusion or papillary muscle malposition. The papillary muscles may be abnormally close together, sometimes so close they merge into a single papillary muscle (the parachute mitral valve). In these patients, the chordae and/or valvular tissue may also be fused. In other patients, mitral annular calcification may build up enough to produce a mitral gradient, most often in the elderly or patients with end-stage renal disease. Calcium in the mitral annulus virtually invades the mitral leaflet from the annulus inward. Mitral valve obstruction may also develop in patients who have had mitral valve repair with a ring that is too small, or in patients who have had a surgical valve replacement.

Clinical Findings

A. Symptoms and Signs

A characteristic finding of rheumatic mitral stenosis is an opening snap following S_2 due to the stiff mitral valve. The interval between the opening snap and aortic closure sound is long when the LA pressure is low but shortens as the LA pressure rises and approaches the aortic diastolic pressure. As mitral stenosis worsens, there is a localized diastolic murmur low in pitch whose duration increases with the severity of the stenosis, and the heart murmur is best heard at the apex with the patient in the left lateral position (Table 10–2). Mitral regurgitation may accompany mitral stenosis. Generally, if a regurgitant murmur is audible, there is too much mitral regurgitation to allow either percutaneous valvuloplasty or surgical commissurotomy and valve replacement is the only alternative when appropriate.

Two clinical syndromes occur with mitral stenosis. In **mild to moderate mitral stenosis,** LA pressure and cardiac output may be essentially normal, and the patient is either asymptomatic or symptomatic only with extreme exertion. The measured valve area is usually between 1.8 cm² and 1.3 cm². In **severe mitral stenosis** (valve area < 1.0 cm²), severe pulmonary hypertension develops due to a "secondary stenosis" of the pulmonary vasculature. In this condition, pulmonary edema is uncommon, but symptoms of low cardiac output and right heart failure predominate.

Paroxysmal or chronic atrial fibrillation develops in 50–80% of patients. Any increase in the heart rate reduces diastolic time and increases the mitral gradient. A sudden increase in heart rate may precipitate pulmonary edema. Therefore, heart rate control is important to maintain, with slow heart rates preferred.

B. Diagnostic Studies

Echocardiography is the most valuable technique for assessing mitral stenosis. A scoring system is used to help define which patients are eligible for percutaneous valvuloplasty. One to four points are assigned to each of four observed parameters, with one being the least involvement and four the greatest: mitral leaflet thickening, mitral leaflet mobility, submitral scarring, and commissural calcium. Patients with a total valve score of 8 or less respond best to balloon valvuloplasty. LA size can also be determined by echocardiography: increased size denotes an increased likelihood of atrial fibrillation and thrombus formation. The effective mitral valve area can be determined by planimetering the smallest mitral orifice or by using the continuous-wave Doppler gradient. Some determination of the pulmonary pressure can also be quantitated by measuring the peak RV pressure from the tricuspid velocity jet signal.

Because echocardiography and careful symptom evaluation provide most of the needed information, cardiac catheterization is used primarily to detect associated valve, coronary, or myocardial disease—usually after the decision to intervene has been made.

Treatment & Prognosis

In most cases, there is a long asymptomatic phase, followed by subtle limitation of activity. Pregnancy and its associated increase in cardiac output results in an increased transmitral pressure gradient that often precipitates symptoms. Toward the end of pregnancy, the cardiac output is also maintained by an increase in heart rate, further increasing the mitral gradient. Patients with moderate to severe mitral should have the condition corrected prior to becoming pregnant if possible. Patients who become symptomatic can undergo successful surgery, preferably in the third trimester, although balloon valvuloplasty is the treatment of choice if the echo score is low enough.

The onset of atrial fibrillation often precipitates more severe symptoms, which usually improve with control of the ventricular rate or restoration of sinus rhythm. Conversion to and subsequent maintenance of sinus rhythm are most commonly successful when the duration of atrial fibrillation is brief (< 6–12 months) and the LA is not severely dilated (diameter < 4.5 cm). Once atrial fibrillation occurs, the patient should receive warfarin anticoagulation therapy even if sinus rhythm is restored, since atrial fibrillation often recurs even with antiarrhythmic therapy and 20–30% of these patients will have systemic embolization if untreated. Systemic embolization in the presence of only mild to moderate disease is not an indication for surgery but should be treated with warfarin anticoagulation.

Indications for intervention focus on symptoms such as an episode of pulmonary edema, a decline in exercise capacity, or any evidence for pulmonary hypertension (peak systolic pulmonary pressure > 50 mm Hg). Some experts believe that the presence of atrial fibrillation should be a consideration for an intervention.

Open mitral commissurotomy is now rarely performed and has given way to percutaneous balloon valvuloplasty. Ten-year follow-up data comparing surgery to balloon valvuloplasty suggest no real difference in outcome between the two modalities. Replacement of the valve is indicated when combined stenosis and regurgitation are present or when the mitral valve echo score is > 8. Percutaneous mitral valvuloplasty has a very low mortality rate (< 0.5%) and low morbidity rate (3–5%). Operative mortality rates are also low: 1–3% in most institutions. Repeat valvuloplasty can be done if the morphology of the valve is suitable. A Maze procedure may be done at the same time to reduce recurrent atrial arrhythmias.

When to Refer

- Patients with mitral stenosis should be monitored with yearly examinations and echocardiograms.
- All patients should initially be seen by a cardiologist, who then decides how often the patient needs follow-up with the cardiologist.

Bonow RO et al. 2008 focused update incorporated into the ACC/AHA 2006 guidelines for the management of patients with valvular heart disease: a report of the American College of Cardiology/American Heart Association Task Force on Practice Guidelines. Endorsed by the Society of Cardiovascular Anesthesiologists, Society for Cardiovascular Angiography and Interventions, and Society of Thoracic Surgeons. J Am Coll Cardiol. 2008 Sep 23;52(13):e1–142. [PMID: 18848134]

MITRAL REGURGITATION (Mitral Insufficiency)

 ESSENTIALS OF DIAGNOSIS

▶ May be asymptomatic for many years (or for life) or may cause left-sided heart failure.

▶ Echocardiographic findings can help decide when to operate.

▶ For primary mitral regurgitation, surgery is indicated for symptoms or when the LV ejection fraction is < 60% or the echocardiographic LV end-systolic diameter is > 4.0 cm.

▶ In patients with mitral prolapse and severe mitral regurgitation, early surgery is indicated if mitral repair can be performed.

▶ General Considerations

Mitral regurgitation places a volume load on the heart (increases preload) but reduces afterload. The result is an enlarged LV with an increased ejection fraction (EF). Over time, the stress of the volume overload weakens the LV; when this occurs, there is a drop in EF and a rise in end-systolic volume.

▶ Clinical Findings

A. Symptoms and Signs

In acute mitral regurgitation, LA pressure rises abruptly, leading to pulmonary edema if severe. When chronic, the LA enlarges progressively and the increased volume can be handled without a major rise in the LA pressure; the pressure in pulmonary veins and capillaries may rise only transiently during exertion. Exertional dyspnea and fatigue progress gradually over many years.

Mitral regurgitation leads to LA enlargement and may cause subsequent atrial fibrillation. Systemic embolization is relatively unusual compared with other conditions causing atrial fibrillation. Mitral regurgitation may predispose to infective endocarditis, although endocarditis prophylaxis is optional.

Clinically, mitral regurgitation is characterized by a pansystolic murmur maximal at the apex, radiating to the axilla and occasionally to the base; a hyperdynamic LV impulse and a brisk carotid upstroke; and a prominent third heart sound due to the increased volume returning to the LV in early diastole (Tables 10–2, 10–3).

B. Diagnostic Studies

Echocardiography is useful in demonstrating the underlying pathologic process (rheumatic, prolapse, flail leaflet, cardiomyopathy), and Doppler techniques provide qualitative and semiquantitative estimates of the severity of mitral regurgitation. It should be noted that a minor degree of retrograde flow from the closing of the mitral valve occurs almost uniformly and echocardiography/Doppler detects this clinically insignificant regurgitation in many normal individuals. Echocardiographic information concerning LV size and function, LA size, PA pressure, and RV function can be invaluable in planning treatment as well as in recognizing associated lesions. TEE may help reveal the cause of regurgitation and is especially useful in patients who have had mitral valve replacement, in suspected endocarditis, and in identifying candidates for valvular repair. Echocardiographic dimensions and measures of systolic function are critical in deciding the timing of surgery. In the past, exercise radionuclide angiography for measurements of exercise EF or determination of myocardial stress–EF relationships was recommended, but this is now rarely done. There is a growing body of evidence of the usefulness of B-type natriuretic peptide (BNP) in the early identification of LV dysfunction in the presence of mitral regurgitation.

Cardiac MRI is occasionally useful, for example, if specific myocardial causes are being sought (such as amyloid or myocarditis) or if myocardial viability is needed prior to deciding whether to add coronary artery bypass grafting to mitral repair in patients with chronic ischemic mitral regurgitation.

Cardiac catheterization provides a further assessment of regurgitation and its hemodynamic impact along with LV function, resting cardiac output, and PA pressure. Coronary angiography is often indicated to determine the presence of CAD prior to valve surgery in patients with risk factors or those older than age 45 years. In the near future, it may be that cardiac multidetector **CT** may be adequate to screen patients with valvular heart disease for asymptomatic CAD.

▶ Treatment & Prognosis

A. Mitral Regurgitation

LA enlargement is at times considerable in chronic mitral regurgitation; the degree of LV enlargement usually reflects the severity of regurgitation. Calcification of the mitral valve is less common than in pure mitral stenosis. Hemodynamically, LV volume overload may ultimately lead to LV failure and reduced cardiac output, but for many years the LV end-diastolic pressure and the cardiac output may be normal at rest. Nonrheumatic mitral regurgitation may develop abruptly, such as with papillary muscle dysfunction following myocardial infarction, valve perforation in infective endocarditis, or ruptured chordae tendineae in mitral valve prolapse.

Acute mitral regurgitation due to endocarditis, myocardial infarction, and ruptured chordae tendineae often requires emergency surgery. Some patients can be stabilized with vasodilators or intra-aortic balloon counterpulsation, which reduce the amount of regurgitant flow by lowering systemic vascular resistance. Patients with chronic lesions may remain asymptomatic for many years. Surgery is necessary when symptoms develop. However, because progressive and irreversible deterioration of LV function may occur prior to the onset of symptoms, early operation is indicated even in asymptomatic patients with a reduced EF (< 60%) or marked LV dilation (end-systolic dimension > 4.0 cm on echocardiography). In some institutions, the calculation of an effective regurgitant orifice area by echocardiogram has

proven useful in helping decide the severity of the mitral regurgitation. Regurgitant orifice areas > 40 mm^2 are considered severe. There is controversy regarding the role of afterload reduction in mitral regurgitation, since the lesion inherently results in a reduction in afterload. A heightened sympathetic state has led some to suggest β-blockade instead. Most clinicians who monitor patients with chronic mitral regurgitation still prescribe medications, eg, angiotensin-converting enzyme (ACE) inhibitors, to reduce afterload, but there are little supportive data.

B. Ischemic Heart Disease

When mitral regurgitation is due to papillary dysfunction, it may subside as the infarction heals or LV dilation diminishes. The cause of the regurgitation in most situations is displacement of the papillary muscles and an enlarged mitral annulus rather than true papillary muscle ischemia. In acute infarction, rupture of the papillary muscle may occur with catastrophic results. Transient—but sometimes severe—mitral regurgitation may occur during episodes of myocardial ischemia and contribute to flash pulmonary edema. Patients with dilated cardiomyopathies of any origin may have **secondary mitral regurgitation** due to papillary muscle displacement or dilation of the mitral annulus. In patients with ischemic cardiomyopathy, ventricular reconstructive surgery to restore the mitral apparatus anatomy is under investigation (eg, the Dor procedure). If mitral valve replacement is performed, preservation of the chordae to the native valve helps prevent further ventricular dilation following surgery. Several groups have reported good results with mitral valve repair in patients with LV EFs greater than 30% and secondary mitral insufficiency. Recent guidelines consider it acceptable to attempt mitral valve repair in patients with an EF < 30% or an LV end systolic dimension > 5.5 cm, or both, as long as repair and preservation of the chordate is possible.

▶ When to Refer

All patients with more than mild mitral regurgitation should be referred to a cardiologist for an evaluation. Serial examinations and echocardiograms (usually yearly) should be obtained, and referral made if there is any increase in the LV end-systolic dimensions or a fall in the EF to less than 60%.

Bonow RO et al. 2008 focused update incorporated into the ACC/AHA 2006 guidelines for the management of patients with valvular heart disease: a report of the American College of Cardiology/American Heart Association Task Force on Practice Guidelines. Endorsed by the Society of Cardiovascular Anesthesiologists, Society for Cardiovascular Angiography and Interventions, and Society of Thoracic Surgeons. J Am Coll Cardiol. 2008 Sep 23;52(13):e1–142. [PMID: 18848134]

Carabello BA. The current therapy for mitral regurgitation. J Am Coll Cardiol. 2008 Jul 29;52(5):319–26. [PMID: 18652937]

Feldman T et al. Prospects for percutaneous valve therapies. Circulation. 2007 Dec 11;116(24):2866–77. [PMID: 18071090]

Yusoff R et al. Utility of plasma N-terminal brain natriuretic peptide as a marker of functional capacity in patients with chronic severe mitral regurgitation. Am J Cardiol. 2006 May 15;97(10):1498–501. [PMID: 16679092]

MITRAL VALVE PROLAPSE

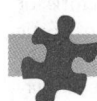

ESSENTIALS OF DIAGNOSIS

▸ Single or multiple mid-systolic clicks often heard on auscultation.

▸ Murmur may be pansystolic or only late in systole.

▸ Often associated with skeletal changes (straight back, pectus, scoliosis) or hyperreflexivity of joints.

▸ Echocardiography is confirmatory with prolapse of mitral leaflets in systole into the LA.

▸ Chest pain and palpitations common symptoms in the young adult.

General Considerations

The significance of **mitral valve prolapse ("floppy" or myxomatous mitral valve)** is in dispute because of the frequency with which it is diagnosed in healthy young women (up to 10%); however, this condition can be problematic in the many patients. A hyperadrenergic syndrome has been described, especially in young females, that may be responsible for some of the noncardiac symptoms observed. Fortunately, this syndrome attenuates with age. Some patients have findings of a systemic collagen abnormality (Marfan or Ehlers-Danlos syndrome). In these conditions, a dilated aortic root and aortic regurgitation may coexist with the mitral valve prolapse.

Patients who have only a mid-systolic click usually have no sequelae, but significant mitral regurgitation may develop, occasionally due to rupture of chordae tendineae (flail leaflet). The need for valve repair or replacement increases with age, so that approximately 2% of patients with clinically significant regurgitation over age 60 years will require surgery.

Clinical Findings

A. Symptoms and Signs

Mitral valve prolapse is usually asymptomatic but may be associated with nonspecific chest pain, dyspnea, fatigue, or palpitations. Most patients are female, many are thin, and some have skeletal deformities such as pectus excavatum or scoliosis. On auscultation, there are characteristic mid-systolic clicks that emanate from the chordae or redundant valve tissue and that may be multiple. If leaflets fail to come together properly, the clicks will be followed by a late systolic murmur. As the mitral regurgitation worsens, the murmur is heard more and more throughout systole. The smaller the LV chamber, the greater the degree of prolapse, and thus auscultatory findings are often accentuated in the standing position.

B. Diagnostic Studies

The diagnosis is primarily clinical but can be confirmed echocardiographically. Mitral prolapse is often associated with aortic root disease, and any evidence for a dilated aorta by chest radiography should prompt either CT or MRI angiography. If palpitations are an issue, an ambulatory monitor is often helpful to distinguish atrial from ventricular tachyarrhythmias.

Treatment

β-Blockers in low doses are used to treat the hyperadrenergic state when present and are usually satisfactory for treatment of arrhythmias. Aspirin has been advocated in the past due to concern regarding systemic emboli, but that practice has been abandoned without evidence for atrial tachyarrhythmias.

Mitral valve repair is favored over valve replacement, and its efficacy has led many to recommend intervention earlier and earlier in the course of the disease process. Mitral repair may include shortening of chordae, chordae transfers, wedge resection of redundant valve tissue, and mitral annular ring to reduce the annular size. Stitching of the leaflets together to create a double orifice mitral valve is also used at times (Alfieri procedure). Mitral repair or replacement can be done through a right minithoracotomy. Robotic devices are also being used to repair these valves. A variety of percutaneous methods for repair of the regurgitant mitral valve are being investigated. These methods include devices to create a double orifice mitral valve by clipping the anterior and posterior leaflets together, devices that are inserted in the coronary sinus to cinch the annulus and make it smaller, and devices that can be inserted onto the annulus from the ventricular side that can pull the annulus inward and reduce annular circumference. Only the mitral clip device has passed phase 2 trials with encouraging results to date. Endocarditis prophylaxis for most situations is no longer recommended.

When to Refer

• All patients with mitral valve prolapse and audible mitral regurgitation should be seen at least once and then periodically by a cardiologist. Those with only mitral clicks need not.

• Periodic echocardiography is warranted to assess LV size (especially end-systolic dimensions) and EF.

Carabello BA. The current therapy for mitral regurgitation. J Am Coll Cardiol. 2008 Jul 29;52(5):319–26. [PMID: 18652937]

Feldman T. Percutaneous mitral valve repair. J Interv Cardiol. 2007 Dec;20(6):488–94. [PMID: 18042054]

AORTIC STENOSIS

ESSENTIALS OF DIAGNOSIS

▸ Congenital bicuspid aortic valve, usually asymptomatic until middle or old age.

▸ "Degenerative" or calcific aortic stenosis; same risk factors as atherosclerosis.

▸ Symptoms likely once the peak echo gradient is > 64 mm Hg.

▶ Echocardiography/Doppler is diagnostic.

▶ Surgery indicated for symptoms. Surgical risk is typically low even in the very elderly.

▶ Surgery considered for asymptomatic patients with severe aortic stenosis.

General Considerations

There are two common clinical scenarios in which aortic stenosis is prevalent. The first is due to a congenitally abnormal **unicuspid** or **bicuspid valve,** rather than tricuspid. Symptoms at times occur in young or adolescent individuals if severe, but more often emerge at age 50–65 years when calcification and degeneration of the valve becomes manifest. A dilated ascending aorta, primarily due to an intrinsic defect in the aortic media, may accompany the bicuspid valve. Coarctation of the aorta is also seen in a number of patients with congenital aortic stenosis. A second group develops what has traditionally been called **degenerative or calcific aortic stenosis,** which is thought to be related to calcium deposition due to processes similar to what occurs in atherosclerotic vascular disease. Approximately 25% of patients over age 65 years and 35% of those over age 70 years have echocardiographic evidence of aortic sclerosis. About 10–20% of these will progress to hemodynamically significant aortic stenosis over a period of 10–15 years. Certain genetic markers are now being discovered that are associated with aortic stenosis (most notably Notch 1), so a genetic component appears likely, at least in some patients.

Thus, aortic stenosis has become the most common surgical valve lesion in developed countries, and many patients are elderly. The risk factors include hypertension, hypercholesterolemia, and smoking. Hypertrophic obstructive cardiomyopathy may also coexist with valvular aortic stenosis.

Clinical Findings

A. Symptoms and Signs

Slightly narrowed, thickened, or roughened valves (aortic sclerosis) or aortic dilation may produce the typical ejection murmur of aortic stenosis. In mild or moderate cases where the valve is still pliable, an ejection click may precede the murmur. The characteristic systolic ejection murmur is heard at the aortic area and is usually transmitted to the neck and apex. In some cases, only the high-pitched components of the murmur are heard at the apex, and the murmur may sound like mitral regurgitation (so-called Gallaverdin phenomenon). In severe aortic stenosis, a palpable LV heave or thrill, a weak to absent aortic second sound, or reversed splitting of the second sound is present (see Table 10–2). When the valve area is less than 0.8–1 cm^2 (normal, 3–4 cm^2), ventricular systole becomes prolonged and the typical carotid pulse pattern of delayed upstroke and low amplitude is present. This may be an unreliable finding, however, in older patients with extensive arteriosclerotic vascular disease. LVH increases progressively, with resulting elevation in ventricular end-diastolic pressure.

Cardiac output is maintained until the stenosis is severe (with a valve area < 0.8 cm^2). LV failure, angina pectoris, or syncope may be presenting symptoms and signs of aortic stenosis; importantly, all occur with exertion.

Symptoms of failure may be sudden in onset or may progress gradually. Angina pectoris frequently occurs in aortic stenosis due to underperfusion of the endocardium. Of patients with calcific aortic stenosis and angina, 50% have significant associated CAD. Syncope is typically exertional and a late finding. Syncope occurs with exertion as the LV pressures rises, stimulating the LV baroreceptors to cause peripheral vasodilation. This vasodilation results in the need for an increase in stroke volume, which increases the LV systolic pressure again, creating a cycle of vasodilation and stimulation of the baroreceptors that eventually results in a drop in BP, as the stenotic valve prevents further increase in stroke volume. Less commonly, syncope may be due to arrhythmias (usually ventricular tachycardia but sometimes AV block as calcific invasion of the conduction system from the aortic valve may occur).

B. Diagnostic Studies

The clinical assessment of the severity of aortic stenosis may be difficult, especially when there is reduced cardiac output or significant associated aortic regurgitation. The ECG reveals LVH or suggestive repolarization changes in most patients, but can be normal in up to 10%. The chest radiograph may show a normal or enlarged cardiac silhouette, calcification of the aortic valve, and dilation and calcification of the ascending aorta. The echocardiogram provides useful data about aortic valve calcification and opening and LV thickness and function, while Doppler can provide an excellent estimate of the aortic valve gradient. The peak Doppler gradient is derived by squaring the maximal flow velocity through the valve orifice and multiplying times 4; thus, a 4 m/s maximum velocity gradient translates into a 64 mm Hg peak Doppler gradient. Valve area estimation by echocardiography is less reliable. Cardiac catheterization mostly provides an assessment of the hemodynamic consequence of the aortic stenosis, and a look at the coronary arteries. In younger patients, and in patients with high aortic gradients the aortic valve need not be crossed at catheterization. If it is crossed, the valve gradient can be measured at catheterization and an estimated valve area calculated; a valve area below 1.0 cm^2 indicates significant stenosis in the newest ACC/AHA guidelines. Aortic regurgitation can be semiquantified by aortic root angiography. In patients with a low EF and both low output and a low valve gradient, it may be unclear if an increased afterload is responsible for the low EF or if there is an associated cardiomyopathy. To sort this out, the patient should be studied at baseline and then during an intervention that increases cardiac output (eg, dobutamine or nitroprusside infusion). If the valve area increases, the flow-limiting problem is not the valve, but rather the cardiomyopathy, and surgery is not warranted. If the valve area remains unchanged at the higher outputs, then the valve is considered flow limiting and surgery is indicated. Recent data have suggested the use of BNP may provide prognostic data in the setting of poor LV function and aortic stenosis. A BNP > 550 pg/mL has been associated with a poor outcome in these patients regardless of the results of dobutamine testing.

Prognosis & Treatment

Following the onset of heart failure, angina, or syncope, the prognosis without surgery is poor (50% 3-year mortality rate). Medical treatment may stabilize patients in heart failure, but surgery is indicated for all symptomatic patients with evidence of significant aortic stenosis. Valve replacement is usually not indicated in asymptomatic individuals, though a class II indication is to operate once the peak valve gradient by Doppler exceeds 64 mm Hg or the mean exceeds 40 mm Hg. Stress testing and perhaps the use of BNP may help identify patients who deny symptoms but are actually compromised from a ventricular function standpoint.

The surgical mortality rate for valve replacement is low, even in the elderly, and ranges from 2% to 5%. This low risk is due to the dramatic hemodynamic improvement that occurs with relief of the increased afterload. Mortality rates are substantially higher when there is an associated ischemic cardiomyopathy. Severe coronary lesions are usually bypassed at the same time. Around one-third to one-half of all patients with aortic stenosis have CAD.

The interventional options in patients with aortic stenosis are variable and dependent on the patient's lifestyle and age. In the young and adolescent patient, percutaneous valvuloplasty still has a role. Balloon valvuloplasty is less effective and is associated with early restenosis in the elderly, and thus is rarely used. Data suggest aortic balloon valvuloplasty has an advantage only in those with preserved LV function, and such patients are usually excellent candidates for surgical aortic valve replacement (AVR). The Ross procedure is generally still considered a viable option in younger patients, and it is performed by moving the patient's own pulmonary valve to the aortic position and replacing the pulmonary valve with a homograft (or rarely a bioprosthetic valve). However, dilation of the pulmonary valve autograft and consequent aortic regurgitation, plus early stenosis of the pulmonary homograft in the pulmonary position, has reduced the enthusiasm for this approach in many institutions. Middle-aged adults generally can take the anticoagulation therapy necessary for the use of mechanical AVR, so most undergo AVR with a bileaflet mechanical valve. If the aortic root is severely dilated as well (> 5.0 cm), then the valve may be housed in a Dacron sheath (Bentall procedure) and the root replaced as well. Alternatively, a human homograft root and valve replacement may be used. In the elderly, bioprosthetic (either porcine or bovine pericardial) valves with a life expectancy of about 10–15 years are routinely used to avoid need for anticoagulation. Recent data favor the bovine pericardial valve over the porcine pericardial valve. If the aortic annulus is small, a bioprosthetic valve with a short sheath can be sewn to the aortic wall (the stentless AVR) rather than sewing the prosthetic annulus to the aortic annulus.

Anticoagulation is required with the use of mechanical valves, and the international normalized ratio (INR) should be maintained between 2.0 and 2.5. Mechanical aortic valves are less subject to thrombosis than mechanical mitral valves.

There is growing interest in developing a percutaneous approach to AVR. Both a retrograde approach (from the aorta) and an antegrade approach (from the ventricles by way of a transseptal catheter across the atrial septum) are being investigated. The devices being tested use either a stent with a trileaflet bovine pericardial valve constructed in it, or a stent with a large valve from a cow's jugular vein mounted inside. Preliminary data are encouraging.

When to Refer

- All patients with an aortic murmur and echocardiographic evidence for aortic stenosis (estimated peak valve gradient > 30 mm Hg) should be referred to a cardiologist for evaluation and to determine the frequency of follow-up.

- Any patients with symptoms suggestive of aortic stenosis should be seen by a cardiologist.

Bossé Y et al. Genomics: the next step to elucidate the etiology of calcific aortic valve stenosis. J Am Coll Cardiol. 2008 Apr 8;51(14):1327–36. [PMID: 18387432]

Carbello BA. Aortic stenosis: two steps forward, one back. Circulation. 2007 Jun 5;115(22):2799–800. [PMID: 17548741]

Feldman T et al. Prospects for percutaneous valve therapies. Circulation. 2007 Dec 11;116(24):2866–77. [PMID: 18071090]

Otto C. Valvular aortic stenosis: disease severity and timing of intervention. J Am Coll Cardiol. 2006 Jun 6;47(11):2141–51. [PMID: 16750677]

AORTIC REGURGITATION (Chronic Regurgitation)

 ESSENTIALS OF DIAGNOSIS

- ▶ Usually asymptomatic until middle age; presents with left-sided failure or chest pain.
- ▶ Wide pulse pressure.
- ▶ Echocardiography/Doppler is diagnostic.
- ▶ Afterload reduction may be beneficial if the LV is dilated (LV end-diastolic dimension > 5.0 cm) or there is evidence for systolic blood pressure elevation.
- ▶ Surgery indicated for symptoms, EF < 55%, or LV end-systolic dimension > 5.0 cm.

General Considerations

Rheumatic aortic regurgitation has become much less common than in the preantibiotic era, and nonrheumatic causes now predominate. These include congenitally bicuspid valves, infective endocarditis, and hypertension. Many patients have aortic regurgitation secondary to aortic root diseases such as cystic medial necrosis, Marfan syndrome, or aortic dissection. Rarely, inflammatory diseases, such as ankylosing spondylitis or Reiter syndrome, may be causative.

Clinical Findings

A. Symptoms and Signs

The clinical presentation is determined by the rapidity with which regurgitation develops. In chronic regurgitation, the only sign for many years may be a soft aortic diastolic murmur. As the severity of the aortic regurgitation increases, diastolic BP falls, and the LV progressively enlarges. Most patients remain asymptomatic even at this point. LV failure is a late event and may be sudden in onset. Exertional dyspnea and fatigue are the most frequent symptoms, but paroxysmal nocturnal dyspnea and pulmonary edema may also occur. Angina pectoris or atypical chest pain may occasionally be present. Associated CAD and presyncope or syncope are less common than in aortic stenosis.

Hemodynamically, because of compensatory LV dilation, patients eject a large stroke volume, which is adequate to maintain forward cardiac output until late in the course of the disease. LV diastolic pressure may rise when heart failure occurs. Abnormal LV systolic function, as manifested by reduced EF (< 55%) and increasing end-systolic LV volume (> 5 cm), is a sign that surgical intervention is warranted.

The major physical findings in **chronic aortic regurgitation** relate to the high stroke volume being ejected into the systemic vascular system with rapid runoff as the regurgitation takes place (see Table 10–2). This results in a wide arterial pulse pressure. The pulse has a rapid rise and fall (water-hammer pulse or Corrigan pulse), with an elevated systolic and low diastolic pressure. The large stroke volume is also responsible for characteristic findings such as Quincke pulses (nailbed capillary pulsations), Duroziez sign (to and fro murmur over a partially compressed peripheral artery, commonly the femoral), and Musset sign (head bob with each pulse). In younger patients, the increased stroke volume may summate with the reflected wave from the periphery and create an even higher systolic pressure in the extremity compared with the central aorta. Since the peripheral bed is much larger in the leg than the arm, the BP in the leg may be over 40 mm Hg higher than in the arm (Hill sign). The apical impulse is prominent, laterally displaced, usually hyperdynamic, and may be sustained. A systolic murmur is usually present and may be quite soft and localized; the aortic diastolic murmur is usually high-pitched and decrescendo. A mid or late diastolic low-pitched mitral murmur (Austin Flint murmur) may be heard in advanced aortic regurgitation, owing to partial obstruction of mitral inflow produced by partial closure of the mitral valve by the regurgitant jet and the rapidly rising LV diastolic pressure.

In **acute aortic regurgitation** (usually from aortic dissection or infective endocarditis), LV failure is manifested primarily as pulmonary edema and may develop rapidly; surgery is urgently required in such cases. Patients with acute aortic regurgitation do not have the dilated LV of chronic aortic regurgitation and the extra volume is handled poorly. For the same reason, the diastolic murmur is shorter and may be minimal in intensity, and the pulse pressure may not be widened, making clinical diagnosis difficult. The mitral valve may close prematurely even before systole has been initiated (pre-closure) due to the rapid rise in the LV diastolic pressure, and the first heart sound is thus diminished or inaudible.

B. Diagnostic Studies

The ECG usually shows moderate to severe LVH. Radiographs show cardiomegaly with LV prominence and sometimes a dilated aorta.

Echocardiography demonstrates the major diagnostic features, including whether the lesion involves the proximal aortic root and what valvular disease is present. Serial assessments of LV size and function are critical in determining the timing for valve replacement. Color Doppler techniques can qualitatively estimate the severity of regurgitation, though some "mild" regurgitation due to aortic valve closure is not uncommon and should not be overinterpreted. Cardiac MRI and CT can estimate aortic root size, particularly when there is concern for an ascending aneurysm. MRI can provide a regurgitant fraction to help confirm severity. Scintigraphic studies are infrequently used but can quantify LV function and functional reserve during exercise. Exercise increases the heart rate and reduces the diastolic time, resulting in less aortic regurgitation per beat; this complicates interpretation of the exercise EF. Cardiac catheterization may be unnecessary in younger patients, particularly those with acute aortic regurgitation, but can help define hemodynamics, aortic root abnormalities, and associated CAD preoperatively in older patients.

Treatment & Prognosis

Aortic regurgitation that appears or worsens during or after an episode of infective endocarditis or aortic dissection may lead to acute severe LV failure or subacute progression over weeks or months. The former usually presents as pulmonary edema; surgical replacement of the valve is indicated even during active infection. These patients may be transiently improved or stabilized by vasodilators.

Chronic regurgitation has a long natural history, but the prognosis without surgery becomes poor when symptoms occur. Since aortic regurgitation places both a volume and afterload increase on the LV, medications that decrease afterload can reduce regurgitation severity. Current recommendations continue to advocate afterload reduction in aortic regurgitation, though the data are derived from very few patients, and its use remains controversial. Most clinicians prescribe ACE inhibitors whenever the LV diastolic size is increased > 5.0 cm on echocardiogram or if there is evidence for systemic hypertension. There are experimental data that suggest ACE-inhibitors may actually be harmful, however. β-Blocker therapy may slow the rate of aortic dilation in Marfan syndrome by reducing the dP/dt, though the slower heart rates that result may theoretically increase the diastolic time and the amount of regurgitation per beat, and increase the volume overload on the heart. Patients with aortic regurgitation need to be monitored serially by echocardiography. Surgery is indicated once symptoms emerge or for any evidence of LV dysfunction. LV dysfunction in this situation can be defined by echocardiography if the EF is < 55% or if the LV end-systolic dimension is > 5.0 cm, even in the asymptomatic patient. In addition, aortic root diameters of > 4.5 cm in Marfan or > 5.0 cm in non-Marfan patients are indications for surgery to avoid rapid expansion. Although the operative mortality rate is higher when LV function is severely impaired, valve replacement or repair is still indicated, since LV function often improves and the long-term prognosis is thereby enhanced even in this situation. The issues with AVR covered in the above section concerning aortic stenosis pertain here. Currently, however, there are no percutaneous approaches to aortic regurgitation. The choice of prosthetic valve for AVR depends on the patient's age and compatibility with warfarin anticoagulation.

The operative mortality rate is usually in the 3–5% range. Aortic regurgitation due to aortic root disease requires repair or replacement of the root. Though valve-sparing operations have improved recently, most patients with root replacement undergo valve replacement at the same time. Root replacement procedures include the Ross procedure (moving the pulmonary valve to the aortic position and replacing the pulmonary valve with a homograft or, less commonly, bioprosthetic valve), the direct homograft for the aortic root and valve, and the Bentall procedure (the use of a Dacron sheath with a mechanical or bioprosthetic valve sewn in place). Root replacement in association with valve replacement requires reanastomosis of the coronary arteries, and thus the procedure is more complex than valve replacement alone. Following surgery, LV size usually decreases and LV function generally improves even when the baseline EF is depressed.

When to Refer

- Patients with audible aortic regurgitation should been seen, at least initially, by a cardiologist and decision made as to how often the patient needs follow-up.
- Patients with a dilated aortic root should be monitored by a cardiologist, since other imaging studies may be required to decide surgical timing.

Carabello BA. What is new in the 2006 ACC/AHA guidelines on valvular heart disease? Curr Cardiol Rep. 2008 Mar;10(2):85–90. [PMID: 18417007]

Inamo J et al. Are vasodilators still indicated in the treatment of severe aortic regurgitation? Curr Cardiol Rep. 2007 Apr;9(2):87–92. [PMID: 17430674]

TRICUSPID STENOSIS

 ESSENTIALS OF DIAGNOSIS

- Female predominance.
- History of rheumatic heart disease. Carcinoid disease more common etiology in the United States.
- Echocardiography/Doppler is key to diagnosis.
- Mean valve gradient > 5 mm Hg by echocardiography indicates severe tricuspid stenosis.

General Considerations

Tricuspid stenosis is usually rheumatic in origin, though in the United States, tricuspid stenosis is more commonly due to tricuspid valve repair or replacement or to the carcinoid syndrome than to rheumatic fever. Tricuspid regurgitation frequently accompanies the lesion. It should be suspected when "right heart failure" appears in the course of mitral valve disease or in the postoperative period after tricuspid valve repair or replacement.

Clinical Findings

A. Symptoms and Signs

Tricuspid stenosis is characterized by right heart failure and hepatomegaly, ascites, and dependent edema. A giant *a* wave is seen in the JVP, which is elevated (Table 10–2). The typical diastolic rumble along the lower left sternal border mimics mitral stenosis, though the rumble increases with inspiration. In sinus rhythm, a presystolic liver pulsation may be found.

B. Diagnostic Studies

In the absence of atrial fibrillation, the ECG reveals RA enlargement. The chest radiograph may show marked cardiomegaly with a normal PA size. A dilated SVC and azygous vein may be evident.

The normal valve area of the tricuspid valve is 10 cm^2, so significant stenosis must be present to produce a gradient. Hemodynamically, a mean diastolic pressure gradient of > 5 mm Hg is considered significant, though even a 2 mm Hg gradient can be considered abnormal. This can be demonstrated by echocardiography or at cardiac catheterization.

Treatment & Prognosis

Tricuspid stenosis may be progressive, eventually causing severe right heart failure. Initial therapy is directed at reducing the fluid congestion, with diuretics the mainstay. When there is considerable bowel edema, torsemide may have an advantage over other loop diuretics, such as furosemide, because it is better absorbed from the gut. Aldosterone inhibitors may also help if there is liver engorgement or ascites. Neither surgical nor percutaneous valvuloplasty is effective for tricuspid stenosis, as residual tricuspid regurgitation is common. Tricuspid valve replacement is clearly the preferred surgical approach. Mechanical tricuspid valve replacement is rarely done because the low flow predisposes to thrombosis and because the mechanical valve cannot be crossed should the need arise for right heart catheterization or pacemaker implantation. Therefore, bioprosthetic valves are almost always used. Often tricuspid valve replacement is done in conjunction with mitral valve replacement for mitral stenosis.

Garcia-Pinilla JM et al. Reversible tricuspid stenosis secondary to massive ascites in hepatic cirrhosis. Ann Intern Med. 2004 Feb 3;140(3):233–4. [PMID: 14757628]

Staicu I et al. Tricuspid stenosis: a rare cause of heart failure in the United States. Congest Heart Fail. 2002 Sep–Oct;8(5):281–3. [PMID: 12368592]

Thatipelli MR et al. Isolated tricuspid stenosis and heart failure: a focus on carcinoid heart disease. Congest Heart Fail. 2003 Sep–Oct;9(5):294–6. [PMID: 14564150]

TRICUSPID REGURGITATION

 ESSENTIALS OF DIAGNOSIS

► Frequently occurs in patients with pulmonary or cardiac disease, especially if pulmonary hypertension is present.

► Systolic c-v wave in jugular venous pulsations.

► Holosystolic murmur along left sternal border, which increases with inspiration.

► Echocardiography useful in determining cause (low- or high-pressure tricuspid regurgitation).

General Considerations

Tricuspid valvular incompetence often occurs whenever there is RV dilation from any cause. As tricuspid regurgitation increases, the RV size increases further, and this in turn worsens the tricuspid regurgitation. The causes of tricuspid regurgitation thus relate to anatomic issues with either the valve itself or to the RV geometry. An enlarged, dilated RV may be present if there is pulmonary hypertension for any reason, in severe pulmonic regurgitation, or in cardiomyopathy. The RV may be injured from myocardial infarction or may be inherently dilated due to infiltrative diseases (RV dysplasia or sarcoidosis). The RV dilation is often secondary to left heart failure. Inherent abnormalities of the tricuspid valve include Ebstein anomaly (displacement of the septal and posterior, but never the anterior, leaflets into the RV), tricuspid valve prolapse, carcinoid plaque formation, collagen disease inflammation, tricuspid endocarditis, or RV pacemaker catheter injury.

Clinical Findings

A. Symptoms and Signs

The symptoms and signs of tricuspid regurgitation are identical to those resulting from RV failure due to any cause. As a generality, the diagnosis can be made by careful inspection of the JVP (Table 10–2). The JVP waveform should decline during ventricular systole (the x descent). The timing of this decline can be observed by palpating the opposite carotid artery. As tricuspid regurgitation worsens, more and more of this valley in the JVP is filled with the regurgitant wave until all of the x descent is obliterated and a positive systolic waveform will be noted in the JVP. An associated tricuspid regurgitation murmur may or may not be present and can be distinguished from mitral regurgitation by the left parasternal

location and increase with inspiration. An S_3 may accompany the murmur and is related to the high flow returning from the RA. Cyanosis may be present if the increased RA pressure stretches the atrial septum and opens a PFO or there is a true ASD (eg, in about 50% of patients with Ebstein anomaly).

B. Diagnostic Studies

The ECG is usually nonspecific, though atrial fibrillation is not uncommon. The chest radiograph may reveal evidence for an enlarged RA or dilated azygous vein and pleural effusion. The echocardiogram helps assess severity of tricuspid regurgitation, PA pressure, and RV size and function. A paradoxically moving interventricular septum may be present. Catheterization confirms the presence of the regurgitant wave in the RA and elevated RA pressures. If the PA or RV systolic pressure is < 40 mm Hg, primary tricuspid regurgitation should be suspected.

Treatment & Prognosis

Minor tricuspid regurgitation is well tolerated. When present, bowel edema may reduce the effectiveness of oral furosemide, and intravenous diuretics should initially be used. Torsemide is better absorbed in this situation. Aldosterone antagonists have a role as well, particularly if ascites is present. At times, the efficacy of loop diuretics can be enhanced by adding a thiazide diuretic.

Definitive treatment usually requires elimination of the cause of the tricuspid regurgitation. If the problem is left heart disease, then treatment of the left heart issues may lower pulmonary pressures, reduce RV size, and resolve the tricuspid regurgitation. Treatment for primary and secondary causes of pulmonary hypertension will generally reduce the tricuspid regurgitation. If surgery is contemplated for other reasons, especially mitral valve disease, then tricuspid annuloplasty is generally performed at the same time with a valvular ring sewn in place. Annuloplasty without insertion of a prosthetic ring (DeVega annuloplasty) may also be effective to reduce the annular dilation. The valve leaflet itself can occasionally be repaired in tricuspid valve endocarditis. In years past, in patients with tricuspid regurgitation due to endocarditis from substance abuse, the tricuspid valve has been temporarily removed to aid in cure of the endocarditis, though it must eventually be replaced (usually by 3–6 months); this practice is less common now. If there is an inherent defect in the tricuspid apparatus that cannot be repaired, then replacement of the tricuspid valve is warranted. Almost always, a bioprosthetic valve, and not a mechanical valve, is used. Anticoagulation is not required for bioprosthetic valves unless there is associated atrial fibrillation.

Bonow RO et al. ACC/AHA 2006 guidelines for the management of patients with valvular heart disease: a report of the American College of Cardiology/American Heart Association Task Force on Practice Guidelines (writing committee to revise the 1998 Guidelines for the Management of Patients With Valvular Heart Disease): developed in collaboration with the Society of Cardiovascular Anesthesiologists: endorsed by the Society for Cardiovascular Angiography and Interventions and the Society of Thoracic Surgeons. Circulation. 2006 Aug 1;114(5):e84–231. [PMID: 16880336]

Shah PM et al. Tricuspid valve disease. Curr Probl Cardiol. 2008 Feb;33(2):47–84. [PMID: 18222317]

PULMONIC REGURGITATION

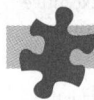 ESSENTIALS OF DIAGNOSIS

► Most cases are due to pulmonary hypertension.
► Echocardiogram is definitive in high-pressure but may be less helpful in low-pressure pulmonic regurgitation.
► Low-pressure pulmonic regurgitation is well tolerated.

General Considerations

Pulmonary valve regurgitation can be divided into **high-pressure causes** (due to pulmonary hypertension) and **low-pressure causes** (usually due to a dilated pulmonary annulus [idiopathic or traumatic] or to plaque from carcinoid disease or following surgical repair). It may be iatrogenic, eg, frequently occurring after repair of tetralogy of Fallot. Because the RV tolerates a volume load better than a pressure load, it tends to tolerate pulmonic regurgitation well.

Clinical Findings

On examination, a hyperdynamic RV can usually be palpated. If the PA is enlarged, it may be palpated along the left sternal border. P_2 will be palpable in pulmonary hypertension and both systolic and diastolic thrills are occasionally noted. On auscultation, the second heart sound may be widely split due to prolonged RV systole. Systolic clicks may be noted as well as a right-sided gallop. In high-pressure pulmonic regurgitation, the pulmonary diastolic (Graham Steell) murmur is readily audible. It is often due to a dilated pulmonary annulus. The murmur increases with inspiration and diminishes with the Valsalva maneuver. In low-pressure pulmonic regurgitation, the PA diastolic pressure may be only a few mm Hg higher than the RV diastolic pressure, and there is little diastolic gradient to produce a murmur or characteristic echocardiography/Doppler findings. At times, only contrast angiography or MRI of the main PA will show the free flowing pulmonic regurgitation in this situation.

The ECG is generally of little value. The chest radiograph may show only the enlarged RV and PA. Echocardiography may demonstrate evidence of RV volume overload (paradoxic septal motion), and Doppler can determine peak systolic RV pressure and reveal any associated tricuspid regurgitation. The size of the main PA can be determined and color flow Doppler can demonstrate the pulmonic regurgitation, particularly in the high-pressure situation. Cardiac MRI and CT can be useful for assessing the size of the PA, for imaging the jet lesion, for excluding other causes of pulmonary hypertension (eg, thromboembolic disease, peripheral PA stenosis), and for evaluating RV function. MRI provides a regurgitant fraction to help quantitate the degree of pulmonic regurgitation.

► Treatment & Prognosis

Pulmonic regurgitation rarely needs specific therapy other than treatment of the primary cause. In low-pressure pulmonic regurgitation due to surgical patch repair of tetralogy of Fallot, pulmonary valve replacement may be indicated if RV enlargement or dysfunction is present. In tetralogy of Fallot, the QRS will widen as RV function declines and the ECG is helpful here. In carcinoid heart disease, pulmonary valve replacement with a porcine bioprosthesis may be undertaken, though the plaque from this disorder eventually covers the prosthetic valve and this tends to limit the lifespan of these valves. In high-pressure pulmonic regurgitation, treatment to control the cause of the pulmonary hypertension is key.

Backer CL. Severe pulmonary valvar insufficiency should be aggressively treated. Cardiol Young. 2005 Feb;15(Suppl 1):64–7. [PMID: 15934694]
Bouzas B et al. Pulmonary regurgitation: not a benign lesion. Eur Heart J. 2005 Mar;26(5):433–9. [PMID: 15640261]
Gaynor JW. Severe pulmonary insufficiency should be conservatively treated. Cardiol Young. 2005 Feb;15(Suppl 1):68–71. [PMID: 15934695]

CHOICE & MANAGEMENT OF PROSTHETIC VALVES

Less invasive surgical procedures for valve replacement have improved over the past few decades. There are now mini-incisional approaches to aortic, mitral, and tricuspid valve replacement and repair. Percutaneous valvuloplasty has replaced surgical commissurotomy for mitral stenosis in most cases. However, percutaneous aortic valvuloplasty is moderately effective only in children and adolescents; it has a very limited role in adults. Neither surgical nor percutaneous tricuspid valvuloplasty is very effective.

Repair of the mitral valve is successful in appropriate patients and has lowered the threshold for intervention in mitral regurgitation. Some experts recommend that all mitral prolapse patients with mitral regurgitation undergo mitral valve repair even when other indications are not present. However, to recommend this option, the surgeon performing the procedure must have extensive experience with excellent results. When tricuspid regurgitation is present and mitral valve repair or replacement is planned, tricuspid repair is now a class I recommendation. Aortic valve sparing procedures are also improving and may obviate the need for AVR, especially in patients undergoing root replacement. Early experience, though, with aortic valve repair is mixed. Direct valvular repair and removal of vegetations are also viable options in some patients with endocarditis.

The choice of prosthetic valve depends on a variety of considerations, such as assessing the expected survival of the patient versus the durability of the valve and the safety of warfarin for the patient. Bioprosthetic valves usually have a life expectancy of 10–15 years, but less in young patients, those on dialysis, or those with hypercalcemia. The lifespan of bovine pericardial valves is somewhat longer than porcine valves, and these are becoming the favorite bioprostheses. Bioprosthetic valves, homografts, and the Ross procedure (replacement of the aortic valve with the patient's own pulmonary valve, then replacement of the removed pulmonary valve with a homograft) do not require anticoagulation with warfarin, though current guidelines suggest warfarin be used for 3 months after valve implantation to allow for endothelial growth over the sewing ring. This latter recommendation is controversial. Mechanical valves have a much longer lifespan, but all require use of warfarin (and frequently aspirin as an adjunct). The long-term risk of warfarin depends on patient compliance and whether there is coexisting disease that may predispose to bleeding.

Mechanical mitral valve prostheses pose a greater risk for thrombosis than mechanical aortic valves. For that reason, the INR should be kept between 2.5 and 3.5 for mechanical mitral prosthetic valves but can be kept between 2.0 and 2.5 for mechanical aortic prosthetic valves. Enteric-coated aspirin (81 mg once daily) is given to patients with both types of mechanical valves but appears to be more important for mitral valve prostheses and for both types of valves when other risk factors are present, such as atrial fibrillation, a reduced EF, a hypercoagulable state, associated CAD, peripheral vascular disease, or a history of CVA.

Warfarin causes fetal skeletal abnormalities in about 2% of women who become pregnant while taking warfarin, so every effort is made to defer valve replacement in women until after childbearing age. However, if a woman with a mechanical valve becomes pregnant while taking warfarin, the risk of stopping warfarin is higher for the mother than the risk of continuing warfarin for the fetus. The risk of warfarin to the fetal skeleton is greatest during the first trimester, so if pregnancy is planned in a woman with a mechanical valve, unfractionated heparin is often used temporarily during the first trimester. After the first trimester, warfarin use is safe again until 2 weeks before planned delivery, when the patient should be switched back to unfractionated heparin. Low-molecular-weight heparin has not been shown to be effective and should not be substituted for unfractionated heparin in the pregnant patient with a mechanical heart valve.

When patients with mechanical valves must undergo noncardiac surgery, the risk of thrombosis from stopping warfarin versus the risk of excessive bleeding from continuing warfarin must be weighed. In general, for bileaflet aortic mechanical valves, warfarin can be stopped 5 days ahead of the surgical procedure and resumed the night of the procedure with no preprocedural "bridging". After the procedure, unfractionated heparin or low-molecular-weight heparin can be used until the INR is 2.0. In patients with a bileaflet mitral valve, warfarin may be stopped 5 days ahead of time and bridging with either unfractionated heparin or low-molecular-weight heparin is often used preoperatively if the INR falls below 2.0. The last dose of low-molecular-weight heparin should be half the therapeutic dose and be given 24 hours before any procedure. If unfractionated heparin is used, it should be stopped 4 hours before the procedure. As with AVR, warfarin is generally started within 24 hours after surgery, but heparin should not be started for 48–72 hours or until hemostasis is secured. Heparin therapy should be continued until the INR is > 2.0.

Hirsh J et al; American College of Chest Physicians. Executive summary: American College of Chest Physicians Evidence-Based Clinical Practice Guidelines (8th Edition). Chest. 2008 Jun;133(6 Suppl):71S–109S. [PMID: 18574259]

Hung L et al. Prosthetic heart valves and pregnancy. Circulation. 2003 Mar 11;107(9):1240–6. [PMID: 12628941]

Rahimtoola SH. Choice of prosthetic heart valve for adult patients. J Am Coll Cardiol. 2003 Mar 19;41(6):893–904. [PMID: 12651032]

CORONARY HEART DISEASE (ATHEROSCLEROTIC CAD, ISCHEMIC HEART DISEASE)

Coronary heart disease, or atherosclerotic CAD, is the number one killer in the United States and worldwide. Every minute, an American dies of coronary heart disease. About 38% of people who experience an acute coronary event, either angina or myocardial infarction, will die of it in the same year. Death rates of coronary heart disease have declined every year since 1968, with about half of the decline from 1980 to 2000 due to treatments and half due to improved risk factors. Coronary heart disease is still responsible for approximately one of five deaths and over 600,000 deaths per year in the United States. Coronary heart disease afflicts nearly 16 million Americans and the prevalence rises steadily with age; thus, the aging of the US population promises to increase the overall burden of coronary heart disease.

▶ Risk Factors for CAD

Most patients with coronary heart disease have some identifiable risk factor. These include a positive family history (the younger the onset in a first-degree relative, the greater the risk), male gender, blood lipid abnormalities, diabetes mellitus, hypertension, physical inactivity, abdominal obesity, and cigarette smoking, psychosocial factors, consumption of too few fruits and vegetables and too much alcohol. Smoking remains the number one preventable cause of cardiovascular disease worldwide. Although smoking rates have declined in the United States in recent decades, 19% of women and 23% of men smoke. According to the World Health Organization, 1 year after quitting, the risk of coronary heart disease decreases by 50%. Various interventions have been shown to increase the likelihood of successful smoking cessation (see Chapter 1).

Hypercholesterolemia and other lipid abnormalities provide an important modifiable risk factor for coronary heart disease. Risk increases progressively with higher levels of low-density lipoprotein (LDL) cholesterol and declines with higher levels of high-density lipoprotein (HDL) cholesterol. Composite risk scores, such as the Framingham score (see Table 28–2), provide estimates of 10-year probability of development of coronary heart disease that can guide primary prevention strategies.

The metabolic syndrome is defined as a constellation of three or more of the following: abdominal obesity, triglycerides ≥ 150 mg/dL, HDL cholesterol < 40 mg/dL for men and < 50 mg/dL for women, fasting glucose ≥ 110 mg/dL, and hypertension. This syndrome is increasing in prevalence at an alarming rate. Related to the metabolic syndrome, the epidemic of obesity in the United States is likewise a major factor contributing to coronary heart disease risk. Data from National Health and Nutrition Examination Survey (NHANES) show that the prevalence of obesity (body mass index [BMI] ≥ 30 kg/m^2) continues to increase at about 2% per year, up to 33% of the adult population in the 2003–2004 survey. Particularly alarming is the rapidly increasing incidence of obesity in adolescents in the United States, such that for children aged 12–19 years, prevalence of obesity increased from 5% (in 1976–1980) to 17%. Increasing physical activity is an important goal to help combat obesity and its consequences. Although the AHA continues to promote a diet based largely on low saturated fat, more information is needed on the health consequences of all diets, especially given the lack of protection from a low-fat diet in the largest randomized study ever done, the Women's Health Initiative trial. Low carbohydrate diets, even when high in saturated fat, may improve the cholesterol profile in overweight men and are as effective at achieving weight loss. Fish, rich in omega-3 fatty acids, may help protect against vascular disease, and it is recommended that it be eaten three times a week by patients at risk.

Markers of inflammation are strong risk factors for CAD. High sensitivity (hs) CRP is the best-characterized inflammatory marker, but others include interleukin-6, CD-40 ligand, myelopyroxidase, and placental growth factor. Although CRP levels > 10 mcg/mL are often found in systemic inflammation, levels < 1, 1–3, and > 3 mcg/mL, respectively, identify patients at low, intermediate, and high risk for future cardiovascular events. The prognostic value of CRP levels is independent and additive to lipid levels. Use of CRP may be helpful in determining which patients at intermediate risk according to the Framingham 10-year risk of coronary heart disease calculation (score of 10–20%) are at high enough risk to warrant more intensive primary prevention, including use of statins to lower LDL cholesterol. HsCRP ≥ 2 mg/L identifies older people without vascular disease and with normal cholesterol who benefit from statins. CRP levels are often elevated in patients who have other conditions associated with accelerated atherosclerosis, such as diabetes, the metabolic syndrome, and obesity. In patients presenting with acute coronary syndromes, the CRP elevation identifies a group that is at high risk for early recurrent events.

▶ Myocardial Hibernation & Stunning

Areas of myocardium that are persistently underperfused but still viable may develop sustained contractile dysfunction. This phenomenon, which is termed "myocardial hibernation," appears to represent an adaptive response that maybe associated with depressed LV function. It is important to recognize this phenomenon, since this form

of dysfunction is reversible following coronary revascularization. Hibernating myocardium can be identified by radionuclide testing, positron emission tomography (PET), contrast-enhanced MRI, or its retained response to inotropic stimulation with dobutamine. A related phenomenon, termed "myocardial stunning," is the occurrence of persistent contractile dysfunction following prolonged or repetitive episodes of myocardial ischemia. Clinically, myocardial stunning is often seen after reperfusion of acute myocardial infarction.

Centers for Disease Control and Prevention. Overweight and Obesity: Home (www.cdc.gov/nccdphp/dnpa/obesity; accessed March 2009)

Gardner CD et al. Comparison of the Atkins, Zone, Ornish, and LEARN diets for change in weight and related risk factors among overweight premenopausal women: the A TO Z Weight Loss Study: a randomized trial. JAMA. 2007 Mar 7;297(9):969–77. [PMID: 17341711]

Howard BV et al. Low-fat dietary pattern and risk of cardiovascular disease: the Women's Health Initiative Randomized Dietary Modification Trial. JAMA. 2006 Feb 8;295(6):655–66. [PMID: 16467234]

Pearson TA et al; Centers for Disease Control and Prevention; American Heart Association. Markers of inflammation and cardiovascular disease: application to clinical and public health practice: A statement for healthcare professionals from the Centers for Disease Control and Prevention and the American Heart Association. Circulation. 2003 Jan 28;107(3):499–511. [PMID: 12551878]

Yusuf S et al; INTERHEART Study Investigators. Effect of potentially modifiable risk factors associated with myocardial infarction in 52 countries (the INTERHEART study): case-control study. Lancet. 2004 Sep 11–17;364(9438):937–52. [PMID: 15364185]

CHRONIC STABLE ANGINA PECTORIS

ESSENTIALS OF DIAGNOSIS

▶ Precordial chest pain, usually precipitated by stress or exertion, relieved rapidly by rest or nitrates.

▶ ECG or scintigraphic evidence of ischemia during pain or stress testing.

▶ Angiographic demonstration of significant obstruction of major coronary vessels.

▶ General Considerations

Angina pectoris is usually due to atherosclerotic heart disease. Coronary vasospasm may occur at the site of a lesion or, less frequently, in apparently normal vessels. Other unusual causes of coronary artery obstruction such as congenital anomalies, emboli, arteritis, or dissection may cause ischemia or infarction. Angina may also occur in the absence of coronary artery obstruction as a result of severe myocardial hypertrophy, severe aortic stenosis or regurgitation, or in response to increased metabolic demands, as in hyperthyroidism, marked anemia, or paroxysmal tachycardias with rapid ventricular rates. Rarely, angina occurs with angiographically normal coronary arteries and without other identifiable causes. This presentation has been labeled **syndrome X** and is most likely due to inadequate flow reserve in the resistance vessels (microvasculature). Syndrome X remains difficult to diagnose. Although treatment is often not very successful in relieving symptoms, the prognosis of syndrome X is good.

► Clinical Findings

A. Symptoms

The diagnosis of angina pectoris depends principally upon the history, which should specifically include the following information: circumstances that precipitate and relieve angina, characteristics of the discomfort, location and radiation, duration of attacks, and effect of nitroglycerin.

1. Circumstances that precipitate and relieve angina— Angina occurs most commonly during activity and is relieved by resting. Patients may prefer to remain upright rather than lie down, as increased preload in recumbency increases myocardial work. The amount of activity required to produce angina may be relatively consistent under comparable physical and emotional circumstances or may vary from day to day. The threshold for angina is usually less after meals, during excitement, or on exposure to cold. It is often lower in the morning or after strong emotion; the latter can provoke attacks in the absence of exertion. In addition, discomfort may occur during sexual activity, at rest, or at night as a result of coronary spasm.

2. Characteristics of the discomfort— Patients often do not refer to angina as "pain" but as a sensation of tightness, squeezing, burning, pressing, choking, aching, bursting, "gas," indigestion, or an ill-characterized discomfort. It is often characterized by clenching a fist over the mid chest. The distress of angina is rarely sharply localized and is not spasmodic.

3. Location and radiation— The distribution of the distress may vary widely in different patients but is usually the same for each patient unless unstable angina or myocardial infarction supervenes. In most cases, the discomfort is felt behind or slightly to the left of the mid sternum. When it begins farther to the left or, uncommonly, on the right, it characteristically moves centrally substernally. Although angina may radiate to any dermatome from C8 to T4, it radiates most often to the left shoulder and upper arm, frequently moving down the inner volar aspect of the arm to the elbow, forearm, wrist, or fourth and fifth fingers. It may also radiate to the right shoulder or arm, the lower jaw, the neck, or even the back.

4. Duration of attacks— Angina is generally of short duration and subsides completely without residual discomfort. If the attack is precipitated by exertion and the patient promptly stops to rest, it usually lasts less than 3 minutes. Attacks following a heavy meal or brought on by anger often last 15–20 minutes. Attacks lasting more than 30 minutes are unusual and suggest the development of unstable angina, myocardial infarction, or an alternative diagnosis.

5. Effect of nitroglycerin— The diagnosis of angina pectoris is strongly supported if sublingual nitroglycerin promptly and invariably shortens an attack and if prophylactic nitrates permit greater exertion or prevent angina entirely.

B. Signs

Examination during angina frequently reveals a significant elevation in systolic and diastolic BP, although hypotension may also occur, and may reflect more severe ischemia or inferior ischemia (especially with bradycardia) due to a Bezold–Jarisch reflex. Occasionally, a gallop rhythm and an apical systolic murmur due to transient mitral regurgitation from papillary muscle dysfunction are present during pain only. Supraventricular or ventricular arrhythmias may be present, either as the precipitating factor or as a result of ischemia.

It is important to detect signs of diseases that may contribute to or accompany atherosclerotic heart disease, eg, diabetes mellitus (retinopathy or neuropathy), xanthelasma, tendinous xanthomas, hypertension, thyrotoxicosis, myxedema, or peripheral vascular disease. Aortic stenosis or regurgitation, hypertrophic cardiomyopathy, and mitral valve prolapse should be sought, since they may produce angina or other forms of chest pain.

C. Laboratory Findings

Other than standard laboratory tests to evaluate for acute coronary syndrome (troponin and CK-MB), factors contributing to ischemia (such as anemia), and to screen for risk factors that may increase the probability of true coronary heart disease (such as hyperlipidemia), blood tests are not helpful to diagnose chronic angina.

D. ECG

The resting ECG is often normal in patients with angina. In the remainder, abnormalities include old myocardial infarction, nonspecific ST–T changes, and changes of LVH. During anginal episodes, as well as during asymptomatic ischemia, the characteristic ECG change is horizontal or downsloping ST-segment depression that reverses after the ischemia disappears. T wave flattening or inversion may also occur. Less frequently, transient ST-segment elevation is observed; this finding suggests severe (transmural) ischemia from coronary occlusion, and it can occur with coronary spasm.

E. Exercise ECG

Exercise testing is the most commonly used noninvasive procedure for evaluating for inducible ischemia in the patient with angina. Exercise testing is often combined with imaging studies (nuclear, echocardiography, or MRI [see below]), but in patients without baseline ST segment abnormalities or in whom anatomic localization is not necessary, the exercise ECG remains the recommended initial procedure because of considerations of cost and convenience.

Exercise testing can be done on a motorized treadmill or with a bicycle ergometer. A variety of exercise protocols are utilized, the most common being the Bruce protocol, which increases the treadmill speed and elevation every 3 minutes until limited by symptoms. At least two ECG leads should be monitored continuously.

1. Precautions and risks—The risk of exercise testing is about one infarction or death per 1000 tests, but individuals who have pain at rest or minimal activity are at higher risk and should not be tested. Many of the traditional exclusions, such as recent myocardial infarction or CHF, are no longer used *if the patient is stable and ambulatory*, but symptomatic aortic stenosis remains a contraindication.

2. Indications—Exercise testing is used (1) to confirm the diagnosis of angina; (2) to determine the severity of limitation of activity due to angina; (3) to assess prognosis in patients with known coronary disease, including those recovering from myocardial infarction, by detecting groups at high or low risk; (4) to evaluate responses to therapy; and (5) less successfully, to screen asymptomatic populations for silent coronary disease. The latter application is controversial. Because false-positive tests often exceed true positives, leading to much patient anxiety and self-imposed or mandated disability, exercise testing of asymptomatic individuals should be done only for those at high risk, those whose occupations place them or others at special risk (eg, airline pilots), and older individuals commencing strenuous activity.

3. Interpretation—The usual ECG criterion for a positive test is 1 mm (0.1 mV) horizontal or downsloping ST-segment depression (beyond baseline) measured 80 milliseconds after the J point. By this criterion, 60–80% of patients with anatomically significant coronary disease will have a positive test, but 10–30% of those without significant disease will also be positive. False positives are uncommon when a 2-mm depression is present. Additional information is inferred from the time of onset and duration of the ECG changes, their magnitude and configuration, BP and heart rate changes, the duration of exercise, and the presence of associated symptoms. In general, patients exhibiting more severe ST-segment depression (> 2 mm) at low workloads (< 6 minutes on the Bruce protocol) or heart rates (< 70% of age-predicted maximum)—especially when the duration of exercise and rise in BP are limited or when hypotension occurs during the test—have more severe disease and a poorer prognosis. Depending on symptom status, age, and other factors, such patients should be referred for coronary arteriography and possible revascularization. On the other hand, less impressive positive tests in asymptomatic patients are often "false positives." Therefore, exercise testing results that do not conform to the clinical picture should be confirmed by stress imaging.

F. Myocardial Stress Imaging

Myocardial stress imaging (scintigraphy, echocardiography, or MRI) is indicated (1) when the resting ECG makes an exercise ECG difficult to interpret (eg, left bundle branch block, baseline ST–T changes, low voltage); (2) for confirmation of the results of the exercise ECG when they are contrary to the clinical impression (eg, a positive test in an asymptomatic patient); (3) to localize the region of ischemia; (4) to distinguish ischemic from infarcted myocardium; (5) to assess the completeness of vascularization following bypass surgery or coronary angioplasty; or (6) as a prognostic indicator in patients with known coronary disease.

1. Myocardial perfusion scintigraphy—This test provides images in which radionuclide uptake is proportionate to blood flow at the time of injection. Thallium-201, technetium-99m sestamibi, and tetrafosmin are most frequently used. If the radiotracer is injected during exercise or dipyridamole- or adenosine-induced coronary vasodilation, scintigraphic defects indicate a zone of hypoperfusion that may represent either ischemia or scar. If the myocardium is viable, as relative blood flow equalizes over time or during a scintigram performed under resting conditions, these defects tend to "fill in" or reverse, indicating reversible ischemia. Defects observed when the radiotracer is injected at rest or still present 3–4 hours after an injection during exercise or pharmacologic vasodilation (intravenous adenosine or dipyridamole) usually indicate myocardial infarction (old or recent) but may be present with severe ischemia. Occasionally, other conditions, including infiltrative diseases (sarcoidosis, amyloidosis), left bundle branch block, and dilated cardiomyopathy, may produce resting or persistent perfusion defects.

Stress imaging is positive in about 75–90% of patients with anatomically significant coronary disease and in 20–30% of those without it. False-positive radionuclide tests may occur as a result of diaphragmatic attenuation or, in women, attenuation through breast tissue. Tomographic imaging (single-photon emission computed tomography, SPECT) can reduce the severity of artifacts. Gated imaging allows for analysis of ventricular size, EF, and regional wall motion.

2. Radionuclide angiography—This procedure images the LV and measures its EF and wall motion. In coronary disease, resting abnormalities usually represent infarction, and those that occur only with exercise usually indicate stress-induced ischemia. Exercise radionuclide angiography has approximately the same sensitivity as thallium-201 scintigraphy, but it is less specific in older individuals and those with other forms of heart disease. The indications are similar to those for thallium-201 scintigraphy.

3. Stress echocardiography—Echocardiograms performed during supine exercise or immediately following upright exercise may demonstrate exercise-induced segmental wall motion abnormalities as an indicator of ischemia. This technique requires considerable expertise; however, in experienced laboratories, the test accuracy is comparable to that obtained with scintigraphy—though a higher proportion of tests is technically inadequate. While exercise is the preferred stress because of other information derived, pharmacologic stress with high-dose dobutamine (20–40 mcg/kg/min) can be used as an alternative to exercise. Echocardiography contrast agents allow for perfusion imaging and may improve the diagnostic accuracy of this form of testing, although these are not commonly used.

G. Other Imaging

1. Positron emission tomography—PET scanning uses positron-emitting agents to demonstrate either perfusion or metabolism of myocardium. PET scanning can accurately distinguish transiently dysfunctional ("stunned") myocardium from scar by showing persistent glycolytic metabolism with the tracer fluorodeoxyglucose (FDG) in regions with reduced blood flow. The newer SPECT camera can provide acceptable images without the more expensive PET technology.

2. CT and MRI scanning—**CT scanning** can image the heart and, with contrast medium and multislice technology, the coronary arteries, with increasing resolution. Excellent coronary artery images can be obtained by 64- and higher slice technology, and, if the images are normal, this technology has high specificity for excluding significant coronary artery disease.

Thus, this technology may be useful in evaluating patients with low likelihood of significant coronary artery disease who would otherwise have undergone coronary angiography. CT angiography may also be useful for evaluating chest pain and suspected acute coronary syndrome. However, the role of CT angiography in routine practice is yet to be established, since it currently requires a relatively large radiation exposure and contrast load.

Electron beam CT (EBCT) can quantify coronary artery calcification, which is highly correlated with atheromatous plaque and has high sensitivity, but low specificity, for obstructive coronary disease. Thus, although this test can stratify patients into lower and higher risk groups, the appropriate management of individual patients with asymptomatic coronary artery calcification—beyond aggressive risk factors modification—is unclear. According to the American Heart Association, persons who are at low risk (< 10% 10-year risk) or at high risk (> 20% 10-year risk) do not benefit from coronary calcium assessment (class III, level of evidence: B) (see Tables 28–2 and 28–3). However, in clinically selected, intermediate-risk patients, it may be reasonable to determine the atherosclerosis burden using EBCT in order to refine clinical risk prediction and to select patients for more aggressive target values for lipid-lowering therapies (class IIb, level of evidence: B).

Cardiac MRI provides high-resolution images of the heart and great vessels without radiation exposure or use of iodinated contrast media. It provides excellent assessment of pericardial disease, neoplastic disease of the heart, myocardial thickness, chamber size, and many congenital heart defects. It is an excellent noninvasive test for nonemergently evaluating dissection of the aorta. Rapid acquisition sequences is a useful alternative when the echocardiogram is suboptimal. Perfusion imaging can be done with gadolinium first pass perfusion using dobutamine or adenosine to produce pharmacologic stress. Advances have been made in imaging the proximal coronary arteries, but this application remains investigational.

H. Ambulatory ECG Monitoring

Ambulatory ECG recorders can monitor for ischemic ST-segment depression. In patients with CAD, these episodes usually signify ischemia, even when asymptomatic ("silent").

In many patients, silent episodes are more frequent than symptomatic ones. In most cases, they occur in patients with other evidence of ischemia, so the role of ambulatory monitoring is limited.

I. Coronary Angiography

Selective coronary arteriography is the definitive diagnostic procedure for CAD. It can be performed with low mortality (about 0.1%) and morbidity (1–5%), but the cost is high, and with currently available noninvasive techniques it is usually not indicated solely for diagnosis.

Coronary arteriography should be performed in the following circumstances if percutaneous transluminal coronary angioplasty or bypass surgery is a consideration:

1. Limiting stable angina despite an adequate medical regimen.
2. Clinical presentation (unstable angina, postinfarction angina, etc) or noninvasive testing suggests high-risk disease (see Indications for Revascularization).
3. Concomitant aortic valve disease and angina pectoris, to determine whether the angina is due to accompanying coronary disease.
4. Asymptomatic older patients undergoing valve surgery so that concomitant bypass may be done if the anatomy is propitious.
5. Recurrence of symptoms after coronary revascularization to determine whether bypass grafts or native vessels are occluded.
6. Cardiac failure where a surgically correctable lesion, such as LV aneurysm, mitral regurgitation, or reversible ischemic dysfunction, is suspected.
7. Survivors of sudden death or symptomatic or life-threatening arrhythmias when CAD may be a correctable cause.
8. Chest pain of uncertain cause or cardiomyopathy of unknown cause.

A narrowing greater than 50% of the luminal diameter is considered hemodynamically (and clinically) significant, although most lesions producing ischemia are associated with narrowing in excess of 70%. In those with strongly positive exercise ECGs or scintigraphic studies, three-vessel or left main disease may be present in 75–95% depending on the criteria used. **Intravascular ultrasound** (IVUS) can be positioned within the artery and image beneath the endothelial surface. This technique is useful when the angiogram is equivocal as well as for assessing the results of angioplasty or stenting. In addition, IVUS is the invasive diagnostic method of choice for ostial left main lesions and coronary dissections.

LV angiography is usually performed at the same time as coronary arteriography. Global and regional LV function are visualized, as well as mitral regurgitation if present. LV function is a major determinant of prognosis in coronary heart disease.

▶ Differential Diagnosis

When atypical features are present—such as prolonged duration (hours or days) or darting, knifelike pains at the apex or over the precordium—ischemia is less likely.

Anterior chest wall syndrome is characterized by sharply localized tenderness of intercostal muscles. Inflammation of the chondrocostal junctions, which may be warm, swollen, and red, may result in diffuse chest pain that is also reproduced by local pressure (Tietze syndrome). Intercostal neuritis (due to herpes zoster, diabetes mellitus, for example) also mimics angina.

Cervical or thoracic spine disease involving the dorsal roots produces sudden sharp, severe chest pain suggesting angina in location and "radiation" but related to specific movements of the neck or spine, recumbency, and straining or lifting. Pain due to cervical or thoracic disk disease involves the outer or dorsal aspect of the arm and the thumb and index fingers rather than the ring and little fingers.

Reflux esophagitis, peptic ulcer, chronic cholecystitis, esophageal spasm, and functional gastrointestinal disease may produce pain suggestive of angina pectoris. The picture may be especially confusing because ischemic pain may also be associated with upper gastrointestinal symptoms, and esophageal motility disorders may be improved by nitrates and calcium channel blockers. Assessment of esophageal motility may be helpful.

Degenerative and inflammatory lesions of the left shoulder and thoracic outlet syndromes may cause chest pain due to nerve irritation or muscular compression; the symptoms are usually precipitated by movement of the arm and shoulder and are associated with paresthesias.

Pneumonia, pulmonary embolism, and spontaneous pneumothorax may cause chest pain as well as dyspnea. Dissection of the thoracic aorta can cause severe chest pain that is commonly felt in the back; it is sudden in onset, reaches maximum intensity immediately, and may be associated with changes in pulses. Other cardiac disorders such as mitral valve prolapse, hypertrophic cardiomyopathy, myocarditis, pericarditis, aortic valve disease, or RVH may cause atypical chest pain or even myocardial ischemia.

► Treatment

Sublingual nitroglycerin is the drug of choice for acute management; it acts in about 1–2 minutes. Nitrates decrease arteriolar and venous tone, reduce preload and afterload, and lower the oxygen demand of the heart. As soon as the attack begins, one fresh tablet is placed under the tongue. This may be repeated at 3- to 5-minute intervals, but current recommendations are that if pain is not relieved or improving after 5 minutes, that the patient call 9-1-1. The dosage (0.3, 0.4, or 0.6 mg) and the number of tablets to be used before seeking further medical attention must be individualized. Nitroglycerin buccal spray is also available as a metered (0.4 mg) delivery system. It has the advantage of being more convenient for patients who have difficulty handling the pills and of being more stable. Nitroglycerin can also be used prophylactically before activities likely to precipitate angina. Pain not responding to three tablets or lasting more than 20 minutes may represent evolving infarction, and the patient should be instructed to seek immediate medical attention.

► Prevention of Further Attacks

A. Aggravating Factors

Angina may be aggravated by hypertension, LV failure, arrhythmia (usually tachycardias), strenuous activity, cold temperatures, and emotional states. These factors should be identified and treated when possible.

B. Nitroglycerin

Nitroglycerin, 0.3–0.6 mg sublingually or 0.4–0.8 mg translingually by spray, should be taken 5 minutes before any activity likely to precipitate angina. Sublingual isosorbide dinitrate (2.5–10 mg) is only slightly longer-acting than sublingual nitroglycerin.

C. Long-Acting Nitrates

Longer-acting nitrate preparations include isosorbide dinitrate, 10–40 mg orally three times daily; isosorbide mononitrate, 10–40 mg orally twice daily or 60–120 mg once daily in a sustained-release preparation; oral sustained-release nitroglycerin preparations, 6.25–12.5 mg two to four times daily; nitroglycerin ointment, 6.25–25 mg applied two to four times daily; and transdermal nitroglycerin patches that deliver nitroglycerin at a predetermined rate (usually 5–20 mg/24 h). The main limitation to long-term nitrate therapy is tolerance, which can be limited by using a regimen that includes a minimum 8- to 10-hour period per day without nitrates. Isosorbide dinitrate can be given three times daily, with the last dose after dinner, or longer-acting isosorbide mononitrate once daily. Transdermal nitrate preparations should be removed overnight in most patients.

Nitrate therapy is often limited by headache. Other side effects include nausea, light-headedness, and hypotension.

D. β-Blockers

β-Blockers are the only antianginal agents that have been demonstrated to prolong life in patients with coronary disease (post-myocardial infarction). They are at least as effective at relieving angina as alternative agents in studies employing exercise testing, ambulatory monitoring, and symptom assessment. β-Blockers should be considered for first-line therapy in most patients with chronic angina.

β-Blockers with intrinsic sympathomimetic activity, such as pindolol, are less desirable because they may exacerbate angina in some individuals and have not been effective in secondary prevention trials. The pharmacology and side effects of the β-blockers are discussed in Chapter 11 (see Table 11–7). The dosages of all these drugs when given for angina are similar. The major contraindications are severe bronchospastic disease, bradyarrhythmias, and decompensated heart failure.

E. Calcium Channel Blocking Agents

Unlike the β-blockers, calcium channel blockers have not been shown to reduce mortality postinfarction and in some cases have increased ischemia and mortality rates.

This appears to be the case with some dihydropyridines and with diltiazem and verapamil in patients with clinical heart failure or moderate to severe LV dysfunction. Meta-analyses have suggested that short-acting nifedipine in moderate to high doses causes an increase in mortality. It is uncertain whether these findings are relevant to longer-acting dihydropyridines. Nevertheless, considering the uncertainties and the lack of demonstrated favorable effect on outcomes, calcium channel blockers should be considered third-line anti-ischemic drugs in the postinfarction patient. Similarly, with the exception of amlodipine, which in the PRAISE trial proved safe in patients with heart failure, these agents should be avoided in patients with CHF or low EFs.

The pharmacologic effects and side effects of the calcium channel blockers are discussed in Chapter 11 and summarized in Table 11–9. Diltiazem and verapamil are preferable because they produce less reflex tachycardia and because the former, at least, may cause fewer side effects. Nifedipine, nicardipine, and amlodipine are also approved agents for angina. Isradipine, felodipine, and nisoldipine are not approved for angina but probably are as effective as the other dihydropyridines.

F. Ranolazine

Ranolazine is the first new antianginal drug to be approved by the FDA in many years, and it is approved as first-line use for chronic angina. It decreases the late sodium current and thereby decreases intracellular calcium overload. Ranolazine has no effect on heart rate and blood pressure, and it has been shown in clinical trials to prolong exercise duration and time to angina, both as monotherapy and when administered with conventional antianginal therapy. It is safe to use with erectile dysfunction drugs. The usual dose is 500 mg orally twice a day. Because it can cause QT prolongation, it is contraindicated in patients with existing QT prolongation; in patients taking QT prolonging drugs, such as class I or III antiarrhythmics (eg, quinidine, dofetilide, sotalol); and in those taking potent and moderate CYP450 3A inhibitors. Of interest, in spite of the QT prolongation, there is a significantly lower rate of ventricular arrhythmias with its use following acute coronary syndromes, shown in the MERLIN trial. It also decreases occurrence of atrial fibrillation and results in a small decrease in Hgb_{A1C}. It is also contraindicated in patients with significant liver and kidney disease. Ranolazine is not to be used for treatment of acute anginal episodes.

G. Alternative and Combination Therapies

Patients who do not respond to one class of antianginal medication often respond to another. It may, therefore, be worthwhile to use an alternative agent before progressing to combinations. If the patient remains symptomatic, a β-blocker and a long-acting nitrate or a β-blocker and a calcium channel blocker (other than verapamil, where the risk of AV block or heart failure is higher) are the most appropriate combinations. A few patients will have a further response to a regimen including all three agents.

H. Platelet-Inhibiting Agents

Several studies have demonstrated the benefit of antiplatelet drugs for patients with stable and unstable vascular disease. Therefore, unless contraindicated, aspirin (81–325 mg daily) should be prescribed for all patients with angina. Clopidogrel, 75 mg daily, reduces vascular events in patients with stable vascular disease (as an alternative to aspirin) and in patients with acute coronary syndromes (in addition to aspirin). Thus, it is also a good alternative in aspirin-intolerant patients. Clopidogrel may rarely induce thrombotic thrombocytopenic purpura.

I. Risk Reduction

Patients with coronary disease should undergo aggressive risk factor modification. This approach, with a particular focus on statin treatment, treating hypertension, stopping smoking, and exercise and weight control (especially for patients with metabolic syndrome or at risk for diabetes), may markedly improve outcome.

J. Revascularization

1. Indications—There is general agreement that otherwise healthy patients in the following groups should undergo revascularization: (1) Patients with unacceptable symptoms despite medical therapy to its tolerable limits. (2) Patients with left main coronary artery stenosis greater than 50% with or without symptoms. (3) Patients with three-vessel disease with LV dysfunction (EF < 50% or previous transmural infarction). (4) Patients with unstable angina who after symptom control by medical therapy continue to exhibit ischemia on exercise testing or monitoring. (5) Postmyocardial infarction patients with continuing angina or severe ischemia on noninvasive testing. The use of revascularization for patients with acute coronary syndromes and acute ST elevation myocardial infarction is discussed below.

In addition, many cardiologists have believed that patients with less severe symptoms should be revascularized if they have two-vessel disease associated with underlying LV dysfunction, anatomically critical lesions (> 90% proximal stenoses, especially of the proximal left anterior descending artery), or physiologic evidence of severe ischemia (early positive exercise tests, large exercise-induced thallium scintigraphic defects, or frequent episodes of ischemia on ambulatory monitoring). Two sources of data have tempered some of the enthusiasm for coronary intervention for stable angina. Drug-eluting stents, widely used because of their benefits in preventing restenosis, have been associated with higher rates of late stent thrombosis. In addition, data from the COURAGE trial have shown that for patients with chronic angina, percutaneous coronary intervention (PCI) offers no mortality benefit beyond excellent medical therapy, and relatively little long-term symptomatic improvement.

2. Type of procedure

A. CORONARY ARTERY BYPASS GRAFTING—Coronary artery bypass grafting (CABG) can be accomplished with a very low mortality rate (1–3%) in otherwise healthy patients with preserved cardiac function. However, the mortality rate of this procedure rises to 4–8% in older individuals and in patients who have had a prior CABG.

Grafts using one or both internal mammary arteries (usually to the left anterior descending artery or its branches) provide the best long-term results in terms of patency and flow. Segments of the saphenous vein (or, less optimally, other veins) or the radial artery interposed between the aorta and the coronary arteries distal to the obstructions are also used. One to five distal anastomoses are commonly performed.

Minimally invasive surgical techniques utilize different approaches to the heart than standard sternotomy and cardiopulmonary bypass. The surgical approach may involve a limited sternotomy, lateral thoracotomy (MIDCAB), or thoracoscopy (port-access). These techniques allow earlier postoperative mobilization and discharge. They are more technically demanding, usually not suitable for more than two grafts, and do not have established durability. Bypass surgery can be performed both on circulatory support (on pump) and without direct circulatory support (off-pump). No evidence to date has demonstrated a clinical difference in outcomes with either technique.

The operative mortality rate is increased in patients with poor LV function (LV EF < 35%) or those requiring additional procedures (valve replacement or ventricular aneurysmectomy). Patients over 70 years of age, patients undergoing repeat procedures, or those with important noncardiac disease (especially chronic kidney disease and diabetes) or poor general health also have higher operative mortality and morbidity rates, and full recovery is slow. Thus, CABG should be reserved for more severely symptomatic patients in this group. Early (1–6 months) graft patency rates average 85–90% (higher for internal mammary grafts), and subsequent graft closure rates are about 4% annually. Early graft failure is common in vessels with poor distal flow, while late closure is more frequent in patients who continue smoking and those with untreated hyperlipidemia. Antiplatelet therapy with aspirin improves graft patency rates. Smoking cessation and vigorous treatment of blood lipid abnormalities (particularly with statins) are necessary. While the most important principle is to use proven doses of statins shown to improve outcomes in large trials, many advocate a goal for LDL cholesterol of 70–100 mg/dL and for HDL cholesterol of 45 mg/dL. Repeat revascularization (see below) may be necessitated because of recurrent symptoms due to progressive native vessel disease and graft occlusions. Reoperation is technically demanding and less often fully successful than the initial operation.

B. Percutaneous coronary intervention including stenting—PCI, including balloon angioplasty and coronary stenting, can effectively open stenotic coronary arteries. Coronary stenting, with either bare metal stents or drug-eluting stents, has substantially reduced restenosis. Stenting can also be used selectively for left main coronary stenosis, particularly when CABG is contraindicated.

PCI is possible but often less successful in bypass graft stenoses. Experienced operators are able to successfully dilate 90% of lesions attempted. The major early complication is intimal dissection with vessel occlusion, although this is rare with coronary stenting. The use of intravenous platelet glycoprotein IIb/IIIa inhibitors (abciximab, eptifibatide, tirofiban) has substantially reduced the rate of periprocedural myocardial infarction, and placement of intracoronary stents has markedly improved initial and long-term angiographic results, especially with complex and long lesions. After percutaneous coronary intervention, all patients should have CK-MB and troponin measured, and a new rise of greater than three times the upper limit of normal constitutes a significant periprocedural myocardial infarction. Acute thrombosis after stent placement can largely be prevented by aggressive antithrombotic therapy (long-term aspirin, 81–325 mg, plus clopidogrel, 300–600 mg loading dose followed by 75 mg daily, for between 30 days and 1 year, and with acute use of platelet glycoprotein IIb/IIIa inhibitors).

A major limitation with PCI has been restenosis, which occurs in the first 6 months in less than 10% of vessels treated with drug-eluting stents, 15–30% of vessels treated with bare metal stents, and 30–40% of vessels without stenting. Factors associated with higher restenosis rates include diabetes, small luminal diameter, longer and more complex lesions, and lesions at coronary ostia or in the left anterior descending coronary artery. Drug-eluting stents that elute antiproliferative agents such as sirolimus, everolimus, zotarolimus, or paclitaxel have substantially reduced restenosis. In-stent restenosis is often treated with either brachytherapy or restenting with drug-eluting stents, and rarely with brachytherapy. The nearly 2 million PCIs performed worldwide per year far exceeds the number of CABG operations, but the justification rationale for many of the procedures performed in patients with stable angina is unclear. The COURAGE trial has confirmed earlier studies in showing that even for patients with moderate anginal symptoms and positive stress tests, PCI provides no benefit over medical therapy with respect to death or with respect to death or myocardial infarction. PCI was more effective at relieving angina, although most patients in the medical group had improvement in symptoms. Thus, in patients with mild or moderate stable symptoms, aggressive lipid-lowering and antianginal therapy may be a preferable initial strategy, reserving PCI for patients with significant and refractory symptoms.

Several studies of PTCA, including with drug-eluting stents, versus CABG in patients with multivessel disease have been reported. The consistent finding has been comparable mortality and infarction rates over follow-up periods of 1–3 years but a high rate (approximately 40%) of repeat procedures following PTCA. Stroke rates are higher with CABG. As a result, the choice of revascularization procedure may depend on details of coronary anatomy and is often a matter of patient preference. However, it should be noted that less than 20% of patients with multivessel disease met the entry criteria for the clinical trials, so these results cannot be generalized to all multivessel disease patients. Outcomes with percutaneous revascularization in diabetics have generally been inferior to those with CABG. However, most of these trials preceded the widespread use of stenting.

K. Mechanical Extracorporeal Counterpulsation

Extracorporeal counterpulsation (ECP) entails repetitive inflation of a high-pressure chamber surrounding the lower half of the body during the diastolic phase of the cardiac cycle for daily 1-hour sessions over a period of 7 weeks. Randomized trials have shown that ECP reduces angina, improves exercise tolerance, and can reduce symptoms of heart failure.

L. Neuromodulation

Spinal cord stimulation can be used to relieve chronic refractory angina. Spinal cord stimulators are subcutaneously implantable via a minimally invasive procedure under local anesthesia.

▶ Prognosis

The prognosis of angina pectoris has improved with development of therapies aimed at secondary prevention. Mortality rates vary depending on the number of vessels diseased, the severity of obstruction, the status of LV function, and the presence of complex arrhythmias. Mortality rates are progressively higher in patients with one-, two-, and three-vessel disease and those with left main coronary artery obstruction (ranging from 1% per year to 25% per year). The outlook in individual patients is unpredictable, and nearly half of the deaths are sudden. Therefore, risk stratification is often attempted. Patients with accelerating symptoms have a poorer outlook. Among stable patients, those whose exercise tolerance is severely limited by ischemia (less than 6 minutes on the Bruce treadmill protocol) and those with extensive ischemia by exercise ECG or scintigraphy have more severe anatomic disease and a poorer prognosis. The Duke Treadmill Score, based on a standard Bruce protocol exercise treadmill test, provides an estimate of risk of death at 1 year. The score uses time on the treadmill, amount of ST-segment depression, and presence of angina (Table 10–4).

▶ Trial Results

Several randomized trials have shown that over follow-up periods of several years, the mortality and infarction rates

Table 10–4. Duke treadmill score: Calculation and interpretation.

Time in minutes on Bruce protocol	=	
-5 × amount of depression (in mm)	=	
-4 × angina index	=	
0 = no angina on test		
1 = angina, not limiting		
2 = limiting angina		

Total Score	Risk Group	Annual Mortality
≥ 5	Low	0.25%
-10 to +4	Intermediate	1.25%
≤ -11	High	5.25%

with percutaneous revascularization and CABG are generally comparable. Exceptions are patients with left main or three-vessel disease with reduced ventricular function, and perhaps diabetic patients, who have had better outcomes with CABG. The increasing popularity of PCI and stenting primarily reflects the lower cost and shorter hospitalization, the perception that CABG is best done only once and can be reserved for later, and the preference of patients for less invasive treatment. These arguments make PCI the procedure of choice for revascularization of single-vessel disease. The situation is less clear with multivessel disease. It should also be noted that the excellent outcome of patients treated medically has made it difficult to show an advantage with either revascularization approach except in patients who remain symptom limited or have left main lesions or three-vessel disease and LV dysfunction. The issue of late stent thrombosis is shifting the balance toward bare metal stents for many patients.

Boden WE et al; COURAGE Trial Research Group. Optimal medical therapy with or without PCI for stable coronary disease. N Engl J Med. 2007 Apr 12;356(15):1503–16. [PMID: 17387127]

Botoman VA. Noncardiac chest pain. J Clin Gastroenterol. 2002 Jan;34(1):6–14. [PMID: 11743240]

Budoff MJ et al. Assessment of coronary artery disease by cardiac computed tomography: a scientific statement from the American Heart Association Committee on Cardiovascular Imaging and Intervention, Council on Cardiovascular Radiology and Intervention, and Committee on Cardiac Imaging, Council on Clinical Cardiology. Circulation. 2006 Oct 17;114(16):1761–91. [PMID: 17015792]

Eagle KA et al. ACC/AHA 2004 guideline update for coronary artery bypass graft surgery: a report of the American College of Cardiology/American Heart Association Task Force on Practice Guidelines (Committee to Update the 1999 Guidelines for Coronary Artery Bypass Graft Surgery). (http://www.acc.org/qualityandscience/clinical/guidelines/cabg/index_rev.pdf; accessed June 2009)

Gibbons RJ et al. ACC/AHA 2002 guideline update for the management of patients with chronic stable angina—summary article: a report of the American College of Cardiology/American Heart Association Task Force on practice guidelines (Committee on the Management of Patients With Chronic Stable Angina). J Am Coll Cardiol. 2003 Jan 1;41(1):159–68. [PMID: 12570960]

Goldstein J et al. A randomized controlled trial of multi-slice coronary computed tomography for evaluation of acute chest pain. J Am Coll Cardiol. 2007 Feb 27;49(8):863–71. [PMID: 17320744]

Grines CL et al. Prevention of premature discontinuation of dual antiplatelet therapy in patients with coronary artery stents: a science advisory from the American Heart Association, American College of Cardiology, Society for Cardiovascular Angiography and Interventions, American College of Surgeons, and American Dental Association, with representation from the American College of Physicians. Circulation. 2007 Feb 13;115(6):813–8. [PMID: 17224480]

Lee TH et al. Clinical practice. Noninvasive tests in patients with stable coronary artery disease. N Engl J Med. 2001 Jun 14;344(24):1840–5. [PMID: 11407346]

Morrow DA et al. Effects of ranolazine on recurrent cardiovascular events in patients with non-ST-elevation acute coronary syndromes: the MERLIN-TIMI 36 randomized trial. JAMA. 2007 Apr 25;297(16):1775–83. [PMID: 17456819]

Paetsch I et al. Comparison of dobutamine stress magnetic resonance, adenosine stress magnetic resonance, and adenosine stress magnetic resonance perfusion. Circulation. 2004 Aug 17;110(7):835–42. [PMID: 15289384]

Patel MR et al. ACCF/SCAI/STS/AATS/AHA/ASNC 2009 Appropriateness Criteria for Coronary Revascularization: a report by the American College of Cardiology Foundation Appropriateness Criteria Task Force, Society for Cardiovascular Angiography and Interventions, Society of Thoracic Surgeons, American Association for Thoracic Surgery, American Heart Association, and the American Society of Nuclear Cardiology Endorsed by the American Society of Echocardiography, the Heart Failure Society of America, and the Society of Cardiovascular Computed Tomography. J Am Coll Cardiol. 2009 Feb 10;53(6):530–53. [PMID: 19195618]

Raff GL et al. Coronary angiography by computed tomography: coronary imaging evolves. J Am Coll Cardiol. 2007 May 8;49(18):1830–3. [PMID: 17481441]

Smith SC Jr et al. ACC/AHA/SCAI 2005 guideline update for percutaneous coronary intervention: a report of the American College of Cardiology/American Heart Association Task Force on Practice Guidelines (ACC/AHA/SCAI Writing Committee to Update the 2001 Guidelines for Percutaneous Coronary Intervention). (http://www.acc.org/qualityandscience/clinical/guidelines/percutaneous/update/index.pdf; accessed June 2009)

CORONARY VASOSPASM & ANGINA WITH NORMAL CORONARY ARTERIOGRAMS

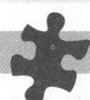 ESSENTIALS OF DIAGNOSIS

► Precordial chest pain, often occurring at rest during stress or without known precipitant, relieved rapidly by nitrates.

► ECG evidence of ischemia during pain, sometime with ST-segment elevation, including by Holter monitor.

► Angiographic demonstration of no significant obstruction of major coronary vessels.

► Angiographic demonstration of coronary spasm that responds to intra-coronary nitroglycerin or calcium channel blockers.

General Considerations

Although most symptoms of myocardial ischemia result from fixed stenosis of the coronary arteries or intraplaque hemorrhage or thrombosis at the site of lesions, some ischemic events may be precipitated or exacerbated by coronary vasoconstriction.

Spasm of the large coronary arteries with resulting decreased coronary blood flow may occur spontaneously or may be induced by exposure to cold, emotional stress, or vasoconstricting medications, such as ergot derivative drugs. Spasm may occur both in normal and in stenosed coronary arteries. Even myocardial infarction may occur as a result of spasm in the absence of visible obstructive coronary heart disease, although most instances of such coronary spasm occur in the presence of coronary stenosis.

Cocaine can induce myocardial ischemia and infarction by causing coronary artery vasoconstriction or by increasing myocardial energy requirements. It also may contribute to accelerated atherosclerosis and thrombosis. The ischemia in **Prinzmetal (variant) angina** usually results from coronary vasoconstriction. It tends to involve the right coronary artery and there may be no fixed stenoses. Myocardial ischemia may also occur in patients with normal coronary arteries as a result of disease of the coronary microcirculation or abnormal vascular reactivity. This has been termed "syndrome X."

Clinical Findings

Ischemia may be silent or result in angina pectoris.

Prinzmetal (variant) angina is a clinical syndrome in which chest pain occurs without the usual precipitating factors and is associated with ST-segment elevation rather than depression. It often affects women under 50 years of age. It characteristically occurs in the early morning, awakening patients from sleep, and is apt to be associated with arrhythmias or conduction defects. It may be diagnosed by challenge with ergonovine (a vasoconstrictor), although the results of such provocation are not specific and it entails risk.

Treatment

Patients with chest pain associated with ST-segment elevation should undergo coronary arteriography to determine whether fixed stenotic lesions are present. If they are, aggressive medical therapy or revascularization is indicated, since this may represent an unstable phase of the disease. If significant lesions are not seen and spasm is suspected, avoidance of precipitants such as cigarette smoking and cocaine is the top priority. Episodes of coronary spasm generally respond well to nitrates, and both nitrates and calcium channel blockers (including long-acting nifedipine, diltiazem, or amlopidine) are effective prophylactically. By allowing unopposed α_1-mediated vasoconstriction, β-blockers have exacerbated coronary vasospasm, but they may have a role in management of patients in whom spasm is associated with fixed stenoses.

Al Suwaidi J et al. Pathophysiology, diagnosis, and current management strategies for chest pain in patients with normal findings on angiography. Mayo Clin Proc. 2001 Aug;76(8):813–22. [PMID: 11499821]

Frishman WH et al. Cardiovascular manifestations of substance abuse part 1: cocaine. Heart Dis. 2003 May–Jun;5(3):187–201. [PMID: 12783633]

Lange RA et al. Cardiovascular complications of cocaine use. N Engl J Med. 2001 Aug 2;345(5):351–8. [PMID: 11484693]

ACUTE CORONARY SYNDROMES WITHOUT ST SEGMENT ELEVATION

 ESSENTIALS OF DIAGNOSIS

► Acute coronary syndromes are classified based on presenting ECG

• Non–ST-segment elevation acute coronary syndrome.

- ST-segment elevation myocardial infarction.
▸ Non–ST-segment elevation acute coronary syndrome is further divided into non–ST-elevation myocardial infarction or unstable angina, based primarily on presence or absence of elevation of cardiac biomarkers.
▸ CK-MB or troponin, or both, may be elevated or normal.
▸ ECG may show ST depression or T wave inversion, or may be normal.

General Considerations

Acute coronary syndromes comprise the spectrum of unstable cardiac ischemia from unstable angina to acute myocardial infarction. Acute coronary syndromes are classified based on the presenting ECG as either "ST segment elevation" (STEMI) or "non-ST segment elevation." This allows for immediate classification and guides determination of whether patients should be considered for acute reperfusion therapy. The evolution of cardiac biomarkers then allows determination of whether myocardial infarction has occurred. The universal definition of myocardial infarction in a rise of cardiac biomarkers with at least one value above the 99th percentile of the upper reference limit together with evidence of myocardial ischemia with at least one of the following: symptoms of ischemia, ECG changes of new ischemia, new Q waves, or imaging evidence of new loss of viable myocardium or new wall motion abnormality.

Acute coronary syndromes represent a dynamic state in which patients frequently shift from one category to another, as new ST elevation can develop after presentation and cardiac biomarkers can become abnormal with recurrent ischemic episodes.

Chest pain is one of the most frequent reasons for emergency department visits. Algorithms have been developed to aid in determining the likelihood that a patient has an acute coronary syndrome, and for those patients who do have an acute coronary syndrome, the risk of ischemic events and death.

Clinical Findings

A. Symptoms and Signs

Patients with acute coronary syndromes generally have symptoms and signs of myocardial ischemia either at rest or with minimal exertion. These symptoms and signs are similar to chronic angina symptoms described above, consisting of substernal chest pain or discomfort that may radiate to the jaw, left shoulder or arm. Dyspnea, nausea, diaphoresis or syncope may either accompany the chest discomfort or may be the only symptom of acute coronary syndrome. About one-third of patients with myocardial infarction have no chest pain per se—these patients tend to be older, female, have diabetes, and be at higher risk for subsequent mortality. Patients with acute coronary syndromes have signs of heart failure in about 10% of cases, and this is also associated with higher risk of death.

Many hospitals have developed **chest pain observation units** to provide a systematic approach toward serial risk stratification to improve the triage process. In many cases, those who have not experienced new chest pain and have insignificant ECG changes and no cardiac biomarker elevation undergo treadmill exercise tests or imaging procedures to exclude ischemia at the end of an 8- to 24-hour period and are discharged directly from the emergency department if these tests are negative.

B. Laboratory Findings

Depending on the time from symptom onset to presentation, initial laboratory findings may be normal. The markers of cardiac myocyte necrosis, myoglobin, CK, CK-MB, and troponin I and T may all be used to identify acute myocardial infarction. These markers have a well-described pattern of release over time in patients with myocardial infarction. In patients with STEMI, these initial markers are often within normal limits as the patient is being rushed to immediate reperfusion. In patients without ST-segment elevation, it is the presence of abnormal CK-MB or troponin values that are associated with myocyte necrosis and the diagnosis of myocardial infarction. Serum creatine is an important determinant of risk, and estimated creatine clearance is important to guide dosing of certain antithrombotics, including eptifibatide and enoxaparin.

C. ECG

Many patients with acute coronary syndromes will exhibit ECG changes during pain—either ST-segment elevation, ST-segment depression, or T wave flattening or inversion. Dynamic ST segment shift is the most specific for acute coronary syndrome. Patients may exhibit signs of LV dysfunction during pain and for a time thereafter.

Treatment

A. General Measures

Treatment of acute coronary syndromes without ST elevation should be multifaceted. Patients who are at medium or high risk should be hospitalized, maintained at bed rest or at very limited activity for the first 24 hours, monitored, and given supplemental oxygen. Sedation with a benzodiazepine agent may help if anxiety is present.

B. Specific Measures

Table 10–5 provides a summary of the ACC/AHA Guideline recommendations for selected medical treatments.

C. Anticoagulation and Antiplatelet Therapy

Patients should receive a combination of antiplatelet and anticoagulant agents. Aspirin, 81–325 mg daily, and an anticoagulant (unfractionated heparin, enoxaparin, fondaparinux, or bivalirudin) should be commenced on presentation. Several trials have shown that low-molecular-weight heparin (enoxaparin 1 mg/kg subcutaneously every 12 hours) is somewhat more effective than unfractionated heparin in preventing recurrent ischemic events in the setting of acute coronary syndromes. However, the SYNERGY trial showed that unfractionated heparin and

Table 10–5. Summary of the current ACC/AHA guideline recommendations for medical management of acute coronary syndromes (ACS) and acute myocardial infarction (AMI).[1]

Medication	Acute Therapies ACS	Acute Therapies AMI	Discharge Therapies
Aspirin (ASA)	IA	IA	IA
Clopidogrel in ASA-allergic patients	IA	IC	IA
Clopidogrel, intended medical management	IA	—	IA
Clopidogrel and IIb/IIIa inhibitor, up front (prior to catheterization)	IIaB		
Clopidogrel, early catheterization/percutaneous coronary intervention (catheterization/percutaneous coronary intervention [cath/PCI])	IA (prior to or at time of PCI)	IB	IA
Heparin (unfractionated or low-molecular-weight)	IA	IC[2]	—
Fondaparinux	IB	IC	
Bivalirudin	IB		
Bivalirudin for early invasive strategy (without IIb/IIIa inhibitor), if clopidogrel at least 300 mg was administered 6 hours before planned catheterization or PCI	IIaB		
β-Blockers (oral)	IB	IA	IB
β-Blockers (intravenous)[3]	IIaB[3]	IIaB[3]	
Angiotensin-converting enzyme (ACE) inhibitors	IB[3]	IA/IIaB[4]	IA/IIaB[5]
GP IIb/IIIa inhibitors for intended early cath/PCI			
Eptifibatide/tirofiban	IA	—	—
Abciximab	IA	IIaB[6]	—
GP IIb/IIIa inhibitors for high-risk patients without intended early cath/PCI			
Eptifibatide/tirofiban	IIaA	—	—
Abciximab	IIIA	—	—
Lipid-lowering agent[7]	—	—	IA
Smoking cessation counseling	—	—	IB
Nonsteroidal anti-inflammatory agents (other than aspirin)	IIIC	IIIC	—

[1]Class I indicates treatment is useful and effective, IIa indicates weight of evidence is in favor of usefulness/efficacy, class IIb indicates weight of evidence is less well established, and class III indicates intervention is not useful/effective and may be harmful. Type A recommendations are derived from large-scale randomized trials, and B recommendations are derived from smaller randomized trials or carefully conducted observational analyses. ACC/AHA = American College of Cardiology/American Heart Association.
[2]Unfractionated heparin, enoxaparin, or fondaparinux have established efficacy and should be used (IC) for a minimum of 48 hours and preferably for the duration of the hospitalization, up to 8 days. Enoxaparin or fondaparinux are preferred if therapy is given for more than 48 hours because of risk of heparin-induced thrombocytopenia (IA). Because of risk of catheter thrombosis, fondaparinux should not be used as the sole anticoagulant to support PCI.
[3]For patients with hypertension and no heart failure, low output state, increased risk of shock, or other contraindications to β-blockers.
[4]For patients with persistent hypertension despite treatment, diabetes mellitus, congestive heart failure, or any left ventricular dysfunction.
[5]IA for patients with congestive heart failure or ejection fraction < 0.40, IIa for others, in absence of hypotension (systolic blood pressure < 100 mm Hg); angiotensin receptor blocker (valsartan or candesartan) for patients with ACE inhibitor intolerance.
[6]As early as possible before primary PCI.
[7]For patients with a low-density lipoprotein cholesterol level > 100 mg/dL.

enoxaparin had similar rates of death or (re)infarction in the setting of frequent early coronary intervention. **Fondaparinux,** a specific factor Xa inhibitor given in a dose of 2.5 mg subcutaneously once a day, was found in the OASIS-5 trial to be equally effective as enoxaparin among 20,000 patients at preventing early death, myocardial infarction, and refractory ischemia, and resulted in a 50% reduction in major bleeding. This reduction in major bleeding translated into a significant reduction in mortality (and in death and/or myocardial infarction) at 30 days. While catheter-related thrombosis was more common during coronary intervention procedures with fondaparinux, it appears that this can be controlled by adding unfractionated heparin (in the dose of approximately 50–70 units/kg) during the procedure. Guidelines recommend fondaparinux, describing it as especially favorable for patients who are initially treated medically and who are at high risk for bleeding, such as the elderly.

The ACUITY trial showed that the direct thrombin inhibitor **bivalirudin** appears to be a reasonable alternative to heparin (unfractionated heparin or enoxaparin) plus a glycoprotein IIb/IIIa antagonist for many patients with acute coronary syndromes who are undergoing early coronary intervention. Bivalirudin (without routine glycoprotein IIb/IIIa inhibitor) is associated with substantially less bleeding than heparin plus glycoprotein IIb/IIIa inhibitor.

The Clopidogrel in Unstable Angina to Prevent Recurrent Events (CURE) trial demonstrated a 20% reduction in the composite end point of cardiovascular death, myocardial infarction, and stroke with the addition of clopidogrel (300 mg loading dose, 75 mg/d for 9–12 months) in patients with non–ST-segment elevation acute coronary syndromes. When treated with clopidogrel, the optimal aspirin dose appears to be 81 mg/d (versus 160 mg/d or 325 mg/d) based on similar thrombotic event rates and lower rates of bleeding, although the ACC/AHA guidelines call for 162–325 mg/d for 1 month after bare metal stents and 3–6 months for drug-eluting stents. ACC/AHA guidelines call for either clopidogrel or glycoprotein IIb/IIIa inhibitor "upfront" prior to coronary angiography as a class IA recommendation. The European Society of Cardiology guidelines provide a stronger recommendation for clopidogrel upfront, as a class IA recommendation for all patients.

Prasugrel is a new thienopyridine that is both more potent and has a faster onset of action than clopidogrel. The TRITON trial compared prasugrel with clopidogrel in patients with STEMI or non-ST elevation MI in whom PCI was planned; prasugrel resulted in a 19% relative reduction in death from cardiovascular causes, myocardial infarction, or stroke, at the expense of a small increase in serious bleeding (including fatal bleeding).

Small molecule inhibitors of the platelet glycoprotein IIb/IIIa receptor are useful adjuncts in high-risk patients (usually defined by fluctuating ST-segment depression or positive biomarkers) with acute coronary syndromes, particularly when they are undergoing PCI. Tirofiban, 0.4 mcg/kg/min for 30 minutes, followed by 0.1 mcg/kg/min, and eptifibatide, 180 mcg/kg bolus followed by a continuous infusion of 2.0 mcg/kg/min, have both been shown to be effective. Downward dose adjustments (1.0 mcg/kg/min) are required in patients with reduced kidney function. For example, if the estimated creatinine clearance is below 50 mL/min, the eptifibatide infusion should be cut in half to 1 mcg/kg/min. The ISAR-REACT 2 trial showed that for patients undergoing PCI with high-risk acute coronary syndrome, especially with elevated troponin, intravenous abciximab (added to clopidogrel 600 mg loading dose) reduces ischemic events by about 25%.

Fibrinolytic therapy should be avoided in patients without ST-segment elevation since they generally have a patent culprit artery, and since the risk of such therapy appears to outweigh the benefit.

D. Nitroglycerin

Nitrates are first-line therapy for patients with acute coronary syndromes presenting with chest pain. Nonparenteral therapy with sublingual or oral agents or nitroglycerin ointment is usually sufficient. If pain persists or recurs, intravenous nitroglycerin should be started. The usual initial dosage is 10 mcg/min. The dosage should be titrated upward by 10–20 mcg/min (to a maximum of 200 mcg/min) until angina disappears or mean arterial pressure drops by 10%. Careful—usually continuous—BP monitoring is required when intravenous nitroglycerin is used. Avoid hypotension (systolic BP < 100 mm Hg). Tolerance to continuous nitrate infusion is common.

E. β-Blockers

β-Blockers are an important part of the initial treatment of unstable angina unless otherwise contraindicated. The pharmacology of these agents is discussed in Chapter 11 and summarized in Table 11–7. Use of agents with intrinsic sympathomimetic activity should be avoided in this setting. Oral medication is adequate in most patients, but intravenous treatment with metoprolol, given as three 5-mg doses 5 minutes apart as tolerated and in the absence of heart failure, achieves a more rapid effect. Oral therapy should be titrated upward as BP permits.

F. Calcium Channel Blockers

Calcium channel blockers have not been shown to favorably affect outcome in unstable angina, and they should be used primarily as third-line therapy in patients with continuing symptoms on nitrates and β-blockers or those who are not candidates for these drugs. In the presence of nitrates and without accompanying β-blockers, diltiazem or verapamil is preferred, since nifedipine and the other dihydropyridines are more likely to cause reflex tachycardia or hypotension. The initial dosage should be low, but upward titration should proceed steadily (see Table 11–9).

G. Statins

The PROVE-IT trial provides evidence for starting a statin in the days immediately following an acute coronary syndrome. In this trial, more intensive therapy with atorvastatin 80 mg a day, regardless of total or LDL cholesterol level, improved outcome compared to pravastatin 40 mg a day, with the curves of death or major cardiovascular event separating as early as 3 months after starting therapy.

▶ Indications for Coronary Angiography

For patients with acute coronary syndrome, including non–ST-segment elevation myocardial infarction, risk stratification is important for determining intensity of care. Several therapies, including glycoprotein IIb/IIIa receptor antagonists, low-molecular-weight heparin, and early invasive catheterization, have been shown to have the greatest benefit in higher-risk patients with acute coronary syndrome. As outlined in the ACC/AHA guidelines, patients with any high-risk feature (Table 10–6) generally warrant an early invasive strategy with catheterization and revascularization. For patients without these high-risk features, either an invasive or noninvasive approach, using exercise (or pharmacologic stress for patients unable to exercise) stress testing to identify patients who have residual ischemia and/or high risk, can be used. Moreover, based on the ICTUS

Table 10–6. Indications for catheterization and percutaneous coronary intervention.[1]

Acute coronary syndromes (unstable angina and non-ST elevation MI)	
Class I	Early invasive strategy for any of the following high-risk indicators:
	Recurrent angina/ischemia at rest or with low-level activity
	Elevated troponin
	ST-segment depression
	Recurrent ischemia with evidence of CHF
	High-risk stress test result
	EF < 0.40
	Hemodynamic instability
	Sustained ventricular tachycardia
	PCI within 6 months
	Prior CABG
	In the absence of these findings, either an early conservative or early invasive strategy
Class IIa	Early invasive strategy for patients with repeated presentations for ACS despite therapy
Class III	Extensive comorbidities in patients in whom benefits of revascularization are not likely to outweigh the risks
	Acute chest pain with low likelihood of ACS
Acute MI after fibrinolytic therapy (2004 ACC/AHA AMI Guideline)	
Class I	Recurrent ischemia (spontaneous or provoked)
	Recurrent MI
	Cardiogenic shock or hemodynamic instability
Class IIa	LV EF ≤ 0.40, CHF (even transient), serious ventricular arrhythmias
Class IIb	Routine PCI as part of invasive strategy after fibrinolytic therapy

[1]Class 1 indicates treatment is useful and effective, IIa indicates weight of evidence is in favor of usefulness/efficacy, class IIb indicates weight of evidence is less well established, and class III indicates intervention is not useful/effective and may be harmful. Type A recommendations are derived from large-scale randomized trials, and B recommendations are derived from smaller randomized trials or carefully conducted observational analyses.
ACC/AHA, American College of Cardiology/American Heart Association; ACS, acute coronary syndrome; AMI, acute myocardial infarction; CABG, coronary artery bypass grafting; CHF, congestive heart failure; EF, ejection fraction; LV EF, left ventricular ejection fraction; MI, myocardial infarction; PCI, percutaneous coronary intervention.

trial, a strategy based on selective coronary angiography and revascularization for instability or inducible ischemia, or both, even for patients with positive troponin, is acceptable (ACC/AHA class IIB recommendation).

The optimal timing of coronary angiography and revascularization is not known, although a recent trial (TIMACS) found better outcomes among high-risk patients (GRACE risk > 140 or > 3% estimated in-hospital risk of death) treated with early coronary angiography, within 24 hours of admission.

Two risk-stratification tools are available that can be used at the bedside, the TIMI Risk Score and the GRACE Risk Score. The TIMI Risk Score includes nine variables: age ≥ 65, three or more cardiac risk factors, prior coronary stenosis ≥ 50%, ST-segment deviation, two anginal events in prior 24 hours, acetylsalicylic acid in prior 7 days, and elevated cardiac markers. The GRACE risk score, which applies to patients with or without ST elevation, includes Killip class, BP, ST-segment deviation, cardiac arrest at presentation, serum creatinine, elevated creatine kinase (CK)-MB or troponin, and heart rate. The TIMI Risk Score is available for PDA download at http://www.timi.org, and the GRACE risk score at http://www.outcomes-umassmed. org/GRACE/acs_risk.cfm.

Anderson JL et al. ACC/AHA 2007 guidelines for the management of patients with unstable angina/non ST-elevation myocardial infarction: a report of the American College of Cardiology/American Heart Association Task Force on Practice Guidelines (Writing Committee to Revise the 2002 Guidelines for the Management of Patients With Unstable Angina/Non ST-Elevation Myocardial Infarction): developed in collaboration with the American College of Emergency Physicians, the Society for Cardiovascular Angiography and Interventions, and the Society of Thoracic Surgeons: endorsed by the American Association of Cardiovascular and Pulmonary Rehabilitation and the Society for Academic Emergency Medicine. Circulation. 2007 Aug 14;116(7):e148–304. [PMID: 17679616]

Bavry AA et al. Benefit of early invasive therapy in acute coronary syndromes: a meta-analysis of contemporary randomized clinical trials. J Am Coll Cardiol. 2006 Oct 3;48(7):1319–25. [PMID: 17010789]

Boersma E et al. Platelet glycoprotein IIb/IIIa inhibitors in acute coronary syndromes: a meta-analysis of all major randomised clinical trials. Lancet. 2002 Jan 19;359(9302):189–98. [PMID: 11812552]

Fox KA et al. Interventional versus conservative treatment for patients with unstable angina or non-ST-elevation myocardial infarction: the British Heart Foundation RITA 3 randomised trial. Lancet. 2002 Sep 7;360(9335):743–51. [PMID: 12241831]

Granger CB et al; Global Registry of Acute Coronary Events Investigators. Predictors of hospital mortality in the global registry of acute coronary events. Arch Intern Med. 2003 Oct 27;163(19):2345–53. [PMID: 14581255]

Hirsch A et al; Invasive versus Conservative Treatment in Unstable coronary Syndromes (ICTUS) investigators. Long-term outcome after an early invasive versus selective invasive treatment strategy in patients with non-ST-elevation acute coronary syndrome and elevated cardiac troponin T (the ICTUS trial): a follow-up study. Lancet. 2007 Mar 10;369(9564):827–35. [PMID: 17350451]

Kastrati A et al; Intracoronary Stenting and Antithrombotic: Regimen Rapid Early Action for Coronary Treatment 2 (ISAR-REACT 2) Trial Investigators. Abciximab in patients with acute coronary syndromes undergoing percutaneous coronary intervention after clopidogrel pretreatment: the ISAR-REACT 2 randomized trial. JAMA. 2006 Apr 5;295(13):1531–8. [PMID: 16533938]

Stone GW; ACUITY Investigators. Bivalirudin for patients with acute coronary syndromes. N Engl J Med. 2006 Nov 23;355 (21):2203–16. [PMID: 17124018]

Task Force for Diagnosis and Treatment of Non-ST-Segment Elevation Acute Coronary Syndromes of European Society of Cardiology; Bassand JP et al. Guidelines for the diagnosis and treatment of non-ST-segment elevation acute coronary syndromes. Eur Heart J. 2007 Jul;28(13):1598–660. [PMID: 17569677]

Thygesen K et al; Joint ESC/ACCF/AHA/WHF Task Force for the Redefinition of Myocardial Infarction. Universal definition of myocardial infarction. Eur Heart J. 2007 Oct;28(20):2525–38. [PMID: 17951287]

Udelson JE et al. Myocardial perfusion imaging for evaluation and triage of patients with suspected acute cardiac ischemia: a randomized controlled trial. JAMA. 2002 Dec 4;288(21): 2693–700. [PMID: 12460092]

Wiviott SD et al; TITRON-TIMI 38 Investigators. Prasugrel versus clopidogrel in patients with acute coronary syndromes. N Engl J Med. 2007 Nov 15;357(20):2001–15. [PMID: 17982182]

Yusuf S et al. Effects of clopidogrel in addition to aspirin in patients with acute coronary syndromes without ST-segment elevation. N Engl J Med. 2001 Aug 16;345(7):494–502. [PMID: 11519503]

Yusuf S et al; Fifth Organization to Assess Strategies in Acute Ischemic Syndromes Investigators. Comparison of fondaparinux and enoxaparin in acute coronary syndromes. N Engl J Med. 2006 Apr 6;354(14):1464–76. [PMID: 16537663]

ACUTE MYOCARDIAL INFARCTION WITH ST SEGMENT ELEVATION

 ESSENTIALS OF DIAGNOSIS

▶ Sudden but not instantaneous development of prolonged (> 30 minutes) anterior chest discomfort (sometimes felt as "gas" or pressure).

▶ Sometimes painless, masquerading as acute CHF, syncope, stroke, or shock.

▶ ECG: ST-segment elevation or left bundle branch block.

▶ Immediate reperfusion treatment is warranted.

▶ Primary PCI within 90 minutes of hospital presentation superior to thrombolysis.

▶ Thrombolysis within 30 minutes of hospital presentation and 6–12 hours of onset of symptoms reduces mortality.

▶ General Considerations

STEMI results, in most cases, from an occlusive coronary thrombus at the site of a preexisting (though not necessarily severe) atherosclerotic plaque. More rarely, infarction may result from prolonged vasospasm, inadequate myocardial blood flow (eg, hypotension), or excessive metabolic demand. Very rarely, myocardial infarction may be caused by embolic occlusion, vasculitis, aortic root or coronary artery dissection, or aortitis. Cocaine is a cause of infarction, which should be considered in young individuals without risk factors. A condition that may mimic STEMI is stress cardiomyopathy (also referred to as Tako-Tsubo or stress cardiomyopathy, or apical ballooning syndrome) (see below).

ST elevation connotes an acute coronary occlusion and thus warrants immediate reperfusion therapy.

▶ Clinical Findings

A. Symptoms

1. Premonitory pain—There is usually a worsening in the pattern of angina preceding the onset of symptoms of myocardial infarction; classically the onset of angina occurs with minimal exertion or at rest.

2. Pain of infarction—Unlike anginal episodes, most infarctions occur at rest, and more commonly in the early morning. The pain is similar to angina in location and radiation but it may be more severe, and it builds up rapidly or in waves to maximum intensity over a few minutes or longer. Nitroglycerin has little effect; even opioids may not relieve the pain.

3. Associated symptoms—Patients may break out in a cold sweat, feel weak and apprehensive, and move about, seeking a position of comfort. They prefer not to lie quietly. Light-headedness, syncope, dyspnea, orthopnea, cough, wheezing, nausea and vomiting, or abdominal bloating may be present singly or in any combination.

4. Painless infarction—One-third of patients with acute myocardial infarction present without chest pain, and these patients tend to be undertreated and have poor outcomes. Older patients, women, and patients with diabetes mellitus are more likely to present without classic chest pain. As many as 25% of infarctions are detected on routine ECG without any recallable acute episode.

5. Sudden death and early arrhythmias—Of all deaths from myocardial infarction, about 50% occur before the patients arrive at the hospital, with death presumably caused by ventricular fibrillation.

B. Signs

1. General—Patients may appear anxious and sometimes are sweating profusely. The heart rate may range from marked bradycardia (most commonly in inferior infarction) to tachycardia, low cardiac output, or arrhythmia. The BP may be high, especially in former hypertensive patients, or low in patients with shock. Respiratory distress usually indicates heart failure. Fever, usually low grade, may appear after 12 hours and persist for several days.

2. Chest—The **Killip classification** is the standard way to classify heart failure in patients with acute myocardial infarction and has powerful prognostic value. Killip Class I is absence of rales and S_3, Class II is rales that do not clear with coughing over one-third or less of the lung fields or presence of an S_3, Class III is rales that do not clear with coughing over more than one-third of the lung fields, and Class IV is cardiogenic shock (rales, hypotension, and signs of hypoperfusion).

3. Heart—The cardiac examination may be unimpressive or very abnormal. Jugular venous distention reflects RA hypertension, and a Kussmaul sign (failure of decrease of jugular venous pressure with inspiration) is suggestive of RV infarction. Soft heart sounds may indicate LV dysfunction. Atrial gallops (S_4) are the rule, whereas ventricular gallops (S_3) are less common and indicate significant LV dysfunction. Mitral regurgitation murmurs are not uncommon and may indicate papillary muscle dysfunction or, rarely, rupture. Pericardial friction rubs are uncommon in the first 24 hours but may appear later.

4. Extremities—Edema is usually not present. Cyanosis and cold temperature indicate low output. The peripheral pulses should be noted, since later shock or emboli may alter the examination.

C. Laboratory Findings

Cardiac-specific markers of myocardial damage include quantitative determinations of CK-MB, troponin I, and troponin T. Normal cut-off levels for troponins depend on the assay used and reference ranges for the laboratory performing the test. Troponins are more sensitive and specific than CK-MB. Each of these tests may become positive as early as 4–6 hours after the onset of a myocardial infarction and should be abnormal by 8–12 hours. Circulating levels of troponins may remain elevated for 5–7 days or longer and therefore are generally not useful for evaluating suspected early reinfarction. Elevated CK-MB generally normalizes within 24 hours, thus being more helpful for evaluation of reinfarction.

D. ECG

The extent of the ECG abnormalities, especially the sum of the total amount of ST-segment deviation, is a good indicator of extent of acute infarction and risk of subsequent adverse events. The classic evolution of changes is from peaked ("hyperacute") T waves, to ST-segment elevation, to Q wave development, to T wave inversion. This may occur over a few hours to several days. The evolution of new Q waves (> 30 milliseconds in duration and 25% of the R wave amplitude) is diagnostic, but Q waves do not occur in 30–50% of acute infarctions (non-Q wave infarctions).

E. Chest Radiography

The chest radiograph may demonstrate signs of CHF, but these changes often lag behind the clinical findings. Signs of aortic dissection, including mediastinal widening, should be sought as a possible alternative diagnosis.

F. Echocardiography

Echocardiography provides convenient bedside assessment of LV global and regional function. This can help with the diagnosis and management of infarction; echocardiography has been used successfully to make judgments about admission and management of patients with suspected infarction, including in patients with ST-segment elevation or left bundle branch block of uncertain significance, since normal wall motion makes an infarction unlikely. Doppler echocardiography is generally the most convenient procedure for diagnosing postinfarction mitral regurgitation or VSD.

G. Other Noninvasive Studies

Diagnosis of myocardial infarction and extent of myocardial infarction can be assessed by various imaging studies in addition to echocardiography. **MRI** with gadolinium contrast enhancement is now the most sensitive test to detect and quantitate extent of infarction, with the ability to detect as little as 2 g of myocardial infarction. **Technetium-99m pyrophosphate scintigraphy,** when injected at least 18 hours postinfarction, complexes with calcium in necrotic myocardium to provide a "hot spot" image of the infarction. This test is insensitive to small infarctions, and false-positive studies occur, so its use is limited to patients in whom the diagnosis by ECG and enzymes is not possible—principally those who present several days after the event or have intraoperative infarctions. **Scintigraphy with thallium-201** or technetium-based perfusion tracers will demonstrate "cold spots" in regions of diminished perfusion, which usually represent infarction when the radiotracer is administered at rest, but abnormalities do not distinguish recent from old damage.

H. Hemodynamic Measurements

These can be helpful in managing the patient with suspected cardiogenic shock. Use of PA catheters, however, has generally not been associated with better outcomes and should be limited to patients with severe hemodynamic compromise (Table 10–7).

Ammann P et al. Characteristics and prognosis of myocardial infarction in patients with normal coronary arteries. Chest. 2000 Feb;117(2):333–8. [PMID: 10669671]

Table 10–7. Hemodynamic subsets in acute myocardial infarction.

Category	CI or SWI	PCWP	Treatment	Comment
Normal	> 2.2, < 30	< 15	None	Mortality rate < 5%.
Hyperdynamic	> 3.0, > 40	< 15	β-Blockers	Characterized by tachycardia; mortality rate < 5%.
Hypovolemic	< 2.5, < 30	< 10	Volume expansion	Hypotension, tachycardia, but preserved left ventricular function by echocardiography; mortality rate 4–8%.
Left ventricular failure	< 2.2, < 30	> 15	Diuretics	Mild dyspnea, rales, normal blood pressure; mortality rate 10–20%.
Severe failure	< 2.0, < 20	> 18	Diuretics, vasodilators	Pulmonary edema, mild hypotension; inotropic agents, IABC may be required; mortality rate 20–40%.
Shock	< 1.8, < 30	> 20	Inotropic agents, IABC	IABC early unless rapid reversal occurs; mortality rate > 60%.

CI, cardiac index (L/min/m²); SWI, stroke work index (g-m/m², calculated as [mean arterial pressure − PCWP] · stroke volume index · 0.0136); PCWP, pulmonary capillary wedge pressure (in mm Hg; pulmonary artery diastolic pressure may be used instead); IABC, intra-aortic balloon counterpulsation.

Ricciardi MJ et al. Visualization of discrete microinfarction after percutaneous coronary intervention associated with mild creatine kinase-MB elevation. Circulation. 2001 Jun 12;103(23):2780–3. [PMID: 11401931]

Thygesen K et al; Joint ESC/ACCF/AHA/WHF Task Force for the Redefinition of Myocardial Infarction. Universal definition of myocardial infarction. Circulation. 2007 Nov 27;116(22):2634–53. [PMID: 17951284]

► Treatment

Table 10–5 provides a summary of the ACC/AHA Guideline recommendations for selected medical treatments.

A. Aspirin, Clopidogrel, and Prasugrel

All patients with definite or suspected myocardial infarction should receive aspirin at a dose of 162 mg or 325 mg at once regardless of whether thrombolytic therapy is being considered or the patient has been taking aspirin. Chewable aspirin provides more rapid blood levels. Patients with a definite aspirin allergy should be treated with clopidogrel; a 300 mg (or 600 mg) loading dose will result in faster onset of action than the standard 75 mg dose.

Clopidogrel, in combination with aspirin, has also been shown to provide important benefits in patients with acute ST elevation myocardial infarction. In the CLARITY trial, a loading dose of 300 mg of clopidogrel given with thrombolytic therapy, followed by 75 mg a day, led to substantial improvement in coronary patency on catheterization 3.5 days following thrombolysis. Moreover, there was no increase in serious bleeding in this population of patients up to 75 years of age. The COMMIT/CCS-2 trial randomized over 45,000 patients in China with acute myocardial infarction to clopidogrel 75 mg a day or placebo, and found a small but statistically significant reduction in early death, myocardial reinfarction, and stroke, with no excess in major bleeding. Thus, guidelines now call for clopidogrel to be added to aspirin to all patients with STEMI, regardless of whether or not reperfusion is given, and continued for at least 14 days, and generally for 1 year. For patients who have received thrombolytic therapy but will undergo angiography in the first day or two, the early benefits of clopidogrel need to be weighed against the necessary delay in bypass surgery for approximately 5 days for those patients found to require surgical revascularization.

Compared with clopidogrel, prasugrel provides further benefit in reducing thrombotic events in the subgroup of patients with STEMI, including a 50% reduction in stent thrombosis.

B. Reperfusion Therapy

The current recommendation is to treat patients with STEMI who seek medical attention within 12 hours of the onset of symptoms with reperfusion therapy, either primary PCI or thrombolytic therapy. Patients without ST-segment elevation (previously labeled "non-Q wave" infarctions) do not benefit, and may derive harm, from thrombolysis.

1. Primary percutaneous coronary intervention— Immediate coronary angiography and primary PCI (including stenting) of the infarct-related artery have been shown to be superior to thrombolysis when done by experienced operators in high-volume centers with rapid time from first medical contact to intervention ("door-to-balloon"). US and European guidelines call for first medical contact or "door-to-balloon" times of less than 90 minutes. Several trials have shown that if efficient transfer systems are in place, transfer of patients with acute myocardial infarction from hospitals without primary PCI capability to hospitals with primary PCI capability can improve outcome compared with thrombolytic therapy at the presenting hospital, although this requires sophisticated systems to ensure rapid identification, transfer, and PCI. Primary PCI is the approach of choice in patients with absolute and many relative contraindications to thrombolytic therapy. The results of this approach in specialized centers are excellent, exceeding those obtainable by thrombolytic therapy even in good candidates, but this experience may not be generalizable to centers and operators with less experience or expertise. Stenting—generally in conjunction with the platelet glycoprotein IIb/IIIa antagonist abciximab—is standard for patients with acute myocardial infarction. Since the rate of late stent thrombosis with drug-eluting stents is not well defined following stenting in the primary PCI setting, bare metal stents are most commonly used. In the subgroup of patients with cardiogenic shock, early catheterization and percutaneous or surgical revascularization are the preferred management and has been shown to reduce mortality. Because an acute interventional approach carries a lower risk of hemorrhagic complications, it may also be the preferred strategy in many older patients (see Tables 10–5 and 10–6 for factors to consider in choosing thrombolytic therapy or primary PCI).

Glycoprotein IIb/IIIa inhibitors, and specifically abcixmab, have been shown to reduce major thrombotic events, and possibly mortality, for patients undergoing primary PCI. The HORIZONS trial showed that compared with unfractionated heparin plus abciximab, bivalirudin (with provisional use of "bail-out" IIb/IIIa inhibitors) results in similar rates of thrombotic events and 40% less bleeding. This appeared to be accompanied by lower mortality at 30 days and 1 year, providing further support for the safety and efficacy of bivalirudin in this setting.

In part because patients in the United States who are transferred for primary PCI tend to have long delays from first hospital arrival to balloon inflation, there has been interest in developing "facilitated" PCI whereby a combination of medications (full or reduced dose fibrinolytic agents with or without glycoprotein IIb/IIIa inhibitors) is given to establish patency followed by immediate PCI. However, recent trials (and overviews of completed trials) have shown either no benefit or harm with this approach. Thus, patients should be treated either with fibrinolytic agents (and immediate rescue PCI for reperfusion failure) or with primary PCI, if it can be done promptly as outlined in the ACC/AHA and European guidelines.

2. Thrombolytic therapy

A. Benefit—Thrombolytic therapy reduces mortality and limits infarct size in patients with acute myocardial infarction associated with ST-segment elevation (defined as ≥ 0.1

mV in two inferior or lateral leads or two contiguous precordial leads), or with left bundle branch block (not known to be old). The greatest benefit occurs if treatment is initiated within the first 3 hours, when up to a 50% reduction in mortality rate can be achieved. The magnitude of benefit declines rapidly thereafter, but a 10% relative mortality reduction can be achieved up to 12 hours after the onset of chest pain. The survival benefit is greatest in patients with large—usually anterior—infarctions.

B. Contraindications—Major bleeding complications occur in 0.5–5% of patients, the most serious of which is intracranial hemorrhage. The major risk factors for intracranial bleeding are older age (greater than 65 years), hypertension at presentation (especially over 180/110 mm Hg), low body weight (< 70 kg), and the use of clot-specific thrombolytic agents (alteplase, reteplase, tenecteplase). Although patients over age 75 years have a much higher mortality rate with acute myocardial infarction and therefore may derive greater benefit, the risk of severe bleeding is also higher, particularly among patients with risk factors for intracranial hemorrhage, such as severe hypertension or recent stroke. Patients presenting more than 12 hours after the onset of chest pain may also derive a small benefit, particularly if pain and ST-segment elevation persist, but rarely does this benefit outweigh the attendant risk.

Contraindications to thrombolytic therapy include previous hemorrhagic stroke, other strokes or cerebrovascular events within 1 year, known intracranial neoplasm, recent head trauma (including minor trauma), active internal bleeding (excluding menstruation), or suspected aortic dissection. Relative contraindications are BP > 180/110 mm Hg at presentation, other intracerebral pathology not listed above as a contraindication, known bleeding diathesis, trauma (including minor head trauma) within 2–4 weeks, major surgery within 3 weeks, prolonged (> 10 minutes) or traumatic cardiopulmonary resuscitation, recent (within 2–4 weeks) internal bleeding, noncompressible vascular punctures, active diabetic retinopathy, pregnancy, active peptic ulcer disease, a history of severe hypertension, current use of anticoagulants (INR > 2.0–3.0), and (for streptokinase) prior allergic reaction or exposure to streptokinase or anistreplase within 2 years.

C. Thrombolytic agents—The following thrombolytic agents are available for acute myocardial infarction and are characterized in Table 10–8.

Streptokinase is not commonly used for treatment of acute myocardial infarction in the United States since it is less effective at opening occluded arteries and less effective at reducing mortality. It is non-fibrin-specific, causes depletion of circulating fibrinogen, and has a tendency to induce hypotension, particularly if infused rapidly. This can be managed by slowing or interrupting the infusion and administering fluids. There is controversy as to whether adjunctive heparin is beneficial in patients given streptokinase, unlike its administration with the more clot-specific agents. Allergic reactions, including anaphylaxis,

Table 10–8. Thrombolytic therapy for acute myocardial infarction.

	Streptokinase	Alteplase; Tissue Plasminogen Activator (t-PA)	Reteplase	Tenecteplase (TNK-t-PA)
Source	Group C streptococcus	Recombinant DNA	Recombinant DNA	Recombinant DNA
Half-life	20 minutes	5 minutes	15 minutes	20 minutes
Usual dose	1.5 million units	100 mg	20 units	40 mg
Administration	750,000 units over 20 minutes followed by 750,000 units over 40 minutes	Initial bolus of 15 mg, followed by 50 mg infused over the next 30 minutes and 35 mg over the following 60 minutes	10 units as a bolus over 2 minutes, repeated after 30 minutes	Single weight-adjusted bolus, 0.5 mg/kg
Anticoagulation after infusion	Aspirin, 325 mg daily; there is no evidence that adjunctive heparin improves outcome following streptokinase	Aspirin, 325 mg daily; heparin, 5000 units as bolus, followed by 1000 units per hour infusion, subsequently adjusted to maintain PTT 1.5–2 times control	Aspirin, 325 mg; heparin as with t-PA	Aspirin, 325 mg daily
Clot selectivity	Low	High	High	High
Fibrinogenolysis	+++	+	+	+
Bleeding	+	+	+	+
Hypotension	+++	+	+	+
Allergic reactions	++	0	0	+
Reocclusion	5–20%	10–30%	—	5–20%
Approximate cost[1]	$562.50	$4378.00	$3475.00	$3005.00

[1]Average wholesale price (AWP, for AB-rated generic when available) for quantity listed. Source: *Red Book Update*, Vol. 28, No. 3, March 2009. AWP may not accurately represent the actual pharmacy cost because wide contractual variations exist among institutions. PTT, partial thromboplastin time.

occur in 1–2% of patients, and this agent should generally not be administered to patients with prior exposure.

Alteplase (recombinant tissue plasminogen activator; t-PA) is a naturally occurring plasminogen activator that is modestly fibrin specific, resulting in about a 50% reduction in circulating fibrinogen. In the first GUSTO trial, which compared a 90-minute dosing of t-PA (with unfractionated heparin) with streptokinase, the 30-day mortality rate with t-PA was one absolute percentage point lower (one additional life saved per 100 patients treated), though there was also a small *increase* in the rate of intracranial hemorrhage. An angiographic substudy confirmed a higher 90-minute patency rate and a higher rate of normal (TIMI grade 3) flow in patients.

Reteplase is a recombinant deletion mutant of t-PA that is slightly less fibrin specific. In comparative trials, it appears to have efficacy similar to that of alteplase, but it has a longer duration of action and can be administered as two boluses 30 minutes apart.

Tenecteplase (TNK-t-PA) is a genetically engineered substitution mutant of native t-PA that has reduced plasma clearance, increased fibrin sensitivity, and increased resistance to plasminogen activator inhibitor-1. It can be given as a single weight-adjusted bolus. In a large comparative trial, this agent was equivalent to t-PA with regard to efficacy and resulted in significantly less noncerebral bleeding.

(1) Selection of a thrombolytic agent—In the United States, most patients are treated with alteplase, reteplase, or tenecteplase. The differences in efficacy between them are small compared with the potential benefit of treating a greater proportion of appropriate candidates in a more prompt manner. The principal objective should be to administer a thrombolytic agent within 30 minutes of presentation—or even during transport. The ability to administer tenecteplase as a single bolus is an attractive feature that may facilitate earlier treatment. The combination of a reduced-dose thrombolytic given with a platelet glycoprotein IIb/IIIa antagonist has been investigated in several trials, with no evidence of reduction in mortality but a modest increase in bleeding complications.

(2) Postthrombolytic management—After completion of the thrombolytic infusion, aspirin (81–325 mg/d) and heparin should be continued. The 2008 ACC/AHA guidelines recommend continued anticoagulation for the duration of the hospital stay (or up to 8 days) with some anticoagulant, with advantages favoring either enoxaparin or fondaparinux.

(a) Unfractionated heparin—Anticoagulation with intravenous heparin (initial dose of 60 units/kg bolus to a maximum of 4000 units, followed by an infusion of 12 units/kg/min to a maximum of 1000 units, then adjusted to maintain an activated partial thromboplastin time [aPTT] of 50–75 seconds beginning with an aPTT drawn 3 hours after thrombolytic) is continued for at least 48 hours after alteplase, reteplase, or tenecteplase, and with continuation of some anticoagulant until revascularization (if performed) or until hospital discharge (or day 8).

(b) Low-molecular-weight heparin—In the EXTRACT trial, enoxaparin significantly reduced death and myocardial infarction at day 30 (compared with unfractionated heparin), at the expense of a modest increase in bleeding. In patients younger than age 75, enoxaparin was given as a 30 mg intravenous bolus and 1 mg/kg every 12 hours; in patients age 75 years and older, it was given with no bolus and 0.75 mg/kg intravenously every 12 hours. This appeared to attenuate the risk of intracranial hemorrhage in the elderly that had been seen with full dose enoxaparin. Another antithrombotic option is fondaparinux, given at a dose of 2.5 mg subcutaneously once a day. In the OASIS-6 trial, it resulted in significant reductions in death and reinfarction when compared with control (unfractionated heparin when indicated, otherwise placebo). Similar to the findings of the OASIS-5 trial, fondaparinux tended to result in less bleeding, despite its longer duration compared with heparin and despite its comparison to placebo in about half of the enrolled patients. There was no benefit of fondaparinux among patients undergoing primary PCI, and fondaparinux is not recommended as a sole anticoagulant during PCI due to risk of catheter thrombosis.

For all patients with acute myocardial infarction treated with intensive antithrombotic therapy, prophylactic treatment with proton pump inhibitors or antacids and an H_2-blocker is advisable.

3. Assessment of myocardial reperfusion, recurrent ischemic pain, reinfarction—Myocardial reperfusion can be recognized clinically by the early cessation of pain and the resolution of ST-segment elevation. Although at least 50% resolution of ST-segment elevation by 90 minutes may occur without coronary reperfusion, ST resolution is a strong predictor of better outcome. Even with anticoagulation, 10–20% of reperfused vessels will reocclude during hospitalization, although reocclusion and reinfarction appear to be reduced following intervention. Reinfarction, indicated by recurrence of pain and ST-segment elevation, can be treated by readministration of a thrombolytic agent or immediate angiography and PCI.

C. General Measures

Cardiac care unit monitoring should be instituted as soon as possible. Patients without complications can be transferred to a telemetry unit after 24 hours. Activity should initially be limited to bed rest but can be advanced within 24 hours. Progressive ambulation should be started after 24–72 hours if tolerated. For patients without complications, discharge by day 4 appears to be appropriate. Low-flow oxygen therapy (2–4 L/min) should be given if oxygen saturation is reduced.

D. Analgesia

An initial attempt should be made to relieve pain with sublingual nitroglycerin. However, if no response occurs after two or three tablets, intravenous opioids provide the most rapid and effective analgesia and may also reduce pulmonary congestion. Morphine sulfate, 4–8 mg, or meperidine, 50–75 mg, should be given. Subsequent small doses can be given every 15 minutes until pain abates.

Nonsteroidal anti-inflammatory agents, other than aspirin, should be avoided during hospitalization for STEMI due to increased risk of mortality, myocardial rupture, hypertension, heart failure, and kidney injury with their use.

E. β-Adrenergic Blocking Agents

Although trials have shown modest short-term benefit from β-blockers given immediately after acute myocardial infarction, it has not been clear that intravenous β-blockers provide an advantage over simply beginning an oral β-blocker, which should be started during the first 24 hours if there are no contraindications. The Chinese COMMIT/CCS-2 trial involving 45,000 patients found no overall benefit to intravenous followed by oral metoprolol; the aggressive dosing (three 5 mg intravenous boluses followed by 200 mg/d orally) appeared to prevent reinfarction at the cost of increasing shock, with overall harm in patients presenting with heart failure. Thus, early β-blockade should be avoided in patients with any degree of heart failure, evidence of low output state, increased risk of cardiogenic shock, or other relative contraindications to β-blockade. The CAPRICORN trial showed the benefits of carvedilol (beginning at 6.25 mg twice a day, titrated to 25 mg twice a day) following the acute phase of large myocardial infarction with contemporary care.

F. Nitrates

Nitroglycerin is the agent of choice for continued or recurrent ischemic pain and is useful in lowering BP or relieving pulmonary congestion. However, routine nitrate administration is not recommended, since no improvement in outcome has been observed in the ISIS-4 or GISSI-3 trials, in which a total of over 70,000 patients were randomized to nitrate treatment or placebo. Nitrates should be avoided in patients who received phosphodiesterase inhibitors (sildenafil, vardenafil, and tadalafil) in the prior 24 hours.

G. ACE Inhibitors

A series of trials (SAVE, AIRE, SMILE, TRACE, GISSI-III, and ISIS-4) have shown both short- and long-term improvement in survival with ACE inhibitor therapy. The benefits are greatest in patients with EF ≤ 40%, large infarctions, or clinical evidence of heart failure. Because substantial amounts of the survival benefit occur on the first day, ACE inhibitor treatment should be commenced early in patients without hypotension, especially patients with large or anterior myocardial infarction. Given the benefits of ACE-inhibitors for patients with vascular disease, it is reasonable to use ACE-inhibitors for all patients following STEMI who do not have contraindications.

H. Angiotensin Receptor Blockers

Although there has been inconsistency in the effects of different angiotensin receptor blockers (ARBs) on mortality for patients post-myocardial infarction with heart failure and/or LV dysfunction, the VALIANT trial showed that valsartan 160 mg twice a day is equivalent to captopril in reducing mortality. Thus, valsartan should be used for all patients with ACE inhibitor intolerance, and is a reasonable, albeit more expensive, alternative to captopril. The combination of captopril and valsartan (at reduced dose) was no better than either agent alone and resulted in more side effects.

I. Aldosterone Antagonists

The RALES trial showed that spironolactone can reduce the mortality rate of patients with advanced heart failure, and the EPHESUS trial showed a 15% relative risk reduction in mortality with eplerenone for patients post-myocardial infarction with LV dysfunction and either heart failure or diabetes. Kidney dysfunction or hyperkalemia are contraindications, and patients must be monitored carefully for development of hyperkalemia.

J. Antiarrhythmic Prophylaxis

The incidence of ventricular fibrillation in hospitalized patients is approximately 5%, with 80% of episodes occurring in the first 12–24 hours. Prophylactic lidocaine infusions (1–2 mg/min) prevent most episodes, but this therapy has not reduced the mortality rate and it increases the risk of asystole, so this approach is no longer recommended except in patients with sustained ventricular tachycardia.

K. Calcium Channel Blockers

There are no studies to support the routine use of calcium channel blockers in most patients with acute myocardial infarction—and indeed, they have the potential to exacerbate ischemia and cause death from reflex tachycardia or myocardial depression. Long-acting calcium channel blockers should generally be reserved for management of hypertension or ischemia as second- or third-line drugs after β-blockers and nitrates.

L. Long-Term Antithrombotic Therapy

Discharge on aspirin, 81–325 mg/d, since it is highly effective, inexpensive, and well tolerated, is a key quality indicator of myocardial infarction care. In the WARIS-II trial, long-term anticoagulation with warfarin post-myocardial infarction was associated with a reduction in the composite of death, reinfarction, and stroke. However, whether the results of this trial are transferable to the United States where anticoagulation services may be less organized and effective than in Norwegian hospitals is unknown. In the CURE trial, clopidogrel, 75 mg/d, (in addition to aspirin) for 3–12 months for non-ST elevation acute coronary syndromes resulted in a similar 20% relative risk reduction in cardiovascular death, myocardial infarction, and stroke, and continuing clopidogrel for 1 year for patients with STEMI is reasonable, regardless of whether they underwent reperfusion therapy. The TRITON trial showed that prasugrel was more beneficial than clopidogrel in reducing ischemic events in patients undergoing PCI.

M. Coronary Angiography

For patients who do not reperfuse based on lack of at least 50% resolution of ST elevation, rescue angioplasty should be performed and has been shown to reduce the composite of death, reinfarction, stroke, or severe heart failure. Many cardiologists advocate routine catheterization and revascularization following acute myocardial infarction, in otherwise suitable candidates, and recent trials suggest that this may improve outcome. Patients with recurrent ischemic pain prior to discharge should undergo catheterization and, if indicated, revascularization. Asymptomatic, clinically stable patients should undergo predischarge stress testing to determine whether residual jeopardized myocardium is present. This can be accomplished by submaximal exercise or pharmacologic stress scintigraphy. Those with significantly positive tests or a low threshold for symptomatic ischemia should undergo angiography and revascularization where feasible. PCI of a totally occluded infarct-related artery greater than 24 hours after STEMI should generally not be performed in asymptomatic patients with one or two vessel disease without evidence of severe ischemia.

Antman EM et al. 2007 focused update of the ACC/AHA 2004 Guidelines for the Management of Patients With ST-Elevation Myocardial Infarction: a report of the American College of Cardiology/American Heart Association Task Force on Practice Guidelines (Writing Group to Review New Evidence and Update the ACC/AHA 2004 Guidelines for the Management of Patients With ST-Elevation Myocardial Infarction). Circulation. 2008 Jan 15;117(2):296–329. [PMID: 18071078]

Antman EM et al. ACC/AHA guidelines for the management of patients with ST-elevation myocardial infarction; A report of the American College of Cardiology/American Heart Association Task Force on Practice Guidelines (Committee to Revise the 1999 Guidelines for the Management of patients with acute myocardial infarction). J Am Coll Cardiol. 2004 Aug 4;44(3):E1–E211. [PMID: 15358047]

Antman EM et al; ExTRACT-TIMI 25 Investigators. Enoxaparin versus unfractionated heparin with fibrinolysis for ST-elevation myocardial infarction. N Engl J Med. 2006 Apr 6;354 (14):1477–88. [PMID: 16537665]

Assessment of the Safety and Efficacy of a New Treatment Strategy with Percutaneous Coronary Intervention (ASSENT-4 PCI) investigators. Primary versus tenecteplase-facilitated percutaneous coronary intervention in patients with ST-segment elevation acute myocardial infarction (ASSENT-4 PCI): randomised trial. Lancet. 2006 Feb 18;367(9510):569–78. [PMID: 16488800]

Chen ZM; COMMIT (Clopidogrel and Metoprolol in Myocardial Infarction Trial) Collaborative Group. Addition of clopidogrel to aspirin in 45,852 patients with acute myocardial infarction: randomised placebo-controlled trial. Lancet. 2005 Nov 5;366(9497):1607–21. [PMID: 16271642]

Chen ZM; COMMIT (Clopidogrel and Metoprolol in Myocardial Infarction Trial) Collaborative Group. Early intravenous then oral metoprolol in 45,852 patients with acute myocardial infarction: randomised placebo-controlled trial. Lancet. 2005 Nov 5;366(9497):1622–32. [PMID: 16271643]

Hochman JS et al; Occluded Artery Trial Investigators. Coronary intervention for persistent occlusion after myocardial infarction. N Engl J Med. 2006 Dec 7;355(23):2395–407. [PMID: 17105759]

Hurlen M et al. Warfarin, aspirin, or both after myocardial infarction. N Engl J Med. 2002 Sep 26;347(13):969–74. [PMID: 12324552]

Keeley EC et al. Comparison of primary and facilitated percutaneous coronary interventions for ST-elevation myocardial infarction: quantitative review of randomised trials. Lancet. 2006 Feb 18;367(9510):579–88. [PMID: 16488801]

Keeley EC et al. Primary coronary intervention for acute myocardial infarction. JAMA. 2004 Feb 11;291(6):736–9. [PMID: 14871919]

Pfeffer MA et al. Valsartan, captopril, or both in myocardial infarction complicated by heart failure, left ventricular dysfunction, or both. N Engl J Med. 2003 Nov 13;349(20):1893–906. [PMID: 14610160]

Sabatine MS et al; CLARITY-TIMI 28 Investigators. Addition of clopidogrel to aspirin and fibrinolytic therapy for myocardial infarction with ST-segment elevation. N Engl J Med. 2005 Mar 24;352(12):1179–89. [PMID: 15758000]

Stone GW et al; HORIZONS-AMI Trial Investigators. Bivalirudin during primary PCI in acute myocardial infarction. N Engl J Med. 2008 May 22;358(21):2218–30. [PMID: 18499566]

Yusuf S et al; OASIS-6 Trial Group: Effects of fondaparinux on mortality and reinfarction in patients with acute ST-segment elevation myocardial infarction: the OASIS-6 randomized trial. JAMA. 2006 Apr 5;295(13):1519–30. [PMID: 16537725]

► **Complications**

A variety of complications can occur after myocardial infarction even when treatment is initiated promptly.

A. Postinfarction Ischemia

In clinical trials of thrombolysis, recurrent ischemia occurred in about one-third of patients, was more common following non–ST elevation myocardial infarction than after STEMI, and had important short- and long-term prognostic implications. Vigorous medical therapy should be instituted, including nitrates and β-blockers as well as aspirin 81–325 mg/d, anticoagulant therapy (unfractionated heparin, enoxaparin, or fondaparinux) and clopidogrel. Most patients with postinfarction angina—and all who are refractory to medical therapy—should undergo early catheterization and revascularization by PCI or CABG.

B. Arrhythmias

Abnormalities of rhythm and conduction are common.

1. Sinus bradycardia—This is most common in inferior infarctions or may be precipitated by medications. Observation or withdrawal of the offending agent is usually sufficient. If accompanied by signs of low cardiac output, atropine, 0.5–1 mg intravenously, is usually effective. Temporary pacing is rarely required.

2. Supraventricular tachyarrhythmias—Sinus tachycardia is common and may reflect either increased adrenergic stimulation or hemodynamic compromise due to hypovolemia or pump failure. In the latter, β-blockade is contraindicated. Supraventricular premature beats are common and may be premonitory for atrial fibrillation. Electrolyte abnormalities and hypoxia should be corrected and causative agents (especially aminophylline) stopped. Atrial fibrillation should be rapidly controlled or converted to sinus rhythm. Intravenous β-blockers such as metoprolol (2.5–5 mg/h) or short-acting esmolol (50–200 mcg/kg/min) are the agents of choice if cardiac function is adequate. Intravenous diltiazem (5–15 mg/h) may be used if β-blockers are contraindicated or ineffective. Digoxin (0.5 mg as initial dose, then 0.25 mg every 90–120 minutes [up to 1–1.25 mg] for a loading dose, followed by 0.25 mg daily if kidney function is normal) is preferable if heart failure is present with atrial fibrillation, but the onset of action is delayed. Electrical cardioversion (commencing with 100 J) may be necessary if atrial fibrillation is complicated by hypotension, heart failure, or ischemia, but the arrhythmia often recurs. Amiodarone (150 mg intravenous bolus and then 15–30 mg/h intravenously, or rapid oral loading with 400 mg three times daily) may be helpful to restore or maintain sinus rhythm.

3. Ventricular arrhythmias—Ventricular arrhythmias are most common in the first few hours after infarction. Ventricular premature beats may be premonitory for ventricular tachycardia or fibrillation but generally should not be treated in the absence of frequent nonsustained ventricular tachycardia (usually more than six consecutive beats). Lidocaine is recommended as a prophylactic measure. Toxicity (tremor, anxiety, confusion, seizures) is common, especially in older patients and those with hypotension, heart failure, or liver disease.

Sustained ventricular tachycardia should be treated with a 1 mg/kg bolus of lidocaine if the patient is stable or by electrical cardioversion (100–200 J) if not. If the arrhythmia cannot be suppressed with lidocaine, procainamide (100 mg boluses over 1–2 minutes every 5 minutes to a cumulative dose of 750–1000 mg) or intravenous amiodarone (150 mg over 10 minutes, which may be repeated as needed, followed by 360 mg over 6 hours and then 540 mg over 18 hours) should be initiated, followed by an infusion of 20–80 mg/kg/min. Ventricular fibrillation is treated electrically (300–400 J). Unresponsive ventricular fibrillation should be treated with additional amiodarone and repeat cardioversion while cardiopulmonary resuscitation (CPR) is administered.

Accelerated idioventricular rhythm is a regular, wide-complex rhythm at a rate of 70–100/min. It may occur with or without reperfusion and should not be treated with antiarrhythmics, which could cause asystole.

4. Conduction disturbances—All degrees of AV block may occur in the course of acute myocardial infarction. Block at the level of the AV node is more common than infranodal block and occurs in approximately 20% of inferior myocardial infarctions. First-degree block is the most common and requires no treatment. Second-degree block is usually of the Mobitz type I form (Wenckebach), is often transient, and requires treatment only if associated with a heart rate slow enough to cause symptoms. Complete AV block occurs in up to 5% of acute inferior infarctions, usually is preceded by Mobitz I second-degree block, and generally resolves spontaneously, though it may persist for hours to several weeks. The escape rhythm originates in the distal AV node or AV junction and hence has a narrow QRS complex and is reliable, albeit often slow (30–50 beats/min). Treatment is often necessary because of resulting hypotension and low cardiac output. Intravenous atropine (1 mg) usually restores AV conduction temporarily, but if the escape complex is wide or if repeated atropine treatments are needed, temporary ventricular pacing is indicated. The prognosis for these patients is only slightly worse than for patients in whom AV block did not develop.

In anterior infarctions, the site of block is distal, below the AV node, and usually a result of extensive damage of the His-Purkinje system and bundle branches. New first-degree block (prolongation of the PR interval) is unusual in anterior infarction; Mobitz type II AV block or complete heart block may be preceded by intraventricular conduction defects or may occur abruptly. The escape rhythm, if present, is an unreliable wide-complex idioventricular rhythm. Urgent ventricular pacing is mandatory, but even with successful pacing, morbidity and mortality are high because of the extensive myocardial damage. New conduction abnormalities such as right or left bundle branch block or fascicular blocks may presage progression, often sudden, to second- or third-degree AV block. Temporary ventricular pacing is recommended for new-onset alternating bilateral bundle branch block, bifascicular block, or bundle branch block with worsening first-degree AV block. Patients with anterior infarction who progress to second- or third-degree block even transiently should be considered for insertion of a prophylactic permanent ventricular pacemaker before discharge.

C. Myocardial Dysfunction

The severity of cardiac dysfunction is proportionate to the extent of myocardial necrosis but is exacerbated by preexisting dysfunction and ongoing ischemia. Persons with hypotension not responsive to fluid resuscitation or refractory heart failure or cardiogenic shock should be considered for urgent echocardiography to assess left and right ventricular function and for mechanical complications, right heart catheterization, and continuous measurements of arterial pressure. These measurements permit the accurate assessment of volume status and may facilitate decisions about volume resuscitation, selective use of pressors and inotropes, and mechanical support. Table 10–7 categorizes patients based on these hemodynamic findings.

1. Acute LV failure—Dyspnea, diffuse rales, and arterial hypoxemia usually indicate LV failure. General measures include supplemental oxygen to increase arterial saturation to above 95% and elevation of the trunk. Diuretics are usually the initial therapy unless RV infarction is present. Intravenous furosemide (10–40 mg) or bumetanide (0.5–1 mg) is preferred because of the reliably rapid onset and short duration of action of these drugs. Higher dosages can be given if an inadequate response occurs. Morphine sulfate (4 mg intravenously followed by increments of 2 mg) is valuable in acute pulmonary edema.

Diuretics are usually effective; however, because most patients with acute infarction are not volume overloaded, the hemodynamic response may be limited and may be associated with hypotension. Vasodilators will reduce PCWP and improve cardiac output by a combination of venodilation (increasing venous capacitance) and arteriolar dilation (reducing afterload and LV wall stress). In mild heart failure, sublingual isosorbide dinitrate (2.5–10 mg every 2 hours) or nitroglycerin ointment (6.25–25 mg every 4 hours) may be adequate to lower PCWP. In more severe failure, especially if cardiac output is reduced and BP is normal or high, sodium nitroprusside may be the preferred agent. It should be initiated only with arterial pressure monitoring; the initial dosage should be low (0.25 mcg/kg/min) to avoid excessive hypotension, but the dosage can be increased by increments of 0.5 mcg/kg/min every 5–10 minutes up to 5–10 mcg/kg/min until the desired hemodynamic response is obtained. Excessive hypotension (mean BP < 65–75 mm Hg) or tachycardia (> 10/min increase) should be avoided.

Intravenous nitroglycerin (starting at 10 mcg/min) also may be effective but may lower PCWP with less hypotension. Oral or transdermal vasodilator therapy with nitrates or ACE inhibitors is often necessary after the initial 24–48 hours (see below).

Inotropic agents should be avoided if possible, because they often increase heart rate and myocardial oxygen requirements and worsen clinical outcomes. Dobutamine has the best hemodynamic profile, increasing cardiac output and modestly lowering PCWP, usually without excessive tachycardia, hypotension, or arrhythmias. The initial dosage is 2.5 mcg/kg/min, and it may be increased by similar increments up to 15–20 mcg/kg/min at intervals of 5–10 minutes. Dopamine is more useful in the presence of hypotension (see below), since it produces peripheral vasoconstriction, but it has a less beneficial effect on PCWP. Digoxin has not been helpful in acute infarction except to control the ventricular response in atrial fibrillation, but it may be beneficial if chronic heart failure persists.

2. Hypotension and shock—Patients with hypotension (systolic BP < 90 mm Hg, individualized depending on prior BP) and signs of diminished perfusion (low urinary output, confusion, cold extremities) that does not respond to fluid resuscitation should be presumed to have cardiogenic shock and should be considered for urgent catheterization and revascularization, intra-aortic balloon pump (IABP) support, and hemodynamic monitoring with a PA catheter. Up to 20% will have findings indicative of intravascular hypovolemia (due to diaphoresis, vomiting, decreased venous tone, medications—such as diuretics, nitrates, morphine, β-blockers, calcium channel blockers, and thrombolytic agents—and lack of oral intake). These should be treated with successive boluses of 100 mL of normal saline until PCWP reaches 15–18 mm Hg to determine whether cardiac output and BP respond. Pericardial tamponade due to hemorrhagic pericarditis (especially after thrombolytic therapy or cardiopulmonary resuscitation) or ventricular rupture should be considered and excluded by echocardiography if clinically indicated. RV infarction, characterized by a normal PCWP but elevated RA pressure, can produce hypotension. This is discussed below.

Most patients with cardiogenic shock will have moderate to severe LV systolic dysfunction, with a mean EF of 30% in the SHOCK trial. If hypotension is only modest (systolic pressure > 90 mm Hg) and the PCWP is elevated, diuretics and an initial trial of nitroprusside (see above for dosing) are indicated. If the BP falls, inotropic support will need to be added or substituted. Such patients should generally also be treated with IABP counterpulsation, which can both reduce myocardial energy requirements (systolic unloading) and improve diastolic coronary blood flow.

Dopamine is the most appropriate pressor for cardiogenic hypotension. It should be initiated at a rate of 2–4 mcg/kg/min and increased at 5-minute intervals to the appropriate hemodynamic end point. At low dosages (< 5 mcg/kg/min), it improves renal blood flow; at intermediate dosages (2.5–10 mcg/kg/min), it stimulates myocardial contractility; at higher dosages (> 8 mcg/kg/min), it is a potent α_1-adrenergic agonist. In general, BP and cardiac index rise, but PCWP does not fall. Dopamine may be combined with nitroprusside or dobutamine (see above for dosing), or the latter may be used in its place if hypotension is not severe. Norepinephrine (0.1–0.5 mcg/kg/min) is the usual pressor of last resort, since isoproterenol and epinephrine produce less vasoconstriction and do not increase coronary perfusion pressure (aortic diastolic pressure), but both tend to worsen the balance between myocardial oxygen delivery and utilization.

Patients with cardiogenic shock not due to hypovolemia have a poor prognosis, with 30-day mortality rates of 50–80%. If they do not respond rapidly, IABP should be instituted to both reduce myocardial energy requirements (systolic unloading) and improve diastolic coronary blood flow. Surgically implanted (or percutaneous) ventricular assist devices may be used in refractory cases. Emergent cardiac catheterization and coronary angiography followed by percutaneous or surgical revascularization offer the best chance of survival, particularly in patients under 75 years of age.

D. RV Infarction

RV infarction is present in one-third of patients with inferior wall infarction but is clinically significant in less than 50% of these. It presents as hypotension with relatively preserved LV function and should be considered whenever patients with inferior infarction exhibit low BP, raised venous pressure, and clear lungs. Hypotension is often exacerbated by medications that decrease intravascular volume or produce venodilation, such as diuretics, nitrates, and narcotics. RA pressure and jugular venous pulsations are high, while PCWP is normal or low and the lungs are clear. The diagnosis is suggested by ST-segment elevation in right-sided anterior chest leads, particularly RV_4. The diagnosis can be confirmed by echocardiography or hemodynamic measurements. Treatment consists of fluid loading to improve LV filling, and inotropic agents if necessary.

E. Mechanical Defects

Partial or complete rupture of a papillary muscle or of the interventricular septum occurs in less than 1% of acute myocardial infarctions and carries a poor prognosis. These complications occur in both anterior and inferior infarctions, usually 3–7 days after the acute event. They are detected by the appearance of a new systolic murmur and clinical deterioration, often with pulmonary edema. The two lesions are distinguished by the location of the murmur (apical versus parasternal) and by Doppler echocardiography. Hemodynamic monitoring is essential for appropriate management and demonstrates an increase in oxygen saturation between the RA and PA in VSD and, often, a large v wave with mitral regurgitation. Treatment by nitroprusside and, preferably, IABC reduces the regurgitation or shunt, but surgical correction is mandatory. In patients remaining hemodynamically unstable or requiring continuous parenteral pharmacologic treatment or counterpulsation, early surgery is recommended, though mortality rates are high (15% to nearly 100%, depending on residual ventricular function and clinical status). Patients who are stabilized medically can have delayed surgery with lower risks (10–25%), although this may be due to the death of sicker patients, some of whom may have been saved by earlier surgery.

F. Myocardial Rupture

Complete rupture of the LV free wall occurs in less than 1% of patients and usually results in immediate death. It occurs 2–7 days postinfarction, usually involves the anterior wall, and is more frequent in older women. Incomplete or gradual rupture may be sealed off by the pericardium, creating a **pseudoaneurysm**. This may be recognized by echocardiography, radionuclide angiography, or LV angiography, often as an incidental finding. It demonstrates a narrow-neck connection to the LV. Early surgical repair is indicated, since delayed rupture is common.

G. LV Aneurysm

An LV aneurysm, a sharply delineated area of scar that bulges paradoxically during systole, develops in 10–20% of patients surviving an acute infarction. This usually follows anterior Q wave infarctions. Aneurysms are recognized by persistent ST-segment elevation (beyond 4–8 weeks), and a wide neck from the LV can be demonstrated by echocardiography, scintigraphy, or contrast angiography. They rarely rupture but may be associated with arterial emboli, ventricular arrhythmias, and CHF. Surgical resection may be performed for these indications if other measures fail. The best results (mortality rates of 10–20%) are obtained when the residual myocardium contracts well and when significant coronary lesions supplying adjacent regions are bypassed.

H. Pericarditis

The pericardium is involved in approximately 50% of infarctions, but pericarditis is often not clinically significant. Twenty percent of patients with Q wave infarctions will have an audible friction rub if examined repetitively. Pericardial pain occurs in approximately the same proportion after 2–7 days and is recognized by its variation with respiration and position (improved by sitting). Often, no treatment is required, but aspirin (650 mg every 4–6 hours) will usually relieve the pain. Indomethacin and corticosteroids can cause impaired infarct healing and predispose to myocardial rupture, and therefore should generally be avoided in the early post-myocardial infarction period. Likewise, anticoagulation should be used cautiously, since hemorrhagic pericarditis may result.

One week to 12 weeks after infarction, Dressler syndrome (post-myocardial infarction syndrome) occurs in less than 5% of patients. This is an autoimmune phenomenon and presents as pericarditis with associated fever, leukocytosis and, occasionally, pericardial or pleural effusion. It may recur over months. Treatment is the same as for other forms of pericarditis. A short course of nonsteroidal agents or corticosteroids may help relieve symptoms.

I. Mural Thrombus

Mural thrombi are common in large anterior infarctions but not in infarctions at other locations. Arterial emboli occur in approximately 2% of patients with known infarction, usually within 6 weeks. Anticoagulation with heparin followed by short-term (3-month) warfarin therapy prevents most emboli and should be considered in all patients with large anterior infarctions. Mural thrombi can be detected by echocardiography or CT scan (MRI has yielded frequent false-positive results) but with only moderate reliability, and only a small percentage (up to 25%) embolize, so these procedures should not be relied upon for determining the need for anticoagulation.

Crenshaw BS et al. Risk factors, angiographic patterns, and outcomes in patients with ventricular septal defect complicating acute myocardial infarction. GUSTO-I (Global Utilization of Streptokinase and TPA for Occluded Coronary Arteries) Trial Investigators. Circulation. 2000 Jan 4–11;101 (1):27–32. [PMID: 10618300]

Hochman JS et al. Early revascularization in acute myocardial infarction complicated by cardiogenic shock. SHOCK Investigators. Should We Emergently Revascularize Occluded Coronaries for Cardiogenic Shock. N Engl J Med. 1999 Aug 26; 341(9):625–34. [PMID: 10460813]

Menon V et al. Management of cardiogenic shock complicating acute myocardial infarction. Heart. 2002 Nov;88(5):531–7. [PMID: 12381652]

Pfisterer M. Right ventricular involvement in myocardial infarction and cardiogenic shock. Lancet. 2003 Aug 2;362(9381): 392–4. [PMID: 12907014]

Rathore SS et al. Acute myocardial infarction complicated by heart block in the elderly: prevalence and outcomes. Am Heart J. 2001 Jan;141(1):47–54. [PMID: 11136486]

▶ Postinfarction Management

After the first 24 hours, the focus of patient management is to prevent recurrent ischemia, improve infarct healing and prevent remodeling, and prevent recurrent vascular events. Patients with hemodynamic compromise, who are at high risk for death, need careful monitoring and management of volume status.

A. Risk Stratification

Risk stratification is important for management of STEMI. GRACE and TIMI risk scores can be helpful tools. The TIMI Risk Score is available for PDA download at http://www.timi.org, and the GRACE risk score at http://www.outcomes-umassmed.org/GRACE/acs_risk.cfm.

Patients with recurrent ischemia (spontaneous or provoked), hemodynamic instability, impaired LV function, heart failure, or serious ventricular arrhythmias should undergo cardiac catheterization (Table 10–6). ACE inhibitor (or ARB) therapy is indicated in patients with clinical heart failure or LV EF ≤ 40%.

For patients not undergoing cardiac catheterization, submaximal exercise (or pharmacologic stress testing for patients unable to exercise) before discharge or a maximal test after 3–

6 weeks (the latter being more sensitive for ischemia) helps patients and clinicians plan the return to normal activity. Imaging in conjunction with stress testing adds additional sensitivity for ischemia and provides localizing information. Both exercise and pharmacologic stress imaging have successfully predicted subsequent outcome. One of these tests should be used prior to discharge in patients who have received thrombolytic therapy as a means of selecting appropriate candidates for coronary angiography.

B. Secondary Prevention

Postinfarction management should begin with identification and modification of risk factors. Treatment of hyperlipidemia and smoking cessation both prevent recurrent infarction and death. LDL cholesterol levels should be lowered below 100 mg/dL, and probably to a goal of 70 mg/dL, with a statin commencing prior to discharge. BP control and cardiac rehabilitation or exercise are also recommended.

β-Blockers improve survival rates, primarily by reducing the incidence of sudden death in high-risk subsets of patients, though their value may be less in patients without complications with small infarctions and normal exercise tests. While a variety of β-blockers have been shown to be beneficial, for patients with LV dysfunction managed with contemporary treatment, carvedilol titrated to 25 mg twice a day has been shown to reduce mortality. β-Blockers with intrinsic sympathomimetic activity have not proved beneficial in postinfarction patients.

Antiplatelet agents are beneficial; aspirin (81–325 mg daily) is recommended, and adding clopidogrel (75 mg daily) has been shown to provide additional benefit short term after STEMI and for up to 1 year after non-ST elevation acute coronary syndromes. Prasugrel provides further reduction in thrombotic outcomes compared with clopidogrel, at the cost of more bleeding. Warfarin anticoagulation for 3 months reduces the incidence of arterial emboli after large anterior infarctions, and according to the results of at least one study it improves long-term prognosis, but these studies were before routine use of aspirin and clopidogrel. An advantage to combining low-dose aspirin and warfarin has not been demonstrated, except perhaps in patients with atrial fibrillation.

Calcium channel blockers have not been shown to improve prognoses overall and should not be prescribed purely for secondary prevention. Antiarrhythmic therapy other than with β-blockers has not been shown to be effective except in patients with symptomatic arrhythmias. Amiodarone has been studied in several trials of postinfarct patients with either LV dysfunction or frequent ventricular ectopy. Although survival was not improved, amiodarone was not harmful—unlike other agents in this setting. Therefore, it is the agent of choice for individuals with symptomatic postinfarction supraventricular arrhythmias. While implantable defibrillators improve survival for patients with postinfarction LV dysfunction and heart failure, the DINAMIT trial found no benefit to implantable defibrillators implanted in the 40 days following acute myocardial infarction.

Cardiac rehabilitation programs and exercise training can be of considerable psychological benefit and appear to improve prognosis.

C. ACE Inhibitors and ARBs in Patients with LV Dysfunction

Patients who sustain substantial myocardial damage often experience subsequent progressive LV dilation and dysfunction, leading to clinical heart failure and reduced long-term survival. In patients with EFs less than 40%, long-term ACE inhibitor (or ARB) therapy prevents LV dilation and the onset of heart failure and prolongs survival. The HOPE trial, as well as an overview of trials of ACE-inhibitors for secondary prevention, also demonstrated a reduction of approximately 20% in mortality rates and the occurrence of nonfatal myocardial infarction and stroke with ramipril treatment of patients with vascular disease and without confirmed LV systolic dysfunction. Therefore, ACE inhibitor therapy should be strongly considered in this broader group of patients—and especially in diabetics and patients with even mild systolic hypertension, in whom the greatest benefit was observed.

D. Revascularization

Postinfarction patients not treated with primary PCI who appear likely to benefit from early revascularization if the anatomy is appropriate are (1) those who have undergone thrombolytic therapy and have residual symptoms or laboratory evidence of ischemia; (2) patients with LV dysfunction (EF < 30–40%) and evidence of ischemia; (3) patients with non–ST elevation MI and high-risk features; and (4) patients with markedly positive exercise tests and multivessel disease. The value of revascularization in the following groups is less clear: (1) patients treated with thrombolytic agents, with little evidence of reperfusion or residual ischemia; (2) patients with LV dysfunction but no detectable ischemia; and (3) patients with preserved LV function who have mild ischemia and are not symptom limited. In general, patients who survive infarctions without complications, have preserved LV function (EF > 50%), and have no exercise-induced ischemia have an excellent prognosis and do not require invasive evaluation.

Ades PA. Cardiac rehabilitation and secondary prevention of coronary heart disease. N Engl J Med. 2001 Sep 20;345(12):892–902. [PMID: 11565523]

Dagenais GR et al. Angiotensin-converting-enzyme inhibitors in stable vascular disease without left ventricular systolic dysfunction or heart failure: a combined analysis of three trials. Lancet. 2006 Aug 12;368(9535):581–8. [PMID: 16905022]

Dargie HJ et al. Effect of carvedilol on outcome after myocardial infarction in patients with left ventricular dysfunction: the CAPRICORN randomized trial. Lancet. 2001 May 5;357 (9266):1385–90. [PMID: 11356434]

Hurlen M et al. Warfarin, aspirin, or both after myocardial infarction. N Engl J Med. 2002 Sep 26;347(13):969–74. [PMID: 12324552]

▼ DISTURBANCES OF RATE & RHYTHM

SINUS ARRHYTHMIA, BRADYCARDIA, & TACHYCARDIA

Sinus arrhythmia is a cyclic increase in normal heart rate with inspiration and decrease with expiration. It results from reflex changes in vagal influence on the normal pacemaker and disappears with breath holding or increase of heart rate. It has no clinical significance. It is common in both the young and the elderly.

Sinus bradycardia is a heart rate slower than 60 beats/min due to increased vagal influence on the normal pacemaker or organic disease of the sinus node. The rate usually increases during exercise or administration of atropine. In healthy individuals, and especially in patients who are in excellent physical condition, sinus bradycardia to rates of 50 beats/min or even lower is a normal finding. However, severe sinus bradycardia (< 45 beats/min) may be an indication of sinus node pathology (see below), especially in elderly patients and individuals with heart disease. It may cause weakness, confusion, or syncope if cerebral perfusion is impaired. Atrial, junctional and ventricular ectopic rhythms are more apt to occur with slow sinus rates. Pacing may be required if symptoms correlate with the bradycardia.

Sinus tachycardia is defined as a heart rate faster than 100 beats/min that is caused by rapid impulse formation from the sinoatrial node; it occurs with fever, exercise, emotion, pain, anemia, heart failure, shock, thyrotoxicosis, or in response to many drugs. Alcohol and alcohol withdrawal are common causes of sinus tachycardia and other supraventricular arrhythmias. The onset and termination are usually gradual, in contrast to paroxysmal supraventricular tachycardia due to reentry. The rate infrequently exceeds 160 beats/min but may reach 180 beats/min in young persons. The rhythm is generally regular, but serial 1-minute counts of the heart rate indicate that it varies five or more beats per minute with changes in position, with breath holding, or with sedation. Rare individuals have persistent or episodic "inappropriate" sinus tachycardia that may be very symptomatic or may lead to LV contractile dysfunction. Pharmacologic agents, such as β-blockers and in some cases flecainide, or catheter-based radiofrequency modification of the sinus node have shown to have varying success in treating this problem.

When to Refer

Patients with symptoms related to bradycardia or tachycardia when reversible etiologies have been excluded.

When to Admit

Patients with bradycardia and recent or recurrent syncope.

Still AM et al. Prevalence, characteristics and natural course of inappropriate sinus tachycardia. Europace. 2005 Mar;7(2):104–12. [PMID: 15763524]
Yusuf S et al. Deciphering the sinus tachycardias. Clin Cardiol. 2005 Jun;28(6):267–76. [PMID: 16028460]

ATRIAL PREMATURE BEATS (Atrial Extrasystoles)

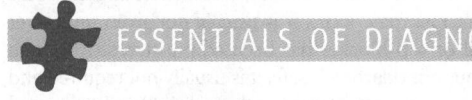

ESSENTIALS OF DIAGNOSIS

► Usually asymptomatic.

► Isolated interruption in regular rhythm.

► Can be harbingers of future development of atrial fibrillation.

► P-wave morphology on ECG usually differs from sinus P-wave morphology.

Atrial premature beats occur when an ectopic focus in the atria fires before the next sinus node impulse or a reentry circuit is established. The contour of the P wave usually differs from the patient's normal complex, unless the ectopic focus is near the sinus node. The subsequent RR cycle length is usually unchanged or only slightly prolonged. Such premature beats occur frequently in normal hearts. Acceleration of the heart rate by any means usually abolishes most premature beats. Early atrial premature beats may cause aberrant QRS complexes (wide and bizarre) or may be nonconducted to the ventricles because the AV node or ventricles are still refractory.

Differentiation of Aberrantly Conducted Supraventricular Beats from Ventricular Beats

This distinction can be very difficult in patients with a wide QRS complex; it is important because of the differing prognostic and therapeutic implications of each type. Findings favoring a ventricular origin include (1) AV dissociation; (2) a QRS duration exceeding 0.14 second; (3) capture or fusion beats (infrequent); (4) left axis deviation with right bundle branch block morphology; (5) monophasic (R) or biphasic (qR, QR, or RS) complexes in V_1; and (6) a qR or QS complex in V_6. Supraventricular origin is favored by (1) a triphasic QRS complex, especially with initial negativity in leads I and V_6; (2) ventricular rates exceeding 170 beats/min; (3) QRS duration longer than 0.12 second but not longer than 0.14 second; and (4) the presence of preexcitation syndrome.

The relationship of the P waves to the tachycardia complex is helpful. A 1:1 relationship usually means a supraventricular origin, except in the case of ventricular tachycardia with retrograde P waves.

PAROXYSMAL SUPRAVENTRICULAR TACHYCARDIA

ESSENTIALS OF DIAGNOSIS

► Frequently associated with palpitations.

► Abrupt onset/offset.

► Rapid, regular rhythm.

► Most commonly seen in young adults.

► Rarely causes frank syncope.

► Usually have a narrow QRS complex on ECG.

► Often responsive to vagal maneuvers, AV nodal blockers, or adenosine.

General Considerations

This is the most common paroxysmal tachycardia and often occurs in patients without structural heart disease. The most common mechanism for paroxysmal supraventricular tachycardia is reentry, which may be initiated or terminated by a fortuitously timed atrial or ventricular premature beat. The reentrant circuit most commonly involves dual pathways (a slow and a fast pathway) within the AV node. This is referred to as AV nodal reentrant tachycardia (AVNRT). Less commonly, reentry is due to an accessory pathway between the atria and ventricles, referred to as AV reentrant tachycardia (AVRT). Approximately one-third of patients with supraventricular tachycardia have accessory pathways to the ventricles. The pathophysiology and management of arrhythmias due to accessory pathways differ in important ways and are discussed separately below.

Clinical Findings

A. Symptoms and Signs

Patients may be asymptomatic except for awareness of rapid heart action, but some experience mild chest pain or shortness of breath, especially when episodes are prolonged, even in the absence of associated cardiac abnormalities. Episodes begin and end abruptly and may last a few seconds to several hours or longer.

B. ECG

The heart rate may be 140–240 beats/min (usually 160–220 beats/min) and is regular (despite exercise or change in position). The P wave usually differs in contour from sinus beats and is often buried in the QRS complex.

Treatment

In the absence of heart disease, serious effects are rare, and most attacks break spontaneously. Particular effort should be made to terminate the attack quickly if cardiac failure, syncope, or anginal pain develops or if there is underlying cardiac or (particularly) coronary disease. Because reentry is the most common mechanism for paroxysmal supraventricular tachycardia, effective therapy requires that conduction be interrupted at some point in the reentry circuit and the vast majority of these circuits involve the AV node.

A. Mechanical Measures

A variety of methods have been used to interrupt attacks, and patients may learn to perform these themselves. These methods result in an acute increase in vagal tone and include the Valsalva maneuver, stretching the arms and body, lowering the head between the knees, coughing, splashing cold water on the face, and breath holding. Carotid sinus massage is often performed by physicians but should be avoided if the patient has carotid bruits or a history of transient cerebral ischemic attacks. Firm but gentle pressure and massage are applied first over the right carotid sinus for 10–20 seconds and, if unsuccessful, then over the left carotid sinus. *Pressure should not be exerted on both sides at the same time!* Continuous ECG or auscultatory monitoring of the heart rate is essential so that pressure can be relieved as soon as the rhythm is broken or if excessive bradycardia occurs. Carotid sinus pressure will interrupt up to half of the attacks, especially if the patient has received a digitalis glycoside or other agent (such as adenosine or a calcium channel blocker) that delays AV conduction. These maneuvers stimulate the vagus nerve, delay AV conduction, and block the reentry mechanism at the level of the AV node, terminating the arrhythmia.

B. Drug Therapy

If mechanical measures fail, two rapidly acting intravenous agents will terminate more than 90% of episodes. Intravenous adenosine has a very brief duration of action and minimal negative inotropic activity (Table 10–9). Initially, a 6 mg bolus is administered. If no response is observed after 1–2 minutes, a second 12 mg bolus should be given, followed by a third if necessary. Because the half-life of adenosine is less than 10 seconds, the drug must be given rapidly (in 1–2 seconds from a peripheral intravenous line); use half the dose if given through a central line. Adenosine causes block of electrical conduction through the AV node. Adenosine is very well tolerated, but nearly 20% of patients will experience transient flushing, and some patients experience severe chest discomfort. Caution must be taken when adenosine is given to elderly patients because the resulting pause can be prolonged. Adenosine must also be used with caution in patients with reactive airways disease because it can promote **bronchospasm**.

Calcium channel blockers also rapidly induce AV block and break many episodes of reentrant supraventricular tachycardia. These agents should be used with caution in patients with heart failure due to their negative inotropic effects. Intravenous verapamil may be given as a 2.5 mg bolus, followed by additional doses of 2.5–5 mg every 1–3 minutes up to a total of 20 mg if BP and rhythm are stable. If the rhythm recurs, further doses can be given. Oral verapamil, 80–120 mg every 4–6 hours, can be used as well in stable patients who are tolerating the rhythm without difficulty, but avoid it if there is any concern that the arrhythmia may be ventricular in origin. Intravenous diltiazem (0.25 mg/kg over 2 minutes, followed by a second bolus of 0.35 mg/kg if necessary and then an infusion of 5–15 mg/h) may cause less hypotension and myocardial depression.

Esmolol, a very short-acting β-blocker, may also be effective; the initial dose is 500 mcg/kg intravenously over 1 minute followed by an infusion of 25–200 mcg/min. Metoprolol is also effective and can be given in 5 mg boluses every 5 minutes and repeated up to two times. If the tachycardia is believed to be mediated by an accessory pathway, intravenous procainamide may terminate supraventricular tachycardia by prolonging refractoriness in the accessory pathway; however, because it facilitates AV conduction and an initial increase in rate may occur, it is usually not given until after verapamil or a β-blocker has been administered. Although intravenous amiodarone is safe, it is usually not required and often ineffective for treatment of these arrhythmias.

Table 10–9. Antiarrhythmic drugs.

Agent	Intravenous Dosage	Oral Dosage	Therapeutic Plasma Level	Route of Elimination	Side Effects
Class Ia: Action: Sodium channel blockers: Depress phase 0 depolarization; slow conduction; prolong repolarization.					
Indications: Supraventricular tachycardia, ventricular tachycardia, prevention of ventricular fibrillation, symptomatic ventricular premature beats.					
Quinidine	6–10 mg/kg (intramuscularly or intravenously) over 20 min (rarely used parenterally)	200–400 mg every 4–6 h or every 8 h (long-acting)	2–5 mg/mL	Hepatic	GI, ↓LVF, ↑Dig
Procainamide	100 mg/1–3 min to 500–1000 mg; maintain at 2–6 mg/min	50 mg/kg/d in divided doses every 3–4 h or every 6 h (long-acting)	4–10 mg/mL; NAPA (active metabolite), 10–20 mcg/mL	Renal	SLE, hypersensitivity, ↓LVF
Disopyramide		100–200 mg every 6–8 h	2–8 mg/mL	Renal	Urinary retention, dry mouth, markedly ↓LVF
Class Ib: Action: Shorten repolarization.					
Indications: Ventricular tachycardia, prevention of ventricular fibrillation, symptomatic ventricular beats.					
Lidocaine	1–2 mg/kg at 50 mg/min; maintain at 1–4 mg/min		1–5 mg/mL	Hepatic	CNS, GI
Mexiletine		100–300 mg every 6–12 h; maximum: 1200 mg/d	0.5–2 mg/mL	Hepatic	CNS, GI, leukopenia
Class Ic: Action: Depress phase 0 repolarization; slow conduction. *Propafenone* is a weak calcium channel blocker and β-blocker and prolongs action potential and refractoriness.					
Indications: Life-threatening ventricular tachycardia or fibrillation, refractory supraventricular tachycardia.					
Flecainide		100–200 mg twice daily	0.2–1 mg/mL	Hepatic	CNS, GI, ↓↓LVF, incessant VT, sudden death
Propafenone		150–300 mg every 8–12 h	***Note:*** Active metabolites	Hepatic	CNS, GI, ↓↓LVF, ↑Dig
Class II: Action: β-blocker, slows AV conduction. *Note:* Other β-blockers may also have antiarrhythmic effects but are not yet approved for this indication in the United States.					
Indications: Supraventricular tachycardia; may prevent ventricular fibrillation.					
Esmolol	500 mcg/kg over 1–2 min; maintain at 25–200 mcg/kg/min	Other β-blockers may be used concomitantly	Not established	Hepatic	↓LVF, bronchospasm
Propranolol	1–5 mg at 1 mg/min	40–320 mg in 1–4 doses daily (depending on preparation)	Not established	Hepatic	↓LVF, bradycardia, AV block, bronchospasm
Metoprolol	2.5–5 mg	50–200 mg daily	Not established	Hepatic	↓LVF, bradycardia, AV block
Class III: Action: Prolong action potential.					
Indications: *Amiodarone:* refractory ventricular tachycardia, supraventricular tachycardia, prevention of ventricular tachycardia, atrial fibrillation, ventricular fibrillation; *dofetilide:* atrial fibrillation and flutter; *sotalol:* ventricular tachycardia, atrial fibrillation; *ibutilide:* conversion of atrial fibrillation and flutter.					
Amiodarone	150–300 mg infused rapidly, followed by 1-mg/min infusion for 6 h (360 mg) and then 0.5 mg/min	800–1600 mg/d for 7–21 days; maintain at 100–400 mg/d (higher doses may be needed)	1–5 mg/mL	Hepatic	Pulmonary fibrosis, hypothyroidism, hyperthyroidism, photosensitivity, corneal and skin deposits, hepatitis, ↑Dig, neurotoxicity, GI

(continued)

Table 10–9. Antiarrhythmic drugs. (continued)

Agent	Intravenous Dosage	Oral Dosage	Therapeutic Plasma Level	Route of Elimination	Side Effects
Sotalol		80–160 mg every 12 h (higher doses may be used for life-threatening arrhythmias)		Renal (dosing interval should be extended if creatinine clearance is < 60 mL/min)	Early incidence of torsades de pointes, ↓LVF, bradycardia, fatigue (and other side effects associated with β-blockers)
Dofetilide		500 mcg every 12 h		Renal (dose must be reduced with kidney dysfunction)	Torsades de pointes in 3%; interaction with cytochrome P-450 inhibitors
Ibutilide	1 mg over 10 min, followed by a second infusion of 0.5–1 mg over 10 min			Hepatic and renal	Torsades de pointes in up to 5% of patients within 3 h after administration; patients must be monitored with defibrillator nearby
Class IV: Action: Slow calcium channel blockers.					
Indications: Supraventricular tachycardia.					
Verapamil	10–20 mg over 2–20 min; maintain at 5 mg/kg/min	80–120 mg every 6–8 h; 240–360 mg once daily with sustained-release preparation	0.1–0.15 mg/mL	Hepatic	↓LVF, constipation, ↑Dig, hypotension
Diltiazem	0.25 mg/kg over 2 min; second 0.35-mg/kg bolus after 15 min if response is inadequate; infusion rate, 5–15 mg/h	180–360 mg daily in 1–3 doses depending on preparation (oral forms not approved for arrhythmias)		Hepatic metabolism, renal excretion	Hypotension, ↓LVF
Miscellaneous: Indications: Supraventricular tachycardia.					
Adenosine	6 mg rapidly followed by 12 mg after 1–2 min if needed; use half these doses if administered via central line			Adenosine receptor stimulation, metabolized in blood	Transient flushing, dyspnea, chest pain, AV block, sinus bradycardia; effect ↓ by theophylline, ↑ by dipyridamole
Digoxin	0.5 mg over 20 min followed by increment of 0.25 or 0.125 mg to 1–1.5 mg over 24 h	1–1.5 mg over 24–36 h in 3 or 4 doses; maintenance, 0.125–0.5 mg/d	0.7–2 mg/mL	Renal	AV block, arrhythmias, GI, visual changes

AV, atrioventricular; CNS, central nervous system; ↑Dig, elevation of serum digoxin level; GI, gastrointestinal (nausea, vomiting, diarrhea); ↓LVF, reduced left ventricular function; NAPA, N-acetylprocainamide; SLE, systemic lupus erythematosus; VT, ventricular tachycardia.

C. Cardioversion

If the patient is hemodynamically unstable or if adenosine and verapamil are contraindicated or ineffective, synchronized electrical cardioversion (beginning at 100 J) is almost universally successful. If digitalis toxicity is present or strongly suspected, as in the case of paroxysmal tachycardia with block, electrical cardioversion should be avoided.

▶ Prevention

A. Catheter Ablation

Because of concerns about the safety and the intolerability of antiarrhythmic medications, radiofrequency ablation is the preferred approach to patients with recurrent symptomatic reentrant supraventricular tachycardia, whether it is due to dual pathways within the AV node or to accessory pathways.

B. Drugs

AV nodal blocking agents are the drugs of choice as first-line medical therapy (Table 10–9). Non-dihydropyridine calcium channel blockers, such as diltiazem and verapamil, or β-blockers are typically used first. Patients who do not respond to agents that increase refractoriness of the AV node may be treated with antiarrhythmics. The class Ic agents (flecainide, propafenone) can be used in patients without underlying structural heart disease. In patients with evidence of structural heart disease, class III agents, such as sotalol or amiodarone, are probably a better choice because of the lower incidence of ventricular proarrhythmia during long-term therapy.

Blomstrom-Lundqvist C et al; European Society of Cardiology Committee, NASPE-Heart Rhythm Society. ACC/AHA/ESC guidelines for the management of patients with supraventricular arrhythmias—executive summary. A report of the American College of Cardiology/American Heart Association task force on practice guidelines and the European Society of Cardiology committee for practice guidelines (writing committee to develop guidelines for the management of patients with supraventricular arrhythmias) developed in collaboration with NASPE-Heart Rhythm Society. J Am Coll Cardiol. 2003 Oct 15;42(8):1493–531. [PMID: 14563598]

Chauhan VS et al. Supraventricular tachycardia. Med Clin North Am. 2001 Mar;85(2):193–223. [PMID: 11233946]

Hebbar AK et al. Management of common arrhythmias: Part I. Supraventricular arrhythmias. Am Fam Physician. 2002 Jun 15;65(12):2479–86. [PMID: 12086237]

SUPRAVENTRICULAR TACHYCARDIAS DUE TO ACCESSORY AV PATHWAYS (Preexcitation Syndromes)

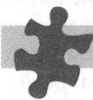 ESSENTIALS OF DIAGNOSIS

► Frequently associated with palpitations.
► Can be associated with syncope.
► Rapid, regular rhythm.
► May have narrow or wide QRS complex on ECG.
► Often have preexcitation (delta wave) on baseline ECG.

General Considerations

Accessory pathways or bypass tracts between the atria and the ventricle bypass the compact AV node predispose to reentrant arrhythmias, such as AVRT and atrial fibrillation. These may be wholly or partly within the node (Mahaim fibers), yielding a short PR interval and normal QRS morphology (**Lown-Ganong-Levine syndrome**). More commonly, they make direct connections between the atria and ventricle through Kent bundles (**Wolff-Parkinson-White syndrome**). This often produces a short PR interval with a delta wave (preexcitation) at the onset of the wide, slurred QRS complex owing to early ventricular depolarization of the region adjacent to the pathway. Although the morphology and polarity of the delta wave can suggest the location of the pathway, mapping by intracardiac recordings is required for precise anatomic localization.

Accessory pathways occur in 0.1–0.3% of the population and facilitate reentrant arrhythmias owing to the disparity in refractory periods of the AV node and accessory pathway. Whether the tachycardia is associated with a narrow or wide QRS complex is frequently determined by whether antegrade conduction is through the node (narrow) or the bypass tract (wide). Some bypass tracts only conduct in a retrograde direction. In these cases, the bypass tract is termed "concealed." Orthodromic tachycardia is a reentrant rhythm that conducts antegrade down the AV node and retrograde up the accessory pathway, resulting in a narrow QRS complex unless an underlying bundle branch block or interventricular conduction delay is present. Antidromic tachycardia conducts antegrade down the accessory pathway and retrograde through the AV node, resulting in a wide QRS complex. Because accessory pathways are often less refractory than specialized conduction tissue, tachycardias proceeding in this direction have the potential to be more rapid. Up to 30% of patients with Wolff-Parkinson-White syndrome will develop atrial fibrillation or flutter with antegrade conduction down the accessory pathway and a rapid ventricular response. If this conduction is very rapid, it can potentially degenerate to ventricular fibrillation.

► Treatment

Some patients have a delta wave found incidentally on ECG. In the absence of palpitations, light-headedness, or syncope, these patients do not require specific therapy. They should be advised to report the onset of any of these symptoms. Occasionally, these patients are referred for exercise treadmill testing to determine if preexcitation is lost at rapid rates. Patients found incidentally to have delta waves who have jobs that could potentially put others at risk (ie, pilot, bus driver, etc) may need to undergo electrophysiologic testing with possible catheter ablation to ensure that they are not at risk for sudden death.

A. Catheter Ablation

As with AVNRT, radiofrequency ablation has become the procedure of choice in patients with accessory pathways and recurrent symptoms. Patients with preexcitation syndromes who have episodes of atrial fibrillation or flutter should be tested by induction of atrial fibrillation in the electrophysiologic laboratory, noting duration of the RR cycle; if it is less than 220 ms, a short refractory period is present. These individuals are at highest risk for sudden death, and prophylactic ablation is indicated. Success rates for ablation of accessory pathways with radiofrequency catheters exceed 90% in appropriate patients.

B. Pharmacologic Therapy

Narrow-complex reentry rhythms involving a bypass tract can be managed as discussed for AVNRT. Atrial fibrillation and flutter with a concomitant antegrade conducting bypass tract must be managed differently, since agents such as digoxin, calcium channel blockers, and even β-blockers may decrease the refractoriness of the accessory pathway or increase that of the AV node, leading to sometimes faster ventricular rates. Therefore, these agents should be avoided. The class Ia, class Ic, and class III antiarrhythmic agents will increase the refractoriness of the bypass tract and are the drugs of choice for wide-complex tachycardias. If hemodynamic compromise is present, electrical cardioversion is warranted.

Long-term therapy often involves a combination of agents that increases refractoriness in the bypass tract (class Ia or Ic agents) and in the AV node (verapamil and β-blockers), provided that atrial fibrillation or flutter with short RR cycle lengths is not present (see above). The class III agents sotalol and amiodarone are effective in refractory cases. Patients who are difficult to manage should undergo electrophysiologic evaluation.

When to Refer

- Patients with an incidental finding of preexcitation and a high-risk job.
- Patients with recurrent symptoms or episodes despite treatment with AV nodal blocking agents.

When to Admit

- Patients with paroxysmal supraventricular tachycardia and syncope.
- Patients with a history of syncope and preexcitation identified on an ECG.

Antz M et al. Risk of sudden death after successful accessory atrioventricular pathway ablation in resuscitated patients with Wolff-Parkinson-White syndrome. J Cardiovasc Electrophysiol. 2002 Mar;13(3):231–6. [PMID: 11942588]

Hamada T et al. Mechanisms for atrial fibrillation in patients with Wolff-Parkinson-White syndrome. J Cardiovasc Electrophysiol. 2002 Mar;13(3):223–9. [PMID: 11942586]

Jezior MR et al. Exercise testing in Wolff-Parkinson-White syndrome: case report with ECG and literature review. Chest. 2005 Apr;127(4):1454–7. [PMID: 15821231]

Pappone C et al. A randomized study of prophylactic catheter ablation in asymptomatic patients with the Wolff-Parkinson-White syndrome. N Engl J Med. 2003 Nov 6;349(19):1803–11. [PMID: 14602878]

ATRIAL FIBRILLATION

ESSENTIALS OF DIAGNOSIS

- ▶ Irregular heart rhythm.
- ▶ Usually tachycardic.
- ▶ Often associated with palpitations (acute onset) or fatigue (chronic).
- ▶ ECG shows erratic atrial activity with irregular ventricular response.
- ▶ High incidence and prevalence in the elderly population.

General Considerations

Atrial fibrillation is the most common chronic arrhythmia, with an incidence and prevalence that rise with age, so that it affects approximately 10% of individuals over age 80 years. It occurs in rheumatic and other forms of valvular heart disease, dilated cardiomyopathy, ASD, hypertension, and coronary heart disease as well as in patients with no apparent cardiac disease; it may be the initial presenting sign in thyrotoxicosis, and this condition should be excluded with the initial episode. The heart rate may range from quite slow to extremely rapid, but is uniformly irregular unless underlying complete heart block and a permanent ventricular pacemaker is in place. The surface ECG typically demonstrates erratic, disorganized atrial activity between discrete QRS complexes occurring in an irregular pattern. The atrial activity may be very fine and difficult to detect on the ECG, or quite course and often mistaken for atrial flutter. Atrial fibrillation often appears paroxysmally before becoming the established rhythm. Pericarditis, chest trauma, thoracic or cardiac surgery, thyroid disorders, or pulmonary disease (as well as medications such as theophylline and β-adrenergic agonists) may cause attacks in patients with normal hearts. Acute alcohol excess and alcohol withdrawal—and, in predisposed individuals, even consumption of small amounts of alcohol—may precipitate atrial fibrillation. This latter presentation, which is often termed "holiday heart," is usually transient and self-limited. Short-term rate control usually suffices as treatment. Perhaps the most serious consequence of atrial fibrillation is the propensity for thrombus formation due to stasis in the atria (particularly the left atrial appendage) and consequent embolization, most devastatingly to the cerebral circulation. Overall, the rate of stroke is approximately 5 events per 100 patient-years of follow-up. However, patients with significant obstructive valvular disease, chronic heart failure or LV dysfunction, diabetes, hypertension, or age over 75 years and those with a history of prior embolic events are at substantially higher risk (up to nearly 20 events per 100 patient-years in patients with multiple risk factors) (Table 10–10).

Clinical Findings

A. Symptoms and Signs

Atrial fibrillation itself is rarely life-threatening; however, it can have serious consequences if the ventricular rate is sufficiently rapid to precipitate hypotension, myocardial ischemia, or tachycardia-induced myocardial dysfunction. Although many patients—particularly older or inactive individuals—have relatively few symptoms if the rate is controlled, some patients are aware of the irregular rhythm and may find it as very uncomfortable. Most patients will complain of fatigue whether they experience other symptoms or not. The heart rate may range from quite slow to extremely rapid, but is uniformly irregular unless underlying complete heart block and a permanent ventricular pacemaker is in place. Atrial fibrillation is the only common arrhythmia in which the ventricular rate is rapid and the rhythm very irregular. Because of the varying stroke

Table 10–10. Risk factors for ischemic stroke and systemic embolism in patients with nonvalvular atrial fibrillation.

Risk Factors[1]	Relative Risk
Previous stroke or TIA	2.5
Diabetes mellitus	1.7
History of hypertension	1.6
Congestive heart failure	1.4
Advanced age (continuous, per decade)	1.4

[1]Data derived from collaborative analysis of five untreated control groups in primary prevention trials. As a group, patients with nonvalvular atrial fibrillation have about a sixfold increased risk of thromboembolism compared with patients in normal sinus rhythm. TIA, transient ischemic attack.
Reproduced, with permission, from ACC/AHA/ESC 2006 guidelines for the management of patients with atrial fibrillation. © 2006, American Heart Association, Inc.

volumes resulting from varying periods of diastolic filling, not all ventricular beats produce a palpable peripheral pulse. The difference between the apical rate and the pulse rate is the "pulse deficit"; this deficit is greater when the ventricular rate is high.

B. ECG

The surface ECG typically demonstrates erratic, disorganized atrial activity between discrete QRS complexes occurring in an irregular pattern. The atrial activity may be very fine and difficult to detect on the ECG, or quite course and often mistaken for atrial flutter.

▶ Treatment

A. Newly Diagnosed Atrial Fibrillation

1. Initial management

A. HEMODYNAMICALLY STABLE PATIENT—If, as is often the case—particularly in older individuals—the patient has no symptoms, hemodynamic instability, or evidence of important precipitating conditions (such as silent myocardial infarction or ischemia, decompensated heart failure, pulmonary embolism, or hemodynamically significant valvular disease), hospitalization is usually not necessary. In most of these cases, atrial fibrillation is an unrecognized chronic or paroxysmal condition and should be managed accordingly (see below). For new onset atrial fibrillation, thyroid function tests and assessment for occult valvular or myocardial disease should be performed.

B. HEMODYNAMICALLY UNSTABLE PATIENT—If the patient is hemodynamically unstable—usually as a result of a rapid ventricular rate or associated cardiac or noncardiac conditions—hospitalization and immediate treatment of atrial fibrillation are required. Urgent cardioversion is usually indicated in patients with shock or severe hypotension, pulmonary edema, or ongoing myocardial infarction or

ischemia. Although there exists a potential risk of thromboembolism with cardioversion if atrial fibrillation has been present for more than 48 hours, in hemodynamically unstable patients the need for immediate rate control outweighs that risk. Electrical cardioversion is usually preferred in unstable patients. An initial shock with 100–200 J is administered in synchrony with the R wave. If sinus rhythm is not restored, an additional attempt with 360 J is indicated. If this fails, cardioversion may be successful after loading with intravenous ibutilide (1 mg over 10 minutes, repeated in 10 minutes if necessary).

In more stable patients or those at particularly high risk for embolism (ie, underlying mitral stenosis, a history of prior embolism, or severe heart failure), a strategy of rate control is appropriate. This is also true when the conditions that precipitated atrial fibrillation are likely to persist (such as following cardiac or noncardiac surgery, respiratory failure, or pericarditis) and when these conditions might resolve spontaneously over a period of hours to days (such as alcohol-induced atrial fibrillation, electrolyte or fluid imbalances, excessive exposure to theophylline or sympathomimetic agents, or some of the same previously cited conditions). The choice of agent is guided by the hemodynamic status of the patient, associated conditions, and the urgency of achieving rate control. Although both hypotension and heart failure may improve when the ventricular rate is slowed, calcium channel blockers and β-blockers may themselves precipitate hemodynamic deterioration. Digoxin is less risky, but even when used aggressively (0.5 mg intravenously over 30 minutes, followed by increments of 0.25 mg every 1–2 hours to a total dose of 1–1.5 mg over 24 hours in patients not previously receiving this agent), rate control is rather slow and may be inadequate, particularly in patients with sympathetic activation. In the setting of myocardial infarction or ischemia, β-blockers are the preferred agent. The most frequently used agents are either metoprolol (administered as a 5 mg intravenous bolus, repeated twice at intervals of 5 minutes and then given as needed by repeat boluses or orally at total daily doses of 50–400 mg) or, in very unstable patients, esmolol (0.5 mg/kg intravenously, repeated if necessary, followed by a titrated infusion of 0.05–0.2 mg/kg/min). If hypertension is present or β-blockers are contraindicated, calcium channel blockers are immediately effective. Diltiazem (20 mg bolus, repeated after 15 minutes if necessary, followed by a maintenance infusion of 5–15 mg/h) is the preferred calcium blocker if hypotension or LV dysfunction is present. Otherwise, verapamil (5–10 mg intravenously over 2–3 minutes, repeated after 30 minutes if necessary) may be used. Amiodarone, even when administered intravenously, has a relatively slow onset but is often a useful adjunct when rate control with the previously cited agents is incomplete or contraindicated or when cardioversion is planned in the near future. However, amiodarone should not be used in this setting if long-term therapy is planned with other antiarrhythmic agents.

If rate control proves unsuccessful or early cardioversion is considered necessary and the duration of atrial fibrillation exceeds 2–3 days or is unknown, a strategy of transesophageal echocardiography-guided cardioversion should be considered. By this approach, the presence of atrial thrombus is excluded and electrical cardioversion can be attempted while the patient remains under sedation. If thrombus is present, the cardioversion is delayed until after a 4-week period of therapeutic anticoagulation. In any case, because atrial contractile activity may not recover for several weeks after restoration of sinus rhythm in patients who have been in atrial fibrillation for more than several days, cardioversion is usually followed by anticoagulation for at least 1 month unless it is contraindicated.

2. Subsequent management—Up to two-thirds of patients experiencing a first episode of atrial fibrillation will spontaneously revert to sinus rhythm within 24 hours. If atrial fibrillation persists or has been present for more than a week, spontaneous conversion is unlikely. In most cases early cardioversion is not required, so management consists of rate control and anticoagulation whether or not the patient has been admitted to hospital. Rate control is usually relatively easy to achieve with β-blockers, rate-slowing calcium blockers and, occasionally, digoxin, used as single agents or more often in combination. Good rate control should consist of a ventricular rate between 50 and 100 beats/min with usual daily activities and a ventricular rate not exceeding 120 beats/min except with moderate to strenuous activity. In older patients, who often have diminished AV nodal function and relatively limited activity, this can often be achieved with a single agent. Most younger or more active individuals require a combination of two agents. Choice of the initial medication is best based on the presence of accompanying conditions: Hypertensive patients should be given β-blockers or calcium blockers; coronary patients should usually receive a β-blocker; and patients with heart failure should be given a β-blocker with consideration of adding digoxin. Adequacy of rate control should be evaluated by recording the apical pulse rate both at rest and with an appropriate level of activity (such as after brisk walking around the corridor or climbing stairs).

A. ANTICOAGULATION—For patients with atrial fibrillation, even when it is paroxysmal or occurs rarely, anticoagulation with warfarin to an INR target of 2.0–3.0 should be established and maintained indefinitely, at least for patients with at least one risk factor for stroke (Table 10–10). Cardioversion, if planned, should be performed after at least 4 weeks of anticoagulation at a therapeutic level. Anticoagulation clinics with systematic management of warfarin dosing and adjustment have been shown to result in better maintenance of target anticoagulation. While there was hope that clopidogrel and aspirin might be reasonable alternatives for warfarin for some patients, the ACTIV-W trial was stopped early because of substantially lower rates of stroke with warfarin compared with the combination of clopidogrel and aspirin. An exception to the need for anticoagulation is the patient with "lone atrial fibrillation" (eg, no evidence of associated heart disease, hypertension, atherosclerotic vascular disease, or diabetes) who is under age 65 years. Such patients should be treated with aspirin 81–325 mg daily or no antithrombotic therapy.

B. RATE CONTROL OR ELECTIVE CARDIOVERSION—Two large randomized controlled trials (the 4060-patient Atrial Fibrillation Follow-up Investigation of Rhythm Management, or AFFIRM trial; and the Rate Control Versus Electrical Cardioversion for Persistent Atrial Fibrillation, or RACE trial) compared strategies of rate control and rhythm control. In both, a strategy of rate control and long-term anticoagulation was associated with no higher rates of death or stroke—both, if anything, favored rate control—and only a modestly increased risk of hemorrhagic events than a strategy of restoring sinus rhythm and maintaining it with antiarrhythmic drug therapy. Of note is that exercise tolerance and quality of life were not significantly better in the rhythm control group. Nonetheless, the decision as to whether to attempt to restore sinus rhythm following the initial episode remains controversial. Elective cardioversion following an appropriate period of anticoagulation is generally recommended for the initial episode in patients in whom atrial fibrillation is thought to be of recent onset and when there is an identifiable precipitating factor. Similarly, cardioversion is appropriate in patients who remain symptomatic from the rhythm despite aggressive efforts to achieve rate control. However, it should be noted that even in patients for whom this is the initial episode of atrial fibrillation, the recurrence rate is sufficiently high that longer-term anticoagulation is generally appropriate until persistence of sinus rhythm can be confirmed for at least 6 months.

In cases in which elective cardioversion is required, it may be accomplished electrically (as described above) or pharmacologically. Intravenous ibutilide may also be used as described above in a setting in which the patient can undergo continuous ECG monitoring for at least 3 hours following administration. In patients in whom a decision has been made to continue antiarrhythmic therapy to maintain sinus rhythm (see next paragraph), cardioversion can be attempted with an agent that is being considered for long-term use. For instance, after therapeutic anticoagulation has been established, amiodarone can be initiated on an outpatient basis (300–400 mg twice daily for 2 weeks, followed by 200 mg twice daily for at least a 2–4 weeks and then a maintenance dose of 200 mg daily). Because amiodarone increases the prothrombin time in patients taking warfarin and increases digoxin levels, careful monitoring of anticoagulation and drug levels is required. Other agents that may be used for both cardioversion and maintenance therapy include propafenone (150–300 mg twice daily; should be avoided in patients with structural heart disease), flecainide (50–150 mg twice daily; should be avoided in patients with structural heart disease and should be used in conjunction with an AV nodal blocking drug if there is a history of atrial flutter), and dofetilide (500 mcg twice daily; downward dose adjustment is required with kidney dysfunction and dosing must be initiated in hospital because of risk of torsades de pointes). Sotalol (80–160 mg twice daily; should be initiated in hospital in patients with structural heart disease because of risk of torsades de pointes) is not very effective for converting atrial fibrillation but can be used to maintain sinus rhythm following cardioversion.

Unfortunately, sinus rhythm will persist in only 25% of patients who have had a sustained (lasting more than several days) or recurrent episode of atrial fibrillation. However, if the patient is treated long-term with an antiarrhythmic agent, sinus rhythm will persist in approximately 50%. The most commonly used medications are amiodarone, sotalol, propafenone, flecainide, and dofetilide, but the latter four agents are associated with a clear risk of proarrhythmia, and amiodarone frequently causes other adverse effects. Therefore, it may be prudent to determine whether atrial fibrillation recurs during a period of 6 months without antiarrhythmic drugs during which anticoagulation is maintained. If it does recur, the decision as to whether to restore sinus rhythm and initiate long-term antiarrhythmic therapy can be based on how well the patient tolerates atrial fibrillation. In such a patient, long-term anticoagulation is probably indicated in any case, because of the high rate of recurrence and the likely occurrence of asymptomatic paroxysmal episodes.

B. Paroxysmal and Refractory Atrial Fibrillation

1. Recurrent paroxysmal atrial fibrillation—It is now well established that patients with recurrent paroxysmal atrial fibrillation are at similar stroke risk as those who are in atrial fibrillation chronically. Although these episodes may be apparent to the patient, many are not recognized and may be totally asymptomatic. Thus, ambulatory ECG monitoring or event recorders are indicated in those in whom paroxysmal atrial fibrillation is suspected. Antiarrhythmic agents are usually not successful in preventing all paroxysmal atrial fibrillation episodes. However, dofetilide has been shown to be as effective as amiodarone in maintaining sinus rhythm in certain patients and does not have as many untoward long-term effects. Long-term anticoagulation is indicated except in those who are under 65–75 years of age and have no additional stroke risk factors (see above).

2. Refractory atrial fibrillation—Because of trial results indicating that important adverse clinical outcomes (death, stroke, hemorrhage, heart failure) are no more common with rate control than rhythm control, atrial fibrillation should generally be considered refractory if it causes persistent symptoms or limits activity. This is much more likely in younger individuals and those who are very active or engage in strenuous exercise. Even in such individuals, two-drug or three-drug combinations of a β-blocker, rate-slowing calcium blocker, and digoxin usually can prevent excessive ventricular rates, though in some cases they are associated with excessive bradycardia during sedentary periods.

If no drug works, radiofrequency AV node ablation and permanent pacing ensure rate control and may facilitate a more physiologic rate response to activity, but this is used only as a last resort. There is growing experience with ablation of foci in and around the pulmonary veins that initiate atrial fibrillation, following which sinus rhythm may be restored or maintained. This therapy has become more widely accepted and is a reasonable second-line therapy for individuals with symptomatic atrial fibrillation that is refractory to pharmacologic therapy. This procedure is routinely performed in the electrophysiology laboratory using a catheter-based approach and can also be performed thorascopically or via thoracotomy or median sternotomy in the operating room by experienced surgeons.

When to Refer

- Symptomatic atrial fibrillation with or without rate control.
- Asymptomatic atrial fibrillation with poor rate control despite AV nodal blockers.

When to Admit

- Atrial fibrillation with rapid ventricular response resulting in hemodynamic compromise.
- Atrial fibrillation resulting in acute heart failure.

Fang MC et al. Anticoagulation for atrial fibrillation. Cardiol Clin. 2004 Feb;22(1):47–62. [PMID: 14994847]

Gage BF et al. Selecting patients with atrial fibrillation for anticoagulation: stroke risk stratification in patients taking aspirin. Circulation. 2004 Oct 19;110(16):2287–92. [PMID: 15477396]

Gillinov AM et al. Advances in the surgical treatment of atrial fibrillation. Cardiol Clin. 2004 Feb;22(1):147–57. [PMID: 14994854]

Joglar JA et al. Electrical cardioversion of atrial fibrillation. Cardiol Clin. 2004 Feb;22(1):101–11. [PMID: 14994851]

Lip GY et al. Management of atrial fibrillation. Lancet. 2007 Aug 18;370(9587):604–18. [PMID: 17707756]

McKeown PP et al; American College of Chest Physicians. Executive summary: American College of Chest Physicians guidelines for the prevention and management of postoperative atrial fibrillation after cardiac surgery. Chest. 2005 Aug; 128(2 Suppl):1S–5S. [PMID: 16167657]

Stevenson WG et al. Management of atrial fibrillation in patients with heart failure. Heart Rhythm. 2007 Mar;4(3 Suppl):S28–30. [PMID: 17336880]

Vassallo P et al. Prescribing amiodarone: an evidence-based review of clinical indications. JAMA. 2007 Sep 19;298(11):1312–22. [PMID: 17878423]

Wazni OM et al. Radiofrequency ablation vs antiarrhythmic drugs as first-line treatment of symptomatic atrial fibrillation: a randomized trial. JAMA. 2005 Jun 1;293(21):2634–40. [PMID: 15928285]

Yamada T et al. Evidence-based approach to ablating atrial fibrillation. Curr Cardiol Rep. 2007 Sep;9(5):366–70. [PMID: 17877931]

ATRIAL FLUTTER

 ESSENTIALS OF DIAGNOSIS

- ▶ Regular heart rhythm.
- ▶ Usually tachycardic (100–150 beats/min).
- ▶ Often associated with palpitations (acute onset) or fatigue (chronic).
- ▶ ECG shows "sawtooth" pattern of atrial activity in leads II, III, and AVF.
- ▶ Often seen in conjunction with structural heart disease or chronic obstructive pulmonary disease.

Atrial flutter is less common than fibrillation. It occurs most often in patients with chronic obstructive pulmonary disease (COPD) but may be seen also in those with rheumatic or coronary heart disease, CHF, ASD, or surgically repaired congenital heart disease. The reentrant circuit generates atrial rates of 250–350 beats/min, usually with transmission of every second, third, or fourth impulse through the AV node to the ventricles. The ECG typically demonstrates a "sawtooth" pattern of atrial activity in the inferior leads (II, III, and AVF).

▶ Treatment

Ventricular rate control is accomplished using the same agents used in atrial fibrillation, but it is much more difficult with atrial flutter than with atrial fibrillation. Conversion of atrial flutter to sinus rhythm with class I antiarrhythmic agents is also difficult to achieve, and administration of these drugs has been associated with slowing of the atrial flutter rate to the point at which 1:1 AV conduction can occur at rates in excess of 200 beats/min, with subsequent hemodynamic collapse. The intravenous class III antiarrhythmic agent ibutilide has been significantly more successful in converting atrial flutter. About 50–70% of patients return to sinus rhythm within 60–90 minutes following the infusion of 1–2 mg of this agent. Electrical cardioversion is also very effective for atrial flutter, with approximately 90% of patients converting following synchronized shocks of as little as 25–50 J.

The persistence of atrial contractile function in this arrhythmia provides some protection against thrombus formation, though the risk of systemic embolization remains increased. Precardioversion anticoagulation is not necessary for atrial flutter of less than 48 hours duration except in the setting of mitral valve disease. However, **anticoagulation** is prudent in chronic atrial flutter, particularly since transient periods of atrial fibrillation are common in these patients.

Chronic atrial flutter is often a difficult management problem, as rate control is difficult. If pharmacologic therapy is chosen, amiodarone and dofetilide are the antiarrhythmics of choice. Dofetilide is often given in conjunction with an AV nodal blocker. Atrial flutter can follow a typical or atypical reentry circuit around the atrium. The anatomy of the typical circuit has been well defined and allows for catheter ablation within the atrium to interrupt the circuit and eliminate atrial flutter. Catheter ablation has become the preferred treatment for recurrent typical atrial flutter.

▶ When to Refer

- Symptomatic atrial flutter with or without rate control.
- Asymptomatic atrial flutter with poor rate control despite AV nodal blockers.

▶ When to Admit

- Atrial flutter with 1:1 conduction resulting in hemodynamic compromise.
- Atrial flutter resulting in acute heart failure.

Da Costa A et al. Results from the Loire-Ardèche-Drôme-Isère-Puy-de-Dôme (LADIP) trial on atrial flutter, a multicentric prospective randomized study comparing amiodarone and radiofrequency ablation after the first episode of symptomatic atrial flutter. Circulation. 2006 Oct 17;114(16):1676–81. [PMID: 17030680]

Ghali WA et al. Atrial flutter and the risk of thromboembolism: a systematic review and meta-analysis. Am J Med. 2005 Feb; 118(2):101–7. [PMID: 15694889]

Lee KW et al. Atrial flutter: a review of its history, mechanisms, clinical features, and current therapy. Curr Probl Cardiol. 2005 Mar;30(3):121–67. [PMID: 15711509]

Sun JL et al. Clinical comparison of ibutilide and propafenone for converting atrial flutter. Cardiovasc Drugs Ther. 2005 Jan;19(1):57–64. [PMID: 15883757]

Wu RC et al. Catheter ablation of atrial flutter and macroreentrant atrial tachycardia. Curr Opin Cardiol. 2002 Jan;17(1): 58–64. [PMID: 11790935]

MULTIFOCAL (Chaotic) ATRIAL TACHYCARDIA

ESSENTIALS OF DIAGNOSIS

- ▶ ECG reveals three or more distinct P-wave morphologies.
- ▶ Often associated with palpitations.
- ▶ Associated with severe COPD.
- ▶ Treatment of the underlying lung disease is the most effective therapy.

This is a rhythm characterized by varying P wave morphology (by definition, three or more foci) and markedly irregular PP intervals. The rate is usually between 100 and 140 beats/min, and AV block is unusual. Most patients have concomitant severe COPD. Treatment of the underlying condition is the most effective approach; verapamil, 240–480 mg daily in divided doses, is also of value in some patients, but this particular arrhythmia is very difficult to manage.

Spodick DH. Multifocal atrial arrhythmia. Am J Geriatr Cardiol. 2005 May–Jun;14(3):162. [PMID: 15886545]

AV JUNCTIONAL RHYTHM

ESSENTIALS OF DIAGNOSIS

- ▶ Regular heart rhythm.
- ▶ Can have wide or narrow QRS complex.
- ▶ Often seen in digitalis toxicity.

The atrial-nodal junction or the nodal-His bundle junctions may assume pacemaker activity for the heart, usually at a rate of 40–60 beats/min. This may occur in patients with myocarditis, CAD, and digitalis toxicity as well as in individuals with normal hearts. The rate responds normally to exercise, and the diagnosis is often an incidental finding on ECG monitoring, but it can be suspected if the jugular venous pulse shows cannon *a* waves. Junctional rhythm is often an escape rhythm because of depressed sinus node function with sinoatrial block or delayed conduction in the AV node. **Nonparoxysmal junctional tachycardia** results from increased automaticity of the junctional tissues in digitalis toxicity or ischemia and is associated with a narrow QRS complex and a rate usually less than 120–130 beats/min. It is usually considered benign when it occurs in acute myocardial infarction, but the ischemia that induces it may also cause ventricular tachycardia and ventricular fibrillation.

VENTRICULAR PREMATURE BEATS (Ventricular Extrasystoles)

Sudden death occurs more frequently (presumably as a result of ventricular fibrillation) when ventricular premature beats occur in the presence of organic heart disease but not in individuals with no known cardiac disease.

▶ Clinical Findings

The patient may or may not sense the irregular beat, usually as a skipped beat. Exercise generally abolishes premature beats in normal hearts, and the rhythm becomes regular. Ventricular premature beats are characterized by wide QRS complexes that differ in morphology from the patient's normal beats. They are usually not preceded by a P wave, although retrograde ventriculoatrial conduction may occur. Unless the latter is present, there is a fully compensatory pause (ie, without change in the PP interval). Bigeminy and trigeminy are arrhythmias in which every second or third beat is premature; these patterns confirm a reentry mechanism for the ectopic beat. Ambulatory ECG monitoring or monitoring during graded exercise may reveal more frequent and complex ventricular premature beats than occur in a single routine ECG. An increased frequency of ventricular premature beats during exercise is associated with a higher risk of cardiovascular mortality, though there is no evidence that specific therapy has a role.

▶ Treatment

If no associated cardiac disease is present and if the ectopic beats are asymptomatic, no therapy is indicated. If they are frequent, electrolyte abnormalities (especially hypokalemia or hyperkalemia and hypomagnesemia), hyperthyroidism, and occult heart disease should be excluded. Pharmacologic treatment is indicated only for patients who are symptomatic. Because of concerns about worsening arrhythmia and sudden death with most antiarrhythmic agents, β-blockers are the agents of first choice. If the underlying condition is mitral prolapse, hypertrophic cardiomyopathy, LVH, or coronary disease—or if the QT interval is prolonged—β-blocker therapy is appropriate. The class I and III agents (see Table 10–9) are all effective in reducing ventricular premature beats but often cause side effects and may exacerbate serious arrhythmias in 5–20% of patients. Therefore, every attempt should be made to avoid using class I or III antiarrhythmic agents in patients without symptoms. Catheter ablation is now a well-established therapy for symptomatic individuals who do not respond to antiarrhythmic drugs or for those patients whose burden of ectopic beats has resulted in a tachycardia-induced cardiomyopathy.

Conti CR. Ventricular arrhythmias: a general cardiologist's assessment of therapies in 2005. Clin Cardiol. 2005 Jul;28(7): 314–6. [PMID: 16075822]

Morshedi-Meibodi A et al. Clinical correlates and prognostic significance of exercise-induced ventricular premature beats in the community: the Framingham Heart Study. Circulation. 2004 May 25;109(20):2417–22. [PMID: 15148273]

O'Neill JO et al. Severe frequent ventricular ectopy after exercise as a predictor of death in patients with heart failure. J Am Coll Cardiol. 2004 Aug 18;44(4):820–6. [PMID: 15312865]

VENTRICULAR TACHYCARDIA

 ESSENTIALS OF DIAGNOSIS

▶ Fast, wide complex rhythm.

▶ Often associated with structural heart disease.

▶ Frequently associated with syncope.

▶ If associated with structural heart disease, the implantable cardioverter-defibrillator is the seminal therapy.

▶ General Considerations

Ventricular tachycardia is defined as three or more consecutive ventricular premature beats. The usual rate is 160–240 beats/min and is moderately regular but less so than atrial tachycardia. The usual mechanism is reentry, but abnormally triggered rhythms occur.

Ventricular tachycardia is a frequent complication of acute myocardial infarction and dilated cardiomyopathy but may occur in chronic coronary disease, hypertrophic cardiomyopathy, mitral valve prolapse, myocarditis, and in most other forms of myocardial disease. However, ventricular tachycardia can also occur in patients with structurally normal hearts. **Torsades de pointes**, a form of ventricular tachycardia in which QRS morphology twists around the baseline, may occur spontaneously in the setting of hypokalemia or hypomagnesemia or after any drug that prolongs the QT interval. In nonacute settings, most patients with ventricular tachycardia have known or easily detectable cardiac disease, and the finding of ventricular tachycardia is an unfavorable prognostic sign.

▶ Clinical Findings

A. Symptoms and Signs

Patients may be asymptomatic or experience syncope or milder symptoms of impaired cerebral perfusion.

B. Laboratory Findings

Ventricular tachycardia can occur in the setting of hypokalemia and hypomagnesemia.

C. Differentiation of Aberrantly Conducted Supraventricular Beats from Ventricular Beats

Ventricular tachycardia is either nonsustained (lasting less than 30 seconds) or sustained. The distinction from aberrant conduction of supraventricular tachycardia may be difficult in patients with a wide QRS complex; it is important because of the differing prognostic and therapeutic implications of each type. Findings favoring a ventricular origin include (1) AV dissociation; (2) a QRS duration exceeding 0.14 second; (3) capture or fusion beats (infrequent); (4) left axis deviation with right bundle branch block morphology; (5) monophasic (R) or biphasic (qR, QR, or RS) complexes in V_1; and (6) a qR or QS complex in V_6. Supraventricular origin is favored by (1) a triphasic QRS complex, especially if there was initial negativity in leads I and V_6; (2) ventricular rates exceeding 170 beats/min; (3) QRS duration longer than 0.12 second but not longer than 0.14 second; and (4) the presence of preexcitation syndrome.

The relationship of the P waves to the tachycardia complex is helpful. A 1:1 relationship usually means a supraventricular origin, except in the case of ventricular tachycardia with retrograde P waves.

▶ Treatment

A. Acute Ventricular Tachycardia

The treatment of acute ventricular tachycardia is determined by the degree of hemodynamic compromise and the duration of the arrhythmia. The management of ventricular tachycardia in acute myocardial infarction has been discussed. In other patients, if ventricular tachycardia causes hypotension, heart failure, or myocardial ischemia, synchronized DC cardioversion with 100–360 J should be performed immediately. If the patient is tolerating the rhythm, lidocaine, 1 mg/kg as an intravenous bolus injection, or amiodarone 150 mg as a slow intravenous bolus over 10 minutes, followed by a slow infusion of 1 mg/min for 6 hours and then a maintenance infusion of 0.5 mg/min for an additional 18–42 hours can be used. If the ventricular tachycardia recurs, supplemental amiodarone infusions of 150 mg over 10 minutes can be given. If the patient is stable, intravenous procainamide, 20 mg/min intravenously (up to 1000 mg), followed by an infusion of 20–80 mcg/kg/min could also be tried. Empiric magnesium replacement (1 g intravenously) may help. Ventricular tachycardia can also be terminated by ventricular overdrive pacing, and this approach is useful when the rhythm is recurrent.

B. Chronic Recurrent Ventricular Tachycardia

1. Sustained ventricular tachycardia—Patients with symptomatic or sustained ventricular tachycardia in the absence of a reversible precipitating cause (acute myocardial infarction or ischemia, electrolyte imbalance, drug toxicity, etc) are at high risk for recurrence. In those with significant LV dysfunction, subsequent sudden death is common. Several trials, including the Antiarrhythmic Drug Versus Implantable Defibrillator (AVID) and the Canadian Implantable Defibrillator trials, strongly suggest that these patients should be managed with implantable cardioverter-defibrillators (ICDs). In those with preserved LV function, the mortality rate is lower and the etiology is often different than in those with depressed ventricular function. Treatment with amiodarone, optimally in combination with a β-blocker,

may be adequate. Sotalol may be an alternative, though there is less supporting evidence. However, many times if ventricular tachycardia occurs in a patient with preserved ventricular function, it is either an outflow tract tachycardia or a fascicular ventricular tachycardia, and these arrhythmias will often respond to AV nodal blockers and can be effectively treated with catheter ablation. The role of electrophysiologic studies in this group is less clear than was previously thought, but they may help identify patients who are candidates for radiofrequency ablation of a ventricular tachycardia focus. This is particularly the case for arrhythmias that originate in the RV outflow tract (appearing as left bundle branch block with inferior axis on the surface ECG), the posterior fascicle (right bundle branch block, superior axis morphology), or sustained bundle branch reentry. Catheter ablation can be used as a palliative therapy for those patients with recurrent tachycardia who receive ICD shocks despite antiarrhythmic therapy.

2. Nonsustained ventricular tachycardia (NSVT)—NSVT is defined as runs of three or more ventricular beats lasting less than 30 seconds. These may be symptomatic (usually experienced as light-headedness) or asymptomatic. In individuals without heart disease, NSVT is not clearly associated with a poor prognosis. However, in patients with structural heart disease, particularly when they have reduced EFs, there is an increased risk of subsequent symptomatic ventricular tachycardia or sudden death. β-Blockers reduce these risks in patients who have coronary disease with significant LV systolic dysfunction (EFs < 35–40%), but if sustained ventricular tachycardia has been induced during electrophysiologic testing, an implantable defibrillator may be indicated. In patients with chronic heart failure and reduced EFs—whether due to coronary disease or primary cardiomyopathy and regardless of the presence of asymptomatic ventricular arrhythmias—β-blockers reduce the incidence of sudden death by 40–50% and should be routine therapy (see section on Heart Failure).

Although there are no definitive data with amiodarone in this group, trends from a number of studies suggest that it may be beneficial. Other antiarrhythmic agents should generally be avoided because their proarrhythmic risk appears to outweigh any benefit, even in patients with inducible arrhythmias that are successfully suppressed in the electrophysiology laboratory.

▶ When to Admit

Any sustained ventricular tachycardia.

Ermis C et al. Comparison of ventricular arrhythmia frequency in patients with ischemic cardiomyopathy versus nonischemic cardiomyopathy treated with implantable cardioverter defibrillators. Am J Cardiol. 2005 Jul 15;96(2):233–8. [PMID: 16018849]
Katritsis DG et al. Nonsustained ventricular tachycardia: where do we stand? Eur Heart J. 2004 Jul;25(13):1093–9. [PMID: 15231366]

VENTRICULAR FIBRILLATION & DEATH

Sudden cardiac death is defined as unexpected nontraumatic death in clinically well or stable patients who die within 1 hour after onset of symptoms. The causative rhythm in most cases is ventricular fibrillation, which is usually preceded by ventricular tachycardia except in the setting of acute ischemia or infarction. Complete heart block and sinus node arrest may also cause sudden death. A disproportionate number of sudden deaths occur in the early morning hours. Over 75% of victims of sudden cardiac death have severe CAD. Many have old infarctions. Sudden death may be the initial manifestation of coronary disease in up to 20% of patients and accounts for approximately 50% of deaths from coronary disease. Other conditions that predispose to sudden death include severe LVH, hypertrophic cardiomyopathy, congestive cardiomyopathy, aortic stenosis, pulmonary stenosis, primary pulmonary hypertension, cyanotic congenital heart disease, atrial myxoma, mitral valve prolapse, hypoxia, electrolyte abnormalities, prolonged QT interval syndrome, the Brugada syndrome and conduction system disease. Late potentials (after the QRS complex) on a signal-averaged surface ECG in patients with prior myocardial infarction may identify a group of patients at risk for ventricular arrhythmias and sudden death.

► Treatment

Unless ventricular fibrillation occurred shortly after myocardial infarction, is associated with ischemia, or is seen with an unusual correctable process (such as an electrolyte abnormality, drug toxicity, or aortic stenosis), surviving patients require evaluation and intervention since recurrences are frequent. Coronary arteriography should be performed to exclude coronary disease as the underlying cause, since revascularization may prevent recurrence. When ventricular fibrillation occurs in the initial 24 hours after infarction, long-term management is no different from that of other patients with acute infarction. Conduction disturbances should be managed as described in the next section. The current consensus is that if myocardial infarction or ischemia, bradyarrhythmias and conduction disturbances or other identifiable and correctable precipitating causes of ventricular fibrillation are not found to be the cause of the sudden death episode, an implantable cardioverter-defibrillator is the treatment of choice. In addition, evidence from the MADIT II study and Sudden Cardiac Death in Heart Failure Trial (SCD-HeFT) suggest that patients with severe LV dysfunction—whether due to an ischemic cause such as a remote myocardial infarction or a nonischemic cause of advanced heart failure—have a reduced risk of death with the prophylactic implantation of an implantable cardioverter-defibrillator. However, the DINAMIT study demonstrated that implanting prophylactic ICDs in patients early after myocardial infarction is associated with a trend toward worse outcomes.

Brodine WN et al; MADIT-II Research Group. Effects of beta-blockers on implantable cardioverter defibrillator therapy and survival in the patients with ischemic cardiomyopathy (from the Multicenter Automatic Defibrillator Implantation Trial-II). Am J Cardiol. 2005 Sep 1;96(5):691–5. [PMID: 16125497]

Eckardt L et al. Long-term prognosis of individuals with right precordial ST-segment-elevation Brugada syndrome. Circulation. 2005 Jan 25;111(3):257–63. [PMID: 15642768]

Hohnloser SH et al; DINAMIT Investigators. Prophylactic use of an implantable cardioverter-defibrillator after acute myocardial infarction. N Engl J Med. 2004 Dec 9;351(24): 2481–8. [PMID: 15590950]

Kadish A et al; Defibrillators in Non-Ischemic Cardiomyopathy Treatment Evaluation (DEFINITE) Investigators. Prophylactic defibrillator implantation in patients with nonischemic dilated cardiomyopathy. N Engl J Med. 2004 May 20;350(21): 2151–8. [PMID: 15152060]

Sanders GD et al. Cost-effectiveness of implantable cardioverter-defibrillators. N Engl J Med. 2005 Oct 6;353(14):1471–80. [PMID: 16207849]

ACCELERATED IDIOVENTRICULAR RHYTHM

Accelerated idioventricular rhythm is a regular wide complex rhythm with a rate of 60–120 beats/min, usually with a gradual onset. Because the rate is often similar to the sinus rate, fusion beats and alternating rhythms are common. Two mechanisms have been invoked: (1) an escape rhythm due to suppression of higher pacemakers resulting from sinoatrial and AV block or from depressed sinus node function; and (2) slow ventricular tachycardia due to increased automaticity or, less frequently, reentry. It occurs commonly in acute infarction and following reperfusion after thrombolytic drugs. The incidence of associated ventricular fibrillation is much less than that of ventricular tachycardia with a rapid rate, and treatment is not indicated unless there is hemodynamic compromise or more serious arrhythmias. This rhythm also is common in digitalis toxicity.

Accelerated idioventricular rhythm must be distinguished from the idioventricular or junctional rhythm with rates less than 40–45 beats/min that occurs in the presence of complete AV block. AV dissociation—where ventricular rate exceeds sinus—but not AV block occurs in most cases of accelerated idioventricular rhythm.

LONG QT SYNDROME

Congenital long QT syndrome is an uncommon disease that is characterized by recurrent syncope, a long QT interval (usually 0.5–0.7 second), documented ventricular arrhythmias, and sudden death. It may occur in the presence (Jervell-Lange-Nielsen syndrome) or absence (Romano-Ward syndrome) of congenital deafness. Inheritance may be autosomal recessive or autosomal dominant (Romano-Ward). Specific genetic mutations affecting membrane potassium and sodium channels have been identified and help delineate the mechanisms of susceptibility to arrhythmia.

Because this is a primary electrical disorder, usually with no evidence of structural heart disease or LV dysfunction, the long-term prognosis is excellent if arrhythmia is controlled. Long-term treatment with β-blockers, permanent pacing, or left cervicothoracic sympathectomy has been shown to be effective. ICD implantation is recommended for patients in whom recurrent syncope, sustained ventricular arrhythmias, or sudden cardiac death occurs despite drug therapy. The ICD should be considered as primary therapy in certain patients, such as those in whom aborted sudden cardiac death is the initial presentation of the long-QT syndrome, when there is a strong family history of sudden cardiac death, or when compliance or intolerance to drugs is a concern.

Acquired long QT interval secondary to use of antiarrhythmic agents or antidepressant drugs, electrolyte abnormalities, myocardial ischemia, or significant bradycardia may result in ventricular tachycardia (particularly torsades de pointes, ie, twisting about the baseline into varying QRS morphology). Notably, many drugs that are in some settings effective for the treatment of ventricular arrhythmias prolong the QT interval. Prudence dictates that drug therapy that prolongs the QT interval beyond 500 ms be discontinued.

The management of **torsades de pointes** differs from that of other forms of ventricular tachycardia. Class I, Ic, or III antiarrhythmics, which prolong the QT interval, should be avoided—or withdrawn immediately if being used. Intravenous β-blockers may be effective, especially in the congenital form; intravenous magnesium should be given acutely. An effective approach is temporary ventricular or atrial pacing, which can both break and prevent the rhythm.

Goldenberg I et al. Sudden cardiac death without structural heart disease: update on the long QT and Brugada syndromes. Curr Cardiol Rep. 2005 Sep;7(5):349–56. [PMID: 16105490]
Monnig G et al. Implantable cardioverter-defibrillator therapy in patients with congenital long-QT syndrome: a long-term follow-up. Heart Rhythm. 2005 May;2(5):497–504. [PMID: 15840474]
Priori SG et al. Association of long QT syndrome loci and cardiac events among patients treated with beta-blockers. JAMA. 2004 Sep 15;292(11):1341–4. [PMID: 15367556]
Roden DM. Clinical practice. Long-QT syndrome. N Engl J Med. 2008 Jan 10;358(2):169–76. [PMID: 18184962]
Welde AA. Is there a role for implantable cardioverter defibrillators in long QT syndrome? J Cardiovasc Electrophysiol. 2002 Jan;13(1 Suppl):S110–3. [PMID: 11852886]

BRADYCARDIAS & CONDUCTION DISTURBANCES

SICK SINUS SYNDROME

 ESSENTIALS OF DIAGNOSIS

▶ Most patients are asymptomatic.

▶ More common in elderly population.

▶ May have recurrent supraventricular arrhythmia and bradyarrhythmia.

▶ Frequently seen in patients with concomitant atrial fibrillation.

▶ Often chronotropically incompetent.

▶ May be caused by drug therapy.

General Considerations

This imprecise diagnosis is applied to patients with sinus arrest, sinoatrial exit block (recognized by a pause equal to a multiple of the underlying PP interval or progressive shortening of the PP interval prior to a pause), or persistent sinus bradycardia. These rhythms are often caused or exacerbated by drug therapy (digitalis, calcium channel blockers, β-blockers, sympatholytic agents, antiarrhythmics), and agents that may be responsible should be withdrawn prior to making the diagnosis. Another presentation is of recurrent supraventricular tachycardias (paroxysmal reentry tachycardias, atrial flutter, and atrial fibrillation), associated with bradyarrhythmias ("tachy-brady syndrome"). The long pauses that often follow the termination of tachycardia cause the associated symptoms.

Sick sinus syndrome occurs most commonly in elderly patients. The pathologic changes are usually nonspecific, characterized by patchy fibrosis of the sinus node and cardiac conduction system. Sick sinus syndrome may be caused by other conditions, including sarcoidosis, amyloidosis, Chagas disease, and various cardiomyopathies. Coronary disease is an uncommon cause.

Clinical Findings

Most patients with ECG evidence of sick sinus syndrome are asymptomatic, but rare individuals may experience syncope, dizziness, confusion, palpitations, heart failure, or angina. Because these symptoms are either nonspecific or are due to other causes, it is essential that they be demonstrated to coincide temporally with arrhythmias. This may require prolonged ambulatory monitoring or the use of an event recorder.

Treatment

Most symptomatic patients will require permanent pacing (see AV block, below). Dual-chamber pacing is preferred because ventricular pacing is associated with a higher incidence of subsequent atrial fibrillation, and subsequent AV block occurs at a rate of 2% per year. In addition, resultant "pacemaker syndrome" can result from loss of AV synchrony. Treatment of associated tachyarrhythmias is often difficult without first instituting pacing, since digoxin and other antiarrhythmic agents may exacerbate the bradycardia. Unfortunately, symptomatic relief following pacing has not been consistent, largely because of inadequate documentation of the etiologic role of bradyarrhythmias in producing the symptom. Furthermore, many of these patients may have associated ventricular arrhythmias that may require treatment; however, carefully selected patients may become asymptomatic with permanent pacing alone.

Adan V et al. Diagnosis and treatment of sick sinus syndrome. Am Fam Physician. 2003 Apr 15;67(8):1725–32. [PMID: 12725451]
Brignole M. Sick sinus syndrome. Clin Geriatr Med. 2002 May; 18(2):211–27. [PMID: 12180244]
Dretzke J et al. Dual chamber versus single chamber ventricular pacemakers for sick sinus syndrome and atrioventricular block. Cochrane Database Syst Rev. 2004;(2):CD003710. [PMID: 15106214]
Sweeney MO et al; Search AV Extension and Managed Ventricular Pacing for Promoting Atrioventricular Conduction (SAVE PACe) Trial. Minimizing ventricular pacing to reduce atrial fibrillation in sinus node disease. N Engl J Med. 2007 Sep 6;357(10):1000–8. [PMID: 17804844]

AV BLOCK

AV block is categorized as first-degree (PR interval > 0.21 second with all atrial impulses conducted), second-degree (intermittent blocked beats), or third-degree (complete heart block, in which no supraventricular impulses are conducted to the ventricles).

Second-degree block is subclassified. In **Mobitz type I (Wenckebach)** AV block, the AV conduction time (PR interval) progressively lengthens, with the RR interval shortening, before the blocked beat; this phenomenon is almost always due to abnormal conduction within the AV node. In **Mobitz type II** AV block, there are intermittently nonconducted atrial beats not preceded by lengthening AV conduction. It is usually due to block within the His bundle system. The classification as Mobitz type I or Mobitz type II is only partially reliable because patients may appear to have both types on the surface ECG, and the site of origin of the 2:1 AV block cannot be predicted from the ECG. The width of the QRS complexes assists in determining whether the block is nodal or infranodal. When they are narrow, the block is usually nodal; when they are wide, the block is usually infranodal. Electrophysiologic studies may be necessary for accurate localization. Management of AV block in acute myocardial infarction has already been discussed. This section deals with patients in the nonischemic setting.

First-degree and **Mobitz type I block** may occur in normal individuals with heightened vagal tone. They may also occur as a drug effect (especially digitalis, calcium channel blockers, β-blockers, or other sympatholytic agents), often superimposed on organic disease. These disturbances also occur transiently or chronically due to ischemia, infarction, inflammatory processes, fibrosis, calcification, or infiltration. The prognosis is usually good, since reliable alternative pacemakers arise from the AV junction below the level of block if higher degrees of block occur.

Mobitz type II block is almost always due to organic disease involving the infranodal conduction system. In the event of progression to complete heart block, alternative pacemakers are not reliable. Thus, prophylactic ventricular pacing is required.

Complete (third-degree) heart block is a more advanced form of block often due to a lesion distal to the His bundle and associated with bilateral bundle branch block. The QRS is wide and the ventricular rate is slower, usually less than 50 beats/min. Transmission of atrial impulses through the AV node is completely blocked, and a ventricular pacemaker maintains a slow, regular ventricular rate, usually less than 45 beats/min. Exercise does not increase the rate. The first heart sound varies in intensity; wide pulse pressure, a changing systolic BP level, and cannon venous pulsations in the neck are also present. Patients may be asymptomatic or may complain of weakness or dyspnea if the rate is less than 35 beats/min; symptoms may occur at higher rates if the left ventricle cannot increase its stroke output. During periods of transition from partial to complete heart block, some patients have ventricular asystole that lasts several seconds to minutes. Syncope occurs abruptly.

Patients with episodic or chronic infranodal complete heart block require permanent pacing, and temporary pacing is indicated if implantation of a permanent pacemaker is delayed.

▶ **Treatment**

The indications for **permanent pacing** have been discussed: symptomatic bradyarrhythmias, asymptomatic Mobitz II AV block, or complete heart block. The versatility of pacemaker generator units has increased markedly, and dual-chamber multiple programmable units are being implanted with increasing frequency. A standardized nomenclature for pacemaker generators is used, usually consisting of four letters. The first letter refers to the chamber that is stimulated (A = atrium, V = ventricle, D = dual, for both). The second letter refers to the chamber in which sensing occurs (also A, V, or D). The third letter refers to the sensory mode (I = inhibition by a sensed impulse, T = triggering by a sensed impulse, D = dual modes of response). The fourth letter refers to the programmability or rate modulation capacity (usually P for programming for two functions, M for programming more than two, and R for rate modulation).

A pacemaker that senses and paces in both chambers is the most physiologic approach to pacing patients who remain in sinus rhythm. AV synchrony is particularly important in patients in whom atrial contraction produces a substantial increment in stroke volume and in those in whom sensing the atrial rate to provide rate-responsive ventricular pacing is useful. Dual-chamber pacing is most useful for individuals with LV systolic or—perhaps more importantly—diastolic dysfunction and for physically active individuals. In patients with single-chamber pacemakers, the lack of an atrial kick may lead to the so-called pacemaker syndrome, in which the patient experiences signs of low cardiac output while upright.

Pulse generators are also available that can increase their rate in response to motion or respiratory rate when the atrial rate is not an indication of the optimal heart rate. These are most useful in active individuals. Follow-up after pacemaker implantation, usually by telephonic monitoring, is essential. All pulse generators and lead systems have an early failure rate that is now below 1% and an expected battery life varying from 4 years to 10 years.

Bourke JP. Atrioventricular block and problems with atrioventricular conduction. Clin Geriatr Med. 2002 May;18(2):229–51. [PMID: 12180245]

Toff WD et al; United Kingdom Pacing and Cardiovascular Events Trial Investigators. Single-chamber versus dual-chamber pacing for high-grade atrioventricular block. N Engl J Med. 2005 Jul 14;353(2):145–55. [PMID: 16014884]

AV DISSOCIATION

When a ventricular pacemaker is firing at a rate faster than or close to the sinus rate (accelerated idioventricular rhythm, ventricular premature beats, or ventricular tachycardia), atrial impulses arriving at the AV node when it is refractory may not be conducted. This phenomenon is AV dissociation but does not necessarily indicate AV block. No treatment is required aside from management of the causative arrhythmia.

INTRAVENTRICULAR CONDUCTION DEFECTS

Intraventricular conduction defects, including bundle branch block, are common in individuals with otherwise normal hearts and in many disease processes, including ischemic heart disease, inflammatory disease, infiltrative disease, cardiomyopathy, and postcardiotomy. Below the AV node and bundle of His, the conduction system trifurcates into a right bundle and anterior and posterior fascicles of the left bundle. Conduction block in each of these fascicles can be recognized on the surface ECG. Although such conduction abnormalities are often seen in normal hearts, they are more commonly due to organic heart disease—either an isolated process of fibrosis and calcification or more generalized myocardial disease. Bifascicular block is present when two of these—right bundle, left anterior and posterior hemibundle—are involved. Trifascicular block is defined as right bundle branch block with alternating left hemiblock, alternating right and left bundle branch block, or bifascicular block with documented prolonged infranodal conduction (long His-ventricular interval).

The prognosis of intraventricular block is generally that of the underlying myocardial process. Patients with no apparent heart disease have an overall survival rate similar to that of matched controls. However, left bundle branch block—but not right—is associated with a higher risk of development of overt cardiac disease and cardiac mortality. Even in bifascicular block, the incidence of occult complete heart block or progression to it is low, and pacing is not usually warranted. In patients with symptoms (eg, syncope) consistent with heart block and intraventricular block, pacing should be reserved for those with documented concomitant complete heart block on monitoring or those with a very prolonged HV interval (> 90 ms) with no other cause for symptoms. Even in the latter group, prophylactic pacing has not improved the prognosis significantly, probably because of the high incidence of ventricular arrhythmias in the same population.

ACC/AHA/NASPE 2002 guideline update for implantation of cardiac pacemakers and antiarrhythmia devices: summary article. J Am Coll Cardiol. 2002 Nov 6;40(9):1703–19. [PMID: 12427427]

Faddis MN et al. Pacing interventions for falls and syncope in the elderly. Clin Geriatr Med. 2002 May;18(2):279–94. [PMID: 12180248]

Gregoratos G. Indications and recommendations for pacemaker therapy. Am Fam Physician. 2005 Apr 15;71(8):1563–70. [PMID: 15864898]

Vlietstra RE et al. Choice of pacemakers in patients aged 75 years and older: ventricular pacing mode vs. dual-chamber pacing mode. Am J Geriatr Cardiol. 2005 Jan–Feb;14(1):35–8. [PMID: 15654152]

SYNCOPE

ESSENTIALS OF DIAGNOSIS

► Transient loss of consciousness and postural tone from vasodepressor or cardiogenic causes.

► Prompt recovery without resuscitative measures.

► Common clinical problem.

► Accounts for 3% of all visits to the emergency department.

► General Considerations

Thirty percent of the adult population will experience at least one episode of syncope. It accounts for approximately 3% of emergency department visits. Syncope may be neurocardiogenic in origin, mediated by excessive vagal stimulation, or an imbalance between sympathetic and parasympathetic autonomic activity. With assumption of upright posture, there is venous pooling in the lower limbs. However, instead of the normal response, which consists of an increase in heart rate and vasoconstriction, a sympathetically mediated increase in myocardial contractility activates mechanoreceptors that trigger reflex bradycardia and vasodilation. A specific cause of syncope is identified in about 50% of cases during the initial evaluation. The prognosis is relatively favorable except when accompanying cardiac disease is present. In many patients with recurrent syncope or near syncope, arrhythmias are not the cause. This is particularly true when the patient has no evidence of associated heart disease by history, examination, standard ECG, or noninvasive testing.

Vasodepressor syncope may be due to excessive vagal tone or impaired reflex control of the peripheral circulation. The most frequent type of vasodepressor syncope is vasovagal hypotension or the "common faint," which is often initiated by a stressful, painful, or claustrophobic experience, especially in young women. Enhanced vagal tone with resulting hypotension is the cause of syncope in carotid sinus hypersensitivity and postmicturition syncope; vagal-induced sinus bradycardia, sinus arrest, and AV block are common accompaniments and may themselves be the cause of syncope.

Orthostatic (postural) hypotension is another common cause of vasodepressor syncope, especially in the elderly; in diabetics or other patients with autonomic neuropathy; in patients with blood loss or hypovolemia; and in patients taking vasodilators, diuretics, and adrenergic-blocking drugs. In addition, a syndrome of chronic idiopathic orthostatic hypotension exists primarily in older men. In most of these conditions, the normal vasoconstrictive response to assuming upright posture, which compensates for the abrupt decrease in venous return, is impaired.

Cardiogenic syncope can occur on a mechanical or arrhythmic basis. There is usually no prodrome; thus, injury secondary to falling is common. Mechanical problems that can cause syncope include aortic stenosis (where syncope may occur from autonomic reflex abnormalities or ventricular tachycardia), pulmonary stenosis, hypertrophic obstructive cardiomyopathy, congenital lesions associated with pulmonary hypertension or right-to-left shunting, and LA myxoma obstructing the mitral valve. Episodes are commonly exertional or postexertional. More commonly, cardiac syncope is due to disorders of automaticity (sick sinus syndrome), conduction disorders (AV block), or tachyarrhythmias (especially ventricular tachycardia and supraventricular tachycardia with rapid ventricular rate).

Clinical Findings

A. Symptoms and Signs

Syncope is characteristically abrupt in onset, often resulting in injury, transient (lasting for seconds to a few minutes), and followed by prompt recovery of full consciousness.

Vasodepressor premonitory symptoms, such as nausea, diaphoresis, tachycardia, and pallor, are usual in the "common faint." Episodes can be aborted by lying down or removing the inciting stimulus. In **orthostatic (postural) hypotension,** a greater than normal decline (20 mm Hg) in BP immediately upon arising from the supine to the standing position is observed, with or without tachycardia depending on the status of autonomic (baroreceptor) function.

B. Diagnostic Tests

The evaluation for syncope depends on findings from the history and physical examination (especially orthostatic BP evaluation, examination of carotid and other arteries, and cardiac examination).

1. ECG—The resting ECG may reveal arrhythmias, evidence of accessory pathways, prolonged QT interval, and other signs of heart disease (such as infarction or hypertrophy). If the history is consistent with syncope, ambulatory ECG monitoring is essential. This may need to be repeated several times, since yields increase with longer periods of monitoring, at least up to 3 days. Event recorder and transtelephone ECG monitoring may be helpful in patients with intermittent presyncopal episodes. Caution is required before attributing a patient's symptom to rhythm or conduction abnormalities observed during monitoring without concomitant symptoms. In many cases, the symptoms are due to a different arrhythmia or to noncardiac causes. For instance, dizziness or syncope in older patients may be unrelated to concomitantly observed bradycardia, sinus node abnormalities, and ventricular ectopy.

2. Autonomic testing—Orthostatic hypotension from autonomic function can be diagnosed with more certainty by observing BP and heart rate responses to Valsalva maneuver and by tilt testing.

Carotid sinus massage in patients who do not have carotid bruits or a history of cerebral vascular disease can precipitate sinus node arrest or AV block in patients with carotid sinus hypersensitivity. **Head-up tilt-table testing** can identify patients whose syncope may be on a vasovagal basis. In older patients, vasoconstrictor abnormalities and autonomic insufficiency are perhaps the most common causes of syncope. Thus, tilt testing should be done before proceeding to invasive studies unless clinical and ambulatory ECG evaluation suggests a cardiac abnormality. Although different testing protocols are used, passive tilting to at least 70 degrees for 10–40 minutes—in conjunction with isoproterenol infusion, if necessary—is typical. Syncope due to bradycardia, hypotension, or both will occur in approximately one-third of patients with recurrent syncope. Some studies have suggested that, at least with some of the more extreme protocols, false-positive responses may occur.

3. Electrophysiologic studies—Electrophysiologic studies to assess sinus node function and AV conduction and to induce supraventricular or ventricular tachycardia are indicated in patients with recurrent episodes, nondiagnostic ambulatory ECGs, and negative autonomic testing if vasomotor syncope is a consideration. Electrophysiologic studies reveal an arrhythmic cause in 20–50% of patients, depending on the study criteria, and are most often diagnostic when the patient has had multiple episodes and has identifiable cardiac abnormalities.

4. Exercise testing—When the symptoms are associated with exertion or stress, exercise testing may be helpful.

Treatment

Treatment consists largely of counseling patients to avoid predisposing situations. Paradoxically, β-blockers have been used in patients with altered autonomic function uncovered by head-up tilt testing but they have provided only minimal benefit. If symptomatic bradyarrhythmias or supraventricular tachyarrhythmias are detected, therapy can usually be initiated without additional diagnostic studies. Permanent pacing has little benefit except in patients with documented severe pauses and bradycardiac responses.

Volume expanders, such as fludrocortisone, or vasoconstrictors, such as midodrine, have also been tried but with minimal benefit. Selective serotonin reuptake inhibitors have shown some benefit in select patients.

See Recommendations for Resumption of Driving, below.

When to Admit

- Patients with recent or recurrent syncope are often monitored in the hospital.
- Those with less ominous symptoms may be monitored as outpatients.

Fitzpatrick AP et al. Tilt methodology in reflex syncope: emerging evidence. J Am Coll Cardiol. 2000 Jul;36(1):179–80. [PMID: 10898431]

Goldschlager N. Etiologic considerations in the patient with syncope and an apparently normal heart. Arch Intern Med. 2003 Jan 27;163(2):151–62. [PMID: 12546605]

Grubb BP. Neurocardiogenic syncope. N Engl J Med. 2005 Mar 10;352(10):1004–10. [PMID: 15758011]

Sheldon R. Tilt testing for syncope: a reappraisal. Curr Opin Cardiol. 2005 Jan;20(1):38–41. [PMID: 15596958]

RECOMMENDATIONS FOR RESUMPTION OF DRIVING

An important management problem in patients who have experienced syncope, symptomatic ventricular tachycardia, or aborted sudden death is to provide recommendations concerning automobile driving. According to a survey published in 1991, only eight states had specific laws dealing with this issue, whereas 42 had laws restricting driving in patients with seizure disorders. Patients with syncope or aborted sudden death thought to have been due to temporary factors (acute myocardial infarction, bradyarrhythmias subsequently treated with permanent pacing, drug effect, electrolyte imbalance) should be strongly advised after recovery not to drive for at least 1 month. Other patients with symptomatic ventricular tachycardia or aborted sudden death, whether treated pharmacologically, with anti-tachycardia devices, or with ablation therapy, should not drive for at least 6 months. Longer restrictions are warranted in these patients if spontaneous arrhythmias persist. The physician should comply with local regulations and consult local authorities concerning individual cases.

Akiyama T et al. Resumption of driving after life-threatening ventricular tachyarrhythmia. N Engl J Med. 2001 Aug 9;345 (6):391–7. [PMID: 11496849]

Baessler C et al; DAVID Investigators. Time to resumption of driving after implantation of an automatic defibrillator (from the Dual chamber and VVI Implantable Defibrillator [DAVID] trial). Am J Cardiol. 2005 Mar 1;95(5):665–6. [PMID: 15721116]

CONGESTIVE HEART FAILURE

 ### ESSENTIALS OF DIAGNOSIS

▶ **LV failure:** Exertional dyspnea, cough, fatigue, orthopnea, paroxysmal nocturnal dyspnea, cardiac enlargement, rales, gallop rhythm, and pulmonary venous congestion.

▶ **RV failure:** Elevated venous pressure, hepatomegaly, dependent edema; usually due to LV failure.

▶ Assessment of LV function is a crucial part of diagnosis and management.

General Considerations

Heart failure is a common syndrome that is increasing in incidence and prevalence. Approximately 5 million patients in the United States have heart failure, and there are nearly 500,000 new cases each year. It is primarily a disease of aging, with over 75% of existing and new cases occurring in individuals over 65 years of age. The prevalence of heart failure rises from < 1% in individuals below 60 years to nearly 10% in those over 80 years of age.

Heart failure may be right sided or left sided (or both). Patients with **left heart failure** have symptoms of low cardiac output and elevated pulmonary venous pressure; dyspnea is the predominant feature. Signs of fluid retention predominate in **right heart failure**. Most patients exhibit symptoms or signs of both right- and left-sided failure, and LV dysfunction is the primary cause of RV failure. Although this section primarily concerns cardiac failure due to systolic LV dysfunction, patients with heart failure with preserved systolic dysfunction, in large part due to **diastolic dysfunction,** experience many of the same symptoms and may be difficult to distinguish clinically.

Diastolic pressures are elevated even though diastolic volumes are normal or small. These pressures are transmitted to the pulmonary and systemic venous systems, resulting in dyspnea and edema. The most frequent cause of diastolic cardiac dysfunction is LVH, commonly resulting from hypertension, but conditions such as hypertrophic or restrictive cardiomyopathy, diabetes, and pericardial disease can produce the same clinical picture. In developed countries, CAD with resulting myocardial infarction and loss of functioning myocardium (ischemic cardiomyopathy) is the most common cause of heart failure. Systemic hypertension remains an important cause of CHF and, even more commonly in the United States, an exacerbating factor in patients with cardiac dysfunction due to other causes such as CAD. Several processes may present with dilated or congestive cardiomyopathy, which is characterized by LV or biventricular dilation and generalized systolic dysfunction. These are discussed elsewhere in this chapter, but the most common are alcoholic cardiomyopathy, viral myocarditis (including infections by HIV), and dilated cardiomyopathies with no obvious underlying cause (idiopathic cardiomyopathy). Rare causes of dilated cardiomyopathy include infiltrative diseases (hemochromatosis, sarcoidosis, amyloidosis, etc), other infectious agents, metabolic disorders, cardiotoxins, and drug toxicity. Valvular heart diseases—particularly degenerative aortic stenosis and chronic aortic or mitral regurgitation—are not infrequent causes of heart failure.

Heart failure is often preventable by early detection of patients at risk and early intervention. The importance of these approaches is emphasized by guidelines that have incorporated a classification of heart failure that includes four stages. Stage A includes patients at risk for developing heart failure (such as patients with hypertension or CAD without current or previous symptoms or identifiable structural abnormalities of the myocardium). In the majority of these patients, development of heart failure can be prevented with interventions such as the aggressive treatment of hypertension, modification of coronary risk factors, and reduction of excessive alcohol intake (Figure 10–1). Stage B includes patients who have structural heart disease but no current or previously recognized symptoms of heart failure. Examples include patients with previous myocardial infarction, other causes of reduced systolic function, LVH, or asymptomatic valvular disease. Both ACE inhibitors and β-blockers prevent heart failure in the first two of these conditions, and more aggressive treatment of hypertension and early surgical intervention are effective in the latter two. Stages C and D include patients with clinical heart failure and the relatively small group of patients that has become refractory to the usual therapies, respectively. These are discussed below.

Clinical Findings

A. Symptoms

The most common complaint of patients with **left heart failure** is shortness of breath, chiefly exertional dyspnea at first and then progressing to orthopnea, paroxysmal noc-

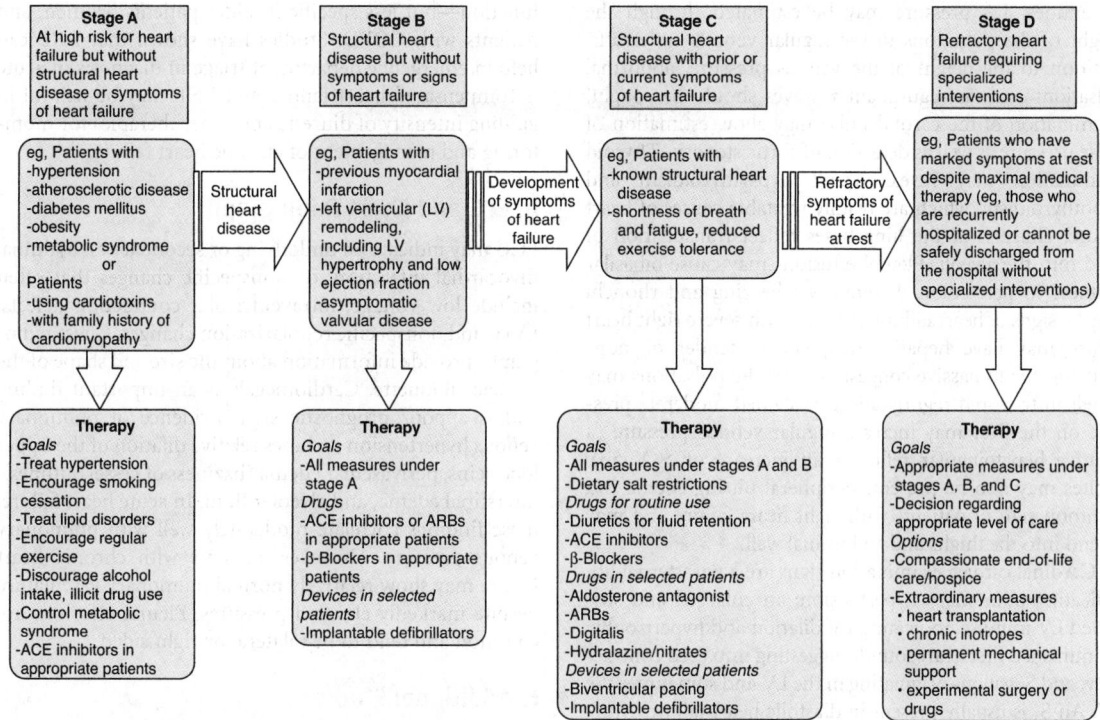

| **Stage A**
At high risk for heart failure but without structural heart disease or symptoms of heart failure | | **Stage B**
Structural heart disease but without symptoms or signs of heart failure | | **Stage C**
Structural heart disease with prior or current symptoms of heart failure | | **Stage D**
Refractory heart failure requiring specialized interventions |

eg, Patients with
-hypertension
-atherosclerotic disease
-diabetes mellitus
-obesity
-metabolic syndrome
or
Patients
-using cardiotoxins
-with family history of cardiomyopathy

→ Structural heart disease →

eg, Patients with
-previous myocardial infarction
-left ventricular (LV) remodeling, including LV hypertrophy and low ejection fraction
-asymptomatic valvular disease

→ Development of symptoms of heart failure →

eg, Patients with
-known structural heart disease
-shortness of breath and fatigue, reduced exercise tolerance

→ Refractory symptoms of heart failure at rest →

eg, Patients who have marked symptoms at rest despite maximal medical therapy (eg, those who are recurrently hospitalized or cannot be safely discharged from the hospital without specialized interventions)

Therapy
Goals
-Treat hypertension
-Encourage smoking cessation
-Treat lipid disorders
-Encourage regular exercise
-Discourage alcohol intake, illicit drug use
-Control metabolic syndrome
-ACE inhibitors in appropriate patients

Therapy
Goals
-All measures under stage A
Drugs
-ACE inhibitors or ARBs in appropriate patients
-β-Blockers in appropriate patients
Devices in selected patients
-Implantable defibrillators

Therapy
Goals
-All measures under stages A and B
-Dietary salt restrictions
Drugs for routine use
-Diuretics for fluid retention
-ACE inhibitors
-β-Blockers
Drugs in selected patients
-Aldosterone antagonist
-ARBs
-Digitalis
-Hydralazine/nitrates
Devices in selected patients
-Biventricular pacing
-Implantable defibrillators

Therapy
Goals
-Appropriate measures under stages A, B, and C
-Decision regarding appropriate level of care
Options
-Compassionate end-of-life care/hospice
-Extraordinary measures
 • heart transplantation
 • chronic inotropes
 • permanent mechanical support
 • experimental surgery or drugs

▲ **Figure 10–1.** Stages in the evolution of heart failure and recommended therapy by stage. ACE, angiotensin-converting enzyme; ARBs, angiotensin receptor blockers. (Reproduced, with permission, from Hunt SA et al. ACC/AHA 2005 Guidelines Update for the evaluation and management of chronic heart failure in the adult: A report of the American College of Cardiology/American Heart Association Task Force on Practice Guidelines [Writing Committee to Update the 2001 Guidelines for the Evaluation and Management of Heart Failure]. ACC/AHA 2005 Guidelines Update for the diagnosis and management of chronic heart failure in the adult. ©2005, American Heart, Inc.)

turnal dyspnea, and rest dyspnea. A more subtle and often overlooked symptom of heart failure is a chronic nonproductive cough, which is often worse in the recumbent position. Nocturia due to excretion of fluid retained during the day and increased renal perfusion in the recumbent position is a common nonspecific symptom of heart failure. Patients also complain of fatigue and exercise intolerance. These symptoms correlate poorly with the degree of cardiac dysfunction. Patients with **right heart failure** have predominate signs of fluid retention, with the patient exhibiting edema, hepatic congestion and, on occasion, loss of appetite and nausea due to edema of the gut or impaired gastrointestinal perfusion and ascites. Surprisingly, some individuals with severe LV dysfunction will display few signs of left heart failure and appear to have isolated right heart failure. Indeed, they may be clinically indistinguishable from patients with cor pulmonale, who have right heart failure secondary to pulmonary disease.

Patients with acute heart failure from myocardial infarction, myocarditis, and acute valvular regurgitation due to endocarditis or other conditions usually present with pulmonary edema. Patients with episodic symptoms may be having LV dysfunction due to intermittent ischemia. Patients may also present with acute exacerbations of chronic, stable heart failure. Exacerbations are usually caused by alterations in therapy (or patient non-compliance), excessive salt and fluid intake, arrhythmias, excessive activity, pulmonary emboli, intercurrent infection, or progression of the underlying disease.

Patients with heart failure are often categorized by the NYHA classification as class I (asymptomatic), class II (symptomatic with mild activity), class III (symptomatic with moderate activity), or class IV (symptomatic at rest). However, this classification has major limitations in that patient reports are highly subjective and in that symptoms vary from day to day. In any case, the classification is insufficiently sensitive to be useful in predicting outcomes or assessing the results of treatment.

B. Signs

Many patients with heart failure, including some with severe symptoms, appear comfortable at rest. Others will be dyspneic during conversation or minor activity, and those with long-standing severe heart failure may appear cachectic or cyanotic. The vital signs may be normal, but tachycardia, hypotension, and reduced pulse pressure may be present. Patients often show signs of increased sympathetic nervous system activity, including cold extremities and diaphoresis. Important peripheral signs of heart failure can be detected by examination of the neck, the lungs, the abdomen, and the extremities. RA pressure may be estimated through the height of the pulsations in the jugular venous system. In addition to the height of the venous pressure, abnormal pulsations such as regurgitant *v* waves should be sought. Examination of the carotid pulse may allow estimation of pulse pressure as well as detection of aortic stenosis. Thyroid examination may reveal occult hyperthyroidism and hypothyroidism, which are readily treatable causes of heart failure. Crackles at the lung bases reflect transudation of fluid into the alveoli. Pleural effusions may cause bibasilar dullness to percussion. Expiratory wheezing and rhonchi may be signs of heart failure. Patients with severe right heart failure may have hepatic enlargement—tender or non-tender—due to passive congestion. Systolic pulsations may be felt in tricuspid regurgitation. Sustained moderate pressure on the liver may increase jugular venous pressure (a positive hepatojugular reflux is an increase of > 1 cm). Ascites may also be present. Peripheral pitting edema is a common sign in patients with right heart failure and may extend into the thighs and abdominal wall.

Cardinal cardiac examination signs are a parasternal lift, indicating pulmonary hypertension; an enlarged and sustained LV impulse, indicating LV dilation and hypertrophy; a diminished first heart sound, suggesting impaired contractility; and S_3 gallops originating in the LV and sometimes the RV. An S_4 is usually present in diastolic heart failure. Murmurs should be sought to exclude primary valvular disease; secondary mitral regurgitation and tricuspid regurgitation murmurs are common in patients with dilated ventricles. In chronic heart failure, many of the expected signs of heart failure may be absent despite markedly abnormal cardiac function and hemodynamic measurements.

C. Laboratory Findings

A blood count may reveal anemia, which is associated with poor prognosis in chronic heart failure through poorly understood mechanisms. Renal function tests can determine whether cardiac failure is associated with prerenal azotemia. Chronic kidney disease is another poor prognostic factor in heart failure and may limit certain treatment options. Serum electrolytes may disclose hypokalemia, which increases the risk of arrhythmias; hyperkalemia, which may limit the use of inhibitors of the renin–angiotensin system; or hyponatremia, an indicator of marked activation of the renin–angiotensin system and a poor prognostic sign. Thyroid function should be assessed to detect occult thyrotoxicosis or myxedema and iron studies test should be checked to test for hemochromatosis. In unexplained cases, appropriate biopsies may lead to a diagnosis of amyloidosis. Myocardial biopsy may exclude specific causes of dilated cardiomyopathy but rarely reveals specific reversible diagnoses.

Serum BNP is a powerful prognostic marker that adds to clinical assessment in differentiating dyspnea due to heart failure from noncardiac causes. Two markers—BNP and N-terminal pro-BNP—provide similar diagnostic and prognostic information. BNP is expressed primarily in the ventricles and is elevated when ventricular filling pressures are high. It is quite sensitive in patients with symptomatic heart failure—whether due to systolic or to diastolic dys-

function—but less specific in older patients, women, and patients with COPD. Studies have shown that BNP can help in emergency department triage in diagnosis of acute decompensated heart failure and BNP may be helpful in guiding intensity of diuretic and other therapies for monitoring and management of chronic heart failure.

D. ECG and Chest Radiography

ECG may indicate an underlying or secondary arrhythmia, myocardial infarction, or nonspecific changes that often include low voltage, intraventricular conduction defects, LVH, and nonspecific repolarization changes. Chest radiographs provide information about the size and shape of the cardiac silhouette. Cardiomegaly is an important finding and is a poor prognostic sign. Evidence of pulmonary venous hypertension includes relative dilation of the upper lobe veins, perivascular edema (haziness of vessel outlines), interstitial edema, and alveolar fluid. In acute heart failure, these findings correlate moderately well with pulmonary venous pressure. However, patients with chronic heart failure may show relatively normal pulmonary vasculature despite markedly elevated pressures. Pleural effusions are common and tend to be bilateral or right sided.

E. Additional Studies

Many studies have indicated that the clinical diagnosis of systolic myocardial dysfunction is often inaccurate. The primary confounding conditions are diastolic dysfunction of the heart with decreased relaxation and filling of the LV (particularly in hypertension and in hypertrophic states) and pulmonary disease. Because patients with heart failure usually have significant resting ECG abnormalities, stress imaging procedures such as perfusion scintigraphy or dobutamine echocardiography are often indicated.

The most useful test is the echocardiogram. This will reveal the size and function of both ventricles and of the atria. It will also allow detection of pericardial effusion, valvular abnormalities, intracardiac shunts, and segmental wall motion abnormalities suggestive of old myocardial infarction as opposed to more generalized forms of dilated cardiomyopathy.

Radionuclide angiography measures LV EF and permits analysis of regional wall motion. This test is especially useful when echocardiography is technically suboptimal, such as in patients with severe pulmonary disease. When myocardial ischemia is suspected as a cause of LV dysfunction, stress testing should be performed.

F. Cardiac Catheterization

In most patients with heart failure, clinical examination and noninvasive tests can determine LV size and function and valve function well enough to confirm the diagnosis. Left heart catheterization may be helpful to define the presence and extent of CAD, although CT angiography may also be appropriate, especially when the likelihood of coronary disease is low. Evaluation for coronary disease is particularly important when LV dysfunction may be partially reversible by revascularization. The combination of angina or noninvasive evidence of significant myocardial ischemia with symptomatic heart failure is often an indication for coronary angiography if the patient is a potential candidate for revascularization. Right heart catheterization may be useful to select and monitor therapy in patients refractory to standard therapy.

Drazner MH et al. Prognostic importance of elevated jugular venous pressure and a third heart sound in patients with heart failure. N Engl J Med. 2001 Aug 23;345(8):574–81. [PMID: 11529211]

Jourdain P et al. Plasma brain natriuretic peptide-guided therapy to improve outcome in heart failure: the STARS-BNP Multicenter Study. J Am Coll Cardiol. 2007 Apr 24;49(16):1733–9. [PMID: 17448376]

Maisel AS et al. Rapid measurement of B-type natriuretic peptide in the emergency diagnosis of heart failure. N Engl J Med. 2002 Jul 18;347(3):161–7. [PMID: 12124404]

Treatment

Although diuretics are often useful in patients with **right heart failure**, the other therapies discussed in this section (digitalis, vasodilators, inotropic agents) may be inappropriate.

A. Correction of Reversible Causes

The major reversible causes of chronic heart failure include valvular lesions, myocardial ischemia, uncontrolled hypertension, arrhythmias (especially persistent tachycardias), alcohol- or drug-induced myocardial depression, intracardiac shunts, and high-output states. Calcium channel blockers, antiarrhythmic drugs, and nonsteroidal anti-inflammatory agents are important causes of worsening heart failure. Some metabolic and infiltrative cardiomyopathies may be partially reversible, or their progression may be slowed; these include hemochromatosis, sarcoidosis, and amyloidosis. Reversible causes of diastolic dysfunction include pericardial disease and LVH due to hypertension. Once it is established that there is no reversible component, the measures outlined below are appropriate.

B. Pharmacologic

See also the following section on Acute Heart Failure & Pulmonary Edema.

1. Diuretic therapy—Diuretics are the most effective means of providing symptomatic relief to patients with moderate to severe CHF. Few patients with symptoms or signs of fluid retention can be optimally managed without a diuretic. However, excessive diuresis can lead to electrolyte imbalance and neurohormonal activation. **A combination of a diuretic and an ACE inhibitor should be the initial treatment in most symptomatic patients.**

When fluid retention is mild, thiazide diuretics or a similar type of agent (hydrochlorothiazide, 25–100 mg; metolazone, 2.5–5 mg; chlorthalidone, 25–50 mg; etc) may be sufficient. Thiazide or related diuretics often provide better control of hypertension than short-acting loop agents. The thiazides are generally ineffective when the glomerular filtration rate falls below 30–40 mL/min, a not infrequent occurrence in patients with severe heart failure. Metolazone

maintains its efficacy down to a glomerular filtration rate of approximately 20–30 mL/min. Adverse reactions include hypokalemia and intravascular volume depletion with resulting prerenal azotemia, skin rashes, neutropenia and thrombocytopenia, hyperglycemia, hyperuricemia, and hepatic dysfunction.

Patients with more severe heart failure should be treated with one of the loop diuretics. These include furosemide (20–320 mg daily), bumetanide (1–8 mg daily), and torsemide (20–200 mg daily). These agents have a rapid onset and a relatively short duration of action. In patients with preserved kidney function, two or more doses are preferable to a single larger dose. In acute situations or when gastrointestinal absorption is in doubt, they should be given intravenously. They are active even in severe kidney disease, but larger doses (up to 500 mg of furosemide or equivalent) may be required. The major adverse reactions include intravascular volume depletion, prerenal azotemia, and hypotension. Hypokalemia, particularly with accompanying digitalis therapy, is a major problem. Less common side effects include skin rashes, gastrointestinal distress, and ototoxicity (the latter more common with ethacrynic acid and possibly less common with bumetanide).

The potassium-sparing agents spironolactone, triamterene, and amiloride are often useful in combination with the loop diuretics and thiazides. Triamterene and amiloride act on the distal tubule to reduce potassium secretion. Their diuretic potency is only mild and not adequate for most patients with heart failure, but they may minimize the hypokalemia induced by more potent agents. Side effects include hyperkalemia, gastrointestinal symptoms, and kidney dysfunction. Spironolactone is a specific inhibitor of aldosterone, which is often increased in CHF and has important effects beyond potassium retention (see below). Its onset of action is slower than the other potassium-sparing agents, and its side effects include gynecomastia. Combinations of potassium supplements or ACE inhibitors and potassium-sparing drugs can produce hyperkalemia but have been used with success in patients with persistent hypokalemia.

Patients with refractory edema may respond to combinations of a loop diuretic and thiazide-like agents. Metolazone, because of its maintained activity with chronic kidney disease, is the most useful agent for such a combination. Extreme caution must be observed with this approach, since massive diuresis and electrolyte imbalances often occur; 2.5 mg of metolazone should be added to the previous dosage of loop diuretic. In many cases this is necessary only once or twice a week, but dosages up to 10 mg daily have been used in some patients.

2. Inhibitors of the renin–angiotensin–aldosterone system—Inhibition of renin–angiotensin–aldosterone system with ACE inhibitors should be considered part of the initial therapy of this syndrome based on their life-saving benefits.

A. ACE INHIBITORS—Many ACE inhibitors are available, and at least seven have been shown to be effective for the treatment of heart failure or the related indication of postinfarction LV dysfunction (see Table 11–8). ACE inhibitors reduce mortality by approximately 20% in patients with symptomatic heart failure and have been shown also to prevent hospitalizations, increase exercise tolerance, and reduce symptoms in these patients. As a result, ACE inhibitors should be part of first-line treatment of patients with symptomatic LV systolic dysfunction (EF < 40%), usually in combination with a diuretic. They are also indicated for the management of patients with reduced EFs without symptoms because they prevent the progression to clinical heart failure.

Because ACE inhibitors may induce significant hypotension, particularly following the initial doses, they must be started with caution. Hypotension is most prominent in patients with already low BPs (systolic pressure < 100 mm Hg), hypovolemia, prerenal azotemia (especially if it is diuretic induced), and hyponatremia (an indicator of activation of the renin–angiotensin system). These patients should generally be started at low dosages (captopril 6.25 mg three times daily, enalapril 2.5 mg daily, or the equivalent), but other patients may be started at twice these dosages. Within several days (for those with the markers of higher risk) or at most 2 weeks, patients should be questioned about symptoms of hypotension, and both kidney function and K^+ levels should be monitored.

ACE inhibitors should be titrated to the dosages proved effective in clinical trials (captopril 50 mg three times daily, enalapril 10 mg twice daily, lisinopril 20 mg daily, or the equivalent) over a period of 1–3 months. Most patients will tolerate these doses. Asymptomatic hypotension is not a contraindication to up-titrating or continuing ACE inhibitors. Some patients exhibit increases in serum creatinine or K^+, but they do not require discontinuation if the levels stabilize—even at values as high as 3 mg/dL and 5.5 mEq/L, respectively. Kidney dysfunction is more frequent in diabetics, older patients, and those with low systolic pressures, and these groups should be monitored more closely. The most common side effects of ACE inhibitors in heart failure patients are dizziness (often not related to the level of BP) and cough, though the latter is often due as much to heart failure or intercurrent pulmonary conditions as to the ACE inhibitor.

B. ANGIOTENSIN II RECEPTOR BLOCKERS—Another approach to inhibiting the renin–angiotensin–aldosterone system is the use of specific ARBs (see Table 11–8), which will block or decrease most of the effects of the system. In addition, because there are alternative pathways of angiotensin II production in many tissues, the receptor blockers may provide more complete system blockade.

However, these agents do not share the effects of ACE inhibitors on other potentially important pathways that produce increases in bradykinin, prostaglandins, and nitric oxide in the heart, blood vessels, and other tissues. The Valsartan in Heart Failure Trial (Val-HeFT) examined the efficacy of adding valsartan (titrated to a dose of 160 mg twice a day) to ACE inhibitor therapy. While the addition of valsartan did not reduce mortality, the composite of death or hospitalization for heart failure was significantly reduced. The CHARM trial randomized 7601 patients with chronic heart failure with or without LV systolic dysfunc-

tion and with or without background ACE inhibitor therapy to candesartan (titrated to 32 mg a day) or placebo. Among patients with an LV EF of < 40%, there was an 18% reduction in cardiovascular death or heart failure hospitalization and a statistically significant 12% reduction in all-cause mortality. The benefits were similar among patients on ACE inhibitors, including among patients on full-dose ACE inhibitors. Thus, ARBs, specifically candesartan or valsartan, provide important benefits as an alternative to, and in addition to, ACE inhibitors in chronic heart failure with reduced LV EF. A large trial of patients with chronic heart failure and preserved LV EF found no benefit from the ARB irbesartan.

C. SPIRONOLACTONE—There is evidence that aldosterone mediates some of the major effects of renin–angiotensin–aldosterone system activation, such as myocardial remodeling and fibrosis, as well as sodium retention and potassium loss at the distal tubules. Thus, spironolactone should be considered as a neurohormonal antagonist rather than narrowly as a potassium-sparing diuretic. The RALES trial compared spironolactone 25 mg daily with placebo in patients with advanced heart failure (current or recent class IV) already receiving ACE inhibitors and diuretics and showed a 29% reduction in mortality as well as similar decreases in other clinical end points. Hyperkalemia was uncommon in this severe heart failure clinical trial population, which was maintained on high doses of diuretic, but hyperkalemia with spironolactone appears to be common in general practice. Potassium levels should be monitored closely during initiation of spironolactone (after 1 and 4 weeks of therapy), particularly for patients with even mild degrees of kidney injury, and in patients receiving ACE inhibitors. Neither the efficacy nor the safety of spironolactone has been established in the large majority of patients with mild or moderate heart failure who are taking low doses of diuretics, though this agent may be considered in patients who require potassium supplementation. It is not known whether the more selective aldosterone inhibitor, eplerenone, is effective in improving outcome in chronic heart failure.

3. β-Blockers—β-Blockers are part of the foundation of care of chronic heart failure based on their life-saving benefits. The mechanism of this benefit remains unclear, but it is likely that chronic elevations of catecholamines and sympathetic nervous system activity cause progressive myocardial damage, leading to worsening LV function and dilation. The primary evidence for this hypothesis is that over a period of 3–6 months, β-blockers produce consistent substantial rises in EF (averaging 10% absolute increase) and reductions in LV size and mass.

Clinical trial results have been reported in nearly 14,000 patients (ranging from asymptomatic post-myocardial infarction LV dysfunction to severe heart failure with LV EFs < 35–40%) receiving ACE inhibitors and diuretics randomized to β-blockers or placebo. Carvedilol, a nonselective β_1- and β_2-receptor blocker with additional weak α-blocking activity, was the first β-blocker approved for heart failure in the United States after showing a reduction in death and hospitalizations in four smaller studies with a total of nearly 1100 patients. Subsequently, trials with two β_1-selective agents, bisoprolol (CIBIS II, with 2647 patients) and sustained-release metoprolol succinate (MERIT, with nearly 4000 patients), showed 35% reductions in mortality as well as fewer hospitalizations. A trial using carvedilol in 2200 patients with severe (NYHA class III/IV) heart failure was terminated ahead of schedule because of a 35% reduction in mortality. The SENIORS trial of 2135 patients found that nebivolol was effective in elderly patients (70 years and older) with chronic heart failure. In these trials, there were reductions in sudden deaths and deaths from worsening heart failure, and benefits were seen in patients with underlying coronary disease and those with primary cardiomyopathies. In all these studies, the β-blockers were generally well tolerated, with similar numbers of withdrawals in the active and placebo groups. This has led to a strong recommendation that *stable* patients (defined as having no recent deterioration or evidence of volume overload) with mild, moderate, and even severe heart failure should be treated with a β-blocker unless there is a noncardiac contraindication. In the COPERNICUS trial, carvedilol was both well tolerated and highly effective in reducing both mortality and heart failure hospitalizations in a group of patients with severe (NYHA class III or IV) symptoms, but care was taken to ensure that they were free of fluid retention at the time of initiation. In this study, one death was prevented for every 13 patients treated for 1 year—as dramatic an effect as has been seen with a pharmacologic therapy in the history of cardiovascular medicine. One trial comparing carvedilol and (short-acting) metoprolol tartrate (COMET) found significant reductions in all-cause mortality and cardiovascular mortality with carvedilol. Thus, patients with chronic heart failure should be treated with extended-release metoprolol, bisoprolol, or carvedilol, but not short-acting metoprolol.

Because even apparently stable patients may deteriorate when β-blockers are initiated, initiation must be done gradually and with great care. Carvedilol is initiated at a dosage of 3.125 mg twice daily and may be increased to 6.25, 12.5, and 25 mg twice daily at intervals of approximately 2 weeks. The protocols for sustained-release metoprolol use were started at 12.5 or 25 mg daily and doubled at intervals of 2 weeks to a target dose of 200 mg daily (using the Toprol XL sustained-release preparation). Bisoprolol was administered at a dosage of 1.25, 2.5, 3.75, 5, 7.5, and 10 mg daily, with increments at 1- to 4-week intervals. More gradual up-titration is often more convenient and may be better tolerated.

Patients should be instructed to monitor their weights at home as an indicator of fluid retention and to report any increase or change in symptoms immediately. Before each dose increase, the patient should be seen and examined to ensure that there has not been fluid retention or worsening of symptoms. If heart failure worsens, this can usually be managed by increasing diuretic doses and delaying further increases in β-blocker doses, though downward adjustments or discontinuation is sometimes required. Carvedilol, because of its α-blocking activity, may cause dizziness or hypotension. This can usually be managed by reducing the doses of other vasodilators and by slowing the pace of dose increases.

4. Digitalis glycosides—Although the digitalis glycosides were once the mainstay of treatment of CHF, their use in patients who are in sinus rhythm has declined because they lack the benefits of the neurohormonal antagonists on prognosis and because safety concerns persist. However, their efficacy in reducing the symptoms of heart failure has been established in at least four multicenter trials that have demonstrated that digoxin withdrawal is associated with worsening symptoms and signs of heart failure, more frequent hospitalizations for decompensation, and reduced exercise tolerance. This was also seen in the 6800-patient Digitalis Investigators Group (DIG) trial, though that study found no benefit (or harm) with regard to survival. A reduction in deaths due to progressive heart failure was balanced by an increase in deaths due to ischemic and arrhythmic events. Based on these results, digoxin should be used for patients who remain symptomatic when taking diuretics and ACE inhibitors as well as for patients with heart failure who are in atrial fibrillation and require rate control.

Digoxin, the only widely used digitalis preparation, has a half-life of 24–36 hours and is eliminated almost entirely by the kidneys. The oral maintenance dose may range from 0.125 mg three times weekly to 0.5 mg daily. It is lower in patients with kidney dysfunction, in older patients, and in those with smaller lean body mass. Although a loading dose of 0.75–1.25 mg (depending primarily on lean body size) over 24–48 hours may be given if an early effect is desired, in most patients with chronic heart failure it is sufficient to begin with the expected maintenance dose (usually 0.125–0.25 mg daily). Amiodarone, quinidine, propafenone, and verapamil are among the drugs that may increase digoxin levels up to 100%. It is prudent to measure a blood level after 7–14 days (and at least 6 hours after the last dose was administered). Most of the positive inotropic effect is apparent with serum digoxin levels between 0.7 ng/mL and 1.2 ng/mL, and levels above this range may be associated with a higher risk of arrhythmias and lower survival rates, though clinically evident toxicity is rare with levels below 1.8 ng/mL. Once an appropriate maintenance dose is established, subsequent levels are usually not indicated unless there is a change in kidney function or medications that affects digoxin levels or a significant deterioration in cardiac status that may be associated with reduced clearance. Digoxin may induce ventricular arrhythmias, especially when hypokalemia or myocardial ischemia is present.

Digoxin toxicity has become less frequent as there has been a better appreciation of its pharmacology, but the therapeutic-to-toxic ratio is quite narrow. Symptoms of digitalis toxicity include anorexia, nausea, headache, blurring or yellowing of vision, and disorientation. Cardiac toxicity may take the form of AV conduction or sinus node depression; junctional, atrial, or ventricular premature beats or tachycardias; or ventricular fibrillation. Potassium administration (following serum potassium measurement, since severe toxicity may be associated with hyperkalemia) is usually indicated for the tachyarrhythmias even when levels are in the normal range, but may worsen conduction disturbances. Lidocaine or phenytoin may be useful for ventricular arrhythmias, as is overdrive pacing, but quinidine, amiodarone, and propafenone should be avoided because they will increase digoxin levels. Electrical cardioversion should be avoided if possible, as it may cause intractable ventricular fibrillation or cardiac standstill. Pacing is indicated for third-degree AV block (complete heart block) and symptomatic or severe block (heart rate < 40 beats/min) if they persist after treatment with atropine. Digoxin immune fab (ovine) is available for life-threatening toxicity or large overdoses, but it should be remembered that its half-life is shorter than that of digoxin and so repeat administration may be required.

5. Vasodilators—Because most patients with moderate to severe heart failure have both elevated preload and reduced cardiac output, the maximum benefit of vasodilator therapy can be achieved by an agent or combination of agents with both actions. Many patients with heart failure have mitral or tricuspid regurgitation; agents that reduce resistance to ventricular outflow tend to redirect regurgitant flow in a forward direction.

Although vasodilators that are also neurohumoral antagonists—specifically, the ACE inhibitors—improve prognosis, such a benefit is less clear with the direct-acting vasodilators. The combination of hydralazine and isosorbide dinitrate has improved survival, but to a lesser extent than ACE inhibitors. The A-HeFT trial studied hydralazine (75 mg) and isosorbide dinitrate (40 mg) three times a day in 1050 African Americans with NYHA class III or IV chronic heart failure, most of whom were treated with ACE inhibitors and β-blockers. The primary endpoint was a clinical composite. The trial was stopped early because of a significant 43% reduction in all-cause mortality with hydralazine and nitrates, although the relatively small sample size limits the confidence in the results. Whether the benefits of this approach are limited to African Americans, who may have a less active renin–angiotensin system is not known, but it is appropriate to use this combination in addition to other effective therapies in African Americans with severe heart failure.

See section on Acute Myocardial Infarction earlier in this chapter for a discussion on the intravenous vasodilating drugs and their dosages.

A. NITRATES—Intravenous vasodilators (sodium nitroprusside or nitroglycerin) are used primarily for acute or severely decompensated chronic heart failure, especially when accompanied by hypertension or myocardial ischemia. If neither of the latter is present, therapy is best initiated and adjusted based on hemodynamic measurements. The starting dosage for nitroglycerin is generally about 10 mcg/min, which is titrated upward by 10–20 mcg/min (to a maximum of 200 mcg/min) until mean arterial pressure drops by 10%. Hypotension (BP < 100 mm Hg systolic) should be avoided. For sodium nitroprusside, the starting dosage is 0.3–0.5 mcg/kg/min with upward titration to a maximum dose of 10 mcg/kg/min.

Isosorbide dinitrate, 20–80 mg orally three times daily, has proved effective in several small studies. Nitroglycerin ointment, 12.5–50 mg (1–4 inches) every 6–8 hours, appears to be equally effective although somewhat inconvenient for long-term therapy. The nitrates are moderately effective in relieving shortness of breath, especially in patients with mild to moderate symptoms, but less successful—probably because they have little effect on cardiac output—in advanced heart failure. Nitrate therapy is generally well tolerated, but headaches and hypotension may limit the dose of all agents. The development of tolerance to long-term nitrate therapy occurs. This is minimized by intermittent therapy, especially if a daily 8- to 12-hour nitrate-free interval is used, but probably develops to some extent in most patients receiving these agents. Transdermal nitroglycerin patches have no sustained effect in patients with heart failure and should not be used for this indication.

B. NESIRITIDE—This agent, a recombinant form of human brain natriuretic peptide, is a potent vasodilator that reduces ventricular filling pressures and improves cardiac output. Its hemodynamic effects resemble those of intravenous nitroglycerin with a more predictable dose–response curve and a longer duration of action. In clinical studies, nesiritide (administered as 2 mcg/kg by intravenous bolus injection followed by an infusion of 0.01 mcg/kg/min, which may be up-titrated if needed) produced a rapid improvement in both dyspnea and hemodynamics. The primary adverse effect is hypotension, which may be symptomatic and sustained. Because most patients with acute heart failure respond well to conventional therapy, the role of nesiritide may be primarily in patients who continue to be symptomatic after initial treatment with diuretics and nitrates. Moreover, concern has been raised about the impact of nesiritide on mortality, the subject of ongoing trials.

C. HYDRALAZINE—Oral hydralazine is a potent arteriolar dilator and markedly increases cardiac output in patients with CHF. However, as a single agent, it has not been shown to improve symptoms or exercise tolerance during long-term treatment. The combination of nitrates and oral hydralazine produces greater hemodynamic effects.

Hydralazine therapy is frequently limited by side effects. Approximately 30% of patients are unable to tolerate the relatively high doses required to produce hemodynamic improvement in heart failure (200–400 mg daily in divided doses). The major side effect is gastrointestinal distress, but headaches, tachycardia, and hypotension are relatively common. ARBs have largely supplanted the use of the hydralazine–isosorbide dinitrate combination in ACE-intolerant patients.

6. Combination of medical therapies—Optimal management of chronic heart failure involves using combinations of proven life-saving therapies. In addition to ACE-inhibitors and β-blockers, patients who remain symptomatic should be considered for additional therapy, in the form of ARBs (best proven in class II–III heart failure), spironolactone (best proven in current or recent class IV heart failure), or hydralazine and isosorbide dinitrate (with evidence of benefit in African Americans).

7. Positive inotropic agents—The digitalis derivatives are the only available oral inotropic agents in the United

States (see above). A number of other oral positive inotropic agents have been investigated for the long-term treatment of heart failure, but all have increased mortality without convincing evidence of improvement in symptoms. Intravenous agents, such as the β_1-agonist dobutamine and the phosphodiesterase inhibitor milrinone, are sometimes used on a long-term or intermittent basis. The limited available data suggest that continuous therapy is also likely to increase mortality; intermittent inotropic therapy has never been evaluated in controlled trials, and its use is largely based on anecdotal experience. A randomized placebo-controlled trial of 950 patients evaluating intravenous milrinone in patients admitted for decompensated heart failure who had no definite indications for inotropic therapy showed no benefit in terms of survival, decreasing length of admission, or preventing readmission—and significantly increased rates of sustained hypotension and atrial fibrillation. Thus, the role of positive inotropic agents appears to be limited to patients with symptoms and signs of low cardiac output (primarily hypoperfusion and deteriorating kidney function) and those who do not respond to intravenous diuretics. In some cases, dobutamine or milrinone may help maintain patients who are awaiting cardiac transplantation.

8. Calcium channel blockers—First-generation calcium channel blockers may accelerate the progression of CHF. However, two trials with amlodipine in patients with severe heart failure showed that this agent was safe, though not superior to placebo. These agents should be avoided unless they need to be utilized to treat associated hypertension or angina, and for these indications amlodipine is the drug of choice.

9. Anticoagulation—Patients with LV failure and reduced EFs are at somewhat increased risk for developing intracardiac thrombi and systemic arterial emboli. However, this risk appears to be primarily in patients who are in atrial fibrillation or who have large recent anterior myocardial infarction, who should generally be anticoagulated with warfarin for 3 months following the MI. Other patients with heart failure have embolic rates of approximately two per 100 patient-years of follow-up, which approximates the rate of major bleeding, and routine anticoagulation does not appear warranted except in patients with prior embolic events or mobile LV thrombi.

10. Antiarrhythmic therapy—Patients with moderate to severe heart failure have a high incidence of both symptomatic and asymptomatic arrhythmias. Although less than 10% of patients have syncope or presyncope resulting from ventricular tachycardia, ambulatory monitoring reveals that up to 70% of patients have asymptomatic episodes of nonsustained ventricular tachycardia. These arrhythmias indicate a poor prognosis independent of the severity of LV dysfunction, but many of the deaths are probably not arrhythmia related. β-Blockers, because of their marked favorable effect on prognosis in general and on the incidence of sudden death specifically, should be initiated in these as well as all other patients with heart failure. Empiric antiarrhythmic therapy with amiodarone did not improve outcome in the SCD-HeFT trial, and most other agents are contraindicated because of their proarrhythmic effects in this population and their adverse effect on cardiac function.

11. Statin therapy—Even though vascular disease is present in many patients with chronic heart failure, the role of statins has not been well defined in the heart failure population. Two trials—the CORONA and the GISSI-HF trials—have failed to show benefits of statins in the chronic heart failure population.

C. Nonpharmacologic Treatment

1. Implantable cardioverter defibrillators—Randomized clinical trials have extended the indications for ICDs beyond patients with symptomatic or asymptomatic arrhythmias to the broad population of patients with chronic heart failure and LV systolic dysfunction after established medical therapy. In the second Multicenter Automatic Defibrillator Implantation Trial (MADIT II), 1232 patients with prior myocardial infarction and an EF < 30% were randomized to an ICD or a control group. Mortality was 31% lower in the ICD group, which translated into nine lives saved for each 100 patients who received a device and were monitored for 3 years. The Sudden Cardiac Death in Heart Failure Trial (SCD-HeFT) reinforced and extended these results, showing a 23% relative (7.2% absolute) reduction in mortality over 5 years with a simple single-lead ICD in a population of patients with symptomatic chronic heart failure and an EF of ≤ 35%. Patients with class II symptoms appeared to have even larger benefits than patients with class III symptoms. These patients were well-managed with contemporary heart failure treatments, including β-blockers. Based on these results, the United States Centers for Medicare and Medicaid Services provides reimbursement coverage to include patients with chronic heart failure and ischemic or nonischemic cardiomyopathy with an EF ≤ 35%.

2. Biventricular pacing (resynchronization)—Many patients with heart failure due to systolic dysfunction have abnormal intraventricular conduction that results in dyssynchronous and hence inefficient contractions. Several studies have evaluated the efficacy of "multisite" pacing, using leads that stimulate the RV from the apex and the LV from the lateral wall via the coronary sinus. Patients with wide QRS complexes (generally ≥ 120 milliseconds), reduced EFs, and moderate to severe symptoms have been evaluated. Results from trials with up to 2 years of follow-up have shown an increase in EF, improvement in symptoms and exercise tolerance, and reduction in death and hospitalization. The COMPANION trial included 1520 patients with NYHA class III or IV heart failure, EF of ≤ 35%, and QRS duration ≥ 120 milliseconds. In addition to optimal medical therapy, resynchronization therapy with biventricular pacing with or without implantable defibrillator capability reduced death and hospitalization from any cause by about 20%. The CARE-HF trial randomized 813 similar patients, who also required mechanical evidence of dyssynchrony if QRS duration was 120–149 milliseconds, to resynchronization therapy. Over a mean follow-up of 29 months, death or hospitalization for cardiac cause was reduced by 37% and mortality was reduced by 36%. Thus, resynchronization therapy is indicated for patients with moderate to severe heart failure, EF ≤ 35%, and prolonged QRS duration.

3. Case management, diet, and exercise training—
Thirty to 50 percent of CHF patients who are hospitalized will be readmitted within 3–6 months. Strategies to prevent clinical deterioration, such as case management, home monitoring of weight and clinical status, and patient adjustment of diuretics, can prevent rehospitalizations and should be part of the treatment regimen of advanced heart failure.

Patients should routinely practice moderate salt restriction (2–2.5 g sodium or 5–6 g salt per day). More severe sodium restriction is usually difficult to achieve and unnecessary because of the availability of potent diuretic agents.

Exercise training improves activity tolerance in significant part by reversing the peripheral abnormalities associated with heart failure and deconditioning. In severe heart failure, restriction of activity may facilitate temporary recompensation. A large trial (HF ACTION, 2331 patients) did not show significant benefits from a structured exercise training program on death or hospitalization. However, in stable patients, a prudent increase in activity or a regular exercise regimen can be encouraged. Indeed, a gradual exercise program is associated with diminished symptoms and substantial increases in exercise capacity.

4. Coronary revascularization—
Since underlying CAD is the cause of heart failure in the majority of patients, coronary revascularization may both improve symptoms and prevent progression. However, trials have not been performed in patients with symptomatic heart failure. Nonetheless, noninvasive testing for ischemic but viable myocardium is an appropriate first step in patients with known coronary disease but no current clinical evidence of ischemia. Patients with angina who are candidates for surgery should be evaluated for revascularization, usually by coronary angiography. In general, bypass surgery is preferable to PTCA in the setting of heart failure because it provides more complete revascularization.

5. Cardiac transplantation—
Because of the poor prognosis of patients with advanced heart failure, cardiac transplantation has become widely used. Many centers now have 1-year survival rates exceeding 80–90%, and 5-year survival rates above 70%. Infections, hypertension and kidney dysfunction caused by cyclosporine, rapidly progressive coronary atherosclerosis, and immunosuppressant-related cancers have been the major complications. The high cost and limited number of donor organs require careful patient selection early in the course.

6. Other surgical treatment options—
Several surgical procedures for severe heart failure have received considerable publicity. Cardiomyoplasty is a procedure in which the latissimus dorsi muscle is wrapped around the heart and stimulated to contract synchronously with it. In ventricular reduction surgery, a large part of the anterolateral wall is resected to make the heart function more efficiently. Both approaches are too risky in end-stage patients and

have not been shown to improve prognosis or symptoms in controlled studies, and for these reasons they have largely been dropped. Externally powered and implantable ventricular assist devices can be used in patients who require ventricular support either to allow the heart to recover or as a bridge to transplantation. The latest generation devices are small enough to allow patients unrestricted mobility and even discharge from the hospital. However, complications are frequent, including bleeding, thromboembolism, and infection, and the cost is very high, exceeding $200,000 in the initial 1–3 months.

Although 1-year survival was improved in the REMATCH randomized trial, all 129 patients died by 26 months.

7. Palliative care—
Despite the technologic advances of recent years, including cardiac resynchronization, implantable defibrillators, LV assist devices, and totally implantable artificial hearts, it should be remembered that many patients with chronic heart failure are elderly and have multiple comorbidities. Many of them will not experience meaningful improvements in survival with aggressive therapy, and the goal of management should be symptomatic improvement and palliation (see Chapter 5).

▶ Prognosis

Once manifest, heart failure carries a poor prognosis. Even with modern treatment, the 5-year mortality is approximately 50%. Mortality rates vary from less than 5% per year in those with no or few symptoms to greater than 30% per year in those with severe and refractory symptoms. These figures emphasize the critical importance of early detection and intervention. Higher mortality is related to older age, lower LV EF, more severe symptoms, chronic kidney disease, and diabetes. The prognosis of heart failure has improved in the past two decades, probably at least in part because of the more widespread use of ACE inhibitors and β-blockers, which markedly improve survival.

Bardy GH; Sudden Cardiac Death in Heart Failure Trial (SCD-HeFT) Investigators. Amiodarone or an implantable cardioverter-defibrillator for congestive heart failure. N Engl J Med. 2005 Jan 20;352(3):225–37. [PMID: 15659722]

Bradley DJ et al. Cardiac resynchronization and death from progressive heart failure: a meta-analysis of randomized controlled trials. JAMA. 2003 Feb 12;289(6):730–40. [PMID: 12585952]

Bristow MR et al; Comparison of Medical Therapy, Pacing, and Defibrillation in Heart Failure (COMPANION) Investigators. Cardiac-resynchronization therapy with or without an implantable defibrillator in advanced chronic heart failure. N Engl J Med. 2004 May 20;350(21):2140–50. [PMID: 15152059]

Cleland JG et al. The effect of cardiac resynchronization on morbidity and mortality in heart failure. N Engl J Med. 2005 Apr 14;352(15):1539–49. [PMID: 15753115]

Cuffe MS et al. Short-term intravenous milrinone for acute exacerbation of chronic heart failure: a randomized controlled trial. JAMA. 2002 Mar 27;287(12):1541–7. [PMID: 11911756]

Gissi-HF Investigators; Tavazzi L et al. Effect of rosuvastatin in patients with chronic heart failure (the GISSI-HF trial): a randomised, double-blind, placebo-controlled trial. Lancet. 2008 Oct 4;372(9645):1231–9. [PMID: 18757089]

Hunt SA et al. ACC/AHA Guidelines for the evaluation and management of chronic heart failure in the adult: executive summary. A report of the American College of Cardiology/American Heart Association Task Force on Practice Guidelines (Committee to Revise the 1995 Guidelines for the Evaluation and Management of Heart Failure). J Am Coll Cardiol. 2001 Dec;38(7): 2101–13. [PMID: 11738322]

Kjekshus J et al; CORONA Group. Rosuvastatin in older patients with systolic heart failure. N Engl J Med. 2007 Nov 29;357(22):2248–61. [PMID: 17984166]

Moss AJ et al. Prophylactic implantation of a defibrillator in patients with myocardial infarction and reduced ejection fraction. N Engl J Med. 2002 Mar 21;346(12):877–83. [PMID: 11907286]

Mueller C et al. Use of B-type natriuretic peptide in the evaluation and management of acute dyspnea. N Engl J Med. 2004 Feb 12;350(7):647–54. [PMID: 14960741]

Pfeffer MA et al. Valsartan, captopril, or both in myocardial infarction complicated by heart failure, left ventricular dysfunction, or both. N Engl J Med. 2003 Nov 13;349(20):1893–906. [PMID: 14610160]

Swedberg K et al. Guidelines for the diagnosis and treatment of chronic heart failure: executive summary (update 2005): The Task Force for the Diagnosis and Treatment of Chronic Heart Failure of the European Society of Cardiology. Eur Heart J. 2005 Jun;26(11):1115–40. [PMID: 15901669]

Taylor AL et al; African-American Heart Failure Trial Investigators. Combination of isosorbide dinitrate and hydralazine in blacks with heart failure. N Engl J Med. 2004 Nov 11;351(20):2049–57. [PMID: 15533851]

Williams M et al. Cardiac assist devices for end-stage heart failure. Heart Dis. 2001 Mar–Apr;3(2):109–15. [PMID: 11975779]

ACUTE HEART FAILURE & PULMONARY EDEMA

 ESSENTIALS OF DIAGNOSIS

- ▶ Acute onset or worsening of dyspnea at rest.
- ▶ Tachycardia, diaphoresis, cyanosis.
- ▶ Pulmonary rales, rhonchi; expiratory wheezing.
- ▶ Radiograph shows interstitial and alveolar edema with or without cardiomegaly.
- ▶ Arterial hypoxemia.

▶ General Considerations

Typical causes of acute cardiogenic pulmonary edema include acute myocardial infarction or severe ischemia, exacerbation of chronic heart failure, acute volume overload of the LV (valvular regurgitation), and mitral stenosis. By far the most common presentation in developed countries is one of acute or subacute deterioration of chronic heart failure, precipitated by discontinuation of medications, excessive salt intake, myocardial ischemia, tachyarrhythmias (especially rapid atrial fibrillation), or intercurrent infection. Often in the latter group, there is preceding volume overload with worsening edema and progressive shortness of breath for which earlier intervention can usually avoid the need for hospital admission.

▶ Clinical Findings

Acute pulmonary edema presents with a characteristic clinical picture of severe dyspnea, the production of pink, frothy sputum, and diaphoresis and cyanosis. Rales are present in all lung fields, as are generalized wheezing and rhonchi. Pulmonary edema may appear acutely or subacutely in the setting of chronic heart failure or may be the first manifestation of cardiac disease, usually acute myocardial infarction, which may be painful or silent. Less severe decompensations usually present with dyspnea at rest and rales and other evidence of fluid retention but without severe hypoxia.

Noncardiac causes of pulmonary edema include intravenous opioids, increased intracerebral pressure, high altitude, sepsis, several medications, inhaled toxins, transfusion reactions, shock, and disseminated intravascular coagulation. These are distinguished from cardiogenic pulmonary edema by the clinical setting, the history, and the physical examination. Conversely, in most patients with cardiogenic pulmonary edema, an underlying cardiac abnormality can usually be detected clinically or by the ECG, chest radiograph, or echocardiogram.

The chest radiograph reveals signs of pulmonary vascular redistribution, blurriness of vascular outlines, increased interstitial markings, and, characteristically, the butterfly pattern of distribution of alveolar edema. The heart may be enlarged or normal in size depending on whether heart failure was previously present. Assessment of cardiac function by echocardiography is important, since a substantial proportion of patients has normal EFs with elevated atrial pressures due to diastolic dysfunction. In cardiogenic pulmonary edema, the PCWP is invariably elevated, usually over 25 mm Hg. In noncardiogenic pulmonary edema, the wedge pressure may be normal or even low.

▶ Treatment

In full-blown pulmonary edema, the patient should be placed in a sitting position with legs dangling over the side of the bed; this facilitates respiration and reduces venous return. Oxygen is delivered by mask to obtain an arterial PO_2 greater than 60 mm Hg. Noninvasive pressure support ventilation may improve oxygenation and prevent severe CO_2 retention while pharmacologic interventions take effect. However, if respiratory distress remains severe, endotracheal intubation and mechanical ventilation may be necessary.

Morphine is highly effective in pulmonary edema and may be helpful in less severe decompensations when the patient is uncomfortable. The initial dosage is 2–8 mg intravenously (subcutaneous administration is effective in milder cases) and may be repeated after 2–4 hours. Morphine increases venous capacitance, lowering LA pressure, and relieves anxiety, which can reduce the efficiency of ventilation. However, morphine may lead to CO_2 retention by reducing the ventilatory drive. It should be avoided in patients with opioid-induced pulmonary edema, who may improve with opioid-antagonists, and in those with neurogenic pulmonary edema.

Intravenous diuretic therapy (furosemide, 40 mg, or bumetanide, 1 mg—or higher doses if the patient has been receiving long-term diuretic therapy) is usually indicated even if the patient has not exhibited prior fluid retention. These agents produce venodilation prior to the onset of diuresis.

Nitrate therapy accelerates clinical improvement by reducing both BP and LV filling pressures. Sublingual nitroglycerin or isosorbide dinitrate, topical nitroglycerin, or intravenous nitrates will ameliorate dyspnea rapidly prior to the onset of diuresis, and these agents are particularly valuable in patients with accompanying hypertension. Intravenous nesiritide (recombinant BNP), when given as a bolus followed by an infusion, improves dyspnea more rapidly than intravenous nitroglycerin, though this may reflect the cautious way in which nitroglycerin is up-titrated by many practitioners. This agent, as well as nitrates, may precipitate hypotension, especially since these agents are used in combination with multiple drugs that lower BP. In patients with low-output states—particularly when hypotension is present—positive inotropic agents are indicated. These approaches to treatment have been discussed previously.

Bronchospasm may occur in response to pulmonary edema and may itself exacerbate hypoxemia and dyspnea. Treatment with inhaled β-adrenergic agonists or intravenous aminophylline may be helpful, but both may also provoke tachycardia and supraventricular arrhythmias.

In most cases, pulmonary edema responds rapidly to therapy. When the patient has improved, the cause or precipitating factor should be ascertained. In patients without prior heart failure, evaluation should include echocardiography and in many cases cardiac catheterization and coronary angiography. Patients with acute decompensation of chronic heart failure should be treated to achieve a euvolemic state and have their medical regimen optimized. Generally, an oral diuretic and an ACE inhibitor should be initiated, with efficacy and tolerability confirmed prior to discharge. In selected patients, early but careful initiation of β-blockers in low doses should be considered.

Fonarow GC. Pharmacologic therapies for acutely decompensated heart failure. Rev Cardiovasc Med. 2002;3(Suppl)4:S18–27. [PMID: 12439427]

Gandhi SK et al. The pathogenesis of acute pulmonary edema associated with hypertension. N Engl J Med. 2001 Jan 4;344(1):17–22. [PMID: 11136955]

Jain P et al. Current medical treatment for the exacerbation of chronic heart failure resulting in hospitalization. Am Heart J. 2003 Feb;145(2 Suppl):S3–17. [PMID: 12594447]

Young JB et al. Intravenous nesiritide vs nitroglycerin for treatment of decompensated congestive heart failure: a randomized controlled trial. JAMA. 2002 Mar 27;287(12):1531–40. [PMID: 11911755]

MYOCARDITIS & THE CARDIOMYOPATHIES

INFECTIOUS MYOCARDITIS

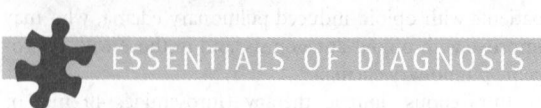

ESSENTIALS OF DIAGNOSIS

▸ Often follows an upper respiratory infection.

▸ May present with chest pain (pleuritic or nonspecific) or signs of heart failure.

▸ Echocardiogram documents cardiomegaly and contractile dysfunction.

▸ Myocardial biopsy, though not sensitive, may reveal a characteristic inflammatory pattern.

▸ General Considerations

Cardiac dysfunction due to primary myocarditis is presumed to be caused by either an acute viral infection or a postviral immune response. Secondary myocarditis is the result of inflammation caused by nonviral pathogens, drugs, chemicals, physical agents, or inflammatory diseases such as systemic lupus erythematosus. The list of infectious causes of myocarditis is extensive and includes viruses with DNA and RNA cores. The coxsackie virus is the predominant agent, but many others have been implicated. Rickettsial myocarditis occurs with scrub typhus, Rocky Mountain spotted fever, and Q fever. Diphtheritic myocarditis is caused by the exotoxin and is often manifested by conduction abnormalities as well as heart failure.

Chagas disease, caused by the insect-borne protozoan *Trypanosoma cruzi*, is a common form of myocarditis in Central and South America; the major clinical manifestations appear after a latent period of more than a decade. At this stage, patients present with cardiomyopathy, conduction disturbances, and sudden death. Associated gastrointestinal involvement (megaesophagus and megacolon) is the rule. Toxoplasmosis causes myocarditis that is usually asymptomatic but can lead to heart failure. Among parasitic infections, trichinosis is the most common cause of cardiac involvement. HIV virus can cause myocarditis, though the prevalence of this complication is not known and it appears related to the level of viral load and CD4 count. In addition, other infectious causes of myocarditis are more common in patients with AIDS. A list of infectious causes of myocarditis is shown in Table 10–11.

Giant cell myocarditis is a rare idiopathic disorder characterized by giant cell and lymphocyte infiltration of the heart muscle. Patients usually die of ventricular arrhythmias or heart failure but occasionally respond to immunosuppressive therapy or early transplantation.

▸ Clinical Findings

A. Symptoms and Signs

Patients may present several days to a few weeks after the onset of an acute febrile illness or a respiratory infection or with heart failure without antecedent symptoms. The onset of heart failure may be gradual or may be abrupt and fulminant. Emboli may occur. Pleural-pericardial chest pain is common. Examination reveals tachycardia, gallop rhythm, and other evidence of heart failure or conduction defect. Many acute infections are subclinical, though they may present later as idiopathic cardiomyopathy or with ventricular arrhythmias. At times, the presentation may mimic an acute myocardial infarction with ST changes, positive cardiac markers, and regional wall motion abnor-

Table 10–11. Major causes of infectious myocarditis.

Viral
Adenovirus, arbovirus (dengue fever, yellow fever), arenavirus (Lassa fever), coxsackie virus, cytomegalovirus, echovirus, encephalomyocarditis virus, Epstein–Barr virus, hepatitis B, herpesvirus, HIV-1, influenza virus, mumps virus, poliomyelitis virus, rabies, respiratory syncytial virus, rubella and rubeola virus, vaccinia virus, varicella virus, variola virus

Bacterial
Brucellosis, clostridia, diphtheria, *Francisella* (tularemia), gonococcus, *Haemophilus*, *Legionella*, meningococcus, *Mycobacterium*, *Mycoplasma*, *Pneumococcus*, psittacosis, *Salmonella*, *Staphylococcus*, *Streptococcus*, Whipple disease

Fungal
Actinomyces, *Aspergillus*, *Blastomyces*, *Candida*, *Cryptococcus*, *Histoplasma*, *Nocardia*, *Sporothrix*

Rickettsial
Rocky Mountain spotted fever, Q fever, scrub typhus, typhus

Spirochetal
Borrelia (Lyme disease and relapsing fever), *Leptospira*, syphilis

Helminthic
Cysticercus, *Echinococcus*, *Schistosoma*, *Toxocara* (visceral larva migrans), *Trichinella*

Protozoal
Entamoeba, *Leishmania*, *Tryponosoma* (Chagas disease), toxoplasmosis

Modified, with permission, from Pisani B et al. Inflammatory myocardial disease and cardiomyopathies. Am J Med. 1997 May;102(5):459–69.

malities despite normal coronaries. Microaneurysms may also occur and may be associated with serious ventricular arrhythmias. Patients may present in a variety of ways with fulminant, subacute, or chronic myocarditis.

B. ECG and Chest Radiography

ECG may show sinus tachycardia, other arrhythmias, nonspecific repolarization changes, and intraventricular conduction abnormalities. Ventricular ectopy may be the initial and only clinical finding. Chest radiograph is nonspecific, but cardiomegaly is frequent, though not universal. Evidence for pulmonary venous hypertension is common and frank pulmonary edema may be present.

C. Diagnostic Studies

There is no specific laboratory study that is consistently present, though the white blood cell count is usually elevated and the sedimentation rate may increase. Troponin I levels are elevated in about one-third of patients, but CK-MB is elevated in only 10%. Echocardiography provides the most convenient way of evaluating cardiac function and can exclude many other processes. Gallium-67 scintigraphy may reveal increased cardiac uptake in acute or subacute myocarditis, but it is not very sensitive. MRI with gadolinium enhancement reveals spotty areas of injury throughout the myocardium. Paired serum viral titers and serologic tests for other agents may indicate the cause.

D. Endomyocardial Biopsy

Pathologic examinations may reveal a lymphocytic inflammatory response with necrosis, but the patchy distribution of abnormalities makes this relatively insensitive. By biopsy, the diagnosis of myocarditis has been established by the 1986 "Dallas" criteria. The diagnosis is dependent on describing the severity of an inflammatory infiltrate with necrosis and degeneration of adjacent myocytes. The type of infiltrate is dependent on the causal agent; usually this is lymphocytic in viral disease, but it may be neutrophilic, eosinophilic, giant cell, granulomatous, or mixed.

► Treatment & Prognosis

Patients with fulminant myocarditis may present with acute cardiogenic shock. Their ventricles are usually not dilated, but thickened (possibly due to myoedema). There is a high death rate, but if the patients recover, they are usually left with no residual cardiomyopathy. Patients who present with subacute disease have a dilated cardiomyopathy and generally make an incomplete recovery. Those who present with chronic disease tend to have only mild dilation of the LV and eventually present with a more restrictive cardiomyopathy.

Specific antimicrobial therapy is indicated when an infecting agent is identified. All patients should receive standard heart failure therapy and have arrhythmias suppressed. Exercise should be limited during the recovery phase. Some believe digoxin should be avoided. Immunosuppressive therapy with corticosteroids and intravenous immunoglobulins may improve the outcome when the process is acute (< 6 months) and if the biopsy suggests ongoing inflammation. However, controlled trials have not been positive, so the value of routine myocardial biopsies in patients presenting with an acute myocarditic picture is uncertain; immunosuppressive therapy without histologic confirmation is clearly unwise, and there are few data to support its use. Patients with fulminant myocarditis require aggressive short-term support including an IABP or an LV assist device. Ongoing studies are addressing whether patients with giant cell myocarditis may be responsive to immunosuppressive agents, as a special case. Overall, if improvement does not occur, many patients may be eventual candidates for cardiac transplantation.

Kindermann I et al. Predictors of outcome in patients with suspected myocarditis. Circulation. 2008 Aug 5;118(6):639–48. [PMID: 18645053]

Magnani JW et al. Myocarditis: current trends in diagnosis and treatment. Circulation. 2006 Feb 14;113(6):876–90. [PMID: 16476862]

DRUG-INDUCED & TOXIC MYOCARDITIS

A variety of medications, illicit drugs, and toxic substances can produce acute or chronic myocardial injury; the clinical presentation varies widely. Doxorubicin and other cytotoxic agents, emetine, and catecholamines (especially with pheochromocytoma) can produce a pathologic picture of inflammation and necrosis together with clinical heart failure and arrhythmias; toxicity of the first two is dose related. The phenothiazines, lithium, chloroquine, disopyramide, antimony-containing compounds, and arsenicals can also cause ECG changes, arrhythmias, or heart failure. Hypersensitivity reactions to sulfonamides, penicillins, and aminosalicylic acid as well as other drugs can result in cardiac dysfunction. Radiation can cause an acute inflammatory reaction as well as a chronic fibrosis of heart muscle, usually in conjunction with pericarditis.

The incidence of cocaine cardiotoxicity has increased markedly. Cocaine can cause coronary artery spasm, myocardial infarction, arrhythmias, and myocarditis. Because many of these processes are believed to be mediated by cocaine's inhibitory effect on norepinephrine reuptake by sympathetic nerves, β-blockers have been used therapeutically. In documented coronary spasm, calcium channel blockers and nitrates may be effective.

Floyd JD et al. Cardiotoxicity of cancer therapy. J Clin Oncol. 2005 Oct 20;23(30):7685–96. [PMID: 16234530]

Gupta S et al. Fulminant myocarditis. Nat Clin Pract Cardiovasc Med. 2008 Nov;5(11):693–706. [PMID: 18797433]

Khakoo AY et al. Therapy Insight: management of cardiovascular disease in patients with cancer and cardiac complications of cancer therapy. Nat Clin Pract Oncol. 2008 Nov;5(11):655–67. [PMID: 18797437]

DILATED CARDIOMYOPATHY

 ESSENTIALS OF DIAGNOSIS

▶ Symptoms and signs of heart failure.

▶ Echocardiogram confirms LV dilation, thinning, and global dysfunction.

▶ General Considerations

The cardiomyopathies are a heterogeneous group of entities affecting the myocardium primarily and not associated with the major causes of cardiac disease, ie, ischemic heart disease, hypertension, pericardial disease, valvular disease, or congenital defects. More recently, two additional entities have been added to the list: a transient cardiomyopathy due to high catecholamine discharge (Tako-Tsubo cardiomyopathy, see below) and an embryologic defect resulting in massive trabeculation in the LV (ventricular noncompaction). Although some have specific causes, many cases are idiopathic. The classification of cardiomyopathies is based on features of presentation and pathophysiology (Table 10–12).

Dilated cardiomyopathies cause about 25% of all cases of CHF. It usually presents with symptoms and signs of CHF (most commonly dyspnea). Occasionally, symptomatic ventricular arrhythmias are the presenting event. LV dilation and systolic dysfunction (EF < 50%) are essential for diagnosis. Dilated cardiomyopathy occurs more often in blacks than whites and in men more than women. A growing number of cardiomyopathies due to genetic abnormalities are being recognized, and these may represent up to 25–30% of cases. Often no cause can be identified, but chronic alcohol abuse and unrecognized myocarditis are probably frequent causes. There is increasing recognition that chronic tachycardia may also precipitate a dilated cardiomyopathy that may improve over time if rate control can be achieved. Amyloidosis, sarcoidosis, hemochromatosis, and diabetes may rarely present as dilated cardiomyopathies, as well as the more classic restrictive picture. The RV may be primarily involved in arrhythmogenic RV dysplasia, an unusual cardiomyopathy with displacement of myocar-

Table 10–12. Classification of the cardiomyopathies.

	Dilated	Hypertrophic	Restrictive
Frequent causes	Idiopathic, alcoholic, major catecholamine discharge, myocarditis, postpartum, doxorubicin, endocrinopathies, genetic diseases	Hereditary syndrome, possibly chronic hypertension	Amyloidosis, post-radiation, post-open heart surgery, diabetes, endomyocardial fibrosis
Symptoms	Left or biventricular congestive heart failure	Dyspnea, chest pain, syncope	Dyspnea, fatigue, right-sided congestive heart failure
Physical examination	Cardiomegaly, S_3, elevated jugular venous pressure, rales	Sustained point of maximal impulse, S_4, variable systolic murmur, bisferiens carotid pulse	Elevated jugular venous pressure, Kussmaul sign
Electrocardiogram	ST-T changes, conduction abnormalities, ventricular ectopy	Left ventricular hypertrophy, exaggerated septal Q waves	ST-T changes, conduction abnormalities, low voltage
Chest radiograph	Enlarged heart, pulmonary congestion	Mild cardiomegaly	Mild to moderate cardiomegaly
Echocardiogram, nuclear studies, MRI	Left ventricular dilation and dysfunction	Left ventricular hypertrophy, asymmetric septal hypertrophy, small left ventricular size, normal or supranormal function, systolic anterior mitral motion, diastolic dysfunction	Small or normal left ventricular size, normal or mildly reduced left ventricular function
Cardiac catheterization	Left ventricular dilation and dysfunction, high diastolic pressures, low cardiac output	Small, hypercontractile left ventricle, dynamic outflow gradient, diastolic dysfunction	High diastolic pressure, "square root" sign, normal or mildly reduced left ventricular function

dial cells by adipose tissue, or in Uhl disease, in which there is extreme thinning of the RV walls.

Dilated cardiomyopathy can now be considered a disease that results from more varied perturbations, including, but not limited to, defects of the cytoskeleton. Positional cloning and candidate gene approaches have been successful in identifying greater than 40 disease loci, many of which have led to disease genes in hypertrophic cardiomyopathy, restrictive cardiomyopathy, dilated cardiomyopathy, and arrhythmogenic right ventricular dysplasia. This exciting area is only now being explored. Since most dilated cardiomyopathies are considered "idiopathic," the potential for discovery of a genetic predisposition seems very promising.

Intraventricular thrombus is not uncommon in dilated cardiomyopathy. Histologically, the picture is one of extensive fibrosis unless a specific diagnosis is established. Myocardial biopsy is rarely useful in establishing the diagnosis, though occasionally the underlying cause (eg, sarcoidosis, hemochromatosis) can be discerned. Biopsy is most useful in transplant rejection.

► Clinical Findings

A. Symptoms and Signs

In most patients, symptoms of heart failure develop gradually. The physical examination reveals rales, an elevated JVP, cardiomegaly, S_3 gallop rhythm, often the murmurs of functional mitral or tricuspid regurgitation, peripheral edema, or ascites. In severe CHF, Cheyne-Stokes breathing, pulsus alternans, pallor, and cyanosis may be present.

B. ECG and Chest Radiography

The major findings are listed in Table 10–12. Sinus tachycardia is common. Other common abnormalities include left bundle branch block and ventricular or atrial arrhythmias. The chest radiograph reveals cardiomegaly, evidence for left and/or right heart failure, and pleural effusions (right > left).

C. Diagnostic Studies

An echocardiogram is indicated to exclude unsuspected valvular or other lesions and confirm the presence of dilated cardiomyopathy and reduced systolic function (as opposed to pure diastolic heart failure). Mitral Doppler inflow patterns also help in the diagnosis of associated diastolic dysfunction. Color flow Doppler can reveal tricuspid or mitral regurgitation, and continuous Doppler can help define PA pressures. Exercise or pharmacologic stress myocardial perfusion imaging may suggest the possibility of underlying coronary disease. Radionuclide ventriculography provides a noninvasive measure of the EF and both RV and LV wall motion. Cardiac MRI is particularly helpful in infiltrative processes, such as sarcoidosis or hemochromatosis, and is the diagnostic study of choice for RV dysplasia. MRI can also help define an ischemic etiology by noting gadolinium enhancement consistent with myocardial scar. Cardiac catheterization is seldom of specific value unless myocardial ischemia or LV aneurysm is suspected. The serum ferritin is an adequate screening study for hemochromatosis. The erythrocyte sedimentation rate may be low due to liver congestion if right heart failure is present. The serum level of BNP or pro-BNP can be used to help quantitate the severity of CHF.

► Treatment

Standard therapy for heart failure should include ACE inhibitor, β-blockers, diuretics, and an aldosterone antagonist. Digoxin is a second-line drug but remains favored as an adjunct by some clinicians. Calcium channel blockers should generally be avoided unless absolutely necessary for rate control in atrial fibrillation. Sodium restriction is helpful, especially in acute CHF. When atrial fibrillation is present, heart rate control is important if sinus rhythm cannot be established or maintained. Many patients may be candidates for cardiac synchronization therapy with biventricular pacing and an implantable defibrillator. Few cases of cardiomyopathy are amenable to specific therapy for the underlying cause. Alcohol use should be discontinued, since there is often marked recovery of cardiac function following a period of abstinence in alcoholic cardiomyopathy. Endocrine causes (thyroid dysfunction, acromegaly, and pheochromocytoma) should be treated. Immunosuppressive therapy is not indicated in chronic dilated cardiomyopathy. The management of CHF is outlined in the section on heart failure.

► Prognosis

The prognosis of dilated cardiomyopathy without clinical heart failure is variable, with some patients remaining stable, some deteriorating gradually, and others declining rapidly. Once heart failure is manifest, the natural history is similar to that of other causes of heart failure, with an annual mortality around 11–13%. Arterial and pulmonary emboli are more common in dilated cardiomyopathy than in ischemic cardiomyopathy. Suitable candidates may benefit from long-term anticoagulation, and all patients with atrial fibrillation should be so treated. Some patients may be candidates for cardiac transplantation.

► When to Refer

- Referral to a cardiologist is warranted when there is any question about the etiology of the reduced systolic function.

- Essentially all patients with a dilated cardiomyopathy need to have a coronary evaluation to exclude an underlying ischemic cause that might be treatable.

- Referral should also be considered when heart failure symptoms emerge, especially if there is a possibility the patient may eventually be a cardiac transplant candidate.

Anderson L et al. The role of endomyocardial biopsy in the management of cardiovascular disease: a scientific statement from the American Heart Association, the American College of Cardiology, and the European Society of Cardiology. Eur Heart J. 2008 Dec;29(13):1696–97. [PMID: 18456711]

Ashrafian H et al. Reviews of translational medicine and genomics in cardiovascular disease: new disease taxonomy and therapeutic implications cardiomyopathies: therapeutics based on molecular phenotype. J Am Coll Cardiol. 2007 Mar 27;49(12):1251–64. [PMID: 17394955]

Marcus F et al. The mystery of arrhythmogenic right ventricular dysplasia/cardiomyopathy: from observation to mechanistic explanation. Circulation. 2006 Oct 24;114(17):1794–5. [PMID: 17060394]

TAKO-TSUBO CARDIOMYOPATHY

 ESSENTIALS OF DIAGNOSIS

► Occurs after a major catecholamine discharge.

► Acute chest pain or shortness of breath.

► Predominately affects postmenopausal women.

► Presents as an acute anterior myocardial infarction, but coronaries normal at cardiac catheterization.

► Imaging reveals apical left ventricular ballooning due to anteroapical stunning of the myocardium.

General Considerations

LV apical ballooning can follow a high catecholamine stress. The resulting shape of the LV suggests a rounded ampulla form similar to a Japanese octopus pot (tako-tsubo pot). Mid-ventricular ballooning is also seen on occasion. The acute myocardial injury is more common in postmenopausal women. It has been described following some stressful event, such as hypoglycemia, lightning strikes, earthquakes, postventricular tachycardia, during alcohol withdrawal, following surgery, during hyperthyroidism, and following emotional stress.

Clinical Findings

A. Symptoms and Signs

The symptoms are similar to any acute coronary syndrome. Typical angina and dyspnea is usually present. Syncope is rare.

B. ECG and Chest Radiography

The ECG reveals ST segment elevation as well as deep anterior T wave inversion. The chest radiograph is either normal or reveals pulmonary congestion. The dramatic T wave inversions gradually resolve over time.

C. Diagnostic Studies

The echocardiogram reveals LV apical dyskinesia. The urgent cardiac catheterization reveals the LV apical ballooning in association with normal coronaries. Initial cardiac enzymes are positive but often taper quickly.

Treatment

Immediate therapy is similar to any acute myocardial infarction. Initiation of long-term therapy depends on whether LV dysfunction persists. Most patients receive aspirin, β-blockers, and ACE-inhibitors until the LV fully recovers.

Prognosis

Prognosis is good unless there is a serious complication (such as mitral regurgitation, ventricular rupture, ventricular tachycardia). Recovery is expected in most cases after a period of weeks to months. At times, the LV function recovers in days.

Singh NK. Apical ballooning syndrome: the emerging evidence of a neurocardiogenic basis. Am Heart J. 2008 Sep;156(3):e33. [PMID: 18760116]

Valente AM et al. Unusual cardiomyopathies: ventricular non-compaction and takotsubo cardiomyopathy. Rev Cardiovasc Med. 2006 Summer;7(3):111–8. [PMID: 17088856]

HYPERTROPHIC CARDIOMYOPATHY

 ESSENTIALS OF DIAGNOSIS

► May present with dyspnea, chest pain, syncope.

► Though LV outflow gradient is classic, symptoms are primarily related to diastolic dysfunction.

► Echocardiogram shows septal hypertrophy, which is usually asymmetric, and enhanced contractility. Systolic anterior motion of the anterior mitral valve is present if there is outflow tract obstruction.

► The highest risk group for sudden death includes those with a marked LVH, with a family history for sudden death, with ventricular ectopy, and with an abnormal BP response to exercise.

General Considerations

Myocardial hypertrophy unrelated to any pressure or volume overload reduces LV systolic stress, increases the EF, and can result in an "empty ventricle" at end-systole. The interventricular septum may be disproportionately involved (asymmetric septal hypertrophy), but in some cases the hypertrophy is localized to mid ventricle or to the apex. The LV outflow tract is often narrowed during systole between the bulging septum and an anteriorly displaced anterior mitral valve leaflet, causing a dynamic obstruction. The obstruction is worsened by factors that increase myocardial contractility (sympathetic stimulation, digoxin, postextrasystolic beat) or that decrease LV filling (Valsalva maneuver, peripheral vasodilators). The amount of obstruction is preload and afterload dependent and can vary from day to day. The consequence of the hypertrophy is elevated diastolic pressures rather than systolic dysfunction. Rarely, systolic dysfunction develops late in the disease. The LV is usually more involved than the RV and the atria are frequently significantly enlarged. It has been increasingly appreciated that hypertrophic obstructive cardiomyopathy (HOCM) is inherited as an autosomal dominant trait with variable penetrance and is caused by mutations of one of a large number of genes, most of which code for myosin heavy chains or proteins regulating calcium handling. The prognosis is related to the specific gene mutation. These patients usually present in early adulthood. Elite athletes may demonstrate considerable hypertrophy that can be confused with HOCM, but generally diastolic dysfunction is not present. The apical variety is particularly common in those of Asian descent. A mid-ventricular obstructive form is also known. A hypertrophic cardiomyopathy in the elderly (usually in association with hypertension) has also been defined as a distinct entity. Mitral annular calcification is often present.

Clinical Findings

A. Symptoms and Signs

The most frequent symptoms are dyspnea and chest pain (Table 10–12). Syncope is also common and is typically postexertional, when diastolic filling diminishes and outflow obstruction increases. Arrhythmias are an important problem. Atrial fibrillation is a long-term consequence of chronically elevated LA pressures and is a poor prognostic sign. Ventricular arrhythmias are also common, and sudden death may occur, often in athletes after extraordinary exertion.

Features on physical examination are a bisferiens carotid pulse, triple apical impulse (due to the prominent atrial filling wave and early and late systolic impulses), and a loud S_4. The JVP may reveal a prominent a wave due to reduced RV compliance. In cases with outflow obstruction, a loud systolic murmur is present along the left sternal border that increases with upright posture or Valsalva maneuver and decreases with squatting. These maneuvers help differentiate the murmur of HOCM from that of aortic stenosis. Mitral regurgitation is frequently present as well.

B. ECG and Chest Radiography

LVH is nearly universal in symptomatic patients, though entirely normal ECGs are present in up to 25%, usually in those with localized hypertrophy. Exaggerated septal Q waves inferolaterally may suggest myocardial infarction. The chest radiograph is often unimpressive. Unlike aortic stenosis, the ascending aorta is not dilated.

C. Diagnostic Studies

The echocardiogram is diagnostic, revealing asymmetric LVH, systolic anterior motion of the mitral valve, early closing followed by reopening of the aortic valve, a small and hypercontractile LV, and delayed relaxation and filling of the LV during diastole. The septum is usually 1.3–1.5 times the thickness of the posterior wall. Septal motion tends to be reduced. Doppler ultrasound reveals turbulent flow and a dynamic gradient in the LV outflow tract and, commonly, mitral regurgitation. Abnormalities in the diastolic filling pattern are present in 80% of patients. Myocardial perfusion imaging may suggest septal ischemia in the presence of normal coronary arteries. Cardiac MRI confirms the hypertrophy and contrast enhancement frequently reveals evidence for scar at the junction of the RV attachment to the septum. Cardiac catheterization confirms the diagnosis and assesses the presence of CAD. Frequently, coronary arterial bridging (squeezing in systole) occurs, especially of the septal arteries.

Treatment

β-Blockers should be the initial drug in symptomatic individuals, especially when dynamic outflow obstruction is noted on the echocardiogram. The resulting slower heart rates assist with diastolic filling of the stiff LV. Dyspnea, angina, and arrhythmias respond in about 50% of patients. Calcium channel blockers, especially verapamil, have also been effective in symptomatic patients. Their effect is due primarily to improved diastolic function, but their vasodilating actions can also increase outflow obstruction and cause hypotension. Disopyramide (Norpace) is also used because of its negative inotropic effects; it is usually used in addition to the other therapies. Diuretics are frequently necessary due to the high diastolic pressure and PCWP. Patients do best in sinus rhythm, and atrial fibrillation should be aggressively treated with antiarrhythmics. Dual-chamber pacing may prevent the progression of hypertrophy and obstruction. Nonsurgical septal ablation has been performed by injection of alcohol into septal branches of the left coronary artery with good results in small series of patients. Patients with malignant ventricular arrhythmias and unexplained syncope in the presence of a positive family history for sudden death are probably best managed with an implantable defibrillator. Excision of part of the outflow myocardial septum (myotomy–myomectomy) by surgeons experienced with the procedure has been successful in patients with severe symptoms. A few surgeons advocate mitral valve replacement, as this results in resolution of the gradient as well, and prevents associated mitral regurgitation.

Prognosis

The natural history of HOCM is highly variable. Several specific mutations are associated with a higher incidence of early malignant arrhythmias and sudden death, and definition of the genetic abnormality provides the best estimate of prognosis. Some patients remain asymptomatic for many years or for life. Sudden death, especially during exercise, may be the initial event. The *highest risk patients* are those with a family history of sudden death, those with marked hypertrophy, and those that do not increase their systemic BP with exercise. HOCM is the pathologic feature most frequently associated with sudden death in athletes. Pregnancy is generally well tolerated. Endocarditis prophylaxis is no longer indicated. A final stage may be a transition into dilated cardiomyopathy in 5–10% of patients due to the long-term effects of LV remodeling.

When to Refer

Patients should be referred to a cardiologist when symptoms are difficult to control, syncope has occurred, or there are any of the high-risk features present as noted above.

Fifer MA et al. Management of symptoms in hypertrophic cardiomyopathy. Circulation. 2008 Jan 22;117(3):429–39. [PMID: 18212300]

Harris KM et al. Prevalence, clinical profile and significance of LV remodeling in the end-stage phase of hypertrophic cardiomyopathy. Circulation. 2006 Jul 18;114(3):216–25. [PMID: 16831987]

Ho CY et al. A contemporary approach to hypertrophic cardiomyopathy. Circulation. 2006 Jun 20;113(24):e858–62. [PMID: 16785342]

Sherrod MV. Pathophysiology and treatment of hypertrophic cardiomyopathy. Prog Cardiovasc Dis. 2006 Sep–Oct;49(2): 123–51. [PMID: 17046437]

Sorajja P et al. Outcome of alcohol septal ablation for obstructive hypertrophic cardiomyopathy. Circulation. 2008 Jul 8;118(2):131–9. [PMID: 18591440]

RESTRICTIVE CARDIOMYOPATHY

ESSENTIALS OF DIAGNOSIS

▸ Right heart failure tends to dominate over left heart failure.

▸ Pulmonary hypertension present.

▸ Amyloidosis is the most common cause.

▸ Echocardiography is key to diagnosis. Rapid early filling is present with diastolic dysfunction. Normal or near normal EF.

▸ MRI and cardiac catheterization are helpful. Myocardial biopsy can confirm.

General Considerations

Restrictive cardiomyopathy is characterized by impaired diastolic filling with reasonably preserved contractile function. The condition is relatively uncommon, with the most frequent cause being amyloidosis. In Africa, endomyocardial fibrosis, a specific entity in which there is severe fibrosis of the endocardium, often with eosinophilia (Löffler syndrome), is seen. Other causes of restrictive cardiomyopathy are infiltrative cardiomyopathies (eg, hemochromatosis, sarcoidosis) and connective tissue diseases (eg, scleroderma).

Clinical Findings

A. Symptoms and Signs

Restrictive cardiomyopathy must be distinguished from constrictive pericarditis (Table 10–12). The key feature is that ventricular interaction is accentuated with respiration in constrictive pericarditis, and that interaction is absent in restrictive cardiomyopathy. Pulmonary pressure is invariably elevated in restrictive cardiomyopathy due to the high pulmonary capillary wedge pressure and is normal in uncomplicated constrictive pericarditis.

B. Diagnostic Studies

Conduction disturbances are frequently present. Low voltage on the ECG combined with ventricular hypertrophy on the echocardiogram is suggestive of disease. Cardiac MRI presents a distinctive pattern of hyper-enhancement of the gadolinium image in amyloidosis and is a useful screening test. The echocardiogram reveals a small thickened LV with bright myocardium, rapid early diastolic filling revealed by the mitral inflow Doppler, and biatrial enlargement. Atrial septal thickening may be evident. Rectal, abdominal fat, or gingival biopsies can confirm systemic involvement, but myocardial involvement may still be present if these are negative, and requires endomyocardial biopsy for the confirmation of cardiac amyloid. Demonstration of tissue infiltration on biopsy specimens using special stains followed by immunohistochemical studies and genetic testing is essential to define which specific protein is involved.

Treatment

Unfortunately, little useful therapy is available for either the causative conditions or the restrictive cardiomyopathy itself. Diuretics can help, but excessive diuresis can produce worsening kidney dysfunction. As with most patients with severe right heart failure, loop diuretics, thiazides, and aldosterone antagonists are all useful. Recently, the use of ultrafiltration devices have allowed for improved diuresis. Digoxin may precipitate arrhythmias and generally should not be used. β-Blockers help slow heart rates and improve filling. Corticosteroids may be helpful in sarcoidosis but they are more effective for the conduction abnormalities than heart failure. In amyloidosis, the therapeutic strategy depends on the characterization of the type of amyloid protein and extent of disease and may include chemotherapy or bone marrow transplantation. In familial amyloidosis liver transplantation may be an option. Cardiac transplantation has also been used in patients with primary cardiac amyloidosis.

When to Refer

All patients with the diagnosis of a restrictive cardiomyopathy should be referred to a cardiologist to decide etiology and plan appropriate treatment. This is especially true if amyloidosis is suspected.

Goldstein JA. Cardiac tamponade, constrictive pericarditis, and restrictive cardiomyopathy. Curr Probl Cardiol. 2004 Sep;29 (9):503–67. [PMID: 15365561]

Selvanayagam JB et al. Evaluation and management of the cardiac amyloidosis. J Am Coll Cardiol. 2007 Nov 27;50(22):2101–10. [PMID: 18036445]

Yazdani K et al. Differentiating constrictive pericarditis from restrictive cardiomyopathy. Rev Cardiovasc Med. 2005 Spring;6(2):61–71. [PMID: 15976729]

ACUTE RHEUMATIC FEVER & RHEUMATIC HEART DISEASE

ESSENTIALS OF DIAGNOSIS

▸ Uncommon in the United States (approximately 2 cases/100,000 population); more common (100 cases/100,000 population) in developing countries.

▸ Peak incidence ages 5–15 years.

▶ Diagnosis based on Jones criteria and confirmation of streptococcal infection.

▶ May involve mitral and other valves acutely, rarely leading to heart failure.

General Considerations

Rheumatic fever is a systemic immune process that is a sequela to β-hemolytic streptococcal infection of the pharynx. Pyodermic infections are not associated with rheumatic fever. Signs of rheumatic fever usually commence 2–3 weeks after infection but may appear as early as 1 week or as late as 5 weeks. In recent years, the disease has become quite uncommon in the United States, except in immigrants; however, there have been reports of new outbreaks in several regions of the United States. The peak incidence is between ages 5 and 15 years; rheumatic fever is rare before age 4 years or after age 40 years. Rheumatic carditis and valvulitis may be self-limited or may lead to slowly progressive valvular deformity. The characteristic lesion is a perivascular granulomatous reaction with vasculitis. The mitral valve is attacked in 75–80% of cases, the aortic valve in 30% (but rarely as the sole valve), and the tricuspid and pulmonary valves in under 5% of cases.

Chronic rheumatic heart disease results from single or repeated attacks of rheumatic fever that produce rigidity and deformity of valve cusps, fusion of the commissures, or shortening and fusion of the chordae tendineae. Stenosis or insufficiency results, and the two often coexist. The mitral valve alone is affected in 50–60% of cases; combined lesions of the aortic and mitral valves occur in 20%; pure aortic lesions are less common. Tricuspid involvement occurs in about 10% of cases but only in association with mitral or aortic disease and is thought to be more common when recurrent infections have occurred. The pulmonary valve is rarely affected. A history of rheumatic fever is obtainable in only 60% of patients with rheumatic heart disease.

Clinical Findings

The diagnostic criteria first described by Jones were updated in 1992. The presence of two major criteria—or one major and two minor criteria—establishes the diagnosis. Echocardiographic studies revealing valvular abnormalities have suggested that subclinical cardiac involvement may be missed using the strick Jones criteria. India, New Zealand, and Australia have all published revised guidelines.

A. Major Criteria

1. Carditis—Carditis is most likely to be evident in children and adolescents. Any of the following suggests the presence of carditis: (1) pericarditis; (2) cardiomegaly, detected by physical signs, radiography, or echocardiography; (3) CHF, right- or left-sided—the former perhaps more prominent in children, with painful liver engorgement due to tricuspid regurgitation; and (4) mitral or aortic regurgitation murmurs, indicative of dilation of a valve ring with or without associated valvulitis. The Carey–Coombs short mid-diastolic mitral murmur may be present.

In the absence of any of the above definitive signs, the diagnosis of carditis depends on the following less specific abnormalities: (1) ECG changes, including changing contour of P waves or inversion of T waves; (2) changing quality of heart sounds; and (3) sinus tachycardia, arrhythmia, or ectopic beats.

2. Erythema marginatum and subcutaneous nodules—Erythema marginatum begins as rapidly enlarging macules that assume the shape of rings or crescents with clear centers. They may be raised, confluent, and either transient or persistent.

Subcutaneous nodules are uncommon except in children. They are small (≤ 2 cm in diameter), firm, and nontender and are attached to fascia or tendon sheaths over bony prominences. They persist for days or weeks, are recurrent, and are indistinguishable from rheumatoid nodules.

3. Sydenham chorea—Sydenham chorea—involuntary choreoathetoid movements primarily of the face, tongue, and upper extremities—may be the sole manifestation; only 50% of cases have other overt signs of rheumatic fever. Girls are more frequently affected, and occurrence in adults is rare. This is the least common (3% of cases) but most diagnostic of the manifestations of rheumatic fever.

4. Polyarthritis—This is a migratory polyarthritis that involves the large joints sequentially. In adults, only a single joint may be affected. The arthritis lasts 1–5 weeks and subsides without residual deformity. Prompt response of arthritis to therapeutic doses of salicylates or nonsteroidal agents is characteristic.

B. Minor Criteria

These include fever, polyarthralgias, reversible prolongation of the PR interval, and an elevated erythrocyte sedimentation rate or CRP. Supporting evidence includes positive throat culture or rapid streptococcal antigen test and elevated or rising streptococcal antibody titer.

C. Laboratory Findings

There is nonspecific evidence of inflammatory disease, as shown by a rapid sedimentation rate. High or increasing titers of antistreptococcal antibodies (antistreptolysin O and anti-DNase B) are used to confirm recent infection; 10% of cases lack this serologic evidence.

Differential Diagnosis

Rheumatic fever may be confused with the following: rheumatoid arthritis, osteomyelitis, endocarditis, chronic meningococcemia, systemic lupus erythematosus, Lyme disease, sickle cell anemia, "surgical abdomen," and many other diseases.

Complications

CHF occurs in severe cases. In the longer term, the development of rheumatic heart disease is the major problem. Other complications include arrhythmias, pericarditis with effusion, and rheumatic pneumonitis.

Treatment

A. General Measures

The patient should be kept at strict bed rest until the temperature returns to normal (without the use of antipyretic medications) and the sedimentation rate, plus the resting pulse rate, and the ECG have all returned to baseline.

B. Medical Measures

1. Salicylates—The salicylates markedly reduce fever and relieve joint pain and swelling. They have no effect on the natural course of the disease. Adults may require large doses of aspirin, 0.6–0.9 g every 4 hours; children are treated with lower doses.

2. Penicillin—Penicillin (benzathine penicillin, 1.2 million units intramuscularly once, or procaine penicillin, 600,000 units intramuscularly daily for 10 days) is used to eradicate streptococcal infection if present. Erythromycin may be substituted (40 mg/kg/d).

3. Corticosteroids—There is no proof that cardiac damage is prevented or minimized by corticosteroids. A short course of corticosteroids (prednisone, 40–60 mg orally daily, with tapering over 2 weeks) usually causes rapid improvement of the joint symptoms and is indicated when response to salicylates has been inadequate.

Prevention of Recurrent Rheumatic Fever

The initial episode of rheumatic fever can usually be prevented by early treatment of streptococcal pharyngitis. (See Chapter 33.) Prevention of recurrent episodes of rheumatic fever is critical. Recurrences of rheumatic fever are most common in patients who have had carditis during their initial episode and in children, 20% of whom will have a second episode within 5 years. The preferred method of prophylaxis is with benzathine penicillin G, 1.2 million units intramuscularly every 4 weeks. Oral penicillin (200,000–250,000 units twice daily) is less reliable.

If the patient is allergic to penicillin, sulfadiazine (or sulfisoxazole), 1 g daily, or erythromycin, 250 mg orally twice daily, may be substituted. The macrolide azithromycin is similarly effective against group A streptococcal infection. If the patient has not had an immediate hypersensitivity (anaphylactic-type) reaction to penicillin, then cephalosporin may also be used.

Recurrences are uncommon after 5 years following the first episode, and in patients over 25 years of age. Prophylaxis is usually discontinued after these times except in groups with a high risk of streptococcal infection—parents or teachers of young children, nurses, military recruits, etc. Secondary prevention of rheumatic fever depends on whether carditis has occurred. If there is no evidence for carditis, preventive therapy can be stopped at age 21 years. If carditis has occurred but there is no residual valvular disease, it can be stopped at 10 years after the episode. If carditis has occurred with residual valvular involvement, it should be continued for 10 years after the last episode or until age 40 years if the patient is in a situation in which reexposure would be expected.

Prognosis

Initial episodes of rheumatic fever may last months in children and weeks in adults. The immediate mortality rate is 1–2%. Persistent rheumatic carditis with cardiomegaly, heart failure, and pericarditis implies a poor prognosis; 30% of children thus affected die within 10 years after the initial attack. After 10 years, two-thirds of patients will have detectable valvular abnormalities (usually thickened valves with limited mobility), but significant symptomatic valvular heart disease or persistent cardiomyopathy occurs in less than 10% of patients with a single episode. In developing countries, acute rheumatic fever occurs earlier in life, recurs more frequently, and the evolution to chronic valvular disease is both accelerated and more severe.

Atatoa-Carr P et al. Rheumatic fever diagnosis, management, and secondary prevention: a New Zealand guideline. N Z Med J. 2008 Apr 4;121(1271):59–69. [PMID: 18392063]

Lee GM et al. Changing epidemiology of acute rheumatic fever in the United States. Clin Infect Dis. 2006 Feb 15;42(4):448–50. [PMID: 16421786]

Saxena A et al; Working Group on Pediatric Acute Rheumatic Fever and Cardiology Chapter of Indian Academy of Pediatrics. Consensus guidelines on pediatric acute rheumatic fever and rheumatic heart disease. Indian Pediatr. 2008 Jul;45(7):565–73. [PMID: 18695275]

Tubridy-Clark M et al. Subclinical carditis in rheumatic fever: a systematic review. Int J Cardiol. 2007 Jun 25;119(1):54–8. [PMID: 17034886]

▼ DISEASES OF THE PERICARDIUM

ACUTE INFLAMMATORY PERICARDITIS

ESSENTIALS OF DIAGNOSIS

► Anterior pleuritic chest pain that is worse supine than upright.

► Pericardial rub.

► Fever common.

► Erythrocyte sedimentation rate usually elevated.

► ECG reveals diffuse ST segment elevation with associated PR depression.

General Considerations

Acute (< 2 weeks) inflammation of the pericardium may be infectious in origin or may be due to systemic diseases (autoimmune syndromes, uremia), neoplasm, radiation, drug toxicity, hemopericardium, postcardiac surgery, or contiguous inflammatory processes in the myocardium or lung. In many of these conditions, the pathologic process involves both the pericardium and the myocardium.

Viral infections (especially infections with coxsackieviruses and echoviruses but also influenza, Epstein–Barr, varicella, hepatitis, mumps, and HIV viruses) are the most common cause of acute pericarditis and probably are responsible for many cases classified as idiopathic. Males—usually under age 50 years—are most commonly affected. The differential diagnosis is primarily with myocardial infarction. **Tuberculous pericarditis** has become rare in developed countries but remains common in other areas. It results from direct lymphatic or hematogenous spread; clinical pulmonary involvement may be absent or minor, although associated pleural effusions are common. **Bacterial pericarditis** has become rare and usually results from direct extension from pulmonary infections. Pneumococci can cause a primary pericardial infection. *Borrelia burgdorferi,* the organism responsible for Lyme disease, can also cause myopericarditis. **Uremic pericarditis** is a common complication of chronic kidney disease. The pathogenesis is uncertain; it occurs both with untreated uremia and in otherwise stable dialysis patients. Spread of adjacent lung cancer as well as invasion by breast cancer, renal cell carcinoma, Hodgkin disease, and lymphomas are the most common **neoplastic processes** involving the pericardium and have become the most frequent causes of pericardial tamponade in many countries. Pericarditis may occur 2–5 days after infarction due to an inflammatory reaction to transmural myocardial necrosis (**postmyocardial infarction or postcardiotomy pericarditis (Dressler syndrome).** **Radiation** can initiate a fibrinous and fibrotic process in the pericardium, presenting as subacute pericarditis or constriction. Radiation pericarditis usually follows treatments of more than 4000 cGy delivered to ports including more than 30% of the heart.

Other causes of pericarditis include connective tissue diseases, such as lupus erythematosus and rheumatoid arthritis, drug-induced pericarditis (minoxidil, penicillins, clozapine), and myxedema.

▶ Clinical Findings

A. Symptoms and Signs

The presentation and course of inflammatory pericarditis depend on its cause, but most syndromes have associated chest pain, which is usually pleuritic and postural (relieved by sitting). The pain is substernal but may radiate to the neck, shoulders, back, or epigastrium. Dyspnea may also be present and the patient is often febrile. A pericardial friction rub is characteristic, with or without evidence of fluid accumulation or constriction (see below). The presentation of **tuberculous pericarditis** tends to be subacute, but nonspecific symptoms (fever, night sweats, fatigue) may be present for days to months. Pericardial involvement develops in 1–8% of patients with pulmonary tuberculosis. Symptoms and signs of **bacterial pericarditis** are similar to those of other types of inflammatory pericarditides, but patients appear toxic and are often critically ill. **Uremic pericarditis** can present with or without symptoms; fever is absent. Often **neoplastic pericarditis** is painless, and the presenting symptoms relate to hemodynamic compromise or the primary disease. **Postmyocardial infarction or postcardiotomy pericarditis (Dressler syndrome)** usually presents as a recurrence of pain with pleural-pericardial features. A rub is often audible, and repolarization changes on the ECG may be confused with

ischemia. Large effusions are uncommon, and spontaneous resolution usually occurs in a few days. Dressler syndrome occurs weeks to several months after myocardial infarction or open heart surgery, may be recurrent, and probably represents an autoimmune syndrome. Patients present with typical pain, fever, malaise, and leukocytosis. Occasionally, the syndrome will occur within days of surgery. Rarely, other symptoms of an autoimmune disorder, such as joint pain and fever, may occur. Tamponade is rare with Dressler syndrome after myocardial infarction but not when it occurs postoperatively. The clinical onset of **radiation pericarditis** is usually within the first year but may be delayed for many years; often a full decade may past before constriction becomes evident.

B. Laboratory Findings and Diagnostic Studies

The diagnosis of **viral pericarditis** is usually clinical, and leukocytosis is often present. Rising viral titers in paired sera may be obtained for confirmation but are rarely done. Cardiac enzymes may be slightly elevated, reflecting an epicardial myocarditis component. The echocardiogram is often normal or reveals only a trivial amount of fluid during the acute inflammatory process. The diagnosis of **tuberculous pericarditis** can be inferred if acid-fast bacilli are found elsewhere. The tuberculous pericardial effusions are usually small or moderate but may be large. The yield of organisms by pericardiocentesis is low; pericardial biopsy has a higher yield but may also be negative, and pericardiectomy may be required. If **bacterial pericarditis** is suspected on clinical grounds, diagnostic pericardiocentesis may be of value. In **uremic patients** not on dialysis, the incidence of pericarditis correlates roughly with the level of blood urea nitrogen (BUN) and creatinine. The pericardium is characteristically "shaggy" in uremic pericarditis, and the effusion is hemorrhagic and exudative. The diagnosis of **neoplastic pericarditis** can occasionally be made by cytologic examination of the effusion or by pericardial biopsy, but it may be difficult to establish clinically if the patient has received mediastinal radiation within the previous year. Neoplastic pericardial effusions develop over a long period of time and may become quite huge (> 2 L). The sedimentation rate is high in **postmyocardial infarction or postcardiotomy pericarditis.** Large pericardial effusions and accompanying pleural effusions are frequent. Myxedema pericardial effusions due to hypothyroidism usually are characterized by the presence of cholesterol crystals.

C. Other Studies

The ECG usually shows generalized ST and T wave changes and may manifest a characteristic progression beginning with diffuse ST elevation, followed by a return to baseline and then to T wave inversion. Atrial injury is often present and manifested by PR depression especially in the limb leads. The chest radiograph is frequently normal, but may show cardiac enlargement if pericardial fluid is present, as well as signs of related pulmonary disease. Mass lesions and enlarged lymph nodes may suggest a neoplastic process. MRI and CT scan can visualize neighboring tumor in neoplastic pericarditis. A screening chest CT or MRI is often recommended to ensure there are no extracardiac diseases contiguous to the pericardium.

► Treatment

Treatment of **viral pericarditis** is generally symptomatic. Aspirin (650 mg every 3–4 hours) or other nonsteroidal agents (eg, indomethacin, 100–150 mg daily in divided doses) are usually effective. Corticosteroids may be beneficial in unresponsive cases. In general, symptoms subside in several days to weeks. The major early complication is tamponade, which occurs in less than 5% of patients. There may be recurrences in the first few weeks or months. Rare patients will continue to experience recurrences chronically. These patients may require long-term anti-inflammatory medications, either corticosteroids or colchicine. Rarely, acute pericarditis may lead to constrictive pericarditis, which may necessitate pericardial resection (see below). Standard antituberculous drug therapy is usually successful for **tuberculous pericarditis** (see Chapter 9), but constrictive pericarditis can occur. **Uremic pericarditis** usually resolves with the institution of—or with more aggressive—dialysis. Tamponade is fairly common, and partial pericardiectomy (pericardial window) may be necessary. Whereas anti-inflammatory agents may relieve the pain and fever associated with uremic pericarditis, indomethacin and systemic corticosteroids do not affect its natural history. The prognosis with **neoplastic effusion** is dismal, with only a small minority surviving 1 year. If it is compromising the clinical comfort of the patient, the effusion is initially drained percutaneously. Early attempts at ballooning the pericardium from a subxiphoid approach have been mostly abandoned in favor of surgical approaches. A pericardial window, either by a subxiphoid approach or via video-assisted thoracic surgery, allows for partial pericardiectomy. Instillation of chemotherapeutic agents or tetracycline may occasionally be used to reduce the recurrence rate. Aspirin or other nonsteroidal anti-inflammatory agents in dosages given for viral pericarditis above for 2–4 weeks are usually effective for the treatment of **postmyocardial infarction or postcardiotomy pericarditis (Dressler syndrome).** In more severe cases, corticosteroids should be given in rapidly tapering doses. Relapses do occur and may require slow withdrawal of anti-inflammatory therapy over several months. Colchicine may be required for months to help prevent recurrences. Symptomatic therapy is the initial approach to **radiation pericarditis,** but recurrent effusions and constriction often require surgery.

Imazio M et al. Management, risk factors, and outcomes in recurrent pericarditis. Am J Cardiol. 2005 Sep 1;96(5):736–9. [PMID: 16125506]

Ross AM et al. Acute pericarditis. Evaluation and treatment of infectious and other causes. Postgrad Med. 2004 Mar;115(3):67–70, 73–5. [PMID: 15038256]

Tingle LE et al. Acute pericarditis. Am Fam Physician. 2007 Nov 15;76(10):1509–14. [PMID: 18052017]

PERICARDIAL EFFUSION

Pericardial effusion can develop during any of the processes previously discussed. The speed of accumulation determines the physiologic importance of the effusion. Because the pericardium stretches, large effusions (> 1000 mL) that develop slowly may produce no hemodynamic effects. Conversely, smaller effusions that appear rapidly can cause tamponade. Tamponade is characterized by elevated intrapericardial pressure (> 15 mm Hg), which restricts venous return and ventricular filling. As a result, the stroke volume and pulse pressure fall, and the heart rate and venous pressure rise. Shock and death may result.

► Clinical Findings

A. Symptoms and Signs

Pericardial effusions may be associated with pain if they occur as part of an acute inflammatory process or may be painless, as is often the case with neoplastic or uremic effusion. Dyspnea and cough are common, especially with tamponade. Other symptoms may result from the primary disease.

A pericardial friction rub may be present even with large effusions. In cardiac tamponade, tachycardia, tachypnea, a narrow pulse pressure, and a relatively preserved systolic pressure are characteristic. Pulsus paradoxus—a greater than 10 mm Hg decline in systolic pressure during inspiration due to further impairment of LV filling—is the classic finding, but it may also occur with obstructive lung disease. Central venous pressure is elevated and there is no evident y descent in the RA, RV, or LV hemodynamic tracings. Edema or ascites are rarely present; these signs favor a more chronic process.

B. Laboratory Findings

Laboratory tests tend to reflect the underlying processes (see causes of pericarditis above).

C. Diagnostic Studies

Chest radiograph can suggest chronic effusion by an enlarged cardiac silhouette with a globular configuration but may appear normal in acute situations. The ECG often reveals nonspecific T wave changes and low QRS voltage. Electrical alternans is present uncommonly but is pathognomonic. It is due to the heart swinging within the large effusion. Echocardiography is the primary method for demonstrating pericardial effusion and is quite sensitive. If tamponade is present, the high intrapericardial pressure may collapse lower pressure cardiac structures, such as the RA and RV. In tamponade, the normal inspiratory reduction in LV filling is accentuated due to RV/LV interaction and there is a > 25% reduction in maximal mitral inflow velocities. Cardiac CT and MRI also demonstrate pericardial fluid and any associated contiguous lesions. Diagnostic pericardiocentesis or biopsy is often indicated for microbiologic and cytologic studies; a pericardial biopsy may be performed relatively simply through a small subxiphoid incision. Unfortunately, the quality of the pericardial fluid rarely leads to a diagnosis, and any type of fluid (serous, serosanguinous, bloody, etc) can be seen in most diseases.

► Treatment

Small effusions can be followed clinically by careful observations of the JVP and by testing for a paradoxical pulse.

Serial echocardiograms are indicated if no intervention is immediately contemplated. When tamponade is present, urgent pericardiocentesis is required. Because the pressure–volume relationship in the pericardial fluid is curvilinear and upsloping, removal of a small amount of fluid often produces a dramatic fall in the intrapericardial pressure and immediate hemodynamic benefit; but complete drainage with a catheter is preferable. Continued or repeat drainage may be indicated, especially in malignant effusions. Pericardial windows via video-assisted thorascopy have been particularly effective in preventing recurrences.

Additional therapy is determined by the nature of the primary process. Recurrent effusion in neoplastic disease and uremia, in particular, may require partial pericardiectomy as noted earlier.

When to Refer

- Any unexplained pericardial effusion should be referred to a cardiologist for a complete evaluation and treatment.
- Trivial pericardial effusions are common, especially in CHF, and need not be referred.
- Hypotension or a paradoxical pulse suggesting the pericardial effusion is hemodynamically compromising the patient should prompt an immediate referral.

Burgess LJ et al. Role of biochemical tests in the diagnosis of large pericardial effusions. Chest. 2002 Feb;121(2):495–9. [PMID: 11834663]

Kühn B et al. Etiology, management, and outcome of pediatric pericardial effusions. Pediatr Cardiol. 2008 Jan;29(1):90–4. [PMID: 17674083]

Roy CL et al. Does this patient with a pericardial effusion have cardiac tamponade? JAMA. 2007 Apr 25;297(16):1810–8. [PMID: 17456823]

CONSTRICTIVE PERICARDITIS

 ESSENTIALS OF DIAGNOSIS

- ▸ Evidence of right heart failure with an elevated JVP, edema, hepatomegaly, and ascites.
- ▸ No fall or an elevation of the JVP with inspiration (Kussmaul sign).
- ▸ Echocardiographic evidence for septal bounce and reduced mitral inflow velocities with inspiration.
- ▸ Catheterization evidence for RV-LV interaction, a "square root" sign, equalization of diastolic pressures, normal pulmonary artery pressure, and narrow RV pressure tracing that increases with inspiration.

General Considerations

Inflammation can lead to a thickened, fibrotic, adherent pericardium that restricts diastolic filling and produces chronically elevated venous pressures. In the past, tuberculosis was the most common cause of constrictive pericarditis, but the process now more often occurs after radiation therapy, cardiac surgery, or viral pericarditis; histoplasmosis is another uncommon cause.

Clinical Findings

A. Symptoms and Signs

The principal symptoms are slowly progressive dyspnea, fatigue, and weakness. Chronic edema, hepatic congestion, and ascites are usually present. Ascites often seems out of proportion to the degree of peripheral edema. The examination reveals these signs and a characteristically elevated jugular venous pressure with a rapid y descent. This can be detected at bedside by careful observation of the jugular pulse and noting an apparent increased pulse wave at the end of systole (due to accentuation of the v wave by the rapid y descent). Kussmaul sign—a failure of the JVP to fall with inspiration—is also a frequent finding. The apex may actually retract with systole and a pericardial "knock" may be heard in early diastole. Pulsus paradoxus is unusual. Atrial fibrillation is common.

B. Diagnostic Studies

At times constrictive pericarditis is extremely difficult to differentiate from restrictive cardiomyopathy. When unclear, the use of noninvasive testing and cardiac catheterization is required to sort out the difference.

1. Radiographic findings—The chest radiograph may show normal heart size or cardiomegaly. Pericardial calcification is best seen on the lateral view and is uncommon. It rarely involves the LV apex, and finding of calcification at the LV apex is more consistent with LV aneurysm. Cardiac CT and MRI are only occasionally helpful. Pericardial thickening of > 4 mm must be present to establish the diagnosis, yet no pericardial thickening is demonstrated in 20–25% of patients with constrictive pericarditis.

2. Echocardiography—Echocardiography rarely demonstrates a thickened pericardium. A septal "bounce" reflecting the rapid early filling is common, though. RV/LV interaction may be demonstrated by a reduction in the mitral inflow pattern of > 25%, much as in tamponade.

3. Cardiac catheterization—As a generality, the pulmonary pressure is low in constriction and there must be signs of RV/LV interaction (reduced LV filling pattern with inspiration) on echocardiography/Doppler. In constrictive pericarditis, because of the need to demonstrate RV/LV interaction, cardiac catheterization should include simultaneous measurement of both the LV and RV. Hemodynamically, patients with constriction have equalization of end-diastolic pressures throughout their cardiac chambers, there is rapid early filling then an abrupt increase in diastolic pressure ("square-root" sign), the RV end-diastolic pressure is more than one-third the systolic pressure, simultaneous measurements of RV and LV systolic pressure reveal a discordance with inspiration (the RV rises as the LV falls), and there is usually a Kussmaul sign (failure of the RA pressure to fall with inspiration). The width (or area) of the RV pressure tracing may also be less in expiration and greater during inspiration, reflecting the variability in filling of the RV with respiration.

In restrictive cardiomyopathy, the LV diastolic pressure is usually greater than the RV diastolic pressure by 5 mm Hg, there is pulmonary hypertension, and simultaneous measurements of the RV and LV systolic pressure reveal a concordant drop in the peak systolic pressure in both with inspiration.

▶ Treatment

Initial treatment consists of diuresis. As in other disorders of right heart failure, the diuresis should be aggressive, using loop diuretics (torsemide if bowel edema is suspected), thiazides, and aldosterone antagonists (especially if ascites is present). At times, aquaphoresis may be of value. Surgical pericardiectomy should be done when diuretics are unable to control symptoms. Pericardiectomy removes the pericardium between the phrenic nerve pathways only, however, and most patients still require diuretics after the procedure, though symptoms are usually dramatically improved. Morbidity and mortality after pericardiectomy are high (up to 15%) and are greatest in those with the most disability prior to the procedure. For that reason, most experts recommend earlier rather than later pericardiectomy if symptoms are present.

▶ When to Refer

If the diagnosis of constrictive pericarditis is unclear or the symptoms resist medical therapy, then referral to a cardiologist is warranted to both establish the diagnosis and recommend therapy.

Nishimura RA. Constrictive pericarditis in the modern era: a diagnostic dilemma. Heart. 2001 Dec;86(6):619–23. [PMID: 11711451]

Talreja DR et al. Constrictive pericarditis in the modern era: novel criteria for diagnosis in the cardiac catheterization laboratory. J Am Coll Cardiol. 2008 Jan 22;51(3):315–9. [PMID: 18206742]

Wang A et al. Clinical problem-solving. Undercover and overlooked. N Engl J Med. 2004 Sep 2;351(10):1014–9. [PMID: 15342810]

PULMONARY HYPERTENSION & PULMONARY HEART DISEASE

IDIOPATHIC PULMONARY HYPERTENSION

 ESSENTIALS OF DIAGNOSIS

▶ Most frequently seen in younger women.

▶ Dyspnea, and often cyanosis, with no evidence of left heart disease.

▶ Enlarged pulmonary arteries on chest radiograph.

▶ Elevated JVP and RV heave.

▶ Echocardiography is often diagnostic.

▶ General Considerations

The normal pulmonary bed offers about one-tenth as much resistance to blood flow as the systemic arterial system.

Pulmonary hypertension is classified as mild if the mean PA pressure is > 20 mm Hg, moderate if > 30 mm Hg, and severe if > 45 mm Hg. As opposed to the systemic circulation, the pulmonary resistance is influenced by local vascular mediators much more than the adrenergic nervous system, even though both α- and β-receptors are present on pulmonary vascular smooth muscle. The normal pulmonary endothelial cell maintains the vascular smooth muscle in a state of relaxation. Pulmonary vasoconstriction is mediated by hypoxia and by endothelin and angiotensin II. Vasodilation can be affected by certain prostaglandins, endothelin receptor blockers, smooth muscle relaxants, and by nitric oxide. Formally called "**primary**" **pulmonary hypertension**, the preferred term now is "idiopathic pulmonary hypertension" and is defined as pulmonary hypertension and elevated PVR in the absence of other disease of the lungs or heart. Its cause is unknown, though there are clear genetic patterns that have been identified, and it likely represents a derangement in one or more of the biologic pathways described above. Pathologically, it is characterized by diffuse narrowing of the pulmonary arterioles. Circumstantial evidence suggests that unrecognized recurrent pulmonary emboli or in situ thrombosis may play a role in some cases. However, the latter may well be an exacerbating factor (precipitated by local endothelial injury) rather than a cause of the syndrome. Idiopathic pulmonary hypertension must be distinguished from other causes of severe secondary pulmonary hypertension, such as systemic sclerosis, HIV-related pulmonary hypertension, cirrhosis, and congenital heart defects (primarily those with a shunt distal to the level of the tricuspid valve). Rarely, pulmonary venous disease (pulmonary veno-occlusive disease) or peripheral PA stenosis may be present. Left heart disease, in particular mitral stenosis, or any reason for an elevated LA pressure must be excluded as well. Table 10–13 includes clinical disorders causing pulmonary hypertension.

▶ Clinical Findings

A. Symptoms and Signs

The clinical picture is similar to that of pulmonary hypertension from other causes. Chronic lung disease, especially sleep apnea, can be overlooked as a cause for pulmonary hypertension. Patients are characteristically young women who have evidence of right heart failure that is usually progressive, leading to death in 2–8 years. This is a decidedly different prognosis than patients with Eisenmenger physiology due to a left-to-right shunt; 40% of patients with Eisenmenger physiology are alive 25 years after the diagnosis has been made. Patients have manifestations of low cardiac output, with weakness and fatigue, as well as edema and ascites as right heart failure advances. Peripheral cyanosis is present, and syncope on effort may occur.

B. Diagnostic Studies

The laboratory evaluation of idiopathic pulmonary hypertension must exclude a secondary cause. A hypercoagulable state should be sought and chronic pulmonary emboli excluded (usually by lung scan or contrast spiral CT). The chest radiograph helps exclude a primary pulmonary etiol-

Table 10–13. Causes of pulmonary hypertension.

Pulmonary arterial hypertension
  Primary pulmonary hypertension
  Persistent pulmonary hypertension of the newborn
  Secondary causes
    Connective tissue disease
    Eisenmenger physiology (congenital heart disease)
    Portal hypertension
    HIV
    Drugs/toxins (especially anorexigens)
Pulmonary venous hypertension
  Left-sided heart disease
  Pulmonary venous obstruction
    Veno-occlusive disease
    Fibrosing mediastinitis (usually related to histoplasmosis or
      radiation)
Disorders of the lung or hypoxemia
  Chronic obstructive pulmonary disease
  Interstitial lung disease
  Sleep apnea
  High altitude (chronic exposure)
  Alveolar-capillary dysplasia
Chronic thromboembolic disease
  Thrombotic obstruction (clot)
  Pulmonary emboli (tumor, foreign material)
Disorders of pulmonary vasculature
  Schistosomiasis
  Sarcoidosis
  Histiocytosis X
  Other

Modified from Rich S (editor). Primary pulmonary hypertension: Executive summary from the World Symposium–Primary Pulmonary Hypertension, 1998.

ogy—evidence for patchy edema may raise the suspicion of pulmonary veno-occlusive disease. A sleep study may be warranted. The ECG is generally consistent with RVH and RA enlargement. Echocardiography/Doppler demonstrates an enlarged RV and RA—at times they may be huge and hypocontractile. Severe pulmonic or tricuspid regurgitation may be present. Septal flattening is consistent with pulmonary hypertension. Doppler interrogation of the tricuspid regurgitation jet helps provide an estimate of RV systolic pressure. Pulmonary function tests help exclude other disorders, though primary pulmonary hypertension may present with a reduced carbon monoxide diffusing capacity of the lung (DL_{CO}) and severe desaturation (particularly if a PFO has been stretched open and a right-to-left shunt is present). Chest CT demonstrates enlarged pulmonary arteries and excludes other causes (such as emphysema or interstitial lung disease). Pulmonary angiography (or MR angiography or CT angiography) reveals loss of the smaller acinar pulmonary vessels and tapering of the larger ones. Catheterization allows measurement of pulmonary pressures and testing for vasoreactivity using a variety of agents, including 100% oxygen, adenosine, epoprostenol, and nitric oxide. A positive response is one that decreases the pulmonary mean pressure by > 20%, and the mean pulmonary pressure is reduced to ≤ 45 mm Hg.

► Treatment

Until recently, the only therapy for idiopathic pulmonary hypertension has been trials of calcium channel blockers, oxygen, and eventually lung transplantation. Currently, a variety of therapeutic options are now available and approved. Many authorities advocate long-term oral anticoagulation and this is given to most patients with idiopathic pulmonary hypertension. Supplemental oxygen, particularly at night, appears to improve symptoms and helps reduce pulmonary pressures. Diuretics help with right heart edema. Calcium channel blockers, at times in large doses, have been used with mixed results. Some patients respond well, especially if the patient has responded to acute vasodilator testing. However, calcium channel blockers can worsen RV function by their negative inotropic effects. Responders should also be considered for phosphodiesterase-5 inhibitors, such as sildenafil.

Other agents are available for treatment of patients who do not respond to vasodilator challenge. Epoprostenol is administered by continuous infusion and has been shown to improve functional capacity and survival. Analogs of epoprostenol are also available, including treprostinil, beraprost, and iloprost. Treprostinil is given by subcutaneous injection, beraprost by mouth, and iloprost by inhalation. Endothelin antagonists are also available orally, such as bosentan and sitaxentan. Pulmonary transplantation is a viable option in selected centers, though the operative mortality is high (around 20–25%) and 2-year survival only about 55%. Women with significant pulmonary hypertension should not get pregnant, and permanent birth control measures should be considered.

► When to Refer

All patients with suspected idiopathic pulmonary hypertension should be referred to either a cardiologist or pulmonologist who specializes in the evaluation and treatment of patients with unexplained pulmonary hypertension (RV systolic > 35 mm Hg as measured by an echocardiogram).

Ghofrani HA et al. Uncertainties in the diagnosis and treatment of pulmonary arterial hypertension. Circulation. 2008 Sep 9;118(11):1195–201. [PMID: 18779455]
Rubin LJ et al. Evaluation and management of the patient with pulmonary arterial hypertension. Ann Intern Med. 2005 Aug 16;143(4):282–92. [PMID: 16103472]

PULMONARY HEART DISEASE (Cor Pulmonale)

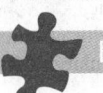

ESSENTIALS OF DIAGNOSIS

► Symptoms and signs of chronic bronchitis and pulmonary emphysema.

► Elevated jugular venous pressure, parasternal lift, edema, hepatomegaly, ascites.

► ECG shows tall, peaked P waves (P pulmonale), right axis deviation, and RVH.

▶ Chest radiograph: Enlarged RV and PA.

▶ Echocardiogram or radionuclide angiography excludes primary LV dysfunction.

General Considerations

The term "cor pulmonale" denotes RV hypertrophy and eventual failure resulting from pulmonary disease and the attendant hypoxia or from pulmonary vascular disease (pulmonary hypertension). Its clinical features depend on both the primary underlying disease and its effects on the heart.

Cor pulmonale is most commonly caused by COPD. Less frequent causes include pneumoconiosis, pulmonary fibrosis, kyphoscoliosis, idiopathic pulmonary hypertension, repeated episodes of subclinical or clinical pulmonary embolization, Pickwickian syndrome, schistosomiasis, and obliterative pulmonary capillary or lymphangitic infiltration from metastatic carcinoma.

Clinical Findings

A. Symptoms and Signs

The predominant symptoms of compensated cor pulmonale are related to the pulmonary disorder and include chronic productive cough, exertional dyspnea, wheezing respirations, easy fatigability, and weakness. When the pulmonary disease causes RV failure, these symptoms may be intensified. Dependent edema and right upper quadrant pain may also appear. The signs of cor pulmonale include cyanosis, clubbing, distended neck veins, RV heave or gallop (or both), prominent lower sternal or epigastric pulsations, an enlarged and tender liver, and dependent edema.

B. Laboratory Findings

Polycythemia is often present in cor pulmonale secondary to COPD. The arterial oxygen saturation is often below 85%; PCO_2 may or may not be elevated.

C. ECG and Chest Radiography

The ECG may show right axis deviation and peaked P waves. Deep S waves are present in lead V_6. Right axis deviation and low voltage may be noted in patients with pulmonary emphysema. Frank RVH is uncommon except in idiopathic pulmonary hypertension. The ECG often mimics myocardial infarction; Q waves may be present in leads II, III, and aVF because of the vertically placed heart, but they are rarely deep or wide, as in inferior myocardial infarction. Supraventricular arrhythmias are frequent and nonspecific.

The chest radiograph discloses the presence or absence of parenchymal disease and a prominent or enlarged RV and PA.

D. Diagnostic Studies

Pulmonary function tests usually confirm the underlying lung disease. The echocardiogram should show normal LV size and function but RV and RA dilation. Perfusion lung scans are rarely of value, but, if negative, they help to exclude chronic pulmonary emboli, an occasional cause of cor pulmonale. Multislice CT has replaced pulmonary angiography as the most specific method of diagnosis for the pulmonary emboli.

Differential Diagnosis

In its early stages, cor pulmonale can be diagnosed on the basis of radiologic, echocardiographic, or ECG evidence. Catheterization of the right heart will establish a definitive diagnosis but is more often performed to exclude left-sided heart failure, which can be an unrecognized cause of right-sided failure in some patients. Differential diagnostic considerations relate primarily to the specific pulmonary disease that has produced RV failure (see above).

Treatment

The details of the treatment of chronic pulmonary disease (chronic respiratory failure) are discussed in Chapter 9. Otherwise, therapy is directed at the pulmonary process responsible for right heart failure. Oxygen, salt and fluid restriction, and diuretics are mainstays, with combination diuretic therapy (loop diuretics, thiazides and spironolactone) often useful, as described above for other causes of right heart failure.

Prognosis

Compensated cor pulmonale has the same prognosis as the underlying pulmonary disease. Once congestive signs appear, the average life expectancy is 2–5 years, but survival is significantly longer when uncomplicated emphysema is the cause.

When to Refer

Patients with unexplained or difficult to manage right heart failure should be referred to a cardiologist or a pulmonologist.

Han MK et al. Pulmonary diseases and the heart. Circulation. 2007 Dec 18;116(25):2992–3005. [PMID: 18086941]

Lehrman S et al. Primary pulmonary hypertension and cor pulmonale. Cardiol Rev. 2002 Sep–Oct;10(5):265–78. [PMID: 12215190]

Morrison LK et al. Utility of a rapid B-natriuretic peptide assay in differentiating congestive heart failure from lung disease in patients presenting with dyspnea. J Am Coll Cardiol. 2002 Jan 16;39(2):202–9. [PMID: 11788208]

NEOPLASTIC DISEASES OF THE HEART

Primary cardiac tumors are rare and constitute only a small fraction of all tumors that involve the heart or pericardium. The most common primary tumor is atrial myxoma; it comprises about 50% of all tumors in adult case series. It is generally attached to the atrial septum and is more likely to affect the LA than the RA. Familial myxomas occur as part of the **Carney complex**—that consists of myxomas, pigmented skin lesions, and endocrine neoplasia. Patients with myxoma can present with the characteristics of a systemic illness, with obstruction of blood flow through the heart, or with signs of peripheral embolization. The characteristics include fever, malaise, weight loss, leukocytosis, elevated sedimentation rate, and emboli (peripheral or pulmonary, depending on the location of the tumor). This is often confused with infective endocarditis, lymphoma, other cancers, or autoimmune diseases. In other cases, the tumor may grow to considerable size and produce symptoms by obstructing mitral flow. Episodic pulmonary edema (classically occurring when an upright posture is assumed) and signs of low output may result. Physical examination may reveal a diastolic sound related to motion of the tumor ("tumor plop") or a diastolic murmur similar to that of mitral stenosis. Right-sided myxomas may cause symptoms of right-sided failure. The diagnosis is established by echocardiography or by pathologic study of embolic material. Cardiac MRI is useful as an adjunct only. Contrast angiography is frequently not necessary. Surgical excision is usually curative, though recurrences do occur and serial echocardiographic follow-up, on at least a yearly basis, is recommended.

The second most common cardiac tumors are valvular papillary fibroelastomas and atrial septal lipomas. These tend to be benign and usually require no therapy. Other primary cardiac tumors include rhabdomyomas (that often appear multiple in both the RV and LV), fibrous histiocytomas, hemangiomas, and a variety of unusual sarcomas. The diagnosis may be supported by an abnormal cardiac contour on radiograph. Echocardiography is usually helpful but may miss tumors infiltrating the ventricular wall. Cardiac MRI is emerging as the diagnostic procedure of choice.

Metastases from malignant tumors can also affect the heart. Most often this occurs in malignant melanoma, but other tumors involving the heart include bronchogenic carcinoma, carcinoma of the breast, the lymphomas, renal cell carcinoma, and, in patients with AIDS, Kaposi sarcoma. These are often clinically silent but may lead to pericardial tamponade, arrhythmias and conduction disturbances, heart failure, and peripheral emboli. The diagnosis is often made by echocardiography, but cardiac MRI and CT scanning are also helpful. ECG may reveal regional Q waves. The prognosis is dismal; effective treatment is not available. On rare occasions, surgical resection or chemotherapy is warranted.

Bennett KR et al. The Carney complex: unusual skin findings and recurrent cardiac myxoma. Arch Dermatol. 2005 Jul;141(7):916–8. [PMID: 16027322]

Butany J et al. Cardiac tumours: diagnosis and management. Lancet Oncol. 2005 Apr;6(4):219–28. [PMID: 15811617]

Restrepo CS et al. CT and MR imaging findings of benign cardiac tumors. Curr Probl Diagn Radiol. 2005 Jan–Feb;34(1):12–21. [PMID: 15644859]

Sun JP et al. Clinical and echocardiographic characteristics of papillary fibroelastomas: a retrospective and prospective study in 162 patients. Circulation. 2001 Jun 5;103(22):2687–93. [PMID: 11390338]

▼ CARDIAC INVOLVEMENT IN MISCELLANEOUS SYSTEMIC DISEASES

The heart may be involved in a number of systemic syndromes. Many of these have been mentioned briefly in this chapter. The pericardium, myocardium, heart valves, and coronary arteries may be involved either singly or in various combinations. In most cases the cardiac manifestations are not the dominant feature, but in some it is the primary cause of symptoms and may be fatal.

The most common type of myocardial involvement is an infiltrative cardiomyopathy, such as systemic amyloidosis, sarcoidosis, hemochromatosis, Fabry or glycogen storage disease. These result in a restrictive cardiomyopathy (see above). Cardiac calcinosis can occur in hyperparathyroidism (usually the secondary form) and in primary oxalosis. A number of muscular dystrophies can cause a cardiomyopathic picture (particularly Duchenne, less frequently myotonic dystrophy, and several rarer forms). Involvement of the heart in Duchenne dystrophy results in a focal cardiomyopathy of the posterior wall; the classic ECG has prominent anterior precordial forces. In addition to LV dysfunction and heart failure, all of these conditions frequently cause conduction abnormalities, which may be the presenting or only feature. The myocardium may also be involved in inflammatory and autoimmune diseases. It is commonly affected in polymyositis and dermatomyositis, but usually this is subclinical. Systemic lupus erythematosus, scleroderma, and mixed connective tissue disease may cause myocarditis, but these more commonly involve the pericardium, coronary arteries, or valves. Several endocrinopathies, including acromegaly, thyrotoxicosis, myxedema, and pheochromocytoma, can produce dilated cardiomyopathies that resolve when the underlying disease is appropriately treated.

Pericardial involvement is quite common in many of the connective tissue diseases. Systemic lupus erythematosus may present with pericarditis, and pericardial involvement is not uncommon (but is less frequently symptomatic) in active rheumatoid arthritis, systemic sclerosis, and mixed connective tissue disease. Endocardial involvement takes the form of patchy fibrous—predominantly on the right side—or inflammatory or sclerotic changes of the heart valves. Carcinoid heart disease results from the layering of plaque-like material over the tricuspid valve, RV endocardium, and pulmonic valve and presents with right heart failure due to tricuspid and pulmonic regurgitation. The hypereosinophilic syndromes involve the endocardium, leading to restrictive cardiomyopathy. A variety of arthritic syndromes are associated with aortic valvulitis or aortitis with resulting aortic regurgitation. These include ankylosing spondylitis, rheumatoid arthritis, and Reiter syndrome. Disorders of collagen (Marfan syndrome is the most frequent, followed by Ehlers–Danlos syndrome) often affect the ascending aorta, with resulting aneurysmal dilation and aortic regurgitation. Mitral valve prolapse is also a common finding in these disorders.

Almost any vasculitic syndrome can involve the coronary arteries, leading to myocardial infarction. This is most common with polyarteritis nodosa and systemic lupus erythematosus. Two vasculitic syndromes have a particular predilection for the coronary arteries—Kawasaki disease and Takayasu disease. Kawasaki disease can result in coronary aneurysms, occasionally of huge size. Takayasu disease affects the great vessels more than the coronaries and smooth, tapering lesions are usually seen, particularly at the vessel ostia. In these, myocardial infarction may be the presenting symptom.

Freeman AF et al. Kawasaki disease: summary of the American Heart Association guidelines. Am Fam Physician. 2006 Oct 1;74(7):1141–8. [PMID: 17039750]

Magnani JW et al. Myocarditis: current trends in diagnosis and treatment. Circulation. 2006 Feb 14;113(6):876–90. [PMID: 16476862]

Riboldi P et al. Cardiac involvement in systemic autoimmune diseases. Clin Rev Allergy Immunol. 2002 Dec;23(3):247–61. [PMID: 12402411]

Strickberger SA et al. AHA/ACCF Scientific Statement on the evaluation of syncope: from the American Heart Association Councils on Clinical Cardiology, Cardiovascular Nursing, Cardiovascular Disease in the Young, and Stroke, and the Quality of Care and Outcomes Research Interdisciplinary Working Group; and the American College of Cardiology Foundation: in collaboration with the Heart Rhythm Society: endorsed by the American Autonomic Society. Circulation. 2006 Jan 17;113(2):316–27. [PMID: 16418451]

TRAUMATIC HEART DISEASE

Penetrating wounds to the heart are, of course, usually lethal unless surgically repaired. Stab wounds to the RV occasionally lead to hemopericardium without progressing to tamponade.

Blunt trauma is a more frequent cause of cardiac injuries, particularly outside of the emergency department setting. This type of injury is quite frequent in motor vehicle accidents and may occur with any form of chest trauma, including CPR efforts. The most common injuries are myocardial contusions or hematomas. Other forms of nonischemic cardiac injury include metabolic injury due to burns, electrical current, or sepsis. These may be asymptomatic (particularly in the setting of more severe injuries) or may present with chest pain of a nonspecific nature or, not uncommonly, with a pericardial component. Elevations of cardiac enzymes are frequent but the levels do not correlate with prognosis. Echocardiography may reveal an akinetic segment or pericardial effusion. Pericardiocentesis is warranted if tamponade is evident. Heart failure is uncommon if there are no associated cardiac or pericardial injuries, and conservative management is usually sufficient.

Severe trauma may also cause cardiac or valvular rupture. Cardiac rupture may involve any chamber, but survival is most likely if injury is to one of the atria or the RV. Hemopericardium or pericardial tamponade is the usual clinical presentation, and surgery is almost always necessary. Mitral and aortic valve rupture may occur during severe blunt trauma—the former presumably if the impact occurs during systole and the latter if during diastole. Patients reach the hospital in shock or severe heart failure. Immediate surgical repair is essential. The same types of injuries may result in transection of the aorta, either at the level of the arch or distal to the takeoff of the left subclavian artery. Transthoracic echocardiography and TEE are the most helpful and immediately available diagnostic techniques.

Blunt trauma may also result in damage to the coronary arteries. Acute or subacute coronary thrombosis is the most common presentation. The clinical syndrome is one of acute myocardial infarction with attendant ECG, enzymatic, and contractile abnormalities. Emergent revascularization is sometimes feasible, either by the percutaneous route or by coronary artery bypass surgery. LV aneurysms are common outcomes of traumatic coronary occlusions. Coronary artery dissection or rupture may also occur in the setting of blunt cardiac trauma.

Embrey R. Cardiac trauma. Thorac Surg Clin. 2007 Feb;17(1):87–93. [PMID: 17650701]

Navid F et al. Great vessel and cardiac trauma: diagnostic and management strategies. Semin Thorac Cardiovasc Surg. 2008 Spring;20(1):31–8. [PMID: 18420124]

▼ THE CARDIAC PATIENT & SURGERY

There are now guidelines to help the physician and patient better define the risk of both cardiac and noncardiac surgery in heart patients. The easiest to use algorithms for cardiac surgery can be found on either of two websites: one includes the euroSCORE (euroSCORE.org/calc.html) and the other the STS (Society of Thoracic Surgeons) database that provides a longitudinal look at the risk of cardiac surgery (www.ctsnet.org/section/stsdatabase).

To assess the risk of noncardiac surgery, the guidelines from the ACC/AHA Task Force provide useful algorithms to help determine risk (www.acc.org or http://content.onlinejacc.org/cgi/content/full/50/17/e59).

▼ THE CARDIAC PATIENT & PREGNANCY

The management of cardiac disease in pregnancy is discussed in detail in the references listed below. Only a few major points can be covered in this brief section.

A comprehensive review of the safety of drugs in pregnancy and during breast-feeding can be found at www.perinatology.com/exposures/druglist.htm.

Elkayam U et al. Valvular heart disease and pregnancy: part I: native valves. J Am Coll Cardiol. 2005 Jul 19;46(2):223–30. [PMID: 16022946]

Elkayam U et al. Valvular heart disease and pregnancy: part II: prosthetic valves. J Am Coll Cardiol. 2005 Aug 2;46(3):403–10. [PMID: 16053950]

Warnes CA et al. ACC/AHA 2008 Guidelines for the Management of Adults With Congenital Heart Disease. A Report of the American College of Cardiology/American Heart Association Task Force on Practice Guidelines. Circulation. 2008 Dec 2;118(23):e714–833. [PMID: 18997169]

CARDIOVASCULAR COMPLICATIONS OF PREGNANCY

Pregnancy-related hypertension (eclampsia and pre-eclampsia) is discussed in Chapter 19.

1. Cardiomyopathy of Pregnancy (Peripartum Cardiomyopathy)

In approximately one of 4000–15,000 patients, dilated cardiomyopathy develops in the final month of pregnancy or within 6 months after delivery. The cause is unclear, but immune and viral causes have been postulated. More recently, it has been noted that the disease may be related to a cathepsin-D cleavage product of the hormone prolactin-suggesting blockage of prolactin may be a potential therapeutic strategy if proven in clinical trials using bromocriptine. The disease occurs more frequently in women over age 30 years, is generally related to the first or second pregnancy, and is associated with gestational hypertension and drugs used to stop uterine contractions. The course of the disease is variable; many cases improve or resolve completely over several months, but others progress to refractory heart failure. About 60% of patients make a complete recovery. Immunosuppressive therapy has been advocated, but few supportive data are available. Recently, β-blockers have been administered judiciously to these patients, with at least anecdotal success. Some advocate anticoagulation because of an increased risk for thrombotic events. Recurrence in subsequent pregnancies is common, particularly if cardiac function has not recovered.

Abboud J et al. Peripartum cardiomyopathy: a comprehensive review. Int J Cardiol. 2007 Jun 12;118(3):295–303. [PMID: 17208320]
Leinwand LA. Molecular events underlying pregnancy-induced cardiomyopathy. Cell. 2007 Feb 9;128(3):437–8. [PMID: 17289564]

2. Coronary Artery & Other Vascular Abnormalities

There have been a number of reports of myocardial infarction during pregnancy. It is known that pregnancy predisposes to dissection of the aorta and other arteries, perhaps because of the accompanying connective tissue changes. The risk may be particularly high in patients with Marfan or Ehlers-Danlos syndromes. However, coronary artery dissection is responsible for only a minority of the infarctions; most are caused by atherosclerotic CAD or coronary emboli. Most of the events occur near term or shortly following delivery, and paradoxical emboli through a PFO has been implicated in some cases. Clinical management is essentially similar to that of other patients with acute infarction, unless there is a connective tissue disorder. If nonatherosclerotic dissection is present, coronary intervention is risky as further dissection can be aggravated. In most instances, conservative management is warranted.

James AH et al. Acute myocardial infarction in pregnancy: a United States population-based study. Circulation. 2006 Mar 28;113(12):1564–71. [PMID: 16534011]

SPECIAL PROBLEMS

▷ Prophylaxis for Infective Endocarditis

The ACC/AHA Task Force addressing adults with congenital heart disease has formulated new guidelines outlining recommendations for pregnant women during labor and delivery.

There are no class 1 indications nor class 3 contraindications. The patients who should be considered for coverage with antibiotics during delivery include those who fall into the class 2A category (level of evidence: B).

In select patients with the highest risk of adverse outcomes, it is reasonable to consider antibiotic prophylaxis against infective endocarditis before vaginal delivery at the time of membrane rupture. This includes patients with the following indications: (1) prosthetic cardiac valve or prosthetic material used for cardiac valve repair, and (2) unrepaired and palliated cyanotic congenital heart disease, including surgically constructed palliative shunts conduits.

Warnes CA et al. ACC/AHA 2008 Guidelines for the Management of Adults With Congenital Heart Disease. A Report of the American College of Cardiology/American Heart Association Task Force on Practice Guidelines. Circulation. 2008 Dec 2;118(23):e714–833. [PMID: 18997169]
Wilson W et al. Prevention of infective endocarditis: guidelines from the American Heart Association: a guideline from the American Heart Association Rheumatic Fever, Endocarditis and Kawasaki Disease Committee, Council on Cardiovascular Disease in the Young, and the Council on Clinical Cardiology, Council on Cardiovascular Surgery and Anesthesia, and the Quality of Care and Outcomes Research Interdisciplinary Working Group. J Am Dent Assoc. 2007 Jun;138(6):739–45, 747–60. [PMID: 17545263]

▷ Management of Labor

Although vaginal delivery is usually well tolerated, unstable patients (including patients with severe hypertension and worsening heart failure) should have planned cesarean section. An increased risk of aortic rupture has been noted during delivery in patients with coarctation of the aorta and severe aortic root dilation with Marfan syndrome, and vaginal delivery should be avoided in these conditions. For most patients, even those with congenital heart disease, vaginal delivery is preferred.

▼ CARDIOVASCULAR SCREENING OF ATHLETES

The sudden death of a competitive athlete inevitably becomes an occasion for local if not national publicity. On each occasion, the public and the medical community ask whether such events could be prevented by more careful or complete screening. Although each event is tragic, it must be appreciated that there are approximately 5 million competitive athletes at the high school level or above in any given year. The number of cardiac deaths occurring during athletic participation is unknown, but estimates at the high school level range from one in 300,000 to one in 100,000 participants. Death rates among more mature athletes increase as the prevalence of CAD rises. These numbers highlight the problem of how to screen individual participants. Even an inexpensive test such as an ECG would generate an enormous cost if required of all athletes, and it is likely that few at-risk individuals would be detected. Echocardiography, either as a routine test or as a follow-up examination for abnormal ECGs, would be prohibitively expensive except for the elite professional athlete. Thus, the most feasible approach is that of a careful medical history and cardiac examination performed by personnel aware of the conditions responsible for most sudden deaths in competitive athletes. In a series of 158 athletic deaths in the United States between 1985 and 1995, hypertrophic cardiomyopathy (36%) and coronary anomalies (19%) were by far the most frequent underlying conditions. LV hypertrophy was present in another 10%, ruptured aorta (presumably due to Marfan syndrome or cystic medial necrosis) in 6%, myocarditis or dilated cardiomyopathy in 6%, aortic stenosis in 4%, and arrhythmogenic RV dysplasia in 3%. In addition, commotio cordis, or sudden death due to direct myocardial injury, may occur. More common in children, it may occur even after a minor direct blow to the heart; it is thought to be due to the precipitation of a premature ventricular contraction just prior to the peak of the T wave on ECG.

It is likely that a careful family and medical history and cardiovascular examination will identify some individuals at risk. A family history of premature sudden death or cardiovascular disease or of any of these predisposing conditions should mandate further workup, including an ECG and echocardiogram. Symptoms of chest pain, syncope, or near-syncope also warrant further evaluation. A Marfan-like appearance, significant elevation of BP or abnormalities of heart rate or rhythm, and pathologic heart murmurs or heart sounds should also be investigated before clearance for athletic participation is given. Such an evaluation is recommended before participation at the high school and college levels and every 2 years during athletic competition.

Stress-induced syncope or chest pressure may be the first clue to an anomalous origin of a coronary artery. Anatomically, this lesion occurs most often when the left anterior descending artery arises from the right coronary cusp and traverses between the aorta and pulmonary trunks. The "slit-like" orifice that results from the angulation at the vessel origin is thought to cause ischemia when the aorta and pulmonary arteries enlarge during rigorous exercise.

The toughest distinction may be in sorting out the healthy athlete with LVH from the athlete with hypertrophic cardiomyopathy. In general, the healthy athlete's heart is *less* likely to have an unusual pattern of LVH, LA enlargement, an abnormal ECG, an LV cavity < 45 mm in diameter at end-diastole, an abnormal diastolic filling pattern, a family history of hypertrophic cardiomyopathy, and the athlete is more likely to be male than the individual with hypertrophic cardiomyopathy.

Selective use of routine ECG and stress testing is recommended in men above age 40 years and women above age 50 years who continue to participate in vigorous exercise and at earlier ages when there is a positive family history for premature CAD, hypertrophic cardiomyopathy, or multiple risk factors.

Hosey RG. Sudden cardiac death. Clin Sports Med. 2003 Jan;22(1):51–66. [PMID: 12613086]

Maron BJ et al; Working Groups of the American Heart Association Committee on Exercise, Cardiac Rehabilitation, and Prevention; Councils on Clinical Cardiology and Cardiovascular Disease in the Young. Recommendations for physical activity and recreational sports participation for young patients with genetic cardiovascular diseases. Circulation. 2004 Jun 8;109(22):2807–16. [PMID: 15184297]

Systemic Hypertension

Michael Sutters, MD, MRCP (UK)

Sixty-six million Americans have elevated blood pressure (systolic blood pressure ≥ 140 mm Hg or diastolic blood pressure ≥ 90 mm Hg); of these, 63% are aware of their diagnosis, but only 45% are receiving treatment and only 34% are under control using a threshold criterion of 140/90 mm Hg. The prevalence of hypertension increases with age and is more common in blacks than in whites. The mortality rates for stroke and coronary heart disease, two of the major complications of hypertension, have declined by 50–60% over the past three decades but have recently leveled off. The numbers of patients with end-stage kidney disease and heart failure—two other conditions in which hypertension plays a major causative role—continue to rise.

Cardiovascular morbidity and mortality increase as both systolic and diastolic blood pressures rise, but in individuals over age 50 years, the systolic pressure and pulse pressure are better predictors of complications than diastolic pressure. Table 11–1 provides a summary of the classification and management of blood pressure in adults from the 7th Report of the U.S. Joint National Commission on Prevention, Detection, Evaluation, and Treatment of High Blood Pressure (JNC 7).

HOW IS BLOOD PRESSURE MEASURED AND HYPERTENSION DIAGNOSED?

Blood pressure should be measured with a well-calibrated sphygmomanometer. The bladder width within the cuff should encircle at least 80% of the arm circumference. Readings should be taken after the patient has been resting comfortably, back supported in the sitting or supine position, for at least 5 minutes and at least 30 minutes after smoking or coffee ingestion. A video demonstrating the correct technique can be found at http://content.nejm.org/cgi/video/360/5/e6/. Hypertension is diagnosed when systolic blood pressure is consistently elevated above 140 mm Hg, or diastolic blood pressure is above 90 mm Hg; a single elevated blood pressure reading is not sufficient to establish the diagnosis of hypertension. The major exceptions to this rule are hypertensive presentations with unequivocal evidence of life-threatening end-organ damage, as seen in hypertensive emergency, or in hypertensive urgency where blood pressure is > 220/125 mm Hg but life-threatening end-organ damage is absent. In less severe cases, the diagnosis of hypertension depends on a series of measurements of blood pressure, since readings can vary and tend to regress toward the mean with time. Patients whose initial blood pressure is in the hypertensive range exhibit the greatest fall toward the normal range between the first and second encounters. Although blood pressure readings may still show variability after the third visit, these later changes are mostly random. However, the concern for diagnostic precision needs to be balanced by an appreciation of the importance of establishing the diagnosis of hypertension as quickly as possible, since a 3-month delay in treatment of hypertension in high-risk patients is associated with a twofold increase in cardiovascular morbidity and mortality. The guidelines of the 2005 Canadian Hypertension Education Program provide an algorithm designed to expedite the diagnosis of hypertension (Figure 11–1). To this end, these guidelines recommend short intervals between the initial office visits and stress the importance of early identification of target organ damage which, if present, obviates the need for protracted confirmation of blood pressure elevation prior to pharmacologic intervention. The Canadian guidelines exploit the less volatile ambulatory and home blood pressure measurements as complements to office-based evaluations. Hypertension is diagnosed at lower levels when based on measurements taken outside the office environment. In addition to avoiding office-induced artifacts, ambulatory blood pressure measurements provide a more integrated view of blood pressure and the response to treatment. There is now evidence that ambulatory measurements are more reliable predictors of cardiovascular risk than measurements taken in the office. Blood pressure is normally lowest at night and the loss of this nocturnal dip is strongly associated with cardiovascular risk, particularly thrombotic stroke. An accentuation of the normal morning increase in blood pressure is associated with increased likelihood of cerebral hemorrhage.

PREHYPERTENSION

Data from the Framingham cohort indicate that blood pressure bears a linear relationship with cardiovascular risk down to a systolic blood pressure of 115 mm Hg; based on

Table 11–1. Classification and management of blood pressure for adults aged 18 years or older.

BP Classification	Systolic BP, mm Hg[1]		Diastolic BP, mm Hg[1]	Management		
					Initial Drug Therapy	
				Lifestyle Modification	Without Compelling Indication	With Compelling Indications[2]
Normal	< 120	and	< 80	Encourage		
Prehypertension	120–139	or	80–89	Yes	No antihypertensive drug indicated	Drug(s) for the compelling indications[3]
Stage 1 hypertension	140–159	or	90–99	Yes	Thiazide-type diuretics for most; may consider ACE inhibitor, ARB, β-blocker, CCB, or combination	Drug(s) for the compelling indications Other antihypertensive drugs (diuretics, ACE inhibitor, ARB, β-blocker, CCB) as needed
Stage 2 hypertension	≥ 160	or	≥ 100	Yes	Two-drug combination for most (usually thiazide-type diuretic and ACE inhibitor or ARB or β-blocker or CCB)[4]	Drug(s) for the compelling indications Other antihypertensive drugs (diuretics, ACE inhibitor, ARB, β-blocker, CCB) as needed

[1]Treatment determined by highest BP category.
[2]See Table 11–4.
[3]Treat patients with chronic kidney disease or diabetes to BP goal of < 130/80 mm Hg.
[4]Initial combined therapy should be used cautiously in those at risk for orthostatic hypotension.
ACE, angiotensin-converting enzyme; ARB, angiotensin receptor blocker; BP, blood pressure; CCB, calcium channel blocker.
Source: Chobanian AV et al. The Seventh Report of the Joint National Committee on Prevention, Detection, Evaluation, and Treatment of High Blood Pressure: the JNC 7 report. JAMA. 2003 May 21;289(19):2560–72.

these data, it is recommended that individuals with blood pressures in the gray area of 120–139/80–89 mm Hg be categorized as having prehypertension (Table 11–1). This demonstrates a trend away from defining hypertension as a simple numerical threshold and toward a more subtle appreciation of blood pressure as a component of overall cardiovascular risk. This trend gains support from increasing evidence for a relationship between blood pressure and disruption of cardiovascular function at levels below the hypertensive threshold. Because prehypertension often develops into hypertension (50% of people within 4 years), even low-risk prehypertensive patients should be monitored annually. Circumspection about labeling patients as hypertensive is warranted since there is evidence that simply telling someone that he or she has hypertension has unintended consequences, transforming a perception of general health into one of general ill-health.

Chobanian AV. Prehypertension revisited. Hypertension. 2006 Nov;48(5):812–4. [PMID: 16982962]
Chobanian AV et al. The Seventh Report of the Joint National Committee on Prevention, Detection, Evaluation, and Treatment of High Blood Pressure: the JNC 7 Report. JAMA. 2003 May 21;289(19):2560–72. [PMID: 12748199]
Dolan E et al. Superiority of ambulatory over clinic blood pressure measurement in predicting mortality: the Dublin outcome study. Hypertension. 2005 Jul;46(1):156–61. [PMID: 15939805]
Metoki H et al. Prognostic significance of night-time, early morning, and daytime blood pressures on the risk of cerebrovascular and cardiovascular mortality: the Ohasama Study. J Hypertens. 2006 Sep;24(9):1841–8. [PMID: 16915034]
Padwal RJ et al. The 2008 Canadian Hypertension Education Program recommendations for the management of hypertension: Part 1 - blood pressure measurement, diagnosis and assessment of risk. Can J Cardiol. 2008 Jun;24(6):455–63. [PMID: 18548142]
Williams B et al; British Hypertension Society. Guidelines for management of hypertension: Report of the Fourth Working Party of the British Hypertension Society, 2004-BHS IV. J Hum Hypertens. 2004 Mar;18(3):139–85. [PMID: 14973512]

APPROACH TO HYPERTENSION

▶ Etiology & Classification

A. Primary (Essential) Hypertension

Primary (essential) hypertension is the term applied to the 95% of cases in which no cause for hypertension can be identified. When there is no identifiable cause of hypertension, it is most often the result of complex interactions between multiple genetic and environmental factors, but the proportion regarded as "primary/essential" will diminish with improved detection of clearly defined secondary causes and with better understanding of pathophysiology. Primary or essential hypertension occurs in 10–15% of white adults and 20–30% of black adults in the United States. The onset is usually between ages 25 and 55 years; it is uncommon before age 20 years. The best understood endogenous and environmental determinants of blood pressure are discussed below.

1. Sympathetic nervous system hyperactivity—This is most apparent in younger persons with hypertension, who

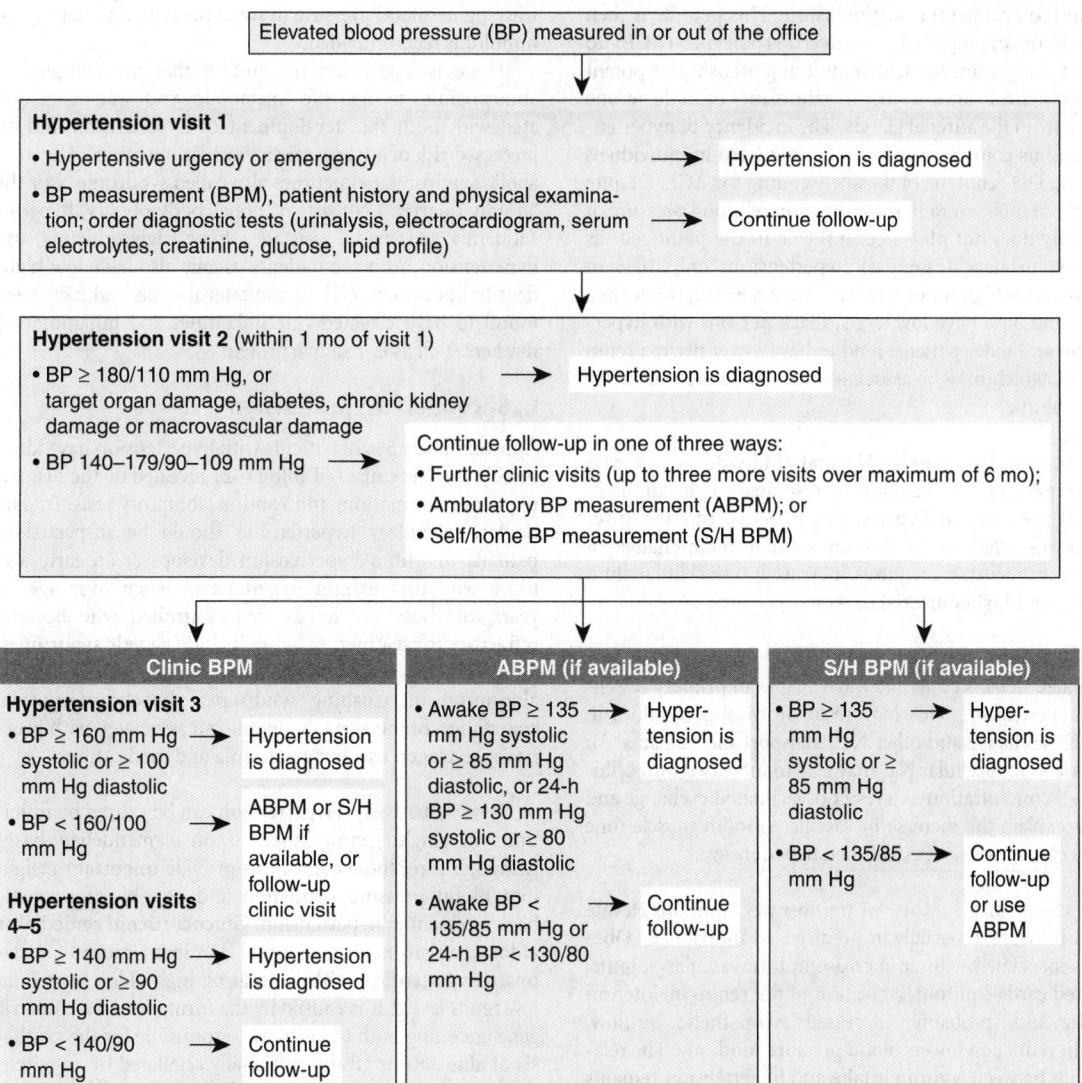

▲ **Figure 11–1.** The 2005 Canadian Hypertension Education Program recommendations for the assessment and diagnosis of hypertension. Patients with an elevated blood pressure measured during visits 4–5 may still have white-coat (office-induced) hypertension. (Applying the 2005 Canadian Hypertension Education Program recommendations: 1. Diagnosis of hypertension—Reprinted, with permission from CMAJ 30-Aug-05; 173(5), Page(s) 480–483. © 2005 CMA Media Inc.)

may exhibit tachycardia and an elevated cardiac output. However, correlations between plasma catecholamines and blood pressure are poor. Insensitivity of the baroreflexes may play a role in the genesis of adrenergic hyperactivity.

2. Abnormal cardiovascular or renal development—
The normal cardiovascular system develops so that elasticity of the great arteries is matched to the resistance in the periphery to optimize large vessel pressure waves. In this way, myocardial oxygen consumption is minimized and coronary flow maximized. Elevated blood pressure later in life could arise from abnormal development of aortic elasticity or reduced development of the microvascular network. This has been postulated as the sequence of events in

low birth weight infants, who have an increased risk of hypertension developing in adulthood. Another hypothesis proposes that the association between low birth weight and hypertension arises from reduced nephron number.

3. Renin–angiotensin system activity—Renin, a proteolytic enzyme, is secreted by cells surrounding glomerular afferent arterioles in response to a number of stimuli, including reduced renal perfusion pressure, diminished intravascular volume, circulating catecholamines, increased sympathetic nervous system activity, increased arteriolar stretch, and hypokalemia. Plasma renin levels are classified in relation to dietary sodium intake or urinary sodium excretion. Renin acts on angiotensinogen to cleave off the ten-amino-acid peptide angiotensin I. This peptide is then acted upon by angiotensin-converting enzyme (ACE) to create the eight-amino-acid peptide angiotensin II, a potent vasoconstrictor and a major stimulant of aldosterone release from the adrenal glands. The incidence of hypertension and its complications may be increased in individuals with the DD genotype of the allele coding for ACE. Despite the role of this system in the regulation of blood pressure, it probably does not play a central role in the pathogenesis of most primary (essential) hypertension; only 10% of patients have high renin activity, whereas 60% have normal levels, and 30% have low levels. Black persons with hypertension and older patients tend to have lower plasma renin activity, which may be associated with expanded intravascular volume.

4. Defect in natriuresis—Normal individuals increase their renal sodium excretion in response to elevations in arterial pressure. In hypertensive patients, this pressure-natriuresis relationship is reset so that maintenance of sodium homeostasis requires increased extracellular fluid volume and higher arterial pressure.

5. Intracellular sodium and calcium—Intracellular Na^+ is elevated in blood cells and other tissues in primary (essential) hypertension. This may result from abnormalities in Na^+–K^+ exchange and other Na^+ transport mechanisms. An increase in intracellular Na^+ may lead to increased intracellular Ca^{2+} concentration as a result of facilitated exchange and might explain the increase in vascular smooth muscle tone that is characteristic of established hypertension.

6. Exacerbating factors—A number of conditions elevate blood pressure, especially in predisposed individuals. **Obesity** is associated with an increase in intravascular volume, elevated cardiac output, activation of the renin-angiotensin system and, probably, increased sympathetic outflow. Weight reduction lowers blood pressure modestly. The relationship between **sodium intake** and hypertension remains controversial, but dietary salt restriction is recommended in patients with elevated blood pressure (see below).

Excessive use of **alcohol** also raises blood pressure, perhaps by increasing plasma catecholamines. Hypertension can be difficult to control in patients who consume more than 40 g of ethanol (two drinks) daily or drink in "binges." **Cigarette smoking** raises blood pressure, again by increasing plasma norepinephrine. Although the long-term effect of smoking on blood pressure is less clear, the synergistic effects of smoking and high blood pressure on cardiovascular risk are well documented. The relationship of **exercise** to hypertension is variable. Aerobic exercise lowers blood pressure in previously sedentary individuals, but increasingly strenuous exercise in already active subjects has less effect. The relationship between stress and hypertension is not established. **Polycythemia,** whether primary or due to diminished plasma volume, increases blood viscosity and may raise blood pressure. **Nonsteroidal anti-inflammatory drugs (NSAIDs)** produce increases in blood pressure averaging 5 mm Hg and are best avoided in patients with borderline or elevated blood pressures. Low **potassium intake** is associated

with higher blood pressure in some patients; an intake of 90 mmol/d is recommended.

There is a growing recognition that the complex of abnormalities termed the "metabolic syndrome" is associated with both the development of hypertension and an increased risk of adverse cardiovascular outcomes. The metabolic syndrome (sometimes also called syndrome X or the "deadly quartet") consists of upper body obesity, hyperinsulinemia and insulin resistance, hypertriglyceridemia, and hypertension. Affected patients usually also have low high-density lipoprotein (HDL) cholesterol levels and have been found to have elevated catecholamines and inflammatory markers such as C-reactive protein.

B. Secondary Hypertension

Approximately 5% of patients with hypertension have identifiable specific causes (Table 11–2) revealed by the history, physical examination, and routine laboratory tests. In particular, secondary hypertension should be suspected in patients in whom hypertension develops at an early age, those who first exhibit hypertension when over age 50 years, or those previously well controlled who become refractory to treatment. Causes include genetic syndromes, kidney disease, renal vascular hypertension, primary hyperaldosteronism, Cushing syndrome, pheochromocytoma, coarctation of the aorta, hypertension associated with pregnancy, estrogen use, hypercalcemia and medications.

1. Genetic causes—Hypertension can be caused by mutations in single genes, inherited on a mendelian basis. Although rare, these conditions provide important insight into blood pressure regulation and possibly the genetic basis of essential hypertension. **Glucocorticoid remediable aldosteronism** is an autosomal dominant cause of early-onset hypertension with normal or high aldosterone and low renin levels. It is caused by the formation of a chimeric gene encoding both the enzyme responsible for the synthesis of aldosterone (transcriptionally regulated by angiotensin II) and an enzyme responsible for synthesis of cortisol (transcriptionally regulated by ACTH). As a consequence, aldosterone synthesis becomes driven by ACTH, which can

Table 11–2. Identifiable causes of hypertension.

Sleep apnea
Drug-induced or drug-related
Chronic kidney disease
Primary aldosteronism
Renovascular disease
Long-term corticosteroid therapy and Cushing syndrome
Pheochromocytoma
Coarctation of the aorta
Thyroid or parathyroid disease

Source: Chobanian AV et al. The Seventh Report of the Joint National Committee on Prevention, Detection, Evaluation, and Treatment of High Blood Pressure: the JNC 7 report. JAMA. 2003 May 21;289(19):2560–72.

be suppressed by exogenous cortisol. In the **syndrome of apparent mineralocorticoid excess**, early-onset hypertension with hypokalemic metabolic alkalosis is inherited on an autosomal recessive basis. Although plasma renin is low and plasma aldosterone level is very low in these patients, aldosterone antagonists are effective in controlling hypertension. This disease is caused by loss of the enzyme, 11β-hydroxysteroid dehydrogenase, which normally metabolizes cortisol and thus protects the otherwise "promiscuous" mineralocorticoid receptor in the distal nephron from inappropriate glucocorticoid activation. Similarly, glycyrrhetinic acid, found in licorice, causes increased blood pressure through inhibition of 11β-hydroxysteroid dehydrogenase. The syndrome of **hypertension exacerbated in pregnancy** is inherited as an autosomal dominant trait. In these patients, a mutation in the mineralocorticoid receptor makes it abnormally responsive to progesterone and, paradoxically, to spironolactone. **Liddle syndrome** is an autosomal dominant condition characterized by early-onset hypertension, hypokalemic alkalosis, low renin and low aldosterone levels. This is caused by a mutation that results in constitutive activation of the epithelial sodium channel of the distal nephron, with resultant unregulated sodium reabsorption and volume expansion.

2. Renal disease—Renal parenchymal disease is the most common cause of secondary hypertension. Hypertension may result from diabetic and inflammatory glomerular diseases, tubular interstitial disease, and polycystic kidneys. Most cases are related to increased intravascular volume or increased activity of the renin–angiotensin–aldosterone system.

3. Renal vascular hypertension—Renal artery stenosis is present in 1–2% of hypertensive patients. Its cause in most younger individuals is fibromuscular hyperplasia, particularly in women under 50 years of age. The remainder of renal vascular disease is due to atherosclerotic stenoses of the proximal renal arteries. The mechanism of hypertension is excessive renin release due to reduction in renal blood flow and perfusion pressure.

Renal vascular hypertension should be suspected in the following circumstances: (1) if the documented onset is before age 20 or after age 50 years, (2) hypertension is resistant to three or more drugs, (3) if there are epigastric or renal artery bruits, (4) if there is atherosclerotic disease of the aorta or peripheral arteries (15–25% of patients with symptomatic lower limb atherosclerotic vascular disease have renal artery stenosis), (5) if there is abrupt deterioration in kidney function after administration of ACE inhibitors, or (6) if episodes of pulmonary edema are associated with abrupt surges in blood pressure. There is no ideal screening test for renal vascular hypertension. If suspicion is sufficiently high and endovascular intervention is a viable option, renal arteriography, the definitive diagnostic test, is the best approach. Renal arteriography is not recommended as a routine adjunct to coronary studies. Where suspicion is moderate to low, noninvasive angiography using magnetic resonance (MR) or CT are reasonable approaches. With improvements in technology, Doppler

sonography may play an increasing role in detection of RAS, providing physiologic indices of stenosis severity and ease of repeated examination to detect progression. However, results of all these modalities vary greatly between institutions. In 2006, a public health advisory was issued regarding the use of gadolinium (a contrast agent used in MRA), warning that it might precipitate nephrogenic systemic fibrosis in patients with advanced kidney disease. Clearly, no diagnostic study should be undertaken without a careful consideration of the risk-benefit ratio. In young patients with fibromuscular disease, angioplasty is very effective, but there is controversy regarding the best approach to the treatment of atheromatous renal artery stenosis. Correction of the stenosis in selected patients might reduce the number of medications required to control blood pressure and could protect kidney function, but the extent of preexisting parenchymal damage to the affected and contralateral kidney has a significant influence on both blood pressure and kidney function outcomes following revascularization. A reasonable approach advocates medical therapy as long as hypertension can be well controlled and there is no progression of kidney disease. The addition of a statin should be considered. Endovascular intervention might be considered in patients with uncontrollable hypertension, progressive kidney disease, or episodic pulmonary edema attributable to the lesion. Angioplasty might also be warranted when progression of stenosis is either demonstrated or is predicted by a constellation of risk factors, including systolic blood pressure > 160 mm Hg, advanced age, diabetes mellitus, and high-grade stenosis (> 60%) at the time of diagnosis. However, conclusive outcomes data to guide management are still awaited. Although ACE inhibitors have improved the success rate of medical therapy of hypertension due to renal artery stenosis, they have been associated with marked hypotension and (usually reversible) kidney dysfunction in individuals with bilateral disease. Thus, kidney function and blood pressure should be closely monitored during the first weeks of therapy in patients in whom this is a consideration.

4. Primary hyperaldosteronism—Over the past decade, studies have suggested that primary hyperaldosteronism might account for some 10% of essential hypertension. However, this could be an overestimate due to sampling bias and problems with the specificity of a screening test based on the measurement of plasma aldosterone concentration (normal: 1–16 ng/dL) and plasma renin activity (normal: 1–2.5 ng/mL/h) and calculation of the plasma aldosterone/renin ratio (normal < 30). This is because "bottoming out" of renin assays leads to exponential increases in the plasma aldosterone/renin ratio even when aldosterone levels are normal. Hence, an elevated plasma aldosterone/renin ratio should probably not be taken as evidence of hyperaldosteronism unless the aldosterone level is actually elevated. The primacy of aldosterone in driving hypertension in low-renin patients has been questioned because spironolactone, which is uniquely potent in hyperaldosteronism, seems to be no more effective at lowering blood pressure than thiazide diuretics in low renin hypertensive patients. The lesion responsible for hyperaldosteronism is an adrenal adenoma or bilateral adrenal hyperplasia and can be demonstrated by CT or MRI scanning. Screening is appropriate in patients with resistant hypertension, (needing more than three drugs for control) and those with spontaneous or thiazide-induced hypokalemia, incidentaloma, or family history of primary hyperaldosteronism.

Medications that alter renin and aldosterone levels, including ACE inhibitors, angiotensin receptor blockers (ARBs), diuretics (especially spironolactone), β-blockers, and clonidine, should be discontinued at least a week before sampling. Calcium channel and α-receptor blockers can be used to control blood pressure during this drug washout period. Based on this approach, patients with aldosterone/renin ratios of ≥ 30 with a plasma aldosterone level > 15 ng/dL might require further evaluation for primary hyperaldosteronism.

5. Cushing syndrome—Among those with spontaneous Cushing syndrome, hypertension occurs in about 75–85% of patients. The exact pathogenesis of the hypertension is unclear. It may be related to salt and water retention from the mineralocorticoid effects of the excess glucocorticoid. Alternatively, it may be due to increased secretion of angiotensinogen. In addition, glucocorticoids exert permissive effects on vascular tone by a variety of mechanisms.

Diagnosis and treatment of Cushing syndrome are discussed in Chapter 26.

6. Pheochromocytoma—Pheochromocytomas are uncommon; they are probably found in less than 0.1% of all patients with hypertension and in approximately two individuals per million population. However, autopsy studies indicate that pheochromocytomas are very often undiagnosed in life. The blood pressure elevation caused by the catecholamine excess results from two mechanisms: α-receptor-mediated vasoconstriction of arterioles, leading to an increase in peripheral resistance, and β_1-receptor-mediated increases in cardiac output and in renin release, leading to increased circulating levels of angiotensin II. The increased total peripheral vascular resistance is probably primarily responsible for the maintenance of high arterial pressures. Chronic vasoconstriction of the arterial and venous beds leads to a reduction in plasma volume and predisposes to postural hypotension. Glucose intolerance develops in some patients. Hypertensive crisis in pheochromocytoma may be precipitated by a variety of drugs, including tricyclic antidepressants, antidopaminergic agents, metoclopramide, and naloxone. The diagnosis and treatment of pheochromocytoma are discussed in Chapter 26.

7. Coarctation of the aorta—This uncommon cause of hypertension is discussed in Chapter 10.

8. Hypertension associated with pregnancy—Hypertension occurring de novo or worsening during pregnancy, including preeclampsia and eclampsia, is one of the most common causes of maternal and fetal morbidity and mortality (see Chapter 19).

9. Estrogen use—A small increase in blood pressure occurs in most women taking oral contraceptives, but considerable increases are noted occasionally. This is caused by volume expansion due to increased hepatic synthesis of renin substrate and consequent activation of the renin–angiotensin–aldosterone system. Five percent of women taking long-term oral contraceptives exhibit a rise in blood pressure above 140/90 mm Hg, twice the expected prevalence. Contraceptive-related hypertension is more common in women over 35 years of age, in those who have taken contraceptives for more than 5 years, and in obese individuals. It is less common in those taking low-dose estrogen tablets. In most, hypertension is reversible by discontinuing the contraceptive, but it may take several weeks. Postmenopausal estrogen does not generally cause hypertension, but rather maintains endothelium-mediated vasodilation.

10. Other causes of secondary hypertension—Hypertension has also been associated with hypercalcemia due to any cause: acromegaly, hyperthyroidism, hypothyroidism, baroreceptor denervation, compression of the rostral ventrolateral medulla, and increased intracranial pressure. A number of medications may cause or exacerbate hypertension—most importantly cyclosporine, tacrolimus, angiogenesis inhibitors, decongestants, and NSAIDs; cocaine and alcohol should also be considered.

▶ **When to Refer**

Referral to a hypertension specialist should be considered in cases of severe, resistant or early/late onset hypertension or when secondary hypertension is suggested by screening.

Gonzaga CC et al. Resistant hypertension and hyperaldosteronism. Curr Hypertens Rep. 2008 Dec;10(6):496–503. [PMID: 18959838]

Hollenberg NK et al. Nonmodulation and essential hypertension. Curr Hypertens Rep. 2006 May;8(2):127–31. [PMID: 16672145]

Hood SJ et al. The spironolactone, amiloride, losartan, and thiazide (SALT) double-blind crossover trial in patients with low-renin hypertension and elevated aldosterone-renin ratio. Circulation. 2007 Jul 17;116(3):268–75. [PMID: 17606839]

Karagiannis A et al. Pheochromocytoma: an update on genetics and management. Endocr Relat Cancer. 2007 Dec;14(4):935–56. [PMID: 18045948]

Messerli FH et al. Essential hypertension. Lancet. 2007 Aug 18;370(9587):591–603. [PMID: 17707755]

Schirpenbach C et al. Primary aldosteronism: current knowledge and controversies in Conn's syndrome. Nat Clin Pract Endocrinol Metab. 2007 Mar;3(3):220–7. [PMID: 17315030]

Textor SC. Renovascular hypertension in 2007: where are we now? Curr Cardiol Rep. 2007 Nov;9(6):453–61. [PMID: 17999870]

▶ **Complications of Untreated Hypertension**

Complications of hypertension are related either to sustained elevations of blood pressure, with consequent changes in the vasculature and heart, or to atherosclerosis that accompanies and is accelerated by long-standing hypertension. Most of the adverse outcomes in hypertension are associated with thrombosis rather than bleeding, possibly because increased vascular shear stress converts the normally anticoagulant endothelium to a prothrombotic state. The excess morbidity and mortality related to hypertension are progressive over the whole range of systolic and diastolic blood pressures; the risk approximately doubles for each 6 mm Hg increase in diastolic blood pressure. However, target-organ damage varies markedly between individuals with similar levels of office hypertension; ambulatory pressures are superior to office readings in the prediction of end-organ damage.

A. Hypertensive Cardiovascular Disease

Cardiac complications are the major causes of morbidity and mortality in primary (essential) hypertension, and preventing them is a major goal of therapy. Electrocardiographic evidence of left ventricular hypertrophy is found in up to 15% of persons with chronic hypertension. For any level of blood pressure, its presence is associated with incremental cardiovascular risk. Echocardiographic left ventricular hypertrophy is a powerful predictor of prognosis. Left ventricular hypertrophy may cause or facilitate many cardiac complications of hypertension, including congestive heart failure, ventricular arrhythmias, myocardial ischemia, and sudden death.

Left ventricular diastolic dysfunction, which may present with all of the symptoms and signs of congestive heart failure, is common in patients with long-standing hypertension. The occurrence of heart failure is reduced by 50% with antihypertensive therapy. Hypertensive left ventricular hypertrophy regresses with therapy and is most closely related to the degree of systolic blood pressure reduction. Diuretics have produced equal or greater reductions of left ventricular mass when compared with other drug classes. β-Blockers are less effective in reducing left ventricular hypertrophy but play a specific role in patients with established coronary artery disease or impaired left ventricular function.

B. Hypertensive Cerebrovascular Disease and Dementia

Hypertension is the major predisposing cause of hemorrhagic and ischemic stroke. Cerebrovascular complications are more closely correlated with systolic than diastolic blood pressure. The incidence of these complications is markedly reduced by antihypertensive therapy. Preceding hypertension is associated with a higher incidence of subsequent dementia of both vascular and Alzheimer types. Effective blood pressure control may reduce the risk of development of cognitive dysfunction later in life, but once cerebral small vessel disease is established, low blood pressure might exacerbate this problem.

C. Hypertensive Kidney Disease

Chronic hypertension leads to nephrosclerosis, a common cause of chronic kidney disease; aggressive blood pressure control attenuates the process. In patients with hypertensive nephropathy, the blood pressure should be 130/80 mm Hg or lower, especially when proteinuria is present. Secondary kidney disease is more common in blacks, particularly when accompanied by diabetes mellitus. Hypertension also plays an important role in accelerating the progression of all forms of kidney disease.

D. Aortic Dissection

Hypertension is a contributing factor in many patients with dissection of the aorta. Its diagnosis and treatment are discussed in Chapter 12.

E. Atherosclerotic Complications

Most Americans with hypertension die of complications of atherosclerosis, but the link between hypertension and atherosclerotic cardiovascular disease is not as clear as that with the previously discussed complications. Effective antihypertensive therapy is thus less successful in preventing complications of coronary heart disease.

Blacher J et al. Large-artery stiffness, hypertension and cardiovascular risk in older patients. Nat Clin Pract Cardiovasc Med. 2005 Sep;2(9):450–5. [PMID: 16265585]

Hill GS. Hypertensive nephrosclerosis. Curr Opin Nephrol Hypertens. 2008 May;17(3):266–70. [PMID: 18408477]

Persu A et al. Recent insights in the development of organ damage caused by hypertension. Acta Cardiol. 2004 Aug;59(4):369–81. [PMID: 15368798]

Qiu C et al. The age-dependent relation of blood pressure to cognitive function and dementia. Lancet Neurol. 2005 Aug;4(8):487–99. [PMID: 16033691]

► Clinical Findings

The clinical and laboratory findings are mainly referable to involvement of the target organs: heart, brain, kidneys, eyes, and peripheral arteries.

A. Symptoms

Mild to moderate primary (essential) hypertension is largely asymptomatic for many years. The most frequent symptom, headache, is also very nonspecific. Accelerated hypertension is associated with somnolence, confusion, visual disturbances, and nausea and vomiting (hypertensive encephalopathy).

Hypertension in patients with pheochromocytomas that secrete predominantly norepinephrine is usually sustained but may be episodic. The typical attack lasts from minutes to hours and is associated with headache, anxiety, palpitation, profuse perspiration, pallor, tremor, and nausea and vomiting. Blood pressure is markedly elevated, and angina or acute pulmonary edema may occur. In primary aldosteronism, patients may have muscular weakness, polyuria, and nocturia due to hypokalemia; malignant hypertension is rare. Chronic hypertension often leads to left ventricular hypertrophy, which can present with exertional and paroxysmal nocturnal dyspnea. Cerebral involvement causes stroke due to thrombosis or hemorrhage from microaneurysms of small penetrating intracranial arteries. Hypertensive encephalopathy is probably caused by acute capillary congestion and exudation with cerebral edema, which is reversible.

B. Signs

Like symptoms, physical findings depend on the cause of hypertension, its duration and severity, and the degree of effect on target organs.

1. Blood pressure—Blood pressure is taken in both arms and, if lower extremity pulses are diminished or delayed, in the legs to exclude coarctation of the aorta. An orthostatic drop is present in pheochromocytoma. Older patients may have falsely elevated readings by sphygmomanometry because of noncompressible vessels. This may be suspected in the presence of Osler sign—a palpable brachial or radial artery when the cuff is inflated above systolic pressure. Occasionally, it may be necessary to make direct measurements of intra-arterial pressure, especially in patients with apparent severe hypertension who do not tolerate therapy.

2. Retinas—Narrowing of arterial diameter to less than 50% of venous diameter, copper or silver wire appearance, exudates, hemorrhages, or papilledema are associated with a worse prognosis.

3. Heart—A left ventricular heave indicates severe or long-standing hypertrophy. Aortic insufficiency may be auscultated in up to 5% of patients, and hemodynamically insignificant aortic insufficiency can be detected by Doppler echocardiography in 10–20%. A presystolic (S4) gallop due to decreased compliance of the left ventricle is quite common in patients in sinus rhythm.

4. Pulses—Radial-femoral delay suggests coarctation of the aorta; loss of peripheral pulses occurs due to atherosclerosis, less commonly aortic dissection, and rarely Takayasu arteritis, all of which can involve the renal arteries.

C. Laboratory Findings

Recommended testing includes the following: hemoglobin; urinalysis and renal function studies, to detect hematuria, proteinuria, and casts, signifying primary kidney disease or nephrosclerosis; fasting blood sugar level, since hypertension is a risk factor for the development of diabetes and hyperglycemia can be a presenting feature of pheochromocytoma; plasma lipids, as an indicator of atherosclerosis risk and an additional target for therapy; serum uric acid which, if elevated, is a relative contraindication to diuretic therapy; and serum electrolytes. Measurement of the plasma aldosterone/renin ratio is indicated to screen for mineralocorticoid excess in hypertensive patients with hypokalemic alkalosis (even if they are taking diuretics), resistant hypertension, or an adrenal incidentaloma (see Primary Hyperaldosteronism, above).

D. Electrocardiography and Chest Radiographs

Electrocardiographic criteria are highly specific but not very sensitive for left ventricular hypertrophy. The "strain" pattern of ST–T wave changes is a sign of more advanced disease and is associated with a poor prognosis. A chest radiograph is not necessary in the workup for uncomplicated hypertension.

E. Echocardiography

The primary role of echocardiography should be to evaluate patients with clinical symptoms or signs of cardiac disease.

F. Diagnostic Studies

Additional diagnostic studies are indicated only if the clinical presentation or routine tests suggest secondary or complicated hypertension. These may include tests such as 24-hour urine free cortisol, plasma metanephrines and the plasma aldosterone/renin ratio for endocrine causes of hypertension, renal ultrasound to diagnose primary kidney disease (polycystic kidneys, obstructive uropathy), and testing for renal artery stenosis. Further evaluation may include abdominal imaging studies (ultrasound, CT scan, or MRI) or renal arteriography.

G. Summary

Since most hypertension is "primary," few studies are necessary beyond those listed above. If conventional therapy is unsuccessful or if symptoms suggest a secondary cause, further studies are indicated.

Wong TY et al. The eye in hypertension. Lancet. 2007 Feb 3;369(9559):425–35. [PMID: 17276782]

▶ Nonpharmacologic Therapy

Lifestyle modification may have an impact on morbidity and mortality. A diet rich in fruits, vegetables, and low-fat dairy foods and low in saturated and total fats (DASH diet) has been shown to lower blood pressure. Additional measures, listed in Table 11–3, can prevent or mitigate hypertension or its cardiovascular consequences.

All patients with high-normal or elevated blood pressures, those who have a family history of cardiovascular complications of hypertension, and those who have multiple coronary risk factors should be counseled about nonpharmacologic approaches to lowering blood pressure. Approaches of proved but modest value include weight reduction, reduced alcohol consumption and, in some patients, reduced salt intake. Gradually increasing activity levels should be encouraged in previously sedentary patients, but strenuous exercise training programs in already active individuals may have less benefit. Calcium and potassium supplements have been advocated, but their ability to lower blood pressure is limited. Smoking cessation will reduce overall cardiovascular risk. Overall, the effects of lifestyle modification on blood pressure are modest. Although all patients should be urged to modify risk factors, medication is likely to be required for optimal blood pressure control in stage 1 hypertension.

Cook NR et al. Trials of Hypertension Prevention Collaborative Research Group. Joint effects of sodium and potassium intake on subsequent cardiovascular disease: the Trials of Hypertension Prevention follow-up study. Arch Intern Med. 2009 Jan 12;169(1):32–40. [PMID: 19139321]

Elmer PJ et al; PREMIER Collaborative Research Group. Effects of comprehensive lifestyle modification on diet, weight, physical fitness, and blood pressure control: 18-month results of a randomized trial. Ann Intern Med. 2006 Apr 4;144(7):485–95. [PMID: 16585662]

Stewart KJ et al. Effect of exercise on blood pressure in older persons: a randomized controlled trial. Arch Intern Med. 2005 Apr 11;165(7):756–62. [PMID: 15824294]

Table 11-3. Lifestyle modifications to manage hypertension.[1]

Modification	Recommendation	Approximate Systolic BP Reduction, Range
Weight reduction	Maintain normal body weight (BMI, 18.5–24.9)	5–20 mm Hg/10-kg weight loss
Adopt DASH eating plan	Consume a diet rich in fruits, vegetables, and low-fat dairy products with a reduced content of saturated fat and total fat	8–14 mm Hg
Dietary sodium reduction	Reduce dietary sodium intake to no more than 100 mEq/d (2.4 g sodium or 6 g sodium chloride)	2–8 mm Hg
Physical activity	Engage in regular aerobic physical activity such as brisk walking (at least 30 minutes per day, most days of the week)	4–9 mm Hg
Moderation of alcohol consumption	Limit consumption to no more than two drinks per day (1 oz or 30 mL ethanol [eg, 24 oz beer, 10 oz wine, or 3 oz 80-proof whiskey]) in most men and no more than one drink per day in women and lighter-weight persons	2–4 mm Hg

[1]For overall cardiovascular risk reduction, stop smoking. The effects of implementing these modifications are dose and time dependent and could be higher for some individuals.
BMI, body mass index calculated as weight in kilograms divided by the square of height in meters; BP, blood pressure; DASH, Dietary Approaches to Stop Hypertension.
Source: Chobanian AV et al. The Seventh Report of the Joint National Committee on Prevention, Detection, Evaluation, and Treatment of High Blood Pressure: the JNC 7 report. JAMA. 2003 May 21;289(19):2560–72.

Swift PA et al. Modest salt reduction reduces blood pressure and urine protein excretion in black hypertensives: a randomized control trial. Hypertension. 2005 Aug;46(2):308–12. [PMID: 15983240]

Who Should Be Treated with Medications?

The decision to initiate drug therapy is relatively straightforward once hypertension has been unequivocally diagnosed (Table 11–1 and Figure 11–1), but less clear in persons with prehypertension (blood pressure of 120–139/80–89 mm Hg). Some experts have suggested that early blood pressure elevation, and perhaps antecedent metabolic abnormalities, lead to vascular damage that propels further blood pressure elevation in an ever accelerating spiral of progression. If so, then interception early in the course might modify the natural history of the disease, leading to diminished requirements for multiple antihypertensive agents and, perhaps, a much more dramatic effect on cardiovascular risk than can be attained with initiation of treatment once hypertension is established. In beginning to address this question, the TROPHY study showed that treatment of prehypertension in a population at no particular risk for cardiovascular events only seemed to delay the onset of hypertension, since blood pressure in the treated group increased toward the placebo group when treatment was discontinued. The situation is a little clearer in nonhypertensive patients at elevated cardiovascular risk, in whom the HOPE and PROGRESS trials indicated improved outcomes with antihypertensive medication (ACE inhibitor and ACE inhibitor plus diuretic, respectively). These observations have prompted some to think in terms of "optimizing" blood pressure to a suggested 120/80 mm Hg. However, the public health consequences of recommendations to treat prehypertension would be enormous. Forty-eight percent of all Americans have hypertension or prehypertension, and much higher proportions fit these categories in a typical family medicine population. The JNC 7 guidelines suggest that antihypertensive medications be offered to persons with prehypertension with compelling indications for treatment such as chronic kidney disease or diabetes mellitus (Table 11–4). According to the British Hypertension Society (BHS) recommendations, risk analysis should be used to target treatment to patients with borderline hypertension who are most likely to benefit, particularly individuals at high combined risk of coronary heart or stroke event (> 20–30% within 10 years) (Figure 11–2). Risk is calculated according to Framingham study criteria (calculated from several of the risk factors listed in Table 11–5). A low-risk patient with blood pressure between 120–139/80–89 mm Hg may be advised to make lifestyle modifications (Table 11–3) and be monitored without receiving an absolute diagnosis of prehypertension. A risk calculation tool can be downloaded from http://www.bhsoc.org/Cardiovascular_Risk_Charts_and_Calculators.stm (in using this tool, convert serum cholesterol from mg/dL to mmol/L by dividing by 38.7). A free PDA-based coronary heart disease risk calculator is available at http://www.statcoder.com/cholesterol.htm. In general, 20% total cardiovascular risk (which includes stroke) is equivalent to 15% coronary heart disease risk.

Goals of Treatment

Treatment should ideally be offered to all persons in whom blood pressure reduction, irrespective of initial blood pressure levels, will reduce overall cardiovascular risk (see above). Blood pressure targets for hypertensive patients at the greatest risk for cardiovascular events, particularly patients with diabetes and those with chronic kidney disease, should be lower (< 130/80 mm Hg) than for individuals at lower total cardiovascular risk (< 140/90 mm Hg). However, since there does not seem to be a blood pressure level below which risk plateaus, these recommendations should be taken

Table 11–4. Clinical trial and guideline basis for compelling indications for individual drug classes.[1]

High-Risk Conditions with Compelling Indication[2]	Recommended Drugs						Clinical Trial Basis
	Diuretic	β-Blockers	ACE Inhibitors	ARB	CCB	Aldosterone Antagonist	
Heart failure	•	•	•	•		•	ACC/AHA Heart Failure Guideline, MERIT-HF, COPERNICUS, CIBIS, SOLVD, AIRE, TRACE, ValHEFT, RALES
Post-myocardial infarction		•	•			•	ACC/AHA Post-MI Guideline, BHAT, SAVE, Capricorn, EPHESUS
High coronary disease risk	•	•	•		•		ALLHAT, HOPE, ANBP2, LIFE, CONVINCE
Diabetes mellitus	•	•	•	•	•		NKF-ADA Guideline, UKPDS, ALLHAT
Chronic kidney disease			•	•			NKF Guideline, Captopril Trial, RENAAL, IDNT, REIN, AASK
Recurrent stroke prevention	•		•				PROGRESS

[1]Compelling indications for antihypertensive drugs are based on benefits from outcome studies or existing clinical guidelines; the compelling indication is managed in parallel with the blood pressure.
[2]Conditions for which clinical trials demonstrate benefit of specific classes of antihypertensive drugs.
AASK, African American Study of Kidney Disease and Hypertension; ACC/AHA, American College of Cardiology/American Heart Association; ACE, angiotensin converting enzyme; AIRE, Acute Infarction Ramipril Efficacy; ALLHAT, Antihypertensive and Lipid-Lowering Treatment to Prevent Heart Attack Trial; ANBP2, Second Australian National Blood Pressure Study; ARB, angiotensin receptor blocker; BHAT, β-Blocker Heart Attack Trial; CCB, calcium channel blocker; CIBIS, Cardiac Insufficiency Bisoprolol Study; CONVINCE, Controlled Onset Verapamil Investigation of Cardiovascular End Points; COPERNICUS, Carvedilol Prospective Randomized Cumulative Survival Study; EPHESUS, Eplerenone Post-Acute Myocardial Infarction Heart Failure Efficacy and Survival Study; HOPE, Heart Outcomes Prevention Evaluation Study; IDNT, Irbesartan Diabetic Nephropathy Trial; LIFE, Losartan Intervention For Endpoint Reduction in Hypertension Study; MERIT-HF, Metoprolol CR/XL Randomized Intervention Trial in Congestive Heart Failure; NKF-ADA, National Kidney Foundation–American Diabetes Association; PROGRESS, Perindopril Protection Against Recurrent Stroke Study; RALES, Randomized Aldactone Evaluation Study; REIN, Ramipril Efficacy in Nephropathy Study; RENAAL, Reduction of Endpoints in Non-Insulin-Dependent Diabetes Mellitus with the Angiotensin II Antagonist Losartan Study; SAVE, Survival and Ventricular Enlargement Study; SOLVD, Studies of Left Ventricular Dysfunction; TRACE, Trandolapril Cardiac Evaluation Study; UKPDS, United Kingdom Prospective Diabetes Study; ValHEFT, Valsartan Heart Failure Trial.
Source: Chobanian AV et al. The Seventh Report of the Joint National Committee on Prevention, Detection, Evaluation, and Treatment of High Blood Pressure: the JNC 7 report. JAMA. 2003 May 21;289(19):2560–72.

as reasonable goals pending further information on optimal targets, which may be even lower. On the other hand, lower may not always be better. The association between cognitive decline and lower blood pressure in the elderly has led to the proposal that hypertension in mid-life gives rise to cerebrovascular small vessel disease that predisposes to hypoperfusion of subcortical white matter and cognitive decline later in life. Similarly, excessive lowering of diastolic pressure, perhaps below 70 mm Hg, should be avoided in patients with coronary artery disease. Overall, however, several studies in older persons with predominantly systolic hypertension have confirmed that antihypertensive therapy prevents fatal and nonfatal myocardial infarction and overall cardiovascular mortality. These trials have also placed the focus on control of systolic blood pressure—in contrast to the historical emphasis on diastolic blood pressures.

There is no clear consensus on blood pressure goals in the management of prehypertension, but pressure should still be treated until it is < 130/80 mm Hg in prehypertensive patients with diabetes or chronic kidney disease and perhaps also in those at high risk for a cardiovascular event.

Large-scale trials in hypertension have focused on discrete end points occurring over relatively short intervals, thereby placing the emphasis on the prevention of cata-strophic events in advanced disease. More recently, in parallel with a new emphasis on hypertension in the context of overall cardiovascular risk, attention is turning to the importance of the long view. Accordingly, treatment of persons with hypertension should focus on comprehensive risk reduction with more careful consideration of the possible long-term adverse consequences of the metabolic derangements linked to some antihypertensives (particularly conventional β-blockers and thiazide diuretics).

Statins should be more widely used. In this respect, there is evidence from the Anglo-Scandinavian Cardiac Outcomes Trial (ASCOT) that statins can significantly improve outcomes in persons with hypertension (with modest background cardiovascular risk) whose total cholesterol is < 250 mg/dL. Furthermore, this effect appeared to be synergistic with calcium channel blocker/ACE inhibitor regimens but not β-blocker/diuretic regimens. The BHS guidelines recommend that statins be offered as secondary prevention to patients whose total cholesterol exceeds 135 mg/dL if they have documented coronary artery disease or a history of ischemic stroke. In addition, statins should be considered as primary prevention in patients with long-standing type 2 diabetes mellitus or in those with type 2 diabetes mellitus who are older than age 50 years, and perhaps in all persons

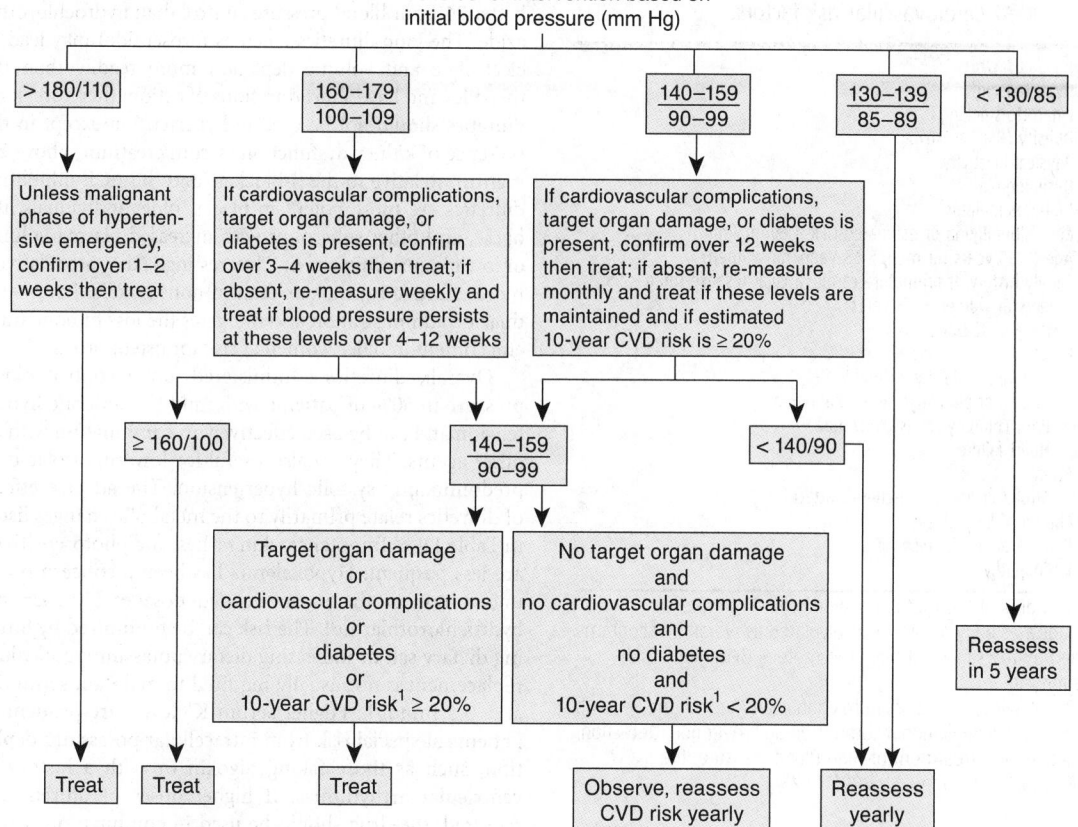

Thresholds for intervention based on
initial blood pressure (mm Hg)

> 180/110

160–179
100–109

140–159
90–99

130–139
85–89

< 130/85

Unless malignant phase of hypertensive emergency, confirm over 1–2 weeks then treat

If cardiovascular complications, target organ damage, or diabetes is present, confirm over 3–4 weeks then treat; if absent, re-measure weekly and treat if blood pressure persists at these levels over 4–12 weeks

If cardiovascular complications, target organ damage, or diabetes is present, confirm over 12 weeks then treat; if absent, re-measure monthly and treat if these levels are maintained and if estimated 10-year CVD risk is ≥ 20%

≥ 160/100

140–159
90–99

< 140/90

Target organ damage
or
cardiovascular complications
or
diabetes
or
10-year CVD risk[1] ≥ 20%

No target organ damage
and
no cardiovascular complications
and
no diabetes
and
10-year CVD risk[1] < 20%

Reassess
in 5 years

Treat   Treat   Treat

Observe, reassess
CVD risk yearly

Reassess
yearly

[1]Assessed with CVD risk chart.

▲ **Figure 11–2.** British Hypertension Society algorithm for diagnosis and treatment of hypertension, incorporating total cardiovascular risk in deciding which "prehypertensive" patients to treat. (CVD, cardiovascular disease.) (Reproduced, with permission, from: Guidelines for management of hypertension: report of the Fourth Working Party of the British Hypertension Society, 2004-BHS IV. J Hum Hypertens. 2004 Mar;18(3):139–185.)

with type 2 diabetes mellitus. Ideally, total and low-density lipoprotein (LDL) cholesterol should be reduced by 30% and 40% respectively, or to approximately < 155 mg/dL and < 77 mg/dL, whichever is the greatest reduction. However, total and LDL cholesterol levels of < 194 mg/dL and < 116 mg/dL respectively, or reductions of 25% and 30% are regarded as clinically acceptable objectives. Primary prevention with statins might also be reasonably extended to all patients with total cholesterol > 135 mg/dL and a total cardiovascular risk > 20% (to similar target cholesterol levels), but trial evidence for this is not currently available. Low-dose aspirin (81 mg/day) is likely to be beneficial in patients older than age 50 with either target organ damage or elevated total cardiovascular risk (> 20–30%). Care should be taken to ensure that blood pressure is controlled to the recommended levels before starting aspirin to minimize the risk of bleeding.

Giles TD. Blood pressure goals for hypertension guidelines: what is wrong with "optimal"? J Clin Hypertens (Greenwich). 2006 Dec;8(12):835–9. [PMID: 17170608]

Julius S et al; Trial of Preventing Hypertension (TROPHY) Study Investigators. Feasibility of treating prehypertension with an angiotensin-receptor blocker. N Engl J Med. 2006 Apr 20;354(16):1685–97. [PMID: 16537662]

Papadopoulos DP et al. Is it time to treat prehypertension? Hypertens Res. 2008 Sep;31(9):1681–6. [PMID: 18971545]

Sever PS et al; ASCOT Investigators. Prevention of coronary and stroke events with atorvastatin in hypertensive patients who have average or lower-than-average cholesterol concentrations, in the Anglo-Scandinavian Cardiac Outcomes Trial—Lipid Lowering Arm (ASCOT-LLA): a multicentre randomised controlled trial. Lancet. 2003 Apr 5;361(9364):1149–58. [PMID: 12686036]

Sever P et al. ASCOT Steering Committee Members. Potential synergy between lipid-lowering and blood-pressure-lowering in the Anglo-Scandinavian Cardiac Outcomes Trial. Eur Heart J. 2006 Dec;27(24):2982–8. [PMID: 17145722]

Turnbull F et al; Blood Pressure Lowering Treatment Trialists' Collaboration. Effects of different blood pressure-lowering regimens on major cardiovascular events in individuals with and without diabetes mellitus: results of prospectively designed overviews of randomized trials. Arch Intern Med. 2005 Jun 27;165(12):1410–9. [PMID: 15983291]

Williams B et al. Systolic pressure is all that matters. Lancet. 2008 Jun 28;371(9631):2219–21. [PMID: 18561995]

Table 11–5. Cardiovascular risk factors.

Major risk factors
  Hypertension[1]
  Cigarette smoking
  Obesity (BMI ≥ 30)[1]
  Physical inactivity
  Dyslipidemia[1]
  Diabetes mellitus[1]
  Microalbuminuria or estimated GFR < 60 mL/min
  Age (> 55 years for men, > 65 years for women)
  Family history of premature cardiovascular disease (men < 55
    years or women < 65 years)
Target-organ damage
  Heart
    Left ventricular hypertrophy
    Angina or prior myocardial infarction
    Prior coronary revascularization
    Heart failure
  Brain
    Stroke or transient ischemic attack
  Chronic kidney disease
  Peripheral arterial disease
  Retinopathy

---

[1]Components of the metabolic syndrome.
BMI indicates body mass index calculated as weight in kilograms divided by the square of height in meters; GFR, glomerular filtration rate.
Reprinted, with permission, from Chobanian AV et al. The Seventh Report of the Joint National Committee on Prevention, Detection, Evaluation, and Treatment of High Blood Pressure: the JNC 7 report. JAMA. 2003 May 21; 289(19):2560–72.

DRUG THERAPY: CURRENT ANTIHYPERTENSIVE AGENTS

There are now many classes of potentially antihypertensive drugs of which six (diuretics, β-blockers, renin inhibitors, ACE inhibitors, calcium channel blockers, and ARBs) are suitable for initial therapy based on efficacy and tolerability. A number of considerations enter into the selection of the initial regimen for a given patient. These include the weight of evidence for beneficial effects on clinical outcomes, the safety and tolerability of the drug, its cost, demographic differences in response, concomitant medical conditions, and lifestyle issues. The specific classes of antihypertensive medications are discussed below, and guidelines for the choice of initial medications are offered.

A. Diuretics

Thiazide diuretics (Table 11–6) are the antihypertensives that have been most extensively studied and most consistently effective in clinical trials. They lower blood pressure initially by decreasing plasma volume (by suppressing tubular reabsorption of sodium, thus increasing the excretion of sodium and water) and cardiac output, but during long-term therapy their major hemodynamic effect is reduction of peripheral vascular resistance. Most of the antihypertensive effect of these agents is achieved at lower dosages than used previously (typically, 12.5 or 25 mg of hydrochlorothiazide or equivalent), but their biochemical and metabolic effects are dose related. Chlorthalidone has the advantage of better 24-hour blood pressure control than hydrochlorothiazide. The loop diuretics (such as furosemide) may lead to electrolyte and volume depletion more readily than the thiazides and have short durations of action; therefore, loop diuretics should not be used in hypertension except in the presence of kidney dysfunction (serum creatinine above 2.5 mg/dL). Relative to the β-blockers and the ACE inhibitors, diuretics are more potent in blacks, older individuals, the obese, and other subgroups with increased plasma volume or low plasma renin activity. Interestingly, they are relatively more effective in smokers than in nonsmokers. Long-term thiazide administration also mitigates the loss of bone mineral content in older women at risk for osteoporosis.

Overall, diuretics administered alone control blood pressure in 50% of patients with mild to moderate hypertension and can be used effectively in combination with all other agents. They are also useful for lowering isolated or predominantly systolic hypertension. The adverse effects of diuretics relate primarily to the metabolic changes listed in Table 11–6. Impotence, skin rashes, and photosensitivity are less frequent. Hypokalemia has been a concern but is uncommon at the recommended dosages (12.5–25 mg hydrochlorothiazide). The risk can be minimized by limiting dietary salt or increasing dietary potassium; potassium replacement is not usually required to maintain serum K^+ at > 3.5 mmol/L. Higher serum K^+ levels are prudent in patients at special risk from intracellular potassium depletion, such as those taking digoxin or with a history of ventricular arrhythmias. If higher doses of diuretic are required, the drug should be used in combination with a potassium-sparing agent or with an ACE inhibitor or ARB. Compared with ACE inhibitors and ARBs, diuretic therapy is associated with a slightly higher incidence of mild new-onset diabetes. Diuretics also increase serum uric acid and may precipitate gout. Increases in blood glucose, triglycerides, LDL cholesterol, and plasma insulin may occur but are relatively minor during long-term low-dose therapy.

B. β-Adrenergic Blocking Agents

These drugs are effective in hypertension because they decrease the heart rate and cardiac output. Even after continued use of β-blockers, cardiac output remains lower and systemic vascular resistance higher with agents that do not have intrinsic sympathomimetic or α-blocking activity. The β-blockers also decrease renin release and are more efficacious in populations with elevated plasma renin activity, such as younger white patients. They neutralize the reflex tachycardia caused by vasodilators and are especially useful in patients with associated conditions that benefit from the cardioprotective effects of these agents. These include individuals with angina pectoris, previous myocardial infarction, and stable congestive heart failure as well as those with migraine headaches and somatic manifestations of anxiety.

Although all β-blockers appear to be similar in antihypertensive potency, controlling approximately 50% of patients, they differ in a number of pharmacologic properties (these differences are summarized in Table 11–7), including specificity to the cardiac β_1-receptors (cardioselec-

Table 11–6. Antihypertensive drugs: Diuretics.

Drugs	Proprietary Names	Initial Oral Doses	Dosage Range	Cost per Unit	Cost of 30 Days Treatment[1] (Average Dosage)	Adverse Effects	Comments
Thiazides and related diuretics							
Hydrochloro-thiazide	Esidrix, Hydro-Diuril	12.5 or 25 mg once daily	12.5–50 mg once daily	$0.08/ 25 mg	$2.40	↓ K⁺, ↓ Mg²⁺, ↑ Ca²⁺, ↓ Na⁺, ↑ uric acid, ↑ glucose, ↑ LDL cholesterol, ↑ triglycerides; rash, erectile dysfunction.	Low dosages effective in many patients without associated metabolic abnormalities; metolazone more effective with concurrent kidney disease; indapamide does not alter serum lipid levels.
Chlorthalidone	Hygroton, Thaliton	12.5 or 25 mg once daily	12.5–50 mg once daily	$0.23/ 25 mg	$6.90		
Metolazone	Zaroxolyn	1.25 or 2.5 mg once daily	1.25–5 mg once daily	$1.48/ 5 mg	$44.40		
Indapamide	Lozol	2.5 mg once daily	2.5–5 mg once daily	$0.83/ 2.5 mg	$24.90		
Loop diuretics							
Furosemide	Lasix	20 mg twice daily	40–320 mg in 2 or 3 doses	$0.16/ 40 mg	$9.60	Same as thiazides, but higher risk of excessive diuresis and electrolyte imbalance. Increases calcium excretion.	Furosemide: Short duration of action a disadvantage; should be reserved for patients with kidney disease or fluid retention. Poor antihypertensive.
Ethacrynic acid	Edecrin	50 mg once daily	50–100 mg once or twice daily	$1.17/ 25 mg	$140.00		
Bumetanide	Bumex	0.25 mg twice daily	0.5–10 mg in 2 or 3 doses	$0.45/ 1 mg	$27.00		
Torsemide	Demadex	2.5 mg once daily	5–10 mg once daily	$0.70/ 10 mg	$21.00		Torsemide: Effective blood pressure medication at low dosage.
Aldosterone receptor blockers							
Spironolactone	Aldactone	12.5 or 25 mg once daily	12.5–100 mg once daily	$0.46/ 25 mg	$13.80	Hyperkalemia, metabolic acidosis, gynecomastia.	Can be useful add-on therapy in patients with refractory hypertension.
Amiloride	Midamor	5 mg once daily	5–10 mg once daily	$1.29/ 5 mg	$38.70		
Eplerenone	Inspra	25 mg once daily	25–100 mg once daily	$4.10/ 25 mg	$123.07		
Combination products							
Hydrochloro-thiazide and triamterene	Dyazide (25/ 50 mg); Maxzide (25/37.5 mg)	1 tab once daily	1 or 2 tabs once daily	$0.34	$10.20	Same as thiazides plus GI disturbances, hyperkalemia rather than hypokalemia, headache; triamterene can cause kidney stones and kidney dysfunction; spironolactone causes gynecomastia. Hyperkalemia can occur if this combination is used in patients with advanced kidney disease or those taking ACE inhibitors.	Use should be limited to patients with demonstrable need for a potassium-sparing agent.
Hydrochloro-thiazide and amiloride	Moduretic (50/5 mg)	¹/₂ tab once daily	1 or 2 tabs once daily	$0.42	$12.60		
Hydrochloro-thiazide and spirono-lactone	Aldactazide (25/25 mg)	1 tab once daily	1 or 2 tabs once daily	$0.50	$15.00		

[1]Average wholesale price (AWP, for AB-rated generic when available) for quantity listed. Source: *Red Book Update,* Vol. 28, No. 3, March 2009. AWP may not accurately represent the actual pharmacy cost because wide contractual variations exist among institutions. ACE, angiotensin-converting enzyme; GI, gastrointestinal; LDL, low-density lipoprotein.

Table 11–7. Antihypertensive drugs: β-Adrenergic blocking agents.

Drug	Proprietary Name	Initial Oral Dosage	Dosage Range	Cost per Unit	Cost of 30 Days Treatment (Based on Average Dosage)[1]	Special Properties					Comments[5]
						β_1 Selectivity[2]	ISA[3]	MSA[4]	Lipid Solubility	Renal vs Hepatic Elimination	
Acebutolol	Sectral	200 mg once daily	200–1200 mg in 1 or 2 doses	$1.34/400 mg	$40.20	+	+	+	+	H > R	Positive ANA; rare LE syndrome; also indicated for arrhythmias. Doses > 800 mg have β_1 and β_2 effects.
Atenolol	Tenormin	25 mg once daily	25–200 mg once daily	$0.85/50 mg	$25.50	+	0	0	0	R	Also indicated for angina pectoris and post-MI. Doses > 100 mg have β_1 and β_2 effects.
Betaxolol	Kerlone	10 mg once daily	10–40 mg once daily	$1.24/10 mg	$37.20	+	0	0	+	H > R	
Bisoprolol and hydrochlorothiazide	Ziac	5 mg/6.25 mg once daily	2.5–10 mg plus 6.25 mg	$1.14/2.5/6.25 mg	$34.20	+	0	0	0	R = H	Low-dose combination approved for initial therapy. Bisoprolol also effective for heart failure.
Carvedilol	Coreg	6.25 mg twice daily	12.5–100 mg in 2 doses	$2.13/25 mg	$127.80 (25 mg twice a day)	0	0	0	+++	H > R	α:β-Blocking activity 1:9; may cause orthostatic symptoms; effective for congestive heart failure.
Labetalol	Normodyne, Trandate	100 mg twice daily	200–1200 mg in 2 doses	$0.71/200 mg	$42.60	0	0/+	0	++	H	α:β-Blocking activity 1:3; more orthostatic hypotension, fever, hepatotoxicity.
Metoprolol	Lopressor	50 mg in 1 or 2 doses	50–200 mg in 1 or 2 doses	$0.55/50 mg	$33.00	+	0	+	+++	H	Also indicated for angina pectoris and post-MI. Approved for heart failure. Doses > 100 mg have β_1 and β_2 effects.

Drug	Proprietary Name	Initial Oral Dosage	Dosage Range	Cost per Unit [1]	Cost of 30 Days Treatment	β1 Selectivity [2]	ISA [3]	MSA [4]	Lipid Solubility	Renal vs Hepatic Elimination	Comments [5]
Toprol XL (SR preparation)		50 mg once daily	50–200 mg once daily	$1.44/100 mg	$43.20						
Nadolol	Corgard	20 mg once daily	20–160 mg once daily	$1.05/40 mg	$31.50	0	0	0	0	R	In adults, 35% renal clearance.
Penbutolol	Levatol	20 mg once daily	20–80 mg once daily	$2.11/20 mg	$63.30	0	+	0	++	R > H	
Pindolol	Visken	5 mg twice daily	10–60 mg in 2 doses	$0.73/5 mg	$43.80	0	++	+	+	H > R	
Propranolol	Inderal	20 mg twice daily	40–320 mg in 2 doses	$0.51/40 mg	$30.60	0	0	++	+++	H	Once-daily SR preparation also available. Also indicated for angina pectoris and post-MI.
Timolol	Blocadren	5 mg twice daily	10–40 mg in 2 doses	$0.50/10 mg	$30.00	0	0	0	++	H > R	Also indicated for post-MI. 80% hepatic clearance.

[1] Average wholesale price (AWP, for AB-rated generic when available) for quantity listed. Source: *Red Book Update*, Vol. 28, No. 3, March 2009. AWP may not accurately represent the actual pharmacy cost because wide contractual variations exist among institutions.

[2] Agents with β1 selectivity are less likely to precipitate bronchospasm and decreased peripheral blood flow *in low doses*, but selectivity is only relative.

[3] Agents with ISA cause less resting bradycardia and lipid changes.

[4] MSA generally occurs at concentrations greater than those necessary for β-adrenergic blockade. The clinical importance of MSA by β-blockers has not been defined.

[5] Adverse effects of all β-blockers: bronchospasm, fatigue, sleep disturbance and nightmares, bradycardia and atrioventricular block, worsening of congestive heart failure, cold extremities, gastrointestinal disturbances, impotence, ↑triglycerides, ↓HDL cholesterol, rare blood dyscrasias.

ANA, antinuclear antibody; ISA, intrinsic sympathomimetic activity; LE, lupus erythematosus; MI, myocardial infarction; MSA, membrane-stabilizing activity; SR, sustained release; 0, no effect; +, some effect; ++, moderate effect; +++, most effect.

tivity) and whether they also block the β_2-receptors in the bronchi and vasculature; at higher dosages, however, all agents are nonselective. The β-blockers also differ in their pharmacokinetics and lipid solubility—which determines whether they cross the blood–brain barrier and affect the incidence of central nervous system side effects—and route of metabolism. Labetalol and carvedilol are combined α- and β-blockers and, unlike most β-blockers, decrease peripheral vascular resistance.

The side effects of all β-blockers include inducing or exacerbating bronchospasm in predisposed patients (eg, those with asthma and some patients with chronic obstructive pulmonary disease [COPD]); sinus node dysfunction and atrioventricular (AV) conduction depression (resulting in bradycardia or AV block); nasal congestion; Raynaud phenomenon; and central nervous system symptoms with nightmares, excitement, depression, and confusion. Fatigue, lethargy, and impotence may occur. All β-blockers tend to increase plasma triglycerides. The nonselective and, to a lesser extent, the cardioselective (β_1-selective) β-blockers tend to depress the protective HDL fraction of plasma cholesterol. As with diuretics, the changes are blunted with time and dietary changes.

β-Blockers have traditionally been considered contraindicated in patients with congestive heart failure. Evolving experience suggests that they have a propitious effect on the natural history of patients with chronic stable heart failure and reduced ejection fraction (see Chapter 10). β-Blockers are used cautiously in patients with type 1 diabetes, since they can mask the symptoms of hypoglycemia and prolong these episodes by inhibiting gluconeogenesis. Although they may increase blood glucose levels in type 2 diabetics, the prognosis of these patients on balance is improved. These drugs should also be used with caution in patients with advanced peripheral vascular disease associated with rest pain or nonhealing ulcers, but they are generally well tolerated in patients with mild claudication. In treatment of pheochromocytoma, β-blockers should not be administered until α-blockade has been established. Otherwise, blockade of vasodilatory β_2-adrenergic receptors will allow unopposed vasoconstrictor α-adrenergic receptor activation with worsening of hypertension. For the same reason, β-blockers should not be used to treat hypertension arising from cocaine use.

Because of the lack of efficacy in prevention of myocardial infarction and inferiority compared with other drugs in prevention of stroke and left ventricular hypertrophy, there is now increasing doubt whether β-blockers should still be regarded as ideal first-line agents in the treatment of hypertension without specific compelling indications (such as active coronary artery disease). In addition to adverse metabolic changes associated with their use (see below), some experts have suggested that the therapeutic shortcomings of β-blockers are the consequence of the particular hemodynamic profile associated with these drugs. Pressure peaks in the aorta are augmented by reflection of pressure waves from the peripheral circulation. These reflected waves are delayed in patients taking ACE inhibitors and thiazide diuretics, resulting in decreased systolic and pulse pressures. By contrast, β-blockers appear to potentiate

reflection of pressure waves, possibly because peripheral resistance vessels are a reflection point and peripheral resistance is not decreased by β-blockers. This might explain why β-blockers are less effective at controlling systolic and pulse pressure.

Despite these concerns, the compelling indications for β-blockers remain, such as active coronary artery disease and impaired left ventricular function. Great care should be exercised if the decision is made, in the absence of compelling indications, to remove β-blockers from the treatment regimen since abrupt withdrawal can precipitate acute coronary events and severe increases in blood pressure.

C. Renin Inhibitors

Since renin cleavage of angiotensinogen is the rate-limiting step in the renin-angiotensin cascade, the most efficient inactivation of this system would be expected with renin inhibition, but this option has only recently become available. Conventional ACE inhibitors and ARBs probably offer incomplete blockade, even in combination. Aliskiren, a renin inhibitor, was recently approved by the FDA for use as monotherapy or combination therapy of hypertension. This drug binds the proteolytic site of renin, thereby preventing cleavage of angiotensinogen. As a consequence, levels of angiotensins I and II are reduced and renin concentration is increased. Aliskiren is synergistic with diuretics, ACE inhibitors, and ARBs in lowering blood pressure. Whether renin inhibition offers real advantages over conventional drugs remains to be demonstrated. As yet there is no clinical trial data with this new drug, so the effect of aliskiren on outcomes in hypertension, diabetes, or cardiovascular disease remains unknown.

D. Angiotensin-Converting Enzyme Inhibitors

ACE inhibitors are being increasingly used as the initial medication in mild to moderate hypertension (Table 11–8). Their primary mode of action is inhibition of the renin–angiotensin–aldosterone system, but they also inhibit bradykinin degradation, stimulate the synthesis of vasodilating prostaglandins and, sometimes, reduce sympathetic nervous system activity. These latter actions may explain why they exhibit some effect even in patients with low plasma renin activity. ACE inhibitors appear to be more effective in younger white patients. They are relatively less effective in blacks and older persons and in predominantly systolic hypertension. Although as single therapy they achieve adequate antihypertensive control in only about 40–50% of patients, the combination of an ACE inhibitor and a diuretic or calcium channel blocker is potent.

ACE inhibitors are the agents of choice in persons with type 1 diabetes with frank proteinuria or evidence of kidney dysfunction because they delay the progression to end-stage kidney disease. Many authorities have expanded this indication to include persons with type 2 diabetes and those who have type 1 diabetes with microalbuminuria, even when they do not meet the usual criteria for antihypertensive therapy. ACE inhibitors may also delay the progression of nondiabetic kidney disease. The Heart Outcomes Prevention Evaluation (HOPE) trial demonstrated

Table 11–8. Antihypertensive drugs: Renin and ACE inhibitors and angiotensin II receptor blockers.

Drug	Proprietary Name	Initial Oral Dosage	Dosage Range	Cost per Unit	Cost of 30 Days Treatment (Average Dosage)[1]	Adverse Effects	Comments
Renin inhibitors							
Aliskiren	Tekturna	150 mg once daily	150–300 mg/d	$2.48/150 mg	$74.41	Angioedema, hypotension, hyperkalemia Contraindicated in pregnancy.	Probably metabolized by CYP3A4. Absorption is inhibited by high fat meal.
Aliskiren/Hydrochlorothiazide	Tekturna HCT	150 mg/12.5 mg once daily	150–300 mg Aliskiren daily	$2.48/150 mg/12.5 mg	$74.41		
ACE inhibitors							
Benazepril	Lotensin	10 mg once daily	5–40 mg in 1 or 2 doses	$1.05/20 mg	$31.50	Cough, hypotension, dizziness, kidney dysfunction, hyperkalemia, angioedema; taste alteration and rash (may be more frequent with captopril); rarely, proteinuria, blood dyscrasia. Contraindicated in pregnancy.	More fosinopril is excreted by the liver in patients with renal dysfunction (dose reduction may or may not be necessary). Captopril and lisinopril are active without metabolism. Captopril, enalapril, lisinopril, and quinapril are approved for congestive heart failure.
Captopril	Capoten	25 mg twice daily	50–300 mg in 2 or 3 doses	$0.76/25 mg	$45.60		
Enalapril	Vasotec	5 mg once daily	5–40 mg in 1 or 2 doses	$1.52/20 mg	$45.60		
Fosinopril	Monopril	10 mg once daily	10–80 mg in 1 or 2 doses	$1.19/20 mg	$35.70		
Lisinopril	Prinivil, Zestril	5–10 mg once daily	5–40 mg once daily	$1.06/20 mg	$31.80		
Moexipril	Univasc	7.5 mg once daily	7.5–30 mg in 1 or 2 doses	$1.39/7.5 mg	$41.70		
Perindopril	Aceon	4 mg once daily	4–16 mg in 1 or 2 doses	$3.11/8 mg	$93.30		
Quinapril	Accupril	10 mg once daily	10–80 mg in 1 or 2 doses	$1.57/20 mg	$47.10		
Ramipril	Altace	2.5 mg once daily	2.5–20 mg in 1 or 2 doses	$1.89/5 mg	$56.70		
Trandolapril	Mavik	1 mg once daily	1–8 mg once daily	$1.24/4 mg	$37.20		
Angiotensin II receptor blockers							
Candesartan cilexitil	Atacand	16 mg once daily	8–32 mg once daily	$2.02/16 mg	$60.68	Hyperkalemia, kidney dysfunction, rare angioedema. Combinations have additional side effects. Contraindicated in pregnancy.	Losartan has a very flat dose-response curve. Valsartan and irbesartan have wider dose-response ranges and longer durations of action. Addition of low-dose diuretic (separately or as combination pills) increases the response.
Candesartan cilexitil/HCTZ	Atacand HCT	16 mg/12.5 mg once daily	8–32 mg of candesartan once daily	$2.74/16 mg/12.5 mg	$82.20		
Eprosartan	Teveten	600 mg once daily	400–800 mg in 1–2 doses	$3.11/600 mg	$93.30		
Eprosartan/HCTZ	Teveten HCT	600 mg/12.5 mg once daily	600 mg/12.5 mg or 600 mg/25 mg once daily	$3.30/600 mg/12.5 mg	$99.00		
Irbesartan	Avapro	150 mg once daily	150–300 mg once daily	$2.27/150 mg	$68.17		
Irbesartan and HCTZ	Avalide	150 mg/12.5 mg once daily	150–300 mg irbesartan daily	$2.75/150 mg	$82.48		

(continued)

Table 11–8. Antihypertensive drugs: Renin and ACE inhibitors and angiotensin II receptor blockers. (continued)

Drug	Proprietary Name	Initial Oral Dosage	Dosage Range	Cost per Unit	Cost of 30 Days Treatment (Average Dosage)[1]	Adverse Effects	Comments
Losartan	Cozaar	50 mg once daily	25–100 mg in 1 or 2 doses	$2.28/50 mg	$68.47	Hyperkalemia, kidney dysfunction, rare angioedema. Combinations have additional side effects. Contraindicated in pregnancy.	Losartan has a very flat dose-response curve. Valsartan and irbesartan have wider dose-response ranges and longer durations of action. Addition of low-dose diuretic (separately or as combination pills) increases the response.
Losartan and hydrochlorothiazide	Hyzaar	50 mg/12.5 mg once daily	One or 2 tablets once daily	$2.50/50 mg/12.5 mg/tablet	$75.07		
Olmesartan	Benicar	20 mg once daily	20–40 mg daily	$2.10/20 mg	$63.00		
Olmesartan and HCTZ	Benicar HCT	20 mg/12.5 mg daily	20–40 mg olmesartan daily	$2.54/20 mg/12.5 mg	$76.32		
Telmisartan	Micardis	40 mg once daily	20–80 mg once daily	$2.30/40 mg	$69.02		
Telmisartan and HCTZ	Micardis HCT	40 mg/12.5 mg once daily	20–80 mg telmisartan daily	$2.46/40 mg/12.5 mg	$73.93		
Valsartan	Diovan	80 mg once daily	80–320 mg once daily	$2.68/160 mg	$80.53		
Valsartan and HCTZ	Diovan HCT	80 mg/12.5 mg once daily	80–320 mg valsartan daily	$3.31/160 mg/12.5 mg	$99.40		

[1]Average wholesale price (AWP, for AB-rated generic when available) for quantity listed. Source: *Red Book Update*, Vol. 28, No. 3, March 2009. AWP may not accurately represent the actual pharmacy cost because wide contractual variations exist among institutions.
ACE, angiotensin-converting enzyme; HCTZ, hydrochlorothiazide.

that the ACE inhibitor ramipril reduced the number of cardiovascular deaths, nonfatal myocardial infarctions, and nonfatal strokes and also reduced the incidence of new-onset heart failure, kidney dysfunction, and new-onset diabetes in a population of patients at high risk for vascular events. Although this was not specifically a hypertensive population, the benefits were associated with a modest reduction in blood pressure, and the results inferentially support the use of ACE inhibitors in similar hypertensive patients. ACE inhibitors are a drug of choice (usually in conjunction with a diuretic and a β-blocker) in patients with congestive heart failure and are indicated also in asymptomatic patients with reduced ejection fraction. An advantage of the ACE inhibitors is their relative freedom from troublesome side effects. Severe hypotension can occur in patients with bilateral renal artery stenosis; acute renal failure may ensue but is usually reversible with discontinuation of ACE inhibition. Hyperkalemia may develop in patients with intrinsic kidney disease and type IV renal tubular acidosis (commonly seen in diabetics) and in the elderly. A chronic dry cough is common, seen in 10% of patients or more, and may require stopping the drug. Skin rashes are observed with any ACE inhibitor. Angioedema is an uncommon but potentially dangerous side effect of all agents of this class because of their inhibition of kininase. Exposure of the fetus to ACE inhibitors during the second and third trimesters of pregnancy has been associated with a variety of defects due to hypotension and reduced renal blood flow.

E. Angiotensin II Receptor Blockers

A growing body of data indicates that ARBs can improve cardiovascular outcomes in patients with hypertension as well as in patients with related conditions such as heart failure and type 2 diabetes with nephropathy. ARBs have not been compared with ACE inhibitors in randomized controlled trials in patients with hypertension, but two trials comparing losartan with captopril in heart failure and post-myocardial infarction left ventricular dysfunction showed trends toward worse outcomes in the losartan group. Whether this suggestion of reduced efficacy is specific to losartan or may also be true for other ARBs is as yet unknown. However, the Losartan Intervention for Endpoints (LIFE) trial in nearly 9000 hypertensive patients with electrocardiographic evidence of left ventricular hypertrophy—comparing losartan with the β-blocker atenolol as initial therapy—demonstrated a significant reduction in stroke with losartan. Of note is that in diabetic patients, death and myocardial infarction were also reduced, and there was a lower occurrence of new-onset diabetes. In this trial, as in the Antihypertensive and Lipid-Lowering Treatment to Prevent Heart Attack Trial (ALL-HAT) with an ACE inhibitor, blacks exhibited less blood pressure reduction and less benefit with regard to clinical end points. ARBs may synergize with ACE inhibitors in protection of heart and kidney, and ARB/ACE inhibitor combinations may also improve control of hypertension.

Unlike ACE inhibitors, the ARBs do not cause cough and are less likely to be associated with skin rashes or angioedema. However, as seen with ACE inhibitors, hyperkalemia can be a problem, and patients with bilateral renal artery stenosis may exhibit hypotension and worsened kidney function.

F. Aldosterone Receptor Antagonists

Spironolactone and eplerenone are natriuretic in sodium-retaining states, such as heart failure and cirrhosis, but only very weakly so in hypertension. These drugs have reemerged in the treatment of hypertension, particularly in resistant patients and are helpful additions to most other antihypertensive medications. Consistent with the increasingly appreciated importance of aldosterone in essential hypertension, the aldosterone receptor blockers are effective at lowering blood pressure in all hypertensive patients regardless of renin level, and are also effective in blacks. Aldosterone plays a central role in target organ damage, including the development of ventricular and vascular hypertrophy and renal fibrosis. Aldosterone receptor antagonists ameliorate these consequences of hypertension, to some extent independently of effects on blood pressure. Spironolactone can cause breast pain and gynecomastia in men through activity at the progesterone receptor, an effect not seen with the more specific eplerenone. Hyperkalemia is a problem with both drugs, chiefly in patients with chronic kidney disease.

G. Calcium Channel Blocking Agents

These agents act by causing peripheral vasodilation but with less reflex tachycardia and fluid retention than other vasodilators. They are effective as single-drug therapy in approximately 60% of patients in all demographic groups and all grades of hypertension (Table 11–9). For these reasons, they may be preferable to β-blockers and ACE inhibitors in blacks and older persons. Verapamil and diltiazem should be combined cautiously with β-blockers because of their potential for depressing AV conduction and sinus node automaticity as well as contractility.

Initial concerns about possible adverse cardiac effects of calcium channel blockers have been convincingly allayed by several subsequent large studies which have demonstrated that calcium channel blockers are equivalent to ACE inhibitors and thiazide diuretics in prevention of coronary heart disease, major cardiovascular events, cardiovascular death, and total mortality. A protective effect against stroke with calcium channel blockers is well established, and in two trials (ALLHAT and the Systolic Hypertension in Europe trial), these agents appeared to be more effective than diuretic-based therapy.

The most common side effects of calcium channel blockers are headache, peripheral edema, bradycardia, and constipation (especially with verapamil in the elderly). The dihydropyridine agents—nifedipine, nicardipine, isradipine, felodipine, nisoldipine, and amlodipine—are more likely to produce symptoms of vasodilation, such as headache, flushing, palpitations, and peripheral edema. Calcium channel blockers have negative inotropic effects and should be used cautiously in patients with cardiac dysfunction.

Table 11-9. Antihypertensive drugs: Calcium channel blocking agents.

Drug	Proprietary Name	Initial Oral Dosage	Dosage Range	Cost of 30 Days Treatment (Average Dosage)[1]	Special Properties			Adverse Effects	Comments
					Peripheral Vasodilation	Cardiac Automaticity and Conduction	Contractility		
Nondihydropyridine agents									
Diltiazem	Cardizem SR	90 mg twice daily	180–360 mg in 2 doses	$74.25 (120 mg twice daily)	++	↓↓	↓↓	Edema, headache, bradycardia, GI disturbances, dizziness, AV block, congestive heart failure, urinary frequency.	Also approved for angina.
	Cardizem CD; Cartia XT	180 mg daily	180–360 mg daily	$61.50 (240 mg daily)					
	Dilacor XR	180 or 240 mg daily	180–480 mg daily	$34.50 (240 mg daily)					
	Tiazac SA	240 mg daily	180–540 mg daily	$73.40 (240 mg daily)					
Verapamil	Calan SR	180 mg daily	180–480 mg in 1 or 2 doses	$46.80 (240 mg daily)	++	↓↓↓	↓↓↓	Same as diltiazem but more likely to cause constipation and congestive heart failure.	Also approved for angina and arrhythmias.
	Isoptin SR								
	Verelan								
	Covera HS			$73.20 (240 mg daily)					
Dihydropyridines									
Amlodipine	Norvasc	2.5 mg daily	2.5–10 mg daily	$71.20 (10 mg daily)	+++	↓/0	↓/0	Edema, dizziness, palpitations, flushing, headache, hypotension, tachycardia, GI disturbances, urinary frequency, worsening of congestive heart failure (may be less common with felodipine, amlodipine).	Amlodipine, nicardipine, and nifedipine also approved for angina.
Felodipine	Plendil	5 mg daily	5–20 mg daily	$81.60 (10 mg daily)	+++	↓/0	↓/0		
Isradipine	DynaCirc	2.5 mg twice daily	2.5–5 mg twice daily	$120.00 (5 mg twice daily)	+++	↓/0	→		
	DynaCirc CR	5 mg daily	5–10 mg daily	$126.12 (10 mg daily)					
Nicardipine	Cardene	20 mg three times daily	20–40 mg three times daily	$36.90 (20 mg three times daily)	+++	↓/0	→		
	Cardene SR	30 mg twice daily	30–60 mg twice daily	$72.31 (30 mg twice daily)					
Nifedipine	Adalat CC	30 mg daily	30–120 mg daily	$65.10 (60 mg daily)	+++	→	→		
	Procardia XL	30 mg daily	30–120 mg daily	$70.80 (60 mg daily)					
Nisoldipine	Sular	20 mg/d	20–60 mg/d	$93.00 (40 mg daily)	+++	↓/0	→		

[1]Average wholesale price (AWP, for AB-rated generic when available) for quantity listed. Source: *Red Book Update*, Vol. 28, No. 3, March 2009. AWP may not accurately represent the actual pharmacy cost because wide contractual variations exist among institutions.
AV, atrioventricular; GI, gastrointestinal.

Amlodipine is the only calcium channel blocker with established safety in patients with severe heart failure. Most calcium channel blockers are now available in preparations that can be administered once daily.

H. α-Adrenoceptor Antagonists

Prazosin, terazosin, and doxazosin (Table 11–10) block postsynaptic α-receptors, relax smooth muscle, and reduce blood pressure by lowering peripheral vascular resistance. These agents are effective as single-drug therapy in some individuals, but tachyphylaxis may appear during long-term therapy and side effects are relatively common. These include marked hypotension and syncope after the first dose which, therefore, should be small and given at bedtime. Post-dosing palpitations, headache, and nervousness may continue to occur during long-term therapy; these symptoms may be less frequent or severe with doxazosin because of its more gradual onset of action. Cataractectomy in patients exposed to α-blockers can be complicated by the floppy iris syndrome, even after discontinuation of the drug, so the ophthalmologist should be alerted that the patient has been taking the drug prior to surgery.

Unlike the β-blockers and diuretics, the α-blockers have no adverse effect on serum lipid levels—in fact, they increase HDL cholesterol while reducing total cholesterol. Whether this is beneficial in the long term has not been established. In ALLHAT, persons receiving doxazosin as initial therapy had a significant increase in heart failure hospitalizations and a higher incidence of stroke relative to the persons receiving diuretics, prompting discontinuation of this arm of the study. To summarize, α-blockers should generally not be used as initial agents to treat hypertension—except perhaps in men with symptomatic prostatism.

I. Drugs with Central Sympatholytic Action

Methyldopa, clonidine, guanabenz, and guanfacine (Table 11–10) lower blood pressure by stimulating α-adrenergic receptors in the central nervous system, thus reducing efferent peripheral sympathetic outflow. These agents are effective as single therapy in some patients, but they are usually used as second- or third-line agents because of the high frequency of drug intolerance, including sedation, fatigue, dry mouth, postural hypotension, and impotence. An important concern is rebound hypertension following withdrawal. Methyldopa also causes hepatitis and hemolytic anemia and is avoided except in individuals who have already tolerated long-term therapy. There is considerable experience with methyldopa in pregnant women, and it is still used for this population. Clonidine is available in patches and may have particular value in patients in whom compliance is a troublesome issue.

J. Arteriolar Dilators

Hydralazine and minoxidil (Table 11–10) relax vascular smooth muscle and produce peripheral vasodilation. When given alone, they stimulate reflex tachycardia, increase myocardial contractility, and cause headache, palpitations, and fluid retention. They are usually given in combination with diuretics and β-blockers in resistant patients. Hydralazine produces frequent gastrointestinal disturbances and may induce a lupus-like syndrome. Minoxidil causes hirsutism and marked fluid retention; this agent is reserved for the most refractory of cases.

K. Peripheral Sympathetic Inhibitors

These agents are now used infrequently and usually in refractory hypertension. Reserpine remains a cost-effective antihypertensive agent (Table 11–10). Its reputation for inducing mental depression and its other side effects—sedation, nasal stuffiness, sleep disturbances, and peptic ulcers—has made it unpopular, though these problems are uncommon at low dosages. Guanethidine and guanadrel inhibit catecholamine release from peripheral neurons but frequently cause orthostatic hypotension (especially in the morning or after exercise), diarrhea, and fluid retention.

▶ Developing an Antihypertensive Regimen

Historically, data from a number of large trials support the overall conclusion that antihypertensive therapy with diuretics and β-blockers has a major beneficial effect on a broad spectrum of cardiovascular outcomes, reducing the incidence of stroke by 30–50% and of congestive heart failure by 40–50%, and halting progression to accelerated hypertension syndromes. The decreases in fatal and nonfatal coronary heart disease and cardiovascular and total mortality have been less dramatic, ranging from 10% to 15%. Similar placebo-controlled data pertaining to the newer agents are generally lacking, except for stroke reduction with the calcium channel blocker nitrendipine in the Systolic Hypertension in Europe trial. However, there is substantial evidence that ACE inhibitors, and to a lesser extent ARBs, reduce adverse cardiovascular outcomes in other related populations (eg, patients with diabetic nephropathy, heart failure, or postmyocardial infarction and individuals at high risk for cardiovascular events). Most large clinical trials that have compared outcomes in relatively unselected patients have failed to show a difference between newer agents—such as ACE inhibitors, calcium channel blockers, and ARBs—and the older diuretic-based regimens with regard to survival, myocardial infarction, and stroke. Where differences have been observed, they have mostly been attributable to subtle asymmetries in blood pressure control rather than to any inherent advantages of one agent over another. Therefore, experts recommend thiazide diuretics as the first-line treatment of older and perhaps all patients with hypertension because these agents are very effective and less expensive than the newer drugs. Exceptions are appropriate for individuals who have specific indications for another class of agent, such as postmyocardial infarction patients (β-blockers, ACE inhibitors), patients with diabetic nephropathy (ACE inhibitors, ARBs), or other comorbid conditions. Table 11–4 provides suggestions for individualizing first-line treatment based on compelling indications.

As discussed above, many experts would suggest that β-blockers no longer be considered ideal first-line drugs in the

Table 11–10. α-Adrenoceptor blocking agents, sympatholytics, and vasodilators.

Drug	Proprietary Names	Initial Dosage	Dosage Range	Cost per Unit	Cost of 30 Days Treatment (Average Dosage)[1]	Adverse Effects	Comments
α-Adrenoceptor blockers							
Prazosin	Minipress	1 mg hs	2–20 mg in 2 or 3 doses	$0.78/5 mg	$46.80 (5 mg twice daily)	Syncope with first dose; postural hypotension, dizziness, palpitations, headache, weakness, drowsiness, sexual dysfunction, anticholinergic effects, urinary incontinence; first-dose effects may be less with doxazosin.	May ↑ HDL and ↓ LDL cholesterol. May provide short-term relief of obstructive prostatic symptoms. Less effective in preventing cardiovascular events than diuretics.
Terazosin	Hytrin	1 mg hs	1–20 mg in 1 or 2 doses	$1.60/1, 2, 5, 10 mg	$48.00 (5 mg daily)		
Doxazosin	Cardura	1 mg hs	1–16 mg daily	$0.97/4 mg	$29.10 (4 mg daily)		
Central sympatholytics							
Clonidine	Catapres	0.1 mg twice daily	0.2–0.6 mg in 2 doses	$0.22/0.1 mg	$13.20 (0.1 mg twice daily)	Sedation, dry mouth, sexual dysfunction, headache, bradyarrhythmias; side effects may be less with guanfacine. Contact dermatitis with clonidine patch. Methyldopa also causes hepatitis, hemolytic anemia, fever.	"Rebound" hypertension may occur even after gradual withdrawal. Methyldopa should be avoided in favor of safer agents.
	Catapres TTS	0.1 mg/d patch weekly	0.1–0.3 mg/d patch weekly	$39.23/0.2 mg	$156.90 (0.2 mg weekly)		
Guanabenz	Wytensin	4 mg twice daily	8–64 mg in 2 doses	$0.98/4 mg	$58.80 (4 mg twice daily)		
Guanfacine	Tenex	1 mg once daily	1–3 mg daily	$0.87/1 mg	$26.10 (1 mg daily)		
Methyldopa	Aldomet	250 mg twice daily	500–2000 mg in 2 doses	$0.63/500 mg	$37.80 (500 mg twice daily)		
Peripheral neuronal antagonists							
Reserpine	Serpasil	0.05 mg once daily	0.05–0.25 mg daily	$0.48/0.1 mg	$14.40 (0.1 mg daily)	Depression (less likely at low dosages, ie, < 0.25 mg), night terrors, nasal stuffiness, drowsiness, peptic disease, gastrointestinal disturbances, bradycardia.	
Direct vasodilators							
Hydralazine	Apresoline	25 mg twice daily	50–300 mg in 2–4 doses	$0.51/25 mg	$30.60 (25 mg twice daily)	GI disturbances, tachycardia, headache, nasal congestion, rash, LE-like syndrome.	May worsen or precipitate angina.
Minoxidil	Loniten	5 mg once daily	5–40 mg once daily	$1.29/10 mg	$38.70 (10 mg once daily)	Tachycardia, fluid retention, headache, hirsutism, pericardial effusion, thrombocytopenia.	Should be used in combination with β-blocker and diuretic.

[1]Average wholesale price (AWP, for AB-rated generic when available) for quantity listed. Source: *Red Book Update,* Vol. 28, No. 3, March 2009. AWP may not accurately represent the actual pharmacy cost because wide contractual variations exist among institutions.
GI, gastrointestinal; LE, lupus erythematosus.

treatment of hypertension without compelling indications for their use. Although theoretical considerations suggest that the newer vasodilator β-blockers may be superior to the older drugs, this possibility remains to be tested.

For the purpose of devising an optimal treatment regimen, drugs can be divided into two complementary groups easily remembered as AB and CD. A and B refer to drugs that interrupt the renin-angiotensin system (**A**CE/ARB and β-**b**lockers) and C and D refer to those that do not (**c**alcium channel blockers and thiazide **d**iuretics). Combinations of drugs between these groups are likely to be more potent in lowering blood pressure than combinations within a group. Drugs A/B are more effective in young, white persons, in whom renins tend to be higher, and drugs C/D are more effective in old or black persons, in whom renin levels are generally lower. It is also important to note that antihypertensive treatment is effective at reducing cardiovascular risk at all ages, including the very elderly.

Figure 11–3 illustrates guidelines established by the BHS for developing a rational antihypertensive regimen. In the BHS guidelines, "B" is placed in parentheses to reflect the increasingly prevalent view that β-blockers should no longer be considered an ideal first-line agent. In trials that include patients with systolic hypertension, most patients require two or more medications and even then a substantial proportion fail to achieve the goal systolic blood pressure of < 140 mm Hg (< 130 mm Hg in high-risk persons).

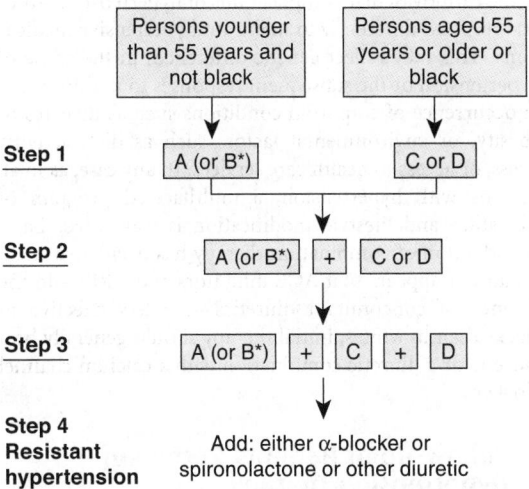

	Persons younger than 55 years and not black		Persons aged 55 years or older or black
Step 1	A (or B*)		C or D
Step 2	A (or B*)	+	C or D
Step 3	A (or B*)	+	C	+	D
Step 4 Resistant hypertension	Add: either α-blocker or spironolactone or other diuretic		

▲ **Figure 11–3.** The British Hypertension Society's recommendations for combining blood pressure lowering drugs. The "ABCD" rule. A, Angiotensin-converting enzyme inhibitor or angiotensin receptor blocker; B, β-blocker (the parentheses indicate that β-blockers should no longer be considered ideal first-line agents); C, calcium channel blockers; D, diuretic (thiazide). (Reprinted, with permission, from Williams B; British Hypertension Society. Guidelines for management of hypertension: report of the Fourth Working Party of the British Hypertension Society, 2004-BHS IV. J Hum Hypertens. 2004 Mar;18(3):139–185.)

In diabetic patients, three or four drugs are usually required to reduce systolic blood pressure to < 140 mm Hg. In many patients, blood pressure cannot be maintained at the recommended goal of < 130 mm Hg with any combination. As a result, debating the appropriate first-line agent is less relevant than determining the most appropriate combinations of agents. This has led many experts and practitioners to reconsider the use of fixed-dose combination antihypertensive agents as first-line therapy in patients with substantially elevated systolic pressures (> 160/100 mm Hg) or difficult-to-control hypertension (which is often associated with diabetes or kidney dysfunction). Based both on antihypertensive efficacy and complementarity, combinations of a diuretic and an ACE inhibitor (or an ARB if patient is intolerant of ACE inhibitor) are recommended. In younger white patients, the best choice is probably a combination of an ACE inhibitor and calcium channel blocker or thiazide. In light of side effect profiles, some experts have expressed the view that calcium channel blockers might be preferable to thiazides in the younger hypertensive patient. Furthermore, based on the results from the ACCOMPLISH trial, a combination of ACE inhibitor and calcium channel blocker may also prove optimal for patients at high risk for cardiovascular events. The initial use of low-dose combinations allows faster blood pressure reduction without substantially higher intolerance rates and is likely to be better accepted by patients. Improved blood pressure control can also be achieved by combining an ACE with an ARB. A suggested approach to treatment, tailored to patient demographics, is outlined in Table 11–11.

When an initial agent is selected, the patient should be informed of common side effects and the need for diligent compliance. Treatment should start at a low dose, and unless the initial blood pressure is very high (> 160/100 mm Hg), follow-up visits should usually be at 4- to 6-week intervals to allow for full medication effects to be established (especially with diuretics) before further titration or adjustment. If, after titration to usual doses, the patient has shown a discernible but incomplete response and a good tolerance of the initial drug, a second medication should be added. As a rule of thumb, a blood pressure reduction of 10 mm Hg can be expected for each antihypertensive agent added to the regimen.

Patients who are compliant with their medications and who do not respond to the combination regimens should usually be evaluated for secondary hypertension before proceeding to more complex regimens.

▶ Special Considerations in the Treatment of Diabetic Hypertensive Patients

Hypertensive patients with diabetes are at particularly high risk for cardiovascular events. More aggressive treatment of hypertension in these patients prevents progressive nephropathy, and a meta-analysis supports the notion that lower treatment goals (perhaps to lowest tolerated levels), are especially effective at reducing cardiovascular risk in diabetics compared with nondiabetics. Because of their beneficial effects in diabetic nephropathy, ACE inhibitors (and ARBs or perhaps renin inhibitors in intolerant

Table 11–11. Choice of antihypertensive agent based on demographic considerations.[1,2]

	Black, All Ages	All Others, Age < 55 Years	All Others, Age > 55 Years
First-line	Diuretic or CCB	ACE or ARB[3,4] or diuretic[5] or CCB	Diuretic[6] or CCB
Second-line	ACE or ARB[3,4] or β-blocker	β-Blocker[5]	ACE or ARB or β-blocker
Alternatives	α-Agonist or α-antagonist[7]	α-Agonist or α-antagonist	α-Agonist or α-antagonist[7]
Resistant hypertension	Spironolactone	Spironolactone	Spironolactone

[1]Compelling indications may alter the selection of an antihypertensive drug.
[2]Start with full dose of one agent, or lower doses of combination therapy.
[3]ACE and ARB can be synergistic in combination.
[4]Women of childbearing age should avoid ACE and ARB or discontinue as soon as pregnancy is diagnosed.
[5]The adverse metabolic effects of thiazide diuretics and β-blockers should be considered in younger patients but may be less important in the older patient.
[6]For patients with significant renal impairment, use loop diuretic instead of thiazide.
[7]α-Antagonists may precipitate or exacerbate orthostatic hypotension in the elderly.
ACE, angiotensin-converting enzyme inhibitor; ARB, angiotensin II receptor blocker; CCB, calcium channel blocker.

patients) should be part of the initial treatment regimen. However, most diabetics require combinations of three to five agents to achieve target blood pressure, usually including a diuretic and a calcium channel blocker or β-blocker. In addition to rigorous blood pressure control, treatment of persons with diabetes should include aggressive treatment of other risk factors and early intervention for coronary disease and left ventricular dysfunction.

▶ Treatment of Hypertension in Chronic Kidney Disease

Hypertension is present in 40% of patients with a glomerular filtration rate (GFR) of 60–90 mL/min, and 75% of patients with a GFR < 30 mL/min. ACE inhibitors and ARBs have been shown to delay progression of kidney disease in persons with type 1 and type 2 diabetes, respectively. It is also likely that inhibition of the renin-angiotensin system protects kidney function in nondiabetic kidney disease associated with significant proteinuria.

As discussed above, hypertension should be treated until blood pressure reaches < 130/80 mm Hg in patients with chronic kidney disease. There is a lack of definitive data to show that this level of blood pressure control slows the decline of GFR in persons with hypertensive chronic kidney disease without high-grade proteinuria. However, since all patients with chronic kidney disease are at high risk for cardiovascular damage, treatment of blood pressure to the < 130/80 mm Hg target is appropriate, and interruption of the renin-angiotensin system would seem a reasonable approach. Transition from thiazide to loop diuretic is often necessary to control volume expansion as kidney function worsens. Evidence has demonstrated that ACE inhibitors remain protective and safe in kidney disease associated with significant proteinuria and serum creatinine as high as 5 mg/dL. Note that such treatment would likely result in acute worsening of kidney function in patients with significant renal artery stenosis, so kidney function and electrolytes should be monitored carefully after introduction of ACE inhibitors. In any event, persis-

tence with ACE inhibitor/ARB therapy in the face of hyperkalemia is probably not warranted, since other antihypertensive medications are renoprotective as long as goal blood pressures are maintained.

▶ Hypertension Management in Blacks

Substantial evidence indicates that blacks are not only more likely to become hypertensive and more susceptible to the cardiovascular complications of hypertension—they also respond differently to many antihypertensive medications. This may reflect genetic differences in the cause of hypertension or the subsequent responses to it, differences in occurrence of comorbid conditions such as diabetes or obesity, or environmental factors such as diet, activity, stress, or access to health care services. In any case, as in all persons with hypertension, a multifaceted program of education and lifestyle modification is warranted. Early introduction of combination therapy has been advocated. Because it appears that ACE inhibitors and ARBs—in the absence of concomitant diuretics—are less effective in blacks than in whites, initial therapy should generally be a diuretic or a diuretic combination with a calcium channel blocker.

▶ Follow-Up of Patients Receiving Hypertension Therapy

Once blood pressure is controlled on a well-tolerated regimen, follow-up visits can be infrequent and laboratory testing limited to tests appropriate for the patient and the medications used. Yearly monitoring of blood lipids is recommended, and an electrocardiogram should be repeated at 2- to 4-year intervals depending on whether initial abnormalities are present, the presence of coronary risk factors, and age. Pharmacy care programs have been shown to improve compliance with medications. Patients who have had excellent blood pressure control for several years, especially if they have lost weight and initiated favorable lifestyle modifications, should be considered for "step-down" of therapy to determine whether lower doses or discontinuation of medications are feasible.

Chobanian AV. Does it matter how hypertension is controlled? N Engl J Med. 2008 Dec 4;359(23):2485–8. [PMID: 19052130]

Cohen JD. Managing hypertension: state of the science. J Clin Hypertens (Greenwich). 2006 Oct;8(10 Suppl 3):5–11. [PMID: 17028478]

Ferdinand KC et al. The management of hypertension in African Americans. Crit Pathw Cardiol. 2007 Jun;6(2):67–71. [PMID: 17667868]

Jamerson K et al; ACCOMPLISH Trial Investigators. Benazepril plus amlodipine or hydrochlorothiazide for hypertension in high-risk patients. N Engl J Med. 2008 Dec 4;359(23):2417–28. [PMID: 19052124]

Khan NA et al. The 2008 Canadian Hypertension Education Program recommendations for the management of hypertension: part 2 - therapy. Can J Cardiol. 2008 Jun;24(6):465–75. [PMID: 18548143]

Major outcomes in high-risk hypertensive patients randomized to angiotensin-converting enzyme inhibitor or calcium channel blocker vs diuretic. The Antihypertensive and Lipid-Lowering Treatment to Prevent Heart Attack Trial (ALLHAT). JAMA. 2002 Dec 18;288(23):2981–97. [PMID: 12479763]

Turnbull F et al; Blood Pressure Lowering Treatment Trialists' Collaboration. Effects of different blood pressure-lowering regimens on major cardiovascular events in individuals with and without diabetes mellitus: results of prospectively designed overviews of randomized trials. Arch Intern Med. 2005 Jun 27;165(12):1410–9. [PMID: 15983291]

RESISTANT HYPERTENSION

Resistant hypertension is defined in JNC 7 as the failure to reach blood pressure control in patients who are adherent to full doses of an appropriate three-drug regimen (including a diuretic). In this situation, the clinician should first exclude identifiable causes of hypertension (Table 11–2), and then carefully explore reasons why the patient might not be at goal blood pressure (Table 11–12). The clinician should pay particular attention to the type of diuretic being used in relation to the patient's kidney function. Aldosterone may play an important role in resistant hypertension and aldosterone receptor blockers can be very useful. If goal blood pressure cannot be achieved by these measures, consultation with a hypertension specialist should be considered.

Chapman N et al. Effect of spironolactone on blood pressure in subjects with resistant hypertension. Hypertension. 2007 Apr;49(4):839–45. [PMID: 17309946]

Epstein M. Resistant hypertension: prevalence and evolving concepts. J Clin Hypertens (Greenwich). 2007 Jan;9(1 Suppl 1):2–6. [PMID: 17215648]

HYPERTENSIVE URGENCIES & EMERGENCIES

Hypertensive emergencies have become less frequent in recent years but still require prompt recognition and aggressive but careful management. A spectrum of urgent presentations exists, and the appropriate therapeutic approach varies accordingly.

Hypertensive urgencies are situations in which blood pressure must be reduced within a few hours. These include patients with asymptomatic severe hypertension

Table 11–12. Causes of resistant hypertension.

Improper blood pressure measurement
Volume overload and pseudotolerance
Excess sodium intake
Volume retention from kidney disease
Inadequate diuretic therapy
Drug-induced or other causes
Nonadherence
Inadequate doses
Inappropriate combinations
Nonsteroidal anti-inflammatory drugs; cyclooxygenase-2 inhibitors
Cocaine, amphetamines, other illicit drugs
Sympathomimetics (decongestants, anorectics)
Oral contraceptives
Adrenal steroids
Cyclosporine and tacrolimus
Erythropoietin
Licorice (including some chewing tobacco)
Selected over-the-counter dietary supplements and medicines (eg, ephedra, ma huang, bitter orange)
Associated conditions
Obesity
Excess alcohol intake
Identifiable causes of hypertension (see Table 11-2)

Source: Chobanian AV et al. The Seventh Report of the Joint National Committee on Prevention, Detection, Evaluation, and Treatment of High Blood Pressure: the JNC 7 report. JAMA. 2003 May 21;289(19):2560–72.

(systolic blood pressure > 220 mm Hg or diastolic pressure > 125 mm Hg that persists after a period of observation) and those with optic disk edema, progressive target organ complications, and severe perioperative hypertension. Elevated blood pressure levels alone—in the absence of symptoms or new or progressive target organ damage—rarely require emergency therapy. Parenteral drug therapy is not usually required, and partial reduction of blood pressure with relief of symptoms is the goal.

Hypertensive emergencies require substantial reduction of blood pressure within 1 hour to avoid the risk of serious morbidity or death. Although blood pressure is usually strikingly elevated (diastolic pressure > 130 mm Hg), the correlation between pressure and end-organ damage is often poor. It is the latter that determines the seriousness of the emergency and the approach to treatment. Emergencies include hypertensive encephalopathy (headache, irritability, confusion, and altered mental status due to cerebrovascular spasm), hypertensive nephropathy (hematuria, proteinuria, and progressive kidney dysfunction due to arteriolar necrosis and intimal hyperplasia of the interlobular arteries), intracranial hemorrhage, aortic dissection, preeclampsia-eclampsia, pulmonary edema, unstable angina, or myocardial infarction. **Malignant hypertension** is by historical definition characterized by encephalopathy or nephropathy with accompanying papilledema. Progressive kidney disease usually ensues if treatment is not provided. The therapeutic approach is identical to that used with other antihypertensive emergencies.

Parenteral therapy is indicated in most hypertensive emergencies, especially if encephalopathy is present. The initial goal in hypertensive emergencies is to reduce the pressure by no more than 25% (within minutes to 1 or 2 hours) and then toward a level of 160/100 mm Hg within 2–6 hours. Excessive reductions in pressure may precipitate coronary, cerebral, or renal ischemia. To avoid such declines, the use of agents that have a predictable, dose-dependent, transient, and not precipitous antihypertensive effect is preferable. In that regard, the use of sublingual or oral fast-acting nifedipine preparations is best avoided.

Acute ischemic stroke is often associated with marked elevation of blood pressure, which will usually fall spontaneously. In such cases, antihypertensives should only be used if the blood pressure exceeds 220/120 mm Hg, and blood pressure should be reduced cautiously by 10–15%. If thrombolytics are to be given, blood pressure should be maintained at < 185/110 mm Hg during treatment and for 24 hours following treatment.

In hemorrhagic stroke, the aim is to minimize bleeding with a target mean arterial pressure of < 130 mm Hg. In acute subarachnoid hemorrhage, as long as the bleeding source remains uncorrected, a compromise must be struck between preventing further bleeding and maintaining cerebral perfusion in the face of cerebral vasospasm. In this situation, blood pressure goals depend on the patient's usual blood pressure. In normotensive patients, the target should be a systolic blood pressure of 110–120 mm Hg; in hypertensive patients, blood pressure should be treated to 20% below baseline pressure. In the treatment of hypertensive emergencies complicated by (or precipitated by) central nervous system injury, labetalol or nicardipine are good choices, since they are nonsedating and do not appear to cause significant increases in cerebral blood flow or intracranial pressure in this setting. In hypertensive emergencies arising from catecholaminergic mechanisms, such as pheochromocytoma or cocaine use, β-blockers can worsen the hypertension because of unopposed peripheral vasoconstriction; phentolamine is a better choice. Labetalol is useful in these patients if the heart rate must be controlled.

▶ **Pharmacologic Management**

A. Parenteral Agents

A growing number of agents are available for management of acute hypertensive problems. (Table 11–13 lists drugs, dosages, and adverse effects.) Sodium nitroprusside is the agent of choice for the most serious emergencies because of its rapid and easily controllable action, but continuous monitoring is essential when this agent is used. In the presence of myocardial ischemia, intravenous nitroglycerin or an intravenous β-blocker, such as labetalol or esmolol, is preferable.

1. Nitroprusside sodium—This agent is given by controlled intravenous infusion gradually titrated to the desired effect. It lowers the blood pressure within seconds by direct arteriolar and venous dilation. Monitoring with an intra-arterial line avoids hypotension. Nitroprusside—in combination with a β-blocker—is especially useful in patients with aortic dissection.

2. Nitroglycerin, intravenous—This agent is a less potent antihypertensive than nitroprusside and should be reserved for patients with accompanying acute ischemic syndromes.

3. Labetalol—This combined β- and α-blocking agent is the most potent adrenergic blocker for rapid blood pressure reduction. Other β-blockers are far less potent. Excessive blood pressure drops are unusual. Experience with this agent in hypertensive syndromes associated with pregnancy has been favorable.

4. Esmolol—This rapidly acting β-blocker is approved only for treatment of supraventricular tachycardia but is often used for lowering blood pressure. It is less potent than labetalol and should be reserved for patients in whom there is particular concern about serious adverse events related to β-blockers.

5. Fenoldopam—Fenoldopam is a peripheral dopamine-1 (DA_1) receptor agonist that causes a dose-dependent reduction in arterial pressure without evidence of tolerance, rebound, or withdrawal or deterioration of kidney function. In higher dosage ranges, tachycardia may occur.

6. Nicardipine—Intravenous nicardipine is the most potent and the longest acting of the parenteral calcium channel blockers. As a primarily arterial vasodilator, it has the potential to precipitate reflex tachycardia, and for that reason it should not be used without a β-blocker in patients with coronary artery disease.

7. Enalaprilat—This is the active form of the oral ACE inhibitor enalapril. The onset of action is usually within 15 minutes, but the peak effect may be delayed for up to 6 hours. Thus, enalaprilat is used primarily as an adjunctive agent.

8. Diuretics—Intravenous loop diuretics can be very helpful when the patient has signs of heart failure or fluid retention, but the onset of their hypotensive response is slow, making them an adjunct rather than a primary agent for hypertensive emergencies. Low dosages should be used initially (furosemide, 20 mg, or bumetanide, 0.5 mg). They facilitate the response to vasodilators, which often stimulate fluid retention.

9. Diazoxide—Diazoxide acts promptly as a vasodilator without decreasing renal blood flow. To avoid hypotension, it should be given in small boluses or as an infusion rather than as the previously recommended large bolus. One use of diazoxide has been in preeclampsia-eclampsia. Hyperglycemia and sodium and water retention may occur. The drug should be used only for short periods and is best combined with a loop diuretic.

10. Hydralazine—Hydralazine can be given intravenously or intramuscularly, but its effect is less predictable than that of other drugs in this group. It produces reflex tachycardia and should not be given without β-blockers in patients with possible coronary disease or aortic dissection. Hydralazine is now used primarily in pregnancy and in children, but even in these situations, newer agents are supplanting it.

11. Trimethaphan—The ganglionic blocking agent trimethaphan is titrated with the patient sitting; its activity

Table 11–13. Drugs for hypertensive emergencies and urgencies.

Agent	Action	Dosage	Onset	Duration	Adverse Effects	Comments
Parenteral agents (intravenous unless noted)						
Nitroprusside (Nipride)	Vasodilator	0.25–10 mcg/kg/min	Seconds	3–5 minutes	GI, CNS; thiocyanate and cyanide toxicity, especially with renal and hepatic insufficiency; hypotension.	Most effective and easily titratable treatment. Use with β-blocker in aortic dissection.
Nitroglycerin	Vasodilator	0.25–5 mcg/kg/min	2–5 minutes	3–5 minutes	Headache, nausea, hypotension, bradycardia.	Tolerance may develop. Useful primarily with myocardial ischemia.
Labetalol (Normodyne, Trandate)	β- and α-blocker	20–40 mg every 10 minutes to 300 mg; 2 mg/min infusion	5–10 minutes	3–6 hours	GI, hypotension, bronchospasm, bradycardia, heart block.	Avoid in congestive heart failure, asthma. May be continued orally.
Esmolol (Brevibloc)	β-Blocker	Loading dose 500 mcg/kg over 1 minute; maintenance, 25–200 mcg/kg/min	1–2 minutes	10–30 minutes	Bradycardia, nausea.	Avoid in congestive heart failure, asthma. Weak antihypertensive.
Fenoldopam (Corlopam)	Dopamine receptor agonist	0.1–1.6 mcg/kg/min	4–5 minutes	< 10 minutes	Reflex tachycardia, hypotension, ↑intraocular pressure.	May protect kidney function.
Nicardipine (Cardene)	Calcium channel blocker	5 mg/h; may increase by 1–2.5 mg/h every 15 minutes to 15 mg/h	1–5 minutes	3–6 hours	Hypotension, tachycardia, headache.	May precipitate myocardial ischemia.
Enalaprilat (Vasotec)	ACE inhibitor	1.25 mg every 6 hours	15 minutes	6 hours or more	Excessive hypotension.	Additive with diuretics; may be continued orally.
Furosemide (Lasix)	Diuretic	10–80 mg	15 minutes	4 hours	Hypokalemia, hypotension.	Adjunct to vasodilator.
Hydralazine (Apresoline)	Vasodilator	5–20 mg intravenously or intramuscularly (less desirable); may repeat after 20 minutes	10–30 minutes	2–6 hours	Tachycardia, headache, GI.	Avoid in coronary artery disease, dissection. Rarely used except in pregnancy.
Diazoxide (Hyperstat)	Vasodilator	50–150 mg repeated at intervals of 5–15 minutes, or 15–30 mg/min by intravenous infusion to a maximum of 600 mg	1–2 minutes	4–24 hours	Excessive hypotension, tachycardia, myocardial ischemia, headache, nausea, vomiting, hyperglycemia. Necrosis with extravasation.	Avoid in coronary artery disease and dissection. Use with β-blocker and diuretic. Mostly obsolete.
Trimethaphan (Arfonad)	Ganglionic blocker	0.5–5 mg/min	1–3 minutes	10 minutes	Hypotension, ileus, urinary retention, respiratory arrest. Liberates histamine; use caution in allergic individuals.	Useful in aortic dissection. Otherwise rarely used.
Oral agents						
Nifedipine (Adalat, Procardia)	Calcium channel blocker	10 mg initially; may be repeated after 30 minutes	15 minutes	2–6 hours	Excessive hypotension, tachycardia, headache, angina, myocardial infarction, stroke.	Response unpredictable.
Clonidine (Catapres)	Central sympatholytic	0.1–0.2 mg initially; then 0.1 mg every hour to 0.8 mg	30–60 minutes	6–8 hours	Sedation.	Rebound may occur.
Captopril (Capoten)	ACE inhibitor	12.5–25 mg	15–30 minutes	4–6 hours	Excessive hypotension.	

ACE, angiotensin-converting enzyme; CNS, central nervous system; GI, gastrointestinal.

depends on this. The patient can be placed supine if the hypotensive effect is excessive. The effect occurs within a few minutes and persists for the duration of the infusion. This agent has largely been replaced by nitroprusside and newer medications.

B. Oral Agents

Patients with less severe acute hypertensive syndromes can often be treated with oral therapy. Abrupt blood pressure lowering is not usually necessary in asymptomatic individuals, and the use of agents such as rapid-acting nifedipine probably causes more adverse effects than benefits.

1. Nifedipine—The effect of fast-acting nifedipine capsules is unpredictable and may be excessive, resulting in hypotension and reflex tachycardia. Because myocardial infarction and stroke have been reported in this setting, the use of sublingual nifedipine is not advised.

2. Clonidine—Clonidine, 0.2 mg orally initially, followed by 0.1 mg every hour to a total of 0.8 mg, will usually lower blood pressure over a period of several hours. Sedation is frequent, and rebound hypertension may occur if the drug is stopped.

3. Captopril—Captopril, 12.5–25 mg orally, will also lower blood pressure in 15–30 minutes. The response is variable and may be excessive.

C. Subsequent Therapy

When the blood pressure has been brought under control, combinations of oral antihypertensive agents can be added as parenteral drugs are tapered off over a period of 2–3 days. Most subsequent regimens should include a diuretic.

Flanigan JS et al. Hypertensive emergency and severe hypertension: what to treat, who to treat, and how to treat. Med Clin North Am. 2006 May;90(3):439–51. [PMID: 16473099]

Migneco A et al. Hypertensive crises: diagnosis and management in the emergency room. Eur Rev Med Pharmacol Sci. 2004 Jul–Aug;8(4):143–52. [PMID: 15636400]

Blood Vessel & Lymphatic Disorders

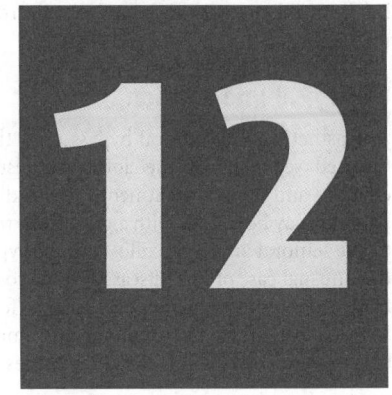

Joseph H. Rapp, MD

Rajabrata Sarkar, MD, PhD

Christopher D. Owens, MD, MSc

ATHEROSCLEROTIC PERIPHERAL VASCULAR DISEASE

OCCLUSIVE DISEASE: AORTA & ILIAC ARTERIES

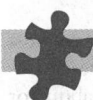

ESSENTIALS OF DIAGNOSIS

▸ Cramping pain or tiredness in the calf, thigh, or hip while walking (claudication).

▸ Diminished femoral pulses.

▸ Tissue loss (ulceration, gangrene) or rest pain.

General Considerations

Occlusive atherosclerotic lesions can develop in the distal aorta and proximal common iliac arteries, often in relatively young men, age 50–60 years. The patient with aortoiliac disease is usually a smoker in whom this is the initial manifestation of systemic atherosclerosis. Disease progression may lead to complete occlusion of one or both common iliac arteries, which can precipitate occlusion of the entire abdominal aorta to the level of the renal arteries. Lesions affecting the external iliac arteries are less common as are lesions isolated to the aorta. Pathologic changes of atherosclerosis may be diffuse, but flow-limiting stenoses occur segmentally. This is particularly true of the aortoiliac segment where patients may have limited or no narrowing of the vessels in the more distal vessels of the lower extremities.

Clinical Findings

A. Symptoms and Signs

Intermittent claudication occurs because blood flow cannot keep up with demand. The pain is severe, cramping, and usually located in the calf muscles. The pain may extend into the thigh and buttocks with continued exercise. It may be unilateral or bilateral if there is bilateral disease. Rarely, patients complain only of weakness in the legs when walking, or simply extreme limb fatigue. The symptoms are relieved with rest. With bilateral common iliac disease, impotence is a common complaint. Femoral pulses are absent or very weak as are the distal pulses. A bruit may be heard over the aorta, iliac, or femoral arteries or over all three arteries.

B. Doppler Findings

The ratio of systolic blood pressure detected by Doppler examination at the ankle compared with the brachial artery is reduced to below 0.9 (normal ratio is 1.0–1.2); this difference is exaggerated by exercise. Segmental waveforms or pulse volume recordings obtained by strain gaze technology through blood pressure cuffs demonstrate blunting of the arterial inflow throughout the lower extremity.

C. Imaging

CT angiography (CTA) and magnetic resonance angiography (MRA) have largely replaced invasive angiography to determine the anatomic location of disease. Imaging is only required when symptoms require intervention, since a history and physical examination with segmental waveform analysis should appropriately identify the involved levels of the arterial tree.

Treatment

A. Conservative Care

A program that includes smoking cessation, risk factor reduction, weight loss, and walking will substantially improve exercise tolerance. A trial of phosphodiesterase inhibitors, such as cilostazol 100 mg orally twice a day, may be beneficial in approximately two-thirds of patients. Antiplatelet agents reduce overall cardiovascular morbidity but do not ameliorate symptoms. Several large trials have failed to show a benefit from warfarin therapy. In the initial stages of a rehabilitation program, simply slowing the cadence of walking will allow patients to walk further without pain.

B. Endovascular Techniques

If the atherosclerotic lesions are truly segmental, they can be effectively treated with angioplasty and stenting. This approach matches the results of surgery for single stenoses but both effectiveness and durability decreases with multiple stenoses.

C. Surgical Intervention

A prosthetic aorto-femoral bypass graft that bypasses the diseased segments of the aortoiliac system is a highly effective and durable treatment for this disease. High-risk patients may be treated with a graft from the axillary artery to the femoral arteries (axillo-femoral bypass graft) or, in the unusual case of iliac disease limited to one side, a graft from the contralateral femoral artery (fem-fem bypass). The axillo-femoral and femoral to femoral grafts have lower operative risk; however, they are less durable.

► Complications

The complications of the aorto-femoral bypass are those of any major abdominal reconstruction in a patient population that has a high prevalence of cardiovascular disease. Mortality should be low, in the range of 2–3%, but morbidity is higher with a 5–10% rate of myocardial infarction. The total complication rate may be over 10%. Complications of endovascular repair include embolization and vessel dissection. These are relatively uncommon and the total complication rate should be below 3% with this technique.

► Prognosis

Without intervention patients with aorto-iliac disease may have a further reduction in walking distance but symptoms rarely progress to rest pain or threatened limb loss. Life expectancy is limited by their attendant cardiac disease with a mortality rate of 25–40% at 5 years.

Symptomatic relief is generally excellent after intervention. After aorto-femoral bypass, a patency rate of 90% at 5 years is common. Patency rates and symptom relief for less extensive procedures are also good with 20–30% symptom return at 3 years.

► When to Refer

Patients with progressive reduction in walking distance and those with limitations in ambulation that interfere with their activities of daily living should be referred for consultation to a vascular surgeon.

Hirsch AT et al. ACC/AHA 2005 Practice Guidelines for the management of patients with peripheral arterial disease (lower extremity, renal, mesenteric, and abdominal aortic): a collaborative report from the American Association for Vascular Surgery/Society for Vascular Surgery, Society for Cardiovascular Angiography and Interventions, Society for Vascular Medicine and Biology, Society of Interventional Radiology, and the ACC/AHA Task Force on Practice Guidelines (Writing Committee to Develop Guidelines for the Management of Patients With Peripheral Arterial Disease): endorsed by the American Association of Cardiovascular and Pulmonary Rehabilitation; National Heart, Lung, and Blood Institute; Society for Vascular Nursing; TransAtlantic Inter-Society Consensus; and Vascular Disease Foundation. Circulation. 2006 Mar 21;113(11):e463–654. [PMID: 16549646]

Sontheimer DL. Peripheral vascular disease: diagnosis and treatment. Am Fam Physician. 2006 Jun 1;73(11):1971–6. [PMID: 16770929]

WAVE Investigators. The effects of oral anticoagulants in patients with peripheral arterial disease: rationale, design, and baseline characteristics of the Warfarin and Antiplatelet Vascular Evaluation (WAVE) trial, including a meta-analysis of trials. Am Heart J. 2006 Jan;151(1):1–9. [PMID: 16368284]

OCCLUSIVE DISEASE: FEMORAL & POPLITEAL ARTERIES

 ESSENTIALS OF DIAGNOSIS

- ► Cramping pain or tiredness in the calf with exercise.
- ► Reduced popliteal or pedal pulses.
- ► Foot pain at rest, relieved by dependency.
- ► Foot gangrene or ulceration.

► General Considerations

The superficial femoral artery (SFA) is the artery most commonly occluded by atherosclerosis. The disease frequently occurs where the SFA passes through the abductor magnis tendon in the distal thigh. The profunda femoris artery and the popliteal artery are relatively spared occlusive lesions except in patients with diabetes. As with atherosclerosis of the aorto-iliac segment, these lesions are closely associated with a history of smoking.

► Clinical Findings

A. Symptoms and Signs

Symptoms of intermittent claudication are confined to the calf. Occlusion or stenosis of the SFA at the abductor canal when the patient has good collaterals from the profunda femoris will cause claudication at approximately 2–4 blocks. However, with concomitant disease of the profunda femoris or the popliteal artery, much shorter distances may trigger symptoms. With short-distance claudication, dependent rubor of the foot with blanching on elevation may be present. Chronic low blood flow states will also cause atrophic changes in the lower leg and foot with loss of hair, thinning of the skin and subcutaneous tissues, and disuse atrophy of the muscles. With segmental occlusive disease of the SFA, the common femoral pulsation is normal, but the popliteal and pedal pulses are reduced.

B. Laboratory Findings

The ankle-brachial index (ABI) is reduced; levels below 0.5 suggest severe reduction in flow. ABI readings depend on arterial compression. Since the vessels may be calcified in diabetic patients and the elderly, ABIs can be misleading and must be accompanied by a waveform analysis. Pulse volume recordings with cuffs placed at the high thigh, mid thigh, calf, and ankle will delineate the levels of obstruction with reduced pressures and blunted waveforms. Angiography, CTA, or MRA all adequately show the anatomic location of the obstructive lesions. Generally, these studies are only done if revascularization is planned.

Treatment

A. Conservative Care

As with aorto-iliac disease, conservative management has an important role for some patients, particularly those individuals with SFA occlusion and good profunda femoris collaterals. For these patients conservative management as noted above can result in excellent outcomes with no intervention required.

B. Surgical Intervention

1. Bypass surgery—Intervention is indicated if intermittent claudication is progressive, incapacitating or interferes significantly with essential daily activities. Intervention is mandatory if there is rest pain or threatened tissue loss of the foot. The most effective and durable treatment for lesions of the SFA is a femoral-popliteal bypass with autogenous saphenous vein. Synthetic material, usually polytetrafluoroethylene (PTFE), can be used, but these grafts do not have the durability of vein bypass.

2. Endovascular surgery—Endovascular techniques are effective for lesions of the SFA. There are several options. Angioplasty may be combined with stenting either with a bare metal stent or a PTFE-covered stent to form an endoluminal bypass. Cryoplasty, angioplasty with balloon cooled to −20 °C, and endoluminal atherectomy also have their proponents. These techniques have lower morbidity than bypass surgery but also have a lower rate of success and durability.

Endovascular therapy is most effective when the lesions are less than 10 cm long and in patients who are undergoing aggressive risk factor modification.

3. Thromboendarterectomy—Removal of the atherosclerotic plaque is limited to the lesions of the common femoral and profunda femoris artery where bypass grafts and endovascular techniques have a more limited role.

Complications

Open surgical procedures of the lower extremity, particularly long bypasses with vein harvest, have a risk of wound infection that is higher than in other areas of the body. Wound infection or seroma can occur in as many as 15–20% of cases. Myocardial infarction rates after open surgery are 5–10%, with a 1–4% mortality rate. Complication rates of endovascular therapy are 1–5%, making these therapies attractive despite their lower durability.

Prognosis

The prognosis for motivated patients with isolated SFA disease is excellent, and surgery is not recommended for mild or moderate claudication in these patients. However, when claudication significantly limits daily activity and undermines quality of life as well as overall cardiovascular

health, intervention may be warranted. All interventions require close postprocedure follow-up with ultrasound surveillance so that any recurrent narrowing can be treated promptly to prevent complete occlusion. The patency rate of bypass grafts of the femoral artery, SFA, and popliteal artery may be as high as 70% at 3 years with patency for endovascular procedures somewhat lower.

Because of the extensive atherosclerotic disease, including associated coronary lesions, 5-year survival among patients with lower extremity disease can be as high as 50%, particularly with involvement of the infrapopliteal vessels (see below). However, with aggressive risk factor modification, substantial improvement in longevity has been reported.

When to Refer

Patients with progressive symptoms, short distance claudication, rest pain, or any ulceration should be referred to a peripheral vascular specialist.

Diehm C. Association of low ankle brachial index with high mortality in primary care. Eur Heart J. 2006 Jul;27(14):1743–9. [PMID: 16782720]
McDermott MM et al. Lower extremity nerve function in patients with lower extremity ischemia. Arch Intern Med. 2006 Oct 9;166(18):1986–92. [PMID: 17030832]
White C. Intermittent claudication. N Engl J Med. 2007 Mar 22;356(12):1241–50. [PMID: 17377162]

OCCLUSIVE DISEASE: LOWER LEG & FOOT ARTERIES

ESSENTIALS OF DIAGNOSIS

▸ Rest pain of the forefoot that is severe and relieved by dependency.

▸ Pain or numbness of the foot with walking.

▸ Ulceration or gangrene of the foot or toes.

▸ Pallor when the foot is elevated.

General Considerations

Occlusive processes of the lower leg and foot primarily involve the tibial vessels with rare involvement the arteries of the foot. There often is extensive calcification of the artery wall. This distribution of atherosclerosis is primarily seen in patients with diabetes mellitus.

Clinical Findings

A. Symptoms and Signs

Unless there are associated lesions in the aorto-iliac or femoral/SFA segments, claudication may not be evident. The gastrocnemius and soleus muscles may receive adequate blood supply from collateral vessels from the popliteal artery; therefore, when disease is isolated to the tibial vessels, there may be foot ischemia without attendant claudication, and rest pain or ulceration may be the first sign of severe vascular insufficiency. Classically, rest pain is confined to the dorsum of the foot at the area of the metatarsal heads and is relieved with dependency. The pain is severe, usually burning in character and will awaken the patient from sleep. Because of the high incidence of neuropathy in these patients, it is important to differentiate rest pain from neuropathic dysesthesia. If the pain is relieved by simply dangling the foot over the edge of the bed, which increases blood flow to the foot, then the rest pain is due to vascular insufficiency. On examination, depending on whether associated proximal disease is present, there may or may not be femoral and popliteal pulses, but the pedal pulses will be absent. Dependent rubor may be prominent with pallor on elevation. The skin of the foot is generally cool, atrophic, and hairless.

B. Laboratory Findings

The ABI may be quite low (in the range of 0.3 or lower), but ABIs may be falsely elevated because of the noncompressability of the calcified tibial vessels. Waveform analysis is important in these patients; a monophasic flow pattern denotes critically low flow. Segmental pulse volume recordings will show a fall-off in blood pressure between the calf and ankle, although pulse volume recordings also may also be affected by tibial vessel calcification.

C. Imaging

CTA, MRA, or angiography, is often needed to delineate the anatomy of the tibial-popliteal segment.

▶ Treatment

Good foot care may avoid ulceration, and most diabetic patients will do well with a conservative regimen. However, if ulcerations appear and there is no significant healing within 2–3 weeks, revascularization will be required. Infrequent rest pain is not an absolute indication for revascularization. However, rest pain occurring nightly with monophasic waveforms requires revascularization to prevent threatened tissue loss.

A. Bypass and Endovascular Techniques

Bypass with vein to the distal tibial or pedal arteries has been shown to be an effective mechanism to treat rest pain and heal gangrene or ischemic ulcerations of the foot. Because the foot often has relative sparing of vascular disease, these bypasses have had adequate patency rates (70% at 3 years). Fortunately, in nearly all series, limb salvage rates are much higher than patency rates.

Endovascular techniques are beginning to be used in the tibial vessels with modest results, but bypass grafting remains the primary technique of revascularization.

B. Amputation

Patients with rest pain and tissue loss are at high risk for amputation, particularly if revascularization cannot be done. It may be necessary to debride necrotic or severely infected tissue. Toe amputations have little or no affect on the mechanics of walking. Removal of the first toe or a transmetatarsal amputation, removing all toes and the heads of the metatarsals, are durable but increase the energy required of walking by 5–10%. Unfortunately, the next level that can be successfully used for a prosthesis is at the below-knee level. The energy expenditure of walking is then increased by 50%. With an above-knee amputation, the energy required to ambulate may be increased as much as 100%. While there are good prosthetic alternatives for these patients, activity levels are limited after amputation, and there are issues relating to self-image. These factors combine to demand revascularization whenever possible to preserve the limb.

▶ Complications

The complications of intervention are similar to those listed for SFA disease with evidence that the overall cardiovascular risk increases with decreasing ABI. The patients with critical limb ischemia require aggressive risk factor modification. Wound infection rates after bypass are higher if there is an open wound in the foot.

▶ Prognosis

Patients with tibial atherosclerosis have extensive atherosclerotic burden and a high prevalence of diabetes. Their prognosis without intervention is poor and complicated by the risk of amputation.

▶ When to Refer

Patients with diabetes should be referred to a vascular specialist for evaluation if there is a reduction in the pedal pulses, even if small. Intervention may not be necessary but the severity of the disease will be quantified, which has implications for future symptom development.

Nguyen LL et al. Prospective multicenter study of quality of life before and after lower extremity vein bypass in 1404 patients with critical limb ischemia. J Vasc Surg. 2006 Nov;44(5):977–83. [PMID: 17098529]

Raghunathan A et al. Postoperative outcomes for patients undergoing elective revascularization for critical limb ischemia and intermittent claudication: a subanalysis of the Coronary Artery Revascularization Prophylaxis (CARP) trial. J Vasc Surg. 2006 Jun;43(6):1175–82. [PMID: 16765234]

ACUTE ARTERIAL OCCLUSION OF A LIMB

 ESSENTIALS OF DIAGNOSIS

▶ Sudden pain in an extremity.

▶ Generally associated with some element of neurologic dysfunction with numbness, weakness, or complete paralysis.

▶ Absent extremity pulses.

General Considerations

Acute occlusion may be due to an embolus or to thrombosis of a diseased atherosclerotic segment. Arterial to arterial emboli such as in the cerebrovascular tree can occur, but emboli large enough to occlude proximal arteries in the lower extremities are almost always from the heart. Over 50% of the emboli from cardiac sources go to the lower extremities, 20% to the cerebrovascular circulation, and the remainder to the upper extremities and mesenteric and renal circulation. Atrial fibrillation is the usual cause of cardiac thrombus formation; other causes are valvular disease or ischemic heart disease where thrombus has formed on the ventricular surface of a transmural myocardial infarct.

Emboli from arterial sources such as arterial ulcerations or calcified excrescences are usually small and go to the distal arterial tree (toes).

The typical patient with **primary** thrombosis has had a history of claudication and now has an acute occlusion. If the stenosis has developed over time, collateral blood vessels will develop, and the resulting occlusion may only cause a minimal increase in symptoms.

Clinical Findings

A. Symptoms and Signs

The sudden onset of extremity pain, with loss or reduction in pulses, is diagnostic of acute arterial occlusion. This often will be accompanied by neurologic dysfunction, such as numbness or paralysis in extreme cases. With popliteal occlusion, symptoms may only affect the foot. With proximal occlusions, the whole leg may be affected. Signs of severe arterial ischemia, such as pallor on elevation, coolness of the extremity, mottling, and impaired neurologic function with hyperesthesia progressing to anesthesia accompanied with paralysis will also occur.

B. Laboratory Findings

There will be little or no flow found with Doppler examination of the distal vessels. Imaging, if done, shows an abrupt cutoff of the vessel involved. Blood work may indicate systemic acidosis.

C. Imaging

Whenever possible, imaging should be done in the operating room because obtaining angiography, MRA, or CTA may delay revascularization and jeopardize the viability of the extremity. However, in cases with only modest symptoms and light touch of the extremity is maintained, imaging may be helpful in planning the revascularization procedure.

Treatment

Immediate revascularization is required in all cases of symptomatic acute arterial thrombosis. Evidence of neurologic injury, including loss of light touch sensation, indicates that collateral flow is inadequate to maintain limb viability and revascularization should be accomplished within 3 hours. Longer delays carry a significant risk of irreversible tissue damage. This risk approaches 100% at 6 hours.

A. Heparin

As soon as the diagnosis is made, unfractionated heparin should be administered (5000–10,000 units) intravenously. This helps prevent clot propagation and may also help relieve associated vessel spasm. There may be some reduction in symptoms with aggressive anticoagulation, but revascularization will still be required. Patients in atrial fibrillation need to continue taking anticoagulants until cardioversion can be attempted.

B. Endovascular Techniques

Chemical thrombolysis with TPA may be done but often requires 24 hours or longer to fully lyse the thrombus. This approach can be taken only in patients with an intact neurologic exam. An echocardiogram should be done first to identify additional clot in the atrium. If an additional clot is found, thrombolysis may be ill advised because of the risk of subsequent emboli from the cardiac clot. Catheter-based mechanical thrombolysis may be an excellent alternative.

C. Surgical Intervention

General anesthesia is usually indicated in these patients; local anesthesia may be used in extremely high-risk patients if the exploration is to be limited to the common femoral artery. In extreme cases, it may be necessary to perform embolectomy from the femoral, popliteal and even the pedal vessels to revascularize the limb. Devices to pulverize and aspirate clot and intraoperative thrombolysis with tissue plasminogen activator (TPA) are being used to improve outcomes.

Complications

Complications of revascularization of an acutely ischemic limb can include severe acidosis and myocardial arrest. In cases where several hours have elapsed but recovery of viable tissue may still possible, significant levels of lactic acid, potassium, and other harmful agents may be released into the circulation during revascularization. Pretreatment of the patient with sodium bicarbonate prior to reestablishing arterial flow is required. Surgery in the presence of thrombolytic agents and heparin carries a high risk of postoperative wound hematoma.

Prognosis

There is a 10–25% risk of amputation with acute arterial occlusion, and a 25% or higher in-hospital mortality rate. Prognosis for acute occlusion of an atherosclerotic segment is generally much better because the collateral flow can maintain extremity viability. The longer term survival reflects the overall condition of the patient. In high-risk patients, an acute arterial occlusion suggests a dismal prognosis.

OCCLUSIVE CEREBROVASCULAR DISEASE

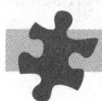 ESSENTIALS OF DIAGNOSIS

► Sudden onset of weakness and numbness of an extremity, aphasia, dysarthria, or unilateral blindness (amaurosis fugax).

► Bruit heard loudest in the mid neck.

General Considerations

Unlike the other vascular territories, symptoms of occlusive cerebrovascular disease are predominantly due to emboli. Transient ischemic attacks (TIAs) are the result of small emboli, and the risk of additional emboli causing permanent deficits is high. One-third of all strokes may be due to emboli. In the absence of atrial fibrillation, approximately 90% of these emboli originate from the proximal internal carotid artery, an area uniquely prone to the development of atherosclerosis. Lesions in the proximal great vessels, the common carotid and the carotid siphon, are far less common.

Clinical Findings

A. Symptoms and Signs

Generally, the symptoms of a TIA last only a few minutes but may continue up to 24 hours. The most common lesions develop in the cortex, and there is usually both motor and sensory involvement. Emboli to the retinal artery cause unilateral blindness which, when transient, is termed "amaurosis fugax." Posterior circulation symptoms referable to the brainstem, cerebellum, and visual regions of the brain are due to atherosclerosis of the vertebral basilar systems and are much less common.

Signs of cerebrovascular disease include bruits in the mid-cervical area with reduced or absent arm pulses. While bruits in the neck in older patients and generalized atherosclerosis are important signs of cerebrovascular disease, they are not specific for narrowing within the vessel. There is poor correlation between the degree of stenosis and the presence of the bruit. Furthermore, absence of a bruit does not exclude the possibility of carotid stenosis. Nonfocal symptoms, such as dizziness and unsteadiness, seldom are related to cerebrovascular atherosclerosis.

B. Imaging

Duplex ultrasonography is the imaging modality of choice with a high specificity and sensitivity for detecting and grading the degree of stenosis at the carotid bifurcation: 50% stenosis in a symptomatic patient and 80% in an asymptomatic patient require intervention. Mild to moderate disease (30–50% stenosis) indicates the need for ongoing surveillance and aggressive risk factor modification.

Excellent depiction of the full anatomy of the cerebrovascular circulation from arch to cranium can be obtained with either MRA or CTA. Each of these modalities may have false-positive or false-negative findings. Since the decision to intervene in cases of carotid stenosis depends on an accurate assessment of the degree of stenosis, it is recommended that at least two modalities be used to confirm the degree of stenosis. Cerebral angiography is reserved for cases that cannot be resolved by these less invasive imaging modalities.

Treatment

A. Asymptomatic Patients

Patients with no neurologic symptoms but with carotid stenosis on imaging will benefit from carotid intervention if they are considered to be at low risk for intervention and their expected survival is greater than 5 years. Recommendation for intervention also presumes that the treating institution has a stroke rate in asymptomatic patients that is acceptable (< 3%). Large studies indicate a reduction in stroke from 11.5% to 5.0% over 5 years with surgical treatment of asymptomatic carotid stenoses of greater than 60%. However, the usual practice is to only treat those patients who have greater than 80% stenosis. Patients with carotid stenosis that suddenly worsens are thought to have an unstable plaque and are at particularly high risk for embolic stroke.

B. Symptomatic Patients

Large randomized trials have shown that patients with TIAs or strokes from which they have completely or nearly completely recovered will benefit from carotid intervention if the ipsilateral carotid stenosis has a stenosis of ≥ 70%, and they are likely to derive benefit with a stenosis of 50–69%. In these situations, carotid endarterectomy has been shown to have a durable effect in preventing further events.

Complications

The primary complication of carotid intervention is stroke due to embolization of plaque material during the procedure. The American Heart Association has recommended upper limits of acceptable combined morbidity and mortality for these interventions: 3% for asymptomatic, 5% for those with TIAs, and 7% for patients with previous stroke. Results that do not match these guidelines will jeopardize the therapeutic benefit of carotid intervention.

A. Carotid Endarterectomy

In addition to stroke risk, carotid endarterectomy carries an 8% risk of transient cranial nerve injury (usually the vagus or hypoglossal nerve) and 1–2% risk of permanent deficits. There is also the risk of postoperative neck hematoma, which can cause acute compromise of the airway. Coronary artery disease exists as a comorbidity in most of these patients. Myocardial infarction rates after carotid endarterectomy are approximately 5%.

B. Angioplasty and Stenting

Carotid angioplasty and stenting has been advocated as an alternative to carotid endarterectomy. Angioplasty and stenting offers the advantage of avoidance of both cranial nerve injury and neck hematoma. However, emboli are more common during angioplasty in spite of the use of embolic protection devices during the procedure. The Carotid Revascularization Endarterectomy versus Stent Trial (CREST), sponsored by the National Institutes of Health, is a randomized trial comparing outcomes of carotid endarterectomy and angioplasty and should determine the role of stenting in carotid disease.

C. Recurrent Carotid Stenosis

Scarring of the arterial wall at the site of the intervention after both angioplasty and endarterectomy may create recurrent stenosis. These lesions tend to be less embologenic, and treatment need not be as aggressive as for primary disease. The cranial nerve risk for these patients may be higher with repeat endarterectomy than with angioplasty of the narrowed segment.

► Prognosis

Prognosis for patients with carotid stenosis who have had a TIA or small stroke is poor without treatment; 25% of these patients will have a stroke with most of the events occurring in the first year of follow-up. Patients with carotid stenosis without symptoms have an annual stroke rate of just over 2% even with risk factor modification and antiplatelet agents. Symptomatic patients most likely have unstable plaques with ulceration or they have had a recent progression of the stenosis; prospective ultrasound screening is recommended in asymptomatic patients. Approximately 10% of asymptomatic patients have evidence of plaque progression in a given year. Concomitant coronary artery disease is common and is an important factor in these patients both for perioperative risk and long-term prognosis. Aggressive risk factor modification should be prescribed for patients with cerebrovascular disease regardless of planned intervention.

► When to Refer

Patients in whom an intervention is indicated should be referred to a vascular specialist.

Mas JL et al; EVA-3S Investigators. Endarterectomy versus stenting in patients with symptomatic severe carotid stenosis. N Engl J Med. 2006 Oct 19;355(16):1660–71. [PMID: 17050890]
Safian RD et al; CREATE Pivotal Trial Investigators. Protected carotid stenting in high-risk patients with severe carotid artery stenosis. J Am Coll Cardiol. 2006 Jun 20;47(12):2384–9. [PMID: 16781363]

VISCERAL ARTERY INSUFFICIENCY (Intestinal Angina)

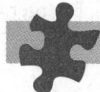

ESSENTIALS OF DIAGNOSIS

► Severe postprandial abdominal pain.

► Weight loss with a "fear of eating."

► Acute mesenteric ischemia: severe abdominal pain yet minimal findings on physical examination.

► General Considerations

Acute visceral artery insufficiency results from either embolic occlusion or primary thrombosis of at least one major mesenteric vessel. Ischemia can also result from non-occlusive mesenteric vascular insufficiency, which is generally seen in patients with low flow states, such as congestive heart failure, or who are in shock. A **chronic syndrome** occurs when there is adequate perfusion for the viscera at rest but ischemia occurs with severe abdominal pain when flow demands increase with feeding. Because of the rich collateral network in the mesentery, generally at least two of the three major visceral vessels (celiac, superior mesenteric, inferior mesenteric arteries) are affected before symptoms develop. **Ischemic colitis,** a variant of mesenteric ischemia, usually occurs in the distribution of the inferior mesenteric artery. The intestinal mucosa is the most sensitive to ischemia and will slough if underperfused. The clinical presentation is similar to inflammatory bowel disease. Ischemic colitis can occur after aortic surgery, particularly aortic aneurysm resection or aorto-femoral bypass for occlusive disease, when there is sudden reduction in blood flow to the inferior mesenteric artery.

► Clinical Findings

A. Symptoms and Signs

1. Acute intestinal ischemia—Patients with primary visceral thrombosis often give an antecedent history consistent with chronic intestinal ischemia. The key finding with acute mesenteric ischemia is severe, steady epigastric and periumbilical pain with minimal or no findings on physical examination of the abdomen because the visceral peritoneum is severely ischemic or infarcted and the parietal peritoneum is not involved. A high white cell count, lactic acidosis, hypotension, and abdominal distention may aid in the diagnosis.

2. Chronic intestinal ischemia—Patients are generally over 45 years of age and may have evidence of atherosclerosis in other vascular beds. Symptoms consist of epigastric or periumbilical postprandial pain lasting 1–3 hours. To avoid the pain, patients limit food intake and may develop a fear of eating. Weight loss is universal.

3. Ischemic colitis—Characteristic symptoms are left lower quadrant pain and tenderness, abdominal cramping, and mild diarrhea, which is often bloody.

B. Imaging and Colonoscopy

In patients with **acute** or **chronic mesenteric ischemia,** a CTA or MRA can demonstrate narrowing of the proximal visceral vessels. In acute mesenteric ischemia from a non-occlusive low flow state, angiography is needed to display the typical "pruned tree" appearance of the distal visceral vascular bed. Ultrasound scanning of the mesenteric vessels may show proximal obstructing lesions in laboratories that have experience with this technique.

In patients with **ischemic colitis,** colonoscopy may reveal segmental ischemic changes, most often in the rectal sigmoid and splenic flexure where collateral circulation may be poor.

Treatment

A high suspicion of **acute mesenteric ischemia** dictates immediate exploration to determine bowel viability. If the bowel remains viable, bypass can be done from the aorta to the celiac and the superior mesentery artery. In cases where bowel viability is questionable or bowel resection will be required, the bypass can be done with autologous vein, or with PTFE. There is a surprisingly low incidence of graft infection in these cases. For the treatment of **nonocclusive mesenteric disease**, vasodilators can be delivered through a catheter in the mesenteric arteries.

In **chronic visceral ischemia**, angioplasty and stenting of the proximal vessel may be beneficial depending on the anatomy of the stenosis. Should an endovascular solution not be available, an aorto-visceral artery bypass is the preferred management. The long-term results are highly durable. Visceral artery endarterectomy is reserved for cases with multiple lesions where bypass would be difficult.

The mainstay of treatment of **ischemic colitis** is maintenance of blood pressure and perfusion until collateral circulation becomes well established.

Prognosis

The combined morbidity and mortality rates are 10–15% from surgical intervention in these debilitated patients. However, without intervention both acute and chronic visceral ischemia are uniformly fatal. Adequate collateral circulation usually develops in those who have ischemic colitis; the prognosis for this entity is better than chronic mesenteric insufficiency.

When to Refer

Any patient in whom there is a suspicion of visceral ischemia should be referred for imaging and possible intervention.

Acosta S et al. Clinical implications for the management of acute thromboembolic occlusion of the superior mesenteric artery: autopsy findings in 213 patients. Ann Surg. 2005 Mar;241(3):516–22. [PMID: 15729076]

Wilson DB et al. Clinical course of mesenteric artery stenosis in elderly Americans. Arch Intern Med. 2006 Oct 23;166(19):2095–100. [PMID: 17060539]

ACUTE MESENTERIC VEIN OCCLUSION

The hallmarks of acute mesenteric vein occlusion are postprandial pain and evidence of a hypercoagulable state. Acute mesenteric vein occlusion presents similarly to the arterial occlusive syndromes but is much less common. Patients at risk include those with a systemic hypercoagulable state, such as that observed with paroxysmal nocturnal hemoglobinuria or protein C, protein S, or antithrombin deficiencies. These lesions are difficult to treat surgically, and thrombolysis is the mainstay of therapy. Aggressive long-term anticoagulation is required for these patients.

NONATHEROSCLEROTIC VASCULAR DISEASE

THROMBOANGIITIS OBLITERANS (Buerger Disease)

 ESSENTIALS OF DIAGNOSIS

- ▶ Typically occurs in young male cigarette smokers.
- ▶ Distal extremities involved with severe circulatory insufficiency.
- ▶ Thrombosis of the superficial veins may occur.
- ▶ Amputation will be necessary unless the patient stops smoking.

General Considerations

Buerger disease is a segmental, inflammatory, and thrombotic process of the distal most arteries and occasionally veins of the extremities. Pathologic examination reveals arteritis in the affected vessels. The cause is not known but it is rarely seen in nonsmokers. Arteries most commonly affected are the plantar and digital vessels of the foot and lower leg. In advanced stages, the fingers and hands may become involved. Fortunately, the incidence of Buerger disease seems to have decreased in the past decade.

Clinical Findings

A. Symptoms and Signs

Buerger disease may be initially difficult to differentiate from routine peripheral vascular disease, but in most cases, the lesions are on the toes and the patient is younger than 40 years old. The observation of superficial thrombophlebitis may aid the diagnosis. Because the distal vessels are usually affected, intermittent claudication is not common with Buerger disease, but rest pain, particularly pain in the distal most extremity (ie, toes), is frequent. This pain often progresses to tissue loss and amputation, unless the patient stops smoking. The progression of the disease seems to be intermittent with acute and dramatic episodes followed by some periods of remission.

B. Imaging

MRA or invasive angiography can demonstrate the obliteration of the distal arterial tree typical of Buerger disease.

Differential Diagnosis

In atherosclerotic peripheral vascular disease, the onset of tissue ischemia tends to be less dramatic than in Buerger disease, and symptoms of proximal arterial involvement, such as claudication, predominate.

Symptoms of Raynaud disease may be difficult to differentiate from Buerger disease. Repetitive atheroemboli may also mimic Buerger disease and may be difficult to differentiate. It may be necessary to image the proximal arterial tree to rule out sources of arterial emboli.

▶ Treatment

Smoking cessation is the mainstay of therapy and will halt the disease in most cases. As the distal arterial tree is occluded, revascularization is not possible. Sympathectomy is rarely effective.

▶ Prognosis

If smoking cessation can be achieved, the outlook for Buerger disease may be better than in patients with premature peripheral vascular disease. If smoking cessation is not achieved, then the prognosis is generally poor, with amputation of both lower and upper extremities the eventual outcome.

Olin JW. Thromboangiitis obliterans (Buerger's disease). N Engl J Med. 2000 Sep 21;343(12):864–9. [PMID: 10995867]

▼ ARTERIAL ANEURYSMS

ABDOMINAL AORTIC ANEURYSMS

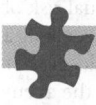

ESSENTIALS OF DIAGNOSIS

▶ Most aortic aneurysms are asymptomatic until rupture.

▶ Abdominal aortic aneurysms measuring 5 cm are palpable in 80% of patients.

▶ Back or abdominal pain with aneurysmal tenderness may precede rupture.

▶ Rupture is catastrophic; hypotension; excruciating abdominal pain that radiates to the back.

▶ General Considerations

Dilatation of the infrarenal aorta is a normal part of aging. The aorta of a healthy young man measures approximately 2 cm. An aneurysm is considered present when the aortic diameter exceeds 3 cm, but aneurysms rarely rupture until their diameter exceeds 5 cm. Abdominal aortic aneurysms are found in 2% of men over 55 years of age; the male to female ratio is 8:1. Ninety percent of abdominal atherosclerotic aneurysms originate below the renal arteries. The aneurysms usually involve the aortic bifurcation and often involve the common iliac arteries.

Inflammatory aneurysms are an unusual variant. These have an inflammatory peel, similar to the inflammation seen with retroperitoneal fibrosis that surrounds the aneurysm and encases adjacent retroperitoneal structures, such as the duodenum and, occasionally, the ureters.

▶ Clinical Findings

A. Symptoms and Signs

1. Asymptomatic—Although 80% of 5-cm infrarenal aneurysms are palpable on routine physical examination, most aneurysms are discovered as incidental findings on ultrasound or CT imaging during the evaluation of unrelated abdominal symptoms.

2. Symptomatic

A. Pain—Aneurysmal expansion may be accompanied by pain that is mild to severe midabdominal discomfort often radiating to the lower back. The pain may be constant or intermittent and is exacerbated by even gentle pressure on the aneurysm sack. Pain may also accompany inflammatory aneurysms.

B. Rupture—The sudden escape of blood into the retroperitoneal space causes severe pain, a palpable abdominal mass, and hypotension. Free rupture into the peritoneal cavity is a lethal event. Most aneurysms have a thick lining of blood clot, which can embolize to a peripheral artery and occlude blood flow. This phenomenon is surprisingly rare.

B. Laboratory Findings

Even with a contained rupture, there may be little change in routine laboratory findings. The hematocrit will be normal, since there has been no opportunity for hemodilution.

Aneurysms are associated with the cardiopulmonary diseases of elderly male smokers, which include coronary artery disease, carotid disease, renal impairment, and emphysema. Preoperative testing may indicate the presence of these comorbid conditions, which may increase the risk of intervention.

C. Imaging

Abdominal ultrasonography is the diagnostic study of choice for initial diagnosis. In approximately three-quarters of patients with aneurysms, curvilinear calcifications outlining portions of the aneurysm wall may be visible on plain films of the abdomen or back. CT scans provide a more reliable assessment of aneurysm diameter and should be done when the aneurysm nears the diameter threshold (5.5 cm) for treatment. Contrast-enhanced CT scans show the arteries above and below the aneurysm. The visualization of this vasculature is essential for planning repair.

▶ Screening

Data support the use of abdominal ultrasound to screen 65- to 74-year-old men, but not women, who have a history of smoking. Repeated screening does not appear to be needed if the aorta shows no enlargement.

▶ Treatment

A. Elective Repair

In general, elective repair is indicated for aortic aneurysms > 5.5 cm in diameter or aneurysms that have undergone rapid expansion (> 5 mm in 6 months). Symptoms such as pain or tenderness may indicate impending rupture. These patients need to undergo aneurysm repair regardless of the aneurysm's diameter. Improving outcomes with endovascular techniques have caused some experts to recommend treatment of smaller aneurysms. Current studies are ongoing to determine whether this may be appropriate with initial findings suggesting that it is not.

B. Aneurysmal Rupture

In approximately one-half of patients, aortic rupture is lethal. In the others, the bleeding is contained in the retroperitoneum, which may arrest the blood loss long enough for the patient to undergo urgent operation. Endovascular repair is available for urgent aneurysm repair in most major vascular centers, although the results offer only slight improvement over open repair for these critically ill patients.

C. Inflammatory Aneurysm

The presence of peri-aortic inflammation (inflammatory aneurysm) is not an indication for surgical treatment, unless there is associated compression of retroperitoneal structures, such as the ureter. Interestingly, the inflammation that encases an inflammatory aneurysm recedes after either endovascular or surgical aneurysm repair.

D. Assessment of Operative Risk

Aneurysms appear to be a variant of systemic atherosclerosis. Patients with aneurysms have a high rate of coronary disease. A 2004 trial demonstrated minimal value in addressing stable coronary artery disease prior to aneurysm resection. However, in patients with significant symptoms of coronary disease, the coronary disease should be treated first. Aneurysm resection should follow shortly thereafter because there is a significant increased risk in aneurysm rupture after the coronary procedures. In patients with concomitant carotid stenosis, there is no benefit in repairing asymptomatic carotid disease prior to aneurysm resection unless it is symptomatic or involves bilateral critical stenoses.

E. Open Surgical Resection versus Endovascular Repair

In open surgical aneurysm repair, a graft is sutured to the non-dilated vessels above and below the aneurysm. This involves an abdominal incision, extensive dissection, and interruption of aortic blood flow. The mortality rate is low in centers that have a high volume for this procedure and when it is performed in good risk patients. Older, sicker patients may not tolerate the cardiopulmonary stresses of the operation. With endovascular repair, a stent-graft is used to line the aorta and exclude the aneurysm. The anatomic requirements to securely achieve aneurysm exclusion vary according to the performance characteristics of the specific stent-graft device. In general, successful attachment requires a segment of non-dilated aorta (neck) between the renal arteries and the aneurysm that is at least 15 mm in length, and device insertion requires the lumen of the iliac arteries to be at least 7 mm in diameter.

▶ Complications

Myocardial infarction, the most common complication, occurs in up to 10% of patients who undergo open aneurysm repair. The incidence of myocardial infarction is substantially lower with endovascular repair. For routine infrarenal aneurysms, renal injury is unusual; however, when it does occur, or if the baseline creatinine is elevated, it is a significant complicating factor in the postoperative period. Respiratory complications are similar to those seen in most major abdominal surgery. Gastrointestinal hemorrhage, even years after aortic surgeries, suggests the possibility of graft enteric fistula; the incidence of this complication is higher when the initial surgery is performed on an emergency basis.

▶ Prognosis

The mortality rate for an open elective surgical resection is 1–5%. Of those who survive surgery, approximately 60% are alive at 5 years; myocardial infarction is the leading cause of death. The decision to repair aneurysms in high-risk patients has been made easier with the reduced perioperative morbidity and mortality of the endovascular approach. In long-term follow up, there is no survival advantage for endovascular repair.

Mortality rates of untreated aneurysms vary with aneurysm diameter. The mortality rate among patients with large aneurysms who have not undergone surgery, has been defined as follows: 12% annual risk of rupture with an aneurysm ≥ 6 cm in diameter and a 25% annual risk of rupture in aneurysms of ≥ 7 cm diameter. In general, a patient with an aortic aneurysm has a threefold greater chance of dying of a consequence of rupture of the aneurysm than of dying of the surgical resection.

At present, endovascular aneurysm repair may be less definitive than open surgical repair and requires close follow up. With complete exclusion of blood from the aneurysm sac, the pressure is lowered, which causes the aneurysm to shrink. An "endoleak" from the top or bottom of the graft (type 1) or through a graft defect (type 3) is associated with a persistent risk of rupture. Indirect leakage of blood through persistent lumbar and inferior mesenteric branches of the aneurysm (endoleak, type 2) produces an intermediate picture with somewhat reduced pressure in the sac, slow shrinkage, and low rupture risk. However, type 2 endoleak warrants close observation because aneurysm dilatation and rupture can occur.

▶ When to Refer

- Any patient with a 4 cm aortic aneurysm or larger should be referred for imaging and assessment by a vascular specialist.

- Urgent referrals should be made if the patient complains of pain and gentle palpation of the aneurysm confirms that it is the source.

▶ When to Admit

Patients with signs of aortic rupture require hospital admission.

Blankensteijn JD et al; Dutch Randomized Endovascular Aneurysm Management (DREAM) Trial Group. Two-year outcomes after conventional or endovascular repair of abdominal aortic aneurysms. N Engl J Med. 2005 Jun 9;352(23):2398–405. [PMID: 15944424]

Fleming C et al. Screening for abdominal aortic aneurysm: a best-evidence systematic review for the U.S. Preventive Services Task Force. Ann Intern Med. 2005 Feb 1;142(3):203–11. [PMID: 15684209]

Hellmann DB et al. Inflammatory abdominal aortic aneurysm. JAMA. 2007 Jan 24;297(4):395–400. [PMID: 17244836]

Kim LG et al. Multicentre Aneurysm Screening Group. A sustained mortality benefit from screening for abdominal aortic aneurysm. Ann Intern Med. 2007 May 15;146(10):699–706. [PMID: 17502630]

McFalls EO et al. Coronary-artery revascularization before elective major vascular surgery. N Engl J Med. 2004 Dec 30;351(27):2795–804. [PMID: 15625331]

Prinssen M et al; Dutch Randomized Endovascular Aneurysm Management (DREAM) Trial Group. A randomized trial comparing conventional and endovascular repair of abdominal aortic aneurysms. N Engl J Med. 2004 Oct 14;351(16):1607–18. [PMID: 15483279]

Schermerhorn ML et al. Endovascular vs. open repair of abdominal aortic aneurysms in the Medicare population. N Engl J Med. 2008 Jan 31;358(5):464–74. [PMID: 18234751]

THORACIC AORTIC ANEURYSMS

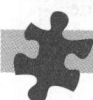 ESSENTIALS OF DIAGNOSIS

► Widened mediastinum on chest radiograph.
► With rupture, sudden onset chest pain radiating to the back.

General Considerations

Most thoracic aortic aneurysms are due to atherosclerosis; syphilis is now a rare cause. Disorders of connective tissue and Ehlers-Danlos and Marfan syndromes also are rare causes but have important therapeutic implications. Traumatic, false aneurysms, caused by partial tearing of the aortic wall with deceleration injuries, may occur just beyond the origin of the left subclavian artery. Less the 10% of aortic aneurysms occur in the thoracic aorta.

Clinical Findings

A. Symptoms and Signs

Most thoracic aneurysms are asymptomatic. When symptoms occur, they depend largely on the size and the position of the aneurysm and its rate of growth. Substernal back or neck pain may occur. Pressure on the trachea, esophagus, or superior vena cava can result in the following symptoms and signs: dyspnea, stridor, or brassy cough; dysphagia; and edema in the neck and arms as well as distended neck veins. Stretching of the left recurrent laryngeal nerve causes hoarseness. With aneurysms of the ascending aorta, aortic regurgitation may be present due to dilation of the aortic valve annulus. Rupture of a thoracic aneurysm is catastrophic because bleeding is rarely contained, so there is not enough time for emergent repair.

B. Imaging

The aneurysm may be diagnosed on chest radiograph by the calcified outline of the dilated aorta. CT scanning is the modality of choice to demonstrate the anatomy and size of the aneurysm and to exclude lesions that can mimic aneurysms, such as neoplasms or substernal goiter. MRI can also be useful. Cardiac catheterization and echocardiography may be required to describe the relationship of the coronary vessels to an aneurysm of the ascending aorta.

Treatment

Indications for repair depend on the location of dilation, rate of growth, associated symptoms, and overall condition of the patient. Aneurysms measuring 6 cm or larger may be considered for repair. Aneurysms of the **descending thoracic aorta** are treated routinely by endovascular grafting. Repair of **arch aneurysms** should be undertaken only if there is a skilled surgical team with an acceptable record of outcomes for these complex procedures. The availability of endografting for descending thoracic aneurysms or experimental branched endovascular reconstructions for arch aneurysms (custom made grafts with branches to the vessels involved in the aneurysm) does not change the indications for aneurysm repair. Aneurysms that involve the proximal aortic arch or ascending aorta represent particularly challenging problems. Open surgery is usually required, which carries substantial risk of morbidity, including stroke, diffuse neurologic injury, and intellectual impairment.

Complications

With the exception of endovascular repair for discrete saccular aneurysms of the descending thoracic aorta, the morbidity and mortality of thoracic repair is considerably higher than that for infra-renal abdominal aortic aneurysm repair. Paraplegia remains a rare, but devastating, complication. Most large series report approximately 4% rate of paraplegia following endovascular repair of thoracic aortic aneurysms. The spinal arterial supply is segmental through intercostal branches of the aorta with variable degrees of intersegmental connection. Therefore, the more extensive the aneurysm, the greater is the risk of paraplegia with resection. Prior to abdominal aortic surgery, compromise of the subclavian or internal iliac arteries and hypotension all increase the paraplegia risk. Involvement of the aortic arch also increases the risk of stroke, even when the aneurysm does not directly affect the carotid artery.

Prognosis

Generally, degenerative aneurysms of the thoracic aorta will enlarge and require repair to prevent death from rupture. However, stable aneurysms can be followed with CT scanning. Saccular aneurysms, particularly those distal to the left subclavian artery and the descending thoracic aorta, have had good results with endovascular repair.

Resection of large complex aneurysms of the aortic arch involves major technical issues and requires a skilled surgical team and should only be attempted in low-risk patients. Experimental branched technology for endovascular grafting holds promise for reduced morbidity and mortality.

When to Refer

Patients who are deemed to have a reasonable surgical risk with a 5–6 cm aneurysm should be considered for repair, particularly if the aneurysm involves the descending thoracic aorta.

When to Admit

Any patient with chest or back pain with a known or suspected thoracic aorta aneurysm must be admitted to the hospital and undergo appropriate imaging studies to rule out the aneurysm as a cause of the pain.

Chuter TA. Branched and fenestrated stent grafts for endovascular repair of thoracic aortic aneurysms. J Vasc Surg. 2006 Feb;43(Suppl A):111A–115A. [PMID: 16473163]

Svensson LG et al; Society of Thoracic Surgeons Endovascular Surgery Task Force. Expert consensus document on the treatment of descending thoracic aortic disease using endovascular stent-grafts. Ann Thorac Surg. 2008 Jan;85(1 Suppl):S1–41. [PMID: 18083364]

AORTIC DISSECTION

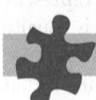

ESSENTIALS OF DIAGNOSIS

- ▶ Sudden searing chest pain with radiation to the back, abdomen, or neck in a hypertensive patient.
- ▶ Widened mediastinum on chest radiograph.
- ▶ Pulse discrepancy in the extremities.
- ▶ Acute aortic regurgitation may develop.

General Considerations

Aortic dissection occurs when a spontaneous intimal tear develops and blood dissects into the media of the aorta. The tear probably results from the repetitive torque applied to the ascending and proximal descending aorta during the cardiac cycle; hypertension is an important component of this disease process. **Type A dissection** involves the arch proximal to the left subclavian artery, and **type B dissection** occurs in the proximal descending thoracic aorta typically just beyond the left subclavian artery. Dissections may occur in the absence of hypertension but abnormalities of smooth muscle, elastic tissue, or collagen are more common in these patients. Pregnancy, bicuspid aortic valve, and coarctation also are associated with increased risk of dissection.

Blood entering the intimal tear may extend the dissection into the abdominal aorta, the lower extremities, the carotid arteries or, less commonly, the subclavian arteries. Both absolute pressure levels and the pulse pressure are important

in propagation of dissection. The aortic dissection is a true emergency and requires immediate control of blood pressure to limit the extent of the dissection. With type A dissection, which has the worse prognosis, death may occur within hours, usually due to rupture of the dissection into the pericardial sac. Rupture into the plural cavity is also possible. The intimal/medial flap of the aortic wall created by the dissection may occlude major aortic branches, resulting in ischemia of the brain, intestines, kidney, or lower extremities. Patients whose blood pressure is controlled and who survive the acute episode without complications may have long-term survival without surgical treatment.

Clinical Findings

A. Symptoms and Signs

Severe persistent chest pain of sudden onset radiating down the back or possibly into the anterior chest is characteristic. Radiation of the pain into the neck may also occur. The patient is usually hypertensive. Syncope, hemiplegia, or paralysis of the lower extremities may occur. Intestinal ischemia or renal insufficiency may develop. Peripheral pulses may be diminished or unequal. A diastolic murmur may develop as a result of a dissection in the ascending aorta close to the aortic valve, causing valvular regurgitation, heart failure, and cardiac tamponade.

B. Electrocardiographic Findings

Left ventricular hypertrophy from long-standing hypertension is often present. Acute changes suggesting myocardial ischemia do not develop unless dissection involves the coronary artery ostium. Classically, inferior wall abnormalities predominate since dissection leads to compromise of the right rather than the left coronary artery. In some patients, the ECG may be completely normal.

C. Imaging

A multiplanar CT scan is the immediate diagnostic imaging modality of choice; clinicians should have a low threshold for obtaining a CT scan in any hypertensive patient with chest pain and equivocal findings on ECG.

The CT scan should include both the chest and abdomen to fully delineate the extent of the dissected aorta. MRI is an excellent imaging modality for chronic dissections, but in the acute situation, the longer imaging time and the difficulty of monitoring patients in the MRI scanner make the CT scan preferable. Chest radiographs may reveal an abnormal aortic contour or widened superior mediastinum. Although transesophageal echocardiography (TEE) is an excellent diagnostic imaging method, it is generally not readily available in the acute setting.

Differential Diagnosis

Aortic dissection is most commonly misdiagnosed as myocardial infarction or other causes of chest pain such as pulmonary embolization. Dissections may occur with minimal pain; branch vessel occlusion of the lower extremity can mimic arterial embolus.

▶ Treatment

A. Medical

Aggressive measures to lower blood pressure should occur when an aortic dissection is suspected, even before the diagnostic studies have been completed. Treatment requires a simultaneous reduction of the systolic blood pressure to 100–120 mm Hg and pulse pressure. β-Blockers have the most desirable effect of reducing the left ventricular ejection force that continues to weaken the arterial wall and should be first-line therapy. Labetalol, both an α- and β-blocker, lowers pulse pressure and achieve rapid blood pressure control. Give 20 mg over 2 minutes by intravenous injection. Additional doses of 40–80 mg intravenously can be given every 10 minutes (maximum dose 300 mg) until the desired blood pressure has been reached. Alternatively, 2 mg/min may be given by intravenous infusion, titrated to desired effect. In patients who have asthma, bradycardia, or other conditions that necessitate the patient's reaction to β-blockers be tested, esmolol is a reasonable choice because of its short half-life. Give a loading dose of esmolol, 0.5 mg/ kg over 1 minute followed by an infusion of .0025–.02 mg/ kg/min. Titrate the infusion to a goal heart rate of 60–70 beats/min. If β-blockade alone does not control the hypertension, nitroprusside may be added as follows: 50 mg of nitroprusside in 1000 mL of 5% dextrose and water, infused at a rate of 0.5 mL/min; the infusion rate is increased by 0.5 mL every 5 minutes until adequate control of the pressure has been achieved. In patients with bronchial asthma, while there are no data supporting the use of the calcium-channel antagonists, diltiazem and verapamil are potential alternatives to treatment with β-blocking drugs. Morphine sulfate is the appropriate drug to use for pain relief. Long-term medical care of patients should include β-blockers in their antihypertensive regimen.

B. Surgical Intervention

Urgent surgical intervention is required for all **type A aneurysms.** If a skilled cardiovascular team is not available, the patient should be transferred to an appropriate facility. The procedure involves grafting and replacing the diseased portion of the arch and brachiocephalic vessels as necessary. Replacement of the aortic valve may be required with reattachment of the coronary arteries.

Urgent surgery is required for **type B aneurysms** if the dissection is continuing or there is aortic branch compromise. Endovascular repair of type B dissections is the treatment of choice if it is anatomically feasible.

▶ Prognosis & Follow-up

The mortality rate for untreated type A dissections is approximately 1% per hour for 72 hours and over 90% at 3 months. Mortality is also extremely high for untreated complicated type B dissections. The surgical and endovascular options for these patients also have significant morbidity and mortality. They are technically demanding and require an experienced team to achieve perioperative mortalities of less than 10%. Patients with uncomplicated type B dissections whose blood pressure is controlled and who survive the acute episode without complications may have long-term survival without surgical treatment. Aneurysmal enlargement of the false lumen may develop in these patients despite adequate antihypertensive therapy. Yearly CT scans are required to monitor the size of the dissecting aneurysm. Indications for repair are similar to undissected thoracic aneurysms. Endovascular covering of the intimal tear in the acute setting may prevent this complication, but initial trials on the routine endovascular treatment of type B dissections have not shown an advantage for early intervention and therefore cannot be widely endorsed at this time. Indications for repair remain similar to those of undissected thoracic aneurysms.

▶ When to Admit

Any dissection involving the aortic arch (type A) should be immediately repaired. Acute type B dissections require repair only when there is evidence of rupture or major branch occlusion.

Ince H et al. Diagnosis and management of patients with aortic dissection. Heart. 2007 Feb;93(2):266–70. [PMID: 17228080]

Shiga T et al. Diagnostic accuracy of transesophageal echocardiography, helical computed tomography, and magnetic resonance imaging for suspected thoracic aortic dissection: systematic review and meta-analysis. Arch Intern Med. 2006 Jul 10;166(13):1350–6. [PMID: 16831999]

▼ VENOUS DISEASES

VARICOSE VEINS

ESSENTIALS OF DIAGNOSIS

▶ Dilated, tortuous superficial veins in the lower extremities.

▶ May be asymptomatic or associated with aching discomfort or pain.

▶ Edema, pigmentation, and stasis ulcers of the skin may develop.

▶ Usually hereditary, with most patients reporting a family member with similar lesions.

▶ Increased frequency after pregnancy.

▶ General Considerations

Varicose veins develop in the lower extremities. Periods of high venous pressure related to prolonged standing or heavy lifting are contributing factors, but the highest incidence occurs in women after pregnancy. Varicosities develop in 15% of all adults.

The greater saphenous vein and its tributaries are most commonly involved, but the short saphenous vein (posterior lower leg) may also be affected. Distention of the vein prevents the valve leaflets from coapting, creating incompetence. Thus, dilation at any point along the vein leads to increased pressure and distention of the vein segment below that valve, which in turn causes progressive failure of the next lower valve and progressive venous reflux. Perforating veins that connect the deep and superficial systems may become incompetent, allowing blood to reflux into the superficial veins from the deep system through the incompetent perforators and increasing venous pressure and distention.

Secondary varicosities can develop as a result of obstructive changes and valve damage in the deep venous system following thrombophlebitis, or rarely as a result of proximal venous occlusion due to neoplasm or fibrosis. Congenital or acquired arteriovenous fistulas or venous malformations are also associated with varicosities.

Clinical Findings

A. Symptoms and Signs

Symptom severity is not correlated with the number and size of the varicosities; extensive varicose veins may produce no subjective symptoms, whereas minimal varicosities may produce many symptoms. Dull, aching heaviness or a feeling of fatigue of the legs brought on by periods of standing is the most common complaint.

Clinicians must be careful to identify symptoms of arteriosclerotic peripheral vascular disease, such as intermittent claudication and coldness of the feet, since occlusive arterial disease is usually a contraindication to the operative treatment of varicosities distal to the knee. Itching from a venous stasis dermatitis may occur either above the ankle or directly overlying large varicosities.

Dilated, tortuous veins beneath the skin in the thigh and leg are generally visible upon standing, although in very obese patients palpation may be necessary to detect their presence and location. Some swelling is common but secondary tissue changes may be absent even in extensive varicosities. However, if the varicosities are of long duration, brownish pigmentation and thinning of the skin above the ankle may be present. The presence of a bruit or a thrill is useful in making the diagnosis of an associated arteriovenous fistula.

B. Imaging

The identification of the source of venous reflux that feeds the symptomatic veins is necessary for effective surgical treatment. Duplex ultrasonography by a technician experienced in the diagnosis and localization of venous reflux is the test of choice for planning therapy. In most cases, reflux will arise from the greater saphenous vein.

Differential Diagnosis

Primary varicose veins should be differentiated from those secondary to chronic venous insufficiency of the deep system of veins with extensive swelling, fibrosis, pigmentation, and ulceration of the distal lower leg (the postphlebitic syndrome). Pain or discomfort secondary to arthritis, radiculopathy, or arterial insufficiency should be distinguished from symptoms associated with coexistent varicose veins. In adolescent patients with varicose veins,

imaging of the deep venous system is important to exclude a congenital malformation or atresia of the deep veins. Surgical treatment of varicose veins in these patients is contraindicated because the varicosities may play a significant role in venous drainage of the limb.

Complications

Thrombophlebitis within a varicose vein is uncommon. This presents as subacute to acute localized pain and palpable hardness at the site of the phlebitis. The process is self-limiting, has a low risk of embolization, and usually resolves within weeks. Rarely, the phlebitis extends to involve the greater saphenous vein.

In older patients, superficial varicosities may bleed with even minor trauma. The amount of bleeding can be alarming as the pressure in the varicosity is high.

Predisposing conditions for thrombophlebitis include pregnancy, local trauma, or prolonged periods of sitting.

Treatment

A. Nonsurgical Measures

Nonsurgical treatment is effective. Elastic graduated compression stockings (medium or heavy weight) give external support to the veins. These stockings may be useful in early varicosities to prevent progression of disease. When elastic stockings worn during standing are combined with elevation of the legs when possible, good control can be maintained and the development of complications can often be avoided. This approach may be used in elderly patients, in those who refuse or wish to defer surgery, and in those with mild asymptomatic varicosities.

B. Surgical Measures

Treatment with endovenous ablation (with either radiofrequency or laser) or, less commonly, with greater saphenous vein stripping is very effective for reflux arising from the greater saphenous vein. Less common sources of reflux include the lesser saphenous vein (for varicosities in the posterior calf), and nonsaphenous incompetent perforator veins arising directly from the deep venous system in the thigh. Correction of reflux is performed at the same time as excision of the symptomatic varicose veins. Phlebectomy without correction of reflux results in a high rate of recurrent varicosities, as the uncorrected reflux progressively dilates adjacent veins. Concurrent reflux detected by ultrasonography in the deep system is not a contraindication to treatment of superficial reflux because the majority of deep vein dilatation is secondary to volume overload in this setting, which will resolve with correction of the superficial reflux.

C. Compression Sclerotherapy

Sclerotherapy to obliterate and produce permanent fibrosis of the involved veins is generally reserved for the treatment of small varicose veins less than 4 mm in diameter. Use of foam sclerotherapy can allow treatment of larger veins, although systemic embolization of the foam sclerosant may be a concern. The injection of the sclerosing solution into the varicosed vein is followed by a period of compression of the segment, resulting in obliteration of the vein. Complications such as phlebitis, tissue necrosis, or infection may occur, and vary in incidence with the skill of the clinician.

Prognosis

Correction of the venous insufficiency and excision of varicose veins provide excellent results. The 5-year success rate (as defined as lack of pain and recurrent varicosities) is 85–90%. Simple excision (phlebectomy) or injection sclerotherapy without correction of reflux is associated with higher rates of recurrence. Even after adequate treatment, secondary tissue changes, such as lipodermosclerosis, may persist.

When to Refer

- Absolute indications for referral for saphenous ablation include phlebitis and bleeding.
- Pain and cosmetic concerns are responsible for the majority of referrals for ablation.

Bergan JJ et al. Chronic venous disease. N Engl J Med. 2006 Aug 3;355(5):488–98. [PMID: 16885552]
Campbell B. Varicose veins and their management. BMJ. 2006 Aug 5;333(7562):287–92. [PMID: 16888305]

SUPERFICIAL VENOUS THROMBOPHLEBITIS

ESSENTIALS OF DIAGNOSIS

- ▶ Induration, redness, and tenderness along a superficial vein, usually the saphenous vein.
- ▶ Induration at the site of a recent intravenous line or trauma.
- ▶ Significant swelling of the extremity may not be seen.

General Considerations

Short-term venous catheterization of superficial arm veins as well as the use of longer term peripherally inserted central catheter (PICC) lines are the most common cause of superficial thrombophlebitis. Intravenous catheter sites should be observed daily for signs of local inflammation and should be removed if a local reaction develops in the vein. Serious thrombotic or septic complications can occur if this policy is not followed.

Superficial thrombophlebitis may occur spontaneously, as in pregnant or postpartum women or in individuals with varicose veins or thromboangiitis obliterans; or it may be associated with trauma, as in the case of a blow to the leg or following intravenous therapy with irritating solutions. It also may be a manifestation of systemic hypercoagulability secondary to abdominal cancer such as carcinoma of the pancreas and may be the earliest sign of these conditions. Superficial thrombophlebitis may be associated with occult deep venous thrombosis (DVT) in about 20% of cases. Pulmonary emboli are exceedingly rare and occur from an associated DVT. (See Chapter 9 for discussion on Deep Venous Thrombosis.)

Clinical Findings

In spontaneous superficial thrombophlebitis, the long saphenous vein is most often involved. The patient usually experiences a dull pain in the region of the involved vein. Local findings consist of induration, redness, and tenderness along the course of a vein. The process may be localized, or it may involve most of the long saphenous vein and its tributaries. The inflammatory reaction generally subsides in 1–2 weeks; a firm cord may remain for a much longer period. Edema of the extremity is uncommon.

Localized redness and induration at the site of a recent intravenous line requires urgent attention. Chills and high fever suggest septic phlebitis and indicate that aggressive debridement of the area is warranted.

Differential Diagnosis

The linear rather than circular nature of the lesion and the distribution along the course of a superficial vein serve to differentiate superficial phlebitis from cellulitis, erythema nodosum, erythema induratum, panniculitis, and fibrositis. Lymphangitis and deep thrombophlebitis must also be considered.

Treatment

If the process is well localized and not near the saphenofemoral junction, local heat, and nonsteroidal anti-inflammatory medications are usually effective in limiting the process. If the induration is extensive or is progressing toward the saphenofemoral junction (leg) or cephaloaxillary junction (arm), ligation and division of the vein at the junction of the deep and superficial veins is indicated.

Anticoagulation therapy is usually not indicated unless the disease is rapidly progressing or there is extension into the deep system.

Septic superficial thrombophlebitis is an intravascular abscess and may require excision of the involved vein in order to control the infection. *Staphylococcus aureus* is the most common pathogen. Because of the lethal nature of this complication, broad-spectrum antibiotics and systemic anticoagulation with heparin should be instituted immediately. If cultures are positive, therapy should be continued for 7–10 days or for 4–6 weeks if complicating endocarditis cannot be excluded. Other organisms, including fungi, may also be responsible.

Prognosis

With spontaneous thrombophlebitis, the course is generally benign and brief. The prognosis depends on the underlying pathologic process. In patients with phlebitis secondary to varicose veins, recurrent episodes are likely unless correction of the underlying venous reflux and excision of varicosities is done. The mortality from septic thrombophlebitis is 20% or higher and requires aggressive treatment. However, if the involvement is localized, the mortality is low and prognosis is excellent with early treatment.

Katz SC et al. Superficial septic thrombophlebitis. J Trauma. 2005 Sep;59(3):750–3. [PMID: 16361925]

van Weert H et al. Spontaneous superficial venous thrombophlebitis: does it increase risk for thromboembolism? A historic follow-up study in primary care. J Fam Pract. 2006 Jan;55(1):52–7. [PMID: 16388768]

CHRONIC VENOUS INSUFFICIENCY

 ESSENTIALS OF DIAGNOSIS

▶ History of prior DVT or leg injury.

▶ Edema, stasis (brawny) skin pigmentation, subcutaneous liposclerosis in the lower leg.

▶ Large ulcerations at or above the ankle are common (stasis ulcers).

General Considerations

Chronic venous insufficiency can result from changes secondary to deep venous thrombophlebitis, although a definite history of phlebitis is not obtainable in about 25% of these patients. There may be a history of leg trauma. Obesity is often a complicating factor. Chronic venous insufficiency also may occur in association with superficial venous reflux and varicose veins or as a result of neoplastic obstruction of the pelvic veins or congenital or acquired arteriovenous fistula.

The basic pathology is caused by valve leaflets that do not coapt because they are either thickened and scarred (the post-thrombotic syndrome) or in a dilated vein and are therefore functionally inadequate. This results in an abnormally high hydrostatic force transmitted to the subcutaneous veins and tissues of the lower leg. The resulting edema results in dramatic and deleterious secondary changes. The stigmata of chronic venous insufficiency include fibrosis of the subcutaneous tissue and skin, pigmentation of skin (hemosiderin taken up by the dermal macrophages) and, later, ulceration which is extremely slow to heal. Itching may precipitate the formation of ulceration or local wound cellulitis. Dilation of the superficial veins may occur, leading to varicosities. Whereas primary varicose veins with no abnormality of the deep venous system may be associated with some similar changes, the edema is more pronounced in the post-thrombotic extremities, and the secondary changes are more extensive and debilitating.

Clinical Findings

A. Symptoms and Signs

Progressive edema of the leg (particularly the lower leg) is the usual initial symptom. Secondary changes in the skin and subcutaneous tissues develop. The usual symptoms are itching, a dull discomfort made worse by periods of stand-ing, and pain if an ulceration is present. The skin at the ankle is usually thin, shiny, and a brownish pigmentation often develops. If the condition is long-standing, the subcutaneous tissues become thick and fibrous. Ulcerations may occur, usually just above the ankle, on the medial or anterior aspect of the leg. Healing results in a thin scar on a fibrotic base that often breaks down with minor trauma or another bout of leg swelling. Varicosities frequently appear that are associated with incompetent perforating veins. Cellulitis, which is often difficult to distinguish from the hemosiderin pigmentation, may be diagnosed by blanching erythema.

B. Imaging

Patients with post-thrombotic syndrome or signs of chronic venous insufficiency should undergo duplex ultrasonography to determine whether superficial reflux is present and to evaluate the degree of deep reflux and obstruction.

Differential Diagnosis

Patients with congestive heart failure, chronic renal disease, or decompensated liver disease may have bilateral edema of the lower extremities. Swelling from lymphedema may be unilateral, and varicosities are absent. Edema from these causes pits easily and brawny discoloration is rare. Lipedema is a disorder of adipose tissue that occurs almost exclusively in women, is bilateral and symmetric, and is characterized by stopping at a distinct line just above the ankles.

Primary varicose veins may be difficult to differentiate from the secondary varicosities that often develop in this condition, as discussed above.

Other conditions associated with chronic ulcers of the leg include autoimmune diseases (eg, Felty syndrome), arterial insufficiency (often very painful with absent pulses), sickle cell anemia, erythema induratum (bilateral and usually on the posterior aspect of the lower part of the leg), and fungal infections (cultures specific: no chronic swelling or varicosities).

Prevention

Irreversible tissue changes and associated complications in the lower legs can be minimized through early and aggressive anticoagulation of acute DVT to minimize the valve damage and by prescribing stockings if chronic edema develops in subsequent years. Catheter-directed thrombolysis or mechanical thrombectomy of acute DVT may be of greater value than simple anticoagulants in preventing post-thrombotic syndrome and chronic venous insufficiency.

Treatment

A. General Measures

Well-fitting, graduated compression stockings worn from the mid foot to just below the knee during the day and evening are the mainstays of treatment. Long periods of sitting or standing should be avoided. During the day, the patient's legs should be elevated intermittently, and at night, the legs should be kept above the level of the heart with pillows under the mattress. Pneumatic compression of the leg, which can pump the fluid out of the leg, is used in cases refractory to the above measures.

B. Ulceration

As the primary pathology is edema, healing of the ulcer will not occur until the edema is controlled. A lesion can often be treated on an ambulatory basis by means of a semi-rigid gauze boot made with Unna paste (Gelocast, Medicopaste) or a multi-layer compression (such as Profore) and applied to the leg after much of the swelling has been reduced by a period of elevation. The pumping action of the calf muscles on the blood flow out of the lower extremity is enhanced by a circumferential nonelastic bandage on the ankle and lower leg. The boot must be changed every 2–3 days, depending on the amount of drainage from the ulcer. The ulcer, tendons, and bony prominences must be adequately padded. As an alternative and after the ulcer has healed, elastic stockings with graduated compression below the knee are used in an effort to prevent recurrent edema and ulceration. If compression stockings are used with ulcers, an absorbent dressing must be applied under the stocking as the wounds can leak large volumes of fluid. Home compression therapy with a pneumatic compression device is also effective at reducing edema but many patients have severe pain with the "milking" action of the pump device. Some patients will require admission for complete bed rest and leg elevation to achieve ulcer healing.

C. Correction of Superficial Reflux

Incompetent (refluxing) perforator veins that feed the area of ulceration can be treated with percutaneous means (radiofrequency ablation or endovenous laser treatment) to help decrease the venous pressure in the area of ulceration and promote healing. Venous valvular reconstructive surgery is under investigation. Where there is substantial obstruction of the deep venous system, superficial varicosities supply the venous return and they should not be removed.

Prognosis

Individuals with chronic venous insufficiency often have recurrent problems, particularly if they do not consistently wear support stockings that have at least 30 mm Hg compression.

When to Refer

- Patients with significant saphenous reflux should be evaluated for ablation as this may reduce the recirculation of blood and return the deep system to competence.
- Patients with ulcers should be monitored in a wound center where these challenging wounds can receive aggressive care.

Bergan JJ et al. Chronic venous disease. N Engl J Med. 2006 Aug 3;355(5):488–98. [PMID: 16885552]

Eberhard RT et al. Chronic venous insufficiency. Circulation. 2005 May 10;111(18):2398–409. [PMID: 15883226]

Grey JE et al. Venous and arterial leg ulcers. BMJ. 2006 Feb 11;332(7537):347–50. [PMID: 16470058]

Patel NP et al. Current management of venous ulceration. Plast Reconstr Surg. 2006 Jun;117(7 Suppl):254S–260S. [PMID: 16799394]

SUPERIOR VENA CAVAL OBSTRUCTION

 ESSENTIALS OF DIAGNOSIS

▶ Swelling of the neck, face and upper extremities.
▶ Dilated veins over the upper chest and neck.

General Considerations

Partial or complete obstruction of the superior vena cava is a relatively rare condition that is usually secondary to neoplastic or inflammatory processes in the superior mediastinum. The most frequent causes are (1) neoplasms, such as lymphomas, primary malignant mediastinal tumors, or carcinoma of the lung with direct extension (over 80%); (2) chronic fibrotic mediastinitis, either of unknown origin or secondary to tuberculosis, histoplasmosis, pyogenic infections, or drugs, especially methysergide; (3) DVT, often by extension of the process from the axillary or subclavian vein into the innominate vein and vena cava associated with catheterization of these veins for dialysis or for hyperalimentation; (4) aneurysm of the aortic arch; and (5) constrictive pericarditis.

Clinical Findings

A. Symptoms and Signs

The onset of symptoms is acute or subacute. Symptoms include swelling of the neck and face, and upper extremities. Symptoms are often perceived as congestion and present as headache, dizziness, visual disturbances, stupor, syncope, or cough. Symptoms are particularly exacerbated when the patient is supine or bends over. There is progressive obstruction of the venous drainage of the head, neck, and upper extremities. The cutaneous veins of the upper chest and lower neck become dilated, and flushing of the face and neck develops. Brawny edema of the face, neck, and arms occurs later, and cyanosis of these areas then appears. Cerebral and laryngeal edema ultimately results in impaired function of the brain as well as respiratory insufficiency. Bending over or lying down accentuates the symptoms; sitting quietly is generally preferred. The manifestations are more severe if the obstruction develops rapidly and if the azygos junction or the vena cava between that vein and the heart is obstructed.

B. Laboratory Findings

The venous pressure is elevated (often > 20 cm of water) in the arm and is normal in the leg. Since lung cancer is a common cause, bronchoscopy is often performed; transbronchial biopsy, however, is relatively contraindicated because of venous hypertension and the risk of bleeding.

C. Imaging

Chest radiographs and a CT scan will define the location and often the nature of the obstructive process, and contrast venography or magnetic resonance venography (MRV) will map out the extent and degree of the venous obstruction and the collateral circulation. Brachial venography or radionuclide scanning following intravenous injection of technetium Tc-99m pertechnetate demonstrates a block to the flow of contrast material into the right heart and enlarged collateral veins. These techniques also allow estimation of blood flow around the occlusion as well as serial evaluation of the response to therapy.

▶ Treatment

Urgent treatment for neoplasm consists of (1) cautious use of intravenous diuretics and (2) mediastinal irradiation, starting within 24 hours, with a treatment plan designed to give a high daily dose but a short total course of therapy to rapidly shrink the local tumor even further. Intensive combined therapy will palliate the process in up to 90% of patients. In patients with a subacute presentation, radiation therapy alone usually suffices. Chemotherapy is added if lymphoma or small-cell carcinoma is diagnosed.

Conservative measures, such as elevation of the head of the bed and lifestyle modification to avoid bending over, are useful. Occasionally, anticoagulation is needed, while thrombolysis is rarely needed. Balloon angioplasty of the obstructed caval segment combined with stent placement provides prompt relief of symptoms and is the procedure of choice. Long-term outcome is complicated by risk of re-occlusion from either thrombosis or further growth of neoplasm. Surgical procedures to bypass the obstruction are complicated by bleeding relating to high venous pressure. In cases where the thrombosis is secondary to an indwelling catheter, thrombolysis may be attempted. Clinical judgment is required since a long-standing clot may be fibrotic and the risk of bleeding will outweigh the potential benefit.

▶ Prognosis

The prognosis depends on the nature and degree of obstruction and its speed of onset. Slowly developing forms secondary to fibrosis may be tolerated for years. A high degree of obstruction of rapid onset secondary to cancer is often fatal in a few days or weeks because of increased intracranial pressure and cerebral hemorrhage, but treatment of the tumor with radiation and chemotherapeutic drugs may result in significant palliation. Balloon angioplasty and stenting provides good relief but may require re-treatment for recurrent symptoms secondary to thrombosis or restenosis.

▶ When to Refer

Referral should occur with any patient with progressive head and neck swelling to rule out superior vena cava syndrome.

▶ When to Admit

Any patient with acute edema of the head and neck or any patient in whom signs and symptoms of airway compromise, such as hoarseness or stridor, develop should be admitted.

Watkinson AF et al. Endovascular stenting to treat obstruction of the superior vena cava. BMJ. 2008 Jun 21;336(7658):1434–7. [PMID: 18566082]

Wilson LD et al. Clinical practice. Superior vena cava syndrome with malignant causes. N Engl J Med. 2007 May 3;356(18):1862–9. [PMID: 17476012]

DISEASES OF THE LYMPHATIC CHANNELS

LYMPHANGITIS & LYMPHADENITIS

ESSENTIALS OF DIAGNOSIS

▶ Red streak from wound or area of cellulitis toward regional lymph nodes, which are usually enlarged and tender.

▶ Chills, fever, and malaise may be present.

▶ General Considerations

Lymphangitis and lymphadenitis are common manifestations of a bacterial infection that is usually caused by hemolytic streptococci or *S aureus* (or by both organisms) and usually arises from the site of an infected wound. The wound may be very small or superficial, or an established abscess may be present, feeding bacteria into the lymphatics. The involvement of the lymphatics is often manifested by a red streak in the skin extending in the direction of the regional lymph nodes, which are, in turn, generally tender and engorged. Systemic manifestations include fever, chills, and malaise. The infection may progress rapidly, often in a matter of hours, and may lead to septicemia and even death.

▶ Clinical Findings

A. Symptoms and Signs

Throbbing pain is usually present in the area of cellulitis at the site of bacterial invasion. Malaise, anorexia, sweating, chills, and fever of 38–40 °C develop rapidly. The red streak, when present may be definite or may be very faint and easily missed, especially in dark-skinned patients. It is usually tender or indurated in the area of cellulitis. The involved regional lymph nodes may be significantly enlarged and are usually quite tender. The pulse is often rapid.

B. Laboratory Findings

Leukocytosis with a left shift is usually present. Blood cultures may be positive, most often for staphylococcal or streptococcal species. Culture and sensitivity studies of the wound exudate or pus may be helpful in treatment of the more severe or refractory infections but are often difficult to interpret because of skin contaminants.

Differential Diagnosis

Lymphangitis may be confused with superficial thrombophlebitis, but the erythema and induration of thrombophlebitis is localized in and around the thrombosed vein. Venous thrombosis is not associated with lymphadenitis, and a wound of entrance with secondary cellulitis is generally absent.

Cat-scratch fever should be considered when lymphadenitis is present; the nodes, though often very large, are relatively nontender. Exposure to cats is common, but the patient may have forgotten about the scratch.

It is extremely important to differentiate cellulitis from acute streptococcal hemolytic gangrene or necrotizing fasciitis. These are deeper infections that may be extensive and are potentially lethal. Patients appear more seriously ill; there may be redness due to leakage of red cells, creating a non-blanching erythema; and subcutaneous crepitus may be palpated or auscultated using the diaphragm with light pressure over the involved area. Immediate wide debridement of all involved deep tissues should be done if these signs are present.

Treatment

A. General Measures

Prompt treatment should include heat (hot, moist compresses or heating pad), elevation when feasible, and immobilization of the infected area. Analgesics may be prescribed for pain.

B. Specific Measures

Antibiotic therapy should always be instituted when local infection becomes invasive, as manifested by cellulitis and lymphangitis. Because such infections are so frequently caused by streptococci, cephalosporins or extended-spectrum penicillins are commonly used. Given the increasing incidence of methicillin-resistant *S aureus* (MRSA) in the community, coverage of this pathogen with appropriate antibiotic therapy should be considered (see Table 30–4).

C. Wound Care

Any wound that is the initiating site of lymphangitis should be treated aggressively. Any necrotic tissue must be debrided and loculated pus drained.

Prognosis

With proper therapy including an antibiotic effective against the invading bacteria, control of the infection can usually be achieved in a few days. Delayed or inadequate therapy can lead to overwhelming infection with septicemia.

LYMPHEDEMA

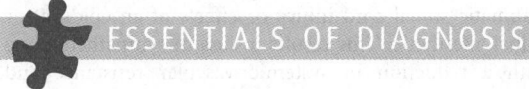

ESSENTIALS OF DIAGNOSIS

▶ Painless persistent edema of one or both lower extremities, primarily in young women.

▶ Pitting edema without ulceration, varicosities, or stasis pigmentation.

▶ There may be episodes of lymphangitis and cellulitis.

General Considerations

When lymphedema is due to congenital developmental abnormalities consisting of hypoplastic or hyperplastic involvement of the proximal or distal lymphatics, it is referred to as the **primary** form. The obstruction may be in the pelvic or lumbar lymph channels and nodes when the disease is extensive and progressive. The **secondary** form of lymphedema involves inflammatory or mechanical lymphatic obstruction from trauma, regional lymph node resection or irradiation, or extensive involvement of regional nodes by malignant disease or filariasis. Secondary dilation of the lymphatics that occurs in both forms leads to incompetence of the valve system, disrupting the orderly flow along the lymph vessels, and results in progressive stasis of a protein-rich fluid. Episodes of acute and chronic inflammation may be superimposed, with further stasis and may create secondary fibrosis. Hypertrophy of the limb results, with markedly thickened and fibrotic skin and subcutaneous tissue in very advanced cases.

Lymphangiography and radioactive isotope studies may identify focal defects in lymph flow but are of little value in planning therapy.

Treatment

Since there is no effective cure for lymphedema, the treatment strategies are designed to control the problem and allow normal activity and function. Most patients can be treated with some of the following measures: (1) The flow of lymph out of the extremity can be aided through intermittent elevation of the extremity, especially during the sleeping hours (foot of bed elevated 15–20 degrees, achieved by placing pillows beneath the mattress); the constant use of graduated elastic compression stockings; and massage toward the trunk—either by hand or by means of pneumatic pressure devices designed to milk edema out of an extremity. (2) Secondary cellulitis in the extremity should be avoided by means of good hygiene and treatment of any trichophytosis of the toes. Once an infection starts, it should be treated by periods of elevation and antibiotic therapy that covers *Staphylococcus* and *Streptococcus* organisms. Infections can be a serious and recurring problem and are often difficult to control. Prophylactic antibiotics have not been shown to be of benefit. (3) Intermittent courses of diuretic therapy, especially in those with premenstrual or seasonal exacerbations, are rarely helpful. (4) Amputation is used only for the rare complication of lymphangiosarcoma in the extremity.

Prognosis

With aggressive treatment, including pneumatic compression devices, good relief of symptoms can be achieved. The long-term outlook is dictated by the associated conditions and avoidance of recurrent cellulitis.

Rockson SG. Diagnosis and management of lymphatic vascular disease. J Am Coll Cardiol. 2008 Sep 2;52(10):799–806. [PMID: 18755341]

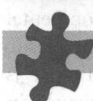

SHOCK

ESSENTIALS OF DIAGNOSIS

▶ Hypotension, tachycardia, oliguria, altered mental status.
▶ Peripheral hypoperfusion and impaired oxygen delivery.

General Considerations

Shock occurs when the rate of arterial blood flow is inadequate to meet tissue metabolic needs. This results in regional hypoxia and subsequent lactic acidosis from anaerobic metabolism in peripheral tissues as well as eventual end-organ damage and failure.

Classification (Table 12–1)

A. Hypovolemic Shock

Hypovolemic shock results from decreased intravascular volume secondary to loss of blood or fluids and electrolytes. The etiology may be suggested by the clinical setting (eg, trauma) or by signs and symptoms of blood loss (eg, gastrointestinal bleeding) or dehydration (eg, vomiting or diarrhea). Compensatory vasoconstriction may transiently maintain the blood pressure but unreplaced losses of over 15% of the intravascular volume can result in hypotension and progressive tissue hypoxia.

B. Cardiogenic Shock

Cardiogenic shock results from pump failure. This may be related to myocardial infarction, cardiomyopathy, myocardial contusion, valvular incompetence or stenosis, or arrhythmias. See Chapter 10.

C. Obstructive Shock

Cardiac tamponade, tension pneumothorax, and massive pulmonary embolism can cause an acute decrease in cardiac output resulting in shock. These are medical emergencies requiring prompt diagnosis and treatment.

D. Distributive Shock

Distributive or vasodilatory shock has many causes including sepsis, anaphylaxis, systemic inflammatory response syndrome (SIRS) produced by severe pancreatitis or burns, or acute adrenal insufficiency. The reduction in systemic vascular resistance results in inadequate cardiac output and tissue hypoperfusion despite normal circulatory volume.

1. Septic shock—Sepsis is the most common cause of distributive shock and carries a high mortality rate of 30–87%. Sepsis is typically secondary to gram-negative bacte-

Table 12–1. Classification of shock by mechanism and common causes.

Hypovolemic shock
Loss of blood (hemorrhagic shock)
External hemorrhage
Trauma
Gastrointestinal tract bleeding
Internal hemorrhage
Hematoma
Hemothorax or hemoperitoneum
Loss of plasma
Burns
Exfoliative dermatitis
Loss of fluid and electrolytes
External
Vomiting
Diarrhea
Excessive sweating
Hyperosmolar states (diabetic ketoacidosis, hyperosmolar nonketotic coma)
Internal ("third spacing")
Pancreatitis
Ascites
Bowel obstruction
Cardiogenic shock
Dysrhythmia
Tachyarrhythmia
Bradyarrhythmia
"Pump failure" (secondary to myocardial infarction or other cardiomyopathy)
Acute valvular dysfunction (especially regurgitant lesions)
Rupture of ventricular septum or free ventricular wall
Obstructive shock
Tension pneumothorax
Pericardial disease (tamponade, constriction)
Disease of pulmonary vasculature (massive pulmonary emboli, pulmonary hypertension)
Cardiac tumor (atrial myxoma)
Left atrial mural thrombus
Obstructive valvular disease (aortic or mitral stenosis)
Distributive shock
Septic shock
Anaphylactic shock
Neurogenic shock
Vasodilator drugs
Acute adrenal insufficiency

Reproduced, with permission, from Stone CK, Humphries RL (editors). *Current Emergency Diagnosis & Treatment*, 5th ed. p. 193. McGraw-Hill, 2004.

remia (such as *Escherichia coli, Klebsiella, Proteus,* and *Pseudomonas*) and less often due to gram-positive cocci and gram-negative anaerobes (*Bacteroides*). Risk factors include extremes of age, diabetes, immunosuppression, and history of a recent invasive procedure.

2. Neurogenic shock—Neurogenic shock is caused by traumatic spinal cord injury or effects of an epidural or spinal anesthetic. This results in loss of sympathetic tone with a reduction in systemic vascular resistance and hypotension without a compensatory tachycardia. Reflex vagal parasympathetic stimulation evoked by pain, gastric dilation, or fright may simulate neurogenic shock, producing hypotension, bradycardia, and syncope.

▶ Clinical Findings

Hypotension is traditionally defined as a systolic blood pressure of 90 mm Hg or less or a mean arterial pressure of less than 60–65 mm Hg but must be evaluated relative to the patient's normal blood pressure. A drop in systolic pressure of more than 10–20 mm Hg and an increase in pulse of more than 15 beats per minute with positional change suggests depleted intravascular volume. However, blood pressure is often not the best indicator of organ perfusion because compensatory mechanisms, such as increased heart rate, contractility, and vasoconstriction can occur to prevent hypotension. Patients often have cool or mottled extremities and weak or thready peripheral pulses. Splanchnic vasoconstriction may lead to oliguria, bowel ischemia, and hepatic dysfunction, which can ultimately result in multiorgan failure. Mentation may be normal or patients may become restless, agitated, confused, lethargic, or comatose as a result of inadequate perfusion of the brain. Consequently, intubation and mechanical ventilation may be required to protect the patient's airway.

Hypovolemic shock is evident when signs of hypoperfusion, such as oliguria, altered mental status, and cool extremities, are present. Jugular venous pressure is low, and there is a narrow pulse pressure indicative of reduced stroke volume. Rapid replacement of fluids restores tissue perfusion. In **cardiogenic shock,** there are also signs of global hypoperfusion with oliguria, altered mental status, and cool extremities. Jugular venous pressure is elevated. There may be evidence of pulmonary edema in the setting of left-sided heart failure. A transthoracic echocardiogram (TTE) or a TEE is an effective diagnostic tool to differentiate hypovolemic shock from cardiogenic shock. In hypovolemic shock, the left ventricle will be small because of decreased filling, but contractility is often preserved. Cardiogenic shock results from pump failure and therefore there will be evidence of a decrease in left ventricular contractility. In some cases, the left ventricle may appear dilated and full because of its inability to eject.

In **obstructive shock,** the central venous pressure may be elevated but the TEE or TTE may show reduced left ventricular filling, a layer of fluid between the pericardium as in the case of tamponade, or thickened pericardium as in the case of pericarditis. Pericardiocentesis or pericardial window, chest tube placement, or catheter-directed thrombolytic therapy can be lifesaving in the case of tamponade.

In **distributive shock,** signs include hyperdynamic heart sounds, warm extremities, and a wide pulse pressure indicative of large stroke volume. The echocardiogram may show hyperdynamic left ventricle. Fluid resuscitation may have little effect on blood pressure, urinary output, or mentation.

Septic shock is diagnosed when there is clinical evidence of infection in the setting of persistent hypotension and evidence of organ hypoperfusion, such as lactic acidosis, decreased urinary output, or altered mental status despite volume resuscitation. Neurogenic shock is diagnosed when there is evidence of central nervous system injury and persistent hypotension despite volume resuscitation.

▶ Treatment

A. General Measures

Treatment depends on prompt diagnosis and an accurate appraisal of inciting conditions. Initial management consists of basic life support with an assessment of the patient's airway, breathing, and circulation. This may entail airway intubation and mechanical ventilation. Ventilatory failure should be anticipated in patients with a severe metabolic acidosis in association with shock. Mechanical ventilation along with sedation and paralysis can decrease the oxygen demand of the respiratory muscles and allow improved oxygen delivery to other hypoperfused tissues. Intravenous access and fluid resuscitation should be instituted along with cardiac monitoring and assessment of hemodynamic parameters such as blood pressure and heart rate. Cardiac monitoring can detect myocardial ischemia requiring cardiac catheterization or malignant arrhythmias, which can be treated by standard advanced cardiac life support (ACLS) protocols.

Unresponsive or minimally responsive patients should immediately be given 1 ampule of **50% dextrose** intravenously and 2 mg of **naloxone** intravenously or intramuscularly. An **arterial line** should be placed for continuous blood pressure measurement, and a **Foley catheter** should be inserted to monitor urinary output. **Blood specimens** should be evaluated for complete blood count, electrolytes, glucose, arterial blood gas determinations, coagulation parameters, typing and cross-matching, and bacterial cultures.

B. Central Venous Pressure or Pulmonary Capillary Wedge Pressure

Early consideration is given to placement of a central line or pulmonary artery catheter for hemodynamic pressure measurements. A pulmonary artery catheter can be helpful in distinguishing cardiogenic and septic shock and in monitoring the effects of volume resuscitation or pressor medications. Pulmonary artery catheter allows measurement of the pulmonary artery pressure, left-sided filling pressure or the pulmonary capillary wedge pressure (PCWP), and cardiac output. Because of the attendant risks associated with pulmonary artery catheters (such as infection, arrhythmias, vein thrombosis, and pulmonary artery rupture), the value of the information they might provide must be carefully weighed in each patient. TTE is a noninvasive alternative to pulmonary artery catheter and can provide information about the pulmonary artery pressure, PCWP, and cardiac output. In addition, TTE can provide information about the function of the heart.

A **central venous pressure (CVP)** under 5 mm Hg suggests hypovolemia, and a CVP over 18 mm Hg suggests volume overload, cardiac failure, tamponade, or pulmonary hypertension. A cardiac index < 2 L/min/m^2 indicates a need for inotropic support. A high cardiac index > 4 L/min/m^2 in a hypotensive patient is consistent with early septic shock. The systemic vascular resistance is low (< 800 dynes.s/cm^{-5}) in sepsis and neurogenic shock and high (> 1500 dynes.s/cm^{-5}) in hypovolemic and cardiogenic shock. Treatment is directed at maintaining a CVP of 8–12 mm Hg, and mean arterial pressure of 65–90 mm Hg, a cardiac index of 2–4 L/min/m^2, and a central venous oxygen saturation of greater than 70%.

C. Volume Replacement

Volume replacement is critical in the initial management of shock. **Hemorrhagic shock** is treated with immediate efforts to achieve hemostasis and rapid infusions of blood substitutes, such as type-specific or type O negative packed red blood cells (PRBC) or whole blood, which also provides extra volume and clotting factors. Each unit of PRBC or whole blood is expected to raise the hematocrit by 3%. **Hypovolemic shock** secondary to dehydration is managed with rapid boluses of isotonic crystalloid, usually in 1 liter increments. **Cardiogenic shock** in the absence of fluid overload requires smaller fluid challenges, usually in increments of 250 mL. **Septic shock** usually requires large volumes of fluid for resuscitation as the associated capillary leak releases fluid to the extravascular space.

Meta-analyses of studies of critically ill heterogenous populations comparing crystalloid and colloid resuscitation (with albumin) indicate no benefit of colloid over crystalloid solutions, and some have suggested a trend toward increased mortality with albumin. Clinical trials and meta-analyses have also found no difference in mortality between trauma patients receiving hypertonic saline (7.5%) and those receiving isotonic crystalloid. More positive results were found with hypertonic saline plus dextran with an increase in survival over patients managed with isotonic saline, particularly in patients with traumatic brain injury.

Large-volume resuscitation with unwarmed fluids produces hypothermia, which must be treated to avoid hypothermia-induced coagulopathy.

D. Early Goal-Directed Therapy

Early goal-directed therapy within the first 6 hours in the treatment of septic shock provides significant benefits. In a randomized, controlled trial, patients were assigned to early goal-directed therapy or usual care. Patients who were assigned to early goal-directed care received fluid resuscitation to achieve a CVP of 8–12 mm Hg; PRBCs to reach a hematocrit of 30%; vasopressors to reach a mean arterial blood pressure of 65 mm Hg; and dobutamine, if necessary, to achieve a central venous oxygen saturation of $> 70\%$. These patients had a significantly lower in-hospital and 60-day mortality rate compared with control patients. A meta-analysis of hemodynamic optimization trials has also suggested that early treatment before the development of organ failure results in improved survival.

Compensated shock can occur in the setting of normalized hemodynamic parameters with ongoing global tissue hypoxia. Traditional endpoints of resuscitation such as blood pressure, heart rate, urinary output, mental status, and skin perfusion can therefore be misleading. Additional endpoints such as lactate levels and base deficit can help guide further resuscitative therapy. Patients who respond well to initial efforts demonstrate a survival advantage over nonresponders.

E. Medications

1. Vasoactive therapy—Vasopressors and inotropic agents are administered only after adequate fluid resuscitation. Choice of vasoactive therapy depends on cardiac output. If there is evidence of low cardiac output with high filling pressures, inotropic support is needed to improve contractility. If there is continued hypotension with evidence of high cardiac output after adequate volume resuscitation, then vasopressor support is needed to improve vasomotor tone.

Dobutamine, a β-adrenergic agonist, is the first-line drug for **cardiogenic shock,** increasing contractility and decreasing afterload. The initial dose is 0.5–1 mcg/kg/min as a continuous intravenous infusion, then titrated every few minutes. The usual dosage range is 2–20 mcg/kg/min intravenously. Tachyphylaxis can occur after 48 hours secondary to the down-regulation of β-adrenergic receptors. Amrinone or milrinone are phosphodiesterase inhibitors that can be substituted for dobutamine. These drugs increase cyclic AMP levels and increase cardiac contractility, bypassing the β-adrenergic receptor. However, vasodilation is a side effect of amrinone and milrinone.

For **vasodilatory shock** when increased vasoconstriction is required to maintain an adequate perfusion pressure, α-adrenergic agonists such as phenylephrine and norepinephrine are generally used. Although **norepinephrine** is both an α-adrenergic and β-adrenergic agonist, it preferentially increases mean arterial pressure over cardiac output. The initial dose is 0.5–1 mcg/min as an intravenous infusion, titrated to maintain the systolic blood pressure to at least 80 mm Hg. The usual maintenance dose is 2–4 mcg/min (maximum dose is 30 mcg/min). Patients with refractory shock may require dosages of 8–30 mcg/min. **Epinephrine,** also with both α-adrenergic and β-adrenergic effects, may be used in severe shock and during acute resuscitation. Initially, give 1 mcg/min as a continuous intravenous infusion; the usual dosage range is 2–10 mcg/min IV.

Dopamine has variable effects according to dosage. At low doses (2–3 mcg/kg/min) stimulation of dopaminergic and β-agonist receptors produces increased glomerular filtration, heart rate, and contractility. At higher doses (> 5 mcg/kg/min), α-adrenergic effects predominate, resulting in peripheral vasoconstriction. Recent studies have suggested some advantages to norepinephrine over dopamine at high doses.

Vasopressin (antidiuretic hormone or ADH) is gaining widespread acceptance in the treatment of **distributive** or **vasodilatory shock.** Vasopressin causes peripheral vasoconstriction via V1 receptors located on smooth muscle cells and attenuation of nitric oxide (NO) synthesis and cGMP, the second messenger of NO. The rationale for using low-dose vasopressin in the management of septic shock include the relative deficiency of vasopressin in late shock and the increased sensitivity of the systemic circulation to the vasopressor effects of vasopressin. Vasopressin also potentiates the effects of catecholamines on the vasculature and stimulates cortisol production. Several small clinical trials have demonstrated improvement in hemodynamic parameters and urinary output with vasopressin use but no clinical study has yet demonstrated improved survival. In addition, some studies have reported reduced catecholamine requirements with vasopressin administration. Infusion of vasopressin at a low dose (0.01–0.04 units/min) may be safe and beneficial in septic patients with hypotension that is refractory to fluid resuscitation and conventional catecholamine vasopressors. Higher doses of vasopressin decrease cardiac output and may put patients at greater risk for splanchnic and coronary artery ischemia. Further recommendations regarding vasopressin use will likely follow the publication of the results from the recent Vasopressin in Septic Shock Trial. Terlipressin is a synthetic long-acting analog of vasopressin that increases blood pressure at the expense of cardiac index and oxygen consumption but may be an effective rescue therapy in patients with catecholamine resistant septic shock.

NO plays an important role in the vasodilatation associated with septic shock. Endotoxin and inflammatory cytokines induce a calcium independent NO synthase that results in a sustained production of NO. The NO pathway is inhibited by methylene blue which, when given to patients with septic shock, has been shown to increase mean arterial pressure and systemic vascular resistance while decreasing vasopressor requirements. However, no improvement in survival has been demonstrated. A large randomized study showed an increased mortality rate in patients with septic shock who received another NO inhibitor N^G-methyl-L-arginine hydrochloride.

2. Corticosteroids—The observation that severe sepsis may be associated with relative adrenal insufficiency or glucocorticoid receptor resistance has led to several trials to evaluate the role of treatment with corticosteroids in septic shock. Early trials where high doses of corticosteroids were administered to patients in septic shock did not show improved survival; rather, some worse outcomes were observed from increased rates of secondary infections. Subsequent trials have studied the use of low-dose corticosteroids in patients who were in septic shock and had relative adrenal insufficiency, defined by a cortisol response of 9 mcg/dL or less after one injection of 250 mcg of corticotropin. Low-dose corticosteroid regimens included hydrocortisone 50 mg every 6 hours and 50 mcg of 9-alpha-fludrocortisone once a day, both for 7 days, or hydrocortisone 50 mg by intravenous bolus, followed by a continuous infusion of 0.18 mg/kg of body weight/hr until cessation of vasopressor support. These trials demonstrated a shorter duration of use of vasopressors, significantly reduced 28-day mortality rates, and no increased adverse effects. There was no benefit from low-dose corticosteroid use in patients who did not have adrenal insufficiency. In 2008, however, the Corticosteroid Therapy of Septic Shock (CORTICUS) study has shown that low-dose hydrocortisone (50 mg every 6 hours for 5 days and then tapered over a 6 day period) did not improve survival in patients with septic shock, either overall or in patients who did not respond to corticotropin. This study was a randomized, double-blinded, placebo-controlled trial that is the largest to date of corticosteroids in septic patients. One limitation of the CORTICUS trial was it was not adequately powered to detect a clinically important difference in mortality. Thus, there is still uncertainty over the role of corticosteroids and corticotropin stimulation testing in patients with septic shock.

3. Activated Protein C (Drotrecogin alpha)—Activated protein C is an endogenous protein that has antithrombotic, profibrinolytic, and anti-inflammatory properties. A large randomized trial demonstrated an improved 28-day mortality rate (from 31% to 25%) in patients with severe sepsis and organ failure when treated with recombinant human activated protein C as a continuous infusion of 24 mcg/kg/h for 96 hours. A retrospective follow up of the persons enrolled in the trial demonstrated that the survival benefit observed in patients with severe sepsis persisted only to hospital discharge. Post hoc analysis, however, suggested that the benefit of activated protein C on long-term survival was greater in patients with APACHE (acute physiology and chronic health evaluation) II scores $\geq$ 25. A randomized, placebo-controlled study evaluating patients with severe sepsis and a low risk of death, as defined by an APACHE II score of < 25 or single organ failure, confirmed the finding of no mortality benefit at 28 days. However, the rate of serious bleeding was greater in the group treated with activated protein C.

4. Antibiotics—Definitive therapy for septic shock includes an early initiation of empiric broad-spectrum antibiotics after appropriate cultures have been obtained. Surgical management may also be necessary if necrotic tissue or loculated infections are present (see Table 30–9).

5. Sodium bicarbonate—For patients with sepsis of any etiology and lactic acidosis, clinical studies have failed to show any hemodynamic benefit from bicarbonate therapy, either in increasing cardiac output or in decreasing the vasopressor requirement even in patients with severe acidemia.

F. Other Treatment Modalities

Cardiac failure may require use of transcutaneous or transvenous pacing or placement of an intra-arterial balloon pump. Emergent revascularization by percutaneous angioplasty or coronary artery bypass surgery appears to improve long-term outcome with increased survival compared with initial medical stabilization. Urgent hemodialysis or continuous venovenous hemofiltration may be indicated for maintenance of fluid and electrolyte balance during acute renal insufficiency resulting in shock.

Alam HB et al. New developments in fluid resuscitation. Surg Clin North Am. 2007 Feb;87(1):55–72. [PMID: 17127123]

Annane D et al; Ger-Inf-05 Study Group. Effect of low doses of corticosteroids in septic shock patients with or without early acute respiratory distress syndrome. Crit Care Med. 2006 Jan;34(1):22–30. [PMID: 16374152]

Fourrier F. Recombinant human activated protein C in the treatment of severe sepsis: an evidence-based review. Crit Care Med. 2004 Nov;32(11 Suppl):S534–41. [PMID: 15542961]

Lange M et al. Vasopressin vs. terlipressin in the treatment of cardiovascular failure in sepsis. Intensive Care Med. 2008 May;34(5):821–32. [PMID: 18066524]

Nguyen HB et al; Emergency Department Sepsis Education Program and Strategies to Improve Survival (ED-SEPSIS) Working Group. Severe sepsis and septic shock: review of the literature and emergency department management guidelines. Ann Emerg Med. 2006 Jul;48(1):28–54. [PMID: 16781920]

Oppert M et al. Low-dose hydrocortisone improves shock reversal and reduces cytokine levels in early hyperdynamic septic shock. Crit Care Med. 2005 Nov;33(11):2457–64. [PMID: 16276166]

Siraux V et al. Relative adrenal insufficiency in patients with septic shock: comparison of low-dose and conventional corticotropin tests. Crit Care Med. 2005 Nov;33(11):2479–86. [PMID: 16276169]

Sprung CL et al. Hydrocortisone therapy for patients with septic shock. N Engl J Med. 2008 Jan;358(2):111–24. [PMID: 18184957]

Blood Disorders

Charles A. Linker, MD

ANEMIAS

General Approach to Anemias

Anemia is present in adults if the hematocrit is less than 41% (hemoglobin < 13.5 g/dL) in males or less than 37% (hemoglobin < 12 g/dL) in females. Congenital anemia is suggested by the patient's personal and family history. Poor diet may result in folic acid deficiency and contribute to iron deficiency, but bleeding is much more commonly the cause of iron deficiency in adults. Physical examination includes attention to signs of primary hematologic diseases (lymphadenopathy, hepatosplenomegaly, or bone tenderness). Mucosal changes such as a smooth tongue suggest megaloblastic anemia.

Anemias are classified according to their pathophysiologic basis, ie, whether related to diminished production or accelerated loss of red blood cells (Table 13–1), or according to cell size (Table 13–2). The diagnostic possibilities in microcytic anemia are iron deficiency, thalassemia, and anemia of chronic disease. A severely microcytic anemia (mean cell volume [MCV] < 70 fL) is due either to iron deficiency or thalassemia. Macrocytic anemia may be due to megaloblastic (folate or vitamin B_{12} deficiency) or nonmegaloblastic causes, in particular myelodysplasia and the use of antiretroviral drugs. A severely macrocytic anemia (MCV > 125 fL) is almost always due to either megaloblastic anemia or myelodysplasia.

IRON DEFICIENCY ANEMIA

 ESSENTIALS OF DIAGNOSIS

- ▶ Serum ferritin < 12 mcg/L.
- ▶ Caused by bleeding unless proved otherwise.
- ▶ Responds to iron therapy.

General Considerations

Iron deficiency is the most common cause of anemia worldwide. The causes are listed in Table 13–3. Aside from circulating red blood cells, the major location of iron in the body is the storage pool as ferritin or as hemosiderin and in macrophages.

The average American diet contains 10–15 mg of iron per day. About 10% of this amount is absorbed. Absorption occurs in the stomach, duodenum, and upper jejunum. Dietary iron present as heme is efficiently absorbed (10–20%) but nonheme iron less so (1–5%), largely because of interference by phosphates, tannins, and other food constituents. Small amounts of iron—approximately 1 mg/d—are normally lost through exfoliation of skin and mucosal cells. There is no physiologic mechanism for increasing normal body iron losses.

Menstrual blood loss plays a major role in iron metabolism. The average monthly menstrual blood loss is approximately 50 mL, or about 0.7 mg/d. However, menstrual blood loss may be five times the average. To maintain adequate iron stores, women with heavy menstrual losses must absorb 3–4 mg of iron from the diet each day. This strains the upper limit of what may reasonably be absorbed, and women with menorrhagia of this degree will almost always become iron deficient without iron supplementation.

In general, iron metabolism is balanced between absorption of 1 mg/d and loss of 1 mg/d. Pregnancy may also upset the iron balance, since requirements increase to 2–5 mg of iron per day during pregnancy and lactation. Normal dietary iron cannot supply these requirements, and medicinal iron is needed during pregnancy and lactation. Repeated pregnancy (especially with breast-feeding) may cause iron deficiency if increased requirements are not met with supplemental medicinal iron. Decreased iron absorption can on very rare occasions cause iron deficiency and usually occurs after gastric surgery, though concomitant bleeding is frequent.

By far the most important cause of iron deficiency anemia is blood loss, especially gastrointestinal blood loss. Prolonged aspirin use, or the use of other anti-inflammatory drugs, may cause it even without a documented structural lesion. Iron deficiency demands a search for a source of gastrointestinal bleeding if other sites of blood loss (menorrhagia, other uterine bleeding, and repeated blood donations) are excluded.

Table 13–1. Classification of anemias by pathophysiology.

Decreased production
  Hemoglobin synthesis lesion: iron deficiency, thalassemia, anemia of chronic disease
  DNA synthesis lesion: megaloblastic anemia
  Stem cell lesion: aplastic anemia, myeloproliferative leukemia
  Bone marrow infiltration: carcinoma, lymphoma
  Pure red cell aplasia
Increased destruction
  Blood loss
  Hemolysis (intrinsic)
    Membrane lesion: hereditary spherocytosis, elliptocytosis
    Hemoglobin lesion: sickle cell, unstable hemoglobin
    Glycolysis: pyruvate kinase deficiency, etc
    Oxidation lesion: glucose-6-phosphate dehydrogenase deficiency
  Hemolysis (extrinsic)
    Immune: warm antibody, cold antibody
    Microangiopathic: thrombotic thrombocytopenic purpura, hemolytic-uremic syndrome, mechanical cardiac valve, paravalvular leak
    Infection: clostridial
  Hypersplenism

Chronic hemoglobinuria may lead to iron deficiency since iron is lost in the urine, but this is uncommon; traumatic hemolysis due to a prosthetic cardiac valve and other causes of intravascular hemolysis (eg, paroxysmal nocturnal hemoglobinuria) should also be considered. Frequent blood donors may also be at risk for iron deficiency.

► Clinical Findings

A. Symptoms and Signs

As a rule, the only symptoms of iron deficiency anemia are those of the anemia itself (easy fatigability, tachycardia, palpitations and tachypnea on exertion). Severe deficiency causes skin and mucosal changes, including a smooth tongue, brittle nails, and cheilosis. Dysphagia because of the formation of esophageal webs (Plummer–Vinson syndrome) also occurs.

Table 13–2. Classification of anemias by mean cell volume.

Microcytic
  Iron deficiency
  Thalassemia
  Anemia of chronic disease
Macrocytic
  Megaloblastic
    Vitamin B_{12} deficiency
    Folate deficiency
  Nonmegaloblastic
  Myelodysplasia, chemotherapy
  Liver disease
  Increased reticulocytosis
  Myxedema
Normocytic
  Many causes

Table 13–3. Causes of iron deficiency.

Deficient diet
Decreased absorption
Increased requirements
  Pregnancy
  Lactation
Blood loss
  Gastrointestinal
  Menstrual
  Blood donation
Hemoglobinuria
Iron sequestration
  Pulmonary hemosiderosis

Many iron-deficient patients develop pica, craving for specific foods (ice chips, etc) often not rich in iron.

B. Laboratory Findings

Iron deficiency develops in stages. The first is depletion of iron stores. At this point, there is anemia and no change in red blood cell size. The serum ferritin will become abnormally low. A ferritin value less than 12 mcg/L is a highly reliable indicator of iron deficiency. Bone marrow biopsy for evaluation of iron stores is now rarely performed because of intraobserver variation in its interpretation.

After iron stores have been depleted, red blood cell formation will continue with deficient supplies of iron. Serum iron values decline to less than 30 mcg/dL and transferrin levels rise, leading to transferring saturation of less than 15%.

In the early stages, the MCV remains normal. Subsequently, the MCV falls and the blood smear shows hypochromic microcytic cells. With further progression, anisocytosis (variations in red blood cell size) and poikilocytosis (variation in shape of red cells) develop. Severe iron deficiency will produce a bizarre peripheral blood smear, with severely hypochromic cells, target cells, hypochromic pencil-shaped cells, and occasionally small numbers of nucleated red blood cells. The platelet count is commonly increased.

► Differential Diagnosis

Other causes of microcytic anemia include anemia of chronic disease, thalassemia, and sideroblastic anemia. Anemia of chronic disease is characterized by normal or increased iron stores in the bone marrow and a normal or elevated ferritin level; the serum iron is low, often drastically so, and the total iron-binding capacity (TIBC) is either normal or low. Thalassemia produces a greater degree of microcytosis for any given level of anemia than does iron deficiency. Red blood cell morphology on the peripheral smear is abnormal earlier in the course of thalassemia.

► Treatment

The diagnosis of iron deficiency anemia can be made either by the laboratory demonstration of an iron-deficient state or by evaluating the response to a therapeutic trial of iron replacement.

Since the anemia itself is rarely life-threatening, the most important part of treatment is identification of the cause—especially a source of occult blood loss.

A. Oral Iron

Ferrous sulfate, 325 mg three times daily, which provides 180 mg of iron daily of which up to 10 mg is absorbed (though absorption may exceed this amount in cases of severe deficiency), is the preferred therapy. Compliance is improved by introducing the medicine more slowly in a gradually escalating dose with food. Alternatively, in cases of poor tolerance, one pill of ferrous sulfate can be taken at bedtime on an empty stomach. It is preferable to prescribe a lower dose of iron or to allow ingestion concurrent with food than to insist on a more rigorous schedule that will not be followed. An appropriate response is a return of the hematocrit level halfway toward normal within 3 weeks with full return to baseline after 2 months. Iron therapy should continue for 3–6 months after restoration of normal hematologic values to replenish iron stores. Failure of response to iron therapy is usually due to noncompliance, although occasional patients may absorb iron poorly, particularly if the stomach is achlorhydric. Such patients may benefit from concomitant administration of ascorbic acid (250 mg daily). Other reasons for failure to respond include incorrect diagnosis (anemia of chronic disease, thalassemia) and ongoing gastrointestinal blood loss that exceeds the rate of new erythropoiesis.

B. Parenteral Iron

The indications are intolerance to oral iron, refractoriness to oral iron, gastrointestinal disease (usually inflammatory bowel disease) precluding the use of oral iron, and continued blood loss that cannot be corrected. Because of the possibility of anaphylactic reactions, parenteral iron therapy has been advocated only for use in cases of persistent anemia after a reasonable course of oral therapy. Sodium ferric gluconate is available and has been shown to result in a lower incidence of severe anaphylaxis, allowing wider use of parenteral therapy.

The dose (total 1.5–2 g) may be calculated by estimating the decrease in volume of red blood cell mass and then supplying 1 mg of iron for each milliliter of volume of red blood cells below normal. Approximately 1 g should then be added for storage iron. Total body iron ranges between 2 g and 4 g: approximately 50 mg/kg in men and 35 mg/kg in women. Most (70–95%) of the iron is present in hemoglobin in circulating red blood cells. One milliliter of packed red blood cells (not whole blood) contains approximately 1 mg of iron. In men, red blood cell volume is approximately 30 mL/kg. A 70-kg man will therefore have approximately 2100 mL of packed red blood cells and consequently 2100 mg of iron in his circulating blood. In women, the red cell volume is about 27 mL/kg; a 50-kg woman will thus have 1350 mg of iron circulating in her red blood cells. Thus, a woman whose hemoglobin is 9 g/dL would be treated with a total of 1315

mg of parenteral iron, 315 mg for the increased red blood cell mass and 1000 mg to provide iron stores. The entire dose may be given as an intravenous infusion over 4–6 hours. A test dose of a dilute solution is given first, and the patient should be observed during the entire infusion for anaphylaxis.

When to Refer

Referral to a hematologist should not generally be necessary. Refer the patient if he or she is not responsive to iron therapy.

Andrews NC. Forging a field: the golden age of iron biology. Blood. 2008 Jul 15;112(2):219–30. [PMID: 18606887]

Chang J et al. Clinical utility of serum soluble transferrin receptor levels and comparison with bone marrow iron stores as an index for iron-deficient erythropoiesis in a heterogeneous group of patients. Pathology. 2007 Jun;39(3):349–53. [PMID: 17558864]

Killip S et al. Iron deficiency anemia. Am Fam Physician. 2007 Mar 1;75(5):671–8. [PMID: 17375513]

Miller HJ et al. Efficacy and tolerability of intravenous ferric gluconate in the treatment of iron deficiency anemia in patients without kidney disease. Arch Intern Med. 2007 Jun 25;167(12):1327–8. [PMID: 17592108]

ANEMIA OF CHRONIC DISEASE

 ESSENTIALS OF DIAGNOSIS

- ▶ Anemia, normocytic, or microcytic.
- ▶ Normal or increased iron stores.
- ▶ Underlying chronic disease.

General Considerations

Many chronic systemic diseases are associated with mild or moderate anemia. Common causes include chronic infection or inflammation, cancer, and liver disease. The anemia of chronic kidney failure is somewhat different in pathophysiology, involving reduced production of erythropoietin, and is usually more severe. Hepcidin has been identified as an important mediator of sequestration of iron within macrophages, and upregulation of hepcidin in response to mediators of inflammation, such as IL-6, is an important cause of anemia of chronic disease.

Clinical Findings

A. Symptoms and Signs

The clinical features are those of the causative condition. The diagnosis should be suspected in patients with known chronic diseases. In cases of significant anemia, coexistent iron deficiency or folic acid deficiency should be suspected. Decreased dietary intake of folate or iron is common in these ill patients, and many will also have ongoing gastrointestinal blood losses. Patients undergoing hemodialysis regularly lose both iron and folate during dialysis.

B. Laboratory Findings

The hematocrit rarely falls below 60% of baseline (except in kidney failure). The MCV is usually normal or slightly reduced. Red blood cell morphology is nondiagnostic, and the reticulocyte count is neither strikingly reduced nor increased. Serum iron values may be low or unmeasurable, and transferrin saturation may be extremely low, leading to an erroneous diagnosis of iron deficiency. In contrast to iron deficiency, serum ferritin values should be normal or increased. A serum ferritin value of less than 30 mcg/L should suggest coexistent iron deficiency.

▶ Treatment

In most cases no treatment is necessary. Purified recombinant erythropoietin (epoetin alfa) is effective for treatment of the anemia of kidney failure and other secondary anemias such as anemia related to cancer or inflammatory disorders (eg, rheumatoid arthritis). In kidney failure, optimal response to epoetin alfa requires adequate intensity of dialysis. Epoetin alfa must be injected subcutaneously and is very expensive. One effective schedule is 30,000 units once weekly, or darbepoetin 300 mcg every 2 to 3 weeks. Because of its cost, erythropoietin should be used only when the patient is transfusion-dependent or when the quality of life is improved by the hematologic response.

▶ When to Refer

Referral to a hematologist is not necessary.

Adamson JW. The anemia of inflammation/malignancy: mechanisms and management. Hematology Am Soc Hematol Educ Porgram. 2008;2008:159–65. [PMID: 19074075]

Benz R et al. Epoetin alfa once every 2 weeks is effective for initiation of treatment of anemia of chronic kidney disease. Clin J Am Soc Nephrol. 2007 Mar;2(2):215–21. [PMID: 17699416]

Ganz T. Hepcidin and its role in regulating systemic iron metabolism. Hematology Am Soc Hematol Educ Program. 2006:29–35. [PMID: 17124036]

Schwartz RN. Anemia in patients with cancer: incidence, causes, impact, management, and use of treatment guidelines and protocols. Am J Health Syst Pharm. 2007 Feb 1;64(3 Suppl 2):S5–13. [PMID: 17244886]

THE THALASSEMIAS

ESSENTIALS OF DIAGNOSIS

▶ Microcytosis disproportionate to the degree of anemia.

▶ Positive family history or lifelong personal history of microcytic anemia.

▶ Abnormal red blood cell morphology with microcytes, acanthocytes, and target cells.

▶ In β-thalassemia, elevated levels of hemoglobin A_2 or F.

▶ General Considerations

The thalassemias are hereditary disorders characterized by reduction in the synthesis of globin chains (α or β). Reduced globin chain synthesis causes reduced hemoglobin synthesis and eventually produces a hypochromic microcytic anemia because of defective hemoglobinization of red blood cells. Thalassemias can be considered among the hypoproliferative anemias, the hemolytic anemias, and the anemias related to abnormal hemoglobin, since all of these factors play a role in pathogenesis.

Normal adult hemoglobin is primarily hemoglobin A, which represents approximately 98% of circulating hemoglobin. Hemoglobin A is formed from a tetramer—two α chains and two β chains—and can be designated $\alpha_2\beta_2$. Two copies of the α-globin gene are located on chromosome 16, and there is no substitute for α-globin in the formation of hemoglobin. The β-globin gene resides on chromosome 11 adjacent to genes encoding the β-like globin chains, δ and γ. The tetramer of $\alpha_2\delta_2$ forms hemoglobin A_2, which normally comprises 1–2% of adult hemoglobin. The tetramer $\alpha_2\gamma_2$ forms hemoglobin F, which is the major hemoglobin of fetal life but which comprises less than 1% of normal adult hemoglobin.

The thalassemias are described as "**trait**" when there are laboratory features without significant clinical impact, "**intermedia**" when there is a red blood cell transfusion requirement or other moderate clinical impact, and "**major**" when the disorder is life-threatening.

α-**Thalassemia** is due primarily to gene deletion causing reduced α-globin chain synthesis (Table 13–4). Since all adult hemoglobins are α containing, α-thalassemia produces no change in the percentage distribution of hemoglobins A, A_2, and F. In severe forms of α-thalassemia, excess β chains may form a β_4 tetramer called hemoglobin H.

β-**Thalassemias** are usually caused by point mutations rather than deletions (Table 13–5). These mutations result in premature chain termination or in problems with transcription of RNA and ultimately result in reduced or absent β-globin chain synthesis. The molecular defects leading to β-thalassemia are numerous and heterogeneous. Defects that result in absent globin chain expression are termed β^0, whereas those causing reduced synthesis are termed β^+. The reduced β-globin chain synthesis in β-thalassemia results in a relative increase in the percentages of hemoglobins A_2 and F compared to hemoglobin A, as the β-like globins (γ and δ) substitute for the missing β chains. In the presence of reduced β chains, the excess α chains are unstable and precipitate, leading to damage of red blood cell membranes. This leads to intramedullary and peripheral hemolysis. The bone marrow becomes hyperplastic under the drive of anemia and ineffective erythropoiesis resulting from the intramedullary destruction of the developing erythroid cells. In cases of severe thalassemia, the marked expansion of the erythroid element in the bone marrow may cause severe bony deformities, osteopenia, and pathologic fractures.

▶ Clinical Findings

A. Symptoms and Signs

The α-**thalassemia** syndromes are seen primarily in persons from southeast Asia and China, and, less commonly, in blacks.

Table 13–4. α-Thalassemia syndromes.

α-Globin Genes	Syndrome	Hematocrit	MCV
4	Normal	Normal	
3	Silent carrier	Normal	
2	Thalassemia minor	28–40%	60–75 fL
1	Hemoglobin H disease	22–32%	60–70 fL
0	Hydrops fetalis		

MCV, mean cell volume.

Normally, adults have four copies of the α-globin chain. When three α-globin genes are present, the patient is hematologically normal (silent carrier). When two α-globin genes are present, the patient is said to have α-thalassemia trait, one form of thalassemia minor. These patients are clinically normal and have a normal life expectancy and performance status, with a mild microcytic anemia. When only one α-globin chain is present, the patient has hemoglobin H disease. This is a chronic hemolytic anemia of variable severity (thalassemia minor or intermedia). Physical examination will reveal pallor and splenomegaly. Although affected individuals do not usually require transfusions, they may do so during periods of hemolytic exacerbation caused by infection or other stresses. When all four α-globin genes are deleted, the affected fetus is stillborn as a result of hydrops fetalis.

β-Thalassemia primarily affects persons of Mediterranean origin (Italian, Greek) and to a lesser extent Chinese, other Asians, and blacks. Patients homozygous for β-thalassemia have thalassemia major. Affected children are normal at birth but after 6 months, when hemoglobin synthesis switches from hemoglobin F to hemoglobin A, develop severe anemia requiring transfusion. Numerous clinical problems ensue, including growth failure, bony deformities (abnormal facial structure, pathologic fractures), hepatosplenomegaly, and jaundice. The clinical course is modified significantly by transfusion therapy, but the transfusional iron overload (hemosiderosis) results in a clinical picture similar to hemochromatosis, with heart failure, cirrhosis, and endocrinopathies, usually after more than 100 units of red blood cells. These problems develop because of the body's inability to excrete the iron (see above) from transfused red

cells. Before the application of allogeneic stem cell transplantation and the development of more effective forms of iron chelation, death from cardiac failure usually occurred between the ages of 20 and 30 years. This has been profoundly changed.

Patients homozygous for a milder form of β-thalassemia (allowing a higher rate of globin gene synthesis) have thalassemia intermedia. These patients have chronic hemolytic anemia but do not require transfusions except under periods of stress. They also may develop iron overload because of periodic transfusion. They survive into adult life but with hepatosplenomegaly and bony deformities. Patients heterozygous for β-thalassemia have thalassemia minor and a clinically insignificant microcytic anemia.

Prenatal diagnosis is available, and genetic counseling should be offered and the opportunity for prenatal diagnosis discussed.

B. Laboratory Findings

1. α-Thalassemia trait—Patients with two α-globin genes have mild anemia, with hematocrits between 28% and 40%. The MCV is strikingly low (60–75 fL) despite the modest anemia, and the red blood count is normal or increased. The peripheral blood smear shows microcytes, hypochromia, occasional target cells, and acanthocytes (cells with irregularly spaced bulbous projections). The reticulocyte count and iron parameters are normal. Hemoglobin electrophoresis will show no increase in the percentage of hemoglobins A_2 or F and no hemoglobin H. α-Thalassemia trait is thus usually diagnosed by exclusion.

Table 13–5. β-Thalassemia syndromes.

	β-Globin Genes	Hb A	Hb A_2	Hb F
Normal	Homozygous β	97–99%	1–3%	< 1%
Thalassemia major	Homozygous $β^0$	0%	4–10%	90–96%
Thalassemia major	Homozygous $β^+$	0–10%	4–10%	90–96%
Thalassemia intermedia	Homozygous $β^+$ (mild)	0–30%	0–10%	6–100%
Thalassemia minor	Heterozygous $β^0$	80–95%	4–8%	1–5%
	Heterozygous $β^+$	80–95%	4–8%	1–5%

Hb, hemoglobin.

Genetic testing to demonstrate α-globin gene deletion is available in research laboratories.

2. Hemoglobin H disease—These patients have a more marked hemolytic anemia, with hematocrits between 22% and 32%. The MCV is remarkably low (60–70 fL) and the peripheral blood smear is markedly abnormal, with hypochromia, microcytosis, target cells, and poikilocytosis. The reticulocyte count is elevated. Hemoglobin electrophoresis will show the presence of a fast migrating hemoglobin (hemoglobin H), which comprises 10–40% of the hemoglobin. A peripheral blood smear can be stained with supravital dyes to demonstrate the presence of hemoglobin H.

3. β-Thalassemia minor—As in α-thalassemia trait, these patients have a modest anemia with hematocrit between 28% and 40%. The MCV ranges from 55 to 75 fL, and the red blood cell count is normal or increased. The peripheral blood smear is mildly abnormal, with hypochromia, microcytosis, and target cells. In contrast to α-thalassemia, basophilic stippling may be present. The reticulocyte count is normal or slightly elevated. Hemoglobin electrophoresis (using quantitative techniques) may show an elevation of hemoglobin A_2 to 4–8% and occasional elevations of hemoglobin F to 1–5%.

4. β-Thalassemia major—β-Thalassemia major produces severe anemia, and without transfusion the hematocrit may fall to less than 10%. The peripheral blood smear is bizarre, showing severe poikilocytosis, hypochromia, microcytosis, target cells, basophilic stippling, and nucleated red blood cells. Little or no hemoglobin A is present. Variable amounts of hemoglobin A_2 are seen, and the major hemoglobin present is hemoglobin F.

▶ Differential Diagnosis

Mild forms of thalassemia must be differentiated from iron deficiency. Compared to iron deficiency anemia, patients with thalassemia have a lower MCV, a more normal red blood count, and a more abnormal peripheral blood smear at modest levels of anemia. Iron studies are normal. Severe forms of thalassemia may be confused with other hemoglobinopathies. The diagnosis is made by hemoglobin electrophoresis.

▶ Treatment

Patients with mild thalassemia (α-thalassemia trait or β-thalassemia minor) require no treatment and should be identified so that they will not be subjected to repeated evaluations and treatment for iron deficiency. Patients with hemoglobin H disease should take folate supplementation and avoid medicinal iron and oxidative drugs such as sulfonamides. Patients with severe thalassemia are maintained on a regular transfusion schedule and receive folate supplementation. Splenectomy is performed if hypersplenism causes a marked increase in the transfusion requirement. Patients with regular transfusion requirements should be treated with iron chelation in order to prevent life-limiting organ damage from iron overload. Subcutaneous infusion of deferoxamine has largely been replaced by the oral agent deferasirox.

Allogeneic bone marrow transplantation is the treatment of choice for β-thalassemia major. Children who have not yet experienced iron overload and chronic organ toxicity do well, with long-term survival in more than 80% of cases.

Borgna-Pignatti C. Modern treatment of thalassaemia intermedia. Br J Haematol. 2007 Aug;138(3):291–304. [PMID: 17565568]

Cohen AR. New advances in iron chelation therapy. Hematology Am Soc Hematol Educ Program. 2006:42–7. [PMID: 17124038]

Cohen AR et al. Effect of transfusional iron intake on response to chelation therapy in beta-thalassemia major. Blood. 2008 Jan 15;111(2):583–7. [PMID: 17951527]

Hershko C. Iron loading and its clinical implications. Am J Hematol. 2007 Dec;82(12 Suppl):1147–8. [PMID: 17963253]

Vento S et al. Infections and thalassaemia. Lancet Infect Dis. 2006 Apr;6(4):226–33. [PMID: 16554247]

SIDEROBLASTIC ANEMIA

ESSENTIALS OF DIAGNOSIS

▶ Presence of ringed sideroblasts in the bone marrow.

▶ Elevated serum iron levels and transferrin saturation.

▶ General Considerations

The sideroblastic anemias are a heterogeneous group of disorders in which hemoglobin synthesis is reduced because of failure to incorporate heme into protoporphyrin to form hemoglobin. Iron accumulates, particularly in the mitochondria. The disorder is usually acquired. Sometimes it represents a stage in evolution of a generalized bone marrow disorder (myelodysplasia) that may ultimately terminate in acute leukemia. Other causes include chronic alcoholism and lead poisoning.

▶ Clinical Findings

Patients have no specific clinical features other than those related to anemia. The anemia is usually moderate, with hematocrits of 20–30%, but transfusions may occasionally be required. Although the MCV is usually normal or slightly increased, it may occasionally be low, leading to confusion with iron deficiency. However, serum iron level is elevated and transferrin saturation is high. The peripheral blood smear characteristically shows a dimorphic population of red blood cells, one normal and one hypochromic. In cases of lead poisoning, coarse basophilic stippling of the red cells is seen and the serum lead levels will be elevated.

The diagnosis is made by examination of the bone marrow. Characteristically, there is marked erythroid hyperplasia, a sign of ineffective erythropoiesis (expansion of the erythroid compartment of the bone marrow that does not result in the production of reticulocytes in the peripheral blood). The Prussian blue iron stain of the bone marrow shows a generalized increase in iron stores and the presence of ringed sideroblasts, which are cells with iron deposits encircling the red cell nucleus. Occasionally, the anemia is so severe that support with transfusion is required. These patients usually do not respond to erythropoietin therapy.

When to Refer

Refer to a hematologist if transfusion support is needed.

Bottomley SS. Congenital sideroblastic anemias. Curr Hematol Rep. 2006 Mar;5(1):41–9. [PMID: 16537045]

Germing U et al. Prospective validation of the WHO proposals for the classification of myelodysplastic syndromes. Haematologica. 2006 Dec;91(12):1596–604. [PMID: 17145595]

VITAMIN B₁₂ DEFICIENCY

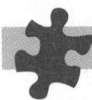

ESSENTIALS OF DIAGNOSIS

▶ Macrocytic anemia.

▶ Macro-ovalocytes and hypersegmented neutrophils on peripheral blood smear.

▶ Serum vitamin B_{12} level less than 100 pg/mL.

General Considerations

Vitamin B_{12} belongs to the family of cobalamins and serves as a cofactor for two important reactions in humans. As methylcobalamin, it is a cofactor for methionine synthetase in the conversion of homocysteine to methionine, and as adenosylcobalamin for the conversion of methylmalonyl-coenzyme A (CoA) to succinyl-CoA. All vitamin B_{12} comes from the diet and is present in all foods of animal origin. The daily absorption of vitamin B_{12} is 5 mcg.

The liver contains 2000–5000 mcg of stored vitamin B_{12}. Since daily losses are 3–5 mcg/d, the body usually has sufficient stores of vitamin B_{12} so that vitamin B_{12} deficiency develops more than 3 years after vitamin B_{12} absorption ceases.

Since vitamin B_{12} is present in all foods of animal origin, dietary vitamin B_{12} deficiency is extremely rare and is seen only in vegans—strict vegetarians who avoid all dairy products as well as meat and fish (Table 13–6). Abdominal surgery may lead to vitamin B_{12} deficiency in several ways. Gastrectomy will eliminate that site of intrinsic factor production; blind loop syndrome will cause competition for vitamin B_{12} by bacterial overgrowth in the lumen of the intestine; and surgical resection of the ileum will eliminate the site of vitamin B_{12} absorption. Rare causes of vitamin B_{12} deficiency include fish tapeworm (*Diphyllobothrium latum*) infection, in which the parasite uses luminal vitamin B_{12}, pancreatic insufficiency (with failure to inactivate competing cobalamin-binding proteins), and severe Crohn disease, causing sufficient destruction of the ileum to impair vitamin B_{12} absorption.

Clinical Findings

A. Symptoms and Signs

The hallmark of symptomatic vitamin B_{12} deficiency is megaloblastic anemia. However, subclinical cobalamin defi-

Table 13–6. Causes of vitamin B_{12} deficiency.

Dietary deficiency (rare)
Decreased production of intrinsic factor
Pernicious anemia
Gastrectomy
Helicobacter pylori infection
Competition for vitamin B_{12} in gut
Blind loop syndrome
Fish tapeworm (rare)
Pancreatic insufficiency
Decreased ileal absorption of vitamin B_{12}
Surgical resection
Crohn disease
Transcobalamin II deficiency (rare)

ciency is an increasingly recognized condition, especially in those with predisposing conditions such as ileal disease or gastric surgery. In advanced cases, the anemia may be severe, with hematocrits as low as 10–15%, and may be accompanied by leukopenia and thrombocytopenia. The megaloblastic state also produces changes in mucosal cells, leading to glossitis, as well as other vague gastrointestinal disturbances such as anorexia and diarrhea. Vitamin B_{12} deficiency also leads to a complex neurologic syndrome. Peripheral nerves are usually affected first, and patients complain initially of paresthesias. The posterior columns next become impaired, and patients complain of difficulty with balance. In more advanced cases, cerebral function may be altered as well, and on occasion dementia and other neuropsychiatric changes may precede hematologic changes.

Patients are usually pale and may be mildly icteric. Neurologic examination may reveal decreased vibration and position sense but is more commonly normal in early stages of the disease.

B. Laboratory Findings

The megaloblastic state produces an anemia of variable severity that on occasion may be very severe. The MCV is usually strikingly elevated, between 110 and 140 fL. However, it is possible to have vitamin B_{12} deficiency with a normal MCV. Occasionally, the normal MCV may be explained by coexistent thalassemia or iron deficiency, but in other cases the reason is obscure. Patients with neurologic symptoms and signs that suggest possible vitamin B_{12} deficiency should be evaluated for that deficiency despite a normal MCV and the absence of anemia. The peripheral blood smear is usually strikingly abnormal, with anisocytosis and poikilocytosis. A characteristic finding is the macro-ovalocyte, but numerous other abnormal shapes are usually seen. The neutrophils are hypersegmented. Typical features include a mean lobe count greater than four or the finding of six-lobed neutrophils. The reticulocyte count is reduced. Because vitamin B_{12} deficiency affects all hematopoietic cell lines, in severe cases the white blood cell count and the platelet count are reduced, and pancytopenia is present.

Bone marrow morphology is characteristically abnormal. Marked erythroid hyperplasia is present as a response to defective red blood cell production (ineffective erythropoiesis). Megaloblastic changes in the erythroid series include abnormally large cell size and asynchronous maturation of the nucleus and cytoplasm—ie, cytoplasmic maturation continues while impaired DNA synthesis causes retarded nuclear development. In the myeloid series, giant metamyelocytes are characteristically seen.

Other laboratory abnormalities include elevated serum lactate dehydrogenase (LDH) and a modest increase in indirect bilirubin. These two findings are a reflection of intramedullary destruction of developing abnormal erythroid cells and are similar to those observed in peripheral hemolytic anemias.

The diagnosis of vitamin B_{12} deficiency is made by finding an abnormally low vitamin B_{12} (cobalamin) serum level. Whereas the normal vitamin B_{12} level is > 240 pg/mL, most patients with overt vitamin B_{12} deficiency will have serum levels < 170 pg/mL, with symptomatic patients usually having levels < 100 pg/mL. A level of 170–240 pg/mL is borderline. When the serum level of vitamin B_{12} is borderline, the diagnosis is best confirmed by finding an elevated level of serum methylmalonic acid (> 1000 nmol/L). However, elevated levels of serum methylmalonic acid can be due to kidney insufficiency.

Differential Diagnosis

Vitamin B_{12} deficiency should be differentiated from folic acid deficiency, the other common cause of megaloblastic anemia, in which red blood cell folate is low while vitamin B_{12} levels are normal. The distinction between vitamin B_{12} deficiency and myelodysplasia (the other common cause of macrocytic anemia with abnormal morphology) is based on the characteristic morphology and the low vitamin B_{12} and elevated methylmalonic acid levels.

Treatment

Patients with pernicious anemia have historically been treated with parenteral therapy. Intramuscular injections of 100 mcg of vitamin B_{12} are adequate for each dose. Replacement is usually given daily for the first week, weekly for the first month, and then monthly for life. It is a lifelong disorder, and if patients discontinue their monthly therapy the vitamin deficiency will recur. Oral cobalamin may be used instead of parenteral therapy and can provide equivalent results. The dose is 1000 mcg/d and must be continued indefinitely.

Patients respond to therapy with an immediate improvement in their sense of well-being. Hypokalemia may complicate the first several days of therapy, particularly if the anemia is severe. A brisk reticulocytosis occurs in 5–7 days, and the hematologic picture normalizes in 2 months. Central nervous system symptoms and signs are reversible if they are of relatively short duration (less than 6 months) but become permanent if treatment is not initiated promptly.

When to Refer

Referral to a hematologist is not usually necessary.

Butler CC et al. Oral vitamin B_{12} versus intramuscular vitamin B_{12} for vitamin B_{12} deficiency: a systematic review of randomized controlled trials. Fam Pract. 2006 Jun;23(3):279–85. [PMID: 16585128]

Headstrom PD et al. Prevalence of and risk factors for vitamin B(12) deficiency in patients with Crohn's disease. Inflamm Bowel Dis. 2008 Feb;14(2):217–23. [PMID: 17886286]

Hvas AM et al. Diagnosis and treatment of vitamin B12 deficiency—an update. Haematologica. 2006 Nov;91(11):1506–12. [PMID: 17043022]

FOLIC ACID DEFICIENCY

 ESSENTIALS OF DIAGNOSIS

▶ Macrocytic anemia.

▶ Macro-ovalocytes and hypersegmented neutrophils on peripheral blood smear.

▶ Normal serum vitamin B_{12} levels.

▶ Reduced folate levels in red blood cells or serum.

▶ General Considerations

Folic acid is the term commonly used for pteroylmonoglutamic acid. Folic acid is present in most fruits and vegetables (especially citrus fruits and green leafy vegetables) and daily requirements of 50–100 mcg/d are usually met in the diet. Total body stores of folate are approximately 5000 mcg, enough to supply requirements for 2–3 months.

By far the most common cause of folate deficiency is inadequate dietary intake (Table 13–7). Alcoholic or anorectic patients, persons who do not eat fresh fruits and vegetables, and those who overcook their food are candidates for folate deficiency. Reduced folate absorption is rarely seen, since absorption occurs from the entire gastrointestinal tract. However, drugs such as phenytoin, trimethoprim-sulfamethoxazole, or sulfasalazine may interfere with folate absorption. Folic acid requirements are increased in pregnancy, hemolytic anemia, and exfoliative skin disease, and in these cases the increased requirements (five to ten times normal) may not be met by a normal diet. Patients with increased folate requirements should receive supplementation with 1 mg/d of folic acid.

Table 13–7. Causes of folate deficiency.

Dietary deficiency
Decreased absorption
Tropical sprue
Drugs: phenytoin, sulfasalazine, trimethoprim-sulfamethoxazole
Increased requirement
Chronic hemolytic anemia
Pregnancy
Exfoliative skin disease
Loss: dialysis
Inhibition of reduction to active form
Methotrexate

Clinical Findings

A. Symptoms and Signs

The features are similar to those of vitamin B_{12} deficiency, with megaloblastic anemia and megaloblastic changes in mucosa. However, there are none of the neurologic abnormalities associated with vitamin B_{12} deficiency.

B. Laboratory Findings

Megaloblastic anemia is identical to anemia resulting from vitamin B_{12} deficiency (see above). However, the serum vitamin B_{12} level is normal. A red blood cell folate level of less than 150 ng/mL is diagnostic of folate deficiency.

Differential Diagnosis

The megaloblastic anemia of folate deficiency should be differentiated from vitamin B_{12} deficiency by the finding of a normal vitamin B_{12} level and a reduced red blood cell folate or serum folate level. Alcoholic patients, who often have folate deficiency, may also have anemia of liver disease. This latter macrocytic anemia does not cause megaloblastic morphologic changes but rather produces target cells in the peripheral blood. Hypothyroidism is associated with mild macrocytosis but also with pernicious anemia.

Treatment

Folic acid deficiency is treated with folic acid, 1 mg/d orally. The response is similar to that seen in the treatment of vitamin B_{12} deficiency, with rapid improvement and a sense of well-being, reticulocytosis in 5–7 days, and total correction of hematologic abnormalities within 2 months. Large doses of folic acid may produce hematologic responses in cases of vitamin B_{12} deficiency but will allow neurologic damage to progress.

When to Refer

Referral to a hematologist is not usually necessary.

Halfdanarson TR et al. Hematologic manifestations of celiac disease. Blood. 2007 Jan 15;109(2):412–21. [PMID: 16973955]
Wickramasinghe SN. Diagnosis of megaloblastic anaemias. Blood Rev. 2006 Nov;20(6):299–318. [PMID: 16716475]

PURE RED CELL APLASIA

Adult acquired pure red cell aplasia is rare. It appears to be an autoimmune disease mediated either by T lymphocytes or (rarely) by an IgG antibody against erythroid precursors. In adults, the disease is usually idiopathic. However, cases have been seen in association with systemic lupus erythematosus, chronic lymphocytic leukemia, lymphomas, or thymoma. Some drugs (phenytoin, chloramphenicol) may cause red cell aplasia. Transient episodes of red cell aplasia are probably common in response to viral infections, especially parvovirus infections. However, these acute episodes will go unrecognized unless the patient has a chronic hemolytic disorder, in which case the hematocrit may fall precipitously.

The only signs are those of anemia unless the patient has an associated autoimmune or lymphoproliferative disorder. The anemia is often severe and normochromic, with low or absent reticulocytes. Red blood cell morphology is normal, and the myeloid and platelet lines are unaffected. The bone marrow is normocellular. All elements present are normal, but erythroid precursors are markedly reduced or absent. In some cases, chest imaging studies will reveal a thymoma.

The disorder is distinguished from aplastic anemia (in which the marrow is hypocellular and all cell lines are affected) and from myelodysplasia. This latter disorder is recognized by the presence of morphologic abnormalities that should not be present in pure red cell aplasia.

Possible offending drugs should be stopped. With thymoma, resection results in amelioration of anemia in some instances. High-dose intravenous immune globulin has produced excellent responses in a small number of cases, especially in parvovirus-related cases. For most cases, the treatment of choice is immunosuppressive therapy with a combination of antithymocyte globulin and cyclosporine (or tacrolimus)—similar to therapy of aplastic anemia. Anti-CD20 monoclonal antibody (rituximab) has also enjoyed some success.

When to Refer

All patients should be referred to a hematologist.

Rossert J; Pure Red Cell Aplasia Global Scientific Advisory Board (GSAB). Erythropoietin-induced, antibody-mediated pure red cell aplasia. Eur J Clin Invest. 2005 Dec;35(Suppl 3):95–9. [PMID: 16281965]
Servey JT et al. Clinical presentations of parvovirus B19 infection. Am Fam Physician. 2007 Feb 1;75(3):373–6. [PMID: 17304869]

HEMOLYTIC ANEMIAS

Hemolytic disorders are generally classified according to whether the defect is intrinsic to the red cell or due to some external factor (Table 13–8). Intrinsic defects have been described in all components of the red blood cell, including the membrane, enzyme systems, and hemoglobin; most of these disorders are hereditary. Hemolytic anemias due to external factors are the immune and microangiopathic hemolytic anemias.

Certain laboratory features are common to all the hemolytic anemias. Haptoglobin, a normal plasma protein that binds and clears hemoglobin released into plasma, may be depressed in hemolytic disorders. However, haptoglobin levels are influenced by many factors and, by themselves, are not a reliable indicator of hemolysis. When intravascular hemolysis occurs, transient hemoglobinemia occurs. Hemoglobin is filtered through the glomerulus and is usually reabsorbed by tubular cells. Hemoglobinuria will be present only when the capacity for reabsorption of hemoglobin by these cells is exceeded. In its absence, evidence for prior intravascular hemolysis is the presence of hemosiderin in shed renal tubular cells (positive urine hemosiderin). With severe intravascular hemolysis, hemo-

Table 13–8. Classification of hemolytic anemias.

Intrinsic
    Membrane defects: hereditary spherocytosis, hereditary elliptocytosis, paroxysmal nocturnal hemoglobinuria
    Glycolytic defects: pyruvate kinase deficiency, severe hypophosphatemia
    Oxidation vulnerability: glucose-6-phosphate dehydrogenase deficiency, methemoglobinemia
    Hemoglobinopathies: sickle cell syndromes, unstable hemoglobins, methemoglobinemia
Extrinsic
    Immune: autoimmune, lymphoproliferative disease, drug toxicity
    Microangiopathic: thrombotic thrombocytopenic purpura, hemolytic-uremic syndrome, disseminated intravascular coagulation, valve hemolysis, metastatic adenocarcinoma, vasculitis
    Infection: *Plasmodium, Clostridium, Borrelia*
    Hypersplenism
    Burns

globinemia and methemalbuminemia may be present. Hemolysis increases the indirect bilirubin, and the total bilirubin may rise to 4 mg/dL. Bilirubin levels higher than this may indicate some degree of hepatic dysfunction. Serum LDH levels are strikingly elevated in cases of microangiopathic hemolysis (thrombotic thrombocytopenic purpura, hemolytic-uremic syndrome) and may be elevated in other hemolytic anemias.

HEREDITARY SPHEROCYTOSIS

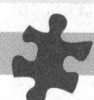

ESSENTIALS OF DIAGNOSIS

▶ Positive family history.

▶ Splenomegaly.

▶ Spherocytes and increased reticulocytes on peripheral blood smear.

▶ Microcytic, hyperchromic indices.

General Considerations

Hereditary spherocytosis is a disorder of the red blood cell membrane, leading to chronic hemolytic anemia.

The membrane defect is an abnormality in spectrin or actin, the proteins providing most of the scaffolding for the red blood cell membranes. The result is a decrease in surface-to-volume ratio that results in a spherical shape of the cell. These spherical cells are less deformable and unable to pass through 2-mcm fenestrations in the splenic red pulp. Hemolysis takes place because of trapping of red blood cells within the spleen.

Clinical Findings

A. Symptoms and Signs

Hereditary spherocytosis is an autosomal dominant disease of variable severity. It is often diagnosed during childhood, but milder cases may be discovered incidentally late in adult

life. Anemia may or may not be present, since the bone marrow may be able to compensate for shortened red cell survival. Severe anemia (aplastic crisis) may occur in folic acid deficiency or when bone marrow compensation is temporarily impaired by infection. Chronic hemolysis causes jaundice and pigment (calcium bilirubinate) gallstones, leading to attacks of cholecystitis. Examination may reveal icterus and a palpable spleen.

B. Laboratory Findings

The anemia is of variable severity, and the hematocrit may be normal. Reticulocytosis is always present. The peripheral blood smear shows the presence of spherocytes, small cells that have lost their central pallor. Spherocytes usually make up only a small percentage of red blood cells on the peripheral smear. Hereditary spherocytosis is the only important disorder associated with microcytosis and an increased mean corpuscular hemoglobin concentration (MCHC), often greater than 36 g/dL. As with other hemolytic disorders, there may be an increase in indirect bilirubin. The Coombs test is negative.

Because spherocytes are red cells that have lost some membrane surface, they are abnormally vulnerable to swelling induced by hypotonic media. Increased osmotic fragility merely reflects the presence of spherocytes and does not distinguish hereditary spherocytosis from other spherocytic hemolytic disorders such as autoimmune hemolytic anemia. In some laboratories, the osmotic fragility test has been supplanted by ektacytometry, which has the advantages of better reliability and the ability to distinguish spherocytes from other red blood cell abnormalities such as elliptocytosis.

Treatment

These patients should receive uninterrupted supplementation with folic acid, 1 mg/d. The treatment of choice is splenectomy, which will correct neither the membrane defect nor the spherocytosis but will eliminate the site of hemolysis. In very mild cases discovered late in adult life, splenectomy may not be necessary.

When to Refer

Patients in whom hereditary spherocytosis is suspected should have the diagnosis confirmed by a hematologist, and decisions regarding splenectomy should be made in consultation with a hematologist.

Delaunay J. The molecular basis of hereditary red cell membrane disorders. Blood Rev. 2007 Jan;21(1):1–20. [PMID: 16730867]
Stoya G et al. Flow cytometry as a diagnostic tool for hereditary spherocytosis. Acta Haematol. 2006;116(3):186–91. [PMID: 17016037]

PAROXYSMAL NOCTURNAL HEMOGLOBINURIA

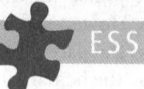

ESSENTIALS OF DIAGNOSIS

▶ Episodic hemoglobinuria.

▶ Thrombosis is common.

▶ Suspect in confusing cases of hemolytic anemia or pancytopenia.

▶ Flow cytometry is best screening test.

General Considerations

Paroxysmal nocturnal hemoglobinuria (PNH) is an acquired clonal stem cell disorder that results in abnormal sensitivity of the red blood cell membrane to lysis by complement. The underlying cause is a defect in the gene for phosphatidylinositol class A (PIG-A), which results in a deficiency of the glycosylphosphatidylinositol (GPI) anchor for cellular membrane proteins. In particular, the complement-regulating proteins CD55 and CD59 are deficient.

Clinical Findings

A. Symptoms and Signs

Classically, patients report episodic hemoglobinuria resulting in reddish brown urine. Hemoglobinuria is most often noticed in the first morning urine, probably because of its increased concentration. In addition to being prone to anemia, these patients are prone to thrombosis, especially mesenteric and hepatic vein thromboses. Other common sites of thrombosis include the central nervous system (saggital vein) and the skin, with formation of painful nodules. This hypercoagulopathy may be related to platelet activation by complement. As this is a stem cell disorder, PNH may progress either to aplastic anemia, to myelodysplasia, or to acute myeloid leukemia.

B. Laboratory Findings

Anemia is of variable severity, and reticulocytosis may or may not be present. Abnormalities on the blood smear are nondiagnostic and may include macro-ovalocytes. Since the episodic hemolysis in PNH is intravascular, the finding of urine hemosiderin is a useful test. Serum LDH is characteristically elevated. Iron deficiency is commonly present and is related to chronic iron loss from hemoglobinuria, since hemolysis is primarily intravascular.

The white blood cell count and platelet count may be decreased. The best screening test is flow cytometry to demonstrate deficiency of CD59 and CD55 on red blood cells. Bone marrow morphology is variable and may show either generalized hypoplasia or erythroid hyperplasia. Flow cytometric assays may confirm the diagnosis by demonstrating the absence of CD59.

Treatment

Iron replacement is often indicated for treatment of iron deficiency. This may improve the anemia but may also cause a transient increase in hemolysis. For unclear reasons, prednisone is effective in decreasing hemolysis, and some patients can be managed effectively with alternate-day steroids. In severe cases and cases of transformation to myelodysplasia, allogeneic bone marrow transplantation has been used to treat the disorder. The anti-complement C5 antibody eculizumab has been shown to be effective in reducing hemolysis and transfusion requirements.

When to Refer

Most patients with PNH should be under the care of a hematologist.

Bessler M et al. The pathophysiology of disease in patients with paroxysmal nocturnal hemoglobinuria. Hematology Am Soc Hematol Educ Program. 2008:104–10. [PMID: 19074066]

Hillmen P. The role of complement inhibition in PNH. Hematology Am Soc Hematol Educ Program. 2008:116–23. [PMID: 19074068]

Richards SJ et al. The role of flow cytometry in the diagnosis of paroxysmal nocturnal hemoglobinuria in the clinical laboratory. Clin Lab Med. 2007 Sep;27(3):577–90, vii. [PMID: 17658408]

Savage WJ et al. New insights into paroxysmal nocturnal hemoglobinuria. Hematology. 2007 Aug;20:1. [PMID: 17852463]

GLUCOSE-6-PHOSPHATE DEHYDROGENASE DEFICIENCY

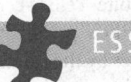 ESSENTIALS OF DIAGNOSIS

▶ X-linked recessive disorder seen commonly in American black men.

▶ Episodic hemolysis in response to oxidant drugs or infection.

▶ Minimally abnormal peripheral blood smear.

▶ Reduced levels of glucose-6-phosphate dehydrogenase between hemolytic episodes.

General Considerations

Glucose-6-phosphate dehydrogenase (G6PD) deficiency is a hereditary enzyme defect that causes episodic hemolytic anemia because of the decreased ability of red blood cells to deal with oxidative stresses. Oxidized hemoglobin denatures and forms precipitants called Heinz bodies. These Heinz bodies cause membrane damage, which leads to removal of these cells by the spleen.

Numerous types of glucose-6-phosphate dehydrogenase deficiency (G6PD) enzymes have been described. The normal type found in whites is designated G6PD-B. Most American blacks have G6PD-A, which is normal in function. Ten to 15 percent of American blacks have the variant G6PD designated A–, in which there is only 15% of normal enzyme activity, and enzyme activity declines rapidly as the red blood cell ages past 40 days, a fact that explains many of the clinical findings in this disorder. Many other G6PD variants have been described, including some Mediterranean variants with extremely low enzyme activity.

Clinical Findings

G6PD deficiency is an X-linked recessive disorder affecting 10–15% of American black males. Female carriers are rarely affected—only when an unusually high percentage of cells producing the normal enzyme is inactivated.

A. Symptoms and Signs

Patients are usually healthy, without chronic hemolytic anemia or splenomegaly. Hemolysis occurs as a result of oxidative stress on the red blood cells, generated either by infection or exposure to certain drugs. Common drugs initiating hemolysis include dapsone, primaquine, quinidine, quinine, sulfonamides, and nitrofurantoin. Even with continuous use of the offending drug, the hemolytic episode is self-limited because older red blood cells (with low enzyme activity) are removed and replaced with a population of young red blood cells with adequate functional levels of G6PD. Severe G6PD deficiency (as in Mediterranean variants) may produce a chronic hemolytic anemia.

B. Laboratory Findings

Between hemolytic episodes, the blood is normal. During episodes of hemolysis, there is reticulocytosis and increased serum indirect bilirubin. The red blood cell smear is not diagnostic but may reveal a small number of "bite" cells—cells that appear to have had a bite taken out of their periphery. This indicates pitting of hemoglobin aggregates by the spleen. Heinz bodies may be demonstrated by staining a peripheral blood smear with cresyl violet; they are not visible on the usual Wright-Giemsa–stained blood smear. Specific enzyme assays for G6PD may reveal a low level but may be misleading if they are performed shortly after a hemolytic episode when the enzyme-deficient cohort of cells has been removed. In these cases, the enzyme assays should be repeated weeks after hemolysis has resolved. In severe cases of G6PD deficiency, enzyme levels are always low.

▶ Treatment

No treatment is necessary except to avoid known oxidant drugs.

Beutler E. Glucose-6-phosphate dehydrogenase deficiency: a historical perspective. Blood. 2008 Jan 1;111(1):16–24. [PMID: 18156501]

Mason PJ et al. G6PD deficiency: the genotype-phenotype association. Blood Rev. 2007 Sep;21(5):267–83. [PMID: 17611006]

Tripathy V et al. Present status of understanding on the G6PD deficiency and natural selection. J Postgrad Med. 2007 Jul–Sep;53(3):193–202. [PMID: 17699998]

SICKLE CELL ANEMIA & RELATED SYNDROMES

ESSENTIALS OF DIAGNOSIS

▶ Recurrent painful episodes.

▶ Positive family history and lifelong history of hemolytic anemia.

▶ Irreversibly sickled cells on peripheral blood smear.

▶ Hemoglobin S is the major hemoglobin seen on electrophoresis.

▶ General Considerations

Sickle cell anemia is an autosomal recessive disorder in which an abnormal hemoglobin leads to chronic hemolytic anemia with numerous clinical consequences. A single DNA base change leads to an amino acid substitution of valine for glutamine in the sixth position on the β-globin chain. The abnormal β chain is designated β^s and the tetramer of $\alpha_2\beta^s_2$ is designated hemoglobin S.

The rate of sickling is influenced by the concentration of hemoglobin S and by the presence of other hemoglobins within the cell. Hemoglobin F cannot participate in polymer formation, and its presence markedly retards sickling. Other factors that increase sickling are red cell dehydration and factors that lead to formation of deoxyhemoglobin S, eg, acidosis and hypoxemia, either systemic or locally in tissues. Hemolytic crises may be related to splenic sequestration of sickled cells (primarily in childhood before the spleen has been infarcted as a result of repeated sickling) or with coexistent disorders such as G6PD deficiency.

The hemoglobin S gene is carried in 8% of American blacks, and 1 of 400 American black children will be born with sickle cell anemia. Prenatal diagnosis is available for couples at risk for producing a child with sickle cell anemia. Genetic counseling should be made available to such couples.

▶ Clinical Findings

A. Symptoms and Signs

The disorder has its onset during the first year of life, when hemoglobin F levels fall as a signal is sent to switch from production of γ-globin to β-globin.

Chronic hemolytic anemia produces jaundice, pigment (calcium bilirubinate) gallstones, splenomegaly, and poorly healing ulcers over the lower tibia. Life-threatening severe anemia can occur during hemolytic or aplastic crises, generally associated with viral or other infection or by folate deficiency.

Acute painful episodes due to acute vaso-occlusion from clusters of sickled red cells may occur spontaneously or be provoked by infection, dehydration, or hypoxia. Common sites of acute painful episodes include the bones (especially the back and long bones) and the chest. These episodes last hours to days and may produce low-grade fever. Acute vaso-occlusion may also cause strokes due to sinus thrombosis and priapism. Vaso-occlusive episodes are not associated with increased hemolysis.

Repeated episodes of vascular occlusion especially affect the heart, lungs, and liver. Ischemic necrosis of bone occurs, rendering the bone susceptible to osteomyelitis due to staphylococci or (less commonly) salmonellae. Infarction of the papillae of the renal medulla causes renal tubular concentrating defects and gross hematuria, more often encountered in sickle cell trait than in sickle cell anemia. Retinopathy similar to that noted in diabetes is often present and may lead to blindness. Pulmonary hypertension may develop and is associated with a poor prognosis.

These patients are prone to delayed puberty. An increased incidence of infection is related to hyposplenism as well as to defects in the alternative pathway of complement.

On examination, patients are often chronically ill and jaundiced. There is hepatomegaly, but the spleen is not palpable in adult life. The heart is enlarged, with a hyperdynamic precordium and systolic murmurs. Nonhealing ulcers of the lower leg and retinopathy may be present.

Sickle cell anemia becomes a chronic multisystem disease, with death from organ failure. With improved supportive care, average life expectancy is now between 40 and 50 years of age.

B. Laboratory Findings

Chronic hemolytic anemia is present. The hematocrit is usually 20–30%. The peripheral blood smear is characteristically abnormal, with irreversibly sickled cells comprising 5–50% of red cells. Other findings include reticulocytosis (10–25%), nucleated red blood cells, and hallmarks of hyposplenism such as Howell–Jolly bodies and target cells. The white blood cell count is characteristically elevated to 12,000–15,000/mcL, and thrombocytosis may occur. Indirect bilirubin levels are high.

After a screening test for sickle cell hemoglobin, the diagnosis of sickle cell anemia is confirmed by hemoglobin electrophoresis (Table 13–9). Hemoglobin S will usually comprise 85–98% of hemoglobin. In homozygous S disease, no hemoglobin A will be present. Hemoglobin F levels are variably increased, and high hemoglobin F levels are associated with a more benign clinical course.

▶ Treatment

No specific treatment is available for the primary disease. Patients are maintained on folic acid supplementation and given transfusions for aplastic or hemolytic crises. Pneumococcal vaccination reduces the incidence of infections with this pathogen.

When acute painful episodes occur, precipitating factors should be identified and infections treated if present. The patient should be kept well hydrated, and oxygen should be given if the patient is hypoxic.

Acute vaso-occlusive crises can be treated with exchange transfusion. These are primarily indicated for the treatment of intractable pain crises, priapism, and stroke. Long-term transfusion therapy has been shown to be effective in reducing the risk of recurrent stroke in children.

Cytotoxic agents increase hemoglobin F levels by stimulating erythropoiesis in more primitive erythroid precursors. Hydroxyurea (500–750 mg/d) reduces the frequency of painful crises in patients whose quality of life is disrupted by frequent pain crises. Although there remains some level of concern about the possibility of secondary malignancies from this type of treatment, substantial data suggest that it is safe. Allogeneic bone marrow transplantation is being studied as a possible curative option for severely affected young patients.

▶ When to Refer

Patients with sickle cell anemia should have their care coordinated with a hematologist and should be referred to a Comprehensive Sickle Cell Center if one is available.

▶ When to Admit

Patients should be admitted for management of chest crises or for painful episodes that do not respond to outpatient care.

Al Hajeri AA et al. Piracetam for reducing the incidence of painful sickle cell disease crises. Cochrane Database Syst Rev. 2007 Apr 18;(2):CD006111. [PMID: 17443614]

Josephson CD et al. Transfusion in the patient with sickle cell disease: a critical review of the literature and transfusion guidelines. Transfus Med Rev. 2007 Apr;21(2):118–33. [PMID: 17397762]

Marti-Carvajal AJ et al. Antibiotics for treating acute chest syndrome in people with sickle cell disease. Cochrane Database Syst Rev. 2007 Apr 18;(2):CD006110. [PMID: 17443613]

Okomo U et al. Fluid replacement therapy for acute episodes of pain in people with sickle cell disease. Cochrane Database Syst Rev. 2007 Apr 18;(2):CD005406. [PMID: 17443589]

Platt OS. Hydroxyurea for the treatment of sickle cell anemia. N Engl J Med. 2008 Mar 27;358(13):1362–9. [PMID: 18367739]

Telen MJ. Role of adhesion molecules and vascular endothelium in the pathogenesis of sickle cell disease. Hematology Am Soc Hematol Educ Program. 2007:84–90. [PMID: 18024614]

SICKLE CELL TRAIT

Patients with the heterozygous genotype (AS) have sickle cell trait. These persons are clinically normal and have acute painful episodes only under extreme conditions such as vigorous exertion at high altitudes (or in unpressurized

Table 13–9. Hemoglobin distribution in sickle cell syndromes.

Genotype	Clinical Diagnosis	Hb A	Hb S	Hb A$_2$	Hb F
AA	Normal	97–99%	0	1–2%	< 1%
AS	Sickle trait	60%	40%	1–2%	< 1%
SS	Sickle cell anemia	0	86–98%	1–3%	5–15%
S β^0-thalassemia	Sickle β-thalassemia	0	70–80%	3–5%	10–20%
S β$^+$-thalassemia	Sickle β-thalassemia	10–20%	60–75%	3–5%	10–20%
AS, α-thalassemia	Sickle trait	70–75%	25–30%	1–2%	< 1%

Hb, hemoglobin.

aircraft). The patients are hematologically normal, with no anemia and normal red blood cells on peripheral blood smear. They may, however, have a defect in renal tubular function, causing an inability to concentrate the urine, and experience episodes of gross hematuria. This appears to be caused by many years of sickling in the sluggish circulation of the renal medulla. A screening test for sickle hemoglobin will be positive, and hemoglobin electrophoresis will reveal that approximately 40% of hemoglobin is hemoglobin S (Table 13–9).

No treatment is necessary. Genetic counseling is a reasonable strategy.

SICKLE THALASSEMIA

Patients with homozygous sickle cell anemia and α-thalassemia have a somewhat milder form of hemolysis because of a slower rate of sickling related to reduced hemoglobin concentration within the red blood cell.

Patients who are double heterozygotes for sickle cell anemia and β-thalassemia are clinically affected with sickle cell syndromes. Sickle β^0-thalassemia is clinically very similar to homozygous SS disease. Vaso-occlusive crises may be somewhat less severe, and the spleen is usually not infarcted. Hematologically, the MCV is usually low, in contrast to the normal MCV of sickle cell anemia. Hemoglobin electrophoresis (Table 13–9) reveals no hemoglobin A but will show an increase in hemoglobin A_2, which is not present in sickle cell anemia.

Sickle β^+-thalassemia is a milder disorder than homozygous SS disease, with fewer crises. The spleen is usually palpable. The hemolytic anemia is less severe, and the hematocrit is usually 30–38%, with reticulocytes of 5–10%. Hemoglobin electrophoresis shows the presence of some hemoglobin A.

HEMOGLOBIN C DISORDERS

Hemoglobin C is formed by a single amino acid substitution at the same site of substitution as in sickle hemoglobin but with lysine instead of valine substituted for glutamine at the β_6 position. Hemoglobin C is nonsickling but may participate in polymer formation in association with hemoglobin S. Homozygous hemoglobin C disease produces a mild hemolytic anemia with splenomegaly, mild jaundice, and pigment (calcium bilirubinate) gallstones. The peripheral blood smear shows generalized red cell targeting and occasional cells with rectangular crystals of hemoglobin C. Persons heterozygous for hemoglobin C are clinically normal.

Patients with hemoglobin SC disease are double heterozygotes for β S and β C. These patients, like those with sickle β^+-thalassemia, have a milder hemolytic anemia and milder clinical course than those with homozygous SS disease. There are fewer vaso-occlusive events, and the spleen remains palpable in adult life. However, persons with hemoglobin SC disease have more retinopathy and more ischemic necrosis of bone than those with SS disease. The hematocrit is usually 30–38%, with 5–10% reticulocytes and few irreversibly sickled cells on the blood smear. Target cells are more numerous than in SS disease. Hemoglobin electro-

phoresis will show approximately 50% hemoglobin C, 50% hemoglobin S, and no increase in hemoglobin F levels.

Nagel RL et al. The paradox of hemoglobin SC disease. Blood Rev. 2003 Sep;17(3):167–78. [PMID: 12818227]

UNSTABLE HEMOGLOBINS

Unstable hemoglobins are prone to oxidative denaturation even in the presence of a normal G6PD system. The disorder is autosomal dominant and of variable severity. Most patients have a mild chronic hemolytic anemia with splenomegaly, mild jaundice, and pigment (calcium bilirubinate) gallstones. Less severely affected patients are not anemic except under conditions of oxidative stress.

The diagnosis is made by the finding of Heinz bodies and a normal G6PD level. Hemoglobin electrophoresis is usually normal, since these hemoglobins characteristically do not have a change in their migration pattern. These hemoglobins precipitate in isopropanol. Usually no treatment is necessary. Patients with chronic hemolytic anemia should receive folate supplementation and avoid known oxidative drugs. In rare cases, splenectomy may be required.

AUTOIMMUNE HEMOLYTIC ANEMIA

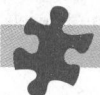

ESSENTIALS OF DIAGNOSIS

▶ Acquired anemia caused by IgG autoantibody.

▶ Spherocytes and reticulocytosis on peripheral blood smear.

▶ Positive Coombs test.

▶ General Considerations

Autoimmune hemolytic anemia is an acquired disorder in which an IgG autoantibody is formed that binds to the red blood cell membrane. The antibody is most commonly directed against a basic component of the Rh system present on most human red blood cells. When IgG antibodies coat the red blood cell, the Fc portion of the antibody is recognized by macrophages present in the spleen and other portions of the reticuloendothelial system. The interaction between splenic macrophage and the antibody-coated red blood cell results in removal of red blood cell membrane and the formation of a spherocyte because of the decrease in surface-to-volume ratio of the red blood cell. These spherocytic cells have decreased deformability and become trapped in the red pulp of the spleen because of their inability to squeeze through the 2-mcm fenestrations. When large amounts of IgG are present on red blood cells, complement may be fixed. Direct lysis of cells is rare, but the presence of C3b on the surface of red blood cells allows Kupffer cells in the liver to participate in the hemolytic process because of the presence of C3b receptors on Kupffer cells.

Approximately 50% of all cases of autoimmune hemolytic anemia are idiopathic. The disorder may also be seen in association with systemic lupus erythematosus, chronic lymphocytic leukemia, or lymphomas. It must be distinguished from drug-induced hemolytic anemia. Penicillin (and other drugs) coats the red blood cell membrane, and the antibody is directed against the membrane–drug complex.

Clinical Findings

A. Symptoms and Signs

Autoimmune hemolytic anemia typically produces an anemia of rapid onset that may be life-threatening in severity. Patients complain of fatigue and may present with angina or congestive heart failure. On examination, jaundice and splenomegaly are usually present.

B. Laboratory Findings

The anemia is of variable severity but may be severe, with hematocrit of less than 10%. Reticulocytosis is usually present, and spherocytes are seen on the peripheral blood smear. In cases of severe hemolysis, the stressed bone marrow may also release nucleated red blood cells. As with other hemolytic disorders, indirect bilirubin is increased. Approximately 10% of patients with autoimmune hemolytic anemia have coincident immune thrombocytopenia (Evans syndrome).

The Coombs antiglobulin test forms the basis for diagnosis. The Coombs reagent is a rabbit IgM antibody raised against human IgG or human complement. The direct Coombs test is performed by mixing the patient's red blood cells with the Coombs reagent and looking for agglutination, which indicates the presence of antibody on the red blood cell surface. The indirect Coombs test is performed by mixing the patient's serum with a panel of type O red blood cells. After incubation of the test serum and panel red blood cells, the Coombs reagent is added. Agglutination in this system indicates the presence of free antibody in the patient's serum.

The direct Coombs test is positive in autoimmune hemolytic anemia, and the indirect Coombs test may or may not be positive. A positive indirect Coombs test indicates the presence of a large amount of autoantibody that has saturated binding sites in the red blood cell and consequently appears in the serum. Because the patient's serum usually contains the autoantibody, it may be difficult to obtain a compatible cross-match with donor's cells.

Treatment

Initial treatment consists of prednisone, 1–2 mg/kg/d in divided doses. Most transfused blood will survive similarly to the patient's own red blood cells. Because of difficulty in performing the cross-match, incompatible blood may be given. Decisions regarding transfusions should be made in consultation with a hematologist. If prednisone is ineffective or if the disease recurs on tapering the dose, splenectomy should be performed. Patients with autoimmune hemolytic anemia refractory to prednisone and splenectomy may be treated with a variety of agents. Treatment with rituximab, a monoclonal antibody against the B cell antigen CD20, is effective in some cases. The suggested dose is 375 mg/m^2 intravenously weekly for 4 weeks. Danazol,

600–800 mg/d, is less often effective than in immune thrombocytopenia but is well suited for long-term use because of its low toxicity. Immunosuppressive agents, including cyclophosphamide, azathioprine, mycophenolate mofetil, or cyclosporine, may also be used. High-dose intravenous immune globulin (1 g daily for 1 or 2 days) may be highly effective in controlling hemolysis. The benefit is short-lived (1–3 weeks), and the drug is very expensive. The long-term prognosis for patients with this disorder is good, especially if there is no underlying autoimmune disorder or lymphoma. Splenectomy is often successful in controlling the disorder.

When to Refer

Patients with autoimmune hemolytic anemia should be referred to a hematologist for confirmation of the diagnosis and subsequent care.

When to Admit

Patients should be hospitalized for symptomatic anemia or rapidly falling hematocrit levels.

Berentsen S et al. Primary chronic cold agglutinin disease: an update on pathogenesis, clinical features and therapy. Hematology. 2007 Oct;12(5):361–70. [PMID: 17891600]

Hamblin TJ. Autoimmune complications of chronic lymphocytic leukemia. Semin Oncol. 2006 Apr;33(2):230–9. [PMID: 16616070]

Packman CH. Hemolytic anemia due to warm autoantibodies. Blood Rev. 2008 Jan;22(1):17–31. [PMID: 17904259]

Stern M et al. Autoimmunity and malignancy in hematology—more than an association. Crit Rev Oncol Hematol. 2007 Aug;63(2):100–10. [PMID: 17391977]

COLD AGGLUTININ DISEASE

ESSENTIALS OF DIAGNOSIS

▶ Increased reticulocytes and spherocytes on peripheral blood smear.

▶ Coombs test positive only for complement.

▶ Positive cold agglutinin test.

General Considerations

Cold agglutinin disease is an acquired hemolytic anemia due to an IgM autoantibody usually directed against the I antigen on red blood cells. These IgM autoantibodies characteristically will not react with cells at 37 °C but only at lower temperatures. Since the blood temperature (even in the most peripheral parts of the body) rarely goes lower than 20 °C, only antibodies active at higher temperatures will produce clinical effects. Hemolysis results indirectly from attachment of IgM, which in the cooler parts of the circulation (fingers, nose, ears) binds and fixes complement. When the red blood cell returns to a warmer temperature, the IgM antibody dissociates, leaving complement on the cell. Lysis of cells rarely occurs. Rather, C3b present on the red cells is recognized by Kupffer cells (which have receptors for C3b), and red blood cell sequestration ensues.

Most cases of chronic cold agglutinin disease are idiopathic. Others occur in association with Waldenström macroglobulinemia, in which a monoclonal IgM paraprotein is produced. Acute postinfectious cold agglutinin disease occurs following mycoplasmal pneumonia or infectious mononucleosis (with antibody directed against antigen i rather than I).

Clinical Findings

A. Symptoms and Signs

In chronic cold agglutinin disease, symptoms related to red blood cell agglutination occur on exposure to cold, and patients may complain of mottled or numb fingers or toes. Hemolytic anemia is rarely severe, but episodic hemoglobinuria may occur on exposure to cold. The hemolytic anemia in acute postinfectious syndromes is rarely severe.

B. Laboratory Findings

Mild anemia is present with reticulocytosis and spherocytes. The direct Coombs test will be positive for complement only. Occasionally, a micro-Coombs test is necessary to reveal bound complement (low-titer cold agglutinin disease). A bedside cold agglutinin test may be performed by placing a glass slide in ice and then putting a few drops of heparinized blood on it. Inspection may reveal small clumps of agglutinated blood.

Treatment

Treatment is largely symptomatic, based on avoiding exposure to cold. Splenectomy and prednisone are usually ineffective since hemolysis takes place in the liver. Rituximab, a monoclonal antibody directed against the CD20 antigen on B lymphocytes, is the treatment of choice. The dose is 375 mg/m^2 intravenously weekly for 4 weeks. Relapses may be effectively re-treated. High-dose intravenous immunoglobulin (2 g/kg) may be effective temporarily, but it is rarely used because of the extreme cost and short duration of benefit. Patients with severe involvement may be treated with alkylating agents, such as cyclophosphamide, or with immunosuppressive agents, such as cyclosporine.

Gertz MA. Cold hemolytic syndrome. Hematology Am Soc Hematol Educ Program. 2006:19–23. [PMID: 17124034]

MICROANGIOPATHIC HEMOLYTIC ANEMIAS

The microangiopathic hemolytic anemias are a group of disorders in which red blood cell fragmentation takes place. The anemia is intravascular, producing hemoglobinemia, hemoglobinuria and, in severe cases, methemalbuminemia. The hallmark of the disorder is the finding of fragmented red blood cells (schistocytes, helmet cells) on the peripheral blood smear.

These fragmentation syndromes can be caused by a variety of disorders (Table 13–8). Thrombotic thrombocytopenic purpura is the most important of these and is discussed below. Clinical features are variable and depend on the underlying disorder. Coagulopathy and thrombocytopenia are variably present.

Chronic microangiopathic hemolytic anemia (such as is present with a malfunctioning cardiac valve prosthesis) may cause iron deficiency anemia because of continuous low-grade hemoglobinuria.

APLASTIC ANEMIA

 ESSENTIALS OF DIAGNOSIS

► Pancytopenia.
► No abnormal cells seen.
► Hypocellular bone marrow.

General Considerations

Aplastic anemia is a condition of bone marrow failure that arises from injury to or abnormal expression of the stem cell. The bone marrow becomes hypoplastic, and pancytopenia develops.

There are a number of causes of aplastic anemia (Table 13–10). Direct stem cell injury may be caused by radiation, chemotherapy, toxins, or pharmacologic agents. Systemic lupus erythematosus may rarely cause suppression of the hematopoietic stem cell by an IgG autoantibody directed against the stem cell. However, the most common pathogenesis of aplastic anemia appears to be autoimmune suppression of hematopoiesis by a T cell-mediated cellular mechanism.

Clinical Findings

A. Symptoms and Signs

Patients come to medical attention because of the consequences of bone marrow failure. Anemia leads to symptoms of weakness and fatigue, neutropenia causes vulnerability to bacterial infections, and thrombocytopenia results in mucosal and skin bleeding. Physical examination may reveal signs of pallor, purpura, and petechiae. Other abnormalities such as hepatosplenomegaly, lymphadenopathy, or bone tenderness should *not* be present, and their presence should lead to questioning the diagnosis.

Table 13–10. Causes of aplastic anemia.

Congenital (rare)
"Idiopathic" (probably autoimmune)
Systemic lupus erythematosus
Chemotherapy, radiotherapy
Toxins: benzene, toluene, insecticides
Drugs: chloramphenicol, phenylbutazone, gold salts, sulfonamides, phenytoin, carbamazepine, quinacrine, tolbutamide
Posthepatitis
Pregnancy
Paroxysmal nocturnal hemoglobinuria

B. Laboratory Findings

The hallmark of aplastic anemia is pancytopenia. However, early in the evolution of aplastic anemia, only one or two cell lines may be reduced.

Anemia may be severe and is always associated with decreased reticulocytes. Red blood cell morphology is unremarkable, but there may be macrocytosis. Neutrophils and platelets are reduced in number, and no immature or abnormal forms are seen. The bone marrow aspirate and the bone marrow biopsy appear hypocellular, with only scant amounts of normal hematopoietic progenitors. No abnormal cells are seen.

Differential Diagnosis

Aplastic anemia must be differentiated from other causes of pancytopenia (Table 13–11). Myelodysplastic disorders, especially hypocellular forms of myelodysplasia, or acute leukemia may occasionally be confused with aplastic anemia. These are differentiated by the presence of morphologic abnormalities or increased blasts, or by the presence of abnormal cytogenetics in bone marrow cells. Hairy cell leukemia has been misdiagnosed as aplastic anemia and should be recognized by the presence of splenomegaly and by abnormal lymphoid cells on the bone marrow biopsy. Pancytopenia with a normocellular bone marrow may be due to systemic lupus erythematosus, disseminated infection, or hypersplenism. Isolated thrombocytopenia may occur early as aplastic anemia develops and be confused with immune thrombocytopenia.

Treatment

Mild cases of aplastic anemia may be treated with supportive care. Red blood cell transfusions and platelet transfusions are given as necessary, and antibiotics are used to treat infections.

Severe aplastic anemia is defined by a neutrophil count of less than 500/mcL, platelets less than 20,000/mcL, reticulocytes less than 1%, and bone marrow cellularity less than 20%. When this constellation of features is present (or three of the four), the median survival without treatment is approximately 3 months, and only 20% of patients survive for 1 year. The treatment of choice for young adults (under

Table 13–11. Causes of pancytopenia.

Bone marrow disorders
  Aplastic anemia
  Myelodysplasia
  Acute leukemia
  Myelofibrosis
  Infiltrative disease: lymphoma, myeloma, carcinoma, hairy cell leukemia
  Megaloblastic anemia
Nonmarrow disorders
  Hypersplenism
  Systemic lupus erythematosus
  Infection: tuberculosis, AIDS, leishmaniasis, brucellosis

age 50 years) who have HLA-matched siblings is allogeneic bone marrow transplantation. Children or young adults may also benefit from allogeneic transplantation using an unrelated donor. The use of reduced-intensity preparative regimens for allogeneic transplantation has reduced the toxicity of transplantation. Because of the increased risks associated with unrelated-donor transplantation, this treatment is usually reserved for patients who have not benefited from immunosuppressive therapy.

For adults over age 50 years or those without HLA-matched donors, the treatment of choice for severe aplastic anemia is immunosuppression with antithymocyte globulin (ATG) plus cyclosporine (or tacrolimus). ATG is given in the hospital in conjunction with transfusion and antibiotic support. A useful regimen is equine ATG 40 mg/kg/d for 4 days in combination with cyclosporine, 6 mg/kg orally twice daily. Rabbit ATG is more immunosuppressive than equine ATG and may also be used in a dose of 3.5 mg/kg for 4 days. ATG must be used in combination with corticosteroids (prednisone 1–2 mg/kg/d initially, followed by a rapid taper) to avoid complications of serum sickness. Responses usually occur in 4–12 weeks and are usually only partial, but the blood counts rise high enough to give patients a safe and transfusion-free life.

High-dose immunosuppression with cyclophosphamide, 200 mg/kg, has produced remissions in refractory cases and should be considered for patients without suitable bone marrow donors. Androgens have been widely used in the past, with a low response rate. However, a few patients can be maintained successfully with this form of treatment. One regimen is oxymetholone, 2–3 mg/kg orally daily.

Course & Prognosis

Patients with severe aplastic anemia have a rapidly fatal illness if left untreated. Allogeneic bone marrow transplantation is highly successful in children and young adults, especially with HLA-matched siblings. For this group of patients, the durable complete response rate exceeds 80%. Advances in the field of unrelated donor transplantation have made this a more attractive option than in the past, with durable responses in more than 50% of cases. ATG treatment leads to partial response in approximately 60% of adults, and the long-term prognosis of responders appears to be good. There is increasing evidence that clonal hematologic disorders, such as PNH or myelodysplasia, may develop in some fraction (as many as 25%) of these nontransplanted patients after many years of follow-up.

When to Refer

All patients should be referred to a hematologist.

When to Admit

Admission is necessary only for treatment of neutropenic infection.

Armand P et al. Allogeneic stem cell transplantation for aplastic anemia. Biol Blood Marrow Transplant. 2007 May;13(5):505–16. [PMID: 17448909]

Bacigalupo A. Aplastic anemia: pathogenesis and treatment. Hematology Am Soc Hematol Educ Program. 2007:23–28. [PMID: 18024605]

Young NS. Pathophysiologic mechanisms in acquired aplastic anemia. Hematology Am Soc Hematol Educ Program. 2006:72–7. [PMID: 17124043]

Young NS et al. Current concepts in the pathophysiology and treatment of aplastic anemia. Blood. 2006 Oct 15;108(8):2509–19. [PMID: 16778145]

NEUTROPENIA

ESSENTIALS OF DIAGNOSIS

► Severe neutropenia if neutrophils < 500/mcL.
► Sharp rise in risk of infection in severe neutropenia.

General Considerations

Neutropenia is present when the neutrophil count is below 1500/mcL, although blacks and other specific population groups may normally have neutrophil counts as low as 1200/mcL. The neutropenic patient is increasingly vulnerable to infection by gram-positive and gram-negative bacteria and by fungi. The risk of infection is related to the severity of neutropenia. The risk of serious infection rises sharply with neutrophil counts below 500/mcL, and neutrophil counts less than 100/mcL ("profound neutropenia") are associated with a high risk of infection within days. Patients with "chronic benign neutropenia" are free of infection for years despite very low stable neutrophil levels. In contrast, the neutrophil count of patients with cyclic neutropenia alternates between normal and low, and the period during which there is a risk of infection is during the nadirs.

A variety of bone marrow disorders and nonmarrow conditions may cause neutropenia (Table 13–12). All the causes of aplastic anemia (Table 13–10) and pancytopenia (Table 13–11) may cause neutropenia. Isolated neutropenia is

Table 13–12. Causes of neutropenia.

Bone marrow disorders
Aplastic anemia
Pure white cell aplasia
Congenital (rare)
Cyclic neutropenia
Drugs: sulfonamides, chlorpromazine, procainamide, penicillin, cephalosporins, cimetidine, methimazole, phenytoin, chlorpropamide, antiretroviral medications
Benign chronic
Peripheral disorders
Hypersplenism
Sepsis
Immune
Felty syndrome
HIV infection
Large granular lymphocytosis

often due to an idiosyncratic reaction to a drug, and agranulocytosis (complete absence of neutrophils in the peripheral blood) is almost always due to a drug reaction. In these cases, examination of the bone marrow shows an almost complete absence of myeloid precursors, with other cell lines undisturbed. **Felty syndrome**—immune neutropenia associated with seropositive nodular rheumatoid arthritis and splenomegaly—is another cause. Neutropenia in the presence of a normal bone marrow may be due to immunologic peripheral destruction, sepsis, or hypersplenism. Severe neutropenia may be associated with clonal disorders of T lymphocytes, often with the morphology of large granular lymphocytes.

Clinical Findings

Neutropenia results in stomatitis and in infections due to gram-positive or gram-negative aerobic bacteria or to fungi such as *Candida* or *Aspergillus*. The most common infections are septicemia, cellulitis, and pneumonia. In the presence of severe neutropenia, the usual signs of inflammatory response to infection may be absent. Nevertheless, fever in the neutropenic patient should always be assumed to be of infectious origin.

Treatment

Potential causative drugs are discontinued. Infections are treated with broad-spectrum antibiotics, but particular attention should be paid to enteric gram-negative bacteria. Effective antibiotics include the quinolones such as levofloxacin, 500 mg orally or intravenously daily, or new cephalosporins such as cefepime, 2 g intravenously every 8 hours. The antifungal agent voriconazole provides both better efficacy and reduced toxicity compared with amphotericin.

Many cases of idiopathic or autoimmune neutropenia respond to myeloid growth factors such as granulocyte colony-stimulating factor (G-CSF). Once-weekly or twice-weekly dosage will often be sufficient to produce a protective neutrophil count.

When Felty syndrome leads to repeated bacterial infections, splenectomy has been the treatment of choice, but it now appears that sustained use of G-CSF is effective and provides a nonsurgical alternative. The prognosis of patients with neutropenia depends on the underlying cause. Most patients with drug-induced agranulocytosis can be supported with broad-spectrum antibiotics and will recover completely. The myeloid growth factor G-CSF (filgrastim) may be useful in shortening the duration of neutropenia associated with chemotherapy. The neutropenia associated with large granular lymphocytes may respond to therapy with either cyclosporine or low-dose methotrexate.

When to Refer

Refer to a hematologist if neutrophils are less than 1000/mcL.

When to Admit

Neutropenia by itself is not an indication for hospitalization. However, most patients with severe neutropenia have a serious underlying disease that may require inpatient treatment.

Klastersky J et al. Outpatient oral antibiotics for febrile neutropenic cancer patients using a score predictive for complications. J Clin Oncol. 2006 Sep 1;24(25):4129–34. [PMID: 16943529]

Kuderer NM et al. Impact of primary prophylaxis with granulo-cyte colony-stimulating factor on febrile neutropenia and mortality in adult cancer patients receiving chemotherapy: a systematic review. J Clin Oncol. 2007 Jul 20;25(21):3158–67. [PMID: 17634496]

LEUKEMIAS & OTHER MYELOPROLIFERATIVE DISORDERS

Myeloproliferative disorders are due to acquired clonal abnormalities of the hematopoietic stem cell. Since the stem cell gives rise to myeloid, erythroid, and platelet cells, qualitative and quantitative changes are seen in all these cell lines. In some disorders (chronic myeloid leukemia), specific characteristic chromosomal changes are seen. In others, no characteristic cytogenetic abnormalities are seen.

Classically, the myeloproliferative disorders produce characteristic syndromes with well-defined clinical and laboratory features (Tables 13–13 and 13–14). However, these disorders are grouped together because the disease may evolve from one form into another and because hybrid disorders are commonly seen. All of the myeloproliferative disorders may progress to acute myeloid leukemia.

POLYCYTHEMIA VERA

ESSENTIALS OF DIAGNOSIS

- JAK2 mutation.
- Increased red blood cell mass.
- Splenomegaly.
- Normal arterial oxygen saturation.
- Usually elevated white blood count and platelet count.

General Considerations

Polycythemia vera is an acquired myeloproliferative disorder that causes overproduction of all three hematopoietic cell lines, most prominently the red blood cells. The hematocrit is elevated (at sea level) when values exceed 54% in males or 51% in females (Table 13–15). True

Table 13–13. Classification of myeloproliferative disorders.

Myeloproliferative syndromes
Polycythemia vera
Myelofibrosis
Essential thrombocytosis
Chronic myeloid leukemia
Myelodysplastic syndromes
Acute myeloid leukemia

erythrocytosis, with an elevated red blood cell mass, is distinguished from spurious erythrocytosis caused by a constricted plasma volume.

Primary polycythemia (polycythemia vera) is a bone marrow disorder characterized by autonomous overproduction of erythroid cells. Erythroid production is independent of erythropoietin, and the serum erythropoietin level is low. A mutation in JAK2, a signaling molecule, has been demonstrated in 95% of cases, and is almost certainly involved in the pathogenesis.

Clinical Findings

A. Symptoms and Signs

Common complaints related to expanded blood volume and increased blood viscosity are headache, dizziness, tinnitus, blurred vision, and fatigue. Generalized pruritus, especially following a warm shower or bath, is related to histamine release from the basophilia. Epistaxis is probably related to engorgement of mucosal blood vessels in combination with abnormal hemostasis due to qualitative abnormalities in platelet function. Sixty percent of patients are men, and the median age at presentation is 60 years. Polycythemia rarely occurs in persons under age 40 years.

Physical examination reveals plethora and engorged retinal veins. The spleen is palpable in 75% of cases but is nearly always enlarged when imaged.

Thrombosis is the most common complication of polycythemia vera and the major cause of morbidity and death in this disorder. Thrombosis appears to be related both to increased blood viscosity and abnormal platelet function. Uncontrolled polycythemia leads to a very high incidence of thrombotic complications of surgery, and elective surgery should be deferred until the condition has been treated. Paradoxically, in addition to thrombosis, increased bleeding also occurs. There is a high incidence of peptic ulcer disease.

Table 13–14. Laboratory features of myeloproliferative disorders.

	White Count	Hematocrit	Platelet Count	Red Cell Morphology
Chronic myeloid leukemia	↑↑	N	N or ↑	N
Myelofibrosis	N or ↓ or ↑	N or ↓	↓ or N or ↑	Abn
Polycythemia vera	N or ↑	↑	N or ↑	N
Essential thrombocytosis	N or ↑	N	↑↑	N

Table 13–15. Causes of polycythemia.

Spurious polycythemia
Secondary polycythemia
Hypoxia: cardiac disease, pulmonary disease, high altitude
Carboxyhemoglobin: smoking
Kidney lesions
Erythropoietin-secreting tumors (rare)
Abnormal hemoglobins (rare)
Polycythemia vera

B. Laboratory Findings

The hallmark of polycythemia vera is a hematocrit above normal, at times greater than 60%. Red blood cell morphology is normal (Table 13–14). By definition, the red blood cell mass is elevated, but this is rarely measured. The white blood count is elevated to 10,000–20,000/mcL and the platelet count is variably increased, sometimes to counts exceeding 1,000,000/mcL. Platelet morphology is usually normal. White blood cells are usually normal, but basophilia and eosinophilia are frequently present. Erythropoietin levels are suppressed and are usually low. The diagnosis should be confirmed with the finding of the JAK2 mutation (JAK2V617F), and the absence of this finding should lead the clinician to question the diagnosis.

The bone marrow is hypercellular, with panhyperplasia of all hematopoietic elements, but bone marrow examination is usually not necessary to establish the diagnosis. Iron stores are usually absent from the bone marrow, having been transferred to the increased circulating red blood cell mass. Iron deficiency may also result from chronic gastrointestinal blood loss. Bleeding may lower the hematocrit to the normal range (or lower), creating diagnostic confusion.

Vitamin B_{12} levels are strikingly elevated because of increased levels of transcobalamin III (secreted by white blood cells). Overproduction of uric acid may lead to hyperuricemia.

Although red blood cell morphology is usually normal at presentation, microcytosis, hypochromia, and poikilocytosis may result from iron deficiency following treatment by phlebotomy (see below). Progressive hypersplenism may also lead to elliptocytosis.

▶ Differential Diagnosis

Spurious polycythemia, in which an elevated hematocrit is due to contracted plasma volume rather than increased red cell mass, may be related to diuretic use or may occur without obvious cause.

A secondary cause of polycythemia should be suspected if splenomegaly is absent and the high hematocrit is not accompanied by increases in other cell lines. Secondary causes of polycythemia include hypoxia and smoking; carboxyhemoglobin levels may be elevated in smokers. A renal CT scan or sonogram may be considered to look for an erythropoietin-secreting cyst or tumor. A positive family history should lead to investigation for congenital high-oxygen-affinity hemoglobin. An absence of a mutation in JAK2 suggests a different diagnosis. However, JAK2 muta-

tions are also commonly found in the myeloproliferative disorders essential thrombocytosis and myelofibrosis.

Polycythemia vera should be differentiated from other myeloproliferative disorders (Table 13–14). Marked elevation of the white blood count (above 30,000/mcL) suggests chronic myeloid leukemia. Abnormal red blood cell morphology and nucleated red blood cells in the peripheral blood are seen in myelofibrosis. Essential thrombocytosis is suggested when the platelet count is strikingly elevated.

▶ Treatment

The treatment of choice is phlebotomy. One unit of blood (approximately 500 mL) is removed weekly until the hematocrit is less than 45%; the hematocrit is maintained at less than 45% by repeated phlebotomy as necessary. Patients for whom phlebotomy is problematic (because of poor venous access or logistical reasons) may be managed primarily with hydroxyurea (see below). Because repeated phlebotomy intentionally produces iron deficiency, the requirement for phlebotomy should gradually decrease. It is important to avoid medicinal iron supplementation, as this can thwart the goals of a phlebotomy program. Maintaining the hematocrit at normal levels has been shown to decrease the incidence of thrombotic complications. A diet low in iron may also increase the intervals between phlebotomies.

Occasionally, myelosuppressive therapy is indicated. Indications include a high phlebotomy requirement, thrombocytosis, and intractable pruritus. There is evidence that reduction of the platelet count to less than 600,000/mcL will reduce the risk of thrombotic complications. Alkylating agents have been shown to increase the risk of conversion of this disease to acute leukemia and should be avoided. Hydroxyurea is now being widely used when myelosuppressive therapy is indicated. The usual dose is 500–1500 mg/d orally, adjusted to keep platelets < 500,000/mcL without reducing the neutrophil count to < 2000/mcL. Anagrelide may be substituted or added when hydroxyurea is not well tolerated, but it is not the preferred initial agent. Low-dose aspirin (75–81 mg daily) has been shown to reduce the risk of thrombosis without excessive bleeding, and should be part of therapy for all patients without contraindications to aspirin.

Allopurinol 300 mg orally daily may be indicated for hyperuricemia. Antihistamine therapy with diphenhydramine or other H_1-blockers may be helpful for control of pruritus, and some reports suggest the efficacy of selective serotonin reuptake inhibitors in refractory cases.

▶ Prognosis

Polycythemia is an indolent disease with median survival of 11–15 years. The major cause of morbidity and mortality is arterial thrombosis. Over time, polycythemia vera may convert to myelofibrosis or to chronic myeloid leukemia. In approximately 5% of cases, the disorder progresses to acute myeloid leukemia, which is usually refractory to therapy.

▶ When to Refer

Patients with polycythemia vera should be referred to a hematologist.

When to Admit

Inpatient care is not required.

Finazzi G et al. How I treat patients with polycythemia vera. Blood. 2007 Jun 15;109(12):5104–11. [PMID: 17264301]

Ruggeri M et al. Post-surgery outcomes in patients with polycythemia vera and essential thrombocythemia: a retrospective survey. Blood. 2008 Jan 15;111(2):666–71. [PMID: 17909074]

Tefferi A. Classification, diagnosis, and management of myeloproliferative disorders in the JAK2V617F era. Hematology Am Soc Hematol Educ Program. 2006:240–5. [PMID: 17124067]

ESSENTIAL THROMBOCYTOSIS

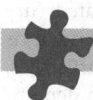 ESSENTIALS OF DIAGNOSIS

- ▶ Elevated platelet count in absence of other causes.
- ▶ Normal red blood cell mass.
- ▶ Absence of Philadelphia chromosome.

General Considerations

Essential thrombocytosis is an uncommon myeloproliferative disorder of unknown cause in which marked proliferation of the megakaryocytes in the bone marrow leads to elevation of the platelet count. As with polycythemia vera, the recent finding of a high frequency of mutations of JAK2 in these patients promises to advance the understanding of this disorder.

Clinical Findings

A. Symptoms and Signs

The median age at presentation is 50–60 years, and there is a slightly increased incidence in women. The disorder is often suspected when an elevated platelet count is found. Less frequently, the first sign is thrombosis, which is the most common clinical problem. The risk of thrombosis rises with age. Venous thromboses may occur in unusual sites such as the mesenteric, hepatic, or portal vein. Some patients experience erythromelalgia, painful burning of the hands accompanied by erythema; this symptom is reliably relieved by aspirin. Bleeding, typically mucosal, is less common and is related to a concomitant qualitative platelet defect. Splenomegaly is present in at least 25% of patients.

B. Laboratory Findings

An elevated platelet count is the hallmark of this disorder, and may be over 2,000,000/mcL (Table 13–14). The white blood cell count is often mildly elevated, usually not above 30,000/mcL, but with some immature myeloid forms. The hematocrit is normal. The peripheral blood smear reveals large platelets, but giant degranulated forms seen in myelofibrosis are not observed. Red blood cell morphology is normal.

The bone marrow shows increased numbers of megakaryocytes but no other morphologic abnormalities. The Philadelphia chromosome is absent but should be assayed by molecular testing of peripheral blood for the *bcr/abl* fusion gene in all suspected cases to differentiate the disorder from chronic myeloid leukemia.

Differential Diagnosis

Essential thrombocytosis must be distinguished from secondary causes of an elevated platelet count. In reactive thrombocytosis, the platelet count seldom exceeds 1,000,000/mcL. Inflammatory disorders such as rheumatoid arthritis and ulcerative colitis cause significant elevations of the platelet count, as may chronic infection. The thrombocytosis of iron deficiency is observed only when anemia is significant. The platelet count is temporarily elevated after splenectomy. JAK2 mutations are found in 50% of cases.

Regarding other myeloproliferative disorders, the lack of erythrocytosis distinguishes it from polycythemia vera. Unlike myelofibrosis, red blood cell morphology is normal, nucleated red blood cells are absent, and giant degranulated platelets are not seen. In chronic myeloid leukemia, the Philadelphia chromosome (or *bcr/abl* by molecular testing) establishes the diagnosis.

Treatment

The risk of thrombosis can be reduced by control of the platelet count, which should be kept at less than 500,000/mcL. The treatment of choice is hydroxyurea in a dose of 0.5–2 g/d. Hydroxyurea has been shown to be more effective than anagrelide in preventing thrombotic events, with no increase in toxicity. In cases in which hydroxyurea is not well tolerated because of anemia, low doses of anagrelide, 1–2 mg/d, may be added. Higher doses of anagrelide are often complicated by headache, peripheral edema, and congestive heart failure.

Vasomotor symptoms such as erythromelalgia and paresthesias respond rapidly to aspirin, and long-term low-dose (81 mg/d) aspirin may reduce the risk of thrombotic complications. In the unusual event of severe bleeding, the platelet count can be lowered rapidly with plateletpheresis.

Course & Prognosis

Essential thrombocytosis is an indolent disorder and allows long-term survival. Average survival is longer than 15 years from diagnosis, and the survival of patients younger than 50 years does not appear different from matched controls. The major source of morbidity—thrombosis—can be reduced by appropriate platelet control. Late in the course of the disease, the bone marrow may become fibrotic, and massive splenomegaly may occur, sometimes with splenic infarction. There is a 10–15% risk of progression to myelofibrosis after 15 years, and a 1–5% risk of transformation to acute leukemia over 20 years.

When to Refer

Patients with essential thrombocytosis should be referred to a hematologist.

Alvarez-Larran A et al. Essential thrombocythemia in young individuals: frequency and risk factors for vascular events and evolution to myelofibrosis in 126 patients. Leukemia. 2007 Jun;21(6):1218–23. [PMID: 17519959]

Levine RL et al. New advances in the pathogenesis and therapy of essential thrombocytosis. Hematology Am Soc Hematol Educ Program. 2008:76–82. [PMID: 19074062]

Vannucchi AM et al. Clinical profile of homozygous JAK2 617V>F mutation in patients with polycythemia vera or essential thrombocythemia. Blood. 2007 Aug 1;110(3):840–6. [PMID: 17379742]

MYELOFIBROSIS

 ESSENTIALS OF DIAGNOSIS

- ▸ Striking splenomegaly.
- ▸ Teardrop poikilocytosis on peripheral smear.
- ▸ Leukoerythroblastic blood picture; giant abnormal platelets.
- ▸ Hypercellular bone marrow with reticulin or collagen fibrosis.

▸ General Considerations

Myelofibrosis (myelofibrosis with myeloid metaplasia, agnogenic myeloid metaplasia) is a myeloproliferative disorder characterized by fibrosis of the bone marrow, splenomegaly, and a leukoerythroblastic peripheral blood picture with teardrop poikilocytosis. It is believed that fibrosis occurs in response to increased secretion of platelet-derived growth factor (PDGF) and possibly other cytokines. In response to bone marrow fibrosis, extramedullary hematopoiesis takes place in the liver, spleen, and lymph nodes. In these sites, mesenchymal cells responsible for fetal hematopoiesis can be reactivated. As with other myeloproliferative diseases, abnormalities of JAK2 signaling pathways may be involved in the pathogenesis.

▸ Clinical Findings

A. Symptoms and Signs

Myelofibrosis develops in adults over age 50 years and is usually insidious in onset. Patients most commonly present with fatigue due to anemia or abdominal fullness related to splenomegaly. Uncommon presentations include bleeding and bone pain. On examination, splenomegaly is almost invariably present and is commonly massive. The liver is enlarged in more than 50% of cases.

Later in the course of the disease, progressive bone marrow failure takes place as it becomes increasingly more fibrotic. Progressive thrombocytopenia leads to bleeding. The spleen continues to enlarge, which leads to early satiety. Painful episodes of splenic infarction may occur. The patient becomes cachectic and may experience severe bone pain, especially in the upper legs. Hematopoiesis in the liver leads to portal hypertension with ascites, esophageal varices, and occasionally transverse myelitis caused by myelopoiesis in the epidural space.

B. Laboratory Findings

Patients are almost invariably anemic at presentation. The white blood count is variable—either low, normal, or elevated—and may be increased to 50,000/mcL. The platelet count is variable. The peripheral blood smear is dramatic, with significant poikilocytosis and numerous teardrop forms in the red cell line. Nucleated red blood cells are present and the myeloid series is shifted, with immature forms including a small percentage of promyelocytes or myeloblasts. Platelet morphology may be bizarre, and giant degranulated platelet forms (megakaryocyte fragments) may be seen. The triad of teardrop poikilocytosis, leukoerythroblastic blood, and giant abnormal platelets is highly suggestive of myelofibrosis.

The bone marrow usually cannot be aspirated (dry tap), though early in the course of the disease it is hypercellular, with a marked increase in megakaryocytes. Fibrosis at this stage is detected by a silver stain demonstrating increased reticulin fibers. Later, biopsy reveals more severe fibrosis, with eventual replacement of hematopoietic precursors by collagen. There is no characteristic chromosomal abnormality.

▸ Differential Diagnosis

A leukoerythroblastic blood picture from other causes may be seen in response to severe infection, inflammation, or infiltrative bone marrow processes. However, teardrop poikilocytosis and giant abnormal platelet forms will not be present. Bone marrow fibrosis may be seen in metastatic carcinoma, Hodgkin disease, and hairy cell leukemia. These disorders are diagnosed by characteristic morphology of involved tissues.

Of the other myeloproliferative disorders, chronic myeloid leukemia is diagnosed when there is marked leukocytosis, normal red blood cell morphology, and the presence of the *bcr/abl* fusion gene. Polycythemia vera is characterized by an elevated hematocrit. Essential thrombocytosis shows predominant platelet count elevations.

▸ Treatment

Patients with mild forms of the disease may require no therapy or occasional transfusion support. Biologic agents have shown some benefit. Thalidomide has produced definite responses with acceptable toxicity, and lenalidomide has at least the same efficacy with less toxicity. Clinical trials testing the effect of JAK2 inhibitors are currently being performed, but it is too early to know the results. Allogeneic bone marrow transplantation has been performed successfully with 50% long-term survival and should be considered in younger patients. The use of less toxic, nonmyeloablative regimens for allogeneic transplantation has produced encouraging results. Anemic patients are supported with transfusion. Erythropoietin may increase red blood cell production and decrease transfusion requirements. Splenectomy is not routinely performed but is indicated for splenic enlargement causing recurrent painful episodes, severe thrombocytopenia, or an unacceptable transfusion requirement.

Course & Prognosis

The median survival from time of diagnosis is approximately 5 years. Therapies with biologic agents, such as thalidomide and lenalidomide, and the application of reduced-intensity allogeneic stem cell transplantation appear to offer the possibility of improving the outcome for many patients. End-stage myelofibrosis is characterized by generalized asthenia liver failure, and bleeding from thrombocytopenia, with some cases terminating in acute myeloid leukemia.

When to Refer

Patients in whom myelofibrosis is suspected should be referred to a hematologist.

When to Admit

Admission is not usually necessary.

Levine RL et al. Role of JAK2 in the pathogenesis and therapy of myeloproliferative disorders. Nat Rev Cancer. 2007 Sep;7(9):673–83. [PMID: 17721432]

Rambaldi A et al. From palliation to epigenetic therapy in myelofibrosis. Hematology Am Soc Hematol Educ Program. 2008:83–91. [PMID: 19074063]

Tefferi A. New insights into the pathogenesis and drug treatment of myelofibrosis. Curr Opin Hematol. 2006 Mar;13(2):87–92. [PMID: 16456374]

CHRONIC MYELOID LEUKEMIA

ESSENTIALS OF DIAGNOSIS

▶ Elevated white blood count.

▶ Markedly left-shifted myeloid series but with a low percentage of promyelocytes and blasts.

▶ Presence of Philadelphia chromosome or *bcr/abl* gene.

General Considerations

Chronic myeloid leukemia (CML) is a myeloproliferative disorder characterized by overproduction of myeloid cells. These myeloid cells retain the capacity for differentiation, and normal bone marrow function is retained during the early phases.

CML is characterized by a specific chromosomal abnormality and specific molecular abnormality. The Philadelphia chromosome is a reciprocal translocation between the long arms of chromosomes 9 and 22. A large portion of 22q is translocated to 9q, and a smaller piece of 9q is moved to 22q. The portion of 9q that is translocated contains *abl*, a protooncogene that is the cellular homolog of the Ableson murine leukemia virus. The *abl* gene is received at a specific site on 22q, the break point cluster (bcr). The fusion gene *bcr/abl* produces a novel protein that differs from the normal transcript of the *abl* gene in that it possesses tyrosine kinase activity (a characteristic activity of transforming genes). Evidence that the *bcr/abl* fusion gene is pathogenic is provided by transgenic mouse models in which introduction of the gene almost invariably leads to leukemia.

Early CML ("chronic phase") does not behave like a malignant disease. Normal bone marrow function is retained, white blood cells differentiate and, despite some qualitative abnormalities, the neutrophils combat infection normally. However, untreated CML is inherently unstable, and without treatment the disease progresses to an accelerated and then acute blast phase, which is morphologically indistinguishable from acute leukemia. In recent years, remarkable advances in therapy have changed the natural history of the disease, and the relentless progression to more advanced stages of disease is at least greatly delayed, if not eliminated.

Clinical Findings

A. Symptoms and Signs

CML is a disorder of middle age (median age at presentation is 55 years). Patients usually complain of fatigue, night sweats, and low-grade fever related to the hypermetabolic state caused by overproduction of white blood cells. Patients may also complain of abdominal fullness related to splenomegaly. In some cases, an elevated white blood count is discovered incidentally. Rarely, the patient will present with a clinical syndrome related to leukostasis with blurred vision, respiratory distress, or priapism. The white blood count in these cases is usually greater than 500,000/mcL.

On examination, the spleen is enlarged (often markedly so), and sternal tenderness may be present as a sign of marrow overexpansion. In cases discovered during routine laboratory monitoring, these findings are often absent.

Acceleration of the disease is often associated with fever in the absence of infection, bone pain, and splenomegaly.

B. Laboratory Findings

CML is characterized by an elevated white blood count; the median white blood count at diagnosis is 150,000/mcL, although in some cases the white blood cell count is only modestly increased (Table 13–14). The peripheral blood is characteristic. The myeloid series is left shifted, with mature forms dominating and with cells usually present in proportion to their degree of maturation. Blasts are usually less than 5%. Basophilia and eosinophilia of granulocytes may be present. At presentation, the patient is usually not anemic. Red blood cell morphology is normal, and nucleated red blood cells are rarely seen. The platelet count may be normal or elevated (sometimes to strikingly high levels).

The bone marrow is hypercellular, with left-shifted myelopoiesis. Myeloblasts comprise less than 5% of marrow cells.

The hallmark of the disease is that the *bcr/abl* gene is detected by the polymerase chain reaction (PCR) test in the peripheral blood. A bone marrow examination is not necessary for diagnosis, although it is useful for prognosis and for detecting additional chromosomal abnormalities in addition to the Philadelphia chromosome.

With progression to the accelerated and blast phases, progressive anemia and thrombocytopenia occur, and the percentage of blasts in the blood and bone marrow increases. Blast phase CML is diagnosed when blasts comprise more than 20% of bone marrow cells.

Differential Diagnosis

Early CML must be differentiated from the reactive leukocytosis associated with infection. In such cases, the white blood count is usually less than 50,000/mcL, splenomegaly is absent, and the *bcr/abl* gene is not present.

CML must be distinguished from other myeloproliferative disease (Table 13–14). The hematocrit should not be elevated, the red blood cell morphology is normal, and nucleated red blood cells are rare or absent. Definitive diagnosis is made by finding the *bcr/abl* gene.

Treatment

Treatment is usually not emergent even with white blood counts over 200,000/mcL, since the majority of circulating cells are mature myeloid cells that are smaller and more deformable than primitive leukemic blasts. In the rare instances in which symptoms result from extreme hyperleukocytosis (priapism, respiratory distress, visual blurring, altered mental status), emergent leukapheresis is performed in conjunction with myelosuppressive therapy.

Imatinib mesylate specifically inhibits the tyrosine kinase activity of the *bcr/abl* oncogene. It is well tolerated and results in nearly universal (98%) hematologic control of chronic phase disease. For patients with the chronic phase of CML, the standard dose is 400 mg orally daily. Higher doses such as 600–800 mg daily may overcome some degree of resistance and may produce more rapid initial responses, but side effects are more prominent with these doses. The most common toxicities are nausea, periorbital swelling, edema, rash, and myalgia, but most of these are modest. Less than 5% of patients discontinue the drug due to unacceptable side effects.

Response is assessed in several ways. First, the patient should enter hematologic complete remission, with normalization of blood counts and splenomegaly. This usually occurs within several weeks, but should occur within 3 months. Second, cytogenetic responses should be achieved, ideally within 6 months but certainly within 12 months. A "major cytogenetic response" is identified when < 35% of metaphases contain the Philadelphia chromosome, and a "complete cytogenetic response" indicates the absence of the abnormal chromosome by standard cytogenetic testing. Quantitative assessment of the *bcr/abl* gene using PCR assays is the standard method of assessment. The current goal of therapy is to achieve a "good molecular response," with at least a 3-log reduction in *bcr/abl* level. This roughly corresponds to a *bcr/abl* ratio (compared to *abl*) of less than 0.03. Patients who achieve this level of molecular response have an excellent prognosis, with 100% of such patients remaining free of progression at 7 years. Furthermore, in this favorable group, the depth of molecular remission appears to increase over time, leading to the hope that this can actually be a curative treatment. Patients with suboptimal molecular responses are best treated by switching from imatinib to an alternative tyrosine kinase inhibitor such as dasatinib (or nilotinib). Dasatinib appears to be a more potent agent and can over-

come approximately 90% of the mutations that can form in *bcr/abl* and limit the effectiveness of imatinib. Dasatinib can be given in a dose of 100 mg/d but is dependent on an acid environment for absorption and cannot be used concurrently with drugs that decrease stomach acidity. Patients who cannot achieve a good molecular response to any of these agents are at increased risk for disease progression and should be considered for treatment with allogeneic transplantation.

Patients with an accelerated phase of CML should initially be treated with imatinib, 600 mg/d, or dasatinib, 100 mg/d, but should be considered for allogeneic transplantation.

The only proven curative therapy for CML is allogeneic bone marrow transplantation. The best results (80% cure rate) are obtained in patients who are under 40 years of age and transplanted within 1 year after diagnosis from HLA-matched siblings. The introduction of imatinib has changed the approach to allogeneic transplant for CML. Allogeneic transplantation is reserved for patients in whom disease is not well controlled, in whom disease progresses after initial control, or for those who have accelerated phase disease. It is too early to judge whether the curative potential from transplantation in patients who are initially treated with imatinib will be compromised compared to using transplantation as initial therapy.

Course & Prognosis

In the era of imatinib therapy (since 2001), and with the development of molecular targeted agents, more than 80% of patients remain alive and without disease progression at 7 years. While allogeneic stem cell transplantation is the only proven curative option, some patients may be cured by well-tolerated oral agents.

When to Refer

All patients with CML should be referred to a hematologist.

When to Admit

Hospitalization is rarely necessary and should be reserved for symptoms of leukostasis at diagnosis or for transformation to acute leukemia.

Goldman JM. How I treat chronic myeloid leukemia in the imatinib era. Blood. 2007 Oct 15;110(8):2828–37. [PMID: 17626839]

Hehlmann R et al; European LeukemiaNet. Chronic myeloid leukaemia. Lancet. 2007 Jul 28;370(9584):342–50. [PMID: 17662883]

Shah N. Medical Management of CML. Hematology Am Soc Hematol Educ Program. 2007;371–375. [PMID: 18024653]

White D et al. Measurement of in vivo BCR-ABL kinase inhibition to monitor imatinib-induced target blockade and predict response in chronic myeloid leukemia. J Clin Oncol. 2007 Oct 1;25(28):4445–51. [PMID: 17906206]

MYELODYSPLASTIC SYNDROMES

ESSENTIALS OF DIAGNOSIS

► Cytopenias with a hypercellular bone marrow.
► Morphologic abnormalities in two or more hematopoietic cell lines.

General Considerations

The myelodysplastic syndromes are a group of acquired clonal disorders of the hematopoietic stem cell. They are characterized by the constellation of cytopenias, a usually hypercellular marrow, and a number of morphologic and cytogenetic abnormalities. The disorders are usually idiopathic but may be seen after cytotoxic chemotherapy. Ultimately, the disorder may evolve into acute myeloid leukemia, and the term "preleukemia" has been used in the past to describe these disorders. Although no single specific chromosomal abnormality is seen in myelodysplasia, there are frequently abnormalities involving the long arm of chromosome 5 (which contains a number of genes encoding both growth factors and receptors involved in myelopoiesis) as well as deletions of chromosomes 5 and 7.

Myelodysplasia encompasses several heterogeneous syndromes. Those without excess bone marrow blasts are termed "refractory anemia," with or without ringed sideroblasts. One important subgroup of the refractory anemia patients are those with the 5q– syndrome, characterized by the cytogenetic finding of loss of part of the long arm of chromosome 5. Those with excess blasts are diagnosed as "refractory anemia with excess blasts" (RAEB 5–19% blasts). Those with a proliferative syndrome including peripheral blood monocytosis greater than 1000/mcL are termed "chronic myelomonocytic leukemia" (CMML). An International Prognostic Scoring System (IPSS) has been developed that classifies patients by risk status based on the percentage of bone marrow blasts, cytogenetics, and the severity of cytopenias.

Clinical Findings

A. Symptoms and Signs

Patients are usually over age 60 years. Many are diagnosed while asymptomatic because of the finding of abnormal blood counts. Patients usually present with fatigue, infection, or bleeding related to bone marrow failure. The course may be indolent, and the disease may present as a wasting illness with fever, weight loss, and general debility. On examination, splenomegaly may be present in combination with pallor, bleeding, and various signs of infection.

B. Laboratory Findings

Anemia may be marked and may require transfusion support. The MCV is normal or increased, and macroovalocytes may be seen on the peripheral blood smear. The white blood cell count is usually normal or reduced, and neutropenia is common. The neutrophils may exhibit morphologic abnormalities, including deficient numbers of granules or deficient segmentation of the nucleus, especially a bilobed nucleus (Pelger–Huet). The myeloid series may be left shifted, and small numbers of promyelocytes or blasts may be seen. The platelet count is normal or reduced, and hypogranular platelets may be present.

The bone marrow is characteristically hypercellular, but may be hypocellular. Erythroid hyperplasia is common, and signs of abnormal erythropoiesis include megaloblastic features, nuclear budding, or multinucleated erythroid precursors. The Prussian blue stain may demonstrate ringed sideroblasts. The myeloid series is often left shifted, with variable increases in blasts. Deficient or abnormal granules may be seen. A characteristic abnormality is the presence of dwarf megakaryocytes with a unilobed nucleus. A variety of cytogenetic abnormalities in the bone marrow are characteristic of myelodysplasia. Some patients with an indolent form of the disease have an isolated partial deletion of chromosome 5 (5q– syndrome). The presence of other abnormalities such as monosomy 7 or complex abnormalities is associated with more aggressive disease.

Differential Diagnosis

In subtle cases, cytogenetic evaluation of the bone marrow may help distinguish this clonal disorder from other causes of cytopenias. As the number of blasts increases in the bone marrow, myelodysplasia is arbitrarily separated from acute myeloid leukemia by the presence of less than 20% blasts.

Treatment

Erythropoietin (epoetin alfa), 30,000 units subcutaneously weekly, reduces the red cell transfusion requirement in some patients. The response rate is 20%, but a 4-week trial of epoetin alfa is reasonable since it will be cost-effective for the subgroup of responders. Patients with low serum erythropoietin (< 100 mU/mL) levels are the most likely to respond to erythropoietin treatment, whereas those with levels > 500 mU/mL almost never respond. Unfortunately, the patients with the highest transfusion requirements are the least likely to respond. Lenalidomide is approved for the treatment of transfusion-dependent anemia due to myelodysplasia. It is the treatment of choice in patients with the 5q– cytogenetic abnormality, with significant responses and freedom from transfusion in 70% of patients, and with responses typically lasting longer than 2 years. In addition, nearly half of these patients enter a cytogenetic remission with clearing of the abnormal 5q– clone, leading to the hope that lenalidomide may change the natural history of the disease. The response rate in patients with transfusion-dependent myelodysplasia lacking 5q– is only 25% and responses usually last less than 1 year, but it is still worth trying. The recommended initial dose is 10 mg orally daily. The most common side effects are neutropenia and thrombocytopenia, but venous thrombosis is also seen and warrants prophylaxis with aspirin. The cost of lenalidomide is extremely high, and it is not usually effective either for cell lines other than red blood cells or for patients with increased blasts. Patients who remain dependent on red blood cell transfusion and who do not have immediately life-threatening disease should receive iron chelation in order to prevent serious iron overload; the dose of oral agent deferasirox is 20 mg/kg/d. Patients affected primarily with severe neutropenia may benefit from the use of myeloid growth factors such as G-CSF. Experimental oral agents (AMG 531) that stimulate platelet production by mimicking the effect of thrombopoietin on the thrombopoietin receptor have shown some effectiveness in raising the platelet count in myelodysplasia.

Azacitidine is approved as an effective treatment based on its ability to improve both symptoms and blood counts and to prolong both overall survival and the time to conversion to acute leukemia. It is the treatment of choice for many patients, especially those with higher risk disease based on increased blasts in the bone marrow. A related agent, decitabine, can produce similar responses. Occasional patients can benefit from immunosuppressive therapy including antithymocyte globulin (ATG). Predictors of response to ATG include age less than 60 years, absence of 5q–, and presence of HLA DR15. Allogeneic stem cell transplantation is the only curative therapy for myelodysplasia, but its role is limited by the advanced age of many patients and the indolent course of disease in some subsets of patients. The optimal use and timing of allogeneic transplantation are controversial, but the use of reduced-intensity preparative regimens for transplantation has expanded the role of this therapy, using both family and matched unrelated donors.

▶ Course & Prognosis

Myelodysplasia is an ultimately fatal disease, and allogeneic transplantation is the only curative therapy, with cure rates of 30–60% depending primarily on the risk status of the disease. Patients most commonly succumb to infections or bleeding. The risk of transformation to acute myeloid leukemia depends on the percentage of blasts in the bone marrow. Patients with refractory anemia may survive many years, and the risk of leukemia is low (< 10%). Those with excess blasts or CMML have short survivals (usually < 2 years) and have a higher (20–50%) risk of developing acute leukemia. The finding of full deletions of chromosomes 5 and 7 is associated with a poor prognosis.

▶ When to Refer

All patients with myelodysplasia should be referred to a hematologist.

▶ When to Admit

Hospitalization is needed only for specific complications, such as severe infection.

Cervantes F et al. A new prognostic scoring system for primary myelofibrosis based on a study of the International Working Group for Myelofibrosis Research and Treatment. Blood. 2009 Mar 26;113(13):2895–901. [PMID: 18988864]

Fenaux P et al. Treatment of 5q– syndrome. Hematology Am Soc Hematol Educ Program. 2006:192–98. [PMID: 17124060]

Garcia-Manero G. Modifying the epigenome as a therapeutic strategy in myelodysplasia. Hematology Am Soc Hematol Educ Program. 2007:405–11. [PMID: 18024658]

Ingram W et al. Allogeneic transplantation for myelodysplastic syndrome (MDS). Blood Rev. 2007 Mar;21(2):61–71. [PMID: 16759774]

Kao JM et al. International MDS risk analysis workshop (IMRAW)/IPSS reanalyzed: impact of cytopenias on clinical outcomes in myelodysplastic syndromes. Am J Hematol. 2008 Oct;83(10):765–70. [PMID: 18645988]

Leone G et al. Therapy-related leukemia and myelodysplasia: susceptibility and incidence. Haematologica. 2007 Oct;92(10:1389–98. [PMID: 17768113]

van de Loosdrecht AA et al. Identification of distinct prognostic subgroups in low and intermediate-1 risk myelodysplastic syndromes by flow cytometry. Blood. 2008 Feb 1;111(3):1067–77. [PMID: 17971483]

ACUTE LEUKEMIA

ESSENTIALS OF DIAGNOSIS

▶ Short duration of symptoms, including fatigue, fever, and bleeding.

▶ Cytopenias or pancytopenia.

▶ More than 20% blasts in the bone marrow.

▶ Blasts in peripheral blood in 90% of patients.

▶ Classify as acute myeloid leukemia (AML) or acute lymphoblastic leukemia (ALL).

▶ General Considerations

Acute leukemia is a malignancy of the hematopoietic progenitor cell. These cells proliferate in an uncontrolled fashion and replace normal bone marrow elements. Most cases arise with no clear cause. However, radiation and some toxins (benzene) are leukemogenic. In addition, a number of chemotherapeutic agents (especially cyclophosphamide, melphalan, other alkylating agents, and etoposide) may cause leukemia. The leukemias seen after toxin or chemotherapy exposure often develop from a myelodysplastic prodrome and are often associated with abnormalities in chromosomes 5 and 7, and those related to etoposide may have abnormalities in chromosome 11q23.

Much has been learned about the molecular biology of the leukemias. One subtype, acute promyelocytic leukemia (APL), is characterized by chromosomal translocation t(15;17), which produces the fusion gene PML-$RAR\alpha$ which interacts with the retinoic acid receptor to produce a block in differentiation that can be overcome with pharmacologic doses of retinoic acid (see below).

Most of the clinical findings in acute leukemia are due to replacement of normal bone marrow elements by the malignant cell. Less common manifestations result from organ infiltration (skin, gastrointestinal tract, meninges). Acute leukemia is potentially curable with combination chemotherapy.

Acute lymphoblastic leukemia (ALL) comprises 80% of the acute leukemias of childhood. The peak incidence is between 3 and 7 years of age. It is also seen in adults, causing approximately 20% of adult acute leukemias. Acute myeloid leukemia (AML) is primarily an adult disease with a median age at presentation of 60 years and an increasing incidence with advanced age.

▶ Clinical Findings

A. Symptoms and Signs

Most patients have been ill only for days or weeks. Bleeding (usually due to thrombocytopenia) occurs in the skin and mucosal surfaces, with gingival bleeding, epistaxis, or menorrhagia. Less commonly, widespread bleeding is seen in patients with disseminated intravascular coagulation (DIC) (in APL and monocytic leukemia). Infection is due to neutropenia, with the risk of infection rising as the neutrophil count falls below 500/mcL; with neutrophil counts less than 100/mcL, infection within days is the rule. The most common pathogens are gram-negative bacteria (*Escherichia coli, Klebsiella, Pseudomonas*) or fungi (*Candida, Aspergillus*). Common presentations include cellulitis, pneumonia, and perirectal infections; death within a few hours may occur if treatment with appropriate antibiotics is delayed.

Patients may also seek medical attention because of gum hypertrophy and bone and joint pain. The most dramatic presentation is hyperleukocytosis, in which a markedly elevated circulating blast count (usually > 200,000/mcL) leads to impaired circulation, presenting as headache, confusion, and dyspnea. Such patients require emergent leukapheresis and chemotherapy.

On examination, patients appear pale and have purpura and petechiae; signs of infection may not be present. Stomatitis and gum hypertrophy may be seen in patients with monocytic leukemia, as may rectal fissures. There is variable enlargement of the liver, spleen, and lymph nodes. Bone tenderness may be present, particularly in the sternum, tibia, and femur.

B. Laboratory Findings

The hallmark of acute leukemia is the combination of pancytopenia with circulating blasts. However, blasts may be absent from the peripheral smear in as many as 10% of cases ("aleukemic leukemia"). The bone marrow is usually hypercellular and dominated by blasts. More than 20% blasts are required to make a diagnosis of acute leukemia.

Hyperuricemia may be seen. If DIC is present, the fibrinogen level will be reduced, the prothrombin time prolonged, and fibrin degradation products or fibrin D-dimers present. Patients with ALL (especially T cell) may have a mediastinal mass visible on chest radiograph. Meningeal leukemia will have blasts present in the spinal fluid, seen in approximately 5% of cases at diagnosis; it is more common in monocytic types of AML.

The Auer rod, an eosinophilic needle-like inclusion in the cytoplasm, is pathognomonic of AML and, if seen, secures the diagnosis. Leukemia cells retain properties of the lineages from which they are derived. Thus, histochemistry will demonstrate peroxidase in myeloid cells and butyrate esterase in monocytic cells, whereas ALL cells will not contain either of these enzymes. The phenotype of leukemia cells is usually demonstrated by flow cytometry. AML cells usually express myeloid antigens such as CD 13 or CD 33. ALL cells of B lineage will express CD19, common to all B cells, and most cases will express CD10, formerly known as the "common ALL antigen." ALL cells of T lineage will usually not express mature T-cell markers, such as CD 3, 4, or 8, but will express some combination of CD 2, 5, and 7 and do not express surface immunoglobulin. Almost all ALL cells express terminal deoxynucleotidyl transferase (TdT). The uncommon Burkitt type of ALL has a "lymphoma"

phenotype, expressing CD19, CD20 and surface immunoglobulin but not TdT.

AML has been characterized in several ways. The "FAB," (French, American, British) classification was based on morphology and histochemistry as follows: acute undifferentiated leukemia (M0), acute myeloblastic leukemia (M1), acute myeloblastic leukemia with differentiation (M2), acute promyelocytic leukemia (APL) (M3), acute myelomonocytic leukemia (M4), acute monoblastic leukemia (M5), erythroleukemia (M6), and megakaryoblastic leukemia (M7). The World Health Organization (WHO) has sponsored a classification of the leukemias and other hematologic malignancies that incorporates cytogenetic, molecular, and immunophenotype information.

ALL is most usefully classified by immunologic phenotype as follows: common, early B lineage, and T cell.

In considering the various types of AML, APL is now considered separately because of its unique biologic features and unique response to non-chemotherapy treatments. APL is characterized by the cytogenetic finding of t(15;17) and the fusion gene *PML-RAR alpha*. Among the other types of AML, cytogenetic studies are the most powerful prognostic factors. Favorable cytogenetics such as t(8;21) and inv(16)(p13;q22) are seen in 15% of cases and are, termed the "core-binding factor" leukemias because of common genetic lesions affecting DNA-binding elements. These patients have a higher chance of achieving both short- and long-term disease control. The majority of cases of AML are of intermediate risk and have either normal cytogenetics or abnormalities that do not confer strong prognostic significance. Within this large subgroup, a relatively favorable group of patients has been defined based on a molecular signature that includes mutations of nucleophosmin 1 (NPM1) and lacks the internal tandem duplication of the *FLT3* gene. A poor prognosis is conferred by the cytogenetics finding of monosomy 5 or 7, or complex cytogenetics with more than three separate abnormalities.

In ALL, the hyperdiploidy (with more than 50 chromosomes) is associated with a better prognosis, but is seldom seen in adults. Unfavorable cytogenetics in ALL are the Philadelphia chromosome t(9;22) and t(4;11), which has fusion genes involving the *MLL* gene at 11q23.

► Differential Diagnosis

AML must be distinguished from other myeloproliferative disorders, chronic myeloid leukemia, and myelodysplastic syndromes. Acute leukemia may also resemble a left-shifted bone marrow recovering from a previous toxic insult. If the question is in doubt, a bone marrow study should be repeated in several days to see if maturation has taken place. ALL must be separated from other lymphoproliferative disease such as chronic lymphocytic leukemia, lymphomas, and hairy cell leukemia. It may also be confused with the atypical lymphocytosis of mononucleosis and pertussis.

► Treatment

Most young patients with acute leukemia are treated with the objective of effecting a cure. The first step in treatment is to obtain complete remission, defined as normal peripheral blood with resolution of cytopenias, normal bone marrow with no excess blasts, and normal clinical status. The type of initial chemotherapy depends on the subtype of leukemia.

1. AML—Most patients with AML are treated with a combination of an anthracycline (daunorubicin or idarubicin) plus cytarabine, either alone or in combination with other agents. This therapy will produce complete remissions in 80% of patients under age 60 years and in 50–60% of older patients (see Tables 39–3 and 39–4). APL is treated differently from other forms of AML. Induction therapy should include an anthracycline plus all-*trans*-retinoic acid. With this approach 90–95% of patients will achieve complete remission. For patients with high-risk APL based on an initial white blood cell count > 10,000/mcL, the addition of arsenic trioxide may be beneficial, and the addition of this biologic agent may be helpful in other cases as well.

Once a patient has entered remission, postremission therapy should be given with curative intent whenever possible. Options include standard chemotherapy and autologous and allogeneic transplantation. The optimal treatment strategy depends on the patient's age and clinical status, and the risk factor profile of the leukemia. Significant advances have been made in the treatment of APL. With the use of all-trans retinoic acid, arsenic trioxide, and chemotherapy, 90% of patients remain in long-term remission. Only the uncommon group of high-risk patients (based on initial white blood cell count > 10,000/mcL) have not shared in this favorable outcome, but studies of the potentially synergistic combination of retinoic acid and arsenic trioxide may improve results here. For intermediate-risk patients with AML, cure rates for postremission therapy are 35–40% for chemotherapy, 40–50% for autologous transplantation, and 50–60% for allogeneic transplantation. Some types of AML whose cytogenetics involved core-binding factors have a more favorable prognosis, with cure rates of 50–60% with chemotherapy and 70–80% with autologous transplantation. Patients who do not enter remission or who have high-risk cytogenetics (such as monosomy 7 and complex cytogenetics) do far more poorly and are rarely cured with chemotherapy. Allogeneic transplantation is the treatment of choice, but cure rates are only 20–30%.

Once leukemia has recurred after initial chemotherapy, the prognosis is much more guarded. For patients in second remission, transplantation (autologous or allogeneic) offers a 20–40% chance of cure. For those patients with APL who relapse, arsenic trioxide can produce second remissions in 90% of cases, and autologous transplant in second remission produces cure rates of 60–70%.

2. ALL—Adults with ALL are treated with combination chemotherapy, including daunorubicin, vincristine, prednisone, and asparaginase. This treatment produces complete remissions in 90% of patients. Those patients with Philadelphia chromosome-positive ALL (or *bcr-abl* plus ALL) should have imatinib (or dasatinib) added to their initial chemotherapy.

Remission induction therapy for ALL is less myelosuppressive than treatment for AML and does not necessarily produce marrow aplasia. After achieving complete remission, patients receive central nervous system prophylaxis so that meningeal sequestration of leukemic cells does not develop. As with AML, patients may be treated with either chemotherapy or high-dose chemotherapy plus bone marrow transplantation. Treatment decisions are made based on patient age and risk factors of the disease. Low-risk patients with ALL may be treated with chemotherapy with a 70% chance of cure. Intermediate-risk patients have a 30–50% chance of cure with chemotherapy, and high-risk patients are rarely cured with chemotherapy alone. High-risk patients with adverse cytogenetics or poor responses to chemotherapy are best treated with allogeneic transplantation. Autologous transplantation is a possibility in high-risk patients who lack a suitable donor.

▶ **Prognosis**

Approximately 70–80% of adults with AML under age 60 years achieve complete remission. High-dose postremission chemotherapy leads to cure in 35–40% of these patients, and high-dose cytarabine has been shown to be superior to therapy with lower doses. Allogeneic bone marrow transplantation (for younger adults with HLA-matched siblings) is curative in 50–60% of cases. Autologous bone marrow transplantation may be superior to nonablative chemotherapy. Older adults with AML achieve complete remission in up to 50% of instances. The cure rates for older patients with AML have been very low (approximately 10–15%) even if they achieve remission and are able to receive postremission chemotherapy. The use of reduced-intensity allogeneic transplantation is being explored in order to improve on these outcomes.

▶ **When to Refer**

All patients should be referred to a hematologist.

▶ **When to Admit**

Most patients with acute leukemia will be admitted for treatment.

Ades L et al. Treatment of newly diagnosed acute promyelocytic leukemia (APL): a comparison of French-Belgian-Swiss and PETHEMA results. Blood. 2008 Feb 1;111(3):1078–84. [PMID: 17975017]

Apostolidou E et al. Treatment of acute lymphoblastic leukaemia: a new era. Drugs. 2007;67(15):2153–71. [PMID: 17927282]

Estey E. Acute myeloid leukemia and myelodysplastic syndromes in older patients. J Clin Oncol. 2007 May 10; 25(14):1908–15. [PMID: 17488990]

Fielding A. The treatment of adults with acute lymphoblastic leukemia. Hematology Am Soc Hematol Educ Program. 2008:381–9. [PMID: 19074114]

Sorror ML et al. Comorbidity and disease status based risk stratification of outcomes among patients with acute myeloid leukemia or myelodysplasia receiving allogeneic hematopoietic cell transplantation. J Clin Oncol. 2007 Sep 20;25(27):4246–54. [PMID: 17724349]

CHRONIC LYMPHOCYTIC LEUKEMIA

ESSENTIALS OF DIAGNOSIS

▶ Lymphocytosis > 5000/mcL.
▶ Coexpression of CD19, CD5 on lymphocytes.

General Considerations

Chronic lymphocytic leukemia (CLL) is a clonal malignancy of B lymphocytes. The disease is usually indolent, with slowly progressive accumulation of long-lived small lymphocytes. These cells are immunoincompetent and respond poorly to antigenic stimulation.

CLL is manifested clinically by immunosuppression, bone marrow failure, and organ infiltration with lymphocytes. Immunodeficiency is also related to inadequate antibody production by the abnormal B cells. With advanced disease, CLL may cause damage by direct tissue infiltration.

Information about CLL is now evolving rapidly, with new findings in biology and new treatment options.

Clinical Findings

A. Symptoms and Signs

CLL is a disease of older patients, with 90% of cases occurring after age 50 years and a median age at presentation of 70 years. Many patients will be incidentally discovered to have lymphocytosis. Others present with fatigue or lymphadenopathy. On examination, 80% of patients will have lymphadenopathy and 50% will have enlargement of the liver or spleen.

The long-standing Rai classification system remains prognostically useful today: stage 0, lymphocytosis only; stage I, lymphocytosis plus lymphadenopathy; stage II, organomegaly; stage III, anemia; stage IV, thrombocytopenia. These stages can be collapsed in to low-risk (stages 0–I), intermediate risk (stage II) and high-risk (stages III–IV).

CLL usually pursues an indolent course, but some subtypes behave more aggressively; a variant, prolymphocytic leukemia, is more aggressive. The morphology of the latter is different, characterized by larger and more immature cells. In 5–10% of cases, CLL may be complicated by autoimmune hemolytic anemia or autoimmune thrombocytopenia. In approximately 5% of cases, while the systemic disease remains stable, an isolated lymph node transforms into an aggressive large cell lymphoma (**Richter syndrome**).

B. Laboratory Findings

The hallmark of CLL is isolated lymphocytosis. The white blood count is usually greater than 20,000/mcL and may be markedly elevated to several hundred thousand. Usually 75–98% of the circulating cells are lymphocytes. Lymphocytes appear small and mature, with condensed nuclear chromatin, and are morphologically indistinguishable from normal small lymphocytes, but smaller numbers of larger and activated lymphocytes may be seen. The hemat-

ocrit and platelet count are usually normal at presentation. The bone marrow is variably infiltrated with small lymphocytes. The immunophenotype of CLL demonstrates coexpression of the B lymphocyte lineage marker CD19 with the T lymphocyte marker CD5; this finding is commonly observed only in CLL and mantle cell lymphoma. CLL is distinguished from mantle cell lymphoma by the expression of CD23, low expression of surface immunoglobulin and CD20, and the absence of overexpression of cyclin D1. Patients whose CLL cells have mutated forms of the immunoglobulin gene (which can currently be tested only in research laboratories) have a more indolent form of disease; these cells typically express low levels of the surface antigen CD38 and do not express the zeta-associated protein (ZAP-70). Conversely, patients whose cells have unmutated IgV genes and high levels of ZAP-70 expression do less well and require treatment sooner. The assessment of genomic changes by fluorescence in-situ hybridization (FISH) provides important prognostic information. The finding of deletions of chromosome 17p or 11q confers a poor prognosis, whereas those whose only genomic change is deletion of 13q have a very favorable outcome.

Hypogammaglobulinemia is present in 50% of patients and becomes more common with advanced disease. In some, a small amount of IgM paraprotein is present in the serum.

Differential Diagnosis

Few syndromes can be confused with CLL. Viral infections producing lymphocytosis should be obvious from the presence of fever and other clinical findings; however, fever may occur in CLL from concomitant bacterial infection. Pertussis may cause a particularly high total lymphocyte count. Other lymphoproliferative diseases such as Waldenström macroglobulinemia, hairy cell leukemia, or lymphoma (especially mantle cell) in the leukemic phase are distinguished on the basis of the morphology and immunophenotype of circulating lymphocytes and bone marrow.

Treatment

Most cases of early indolent CLL require no specific therapy, and the standard of care for early stage disease has been observation. Indications for treatment include progressive fatigue, symptomatic lymphadenopathy, or anemia or thrombocytopenia. These patients have either symptomatic and progressive Rai stage II disease or stage III/IV disease. The initial treatment of choice is the combination of the chemotherapeutic agent fludarabine plus the antibody rituximab, with or without the addition of the chemotherapeutic drug cyclophosphamide. The addition of cyclophosphamide appears to have greater anti-leukemic effectiveness but also increases the risk of treatment-related infection. The question of whether this increase in toxicity is warranted by improved anti-leukemic effectiveness is currently being studied. Chlorambucil, 0.6–1 mg/kg orally every 3 weeks for approximately 6 months, was the standard treatment prior to the development of fludarabine. This treatment is convenient, well tolerated, and remains a reasonable first choice for elderly patients for whom frequent trips to the clinician's office is a hardship. The monoclonal antibody alemtuzumab is approved for treatment of refractory CLL and can be especially useful in clearing the blood and bone marrow of disease. However, it produces significant immunosuppression, and its role in primary therapy has been limited due to the risk of severe and fatal infections. Lenalidomide has been shown to have effectiveness in refractory cases of CLL, and its role in primary therapy is being studied. The investigational agent flavopiridol has produced encouraging results in types of CLL (such as those with deletions of 17p) that have not responded to other treatments.

Associated autoimmune hemolytic anemia or immune thrombocytopenia may require treatment with rituximab, prednisone, or splenectomy. Fludarabine should be avoided in patients with autoimmune hemolytic anemia since it may exacerbate this condition. Patients with recurrent bacterial infections and hypogammaglobulinemia benefit from prophylactic infusions of gamma globulin 0.4 g/kg/month), but this treatment is very expensive and can be justified only when these infections are severe.

Allogeneic transplantation offers potentially curative treatment for patients with CLL, but it should be used only in patients whose disease cannot be controlled by standard therapies. Nonmyeloablative allogeneic transplant has produced encouraging results and may expand the role of transplant in CLL. Some subtypes of CLL with genomic abnormalities such as 17p deletions have a sufficiently poor prognosis with standard therapies that early intervention with allogeneic transplant is being studied to assess whether it can improve outcomes.

Prognosis

New therapies are changing the prognosis of CLL. In the past, median survival was approximately 6 years, and only 25% of patients lived more than 10 years. Patients with stage 0 or stage I disease have a median survival of 10–15 years, and these patients may be reassured that they can live a normal life for many years. Patients with stage III or stage IV disease had a median survival of less than 2 years in the past, but with fludarabine-based combination therapies, 2-year survival is now greater than 90% and the long-term outlook appears to be substantially changed. For patients with high-risk and resistant forms of CLL, there is evidence that allogeneic transplantation can overcome risk factors and lead to long-term disease control.

When to Refer

All patients with CLL should be referred to a hematologist.

When to Admit

Hospitalization is rarely needed.

Flinn IW et al. Phase III trial of fludarabine plus cyclophosphamide compared with fludarabine for patients with previously untreated chronic lymphocytic leukemia: US Intergroup Trial E2997. J Clin Oncol. 2007 Mar 1;25(7):793–8. [PMID: 17283364]

Hallek M et al. Guidelines for the diagnosis and treatment of chronic lymphocytic leukemia: a report from the International Workshop on Chronic Lymphocytic Leukemia updating the National Cancer Center Institute-Working Group 1996 guidelines. Blood. 2008 Jun 15;111(12):5446–56. [PMID: 18216293]

Tam CS et al. Long-term results of the fludarabine, cyclophosphamide, and rituximab regimen as initial therapy of chronic lymphocytic leukemia. Blood. 2008 Aug 15;112(4):975–80. [PMID: 18411418]

HAIRY CELL LEUKEMIA

ESSENTIALS OF DIAGNOSIS

► Pancytopenia.
► Splenomegaly, often massive.
► Hairy cells present on blood smear and especially in bone marrow biopsy.

► General Considerations

Hairy cell leukemia, an uncommon form of leukemia, is an indolent cancer of B lymphocytes.

► Clinical Findings

A. Symptoms and Signs

The disease characteristically presents in middle-aged men. The median age at presentation is 55 years, and there is a striking 5:1 male predominance. Most patients present with gradual onset of fatigue, others complain of symptoms related to markedly enlarged spleen, and some come to attention because of infection.

Splenomegaly is almost invariably present and may be massive. The liver is enlarged in 50% of cases; lymphadenopathy is uncommon.

Hairy cell leukemia is usually an indolent disorder whose course is dominated by pancytopenia and recurrent infections, including mycobacterial infections.

B. Laboratory Findings

The hallmark of hairy cell leukemia is pancytopenia. Anemia is nearly universal, and 75% of patients have thrombocytopenia and neutropenia. Nearly all patients have striking monocytopenia, which is encountered in almost no other condition. The "hairy cells" are usually present in small numbers on the peripheral blood smear and have a characteristic appearance with numerous cytoplasmic projections. The bone marrow is usually inaspirable (dry tap), and the diagnosis is made by characteristic morphology on bone marrow biopsy. The hairy cells have a characteristic histochemical staining pattern, with tartrate-resistant acid phosphatase (TRAP). On immunophenotyping, the cells coexpress the antigens CD11c and CD22. Pathologic examination of the spleen shows marked infiltration of the red pulp with hairy cells. This is in contrast to the usual predilection of lymphomas to involve the white pulp of the spleen.

Differential Diagnosis

Hairy cell leukemia should be distinguished from other lymphoproliferative diseases such as Waldenström macroglobulinemia and non-Hodgkin lymphomas. It also may be confused with other causes of pancytopenia, including hypersplenism due to any cause, aplastic anemia, and paroxysmal nocturnal hemoglobinuria.

Treatment

The treatment of choice is intravenous cladribine (2-chlorodeoxyadenosine; CdA), 0.14 mg/kg daily for 7 days. This is a relatively nontoxic drug that produces benefit in 95% of cases and complete remission in more than 80%. Responses are long-lasting, with few patients relapsing in the first few years. Treatment with pentostatin produces similar results, but that drug is more cumbersome to administer.

Course & Prognosis

The development of new therapies has changed the prognosis of this disease. Formerly, median survival was 6 years, and only one-third of patients survived longer than 10 years. More than 95% of patients with hairy cell leukemia will live longer than 10 years.

Ravandi F et al. Eradication of minimal residual disease in hairy cell leukemia. Blood. 2006 Jun 15;107(12):4658–62. [PMID: 16497968]

Robak T et al. Cladribine in a weekly versus daily schedule for untreated active hairy cell leukemia: final report from the Polish Adult Leukemia Group (PALG) of a prospective, randomized, multicenter trial. Blood. 2007 May 1;109(9):3672–5. [PMID: 17209059]

Swords R et al. Hairy cell leukemia. Med Oncol. 2007;24(1):7–15. [PMID: 17673807]

LYMPHOMAS

NON-HODGKIN LYMPHOMAS

ESSENTIALS OF DIAGNOSIS

▸ Often presents with painless lymphadenopathy.

▸ Pathologic diagnosis of lymphoma is made by pathologic examination of tissue.

General Considerations

The non-Hodgkin lymphomas are a heterogeneous group of cancers of lymphocytes. The disorders vary in clinical presentation and course from indolent to rapidly progressive.

Molecular biology has provided clues to the pathogenesis of these disorders. The best-studied example is Burkitt lymphoma, in which a characteristic cytogenetic abnormality of translocation between the long arms of chromosomes 8 and 14 has been identified. The protooncogene c-myc is translocated from its normal position on chromosome 8 to the heavy chain locus on chromosome 14. Cells committed to B cell differentiation are likely to have enhanced expression of this heavy chain locus, and it is likely that overexpression of c-myc (in its new anomalous position) is related to malignant transformation. In the follicular lymphomas, the t(14,18) translocation is characteristic and results in overexpression of bcl-2, resulting in protection against apoptosis, the usual mechanism of cell death.

Classification of the lymphomas is a controversial area still undergoing evolution. The most recent grouping (Table 13–16) separates diseases based on both clinical and pathologic features.

Clinical Findings

A. Symptoms and Signs

Patients with indolent lymphomas usually present with painless lymphadenopathy, which may be isolated or widespread. Involved lymph nodes may be present in the retroperitoneum, mesentery, and pelvis. The indolent lymphomas are usually disseminated at the time of diagnosis, and bone marrow involvement is frequent. Patients with intermediate and high-grade lymphomas may have constitutional symptoms such as fever, drenching night sweats, or weight loss.

On examination, lymphadenopathy may be isolated, or extranodal sites of disease (skin, gastrointestinal tract) may be found. Patients with Burkitt lymphoma are noted to have abdominal pain or abdominal fullness because of the predilection of the disease for the abdomen.

Once a pathologic diagnosis is established, the patient is staged. Chest radiograph and CT scan of the abdomen and pelvis, bone marrow biopsy, and—in selected cases with high-risk morphology—a lumbar puncture are performed.

Table 13-16. World Health Organization proposed classification of non-Hodgkin lymphomas.

Precursor B
B cell lymphoblastic lymphoma
Mature B
Diffuse large B cell lymphoma
Mediastinal large B cell lymphoma
Follicular lymphoma
Small lymphocytic lymphoma
Lymphoplasmacytic lymphoma
Mantle cell lymphoma
Burkitt lymphoma
Marginal zone lymphoma
MALT type
Nodal
Splenic
Mucosal tissue associated
Precursor T
T cell lymphoblastic lymphoma
Mature T (and NK cell)
Anaplastic T cell lymphoma
Peripheral T cell lymphoma

B. Laboratory Findings

The peripheral blood is usually normal, but a number of lymphomas may present in a leukemic phase.

Bone marrow involvement is manifested as paratrabecular lymphoid aggregates. In some high-grade lymphomas, the meninges are involved and malignant cells are found with cerebrospinal fluid cytology. The chest radiograph may show a mediastinal mass in lymphoblastic lymphoma. The serum LDH has been shown to be a useful prognostic marker and is now incorporated in risk stratification of treatment.

The diagnosis of lymphoma is made by tissue biopsy. Needle aspiration may yield suspicious results, but a lymph node biopsy (or biopsy of involved extranodal tissue) is required for diagnosis and staging.

Molecular profiling based on the examination of gene expression may lead to a new classification of the lymphomas.

▶ Treatment

The treatment of indolent lymphoma depends on the stage of disease and the clinical status of the patient. A small number of patients have limited disease with only one abnormal lymph node and may be treated with localized irradiation with curative intent. Most patients with indolent lymphoma have disseminated disease at the time of diagnosis. If the disease is not bulky and the patient not symptomatic, no initial therapy may be required. Some patients will have spontaneous remissions and may defer treatment for 1–3 years. There are an increasing number of reasonable treatment options for low-grade lymphomas, but no clear consensus has emerged on the best strategy. Treatment with the anti-CD20 antibody rituximab is a commonly used treatment because of its very low toxicity and avoidance of chemotherapy. Combinations of rituximab with chemotherapy may also be used. Common chemotherapy regimens include fludarabine; the combination of cyclophosphamide, vincristine, and prednisone (R-CVP); and cyclophosphamide, doxorubicin, vincristine, prednisone (R-CHOP). Radioimmunoconjugates that fuse anti-B cell antibodies with radiation may produce improved results with modest increases in toxicity compared with antibody alone, and one such agent (yttrium-90 ibritumomab tiuxetan) is in use. Some patients with clinically aggressive low-grade lymphomas may be appropriate candidates for allogeneic transplantation. As in other hematologic malignancies, the use of less toxic nonmyeloablative regimens for allogeneic transplant may expand the role of transplant in this disease. The role of autologous transplantation for follicular lymphoma remains uncertain, but some patients with recurrent disease appear to have prolonged remissions.

Patients with diffuse large B-cell lymphoma are treated with curative intent. Those with localized disease receive either short-course chemo-immunotherapy (such as three courses of R-CHOP) plus localized radiation or six courses of chemotherapy without radiation. Most patients who have more advanced disease are treated with six to eight cycles of chemotherapy such as R-CHOP. Individuals with very high-risk lymphoma may benefit from autologous stem cell transplantation early in the course. Patients with diffuse large B-cell lymphoma who relapse after initial chemotherapy may still be cured by autologous stem cell transplantation if their disease remains responsive to chemotherapy.

Persons with **special forms of lymphoma** require individualized therapy. Burkitt lymphoma is treated with intensive regimens specifically tailored for this histologic type. Those with lymphoblastic lymphoma receive regimens similar to those used for T cell ALL. Mantle cell lymphoma is not effectively treated with standard chemotherapy regimens. Intensive initial therapy including autologous stem cell transplantation has been shown to improve outcomes and is now the standard of care. Reduced-intensity allogeneic stem cell transplantation offers curative potential. Patients with mucosal associated lymphoid tumors (MALT lymphomas) of the stomach may be appropriately treated with combination antibiotics directed against *Helicobacter pylori* but require frequent endoscopic monitoring.

▶ Prognosis

The median survival of patients with indolent lymphomas has been 6–8 years, but this appears to be improving. These diseases ultimately become refractory to chemotherapy. This often occurs at the time of histologic progression of the disease to a more aggressive form of lymphoma.

The International Prognostic Index is widely used to categorize patients with intermediate-grade lymphoma into risk groups. Factors that confer adverse prognosis are age over 60 years, elevated serum LDH, stage III or stage IV disease, and poor performance status. Patients with no risk factors or one risk factor have high complete response rates (80%) to standard chemotherapy, and most responses (80%) are durable. Patients with two risk factors have a 70% complete response rate, 70% being long-lasting. Patients with higher-risk disease have lower response rates and poor survival with standard regimens, and alternative treatments are needed. Early treatment with high-dose therapy and autologous stem cell transplantation improves the outcome.

For patients who relapse after initial chemotherapy, the prognosis depends on whether the lymphoma is still partially sensitive to chemotherapy. If it is, autologous transplantation offers a 50% chance of long-term salvage.

The treatment of older patients with lymphoma has been difficult because of poorer tolerance of aggressive chemotherapy. The use of myeloid growth factors and prophylactic antibiotics to reduce neutropenic complications may improve outcomes.

Molecular profiling techniques using gene array technology are being studied to better define subsets of lymphomas with different biologic features and prognoses.

▶ When to Refer

All patients with lymphoma should be referred to a hematologist or an oncologist.

▶ When to Admit

Admission is necessary only for specific complications.

Fanale MA et al. Monoclonal antibodies in the treatment of non-Hodgkin's lymphoma. Drugs. 2007;67(3):333–50. [PMID: 17335294]

Jaffe ES et al. Classification of lymphoid neoplasms: the microscope as a tool for disease discovery. Blood. 2008 Dec 1;112(12):4384–99. [PMID: 19029456]

Sparano JA. HIV-associated lymphoma: the evidence for treating aggressively but with caution. Curr Opin Oncol. 2007 Sep;19(5):458–63. [PMID: 17762571]

HODGKIN DISEASE

 ESSENTIALS OF DIAGNOSIS

▶ Painless lymphadenopathy.

▶ Constitutional symptoms may or may not be present.

▶ Pathologic diagnosis by lymph node biopsy.

General Considerations

Hodgkin disease is a group of cancers characterized by Reed–Sternberg cells in an appropriate reactive cellular background. The malignant cell is derived from B lymphocytes of germinal center origin.

Clinical Findings

There is a bimodal age distribution, with one peak in the 20s and a second over age 50 years. Most patients seek medical attention because of a painless mass, commonly in the neck. Others may seek medical attention because of constitutional symptoms such as fever, weight loss, or drenching night sweats, or because of generalized pruritus. An unusual symptom of Hodgkin disease is pain in an involved lymph node following alcohol ingestion.

An important feature of Hodgkin disease is its tendency to arise within single lymph node areas and spread in an orderly fashion to contiguous areas of lymph nodes. Only late in the course of the disease will vascular invasion lead to widespread hematogenous dissemination.

Hodgkin disease is divided into several subtypes: lymphocyte predominance, nodular sclerosis, mixed cellularity, and lymphocyte depletion. Hodgkin disease should be distinguished pathologically from other malignant lymphomas and may occasionally be confused with reactive lymph nodes seen in infectious mononucleosis, cat-scratch disease, or drug reactions (eg, phenytoin).

Patients undergo a staging evaluation to determine the extent of disease. The staging nomenclature (Ann Arbor) is as follows: stage I, one lymph node region involved; stage II, involvement of two lymph node areas on one side of the diaphragm; stage III, lymph node regions involved on both sides of the diaphragm; and stage IV, disseminated disease with bone marrow or liver involvement. In addition, patients are designated stage A if they lack constitutional symptoms and stage B if 10% weight loss over 6 months, fever, or night sweats are present. If symptoms indicate careful evaluation for higher numerical stage, clinical stage IB (for example) is highly likely to emerge as stage II or stage IIIB.

Treatment

The treatment of Hodgkin disease has evolved, with radiation therapy used as initial treatment only for patients with low-risk stage IA and IIA disease. The addition of limited chemotherapy for some patients treated with radiation appears promising.

Most patients with Hodgkin disease (including all with stage IIIB and IV disease) are best treated with combination chemotherapy using doxorubicin (Adriamycin), bleomycin, vincristine, and dacarbazine (ABVD). New shorter and more intensive regimens are being studied, but have not yet proved superior to ABVD.

Prognosis

All patients with both localized and disseminated disease should be treated with curative intent. The prognosis of patients with stage IA or IIA disease treated by radiotherapy is excellent, with 10-year survival rates in excess of 80%. Patients with disseminated disease (IIIB, IV) have 5-year survival rates of 50–60%. Poorer results are seen in patients who are older, those who have bulky disease, and those with lymphocyte depletion or mixed cellularity on histologic examination. The prognosis of those with the lymphocyte-predominant form of the disease is better than in other subtypes, with cure seen in > 70% of those with disseminated disease and with limited treatment needed for those with early-stage disease. Others whose disease recurs after initial radiotherapy treatment may still be curable with chemotherapy. The treatment of choice for patients who relapse after initial chemotherapy is high-dose chemotherapy with autologous stem cell transplantation. This offers a 35–50% chance of cure when disease is still chemotherapy sensitive.

Byrne BJ et al. Salvage therapy in Hodgkin's lymphoma. Oncologist. 2007 Feb;12(2):156–67. [PMID: 17296811]

Engert A et al. Two cycles of doxorubicin, bleomycin, vinblastine, and dacarbazine plus extended-field radiotherapy is superior to radiotherapy alone in early favorable Hodgkin's lymphoma: final results of the GHSG HD7 trial. J Clin Oncol. 2007 Aug 10;25(23):3495–502. [PMID: 17606976]

Fermé C et al; EORTC-GELA H8 Trial. Chemotherapy plus involved-field radiation in early-stage Hodgkin's disease. N Engl J Med. 2007 Nov 8;357(19):1916–27. [PMID: 17989384]

Franklin J et al. Second malignancy risk associated with treatment of Hodgkin's lymphoma: meta-analysis of the randomised trials. Ann Oncol. 2006 Dec;17(12):1749–60. [PMID: 16984979]

Grulich AE et al. Incidence of cancers in people with HIV/AIDS compared with immunosuppressed transplant recipients: a meta-analysis. Lancet. 2007 Jul 7;370(9581):59–67. [PMID: 17617273]

MULTIPLE MYELOMA

 ESSENTIALS OF DIAGNOSIS

▶ Bone pain, often in the lower back.

▶ Monoclonal paraprotein by serum or urine protein electrophoresis or immunofixation.

▶ Abnormal plasma cells ≥ 20% of bone marrow.

General Considerations

Multiple myeloma is a malignancy of plasma cells characterized by replacement of the bone marrow, bone destruction, and paraprotein formation.

Malignant plasma cells can form tumors (plasmacytomas) that may cause spinal cord compression. The pathogenesis of osteoclast activation in myeloma appears to involve osteoprotegerin ligand, and the decoy receptor osteoprotegerin may be able to interfere with this pathway.

The paraproteins secreted by the malignant plasma cells may cause problems in their own right. Very high paraprotein levels (either IgG or IgA) may cause hyperviscosity, though this is more often caused by IgM in Waldenström macroglobulinemia. The light chain component of the immunoglobulin often leads to kidney failure (often aggravated by hypercalcemia). Light chain components may be deposited in tissues as amyloid, worsening kidney failure with albuminuria and causing a vast array of systemic symptoms.

Myeloma patients are prone to recurrent infections for a number of reasons, including neutropenia and the immunosuppressive effects of chemotherapy. More often, there is a failure of antibody production in response to antigen challenge, and myeloma patients are especially prone to infections with encapsulated organisms such as *Streptococcus pneumoniae* and *Haemophilus influenzae*.

Clinical Findings

A. Symptoms and Signs

Myeloma is a disease of older adults (median age at presentation, 65 years). The most common presenting complaints are those related to anemia, bone pain, and infection. Bone pain is most common in the back or ribs or may present as a pathologic fracture, especially of the femoral neck. Patients may also come to medical attention because of kidney failure, spinal cord compression, or the hyperviscosity syndrome (mucosal bleeding, vertigo, nausea, visual disturbances, alterations in mental status). Equally as often, patients are diagnosed because of laboratory findings of hypercalcemia, proteinuria, elevated sedimentation rate, or abnormalities on serum protein electrophoresis obtained for symptoms or in routine screening studies. A few patients come to medical attention because of amyloidosis.

Examination may reveal pallor, bone tenderness, and soft tissue masses. Patients may have neurologic signs related to neuropathy and spinal cord compression. Patients with amyloidosis may have an enlarged tongue, neuropathy, congestive heart failure, or hepatomegaly. Splenomegaly is absent unless amyloidosis is present. Fever occurs only with infection.

B. Laboratory Findings

Anemia is nearly universal. Red blood cell morphology is normal, but rouleau formation is common and may be marked. The neutrophil and platelet counts are usually normal at presentation. Only rarely will plasma cells be visible on peripheral smear (plasma cell leukemia).

The hallmark of myeloma is the finding of a paraprotein on serum protein electrophoresis (SPEP). The majority of patients will have a monoclonal spike visible in the β- or γ-globulin region. Immunofixation (IF) will reveal this to be a monoclonal protein. Approximately 15% of patients will have no demonstrable paraprotein in the serum because their myeloma cells produce only light chains and not intact immunoglobulin, and the light chains pass through the glomerulus into the urine. The paraprotein will be demonstrated by electrophoresis and immunofixation of the urine. A recently developed assay for serum free light chains will similarly demonstrate the abnormality. Overall, approximately 60% of patients with myeloma will have an IgG paraprotein, 25% an IgA, and 15% light chains only. In sporadic cases, no paraprotein is present ("nonsecretory myeloma"); these patients have particularly aggressive disease.

The bone marrow will be infiltrated by variable numbers of plasma cells ranging from 20% to 100%. The plasma cells will occasionally appear normal but more commonly are morphologically abnormal. The plasma cells will display marked skewing of the ratio of kappa to lambda light chain, which will indicate their clonality. Many benign processes can result in plasmacytosis, but the presence of atypical plasma cells, light chain skewing, or effacement of normal bone marrow elements helps distinguish myeloma. Bone radiographs are important in establishing the diagnosis of myeloma. Lytic lesions are most commonly seen in the axial skeleton: skull, spine, proximal long bones, and ribs. At other times, only generalized osteoporosis is seen. The radionuclide bone scan is not useful in detecting bone lesions in myeloma, as there is usually no osteoblastic component. Positron emission tomography (PET) scans will demonstrate significantly more disease than is shown in plain radiographs, but their use has not yet become standard. The International Staging System for myeloma relies on two factors, β_2-microglobulin and albumin. Stage 1 patients have both β_2-microglobulin < 3.5 mg/L and albumin ≥ 3.5; Stage 3 is diagnosed when β_2-microglobulin > 5.5 mg/L, and stage 2 is diagnosed with values in between. The other laboratory finding of important prognostic significance is genetic abnormalities diagnosed by FISH involving the immunoglobulin heavy chain locus at chromosome 14q32. The translocations involved are usually t(4;14) and less commonly t(14;16). The previous finding of the adverse prognostic effect of deletions of chromosome 13 now appear to be due to the linkage between 13q deletions and 14q32 abnormalities. Abnormalities of chromosome 17p also appear to confer a poor prognosis. Hypercalcemia is an important laboratory finding in myeloma and is associated with kidney failure.

Differential Diagnosis

When a patient is discovered to have a monoclonal paraprotein, the distinction between myeloma and monoclonal gammopathy of unknown significance (MGUS) must be made. MGUS is present in 1% of all adults and 3% of adults over age 70 years. Thus, among all patients with paraproteins, MGUS is far more common than myeloma.

Most commonly, patients with MGUS will have a monoclonal IgG spike less than 2.5 g/dL, and the height of the spike remains stable. In approximately 25% of cases, MGUS progresses to overt malignant disease, but this may take many years.

Myeloma is distinguished from MGUS by findings of replacement of the bone marrow, bone destruction, and progression. Although the height of the paraprotein spike should not be used by itself to distinguish benign from malignant disease, nearly all patients with IgG spikes greater than 3.5 g/dL prove to have myeloma; an IgA spike of > 2 g/dL is similarly suggestive. If there is doubt about whether paraproteinemia is benign or malignant, the patient should be observed without therapy, since there is no advantage to early treatment of asymptomatic multiple myeloma.

Myeloma must be distinguished from reactive polyclonal hypergammaglobulinemia. Myeloma may also be similar to other malignant lymphoproliferative diseases such as Waldenström macroglobulinemia, lymphomas, and primary amyloidosis (with which it is commonly associated).

Treatment

Patients with minimal disease or in whom the diagnosis of malignancy is in doubt should be observed without treatment. Most commonly, patients require treatment at diagnosis because of bone pain or other symptoms related to the disease. The initial step in treatment, referred to as "**induction**," has changed from being based on cytotoxic chemotherapy to being based on other biologic agents. The immunomodulatory agents (IMIDs) have significant activity in myeloma; the second-generation agent lenalidomide is both more active and less toxic than thalidomide and has replaced the older drug in treatment. It is given orally and is generally well tolerated. The major side effect of lenalidomide is cumulative myelosuppression, and some type of prophylaxis is needed to prevent deep venous thrombosis. Bortezomib, a proteosome inhibitor, is also highly active and has the advantages of producing rapid responses and of being effective in poor-prognosis myeloma. The major side effect of bortezomib is neuropathy (both peripheral and autonomic), and it has the disadvantage of requiring frequent intravenous administration. At the present time, induction therapy should include dexamethasone and either lenalidomide or bortezomib or both. The combination of bortezomib, dexamethasone, and the chemotherapeutic agent doxorubicin liposomal is also highly successful.

After induction therapy, the optimal **consolidation therapy** for patients under age 70 years with myeloma is autologous stem cell transplantation. Early aggressive treatment prolongs both duration of remission and overall survival, and has the advantage of providing long treatment-free intervals. Clinical trials are evaluating the role of posttransplant maintenance therapy with agents such as lenalidomide. For young patients with aggressive disease, autologous transplant followed by a reduced-intensity allogeneic transplant is under active investigation.

Allogeneic transplantation is potentially curative in myeloma, but its role has been limited because of the unusually high mortality rate (40–50%) in myeloma patients.

Newer and less toxic forms of allogeneic transplantation using nonmyeloablative regimens have produced encouraging results, especially when performed early in the course of disease, such as the minimal disease state following autologous stem cell transplantation.

Localized radiotherapy may be useful for palliation of bone pain or for eradicating tumor at the site of pathologic fracture. Hypercalcemia should be treated aggressively and immobilization and dehydration avoided. The bisphosphonates (pamidronate 90 mg or zoledronic acid 4 mg intravenously monthly) reduce pathologic fractures in patients with significant bony disease and are an important adjunct in this subset of patients. However, long-term zoledronate has been associated with a risk of osteonecrosis of the jaw, and patients must be monitored for this complication.

Prognosis

The outlook for patients with myeloma has been steadily improving for the past decade. The median survival of patients is now between 4 and 6 years, and it is possible that the use of newly approved agents will result in further survival gains. Patients with low-stage disease (low β_2-microglobulin and normal albumin) who lack the high-risk genomic changes involving chromosome 14q32 respond very well to treatment and derive significant benefit from autologous stem cell transplantation as part of initial therapy. With modern treatment, expected survivals for such patients are in excess of 6 years. Novel approaches, possibly involving allogeneic stem cell transplantation, are being studied to try to improve the outlook for patients with high-risk disease.

When to Refer

All patients with myeloma should be referred to a hematologist or an oncologist.

When to Admit

Hospitalization is indicated for treatment of acute kidney failure, hypercalcemia, or suspicion of spinal cord compression.

Attal M et al; Inter-Groupe Francophone du Myelome (IFM). Maintenance therapy with thalidomide improves survival in patients with multiple myeloma. Blood. 2006 Nov 15; 108(10):3289–94. [PMID: 16873668]

Facon T et al; Intergroupe Francophone du Myelome. Melphalan and prednisone plus thalidomide versus melphalan and prednisone alone or reduced-intensity autologous stem cell transplantation in elderly patients with multiple myeloma (IFM 99-06): a randomised trial. Lancet. 2007 Oct 6;370 (9594):1209–18. [PMID: 17920916]

Manochakian R et al. Clinical impact of bortezomib in frontline regimens for patients with multiple myeloma. Oncologist. 2007 Aug;12(8):978–90. [PMID: 17766658]

Orlowski RZ et al. Randomized phase III study of pegylated liposomal doxorubicin plus bortezomib compared with bortezomib alone in relapsed or refractory multiple myeloma: combination therapy improves time to progression. J Clin Oncol. 2007 Sep 1;25(25):3892–901. [PMID: 17679727]

WALDENSTRÖM MACROGLOBULINEMIA

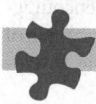

ESSENTIALS OF DIAGNOSIS

▸ Monoclonal IgM paraprotein.

▸ Infiltration of bone marrow by plasmacytic lymphocytes.

▸ Absence of lytic bone disease.

General Considerations

Waldenström macroglobulinemia is a malignant disease of B cells that appear to be a hybrid of lymphocytes and plasma cells. These cells characteristically secrete an IgM paraprotein, and many clinical manifestations of the disease are related to this macroglobulin.

Clinical Findings

A. Symptoms and Signs

This disease characteristically develops insidiously in patients in their 60s or 70s. Patients usually present with fatigue related to anemia. Hyperviscosity of serum may be manifested in a number of ways. Mucosal and gastrointestinal bleeding are related to engorged blood vessels and platelet dysfunction. Other complaints include nausea, vertigo, and visual disturbances. Alterations in consciousness vary from mild lethargy to stupor and coma. The IgM paraprotein may also cause symptoms of cold agglutinin disease or peripheral neuropathy.

On examination, there may be hepatosplenomegaly or lymphadenopathy. The retinal veins are engorged. Purpura may be present. There should be no bone tenderness.

B. Laboratory Findings

Anemia is nearly universal, and rouleau formation is common. The anemia is related in part to expansion of the plasma volume by 50–100% due to the presence of the paraprotein. Other blood counts are usually normal. The abnormal plasmacytic lymphocytes usually appear in small numbers on the peripheral blood smear. The bone marrow is characteristically infiltrated by the plasmacytic lymphocytes.

The hallmark of macroglobulinemia is the presence of a monoclonal IgM spike seen on SPEP in the β- or γ-globulin region. The serum viscosity is usually increased above the normal of 1.4–1.8 times that of water. Symptoms of hyperviscosity usually develop when the serum viscosity is over four times that of water, and marked symptoms usually arise when the viscosity is over six times that of water. Because paraproteins vary in their physicochemical properties, there is no strict correlation between the concentration of paraprotein and serum viscosity.

The IgM paraprotein may cause a positive Coombs test or have cold agglutinin or cryoglobulin properties. If macroglobulinemia is suspected but the SPEP shows only hypogammaglobulinemia, the test should be repeated while taking special measures to maintain the blood at 37 °C, since the paraprotein may precipitate out at room temperature if it is cryoprecipitable.

Bone radiographs are normal, and there is no evidence of kidney failure.

Differential Diagnosis

Waldenström macroglobulinemia is differentiated from monoclonal gammopathy of unknown significance by the finding of bone marrow infiltration. It is distinguished from chronic lymphocytic leukemia and multiple myeloma by bone marrow morphology and the finding of the characteristic IgM spike, and also on clinical grounds.

Treatment

Patients with marked hyperviscosity syndrome (stupor or coma) should be treated on an emergency basis with plasmapheresis. On a chronic basis, some patients can be managed with periodic plasmapheresis alone. As with other indolent lymphoid diseases, fludarabine and rituximab have replaced alkylator-based chemotherapy for initial therapy.

As with multiple myeloma, autologous stem cell transplantation is playing a more important role in management and is considered in younger patients with more aggressive disease.

Prognosis

Waldenström macroglobulinemia is an indolent disease with a median survival rate of 3–5 years. However, patients may survive 10 years or longer.

When to Refer

All patients should be referred to a hematologist or an oncologist.

When to Admit

Patients should be admitted for treatment of hyperviscosity syndrome.

Dimopoulos MA et al. Primary treatment of Waldenström macroglobulinemia with dexamethasone, rituximab, and cyclophosphamide. J Clin Oncol. 2007 Aug 1;25(22):3344–9. [PMID: 17577016]

Vijay A et al. Waldenström macroglobulinemia. Blood. 2007 Jun 15;109(12):5096–103. [PMID: 17303694]

STEM CELL TRANSPLANTATION

Stem cell transplantation using hematopoietic stem cells is an extremely valuable treatment for a variety of hematologic malignancies and is also used in a few non-hematologic cancers and some nonmalignant conditions. In many cases, stem cell transplantation offers the only curative option for some types of cancer and can be a life-saving procedure.

The basis of treatment with stem cell transplantation is the ability of the hematopoietic stem cell to completely restore bone marrow function and formation of all blood components, as well as the ability to re-form the immune system. These hematopoietic stem cells were formerly collected from the bone marrow but are now more commonly collected from the peripheral blood after maneuvers to mobilize them from the bone marrow into the blood.

In the field of cancer chemotherapy, the dose-limiting toxicity of almost all chemotherapy has been myelosuppression, that is, damage to the bone marrow. It is typical during the administration of chemotherapy for blood counts to be transiently suppressed and to have to wait for recovery of the blood in order to safely give the next treatment. However, if too high a dose of chemotherapy is given, it is possible to damage the bone marrow beyond recovery, and for the blood counts to never return to within normal ranges. For cancers for which there is a dose-response relationship, that is, a relationship between the dose of chemotherapy administered and the number of cancer cells killed, the limits placed on the allowable dose of chemotherapy can make the difference between cure and failure to cure. In stem cell transplantation, the limit placed on the allowable dose of chemotherapy by the risks of permanent bone marrow damage is eliminated and much higher doses of chemotherapy can be given, since re-infusion of hematopoietic stem cells can completely restore the bone marrow.

AUTOLOGOUS STEM CELL TRANSPLANTION

Autologous stem cell transplantation is a treatment in which hematopoietic stem cells are collected from the patient and then re-infused after chemotherapy. Therefore, autologous stem cell transplantation relies solely for its effectiveness on the ability to give much higher doses of chemotherapy than would otherwise be possible. In this procedure, the hematopoietic stem cells are usually collected from the patient's peripheral blood. First, the hematopoietic stem cells are mobilized from the bone marrow into the blood. This can be accomplished by a variety of techniques, most commonly the use of myeloid growth factors such as filgrastim (granulocyte-colony stimulating factor, G-CSF) either alone or in combination with chemotherapy. The investigational agent plerixafor can also mobilize these cells into the blood. During the process of leukopheresis the patient's blood is centrifuged into layers of different densities; the hematopoietic stem cells are collected from the appropriate layer while the remainder of the blood elements are returned unchanged to the patient. After collection, these autologous hematopoietic stem cells are frozen and cryopreserved for later use. Treatment with autologous stem cell transplantation involves administration of high-dose chemotherapy (referred to as the "preparative regimen") followed, after clearance of the chemotherapy out of the patient's system, by intravenous re-infusion of the thawed autologous hematopoietic stem cells. The hematopoietic stem cells home to the bone marrow and grow into new bone marrow cells.

With the autologous stem cell transplantation treatment, there is a period of severe pancytopenia during the gap between myelosuppression caused by the chemotherapy and the recovery produced from the new bone marrow derived from the infused hematopoietic stem cells. This period of pancytopenia typically lasts 7–10 days and requires support with transfusions of red blood cells and platelets as well as antibiotics. Hospitalization to receive such treatment usually lasts 2–3 weeks. The morbidity of such a treatment varies according to the type of chemotherapy used, and the chance of fatal treatment-related complications is between 1% and 4%.

Autologous stem cell transplantation has the potential to cure cancers that would otherwise be fatal. Autologous stem cell transplantation is the treatment of choice for lymphomas such as diffuse large B-cell lymphomas that have recurred after initial chemotherapy but are still responsive to chemotherapy. It is similarly also the treatment of choice for relapsed Hodgkin lymphoma that still responds to chemotherapy, and for testicular germ cell cancers that have recurred. Autologous stem cell transplantation is also the treatment of choice for mantle cell lymphomas in first remission. Autologous stem cell transplantation also plays an important role in the treatment of AML in both first and second remission and is potentially curative in these settings. Autologous stem cell transplantation is currently part of the standard of care for the treatment of multiple myeloma, based not on curative potential, but the prolongation of remission.

ALLOGENEIC STEM CELL TRANSPLANTATION

Allogeneic stem cell transplantation is a treatment in which the source of hematopoietic stem cells to restore bone marrow and immune function are derived, not from the patient, but from a different donor. Initially allogeneic stem cell transplantation was thought to derive its effectiveness from the high-dose chemotherapy (or radiation plus chemotherapy) that forms the "preparative regimen" in a manner similar to autologous stem cell transplantation. However, it is now known that there is a second type of effector mechanism in allogeneic stem cell transplantation, the allo-immune graft-versus-malignancy (GVM) effect derived from the donor immune system. In some cases, this GVM effect can be more important than the chemotherapy in producing a cure of disease.

In order to perform an allogeneic stem cell transplantation, an appropriate donor of hematopoietic stem cells must be located. At the present time, it is important that the donor be matched with the patient (recipient) at the HLA loci (HLA A, B, C, DR) that specify major histocompatibility antigens. These donors may be full siblings or unrelated donors recruited from a large panel of anonymous volunteer donors through the National Marrow Donor Program (NMDP). Cells derived from umbilical cord blood units may also be used. The hematopoietic stem cells are collected from the donor either from the bone marrow, or, more commonly through leukopheresis of the blood after mobilizing hematopoietic stem cells from the bone marrow with filgrastim (G-CSF). They are infused intravenously into the recipient and may be given either fresh or after cryopreservation and thawing. The hematopoietic stem cells home to the bone marrow and start to grow.

In the allogeneic stem cell transplantation procedure, the patient is treated with the "preparative regimen" with two purposes: to treat the underlying cancer and to sufficiently suppress the patient's immune system so that the hematopoietic stem cells from the donor will not be rejected. As with autologous stem cell transplantation, the hematopoietic stem cells are infused after the preparative chemotherapy has been given and has had a chance to clear from the body. There is a period of pancytopenia in the gap between the effect of the chemotherapy given to the patient and the time it takes the infused hematopoietic stem cells to grow into bone marrow, usually 10–14 days.

A major difference between autologous and allogeneic SCT is that in the allogeneic setting, the patient becomes a "chimera", that is, a mixture of self and non-self. In allogeneic stem cell transplantation, the infused cells contain mature cells of the donor immune system, and the infused hematopoietic stem cells will grow into bone marrow and blood cells as well as cells of the new immune system. Unless the donor is an identical twin (called a "syngeneic transplant"), the donor's immune system will recognize the patient's tissues as foreign and initiate the "graft-versus-host" (GVH) reaction, the graft from the donor reacting against the patient (host). This GVH is the major cause of morbidity and mortality during an allogeneic SCT. Immunosuppression must be given during allogeneic stem cell transplantation to reduce the incidence and severity of GVH reaction. The most common regimen used for GVH prophylaxis is a combination of a calcineurin inhibitor (cyclosporine or tacrolimus) plus methotrexate. In contrast to the experience with solid organ transplant in which life-long immunosuppression is required to prevent rejection of the transplanted organ, in most cases of allogeneic stem cell transplantation, the immunosuppression can be tapered and discontinued 6 or more months after transplantation.

However, there is an important and positive side to the allo-immune reaction of the donor against the host. If there are residual cancer cells present in the patient that have survived the high-dose chemoradiotherapy of the preparative regimen, these residual cancer cells can be recognized as foreign by the donor immune system and killed in the GVM effect. Even cells that are resistant to chemotherapy may not be resistant to killing through the immune system. Depending on the type of cancer cell, this can be a highly effective mechanism of long-term cancer control. Based on the understanding of how important GVM can be, the allogeneic stem cell transplantation procedure can be modified by reducing the intensity of the preparative regimen, relying for cure more on the GVM effect and less on the high-dose chemotherapy. In these "reduced-intensity" allogeneic stem cell transplantation procedures, the preparative regimen still has to suppress the patient's immune system enough to avoid rejection of the donor hematopoietic stem cells, but these types of transplants can be far less toxic than full-dose transplants. Based on this greatly reduced short-term toxicity, the potential benefits of allogeneic stem cell transplantation have been extended to older adults (age 60–75) and to those with comorbid conditions that would have been a contraindication to standard full-dose stem cell transplantation.

Allogeneic stem cell transplantation is the treatment of choice for high-risk acute leukemias, and in many cases will be the only potentially curative treatment. Allogeneic stem cell transplantation is the only curative treatment for myelodysplasia and for CML, although its use in CML has been greatly curtailed based on the effectiveness of imatinib and related tyrosine kinase inhibitors. Allogeneic stem cell transplantation is also the only definitive treatment for most cases of severe aplastic anemia. The use of reduced-intensity allogeneic stem cell transplantation has led to its exploration in the management of difficult cases of CLL and follicular lymphoma, and it will likely play a major role in these diseases. Given the age of many patients with AML and myelodysplasia, this procedure will likely play an important role in these diseases as well.

Antin JH. Reduced-Intensity Stem Cell Transplantation: "...whereof a little More than a little is by much too much." King Henry IV, part 1, I, 2. Hematology Am Soc Hematol Educ Program. 2007:47–54. [PMID: 18024608]
Kolb HJ. Graft-versus-leukemia effects of transplantation and donor lymphocytes. Blood. 2008 Dec 1;112(12):4371–83. [PMID: 19029455]

BLOOD TRANSFUSIONS

RED BLOOD CELL TRANSFUSIONS

Red blood cell transfusions are given to raise the hematocrit levels in patients with anemia or to replace losses after acute bleeding episodes.

▶ Preparations of Red Cells for Transfusion

Several types of preparations containing red blood cells are available.

A. Fresh Whole Blood

The advantage of whole blood for transfusion is the simultaneous presence of red blood cells, plasma, and fresh platelets. Fresh whole blood is never absolutely necessary, since all the above components are available separately. The major indications for use of whole blood are cardiac surgery or massive hemorrhage when more than 10 units of blood is required in a 24-hour period.

B. Packed Red Blood Cells

Packed red cells are the component most commonly used to raise the hematocrit. Each unit has a volume of about 300 mL, of which approximately 200 mL consists of red blood cells. One unit of packed red cells will usually raise the hematocrit by approximately 4%. The expected rise in hematocrit can be calculated using an estimated red blood cell volume of 200 mL/unit and a total blood volume of about 70 mL/kg. For example, a 70-kg man will have a total blood volume of 4900 mL, and each unit of packed red blood cells will raise the hematocrit by 200 ÷ 4900, or 4%.

C. Leukocyte-Poor Blood

Patients with severe leukoagglutinin reactions to packed red blood cells may require depletion of white blood cells and platelets from transfused units. White blood cells can be removed either by centrifugation or by washing. Preparation of leukocyte-poor blood is expensive and leads to some loss of red cells.

D. Frozen Blood

Red blood cells can be frozen and stored for up to 3 years, but the technique is cumbersome and expensive, and frozen blood should be used sparingly. The major application is for the purpose of maintaining a supply of rare blood types. Patients with such types may donate units for autologous transfusion should the need arise. Frozen red cells are also occasionally needed for patients with severe leukoagglutinin reactions or anaphylactic reactions to plasma proteins, since frozen blood has essentially all white blood cells and plasma components removed.

E. Autologous Packed Red Blood Cells

Patients scheduled for elective surgery may donate blood for autologous transfusion. These units may be stored for up to 35 days.

▶ Compatibility Testing

Before transfusion, the recipient's and the donor's blood are cross-matched to avoid hemolytic transfusion reactions. Although many antigen systems are present on red blood cells, only the ABO and Rh systems are specifically tested prior to all transfusions. The A and B antigens are the most important, because everyone who lacks one or both red cell antigens has isoantibodies against the missing antigen or antigens in his or her plasma. These antibodies activate complement and can cause rapid intravascular lysis of the incompatible red cells. In emergencies, type O blood can be given to any recipient, but only packed cells should be given to avoid transfusion of donor plasma containing anti-A or anti-B antibodies.

The other important antigen routinely tested for is the D antigen of the Rh system. Approximately 15% of the population lack this antigen. In patients lacking the antigen, anti-D antibodies are not naturally present, but the antigen is highly immunogenic. A recipient whose red cells lack D and who receives D-positive blood may develop anti-D antibodies that can cause severe lysis of subsequent transfusions of D-positive red cells.

Blood typing includes assay of recipient serum for unusual antibodies by mixing the serum with panels of red cells representing commonly occurring weak antigens. The screening is particularly important if the recipient has had previous transfusions.

▶ Hemolytic Transfusion Reactions

The most severe reactions are those involving mismatches in the ABO system. Most of these cases are due to clerical errors and mislabeled specimens. Hemolysis is rapid and intravascular, releasing free hemoglobin into the plasma. The severity of these reactions depends on the dose of red blood cells given. The most severe reactions are those seen in surgical patients under anesthesia.

Hemolytic transfusion reactions caused by minor antigen systems are typically less severe. The hemolysis usually takes place at a slower rate and is extravascular. Sometimes these transfusion reactions may be delayed for 5–10 days after transfusion. In such cases, the recipient has received blood containing an immunogenic action, and in the time since transfusion, a new alloantibody has been formed. The most common antigens involved in such reactions are Duffy, Kidd, Kell, and C and E loci of the Rh system.

A. Symptoms and Signs

Major hemolytic transfusion reactions cause fever and chills, with backache and headache. In severe cases, there may be apprehension, dyspnea, hypotension, and vascular collapse. *The transfusion must be stopped immediately.* In severe cases, DIC, acute kidney failure from tubular necrosis, or both can occur.

Patients under general anesthesia will not manifest such signs, and the first indication may be generalized bleeding and oliguria.

B. Laboratory Findings

Identification of the recipient and of the blood should be checked. The donor transfusion bag with its pilot tube must be returned to the blood bank, and a fresh sample of the recipient's blood must accompany the donor bag for retyping of donor and recipient blood samples and for repeat of the cross-match.

The hematocrit will fail to rise by the expected amount. Coagulation studies may reveal evidence of kidney failure and DIC. Hemoglobinemia will turn the plasma pink and eventually result in hemoglobinuria. In cases of delayed hemolytic reactions, the hematocrit will fall and the indirect bilirubin will rise. In these cases, the new offending alloantibody is easily detected in the patient's serum.

C. Treatment

If a hemolytic transfusion reaction is suspected, the transfusion should be stopped at once. A sample of anticoagulated blood from the recipient should be centrifuged to detect free hemoglobin in the plasma. If hemoglobinemia is present, the patient should be vigorously hydrated to prevent acute tubular necrosis. Forced diuresis with mannitol may help prevent kidney damage.

▶ Leukoagglutinin Reactions

Most transfusion reactions are not hemolytic but represent reactions to antigens present on white blood cells in patients who have been sensitized to the antigens through previous transfusions or pregnancy. Most commonly, patients will develop fever and chills within 12 hours after transfusion. In severe cases, cough and dyspnea may occur and the chest radiograph may show transient pulmonary infiltrates. Because no hemolysis is involved, the hematocrit rises by the expected amount despite the reaction.

Leukoagglutinin reactions may respond to acetaminophen and diphenhydramine; corticosteroids are also of value. Removal of leukocytes by filtration before blood storage will reduce the incidence of these reactions.

Anaphylactic Reactions

Rarely, patients will develop urticaria or bronchospasm during a transfusion. These reactions are almost always due to plasma proteins rather than white blood cells. Patients who are IgA deficient may develop these reactions because of antibodies to IgA. Patients with such reactions may require transfusion of washed or even frozen red blood cells to avoid future severe reactions.

Contaminated Blood

Rarely, blood is contaminated with gram-negative bacteria. Transfusion can lead to septicemia and shock from endotoxin. If this is suspected, the offending unit should be cultured and the patient treated with antibiotics as indicated.

Diseases Transmitted Through Transfusion

Despite the use of only volunteer blood donors and the routine screening of blood, transfusion-associated viral diseases remain a problem. All blood products (red blood cells, platelets, plasma, cryoprecipitate) can transmit viral diseases. All blood donors are screened with questionnaires designed to detect donors at high risk of transmitting diseases. All blood is now screened for hepatitis B surface antigen, antibody to hepatitis B core antigen, syphilis, p24 antigen and antibody to HIV, antibody to hepatitis C virus (HCV), antibody to human T cell lymphotropic/leukemia virus (HTLV), and antibody to West Nile virus.

With improved screening, the risk of posttransfusion hepatitis has steadily decreased. The risk of hepatitis B is 1:200,000 per unit and of HIV 1:250,000 per unit. The risk of seroconversion to HTLV is 1:70,000, but clinical sequelae when this occurs are rare. The major infectious risk of blood products is hepatitis C, with a seroconversion rate of 1:3300 per unit transfused. Most of these cases are clinically silent, but there is a high incidence of chronic hepatitis.

PLATELET TRANSFUSION

Platelet transfusions are indicated in cases of thrombocytopenia due to decreased platelet production. They are not useful in immune thrombocytopenia, since transfused platelets will last no longer than the patient's endogenous platelets. The risk of spontaneous bleeding rises when the platelet count falls to less than 10,000/mcL, and the risk of life-threatening bleeding increases when the platelet count is less than 5000/mcL. Because of this, prophylactic platelet transfusions are often given at these very low levels. Platelet transfusions are also given prior to invasive procedures or surgery, and the goal should be to raise the platelet count to over 50,000/mcL.

Platelets are most commonly derived from donated blood units. One unit of platelets (derived from 1 unit of blood) usually contains $5–7 \times 10^{10}$ platelets suspended in

35 mL of plasma. Ideally, 1 platelet unit will raise the recipient's platelet count by 10,000/mcL, and transfused platelets will last for 2 or 3 days. However, responses are often suboptimal, with poor platelet increments and short survival times. This may be due to sepsis, splenomegaly, or alloimmunization. Most alloantibodies causing platelet destruction are directed at HLA antigens. Patients requiring long periods of platelet transfusion support should be monitored to document adequate responses to transfusions so that the most appropriate product can be used. Patients may benefit from HLA-matched platelets derived from either volunteer donors or family members, with platelets obtained by plateletpheresis. Techniques of cross-matching platelets have been developed and appear to identify suitable platelet donors (nonreactive with the patient's serum) without the need for HLA typing. Such single-donor platelets usually contain the equivalent of six units of random platelets, or $30–50 \times 10^{10}$ platelets suspended in 200 mL of plasma. Ideally, these platelet concentrates will raise the recipient's platelet count by 60,000/mcL. Leukocyte depletion of platelets has been shown to delay the onset of alloimmunization.

GRANULOCYTE TRANSFUSIONS

Granulocyte transfusions are seldom indicated and have largely been replaced by the use of myeloid growth factors (G-CSF and GM-CSF) that speed neutrophil recovery. However, they may be beneficial in patients with profound neutropenia (< 100/mcL) who have gram-negative sepsis or progressive soft tissue infection despite optimal antibiotic therapy. In these cases, it is clear that progressive infection is due to failure of host defenses. In such situations, daily granulocyte transfusions should be given and continued until the neutrophil count rises to above 500/mcL. Such granulocytes must be derived from ABO-matched donors. Although HLA matching is not necessary, it is preferred, since patients with alloantibodies to donor white blood cells will have severe reactions and no benefit.

The donor cells usually contain some immunocompetent lymphocytes capable of producing graft-versus-host disease in HLA-incompatible hosts whose immunocompetence may be impaired. Irradiation of the units of cells with 1500 cGy will destroy the lymphocytes without harm to the granulocytes or platelets.

Alter HJ et al. The hazards of blood transfusion in historical perspective. Blood. 2008 Oct 1;112(7):2617–26. [PMID: 18809775]

Blajchman MA et al. New strategies for the optimal use of platelet transfusions. Hematology Am Soc Hematol Educ Program. 2008:198–204. [PMID: 19074082]

Triulzi DJ. Transfusion-related acute lung injury: an update. Hematology Am Soc Hematol Educ Program. 2006:497–501. [PMID: 17124105]

TRANSFUSION OF PLASMA COMPONENTS

Fresh-frozen plasma is available in units of approximately 200 mL. Fresh plasma contains normal levels of all coagulation factors (about 1 unit/mL). Fresh frozen plasma is used to correct coagulation factor deficiencies and to treat TTP. The risk of transmitting viral disease is comparable to that associated with transfusion of red blood cells.

Cryoprecipitate is made from fresh plasma. One unit has a volume of approximately 20 mL and contains approximately 250 mg of fibrinogen and between 80 and 100 units of factor VIII and vWF. Cryoprecipitate is used to supplement fibrinogen in cases of congenital deficiency of fibrinogen or DIC. One unit of cryoprecipitate will raise the fibrinogen level by about 8 mg/dL.

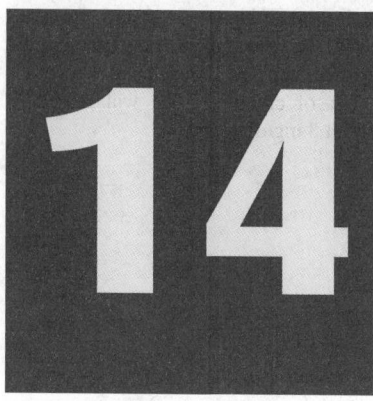

Disorders of Hemostasis, Thrombosis, & Antithrombotic Therapy

Patrick F. Fogarty, MD
Tracy Minichiello, MD

In assessing patients for defects of hemostasis, the clinical context must be considered carefully (Table 14–1). Heritable defects are suggested by bleeding that begins in infancy or childhood, is recurrent, and occurs at multiple anatomic sites, although many other patterns of presentation are possible. Acquired disorders of hemostasis more typically are associated with bleeding that begins later in life and may be relatable to introduction of medications (eg, agents that affect platelet activity) or to onset of underlying medical conditions (such as renal failure or myelodysplasia), or may be idiopathic. Importantly, however, a sufficient hemostatic challenge (such as major trauma) may produce excessive bleeding even in individuals with completely normal hemostasis.

Fogarty PF et al. Disorders of Hemostasis I: Coagulation. In: *The Bethesda Handbook of Clinical Hematology.* Rodgers GP, Young NS (editors). Philadelphia: Lippincott Williams and Wilkins; 2005.

PLATELET DISORDERS

THROMBOCYTOPENIA

The causes of thrombocytopenia are shown in Table 14–2. The age of the patient and presence of any comorbid conditions may help direct the diagnostic work-up.

The risk of spontaneous bleeding (including petechial hemorrhage and bruising) does not typically increase appreciably until the platelet count falls below 10,000–20,000/mcL, although patients with dysfunctional platelets may bleed with higher platelet counts. Suggested platelet counts to prevent spontaneous bleeding or to provide adequate hemostasis around the time of invasive procedures are found in Table 14–3.

DECREASED PLATELET PRODUCTION

1. Bone Marrow Failure

 ESSENTIALS OF DIAGNOSIS

► Bone marrow failure states may be congenital or acquired.

► Most congenital marrow failure disorders present in childhood.

► General Considerations

Congenital conditions that cause thrombocytopenia include amegakaryocytic thrombocytopenia, the thrombocytopenia-absent radius (TAR) syndrome, and Wiskott-Aldrich syndrome; these disorders usually feature isolated thrombocytopenia, whereas patients with Fanconi anemia and dyskeratosis congenita typically have depressions in other blood cell counts as well.

Acquired causes of bone marrow failure leading to thrombocytopenia include acquired aplastic anemia, myelodysplastic syndrome (MDS), and acquired amegakaryocytic thrombocytopenia. Unlike aplastic anemia, MDS is more common among older patients.

► Clinical Findings

Acquired **aplastic anemia** typically presents with reductions in multiple blood cell lines; a bone marrow biopsy subsequently reveals hypocellularity. **Myelodysplasia** may also present as cytopenias with variable marrow cellularity, at times mimicking aplastic anemia; however, the presence of macrocytosis, ringed sideroblasts on iron staining of the bone marrow aspirate, dysplasia of hematopoietic ele-

Table 14–1. Evaluation of the bleeding patient.

Necessary Component of Evaluation	Diagnostic Correlate
Location	
Mucocutaneous (bruises, petechiae, gingival, nosebleeds)	Likely qualitative/quantitative platelet defects
Joints, soft tissue	Likely disorders of coagulation factors
Onset	
Infancy/childhood	Suggests heritable condition
Adulthood	Suggests milder heritable condition or acquired defect of hemostasis (eg, ITP, medication-related)
Clinical context	
Postsurgical	Anatomic/surgical defect must be ruled out
Pregnancy	vWD, HELLP syndrome, ITP, acquired factor VIII inhibitor
Sepsis	May indicate DIC
Patient taking anticoagulants	Rule out excessive anticoagulation
Personal history[1]	
Absent	Suggests acquired rather than congenital defect, or anatomic/surgical defect (if applicable)
Present	Suggests established acquired defect or congenital disorder
Family history	
Absent	Suggests acquired defect or no defect of hemostasis
Present	May signify hemophilia A or B, vWD, other heritable bleeding disorders

[1]Includes evaluation of prior spontaneous bleeding, as well as excessive bleeding with circumcision, menses, dental extractions, trauma, minor procedures (eg, endoscopy, biopsies) and major procedures (surgery).
DIC, disseminated intravascular coagulation; HELLP, hemolysis, elevated liver enzymes, low platelets; ITP, immune thrombocytopenic purpura; vWD, von Willebrand disease.

Table 14–2. Causes of thrombocytopenia.

Decreased production of platelets
  Congenital bone marrow failure (eg, Fanconi anemia, Wiskott-Aldrich syndrome)
  Acquired bone marrow failure (eg, aplastic anemia, myelodysplasia)
  Exposure to chemotherapy, irradiation
  Marrow infiltration (neoplastic, infectious)
  Nutritional (deficiency of vitamin B_{12}, folate, iron; alcohol)
Increased destruction of platelets
  Immune thrombocytopenic purpura (including hepatitis C virus- and HIV-related,[1] and drug-induced)
  Heparin-induced thrombocytopenia
  Thrombotic microangiopathy
  Disseminated intravascular coagulation
  Posttransfusion purpura
  Neonatal alloimmune thrombocytopenia
  Mechanical (aortic valvular dysfunction; extracorporeal bypass)
  von Willebrand disease, type 2B
  Hemophagocytosis
Increased sequestration of platelets
  Hypersplenism (eg, related to cirrhosis, myeloproliferative disorders, lymphoma)
Other conditions causing thrombocytopenia
  Gestational thrombocytopenia
  Bernard-Soulier syndrome, gray platelet syndrome, May-Hegglin anomaly
  Pseudothrombocytopenia

[1]HIV-related thrombocytopenia as well as disorders such as some cases of immune thrombocytopenia and cyclic thrombocytopenia may feature both decreased production and increased clearance of platelets.

▶ **Treatment**

A. Congenital Conditions

Treatment is varied but may include blood product support, blood cell growth factors, androgens, and (some cases) allogeneic hematopoietic progenitor cell transplantation.

B. Acquired Conditions

Patients with severe aplastic anemia are treated with allogeneic hematopoietic progenitor cell transplantation,

ments, or cytogenetic abnormalities (especially monosomy 5 or 7, and trisomy 8) are more suggestive of MDS. Thrombocytopenia in patients with MDS is usually mild to moderate, rather than severe.

▶ **Differential Diagnosis**

Adult patients with acquired amegakaryocytic thrombocytopenia have isolated thrombocytopenia and reduced or absent megakaryocytes in the bone marrow, which (along with failure to respond to immunomodulatory regimens typically administered in immune thrombocytopenic purpura [ITP]) distinguishes them from patients with ITP.

Table 14–3. Desired platelet count ranges.

Clinical Scenario	Platelet count (/mcL)
Prevention of spontaneous mucocutaneous bleeding	> 10,000–20,000
Insertion of central venous catheters	> 20,000–50,000[1]
Administration of therapeutic anticoagulation	> 30,000–50,000
Minor surgery and selected invasive procedures[2]	> 50,000–80,000
Major surgery	> 80,000–100,000

[1]A platelet target within the higher range of the reference is required for tunneled catheters.
[2]Such as endoscopy with biopsy.

which is the preferred therapy for patients younger than age 40 who have an HLA-matched sibling donor (see Chapter 13), or with immunosuppression, which is the preferred therapy for older patients and those who lack an HLA-matched sibling donor.

Treatments of thrombocytopenia due to MDS, if clinically significant bleeding is present or if the risk of bleeding is high, is limited to chronic transfusion of platelets in most instances (Table 14–3). Newer immunomodulatory agents such as lenalidomide do not produce increases in the platelet count in most patients.

Kantarjian H et al. The incidence and impact of thrombocytopenia in myelodysplastic syndromes. Cancer. 2007 May 1;109(9):1705–14. [PMID: 17366593]

2. Bone Marrow Infiltration

Massive replacement of the bone marrow by leukemic cells, myeloma, lymphoma, or other tumors may cause thrombocytopenia; however, abnormalities in other blood cell lines are also usually present. The same is true for infectious causes leading to marrow infiltration (mycobacterial disease, ehrlichiosis). These entities are easily diagnosed after examining the bone marrow biopsy and aspirate or determining the infecting organism from an aspirate specimen. Treatment of thrombocytopenia is directed at eradication of the underlying infiltrative disorder, but platelet transfusion may be required if clinically significant bleeding is present.

3. Chemotherapy & Irradiation

Chemotherapeutic agents and irradiation may lead to thrombocytopenia by direct toxicity to megakaryocytes, hematopoietic progenitor cells, or both. The severity and duration of chemotherapy-induced depressions in the platelet count are determined by the specific regimen used, although the platelet count typically resolves more slowly following a chemotherapeutic insult than does neutropenia or anemia, especially if multiple cycles of treatment have been given. Until recovery occurs, patients may be supported with transfused platelets if bleeding is present or the risk of bleeding is high (Table 14–3). Drug applications of novel platelet growth factors (eltrombopag, romiplostim) are underway for the treatment of chemotherapy-induced thrombocytopenia, whereas use of an existing recombinant IL-11-like cytokine (oprelvekin) has been limited by significant drug-related toxicities.

4. Nutritional Deficiencies

Thrombocytopenia, typically in concert with anemia, may be observed when a deficiency of folate (that may accompany alcoholism) or vitamin B_{12} is present (concomitant neurologic findings are common). In addition, thrombocytopenia rarely can occur in very severe iron deficiency. Replacing the deficient vitamin or mineral results in improvement in the platelet count.

5. Cyclic Thrombocytopenia

Cyclic thrombocytopenia is a very rare disorder that produces cyclic oscillations of the platelet count, usually with a periodicity of 3–6 weeks. The exact pathophysiologic mechanisms responsible for the condition may vary from patient to patient. Severe thrombocytopenia and bleeding typically occur at the platelet nadir. Identification of the endogenous cyclic phenomenon may be difficult because of the usual practice of providing treatment (platelet transfusion or otherwise) at times of very low platelet counts. Oral contraceptive medications, androgens, azathioprine, and thrombopoietic growth factors have been used successfully in the management of cyclic thrombocytopenia.

Bussel JB et al. Eltrombopag for the treatment of chronic idiopathic thrombocytopenic purpura. N Engl J Med. 2007 Nov 29;357(22):2237–47. [PMID: 18046028]

Fogarty PF et al. Large granular lymphocytic proliferation-associated cyclic thrombocytopenia. Am J Hematol. 2005 Aug;79(4):334–6. [PMID: 16044437]

INCREASED PLATELET DESTRUCTION

1. Immune Thrombocytopenic Purpura

 ESSENTIALS OF DIAGNOSIS

► Isolated thrombocytopenia.

► Assess for any new causative medications and HIV and hepatitis C infections.

► ITP is a diagnosis of exclusion.

► General Considerations

ITP is an autoimmune condition in which pathogenic antibodies bind platelets, resulting in accelerated platelet clearance. The disorder is primary and idiopathic in most adult patients, although it can be associated with connective tissue disease (such as lupus), lymphoproliferative disease (such as lymphoma), medications, and infections (such as hepatitis C virus and HIV infections). Targets of antiplatelet antibodies include glycoproteins IIb/IIIa and Ib/IX on the platelet membrane, although antibodies are demonstrable in only two-thirds of patients. The mechanisms underlying drug-induced thrombocytopenia are thought in most cases to be immune, although exceptions exist (such as chemotherapy). Table 14–4 lists medications associated with thrombocytopenia. HIV and hepatitis C virus both are associated with thrombocytopenia that has immune-mediated underpinnings and can respond to immunomodulation, although both also may lead to thrombocytopenia through additional mechanisms (for instance, by direct suppression of platelet production [HIV] and cirrhosis-related splenomegaly [hepatitis C virus]).

► Clinical Findings

A. Symptoms and Signs

Mucocutaneous bleeding manifestations may be present, depending on the platelet count. The typical presentation of **drug-induced thrombocytopenia** is severe thrombocytopenia and mucocutaneous bleeding 7–14 days after

Table 14–4. Medications causing drug-associated thrombocytopenia.

Class	Examples
Chemotherapy	Most agents
Antiplatelet agents	Anagrelide Abciximab Eptifibatide Tirofiban Ticlopidine
Antimicrobial agents	Penicillins Isoniazid Rifampin Sulfa drugs Vancomycin Adefovir Indinavir Ritonavir Fluconazole Linezolid
Cardiovascular agents	Digoxin Amiodarone Captopril Hydrochlorothiazide Procainamide Atorvastatin Simvastatin
Gastrointestinal agents	Cimetidine Ranitidine Famotidine
Neuropsychiatric agents	Haloperidol Carbamazepine Methyldopa Phenytoin
Analgesic agents	Acetaminophen Ibuprofen Sulindac Diclofenac Naproxen
Anticoagulant agents	Heparin Low-molecular-weight heparin
Immunomodulator agents	Interferon-α Gold Rituximab
Immunosuppressant agents	Mycophenolate mofetil Tacrolimus
Other agents	Iodinated contrast dye Immunizations

exposure to a new drug, although a range of presentations is possible.

B. Laboratory Findings

Typically, patients have isolated thrombocytopenia. If bleeding has occurred, anemia may also be present. Hepa-titis virus B and C and HIV infections should be excluded by serologic testing.

Bone marrow should be examined in patients with unexplained cytopenias, in patients older than 60 years, or in those who did not respond to primary ITP-specific therapy. Megakaryocyte abnormalities and hypocellularity or hypercellularity are not characteristic of ITP. If there are clinical findings suggestive of a lymphoproliferative malignancy, a CT scan should be performed. In the absence of such findings, otherwise asymptomatic patients with unexplained isolated thrombocytopenia of recent onset may be considered to have ITP.

▶ Treatment

Discontinuation of the offending agent leads to resolution of drug-induced thrombocytopenia within 7–10 days in most cases, but patients with severe hemorrhage should be given platelet transfusions or intravenous immunoglobulin (IVIG), or both. For other etiologies of ITP, only individuals with platelet counts < 20,000–30,000/mcL or those with significant bleeding should be treated; the remainder may be monitored serially for progression. The mainstay of initial treatment is a short course of corticosteroids with or without IVIG or anti-D (WinRho) (Figure 14–1). Responses are generally seen within 3–5 days of initiating treatment. Platelet transfusions may be given concomitantly if active bleeding is present.

Although over two-thirds of patients with ITP respond to initial treatment, most relapse following reduction of the corticosteroid dose. Patients with a persistent platelet count < 30,000/mcL or clinically significant bleeding are appropriate candidates for treatment. To bring the platelet count into a safe range quickly, an increased dose of corticosteroids can be administered initially, with the goal of rapid taper once the response has been regained. Then, anti-D (WinRho) or IVIG may be administered once every 2–3 weeks as directed by platelet counts < 30,000/mcL; serial anti-D treatment may allow adult patients to delay or avoid splenectomy. The monoclonal anti-B cell antibody **rituximab** leads to initial responses in about 50% of adults with corticosteroid-refractory chronic ITP.

In clinical trials, the novel thrombopoietin receptor agonists romiplostim (administered subcutaneously weekly) and eltrombopag (taken orally daily) led to improvement in platelet counts in most patients with prednisone-refractory ITP; furthermore, these agents were well-tolerated and, importantly, did not show evidence of suppressing the immune system, distinguishing them from other agents. Romiplostim and eltrombopag are indicated in adult patients with chronic ITP who have not responded durably to corticosteroids, IVIG, or splenectomy.

Splenectomy has a durable response rate of over 60%, but usually is reserved for cases of severe thrombocytopenia that is refractory to second-line agents; patients should receive pneumococcal, *Haemophilus influenzae* type b, and meningococcal vaccination at least 2 weeks before the procedure. If available, laparoscopic splenectomy is preferred, in light of decreased morbidity and shorter hospi-

INITIAL TREATMENT	**Prednisone,** 1 mg/kg/d PO for 7–10 days followed by rapid taper *or* **Dexamethasone,** 40 mg/d PO for 4 days monthly for 6 months	±	**IVIG,** 1 g/kg/d IV for 2 days *or* **anti-D,** 75 mcg/kg IV for 1 dose[1]	± **Platelets,** if bleeding

RELAPSED OR PERSISTENT ITP

> **Prednisone,** 1 mg/kg/d PO for 7–10 days followed by rapid taper
> *or*
> **Dexamethasone,** 40 mg/d PO for 4 days monthly for 6 months

and

Rituximab, 375 mg/m² IV weekly for 4 weeks	*or*	**anti-D,** 75 mcg/kg IV serially prn platelets < 30,000/mcL[1]	*or*	**IVIG,** 1 g/kg/d IV for 2 days serially prn platelets < 30,000/mcL	*or*	**Thrombopoietin receptor agonist** (see text)

or

> **Splenectomy** (laparoscopic)

PERSISTENT OR WORSENING ITP

> **Trial of additional agent(s) above**
> *or*

> **Mycophenolate mofetil · Azathioprine/danazol · Cyclosporine · Chemotherapy[2]**
> **Enrollment in clinical trial · Autologous transplantation**

or

> **Splenectomy** (laparoscopic)

[1] Use in non-splenectomized, Rh blood type-positive, non-anemic patients only.
[2] Both lymphoma-type chemotherapy and single-agent vincristine have been used successfully in refractory cases of ITP.

▲ **Figure 14–1.** Management of immune thrombocytopenia (ITP).

talizations when compared with the traditional approach. Additional treatments for ITP are found in Figure 14–1.

The goal of management of **pregnancy-associated ITP** is a platelet count > 10,000/mcL in the first trimester, > 30,000/mcL during the second or third trimester, or > 50,000/mcL prior to cesarean section or vaginal delivery. Moderate-dose oral prednisone or intermittent infusions of IVIG are standard. Splenectomy is reserved for failure to respond to these therapies and may be performed in the first or second trimester.

For thrombocytopenia associated with HIV or hepatitis C virus, treatment of either infection leads to an amelioration in the platelet count in most cases, whereas refractory thrombocytopenia may be treated with infusion of IVIG or anti-D (HIV and hepatitis C virus), splenectomy (HIV), or interferon-alpha (hepatitis C virus). Clinical trials of eltrombopag in treatment of HCV-associated thrombocytopenia have shown promising results. Treatment with corticosteroids is not recommended in hepatitis C virus infection.

When to Refer

Chronic thrombocytopenia will develop in most patients with newly diagnosed ITP; therefore, all patients with ITP should be referred to a subspecialist for evaluation at the time of diagnosis.

Arnold DM et al. Systematic review: efficacy and safety of rituximab for adults with idiopathic thrombocytopenic purpura. Ann Intern Med. 2007 Jan 2;146(1):25–33. [PMID: 17200219]

Bussel JB et al. Eltrombopag for the treatment of chronic idiopathic thrombocytopenic purpura. N Engl J Med. 2007 Nov 29;357(22):2237–47. [PMID: 18046028]

Fogarty PF et al. The epidemiology of immune thrombocytopenic purpura. Curr Opin Hematol. 2007 Sep;14(5):515–9. [PMID: 17934361]

Kuter DJ et al. Efficacy of romiplostim in patients with chronic immune thrombocytopenic purpura: a double-blind randomised controlled trial. Lancet. 2008 Feb 2;371(9610):395–403. [PMID: 18242413]

2. Thrombotic Microangiopathy

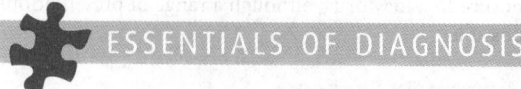

ESSENTIALS OF DIAGNOSIS

► Microangiopathic hemolytic anemia and thrombocytopenia, in the absence of another plausible explanation, are sufficient for the diagnosis of TMA.

- Fever, neurologic abnormalities, and renal insufficiency may occur concurrently but are not required for diagnosis.
- Renal insufficiency occurs in hemolytic-uremic syndrome.

General Considerations

The thrombotic microangiopathies (TMAs) include thrombotic thrombocytopenic purpura (TTP) and the hemolytic-uremic syndrome (HUS). These disorders are characterized by thrombocytopenia, due to the incorporation of platelets into thrombi in the microvasculature, and microangiopathic hemolytic anemia, which results from shearing of erythrocytes in the microcirculation.

In idiopathic TTP, autoantibodies against the ADAMTS-13 (A disintegrin and metalloproteinase with thrombospondin type 1 repeat, member 13) molecule, also known as the von Willebrand factor cleaving protease (vWFCP), leads to accumulation of ultra-large von Willebrand factor (vWF) multimers that bridge platelets and facilitate excessive platelet aggregation, leading to TTP. In some cases of pregnancy-associated TMA, an antibody to vWFCP is present. In contrast, the activity of the vWFCP in congenital TTP is decreased due to a mutation in the gene encoding for the molecule. Damage to endothelial cells—such as the damage that occurs in endemic HUS due to presence of toxins from *Escherichia coli* (especially type O157:H7) or in the setting of cancer, hematopoietic stem cell transplantation, or HIV infection—may also lead to TMA. Certain drugs (eg, cyclosporine, quinine, ticlopidine, clopidogrel, mitomycin C, and bleomycin) have been associated with the development of TMA, possibly by promoting injury to endothelial cells, although inhibitory antibodies to ADAMTS-13 also have been demonstrated in some cases.

Clinical Findings

A. Symptoms and Signs

Microangiopathic hemolytic anemia and thrombocytopenia are presenting signs in all patients with TTP and most patients with HUS; in a subset of patients with HUS, the platelet count remains in the normal range. Only approximately 25% of patients with TMA manifest all components of the so-called pentad of findings (microangiopathic hemolytic anemia, thrombocytopenia, fever, renal insufficiency, and neurologic system abnormalities) (Table 14–5). Most patients (especially children) with HUS have a recent or current diarrheal illness. Neurologic manifestations, including headache, somnolence, delirium, seizures, paresis, and coma, may result from deposition of microthrombi in the cerebral vasculature.

B. Laboratory Findings

Laboratory features of TMA include those associated with microangiopathic hemolytic anemia (anemia, elevated lactate dehydrogenase (LD), elevated indirect bilirubin, decreased haptoglobin, reticulocytosis, negative direct antiglobulin test, and schistocytes on the blood smear); thrombocytopenia; elevated creatinine; positive stool culture for *E coli* O157:H7 or assays for Shiga-like toxins (cases of HUS only); and reductions in vWFCP activity. Notably, routine coagulation studies are within the normal range in most patients with TMA.

Treatment

Immediate administration of plasma exchange is essential in most cases due to the mortality rate of > 95% without treatment. With the exception of children or adults with endemic diarrhea-associated HUS, who generally recover with supportive care only, plasma exchange must be initiated as soon as the diagnosis of TMA is suspected. Plasma exchange usually is administered once daily until the platelet count and LD have returned to normal for at least 2 days, after which the frequency of treatments may be tapered slowly while the platelet count and LD are monitored for relapse. In cases of insufficient response to once-daily plasma exchange, twice-daily treatments should be given. Fresh frozen plasma may be administered if immediate access to plasma exchange is not available or in cases of familial TMA. *Platelet transfusions are contraindicated* in the

Table 14–5. Clinical features of thrombotic microangiopathy.

Parameter	Thrombotic Thrombocytopenic Purpura	Hemolytic-Uremic Syndrome
Microangiopathic hemolytic anemia	All patients	All patients
Thrombocytopenia	All patients	Most patients (may be mild/absent in a subset of patients)
Fever	75% of patients	Usually absent
Renal insufficiency	Mild/absent in some patients	All patients
Neurologic defects	Most patients	Present in less than half
Epidemiologic	Most cases in adults	Most cases in children
Historical	Idiopathic (minority of cases: antecedent viral illness or familial)	Antecedent hemorrhagic enteritis in most patients
Laboratory findings	Decreased activity of ADAMTS-13	Positive stool culture for *Escherichia coli* O157:H7; ADAMTS-13 activity usually normal

ADAMTS-13, a disintegrin and metalloproteinase with a thrombospondin type 1 repeat, member 13 (von Willebrand factor cleaving protease).

treatment of TMAs due to reports of worsening thrombotic microangiopathy, possibly due to propagation of platelet-rich microthrombi. In cases of documented life-threatening bleeding, however, platelet transfusions may be given slowly and after plasma exchange is underway. Red blood cell transfusions may be administered in cases of clinically significant anemia. Hemodialysis should be considered for patients with significant renal impairment.

In cases of relapse following initial treatment, plasma exchange should be reinstituted. If ineffective, or in cases of primary refractoriness, second-line treatments may be considered including rituximab, corticosteroids, IVIG, vincristine, cyclophosphamide, and splenectomy.

When to Refer

Consultation by a hematologist or transfusion medicine specialist familiar with plasma exchange is required at the time of presentation. Patients with refractory or relapsing TMA require ongoing care by a subspecialist.

When to Admit

All patients with newly suspected or diagnosed TMA should be hospitalized initially.

Moake JL. Thrombotic thrombocytopenic purpura and the hemolytic uremic syndrome. Arch Pathol Lab Med. 2002 Nov;126(11):1430–3. [PMID: 12421153]

3. Heparin-Induced Thrombocytopenia

ESSENTIALS OF DIAGNOSIS

▶ Thrombocytopenia within 5–10 days of exposure to heparin.

▶ Decline in baseline platelet count of 50% or greater.

▶ Thrombosis occurs in 50% of cases; bleeding is uncommon.

General Considerations

Heparin-induced thrombocytopenia (HIT) is an acquired disorder that affects approximately 3% of patients who are exposed to unfractionated heparin and 0.6% of patients who are exposed to low molecular-weight heparin (LMWH). The condition results from formation of IgG antibodies to heparin-platelet factor 4 (PF4) complexes; the antibodies then bind platelets, which activates them. Platelet activation leads to both thrombocytopenia and a pro-thrombotic state.

Clinical Findings

A. Symptoms and Signs

Due to the paradoxical pro-thrombotic nature of HIT, bleeding usually does not occur. Thrombosis subsequently is detected in about 50% of patients, which may include thromboses at any venous or arterial site.

B. Laboratory Findings

A presumptive diagnosis of HIT is made when new-onset thrombocytopenia is detected in a patient (frequently a hospitalized patient) within 5–10 days of exposure to heparin. A decline of 50% or more from the baseline platelet count is regarded as compatible with the diagnosis. Occasionally, rapid-onset HIT occurs in a patient with preexisting heparin-PF4 antibodies, due to exposure within the past 100 days; in these cases, the platelet count decline occurs within 1–4 days of reexposure. Confirmation of the diagnosis can be obtained through a positive PF4-heparin antibody enzyme-linked immunosorbent assay (ELISA) or functional assay (such as serotonin release assay), or both.

Treatment

Treatment should be initiated as soon as the diagnosis of HIT is suspected, before results of laboratory testing is available.

Management of HIT (Table 14–6) involves the immediate discontinuation of all forms of heparin.

If thrombosis has not already been detected, duplex Doppler ultrasound of the lower extremities should be per-

Table 14–6. Management of suspected or proven HIT.

I. Discontinue all forms of heparin. Send PF4-heparin ELISA (if indicated).		
II. Begin treatment with direct thrombin inhibitor.		
Agent	**Indication**	**Dosing**
Argatroban	Prophylaxis or treatment of HIT	Continuous IV infusion of 0.5 – 1.2 mcg/kg/min, titrate to aPTT = 1.5 to 3 × the baseline value.[1] Max infusion rate ≤ 10 mcg/kg/min.
Lepirudin	Treatment of HITT	Bolus of 0.4 mg/kg[2] slowly IV followed by continuous IV infusion of 0.15 mg/kg/h. Titrate to aPTT = 1.5 – 2.5 × baseline value.
Bivalirudin	Percutaneous coronary intervention[3]	Bolus of 0.75 mg/kg IV followed by initial continuous IV infusion of 1.75 mg/kg/h. Manufacturer indicates monitoring should be by ACT.

III. Perform Doppler ultrasound of lower extremities to rule out subclinical thrombosis (if indicated).
IV. Follow platelet counts daily until recovery occurs.
V. When platelet count has recovered, transition anticoagulation to warfarin; treat for 30 days (HIT) or 3-6 months (HITT).
VI. Document heparin allergy in medical record (confirmed cases).

[1]Hepatic insufficiency: initial infusion rate = 0.5 mcg/kg/min.
[2]Renal insufficiency: initial bolus = 0.2 mg/kg.
[3]Not approved for HIT/HITT.
ACT, activated clotting time; aPTT, activated partial thromboplastin time; ELISA, enzyme-linked immunosorbent assay; HIT, heparin-induced thrombocytopenia; HITT, heparin-induced thrombocytopenia and thrombosis; PF4, platelet factor 4.

formed to rule out subclinical deep venous thrombosis. Despite thrombocytopenia, platelet transfusions are rarely necessary. Due to the substantial frequency of thrombosis among HIT patients, an alternative anticoagulant, typically a direct thrombin inhibitor (DTI) such as argatroban or lepirudin should be administered immediately. The DTI should be continued until the platelet count has recovered to at least 100,000/mcL, at which point treatment with a vitamin K antagonist (warfarin) may be initiated. The DTI should be continued until therapeutic anticoagulation with the vitamin K antagonist has been achieved (international normalized ratio [INR] of 2.0–3.0) due to the warfarin effect; the infusion of argatroban must be temporarily discontinued for 2 hours before the INR is obtained so that it reflects the anticoagulant effect of warfarin alone. Warfarin is contraindicated as initial treatment of HIT because of its potential to transiently worsen hypercoagulability. In all patients with HIT, warfarin subsequently should be continued for at least 30 days, due to a persistent risk of thrombosis even after the platelet count has recovered, whereas in patients in whom thrombosis has been documented, anticoagulation with warfarin should continue for at least 3 months.

Bivalirudin, another DTI, is not approved for the treatment of HIT but may be considered when hepatic or renal failure prevents use of argatroban or lepirudin.

Subsequent exposure to heparin should be avoided in all patients with a prior history of HIT, if possible. If its use is regarded as necessary for a procedure, it should not be given until PF4-heparin antibodies are no longer detectable by ELISA (usually as of 100 days following an episode of HIT), and exposure should be limited to the shortest time period possible.

When to Refer

Due to the tremendous thrombotic potential of the disorder and the complexity of use of the DTI, all patients with HIT should be evaluated by a hematologist as soon as the thrombocytopenia is detected.

When to Admit

Most patients with HIT are hospitalized at the time of detection of thrombocytopenia. Any outpatient in whom HIT is suspected should be admitted because the DTIs must be administered by continuous intravenous infusion.

Linkins LA et al. The approach to heparin-induced thrombocytopenia. Semin Respir Crit Care Med. 2008 Feb;29(1):66–74. [PMID: 18302088]
Warkentin TE. Heparin-induced thrombocytopenia. Hematol Oncol Clin North Am. 2007 Aug;21(4):589–607. [PMID: 17666280]

4. Disseminated Intravascular Coagulation

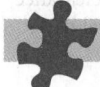 ESSENTIALS OF DIAGNOSIS

► A frequent cause of thrombocytopenia in hospitalized patients.

► Prolonged activated partial thromboplastin time and prothrombin time.

► Thrombocytopenia and decreased fibrinogen levels.

General Considerations

Disseminated intravascular coagulation (DIC) results from uncontrolled local or systemic activation of coagulation, which leads to depletion of coagulation factors and fibrinogen and to thrombocytopenia as platelets are activated and consumed.

The numerous disorders that are associated with DIC include sepsis (in which coagulation is activated by presence of lipopolysaccharide) as well as cancer, trauma, burns, or pregnancy-associated morbidity (in which tissue factor is released). Aortic aneurysm and cavernous hemangiomas may promote DIC by leading to vascular stasis, and snake bites may result in DIC due to the introduction of exogenous toxins.

Clinical Findings

A. Symptoms and Signs

Bleeding in DIC usually occurs at multiple sites, such as intravenous catheters or incisions, and may be widespread (**purpura fulminans**). Malignancy-related DIC may manifest principally as thrombosis (Trousseau syndrome).

B. Laboratory Findings

Frequently, there are acute and progressive prolongations in coagulation studies or thrombocytopenia is found in a patient who is being treated for a separate disorder. In early DIC, the platelet count and fibrinogen levels may remain within the normal range, albeit reduced from baseline levels. There is progressive thrombocytopenia (rarely severe), prolongation of the activated partial thromboplastin time (aPTT) and prothrombin time (PT), and low levels of fibrinogen. D-dimer levels typically are elevated due to the activation of coagulation and diffuse cross-linking of fibrin. Schistocytes on the blood smear, due to shearing of red cells through the microvasculature, are present in 10-20% of patients. Laboratory abnormalities in the HELLP syndrome (hemolysis, elevated liver enzymes, low platelets), a severe form of DIC with a particularly high mortality rate that occurs in peripartum women, include elevated liver transaminases and (many cases) renal dysfunction due to gross hemoglobinuria and pigment nephropathy. Malignancy-related DIC may feature normal platelet counts and coagulation studies.

Treatment

The underlying causative disorder must be treated (eg, antimicrobials, chemotherapy, surgery, or delivery of conceptus [see below]). If clinically significant bleeding is present, hemostasis must be achieved (Table 14–7).

Blood products should be administered only if clinically significant hemorrhage has occurred or is thought likely to occur without intervention (Table 14–7). The goal

Table 14–7. Management of DIC.

I. Assess for underlying cause of DIC and treat.	
II. Establish baseline platelet count, PT, aPTT, D-dimer, fibrinogen.	
III. Transfuse blood products only if ongoing bleeding or high risk of bleeding:	Platelets: goal > 20,000/mcL (most patients) or > 50,000/mcL (severe bleeding, eg, intracranial hemorrhage)
	Cryoprecipitate: goal fibrinogen level > 80–100 mg/dL
	Fresh frozen plasma: goal PT and aPTT < 1.5 × normal
	Packed red blood cells: goal hemoglobin > 8 g/dL or improvement in symptomatic anemia
IV. Follow platelets, aPTT/PT, fibrinogen every 4–6 hours or as clinically indicated.	
V. If persistent bleeding, consider use of heparin[1] (initial infusion, 5–10 units/kg/h); do not administer bolus.	
VI. Follow laboratory parameters every 4–6 hours until DIC resolved and underlying condition successfully treated	

[1]Contraindicated if platelets cannot be maintained at > 50,000/mcL, in cases of gastrointestinal or central nervous system bleeding, in conditions that may require surgical management, or placental abruption.

aPTT, activated partial thromboplastin time; DIC, disseminated intravascular coagulation; PT, prothrombin time.

of platelet therapy for most cases is > 20,000–30,000/mcL or > 50,000/mcL for serious bleeding, such as intracranial bleeding. Fresh frozen plasma should be given only to patients with a prolonged aPTT and PT and significant bleeding; 4 units typically are administered at a time, and the posttransfusion platelet count should be documented. Cryoprecipitate may be given for bleeding and fibrinogen levels < 80–100 mg/dL. The PT, aPTT, fibrinogen, and platelet count should be monitored at least every 6 hours in acutely ill patients with DIC.

In some cases of **refractory bleeding** despite replacement of blood products, administration of low doses of heparin can be considered; it may help interfere with thrombin generation, which then could lead to a lessened consumption of coagulation proteins and platelets. An infusion of 6–10 units/kg/h (no bolus) may be used. Heparin, however, is contraindicated if the platelet count cannot be maintained at ≥ 50,000/mcL and in cases of central nervous system/gastrointestinal bleeding, placental abruption, and any other condition that is likely to require imminent surgery. Fibrinolysis inhibitors may be considered in some patients with refractory DIC.

The treatment of **HELLP syndrome** must include evacuation of the uterus (eg, delivery of a term or near-term infant or removal of retained placental or fetal fragments). Patients with **Trousseau syndrome** require treatment of the underlying malignancy or administration of unfractionated heparin or subcutaneous therapeutic-dose LMWH as treatment of thrombosis, since warfarin typically is ineffective at secondary prevention of thromboembolism in the disorder. Immediate initiation of chemotherapy (usually within 24 hours of diagnosis) is required for patients with **acute**

promyelocytic leukemia (APL)–associated DIC, along with administration of blood products as clinically indicated.

▶ **When to Refer**

Patients with diffuse bleeding that is unresponsive to administration of blood products should be evaluated by a hematologist.

▶ **When to Admit**

Most patients with DIC are hospitalized when DIC is detected.

Bick RL. Disseminated intravascular coagulation current concepts of etiology, pathophysiology, diagnosis, and treatment. Hematol Oncol Clin North Am. 2003 Feb;17(1):149–76. [PMID: 12627667]

Harzstark A et al. Disseminated intravascular coagulation. In: Parsons PE, Weiner-Kronish JP (editors.) *Critical Care Secrets*, 4th ed. Philadelphia: Mosby; 2007.

Sibai BM. Diagnosis, controversies, and management of the syndrome of hemolysis, elevated liver enzymes, and low platelet count. Obstet Gynecol. 2004 May;103(5 Pt 1):981–91. [PMID: 15121574]

OTHER CONDITIONS CAUSING THROMBOCYTOPENIA

1. Posttransfusion Purpura (PTP)

Posttransfusion purpura (PTP) is a rare disorder that features sudden-onset thrombocytopenia in an individual who recently has received transfusion of red cells, platelets, or plasma within 1 week prior to detection of thrombocytopenia. Antibodies against the human platelet antigen Pl^{A1} are detected in most individuals with PTP. Patients with PTP almost universally are either multiparous women or persons who have received transfusions previously. Severe thrombocytopenia and bleeding is typical. Initial treatment consists of administration of IVIG (1 g/kg/d for 2 days) should be administered as soon as the diagnosis is suspected. Platelets are not indicated unless severe bleeding is present, but if they are to be administered, HLA-matched platelets are preferred. A second course or IVIG, plasma exchange, corticosteroids, or splenectomy may be used in case of refractoriness. Pl^{A1}-negative or washed blood products are preferred for subsequent transfusions.

2. von Willebrand Disease Type 2B

von Willebrand disease (vWD) type 2B leads to chronic, characteristically mild to moderate thrombocytopenia via an abnormal vWF molecule that binds platelets with increased affinity, resulting in aggregation and clearance. Passage of the blood for prolonged periods outside the body in an artificial circuit (such as occurs with extracorporeal circulation) also can result in platelet clearance; thrombocytopenia typically resolves within several days.

3. Platelet Sequestration

At any given time, one-third of the platelet mass is sequestered in the spleen. Splenomegaly, due to a variety of

Table 14–8. Selected causes of splenomegaly.

Lymphoproliferative/myeloproliferative disease
Lymphoma
Chronic lymphocytic leukemia
Chronic myeloid leukemia
Polycythemia vera
Essential thrombocythemia
Vascular congestion
Congestive heart failure
Cirrhosis
Hematologic defects
Hereditary spherocytosis
Paroxysmal nocturnal hemoglobinuria
Thalassemia
Autoimmunity
Collagen vascular disease
Felty syndrome, lupus
Autoimmune lymphoproliferative disorder
Infection
Infectious hepatitis
Cytomegalovirus
Malaria
Babesiosis
Inborn errors of metabolism
Gaucher disease
Niemann-Pick disease

conditions (Table 14–8), may lead to thrombocytopenia of variable severity. Whenever possible, treatment of the underlying disorder should be pursued, but splenectomy, splenic embolization, or splenic irradiation may be considered in selected cases.

4. Pregnancy

Gestational thrombocytopenia results from progressive expansion of the blood volume that typically occurs during pregnancy, leading to hemodilution. Cytopenias result, although production of blood cells is normal or increased. Platelet counts < 100,000/mcL, however, are observed in less than 10% of pregnant women in the third trimester; decreases to less than 70,000/mcL should prompt consideration of pregnancy-related ITP (see above) as well as preeclampsia or a pregnancy-related thrombotic microangiopathy.

5. Infection or Sepsis

Both immune- and platelet production–mediated defects are possible, and there may be significant overlap with concomitant DIC (see above). In either case, the platelet count typically improves with effective antimicrobial treatment or after the infection has resolved. In some critically ill patients, a defect in immunomodulation may lead to bone marrow macrophages (histiocytes) engulfing cellular components of the marrow in a process also called hemophagocytosis. The phenomenon typically resolves with resolution of the infection, but with certain infections (Epstein Barr virus) immunosuppression may be required. Hemophagocytosis also may arise in the setting of malignancy, in which case the disorder is usually unresponsive to treatment with immunosuppression.

6. Pseudothrombocytopenia

Pseudothrombocytopenia results from EDTA anticoagulant-induced platelet clumping; the phenomenon typically disappears when blood is collected in a tube containing citrate anticoagulant.

QUALITATIVE PLATELET DISORDERS

CONGENITAL DISORDERS OF PLATELET FUNCTION

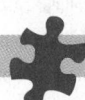 ESSENTIALS OF DIAGNOSIS

▸ Usually diagnosed in childhood.
▸ May be diagnosed in adulthood when there is excessive bleeding.

▸ General Considerations

Heritable qualitative platelet disorders are far less common than acquired disorders of platelet function (see below) and lead to variably severe bleeding, often beginning in childhood. Occasionally, however, disorders of platelet function may go undetected until later in life when excessive bleeding occurs following a sufficient hemostatic insult. Thus, the true incidence of hereditary qualitative platelet disorders is unknown.

Bernard-Soulier syndrome (BSS) is a rare, autosomal recessive bleeding disorder that is due to reduced or abnormal platelet membrane expression of glycoprotein Ib/IX (vWF receptor).

Glanzmann thrombasthenia results from a qualitative or quantitative abnormality in glycoprotein IIb/IIIa receptors on the platelet membrane, which are required to bind fibrinogen and vWF, both of which bridge platelets during aggregation. Inheritance is autosomal recessive.

Under normal circumstances, activated platelets release the contents of platelet granules to reinforce the aggregatory response. **Storage pool disease** is caused by defects in release of alpha or dense (delta) platelet granules, or both (alpha-delta storage pool disease).

▸ Clinical Findings
A. Symptoms and Signs

In patients with **Glanzmann thrombasthenia**, the onset of bleeding is usually in infancy or childhood. The degree of deficiency in IIb/IIIa may not correlate well with bleeding symptoms. Patients with **storage pool disease** are affected by variable bleeding, ranging from mild and trauma-related to spontaneous.

B. Laboratory Findings

In **Bernard-Soulier syndrome**, there are abnormally large platelets (approaching the size of red cells), moderate

Table 14–9. Causes of acquired platelet dysfunction.

Cause	Mechanism(s)	Treatment of Bleeding
Drug-induced		
Salicylates (eg, aspirin)	Irreversible inhibition of platelet cyclooxygenase	Discontinuation of drug; platelet transfusion
NSAIDs (eg, ibuprofen)	Reversible inhibition of cyclooxygenase	
Glycoprotein IIb/IIIa inhibitors (eg, abciximab, tirofiban, eptifibatide	↓ Binding of fibrinogen to PM IIb/IIIa receptor	
Thienopyridines (eg, clopidogrel, ticlopidine)	↓ ADP binding to PM receptor	
Dipyridamole	↓ Intracellular cAMP metabolism	
SSRIs (eg, paroxetine, fluoxetine)	↓ Serotonin in dense-granules	
Omega-3 fatty acids (eg, DHA, EHA)	Disruption of PM phospholipid	
Antibiotics, (eg, high-dose penicillin, nafcillin, ticarcillin, cephalothin, moxalactam)	Not fully elucidated; PM binding may interfere with receptor-ligand interactions	
Alcohol	↓ TXA2 release	
Uremia	↑ Nitric oxide; ↓ release of granules	DDAVP, high-dose estrogens; platelet transfusion, dialysis
Myeloproliferative disorder/myelodysplastic syndrome	Abnormal PM receptors, signal transduction, and/or granule release	Platelet transfusion; myelosuppressive treatment (myeloproliferative disorder)
Cardiac bypass	Platelet activation in bypass circuit	Platelet transfusion

ADP, adenosine diphosphate; cAMP, cyclic adenosine monophosphate; DDAVP, desmopressin acetate; DHA, docosahexaenoic acid; EHA, eicosahexaenoic acid; NSAIDs, nonsteroidal anti-inflammatory drugs; PM, platelet membrane; SSRIs, selective serotonin release inhibitors; TXA2, thromboxane A2.

thrombocytopenia, and a prolonged bleeding time. Platelet aggregation studies show a marked defect in response to ristocetin, whereas aggregation in response to other agonists is normal; the addition of normal platelets corrects the abnormal aggregation. The diagnosis can be confirmed by platelet flow cytometry.

In **Glanzmann thrombasthenia**, platelet aggregation studies show marked impairment of aggregation in response to stimulation with typical agonists.

There are several presentations of **storage pool disease**. Patients have a prolonged bleeding time. Platelet aggregation studies characteristically show platelet dissociation following an initial aggregatory response, and electron microscopy confirms the diagnosis.

▶ **Treatment**

The mainstay of treatment (including periprocedural prophylaxis) is transfusion of normal platelets, although desmopressin acetate (DDAVP), antifibrinolytic agents, and recombinant human activated factor VII also have been used successfully.

Roberts HR et al. The use of recombinant factor VIIa in the treatment of bleeding disorders. Blood. 2004 Dec 15; 104(13):3858–64. [PMID: 15328151]

Toogeh G et al. Presentation and pattern of symptoms in 382 patients with Glanzmann thrombasthenia in Iran. Am J Hematol. 2004 Oct;77(2):198–9. [PMID: 15389911]

ACQUIRED DISORDERS OF PLATELET FUNCTION

Platelet dysfunction is more commonly acquired than inherited; the widespread use of platelet-active medications accounts for most of the cases of qualitative defects (Table 14–9). In these cases, platelet inhibition typically declines within 5–10 days following discontinuation of the drug, and transfusion of platelets may be required if clinically significant bleeding is present.

Laboratory manifestations of aspirin toxicity include a prolonged epinephrine cartridge closure time in the platelet function analyzer (PFA)-100 system, or a decreased aggregation to low-dose collagen and thrombin (and preserved aggregation in response to high-dose collagen and thrombin) on platelet aggregation studies.

▼ DISORDERS OF COAGULATION

CONGENITAL DISORDERS OF COAGULATION
1. Hemophilia A & B

 ESSENTIALS OF DIAGNOSIS

▶ Hemophilia A: congenital deficiency of coagulation factor VIII.

- Hemophilia B: congenital deficiency of coagulation factor IX.
- Symptomatic in males.
- Recurrent hemarthroses and arthropathy.
- Infection with HIV or hepatitis C virus from receipt of contaminated blood products.

General Considerations

The frequency of hemophilia A is 1 per 5000 live male births, whereas hemophilia B occurs in approximately 1 in 25,000 live male births. Inheritance is X-linked recessive, leading to affected males and carrier females. There is no race predilection. Testing is indicated for asymptomatic male infants with a hemophilic pedigree, for male infants with a family history of hemophilia who experience excessive bleeding, or for an otherwise asymptomatic adolescent or adult who experiences unexpected excessive bleeding with trauma or invasion.

Inhibitors to factor VIII will develop in approximately 25% of patients with hemophilia A, and inhibitors to factor IX will develop in less than 5% of patients with hemophilia B.

The prevalence of hepatitis C virus infection is highest among individuals with severe disease who received plasma-derived clotting factor concentrates or blood products in the pre-mid-1980s, and approaches a 100% exposure rate in this population. New infection is now rare, given current methodology for screening of blood products, viral inactivation of plasma-derived factor, and use of recombinant products. Many patients infected with hepatitis C virus have undergone eradication treatment successfully. New HIV infection related to the treatment of hemophilia, too, is rare in the modern era, although a large number of patients with hemophilia were exposed to HIV through contaminated blood products of factor concentrates in the 1980s.

Clinical Findings

A. Symptoms and Signs

Severe hemophilia presents in infant males or in early childhood with spontaneous bleeding into joints, soft tissues, or other locations. Spontaneous bleeding is rare in patients with mild hemophilia, but bleeding may occur with a significant hemostatic challenge (eg, surgery, trauma). Intermediate clinical symptoms are seen in patients with moderate hemophilia. Female carriers of hemophilia are usually asymptomatic.

Significant hemophilic arthropathy is usually avoided in patients who have received long-term prophylaxis with factor concentrate in childhood, whereas severe arthritis and limited range of motion in affected joints are common in adults who received episodic or little treatment during childhood and experienced recurrent hemarthroses.

Inhibitor development to factor VIII or factor IX is characterized by bleeding episodes that are resistant to treatment and new or unusual bleeding.

B. Laboratory Findings

Hemophilia is diagnosed by demonstration of an isolated reproducibly low factor VIII or factor IX activity level, in the absence of other conditions. If the aPTT is prolonged, it typically corrects upon mixing with normal plasma. A variety of mutations, including inversions, large and small deletions, insertions, missense mutations, and nonsense mutations may be causative. Depending on the level of residual factor VIII or factor IX activity and the sensitivity of the thromboplastin used in the aPTT coagulation reaction, the aPTT may or may not be prolonged (although it typically is markedly prolonged in severe hemophilia). Hemophilia is classified according to the level of factor activity in the plasma. Severe hemophilia is characterized by less than 1% factor activity, mild hemophilia features greater than 5% factor activity, and moderate hemophilia features 1–5% factor activity. Female carriers may become symptomatic if significant lyonization has occurred favoring the defective factor VIII or factor IX gene, leading to factor VIII or factor IX activity level markedly less than 50%.

In the presence of an inhibitor to factor VIII or factor IX, there is accelerated clearance of and suboptimal or absent rise in measured activity of infused factor, and the aPTT does not correct on mixing. The Bethesda assay measures the potency of the inhibitor.

Treatment

Plasma-derived or recombinant factor concentrates are the mainstay of treatment. By the age of 4 years, children with severe hemophilia typically receive long-term, prophylactic, twice- or thrice-weekly infusions of factor to prevent the recurrent joint bleeding that otherwise would characterize the disorder, leading to severe morbidity. Adults generally do not use intensive, long-term prophylaxis, and instead treat with factor concentrate as needed for bleeding episodes or prior to high-risk activities (Table 14–10). Patients with mild hemophilia A may respond to as-needed intravenous or intranasal treatment with DDAVP. Antifibrinolytic agents may be useful in cases of mucosal bleeding and are commonly used adjunctively, such as following dental procedures. Thus far, early trials of gene therapy (delivery of normal factor VIII or factor IX genes via viral vectors) have not shown increases in factor activity levels of both adequate magnitude and duration.

The cyclooxygenase (COX)-2 selective nonsteroidal anti-inflammatory drug celecoxib may be used to treat arthritis symptoms; generally, other NSAIDs and aspirin should be avoided due to the increased risk of bleeding from inhibition of platelet function. Oral opioid medications are commonly used to control pain, and surgery, including total joint replacement, is often required.

It may be possible to overcome low-titer inhibitors (< 5 Bethesda units, BU) by giving larger doses of factor, whereas treatment of bleeding in the presence of a high-titer inhibitor (> 5 BU) requires infusion of an activated prothrombin complex concentrate or recombinant activated factor VII. Inhibitor tolerance induction, achieved by giving large doses (50–300 units/kg intravenously of

Table 14–10. Treatment of selected inherited bleeding disorders.

Disorder	Subtype	Treatment for Minor Bleeding	Treatment for Major Bleeding	Comment
Hemophilia A	Mild	DDAVP[1]	DDAVP[1] or factor VIII concentrate	Treat for 3–10 days for major bleeding or following surgery, keeping factor activity level ≥ 50–80% initially. Adjunctive aminocaproic acid may be useful for mucosal bleeding or procedures
	Moderate or severe	Factor VIII concentrate	Factor VIII concentrate	
Hemophilia B	Mild, moderate, or severe	Factor IX concentrate	Factor IX concentrate	
von Willebrand disease	Type 1	DDAVP	DDAVP, vWF concentrate	
	Type 2	DDAVP,[1] vWF concentrate	vWF concentrate	
	Type 3	vWF concentrate	vWF concentrate	
Factor XI deficiency	—	FFP or aminocaproic acid	FFP	Adjunctive aminocaproic acid should be used for mucosal bleeding or procedures

[1]Mild hemophilia A and type 2A or 2B vWD patients: therapeutic trial must have previously confirmed an adequate response (i.e., elevation of factor VIII or vWF activity level into the normal range) and (for type 2B) no exacerbation of thrombocytopenia. DDAVP is not typically effective for type 2M vWD. A vWF-containing factor VIII concentrate is preferred for treatment of type 2N vWD.

Notes:
DDAVP dose is 0.3 mcg/kg IV in 50 mL saline over 20 minutes, or nasal spray 300 mcg for weight > 50 kg or 150 mcg for < 50 kg, every 12–24 hours, maximum of three doses in a 48-hour period. If more than two doses are used in a 12–24 hour period, free water restriction and/or monitoring for hyponatremia is essential.
EACA dose is 50 mg/kg PO four times daily for 3–5 d; maximum 24 g/d, useful for mucosal bleeding/dental procedures.
Factor VIII concentrate dose is 50 units/kg IV initially followed by 25 units/kg every 8 hours followed by lesser doses at longer intervals once hemostasis has been established.
Factor IX concentrate dose is 100 units/kg (120 units/kg if using Benefix) IV initially followed by 50 units/kg (60 units/kg if using Benefix) every 8 hours followed by lesser doses at longer intervals once hemostasis has been established.
vWF-containing factor VIII concentrate dose is 60–80 RCoF units/kg IV every 12 hours initially followed by lesser doses at longer intervals once hemostasis has been established.
FFP is typically administered in 4-unit boluses and may not need to be re-bolused after the initial administration due to the long half-life of factor XI.
DDAVP, desmopressin acetate; FFP, fresh frozen plasma; vWF, von Willebrand factor.

factor VIII daily) for 6–18 months, succeeds in eradicating the inhibitor in 70% of patients with hemophilia A and in 30% of patients with hemophilia B; hemophilia B patients who receive inhibitor tolerance induction, however, are at risk for development of nephrotic syndrome and anaphylactic reactions, making eradication of their inhibitors less feasible.

Highly active antiretroviral treatment is almost universally administered to individuals with HIV infection.

When to Refer

All patients with hemophilia should be seen regularly in a comprehensive hemophilia treatment center staffed by a hematologist.

When to Admit

- Most bleeding events can be treated as an outpatient.
- Some invasive procedures that could otherwise be performed as an outpatient require admission in a patient with hemophilia due to the need for serial infusions of clotting factor concentrate.
- Patients with hemophilia and inhibitors who experience bleeding that is unresponsive to bypassing agents typically require admission.

Hay CR et al. The diagnosis and management of factor VIII and IX inhibitors: a guideline from the United Kingdom Haemophilia Centre Doctors Organisation. Br J Haematol. 2006 Jun;133(6):591–605. [PMID: 16704433]
Mannucci PM et al. The hemophiliac–from royal genes to gene therapy. N Engl J Med. 2001 Jun 7;344(23):1773–9. [PMID: 11396445]

2. von Willebrand Disease

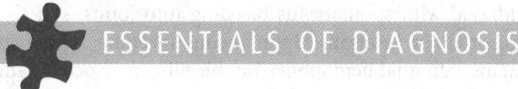 ESSENTIALS OF DIAGNOSIS

- ▶ The most common inherited bleeding disorder.
- ▶ von Willebrand factor aggregates platelets and prolongs the half-life of factor VIII.

General Considerations

Up to 1% of the population have depressed vWF levels. vWF is an unusually large multimeric glycoprotein that binds to its receptor, platelet glycoprotein Ib, bridging platelets together and tethering them to the subendothelial matrix at the site of vascular injury. vWF also has a binding site for factor VIII, prolonging its half-life in the circulation.

Between 75% and 80% of patients with vWD have type 1. It is a quantitative abnormality of the vWF molecule that usually does not feature an identifiable causal mutation in the vWF gene.

Type 2 vWD is seen in 15–20% of patients with vWD. In type 2A or 2B vWD, a qualitative defect in the vWF molecule is causative. Type 2N and 2M vWD are due to defects in vWF that decrease binding to factor VIII or to platelets, respectively. Importantly, type 2N vWD clinically resembles hemophilia A, with the exception of a family history that shows affected females. Factor VIII activity levels are markedly decreased, and vWF activity and antigen (Ag) are normal. Type 2M vWD features a normal multimer pattern. Type 3 vWD is rare, and mutational homozygosity or double heterozygosity leads to undetectable levels of vWF and severe bleeding in infancy or childhood.

Clinical Findings

A. Symptoms and Signs

Patients with type 1 vWD usually have mild or moderate platelet-type bleeding (especially involving the integument and mucous membranes). Patients with type 2 vWD usually have moderate to severe bleeding that presents in childhood or adolescence.

B. Laboratory Findings

In type 1 vWD, the vWF activity (by ristocetin co-factor assay) and Ag are mildly depressed, whereas the vWF multimer pattern is normal (Table 14–11). Laboratory testing of type 2A or 2B vWD typically shows a ratio of vWF Ag:vWF activity of approximately 2:1 and a multimer pattern that lacks the highest molecular weight multimers. Thrombocytopenia is common in type 2B vWD due to a gain-of-function mutation of the vWF molecule, which leads to increased binding to its receptor on platelets, resulting in clearance; a ristocetin-induced platelet aggregation (RIPA) study shows an increase in platelet aggregation in response to low concentrations of ristocetin. Except in the more severe forms of vWD that feature

a significantly decreased factor VIII activity, the aPTT and PT in vWD are usually normal.

Treatment

The treatment of vWD is summarized in Table 14–10. DDAVP is useful in the treatment of mild bleeding in most cases of type 1 and some cases of type 2 vWD. DDAVP causes release of vWF and factor VIII from storage sites, leading to increases in vWF and factor VIII twofold to sevenfold that of baseline levels. A therapeutic trial to document sufficient vWF levels posttreatment is recommended. Due to tachyphylaxis and the risk of significant hyponatremia secondary to fluid retention, more than two doses should not be given in a 48-hour period. Intermediate-purity vWF-containing factor VIII concentrates are used in all other clinical scenarios, and when bleeding is not controlled with DDAVP. Cryoprecipitate should not be given due to lack of viral inactivation. Antifibrinolytic agents (eg, aminocaproic acid) may be used adjunctively for mucosal bleeding or procedures. Pregnant patients with vWD usually do not require treatment because of the natural physiologic increase in vWF levels (up to threefold that of baseline) that are observed by the time of delivery; however, if excessive bleeding is encountered, DDAVP may be given to patients with mild disease or vWF-containing factor VIII concentrates may be given to patients with more severe disease.

Federici AB et al. Biologic response to desmopressin in patients with severe type 1 and type 2 von Willebrand disease: results of a multicenter European study. Blood. 2004 Mar 15;103(6):2032–8. [PMID: 14630825]
The Diagnosis, Evaluation and Management of von Willebrand Disease. National Heart, Lung, and Blood Institute, NIH Pub. No. 08-5832. December 2007. (http://www.nhlbi.nih.gov/guidelines/vwd/index.htm)

3. Factor XI Deficiency

Factor XI deficiency (sometimes referred to as **hemophilia C**) is inherited in an autosomal recessive manner, leading to heterozygous or homozygous defects. It is most prevalent among individuals of Ashkenazi Jewish descent. Levels of factor XI, while variably reduced, do not correlate well with bleeding symptoms. Mild bleeding is most common,

Table 14–11. Laboratory diagnosis of von Willebrand disease.

Type		vWF Activity	vWF Antigen	FVIII	RIPA	Multimer Analysis
1		↓	↓	Nl or ↓	↓	Uniform ↓ in intensity
2	A	↓↓	↓	↓	↓	Large and intermediate multimers decreased or absent.
	B	↓↓	↓	↓	↑	Large multimers decreased or absent
	M	↓	↓	↓	↓	Nl
	N	Nl	Nl	↓↓	Nl	Nl
3		↓↓↓	↓↓↓	↓↓↓	↓↓↓	Absent

Nl, normal; RIPA, ristocetin-induced platelet aggregation; vWF, von Willebrand factor.

and surgery or trauma may expose or worsen the bleeding tendency. Fresh frozen plasma (FFP) is the mainstay of treatment, since no factor XI concentrate is available in the United States. Administration of adjunctive aminocaproic acid is regarded as mandatory for procedures or bleeding episodes involving the mucosa (Table 14–10).

4. Less Common Heritable Disorders of Coagulation

Congenital deficiencies of clotting factors II, V, VII, and X are rare and typically are inherited in an autosomal recessive pattern. A prolongation in the PT (and aPTT for factor X and factor II deficiency) that corrects upon mixing with normal plasma is typical.

Deficiency of factor XIII, a transglutamase that cross-links fibrin, characteristically leads to delayed bleeding that occurs hours to days after a hemostatic challenge (such as surgery or trauma). Cryoprecipitate or infusion of a plasma-derived factor XIII concentrate (available through a research study; appropriate for patients with A-subunit deficiency only) is the treatment of choice for bleeding or surgical prophylaxis.

Congenital deficiencies of factor XII, prekallikrein, high molecular-weight kininogen may lead to a prolonged aPTT that corrects with extended incubation but do not lead to bleeding.

ACQUIRED DISORDERS OF COAGULATION

1. Acquired Antibodies to Factor VIII

Spontaneous antibodies to factor VIII occasionally occur in adults without a prior history of hemophilia; the elderly and patients with lymphoproliferative malignancy or connective tissue disease, who are postpartum, or postsurgical are at highest risk. The clinical presentation typically includes extensive soft-tissue ecchymoses, hematomas, and mucosal bleeding, as opposed to hemarthrosis in congenital hemophilia A. The aPTT is typically prolonged and does not correct upon mixing; factor VIII activity is found to be low and a Bethesda assay reveals the titer of the inhibitor. Inhibitors of low titer (< 5 BU) may often be overcome by infusion of high doses of factor VIII concentrates, whereas high-titer inhibitors (> 5 BU) must be treated with serial infusions of activated prothrombin complex concentrates or recombinant human activated factor VII. Along with establishment of hemostasis by one of these measures, immunosuppressive treatment with corticosteroids and oral cyclophosphamide should be instituted; treatment with IVIG, rituximab, or plasmapheresis can be considered in refractory cases.

Stasi R et al. Selective B-cell depletion with rituximab for the treatment of patients with acquired hemophilia. Blood. 2004 Jun 15;103(12):4424–8. [PMID: 14996701]

2. Acquired Antibodies to Factor II

Patients with antiphospholipid antibodies occasionally manifest specificity to coagulation factor II (prothrombin), leading typically to a severe hypoprothrombinemia and bleeding. Mixing studies may or may not reveal presence of an inhibitor, as the antibody typically binds a non-enzymatically active portion of the molecule that leads to accelerated clearance, but characteristically the PT is prolonged and levels of factor II are low. FFP should be administered for treatment of bleeding. Treatment is immunosuppressive.

3. Acquired Antibodies to Factor V

Products containing bovine factor V (such as topical thrombin or fibrin glue, frequently used in surgical procedures) can lead to formation of an anti-factor V antibody that has specificity for human factor V. Clinicopathologic manifestations range from a prolonged PT in an otherwise asymptomatic individual to severe bleeding. Mixing studies suggest the presence of an inhibitor, and the factor V activity level is low. In cases of serious or life-threatening bleeding, IVIG or platelet transfusions, or both, should be administered, and immunosuppression (as for acquired inhibitors to factor VIII) may be offered.

4. Vitamin K Deficiency

Vitamin K deficiency may occur as a result of deficient dietary intake of vitamin K (from green leafy vegetables, soybeans, and other sources), malabsorption, or decreased production by intestinal bacteria (due to treatment with chemotherapy or antibiotics). Vitamin K normally participates in activity of the vitamin K epoxide reductase that assists in posttranslational gamma-carboxylation of the coagulation factors II, VII, IX, and X that is necessary for their activity. Thus, vitamin K deficiency typically features a prolonged PT (in which the activity of the vitamin K–dependent factors is more reflected than in the aPTT) that corrects upon mixing; levels of individual clotting factors II, VII, IX, and X typically are low. Importantly, a concomitantly low factor V activity level is not indicative of isolated vitamin K deficiency, and may indicate an underlying defect in liver synthetic function (see below).

For treatment, vitamin K_1 (phytonadione) may be administered via intravenous or oral routes; the subcutaneous route is not recommended due to erratic absorption. Oral absorption is typically excellent and at least partial improvement in the PT should be observed within 1 day of administration. Intravenous administration (1 mg/d) results in even faster normalization of a prolonged PT than oral administration (5–10 mg/d); due to descriptions of anaphylaxis, parenteral doses should be administered at lower doses and slowly (eg, over 30 minutes) with concomitant monitoring.

5. Coagulopathy of Liver Disease

Impaired hepatic function due to cirrhosis or other causes leads to decreased synthesis of clotting factors, including factors II, VII, V, VIII, and fibrinogen, whereas factor VIII levels may be elevated in spite of depressed levels of other coagulation factors. The PT (and with advanced disease, the aPTT) is typically prolonged and corrects on mixing with normal plasma. A normal factor V level, in spite of decreases in the activity of factors II, VII, IX, and X, however, suggests vitamin K deficiency rather than liver disease (see above). Qualitative and quantitative deficiencies of fibrinogen also are prevalent among patients with advanced liver disease, typically leading to a prolonged PT, thrombin time, and reptilase time.

The coagulopathy of liver disease usually does not require hemostatic treatment until bleeding complications occur. Infusion of FFP may be considered if active bleeding is present and the aPTT and PT are markedly prolonged; however, the effect is transient and concern for volume overload may limit infusions. Patients with bleeding and a fibrinogen level consistently below 80 mg/dL should receive cryoprecipitate. Liver transplantation, if feasible, results in production of coagulation factors at normal levels. The appropriateness of use of recombinant human activated factor VII in patients with bleeding varices is controversial, although some patient subgroups may experience benefit.

Thabut D et al. Efficacy of activated recombinant factor VII in cirrhotic patients with upper gastrointestinal bleeding: a randomized placebo-controlled double-blind multicenter trial. Critical Care. 2004;8(Suppl 1):P136.
Youssef WI et al. Role of fresh frozen plasma infusion in correction of coagulopathy of chronic liver disease: a dual phase study. Am J Gastroenterol. 2003 Jun;98(6):1391–4. [PMID: 12818286]

6. Warfarin Ingestion

See Antithrombotic Therapy section below.

7. Heparin Use or Contamination

The presence of heparin in the coagulation reaction system (whether by contamination or intentional administration to the patient) may prolong the aPTT. The thrombin time is dramatically prolonged in the presence of heparin. If contamination is suspected, use of a heparin neutralizing agent on the sample will result in normalization of the aPTT; alternatively, a fresh sample from a peripheral site can be obtained and tested. Patients who are receiving heparin and who have bleeding should be managed by discontinuation of the heparin and (some cases) administration of protamine sulfate; 1 mg of protamine neutralizes approximately 100 units of heparin sulfate, and the maximum dose is 50 mg intravenously. LMWHs typically do not prolong clotting times and are poorly reversible with protamine.

8. Disseminated Intravascular Coagulation

The consumptive coagulopathy of DIC results in decreases in the activity of clotting factors, leading to bleeding in most patients (see above). The aPTT and PT are characteristically prolonged, and platelets and fibrinogen levels are reduced from baseline.

9. Lupus Anticoagulants

Lupus anticoagulants prolong clotting times by binding proteins associated with phospholipid, which is a necessary component of coagulation reactions. Lupus anticoagulants were so named because of their increased prevalence among patients with connective tissue disease, although they may occur with increased frequency in individuals with underlying infection, inflammation, or malignancy, and they also can occur in asymptomatic individuals in the general population. Importantly, lupus anticoagulants do not cause bleeding.

A prolongation in the aPTT is observed that does not correct completely on mixing. Specialized testing such as the hexagonal phase phospholipid neutralization assay, the dilute Russel viper venom time, and platelet neutralization assays can confirm the presence of a lupus anticoagulant.

CONDITIONS CAUSING BLEEDING DESPITE NORMAL HEMOSTASIS

Occasionally, abnormalities of the vasculature and integument may lead to bleeding despite normal hemostasis; congenital or acquired disorders may be causative. These abnormalities include Ehlers-Danlos syndrome, osteogenesis imperfecta, Osler-Weber-Rendu disease, and Marfan syndrome (heritable defects) and integumentary thinning due to prolonged corticosteroid administration or normal aging, amyloidosis, vasculitis, and scurvy (acquired defects). The bleeding time often is prolonged. If possible, treatment of the underlying condition should be pursued, but if this is not possible or feasible (ie, congenital syndromes), globally hemostatic agents such as DDAVP can be considered for treatment of bleeding.

Yasui H et al. Combination therapy of DDAVP and conjugated estrogens for a recurrent large subcutaneous hematoma in Ehlers-Danlos syndrome. Am J Hematol. 2003 Jan;72(1):71–2. [PMID: 12508273]

▼ ANTITHROMBOTIC THERAPY

▶ Prevention of Venous Thromboembolic Disease

The frequency of venous thromboembolic disease (VTE) among hospitalized patients ranges widely; up to 20% of low-risk medical patients and 80% of critical care patients and high-risk surgical patients have been reported to experience this complication, which includes deep venous thrombosis (DVT) and pulmonary embolism (PE).

Avoidance of fatal PE, which occurs in up to 5% of high-risk inpatients, as a consequence of hospitalization or surgery is a major goal of pharmacologic prophylaxis. Standard regimens are listed in Table 14–12. In medical patients, 5000 units of subcutaneous unfractionated heparin three times daily resulted in a trend toward decreased proximal DVT and PE but increased risk of major bleeding when compared with 5000 units of unfractionated heparin twice daily. Compared with unfractionated heparin taken three times daily, LMWH appears more effective at preventing DVT without increased bleeding risk.

If bleeding is present or the risk of bleeding is high, some measure of thromboprophylaxis may be provided through use of graduated compression stockings or intermittent pneumatic compression devices, which have been

Table 14–12. Pharmacologic prophylaxis of VTE in selected clinical scenarios.[1]

Anticoagulant	Dose	Frequency	Clinical Scenario	Comment
Enoxaparin	40 mg	Once daily	Most medical inpatients and critical care patients	—
			Surgical patients (moderate risk for VTE)	—
			Abdominal/pelvic cancer surgery	Continue for 4 weeks total duration
		Twice daily	Bariatric surgery	Higher doses may be required
	30 mg	Twice daily	Orthopedic surgery[2]	Give for at least 10 days. For THR, TKA, or HFS, continue up to 35 days after surgery
			Major trauma	Not applicable to patients with isolated lower extremity trauma
			Acute spinal cord injury	—
Dalteparin	2500 units	Once daily	Most medical inpatients	—
			Abdominal surgery (moderate risk for VTE)	Give for 5–10 days
	5000 units	Once daily	Orthopedic surgery[2]	First dose = 2500 units. Give for at least 10 days. For THR, TKA, or HFS, continue up to 35 days after surgery
			Abdominal surgery (higher-risk for VTE)	Give for 5–10 days
			Medical inpatients	—
Fondaparinux	2.5mg	Once daily	Orthopedic surgery[2]	Give for at least 10 days. For THR, TKA or HFS, continue up to 35 days after surgery
Unfractionated heparin	5000 units	Three times daily	Patients with severe renal insufficiency[3]	LMWHs contraindicated
			Patients with epidural catheters	LMWHs contraindicated
			Surgical patients (higher risk for VTE)	Includes gynecologic surgery for malignancy and urologic surgery, neurosurgery in high-risk patients
	5000 units	Twice daily	Surgical patients (moderate risk)	Includes gynecologic surgery (moderate risk)
Warfarin	(variable)	Once daily	Orthopedic surgery[2]	Titrate to goal INR = 2.5. Give for at least 10 days. For THR, TKA, or HFS, continue up to 35 days after surgery

[1]All regimens administered subcutaneously, except for warfarin.
[2]Includes TKA, THR, and HFS.
[3]Defined as creatinine clearance < 30 mL/min.
HFS, hip fracture surgery; LMWH, low-molecular-weight heparin; THR, total hip replacement; TKA, total knee arthroplasty; VTE, venous thromboembolic disease.

shown to reduce the incidence of VTE among select patient groups and can be a valuable adjunctive measure in patients who already are receiving pharmacologic prophylaxis and are at particularly high risk for VTE.

Geerts WH et al. Prevention of venous thromboembolism: American College of Chest Physicians Evidence-Based Clinical Practice Guidelines (8th Edition). Chest. 2008 Jun;133(6 Suppl):381S–453S. [PMID: 18574271]

King CS et al. Twice vs three times daily heparin dosing for thromboembolism prophylaxis in the general medical population: A metaanalysis. Chest. 2007 Feb;131(2):507–16. [PMID: 17296655]

Wein L et al. Pharmacological venous thromboembolism prophylaxis in hospitalized medical patients: a meta-analysis of randomized controlled trials. Arch Intern Med. 2007 Jul 23;167(14):1476–86. [PMID: 17646601]

▶ Treatment of Venous Thromboembolic Disease

A. Anticoagulant Therapy

Treatment for VTE should be offered to patients with objectively confirmed DVT or PE, or to those in whom the clinical suspicion is high for the disorder yet have not yet undergone diagnostic testing (see Chapter 9). The management of VTE primarily involves administration of anticoagulants, which initially are given parenterally followed by long-term oral therapy; the goal is the secondary prevention of additional thrombi. Suggested anticoagulation regimens are found in Table 14–13. Table 14–14 outlines the selection criteria for outpatient treatment of DVT. Most patients with DVT alone may be treated as outpatients, provided that their risk of bleeding is low, they are candi-

Table 14–13. Initial anticoagulation for VTE.[1]

Anticoagulant	Dose/Frequency	Clinical Scenario					Comment
		DVT, Lower Extremity	DVT, Upper Extremity	PE	VTE, with Concomitant Severe Renal Impairment[2]	VTE, Cancer-Related	
Unfractionated heparin	80 units/kg IV bolus then continuous IV infusion of 18 units/kg/h	×	×	×	×		Bolus may be omitted if risk of bleeding is perceived to be elevated. Maximum bolus, 10,000 units. Requires aPTT monitoring. Most patients: begin warfarin at time of initiation of heparin
	17,500 units SC q12h (initial dose)	×					aPTT monitoring required with dose adjustment
	330 units/kg SC × 1 then 250 units/kg SC q12h	×					Fixed-dose; no aPTT monitoring required
Enoxaparin[3]	1 mg/kg SC q12h	×	×	×			Most patients: begin warfarin at time of initiation of LMWH
	1.5 mg/kg SC once daily		×				
Tinzaparin[3]	175 units/kg SC once daily	×	×	×		×	Cancer: administer LMWH for ≥ 3–6 months
Dalteparin[3]	200 units/kg SC once daily	×	×	×		×	Cancer: administer LMWH for ≥ 3–6 months; reduce dose to 150 units/kg after first month of treatment
Fondaparinux	5–10 mg SC once daily (see Comment)	×	×	×			Use 7.5 mg for body weight 50–100 kg. 10 mg for body weight > 100 kg

Note: An "×" denotes appropriate use of the anticoagulant.
[1]Obtain baseline hemoglobin, platelet count, aPTT PT/INR, creatinine, urinalysis, and hemoccult prior to initiation of anticoagulation. *Anticoagulation is contraindicated in the setting of active bleeding.*
[2]Defined as creatinine clearance < 30 mL/min.
[3]Body weight < 50 kg: reduce dose and monitor anti-Xa levels.
DVT, deep venous thrombosis; IV, intravenously; PE, pulmonary embolism; SC, subcutaneously; VTE, venous thromboembolic disease (includes DVT and PE).

dates for injectable anticoagulants, and they have good follow-up. Risk stratification in patients with PE should be done at time of diagnosis to identify patients at higher risk for mortality and complications. These patients may benefit from a higher level of care, prolonged hospitalization, or treatment with thrombolysis.

1. Heparin—Selection of a parenteral anticoagulant should be determined by patient characteristics (renal function, immediate bleeding risk, weight) and clinical scenario (if thrombolysis is being considered). LMWHs are as efficacious as unfractionated heparin in the immediate treatment of DVT and PE. LMWHs are preferred over unfractionated heparin as initial treatment because of predictable pharmacokinetics, which allow for subcutaneous, once- or twice-daily dosing with no requirement for monitoring in most patients. Monitoring of the therapeutic effect of LMWH may be indicated in pregnancy, compromised renal func-

tion, and extremes of weight. Accumulation of the LMWH and increased rates of bleeding have been observed among patients with severe renal insufficiency (creatinine clearance < 30 mL/min), leading to a recommendation to use intravenous unfractionated heparin in the place of LMWH in these higher-risk patients. If concomitant thrombolysis is being considered, unfractionated heparin is indicated. In addition, patients with VTE and a perceived higher risk of bleeding (ie, post-surgery) may be better candidates for treatment with unfractionated heparin than LMWH given its shorter half-life and reversibility.

Weight-based, fixed-dose daily subcutaneous fondaparinux (a synthetic factor Xa inhibitor) may also be used for the initial treatment of DVT and PE, with no increase in bleeding over that observed with LMWH. Its lack of reversibility, long half-life, and primarily renal clearance limits its use in patients with an increased risk of bleeding or renal failure.

Table 14–14. Patient selection for outpatient treatment of DVT.

Patients considered appropriate for outpatient treatment
No clinical signs or symptoms of PE and pain controlled
Motivated and capable of self-administration of injections
Confirmed prescription insurance that covers injectable medication or patient can pay out-of-pocket for injectable agents
Capable and willing to comply with frequent follow-up
Initially, patients may need to be seen daily to weekly
Potential contraindications for outpatient treatment
DVT involving inferior vena cava, iliac, common femoral, or upper extremity vein (these patients might benefit from vascular intervention)
Comorbid conditions
Active peptic ulcer disease, GI bleeding in past 14 days, liver synthetic dysfunction:
Brain metastases, current or recent CNS or spinal cord injury/ surgery in the last 10 days, CVA ≤ 4–6 weeks
Familial bleeding diathesis
Active bleeding from source other than GI
Thrombocytopenia
Creatinine clearance < 30 mL/min
Patient weighs < 55 kg (male) or 45 kg (female)
Recent surgery, spinal or epidural anesthesia in the past 3 days
History of heparin-induced thrombocytopenia
Inability to inject medication at home, reliably follow medication schedule, recognize changes in health status, understand or follow directions

2. Warfarin—Patients with DVT with or without PE require a minimum of 3 months of anticoagulation in order to reduce the risk of recurrence of thrombosis. An oral vitamin K antagonist, such as warfarin, is usually initiated along with the parenteral anticoagulant, although patients with cancer-related thrombosis may benefit from ongoing treatment with LMWH alone. Most patients require 5 mg of warfarin daily for initial treatment, but lower doses (2.5 mg daily) should be considered for patients of Asian descent, the elderly, and those with hyperthyroidism, congestive heart failure, liver disease, recent major surgery, malnutrition, certain polymorphisms for the CYP2C9 or the VKORC1 genes or who are receiving concurrent medications that increase sensitivity to warfarin (Table 14–15). Conversely, individuals of African descent, those with larger body mass index or hypothyroidism, and those who are receiving medications that increase warfarin metabolism may require higher initial doses (7.5 mg daily). Daily INR results should guide dosing adjustments (Table 14–16). Web-based warfarin dosing calculators that consider these clinical and genetic factors are available to help clinicians choose the appropriate starting dose (www.warfarindosing.org and http://warfdocs.ucdavis.edu/). Because an average of 5 days is required to achieve a steady-state reduction in the activity of vitamin K–dependent coagulation factors, the parenteral anticoagulant should be continued for at least 5 days and until the INR is > 2.0 on 2 consecutive days. Meticulous follow-up should be arranged for all patients taking warfarin because of the bleeding risk that is associated with initiation of therapy (Table 14–17). INR monitoring should occur at

Table 14–15. Commonly used agents and their potential effect on the INR.

Tendency to Increase INR	Tendency to Decrease INR
Phenytoin	Phenytoin
Erythromycin	Rifampin/rifabutin
Metronidazole	Carbamazepine
Ketoconazole	Vitamin K
Trimethoprim-sulfamethoxazole	Phenobarbital
Amiodarone	Sucralfate
Cimetidine	Ginseng
Alcohol	Alcohol
Fluconazole	
Itraconazole	
Statins	

INR, international normalized ratio.

least twice weekly during initiation. Once stabilized, the INR should be checked at an interval no longer than every 4 weeks. Supratherapeutic INRs should be managed according to evidence-based guidelines (Table 14–18).

3. New investigational oral anticoagulants—The vitamin K antagonists have been the only oral anticoagulants available for nearly 7 decades. Now, a number of novel oral anticoagulant agents that promise more predictable dose effect and ease of administration than warfarin are under investigation. Rivaroxaban, a direct factor Xa inhibitor, has a

Table 14–16. Warfarin adjustment guidelines for patients newly starting therapy.

	INR	Action
Day 1		5 mg (2.5 or 7.5 mg in select populations[1])
Day 2	< 1.5	Continue dose
	≥ 1.5	Decrease or hold dose[2]
Day 3	≤ 1.2	Increase dose[2]
	> 1.2 and < 1.7	Continue dose
	≥ 1.7	Decrease dose[2]
Day 4 until therapeutic	Daily increase is < 0.2 units	Increase dose[2]
	Daily increase 0.2–0.3 units	Continue dose
	Daily increase 0.4–0.6 units	Decrease dose[2]
	Daily increase ≥ 0.7 units	Hold dose

[1]See text
[2]In general, dosage adjustments should not exceed 2.5 mg or 50%.

Table 14–17. Warfarin dosing adjustment guidelines for patients receiving long-term therapy.[1]

Patient INR	Weekly Dosing Change		
	1.5–2.0 INR	2.0–3.0 INR	2.5–3.5 INR
< 1.5	↑ 5–10%	↑ 5–20%	↑ 15–20%
1.5–2.0	Therapeutic	↑ 5–10%	↑ 5–20%
2.0–2.5	↓ 5–10%	Therapeutic	↑ 5–10%
2.5–3.0	↓ 5–15%	Therapeutic	Therapeutic
3.0–3.5	(May hold) ↓ 10–20%	↓ 5–10% Or may stay same if just at or above 3.0	Therapeutic
3.5–4.0	HOLD dose ↓ 20–50%	(May hold) ↓ 5–10%	↓ 5–10% Or may stay same if just at or above 3.5
4.0–5.0	HOLD 2–3 days ↓ 20–50%	HOLD 1–2 days ↓ 10–20%	(May hold) ↓ 5–15%

[1]Adapted from Guidelines used at the VA Medical Center, Reno NV.

predictable dose effect, minimal drug interactions, and does not require laboratory monitoring. It has been found to be effective in prevention of VTE in orthopedic surgery in phase III trials. Dabigatran, a DTI, was recently approved for use in Europe for prevention of VTE in orthopedic surgery. It requires an acid environment for absorption and cannot be used in renal failure; however, it can be taken once daily and does not require monitoring. Phase III trials for treatment of VTE and stroke prevention in atrial fibrillation are ongoing.

4. Duration of anticoagulation therapy—The clinical scenario in which the thrombosis occurred is the strongest predictor of recurrence and, in most cases, guides duration of anticoagulation (Table 14–19). In the first year after discontinuation of anticoagulation therapy, the frequency of recurrence of VTE among individuals whose thrombosis occurred in the setting of a transient, major, reversible risk factor (such as surgery) is approximately 3%, compared with 8% for individuals whose thrombosis was unprovoked, and > 20% in patients with cancer. Patients with provoked VTE are generally treated with a 3-month course of anticoagulation, whereas unprovoked VTE should prompt consideration of indefinite anticoagulation. Both normal D-dimer levels and lack of residual vein thrombosis

Table 14–18. American College of Chest Physicians' evidence-based clinical practice guidelines for the management of supratherapeutic INR.

Clinical Situation	INR	Recommendations
No significant bleed	Above therapeutic range but < 5.0	• Lower dose or omit dose • Monitor more frequently and resume at lower dose when INR falls within therapeutic range (if INR slightly above range, may not be necessary to decrease dose)
	≥ 5.0 but < 9.0	• Hold next 1–2 doses • Monitor more frequently and resume therapy at lower dose when INR falls within therapeutic range • *Patients at high risk for bleeding*[1]: Hold warfarin PLUS give vitamin K₁ ≤ 2.5 mg PO, check INR in 24–48 h to ensure response to therapy
	≥ 9.0	• Hold warfarin • Vitamin K₁ 2.5–5 mg PO × 1; may repeat • Monitor frequently and resume therapy at lower dose when INR within therapeutic range
Serious/life-threatening bleed		• Hold warfarin and give 10 mg vitamin K by slow IV infusion supplemented by FFP, PCC, or recombinant factor VIIa

[1]Patients at higher risk for bleeding include the elderly; conditions that increase the risk of bleeding include renal failure, hypertension, falls, liver disease, and history of gastrointestinal or genitourinary bleeding.
FFP, fresh frozen plasma; PCC, prothrombin complex concentrate.
(Ansell J et al. Pharmacology and management of the vitamin K antagonists: American College of Chest Physicians Evidence-Based Clinical Practice Guidelines (8th Edition) Chest. 2008 Jun;133(6 Suppl):160S–198S.)

Table 14–19. Long-term treatment of VTE.

Scenario	Suggested Duration of Therapy	Comments
Major transient risk factor (eg, immobilization, major surgery, major trauma, major hospitalization)	3 months	VTE prophylaxis required upon future exposure to transient risk factors
Minor transient risk factor (eg, exposure to exogenous estrogens/progestins, pregnancy, airline travel lasting more than 6 hours)	3 months	VTE prophylaxis required upon future exposure to transient risk factors
Cancer-related VTE	≥ 3–6 months or as long as cancer active, whichever is longer	LMWH recommended for initial treatment (see Table 14–13)
Unprovoked thrombosis	Minimum of 3 months, consider indefinite if bleeding risk allows	May risk-stratify for recurrence based on presence of residual venous occlusion, D-dimer levels
Underlying significant thrombophilia (eg, antiphospholipid antibody syndrome, antithrombin deficiency, protein C deficiency, protein S deficiency, ≥ two concomitant thrombophilic conditions)	Indefinite	Delay investigation for laboratory thrombophilia until 3 months after event to avoid false positivity

LMWH, low-molecular-weight heparin; VTE, venous thromboembolic disease.

3-6 months after cessation of warfarin therapy are associated with lower recurrence risk, potentially identifying a cohort of patients with unprovoked VTE in whom anticoagulation does not need to be continued indefinitely. Risk-stratification schemas have not been standardized and remain an area of active research. The benefit of anticoagulation must be weighed against the bleeding risks posed by this therapy and should be assessed at the initiation of therapy and then at least annually in any patient receiving prolonged therapy. Bleeding risk scores have been developed to help clinicians in this process.

Aspinall SL et al. Bleeding Risk Index in an anticoagulation clinic. Assessment by indication and implications for care. J Gen Intern Med. 2005 Nov;20(11):1008–13. [PMID: 16307625]

Gage BF. Pharmacogenetics-based coumarin therapy. Hematology Am Soc Hematol Educ Program. 2006:467–73. [PMID: 17124101]

Gage BF et al. Clinical classification schemes for predicting hemorrhage: results from the National Registry of Atrial Fibrillation (NRAF). Am Heart J. 2006 Mar;151(3):713–9. [PMID: 16504638]

Kearon C et al. Antithrombotic therapy for venous thromboembolic disease: American College of Chest Physicians Evidence-Based Clinical Practice Guideline (8th Edition). Chest. 2008 Jun;133(6 Suppl):454S–545S. [PMID: 18574272]

Palareti G et al. D-dimer testing to determine the duration of anticoagulation therapy. N Engl J Med. 2006 Oct 26;355 (17):1780–9. [PMID: 17065639]

Ruiz-Gimenez N et al. Predictive variables for major bleeding events in patients presenting with documented acute venous thromboembolism. Findings from the RIETE Registry. Thromb Haemost. 2008 Jul;100(1):26–31. [PMID: 18612534]

Siragusa S et al. Residual vein thrombosis to establish duration of anticoagulation after a first episode of deep vein thrombosis: the Duration of Anticoagulation based on Compressive UltraSonography (DACUS) study. Blood. 2008 August 1;112(3):511–5. [PMID: 18497320]

Verhovsek M et al. Systematic review: D-dimer to predict recurrent disease after stopping anticoagulant therapy for unprovoked venous thromboembolism. Ann Intern Med. 2008 Oct 7;149(7):481–90. [PMID: 18838728]

Weitz J et al. New antithrombotic drugs: American College of Chest Physicians Evidence-Based Clinical Practice Guideline (8th Edition). Chest. 2008 Jun;133(6 Suppl):234S–256S. [PMID: 18574267]

B. Thrombolytic Therapy

Anticoagulation alone is appropriate treatment for most patients with PE; however, those with massive PE, defined as PE with persistent hemodynamic instability, have an in-hospital mortality rate that approaches 30% and require immediate thrombolysis in combination with anticoagulation (Table 14–20). Thrombolytic therapy also has been used in selected patients with submassive PE, defined as PE with hemodynamic stability and evidence of right ventricular compromise. A single, randomized, controlled trial comparing thrombolytics plus heparin with heparin alone in this population showed a statistically significant decrease in the combined end point of mortality and escalation of care in patients who underwent thrombolysis. However, selection of patients with submassive PE remains controversial, and clinical investigation into this issue is in progress.

Limited data suggest that patients with large proximal iliofemoral DVT may also benefit from catheter-directed thrombolysis in addition to treatment with anticoagulation. However, standardized guidelines are lacking, and use of the intervention may be limited by institutional availability and provider experience. Importantly, thrombolytics should be considered only in patients who have a low risk of bleeding, as rates of bleeding are increased in patients who receive these products compared with rates of hemorrhage in those who are treated with anticoagulation alone.

Kearon C et al. Antithrombotic therapy for venous thromboembolic disease: American College of Chest Physicians Evidence-Based Clinical Practice Guideline (8th Edition). Chest. 2008 Jun;133(6 Suppl):454S–545S. [PMID: 18574272]

Table 14-20. Thrombolytic therapies for acute massive pulmonary embolism.

Thrombolytic Agent	Dose	Frequency	Comment
Alteplase	100 mg	Continuous IV infusion over 2 hours	Follow with continuous IV infusion of unfractionated heparin
	100 mg	IV bolus × 1	Appropriate for acute management of cardiac arrest and suspected pulmonary embolism
Urokinase	4400 international units/kg	IV bolus × 1 followed by 4400 international units/kg continuous IV infusion for 12 hours	Unfractionated heparin should be administered concurrently

Konstantinides S et al. Heparin plus alteplase compared with heparin alone in patients with submassive pulmonary embolism. N Engl J Med. 2002 Oct 10;347(15):1143–50. [PMID: 12374874]

Ramakrishnan N. Thrombolysis is not warranted in submassive pulmonary embolism: a systematic and meta-analysis. Crit Care Resusc. 2007 Dec;9(4):357–63. [PMID: 18052901]

Vedantham S. Interventional approaches to acute venous thromboembolism. Semin Respir Crit Care Med. 2008 Feb;29(1):56–65. [PMID: 18302087]

C. Nonpharmacologic Therapy

1. Graduated compression stockings—In order to reduce the likelihood of the post-thrombotic syndrome, which is characterized by swelling, pain, and skin ulceration, all patients with DVT should wear a graduated compression stocking with 30–40 mm Hg pressure at the ankle on the affected lower extremity for 1–2 years. Stockings should be provided immediately to have the most impact on post-thrombotic syndrome; however, they are contraindicated in patients with peripheral vascular disease.

Kolbach DN et al. Non-pharmacologic measures for prevention of post-thrombotic syndrome. Cochrane Database Syst Rev. 2004;(1):CD004174. [PMID: 14974060]

2. Inferior vena caval (IVC) filters—There is a paucity of data to support the use of IVC filters for the prevention of PE in any clinical scenario. A single, randomized, controlled trial of IVC filter placement and PE prevention in patients with documented DVT involved concurrent administration of anticoagulation and showed mixed results of a reduction in the rate of nonfatal PE and an increase in the rate of DVT (20% at 2 years) in patients who had received permanent filters. Most experts agree with placing a device in patients with acute proximal DVT and an absolute contraindication to anticoagulation. The remainder of the indications (submassive PE, free-floating iliofemoral DVT, perioperative risk reduction) are controversial. If the contraindication to anticoagulation is temporary (eg, perisurgical patients), placement of a retrievable IVC filter should be considered so that the device can be removed once anticoagulation has been started and has been shown to be tolerated.

Complications of IVC filters include local thrombosis, tilting, migration, and inability to retrieve the device. When considering placement of an IVC filter, it is best to consider both short- and long-term complications, since even devices intended for removal may become permanent.

Barral FG. Vena cava filters: why, when, what and how? J Cardiovasc Surg (Torino). 2008 Feb;49(1):35–49. [PMID: 18212686]

PREPIC Study Group. Eight-year follow-up of patients with permanent vena cava filters in the prevention of pulmonary embolism: the PREPIC (Prévention du Risque d'Embolie Pulmonaire par Interruption Cave) randomized study. Circulation. 2005 Jul 19;112(3):416–22. [PMID: 16009794]

▶ When to Refer

- Presence of large iliofemoral VTE, IVC thrombosis, or Budd-Chiari syndrome for consideration of catheter-directed thrombolysis.
- Massive PE for urgent embolectomy.
- History of HIT or prolonged PTT plus renal failure for alternative anticoagulation regimens.
- Need for IVC filter placement.

▶ When to Admit

- Documented or suspected PE.
- DVT with poorly controlled pain, high bleeding risk, contraindications to LMWH or fondaparinux.
- Large iliofemoral DVT for consideration of thrombolysis.
- Acute DVT and absolute contraindication to anticoagulation for IVC filter placement.

Gastrointestinal Disorders

Kenneth R. McQuaid, MD

▼ **SYMPTOMS & SIGNS OF GASTROINTESTINAL DISEASE**

DYSPEPSIA

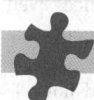 **ESSENTIALS OF DIAGNOSIS**

▶ Epigastric pain or burning, early satiety, or postprandial fullness.

▶ Endoscopy is warranted in patients with alarm features or in those older than 55 years.

▶ All other patients should first undergo testing for *Helicobacter pylori* or a trial of empiric proton pump inhibitor.

▶ General Considerations

Dyspepsia refers to acute, chronic, or recurrent pain or discomfort centered in the upper abdomen. An international committee of clinical investigators (Rome III Committee) has defined dyspepsia as epigastric pain or burning, early satiety, or postprandial fullness. Heartburn (retrosternal burning) should be distinguished from dyspepsia. When heartburn is the dominant complaint, gastroesophageal reflux is nearly always present. Dyspepsia occurs in 25% of the adult population and accounts for 3% of general medical office visits.

▶ Etiology

A. Food or Drug Intolerance

Acute, self-limited "indigestion" may be caused by overeating, eating too quickly, eating high-fat foods, eating during stressful situations, or drinking too much alcohol or coffee. Many medications cause dyspepsia, including aspirin, nonsteroidal anti-inflammatory drugs (NSAIDs), antibiotics (metronidazole, macrolides), diabetes drugs (metformin, α-glucosidase inhibitors, amylin analogs, GLP-1 receptor antagonists), antihypertensive medications (angiotensin-converting enzyme [ACE] inhibitors, angiotensin-receptor blockers), cholesterol-lowering agents (niacin, fibrates), neuropsychiatric medications (cholinesterase inhibitors [donepezil, rivastigmine]), SSRIs (fluoxetine, sertraline), serotonin-norepinephrine-reuptake inhibitors (venlafaxine, duloxetine), Parkinson's drugs (dopamine agonists, monoamine oxidase [MAO]-B inhibitors), corticosteroids, estrogens, digoxin, iron, and opioids.

B. Luminal Gastrointestinal Tract Dysfunction

Peptic ulcer disease is present in 5–15% of patients with dyspepsia. Gastroesophageal reflux disease (GERD) is present in up to 20% of patients with dyspepsia, even without significant heartburn. Gastric cancer is identified in 1% but is extremely rare in persons under age 55 years with uncomplicated dyspepsia. Other causes include gastroparesis (especially in diabetes mellitus), lactose intolerance or malabsorptive conditions, and parasitic infection (*Giardia, Strongyloides*).

C. *Helicobacter pylori* Infection

Although chronic gastric infection with *H pylori* is an important cause of peptic ulcer disease, it is an uncommon cause of dyspepsia in the absence of peptic ulcer disease. The prevalence of *H pylori*-associated chronic gastritis in patients with dyspepsia without peptic ulcer disease is 20–50%, the same as in the general population.

D. Pancreatic Disease

Pancreatic carcinoma and chronic pancreatitis may present with dyspepsia.

E. Biliary Tract Disease

The abrupt onset of epigastric or right upper quadrant pain due to cholelithiasis or choledocholithiasis should be readily distinguished from dyspepsia.

F. Other Conditions

Diabetes mellitus, thyroid disease, chronic kidney disease, myocardial ischemia, intra-abdominal malignancy, gastric volvulus or paraesophageal hernia, and pregnancy are sometimes accompanied by dyspepsia.

G. Functional Dyspepsia

This is the most common cause of chronic dyspepsia. Up to two-thirds of patients have no obvious organic cause for their symptoms after evaluation. Symptoms may arise from a complex interaction of increased visceral afferent sensitivity, gastric delayed emptying or impaired accommodation to food, or psychosocial stressors. Although benign, these symptoms may be chronic and difficult to treat.

▶ Clinical Findings

A. Symptoms and Signs

Given the nonspecific nature of dyspeptic symptoms, the history has limited diagnostic utility. It should clarify the chronicity, location, and quality of the discomfort, and its relationship to meals. The discomfort may be characterized by one or more upper abdominal symptoms including epigastric pain or burning, early satiety, postprandial fullness, bloating, nausea, or vomiting. Concomitant weight loss, persistent vomiting, constant or severe pain, dysphagia, hematemesis, or melena warrants endoscopy or abdominal imaging. Potentially offending medications and excessive alcohol use should be identified and discontinued if possible. The patient's reason for seeking care should be determined. Recent changes in employment, marital discord, physical and sexual abuse, anxiety, depression, and fear of serious disease may all contribute to the development and reporting of symptoms. Patients with functional dyspepsia often are younger, report a variety of abdominal and extra-gastrointestinal complaints, show signs of anxiety or depression, or have a history of use of psychotropic medications.

The symptom profile alone does not differentiate between functional dyspepsia and organic gastrointestinal disorders. Based on the clinical history alone, primary care physicians misdiagnose nearly half of patients with peptic ulcers or gastroesophageal reflux and have < 25% accuracy in diagnosing functional dyspepsia.

The physical examination is rarely helpful. Signs of serious organic disease such as weight loss, organomegaly, abdominal mass, or fecal occult blood are further evaluated. In patients older than age of 50 years, initial laboratory work should include a blood count, electrolytes, liver enzymes, calcium, and thyroid function tests.

B. Laboratory Findings

In patients younger than 55 years with uncomplicated dyspepsia (in whom gastric cancer is rare), initial noninvasive management strategies should be pursued (see below). In most clinical settings, a noninvasive test for H pylori (urea breath test, fecal antigen test, or IgG serology) should be performed first. Although serologic tests are inexpensive, performance characteristics are poor in low-prevalence populations. If breath test or fecal antigen test results are negative in a patient not taking NSAIDs, peptic ulcer disease is virtually excluded.

C. Upper Endoscopy

Upper endoscopy is indicated to look for gastric cancer or other serious organic disease in all patients over age 55 years

with new-onset dyspepsia and in all patients with "alarm" features, such as weight loss, dysphagia, recurrent vomiting, evidence of bleeding, or anemia. Upper endoscopy is the study of choice to diagnose gastroduodenal ulcers, erosive esophagitis, and upper gastrointestinal malignancy. It is also helpful for patients who are concerned about serious underlying disease. For patients born in regions in which there is a higher incidence of gastric cancer, an age threshold of 45 years may be appropriate.

Endoscopic evaluation is also warranted when symptoms fail to respond to initial empiric management strategies or when frequent symptom relapse occurs after discontinuation of antisecretory therapy.

D. Other Tests

Abdominal imaging (ultrasonography or CT scanning) is performed only when pancreatic or biliary tract disease is suspected. Gastric emptying studies are valuable only in patients with recurrent vomiting. Ambulatory esophageal pH testing may be of value when atypical gastroesophageal reflux is suspected.

▶ Treatment

Initial empiric treatment is warranted for patients who are less than 55 years and who have no alarm features (defined above). All other patients as well as patients whose symptoms fail to respond or relapse after empiric treatment should undergo upper endoscopy with subsequent treatment directed at the specific disorder (eg, peptic ulcer, gastroesophageal reflux, cancer). Most patients will have no significant findings on endoscopy and will be given a diagnosis of functional dyspepsia.

A. Empiric Therapy

H pylori–negative patients most likely have functional dyspepsia or atypical GERD and can be treated with an antisecretory agent (proton pump inhibitor) for 4 weeks. For patients who have symptom relapse after discontinuation of the proton pump inhibitor, intermittent or long-term proton pump inhibitor therapy may be considered.

For patients in whom test results are positive for H pylori, antibiotic therapy proves definitive for over 90% of peptic ulcers and may improve symptoms in a small subset (< 10%) of infected patients with functional dyspepsia. Patients with persistent dyspepsia after H pylori eradication can be given a trial of proton pump inhibitor therapy. In clinical settings in which the prevalence of H pylori infection in the population is low (< 10%), it may be more cost-effective to initially treat all young patients with uncomplicated dyspepsia with a 4-week trial of a proton pump inhibitor. Patients who have symptom relapse after discontinuation of the proton pump inhibitor should be tested for H pylori and treated if positive.

B. Treatment of Functional Dyspepsia

1. General measures—Most patients have mild, intermittent symptoms that respond to reassurance and lifestyle changes. Alcohol, caffeine, and fatty foods should be reduced or discontinued. A food diary, in which patients record their food intake, symptoms, and daily events, may reveal dietary or psychosocial precipitants of pain.

2. Pharmacologic agents—Drugs have demonstrated limited efficacy in the treatment of functional dyspepsia. One-third of patients derive relief from placebo. Antisecretory therapy for 4–8 weeks with proton pump inhibitors (omeprazole, esomeprazole, or rabeprazole 20 mg, lansoprazole 30 mg, or pantoprazole 40 mg) may benefit 10–15% of patients, particularly those with dyspepsia characterized as epigastric pain ("ulcer-like dyspepsia") or dyspepsia and heartburn ("reflux-like dyspepsia"). Low doses of antidepressants (eg, desipramine or nortriptyline, 10–50 mg at bedtime) are believed to benefit some patients, possibly by moderating visceral afferent sensitivity. However, side effects are common and response is patient-specific. Doses should be increased slowly. The prokinetic agent metoclopramide (5–10 mg three times daily) may improve symptoms, but improvement does not correlate with the presence or absence of gastric emptying delay. In 2009, the FDA issued a black box warning that metoclopramide use for more than 3 months is associated with a high incidence of tardive dyskinesia and should be avoided. The elderly, particularly elderly women, are most at risk. Recently, a randomized, placebo-controlled study has demonstrated efficacy of the novel prokinetic agent itopride in the treatment of functional dyspepsia. This agent enhances the release of gastric acetylcholine through dual inhibition of D_2 receptors and acetylcholinesterase. This agent is not yet available in the United States.

3. Anti-H pylori treatment—Meta-analyses have suggested that a small number of patients with functional dyspepsia (< 10%) derive benefit from *H pylori* eradication therapy. Therefore, patients with functional dyspepsia should be tested and treated for H pylori.

4. Alternative therapies—Psychotherapy and hypnotherapy may be of benefit in selected motivated patients with functional dyspepsia. Herbal therapies (peppermint, caraway) may offer benefit with little risk of adverse effects.

Ford AC et al. Current guidelines for dyspepsia management. Dig Dis. 2008;26(3):225–30. [PMID: 18463440]

Ford AC et al. Meta-analysis: *Helicobacter pylori* 'test and treat' compared with empirical acid suppression for managing dyspepsia. Aliment Pharmamacol Ther. 2008 Sep 1;28(5):534–44. [PMID: 18616641]

McColl KM. CON: Endoscopy is not necessary before treating *Helicobacter pylori* in patients with uncomplicated dyspepsia. Am J Gastroenterol. 2007 Mar;102(3):474–6. [PMID: 17335440]

Shah R. Dyspepsia and *Helicobacter pylori*. BMJ. 2007 Jan 6;334(7583):41–3. [PMID: 17204803]

Talley NJ et al. Randomized-controlled trial of esomeprazole in functional dyspepsia patients with epigastric pain or burning: does a 1-week trial of acid suppression predict symptom response? Aliment Pharmacol Ther. 2007 Sep 1;26(5):673–82. [PMID: 17697201]

Van Zanten SV et al. One-week acid suppression trial in uninvestigated dyspepsia patients with epigastric pain or burning to predict response to 8 weeks' treatment with esomeprazole: a randomized, placebo-controlled study. Aliment Pharmacol Ther. 2007 Sep 1;26(5):665–72. [PMID: 17697200]

Wang WH et al. Effects of proton-pump inhibitors on functional dyspepsia: a meta-analysis of randomized placebo-controlled trials. Clin Gastroenterol Hepatol. 2007 Feb;5(2):178–85. [PMID: 17174612]

NAUSEA & VOMITING

Nausea is a vague, intensely disagreeable sensation of sickness or "queasiness" and is distinguished from anorexia. Vomiting often follows, as does retching (spasmodic respiratory and abdominal movements). Vomiting should be distinguished from regurgitation, the effortless reflux of liquid or food stomach contents; and from rumination, the chewing and swallowing of food that is regurgitated volitionally after meals.

The brainstem vomiting center is composed of a group of neuronal areas (area postrema, nucleus tractus solitarius, and central pattern generator) within the medulla that coordinate emesis. It may be stimulated by four different sources of afferent input: (1) Afferent vagal fibers from the gastrointestinal viscera are rich in serotonin 5-HT_3 receptors; these may be stimulated by biliary or gastrointestinal distention, mucosal or peritoneal irritation, or infections. (2) Fibers of the vestibular system, which have high concentrations of histamine H_1 and muscarinic cholinergic receptors. (3) Higher central nervous system centers (amygdala); here, certain sights, smells, or emotional experiences may induce vomiting. For example, patients receiving chemotherapy may start vomiting in anticipation of its administration. (4) The chemoreceptor trigger zone, located outside the blood-brain barrier in the area postrema of the medulla, which is rich in opioid, serotonin 5-HT_3, neurokinin 1 (NK_1) and dopamine D_2 receptors. This region may be stimulated by drugs and chemotherapeutic agents, toxins, hypoxia, uremia, acidosis, and radiation therapy. Although the causes of vomiting are many, a simplified list is provided in Table 15–1.

▶ **Clinical Findings**

A. Symptoms and Signs

Acute symptoms without abdominal pain are typically caused by food poisoning, infectious gastroenteritis, drugs, or systemic illness. Inquiry should be made into recent changes in medications, diet, other intestinal symptoms, or similar illnesses in family members. The acute onset of severe pain and vomiting suggests peritoneal irritation, acute gastric or intestinal obstruction, or pancreaticobiliary disease. Persistent vomiting suggests pregnancy, gastric outlet obstruction, gastroparesis, intestinal dysmotility, psychogenic disorders, and central nervous system or systemic disorders. Vomiting that occurs in the morning before breakfast is common with pregnancy, uremia, alcohol intake, and increased intracranial pressure. Vomiting immediately after meals strongly suggests bulimia or psychogenic causes. Vomiting of undigested food one to several hours after meals is characteristic of gastroparesis or a gastric outlet obstruction; physical examination may reveal a succussion splash. Patients with acute or chronic symptoms should be asked about neurologic symptoms that

Table 15–1. Causes of nausea and vomiting.

Visceral afferent stimulation	**Infections**
	Mechanical obstruction
	Gastric outlet obstruction: peptic ulcer disease, malignancy, gastric volvulus
	Small intestinal obstruction: adhesions, hernias, volvulus, Crohn disease, carcinomatosis
	Dysmotility
	Gastroparesis: diabetic, postviral, postvagotomy
	Small intestine: scleroderma, amyloidosis, chronic intestinal pseudo-obstruction, familial myoneuropathies
	Peritoneal irritation
	Peritonitis: perforated viscus, appendicitis, spontaneous bacterial peritonitis
	Viral gastroenteritis: Norwalk agent, rotavirus
	"Food poisoning": toxins from *Bacillus cereus, Staphylococcus aureus, Clostridium perfringens*
	Hepatitis A or B
	Acute systemic infections
	Hepatobiliary or pancreatic disorders
	Acute pancreatitis
	Cholecystitis or choledocholithiasis
	Topical gastrointestinal irritants
	Alcohol, NSAIDs, oral antibiotics
	Postoperative
	Other
	Cardiac disease: acute myocardial infarction, congestive heart failure
	Urologic disease: stones, pyelonephritis
CNS disorders	**Vestibular disorders**
	Labyrinthitis, Meniere syndrome, motion sickness
	Increased intracranial pressure
	CNS tumors, subdural or subarachnoid hemorrhage
	Migraine
	Infections
	Meningitis, encephalitis
	Psychogenic
	Anticipatory vomiting, bulimia, psychiatric disorders
Irritation of chemoreceptor trigger zone	**Antitumor chemotherapy**
	Drugs and medications
	Opioids
	Anticonvulsants
	Antiparkinsonism drugs
	β-blockers, antiarrhythmics, digoxin
	Nicotine
	Oral contraceptives
	Cholinesterase inhibitors
	Diabetes medications (metformin, acarbose, pramlintide, exenatide)
	Radiation therapy
	Systemic disorders
	Diabetic ketoacidosis
	Uremia
	Adrenocortical crisis
	Parathyroid disease
	Hypothyroidism
	Pregnancy
	Paraneoplastic syndrome

CNS, central nervous system; NSAIDs, nonsteroidal anti-inflammatory drugs.

suggest a central nervous system cause such as headache, stiff neck, vertigo, and focal paresthesias or weakness.

B. Special Examinations

With vomiting that is severe or protracted, serum electrolytes should be obtained to look for hypokalemia, azotemia, or metabolic alkalosis resulting from loss of gastric contents. Flat and upright abdominal radiographs or abdominal CT are obtained in patients with severe pain or suspicion of mechanical obstruction to look for free intraperitoneal air or dilated loops of small bowel. If mechanical small intestinal or gastric obstruction is thought likely, a nasogastric tube is placed for relief of symptoms. The cause of gastric outlet obstruction is best demonstrated by upper endoscopy, and the cause of small intestinal obstruction is best demonstrated with abdominal CT imaging. Gastroparesis is confirmed by nuclear scintigraphic studies or ^{13}C-octanoic acid breath tests, which show delayed gastric emptying and either upper endoscopy or barium upper gastrointestinal series showing no evidence of mechanical gastric outlet obstruction. Abnormal liver function tests or elevated amylase or lipase suggest pancreaticobiliary disease, which may be investigated with an abdominal sonogram or CT scan. Central nervous system causes are best evaluated with either head CT or MRI.

▶ Complications

Complications include dehydration, hypokalemia, metabolic alkalosis, aspiration, rupture of the esophagus (Boerhaave syndrome), and bleeding secondary to a mucosal tear at the gastroesophageal junction (Mallory-Weiss syndrome).

▶ Treatment

A. General Measures

Most causes of acute vomiting are mild, self-limited, and require no specific treatment. Patients should ingest clear liquids (broths, tea, soups, carbonated beverages) and small quantities of dry foods (soda crackers). For more severe acute vomiting, hospitalization may be required. Patients unable to eat and losing gastric fluids may become dehydrated, resulting in hypokalemia with metabolic alkalosis. Intravenous 0.45% saline solution with 20 mEq/L of potassium chloride is given in most cases to maintain hydration. A nasogastric suction tube for gastric decompression improves patient comfort and permits monitoring of fluid loss.

B. Antiemetic Medications

Medications may be given either to prevent or to control vomiting (see above). Combinations of drugs from different classes may provide better control of symptoms with less toxicity in some patients. All of these medications should be avoided in pregnancy. (For dosages, see Table 15–2.)

1. Serotonin 5-HT$_3$-receptor antagonists—Ondansetron, granisetron, dolasetron, and palonosetron are effective in preventing chemotherapy- and radiation-induced emesis when initiated prior to treatment. Single-dose administration schedules are as effective as multiple-dose regimens. Although serotonin antagonists are effective for the prevention of postoperative nausea and vomiting, less expensive alternatives (eg, dexamethasone or droperidol) are equally effective.

2. Corticosteroids—Corticosteroids (eg, dexamethasone) have antiemetic properties, but the basis for these effects is unknown. These agents enhance the efficacy of serotonin receptor antagonists for preventing acute and delayed nausea and vomiting in patients receiving moderately to highly emetogenic chemotherapy regimens. For the prevention of postoperative nausea and vomiting, corticosteroids, serotonin antagonists, and droperidol have efficacy; however, combinations of these agents have additive benefit.

3. Neurokinin receptor antagonists—Aprepitant (125 mg orally) and fosaprepitant (115 mg intravenously) are highly selective antagonists for NK$_1$-receptors in the area postrema. They are used in combination with corticosteroids and serotonin antagonists for the prevention of acute and delayed nausea and vomiting with highly emetogenic chemotherapy regimens. Combined therapy with a neurokinin1 receptor antagonist prevents acute emesis in 80–90% and delayed emesis in > 70% of patients treated with highly emetogenic regimens.

4. Dopamine antagonists—The phenothiazines, butyrophenones, and substituted benzamides have antiemetic properties that are due to dopaminergic blockade as well as to their sedative effects. High doses of these agents are associated with antidopaminergic side effects, including extrapyramidal reactions and depression. These agents are used in a variety of situations. Cases of QT prolongation leading to ventricular tachycardia (torsades de pointes) have been reported in several patients receiving droperidol, hence electrocardiographic monitoring is recommended before and after administration.

Table 15–2. Common antiemetic dosing regimens.

	Dosage	Route
Serotonin 5-HT$_3$ antagonists		
Ondansetron	Doses vary: 8 mg once or twice daily to 24–32 mg once daily	IV
	8 mg twice daily	PO
Granisetron	1 mg or 0.01 mg/kg once daily	IV
	2 mg once daily	PO
Dolasetron	100 mg or 1.8 mg/kg once daily	IV
	100 mg once daily	PO
Palonosetron	0.25 mg once as a single dose 30 min before start of chemotherapy	IV
Corticosteroids		
Dexamethasone	8–20 mg once daily	IV
	4–20 mg once or twice daily	PO
Methylprednisolone	40–100 mg once daily	IV
Dopamine receptor antagonists		
Metoclopramide	10–20 mg or 0.5 mg/kg every 6–8 hours	IV
	10–20 mg every 6–8 hours	PO
Prochlorperazine	5–10 mg every 4–6 hours	PO, IM, IV
	25 mg suppository every 6 hours	PR
Promethazine	25 mg every 4–6 hours	PO, PR, IM, IV
Trimethobenzamide	250 mg every 6–8 hours	PO
	200 mg every 6–8 hours	IM, PR
Sedatives		
Diazepam	2–5 mg every 4–6 hours	PO, IV
Lorazepam	1–2 mg every 4–6 hours	PO, IV

IM, intramuscularly; IV, intravenously; PO, orally; PR, per rectum.

5. Antihistamines and anticholinergics—These drugs (eg, meclizine, dimenhydrinate, transdermal scopolamine) may be valuable in the prevention of vomiting arising from stimulation of the labyrinth, ie, motion sickness, vertigo, and migraines. They may induce drowsiness.

6. Sedatives—Benzodiazepines are used in psychogenic and anticipatory vomiting.

7. Cannabinoids—Marijuana has been used widely as an appetite stimulant and antiemetic. Pure Δ^9-tetrahydrocannabinol (THC) is the major active ingredient in marijuana and is available by prescription as dronabinol. In doses of $5–15 \text{ mg/m}^2$, oral dronabinol is effective in treating nausea associated with chemotherapy, but it is associated with central nervous system side effects in most patients.

Hesketh PJ. Chemotherapy-induced nausea and vomiting. N Engl J Med. 2008 June 5;358(23):2482–94. [PMID: 18525044]
Scorza K et al. Evaluation of nausea and vomiting. Am Fam Physician. 2007 Jul 1;76(1):76–84. [PMID 17668843]

HICCUPS (Singultus)

Though usually a benign and self-limited annoyance, hiccups may be persistent and a sign of serious underlying illness. In patients on mechanical ventilation, hiccups can trigger a full respiratory cycle and result in respiratory alkalosis.

Causes of benign, self-limited hiccups include gastric distention (carbonated beverages, air swallowing, overeating), sudden temperature changes (hot then cold liquids, hot then cold shower), alcohol ingestion, and states of heightened emotion (excitement, stress, laughing). There are over 100 causes of recurrent or persistent hiccups, grouped into the following categories:

Central nervous system: Neoplasms, infections, cerebrovascular accident, trauma.

Metabolic: Uremia, hypocapnia (hyperventilation).

Irritation of the vagus or phrenic nerve: (1) Head, neck: Foreign body in ear, goiter, neoplasms. (2) Thorax: Pneumonia, empyema, neoplasms, myocardial infarction, pericarditis, aneurysm, esophageal obstruction, reflux esophagitis. (3) Abdomen: Subphrenic abscess, hepatomegaly, hepatitis, cholecystitis, gastric distention, gastric neoplasm, pancreatitis, or pancreatic malignancy.

Surgical: General anesthesia, postoperative.

Psychogenic and **idiopathic.**

▶ Clinical Findings

Evaluation of the patient with persistent hiccups should include a detailed neurologic examination, serum creatinine, liver chemistry tests, and a chest radiograph. When the cause remains unclear, CT of the head, chest, and abdomen, echocardiography, bronchoscopy, and upper endoscopy may help. On occasion, hiccups may be unilateral; chest fluoroscopy will make the diagnosis.

▶ Treatment

A number of simple remedies may be helpful in patients with acute benign hiccups. (1) Irritation of the nasopharynx by tongue traction, lifting the uvula with a spoon, catheter stimulation of the nasopharynx, or eating 1 tsp of dry granulated sugar. (2) Interruption of the respiratory cycle by breath holding, Valsalva maneuver, sneezing, gasping (fright stimulus), or rebreathing into a bag. (3) Stimulation of the vagus, carotid massage. (4) Irritation of the diaphragm by holding knees to chest or by continuous positive airway pressure during mechanical ventilation. (5) Relief of gastric distention by belching or insertion of a nasogastric tube.

A number of drugs have been promoted as being useful in the treatment of hiccups. Chlorpromazine, 25–50 mg orally or intramuscularly, is most commonly used. Other agents reported to be effective include anticonvulsants (phenytoin, carbamazepine), benzodiazepines (lorazepam, diazepam), metoclopramide, baclofen, gabapentin, and occasionally general anesthesia.

Schuchmann JA et al. Persistent hiccups during rehabilitation hospitalization: three case reports and review of the literature. Am J Phys Med Rehabil. 2007 Dec;86(12):1013–8. [PMID: 18090442]
Turkyilmaz A et al. Use of baclofen in the treatment of esophageal stent-related hiccups. Ann Thorac Surg. 2008 Jan;85(1):328–30. [PMID: 18154840]

CONSTIPATION

Constipation occurs in 10–15% of adults and is a common reason for seeking medical attention. It is more common in women. The elderly are predisposed due to comorbid medical conditions, medications, poor eating habits, decreased mobility and, in some cases, inability to sit on a toilet (bed-bound patients). The first step in evaluating the patient is to determine what is meant by "constipation." Patients may define constipation as infrequent stools (fewer than three in a week), hard stools, excessive straining, or a sense of incomplete evacuation. Table 15–3 summarizes the many causes of constipation, which are discussed below.

▶ Etiology

A. Primary Constipation

Most patients have constipation that cannot be attributed to any structural abnormalities or systemic disease. Some of these patients have normal colonic transit time; however, a subset have slow colonic transit or anorectal dysfunction. Normal colonic transit time is approximately 35 hours; more than 72 hours is significantly abnormal. Slow colonic transit is commonly idiopathic but may be part of a generalized gastrointestinal dysmotility syndrome. Patients may complain of infrequent bowel movements and abdominal bloating. Slow transit is more common in women, some of whom have a history of psychosocial problems (depression, anxiety, eating disorder, childhood trauma) or sexual abuse. Normal defecation requires coordination between relaxation of the anal sphincter and pelvic floor musculature while abdominal pressure is increased. Patients with dyssynergic defecation (also known as anismus or pelvic floor dyssynergia)—women more often than men—have impaired relaxation or paradoxical contraction of the anal sphincter and/or pelvic floor muscles during attempted

Table 15–3. Causes of constipation in adults.

Most common
Inadequate fiber or fluid intake
Poor bowel habits
Systemic disease
Endocrine: hypothyroidism, hyperparathyroidism, diabetes mellitus
Metabolic: hypokalemia, hypercalcemia, uremia, porphyria
Neurologic: Parkinson disease, multiple sclerosis, sacral nerve damage (prior pelvic surgery, tumor), paraplegia, autonomic neuropathy
Medications
Opioids
Diuretics
Calcium channel blockers
Anticholinergics
Psychotropics
Calcium and iron supplements
NSAIDs
Clonidine
Cholestyramine
Structural abnormalities
Anorectal: rectal prolapse, rectocele, rectal intussusception, anorectal stricture, anal fissure, solitary rectal ulcer syndrome
Perineal descent
Colonic mass with obstruction: adenocarcinoma
Colonic stricture: radiation, ischemia, diverticulosis
Hirschsprung disease
Idiopathic megarectum
Slow colonic transit
Idiopathic: isolated to colon
Psychogenic
Eating disorders
Chronic intestinal pseudo-obstruction
Pelvic floor dyssynergia
Irritable bowel syndrome

NSAIDs, nonsteroidal anti-inflammatory drugs.

defecation that impedes the bowel movement. This problem may be acquired during childhood or adulthood. Patients may complain of excessive straining, sense of incomplete evacuation, or need for digital manipulation. Patients with primary complaints of abdominal pain or bloating with alterations in bowel habits (constipation, or alternating constipation and diarrhea) may have irritable bowel syndrome (see below).

B. Secondary Constipation

Constipation may be caused by systemic disorders, medications, or obstructing colonic lesions. Systemic disorders can cause constipation because of neurologic gut dysfunction, myopathies, endocrine disorders, or electrolyte abnormalities (eg, hypercalcemia or hypokalemia); medication side effects are sometimes responsible (eg, anticholinergics or opioids). Colonic lesions that obstruct fecal passage, such as neoplasms and strictures, are an uncommon cause but important in new-onset constipation. Such lesions should be excluded in patients older than 45–50 years, in patients with "alarm" symptoms or signs (hematochezia, weight loss, anemia, or positive fecal occult blood tests [FOBT] or fecal immunochemical tests [FIT]), and in patients with a family history of colon cancer or inflammatory bowel disease. Defecatory difficulties also can be due to a variety of anorectal problems that impede or obstruct flow (perineal descent, rectal prolapse, rectocele), some of which may require surgery, and Hirschsprung disease (usually suggested by lifelong constipation).

▶ **Clinical Findings**

A. Symptoms and Signs

All patients should undergo a history and physical examination to distinguish primary from secondary causes of constipation. Physical examination should include digital rectal examination with assessment for anatomic abnormalities, such as anal stricture, rectocele, rectal prolapse, or perineal descent during straining. Further diagnostic tests should be performed in patients with any of the following: age 50 years or older, severe constipation, signs of an organic disorders, alarm symptoms (hematochezia, weight loss, positive FOBT or FIT), or a family history of colon cancer or inflammatory bowel disease. These tests should include laboratory studies (complete blood count; serum electrolytes, calcium, glucose, and thyroid-stimulating hormone); and a colonoscopy or flexible sigmoidoscopy.

B. Special Examinations

Patients with refractory constipation not responding to routine medical management warrant further diagnostic studies, including colonic transit and pelvic floor function studies, in order to distinguish slow colonic transit from anorectal dysfunction. Colon transit time is most commonly measured by performing an abdominal radiograph 120 hours after ingestion of 24 radiopaque markers. Retention of greater than 20% of the markers indicates prolonged transit. Dyssynergic defecation is assessed with balloon expulsion testing, anal manometry, and defecography.

▶ **Treatment**

A. Chronic Constipation

1. Dietary and lifestyle measures—Adverse psychosocial issues should be identified and addressed. Patients should be instructed on normal defecatory function and optimal toileting habits, including regular timing, proper positioning, and abdominal pressure. Proper dietary fiber intake should be emphasized. A trial of fiber supplements is recommended (Table 15–4). Increased dietary fiber may cause distention or flatulence, which often diminishes over several days. Response to fiber therapy is not immediate, and increases in dosage should be made gradually over 7–10 days. Fiber is most likely to benefit patients with normal colonic transit, but it may not benefit patients with colonic inertia, anorectal dysfunction, or irritable bowel syndrome; it may even exacerbate symptoms in these patients. Regular exercise is associated with a decreased risk of constipation. When possible, discontinue medications that may be causing constipation.

2. Laxatives—Laxatives may be given on an intermittent or chronic basis for constipation that does not respond to

Table 15–4. Pharmacologic management of constipation.

Agent	Dosage	Onset of Action	Comments
Fiber laxatives			
Bran powder	1–4 tbsp orally twice daily	Days	Inexpensive; may cause gas, flatulence
Psyllium	1 tsp once or twice daily	Days	(Metamucil; Perdiem)
Methylcellulose	1 tsp once or twice daily	Days	(Citrucel) Less gas, flatulence
Calcium polycarbophil	1 or 2 tablets once or twice daily	12–24 hours	(FiberCon) Does not cause gas; pill form
Guargum	1 tbsp once or twice daily	Days	(Benefiber) Non-gritty, tasteless, less gas
Stool surfactants			
Docusate sodium	100 mg once or twice daily	12–72 hours	(Colace) Marginal benefit
Mineral oil	15–45 mL once or twice daily	6–8 hours	May cause lipoid pneumonia if aspirated
Osmotic laxatives			
Magnesium hydroxide	15–30 mL orally once or twice daily	6–24 hours	(Milk of magnesia; Epsom salts)
Lactulose or 70% sorbitol	15–60 mL orally once daily to three times daily	6–48 hours	Cramps, bloating, flatulence
Polyethylene glycol (PEG 3350)	17 g in 8 oz liquid once or twice daily	6–24 hours	(Miralax) Less bloating than lactulose, sorbitol
Stimulant laxatives			
Bisacodyl	5–20 mg orally as needed	6–8 hours	May cause cramps; avoid daily use if possible
Bisacodyl	10 mg per rectum as needed	1 hour	
Cascara	4–8 mL or 2 tablets as needed	8–12 hours	(Nature's Remedy) May cause cramps; avoid daily use if possible
Senna	8.6–17.2 mg orally as needed	8–12 hours	(ExLax; Senekot) May cause cramps; avoid daily use if possible
Lubiprostone	24 mcg orally twice daily	12–48 hours	Expensive; may cause nausea. Contraindicated in pregnancy
Enemas			
Tap water	500 mL per rectum	5–15 minutes	
Sodium phosphate enema	120 mL per rectum	5–15 minutes	Commonly used for acute constipation or to induce movement prior to medical procedures
Soapsuds enema	Up to 1500 mL per rectum	5–15 minutes	Impaction
Mineral oil enema	100–250 mL per rectum		To soften and lubricate fecal impaction
Agents used for acute purgative or to clean bowel prior to medical procedures			
Polyethylene glycol (PEG 3350)	4 L orally administered over 2–4 hours	< 4 hours	(GoLYTELY; CoLYTE; NuLYTE, MoviPrep) Used to cleanse bowel before colonoscopy
Sodium phosphate	As directed with total of 2–4 L of clear liquids	1–6 hours	(OsmoPrep, Visicol, Fleets) Used before colonoscopy
Magnesium citrate	10 oz orally	3–6 hours	Lemon-flavored

dietary and lifestyle changes (Table 15–4). There is no evidence that long-term use of these agents is harmful.

A. OSMOTIC LAXATIVES—Nonabsorbable osmotic agents increase secretion of water into the intestinal lumen, thereby softening stools and promoting defecation. Magnesium hydroxide, non-digestible carbohydrates (sorbitol, lactulose), and polyethylene glycol are all efficacious and safe for treating acute and chronic cases. The dosages are adjusted to achieve soft to semi-liquid movements. Magnesium-con-

taining saline laxatives should not be given to patients with chronic renal insufficiency. Non-digestible carbohydrates may induce bloating, cramps, and flatulence. Polyethylene glycol 3350 (Miralax) is a component of solutions traditionally used for colonic lavage prior to colonoscopy and does not cause flatulence. When used in conventional doses, the onset of action of these osmotic agents is generally within 24 hours. For more rapid treatment of acute constipation or as a purgative prior to surgical, endoscopic, or radiographic procedures, polyethylene glycol solutions (GoLYTELY,

CoLYTE, NuLYTE, MoviPrep) may be used. Polyethylene glycol solutions (2–4 L administered over 2–4 hours) are balanced osmotic and electrolyte solutions that do not cause any significant fluid or electrolyte shifts and may be used safely in almost all patients. Alternatively, potent, hyperosmolar saline purgatives may administered. These hyperosmolar agents draw significant fluid into the intestine and must be given with substantial oral fluids (2–4 L) to minimize fluid shifts that can result in dehydration or acute kidney injury. They should be avoided in patients with chronic kidney disease or congestive heart failure. Magnesium citrate may cause hypermagnesemia. Oral sodium phosphate preparations (Visicol, OsmoPrep, and Fleets Phospho-soda) can cause hypocalcemia, hyperphosphatemia, hypokalemia and, rarely, acute kidney injury due to acute phosphate nephropathy. The FDA has issued a warning that sodium phosphate should be avoided in people over age 55, people with known kidney disease, or people taking medications that affect kidney function (diuretics, NSAIDs, ACE inhibitors, angiotensin-receptor blockers). Patients taking sodium phosphate should be advised to ingest sufficient oral fluids (2–4 L).

B. Stimulant laxatives—These agents stimulate fluid secretion and colonic contraction, resulting in a bowel movement within 6–12 hours after oral ingestion or 15–60 minutes after rectal administration. Oral agents are usually administered once daily at bedtime. Common preparations include bisacodyl, senna, and cascara (Table 15–4).

Lubiprostone is an oral cyclic fatty acid that activates intestinal chloride channels, increasing fluid secretion and secondarily increasing peristalsis. In large, multicenter controlled trials, patients treated with lubiprostone 24 mcg orally twice daily increased the number of bowel movements to approximately four to five per week, compared with two to three per week in patients treated with placebo. Lubiprostone is associated with nausea in up to one-third of patients and should not be given to women who may be pregnant (category C). Because lubiprostone is expensive, it should be reserved for patients who have suboptimal response or side effects with less expensive agents.

C. Opioid-receptor antagonists—Long-term use of opioids can cause constipation by inhibiting peristalsis and increasing intestinal fluid absorption. Methylnaltrexone is mu-opioid receptor antagonist that blocks peripheral opioid receptors (including the gastrointestinal tract) without affecting central analgesia. In 2008, it was approved for the treatment of opioid-induced constipation in patients receiving palliative care for advanced illness who had not responded to conventional laxative regimens. In controlled trials, methylnaltrexone subcutaneously (8 mg [38–62 kg], 12 mg [62–114 kg], or 0.15 mg/kg [less 38 kg] every other day) achieves laxation in 50% of patients compared with 15% of patients who received placebo. Its role for other patients with opioid-induced constipation is under investigation.

B. Fecal Impaction

Severe impaction of stool in the rectal vault may result in obstruction to further fecal flow, leading to partial or complete large bowel obstruction. Predisposing factors include medications (eg, opioids), severe psychiatric disease, prolonged bed rest, neurogenic disorders of the colon, and spinal cord disorders. Clinical presentation includes decreased appetite, nausea, and vomiting, and abdominal pain and distention. There may be paradoxical "diarrhea" as liquid stool leaks around the impacted feces. Firm feces are palpable on digital examination of the rectal vault. Initial treatment is directed at relieving the impaction with enemas (saline, mineral oil, or diatrizoate) or digital disruption of the impacted fecal material. Long-term care is directed at maintaining soft stools and regular bowel movements (as above).

▶ **When to Refer**

- Patients with refractory constipation for anorectal testing.
- Patients with dyssynergic defecation may benefit from biofeedback therapy.
- Patients with alarm symptoms or who are over age 50 should be referred for colonoscopy.
- Rarely, surgery (subtotal colectomy) is required for patients with severe colonic inertia.

DiPalma JA et al. A randomized, multicenter, placebo-controlled trial of polyethylene glycol laxative for chronic treatment of chronic constipation. Am J Gastroenterol. 2007 Jul;102(7):1436–41. [PMID: 17403074]

Johanson JF et al. Multicenter, 4-week, double-blind, randomized, placebo-controlled trial of lubiprostone, a locally-acting type-2 chloride channel activator, in patients with chronic constipation. Am J Gastroenterol. 2008 Jan;103(1):170–7. [PMID: 17916109]

Rao SS. Constipation: evaluation and treatment of colonic and anorectal motility disorders. Gastroenterol Clin North Am. 2007 Sep;36(3):687–711. [PMID: 17950444]

Rao SS et al. Randomized controlled trial of biofeedback, sham feedback, and standard therapy for dyssynergic defecation. Clin Gastroenterol Hepatol. 2007 Mar;5(3):331–8. [PMID: 17368232]

Shah ND et al. Ambulatory care for constipation in the United States 1993–2004. Am J Gastroenterol. 2008 Jul;103(7):1746–53. [PMID: 18557708]

Thomas J et al. Methylnaltrexone for opioid-induced constipation in advanced illness. N Engl J Med. 2008 May 29;358(22):2332–43. [PMID: 18509120]

GASTROINTESTINAL GAS

▶ **Belching**

Belching (eructation) is the involuntary or voluntary release of gas from the stomach or esophagus. It occurs most frequently after meals, when gastric distention results in transient lower esophageal sphincter (LES) relaxation. Belching is a normal reflex and does not itself denote gastrointestinal dysfunction. Virtually all stomach gas comes from swallowed air. With each swallow, 2–5 mL of air is ingested, and excessive amounts may result in distention, flatulence, and abdominal pain. This may occur with rapid eating, gum chewing, smoking, and the ingestion of carbonated beverages. Chronic excessive belching is almost always caused by aerophagia, common in anxious individuals and institutionalized patients. Evaluation should be restricted to patients with other complaints such as dysphagia, heartburn, early satiety, or vomiting.

Once patients understand the relationship between aerophagia and belching, most can deal with the problem by behavioral modification. Physical defects that hamper normal swallowing (ill-fitting dentures, nasal obstruction) should be corrected. Antacids and simethicone are of no value.

Flatus

The rate and volume of expulsion of flatus is highly variable. Flatus is derived from two sources: swallowed air and bacterial fermentation of undigested carbohydrate. The majority of swallowed air not belched passes through the gut and leaves as flatus. Swallowed air may contribute up to 500 mL of flatus per day (primarily nitrogen). Bacterial fermentation of undigested carbohydrates leads to the additional production of gas, particularly H_2, CO_2, and methane. The majority of this fermentation takes place in the colon. Under normal circumstances, a small substrate of fermentable substances reaches the colon. These substances include fructose, lactose, sorbitol, trehalose (mushrooms), raffinose, and stachyose (legumes, cruciferous vegetables). Complex starches and fiber may also cause gas. Gas production may be increased with ingestion of these carbohydrates or with malabsorption.

Determining abnormal from normal amounts of flatus is difficult. An initial trial of a lactose-free diet is recommended. Common gas-producing foods should be reviewed and the patient given an elimination trial. These include beans of all kinds, peas, lentils, brussels sprouts, cabbage, parsnips, leeks, onions, beer, and coffee. Fructose intolerance is common. Fructose is present not only in many fruits but is also used commonly as a sweetener or as fructose corn syrup in candy, fruit juices, and soda. Foul odor may be caused by garlic, onion, eggplant, mushrooms, and certain herbs and spices. For patients with persistent complaints, complex starches, and fiber may be eliminated, but such restrictive diets are unacceptable to most patients. Of refined flours, only rice flour is gas-free.

The nonprescription agent Beano (α-d-galactosidase enzyme) reduces gas caused by foods containing raffinose and stachyose, ie, cruciferous vegetables, legumes, nuts, and some cereals. Activated charcoal may afford relief. Simethicone is of no proved benefit.

Complaints of chronic abdominal distention or bloating are common. Some of these patients may produce excess gas. However, many patients have impaired small bowel gas propulsion or enhanced visceral sensitivity to gas distention. Many of these patients have an underlying functional gastrointestinal disorder such as irritable bowel syndrome or functional dyspepsia. Reduction of dietary fat, which delays intestinal gas clearance, may be helpful. Rifaximin, 400 mg twice daily, a nonabsorbable oral antibiotic with high activity against enteric bacteria, has been shown to reduce abdominal bloating and flatulence in approximately 40% of treated patients compared with 20% of controls. Symptom improvement may be attributable to

suppression of gas-producing colonic bacteria; however, relapse occurs within days after stopping the antibiotic. Further trials are needed to clarify the role of nonabsorbable antibiotics in symptom management.

Perez F et al. Gas distribution within the human gut: effect of meals. Am J Gastroenterol. 2007 Apr;102(4):842–9. [PMID: 17397409]

Rao SC et al. Ability of the normal human small intestine to absorb fructose: evaluation by breath testing. Clin Gastroenterol Hepatol. 2007 Aug;5(8):959–963. [PMID: 17625977]

Sharara A et al. A randomized double-blind placebo-controlled trial of rifaximin in patients with abdominal bloating and flatulence. Am J Gastroenterol. 2006 Feb;101(2):326–33. [PMID: 16454838]

DIARRHEA

Diarrhea can range in severity from an acute self-limited episode to a severe, life-threatening illness. To properly evaluate the complaint, the physician must determine the patient's normal bowel pattern and the nature of the current symptoms.

Approximately 10 L of fluid enter the duodenum daily, of which all but 1.5 L are absorbed by the small intestine. The colon absorbs most of the remaining fluid, with < 200 mL lost in the stool. Although diarrhea sometimes is defined as a stool weight of more than 200–300 g/24 h, quantification of stool weight is necessary only in some patients with chronic diarrhea. In most cases, the physician's working definition of diarrhea is increased stool frequency (more than three bowel movements per day) or liquidity of feces.

The causes of diarrhea are myriad. In clinical practice, it is helpful to distinguish acute from chronic diarrhea, as the evaluation and treatment are entirely different (Tables 15–5 and 15–6).

1. Acute Diarrhea

Etiology & Clinical Findings

Diarrhea acute in onset and persisting for less than 2 weeks is most commonly caused by infectious agents, bacterial toxins (either preformed or produced in the gut), or drugs. Community outbreaks (including nursing homes, schools, cruise ships) suggest a viral etiology or a common food source. Similar recent illnesses in family members suggest an infectious origin. Ingestion of improperly stored or prepared food implicates food poisoning. Day care attendance or exposure to unpurified water (camping, swimming) may result in infection with *Giardia* or *Cryptosporidium*. Large *Cyclospora* outbreaks have been traced to contaminated produce. Recent travel abroad suggests "traveler's diarrhea" (see Chapter 30). Antibiotic administration within the preceding several weeks increases the likelihood of *Clostridium difficile* colitis. Finally, risk factors for HIV infection or sexually transmitted diseases should be determined. (AIDS-associated diarrhea is discussed in Chapter 31; infectious proctitis is discussed in this chapter under Anorectal Disorders.) Persons engaging in anal intercourse or oral-anal sexual activities are at risk

Table 15–5. Causes of acute infectious diarrhea.

Noninflammatory Diarrhea	Inflammatory Diarrhea
Viral Noroviruses Rotavirus	**Viral** Cytomegalovirus
Protozoal *Giardia lamblia* *Cryptosporidium* *Cyclospora*	**Protozoal** *Entamoeba histolytica*

Bacterial
1. Preformed enterotoxin production
  Staphylococcus aureus
  Bacillus cereus
  Clostridium perfringens
2. Enterotoxin production
  Enterotoxigenic *Escherichia coli* (ETEC)
  Vibrio cholerae
	Bacterial
	1. Cytotoxin production
	  Enterohemorrhagic *E coli* O157:H5 (EHEC)
	  Vibrio parahaemolyticus
	  Clostridium difficile
	2. Mucosal invasion
	  Shigella
	  Campylobacter jejuni
	  Salmonella
	  Enteroinvasive *E coli* (EIEC)
	  Aeromonas
	  Plesiomonas
	  Yersinia enterocolitica
	  Chlamydia
	  Neisseria gonorrhoeae
	  Listeria monocytogenes

for a variety of infections that cause proctitis, including gonorrhea, syphilis, lymphogranuloma venereum, and herpes simplex.

The nature of the diarrhea helps distinguish among different infectious causes (Table 15–5).

A. Noninflammatory Diarrhea

Watery, nonbloody diarrhea associated with periumbilical cramps, bloating, nausea, or vomiting suggests a small bowel source caused by either a toxin-producing bacterium (enterotoxigenic *Escherichia coli* [ETEC], *Staphylococcus aureus*, *Bacillus cereus*, *Clostridium perfringens*) or other agents (viruses, *Giardia*) that disrupt normal absorption and secretory process in the small intestine. Prominent vomiting suggests viral enteritis or *S aureus* food poisoning. Although typically mild, the diarrhea (which originates in the small intestine) can be voluminous and result in dehydration with hypokalemia and metabolic acidosis (eg, cholera). Because tissue invasion does not occur, fecal leukocytes are not present.

B. Inflammatory Diarrhea

The presence of fever and bloody diarrhea (dysentery) indicates colonic tissue damage caused by invasion (shigellosis, salmonellosis, *Campylobacter* or *Yersinia* infection, amebiasis) or a toxin (*C difficile*, *E coli* O157:H7). Because these organisms involve predominantly the colon,

Table 15–6. Causes of chronic diarrhea.

Osmotic diarrhea
  CLUES: Stool volume decreases with fasting; increased stool osmotic gap
    1. Medications: antacids, lactulose, sorbitol
    2. Disaccharidase deficiency: lactose intolerance
    3. Factitious diarrhea: magnesium (antacids, laxatives)
Secretory diarrhea
  CLUES: Large volume (> 1 L/d); little change with fasting; normal stool osmotic gap
    1. Hormonally mediated: VIPoma, carcinoid, medullary carcinoma of thyroid (calcitonin), Zollinger-Ellison syndrome (gastrin)
    2. Factitious diarrhea (laxative abuse); phenolphthalein, cascara, senna
    3. Villous adenoma
    4. Bile salt malabsorption (idiopathic, ileal resection; Crohn ileitis; postcholecystectomy)
    5. Medications
Inflammatory conditions
  CLUES: Fever, hematochezia, abdominal pain
    1. Ulcerative colitis
    2. Crohn disease
    3. Microscopic colitis
    4. Malignancy: lymphoma, adenocarcinoma (with obstruction and pseudodiarrhea)
    5. Radiation enteritis
Medications
  Common offenders: SSRIs, cholinesterase inhibitors, NSAIDs, proton pump inhibitors, angiotensin II receptor blockers, metformin, allopurinol

Malabsorption syndromes
  CLUES: Weight loss, abnormal laboratory values; fecal fat > 10 g/24h
    1. Small bowel mucosal disorders: celiac sprue, tropical sprue, Whipple disease, eosinophilic gastroenteritis, small bowel resection (short bowel syndrome), Crohn disease
    2. Lymphatic obstruction: lymphoma, carcinoid, infectious (tuberculosis, MAI), Kaposi sarcoma, sarcoidosis, retroperitoneal fibrosis
    3. Pancreatic disease: chronic pancreatitis, pancreatic carcinoma
    4. Bacterial overgrowth: motility disorders (diabetes, vagotomy), scleroderma, fistulas, small intestinal diverticula
Motility disorders
  CLUES: Systemic disease or prior abdominal surgery
    1. Postsurgical: vagotomy, partial gastrectomy, blind loop with bacterial overgrowth
    2. Systemic disorders: scleroderma, diabetes mellitus, hyperthyroidism
    3. Irritable bowel syndrome
Chronic infections
    1. Parasites: *Giardia lamblia, Entamoeba histolytica, Strongyloidiasis stercoralis, Capillaria philippinensis*
    2. AIDS-related:
      Viral: Cytomegalovirus, HIV infection (?)
      Bacterial: *Clostridium difficile, Mycobacterium avium* complex
      Protozoal: Microsporida *(Enterocytozoon bieneusi), Cryptosporidium, Isospora belli*
Factitious
  See Osmotic and Secretory diarrhea above.

MAI, *Mycobacterium avium-intracellulare.*

the diarrhea is small in volume (< 1 L/d) and associated with left lower quadrant cramps, urgency, and tenesmus. Fecal leukocytes or lactoferrin usually are present in infections with invasive organisms. *E coli* O157:H7 is a Shiga toxin-producing noninvasive organism most commonly acquired from contaminated meat that has resulted in several outbreaks of an acute, often severe hemorrhagic colitis. In immunocompromised and HIV-infected patients, cytomegalovirus (CMV) can cause intestinal ulceration with watery or bloody diarrhea.

Infectious dysentery must be distinguished from acute ulcerative colitis, which may also present acutely with fever, abdominal pain, and bloody diarrhea. Diarrhea that persists for more than 14 days is not attributable to bacterial pathogens (except for *C difficile*) and should be evaluated as chronic diarrhea.

▶ Evaluation

In over 90% of patients with acute noninflammatory diarrhea, the illness is mild and self-limited, responding within 5 days to simple rehydration therapy or antidiarrheal agents; diagnostic investigation is unnecessary.

The isolation rate of bacterial pathogens from stool cultures in patients with acute noninflammatory diarrhea is under 3%. Thus, the goal of initial evaluation is to distinguish patients with mild disease from those with more serious illness. If diarrhea worsens or persists for more than 7 days, stool should be sent for fecal leukocyte or lactoferrin determination, ovum and parasite evaluation, and bacterial culture.

Prompt medical evaluation is indicated in the following situations (Figure 15–1): (1) Signs of inflammatory diarrhea manifested by any of the following: fever (> 38.5 °C), bloody diarrhea, or abdominal pain. (2) The passage of six or more unformed stools in 24 hours. (3) Profuse watery diarrhea and dehydration. (4) Frail older patients. (5) Immunocompromised patients (AIDS, posttransplantation). (6) Hospital-acquired diarrhea (onset > 3 days after hospitalization).

Physical examination pays note to the patient's level of hydration, mental status, and the presence of abdominal tenderness or peritonitis. Peritoneal findings may be present in infection with *C difficile* or enterohemorrhagic *E coli*. Hospitalization is required in patients with severe dehydration, toxicity, or marked abdominal pain. Stool specimens should be sent for examination for bacterial cultures.

The rate of positive bacterial cultures in such patients is 60–75%. For bloody stools, the laboratory should be directed to perform serotyping for Shiga-producing *E coli* O157:H7. Special culture media are required for *Yersinia, Vibrio,* and *Aeromonas.* In patients who are hospitalized or who have a history of antibiotic exposure, a stool sample should be tested for *C difficile* toxin. In patients with diar-

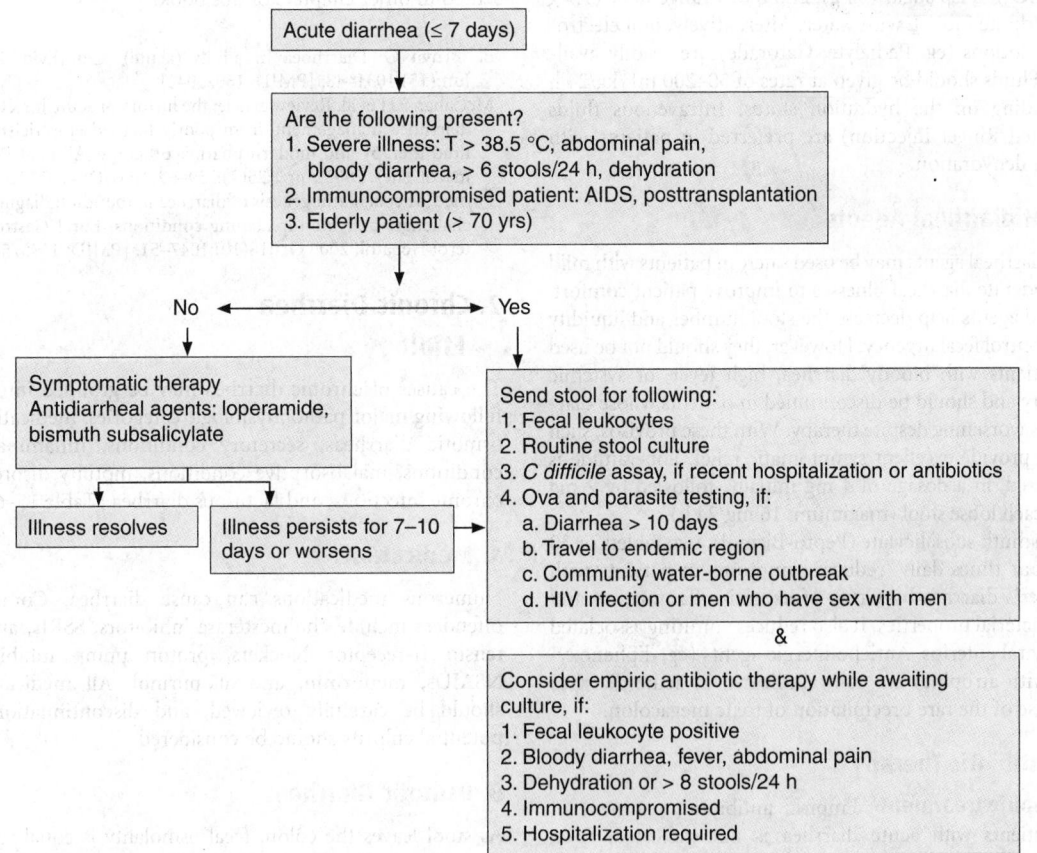

▲ Figure 15–1. Evaluation of acute diarrhea.

rhea that persists for more than 10 days, who have a history of travel to areas where amebiasis is endemic, or who engage in oral-anal sexual practices, three stool examinations for ova and parasites should also be performed. The stool antigen detection tests for both *Giardia* and *Entamoeba histolytica* are more sensitive than stool microscopy for detection of these organisms. A serum antigen detection test for *E histolytica* is also available. *Cyclospora* and *Cryptosporidium* are detected by fecal acid-fast staining.

▶ Treatment

A. Diet

Most mild diarrhea will not lead to dehydration provided the patient takes adequate oral fluids containing carbohydrates and electrolytes. Patients find it more comfortable to rest the bowel by avoiding high-fiber foods, fats, milk products, caffeine, and alcohol. Frequent feedings of tea, "flat" carbonated beverages, and soft, easily digested foods (eg, soups, crackers, bananas, applesauce, rice, toast) are encouraged.

B. Rehydration

In more severe diarrhea, dehydration can occur quickly, especially in children, the frail, and the elderly. Oral rehydration with fluids containing glucose, Na^+, K^+, Cl^-, and bicarbonate or citrate is preferred when feasible. A convenient mixture is $^1/_2$ tsp salt (3.5 g), 1 tsp baking soda (2.5 g $NaHCO_3$), 8 tsp sugar (40 g), and 8 oz orange juice (1.5 g KCl), diluted to 1 L with water. Alternatively, oral electrolyte solutions (eg, Pedialyte, Gatorade) are readily available. Fluids should be given at rates of 50–200 mL/kg/24 h depending on the hydration status. Intravenous fluids (lactated Ringer injection) are preferred in patients with severe dehydration.

C. Antidiarrheal Agents

Antidiarrheal agents may be used safely in patients with mild to moderate diarrheal illnesses to improve patient comfort. Opioid agents help decrease the stool number and liquidity and control fecal urgency. However, they should not be used in patients with bloody diarrhea, high fever, or systemic toxicity and should be discontinued in patients whose diarrhea is worsening despite therapy. With these provisos, such drugs provide excellent symptomatic relief. Loperamide is preferred, in a dosage of 4 mg initially, followed by 2 mg after each loose stool (maximum: 16 mg/24 h).

Bismuth subsalicylate (Pepto-Bismol), two tablets or 30 mL four times daily, reduces symptoms in patients with traveler's diarrhea by virtue of its anti-inflammatory and antibacterial properties. It also reduces vomiting associated with viral enteritis. Anticholinergic agents (eg, diphenoxylate with atropine) are contraindicated in acute diarrhea because of the rare precipitation of toxic megacolon.

D. Antibiotic Therapy

1. Empiric treatment—Empiric antibiotic treatment of all patients with acute diarrhea is not indicated. Even patients with inflammatory diarrhea caused by invasive pathogens usually have symptoms that will resolve within several days without antimicrobials. Empiric treatment may be considered in patients with non–hospital-acquired diarrhea with moderate to severe fever, tenesmus, or bloody stools or the presence of fecal lactoferrin while the stool bacterial culture is incubating, provided that infection with *E coli* O157:H7 is not suspected. The drugs of choice for empiric treatment are the fluoroquinolones (eg, ciprofloxacin 500 mg, ofloxacin 400 mg, or norfloxacin 400 mg, twice daily, or levofloxacin 500 mg once daily) for 5–7 days. Alternatives include trimethoprim-sulfamethoxazole, 160/800 mg twice daily; or doxycycline, 100 mg twice daily. Macrolides and penicillins are no longer recommended because of widespread microbial resistance to these agents. Rifaximin, a nonabsorbed oral antibiotic, 200 mg three times daily for 3 days, is approved for empiric treatment of noninflammatory traveler's diarrhea (see Chapter 30).

2. Specific antimicrobial treatment—Antibiotics are not recommended in patients with nontyphoid *Salmonella, Campylobacter, E coli* O157:H7, *Aeromonas,* or *Yersinia,* except in severe disease, because they do not hasten recovery or reduce the period of fecal bacterial excretion. The infectious diarrheas for which treatment is recommended are shigellosis, cholera, extraintestinal salmonellosis, traveler's diarrhea, *C difficile* infection, giardiasis, and amebiasis. Therapy for traveler's diarrhea, infectious (sexually transmitted) proctitis, and AIDS-related diarrhea is presented in other chapters of this book.

de Bruyn G. Diarrhoea in adults (acute). Clin Evid. 2006 Jun;(15):1031–48. [PMID: 16973042]

McCahan ZH et al. Review article: the history of acute infectious diarrhoea management—from poorly focused empiricism to fluid therapy and modern pharmacotherapy. Aliment Pharmacol Ther. 2007 Apr 1;25(7):759–69. [PMID: 17373914]

Payne CM et al. Pathogenesis of diarrhea in the adult: diagnostic challenges and life-threatening conditions. Eur J Gastroenterol Hepatol. 2006 Oct;18(10):1047–51. [PMID: 16957509]

2. Chronic Diarrhea

▶ Etiology

The causes of chronic diarrhea may be grouped into the following major pathophysiologic categories: medications, osmotic diarrheas, secretory conditions, inflammatory conditions, malabsorptive conditions, motility disorders, chronic infections, and factitious diarrhea (Table 15–6).

A. Medications

Numerous medications can cause diarrhea. Common offenders include cholinesterase inhibitors, SSRIs, angiotensin II-receptor blockers, proton pump inhibitors, NSAIDs, metformin, and allopurinol. All medications should be carefully reviewed, and discontinuation of potential culprits should be considered.

B. Osmotic Diarrheas

As stool leaves the colon, fecal osmolality is equal to the serum osmolality, ie, approximately 290 mosm/kg. Under normal circumstances, the major osmoles are Na^+, K^+, Cl^-, and HCO_3^-. The stool osmolality may be estimated by multiplying the stool $(Na^+ + K^+) \times 2$. The **osmotic gap** is the difference between the *measured* osmolality of the stool (or serum) and the *estimated* stool osmolality and is normally less than 50 mosm/kg. An increased osmotic gap (> 125 mosm/kg) implies that the diarrhea is caused by ingestion or malabsorption of an osmotically active substance. The most common causes are carbohydrate malabsorption (lactose, fructose, sorbitol), laxative abuse, and malabsorption syndromes (see below). Osmotic diarrheas resolve during fasting. Those caused by malabsorbed carbohydrates are characterized by abdominal distention, bloating, and flatulence due to increased colonic gas production.

Carbohydrate malabsorption is common and should be considered in all patients with chronic diarrhea. Lactase deficiency occurs in 75% of nonwhite adults and up to 25% of whites. It may also be acquired after an episode of viral gastroenteritis, medical illness, or gastrointestinal surgery. Fructose and sorbitol are present in many fruits, and are commonly used as a sweetener in gums, candies, and some medications. The diagnosis of carbohydrate malabsorption may be established by an elimination trial for 2–3 weeks or by hydrogen breath tests.

Ingestion of magnesium- or phosphate-containing compounds (laxatives, antacids) should be considered in enigmatic chronic diarrhea. The fat substitute olestra also causes diarrhea and cramps in occasional patients.

C. Secretory Conditions

Increased intestinal secretion or decreased absorption results in a high-volume watery diarrhea with a normal osmotic gap. There is little change in stool output during the fasting state, and dehydration and electrolyte imbalance may develop. Causes include endocrine tumors (stimulating intestinal or pancreatic secretion) and bile salt malabsorption (stimulating colonic secretion).

D. Inflammatory Conditions

Diarrhea is present in most patients with inflammatory bowel disease (ulcerative colitis, Crohn disease, microscopic colitis). A variety of other symptoms may be present, including abdominal pain, fever, weight loss, and hematochezia. (See Inflammatory Bowel Disease, below.)

E. Malabsorptive Conditions

The major causes of malabsorption are small mucosal intestinal diseases, intestinal resections, lymphatic obstruction, small intestinal bacterial overgrowth, and pancreatic insufficiency. Its characteristics are weight loss, osmotic diarrhea, steatorrhea, and nutritional deficiencies. Significant diarrhea in the absence of weight loss is not likely to be due to malabsorption. The physical and laboratory abnormalities related to deficiencies of vitamins or minerals are discussed in Chapter 29.

F. Motility Disorders

Abnormal intestinal motility secondary to systemic disorders or surgery may result in diarrhea due to rapid transit or to stasis of intestinal contents with bacterial overgrowth, resulting in malabsorption. Probably the most common cause of chronic diarrhea is irritable bowel syndrome (see Irritable Bowel Syndrome, below).

G. Chronic Infections

Chronic parasitic infections may cause diarrhea through a number of mechanisms. Pathogens most commonly associated with diarrhea include the protozoans *Giardia*, *E histolytica*, and *Cyclospora* as well as the intestinal nematodes. Strongyloidiasis and capillariasis should be excluded in patients from endemic regions, especially in the presence of eosinophilia. Bacterial infections with *Aeromonas* and *Plesiomonas* may uncommonly be a cause of chronic diarrhea.

Immunocompromised patients are susceptible to infectious organisms that can cause acute or chronic diarrhea (see Chapter 31), including Microsporida, *Cryptosporidium*, CMV, *Isospora belli*, *Cyclospora*, and *Mycobacterium avium* complex.

H. Factitious Diarrhea

Fifteen percent of patients have factitious diarrhea caused by surreptitious laxative abuse or dilution of stool. This should especially be considered in patients with a long history of undiagnosed medical ailments or employment in the medical field.

▶ Clinical Findings

The history and physical examination commonly suggest the underlying pathophysiology that guides the subsequent diagnostic workup (Figure 15–2). Important tests are described here. AIDS-associated diarrhea is discussed in Chapter 31.

A. Stool Analysis

1. Twenty-four-hour stool collection for weight and quantitative fecal fat—A stool weight of more than 200 g/24 h confirms diarrhea. A weight > 500 g excludes irritable bowel syndrome, whereas a weight > 1000–1500 g suggests a secretory process. A fecal fat determination in excess of 10 g/24 h indicates a malabsorptive disorder. (See Celiac Sprue and specific tests for malabsorption, below.)

2. Stool osmolality—Stool osmolality less than serum osmolality implies that water or urine has been added to the specimen (factitious diarrhea). A stool pH < 5.6 is consistent with carbohydrate malabsorption.

3. Stool laxative screen—In cases of suspected laxative abuse, stool magnesium, phosphate, and sulfate levels may be measured. Phenolphthalein and bisacodyl can be analyzed in stool water, using chromatographic techniques. Anthraquinones and bisacodyl are sought for in the urine.

4. Fecal leukocytes—The presence of fecal leukocytes or lactoferrin implies inflammatory diarrhea.

5. Stool for ova and parasites—The presence of *Giardia* and *E histolytica* may be detected in wet mounts. However, fecal antigen detection tests for *Giardia* and *E histolytica* may be a more sensitive and specific method of

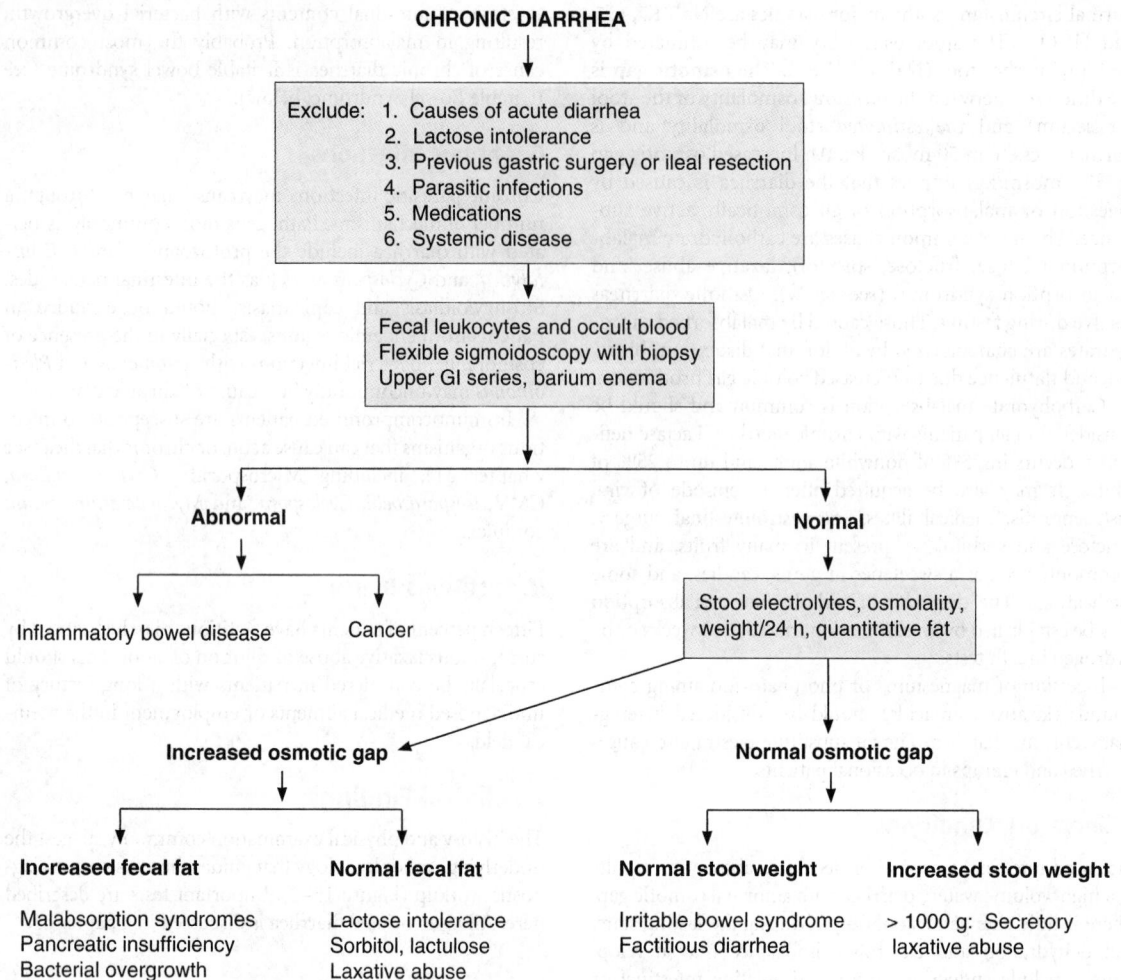

CHRONIC DIARRHEA

Exclude:
1. Causes of acute diarrhea
2. Lactose intolerance
3. Previous gastric surgery or ileal resection
4. Parasitic infections
5. Medications
6. Systemic disease

Fecal leukocytes and occult blood
Flexible sigmoidoscopy with biopsy
Upper GI series, barium enema

Abnormal

Inflammatory bowel disease   Cancer

Normal

Stool electrolytes, osmolality, weight/24 h, quantitative fat

Increased osmotic gap

Increased fecal fat

Malabsorption syndromes
Pancreatic insufficiency
Bacterial overgrowth

Normal fecal fat

Lactose intolerance
Sorbitol, lactulose
Laxative abuse

Normal osmotic gap

Normal stool weight

Irritable bowel syndrome
Factitious diarrhea

Increased stool weight

> 1000 g: Secretory
laxative abuse

▲ **Figure 15-2.** Decision diagram for diagnosis of causes of chronic diarrhea.

detection. *Cryptosporidium* and *Cyclospora* are found with modified acid-fast staining.

B. Diagnostic Tests

1. Routine laboratory tests—Complete blood count, serum electrolytes, liver function tests, calcium, phosphorus, albumin, TSH, vitamin A and D levels, and prothrombin time may be of value. Anemia occurs in malabsorption syndromes (folate, iron deficiency, or vitamin B_{12}) as well as inflammatory conditions. Hypoalbuminemia is present in malabsorption, protein-losing enteropathies, and inflammatory diseases. Hyponatremia and nonanion gap metabolic acidosis occur in secretory diarrheas.

2. Other laboratory tests—In patients with suspected malabsorption, serologic testing for celiac sprue includes IgA tissue transglutaminase (tTG) antibody tests. Secretory diarrheas due to neuroendocrine tumors are rare. When this is suspected, serum chromogranin A, vasoactive intestinal peptide (VIP) (VIPoma), calcitonin (medullary thy-

roid carcinoma), gastrin (Zollinger-Ellison syndrome), and glucagon determinations may be diagnostic, and urine should be sent for 5-hydroxyindoleacetic acid (5-HIAA) (carcinoid).

3. Endoscopic examination and mucosal biopsy—Colonoscopy with terminal ileum inspection mucosal biopsy is helpful in the detection of inflammatory bowel disease (including Crohn disease, ulcerative colitis, and microscopic colitis) and melanosis coli (indicative of chronic anthraquinone laxative use). Upper endoscopy with small bowel biopsy is performed when a small intestinal malabsorptive disorder is suspected (celiac sprue, Whipple disease) and less commonly to diagnose severe helminthic infections (strongyoidiasis, capillariasis); it may also be done in patients with advanced AIDS to document *Cryptosporidium*, Microsporida, and *M avium-intracellulare* infection. If bacterial overgrowth is suspected, the diagnosis is confirmed with noninvasive breath tests (d-[^{14}C]xylose, glucose, or lactulose) or by obtaining an aspirate of small intestinal contents for quantitative aerobic and anaerobic bacterial culture.

4. Other imaging studies—Calcification on a plain abdominal radiograph confirms a diagnosis of chronic pancreatitis, although abdominal CT and endoscopic ultrasonography are more sensitive for the diagnosis of chronic pancreatitis as well as pancreatic cancer. Small intestinal imaging with barium, CT, or MRI is helpful in the diagnosis of Crohn disease, small bowel lymphoma, carcinoid, and jejunal diverticula. Neuroendocrine tumors may be localized using somatostatin receptor scintigraphy. Retention of < 11% at 7 days of intravenous 75Se-homotaurocholate on scintigraphy suggests bile salt malabsorption.

▶ Treatment

A number of antidiarrheal agents may be used in certain patients with chronic diarrheal conditions and are listed below. Opioids are safe in most patients with chronic, stable symptoms.

Loperamide: 4 mg initially, then 2 mg after each loose stool (maximum: 16 mg/d).

Diphenoxylate with atropine: One tablet three or four times daily as needed.

Codeine and deodorized tincture of opium: Because of potential habituation, these drugs are avoided except in cases of chronic, intractable diarrhea. Codeine may be given in a dosage of 15–60 mg every 4 hours; tincture of opium, 0.3–1.2 mL every 6 hours as needed.

Clonidine: α_2-Adrenergic agonists inhibit intestinal electrolyte secretion. Clonidine, 0.1–0.6 mg twice daily, or a clonidine patch, 0.1–0.2 mg/d, may help in some patients with secretory diarrheas, diabetic diarrhea, or cryptosporidiosis.

Octreotide: This somatostatin analog stimulates intestinal fluid and electrolyte absorption and inhibits intestinal fluid secretion and the release of gastrointestinal peptides. It is given for secretory diarrheas due to neuroendocrine tumors (VIPomas, carcinoid) and in some cases of AIDS-related diarrhea. Effective doses range from 50 to 250 mcg subcutaneously three times daily.

Cholestyramine: This bile salt-binding resin may be useful in patients with bile salt-induced diarrhea, which may be idiopathic or secondary to intestinal resection or ileal disease. A dosage of 4 g once to three times daily is recommended.

Fan E et al. Clinical problem-solving. A gut feeling. N Engl J Med. 2008 Jul 3;359(1):75–80. [PMID: 18596276]

Fernández-Bañares F et al. Systematic evaluation of the causes of chronic watery diarrhea with functional characteristics. Am J Gastroenterol. 2007 Nov;102(11):2530–8. [PMID: 17680846]

Headstrom PD et al. Chronic diarrhea. Clin Gastroenterol Hepatol. 2005 Aug;3(8):734–7. [PMID: 16234000]

Pilotto A et al; SOFIA Project Investigators. The prevalence of diarrhea and its association with drug use in elderly outpatients: a multicenter study. Am J Gastroenterol. 2008 Nov;103(11):2816–23. [PMID: 18721240]

Schiller L. Management of diarrhea in clinical practice: strategies for primary care physicians. Rev Gastroenterol Dis. 2007;7(Suppl 3):S27–38. [PMID: 18192963]

GASTROINTESTINAL BLEEDING

1. Acute Upper Gastrointestinal Bleeding

ESSENTIALS OF DIAGNOSIS

▶ Hematemesis (bright red blood or "coffee grounds").

▶ Melena in most cases; hematochezia in massive upper gastrointestinal bleeds.

▶ Volume status to determine severity of blood loss; hematocrit is a poor early indicator of blood loss.

▶ Endoscopy diagnostic and may be therapeutic.

▶ General Considerations

There are over 250,000 hospitalizations a year in the United States for acute upper gastrointestinal bleeding, with a mortality rate of 4–10%. Approximately half of patients are over 60 years of age, and in this age group the mortality rate is even higher. Patients seldom die of exsanguination but rather from complications of an underlying disease.

The most common presentation of upper gastrointestinal bleeding is hematemesis or melena. Hematemesis may be either bright red blood or brown "coffee grounds" material. Melena develops after as little as 50–100 mL of blood loss in the upper gastrointestinal tract, whereas hematochezia requires a loss of more than 1000 mL. Although hematochezia generally suggests a lower bleeding source (eg, colonic), upper gastrointestinal bleeding may present with hematochezia in 10% of cases.

Upper gastrointestinal bleeding is self-limited in 80% of patients; urgent medical therapy and endoscopic evaluation are obligatory in the rest. Patients with bleeding more than 48 hours prior to presentation have a low risk of recurrent bleeding.

▶ Etiology

Acute upper gastrointestinal bleeding may originate from a number of sources. These are listed in order of the frequency and discussed in detail below.

A. Peptic Ulcer Disease

Peptic ulcers account for half of major upper gastrointestinal bleeding with an overall mortality rate of 4%. However, in North America the incidence of bleeding from ulcers is declining, perhaps due to eradication of H pylori, use of safer NSAIDs, and prophylaxis with proton pump inhibitors in high-risk patients.

B. Portal Hypertension

Portal hypertension accounts for 10–20% of upper gastrointestinal bleeding. Bleeding usually arises from esophageal varices and less commonly gastric or duodenal varices or portal hypertensive gastropathy. Approximately 25% of patients with cirrhosis have medium to large esophageal varices, of whom 30% experience acute variceal bleeding within a 2-year period. Due to improved care, the hospital mortality rate has declined over the past 20 years from 40% to 15%. Nevertheless, a mortality rate of 60–80% is expected at 1–4 years due to recurrent bleeding or other complications of chronic liver disease.

C. Mallory-Weiss Tears

Lacerations of the gastroesophageal junction cause 5–10% of cases of upper gastrointestinal bleeding. Many patients report a history of heavy alcohol use or retching. Less than 10% have continued or recurrent bleeding.

D. Vascular Anomalies

Vascular anomalies are found throughout the gastrointestinal tract and may be the source of chronic or acute gastrointestinal bleeding. They account for 7% of cases of acute upper tract bleeding. **Vascular ectasias** (angiodysplasias) have a bright red stellate appearance. They may be part of systemic conditions (hereditary hemorrhagic telangiectasia, CREST syndrome) or may occur sporadically. There is an increased incidence in patients with chronic renal failure. The Dieulafoy lesion is an aberrant, large-caliber submucosal artery, most commonly in the proximal stomach that causes recurrent, intermittent bleeding.

E. Gastric Neoplasms

Gastric neoplasms result in 1% of upper gastrointestinal hemorrhages.

F. Erosive Gastritis

Because this process is superficial, it is a relatively unusual cause of severe gastrointestinal bleeding (< 5% of cases) and more commonly results in chronic blood loss. Gastric mucosal erosions are due to NSAIDs, alcohol, or severe medical or surgical illness (stress-related mucosal disease).

G. Erosive Esophagitis

Severe erosive esophagitis due to chronic gastroesophageal reflux may rarely cause significant upper gastrointestinal bleeding, especially in patients who are bed bound long-term.

H. Others

An aortoenteric fistula complicates 2% of abdominal aortic grafts or can occur as the initial presentation of a previously untreated aneurysm. Usually located between the graft or aneurysm and the third portion of the duodenum, these fistulas characteristically present with a herald nonexsanguinating initial hemorrhage, with melena and hematemesis, or with chronic intermittent bleeding. The diagnosis may be suspected by upper endoscopy or abdominal CT. Surgery is mandatory to prevent exsanguinating hemorrhage. Unusual causes of upper gastrointestinal bleeding include hemobilia (from hepatic tumor, angioma, penetrating trauma), pancreatic malignancy, and pseudoaneurysm (hemosuccus pancreaticus).

▶ Initial Evaluation & Treatment

A. Stabilization

The initial step is assessment of the hemodynamic status. A systolic blood pressure less than 100 mm Hg identifies a high-risk patient with severe acute bleeding. A heart rate over 100 beats/min with a systolic blood pressure over 100 mm Hg signifies moderate acute blood loss. A normal systolic blood pressure and heart rate suggest relatively minor hemorrhage. Postural hypotension and tachycardia are useful when present but may be due to causes other than blood loss. Because the hematocrit may take 24–72 hours to equilibrate with the extravascular fluid, it is not a reliable indicator of the severity of acute bleeding.

In patients with significant bleeding, two 18-gauge or larger intravenous lines should be started prior to further diagnostic tests. Blood is sent for complete blood count, prothrombin time with international normalized ratio (INR), serum creatinine, liver enzymes, and blood typing and screening (in anticipation of need for possible transfusion). In patients without hemodynamic compromise or overt active bleeding, aggressive fluid repletion can be delayed until the extent of the bleeding is further clarified. Patients with evidence of hemodynamic compromise are given 0.9% saline or lactated Ringer injection and cross-matched for 2–4 units of packed red blood cells. It is rarely necessary to administer type-specific or O-negative blood. Central venous pressure monitoring is desirable in some cases, but line placement should not interfere with rapid volume resuscitation.

A nasogastric tube should be placed in all patients with suspected active upper tract bleeding. The aspiration of red blood or "coffee grounds" confirms an upper gastrointestinal source of bleeding, though 10% of patients with confirmed upper tract sources of bleeding have nonbloody aspirates—especially when bleeding originates in the duodenum. An aspirate of bright red blood indicates active bleeding and is associated with the highest risk of further bleeding, and complications, while a clear aspirate identifies patients at lower initial risk. Erythromycin (250 mg) administered intravenously 30 minutes prior to upper endoscopy promotes gastric emptying of clots and improves quality of endoscopic examination. Efforts to stop or slow bleeding by gastric lavage with large volumes of fluid are of no benefit and expose the patient to an increased risk of aspiration. Periodic reaspiration of the nasogastric tube serves as an indicator of ongoing bleeding or rebleeding.

B. Blood Replacement

The amount of fluid and blood products required is based on assessment of vital signs, evidence of active bleeding from nasogastric aspirate, and laboratory tests. Sufficient packed red blood cells should be given to maintain a hematocrit of 25–30%. In the absence of continued bleeding, the hematocrit should rise 4% for each unit of transfused packed red cells. Transfusion of blood should not be withheld from patients with brisk active bleeding regardless of the hematocrit. It is desirable to transfuse blood in anticipation of the nadir hematocrit. In actively bleeding patients, platelets are transfused if the platelet count is under 50,000/mcL and considered if there is impaired platelet function due to aspirin or clopidogrel use (regardless of the platelet count). Uremic patients (who also have dysfunctional platelets) with active bleeding are given three doses of desmopressin (DDAVP), 0.3 mcg/kg intravenously, at 12-hour intervals. Fresh frozen plasma is administered for actively bleeding patients with a coagulopathy and an INR > 1.5. In the face of massive bleeding, 1 unit of fresh frozen plasma should be given for each 5 units of packed red blood cells transfused.

C. Initial Triage

A preliminary assessment of risk based on several clinical factors aids in the resuscitation as well as the rational triage of the patient. Clinical predictors of increased risk of rebleeding and death include age > 60 years, comorbid illnesses, systolic blood pressure < 100 mm Hg, pulse > 100 beats/min, and bright red blood in the nasogastric aspirate or on rectal examination.

1. High risk—Patients with active bleeding manifested by hematemesis or bright red blood on nasogastric aspirate, shock, persistent hemodynamic derangement despite fluid resuscitation, serious comorbid medical illness, or evidence of advanced liver disease require admission to an intensive care unit (ICU). Emergent endoscopy should be performed after adequate resuscitation, usually within 12 hours.

2. Low to moderate risk—All other patients are admitted to a step-down unit or medical ward after appropriate stabilization for further evaluation and treatment. Patients without evidence of active bleeding undergo nonemergent endoscopy usually within 12–24 hours.

▶ Subsequent Evaluation & Treatment

Specific treatment of the various causes of upper gastrointestinal bleeding is discussed elsewhere in this chapter. The following general comments apply to most patients with bleeding.

The physician's impression of the bleeding source is correct in only 40% of cases. Signs of chronic liver disease implicate bleeding due to portal hypertension, but a different lesion is identified in 25% of patients with cirrhosis. A history of dyspepsia, NSAID use, or peptic ulcer disease suggests peptic ulcer. Acute bleeding preceded by heavy alcohol ingestion or retching suggests a Mallory-Weiss tear, though most of these patients have neither.

A. Upper Endoscopy

Virtually all patients with upper tract bleeding should undergo upper endoscopy within 6–24 hours of arriving in the emergency department. The benefits of endoscopy in this setting are threefold.

1. To identify the source of bleeding—The appropriate acute and long-term medical therapy is determined by the cause of bleeding. Patients with portal hypertension will be treated differently from those with ulcer disease. If

surgery is required for uncontrolled bleeding, the source of bleeding as determined at endoscopy will determine the approach.

2. To determine the risk of rebleeding and guide triage—Patients with a nonbleeding Mallory-Weiss tear, esophagitis, gastritis, and ulcers that have a clean, white base have a very low risk (< 5%) of rebleeding. Patients with one of these findings who are < age 60 years, without hemodynamic instability or transfusion requirement, without serious coexisting illness, and who have stable social support may be discharged from the emergency department or medical ward after endoscopy with outpatient follow-up. All others with one of these low-risk lesions should be observed on a medical ward for 24–48 hours. Patients with ulcers that are actively bleeding or have a visible vessel or adherent clot, or who have variceal bleeding usually require at least a 3-day hospitalization with closer initial observation in an ICU or step down unit.

3. To render endoscopic therapy—Hemostasis can be achieved in actively bleeding lesions with endoscopic modalities such as cautery, injection, or endoclips. About 90% of bleeding or nonbleeding varices can be effectively treated immediately with injection of a sclerosant or application of rubber bands to the varices. Similarly, 90% of bleeding ulcers, angiomas, or Mallory-Weiss tears can be controlled with either injection of epinephrine, direct cauterization of the vessel by a heater probe or multipolar electrocautery probe, or application of an endoclip. Certain nonbleeding lesions such as ulcers with visible blood vessels, and angiomas are also treated with these therapies. Specific endoscopic therapy of varices, peptic ulcers, and Mallory-Weiss tears is dealt with elsewhere in this chapter.

B. Acute Pharmacologic Therapies

1. Acid inhibitory therapy—Intravenous **proton pump inhibitors** (esomeprazole or pantoprazole, 80 mg bolus, followed by 8 mg/h continuous infusion for 72 hours) reduce the risk of rebleeding in patients with peptic ulcers with high-risk features (active bleeding, visible vessel, or adherent clot) after endoscopic treatment. High doses of **oral proton pump inhibitors** (esomeprazole 40 mg or lansoprazole 60 mg, twice daily for 5 days) may also be effective.

A randomized, placebo-controlled clinical trial demonstrated that a continuous intravenous infusion of omeprazole *before* endoscopy resulted in an increased number of clean-based peptic ulcers (which do not require endoscopic therapy) and a decreased number of ulcers that were actively bleeding or had a visible vessel (resulting in a decreased need for endoscopic therapy) *during* endoscopy. It has become standard clinical practice at many institutions to administer either an intravenous or a high-dose oral proton pump inhibitor prior to endoscopy in patients with significant upper gastrointestinal bleeding. Based on the findings during endoscopy, the proton pump inhibitor may be continued or discontinued.

2. Octreotide—Continuous intravenous infusion of octreotide (100 mcg bolus, followed by 50–100 mcg/h) reduces splanchnic blood flow and portal blood pressures and is effective in the initial control of bleeding related to portal hypertension. It is administered promptly to all patients with active upper gastrointestinal bleeding and evidence of liver disease or portal hypertension until the source of bleeding can be determined by endoscopy.

3. Vasoactive agents—Intravenous vasopressin is no longer used in the treatment of upper gastrointestinal bleeding. In countries where it is available, terlipressin may be preferred to octreotide for the treatment of bleeding related to portal hypertension because of its sustained reduction of portal and variceal pressures and its proven reduction in mortality.

C. Other Treatment

1. Intra-arterial embolization—Angiographic treatment is used rarely in patients with persistent bleeding from ulcers, angiomas, or Mallory-Weiss tears who have failed endoscopic therapy and are poor operative risks.

2. Transvenous intrahepatic portosystemic shunts (TIPS)—Placement of a wire stent from the hepatic vein through the liver to the portal vein provides effective decompression of the portal venous system and control of acute variceal bleeding. It is indicated in patients in whom endoscopic modalities have failed to control acute variceal bleeding.

Capell MS et al. Initial management of acute gastrointestinal bleeding: from initial evaluation up to gastrointestinal endoscopy. Med Clin North Am. 2008 May;92(3):491–509. [PMID: 18387374]

Gralnek I et al. Management of acute bleeding from a peptic ulcer. N Engl J Med. 2008 Aug 28;359(9):928–37. [PMID: 18753649]

Lau JY et al. Omeprazole before endoscopy in patients with gastrointestinal bleeding. N Engl J Med. 2007 Apr 19;356(16):1631–40. [PMID: 17442905]

Leontiadis GI et al. Proton pump inhibitor treatment for acute peptic ulcer bleeding. Cochrane Database Syst Rev. 2006 Jan 25;(1):CD002094. [PMID: 16437441]

2. Acute Lower Gastrointestinal Bleeding

ESSENTIALS OF DIAGNOSIS

- ▶ Hematochezia usually present.
- ▶ Ten percent of cases of hematochezia due to upper gastrointestinal source.
- ▶ Evaluation with colonoscopy in stable patients.
- ▶ Massive active bleeding calls for evaluation with sigmoidoscopy, upper endoscopy, angiography, or nuclear bleeding scan.

▶ General Considerations

Lower gastrointestinal bleeding is defined as that arising below the ligament of Treitz, ie, the small intestine or colon; however, up to 95% of cases arise from the colon.

The severity of lower gastrointestinal bleeding ranges from mild anorectal bleeding to massive, large-volume hematochezia. Bright red blood that drips into the bowl after a bowel movement or is mixed with solid brown stool signifies mild bleeding, usually from an anorectosigmoid source, and can be evaluated in the outpatient setting. Serious lower gastrointestinal bleeding is more common in older men. In patients hospitalized with gastrointestinal bleeding, lower tract bleeding is one-fourth as common as upper gastrointestinal hemorrhage and tends to have a more benign course. Patients hospitalized with lower gastrointestinal tract bleeding are less likely to present with shock or orthostasis (< 20%) or to require transfusions (< 40%). Spontaneous cessation of bleeding occurs in over 85% of cases, and hospital mortality is less than 4%.

▶ Etiology

The cause of these lesions depends on both the age of the patient and the severity of the bleeding. In patients under 50 years of age, the most common causes are infectious colitis, anorectal disease, and inflammatory bowel disease. In older patients, significant hematochezia is most often seen with diverticulosis, vascular ectasias, malignancy, or ischemia. In 20% of acute bleeding episodes, no source of bleeding can be identified.

A. Diverticulosis

Hemorrhage occurs in 3–5% of all patients with diverticulosis and is the most common cause of major lower tract bleeding, accounting for 50% of cases. A significant percentage of cases are associated with the use of nonsteroidal anti-inflammatory agents. Although diverticula are more prevalent on the left side of the colon, bleeding more commonly originates on the right side. Diverticular bleeding usually presents as acute, painless, large-volume maroon or bright red hematochezia in patients over age 50 years. More than 95% of cases require less than 4 units of blood transfusion. Bleeding subsides spontaneously in 80% but may recur in up to 25% of patients.

B. Vascular Ectasias

Vascular ectasias (or angiodysplasias) occur throughout the upper and lower intestinal tracts and cause painless bleeding ranging from melena or hematochezia to occult blood loss. They are responsible for 3% of cases of lower gastrointestinal bleeding, where they are most often seen in the cecum and ascending colon. They are flat, red lesions (2–10 mm) with ectatic peripheral vessels radiating from a central vessel, and are most common in patients over 70 years and in those with chronic renal failure. Bleeding in younger patients more commonly arises from the small intestine.

Most colonic ectasias are degenerative lesions that are believed to arise from chronic colonic mucosal contraction obstructing venous mucosal drainage. The cause of gastric and small intestinal ectasias is unknown. Some are congenital, part of an inherited syndrome such as hereditary hemorrhagic telangiectasia, or related to autoimmune disorders, typically scleroderma. Ectasias can be identified in up to 6% of subjects over age 60 years, so their mere presence does not prove that the lesion is the source of bleeding, as active bleeding is seldom seen.

C. Neoplasms

Benign polyps and carcinoma are associated with chronic occult blood loss or intermittent anorectal hematochezia. Furthermore, they may cause up to 7% of acute lower gastrointestinal hemorrhage. After endoscopic removal of colonic polyps, important bleeding may occur up to 2 weeks later in 0.3% of patients. In general, prompt colonoscopy is recommended to treat postpolypectomy hemorrhage and minimize the need for transfusions.

D. Inflammatory Bowel Disease

Patients with inflammatory bowel disease (especially ulcerative colitis) often have diarrhea with variable amounts of hematochezia. Bleeding varies from occult blood loss to recurrent hematochezia usually mixed with stool. Symptoms of abdominal pain, tenesmus, and urgency are often present.

E. Anorectal Disease

Anorectal disease (hemorrhoids, fissures) usually results in small amounts of bright red blood noted on the toilet paper, streaking of the stool, or dripping into the toilet bowl; clinically significant blood loss can sometimes occur. Hemorrhoids are the source in 10% of patients admitted with lower bleeding. Rectal ulcers may account for up to 9% of lower bleeding, usually in elderly or debilitated patients with constipation.

F. Ischemic Colitis

This condition is seen commonly in older patients, most of whom have atherosclerotic disease. Most cases occur spontaneously due to transient episodes of nonocclusive ischemia. Ischemic colitis may also occur in 5% of patients after surgery for ileoaortic or abdominal aortic aneurysm. In young patients, colonic ischemia may develop due to vasculitis, coagulation disorders, estrogen therapy, and long distance running. Ischemic colitis results in hematochezia or bloody diarrhea associated with mild cramps. In most patients, the bleeding is mild and self-limited.

G. Others

Radiation-induced proctitis causes anorectal bleeding that may develop months to years after pelvic radiation. Endoscopy reveals multiple rectal telangiectasias. Acute infectious colitis (see Acute Diarrhea, above) commonly causes bloody diarrhea. Rare causes of lower tract bleeding include vasculitic ischemia, solitary rectal ulcer, NSAID-induced ulcers in the small bowel or right colon, small bowel diverticula, and colonic varices.

▶ Clinical Findings

A. Symptoms and Signs

The color of the stool helps distinguish upper from lower gastrointestinal bleeding, especially when observed by the clinician. Brown stools mixed or streaked with blood predict a source in the rectosigmoid or anus. Large volumes of bright red blood suggest a colonic source; maroon stools imply a lesion in the right colon or small intestine; and black stools (melena) predict a source proximal to the ligament of Treitz. Although 10% of patients admitted with self-reported hematochezia have an upper gastrointestinal source of bleeding (eg, peptic ulcer), this almost always occurs in the setting of massive hemorrhage with hemodynamic instability. Painless large-volume bleeding usually suggests diverticular bleeding. Bloody diarrhea associated with cramping abdominal pain, urgency, or tenesmus is characteristic of inflammatory bowel disease, infectious colitis, or ischemic colitis.

B. Diagnostic Tests

Important considerations in management include exclusion of an upper tract source, anoscopy and sigmoidoscopy, colonoscopy, nuclear bleeding scans and angiography, and small intestine push enteroscopy or capsule imaging.

1. Exclusion of an upper tract source—A nasogastric tube with aspiration should be considered, especially in patients with hemodynamic compromise. Aspiration of red blood or dark brown ("coffee grounds") guaiac-positive material strongly implicates an upper gastrointestinal source of bleeding. If blood is not seen and bile is aspirated, an upper source is found in only 1% of patients.

2. Anoscopy and sigmoidoscopy—In otherwise healthy patients without anemia under age 45 years with small-volume bleeding, anoscopy and sigmoidoscopy are performed to look for evidence of anorectal disease, inflammatory bowel disease, or infectious colitis. If a lesion is found, no further evaluation is needed immediately unless the bleeding persists or is recurrent. In patients over age 45 years with small-volume hematochezia, the entire colon must be evaluated with colonoscopy to exclude tumor.

3. Colonoscopy—In patients with acute, large-volume bleeding requiring hospitalization, colonoscopy is the preferred initial study in most cases. The bowel first is purged rapidly by administration of a high-volume colonic lavage solution, given until the effluent is clear of blood and clots (4–10 L of GoLYTELY, CoLYTE, NuLYTE given orally or 1 L every 30 minutes over 2–5 hours by nasogastric tube). For patients with stable vital signs and whose lower gastrointestinal bleeding appears to have stopped, colonoscopy can be performed electively within 24 hours of admission. For patients with signs of hemodynamically significant bleeding (unstable vital signs) or who have signs of continued active bleeding during bowel preparation, urgent colonoscopy should be performed within 1–2 hours of completing the bowel purgative, when the bowel discharge is without clots. The probable site of bleeding can be identified in 70–85% of patients, and a high-risk lesion can be identified and treated in up to 20%.

4. Nuclear bleeding scans and angiography—Technetium-labeled red blood cell scanning can detect significant active bleeding and, in some cases, can localize the source to the small intestine, right colon, or left colon. Thus, some physicians obtain a nuclear bleeding scan to guide initial decision-making. If no bleeding is detected on scintigraphy, an "elective" colonoscopy is performed within 24 hours after conventional bowel preparation. If bleeding is detected on scintigraphy, urgent angiography is performed instead of colonoscopy. Nuclear studies are more apt to be positive in patients who are passing bright red or maroon stools at the time of the scan. Because most bleeding is slow or intermittent, less than half of nuclear studies are diagnostic and the accuracy of localization is poor. Thus, the main utility of scintigraphy is to determine whether bleeding is ongoing in order to determine whether angiography should be pursued. Less than half of patients with a positive nuclear study have positive angiography. Accordingly, angiograms are performed only in patients with positive technetium scans believed to have significant, ongoing bleeding.

In patients with massive lower gastrointestinal bleeding manifested by continued hemodynamic instability and hematochezia, urgent angiography should be performed without attempt at colonoscopy or scintigraphy.

5. Small intestine push enteroscopy or capsule imaging—Up to 5% of acute episodes of lower gastrointestinal bleeding arise from the small intestine, eluding diagnostic evaluation with upper endoscopy and colonoscopy. Because of the difficulty of examining the small intestine and its relative rarity as a source of acute bleeding, evaluation of the small bowel is not usually pursued in patients during the initial episode of acute lower gastrointestinal bleeding. However, the small intestine is investigated in patients with unexplained recurrent hemorrhage of obscure origin. (See Obscure Gastrointestinal Bleeding below.)

▶ Treatment

Initial stabilization, blood replacement, and triage are managed in the same manner as described above for Acute Upper Gastrointestinal Bleeding.

A. Therapeutic Colonoscopy

High-risk lesions (eg, angioectasias or diverticulum, rectal ulcer with active bleeding, or a visible vessel) may be treated endoscopically with epinephrine injection, cautery (bipolar or heater probe), or application of metallic endoclips or bands. In diverticular hemorrhage with high-risk lesions identified at colonoscopy, rebleeding occurs in half of untreated patients compared with virtually no rebleeding in patients treated endoscopically. Radiation proctitis is effectively treated with applications of cautery therapy to the rectal telangiectasias, preferably with an argon plasma coagulator.

B. Intra-arterial Embolization

When a bleeding lesion is identified, angiography with selective embolization achieves immediate hemostasis in more than 95% of patients. Major complications occur in 5% (mainly ischemic colitis) and rebleeding occurs in up to 25%.

C. Surgical Treatment

Emergency surgery is required in less than 5% of patients with acute lower gastrointestinal bleeding due to the efficacy of colonoscopic and angiographic therapies. It is indicated in patients with ongoing bleeding that requires more than 4–6 units of blood within 24 hours or more than 10 total units in whom attempts at endoscopic or angiographic therapy failed. Most such hemorrhages are caused by a bleeding diverticulum or vascular ectasia. Preoperative localization of the bleeding site by nuclear scan or angiography allows limited resection of the bleeding segment of small intestine or colon. When accurate localization is not possible or when emergency surgery is required for massive hemorrhage, total abdominal colectomy with ileorectal anastomosis is required—with significantly higher morbidity and mortality than limited resections.

Surgery may also be indicated in patients with two or more hospitalizations for diverticular hemorrhage depending on the severity of bleeding and the patient's other comorbid conditions.

Bounds BC et al. Lower gastrointestinal bleeding. Gastrointest Endosc Clin North Am. 2007 Apr;17(2):237–88. [PMID: 17556148]

Strate L et al. Risk factors for mortality in lower intestinal bleeding. Clin Gastroenterol Hepatol. 2008 Sept;6(9):1004–10. [PMID: 18558513]

Wong Kee Song LM et al. Endoscopic management of acute lower gastrointestinal bleeding. Am J Gastroenterol. 2008 Aug;103(8):1881–7. [PMID: 18796089]

3. Occult Gastrointestinal Bleeding

Occult gastrointestinal bleeding refers to bleeding that is not apparent to the patient. Chronic gastrointestinal blood loss of less than 100 mL/d may cause no appreciable change in stool appearance. Thus, occult bleeding in an adult is identified by a positive FOBT, FIT, or iron deficiency anemia in the absence of visible blood loss. FOBT or FIT may be performed in patients with gastrointestinal symptoms or as a screening test for colorectal neoplasia (see Chapter 39). From 2% to 6% of patients in screening programs have a positive FOBT or FIT.

In the United States, 2% of men and 5% of women have iron deficiency anemia (serum ferritin < 30–45 mcg/L). In premenopausal women, iron deficiency anemia is most commonly attributable to menstrual and pregnancy-associated iron loss; however, a gastrointestinal source of chronic blood loss is present in 10%. Occult blood loss may arise from anywhere in the gastrointestinal tract. Among men and postmenopausal women, a potential gastrointestinal cause of blood loss can be identified in the colon in 15–30% and in the upper gastrointestinal tract in 35–55%; a malignancy is present in 10%. Iron deficiency on rare occasions is caused by malabsorption (especially celiac disease) or malnutrition. The most common causes are: (1) neoplasms; (2) vascular abnormalities (vascular ectasias); (3) acid-peptic lesions (esophagitis, peptic ulcer disease, erosions in hiatal hernia); (4) infections (nematodes, especially hookworm; tuberculosis); (5) medications (especially NSAIDs or aspirin); and (6) other causes such as inflammatory bowel disease.

▶ **Evaluation of Occult Bleeding**

Asymptomatic adults with positive FOBTs or FITs that are performed for routine colorectal cancer screening should undergo colonoscopy (see Chapter 39). All symptomatic adults with positive FOBTs or FITs or iron deficiency anemia should undergo evaluation of the upper and lower gastrointestinal tract with colonoscopy and upper endoscopy, unless the anemia can be definitively ascribed to a nongastrointestinal source (eg, menstruation, blood donation, or recent surgery). The presence and nature of gastrointestinal symptoms help guide the choice of initial study. After evaluation of the upper and lower gastrointestinal tract with upper endoscopy and colonoscopy, the origin of occult bleeding remains unexplained in 30–50% of patients. Patients with occult bleeding who have a negative initial endoscopic evaluation may be given a trial of iron supplementation and closely observed. Although many older patients require no further evaluation, it is reasonable in younger patients with unexplained iron deficiency anemia to pursue further evaluation of the small intestine for a source of bleeding (as described below). When possible, antiplatelet agents (aspirin, NSAIDs, clopidogrel) should be discontinued. For recurrent or persistent chronic gastrointestinal blood loss or anemia that responds poorly to iron supplementation, further evaluation is pursued for a source of obscure bleeding (as described below).

4. Obscure Gastrointestinal Bleeding

Obscure gastrointestinal bleeding refers to bleeding of unknown origin that persists or recurs after initial endoscopic evaluation with upper endoscopy and colonoscopy. Obscure-occult bleeding refers to bleeding that is not apparent to the patient. It is manifested by recurrent positive FOBTs or FITs or recurrent iron deficiency anemia, or both in the absence of visible blood loss. Obscure-overt bleeding is manifested by persistent or recurrent visible evidence of gastrointestinal bleeding (hematemesis, hematochezia, or melena). Up to 5% of patients admitted to hospitals with clinically overt gastrointestinal bleeding do not have a cause identified on upper endoscopy or colonoscopy (and therefore have obscure-overt bleeding).

Obscure bleeding (either occult or overt) most commonly arises from lesions in the small intestine. In up to one-third of cases, however, a source of bleeding has been overlooked in the upper or lower tract on prior endoscopic studies. Hematemesis or melena suggests an overlooked source proximal to the ligament of Treitz (ie, within the esophagus, stomach, or duodenum): erosions in a hiatal hernia ("Cameron erosions"), peptic ulcer, vascular ectasias, Dieulafoy vascular malformation, portal hypertensive gastropathy, gastroduodenal varices, duodenal neoplasms, aortoenteric fistula, or hepatic and pancreatic lesions. In the colon, the most commonly overlooked lesions are vascular ectasias and neoplasms. The etiology of obscure bleeding that arises from the small intestine depends on the age of the patient. The most common causes of small intestinal bleeding in patients younger than 40 years are neoplasms (stromal tumors, lymphomas, adenocarcinomas, carcinoids), Crohn disease, celiac disease, and Meckel diverticulum. These disorders also occur in patients over age 40; however, vascular ectasias and NSAID-induced ulcers are far more common.

Evaluation of Obscure Bleeding

The evaluation of obscure bleeding depends on the age and overall health status of the patient, associated symptoms, and severity of the bleeding. In an older patient with significant comorbid illnesses, no gastrointestinal symptoms, and occult or obscure bleeding in whom the suspected source of bleeding is vascular ectasias, it may be reasonable to limit diagnostic evaluations, provided the anemia can be managed with long-term iron therapy or occasional transfusions. On the other hand, aggressive diagnostic evaluation is warranted in younger patients with obscure bleeding (in whom small bowel tumors are the most common cause) and symptomatic older patients with overt or obscure bleeding. Upper endoscopy and colonoscopy should be repeated to ascertain that a lesion in these regions has not been overlooked. If these studies are unrevealing, capsule endoscopy should be performed to evaluate the small intestine. Capsule endoscopy is superior to radiographic studies (standard small bowel follow through, enteroclysis, or CT enterography) and standard push enteroscopy for the detection of small bowel abnormalities, demonstrating possible sources of occult bleeding in 60–70% of patients, most commonly vascular abnormalities (25–35%), ulcers (25%), and neoplasms (10%). Further management depends on the capsule endoscopic findings. Laparotomy is warranted if a small bowel tumor is identified by capsule endoscopy or radiographic studies. Most other lesions identified by capsule imaging can be further evaluated with one of several new enteroscopes that use balloons or spiral overtubes to advance the scope through most of the small intestine in a forward and retrograde direction. Neoplasms can be biopsied or resected, and vascular ectasias may be cauterized. For patients with overt obscure bleeding, it may be more cost-effective to proceed directly with deep enteroscopy rather than capsule endoscopy. For hemodynamically significant acute bleeding, angiography may be superior to enteroscopy for localization and embolization of a bleeding vascular abnormality. Abdominal CT may be considered to exclude a hepatic or pancreatic source of bleeding. With the advent of capsule imaging and advanced endoscopic technologies for evaluating and treating bleeding lesions in the small intestine, intraoperative enteroscopy of the small bowel is seldom required.

Concha R et al. Obscure gastrointestinal bleeding: diagnostic and therapeutic approach. J Clin Gastroenterol. 2007 Mar;41(3):242–51. [PMID: 17426461]

De Leusse A et al. Capsule endoscopy or push enteroscopy for first-line exploration of obscure gastrointestinal bleeding? Gastroenterology. 2007 Mar;132(3):855–62. [PMID: 17324401]

Gerson L et al. Cost-effectiveness analysis of management strategies for obscure GI bleeding. Gastrointest Endosc. 2008 Nov;68(5):920–36. [PMID: 18407270]

Kaffes AJ et al. Clinical outcomes after double-balloon enteroscopy in patients with obscure GI bleeding and a positive capsule endoscopy. Gastrointest Endosc. 2007 Aug;66(2):304–9. [PMID: 17643704]

Mishkin D et al. ASGE technology status evaluation report: wireless capsule endoscopy. Gastrointest Endosc. 2006 Apr; 63(4):539–45. [PMID: 16564850]

Pasha SF et al. Double-balloon enteroscopy and capsule endoscopy have comparable diagnostic yield in small-bowel disease: a meta-analysis. Clin Gastroenterol Hepatol. 2008 Jun;6(6):671–6. [PMID: 18356113]

Raju GS et al. American Gastroenterological Association (AGA) Institute medical position statement on obscure gastrointestinal bleeding. Gastroenterology. 2007 Nov;133(5):1694–6. [PMID: 17983811]

Raju GS et al. American Gastroenterological Association (AGA) Institute technical review on obscure gastrointestinal bleeding. Gastroenterology. 2007 Nov;133(5):1697–717. [PMID: 17983812]

Somsouk M et al. Management of obscure occult gastrointestinal bleeding: a cost-minimization analysis. Clin Gastroenterol Hepatol. 2008 Jun;6(6):661–70. [PMID: 18550005]

▼ DISEASES OF THE PERITONEUM

ASSESSMENT OF THE PATIENT WITH ASCITES

▶ Etiology of Ascites

The term "ascites" denotes the pathologic accumulation of fluid in the peritoneal cavity. Healthy men have little or no intraperitoneal fluid, but women normally may have up to 20 mL depending on the phase of the menstrual cycle. The causes of ascites may be classified into two broad pathophysiologic categories: that which is associated with a normal peritoneum and that which occurs due to a diseased peritoneum (Table 15–7). The most common cause of ascites is portal hypertension secondary to chronic liver disease, which accounts for over 80% of patients with ascites. The management of portal hypertensive ascites is discussed in Chapter 16. The most common causes of nonportal hypertensive ascites include infections (tuberculous peritonitis), intra-abdominal malignancy, inflammatory disorders of the peritoneum, and ductal disruptions (chylous, pancreatic, biliary).

▶ Clinical Findings

A. Symptoms and Signs

The history usually is one of increasing abdominal girth, with the presence of abdominal pain depending on the cause. Because most ascites is secondary to chronic liver disease with portal hypertension, patients should be asked about risk factors for liver disease, especially alcohol consumption, transfusions, tattoos, injection drug use, a history of viral hepatitis or jaundice, and birth in an area endemic for hepatitis. A history of cancer or marked weight loss arouses suspicion of malignant ascites. Fevers may suggest infected peritoneal fluid, including bacterial peritonitis (spontaneous or secondary). Patients with chronic liver disease and ascites are at greatest risk for developing spontaneous bacterial peritonitis. In immigrants, immunocompromised hosts, or severely malnourished alcoholics, tuberculous peritonitis should be considered.

Physical examination should emphasize signs of portal hypertension and chronic liver disease. Elevated jugular

Table 15–7. Causes of ascites.

Normal Peritoneum
Portal hypertension (SAAG ≥ 1.1 g/dL)
1. Hepatic congestion[1]
Congestive heart failure
Constrictive pericarditis
Tricuspid insufficiency
Budd-Chiari syndrome
Veno-occlusive disease
2. Liver disease[2]
Cirrhosis
Alcoholic hepatitis
Fulminant hepatic failure
Massive hepatic metastases
Hepatic fibrosis
Acute fatty liver of pregnancy
3. Portal vein occlusion
Hypoalbuminemia (SAAG < 1.1 g/dL)
Nephrotic syndrome
Protein-losing enteropathy
Severe malnutrition with anasarca
Miscellaneous conditions (SAAG < 1.1 g/dL)
Chylous ascites
Pancreatic ascites
Bile ascites
Nephrogenic ascites
Urine ascites
Myxedema (SAAG ≥ 1.1 g/dL)
Ovarian disease
Diseased Peritoneum (SAAG < 1.1 g/dL)[2]
Infections
Bacterial peritonitis
Tuberculous peritonitis
Fungal peritonitis
HIV-associated peritonitis
Malignant conditions
Peritoneal carcinomatosis
Primary mesothelioma
Pseudomyxoma peritonei
Massive hepatic metastases
Hepatocellular carcinoma
Other conditions
Familial Mediterranean fever
Vasculitis
Granulomatous peritonitis
Eosinophilic peritonitis

[1]Hepatic congestion usually associated with SAAG ≥ 1.1 g/dL and ascitic fluid total protein > 2.5 g/dL.
[2]There may be cases of "mixed ascites" in which portal hypertensive ascites is complicated by a secondary process such as infection. In these cases, the SAAG is ≥ 1.1 g/dL.
SAAG, serum-ascites albumin gradient.

venous pressure may suggest right-sided congestive heart failure or constrictive pericarditis. A large tender liver is characteristic of acute alcoholic hepatitis or Budd-Chiari syndrome. The presence of large abdominal wall veins with cephalad flow also suggests portal hypertension; inferiorly directed flow implies hepatic vein obstruction. Signs of chronic liver disease include palmar erythema, cutaneous spider angiomas, gynecomastia, and Dupuytren contracture. Asterixis secondary to hepatic encephalopathy may be present. Anasarca results from cardiac failure or nephrotic syndrome with hypoalbuminemia. Finally, firm lymph nodes in the left supraclavicular region or umbilicus may suggest intra-abdominal malignancy.

The physical examination is relatively insensitive for detecting ascitic fluid. In general, patients must have at least 1500 mL of fluid to be detected reliably by this method. Even the experienced clinician may find it difficult to distinguish between obesity and small-volume ascites. Abdominal ultrasound establishes the presence of fluid.

B. Laboratory Testing

1. Abdominal paracentesis—Abdominal paracentesis is performed as part of the diagnostic evaluation in all patients with new onset of ascites to help determine the cause. It should also be performed to diagnose bacterial peritonitis in all patients admitted to the hospital with cirrhosis and ascites (in whom the prevalence of bacterial peritonitis is 10–30%) and when patients with known ascites develop clinical deterioration (fever, abdominal pain, rapid worsening of renal function, or worsened hepatic encephalopathy).

A. INSPECTION—Cloudy fluid suggests infection. Milky fluid is seen with chylous ascites due to high triglyceride levels. Bloody fluid is most commonly attributable to a traumatic paracentesis, but up to 20% of cases of malignant ascites are bloody.

B. ROUTINE STUDIES

(1) Cell count—A white blood cell count with differential is the most important test. Normal ascitic fluid contains < 500 leukocytes/mcL and < 250 polymorphonuclear neutrophils (PMNs)/mcL. Any inflammatory condition can cause an elevated ascitic white count. A PMN count of > 250/mcL (neutrocytic ascites) with a percentage of > 75% of all white cells is highly suggestive of bacterial peritonitis, either spontaneous primary peritonitis or secondary peritonitis (ie, caused by an intra-abdominal source of infection, such as a perforated viscus or appendicitis). An elevated white count with a predominance of lymphocytes arouses suspicion of tuberculosis or peritoneal carcinomatosis.

(2) Albumin and total protein—The serum-ascites albumin gradient (SAAG) is the best single test for the classification of ascites into portal hypertensive and nonportal hypertensive causes (Table 15–7). Calculated by subtracting the ascitic fluid albumin from the serum albumin, the gradient correlates directly with the portal pressure. An SAAG ≥ 1.1 g/dL suggests underlying portal hypertension, while gradients < 1.1 g/dL implicate nonportal hypertensive causes.

The accuracy of the SAAG exceeds 95% in classifying ascites. It should be recognized, however, that approximately 4% of patients have "mixed ascites," ie, underlying cirrhosis with portal hypertension complicated by a second cause for ascites formation (such as malignancy or tuberculosis). Thus, a high SAAG is indicative of portal hypertension but does not exclude concomitant malignancy.

The ascitic fluid total protein provides some additional clues to the cause. An elevated SAAG and a high protein level (> 2.5 g/dL) are seen in most cases of hepatic congestion secondary to cardiac disease or Budd-Chiari syndrome. However, an increased ascitic fluid protein is also found in up to 20% of cases of uncomplicated cirrhosis. Two-thirds of patients with malignant ascites have a total protein level > 2.5 g/dL.

(3) Culture and Gram stain—The best technique consists of the inoculation of aerobic and anaerobic blood culture bottles with 5–10 mL of ascitic fluid at the patient's bedside, which increases the sensitivity for detecting bacterial peritonitis to over 85% in patients with neutrocytic ascites (> 250 PMNs/mcL), compared with approximately 50% sensitivity by conventional agar plate or broth cultures.

C. OPTIONAL STUDIES—Other laboratory tests are of utility in some specific clinical situations. Glucose and lactate dehydrogenase (LDH) may be helpful in distinguishing spontaneous from secondary bacterial peritonitis (see below). An elevated amylase may suggest pancreatic ascites or a perforation of the gastrointestinal tract with leakage of pancreatic secretions into the ascitic fluid. Perforation of the biliary tree is suspected with an ascitic bilirubin concentration that is greater than the serum bilirubin. An elevated ascitic creatinine suggests leakage of urine from the bladder or ureters. Ascitic fluid cytologic examination is ordered if peritoneal carcinomatosis is suspected. Adenosine deaminase may be useful for the diagnosis of tuberculous peritonitis.

C. Imaging

Abdominal ultrasound is useful in confirming the presence of ascites and in the guidance of paracentesis. Both ultrasound and CT imaging are useful in distinguishing between causes of portal and nonportal hypertensive ascites. Doppler ultrasound and CT can detect thrombosis of the hepatic veins (Budd-Chiari syndrome) or portal veins. In patients with nonportal hypertensive ascites, these studies are useful in detecting lymphadenopathy and masses of the mesentery and of solid organs such as the liver, ovaries, and pancreas. Furthermore, they permit directed percutaneous needle biopsies of these lesions. Ultrasound and CT are poor procedures for the detection of peritoneal carcinomatosis; the role of positron emission tomography (PET) imaging is unclear.

D. Laparoscopy

Laparoscopy is an important test in the evaluation of some patients with nonportal hypertensive ascites (low SAAG) or mixed ascites. It permits direct visualization and biopsy of the peritoneum, liver, and some intra-abdominal lymph nodes. Cases of suspected peritoneal tuberculosis or suspected malignancy with nondiagnostic CT imaging and ascitic fluid cytology are best evaluated by this method.

Kuiper JJ et al. Management of ascites and associated complications in patients with cirrhosis. Aliment Pharmacol Ther. 2007 Dec;26(Suppl 2):183–93. [PMID: 18081661]

McGibbon A et al. An evidence-based manual for abdominal paracentesis. Dig Dis Sci. 2007 Dec;52(12):3307–15. [PMID: 17393312]

Wong CL et al. Does this patient have bacterial peritonitis or portal hypertension? How do I perform a paracentesis and analyze the results? JAMA. 2008 Mar 12;299(10):1166–78. [PMID: 18334692]

SPONTANEOUS BACTERIAL PERITONITIS

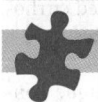

▶ A history of chronic liver disease and ascites.

▶ Fever and abdominal pain.

▶ Peritoneal signs uncommonly encountered on examination.

▶ Neutrocytic ascites (> 250 white blood cells/mcL) with neutrophilic predominance.

General Considerations

"Spontaneous" bacterial infection of ascitic fluid occurs in the absence of an apparent intra-abdominal source of infection. It is seen with few exceptions in patients with ascites caused by chronic liver disease. Translocation of enteric bacteria across the gut wall or mesenteric lymphatics leads to seeding of the ascitic fluid, as may bacteremia from other sites. Approximately 20–30% of cirrhotic patients with ascites develop spontaneous peritonitis; however, the incidence is greater than 40% in patients with ascitic fluid total protein < 1 g/dL, probably due to decreased ascitic fluid opsonic activity.

Virtually all cases of spontaneous bacterial peritonitis are caused by a monomicrobial infection. The most common pathogens are enteric gram-negative bacteria (*E coli, Klebsiella pneumoniae*) or gram-positive bacteria (*Streptococcus pneumoniae*, viridans streptococci, *Enterococcus* species). Anaerobic bacteria are not associated with spontaneous bacterial peritonitis.

Clinical Findings

A. Symptoms and Signs

Eighty to 90 percent of patients with spontaneous bacterial peritonitis are symptomatic; in many cases the presentation is subtle. Spontaneous bacterial peritonitis may be present in 20% of patients hospitalized with chronic liver disease in the absence of any suggestive symptoms or signs.

The most common symptoms are fever and abdominal pain, present in two-thirds of patients. Spontaneous bacterial peritonitis may also present with a change in mental status due to exacerbation or precipitation of hepatic encephalopathy, or sudden worsening of renal function. Physical examination typically demonstrates signs of chronic liver disease with ascites. Abdominal tenderness is present in less than 50% of patients, and its presence suggests other processes.

B. Laboratory Findings

The most important diagnostic test is abdominal paracentesis. Ascitic fluid should be sent for cell count with differential, and blood culture bottles should be inoculated at the bedside; Gram stain is insensitive.

In the proper clinical setting, an ascitic fluid PMN count of > 250 cells/mcL (neutrocytic ascites) is presumptive evidence of bacterial peritonitis. The percentage of PMNs is greater than 50–70% of the ascitic fluid white blood cells and commonly approximates 100%. Patients with neutrocytic ascites are presumed to be infected and should be started—regardless of symptoms—on antibiotics. Although 10–30% of patients with neutrocytic ascites have negative ascitic bacterial cultures ("culture-negative neutrocytic ascites"), it is presumed that these patients have bacterial peritonitis and should be treated empirically. Occasionally, a positive blood culture identifies the organism when ascitic fluid is sterile.

Differential Diagnosis

Spontaneous bacterial peritonitis must be distinguished from secondary bacterial peritonitis, in which ascitic fluid has become secondarily infected by an intra-abdominal infection. Even in the presence of perforation, clinical symptoms and signs of peritonitis may be lacking owing to the separation of the visceral and parietal peritoneum by the ascitic fluid. Causes of secondary bacterial peritonitis include appendicitis, diverticulitis, perforated peptic ulcer, and perforated gallbladder. Secondary bacterial infection accounts for 3% of cases of infected ascitic fluid.

Ascitic fluid total protein, LDH, and glucose are useful in distinguishing spontaneous bacterial peritonitis from secondary infection. Up to two-thirds of patients with secondary bacterial peritonitis have at least two of the following: decreased glucose level (< 50 mg/dL), an elevated LDH level (greater than serum), and total protein > 1 g/dL. Ascitic neutrophil counts > 10,000/mcL also are suspicious; however, most patients with secondary peritonitis have neutrophil counts within the range of spontaneous peritonitis. The presence of multiple organisms on ascitic fluid Gram stain or culture is diagnostic of secondary peritonitis.

If secondary bacterial peritonitis is suspected, abdominal CT imaging of the upper and lower gastrointestinal tracts should be obtained to look for evidence of an intra-abdominal source of infection. If these studies are negative and secondary peritonitis still is suspected, repeat paracentesis should be performed after 48 hours of antibiotic therapy to confirm that the PMN count is decreasing. Secondary bacterial peritonitis should be suspected in patients in whom the PMN count is not below the pretreatment value at 48 hours.

Neutrocytic ascites may also be seen in some patients with peritoneal carcinomatosis, pancreatic ascites, or tuberculous ascites. In these circumstances, however, PMNs account for less than 50% of the ascitic white blood cells.

Prevention

Up to 70% of patients who survive an episode of spontaneous bacterial peritonitis will have another episode within 1 year. Prophylactic therapy—with norfloxacin, 400 mg/d; ciprofloxacin, 750 mg weekly; or trimethoprim-sulfamethoxazole, one double-strength tablet daily—has been shown to reduce the rate of recurrent infections to less than 20% and is recommended. Prophylaxis should be considered also in patients who have not had prior bacterial peritonitis but are at increased risk of infection due to low-protein ascites (total ascitic protein < 1 g/dL). Although improvement in survival in cirrhotic patients with ascites treated with prophylactic antibiotics has not been shown, decision analytic modeling suggests that in patients with prior bacterial peritonitis or low ascitic fluid protein, the use of prophylactic antibiotics is a cost-effective strategy.

▶ **Treatment**

Empiric therapy for spontaneous bacterial peritonitis should be initiated with a third-generation cephalosporin such as cefotaxime (dosage: 2 g intravenously every 8–12 hours depending on renal function), which covers 98% of causative agents of this disorder. If enterococcus infection is suspected, ampicillin may be added. Because of a high risk of nephrotoxicity in patients with chronic liver disease, aminoglycosides should not be used. Although the optimal duration of therapy is unknown, a course of 5–10 days is sufficient in most patients, or until the ascites fluid PMN count decreases to < 250 cells/mcL. Renal failure develops in up to 40% of patients and is a major cause of death. In patients given intravenous albumin, 1.5 g/kg on day 1 and 1 g/kg on day 3, the incidence of renal failure and mortality are reduced both during hospitalization and at follow-up. Patients with suspected secondary bacterial peritonitis should be given broad-spectrum coverage for enteric aerobic and anaerobic flora with a third-generation cephalosporin and metronidazole pending identification and definitive (usually surgical) treatment of the cause. In fact, the most effective treatment for spontaneous bacterial peritonitis is liver transplant.

▶ **Prognosis**

The mortality rate of spontaneous bacterial peritonitis exceeds 30%. However, if the disease is recognized and treated early, the rate is less than 10%. As the majority of patients have underlying severe liver disease, many may die of liver failure, hepatorenal syndrome, or bleeding complications from portal hypertension.

Christou L et al. Bacterial infection-related morbidity and mortality in cirrhosis. Am J Gastroenterol. 2007 Jul;102(7):1510–7. [PMID: 17509025]

Fernández J et al. Primary prophylaxis of spontaneous bacterial peritonitis delays hepatorenal syndrome and improves survival in cirrhosis. Gastroenterology. 2007 Sep;133(3):818–24. [PMID: 17854593]

Ghassemi S et al. Prevention and treatment of infections in patients with cirrhosis. Best Pract Res Clin Gastroenterol. 2007;21(1):77–93. [PMID: 17223498]

Koulaouzidis A et al. Spontaneous bacterial peritonitis. Postgrad Med J. 2007 Jun;83(980):379–83. [PMID: 17551068]

Parsi MA et al. Ascitic fluid lactoferrin for diagnosis of spontaneous bacterial peritonitis. Gastroenterology. 2008 Sept;135(3):803–7. [PMID: 18590731]

Sigal SH et al. Restricted use of albumin for spontaneous bacterial peritonitis. Gut. 2007 Apr;56(4):597–9. [PMID: 17369392]

TUBERCULOUS PERITONITIS

Tuberculosis occurs in extrapulmonary sites in 20% of non–HIV-infected people and up to 70% of those infected with HIV. Although tuberculous involvement of the peritoneum accounts for less than 2% of all causes of ascites in the United States, it remains a significant problem in the developing world. In Western countries, its incidence is higher among those with uncontrolled HIV disease, immigrants from underdeveloped countries, the urban poor, patients with cirrhosis, and nursing home residents.

The presenting symptoms include low-grade fever, abdominal pain, anorexia, and weight loss. Most patients have symptoms for months before the diagnosis is established. On physical examination, patients may have generalized abdominal tenderness and distention. There may be clinically evident ascites or suggestion of an abdominal mass. Ultrasonography or CT imaging of the abdomen reveals free or loculated ascites in > 80% of patients and also may demonstrate lymphadenopathy or peritoneal, mesenteric, or omental thickening.

The diagnosis thus can be difficult to establish, particularly in patients with underlying cirrhosis with ascites and in patients without ascites (in whom the diagnosis may not be suspected). Chest radiographs are abnormal in over 70%, but active tuberculous pulmonary disease is evident in less than 20% of patients. Skin tests are positive in 50%. Smears of ascitic fluid for acid-fast bacilli are usually negative, and cultures are positive in only 35%. Other findings are an ascitic fluid total protein > 3.0 g/dL, LDH > 90 units/L, or mononuclear cell-predominant leukocytosis > 500/mcL—each has a sensitivity of 70–80% but limited specificity. Meta-analysis of four international studies reports that ascites adenosine deaminase activity ≥ 36–40 international unit/L has a sensitivity of 100% and a specificity of 97% for the diagnosis of tuberculous peritonitis; however, the accuracy of this method may be lower in patients in the United States who have cirrhotic ascites or HIV disease.

In patients with suspected tuberculous peritonitis, laparoscopy establishes the diagnosis. In over 90% of patients, characteristic peritoneal nodules are visible, and granulomas are seen on peritoneal biopsy. Peritoneal cultures require at least 4–6 weeks and are positive in less than two-thirds of patients.

Treatment of tuberculosis is discussed in Chapter 9.

Jacob JT et al. Acute forms of tuberculosis in adults. Am J Med. 2009 Jan;122(1):12–7. [PMID: 19114163]

Riquelme A et al. Value of adenosine deaminase (ADA) in ascitic fluid for the diagnosis of tuberculous peritonitis: a meta-analysis. J Clin Gastroenterol. 2006 Sep;40(8):705–10. [PMID: 16940883]

MALIGNANT ASCITES

Two-thirds of cases of malignant ascites are caused by peritoneal carcinomatosis. The most common tumors causing carcinomatosis are primary adenocarcinomas of the ovary, uterus, pancreas, stomach, colon, lung, or breast. The remaining one-third is due to lymphatic obstruction or portal hypertension due to hepatocellular carcinoma or diffuse hepatic metastases. Patients present with nonspecific abdominal discomfort and weight loss associated with increased abdominal girth. Nausea or vomiting may be caused by partial or complete intestinal obstruction.

Abdominal CT may be useful to demonstrate the primary malignancy or hepatic metastases but seldom confirms the diagnosis of peritoneal carcinomatosis. In patients with carcinomatosis, paracentesis demonstrates a low serum ascites-albumin gradient (< 1.1 mg/dL), an increased total protein (> 2.5 g/dL), and an elevated white cell count (often both neutrophils and mononuclear cells) but with a lymphocyte predominance. Cytology is positive in over 95%, but laparoscopy may be required in patients with negative cytology to confirm the diagnosis and to exclude tuberculous peritonitis, with which it may be confused. Malignant ascites attributable to portal hypertension usually is associated with an increased serum ascites-albumin gradient (> 1.1 g/dL), a variable total protein, and negative ascitic cytology. Ascites caused by peritoneal carcinomatosis does not respond to diuretics.

Patients may be treated with periodic large-volume paracentesis for symptomatic relief. Intraperitoneal chemotherapy is sometimes used to shrink the tumor, but the overall prognosis is extremely poor, with only 10% survival at 6 months. Ovarian cancers represent an exception to this rule. With newer treatments consisting of surgical debulking and intraperitoneal chemotherapy, long-term survival from ovarian cancer is possible.

Becker G. Medical and palliative management of malignant ascites. Cancer Treat Res. 2007;134:459–67. [PMID: 17633074]
Tamsma J. The pathogenesis of malignant ascites. Cancer Treat Res. 2007;134:109–18. [PMID: 17633049]

FAMILIAL MEDITERRANEAN FEVER

This is a rare autosomal recessive disorder of unknown pathogenesis that almost exclusively affects people of Mediterranean ancestry, especially Sephardic Jews, Armenians, Turks, and Arabs. Patients lack a protease in serosal fluids that normally inactivates interleukin-8 and the chemotactic complement factor 5A. Symptoms present in most patients before the age of 20 years. It is characterized by episodic bouts of acute peritonitis that may be associated with serositis involving the joints and pleura. Peritoneal attacks are marked by the sudden onset of fever, severe abdominal pain, and abdominal tenderness with guarding or rebound tenderness. If left untreated, attacks resolve within 24–48 hours. Because symptoms resemble those of surgical peritonitis, patients may undergo unnecessary exploratory laparotomy. Colchicine, 0.6 mg two or three times daily, has been shown to decrease the frequency and severity of attacks. Secondary amyloidosis (AA protein) with renal or hepatic involvement may occur in 25% of cases and is the main cause of death. Colchicine prevents or arrests further progression of amyloidosis development. In the absence of amyloidosis, the prognosis is excellent. The diagnosis of familial Mediterranean fever still is based on clinical criteria. Although the gene responsible for familial Mediterranean fever (MEFV) has been identified, commercial genetic tests fail to identify one of the known gene mutations in up to one-third of patients. Genetic testing is most useful to confirm the diagnosis in patients with atypical symptoms.

Bhat A et al. Genetics and new treatment modalities for familial Mediterranean fever. Ann N Y Acad Sci. 2007 Sep;1110:201–8. [PMID: 17911435]
Samuels J et al. Familial Mediterranean fever and other autoinflammatory syndromes: evaluation of the patient with recurrent fever. Curr Opin Rheumatol. 2006 Jan;18(1):108–17. [PMID: 16344627]

MESOTHELIOMA

Primary malignant mesothelioma is a rare tumor. Over 70% of cases have a history of asbestos exposure. Presenting symptoms and signs include abdominal pain or bowel obstruction, increased abdominal girth, and small to moderate ascites. The chest radiograph reveals pulmonary asbestosis in over 50%. The ascitic fluid is hemorrhagic, with a low serum-ascites albumin gradient. Cytology is often negative. Abdominal CT or PET-CT may reveal sheet-like masses involving the mesentery and omentum. Diagnosis is made at laparotomy or laparoscopy. The prognosis is extremely poor, but long-term survivors have been described with a combination of surgical debulking of tumor followed by heated intraoperative intraperitoneal chemotherapy and early postoperative intraperitoneal chemotherapy. Postoperative radiotherapy or combination chemotherapy may be helpful. Multicystic and well-differentiated papillary mesotheliomas are associated with a long survival with surgical treatment alone. (**See Chapter 39 for Mesothelioma.**)

Bridda A et al. Peritoneal mesothelioma: a review. MedGenMed. 2007 May 10;9(2):32. [PMID: 17955087]

MISCELLANEOUS PERITONEAL DISEASES

Chylous ascites is the accumulation of lipid-rich lymph in the peritoneal cavity. The ascitic fluid is characterized by a milky appearance with a triglyceride level > 1000 mg/dL. The usual cause in adults is lymphatic obstruction or leakage caused by malignancy, especially lymphoma. Nonmalignant causes include postoperative trauma, cirrhosis, tuberculosis, pancreatitis, and filariasis.

Pancreatic ascites is the intraperitoneal accumulation of massive amounts of pancreatic secretions due either to disruption of the pancreatic duct or to a pancreatic pseudocyst. It is most commonly seen in patients with chronic pancreatitis and complicates up to 3% of cases of acute pancreatitis. Because the pancreatic enzymes are not activated, pain often is absent. The ascitic fluid is characterized by a high protein level (> 2.5 g/dL) but a low SAAG. Ascitic fluid amylase levels are in excess of 1000 units/L. In nonsurgical cases, initial treatment consists of bowel rest, total parenteral nutrition (TPN), and octreotide to decrease pancreatic secretion. Persistent leakage requires treatment with either endoscopic placement of stents into the pancreatic duct or surgical drainage.

Bile ascites is caused most commonly by complications of biliary tract surgery, percutaneous liver biopsy, or abdominal trauma. Unless the bile is infected, bile ascites usually does not cause abdominal pain, fever, or leukocytosis. Paracentesis reveals yellow fluid with a ratio of ascites bilirubin to serum bilirubin greater than 1.0. Treatment depends on the location and rate of bile leakage. Postcholecystectomy cystic duct leaks may be treated with endoscopic sphincterotomy or biliary stent placement to facilitate bile flow across the sphincter of Oddi. Other leaks may be treated with percutaneous drainage by interventional radiologists or with surgical closure.

Al-Ghamdi MY et al. Chylous ascites secondary to pancreatitis: management of an uncommon entity using parenteral nutrition and octreotide. Dig Dis Sci. 2007 Sep;52(9):2261–4. [PMID: 17436089]

Baron TH. Treatment of pancreatic pseudocysts, pancreatic necrosis, and pancreatic duct leaks. Gastrointest Endosc Clin N Am. 2007 Jul;17(3):559–79. [PMID: 17640583]

▼ DISEASES OF THE ESOPHAGUS

▷ Symptoms

Heartburn, dysphagia, and odynophagia almost always indicate a primary esophageal disorder.

A. Heartburn

Heartburn (pyrosis) is the feeling of substernal burning, often radiating to the neck. Caused by the reflux of acidic (or, rarely, alkaline) material into the esophagus, it is highly specific for GERD.

B. Dysphagia

Difficulties in swallowing may arise from problems in transferring the food bolus from the oropharynx to the upper esophagus (oropharyngeal dysphagia) or from impaired transport of the bolus through the body of the esophagus (esophageal dysphagia). The history usually leads to the correct diagnosis.

1. Oropharyngeal dysphagia—The oropharyngeal phase of swallowing is a complex process requiring elevation of the tongue, closure of the nasopharynx, relaxation of the upper esophageal sphincter, closure of the airway, and pharyngeal peristalsis. A variety of mechanical and neuromuscular conditions can disrupt this process (Table 15–8). Problems with the oral phase of swallowing cause drooling or spillage of food from the mouth, inability to chew or initiate swallowing, or dry mouth. Pharyngeal dysphagia is characterized by an immediate sense of the bolus catching in the neck, the need to swallow repeatedly to clear food from the pharynx, or coughing or choking during meals. There may be associated dysphonia, dysarthria, or other neurologic symptoms.

2. Esophageal dysphagia—Esophageal dysphagia may be caused by **mechanical lesions** obstructing the esophagus or by **motility disorders** (Table 15–9). Patients with mechanical obstruction experience dysphagia, primarily for solids. This is recurrent, predictable, and, if the lesion progresses, will worsen as the lumen narrows. Patients with **motility disorders** have dysphagia for both solids and liquids. It is episodic, unpredictable, and can be progressive.

Table 15–8. Causes of oropharyngeal dysphagia.

Neurologic disorders
  Brainstem cerebrovascular accident, mass lesion
  Amyotrophic lateral sclerosis, multiple sclerosis, pseudobulbar palsy, post-polio syndrome, Guillain-Barré syndrome
  Parkinson disease, Huntington disease, dementia
  Tardive dyskinesia
Muscular and rheumatologic disorders
  Myopathies, polymyositis
  Oculopharyngeal dystrophy
  Sjögren syndrome
Metabolic disorders
  Thyrotoxicosis, amyloidosis, Cushing disease, Wilson disease
  Medication side effects: anticholinergics, phenothiazines
Infectious disease
  Polio, diphtheria, botulism, Lyme disease, syphilis, mucositis (Candida, herpes)
Structural disorders
  Zenker diverticulum
  Cervical osteophytes, cricopharyngeal bar, proximal esophageal webs
  Oropharyngeal tumors
  Postsurgical or radiation changes
  Pill-induced injury
Motility disorders
  Upper esophageal sphincter dysfunction

C. Odynophagia

Odynophagia is sharp substernal pain on swallowing that may limit oral intake. It usually reflects severe erosive disease. It is most commonly associated with infectious esophagitis due to Candida, herpesviruses, or CMV, especially in immunocompromised patients. It may also be caused by corrosive injury due to caustic ingestions and by pill-induced ulcers.

Table 15–9. Causes of esophageal dysphagia.

Cause	Clues
Mechanical obstruction	**Solid foods worse than liquids**
Schatzki ring	Intermittent dysphagia; not progressive
Peptic stricture	Chronic heartburn; progressive dysphagia
Esophageal cancer	Progressive dysphagia; age over 50 years
Eosinophilic esophagitis	Young adults; small-caliber lumen, proximal stricture, corrugated rings, or white papules
Motility disorder	**Solid and liquid foods**
Achalasia	Progressive dysphagia
Diffuse esophageal spasm	Intermittent; not progressive; may have chest pain
Scleroderma	Chronic heartburn; Raynaud phenomenon

Diagnostic Studies

A. Upper Endoscopy

Endoscopy is the study of choice for evaluating persistent heartburn, dysphagia, odynophagia, and structural abnormalities detected on barium esophagography. In addition to direct visualization, it allows biopsy of mucosal abnormalities and of normal mucosa (to evaluate for eosinophilic esophagitis) as well as dilation of strictures.

B. Videoesophagography

Oropharyngeal dysphagia is best evaluated with rapid-sequence videoesophagography.

C. Barium Esophagography

Patients with esophageal dysphagia often are evaluated first with a radiographic barium study to differentiate between mechanical lesions and motility disorders, providing important information about the latter in particular. In patients with esophageal dysphagia and a suspected motility disorder, barium esophagoscopy should be obtained first. In patients in whom there is a high suspicion of a mechanical lesion, many clinicians will proceed first to endoscopic evaluation because it better identifies mucosa lesions (eg, erosions) and permits mucosal biopsy and dilation. However, barium study is more sensitive for detecting subtle esophageal narrowing due to rings, achalasia, and proximal esophageal lesions.

D. Esophageal Manometry

Esophageal motility may be assessed using manometric techniques. They are indicated: (1) to determine the location of the LES to allow precise placement of a conventional electrode pH probe; (2) to establish the etiology of dysphagia in patients in whom a mechanical obstruction cannot be found, especially if a diagnosis of achalasia is suspected by endoscopy or barium study; (3) for the preoperative assessment of patients being considered for antireflux surgery to exclude an alternative diagnosis (eg, achalasia) or possibly to assess peristaltic function in the esophageal body. High-resolution manometry may be superior to conventional manometry for distinguishing motility disorders.

E. Esophageal pH Recording and Impedance Testing

The pH within the esophageal lumen may be monitored continuously for 24–48 hours. There are two kinds of systems in use: catheter-based and wireless. Traditional systems use a long transnasal catheter that is connected directly to the recording device. Wireless systems are increasingly used; in these systems, a capsule is attached directly to the esophageal mucosa under endoscopic visualization and data are transmitted by radiotelemetry to the recording device. The recording provides information about the amount of esophageal acid reflux and the temporal correlations between symptoms and reflux.

Esophageal pH monitoring devices provide information about the amount of esophageal acid reflux but not nonacid reflux. New techniques using multichannel intraluminal impedance allow assessment of gas and nonacid liquid reflux. Although not yet widely available, they may be useful in evaluation of patients with atypical reflux symptoms or persistent symptoms despite therapy with proton pump inhibitors to diagnose hypersensitivity, functional symptoms, and symptoms caused by non-acid reflux.

Cook IJ. Diagnostic evaluation of dysphagia. Nat Clin Pract Gastroenterol Hepatol. 2008 Jul;5(7):393–403. [PMID: 18542115]

Hirano I et al. ACG practice guidelines: esophageal reflux testing. Am J Gastroenterol. 2007 Mar;102(3):668–85. [PMID: 17335450]

Katz PO et al. Utility and standards in esophageal manometry. J Clin Gastroenterol. 2008 May–Jun;42(5):620–6. [PMID: 18364580]

Levine MS et al. Barium esophagography: a study for all seasons. Clin Gastroenterol Hepatol. 2008 Jan;6(1):11–25. [PMID: 18083069]

GASTROESOPHAGEAL REFLUX DISEASE

 ESSENTIALS OF DIAGNOSIS

▶ Heartburn; may be exacerbated by meals, bending, or recumbency.

▶ Typical uncomplicated cases do not require diagnostic studies.

▶ Endoscopy demonstrates abnormalities in one-third of patients.

General Considerations

GERD is defined by a recent consensus as a condition that develops when the reflux of stomach contents causes troublesome symptoms or complications. GERD affects 20% of adults, who report at least weekly episodes of heartburn, and up to 10% complain of daily symptoms. Although most patients have mild disease, esophageal mucosal damage (reflux esophagitis) develops in up to one-third and more serious complications develop in a few others. Several factors may contribute to GERD.

A. Impaired Lower Esophageal Sphincter Function

The antireflux barrier at the gastroesophageal junction depends on LES pressure, the intra-abdominal location of the sphincter, and the extrinsic compression of the sphincter by the crural diaphragm. In most patients with GERD, baseline LES pressures are normal (10–30 mm Hg). In these patients, most reflux episodes occur during transient relaxations of the LES that are triggered by gastric distention by a vagovagal reflex. A subset of patients with GERD have an incompetent (< 10 mm Hg) LES that results in increased acid reflux, especially when supine or when intra-abdominal pressures are increased by lifting or bending. A hypotensive sphincter is present in up to 50% of patients with severe erosive GERD.

B. Hiatal Hernia

Hiatal hernias are common and usually cause no symptoms. In patients with gastroesophageal reflux, however, they are associated with higher amounts of acid reflux and delayed esophageal acid clearance leading to more severe esophagitis, especially Barrett esophagus. Increased reflux episodes occur during normal swallowing-induced relaxation, transient LES relaxations, and straining due to reflux of acid from the hiatal hernia sac into the esophagus. Hiatal hernias are found in one-fourth of patients with nonerosive GERD, three-fourths of patients with severe erosive esophagitis, and over 90% of patients with Barrett esophagus.

C. Irritant Effects of Refluxate

Esophageal mucosal damage is related to the potency of the refluxate and the amount of time it is in contact with the mucosa. Acidic gastric fluid (pH < 4.0) is extremely caustic to the esophageal mucosa and is the major injurious agent in the majority of cases. In some patients, reflux of bile or alkaline pancreatic secretions may be contributory.

D. Abnormal Esophageal Clearance

Acid refluxate normally is cleared and neutralized by esophageal peristalsis and salivary bicarbonate. During sleep, swallowing-induced peristalsis is infrequent, prolonging acid exposure to the esophagus. One-half of patients with severe GERD also have diminished peristaltic clearance. Certain medical conditions such as scleroderma are associated with diminished peristalsis. Sjögren syndrome, anticholinergic medications, and oral radiation therapy may exacerbate GERD due to impaired salivation.

E. Delayed Gastric Emptying

Impaired gastric emptying due to gastroparesis or partial gastric outlet obstruction potentiates GERD.

▶ Clinical Findings

A. Symptoms and Signs

The typical symptom is heartburn. This most often occurs 30–60 minutes after meals and upon reclining. Patients often report relief from taking antacids or baking soda. When this symptom is dominant, the diagnosis is established with a high degree of reliability. Many patients, however, have less specific dyspeptic symptoms with or without heartburn. Overall, a clinical diagnosis of gastroesophageal reflux has a sensitivity of 80% but a specificity of only 70%. Severity is not correlated with the degree of tissue damage. In fact, some patients with severe esophagitis are only mildly symptomatic. Patients may complain of regurgitation—the spontaneous reflux of sour or bitter gastric contents into the mouth. Dysphagia occurs in one-third of patients and may be due to erosive esophagitis, abnormal esophageal peristalsis, or the development of an esophageal stricture.

"Atypical" or "extraesophageal" manifestations of gastroesophageal disease may occur, including asthma, chronic cough, chronic laryngitis, sore throat, and noncardiac chest pain. Gastroesophageal reflux may be either a causative or an exacerbating factor in up to 50% of these patients, especially those with refractory symptoms. In the absence of heartburn or regurgitation, atypical symptoms are unlikely to be related to gastroesophageal reflux.

Physical examination and laboratory data are normal in uncomplicated disease.

B. Special Examinations

Initial diagnostic studies are not warranted for patients with typical GERD symptoms suggesting uncomplicated reflux disease. Patients with typical symptoms of heartburn and regurgitation should be treated empirically with a once- or twice-daily proton pump inhibitor for 4–8 weeks. Further investigation is required in patients with "alarm features" (troublesome dysphagia, odynophagia, weight loss, iron deficiency anemia) and in patients with troublesome symptoms that persist despite empiric proton pump inhibitor therapy in order to identify complications of reflux disease and to diagnose other conditions with similar symptoms.

1. Upper endoscopy—Upper endoscopy with biopsy is excellent for documenting the type and extent of tissue damage in gastroesophageal reflux; for detecting other gastroesophageal lesions that may mimic GERD; and for detecting GERD complications, including esophageal stricture, Barrett metaplasia, and esophageal adenocarcinoma. In the absence of prior antisecretory therapy, up to one-third of patients with GERD have visible mucosal damage (known as reflux esophagitis), characterized by single or multiple erosions or ulcers in the distal esophagus at the squamocolumnar junction. In patients treated with a proton pump inhibitor prior to endoscopy, preexisting reflux esophagitis may be partially or completely healed. The Los Angeles classification grades reflux esophagitis on a scale of A (one or more isolated mucosal breaks ≤ 5 mm that do not extend between the tops of two mucosal folds) to D (one or more mucosal breaks that involve at least 75% of the esophageal circumference).

2. Barium esophagography—This study plays a limited role. In patients with severe dysphagia, it is sometimes obtained prior to endoscopy to identify a stricture.

3. Manometry and esophageal pH monitoring—Esophageal manometry and pH monitoring are unnecessary in most patients but may be indicated in a small percentage who have persistent troublesome symptoms despite empiric twice-daily proton pump inhibitor therapy and who have normal findings on endoscopy. Esophageal manometry may be useful to diagnose motility disorders presenting with atypical GERD-like symptoms such as achalasia or diffuse esophageal spasm. Ambulatory or impedance pH monitoring may be indicated under the following circumstances: (1) to document abnormal esophageal acid exposure in a patient being considered for antireflux surgery who has a normal endoscopy (ie, no evidence of reflux esophagitis); and (2) to determine the correlation between symptoms and acid and non-acid reflux episodes.

▶ Differential Diagnosis

Symptoms of GERD may be similar to those of other diseases such as esophageal motility disorders, peptic ulcer, functional dyspepsia, and angina pectoris. Reflux erosive esophagitis may be confused with pill-induced damage, eosinophilic esophagitis, or infections (CMV, herpes, *Candida*).

▶ Complications

A. Barrett Esophagus

This is a condition in which the squamous epithelium of the esophagus is replaced by metaplastic columnar epithelium containing goblet and columnar cells (specialized intestinal metaplasia). Present in up to 10% of patients with chronic reflux, it arises from chronic reflux-induced injury to the esophageal squamous epithelium. Barrett esophagus is suspected at endoscopy from the presence of orange, gastric type epithelium that extends upward from the stomach into the distal tubular esophagus in a tongue-like or circumferential fashion. Biopsies obtained at endoscopy confirm the diagnosis. Three types of columnar epithelium may be identified: gastric cardiac, gastric fundic, and specialized intestinal metaplasia. Only the latter is believed to carry an increased risk of neoplasia.

Barrett esophagus does not provoke specific symptoms but gastroesophageal reflux does. Most patients have a long history of reflux symptoms, such as heartburn and regurgitation. Paradoxically, one-third of patients report minimal or no symptoms of GERD, suggesting decreased acid sensitivity of Barrett epithelium. Indeed, over 90% of individuals with Barrett esophagus in the general population do not seek medical attention.

Barrett esophagus should be treated with long-term proton pump inhibitors. Medical therapy may prevent progression, but there is no convincing evidence that regression occurs in most patients.

The most serious complication of Barrett esophagus is esophageal adenocarcinoma. It is believed that most adenocarcinomas of the esophagus and many such tumors of the gastric cardia arise from dysplastic epithelium in Barrett esophagus. The incidence of adenocarcinoma in patients with Barrett esophagus is 0.5%/year. Although this is a 40-fold increased risk compared with patients without Barrett esophagus, adenocarcinoma of the esophagus remains a relatively uncommon malignancy in the United States (7000 cases/year). Some clinical guidelines recommend endoscopic screening for Barrett esophagus and dysplasia in adults 50 years or older with more than 5–10 years of heartburn. However, given the large number of adults with chronic GERD relative to the small number in whom adenocarcinoma develops, it is unclear whether screening for Barrett esophagus is cost-effective.

A number of endoscopic therapies (multipolar electrocoagulation, argon plasma coagulation, and photodynamic therapy using photosensitizers and laser energy) have been used to ablate the Barrett columnar epithelium in an effort to reduce the risk of progression to neoplasia. When high-dose proton pump inhibitors are administered to normalize intraesophageal pH, ablation of Barrett columnar epithelium may be followed by healing with normal squamous epithelium. These techniques are often incompletely effective, have a significant risk of complications (bleeding, perforation, strictures), and may result in mucosal healing in which residual metaplastic tissue is buried beneath reconstituted squamous epithelium. The FDA has recently approved a bipolar probe (HALO) that uses radiofrequency wave energy for thermal ablative therapy. Preliminary studies with this probe demonstrate complete eradication of Barrett epithelium in up to 70% of patients without significant complications. Further long-term studies are needed to establish the role of ablative therapy in patients with Barrett esophagus without dysplasia.

In patients known to have Barrett esophagus, surveillance endoscopy every 3 years to look for dysplasia or adenocarcinoma generally is recommended. Patients with low-grade dysplasia require repeat endoscopic surveillance in 6 months to screen for coexisting high-grade dysplasia or cancer. If low-grade dysplasia persists (which occurs in < 25% of patients), endoscopic surveillance should be repeated yearly. The treatment of patients with high-grade dysplasia or superficial mucosal cancers is controversial and evolving rapidly. Approximately 40% of patients may progress to (or already have) adenocarcinoma, of which 28% are intramucosal but 12% have tumor that invades the submucosal or lymph nodes. Until recently, esophagectomy has been recommended for all patients deemed to have a low operative risk. However, esophagectomy is associated with high morbidity and mortality rates (40% and 2–9%, respectively). Therefore, other options should be considered for patients with high-grade dysplasia, especially those who are deemed to be at high risk for esophagectomy.

Patients with a visible esophageal nodule containing high-grade dysplasia or intramucosal cancer should undergo endoscopic ultrasound evaluation to look for invasive cancer. For patients with disease that appears to be limited to the mucosa, endoscopic mucosal snare resection may be performed. If pathologic assessment of the tissue specimen demonstrates submucosal invasion, esophagectomy should be recommended; however, if the cancer is intramucosal, the risk of esophagectomy may exceed the risk of developing metastatic disease (< 5%). Photodynamic therapy or radiofrequency wave electrocautery (HALO) may be used to ablate Barrett tissue in patients with high-grade dysplasia without a visible esophageal nodule and to ablate Barrett tissue after endoscopic mucosal resection of a nodule with high-grade dysplasia or intramucosal cancer. An uncontrolled prospective US endoscopic study of radiofrequency wave ablation of Barrett tissue with high-grade dysplasia has shown complete resolution of dysplasia in 80% of patients. Alternatively, patients with high-grade dysplasia without visible lesions may undergo close endoscopic surveillance with biopsy every 3–6 months, reserving surgery or photodynamic therapies for approximately 7% of patients per year during follow-up in whom adenocarcinoma develops.

B. Peptic Stricture

Stricture formation occurs in about 5% of patients with esophagitis. It is manifested by the gradual development of solid food dysphagia progressive over months to years. Often there is a reduction in heartburn because the stricture acts as a barrier to reflux. Most strictures are located at the gastroesophageal junction. Endoscopy with biopsy is mandatory in all cases to differentiate peptic stricture from malignant causes of esophageal stricture (esophageal carcinoma). Active erosive esophagitis is often present. Up to 90% of symptomatic patients are effectively treated with dilation with graduated polyvinyl catheters passed over a wire placed at the time of endoscopy or fluoroscopically, or balloons passed fluoroscopically or through an endoscope. Dilation is continued over one to several sessions. A luminal diameter of 13–17 mm is usually sufficient to relieve dysphagia. Long-term therapy with a proton pump inhibitor is required to decrease the likelihood of stricture recurrence. Some patients require intermittent dilation to maintain luminal patency, but operative management for strictures that do not respond to dilation is seldom required. Refractory strictures may benefit from endoscopic injection of triamcinolone into the stricture.

▶ Treatment

A. Medical Treatment

The goal of treatment is to provide symptomatic relief, to heal esophagitis (if present), and to prevent complications. In the majority of patients with uncomplicated disease, empiric treatment is initiated based on a compatible history without the need for further confirmatory studies. Patients not responding and those with suspected complications undergo further evaluation with upper endoscopy or esophageal manometry and pH recording (see above).

1. Mild, intermittent symptoms—Patients with mild or intermittent symptoms that do not impact adversely on quality of life may benefit from lifestyle modifications with medical interventions taken as needed. Patients may find that eating smaller meals and elimination of acidic foods (citrus, tomatoes, coffee, spicy foods) and foods that precipitate reflux (fatty foods, chocolate, peppermint, alcohol, cigarettes) may reduce symptoms. Weight loss should be recommended for overweight patients. Patients with nocturnal symptoms should be advised to avoid lying down within 3 hours after meals, the period of greatest reflux, and to elevate the head of the bed on 6-inch blocks or a foam wedge to reduce reflux and enhance esophageal clearance.

Antacids are the mainstay for rapid relief of occasional heartburn; however, their duration of action is less than 2 hours. Many are available over the counter. Those containing magnesium should not be used in renal failure, and patients with this condition should be cautioned appropriately.

All H_2-receptor antagonists are available in over-the-counter formulations: cimetidine 200 mg, ranitidine and nizatidine 75 mg, famotidine 10 mg—all of which are half of the typical prescription strength. When taken for active heartburn, these agents have a delay in onset of at least 30 minutes; antacids provide more immediate relief. However, once these agents take effect, they provide heartburn relief for up to 8 hours. When taken before meals known to provoke heartburn, these agents reduce the symptom. A combination agent containing famotidine 10 mg and antacid (calcium carbonate and magnesium hydroxide) is available.

2. Troublesome symptoms

A. INITIAL THERAPY—Patients with troublesome reflux symptoms and patients with known complications of GERD should be treated with a once-daily oral proton pump inhibitor (omeprazole or rabeprazole, 20 mg; omeprazole with sodium bicarbonate, 40 mg; lansoprazole, 30 mg; esomeprazole or pantoprazole, 40 mg) taken 30 minutes before breakfast for 4–8 weeks. Because there appears to be little difference between these agents in efficacy or side effect profiles, the choice of agent is determined by cost. Omeprazole, 20 mg, is now available both as an over-the-counter formulation and as a generic formulation available by prescription. Once-daily proton pump inhibitors achieve adequate control of heartburn in 80–90% of patients, complete heartburn resolution in over 50%, and healing of erosive esophagitis (when present) in over 80%. Because of their superior efficacy and ease of use, proton pump inhibitors are preferred to H_2-receptor antagonists for the treatment of acute and chronic GERD. Approximately 10–20% of patients do not achieve symptom relief with a once-daily dose within 2–4 weeks and require a twice-daily proton pump inhibitor (taken 30 minutes before breakfast and dinner). Patients with inadequate symptom relief with empiric twice-daily proton pump inhibitor therapy should undergo evaluation with upper endoscopy. Many providers prefer to prescribe initial twice-daily proton pump inhibitor therapy for patients who have documented severe erosive esophagitis (LA Grade C or D), Barrett esophagus, or peptic stricture.

B. LONG-TERM THERAPY—In those who achieve good symptomatic relief with a course of empiric once-daily proton pump inhibitor, therapy may be discontinued after 8–12 weeks. Most patients (over 80%) will experience relapse of GERD symptoms, usually within 3 months. Patients whose symptoms relapse may be treated with either continuous proton pump inhibitor therapy, intermittent 2–4 week courses, or "on demand" therapy (ie, drug taken until symptoms abate) depending on symptom frequency and patient preference. Patients who required twice-daily proton pump inhibitor therapy for initial symptom control and patients with complications of GERD, including severe erosive esophagitis, Barrett esophagus, or peptic stricture, should be maintained on long-term therapy with a once- or twice-daily proton pump inhibitor titrated to the lowest effective dose to achieve satisfactory symptom control.

Side effects of proton pump inhibitors are uncommon. Headache, diarrhea, and abdominal pain may occur with any of the agents but generally resolve when another formulation is tried. Potential risks of long-term use of proton pump inhibitors include an increased risk of infectious gastroenteritis (including *C difficile*), hip fractures (possibly due to impaired calcium absorption), and fundic gland polyps (which appear to be of no clinical significance).

3. Extraesophageal reflux manifestations—Establishing a causal relationship between gastroesophageal reflux and extraesophageal symptoms (eg, asthma, hoarseness, cough) is difficult. Gastroesophageal reflux seldom is the sole cause of extraesophageal disorders but may be a contributory factor. Although ambulatory esophageal pH testing can document the presence of increased acid esophageal reflux, it does not prove a causative connection. Current guidelines recommend that a trial of a twice-daily proton pump inhibitor be administered for 3 months in patients with suspected extraesophageal GERD syndromes who also have typical GERD symptoms. Improvement of extraesophageal symptoms suggests but does not prove that acid reflux is the causative factor. Esophageal pH testing should be performed in patients whose symptoms persist after 3 months of twice-daily proton pump inhibitor therapy. The pH study is performed on therapy if the suspicion for GERD is high (to determine whether therapy has adequately suppressed acid esophageal reflux) and off therapy if the suspicion for GERD is low (to determine whether the patient has reflux disease). Combined esophageal pH monitoring with impedance monitoring may be considered to look for nonacid reflux events in patients with persistent reflux symptoms who are receiving prolonged proton pump inhibitor therapy.

4. Unresponsive disease—Approximately 5% do not respond to twice-daily proton pump inhibitors or a change to a different proton pump inhibitor. These patients undergo endoscopy prior for detection of severe, inadequately treated reflux esophagitis and for other gastroesophageal lesions that may mimic GERD. The presence of active erosive esophagitis usually is indicative of inadequate acid suppression and can almost always be treated successfully with higher proton pump inhibitor doses (eg, omeprazole 40 mg twice daily). Truly refractory esophagitis may be caused by gastrinoma with gastric acid hypersecretion (Zollinger-Ellison syndrome), pill-induced esophagitis, resistance to proton pump inhibitors, and medical noncompliance. Patients without endoscopically visible esophagitis should undergo esophageal manometry followed by ambulatory pH or impedance pH and to determine the correlation between symptoms and acid and nonacid reflux episodes. If the pH study shows a normal amount of acid reflux, treatment with a low-dose tricyclic antidepressant (eg, imipramine or nortriptyline 25 mg at bedtime) may be beneficial.

B. Surgical Treatment

Surgical fundoplication affords good to excellent relief of symptoms and healing of esophagitis in over 85% of properly selected patients and can be performed laparoscopically with low complication rates in most instances. Cost-effectiveness studies suggest that aggregate medical costs exceed surgical costs after 10 years. Although patient satisfaction is high, over 50% of patients require intermittent or continuous acid-suppression medication after fundoplication. Furthermore, new symptoms of dysphagia, bloating, increased flatulence, dyspepsia, or diarrhea develop in over 30% of patients. Within 5–10 years after surgery, typical reflux symptoms occur in 10–30% of patients. Surgical treatment is not recommended for patients who are well controlled with medical therapies but should be considered for: (1) otherwise healthy, carefully selected patients with extraesophageal manifestations of reflux, as these symptoms often require high doses of proton pump inhibitors and may be more effectively controlled with antireflux surgery; (2) those with severe reflux disease who are unwilling to accept lifelong medical therapy due to its expense, inconvenience, or theoretical risks; and (3) patients with large hiatal hernias and persistent regurgitation despite proton pump inhibitor therapy.

▶ When to Refer

- Patients with typical GERD whose symptoms do not resolve with empiric management with a twice-daily proton pump inhibitor.

- Patients with suspected extraesophageal GERD symptoms that do not resolve with 3 months of twice-daily proton pump inhibitor therapy.

- Patients with significant dysphagia or other alarm symptoms for upper endoscopy.

- Patients with Barrett esophagus for endoscopic surveillance.

- Patients who have Barrett esophagus with dysplasia or early mucosal cancer.

- Surgical fundoplication is considered.

ASGE Standards of Practice Committee; Lichtenstein DR et al. Role of endoscopy in the management of GERD. Gastrointest Endosc. 2007 Aug;66(2):219–24. [PMID: 17643692]

Boeckxstaens GE. Review article: the pathophysiology of gastro-oesophageal reflux disease. Aliment Pharmacol Ther. 2007 Jul 15;26(2):149–60. [PMID: 17593062]

Das A et al. A comparison of endoscopic treatment and surgery in early esophageal cancer: an analysis of Surveillance Epidemiology and End Results data. Am J Gastroenterol. 2008 Jun;103(6):1340–5. [PMID: 18510606]

Egan JV et al. ASGE Guideline: esophageal dilation. Gastrointest Endosc. 2006 May;63(6):755–60. [PMID: 16650533]

Fass R. Persistent heartburn in a patient on proton-pump inhibitor. Clin Gastroenterol Hepatol. 2008 Apr;6(4):393–400. [PMID: 18387497]

Fleischer DE et al. Endoscopic ablation of Barrett's esophagus: a multicenter study with 2.5 year follow up. Gastrointest Endosc. 2008 Nov;68(5):867–76. [PMID: 18561930]

Galmiche JP et al. Respiratory manifestations of gastro-oesophageal reflux disease. Aliment Pharmacol Ther. 2008 Mar 15;27(6):449–64. [PMID: 18194498]

Ganz R et al. Circumferential ablation of Barrett's esophagus that contains high-grade dysplasia: a U.S. multicenter registry. Gastrointest Endosc. 2008 Jul;68(1):35–40. [PMID: 18355819]

Kahrilas PJ. Clinical practice. Gastroesophageal reflux disease. N Engl J Med. 2008 Oct 16;359(16):1700–7. [PMID: 18923172]

Kahrilas PJ et al. American Gastroenterological Association Medical Position Statement on the management of gastroesophageal reflux disease. Gastroenterology. 2008 Oct;135(4):1383–91. [PMID: 18789939]

Konda VJ et al. Is the risk of concomitant invasive esophageal cancer in high-grade dysplasia in Barrett's esophagus overestimated? Clin Gastroenterol Hepatol. 2008 Feb;6(2):159–64. [PMID: 18096439]

Metz DC et al. On-demand therapy for gastroesophageal reflux disease. Am J Gastroenterol. 2007 Mar;102(3):642–53. [PMID: 17156134]

Prassad G et al. Long-term survival following endoscopic and surgical treatment of high-grade dysplasia in Barrett's esophagus. Gastroenterology. 2007 Apr;132(4):1226–33. [PMID: 17408660]

Rastogi A et al. Incidence of esophageal adenocarcinoma in patients with Barrett's esophagus and high-grade dysplasia: a meta-analysis. Gastrointest Endosc. 2008 Mar;67(3):394–8. [PMID: 18045592]

Sharma P et al. Endoscopic therapy for high-grade dysplasia in Barrett's esophagus: ablate, resect, or both? Gastrointest Endosc. 2007 Sep;66(3):469–74. [PMID: 17725936]

Sharma VK et al. Balloon-based, circumferential, endoscopic radiofrequency ablation of Barrett's esophagus: 1-year follow-up of 100 patients. Gastrointest Endosc. 2007 Feb;65(2):185–95. [PMID: 17258973]

Sontag S. Con: surgery for Barrett's with flat HGD—no! Am J Gastroenterol. 2006 Oct;101(10):2180–3. [PMID: 17032179]

Vakil N. Review article: the role of surgery in gastro-oesophageal reflux disease. Aliment Pharmacol Ther. 2007 Jun 15;25(12):1365–72. [PMID: 17539976]

Wang K et al. Updated guidelines 2008 for the diagnosis, surveillance and therapy of Barrett's esophagus. Am J Gastroenterol. 2008 Mar;103(3):788–97. [PMID: 18341497]

INFECTIOUS ESOPHAGITIS

ESSENTIALS OF DIAGNOSIS

▸ Immunosuppressed patient.

▸ Odynophagia, dysphagia, and chest pain.

▸ Endoscopy with biopsy establishes diagnosis.

General Considerations

Infectious esophagitis occurs most commonly in immunosuppressed patients. Patients with AIDS, solid organ transplants, leukemia, lymphoma, and those receiving immunosuppressive drugs are at particular risk for opportunistic infections. *Candida albicans*, herpes simplex, and CMV are the most common pathogens. *Candida* infection may occur also in patients who have uncontrolled diabetes and those being treated with systemic corticosteroids, radiation therapy, or systemic antibiotic therapy. Herpes simplex can affect normal hosts, in which case the infection is generally self-limited.

Clinical Findings

A. Symptoms and Signs

The most common symptoms are odynophagia and dysphagia. Substernal chest pain occurs in some patients. Patients with candidal esophagitis are sometimes asymptomatic. Oral thrush is present in only 75% of patients with candidal esophagitis and 25–50% of patients with viral esophagitis and is therefore an unreliable indicator of the cause of esophageal infection. Patients with esophageal CMV infection may have infection at other sites such as the colon and retina. Oral ulcers (herpes labialis) are often associated with herpes simplex esophagitis.

B. Special Examinations

Treatment may be empiric. For diagnostic certainty, endoscopy with biopsy and brushings (for microbiologic and histopathologic analysis) is preferred because of its high diagnostic accuracy. The endoscopic signs of candidal esophagitis are diffuse, linear, yellow-white plaques adherent to the mucosa. CMV esophagitis is characterized by one to several large, shallow, superficial ulcerations. Herpes esophagitis results in multiple small, deep ulcerations.

Treatment

A. Candidal Esophagitis

Initial episodes of oropharyngeal candidiasis may be treated with clotrimazole troches (10 mg dissolved in mouth five times daily) or nystatin suspension (500,000 units five times daily), but systemic therapy is required for esophageal candidiasis. An empiric trial of antifungal therapy is often administered without performing diagnostic endoscopy. Initial therapy is generally with fluconazole, 100 mg/d orally for 14–21 days. Patients not responding to empiric therapy within 7–14 days should undergo endoscopy with brushings, biopsy, and culture to distinguish resistant fungal infection from other infections (eg, CMV, herpes). Esophageal candidiasis not responding to fluconazole therapy may be treated with itraconazole suspension (not capsules), 200 mg/d orally, or voriconazole, 200 mg twice daily. Refractory infection may be treated intravenously with caspofungin, 50 mg daily or amphotericin B, 0.3–0.7 mg/kg/d.

B. Cytomegalovirus Esophagitis

In patients with HIV infection, immune restoration with highly active antiretroviral therapy (HAART) is the most effective means of controlling CMV disease. Initial therapy is with ganciclovir, 5 mg/kg intravenously every 12 hours for 3–6 weeks. Neutropenia is a frequent dose-limiting side effect. Once resolution of symptoms occurs, it may be possible to complete the course of therapy with oral valganciclovir, 900 mg once daily. Patients who either do not respond to or cannot tolerate ganciclovir are treated acutely with foscarnet, 90 mg/kg intravenously every 12 hours for 3–6 weeks. The principal toxicity is renal failure, hypocalcemia, and hypomagnesemia.

C. Herpetic Esophagitis

Immunocompetent patients may be treated symptomatically and generally do not require specific antiviral therapy. Immunosuppressed patients may be treated with oral acyclovir, 400 mg orally five times daily, or 250 mg/m^2 intravenously every 8–12 hours, usually for 7–10 days. Famciclovir, 250 mg three times daily, and valacyclovir, 1 g twice daily, are effective but significantly more expensive than generic acyclovir. Nonresponders require therapy with foscarnet, 40 mg/kg intravenously every 8 hours for 21 days.

Prognosis

Most patients with infectious esophagitis can be effectively treated with complete symptom resolution. Depending on the patient's underlying immunodeficiency, relapse of symptoms off therapy can raise difficulties. Long-term suppressive therapy is sometimes required.

Lavery EA et al. Herpes simplex virus and the alimentary tract. Curr Gastroenterol Rep. 2008 Aug;10(4):417–23. [PMID: 18627656]

Pace F et al. Nongastroesophageal reflux disease-related infectious, inflammatory and injurious disorders of the esophagus. Curr Opin Gastroenterol. 2007 Jul;23(4):446–51. [PMID: 17545784]

Weerasuriya N et al. Oesophageal candidiasis in elderly patients: risk factors, prevention and management. Drugs Aging. 2008;25(2):119–30. [PMID: 18257599]

PILL-INDUCED ESOPHAGITIS

A number of different medications may injure the esophagus, presumably through direct, prolonged mucosal contact. The most commonly implicated are the NSAIDs, potassium chloride pills, quinidine, zalcitabine, zidovudine, alendronate and risedronate, emepronium bromide, iron, vitamin C, and antibiotics (doxycycline, tetracycline, clindamycin, trimethoprim-sulfamethoxazole). Because injury is most likely to occur if pills are swallowed without water or while supine, hospitalized or bed-bound patients are at greater risk. Symptoms include severe retrosternal chest pain, odynophagia, and dysphagia, often beginning several hours after taking a pill. These may occur suddenly and persist for days. Some patients (especially the elderly) have relatively little pain, presenting with dysphagia. Endoscopy may reveal one to several discrete ulcers that may be shallow or deep. Chronic injury may result in severe esophagitis with stricture, hemorrhage, or perforation. Healing occurs rapidly when the offending agent is eliminated. To prevent pill-induced damage, patients should take pills with 4 oz of water and remain upright for 30 minutes after ingestion. Known offending agents should not be given to patients with esophageal dysmotility, dysphagia, or strictures.

Abid S et al. Pill-induced esophageal injury: endoscopic features and clinical outcomes. Endoscopy. 2005 Aug;37(8):740–4. [PMID: 16032493]

CAUSTIC ESOPHAGEAL INJURY

Caustic esophageal injury occurs from accidental (usually children) or deliberate (suicidal) ingestion of liquid or crystalline alkali (drain cleaners, etc) or acid. Ingestion is followed almost immediately by severe burning and varying degrees of chest pain, gagging, dysphagia, and drooling. Aspiration results in stridor and wheezing. Initial examination should be directed to circulatory status as well as assessment of airway patency and the oropharyngeal mucosa, including laryngoscopy. Patients without major symptoms (dyspnea, dysphagia, drooling, hematemesis) or oropharyngeal lesions have a very low likelihood of having severe gastroesophageal injury. Subsequently, chest and abdominal radiographs are obtained looking for pneumonitis or free perforation. Initial treatment is supportive, with intravenous fluids and analgesics. Nasogastric lavage and oral antidotes may be dangerous and should generally not be administered. Most patients may be managed medically. Endoscopy is usually performed within the first 12–24 hours to assess the extent of injury, especially in patients with significant symptoms or oropharyngeal lesions. Many patients are discovered to have no mucosal injury to the esophagus or stomach, allowing prompt discharge and psychiatric referral. Patients with evidence of mild damage (edema, erythema, exudates or superficial ulcers) recover quickly, have low risk of developing stricture, and may be advanced from liquids to a regular diet over 24–48 hours. Patients with signs of severe injury—deep or circumferential ulcers or necrosis (black discoloration) have a high risk (up to 65%) of acute complications, including perforation with mediastinitis or peritonitis, bleeding, stricture, or esophageal-tracheal fistulas. These patients must be kept fasting and monitored closely for signs of deterioration that warrant emergency surgery with possible esophagectomy and colonic or jejunal interposition. A nasoenteric feeding tube is placed after 24 hours. Oral feedings of liquids may be initiated after 2–3 days if the patient is able to tolerate secretions. Neither corticosteroids nor antibiotics are recommended. Esophageal strictures develop in up to 70% of patients with serious esophageal injury weeks to months after the initial injury, requiring recurrent dilations. Endoscopic injection of intralesional corticosteroids (triamcinolone 40 mg) increases the interval between dilations. The risk of esophageal squamous carcinoma is 2–3%, warranting endoscopic surveillance 15–20 years after the caustic ingestion.

Betalli P et al. Caustic ingestion in children: is endoscopy always indicated? The results of an Italian multicenter observational study. Gastrointest Endosc. 2008 Sept;68(3):434–9. [PMID: 18448103]

BENIGN ESOPHAGEAL LESIONS

1. Mallory-Weiss Syndrome (Mucosal Laceration of Gastroesophageal Junction)

 ESSENTIALS OF DIAGNOSIS

► Hematemesis; usually self-limited.
► Prior history of vomiting, retching in 50%.
► Endoscopy establishes diagnosis.

General Considerations

Mallory-Weiss syndrome is characterized by a nonpenetrating mucosal tear at the gastroesophageal junction that is hypothesized to arise from events that suddenly raise transabdominal pressure, such as lifting, retching, or vomiting. Alcoholism is a strong predisposing factor. Mallory-Weiss tears are responsible for approximately 5% of cases of upper gastrointestinal bleeding.

Clinical Findings

A. Symptoms and Signs

Patients usually present with hematemesis with or without melena. A history of retching, vomiting, or straining is obtained in about 50% of cases.

B. Special Examinations

As with other causes of upper gastrointestinal hemorrhage, upper endoscopy should be performed after the patient has been appropriately resuscitated. The diagnosis is established by identification of a 0.5- to 4-cm linear mucosal tear usually located either at the gastroesophageal junction or, more commonly, just below the junction in the gastric mucosa.

Differential Diagnosis

At endoscopy, other potential causes of upper gastrointestinal hemorrhage are found in over 35% of patients with Mallory-Weiss tears, including peptic ulcer disease, erosive gastritis, arteriovenous malformations, and esophageal varices. Patients with underlying portal hypertension are at higher risk of continued or recurrent bleeding.

Treatment

Patients are initially treated as needed with fluid resuscitation and blood transfusions. Most patients stop bleeding spontaneously and require no therapy. Endoscopic hemostatic therapy is employed in patients who have continuing active bleeding. Injection with epinephrine (1:10,000), cautery with a bipolar or heater probe coagulation device, or mechanical compression of the artery by application of an endoclip or band is effective in 90–95% of cases. Angiographic arterial embolization or operative intervention is required in patients who fail endoscopic therapy.

Cho YS et al. Endoscopic band ligation and endoscopic hemoclip placement for patients with Mallory-Weiss syndrome and active bleeding. World J Gastroenterol. 2008 Apr 7;14(13):2080–4. [PMID: 18395910]

2. Eosinophilic Esophagitis

General Considerations

Eosinophilic esophagitis is an entity that previously was recognized in children but is increasingly identified in young or middle-aged adults, predominantly men (75%). A history of allergies or atopic conditions (asthma, eczema, hayfever) is present in over half of patients.

Clinical Findings

Most adults have a long history of dysphagia for solid-foods or with an episode of food impaction. Heartburn may be present. Children may have abdominal pain, vomiting, chest pain, or failure to thrive. On laboratory tests, a few have eosinophilia or elevated IgE levels. Barium swallow studies may demonstrate a small-caliber esophagus, long and tapered strictures, or multiple concentric rings. However, endoscopy with esophageal biopsy and histologic evaluation is required to establish the diagnosis. Endoscopic appearances include multiple fine concentric rings, vertical furrowing or shearing, and whitish papules or exudates; however, the esophagus is grossly normal in one-third of patients. Multiple biopsies (at least 5) from the proximal and distal esophagus should be obtained to demonstrate multiple (> 15/high-powered field) eosinophils in the mucosa. GERD may cause increased eosinophils in the distal esophageal mucosa and must be excluded. Most children have other coexisting atopic disorders. Skin testing for food allergies may be helpful to identify causative factors, especially in children.

Treatment

The optimal treatment of eosinophilic esophagitis is uncertain. Referral to an allergist for evaluation of coexisting atopic disorders and for skin prick testing for food and environmental allergens is recommended. In children, food elimination or elemental diets lead to clinical and histologic improvement in 75%; however, the effectiveness of dietary therapy in adults is not established. The most common allergenic foods are dairy, eggs, wheat, soy, peanuts, and shellfish. To exclude GERD, all patients should be given an empiric trial of a proton pump inhibitor (eg, omeprazole, lansoprazole, pantoprazole, esomeprazole, rabeprazole) orally twice daily or undergo esophageal pH testing. Topical corticosteroids (eg, use of fluticasone 220 mcg/puff inhaler without a spacer, swallowing two to four puffs after inspiration, twice daily after meals) led to symptom resolution in 75% of adults in uncontrolled trials. Symptomatic relapse is common after discontinuation of therapy. Graduated dilation of strictures should be conducted cautiously because there is an increased risk of perforation and postprocedural chest pain.

Furuta G et al. Eosinophilic esophagitis in children and adults: a systematic review and consensus recommendations for diagnosis and treatment. Gastroenterology. 2007 Oct;133(4):1342–63. [PMID: 17919504]
Kapel RC et al. Eosinophilic esophagitis: a prevalent disease in the United States that affects all age groups. Gastroenterology. 2008 May;134(5):1316–21. [PMID: 18471509]

3. Esophageal Webs & Rings

Esophageal webs are thin, diaphragm-like membranes of squamous mucosa that typically occur in the mid or upper esophagus and may be multiple. They may be congenital but also occur with graft-versus-host disease, pemphigoid, epidermolysis bullosa, pemphigus vulgaris, and, rarely, in association with iron deficiency anemia (Plummer-Vinson syndrome). Esophageal "Schatzki" rings are smooth, circumferential, thin (< 4 mm in thickness) mucosal structures located in the distal esophagus at the squamocolumnar junction. Their pathogenesis is controversial. They are associated in nearly all cases with a hiatal hernia, and reflux symptoms are common, suggesting that acid gastroesophageal reflux may be contributory in many cases. Most webs and rings are over 20 mm in diameter and are asymptomatic. Solid food dysphagia most often occurs with rings less than 13 mm in diameter. Characteristically, dysphagia is intermittent and not progressive. Large poorly chewed food boluses such as beefsteak are most likely to cause symptoms. Obstructing boluses may pass by drinking extra liquids or after regurgitation. In some cases, an impacted bolus must be extracted endoscopically. Esophageal webs and rings are best visualized using a barium esophagogram with full esophageal distention. Endoscopy is less sensitive than barium esophagography.

The majority of symptomatic patients with a single ring or web can be effectively treated with the passage of a large (> 16-mm-diameter) bougie dilator to disrupt the lesion or endoscopic electrosurgical incision of the ring. A single dilation may suffice, but repeat dilations are required in many patients. Patients who have heartburn or who require repeated dilation should receive long-term acid suppressive therapy with a proton pump inhibitor.

Sgouros SN et al. Long-term acid suppressive therapy may prevent the relapse of esophageal (Schatzki's) rings: a prospective, randomized, placebo-controlled study. Am J Gastroenterol. 2005 Sep;100(9):1929–34. [PMID: 16128935]
Wills JC et al. A randomized, prospective trial of electrosurgical incision followed by rabeprazole versus bougie dilation followed by rabeprazole of symptomatic esophageal (Schatzki's) rings. Gastrointest Endosc. 2008 May;67(6):808–13. [PMID: 18313671]

4. Esophageal Diverticula

Diverticula may occur in the proximal, mid, or distal esophagus. These may arise secondary to motility disorders (diffuse esophageal spasm, achalasia) or may develop above esophageal strictures. Diverticula are seldom symptomatic. For patients with severe symptoms or pulmonary complications, surgical myotomy with or without diverticulectomy is the optimal treatment.

▷ Zenker Diverticulum

Zenker diverticulum is a protrusion of pharyngeal mucosa that develops at the pharyngoesophageal junction between the inferior pharyngeal constrictor and the cricopharyngeus. The cause is believed to be loss of elasticity of the upper esophageal sphincter, resulting in restricted opening during swallowing. Symptoms of dysphagia and regurgitation tend to develop insidiously over years in older patients. Initial symptoms include vague oropharyngeal dysphagia with coughing or throat discomfort. As the diverticulum enlarges and retains food, patients may note halitosis, spontaneous regurgitation of undigested food, nocturnal choking, gurgling in the throat, or a protrusion in the neck. Complications include aspiration pneumonia, bronchiectasis, and lung abscess. The diagnosis is best established by a barium esophagogram.

Symptomatic patients require upper esophageal myotomy and, in most cases, surgical diverticulectomy. An intraluminal approach has been developed in which the septum between the esophagus and diverticulum is incised using a rigid or flexible endoscope. Significant improvement occurs in over 90% of patients treated surgically. Small asymptomatic diverticula may be observed.

Cassivi SD et al. Diverticula of the esophagus. Surg Clin North Am. 2005 Jun;85(3):495–503. [PMID: 15927646]
Ferreira LE et al. Zenker's diverticula: pathophysiology, clinical presentation, and flexible endoscopic management. Dis Esophagus. 2008;21(1):1–8. [PMID: 18197932]

Seaman DL et al. A new device to simplify flexible endoscopic treatment of Zenker's diverticulum. Gastrointest Endosc. 2008 Jan;67(1):112–5. [PMID: 18155432]

5. Benign Esophageal Neoplasms

Benign tumors of the esophagus are quite rare. They are submucosal, the most common being leiomyoma. Most are asymptomatic and picked up incidentally on endoscopy or barium esophagography. Larger lesions can cause dysphagia, pain, and rarely ulceration with bleeding. The risk of malignant transformation is low. Therefore, the major clinical importance of these lesions is to distinguish them from malignant neoplasms. At endoscopy, a smooth, sessile nodule is observed with normal overlying mucosa. Because the lesion is submucosal, endoscopic biopsies are generally nonrevealing. Endoscopic ultrasonography is extremely helpful to confirm the submucosal origin of the tumor and to help distinguish benign leiomyomas from malignant leiomyosarcomas. Surgical (or in selected cases endoscopic) resection is indicated for lesions that are symptomatic, ulcerated, or increasing in size. (**See Chapter 39 for Esophageal Cancer.**)

Jiang G et al. Thoroscopic enucleation of esophageal leiomyoma: a retrospective study on 40 cases. Dis Esophagus. 2009;22(3):279–83. [PMID: 19021682]

6. Esophageal Varices

 ESSENTIALS OF DIAGNOSIS

- ▷ Develop secondary to portal hypertension.
- ▷ Found in 50% of patients with cirrhosis.
- ▷ One-third of patients with varices develop upper gastrointestinal bleeding.
- ▷ Diagnosis established by upper endoscopy.

▷ General Considerations

Esophageal varices are dilated submucosal veins that develop in patients with underlying portal hypertension and may result in serious upper gastrointestinal bleeding. The causes of portal hypertension are discussed in Chapter 16. Under normal circumstances, there is a 2–6 mm Hg pressure gradient between the portal vein and the inferior vena cava. When the gradient exceeds 10–12 mm Hg, significant portal hypertension exists. Esophageal varices are the most common cause of important gastrointestinal bleeding due to portal hypertension, though gastric varices and, rarely, intestinal varices may also bleed. Bleeding from esophageal varices most commonly occurs in the distal 5 cm of the esophagus.

The most common cause of portal hypertension is cirrhosis. Approximately 50% of patients with cirrhosis have esophageal varices. Bleeding from varices occurs in 30% of patients with esophageal varices. In the absence of any treatment, variceal bleeding spontaneously stops in about 50% of patients. Patients surviving this bleeding episode have a 60% chance of recurrent variceal bleeding, usually within the first 6 weeks. With current therapies, the in-hospital mortality rate associated with bleeding esophageal varices is 15%.

A number of factors have been identified that may portend an increased risk of bleeding from esophageal varices. The most important are: (1) the size of the varices; (2) the presence at endoscopy of red wale markings on the varix; (3) the severity of liver disease (as assessed by Child scoring); and (4) active alcohol abuse—alcoholic cirrhotics who continue to drink have an extremely high risk of bleeding.

► Clinical Findings

A. Symptoms and Signs

Patients with bleeding esophageal varices present with symptoms and signs of acute gastrointestinal hemorrhage. (See Acute Upper Gastrointestinal Bleeding, above.) In some cases, there may be preceding retching or dyspepsia attributable to alcoholic gastritis or withdrawal. Varices per se do not cause symptoms of dyspepsia, dysphagia, or retching. Variceal bleeding usually is severe, resulting in hypovolemia manifested by postural vital signs or shock. Twenty percent of patients with chronic liver disease in whom bleeding develops have a nonvariceal source of bleeding.

B. Laboratory Findings

These are identical to those listed above in the section on acute upper gastrointestinal tract bleeding.

► Initial Management

A. Acute Resuscitation

The initial management of patients with acute upper gastrointestinal bleeding is also discussed in the section on acute upper gastrointestinal bleeding (see above). Variceal hemorrhage is life-threatening; rapid assessment and resuscitation with fluids or blood products are essential. Overtransfusion should be avoided as it leads to increased central and portal venous pressures, increasing the risk of rebleeding. Many patients with bleeding esophageal varices have coagulopathy due to underlying cirrhosis; fresh frozen plasma (20 mL/kg loading dose, then 10 mg/kg every 6 hours) or platelets should be administered to patients with INRs > 1.8–2.0 or with platelet counts < 50,000/mcL in the presence of active bleeding. Patients with advanced liver disease are at high risk for poor outcome regardless of the bleeding source and should be transferred to an ICU.

B. Pharmacologic Therapy

1. Antibiotic prophylaxis—Cirrhotic patients admitted with upper gastrointestinal bleeding have a greater than 50% chance of developing a severe bacterial infection during hospitalization—such as bacterial peritonitis, pneumonia, or urinary tract infection. Most infections are caused by gram-negative organisms of gut origin. Prophylactic administration of antibiotics reduces the risk of serious infection to 10–20% as well as hospital mortality. Antibiotic treatment with an oral poorly absorbed quinolone antibiotic (norfloxacin 400 mg twice daily) for 5–7 days has been recommended; however, a controlled trial found that patients who had decompensated cirrhosis with gastrointestinal bleeding had a significantly higher probability of developing infections when treated with norfloxacin 400 mg orally twice daily (26%) than those who were treated with ceftriaxone 1 g/d intravenously for 7 days (11%). Because of a rising incidence of infections caused by gram-positive organisms as well as fluoroquinolone-resistant organisms, intravenous third-generation cephalosporins may be preferred.

2. Vasoactive drugs—Somatostatin and octreotide infusions reduce portal pressures in ways that are poorly understood. Somatostatin (250 mcg/h)—not available in the United States—or octreotide (50 mcg intravenous bolus followed by 50 mcg/h) reduces splanchnic and hepatic blood flow and portal pressures in cirrhotic patients. Both agents appear to provide acute control of variceal bleeding in up to 80% of patients although neither has been shown to reduce mortality. Data about the absolute efficacy of both are conflicting, but they may be comparable in efficacy to endoscopic therapy. Combined treatment with octreotide or somatostatin infusion and endoscopic therapy (band ligation or sclerotherapy) is superior to either modality alone in controlling acute bleeding and early rebleeding, and it may improve survival. In patients with advanced liver disease and upper gastrointestinal hemorrhage, it is reasonable to initiate therapy with octreotide or somatostatin on admission and continue for 3–5 days. If bleeding is determined by endoscopy not to be secondary to portal hypertension, the infusion can be discontinued.

Terlipressin, 1–2 mg intravenous every 4 hours, (not available in the United States) is a synthetic vasopressin analog that causes a significant and sustained reduction in portal and variceal pressures while preserving renal perfusion. It is superior to placebo in the control of acute variceal hemorrhage and reduces mortality by 34%. Where available, terlipressin may be preferred to somatostatin or octreotide. Terlipressin is contraindicated in patients with significant coronary, cerebral, or peripheral vascular disease.

3. Vitamin K—In cirrhotic patients with an abnormal prothrombin time, vitamin K (10 mg) should be administered subcutaneously.

4. Lactulose—Encephalopathy may complicate an episode of gastrointestinal bleeding in patients with severe liver disease. In patients with encephalopathy, lactulose should be administered in a dosage of 30–45 mL/h orally until evacuation occurs, then reduced to 15–45 mL/h every 8–12 hours as needed to promote two or three bowel movements daily. (See Chapter 16.)

C. Emergent Endoscopy

Emergent endoscopy is performed after the patient's hemodynamic status has been appropriately stabilized (usually within 2–12 hours). In patients with active bleeding, endotracheal intubation is commonly performed to protect against aspiration during endoscopy. An endoscopic examination is performed to exclude other or associated causes of upper gastrointestinal bleeding such as Mallory-Weiss tears, peptic ulcer disease, and portal hypertensive gastropathy. In many patients, variceal bleeding has stopped spontaneously by the time of endoscopy, and the diagnosis of variceal bleeding is made presumptively. Acute endoscopic treatment of the varices is performed with either banding or sclerotherapy. These techniques arrest active bleeding in 80–90% of patients and reduce the chance of in-hospital recurrent bleeding to about 20%.

If banding is chosen, repeat sessions are scheduled at intervals of 1–3 weeks until the varices are obliterated or reduced to a small size. Banding achieves lower rates of rebleeding, complications, and death than sclerotherapy and should be considered the endoscopic treatment of choice.

Sclerotherapy is still preferred by some endoscopists in the actively bleeding patient (in whom visualization for banding may be difficult). Sclerotherapy is performed by injecting the variceal trunks with a sclerosing agent (eg, ethanolamine, tetradecyl sulfate). Complications occur in 20–30% of patients and include chest pain, fever, bacteremia, esophageal ulceration, stricture, and perforation. After initial treatment, band ligation therapy should be performed.

D. Balloon Tube Tamponade

Mechanical tamponade with specially designed nasogastric tubes containing large gastric and esophageal balloons (Minnesota or Sengstaken-Blakemore tubes) provides initial control of active variceal hemorrhage in 60–90% of patients; rebleeding occurs in 50%. The gastric balloon is inflated first, followed by the esophageal balloon if bleeding continues. After balloon inflation, tension is applied to the tube to directly tamponade the varices. Complications of prolonged balloon inflation include esophageal and oral ulcerations, perforation, aspiration, and airway obstruction (due to a misplaced balloon). Endotracheal intubation is recommended before placement. Given its high rate of complications, mechanical tamponade is used as a temporizing measure only in patients with bleeding that cannot be controlled with pharmacologic or endoscopic techniques until more definitive decompressive therapy (eg, TIPS; see below) can be provided.

E. Portal Decompressive Procedures

In patients with variceal bleeding that cannot be controlled with pharmacologic or endoscopic therapy, emergency portal decompression may be considered.

1. Transvenous intrahepatic portosystemic shunts (TIPS)—Over a wire that is passed through a catheter inserted in the jugular vein, an expandable wire mesh stent (8–12 mm in diameter) is passed through the liver parenchyma, creating a portosystemic shunt from the portal vein to the hepatic vein. TIPS can control acute hemorrhage in over 90% of patients actively bleeding from gastric or esophageal varices. However, when TIPS is performed in the actively bleeding patient, the mortality approaches

40%, especially in patients requiring ventilatory support or blood pressure support and patients with renal insufficiency, bilirubin > 3.0 mg/dL, or encephalopathy. Therefore, TIPS should be considered in the 10–20% of patients with acute variceal bleeding that cannot be controlled with pharmacologic and endoscopic therapy, but it may not be warranted in patients with a poor prognosis.

2. Emergency portosystemic shunt surgery—Emergency portosystemic shunt surgery is associated with a 40–60% mortality rate. At centers where TIPS is available, that procedure has become the preferred means of providing emergency portal decompression.

▶ Prevention of Rebleeding

Once the initial bleeding episode has been controlled, therapy is warranted to reduce the high risk (60%) of rebleeding.

A. β-Blockers and Variceal Band Ligation

Long-term treatment with band ligation reduces the incidence of rebleeding to about 30%; the mortality rate may also be reduced. In most patients, two to six treatment sessions (performed at 7–14 day intervals) are needed to eradicate the varices.

Nonselective β-adrenergic blockers (propranolol, nadolol) reduce the risk of rebleeding from esophageal varices to about 40%. Some—but not all—studies demonstrate a lower incidence of rebleeding with band ligation than with β-adrenergic blockers. However, a combination of band ligation plus β-blockers is superior to either variceal band ligation or β-blockers alone. In randomized clinical trials, combination therapy markedly reduced the rate of recurrent bleeding (25%) compared with endoscopic therapy alone (37%). Therefore, combination therapy is recommended for patients without contraindications to β-blockers. Propranolol, 20–60 mg twice daily, long-acting propranolol, 60–80 mg once daily, or nadolol, 40 mg once daily may be used, with gradual increases in the dosage every 1–2 weeks until the heart rate falls by 25% or reaches 55 beats/min, provided the systolic blood pressure remains above 90 mm Hg and the patient has no side effects. The average dosage of long-acting propranolol is 120 mg once daily and for nadolol, 80 mg once daily. One-third of patients with cirrhosis are intolerant of β-blockers, experiencing fatigue or hypotension. Drug administration at bedtime may reduce the frequency and severity of side effects.

B. Transvenous Intrahepatic Portosystemic Shunt

TIPS has resulted in a significant reduction in recurrent bleeding compared with endoscopic sclerotherapy or band ligation—either alone or in combination with β-blocker therapy. At 1 year, rebleeding rates in patients treated with TIPS versus various endoscopic therapies average 20% and 40%, respectively. However, TIPS was also associated with a higher incidence of encephalopathy (35% versus 15%) and did not result in a decrease in mortality. Another limitation of TIPS is that stenosis and thrombosis of the stents occur in the majority of patients over time with a consequent risk of rebleeding. Therefore, periodic monitoring with Doppler ultrasonography or hepatic venography is required. Stent patency usually can be maintained by balloon angioplasty or additional stent placement. Given these problems, TIPS should be reserved for patients who have recurrent (two or more) episodes of variceal bleeding that have failed endoscopic or pharmacologic therapies. TIPS is also useful in patients with recurrent bleeding from gastric varices or portal hypertensive gastropathy (for which endoscopic therapies cannot be used). TIPS is likewise considered in patients who are noncompliant with other therapies or who live in remote locations (without access to emergency care).

C. Surgical Portosystemic Shunts

Shunt surgery has a significantly lower rate of rebleeding compared with endoscopic therapy but also a higher incidence of encephalopathy. With the advent and widespread adoption of TIPS, surgical shunts are seldom performed.

D. Liver Transplantation

Candidacy for orthotopic liver transplantation should be assessed in all patients with chronic liver disease and bleeding due to portal hypertension. Transplant candidates should be treated with band ligation or TIPS to control bleeding pretransplant.

▶ Prevention of First Episodes of Variceal Bleeding

Because of the high mortality rate associated with variceal hemorrhage, prevention of the initial bleeding episode is desirable. Therefore, patients with cirrhosis should undergo diagnostic endoscopy or capsule endoscopy to determine whether varices are present as well as their size and whether they have red wale markings. Varices are present in 40% of patients with Child-Turcotte-Pugh class A cirrhosis and in 85% with Child-Turcotte-Pugh class C cirrhosis. Approximately 25% of patients have large varices (> 5 mm in size). Patients with varices have a higher risk of bleeding if they have Childs-Turcotte-Pugh class B or C cirrhosis or varices with red wale markings, or both. The risk of bleeding in patients with small varices (< 5 mm) is 5% per year and with large varices is 15–20% per year. Nonselective β-adrenergic blockers are recommended to reduce the risk of first variceal hemorrhage in patients with large varices and patients with small varices who either have variceal red wale marks or advanced cirrhosis (Child-Turcotte-Pugh class B or C). For patients with contraindications to or intolerance of β-blockers and for higher risk patients with large varices (Childs-Turcotte-Pugh class B or C or red wale markings), prophylactic treatment with band ligation should be considered. For patients with small varices (without red wale marks) and compensated (Child-Turcotte-Pugh class A) cirrhosis, no prophylaxis is necessary, but endoscopy should be repeated in 1–2 years. In patients without varices on screening endoscopy, a repeat endoscopy is recommended in 3 years, since varices develop in 8% of patients per year.

▶ When to Refer

- All patients with upper gastrointestinal bleeding and suspected varices should be evaluated by a physician skilled in therapeutic endoscopy.
- Patients being considered for TIPS procedures or liver transplantation.

▶ When to Admit

All patients with acute upper gastrointestinal bleeding and suspected cirrhosis should be admitted to an ICU.

Abraldes JG et al. The treatment of acute variceal bleeding. J Clin Gastroenterol. 2007 Nov–Dec;41(Suppl 3):S312–7. [PMID: 17975482]

Garcia-Pagan JC et al. The modern management of portal hypertension—primary and secondary prophylaxis of variceal bleeding in cirrhotic patients. Aliment Pharmacol Ther. 2008 Jul;28(2):178–86. [PMID: 18462268]

Garcia-Tsao G et al; Practice Guidelines Committee of the American Association for the Study of Liver Diseases; Practice Parameters Committee of the American College of Gastroenterology. Prevention and management of gastroesophageal varices and variceal hemorrhage in cirrhosis. Hepatology. 2007 Sep;46(3):922–38. [PMID: 17879356]

Gluud LL et al. Banding ligation versus beta-blockers as primary prophylaxis in esophageal varices: systematic review of randomized trials. Am J Gastroenterol. 2007 Dec;102(12):2842–8. [PMID: 18042114]

Habib A et al. Acute variceal hemorrhage. Gastrointest Endosc Clin N Am. 2007 Apr;17(2):223–52. [PMID: 17556146]

Sanyal AJ et al. Portal hypertension and its complications. Gastroenterology. 2008 May;134(6):1715–28. [PMID: 18471549]

ESOPHAGEAL MOTILITY DISORDERS

1. Achalasia

 ESSENTIALS OF DIAGNOSIS

- ▶ Gradual, progressive dysphagia for solids and liquids.
- ▶ Regurgitation of undigested food.
- ▶ Barium esophagogram with "bird's beak" distal esophagus.
- ▶ Esophageal manometry confirms diagnosis.

▶ General Considerations

Achalasia is an idiopathic motility disorder characterized by loss of peristalsis in the distal two-thirds (smooth muscle) of the esophagus and impaired relaxation of the LES. There appears to be denervation of the esophagus resulting primarily from loss of nitric oxide-producing inhibitory neurons in the myenteric plexus. The cause of the neuronal degeneration is unknown.

Clinical Findings

A. Symptoms and Signs

There is a steady increase in the incidence of achalasia with age; however, it can be seen in individuals as young as 25 years. Patients complain of the gradual onset of dysphagia for solid foods and, in the majority, of liquids also. Symptoms at presentation may have persisted for months to years. Substernal discomfort or fullness may be noted after eating. Many patients eat more slowly and adopt specific maneuvers such as lifting the neck or throwing the shoulders back to enhance esophageal emptying. Regurgitation of undigested food is common and may occur during meals or up to several hours later. Nocturnal regurgitation can provoke coughing or aspiration. Up to 50% of patients report substernal chest pain that is unrelated to meals or exercise and may last up to hours. Weight loss is common. Physical examination is unhelpful.

B. Imaging

Chest radiographs may show an air-fluid level in the enlarged, fluid-filled esophagus. Barium esophagography discloses characteristic findings, including esophageal dilation, loss of esophageal peristalsis, poor esophageal emptying, and a smooth, symmetric "bird's beak" tapering of the distal esophagus. Without treatment, the esophagus may become markedly dilated ("sigmoid esophagus").

C. Special Examinations

After esophagography, endoscopy is always performed to evaluate the distal esophagus and gastroesophageal junction to exclude a distal stricture or a submucosal infiltrating carcinoma. The diagnosis is confirmed by esophageal manometry. The typical manometric features are as follows: (1) Complete absence of peristalsis; swallowing results in simultaneous waves that are usually of low amplitude. (2) Incomplete lower esophageal sphincteric relaxation with swallowing. Whereas the normal sphincter relaxes by over 90%, relaxation with most swallows in patients with achalasia is less than 50%. In many patients, the baseline lower esophageal sphincteric pressure is quite elevated. (3) Intraesophageal pressures are greater than gastric pressures due to a fluid- and food-filled esophagus.

Differential Diagnosis

Chagas disease is associated with esophageal dysfunction that is indistinguishable from idiopathic achalasia and should be considered in patients from endemic regions (Central and South America); it is becoming more common in the southern United States. Primary or metastatic tumors can invade the gastroesophageal junction, resulting in a picture resembling that of achalasia, called "pseudoachalasia." Endoscopic ultrasonography and chest CT may be required to examine the distal esophagus in suspicious cases. Tumors such as small cell lung cancer can cause a paraneoplastic syndrome resembling achalasia due to secretion of antineuronal nuclear antibodies (ANNA-1 or Anti-Hu) that affect the myenteric plexus. Achalasia must be distinguished from other motility disorders such as diffuse esophageal spasm and scleroderma esophagus with a peptic stricture.

Treatment

A. Botulinum Toxin Injection

Endoscopically guided injection of botulinum toxin directly into the LES results in a marked reduction in LES pressure with initial improvement in symptoms in 65–85% of patients. However, symptom relapse occurs in over 50% of patients within 6–9 months and in all patients within 2 years. Three-fourths of initial responders who relapse have improvement with repeated injections. Because it is inferior to pneumatic dilation therapy and surgery in producing sustained symptomatic relief, this therapy is most appropriate for patients with comorbidities who are poor candidates for more invasive procedures. Botulinum injection may cause submucosal scarring that may make subsequent surgical myotomy more difficult.

B. Pneumatic Dilation

Between 75% and 85% of patients derive good to excellent relief of dysphagia after one to three sessions of pneumatic dilation of the LES. Approximately 15% of patients respond poorly to dilation and require surgical myotomy. Dilation is less effective in patients who are younger than age 50 or have spastic esophageal contractions ("vigorous achalasia"). Symptoms recur in up to 60% within 10 years but usually respond to repeated dilation. Perforations occur in less than 3% of dilations and may require operative repair. The success of laparoscopic myotomy is not compromised by prior pneumatic dilation.

C. Surgical Myotomy

A modified Heller cardiomyotomy of the LES and cardia results in good to excellent symptomatic improvement in over 85% of patients. Because gastroesophageal reflux develops in up to 20% of patients after myotomy, most surgeons also perform an antireflux procedure (fundoplication), and all patients are prescribed a once-daily proton pump inhibitor. Myotomy is now performed with a laparoscopic approach and is preferred to the open surgical approach. The low morbidity of laparoscopic surgery has led some experts to recommend it for initial treatment, especially for young patients. In experienced hands, however, the initial efficacies of pneumatic dilation and laparoscopic myotomy are nearly equivalent.

Ferulano GP et al. Short and long term results of the laparoscopic Heller-Dor myotomy. The influence of age and previous conservative therapies. Surg Endosc. 2007 Nov;21(11):2017–23. [PMID: 17705085]

Pandolfino JE et al. Achalasia: a new clinically relevant classification by high-resolution manometry. Gastroenterology. 2008 Nov;135(5):1526–33. [PMID: 18722376]

Richter JE. A young man with new diagnosis of achalasia. Clin Gastroenterol Hepatol. 2008 Aug;6(8):859–63. [PMID: 18456570]

2. Other Primary Esophageal Motility Disorders

Abnormalities in esophageal motility may cause dysphagia or chest pain. Dysphagia for liquids as well as solids tends to be intermittent and nonprogressive. Periods of normal swallowing may alternate with periods of dysphagia, which usually is mild though bothersome—rarely severe enough to result in significant alterations in lifestyle or weight loss. Dysphagia may be provoked by stress, large boluses of food, or hot or cold liquids. Some patients may experience anterior chest pain that may be confused with angina pectoris but usually is nonexertional. The pain generally is unrelated to eating. (See Chest Pain of Undetermined Origin, below.)

The evaluation of suspected esophageal motility disorders includes barium esophagography, upper endoscopy, and, in some cases, esophageal manometry. Barium esophagography is useful to exclude mechanical obstruction and to evaluate esophageal motility. The presence of simultaneous contractions (spasm), disordered peristalsis, or failed peristalsis supports a diagnosis of esophageal dysmotility. Upper endoscopy also is performed to exclude a mechanical obstruction (as a cause of dysphagia) and to look for evidence of erosive reflux esophagitis (a common cause of chest pain) or eosinophilic esophagitis (confirmed by esophageal biopsy).

The further evaluation of noncardiac chest pain is discussed in a subsequent section. For patients with mild symptoms of dysphagia, therapy is directed at symptom reduction and reassurance. Patients should be instructed to eat more slowly and take smaller bites of food. In some cases, a warm liquid at the start of a meal may facilitate swallowing. Because unrecognized gastroesophageal reflux may cause dysphagia, a trial of a proton pump inhibitor (esomeprazole 40 mg, lansoprazole 30 mg) orally twice daily should be administered for 4–8 weeks. Manometry is not routinely used for mild to moderate symptoms because the findings seldom influence further medical management, but it may be useful in patients with persistent, disabling dysphagia to exclude achalasia and to look for other disorders of esophageal motility. These include spastic disorders (diffuse esophageal spasm, nutcracker esophagus, and hypertensive LES) and findings of ineffective esophageal peristalsis (failed or low-amplitude esophageal contractions).

Treatment of patients with severe dysphagia is empiric. Suspected spastic disorders may be treated with nitrates (isosorbide, 10–20 mg four times daily) or nitroglycerin (0.4 mg sublingually as needed) and calcium channel blockers (nifedipine 10 mg or diltiazem 60–90 mg, 30–45 minutes before meals) may be tried; their efficacy is unproved. Phosphodiesterase type 5 inhibitors (eg, sildenafil) promote smooth muscle relaxation and improve esophageal motility in small numbers of patients with spastic disorders but require further clinical study before they can be recommended. Injection of botulinum toxin into the lower esophagus may improve chest pain and dysphagia in some patients for a limited time. For unclear reasons, esophageal dilation provides symptomatic relief in some cases. Debilitated patients with severe dysphagia and proven esophageal spasm may be treated with a long surgical myotomy.

Grubel C et al. Diffuse esophageal spasm. Am J Gastroenterol. 2008 Feb;103(2):450–7. [PMID: 18005367]

Konturek T et al. Spasm, nutcracker, and IEM: real or manometry findings? J Clin Gastroenterol. 2008 May–Jun;42(5):647–51. [PMID: 18364582]

Lacy BE et al. Esophageal motility disorders: medical Therapy. J Clin Gastroenterol. 2008 May–Jun;42(5):652–8. [PMID: 18364589]

CHEST PAIN OF UNDETERMINED ORIGIN

One-third of patients with chest pain undergo negative cardiac evaluation. Patients with recurrent noncardiac chest pain thus pose a difficult clinical problem. Because coronary artery disease is common and can present atypically, it must be excluded prior to evaluation for other causes.

Causes of noncardiac chest pain may include the following.

A. Chest Wall and Thoracic Spine Disease

These are easily diagnosed by history and physical examination.

B. Gastroesophageal Reflux

Up to 50% of patients have increased amounts of gastroesophageal acid reflux or a correlation between acid reflux episodes and chest pain demonstrated on esophageal pH testing. An empiric 4-week trial of acid-suppressive therapy with a high-dose proton pump inhibitor is recommended (eg, omeprazole or rabeprazole, 40 mg orally twice daily; lansoprazole, 30–60 mg orally twice daily; or esomeprazole or pantoprazole, 40 mg orally twice daily), especially in patients with reflux symptoms. In patients with persistent symptoms, ambulatory esophageal pH or impedance and pH study may be useful to exclude definitively a relationship between acid and nonacid reflux episodes and chest pain events.

C. Esophageal Dysmotility

Esophageal motility abnormalities such as diffuse esophageal spasm or nutcracker esophagus are uncommon causes of noncardiac chest pain. In patients with chest pain and dysphagia, a barium swallow radiograph should be obtained to look for evidence of achalasia or diffuse esophageal spasm. Esophageal manometry is not routinely performed because of low specificity and the unlikelihood of finding a clinically significant disorder, but it may be recommended in patients with frequent symptoms.

D. Heightened Visceral Sensitivity

Some patients with noncardiac chest pain report pain in response to a variety of minor noxious stimuli such as physiologically normal amounts of acid reflux, inflation of balloons within the esophageal lumen, injection of intravenous edrophonium (a cholinergic stimulus), or intracardiac catheter manipulation. Low doses of antidepressants such as trazodone 50 mg or imipramine 50 mg reduce chest pain symptoms and are thought to reduce visceral afferent awareness.

E. Psychological Disorders

A significant number of patients have underlying depression, anxiety, and panic disorder. Patients reporting dyspnea, sweating, tachycardia, suffocation, or fear of dying should be evaluated for panic disorder.

Fass R et al. Noncardiac chest pain. J Clin Gastroenterol. 2008 May–Jun;42(5):636–46. [PMID: 18364579]

▼ DISEASES OF THE STOMACH & DUODENUM

GASTRITIS & GASTROPATHY

The term "gastropathy" should be used to denote conditions in which there is epithelial or endothelial damage without inflammation, and "gastritis" should be used to denote conditions in which there is histologic evidence of inflammation. In clinical practice, the term "gastritis" is commonly applied to three categories: (1) erosive and hemorrhagic "gastritis" (gastropathy); (2) nonerosive, nonspecific (histologic) gastritis; and (3) specific types of gastritis, characterized by distinctive histologic and endoscopic features diagnostic of specific disorders.

1. Erosive & Hemorrhagic "Gastritis" (Gastropathy)

ESSENTIALS OF DIAGNOSIS

▶ Most commonly seen in alcoholics, critically ill patients, or patients taking NSAIDs.

▶ Often asymptomatic; may cause epigastric pain, nausea, and vomiting.

▶ May cause hematemesis; usually not significant bleeding.

▶ General Considerations

The most common causes of erosive gastropathy are drugs (especially NSAIDs), alcohol, stress due to severe medical or surgical illness, and portal hypertension ("portal gastropathy"). Uncommon causes include caustic ingestion and radiation. Erosive and hemorrhagic gastropathy typically are diagnosed at endoscopy, often being performed because of dyspepsia or upper gastrointestinal bleeding. Endoscopic findings include subepithelial hemorrhages, petechiae, and erosions. These lesions are superficial, vary in size and number, and may be focal or diffuse. There usually is no significant inflammation on histologic examination.

Major risk factors for stress gastritis include mechanical ventilation, coagulopathy, trauma, burns, shock, sepsis, central nervous system injury, liver failure, kidney disease, and multiorgan failure. The use of enteral nutrition reduces the risk of stress-related bleeding.

▶ Clinical Findings

A. Symptoms and Signs

Erosive gastropathy is usually asymptomatic. Symptoms, when they occur, include anorexia, epigastric pain, nausea, and vomiting. There is poor correlation between symptoms and the number or severity of endoscopic abnormalities. The most common clinical manifestation of erosive gastritis is upper gastrointestinal bleeding, which presents as hematemesis, "coffee grounds" emesis, or bloody aspirate in a patient receiving nasogastric suction, or as melena. Because erosive gastritis is superficial, hemodynamically significant bleeding is rare.

B. Laboratory Findings

The laboratory findings are nonspecific. The hematocrit is low if significant bleeding has occurred; iron deficiency may be found.

C. Special Examinations

Upper endoscopy is the most sensitive method of diagnosis. Although bleeding from gastritis is usually insignificant, it cannot be distinguished on clinical grounds from more serious lesions such as peptic ulcers or esophageal varices. Hence, endoscopy is generally performed within 24 hours in patients with upper gastrointestinal bleeding to identify the source. An upper gastrointestinal series is sometimes obtained in lieu of endoscopy in patients with hemodynamically insignificant upper gastrointestinal bleeds to exclude serious lesions but is insensitive for the detection of gastritis.

▶ Differential Diagnosis

Epigastric pain may be due to peptic ulcer, gastroesophageal reflux, gastric cancer, biliary tract disease, food poisoning, viral gastroenteritis, and functional dyspepsia. With severe pain, one should consider a perforated or penetrating ulcer, pancreatic disease, esophageal rupture, ruptured aortic aneurysm, gastric volvulus, and myocardial colic. Causes of upper gastrointestinal bleeding include peptic ulcer disease, esophageal varices, Mallory-Weiss tear, and arteriovenous malformations.

▶ Specific Causes & Treatment

A. Stress Gastritis

1. Prophylaxis—Stress-related mucosal erosions and subepithelial hemorrhages develop within 72 hours in the majority of critically ill patients. Clinically overt bleeding occurs in 6%, but clinically important bleeding in less than 3%. Bleeding is associated with a higher mortality rate but is seldom the cause of death.

In critically ill patients, pharmacologic prophylaxis with intravenous H_2-receptor antagonists, sucralfate, and an oral, rapid-release suspension of omeprazole plus sodium bicarbonate (Zegerid) has been shown to reduce the incidence of clinically overt and significant bleeding by 50%. At this time, the optimal, cost-effective regimen for the reduction of stress-related mucosal bleeding is uncertain. Prophylaxis should be routinely administered upon admission to critically ill patients with risk factors for significant bleeding. Two of the most important risk factors are coagulopathy (platelets < 50,000/mcL or INR greater than 1.5) and respiratory failure with the need for mechanical ventilation for over 48 hours. When these two risk factors are absent, the risk of significant bleeding is only 0.1%.

Although most critically ill patients have normal or decreased acid secretion, numerous studies have shown that maintaining intragastric pH > 4 reduces the incidence of clinically significant stress-related bleeding. Continuous infusions of H_2-receptor antagonists provide adequate control of intragastric pH in most patients in the following doses over 24 hours: cimetidine (900–1200 mg), ranitidine (150 mg), or famotidine (20 mg). After 4 hours of infusion, the pH should be checked by nasogastric aspirate and the dose doubled if the pH is under 4.0. For patients with nasoenteric tubes, immediate-release omeprazole (40 mg at 1 and 6 hours on day 1; then 40 mg once daily beginning on day 2) may be preferred to intravenous H_2-receptor antagonists because of lower cost, ease of administration, and comparable efficacy. Although intravenous proton pump inhibitors also are widely used for this indication, their efficacy and optimal dosing have not been established in controlled trials.

Sucralfate suspension (1 g orally every 4–6 hours) is effective also for the prevention of stress-related bleeding, and a reduction of nosocomial pneumonia had been observed compared with H_2-receptor antagonists. However, there is a higher incidence of clinically important upper gastrointestinal bleeding with sucralfate (4%) versus H_2-receptor antagonists (2%) with no difference in nosocomial pneumonia in more recent studies. In most ICUs, intravenous H_2-receptor antagonists or proton pump inhibitors are preferred because of their ease of administration.

2. Treatment—Once bleeding occurs, patients should receive continuous infusions of a proton pump inhibitor (esomeprazole or pantoprazole, 80 mg intravenous bolus, followed by 8 mg/h continuous infusion) as well as sucralfate suspension. Endoscopy should be performed in patients with clinically significant bleeding to look for treatable causes, especially stress-related peptic ulcers with active bleeding or visible vessels. When bleeding arises from diffuse gastritis, endoscopic hemostasis techniques are not helpful.

B. NSAID Gastritis

Of patients receiving NSAIDs in clinical trials, 25–50% have gastritis and 10–20% have ulcers at endoscopy; however, symptoms of significant dyspepsia develop in about 5%. In population surveys, the rate of dyspepsia is increased 1.5- to 2-fold with NSAID use. However, dyspeptic symptoms correlate poorly with significant mucosal abnormalities or the development of adverse clinical events (ulcer bleeding or perforation). Given the frequency of dyspeptic symptoms in patients taking NSAIDs, it is neither feasible nor desirable to investigate all such cases. Patients with alarm symptoms or signs, such as severe pain, weight loss, vomiting, gastrointestinal bleeding, or anemia, should undergo diagnostic upper endoscopy. For other patients, symptoms may improve with discontinuation of the agent, reduction to the lowest effective dose, or administration with meals. Proton pump inhibitors have demonstrated efficacy in controlled trials for the treatment NSAID-related dyspepsia. Although superiority to H_2-receptor antagonists for relief of NSAID-related dyspepsia has not been established, proton pump inhibitors have demonstrated superiority for healing of NSAID-related ulcers in the setting of continued NSAID use. Therefore, an empiric 2–4 week trial of an oral proton pump inhibitor (omeprazole, rabeprazole, or esomeprazole 20–40 mg/d; lansoprazole, 30 mg/d; pantoprazole, 40 mg/d) is recommended for patients with NSAID-related dyspepsia, especially those in whom continued NSAID treatment is required. If symptoms do not improve, diagnostic upper endoscopy should be conducted.

C. Alcoholic Gastritis

Excessive alcohol consumption may lead to dyspepsia, nausea, emesis, and minor hematemesis—a condition sometimes labeled "alcoholic gastritis." However, it is not proven that alcohol alone actually causes significant erosive gastritis. Therapy with H_2-receptor antagonists, proton pump inhibitors, or sucralfate for 2–4 weeks often is empirically prescribed.

D. Portal Hypertensive Gastropathy

Portal hypertension commonly results in gastric mucosal and submucosal congestion of capillaries and venules, which is correlated with the severity of the portal hypertension and underlying liver disease. Usually asymptomatic, it may cause chronic gastrointestinal bleeding in 10% of patients and, less commonly, clinically significant bleeding with hematemesis. Treatment with propranolol or nadolol reduces the incidence of recurrent acute bleeding by lowering portal pressures. Patients who fail propranolol therapy may be successfully treated with portal decompressive procedures (see section on treatment of esophageal varices).

Hawkey CJ et al. Efficacy of esomeprazole for resolution of symptoms of heartburn and acid regurgitation in continuous users of non-steroidal anti-inflammatory drugs. Aliment Pharmacol Ther. 2007 Apr 1;25(7):813–21. [PMID: 17373920]

Klebl FH et al. Therapy insight: prophylaxis of stress-induced gastrointestinal bleeding in critically ill patients. Nat Clin Pract Gastroenterol Hepatol. 2007 Oct;4(10):562–70. [PMID: 17909533]

Sesler JM. Stress-related mucosal disease in the intensive care unit: an update on prophylaxis. AACN Adv Crit Care. 2007 Apr–Jun;18(2):119–26. [PMID: 17473539]

2. Nonerosive, Nonspecific Gastritis

The diagnosis of nonerosive gastritis is based on histologic assessment of mucosal biopsies. Endoscopic findings are normal in many cases and do not reliably predict the presence of histologic inflammation. The main types of nonerosive gastritis are those due to *H pylori* infection, those associated with pernicious anemia, and lymphocytic gastritis. (See Specific Types of Gastritis below.)

Helicobacter pylori Gastritis

H pylori is a spiral gram-negative rod that resides beneath the gastric mucous layer adjacent to gastric epithelial cells. Although not invasive, it causes gastric mucosal inflammation with PMNs and lymphocytes. The mechanisms of injury and inflammation may in part be related to the products of two genes, *vacA* and *cagA*.

In developed countries the prevalence of *H pylori* is rapidly declining. In the United States, the prevalence rises from less than 10% in non-immigrants under age 30 years to over 50% in those over age 60 years. The prevalence is higher in non-whites and immigrants from developing countries and is correlated inversely with socioeconomic status. Transmission is from person to person, mainly during infancy and childhood; however, the mode of transmission is unknown.

Acute infection with *H pylori* may cause a transient clinical illness characterized by nausea and abdominal pain that may last for several days and is associated with acute histologic gastritis with PMNs. After these symptoms resolve, the majority progress to chronic infection with chronic, diffuse mucosal inflammation (gastritis) characterized by PMNs and lymphocytes. Although chronic *H pylori* infection with gastritis is present in 30–50% of the population, most persons are asymptomatic and suffer no sequelae. Three gastritis phenotypes occur which determine clinical outcomes. Most infected people have a mild, diffuse gastritis that does not disrupt acid secretion and seldom causes clinically important outcomes. About 15% of infected people have inflammation that predominates in the gastric antrum but spares the gastric body (where acid is secreted). People with this phenotype tend to have increased gastrin; increased acid production; and increased risk of developing peptic ulcers, especially duodenal ulcers. About 1% of infected adults have inflammation that predominates in the gastric body. Over time, this may lead to destruction of acid-secreting glands with resultant mucosal atrophy, decreased acid secretion, and intestinal metaplasia. This phenotype is associated with an increased risk of gastric ulcers and gastric cancer. Chronic *H pylori* gastritis is associated with a 3.5- to 20-fold increased risk of gastric adenocarcinoma and low-grade B cell gastric lymphoma (mucosa-associated lymphoid tissue lymphoma; MALToma).

Eradication of *H pylori* may be achieved with antibiotics in over 85% of patients and leads to resolution of the chronic gastritis (see section on Peptic Ulcer Disease). Testing for H pylori is indicated for patients with either active or a past history of documented peptic ulcer disease or gastric MALToma and for patients with a family history of gastric carcinoma. Testing and empiric treatment is cost-effective in young patients (< 55 years of age) with uncomplicated dyspepsia prior to further medical evaluation. The role of testing and treating *H pylori* in patients with functional dyspepsia remains controversial (see Dyspepsia, above). Some groups recommend population-based screening of all asymptomatic persons in regions in which there is a high prevalence of *H pylori* and gastric cancer (such as Japan, Korea, and China) to reduce the incidence of gastric cancer. Population-based screening of asymptomatic individuals is not recommended in western countries, in which the incidence of gastric cancer is low, but should be performed in immigrants from high-prevalence regions.

1. Noninvasive Testing for *H pylori*—Although serologic tests are easily obtained and widely available, most clinical guidelines no longer endorse their use for testing for *H pylori* infection because they are less accurate than other noninvasive tests that measure active infection. Laboratory-based quantitative serologic ELISA tests have an overall accuracy of only 80%. In comparison, the fecal antigen immunoassay and [^{13}C] urea breath test have excellent sensitivity and specificity (> 95%) at a cost of less than $60. Although more expensive and cumbersome to perform, these tests of active infection are more cost-effective in most clinical settings because they reduce unnecessary treatment for patients without active infection.

Recent proton pump inhibitors or antibiotics significantly reduce the sensitivity of urea breath tests and fecal antigen assays (but not serologic tests). Prior to testing, proton pump inhibitors should be discontinued 7–14 days and antibiotics for at least 28 days.

2. Endoscopic Testing for *H pylori*—Endoscopy is not indicated to diagnose *H pylori* infection in most circumstances. However, when it is performed for another reason, gastric biopsy specimens can be obtained for detection of *H pylori* and tested for active infection by urease production. This simple, inexpensive ($10) test has excellent sensitivity and specificity (90%). In patients with active upper gastrointestinal bleeding or patients recently taking proton pump inhibitors or antibiotics, histologic assessment for *H pylori* is preferred. Histologic assessment of biopsies from the gastric antrum and body is more definitive but more expensive ($150–$250) than a rapid urease test. Histologic assessment is also indicated in patients with suspected MALTomas and, possibly, in patients with suspected infection whose rapid urease test is negative. However, serologic testing is the most cost-effective means of confirming *H pylori* infection in patients with a negative rapid urease test.

Amieva MR et al. Host-bacterial interactions in *Helicobacter pylori* infection. Gastroenterology. 2008 Jan;134(1):306–23. [PMID: 18166359]

Chey WD et al. American College of Gastroenterology guideline on the management of *Helicobacter pylori* infection. Am J Gastroenterol. 2007 Aug;102(8):1808–25. [PMID: 17608775]

Makola D et al. *Helicobacter pylori* infection and related gastrointestinal diseases. J Clin Gastroenterol. 2007 Jul;41(6):548–58. [PMID: 17577110]

Talley NJ et al. Gastric cancer consensus conference recommends Helicobacter pylori screening and treatment in asymptomatic persons from high-risk populations to prevent gastric cancer. Am J Gastroenterol. 2008 Mar;103(3):510–4. [PMID: 18341483]

Pernicious Anemia Gastritis

Pernicious anemia gastritis is an autoimmune disorder involving the fundic glands with resultant achlorhydria and vitamin B_{12} malabsorption. Of patients with B_{12} deficiency, less than half have pernicious anemia. Most patients have malabsorption secondary to aging or chronic *H pylori* infection that results in atrophic gastritis, hypochlorhydria, and impaired release of B_{12} from food. Fundic histology in pernicious anemia is characterized by severe gland atrophy and intestinal metaplasia caused by autoimmune destruction of the gastric fundic mucosa. Parietal cell antibodies directed against the H^+-K^+-ATPase pump are present in 90% of patients. Inflammation and autoimmune destruction of the acid-secreting parietal cells leads to secondary loss of fundic zymogen cells, which secrete intrinsic factor. Achlorhydria leads to pronounced hypergastrinemia (> 1000 pg/mL) due to loss of acid inhibition of gastrin G cells. Hypergastrinemia may induce hyperplasia of gastric enterochromaffin-like cells that may lead to the development of small, multicentric carcinoid tumors in 5% of patients. Metastatic spread is uncommon in lesions smaller than 2 cm. The risk of gastric adenocarcinoma is increased threefold, with a prevalence of 1–3%. Endoscopy with biopsy is indicated in patients with pernicious anemia at the time of diagnosis. Patients with dysplasia or small carcinoids require periodic endoscopic surveillance. Pernicious anemia is discussed in detail in Chapter 13.

Malizia RW et al. Ambulatory dysfunction due to unrecognized pernicious anemia. J Emerg Med. 2007 Nov 30; [Epub ahead of print]. [PMID: 18061389]

3. Specific Types of Gastritis

A number of disorders are associated with specific mucosal histologic features.

Infections

Acute bacterial infection of the gastric submucosa and muscularis with a variety of aerobic or anaerobic organisms produces a rare, rapidly progressive, life-threatening condition known as phlegmonous or necrotizing gastritis, which requires broad-spectrum antibiotic therapy and, in many cases, emergency gastric resection. Viral infection with CMV is commonly seen in patients with AIDS and after bone marrow or solid organ transplantation. Endoscopic findings include thickened gastric folds and ulcerations. Fungal infection with mucormycosis and *Candida* may occur in immunocompromised and diabetic patients. Larvae of *Anisakis marina* ingested in raw fish or sushi may become embedded in the gastric mucosa, producing severe abdominal pain. Pain persists for several days until the larvae die. Endoscopic removal of the larvae provides rapid symptomatic relief.

Jung JH et al. Emphysematous gastritis associated with invasive gastric mucormycosis: a case report. J Korean Med Sci. 2007 Oct;22(5):923–7. [PMID: 17982248]

Ugenti I et al. Acute gastric anisakiasis: an Italian experience. Minerva Chir. 2007 Feb;62(1):51–60. [PMID: 17287696]

Eosinophilic Gastritis

This is a rare disorder in which eosinophils infiltrate the antrum and sometimes the proximal intestine. Infiltration may involve the mucosa, muscularis, or serosa. Peripheral eosinophilia is prominent. Symptoms include anemia from mucosal blood loss, abdominal pain, early satiety, and postprandial vomiting. Treatment with corticosteroids is beneficial in the majority of patients.

Ménétrier Disease (Hypertrophic Gastropathy)

This is an idiopathic entity characterized by giant thickened gastric folds involving predominantly the body of the stomach. Patients complain of nausea, epigastric pain, weight loss, and diarrhea. Because of chronic protein loss, patients may develop severe hypoproteinemia and anasarca. The cause is unknown. There are case reports of resolution of symptoms and improvement in histologic appearance after *H pylori* eradication. Dramatic improvement has been reported in a small number of patients with cetuximab, an antibody that binds epidermal growth factor receptor (EGFR). Gastric resection is required in severe cases.

Coffey RJ et al. Ménétrier disease and gastrointestinal stromal tumors: hyperproliferative disorders of the stomach. J Clin Invest. 2007 Jan;117(1):70–80. [PMID: 17200708]

PEPTIC ULCER DISEASE

 ESSENTIALS OF DIAGNOSIS

► History of dyspepsia present in 80–90% of patients with variable relationship to meals.

► Ulcer symptoms characterized by rhythmicity and periodicity.

► Ten to 20 percent of patients present with ulcer complications without antecedent symptoms.

► Most NSAID-induced ulcers are asymptomatic.

► Upper endoscopy with gastric biopsy for *H pylori* is the diagnostic procedure of choice in most patients.

► Gastric ulcer biopsy or documentation of complete healing necessary to exclude gastric malignancy.

General Considerations

Peptic ulcer is a break in the gastric or duodenal mucosa that arises when the normal mucosal defensive factors are impaired or are overwhelmed by aggressive luminal factors such as acid and pepsin. By definition, ulcers extend through the muscularis mucosae and are usually over 5 mm in diameter. In the United States, there are about 500,000 new cases per year of peptic ulcer and 4 million ulcer recurrences; the lifetime prevalence of ulcers in the adult population is approximately 10%. Ulcers occur five times more commonly in the duodenum, where over 95% are in the bulb or pyloric channel. In the stomach, benign ulcers are located most commonly in the antrum (60%) and at the junction of the antrum and body on the lesser curvature (25%).

Ulcers occur slightly more commonly in men than in women (1.3:1). Although ulcers can occur in any age group, duodenal ulcers most commonly occur in patients between the ages of 30 and 55 years, whereas gastric ulcers are more common in patients between the ages of 55 and 70 years. Ulcers are more common in smokers and in patients taking NSAIDs on a long-term basis (see below). Alcohol, dietary factors, and stress do not appear to cause ulcer disease. The incidence of duodenal ulcer disease has been declining dramatically for the past 30 years, but the incidence of gastric ulcers appears to be increasing as a result of the widespread use of NSAIDs and low-dose aspirin.

▶ Etiology

There are three major causes of peptic ulcer disease: NSAIDs, chronic *H pylori* infection, and acid hypersecretory states such as Zollinger-Ellison syndrome. Evidence of *H pylori* infection or NSAID ingestion should be sought in all patients with peptic ulcer. NSAID- and *H pylori*–associated ulcers will be considered in the present section; Zollinger-Ellison syndrome will be discussed subsequently. Uncommon causes of ulcer disease include CMV (especially in transplant recipients), systemic mastocytosis, Crohn disease, lymphoma, and medications (eg, alendronate). Up to 10% of ulcers are idiopathic.

A. *H pylori*–Associated Ulcers

H pylori appears to be a necessary cofactor for the majority of duodenal and gastric ulcers not associated with NSAIDs. Overall, it is estimated that one in six infected patients will develop ulcer disease. The prevalence of *H pylori* infection in duodenal ulcer patients is 75–90%. Most *H pylori*–infected duodenal ulcer patients have infection predominantly in the gastric antrum, which is associated with increased gastric acid secretion. It is hypothesized that increased acid exposure can give rise to small islands of gastric metaplasia in the duodenal bulb. Colonization of these islands by *H pylori* may lead to duodenitis or duodenal ulcer. The association with gastric ulcers is lower, but *H pylori* is found in the majority of patients in whom NSAIDs cannot be implicated. *H pylori*–associated gastric ulcers tend to form at the junction of the gastric body and antrum—the site of transition from oxyntic to pyloric epithelium. Most *H pylori*–infected gastric ulcer patients have infection that predominates in the gastric body and is associated with decreased acid secretion. It is hypothesized that chronic inflammation overwhelms the gastric mucosal defense mechanisms.

The natural history of *H pylori*–associated peptic ulcer disease is well defined. In the absence of specific antibiotic treatment to eradicate the organism, 85% of patients will have an endoscopically visible recurrence within 1 year. Half of these will be symptomatic. After successful eradication of *H pylori* with antibiotics, ulcer recurrence rates are reduced dramatically to 5–20% at 1 year. Some of these ulcer recurrences may be due to NSAID use or reinfection with *H pylori*.

B. NSAID-Induced Ulcers

There is a 10–20% prevalence of gastric ulcers and a 2–5% prevalence of duodenal ulcers in long-term NSAID users. Approximately 2–5%/year of long-term NSAID users will have an ulcer that causes clinically significant dyspepsia or a serious complication. The incidence of serious gastrointestinal complications (hospitalization, bleeding, perforation) is 0.2–1.9%/year. The risk of NSAID complications is greater within the first 3 months of therapy and in patients who are older than 60 years; who have a prior history of ulcer disease; or who take NSAIDs in combination with aspirin, corticosteroids, or anticoagulants.

Traditional nonselective NSAIDs (nsNSAIDs) inhibit prostaglandins through reversible inhibition of both cyclooxygenase (COX)-1 and COX-2 enzymes. Aspirin causes irreversible inhibition of COX-1 and COX-2 as well as of platelet aggregation. Coxibs (or selective NSAIDs) preferentially inhibit COX-2—the principal enzyme involved in prostaglandin production at sites of inflammation—while providing relative sparing of COX-1, the principal enzyme involved with mucosal cytoprotection in the stomach and duodenum. Celecoxib is the only coxib currently available in the United States, although other older NSAIDs (etodolac, meloxicam) may have similar COX-2/COX-1 selectivity.

Coxibs decrease the incidence of endoscopically visible ulcers by approximately 75% compared with nsNSAIDs. Of greater clinical importance, the risk of significant clinical events (obstruction, perforation, bleeding) is reduced by up to 50% in patients taking coxibs versus nsNSAIDs. However, a twofold increase in the incidence in cardiovascular complications (myocardial infarction, cerebrovascular infarction, and death) has been detected in patients taking coxibs compared with placebo, prompting the voluntary withdrawal of two coxibs (rofecoxib and valdecoxib) from the market by the manufacturers. It is hypothesized that selective inhibition of COX-2 leads to decreased vascular prostacyclin, reduced arterial vasodilation, hypertension, enhanced atherogenesis, and enhanced platelet adhesion. In two large, prospective, randomized controlled trials testing the efficacy of coxibs on polyp prevention, celecoxib was associated with a 1.3- to 3.4-fold increased risk of cardiovascular complications versus placebo; the risk was greatest in patients taking higher doses of celecoxib. A review by an FDA panel suggested that all NSAIDs (other than aspirin and, possibly, naproxen) may be associated with an increased risk of cardiovascular complications, but concluded that celecoxib, which has less COX-2 selectivity than rofecoxib and valdecoxib, does not have higher risk than other nsNSAIDs when used in currently recommended doses (200 mg/day).

Use of even low-dose aspirin (81–325 mg/d) leads to a twofold increased risk of gastrointestinal bleeding complications. In randomized controlled trials, the absolute annual increase of gastrointestinal bleeding attributable to low-dose aspirin is only 0.12% higher than with placebo therapy. However, in population studies, gastrointestinal bleeding occurs in 1.2% of patients each year. Patients with a prior history of peptic ulcers or gastrointestinal bleeding have a markedly increased risk of complications on low-dose aspirin. It should be noted that low-dose aspirin in combination with NSAIDs or coxibs increases the risk of ulcer complications by up to 10-fold compared with NSAIDs or low-dose aspirin alone.

H pylori infection increases the risk of ulcer disease and complications over 3-fold in patients taking NSAIDs or low-dose aspirin. It is hypothesized that NSAID initiation may potentiate or aggravate ulcer disease in susceptible infected individuals.

► Clinical Findings

A. Symptoms and Signs

Epigastric pain (dyspepsia), the hallmark of peptic ulcer disease, is present in 80–90% of patients. However, this complaint is not sensitive or specific enough to serve as a reliable diagnostic criterion for peptic ulcer disease. The clinical history cannot accurately distinguish duodenal from gastric ulcers. Less than 25% of patients with dyspepsia have ulcer disease at endoscopy. Twenty percent of patients with ulcer complications such as bleeding have no antecedent symptoms ("silent ulcers"). Nearly 60% of patients with NSAID-related ulcer complications do not have prior symptoms.

Pain is typically well localized to the epigastrium and not severe. It is described as gnawing, dull, aching, or "hunger-like." Approximately 50% of patients report relief of pain with food or antacids (especially duodenal ulcers) and a recurrence of pain 2–4 hours later. However, many patients deny any relationship to meals or report worsening of pain. Two-thirds of duodenal ulcers and one-third of gastric ulcers cause nocturnal pain that awakens the patient. A change from a patient's typical rhythmic discomfort to constant or radiating pain may reflect ulcer penetration or perforation. Most patients have symptomatic periods lasting up to several weeks with intervals of months to years in which they are pain free (periodicity).

Nausea and anorexia may occur with gastric ulcers. Significant vomiting and weight loss are unusual with uncomplicated ulcer disease and suggest gastric outlet obstruction or gastric malignancy.

The physical examination is often normal in uncomplicated peptic ulcer disease. Mild, localized epigastric tenderness to deep palpation may be present. FOBT or FIT is positive in one-third of patients.

B. Laboratory Findings

Laboratory tests are normal in uncomplicated peptic ulcer disease but are ordered to exclude ulcer complications or confounding disease entities. Anemia may occur with acute blood loss from a bleeding ulcer or less commonly from chronic blood loss. Leukocytosis suggests ulcer penetration or perforation. An elevated serum amylase in a patient with severe epigastric pain suggests ulcer penetration into the pancreas. A fasting serum gastrin level to screen for Zollinger-Ellison syndrome is obtained in some patients (see below).

C. Endoscopy

Upper endoscopy is the procedure of choice for the diagnosis of duodenal and gastric ulcers. Duodenal ulcers are virtually never malignant and do not require biopsy. Three to 5 percent of benign-appearing gastric ulcers prove to be malignant. Hence, biopsies of the ulcer margin are almost always performed. Provided that the gastric ulcer appears benign to the endoscopist and adequate biopsy specimens reveal no evidence of cancer, dysplasia, or atypia, the patient may be monitored without further endoscopy. If these conditions are not fulfilled, follow-up endoscopy should be performed 12 weeks after the start of therapy to document complete healing; nonhealing ulcers are suspicious for malignancy.

D. Imaging

Because barium upper gastrointestinal series is less sensitive for detection of ulcers and less accurate for distinguishing benign from malignant ulcers, it has been supplanted by upper endoscopy in most settings. Abdominal CT imaging is obtained in patients with suspected complications of peptic ulcer disease (perforation, penetration, or obstruction).

E. Testing for *H pylori*

In patients in whom an ulcer is diagnosed by endoscopy, gastric mucosal biopsies should be obtained both for a rapid urease test and for histologic examination. The specimens for histology are discarded if the urease test is positive.

In patients with a history of peptic ulcer or when an ulcer is diagnosed by upper gastrointestinal series, noninvasive assessment for *H pylori* with fecal antigen assay or urea breath testing should be done. Proton pump inhibitors may cause false-negative urea breath tests and fecal antigen tests and should be withheld for at least 7 days before testing. Because of its lower sensitivity and specificity, serologic testing should not be performed unless fecal antigen testing or urea breath testing is unavailable.

► Differential Diagnosis

Peptic ulcer disease must be distinguished from other causes of epigastric distress (dyspepsia). Over 50% of patients with dyspepsia have no obvious organic explanation for their symptoms and are classified as having functional dyspepsia (see sections above on Dyspepsia and Functional Dyspepsia). Atypical gastroesophageal reflux may be manifested by epigastric symptoms. Biliary tract disease is characterized by discrete, intermittent episodes of pain that should not be confused with other causes of dyspepsia. Severe epigastric pain is atypical for peptic ulcer disease unless complicated by a perforation or penetration. Other causes include acute pancreatitis, acute cholecystitis or choledocholithiasis, esophageal rupture, gastric volvulus, and ruptured aortic aneurysm.

► Pharmacologic Agents

The pharmacology of several agents that enhance the healing of peptic ulcers is briefly discussed here. They may be divided into three categories: (1) acid-antisecretory agents, (2) mucosal protective agents, and (3) agents that promote healing through eradication of *H pylori*. Recommendations for their use are provided in subsequent sections.

A. Acid-Antisecretory Agents

1. Proton pump inhibitors—Proton pump inhibitors covalently bind the acid-secreting enzyme H^+-K^+-ATPase, or "proton pump," permanently inactivating it. Restoration of acid secretion requires synthesis of new pumps, which have a half-life of 18 hours. Thus, although these agents have a serum half-life of less than 60 minutes, their duration of action exceeds 24 hours. The available oral agents—omeprazole or rabeprazole 20 mg, lansoprazole 30 mg, esomeprazole or pantoprazole 40 mg—inhibit over 90% of 24-hour acid secretion, compared with under 65% for H_2-receptor antagonists in standard dosages. Proton pump inhibitors should be administered 30 minutes before meals (usually breakfast).

Each of the proton pump inhibitors results in over 90% healing of duodenal ulcers after 4 weeks and 90% of gastric ulcers after 8 weeks when given once daily. Compared with H_2-receptor antagonists, proton pump inhibitors provide faster pain relief and more rapid ulcer healing. However, nearly equivalent overall healing rates may be achieved with longer courses of H_2-receptor antagonists.

The proton pump inhibitors are remarkably safe in short- and long-term therapy. Serum gastrin levels rise significantly (> 500 pg/mL) in 3% of patients receiving long-term therapy. Clinical experience with these agents for over 15 years has not detected any significant toxicity in humans. Long-term use may lead to mild decreases in vitamin B_{12}, iron, and calcium absorption of unclear significance. Observational studies suggest a twofold increased risk of enteric infections including *C difficile* and bacterial gastroenteritis. A case-control study reported a 1.4-fold higher risk of hip fracture among patients taking long-term proton pump inhibitors.

2. H_2-receptor antagonists—Although H_2-receptor antagonists are effective in the treatment of peptic ulcer disease, proton pump inhibitors are now the preferred agents because of their ease of use and superior efficacy. Four H_2-receptor antagonists are available: cimetidine, ranitidine, famotidine, and nizatidine. All four agents effectively inhibit nocturnal acid output, but they are less effective at inhibiting meal-stimulated acid secretion. For uncomplicated peptic ulcers, H_2-receptor antagonists may be administered once daily at bedtime as follows: ranitidine and nizatidine 300 mg, famotidine 40 mg, and cimetidine 800 mg. Duodenal and gastric ulcer healing rates of 85–90% are obtained within 6 weeks and 8 weeks, respectively. All four agents are well tolerated, and serious adverse effects are rare. Cimetidine is rarely used because it inhibits hepatic cytochrome P450 metabolism (raising the serum concentration of theophylline, warfarin, lidocaine, and phenytoin) and may cause gynecomastia or impotence.

B. Agents Enhancing Mucosal Defenses

Bismuth, misoprostol, and antacids all have been shown to promote ulcer healing through the enhancement of mucosal defensive mechanisms. Given the greater efficacy and safety of antisecretory agents and better compliance of patients, these other agents are no longer used as first-line therapy for active ulcers in most clinical settings. Because of the rapid relief of ulcer symptoms they provide, antacids are commonly used as needed to supplement antisecretory agents during the first few days of treatment. Bismuth has direct antibacterial action against *H pylori* and may be used in combination with antibiotics for eradication (see below). Misoprostol is a prostaglandin analog that stimulates gastroduodenal mucus and bicarbonate secretion. It is effective as a prophylactic agent in reducing the incidence of gastroduodenal ulcers in patients taking nsNSAIDs but must be given four times daily and causes diarrhea in 10–20% of patients.

C. *H pylori* Eradication Therapy

Eradication of *H pylori* has proved difficult. Combination regimens that use two antibiotics with a proton pump inhibitor or bismuth are required to achieve adequate rates of eradication and to reduce the number of failures due to antibiotic resistance. In the United States, up to 50% of strains are resistant to metronidazole and 13% are resistant to clarithromycin. It is advisable to include amoxicillin in first-line therapy in most patients, reserving metronidazole for penicillin-allergic patients. Recommended regimens are listed in Table 15–10. All currently recommended regimens achieve rates of eradication greater than 80% after 10–14 days of treatment. In most centers in the United States, the preferred regimen is with a 14-day course of treatment with an oral proton pump inhibitor—omeprazole or rabeprazole 20 mg twice daily, lansoprazole 30 mg twice daily, pantoprazole 40 mg twice daily, or esomeprazole 40 mg once daily—plus amoxicillin 1 g twice daily and clarithromycin 500 mg twice daily. In patients who are allergic to penicillin, who have previously been treated with a macrolide antibiotic, or whose infection persists after an initial course of antibiotic therapy, the optimal regimen may be quadruple therapy with a proton pump inhibitor, bismuth subsalicylate, tetracycline, and metronidazole for 14 days (Table 15–10). Several international studies report eradication rates of > 90% using a novel 10-day sequential regimen consisting of a proton pump inhibitor and amoxicillin for 5 days, followed by a proton pump inhibitor, clarithromycin, and tinidazole for 5 days; however, corroboration by studies in North America are needed before this can be accepted as first-line therapy.

► Medical Treatment

Patients should be encouraged to eat balanced meals at regular intervals. There is no justification for bland or restrictive diets. Moderate alcohol intake is not harmful. Smoking retards the rate of ulcer healing and increases the frequency of recurrences and should be discouraged.

A. Treatment of *H pylori*–Associated Ulcers

1. Treatment of active ulcer—The goals of treatment of active *H pylori*–associated ulcers are to relieve dyspeptic symptoms, to promote ulcer healing, and to eradicate *H pylori* infection. Uncomplicated *H pylori*–associated ulcers should be treated for 10–14 days with one of the proton

Table 15–10. Treatment options for peptic ulcer disease.

Active *Helicobacter pylori*-associated ulcer

1. Treat with anti-*H pylori* regimen for 10–14 days. Treatment options:

   - Proton pump inhibitor orally twice daily[1]
     Clarithromycin 500 mg orally twice daily[2]
     Amoxicillin 1 g orally twice daily (OR metronidazole 500 mg orally twice daily, if penicillin allergic[3])

   - Proton pump inhibitor orally twice daily[1,4]
     Bismuth subsalicylate two tablets orally four times daily
     Tetracycline 500 mg orally four times daily
     Metronidazole 250 mg orally four times daily
     (OR bismuth subcitrate potassium 140 mg/metronidazole 125 mg/tetracycline 125 mg [Pylera] three capsules orally four times daily)[5]

   - Proton pump inhibitor orally twice daily[1,6]
     Days 1–5: amoxicillin 1 g orally twice daily
     Days 6–10: clarithromycin 500 mg and metronidazole 500 mg, both orally twice daily

2. After completion of course of *H pylori* eradication therapy, continue treatment with proton pump inhibitor[1] once daily for 4–6 weeks if ulcer is large (> 1 cm) or complicated.

3. Confirm successful eradication of *H pylori* with urea breath test, fecal antigen test, or endoscopy with biopsy at least 4 weeks after completion of antibiotic treatment and 1–2 weeks after proton pump inhibitor treatment.

Active ulcer not attributable to *H pylori*

1. Consider other causes: NSAIDs, Zollinger-Ellison syndrome, gastric malignancy. Treatment options:

   - Proton pump inhibitors[1]:
     Uncomplicated duodenal ulcer: treat for 4 weeks
     Uncomplicated gastric ulcer: treat for 8 weeks

   - H_2-receptor antagonists:
     Uncomplicated duodenal ulcer: cimetidine 800 mg, ranitidine or nizatidine 300 mg, famotidine 40 mg, orally once daily at bedtime for 6 weeks
     Uncomplicated gastric ulcer: cimetidine 400 mg, ranitidine or nizatidine 150 mg, famotidine 20 mg, orally twice daily for 8 weeks
     Complicated ulcers: proton pump inhibitors are the preferred drugs

Prevention of ulcer relapse

1. NSAID-induced ulcer: prophylactic therapy for high-risk patients (prior ulcer disease or ulcer complications, use of corticosteroids or anticoagulants, age > 60 years, serious comorbid illnesses).

   Treatment options:

   Proton pump inhibitor once daily[1]
   COX-2 selective NSAID (celecoxib) (contraindicated in patients with increased risk of cardiovascular disease)
   Misoprostol 200 mcg orally 4 times daily

2. Long-term "maintenance" therapy indicated in patients with recurrent ulcers who either are *H pylori*-negative or who have failed attempts at eradication therapy: once-daily oral proton pump inhibitor[1] or oral H_2-receptor antagonist at bedtime (cimetidine 400–800 mg, nizatidine or ranitidine 150–300 mg, famotidine 20–40 mg)

---

[1]Oral proton pump inhibitors: omeprazole 20 mg, rabeprazole 20 mg, lansoprazole 30 mg, pantoprazole 40 mg, esomeprazole 40 mg. Proton pump inhibitors are administered before meals. Esomeprazole may be given as 40 mg orally once daily.
[2]If patient has previously been treated with macrolide antibiotic, choose another regimen.
[3]Avoid in areas of known high metronidazole resistance or in patients who have failed a course of treatment that included metronidazole.
[4]Preferred regimen in patients who have previously received a macrolide antibiotic or are penicillin allergic. Effective against metronidazole-resistant organisms.
[5]Pylera is an FDA-approved formulation containing: bismuth subcitrate 140 mg/tetracycline 125 mg/metronidazole 125 mg per capsule.
[6]Regimen requires validation in US studies. Appears effective against clarithromycin-resistant organisms.
COX-2, cyclooxygenase-2; NSAIDs, nonsteroidal anti-inflammatory drugs.

pump inhibitor-based *H pylori* eradication regimens listed in Table 15–10. At that point, no further antisecretory therapy is needed, provided the ulcer was small (< 1 cm) and dyspeptic symptoms have resolved. For patients with large or complicated ulcers, an antisecretory agent should be continued for an additional 2–4 weeks (duodenal ulcer) or 4–6 weeks (gastric ulcer) after completion of the antibiotic

regimen to ensure complete ulcer healing. A once-daily oral proton pump inhibitor (omeprazole or rabeprazole 20 mg, lansoprazole 30 mg, pantoprazole or esomeprazole 40 mg) is recommended. Confirmation of *H pylori* eradication is recommended for all patients > 4 weeks after completion of therapy either with noninvasive tests (urea breath test, fecal antigen test) or endoscopy with biopsy for histology.

2. Therapy to prevent recurrence—Successful eradication reduces ulcer recurrences to less than 20% after 1–2 years. The most common cause of recurrence after antibiotic therapy is failure to achieve successful eradication. Once cure has been achieved, reinfection rates are less than 0.5% per year. Although *H pylori* eradication has reduced the need for long-term maintenance antisecretory therapy to prevent ulcer recurrences, there remains a subset of patients who require long-term therapy with either a proton pump inhibitor once daily or an H_2-receptor antagonist at bedtime. This subset includes patients with *H pylori*–positive ulcers who have not responded to repeated attempts at eradication therapy, patients with a history of *H pylori*–positive ulcers who have recurrent ulcers despite successful eradication, and patients with idiopathic ulcers (ie, *H pylori*–negative and not taking NSAIDs). In all patients with recurrent ulcers, NSAID usage (unintentional or surreptitious) and hypersecretory states (including gastrinoma) should be excluded.

B. Treatment of NSAID-Associated Ulcers

1. Treatment of active ulcers—In patients with NSAID-induced ulcers, the offending agent should be discontinued whenever possible. Both gastric and duodenal ulcers respond rapidly to therapy with H_2-receptor antagonists or proton pump inhibitors (Table 15–10) once NSAIDs are eliminated. In some patients with severe inflammatory diseases, it may not be feasible to discontinue NSAIDs. These patients should be treated with proton pump inhibitors once daily, which results in ulcer healing rates of approximately 80% at 8 weeks in patients continuing to take NSAIDs. All patients with NSAID-associated ulcers should undergo testing for *H pylori* infection. Antibiotic eradication therapy should be given if *H pylori* tests are positive.

2. Prevention of NSAID-induced ulcers—Clinicians should carefully weigh the benefits of NSAID therapy with the risks of cardiovascular and gastrointestinal complications. For all patients, NSAIDs should be prescribed at the lowest effective dose and for the shortest period possible. Both COX-2 selective NSAIDs ("coxibs") and nonselective NSAIDs (nsNSAIDS) with the possible exception of naproxen increase the risk of cardiovascular complications. Ulcer complications occur in up to 2% of all nsNSAID-treated patients per year but in up to 10–20% per year of patients with multiple risk factors. These include age over 60 years, history of ulcer disease or complications, concurrent use of antiplatelet therapy (low-dose aspirin or clopidogrel, or both), concurrent therapy with anticoagulants or corticosteroids, and serious underlying medical illness. After considering the patient's risk of cardiovascular and gastrointestinal complications due to NSAID use, the clinician can decide what type of NSAID (nsNSAID vs coxib) is appropriate and what strategies should be used to reduce the risk of such complications.

A. Test for and treat *H pylori* infection—All patients with a known history of peptic ulcer disease who are treated with NSAIDs or antiplatelet agents (aspirin, clopidogrel) should be tested for *H pylori* infection and treated, if

positive. Although *H pylori* eradication may decrease the risk of NSAID-related complications, cotherapy with a proton pump inhibitor or misoprostol therapy is still required in high-risk patients.

B. Proton pump inhibitor—Treatment with an oral proton pump inhibitor given once daily (omeprazole or rabeprazole 20 mg, lansoprazole 30 mg, or pantoprazole or esomeprazole 20–40 mg) is effective in the prevention of NSAID-induced gastric and duodenal ulcers and is approved by the FDA for this indication. Among high-risk patients taking nsNSAIDs or coxibs, the incidence of endoscopically visible gastric and duodenal ulcers after 6 months of therapy in patients treated with esomeprazole 20–40 mg/d was 5%, compared with 17% who were given placebo. Nonetheless, proton pump inhibitors are not fully protective in high-risk patients in preventing NSAID-related complications. In prospective, controlled trials of patients with a prior history of NSAID-related ulcer complications, the incidence of recurrent bleeding was almost 5% after 6 months in patients taking nsNSAIDs and a proton pump inhibitor. In prospective, controlled trials of patients with a prior history of ulcer complications related to low-dose aspirin, the incidence of recurrent ulcer bleeding in patients taking low-dose aspirin alone is approximately 15% per year, compared with 0–2% per year in patients taking low-dose aspirin and proton pump inhibitor and 9–14% per year in patients taking clopidogrel. Thus, proton pump inhibitors are highly effective in preventing complications related to low-dose aspirin, even in high-risk patients.

C. Misoprostol—The prostaglandin analog misoprostol reduces the incidence of NSAID-induced gastric and duodenal ulcers by 50–75% when given at a dosage of 100–200 mcg four times daily. In a large, prospective study, misoprostol reduced the incidence of NSAID-associated complications by 40% compared with placebo. However, misoprostol is less commonly used as a prophylactic agent against NSAID-induced complications than either concurrent therapy with a proton pump inhibitor or COX-2 selective agent because of its high side-effect profile and the need for dosing four times daily.

3. Recommendations for use of nsNSAIDs and coxibs—For patients with a low-risk of cardiovascular disease who have no risk factors for gastrointestinal complications, an nsNSAID alone may be given. For patients with 1-2 gastrointestinal risk factors, a coxib alone or an nsNSAID should be given with a proton pump inhibitor once daily (omeprazole or rabeprazole 20 mg, lansoprazole 30 mg, or pantoprazole or esomeprazole 20–40 mg) or misoprostol to reduce the risk of gastrointestinal complications. NSAIDs should be avoided if possible in patients with multiple risk factors. If required, combination therapy with a coxib or one of the "safer" nsNSAIDs (etodolac, meloxicam) and a proton pump inhibitor once daily is recommended.

For patients with an increased risk of cardiovascular complications, it is preferable to avoid NSAIDs, if possible. If an NSAID is required, naproxen is preferred because it appears to have reduced risk of cardiovascular complications compared with other nsNSAIDs. Coxibs should not be prescribed in patients with increased cardiovascular risk. Almost all patients with increased cardiovascular risk also will be taking antiplatelet therapy with low-dose aspirin or clopidogrel, or both. Because combination therapy with an nsNSAID and antiplatelet therapy increases the risks of gastrointestinal complications, these patients should all receive cotherapy with a proton pump inhibitor once daily or misoprostol.

4. Recommendations for use of antiplatelet agents— The risk of significant gastrointestinal complications in persons taking Low-dose aspirin (81–325 mg/d) or clopidogrel, or both, for cardiovascular prophylaxis is 0.5%/year. Aspirin, 81 mg/d, is recommended in most patients because it has a lower risk of gastrointestinal complications but equivalent cardiovascular protection compared with higher aspirin doses. Complications are increased with combinations of aspirin and clopidogrel or aspirin and anticoagulants. Patients with dyspepsia or prior ulcer disease should be tested for *H pylori* infection and treated, if positive. Patients younger than age 60 who have no other risk factors for gastrointestinal complications may be treated with low-dose aspirin alone without a proton pump inhibitor or misoprostol. Virtually all other patients who require low-dose aspirin, dual antiplatelet therapy (aspirin and clopidogrel), or aspirin and anticoagulant therapy should receive a proton pump inhibitor once daily. Recent studies suggest that proton pump inhibitors that are metabolized by CYP2C19 may inhibit activation of clopidogrel, reducing its antiplatelet effects.

C. Refractory Ulcers

Ulcers that are truly refractory to medical therapy are now uncommon. Less than 5% of ulcers are unhealed after 8 weeks of therapy with proton pump inhibitors. Noncompliance is the most common cause of ulcer nonhealing. Cigarettes retard ulcer healing and should be proscribed. NSAID and aspirin use, sometimes surreptitious, are commonly implicated in refractory ulcers and must be stopped. *H pylori* infection should be sought and the infection treated, if present, in all refractory ulcer patients. Fasting serum gastrin levels should be obtained to exclude gastrinoma with acid hypersecretion (Zollinger-Ellison syndrome). Nonhealing gastric ulcers raise concerns that an undiagnosed gastric malignancy may be masquerading as a benign gastric ulcer. Repeat ulcer biopsies are mandatory after 2–3 months of therapy in all nonhealed gastric ulcers, and they should be followed with serial endoscopies to verify complete healing. Almost all benign refractory ulcers heal within 8 weeks with an oral proton pump inhibitor twice daily (omeprazole or rabeprazole 20 mg, lansoprazole 30 mg). Patients with persistent nonhealing ulcers are referred for surgical therapy after exclusion of NSAID use and persistent *H pylori* infection.

Bhatt DL et al. ACCF/ACG/AHA 2008 expert consensus document on reducing the gastrointestinal risks of antiplatelet therapy and NSAID use. Am J Gastroenterol. 2008 Nov;103(11):2890-2907. [PMID: 18853965]

Chan FK. Use of nonsteroidal antiinflammatory drugs in a COX-2 restricted environment. Am J Gastroenterol. 2008 Jan;103(1):221–7. [PMID: 17900323]

Chey WD et al. American College of Gastroenterology guideline on the management of *Helicobacter pylori* infection. Am J Gastroenterol. 2007 Aug;102(8):1808–25. [PMID: 17608775]

García Rodríguez LA et al. Risk of upper gastrointestinal complications among users of traditional NSAIDs and COXIBs in the general population. Gastroenterology. 2007 Feb;132(2):498–506. [PMID: 17258728]

Gilard M et al. Influence of omeprazole on the antiplatelet action of clopidogrel associated with aspirin: the randomized, double-blind OCLA (Omeprazole Clopidogrel Aspirin) study. J Am Coll Cardiol. 2008 Jan;51(3):256–60. [PMID: 18206732]

Jafri NS et al. Meta-analysis: sequential therapy appears superior to standard therapy for *Helicobacter pylori* infection in patients naïve to treatment. Ann Intern Med. 2008 Jun 17;148(12):923–31. [PMID: 18490667]

Leonard J et al. Systematic review of the risk of enteric infection in patients taking acid suppression. Am J Gastroenterol. 2007 Sep;102(9):2047–56. [PMID: 17509031]

Moayyedi P et al. Hip fracture and proton pump inhibitor therapy: balancing the evidence for benefit and harm. Am J Gastroenterol. 2008 Oct;103(10):2428–31. [PMID: 18855852]

Ray WA et al. Risk of peptic ulcer hospitalizations in users of NSAIDs with gastroprotective cotherapy versus coxibs. Gastroenterology. 2007 Sep;133(3):790–8. [PMID: 17854591]

Rostom A et al. Gastrointestinal safety of cyclooxygenase-2 inhibitors: a Cochrane Collaboration systematic review. Clin Gastroenterol Hepatol. 2007 Jul;5(7):818–28. [PMID: 17556027]

Saad RJ et al. Persistent *Helicobacter pylori* infection after a course of antimicrobial therapy—what's next? Clin Gastroenterol Hepatol. 2008 Oct;6(10):1086–90. [PMID: 18639497]

Vakil N et al. Eradication therapy for *Helicobacter pylori*. Gastroenterology. 2007 Sep;133(3):985–1001. [PMID: 17854602]

COMPLICATIONS OF PEPTIC ULCER DISEASE

1. Gastrointestinal Hemorrhage

 ESSENTIALS OF DIAGNOSIS

▶ "Coffee grounds" emesis, hematemesis, melena, or hematochezia.

▶ Emergent upper endoscopy is diagnostic and therapeutic.

▶ General Considerations

Approximately 50% of all episodes of upper gastrointestinal bleeding are due to peptic ulcer. Clinically significant bleeding occurs in 10% of ulcer patients. About 80% of patients stop bleeding spontaneously and generally have an uneventful recovery; the remaining 20% have more severe bleeding. The overall mortality rate for ulcer bleeding is 4%, but it is higher in the elderly, in patients with comorbid medical problems, and in patients with hospital-associated bleeding. Mortality is also higher in patients who present with persistent hypotension or shock, bright red blood in the vomitus or nasogastric lavage fluid, or severe coagulopathy.

Clinical Findings

A. Symptoms and Signs

Up to 20% of patients have no antecedent symptoms of pain; this is particularly true of patients receiving NSAIDs. Common presenting signs include melena and hematemesis. Massive upper gastrointestinal bleeding or rapid gastrointestinal transit may result in hematochezia rather than melena; this may be misinterpreted as signifying a lower tract bleeding source. Nasogastric lavage that demonstrates "coffee grounds" or bright red blood confirms an upper tract source. Recovered nasogastric lavage fluid that is negative for blood does not exclude active bleeding from a duodenal ulcer.

B. Laboratory Findings

The hematocrit may fall as a result of bleeding or expansion of the intravascular volume with intravenous fluids. The blood urea nitrogen (BUN) may rise as a result of absorption of blood nitrogen from the small intestine and prerenal azotemia.

Treatment

The assessment and initial management of upper gastrointestinal tract bleeding are discussed elsewhere in this chapter. Specific issues pertaining to peptic ulcer bleeding are described below.

A. Medical Therapy

1. Antisecretory agents—Intravenous proton pump inhibitors or high-dose oral proton pump inhibitors should be administered for 3 days in patients with ulcers whose endoscopic appearance suggests a high risk of rebleeding after endoscopic therapy. Intravenous or high-dose proton pump inhibitors have been associated with a reduction in rebleeding, transfusions, the need for further endoscopic therapy, and surgery in the subset of patients with high-risk ulcers, ie, an ulcer with active bleeding, visible vessel, or adherent clot (see below). After initial successful endoscopic treatment of ulcer hemorrhage, intravenous omeprazole (80 mg bolus injection, followed by 8 mg/h continuous infusion for 72 hours) reduces the rebleeding rate from approximately 20% to < 10%; however, intravenous omeprazole is not available in the United States. In the United States, intravenous esomeprazole and pantoprazole are available and commonly used at comparable dosing (80 mg bolus injection, followed by 8 mg/h) for this indication, although published data confirming their efficacy are unavailable.

High-dose oral proton pump inhibitors (omeprazole 40 mg twice daily) also appear to be effective in reducing rebleeding but have not been compared with the intravenous regimen. Many physicians choose to administer a high-dose proton pump inhibitor prior to endoscopy in all patients admitted to the hospital with gastrointestinal bleeding suspected to be due to peptic ulcer, discontinuing therapy after endoscopy in patients with ulcers deemed to be at low risk of rebleeding. Intravenous H$_2$-receptor antagonists have not been demonstrated to be of any benefit in the treatment of acute ulcer bleeding.

2. Long-term prevention of rebleeding—Recurrent ulcer bleeding develops within 3 years in one-third of patients if no specific therapy is given. In patients with bleeding ulcers who are *H pylori*-positive, successful eradication effectively prevents recurrent ulcer bleeding in almost all cases. It is therefore recommended that all patients with bleeding ulcers be tested for *H pylori* infection and treated if positive. Four to 8 weeks after completion of antibiotic therapy, a urea breath or fecal antigen test for *H pylori* should be administered or endoscopy performed with biopsy for histologic confirmation of successful eradication. In patients in whom *H pylori* persists or the small subset of patients whose ulcers are not associated with NSAIDs or *H pylori*, long-term acid suppression with a once-daily proton pump inhibitor should be prescribed to reduce the likelihood of recurrence of bleeding.

B. Endoscopy

Endoscopy is the preferred diagnostic procedure in almost all cases of upper gastrointestinal bleeding because of its high diagnostic accuracy, its ability to predict the likelihood of recurrent bleeding, and its availability for therapeutic intervention in high-risk lesions. Endoscopy should be performed within 12–24 hours in most cases. In cases of severe active bleeding, endoscopy is performed as soon as patients have been appropriately resuscitated and are hemodynamically stable.

On the basis of clinical and endoscopic criteria, it is possible to predict which patients are at a higher risk of rebleeding and therefore to make more rational use of hospital resources. Nonbleeding ulcers under 2 cm in size with a base that is clean have a less than 5% chance of rebleeding. Most young (under age 60 years), otherwise healthy patients with clean-based ulcers may be safely discharged from the emergency department or hospital after endoscopy. Ulcers that have a flat red or black spot have a less than 10% chance of significant rebleeding. Patients who are hemodynamically stable with these findings should be admitted to a hospital ward for 24–72 hours and may begin immediate oral feedings and antiulcer (or anti-*H pylori*) medication.

By contrast, the risk of rebleeding or continued bleeding in ulcers with a firmly adherent clot is 12–33%, with a nonbleeding visible vessel is 50%, and with active bleeding it is 80–90%. Endoscopic therapy with thermocoagulation (bipolar or heater probes) or application of endoscopic clips (akin to a staple) is the standard of care for such lesions because it reduces the risk of rebleeding, the number of transfusions, and the need for subsequent surgery. For actively bleeding ulcers, a combination of epinephrine injection followed by thermocoagulation or clip application commonly is used. These techniques achieve successful hemostasis of actively bleeding lesions in 90% of patients. Significant rebleeding occurs in 10–20% of cases, of which over 70% can be managed successfully with repeat endoscopic treatment. After endoscopic treatment, high-risk patients should be monitored in an ICU setting for at least 24 hours and should remain hospitalized for at least 72 hours, when the risk of rebleeding is less than 3%.

C. Surgical Treatment

Patients with recurrent bleeding or bleeding that cannot be controlled by endoscopic techniques should be evaluated by a surgeon. However, less than 5% of patients treated with hemostatic therapy require surgery for continued or recurrent bleeding. Overall surgical mortality for emergency ulcer bleeding is less than 6%. The prognosis is poorer for patients over age 60 years, those with serious underlying medical illnesses or chronic renal failure, and those who require more than 10 units of blood transfusion.

2. Ulcer Perforation

Perforations develop in less than 5% of ulcer patients, usually from ulcers on the anterior wall of the stomach or duodenum. The incidence of perforations may be increasing, perhaps as a consequence of using NSAIDs or crack cocaine. Perforation results in a chemical peritonitis that causes sudden, severe generalized abdominal pain that prompts most patients to seek immediate attention. Elderly or debilitated patients and those receiving long-term corticosteroid therapy may experience minimal initial symptoms, presenting late with bacterial peritonitis, sepsis, and shock. On physical examination, patients appear ill, with a rigid, quiet abdomen and rebound tenderness. Hypotension develops later after bacterial peritonitis has developed. If hypotension is present early with the onset of pain, other abdominal emergencies should be considered such as a ruptured aortic aneurysm, mesenteric infarction, or acute pancreatitis. Leukocytosis is almost always present. A mildly elevated serum amylase (less than twice normal) is sometimes seen. Abdominal CT usually establishes the diagnosis without need for further studies. The absence of free air may lead to a misdiagnosis of pancreatitis, cholecystitis, or appendicitis.

Traditional surgical dogma held that the majority of patients with perforated ulcers should undergo emergency laparotomy. Closure of the perforation was performed with an omental ("Graham") patch and, in stable patients, a proximal gastric vagotomy was performed to decrease the chance of ulcer recurrence. This approach has changed for two reasons. The first is minimally invasive surgical technique. Laparoscopic perforation closure can be performed in many centers, significantly reducing operative morbidity. Second is the recognition that H pylori infection is associated with most ulcers and ulcer perforations. Postoperative treatment of H pylori reduces the risk of ulcer recurrence, obviating the need for intraoperative vagotomy. The overall mortality rate in patients treated surgically is 5%.

Up to 40% of ulcer perforations seal spontaneously by the adherence of omentum or adjacent organs to the lesion and do not have significant intraperitoneal spillage. Thus, initial nonoperative management may be suitable for patients whose onset of symptoms is less than 12 hours and whose upper gastrointestinal series with water-soluble contrast medium does not demonstrate leakage. Such conservative therapy is most appropriate for patients who are poor operative candidates. Patients should be monitored closely while receiving fluids, nasogastric suction, intravenous proton pump inhibitors, and broad-spectrum antibiotics. If their condition deteriorates over the first 12 hours (as evidenced by increasing pain, rising pulse or temperature, or worsening peritonitis), they should be taken to the operating room.

3. Ulcer Penetration

An ulcer located along the posterior wall of the duodenum or stomach may perforate into contiguous structures such as the pancreas, liver, or biliary tree. Patients complain of a change in the intensity and rhythmicity of their ulcer symptoms. The pain becomes more severe and constant, may radiate to the back, and is unresponsive to antacids or food. Physical examination and laboratory tests are nonspecific. Mild amylase elevations may sometimes occur. Endoscopy and barium x-ray studies confirm the ulceration but are not diagnostic of an actual penetration. Patients should be given intravenous proton pump inhibitors and monitored closely. Those who do not improve should be considered for surgery.

4. Gastric Outlet Obstruction

Gastric outlet obstruction occurs in < 2% of patients with ulcer disease and is due to edema or cicatricial narrowing of the pylorus or duodenal bulb. With the advent of potent antisecretory therapy with proton pump inhibitors and the eradication of H pylori, obstruction now is less commonly caused by peptic ulcers than by gastric neoplasms or extrinsic duodenal obstruction by intra-abdominal neoplasms. The most common symptoms are early satiety, vomiting, and weight loss. Early symptoms are epigastric fullness or heaviness after meals. Later, vomiting may develop that typically occurs one to several hours after eating and consists of partially digested food contents. Chronic obstruction may result in a grossly dilated, atonic stomach, severe weight loss, and malnutrition. Patients may develop dehydration, metabolic alkalosis, and hypokalemia. On physical examination, a succussion splash may be heard in the epigastrium. In most cases, nasogastric aspiration will result in evacuation of a large amount (> 200 mL) of foul-smelling fluid, which establishes the diagnosis. Patients are treated initially with intravenous isotonic saline and KCl to correct fluid and electrolyte disorders, an intravenous proton pump inhibitor, and nasogastric decompression of the stomach. Upper endoscopy is performed after 24–72 hours to define the nature of the obstruction and to exclude gastric neoplasm. In patients with gastric outlet obstruction caused by peptic ulcer disease, dilation of the gastric obstruction by hydrostatic balloons passed through the endoscope improves symptoms in up to two-thirds of patients; repeat dilations may be necessary. Surgical treatment with vagotomy and either pyloroplasty or antrectomy is required in patients with inadequate response or symptom relapse after endoscopic dilation.

Andriulli A et al. High- versus low-dose proton pump inhibitors after endoscopic hemostasis in patients with peptic ulcer bleeding: a multicentre, randomized study. Am J Gastroenterol. 2008 Dec;103(12):3011–8. [PMID: 19086953]

Cherian PT et al. Long-term follow-up of patients with gastric outlet obstruction related to peptic ulcer disease treated with endoscopic balloon dilatation and drug therapy. Gastrointest Endosc. 2007 Sep;66(3):491–7. [PMID: 17640640]

Gralnek IM et al. Management of acute bleeding from a peptic ulcer. N Engl J Med. 2008 Aug 28;359(9):928–37. [PMID: 18753649]

Laine L et al. Endoscopic therapy for bleeding ulcers: an evidence-based approach based on meta-analyses of randomized controlled trials. Clin Gastroenterol Hepatol. 2009 Jan;7(1):33–47. [PMID: 18986845]

Lau JY et al. Omeprazole before endoscopy in patients with gastrointestinal bleeding. N Engl J Med. 2007 Apr 19;356(16):1631–40. [PMID: 17442905]

Vergara M et al. Epinephrine injection versus epinephrine injection and a second endoscopic method in high risk bleeding ulcers. Cochrane Database Syst Rev. 2007 Apr 18;(2):CD005584. [PMID: 17443601]

Yuan Y et al. Endoscopic clipping for acute nonvariceal upper-GI bleeding: a meta-analysis and critical appraisal of randomized controlled trials. Gastrointest Endosc. 2008 Aug;68(2):339–51. [PMID: 18656600]

ZOLLINGER-ELLISON SYNDROME (Gastrinoma)

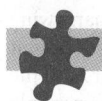 ESSENTIALS OF DIAGNOSIS

▶ Peptic ulcer disease; may be severe and atypical.

▶ Gastric acid hypersecretion.

▶ Diarrhea common, relieved by nasogastric suction.

▶ Most cases are sporadic; 25% with multiple endocrine neoplasia type 1 (MEN 1).

▶ General Considerations

Zollinger-Ellison syndrome is caused by gastrin-secreting gut neuroendocrine tumors (gastrinomas), which result in hypergastrinemia and acid hypersecretion. Less than 1% of peptic ulcer disease is caused by gastrinomas. Primary gastrinomas may arise in the pancreas (25%), duodenal wall (45%), or lymph nodes (5–15%), and in other locations or of unknown primary in 20%. Approximately 80% arise within the "gastrinoma triangle" bounded by the porta hepatis, the neck of the pancreas, and the third portion of the duodenum. Most gastrinomas are solitary or multifocal nodules that are potentially resectable. Over two-thirds of gastrinomas are malignant, and one-third have already metastasized to the liver at initial presentation. Approximately 25% of patients have small multicentric gastrinomas associated with MEN 1 that are more difficult to resect.

▶ Clinical Findings

A. Symptoms and Signs

Over 90% of patients with Zollinger-Ellison syndrome develop peptic ulcers. In most cases, the symptoms are indistinguishable from other causes of peptic ulcer disease and therefore may go undetected for years. Ulcers usually are solitary and located in the duodenal bulb, but they may be multiple or occur more distally in the duodenum. Isolated gastric ulcers do not occur. Gastroesophageal reflux symptoms occur often. Diarrhea occurs in one-third of patients, in some cases in the absence of peptic symptoms. Gastric acid hypersecretion can cause direct intestinal mucosal injury and pancreatic enzyme inactivation, resulting in diarrhea, steatorrhea, and weight loss; nasogastric aspiration of stomach acid stops the diarrhea. Screening for Zollinger-Ellison syndrome with fasting gastrin levels should be obtained in patients with ulcers that are refractory to standard therapies, giant ulcers (> 2 cm), ulcers located distal to the duodenal bulb, multiple duodenal ulcers, frequent ulcer recurrences, ulcers associated with diarrhea, ulcers occurring after ulcer surgery, and patients with ulcer complications. Ulcer patients with hypercalcemia or family histories of ulcers (suggesting MEN 1) should also be screened. Finally, patients with peptic ulcers who are *H pylori* negative and who are not taking NSAIDs should be screened.

B. Laboratory Findings

The most sensitive and specific method for identifying Zollinger-Ellison syndrome is demonstration of an increased fasting serum gastrin concentration (> 150 pg/mL). Levels should be obtained with patients not taking H_2-receptor antagonists for 24 hours or proton pump inhibitors for 6 days. The median gastrin level is 500–700 pg/mL, and 60% of patients have levels less than 1000 pg/mL. Hypochlorhydria with increased gastric pH is a much more common cause of hypergastrinemia than is gastrinoma. Therefore, a measurement of gastric pH (and, where available, gastric secretory studies) is performed in patients with fasting hypergastrinemia. Most patients have a basal acid output of over 15 mEq/h. A gastric pH of > 3.0 implies hypochlorhydria and excludes gastrinoma. In a patient with a serum gastrin level of > 1000 pg/mL and acid hypersecretion, the diagnosis of Zollinger-Ellison syndrome is established. With lower gastrin levels (150–1000 pg/mL) and acid secretion, a secretin stimulation test is performed to distinguish Zollinger-Ellison syndrome from other causes of hypergastrinemia. Intravenous secretin (2 units/kg) produces a rise in serum gastrin of over 200 pg/mL within 2–30 minutes in 85% of patients with gastrinoma. An elevated serum calcium suggests hyperparathyroidism and MEN 1 syndrome. In all patients with Zollinger-Ellison syndrome, a serum parathyroid hormone (PTH), prolactin, luteinizing hormone-follicle-stimulating hormone (LH-FSH), and growth hormone (GH) level should be obtained to exclude MEN 1.

C. Imaging

Imaging studies are obtained in an attempt to determine whether there is metastatic disease and, if not, to identify the site of the primary tumor. Gastrinomas express somatostatin receptors that bind radiolabeled octreotide. Somatostatin receptor scintigraphy (SRS) with single photon emission computed tomography (SPECT) allows total body imaging for detection of primary gastrinomas in the pancreas and lymph nodes, primary gastrinomas in unusual locations, and metastatic gastrinomas (liver and bone). SRS has a sensitivity (> 80%) for tumor detection that exceeds all other imaging studies combined. If SRS is positive for tumor localization, further imaging studies are not necessary. In patients with negative SRS, endoscopic ultrasonography (EUS) may be useful to detect small gastrinomas in the duodenal wall, pancreas, or peripancreatic lymph nodes. CT and MRI scans are commonly obtained to look for large hepatic metastases and primary lesions, but they have low sensitivity for small lesions. With a combination of SRS and EUS, more than 90% of primary gastrinomas can be localized preoperatively.

▶ Differential Diagnosis

Gastrinomas are one of several gut neuroendocrine tumors that have similar histopathologic features and arise either from the gut or pancreas. These include carcinoid, insulinoma, VIPoma, glucagonoma, and somatostatinoma. These tumors usually are differentiated by the gut peptides that they secrete; however, poorly differentiated neuroendocrine tumors may not secrete any hormones. Patients may present with symptoms caused by tumor metastases (jaundice, hepatomegaly) rather than functional symptoms. Once a diagnosis of a neuroendocrine tumor is established from the liver biopsy, the specific type of tumor can subsequently be determined. Both carcinoids and gastrinomas may be detected incidentally during endoscopy after biopsy of a submucosal nodule and must be distinguished by subsequent studies.

Hypergastrinemia due to gastrinoma must be distinguished from other causes of hypergastrinemia. Atrophic gastritis with decreased acid secretion is detected by gastric secretory analysis. Other conditions associated with hypergastrinemia (eg, gastric outlet obstruction, vagotomy, chronic renal failure) are associated with a negative secretin stimulation test.

▶ Treatment

A. Metastatic Disease

The most important predictor of survival is the presence of hepatic metastases. In patients with multiple hepatic metastases, initial therapy should be directed at controlling hypersecretion. Oral proton pump inhibitors (omeprazole, esomeprazole, rabeprazole, pantoprazole, or lansoprazole) are given at a dose of 40–120 mg/d, titrated to achieve a basal acid output of < 10 mEq/h. At this level, there is complete symptomatic relief and ulcer healing. In patients with isolated hepatic metastases, surgical resection or cryoablation may decrease the need for antisecretory medications and may prolong survival. Owing to the slow growth of these tumors, 30% of patients with hepatic metastases have a survival of 10 years.

B. Localized Disease

Cure can be achieved only if the gastrinoma can be resected before hepatic metastatic spread has occurred. Lymph node metastases do not adversely affect prognosis. Laparotomy should be considered in all patients in whom preoperative studies fail to demonstrate hepatic or other distant metastases. A combination of preoperative studies, duodenotomy with careful duodenal inspection, and intraoperative palpation and sonography allows successful localization and resection in the majority of cases. The 15-year survival of patients who do not have liver metastases at initial presentation is over 95%. The role of surgery in patients with MEN 1 is controversial. Surgical cure in patients with MEN 1 rarely occurs, and long-term survival is common in the absence of surgery. Some experts recommend surgery only in patients with MEN 1 whose tumors are larger than 2 cm, in whom the risk of hepatic metastases is increased.

Ellison EC et al. The Zollinger-Ellison syndrome: a comprehensive review of historical, scientific, and clinical considerations. Curr Probl Surg. 2009 Jan;46(1):13–106. [PMID: 19059523]

BENIGN TUMORS OF THE STOMACH

Gastric epithelial polyps are usually detected incidentally at endoscopy. The majority are fundic gland polyps or hyperplastic polyps, which are small, single or multiple, have no malignant potential, and do not require removal or endoscopic surveillance. Adenomatous polyps account for 10–20% of gastric polyps. They are usually solitary lesions. In rare instances they ulcerate, causing chronic blood loss. Because of their premalignant potential, endoscopic removal is indicated. Annual endoscopic surveillance is recommended to screen for further polyp development. Submucosal gastric polypoid lesions include benign gastric stromal tumors (commonly misclassified as leiomyomas) and pancreatic rests. (**See Chapter 39 for Gastric Adenocarcinoma, Lymphoma, Carcinoid Tumors, and Mesenchymal Tumors.**)

Hirota WK et al. ASGE Guideline: the role of endoscopy in the surveillance of premalignant conditions of the upper GI tract. Gastrointest Endosc. 2006 Apr;63(4):570–80. [PMID: 16564854]
Jalving M et al; Standards of Practice Committee, American Society for Gastrointestinal Endoscopy. Increased risk of fundic gland polyps during long-term proton pump inhibitor therapy. Aliment Pharmacol Ther. 2006 Nov 1;24(9):1341–8. [PMID: 17059515]

▼ DISEASES OF THE SMALL INTESTINE

MALABSORPTION

The term "malabsorption" denotes disorders in which there is a disruption of digestion and nutrient absorption. The clinical and laboratory manifestations of malabsorption are summarized in Table 15–11.

▶ Pathogenesis

Normal digestion and absorption may be divided into three phases: intraluminal, mucosal, and absorptive.

A. Intraluminal Phase

Dietary fats, proteins, and carbohydrates are hydrolyzed and solubilized by pancreatic and biliary secretions. Fats

Table 15–11. Clinical manifestations and laboratory findings in malabsorption of various nutrients.

Manifestations	Laboratory Findings	Malabsorbed Nutrients
Steatorrhea (bulky, light-colored stools)	Increased fecal fat; decreased serum cholesterol; decreased serum carotene, vitamin A, vitamin D	Triglycerides, fatty acids, phospholipids, cholesterol. Fat soluble vitamins: A, D, E, K
Diarrhea (increased fecal water)	Increased stool volume and weight; increased fecal fat; increased stool osmolality gap	Fats; carbohydrates
Weight loss; muscle wasting	Increased fecal fat; decreased carbohydrate (D-xylose) absorption	Fat, protein, carbohydrates
Microcytic anemia	Low serum iron	Iron
Macrocytic anemia	Decreased serum vitamin B_{12} or red blood cell folate	Vitamin B_{12} or folic acid
Paresthesia; tetany; positive Trousseau and Chvostek signs	Decreased serum calcium or magnesium	Calcium, vitamin D, magnesium
Bone pain; pathologic fractures; skeletal deformities	Osteopenia on radiograph; osteoporosis (adults); osteomalacia (children)	Calcium, vitamin D
Bleeding tendency (ecchymoses, epistaxis)	Prolonged prothrombin time or INR	Vitamin K
Edema	Decreased serum total protein and albumin; increased fecal loss of α_1-antitrypsin	Protein
Milk intolerance (cramps, bloating, diarrhea)	Abnormal lactose tolerance test	Lactose

INR, international normalized ratio.

are broken down by pancreatic lipase to monoglycerides and fatty acids that form micelles with bile salts. Micelles are important for the solubilization and absorption of fat-soluble vitamins (A, D, E, K). Proteins are hydrolyzed by pancreatic proteases to di- and tripeptides and amino acids. Impaired intraluminal digestion may be caused by insufficient intraluminal concentrations of pancreatic enzymes or bile salts. These conditions will not be covered in detail here (see Chapter 16).

Pancreatic insufficiency may be caused by chronic pancreatitis, cystic fibrosis, or pancreatic cancer. Pancreatic enzymes may also be inactivated within the intestinal lumen by acid hypersecretion (Zollinger-Ellison syndrome). Significant pancreatic enzyme insufficiency generally results in significant steatorrhea (due to malabsorption of triglycerides)—often more than 20–40 g/24 h—resulting in weight loss, gaseous distention and flatulence, and large, greasy, foul-smelling stools. The digestion of proteins and carbohydrates is affected to a far lesser degree and is generally not clinically significant. Because micellar function and intestinal absorption are normal, signs of other nutrient or vitamin deficiencies are rare.

Decreased bile salt concentrations may be due to biliary obstruction or cholestatic liver diseases. Because bile salts are resorbed in the terminal ileum, resection or disease of this area (eg, Crohn disease) can lead to insufficient intraluminal bile salts. Finally, destruction or loss of bile salts may be caused by bacterial overgrowth, massive acid hypersecretion, or medications that bind bile salts (eg, cholestyramine). (Bacterial overgrowth is discussed below.)

Insufficient concentrations of intraluminal bile salts lead to mild steatorrhea (due to malabsorption of fatty acids and monoglycerides), though generally less than 20 g/d. Weight

loss is minimal. Impaired absorption of fat-soluble vitamins (A, D, E, K) is common, resulting in bleeding tendencies, osteoporosis, and hypocalcemia (Table 15–11). Other nutrient absorption is intact. Intestinal loss of bile salts into the colon may cause a watery secretory diarrhea.

B. Mucosal Phase

The mucosal phase requires a sufficient surface area of intact small intestinal epithelium. Brush border enzymes are important in the hydrolysis of disaccharides and di- and tripeptides. Malabsorption of specific nutrients may occur as a result of deficiency in an isolated brush border enzyme. With the exception of lactase deficiency, these are rare congenital disorders that are evident in childhood. Malabsorption due to primary mucosal diseases, extensive intestinal resections (short bowel syndrome), or lymphoma is discussed below. These disorders result in malabsorption of all nutrients: fats, proteins, and amino acids. Depending on the severity of malabsorption, patients may manifest a number of symptoms and signs, as outlined in Table 15–11.

C. Absorptive Phase

Obstruction of the lymphatic system results in impaired absorption of chylomicrons and lipoproteins. This may lead to steatorrhea and significant enteric protein losses or "protein-losing enteropathy," discussed below.

Holt PR. Intestinal malabsorption in the elderly. Dig Dis. 2007;25(2):144–50. [PMID: 17468550]

Montalto M et al. Classification of malabsorption syndromes. Dig Dis. 2008;26(2):104–11. [PMID: 18431059]

1. Celiac Disease

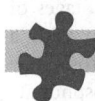

▶ Typical symptoms: weight loss, chronic diarrhea, abdominal distention, growth retardation.

▶ Atypical symptoms: dermatitis herpetiformis, iron deficiency anemia, osteoporosis.

▶ Abnormal serologic test results.

▶ Abnormal small bowel biopsy.

▶ Clinical improvement on gluten-free diet.

▶ General Considerations

Celiac disease is a permanent dietary disorder caused by an immunologic response to gluten, a storage protein found in certain grains, that results in diffuse damage to the proximal small intestinal mucosa with malabsorption of nutrients. Although symptoms may manifest between 6 months and 24 months of age after the introduction of weaning foods, the majority of cases present in childhood or adulthood. Population screening with serologic tests suggests that the disease is present in 1:100 whites of Northern European ancestry, in whom a clinical diagnosis of celiac disease is made in only 10%, suggesting that most cases are undiagnosed or asymptomatic. Celiac disease only develops in people with the HLA-DQ2 (95%) or -DQ8 (5%) class II molecules, which are present in 40% of the population. Although the precise pathogenesis is unclear, celiac disease arises in a small subset of genetically susceptible (-DQ2 or -DQ8) individuals when dietary gluten stimulates an inappropriate immunologic response. Glutens are partially digested in the intestinal lumen into glutamine-rich peptides. Some of the glutamines are deamidated by the enzyme tTG, generating negatively charged glutamic acid residues. If these peptides are able to bind to HLA-DQ2 or -DQ8 molecules on antigen-presenting cells, they may stimulate an inappropriate T cell–mediated activation in the intestinal submucosa that results in destruction of mucosal enterocytes as well as a humoral immune response that results in antibodies to gluten, tTG, and other autoantigens.

▶ Clinical Findings

The most important step in diagnosing celiac disease is to consider the diagnosis. Symptoms are present for more than 10 years in most adults before the correct diagnosis is established. Because of its protean manifestations, celiac disease is grossly underdiagnosed in the adult population.

A. Symptoms and Signs

The gastrointestinal symptoms and signs of celiac disease depend on the length of small intestine involved and the patient's age when the disease presents. "Classic" symptoms of malabsorption, including diarrhea, steatorrhea, weight loss, abdominal distention, weakness, muscle wasting, or growth retardation, more commonly present in infants (< 2 years). Older children and adults are less likely to manifest signs of serious malabsorption. They may report chronic diarrhea, dyspepsia, or flatulence due to colonic bacterial digestion of malabsorbed nutrients, but the severity of weight loss is variable. Many adults have minimal or no gastrointestinal symptoms but present with extraintestinal "atypical" manifestations, including fatigue, depression, iron-deficiency anemia, osteoporosis, short stature, delayed puberty, amenorrhea, or reduced fertility. Approximately 40% of patients with positive serologic tests consistent with sprue have no symptoms of disease; the natural history of these patients with "silent" sprue is unclear.

Physical examination may be normal in mild cases or may reveal signs of malabsorption such as loss of muscle mass or subcutaneous fat, pallor due to anemia, easy bruising due to vitamin K deficiency, hyperkeratosis due to vitamin A deficiency, bone pain due to osteomalacia, or neurologic signs (peripheral neuropathy, ataxia) due to vitamin B_{12} or vitamin E deficiency. Abdominal examination may reveal distention with hyperactive bowel sounds.

Dermatitis herpetiformis is regarded as a cutaneous variant of celiac disease. It is a characteristic skin rash consisting of pruritic papulovesicles over the extensor surfaces of the extremities and over the trunk, scalp, and neck. Dermatitis herpetiformis occurs in less than 10% of patients with celiac disease; however, almost all patients who present with dermatitis herpetiformis have evidence of celiac disease on intestinal mucosal biopsy, though it may not be clinically evident.

B. Laboratory Findings

1. Routine laboratory tests—Depending on the severity of illness and the extent of intestinal involvement, nonspecific laboratory abnormalities may be present that may raise the suspicion of malabsorption and celiac disease. Limited proximal involvement may result only in microcytic anemia due to iron deficiency. Up to 5% of adults with iron deficiency not due to gastrointestinal blood loss have undiagnosed celiac disease. More extensive involvement results in a megaloblastic anemia due to folate or vitamin B_{12} deficiency. Low serum calcium or elevated alkaline phosphatase may reflect impaired calcium or vitamin D absorption with osteomalacia or osteoporosis. Dual-energy x-ray densitometry scanning is recommended for all patients with sprue to screen for osteoporosis. Elevations of prothrombin time, or decreased vitamin A or D levels reflect impaired fat-soluble vitamin absorption. A low serum albumin may reflect small intestine protein loss or poor nutrition. Severe diarrhea may result in a nonanion gap acidosis and hypokalemia. Mild elevations of aminotransferases are found in up to 40%.

2. Serologic tests—Serologic tests should be performed in all patients in whom there is a suspicion of celiac disease. The two tests with the highest diagnostic accuracy are the IgA endomysial antibody and IgA tTG antibody tests, both of which have a ≥ 90% sensitivity and ≥ 95% specificity for the diagnosis of celiac disease. A negative test reliably excludes the diagnosis of celiac disease. Antigliadin antibodies are no longer recommended because of their lower sensitivity and specificity. Because up to 3% of patients with celiac disease have IgA deficiency, an IgA level should be obtained in patients with a negative IgA endomysial antibody or tTG antibody when celiac disease is strongly suspected. For the subset of patients with IgA deficiency, IgG tTG or endomysial antibodies can be obtained. Levels of all antibodies become undetectable after 6–12 months of dietary gluten withdrawal and may be used to monitor dietary compliance, especially in patients whose symptoms fail to resolve after institution of a gluten-free diet.

C. Mucosal Biopsy

Endoscopic mucosal biopsy of the distal duodenum or proximal jejunum is the standard method for confirmation of the diagnosis in patients with a positive serologic test for celiac disease. Rarely, mucosal biopsy may be pursued in patients with negative serologies when symptoms and laboratory studies are suggestive of celiac disease. At endoscopy, atrophy or scalloping of the duodenal folds may be observed. Histology reveals loss or blunting of intestinal villi, hypertrophy of the intestinal crypts, and extensive infiltration of the lamina propria with lymphocytes and plasma cells. An adequate normal biopsy excludes the diagnosis. Partial or complete reversion of these abnormalities on repeat biopsy after a patient is placed on a gluten-free diet establishes the diagnosis. However, if a patient with a compatible biopsy demonstrates prompt clinical improvement on a gluten-free diet and a decrease in antigliadin antibodies, a repeat biopsy is unnecessary.

▶ Differential Diagnosis

Many patients with chronic diarrhea or flatulence are erroneously diagnosed as having irritable bowel syndrome. Celiac sprue must be distinguished from other causes of malabsorption, as outlined above. Severe panmalabsorption of multiple nutrients is almost always caused by mucosal disease. The histologic appearance of celiac sprue may resemble other mucosal diseases such as tropical sprue, bacterial overgrowth, cow's milk intolerance, viral gastroenteritis, eosinophilic gastroenteritis, and mucosal damage caused by acid hypersecretion associated with gastrinoma. Documentation of clinical response to gluten withdrawal therefore is essential to the diagnosis.

▶ Treatment

Removal of all gluten from the diet is essential to therapy—all wheat, rye, and barley must be eliminated. Although oats appear to be safe, commercial products may be contaminated with wheat or barley during processing. Because of the pervasive use of gluten products in manufactured foods and additives, in medications, and by restaurants, it is imperative that patients and their families confer with a knowledgeable dietitian to comply satisfactorily with this lifelong diet. Several excellent dietary guides and patient support groups are available. Most patients with celiac disease also have lactose intolerance either temporarily or permanently and should avoid dairy products until the intestinal symptoms have improved on the gluten-free diet.

Dietary supplements (folate, iron, calcium, and vitamins A, B_{12}, D, and E) should be provided in the initial stages of therapy but usually are not required long-term with a gluten-free diet. Patients with confirmed osteoporosis may require long-term calcium, vitamin D, and bisphosphonate therapy.

Improvement in symptoms should be evident within a few weeks on the gluten-free diet. The most common reason for treatment failure is incomplete removal of gluten.

▶ Prognosis & Complications

If appropriately diagnosed and treated, patients with celiac disease have an excellent prognosis. Celiac disease may be associated with other autoimmune disorders, including Addison disease, Graves disease, type 1 diabetes mellitus, myasthenia gravis, scleroderma, Sjögren syndrome, atrophic gastritis, and pancreatic insufficiency. In some patients, celiac disease may evolve and become refractory to the gluten-free diet. The most common cause is intentional or unintentional dietary noncompliance, which may be suggested by positive serologic tests. Celiac disease that is truly refractory to gluten withdrawal generally carries a poor prognosis. It may be caused by the development of enteropathy-associated T cell lymphoma. This diagnosis should be considered in patients previously responsive to the gluten-free diet in whom new weight loss, abdominal pain, and malabsorption develop. Many other patients with refractory symptoms have a "cryptic" intestinal lymphoma, ie, a monoclonal expansion of the intraepithelial T lymphocyte that may or may not progress. Patients with refractory sprue who do not have intestinal T cell lymphoma may respond to corticosteroids or immunosuppression with azathioprine or cyclosporine.

Barton SH et al. Nutritional deficiencies in celiac disease. Gastroenterol Clin North Am. 2007 Mar;36(1):93–108, vi. [PMID: 17472877]

Celiac Disease Foundation, 13251 Ventura Blvd, Suite #1, Studio City, CA 91604-1838; http://www.celiac.org

Celiac Disease and Gluten-Free Support Page: http://www.celiac.com

Gasbarrini G et al. Celiac disease: what's new about it? Dig Dis. 2008;26(2):121–7. [PMID: 18431061]

Green PH et al. Celiac disease. N Engl J Med. 2007 Oct 25;357(17):1731–43. [PMID: 17960014]

Hopper AD et al. Adult coeliac disease. BMJ. 2007 Sep 15;335(7619):558–62. [PMID: 17855325]

2. Whipple Disease

ESSENTIALS OF DIAGNOSIS

- ▶ Multisystemic disease.
- ▶ Fever, lymphadenopathy, arthralgias.
- ▶ Weight loss, malabsorption, chronic diarrhea.
- ▶ Duodenal biopsy with periodic acid-Schiff (PAS)-positive macrophages with characteristic bacillus.

General Considerations

Whipple disease is a rare multisystemic illness caused by infection with the bacillus *Tropheryma whippelii*. It may occur at any age but most commonly affects white men in the fourth to sixth decades. The source of infection is unknown, but no cases of human-to-human spread have been documented.

Clinical Findings

A. Symptoms and Signs

The clinical manifestations are protean. Arthralgias or a migratory, nondeforming arthritis occurs in 80% and is typically the first symptom experienced. Gastrointestinal symptoms occur in approximately 75% of cases. They include abdominal pain, diarrhea, and some degree of malabsorption with distention, flatulence, and steatorrhea. Weight loss is the most common presenting symptom—seen in almost all patients. Loss of protein due to intestinal or lymphatic involvement may result in protein-losing enteropathy with hypoalbuminemia and edema. In the absence of gastrointestinal symptoms, the diagnosis often is delayed for several years. Intermittent low-grade fever occurs in over 50% of cases. Chronic cough is common. There may be generalized lymphadenopathy that resembles sarcoidosis. Myocardial or valvular involvement may lead to congestive failure or valvular regurgitation. Ocular findings include uveitis, vitreitis, keratitis, retinitis, and retinal hemorrhages. Central nervous system involvement is manifested by a variety of findings such as dementia, lethargy, coma, seizures, myoclonus, or hypothalamic signs. Cranial nerve findings include ophthalmoplegia or nystagmus.

Physical examination may reveal hypotension (a late finding), low-grade fever, and evidence of malabsorption (see Table 15–11). Lymphadenopathy is present in 50%. Heart murmurs due to valvular involvement may be evident. Peripheral joints may be enlarged or warm, and peripheral edema may be present. Neurologic findings are cited above. Hyperpigmentation on sun-exposed areas is evident in up to 40%.

B. Laboratory Findings

If significant malabsorption is present, patients may have laboratory abnormalities as outlined in Table 15–11. There may be steatorrhea.

C. Histologic Evaluation

In most cases, the diagnosis of Whipple disease is established by endoscopic biopsy of the duodenum with histologic evaluation, which demonstrates infiltration of the lamina propria with PAS-positive macrophages that contain gram-positive bacilli (which are not acid-fast) and dilation of the lacteals. The Whipple bacillus has a characteristic trimellar wall appearance on electron microscopy. In some patients who present with nongastrointestinal symptoms, the duodenal biopsy may be normal, and biopsy of other involved organs or lymph nodes may be necessary. Because the PAS stain is less sensitive and specific for extraintestinal Whipple disease, polymerase chain reaction (PCR) is used to confirm the diagnosis by demonstrating the presence of 16S ribosomal RNA of *T whippelii* in blood, cerebrospinal fluid, vitreous fluid, synovial fluid, or cardiac valves. The sensitivity of PCR is 97% and the specificity 100%.

Differential Diagnosis

Whipple disease should be considered in patients who present with signs of malabsorption, fever of unknown origin, lymphadenopathy, seronegative arthritis, culture-negative endocarditis, or multisystemic disease. Small bowel biopsy readily distinguishes Whipple disease from other mucosal malabsorptive disorders, such as celiac sprue. Patients with AIDS and infection of the small intestine with *Mycobacterium avium* complex (MAC) may have a similar clinical and histologic picture; although both conditions are characterized by PAS-positive macrophages, they may be distinguished by the acid-fast stain, which is positive for MAC and negative for the Whipple bacillus. Other conditions that may be confused with Whipple disease include sarcoidosis, Reiter syndrome, familial Mediterranean fever, systemic vasculitides, Behçet disease, intestinal lymphoma, and subacute infective endocarditis.

Treatment

Antibiotic therapy results in a dramatic clinical improvement within several weeks, even in some patients with neurologic involvement. The optimal regimen is unknown. Complete clinical response usually is evident within 1–3 months; however, relapse may occur in up to one-third of patients after discontinuation of treatment. Therefore, prolonged treatment for at least 1 year is required. Drugs that cross the blood-brain barrier are preferred. In severely ill patients, treatment should be initiated with intravenous ceftriaxone (2 g daily) for 2 weeks. Thereafter, trimethoprim-sulfamethoxazole (one double-strength tablet twice daily for 1 year) is recommended as first-line therapy. In patients allergic to sulfonamides or resistant to therapy, long-term treatment with doxycycline and hydroxychloroquine has been proposed. After treatment, repeat duodenal biopsies may be obtained at 6 and 12 months for histologic evaluation. The absence of PAS-positive material predicts a low likelihood of clinical relapse.

Prognosis

If untreated, the disease is fatal. Because some neurologic signs may be permanent, the goal of treatment is to prevent this progression. Patients must be followed closely after treatment for signs of symptom recurrence.

Schneider T et al. Whipple's disease: new aspects of pathogenesis and treatment. Lancet Infect Dis. 2008 Mar;8(3):179–90. [PMID: 18291339]

3. Bacterial Overgrowth

The small intestine normally contains a small number of bacteria. Bacterial overgrowth in the small intestine of whatever cause may result in malabsorption via a number of mechanisms. Bacterial deconjugation of bile salts may lead to inadequate micelle formation, resulting in decreased fat absorption with steatorrhea. Microbial uptake of specific nutrients reduces absorption of vitamin B_{12} and carbohydrates. Bacterial proliferation also causes direct damage to intestinal epithelial cells and the brush border, further impairing absorption of proteins and carbohydrates. Passage of the malabsorbed bile acids and carbohydrates into the colon leads to an osmotic and secretory diarrhea.

Causes of bacterial overgrowth include: (1) gastric achlorhydria (including proton pump inhibitor therapy); (2) anatomic abnormalities of the small intestine with stagnation (afferent limb of Billroth II gastrojejunostomy, resection of ileocecal valve, small intestine diverticula, obstruction, blind loop); (3) small intestine motility disorders (scleroderma, diabetic enteropathy, chronic intestinal pseudo-obstruction); (4) gastrocolic or coloenteric fistula (Crohn disease, malignancy, surgical resection); and (5) miscellaneous disorders. Bacterial overgrowth is an important cause of malabsorption in the elderly, perhaps because of decreased gastric acidity or impaired intestinal motility.

Clinical Findings

Many patients with bacterial overgrowth are asymptomatic. Patients with severe overgrowth have symptoms and signs of malabsorption, including distention, weight loss, and steatorrhea (Table 15–11). Watery diarrhea is common. Megaloblastic anemia or neurologic signs due to vitamin B_{12} deficiency are common findings and may be manifest at presentation. Qualitative or quantitative fecal fat assessment typically is abnormal. D-Xylose absorption is also abnormal due to bacterial uptake of the carbohydrate.

Bacterial overgrowth should be considered in any patient with diarrhea, steatorrhea, weight loss, or macrocytic anemia, especially if the patient has a predisposing cause (such as prior gastrointestinal surgery). A stool collection should be obtained to corroborate the presence of steatorrhea. A small bowel barium radiography or CT enterography study should be obtained to look for mechanical factors predisposing to intestinal stasis. A small intestinal biopsy may be necessary to exclude other mucosal malabsorptive conditions and to detect intestinal inflammation, commonly present with symptomatic bacterial overgrowth. A specific diagnosis can be established firmly only by an aspirate and culture of proximal jejunal secretion that demonstrates over 10^5 organisms/mL. However, this is an invasive and laborious test that requires careful collection and culturing techniques and therefore is not available in many clinical settings. Noninvasive breath tests have been developed that are easier to perform and have a sensitivity of 60–90% and specificity of 85% compared with jejunal cultures. Breath hydrogen tests with glucose or lactulose as substrate are commonly done because of their ease of use.

Owing to the lack of an optimal test for bacterial overgrowth, many clinicians use an empiric antibiotic trial as a diagnostic and therapeutic maneuver in patients with predisposing conditions for bacterial overgrowth in whom unexplained diarrhea or steatorrhea develops.

Treatment

Where possible, the anatomic defect that has potentiated bacterial overgrowth should be corrected. Otherwise, treatment as follows for 1–2 weeks with broad-spectrum antibiotics effective against enteric aerobes and anaerobes usually leads to dramatic improvement: twice daily ciprofloxacin 500 mg, norfloxacin 400 mg, or amoxicillin clavulanate 875 mg, or a combination of metronidazole 250 mg three times daily plus either trimethoprim-sulfamethoxazole (one double-strength tablet) twice daily or cephalexin 250 mg four times daily. Rifaximin 400 mg three times daily is a nonabsorbable antibiotic that also appears to be effective but has fewer side effects than the other systemically absorbed antibiotics.

In patients in whom symptoms recur off antibiotics, cyclic therapy (eg, 1 week out of 4) may be sufficient. Continuous antibiotics should be avoided, if possible, to avoid development of bacterial antibiotic resistance.

In patients with severe intestinal dysmotility, treatment with small doses of octreotide may prove to be of benefit.

Lauritano E et al. Small intestinal bacterial overgrowth recurrence after antibiotic therapy. Am J Gastroenterol. 2008 Aug;103(8):2031–5. [PMID: 18802998]

Scarpellini E et al. High dosage rifaximin for the treatment of small intestinal bacterial overgrowth. Aliment Pharmacol Ther. 2007 Apr 1;25(7):781–6. [PMID: 17373916]

4. Short Bowel Syndrome

Short bowel syndrome is the malabsorptive condition that arises secondary to removal of significant segments of the small intestine. The most common causes in adults are Crohn disease, mesenteric infarction, radiation enteritis, volvulus, tumor resection, and trauma. The type and degree of malabsorption depend on the length and site of the resection and the degree of adaptation of the remaining bowel.

Terminal Ileal Resection

Resection of the terminal ileum results in malabsorption of bile salts and vitamin B_{12}, which are normally absorbed in this region. Patients with low serum vitamin B_{12} levels, an abnormal Schilling test, or resection of over 50 cm of ileum require monthly intramuscular vitamin B_{12} injections. In patients with less than 100 cm of ileal resection, bile salt malabsorption stimulates fluid secretion from the colon, resulting in watery diarrhea. This may be treated with bile salt binding resins (cholestyramine, 2–4 g three times daily with meals). Resection of over 100 cm of ileum leads to a reduction in the bile salt pool that results in steatorrhea and malabsorption of fat-soluble vitamins. Treatment is with a low-fat diet and vitamins supplemented with medium-chain triglycerides, which do not require micellar solubilization. Unabsorbed fatty acids bind with calcium, reducing its absorption and enhancing the absorption of oxalate. Oxalate kidney stones may develop. Calcium supplements should be administered to bind oxalate and increase serum calcium. Cholesterol gallstones due to decreased bile salts are common also. In patients with resection of the ileocolonic valve, bacterial overgrowth may occur in the small intestine, further complicating malabsorption (as outlined above).

Extensive Small Bowel Resection

Resection of 40–50% of the total length of small intestine usually is well tolerated. A more massive resection may result in "short-bowel syndrome," characterized by weight loss and diarrhea due to nutrient, water, and electrolyte malabsorption. After resection, the remaining small intestine has a remarkable ability to adapt, gradually increasing its absorptive capacity up to fourfold over 1 year. The colon also plays an important role in absorption of fluids, electrolytes, and digestion of complex carbohydrates (through bacterial fermentation to short-chain fatty acids) after small bowel resection. If the colon is preserved, 100 cm of proximal jejunum may be sufficient to maintain adequate oral nutrition with a low-fat, high complex-carbohydrate diet, though fluid and electrolyte losses may still be significant. In patients in whom the colon has been removed, at least 200 cm of proximal jejunum is typically required to maintain oral nutrition. Duodenal resection may result in folate, iron, or calcium malabsorption. Levels of other minerals such as zinc, selenium, and magnesium should be monitored. Parenteral vitamin supplementation may be necessary. Antidiarrheal agents (loperamide, 2–4 mg three times daily) slow transit and reduce diarrheal volume. Octreotide reduces intestinal transit time and fluid and electrolyte secretion. Gastric hypersecretion initially complicates intestinal resection and should be treated with proton pump inhibitors.

Patients with less than 100–200 cm of proximal jejunum remaining almost always require parenteral nutrition. Of patients who do, the estimated annual mortality rate is 2–5% per year. Death is most commonly due to TPN-induced liver disease, sepsis, or loss of venous access. Small intestine transplantation is now being performed with reported 5-year graft survival rates of 40%. Currently, it is performed chiefly in patients who develop serious problems due to parenteral nutrition.

DeLegge M et al. Short bowel syndrome: parenteral nutrition versus intestinal transplantation. Where are we today? Dig Dis Sci. 2007 Apr;52(4):876–92. [PMID: 17380398]

Misiakos EP et al. Short bowel syndrome: current medical and surgical trends. J Clin Gastroenterol. 2007 Jan;41(1):5–18. [PMID: 17198059]

5. Lactase Deficiency

Lactase is a brush border enzyme that hydrolyzes the disaccharide lactose into glucose and galactose. The concentration of lactase enzyme levels is high at birth but declines steadily in most people of non-European ancestry during childhood and adolescence and into adulthood. Thus, approximately 50 million people in the United States have partial to complete lactose intolerance. As many as 90% of Asian-Americans, 70% of African-Americans, 95% of Native Americans, 50% of Mexican-Americans, and 60% of Jewish Americans are lactose intolerant compared with less than 25% of white adults. Lactase deficiency may also arise secondary to other gastrointestinal disorders that affect the proximal small intestinal mucosa. These include Crohn disease, sprue, viral gastroenteritis, giardiasis, short bowel syndrome, and malnutrition. Malabsorbed lactose is fermented by intestinal bacteria, producing gas and organic acids. The nonmetabolized lactose and organic acids result in an increased stool osmotic load with an obligatory fluid loss.

Clinical Findings

A. Symptoms and Signs

Patients have great variability in clinical symptoms, depending both on the severity of lactase deficiency and the amount of lactose ingested. Because of the nonspecific nature of these symptoms, there is a tendency for both lactose-intolerant and lactose-tolerant individuals to mistakenly attribute a variety of abdominal symptoms to lactose intolerance. Most patients with lactose intolerance can drink one or two 8 oz glasses of milk daily without symptoms if taken with food at wide intervals, though rare patients have almost complete intolerance. With mild to moderate amounts of lactose malabsorption, patients may experience bloating, abdominal cramps, and flatulence. With higher lactose ingestions, an osmotic diarrhea will result. Isolated lactase deficiency does not result in other signs of malabsorption or weight loss. If these findings are present, other gastrointestinal disorders should be pursued. Diarrheal specimens reveal an increased osmotic gap and a pH of less than 6.0.

B. Laboratory Findings

The most widely available test for the diagnosis of lactase deficiency is the hydrogen breath test. After ingestion of 50 g of lactose, a rise in breath hydrogen of greater than 20 ppm within 90 minutes is a positive test, indicative of bacterial carbohydrate metabolism. In clinical practice, many physicians prescribe an empiric trial of a lactose-free diet for 2 weeks. Resolution of symptoms (bloating, flatulence, diarrhea) is highly suggestive of lactase deficiency (though a placebo response cannot be excluded) and may be confirmed, if necessary, with a breath hydrogen study.

Differential Diagnosis

The symptoms of late-onset lactose intolerance are nonspecific and may mimic a number of gastrointestinal disorders, such as inflammatory bowel disease, mucosal malabsorptive disorders, irritable bowel syndrome, and pancreatic insufficiency. Furthermore, lactase deficiency frequently develops secondary to other gastrointestinal disorders (as listed above). Concomitant lactase deficiency should always be considered in these gastrointestinal disorders.

Treatment

The goal of treatment in patients with isolated lactase deficiency is achieving patient comfort. Patients usually find their "threshold" of intake at which symptoms will occur. Foods that are high in lactose include milk (12 g/cup), ice cream (9 g/cup), and cottage cheese (8 g/cup). Aged cheeses have a lower lactose content (0.5 g/oz). Unpasteurized yogurt contains bacteria that produce lactase and is generally well tolerated.

Many patients will choose simply to restrict or eliminate milk products. By spreading dairy product intake throughout the day in quantities of less than 12 g of lactose (one cup of milk), most patients can take dairy products without symptoms and do not require lactase supplements. Calcium supplementation should be considered in susceptible patients to prevent osteoporosis. Most food markets provide milk that has been pretreated with lactase, rendering it 70–100% lactose free. Lactase enzyme replacement is commercially available as a nonprescription formulation (Lactaid). Caplets of lactase may be taken with milk products, improving lactose absorption and eliminating symptoms. The number of caplets ingested depends on the degree of lactose intolerance.

Montalto M et al. Management and treatment of lactose malabsorption. World J Gastroenterol. 2006 Jan 14;12(2):187–91. [PMID: 16482616]

INTESTINAL MOTILITY DISORDERS

1. Acute Paralytic Ileus

 ESSENTIALS OF DIAGNOSIS

▶ Precipitating factors: surgery, peritonitis, electrolyte abnormalities, medications, severe medical illness.

▶ Nausea, vomiting, obstipation, distention.

▶ Minimal abdominal tenderness; decreased bowel sounds.

▶ Plain abdominal radiography with gas and fluid distention in small and large bowel.

General Considerations

Ileus is a condition in which there is neurogenic failure or loss of peristalsis in the intestine in the absence of any mechanical obstruction. It is commonly seen in hospitalized patients as a result of: (1) intra-abdominal processes such as recent gastrointestinal or abdominal surgery or peritoneal irritation (peritonitis, pancreatitis, ruptured viscus, hemorrhage); (2) severe medical illness such as pneumonia, respiratory failure requiring intubation, sepsis or severe infections, uremia, diabetic ketoacidosis, and electrolyte abnormalities (hypokalemia, hypercalcemia, hypomagnesemia, hypophosphatemia); and (3) medications that affect intestinal motility (opioids, anticholinergics, phenothiazines). Following surgery, small intestinal motility usually normalizes first (often within hours), followed by the stomach (24–48 hours), and the colon (48–72 hours).

Clinical Findings

A. Symptoms and Signs

Patients who are conscious report mild diffuse, continuous abdominal discomfort with nausea and vomiting. Generalized abdominal distention is present with minimal abdominal tenderness but no signs of peritoneal irritation (unless due to the primary disease). Bowel sounds are diminished to absent.

B. Laboratory Findings

The laboratory abnormalities are attributable to the underlying condition. Serum electrolytes, including potassium, magnesium, phosphorus, and calcium, should be obtained to exclude abnormalities as contributing factors.

C. Imaging

Plain film radiography of the abdomen demonstrates distended gas-filled loops of small and large intestine. Air-fluid levels may be seen. Under some circumstances, it may be difficult to distinguish ileus from partial small bowel obstruction. A CT scan may be useful in such instances to exclude mechanical obstruction, especially in postoperative patients.

Differential Diagnosis

Ileus must be distinguished from mechanical obstruction of the small bowel or proximal colon. Pain from small bowel mechanical obstruction is usually intermittent, cramping, and associated initially with profuse vomiting. Acute gastroenteritis, acute appendicitis, and acute pancreatitis may all present with ileus.

Treatment

The primary medical or surgical illness that has precipitated adynamic ileus should be treated. Most cases of ileus respond to restriction of oral intake with gradual liberalization of diet as bowel function returns. Severe or prolonged ileus requires nasogastric suction and parenteral administration of fluids and electrolytes. Alvimopan is a new peripherally acting mu-opioid receptor antagonist with limited absorption or systemic activity that reverses opioid-induced inhibition of intestinal motility. In five randomized controlled trials, it reduced the time to first flatus, bowel movement, solid meal, and hospital discharge compared with placebo in postoperative patients. Alvimopan may be considered in patients undergoing partial large or small bowel resection when postoperative opioid therapy is anticipated.

Batke M et al. Adynamic ileus and acute colonic pseudoobstruction. Med Clin North Am. 2008 May;92(3):649–70. [PMID: 18387380]

Tan EK et al. Meta-analysis: alvimopan vs. placebo in the treatment of post-operative ileus. Aliment Pharmacol Ther. 2007 Jan 1;25(1):47–57. [PMID: 17042776]

2. Acute Colonic Pseudo-obstruction (Ogilvie Syndrome)

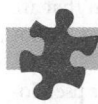

ESSENTIALS OF DIAGNOSIS

▸ Severe abdominal distention.

▸ Arises in postoperative state or with severe medical illness.

▸ May be precipitated by electrolyte imbalances, medications.

▸ Absent to mild abdominal pain; minimal tenderness.

▸ Massive dilation of cecum or right colon.

General Considerations

Spontaneous massive dilation of the cecum and proximal colon may occur in a number of different settings in hospitalized patients. Progressive cecal dilation may lead to spontaneous perforation with dire consequences. The risk of perforation correlates poorly with absolute cecal size and duration of colonic distention. Early detection and management are important to reduce morbidity and mortality. Colonic pseudo-obstruction is most commonly detected in postsurgical patients (mean 3–5 days), after trauma, and in medical patients with respiratory failure, metabolic imbalance, malignancy, myocardial infarction, congestive heart failure, pancreatitis, or a recent neurologic event (stroke, subarachnoid hemorrhage, trauma). Liberal use of opioids or anticholinergic agents may precipitate colonic pseudo-obstruction in susceptible patients. It may also occur as a manifestation of colonic ischemia. The etiology of colonic pseudo-obstruction is unknown, but either an increase in gut sympathetic activity or a decrease in sacral parasympathetic activity of the distal colon, or both, is hypothesized to impair colonic motility.

Clinical Findings

A. Symptoms and Signs

Many patients are on ventilatory support or are unable to report symptoms due to altered mental status. Abdominal distention is frequently noted by the clinician as the first sign, often leading to a plain film radiograph that demonstrates colonic dilation. Some patients are asymptomatic, although most report constant but mild abdominal pain. Nausea and vomiting may be present. Bowel movements may be absent, but up to 40% of patients continue to pass flatus or stool. Abdominal tenderness with some degree of guarding or rebound tenderness may be detected; however, signs of peritonitis are absent unless perforation has occurred. Bowel sounds may be normal or decreased.

B. Laboratory Findings

Laboratory findings reflect the underlying medical or surgical problems. Serum sodium, potassium, magnesium, phosphorus, and calcium should be obtained. Significant fever or leukocytosis raises concern for colonic ischemia or perforation.

C. Imaging

Radiographs demonstrate colonic dilation, usually confined to the cecum and proximal colon. The upper limits of normal for cecal size is 9 cm. A cecal diameter greater than 10–12 cm is associated with an increased risk of colonic perforation. Varying amounts of small intestinal dilation and air-fluid levels due to adynamic ileus may be seen. Because the dilated appearance of the colon may raise concern that there is a distal colonic mechanical obstruction due to malignancy, volvulus, or fecal impaction, a CT scan or water-soluble (diatrizoate meglumine) enema may sometimes be performed.

Differential Diagnosis

Colonic pseudo-obstruction should be distinguished from distal colonic mechanical obstruction (as above) and toxic megacolon, which is acute dilation of the colon due to inflammation (inflammatory bowel disease) or infection (C difficile–associated colitis, CMV). Patients with toxic megacolon manifest fever; dehydration; significant abdominal pain; leukocytosis; and diarrhea, which is often bloody.

Treatment

Conservative treatment is the appropriate first step for patients with no or minimal abdominal tenderness, no fever, no leukocytosis, and a cecal diameter less than 12 cm. The underlying illness is treated appropriately. A nasogastric tube and a rectal tube should be placed. Patients should be ambulated or periodically rolled from side to side and to the knee-chest position in an effort to promote expulsion of colonic gas. All drugs that reduce intestinal motility, such as opioids, anticholinergics, and calcium channel blockers, are discontinued if possible. Enemas may be administered judiciously if large amounts of stool are evident on radiography. Oral laxatives are not helpful and may cause perforation, pain, or electrolyte abnormalities.

Conservative treatment is successful in over 80% of cases within 1–2 days. Patients must be watched for signs of worsening distention or abdominal tenderness. Cecal size should be assessed by abdominal radiographs every 12 hours. Intervention should be considered in patients with any of the following: (1) no improvement or clinical deterioration after 24–48 hours of conservative therapy; (2) cecal dilation > 10 cm for a prolonged period (> 3–4 days); (3) patients with cecal dilation > 12 cm. Neostigmine injection should be given unless contraindicated. A single dose (2 mg intravenously) results in rapid (within 30 minutes) colonic decompression in 75–90% of patients. Cardiac monitoring during neostigmine infusion is indicated for possible bradycardia that may require atropine administration. Colonoscopic decompression is indicated in patients who fail to respond to neostigmine. Colonic decompression with aspiration of air or placement of a decompression tube is successful in 70% of patients. However, the procedure is technically difficult in an unprepared bowel and has been associated with perforations in the distended colon. Dilation recurs in up to 50% of patients. In patients in whom colonoscopy is unsuccessful, a tube cecostomy can be created through a small laparotomy or with percutaneous radiologically guided placement.

► Prognosis

In most cases, the prognosis is related to the underlying illness. The risk of perforation or ischemia is increased with cecal diameter > 12 cm and when distention has been present for more than 6 days. With aggressive therapy, the development of perforation is unusual.

Saunders MD. Acute colonic pseudo-obstruction. Gastrointest Endosc Clin N Am. 2007 Apr;17(2):341–60. [PMID: 17556152]

3. Chronic Intestinal Pseudo-obstruction & Gastroparesis

Gastroparesis and chronic intestinal pseudo-obstruction are chronic conditions characterized by intermittent, waxing and waning symptoms and signs of gastric or intestinal obstruction in the absence of any mechanical lesions to account for the findings. They are caused by a heterogeneous group of endocrine disorders (diabetes mellitus, hypothyroidism, cortisol deficiency), postsurgical conditions (vagotomy, partial gastric resection, fundoplication, gastric bypass, Whipple procedure), neurologic conditions (Parkinson disease, muscular and myotonic dystrophy, autonomic dysfunction, multiple sclerosis, postpolio syndrome, porphyria), rheumatologic syndromes (progressive systemic sclerosis), infections (postviral, Chagas disease), amyloidosis, paraneoplastic syndromes, medications, and eating disorders (anorexia); a cause may not always be identified.

Gastric involvement leads to chronic or intermittent symptoms of gastroparesis with postprandial fullness (early satiety), nausea, and vomiting (1–3 hours after meals). Patients with predominantly small bowel involvement may have abdominal distention, vomiting, diarrhea, and varying degrees of malnutrition. Abdominal pain is not common and should prompt investigation for structural causes of obstruction. Bacterial overgrowth in the stagnant intestine may result in malabsorption. Colonic involvement may result in constipation or alternating diarrhea and constipation.

Plain film radiography may demonstrate dilation of the esophagus, stomach, small intestine, or colon resembling ileus or mechanical obstruction. Mechanical obstruction of the stomach, small intestine, or colon is much more common than gastroparesis or intestinal pseudo-obstruction and must be excluded with endoscopy, barium radiography (upper gastrointestinal series with small bowel follow-through), or CT enterography, especially in patients with prior surgery, recent onset of symptoms, or abdominal pain. In cases of unclear origin, studies based on the clinical picture are obtained to exclude underlying systemic disease. Gastric scintigraphy with a low-fat solid meal is the optimal means for assessing gastric emptying. Gastric retention of 60% after 2 hours or more than 10%

after 4 hours is abnormal. Small bowel manometry is useful for distinguishing visceral from myopathic disorders and for excluding cases of mechanical obstruction that are otherwise difficult to diagnose by endoscopy or radiographic studies.

There is no specific therapy for gastroparesis or pseudo-obstruction. Acute exacerbations are treated with nasogastric suction and intravenous fluids. Long-term treatment is directed at maintaining nutrition. Patients should eat small, frequent meals that are low in fiber, milk, gas-forming foods, and fat. Some patients may require liquid enteral supplements. Agents that reduce gastrointestinal motility (opioids, anticholinergics, calcium channel blockers) should be avoided. In diabetics, glucose levels should be maintained below 200 mg/dL, as hyperglycemia may slow gastric emptying even in the absence of diabetic neuropathy, and amyline analogs (exenatide or pramlintide) should be discontinued. Metoclopramide (5–20 mg orally or 5–10 mg intravenously or subcutaneously four times daily) and erythromycin (50–125 mg orally three times daily) before meals is of benefit in treatment of gastroparesis but not small bowel dysmotility. The FDA issued a black box warning in 2009 that use of metoclopramide for more than 3 months is associated with an increased risk of tardive dyskinesia and should be avoided. The elderly are at greatest risk. Unblinded studies in small numbers of patients with diabetic or idiopathic gastroparesis report improvement in symptoms and gastric emptying after injection of botulinum toxin into the pylorus, which is hypothesized to reduce pyloric spasm; however, a controlled trial showed no efficacy. Gastric electrical stimulation with internally implanted neurostimulators has shown reduction in vomiting in small studies of patients with severe gastroparesis; however, no randomized studies have been conducted and the mechanism of action is uncertain. Bacterial overgrowth should be treated with intermittent antibiotics (see above). Patients with predominant small bowel distention may require a venting gastrostomy to relieve distress. Some patients may require placement of a jejunostomy for long-term enteral nutrition. Patients unable to maintain adequate enteral nutrition require TPN or small bowel transplantation. Difficult cases should be referred to centers with expertise in this area.

Abrahamsson H. Treatment options for patients with severe gastroparesis. Gut. 2007 Jun;56(6):877–83. [PMID: 17519490]

Camilleri M. Clinical practice. Diabetic gastroparesis. N Engl J Med. 2007 Feb 22;356(8):820–9. [PMID: 17314341]

Friedenberg FK et al. Persistent nausea and abdominal pain in a patient with delayed gastric emptying. Clin Gastroenterol Hepatol. 2008 Dec;6(12):1309–14. [PMID: 18829390]

Patrick A. Gastroparesis. Aliment Pharmacol Ther. 2008 May;27(9):724–40. [PMID: 18248660]

Yin J et al. Implantable gastric electrical stimulation: ready for prime time? Gastroenterology. 2008 Mar;134(3):665–7. [PMID: 18325383]

BENIGN TUMORS OF THE SMALL INTESTINE

Benign and malignant tumors (**see Chapter 39 for Malignant Tumors**) of the small intestine are rare. They often cause no symptoms or signs. However, they may cause acute gastrointestinal bleeding with hematochezia or melena or chronic gastrointestinal blood loss resulting in fatigue and iron deficiency anemia. Small bowel tumors may cause obstruction due to luminal narrowing or intussusception of a polypoid mass. Small bowel tumors usually are identified by barium radiographic studies, either enteroclysis or a small bowel series. Visualization and biopsy of duodenal and proximal jejunal mass lesions are performed with a long upper endoscope known as an enteroscope.

Benign polyps may be symptomatic or may be incidental findings detected on endoscopy or radiographic study. Most occur singly, and the presence of multiple polyps is suggestive of hereditary polyposis syndrome (discussed under Diseases of the Colon and Rectum). With the exception of lipomas, surgical or endoscopic excision usually is recommended.

Adenomatous polyps are the most common benign mucosal tumor. The majority are asymptomatic, though acute or chronic bleeding may occur. Because malignant transformation does occur, endoscopic or surgical resection is warranted. Villous adenomas occur most commonly in the periampullary region of the duodenum (especially in patients with familial adenomatous polyposis) and carry a high risk for development of invasive cancer. Periodic endoscopic surveillance to detect early ampullary neoplasms is recommended in patients with familial adenomatous polyposis. Evaluation with endoscopic retrograde cholangiopancreatography (ERCP) and endoscopic ultrasound is required to exclude invasive carcinoma. Ampullary adenomas may be removed by endoscopic or surgical techniques. Lipomas occur commonly in the ileum. Most are asymptomatic and identified incidentally at endoscopy or radiography; however, they rarely may cause obstruction with intussusception.

Benign stromal tumors (formerly called leiomyomas) are found at all levels of the intestine. These submucosal mesenchymal lesions may be intraluminal, intramural, or extraluminal. Although most are asymptomatic, they may ulcerate and cause acute or chronic bleeding or obstruction. It is difficult to distinguish benign from malignant stromal tumors (leiomyosarcomas) except by excision.

Adler DG et al. ASGE Guideline: the role of endoscopy in ampullary and duodenal adenomas. Gastrointest Endosc. 2006 Dec;64(6):849–54. [PMID: 17140885]
Gore RM et al. Diagnosis and staging of small bowel tumours. Cancer Imaging. 2006 Dec 29;6:209–12. [PMID: 17208678]

APPENDICITIS

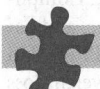 ESSENTIALS OF DIAGNOSIS

▶ Early: periumbilical pain; later: right lower quadrant pain and tenderness.

▶ Anorexia, nausea and vomiting, obstipation.

▶ Tenderness or localized rigidity at McBurney point.

▶ Low-grade fever and leukocytosis.

General Considerations

Appendicitis is the most common abdominal surgical emergency, affecting approximately 10% of the population. It occurs most commonly between the ages of 10 and 30 years. It is initiated by obstruction of the appendix by a fecalith, inflammation, foreign body, or neoplasm. Obstruction leads to increased intraluminal pressure, venous congestion, infection, and thrombosis of intramural vessels. If untreated, gangrene and perforation develop within 36 hours.

Clinical Findings

A. Symptoms and Signs

Appendicitis usually begins with vague, often colicky periumbilical or epigastric pain. Within 12 hours the pain shifts to the right lower quadrant, manifested as a steady ache that is worsened by walking or coughing. Almost all patients have nausea with one or two episodes of vomiting. Protracted vomiting or vomiting that begins before the onset of pain suggests another diagnosis. A sense of constipation is typical, and some patients administer cathartics in an effort to relieve their symptoms—though some report diarrhea. Low-grade fever (< 38 °C) is typical; high fever or rigors suggest another diagnosis or appendiceal perforation.

On physical examination, localized tenderness with guarding in the right lower quadrant can be elicited with gentle palpation with one finger. When asked to cough, patients may be able to precisely localize the painful area, a sign of peritoneal irritation. Light percussion may also elicit pain. Although rebound tenderness is also present, it is unnecessary to elicit this finding if the above signs are present. The psoas sign (pain on passive extension of the right hip) and the obturator sign (pain with passive flexion and internal rotation of the right hip) are indicative of adjacent inflammation and strongly suggestive of appendicitis.

B. Laboratory Findings

Moderate leukocytosis (10,000–20,000/mcL) with neutrophilia is common. Microscopic hematuria and pyuria are present in 25% of patients.

C. Imaging

Both abdominal ultrasound and CT scanning are useful in diagnosing appendicitis as well as excluding other diseases presenting with similar symptoms, including adnexal disease in younger women. However, CT scanning appears to be more accurate (sensitivity 94%, specificity 95%, positive likelihood ratio 13.3, negative likelihood ratio 0.09). Abdominal CT scanning is also useful in cases of suspected appendiceal perforation to diagnose a periappendiceal abscess. In patients in whom there is a clinically high suspicion of appendicitis, some surgeons feel that preoperative diagnostic imaging is unnecessary. However, studies suggest that even in this group, imaging studies suggest an alternative diagnosis in up to 15%.

1. Atypical Presentations of Appendicitis

Owing to the variable location of the appendix, there are a number of "atypical" presentations. Because the retrocecal appendix does not touch the anterior abdominal wall, the pain remains less intense and poorly localized; abdominal tenderness is minimal and may be elicited in the right flank. The psoas sign may be positive. With pelvic appendicitis there is pain in the lower abdomen, often on the left, with an urge to urinate or defecate. Abdominal tenderness is absent, but tenderness is evident on pelvic or rectal examination; the obturator sign may be present. In the elderly, the diagnosis of appendicitis is often delayed because patients present with minimal, vague symptoms and mild abdominal tenderness. Appendicitis in pregnancy may present with pain in the right lower quadrant, periumbilical area, or right subcostal area owing to displacement of the appendix by the uterus.

▶ Differential Diagnosis

Given its frequency and myriad presentations, appendicitis should be considered in the differential diagnosis of all patients with abdominal pain. It is difficult to reliably diagnose the disease in some cases. A several-hour period of close observation with reassessment usually clarifies the diagnosis. Absence of the classic migration of pain (from the epigastrium to the right lower abdomen), right lower quadrant pain, fever, or guarding makes appendicitis less likely. Ten to 20 percent of patients with suspected appendicitis have either a negative examination at laparotomy or an alternative surgical diagnosis. The widespread use of ultrasonography and CT has reduced the number of incorrect diagnoses. Still, in some cases diagnostic laparotomy or laparoscopy is required. The most common causes of diagnostic confusion are gastroenteritis and gynecologic disorders. Viral gastroenteritis presents with nausea, vomiting, low-grade fever, and diarrhea and can be difficult to distinguish from appendicitis. The onset of vomiting before pain makes appendicitis less likely. As a rule, the pain of gastroenteritis is more generalized and the tenderness less well localized. Acute salpingitis or tubo-ovarian abscess should be considered in young, sexually active women with fever and bilateral abdominal or pelvic tenderness. A twisted ovarian cyst may also cause sudden severe pain. The sudden onset of lower abdominal pain in the middle of the menstrual cycle suggests mittelschmerz. Sudden severe abdominal pain with diffuse pelvic tenderness and shock suggests a ruptured ectopic pregnancy. A positive pregnancy test and pelvic ultrasonography are diagnostic. Retrocecal or retroileal appendicitis (often associated with pyuria or hematuria) may be confused with ureteral colic or pyelonephritis. Other conditions that may resemble appendicitis are diverticulitis, Meckel diverticulitis, carcinoid of the appendix, perforated colonic cancer, Crohn ileitis, perforated peptic ulcer, cholecystitis, and mesenteric adenitis. It is virtually impossible to distinguish appendicitis from Meckel diverticulitis, but both require surgical treatment.

▶ Complications

Perforation occurs in 20% of patients and should be suspected in patients with pain persisting for over 36 hours, high fever, diffuse abdominal tenderness or peritoneal findings, a palpable abdominal mass, or marked leukocytosis. Localized perforation results in a contained abscess, usually in the pelvis. A free perforation leads to suppurative peritonitis with toxicity. Septic thrombophlebitis (pylephlebitis) of the portal venous system is rare and suggested by high fever, chills, bacteremia, and jaundice.

▶ Treatment

The treatment of uncomplicated appendicitis is surgical appendectomy. This may be performed through a laparotomy or by laparoscopy. Prior to surgery, patients should be given systemic antibiotics, which reduce the incidence of postoperative wound infections. Emergency appendectomy is also required in patients with perforated appendicitis with generalized peritonitis.

The optimal treatment of stable patients with perforated appendicitis and a contained abscess is controversial. Surgery in this setting can be difficult. Many recommend percutaneous CT-guided drainage of the abscess with intravenous fluids and antibiotics to allow the inflammation to subside. An interval appendectomy may be performed after 6 weeks to prevent recurrent appendicitis.

▶ Prognosis

The mortality rate from uncomplicated appendicitis is extremely low. Even with perforated appendicitis, the mortality rate in most groups is only 0.2%, though it approaches 15% in the elderly.

Van Randen A et al. Acute appendicitis: meta-analysis of diagnostic performance of CT and graded compression US related to prevalence of disease. Radiology. 2008 Oct;249(1):97–106. [PMID: 18682583]

INTESTINAL TUBERCULOSIS

Intestinal tuberculosis is common in underdeveloped countries. Previously rare in the United States, its incidence has been rising in immigrant groups and patients with AIDS. It is caused by both *Mycobacterium tuberculosis* and *M bovis*. Active pulmonary disease is present in less than 50% of patients. The most frequent site of involvement is the ileocecal region; however, any region of the gastrointestinal tract may be involved. Intestinal tuberculosis may cause mucosal ulcerations or scarring and fibrosis with narrowing of the lumen. Patients may be without symptoms or complain of chronic abdominal pain, obstructive symptoms, weight loss, and diarrhea. An abdominal mass may be palpable. Complications include intestinal obstruction, hemorrhage, and fistula formation. The purified protein derivative (PPD) skin test may be negative, especially in patients with weight loss or AIDS. Barium radiography may demonstrate mucosal ulcerations, thickening, or stricture formation. Colonoscopy may demonstrate an ulcerated mass, multiple ulcers with steep edges and adjacent small sessile polyps, small ulcers or erosions, or small diverticula, most commonly in the ileocecal region. The differential diagnosis includes Crohn disease, carcinoma, and intestinal amebiasis. The diagnosis is established by either endoscopic or surgical biopsy revealing acid-fast bacilli, caseating granuloma, or positive cultures from the organism. Detection of tubercle bacilli in biopsy specimens by PCR is now the most sensitive means of diagnosis.

Treatment with standard antituberculous regimens is effective.

Rasheed S et al. Intra-abdominal and gastrointestinal tuberculosis. Colorectal Dis. 2007 Nov;9(9):773–83. [PMID: 17868413]

PROTEIN-LOSING ENTEROPATHY

Protein-losing enteropathy comprises a number of conditions that result in excessive loss of serum proteins into the gastrointestinal tract. The essential diagnostic features are hypoalbuminemia and an elevated fecal α_1-antitrypsin level.

The normal intact gut epithelium prevents the loss of serum proteins. Proteins may be lost through one of three mechanisms: (1) mucosal disease with ulceration, resulting in the loss of proteins across the disrupted mucosal surface, such as in chronic gastric ulcer, gastric carcinoma, or inflammatory bowel disease; (2) lymphatic obstruction, resulting in the loss of protein-rich chylous fluid from mucosal lacteals, such as in primary intestinal lymphangiectasia, constrictive pericarditis or congestive heart failure, Whipple disease or tuberculosis, Kaposi sarcoma or lymphoma, retroperitoneal fibrosis, or sarcoidosis; and (3) idiopathic change in permeability of mucosal capillaries and conductance of interstitium, resulting in "weeping" of protein-rich fluid from the mucosal surface, such as in Ménétrier disease, Zollinger-Ellison syndrome, viral or eosinophilic gastroenteritis, celiac disease, giardiasis or hookworm, common variable immunodeficiency, systemic lupus erythematosus, amyloidosis, or allergic protein-losing enteropathy.

Hypoalbuminemia is the sine qua non of protein-losing enteropathy. However, a number of other serum proteins such as α_1-antitrypsin also are lost from the gut epithelium. In protein-losing enteropathy caused by lymphatic obstruction, loss of lymphatic fluid commonly results in lymphocytopenia (< 1000/mcL), hypoglobulinemia, and hypocholesterolemia.

In most cases, protein-losing enteropathy is recognized as a sequela of a known gastrointestinal disorder. In patients in whom the cause is unclear, evaluation is indicated and is guided by the clinical suspicion. Protein-losing enteropathy must be distinguished from other causes of hypoalbuminemia, which include liver disease and nephrotic syndrome; and from congestive heart failure. Protein-losing enteropathy is confirmed by determining the gut α_1-antitrypsin clearance (24-hour volume of feces × stool concentration of α_1-antitrypsin ÷ serum α_1-antitrypsin concentration). A clearance of more than 13 mL/24 h is abnormal.

Laboratory evaluation of protein-losing enteropathy includes serum protein electrophoresis, lymphocyte count, and serum cholesterol to look for evidence of lymphatic obstruction. Serum ANA and C3 levels are useful to screen for autoimmune disorders. Stool samples should be examined for ova and parasites. Evidence of malabsorption is evaluated by means of a stool qualitative fecal fat determi-

nation. Intestinal imaging is performed with small bowel enteroscopy biopsy, CT enterography, or wireless capsule endoscopy of the small intestine. Colonic diseases are excluded with colonoscopy. A CT scan of the abdomen is performed to look for evidence of neoplasms or lymphatic obstruction. Rarely, lymphangiography is helpful. In some situations, laparotomy with full-thickness intestinal biopsy is required to establish a diagnosis.

Treatment is directed at the underlying cause. Patients with lymphatic obstruction benefit from low-fat diets supplemented with medium-chain triglycerides. Case reports suggest that octreotide may lead to symptomatic and nutritional improvement in some patients.

Pungpapong S et al. Protein-losing enteropathy from eosinophilic enteritis diagnosed by wireless capsule endoscopy and double-balloon enteroscopy. Gastrointest Endosc. 2007 May;65(6):917–8. [PMID: 17208236]

DISEASES OF THE COLON & RECTUM

IRRITABLE BOWEL SYNDROME

 ESSENTIALS OF DIAGNOSIS

▶ Chronic functional disorder characterized by abdominal pain or discomfort with alterations in bowel habits.

▶ Symptoms usually begin in late teens to early twenties.

▶ Limited evaluation to exclude organic causes of symptoms.

▶ General Considerations

The functional gastrointestinal disorders are characterized by a variable combination of chronic or recurrent gastrointestinal symptoms *not explicable by the presence of structural or biochemical abnormalities*. Several clinical entities are included under this broad rubric, including chest pain of unclear origin (noncardiac chest pain), functional dyspepsia, and biliary dyskinesia (sphincter of Oddi dysfunction). There is a large overlap among these entities. For example, over 50% of patients with noncardiac chest pain and over one-third with functional dyspepsia also have symptoms compatible with irritable bowel syndrome. In none of these disorders is there a definitive diagnostic study. Rather, the diagnosis is a subjective one based on the presence of a compatible profile and the exclusion of similar disorders.

Irritable bowel syndrome can be defined, therefore, as an idiopathic clinical entity characterized by chronic (more than 3 months) abdominal pain or discomfort that occurs in association with altered bowel habits. These symptoms may be continuous or intermittent. Consensus definition of irritable bowel syndrome is abdominal discomfort or pain that has two of the following three features: (1) relieved with defecation, (2) onset associated with a change in frequency of stool, or (3) onset associated with a change in form (appearance) of stool. Other symptoms supporting the diagnosis include abnormal stool frequency; abnormal stool form (lumpy or hard; loose or watery); abnormal stool passage (straining, urgency, or feeling of incomplete evacuation); passage of mucus; and bloating or a feeling of abdominal distention.

Patients may have other somatic or psychological complaints such as dyspepsia, heartburn, chest pain, headaches, fatigue, myalgias, urologic dysfunction, gynecologic symptoms, anxiety, or depression.

The disorder is a common problem presenting to both gastroenterologists and primary care physicians. Up to 10% of the adult population have symptoms compatible with the diagnosis, but most never seek medical attention. Approximately two-thirds of patients with irritable bowel syndrome are women.

► Pathogenesis

A number of pathophysiologic mechanisms have been identified and may have varying importance in different individuals.

A. Abnormal Motility

A variety of abnormal myoelectrical and motor abnormalities have been identified in the colon and small intestine. In some cases, these are temporally correlated with episodes of abdominal pain or emotional stress. Whether they represent a primary motility disorder or are secondary to psychosocial stress is debated. Differences between patients with constipation-predominant and diarrhea-predominant syndromes are reported.

B. Visceral Hypersensitivity

Patients often have a lower visceral pain threshold, reporting abdominal pain at lower volumes of colonic gas insufflation or colonic balloon inflation than controls. Although many patients complain of bloating and distention, their absolute intestinal gas volume is normal. Many patients report rectal urgency despite small rectal volumes of stool.

C. Enteric Infection

Symptoms compatible with irritable bowel syndrome develop within 1 year in up to 10% of patients after an episode of bacterial gastroenteritis compared with less than 2% of controls. Women and patients with increased life stressors at the onset of gastroenteritis appear to be at increased risk for developing "postinfectious" irritable bowel syndrome. Increased inflammatory cells have been found in the mucosa, submucosa, and muscularis of some patients with irritable bowel syndrome, but their importance is unclear. Chronic inflammation is postulated by some investigators to contribute to alterations in motility or visceral hypersensitivity. Some investigators suggest that alterations in the numbers and distribution of bacterial species (estimated 30,000 different species) may affect bowel transit time, gas production, and sensitivity. An increase in breath hydrogen or methane excretion after lactulose inges-

tion in up to 80% of patients with irritable bowel syndrome has been reported, believed to be suggestive of small intestinal bacterial overgrowth, although several investigators dispute these findings. Small bowel bacterial overgrowth may be more likely in patients with bloating, postprandial discomfort, and loose stools. It is hypothesized that bacterial overgrowth may lead to alterations in immune alterations that affect motility or visceral sensitivity or to degradation of carbohydrates in the small intestine could cause increased postprandial gas, bloating, and distention.

D. Psychosocial Abnormalities

More than 50% of patients with irritable bowel who seek medical attention have underlying depression, anxiety, or somatization. By contrast, those who do not seek medical attention are similar psychologically to normal individuals. Psychological abnormalities may influence how the patient perceives or reacts to illness and minor visceral sensations. Chronic stress may alter intestinal motility or modulate pathways that affect central and spinal processing of visceral afferent sensation.

► Clinical Findings

A. Symptoms and Signs

Irritable bowel is a chronic condition. Symptoms usually begin in the late teens to twenties. Symptoms should be present for at least 3 months before the diagnosis can be considered. The diagnosis is established in the presence of compatible symptoms and the judicious use of tests to exclude organic disease.

Abdominal pain usually is intermittent, crampy, and in the lower abdominal region. As previously stated, the onset of pain typically is associated with a change in stool frequency or form and commonly is relieved by defecation. It does not usually occur at night or interfere with sleep. Patients with irritable bowel syndrome may be classified into one of three categories based on the predominant bowel habit: irritable bowel syndrome with diarrhea; irritable bowel syndrome with constipation; or irritable bowel syndrome with mixed constipation and diarrhea. It is important to clarify what the patient means by these complaints. Patients with irritable bowel and constipation report infrequent bowel movements (less than three per week), hard or lumpy stools, or straining. Patients with irritable bowel syndrome with diarrhea refer to loose or watery stools, frequent stools (more than three per day), urgency, or fecal incontinence. Many patients report that they have a firm stool in the morning followed by progressively looser movements. Complaints of visible distention and bloating are common, though these are not always clinically evident.

The patient should be asked about "alarm symptoms" that suggest a diagnosis other than irritable bowel syndrome and warrant further investigation. The acute onset of symptoms raises the likelihood of organic disease, especially in patients aged > 40–50 years. Nocturnal diarrhea, severe constipation or diarrhea, hematochezia, weight loss, and fever are incompatible with a diagnosis of irritable bowel syndrome and warrant investigation for underlying disease.

Patients who have a family history of cancer, inflammatory bowel disease, or celiac disease should undergo additional evaluation.

A physical examination should be performed to look for evidence of organic disease and to allay the patient's anxieties. The physical examination usually is normal. Abdominal tenderness, especially in the lower abdomen, is common but not pronounced. A new onset of symptoms in a patient over age 40 years warrants further examination.

B. Laboratory Findings and Special Examinations

In patients whose symptoms fulfill the diagnostic criteria for irritable bowel syndrome and who have no other alarm symptoms, evidence-based consensus guidelines do not support further diagnostic testing, as the likelihood of serious organic diseases does not appear to be increased. Although the vague nature of symptoms and patient anxiety may prompt clinicians to consider a variety of diagnostic studies, overtesting should be avoided. The use of routine blood tests (complete blood count, chemistry panel, serum albumin, thyroid function tests, erythrocyte sedimentation rate) is unnecessary in most patients. Stool specimen examinations for ova and parasites should be obtained only in patients with increased likelihood of infection (eg, day care workers, campers, foreign travelers). Routine sigmoidoscopy or colonoscopy also are not recommended in young patients with symptoms of irritable bowel syndrome without alarm symptoms but should be considered in patients who do not improve with conservative management. In all patients age 50 years or older who have not had a previous evaluation, colonoscopy should be obtained to exclude malignancy. When colonoscopy is performed, random mucosal biopsies should be obtained to look for evidence of microscopic colitis (which may have similar symptoms). In patients with irritable bowel syndrome with diarrhea, serologic tests for celiac disease may be performed. Pending further clinical studies, routine testing for bacterial overgrowth with hydrogen breath tests are not recommended.

▶ Differential Diagnosis

A number of disorders may present with similar symptoms. Examples include colonic neoplasia, inflammatory bowel disease (ulcerative colitis, Crohn disease, microscopic colitis), hyperthyroidism or hypothyroidism, parasites, malabsorption (especially celiac disease, bacterial overgrowth, lactase deficiency), causes of chronic secretory diarrhea (carcinoid), and endometriosis. Psychiatric disorders such as depression, panic disorder, and anxiety must be considered as well. Women with refractory symptoms have an increased incidence of prior sexual and physical abuse. These diagnoses should be excluded in patients with presumed irritable bowel syndrome who do not improve within 2–4 weeks of empiric treatment or in whom subsequent alarm symptoms develop.

▶ Treatment

A. General Measures

As with other functional disorders, the most important interventions the clinician can offer are reassurance, educa-

tion, and support. This includes identifying and responding to the patient's concerns, careful explanation of the pathophysiology and natural history of the disorder, setting realistic treatment goals, and involving the patient in the treatment process. Because irritable bowel symptoms are chronic, the patient's reasons for seeking consultation at this time should be determined. These may include major life events or recent psychosocial stressors, dietary or medication changes, concerns about serious underlying disease, or reduced quality of life and impairment of daily activities. In discussing with the patient the importance of the mind-gut interaction, it may be helpful to explain that alterations in visceral motility and sensitivity may be exacerbated by environmental, social, or psychological factors such as foods, medications, hormones, and stress. Symptoms such as pain, bloating, and altered bowel habits may lead to anxiety and distress, which in turn may further exacerbate bowel disturbances due to disordered communication between the gut and the central nervous system. A symptom diary in which patients record the time and severity of symptoms, food intake, and life events may help uncover aggravating dietary or psychosocial factors. Fears that the symptoms will progress, require surgery, or degenerate into serious illness should be allayed. The patient should understand that irritable bowel syndrome is a chronic disorder characterized by periods of exacerbation and quiescence. The emphasis should be shifted from finding the cause of the symptoms to finding a way to cope with them. Clinicians must resist the temptation to chase chronic complaints with new or repeated diagnostic studies.

B. Dietary Therapy

Patients commonly report dietary intolerances, although a role for dietary triggers in irritable bowel syndrome has never been convincingly demonstrated. Fatty foods and caffeine are poorly tolerated by many patients with irritable bowel syndrome. In patients with diarrhea, bloating, and flatulence, lactose intolerance should be excluded with a breath hydrogen test or a trial of a lactose-free diet. A host of poorly absorbed, fermentable, short-chain carbohydrates may exacerbate bloating, flatulence, and diarrhea in some patients. These include fructose (corn syrups, apples, pears, watermelon, raisins), fructans (onions, leeks, asparagus, artichokes), wheat-based products (breads, pasta, cereals, cakes) sorbitol (stone fruits), and raffinose (legumes, lentils, brussel sprouts, cabbage).

A high-fiber diet and fiber supplements appears to be of little value in patients with irritable bowel syndrome. Many patients report little change in bowel frequency but increased gas and distention.

C. Pharmacologic Measures

More than two-thirds of patients with irritable bowel syndrome have mild symptoms that respond readily to education, reassurance, and dietary interventions. Drug therapy should be reserved for patients with moderate to severe symptoms that do not respond to conservative measures. These agents should be viewed as being adjunctive rather than curative. Given the wide spectrum of symptoms, no single agent is expected to provide relief in all or even most patients. Nevertheless, therapy targeted at the specific dominant symptom (pain, constipation, or diarrhea) may be beneficial.

1. Antispasmodic agents—Anticholinergic agents are used by some practitioners for treatment of acute episodes of pain or bloating despite a lack of well-designed trials demonstrating efficacy. Available agents include hyoscyamine, 0.125 mg orally (or sublingually as needed) or sustained-release, 0.037 mg or 0.75 mg orally twice daily; dicyclomine, 10–20 mg orally; or methscopolamine 2.5–5 mg orally before meals and at bedtime. Anticholinergic side effects are common, including urinary retention, constipation, tachycardia, and dry mouth. Hence, these agents should be used with caution in the elderly and in patients with constipation. Peppermint oil formulations (which relax smooth muscle) may be helpful.

2. Antidiarrheal agents—Loperamide (2 mg orally three or four times daily) is effective for the treatment of patients with diarrhea, reducing stool frequency, liquidity, and urgency. It may best be used "prophylactically" in situations in which diarrhea is anticipated (such as stressful situations) or would be inconvenient (social engagements).

3. Anticonstipation agents—Treatment with osmotic laxatives (milk of magnesia or polyethylene glycol) may increase stool frequency, improve stool consistency, and reduce straining. Lactulose or sorbitol produces increased flatus and distention, which are poorly tolerated in patients with irritable bowel syndrome. Lubiprostone is a selective chloride C-2 activator that stimulates increased intestinal chloride secretion, which leads to increased stool frequency. Lubiprostone is approved for the treatment of chronic constipation (24 mcg twice daily) as well as for the treatment of women with irritable bowel with constipation (8 mcg twice daily). In clinical trials of patients with irritable bowel syndrome and constipation, lubiprostone led to global symptom improvement in 18% of patients compared with 10% of patients who received placebo. Patients with intractable constipation should undergo further assessment for slow colonic transit and pelvic floor dysfunction (see Constipation, above).

4. Psychotropic agents—Patients with predominant symptoms of pain or bloating may benefit from low doses of tricyclic antidepressants, which are believed to have effects on motility, visceral sensitivity, and central pain perception that are independent of their psychotropic effects. Because of their anticholinergic effects, these agents may be more useful in patients with diarrhea-predominant than constipation-predominant symptoms. Nortriptyline, desipramine, or imipramine, may be started at a low dosage of 10 mg at bedtime and increased gradually to 50–150 mg as tolerated. Response rates do not correlate with dosage, and many patients respond to doses of ≤ 50 mg daily. Side effects are common, and lack of efficacy with one agent does not preclude benefit from another. Improvement should be evident within 4 weeks. The serotonin reuptake inhibitors (sertraline, 50–150 mg daily; citalopram 5–20 mg; paroxetine 10–20 mg daily; or fluoxetine, 20–40 mg daily) may lead

to improvement in overall sense of well-being but have little impact on abdominal pain or bowel symptoms. Anxiolytics should not be used chronically in irritable bowel syndrome because of their habituation potential. Patients with major depression or anxiety disorders should be identified and treated with therapeutic doses of appropriate agents.

5. Serotonin receptor agonists and antagonists—Serotonin is an important mediator of gastrointestinal motility and sensation. Alosetron and tegaserod modulate serotonin pathways. However, in 2007, tegaserod was withdrawn by the FDA from the US market after an analysis of safety data from over 18,000 patients in 29 clinical trials showed an excessive number of serious cardiovascular side effects.

Alosetron is a 5-HT$_3$ antagonist that is FDA-approved for the treatment of women with severe irritable bowel syndrome with predominant diarrhea. It appears to alter visceral sensation through blockade of peripheral 5-HT$_3$-receptors on enteric afferent neurons and inhibits enteric cholinergic motor neurons, resulting in inhibition of colonic motility. Alosetron (0.5–1 mg twice daily) reduces symptoms of pain, cramps, urgency, and diarrhea in 50–60% of women compared with 30–40% treated with placebo. Efficacy in men has not been demonstrated. In contrast to the excellent safety profile of other 5-HT$_3$ antagonists (eg, ondansetron), alosetron may cause constipation (sometimes severe) in 30% of patients or ischemic colitis in 4:1000 patients. Given the seriousness of these side effects, alosetron is restricted to women with severe irritable bowel syndrome with diarrhea who have not responded to conventional therapies and who have been educated about the relative risks and benefits of the agent. It should not be used in patients with constipation.

6. Nonabsorbable antibiotics—A randomized controlled study reported symptom improvement in 40% of patients treated with the nonabsorbable antibiotic rifaximin, 400 mg three times daily for 10 days, compared with a 25% improvement in placebo-treated patients. Improvement persisted over a 10-week follow-up period. Symptom improvement may be attributable to suppression of bacteria in either the small intestine or colon. At this time, the pathologic importance of small intestinal bacterial overgrowth and the therapeutic role of antibiotics in irritable bowel syndrome are controversial. If bacterial overgrowth is suspected, some clinicians may order a lactulose hydrogen breath test to confirm the diagnosis. Others may administer an empiric trial of rifaximin therapy. Still others may choose to defer evaluation or treatment pending further clinical studies.

7. Probiotics—Small controlled clinical trials report improved symptoms in some patients treated with one probiotic, *Bifidobacterium infantis*, but not with another probiotic, *Lactobacillus salivarius*, or placebo. It is hypothesized that alterations in gut flora may reduce symptoms through suppression of inflammation or reduction of bacterial gas production, resulting in reduced distention, flatus, and visceral sensitivity. Such therapy is attractive because it is safe, well tolerated, and inexpensive. A randomized, controlled trial confirmed global symptom improvement in approximately 60% of patients treated with *B infantis* (10^8

bacteria/capsule once daily), compared with 40% treated with placebo. Although promising, further study is needed to define the efficacy and optimal formulations of probiotic therapy.

D. Psychological Therapies

Cognitive-behavioral therapies, relaxation techniques, and hypnotherapy appear to be beneficial in some patients. Patients with underlying psychological abnormalities may benefit from evaluation by a psychiatrist or psychologist. Patients with severe disability should be referred to a pain treatment center.

▶ Prognosis

The majority of patients with irritable bowel syndrome learn to cope with their symptoms and lead productive lives.

American College of Gastroenterology IBS Task Force. An evidence-based position statement on the management of irritable bowel syndrome. Am J Gastroenterol. 2009 Jan;104(Suppl 1):S8–35.

Lackner JM et al. How does cognitive behavior therapy for irritable bowel syndrome work? A mediational analysis of a randomized clinical trial. Gastroenterology. 2007 Aug;133 (2):433–44. [PMID: 17681164]

Mayer EA. Clinical practice. Irritable bowel syndrome. N Engl J Med. 2008 Apr 17;358(16):1692–9. [PMID: 18420501]

Parkes GC et al. Gastrointestinal microbiota in irritable bowel syndrome: their role in pathogenesis and treatment. Am J Gastroenterol. 2008 Jun;103(6):1557–67. [PMID: 18513268]

Quigley EM. A 51-year old with irritable bowel syndrome: test or treat for bacterial overgrowth? Clin Gastroenterol Hepatol. 2007 Oct;5(10):1140–3. [PMID: 17916541]

ANTIBIOTIC-ASSOCIATED COLITIS

ESSENTIALS OF DIAGNOSIS

▶ Most cases of antibiotic-associated diarrhea are not attributable to *C difficile* and are usually mild and self-limited.

▶ Symptoms of antibiotic-associated colitis vary from mild to fulminant; almost all colitis is attributable to *C difficile*.

▶ Diagnosis in mild to moderate cases established by stool toxin assay.

▶ Flexible sigmoidoscopy provides most rapid diagnosis in severe cases.

▶ General Considerations

Antibiotic-associated diarrhea is a common clinical occurrence. Characteristically, the diarrhea occurs during the period of antibiotic exposure, is dose related, and resolves spontaneously after discontinuation of the antibiotic. In most cases, this diarrhea is mild, self-limited, and does not require any specific laboratory evaluation or treatment. Stool examination usually reveals no fecal leukocytes, and stool cultures reveal no pathogens. Although *C difficile* is identified in the stool of 15–25% of cases of antibiotic-associated diarrhea, it is also identified in 5–10% of patients treated with antibiotics who do not have diarrhea. Most cases of antibiotic-associated diarrhea are due to changes in colonic bacterial fermentation of carbohydrates and are not due to *C difficile*.

Antibiotic-associated colitis is a significant clinical problem almost always caused by *C difficile* infection. Hospitalized patients are most susceptible, especially those who are severely ill or malnourished or who are receiving chemotherapy. *C difficile*–colitis is the major cause of diarrhea in patients hospitalized for more than 3 days, affecting 22 patients of every 1000. This anaerobic bacterium colonizes the colon of 3% of healthy adults. It is acquired by fecal-oral transmission. Found throughout hospitals in patient rooms and bathrooms, it is readily transmitted from patient to patient by hospital personnel. Fastidious hand washing and use of disposable gloves are helpful in minimizing transmission. *C difficile* is acquired in approximately 20% of hospitalized patients, most of whom have received antibiotics that disrupt the normal bowel flora and thus allow the bacterium to flourish. Although almost all antibiotics have been implicated, colitis most commonly develops after use of ampicillin, clindamycin, third-generation cephalosporins, and fluoroquinolones. *C difficile*–colitis will develop in approximately one-third of infected patients. Symptoms usually begin during or shortly after antibiotic therapy but may be delayed for up to 8 weeks. All patients with acute diarrhea should be asked about recent antibiotic exposure. Patients who are elderly, debilitated, immunocompromised, receiving multiple antibiotics or prolonged (> 10 days) antibiotic therapy, receiving enteral tube feedings or proton pump inhibitors, or who have gastrointestinal tract disease or surgery have a higher risk of acquiring *C difficile* and developing *C difficile*–associated diarrhea.

The incidence and severity of *C difficile*–colitis in hospitalized patients appear to be increasing, which is attributable to the emergence of a more virulent strain of *C difficile* (BI/ NAP1) that contains an 18-base pair deletion of the tcdC gene, resulting in 10-fold higher toxin A and B production. This toxin-gene variant strain has been associated with several hospital outbreaks. The 30-day mortality attributed to infection with this strain is 7% but is 14% in the elderly. A recent placebo-controlled study demonstrated that prophylactic administration of probiotics (containing *Lactobacillus casei*, *Lactobacillus bulgaricus*, and *Streptococcus thermophilus*) to hospitalized patients who are receiving antibiotics reduced the incidence of *C difficile*–associated diarrhea from 34% to 12%.

▶ Clinical Findings

A. Symptoms and Signs

Most patients report mild to moderate greenish, foul-smelling watery diarrhea with lower abdominal cramps. Physical examination is normal or reveals mild left lower quadrant tenderness. With more serious illness, there is abdominal pain and profuse watery diarrhea with up to 30 stools per day. The stools may have mucus but seldom gross blood. There may be fever up to 40 °C, abdominal tenderness, and leukocytosis as high as 50,000/mcL. *C difficile*–colitis should be considered in all hospitalized patients with unexplained leukocytosis. In most patients, colitis is most severe in the distal colon and rectum. When colitis is more severe in the right side of the colon, there may be little or no diarrhea. In such cases, fever, abdominal distention, pain and tenderness, and leukocytosis suggest the presence of infection.

B. Special Examinations

1. Stool studies—Pathogenic strains of *C difficile* produce two toxins: toxin A is an enterotoxin and toxin B is a cytotoxin. In most patients, the diagnosis of antibiotic-associated colitis is established by the demonstration of *C difficile* toxins in the stool. A cytotoxicity assay (toxin B) performed in cell cultures has a specificity of 90% and a sensitivity of 95%. This is the definitive test, but it is expensive and results are not available for 24–48 hours. Rapid enzyme immunoassays (EIA) (2–4 hours) for toxins A and B are now widely used and have an 80–90% sensitivity with a single stool specimen but > 90% with two specimens. Some toxic strains of *C difficile* do not produce a functional toxin A (and therefore have a negative EIA); therefore, testing for toxin A and B is preferred. When *C difficile* is suspected but the EIA is negative, a cytotoxicity assay should be performed. Culture for *C difficile* is the most sensitive test, but 25% of isolates are not pathogenic. Because it is slower (2–3 days), more costly, and less specific than toxin assays, it is not used in most clinical settings. Fecal leukocytes are present in only 50% of patients with colitis.

2. Flexible sigmoidoscopy—Flexible sigmoidoscopy is performed in patients with more severe symptomatology when a rapid diagnosis is desired so that therapy can be initiated. In patients with mild to moderate symptoms, there may be no abnormalities or only patchy or diffuse, nonspecific colitis indistinguishable from other causes. In patients with severe illness, true **pseudomembranous colitis** is seen. This has a characteristic appearance, with yellow adherent plaques 2–10 mm in diameter scattered over the colonic mucosa interspersed with hyperemic mucosa. Biopsies reveal epithelial ulceration with a classic "volcano" exudate of fibrin and neutrophils. In 10% of cases, pseudomembranous colitis is confined to the proximal colon and may be missed at sigmoidoscopy.

3. Imaging studies—Abdominal radiographs are obtained in patients with fulminant symptoms to look for evidence of toxic dilation or megacolon but are of no value in mild disease. Mucosal edema or "thumbprinting" may be evident. Abdominal CT scan may be very useful in detecting colonic edema, especially in patients with predominantly right-sided colitis or abdominal pain without significant diarrhea (in whom the diagnosis may be unsuspected). CT scanning is also useful in the evaluation of possible complications.

▶ Differential Diagnosis

In the hospitalized patient in whom acute diarrhea develops after admission, the differential diagnosis includes simple antibiotic-associated diarrhea (not related to *C difficile*), enteral feedings, medications, and ischemic colitis. Other infectious causes are unusual in hospitalized patients in whom diarrhea develops more than 72 hours after admission, and it is not cost-effective to obtain stool cultures unless tests for *C difficile* are negative. Rarely, other organisms (staphylococci, *Clostridium perfringens*) have been associated with pseudomembranous colitis. *Klebsiella oxytoca* may cause a distinct form of antibiotic-associated hemorrhagic colitis that is segmental (usually in the right or transverse colon); spares the rectum; and is more common in younger, healthier outpatients.

▶ Complications

Fulminant disease may result in dehydration, electrolyte imbalance, toxic megacolon, perforation, and death. Chronic untreated colitis may result in weight loss and protein-losing enteropathy.

▶ Treatment

A. Immediate Treatment

If possible, antibiotic therapy should be discontinued and therapy with metronidazole or vancomycin should be initiated. For patients with mild disease, metronidazole, 500 mg orally three times daily or 250 mg orally four times daily, or vancomycin, 125 mg orally four times daily, are equally effective for initial treatment. Vancomycin is significantly more expensive than metronidazole and promotes the emergence of vancomycin-resistant hospital-associated infections. Therefore, metronidazole remains the preferred first-line therapy in most patients, while vancomycin should be reserved for patients who are intolerant of metronidazole, pregnant women, children, and patients who do not respond to metronidazole. The duration of initial therapy is usually 10–14 days. However, in patients requiring long-term systemic antibiotics, it may be appropriate to continue therapy until the antibiotics can be discontinued. Symptomatic improvement occurs in most patients within 72 hours.

For patients with severe disease, vancomycin, 125 mg orally four times daily, is the preferred agent because it achieves significantly higher response rates (97%) than metronidazole (76%). In patients who are unable to take oral medications due to ileus or who do not respond to oral vancomycin and in severely ill patients (marked leukocytosis, acute kidney injury, hypotension), intravenous metronidazole, 500 mg every 6 hours, should be given—supplemented by oral vancomycin administered per nasoenteric tube or enema. Intravenous vancomycin does not penetrate the bowel and should not be used. Total abdominal colectomy may be required in patients with toxic megacolon, perforation, sepsis, or hemorrhage.

B. Treatment of Relapse

Up to 20% of patients have a relapse of diarrhea from *C difficile* within 1 or 2 weeks after stopping initial therapy. This may be due to reinfection or failure to eradicate the organism. Most relapses respond promptly to a second course of metronidazole therapy. Some patients have recurrent relapses that can be difficult to treat. The optimal treatment regimen for recurrent relapses is unknown. Many authorities recommend a 7-week tapering regimen of vancomycin (125 mg orally four times daily for 14 days; twice daily for 7 days; once daily for 7 days; every other day for 7 days; and every third day for 14 days). Controlled trials show that oral administration of a live yeast, *Saccharomyces boulardii*, 500 mg twice daily, reduces the incidence of relapse by 50%. Probiotic therapy with this agent is recommended as adjunctive therapy in patients with relapsing disease.

Hickson M et al. Use of probiotic *Lactobacillus* preparation to prevent diarrhoea associated with antibiotics: randomised double blind placebo controlled trial. BMJ. 2007 Jul 14;335(7610):80. [PMID: 17604300]

Jaber MR et al. Clinical review of the management of fulminant *Clostridium difficile* infection. Am J Gastroenterol. 2008 Dec;103(12):3195–3203. [PMID: 18853982]

Kelly CP et al. *Clostridium difficile*—more difficult than ever. N Engl J Med. 2008 Oct 30;359(18):1932–40. [PMID: 18971494]

Nelson R. Antibiotic treatment for *Clostridium difficile*-associated diarrhea in adults. Cochrane Database Syst Rev. 2007 Jul 18;(3):CD004610. [PMID: 17636768]

INFLAMMATORY BOWEL DISEASE

The term "inflammatory bowel disease" includes ulcerative colitis and Crohn disease. Ulcerative colitis is a chronic, recurrent disease characterized by diffuse mucosal inflammation involving only the colon. Ulcerative colitis invariably involves the rectum and may extend proximally in a continuous fashion to involve part or all of the colon. Crohn disease is a chronic, recurrent disease characterized by patchy transmural inflammation involving any segment of the gastrointestinal tract from the mouth to the anus.

Crohn disease and ulcerative colitis may be associated in 50% of patients with a number of extraintestinal manifestations, including oral ulcers, oligoarticular or polyarticular nondeforming peripheral arthritis, spondylitis or sacroiliitis, episcleritis or uveitis, erythema nodosum, pyoderma gangrenosum, hepatitis and sclerosing cholangitis, and thromboembolic events.

▶ Drug Therapy

Although ulcerative colitis and Crohn disease appear to be distinct entities, the same pharmacologic agents are used to treat both. Despite extensive research, there are still no specific therapies for these diseases. The mainstays of therapy are 5-aminosalicylic acid derivatives, corticosteroids, immunomodulating agents (such as mercaptopurine or azathioprine), methotrexate, and biologic agents.

A. 5-Aminosalicylic Acid (5-ASA)

5-ASA is a topically active agent that has a variety of anti-inflammatory effects. It is used in the active treatment of ulcerative colitis and Crohn disease and during disease inactivity to maintain remission. It is readily absorbed from the small intestine but demonstrates minimal colonic absorption. A number of oral and topical compounds have been designed to target delivery of 5-ASA to the colon or small intestine while minimizing absorption. Commonly used formulations of 5-ASA are sulfasalazine, mesalamine, and azo compounds. Side effects of these compounds are uncommon but include nausea, rash, diarrhea, pancreatitis, and acute interstitial nephritis.

1. Oral mesalamine agents—These 5-ASA agents are coated in various pH-sensitive resins (Asacol and Lialda) or packaged in timed-release capsules (Pentasa). Pentasa releases 5-ASA slowly throughout the small intestine and colon. Asacol and Lialda tablets dissolve at pH 7.0, releasing 5-ASA in the terminal small bowel and proximal colon. Lialda has a multi-matrix system that gradually releases 5-ASA throughout the colon.

2. Azo compounds—Sulfasalazine, balsalazide and olsalazine contain 5-ASA linked by an azo bond that requires cleavage by colonic bacterial azoreductases to release 5-ASA. Absorption of these drugs from the small intestine is negligible. After release within the colon, the 5-ASA works topically and is largely unabsorbed. Olsalazine contains two 5-ASA molecules connected by the azo bond. Balsalazide contains 5-ASA linked to an inert carrier (4-aminobenzoyl-β-alanine).

Sulfasalazine contains 5-ASA linked to a sulfapyridine moiety. It is unclear whether the sulfapyridine group has any anti-inflammatory effects. One gram of sulfasalazine contains 400 mg of 5-ASA. The sulfapyridine group, however, is absorbed and may cause side effects in 15–30% of patients—much higher than with other 5-ASA compounds. Dose-related side effects include nausea, headaches, leukopenia, oligospermia, and impaired folate metabolism. Allergic and idiosyncratic side effects are fever, rash, hemolytic anemia, neutropenia, worsened colitis, hepatitis, pancreatitis, and pneumonitis. Because of its side effects, sulfasalazine is less frequently used than other 5-ASA agents. It should always be administered in conjunction with folate. Eighty percent of patients intolerant of sulfasalazine can tolerate mesalamine.

3. Topical mesalamine—5-ASA is provided in the form of suppositories (Canasa; 1000 mg) and enemas (Rowasa; 4 g/60 mL). These formulations can deliver much higher concentrations of 5-ASA to the distal colon than oral compounds. Side effects are uncommon.

B. Corticosteroids

A variety of intravenous, oral, and topical corticosteroid formulations have been used in inflammatory bowel disease. They have utility in the short-term treatment of moderate to severe disease. However, long-term use is associated with serious, potentially irreversible side effects and is to be avoided. The agents, route of administration, duration of use, and tapering regimens used are based more on personal bias and experience than on data from rigorous clinical trials. The most commonly used intravenous formulations have been hydrocortisone or methylprednisolone, which are given by continuous infusion or every 6 hours. Oral formulations are prednisone or methylprednisolone. Adverse events commonly occur during short-term systemic corticosteroid therapy, including mood changes, insomnia, dyspepsia, weight gain, edema, elevated serum glucose levels, acne, and moon facies. Side effects of long-term use include osteoporosis, osteonecrosis of the femoral head, myopathy, cataracts, and susceptibility to infections. Calcium and vitamin D supplementation should be administered to all patients receiving long-term corticosteroid therapy. Bone densitometry should be considered in patients with inflammatory bowel disease with other risk factors for osteoporosis and in all patients requiring long-term corticosteroids. Topical preparations are provided as hydrocortisone suppositories (100 mg), foam (90 mg), and enemas (100 mg). Budesonide is an oral glucocorticoid with high topical anti-inflammatory activity but low systemic activity due to high first-pass hepatic metabolism. A controlled-release formulation is available (Entocort) that targets delivery to the terminal ileum and proximal colon. It produces less suppression of the hypothalamic-pituitary-adrenal axis and fewer steroid-related side effects than hydrocortisone or prednisone.

C. Immunomodulating Drugs: Mercaptopurine, Azathioprine, or Methotrexate

Mercaptopurine and azathioprine are thiopurine drugs that are used in many patients with Crohn disease and ulcerative colitis who are corticosteroid-dependent in an attempt to reduce or withdraw the corticosteroids and to maintain patients in remission. Azathioprine is converted in vivo to mercaptopurine. It is believed that the active metabolite of mercaptopurine is 6-thioguanine. Monitoring of 6-thioguanine levels is performed in some clinical settings but is of unproven value in the management of most patients. Side effects of mercaptopurine and azathioprine, including allergic reactions (fever, rash, or arthralgias) and nonallergic reactions (nausea, vomiting, pancreatitis, hepatotoxicity, bone marrow suppression, infections, and a higher risk of lymphoma), occur in 15% of patients.

Three competing enzymes are involved in the metabolism of mercaptopurine to its active (6-thioguanine) and inactive metabolites. About 1 person in 300 has a homozygous mutation of one of the enzymes that metabolizes thiopurine methyltransferase (TPMT), placing them at risk for profound immunosuppression; 1 person in 9 is heterozygous for TPMT, resulting in intermediate enzyme activity. Measurement of TPMT functional activity is recommended prior to initiation of therapy. Treatment should be withheld in patients with absent TPMT activity. The most effective dose of mercaptopurine is 1–1.5 mg/kg or of azathioprine is 2–3 mg/kg daily. For patients with normal TPMT activity, both drugs may be initiated at the weight-calculated dose. A complete blood count should be obtained weekly for 4 weeks, biweekly for 4 weeks, and then every 1–3 months for the duration of therapy. Liver function tests should be measured periodically. Some clinicians prefer gradual dose-escalation, especially for patients with intermediate TPMT activity or in whom TPMT measurement is not available; both drugs may be started at 25 mg/d and increased by 25 mg every 1–2 weeks while monitoring

for myelosuppression until the target dose is reached. If the white blood count falls below 3000–4000/mcL or the platelet count falls below 100,000/mcL, the medication should be held for at least 1 week before reducing the daily dose by 25–50 mg.

Methotrexate is used in the treatment of patients with inflammatory bowel disease, especially patients with Crohn disease who are intolerant of mercaptopurine. Methotrexate is an analog of dihydrofolic acid. Although at high doses it interferes with cell proliferation through inhibition of nucleic acid metabolism, at low doses it has anti-inflammatory properties, including inhibition of expression of tumor necrosis factor-α (TNF-α) in monocytes and macrophages. Methotrexate may be given intramuscularly, subcutaneously, or orally. Side effects of methotrexate include nausea, vomiting, stomatitis, infections, bone marrow suppression, hepatic fibrosis, and life-threatening pneumonitis. A complete blood count and liver function tests should be monitored every 1–3 months. Folate supplementation (1 mg/d) should be administered.

D. Biologic Therapies

Although the etiology of inflammatory bowel disorders is uncertain, it appears that an abnormal response of the mucosal innate immune system to luminal bacteria may trigger inflammation, which is perpetuated by dysregulation of cellular immunity. A number of biologic therapies are available or in clinical testing that more narrowly target various components of the immune system. Biologic agents are highly effective for patients with corticosteroid-dependent or refractory disease and potentially may improve the natural history of disease. The potential benefits of these agents, however, must be carefully weighed with their high cost and risk of serious and potentially life-threatening side effects.

1. Anti-TNF therapies—A dysregulation of the T_H1 T cell response is present in some patients with inflammatory bowel disease, especially Crohn disease. TNF is one of the key proinflammatory cytokines in the T_H1 response. TNF exists in two biologically active forms: a soluble form (sTNF), which is enzymatically cleaved from its cell surface, and membrane-bound precursor (tmTNF). When either form binds to the TNF-receptors on effector cells, they initiate a variety of signaling pathways that lead to inflammatory gene activation. Three monoclonal antibodies to TNF currently are available for the treatment of inflammatory bowel disease: infliximab, adalimumab, and certolizumab. All three agents bind and neutralize soluble as well as membrane-bound TNF on macrophages and activated T lymphocytes, thereby preventing TNF stimulation of effector cells. When bound to membrane-associated TNF, infliximab and adalimumab may also cause apoptosis and cell lysis of TNF-producing cells.

Infliximab is a chimeric (75% human/25% mouse) IgG$_1$ antibody that is administered by intravenous infusion. A three-dose regimen of 5 mg/kg administered at 0, 2, and 6 weeks is recommended for acute induction, followed by infusions every 8 weeks for maintenance therapy. Acute infusion reactions occur in 5–10% of infusions but occur less commonly in patients receiving regularly scheduled infusions or concomitant immunomodulators (ie, azathioprine or methotrexate). Most reactions are mild or moderate (nausea; headache; dizziness; urticaria; diaphoresis; or mild cardiopulmonary symptoms that include chest tightness, dyspnea, or palpitations) and can be treated by slowing the infusion rate and administering acetaminophen and diphenhydramine. Severe reactions (hypotension, severe shortness of breath, rigors, severe chest discomfort) occur in less than 1% and may require oxygen, diphenhydramine, hydrocortisone, and epinephrine. Delayed serum sickness-like reactions occur in 1%. With repeated, intermittent intravenous injections, antibodies to infliximab develop in up to 40% of patients, which are associated with a shortened duration or loss of response and increased risk of acute or delayed infusion reactions. Giving infliximab in a regularly scheduled maintenance therapy (eg, every 8 weeks), concomitant use of infliximab with other immunomodulating agents (azathioprine, mercaptopurine, or methotrexate), or preinfusion treatment with corticosteroids (intravenous hydrocortisone 200 mg) significantly reduces the development of antibodies to approximately 10%.

Adalimumab is a fully human IgG$_1$ antibody that is administered by subcutaneous injection. A dose of 160 mg at week 0 and 80 mg at week 2 is recommended for acute induction, followed by maintenance therapy with 40 mg subcutaneously every other week. Certolizumab is a fusion compound in which the Fab1 portion of a chimeric (95% human/5% mouse) TNF-antibody is bound to polyethylene glycol in order to prolong the drug half-life. Because it lacks an Fc portion, it does not induce apoptosis, complement activation, or lysis of macrophages and activated T lymphocytes. A dose of 400 mg at weeks 0, 2, and 4 is recommended for acute induction, followed by maintenance therapy every 4 weeks with 400 mg. Both adalimumab and certolizumab are administered subcutaneously. Injection site reactions (burning, pain, redness, itching) are relatively common but are usually minor and self-limited. Because of their subcutaneous route of injection, acute and delayed hypersensitivity reactions are rare. Antibodies to adalimumab develop in 5% of patients and to certolizumab in 10%, which may lead to shortened duration or loss of response to the drug.

Serious infections with anti-TNF therapies may occur in 2–5% of patients, including sepsis, pneumonia, abscess, and cellulitis; however, controlled studies suggest the increased risk may be attributable to increased severity of disease and concomitant use of corticosteroids. Patients treated with anti-TNF therapies are at increased risk for the development of bacterial infections, tuberculosis, mycoses (candidiasis, histoplasmosis, coccidiomycosis, nocardiosis), reactivation of hepatitis B, and other opportunistic infections. Prior to use of these agents, patients should be screened for latent tuberculosis with PPD testing and a chest radiograph. Antinuclear and anti-DNA antibodies occur in a large percentage of patients; however, the development of drug-induced lupus is rare. All agents may cause severe hepatic reactions leading to acute hepatic failure; liver enzymes should be monitored routinely dur-

ing therapy. Although there are conflicting data, some studies suggest that anti-TNF therapies increase the risk of malignancies, especially non-Hodgkin lymphoma and nonmelanoma skin cancer. Rare cases of optic neuritis and demyelinating diseases, including multiple sclerosis have been reported. Anti-TNF therapies may worsen congestive heart failure in patients with cardiac disease.

2. Anti-Integrins—Natalizumab is a humanized monoclonal antibody targeted against α_4-integrins, heterodimeric glycoproteins on circulating immune cells that are involved with adhesion to and migration through the vascular endothelium into sites of inflammation. By binding to α_4-integrins, natalizumab may decrease the trafficking of circulating leukocytes through the vasculature and reduce chronic inflammation. In clinical trials, natalizumab was efficacious for the induction and maintenance of response and remission in patients with Crohn disease. Natalizumab was approved in 2008 for the treatment of patients with Crohn disease who had not responded to other therapies. However, due to an increased incidence of progressive multifocal leukoencephalopathy caused by reactivation of the JC virus, it is no longer available from the manufacturer for the treatment of Crohn disease.

Ansari A et al. Prospective evaluation of the pharmacogenetics of azathioprine in the treatment of inflammatory bowel disease. Aliment Pharmacol Ther. 2008 Oct 15;28(8):973–83. [PMID: 18616518]

Clark M et al. American Gastroenterological Association consensus development conference on the use of biologics in the treatment of inflammatory bowel disease, June 21–23, 2006. Gastroenterology. 2007 Jul;133(1):312–39. [PMID: 17631151]

Nielsen OH et al. Drug insight: aminosalicylates for the treatment of IBD. Nat Clin Pract Gastroenterol Hepatol. 2007 Mar;4(3):160–70. [PMID: 17339853]

▶ **Social Support for Patients**

Inflammatory bowel disease is a lifelong illness that can have profound emotional and social impacts on the individual. Patients should be encouraged to become involved in the Crohn's and Colitis Foundation of America (CCFA). National headquarters may be contacted at 444 Park Avenue South, 11th Floor, New York, NY 10016-7374; phone 212-685-3440. Internet address: http://www.ccfa.org.

1. Crohn Disease

ESSENTIALS OF DIAGNOSIS

▶ Insidious onset.

▶ Intermittent bouts of low-grade fever, diarrhea, and right lower quadrant pain.

▶ Right lower quadrant mass and tenderness.

▶ Perianal disease with abscess, fistulas.

▶ Radiographic evidence of ulceration, stricturing, or fistulas of the small intestine or colon.

General Considerations

One-third of cases of Crohn disease involve the small bowel only, most commonly the terminal ileum (ileitis). Half of all cases involve the small bowel and colon, most often the terminal ileum and adjacent proximal ascending colon (ileocolitis). In 20% of cases, the colon alone is affected. One-third of patients have associated perianal disease (fistulas, fissures, abscesses). Less than 5% patients have symptomatic involvement of the upper intestinal tract. Unlike ulcerative colitis, Crohn disease is a transmural process that can result in mucosal inflammation and ulceration, stricturing, fistula development, and abscess formation. Cigarette smoking is strongly associated with the development of Crohn disease, resistance to medical therapy, and early disease relapse.

Clinical Findings

A. Symptoms and Signs

Because of the variable location of involvement and severity of inflammation, Crohn disease may present with a variety of symptoms and signs. In eliciting the history, the clinician should take particular note of fevers, the patient's general sense of well-being, weight loss, the presence of abdominal pain, the number of liquid bowel movements per day, and prior surgical resections. Physical examination should focus on the patient's temperature, weight, and nutritional status, the presence of abdominal tenderness or an abdominal mass, rectal examination, and extraintestinal manifestations (described below). Most commonly, there is one or a combination of the following clinical constellations.

1. Chronic inflammatory disease—This is the most common presentation and is often seen in patients with ileitis or ileocolitis. Patients report low-grade fever, malaise, weight loss, and loss of energy. In patients with ileitis or ileocolitis, there may be diarrhea, which is usually nonbloody and often intermittent. In patients with colitis involving the rectum or left colon, there may be bloody diarrhea and fecal urgency, which may mimic the symptoms of ulcerative colitis. Cramping or steady right lower quadrant or periumbilical pain is common. Physical examination reveals focal tenderness, usually in the right lower quadrant. A palpable, tender mass that represents thickened or matted loops of inflamed intestine may be present in the lower abdomen.

2. Intestinal obstruction—Narrowing of the small bowel may occur as a result of inflammation, spasm, or fibrotic stenosis. Patients report postprandial bloating, cramping pains, and loud borborygmi. This may occur in patients with active inflammatory symptoms (as above) or later in the disease from chronic fibrosis without other systemic symptoms or signs of inflammation.

3. Penetrating disease and fistulae—Sinus tracts that penetrate through the bowel, where they may be contained or form fistulas to adjacent structures, develop in a subset of patients. Penetration through the bowel can result in an intra-abdominal or retroperitoneal phlegmon or abscess manifested by fevers, chills, a tender abdominal mass, and leukocytosis. Fistulas between the small intestine and colon commonly are asymptomatic but can result in diarrhea, weight loss, bacterial overgrowth, and malnutrition. Fistulas to the bladder produce recurrent infections. Fistulas to the vagina result in malodorous drainage and problems with personal hygiene. Fistulas to the skin usually occur at the site of surgical scars.

4. Perianal disease—One-third of patients with either large or small bowel involvement develop perianal disease manifested by large painful skin tags, anal fissures, perianal abscesses, and fistulas.

5. Extraintestinal manifestations—Extraintestinal manifestations may be seen with both Crohn disease and ulcerative colitis. These include arthralgias, arthritis, iritis or uveitis, pyoderma gangrenosum (Plate 68), or erythema nodosum. Oral aphthous lesions are common. There is an increased prevalence of gallstones due to malabsorption of bile salts from the terminal ileum. Nephrolithiasis with urate or calcium oxalate stones may occur.

B. Laboratory Findings

There is a poor correlation between laboratory studies and the patient's clinical picture. Laboratory values may reflect inflammatory activity or nutritional complications of disease. A complete blood count and serum albumin should be obtained in all patients. Anemia may reflect chronic inflammation, mucosal blood loss, iron deficiency, or vitamin B_{12} malabsorption secondary to terminal ileal inflammation or resection. Leukocytosis may reflect inflammation or abscess formation or may be secondary to corticosteroid therapy. Hypoalbuminemia may be due to intestinal protein loss (protein-losing enteropathy), malabsorption, bacterial overgrowth, or chronic inflammation. The sedimentation rate or C-reactive protein level is elevated in many patients during active inflammation. Fecal lactoferrin or calprotectin levels also are increased in patients with intestinal inflammation. Stool specimens are sent for examination for routine pathogens, ova and parasites, leukocytes, fat, and *C difficile* toxin.

C. Special Diagnostic Studies

In most patients, the initial diagnosis of Crohn disease is based on a compatible clinical picture with supporting endoscopic, pathologic, and radiographic findings. Colonoscopy usually is performed first to evaluate the colon and terminal ileum and to obtain mucosal biopsies. Typical endoscopic findings include aphthoid, linear or stellate ulcers, strictures, and segmental involvement with areas of normal-appearing mucosa adjacent to inflamed mucosa. In 10% of cases, it may be difficult to distinguish ulcerative colitis from Crohn disease. Granulomas on biopsy are present in less than 25% of patients but are highly suggestive of Crohn disease. CT or MR enterography or a barium upper gastrointestinal series with small bowel follow-through often is obtained in patients with suspected small bowel involvement. Suggestive findings include ulcerations, strictures, and fistulas; in addition, CT or MR enterography may identify bowel wall thickening and vascularity, mucosal enhancement, and fat stranding. Capsule imaging may help establish a diagnosis when clinical suspicion for small bowel involvement is high but radiographs are normal or nondiagnostic. When the diagnosis remains uncertain, a panel of seven tests that measure autoantibodies to P-ANCA as well as antibodies to the yeast *Saccharomyces cerevisiae*, to the outer membrane porin C of *E coli*, and to the bacterial flagellin Cbir1 (Prometheus IBD Serology 7) is marketed as being 92% accurate for diagnosing inflammatory bowel disease and for distinguishing between Crohn disease and ulcerative colitis. While intriguing, the data supporting these claims are unpublished and independent confirmation is needed before this panel can be recommended in routine clinical practice.

► Complications

A. Abscess

The presence of a tender abdominal mass with fever and leukocytosis suggests an abscess. Emergent CT of the abdomen is necessary to confirm the diagnosis. Patients should be given broad-spectrum antibiotics. Percutaneous drainage or surgery is usually required.

B. Obstruction

Small bowel obstruction may develop secondary to active inflammation or chronic fibrotic stricturing and is often acutely precipitated by dietary indiscretion. Patients should be given intravenous fluids with nasogastric suction. Systemic corticosteroids are indicated in patients with symptoms or signs of active inflammation but are unhelpful in patients with inactive, fixed disease. Patients unimproved on medical management require surgical resection of the stenotic area or stricturoplasty.

C. Abdominal and Rectovaginal Fistulas

Many fistulas are asymptomatic and require no specific therapy. Most symptomatic fistulas eventually require surgical therapy; however, medical therapy is effective in a subset of patients and is usually tried first in outpatients who otherwise are stable. Large abscesses associated with fistulas require percutaneous or surgical drainage. After percutaneous drainage, long-term antibiotics are administered in order to reduce recurrent infections until the fistula is closed or surgically resected. Fistulas may close temporarily in response to TPN or oral elemental diets but recur when oral feedings are resumed. Immunomodulating agents heal fistulas in one-third of patients within 3–6 months. For fistulas that do not close with immunomodulators, anti-TNF agents may promote closure in up to 60% within 10 weeks; however, relapse occurs in over one-half of patients within 1 year despite continued therapy. Surgical therapy is required for symptomatic fistulas that do not respond to medical therapy. Fistulas that arise above (proximal to) areas of intestinal stricturing commonly require surgical treatment.

D. Perianal Disease

Patients with fissures, fistulas, and skin tags commonly have perianal discomfort. Successful treatment of active intestinal disease also may improve perianal disease. Specific treatment of perianal disease can be difficult and is best approached jointly with a surgeon with an expertise in colorectal disorders. Pelvic MRI and endoscopic ultrasonography are the best noninvasive studies for evaluating perianal fistulas. Patients should be instructed on proper perianal skin care, including gentle wiping with a premoistened pad (baby wipes) followed by drying with a cool hair dryer, daily cleansing with sitz baths or a water wash, and use of perianal cotton balls or pads to absorb drainage. Oral antibiotics (metronidazole, 250 mg three times daily, or ciprofloxacin, 500 mg twice daily) may promote symptom improvement or healing in patients with fissures or uncomplicated fistulas; however, recurrent symptoms are common. Refractory fissures may benefit from mesalamine suppositories or topical 0.1% tacrolimus ointment. Immunomodulators or anti-TNF agents or both promote short-term symptomatic improvement from anal fistulas in two-thirds of patients and complete closure in up to one-half of patients; however, less than one-third maintain symptomatic remission during long-term maintenance treatment.

Anorectal abscesses should be suspected in patients with severe, constant perianal pain, or perianal pain in association with fever. Superficial abscesses are evident on perianal examination, but deep perirectal abscesses may be detected by digital examination or pelvic CT scan. Depending on the abscess location, surgical drainage may be achieved by incision, or catheter or seton placement. Surgery should be considered for patients with severe, refractory symptoms but is best approached after medical therapy of the Crohn disease has been optimized.

E. Carcinoma

Patients with colonic Crohn disease are at increased risk for developing colon carcinoma; hence, screening colonoscopy to detect dysplasia or cancer is recommended for patients with a history of 8 or more years of Crohn colitis. Patients with Crohn disease have an increased risk of lymphoma and of small bowel adenocarcinoma; however, both are rare.

F. Hemorrhage

Unlike ulcerative colitis, severe hemorrhage is unusual in Crohn disease.

G. Malabsorption

Malabsorption may arise after extensive surgical resections of the small intestine and from bacterial overgrowth in patients with enterocolonic fistulas, strictures, and stasis resulting in bacterial overgrowth.

► Differential Diagnosis

Chronic cramping abdominal pain and diarrhea are typical of both irritable bowel syndrome and Crohn disease, but x-ray examinations are normal in the former. Acute fever and right lower quadrant pain may resemble appendicitis or *Yersinia enterocolitica* enteritis. Intestinal lymphoma causes fever, pain, weight loss, and abnormal small bowel radiographs that may mimic Crohn disease. Patients with undiagnosed AIDS may present with fever and diarrhea. Segmental colitis may be caused by tuberculosis, *E histolytica*, *Chlamydia*, or ischemic colitis. *C difficile* or CMV infection may develop in patients with inflammatory bowel disease, mimicking disease recurrence. Diverticulitis with abscess formation may be difficult to distinguish acutely from Crohn disease. NSAIDs may exacerbate inflammatory bowel disease and may also cause NSAID-induced colitis characterized by small bowel or colonic ulcers, erosion, or strictures that tend to be most severe in the terminal ileum and right colon.

▶ Treatment of Active Disease

Crohn disease is a chronic lifelong illness characterized by exacerbations and periods of remission. As no specific therapy exists, current treatment is directed toward symptomatic improvement and controlling the disease process. The treatment must address the specific problems of the individual patient. All patients with Crohn disease should be counseled to discontinue cigarettes.

A. Nutrition

1. Diet—Patients should eat a well-balanced diet with as few restrictions as possible. Eating smaller but more frequent meals may be helpful. Patients with diarrhea should be encouraged to drink fluids to avoid dehydration. Many patients report that certain foods worsen symptoms, especially fried or greasy foods. Because lactose intolerance is common, a trial off dairy products is warranted if flatulence or diarrhea is a prominent complaint. Patients with obstructive symptoms should be placed on a low-roughage diet, ie, no raw fruits or vegetables, popcorn, nuts, etc. Resection of more than 100 cm of terminal ileum results in fat malabsorption for which a low-fat diet is recommended. Parenteral vitamin B_{12} (100 mcg intramuscularly per month) commonly is needed for patients with previous ileal resection or extensive terminal ileal disease.

2. Enteral therapy—Supplemental enteral therapy via nasogastric tube may be required for children and adolescents with poor intake and growth retardation.

3. Total parenteral nutrition—TPN is used short term in patients with active disease and progressive weight loss or those awaiting surgery who have malnutrition but cannot tolerate enteral feedings because of high-grade obstruction, high-output fistulas, severe diarrhea, or abdominal pain. It is required long term in a small subset of patients with extensive intestinal resections resulting in short bowel syndrome with malnutrition.

B. Symptomatic Medications

There are several potential mechanisms by which diarrhea may occur in Crohn disease in addition to active Crohn disease. A rational empiric treatment approach often yields therapeutic improvement that may obviate the need for corticosteroids or immunosuppressive agents. Involvement of the terminal ileum with Crohn disease or prior ileal resection may lead to reduced absorption of bile acids that may induce secretory diarrhea from the colon. This diar-

rhea commonly responds to cholestyramine 2–4 g, colestipol 5 g, or colesevelam 625 mg one to two times daily before meals to bind the malabsorbed bile salts. Patients with extensive ileal disease of more than 100 cm of ileal resection have such severe bile salt malabsorption that steatorrhea may arise. Such patients may benefit from a low-fat diet; bile salt-binding agents will exacerbate the diarrhea and should not be given. Patients with Crohn disease are at risk for the development of small intestinal bacterial overgrowth due to enteral fistulas, ileal resection, and impaired motility and may benefit from a course of broad-spectrum antibiotics (see Bacterial Overgrowth, above). Other causes of diarrhea include lactase deficiency and short bowel syndrome (described in other sections). Use of antidiarrheals may provide benefit in some patients. Loperamide (2–4 mg), diphenoxylate with atropine (one tablet), or tincture of opium (5–15 drops) may be given as needed up to four times daily. Because of the risk of toxic megacolon, these drugs should not be used in patients with active severe colitis.

C. Specific Drug Therapy

1. 5-Aminosalicylic acid agents—Mesalamine (Asacol 2.4–4.8 g/d; Pentasa 4 g/d) has long been used as initial therapy for the treatment of mild to moderately active colonic and ileocolonic Crohn disease. However, meta-analyses of published and unpublished trial data suggest that mesalamine is of little or no value in either the treatment of active Crohn disease or the maintenance of remission. Notwithstanding these data, many clinicians continue to use mesalamine as first-line therapy for patients with mild disease because of its safety relative to other agents.

2. Antibiotics—Antibiotics also are widely used by clinicians for the treatment of active luminal Crohn disease, although meta-analyses of controlled trials suggest that they have little or no efficacy. It is hypothesized that antibiotics may reduce inflammation through alteration of gut flora, reduction of bacterial overgrowth, or treatment of microperforations. Oral metronidazole (10 mg/kg/d) or ciprofloxacin (500 mg twice daily), or rifaximin (400 mg three times daily) are commonly administered for 6–12 weeks.

3. Corticosteroids—Approximately one-half of patients with Crohn disease require corticosteroids at some time in their illness. Corticosteroids dramatically suppress the acute clinical symptoms or signs in most patients with both small and large bowel disease; however, they do not alter the underlying disease. An ileal-release budesonide preparation (Entocort), 9 mg once daily for 8–16 weeks, induces remission in 50–70% of patients with mild to moderate Crohn disease involving the terminal ileum or ascending colon. After initial treatment, budesonide is tapered over 2–4 weeks in 3 mg increments. In some patients, low-dose budesonide (6 mg/d) may be used for up to 1 year to maintain remission. Budesonide is superior to mesalamine but somewhat less effective than prednisone. However, because budesonide has markedly reduced acute and chronic steroid-related adverse effects, including smaller reductions of bone mineral density, it is preferred to other systemic corticosteroids for the treatment of mild to moderate Crohn disease involving the terminal ileum or ascending colon.

Prednisone or methylprednisolone, 40–60 mg/d, is generally administered to patients with Crohn disease that is severe, that involves the distal colon or proximal small intestine, or that has failed treatment with budesonide. Remission or significant improvement occurs in greater than 80% of patients after 8–16 weeks of therapy. After improvement at 2 weeks, tapering proceeds at 5 mg/wk until a dosage of 20 mg/d is being given. Thereafter, slow tapering by 2.5 mg/wk is recommended. Approximately 20% of patients cannot be completely withdrawn from corticosteroids without experiencing a symptomatic flare-up. Furthermore, more than 50% of patients who achieve initial remission on corticosteroids will experience a relapse within 1 year. Use of long-term low corticosteroid doses (2.5–10 mg/d) should be avoided, because of associated complications (see above). Patients requiring long-term corticosteroid treatment should be given immunomodulatory drugs (as described below) in an effort to wean them from corticosteroids.

Patients with persisting symptoms despite oral corticosteroids or those with high fever, persistent vomiting, evidence of intestinal obstruction, severe weight loss, severe abdominal tenderness, or suspicion of an abscess should be hospitalized. In patients with a tender, palpable inflammatory abdominal mass, CT scan of the abdomen should be obtained prior to administering corticosteroids to rule out an abscess. If no abscess is identified, parenteral corticosteroids should be administered (as described for ulcerative colitis).

4. Immunomodulating drugs: Azathioprine, mercaptopurine, or methotrexate—Immunomodulating agents are used in approximately two-thirds of patients with Crohn disease who have not responded to corticosteroids or who require repeated courses of long-term corticosteroids to control symptoms. These agents permit elimination or reduction of corticosteroids in over 75% and fistula closure in 30% of patients. In the United States, mercaptopurine or azathioprine are more commonly used than methotrexate. The mean time to symptomatic response is 2–4 months, so these agents are not useful for acute exacerbations. Meta-analyses of controlled trials suggest that patients with Crohn disease treated with immunomodulating agents are three times as likely to achieve remission and 2.25 times as likely to maintain remission as those treated with corticosteroids. Once patients achieve remission, immunomodulating drugs reduce the 3-year relapse rate from over 60% to less than 25%. Methotrexate (25 mg intramuscularly or subcutaneously weekly for 12 weeks, followed by 12.5–15 mg once weekly) is used in patients who are unresponsive to or intolerant of mercaptopurine or azathioprine. Because oral absorption may be erratic, parenteral administration is preferred. Other immunosuppressive agents have been investigated in the treatment of Crohn disease, including cyclosporine and thalidomide; however, efficacy has been modest and toxicity greater than with the thiopurines.

5. Anti-TNF therapies—Infliximab, adalimumab, and certolizumab are used for the treatment of patients with moderate to severe Crohn disease (including fistulizing disease) with an inadequate response to mesalamine, antibiotics, corticosteroids or immunomodulators. These agents are also used to treat severe disease in hospitalized patients and extraintestinal manifestations of Crohn disease (except optic neuritis). The doses for acute induction therapy are described above. Up to two-thirds of patients have significant clinical improvement during acute induction therapy. After initial clinical response, symptom relapse occurs in greater than 80% of patients within 1 year in the absence of further maintenance therapy. Therefore, scheduled maintenance therapy is usually recommended (infliximab, 5 mg/kg infusion every 8 weeks; adalimumab, 40 mg subcutaneous injection every 2 weeks; certolizumab, 400 mg subcutaneous injection every 4 weeks). With long-term maintenance therapy, approximately two-thirds have continued clinical response and up to one-half have complete symptom remission. A gradual or complete loss of efficacy occurs over time in some patients, necessitating increased dosing (infliximab 10 mg/kg; adalimumab 80 mg), decreased dosing intervals (infliximab every 6 weeks; adalimumab every week), changing to the alternative agent, or discontinuation of anti-TNF therapy. In some cases, loss of efficacy is due to the development of antibodies to the anti-TNF agent (ATAs). Scheduled maintenance therapy is associated with a lower likelihood of developing ATA and an increased likelihood of sustained response. Concomitant therapy with anti-TNF agents and immunomodulating agents (azathioprine, mercaptopurine, or methotrexate) reduces the risk of development of ATA but may increase the risk of complications from anti-TNF agents, including the development of hepatosplenic T-cell lymphoma. One 2008 trial comparing infliximab alone to combination infliximab and methotrexate found no difference in disease remission rates after 1 year. However, the 2008 interim 6-month analysis of a trial comparing infliximab alone to combination infliximab and azathioprine found higher disease remission rates with combination therapy. Pending further analysis of the outcomes of these trials (including remission rates, complications, and incidence of ATA), it remains controversial whether anti-TNF agents should be used alone or in combination with immunomodulators.

There is also controversy about to whether anti-TNF agents should continue to be reserved as second-line therapy in patients with moderate to severe Crohn disease who have not responded to prior therapy with corticosteroids and immunomodulators ("step-up" therapy) or whether it should be used early in the course of illness ("step-down" therapy) with the goal of inducing early remission and altering the natural history of the disease. A 2008 study of patients with moderate to severe Crohn disease of less than 4 years duration, compared step-down therapy (infliximab for induction followed by azathioprine for maintenance) with step-up therapy (corticosteroids, followed by azathioprine, followed by infliximab). After 1-year, 61% of patients who received step-down therapy were in clinical remission compared with 42% who received step-up therapy. Further investigation of the role up step-down therapy is needed.

Indications for Surgery

Over 50% of patients will require at least one surgical procedure. The main indications for surgery are intractability to medical therapy, intra-abdominal abscess, massive bleeding, symptomatic refractory internal or perianal fistulas, and intestinal obstruction. Patients with chronic obstructive symptoms due to a short segment of ileal stenosis are best treated with resection or strictureplasty (rather than long-term medical therapy), which promotes rapid return of well-being and elimination of corticosteroids. After surgery, endoscopic evidence of recurrence occurs in 60% within 1 year. Clinical recurrence occurs in 20% of patients within 1 year and 80% within 10–15 years. Therapy with metronidazole, 250 mg three times daily for 3 months, or long-term therapy with immunomodulators (mercaptopurine or azathioprine), or both, may be modestly effective in preventing clinical and endoscopic recurrence after ileocolic resection and is recommended for high-risk patients.

Prognosis

With proper medical and surgical treatment, the majority of patients are able to cope with this chronic disease and its complications and lead productive lives. Few patients die as a direct consequence of the disease.

When to Refer

- For expertise in endoscopic procedures or capsule endoscopy.
- Any patient requiring hospitalization for follow-up.
- Patients with moderate to severe disease for whom therapy with immunomodulators or biologic agents is being considered.
- When surgery may be necessary.

When to Admit

- An intestinal obstruction is suspected.
- An intra-abdominal or perirectal abscess is suspected.
- A serious infectious complication is suspected, especially in patients who are immunocompromised due to concomitant use of corticosteroids, immunomodulators, or anti-TNF agents.
- Patients with severe symptoms of diarrhea, dehydration, weight loss, or abdominal pain.
- Patients with severe or persisting symptoms despite treatment with corticosteroids.

Austin GL et al. A critical evaluation of serologic markers for inflammatory bowel disease. Clin Gastrenterol Hepatol. 2007 May 5;5(5):545–7. [PMID: 17433787]

Caspersen S et al. Infliximab for inflammatory bowel disease in Denmark 1999–2005: clinical outcome and follow-up evaluation of malignancy and mortality. Clin Gastroenterol Hepatol. 2008 Nov;6(11):1212–7. [PMID: 18848503]

Colombel JF et al. Adalimumab for maintenance of clinical response and remission in patients with Crohn's disease: the CHARM trial. Gastroenterology. 2007 Jan;132(1):52–65. [PMID: 17241859]

D'Haens G et al. Early combined immunosuppression or conventional management in patients with newly diagnosed Crohn's disease: an open randomized trial. Lancet. 2008 Feb 23;371(9613):660–7. [PMID: 18295023]

D'Haens G et al. Therapy of metronidazole with azathioprine to prevent postoperative recurrence of Crohn's disease: a controlled randomized trial. Gastroenterology. 2008 Oct;135(4):1123–9. [PMID: 18727929]

Feagan BG et al. Effects of adalimumab therapy on hospitalization and surgery in Crohn's disease: results from the CHARM study. Gastroenterology. 2008 Nov;135(5):1493–9. [PMID: 18848553]

Irving PM et al. Review article: appropriate use of corticosteroids in Crohn's disease. Aliment Pharmacol Ther. 2007 Aug 1;26(3):313–29. [PMID: 17635367]

Jones J et al. Relationships between disease activity and serum and fecal biomarkers in patients with Crohn's disease. Clin Gastroenterol Hepatol. 2008 Nov;6(11):1218–24. [PMID: 18799360]

Nikolaus S et al. Diagnostics of inflammatory bowel disease. Gastroenterology. 2007 Nov;133(5):1670–89. [PMID: 17983810]

Peyrin-Biroulet L et al. Efficacy and safety of tumor necrosis factor antagonists in Crohn's disease: meta-analysis of placebo-controlled trials. Clin Gastroenterol Hepatol. 2008 Jun;6(6):644–53. [PMID: 18550004]

Sandborn WJ. Current directions in IBD therapy: what goals are feasible with biological modifiers? Gastroenterology. 2008 Nov;135(5):1442–7. [PMID: 18848556]

Solem CA et al. Small-bowel imaging in Crohn's disease: a prospective, blinded, 4-way comparison. Gastrointest Endosc. 2008 Aug;68(2):255–66. [PMID: 18513722]

Terdiman JP. Prevention of postoperative recurrence in Crohn's disease. Clin Gastroenterol Hepatol. 2008 Jun;6(6):616–20. [PMID: 17967564]

Van Assche G et al. Withdrawal of immunosuppression in Crohn's disease treated with scheduled infliximab maintenance: a randomized trial. Gastroenterology. 2008 Jun;134(7):1861–8. [PMID: 18440315]

2. Ulcerative Colitis

ESSENTIALS OF DIAGNOSIS

- ▶ Bloody diarrhea.
- ▶ Lower abdominal cramps and fecal urgency.
- ▶ Anemia, low serum albumin.
- ▶ Negative stool cultures.
- ▶ Sigmoidoscopy is the key to diagnosis.

General Considerations

Ulcerative colitis is an idiopathic inflammatory condition that involves the mucosal surface of the colon, resulting in diffuse friability and erosions with bleeding. Approximately one-third of patients have disease confined to the rectosigmoid region (proctosigmoiditis); one-third have disease that extends to the splenic flexure (left-sided colitis); and one-third have disease that extends more proximally (extensive colitis). There is some correlation between disease extent and symptom severity. In the majority of patients, the extent of colonic involvement does not progress over time. In most patients, the disease is characterized by periods of symptomatic flare-ups and remissions. Ulcerative colitis is more common in nonsmokers and former smokers. Disease severity may be lower in active smokers and may worsen in patients who stop smoking. Appendectomy before the age of 20 years for acute appendicitis is associated with a reduced risk of developing ulcerative colitis.

Clinical Findings

A. Symptoms and Signs

The clinical profile in ulcerative colitis is highly variable. Bloody diarrhea is the hallmark. On the basis of several clinical and laboratory parameters, it is clinically useful to classify patients as having mild, moderate, or severe disease (Table 15–12). Patients should be asked about stool frequency, the presence and amount of rectal bleeding, cramps, abdominal pain, fecal urgency, and tenesmus. Physical examination should focus on the patient's volume status as determined by orthostatic blood pressure and pulse measurements and by nutritional status. On abdominal examination, the clinician should look for tenderness and evidence of peritoneal inflammation. Red blood may be present on digital rectal examination.

1. Mild to moderate disease—Patients with mild disease have a gradual onset of infrequent diarrhea (less than five movements per day) with intermittent rectal bleeding and mucus. Stools may be formed or loose in consistency. Because of rectal inflammation, there is fecal urgency and tenesmus. Left lower quadrant cramps relieved by defecation are common, but there is no significant abdominal tenderness. Patients with moderate disease have more severe diarrhea with frequent bleeding. Abdominal pain and tenderness may be present but are not severe. There may be mild fever, anemia, and hypoalbuminemia.

2. Severe disease—Patients with severe disease have more than six to ten bloody bowel movements per day, resulting in severe anemia, hypovolemia, and impaired nutrition with hypoalbuminemia. Abdominal pain and tenderness are present. "Fulminant colitis" is a subset of severe disease characterized by rapidly worsening symptoms with signs of toxicity.

B. Laboratory Findings

The degree of abnormality of the hematocrit, sedimentation rate, and serum albumin reflects disease severity.

C. Endoscopy

In acute colitis, the diagnosis is readily established by sigmoidoscopy. The mucosal appearance is characterized by edema, friability, mucopus, and erosions. Colonoscopy should not be performed in patients with fulminant disease because of the risk of perforation. After patients have demonstrated improvement on therapy, colonoscopy is performed to determine the extent of disease.

D. Imaging

Plain abdominal radiographs are obtained in patients with severe colitis to look for significant colonic dilation. Barium enemas are of little utility in the evaluation of acute ulcerative colitis and may precipitate toxic megacolon in patients with severe disease.

Differential Diagnosis

The initial presentation of ulcerative colitis is indistinguishable from other causes of colitis, clinically as well as endoscopically. Thus, the diagnosis of idiopathic ulcerative colitis is reached after excluding other known causes of colitis. Infectious colitis should be excluded by sending stool specimens for routine bacterial cultures (to exclude *Salmonella, Shigella,* and *Campylobacter,* as well as specific assays for *E coli* O157), ova and parasites (to exclude amebiasis), and stool toxin assay for *C difficile.* Mucosal biopsy can distinguish amebic colitis from ulcerative colitis. CMV colitis occurs in immunocompromised patients and is diagnosed on mucosal biopsy. Gonorrhea, chlamydial infection, herpes, and syphilis are considerations in sexually active patients with proctitis. In elderly patients with cardiovascular disease, ischemic colitis may involve the rectosigmoid. A history of radiation to the pelvic region can result in proctitis months to years later. Crohn disease involving the colon but not the small intestine may be confused with ulcerative colitis. In 10% of patients, a distinction between Crohn disease and ulcerative colitis may not be possible. The possible utility of serologic testing (Prometheus IBD Serology 7 panel) in patients with indeterminate colitis requires further clinical study (see discussion in the section on Crohn disease).

Treatment

There are two main treatment objectives: (1) to terminate the acute, symptomatic attack and (2) to prevent recurrence of attacks. The treatment of acute ulcerative colitis depends on the extent of colonic involvement and the severity of illness.

Patients with mild to moderate disease should eat a regular diet but limit their intake of caffeine and gas-

Table 15–12. Ulcerative colitis: Assessment of disease activity.

	Mild	Moderate	Severe
Stool frequency (per day)	< 4	4–6	> 6 (mostly bloody)
Pulse (beats/min)	< 90	90–100	> 100
Hematocrit (%)	Normal	30–40	< 30
Weight loss (%)	None	1–10	> 10
Temperature (°F)	Normal	99–100	> 100
ESR (mm/h)	< 20	20–30	> 30
Albumin (g/dL)	Normal	3–3.5	< 3

ESR, erythrocyte sedimentation rate.

producing vegetables. Antidiarrheal agents should not be given in the acute phase of illness but are safe and helpful in patients with mild chronic symptoms. Loperamide (2 mg) or diphenoxylate with atropine (one tablet) may be given up to four times daily. Such remedies are particularly useful at nighttime and when taken prophylactically for occasions when patients may not have reliable access to toilet facilities.

A. Distal Colitis

Patients with disease confined to the rectum or rectosigmoid region generally have mild but distressing symptoms. Patients may be treated with topical mesalamine, topical corticosteroids, or oral aminosalicylates (5-ASA) according to patient preference and cost considerations. Topical mesalamine is the drug of choice and is superior to topical corticosteroids and 5-ASA. Mesalamine is administered as a suppository, 1000 mg once daily at bedtime for proctitis, and as an enema, 4 g at bedtime for proctosigmoiditis, for 4–12 weeks, with 75% of patients improving (Table 15–13). Topical corticosteroids are a less expensive alternative to mesalamine but are also less effective. Hydrocortisone suppository or foam is prescribed for proctitis and hydrocortisone enema (80–100 mg) for proctosigmoiditis. Systemic effects from short-term use are very slight. Patients who either decline or are unable to manage topical therapy may be treated with oral 5-ASA, as discussed below. For patients with distal disease who do not improve with once daily topical therapy, the following options may be considered: (1) combination topical therapy with a 5-ASA suppository or enema at bedtime and a corticosteroid enema or foam in the morning, or (2) a combination of a topical agent with an oral 5-ASA agent.

Patients whose acute symptoms resolve rapidly with immediate therapy may have prolonged periods of remission that are treated successfully with intermittent courses of therapy. Patients with early or frequent relapse should be treated with maintenance therapy with mesalamine suppositories (1000 mg) or enemas (4 g) nightly or every

---

Table 15–13. Treatment of ulcerative colitis.

Distal colitis
  Proctitis
    Mesalamine suppositories, 1000 mg per rectum once daily, or—
    Hydrocortisone foam, 90 mg per rectum daily, or—
    Hydrocortisone suppositories, 100 mg per rectum daily
  Proctosigmoiditis
    Mesalamine enema, 4 g per rectum daily, or—
    Hydrocortisone enema, 100 mg per rectum daily
Extensive colitis
  Mild to moderate
    Sulfasalazine, 1–1.5 g orally twice daily, or—
    Mesalamine tablets (delayed-release), 2.0–4.8 g orally daily, or—
    Balsalazide, 2.25 g orally three times a day
    If no response after 2–4 weeks, add mesalamine enema 4 g orally daily or prednisone, 40–60 mg orally daily (taper by 5 mg/wk)
  Severe
    Methylprednisolone, 48–60 mg IV daily

---

other night. For patients who have difficulty complying with topical therapies, oral 5-ASA agents are an acceptable, though possibly less effective, alternative (see below).

B. Mild to Moderate Colitis

1. 5-ASA Agents—Disease extending above the sigmoid colon is best treated with 5-ASA agents (mesalamine, balsalazide, or sulfasalazine), which result in symptomatic improvement in 50–75% of patients. Most patients improve within 3–6 weeks, though some require 2–3 months. Mesalamine (Asacol 0.8–1.6 g three times daily; Lialda 1.2 g once or twice daily; Pentasa 0.5–1 g four times daily) and balsalazide, 2.25 g three times daily, are approved for active disease (Table 15–13). These agents achieve clinical improvement in 50–70% of patients and remission in 20–30%. Total doses of mesalamine above 2.0–2.4 g/d result in marginal increases in remission. Sulfasalazine is comparable in efficacy to mesalamine and because of its low cost is still commonly used as a first-line agent by many providers, though it is associated with greater side effects. To minimize side effects, sulfasalazine is begun at a dosage of 500 mg twice daily and increased gradually over 1–2 weeks to 2 g twice daily (Table 15–13). Total doses of 5–6 g/d may have greater efficacy but are poorly tolerated. Folic acid, 1 mg/d, should be administered to all patients taking sulfasalazine.

2. Corticosteroids—Patients with mild to moderate disease who do not improve after 4–8 weeks of 5-ASA therapy should have the addition of corticosteroid therapy. The addition of topical therapy with 5-ASA enemas (4 g once daily) or hydrocortisone foam or enemas (80–100 mg once or twice daily) may be tried first. Patients who do not improve after 2 more weeks require systemic corticosteroid therapy. Prednisone and methylprednisolone are most commonly used. Depending on the severity of illness, the initial oral dose of prednisone is 40–60 mg daily. Rapid improvement is observed in most cases within 2 weeks. Thereafter, tapering of prednisone should proceed by 5–10 mg/wk. After tapering to 20 mg/d, slower tapering (2.5 mg/week) is sometimes required. Complete tapering without symptomatic flare-ups is possible in the majority of patients.

3. Immunomodulating agents—A subset of patients either does not respond to aminosalicylates or corticosteroids or has symptomatic flares during attempts at corticosteroid tapering. Although surgical resection is traditionally recommended for patients with refractory disease, many patients may wish to avoid surgery and others have moderately severe disease for which surgery might not otherwise be warranted. Immunomodulating agents are used for the treatment of ulcerative colitis; however, the risks of these drugs from chronic immunosuppression must be weighed against the certainty of cure with surgical resection. Limited trials suggest mercaptopurine or azathioprine is of benefit in 60% of patients, allowing tapering of corticosteroids and maintenance of remission. There is less evidence that methotrexate is effective.

Infliximab is approved in the United States for the treatment of patients with moderate to severe ulcerative colitis who have had an inadequate response to conventional therapies (oral corticosteroids, mercaptopurine or azathioprine, and mesalamine). Following a three-dose induction regimen of 5 mg/kg administered at 0, 2, and 6 weeks, clinical response occurs in 65% and clinical remission in 35%. Other anti-TNF agents (ie, adalimumab) have not been approved for treatment of ulcerative colitis.

C. Severe Colitis

About 15% of patients with ulcerative colitis have a more severe course. Because they may progress to fulminant colitis or toxic megacolon, hospitalization is generally required.

1. General measures—Discontinue all oral intake for 24–48 hours or until the patient demonstrates clinical improvement. TPN is indicated only in patients with poor nutritional status or if feedings cannot be reinstituted within 7–10 days. All opioid or anticholinergic agents should be discontinued. Restore circulating volume with fluids, correct electrolyte abnormalities, and consider transfusion for significant anemia (hematocrit < 25–28%). Abdominal examinations should be repeated to look for evidence of worsening distention or pain. A plain abdominal radiograph should be ordered on admission to look for evidence of colonic dilation. Send stools for bacterial culture, *C difficile* toxin assay, and examination for ova and parasites. CMV superinfection should be considered in patients receiving long-term immunosuppressive therapy who are unresponsive to corticosteroid therapy. Surgical consultation should be sought for all patients with severe disease.

2. Corticosteroid therapy—Methylprednisolone, 48–64 mg, or hydrocortisone, 300 mg, is administered in four divided doses or by continuous infusion over 24 hours. Higher or "pulse" doses are of no benefit. Hydrocortisone enemas (100 mg) may also be administered twice daily for treatment of urgency or tenesmus. Approximately 50–75% of patients achieve remission with systemic corticosteroids within 7–10 days. Once symptomatic improvement has occurred, oral fluids are reinstituted. If fluids are well tolerated, intravenous corticosteroids are discontinued and the patient is started on oral prednisone (as described for moderate disease).

3. Anti-TNF therapies—A single infusion of infliximab, 5 mg/kg, has been shown in recent controlled and uncontrolled studies to be effective in treating severe colitis in patients who did not improve within 4–7 days of intravenous corticosteroid therapy. In a controlled study of patients hospitalized for ulcerative colitis, colectomy was required within 3 months in 69% who received placebo therapy, compared with 47% who received infliximab. Although further studies are needed, infliximab therapy should be considered in patients with severe ulcerative colitis who have not improved with intravenous corticosteroid therapy.

4. Cyclosporine—Intravenous cyclosporine (2–4 mg/kg/d as a continuous infusion) benefits 60–75% of patients with severe colitis who have not improved after 7–10 days of corticosteroids. In patients with severe steroid-resistant colitis who are reluctant to undergo colectomy, intravenous cyclosporine may be considered as a "bridge" therapy

while mercaptopurine or azathioprine therapy (which take 2–4 months for full efficacy) is initiated. Up to two-thirds of responders may be maintained in remission with a combination of oral cyclosporine for 3 months and long-term therapy with mercaptopurine or azathioprine. The relative role of infliximab versus cyclosporine in the treatment of severe colitis requires further clinical study.

5. Surgical therapy—Patients with severe disease who fail to improve after 7–10 days of corticosteroid, infliximab or cyclosporine therapy are unlikely to respond to further medical therapy, and surgery is recommended.

D. Fulminant Colitis and Toxic Megacolon

A subset of patients with severe disease has a more fulminant course with rapid progression of symptoms over 1–2 weeks and signs of severe toxicity. These patients appear quite ill, with fever, prominent hypovolemia, hemorrhage requiring transfusion, and abdominal distention with tenderness. They are at a higher risk of perforation or development of toxic megacolon and must be followed closely. Broad-spectrum antibiotics should be administered to cover anaerobes and gram-negative bacteria.

Toxic megacolon develops in less than 2% of cases of ulcerative colitis. It is characterized by colonic dilation of more than 6 cm on plain films with signs of toxicity. In addition to the therapies outlined above, nasogastric suction should be initiated. Patients should be instructed to roll from side to side and onto the abdomen in an effort to decompress the distended colon. Serial abdominal plain films should be obtained to look for worsening dilation or ischemia. Patients with fulminant disease or toxic megacolon who worsen or fail to improve within 48–72 hours should undergo surgery to prevent perforation. If the operation is performed before perforation, the mortality rate should be low.

▶ Maintenance of Remission

Without long-term therapy, 75% of patients who initially go into remission on medical therapy will experience a symptomatic relapse within 1 year. Long-term maintenance therapy with sulfasalazine, 1–1.5 g twice daily, and mesalamine, 800 mg 2–3 times daily or 500 mg four times daily, has been shown to reduce relapse rates to less than 35%. Mercaptopurine and azathioprine are useful in patients with frequent disease relapses (more than two per year) or corticosteroid-dependent disease to maintain remission. The role of long-term infliximab therapy in the maintenance of remission is evolving. In two, large, controlled studies of patients with active moderate to severe colitis, initial induction therapy was followed by infliximab maintenance infusions (5 mg/kg) administered every 8 weeks for 30–54 weeks. At the end of the study (30 or 54 weeks), 35% were in clinical remission, (21% in corticosteroid-free remission), a modest but impressive response in patients with more refractory disease. In considering long-term infliximab therapy, patients and clinicians need to weigh the long-term risks of immunosuppression against colectomy.

Risk of Colon Cancer

In patients with ulcerative colitis with disease proximal to the rectum and in patients with Crohn colitis, there is a markedly increased risk of developing colon carcinoma. A large meta-analysis of observational studies reported a cumulative incidence of 2% at 10 years, 8% at 20 years, and 18% after 30 years of disease. Retrospective studies suggest that the risk of colon cancer may be reduced in patients treated with long-term 5-ASA therapy. Ingestion of folic acid, 1 mg/d, also is associated with a decreased risk of cancer development. Colonoscopies are recommended every 1–2 years in patients with colitis, beginning 8–10 years after diagnosis. At colonoscopy, multiple (at least 32) random mucosal biopsies are taken throughout the colon at 10-cm intervals as well as biopsies of mass lesions to look for dysplasia or carcinoma. Because of the relatively high incidence of concomitant carcinoma in patients with dysplasia (either low or high grade) in flat mucosa or mass lesions, colectomy is recommended. Several prospective studies demonstrate that dye spraying with methylene blue or indigo carmine ("chromoendoscopy") enhances the detection of subtle mucosal lesions, thereby significantly increasing the detection of dysplasia compared with standard colonoscopy. Although surveillance colonoscopy appears to be effective in reducing the incidence of colon cancer, patients must understand that approximately one-third of detected cancers are advanced, despite compliance with routine colonoscopy surveillance.

Surgery in Ulcerative Colitis

Surgery is required in 25% of patients. Severe hemorrhage, perforation, and documented carcinoma are absolute indications for surgery. Surgery is indicated also in patients with fulminant colitis or toxic megacolon that does not improve within 48–72 hours, in patients with dysplasia on surveillance colonoscopy, and in patients with refractory disease requiring long-term corticosteroids to control symptoms.

Although total proctocolectomy (with placement of an ileostomy) provides complete cure of the disease, most patients seek to avoid it out of concern for the impact it may have on their bowel function, their self-image, and their social interactions. After complete colectomy, patients may have a standard ileostomy with an external appliance, a continent ileostomy, or an internal ileal pouch that is anastomosed to the anal canal (ileal pouch-anal anastomosis). The latter maintains intestinal continuity, thereby obviating an ostomy. Under optimal circumstances, patients have five to seven loose bowel movements per day without incontinence. Endoscopic or histologic inflammation in the ileal pouch ("pouchitis") develops in over 40% of patients, resulting in increased stool frequency, fecal urgency, cramping, and bleeding, but usually resolves with a 2-week course of metronidazole (10 mg/kg/d) or ciprofloxacin (500 mg twice daily). Patients with frequently relapsing pouchitis may need continuous antibiotics. Probiotics containing nonpathogenic strains of lactobacilli, bifidobacteria, and streptococci (VSL#3) are effective in the maintenance of remission in patients with recurrent pouchitis. Bismuth subsalicylate (Pepto Bismol, 262 mg, two tablets four times daily) has demonstrated benefit in some series. Some clinicians report that topical corticosteroids or oral budesonide 9 mg/d are of benefit. Refractory cases of proctitis can be disabling and may require conversion to a standard ileostomy.

Prognosis

Ulcerative colitis is a lifelong disease characterized by exacerbations and remissions. For most patients, the disease is readily controlled by medical therapy without need for surgery. The majority never require hospitalization. A subset of patients with more severe disease will require surgery, which results in complete cure of the disease. Properly managed, most patients with ulcerative colitis lead close to normal productive lives.

When to Refer

- Colonoscopy: for evaluation of activity and extent of active disease and for surveillance for neoplasia in patients with quiescent disease for more than 8–10 years.
- When hospitalization is required.
- When surgical colectomy is indicated.

When to Admit

- Patients with severe disease manifested by frequent bloody stools, anemia, weight loss, and fever.
- Patients with fulminant disease manifested by rapid progression of symptoms, worsening abdominal pain, distention, high fever, tachycardia.
- Patients with moderate to severe symptoms that do not respond to oral corticosteroids and require a trial of bowel rest and intravenous corticosteroids.

Bergman R et al. Systematic review: the use of mesalazine in inflammatory bowel disease. Aliment Pharmacol Ther. 2006 Apr 1;23(7):841–55. [PMID: 16573787]

Bossa F et al. Continuous infusion versus bolus administration of steroids in severe attacks of ulcerative colitis: a randomized, double-blind trial. Am J Gastroenterol. 2007 Mar;102(3):601–8. [PMID: 17156148]

Caprilli R et al. Current management of severe ulcerative colitis. Nat Clin Pract Gastroenterol Hepatol. 2007 Feb;4(2):92–101. [PMID: 17268544]

Gisbert JP et al. Systematic review: infliximab therapy in ulcerative colitis. Aliment Pharmacol Ther. 2007 Jan 1;25(1):19–37. [PMID: 17229218]

Kamm MA et al. Once-daily, high-concentration MMX mesalamine in active ulcerative colitis. Gastroenterology. 2007 Jan;132(1):66–75. [PMID: 17241860]

Kiesslich R et al. Endoscopic surveillance in ulcerative colitis: smart biopsies do it better. Gastroenterology. 2007 Sep;133(3):742–5. [PMID: 17854587]

Kohn A et al. Infliximab in severe ulcerative colitis: short-term results of different infusion regimens and long-term follow-up. Aliment Pharmacol Ther. 2007 Sep 1;26(5):747–56. [PMID: 17697208]

Marion JF et al. Chromoendoscopy-targeted biopsies are superior to standard colonoscopic surveillance for detecting dysplasia in inflammatory bowel disease patients: a prospective endoscopic trial. Am J Gastroenterol. 2008 Sep;103(9):2342–9. [PMID: 18844620]

Maser EA et al. Cyclosporine and infliximab as rescue therapy for each other in patients with steroid-refractory ulcerative colitis. Clin Gastroenterol Hepatol. 2008 Oct;6(10):1112–6. [PMID: 18928936]

McLaughlin SD et al. Restorative proctocolectomy, indications, management of complications and follow-up—a guide for gastroenterologists. Aliment Pharmacol Ther. 2008 May;27(1):895–909. [PMID: 18266993]

Oussalah A et al. Long-term outcome of adalimumab therapy for ulcerative colitis with intolerance or lost response to infliximab: a single-centre experience. Aliment Pharmacol Ther. 2008 Oct 15;28(8):966–72. [PMID: 18652603]

Sternthal MB et al. Adverse events associated with the use of cyclosporine in patients with inflammatory bowel disease. Am J Gastroenterol. 2008 Apr;103(4):937–43. [PMID: 18177449]

Tremaine WJ. Inflammatory bowel disease and *Clostridium difficile*-associated diarrhea: a growing problem. Clin Gastroenterol Hepatol. 2007 Mar;5(3):310–1. [PMID: 17368229]

Turner D et al. Response to corticosteroids in severe ulcerative colitis: a systematic review of the literature and a meta-regression. Clin Gastroenterol Hepatol. 2007 Jan;5(1):103–10. [PMID: 17142106]

3. Microscopic Colitis

Microscopic colitis is an idiopathic condition that is found in up to 15% of patients who have chronic or intermittent watery diarrhea with normal-appearing mucosa at endoscopy. There appear to be two subtypes—lymphocytic colitis and collagenous colitis. In both, histologic evaluation of mucosal biopsies reveals chronic inflammation (lymphocytes, plasma cells) in the lamina propria and increased intraepithelial lymphocytes. Collagenous colitis is further characterized by the presence of a thickened band (> 10 mcm) of subepithelial collagen. Both forms occur more commonly in women, especially in the fifth to sixth decades. Symptoms tend to be chronic or recurrent but may remit in most patients after several years. A more severe illness characterized by abdominal pain, fatigue, dehydration, and weight loss may develop in a subset of patients. The cause of microscopic colitis usually is unknown. Several medications have been implicated as etiologic agents, including NSAIDs, sertraline, paroxetine, lansoprazole, lisinopril, and simvastatin. Diarrhea usually abates within 30 days of stopping the offending medication. Celiac sprue may be present in a small subset of patients and should be excluded with serologic testing (anti-tissue transglutaminase or anti-endomysial antibody). Treatment is largely empiric since there are few well-designed, controlled treatment trials. Mild disease may be treated with antidiarrheal agents (loperamide, cholestyramine). In uncontrolled studies, treatment with 5-ASAs (sulfasalazine, mesalamine) or bile-salt binding agents (cholestyramine, colestipol) is reported to be effective in many patients. A small unpublished controlled trial demonstrated efficacy for bismuth subsalicylate (two tablets four times daily) for 2 months; however, clinical experience has yielded only modest benefit. Delayed release budesonide (Entocort) 9 mg/d for 6–8 weeks has been shown in three prospective controlled studies to induce clinical improvement in 81% of patients compared with 17% treated with placebo; however, clinical relapse is common after cessation of therapy. Patients with refractory or severe symptoms may be treated with systemic corticosteroids or, rarely, azathioprine. After entering remission, clinical relapse occurs in 20–30% of patients within 3 years.

Chande N et al. Interventions for treating lymphocytic colitis. Cochrane Database Syst Rev. 2007 Jan 24;(1):CD006096. [PMID: 17253579]

Miehlke S et al. Oral budesonide for maintenance treatment of collagenous colitis: a randomized, double-blind, placebo-controlled trial. Gastroenterology. 2008 Nov;135(5):1510–6. [PMID: 18926826]

DIVERTICULAR DISEASE OF THE COLON

Colonic diverticulosis increases with age, ranging from 5% in those under age 40, to 30% at age 60, to more than 50% over age 80 years in Western societies. In contrast, it is very uncommon in developing countries with much lower life expectancies. Most are asymptomatic, discovered incidentally at endoscopy or on barium enema. Complications in one-third include lower gastrointestinal bleeding and diverticulitis.

Colonic diverticula may vary in size from a few millimeters to several centimeters and in number from one to several dozen. Almost all patients with diverticulosis have involvement in the sigmoid and descending colon; however, only 15% have proximal colonic disease.

In most patients, diverticulosis is believed to arise after many years of a diet deficient in fiber. The undistended, contracted segments of colon have higher intraluminal pressures. Over time, the contracted colonic musculature, working against greater pressures to move small, hard stools, develops hypertrophy, thickening, rigidity, and fibrosis. Diverticula may develop more commonly in the sigmoid because intraluminal pressures are highest in this region. The extent to which abnormal motility and hereditary factors contribute to diverticular disease is unknown. Patients with diffuse diverticulosis may have an inherent weakness in the colonic wall. Patients with abnormal connective tissue are also disposed to development of diverticulosis, including Ehlers-Danlos syndrome, Marfan syndrome, and scleroderma.

1. Uncomplicated Diverticulosis

More than two-thirds of patients with diverticulosis have uncomplicated disease and no specific symptoms. In some, diverticulosis may be an incidental finding detected during colonoscopic examination or barium enema examination. Some patients have nonspecific complaints of chronic constipation, abdominal pain, or fluctuating bowel habits. It is unclear whether these symptoms are due to alterations in the colonic musculature or underlying irritable bowel syndrome. Physical examination is usually normal but may reveal mild left lower quadrant tenderness with a thickened, palpable sigmoid and descending colon. Screening laboratory studies should be normal in uncomplicated diverticulosis.

There is no reason to perform imaging studies for the purpose of diagnosing uncomplicated disease. Diverticula are best seen on barium enema. Involved segments of colon may also be narrowed and deformed. Colonoscopy is a less sensitive means of detecting diverticula.

Asymptomatic patients in whom diverticulosis is discovered and patients with a history of complicated disease (see below) should be treated with a high-fiber diet or fiber supplements (bran powder, 1–2 tbsp twice daily; psyllium or methylcellulose) (see section on constipation). Retrospective studies suggest that such treatment may decrease the likelihood of subsequent complications.

Brian West A. The pathology of diverticulosis: classical concepts and mucosal changes in diverticula. J Clin Gastroenterol. 2006 Aug;40(7 Suppl 3):S126–31. [PMID: 16885695]
Petruzziello L et al. Review article: uncomplicated diverticular disease of the colon. Aliment Pharmacol Ther. 2006 May 15;23(10):1379–91. [PMID: 16669953]

2. Diverticulitis

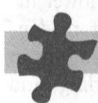 ESSENTIALS OF DIAGNOSIS

▶ Acute abdominal pain and fever.
▶ Left lower abdominal tenderness and mass.
▶ Leukocytosis.

▶ Clinical Findings

A. Symptoms and Signs

Perforation of a colonic diverticulum results in an intra-abdominal infection that may vary from microperforation (most common) with localized paracolic inflammation to macroperforation with either abscess or generalized peritonitis. Thus, there is a range from mild to severe disease. Most patients with localized inflammation or infection report mild to moderate aching abdominal pain, usually in the left lower quadrant. Constipation or loose stools may be present. Nausea and vomiting are frequent. In many cases, symptoms are so mild that the patient may not seek medical attention until several days after onset. Physical findings include a low-grade fever, left lower quadrant tenderness, and a palpable mass. Stool occult blood is common, but hematochezia is rare. Leukocytosis is mild to moderate. Patients with free perforation present with a more dramatic picture of generalized abdominal pain and peritoneal signs.

B. Imaging

In patients with mild symptoms and a presumptive diagnosis of diverticulitis, empiric medical therapy is started without further imaging in the acute phase. Patients who respond to acute medical management should undergo complete colonic evaluation with colonoscopy or barium enema after resolution of clinical symptoms to corroborate the diagnosis or exclude other disorders such as colonic neoplasms. In patients who do not improve rapidly after 2–4 days of empiric therapy and in those with severe disease, CT scan of the abdomen is obtained to look for evidence of diverticulitis and determine its severity, and to exclude other disorders that may cause lower abdominal pain. The presence of colonic diverticula and wall thickening, pericolic fat infiltration, abscess formation, or extraluminal air or contrast suggest diverticulitis. Endoscopy and barium enema are contraindicated during the initial stages of an acute attack because of the risk of free perforation.

▶ Differential Diagnosis

Diverticulitis must be distinguished from other causes of lower abdominal pain, including perforated colonic carcinoma, Crohn disease, appendicitis, ischemic colitis, C difficile–associated colitis, and gynecologic disorders (ectopic pregnancy, ovarian cyst or torsion) by abdominal CT scan, pelvic ultrasonography, or radiographic studies of the distal colon that use water-soluble contrast enemas.

▶ Complications

Fistula formation may involve the bladder, ureter, vagina, uterus, bowel, and abdominal wall. Diverticulitis may result in stricturing of the colon with partial or complete obstruction.

▶ Treatment

A. Medical Management

Most patients can be managed with conservative measures. Patients with mild symptoms and no peritoneal signs may be managed initially as outpatients on a clear liquid diet and broad-spectrum oral antibiotics with anaerobic activity. Reasonable regimens include amoxicillin and clavulanate potassium (875 mg/125 mg) twice daily; or metronidazole, 500 mg three times daily; plus either ciprofloxacin, 500 mg twice daily, or trimethoprim-sulfamethoxazole, 160/800 mg twice daily orally, for 7–10 days or until the patient is afebrile for 3–5 days. Symptomatic improvement usually occurs within 3 days, at which time the diet may be advanced. Patients with increasing pain, fever, or inability to tolerate oral fluids require hospitalization. Patients with severe diverticulitis (high fevers, leukocytosis, or peritoneal signs) and patients who are elderly or immunosuppressed or who have serious comorbid disease require hospitalization acutely. Patients should be given nothing by mouth and should receive intravenous fluids. If ileus is present, a nasogastric tube should be placed. Intravenous antibiotics should be given to cover anaerobic and gram-negative bacteria. Single-agent therapy with either a second-generation cephalosporin (eg, cefoxitin), piperacillin-tazobactam, or ticarcillin clavulanate appears to be as effective as combination therapy (eg, metronidazole or clindamycin plus an aminoglycoside or third-generation cephalosporin [eg, ceftazidime, cefotaxime]). Symptomatic improvement should be evident within 2–3 days. Intravenous antibiotics should be continued for 5–7 days, before changing to oral antibiotics. Colonoscopy or barium enema should be performed approximately 6 weeks after the acute episode has resolved in order to exclude unsuspected colon carcinoma or inflammatory bowel disease.

B. Surgical Management

Surgical consultation and repeat abdominal CT imaging should be obtained on all patients with severe disease or those who do not improve after 72 hours of medical management.

Patients with a localized abdominal abscess greater than or equal to 4 cm in size are usually treated urgently with a percutaneous catheter drain placed by an interventional radiologist. This permits control of the infection and resolution of the immediate infectious inflammatory process. In this manner, a subsequent elective one-stage surgical operation can be performed (if deemed necessary) in which the diseased segment of colon is removed and primary colonic anastomosis performed. Patients with chronic disease resulting in fistulas or colonic obstruction will also require elective surgical resection.

Indications for emergent surgical management include generalized peritonitis, large undrainable abscesses, and clinical deterioration despite medical management and percutaneous drainage. Surgery may be performed in one- or two-stage operations depending on the patient's nutritional status, severity of illness, and extent of intra-abdominal peritonitis and abscess formation. In a two-stage operation, the diseased colon is resected and the proximal colon brought out to form a temporary colostomy. The distal colonic stump is either closed (forming a Hartmann pouch) or exteriorized as a mucous fistula. Weeks later, after inflammation and infection have completely subsided, the colon can be reconnected electively.

Prognosis

Diverticulitis recurs in 10–30% of patients treated with medical management. Recurrent attacks warrant elective surgical resection, which carries a lower morbidity and mortality risk than emergency surgery.

When to Refer

- Failure to improve within 72 hours of medical management.
- Presence of significant peridiverticular abscesses (≥ 4 cm) requiring possible percutaneous or surgical drainage.
- Generalized peritonitis or sepsis.
- Recurrent attacks.
- Chronic complications including colonic strictures or fistulas.

When to Admit

- Severe pain or inability to tolerate oral intake.
- Signs of sepsis or peritonitis.
- CT scan showing signs of complicated disease (abscess, perforation).
- Failure to improve with outpatient management.
- Immunocompromised or frail, elderly patient.

Jacobs DO. Clinical practice. Diverticulitis. N Engl J Med. 2007 Nov 15;357(20):2057–66. [PMID: 18003962]
Liljegren G et al. Acute colonic diverticulitis: a systematic review of diagnostic accuracy. Colorectal Dis. 2007 Jul;9(6):480–8. [PMID: 17573739]

3. Diverticular Bleeding

Half of all cases of acute lower gastrointestinal bleeding are attributable to diverticulosis. For a full discussion, see the section on Acute Lower Gastrointestinal Bleeding.

POLYPS OF THE COLON & SMALL INTESTINE

Polyps are discrete mass lesions that protrude into the intestinal lumen. Although most commonly sporadic, they may be inherited as part of a familial polyposis syndrome. Polyps may be divided into three major pathologic groups: mucosal neoplastic (adenomatous) polyps, mucosal nonneoplastic polyps (hyperplastic, juvenile polyps, hamartomas, inflammatory polyps), and submucosal lesions (lipomas, lymphoid aggregates, carcinoids, pneumatosis cystoides intestinalis). The nonneoplastic mucosal polyps have no malignant potential and usually are discovered incidentally at colonoscopy or barium enema. Only the adenomatous polyps have significant clinical implications and will be considered further here. Of polyps removed at colonoscopy, over 70% are adenomatous; most of the remainder are hyperplastic. Small hyperplastic polyps (< 5 mm) located in the rectosigmoid region are of no consequence, except that they cannot reliably be distinguished from adenomatous lesions other than by biopsy. Large hyperplastic polyps located in the proximal colon may evolve into a unique type of premalignant lesion called a "serrated adenoma."

NONFAMILIAL ADENOMATOUS POLYPS

Histologically, adenomas are classified as tubular, villous, tubulovillous, or serrated. Adenomas may be flat, sessile or pedunculated (containing a stalk). They are present in 30% of adults over 50 years of age. Their significance is that over 95% of cases of adenocarcinoma of the colon are believed to arise from adenomas. It is proposed that there is an adenoma → carcinoma sequence whereby colorectal cancer develops through a continuous process from normal mucosa to adenoma to carcinoma. Most adenomas are small (< 1 cm) and have a low risk of becoming malignant; less than 5% of these enlarge with time. Adenomas are classified as "advanced" if they are ≥ 1 cm, or contain villous features or high-grade dysplasia. Advanced adenomas are believed to have a higher risk of harboring or progressing to malignancy. It has been estimated from longitudinal studies that it takes an average of 5 years for a medium-sized polyp to develop from normal-appearing mucosa and 10 years for a gross cancer to arise. In an asymptomatic population of male veterans over age 50 years undergoing screening with colonoscopy, invasive cancer was detected in 1%, adenomas containing high-grade dysplasia in 1.7%, and other adenomas ≥ 1 cm in size in 7.2%. The role of aspirin and NSAIDs for the chemoprevention of adenomatous polyps is discussed in Chapter 39, in the section on Colorectal Cancer.

Clinical Findings

A. Symptoms and Signs

Most patients with adenomatous polyps are completely asymptomatic. Chronic occult blood loss may lead to iron deficiency anemia. Large polyps may ulcerate, resulting in intermittent hematochezia.

B. Fecal Occult Blood or Multitarget DNA Tests

FOBT, FIT, and, more recently, fecal DNA tests are available as part of colorectal cancer screening programs (see

Chapter 39). FIT is a new fecal blood test (an immunochemical test for hemoglobin) that is more sensitive than prior guaiac-based tests for the detection of colorectal cancer and advanced adenomas. In two recent prospective studies, the FIT and other new fecal tests detected 40–60% of advanced noncancerous adenomas.

C. Radiologic Tests

Polyps are identified by means of barium enema examinations or CT colonography. Barium enema examinations as currently performed detect < 50% of colorectal polyps ≥ 1 cm in size. CT colonography ("virtual colonoscopy") uses data from helical CT imaging with computer-enabled luminal image reconstruction to generate two-dimensional and three-dimensional images of the colon. Using optimal imaging software with multidetector helical CT scanners, several studies report a sensitivity of ≥ 90% for the detection of polyps > 10 mm in size. However, the accuracy for detection of polyps 5–9 mm in size is significantly lower (sensitivity 50%). A small proportion of these small polyps harbor advanced histology (3-7%) or carcinoma (< 1%). Abdominal CT imaging results in a radiation exposure that may lead to a small risk of cancer. CT colonography has been endorsed by US Multisociety Task Force as an acceptable option for screening for colorectal adenomatous polyps and cancer in average risk asymptomatic adults.

D. Endoscopic Tests

Flexible sigmoidoscopy is commonly performed as part of colorectal screening programs. Approximately one-half to two-thirds of colonic adenomas are within the reach of a flexible sigmoidoscope. Polyps are seen in 10–20% of patients undergoing screening sigmoidoscopy, and polyps less than 8 mm in size should be removed by excisional biopsy to assess histology. Patients in whom no adenomas are detected or in whom hyperplastic polyps only are detected on sigmoidoscopy require no further evaluation. In such patients, the prevalence of an undetected advanced proximal adenoma is only 1–3%. Patients with an advanced adenoma (as defined above) or multiple small (< 1 cm) adenomas in the distal colon have an increased risk (12%) of harboring other advanced neoplasms in the proximal colon and should undergo colonoscopy. Opinions are conflicting about whether the presence of one or two small adenomas found on sigmoidoscopy is predictive of finding an increased prevalence of advanced neoplasms at colonoscopy. However, several studies suggest that among patients with a distal adenoma less than 10 mm in size, the prevalence of advanced neoplasia at colonoscopy is 5–7%. Therefore, professional guidelines recommend colonoscopy for all patients with adenomas found in the distal colon at sigmoidoscopy irrespective of size.

Colonoscopy allows evaluation of the entire colon and is the best means of detecting and removing adenomatous polyps (Plate 69). It should be performed in all patients who have positive FOBT, FIT, fecal, or DNA tests or iron deficiency anemia (see Occult Gastrointestinal Bleeding and Obscure Gastrointestinal Bleeding, above), as the prevalence of colonic neoplasms is increased in these patients. Colonoscopy should also be performed in patients with polyps detected on radiologic imaging studies (barium enema or CT colonography) or adenomas detected on flexible sigmoidoscopy to remove these polyps and to fully evaluate the entire colon.

▶ Treatment

A. Colonoscopic Polypectomy

Most adenomatous polyps are amenable to colonoscopic removal with biopsy forceps or snare cautery. Large sessile polyps (> 2–3 cm) may be removed in piecemeal fashion or may require surgical resection. Patients with large sessile polyps removed in piecemeal fashion should undergo repeated colonoscopy in 2–6 months to verify complete polyp removal. Complications after colonoscopic polypectomy include perforation in 0.2% and clinically significant bleeding in 0.3–1% of patients.

A malignant polyp is an adenoma that appears grossly benign at endoscopy but on histologic assessment is found to contain cancer that has penetrated through the muscularis mucosae into the submucosa. Malignant polyps may be considered to be adequately treated by polypectomy alone if: (1) the polyp is completely excised and submitted for pathologic examination, (2) it is well differentiated, (3) the margin is not involved, and (4) there is no tumor budding vascular invasion. The risk of residual cancer or nodal metastasis with favorable histologic features is < 1%. The excision site of these "favorable" malignant polyps should be checked in 3 months for residual tissue. In patients with malignant polyps that have unfavorable histologic features, cancer resection is advisable if the patient is a good operative candidate.

B. Postpolypectomy Surveillance

Adenomas can be found in 30–40% of patients when another colonoscopy is performed within 3–5 years after the initial examination. Periodic colonoscopic surveillance is therefore recommended to detect these "metachronous" adenomas, which either may be new or may have been overlooked during the initial examination. Most of these adenomas are small, without high-risk features and of little immediate clinical significance. The probability of detecting advanced neoplasms at surveillance colonoscopy depends on the number, size, and histologic features of the polyps removed on initial (index) colonoscopy. Patients with 1–2 small (< 1 cm) tubular adenomas (without villous features or high-grade dysplasia) should have their next colonoscopy in 5–10 years. Patients with 3–10 adenomas, an adenoma > 1 cm, or an adenoma with villous features or high-grade dysplasia should have their next colonoscopy at 3 years. Patients with more than 10 adenomas should have a repeat colonoscopy at 1–2 years and may be considered for evaluation for a familial polyposis syndrome (see below).

Allison JE et al. Screening for colorectal neoplasms with new fecal occult blood tests: update on performance characteristics. J Natl Cancer Institute. 2007 Oct 3;99(19):1462–70. [PMID: 17895475]

Butterly LF et al. Prevalence of clinically important histology on small adenomas. Clin Gastroenterol Hepatol. 2006 Mar; 4(3):343–8. [PMID: 16527698]

Kim DH et al. CT colonography versus colonoscopy for the detection of advanced neoplasia. N Engl J Med. 2007 Oct 4;357(14):1403–12. [PMID: 17914041]

Levin B et al. Screening and surveillance for the early detection of colorectal cancer and adenomatous polyps 2008: a joint guideline from the American Cancer Society, the US Multi-Society Task Force on Colorectal Cancer, and the American College of Radiology. Gastroenterology. 2008 May;134(5):1570–95. [PMID: 18384785]

Lieberman D. Eighty-year-old patient with a history of a twelve millimeter adenomatous polyp resected at age of seventy-five years. Clin Gastroenterol Hepatol. 2007 Feb;5(2):166–9. [PMID: 17296526]

Winawer SJ et al. Guidelines for colonoscopy surveillance after polypectomy: a consensus update by the US Multi-Society Task Force on Colorectal Cancer and the American Cancer Society. Gastroenterology. 2006 May;130(6):1872–85. [PMID: 16697750]

HEREDITARY COLORECTAL CANCER & POLYPOSIS SYNDROMES

Up to 4% of all colorectal cancers are caused by germline genetic mutations that impose on carriers a high lifetime risk of developing colorectal cancer (see Chapter 39). Because the diagnosis of these disorders has important implications for treatment of affected members and for screening of family members, it is important to consider these disorders in patients with a family history of colorectal cancer that has affected more than one family member, those with a personal or family history of colorectal cancer developing at an early age ($\geq$ 50 years), those with a personal or family history of multiple polyps (> 20), and those with a personal or family history of multiple extracolonic malignancies.

1. Familial Adenomatous Polyposis

Familial adenomatous polyposis (FAP) is a syndrome affecting 1:10,000 people and accounts for approximately 0.5% of colorectal cancer. The classic form of FAP is characterized by the development of hundreds to thousands of colonic adenomatous polyps and a variety of extracolonic manifestations. An attenuated variant of FAP also has been recognized in which an average of only 25 polyps (range of 0–500) develop. FAP is most commonly caused by autosomally dominant inherited mutations in the adenomatous polyposis coli (*APC*) gene on chromosome 5q21. FAP arises de novo in 15% of patients in the absence of genetic mutations in the parents. Recently, mutations in the *MYH* gene, a gene involved with base excision repair, have been identified in patients with the classic and attenuated forms of FAP who do not have mutations of the *APC* gene. FAP due to *MYH* mutation is inherited in an autosomal recessive fashion, hence a family history of colorectal cancer may not be evident. Of patients with classic FAP, approximately 90% have a mutation in the *APC* gene and 8% in the *MYH* gene. In contrast, among patients with 10–100 adenomatous polyps and suspected attenuated FAP, *APC* mutations are identified in 15% but *MYH* mutations in 25%.

Colorectal polyps develop by a mean age of 15 years and cancer at 40 years. Unless prophylactic colectomy is performed, colorectal cancer is inevitable by age 50 years. In attenuated FAP, the mean age for development of cancer is about 56 years.

Adenomatous polyps of the duodenum and periampullary area develop in over 90% of patients, resulting in a 5–8% lifetime risk of adenocarcinoma. Adenomas occur less frequently in the gastric antrum and small bowel and in those locations have a lower risk of malignant transformation. Gastric fundus gland polyps occur in over 50% but have an extremely low (0.6%) malignant potential.

A variety of other benign extraintestinal manifestations, including soft tissue tumors of the skin, desmoid tumors, osteomas, and congenital hypertrophy of the retinal pigment, develop in some patients with FAP. These extraintestinal manifestations vary among families, depending in part on the type or site of mutation in the *APC* gene. Desmoid tumors are locally invasive fibromas, most commonly intra-abdominal, that may cause bowel obstruction, ischemia, or hemorrhage. They occur in 15% of patients and are the second leading cause of death in FAP. Malignancies of the central nervous system (Turcot syndrome) and tumors of the thyroid and liver (hepatoblastomas) may also develop in patients with FAP.

Genetic counseling and testing should be offered to patients with a diagnosis of FAP established by endoscopy and to first-degree family members of patients with the disease; testing should be done also to confirm a diagnosis of attenuated disease in patients with 20 or more adenomas. Genetic testing is best performed by sequencing the *APC* gene to identify disease-associated mutations, which are identified in approximately 90% of cases of typical FAP. Mutational assessment of *MYH* should be considered in patients with negative test results and in patients with suspected attenuated FAP. First-degree relatives of patients with FAP should undergo genetic screening after age 10 years. If the assay cannot be done or is not informative, family members at risk should undergo yearly sigmoidoscopy beginning at 12 years of age. Once the diagnosis has been established, complete proctocolectomy with ileoanal anastomosis or colectomy with ileorectal anastomosis is recommended, usually before age 20 years. Ileorectal anastomosis affords superior bowel function but has a 5% risk of development of rectal cancer, and for that reason frequent sigmoidoscopy with fulguration of polyps is required. Sulindac and COX-2 selective agents (celecoxib) have been shown to decrease the number and size of polyps in the rectal stump but not the duodenum. Upper endoscopic evaluation of the stomach, duodenum, and periampullary area should be performed every 1–3 years to look for adenomas or carcinoma. Large (> 2 cm) periampullary adenomas require surgical resection.

Vasen HF et al. Guidelines for the clinical management of familial adenomatous polyposis (FAP). Gut. 2008 May;57(5):704–13. [PMID: 18194984]

2. Hamartomatous Polyposis Syndromes

Hamartomatous polyposis syndromes are rare and account for less than 0.1% of colorectal cancers.

Peutz-Jeghers syndrome is an autosomal dominant condition characterized by hamartomatous polyps throughout the gastrointestinal tract (most notably in the small intestine) as well as mucocutaneous pigmented macules on the lips, buccal mucosa, and skin. The hamartomas may become large, leading to bleeding, intussusception, or obstruction. Although hamartomas are not malignant, gastrointestinal malignancies (stomach, small bowel, and colon) develop in 40%, breast cancer in 50%, as well as a host of other malignancies of nonintestinal organs (gonads, pancreas). The defect has been localized to the serine threonine kinase 11 gene, and genetic testing is available.

Familial juvenile polyposis is also autosomal dominant and is characterized by several (more than ten) juvenile hamartomatous polyps located most commonly in the colon. There is an increased risk (up to 50%) of adenocarcinoma due to synchronous adenomatous polyps or mixed hamartomatous-adenomatous polyps. Genetic defects have been identified to loci on 18q and 10q (*MADH4* and *BMPR1A*). Genetic testing is available.

PTEN multiple hamartoma syndrome (Cowden disease) is characterized by hamartomatous polyps and lipomas throughout the gastrointestinal tract, trichilemmomas, and cerebellar lesions. An increased rate of malignancy is demonstrated in the thyroid, breast, and urogenital tract.

Giardiello FM et al. Peutz-Jeghers syndrome and management recommendations. Clin Gastroenterol Hepatol. 2006 Apr;4 (4):408–15. [PMID: 16616343]

Zbuk KM et al. Hamartomatous polyposis syndromes. Nat Clin Pract Gastroenterol Hepatol. 2007 Sep;4(9):492–502. [PMID: 17768394]

3. Hereditary Nonpolyposis Colorectal Cancer (HNPCC)

HNPCC (also known as Lynch syndrome) is an autosomal dominant condition in which there is a markedly increased risk of developing colorectal cancer as well as a host of other cancers, including endometrial, ovarian, renal or vesical, hepatobiliary, gastric, and small intestinal cancers. It is estimated to account for up to 3% of all colorectal cancers. Affected individuals have a 50–80% lifetime risk of developing colorectal carcinoma and a 30–60% lifetime risk of endometrial cancer. Unlike individuals with familial adenomatous polyposis, patients with HNPCC develop only a few adenomas, which may be flat and more often contain villous features or high-grade dysplasia. In contrast to the traditional polyp → cancer progression (which may take over 10 years), these polyps are believed to undergo rapid transformation from normal tissue → adenoma → cancer. HNPCC and endometrial cancer tend to develop at an earlier age than sporadic, nonhereditary cancers (mean age 45–50 years). Compared with patients with sporadic tumors of similar pathologic stage, those with HNPCC tumors have improved survival. Synchronous or metachronous cancers occur within 10 years in up to 45% of patients.

HNPCC is caused by a defect in one of several genes that are important in the detection and repair of DNA base-pair mismatches: *MLH1*, *MSH2*, *MSH6*, and *PMS2*. Germline mutations in *MLH1* and *MSH2* account for more than 90% of the known mutations in families with HNPCC. Mutations in any of these mismatch repair genes result in a characteristic phenotypic DNA abnormality known as microsatellite instability. In over 90% of cancers in patients with HNPCC, microsatellite instability is readily demonstrated by expansion or contraction of DNA microsatellites (short, repeated DNA sequences). Microsatellite instability also occurs in 15% of sporadic colorectal cancers, usually due to aberrant methylation of the *MLH1* promoter resulting in decreased gene expression.

A thorough family cancer history is essential to identify families that may be affected with HNPCC so that appropriate genetic and colonoscopic screening can be offered. Owing to the limitations of genetic testing for HNPCC and the medical, psychological, and social implications that such testing may have, families with suspected HNPCC should be evaluated first by a genetic counselor and should give informed consent in writing before genetic testing is performed. Patients whose families meet any of the revised "Bethesda criteria" have an increased likelihood of harboring a germline mutation in one of the mismatch repair genes and should be considered for genetic testing: (1) colorectal cancer under age 50; (2) synchronous or metachronous colorectal or HNPCC-associated tumor regardless of age (endometrial, stomach, ovary, pancreas, ureter and renal pelvis, biliary tract, brain); (3) colorectal cancer with one or more first-degree relatives with colorectal or HNPCC-related cancer, with one of the cancers occurring before age 50; (4) colorectal cancer with two or more second-degree relatives with colorectal or HNPCC cancer, regardless of age; (5) tumors with infiltrating lymphocytes, mucinous/signet ring differentiation, or medullary growth pattern in patients younger than 60 years. These criteria will identify greater than 90% of mutation-positive HNPCC families. Tumor tissues of affected individuals or family members meeting the revised Bethesda criteria should undergo immunohistochemical staining for *MLH1*, *MSH2*, *MSH6*, and *PMS2* (using commercially available assays) or testing for microsatellite instability (PCR amplification of a panel of DNA markers) or both. Individuals whose tumors have normal immunohistochemical staining or do not have microsatellite instability are unlikely to have germline mutations in mismatch repair genes, do not require further genetic testing, and do not require intensive cancer surveillance. Germline testing for gene mutations is positive in > 90% of individuals whose tumors show absent histochemical staining of one of the mismatch repair genes and in 50% of those whose tumors have a high level of microsatellite instability. Germline testing is also warranted in families with a strong history consistent with HNPCC when tumors from affected members are unavailable for assessment. If a mutation is detected in a patient with cancer in one of the known mismatch genes, genetic testing of other first-degree family members is indicated.

If genetic testing documents an HNPCC gene mutation, affected relatives should be screened with colonoscopy every 1–2 years beginning at age 25 (or at age 5 years younger than the age at diagnosis of the youngest affected family member). If cancer is found, subtotal colectomy with ileorectal anastomosis (followed by annual surveillance of the rectal stump) should be performed. Women should undergo screening for endometrial and ovarian cancer beginning at age 25–35 years with pelvic examination, CA-125 assay, endometrial aspiration, and transvaginal ultrasound. Prophylactic hysterectomy and oophorectomy may be considered, especially in women of postchildbearing age. Similarly, consideration should be given for increased cancer surveillance in family members in proven or suspected HNPCC families who do not wish to undergo germline testing. (**See Chapter 39 for Colorectal Cancer.**)

Jenkins MA et al. Pathology features in Bethesda guidelines predict colorectal cancer microsatellite instability: a population-based study. Gastroenterology. 2007 Jul;133(1):48–56. [PMID: 17631130]

Julie C et al. Identification in daily practice of patients with Lynch syndrome (hereditary nonpolyposis colorectal cancer): revised Bethesda guidelines-based approach versus molecular screening. Am J Gastroenterol. 2008 Nov;103(11):2825–35. [PMID: 18759827]

Ramsoekh D et al. Detection and management of hereditary nonpolyposis colorectal cancer (Lynch syndrome). Aliment Pharmacol Ther. 2007 Dec;26(Suppl 2):101–11. [PMID: 18081654]

Vasen HF. The Lynch syndrome (hereditary nonpolyposis colorectal cancer). Aliment Pharmacol Ther. 2007 Dec;26(Suppl 2):113–26. [PMID: 18081655]

ANORECTAL DISEASES

HEMORRHOIDS

ESSENTIALS OF DIAGNOSIS

▶ Bright red blood per rectum.

▶ Protrusion, discomfort.

▶ Characteristic findings on external anal inspection and anoscopic examination.

General Considerations

Internal hemorrhoids are subepithelial vascular cushions consisting of connective tissue, smooth muscle fibers, and arteriovenous communications between terminal branches of the superior rectal artery and rectal veins. They are a normal anatomic entity, occurring in all adults, that contribute to normal anal pressures and ensure a water-tight closure of the anal canal. They commonly occur in three primary locations—right anterior, right posterior, and left lateral. External hemorrhoids arise from the inferior hemorrhoidal veins located below the dentate line and are covered with squamous epithelium of the anal canal or perianal region.

Hemorrhoids may become symptomatic as a result of activities that increase venous pressure, resulting in distention and engorgement. Straining at stool, constipation, prolonged sitting, pregnancy, obesity, and low-fiber diets all may contribute. With time, redundancy and enlargement of the venous cushions may develop and result in bleeding or protrusion.

Clinical Findings

A. Symptoms and Signs

Patients often attribute a variety of perianal complaints to "hemorrhoids." However, the principal problems attributable to internal hemorrhoids are bleeding, prolapse, and mucoid discharge. Bleeding is manifested by bright red blood that may range from streaks of blood visible on toilet paper or stool to bright red blood that drips into the toilet bowl after a bowel movement. Rarely is bleeding severe enough to result in anemia. Initially, internal hemorrhoids are confined to the anal canal (stage I). Over time, the internal hemorrhoids may gradually enlarge and protrude from the anal opening. At first, this mucosal prolapse occurs during straining and reduces spontaneously (stage II). With progression over time, the prolapsed hemorrhoids may require manual reduction after bowel movements (stage III) or may remain chronically protruding (stage IV). Chronically prolapsed hemorrhoids may result in a sense of fullness or discomfort and mucoid perianal discharge, resulting in irritation and soiling of underclothes. Pain is unusual with internal hemorrhoids, occurring only when there is extensive inflammation and thrombosis of irreducible tissue or with thrombosis of an external hemorrhoid (see below).

B. Examination

External hemorrhoids are readily visible on perianal inspection. Nonprolapsed internal hemorrhoids are not visible but may protrude through the anus with gentle straining while the physician spreads the buttocks. Prolapsed hemorrhoids are visible as protuberant purple nodules covered by mucosa. The perianal region should also be examined for other signs of disease such as fistulas, fissures, skin tags, or dermatitis. On digital examination, uncomplicated internal hemorrhoids are neither palpable nor painful. Anoscopic evaluation, best performed in the prone jackknife position, provides optimal visualization of internal hemorrhoids.

Differential Diagnosis

Small volume rectal bleeding may be caused by anal fissure or fistula, neoplasms of the distal colon or rectum, ulcerative colitis or Crohn colitis, infectious proctitis, or rectal ulcers. Rectal prolapse, in which a full thickness of rectum protrudes concentrically from the anus, is readily distinguished from mucosal hemorrhoidal prolapse. Proctosigmoidoscopy or colonoscopy should be performed in all patients with hematochezia to exclude disease in the rectum or sigmoid colon that could be misinterpreted in the presence of hemorrhoidal bleeding.

Treatment

A. Conservative Measures

Most patients with early (stage I and stage II) disease can be managed with conservative treatment. To decrease straining with defecation, patients should be given instructions for a high-fiber diet and told to increase fluid intake with meals. Dietary fiber may be supplemented with bran powder (1–2 tbsp twice daily added to food or in 8 oz of liquid) or with commercial bulk laxatives (eg, Benefiber, Metamucil, Citrucel). Suppositories and rectal ointments have no demonstrated utility in the management of mild disease. Mucoid discharge may be treated effectively by the local application of a cotton ball tucked next to the anal opening after bowel movements. For edematous, prolapsed hemorrhoids, gentle manual reduction may be supplemented by suppositories (eg, Anusol with or without hydrocortisone) or topical pads containing witch hazel (eg, Tucks) that have anesthetic and astringent properties and by warm sitz baths.

B. Medical Treatment

Patients with stage I, stage II, and stage III hemorrhoids and recurrent bleeding despite conservative measures may be treated without anesthesia with injection sclerotherapy, rubber band ligation, or application of electrocoagulation (bipolar cautery or infrared photocoagulation). The choice of therapy is dictated by operator preference, but rubber band ligation increasingly is preferred due to its ease of use and high rate of efficacy. Major complications occur in < 2%, including pelvic sepsis, pelvic abscess, urinary retention, and bleeding. Recurrence is common unless patients alter their dietary habits.

C. Surgical Treatment

Surgical excision (hemorrhoidectomy) is reserved for < 5–10% of patients with chronic severe bleeding due to stage III or stage IV hemorrhoids or patients with acute thrombosed stage IV hemorrhoids. Complications of surgical hemorrhoidectomy include postoperative pain (which may persist for 2–4 weeks) and impaired continence.

Thrombosed External Hemorrhoid

Thrombosis of the external hemorrhoidal plexus results in a perianal hematoma. It most commonly occurs in otherwise healthy young adults and may be precipitated by coughing, heavy lifting, or straining at stool. The condition is characterized by the relatively acute onset of an exquisitely painful, tense and bluish perianal nodule covered with skin that may be up to several centimeters in size. Pain is most severe within the first few hours but gradually eases over 2–3 days as edema subsides. Symptoms may be relieved with warm sitz baths, analgesics, and ointments. If the patient is evaluated in the first 24–48 hours, removal of the clot may hasten symptomatic relief. With the patient in the lateral position, the skin around and over the lump is injected subcutaneously with 1% lidocaine using a tuberculin syringe with a 30-gauge needle. An ellipse of skin is then excised and the clot evacuated. A dry gauze dressing is applied for 12–24 hours, and daily sitz baths are then begun.

▶ When to Refer

- Stage I, II, or III: When conservative measures fail and expertise in medical procedures is needed (injection, banding, thermocoagulation).
- Stage III or IV: When surgical excision is required.

Chong PS et al. Hemorrhoids and fissure in ano. Gastroenterol Clin North Am. 2008 Sep;37(3):627–44. [PMID: 18794000]

ANORECTAL INFECTIONS

A number of organisms can cause inflammation of the anal and rectal mucosa. Proctitis is characterized by anorectal discomfort, tenesmus, constipation, and mucus or bloody discharge. Most cases of proctitis are sexually transmitted, especially by anal-receptive intercourse. Infectious proctitis must be distinguished from noninfectious causes of anorectal symptoms, including anal fissures or fistulae, perirectal abscesses, anorectal carcinomas, and inflammatory bowel disease (ulcerative colitis or Crohn disease).

▶ Etiology & Management

Several organisms may cause infectious proctitis.

A. *Neisseria gonorrhoeae*

Gonorrhea may cause itching, burning, tenesmus, and a mucopurulent discharge, although many anorectal infections are asymptomatic. Rectal swab specimens should be taken during anoscopy for culture; Gram staining is unreliable. Cultures should also be taken from the urethra and pharynx in men and from the cervix in women. Complications of untreated infections include strictures, fissures, fistulas, and perirectal abscesses.

B. *Treponema pallidum*

Anal syphilis may be asymptomatic or may lead to perianal pain and discharge. With primary syphilis, the chancre may be at the anal margin or within the anal canal and may mimic a fissure, fistula, or ulcer. Proctitis or inguinal lymphadenopathy may be present. With secondary syphilis, condylomata lata (pale-brown, flat verrucous lesions) may be seen, with secretion of foul-smelling mucus. Although the diagnosis may be established with dark-field microscopy or fluorescent antibody testing of scrapings from the chancre or condylomas, this requires proper equipment and trained personnel. The VDRL or RPR test is positive in 75% of primary cases and in 99% of secondary cases.

C. *Chlamydia trachomatis*

Chlamydial infection may cause proctitis similar to gonorrheal proctitis; however, some infections are asymptomatic. It also may cause lymphogranuloma venereum, characterized by proctocolitis with fever and bloody diarrhea, painful perianal ulcerations, anorectal strictures and fistulas, and inguinal adenopathy (buboes); however, this is rare in developed countries. The diagnosis is established by serology and culture of rectal discharge or rectal biopsy.

D. Herpes Simplex Type 2

Herpes simplex virus is a common cause of anorectal infection. Symptoms occur 4–21 days after exposure and include severe pain, itching, constipation, tenesmus, urinary retention, and radicular pain from involvement of lumbar or sacral nerve roots. Small vesicles or ulcers may be seen in the perianal area or anal canal. Sigmoidoscopy is not usually necessary but may reveal vesicular or ulcerative lesions in the distal rectum. Diagnosis is established by viral culture, PCR, or antigen detection assays of vesicular fluid. Symptoms resolve within 2 weeks, but viral shedding may continue for several weeks. Patients may remain asymptomatic with or without viral shedding or may have recurrent mild relapses. Treatment of acute infection for 7–10 days with acyclovir, 400 mg or famciclovir 250 mg orally three times daily or valacyclovir 1 g twice daily, has been shown to reduce the duration of symptoms and viral shedding. Patients with AIDS and recurrent relapses may benefit from long-term suppressive therapy (see Chapter 31).

E. Condylomata Acuminata

Condylomata acuminata (warts) are a significant cause of anorectal symptoms. Caused by the human papillomavirus (HPV), they may occur in the perianal area, the anal canal, or the genitals. Perianal or anal warts are seen in up to 25% of men who have sex with men. HIV-positive individuals with condylomas have a higher relapse rate after therapy and a higher rate of progression to high-grade dysplasia or anal cancer. The warts are located on the perianal skin and extend within the anal canal up to 2 cm above the dentate line (Plate 35). Patients may have no symptoms or may report itching, bleeding, and pain. The warts may be small and flat or verrucous, or may form a confluent mass that may obscure the anal opening. Warts must be distinguished from condyloma lata (secondary syphilis) or anal cancer. Biopsies should be obtained from large or suspicious lesions. Treatment can be difficult. Sexual partners should also be examined and treated. The treatment of anogenital warts is discussed in Chapter 30. HPV vaccines have demonstrated efficacy in preventing anogenital warts and routine vaccination is now recommended for all girls and women ages 9–26 years. The role of HPV vaccination in boys and men is under investigation (see Chapters 1 and 30). HIV-positive individuals with condylomas who have detectable serum HIV RNA levels should have anoscopic surveillance every 3–6 months.

Jutchinson DJ et al. Human papillomavirus disease and vaccines. Am J Health Syst Pharm. 2008 Nov 15;65(22):2105–12. [PMID: 18997137]

Tinmouth J et al. Lymphogranuloma venereum in North America: case reports and an update for gastroenterologists. Clin Gastroenterol Hepatol. 2006 Apr;4(4):469–73. [PMID: 16616352]

Workowski KA et al. Sexually transmitted diseases treatment guidelines 2006. Centers for Disease Control and Prevention. MMWR Recomm Rep. 2006 Aug 4;55(RR-11):1–94. (Available at http://www.cdc.gov/mmwr/preview/mmwrhtml/rr5511a1.htm) [PMID: 16888612]

FECAL INCONTINENCE

There are five general requirements for bowel continence: (1) solid or semisolid stool (even healthy young adults have difficulty maintaining continence with liquid rectal contents); (2) a distensible rectal reservoir (as sigmoid contents empty into the rectum, the vault must expand to accommodate); (3) a sensation of rectal fullness (if the patient cannot sense this, overflow may occur before the patient can take appropriate action); (4) intact pelvic nerves and muscles; and (5) the ability to reach a toilet in a timely fashion.

▶ Minor Incontinence

Many patients complain of inability to control flatus or slight soilage of undergarments that tends to occur after bowel movements or with straining or coughing. This may be due to local anal problems such as prolapsed hemorrhoids that make it difficult to form a tight anal seal or isolated weakness of the internal anal sphincter, especially if stools are somewhat loose. Patients should be treated with fiber supplements to provide greater stool bulk. Coffee and other caffeinated beverages should be eliminated. The perianal skin should be cleansed with moist, lanolin-coated tissue (baby wipes) to reduce excoriation and infection. After wiping, loose application of a cotton ball near the anal opening may absorb small amounts of fecal leakage. Prolapsing hemorrhoids may be treated with band ligation or surgical hemorrhoidectomy. Control of flatus and seepage may be improved by Kegel perineal exercises. Conditions such as ulcerative proctitis that cause tenesmus and urgency, chronic diarrheal conditions, and irritable bowel syndrome may result in difficulty in maintaining complete continence, especially if a toilet is not readily available. Loperamide may be helpful to reduce urge incontinence in patients with loose stools and may be taken in anticipation of situations in which a toilet may not be readily available. The elderly may require more time or assistance to reach a toilet, which may lead to incontinence. Scheduled toileting and the availability of a bedside commode are helpful. Elderly patients with chronic constipation may develop stool impaction leading to "overflow" incontinence.

▶ Major Incontinence

Complete uncontrolled loss of stool reflects a significant problem with central perception or neuromuscular function. Incontinence that occurs without awareness suggests a loss of central awareness (eg, dementia, cerebrovascular accident, multiple sclerosis) or peripheral nerve injury (eg, spinal cord injury, cauda equina syndrome, pudendal nerve damage due to obstetric trauma or pelvic floor prolapse, aging, or diabetes mellitus). Incontinence that occurs despite awareness and active efforts to retain stool suggests sphincteric damage, which may be caused by traumatic childbirth (especially forceps delivery), episiotomy, prolapse, prior anal surgery, and physical trauma.

Physical examination should include careful inspection of the perianal area for hemorrhoids, rectal prolapse, fissures, fistulas, and either gaping or a keyhole defect of the anal sphincter (indicating severe sphincteric injury or neurologic disorder). The perianal skin should be stimulated to confirm an intact anocutaneous reflex. Digital examination during relaxation gives valuable information about resting tone (due mainly to the internal sphincter) and contraction of the external sphincter and pelvic floor during squeezing. It also excludes fecal impaction. Anoscopy is required to evaluate for hemorrhoids, fissures, and fistulas. Proctosigmoidoscopy is useful to exclude rectal carcinoma or proctitis. Anal ultrasonography or pelvic MRI is the most reliable test for definition of anatomic defects in the external and internal anal sphincters. Anal manometry may also be useful to define the severity of weakness, to assess sensation, and to predict response to biofeedback training. In special circumstances, surface electromyography is useful to document sphincteric denervation and proctography to document perineal descent or rectal intussusception.

Patients who are incontinent only of loose or liquid stools are treated with bulking agents and antidiarrheal drugs (eg, loperamide, 2 mg before meals and prophylactically before social engagements, shopping trips, etc). Patients with incontinence of solid stool benefit from scheduled toilet use after glycerin suppositories or tap water enemas. Biofeedback training with anal sphincteric strengthening (Kegel) exercises (alternating 5-second squeeze and 10-second rest for 10 minutes twice daily) may be helpful in motivated patients to lower the threshold for awareness of rectal filling—or to improve anal sphincter squeeze function—or both. Operative management is seldom needed but should be considered in patients with major incontinence due to prior injury to the anal sphincter who have not responded to medical therapy.

▶ When to Refer

- Conservative measures fail.
- Anorectal tests are deemed necessary (manometry, ultrasonography, electromyography).
- A surgically correctable lesion is suspected.

Bharucha AE et al. Relation of bowel habits to fecal incontinence in women. Am J Gastroenterol. 2008 Jun;103(6):1470–5. [PMID: 18510612]

Rao SS. Fecal incontinence in a 56-year-old female executive. Clin Gastroenterol Hepatol. 2007 Apr;5(4):422–6. [PMID: 17445749]

Wald A. Fecal incontinence in adults. N Engl J Med. 2007 Apr 19;356(16):1648–55. [PMID: 17442907]

OTHER ANAL CONDITIONS

▶ Anal Fissures

Anal fissures are linear or rocket-shaped ulcers that are usually less than 5 mm in length. Most fissures are believed to arise from trauma to the anal canal during defecation, perhaps caused by straining, constipation, or high internal sphincter tone. They occur most commonly in the posterior midline, but 10% occur anteriorly. Fissures that occur off the midline should raise suspicion for Crohn disease, HIV/ AIDS, tuberculosis, syphilis, or anal carcinoma. Patients complain of severe, tearing pain during defecation followed by throbbing discomfort that may lead to constipation due to fear of recurrent pain. There may be mild associated hematochezia, with blood on the stool or toilet paper. Anal fissures are confirmed by visual inspection of the anal verge while gently separating the buttocks. Acute fissures look like

cracks in the epithelium. Chronic fissures result in fibrosis and the development of a skin tag at the outermost edge (sentinel pile). Digital and anoscopic examinations may cause severe pain and may not be possible. Medical management is directed at promoting effortless, painless bowel movements. Fiber supplements and sitz baths should be prescribed. Topical anesthetics (EMLA cream) may provide temporary relief. Healing occurs within 2 months in up to 45% of patients with conservative management. Chronic fissures may be treated with topical 0.2–0.4% nitroglycerin or diltiazem 2% ointment (1 cm of ointment) applied twice daily just inside the anus with the tip of a finger for 4–8 weeks or injection of botulinum toxin (20 units) into the anal sphincter. All of these treatments result in healing in 50–80% of patients with chronic anal fissure, but headaches occur in up to 40% of patients treated with nitroglycerin. Fissures recur in up to 40% of patients after treatment. Chronic or recurrent fissures benefit from lateral internal sphincterotomy; however, minor incontinence may complicate this procedure.

Brisinda G et al. Botulinum toxin for recurrent anal fissure following lateral internal sphincterotomy. Br J Surg. 2008 Jun;95(6):774–8. [PMID: 18425796]

Dhawan S et al. Nonsurgical approaches for the treatment of anal fissures. Am J Gastroenterol. 2007 Jun;102(6):1312–21. [PMID: 17531031]

▶ Perianal Abscess & Fistula

The anal glands located at the base of the anal crypts at the dentate line may become infected, leading to abscess formation. Other causes of abscess include anal fissure and Crohn disease. Abscesses may extend upward or downward through the intersphincteric plane. Symptoms of perianal abscess are throbbing, continuous perianal pain. Erythema, fluctuance, and swelling may be found in the perianal region on external examination or in the ischiorectal fossa on digital rectal examination. Perianal abscesses are treated with local incision and drainage, while ischiorectal abscesses require drainage in the operating room. After drainage of an abscess, most patients are found to have a fistula in ano.

Fistula in ano most often arises in an anal crypt and is usually preceded by an anal abscess. In patients with fistulas that connect to the rectum, other disorders such as Crohn disease, lymphogranuloma venereum, rectal tuberculosis, and cancer should be considered. Fistulas are associated with purulent discharge that may lead to itching, tenderness, and pain. The treatment of Crohn-related fistula is discussed elsewhere in this chapter. Treatment of idiopathic fistula in ano is by surgical incision or excision under anesthesia. Care must be taken to preserve the anal sphincters.

▶ Perianal Pruritus

Perianal pruritus is characterized by perianal itching and discomfort. It may be caused by poor anal hygiene associated with fistulas, fissures, prolapsed hemorrhoids, skin tags, and minor incontinence. Conversely, overzealous cleansing with soaps may contribute to local irritation or contact dermatitis. Contact dermatitis, atopic dermatitis, bacterial infections (*Staphylococcus* or *Streptococcus*), parasites (pinworms, scabies), candidal infection (especially in diabetics), sexually transmitted disease (condylomata acuminata, herpes, syphilis, molluscum contagiosum), and other skin conditions (psoriasis, Paget, lichen sclerosis) must be excluded. In patients with idiopathic perianal pruritus, examination may reveal erythema, excoriations, or lichenified, eczematous skin. Education is vital to successful therapy. Spicy foods, coffee, chocolate, and tomatoes may cause irritation and should be eliminated. After bowel movements, the perianal area should be cleansed with nonscented wipes premoistened with lanolin followed by gentle drying. A piece of cotton ball should be tucked next to the anal opening to absorb perspiration or fecal seepage. Anal ointments and lotions may exacerbate the condition and should be avoided. A short course of high-potency topical corticosteroid may be tried, although efficacy has not been demonstrated. Diluted capsaicin cream (0.006%) led to symptomatic relief in 75% of patients in a double-blind crossover study. (**See Chapter 39 for Carcinoma of the Anus.**)

Siddiqi S et al. Pruritus ani. Ann R Coll Surg Engl. 2008 Sep;90(6):457–63. [PMID: 18765023]

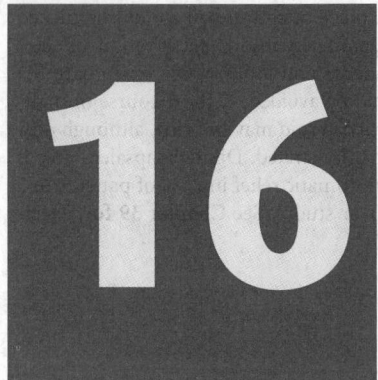

Liver, Biliary Tract, & Pancreas Disorders

Lawrence S. Friedman, MD

JAUNDICE

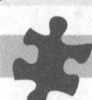

ESSENTIALS OF DIAGNOSIS

▶ Results from accumulation of bilirubin in the body tissues; cause may be hepatic or nonhepatic.

▶ Hyperbilirubinemia may be due to abnormalities in the formation, transport, metabolism, and excretion of bilirubin.

▶ Total serum bilirubin is normally 0.2–1.2 mg/dL; jaundice may not be recognizable until levels are about 3 mg/dL.

▶ Evaluation of obstructive jaundice begins with ultrasonography and is usually followed by cholangiography.

▶ General Considerations

Jaundice (icterus) results from the accumulation of bilirubin—a product of heme metabolism—in the body tissues. Hyperbilirubinemia may be due to abnormalities in the formation, transport, metabolism, and excretion of bilirubin. Total serum bilirubin is normally 0.2–1.2 mg/dL (mean levels are higher in men than women and higher in whites and Hispanics than blacks and correlate inversely with the risk of stroke, suggesting that bilirubin is somehow neuroprotective). Jaundice may not be recognizable until levels are about 3 mg/dL.

Jaundice is caused by predominantly unconjugated or conjugated bilirubin in the serum (Table 16–1). Unconjugated hyperbilirubinemia may result from overproduction of bilirubin because of hemolysis; impaired hepatic uptake of bilirubin due to certain drugs; or impaired conjugation of bilirubin by glucuronide, as in Gilbert syndrome, due to mild decreases in glucuronyl transferase, or Crigler–Najjar syndrome, caused by moderate decreases or absence of glucuronyl transferase. Hemolysis alone rarely elevates the serum bilirubin level to more than 7 mg/dL. Predominantly conjugated hyperbilirubinemia may result from impaired excretion of bilirubin from the liver due to hepatocellular disease, drugs, sepsis, hereditary hepatocanalicular transport defects

(such as Dubin–Johnson syndrome, progressive familial intrahepatic cholestasis syndromes, and some cases of intrahepatic cholestasis of pregnancy), or extrahepatic biliary obstruction. Features of some hyperbilirubinemic syndromes are summarized in Table 16–2. The term "cholestasis" denotes retention of bile in the liver, and the term "cholestatic jaundice" is often used when conjugated hyperbilirubinemia results from impaired bile flow.

▶ Clinical Findings

A. Unconjugated Hyperbilirubinemia

Stool and urine color are normal, and there is mild jaundice and indirect (unconjugated) hyperbilirubinemia with no bilirubin in the urine. Splenomegaly occurs in hemolytic disorders except in sickle cell anemia.

B. Conjugated Hyperbilirubinemia

1. Hereditary cholestatic syndromes or intrahepatic cholestasis—The patient may be asymptomatic; cholestasis is often accompanied by pruritus, light-colored stools, and jaundice.

2. Hepatocellular disease—Malaise, anorexia, low-grade fever, and right upper quadrant discomfort are frequent. Dark urine, jaundice, and, in women, amenorrhea occur. An enlarged tender liver, vascular spiders, palmar erythema, ascites, gynecomastia, sparse body hair, fetor hepaticus, and asterixis may be present, depending on the cause, severity, and chronicity of liver dysfunction.

C. Biliary Obstruction

There may be right upper quadrant pain, weight loss (suggesting carcinoma), jaundice, dark urine, and light-colored stools. Symptoms and signs may be intermittent if caused by stone, carcinoma of the ampulla, or cholangiocarcinoma. Pain may be absent early in pancreatic cancer. Occult blood in the stools suggests cancer of the ampulla. Hepatomegaly and a palpable gallbladder (Courvoisier sign) are characteristic, but neither specific nor sensitive, of a pancreatic head tumor. Fever and chills are more common in benign obstruction with associated cholangitis.

Table 16–1. Classification of jaundice.

Type of Hyperbilirubinemia	Location and Cause
Unconjugated hyperbilirubinemia (predominant indirect-reacting bilirubin)	Increased bilirubin production (eg, hemolytic anemias, hemolytic reactions, hematoma, pulmonary infarction)
	Impaired bilirubin uptake and storage (eg, posthepatitis hyperbilirubinemia, Gilbert syndrome, Crigler-Najjar syndrome, drug reactions)
Conjugated hyperbilirubinemia (predominant direct-reacting bilirubin)	**HEREDITARY CHOLESTATIC SYNDROMES**
	Faulty excretion of bilirubin conjugates (eg, Dubin-Johnson syndrome, Rotor syndrome) or mutation in genes coding for bile salt transport proteins (eg, progressive familial intrahepatic cholestasis syndromes, benign recurrent intrahepatic cholestasis, and some cases of intrahepatic cholestasis of pregnancy)
	HEPATOCELLULAR DYSFUNCTION
	Biliary epithelial and hepatocyte damage (eg, hepatitis, hepatic cirrhosis)
	Intrahepatic cholestasis (eg, certain drugs, biliary cirrhosis, sepsis, postoperative jaundice)
	Hepatocellular damage or intrahepatic cholestasis resulting from miscellaneous causes (eg, spirochetal infections, infectious mononucleosis, cholangitis, sarcoidosis, lymphomas, industrial toxins)
	BILIARY OBSTRUCTION
	Choledocholithiasis, biliary atresia, carcinoma of biliary duct, sclerosing cholangitis, choledochal cyst, external pressure on common duct, pancreatitis, pancreatic neoplasms

Table 16–2. Hyperbilirubinemic disorders.

	Nature of Defect	Type of Hyperbilirubinemia	Clinical and Pathologic Characteristics
Gilbert syndrome	Reduced activity of glucuronyl transferase	Unconjugated (indirect) bilirubin	Benign, asymptomatic hereditary jaundice. Hyperbilirubinemia increased by 24- to 36-hour fast. No treatment required. Prognosis excellent.
Dubin-Johnson syndrome[1]	Faulty excretory function of hepatocytes	Conjugated (direct) bilirubin	Benign, asymptomatic hereditary jaundice. Gallbladder does not visualize on oral cholecystography. Liver darkly pigmented on gross examination. Biopsy shows centrilobular brown pigment. Prognosis excellent.
Rotor syndrome			Similar to Dubin-Johnson syndrome, but liver is not pigmented and the gallbladder is visualized on oral cholecystography. Prognosis excellent.
Recurrent intrahepatic cholestasis[2]	Cholestasis, often on a familial basis	Unconjugated plus conjugated (total) bilirubin	Episodic attacks of jaundice, itching, and malaise. Onset in early life and may persist for a lifetime. Alkaline phosphatase increased. Cholestasis found on liver biopsy. (Biopsy may be normal during remission.) Prognosis is generally excellent for "benign" recurrent intrahepatic cholestasis but may not be for familial forms.
Intrahepatic cholestasis of pregnancy[3]			Benign cholestatic jaundice, usually occurring in the third trimester of pregnancy. Itching, gastrointestinal symptoms, and abnormal liver excretory function tests. Cholestasis noted on liver biopsy. Prognosis excellent, but recurrence with subsequent pregnancies or use of birth control pills is characteristic.

[1]The Dubin-Johnson syndrome is caused by a point mutation in the gene coding for an organic anion transporter in bile canaliculi on chromosome 10q23–24.
[2]Mutations in genes that control hepatocellular transport systems that are involved in the formation of bile and inherited as autosomal recessive traits are on chromosomes 18q21–22, 2q24, and 7q21 in families with progressive familial intrahepatic cholestasis. Gene mutations on chromosome 18q21–22 alter a P-type ATPase expressed in the small intestine and liver and others on chromosome 2q24 alter the bile acid export pump and cause benign recurrent intrahepatic cholestasis.
[3]Mutations in the *MDR3* gene on chromosome 7q 21 that are responsible for progressive familial intrahepatic cholestasis type 3 account for some cases of intrahepatic cholestasis of pregnancy.

▶ Diagnostic Methods for Evaluation of Liver Disease & Jaundice (Tables 16–3, 16–4)

A. Laboratory Studies

Serum alanine and aspartate aminotransferase (ALT and AST) levels vary with age and correlate with body mass index, coronary artery disease, and mortality from liver disease and inversely with caffeine consumption. Normal reference values for ALT and AST may be lower than generally reported when persons with risk factors for fatty liver are excluded. Early-onset paternal obesity is a risk factor for increased ALT levels. Elevated ALT and AST levels result from hepatocellular

Table 16–3. Liver biochemical tests: Normal values and changes in two types of jaundice.

Tests	Normal Values	Hepatocellular Jaundice	Uncomplicated Obstructive Jaundice
Bilirubin			
Direct	0.1–0.3 mg/dL	Increased	Increased
Indirect	0.2–0.7 mg/dL	Increased	Increased
Urine bilirubin	None	Increased	Increased
Serum albumin/total protein	Albumin, 3.5–5.5 g/dL	Albumin decreased Total protein, 6.5–8.4 g/dL	Unchanged
Alkaline phosphatase	30–115 units/L	Increased (+)	Increased (++++)
Prothrombin time	INR of 1.0–1.4. After vitamin K, 10% increase in 24 hours	Prolonged if damage severe and does not respond to parenteral vitamin K	Prolonged if obstruction marked, but responds to parenteral vitamin K
ALT, AST	ALT, 5–35 units/L; AST, 5–40 units/L	Increased in hepatocellular damage, viral hepatitis	Minimally increased

ALT, alanine aminotransferase; AST, aspartate aminotransferase; INR, international normalized ratio.

necrosis or inflammation. Levels are frequently elevated in persons with untreated celiac disease and often rise transiently in healthy persons who begin taking 4 g of acetaminophen per day or experience rapid weight gain on a fast-food diet. Elevated alkaline phosphatase levels are seen

Table 16–4. Causes of serum aminotransferase elevations.[1]

Mild Elevations (< 5× normal)	Severe Elevations (> 15× normal)
Hepatic: ALT-predominant	Acute viral hepatitis (A-E, herpes)
Chronic hepatitis B, C, and D	Medications/toxins
Acute viral hepatitis (A-E, EBV, CMV)	Ischemic hepatitis
Steatosis/steatohepatitis	Autoimmune hepatitis
Hemochromatosis	Wilson disease
Medications/toxins	Acute bile duct obstruction
Autoimmune hepatitis	Acute Budd-Chiari syndrome
α_1-Antitrypsin (α_1-antiprotease) deficiency	Hepatic artery ligation
Wilson disease	
Celiac disease	
Hepatic: AST-predominant	
Alcohol-related liver injury (AST:ALT > 2:1)	
Cirrhosis	
Nonhepatic	
Strenuous exercise	
Hemolysis	
Myopathy	
Thyroid disease	
Macro-AST	

[1]Almost any liver disease can cause moderate aminotransferase elevations (5–15× normal)

ALT, alanine aminotransferase; AST, aspartate aminotransferase; CMV, cytomegalovirus; EBV, Epstein-Barr virus.

Adapted with permission from Green RM et al. AGA technical review on the evaluation of liver chemistry tests. Gastroenterology. 2002 Oct;123(4):1367–84.

in cholestasis or infiltrative liver disease (such as tumor or granuloma). Alkaline phosphatase elevations of hepatic rather than bone, intestinal, or placental origin are confirmed by concomitant elevation of γ-glutamyl transpeptidase or 5'-nucleotidase levels. The differential diagnosis of any liver test elevation includes toxicity caused by drugs, herbal remedies, and toxins.

B. Liver Biopsy

Percutaneous liver biopsy is the definitive study for determining the cause and histologic severity of hepatocellular dysfunction or infiltrative liver disease. In patients with suspected metastatic disease or a hepatic mass, it is performed under ultrasound or CT guidance. A transjugular route can be used in patients with coagulopathy or ascites. Panels of blood tests (eg, FibroSure) and transient or magnetic resonance elastography (ultrasonographic and magnetic resonance techniques, respectively, to measure liver stiffness) are emerging approaches for estimating the degree of liver fibrosis without the need for liver biopsy.

C. Imaging

Demonstration of dilated bile ducts by ultrasonography or CT scan indicates biliary obstruction (90–95% sensitivity). Ultrasonography, CT scan, and MRI may also demonstrate hepatomegaly, intrahepatic tumors, and portal hypertension. Multiphasic helical or multislice CT, CT arterial portography, in which imaging follows intravenous contrast infusion via a catheter placed in the superior mesenteric artery, MRI with use of gadolinium or ferumoxides as contrast agents, and intraoperative ultrasonography are the most sensitive techniques for detection of individual small hepatic lesions in patients eligible for resection of metastases. Use of color Doppler ultrasound or contrast agents that produce microbubbles increases the sensitivity of transcutaneous ultrasound for detecting small neoplasms. MRI is the most accurate technique for identifying isolated liver lesions such as hemangiomas, focal nodular hyperplasia, or focal fatty infiltration and for detecting hepatic iron overload. Dynamic gadolinium-enhanced MRI and administration of superparamagnetic iron oxide show promise in visualizing hepatic fibrosis. Because of its much lower cost (amount charged), ultrasonography ($300–$1000) is preferable to CT ($1700) or MRI ($2100) as a screening test. Ultrasonography can detect gallstones with a sensitivity of 95%.

Magnetic resonance cholangiopancreatography (MRCP) is a sensitive, noninvasive method of detecting bile duct stones, strictures, and dilation; however, it is less reliable than endoscopic retrograde cholangiopancreatography (ERCP) for distinguishing malignant from benign strictures. ERCP requires a skilled endoscopist and may be used to demonstrate pancreatic or ampullary causes of jaundice, to carry out papillotomy and stone extraction, or to insert a stent through an obstructing lesion or to facilitate direct cholangiopancreatoscopy. Complications of ERCP include pancreatitis (5%) and, less commonly, cholangitis, bleeding, or duodenal perforation after papillotomy. Risk factors for post-ERCP pancreatitis include female gender, prior post-ERCP pancreatitis, suspected sphincter of Oddi dysfunction, and a difficult or failed cannulation. Percutaneous transhepatic cholangiography (PTC) is an alternative approach to evaluating the anatomy of the biliary tree. Severe complications of PTC occur in 3% and include fever, bacteremia, bile peritonitis, and intraperitoneal hemorrhage. Endoscopic ultrasonography is the most sensitive test for detecting small lesions of the ampulla or pancreatic head and for detecting portal vein invasion by pancreatic cancer. It is also accurate in detecting or excluding bile duct stones.

When to Refer

Patients with jaundice should be referred for diagnostic procedures.

When to Admit

Patients with liver failure should be hospitalized.

Castera L et al. Non-invasive evaluation of liver fibrosis using transient elastography. J Hepatol. 2008 May;48(5):835–47. [PMID: 18334275]

Friedrich-Rust M et al. Performance of transient elastography for the staging of liver fibrosis: a meta-analysis. Gastroenterology. 2008 Apr;134(4):960–74. [PMID: 18395077]

Kechagias S et al. Fast-food-based hyperalimentation can induce rapid and profound elevation of serum alanine aminotransferase in healthy subjects. Gut. 2008 May;57(5):568–70. [PMID: 18276725]

Kim WR et al; Public Policy Committee of the American Association for the Study of Liver Disease. Serum activity of alanine aminotransferase (ALT) as an indicator of health and disease. Hepatology. 2008 Apr;47(4):1363–70. [PMID: 18366115]

Loomba R et al. Parental obesity and offspring serum alanine and aspartate aminotransferase levels: the Framingham Heart Study. Gastroenterology. 2008 Apr;134(4):953–9. [PMID: 18395076]

Perlstein TS et al. Serum total bilirubin level, prevalent stroke, and stroke outcomes: NHANES 1999–2004. Am J Med. 2008 Sep;121(9):781–8. [PMID: 18724968]

DISEASES OF THE LIVER

ACUTE VIRAL HEPATITIS

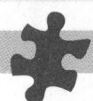

ESSENTIALS OF DIAGNOSIS

▶ Prodrome of anorexia, nausea, vomiting, malaise, aversion to smoking.

▶ Fever, enlarged and tender liver, jaundice.

▶ Normal to low white cell count; abnormal liver tests, especially markedly elevated aminotransferases early in the course.

▶ Liver biopsy shows hepatocellular necrosis and mononuclear infiltrate but is rarely indicated.

▶ General Considerations

Hepatitis can be caused by many drugs and toxic agents as well as by numerous viruses, the clinical manifestations of which may be quite similar. Viruses causing hepatitis are (1) hepatitis A virus (HAV), (2) hepatitis B virus (HBV), (3) hepatitis C virus (HCV), (4) hepatitis D virus (HDV) (delta agent), and (5) hepatitis E virus (HEV) (an enterically transmitted hepatitis seen in epidemic form in Asia, the Middle East, and North Africa). Hepatitis G virus (HGV) rarely, if ever, causes frank hepatitis. A DNA virus designated the TT virus (TTV) has been identified in up to 7.5% of blood donors and found to be transmitted readily by blood transfusions, but an association between this virus and liver disease has not been established. A related virus known as SEN-V has been found in 2% of US blood donors, is transmitted by transfusion, and may account for some cases of transfusion-associated non-ABCDE hepatitis. In immunocompromised and rare immunocompetent persons, cytomegalovirus, Epstein–Barr virus, and herpes simplex virus should be considered in the differential diagnosis of hepatitis. Severe acute respiratory syndrome (SARS) may be associated with marked serum aminotransferase elevations. Unidentified pathogens account for a small percentage of cases of acute viral hepatitis.

A. Hepatitis A

Figure 16–1 shows the typical course of HAV infection. HAV is a 27-nm RNA hepatovirus (in the picornavirus family) that causes epidemics or sporadic cases of hepatitis. The virus is transmitted by the fecal–oral route, and its spread is favored by crowding and poor sanitation. Since introduction of the HAV vaccine in the United States in 1995, the incidence rate of HAV infection has declined by over 76%, with a corresponding decline in the mortality rate of 32%. Common source outbreaks result from contaminated water or food, including inadequately cooked shellfish. A large outbreak among patrons of a restaurant in Monaca, Pennsylvania, in 2003 was traced to contaminated green onions from Mexico. Outbreaks among injection drug users and cases among international adoptees and their contacts have been reported.

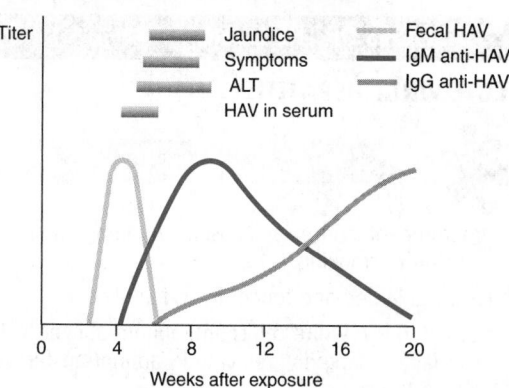

▲ **Figure 16–1.** The typical course of acute type A hepatitis. (HAV, hepatitis A virus; anti-HAV, antibody to hepatitis A virus; ALT, alanine aminotransferase.)
(Reprinted with permission from Koff RS. Acute viral hepatitis. In: *Handbook of Liver Disease.* Friedman LS, Keeffe EB [editors], 2nd ed. ©Elsevier, 2004.)

The incubation period averages 30 days. HAV is excreted in feces for up to 2 weeks before clinical illness but rarely after the first week of illness. The mortality rate for hepatitis A is low, and fulminant hepatitis A is uncommon except for rare instances in which it occurs in a patient with chronic hepatitis C. There is no chronic carrier state. Clinical illness is more severe in adults than in children, in whom it is typically asymptomatic.

Antibody to hepatitis A (anti-HAV) appears early in the course of the illness. Both IgM and IgG anti-HAV are detectable in serum soon after the onset. Peak titers of IgM anti-HAV occur during the first week of clinical disease and disappear within 3–6 months. Detection of IgM anti-HAV is an excellent test for diagnosing acute hepatitis A but is not recommended for the evaluation of asymptomatic persons with persistently elevated serum aminotransferase levels because false-positive results occur. Titers of IgG anti-HAV rise after 1 month of the disease and may persist for years. IgG anti-HAV indicates previous exposure to HAV, noninfectivity, and immunity. In the United States, about 30% of the population have serologic evidence of previous infection.

B. Hepatitis B

Figure 16–2 shows the typical course of HBV infection. HBV is a 42-nm hepadnavirus with a partially double-stranded DNA genome, inner core protein (hepatitis B core antigen, HBcAg), and outer surface coat (hepatitis B surface antigen, HBsAg). There are eight different genotypes (A–H), which may influence the course of infection and responsiveness to antiviral therapy. HBV is usually transmitted by inoculation of infected blood or blood products or by sexual contact and is present in saliva, semen, and vaginal secretions. HBsAg-positive mothers may transmit HBV at delivery; the risk of chronic infection in the infant is as high as 90%.

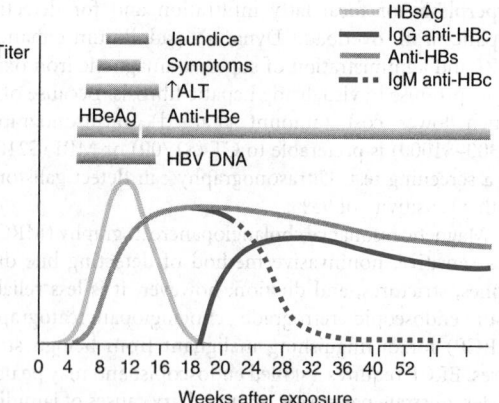

▲ **Figure 16–2.** The typical course of acute type B hepatitis. (HBsAg, hepatitis B surface antigen; anti-HBs, antibody to HBsAg; HBeAg, hepatitis Be antigen; anti-HBe, antibody to HBeAg; anti-HBc, antibody to hepatitis B core antigen; ALT, alanine aminotransferase.)
(Reprinted with permission from Koff RS. Acute viral hepatitis. In: *Handbook of Liver Disease.* Friedman LS, Keeffe EB [editors], 2nd ed. ©Elsevier, 2004.)

HBV is prevalent in men who have sex with men and in injection drug users (about 7% of HIV-infected persons are coinfected with HBV), but the greatest number of cases results from heterosexual transmission; the incidence has decreased by over 75% since the 1980s. Groups at risk include patients and staff at hemodialysis centers, physicians, dentists, nurses, and personnel working in clinical and pathology laboratories and blood banks. Half of all patients with acute hepatitis B in the United States have previously been incarcerated or treated for a sexually transmitted disease. The risk of HBV infection from a blood transfusion is less than 1 in 60,000 units transfused in the United States.

The incubation period of hepatitis B is 6 weeks to 6 months (average 12–14 weeks). The onset of hepatitis B is more insidious and the aminotransferase levels are higher than in HAV infection. Fulminant hepatitis occurs in less than 1%, with a mortality rate of up to 60%. Following acute hepatitis B, HBV infection persists in 1–2% of immunocompetent adults but in a higher percentage of immunocompromised adults or children. Persons with chronic hepatitis B, particularly when HBV infection is acquired early in life and viral replication persists, are at substantial risk of cirrhosis and hepatocellular carcinoma (up to 25–40%). Men are at greater risk than women. Infection caused by HBV may be associated with serum sickness, glomerulonephritis, and polyarteritis nodosa.

There are three distinct antigen–antibody systems that relate to HBV infection and circulating markers that are useful in diagnosis. Interpretation of common serologic patterns is shown in Table 16–5.

1. HBsAg—The appearance of HBsAg is the first evidence of infection, appearing before biochemical evidence of

Table 16–5. Common serologic patterns in hepatitis B virus infection and their interpretation.

HBsAg	Anti-HBs	Anti-HBc	HBeAg	Anti-HBe	Interpretation
+	–	IgM	+	–	Acute hepatitis B
+	–	IgG[1]	+	–	Chronic hepatitis B with active viral replication
+	–	IgG	–	+	Chronic hepatitis B with low viral replication
+	+	IgG	+ or –	+ or –	Chronic hepatitis B with heterotypic anti-HBs (about 10% of cases)
–	–	IgM	+ or –	–	Acute hepatitis B
–	+	IgG	–	+ or –	Recovery from hepatitis B (immunity)
–	+	–	–	–	Vaccination (immunity)
–	–	IgG	–	–	False-positive; less commonly, infection in remote past

[1]Low levels of IgM anti-HBc may also be detected.

liver disease, and persists throughout the clinical illness. Persistence of HBsAg more than 6 months after the acute illness signifies chronic hepatitis B.

2. Anti-HBs—Specific antibody to HBsAg (anti-HBs) appears in most individuals after clearance of HBsAg and after successful vaccination against hepatitis B. Disappearance of HBsAg and the appearance of anti-HBs signal recovery from HBV infection, noninfectivity, and immunity.

3. Anti-HBc—IgM anti-HBc appears shortly after HBsAg is detected. (HBcAg alone does not appear in serum.) Its presence in the setting of acute hepatitis indicates a diagnosis of acute hepatitis B, and it fills the serologic gap in rare patients who have cleared HBsAg but do not yet have detectable anti-HBs. IgM anti-HBc can persist for 3–6 months or longer. IgM anti-HBc may also reappear during flares of previously inactive chronic hepatitis B. IgG anti-HBc also appears during acute hepatitis B but persists indefinitely, whether the patient recovers (with the appearance of anti-HBs in serum) or chronic hepatitis B develops (with persistence of HBsAg). In asymptomatic blood donors, an isolated anti-HBc with no other positive HBV serologic results may represent a falsely positive result or latent infection in which HBV DNA is detectable only by polymerase chain reaction testing.

4. HBeAg—HBeAg is a secretory form of HBcAg that appears in serum during the incubation period shortly after the detection of HBsAg. HBeAg indicates viral replication and infectivity. Persistence of HBeAg beyond 3 months indicates an increased likelihood of chronic hepatitis B. Its disappearance is often followed by the appearance of anti-HBe, generally signifying diminished viral replication and decreased infectivity.

5. HBV DNA—The presence of HBV DNA in serum generally parallels the presence of HBeAg, although HBV DNA is a more sensitive and precise marker of viral replication and infectivity. Very low levels of HBV DNA, detectable only by polymerase chain reaction testing, may persist in serum and liver long after a patient has recovered from acute hepatitis B, but the HBV DNA in serum is bound to IgG and is rarely infectious. In some patients with chronic hepatitis B, HBV

DNA is present at high levels without HBeAg in serum because of development of a mutation in the core promoter or precore region of the gene that codes HBcAg; these mutations prevent synthesis of HBeAg in infected hepatocytes. When additional mutations in the core gene are present, the pre-core mutant enhances the severity of HBV infection and increases the risk of cirrhosis.

C. Hepatitis D (Delta Agent)

HDV is a defective RNA virus that causes hepatitis only in association with hepatitis B infection and specifically only in the presence of HBsAg; it is cleared when the latter is cleared.

HDV may coinfect with HBV or may superinfect a person with chronic hepatitis B, usually by percutaneous exposure. When acute hepatitis D is coincident with acute HBV infection, the infection is generally similar in severity to acute hepatitis B alone. In chronic hepatitis B, superinfection by HDV appears to carry a worse short-term prognosis, often resulting in fulminant hepatitis or severe chronic hepatitis that progresses rapidly to cirrhosis.

In the 1970s and early 1980s, HDV was endemic in some areas, such as the Mediterranean countries (and later in central and Eastern Europe), where up to 80% of HBV carriers were superinfected with it. In the United States, HDV occurred primarily among injection drug users. However, new cases of hepatitis D are now infrequent in the United States, and cases seen today are usually from cohorts infected years ago who survived the initial impact of hepatitis D and now have inactive cirrhosis. These patients have a threefold increased risk of hepatocellular carcinoma. Diagnosis is made by detection of antibody to hepatitis D antigen (anti-HDV) or, where available, hepatitis D antigen (HDAg) or HDV RNA in serum.

D. Hepatitis C

Figure 16–3 shows the typical course of HCV infection. HCV is a single-stranded RNA virus (hepacivirus) with properties similar to those of flavivirus. At least six major genotypes of HCV have been identified. In the past, HCV was responsible for over 90% of cases of posttransfusion

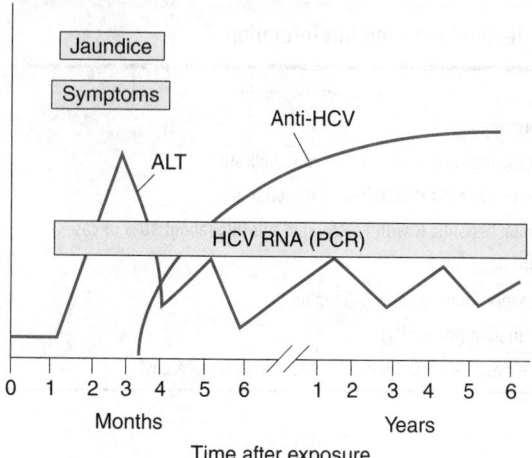

▲ **Figure 16–3.** The typical course of acute and chronic hepatitis C. (ALT, alanine aminotransferase; Anti-HCV, antibody to hepatitis C virus by enzyme immunoassay; HCV RNA [PCR], hepatitis C viral RNA by polymerase chain reaction.)

hepatitis, yet only 4% of cases of hepatitis C were attributable to blood transfusions. Over 50% of cases are transmitted by injection drug use. Body piercing, tattoos, and hemodialysis are risk factors. The risk of sexual and maternal–neonatal transmission is low and may be greatest in a subset of patients with high circulating levels of HCV RNA. Having multiple sexual partners may increase the risk of HCV infection, and HIV coinfection increases the risk of HCV transmission in men who have sex with men. Transmission via breast-feeding has not been documented. An outbreak of hepatitis C in patients with immune deficiencies occurred in some recipients of intravenous immune globulin. Hospital-acquired transmission has occurred via multidose vials of saline used to flush Portacaths; through reuse of disposable syringes; through contamination of shared saline, radiopharmaceutical, and sclerosant vials; and between hospitalized patients on a liver unit. In the developing world, unsafe medical practices lead to a substantial number of cases of HCV infection. Covert transmission during bloody fisticuffs has even been reported. In many patients, the source of infection is unknown. Coinfection with HCV is found in at least 30% of persons infected with HIV; HIV infection leads to an increased risk of acute hepatic failure and more rapid progression of chronic hepatitis C to cirrhosis; in addition, HCV increases the hepatotoxicity of highly active antiretroviral therapy. There are more than 2.7 million HCV carriers in the United States and another 1.3 million previously exposed persons who have cleared the virus.

The incubation period averages 6–7 weeks, and clinical illness is often mild, usually asymptomatic, and characterized by waxing and waning aminotransferase elevations and a high rate (> 80%) of chronic hepatitis. In pregnant patients, serum aminotransferase levels frequently normalize despite persistence of viremia, only to increase again after delivery. HCV is a pathogenetic factor in mixed cryoglobulinemia and

membranoproliferative glomerulonephritis and may be related to lichen planus, autoimmune thyroiditis, lymphocytic sialadenitis, idiopathic pulmonary fibrosis, sporadic porphyria cutanea tarda, and monoclonal gammopathies. HCV infection confers a 20–30% increased risk of non-Hodgkin lymphoma. Hepatitis C may induce insulin resistance (which in turn increases the risk of hepatic fibrosis), and the risk of type 2 diabetes mellitus is increased in persons with chronic hepatitis C. Hepatic steatosis is a particular feature of infection with HCV genotype 3 and may also occur in patients with risk factors for fatty liver (see below).

Diagnosis of hepatitis C is based on an enzyme immunoassay that detects antibodies to HCV. Anti-HCV is not protective, and in patients with acute or chronic hepatitis its presence in serum generally signifies that HCV is the cause. Limitations of the enzyme immunoassay include moderate sensitivity (false-negatives) for the diagnosis of acute hepatitis C early in the course and low specificity (false-positives) in some persons with elevated γ-globulin levels. In these situations, a diagnosis of hepatitis C may be confirmed by using an assay for HCV RNA. Occasional persons are found to have anti-HCV in serum, confirmed by a recombinant immunoblot assay (RIBA), without HCV RNA in serum, suggesting recovery from HCV infection in the past. Testing donated blood for HCV has helped reduce the risk of transfusion-associated hepatitis C from 10% in 1990 to about 1 case per 2 million units today.

E. Hepatitis E

HEV is a 29- to 32-nm RNA hepevirus (in the Hepeviridae family) that is a major cause of acute hepatitis throughout Central and Southeast Asia, the Middle East, and North Africa, where it is responsible for waterborne hepatitis outbreaks. It is rare in the United States but should be considered in patients with acute hepatitis after a trip to an endemic area. In industrialized countries, it may be spread by swine. Illness generally is self-limited (no carrier state), but instances of chronic hepatitis attributed to HEV have been reported in transplant recipients. The mortality rate is high (10–20%) in pregnant women, and the risk of hepatic decompensation is increased in patients with underlying chronic liver disease.

F. Hepatitis G

HGV is a flavivirus that is percutaneously transmitted and associated with chronic viremia lasting at least 10 years. HGV has been detected in 1.5% of blood donors, 50% of injection drug users, 30% of hemodialysis patients, 20% of hemophiliacs, and 15% of patients with chronic hepatitis B or C, but it does not appear to cause important liver disease or affect the response of patients with chronic hepatitis B or C to antiviral therapy. HGV coinfection may improve survival in patients with HIV infection and reduce the degree of fibrosis in patients with HCV-HIV coinfection.

► Clinical Findings

The clinical picture of viral hepatitis is extremely variable, ranging from asymptomatic infection without jaundice to a fulminating disease and death in a few days.

A. Symptoms

The onset may be abrupt or insidious, with general malaise, myalgia, arthralgia, easy fatigability, upper respiratory symptoms, and anorexia. A distaste for smoking, paralleling anorexia, may occur early. Nausea and vomiting are frequent, and diarrhea or constipation may occur. Serum sickness may be seen early in acute hepatitis B. Fever is generally present but is low-grade except in occasional cases of hepatitis A. Defervescence and a fall in pulse rate often coincide with the onset of jaundice.

Abdominal pain is usually mild and constant in the right upper quadrant or epigastrium, often aggravated by jarring or exertion, and rarely may be severe enough to simulate cholecystitis.

Jaundice occurs after 5–10 days but may appear at the same time as the initial symptoms. In many patients, jaundice never develops. With the onset of jaundice, prodromal symptoms often worsen, followed by progressive clinical improvement. Stools may be acholic during this phase.

The acute illness usually subsides over 2–3 weeks with complete clinical and laboratory recovery by 9 weeks in hepatitis A and by 16 weeks in hepatitis B. In 5–10% of cases, the course may be more protracted, but less than 1% will have a fulminant course. In some cases of acute hepatitis A, clinical, biochemical, and serologic recovery may be followed by one or two relapses, but recovery is the rule. A protracted course of hepatitis A has been reported to be associated with HLA *DRB1*1301*. Acute cholecystitis occasionally complicates the course of acute hepatitis A. Hepatitis B, D, and C (and G) may become chronic (see below).

B. Signs

Hepatomegaly—rarely marked—is present in over half of cases. Liver tenderness is usually present. Splenomegaly is reported in 15% of patients, and soft, enlarged lymph nodes—especially in the cervical or epitrochlear areas—may occur. Systemic toxicity is most often encountered in hepatitis A. Slight neurocognitive impairment has been described in patients with chronic hepatitis C.

C. Laboratory Findings

The white blood cell count is normal to low, especially in the preicteric phase. Large atypical lymphocytes may occasionally be seen. Rarely, aplastic anemia follows an episode of acute hepatitis not caused by any of the known hepatitis viruses. Mild proteinuria is common, and bilirubinuria often precedes the appearance of jaundice. Strikingly elevated AST or ALT occurs early, followed by elevations of bilirubin and alkaline phosphatase; in a minority of patients, the latter persist after aminotransferase levels have normalized. Cholestasis is occasionally marked in acute hepatitis A. Marked prolongation of the prothrombin time in severe hepatitis correlates with increased mortality.

▶ Differential Diagnosis

The differential diagnosis includes other viral diseases such as infectious mononucleosis, cytomegalovirus infection, and herpes simplex virus infection; spirochetal diseases such as leptospirosis and secondary syphilis; brucellosis; rickettsial diseases such as Q fever; drug-induced liver disease; and shock liver (ischemic hepatitis). Occasionally, autoimmune hepatitis (see below) may have an acute onset mimicking acute viral hepatitis. Rarely, metastatic cancer of the liver may present with a hepatitis-like picture.

The prodromal phase of viral hepatitis must be distinguished from other infectious disease such as influenza, upper respiratory infections, and the prodromal stages of the exanthematous diseases. Cholestasis may mimic obstructive jaundice.

▶ Prevention

Strict isolation of patients is not necessary, but hand washing after bowel movements is required. Thorough hand washing by medical staff who may contact contaminated utensils, bedding, or clothing is essential. Medical staff should handle disposable needles carefully and not recap them. Screening of donated blood for HBsAg, anti-HBc, and anti-HCV has reduced the risk of transfusion-associated hepatitis markedly. All pregnant women should undergo testing for HBsAg. HBV- and HCV-infected persons should practice safe sex, but there is little evidence that HCV is spread easily by sexual contact, and no precautions are recommended for persons in a monogamous relationship. Vaccination against HAV (after prescreening for prior immunity) and HBV is recommended for patients with chronic hepatitis C, and vaccination against HAV is recommended for patients with chronic hepatitis B. Improved public hygiene reduces the risk of HEV infection in endemic areas. A recombinant vaccine against HEV has shown promise in clinical trials.

A. Hepatitis A

Unvaccinated persons who are exposed to HAV are advised to receive postexposure prophylaxis with a single dose of HAV vaccine or immune globulin (0.02 mL/kg) as soon as possible. The vaccine is preferred in healthy persons ages 1 year to 40 years, whereas immune globulin is preferred in those older than 40 years or younger than 1 year or who are immunocompromised or have chronic liver disease.

Two effective inactivated hepatitis A vaccines are available and recommended for persons living in or traveling to endemic areas (including military personnel), patients with chronic liver disease upon diagnosis, persons with clotting-factor disorders who are treated with concentrates, men who have sex with men, men who have sex with both men and women, animal handlers, illicit drug users, sewage workers, food handlers, and children and caregivers in day care centers and institutions. For healthy travelers, a single dose of vaccine at any time before departure can provide adequate protection. Routine vaccination is advised for all children in states with an incidence of hepatitis A at least twice the national average and has been recommended by the Advisory Committee on Immunization Practices of the Centers for Disease Control and Prevention (CDC) for all children between ages 1 and 2 in the United States. HAV vaccine is also effective in the prevention of secondary spread to household contacts of primary cases. The recommended dose for adults is 1 mL (1440 ELISA units) of Havrix (GlaxoSmithKline) or 1 mL (50 units) of Vaqta (Merck) intramuscularly, followed by a booster dose at 6–18 months. A combined hepatitis A and B vaccine (Twinrix, GlaxoSmithKline) is available. HIV infection impairs the response to the HAV vaccine, especially in persons with a CD4 count less than 200/mcL.

B. Hepatitis B

Hepatitis B immune globulin (HBIG) may be protective—or may attenuate the severity of illness—if given in large doses within 7 days after exposure (adult dose is 0.06 mL/kg body weight) followed by initiation of the HBV vaccine series (see below). This approach is currently recommended for persons exposed to HBsAg-contaminated material via mucous membranes or through breaks in the skin and for individuals who have had sexual contact with a person with HBV infection (irrespective of the presence or absence of HBeAg in the source). HBIG is also indicated for newborn infants of HBsAg-positive mothers followed by initiation of the vaccine series (see below).

The currently used vaccines are recombinant-derived. Initially, the vaccine was targeted to persons at high risk, including renal dialysis patients and attending personnel, patients requiring repeated transfusions, spouses of HBsAg-positive persons, men who have sex with men, injection drug users, newborns of HBsAg-positive mothers, beginning medical and nursing students, and all medical technologists. Because this strategy failed to lower the incidence of hepatitis B, the CDC recommends vaccination of all infants and children in the United States and all adults who are at risk for hepatitis B or request vaccination. Over 90% of recipients of the vaccine mount protective antibody to hepatitis B; immunocompromised persons respond poorly. Reduced response to the vaccine may have a genetic basis in some cases and has also been associated with age over 40 years and celiac disease. The standard regimen for adults is 10–20 mcg initially (depending on the formulation) repeated again at 1 and 6 months, but alternative schedules have been approved, including accelerated schedules of 0, 1, 2, and 12 months and of 0, 7, and 21 days plus 12 months. For greatest reliability of absorption, the deltoid muscle is the preferred site. Vaccine formulations free of the mercury-containing preservative thimerosal are given to infants less than 6 months of age. When documentation of seroconversion is considered desirable, postimmunization anti-HBs titers may be checked. Protection appears to be excellent even if the titer wanes—at least for 20 years—and booster reimmunization is not routinely recommended but is advised for immunocompromised persons in whom anti-HBs titers fall below 10 milli-international units/mL. For vaccine nonresponders, three additional vaccine doses may elicit seroprotective anti-HBs levels in 30–50% of persons. Universal vaccination of neonates in countries endemic for HBV has reduced the incidence of hepatocellular carcinoma.

▶ Treatment

Bed rest is recommended only if symptoms are marked. If nausea and vomiting are pronounced or if oral intake is substantially decreased, intravenous 10% glucose is indicated. Encephalopathy or severe coagulopathy indicates impending acute hepatic failure, and hospitalization at a liver transplant center is mandatory (see below).

Dietary management consists of palatable meals as tolerated, without overfeeding; breakfast is usually tolerated best. Strenuous physical exertion, alcohol, and hepatotoxic agents are avoided. Small doses of oxazepam are safe, as metabolism is not hepatic; morphine sulfate is avoided.

Corticosteroids have no benefit in patients with viral hepatitis, including those with fulminant disease. Treatment of patients with acute hepatitis C with peginterferon (see later) for 6–24 weeks appreciably decreases the risk of chronic hepatitis. In general, patients infected with HCV genotype 1 require a 24-week course of treatment, but a 12-week course is adequate if HCV RNA is undetectable in serum by 4 weeks. Those infected with genotypes 2, 3, or 4 generally require 8–12 weeks of therapy. Because 20% of patients with acute hepatitis C, particularly those who are symptomatic, clear the virus without such treatment, reserving it for patients in whom serum HCV RNA levels fail to clear after 3 months may be advisable. Ribavirin may be added if HCV RNA fails to clear after 3 months of peginterferon. Antiviral therapy is generally unnecessary in patients with acute hepatitis B.

▶ Prognosis

In most patients, clinical recovery is complete in 3–6 months. Laboratory evidence of liver dysfunction may persist for a longer period, but most patients recover completely. The overall mortality rate is less than 1%, but the rate is reportedly higher in older people.

Hepatitis A does not cause chronic liver disease, although it may persist for up to 1 year, and clinical and biochemical relapses may occur before full recovery. The mortality rate is less than 0.2%. The mortality rate for acute hepatitis B is 0.1–1%, but is higher with superimposed hepatitis D. Fulminant hepatitis C is rare in the United States. For unknown reasons, the mortality rate for hepatitis E is especially high in pregnant women (10–20%).

Chronic hepatitis, characterized by elevated aminotransferase levels for more than 6 months, develops in 1–2% of immunocompetent adults with acute hepatitis B but in as many as 90% of infected neonates and infants and a substantial proportion of immunocompromised adults. Chronic hepatitis, which progresses very slowly in many cases, develops in as many as 80% of all persons with acute hepatitis C. Ultimately, cirrhosis develops in up to 30% of those with chronic hepatitis C and 40% of those with chronic hepatitis B; the risk of cirrhosis is even higher in patients coinfected with both viruses or with HIV. Patients with cirrhosis are at risk for hepatocellular carcinoma at a rate of 3–5% per year. Even in the absence of cirrhosis, patients with chronic hepatitis B—particularly those with active viral replication—are at increased risk.

▶ When to Refer

Refer patients with acute hepatitis who require liver biopsy for diagnosis.

When to Admit

- Encephalopathy is present.
- INR > 1.6.
- The patient is unable to maintain hydration.

Cardell K et al. Excellent response rate to a double dose of the combined hepatitis A and B vaccine in previous nonresponders to hepatitis B vaccine. J Infect Dis. 2008 Aug 1;198(3):299–304. [PMID: 18544037]

Fischer GE et al. Hepatitis A among international adoptees and their contacts. Clin Infect Dis. 2008 Sep 15;47(6):812–4. [PMID: 18684098]

Kamar N et al. Hepatitis E virus and chronic hepatitis in organ-transplant recipients. N Engl J Med. 2008 Feb 21;358(8):811–7. [PMID: 18287603]

Maheshwari A et al. Acute hepatitis C. Lancet. 2008 Jul 26;372(9635):321–32. [PMID: 18657711]

Perry W et al. Cognitive dysfunction in chronic hepatitis C: a review. Dig Dis Sci. 2008 Feb;53(2):307–21. [PMID: 17703362]

Purcell RH et al. Hepatitis E: an emerging awareness of an old disease. J Hepatol. 2008 Mar;48(3):494–503. [PMID: 18192058]

Santantonio T et al. Acute hepatitis C: current status and remaining challenges. J Hepatol. 2008 Oct;49(4):625–33. [PMID: 18706735]

Thompson MS et al. Nonhospital health care—associated hepatitis B and C virus transmission: United States, 1998–2008. Ann Intern Med. 2009 Jan 6;150(1):33–9. [PMID: 19124818]

Vogt TM et al. Declining hepatitis A mortality in the United States during the era of hepatitis A vaccination. J Infect Dis. 2008 May 1;197(9):1282–8. [PMID: 18422440]

ACUTE HEPATIC FAILURE

ESSENTIALS OF DIAGNOSIS

- ▶ May be fulminant or subfulminant; both forms carry a poor prognosis.
- ▶ Acetaminophen and idiosyncratic drug reactions are the most common causes.

General Considerations

Acute hepatic failure may be fulminant or subfulminant. Fulminant hepatic failure is characterized by the development of hepatic encephalopathy within 8 weeks after the onset of acute liver disease. Coagulopathy (international normalized ratio [INR] ≥ 1.5) is invariably present. Subfulminant hepatic failure occurs when these findings appear between 8 weeks and 6 months after the onset of acute liver disease and carries an equally poor prognosis.

An estimated 1600 cases of acute hepatic failure occur each year in the United States. Acetaminophen toxicity is the most common cause, accounting for at least 45% of cases. Suicide attempts account for 44% of cases of acetaminophen-induced hepatic failure, and unintentional overdoses ("therapeutic misadventures"), which are often a result of a decrease in the threshold toxic dose because of chronic alcohol use or fasting, account for at least 48%. Other causes include idiosyncratic drug reactions (now the second most common cause), viral hepatitis, poisonous mushrooms (*Amanita phylloides*), shock, hyperthermia or

hypothermia, Budd–Chiari syndrome, malignancy (most commonly lymphomas), Wilson disease, Reye syndrome, fatty liver of pregnancy and other disorders of fatty acid oxidation, autoimmune hepatitis, parvovirus B19 infection and, rarely, grand mal seizures. The risk of acute hepatic failure is increased in patients with diabetes mellitus, and outcome is worsened by obesity. Herbal and dietary supplements are thought to be contributory to acute hepatic failure in a substantial portion of cases, regardless of cause.

Viral hepatitis now accounts for only 12% of all cases of acute hepatic failure. The decline of viral hepatitis as the principal cause of acute hepatic failure is due to universal vaccination of infants and children against hepatitis B and the availability of the hepatitis A vaccine. In endemic areas, hepatitis E is an important cause of acute hepatic failure. Hepatitis C is a rare cause of acute hepatic failure in the United States, but acute hepatitis A or B superimposed on chronic hepatitis C may cause fulminant hepatitis.

Clinical Findings

Gastrointestinal symptoms, systemic inflammatory response, and hemorrhagic phenomena are common. Adrenal insufficiency and subclinical myocardial injury manifesting as an elevated serum troponin I level often complicate acute hepatic failure. Jaundice may be absent or minimal early, but laboratory tests show severe hepatocellular damage. In acetaminophen toxicity, serum aminotransferase levels are often towering (> 5000 units/L), and diagnosis is aided by the detection of acetaminophen-protein adducts in serum. In acute hepatic failure due to microvesicular steatosis (eg, fatty liver of pregnancy), serum aminotransferase elevations may be modest (< 300 units/L). The blood ammonia level is typically elevated and correlates (along with the Model for End-Stage Liver Disease [MELD] score) with the development of encephalopathy and intracranial hypertension.

Treatment

The treatment of acute hepatic failure is directed toward correcting metabolic abnormalities. These include coagulation defects, electrolyte and acid-base disturbances, advanced chronic kidney disease, hypoglycemia, and encephalopathy. Cerebral edema and sepsis are the leading causes of death. Prophylactic antibiotic therapy decreases the risk of infection, observed in up to 90%, but has no effect on survival and is not routinely recommended. For suspected sepsis, broad coverage is indicated. Despite a high rate of adrenal insufficiency, corticosteroids are of uncertain value. Stress gastropathy prophylaxis with an H_2-receptor blocker or proton pump inhibitor is recommended. Administration of acetylcysteine (140 mg/kg orally followed by 70 mg/kg orally every 4 hours for an additional 17 doses or 150 mg/kg in 5% dextrose intravenously over 15 minutes followed by 50 mg/kg over 4 hours and then 100 mg/kg over 16 hours) is indicated for acetaminophen toxicity up to 72 hours after ingestion and improves cerebral blood flow and oxygenation as well as survival in patients with stage 1 or 2 encephalopathy due to fulminant hepatic failure of any cause. (Acetylcysteine treatment can prolong the prothrombin time, leading to the erroneous assumption that liver failure is worsening.) Penicillin G (300,000 to 1 million units/kg/day) or silibinin (silymarin or milk thistle), which is not licensed in the United States, is administered to patients with mushroom poisoning. Nucleoside analogs are recommended for patients with fulminant hepatitis B (see Chronic Hepatitis). Subclinical seizure activity is common in patients with acute liver failure, but the value of prophylactic phenytoin is uncertain.

Early transfer to a liver transplantation center is essential. Extradural sensors may be placed to monitor intracranial pressure for impending cerebral edema. Lactulose is administered for encephalopathy (see Cirrhosis). Mannitol, 100–200 mL of a 20% solution by intravenous infusion over 10 minutes, may decrease cerebral edema but should be used with caution in patients with advanced chronic kidney disease. Preliminary experience suggests that intravenously administered hypertonic saline to induce hypernatremia also may reduce intracranial hypertension. Hypothermia to a temperature of 33.1 °C may reduce intracranial pressure when other measures have failed and may improve survival long enough to permit liver transplantation. The value of hyperventilation and intravenous prostaglandin E_1 is uncertain. Short-acting barbiturates are considered for refractory intracranial hypertension. Nonbiologic liver support (eg, molecular adsorbent recirculating system [MARS], an albumin dialysis system) and hepatic-assist devices using living hepatocytes, extracorporeal whole liver perfusion, hepatocyte transplantation, and liver xenografts have shown promise experimentally but have not been shown conclusively to reduce mortality in patients with acute hepatic failure. They may serve as a "bridge" to liver transplantation.

Prognosis

The mortality rate of fulminant hepatic failure with severe encephalopathy is as high as 80%, except for acetaminophen hepatotoxicity, in which the transplant-free survival is 65% and only 8% of patients undergo liver transplantation. For patients with fulminant hepatic failure of other causes, the outlook is especially poor in patients younger than 10 and older than 40 years of age and in those with an idiosyncratic drug reaction but appears to be improved when acetylcysteine is administered to patients with stage 1 or 2 encephalopathy. Spontaneous recovery is less likely for hepatitis B than for hepatitis A. Other adverse prognostic factors are a serum bilirubin level > 18 mg/dL, INR > 6.5, onset of encephalopathy more than 7 days after the onset of jaundice, and a low factor V level (< 20% of normal). For acetaminophen-induced fulminant hepatic failure, indicators of a poor outcome are acidosis (pH < 7.3), INR > 6.5, and azotemia (serum creatinine ≥ 3.4 mg/dL), whereas a rising serum α-fetoprotein level predicts a favorable outcome. An elevated blood lactate level (> 3.5 mmol/L), blood ammonia level (> 124 mcmol/L), and possibly hyperphosphatemia (> 1.2 mmol/L) also predict poor survival outcomes. A prognostic ("BiLE") score based on the serum bilirubin, serum lactate, and etiology has been proposed. Emergency liver transplantation is considered for patients with stage 2 to stage 3 encephalopathy (see

later) and is associated with a 70% survival rate at 5 years. For mushroom poisoning, liver transplantation should be considered when the interval between ingestion and the onset of diarrhea is < 8 hours or the INR is ≥ 6.0, even in the absence of encephalopathy.

▶ When to Admit

All patients with acute hepatic failure should be hospitalized.

Hadem J et al. Prognostic implications of lactate, bilirubin, and etiology in German patients with acute liver failure. Clin Gastroenterol Hepatol. 2008 Mar;6(3):339–45. [PMID: 18328438]

Lee WM (guest ed). Liver failure and liver support. Semin Liver Dis. 2008;28:135–225.

Lee WM et al. Acute liver failure: summary of a workshop. Hepatology. 2008 Apr;47(4):1401–15. [PMID: 18318440]

Myers RP et al. Impact of liver disease, alcohol abuse, and unintentional ingestions on the outcomes of acetaminophen overdose. Clin Gastroenterol Hepatol. 2008 Aug;6(8):918–25. [PMID: 18486561]

CHRONIC VIRAL HEPATITIS

 ESSENTIALS OF DIAGNOSIS

▶ Defined by chronic infection (HBV, HCV, HDV) for greater than 6 months.

▶ Diagnosis is usually made by antibody tests and viral nucleic acid in serum.

▶ General Considerations

Chronic hepatitis is defined as chronic necroinflammation of the liver of more than 3–6 months' duration, demonstrated by persistently abnormal serum aminotransferase levels or characteristic histologic findings. In many cases, the diagnosis of chronic hepatitis may be made on initial presentation. The causes of chronic hepatitis include HBV, HCV, and HDV as well as autoimmune hepatitis; alcoholic and nonalcoholic steatohepatitis; certain medications, such as isoniazid and nitrofurantoin; Wilson disease; α_1-antiprotease deficiency; and, rarely, celiac disease. Chronic hepatitis is categorized on the basis of etiology; the grade of portal, periportal, and lobular inflammation (minimal, mild, moderate, or severe); and the stage of fibrosis (none, mild, moderate, severe, cirrhosis). In the absence of advanced cirrhosis, patients are often asymptomatic or have mild nonspecific symptoms.

▶ Clinical Findings & Diagnosis

A. Chronic Hepatitis B

Chronic hepatitis B afflicts nearly 400 million people worldwide (endemic areas include Asia and sub-Saharan Africa) and 1.25 million (predominantly males) in the United States. It may be noted as a continuum of acute hepatitis B or diagnosed because of persistence of HBsAg in serum, often with elevated aminotransferase levels.

Four phases of HBV infection are recognized. Early in the course, HBeAg and HBV DNA are present in serum, indicative of active viral replication. When HBV infection is acquired in infancy or early childhood, serum aminotransferase levels often are normal and little necroinflammation is present in the liver (*immune tolerant phase*). These persons, like those who acquire HBV infection later in life, may enter an *immune clearance phase*, in which aminotransferase levels are elevated and necroinflammation is present in the liver, with a risk of progression to cirrhosis (at a rate of 2–5.5% per year) and for hepatocellular carcinoma (at a rate of > 2% per year in those with cirrhosis); low-level IgM anti-HBc is present in about 70%. Immune clearance may ultimately be followed by biochemical improvement, which coincides with disappearance of HBeAg and reduced HBV DNA levels (< 10^5 copies/mL, or < 20,000 international units/mL) in serum, appearance of anti-HBe, and integration of the HBV genome into the host genome in infected hepatocytes. If cirrhosis has not yet developed, such persons enter the *inactive HBsAg carrier state* and are at a low risk for cirrhosis and hepatocellular carcinoma. As noted, infection by a pre-core mutant of HBV or spontaneous mutation of the pre-core or core promoter region of the HBV genome during the course of chronic hepatitis caused by wild-type HBV (HBeAg-negative chronic hepatitis B) may result in *reactivated chronic hepatitis B* with a rise in serum HBV DNA levels and possible progression to cirrhosis (at a rate of 8–10% per year), particularly when additional mutations in the core gene of HBV are present. Risk factors for reactivation include male sex and HBV genotype C. In patients with either HBeAg-positive or HBeAg-negative chronic hepatitis B, the risk of cirrhosis and of hepatocellular carcinoma correlates with the serum HBV DNA level. Other risk factors include male sex, advanced age, alcohol use, cigarette smoking, and coinfection with HCV or HDV. HIV coinfection is also associated with an increased frequency of cirrhosis when the CD4 count is low.

B. Hepatitis D

Acute hepatitis D infection superimposed on chronic HBV infection may result in severe chronic hepatitis, which may progress rapidly to cirrhosis and may be fatal. Patients with long-standing chronic hepatitis D and B often have inactive cirrhosis. The diagnosis is confirmed by detection of anti-HDV or HDAg in serum.

C. Chronic Hepatitis C

Chronic hepatitis C develops in up to 85% of patients with acute hepatitis C. It is clinically indistinguishable from chronic hepatitis due to other causes and may be the most common. Worldwide, 170 million people are infected with HCV, with 1.8% of the US population infected. Peak prevalence in the United States (about 4%) is in persons born between 1945 and 1964. In approximately 40% of cases, serum aminotransferase levels are persistently normal. The diagnosis is confirmed by detection of anti-HCV by enzyme immunoassay (EIA). In rare cases of suspected chronic hepatitis C but a negative EIA, HCV RNA is detected by polymerase chain reaction testing. Progression to cirrhosis occurs in 20% of affected patients after 20 years, with an increased risk in men, those who drink more than 50 g of alcohol daily, and those who acquire HCV infection after age 40 years. The rate of fibrosis progression accelerates after age 50. African Americans have a higher rate of chronic hepatitis C but lower rates of fibrosis progression and response to therapy than whites. Immunosuppressed persons—including patients with hypogammaglobulinemia, HIV infection with a low CD4 count, or those receiving immunosuppressants—appear to progress more rapidly to cirrhosis than immunocompetent persons with chronic hepatitis C. Tobacco and cannibis smoking and hepatic steatosis also appear to promote progression of fibrosis. Persons with chronic hepatitis C and persistently normal serum aminotransferase levels usually have mild chronic hepatitis with slow or absent progression to cirrhosis; however, cirrhosis is present in 10% of these patients.

▶ Treatment

A. Chronic Hepatitis B

Patients with active viral replication (HBeAg and HBV DNA [≥ 10^5 copies/mL, or ≥ 20,000 international units/mL] in serum; elevated aminotransferase levels) may be treated with pegylated interferon or a nucleoside or nucleotide analog. For patients who are HBeAg-negative, the threshold for treatment is a serum HBV DNA level ≥ 10^4 copies/mL, or ≥ 2000 international units/mL. If the threshold HBV DNA level for treatment is met but the serum ALT level is normal, treatment may still be considered in patients over age 35–40 if liver biopsy demonstrates a fibrosis stage of 2 (moderate) or higher. Therapy is aimed at reducing and maintaining the serum HBV DNA level to the lowest possible levels, thereby leading to normalization of the ALT level and histologic improvement. An additional goal in HBeAg-positive patients is seroconversion to anti-HBe, which signifies a high likelihood that the benefit will be sustained after discontinuation of treatment. Nucleoside and nucleotide analogs generally are discontinued 6-12 months after HBeAg-to-anti-HBe seroconversion but must be continued long-term when seroconversion does not occur as well as in HBeAg-negative patients.

Peginterferon alfa-2a, 180 mcg subcutaneously once weekly for 48 weeks, leads to sustained normalization of aminotransferase levels, disappearance of HBeAg and HBV DNA from serum, appearance of anti-HBe, and improved survival in up to 40% of treated patients. A response is most likely in patients with a low baseline HBV DNA level and high aminotransferase levels and is more likely in those infected with HBV genotype A than with other genotypes. Moreover, some responders may eventually clear HBsAg from serum and liver and develop anti-HBs in serum, and are thus cured. Relapses are uncommon in complete responders who seroconvert from HBeAg to anti-HBe. Patients with HBeAg-negative chronic hepatitis B have a response rate of 60% after 48 weeks of therapy with peginterferon, but the response may not be durable. The response to interferon is poor in patients with HIV coinfection.

Nucleoside and nucleotide analogs may be used instead of interferon for the treatment of chronic hepatitis B; they are much better tolerated and are often preferred because they can be taken orally. The available drugs differ in efficiency and rates of resistance. The first available nucleoside analog was lamivudine, 100 mg orally daily, which reliably suppresses HBV DNA in serum, improves liver histology in 60% of patients, and leads to normal ALT levels in over 40% and HBeAg seroconversion in 20% of patients after 1 year of therapy. Rates of complete response increase with longer duration of therapy. However, by the end of 1 year, 15–30% of responders experience a relapse (and occasionally frank decompensation) as a result of a mutation in the polymerase gene (the YMDD motif) of HBV DNA that confers resistance to lamivudine. The rate of resistance reaches 70% by 5 years of therapy, and the drug is no longer considered first-line therapy. In patients with advanced fibrosis or cirrhosis, treatment with lamivudine reduces the risk of hepatic decompensation and hepatocellular carcinoma.

Adefovir dipivoxil, a nucleotide analog, has activity against wild-type and lamivudine-resistant HBV. The standard dose is 10 mg orally once a day for at least 1 year. Adding the drug may be effective in patients who have become resistant to lamivudine. As with lamivudine, only a small number of patients achieve sustained suppression of HBV replication with adefovir, and long-term suppressive therapy is often required. Resistance to adefovir is less frequent than with lamivudine but is seen in up to 29% of patients treated for 5 years. Patients with underlying kidney dysfunction are at risk for nephrotoxicity from adefovir.

Telbivudine, given in a daily dose of 600 mg orally, is more potent than either lamivudine or adefovir. Resistance to this drug may develop, particularly in patients who are resistant to lamivudine, and elevated creatine kinase levels are common in patients treated with telbivudine.

Entecavir, another nucleoside analog, has become a preferred first-line treatment for chronic hepatitis B. It is not nephrotoxic, and it is infrequently associated with resistance unless a patient is already resistant to lamivudine. The daily dose is 0.5 mg orally for patients not resistant to lamivudine and 1 mg for patients who have become resistant to lamivudine. Entecavir is more effective than lamivudine and adefovir, with histologic improvement observed in 70% of treated patients and suppression of HBV DNA in serum in up to 80%.

Tenofovir, a nucleotide analog used for HIV infection approved for HBV infection in 2008, has substantial activity against HBV and is used when resistance to a nucleoside analog has developed. Like entecavir, tenofovir has emerged as a first-line agent because of its potency and low rate of resistance.

Other antiviral agents such as emtricitabine and clevudine are under study but are unlikely to offer advantages over available drugs. Strategies using multiple drugs are being investigated.

Nucleoside and nucleotide analogs are well tolerated even in patients with decompensated cirrhosis (for whom the treatment threshold may be an HBV DNA level < 10^4 copies/mL) and may be effective in patients with rapidly progressive hepatitis B ("fibrosing cholestatic hepatitis") following organ transplantation. Although therapy with these agents leads to biochemical, virologic, and histologic improvement in patients with HBeAg-negative chronic hepatitis B and baseline HBV DNA levels ≥ 10^4 copies/mL (≥ 2000 international units/mL), relapse is frequent when therapy is stopped, and long-term treatment is often required. Resistance is most likely to develop to lamivudine and may develop to adefovir and telbivudine. The development of resistance occasionally results in hepatic decompensation. Sequential addition of a second antiviral agent is usually effective after resistance to the first agent has developed. Combined use of peginterferon or interferon and a nucleoside or nucleotide analog has not been shown convincingly to have a substantial advantage over the use of either type of drug alone.

Nucleoside analogs are also recommended for inactive HBV carriers prior to the initiation of immunosuppressive therapy or cancer chemotherapy to prevent reactivation. In patients infected with both HBV and HIV, antiretroviral therapy, including two drugs active against both viruses (eg, tenofovir plus lamivudine or emtricitabine), has been recommended when treatment of HIV infection is indicated. Telbivudine and tenofovir are classified as pregnancy category B drugs, and lamivudine, a category C drug, has been shown to be safe in pregnant women with HIV infection.

B. Chronic Hepatitis C

Treatment of chronic hepatitis C is generally considered in patients under age 70 with more than minimal fibrosis on liver biopsy. Because of high response rates to treatment in patients infected with HCV genotype 2 or 3, treatment may be initiated in these patients without a liver biopsy.

Two formulations of pegylated interferon are approved for HCV infection: peginterferon alfa-2b, with a 12-kDa polyethylene glycol (PEG), 1.5 mcg/kg, and peginterferon alfa-2a, with a 40-kDa PEG, 180 mcg, both given subcutaneously once per week. Whether there are clinically important differences between the two formulations is unclear. Addition of the nucleoside analog ribavirin, 800–1400 mg orally daily in two divided doses, results in higher sustained response rates than peginterferon alone in previously untreated patients with chronic hepatitis C or patients who have had a relapse after an initial response to interferon alfa (no longer available in the United States) and ribavirin.

Sustained response rates with a combination of peginterferon and ribavirin are as high as 55% (and up to 80% for HCV genotypes 2 or 3). Low levels of HCV RNA may persist in the liver, lymphocytes, and macrophages of successfully treated ("cured") patients, but the significance of this finding is uncertain. Response rates are lower in patients with advanced fibrosis, high levels of viremia, alcohol consumption, HIV coinfection, obesity, insulin resistance, and severe steatosis; they are also lower in blacks and Latinos than in whites, in part because of a higher rate of genotype 1 among infected black patients and in part because of intrinsic resistance to therapy. For prior nonresponders to standard interferon and ribavirin, sustained response rates to retreatment with peginterferon alfa and ribavirin are only 10–15%. When used with peginterferon alfa-2b, the dose of ribavirin in patients infected with genotype 1 is based on the patient's weight and may range from 800 mg to 1400 mg daily in two divided doses. When used with peginterferon alfa-2a, the daily ribavirin dose is 1000 mg or 1200 mg depending on whether the patient's weight is less than or greater than 75 kg. Patients infected with genotype 1 are generally treated for 48 weeks. If there has been a decrease in the serum HCV RNA level to < 50 international units/mL by 4 weeks (rapid virologic response), treatment for at least 24 weeks results in a sustained virologic response rate of 90%. For those who do not achieve a rapid virologic response but have a serum HCV RNA level < 50 international units/mL by 12 weeks (complete early virologic response), treatment is continued for the full 48 weeks. If serum HCV RNA levels decline by at least 2 logs by 12 weeks (partial early virologic response) and become undetectable by 24 weeks (slow response), treatment may be extended to 72 weeks. If none of the aforementioned targets is reached, treatment is discontinued. Patients infected with genotype 2 or 3 (without cirrhosis and with low levels of viremia) are treated for 24 weeks and require a ribavirin total daily dose of only 800 mg. For patients infected with these genotypes who clear the virus within 4 weeks (rapid virologic response), a total treatment duration of only 16 weeks may be sufficient, if the baseline HCV RNA level is < 400,000 international units/mL; however, such a short course is not routinely recommended. For patients with cirrhosis or a high viral level (> 400,000 international units/mL), 48 weeks of treatment may be preferred. For patients infected with HCV genotype 1 and without any hepatic fibrosis, expectant management and a repeat assessment of hepatic fibrosis (usually by liver biopsy) in 3–5 years are often recommended.

Peginterferon alfa with ribavirin may be beneficial in the treatment of cryoglobulinemia associated with chronic hepatitis C. "Chronic HCV carriers" with normal serum aminotransferase levels respond just as well to treatment as do patients with elevated aminotransferase levels. Patients with both HCV and HIV infections may benefit from treatment of HCV. Moreover, in HCV/HIV-coinfected persons, long-term liver-related mortality increases as mortality from HIV infection is reduced by highly active antiretroviral therapy.

Treatment with peginterferon alfa plus ribavirin is costly (up to $20,000 for a 24-week supply), and side effects, which include flu-like symptoms, psychiatric symptoms (irritability, depression), thyroid dysfunction, and bone marrow suppression, are common. Discontinuation rates are 15–30% and higher in persons over age 60 years than in younger patients. Sustained response rates decline if less than 60% of the cumulative dose is taken. A blood count is obtained at weeks 1, 2, and 4 after therapy is started and monthly thereafter. Peginterferon alfa is contraindicated in pregnant or breast-feeding patients and those with decompensated cirrhosis, prior solid organ transplants (except liver), profound cytopenias, severe psychiatric disorders, autoimmune diseases, or an inability to self-administer treatment. HCV treatment can be successful in carefully selected persons who continue to inject illicit drugs if they are managed by a multidisciplinary team. Patients taking ribavirin must be monitored for hemolysis, and men and women taking the drug must practice strict contraception until 6 months after conclusion of therapy because of teratogenic effects in animals. Ribavirin should be avoided in persons over age 65 years and in others in whom hemolysis could pose a risk of angina or stroke. Rash, itching, headache, cough, and shortness of breath also occur with the drug. Lactic acidosis is a concern in patients also taking highly active antiretroviral therapy for HIV infection. Erythropoietin (epoetin alfa) and granulocyte colony-stimulating factor (filgrastim) may be used to treat therapy-induced anemia and leukopenia. Peginterferon alfa is generally contraindicated in heart, lung, and kidney transplant recipients because of an increased risk of organ rejection. Selected liver transplant recipients with recurrent hepatitis C may be treated with peginterferon and ribavirin, but response rates are low.

In patients with advanced fibrosis who are nonresponders to interferon-based therapy, long-term maintenance treatment with peginterferon as a strategy to prevent histologic progression and reduce the risk of cirrhosis and hepatocellular carcinoma has been shown in a 3.5-year randomized, controlled trial to be ineffective. Several approaches have been proposed for the treatment of prior nonresponders, but no interferon-based approach achieves response rates exceeding 10–20% in patients who are truly resistant to peginterferon and ribavirin. New approaches to antiviral therapy for hepatitis C include the development of direct antiviral agents, such as protease and polymerase inhibitors. In early clinical trials, when the protease inhibitors telaprevir (phase III trials) and boceprevir (phase II trials) were used with peginterferon and ribavirin, a sustained virologic response rate of ~60% was achieved after total treatment courses of 24 weeks in patients infected with HCV genotype 1.

C. Chronic Hepatitis D

Peginterferon alfa-2b (1.5 mcg/kg/week for 48 weeks) may lead to normalization of serum aminotransferase levels, histologic improvement, and elimination of HDV RNA from serum in 20–50% of patients with chronic hepatitis D, but patients may relapse and tolerance is poor. Nucleoside and nucleotide analogs are not effective in treating chronic hepatitis D.

► Prognosis

The course of chronic viral hepatitis is variable. The sequelae of chronic hepatitis secondary to hepatitis B include cirrhosis, liver failure, and hepatocellular carcinoma. The 5-year mortality rate is 0–2% in those without cirrhosis, 14–20% in those with compensated cirrhosis, and 70–86% following decompensation. The risk of cirrhosis and hepatocellular carcinoma correlates with serum HBV DNA levels, and a focus of therapy is to suppress HBV DNA levels below 300 copies/mL (60 international units/mL). There is some evidence that HBV genotype C is associated with a higher risk of cirrhosis and hepatocellular carcinoma than other genotypes. Antiviral treatment improves the prognosis in responders.

Chronic hepatitis C is an indolent, often subclinical disease that may lead to cirrhosis and hepatocellular carcinoma after decades. The overall mortality rate in patients with transfusion-associated hepatitis C may be no different from that of an age-matched control population. Nevertheless, mortality rates clearly rise once cirrhosis develops, and mortality from cirrhosis and hepatocellular carcinoma due to hepatitis C is clearly rising. There is some evidence that HCV genotype 1b is associated with a higher risk of hepatocellular carcinoma than other genotypes. Peginterferon plus ribavirin appears to have a beneficial effect on survival and quality of life, is cost-effective, appears to retard and even reverse fibrosis, and in responders may reduce the risk of hepatocellular carcinoma. The risk of mortality from drug addiction is higher than that for liver disease in patients with chronic hepatitis C.

▶ When to Refer

- For liver biopsy.
- For antiviral therapy.

▶ When to Admit

- Hepatic encephalopathy.
- INR > 1.6.

Andriulli A et al. Meta-analysis: the outcome of anti-viral therapy in HCV genotype 2 and genotype 3 infected patients with chronic hepatitis. Aliment Ther Pharm. 2008 Aug 15;28(4):397–404. [PMID: 18549461]

Di Bisceglie AM et al. Prolonged therapy of advanced chronic hepatitis C with low-dose peginterferon. N Engl J Med. 2008 Dec 4;359(23):2429–41. [PMID: 19052125]

Dienstag JL. Hepatitis B virus infection. N Engl J Med. 2008 Oct 2;359(14):1486–500. [PMID: 18832247]

Dusheiko G et al. Current treatment of hepatitis B. Gut. 2008 Jan;57(1):105–24. [PMID: 17502343]

European Association for the Study of the Liver. EASL Clinical Practice Guidelines: Management of chronic hepatitis B. J Hepatol. 2009 Feb;50(2):227–42. [PMID: 19054588]

Fattovich G et al. Natural history of chronic hepatitis B: special emphasis on disease progression and prognostic factors. J Hepatol. 2008 Feb;48(2):335–52. [PMID: 18096267]

Ferenci P et al; Austrian Hepatitis Study Group. Peginterferon alfa-2a and ribavirin for 24 weeks in hepatitis C type 1 and 4 patients with rapid virological response. Gastroenterology. 2008 Aug;135(2):451–8. [PMID: 18503773]

Keeffe EB et al. A treatment algorithm for the management of chronic hepatitis B virus infection in the United States: 2008 update. Clin Gastroenterol Hepatol. 2008 Dec;6(12):1315–41. [PMID: 18845489]

Loomba R et al. Systematic review: the effect of preventive lamivudine on hepatitis B reactivation during chemotherapy. Ann Intern Med. 2008 Apr 1;148(7):519–28. [PMID: 18378948]

Mallat A et al. Environmental factors as disease accelerators during chronic hepatitis C. J Hepatol. 2008 Apr;48(4):657–65. [PMID: 18279998]

Marcellin P et al. Tenofovir disoproxil fumarate versus adefovir dipivoxil for chronic hepatitis B. N Engl J Med. 2008 Dec 4;359(23):2442–55. [PMID: 19052126]

Okoh EJ et al. HCV in patients with end-stage renal disease. Am J Gastroenterol. 2008 Aug;103(8):2123–34. [PMID: 18796105]

Pawlotsky JM et al. Virologic monitoring of hepatitis B virus therapy in clinical trials and practice: recommendations for a standardized approach. Gastroenterology. 2008 Feb;134(2):405–15. [PMID: 18242209]

Sorrell MF et al. National Institutes of Health Consensus Development Conference Statement: Management of Hepatitis B. Ann Intern Med. 2009 Jan 20;150(2):104–110. [PMID: 19124811]

Sulkowski MS. Viral hepatitis and HIV coinfection. J Hepatol. 2008 Feb;48(2):353–67. [PMID: 18155314]

Weinbaum CM et al; Centers for Disease Control and Prevention (CDC). Recommendations for identification and public health management of persons with chronic hepatitis B virus infection. MMWR Recomm Rep. 2008 Sep 19;57(RR-8):1–20. [PMID: 18802412]

Wise M et al. Changing trends in hepatitis C-related mortality in the United States, 1995–2004. Hepatology. 2008 Apr;47(4):1128–35. [PMID: 18318441]

Zeuzem S. Interferon-based therapy for chronic hepatitis C: current and future perspectives. Nat Clin Pract Gastroenterol Hepatol. 2008 Nov;5(11):610–22. [PMID: 18838975]

AUTOIMMUNE HEPATITIS

 ESSENTIALS OF DIAGNOSIS

- ▶ Usually young to middle-aged women.
- ▶ Chronic hepatitis with high serum globulins.
- ▶ Positive antinuclear antibody (ANA) and/or smooth muscle antibody in most common type.
- ▶ Responds to corticosteroids.

▶ Clinical Findings

A. Symptoms and Signs

Although autoimmune hepatitis is usually seen in young women, it can occur in either sex at any age. Affected younger persons are often positive for HLA-B8 and HLA-DR3; older patients are often positive for HLA-DR4. The principal susceptibility allele among white Americans and northern Europeans is HLA *DRB1*0301*; HLA *DRB1*0401* is a secondary but independent risk factor. The onset is usually insidious, but up to 40% present with an acute (occasionally fulminant) attack of hepatitis and some cases follow a viral illness such as hepatitis A, Epstein-Barr infection, or measles or exposure to a drug or toxin such as nitrofurantoin. Exacerbations may occur postpartum. Thirty-four percent of patients are asymptomatic. Typically, examination reveals a healthy-appearing young woman with multiple spider nevi, cutaneous striae, acne, hirsutism, and hepatomegaly. Amenorrhea may be a presenting feature. Extrahepatic features include arthritis, Sjögren syndrome, thyroiditis, nephritis, ulcerative colitis, and Coombs-positive hemolytic anemia. Patients with autoimmune hepatitis are at increased risk for cirrhosis which, in turn, increases the risk of hepatocellular carcinoma (at a rate of about 1% per year).

B. Diagnostic Tests

Serum aminotransferase levels may be > 1000 units/L, and the total bilirubin is usually increased. In type I (classic) autoimmune hepatitis, ANA or smooth muscle antibody (either or both) is detected in serum. Serum γ-globulin levels are typically elevated (up to 5-6 g/dL). In patients with the latter, the EIA for antibody to HCV may be falsely positive. Other antibodies, including atypical perinuclear antineutrophil cytoplasmic antibodies (ANCA) and antibodies to histones, may be found. Antibodies to soluble liver antigen–liver pancreas (anti-SLA/LP) characterize a variant of type I that is marked by severe disease, a high relapse rate after treatment, and absence of the usual antibodies (ANA and smooth muscle antibody). Anti-SLA/LP is directed against a transfer RNA complex responsible for incorporating selenocysteine into peptide chains (Sep tRNA:Sec tRNA synthase). Type II, seen more often in girls under age 14 in Europe, is characterized by circulating antibody to liver-kidney microsomes (anti-LKM1)—directed against cytochrome P450 2D6—without anti-smooth muscle antibody or ANA. In some cases, anti-liver cytosol type 1, directed against formiminotransferase cyclodeaminase, is detected. This type of autoimmune hepatitis can be seen in patients with autoimmune polyglandular syndrome type 1. Concurrent primary biliary cirrhosis or primary sclerosing cholangitis has been recognized in 11% and 5% of patients with autoimmune hepatitis, respectively. Liver biopsy is indicated to help establish the diagnosis, evaluate disease severity, and determine the need for treatment.

Simplified diagnostic criteria based on the detection of autoantibodies (1 or 2 points depending on titers), elevated IgG levels (1 or 2 points depending on levels), and characteristic histologic features (1 or 2 points depending on how typical the features are) and exclusion of viral hepatitis (2 points) can be useful for diagnosis; a score of 6 indicates probable and a score of 7 indicates definite autoimmune hepatitis.

▶ Treatment

Prednisone with or without azathioprine improves symptoms; decreases the serum bilirubin, aminotransferase, and γ-globulin levels; and reduces hepatic inflammation. Symptomatic patients with aminotransferase levels elevated tenfold (or fivefold if the serum globulins are elevated at least twofold) are optimal candidates for therapy, and asymptomatic patients with modest enzyme elevations may be considered for therapy depending on the clinical circumstances and histologic severity; however, asymptomatic patients usually remain asymptomatic, have either mild hepatitis or inactive cirrhosis on liver biopsy specimens, and have a good long-term prognosis without therapy.

Prednisone is given initially in a dose of 30 mg orally daily with azathioprine, 50 mg orally daily, which is generally well tolerated and permits the use of lower corticosteroid doses than a regimen beginning with prednisone 60 mg orally daily alone. Whether patients should undergo testing for the genotype or level of thiopurine methyltransferase prior to treatment with azathioprine to predict toxicity is still a matter of debate. Blood counts are monitored weekly for the first 2 months of therapy and monthly thereafter because of the small risk of bone marrow suppression. The dose of prednisone is lowered from 30 mg/d after 1 week to

20 mg/d and again after 2 or 3 weeks to 15 mg/d. Ultimately, a maintenance dose of 10 mg/d is achieved. While symptomatic improvement is often prompt, biochemical improvement is more gradual, with normalization of serum aminotransferase levels after several months in many cases. Histologic resolution of inflammation may require 18–24 months, the time at which repeat liver biopsy is recommended. Failure of aminotransferase levels to normalize invariably predicts lack of histologic resolution.

The response rate to therapy with prednisone and azathioprine is 80%. Older patients (and those with HLA genotype *DRB1*04*) are more likely to respond than younger patients and those with HLA *DRB1*03* or hyperbilirubinemia. Fibrosis may reverse with therapy and rarely progresses after apparent biochemical and histologic remission. Once remission is achieved, therapy may be withdrawn, but the subsequent relapse rate is 20–90%. Relapses may again be treated in the same manner as the initial episode, with the same remission rate. After successful treatment of a relapse, the patient may continue taking azathioprine (up to 2 mg/kg) indefinitely or the lowest dose of prednisone needed to maintain aminotransferase levels as close to normal as possible—although another attempt at withdrawing therapy may be considered in patients remaining in remission long term (eg, ≥ 4 years). Budesonide, a corticosteroid with less toxicity than prednisone, does not appear to be effective in maintaining remission. Prednisone can be used to treat rare flares during pregnancy, and maintenance azathioprine does not have to be discontinued.

Nonresponders to prednisone and azathioprine (failure of serum aminotransferase levels to decrease by 50% after 6 months) may be considered for a trial of cyclosporine, tacrolimus, methotrexate, or rituximab. Mycophenolate mofetil is an effective alternative to azathioprine in patients who cannot tolerate or do not respond to it. Bone density should be monitored—particularly in patients receiving maintenance corticosteroid therapy—and measures undertaken to prevent or treat osteoporosis (see Chapter 26). Liver transplantation may be required for treatment failures and patients with a fulminant presentation, but the disease has been recognized to recur in up to 40% of transplanted livers (and rarely to develop de novo) as immunosuppression is reduced; sirolimus can be effective in such cases.

▶ When to Refer

- For liver biopsy.
- For immunosuppressive therapy.

▶ When to Admit

- Hepatic encephalopathy.
- INR > 1.6.

Czaja AJ. Genetic factors affecting the occurrence, clinical phenotype, and outcome of autoimmune hepatitis. Clin Gastroenterol Hepatol. 2008 Apr;6(4):379–88. [PMID: 18328791]

Hennes EM et al; International Autoimmune Hepatitis Group. Simplified criteria for the diagnosis of autoimmune hepatitis. Hepatology. 2008 Jul;48(1):169–76. [PMID: 18537184]

Yeoman AD et al. Evaluation of risk factors in the development of hepatocellular carcinoma in autoimmune hepatitis: implications for follow-up and screening. Hepatology. 2008 Sep;48(3):863–70. [PMID: 18752332]

ALCOHOLIC LIVER DISEASE

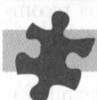 ESSENTIALS OF DIAGNOSIS

► Chronic alcohol intake usually exceeds 80 g/d in men and 30–40 g/d in women with alcoholic hepatitis or cirrhosis.

► Fatty liver is often asymptomatic.

► Fever, right upper quadrant pain, tender hepatomegaly, and jaundice characterize alcoholic hepatitis, but the patient may be asymptomatic.

► AST is usually elevated but rarely above 300 units/L; AST is greater than ALT, usually by a factor of 2 or more.

► Alcoholic hepatitis is often reversible but it is the most common precursor of cirrhosis in the United States.

► General Considerations

Excessive alcohol intake can lead to fatty liver, hepatitis, and cirrhosis. Alcoholic hepatitis is characterized by acute or chronic inflammation and parenchymal necrosis of the liver induced by alcohol. Alcoholic hepatitis is often a reversible disease, is the most common precursor of cirrhosis in the United States, and is associated with four to five times the number of hospitalizations and deaths as hepatitis C, which is the second most common cause of cirrhosis.

The frequency of alcoholic cirrhosis is estimated to be 10–15% among persons who consume over 50 g of alcohol (4 oz of 100-proof whiskey, 15 oz of wine, or four 12-oz cans of beer) daily for over 10 years (although the risk of cirrhosis may be lower for wine than for a comparable intake of beer or spirits). The risk of cirrhosis is lower (5%) in the absence of other cofactors such as chronic viral hepatitis and obesity. Genetic factors, including polymorphisms of the genes encoding for tumor necrosis factor-α and cytochrome P450 2E1, may also account for differences in susceptibility. Women appear to be more susceptible than men, in part because of lower gastric mucosal alcohol dehydrogenase levels. Over 80% of patients with alcoholic hepatitis have been drinking 5 years or more before symptoms that can be attributed to liver disease develop; the longer the duration of drinking (10–15 or more years) and the larger the alcoholic consumption, the greater the probability of developing alcoholic hepatitis and cirrhosis. In individuals who drink alcohol excessively, the rate of ethanol metabolism can be sufficiently high to permit the consumption of large quantities without raising the blood alcohol level over 80 mg/dL.

Deficiencies in vitamins and calories probably contribute to the development of alcoholic hepatitis or its progression to cirrhosis. Many adverse effects of alcohol on the liver are thought to be mediated by tumor necrosis factor-α and by the oxidative metabolite acetaldehyde, which contributes to lipid peroxidation and induction of an immune response following covalent binding to proteins in the liver.

► Clinical Findings

A. Symptoms and Signs

The clinical presentation of alcoholic liver disease can vary from an asymptomatic hepatomegaly to a rapidly fatal acute illness or end-stage cirrhosis. A recent period of heavy drinking, complaints of anorexia and nausea, and the demonstration of hepatomegaly and jaundice strongly suggest the diagnosis. Abdominal pain and tenderness, splenomegaly, ascites, fever, and encephalopathy may be present.

B. Laboratory Findings

In patients with steatosis, mild liver enzyme elevations may be the only laboratory abnormality. Anemia (usually macrocytic) may be present. Leukocytosis with shift to the left is common in patients with severe alcoholic hepatitis. Leukopenia is occasionally seen and resolves after cessation of drinking. About 10% of patients have thrombocytopenia related to a direct toxic effect of alcohol on megakaryocyte production or to hypersplenism.

AST is usually elevated but rarely above 300 units/L. AST is greater than ALT, usually by a factor of 2 or more. Serum alkaline phosphatase is generally elevated, but seldom more than three times the normal value. Serum bilirubin is increased in 60–90% of patients with alcoholic hepatitis.

Serum bilirubin levels greater than 10 mg/dL and marked prolongation of the prothrombin time (≥ 6 seconds above control) indicate severe alcoholic hepatitis with a mortality rate as high as 50%. The serum albumin is depressed, and the γ-globulin level is elevated in 50–75% of individuals, even in the absence of cirrhosis. Increased transferrin saturation, hepatic iron stores, and sideroblastic anemia are found in many alcoholic patients. Folic acid deficiency may coexist.

C. Liver Biopsy

Liver biopsy, if done, demonstrates macrovesicular fat and, in patients with alcoholic hepatitis, polymorphonuclear infiltration with hepatic necrosis, Mallory bodies (alcoholic hyaline), and perivenular and perisinusoidal fibrosis. Micronodular cirrhosis may be present as well. The findings are identical to those of nonalcoholic steatohepatitis.

D. Other Studies

Imaging studies are used to exclude other diagnoses; they can detect moderate to severe hepatic steatosis reliably but not inflammation or fibrosis. Ultrasound helps exclude biliary obstruction and identifies subclinical ascites. CT scanning with intravenous contrast or MRI may be indicated in selected cases to evaluate patients for collateral vessels, space-occupying lesions of the liver, or concomitant disease of the pancreas.

Differential Diagnosis

Alcoholic hepatitis may be closely mimicked by cholecystitis and cholelithiasis and by drug toxicity. Other causes of hepatitis or chronic liver disease may be excluded by serologic or biochemical testing, by imaging studies, or by liver biopsy. A formula based on the AST/ALT ratio, body mass index, mean corpuscular volume, and gender has been reported to reliably distinguish alcoholic liver disease from nonalcoholic fatty liver disease (NAFLD).

Treatment

A. General Measures

Abstinence from alcohol is essential. Fatty liver is quickly reversible with abstinence. Every effort should be made to provide sufficient amounts of carbohydrates and calories in anorectic patients to reduce endogenous protein catabolism, promote gluconeogenesis, and prevent hypoglycemia. Nutritional support (40 kcal/kg with 1.5–2 g/kg as protein) improves survival in patients with malnutrition. Use of liquid formulas rich in branched-chain amino acids does not improve survival beyond that achieved with less expensive caloric supplementation. The administration of vitamins, particularly folic acid and thiamine, is indicated, especially when deficiencies are noted; glucose administration increases the vitamin B_1 requirement and can precipitate Wernicke–Korsakoff syndrome if thiamine is not coadministered.

B. Pharmacologic Measures

Methylprednisolone, 32 mg/d orally or the equivalent for 1 month, may reduce short-term mortality in patients with alcoholic hepatitis and either encephalopathy or a discriminant function (defined by the patient's prothrombin time minus the control prothrombin time times 4.6 plus the total bilirubin in mg/dL is > 32). Failure of the serum bilirubin level to decline after 7 days of treatment predicts nonresponse and poor long-term survival, as does a model that includes age, advanced chronic kidney disease, serum albumin, prothrombin time, serum bilirubin on admission, and serum bilirubin on day 7. No benefit has been demonstrated in patients with concomitant gastrointestinal bleeding.

Pentoxifylline—an inhibitor of tumor necrosis factor—400 mg orally three times daily for 4 weeks, may reduce 1-month mortality rates in patients with severe alcoholic hepatitis, primarily by decreasing the risk of hepatorenal syndrome. Other experimental therapies include propylthiouracil, oxandrolone, S-adenosyl-L-methionine, infliximab, antioxidants, and extracorporeal liver support. Colchicine does not reduce mortality in patients with alcoholic cirrhosis, and etanercept may increase mortality after 6 months.

Prognosis

A. Short-Term

When the prothrombin time is short enough to permit liver biopsy (< 3 seconds above control), the 1-year mortality rate is 7%, rising to 20% if there is progressive prolongation of the prothrombin time during hospitalization. Individuals in whom the prothrombin time prohibits liver biopsy have a 42% mortality rate at 1 year. Other unfavorable prognostic factors are a serum bilirubin greater than 10 mg/dL, hepatic encephalopathy, azotemia, leukocytosis, lack of response to corticosteroid therapy, and possibly little steatosis on a liver biopsy specimen and reversal of portal blood flow by Doppler ultrasound. In addition to the discriminant function discussed above, the MELD score used for cirrhosis (see later) and the Glasgow alcoholic hepatitis score (based on age, white blood cell count, blood urea nitrogen, prothrombin time ratio, and bilirubin level) correlate with mortality from alcoholic hepatitis and have higher specificities. A scoring system based on age, serum bilirubin, INR, and serum creatinine (ABIC) has been proposed.

B. Long-Term

In the United States, the 3-year mortality rate of persons who recover from acute alcoholic hepatitis is ten times greater than that of control individuals of comparable age. Histologically severe disease is associated with continued excessive mortality rates after 3 years, whereas the death rate is not increased after the same period in those whose liver biopsies show only mild alcoholic hepatitis. Complications of portal hypertension (ascites, variceal bleeding, hepatorenal syndrome), coagulopathy, and severe jaundice following recovery from acute alcoholic hepatitis also suggest a poor long-term prognosis. Alcoholic cirrhosis is a risk factor for hepatocellular carcinoma, and the risk is highest in carriers of the C282Y mutation for hemochromatosis or with increased hepatic iron.

The most important prognostic consideration is continued excessive drinking. A 6-month period of abstinence is generally required before liver transplantation is considered, although this requirement has been questioned. Optimal candidates have adequate social support, do not smoke, have no psychosis or personality disorder, are adherent to therapy, and have regular appointments with a psychiatrist or psychologist who specializes in addiction treatment.

When to Refer

Refer patients with alcoholic hepatitis who require liver biopsy for diagnosis.

When to Admit

- Hepatic encephalopathy.
- INR > 1.6.
- Total bilirubin ≥ 10 mg/dL.
- Inability to maintain hydration.

Barve A et al. Treatment of alcoholic liver disease. Ann Hepatol. 2008 Jan–Mar;7(1):5–15. [PMID: 18376362]

Dominguez M et al. A new scoring system for prognostic stratification of patients with alcoholic hepatitis. Am J Gastroenterol. 2008 Nov;103(11):2747–56. [PMID: 18721242]

Kotlyar DS et al. A critical review of candidacy for orthotopic liver transplantation in alcoholic liver disease. Am J Gastroenterol. 2008 Mar;103(3):734–43. [PMID: 18081918]

Louvet et al. Early switch to pentoxifylline in patients with severe alcoholic hepatitis is inefficient in non-responders to corticosteroids. J Hepatol. 2008 Mar;48(3):465–70. [PMID: 18164508]

Rambaldi A et al. Systematic review: glucocorticosteroids for alcoholic hepatitis—a Cochrane Hepato-Biliary Group systematic review with meta-analyses and trial sequential analyses of randomized clinical trials. Aliment Pharmacol Ther. 2008 Jun;27(12):1167–78. [PMID: 18363896]

Yang AL et al. Epidemiology of alcohol-related liver and pancreatic disease in the United States. Arch Intern Med. 2008 Mar 24;168(6):649–56. [PMID: 18362258]

DRUG- & TOXIN-INDUCED LIVER DISEASE

 ESSENTIALS OF DIAGNOSIS

▸ Drug-induced liver disease can mimic viral hepatitis, biliary tract obstruction, or other types of liver disease.

▸ Clinicians must inquire about the use of many widely used therapeutic agents, including over-the-counter "natural" and "herbal" products, in any patient with liver disease.

▶ General Considerations

Many therapeutic agents may cause hepatic injury. The medications most commonly implicated are nonsteroidal anti-inflammatory drugs and antibiotics because of their widespread use. Drug-induced liver disease can mimic viral hepatitis, biliary tract obstruction, or other types of liver disease. In any patient with liver disease, the clinician must inquire carefully about the use of potentially hepatotoxic drugs or exposure to hepatotoxins, including over-the-counter "natural" and herbal products. In some cases, coadministration of a second agent may increase the toxicity of the first (eg, isoniazid and rifampin, acetaminophen and alcohol). Drug toxicity may be categorized on the basis of pathogenesis or histologic appearance.

1. Direct Hepatotoxic Group

The liver lesion caused by this group of drugs is characterized by: (1) dose-related severity, (2) a latent period following exposure, and (3) susceptibility in all individuals. Examples include acetaminophen (toxicity is enhanced by fasting and chronic alcohol use because of depletion of glutathione and induction of cytochrome P450 2E1), alcohol, carbon tetrachloride, chloroform, heavy metals, mercaptopurine, niacin, plant alkaloids, phosphorus, pyrazinamide, tetracyclines, tipranavir, valproic acid, and vitamin A. Statins, like all cholesterol-lowering agents, may cause serum aminotransferase elevations but rarely cause true hepatitis and are no longer considered contraindicated in patients with liver disease.

2. Idiosyncratic Reactions

Except for acetaminophen, most severe hepatotoxicity is idiosyncratic. Reactions of this type are: (1) sporadic, (2) not related to dose, and (3) occasionally associated with features suggesting an allergic reaction, such as fever and eosinophilia, which may be associated with a favorable outcome. In some patients, toxicity results directly from a metabolite that is produced only in certain individuals on a genetic basis. Toxicity may be observed only on postmarketing surveillance and not during preclinical trials. Examples include abacavir, amiodarone, aspirin, carbamazepine, chloramphenicol, diclofenac, disulfiram, duloxetine, ezetimibe, flutamide, halothane, isoniazid, ketoconazole, lamotrigine, methyldopa, nevirapine, oxacillin, phenytoin, pyrazinamide, quinidine, streptomycin, rofecoxib and troglitazone (both withdrawn from the market in the United States), and less commonly other thiazolidinediones, and perhaps tacrine.

3. Cholestatic Reactions

A. Noninflammatory

Drug-induced cholestasis results from inhibition or genetic deficiency of various hepatobiliary transporter systems. The following drugs cause cholestasis: anabolic steroids containing an alkyl or ethinyl group at carbon 17, azathioprine, diclofenac, indinavir (increased risk of indirect hyperbilirubinemia in patients with Gilbert syndrome), cyclosporine, estrogens, mercaptopurine, methyltestosterone, and ticlopidine.

B. Inflammatory

The following drugs cause inflammation of portal areas with bile duct injury (cholangitis), often with allergic features such as eosinophilia: amoxicillin-clavulanic acid (among most common causes of drug-induced liver injury), azathioprine, azithromycin, captopril, cephalosporins, chlorothiazide, chlorpromazine, chlorpropamide, erythromycin, mercaptopurine, penicillamine, prochlorperazine, semisynthetic penicillins (eg, cloxacillin), and sulfadiazine. Cholestatic and mixed cholestatic hepatocellular toxicity is more likely than pure hepatocellular toxicity to lead to chronic liver disease.

4. Acute or Chronic Hepatitis

Medications that may result in acute or chronic hepatitis that is histologically—and in some cases clinically—indistinguishable from autoimmune hepatitis include aspirin, isoniazid (increased risk in HBV and HCV carriers), methyldopa, minocycline, nitrofurantoin, nonsteroidal anti-inflammatory drugs, propylthiouracil, and terbinafine. Hepatitis also can occur in patients taking cocaine, diclofenac, methylenedioxymethamphetamine (MDMA; Ecstasy), efavirenz, imatinib mesylate, nevirapine (like other protease inhibitors, increased risk in HBV and HCV carriers), ritonavir (greater rate than other protease inhibitors), saquinavir, sulfonamides, telithromycin, troglitazone (withdrawn from the market in the United States), and zafirlukast as well as a variety of alternative remedies (eg, black cohosh, chaparral, germander, green tea extracts, Herbalife products, jin bu huan, kava, skullcap). In patients with jaundice due to drug-induced hepatitis, the mortality rate without liver transplantation is at least 10%.

5. Other Reactions

A. Fatty Liver

1. Macrovesicular—This type of liver injury may be produced by alcohol, amiodarone, corticosteroids, methotrexate, irinotecan, tamoxifen, zalcitabine, and possibly oxaliplatin.

2. Microvesicular—Often resulting from mitochondrial injury, this condition is associated with didanosine, stavudine, tetracyclines, valproic acid, and zidovudine.

B. Granulomas

Allopurinol, quinidine, quinine, phenylbutazone, and phenytoin can lead to granulomas.

C. Fibrosis and Cirrhosis

Methotrexate and vitamin A are associated with fibrosis and cirrhosis.

D. Sinusoidal Obstruction Syndrome (Veno-occlusive Disease)

This disorder may result from treatment with antineoplastic agents (eg, pre-bone marrow transplant, oxaliplatin), and pyrrolizidine alkaloids (eg, Comfrey).

E. Peliosis Hepatis (Blood-Filled Cavities)

Peliosis hepatis may be caused by anabolic steroids and oral contraceptive steroids as well as azathioprine and mercaptopurine, which may also cause nodular regenerative hyperplasia.

F. Neoplasms

Neoplasms may result from therapy with oral contraceptive steroids, including estrogens (hepatic adenoma but not focal nodular hyperplasia); and vinyl chloride (angiosarcoma).

▶ When to Refer

Refer patients with drug- and toxin-induced hepatitis who require liver biopsy for diagnosis.

▶ When to Admit

Patients with liver failure should be hospitalized.

Argo CK et al. Statins in liver disease: a molehill, an iceberg, or neither? Hepatology. 2008 Aug;48(2):662–9. [PMID: 18666246]

Chalasani N et al; Drug Induced Liver Injury Network (DILIN). Causes, clinical features, and outcomes from a prospective study of drug-induced liver injury in the United States. Gastroenterology. 2008 Dec;135(6):1924–34. [PMID: 18955056]

Chitturi S et al. Hepatotoxic slimming aids and other herbal hepatotoxins. J Gastroenterol Hepatol. 2008 Mar;23(3):366–73. [PMID: 18318821]

Gupta NK et al. Review article: the use of potentially hepatotoxic drugs in patients with liver disease. Aliment Pharmacol Ther. 2008 Nov 1;28(9):1021–41. [PMID: 18671777]

Fontana RJ. Acute liver failure due to drugs. Semin Liver Dis. 2008 May;28(2):175–87. [PMID: 18452117]

Inductivo-Yu I et al. Highly active antiretroviral therapy-induced liver injury. Curr Drug Saf. 2008 Jan;3(1):4–13. [PMID: 18690975]

Lee WM (guest ed). Drug-induced liver disease. Clin Liver Dis. 2007 Aug;11(3):459–683.

NONALCOHOLIC FATTY LIVER DISEASE

 ESSENTIALS OF DIAGNOSIS

▶ Often asymptomatic.

▶ Elevated aminotransferase levels and/or hepatomegaly.

▶ Macrovesicular and/or microvesicular steatosis with or without inflammation and fibrosis on liver biopsy.

▶ General Considerations

Nonalcoholic fatty liver disease (NAFLD) is estimated to affect 20–30% of the US population. Causes of NAFLD are obesity (present in ≥ 40%), diabetes mellitus (in ≥ 20%), hypertriglyceridemia (in ≥ 20%), corticosteroids, amiodarone, diltiazem, tamoxifen, irinotecan, oxaliplatin, highly active antiretroviral therapy, poisons (carbon tetrachloride and yellow phosphorus), endocrinopathies such as Cushing syndrome and hypopituitarism, polycystic ovary syndrome, hypobetalipoproteinemia and other metabolic disorders, obstructive sleep apnea, starvation and refeeding syndrome, and total parenteral nutrition. Steatosis is nearly universal in obese alcoholic patients and is a hallmark of insulin resistance (metabolic syndrome), which is characterized by obesity, diabetes, hypertriglyceridemia, and hypertension. The risk of fatty liver in persons with metabolic syndrome is 4 to 11 times higher than that of persons without insulin resistance. Physical activity protects against the development of NAFLD. In addition to macrovesicular steatosis, histologic features may include focal infiltration by polymorphonuclear neutrophils and Mallory hyalin, a picture indistinguishable from that of alcoholic hepatitis and referred to as nonalcoholic steatohepatitis (NASH), which affects 3–5% of the US population. In patients with NAFLD, older age, obesity, and diabetes are risk factors for advanced hepatic fibrosis and cirrhosis. Cirrhosis caused by NASH appears to be uncommon in African Americans.

Microvesicular steatosis is seen with Reye syndrome, valproic acid toxicity, high-dose tetracycline, or acute fatty liver of pregnancy and may result in fulminant hepatic failure. Women in whom fatty liver of pregnancy develops often have a defect in fatty acid oxidation due to reduced long-chain 3-hydroxyacyl-CoA dehydrogenase activity.

▶ Clinical Findings

A. Symptoms and Signs

Most patients with NAFLD are asymptomatic or have mild right upper quadrant discomfort. Hepatomegaly is present in up to 75% of patients, but the stigmas of chronic liver disease are uncommon. Rare instances of subacute liver failure caused by previously unrecognized NASH have been described.

B. Laboratory Findings

Laboratory studies may show mildly elevated aminotransferase and alkaline phosphatase levels; however, laboratory values may be normal in up to 80% of persons with hepatic steatosis. In contrast to alcoholic liver disease, the ratio of ALT to AST is almost always greater than 1 in NAFLD, but it decreases to less than 1 as advanced fibrosis and cirrhosis develop. Antinuclear or smooth muscle antibodies and an elevated serum ferritin level may each be detected in one-fourth of patients with NASH.

C. Imaging

Macrovascular steatosis may be demonstrated on ultrasound, CT, or MRI. However, imaging does not distinguish steatosis from steatohepatitis.

D. Liver Biopsy

Percutaneous liver biopsy is diagnostic and is the standard approach to assessing the degree of inflammation and fibrosis. The risks of the procedure must be balanced against the impact of the added information on management decisions and assessment of prognosis. The histologic spectrum includes fatty liver, isolated portal fibrosis, steatohepatitis, and cirrhosis. A risk score for predicting advanced fibrosis, known as BARD for the first letter of the terms defining it, is based on body mass index > 28, AST/ALT ratio ≥ 0.8, and diabetes mellitus; it has a 96% negative predictive value (ie, a low score reliably excludes advanced fibrosis). Another risk score for advanced fibrosis based on age, hyperglycemia, body mass index, platelet count, albumin, and AST/ALT ratio has a positive predictive value of over 80%. A clinical scoring system to predict the likelihood of NASH in morbidly obese persons includes six predictive factors: hypertension, type 2 diabetes mellitus, sleep apnea, AST > 27 units/L, ALT > 27 units/L, and non-black race.

▶ Treatment

Treatment consists of removing or modifying the offending factors. Weight loss, dietary fat restriction, and exercise (through reduction of abdominal obesity) often lead to improvement in liver tests and steatosis in obese patients with NAFLD. Various drugs are under study. Thiazolidinediones reverse insulin resistance and improve both serum aminotransferase levels and histologic features of steatohepatitis but lead to weight gain. Vitamin E (to reduce oxidative stress) is of uncertain benefit. Betaine (a methyl donor) may have some benefit and is under study. Metformin, which reduces insulin resistance, improves abnormal liver chemistries but may not reliably improve liver histology. Pentoxifylline, which inhibits tumor necrosis factor-α, improves liver biochemical test levels but is associated with a high rate of side effects, particularly nausea. Ursodeoxycholic acid, 12–15 mg/kg/d, has not consistently

resulted in biochemical and histologic improvement in patients with NASH but may be effective when given in combination with vitamin E. Hepatic steatosis due to total parenteral nutrition may be ameliorated—and perhaps prevented—with supplemental choline. Other agents under study include orlistat, an inhibitor of gastrointestinal lipases; recombinant human leptin; glucagon-like protein-1-receptor agonists, which promote insulin secretion; rimonobant, a selective inhibitor of cannabinoid type 1 receptors that decreases hepatic lipogenesis and increases satiety; and losartan, an angiotensin antagonist. Statins are not contraindicated in persons with NAFLD. Gastric bypass may be considered in patients with a body mass index > 35.

▶ Prognosis

Fatty liver often has a benign course and is readily reversible with discontinuation of alcohol (or no more than one glass of wine per day) or treatment of other underlying conditions; if untreated, cirrhosis develops in 1-3% of patients. In patients with NAFLD, the likelihood of NASH is increased by the following factors: obesity, older age, non–African American ethnicity, female sex, diabetes, hypertension, higher AST level, higher AST/ALT ratio, and low platelet count. NASH may be associated with hepatic fibrosis in 40% of cases; cirrhosis develops in 9–25%; and decompensated cirrhosis occurs in 30–50% of cirrhotic patients over 10 years. The course may be more aggressive in diabetic persons than in nondiabetic persons. Mortality is increased in patients with NAFLD and is more likely to be the result of malignancy and ischemic heart disease than liver disease. Risk factors for mortality are older age, male gender, white race, higher body mass index, hypertension, diabetes, and cirrhosis. Steatosis is a cofactor for the progression of fibrosis in patients with other causes of chronic liver disease, such as hepatitis C. Hepatocellular carcinoma is a complication of cirrhosis caused by NASH as it is for other causes of cirrhosis. NASH accounts for a substantial percentage of cases labeled as cryptogenic cirrhosis and can recur following liver transplantation. Central obesity is an independent risk factor for death from cirrhosis of any cause.

▶ When to Refer

Refer patients with non-alcoholic fatty liver disease who require liver biopsy for diagnosis.

Aithal GP et al. Randomized, placebo-controlled trial of pioglitazone in nondiabetic subjects with nonalcoholic steatohepatitis. Gastroenterology. 2008 Oct;135(4):1176–84. [PMID: 18718471]

Campos GM et al. A clinical scoring system for predicting nonalcoholic steatohepatitis in morbidly obese patients. Hepatology. 2008 Jun;47(6):1916–23. [PMID: 18433022]

Harrison SA et al. Development and validation of a simple NAFLD clinical scoring system for identifying patients without advanced disease. Gut. 2008 Oct;57(10):1441–7. [PMID: 18390575]

Harrison SA et al. Orlistat for overweight subjects with nonalcoholic steatohepatitis: a randomized, prospective trial. Hepatology. 2009 Jan;49(1):80–6. [PMID: 19053049]

Oh MK et al. Review article: diagnosis and treatment of nonalcoholic fatty liver disease. Aliment Pharmacol Ther. 2008 Sep 1;28(5):503–22. [PMID: 18532991]

Ong JP et al. Increased overall mortality and liver-related mortality in non-alcoholic fatty liver disease. J Hepatol. 2008 Oct;49(4):608–12. [PMID: 18682312]

Ratziu V et al. Rosiglitazone for nonalcoholic steatohepatitis: one-year results of the randomized placebo-controlled Fatty Liver Improvement with Rosiglitazone Therapy (FLIRT) Trial. Gastroenterology. 2008 Jul;135(1):100–10. [PMID: 18503774]

Sanyal AJ. Fatty liver disease. Semin Liver Dis. 2008 Nov;28(4):337–439. [PMID: 18956289]

Torres DM et al. Diagnosis and therapy of nonalcoholic steatohepatitis. Gastroenterology. 2008 May;134(6):1682–98. [PMID: 18471547]

Younossi ZM. Review article: current management of non-alcoholic fatty liver disease and non-alcoholic steatohepatitis. Aliment Pharmacol Ther. 2008 Jul;28(1):2–12. [PMID: 18410557]

CIRRHOSIS

ESSENTIALS OF DIAGNOSIS

▶ End result of injury that leads to both fibrosis and nodular regeneration.

▶ May be reversible if cause is removed.

▶ The clinical features result from hepatic cell dysfunction, portosystemic shunting, and portal hypertension.

General Considerations

Cirrhosis, the twelfth leading cause of death in the United States, is the end result of hepatocellular injury that leads to both fibrosis and nodular regeneration throughout the liver. Mexican Americans and African Americans have a higher frequency of cirrhosis than whites because of a higher rate of risk factors. Causes include chronic viral hepatitis, alcohol, drug toxicity, autoimmune and metabolic liver diseases, and miscellaneous disorders. Many patients have more than one risk factor (eg, chronic hepatitis and alcohol use). In patients at increased risk for liver injury (eg, heavy alcohol use, obesity, iron overload), higher coffee and tea consumption has been reported to reduce the risk of cirrhosis. Hospitalization rates for cirrhosis and portal hypertension are rising in the United States.

The most common histologic classification divides cirrhosis into micronodular, macronodular, and mixed forms. These are descriptive terms rather than separate diseases, and each form may be seen in the same patient at different stages of the disease. In micronodular cirrhosis—typical of alcoholic liver disease (Laennec cirrhosis)—the regenerating nodules are no larger than the original lobules, ie, approximately 1 mm in diameter or less. Macronodular cirrhosis is characterized by larger nodules, which can measure several centimeters in diameter and may contain central veins. This form corresponds more or less to postnecrotic (posthepatitic) cirrhosis but does not necessarily follow episodes of massive necrosis and stromal collapse.

▶ Clinical Findings

A. Symptoms and Signs

The clinical features of cirrhosis result from hepatic cell dysfunction, portosystemic shunting, and portal hypertension. Patients may have no symptoms for long periods. The onset of symptoms may be insidious or, less often, abrupt. Weakness, fatigability, disturbed sleep, muscle cramps, and weight loss are common. In advanced cirrhosis, anorexia is usually present and may be extreme, with associated nausea and occasional vomiting. Abdominal pain may be present and is related either to hepatic enlargement and stretching of Glisson capsule or to the presence of ascites. Menstrual abnormalities (usually amenorrhea), impotence, loss of libido, sterility, and gynecomastia in men may occur. Hematemesis is the presenting symptom in 15–25%.

Skin manifestations consist of spider angioma (invariably on the upper half of the body), palmar erythema (mottled redness of the thenar and hypothenar eminences), and Dupuytren contractures. Evidence of vitamin deficiencies (glossitis and cheilosis) is common. Weight loss, wasting, and the appearance of chronic illness are present. Jaundice—usually not an initial sign—is mild at first, increasing in severity during the later stages of the disease. In 70% of cases, the liver is enlarged, palpable, and firm if not hard and has a sharp or nodular edge; the left lobe may predominate. Splenomegaly is present in 35–50% of cases and is associated with an increased risk of complications of portal hypertension. The superficial veins of the abdomen and thorax are dilated, reflecting the intrahepatic obstruction to portal blood flow, as do rectal varices (hemorrhoids). The abdominal wall veins fill from below when compressed. Ascites, pleural effusions, peripheral edema, and ecchymoses are late findings. Encephalopathy characterized by day–night reversal, asterixis, tremor, dysarthria, delirium, drowsiness, and ultimately coma also occurs late except when precipitated by an acute hepatocellular insult or an episode of gastrointestinal bleeding. Fever may be a presenting symptom in up to 35% of patients and usually reflects associated alcoholic hepatitis, spontaneous bacterial peritonitis, or intercurrent infection.

B. Laboratory Findings

Laboratory abnormalities are either absent or minimal in early or compensated cirrhosis. Anemia, a frequent finding, is often macrocytic; causes include suppression of erythropoiesis by alcohol as well as folate deficiency, hemolysis, hypersplenism, and occult or overt blood loss from the gastrointestinal tract. The white blood cell count may be low, reflecting hypersplenism, or high, suggesting infection; thrombocytopenia is secondary to alcoholic marrow suppression, sepsis, folate deficiency, or splenic sequestration. Prolongation of the prothrombin time may result from reduced levels of clotting factors (except factor VIII). However, bleeding risk correlates poorly with results of conventional coagulation parameters because of concomitant abnormalities of fibrinolysis.

Blood chemistries reflect hepatocellular injury and dysfunction, manifested by modest elevations of AST and alkaline phosphatase and progressive elevation of the bilirubin. Serum albumin is low; γ-globulin is increased and may be as high as in autoimmune hepatitis. The risk of diabetes mellitus is increased in patients with cirrhosis, particularly when associated with HCV infection, alcoholism, hemochromatosis, and NAFLD. Vitamin D deficiency has been reported in as many as 91% of patients with cirrhosis. Patients with alcoholic cirrhosis may have elevated serum cardiac troponin I and brain natriuretic peptide levels. Blunted cardiac inotropic and chronotropic responses to exercise, stress, and drugs, as well as systolic and diastolic ventricular dysfunction ("cirrhotic cardiomyopathy") and prolongation of the QT interval in the setting of a hyperkinetic circulation, are common in cirrhosis of all causes, but overt heart failure is rare in the absence of alcoholism. Relative adrenal insufficiency appears to be common in patients with advanced cirrhosis, even in the absence of sepsis.

Liver biopsy may show inactive cirrhosis (fibrosis with regenerative nodules) with no specific features to suggest the underlying cause. Alternatively, there may be additional features of alcoholic liver disease, chronic hepatitis, NASH, or other specific causes of cirrhosis. Combinations of routine blood tests (eg, AST, platelet count), including a commercially available panel of five tests called FibroSure, and serum markers of hepatic fibrosis (eg, hyaluronic acid, amino-terminal propeptide of type III collagen, tissue inhibitor of matrix metalloproteinase 1) are potential alternatives to liver biopsy for the diagnosis or exclusion of cirrhosis. In persons with chronic hepatitis C, for example, a low FibroSure score reliably excludes advanced fibrosis, a high score reliably predicts advanced fibrosis, and intermediate scores are inconclusive.

C. Imaging

Ultrasound is helpful for assessing liver size and detecting ascites or hepatic nodules, including small hepatocellular carcinomas. Together with a Doppler study, it may establish patency of the splenic, portal, and hepatic veins. Hepatic nodules are characterized further by contrast-enhanced CT scan or MRI. Nodules suspicious for malignancy may be biopsied under ultrasound or CT guidance.

D. Special Examinations

Esophagogastroduodenoscopy confirms the presence of varices and detects specific causes of bleeding in the esophagus, stomach, and proximal duodenum. Liver biopsy may be performed by laparoscopy or, in patients with coagulopathy and ascites, by a transjugular approach. In selected cases, wedged hepatic vein pressure measurement may establish the presence and cause of portal hypertension. Transient elastography, which uses ultrasonography to determine liver stiffness, and magnetic resonance elastography are under study as noninvasive tests for cirrhosis and portal hypertension.

▶ Differential Diagnosis

The most common causes of cirrhosis in the United States are alcohol and chronic hepatitis C. NAFLD and hepatitis

B are also common causes. Hemochromatosis is the most commonly identified genetic disorder that causes cirrhosis. Other metabolic diseases that may lead to cirrhosis include Wilson disease and α_1-antitrypsin (α_1-antiprotease) deficiency. Primary biliary cirrhosis occurs more frequently in women than men. Secondary biliary cirrhosis may result from chronic biliary obstruction due to a stone, stricture, or neoplasm. Congestive heart failure and constrictive pericarditis may lead to hepatic fibrosis ("cardiac cirrhosis") complicated by ascites and may be mistaken for other causes of cirrhosis. Hereditary hemorrhagic telangiectasia can lead to portal hypertension because of portosystemic shunting and nodular transformation of the liver as well as high-output heart failure. Many cases of cirrhosis are "cryptogenic," in which unrecognized NAFLD may play a role. Mutations in the gene encoding cytokeratin 8 have been associated with some cases of cryptogenic cirrhosis.

▶ Complications

Upper gastrointestinal tract bleeding may occur from varices, portal hypertensive gastropathy, or gastroduodenal ulcer (see Chapter 15). Varices may also result from portal vein thrombosis, which may complicate cirrhosis. Liver failure may be precipitated by alcoholism, surgery, and infection. The risk of carcinoma of the liver is increased greatly in patients with cirrhosis. Hepatic Kupffer cell (reticuloendothelial) dysfunction and decreased opsonic activity lead to an increased risk of systemic infection. Osteoporosis occurs in 12–55% of patients with cirrhosis.

▶ Treatment

A. General Measures

The most important principle of treatment is abstinence from alcohol. The diet should be palatable, with adequate calories (25–35 kcal/kg body weight per day in those with compensated cirrhosis and 35–40 kcal/kg/d in those with malnutrition) and protein (1–1.2 g/kg/d in those with compensated cirrhosis and 1.5 g/kg/d in those with malnutrition) and, if there is fluid retention, sodium restriction. In the presence of hepatic encephalopathy, protein intake should be reduced to no less than 60–80 g/d. The benefit of using specialized supplements containing branched-chain amino acids to prevent or treat hepatic encephalopathy or delay progressive liver failure is uncertain. Vitamin supplementation is desirable. Patients with cirrhosis should receive the HAV, HBV, and pneumococcal vaccines and a yearly influenza vaccine. Liver transplantation in appropriate candidates is curative, and pharmacologic treatments to halt progression of or even reverse cirrhosis are being developed.

B. Treatment of Complications

1. Ascites and edema—Diagnostic paracentesis is indicated for new ascites. It is rarely associated with serious complications such as bleeding, infection, or bowel perforation even in patients with severe coagulopathy. In addition to a cell count and culture, the ascitic albumin level should be determined; a serum-ascites albumin gradient (serum albumin minus ascitic albumin) ≥ 1.1 suggests portal hypertension. An elevated ascitic adenosine deaminase level is suggestive of tuberculous peritonitis, but the sensitivity of the test is reduced in patients with portal hypertension. Occasionally, cirrhotic ascites is chylous (rich in triglycerides); other causes of chylous ascites are malignancy, tuberculosis, and recent abdominal surgery or trauma.

Ascites in patients with cirrhosis results from portal hypertension (increased hydrostatic pressure); hypoalbuminemia (decreased oncotic pressure); peripheral vasodilation, perhaps mediated by endotoxin-induced release of nitric oxide from splanchnic and systemic vasculature, with resulting increases in renin and angiotensin levels and sodium retention by the kidneys; impaired liver inactivation of aldosterone; and increased aldosterone secretion secondary to increased renin production. In individuals with ascites, the urinary excretion of sodium is often less than 10 mEq/L. Free water excretion is also impaired in cirrhosis, and hyponatremia may develop.

In all patients with cirrhotic ascites, dietary sodium intake may initially be restricted to 2000 mg/d; the intake of sodium may be liberalized slightly after diuresis ensues. In some patients, ascites diminishes promptly with bed rest and dietary sodium restriction alone. Fluid intake (800–1000 mL/d) is often restricted in patients with hyponatremia (serum sodium < 125 mEq/L). Treatment of severe hyponatremia with vasopressin receptor antagonists (vaptans) is under study.

A. DIURETICS—Spironolactone, generally in combination with furosemide, should be used in patients who do not respond to salt restriction. An initial trial of furosemide 80 mg intravenously demonstrating a rise in urine sodium to 750 mmol in 8 hours may predict response to diuretic therapy. The dose of spironolactone is initially 100 mg orally daily and may be increased by 100 mg every 3–5 days (up to a maximal conventional daily dose of 400 mg/d, although higher doses have been used) until diuresis is achieved, typically preceded by a rise in the urinary sodium concentration. Monitoring for hyperkalemia is important. In patients who cannot tolerate spironolactone because of side effects, such as painful gynecomastia, amiloride (another potassium-sparing diuretic) may be used in a dose of 5–10 mg orally daily. Diuresis is augmented by the addition of a loop diuretic such as furosemide. This potent diuretic, however, will maintain its effect even with a falling glomerular filtration rate, with resulting prerenal azotemia. The dose of oral furosemide ranges from 40 mg/d to 160 mg/d, and the drug should be administered while blood pressure, urinary output, mental status, and serum electrolytes (especially potassium) are monitored.

The goal of weight loss in the ascitic patient without associated peripheral edema should be no more than 1–1.5 lb/d (0.5–0.7 kg/d).

B. LARGE-VOLUME PARACENTESIS—In patients with massive ascites and respiratory compromise, ascites refractory to diuretics, or intolerable diuretic side effects, large-volume paracentesis (4–6 L) is effective. Intravenous albumin concomitantly at a dosage of 10 g/L of ascites fluid removed protects the intravascular volume and may prevent postparacentesis circulatory dysfunction, although

the usefulness of this practice is debated. Moreover, use of albumin adds considerable expense. Large-volume paracentesis can be repeated daily until ascites is largely resolved and may decrease the need for hospitalization. If possible, diuretics should be continued in the hope of preventing recurrent ascites.

C. TRANSJUGULAR INTRAHEPATIC PORTOSYSTEMIC SHUNT (TIPS)—TIPS is an effective treatment of variceal bleeding refractory to standard therapy (eg, endoscopic band ligation or sclerotherapy) and has shown benefit in the treatment of severe refractory ascites. The technique involves insertion of an expandable metal stent between a branch of the hepatic vein and portal vein over a catheter inserted via the internal jugular vein. Increased renal sodium excretion and control of ascites refractory to diuretics can be achieved in about 75% of selected cases. The success rate is lower in patients with underlying chronic kidney disease. TIPS appears to be the treatment of choice for refractory hepatic hydrothorax (translocation of ascites across the diaphragm to the pleural space); video-assisted thoracoscopy with pleurodesis using talc may be effective when TIPS is contraindicated. Complications of TIPS include hepatic encephalopathy in 20–30% of cases, infection, shunt stenosis in up to 60% of cases, and shunt occlusion in up to 30% of cases when bare stents are used but lower rates when covered stents are used. Long-term patency usually requires periodic shunt revisions. In most cases, patency can be maintained by balloon dilation, local thrombolysis, or placement of an additional stent. TIPS is particularly useful in patients who require short-term control of variceal bleeding or ascites until liver transplantation can be performed. In patients with refractory ascites, TIPS results in lower rates of ascites recurrence and hepatorenal syndrome but a higher rate of hepatic encephalopathy than occurs with repeated large-volume paracentesis; a benefit in survival has been demonstrated in one study and a meta-analysis. Chronic kidney disease, refractory encephalopathy, and hyperbilirubinemia are associated with mortality after TIPS.

D. PERITONEOVENOUS SHUNTS—Peritoneovenous shunts are sometimes placed in patients with malignant ascites but are no longer used for refractory cirrhotic ascites because of a considerable complication rate: disseminated intravascular coagulation in 65% of patients (25% symptomatic; 5% severe), bacterial infections in 4–8%, congestive heart failure in 2–4%, and variceal bleeding from sudden expansion of intravascular volume. TIPS is now preferred for refractory ascites.

2. Spontaneous bacterial peritonitis—Spontaneous bacterial peritonitis is heralded by abdominal pain, increasing ascites, fever, and progressive encephalopathy in a patient with cirrhotic ascites; symptoms are typically mild. Paracentesis reveals an ascitic fluid with, most commonly, a total white cell count of up to 500 cells/mcL with a high percentage of polymorphonuclear cells (PMNs) (> 250/mcL) and a protein concentration of 1 g/dL or less, corresponding to decreased ascitic opsonic activity. Rapid diagnosis of bacterial peritonitis can be made with a high degree of specificity with rapid reagent strips ("dipsticks") that detect leukocyte esterase in ascitic fluid, but the sensitivity is too low for routine use. Cultures of ascites give the highest yield—80–90% positive—using blood culture bottles inoculated at the bedside. Common isolates are *Escherichia coli* and pneumococci. (Gram-positive cocci are the most common isolates in patients who have undergone invasive procedures such as central venous line placement.) Anaerobes are rare. Pending culture results, if there are 250 or more PMN/mcL, intravenous antibiotic therapy should be initiated with cefotaxime, 2 g every 8–12 hours for at least 5 days. Ceftriaxone and amoxicillin-clavulanic acid are alternatives. Oral ofloxacin, 400 mg twice daily, or a 2-day course of intravenous ciprofloxacin, 200 mg twice daily, followed by oral ciprofloxacin, 500 mg twice daily for 5 days, may be effective in selected patients. Supplemental administration of intravenous albumin appears to reduce mortality. Response to therapy can be documented, if necessary, by a decrease in the PMN count of at least 50% on repeat paracentesis 48 hours after initiation of therapy. The overall mortality rate is high—up to 30% during hospitalization and up to 70% by 1 year. Patients with cirrhosis and septic shock have a high frequency of relative adrenal insufficiency, which if present requires administration of hydrocortisone. In survivors of bacterial peritonitis, the risk of recurrent peritonitis may be decreased by long-term norfloxacin, 400 mg orally daily (although in recurrence the causative organism is often resistant to fluoroquinolones). In high-risk cirrhotic patients (eg, those with ascitic protein < 1.5 g/dL, serum bilirubin > 3.0 mg/dL), the risk of peritonitis, hepatorenal syndrome, and mortality for at least 1 year may be reduced by prophylactic norfloxacin, ciprofloxacin (500 mg orally once or twice a day), or trimethoprim-sulfamethoxazole (one double-strength tablet five times a week). Oral norfloxacin or intravenous ceftriaxone (1 g per day) for 7 days reduces the risk of bacterial peritonitis in patients with acute variceal bleeding).

3. Hepatorenal syndrome—Hepatorenal syndrome occurs in up to 10% of patients with advanced cirrhosis and ascites and is characterized by azotemia (serum creatinine > 1.5 mg/dL) in the absence of parenchymal kidney disease or shock and by failure of kidney function to improve following 2 days of diuretic withdrawal and volume expansion with albumin, 1 g/kg up to a maximum of 100 g/d. Oliguria, hyponatremia, and low urinary sodium are typical features. Hepatorenal syndrome is diagnosed only when other causes of acute kidney injury (including prerenal azotemia and acute tubular necrosis) have been excluded. Type I hepatorenal syndrome is characterized by doubling of the serum creatinine to a level greater than 2.5 mg/dL or by halving of the creatinine clearance to less than 20 mL/min in less than 2 weeks. Type II hepatorenal syndrome is more slowly progressive and chronic. The pathogenesis involves intense renal vasoconstriction, possibly because of impaired synthesis of renal vasodilators such as prostaglandin E_2 and decreased total renal blood flow; histologically, the kidneys are normal. An acute decrease in cardiac output is often the precipitating event. Improvement may follow intravenous infusion of albumin in combination with one of the following vasoconstrictor regimens for 7–14 days: intravenous vasopressin or ornipressin (but with a high rate of ischemic side effects); intravenous ornipressin plus dopamine; intravenous terlipressin (a long-acting vasopressin analog that is not available in the United States but that may be the preferred agent); intravenous norepinephrine; or oral midodrine, an α-adrenergic drug, plus the somatostatin analog octreotide, subcutaneously or intravenously. Prolongation of survival has been associated with use of MARS, a modified dialysis method that selectively removes albumin-bound substances. Improvement and sometimes normalization of kidney function may also follow placement of a TIPS. Liver transplantation is the treatment of choice, but many patients die before a donor liver can be obtained. Mortality correlates with the MELD score and presence of a systemic inflammatory response.

4. Hepatic encephalopathy—Hepatic encephalopathy is a state of disordered central nervous system function resulting from failure of the liver to detoxify noxious agents of gut origin because of hepatocellular dysfunction and portosystemic shunting. The clinical spectrum ranges from day-night reversal and mild intellectual impairment to coma. Patients with minimal hepatic encephalopathy have no recognizable clinical symptoms but demonstrate mild cognitive and psychomotor deficits and attention deficit on standardized tests and an increased rate of traffic accidents. The stages of overt encephalopathy are: (1) mild confusion, (2) drowsiness, (3) stupor, and (4) coma. Ammonia is the most readily identified and measurable toxin but is not solely responsible for the disturbed mental status. Central to the pathogenesis is low-grade cerebral edema and astrocyte swelling accompanied by increased production of reactive oxygen and nitrogen oxide species that trigger RNA and protein modifications and thereby affect brain function. Factors that contribute to cerebral edema are ammonia, hyponatremia, cytokines, and benzodiazepines. Bleeding into the intestinal tract may significantly increase the amount of protein in the bowel and precipitate encephalopathy. Other precipitants include constipation, alkalosis, and potassium deficiency induced by diuretics, opioids, hypnotics, and sedatives; medications containing ammonium or amino compounds; paracentesis with attendant hypovolemia; hepatic or systemic infection; and portosystemic shunts (including TIPS). The diagnosis is based primarily on detection of characteristic symptoms and signs, including asterixis. The role of neuroimaging studies (eg, cerebral positron emission tomography, magnetic resonance spectroscopy) in the diagnosis of hepatic encephalopathy is evolving.

Dietary protein should be withheld during acute episodes if the patient cannot eat. When the patient resumes oral intake, protein intake should be 60–80 g/d as tolerated; vegetable protein is better tolerated than meat protein. Gastrointestinal bleeding should be controlled and blood purged from the gastrointestinal tract. This can be accomplished with 120 mL of magnesium citrate by mouth or nasogastric tube every 3–4 hours until the stool is free of gross blood, or by administration of lactulose. The value of treating patients with minimal hepatic encephalopathy is uncertain; probiotic agents may have some benefit.

Lactulose, a nonabsorbable synthetic disaccharide syrup, is digested by bacteria in the colon to short-chain fatty acids, resulting in acidification of colon contents. This acidification favors the formation of ammonium ion in the $NH_4^+ \leftrightarrow NH_3 + H^+$ equation; NH_4^+ is not absorbable, whereas NH_3 is absorbable and thought to be neurotoxic. Lactulose also leads to a change in bowel flora so that fewer ammonia-forming organisms are present. When given orally, the initial dose of lactulose for acute hepatic encephalopathy is 30 mL three or four times daily. The dose should then be titrated so that two or three soft stools per day are produced. When rectal use is indicated because of the patient's inability to take medicines orally, the dose is 300 mL of lactulose in 700 mL of saline or sorbitol as a retention enema for 30–60 minutes; it may be repeated every 4–6 hours. Lactilol is a less sweet disaccharide alternative available as a powder in some countries.

The ammonia-producing intestinal flora may also be controlled with an oral antibiotic. Traditionally, neomycin sulfate, 0.5–1 g orally every 6 or 12 hours for 7 days, has been used, but side effects (including diarrhea, malabsorption, superinfection, ototoxicity, and nephrotoxicity) are frequent, especially after prolonged use. The nonabsorbable agent rifaximin, 400 mg orally three times daily, is preferred. Metronidazole, 250 mg orally three times daily, has also shown benefit. Patients who do not respond to lactulose alone may improve with a course of an antibiotic in addition to lactulose.

Opioids and sedatives metabolized or excreted by the liver should be avoided. If agitation is marked, oxazepam, 10–30 mg, which is not metabolized by the liver, may be given cautiously by mouth or by nasogastric tube. Zinc deficiency should be corrected, if present, with oral zinc sulfate, 600 mg/d in divided doses. Sodium benzoate, 5 g orally twice daily, ornithine aspartate, 9 g orally three times daily, and L-acyl-carnitine, 4 g orally daily, may lower blood ammonia levels, but there is less experience with these drugs than with lactulose. The benzodiazepine competitive antagonist flumazenil is effective in about 30% of patients with severe hepatic encephalopathy, but the drug is short-acting and intravenous administration is required. Use of special dietary supplements enriched with branched-chain amino acids is usually unnecessary except in occasional patients who are intolerant of standard protein supplements. Treatment with acarbose (an α–glucosidase inhibitor) and L-carnitine (an essential factor in the mitochondrial transport of long-chain fatty acids) is under study; other therapies being evaluated include modulating the gut flora with prebiotic and probiotic agents and the use of extracorporeal albumin dialysis (MARS).

5. Anemia—For iron deficiency anemia, ferrous sulfate, 0.3-g enteric-coated tablets, one tablet orally three times daily after meals, is effective. Folic acid, 1 mg/d orally, is indicated in the treatment of macrocytic anemia associated with alcoholism. Transfusions with packed red blood cells may be necessary to replace blood loss.

6. Coagulopathy—Severe hypoprothrombinemia may be treated with vitamin K (eg, phytonadione, 5 mg orally or subcutaneously daily). This treatment is ineffective when synthesis of coagulation factors is impaired because of severe hepatic disease. In such cases, correcting the prolonged prothrombin time requires large volumes of fresh frozen plasma (see Chapter 13). Because the effect is transient, plasma infusions are not indicated except for active bleeding or before an invasive procedure. Use of recombinant activated factor VII may be an alternative, but it is expensive and poses a 1–2% risk of thrombotic complications. Eltrombopag, an oral thrombopoietin-receptor agonist, has shown promise in patients with cirrhosis and severe thrombocytopenia.

7. Hemorrhage from esophageal varices—See Chapter 15.

8. Hepatopulmonary syndrome and portopulmonary hypertension—Shortness of breath in patients with cirrhosis may result from pulmonary restriction and atelectasis caused by massive ascites. The hepatopulmonary syndrome is the triad of chronic liver disease, an increased alveolar-arterial gradient while the patient is breathing room air, and intrapulmonary vascular dilations or arteriovenous communications that result in a right-to-left intrapulmonary shunt and occurs in 5–32% of patients with cirrhosis. The syndrome is presumed to result from enhanced pulmonary production of nitric oxide but does not correlate with the degrees of hepatic dysfunction and portal hypertension. Patients often have greater dyspnea (platypnea) and arterial deoxygenation (orthodeoxia) in the upright than in the recumbent position. The diagnosis should be suspected in a cirrhotic patient with a pulse oximetry level $\leq 96\%$.

Contrast-enhanced echocardiography is a sensitive screening test for detecting pulmonary vascular dilations, whereas macroaggregated albumin lung perfusion scanning is more specific and is used to confirm the diagnosis. High-resolution CT may be useful for detecting dilated pulmonary vessels that may be amenable to embolization in patients with severe hypoxemia ($PO_2 < 60$ mm Hg) who respond poorly to supplemental oxygen.

Medical therapy has been disappointing; experimentally, intravenous methylene blue, oral garlic powder, and oral norfloxacin may improve oxygenation by inhibiting nitric oxide-induced vasodilation, and pentoxifylline may prevent hepatopulmonary syndrome by inhibiting production of tumor necrosis factor-α. Long-term oxygen therapy is recommended for severely hypoxemic patients. The syndrome may reverse with liver transplantation, although postoperative mortality is increased in patients with a preoperative arterial oxygen tension < 50 mm Hg or with substantial intrapulmonary shunting. TIPS may provide palliation in patients with hepatopulmonary syndrome awaiting transplantation.

Portopulmonary hypertension occurs in 0.7% of patients with cirrhosis and is thought to result from an excess of circulating vasoconstrictors, particularly endothelin-1.

Female gender and autoimmune hepatitis have been reported to be risk factors. In cases confirmed by right-sided heart catheterization, treatment with epoprostenol or bosentan may reduce pulmonary hypertension and thereby facilitate liver transplantation; β-blockers worsen exercise capacity and are contraindicated. Liver transplantation is contraindicated in patients with moderate to severe pulmonary hypertension (mean pulmonary pressure > 35 mm Hg).

C. Liver Transplantation

Liver transplantation is indicated in selected cases of irreversible, progressive chronic liver disease, acute hepatic failure, and certain metabolic diseases in which the metabolic defect is in the liver. Absolute contraindications include malignancy (except relatively small hepatocellular carcinomas in a cirrhotic liver), advanced cardiopulmonary disease (except hepatopulmonary syndrome), and sepsis. Relative contraindications include age over 70 years, morbid obesity, portal and mesenteric vein thrombosis, active alcohol or drug abuse, severe malnutrition, and lack of patient understanding. With the emergence of effective antiretroviral therapy for HIV disease, a major cause of mortality in these patients has shifted to liver disease caused by HCV and HBV infection; preliminary experience suggests that the outcome of liver transplantation is comparable to that for non–HIV-infected liver transplant recipients. Alcoholics should be abstinent for 6 months. Liver transplantation should be considered in patients with worsening functional status, rising bilirubin, decreasing albumin, worsening coagulopathy, refractory ascites, recurrent variceal bleeding, or worsening encephalopathy. The major impediment to more widespread use of liver transplantation is a shortage of donor organs. Increasingly, adult living donor liver transplantation is an option for some patients. Five-year survival rates as high as 80% are now reported. Hepatocellular carcinoma, hepatitis B and C, and some cases of Budd-Chiari syndrome and autoimmune liver disease may recur in the transplanted liver. The incidence of recurrence of hepatitis B can be reduced by preoperative and postoperative treatment with a nucleoside analog and perioperative administration of HBIG. Immunosuppression is achieved with combinations of cyclosporine, tacrolimus or sirolimus, corticosteroids, azathioprine, and mycophenolate mofetil and may be complicated by infections, advanced chronic kidney disease, neurologic disorders, and drug toxicity as well as graft rejection, vascular occlusion, or bile leaks. Patients are at risk for obesity, diabetes mellitus, and hyperlipidemia.

▶ Prognosis

Factors determining survival include the patient's ability to stop the intake of alcohol as well as the Child-Turcotte-Pugh class (Table 16–6). The MELD score, which incorporates the serum bilirubin and creatinine levels and the INR, is also a measure of mortality risk in patients with end-stage liver disease and is particularly useful for predicting short- and intermediate-term survival and complications of cirrhosis (eg, bacterial peritonitis) and determining allocation priorities for donor livers. The consistency of the MELD score among different hospitals may be improved when the INR is calibrated based on prothrombin time control samples that include patients with liver disease

Table 16–6. Child-Turcotte-Pugh and Model for End-Stage Liver Disease (MELD) scoring systems for staging cirrhosis.

Child-Turcotte-Pugh scoring system			
		Numerical Score	
Parameter	1	2	3
Ascites	None	Slight	Moderate to severe
Encephalopathy	None	Slight to moderate	Moderate to severe
Bilirubin (mg/dL)	< 2.0	2–3	> 3.0
Albumin (g/dL)	> 3.5	2.8–3.5	< 2.8
Prothrombin time (seconds increased)	1–3	4–6	> 6.0

Total Numerical Score and Corresponding Child-Turcotte-Pugh Class	
Score	Class
5–6	A
7–9	B
10–15	C

MELD scoring system

MELD = 11.2 $\log_e$ (INR) + 3.78 $\log_e$ (bilirubin [mg/dL]) + 9.57 $\log_e$ (creatinine [mg/dL]) + 6.43. (Range 6–40).

INR, international normalized ratio.

rather than those taking oral anticoagulants. In patients with a relatively low MELD score (< 21) and a low priority for liver transplantation, a low serum sodium concentration (< 130 mEq/L), an elevated hepatic venous pressure gradient, and persistent ascites appear to be additional independent predictors of mortality, and a modification of the MELD score that incorporates the serum sodium (MELDNa) is under study. Only 50% of patients with severe hepatic dysfunction (serum albumin < 3 g/dL, bilirubin > 3 mg/dL, ascites, encephalopathy, cachexia, and upper gastrointestinal bleeding) survive 6 months. The risk of death in this subgroup of patients with advanced cirrhosis is associated with chronic kidney disease, cognitive dysfunction, ventilatory insufficiency, age ≥ 65 years, and prothrombin time ≥ 16 seconds. Obesity appears to be a risk factor for cirrhosis-related death or hospitalization in nonalcoholic patients, and diabetes mellitus increases the risk of complications and mortality in patients with cirrhosis. Patients with cirrhosis are at risk for the development of hepatocellular carcinoma, with rates of 3–5% per year for alcoholic and viral hepatitis-related cirrhosis. Liver transplantation has markedly improved the outlook for patients with cirrhosis who are acceptable candidates and are referred for evaluation early. Patients with compensated cirrhosis are given additional priority for liver transplantation if they are found to have a lesion > 2 cm in diameter consistent with hepatocellular carcinoma. In-hospital mortality from variceal bleeding in patients with cirrhosis has declined from over 40% in 1980 to 15% in 2000. Medical treatments to reverse hepatic fibrosis are under investigation.

When to Refer

- For liver biopsy.
- Child-Turcotte-Pugh score ≥ 7.
- MELD score ≥ 10.
- For upper endoscopy to screen for gastroesophageal varices.

When to Admit

- Gastrointestinal bleeding.
- Stage 3–4 hepatic encephalopathy.
- Worsening kidney function.
- Severe hyponatremia.
- Profound hypoxia.

Bell BP et al. The epidemiology of newly diagnosed chronic liver disease in gastroenterology practices in the United States: results from population-based surveillance. Am J Gastroenterol. 2008 Nov;103(11):2727–36. [PMID: 18684170]

Bonekamp S et al. Can imaging modalities diagnose and stage hepatic fibrosis and cirrhosis accurately? J Hepatol. 2009 Jan;50(1):17–35. [PMID: 19022517]

Fairbanks KD et al. Liver disease in alpha 1-antitrypsin deficiency: a review. Am J Gastroenterol. 2008 Aug;103(8):2136–41. [PMID: 18796107]

Häussinger D et al. Pathogenetic mechanisms of hepatic encephalopathy. Gut. 2008 Aug;57(8):1156–65. [PMID: 18628377]

Kim WR et al. Hyponatremia and mortality among patients on the liver-transplant waiting list. N Engl J Med. 2008 Sep 4;359(10):1018–26. [PMID: 18768945]

Møller S et al. Cardiovascular complications of cirrhosis. Gut. 2008 Feb;57(2):268–78. [PMID: 18192456]

Rodríguez-Roisin R et al. Hepatopulmonary syndrome—a liver-induced lung vascular disorder. N Engl J Med. 2008 May 29;358(22):2378–87. [PMID: 18509123]

Sanyal AJ et al. Portal hypertension and its complications. Gastroenterology. 2008 May;134(6):1715–28. [PMID: 18471549]

Schuppan D et al. Liver cirrhosis. Lancet. 2008 Mar 8;371(9615):838–51. [PMID: 18328931]

PRIMARY BILIARY CIRRHOSIS

ESSENTIALS OF DIAGNOSIS

- ▶ Occurs in middle-aged women.
- ▶ Often asymptomatic.
- ▶ Elevation of alkaline phosphatase, positive antimitochondrial antibody, elevated IgM, increased cholesterol.
- ▶ Characteristic liver biopsy.
- ▶ In later stages, can present with fatigue, jaundice, features of cirrhosis, xanthelasma, xanthoma, steatorrhea.

General Considerations

Primary biliary cirrhosis is a chronic disease of the liver characterized by autoimmune destruction of small intrahepatic bile ducts and cholestasis. It is insidious in onset, occurs usually in women aged 40–60 years, and is often detected by the chance finding of elevated alkaline phosphatase levels. Estimated incidence and prevalence rates in the United States are 4.5 and 65.4 per 100,000, respectively, in women, and 0.7 and 12.1 per 100,000, respectively, in men. The frequency of the disease among first-degree relatives of affected persons is 1.3–6%, and the concordance rate in identical twins is high. The disease is associated with HLA *DRB1*08*. The disease may be associated with Sjögren syndrome, autoimmune thyroid disease, Raynaud syndrome, scleroderma, hypothyroidism, and celiac disease. Infection with *Novosphingobium aromaticivorans* or *Chlamydophila pneumoniae* may be triggering or causative in primary biliary cirrhosis; other triggers, including viruses (such as human betaretrovirus), lactobacillus vaccination to prevent recurrent vaginitis, and xenobiotics, are also suspected. X-chromosome monosomy may be a predisposing factor. A history of urinary tract infections (caused by *E coli*) and smoking and use of hormone replacement therapy are risk factors.

Clinical Findings

A. Symptoms and Signs

Many patients are asymptomatic for years. The onset of clinical illness is insidious and is heralded by fatigue (excessive daytime somnolence) and pruritus. With progression, physical examination reveals hepatosplenomegaly. Xanthomatous lesions may occur in the skin and tendons and around the eyelids. Jaundice, steatorrhea, and signs of portal hypertension are late findings. Autonomic dysfunction, including orthostatic hypotension, and cognitive dysfunction appear to be common. The risk of low bone density, osteoporosis, and fractures is increased in patients with primary biliary cirrhosis (who tend to be older women) possibly due in part to polymorphisms of the vitamin D receptor.

B. Laboratory Findings

Blood counts are normal early in the disease. Liver biochemical tests reflect cholestasis with elevation of alkaline phosphatase, cholesterol (especially high-density lipoproteins), and, in later stages, bilirubin. Antimitochondrial antibodies (directed against the dihydrolipoamide acetyltransferase component of pyruvate dehydrogenase or other 2-oxo-acid enzymes in mitochondria) are present in 95% of patients, and serum IgM levels are elevated. ANAs directed against the nuclear pore complex (eg, against gp210 in the nuclear envelope) may be detected in specialized laboratories.

Diagnosis

The diagnosis of primary biliary cirrhosis is based on the detection of cholestatic liver chemistries (often initially an isolated elevation of the alkaline phosphatase) and antimitochondrial antibodies in serum. Liver biopsy is not essential for diagnosis but permits histologic staging: I, portal inflammation with granulomas; II, bile duct proliferation, periportal inflammation; III, interlobular fibrous septa; and IV, cirrhosis. Estimation of histologic stage by an "enhanced liver fibrosis assay" that incorporates serum levels of hyaluronic acid, tissue inhibitor of metalloproteinase-1, and procollagen III aminopeptide has shown promise.

Differential Diagnosis

The disease must be differentiated from chronic biliary tract obstruction (stone or stricture), carcinoma of the bile ducts, primary sclerosing cholangitis, sarcoidosis, cholestatic drug toxicity (eg, chlorpromazine), and in some cases chronic hepatitis. Patients with a clinical and histologic picture of primary biliary cirrhosis but no antimitochondrial antibodies are said to have antimitochondrial antibody-negative primary biliary cirrhosis ("autoimmune cholangitis"), which has been associated with lower serum IgM levels and a greater frequency of smooth muscle and ANAs. Many such patients are found to have antimitochondrial antibodies by immunoblot against recombinant proteins (rather than standard immunofluorescence). Some patients have overlapping features of primary biliary cirrhosis and autoimmune hepatitis.

Treatment

Cholestyramine (4 g) or colestipol (5 g) in water or juice three times daily may be beneficial for pruritus. Rifampin, 150–300 mg orally twice daily, is inconsistently beneficial. Opioid antagonists (eg, naloxone, 0.2 mcg/kg/min by intravenous infusion, or naltrexone, 50 mg/d by mouth) show promise in the treatment of pruritus. The 5-hydroxytryptamine (5-HT$_3$) serotonin receptor antagonist ondansetron, 4 mg orally three times a day as needed, and the selective serotonin uptake inhibitor sertraline, 75–100 mg/d orally, may also provide some benefit. For refractory pruritus, plasmapheresis or extracorporeal albumin dialysis may be needed. Modafinil, 100–200 mg/d orally, may improve daytime somnolence. Deficiencies of vitamins A, K, and D may occur if steatorrhea is present and are aggravated when cholestyramine or colestipol is administered. See Chapter 26 for discussion of prevention and treatment of osteoporosis.

Because of its lack of toxicity, ursodeoxycholic acid (13–15 mg/kg/d in one or two doses) is the preferred medical treatment (and only treatment approved by the US FDA) for primary biliary cirrhosis and has been shown to slow the progression of disease (particularly in early-stage disease), stabilize histology, improve long-term survival, reduce the risk of developing esophageal varices, and delay (and possibly prevent) the need for liver transplantation, although the benefit of the drug has been questioned. Complete normalization of liver tests occurs in 20% of treated patients within 2 years and 40% within 5 years, and survival is similar to that of healthy controls when the drug is given to patients with stage 1 or 2 primary biliary cirrhosis. Ursodeoxycholic acid therapy has also been reported to reduce the risk of recurrent colorectal adenomas in patients with primary

biliary cirrhosis. Side effects include weight gain and rarely loose stools. Colchicine (0.6 mg orally twice daily) and methotrexate (15 mg/wk orally) have had some reported benefit in improving symptoms and serum levels of alkaline phosphatase and bilirubin. Methotrexate may also improve liver histology in some patients, but overall response rates have been disappointing. Penicillamine, prednisone, and azathioprine have proved to be of no benefit. Budesonide may improve liver histology but worsens bone density. Mycophenolate mofetil is under study. For patients with advanced disease, liver transplantation is the treatment of choice.

Prognosis

Without liver transplantation, survival averages 7–10 years once symptoms develop but has improved for younger women since the introduction of ursodeoxycholic acid. Progression to liver failure and portal hypertension is associated with the presence of anti-gp210 and anticentromere antibodies, respectively, and may be accelerated by smoking. Patients in whom the alkaline phosphatase is less than three times normal, AST is less than two times normal, and bilirubin is less than or equal to 1 mg/dL after 1 year of therapy with ursodeoxycholic acid have a 10-year transplant-free survival rate of 90%. In advanced disease, adverse prognostic markers are a high Mayo risk score that includes older age, high serum bilirubin, edema, low serum albumin, and prolonged prothrombin time as well as variceal hemorrhage. Fatigue is associated with an increased risk of cardiac mortality. Among asymptomatic patients, at least one-third will become symptomatic within 15 years. The risk of hepatobiliary malignancies appears to be increased in patients with primary biliary cirrhosis; risk factors include older age, male sex, prior blood transfusions, and signs of cirrhosis or portal hypertension. Liver transplantation for advanced primary biliary cirrhosis is associated with a 1-year survival rate of 85–90%. The disease recurs in the graft in 20% of patients by 3 years, but this does not seem to affect survival.

When to Refer

- For liver biopsy.
- For liver transplant evaluation.

When to Admit

- Gastrointestinal bleeding.
- Stage 3–4 hepatic encephalopathy.
- Worsening kidney function.
- Severe hyponatremia.
- Profound hypoxia.

Corpechot C et al. Biochemical response to ursodeoxycholic acid and long-term prognosis in primary biliary cirrhosis. Hepatology. 2008 Sep;48(3):871–7. [PMID: 18752324]

Mayo MJ et al. Prediction of clinical outcomes in primary biliary cirrhosis by serum enhanced liver fibrosis assay. Hepatology. 2008 Nov;48(5):1549–57. [PMID: 18846542]

Mendes FD et al. Mortality attributable to cholestatic liver disease in the United States. Hepatology. 2008 Apr;47(4):1241–7. [PMID: 18318437]

Selmi C et al. The unfinished business of primary biliary cirrhosis. J Hepatol. 2008 Sep;49(3):451–60. [PMID: 18640737]

Silveira MG et al. Surveillance for hepatocellular carcinoma in patients with primary biliary cirrhosis. Hepatology. 2008 Oct;48(4):1149–56. [PMID: 18785621]

Silveira MG et al. Treatment of primary biliary cirrhosis: therapy with choleretic and immunosuppressive agents. Clin Liver Dis. 2008 May;12(2):425–43. [PMID: 18456189]

HEMOCHROMATOSIS

 ESSENTIALS OF DIAGNOSIS

- ▸ Usually diagnosed because of elevated iron saturation or serum ferritin or a family history.
- ▸ Most patients are asymptomatic; the disease is rarely recognized clinically before the fifth decade.
- ▸ Hepatic abnormalities and cirrhosis, congestive heart failure, hypogonadism, and arthritis.
- ▸ *HFE* gene mutation (usually *C282Y/C282Y*) is found in most cases.

▸ General Considerations

Hemochromatosis is an autosomal recessive disease caused in many cases by a mutation in the *HFE* gene on chromosome 6. The HFE protein is thought to play an important role in the process by which duodenal crypt cells sense body iron stores, leading in turn to increased iron absorption from the duodenum. A decrease in the synthesis or expression of hepcidin, the principal iron regulatory hormone, is thought to be a principal pathogenic factor in all forms of hemochromatosis. About 85% of persons with well-established hemochromatosis are homozygous for the *C282Y* mutation. The frequency of the gene mutation averages 7% in Northern European and North American white populations, resulting in a 0.5% frequency of homozygotes (of whom up to 88% will develop biochemical evidence of iron overload but only 28% of men and 1% of women will develop clinical symptoms). By contrast, the gene mutation and hemochromatosis are uncommon in blacks and Asian-American populations. A second genetic mutation (*H63D*) may contribute to the development of hemochromatosis in a small percentage (1.5%) of persons who are compound heterozygotes for *C282Y* and *H63D* and have a comorbidity such as diabetes mellitus and fatty liver. *H63D* homozygotes do not develop hemochromatosis but may be at increased risk for amyotrophic lateral sclerosis. Rare instances of hemochromatosis result from mutations in the genes that encode transferrin receptor 2 and ferroprotein. A juvenile-onset variant that is characterized by severe iron overload, cardiac dysfunction, hypogonadotropic hypogonadism, and a high mortality rate is usually linked to a mutation of a gene on chromosome 1q designated *HJV* that produces a protein called hemojuvelin or, rarely, to a mutation in the

HAMP gene on chromosome 19 that encodes hepcidin but not to the *C282Y* mutation.

Hemochromatosis is characterized by increased accumulation of iron as hemosiderin in the liver, pancreas, heart, adrenals, testes, pituitary, and kidneys. Cirrhosis is more likely to develop in affected persons who drink alcohol excessively or have obesity-related steatosis than in those who do not. Eventually, hepatic and pancreatic insufficiency, congestive heart failure, and hypogonadism may develop. Heterozygotes do not develop cirrhosis in the absence of associated disorders such as viral hepatitis or NAFLD.

▸ Clinical Findings

A. Symptoms and Signs

The onset of clinical disease is usually after age 50 years—earlier in men than in women; however, because of widespread liver biochemical testing and iron screening, the diagnosis is usually made long before symptoms develop. Early symptoms are nonspecific (eg, fatigue, arthralgias). Later clinical manifestations include arthropathy, hepatomegaly and evidence of hepatic insufficiency (late finding), skin pigmentation (combination of slate-gray due to iron and brown due to melanin, sometimes resulting in bronze color), cardiac enlargement with or without heart failure or conduction defects, diabetes mellitus with its complications, and impotence in men. Interestingly, population studies have shown an increased prevalence of liver disease but not of diabetes, arthritis, or heart disease in *C282Y* homozygotes. Bleeding from esophageal varices may occur, and in patients in whom cirrhosis develops, there is a 15–20% frequency of hepatocellular carcinoma. Affected patients are at increased risk of infection with *Vibrio vulnificus*, *Listeria monocytogenes*, *Yersinia enterocolitica*, and other siderophilic organisms. The risk of porphyria cutanea tarda is increased in persons with the *C282Y* or *H63D* mutation.

B. Laboratory Findings

Laboratory findings include mildly abnormal liver tests (AST, alkaline phosphatase), an elevated plasma iron with greater than 50% transferrin saturation in men and 45% in women (after an overnight fast), and an elevated serum ferritin (although a normal iron saturation and a normal ferritin do not exclude the diagnosis). Affected men are more likely than affected women to have an elevated ferritin level.

C. Imaging

MRI and CT may show changes consistent with iron overload of the liver, and MRI can quantitate hepatic iron stores. There is also an emerging role for MRI for assessment of the degree of hepatic fibrosis. Testing for *HFE* mutations is indicated in any patient with evidence of iron overload and in siblings of patients with confirmed hemochromatosis.

D. Liver Biopsy

In patients who are homozygous for *C282Y*, liver biopsy is often indicated to determine whether cirrhosis is present.

Biopsy can be deferred, however, in patients in whom the serum ferritin level is < 1000 mcg/L, serum AST level is normal, and hepatomegaly is absent; the likelihood of cirrhosis is low in these persons. Liver biopsy is also indicated when iron overload is suspected even though the patient is not homozygous for *C282Y*. In patients with hemochromatosis, the liver biopsy characteristically shows extensive iron deposition in hepatocytes and in bile ducts and the hepatic iron index—hepatic iron content per gram of liver converted to micromoles and divided by the patient's age—is generally greater than 1.9. Only 5% of patients with hereditary hemochromatosis identified by screening in a primary care setting have cirrhosis.

Screening

Genetic testing is recommended for all first-degree family members of the proband; children of an affected person (*C282Y* homozygote) need to be screened only if the patient's spouse carries the *C282Y* or *H63D* mutation. Screening all men of Northern European ancestry over age 25 years by measurement of the transferrin saturation or the unbound iron-binding capacity has been recommended by some experts, but the value of screening has been questioned because morbidity and mortality from hemochromatosis are low. Patients with otherwise unexplained chronic liver disease, arthritis, impotence, and late-onset type 1 (and possibly type 2) diabetes mellitus should be screened for iron overload.

Treatment

Affected patients should avoid foods rich in iron (such as red meat), alcohol, vitamin C, raw shellfish, and supplemental iron. Weekly phlebotomies of 1 or 2 units (250–500 mL) of blood (each containing about 250 mg of iron) is indicated in all symptomatic patients, those with a serum ferritin level of at least 1000 mcg/L, and those with an increased fasting iron saturation and should be continued for up to 2–3 years to achieve depletion of iron stores. The hematocrit and serum iron values should be monitored. When iron store depletion is achieved (iron saturation < 50% and serum ferritin level < 50 mcg/L), maintenance phlebotomies (every 2–4 months) are continued, although compliance has been reported to decrease with time; administration of a proton pump inhibitor, which reduces intestinal iron absorption, appears to decrease the maintenance phlebotomy blood volume requirement. The chelating agent deferoxamine is indicated for patients with hemochromatosis and anemia or in those with secondary iron overload due to thalassemia who cannot tolerate phlebotomies. The drug is administered intravenously or subcutaneously in a dose of 20–40 mg/kg/d infused over 24 hours and can mobilize 30 mg of iron per day. However, treatment is painful and time-consuming. An oral chelator, deferasirox, 20 mg/kg once daily, has been approved for treatment of iron overload due to blood transfusions. Complications of hemochromatosis—arthropathy, diabetes, heart disease, portal hypertension, and hypopituitarism—also require treatment.

The course of the disease is favorably altered by phlebotomy therapy. Fibrosis may regress, and in precirrhotic

patients, cirrhosis may be prevented. Cardiac conduction defects and insulin requirements improve with treatment. In patients with cirrhosis, varices may reverse, and the risk of variceal bleeding declines, although the risk of hepatocellular carcinoma persists. In the past, liver transplantation for advanced cirrhosis associated with severe iron overload, including hemochromatosis, was reported to lead to survival rates that were lower than those for other types of liver disease because of cardiac complications and an increased risk of infections, but since 1997, posttransplant survival rates have been excellent.

▶ When to Refer

- For liver biopsy.
- For initiation of therapy.

Acton RT et al. Accuracy of family history of hemochromatosis or iron overload: the hemochromatosis and iron overload screening study. Clin Gastroenterol Hepatol. 2008 Aug;6(8):934–8. [PMID: 18585964]

Allen KJ et al. Iron-overload-related disease in HFE hereditary hemochromatosis. N Engl J Med. 2008 Jan 17;358(3):221–30. [PMID: 18199861]

Brissot P et al. Current approach to hemochromatosis. Blood Rev. 2008 Jul;22(4):195–210. [PMID: 18430498]

Crooks CJ et al. The epidemiology of haemochromatosis: a population-based study. Aliment Pharmacol Ther. 2009 Jan 15;29(2):183–92. [PMID: 18945251]

Deugnier Y et al. Iron and the liver: update 2008. J Hepatol. 2008;48(Suppl 1):S113–23. [PMID: 18304682]

Olynyk JK et al. Hereditary hemochromatosis in the post-HFE era. Hepatology. 2008 Sep;48(3):991–1001. [PMID: 18752323]

Phatak PD et al. Hereditary hemochromatosis: time for targeted screening. Ann Intern Med. 2008 Aug 19;149(4):270–2. [PMID: 18711158]

WILSON DISEASE

 ESSENTIALS OF DIAGNOSIS

▶ Excessive deposition of copper in the liver and brain.

▶ Rare autosomal recessive disorder that usually occurs in persons under age 40.

▶ Serum ceruloplasmin, the plasma copper-carrying protein, is low.

▶ Urinary excretion of copper and hepatic copper concentration are high.

▶ General Considerations

Wilson disease (hepatolenticular degeneration) is a rare autosomal recessive disorder that usually occurs in persons under age 40. The worldwide prevalence is about 30 per million population. The condition is characterized by excessive deposition of copper in the liver and brain. The genetic defect, localized to chromosome 13, has been shown to affect a copper-transporting adenosine triphosphatase (*ATP7B*) in the liver and leads to copper accumulation in the liver and oxidative damage of hepatic mitochondria. Most patients are compound heterozygotes (ie, carry two different mutations). Approximately 300 different mutations in the Wilson disease gene have been identified, making genetic diagnosis impractical except within families in which the mutation has been identified in the index case. The *H1069Q* mutation accounts for 37–63% of disease alleles in populations of Northern European descent.

The major physiologic aberration in Wilson disease is excessive absorption of copper from the small intestine and decreased excretion of copper by the liver, resulting in increased tissue deposition, especially in the liver, brain, cornea, and kidney.

▶ Clinical Findings

Wilson disease tends to present as liver disease in adolescents and neuropsychiatric disease in young adults, but there is great variability, and onset of symptoms after age 40 is more common than previously thought. The diagnosis should always be considered in any child or young adult with hepatitis, splenomegaly with hypersplenism, Coombs-negative hemolytic anemia, portal hypertension, and neurologic or psychiatric abnormalities. Wilson disease should also be considered in persons under 40 years of age with chronic or fulminant hepatitis.

Hepatic involvement may range from elevated liver tests (although the alkaline phosphatase may be low) to cirrhosis and portal hypertension. In a patient with acute liver failure, the diagnosis of Wilson disease is suggested by an alkaline phosphatase-to-total bilirubin ratio < 4 and an AST-to-ALT ratio > 2.2. The neurologic manifestations of Wilson disease are related to basal ganglia dysfunction and include an akinetic-rigid syndrome similar to parkinsonism, pseudosclerosis with tremor, ataxia, and a dystonic syndrome. Dysarthria, dysphagia, incoordination, and spasticity are common. Migraines, insomnia, and seizures have been reported. Psychiatric features include behavioral and personality changes and emotional lability and may precede characteristic neurologic features. The pathognomonic sign of the condition is the brownish or gray-green Kayser-Fleischer ring, which represents fine pigmented granular deposits in Descemet membrane in the cornea (Plate 70). The ring is usually most marked at the superior and inferior poles of the cornea. It is sometimes seen with the naked eye and is readily detected by slit-lamp examination. It may be absent in patients with hepatic manifestations only but is usually present in those with neuropsychiatric disease. Renal calculi, aminoaciduria, renal tubular acidosis, hypoparathyroidism, infertility, and hemolytic anemia may occur in patients with Wilson disease.

▶ Diagnosis

The diagnosis can be challenging and is generally based on demonstration of increased urinary copper excretion (> 40 mcg/24 h and usually > 100 mcg/24 h) or low serum ceruloplasmin levels (< 20 mg/dL; < 5 mg/dL is diagnostic), and elevated hepatic copper concentration (> 250 mcg/g of dry liver). However, increased urinary copper and low serum ceruloplasmin levels are neither completely sensitive nor specific for Wilson disease. In equivocal cases (when the serum ceruloplasmin level is normal), the diagnosis may require demonstration of a rise in urinary copper determination after a penicillamine challenge, although the test has been validated only in children. Liver biopsy may show acute or chronic hepatitis or cirrhosis. MRI of the brain may show evidence of increased basal ganglia, brainstem, and cerebellar copper even early in the course of the disease. If available, molecular analysis of *ATP78* mutations can be diagnostic.

▶ Treatment

Early treatment to remove excess copper is essential before it can produce hepatic or neurologic damage. Early in the treatment phase, restriction of dietary copper (shellfish, organ foods, nuts, mushrooms, and chocolate) may be of value. Oral penicillamine (0.75–2 g/d in divided doses taken 1 h before or 2 h after food) is the drug of choice and enhances urinary excretion of chelated copper. Oral pyridoxine, 50 mg per week, is added, since penicillamine is an antimetabolite of this vitamin. If penicillamine treatment cannot be tolerated because of gastrointestinal intolerance, hypersensitivity, autoimmune reactions, nephrotoxicity, or bone marrow toxicity, consider the use of another chelating agent—trientine, 250–500 mg three times a day. Oral zinc acetate or zinc gluconate, 50 mg three times a day, interferes with intestinal absorption of copper, promotes fecal copper excretion, and may be used as maintenance therapy after decoppering with a chelating agent or as first-line therapy in presymptomatic or pregnant patients. Ammonium tetrathiomolybdate, which complexes copper in the intestinal tract, has shown promise as initial therapy for neurologic Wilson disease.

Treatment should continue indefinitely. The doses of penicillamine and trientine should be reduced during pregnancy. Supplemental vitamin E, an antioxidant, has been recommended but not rigorously studied. Once the serum nonceruloplasmin copper level is within the normal range (50–150 mcg/L), the dose of chelating agent can be reduced to the minimum necessary for maintaining that level. The prognosis is good in patients who are effectively treated before liver or brain damage has occurred. Liver transplantation is indicated for fulminant hepatitis (often after plasma exchange or dialysis with MARS as a stabilizing measure), end-stage cirrhosis, and, in selected cases, intractable neurologic disease, although survival is lower when liver transplantation is undertaken for neurologic disease than for liver disease. Family members, especially siblings, require screening with serum ceruloplasmin, liver biochemical tests, and slit-lamp examination or, if the causative mutation is known, with mutation analysis.

▶ When to Refer

All patients with Wilson disease should be referred for diagnosis and treatment.

▶ When to Admit

- Acute liver failure.

- Gastrointestinal bleeding.
- Stage 3–4 hepatic encephalopathy.
- Worsening kidney function.
- Severe hyponatremia.
- Profound hypoxia.

Chiu A et al. Use of the molecular adsorbents recirculating system as a treatment for acute decompensated Wilson disease. Liver Transpl. 2008 Oct;14(10):1512–6. [PMID: 18825711]

Korman JD et al. Screening for Wilson disease in acute liver failure: a comparison of currently available diagnostic tests. Hepatology. 2008 Oct;48(4):1167–74. [PMID: 18798336]

Mak CM et al. Diagnosis of Wilson's disease: a comprehensive review. Crit Rev Clin Lab Sci. 2008;45(3):263–90. [PMID: 18568852]

Roberts EA et al. Diagnosis and treatment of Wilson disease: an update. Hepatology. 2008 Jun;47(6):2089–111. [PMID: 18506894]

HEPATIC VEIN OBSTRUCTION (Budd-Chiari Syndrome)

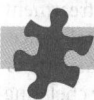 ESSENTIALS OF DIAGNOSIS

▶ Right upper quadrant pain and tenderness.

▶ Ascites.

▶ Imaging studies show occlusion/absence of flow in the hepatic vein(s) or inferior vena cava.

▶ Clinical picture is similar in veno-occlusive disease but major hepatic veins are patent.

General Considerations

Factors that predispose patients to hepatic vein obstruction, or Budd-Chiari syndrome, including hereditary and acquired hypercoagulable states, can be identified in 75% of affected patients; multiple disorders are found in 25%. Up to 50% of cases are associated with polycythemia vera or other myeloproliferative disease (which has a risk of Budd-Chiari syndrome of 1%). These cases are often associated with a specific mutation (*V617F*) in the gene that codes for JAK2 tyrosine kinase and may be subclinical. In some cases, an underlying predisposition to thrombosis (eg, activated protein C resistance [factor V Leiden mutation] [25% of cases], protein C or S or antithrombin deficiency, hyperprothrombinemia [factor II G20210A mutation], the methylenetetrahydrofolate reductase TT677 mutation, antiphospholipid antibodies) can be identified. Hepatic vein obstruction may be associated with caval webs, right-sided heart failure or constrictive pericarditis, neoplasms that cause hepatic vein occlusion, paroxysmal nocturnal hemoglobinuria, Behçet syndrome, blunt abdominal trauma, use of oral contraceptives, and pregnancy. Some cytotoxic agents and pyrrolizidine alkaloids ("bush teas") may cause sinusoidal obstruction syndrome (previously known as veno-occlusive disease because the terminal venules are often occluded), which mimics Budd-Chiari syndrome clinically. Sinusoidal obstruction syndrome is common in patients who have undergone bone marrow transplantation, particularly those with pretransplant aminotransferase elevations or fever during cytoreductive therapy with cyclophosphamide, azathioprine, carmustine, busulfan, or etoposide or those receiving high-dose cytoreductive therapy or high-dose total body irradiation. In India, China, and South Africa, Budd-Chiari syndrome is associated with a poor standard of living and often the result of occlusion of the hepatic portion of the inferior vena cava, presumably due to prior thrombosis. The clinical presentation is mild but the course is frequently complicated by hepatocellular carcinoma.

Clinical Findings

A. Symptoms and Signs

The presentation may be fulminant, acute, subacute, or chronic. An insidious (subacute) onset is most common. Clinical manifestations generally include tender, painful hepatic enlargement, jaundice, splenomegaly, and ascites. With chronic disease, bleeding varices and hepatic coma may be evident; hepatopulmonary syndrome may occur.

B. Imaging

Hepatic imaging studies may show a prominent caudate lobe, since its venous drainage may not be occluded. The screening test of choice is contrast-enhanced, color, or pulsed-Doppler ultrasonography, which has a sensitivity of 85% for detecting evidence of hepatic venous or inferior vena caval thrombosis. MRI with spin-echo and gradient-echo sequences and intravenous gadolinium injection allows visualization of the obstructed veins and collateral vessels. Direct venography can delineate caval webs and occluded hepatic veins ("spider-web" pattern) most precisely.

C. Liver Biopsy

Percutaneous or transjugular liver biopsy frequently shows a characteristic centrilobular congestion and fibrosis and often multiple large regenerating nodules. Liver biopsy is often contraindicated in sinusoidal obstruction syndrome because of thrombocytopenia, and the diagnosis is based on clinical findings.

Treatment

Ascites should be treated with fluid and salt restriction and diuretics. Treatable causes of Budd-Chiari syndrome should be sought. Prompt recognition and treatment of an underlying hematologic disorder may avoid the need for surgery, but the optimal anticoagulation regimen is uncertain. Low-molecular weight heparins are preferred over unfractionated heparin because of a high rate of heparin-induced thrombocytopenia with the latter. Infusion of a thrombolytic agent into recently occluded veins has been attempted with success. In patients with sinusoidal obstruction syndrome, defibrotide, an adenosine receptor agonist that increases endogenous tissue plasminogen activator levels, has shown promise. TIPS placement may be attempted in patients with persistent hepatic congestion or failed thrombolytic therapy, although late TIPS dysfunction is common. TIPS is now preferred over surgical decompression (side-to-side porta-caval, mesocaval, or mesoatrial shunt) which, in contrast to TIPS, has not been proven to improve long-term survival. Older age, higher serum bilirubin level, and greater INR predict a poor outcome with TIPS. Balloon angioplasty, in some cases with placement of an intravascular metallic stent, is preferred in patients with an inferior vena caval web and is being performed increasingly in patients with a short segment of thrombosis in the hepatic vein. Liver transplantation is considered in patients with fulminant hepatic failure, cirrhosis and hepatocellular dysfunction, and failure of a portosystemic shunt, and outcomes have improved with the advent of patient selection based on the MELD score. Patients often require lifelong anticoagulation and treatment of the underlying myeloproliferative disease; antiplatelet therapy with aspirin and hydroxyurea has been suggested as an alternative to warfarin in patients with a myeloproliferative disorder. The overall 5-year survival rate is 50–90% with treatment (but < 10% without intervention). Adverse prognostic factors in patients with Budd-Chiari syndrome are older age, high Child-Turcotte-Pugh score, ascites, encephalopathy, elevated total bilirubin, prolonged prothrombin time, elevated serum creatinine, concomitant portal vein thrombosis, and histologic features of acute liver disease superimposed on chronic liver injury.

▶ **When to Admit**

All patients with hepatic vein obstruction should be hospitalized.

Garcia-Pagán JC et al. TIPS for Budd-Chiari syndrome: long-term results and prognostics factors in 124 patients. Gastroenterology. 2008 Sep;135(3):808–15. [PMID: 18621047]
Plessier A et al. Budd-Chiari syndrome. Semin Liver Dis. 2008 Aug;28(3):259–69. [PMID: 18814079]
Ulrich F et al. Eighteen years of liver transplantation experience in patients with advanced Budd-Chiari syndrome. Liver Transpl. 2008 Feb;14(2):144–50. [PMID: 18236386]
Valla DC. Budd-Chiari syndrome and veno-occlusive disease/sinusoidal obstruction syndrome. Gut. 2008 Oct;57(10):1469–78. [PMID: 18583397]
Valla DC. Primary Budd-Chiari syndrome. J Hepatol. 2009 Jan;50(1):195–203. [PMID: 19012988]

THE LIVER IN HEART FAILURE

Shock liver, or ischemic hepatopathy, results from an acute fall in cardiac output due, for example, to acute myocardial infarction or arrhythmia, usually in a patient with passive congestion of the liver. Clinical hypotension may be absent (or unwitnessed). In some cases, the precipitating event is arterial hypoxemia due to respiratory failure, sleep apnea, septic shock, severe anemia, heat stroke, carbon monoxide poisoning, cocaine use, or bacterial endocarditis. The hallmark is a rapid and striking elevation of serum aminotransferase levels (often > 5000 units/L); an early rapid rise in the serum lactate dehydrogenase level is also typical, but elevations of serum alkaline phosphatase and bilirubin are usually mild. The prothrombin time may be prolonged, and encephalopathy or hepatopulmonary syndrome may develop. The mortality rate due to the underlying disease is high, but in patients who recover, the aminotransferase levels return to normal quickly, usually within 1 week—in contrast to viral hepatitis.

In patients with passive congestion of the liver due to right-sided heart failure, the serum bilirubin level may be elevated, occasionally as high as 40 mg/dL, due in part to hypoxia of perivenular hepatocytes. Serum alkaline phosphatase levels are normal or slightly elevated. Hepatojugular reflux is present, and with tricuspid regurgitation the liver may be pulsatile. Ascites may be out of proportion to peripheral edema, with a high serum ascites-albumin gradient (≥ 1.1) and a protein content of more than 2.5 g/dL. In severe cases, signs of encephalopathy may develop.

Malnick S et al. The involvement of the liver in systemic diseases. J Clin Gastroenterol. 2008 Jan;42(1):69–80. [PMID: 18097294]
Norman D et al. Serum aminotransferase levels are associated with markers of hypoxia in patients with obstructive sleep apnea. Sleep. 2008 Jan 1;31(1):121–6. [PMID: 18220085]

NONCIRRHOTIC PORTAL HYPERTENSION

Noncirrhotic portal hypertension must be considered in the differential diagnosis of splenomegaly or upper gastrointestinal bleeding due to esophageal or gastric varices in patients with little if any liver dysfunction. This syndrome may be due to extrahepatic portal vein obstruction (portal vein thrombosis often with cavernous transformation [portal cavernoma]), splenic vein obstruction (presenting as gastric varices without esophageal varices), schistosomiasis, noncirrhotic portal fibrosis (hepatoportal sclerosis), nodular regenerative hyperplasia, or arterial-portal vein fistula. Acute portal vein thrombosis usually causes abdominal pain. Aside from splenomegaly, the physical findings are not remarkable, although hepatic decompensation can follow severe gastrointestinal bleeding or a concurrent hepatic disorder, and intestinal infarction may occur when portal vein thrombosis is associated with mesenteric venous thrombosis. Minimal hepatic encephalopathy is reported to be common in patients with noncirrhotic portal vein thrombosis. Endoscopy shows esophageal or gastric varices. The liver tests are usually normal, but there may be findings of hypersplenism. Color Doppler ultrasound and contrast-enhanced CT are usually the initial diagnostic tests for portal vein thrombosis. Magnetic resonance angiography (MRA) of the portal system is generally confirmatory. Endoscopic ultrasound may be helpful in some cases. In patients with jaundice, magnetic resonance cholangiography may demonstrate compression of the bile duct by a large portal cavernoma. Needle biopsy of the liver may be indicated to diagnose schistosomiasis, nodular regenerative hyperplasia, and noncirrhotic intrahepatic portal sclerosis and may demonstrate sinusoidal dilatation. An underlying hypercoagulable state is found in many patients with portal vein thrombosis; this includes myeloproliferative disorders (often associated with a specific mutation [*V617F*] in the gene coding for JAK2 tyrosine kinase), mutation G20210A of prothrombin, factor V Leiden mutation, protein C and S deficiency, antiphospholipid syndrome, mutation TT677 of methylenetetrahydrofolate reductase, elevated factor VIII levels, hyperhomocysteinemia, and a mutation in the gene that codes for thrombin-activatable fibrinolysis inhibitor. It is possible, however, that deficiency of protein C and S—as well as of antithrombin—is a secondary phenomenon due to portosystemic shunting and reduced hepatic blood flow. Portal vein thrombosis may occur in up to 15% of patients with cirrhosis and may be associated with hepatocellular carcinoma. Other risk factors are oral contraceptives, pregnancy, chronic inflammatory diseases, and other malignancies. Splenic vein thrombosis may complicate pancreatitis or pancreatic cancer. Pylephlebitis (septic thrombophlebitis of the portal vein) may complicate intra-abdominal inflammatory disorders such as appendicitis or diverticulitis, particularly when anaerobic organisms are involved. Nodular regenerative hyperplasia results from altered hepatic perfusion and can be associated with collagen vascular diseases, myeloproliferative disorders, and drugs, including azathioprine, 5-fluorouracil, and oxaliplatin. In patients infected with HIV, exposure to didanosine has been reported to account for some cases of noncirrhotic portal hypertension due to nodular regenerative hyperplasia.

If splenic vein thrombosis is the cause of variceal bleeding, splenectomy is curative. For other causes of noncirrhotic portal hypertension, band ligation or sclerotherapy followed by β-blockers to reduce portal pressure is initiated for variceal bleeding, and portosystemic shunting (including TIPS) is reserved for failures of endoscopic therapy; rarely progressive liver dysfunction requires liver transplantation. Anticoagulation or thrombolytic therapy may be indicated for isolated acute portal vein and possibly acute splenic vein thrombosis if a hypercoagulable disorder is identified. Long-term anticoagulation may be considered for affected patients with a hypercoagulable state.

When to Refer

All patients with noncirrhotic portal hypertension should be referred.

Garcia-Pagán JC et al. Extrahepatic portal vein thrombosis. Semin Liver Dis. 2008 Aug;28(3):282–92. [PMID: 18814081]
P'ng S et al. Undiagnosed myeloproliferative disease in cases of intra-abdominal thrombosis: the utility of the JAK2 617F mutation. Clin Gastroenterol Hepatol. 2008 Apr;6(4):472–5. [PMID: 18328792]
Saifee S et al. Noncirrhotic portal hypertension in patients with human immunodeficiency virus-1 infection. Clin Gastroenterol Hepatol. 2008 Oct;6(10):1167–9. [PMID: 18639498]

PYOGENIC HEPATIC ABSCESS

 ESSENTIALS OF DIAGNOSIS

▶ Fever, right upper quadrant pain, jaundice.

▶ Often in setting of biliary disease but up to 40% are "cryptogenic" in origin.

▶ Detected by imaging studies.

General Considerations

The liver can be invaded by bacteria via (1) the common duct (ascending cholangitis); (2) the portal vein (pylephlebitis); (3) the hepatic artery, secondary to bacteremia; (4) direct extension from an infectious process; and (5) traumatic implantation of bacteria through the abdominal wall. Risk factors for liver abscess include older age and male gender. Predisposing conditions include malignancy, diabetes mellitus, inflammatory bowel disease, cirrhosis, and liver transplantation.

Ascending cholangitis resulting from biliary obstruction due to a stone, stricture, or neoplasm is the most common identifiable cause of hepatic abscess in the United States. In 10% of cases, liver abscess is secondary to appendicitis or diverticulitis. At least 40% of abscesses have no demonstrable cause and are classified as cryptogenic. A dental source is identified in some cases. The most frequently encountered organisms are *E coli*, *Klebsiella pneumoniae*, *Proteus vulgaris*, *Enterobacter aerogenes*, and multiple microaerophilic and anaerobic species (eg, *Streptococcus milleri*). Liver abscess caused by virulent strains of *K pneumoniae* may be associated with septic ocular or central nervous system complications. *Staphylococcus aureus* is usually the causative organism in patients with chronic granulomatous disease. Unusual causative organisms include *Salmonella*, *Haemophilus*, and *Yersinia*. Hepatic candidiasis, tuberculosis, and actinomycosis are seen in immunocompromised patients and those with hematologic malignancies. Rarely, hepatocellular carcinoma can present as a pyogenic abscess because of tumor necrosis, biliary obstruction, and superimposed bacterial infection (see Chapter 39). The possibility of an amebic liver abscess must always be considered (see Chapter 35).

Clinical Findings

A. Symptoms and Signs

The presentation is often insidious. Fever is almost always present and may antedate other symptoms or signs. Pain may be a prominent complaint and is localized to the right hypochondrium or epigastric area. Jaundice, tenderness in the right upper abdomen, and either steady or swinging fever are the chief physical findings.

B. Laboratory Findings

Laboratory examination reveals leukocytosis with a shift to the left. Liver biochemical tests are nonspecifically abnormal. Blood cultures are positive in 50–100% of cases.

C. Imaging

Chest roentgenograms usually reveal elevation of the diaphragm if the abscess is on the right side. Ultrasound, CT, or MRI may reveal the presence of intrahepatic defects. On MRI, characteristic findings include high signal intensity on T2-weighted images and rim enhancement. The characteristic CT appearance of hepatic candidiasis, usually seen in the setting of systemic candidiasis, is that of multiple "bull's-eyes," but imaging studies may be negative in neutropenic patients.

Treatment

Treatment should consist of antimicrobial agents (generally a third-generation cephalosporin such as cefoperazone 1-2 g intravenously every 12 hours and metronidazole 500 mg intravenously every 6 hours) that are effective against coliform organisms and anaerobes. Antibiotics are administered for 2–3 weeks, and sometimes up to 6 weeks. If the abscess is at least 5 cm in diameter or the response to antibiotic therapy is not rapid, intermittent needle aspiration or catheter or surgical (eg, laparoscopic) drainage should be done. Other suggested indications for abscess drainage are patient age of at least 55 years, symptom duration of at least 7 days, and involvement of both lobes of the liver. The underlying source (eg, biliary disease, dental infection) should be identified and treated. The mortality rate is still substantial ($\geq 8\%$ in most studies) and is highest in patients with underlying biliary malignancy or severe multiorgan dysfunction. Hepatic candidiasis often responds to intravenous amphotericin B (total dose of 2–9 g). Fungal abscesses are associated with mortality rates of up to 50% and are treated with intravenous amphotericin B and drainage.

When to Admit

Nearly all patients with pyogenic hepatic abscess should be hospitalized.

Hope WW et al. Optimal treatment of hepatic abscess. Am Surg. 2008 Feb;74(2):178–82. [PMID: 18306874]

Khan R et al. Predictive factors for early aspiration in liver abscess. World J Gastroenterol. 2008 Apr 7;14(13):2089–93. [PMID: 18395912]

Lee SS-J. Predictors of septic metastatic infection and mortality among patients with *Klebsiella pneumoniae* liver abscess. Clin Infect Dis. 2008 Sep 1;47(5):642–50. [PMID: 18643760]

BENIGN LIVER NEOPLASMS

Benign hepatic neoplasms must be distinguished from hepatocellular carcinoma and metastases (see Chapter 39). The most common benign neoplasm of the liver is the **cavernous hemangioma,** often an incidental finding on ultrasound or CT scan. This lesion may enlarge in women who take hormonal therapy and must be differentiated from other space-occupying intrahepatic lesions, usually by contrast-enhanced MRI, CT, or ultrasound. Rarely, fine-needle biopsy is necessary to differentiate these lesions and does not appear to carry an increased risk of bleeding. Surgical resection of cavernous hemangiomas is rarely necessary but may be required for abdominal pain or rapid enlargement, to exclude malignancy, or to treat Kasabach-Merritt syndrome (consumptive coagulopathy complicating a hemangioma).

In addition to rare instances of sinusoidal dilatation and peliosis hepatis, two distinct benign lesions with characteristic clinical, radiologic, and histopathologic features have been described in women taking oral contraceptives—focal nodular hyperplasia and hepatic adenoma. **Focal nodular hyperplasia** occurs at all ages and is probably not caused by the oral contraceptives. It is often asymptomatic and appears as a hypervascular mass, often with a central hypodense "stellate" scar on CT scan or MRI. Microscopically, focal nodular hyperplasia consists of hyperplastic units of hepatocytes with a central stellate scar containing proliferating bile ducts. It is not a true neoplasm but a nonspecific reaction to altered blood flow is associated with an elevated angiopoietin 1/angiopoietin 2 mRNA ratio and may also occur in patients with cirrhosis, with exposure to certain drugs such as azathioprine, and in antiphospholipid syndrome. The prevalence of hepatic hemangiomas is increased in patients with focal nodular hyperplasia.

Hepatic adenoma occurs most commonly in the third and fourth decades of life and is usually caused by oral contraceptives; acute abdominal pain may occur if the tumor undergoes necrosis or hemorrhage. The tumor may be associated with mutations in: (1) the gene coding for hepatocyte nuclear factor α (*HNF1α*) (characterized by steatosis and a low risk of malignant transformation); (2) the gene coding for β-catenin (characterized by a high rate of malignant transformation); or (3) neither gene (designated inflammatory adenoma [previously termed "telangiectatic focal nodular hyperplasia"], which is associated with a high body mass index and serum biomarkers of inflammation such as C-reactive protein). Rare instances of multiple hepatic adenomas in association with maturity-onset diabetes of the young occur in families with a germline mutation in *HNF1α*. Hepatic adenomas also occur in patients with glycogen storage disease and familial adenomatous polyposis. The tumor is hypovascular and reveals a cold defect on liver scan. Grossly, the cut surface appears structureless. As seen microscopically, the hepatic adenoma consists of sheets of hepatocytes without portal tracts or central veins.

The only physical finding in focal nodular hyperplasia or hepatic adenoma is a palpable abdominal mass in a minority of cases. Liver function is usually normal. Arterial phase helical CT and MRI with contrast can distinguish an adenoma from focal nodular hyperplasia in 80–90% of cases and may suggest a specific subtype of adenoma (eg, homogeneous fat pattern in *HNF1α*-mutated adenomas and marked and persistent arterial enhancement in inflammatory adenomas).

Cystic neoplasms of the liver, such as cystadenoma and cystadenocarcinoma, must be distinguished from simple and echinococcal cysts and von Meyenburg complexes (hamartomas).

Treatment of focal nodular hyperplasia is resection only in the symptomatic patient. The prognosis is excellent. Hepatic adenoma often undergoes necrosis and rupture, and resection is advised if the tumor is > 5 cm in diameter, even in asymptomatic persons, or if symptomatic. In selected cases, laparoscopic resection or percutaneous radiofrequency ablation may be feasible. Regression of benign hepatic tumors may follow cessation of oral contraceptives.

When to Refer

- Diagnostic uncertainty.
- For surgery.

When to Admit

- Severe pain.
- Rupture.

Bahirwani R et al. Review article: the evaluation of solitary liver masses. Aliment Pharmacol Ther. 2008 Oct 15;28(8):953–65. [PMID: 18643922]

Laumonier H et al. Hepatocellular adenomas: magnetic resonance imaging features as a function of molecular pathological classification. Hepatology. 2008 Sep;48(3):808–18. [PMID: 18688875]

DISEASES OF THE BILIARY TRACT

See Chapter 39 for Carcinoma of the Biliary Tract.

CHOLELITHIASIS (Gallstones)

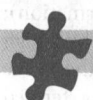

ESSENTIALS OF DIAGNOSIS

- ▶ Often asymptomatic.
- ▶ Classic biliary pain characterized by infrequent episodes of steady severe pain in epigastrium or right upper quadrant with radiation to right scapula.
- ▶ Detected on ultrasound.

General Considerations

Gallstones are more common in women than in men and increase in incidence in both sexes and all races with aging. In the United States, the prevalence of gallstones is 5.5% in men and 8.6% in women, with the highest rates in persons over age 60 and higher rates in Mexican-Americans than in non-Hispanic whites and African Americans. Although cholesterol gallstones are less common in black people, cholelithiasis attributable to hemolysis occurs in over a third of individuals with sickle cell anemia. Native Americans of both the Northern and Southern Hemispheres have a high rate of cholesterol cholelithiasis, probably because of a predisposition resulting from "thrifty" (LITH) genes that promote efficient calorie utilization and fat storage. As many as 75% of Pima and other American Indian women over the age of 25 years have cholelithiasis. Other genetic mutations that predispose persons to gallstones have been identified. Obesity is a risk factor for gallstones, especially in women. Rapid weight loss, as occurs after bariatric surgery, also increases the risk of symptomatic gallstone formation. There is evidence that glucose intolerance and elevated serum insulin levels (insulin resistance) are risk factors for gallstones, and a high intake of carbohydrate and high dietary glycemic load increase the risk of cholecystectomy in women. The incidence of cholelithiasis is increased in patients with diabetes mellitus, and the prevalence of gallbladder disease is increased in men (but not women) with cirrhosis and hepatitis C virus infection. A low-carbohydrate diet, physical activity, and cardiorespiratory fitness may help prevent gallstones. Consumption of caffeinated coffee appears to protect against gallstones in women, and a high intake of magnesium and of polyunsaturated and monounsaturated fats reduces the risk of gallstones in men. A diet high in fiber, as well as fruits and vegetables, reduces the risk of cholecystectomy in women. Hypertriglyceridemia may promote gallstone formation by impairing gallbladder motility. The incidence of gallstones is high in individuals with Crohn disease; approximately one-third of those with inflammatory involvement of the terminal ileum have gallstones due to disruption of bile salt resorption that results in decreased solubility of the bile. Drugs such as clofibrate, octreotide, and ceftriaxone can cause gallstones. In contrast, aspirin and other nonsteroidal anti-inflammatory drugs may protect against gallstones. Prolonged fasting (over 5–10 days) can lead to formation of biliary "sludge" (microlithiasis), which usually resolves with refeeding but can lead to gallstones or biliary symptoms. Pregnancy, particularly in obese women and those with insulin resistance, is associated with an increased risk of gallstones and of symptomatic gallbladder disease. Hormone replacement therapy appears to increase the risk of gallbladder disease and need for cholecystectomy; the risk is lower with transdermal than oral therapy.

Gallstones are classified according to their predominant chemical composition as cholesterol or calcium bilirubinate stones. The latter comprise less than 20% of the stones found in Europe or the United States but 30–40% of stones found in Japan.

Clinical Findings

Table 16–7 lists the clinical and laboratory features of several diseases of the biliary tract as well as their treatment. Cholelithiasis is frequently asymptomatic and is discovered in the course of routine radiographic study, operation, or autopsy. There is generally no need for prophylactic cholecystectomy in an asymptomatic person unless the gallbladder is calcified, gallstones are over 3 cm in diameter, or the patient is a Native American or a candidate for bariatric surgery or cardiac transplantation. Symptoms (biliary pain) develop in 10–25% of patients (1-4% annually), and acute cholecystitis develops in 20% of these symptomatic persons over time. Occasionally, small intestinal obstruction due to "gallstone ileus" (known as Bouveret syndrome when the obstructing stone is in pylorus or duodenum) presents as the initial manifestation of cholelithiasis.

Treatment

Laparoscopic cholecystectomy is the treatment of choice for symptomatic gallbladder disease. Patients may go home within 1 day of the procedure and return to work within days (instead of weeks for those undergoing standard open cholecystectomy). The procedure is often performed on an outpatient basis and is suitable for most patients, including those with acute cholecystitis. Conversion to a conventional open cholecystectomy may be necessary in 2–8% of cases (higher for acute cholecystitis than for uncomplicated cholelithiasis). Bile duct injuries occur in 0.1% of cases done by experienced surgeons. Cholecystectomy may increase the risk of esophageal, proximal small intestinal,

Table 16–7. Diseases of the biliary tract.

	Clinical Features	Laboratory Features	Diagnosis	Treatment
Gallstones	Asymptomatic	Normal	Ultrasound	None
Gallstones	Biliary pain	Normal	Ultrasound	Laparoscopic cholecystectomy
Cholesterolosis of gallbladder	Usually asymptomatic	Normal	Oral cholecystography	None
Adenomyomatosis	May cause biliary pain	Normal	Oral cholecystography	Laparoscopic cholecystectomy if symptomatic
Porcelain gallbladder	Usually asymptomatic, high risk of gallbladder cancer	Normal	Radiograph or CT	Laparoscopic cholecystectomy
Acute cholecystitis	Epigastric or right upper quadrant pain, nausea, vomiting, fever, Murphy sign	Leukocytosis	Ultrasound, HIDA scan	Antibiotics, laparoscopic cholecystectomy
Chronic cholecystitis	Biliary pain, constant epigastric or right upper quadrant pain, nausea	Normal	Ultrasound (stones), oral cholecystography (nonfunctioning gallbladder)	Laparoscopic cholecystectomy
Choledocholithiasis	Asymptomatic or biliary pain, jaundice, fever; gallstone pancreatitis	Cholestatic liver function tests; leukocytosis and positive blood cultures in cholangitis; elevated amylase and lipase in pancreatitis	Ultrasound (dilated ducts), endoscopic ultrasound, MRCP, ERCP	Endoscopic sphincterotomy and stone extraction; antibiotics for cholangitis

ERCP, endoscopic retrograde cholangiopancreatography; HIDA, hepatic iminodiacetic acid; MRCP, magnetic resonance cholangiopancreatography.

and colonic adenocarcinomas because of increased duodenogastric reflux and changes in intestinal exposure to bile. In pregnant patients a conservative approach to biliary pain is advised, but for patients with repeated attacks of biliary pain or acute cholecystitis, cholecystectomy can be performed—even by the laparoscopic route—preferably in the second trimester. Enterolithotomy alone is considered adequate treatment in most patients with gallstone ileus.

Cheno- and ursodeoxycholic acids are bile salts that when given orally for up to 2 years dissolve some cholesterol stones and may be considered in occasional, selected patients who refuse cholecystectomy. The dose is 7 mg/kg/d of each or 8–13 mg/kg of ursodeoxycholic acid in divided doses daily. They are most effective in patients with a functioning gallbladder, as determined by gallbladder visualization on oral cholecystography, and multiple small "floating" gallstones (representing not more than 15% of patients with gallstones). In half of patients, gallstones recur within 5 years after treatment is stopped. Ursodeoxycholic acid, 500–600 mg daily, reduces the risk of gallstone formation with rapid weight loss.

Lithotripsy in combination with bile salt therapy for single radiolucent stones less than 20 mm in diameter was an option in the past but is no longer generally used in the United States.

▶ When to Refer

Patients should be referred when they require surgery.

Keus F et al. Systematic review: open, small-incision or laparoscopic cholecystectomy for symptomatic cholecystolithiasis. Aliment Pharmacol Ther. 2009 Feb 15;29(4):359–78. [PMID: 19035965]

Liu B et al. Gallbladder disease and use of transdermal versus oral hormone replacement therapy in postmenopausal women: prospective cohort study. BMJ. 2008 Jul 10;337:a386. [PMID: 18617493]

Tsai CJ et al. Long-term effect of magnesium consumption on the risk of symptomatic gallstone disease among men. Am J Gastroenterol. 2008 Feb;103(2):375–82. [PMID: 18076730]

Williams PT. Independent effects of cardiorespiratory fitness, vigorous physical activity, and body mass index on clinical gallbladder disease risk. Am J Gastroenterol. 2008 Sep;103(9):2239–47. [PMID: 18637096]

ACUTE CHOLECYSTITIS

 ESSENTIALS OF DIAGNOSIS

▶ Steady, severe pain and tenderness in the right hypochondrium or epigastrium.

▶ Nausea and vomiting.

▶ Fever and leukocytosis.

▶ General Considerations

Cholecystitis is associated with gallstones in over 90% of cases. It occurs when a stone becomes impacted in the cystic duct and inflammation develops behind the obstruction. Acalculous cholecystitis should be considered when unexplained fever or right upper quadrant pain occurs within 2–4 weeks of major surgery or in a critically ill patient who has had no oral intake for a prolonged period; multiorgan failure is often present. Acute cholecystitis caused by infectious agents (eg, cytomegalovirus, cryptosporidiosis, or microsporidiosis) may occur in patients with AIDS.

▶ Clinical Findings

A. Symptoms and Signs

The acute attack is often precipitated by a large or fatty meal and is characterized by the sudden appearance of steady pain localized to the epigastrium or right hypochondrium, which may gradually subside over a period of 12–18 hours. Vomiting occurs in about 75% of patients and in half of instances affords variable relief. Right upper quadrant abdominal tenderness (often with Murphy sign, or inhibition of inspiration by pain on palpation of the right upper quadrant) is almost always present and is usually associated with muscle guarding and rebound tenderness. A palpable gallbladder is present in about 15% of cases. Jaundice is present in about 25% of cases and, when persistent or severe, suggests the possibility of choledocholithiasis. Fever is typical.

B. Laboratory Findings

The white blood cell count is usually high (12,000–15,000/mcL). Total serum bilirubin values of 1–4 mg/dL may be seen even in the absence of bile duct obstruction. Serum aminotransferase and alkaline phosphatase are often elevated—the former as high as 300 units/mL, or even higher when associated with ascending cholangitis. Serum amylase may also be moderately elevated.

C. Imaging

Plain films of the abdomen may show radiopaque gallstones in 15% of cases. ^{99m}Tc hepatobiliary imaging (using iminodiacetic acid compounds), also known as the hepatic iminodiacetic acid (HIDA) scan, is useful in demonstrating an obstructed cystic duct, which is the cause of acute cholecystitis in most patients. This test is reliable if the bilirubin is under 5 mg/dL (98% sensitivity and 81% specificity for acute cholecystitis). False-positive results can occur with prolonged fasting, liver disease, and chronic cholecystitis, and the specificity can be improved by intravenous administration of morphine, which induces spasm of the sphincter of Oddi. Right upper quadrant abdominal ultrasound, which is often performed first, may show the presence of gallstones but is not as sensitive for acute cholecystitis (67% sensitivity, 82% specificity); findings suggestive of acute cholecystitis are gallbladder wall thickening, pericholecystic fluid, and sonographic Murphy sign.

▶ Differential Diagnosis

The disorders most likely to be confused with acute cholecystitis are perforated peptic ulcer, acute pancreatitis, appendicitis in a high-lying appendix, perforated colonic carcinoma or diverticulum of the hepatic flexure, liver abscess, hepatitis, pneumonia with pleurisy on the right side, and even myocardial ischemia. Definite localization of pain and tenderness in the right hypochondrium, with radiation around to the infrascapular area, strongly favors the diagnosis of acute cholecystitis. True cholecystitis without stones suggests the rare possibility of polyarteritis nodosa affecting the cystic artery.

▶ Complications

A. Gangrene of the Gallbladder

Continuation or progression of right upper quadrant abdominal pain, tenderness, muscle guarding, fever, and leukocytosis after 24–48 hours suggests severe inflammation and possible gangrene of the gallbladder, resulting from ischemia due to splanchnic vasoconstriction and intravascular coagulation. Necrosis may occasionally develop without definite signs in the obese, diabetic, elderly, or immunosuppressed patient. Gangrene may lead to gallbladder perforation, usually with formation of a pericholecystic abscess and rarely to generalized peritonitis. Other serious acute complications include emphysematous cholecystitis (secondary infection with a gas-forming organism) and empyema.

B. Chronic Cholecystitis and Other Complications

Chronic cholecystitis results from repeated episodes of acute cholecystitis or chronic irritation of the gallbladder wall by stones and is characterized pathologically by varying degrees of chronic inflammation of the gallbladder. Calculi are usually present. In about 4–5% of cases, the villi of the gallbladder undergo polypoid enlargement due to deposition of cholesterol that may be visible to the naked eye ("strawberry gallbladder," cholesterolosis). In other instances, hyperplasia of all or part of the gallbladder wall may be so marked as to give the appearance of a myoma (adenomyomatosis). Hydrops of the gallbladder results when acute cholecystitis subsides but cystic duct obstruction persists, producing distention of the gallbladder with a clear mucoid fluid. Occasionally, a stone in the neck of the gallbladder may compress the bile duct and cause jaundice (Mirizzi syndrome). Xanthogranulomatous cholecystitis is a rare variant of chronic cholecystitis characterized by grayish-yellow nodules or streaks, representing lipid-laden macrophages, in the wall of the gallbladder.

Cholelithiasis with chronic cholecystitis may be associated with acute exacerbations of gallbladder inflammation, bile duct stone, fistulization to the bowel, pancreatitis and, rarely, carcinoma of the gallbladder. Calcified (porcelain) gallbladder has generally been thought to have a high association with gallbladder carcinoma and to be an indication for cholecystectomy, although the risk of gallbladder cancer may be higher when calcification is mucosal rather than intramural.

▶ Treatment

Acute cholecystitis will usually subside on a conservative regimen (withholding of oral feedings, intravenous alimentation, analgesics, and intravenous antibiotics—generally a second- or third-generation cephalosporin such as cefoperazone, 1-2 g intravenously every 12 hours, with the addition of metronidazole, 500 mg intravenously every 6 hours); in severe cases, a fluoroquinolone such as ciprofloxacin, 250 mg intravenously every 12 hours, plus metronidazole may be given) Morphine or meperidine may be administered for pain. Because of the high risk of recurrent attacks (up to 10% by 1 month and over 30% by 1 year), cholecystectomy—generally laparoscopically—should generally be performed within 2–4 days after hospitalization. If nonsurgical treatment has been elected, the patient (especially if diabetic or elderly) should be watched carefully for recurrent symptoms, evidence of gangrene of the gallbladder, or cholangitis. In high-risk patients, ultrasound-guided aspiration of the gallbladder, if feasible, percutaneous cholecystostomy, or endoscopic insertion of a stent into the gallbladder may postpone or even avoid the need for surgery. Immediate cholecystectomy is mandatory when there is evidence of gangrene or perforation.

Surgical treatment of chronic cholecystitis is the same as for acute cholecystitis. If indicated, cholangiography can be performed during laparoscopic cholecystectomy. Choledocholithiasis can also be excluded by either preoperative or postoperative ERCP or MRCP.

► Prognosis

The overall mortality rate of cholecystectomy is less than 0.2%, but hepatobiliary tract surgery is a more formidable procedure in the elderly, in whom mortality rates are higher. A technically successful surgical procedure in an appropriately selected patient is generally followed by complete resolution of symptoms.

► When to Admit

All patients with acute cholecystitis should be hospitalized.

Hirota M et al. Diagnostic criteria and severity assessment of acute cholecystitis: Tokyo Guidelines. J Hepatobiliary Pancreat Surg. 2007;14(1):78–82. [PMID: 17252300]

Siddiqui T et al. Early versus delayed laparoscopic cholecystectomy for acute cholecystitis: a meta-analysis of randomized clinical trials. Am J Surg. 2008 Jan;195(1):40–7. [PMID: 18070735]

Strasberg SM. Clinical practice. Acute calculous cholecystitis. N Engl J Med. 2008 Jun 26;358(26):2804–11. [PMID: 18579815]

Takada T et al. Background: Tokyo Guidelines for the management of acute cholangitis and cholecystitis. J Hepatobiliary Pancreat Surg. 2007;14(1):1–10. [PMID: 17252291]

PRE- & POSTCHOLECYSTECTOMY SYNDROMES

1. Precholecystectomy

In a small group of patients (mostly women) with biliary pain, conventional radiographic studies of the upper gastrointestinal tract and gallbladder—including cholangiography—are unremarkable. In some such cases, emptying of the gallbladder may be markedly reduced on gallbladder scintigraphy following injection of cholecystokinin; cholecystectomy may be curative. Histologic examination of the resected gallbladder may show chronic cholecystitis or microlithiasis. An additional diagnostic consideration is sphincter of Oddi dysfunction (see below).

2. Postcholecystectomy

Following cholecystectomy, some patients complain of continuing symptoms, ie, right upper quadrant pain, flatulence, and fatty food intolerance. The persistence of symptoms in this group of patients suggests the possibility of an incorrect diagnosis prior to cholecystectomy, eg, esophagitis, pancreatitis, radiculopathy, or functional bowel disease. Choledocholithiasis or bile duct stricture should be ruled out. Pain may also be associated with dilation of the cystic duct remnant, neuroma formation in the ductal wall, foreign body granuloma, or traction on the bile duct by a long cystic duct.

The clinical presentation of right upper quadrant pain, chills, fever, or jaundice suggests biliary tract disease. Endoscopic ultrasonography or retrograde cholangiography may be necessary to demonstrate a stone or stricture. Biliary pain associated with elevated liver tests or a dilated bile duct in the absence of an obstructing lesion suggests sphincter of Oddi dysfunction. Biliary manometry may be useful for documenting elevated baseline sphincter of Oddi pressures typical of sphincter dysfunction when biliary pain is associated with elevated liver tests (twofold) or a dilated bile duct (> 12 mm) (type II sphincter of Oddi dysfunction) but is not necessary when both are present (type I sphincter of Oddi dysfunction) and is associated with a high risk of pancreatitis. In the absence of either elevated liver tests or a dilated bile duct (type III sphincter of Oddi dysfunction), a nonbiliary source of symptoms should be suspected. (Analogous criteria have been developed for pancreatic sphincter dysfunction.) Biliary scintigraphy after intravenous administration of morphine and MRCP following intravenous administration of secretin are under study as screening tests for sphincter dysfunction. Endoscopic sphincterotomy is most likely to relieve symptoms in patients with types I or II sphincter of Oddi dysfunction or an elevated sphincter of Oddi pressure, although many patients continue to have some pain. In some cases, treatment with calcium channel blockers, long-acting nitrates, or possibly injection of the sphincter with botulinum toxin may be beneficial. In refractory cases, surgical sphincteroplasty or removal of the cystic duct remnant may be considered.

► When to Refer

Patients with sphincter of Oddi dysfunction should be referred for diagnostic procedures.

Bosch A et al. The sphincter of Oddi. Dig Dis Sci. 2007 May;52(5):1211-8. [PMID: 17356921]

Saad AM et al. Pancreatic duct stent placement prevents post-ERCP pancreatitis in patients with suspected sphincter of Oddi dysfunction but normal manometry results. Gastrointest Endosc. 2008 Feb;67(2):255–61. [PMID: 18028920]

CHOLEDOCHOLITHIASIS & CHOLANGITIS

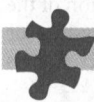

ESSENTIALS OF DIAGNOSIS

▶ Often a history of biliary pain or jaundice.

▶ Sudden onset of severe right upper quadrant or epigastric pain, which may radiate to the right scapula or shoulder.

▶ Occasional patients present with painless jaundice.

▶ Nausea and vomiting.

▶ Fever, which may be followed by hypothermia and gram-negative shock, jaundice, and leukocytosis.

▶ Stones in bile duct most reliably detected by ERCP or endoscopic ultrasound.

General Considerations

About 15% of patients with gallstones have choledocholithiasis (bile duct stones). The percentage rises with age, and the frequency in elderly people with gallstones may be as high as 50%. Bile duct stones usually originate in the gallbladder but may also form spontaneously in the bile duct after cholecystectomy. The risk is increased twofold in persons with a juxtapapillary duodenal diverticulum. Symptoms result if there is obstruction.

Clinical Findings

A. Symptoms and Signs

A history of biliary pain or prior jaundice may be obtained. Biliary pain results from rapid increases in bile duct pressure due to obstructed bile flow. The features that suggest the presence of a bile duct stone are: (1) frequently recurring attacks of right upper abdominal pain that is severe and persists for hours; (2) chills and fever associated with severe pain; and (3) a history of jaundice associated with episodes of abdominal pain. The combination of pain, fever (and chills), and jaundice represents **Charcot triad** and denotes the classic picture of cholangitis. The addition of altered mental status and hypotension (Reynold pentad) signifies acute suppurative cholangitis and is an endoscopic emergency.

Hepatomegaly may be present in calculous biliary obstruction, and tenderness is usually present in the right upper quadrant and epigastrium. Bile duct obstruction lasting longer than 30 days results in liver damage leading to cirrhosis. Hepatic failure with portal hypertension occurs in untreated cases.

B. Laboratory Findings

Acute obstruction of the bile duct typically produces a transient albeit striking increase in serum aminotransferase levels (often > 1000 units/L). Bilirubinuria and elevation of serum bilirubin are present if the bile duct remains obstructed; levels commonly fluctuate. Serum alkaline phosphatase levels rise more slowly. Not uncommonly,

serum amylase elevations are present because of secondary pancreatitis. When extrahepatic obstruction persists for more than a few weeks, differentiation of obstruction from chronic cholestatic liver disease becomes more difficult. Leukocytosis is present in patients with cholangitis. Prolongation of the prothrombin time can result from the obstructed flow of bile to the intestine. In contrast to hepatocellular dysfunction, hypoprothrombinemia due to obstructive jaundice will respond to 10 mg of parenteral vitamin K or water-soluble oral vitamin K (phytonadione, 5 mg) within 24–36 hours.

C. Imaging

Ultrasonography and CT scan may demonstrate dilated bile ducts, and radionuclide imaging may show impaired bile flow. Endoscopic ultrasonography, helical CT, and magnetic resonance cholangiography are accurate in demonstrating bile duct stones and may be used in patients thought to be at low or intermediate risk for choledocholithiasis. ERCP (occasionally with intraductal ultrasound) or percutaneous transhepatic cholangiography provides the most direct and accurate means of determining the cause, location, and extent of obstruction. If the likelihood that obstruction is caused by a stone or that cholangitis is present is high, ERCP is the procedure of choice because it permits sphincterotomy with stone extraction or stent placement.

Differential Diagnosis

The most common cause of obstructive jaundice is a bile duct stone. Next in frequency are neoplasms of the pancreas, ampulla of Vater, or bile duct. Extrinsic compression of the bile duct may result from metastatic carcinoma (usually from the gastrointestinal tract or breast) involving porta hepatis lymph nodes or, rarely, from a large duodenal diverticulum. Gallbladder cancer extending into the bile duct often presents as obstructive jaundice. Chronic cholestatic liver diseases (primarily biliary cirrhosis, sclerosing cholangitis, drug-induced) must be considered. Hepatocellular jaundice can usually be differentiated by the history, clinical findings, and liver tests, but liver biopsy is necessary on occasion. Recurrent pyogenic cholangitis should be considered in persons from Asia (and occasionally elsewhere) with intrahepatic biliary stones (particularly in the left ductal system) and with recurrent cholangitis.

Treatment

Bile duct stone in a patient with cholelithiasis or cholecystitis is usually treated by endoscopic sphincterotomy and stone extraction followed by laparoscopic cholecystectomy. For the elderly (> 70 years) or poor-risk patient with cholelithiasis and choledocholithiasis, however, cholecystectomy may be deferred after endoscopic sphincterotomy because the risk of subsequent cholecystitis is low. ERCP with sphincterotomy should be performed before cholecystectomy in patients with gallstones and jaundice (serum total bilirubin > 5 mg/dL), a dilated bile duct (> 7 mm), or stones in the bile duct seen on ultrasound or CT scan. (Stones may ultimately recur in up to 12% of patients, particularly in the elderly, when the bile duct diameter is ≥ 15 mm, or when brown pigment stones are found at time of the initial sphincterotomy.) Endoscopic balloon dilation of the sphincter of Oddi may be associated with a higher rate of pancreatitis than endoscopic sphincterotomy and is generally reserved for patients with coagulopathy, in whom the risk of bleeding is lower with balloon dilation than with sphincterotomy. In patients with biliary pancreatitis that resolves rapidly, the stone usually passes into the intestine, and ERCP prior to cholecystectomy is not necessary if an intraoperative cholangiogram is done.

Choledocholithiasis discovered at laparoscopic cholecystectomy may be managed via laparoscopic or, if necessary, open bile duct exploration or by postoperative endoscopic sphincterotomy. Operative findings of choledocholithiasis are palpable stones in the bile duct, dilation or thickening of the wall of the bile duct, or stones in the gallbladder small enough to pass through the cystic duct. Laparoscopic intraoperative cholangiography (or intraoperative ultrasonography) should be done at the time of cholecystectomy in patients with liver enzyme elevations but a bile duct diameter of less than 5 mm; if a ductal stone is found, the duct is explored. In the postcholecystectomy patient with choledocholithiasis, endoscopic sphincterotomy with stone extraction is preferable to transabdominal surgery. Lithotripsy (endoscopic or external), direct choledoscopy (cholangioscopy), or biliary stenting may be a therapeutic consideration for large stones. For the patient with a T tube and bile duct stone, the stone may be extracted via the T tube.

Postoperative antibiotics are not administered routinely after biliary tract surgery. Cultures of the bile are always taken at operation. If biliary tract infection was present preoperatively or is apparent at operation, ampicillin (500 mg every 6 hours intravenously) with gentamicin (1.5 mg/kg intravenously every 8 hours) and metronidazole (500 mg intravenously every 6 hours) or ciprofloxacin (250 mg intravenously every 12 hours) or a third-generation cephalosporin (eg, cefoperazone, 1–2 g intravenous every 12 hours) is administered postoperatively until the results of sensitivity tests on culture specimens are available. A T-tube cholangiogram should be done before the tube is removed, usually about 3 weeks after surgery. A small amount of bile frequently leaks from the tube site for a few days.

Urgent ERCP with sphincterotomy and stone extraction is generally indicated for choledocholithiasis complicated by ascending cholangitis and is preferred to surgery. Before ERCP, liver function should be evaluated thoroughly. Prothrombin time should be restored to normal by parenteral administration of vitamin K (see above). Ciprofloxacin, 250 mg intravenously every 12 hours, penetrates well into bile and is effective treatment for cholangitis. Alternative regimens in severely ill patients include mezlocillin, 3 g intravenously every 4 hours, plus either metronidazole or gentamicin (or both). The dose of metronidazole is 500 mg intravenously every 6 hours (if there has been no prior manipulation of the duct); the dose of gentamicin is 2 mg/kg intravenously as loading dose, plus 1.5 mg/kg every 8 hours adjusted for kidney function. Aminoglycosides should not be given for more than a few days because the risk of aminoglycoside nephrotoxicity is increased in patients with cholestasis. Emergent decompression of the bile duct, generally by ERCP, is required for patients who are septic or fail to improve on antibiotics within 12–24 hours. Medical therapy alone is most likely to fail in patients with tachycardia, serum albumin < 3 g/dL, marked hyperbilirubinemia, and prothrombin time > 14 seconds on admission. If sphincterotomy cannot be performed, decompression by a biliary stent or nasobiliary catheter can be done. Once decompression is achieved, antibiotics are generally continued for at least another three days. Elective cholecystectomy can be undertaken after resolution of cholangitis, unless the patient remains unfit for surgery.

▶ When to Refer

All symptomatic patients with choledocholithiasis should be referred.

▶ When to Admit

Patients with sepsis due to cholangitis should be hospitalized.

Attasaranya S et al. Choledocholithiasis, ascending cholangitis, and gallstone pancreatitis. Med Clin North Am. 2008 Jul;92(4):925–60. [PMID: 18570948]

Ledro-Cano D. Suspected choledocholithiasis: endoscopic ultrasound or magnetic resonance cholangio-pancreatography? A systematic review. Eur J Gastroenterol Hepatol. 2007 Nov;19(11):1007–11. [PMID: 18049172]

Lee YT et al. Comparison of EUS and ERCP in the investigation with suspected biliary obstruction caused by choledocholithiasis: a randomized study. Gastrointest Endosc. 2008 Apr;67(4):660–8. [PMID: 18155205]

Rhim AD et al. A young woman with gallstone pancreatitis and abnormal liver tests: when is endoscopic retrograde cholangiopancreatography needed? Clin Gastroenterol Hepatol. 2008 Jul;6(7):741–5. [PMID: 18547871]

Williams EJ et al. Guidelines on the management of common bile duct stones (CBDS). Gut. 2008 Jul;57(7):1004–21. [PMID: 18321943]

BILIARY STRICTURE

Benign biliary strictures are the result of surgical (including liver transplantation) anastomosis or injury in about 95% of cases. The remainder of cases are caused by blunt external injury to the abdomen, pancreatitis, erosion of the duct by a gallstone, or prior endoscopic sphincterotomy.

Signs of injury to the duct may or may not be recognized in the immediate postoperative period. If complete occlusion has occurred, jaundice will develop rapidly; more often, however, a tear has been accidentally made in the duct, and the earliest manifestation of injury may be excessive or prolonged loss of bile from the surgical drains. Bile leakage resulting in a bile collection (biloma) may predispose to localized infection, which in turn accentuates scar formation and the ultimate development of a fibrous stricture.

Cholangitis is the most common complication of stricture. Typically, the patient experiences episodes of pain, fever, chills, and jaundice within a few weeks to months after cholecystectomy. Physical findings may include jaundice during an attack of cholangitis and right upper quadrant abdominal tenderness. Serum alkaline phosphatase is usually elevated. Hyperbilirubinemia is variable, fluctuating during exacerbations and usually remaining in the range of 5–10 mg/dL. Blood cultures may be positive during an episode of cholangitis. Secondary biliary cirrhosis will inevitably develop if a stricture is not treated.

MRCP can be valuable in demonstrating the stricture, whereas ERCP permits biopsy and cytologic specimens to exclude malignancy and allows sphincterotomy to allow closure of a bile leak and dilation and stent placement for a stricture, thereby avoiding surgical repair in some cases. When ERCP is unsuccessful, dilation of a stricture may be accomplished by PTC. Placement of multiple plastic stents appears to be more effective than placement of a single stent. Metal stents, which often cannot be removed endoscopically, are generally avoided in benign strictures unless life expectancy is less than 2 years. The use of covered metal stents, which are more easily removed endoscopically than uncovered metal stents, as well as bioabsorbable stents, is under study. Strictures related to chronic pancreatitis are more difficult to treat endoscopically than postsurgical strictures, and preliminary reports suggest that they may be best managed with a temporary covered metal stent. Following liver transplantation, endoscopic management is more successful for anastomotic than for nonanastomotic strictures, and results are disappointing for biliary strictures after live liver donor liver transplantation. When malignancy cannot be excluded with certainty, additional endoscopic diagnostic approaches may be considered—if available—including endoscopic ultrasonography, intraductal ultrasound, and direct choledoscopy (cholangioscopy). Differentiation from cholangiocarcinoma may ultimately require surgical exploration. Operative treatment of a stricture frequently necessitates performance of an end-to-end ductal repair, choledochojejunostomy, or hepaticojejunostomy to reestablish bile flow into the intestine.

When to Refer

All patients with biliary stricture should be referred.

When to Admit

Patients with cholangitis should be hospitalized.

Farah M et al. Endoscopic retrograde cholangiopancreatography in the management of benign biliary strictures. Curr Gastroenterol Rep. 2008 Apr;10(2):150–6. [PMID: 18462601]

Kahaleh M et al. Temporary placement of covered self-expandable metal stents in benign biliary strictures: a new paradigm? Gastrointest Endosc. 2008 Mar;67(3):446–54. [PMID: 18294506]

Larghi A et al. Management of hilar biliary strictures. Am J Gastroenterol. 2008 Feb;103(2):458–73. [PMID: 18028506]

Sharma S et al. Biliary strictures following liver transplantation: past, present and preventive strategies. Liver Transpl. 2008 Jun;14(6):759–69. [PMID: 18508368]

PRIMARY SCLEROSING CHOLANGITIS

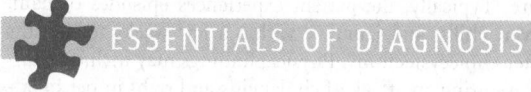
ESSENTIALS OF DIAGNOSIS

► Most common in men aged 20–50 years.

► Often associated with ulcerative colitis.

► Progressive jaundice, itching, and other features of cholestasis.

► Diagnosis based on characteristic cholangiographic findings.

► 10% risk of cholangiocarcinoma.

General Considerations

Primary sclerosing cholangitis is an uncommon disease characterized by a diffuse inflammation of the biliary tract leading to fibrosis and strictures of the biliary system. The disease is most common in men aged 20–50 years, with an incidence rate of 1 per 100,000 and a prevalence rate of 21 per 100,000 men and 6 per 100,000 women in the United States. The disease is closely associated with ulcerative colitis (and in some cases with Crohn colitis), which is present in approximately two-thirds of patients with primary sclerosing cholangitis; however, clinically significant sclerosing cholangitis develops in only 1–4% of patients with ulcerative colitis. As in ulcerative colitis, smoking is associated with a decreased risk of primary sclerosing cholangitis. Primary sclerosing cholangitis is associated with the histocompatible antigens HLA-B8 and -DR3 or -DR4, and first-degree relatives of patients with primary sclerosing cholangitis have a fourfold increased risk of primary sclerosing cholangitis and a threefold increased risk of ulcerative colitis. The diagnosis of primary sclerosing cholangitis may be difficult to make after biliary surgery.

Clinical Findings

A. Symptoms and Signs

Primary sclerosing cholangitis presents as progressive obstructive jaundice, frequently associated with fatigue, pruritus, anorexia, and indigestion. Patients may be diagnosed in the presymptomatic phase because of an elevated alkaline phosphatase level. Complications of chronic cholestasis, such as osteoporosis and malabsorption of fat-soluble vitamins, may occur late in the course. Esophageal varices are most likely in patients with a platelet count below 150,000/mcL, low serum albumin, and advanced histologic stage. In patients with primary sclerosing cholangitis, ulcerative colitis is frequently characterized by rectal sparing and backwash ileitis.

B. Diagnostic Findings

The diagnosis of primary sclerosing cholangitis is increasingly made by magnetic resonance cholangiography, the sensitivity of which approaches that of ERCP. Characteristic cholangiographic findings are segmental fibrosis of bile ducts with saccular dilatations between strictures. Biliary obstruction by a stone or tumor should be excluded. The disease may be confined to small intrahepatic bile ducts, in which case MRCP and ERCP are normal and the diagnosis is suggested by liver biopsy. These patients have a longer survival than patients with involvement of the large ducts and do not appear to be at increased risk for cholangiocarcinoma unless large-duct sclerosing cholangitis develops. Liver biopsy may show characteristic periductal fibrosis ("onion-skinning") and allows staging, which is based on the degree of fibrosis. Perinuclear ANCA (directed against myeloid-specific tubulin-beta isotype 5) as well as antinuclear, anticardiolipin, antithyroperoxidase, and anti-*Saccharomyces cerevisiae* antibodies, and rheumatoid factor are frequently detected in serum. Occasional patients have clinical and histologic features of both sclerosing cholangitis and autoimmune hepatitis. An association with autoimmune pancreatitis (IgG$_4$-associated cholangitis or sclerosing pancreaticocholangitis) is also seen, and this entity is often responsive to corticosteroids. Primary sclerosing cholangitis must be distinguished from idiopathic adulthood ductopenia (a rare disorder affecting young to middle-aged adults who manifest cholestasis resulting from loss of interlobular and septal bile ducts yet who have a normal cholangiogram and caused in some cases by a mutation in the canalicular phospholipid transporter gene *ABCB4*) and from other cholangiopathies (including primary biliary cirrhosis, cystic fibrosis, eosinophilic cholangitis, AIDS cholangiopathy, allograft rejection, graft-versus-host disease, ischemic damage (often with biliary "casts") caused by hepatic artery thrombosis, shock, respiratory failure, or drugs, intra-arterial chemotherapy, and sarcoidosis).

▶ Complications

Cholangiocarcinoma may complicate the course of primary sclerosing cholangitis in up to 20% of cases (1.2% per year) and may be difficult to diagnose by cytologic examination or biopsy because of false-negative results. A serum CA 19-9 level > 100 units/mL is suggestive but not diagnostic of cholangiocarcinoma. Annual ultrasound and serum CA 19-9 testing are recommended for surveillance, with CT or MRI with MRCP and biliary cytology if the results are abnormal. Positron emission tomography and choledochoscopy may play roles in the early detection of cholangiocarcinoma. Extensive surgical resection may result in 5-year survival rates of > 50%. Patients with ulcerative colitis and primary sclerosing cholangitis are at high risk for colorectal neoplasia. The risk of gallstones, cholecystitis, gallbladder polyps, and gallbladder carcinoma appears to be increased in patients with primary sclerosing cholangitis.

▶ Treatment

Episodes of acute bacterial cholangitis may be treated with ciprofloxacin (750 mg twice daily orally or intravenously). Ursodeoxycholic acid in standard doses (10–15 mg/kg/d orally) may improve liver biochemical test results but does not appear to alter the natural history. High-dose ursodeoxycholic acid (25–30 mg/kg/d) also has been shown not to reduce cholangiographic progression and liver fibrosis, nor to improve survival or prevent cholangiocarcinoma. Other drugs such as cyclosporine, tacrolimus, and minocycline are under study. Careful endoscopic evaluation of the biliary tree may permit balloon dilation of localized strictures, and repeated dilation of a dominant stricture may improve survival. Short-term placement of a stent in a major stricture also may relieve symptoms and improve biochemical abnor-

malities, with sustained improvement after the stent is removed. However, long-term stenting may increase the rate of complications such as cholangitis. In patients without cirrhosis, surgical resection of a dominant bile duct stricture may lead to longer survival than endoscopic therapy by decreasing the subsequent risk of cholangiocarcinoma. In patients with ulcerative colitis, primary sclerosing cholangitis is an independent risk factor for the development of colorectal dysplasia and cancer, and strict adherence to a colonoscopic surveillance program is recommended. Treatment with ursodeoxycholic acid has been reported to reduce the risk of colorectal dysplasia and carcinoma in patients with ulcerative colitis and primary sclerosing cholangitis. For patients with cirrhosis and clinical decompensation, liver transplantation is the procedure of choice.

▶ Prognosis

Survival of patients with primary sclerosing cholangitis averages 12–17 years. Adverse prognostic markers are older age, hepatosplenomegaly, higher serum bilirubin and AST levels, lower albumin levels, a history of variceal bleeding, a dominant bile duct stricture, and extrahepatic duct changes. Variceal bleeding is also a risk factor for cholangiocarcinoma. Actuarial survival rates with liver transplantation are as high as 85% at 3 years, but rates are much lower once cholangiocarcinoma has developed. Following transplantation, patients have an increased risk of nonanastomotic biliary strictures and—in those with ulcerative colitis—colon cancer. The retransplantation rate is higher than that for primary biliary cirrhosis. Those patients who are unable to undergo liver transplantation will ultimately require high-quality palliative care (see Chapter 5).

Charatcharoenwitthaya P et al. Utility of serum tumor markers, imaging, and biliary cytology for detecting cholangiocarcinoma in primary sclerosing cholangitis. Hepatology. 2008 Oct;48(4):1106–17. [PMID: 18785620]

Ghazale A et al. Immunoglobulin G4-associated cholangitis: clinical profile and response to therapy. Gastroenterology. 2008 Mar;134(3):706–15. [PMID: 18222442]

Said K et al. Gallbladder disease in patients with primary sclerosing cholangitis. J Hepatol. 2008 Apr;48(4):598–605. [PMID: 18222013]

Tischendorf JJ et al. Current diagnosis and management of primary sclerosing cholangitis. Liver Transpl. 2008 Jun;14(6):735–46. [PMID: 18508363]

▼ DISEASES OF THE PANCREAS

See Chapter 39 for Carcinoma of the Pancreas and Periampullary Area.

ACUTE PANCREATITIS

ESSENTIALS OF DIAGNOSIS

▶ Abrupt onset of deep epigastric pain, often with radiation to the back.

- History of previous episodes, often related to alcohol intake.
- Nausea, vomiting, sweating, weakness.
- Abdominal tenderness and distention and fever.
- Leukocytosis, elevated serum amylase, elevated serum lipase.

General Considerations

Most cases of acute pancreatitis are related to biliary tract disease (a passed gallstone, usually < 5 mm in diameter) or heavy alcohol intake. The exact pathogenesis is not known but may include edema or obstruction of the ampulla of Vater, reflux of bile into pancreatic ducts, and direct injury of pancreatic acinar cells by prematurely activated pancreatic enzymes. Among the numerous other causes or associations are hypercalcemia, hyperlipidemias (chylomicronemia, hypertriglyceridemia, or both), abdominal trauma (including surgery), drugs (including azathioprine, mercaptopurine, asparaginase, pentamidine, didanosine, valproic acid, tetracyclines, dapsone, isoniazid, metronidazole, estrogen and tamoxifen [by raising serum triglycerides], sulfonamides, mesalamine, sulindac, thiazides, enalapril, methyldopa, procainamide, and possibly glucocorticoids and others), vasculitis, infections (eg, mumps, cytomegalovirus, *Mycobacterium avium* complex), peritoneal dialysis, cardiopulmonary bypass, ERCP, and genetic mutations that also predispose to chronic pancreatitis (see below). In patients with pancreas divisum, a congenital anomaly in which the dorsal and ventral pancreatic ducts fail to fuse, acute pancreatitis may result from stenosis of the minor papilla with obstruction to flow from the accessory pancreatic duct, although concomitant mutations in the cystic fibrosis transmembrane conductance regulator (*CFTR*) gene have also been reported to account for acute pancreatitis in some patients with pancreas divisum. Acute pancreatitis may also result from anomalous union of the pancreaticobiliary duct. Rarely, acute pancreatitis may be the presenting manifestation of a pancreatic or ampullary neoplasm. Celiac disease appears to be associated with an increased risk of acute and chronic pancreatitis. Apparently "idiopathic" acute pancreatitis is often caused by occult biliary microlithiasis and may be caused by sphincter of Oddi dysfunction involving the pancreatic duct. Between 15% and 25% of cases are truly idiopathic. Smoking may increase the risk of alcoholic and idiopathic pancreatitis, and older age and obesity increase the risk of a severe course. The incidence of pancreatitis has increased since 1990.

Clinical Findings

A. Symptoms and Signs

Epigastric abdominal pain, generally abrupt in onset, is steady, boring, and severe and often made worse by walking and lying supine and better by sitting and leaning forward. The pain usually radiates into the back but may radiate to the right or left. Nausea and vomiting are usually present. Weakness, sweating, and anxiety are noted in severe attacks. There may be a history of alcohol intake or a heavy meal immediately preceding the attack, or a history of milder similar episodes or biliary pain in the past.

The abdomen is tender mainly in the upper part, most often without guarding, rigidity, or rebound. The abdomen may be distended, and bowel sounds may be absent with associated ileus. Fever of 38.4–39 °C, tachycardia, hypotension (even true shock), pallor, and cool clammy skin are often present. Mild jaundice is common. Occasionally, an upper abdominal mass due to the inflamed pancreas or a pseudocyst may be palpated. Acute kidney injury (usually due to prerenal cause) may occur early in the course of acute pancreatitis.

B. Assessment of Severity

The severity of acute alcoholic pancreatitis can be assessed using **Ranson criteria** (Table 16–8). The Sequential Organ Failure Assessment (SOFA) score can be used to assess injury to other organs, and the Acute Physiology and Chronic Health Evaluation (APACHE II) score is another tool for assessing severity. A simple 5-point clinical scoring system based on blood urea nitrogen > 25 mg/dL, impaired mental status, systemic inflammatory response syndrome, age > 60 years, and pleural effusion (BISAP) during the first 24 hours (before the onset of organ failure) has been proposed.

C. Laboratory Findings

Serum amylase and lipase are elevated—usually more than three times the upper limit of normal—within 24 hours in

Table 16–8. Ranson criteria for assessing the severity of acute pancreatitis.

Three or more of the following predicts a severe course complicated by pancreatic necrosis with a sensitivity of 60–80%
Age over 55 years
White blood cell count > 16,000/mcL
Blood glucose > 200 mg/dL
Serum lactic dehydrogenase > 350 units/L
Aspartate aminotransferase > 250 units/L

Development of the following in the first 48 hours indicates a worsening prognosis
Hematocrit drop of more than 10 percentage points
Blood urea nitrogen rise > 5 mg/dL
Arterial P_{O_2} of < 60 mm Hg
Serum calcium of < 8 mg/dL
Base deficit over 4 mEq/L
Estimated fluid sequestration of > 6 L

Mortality rates correlate with the number of criteria present[1]	
Number of Criteria	**Mortality Rate**
0–2	1%
3–4	16%
5–6	40%
7–8	100%

[1]An APACHE II score ≥ 8 also correlates with mortality.

90% of cases; their return to normal is variable depending on the severity of disease. Lipase remains elevated longer than amylase and is slightly more accurate for the diagnosis of acute pancreatitis. Leukocytosis (10,000–30,000/mcL), proteinuria, granular casts, glycosuria (10–20% of cases), hyperglycemia, and elevated serum bilirubin may be present. Blood urea nitrogen and serum alkaline phosphatase may be elevated and coagulation tests abnormal. An elevated serum creatinine level (> 1.8 mg/dL) at 48 hours is associated with the development of pancreatic necrosis. In patients with clear evidence of acute pancreatitis, a serum ALT level of more than 150 units/L suggests biliary pancreatitis. Decrease in serum calcium may reflect saponification and correlates with severity of disease. Levels lower than 7 mg/dL (when serum albumin is normal) are associated with tetany and an unfavorable prognosis. Patients with acute pancreatitis caused by hypertriglyceridemia generally have fasting triglyceride levels above 1000 mg/dL. An early rise in the hematocrit value above 44% suggests hemoconcentration and predicts pancreatic necrosis. An elevated C-reactive protein (> 150 mg/L) concentration at 48 hours suggests severe disease.

Other tests that offer the possibility of simplicity, rapidity, ease of use, and low cost—including urinary trypsinogen-2, trypsinogen activation peptide, and carboxypeptidase B—are not widely available. In patients in whom ascites or left pleural effusions develop, fluid amylase content is high. Electrocardiography may show ST–T wave changes.

D. Imaging

Plain radiographs of the abdomen may show gallstones, a "sentinel loop" (a segment of air-filled small intestine most commonly in the left upper quadrant), the "colon cutoff sign"—a gas-filled segment of transverse colon abruptly ending at the area of pancreatic inflammation—or linear focal atelectasis of the lower lobe of the lungs with or without pleural effusion. Ultrasound is often not helpful in diagnosing acute pancreatitis because of intervening bowel gas but may identify gallstones in the gallbladder. Unenhanced CT scan is useful in demonstrating an enlarged pancreas when the diagnosis of pancreatitis is uncertain, in detecting pseudocysts, in differentiating pancreatitis from

other possible intra-abdominal catastrophes, and in providing an initial assessment of prognosis (Table 16–9). Rapid-bolus intravenous contrast-enhanced CT following aggressive volume resuscitation is of particular value after the first 3 days of severe acute pancreatitis to identify areas of necrotizing pancreatitis and to assess the degree of necrosis, although the use of intravenous contrast may increase the risk of complications of pancreatitis and of acute kidney injury and should be avoided when the serum creatinine level is greater than 1.5 mg/dL. MRI appears to be a suitable alternative to CT. Perfusion CT on day 3 demonstrating areas of ischemia in the pancreas has been reported to predict the development of pancreatic necrosis. The presence of a fluid collection in the pancreas correlates with an increased mortality rate. CT-guided needle aspiration of areas of necrotizing pancreatitis after the third day may disclose infection, usually by enteric organisms, which invariably leads to death unless surgical debridement is ultimately performed. The presence of gas bubbles on CT scan implies that infection by gas-forming organisms is present. Endoscopic ultrasonography is useful in identifying occult biliary disease (eg, small stones, sludge), which, including microlithiasis, is present in a majority of patients with apparently idiopathic acute pancreatitis, and is indicated in persons over age 40 to exclude malignancy. ERCP is generally not indicated after a first attack of acute pancreatitis unless there is associated cholangitis or jaundice or a bile duct stone is known to be present, but endoscopic ultrasonography or MRCP should be considered, especially after repeated attacks of idiopathic acute pancreatitis. In selected cases, aspiration of bile for crystal analysis may confirm the suspicion of microlithiasis, and manometry of the pancreatic duct sphincter may detect sphincter of Oddi dysfunction as a cause of recurrent pancreatitis.

▶ Differential Diagnosis

Acute pancreatitis must be differentiated from an acutely perforated duodenal ulcer, acute cholecystitis, acute intestinal obstruction, leaking aortic aneurysm, renal colic, and acute mesenteric ischemia. Serum amylase may also be elevated in high intestinal obstruction, in gastroenteritis, in

Table 16–9. Severity index for acute pancreatitis.

	CT Grade	Points	Pancreatic Necrosis	Additional Points	Severity Index[1]	Mortality Rate[2]
A	Normal pancreas	0	0%	0	0	0%
B	Pancreatic enlargement	1	0%	0	1	0%
C	Pancreatic inflammation and/or peripancreatic fat	2	< 30%	2	4	< 3%
D	Single acute peripancreatic fluid collection	3	30–50%	4	7	6%
E	Two or more acute peripancreatic fluid collections or retroperitoneal air	4	> 50%	6	10	> 17%

[1]Severity index = CT Grade Points + Additional Points.
[2]Based on the severity index.
Adapted with permission from Balthazar EJ. Acute pancreatitis: assessment of severity with clinical and CT evaluation. Radiology. 2002 Jun;223(3):603–13.

mumps not involving the pancreas (salivary amylase), in ectopic pregnancy, after administration of opioids, and after abdominal surgery. Serum lipase may also be elevated in many of these conditions.

▶ **Complications**

Intravascular volume depletion secondary to leakage of fluids in the pancreatic bed and ileus with fluid-filled loops of bowel may result in prerenal azotemia and even acute tubular necrosis without overt shock. This usually occurs within 24 hours of the onset of acute pancreatitis and lasts 8–9 days. Some patients require peritoneal dialysis or hemodialysis.

Sterile or infected necrotizing pancreatitis may complicate the course of 5–10% of cases and accounts for most of the deaths. The risk of infection does not correlate with the extent of necrosis. Pancreatic necrosis is often associated with fever, leukocytosis, and, in some cases, shock and is associated with organ failure (eg, pulmonary, renal, gastrointestinal bleeding) in 50% of cases. Because infected pancreatic necrosis is almost always an indication for operative treatment, fine-needle aspiration of necrotic tissue under CT guidance should be performed (if necessary, repeatedly) for Gram stain and culture.

A serious complication of acute pancreatitis is acute respiratory distress syndrome (ARDS); cardiac dysfunction may be superimposed. It usually occurs 3–7 days after the onset of pancreatitis in patients who have required large volumes of fluid and colloid to maintain blood pressure and urinary output. Most patients with ARDS require intubation and mechanical ventilation with positive end-expiratory pressure.

Pancreatic abscess (also referred to as infected or suppurative pseudocyst) is a suppurative process characterized by rising fever, leukocytosis, and localized tenderness and epigastric mass usually 6 or more weeks into the course of acute pancreatitis. This may be associated with a left-sided pleural effusion or an enlarging spleen secondary to splenic vein thrombosis. In contrast to infected necrosis, the mortality rate is low following drainage.

Pseudocysts, encapsulated fluid collections with high enzyme content, commonly appear in pancreatitis when CT scans are used to monitor the evolution of an acute attack. Pseudocysts that are smaller than 6 cm in diameter often resolve spontaneously. They most commonly are within or adjacent to the pancreas but can present anywhere (eg, mediastinal, retrorectal), by extension along anatomic planes. Multiple pseudocysts are seen in 14% of cases. Pseudocysts may become secondarily infected, necessitating drainage as for an abscess. Erosion of the inflammatory process into a blood vessel can result in a major hemorrhage into the cyst.

Pancreatic ascites may present after recovery from acute pancreatitis as a gradual increase in abdominal girth and persistent elevation of the serum amylase level in the absence of frank abdominal pain. Marked elevations in the ascitic protein (> 3 g/dL) and amylase (> 1000 units/L) concentrations are typical. The condition results from rupture of the pancreatic duct or drainage of a pseudocyst into the peritoneal cavity.

Rare complications of acute pancreatitis include hemorrhage caused by erosion of a blood vessel to form a pseudoaneurysm and colonic necrosis. Chronic pancreatitis develops in about 10% of cases. Permanent diabetes mellitus and exocrine pancreatic insufficiency occur uncommonly after a single acute episode.

▶ **Treatment**

A. Management of Acute Disease

In most patients, acute pancreatitis is a mild disease ("nonsevere acute pancreatitis") that subsides spontaneously within several days. The pancreas is "rested" by a regimen of withholding food and liquids by mouth, bed rest, and, in patients with moderately severe pain or ileus and abdominal distention or vomiting, nasogastric suction. Pain is controlled with meperidine, up to 100–150 mg intramuscularly every 3–4 hours as necessary. In those with severe liver or kidney dysfunction, the dose may need to be reduced. Morphine has been thought to cause sphincter of Oddi spasm but is now considered an acceptable alternative, and given the potential side effects of meperidine, may even be preferable. Oral intake of fluid and foods can be resumed when the patient is largely free of pain and has bowel sounds (even if the serum amylase is still elevated). Clear liquids are given first (this step may be skipped in patients with mild acute pancreatitis), followed by gradual advancement to a low-fat diet, guided by the patient's tolerance and by the absence of pain. Pain may recur on refeeding in 20% of patients. Following recovery from acute biliary pancreatitis, laparoscopic cholecystectomy is generally performed, although in selected cases endoscopic sphincterotomy alone may be done. In patients with recurrent pancreatitis associated with pancreas divisum, insertion of a stent in the minor papilla (or minor papilla sphincterotomy) may reduce the frequency of subsequent attacks, although complications of such therapy are frequent.

In more severe pancreatitis—particularly necrotizing pancreatitis—there may be considerable leakage of fluids, necessitating large amounts of intravenous fluids (eg, 500–1000 mL/h for several hours, then 250–300 mL/h) to maintain intravascular volume. Monitoring in an intensive care unit is required, and the importance of aggressive intravenous hydration cannot be overemphasized. Calcium gluconate must be given intravenously if there is evidence of hypocalcemia with tetany. Infusions of fresh frozen plasma or serum albumin may be necessary in patients with coagulopathy or hypoalbuminemia. With colloid solutions, there may be an increased risk of developing ARDS. If shock persists after adequate volume replacement (including packed red cells), pressors may be required. For the patient requiring a large volume of parenteral fluids, central venous pressure and blood gases should be monitored at regular intervals. Parenteral nutrition (including lipids) should be considered in patients who have severe pancreatitis and ileus and will be without oral nutrition for at least 7–10 days. Enteral nutrition via a nasojejunal or possibly nasogastric feeding tube is preferable but may not be tolerated in some patients with an ileus. The routine use of antibiotics to prevent conversion of sterile pancreatic necrosis to infected necrosis is still controversial and is not indicated in those with < 30% pancreatic necrosis. Imipenem (500 mg every 8 hours intravenously) and possibly cefuroxime (1.5 g intravenously three times daily, then 250 mg orally twice daily) administered for no more than 14 days to patients with sterile pancreatic necrosis has been reported in some studies to reduce the risk of pancreatic infection and mortality; meropenem and the combination of ciprofloxacin and metronidazole do not appear to reduce the frequency of infected necrosis, multiorgan failure, or mortality. When infected necrosis is confirmed, imipenem or meropenem should be continued. The role of intravenous somatostatin in severe acute pancreatitis is uncertain, and octreotide is thought to have no benefit. To date, probiotic agents have not been shown to reduce infectious complications of severe pancreatitis and may increase mortality. There is conflicting evidence as to whether the risk of pancreatitis after ERCP can be reduced by the administration of somatostatin or gabexate mesilate, a protease inhibitor. Allopurinol, nonsteroidal anti-inflammatory drugs (administered rectally), and ulinastatin, another protease inhibitor, have been reported to reduce the frequency and severity of post-ERCP pancreatitis. Lexipafant, an antagonist of platelet-activating factor, appears to be of no benefit. Placement of a stent across the pancreatic duct or orifice has been shown to reduce the risk of post-ERCP pancreatitis and is an increasingly common practice.

B. Treatment of Complications and Follow-Up

A surgeon should be consulted in all cases of severe acute pancreatitis. If the diagnosis is in doubt and investigation indicates a strong possibility of a serious surgically correctable lesion (eg, perforated peptic ulcer), exploratory laparotomy is indicated. When acute pancreatitis is unexpectedly found, it is usually wise to close without intervention. If the pancreatitis appears mild and cholelithiasis or microlithiasis is present, cholecystectomy or cholecystostomy may be justified. When severe pancreatitis results from choledocholithiasis—particularly if jaundice (serum total bilirubin > 5 mg/dL) or cholangitis is present—ERCP with endoscopic sphincterotomy and stone extraction is indicated. MRCP may be useful in selecting patients for therapeutic ERCP. Endoscopic sphincterotomy does not appear to improve the outcome of severe pancreatitis in the absence of cholangitis or jaundice.

Operation may improve survival in patients with necrotizing pancreatitis and clinical deterioration with multiorgan failure or lack of resolution by 4 weeks. Surgery is nearly always indicated for infected necrosis. The goal of surgery is to debride necrotic pancreas and surrounding tissue and establish adequate drainage. Outcomes are best if surgery is delayed until the necrosis has organized, usually about 4 weeks after disease onset. In selected cases, nonsurgical drainage of walled-off pancreatic necrosis under radiologic, endoscopic (transgastric or transduodenal), or laparoscopic guidance may be feasible, at least as a temporizing measure, depending on local expertise. Peritoneal lavage has not been shown to improve survival in severe acute pancreatitis, in part because the risk of late septic complications is not reduced.

The development of a pancreatic abscess is an indication for prompt percutaneous or surgical drainage. Chronic pseudocysts require endoscopic, percutaneous catheter, or surgical drainage when infected or associated with persisting pain, pancreatitis, or common duct obstruction. For pancreatic infections, imipenem, 500 mg every 8 hours intravenously, is a good choice of antibiotic because it achieves bactericidal levels in pancreatic tissue for most causative organisms. Pancreatic duct leaks and fistulas may require endoscopic or surgical therapy.

▶ Prognosis

Mortality rates for acute pancreatitis have declined from at least 10% to around 5% since the 1980s, but the mortality rate for severe acute pancreatitis (more than three Ranson criteria; Table 16–8) remains at least 20%, with rates of 10% and 25% in those with sterile and infected necrosis, respectively. Half of the deaths occur within the first 2 weeks, usually from multiorgan failure. Multiorgan failure that persists beyond the first 48 hours is associated with a mortality rate of over 50%. Later deaths occur because of complications of infected necrosis. Hospital-acquired infections increase the mortality of acute pancreatitis, independent of severity. Recurrences are common in alcoholic pancreatitis.

▶ When to Admit

Nearly all patients with acute pancreatitis should be hospitalized.

Bai Y et al. Prophylactic antibiotics cannot reduce infected pancreatic necrosis and mortality in acute necrotizing pancreatitis: evidence from a meta-analysis of randomized controlled trials. Am J Gastroenterol. 2008 Jan;103(1):104–10. [PMID: 17925000]

Baillie J. Endoscopic therapy in acute recurrent pancreatitis. World J Gastroenterol. 2008 Feb 21;14(7):1034–7. [PMID: 18286684]

Bollen TL et al. The Atlanta Classification of acute pancreatitis revisited. Br J Surg. 2008 Jan;95(1):6–21. [PMID: 17985333]

Frossard JL et al. Acute pancreatitis. Lancet. 2008 Jan 12;371(9607):143–52. [PMID: 18191686]

Gardner TB et al. Fluid resuscitation in acute pancreatitis. Clin Gastroenterol Hepatol. 2008 Oct;6(10):1070–6. [PMID: 18619920]

Morgan DE. Imaging of acute pancreatitis and its complications. Clin Gastroenterol Hepatol. 2008 Oct;6(10):1077–85. [PMID: 18928934]

Wu BU et al. The early prediction of mortality in acute pancreatitis: a large population-based study. Gut. 2008 Dec;57(12):1698–703. [PMID: 18519429]

Wu BU et al. The impact of hospital-acquired infection on outcome in acute pancreatitis. Gastroenterology. 2008 Sep;135(3):816–20. [PMID: 18616944]

CHRONIC PANCREATITIS

 ESSENTIALS OF DIAGNOSIS

▶ Chronic or intermittent epigastric pain, steatorrhea, weight loss, abnormal pancreatic imaging.

▶ A mnemonic for the predisposing factors of chronic pancreatitis is TIGAR-O: toxic-metabolic, idiopathic, genetic, autoimmune, recurrent and severe acute pancreatitis, or obstructive.

General Considerations

Chronic pancreatitis occurs most often in patients with alcoholism (70–80% of all cases). The risk of chronic pancreatitis increases with the duration and amount of alcohol consumed, but pancreatitis develops in only 5–10% of heavy drinkers. Tobacco smoking has been reported to accelerate progression of alcoholic chronic pancreatitis. About 2% of patients with hyperparathyroidism develop pancreatitis. In tropical Africa and Asia, tropical pancreatitis, related in part to malnutrition, is the most common cause of chronic pancreatitis. A stricture, stone, or tumor obstructing the pancreas can lead to obstructive chronic pancreatitis. Autoimmune pancreatitis is associated with hypergammaglobulinemia (IgG₄ in particular) and often with autoantibodies and other autoimmune diseases and is responsive to corticosteroids. About 10–20% of cases are idiopathic, with either early onset (median age 23) or late onset (median age 62). Genetic factors may predispose to chronic pancreatitis in some of these cases, including mutations of the cystic fibrosis transmembrane conductance regulator (*CFTR*) gene, the pancreatic secretory trypsin inhibitory gene (*PSTI*, serine protease inhibitor, *SPINK1*), and possibly the gene for uridine 5′-diphosphate glucuronosyltransferase. Mutation of the cationic trypsinogen gene on chromosome 7 (*serine protease 1, PRSS1*) is associated with hereditary pancreatitis, transmitted as an autosomal dominant trait with variable penetrance. A useful mnemonic for the predisposing factors to chronic pancreatitis is TIGAR-O: toxic-metabolic, idiopathic, genetic, autoimmune, recurrent and severe acute pancreatitis, or obstructive.

The pathogenesis of chronic pancreatitis may be explained by the SAPE (sentinel acute pancreatitis event) hypothesis by which the first (sentinel) acute pancreatitis event initiates an inflammatory process that results in injury and later fibrosis ("necrosis-fibrosis"). In many cases, chronic pancreatitis is a self-perpetuating disease characterized by chronic pain or recurrent episodes of acute pancreatitis and ultimately by pancreatic exocrine or endocrine insufficiency (sooner in alcoholic pancreatitis than in other types). After many years, chronic pain may resolve spontaneously or as a result of surgery tailored to the cause of pain. Over 80% of adults develop diabetes mellitus 25 years after the clinical onset of chronic pancreatitis.

Clinical Findings

A. Symptoms and Signs

Persistent or recurrent episodes of epigastric and left upper quadrant pain with referral to the upper left lumbar region are typical. Anorexia, nausea, vomiting, constipation, flatulence, and weight loss are common. During attacks tenderness over the pancreas, mild muscle guarding, and ileus

may be noted. Attacks may last only a few hours or as long as 2 weeks; pain may eventually be almost continuous. Steatorrhea (as indicated by bulky, foul, fatty stools) may occur late in the course.

B. Laboratory Findings

Serum amylase and lipase may be elevated during acute attacks; however, a normal amylase does not exclude the diagnosis. Serum alkaline phosphatase and bilirubin may be elevated owing to compression of the common duct. Glycosuria may be present. Excess fecal fat may be demonstrated on chemical analysis of the stool. Pancreatic insufficiency generally is confirmed by response to therapy with pancreatic enzyme supplements; the secretin stimulation test can be used if available, as can detection of decreased fecal chymotrypsin or elastase levels, although the latter tests lack sensitivity and specificity. Vitamin B₁₂ malabsorption is detectable in about 40% of patients, but clinical deficiency of vitamin B₁₂ and fat-soluble vitamins is rare. Accurate diagnostic tests are available for the major trypsinogen gene mutations, but because of uncertainty about the mechanisms linking heterozygous *CFTR* and *PSTI* mutations with pancreatitis, genetic testing for mutations in these two genes is not currently recommended. Elevated IgG₄ levels, ANA, and antibodies to lactoferrin and carbonic anhydrase II are often found in patients with autoimmune pancreatitis; pancreatic biopsy shows a lymphoplasmacytic inflammatory infiltrate with characteristic IgG4 immunostaining, which is also found in biopsy specimens of the major papilla, bile duct, and salivary glands.

C. Imaging

Plain films show calcifications due to pancreaticolithiasis in 30% of affected patients. CT may show calcifications not seen on plain films as well as ductal dilation and heterogeneity or atrophy of the gland. Occasionally, the findings raise suspicion of pancreatic cancer ("tumefactive chronic pancreatitis"). ERCP is the most sensitive imaging study for chronic pancreatitis and may show dilated ducts, intraductal stones, strictures, or pseudocyst, but the results may be normal in patients with so-called minimal change pancreatitis. MRCP and endoscopic ultrasonography (with pancreatic tissue sampling) are less invasive alternatives to ERCP. Characteristic imaging features of autoimmune pancreatitis include diffuse enlargement of the pancreas, a peripheral rim of hypoattenuation, and irregular narrowing of the main pancreatic duct.

Complications

Opioid addiction is common. Other frequent complications include often brittle diabetes mellitus, pancreatic pseudocyst or abscess, cholestatic liver enzymes with or without jaundice, bile duct stricture, steatorrhea, malnutrition, and peptic ulcer. Pancreatic cancer develops in 4% of patients after 20 years; the risk may relate to tobacco and alcohol use. In patients with hereditary pancreatitis, the risk of pancreatic cancer rises after age 50 years and reaches 19% by age 70 years (see Chapter 39).

Table 16–10. Selected pancreatic enzyme preparations.

Product	Enzyme Content in Units per Dose		
	Lipase	Amylase	Protease
Conventional preparations			
Viokase 8	8000	30,000	30,000
Viokase 16	16,000	60,000	60,000
Pancrelipase	8000	30,000	30,000
Enteric-coated microencapsulated preparations			
Creon 10	10,000	33,200	37,500
Creon 20	20,000	66,400	75,000
Lipram PN10	10,000	30,000	30,000
Lipram UL12	12,000	39,000	39,000
Lipram PN16	16,000	48,000	48,000
Lipram UL18	18,000	58,500	58,500
Lipram UL20	20,000	65,000	65,000
Pancrease MT 10	10,000	30,000	30,000
Pancrease MT 16	16,000	48,000	48,000
Pancrease MT 20	20,000	56,000	44,000
Pangestyme CN 10	10,000	33,200	37,500
Pangestyme UL 12	12,000	39,000	39,000
Pangestyme MT 16	16,000	48,000	48,000
Pangestyme UL 20	20,000	65,000	65,000
Ultrase MT 12	12,000	39,000	39,000
Ultrase MT 20	20,000	65,000	65,000

Source: American Society of Health System Pharmacists, *Drug Information*, 2008.

▶ Treatment

Correctable coexistent biliary tract disease should be treated surgically.

A. Medical Measures

A low-fat diet should be prescribed. Alcohol is forbidden because it frequently precipitates attacks. Opioids should be avoided if possible. Preferred agents for pain are acetaminophen, nonsteroidal anti-inflammatory drugs, and tramadol, along with pain-modifying agents such as tricyclic antidepressants, selective serotonin uptake inhibitors, and gabapentin. Steatorrhea is treated with pancreatic supplements that are selected on the basis of their high lipase activity. A total dose of 30,000 units of lipase in capsules is given with meals (Table 16–10). Higher doses may be required in some cases. The tablets should be taken at the start of, during, and at the end of a meal. Concurrent administration of a H_2-receptor antagonist (eg, ranitidine, 150 mg orally twice daily), a proton pump inhibitor (eg, omeprazole, 20–60 mg orally daily), or sodium bicarbonate, 650 mg orally before and after meals, decreases the inactivation of lipase by acid and may thereby further decrease steatorrhea. In selected cases of alcoholic pancreatitis and in cystic fibrosis, enteric-coated microencapsulated preparations may offer an advantage. However, in patients with cystic fibrosis, high-dose pancreatic enzyme therapy has been associated with strictures of the ascending colon. Pain secondary to idiopathic chronic pancreatitis may be alleviated in some cases by the use of pancreatic enzymes (not enteric-coated) or octreotide, 200 mcg subcutaneously three times daily. Associated diabetes mellitus should be treated (see Chapter 27). Autoimmune pancreatitis is treated with prednisone 40 mg/d orally for 1–2 months, followed by a taper of 5 mg every 2–4 weeks. Other immunosuppressive therapies are under study.

B. Surgical and Endoscopic Treatment

Endoscopic therapy or surgery may be indicated in chronic pancreatitis to treat underlying biliary tract disease, ensure free flow of bile into the duodenum, drain persistent pseudocysts, treat other complications, eliminate obstruction of the pancreatic duct, attempt to relieve pain, or exclude pancreatic cancer. Liver fibrosis may regress after biliary drainage. Distal bile duct obstruction may be relieved by endoscopic placement of multiple bile duct stents. When obstruction of the duodenal end of the pancreatic duct can be demonstrated by ERCP, dilation or placement of a stent in the duct or resection of the tail of the pancreas with implantation of the distal end of the duct by pancreaticojejunostomy may be successful. When the pancreatic duct is diffusely dilated, anastomosis between the duct after it is split longitudinally and a defunctionalized limb of jejunum (modified Puestow procedure), in some cases combined with resection of the head of the pancreas, is associated with relief of pain in 80% of cases. In advanced cases, subtotal or total pancreatectomy may be considered as a last resort but has variable efficacy and causes pancreatic insufficiency and diabetes mellitus. Perioperative administration of somatostatin or octreotide may reduce the risk of postoperative pancreatic fistulas. Endoscopic or surgical drainage is indicated for symptomatic pseudocysts and, in many cases, those over 6 cm in diameter. Endoscopic ultrasonography may facilitate selection of an optimal site for endoscopic drainage. Pancreatic ascites or pancreaticopleural fistulas due to a disrupted pancreatic duct can be managed by endoscopic placement of a stent across the disrupted duct. Pancreatic sphincterotomy or fragmentation of stones in the pancreatic duct by lithotripsy and endoscopic removal of stones from the duct, may relieve pain in selected patients. For patients with chronic pain and nondilated ducts, a percutaneous celiac plexus nerve block may be considered under either CT or endoscopic ultrasound guidance, with pain relief (albeit often short-lived) in approximately 50% of patients.

▶ Prognosis

Chronic pancreatitis often leads to disability. The prognosis is best in patients with recurrent acute pancreatitis caused by a remediable condition such as cholelithiasis, choledocholithiasis, stenosis of the sphincter of Oddi, or hyperparathyroidism. Medical management of the hyperlipidemia frequently associated with the condition may also prevent recurrent attacks of pancreatitis. In alcoholic pancreatitis, pain relief is most likely when a dilated pancreatic duct can be decompressed. In patients with disease not amenable to decompressive surgery, addiction to narcotics is a frequent outcome of treatment.

▶ When to Refer

All patients with chronic pancreatitis should be referred for diagnostic and therapeutic procedures.

▶ When to Admit

- Severe pain.
- New jaundice.
- New fever.

Aghdassi A et al. Diagnosis and treatment of pancreatic pseudocysts in chronic pancreatitis. Pancreas. 2008 Mar;36(2):105–12. [PMID: 18376299]

Callery MP et al. A 21-year-old man with chronic pancreatitis. JAMA. 2008 Apr 2;299(13):1588–94. [PMID: 18319401]

Devière J et al. Treatment of chronic pancreatitis with endotherapy or surgery: critical review of randomized control trials. J Gastrointest Surg. 2008 Apr;12(4):640–4. [PMID: 18247099]

Kamisawa T. Diagnostic criteria for autoimmune pancreatitis. J Clin Gastroenterol. 2008 Apr;42(4):404–7. [PMID: 18277897]

Rebours V et al. The natural history of hereditary pancreatitis: a national series. Gut. 2009 Jan;58(1):97–103. [PMID: 18755888]

Strate T et al. Resection vs drainage in treatment of chronic pancreatitis: long-term results of a randomized trial. Gastroenterology. 2008 May;134(5):1406–11. [PMID: 18471517]

Breast Disorders

Armando E. Giuliano, MD
Sara A. Hurvitz, MD

BENIGN BREAST DISORDERS

FIBROCYSTIC CONDITION

ESSENTIALS OF DIAGNOSIS

- Painful, often multiple, usually bilateral masses in the breast.
- Rapid fluctuation in the size of the masses is common.
- Frequently, pain occurs or worsens and size increases during premenstrual phase of cycle.
- Most common age is 30–50. Rare in postmenopausal women not receiving hormonal replacement.

General Considerations

Fibrocystic condition is the most frequent lesion of the breast. Although commonly referred to as "fibrocystic disease," it does not, in fact, represent a pathologic or anatomic disorder. It is common in women 30–50 years of age but rare in postmenopausal women who are not taking hormonal replacement. Estrogen is considered a causative factor. There may be an increased risk in women who drink alcohol, especially women between 18 and 22 years of age. Fibrocystic condition encompasses a wide variety of benign histologic changes in the breast epithelium, some of which are found so commonly in normal breasts that they are probably variants of normal but have nonetheless been termed a "condition" or "disease."

The microscopic findings of fibrocystic condition include cysts (gross and microscopic), papillomatosis, adenosis, fibrosis, and ductal epithelial hyperplasia. Although fibrocystic condition has generally been considered to increase the risk of subsequent breast cancer, only the variants with a component of epithelial proliferation (especially with atypia) represent true risk factors.

Clinical Findings

A. Symptoms and Signs

Fibrocystic condition may produce an asymptomatic mass in the breast that is discovered by accident, but pain or tenderness often calls attention to it. Discomfort often occurs or worsens during the premenstrual phase of the cycle, at which time the cysts tend to enlarge. Fluctuations in size and rapid appearance or disappearance of a breast mass are common with this condition as are multiple or bilateral masses and serous nipple discharge. Patients will give a history of a transient lump in the breast or cyclic breast pain.

B. Diagnostic Tests

Mammography and ultrasonography should be used to evaluate a mass in a patient with fibrocystic condition. Ultrasonography alone may be used in women under 30 years of age. Because a mass due to fibrocystic condition is difficult to distinguish from carcinoma on the basis of clinical findings, suspicious lesions should be biopsied. Fine-needle aspiration (FNA) cytology may be used, but if a suspicious mass that is nonmalignant on cytologic examination does not resolve over several months, it should be excised. Surgery should be conservative, since the primary objective is to exclude cancer. Occasionally, core needle biopsy or FNA cytology will suffice. Simple mastectomy or extensive removal of breast tissue is rarely, if ever, indicated for fibrocystic condition.

Differential Diagnosis

Pain, fluctuation in size, and multiplicity of lesions are the features most helpful in differentiating fibrocystic condition from carcinoma. If a dominant mass is present, the diagnosis of cancer should be assumed until disproven by biopsy. Mammography may be helpful, but the breast tissue in these young women is usually too radiodense to permit a worthwhile study. Sonography is useful in differentiating a cystic mass from a solid mass, especially in women with dense breasts. Final diagnosis, however, depends on analysis of the excisional biopsy specimen or needle biopsy.

Treatment

When the diagnosis of fibrocystic condition has been established by previous biopsy or is likely because the history is classic, aspiration of a discrete mass suggestive of a cyst is indicated to alleviate pain and, more importantly, to confirm the cystic nature of the mass. The patient is reexamined at intervals thereafter. If no fluid is obtained by aspiration, if fluid is bloody, if a mass persists after aspiration, or if at any time during follow-up a persistent or recurrent mass is noted, biopsy should be performed.

Breast pain associated with generalized fibrocystic condition is best treated by avoiding trauma and by wearing a good supportive brassiere during the night and day. Hormone therapy is not advisable, because it does not cure the condition and has undesirable side effects. Danazol (100–200 mg orally twice daily), a synthetic androgen, is the only treatment approved by the US Food and Drug Administration (FDA) for patients with severe pain. This treatment suppresses pituitary gonadotropins, but androgenic effects (acne, edema, hirsutism) usually make this treatment intolerable; in practice, it is rarely used. Similarly, tamoxifen reduces some symptoms of fibrocystic condition, but because of its side effects, it is not useful for young women unless it is given to reduce the risk of cancer. Postmenopausal women receiving hormone replacement therapy may stop or change doses of hormones to reduce pain. Oil of evening primrose (OEP), a natural form of gamolenic acid, has been shown to decrease pain in 44–58% of users. The dosage of gamolenic acid is six capsules of 500 mg orally twice daily. Studies have also demonstrated a low-fat diet or decreasing dietary fat intake may reduce the painful symptoms associated with fibrocystic condition. Further research is being done to determine the effects of topical treatments such as nonsteroidal anti-inflammatory drugs as well as topical hormonal drugs such as tamoxifen.

The role of caffeine consumption in the development and treatment of fibrocystic condition is controversial. Some studies suggest that eliminating caffeine from the diet is associated with improvement while other studies refute the benefit entirely. Many patients are aware of these studies and report relief of symptoms after giving up coffee, tea, and chocolate. Similarly, many women find vitamin E (400 international units daily) helpful; however, these observations remain anecdotal.

Prognosis

Exacerbations of pain, tenderness, and cyst formation may occur at any time until menopause, when symptoms usually subside, except in patients receiving hormonal replacement. The patient should be advised to examine her own breasts regularly just after menstruation and to inform her practitioner if a mass appears. The risk of breast cancer developing in women with fibrocystic condition with a proliferative or atypical component in the epithelium is higher than that of the general population. These women should be monitored carefully with physical examinations and imaging studies.

Guray M et al. Benign breast diseases: classification, diagnosis, and management. Oncologist. 2006 May;11(5):435–49. [PMID: 16720843]

Mannello F et al. Human gross cyst breast disease and cystic fluid: bio-molecular, morphological, and clinical studies. Breast Cancer Res Treat. 2006 May;97(2):115–29. [PMID: 16331347]

Qureshi S et al. Topical nonsteroidal anti-inflammatory drugs versus oil of evening primrose in the treatment of mastalgia. Surgeon. 2005 Feb;3(1):7–10. [PMID: 15789786]

Rosolowich V et al. Mastalgia. J Obstet Gynaecol Can. 2006 Jan;28(1):49–71. [PMID: 16533457]

FIBROADENOMA OF THE BREAST

This common benign neoplasm occurs most frequently in young women, usually within 20 years after puberty. It is somewhat more frequent and tends to occur at an earlier age in black women. Multiple tumors are found in 10–15% of patients.

The typical fibroadenoma is a round or ovoid, rubbery, discrete, relatively movable, nontender mass 1–5 cm in diameter. It is usually discovered accidentally. Clinical diagnosis in young patients is generally not difficult. In women over 30 years, fibrocystic condition of the breast and carcinoma of the breast must be considered. Cysts can be identified by aspiration or ultrasonography. Fibroadenoma does not normally occur after menopause but may occasionally develop after administration of hormones.

No treatment is usually necessary if the diagnosis can be made by needle biopsy or cytologic examination. Excision or vacuum-assisted core needle removal with pathologic examination of the specimen is performed if the diagnosis is uncertain. In a 2005 study, cryoablation, or freezing of the fibroadenoma, appears to be a safe procedure if the lesion is consistent with fibroadenoma on histology prior to ablation. Cryoablation is not appropriate for all fibroadenomas because some are too large to freeze or the diagnosis may not be certain. The advantages of cryoablation over observation are not clear. It is usually not possible to distinguish a large fibroadenoma from a phyllodes tumor on the basis of needle biopsy results or imaging alone.

Phyllodes tumor is a fibroadenoma-like tumor with cellular stroma that grows rapidly. It may reach a large size and, if inadequately excised, will recur locally. The lesion can be benign or malignant. If benign, phyllodes tumor is treated by local excision with a margin of surrounding breast tissue. The treatment of malignant phyllodes tumor is more controversial, but complete removal of the tumor with a rim of normal tissue avoids recurrence. Because these tumors may be large, simple mastectomy is sometimes necessary. Lymph node dissection is not performed, since the sarcomatous portion of the tumor metastasizes to the lungs and not the lymph nodes.

Bode MK et al. Ultrasonography and core needle biopsy in the differential diagnosis of fibroadenoma and tumor phyllodes. Acta Radiol. 2007 Sep;48(7):708–13. [PMID: 17728999]

Jacklin RK et al. Optimising preoperative diagnosis in phyllodes tumour of the breast. J Clin Pathol. 2006 May;59(5):454–9. [PMID: 16461806]

Lee AH et al. Histological features useful in the distinction of phyllodes tumour and fibroadenoma on needle core biopsy of the breast. Histopathology. 2007 Sep;51(3):336–44. [PMID: 17727475]

Telli ML et al. Phyllodes tumors of the breast: natural history, diagnosis, and treatment. J Natl Compr Canc Netw. 2007 Mar;5(3):324–30. [PMID: 17439760]

NIPPLE DISCHARGE

In order of decreasing frequency, the following are the most common causes of nipple discharge in the nonlactating breast: duct ectasia, intraductal papilloma, and carcinoma. The important characteristics of the discharge and some other factors to be evaluated by history and physical examination are as follows:

1. Nature of the discharge (serous, bloody, or other).
2. Association with a mass.
3. Unilateral or bilateral.
4. Single or multiple duct discharge.
5. Discharge is spontaneous (persistent or intermittent) or must be expressed.
6. Discharge is produced by pressure at a single site or by general pressure on the breast.
7. Relation to menses.
8. Premenopausal or postmenopausal.
9. Patient is taking contraceptive pills or estrogen.

Spontaneous, unilateral, serous or serosanguineous discharge from a single duct is usually caused by an intraductal papilloma or, rarely, by an intraductal cancer. A mass may not be palpable. The involved duct may be identified by pressure at different sites around the nipple at the margin of the areola. Bloody discharge is suggestive of cancer but is more often caused by a benign papilloma in the duct. Cytologic examination may identify malignant cells, but negative findings do not rule out cancer, which is more likely in women over age 50 years. In any case, the involved duct—and a mass if present—should be excised. A ductogram (a mammogram of a duct after radiopaque dye has been injected) is of limited value since excision of the suspicious ductal system is indicated regardless of findings. Ductoscopy, evaluation of the ductal system with a small scope inserted through the nipple, has been attempted but is not effective management.

In premenopausal women, spontaneous multiple duct discharge, unilateral or bilateral, most noticeable just before menstruation, is often due to fibrocystic condition. Discharge may be green or brownish. Papillomatosis and ductal ectasia are usually detected only by biopsy. If a mass is present, it should be removed.

A milky discharge from multiple ducts in the nonlactating breast may occur from hyperprolactinemia. Serum prolactin levels should be obtained to search for a pituitary tumor. Thyroid-stimulating hormone (TSH) helps exclude causative hypothyroidism. Numerous antipsychotic drugs and other drugs may also cause a milky discharge that ceases on discontinuance of the medication.

Oral contraceptive agents or estrogen replacement therapy may cause clear, serous, or milky discharge from a single duct, but multiple duct discharge is more common. In the premenopausal woman, the discharge is more evident just before menstruation and disappears on stopping the medication. If it does not stop, is from a single duct, and is copious, exploration should be performed since this may be a sign of cancer.

A purulent discharge may originate in a subareolar abscess and require removal of the abscess and the related lactiferous sinus.

When localization is not possible, no mass is palpable, and the discharge is nonbloody, the patient should be reexamined every 3 or 4 months for a year, and a mammogram and an ultrasound should be performed. Although most discharge is from a benign process, patients may find it annoying or disconcerting. Cytologic examination of the nipple discharge for exfoliated cancer cells is rarely helpful in determining a diagnosis. To eliminate the discharge, proximal duct excision can be performed both for treatment and diagnosis.

Barghav RK et al. The value of clinical characteristics and breast imaging studies in predicting a histopathologic diagnosis of cancer or high-risk lesion in patients with spontaneous nipple discharge. Am J Surg. 2007 Jan;193(1):141–2. [PMID: 17188113]

Escobar PF et al. The clinical applications of mammary ductoscopy. Am J Surg. 2006 Feb;191(2):211–5. [PMID: 16442948]

Hussain AN et al. Evaluating nipple discharge. Obstet Gynecol Surv. 2006 Apr;61(4):278–83. [PMID: 16551379]

Louie LD et al. Identification of breast cancer in patients with pathologic nipple discharge: does ductoscopy predict malignancy? Am J Surg. 2006 Oct;192(4):530–3. [PMID: 16978968]

FAT NECROSIS

Fat necrosis is a rare lesion of the breast but is of clinical importance because it produces a mass (often accompanied by skin or nipple retraction) that is indistinguishable from carcinoma even with imaging studies. Trauma is presumed to be the cause, though only about 50% of patients give a history of injury. Ecchymosis is occasionally present. If untreated, the mass effect gradually disappears. The safest course is to obtain a biopsy. Needle biopsy is often adequate, but frequently the entire mass must be excised, primarily to exclude carcinoma. Fat necrosis is common after segmental resection, radiation therapy, or flap reconstruction after mastectomy.

Li S et al. Surgical management of recurrent subareolar breast abscesses: Mayo Clinic experience. Am J Surg. 2006 Oct;192(4):528–9. [PMI: 16978967]

Tan PH et al. Fat necrosis of the breast—A review. Breast. 2006 Jun;15(3):313–8. [PMID: 16198567]

BREAST ABSCESS

During nursing, an area of redness, tenderness, and induration may develop in the breast. The organism most commonly found in these abscesses is *Staphylococcus aureus* (see Puerperal Mastitis, Chapter 19).

Infection in the nonlactating breast is rare. A subareolar abscess may develop in young or middle-aged women who are not lactating (Plate 71). These infections tend to recur after incision and drainage unless the area is explored during a quiescent interval, with excision of the involved lactiferous duct or ducts at the base of the nipple. In the nonlactating breast, inflammatory carcinoma must always be considered. Thus, incision and biopsy of any indurated tissue with a small piece of erythematous skin is indicated when suspected abscess or cellulitis in the nonlactating breast does not resolve promptly with antibiotics. Often needle or catheter drainage is adequate to treat an abscess, but surgical incision and drainage may be necessary.

Scott BG et al. Rate of malignancies in breast abscesses and argument for ultrasound drainage. Am J Surg. 2006 Dec;192(6):869–72. [PMID: 17161110]

DISORDERS OF THE AUGMENTED BREAST

At least 4 million American women have had breast implants. Breast augmentation is performed by placing implants under the pectoralis muscle or, less desirably, in the subcutaneous tissue of the breast. Most implants are made of an outer silicone shell filled with a silicone gel, saline, or some combination of the two. Capsule contraction or scarring around the implant develops in about 15–25% of patients, leading to a firmness and distortion of the breast that can be painful. Some require removal of the implant and surrounding capsule. In 2006, the FDA reapproved silicone implants for augmentation cosmetic surgery.

Implant rupture may occur in as many as 5–10% of women, and bleeding of gel through the capsule is noted even more commonly. Although silicone gel may be an immunologic stimulant, there is no increase in autoimmune disorders in patients with such implants. The FDA has advised symptomatic women with ruptured implants to discuss possible surgical removal with their clinicians. However, women who are asymptomatic and have no evidence of rupture of a silicone gel prosthesis should probably not undergo removal of the implant. Women with symptoms of autoimmune illnesses should consider removal.

Studies have failed to show any association between implants and an increased incidence of breast cancer. However, breast cancer may develop in a patient with an augmentation prosthesis, as it does in women without them. Detection in patients with implants is more difficult because mammography is less able to detect early lesions. Mammography is better if the implant is subpectoral rather than subcutaneous. The prosthesis should be placed retropectorally after mastectomy to facilitate detection of a local recurrence of cancer, which is usually cutaneous or subcutaneous and is easily detected by palpation.

If a cancer develops in a patient with implants, it should be treated in the same manner as in women without implants. Such women should be offered the option of mastectomy or breast-conserving therapy, which may require removal or replacement of the implant. Radiotherapy of the augmented breast often results in marked capsular contracture. Adjuvant treatments should be given for the same indications as for women who have no implants.

Fryzek JP et al. Silicone breast implants. J Rheumatol. 2005 Jan;32(1):201. [PMID: 15700387]

McCarthy CM et al. Breast cancer in the previously augmented breast. Plast Reconstr Surg. 2007 Jan;119(1):49–58. [PMID: 17255656]

McIntosh SA et al. Breast cancer following augmentation mammoplasty—a review of its impact on prognosis and management. J Plast Reconstr Aesthet Surg. 2007;60(10):1127–35. [PMID: 17613294]

CARCINOMA OF THE FEMALE BREAST

ESSENTIALS OF DIAGNOSIS

▶ Most women with breast cancer do not have identifiable risk factors.

▶ Risk factors include delayed childbearing, positive family history of breast cancer or genetic mutations (*BRCA1*, *BRCA2*), and personal history of breast cancer or some types of proliferative conditions.

▶ *Early findings:* Single, nontender, firm to hard mass with ill-defined margins; mammographic abnormalities and no palpable mass.

▶ *Later findings:* Skin or nipple retraction; axillary lymphadenopathy; breast enlargement, erythema, edema, pain; fixation of mass to skin or chest wall (Plate 72).

Incidence & Risk Factors

Breast cancer will develop in one of eight American women. Next to skin cancer, breast cancer is the most common cancer in women; it is second only to lung cancer as a cause of death. The probability of developing breast cancer increases throughout life. The mean age and the median age of women with breast cancer is 61 years.

In 2008, it is estimated there will be approximately 182,500 new cases of breast cancer annually and about 41,000 deaths from this disease in women in the United States. An additional 68,000 cases of ductal carcinoma in situ (DCIS) will be detected, principally by screening mammography. The incidence of breast cancer has slightly decreased, presumably because of decreased use of postmenopausal hormone replacement therapy. Mortality has also decreased slightly due to early detection and increased use of systemic therapy.

Although more than 75% of women in whom breast cancer has been diagnosed do not have an obvious risk factor, there are several that play a role in breast cancer development. Breast cancer is three to four times more likely to develop in women with a first-degree relative (mother, daughter, or sister) who had breast cancer than in those without a family history. Risk is further increased in patients whose mothers' or sisters' breast cancers occurred before menopause or were bilateral and in those with a family history of breast cancer in two or more first-degree relatives as well as in women of Ashkenazi Jewish descent.

Nulliparous women and women whose first full-term pregnancy was after age 35 have a 1.5 times higher incidence of breast cancer than multiparous women. Late menarche and artificial menopause are associated with a lower incidence, whereas early menarche (under age 12) and late natural menopause (after age 50) are associated with a slight increase in risk. Fibrocystic condition, when accompanied by proliferative changes, papillomatosis, or atypical epithelial hyperplasia, and increased breast density on mammogram are also associated with an increased incidence. A woman who had cancer in one breast is at increased risk for cancer developing in the other breast. In these women, a contralateral cancer develops at the rate of 1% or 2% per year. Women with cancer of the uterine corpus have a risk of breast cancer significantly higher than that of the general population, and women with breast cancer have a comparably increased risk for endometrial cancer. In the United States, breast cancer is more common in white women. The incidence of the disease among nonwhite (mostly black) women is increasing, especially in younger women. In general, rates reported from developing countries are low, whereas rates are high in developed countries, with the notable exception of Japan. Some of the variability may be due to underreporting in the developing countries, but a real difference probably exists. Dietary factors, particularly increased fat consumption, may account for some differences in incidence. Oral contraceptives do not appear to increase the risk of breast cancer. There is evidence that administration of estrogens to postmenopausal women may result in a slightly increased risk of breast cancer, but only with higher, long-term doses of estrogens. Concomitant administration of progesterone and estrogen may markedly increase the incidence of breast cancer compared with the use of estrogen alone. The Women's Health Initiative prospective randomized study of hormone replacement therapy stopped treatment with estrogen and progesterone early because of an increased risk of breast cancer compared with untreated controls or women treated with estrogen alone. With decreasing use of these hormones, breast cancer rates may continue to decrease. Alcohol consumption increases the risk very slightly.

Some inherited breast cancers have been found to be associated with a gene on chromosome 17. This gene, *BRCA1*, is mutated in families with early-onset breast and ovarian cancer. Breast cancer will develop in approximately 85% of women with *BRCA1* gene mutations during their lifetime. Other genes are associated with increased risk of breast and other cancers, such as *BRCA2* (associated with a gene on chromosome 13); ataxia-telangiectasia mutation; and mutation of *p53*, the tumor suppressor gene. Mutations to *p53* have been found in approximately 1% of breast cancers in women under 40 years of age. Genetic testing is commercially available for women at high risk for breast cancer. Women with genetic mutations in whom breast cancer develops may be treated in the same way as women who do not have mutations (ie, lumpectomy), though there is an increased ipsilateral and contralateral recurrence rate after lumpectomy for these women. Such women with mutations often elect bilateral mastectomy as treatment. Some states have enacted legislation to prevent insurance

Table 17–1. Factors associated with increased risk of breast cancer.

Race	White
Age	Older
Family history	Breast cancer in mother, sister, or daughter (especially bilateral or premenopausal)
Genetics	*BRCA1* or *BRCA2* mutation
Previous medical history	Endometrial cancer Proliferative forms of fibrocystic disease Cancer in other breast
Menstrual history	Early menarche (under age 12) Late menopause (after age 50)
Reproductive history	Nulliparous or late first pregnancy

companies from considering mutations as "preexisting conditions," preventing insurability.

Women at greater than normal risk for developing breast cancer (Table 17–1) should be identified by their practitioners and monitored carefully. Those with an exceptional family history should be counseled about the option of genetic testing. Some of these high-risk women may consider prophylactic mastectomy, oophorectomy, or tamoxifen, an FDA-approved preventive agent.

▶ Prevention

The National Surgical Adjuvant Breast Project (NSABP) conducted the first Breast Cancer Prevention Trial (BCPT) P-1, which evaluated tamoxifen as a preventive agent in women with no personal history of breast cancer but at high risk for developing the disease. Women who received tamoxifen for 5 years had about a 50% reduction in noninvasive and invasive cancers compared with women taking placebo. However, women over age 50 who received the drug had an increased incidence of endometrial cancer and deep venous thrombosis. Unfortunately, no survival data will be produced from this trial because it was stopped.

The selective estrogen receptor modulator (SERM) raloxifene, effective in preventing osteoporosis, is also effective in preventing breast cancer. The initial study, Multiple Outcomes of Raloxifene Evaluations (MORE) trial, aimed at determining the effect of raloxifene on bone, demonstrated that raloxifene also reduced breast cancer risk in women being given the drug. After 8 years, raloxifene demonstrated an overall reduction of invasive breast cancer of 66%. Because this study was designed to determine the effect of raloxifene on bone density, it was conducted in women at lower risk for breast cancer. To better understand the preventive effect of raloxifene in the high-risk population, a randomized study comparing raloxifene with tamoxifen was conducted.

The Study of Tamoxifen and Raloxifene (STAR) P-2 trial, conducted by the National Surgical Adjuvant Breast and Bowel Project (NSABP) and completed in 2006, demonstrated that raloxifene and tamoxifen are equivalent in preventing invasive breast cancer in the high-risk population. Many of the side effects of raloxifene are the same as tamoxifen with a slight decrease in cataracts and thromboembolic events in the raloxifene group. Surprisingly, noninvasive cancer (DCIS) occurred more commonly in women treated with raloxifene.

Similar to SERMs, aromatase inhibitors (AI) have shown great success in treating breast cancer with fewer side effects, although bone loss is a significant side effect of this long-term treatment. Several large multicenter studies (eg, International Breast Cancer Intervention Study II [IBIS-II] and National Cancer Institute of Canada Clinical Trials Group [NCIC CTG]) are underway to determine whether AIs have a role in preventing breast cancer.

In addition to pharmaceutical therapy, patients continue to seek a way to prevent breast cancer. There has been considerable research on incorporating diet and exercise into the lifestyle of women who may be at risk for cancer. The Women's Intervention Nutrition Study was conducted to determine whether decreasing dietary fat intake would reduce the incidence of breast cancer recurrence after initial treatment. Although the trial demonstrated a decrease in recurrence in the follow-up period, it did not reach statistical significance.

Bao T et al. Chemoprevention of breast cancer: tamoxifen, raloxifene, and beyond. Am J Ther. 2006 Jul–Aug;13(4):337–48. [PMID: 16858170]

Boyd NF et al. Mammographic density and the risk and detection of breast cancer. N Engl J Med. 2007 Jan 18;356(3):227–36. [PMID: 17229950]

Chan K et al. Chemoprevention of breast cancer for women at high risk. Semin Oncol. 2006 Dec;33(6):642–6. [PMID: 17145342]

Chlebowski RT et al. Dietary fat reduction and breast cancer outcome: interim efficacy results from the Women's Intervention Nutrition Study. J Natl Cancer Inst. 2006 Dec 20; 98(24):1767–76. [PMID: 17179478]

Jemal A et al. Cancer Statistics, 2008. CA Cancer J Clin. 2008 Mar–Apr;58(2):71–96. [PMID: 18287387]

Jordan VC. Chemoprevention of breast cancer with selective estrogen-receptor modulators. Nat Rev Cancer. 2007 Jan; 7(1):46–53. [PMID: 17186017]

Linos E et al. Diet and breast cancer. Curr Oncol Rep. 2007 Jan;9(1):31–41. [PMID: 17164045]

Lynch HT et al. Hereditary breast cancer: part I. Diagnosing hereditary breast cancer syndromes. Breast J. 2008 Jan–Feb;14(1):3–13. [PMID: 18086272]

Newman LA et al. Breast cancer risk assessment and risk reduction. Surg Clin North Am. 2007 Apr;87(2):307–16. [PMID: 17498528]

Palma M et al. *BRCA1* and *BRCA2*: the genetic testing and the current management options for mutation carriers. Crit Rev Oncol Hematol. 2006 Jan;57(1):1–23. [PMID: 16337408]

Patel RR et al. Optimizing the antihormonal treatment and prevention of breast cancer. Breast Cancer. 2007;14(2):113–22. [PMID: 17485895]

Prentice RL et al. Low-fat dietary pattern and risk of invasive breast cancer: the Women's Health Initiative Randomized Controlled Dietary Modification Trial. JAMA. 2006 Feb 8;295(6):629–42. [PMID: 16467232]

Pruthi S et al. A multidisciplinary approach to the management of breast cancer, part 1: prevention and diagnosis. Mayo Clin Proc. 2007 Aug;82(8):999–1012. [PMID: 17673070]

Vogel VG et al; National Surgical Adjuvant Breast and Bowel Project (NSABP). Effects of tamoxifen vs raloxifene on the risk of developing invasive breast cancer and other disease outcomes: the NSABP Study of Tamoxifen and Raloxifene (STAR) P-2 trial. JAMA. 2006 Jun 21;295(23):2727–41. [PMID: 16754727]

► Early Detection of Breast Cancer

A. Screening Programs

There have been a number of large screening programs conducted over the years. Such programs, consisting of physical and mammographic examination of asymptomatic women, identify about 10 cancers per 1000 women over the age of 50 and about 2 cancers per 1000 women under the age of 50. These studies show the increased survival benefit of screening programs, as screening detects cancer before it has spread to the lymph nodes in about 80% of the women evaluated. This increases the chance of survival to about 85% at 5 years.

Both physical examination and mammography are necessary for maximum yield in screening programs, since about 35–50% of early breast cancers can be discovered only by mammography and another 40% can be detected only by palpation. About one-third of the abnormalities detected on screening mammograms will be found to be malignant when biopsy is performed. The probability of cancer on a screening mammogram is directly related to the Breast Imaging and Reporting Data System (BIRADS) assessment, and work-up should be performed based on this classification. Women 20–40 years of age should have a breast examination as part of routine medical care every 2–3 years. Women over age 40 years should have annual breast examinations. The sensitivity of mammography varies from approximately 60% to 90%. This sensitivity depends on several factors, including patient age (breast density) and tumor size, location, and mammographic appearance. In young women with dense breasts, mammography is less sensitive than in older women with fatty breasts, in whom mammography can detect at least 90% of malignancies. Smaller tumors, particularly those without calcifications, are more difficult to detect, especially in dense breasts. The lack of sensitivity and the low incidence of breast cancer in young women have led to questions concerning the value of mammography for screening in women 40–50 years of age. The specificity of mammography in women under 50 years varies from about 30% to 40% for nonpalpable mammographic abnormalities to 85% to 90% for clinically evident malignancies.

Screening recommendations for women in their 40s are based, in part, on trials from Sweden. Two trials showed a statistical advantage for screening women in their 40s, and a meta-analysis similarly revealed a statistical survival advantage for screened women with longer follow-up. The National Cancer Advisory Board recommended that women in their 40s with average risk factors have screening mammography every 1–2 years and that women at higher risk seek medical advice on when to begin screening. Studies continue to support the value of screening mammography in women over 40 years (see Table 1–9). Such women should have annual mammography and physical examination.

The beneficial effect of screening in women aged 50–69 years is undisputed and has been confirmed by all clinical trials. The efficacy of screening in older women—those older than 70 years—is inconclusive and is difficult to determine because few studies have examined this population.

B. Self-Examination

Breast self-exam (BSE) has not been shown to improve survival. Because of the lack of strong evidence demonstrating value, the American Cancer Society no longer recommends monthly BSE beginning at age 20 years. The recommendation is that patients be made aware of the potential benefits, limitations, and harms (increased biopsies or false-positive results) associated with BSE. Women who choose to perform BSE should be advised regarding the proper technique. Premenopausal women should perform the examination 7–8 days after the start of the menstrual period. First, breasts should be inspected before a mirror with the hands at the sides, overhead, and pressed firmly on the hips to contract the pectoralis muscles causing masses, asymmetry of breasts, and slight dimpling of the skin to become apparent. Next, in a supine position, each breast should be carefully palpated with the fingers of the opposite hand. Some women discover small breast lumps more readily when their skin is moist while bathing or showering. While BSE is not a recommended practice, patients should recognize and report any breast changes to their practitioners as it remains an important facet of proactive care.

C. Imaging

Mammography is the most reliable means of detecting breast cancer before a mass can be palpated. Slowly growing cancers can be identified by mammography at least 2 years before reaching a size detectable by palpation. Film screen mammography delivers less than 0.4 cGy to the mid breast per view. Although full-field digital mammography provides an easier method to maintain and review mammograms, it has not been proven that it provides better images or increases detection rates more than film mammography. In subset analysis of a large study, digital mammography seemed slightly superior in women with dense breasts. Computer-assisted detection (CAD) has not shown any increase in detection of cancers and is not routinely performed at centers with experienced mammographers.

Calcifications are the most easily recognized mammographic abnormality. The most common findings associated with carcinoma of the breast are clustered polymorphic microcalcifications. Such calcifications are usually at least five to eight in number, aggregated in one part of the breast and differing from each other in size and shape, often including branched or V- or Y-shaped configurations. There may be an associated mammographic mass density or, at times, only a mass density with no calcifications. Such a density usually has irregular or ill-defined borders and may lead to architectural distortion within the breast but may be subtle and difficult to detect.

Indications for mammography are as follows: (1) to screen at regular intervals asymptomatic women at high risk for developing breast cancer (see above); (2) to evaluate each breast when a diagnosis of potentially curable breast cancer has been made, and at yearly intervals thereafter; (3) to evaluate a questionable or ill-defined breast mass or other suspicious change in the breast; (4) to search for an occult breast cancer in a woman with metastatic disease in axillary nodes or elsewhere from an unknown primary; (5) to screen women prior to cosmetic operations or prior to biopsy of a mass, to examine for an unsuspected cancer; (6) to monitor those women with breast cancer who have been treated with breast-conserving surgery and radiation; and (7) to monitor the contralateral breast in those women with breast cancer treated with mastectomy.

Patients with a dominant or suspicious mass must undergo biopsy despite mammographic findings. The mammogram should be obtained prior to biopsy so that other suspicious areas can be noted and the contralateral breast can be evaluated. Mammography is never a substitute for biopsy because it may not reveal clinical cancer, especially in a very dense breast, as may be seen in young women with fibrocystic changes, and may not reveal medullary cancers.

Communication and documentation among the patient, the referring practitioner, and the interpreting physician are critical for high-quality screening and diagnostic mammography. The patient should be told about *how* she will receive timely results of her mammogram; that mammography does not "rule out" cancer; and that she may receive a correlative examination such as ultrasound at the mammography facility if referred for a suspicious lesion. She should also be aware of the technique and need for breast compression and that this may be uncomfortable. The mammography facility should be informed *in writing by the clinician* of abnormal physical examination findings. The Agency for Health Care Policy and Research (AHCPR) Clinical Practice Guidelines strongly recommend that all mammography reports be communicated in writing to the patient and referring practitioner. MRI and ultrasound may be useful screening modalities in women who are at high risk for breast cancer but not for the general population. The sensitivity of MRI is much higher than mammography; however, the specificity is significantly lower and this results in multiple unnecessary biopsies. The increased sensitivity despite decreased specificity may be considered a reasonable trade-off for those at increased risk for developing breast cancer but not for normal-risk population. MRI is useful in women with breast implants to determine the character of a lesion present in the breast and to search for implant rupture and at times is helpful in patients with prior lumpectomy and radiation. In addition, positron emission tomography (PET) may play a role in imaging atypical lesions but is less sensitive for early breast cancer than is MRI or mammography. The primary role remains evaluation of metastatic deposits.

Armstrong K et al. Screening mammography in women 40 to 49 years of age: a systematic review for the American College of Physicians. Ann Intern Med. 2007 Apr 3;146(7):516–26. [PMID: 17404354]

Bartella L et al. Imaging breast cancer. Radiol Clin North Am. 2007 Jan;45(1):45–67. [PMID: 17157623]

Budakoglu II et al. The effectiveness of training for breast cancer and breast self-examination in women aged 40 and over. J Cancer Educ. 2007 Summer;22(2):108–11. [PMID: 17605625]

Feig SA. Screening mammography: a successful public health initiative. Rev Panam Salud Publica. 2006 Aug–Sep;20(2-3):125–33. [PMID: 17199907]

Knutson D et al. Screening for breast cancer: current recommendations and future directions. Am Fam Physician. 2007 Jun 1;75(11):1660–6. [PMID: 17575656]

Kuhl C. The current status of breast MR imaging. Part I. Choice of technique, image interpretation, diagnostic accuracy, and transfer to clinical practice. Radiology. 2007 Aug;244(2):356–78. [PMID: 17641361]

Lord SJ et al. A systematic review of the effectiveness of magnetic resonance imaging (MRI) as an addition to mammography and ultrasound in screening young women at high risk of breast cancer. Eur J Cancer. 2007 Sep;43(13):1905–17. [PMID: 17681781]

Saslow D et al. American Cancer Society guidelines for breast screening with MRI as an adjunct to mammography. CA Cancer J Clin. 2007 Mar–Apr;57(2):75–89. [PMID: 17392385]

Skaane P. Studies comparing screen-film mammography and full-field digital mammography in breast center screening: updated review. Acta Radiol. 2009 Jan;50(1):3–14. [PMID: 19037825]

Terry MB et al. Lifetime alcohol intake and breast cancer risk. Ann Epidemiol. 2006 Mar;16(3):230–40. [PMID: 16230024]

Warner E et al. Systematic review: using magnetic resonance imaging to screen women at high risk for breast cancer. Ann Intern Med. 2008 May 6;148(9):671–9. [PMID: 18458280]

Weaver DL et al. Pathologic findings from the Breast Cancer Surveillance Consortium: population-based outcomes in women undergoing biopsy after screening mammography. Cancer. 2006 Feb 15;106(4):732–42. [PMID: 16411214]

Van Ongeval Ch. Digital mammography for screening and diagnosis of breast cancer: an overview. JBR-BTR. 2007 May–Jun;90(3):163–6. [PMID: 17696081]

► Clinical Findings Associated with Early Detection of Breast Cancer

A. Symptoms and Signs

The presenting complaint in about 70% of patients with breast cancer is a lump (usually painless) in the breast. About 90% of these breast masses are discovered by the patient. Less frequent symptoms are breast pain; nipple discharge; erosion, retraction, enlargement, or itching of the nipple; and redness, generalized hardness, enlargement, or shrinking of the breast. Rarely, an axillary mass or swelling of the arm may be the first symptom. Back or bone pain, jaundice, or weight loss may be the result of systemic metastases, but these symptoms are rarely seen on initial presentation.

The relative frequency of carcinoma in various anatomic sites in the breast is shown in Figure 17–1.

Inspection of the breast is the first step in physical examination and should be carried out with the patient sitting, arms at her sides and then overhead. Abnormal variations in breast size and contour, minimal nipple retraction, and slight edema, redness, or retraction of the skin can be identified. Asymmetry of the breasts and retraction or dimpling of the skin can often be accentuated by having the patient raise her arms overhead or press her

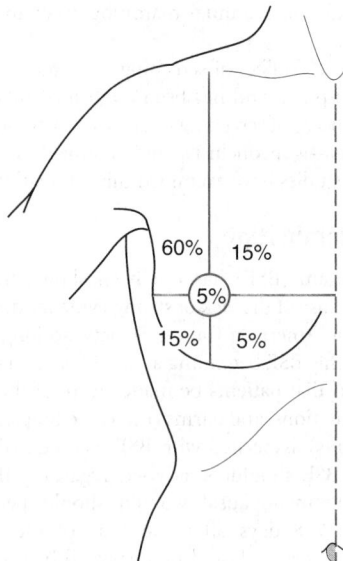

▲ **Figure 17-1.** Frequency of breast carcinoma at various anatomic sites.

hands on her hips to contract the pectoralis muscles. Axillary and supraclavicular areas should be thoroughly palpated for enlarged nodes with the patient sitting (Figure 17–2). Palpation of the breast for masses or other changes should be performed with the patient both seated and supine with the arm abducted (Figure 17–3). Palpation with a rotary motion of the examiner's fingers as well as a horizontal stripping motion has been recommended.

Breast cancer usually consists of a nontender, firm or hard mass with poorly delineated margins (caused by local infiltration). Very small (1–2 mm) erosions of the nipple

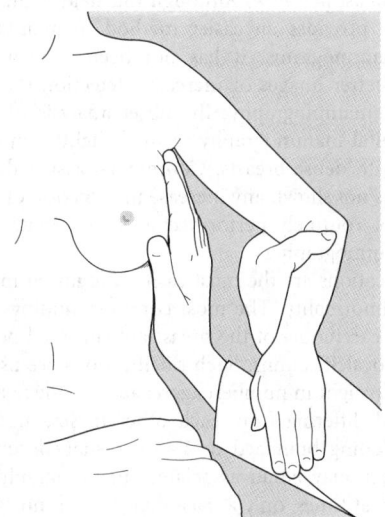

▲ **Figure 17-2.** Palpation of axillary region for enlarged lymph nodes.

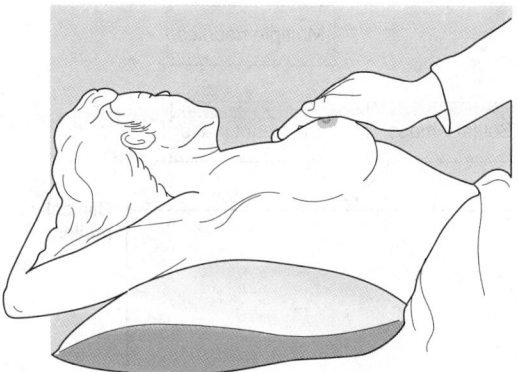

▲ **Figure 17–3.** Palpation of breasts. Palpation is performed with the patient supine and arm abducted.

epithelium may be the only manifestation of Paget carcinoma. Watery, serous, or bloody discharge from the nipple is an occasional early sign but is more often associated with benign disease.

A small lesion, less than 1 cm in diameter, may be difficult or impossible for the examiner to feel but may be discovered by the patient. She should always be asked to demonstrate the location of the mass; if the practitioner fails to confirm the patient's suspicions and imaging studies are normal, the examination should be repeated in 2–3 months, preferably 1–2 weeks after the onset of menses. During the premenstrual phase of the cycle, increased innocuous nodularity may suggest neoplasm or may obscure an underlying lesion. If there is any question regarding the nature of an abnormality under these circumstances, the patient should be asked to return after her period. Ultrasound is often valuable and mammography essential when an area is felt by the patient to be abnormal but the physician feels no mass. MRI may be considered, but the lack of specificity should be discussed by the practitioner and the patient. MRI should not be used to rule out cancer because MRI has a false-negative rate of about 3–5%. Although lower than mammography, this false-negative rate cannot permit safe elimination of the possibility of cancer. False negatives are more likely seen in infiltrating lobular carcinomas and DCIS.

Metastases tend to involve regional lymph nodes, which may be palpable. One or two movable, nontender, not particularly firm axillary lymph nodes 5 mm or less in diameter are frequently present and are generally of no significance. Firm or hard nodes larger than 1 cm are typical of metastases. Axillary nodes that are matted or fixed to skin or deep structures indicate advanced disease (at least stage III). On the other hand, if the examiner thinks that the axillary nodes are involved, that impression will be borne out by histologic section in about 85% of cases. The incidence of positive axillary nodes increases with the size of the primary tumor. Noninvasive cancers (in situ) do not metastasize. Metastases are present in about 30% of patients with clinically negative nodes.

In most cases, no nodes are palpable in the supraclavicular fossa. Firm or hard nodes of any size in this location or just beneath the clavicle are suggestive of metastatic cancer and should be biopsied. Ipsilateral supraclavicular or infraclavicular nodes containing cancer indicate that the tumor is in an advanced stage (stage III or IV). Edema of the ipsilateral arm, commonly caused by metastatic infiltration of regional lymphatics, is also a sign of advanced cancer.

B. Laboratory Findings

A consistently elevated sedimentation rate may be the result of disseminated cancer. Liver or bone metastases may be associated with elevation of serum alkaline phosphatase. Hypercalcemia is an occasional important finding in advanced cancer of the breast. Carcinoembryonic antigen (CEA) and CA 15-3 or CA 27-29 may be used as markers for recurrent breast cancer but are not helpful in diagnosing early lesions. Many scientists are further investigating breast cancer markers through proteomics and hormone assays. These studies are ongoing and may prove to be helpful in early detection or evaluation of prognosis.

C. Imaging for Metastases

Chest radiographs may show pulmonary metastases. CT scanning of the liver and brain is of value only when metastases are suspected in these areas. Bone scans utilizing ^{99m}Tc-labeled phosphates or phosphonates are more sensitive than skeletal radiographs in detecting metastatic breast cancer. Bone scanning has not proved to be of clinical value as a routine preoperative test in the absence of symptoms, physical findings, or abnormal alkaline phosphatase or calcium levels. The frequency of abnormal findings on bone scan parallels the status of the axillary lymph nodes on pathologic examination. PET scanning is less useful than a bone scan to identify metastatic bone lesions. It is effective in soft tissue or visceral metastases in patients with signs or symptoms of metastatic disease. PET scanning combined with CT (PET-CT) is an effective screening method for detecting soft tissue metastases and is replacing CT scans.

D. Diagnostic Tests

1. Biopsy—The diagnosis of breast cancer depends ultimately on examination of tissue or cells removed by biopsy. Treatment should never be undertaken without an unequivocal histologic or cytologic diagnosis of cancer. The safest course is biopsy examination of all suspicious lesions found on physical examination or mammography, or both. About 60% of lesions clinically thought to be cancer prove on biopsy to be benign, while about 30% of clinically benign lesions are found to be malignant. These findings demonstrate the fallibility of clinical judgment and the necessity for biopsy.

All breast masses require a histologic diagnosis with one probable exception, a nonsuspicious, presumably fibrocystic mass, in a premenopausal woman. Rather, these masses can be observed through one or two menstrual cycles. However, if the mass is not cystic and does not completely resolve during this time, it must be biopsied. Figures 17–4 and 17–5 present algorithms for management of breast masses in premenopausal and postmenopausal patients.

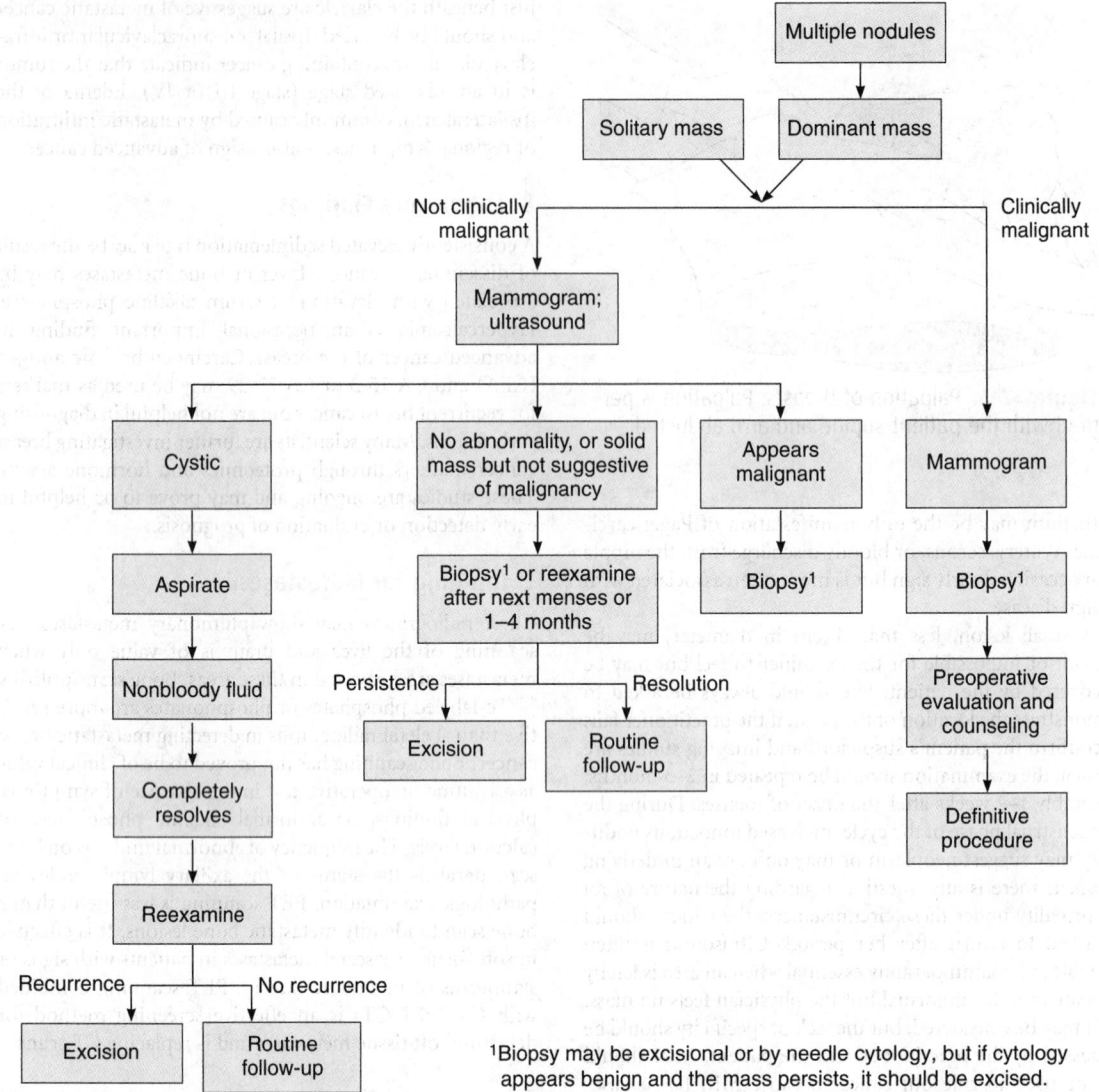

▲ **Figure 17–4.** Evaluation of breast masses in premenopausal women. (Adapted, with permission, from Chang S, Haigh PI, Giuliano AE. Breast disease. In: Berek JS, Hacker NF [editors], Practical Gynecologic Oncology, 4th edition, LWW, 2004.)

The simplest biopsy method is needle biopsy, either by aspiration of tumor cells (FNA cytology) or by obtaining a small core of tissue with a hollow needle (core biopsy).

FNA cytology is a useful technique whereby cells are aspirated with a small needle and examined cytologically. This technique can be performed easily with virtually no morbidity and is much less expensive than excisional or open biopsy. The main disadvantages are that it requires a pathologist skilled in the cytologic diagnosis of breast cancer and that it is subject to sampling problems, particularly because deep lesions may be missed. Furthermore, noninvasive cancers usually cannot be distinguished from invasive cancers. The incidence of false-positive diagnoses is extremely low, perhaps 1–2%. The false-negative rate is as high as 10%. Most experienced clinicians would not leave a suspicious dominant mass in the breast even when

FNA cytology is negative unless the clinical diagnosis, breast imaging studies, and cytologic studies were all in agreement, such as a fibrocystic lesion or fibroadenoma.

Large-needle (core needle) biopsy removes a core of tissue with a large cutting needle. Hand-held biopsy devices make large-core needle biopsy of a palpable mass easy and cost effective in the office with local anesthesia. As in the case of any needle biopsy, the main problem is sampling error due to improper positioning of the needle, giving rise to a false-negative test result. Core biopsy has the advantage that tumor markers, such as estrogen receptor (ER), progesterone receptor (PR) and *HER-2/neu* over-expression can be performed on cores of tissue.

Open biopsy under local anesthesia as a separate procedure prior to deciding upon definitive treatment is the most reliable means of diagnosis. Needle biopsy or aspira-

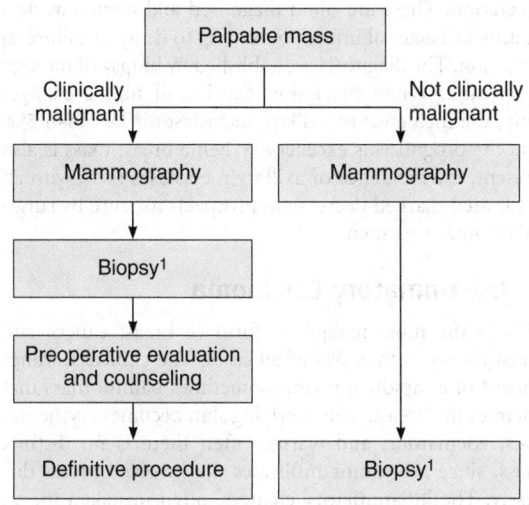

¹Biopsy may be excisional or by needle cytology, but if cytology appears benign and the mass persists, it should be excised.

▲ **Figure 17–5.** Evaluation of breast masses in post-menopausal women. (Adapted, with permission, from Chang S, Haigh PI, Giuliano AE. Breast disease. In: Berek JS, Hacker NF [editors], Practical Gynecologic Oncology, 4th edition, LWW, 2004.)

tion, when positive, offers a more rapid approach with less expense and morbidity, but when nondiagnostic it must be followed by open biopsy. It generally consists of an excisional biopsy, which is done through an incision with the intent to remove the entire abnormality, not simply a sample. Additional evaluation for metastatic disease and therapeutic options can be discussed with the patient after the histologic or cytologic diagnosis of cancer has been established. In situ cancers are not easily diagnosed cytologically and usually require excisional biopsy.

As an alternative in highly suspicious circumstances, the diagnosis may be made on frozen section of tissue obtained by open biopsy under general anesthesia. If the frozen section is positive, the surgeon can proceed immediately with the definitive operation. This one-step method is rarely used today except when a cytologic study has suggested cancer but is not diagnostic and there is a high clinical suspicion of malignancy in a patient well prepared for the diagnosis of cancer and its treatment options.

In general, the two-step approach—outpatient biopsy followed by definitive operation at a later date—is preferred in the diagnosis and treatment of breast cancer, because patients can be given time to adjust to the diagnosis of cancer, can consider alternative forms of therapy, and can seek a second opinion if they wish. There is no adverse effect from the short delay of the two-step procedure.

2. Ultrasonography—Ultrasonography is performed primarily to differentiate cystic from solid lesions but may show signs suggestive of carcinoma. Ultrasonography may show an irregular mass within a cyst in the rare case of

intracystic carcinoma. If a tumor is palpable and feels like a cyst, an 18-gauge needle can be used to aspirate the fluid and make the diagnosis of cyst. If a cyst is aspirated and the fluid is nonbloody, it does not have to be examined cytologically. If the mass does not recur, no further diagnostic test is necessary. Nonpalpable mammographic densities that appear benign should be investigated with ultrasound to determine whether the lesion is cystic or solid. These may even be needle biopsied with ultrasound guidance.

3. Mammography—When a suspicious abnormality is identified by mammography alone and cannot be palpated by the clinician, the lesion should be biopsied under mammographic guidance. In the **computerized stereotactic guided core needle** technique, a biopsy needle is inserted into the lesion with mammographic guidance, and a core of tissue for histologic examination can then be examined. Vacuum assistance increases the amount of tissue obtained and improves diagnosis.

Mammographic localization biopsy is performed by obtaining a mammogram in two perpendicular views and placing a needle or hook-wire near the abnormality so that the surgeon can use the metal needle or wire as a guide during operation to locate the lesion. After mammography confirms the position of the needle in relation to the lesion, an incision is made and the subcutaneous tissue is dissected until the needle is identified. Often, the abnormality cannot even be palpated through the incision—as is the case with microcalcifications—and thus it is essential to obtain a mammogram of the specimen to document that the lesion was excised. At that time, a second marker needle can further localize the lesion for the pathologist. Stereotactic core needle biopsies have proved equivalent to mammographic localization biopsies. Core biopsy is preferable to mammographic localization for accessible lesions since an operation can be avoided. A metal clip should be placed after any image-guided core biopsy to facilitate finding the site of the lesion if subsequent treatment is necessary.

4. Other imaging modalities—Other modalities of breast imaging have been investigated for diagnostic purposes. Automated breast ultrasonography is useful in distinguishing cystic from solid lesions but should be used only as a supplement to physical examination and mammography. Ductography may be useful to define the site of a lesion causing a bloody discharge, but since biopsy is almost always indicated, ductography may be omitted and the blood-filled nipple system excised. Ductoscopy has shown some promise in identifying intraductal lesions, especially in the case of pathologic nipple discharge, but in practice, this technique is rarely used. MRI is highly sensitive but not specific and should not be used for screening except in highly selective cases. For example, MRI is useful in differentiating scar from recurrence postlumpectomy and may be valuable to screen high-risk women (eg, women with *BRCA* mutations). It may also be of value to examine for multicentricity when there is a known primary cancer; to examine the contralateral breast in women with cancer; to examine the extent of cancer, especially lobular carcinomas; or to determine the response to neoadjuvant chemotherapy. PET scanning does not appear useful in evaluating the breast itself but is valuable to examine regional lymphatics and distant metastases.

5. Cytology—Cytologic examination of nipple discharge or cyst fluid may be helpful on rare occasions. As a rule, mammography (or ductography) and breast biopsy are required when nipple discharge or cyst fluid is bloody or cytologically questionable. Ductal lavage, a technique that washes individual duct systems with saline and loosens epithelial cells for cytologic evaluation, is being evaluated as a risk assessment tool but appears to be of little value.

▶ Differential Diagnosis

The lesions to be considered most often in the differential diagnosis of breast cancer are the following, in descending order of frequency: fibrocystic condition of the breast, fibroadenoma, intraductal papilloma, lipoma, and fat necrosis.

▶ Staging

The American Joint Committee on Cancer and the International Union Against Cancer have agreed on a TNM (tumor, regional lymph nodes, distant metastases) staging system for breast cancer. Using the TNM staging system enhances communication between researchers and clinicians. Table 17–2 outlines the TNM classification.

▶ Pathologic Types

Numerous pathologic subtypes of breast cancer can be identified histologically (Table 17–3).

Except for the in situ cancers, the histologic subtypes have only a slight bearing on prognosis when outcomes are compared after accurate staging. Various histologic parameters, such as invasion of blood vessels, tumor differentiation, invasion of breast lymphatics, and tumor necrosis have been examined, but other than tumor grade these have little prognostic value. Genetic analysis for certain high-risk genes in the primary tumor appears to offer prognostic and therapeutic information.

The noninvasive cancers by definition are confined by the basement membrane of the ducts and lack the ability to spread. However, in patients whose biopsies show noninvasive intraductal cancer, associated invasive ductal cancers metastasize to lymph nodes in about 1–3% of cases.

▶ Special Clinical Forms of Breast Cancer

1. Paget Carcinoma

Paget carcinoma is not common (about 1% of all breast cancers). It affects the nipple and may or may not be associated with a breast mass. The basic lesion is usually a well differentiated infiltrating ductal carcinoma or a ductal carcinoma in situ (DCIS). The ducts of the nipple epithelium are infiltrated, but gross nipple changes are often minimal, and a tumor mass may not be palpable.

Because the nipple changes appear innocuous, the diagnosis is frequently missed. The first symptom is often itching or burning of the nipple, with superficial erosion or

ulceration. These are often diagnosed and treated as dermatitis or bacterial infection, leading to delay or failure in detection. The diagnosis is established by biopsy of the area of erosion. When the lesion consists of nipple changes only, the incidence of axillary metastases is less than 5%, and the prognosis is excellent. When a breast mass is also present, the incidence of axillary metastases rises, with an associated marked decrease in prospects for cure by surgical or other treatment.

2. Inflammatory Carcinoma

This is the most malignant form of breast cancer and constitutes less than 3% of all cases. The clinical findings consist of a rapidly growing, sometimes painful mass that enlarges the breast. The overlying skin becomes erythematous, edematous, and warm. Often there is no distinct mass, since the tumor infiltrates the involved breast diffusely. The inflammatory changes, often mistaken for an infection, are caused by carcinomatous invasion of the subdermal lymphatics, with resulting edema and hyperemia. If the practitioner suspects infection but the lesion does not respond rapidly (1–2 weeks) to antibiotics, biopsy should be performed. The diagnosis should be made when the redness involves more than one-third of the skin over the breast and biopsy shows infiltrating carcinoma with invasion of the subdermal lymphatics. Metastases tend to occur early and widely, and for this reason inflammatory carcinoma is rarely curable. Radiation, hormone therapy, and chemotherapy are the measures most likely to be of value rather than operation. Mastectomy is indicated when chemotherapy and radiation have resulted in clinical remission with no evidence of distant metastases. In these cases, residual disease in the breast may be eradicated.

▶ Breast Cancer Occurring during Pregnancy or Lactation

Breast cancer complicates approximately one in 3000 pregnancies. The diagnosis is frequently delayed, because physiologic changes in the breast may obscure the lesion. When the cancer is confined to the breast, the 5-year survival rate is about 70%. In 60–70% of patients, axillary metastases are already present, conferring a 5-year survival rate of 30–40%. Pregnancy (or lactation) is not a contraindication to operation or treatment, and therapy should be based on the stage of the disease as in the nonpregnant (or nonlactating) woman. Overall survival rates have improved, since cancers are now diagnosed in pregnant women earlier than in the past and treatment has improved. Breast-conserving surgery may be performed—and radiation and chemotherapy given—even during the pregnancy.

▶ Bilateral Breast Cancer

Bilateral breast cancer occurs in less than 5% of cases, but there is as high as a 20–25% incidence of later occurrence of cancer in the second breast. Bilaterality occurs more often in familial breast cancer, in women under age 50 years, and when the tumor in the primary breast is lobular. The incidence of second breast cancers increases directly

Table 17–2. TNM staging for breast cancer.

Primary Tumor (T)	
Definitions for classifying the primary tumor (T) are the same for clinical and for pathologic classification. If the measurement is made by physical examination, the examiner will use the major headings (T1, T2, or T3). If other measurements, such as mammographic or pathologic measurements, are used, the subsets of T1 can be used. Tumors should be measured to the nearest 0.1 cm increment.	
TX	Primary tumor cannot be assessed
T0	No evidence of primary tumor
Tis	Carcinoma in situ
Tis (DCIS)	Ductal carcinoma in situ
Tis (LCIS)	Lobular carcinoma in situ
Tis (Paget)	Paget disease of the nipple with no tumor
	Note: Paget disease associated with a tumor is classified according to the size of the tumor.
T1	Tumor 2 cm or less in greatest dimension
T1mic	Microinvasion 0.1 cm or less in greatest dimension
T1a	Tumor more than 0.1 cm but not more than 0.5 cm in greatest dimension
T1b	Tumor more than 0.5 cm but not more than 1 cm in greatest dimension
T1c	Tumor more than 1 cm but not more than 2 cm in greatest dimension
T2	Tumor more than 2 cm but not more than 5 cm in greatest dimension
T3	Tumor more than 5 cm in greatest dimension
T4	Tumor of any size with direct extension to (a) chest wall or (b) skin, only as described below
T4a	Extension to chest wall, not including petoralis muscle
T4b	Edema (including peau d'orange) or ulceration of the skin of the breast, or satellite skin nodules confined to the same breast
T4c	Both T4a and T4b
T4d	Inflammatory carcinoma
Regional Lymph Nodes (N)	
Clinical	
NX	Regional lymph nodes cannot be assessed (eg, previously removed)
N0	No regional lymph node metastasis
N1	Metastasis to movable ipsilateral axillary lymph node(s)
N2	Metastases in ipsilateral axillary lymph nodes fixed or matted, or in clinically apparent ipsilateral internal mammary nodes in the *absence* of clinically evident axillary lymph node metastasis

N2a	Metastasis in ipsilateral axillary lymph nodes fixed to one another (matted) or to other structures
N2b	Metastasis only in clinically apparent[1] ipsilateral internal mammary nodes and in the *absence* of clinically evident axillary lymph node metastasis
N3	Metastasis in ipsilateral infraclavicular lymph node(s) with or without axillary lymph node involvement, or in clinically apparent[1] ipsilateral internal mammary lymph node(s) and in the *presence* of clinically evident axillary lymph node metastasis; or metastasis in ipsilateral supraclavicular lymph node(s) with or without axillary or internal mammary lymph node involvement
N3a	Metastasis in ipsilateral infraclavicular lymph node(s)
N3b	Metastasis in ipsilateral internal mammary lymph node(s) and axillary lymph node(s)
N3c	Metastasis in ipsilateral supraclavicular lymph node(s)
Pathologic (pN)[2]	
pNX	Regional lymph nodes cannot be assessed (eg, previously removed, or not removed for pathologic study)
pN0	No regional lymph node metastasis histologically, no additional examination for isolated tumor cells
	Note: Isolated tumor cells (ITC) are defined as single tumor cells or small cell clusters not greater than 0.2 mm, usually detected only by immunohistochemical (IHC) or molecular methods but which may be verified on hematoxylin and eosin stains. ITCs do not usually show evidence of malignant activity, eg, proliferation or stromal reaction.
pN0(i–)	No regional lymph node metastasis histologically, negative IHC
pN0(i+)	No regional lymph node metastasis histologically, positive IHC, no IHC cluster greater than 0.2 mm
pN0(mol–)	No regional lymph node metastasis histologically, negative molecular findings (RT-PCR)
pN0(mol+)	No regional lymph node metastasis histologically, positive molecular findings (RT-PCR)
pN1	Metastasis in one to three axillary lymph nodes, and/or in internal mammary nodes with microscopic disease detected by sentinel lymph node dissection but not clinically apparent[1]
pN1mi	Micrometastasis (greater than 0.2 mm, none greater than 2.0 mm)
pN1a	Metastasis in one to three axillary lymph nodes
pN1b	Metastasis in internal mammary nodes with microscopic disease detected by sentinel lymph node dissection but not clinically apparent[1]
pN1c	Metastasis in one to three axillary lymph nodes and in internal mammary lymph nodes with microscopic disease detected by sentinel lymph node dissection but not clinically apparent.[1] (If associated with greater than three positive axillary lymph nodes, the internal mammary nodes are classified as pN3b to reflect increased tumor burden)

(continued)

Table 17–2. TNM staging for breast cancer. (continued)

		Distant Metastasis (M)	
pN2	Metastasis in four to nine axillary lymph nodes, or in clinically apparent[1] internal mammary lymph nodes in the *absence* of axillary lymph node metastasis	MX	Distant metastasis cannot be assessed
		M0	No distant metastasis
pN2a	Metastasis in four to nine axillary lymph nodes (at least one tumor deposit greater than 2.0 mm)	M1	Distant metastasis

		Stage Grouping		
pN2b	Metastasis in clinically apparent[1] internal mammary lymph nodes in the *absence* of axillary lymph node metastasis	Stage 0	Tis	N0	M0
pN3	Metastasis in 10 or more axillary lymph nodes, or in infraclavicular lymph nodes, or in clinically apparent[1] ipsilateral internal mammary lymph nodes in the *presence* of one or more positive axillary lymph nodes; or in more than three axillary lymph nodes with clinically negative microscopic metastasis in internal mammary lymph nodes; or in ipsilateral supraclavicular lymph nodes	Stage 1	T1[3]	N0	M0
		Stage IIA	T0	N1	M0
			T1[3]	N1	M0
			T2	N0	M0
		Stage IIB	T2	N1	M0
			T3	N0	M0
		Stage IIIA	T0	N2	M0
			T1[3]	N2	M0
pN3a	Metastasis in 10 or more axillary lymph nodes (at least one tumor deposit greater than 2.0 mm), or metastasis to the infraclavicular lymph nodes		T2	N2	M0
			T3	N1	M0
			T3	N2	M0
pN3b	Metastasis in clinically apparent[1] ipsilateral internal mammary lymph nodes in the *presence* of one or more positive axillary lymph nodes; or in more than three axillary lymph nodes and in internal mammary lymph nodes with microscopic disease detected by sentinel lymph node dissection but not clinically apparent[1]	Stage IIIB	T4	N0	M0
			T4	N1	M0
			T4	N2	M0
		Stage IIIC	Any T	N3	M0
pN3c	Metastasis in ipsilateral supraclavicular lymph nodes	Stage IV	Any T	Any N	M1

Note: Stage designation may be changed if postsurgical imaging studies reveal the presence of distant metastases, provided that the studies are carried out within 4 months of diagnosis in the absence of disease progression and provided that the patient has not received neoadjuvant therapy.

[1]*Clinically apparent* is defined as detected by imaging studies (excluding lymphoscintigraphy) or by clinical examination or grossly visible pathologically. *Not clinically apparent* is defined as not detected by imaging studies (excluding lymphoscintigraphy) or by clinical examination.
[2]Classification is based on axillary lymph node dissection with or without sentinel lymph node dissection. Classification based solely on sentinel lymph node dissection without subsequent axillary lymph node dissection is designated (sn) for "sentinel node," eg, pN0(i+)(sn).
[3]T1 includes T1mic.
RT-PCR, reverse transcriptase/polymerase chain reaction.
Reproduced, with permission, of the American Joint Committee on Cancer (AJCC), Chicago, Illinois. *AJCC Cancer Staging Manual*, 6th edition, Springer Science and Business Media, LLC, 2002. www.springerlink.com.

with the length of time the patient is alive after her first cancer—about 1–2% per year.

In patients with breast cancer, mammography should be performed before primary treatment and at regular intervals thereafter, to search for occult cancer in the opposite breast or conserved ipsilateral breast. MRI may be useful in this high-risk group.

► Noninvasive Cancer

Noninvasive cancer can occur within the ducts (DCIS) or lobules (lobular carcinoma in situ, LCIS). LCIS, although thought to be a premalignant lesion or a risk factor for breast cancer, in fact may behave like DCIS. In a 2004 analysis of multiple NSABP studies, invasive lobular breast

cancer not only developed in patients with LCIS but it developed in the same breast and indexed location as the original LCIS. Although more research needs to be done in this area, the invasive potential of LCIS is being reconsidered. The subtype pleomorphic LCIS may behave more like DCIS. DCIS tends to be unilateral and most often progresses to invasive cancer if untreated. In approximately 40–60% of women who have DCIS treated with biopsy alone, invasive cancer develops within the same breast.

The treatment of intraductal lesions is controversial. DCIS can be treated by wide excision with or without radiation therapy or with total mastectomy. Conservative management is advised in patients with small lesions amenable to lumpectomy. Although research is defining the malignant potential of LCIS, it can be managed with

Table 17–3. Histologic types of breast cancer.

Type	Frequency of Occurence
Infiltrating ductal (not otherwise specified)	80–90%
Medullary	5–8%
Colloid (mucinous)	2–4%
Tubular	1–2%
Papillary	1–2%
Invasive lobular	6–8%
Noninvasive	4–6%
Intraductal	2–3%
Lobular in situ	2–3%
Rare cancers	< 1%
Juvenile (secretory)	
Adenoid cystic	
Epidermoid	
Sudoriferous	

observation. Patients unwilling to accept the increased risk of breast cancer may be offered surgical excision of the area in question or bilateral total mastectomy. Currently, the accepted standard of care offers the alternative of chemoprevention, which is effective in preventing invasive breast cancer in both LCIS and DCIS that has been completely excised. Axillary metastases from in situ cancers should not occur unless there is an occult invasive cancer. Sentinel node biopsy may be indicated in large DCIS treated with mastectomy.

Barnes DM et al. Pregnancy-associated breast cancer: a literature review. Surg Clin North Am. 2007 Apr;87(2):417–30. [PMID: 17498535]

Barni S et al. Locally advanced breast cancer. Curr Opin Obstet Gynecol. 2006 Feb;18(1):47–52. [PMID: 16493260]

Bodner-Adler B et al. Breast cancer diagnosed during pregnancy. Anticancer Res. 2007 May–Jun;27(3B):1705–7. [PMID: 17595801]

Chen CY et al. Paget disease of the breast: changing patterns of incidence, clinical presentation, and treatment in the U.S. Cancer. 2006 Oct 1;107(7):1448–58. [PMID: 16933329]

Cristofanilli M et al. Inflammatory breast cancer (IBC) and patterns of recurrence: understanding the biology of a unique disease. Cancer. 2007 Oct 1;110(7):1436–44. [PMID: 17694554]

Daly MB. Tamoxifen in ductal carcinoma in situ. Semin Oncol. 2006 Dec;33(6):647–9. [PMID: 17145343]

Dawood S et al. What progress have we made in managing inflammatory breast cancer? Oncology (Williston Park). 2007 May;21(6):673–9. [PMID: 17564325]

Erbas B et al. The natural history of ductal carcinoma in situ of the breast: a review. Breast Cancer Res Treat. 2006 May;97(2):135–44. [PMID: 16319971]

Habel KL et al. A population-based study of tumor gene expression and risk of breast cancer death among lymph node-negative patients. Breast Cancer Res. 2006;8(3):R25. [PMID: 16737553]

Hansen NM et al. Breast cancer: pre- and postoperative imaging for staging. Surg Oncol Clin N Am. 2007 Apr;16(2):447–63. [PMID: 17560522]

Irvine T et al. Biology and treatment of ductal carcinoma in situ. Expert Rev Anticancer Ther. 2007 Feb;7(2):135–45. [PMID: 17288525]

Lakhani SR et al. The management of lobular carcinoma in situ (LCIS). Is LCIS the same as ductal carcinoma in situ (DCIS)? Eur J Cancer. 2006 Sep;42(14):2205–11. [PMID: 16876991]

Ring AE et al. Breast cancer and pregnancy. Ann Oncol. 2005 Dec;16(12):1855–60. [PMID: 16030024]

Schirrmeister H. Detection of bone metastases in breast cancer by positron emission tomography. Radiol Clin North Am. 2007 Jul;45(4):669–76. [PMID: 17706531]

Theriault R et al. Management of breast cancer in pregnancy. Curr Oncol Rep. 2007 Jan;9(1):17–21. [PMID: 17164043]

Tohno E et al. Ultrasound screening of breast cancer. Breast Cancer. 2009;16(1):18–22. [PMID: 19009372]

West JG et al. Multidisciplinary management of ductal carcinoma in situ: a 10-year experience. Am J Surg. 2007 Oct;194(4):532–4. [PMID: 17826074]

BIOMARKERS

The ER and PR status and *HER-2/neu* status of the tumor should be determined at the time of initial biopsy. Other studies such as proliferation indices may be performed. These markers may be obtained on core biopsy specimens, which will be necessary to institute neoadjuvant therapy.

The presence or absence of ER and PR is a critical element of breast cancer management. Patients whose primary tumors are receptor-positive have a more favorable course than those whose tumors are receptor-negative. Up to 60% of patients with metastatic breast cancer will respond to hormonal manipulation if their tumors are ER-positive. Less than 5% of patients with metastatic, ER-negative tumors can be treated successfully in this fashion. Adjuvant hormonal therapy, with or without chemotherapy, in receptor-positive tumors and adjuvant chemotherapy alone in receptor-negative tumors improve survival rates even in the absence of lymph node metastases. Hormone receptors have no relationship to response to chemotherapy (see Adjuvant Therapy, below).

PR status may be more sensitive than ER status in determining which patients are likely to respond to hormonal manipulation. Up to 80% of patients with metastatic PR-positive tumors improve with hormonal manipulation.

In addition to ER status and PR status, the rate at which tumor divides and the differentiation of the cells (proliferative indices) are important. In order to establish the rate of growth and differentiation, the amount and type of DNA is measured with flow cytometry.

Another key element in determining treatment and prognosis is the amount of the *HER-2/neu* oncogene present in the cancer. *HER-2/neu* overexpression is scored using a numerical system: 1+ is not an overexpressor, 2+ is borderline, and 3+ is an overexpressor. In the case of 2+ expression, fluorescence in situ hybridization (FISH) is recommended to more accurately assess *HER-2/neu* amplification and provide better prognostic information. The presence of *HER-2/neu* amplification predicts the response to trastuzumab.

While individually these biomarkers provide insight to appropriate adjuvant therapy, when combined they provide a great deal of information regarding risk of recurrence. Several tests now predict relapse rates for patients treated with tamoxifen or chemotherapy. Oncotype DX combines 21 genetic markers, including ER, PR, and *HER-2/neu* expression in a tumor specimen to categorize risk of recurrence into three groups: high risk, intermediate risk, and low risk. In addition, the test is able to identify that the high-risk group was more likely to benefit from chemotherapy in addition to tamoxifen while the low risk group did not. This type of test is quite helpful when the survival advantage of therapy is difficult to determine. It has been most used for ER-positive node-negative tumors but now may apply to node-positive tumors as well.

Another promising biomarker being studied is vascular endothelial growth factor (VEGF), a protein that stimulates the growth of blood vessels. Elevated levels of VEGF may be a marker for a tumor that is more aggressive since it has the ability to develop blood vessels and grow. While researchers look for more specific markers to determine the presence of breast cancer, these markers also provide insight to targeted methods of treatment. Other markers being evaluated are *p53*, nm23, DNA 5c exceeding rate (DNA 5cER), G-actin, urokinase-type plasminogen activator (u-PA), and its type-1 inhibitor (PAI-1).

Badve S et al. Oestrogen-receptor-positive breast cancer: toward bridging histopathological and molecular classifications. J Clin Pathol. 2009 Jan;62(1):6–12. [PMID: 18794199]

Ferretti G et al. HER2/neu role in breast cancer: from a prognostic foe to a predictive friend. Curr Opin Obstet Gynecol. 2007 Feb;19(1):56–62. [PMID: 17218853]

Luadido J et al. HER2 testing: a review of detection methodologies and their clinical performance. Expert Rev Mol Diagn. 2007 Jan;7(1):53–64. [PMID: 17187484]

Nicolini A et al. Biomolecular markers of breast cancer. Front Biosci. 2006 May 1;11:1818–43. [PMID: 16368559]

Retèl VP et al. Constructive Technology Assessment (CTA) as a tool in coverage with evidence development: the case of the 70-gene prognosis signature for breast cancer diagnostics. Int J Technol Assess Health Care. 2009 Jan;25(1):73–83. [PMID: 19126254]

▶ Treatment: Curative

Clearly, not all breast cancer is systemic at the time of diagnosis. For this reason, a pessimistic attitude concerning the management of breast cancer is unwarranted. Most patients with early breast cancer can be cured.

Treatment may be curative or palliative. Curative treatment is advised for clinical stage I, II, and III disease (see Tables 17–2, 39–3, 39–4). Patients with locally advanced (T3, T4) and even inflammatory tumors may be cured with multimodality therapy, but in most, palliation is all that can be expected. Palliative treatment is appropriate for all patients with stage IV disease and for previously treated patients in whom distant metastases develop or who have unresectable local cancers (see Palliative section below).

A. Choice of Primary Therapy

The extent of disease and its biologic aggressiveness are the principal determinants of the outcome of primary therapy. Clinical and pathologic staging help in assessing extent of disease (see Table 17–2), but each is to some extent

imprecise. Other factors such as DNA flow cytometry, tumor grade, hormone receptor assays, and oncogene amplification may be of prognostic value but are not important in determining the type of local therapy.

Controversy has surrounded the choice of primary therapy of stage I, II, and III breast carcinoma. A number of states require physicians to inform patients of alternative treatment methods in the management of breast cancer. Currently, the standard of care for stage I, stage II, and most stage III cancer is surgical resection followed by adjuvant radiation or systemic therapy, or both, when indicated. Neoadjuvant therapy is becoming more popular since large tumors may be shrunk by chemotherapy prior to surgery, making some patients who require mastectomy candidates for lumpectomy.

B. Surgical Resection

1. Breast-conserving therapy—Multiple, large, randomized studies including the Milan and NSABP trials show that disease-free and overall survival rates are similar for patients treated with partial mastectomy plus axillary dissection followed by radiation therapy and for those treated by modified radical mastectomy (total mastectomy plus axillary dissection).

Twenty years of follow-up of the NSABP trial has shown that lumpectomy with axillary dissection followed by postoperative radiation therapy is as effective as modified radical mastectomy for the management of patients with stage I and stage II breast cancer.

Tumor size is a major consideration in determining the feasibility of breast conservation. The lumpectomy trial of the NSABP randomized patients with tumors as large as 4 cm. To achieve an acceptable cosmetic result, the patient must have a breast of sufficient size to enable excision of a 4-cm tumor without considerable deformity. Therefore, large size is only a relative contraindication. Subareolar tumors, also difficult to excise without deformity, are not contraindications to breast conservation. Clinically detectable multifocality is a relative contraindication to breast-conserving surgery, as is fixation to the chest wall or skin or involvement of the nipple or overlying skin. The patient—not the surgeon—should be the judge of what is cosmetically acceptable.

Axillary dissection is valuable in preventing axillary recurrences, in staging cancer, and in planning therapy. Intraoperative lymphatic mapping and sentinel node biopsy identify lymph nodes most likely to harbor metastases if present in the axillary nodes (Plate 73). Sentinel node biopsy is a reasonable alternative to axillary dissection in selected patients with invasive cancer.

Breast-conserving surgery with radiation is the preferred form of treatment for patients with **early-stage breast cancer**. Despite the numerous randomized trials showing no survival benefit of mastectomy over breast-conserving partial mastectomy and irradiation, breast-conserving surgery still appears underutilized.

2. Mastectomy—Modified radical mastectomy was the standard therapy for most patients with early-stage breast cancer. This operation removes the entire breast, overlying skin, nipple, and areolar complex as well as the underlying pectoralis fascia with the axillary lymph nodes in continuity. The major advantage of modified radical mastectomy is that radiation therapy may not be necessary, although radiation may be used when multiple lymph nodes are involved with cancer. The disadvantage of mastectomy is the cosmetic and psychological impact associated with breast loss. Radical mastectomy, which removes the underlying pectoralis muscle, should be performed rarely, if at all. Axillary node dissection is not indicated for noninfiltrating cancers because nodal metastases are rarely present. Skin-sparing mastectomy is currently gaining favor but is not appropriate for all patients. Breast-conserving surgery and radiation should be offered whenever possible, since most patients would prefer to save the breast. Breast reconstruction, immediate or delayed, should be discussed with patients who choose or require mastectomy. Patients should have an interview with a reconstructive plastic surgeon to discuss options prior to making a decision regarding reconstruction. Time is well spent preoperatively in educating the patient and family about these matters.

Radiotherapy after partial mastectomy consists of 5–7 weeks of five daily fractions to a total dose of 5000–6000 cGy. Most radiation oncologists use a boost dose to the cancer location. Several studies are underway examining the utility and recurrence rates after intraoperative radiation or dose dense radiation in which the time course of radiation is shortened. Accelerated partial breast irradiation, in which only the portion of the breast from which the tumor was resected is irradiated for 1–2 weeks, appears effective in achieving local control. A prospective randomized trial to examine the efficacy of this technique is underway. Accrual should be completed this year, but long-term follow-up will be necessary. Current studies suggest that radiotherapy after mastectomy may improve survival in a subset of patients and is being further researched in a large cooperative trial to better identify which subgroups will benefit. Researchers are also examining the utility of axillary irradiation as an alternative to axillary dissection in the clinically node-negative patient with sentinel node micrometastases.

C. Adjuvant Systemic Therapy

The goal of systemic therapy, including hormone modulating drugs and cytotoxic chemotherapy, is to kill cancer cells that have escaped the breast and axillary lymph nodes as micrometastases. In practice, most medical oncologists are currently using adjuvant chemotherapy for patients with either node-positive or higher-risk node-negative breast cancer and using hormonal therapy for all hormone receptor–positive invasive breast cancer unless contraindicated. Prognostic factors other than nodal status that are used to determine the patient's risks are tumor size, ER and PR status, nuclear grade, histologic type, proliferative rate, and oncogene expression (Table 17–4). In general, systemic chemotherapy decreases the chance of recurrence by about 30% and hormonal modulation decreases the risk of recurrence by 40–50% (for hormone receptor–positive cancer). In general, chemotherapy is given before

Table 17–4. Prognostic factors in node-negative breast cancer.

Prognostic Factors	Increased Recurrence	Decreased Recurrence
Size	T3, T2	T1, T0
Hormone receptors	Negative	Positive
DNA flow cytometry	Aneuploid	Diploid
Histologic grade	High	Low
Tumor labeling index	< 3%	> 3%
S phase fraction	> 5%	< 5%
Lymphatic or vascular invasion	Present	Absent
Cathepsin D	High	Low
HER-2/neu oncogene	High	Low
Epidermal growth factor receptor	High	Low

radiation therapy and endocrine therapy is started after radiation therapy.

1. Chemotherapy—Systemic therapy improves survival and is advocated for most patients with curable breast cancer. In addition, chemotherapy may decrease local recurrence in patients treated with breast conservation, whereas hormonal manipulation decreases contralateral breast cancer occurrence as well as ipsilateral recurrence.

On the basis of the superiority of anthracycline-containing regimens in metastatic breast cancer, both doxorubicin and epirubicin have been studied extensively in the adjuvant setting. Studies comparing Adriamycin (doxorubicin) and cyclophosphamide (AC) or epirubicin and cyclophosphamide (EC) with cyclophosphamide-methotrexate-5-fluorouracil (CMF) have shown that treatments with anthracycline-containing regimens are at least as effective, and perhaps more effective, than treatment with CMF. A meta-analysis (Oxford Overview Early Breast Cancer Trialists' Collaborative Group), including over 14,000 patients enrolled in trials comparing anthracycline-based regimens to CMF, showed a small but statistically significant improved disease-free and overall survival with the use of anthracycline-based regimens. It should be noted, however, that most of these studies included a mixed population of *HER-2/neu*-positive and *HER-2/neu*-negative breast cancer patients and were performed before the development of trastuzumab. Retrospective analyses of a number of these studies (CALGB 8541, NSABP B11, MA-5, and others) suggest that anthracyclines may be primarily effective in tumors with *HER-2/neu* overexpression or alteration in the expression of topoisomerase IIa (the target of anthracyclines and close to the *HER-2/neu* gene). Given this, for *HER-2/neu*-negative, node-negative breast cancer, four cycles of AC or six cycles of CMF are probably equally effective.

When taxanes (T=paclitaxel and docetaxel) emerged in the 1990s, trials were conducted to evaluate their use in combination with anthracycline-based regimens. Initial studies demonstrated a 20% proportional reduction in recurrence and a 4% absolute improvement in disease-free survival with the addition of paclitaxel to an AC (AC-T) regimen. A trial comparing six cycles of FAC to six cycles of docetaxel, doxorubicin, and cyclophosphamide (TAC) showed an improvement in disease-free and overall survival for patients receiving TAC. This benefit was most marked for patients with positive nodes and was seen in both ER-negative and ER-positive tumors. Results from CALGB 9741 showed that compared with a standard dose regimen, administration of "dose-dense" AC-P chemotherapy (that is, in an accelerated fashion, in which the frequency of administration is increased without changing total dose or duration) with filgrastim support led to improved both disease-free (82% vs 75% at 4 years) and overall survival (92% vs 90%). Exploratory subset analysis suggested that patients with hormone receptor–negative tumors derived the most benefit from the dose-dense approach.

Recently, the US Oncology trial 9735 compared four cycles of AC with four cycles of Taxotere (docetaxel) and cyclophosphamide (TC) and showed a statistically significantly improved disease-free survival and overall survival in the patients who received TC. Until this, no trial had compared a non-anthracycline, taxane-based regimen to an anthracycline-based regimen.

An important ongoing study (US Oncology 06090) is prospectively evaluating whether anthracyclines add any incremental benefit to a taxane-based regimen by comparing six cycles of TAC to six cycles of TC in *HER-2/neu* negative breast cancer patients. While awaiting the results of this trial, oncologists are faced with choosing between the above treatment regimens for *HER-2/neu*-negative breast cancer.

The overall duration of adjuvant chemotherapy still remains uncertain. However, based on the meta-analysis performed in the Oxford Overview (Early Breast Cancer Trialists' Collaborative Group), the current recommendation is for 3–6 months of the commonly used regimens. Although it is clear that dose intensity to a specific threshold is essential, there is little, if any, evidence to support the long-term survival benefit of high-dose chemotherapy with stem cell support.

Chemotherapy side effects are now generally well controlled. Nausea and vomiting are abated with drugs that directly affect the central nervous system, such as ondansetron and granisetron. Life-threatening neutropenia associated with chemotherapy can be prevented by use of growth factors such as pegfilgrastim and filgrastim (granulocyte colony-stimulating factor; G-CSF), which stimulate proliferation and differentiation of hematopoietic cells. These agents greatly diminish the incidence of infections that may complicate the use of myelosuppressive chemotherapy. Long-term toxicities from chemotherapy, including cardiomyopathy (anthracyclines) and leukemia/myelodysplasia (anthracyclines and alkylating agents), remain a small but significant risk.

2. Targeted therapy

A. HER-2/NEU OVEREXPRESSION—Trastuzumab (Herceptin [H]), a monoclonal antibody that binds to *HER-2/neu*

receptors, has proved effective in combination with chemotherapy in patients with *HER-2/neu* overexpressing metastatic and early breast cancer and has been FDA-approved for both of these patient populations. In the adjuvant setting, the first and most commonly studied chemotherapy backbone used with trastuzumab is AC-T. More recently, the BCIRG006 study showed equivalent efficacy for AC-TH versus TCH (docetaxel, carboplatin, trastuzumab). Both AC-TH and TCH are now FDA-approved for early, *HER-2/neu*-positive breast cancer. In these regimens, trastuzumab is given with chemotherapy and then continues beyond the course of chemotherapy to complete a full year. Other studies have evaluated use of a shorter course of trastuzumab (Finland Herceptin or FinHer trial) and use of trastuzumab sequentially (not concurrently) with chemotherapy (Herceptin Adjuvant or HERA trial). Although both of these studies showed benefits of adding trastuzumab to chemotherapy, the current standard remains 1 full year of trastuzumab for adjuvant therapy.

A small, but significant, percentage (1–4%) of patients who receive trastuzumab-based regimens develop cardiomyopathy. For this reason, anthracyclines and trastuzumab are never given concurrently and cardiac function is monitored periodically throughout therapy.

B. HORMONAL THERAPY—Adjuvant hormonal therapy is highly effective in decreasing recurrence and mortality by 25% in women with ER-positive tumors regardless of menopausal status. The standard regimen has been tamoxifen for 5 years, and this remains the standard for premenopausal women. Ovarian ablation in premenopausal patients with ER-positive tumors may produce a benefit similar to that of adjuvant systemic chemotherapy. Whether the use of ovarian ablation plus tamoxifen (or ovarian ablation plus an AI) is more effective than either measure alone is unclear and is currently being addressed in ongoing clinical trials (Suppression of Ovarian Function Trial [SOFT] and Tamoxifen and Exemestane Trial [TEXT]). AIs, including anastrozole, letrozole, and exemestane, are also effective in the adjuvant setting for postmenopausal women. Approximately seven large randomized trials enrolling more than 24,000 patients have compared the use of AIs with tamoxifen or placebo as adjuvant therapy. All of these studies have shown small but statistically significant improvements in disease-free survival (absolute benefits of 2–6%) with the use of AIs. In addition, AIs have been shown to reduce the risk of contralateral breast cancers and to have fewer associated side effects (such as endometrial cancers and thromboembolic events) than tamoxifen. However, they are associated with accelerated bone loss and an increased risk of fractures. The American Society of Clinical Oncology and National Comprehensive Cancer Network have recommended that postmenopausal women with hormone receptor–positive breast cancer be offered an AI either initially or after tamoxifen therapy. *HER-2/neu* status should not affect the use or choice of hormone therapy.

The long-term advantage of systemic therapy has been well established. Selection of patients for adjuvant treatment should be based on the patient's axillary nodal status, tumor size and grade, hormone receptor status, *HER-2/neu* status, and age. The value of *p53*, angiogenesis factors, and vascular invasion is being investigated, but they remain to be proven prognostic factors. In general, adjuvant systemic chemotherapy should not be given to women who have small node-negative breast cancers with favorable histologic findings and tumor markers. The ability to predict more accurately which patients with *HER-2/neu*-negative, hormone receptor–positive, lymph node–negative tumors should receive chemotherapy is improving with the advent of prognostic tools, such as Oncotype DX and Mammaprint, which evaluate the gene expression profile of a given tumor and can stratify it into low or high risk types. These tests are now undergoing prospective evaluation in two clinical trials (TAILORx and MINDACT). All patients with invasive hormone receptor–positive tumors should consider the use of hormone-modulating therapy. Most patients with *HER-2/neu*-positive tumors receive trastuzumab-containing chemotherapy regimens.

D. Neoadjuvant Therapy

The use of chemotherapy or hormonal therapy prior to resection of the primary tumor (neoadjuvant) is gaining popularity. This enables the assessment of in vivo chemosensitivity. A complete pathologic response at the time of operation is associated with improvement in survival. Neoadjuvant chemotherapy also permits breast conservation by shrinking the primary tumor in women who would otherwise need mastectomy for local control. Survival after neoadjuvant chemotherapy has not been shown to be superior to that seen with postoperative adjuvant chemotherapy but is certainly no worse. There is considerable concern as to the timing of sentinel lymph node biopsy (SLNB), since the chemotherapy may affect any cancer present in the lymph nodes. Several studies have shown that sentinel node biopsy can be done after neoadjuvant therapy. However, a large multicenter study, NSABP B-27, demonstrated a false-negative rate of 10.7%, well above the false-negative rate outside the neoadjuvant setting (< 1–5%). Many physicians recommend performing SLNB before administering the chemotherapy in order to avoid a false-negative result and to aid in planning subsequent radiation therapy. If a complete dissection is necessary, this can be performed at the time of the definitive breast surgery.

Important questions remaining to be answered are the timing and duration of adjuvant and neoadjuvant chemotherapy, which chemotherapeutic agents should be applied for which subgroups of patients, the use of combinations of hormonal therapy and chemotherapy as well as possibly targeted therapy, and the value of prognostic factors other than hormone receptors in predicting response to therapy.

▶ Treatment: Palliative

A. Radiotherapy

Palliative radiotherapy may be advised for primary treatment of locally advanced cancers with distant metastases to control ulceration, pain, and other manifestations in the breast and regional nodes. Irradiation of the breast and chest wall and the axillary, internal mammary, and supraclavicular nodes should be undertaken in an attempt to cure locally advanced and inoperable lesions when there is no evidence of distant metastases. A small number of patients in this group are cured in spite of extensive breast and regional node involvement.

Palliative irradiation is of value also in the treatment of certain bone or soft-tissue metastases to control pain or avoid fracture. Radiotherapy is especially useful in the treatment of isolated bony metastases, chest wall recurrences, brain metastases, and acute spinal cord compression.

B. Targeted Therapy

Targeted therapy refers to agents that are directed specifically against a protein or molecule expressed uniquely on tumor cells or in the tumor microenvironment. The first targeted therapy was the use of antiestrogen therapy in hormone receptor–positive breast cancer. The administration of hormones (eg, estrogens, androgens, progestins; see Table 17–5); ablation of the ovaries, adrenals, or pituitary; administration of drugs that block hormone receptors (eg, antiestrogens such as tamoxifen) or drugs that block the synthesis of hormones (eg, AIs) have all been shown to be effective in hormone receptor–positive metastatic breast cancer. Palliative treatment of metastatic cancer should be based on the ER status of the primary tumor or the metastases. Because only 5–10% of women with ER-negative tumors respond, they should not receive hormonal therapy except in unusual circumstances, eg, in an older patient who cannot tolerate chemotherapy. The rate of response is nearly equal in premenopausal and postmenopausal women with ER-positive tumors. A favorable response to hormonal manipulation occurs in about one-third of patients with metastatic breast cancer. Of those whose tumors contain ER, the response is about 60% and perhaps as high as 80% for patients whose tumors contain PR as well. The choice of endocrine therapy depends on the menopausal status of the patient. Women within 1 year of their last menstrual period are arbitrarily considered to be premenopausal and should receive tamoxifen therapy or ovarian ablation, whereas women whose menses ceased more than a year before are postmenopausal and may receive an AI. Women with ER-positive tumors who do not respond to hormone therapy or experience progression should be given a different form of hormonal manipulation. The initial endocrine treatment used is referred to as primary hormonal manipulation; subsequent endocrine treatment is called secondary or tertiary hormonal manipulation.

Because the quality of life during endocrine manipulation is usually superior to that during cytotoxic chemotherapy, it is best to try endocrine manipulation whenever possible. However, when receptor status is unknown, disease is progressing rapidly or involves visceral organs, chemotherapy should be used as first-line treatment.

In addition to radiotherapy, bisphosphonate therapy has shown excellent results in delaying and reducing skeletal events in women with bony metastases. Bisphosphonates are also sometimes used in conjunction with AIs to decrease the potential bony events associated with AIs.

Table 17–5. Agents commonly used for hormonal management of metastatic breast cancer.

Drug	Action	Dose, Route, Frequency	Major Side Effects
Tamoxifen citrate (Nolvadex)	SERM	20 mg orally daily	Hot flushes, uterine bleeding, thrombophlebitis, rash
Fulvestrant (Faslodex)	Steroidal estrogen receptor antagonist	250 mg intramuscularly monthly	Gastrointestinal upset, headache, back pain, hot flushes, pharyngitis
Toremifene citrate (Fareston)	SERM	40 mg orally daily	Hot flushes, sweating, nausea, vaginal discharge, dry eyes, dizziness
Diethylstilbestrol (DES)	Estrogen	5 mg orally three times daily	Fluid retention, uterine bleeding, thrombophlebitis, nausea
Goserelin (Zoladex)	Synthetic luteinizing hormone releasing analogue	3.6 mg subcutaneously monthly	Arthralgias, blood pressure changes, hot flushes, headaches, vaginal dryness
Megestrol acetate (Megace)	Progestin	40 mg orally four times daily	Fluid retention
Letrozole (Femara)	AI	2.5 mg orally daily	Hot flushes, arthralgia/arthritis, myalgia
Anastrozole (Arimidex)	AI	1 mg orally daily	Hot flushes, skin rashes, nausea and vomiting
Exemestane (Aromasin)	AI	25 mg orally daily	Hot flushes, increased arthralgia/arthritis, myalgia, and alopecia

AI, aromatase inhibitor; SERM, selective estrogen receptor modulator.

Bisphosphonates are routinely given with AIs to patients with bone metastases.

In general, only one type of therapy should be given at a time unless it is necessary to irradiate a destructive lesion of weight-bearing bone while the patient is receiving another regimen. The regimen should be changed only if the disease is clearly progressing. This is especially important for patients with destructive bone metastases, since changes in the status of these lesions are difficult to determine radiographically.

For patients with *HER-2/neu* overexpressing tumors, trastuzumab plus chemotherapy has been shown to increase survival. Lapatinib is a newer oral targeted drug that works by inhibiting the intracellular tyrosine kinases of the EGF and *HER-2/neu* receptors. It was recently approved by the FDA for treatment of trastuzumab-resistant *HER-2/neu*-positive metastatic breast cancer in combination with capecitabine.

Bevacizumab is a monoclonal antibody directed against VEGF. This growth factor stimulates endothelial proliferation and neoangiogenesis in cancer. A phase III randomized trial in women with metastatic breast cancer showed increased response rate and progression-free survival rate with the combination of bevacizumab and paclitaxel as first-line treatment compared with paclitaxel alone; however, there was no significant overall survival benefit. This study led to the FDA approval of bevacizumab in early 2008. While these initial results are promising, studies are now underway to define which patients and tumor types are most likely to benefit from anti-angiogenic agents.

1. The Premenopausal Patient

A. PRIMARY HORMONAL THERAPY—The potent SERM tamoxifen is by far the most common and preferred method of hormonal manipulation in the premenopausal patient, in large part because it can be given with less morbidity and fewer side effects than cytotoxic chemotherapy. Tamoxifen is given orally in a dose of 20 mg daily. The average remission associated with tamoxifen lasts about 12 months.

There is no significant difference in survival or response between tamoxifen therapy and bilateral oophorectomy. Bilateral oophorectomy is less desirable than tamoxifen in premenopausal women because tamoxifen is so well tolerated. However, oophorectomy can be achieved rapidly and safely either by surgery, by irradiation of the ovaries if the patient is a poor surgical candidate, or by chemical ovarian ablation using a gonadotropin-releasing hormone (GnRH) analog. Oophorectomy presumably works by eliminating estrogens, progestins, and androgens, which stimulate growth of the tumor. AIs should not be used in a patient with functioning ovaries since they do not block ovarian production of estrogen.

B. SECONDARY OR TERTIARY HORMONAL THERAPY—Although patients who do not respond to tamoxifen or oophorectomy should be treated with cytotoxic drugs, those who respond and then relapse may subsequently respond to another form of endocrine treatment (Table 17–5). The initial choice for secondary endocrine manipulation has not been clearly defined.

Patients who improve after oophorectomy but subsequently relapse should receive tamoxifen or an AI; if one fails, the other may be tried but is not likely to succeed. Megestrol acetate, a progesterone agent, may be considered. Tamoxifen, AIs, or megestrol cause less morbidity and mortality than surgical adrenalectomy, can be discontinued once the patient improves, and are not associated with the many problems of postsurgical adrenal insufficiency, so that patients who require chemotherapy are more easily managed. Adrenalectomy or hypophysectomy, procedures rarely done today, induced regression in 30–50% of patients who previously responded to oophorectomy. Pharmacologic hormonal manipulation has replaced these invasive procedures. AIs are of value when a tumor responded to tamoxifen or oophorectomy but then progresses.

2. The Postmenopausal Patient

A. PRIMARY HORMONAL THERAPY—For postmenopausal women with metastatic breast cancer amenable to endocrine manipulation, tamoxifen, 20 mg orally daily, or an AI is the initial therapy of choice. AIs have fewer side effects than tamoxifen and may be more effective. The main side effects of tamoxifen are nausea, skin rash, and hot flushes. Rarely, tamoxifen induces hypercalcemia in patients with bony metastases. The main side effects of AIs include hot flushes, vaginal dryness, and joint stiffness; however, osteoporosis and bone fractures are significantly higher than tamoxifen. Tamoxifen therapy is also associated with a higher risk of uterine cancer and venous thromboembolic events compared with AIs.

B. SECONDARY OR TERTIARY HORMONAL THERAPY—AIs are also used for the treatment of advanced breast cancer in postmenopausal women after tamoxifen treatment. In the event that the patient responds to AI but then has progression of disease, an antiestrogen, fulvestrant, has shown efficacy with about 20–30% of women benefiting from use. Postmenopausal patients who do not respond to SERM or AI should be given cytotoxic drugs. Postmenopausal women who respond initially to a SERM or AI but later manifest progressive disease may be crossed over to another hormonal therapy. If they do not respond they should receive cytotoxic drugs. Androgens have many toxicities and should rarely be used. As in premenopausal patients, neither hypophysectomy nor adrenalectomy should be performed.

C. Chemotherapy

Cytotoxic drugs should be considered for the treatment of metastatic breast cancer (1) if visceral metastases are present (especially brain, liver, or lymphangitic pulmonary), (2) if hormonal treatment is unsuccessful or the disease has progressed after an initial response to hormonal manipulation, or (3) if the tumor is ER-negative. Prior adjuvant chemotherapy does not seem to alter response rates in patients who relapse. A number of chemotherapy drugs (including vinorelbine, paclitaxel, docetaxel, gemcitabine, ixabepilone, carboplatin, cisplatin, capecitabine, albumin-bound paclitaxel, and liposomal doxorubicin) may be used as single agents with first-line objective response rates ranging from 30% to 50%.

Combination chemotherapy yields statistically significantly higher response rates and progression-free survival rates, but has not been conclusively shown to improve overall survival rates compared with sequential single-agent therapy. Combinations that have been tested in phase III studies and have proven efficacy compared with single-agent therapy include capecitabine/docetaxel, gemcitabine/paclitaxel, capecitabine/ixabepilone, and bevacizumab/paclitaxel (see Tables 39–10 and 39–11). Various other combinations of drugs have been tested in phase II studies, and a number of clinical trials are ongoing to identify effective combinations. For patients whose tumors have progressed after several lines of therapy and who are considering additional therapy, clinical trial participation with experimental drugs in phase I, II, or III testing should be encouraged.

In the past, high-dose chemotherapy and autologous bone marrow or stem cell transplantation aroused widespread interest for the treatment of metastatic breast cancer. However, multiple clinical trials failed to show any improvement in survival with high-dose chemotherapy with stem cell transplant over conventional chemotherapy and the procedure is now rarely, if ever, performed for stage IV breast cancer.

Albain KS et al. Gemcitabine plus paclitaxel versus paclitaxel monotherapy in patients with metastatic breast cancer and prior anthracycline treatment. J Clin Oncol. 2008 Aug 20;26(24):3950–7. [PMID: 18711184]

American College of Radiology. Practice guideline for the breast conservation therapy in the management of invasive breast carcinoma. J Am Coll Surg. 2007 Aug;205(2):362–376. [PMID: 17660085]

Arimidex, Tamoxifen, Alone or in Combination (ATAC) Trialists' Group; Forbes JF et al. Effect of anastrozole and tamoxifen as adjuvant treatment for early-stage breast cancer: 100-month analysis of the ATAC trial. Lancet Oncol. 2008 Jan;9(1):45–53. [PMID: 18083636]

Bhatnagar AS. Review of the development of letrozole and its use in advanced breast cancer and in the neoadjuvant setting. Breast. 2006 Feb;15(Suppl 1):S3–13. [PMID: 16500235]

Carlson RW et al; National Comprehensive Cancer Network. NCCN Task Force Report: adjuvant therapy for breast cancer. J Natl Compr Canc Netw. 2006 Mar;4(Suppl 1):S1–26. [PMID: 16507275]

Chu QD et al. Adjuvant therapy for patients who have node-positive breast cancer. Adv Surg. 2006;40:77–98. [PMID: 17163096]

Citron ML et al. Randomized trial of dose-dense versus conventionally scheduled and sequential versus concurrent combination chemotherapy as postoperative adjuvant treatment of node-positive primary breast cancer: first report of Intergroup Trial C9741/Cancer and Leukemia Group B Trial 9741. J Clin Oncol. 2003 Apr 15;21(8):1431–9. [PMID: 12668651]

Coates AS et al. Five years of letrozole compared with tamoxifen as initial adjuvant therapy for postmenopausal women with endocrine-responsive early breast cancer: update of study BIG 1-98. J Clin Oncol. 2007 Feb 10;25(5):486–92. [PMID: 17200148]

Coombes RC et al; Intergroup Exemestane Study. Survival and safety of exemestane versus tamoxifen after 2-3 years' tamoxifen treatment: a randomised controlled trial. Lancet. 2007 Feb 17;369(9561):559–70. [PMID: 17307102]

Dienstmann R et al. Evidence-based neoadjuvant endocrine therapy for breast cancer. Clin Breast Cancer. 2006 Oct;7(4):315–20. [PMID: 17092398]

Early Breast Cancer Trialists' Collaborative Group (EBCTCG). Effects of chemotherapy and hormonal therapy for early breast cancer on recurrence and 15-year survival: an overview of the randomised trials. Lancet. 2005 May 14–20;365(9472):1687–717. [PMID: 15894097]

Fitzal F et al. Breast conservation: evolution of surgical strategies. Breast J. 2006 Sep–Oct;12(5 Suppl 2):S165–73. [PMID: 16958997]

Gennari A et al. HER2 status and efficacy of adjuvant anthracyclines in early breast cancer: a pooled analysis of randomized trials. J Natl Cancer Inst. 2008 Jan 2;100(1):14–20. [PMID: 18159072]

Goss PE et al. Randomized trial of letrozole following tamoxifen as extended adjuvant therapy in receptor-positive breast cancer: updated findings from NCIC CTG MA.17. J Natl Cancer Inst. 2005 Sep 7;97(17):1262–71. [PMID: 16145047]

Howell A et al; ATAC Trialists' Group. Results of the ATAC (Arimidex, Tamoxifen, Alone or in Combination) trial after completion of 5 years' adjuvant treatment for breast cancer. Lancet. 2005 Jan 1–7;365(9453):60–2. [PMID: 15639680]

Ingle JN et al. Fulvestrant in women with advanced breast cancer after progression on prior aromatase inhibitor therapy: North Central Cancer Treatment Group Trial N0032. J Clin Oncol. 2006 Mar 1;24(7):1052–6. [PMID: 16505423]

Joensuu H et al; FinHer Study Investigators. Adjuvant docetaxel or vinorelbine with or without trastuzumab for breast cancer. N Engl J Med. 2006 Feb 23;354(8):809–20. [PMID: 16495393]

Jones SE et al. Phase III trial comparing doxorubicin plus cyclophosphamide with docetaxel plus cyclophosphamide as adjuvant therapy for operable breast cancer. J Clin Oncol. 2006 Dec 1;24(34):5381–7. [PMID: 17135639]

Kim T et al. Lymphatic mapping and sentinel lymph node biopsy in early-stage breast carcinoma: a metaanalysis. Cancer. 2006 Jan 1;106(1):4–16. [PMID: 16329134]

Lee MC et al. Management of patients with locally advanced breast cancer. Surg Clin North Am. 2007 Apr;87(2):379–98. [PMID: 17498533]

Leonard C et al. Prospective trial of accelerated partial breast intensity-modulated radiotherapy. Int J Radiat Oncol Biol Phys. 2007 Apr 1;67(5):1291–8. [PMID: 17234359]

Mieog JS et al. Preoperative chemotherapy for women with operable breast cancer. Cochrane Database Syst Rev. 2007 Apr 18;(2):CD005002. [PMID: 17443564]

Miller K et al. Paclitaxel plus bevacizumab versus paclitaxel alone for metastatic breast cancer. N Engl J Med. 2007 Dec 27;357(26):2666–76. [PMID: 18160686]

Nielsen KV et al. The value of TOP2A gene copy number variation as a biomarker in breast cancer: update of DBCG trial 89D. Acta Oncol. 2008;47(4):725–34. [PMID: 18465341]

Orlando L et al. Management of advanced breast cancer. Ann Oncol. 2007 Jun;18(Suppl 6):vi74–6. [PMID: 17591838]

Perez EA et al. Cardiac safety analysis of doxorubicin and cyclophosphamide followed by paclitaxel with or without trastuzumab in the North Central Cancer Treatment Group N9831 adjuvant breast cancer trial. J Clin Oncol. 2008 Mar 10;26(8):1231–8. [PMID: 18250349]

Piccart-Gebhart MJ et al; Herceptin Adjuvant (HERA) Trial Study Team. Trastuzumab after adjuvant chemotherapy in HER2-positive breast cancer. N Engl J Med. 2005 Oct 20;353(16):1659–72. [PMID: 16236737]

Pritchard KI et al; National Cancer Institute of Canada Clinical Trials Group. HER2 and responsiveness of breast cancer to adjuvant chemotherapy. N Engl J Med. 2006 May 18;354(20):2103–11. [PMID: 16707747]

Pruthi S et al. A multidisciplinary approach to the management of breast cancer, part 2: therapeutic considerations. Mayo Clin Proc. 2007 Sep;82(9):1131–40. [PMID: 17803883]

Romond EH et al. Trastuzumab plus adjuvant chemotherapy for operable HER2-positive breast cancer. N Engl J Med. 2005 Oct 20;353(16):1673–84. [PMID: 16236738]

Seidman AD. Systemic treatment of breast cancer. Two decades of progress. Oncology (Williston Park). 2006 Aug;20(9):983–90. [PMID: 16986346]

Slamon DJ et al. Advances in adjuvant therapy for breast cancer. Clin Adv Hematol Oncol. 2006 Mar;4(3 Suppl 7):suppl 1, 4–9. [PMID: 16736568]

Smith I et al. 2-year follow-up of trastuzumab after adjuvant chemotherapy in HER2-positive breast cancer: a randomised controlled trial. Lancet. 2007 Jan 6;369(9555):29–36. [PMID: 17208639]

The National Institutes of Health Consensus Development Conference: Adjuvant Therapy for Breast Cancer. Bethesda, Maryland, USA. November 1–3, 2000. Proceedings. J Natl Cancer Inst Monogr. 2001;(30):1–152. [PMID: 12083020]

Thomas ES et al. Ixabepilone plus capecitabine for metastatic breast cancer progressing after anthracycline and taxane treatment. J Clin Oncol. 2007 Nov 20;25(33):5210–7. [PMID: 17968020]

Veronesi U et al. Lessons from the initial adjuvant cyclophosphamide, methotrexate, and fluorouracil studies in operable breast cancer. J Clin Oncol. 2008 Jan;26(3):342–4. [PMID: 18202404]

Veronesi U et al. Breast conservation: current results and future perspectives at the European Institute of Oncology. Int J Cancer. 2007 Apr 1;120(7):1381–6. [PMID: 17211883]

Voogd AC et al. Prognosis of patients with locally recurrent breast cancer. Am J Surg. 2007 Jan;193(1):138. [PMID: 17188110]

Waljee JF et al. Neoadjuvant systemic therapy and the surgical management of breast cancer. Surg Clin North Am. 2007 Apr;87(2):399–415. [PMID: 17498534]

Prognosis

Stage of breast cancer is the most reliable indicator of prognosis (Table 17–6). Patients with disease localized to the breast with no evidence of pathologic involvement of the lymph nodes have the most favorable prognosis. Axillary lymph node status is the best-analyzed prognostic factor and correlates with survival at all tumor sizes. In addition, increased number of axillary nodes involved correlates directly with lower survival rates. Increasingly, the use of biologic marker status, such as ER, PR, grade, and HER-2/neu, is helping to identify high-risk tumor types as well as direct treatment used (see Biomarkers). The histologic subtype of breast cancer (eg, medullary, lobular, colloid) seems to have little significance in prognosis of invasive carcinomas. Tumors with marked aneuploidy have a poor prognosis (see Table 17–4). Gene analysis studies, such as Oncotype Dx, can predict disease-free survival for some subsets of patients.

The mortality rate of breast cancer patients exceeds that of age-matched normal controls for nearly 20 years. Thereafter, the mortality rates are equal, though deaths that occur among breast cancer patients are often directly the result of tumor. Five-year statistics do not accurately reflect the final outcome of therapy.

Table 17–6. Approximate survival (%) of patients with breast cancer by TNM stage.

TNM Stage	Five Years	Ten Years
0	95	90
I	85	70
IIA	70	50
IIB	60	40
IIIA	55	30
IIIB	30	20
IV	5–10	2
All	65	30

When cancer is localized to the breast, with no evidence of regional spread after pathologic examination, the clinical cure rate with most accepted methods of therapy is 75% to greater than 90%. Variations to this generalization may be related to the hormonal receptor content of the tumor, genetic markers, tumor size, host resistance, or associated illness. Patients with small mammographically detected biologically favorable tumors and no evidence of axillary spread have a 5-year survival rate greater than 95%. When the axillary lymph nodes are involved with tumor, the survival rate drops to 50–70% at 5 years and probably around 25–40% at 10 years. In general, breast cancer appears to be somewhat more malignant in younger than in older women, and this may be related to the fact that fewer younger women have ER-positive tumors. Adjuvant systemic chemotherapy, in general, improves survival by about 30% and adjuvant hormonal therapy by about 25%.

For those patients whose disease progresses despite treatment, studies suggest supportive group therapy may improve survival. As they approach the end of life, such patients will require meticulous efforts at palliative care (see Chapter 5).

Stuart K et al. Life after breast cancer. Aust Fam Physician. 2006 Apr;35(4):219–24. [PMID: 16642238]

Follow-up Care

After primary therapy, patients with breast cancer should be monitored for life in order to detect recurrences and to observe the opposite breast for a second primary carcinoma. Local and distant recurrences occur most frequently within the first 2–5 years. During the first 2 years, most patients should be examined every 6 months, then annually thereafter. The patient should examine her own breasts monthly, and a mammogram should be obtained annually. Special attention is paid to the contralateral breast because a new primary breast malignancy will develop in 20–25% of patients. In some cases, metastases are dormant for long periods and may appear 10–15 years or longer after removal of the primary tumor. Although studies have failed to show an adverse effect of hormonal replacement in disease-free patients, it is rarely used after breast cancer treatment, particularly if the tumor was hormone receptor positive. Even pregnancy has not been clearly associated with shortened survival of patients rendered disease free—yet most oncologists are reluctant to advise a young patient with breast cancer that she may become pregnant, and most are less than enthusiastic about prescribing hormone replacement for the postmenopausal breast cancer patient. The use of estrogen replacement for conditions such as osteoporosis and hot flushes may be considered for a woman with a history of breast cancer after discussion of the benefits and risks, but it is not recommended.

A. Local Recurrence

The incidence of local recurrence correlates with tumor size, the presence and number of involved axillary nodes, the histologic type of tumor, the presence of skin edema or skin and fascia fixation with the primary tumor, and the type of definitive surgery and local irradiation. Local recurrence on the chest wall after total mastectomy and axillary dissection develops in as many as 8% of patients. When the axillary nodes are not involved, the local recurrence rate is less than 5%, but the rate is as high as 25% when they are heavily involved. A similar difference in local recurrence rate was noted between small and large tumors. Factors such as multifocal cancer, in situ tumors, positive resection margins, chemotherapy, and radiotherapy have an effect on local recurrence in patients treated with breast-conserving surgery.

Chest wall recurrences usually appear within the first several years but may occur as late as 15 or more years after mastectomy. All suspicious nodules and skin lesions should be biopsied. Local excision or localized radiotherapy may be feasible if an isolated nodule is present. If lesions are multiple or accompanied by evidence of regional involvement in the internal mammary or supraclavicular nodes, the disease is best managed by radiation treatment of the entire chest wall including the parasternal, supraclavicular, and axillary areas and usually by systemic therapy.

Local recurrence after mastectomy usually signals the presence of widespread disease and is an indication for studies to search for evidence of metastases. Distant metastases will develop within a few years in most patients with locally recurrent tumor after mastectomy. When there is no evidence of metastases beyond the chest wall and regional nodes, irradiation for cure after complete local excision should be attempted. Patients with local recurrence may be cured with local resection and radiation. After partial mastectomy, local recurrence does not have as serious a prognostic significance as after mastectomy. However, those patients in whom a recurrence develops have a worse prognosis than those who do not. It is speculated that the ability of a cancer to recur locally after radiotherapy is a sign of aggressiveness and resistance to therapy. Completion of the mastectomy should be done for local recurrence after partial mastectomy; some of these patients will survive for prolonged periods, especially if the breast recurrence is DCIS or occurs more than 5 years after initial treatment. Systemic chemotherapy or hormonal treatment should be used for women in whom disseminated disease develops or those in whom local recurrence occurs.

B. Edema of the Arm

Significant edema of the arm occurs in about 10–30% of patients after axillary dissection with or without mastectomy. It occurs more commonly if radiotherapy has been given or if there was postoperative infection. Partial mastectomy with radiation to the axillary lymph nodes is followed by chronic edema of the arm in 10–20% of patients. Sentinel lymph node dissection has proved to be a more accurate form of axillary staging without the side effects of edema or infection. It does not replace axillary dissection if the sentinel lymph nodes are involved with metastases. Judicious use of radiotherapy, with treatment fields carefully planned to spare the axilla as much as possible, can greatly diminish the incidence of edema, which will occur in only 5% of patients if no radiotherapy is given to the axilla after a partial mastectomy and lymph node dissection.

Late or secondary edema of the arm may develop years after treatment, as a result of axillary recurrence or infection in the hand or arm, with obliteration of lymphatic channels. When edema develops, a careful examination of the axilla for recurrence or infection is performed. Infection in the arm or hand on the dissected side should be treated with antibiotics, rest, and elevation. If there is no sign of recurrence or infection, the swollen extremity should be treated with rest and elevation. A mild diuretic may be helpful. If there is no improvement, a compressor pump or manual compression decreases the swelling, and the patient is then fitted with an elastic glove or sleeve. Most patients are not bothered enough by mild edema to wear an uncomfortable glove or sleeve and will treat themselves with elevation or manual compression alone. Benzopyrones have been reported to decrease lymphedema but are not approved for this use in the United States. Rarely, edema may be severe enough to interfere with use of the limb.

C. Breast Reconstruction

Breast reconstruction is usually feasible after total or modified radical mastectomy. Reconstruction should be discussed with patients prior to mastectomy, because it offers an important psychological focal point for recovery. Reconstruction is not an obstacle to the diagnosis of recurrent cancer. The most common breast reconstruction has been implantation of a silicone gel or saline prosthesis in the subpectoral plane between the pectoralis minor and pectoralis major muscles. Alternatively, autologous tissue can be used for reconstruction.

Autologous tissue flaps are aesthetically superior to implant reconstruction in most patients. They also have the advantage of not feeling like a foreign body to the patient. The most popular autologous technique currently is the trans-rectus abdominis muscle flap (TRAM flap), which is done by rotating the rectus abdominis muscle with attached fat and skin cephalad to make a breast mound. The free TRAM flap is done by completely removing a small portion of the rectus with overlying fat and skin and using microvascular surgical techniques to reconstruct the vascular supply on the chest wall. A latissimus dorsi flap can be swung from the back but offers less fullness than the TRAM flap and is therefore less acceptable cosmetically. An implant often is used to increase the fullness with a latissimus dorsi flap. Reconstruction may be performed immediately (at the time of initial mastectomy) or may be delayed until later, usually when the patient has completed adjuvant therapy. When considering reconstructive options, concomitant illnesses should be considered, since the ability of an autologous flap to survive depends on medical comorbidities. In addition, the need for radiotherapy may affect the choice of reconstruction as radiation may increase fibrosis around an implant or decrease the volume of a flap.

D. Risks of Pregnancy

Data are insufficient to determine whether interruption of pregnancy improves the prognosis of patients who are identified to have potentially curable breast cancer and who receive definitive treatment during pregnancy. Theoretically, the increasingly high levels of estrogen produced by the placenta as the pregnancy progresses could be detrimental to the patient with occult metastases of hormone-sensitive breast cancer. Moreover, occult metastases are present in most patients with positive axillary nodes, and treatment by adjuvant chemotherapy could be potentially harmful to the fetus early in gestation, although chemotherapy may be given to pregnant women later. Under these circumstances, interruption of early pregnancy seems reasonable, with progressively less rationale for the procedure as term approaches. The decision is affected by many factors, including the patient's desire to have the baby and the prognosis especially when axillary nodes are involved.

Equally important is the advice regarding future pregnancy (or abortion in case of pregnancy) to be given to women of child-bearing age who have had definitive treatment for breast cancer. It is assumed that pregnancy will be harmful if occult metastases are present, though this has not been demonstrated. Patients whose tumors are ER negative (most younger women) may not be affected by pregnancy. To date, no adverse effect of pregnancy on survival of pregnant women who have had breast cancer has been demonstrated, though most oncologists advise against it.

In patients with inoperable or metastatic cancer (stage IV disease), induced abortion is usually advisable because of the possible adverse effects of hormonal treatment, radiotherapy, or chemotherapy upon the fetus.

Banks E et al. Pregnancy in women with a history of breast cancer. BMJ. 2007 Jan 27;334(7586):166–7. [PMID: 17255571]

Dian D et al. Quality of life among breast cancer patients undergoing autologous breast reconstruction versus breast conserving therapy. J Cancer Res Clin Oncol. 2007 Apr;133 (4):247–52. [PMID: 17096124]

Hayes DF. Prognostic and predictive factors for breast cancer: translating technology to oncology. J Clin Oncol. 2005 Mar 10;23(8):1596–7. [PMID: 15755959]

Hu E et al. Breast reconstruction. Surg Clin North Am. 2007 Apr;87(2):453–67. [PMID: 17498537]

Kronowitz SJ et al. Advances and surgical decision-making for breast reconstruction. Cancer. 2006 Sep 1;107(5):893–907. [PMID: 16862569]

Moseley AL et al. A systematic review of common conservative therapies for arm lymphoedema secondary to breast cancer treatment. Ann Oncol. 2007 Apr;18(4):639–46. [PMID: 17018707]

Pomahac B et al. New trends in breast cancer management: is the era of immediate breast reconstruction changing? Ann Surg. 2006 Aug;244(2):282–8. [PMID: 16858192]

Sakorafas GH et al. Lymphedema following axillary lymph node dissection for breast cancer. Surg Oncol. 2006 Nov;15(3):153–65. [PMID: 17187979]

Salhab M et al. Skin-sparing mastectomy and immediate breast reconstruction: patient satisfaction and clinical outcome. Int J Clin Oncol. 2006 Feb;11(1):51–4. [PMID: 16508729]

Soran A et al. Breast cancer-related lymphedema—what are the significant predictors and how they affect the severity of lymphedema? Breast J. 2006 Nov–Dec;12(6):536–43. [PMID: 17238983]

CARCINOMA OF THE MALE BREAST

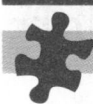

ESSENTIALS OF DIAGNOSIS

▸ A painless lump beneath the areola in a man usually over 50 years of age.

▸ Nipple discharge, retraction, or ulceration may be present.

▸ Generally poorer prognosis than in women.

General Considerations

Breast cancer in men is a rare disease; the incidence is only about 1% of that in women. The average age at occurrence is about 60—somewhat older than the most common presenting age in women. There may be an increased incidence of breast cancer in men with prostate cancer. As in women, hormonal influences are probably related to the development of male breast cancer. There is a high incidence of both breast cancer and gynecomastia in Bantu men, theoretically owing to failure of estrogen inactivation by a liver damaged by associated liver disease. It is important to note that first-degree relatives of men with breast cancer are considered to be at high risk. This risk should be taken into account when discussing options with the patient and family. In addition, *BRCA2* mutations are common in men with breast cancer. Men with breast cancer, especially with a history of prostate cancer, should receive genetic counseling. The prognosis, even in stage I cases, is worse in men than in women. Blood-borne metastases are commonly present when the male patient appears for initial treatment. These metastases may be latent and may not become manifest for many years.

Clinical Findings

A painless lump, occasionally associated with nipple discharge, retraction, erosion, or ulceration, is the primary complaint. Examination usually shows a hard, ill-defined, nontender mass beneath the nipple or areola. Gynecomastia not uncommonly precedes or accompanies breast cancer in men. Nipple discharge is an uncommon presentation for breast cancer in men but is an ominous finding associated with carcinoma in nearly 75% of cases.

Breast cancer staging is the same in men as in women. Gynecomastia and metastatic cancer from another site (eg, prostate) must be considered in the differential diagnosis. Benign tumors are rare, and biopsy should be performed on all males with a defined breast mass.

Treatment

Treatment consists of modified radical mastectomy in operable patients, who should be chosen by the same criteria as women with the disease. Breast conserving therapy is rarely performed. Irradiation is the first step in treating localized metastases in the skin, lymph nodes, or skeleton that are causing symptoms. Examination of the cancer for hormone receptor proteins is of value in predicting response to endocrine ablation. Men commonly have ER-positive tumors and rarely have overexpression of *HER-2/neu*. Adjuvant systemic therapy and radiation is used for the same indications as in breast cancer in women.

Because breast cancer in men is frequently a disseminated disease, endocrine therapy is of considerable importance in its management. Tamoxifen is the main drug for management of advanced breast cancer in men. Tamoxifen (20 mg orally daily) should be the initial treatment. There is little experience with AIs though they should be effective. Castration in advanced breast cancer is a successful measure and more beneficial than the same procedure in women but is rarely used. Objective evidence of regression may be seen in 60–70% of men with hormonal therapy for metastatic disease—approximately twice the proportion in women. The average duration of tumor growth remission is about 30 months, and life is prolonged. Bone is the most frequent site of metastases from breast cancer in men (as in women), and hormonal therapy relieves bone pain in most patients so treated. The longer the interval between mastectomy and recurrence, the longer the remission following treatment is likely. As in women, there is correlation between ERs of the tumor and the likelihood of remission following hormonal therapy.

AIs should replace adrenalectomy in men as they have in women. Corticosteroid therapy alone has been considered to be efficacious but probably has no value when compared with major endocrine ablation. Either tamoxifen or AIs may be primary or secondary hormonal manipulation.

Estrogen therapy—5 mg of diethylstilbestrol three times daily orally—may be effective hormonal manipulation after others have been successful and failed, just as in women. Androgen therapy may exacerbate bone pain. Chemotherapy should be administered for the same indications and using the same dosage schedules as for women with metastatic disease or for adjuvant treatment.

Prognosis

The prognosis of breast cancer is poorer in men than in women. The crude 5- and 10-year survival rates for clinical stage I breast cancer in men are about 58% and 38%, respectively. For clinical stage II disease, the 5- and 10-year survival rates are approximately 38% and 10%. The survival rates for all stages at 5 and 10 years are 36% and 17%. For those patients whose disease progresses despite treatment, meticulous efforts at palliative care are essential (see Chapter 5).

Agrawal A et al. Male breast cancer: a review of clinical management. Breast Cancer Res Treat. 2007 May;103(1):11–21. [PMID: 17033919]

Fentiman IS et al. Male breast cancer. Lancet. 2006 Feb 18;367 (9510):595–604. [PMID: 16488803]

Karhu R et al. Large genomic BRCA2 rearrangements and male breast cancer. Cancer Detect Prev. 2006;30(6):530–4. [PMID: 17113724]

Nahleh ZA. Hormonal therapy for male breast cancer: a different approach for a different disease. Cancer Treat Rev. 2006 Apr;32(2):101–5. [PMID: 16472925]

Gynecologic Disorders

H. Trent MacKay, MD, MPH

ABNORMAL PREMENOPAUSAL BLEEDING

 ESSENTIALS OF DIAGNOSIS

▶ Blood loss of over 80 mL per cycle.

▶ Excessive bleeding, often with the passage of clots, may occur at regular menstrual intervals (menorrhagia) or irregular intervals (dysfunctional uterine bleeding).

▶ Etiology most commonly dysfunctional uterine bleeding on a hormonal basis.

▶ General Considerations

Normal menstrual bleeding lasts an average of 4 days (range, 2–7 days), with a mean blood loss of 40 mL. Blood loss of over 80 mL per cycle is abnormal and frequently produces anemia. When there are less than 21 days between the onset of bleeding episodes, the cycles are likely to be anovular. Ovulation bleeding, a single episode of spotting between regular menses, is quite common. Heavier or irregular intermenstrual bleeding warrants investigation.

Dysfunctional uterine bleeding is usually caused by overgrowth of endometrium due to estrogen stimulation without adequate progesterone to stabilize growth; this occurs in anovular cycles. Anovulation commonly occurs in teenagers, in women aged late 30s to late 40s, and in extremely obese women or those with polycystic ovary syndrome.

▶ Clinical Findings

A. Symptoms and Signs

The diagnosis usually depends on the following: (1) A careful description of the duration and amount of flow, related pain, and relationship to the last menstrual period (LMP). The presence of blood clots or the degree of inconvenience caused by the bleeding may be more useful indicators. (2) A history of pertinent illnesses or weight change. (3) A history of medications taken in the past month. (4) A history of coagulation disorders in the patient or family members. (5) A careful pelvic examination to look for vaginal or cervical lesions, pregnancy, uterine myomas, adnexal masses, or infection.

B. Laboratory Studies

Cervical smears should be obtained as needed for cytologic and culture studies. Blood studies should include a complete blood count, sedimentation rate, and glucose level to rule out diabetes. Diabetes may occasionally initially present with abnormal bleeding. A pregnancy test and studies of thyroid function and coagulation disorders should be considered in the clinical evaluation. Up to 18% of women with severe menorrhagia may have a coagulopathy. Tests for ovulation in cyclic menorrhagia include basal body temperature records, serum progesterone measured 1 week before the expected onset of menses, or an endometrial biopsy specimen for secretory activity shortly before the onset of menstruation.

C. Imaging

Ultrasound may be useful to evaluate endometrial thickness or to diagnose intrauterine or ectopic pregnancy or adnexal masses. Endovaginal ultrasound with saline infusion sonohysterography may be used to diagnose endometrial polyps or subserous myomas. MRI can definitively diagnose submucous myomas and adenomyosis.

D. Cervical Biopsy and Endometrial Curettage

Biopsy, curettage, or aspiration of the endometrium and curettage of the endocervix may be necessary to diagnose the cause of bleeding. These and other invasive gynecologic diagnostic procedures are described in Table 18–1. Polyps, endometrial hyperplasia, and submucous myomas are commonly identified in this way. If cancer of the cervix is suspected, colposcopically directed biopsies and endocervical curettage are indicated as first steps.

E. Hysteroscopy

Hysteroscopy can visualize endometrial polyps, submucous myomas, and exophytic endometrial cancers, fol-

Table 18–1. Common gynecologic diagnostic procedures.

Colposcopy
Visualization of cervical, vaginal, or vulvar epithelium under 5–50× magnification with and without dilute acetic acid to identify abnormal areas requiring biopsy. An office procedure.

D&C
Dilation of the cervix and curettage of the entire endometrial cavity, using a metal curette or suction cannula and often using forceps for the removal of endometrial polyps. Can usually be done in the office under local anesthesia.

Endometrial biopsy
Removal of one or more areas of the endometrium by means of a curette or small aspiration device without cervical dilation. Diagnostic accuracy similar to D&C. An office procedure performed under local anesthesia.

Endocervical curettage
Removal of endocervical epithelium with a small curette for diagnosis of cervical dysplasia and cancer. An office procedure performed under local anesthesia.

Hysteroscopy
Visual examination of the uterine cavity with a small fiberoptic endoscope passed through the cervix. Biopsies, and excision of myomas can be performed. Can be done in the office under local anesthesia or in the operating room under general anesthesia.

Saline infusion sonohysterography
Introduction of saline solution into endometrial cavity with catheter to visualize submucous myomas or endometrial polyps by transvaginal ultrasound. May be performed in the office with oral analgesia.

Hysterosalpingography
Injection of radiopaque dye through the cervix to visualize the uterine cavity and oviducts. Mainly used in investigation of infertility.

Laparoscopy
Visualization of the abdominal and pelvic cavity through a small fiberoptic endoscope passed through a subumbilical incision. Permits diagnosis, tubal sterilization, and treatment of many conditions previously requiring laparotomy. General anesthesia is usually used.

lowed by removal of the polyp or myoma and endometrial sampling.

▶ **Treatment**

Premenopausal patients with abnormal uterine bleeding include those with submucosal myomas, infection, early abortion, thrombophilias, or pelvic neoplasms. The history, physical examination, laboratory findings, and endometrial sampling should identify such patients, who require definitive therapy. A large group of patients remain, most of whom have dysfunctional uterine bleeding on the basis of anovulation.

Dysfunctional uterine bleeding can usually be treated hormonally. Women over the age of 35 should routinely have endometrial sampling to rule out endometrial hyperplasia or carcinoma prior to initiation of hormonal therapy. Progestins, which limit and stabilize endometrial growth, are generally effective. Medroxyprogesterone acetate, 10 mg/d orally, or norethindrone acetate, 5 mg/d orally, should be given for 10–14 days starting on day 15 of

the cycle, following which withdrawal bleeding (so-called medical curettage) will occur. The treatment is repeated for several cycles; it can be reinstituted if amenorrhea or dysfunctional bleeding recurs. In women who are bleeding actively, any of the combination oral contraceptives can be given four times daily for 1 or 2 days followed by two pills daily through day 5 and then one pill daily through day 20; after withdrawal bleeding occurs, pills are taken in the usual dosage for three cycles. In cases of intractable heavy bleeding, danazol, 200 mg orally four times daily, is sometimes used to create an atrophic endometrium. Alternatively, a GnRH agonist such as depot leuprolide, 3.75 mg intramuscularly monthly, or nafarelin, 0.2–0.4 mg intranasally twice daily, can be used for up to 6 months to create a temporary cessation of menstruation by ovarian suppression.

In cases of heavy bleeding, intravenous conjugated estrogens, 25 mg every 4 hours for three or four doses, can be used, followed by oral conjugated estrogens, 2.5 mg daily, or ethinyl estradiol, 20 mcg orally daily, for 3 weeks, with the addition of medroxyprogesterone acetate, 10 mg orally daily for the last 10 days of treatment, or a combination oral contraceptive daily for 3 weeks. This will thicken the endometrium and control the bleeding. Nonsteroidal anti-inflammatory drugs (NSAIDs), such as naproxen or mefenamic acid, in the usual anti-inflammatory doses will often reduce blood loss in menorrhagia—even that associated with a copper intrauterine device (IUD).

If the abnormal bleeding is not controlled by hormonal treatment, hysteroscopy, saline infusion sonohysterography, or a D&C is necessary to check for polyps, submucous myomas, or endometrial cancer. In the absence of specific pathology, bleeding unresponsive to medical therapy may be treated with endometrial ablation, levonorgestrel-releasing IUD, or hysterectomy. While hysterectomy was used commonly in the past for bleeding unresponsive to medical therapy, the low risk of complications and the good short-term results of both endometrial ablation and levonorgestrel-releasing IUD make them attractive alternatives to hysterectomy. Endometrial ablation may be performed through the hysteroscope with laser photocoagulation or electrocautery. Newer, nonhysteroscopic techniques include balloon thermal ablation, cryoablation, free-fluid thermal ablation, impedence bipolar radiofrequency ablation, and microwave ablation. The latter methods are well-adapted to outpatient therapy under local anesthesia.

The levonorgestrel-releasing IUD markedly reduces menstrual blood loss and may be a good alternative to other therapies. However, while short-term results with endometrial ablation and levonorgestrel-releasing IUD are satisfactory, at 5 years after either the endometrial ablation procedure or placement of the levonorgestrel IUD, up to 40% of women will have had either repeat ablation procedures or a hysterectomy.

▶ **When to Refer**

• If bleeding is not controlled with first-line therapy.
• If expertise is needed for a surgical procedure.

When to Admit

If bleeding is uncontrollable with first-line therapy and the patient is not hemodynamically stable.

Casablanca Y. Management of dysfunctional uterine bleeding. Obstet Gynecol Clin N Am. 2008 Jun;35(2):219–34. [PMID: 18486838]

Istre O et al. Current treatment options for abnormal uterine bleeding: an evidenced-based approach. Best Prac Res Clin Obstet Gynecol. 2007 Dec;21(6):905–13. [PMID: 1749953]

Mansour D. Modern management of abnormal uterine bleeding: the levonorgestrel intra-uterine system. Best Prac Res Clin Obstet Gynecol. 2007;21(6):1007–21. [PMID: 17544330]

POSTMENOPAUSAL VAGINAL BLEEDING

ESSENTIALS OF DIAGNOSIS

▶ Vaginal bleeding that occurs 6 months or more following cessation of menstrual function.

▶ Bleeding is usually painless.

▶ Bleeding may be a single episode of spotting or profuse bleeding for days or months.

General Considerations

Vaginal bleeding that occurs 6 months or more following cessation of menstrual function should be investigated. The most common causes are atrophic endometrium, endometrial proliferation or hyperplasia, endometrial or cervical cancer, and administration of estrogens with or without added progestin. Other causes include atrophic vaginitis, trauma, endometrial polyps, friction ulcers of the cervix associated with prolapse of the uterus, and blood dyscrasias. Uterine bleeding is usually painless, but pain will be present if the cervix is stenotic, if bleeding is severe and rapid, or if infection or torsion or extrusion of a tumor is present. The patient may report a single episode of spotting or profuse bleeding for days or months.

Diagnosis

The vulva and vagina should be inspected for areas of bleeding, ulcers, or neoplasms. A cytologic smear of the cervix and vaginal pool should be taken. If available, transvaginal sonography should be used to measure endometrial thickness. A measurement of 5 mm or less indicates a low likelihood of hyperplasia or endometrial cancer, although up to 4% of endometrial cancers may be missed with sonography. If the thickness is greater than 5 mm or there is a heterogeneous appearance to the endometrium, endocervical curettage and endometrial biopsy or D&C, preferably with hysteroscopy, should be performed.

Treatment

Endometrial biopsy or D&C may be curative. Simple endometrial hyperplasia calls for cyclic progestin therapy (medroxyprogesterone acetate, 10 mg/d orally, or norethin-drone acetate, 5 mg/d orally) for 21 days of each month for 3 months. A repeat endometrial biopsy should be performed. If endometrial hyperplasia with atypical cells or carcinoma of the endometrium is found, hysterectomy is necessary.

When to Refer

• Complex endometrial hyperplasia with atypia is present.

• Hysteroscopy is indicated.

Clark TJ et al. Investigating postmenopausal bleeding for endometrial cancer: cost-effectiveness of initial diagnostic strategies. BJOG. 2006 May;113(5):502–10. [PMID: 16637894]

PREMENSTRUAL SYNDROME (Premenstrual Tension)

The premenstrual syndrome (PMS) is a recurrent, variable cluster of troublesome physical and emotional symptoms that develop during the 7–14 days before the onset of menses and subside when menstruation occurs. PMS intermittently affects about 40% of all premenopausal women, primarily those 25–40 years of age. In about 5–8% of affected women, the syndrome may be severe. Although not every woman experiences all the symptoms or signs at one time, many describe bloating, breast pain, ankle swelling, a sense of increased weight, skin disorders, irritability, aggressiveness, depression, inability to concentrate, libido change, lethargy, and food cravings. When emotional or mood symptoms predominate, along with physical symptoms, and there is a clear functional impairment, the term "premenstrual dysphoric disorder" (PMDD) may be applied. The pathogenesis of PMS/PMDD is still uncertain, and current treatment methods are mainly empiric. The clinician should provide support for both the patient's emotional and physical distress. This includes the following:

1. Careful evaluation of the patient, with understanding, explanation, and reassurance.

2. Advise the patient to keep a daily diary of all symptoms for 2–3 months, to evaluate the timing and characteristics of her symptoms. If her symptoms occur throughout the month rather than in the 2 weeks before menses, she may have depression or other emotional problems in addition to PMS.

3. For mild to moderate symptoms, a program of aerobic exercise; reduction of caffeine, salt, and alcohol intake; and an increase in dietary calcium (to 1200 mg per day), vitamin D (to 800 international units per day), and complex carbohydrates in the diet may be helpful.

4. When physical symptoms predominate, spironolactone, 100 mg orally daily during the luteal phase, is effective for reduction of bloating and breast tenderness. Oral contraceptives or injectable progestin medroxyprogesterone acetate (DMPA) will decrease breast pain and cramping. NSAIDs, such as mefenamic acid, 500 mg orally three times a day, will reduce a number of symptoms but not breast pain.

5. When mood disorders predominate, serotonin reuptake inhibitors such as fluoxetine, 20 mg orally, either

daily or only on symptom days, are effective in relieving tension, irritability, and dysphoria with few side effects.

6. When the above regimens are not effective, ovarian function can be suppressed with continuous high-dose progestin (20–30 mg/d of oral medroxyprogesterone acetate [MPA] or 150 mg of DMPA orally every 3 months or GnRH agonist with add-back therapy, such as conjugated equine estrogen, 0.625 mg orally daily with medroxyprogesterone acetate, 2.5–5.0 mg orally daily.

Yonkers KA et al. Premenstrual syndrome. Lancet. 2008 Apr 5;371(9619):1200–10. [PMID: 18395582]

DYSMENORRHEA

1. Primary Dysmenorrhea

Primary dysmenorrhea is menstrual pain associated with ovulatory cycles in the absence of pathologic findings. The pain usually begins within 1–2 years after the menarche and may become more severe with time. The frequency of cases increases up to age 20 and then decreases with age and markedly with parity. Fifty to 75 percent of women are affected at some time and 5–6% have incapacitating pain.

▶ Clinical Findings

Primary dysmenorrhea is low, midline, wave-like, cramping pelvic pain often radiating to the back or inner thighs. Cramps may last for 1 or more days and may be associated with nausea, diarrhea, headache, and flushing. The pain is produced by uterine vasoconstriction, anoxia, and sustained contractions mediated by prostaglandins. The pelvic examination is normal between menses; examination during menses may produce discomfort, but there are no pathologic findings.

▶ Treatment

NSAIDs (ibuprofen, ketoprofen, mefenamic acid, naproxen) and the cyclooxygenase (COX)-2 inhibitor celecoxib are generally helpful. The medication should be started 1–2 days before expected menses. Ovulation can be suppressed and dysmenorrhea usually prevented by oral contraceptives, depot-medroxyprogesterone acetate, or levonorgestrel-releasing IUD. For women who do not wish to use hormonal contraception, other therapies that have shown at least some benefit include local heat; thiamine, 100 mg/d orally; vitamin E, 200 units/d orally from 2 days prior to and for the first 3 days of menses; and high-frequency transcutaneous electrical nerve stimulation.

2. Secondary Dysmenorrhea

Secondary dysmenorrhea is menstrual pain for which an organic cause exists. It usually begins well after menarche, sometimes even as late as the third or fourth decade of life.

▶ Clinical Findings

The history and physical examination commonly suggest endometriosis or pelvic inflammatory disease (PID). Other causes may be submucous myoma, IUD use, cervical stenosis with obstruction, or blind uterine horn (rare).

▶ Diagnosis

Laparoscopy is often needed to differentiate endometriosis from PID. Submucous myomas can be detected most reliably by MRI but also by hysterogram, by hysteroscopy, or by passing a sound or curette over the uterine cavity during D&C. Cervical stenosis may result from induced abortion, creating crampy pain at the time of expected menses with no blood flow; this is easily cured by passing a sound into the uterine cavity after administering a paracervical block.

▶ Treatment

A. Specific Measures

Periodic use of analgesics, including the NSAIDs given for primary dysmenorrhea, may be beneficial, and oral contraceptives may give relief, particularly in endometriosis. Danazol and GnRH agonists are effective in the treatment of endometriosis (see below).

B. Surgical Measures

If disability is marked or prolonged, laparoscopy or exploratory laparotomy is usually warranted. Definitive surgery depends on the degree of disability and the findings at operation.

▶ When to Refer

- Standard therapy fails to relieve pain.
- Suspicion of pelvic pathology, such as endometriosis.

Proctor M et al. Diagnosis and management of dysmenorrhoea. BMJ. 2006 May 13;332(7550):1134–8. [PMID: 16690671]
Sanfilippo J et al. Evaluation and management of dysmenorrhea in adolescents. Clin Obstet Gynecol. 2008 Jun;51(2):257–67. [PMID: 18463457]

VAGINITIS

ESSENTIALS OF DIAGNOSIS

▶ Vaginal irritation.
▶ Pruritus.
▶ Pain.
▶ Unusual discharge.

▶ General Considerations

Inflammation and infection of the vagina are common gynecologic problems, resulting from a variety of pathogens, allergic reactions to vaginal contraceptives or other products, or the friction of coitus. The normal vaginal pH is 4.5 or less, and *Lactobacillus* is the predominant organism. At the time of the midcycle estrogen surge, clear, elastic, mucoid secretions from the cervical os are often profuse. In the luteal phase and during pregnancy, vaginal secretions are thicker, white, and sometimes adherent to the vaginal walls. These normal secretions can be confused with vaginitis by concerned women.

▶ Clinical Findings

When the patient complains of vaginal irritation, pain, or unusual discharge, a history should be taken, noting the onset of the LMP; recent sexual activity; use of contraceptives, tampons, or douches; and the presence of vaginal burning, pain, pruritus, or unusually profuse or malodorous discharge. The physical examination should include careful inspection of the vulva and speculum examination of the vagina and cervix. The cervix is sampled for gonococcus or *Chlamydia* if applicable. A specimen of vaginal discharge is examined under the microscope in a drop of 0.9% saline solution to look for trichomonads or clue cells and in a drop of 10% potassium hydroxide to search for *Candida*. The vaginal pH should be tested; it is frequently greater than 4.5 in infections due to trichomonads and bacterial vaginosis. A bimanual examination to look for evidence of pelvic infection should follow.

A. Vulvovaginal Candidiasis

Pregnancy, diabetes, and use of broad-spectrum antibiotics or corticosteroids predispose patients to *Candida* infections. Heat, moisture, and occlusive clothing also contribute to the risk. Pruritus, vulvovaginal erythema, and a white curd-like discharge that is not malodorous are found (Plate 74). Microscopic examination with 10% potassium hydroxide reveals filaments and spores. Cultures with Nickerson medium may be used if *Candida* is suspected but not demonstrated.

B. *Trichomonas vaginalis* Vaginitis

This protozoal flagellate infects the vagina, Skene ducts, and lower urinary tract in women and the lower genitourinary tract in men. It is sexually transmitted. Pruritus and a malodorous frothy, yellow-green discharge occur, along with diffuse vaginal erythema and red macular lesions on the cervix in severe cases (Plate 75). Motile organisms with flagella are seen by microscopic examination of a wet mount with saline solution.

C. Bacterial Vaginosis

This condition is considered to be a polymicrobial disease that is not sexually transmitted. An overgrowth of *Gardnerella* and other anaerobes is often associated with increased malodorous discharge without obvious vulvitis or vaginitis. The discharge is grayish and sometimes frothy, with a pH of 5.0–5.5. An amine-like ("fishy") odor is present if a drop of discharge is alkalinized with 10% potassium hydroxide. On wet mount in saline, epithelial cells are covered with bacteria to such an extent that cell borders are obscured (clue cells, Plate 76). Vaginal cultures are generally not useful in diagnosis.

D. Condylomata Acuminata (Genital Warts)

Warty growths on the vulva, perianal area, vaginal walls, or cervix are caused by various types of the human papilloma-

virus (HPV). They are sexually transmitted. Pregnancy and immunosuppression favor growth. Vulvar lesions may be obviously wart-like or may be diagnosed only after application of 4% acetic acid (vinegar) and colposcopy, when they appear whitish, with prominent papillae. Fissures may be present at the fourchette. Vaginal lesions may show diffuse hypertrophy or a cobblestone appearance. Cervical lesions may be visible only by colposcopy after pretreatment with 4% acetic acid. These lesions may be related to dysplasia and cervical cancer. Vulvar cancer is also currently considered to be associated with HPV infection.

▶ Treatment

A. Vulvovaginal Candidiasis

A variety of regimens are available to treat vulvovaginal candidiasis. Women with uncomplicated vulvovaginal candidiasis will usually respond to a 1- to 3-day regimen of a topical azole. Women with complicated infection (including four or more episodes in 1 year, severe signs and symptoms, non-albicans species, uncontrolled diabetes, HIV infection, corticosteroid treatment, or pregnancy) should receive 7–14 days of a topical regimen or two doses of fluconazole 3 days apart. (Pregnant women should use only topical azoles.)

1. Single-dose regimens—Effective single-dose regimens include miconazole, 1200-mg vaginal suppository; tioconazole, 6.5%, 5 g vaginally; or sustained-release butoconazole, 2% cream, 5 g vaginally.

2. Three-day regimens—Effective 3-day regimens include butoconazole (2% cream, 5 g once daily), clotrimazole (two 100-mg vaginal tablets once daily), terconazole (0.8% cream, 5 g, or 80-mg suppository once daily), or miconazole (200 mg vaginal suppository once daily).

3. Seven-day regimens—The following regimens are given once daily: clotrimazole (1% cream or 100-mg vaginal tablet), miconazole (2% cream, 5 g, or 100-mg vaginal suppository), or terconazole (0.4% cream, 5 g).

4. Fourteen-day regimen—An effective 14-day regimen is nystatin (100,000-unit vaginal tablet once daily).

5. Recurrent vulvovaginitis (maintenance therapy)—Clotrimazole (500-mg vaginal suppository once weekly or 200 mg cream twice weekly) or fluconazole (100, 150, or 200 mg orally once weekly) are effective regimens for maintenance therapy for up to 6 months.

B. *Trichomonas vaginalis* Vaginitis

Treatment of both partners simultaneously is recommended; metronidazole or tinidazole, 2 g orally as a single dose or 500 mg orally twice a day for 7 days, is usually used.

In the case of treatment failure with metronidazole in the absence of reexposure, the patient should be re-treated with metronidazole, 500 mg orally twice a day for 7 days, or tinidazole 2 g orally as a single dose. If treatment failure occurs again, give metronidazole or tinidazole, 2 g orally once daily for 5 days. If this is not effective in eradicating the organisms, metronidazole and tinidazole susceptibility testing can be arranged with the CDC at 770-488-4115 or at http://www.cdc.gov/std.

C. Bacterial Vaginosis

The recommended regimens are metronidazole, 500 mg orally twice daily for 7 days, clindamycin vaginal cream (2%, 5 g), once daily for 7 days, or metronidazole gel (0.75%, 5 g), twice daily for 5 days. Alternative regimens include clindamycin, 300 mg orally twice daily for 7 days, or clindamycin ovules, 100 g intravaginally at bedtime for 3 days.

D. Condylomata Acuminata

Recommended treatments for vulvar warts include podophyllum resin 10–25% in tincture of benzoin (do not use during pregnancy or on bleeding lesions) or 80–90% trichloroacetic or bichloroacetic acid, carefully applied to avoid the surrounding skin. The pain of bichloroacetic or trichloroacetic acid application can be lessened by a sodium bicarbonate paste applied immediately after treatment. Podophyllum resin must be washed off after 2–4 hours. Freezing with liquid nitrogen or a cryoprobe and electrocautery are also effective. Patient-applied regimens include podofilox 0.5% solution or gel and imiquimod 5% cream. Vaginal warts may be treated with cryotherapy with liquid nitrogen, trichloroacetic acid, or podophyllum resin. Extensive warts may require treatment with CO_2 laser under local or general anesthesia. Interferon is not recommended for routine use because it is very expensive, associated with systemic side effects, and no more effective than other therapies. Routine examination of sex partners is not necessary for the management of genital warts since the risk of reinfection is probably minimal and curative therapy to prevent transmission is not available. However, partners may wish to be examined for detection and treatment of genital warts and other sexually transmitted diseases. While condom use does not appear to prevent HPV transmission, it may result in accelerated regression of associated lesions, including untreated cervical intraepithelial neoplasia (CIN) and in accelerated clearance of genital HPV infection in women.

Mashburn J. Etiology, diagnosis, and management of vaginitis. J Midwifery Womens Health 2006 Nov–Dec;51(6):423–30. [PMID: 17081932]
Sexually transmitted disease treatment guidelines 2006. Centers for Disease Control and Prevention. MMWR Recomm Rep. 2006 Aug 4;55(RR-11):1–94. [PMID: 16888612]

CERVICAL POLYPS

Cervical polyps commonly occur after menarche and are occasionally noted in postmenopausal women. The cause is not known, but inflammation may play an etiologic role. The principal symptoms are discharge and abnormal vaginal bleeding. However, abnormal bleeding should not be ascribed to a cervical polyp without sampling the endocervix and endometrium. The polyps are visible in the cervical os on speculum examination.

Cervical polyps must be differentiated from polypoid neoplastic disease of the endometrium, small submucous pedunculated myomas, and endometrial polyps. Cervical polyps rarely contain dysplasia (0.5%) or malignant (0.5%) foci.

▶ Treatment

Cervical polyps can generally be removed in the office by avulsion with a uterine packing forceps or ring forceps. If the cervix is soft, patulous, or definitely dilated and the polyp is large, surgical D&C is required (especially if the pedicle is not readily visible). Hysteroscopy may aid removal and lead to identification of concomitant endometrial disease. Because of the possibility of endometrial disease, cervical polypectomy should routinely be accompanied by endometrial sampling.

▶ When to Refer

- Polyp with a wide base is present.
- Inability to differentiate endocervical from endometrial polyp.

Berzolla CF et al. Dysplasia and malignancy in endometrial polyps. J Womens Health (Larchmt). 2007;16(9):1317–21. [PMID: 18001188]

CYST & ABSCESS OF BARTHOLIN DUCT

Trauma or infection may involve Bartholin duct, causing obstruction of the gland. Drainage of secretions is prevented, leading to pain, swelling, and abscess formation (Plate 77). The infection usually resolves and pain disappears, but stenosis of the duct outlet with distention often persists. Reinfection causes recurrent tenderness and further enlargement of the duct.

The principal symptoms are periodic painful swelling on either side of the introitus and dyspareunia. A fluctuant swelling 1–4 cm in diameter in the inferior portion of either labium minus is a sign of occlusion of Bartholin duct. Tenderness is evidence of active infection.

Pus or secretions from the gland should be cultured for *Chlamydia* and other pathogens and treated accordingly (see Chapter 33); frequent warm soaks may be helpful. If an abscess develops, aspiration or incision and drainage are the simplest forms of therapy, but the problem may recur. Marsupialization (in the absence of an abscess), incision and drainage with the insertion of an indwelling Word catheter, or laser treatment will establish a new duct opening. Antibiotics are unnecessary unless cellulitis is present. An asymptomatic cyst does not require therapy.

▶ When to Refer

Surgical therapy (marsupialization) is indicated.

Pundir J et al. A review of the management of diseases of the Bartholin's gland. J Obstet Gynaecol. 2008 Feb;28(2):161–5. [PMID: 18393010]

EFFECTS OF EXPOSURE TO DIETHYLSTILBESTROL IN UTERO

Between 1947 and 1971, diethylstilbestrol (DES) was widely used in the United States for diabetic women during pregnancy and to treat threatened abortion. It is estimated that at least 2–3 million fetuses were exposed. A relationship between fetal DES exposure and clear cell carcinoma of the vagina was later discovered, and a number of other related anomalies have since been noted. In one-third of all exposed women, there are changes in the vagina (adenosis, septa), cervix (deformities and hypoplasia of the vaginal portion of the cervix), or uterus (T-shaped cavity).

All women known to be exposed prenatally are advised to have an initial colposcopic examination to outline vaginal and cervical areas of abnormal epithelium, followed by cytologic examination of the vagina (all four quadrants of the upper half of the vagina) and cervix at yearly intervals. Lugol iodine stain of the vagina and cervix will also outline areas of metaplastic squamous epithelium.

Many women are not aware of having been exposed to DES. Therefore, in the age groups at risk (37–61 years), examiners should pay attention to structural changes of the vagina and cervix that may signal the possibility of DES exposure and indicate the need for follow-up.

The incidence of clear cell carcinoma is approximately 1 in 1000 exposed women, and the incidence of cervical and vaginal intraepithelial neoplasia (dysplasia and carcinoma in situ) is twice as high as in unexposed women. DES daughters have more difficulty conceiving and have an increased incidence of early abortion, ectopic pregnancy, and premature births. In addition, mothers treated with DES in pregnancy appear to have a small increase in the incidence of breast cancer, beginning 20 years after exposure.

▶ When to Refer

All patients with a history of DES exposure should be monitored by an experienced colposcopist.

Rubin M. Antenatal exposure to DES: lessons learned…future concerns. Obstet Gynecol Surv. 2007 Aug;62(8):548–55. [PMID: 17634156]

CERVICAL INTRAEPITHELIAL NEOPLASIA (Dysplasia of the Cervix)

ESSENTIALS OF DIAGNOSIS

▸ The presumptive diagnosis is made by an abnormal Pap smear of an asymptomatic woman with no grossly visible cervical changes.

▸ Diagnose by colposcopically directed biopsy.

▸ Increased in women with HIV.

▶ General Considerations

The squamocolumnar junction of the cervix is an area of active squamous cell proliferation. In childhood, this junction is located on the exposed vaginal portion of the cervix. At puberty, because of hormonal influence and possibly because of changes in the vaginal pH, the squamous margin begins to encroach on the single-layered, mucus-secreting epithelium, creating an area of metaplasia (transformation zone). Factors associated with coitus (see Pre-

Table 18–2. Classification systems for Papanicolaou smears.

Numerical	Dysplasia	CIN	Bethesda System
1	Benign	Benign	Normal
2	Benign with inflammation	Benign with inflammation	Normal, ASC-US
3	Mild dysplasia	CIN I	Low-grade SIL
3	Moderate dysplasia	CIN II	High-grade SIL
3	Severe dysplasia	CIN III	
4	Carcinoma in situ		
5	Invasive cancer	Invasive cancer	Invasive cancer

ASC-US, atypical squamous cells of undetermined significance; CIN, cervical intraepithelial neoplasia; SIL, squamous intraepithelial lesion.

vention, below) may lead to cellular abnormalities, which over a period of time can result in the development of squamous cell dysplasia or cancer. There are varying degrees of dysplasia (Table 18–2), defined by the degree of cellular atypia; all types must be observed and treated if they persist or become more severe.

▶ Clinical Findings

There are no specific symptoms or signs of CIN. The presumptive diagnosis is made by cytologic screening of an asymptomatic population with no grossly visible cervical changes. All visibly abnormal cervical lesions should be biopsied (Plate 78).

▶ Diagnosis

A. Cytologic Examination (Papanicolaou Smear)

Screening should begin within 3 years of the onset of sexually activity or at age 21. Testing should be done annually for 3 years and then at least every 3 years if no abnormality is detected. After age 65 or 70, if there have been no abnormalities on the last 3 cytologic tests, screening may be discontinued. With liquid-based cytology (LBC), the initial interval may be increased to every 2 years. Specimens should be taken from a nonmenstruating patient, spread on a single slide, and fixed or rinsed directly into preservative solution if LBC is to be used. A specimen should be obtained from the squamocolumnar junction with a wooden or plastic spatula and from the endocervix with a cotton swab or nylon brush.

Cytologic reports from the laboratory may describe findings in one of several ways (see Table 18–2). The Bethesda System uses the terminology "atypical squamous cells of unknown significance" (ASC-US) and "squamous intraepithelial lesions," either low-grade (LSIL) or high-grade (HSIL). Cytopathologists consider a Pap smear to be a medical consultation and will recommend further diagnostic procedures, treatment for infection, and comments on factors preventing adequate evaluation of the specimen. Either immediate colposcopy or triage with reflex testing for high-risk HPV types with thin layer cytologic smears can be used for ASC-US in premenopausal women age 21 years or older. Women younger than 21 years with ASC-US should have repeat cytology at 12 months and be referred for colposcopy if ASC-US is present. The routine use of combined cytologic screening and reflex high-risk HPV testing is appropriate in women over the age of 30 who are being screened no more frequently than every 3 years. Women who have undergone complete hysterectomy for benign disease do not need to be screened.

B. Colposcopy

Women with ASC-US and a negative HPV screening may be followed-up in 1 year. If the HPV screen is positive, colposcopy should be performed. If HPV screening is unavailable, repeat cytology may be done at 4- to 6-month intervals until two consecutive normal results, or the patient may be referred directly for colposcopy. All patients with SIL or atypical glandular cells should undergo colposcopy. Viewing the cervix with 10–20× magnification allows for assessment of the size and margins of an abnormal transformation zone and determination of extension into the endocervical canal. The application of 3–5% acetic acid (vinegar) dissolves mucus, and the acid's desiccating action sharpens the contrast between normal and actively proliferating squamous epithelium. Abnormal changes include white patches and vascular atypia, which indicate areas of greatest cellular activity. Paint the cervix with Lugol solution (strong iodine solution [Schiller test]). Normal squamous epithelium will take the stain; nonstaining squamous epithelium should be biopsied. (The single-layered, mucus-secreting endocervical tissue will not stain either but can readily be distinguished by its darker pink, shinier appearance.)

C. Biopsy

Colposcopically directed punch biopsy and endocervical curettage are office procedures. If colposcopy is not available, the normal-appearing cervix shedding atypical cells can be evaluated by endocervical curettage and multiple punch biopsies of nonstaining squamous epithelium or biopsies from each quadrant of the cervix. Data from both cervical biopsy and endocervical curettage are important in deciding on treatment.

▶ Prevention

Cervical infection with the HPV is associated with a high percentage of all cervical dysplasias and cancers. There are over 70 recognized HPV subtypes, of which types 6 and 11 tend to cause genital warts and mild dysplasia, while types 16, 18, 31, and others cause higher-grade cellular changes. In 2006, the FDA approved a vaccine to prevent cervical cancer and vaginal and vulvar pre-cancers caused by HPV types 16 and 18, and to protect against low-grade and pre-cancerous

lesions and genital warts caused by HPV types 6, 11, 16, and 18. The quadrivalent HPV 6/11/16/18 L1 virus-like-particle vaccine (known as Gardisil) is recommended for all girls and women aged 11 to 26. Girls as young as 9 years should receive the vaccine at the judgment of the practitioner.

In addition to vaccination, measures to prevent cervical cancer include regular cytologic screening to detect abnormalities, limiting the number of sexual partners, using a diaphragm or condom for coitus, and stopping smoking or exposure to second-hand smoke.

Women with HIV infection appear to be at increased risk for the disease and for recurrent disease after treatment. Women with HIV infection should receive regular cytologic screening and should be monitored closely after treatment for CIN.

▶ Treatment

Treatment varies depending on the degree and extent of CIN. Biopsies should always precede treatment.

A. Cauterization or Cryosurgery

The use of either hot cauterization or freezing (cryosurgery) is effective for noninvasive small lesions visible on the cervix without endocervical extension.

B. CO$_2$ Laser

This well-controlled method minimizes tissue destruction. It is colposcopically directed and requires special training. It may be used with large visible lesions. In current practice, it involves the vaporization of the transformation zone on the cervix and the distal 5–7 mm of endocervical canal.

C. Loop Excision

When the CIN is clearly visible in its entirety, a wire loop can be used for excisional biopsy. Cutting and hemostasis are effected with a low-voltage electrosurgical machine. This office procedure with local anesthesia is quick and uncomplicated.

D. Conization of the Cervix

Conization is surgical removal of the entire transformation zone and endocervical canal. It should be reserved for cases of severe dysplasia or cancer in situ (CIN III), particularly those with endocervical extension. The procedure can be performed with the scalpel, the CO$_2$ laser, the needle electrode, or by large-loop excision.

E. Follow-Up

Because recurrence is possible—especially in the first 2 years after treatment—and because the false-negative rate of a single cervical cytologic test is 20%, close follow-up after colposcopy and biopsy is imperative. For CIN II or III, cytologic examination or cytology and colposcopy should be repeated at 4- to 6-month intervals for up to 2 years. For CIN I, cytology should be performed at 6 and 12 months or HPV DNA testing can be done at 12 months. If testing is normal, then annual cytologic examination can be resumed.

When to Refer

- Patients with CIN II/III should be referred to an experienced colposcopist.
- Patients requiring conization biopsy should be referred to a gynecologist.

American College of Obstetricians-Gynecologists. ACOG Practice Bulletin No. 99: management of abnormal cervical cytology and histology. Obstet Gynecol. 2008 Dec;112(6):1419–44. [PMID: 19037054]

Markowitz LE et al; Centers for Disease Control and Prevention (CDC); Advisory Committee on Immunization Practices (ACIP). Quadrivalent Human Papillomavirus Vaccine: Recommendations of the Advisory Committee on Immunization Practices (ACIP). MMWR Recomm Rep. 2007 Mar 23;56(RR-2):1–24. [PMID: 17380109]

CARCINOMA OF THE CERVIX

ESSENTIALS OF DIAGNOSIS

- ▶ Abnormal uterine bleeding and vaginal discharge.
- ▶ Cervical lesion may be visible on inspection as a tumor or ulceration.
- ▶ Vaginal cytology usually positive; must be confirmed by biopsy.

General Considerations

Cervical cancer can be considered a sexually transmitted disease. Both squamous cell and adenocarcinoma of the cervix are etiologically related to infection with HPV, primarily types 16 and 18. Smoking and possibly dietary factors such as decreased circulating vitamin A appear to be cofactors. While squamous cell carcinoma (SCC) accounts for 85% of cervical cancers, the incidence of SCC is decreasing while the incidence of adenocarcinoma of the cervix is increasing.

SCC appears first in the intraepithelial layers (the preinvasive stage, or carcinoma in situ). Preinvasive cancer (CIN III) is a common diagnosis in women 25–40 years of age. Two to 10 years are required for carcinoma to penetrate the basement membrane and invade the tissues. After invasion, death usually occurs within 3–5 years in untreated or unresponsive patients.

Clinical Findings

A. Symptoms and Signs

The most common signs are metrorrhagia, postcoital spotting, and cervical ulceration. Bloody or purulent, odorous, nonpruritic discharge may appear after invasion. Bladder and rectal dysfunction or fistulas and pain are late symptoms.

B. Cervical Biopsy and Endocervical Curettage, or Conization

These procedures are necessary steps after a positive Papanicolaou smear to determine the extent and depth of invasion of the cancer. Even if the smear is positive, treatment is never justified until definitive diagnosis has been established through biopsy.

C. "Staging," or Estimate of Gross Spread of Cancer of the Cervix

The depth of penetration of the malignant cells beyond the basement membrane is a reliable clinical guide to the extent of primary cancer within the cervix and the likelihood of metastases. It is customary to stage cancers of the cervix under anesthesia. Further assessment may be carried out by abdominal and pelvic CT scanning or MRI.

Complications

Metastases to regional lymph nodes occur with increasing frequency from stage I to stage IV. Paracervical extension occurs in all directions from the cervix. The ureters are often obstructed lateral to the cervix, causing hydroureter and hydronephrosis and consequently impaired kidney function. Almost two-thirds of patients with untreated carcinoma of the cervix die of uremia when ureteral obstruction is bilateral. Pain in the back, in the distribution of the lumbosacral plexus, is often indicative of neurologic involvement. Gross edema of the legs may be indicative of vascular and lymphatic stasis due to tumor.

Vaginal fistulas to the rectum and urinary tract are severe late complications. Hemorrhage is the cause of death in 10–20% of patients with extensive invasive carcinoma.

Prevention

In 2006, the FDA approved a quadrivalent HPV 6/11/16/18 L1 virus-like-particle vaccine, known as Gardisil, to prevent cervical cancer caused by HPV types 16 and 18, and to protect against low-grade and precancerous lesions and genital warts caused by HPV types 6, 11, 16, and 18 (see Cervical Intraepithelial Neoplasia, above).

Treatment

A. Emergency Measures

Vaginal hemorrhage originates from gross ulceration and cavitation in stage II–IV cervical carcinoma. Ligation and suturing of the cervix are usually not feasible, but ligation of the uterine or hypogastric arteries may be lifesaving when other measures fail. Styptics such as Monsel solution or acetone are effective, although delayed sloughing may result in further bleeding. Wet vaginal packing is helpful. Emergency irradiation usually controls bleeding.

B. Specific Measures

1. Carcinoma in situ (stage 0)—In women who have completed childbearing, total hysterectomy is the treatment of choice. In women who wish to retain the uterus, acceptable alternatives include cervical conization or ablation of the lesion with cryotherapy or laser. Close follow-up with Papanicolaou smears every 3 months for 1 year and every 6 months for another year is necessary after cryotherapy or laser.

2. Invasive carcinoma—Microinvasive carcinoma (stage IA1) is treated with simple, extrafascial hysterectomy. Stages IA2, IB1, and IIA cancers may be treated with either radical hysterectomy with concomitant radiation and chemotherapy or with radiation plus chemotherapy alone. Stages IB2, IIB, III and IV cancers are treated with radiation therapy plus concurrent cisplatin-based chemotherapy.

▶ Prognosis

The overall 5-year relative survival rate for carcinoma of the cervix is 68% in white women and 55% in black women in the United States. Survival rates are inversely proportionate to the stage of cancer: stage 0, 99–100%; stage IA, > 95%; stage IB–IIA, 80–90%; stage IIB, 65%; stage III, 40%; and stage IV, < 20%.

▶ When to Refer

All patients with invasive cervical carcinoma (stage 1A or higher) should be referred to a gynecologic oncologist.

Petignat P et al. Diagnosis and management of cervical cancer. BMJ. 2007 Oct 13;335(7623):765–8. [PMID: 17932207]
Villa LL et al. High sustained efficacy of a prophylactic quadrivalent human papillomavirus types 6/11/16/18 L1 virus-like particle vaccine through 5 years of follow-up. Br J Cancer. 2006 Dec 4;95(11):1459–66. [PMID: 17117182]
Whitcomb BP. Gynecologic malignancies. Surg Clin North Am. 2008 Apr;88(2):301–17. [PMID: 18381115]

LEIOMYOMA OF THE UTERUS (Fibroid Tumor)

ESSENTIALS OF DIAGNOSIS

▶ Irregular enlargement of the uterus (may be asymptomatic).

▶ Heavy or irregular vaginal bleeding, dysmenorrhea.

▶ Acute and recurrent pelvic pain if the tumor becomes twisted on its pedicle or infarcted.

▶ Symptoms due to pressure on neighboring organs (large tumors).

▶ General Considerations

Uterine leiomyoma is the most common benign neoplasm of the female genital tract. It is a discrete, round, firm, often multiple uterine tumor composed of smooth muscle and connective tissue. The most convenient classification is by anatomic location: (1) intramural, (2) submucous, (3) subserous, (4) intraligamentous, (5) parasitic (ie, deriving its blood supply from an organ to which it becomes

attached), and (6) cervical. A submucous myoma may become pedunculated and descend through the cervix into the vagina.

▶ Clinical Findings

A. Symptoms and Signs

In nonpregnant women, myomas are frequently asymptomatic. However, they can cause urinary frequency, dysmenorrhea, heavy bleeding (often with anemia), or other complications due to the presence of an abdominal mass. Occasionally, degeneration occurs, causing intense pain. Infertility may be due to a myoma that significantly distorts the uterine cavity.

B. Laboratory Findings

Iron-deficiency anemia may result from blood loss; in rare cases, polycythemia is present, presumably as a result of the production of erythropoietin by the myomas.

C. Imaging

Ultrasonography will confirm the presence of uterine myomas and can be used sequentially to monitor growth. When multiple subserous or pedunculated myomas are being followed, ultrasonography is important to exclude ovarian masses. MRI can delineate intramural and submucous myomas accurately. Hysterography or hysteroscopy can also confirm cervical or submucous myomas.

▶ Differential Diagnosis

Irregular myomatous enlargement of the uterus must be differentiated from the similar but symmetric enlargement that may occur with pregnancy or adenomyosis (the presence of endometrial glands and stroma in the myometrium). Subserous myomas must be distinguished from ovarian tumors. Leiomyosarcoma is an unusual tumor occurring in 0.5% of women operated on for symptomatic myoma. It is very rare under the age of 40 and increases in incidence thereafter.

▶ Treatment

A. Emergency Measures

If the patient is markedly anemic as a result of long, heavy menstrual periods, preoperative treatment with depot medroxyprogesterone acetate, 150 mg intramuscularly every 28 days, or danazol, 400–800 mg orally daily, will slow or stop bleeding, and medical treatment of anemia can be given prior to surgery. Emergency surgery is required for acute torsion of a pedunculated myoma. The only emergency indication for myomectomy during pregnancy is torsion; abortion is not an inevitable result.

B. Specific Measures

Women who have small asymptomatic myomas should be examined at 6-month intervals. If necessary, elective myomectomy can be done to preserve the uterus. Myomas do not require surgery on an urgent basis unless they cause significant pressure on the ureters, bladder, or bowel or severe bleeding leading to anemia or unless they are undergoing rapid growth. Cervical myomas larger than 3–4 cm in diameter or pedunculated myomas that protrude through the cervix must be removed. Submucous myomas can be removed using a hysteroscope and laser or resection instruments.

Because the risk of surgical complications increases with the increasing size of the myoma, preoperative reduction of myoma size is desirable. GnRH analogs such as depot leuprolide, 3.75 mg intramuscularly monthly, or nafarelin, 0.2–0.4 mg intranasally twice a day, are used preoperatively for 3- to 4-month periods to induce reversible hypogonadism, which temporarily reduces the size of myomas, suppresses their further growth, and reduces surrounding vascularity.

C. Surgical Measures

Surgical measures available for the treatment of myoma are laparoscopic or abdominal myomectomy and total or subtotal abdominal, vaginal, or laparoscopy-assisted vaginal hysterectomy. Myomectomy is the treatment of choice for women who wish to preserve fertility. Transcatheter bilateral uterine artery embolization appears to be a safe and effective alternative to myomectomy, although comparative data on subsequent pregnancy outcomes is lacking. Myolysis with MRI-guided high frequency focused ultrasound is another alternative, but long-term outcome data, particularly on pregnancy outcomes, are lacking.

▶ Prognosis

Surgical therapy is curative. Future pregnancies are not endangered by myomectomy, although cesarean delivery may be necessary after wide dissection with entry into the uterine cavity.

▶ When to Refer

Refer to a gynecologist for treatment of symptomatic leiomyomata.

▶ When to Admit

For acute abdomen associated with an infarcted leiomyoma.

American College of Obstetricians and Gynecologists. ACOG Practice Bulletin. Alternatives to hysterectomy in the management of leiomyomas. Obstet Gynecol. 2008 Aug;112(2 Pt 1):387–400. [PMID: 18669742]

Edwards RD et al. Uterine-artery embolization versus surgery for symptomatic uterine fibroids. N Engl J Med. 2007 Jan 25;356(4):360–70. [PMID: 17251532]

CARCINOMA OF THE ENDOMETRIUM

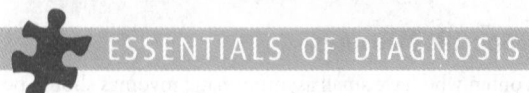

ESSENTIALS OF DIAGNOSIS

▶ Abnormal bleeding is the presenting sign in 80% of cases.

▶ Pap smear is frequently negative.

▶ After a negative pregnancy test, endometrial tissue is required to confirm the diagnosis.

▶ General Considerations

Adenocarcinoma of the endometrium is the second most common cancer of the female genital tract. It occurs most often in women 50–70 years of age. Some patients will have taken unopposed estrogen in the past; their increased risk appears to persist for 10 or more years after stopping the drug. Obesity, nulliparity, diabetes, and polycystic ovaries with prolonged anovulation and the extended use of tamoxifen for the treatment of breast cancer are also risk factors. Women with a family history of colon cancer (hereditary nonpolyposis colorectal cancer, Lynch syndrome) are at significantly increased risk, with a lifetime incidence as high as 30%.

Abnormal bleeding is the presenting sign in 80% of cases. Endometrial carcinoma may cause obstruction of the cervix with collection of pus (pyometra) or blood (hematometra) causing lower abdominal pain. However, pain generally occurs late in the disease, with metastases or infection.

Papanicolaou smears of the cervix occasionally show atypical endometrial cells but are an insensitive diagnostic tool. Endocervical and endometrial sampling is the only reliable means of diagnosis. Simultaneous hysteroscopy can be a valuable addition in order to localize polyps or other lesions within the uterine cavity. Vaginal ultrasonography may be used to determine the thickness of the endometrium as an indication of hypertrophy and possible neoplastic change.

Pathologic assessment is important in differentiating hyperplasias, which often can be treated with cyclic oral progestins.

▶ Prevention

Prompt endometrial sampling for patients who report abnormal menstrual bleeding or postmenopausal uterine bleeding will reveal many incipient as well as clinical cases of endometrial cancer. Younger women with chronic anovulation are at risk for endometrial hyperplasia and subsequent endometrial cancer. They can reduce the risk of hyperplasia almost completely with the use of oral contraceptives or cyclic progestin therapy.

▶ Staging

Examination under anesthesia, endometrial and endocervical sampling, chest radiography, intravenous urography, cystoscopy, sigmoidoscopy, transvaginal sonography, and MRI will help determine the extent of the disease and its appropriate treatment. The staging is based on the surgical and pathologic evaluation.

▶ Treatment

Treatment consists of total hysterectomy and bilateral salpingo-oophorectomy. Peritoneal material for cytologic examination is routinely taken and lymph node sampling may be done. If invasion deep into the myometrium has occurred or if sampled lymph nodes are positive for tumor, postoperative irradiation is indicated. The role of adjuvant chemotherapy alone or with irradiation is currently under investigation, although one study has shown a modest increase in survival with chemotherapy alone versus whole abdominal radiation alone in women with stage III–IV disease. Palliation of advanced or metastatic endometrial adenocarcinoma may be accomplished with large doses of progestins, eg, medroxyprogesterone, 400 mg intramuscularly weekly, or megestrol acetate, 80–160 mg daily orally.

Prognosis

With early diagnosis and treatment, the overall 5-year survival is 80–85%. With stage I disease, the depth of myometrial invasion is the strongest predictor of survival, with a 98% 5-year survival with less than 66% depth of invasion and 78% survival with 66% or greater invasion.

When to Refer

All patients with endometrial carcinoma should be referred to a gynecologist.

Amant F et al. Treatment modalities in endometrial cancer. Curr Opin Oncol. 2007 Sep;19(5):479–85. [PMID: 17762575]
Sorosky JI. Endometrial cancer. Obstet Gynecol. 2008 Feb;111(2 Pt 1):436–47. [PMID: 18238985]

CARCINOMA OF THE VULVA

 ESSENTIALS OF DIAGNOSIS

▶ History of genital warts.
▶ History of prolonged vulvar irritation, with pruritus, local discomfort, or slight bloody discharge.
▶ Early lesions may suggest or include nonneoplastic epithelial disorders.
▶ Late lesions appear as a mass, an exophytic growth, or a firm, ulcerated area in the vulva.
▶ Biopsy is necessary to make the diagnosis.

General Considerations

The majority of cancers of the vulva are squamous lesions that classically have occurred in women over 50 years of age. Several subtypes (particularly 16, 18, and 31) of HPV have been identified in some but not all vulvar cancers. As with squamous cell lesions of the cervix, a grading system of vulvar intraepithelial neoplasia (VIN) from mild dysplasia to carcinoma in situ has been established.

Differential Diagnosis

Biopsy is essential for the diagnosis of VIN and vulvar cancer and should be performed with any localized atypical

vulvar lesion, including white patches. Multiple skin-punch specimens can be taken in the office under local anesthesia, with care to include tissue from the edges of each lesion sampled.

Benign vulvar disorders that must be excluded in the diagnosis of carcinoma of the vulva include chronic granulomatous lesions (eg, lymphogranuloma venereum, syphilis), condylomas, hidradenoma, or neurofibroma. Lichen sclerosus and other associated leukoplakic changes in the skin should be biopsied. The likelihood that a superimposed vulvar cancer will develop in a woman with a nonneoplastic epithelial disorder (vulvar dystrophy) ranges from 1% to 5%.

Treatment

A. General Measures

Early diagnosis and treatment of irritative or other predisposing causes, such as lichen sclerosis and VIN, should be pursued. A 7:3 combination of betamethasone and crotamiton is particularly effective for itching. After an initial response, fluorinated steroids should be replaced with hydrocortisone because of their skin atrophying effect. For lichen sclerosus, recommended treatment is clobetasol propionate cream 0.05% twice daily for 2–3 weeks, then once daily until symptoms resolve. Application one to three times a week can be used for long-term maintenance therapy.

B. Surgical Measures

High-grade VIN may be treated with a variety of approaches including topical chemotherapy, laser ablation, wide local excision, skinning vulvectomy, and simple vulvectomy. Small, invasive basal cell carcinoma of the vulva should be excised with a wide margin. If the VIN is extensive or multicentric, laser therapy or superficial surgical removal of vulvar skin may be required. In this way, the clitoris and uninvolved portions of the vulva may be spared.

Invasive carcinoma confined to the vulva without evidence of spread to adjacent organs or to the regional lymph nodes is treated with wide local excision and inguinal lymphadenectomy or wide local excision alone if invasion is less than 1 mm. Patients with more advanced disease may receive preoperative radiation, chemotherapy, or both.

Prognosis

Basal cell carcinomas very seldom metastasize, and carcinoma in situ by definition has not metastasized. With adequate excision, the prognosis for both lesions is excellent. Patients with invasive vulvar squamous cell carcinoma 2 cm in diameter or less, without inguinal lymph node metastases, have an 85–90% chance of a 5-year survival. If the lesion is greater than 2 cm and lymph node involvement is present, the likelihood of 5-year survival is approximately 40%.

When to Refer

All patients with invasive vulvar carcinoma should be referred to a gynecologic oncologist.

American College of Obstetricians and Gynecologists. ACOG Practice Bulletin No. 93: diagnosis and management of vulvar skin disorders. Obstet Gynecol. 2008 May;111(5):1243–53. [PMID: 18448767]

Duong TH et al. Vulvo-vaginal cancers: risks, evaluation, prevention and early detection. Obstet Gynecol Clin North Am. 2007 Dec;34(4):783–802. [PMID: 18061869]

ENDOMETRIOSIS

 ESSENTIALS OF DIAGNOSIS

▸ Pelvic pain related to menstrual cycle.

▸ Dysmenorrhea.

▸ Dyspareunia.

▸ Increased frequency among infertile women.

▸ General Considerations

Endometriosis is an aberrant growth of endometrium outside the uterus, particularly in the dependent parts of the pelvis and in the ovaries and is the most common cause of secondary dysmenorrhea. While retrograde menstruation is the most widely accepted cause, its pathogenesis and natural course are not fully understood. The overall prevalence in the United States is 6–10% and is fourfold to fivefold greater among infertile women.

▸ Clinical Findings

Women with endometriosis will complain of pelvic pain, which may be associated with infertility, dyspareunia, or rectal pain with bleeding. Initially, pain tends to start 2–7 days before the onset of menses and becomes increasingly severe until flow slackens. With increasing duration of disease, pain may become continuous. Pelvic examination may disclose tender nodules in the cul-de-sac or rectovaginal septum, uterine retroversion with decreased uterine mobility, cervical motion tenderness, or an adnexal mass or tenderness. However, most women with endometriosis have a normal pelvic examination.

Endometriosis must be distinguished from PID, ovarian neoplasms, and uterine myomas. Bowel invasion by endometrial tissue may produce blood in the stool that must be distinguished from bowel neoplasm. Paradoxically, the severity of pain associated with endometriosis may be inversely related to the anatomic extent of the disease.

Imaging is of limited value. Ultrasound examination will often reveal complex fluid-filled masses that cannot be distinguished from neoplasms. MRI is more sensitive and specific than ultrasound, particularly in the diagnosis of retroperitoneal lesions. However, the clinical diagnosis of endometriosis is presumptive and usually confirmed by laparoscopy.

▸ Treatment

A. Medical Treatment

Medical treatment, using a variety of hormonal therapies, is effective in the amelioration of pain associated with endometriosis. However, there is no evidence that any of these agents increase the likelihood of pregnancy. Their preoperative use is of questionable value in reducing the difficulty of surgery. Most of these regimens are designed to inhibit ovulation over 4–9 months and lower hormone levels, thus preventing cyclic stimulation of endometriotic implants and inducing atrophy. The optimum duration of therapy is not clear, and the relative merits in terms of side effects and long-term risks and benefits show insignificant differences when compared with each other and, in mild cases, with placebo. Current research for more effective and acceptable long-term medical therapy is focusing on aromatase inhibitors and selective progesterone receptor modulators. Commonly used medical regimens include the following:

1. The GnRH analogs such as nafarelin nasal spray, 0.2–0.4 mg twice daily, or long-acting injectable leuprolide acetate, 3.75 mg intramuscularly monthly, used for 6 months, suppress ovulation. Side effects of vasomotor symptoms and bone demineralization may be relieved by "add-back" therapy such as conjugated equine estrogen, 0.625 mg and norethindrone, 5 mg orally daily.

2. Danazol is used for 4–6 months in the lowest dose necessary to suppress menstruation, usually 200–400 mg orally twice daily. Danazol has a high incidence of androgenic side effects, including decreased breast size, weight gain, acne, and hirsutism.

3. Any of the combination oral contraceptives, the contraceptive patch, or vaginal ring may be used continuously for 6–12 months. Breakthrough bleeding can be treated with conjugated estrogens, 1.25 mg orally daily for 1 week, or estradiol, 2 mg daily orally for 1 week.

4. Medroxyprogesterone acetate, 100 mg intramuscularly every 2 weeks for four doses and then 100 mg every 4 weeks; add oral estrogen or estradiol valerate, 30 mg intramuscularly, for breakthrough bleeding. Use for 6–9 months.

5. Low-dose oral contraceptives can also be given cyclically; prolonged suppression of ovulation will often inhibit further stimulation of residual endometriosis, especially if taken after one of the therapies mentioned above.

6. Aromatase inhibitors, such as letrozole, 2.5 mg orally daily, have been shown, on an investigational basis, to be useful in the treatment of endometriosis resistant to other therapies.

7. Analgesics, with or without codeine, may be needed during menses. NSAIDs may be helpful.

B. Surgical Measures

Surgical treatment of endometriosis—particularly extensive disease—is effective both in reducing pain and in promoting fertility. Laparoscopic ablation of endometrial implants along with uterine nerve ablation significantly reduces pain. Ablation of implants and, if necessary, removal of ovarian endometriomas enhance fertility, although subsequent pregnancy rates are related to the severity of disease. Women with disabling pain who no longer desire childbearing can be treated definitively with total abdominal hysterectomy and bilateral salpingo-oophorectomy (TAH-BSO).

Prognosis

The prognosis for reproductive function in early or moderately advanced endometriosis is good with conservative therapy. TAH-BSO is curative for patients with severe and extensive endometriosis with pain.

When to Refer

Refer to a gynecologist for laparoscopic diagnosis or treatment.

When to Admit

Rarely necessary except for acute abdomen associated with ruptured or bleeding endometrioma.

Atar E et al. Aromatase inhibitors: the next generation of therapeutics for endometriosis? Fertil Steril. 2006 May;85(5):1307–18. [PMID: 16647373]
Kinkel K et al. Diagnosis of endometriosis with imaging: a review. Eur Radiol. 2006 Feb;16(2):285–98. [PMID: 16155722]
Rodgers AK et al. Treatment strategies for endometriosis. Expert Opin Pharmacother. 2008 Feb;9(2):243–55. [PMID: 18201147]

PELVIC ORGAN PROLAPSE

General Considerations

Cystocele, rectocele, and enterocele are vaginal hernias commonly seen in multiparous women. Cystocele is a hernia of the bladder wall into the vagina, causing a soft anterior fullness. Cystocele may be accompanied by urethrocele, which is not a hernia but a sagging of the urethra following its detachment from the pubic symphysis during childbirth. Rectocele is a herniation of the terminal rectum into the posterior vagina, causing a collapsible pouch-like fullness. Enterocele is a vaginal vault hernia containing small intestine, usually in the posterior vagina and resulting from a deepening of the pouch of Douglas. Two or all three types of hernia may occur in combination. Risk factors may include vaginal birth, genetic predisposition, advancing age, prior pelvic surgery, connective tissue disorders, and increased intra-abdominal pressure associated with obesity or straining associated with chronic constipation.

Classification

A simple classification system, the Baden-Walker System, standardizes the degree of descent of the anterior vaginal wall, cervix or vaginal apex, and the posterior vaginal wall. The degree of prolapse can be evaluated by having the woman perform the Valsalva maneuver while in the lithotomy position. In stage I prolapse, the presenting anatomy descends halfway to the hymen; in stage II prolapse, to the hymen; in stage III prolapse, halfway past the hymen; and in stage IV prolapse, there is the maximum possible descent. Evaluation of the ability to empty the bladder should be evaluated by measuring postvoid residual. If stress incontinence is not present on Valsalva, the prolapse should be reduced to evaluate the possibility of potential post-repair incontinence.

Clinical Findings

Symptoms of pelvic organ prolapse may include sensation of a bulge or protrusion in the vagina, urinary or fecal incontinence, a sense of incomplete bladder emptying, and dyspareunia. The cause of pelvic organ prolapse, including prolapse of the uterus, vaginal apex, and anterior or posterior vaginal walls, is likely multifactorial.

Treatment

The type of therapy depends on the extent of prolapse and the patient's age and her desire for menstruation, pregnancy, and coitus.

A. General Measures

Supportive measures include a high-fiber diet. Weight reduction in obese patients and limitation of straining and lifting are helpful. Pessaries may reduce cystocele, rectocele, or enterocele temporarily and are helpful in women who do not wish to undergo surgery or who are chronically ill.

B. Surgical Measures

The only cure for symptomatic cystocele, rectocele, enterocele, or stress urinary incontinence is corrective surgery.

The most common surgical procedure is vaginal or abdominal hysterectomy with vaginal vault suspension by either uterosacral or sacrospinous fixation vaginally or abdominal sacral colpopexy. Since stress incontinence is common after vault suspension procedures, an anti-incontinence procedure should be considered. If the patient desires pregnancy, a partial resection of the cervix with plication of the cardinal ligaments can be attempted. For elderly women who do not desire coitus, colpocleisis, the partial obliteration of the vagina, is surgically simple and effective. Uterine suspension with sacrospinous cervicocolpopexy may be an effective approach in older women who wish to avoid hysterectomy but preserve coital function.

When to Refer

- Refer to urogynecologist or gynecologist for stress urinary incontinence or stage III prolapse.
- Refer if nonsurgical therapy is ineffective.

ACOG Committee on Practice Bulletins–Gynecology. ACOG Practice Bulletin No. 85: Pelvic organ prolapse. Obstet Gynecol. 2007 Sep;110(3):717–29. [PMID: 17766624]
Doshani A et al. Uterine prolapse. BMJ. 2007 Oct 20;335(7624):819–23. [PMID: 17947787]

PELVIC INFLAMMATORY DISEASE (Salpingitis, Endometritis)

ESSENTIALS OF DIAGNOSIS

- Uterine, adnexal, or cervical motion tenderness.
- Absence of a competing diagnosis.

General Considerations

PID is a polymicrobial infection of the upper genital tract associated with the sexually transmitted organisms *N gonorrhoeae* and *Chlamydia trachomatis* as well as endogenous organisms, including anaerobes, *Haemophilus influenzae*, enteric gram-negative rods, and streptococci. It is most common in young, nulliparous, sexually active women with multiple partners. Other risk markers include non-white race, douching, and smoking. The use of oral contraceptives or barrier methods of contraception may provide significant protection.

Tuberculous salpingitis is rare in the United States but more common in developing countries; it is characterized by pelvic pain and irregular pelvic masses not responsive to antibiotic therapy. It is not sexually transmitted.

Clinical Findings

A. Symptoms and Signs

Patients with PID may have lower abdominal pain, chills and fever, menstrual disturbances, purulent cervical discharge, and cervical and adnexal tenderness. Right upper quadrant pain (Fitz-Hugh and Curtis syndrome) may indicate an associated perihepatitis. However, diagnosis of PID is complicated by the fact that many women may have subtle or mild symptoms that are not readily recognized as PID.

B. Minimum Diagnostic Criteria

Women with uterine adnexal or cervical motion tenderness should be considered to have PID and be treated with antibiotics unless there is a competing diagnosis such as ectopic pregnancy or appendicitis.

C. Additional Criteria

The following criteria may be used to enhance the specificity of the diagnosis: (1) oral temperature greater than 38.3 °C, (2) abnormal cervical or vaginal discharge with white cells on saline microscopy, (3) elevated erythrocyte sedimentation rate, (4) elevated C-reactive protein, and (5) laboratory documentation of cervical infection with *N gonorrhoeae* or *C trachomatis*. Endocervical culture should be performed routinely, but treatment should not be delayed while awaiting results.

D. Definitive Criteria

In selected cases where the diagnosis based on clinical or laboratory evidence is uncertain, the following criteria may be used: (1) histopathologic evidence of endometritis on endometrial biopsy, (2) transvaginal sonography or MRI showing thickened fluid-filled tubes with or without free pelvic fluid or tubo-ovarian complex, and (3) laparoscopic abnormalities consistent with PID.

Differential Diagnosis

Appendicitis, ectopic pregnancy, septic abortion, hemorrhagic or ruptured ovarian cysts or tumors, twisted ovarian cyst, degeneration of a myoma, and acute enteritis must be considered. PID is more likely to occur when there is a history of PID, recent sexual contact, recent onset of menses, or an IUD in place or if the partner has a sexually transmitted disease. Acute PID is highly unlikely when recent intercourse has not taken place or an IUD is not being used. A sensitive serum pregnancy test should be obtained to rule out ectopic pregnancy. Culdocentesis will differentiate hemoperitoneum (ruptured ectopic pregnancy or hemorrhagic cyst) from pelvic sepsis (salpingitis, ruptured pelvic abscess, or ruptured appendix). Pelvic and vaginal ultrasonography is helpful in the differential diagnosis of ectopic pregnancy of over 6 weeks. Laparoscopy is often used to diagnose PID, and it is imperative if the diagnosis is not certain or if the patient has not responded to antibiotic therapy after 48 hours. The appendix should be visualized at laparoscopy to rule out appendicitis. Cultures obtained at the time of laparoscopy are often specific and helpful.

Treatment

A. Antibiotics

Early treatment with appropriate antibiotics effective against *N gonorrhoeae*, *C trachomatis*, and the endogenous organisms listed above is essential to prevent long-term sequelae. The sexual partner should be examined and treated appropriately.

Two inpatient regimens have been shown to be effective in the treatment of acute PID: (1) Cefoxitin, 2 g intravenously every 6 hours, or cefotetan, 2 g intravenously every 12 hours, plus doxycycline, 100 mg intravenously or orally every 12 hours. This regimen is continued for at least 24 hours after the patient shows significant clinical improvement. Doxycycline, 100 mg twice daily, should be continued to complete a total of 14 days therapy. If a tubo-ovarian abscess is present, it is advisable to add clindamycin, 450 mg orally four times daily, or metronidazole, 500 mg orally twice daily, for 14 days to the doxycycline to provide more effective anaerobic coverage. (2) Clindamycin, 900 mg intravenously every 8 hours, plus gentamicin intravenously in a loading dose of 2 mg/kg followed by 1.5 mg/kg every 8 hours. This regimen is continued for at least 24 hours after the patient shows significant clinical improvement and is followed by either clindamycin, 450 mg four times daily, or doxycycline, 100 mg twice daily, to complete a total of 14 days of therapy. When a tubo-ovarian abscess is present, clindamycin, rather than doxycycline, should be given.

Data on the role of ampicillin-sulbactam, 3 g intravenously every 6 hours, plus doxycycline, 100 mg intravenously or orally every 12 hours, are limited.

The recommended outpatient regimen is either a single dose of cefoxitin, 2 g intramuscularly, with probenecid, 1 g orally, ceftriaxone, 250 mg intramuscularly, or a single dose of another parenteral third-generation cephalosporin plus doxycycline, 100 mg orally twice daily, for 14 days. If parenteral cephalosporin cannot be used, levofloxacin (500 mg orally once daily) or ofloxacin (400 mg twice daily) for 14 days with or without metronidazole (500 mg twice daily) for 14 days may be used if the community prevalence and the individual risk of gonorrhea is low (see Chapter 33).

B. Surgical Measures

Tubo-ovarian abscesses may require surgical excision or transcutaneous or transvaginal aspiration. Unless rupture is suspected, institute high-dose antibiotic therapy in the hospital, and monitor therapy with ultrasound. In 70% of cases, antibiotics are effective; in 30%, there is inadequate response in 48–72 hours, and surgical intervention is required. Unilateral adnexectomy is acceptable for unilateral abscess. Hysterectomy and bilateral salpingo-oophorectomy may be necessary for overwhelming infection or in cases of chronic disease with intractable pelvic pain.

▶ Prognosis

In spite of treatment, long-term sequelae, including repeated episodes of infection, chronic pelvic pain, dyspareunia, ectopic pregnancy, or infertility, develop in one-fourth of women with acute disease. The risk of infertility increases with repeated episodes of salpingitis: it is estimated at 10% after the first episode, 25% after a second episode, and 50% after a third episode.

▶ When to Admit

The following patients with acute PID should be admitted for intravenous antibiotic therapy:

- The patient has a tubo-ovarian abscess.
- The patient is pregnant.
- The patient is unable to follow or tolerate an outpatient regimen.
- The patient has not responded clinically to outpatient therapy.
- The patient has severe illness, nausea and vomiting, or high fever.
- Another surgical emergency such as appendicitis cannot be ruled out.

Centers for Disease Control and Prevention; Workowski KA et al. Sexually transmitted disease treatment guidelines 2006. Centers for Disease Control and Prevention. MMWR Recomm Rep. 2006 Aug 4;55(RR-11):1–94. [PMID: 16888612]

Centers for Disease Control and Prevention. Updated recommended treatment regimens for gonococcal infections and associated conditions–United States, April 2007. http://www.cdc.gov/std/treatment/

Crossman SH. The challenge of pelvic inflammatory disease. Am Fam Physician. 2006 Mar 1;73(5):859–64. [PMID: 16529095]

OVARIAN CANCER & OVARIAN TUMORS

ESSENTIALS OF DIAGNOSIS

- ▶ Vague gastrointestinal discomfort.
- ▶ Pelvic pressure and pain.
- ▶ Many cases of early-stage cancer are asymptomatic.
- ▶ Pelvic examination, serum CA 125, and ultrasound are mainstays of diagnosis.

▶ General Considerations

Ovarian tumors are common. Most are benign, but malignant ovarian tumors are the leading cause of death from reproductive tract cancer. The wide range of types and patterns of ovarian tumors is due to the complexity of ovarian embryology and differences in tissues of origin.

In women with no family history of ovarian cancer, the lifetime risk is 1.6%, whereas a woman with one affected first-degree relative has a 5% lifetime risk. With two or more affected first-degree relatives, the risk is 7%. Approximately 3% of women with two or more affected first-degree relatives will have a hereditary ovarian cancer syndrome with a lifetime risk of 40%. Women with a *BRCA1* gene mutation have a 45% lifetime risk of ovarian cancer and those with a *BRCA2* mutation a 25% risk. These women should be screened annually with transvaginal sonography and serum CA 125 testing, and prophylactic oophorectomy is recommended by age 35 or whenever childbearing is completed because of the high risk of disease. The benefits of such screening for women with one or no affected first-degree relatives are unproved, and the risks associated with unnecessary surgical procedures may outweigh the benefits in low-risk women.

▶ Clinical Findings

A. Symptoms and Signs

Unfortunately, most women with both benign and malignant ovarian neoplasms are either asymptomatic or experience only mild nonspecific gastrointestinal symptoms or pelvic pressure. Women with early disease are typically detected on routine pelvic examination. Women with advanced malignant disease may experience abdominal pain and bloating, and a palpable abdominal mass with ascites is often present.

B. Laboratory Findings

An elevated serum CA 125 (> 35 units) indicates a greater likelihood that an ovarian tumor is malignant. CA 125 is elevated in 80% of women with epithelial ovarian cancer overall but in only 50% of women with early disease. Furthermore, serum CA 125 may be elevated in premenopausal women with benign disease such as endometriosis.

C. Imaging Studies

Transvaginal sonography is useful for screening high-risk women but has inadequate sensitivity for screening low-risk women. Ultrasound is helpful in differentiating ovarian masses that are benign and likely to resolve spontaneously from those with malignant potential. Color Doppler imaging may further enhance the specificity of ultrasound diagnosis.

▶ Differential Diagnosis

Once an ovarian mass has been detected, it must be categorized as functional, benign neoplastic, or potentially malignant. Predictive factors include age, size of the mass, ultrasound configuration, CA 125 levels, the presence of symptoms, and whether the mass is unilateral or bilateral. In a premenopausal woman, an asymptomatic, mobile, unilateral, simple cystic mass less than 7.5 cm may be observed for 4–6 weeks. Most will resolve spontaneously. If the mass is larger or unchanged on repeat pelvic examination and transvaginal sonography, surgical evaluation is required.

Most ovarian masses in postmenopausal women require surgical evaluation. However, a postmenopausal woman with an asymptomatic unilateral simple cyst less than 5 cm in diameter and a normal CA 125 level may be followed closely with transvaginal sonography. All others require surgical evaluation.

Laparoscopy may be used when an ovarian mass is small enough to be removed with a laparoscopic approach. If malignancy is suspected, preoperative workup should include chest radiograph, evaluation of liver and kidney function, and hematologic indices.

Treatment

If a malignant ovarian mass is suspected, surgical evaluation should be performed by a gynecologic oncologist. For benign neoplasms, tumor removal or unilateral oophorectomy is usually performed. For ovarian cancer in an early stage, the standard therapy is complete surgical staging followed by abdominal hysterectomy and bilateral salpingo-oophorectomy with omentectomy and selective lymphadenectomy. With more advanced disease, aggressive removal of all visible tumor improves survival. Except for women with low-grade ovarian cancer in an early stage, postoperative chemotherapy is indicated (Table 39–10). Several chemotherapy regimens are effective, such as the combination of cisplatin or carboplatin with paclitaxel, with clinical response rates of up to 60–70% (Table 39–11).

Prognosis

Unfortunately, approximately 75% of women with ovarian cancer are diagnosed with advanced disease after regional or distant metastases have become established. The overall 5-year survival is approximately 17% with distant metastases, 36% with local spread, and 89% with early disease.

When to Refer

If a malignant mass is suspected, surgical evaluation should be performed by a gynecologic oncologist.

American College of Obstetricians and Gynecologists Practice Bulletin. ACOG Practice Bulletin No. 89. Elective and risk-reducing salpingo-oophorectomy. Obstet Gynecol. 2008 Jan;111(1):231–41. [PMID: 18165419]
Chobanian N et al. Ovarian cancer. Surg Clin North Am. 2008 Apr;88(2):285–99. [PMID: 18381114]

POLYCYSTIC OVARY SYNDROME

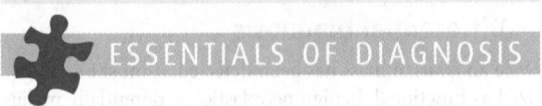

ESSENTIALS OF DIAGNOSIS

► Clinical or biochemical evidence of hyperandrogenism.

► Oligoovulation or anovulation.

► Polycystic ovaries on ultrasonography.

General Considerations

Polycystic ovary syndrome (PCOS) is a common endocrine disorder affecting 5–10% of women of reproductive age and is a common source of chronic anovulation. The underlying etiology is unknown, although most of these women have an aberration of gonadotropin stimulation. This is manifested by an increased release of luteinizing hormone (LH) relative to follicle-stimulating hormone (FSH), resulting in an increased production of androstenedione and testosterone by ovarian theca cells. The androstenedione undergoes aromatization to estrone and converted to estradiol in the ovarian granulosa cells. The high estrone levels are believed to cause suppression of pituitary FSH and constant LH stimulation of the ovary results in anovulation, multiple cysts, and theca cell hyperplasia with excess androgen output.

Women with Cushing syndrome, congenital adrenal hyperplasia, and androgen-secreting adrenal tumors also tend to have high circulating androgen levels and anovulation with polycystic ovaries; these disorders must be ruled out in women with presumed PCOS.

Clinical Findings

PCOS is manifested by hirsutism (50% of cases), obesity (40%), and virilization (20%). Fifty percent of patients have amenorrhea, 30% have abnormal uterine bleeding, and 20% have normal menstruation. In addition, they show insulin resistance and hyperinsulinemia, and these women are at increased risk for early-onset type 2 diabetes. The patients are generally infertile, although they may ovulate occasionally. They have an increased long-term risk of cancer of the endometrium because of unopposed estrogen secretion.

Differential Diagnosis

Anovulation in the reproductive years may also be due to: (1) premature menopause (high FSH and LH levels); (2) rapid weight loss, extreme physical exertion (normal FSH and LH levels for age), or obesity; (3) discontinuation of hormonal contraceptives (anovulation for 6 months or more occasionally occurs); (4) pituitary adenoma with elevated prolactin (galactorrhea may or may not be present); and (5) hyperthyroidism or hypothyroidism. When amenorrhea has persisted for 6 months or more without a diagnosis, FSH, LH, prolactin, and TSH should be checked. Women with clinical evidence of androgen excess should have total testosterone, DHEA-S, and 17-hydroxyprogesterone measured. A 10-day course of progestin (eg, medroxyprogesterone acetate, 10 mg/d orally) will cause withdrawal bleeding if estrogen levels are high. This will aid in the diagnosis and prevent endometrial hyperplasia. Because of the high risk of insulin resistance and dyslipidemia, all women with PCOS should have a 2-hour glucose determination after a 75-g glucose load and a lipoprotein profile.

▶ Treatment

In obese patients with PCOS, weight reduction is often effective. If the patient wishes to become pregnant, clomiphene or other drugs can be used for ovulatory stimulation. (See Infertility, this chapter.) The addition of dexamethasone, 0.5 mg orally at bedtime, to a clomiphene regimen may increase the likelihood of ovulation by suppression of ACTH and any circulating adrenal androgens. For women who are unresponsive to clomiphene, 3- to 6-month courses of the oral hypoglycemic agents, metformin, 500 mg three times daily, or pioglitazone, 30–45 mg daily, may bring resumption of regular cycles and ovulation. These agents reduce the hyperinsulinemia and hyperandrogenemia in PCOS.

If the patient does not desire pregnancy, medroxyprogesterone acetate, 10 mg/d orally for the first 10 days of each month, should be given to ensure regular shedding of the endometrium and avoid hyperplasia. If contraception is desired, a low-dose combination oral contraceptive can be used; this is also useful in controlling hirsutism, for which treatment must be continued for 6–12 months before results are seen.

Hirsutism may be managed with epilation and electrolysis. Dexamethasone, 0.5 mg orally each night, is helpful in women with excess adrenal androgen secretion. Spironolactone, an aldosterone antagonist, is also useful for hirsutism in doses of 25 mg three or four times daily. Flutamide, 250 mg orally daily, and finasteride, 5 mg orally daily, are also effective for treating hirsutism. Because these three agents are potentially teratogenic, they should be used only in conjunction with secure contraception.

▶ When to Refer

- If expertise in diagnosis is needed.
- If patient is infertile.

Magnotti M et al. Obesity and the polycystic ovary syndrome. Med Clin North Am. 2007 Nov;91(6):1151–68. [PMID: 17964914]

Nestler JE. Metformin for the treatment of the polycystic ovarian syndrome. N Engl J Med. 2008 Jan 3;358(1):47–54. [PMID: 18172174]

FEMALE SEXUAL DYSFUNCTION

▶ General Considerations

Female sexual dysfunction is a common problem. Depending on the questions asked, surveys have shown that from 35% to 98% of women report sexual concerns. Questions related to sexual functioning should be asked as part of the routine medical history. Three helpful questions are, "Are you currently involved in a sexual relationship?" "With men, women, or both?" and "Are there any sexual concerns or pain with sex?". If the woman is not involved in a sexual relationship, she should be asked about any concerns that are contributing to a lack of sexual behavior. If a history of sexual dysfunction is elicited, a complete history of factors that may affect sexual function should be taken. These factors include her reproductive history (including pregnancies and mode of delivery) as well as history of infertility, sexually transmitted diseases, rape, gynecologic or urologic disorders, endocrine abnormalities (such as diabetes mellitus or thyroid disease), neurologic problems, cardiovascular disease, psychiatric disease, and current prescription and over-the-counter drug use. A detailed history of the specific sexual dysfunction should be elicited, and a gynecologic examination should focus on findings that may contribute to her sexual complaints.

▶ Etiology

A. Disorders of Sexual Desire

Sexual desire in women is a complex and poorly understood phenomenon. Emotion is a key factor in sexual desire. Anger toward a partner, fear or anxiety related to previous sexual encounters, or history of sexual abuse may contribute. Physical factors, such as chronic illness, fatigue, depression, and specific medical disorders (such as diabetes mellitus, thyroid disease, or adrenal insufficiency) may contribute to a lack of desire. Attitudes toward aging and menopause may play a role. In addition, sexual desire may be influenced by other sexual dysfunctions, such as arousal disorders, dyspareunia, or anorgasmia.

B. Sexual Arousal Disorders

Sexual arousal disorders may be both subjective and objective. Sexual stimulation normally leads to genital vasocongestion and lubrication. Some women may have a physiologic response to sexual stimuli but may not subjectively feel aroused because of factors such as distractions; negative expectations; anxiety; fatigue; depression; or medications, such as selective serotonin reuptake inhibitors (SSRIs) or oral contraceptives. Other women may lack both a subjective and physiologic response to sexual stimuli related to vaginal atrophy.

C. Orgasmic Disorders

In spite of subjective and physiologic arousal, women may experience a marked delay in orgasm, diminished sensation of an orgasm, or anorgasmia. The etiology is complex and typically multifactorial, but the disorder is usually amenable to treatment.

D. Dyspareunia

Dyspareunia may be caused by vulvovaginitis, pelvic disease (such as endometriosis or chronic pelvic inflammatory disease), vulvodynia, vaginal atrophy, or vaginismus. Vulvodynia is the most frequent cause of dyspareunia in premenopausal women. It is characterized by a sensation of burning along with other symptoms, including pain, itching, stinging, irritation, and rawness. The discomfort may be constant or intermittent, focal or diffuse, and experienced as either deep or superficial. There are generally no physical findings except minimal erythema that may be associated in a subset of patients with vulvodynia, those with vulvar vestibulitis. Vulvar vestibulitis is normally asymptomatic, but pain is associated with touching or pressure on the vestibule, such as with vaginal entry or insertion of a tampon. Pain occurring with deep thrusting during coitus is usually due to acute or chronic infection of the cervix, uterus, or adnexa; endometriosis; adnexal tumors; or adhesions resulting from prior pelvic disease or operation. Vaginismus is voluntary or involuntary contraction of the muscles around the introitus. It results from fear, pain, sexual trauma, or a negative attitude toward sex, often learned in childhood.

▶ Treatment

A. Disorders of Sexual Desire

In the absence of specific medical disorders, arousal or orgasmic disorders or dyspareunia, the focus of therapy is psychological. Cognitive behavioral therapy, sexual therapy, and marital therapy may all play a role. Success with pharmacologic therapy, particularly the use of dopamine agonists or testosterone with estrogen has been reported, but data from large long-term clinical trials are lacking.

B. Sexual Arousal Disorders

As with disorders of sexual desire, arousal disorders may respond to psychological therapy. Specific pharmacologic therapy is lacking. The use of the phosphodiesterase inhibitors used in men does not appear to benefit the majority of women with sexual arousal disorders.

C. Orgasmic Disorders

For many women, brief sexual counseling along with the use of educational books (such as *For Yourself*, by Lonnie Barbach) may be adequate therapy. Also, the FDA has approved a vacuum device, the EROS-CTD, that increases clitoral enlargement and improves the likelihood of orgasm.

D. Dyspareunia

Specific medical disorders, such as endometriosis, vulvovaginitis, or vaginal atrophy, should be treated as outlined in other sections of this chapter. Vaginismus may be treated initially with sexual counseling and education on anatomy and sexual functioning. The patient can be instructed in self-dilation, using a lubricated finger or test tubes of graduated sizes. Before coitus (with adequate lubrication) is attempted, the patient—and then her partner—should be able to easily and painlessly introduce two fingers into the vagina. Penetration should never be forced, and the woman should always be the one to control the depth of insertion during dilation or intercourse. Injection of botulinum toxin has been used successfully in refractory cases.

Since the cause of vulvodynia is unknown, management is difficult. Few treatment approaches have been subjected to methodologically rigorous trials. A variety of topical agents have been tried, although only topical anesthetics (eg, estrogen cream and a compounded mixture of topical amitriptyline 2% and baclofen 2% in a water washable base) have been useful in relieving vulvodynia. Useful oral medications include tricyclic antidepressants,

such as amitriptyline in gradually increasing doses from 10 mg/d to 75–100 mg/d; various SSRIs; and anticonvulsants, such as gabapentin, starting at 300 mg three times daily and increasing to 1200 mg three times daily. Biofeedback and physical therapy, with a physical therapist experienced with the treatment of vulvar pain, have been shown to be helpful. Surgery—usually consisting of vestibulectomy—has been useful for women with introital dyspareunia.

▶ When to Refer

- When symptoms or concerns persist despite first-line therapy.
- For expertise in surgical procedures.

Frank JE et al. Diagnosis and treatment of female sexual dysfunction. Am Fam Physician. 2008 Mar 1;77(5):635–42. [PMID: 18350761]

Kammerer-Doak D et al. Female sexual function and dysfunction. Obstet Gynecol Clin North Am. 2008 Jun;35(2):169–83. [PMID: 18486835]

INFERTILITY

A couple is said to be infertile if pregnancy does not result after 1 year of normal sexual activity without contraceptives. About 25% of couples experience infertility at some point in their reproductive lives; the incidence of infertility increases with age. The male partner contributes to about 40% of cases of infertility, and a combination of factors is common.

A. Initial Testing

During the initial interview, the clinician can present an overview of infertility and discuss a plan of study. Separate private consultations are then conducted, allowing appraisal of psychosexual adjustment without embarrassment or criticism. Pertinent details (eg, sexually transmitted disease or prior pregnancies) must be obtained. The ill effects of cigarettes, alcohol, and other recreational drugs on male fertility should be discussed. Prescription drugs that impair male potency should be discussed as well. The gynecologic history should include queries regarding the menstrual pattern. The present history includes use and types of contraceptives, douches, libido, sex techniques, frequency and success of coitus, and correlation of intercourse with time of ovulation. Family history includes repeated spontaneous abortions and maternal DES use.

General physical and genital examinations are performed on the female partner, including screening pelvic ultrasound and hysterosalpingography if there is a history suggestive of pelvic disease. Basic laboratory studies include complete blood count, urinalysis, cervical culture for *Chlamydia*, rubella antibody determination, and thyroid function tests. Tay-Sachs screening should be offered if both parents are Ashkenazi Jews as well as couples of French-Canadian or Cajun ancestry; sickle cell screening should be offered if both parents are black.

If the woman has regular menses, the likelihood of ovulatory cycles is very high. A luteal phase serum progesterone above 3 ng/mL establishes ovulation. Couples should be advised that coitus resulting in conception occurs during the 6-day period ending with the day of ovulation. Self-performed urine tests for the midcycle LH surge at ovulation can enhance basal temperature charting. Semen analysis is recommended; the male partner is instructed to bring a complete ejaculate for analysis. Men must abstain from sexual activity for at least 3 days before the semen is obtained. A clean, dry, wide-mouthed bottle for collection is preferred. Semen should be examined within 1–2 hours after collection. Semen is considered normal with the following minimum values: volume, 2.0 mL; concentration, 20 million sperm per milliliter; motility, $\geq$ 50% forward progression, $\geq$ 25% rapid progression; and normal forms, 30%. If the sperm count is abnormal, further evaluation includes physical examination of the male partner and a search for exposure to environmental and workplace toxins, alcohol or drug abuse.

B. Further Testing

1. Gross deficiencies of sperm (number, motility, or appearance) require repeat analysis. Zona-free hamster egg penetration tests are available to evaluate the ability of human sperm to fertilize an egg.

2. Obvious obstruction of the uterine tubes requires assessment for microsurgery or in vitro fertilization.

3. Absent or infrequent ovulation requires additional laboratory evaluation. Elevated FSH and LH levels indicate ovarian failure causing premature menopause. Elevated LH levels in the presence of normal FSH levels confirm the presence of polycystic ovaries. Elevation of blood prolactin (PRL) levels suggests pituitary microadenoma.

4. Ultrasound monitoring of folliculogenesis may reveal the occurrence of unruptured luteinized follicles.

5. Endometrial biopsy in the luteal phase associated with simultaneous serum progesterone levels will rule out luteal phase deficiency.

6. Hysterosalpingography using an oil dye is performed within 3 days following the menstrual period if structural abnormalities are suspected. This radiographic study will demonstrate uterine abnormalities (septa, polyps, submucous myomas) and tubal obstruction. A repeat radiograph 24 hours later will confirm tubal patency if there is wide pelvic dispersion of the dye. This test has been associated with an increased pregnancy rate if an oil-based rather than water-soluble contrast medium is used. If the woman has had prior pelvic inflammation, one should give doxycycline, 100 mg orally twice daily, beginning immediately before and for 7 days after the radiographic study.

7. If hysterosalpingography or history suggests tubal disease, and in vitro fertilization (IVF) is recommended as the primary treatment option, laparoscopy is indicated. In unexplained infertility, approximately 25% of women whose basic evaluation is normal will have abnormal findings on laparoscopy that explain their infertility (eg, peritubal adhesions, endometriotic implants).

▶ Treatment

A. Medical Measures

Fertility may be restored by treatment of endocrine abnormalities, particularly hypothyroidism or hyperthyroidism. Antibiotic treatment of cervicitis is of value. Women who engage in vigorous athletic training often have low sex hormone levels; fertility improves with reduced exercise and some weight gain.

B. Surgical Measures

Excision of ovarian tumors or ovarian foci of endometriosis can improve fertility. Microsurgical relief of tubal obstruction due to salpingitis or tubal ligation will reestablish fertility in a significant number of cases, although with severe disease or proximal obstruction, IVF is preferable. Peritubal adhesions or endometriotic implants often can be treated via laparoscopy.

In a male with a varicocele, sperm characteristics are often improved following surgical treatment.

C. Induction of Ovulation

1. Clomiphene citrate—Clomiphene citrate stimulates gonadotropin release, especially LH. Consequently, plasma estrone (E_1) and estradiol (E_2) also rise, reflecting ovarian follicle maturation. If E_2 rises sufficiently, an LH surge occurs to trigger ovulation.

After a normal menstrual period or induction of withdrawal bleeding with progestin, one should give 50 mg of clomiphene orally daily for 5 days. If ovulation does not occur, the dosage is increased to 100 mg daily for 5 days. If ovulation still does not occur, the course is repeated with 150 mg daily and then 200 mg daily for 5 days, with the addition of chorionic gonadotropin, 10,000 units intramuscularly, 7 days after clomiphene.

The rate of ovulation following this treatment is 90% in the absence of other infertility factors. The pregnancy rate is high. Twinning occurs in 5% of these patients, and three or more fetuses are found in rare instances (< 0.5% of cases).

In the presence of increased androgen production (DHEA-S > 200 mcg/dL), the addition of dexamethasone, 0.5 mg orally, or prednisone, 5 mg orally, at bedtime, improves the response to clomiphene. Dexamethasone should be discontinued after pregnancy is confirmed.

2. Bromocriptine—Bromocriptine is used only if PRL levels are elevated and there is no withdrawal bleeding following progesterone administration (otherwise, clomiphene is used). To minimize side effects (nausea, diarrhea, dizziness, headache, fatigue), bromocriptine should be taken with meals. The initial dosage is 2.5 mg orally once daily, increased to two or three times daily in increments of 1.25 mg. The drug is discontinued once pregnancy has occurred.

3. Human menopausal gonadotropins (hMG)—hMG or recombinant FSH is indicated in cases of hypogonadotropism and most other types of anovulation (exclusive of ovarian failure). Because of the complexities, laboratory tests, and expense associated with this treatment, these patients should be referred to an infertility specialist.

D. Treatment of Endometriosis

See above.

E. Artificial Insemination in Azoospermia

If azoospermia is present, artificial insemination by a donor usually results in pregnancy, assuming female function is normal. The use of frozen sperm is currently preferable to fresh sperm because the frozen specimen can be held pending cultures and blood test results for sexually transmitted diseases, including HIV infection.

F. Assisted Reproductive Technologies (ART)

Couples who have not responded to traditional infertility treatments, including those with tubal disease, severe endometriosis, oligospermia, and immunologic or unexplained infertility, may benefit from IVF, gamete intrafallopian transfer (GIFT), and zygote intrafallopian transfer (ZIFT). These techniques are complex and require a highly organized team of specialists. All of the procedures involve ovarian stimulation to produce multiple oocytes, oocyte retrieval by transvaginal sonography–guided needle aspiration, and handling of the oocytes outside the body. With IVF, the eggs are fertilized in vitro and the embryos transferred to the uterine fundus. Intracytoplasmic sperm injection (ICSI) allows fertilization with a single sperm. It was originally intended for couples with male factor infertility, but it is now used in more than half of all IVF procedures in the United States.

GIFT involves the placement of sperm and eggs in the uterine tube by laparoscopy or minilaparotomy. With ZIFT, fertilization occurs in vitro, and the early development of the embryo occurs in the uterine tube after transfer by laparoscopy or minilaparotomy. The latter two procedures are used infrequently.

▶ Prognosis

The prognosis for conception and normal pregnancy is good if minor (even multiple) disorders can be identified and treated; it is poor if the causes of infertility are severe, untreatable, or of prolonged duration (over 3 years).

It is important to remember that in the absence of identifiable causes of infertility, 60% of couples will achieve a pregnancy within 3 years. Couples with unexplained infertility who do not achieve pregnancy within 3 years may be offered ovulation induction or assisted reproductive technology. Also, offering appropriately timed information about adoption is considered part of a complete infertility regimen.

▶ When to Refer

Refer to reproductive endocrinologist if ART are indicated.

Balen AH et al. Management of infertility. BMJ. 2007 Oct 22;335:608–11. [PMID: 17884905]

Sutter P. Rational diagnosis and treatment in infertility. Best Pract Res Clin Obstet Gynecol. 2006 Oct;20(5):647–64. [PMID: 16769249]

CONTRACEPTION

Voluntary control of childbearing benefits women, men, and their children. Contraception should be available to all women and men of reproductive ages. Education about contraception and access to contraceptive pills or devices are especially important for sexually active teenagers and for women following childbirth or abortion.

1. Oral Contraceptives

A. Combined Oral Contraceptives

1. Efficacy and methods of use—Oral contraceptives have a perfect use failure rate of 0.3% and a typical use failure rate of 8%. Their primary mode of action is suppression of ovulation. The pills can be initially started on the first day of the menstrual cycle, the first Sunday after the onset of the cycle or on any day of the cycle. If started on any day other than the first day of the cycle, a backup method should be used. There are also pills packaged to be taken continuously for 84 days, followed by 7 days of placebos. If an active pill is missed at any time, and no intercourse occurred in the past 5 days, two pills should be taken immediately and a backup method should be used for 7 days. If intercourse occurred in the previous 5 days, emergency contraception should be used immediately, and the pills restarted the following day. A backup method should be used for 5 days.

2. Benefits of oral contraceptives—Noncontraceptive benefits of oral contraceptives include lighter menses, reducing the likelihood of anemia. Dysmenorrhea is relieved for most women. Functional ovarian cysts are less likely with oral contraceptive use. The risk of ovarian and endometrial cancer is decreased. The risks of salpingitis and ectopic pregnancy may be diminished. Acne is usually improved. The frequency of developing myomas is lower in long-term users (> 4 years). There is a beneficial effect on bone mass.

3. Selection of an oral contraceptive—Any of the combination oral contraceptives containing 35 mcg or less of estrogen are suitable for most women. There is some variation in potency of the various progestins in the pills, but there are essentially no clinically significant differences for most women among the progestins in the low-dose pills. Women who have acne or hirsutism may benefit from use of one of the pills containing the third-generation progestins, desogestrel, drospirenone, or norgestimate, as they are the least androgenic. A combination regimen with 84 active and 7 inert pills that results in only four menses per year is available. There is also a combination regimen that is taken continuously with no regular menses. At the end of one years' use, 58% of the women had amenorrhea, and nearly 80% reported no bleeding requiring sanitary protection. The low-dose oral contraceptives commonly used in the United States are listed in Table 18–3.

4. Drug interactions—Several drugs interact with oral contraceptives to decrease their efficacy by causing induction of microsomal enzymes in the liver, or by other

Table 18–3. Commonly used low-dose oral contraceptives.

Name	Progestin	Estrogen (Ethinyl Estradiol)	Cost per Month[1]
COMBINATION			
Alesse[2,3]	0.1 mg levonorgestrel	20 mcg	$35.16
Loestrin 1/20[2]	1 mg norethindrone acetate	20 mcg	$28.66
Mircette[2]	0.15 mg desogestrel	20 mcg	$59.98
Yaz	3 mg drospirenone	20 mcg	$56.70
Loestrin 1.5/30[2]	1.5 mg norethindrone acetate	30 mcg	$28.94
Lo-Ovral[2]	0.3 mg norgestrel	30 mcg	$61.25
Levlen[2]	0.15 mg levonorgestrel	30 mcg	$36.50
Ortho-Cept[2] Desogen[2]	0.15 mg desogestrel	30 mcg	$30.52 $30.52
Yasmin	3 mg drospirenone	30 mcg	$62.26
Brevicon[2] Modicon[2]	0.5 mg norethindrone	35 mcg	$50.41 $50.41
Demulen 1/35[2]	1 mg ethynodiol diacetate	35 mcg	$42.06
Ortho-Novum 1/35[2]	1 mg norethindrone	35 mcg	$53.11
Ortho-Cyclen[2]	0.25 mg norgestimate	35 mcg	$31.51
Ovcon 35[2]	0.4 mg norethindrone	35 mcg	$66.58
COMBINATION: EXTENDED-CYCLE			
Seasonale	0.15 mg levonorgestrel	30 mcg	$75.83
Seasonique	0.15 mg levonorgestrel (days 1–84)/ 0 mg levonorgestrel (days 85–91)	30 mcg (84 days)/10 mcg (7 days)	$59.59
LoSeasonique	0.10 mg levonorgestrel (days 1–84)/ 0 mg levonorgestrel (days 85–91)	20 mcg (84 days)/10 mcg (7 days)	Cost not yet published
Lybrel	90 mcg levonorgestrel	20 mcg	$52.80
TRIPHASIC			
Estrostep	1.0 mg norethindrone acetate (days 1–5) 1.0 mg norethindrone acetate (days 6–12) 1.0 mg norethindrone acetate (days 13–21)	20 mcg 30 mcg 35 mcg	$65.41
Cyclessa[2]	0.1 mg desogestrel (days 1–7) 0.125 mg desogestrel (days 8–14) 0.15 mg desogestrel (days 15–21)	25 mcg	$47.12
Ortho-Tri-Cyclen Lo	0.18 norgestimate (days 1–7) 0.21 norgestimate (days 8–14) 0.25 norgestimate (days 15–21)	25 mcg	$62.14
Triphasil[2,3]	0.05 mg levonorgestrel (days 1–6) 0.075 mg levonorgestrel (days 7–11) 0.125 mg levonorgestrel (days 12–21)	30 mcg 40 mcg 30 mcg	$42.01
Ortho-Novum 7/7/7[2,3]	0.5 mg norethindrone (days 1–7) 0.75 mg norethindrone (days 8–14) 1 mg norethindrone (days 15–21)	35 mcg	$28.57
Ortho-Tri-Cyclen[2,3]	0.18 mg norgestimate (days 1–7) 0.215 mg norgestimate (days 8–14) 0.25 mg norgestimate (days 15–21)	35 mcg	$31.51
Tri-Norinyl[2,3]	0.5 mg norethindrone (days 1–7) 1 mg norethindrone (days 8–16) 0.5 mg norethindrone (days 17–21)	35 mcg	$52.20

(continued)

Table 18–3. Commonly used low-dose oral contraceptives. (continued)

Name	Progestin	Estrogen (Ethinyl Estradiol)	Cost per Month[1]
PROGESTIN-ONLY MINIPILL			
Ortho Micronor[2,3]	0.35 mg norethindrone to be taken continuously	None	$34.48
Ovrette	0.075 mg norgestrel to be taken continuously	None	$37.54

[1]Average wholesale price (AWP, for AB-rated generic when available) for quantity listed. Source: *Red Book Update,* Vol. 28, No. 3, March 2009. AWP may not accurately represent the actual pharmacy cost because wide contractual variations exist among institutions.
[2]Generic equivalent available.
[3]Multiple other brands available.

mechanisms. Some commonly prescribed drugs in this category are phenytoin, phenobarbital (and other barbiturates), primidone, topiramate, carbamazepine, and rifampin and St. John's Wort. Women taking these drugs should use another means of contraception for maximum safety.

5. Contraindications and adverse effects—Oral contraceptives have been associated with many adverse effects; they are contraindicated in some situations and should be used with caution in others (Table 18–4).

A. MYOCARDIAL INFARCTION—The risk of heart attack is higher with use of oral contraceptives, particularly with pills containing 50 mcg of estrogen or more. Cigarette smoking, obesity, hypertension, diabetes, or hypercholesterolemia increases the risk. Young nonsmoking women have minimal increased risk. Smokers over age 35 and women with other cardiovascular risk factors should use other methods of birth control.

Table 18–4. Contraindications to use of oral contraceptives.

Absolute contraindications
Pregnancy
Thrombophlebitis or thromboembolic disorders (past or present)
Stroke or coronary artery disease (past or present)
Cancer of the breast (known or suspected)
Undiagnosed abnormal vaginal bleeding
Estrogen-dependent cancer (known or suspected)
Benign or malignant tumor of the liver (past or present)
Uncontrolled hypertension
Diabetes mellitus with vascular disease
Age over 35 and smoking > 15 cigarettes daily
Known thrombophilia
Migraine with aura
Active hepatitis
Surgery or orthopedic injury requiring prolonged immobilization
Relative contraindications
Migraine without aura
Hypertension
Heart or kidney disease
Diabetes mellitus
Gallbladder disease
Cholestasis during pregnancy
Sickle cell disease (S/S or S/C type)
Lactation

B. THROMBOEMBOLIC DISEASE—An increased rate of venous thromboembolism is found in oral contraceptive users, especially if the dose of estrogen is 50 mcg or more. While the overall risk is very low (15 per 100,000 woman-years), several studies have reported a twofold increased risk in women using oral contraceptives containing the progestins gestodene (not available in the United States) or desogestrel compared with women using oral contraceptives with levonorgestrel and norethindrone. Women in whom thrombophlebitis develops should stop using this method, as should those at risk for thrombophlebitis because of surgery, fracture, serious injury, or immobilization. Women with a known thrombophilia should not use oral contraceptives.

C. CEREBROVASCULAR DISEASE—Overall, a small increased risk of hemorrhagic stroke and subarachnoid hemorrhage and a somewhat greater increased risk of thrombotic stroke has been found; smoking, hypertension, and age over 35 years are associated with increased risk. Women should stop using contraceptives if such warning symptoms as severe headache, blurred or lost vision, or other transient neurologic disorders develop.

D. CARCINOMA—A relationship between long-term (3–4 years) oral contraceptive use and occurrence of cervical dysplasia and cancer has been found in various studies. A 2002 study showed that there is no increased risk of breast cancer in women aged 35–64 who are current or former users of oral contraceptives. Women with a family history of breast cancer or women who started oral contraceptive use at a young age are not at increased risk. Combination oral contraceptives reduce the risk of endometrial carcinoma by 40% after 2 years of use and 60% after 4 or more years of use. The risk of ovarian cancer is reduced by 30% with pill use for less than 4 years, by 60% with use for 5–11 years, and by 80% after 12 or more years. Rarely, oral contraceptives have been associated with the development of benign or malignant hepatic tumors; this may lead to rupture of the liver, hemorrhage, and death. The risk increases with higher dosage, longer duration of use, and older age.

E. HYPERTENSION—Oral contraceptives may cause hypertension in some women; the risk is increased with longer duration of use and older age. Women in whom hypertension develops while using oral contraceptives should use other contraceptive methods. However, with regular blood pressure monitoring, nonsmoking women under the age of 40 with well-controlled mild hypertension may use oral contraceptives.

F. HEADACHE—Migraine or other vascular headaches may occur or worsen with pill use. If severe or frequent headaches develop while using this method, it should be discontinued. Women with migraine headaches with an aura should not use oral contraceptives.

G. LACTATION—Combined oral contraceptives can impair the quantity and quality of breast milk. While it is preferable to avoid the use of combination oral contraceptives during lactation, the effects on milk quality are small and are not associated with developmental abnormalities in infants. Combination oral contraceptives should be started no earlier than 6 weeks postpartum to allow for establishment of lactation. Progestin-only pills, levonorgestrel implants, and depot medroxyprogesterone acetate are alternatives with no adverse effects on milk quality.

H. OTHER DISORDERS—Depression may occur or be worsened with oral contraceptive use. Fluid retention may occur. Patients who had cholestatic jaundice during pregnancy may develop it while taking birth control pills.

6. Minor side effects—Nausea and dizziness may occur in the first few months of pill use. A weight gain of 2–5 lb commonly occurs. Spotting or breakthrough bleeding between menstrual periods may occur, especially if a pill is skipped or taken late; this may be helped by switching to a pill of slightly greater potency (see section C, above). Missed menstrual periods may occur, especially with low-dose pills. A pregnancy test should be performed if pills have been skipped or if two or more menstrual periods are missed. Depression, fatigue, and decreased libido can occur. Chloasma may occur, as in pregnancy, and is increased by exposure to sunlight.

B. Progestin Minipill

1. Efficacy and methods of use—Formulations containing 0.35 mg of norethindrone or 0.075 mg of norgestrel are available in the United States. Their efficacy is similar to that of combined oral contraceptives. The minipill is believed to prevent conception by causing thickening of the cervical mucus to make it hostile to sperm, alteration of ovum transport (which may account for the higher rate of ectopic pregnancy with these pills), and inhibition of implantation. Ovulation is inhibited inconsistently with this method. The minipill is begun on the first day of a menstrual cycle and then taken continuously for as long as contraception is desired.

2. Advantages—The low dose and absence of estrogen make the minipill safe during lactation; it may increase the flow of milk. It is often tried by women who want minimal doses of hormones and by patients who are over age 35. They lack the cardiovascular side effects of combination pills. The minipill can be safely used by women with sickle cell disease (S/S or S/C).

3. Complications and contraindications—Minipill users often have bleeding irregularities (eg, prolonged flow,

spotting, or amenorrhea); such patients may need regular pregnancy tests. Ectopic pregnancies are more frequent, and complaints of abdominal pain should be investigated with this in mind. The absolute contraindications and many of the relative contraindications listed in Table 18–4 apply to the minipill. Minor side effects of combination oral contraceptives such as weight gain and mild headache may also occur with the minipill.

ACOG Committee on Practice Bulletins—Gynecology. ACOG practice bulletin. No. 73: Use of hormonal contraception in women with coexisting medical conditions. Obstet Gynecol. 2006 Jun;107(6):1453–72. [PMID: 16738183]
Kiley J et al. Combined oral contraceptives: a comprehensive review. Clin Obstet Gynecol. 2007 Dec;50(4):868–77. [PMID: 17982329]
Lin K et al. The clinical rationale for menses-free contraception. J Womens Health (Larchmt). 2007 Oct;16(8):1171–80. [PMID: 17937570]

2. Contraceptive Injections & Implants (Long-Acting Progestins)

The injectable progestin medroxyprogesterone acetate (DMPA) is approved for contraceptive use in the United States. There is extensive worldwide experience with this method over the past 3 decades. The medication is given as a deep intramuscular injection of 150 mg every 3 months and has a contraceptive efficacy of 99.7%. A subcutaneous preparation, containing 104 mg of DMPA is available in the United States. Common side effects include irregular bleeding, amenorrhea, weight gain, and headache. It is associated with bone mineral loss that is usually reversible after discontinuation of the method. Users commonly have irregular bleeding initially and subsequently develop amenorrhea. Ovulation may be delayed after the last injection. Contraindications are similar to those for the minipill.

A single-rod, subdermal progestin implant, Implanon, is approved for use in the United States. Implanon is a 40-mm by 2-mm rod containing 68 mg of the progestin etonogestrel that is inserted in the inner aspect of the nondominant arm. Insertion and removal are much simpler and faster than with Norplant. Hormone levels drop rapidly after removal, and there is no delay in the return of fertility. In clinical trials, the pregnancy rate was 0.0% with 3 years of use. The side effect profile is similar to minipills, Depo-Provera, and Norplant. Irregular bleeding has been the most common reason for discontinuation.

Haider S et al. Injectable contraception. Clin Obstet Gynecol. 2007 Dec;50(4)898–906. [PMID: 17982332]
Isley MM et al. Contraceptive implants: an overview and update. Obstet Gynecol Clin North Am. 2007 Mar;34(1):73–90. [PMID: 17472866]

3. Other Hormonal Methods

A transdermal contraceptive patch containing 150 mcg norelgestromin and 20 mcg ethinyl estradiol and measuring 20 cm^2 is available. The patch is applied to the lower abdomen, upper torso, or buttock once a week for 3 consecutive weeks, followed by 1 week without the patch. It appears that the average steady-state concentration of ethinyl estradiol with the patch is approximately 60% higher than with a 35 mcg pill. However, there is currently no evidence for an increased incidence of estrogen-related side effects. The mechanism of action, side effects, and efficacy are similar to those associated with oral contraceptives, although compliance may be better.

A contraceptive vaginal ring that releases 120 mcg of etonogestrel and 15 mcg of ethinyl estradiol daily is available. The ring is soft and flexible and is placed in the upper vagina for 3 weeks, removed, and replaced 1 week later. The efficacy, mechanism of action, and systemic side effects are similar to those associated with oral contraceptives. In addition, users may experience an increased incidence of vaginal discharge.

4. Intrauterine Devices

IUDs available in the United States include the Mirena (which releases levonorgestrel) and the copper-bearing TCu380A. The mechanism of action of IUDs is thought to involve either spermicidal or inhibitory effects on sperm capacitation and transport. IUDs are not abortifacients.

The Mirena is effective for 5 years, and the TCu380A for 10 years. The hormone-containing IUDs have the advantage of reducing cramping and menstrual flow.

The IUD is an excellent contraceptive method for most women. The devices are highly effective, with failure rates similar to those achieved with surgical sterilization. Nulliparity is not a contraindication to IUD use. Women who are not in mutually monogamous relationships should use condoms for protection from sexually transmitted diseases. The Mirena may have a protective effect against upper tract infection similar to that of the oral contraceptives.

A. Insertion

Insertion can be performed during or after the menses, at midcycle to prevent implantation, or later in the cycle if the patient has not become pregnant. Most clinicians wait for 6–8 weeks postpartum before inserting an IUD. When insertion is performed during lactation, there is greater risk of uterine perforation or embedding of the IUD. Insertion immediately following abortion is acceptable if there is no sepsis and if follow-up insertion a month later will not be possible; otherwise, it is wise to wait until 4 weeks post-abortion.

B. Contraindications & Complications

Contraindications to use of IUDs are outlined in Table 18–5.

1. Pregnancy—A copper-containing IUD can be inserted within 5 days following a single episode of unprotected midcycle coitus as a postcoital contraceptive. An IUD should not be inserted into a pregnant uterus. If pregnancy occurs as an IUD failure, there is a greater chance of spontaneous abortion if the IUD is left in situ (50%) than if it is removed (25%). Spontaneous abortion with an IUD in place is associated with a high risk of severe sepsis, and death can occur rapidly. Women using an IUD who become pregnant should have the IUD removed if the string is visible. It can be removed at the time of abortion if this is desired. If the

Table 18–5. Contraindications to IUD use.

Absolute contraindications
Pregnancy
Acute or subacute pelvic inflammatory disease or purulent cervicitis
Significant anatomic abnormality of uterus
Unexplained uterine bleeding
Active liver disease (Mirena only)
Relative contraindications
History of pelvic inflammatory disease since the last pregnancy
Lack of available follow-up care
Menorrhagia or severe dysmenorrhea (copper IUD)
Cervical or uterine neoplasia

IUD, intrauterine device.

string is not visible and the patient wants to continue the pregnancy, she should be informed of the serious risk of sepsis and, occasionally, death with such pregnancies. She should be informed that any flu-like symptoms such as fever, myalgia, headache, or nausea warrant immediate medical attention for possible septic abortion.

Since the ratio of ectopic to intrauterine pregnancies is increased among IUD wearers, clinicians should search for adnexal masses in early pregnancy and should always check the products of conception for placental tissue following abortion.

2. Pelvic infection—There is an increased risk of pelvic infection during the first month following insertion. The subsequent risk of pelvic infection appears to be primarily related to the risk of acquiring sexually transmitted infections. Infertility rates do not appear to be increased among women who have previously used the currently available IUDs. At the time of insertion, women with an increased risk of sexually transmitted diseases should be screened for gonorrhea and *Chlamydia*. Women with a history of recent or recurrent pelvic infection are not good candidates for IUD use.

3. Menorrhagia or severe dysmenorrhea—The copper IUD can cause heavier menstrual periods, bleeding between periods, and more cramping, so it is generally not suitable for women who already suffer from these problems. However, hormone-releasing IUDs can be tried in these cases, as they often cause decreased bleeding and cramping with menses. NSAIDs are also helpful in decreasing bleeding and pain in IUD users.

4. Complete or partial expulsion—Spontaneous expulsion of the IUD occurs in 10–20% of cases during the first year of use. Any IUD should be removed if the body of the device can be seen or felt in the cervical os.

5. Missing IUD strings—If the transcervical tail cannot be seen, this may signify unnoticed expulsion, perforation of the uterus with abdominal migration of the IUD, or simply retraction of the string into the cervical canal or uterus owing to movement of the IUD or uterine growth with pregnancy. Once pregnancy is ruled out, one should probe for the IUD with a sterile sound or forceps designed for

IUD removal, after administering a paracervical block. If the IUD cannot be detected, pelvic ultrasound will demonstrate the IUD if it is in the uterus. Alternatively, obtain anteroposterior and lateral x-rays of the pelvis with another IUD or a sound in the uterus as a marker, to confirm an extrauterine IUD. If the IUD is in the abdominal cavity, it should generally be removed by laparoscopy or laparotomy. Perforations of the uterus are less likely if insertion is performed slowly, with meticulous care taken to follow directions applicable to each type of IUD.

ESHRE Capri Workshop Group. Intrauterine devices and intrauterine systems. Hum Reprod Update. 2008 May–Jun;14(3):197–208. [PMID: 18400840]

Thonneau PF et al. Contraceptive efficacy of intrauterine devices. Am J Obstet Gynecol. 2008 Mar;198(3):248–53. [PMID: 18221924]

5. Diaphragm & Cervical Cap

The diaphragm (with contraceptive jelly) is a safe and effective contraceptive method with features that make it acceptable to some women and not others. Failure rates range from 6% to 16%, depending on the motivation of the woman and the care with which the diaphragm is used. The advantages of this method are that it has no systemic side effects and gives significant protection against pelvic infection and cervical dysplasia as well as pregnancy. The disadvantages are that it must be inserted near the time of coitus and that pressure from the rim predisposes some women to cystitis after intercourse.

The cervical cap (with contraceptive jelly) is similar to the diaphragm but fits snugly over the cervix only (the diaphragm stretches from behind the cervix to behind the pubic symphysis). The cervical cap is more difficult to insert and remove than the diaphragm. The main advantages are that it can be used by women who cannot be fitted for a diaphragm because of a relaxed anterior vaginal wall or by women who have discomfort or develop repeated bladder infections with the diaphragm. However, failure rates are 9% (perfect use) and 16% (typical use) in nulliparous women and 26% (perfect use) and 32% (typical use) in parous women.

Because of the small risk of toxic shock syndrome, a cervical cap or diaphragm should not be left in the vagina for over 12–18 hours, nor should these devices be used during the menstrual period.

6. Contraceptive Foam, Cream, Film, Sponge, Jelly, & Suppository

These products are available without prescription, are easy to use, and are fairly effective, with typical failure rates of 10–22%. All contain the spermicide nonoxynol-9, which also has some virucidal and bactericidal activity. Nonoxynol-9 does not appear to adversely affect the vaginal colonization of hydrogen peroxide-producing lactobacilli. A 2002 study suggests that nonoxynol-9 is not protective against HIV infection, particularly in women who have frequent intercourse. The FDA now requires products containing nonoxynol-9 to include a warning that the products do not protect against HIV or other sexually transmitted diseases and that use of these products can irritate the vagina and rectum and may increase the risk of getting the AIDS virus from an infected partner. Recent data suggest that low-risk women using a nonoxynol-9 product, with coital activity two to three times per week, are not at increased risk for epithelial disruption, compared with couples using condoms alone.

Harwood B et al. Cervicovaginal colposcopic lesions associated with 5 nonoxynol-9 spermicide formulations. Am J Obstet Gynecol. 2008 Jan;198(1):32.e1–7. [PMID: 18166301]

7. Condom

The male condom of latex or animal membrane affords good protection against pregnancy—equivalent to that of a diaphragm and spermicidal jelly; latex (but not animal membrane) condoms also offer protection against many sexually transmitted diseases, including HIV. When a spermicide, such as vaginal foam, is used with the condom, the failure rate approaches that of oral contraceptives. The disadvantages of condoms are dulling of sensation and spillage of semen due to tearing, slipping, or leakage with detumescence of the penis.

A female condom made of polyurethane is available in the United States. The reported failure rates range from 5% to 21%; the efficacy is comparable to that of the diaphragm. This is the only female-controlled method that offers significant protection from both pregnancy and sexually transmitted diseases.

8. Contraception Based on Awareness of Fertile Periods

These methods are most effective when the couple restricts intercourse to the postovular phase of the cycle or uses a barrier method at other times. Well-instructed, motivated couples may be able to achieve low pregnancy rates with fertility awareness methods. However, properly done randomized clinical trials comparing the efficacy of most of these methods with other contraceptive methods do not exist.

Grimes DA et al. Fertility awareness-based methods for contraception: systematic review of randomized controlled trials. Contraception. 2005 Aug;72(2):85–90. [PMID: 16022845]

A. "Symptothermal" Natural Family Planning

The basis for this approach is patient-observed increase in clear elastic cervical mucus, brief abdominal midcycle discomfort ("mittelschmerz"), and a sustained rise of the basal body temperature about 2 weeks after onset of menstruation. Unprotected intercourse is avoided from shortly after the menstrual period, when fertile mucus is first identified, until 48 hours after ovulation, as identified by a sustained rise in temperature and the disappearance of clear elastic mucus.

B. Calendar Method

After the length of the menstrual cycle has been observed for at least 8 months, the following calculations are made:

(1) The first fertile day is determined by subtracting 18 days from the shortest cycle, and (2) the last fertile day is determined by subtracting 11 days from the longest cycle. For example, if the observed cycles run from 24 to 28 days, the fertile period would extend from the sixth day of the cycle (24 minus 18) through the 17th day (28 minus 11). Day 1 of the cycle is the first day of menses.

C. Basal Body Temperature Method

This method indicates the safe time for intercourse after ovulation has passed. The temperature must be taken immediately upon awakening, before any activity. A slight drop in temperature often occurs 12–24 hours before ovulation, and a rise of about 0.4 °C occurs 1–2 days after ovulation. The elevated temperature continues throughout the remainder of the cycle. Data suggest that the risk of pregnancy increases starting 5 days prior to the day of ovulation, peaks on the day of ovulation, and then rapidly decreases to zero by the day after ovulation.

D. Standard Days Method

This fertility awareness method requires the use of a set of beads that reminds the couple to avoid intercourse (or use a barrier method of contraception) during days 8 through 19 of the menstrual cycle. The beads are in a circle and color-coded to show the days when a woman is likely to become pregnant and the days that are "safe" during the cycle. A movable ring is repositioned to a new bead each day starting on the first day of menses. In a small multicenter trial, the perfect use failure rate was 5% and the typical use failure rate was 12%. The method is applicable to women with a history of menstrual cycles between 29 and 32 days.

E. TwoDay Method

The TwoDay method requires that women be able to identify cervical secretions by observation or touching them in underwear or toilet paper, by touching the genitals, or by the sensation of wetness in the genital area or on underwear. The woman then uses a two-question algorithm to determine whether she is fertile. She asks herself: (1) Did I note secretions today? and (2) Did I note secretions yesterday? If the answer to either of these questions is "yes," she should consider herself fertile. In a multicenter study of 450 women, effectiveness with perfect use was 96.5% and with typical use 76.3%.

Germano E et al. New approaches to fertility awareness-based methods: incorporating the Standard Days and TwoDay Methods into practice. J Midwifery Womens Health. 2006 Nov–Dec;51(6):471–7. [PMID: 17081938]

9. Emergency Contraception

If unprotected intercourse occurs in midcycle and if the woman is certain she has not inadvertently become pregnant earlier in the cycle, the following regimens are effective in preventing implantation. These methods should be started as soon as possible and within 120 hours after unprotected coitus. (1) Levonorgestrel, 1.5 mg orally as a single dose (available in the United States prepackaged as Plan B and available over-the-counter for women aged 17 years and above), has a 1% failure rate, when taken within 72 hours. It remains efficacious up to 120 hours after intercourse, though less so compared with earlier use. (2) If the levonorgestrel regimen is not available, a combination oral contraceptive containing ethinyl estradiol and levonorgestrel given in a regimen of two to six tablets initially, followed by two to six tablets 12 hours later my be used. At least 20 brands of pills may be used in this way. For specific instructions for each pill brand, consult www.not-2-late.com. Used within 72 hours, the failure rate of these regimens is approximately 3%, and antinausea medication is often necessary. (3) Mifepristone, 10 mg orally as a single dose, has been shown to have the same failure rate as the levonorgestrel regimen. It is not currently available at this dose in the United States. (4) IUD insertion within 5 days after one episode of unprotected midcycle coitus will also prevent pregnancy; copper-bearing IUDs have been tested for this purpose.

Information on clinics or individual clinicians providing emergency contraception in the United States may be obtained by calling 1-888-668-2528.

Allen RH et al. Emergency contraception: a clinical review. Clin Obstet Gynecol. 2007 Dec;50(4):927–36. [PMID: 17982335]

10. Abortion

Since the legalization of abortion in the United States in 1973, the related maternal mortality rate has fallen markedly, because illegal and self-induced abortions have been replaced by safer medical procedures. Abortions in the first trimester of pregnancy are performed by vacuum aspiration under local anesthesia or with medical regimens. Dilation and evacuation, a variation of vacuum aspiration is generally used in the second trimester. Techniques utilizing intra-amniotic instillation of hypertonic saline solution or various prostaglandins regimens, along with medical or osmotic dilators are occasionally used after 18 weeks. Several medical abortion regimens utilizing mifepristone and multiple doses of misoprostol have been reported as being effective in the second trimester. Overall, legal abortion in the United States has a mortality rate of less than 1:100,000. Rates of morbidity and mortality rise with length of gestation. Currently in the United States, 88% of abortions are performed before 13 weeks' gestation and only 1.3% are performed after 20 weeks. If abortion is chosen, every effort should be made to encourage the patient to seek an early procedure. While numerous state laws limiting access to abortion and a federal law banning a rarely-used variation of dilation and evacuation have been enacted, abortion remains legal and available until fetal viability under Roe v. Wade.

Complications resulting from abortion include retained products of conception (often associated with infection and heavy bleeding) and unrecognized ectopic pregnancy. Immediate analysis of the removed tissue for placenta can exclude or corroborate the diagnosis of ectopic pregnancy. Women who have fever, bleeding, or abdominal pain after abortion should be examined; use of broad-spectrum antibiotics and reaspiration of the uterus are frequently necessary. Hospitalization is advisable if acute salpingitis requires intravenous administration of antibiotics. Complications following illegal abortion often need emergency care for hemorrhage, septic shock, or uterine perforation.

Rh immune globulin should be given to all Rh-negative women following abortion. Prophylactic antibiotics are indicated for surgical abortion; for example a one-dose regimen of doxycycline, 200 mg orally 1 hour before the procedure. Many clinics prescribe tetracycline, 500 mg orally four times daily for 5 days after the procedure, as presumptive treatment for *Chlamydia*.

Mifepristone (RU 486) is approved by the FDA as an oral abortifacient at a dose of 600 mg on day 1, followed by 400 mcg orally of misoprostol on day 3. This combination is 95% successful in terminating pregnancies of up to 9 weeks' duration with minimum complications. A more commonly used, evidence-based regimen is mifepristone, 200 mg orally on day 1, followed by misoprostol, 800 mcg vaginally either immediately or within 6–8 hours. Although not approved by the FDA for this indication, a combination of intramuscular methotrexate, 50 mg/m^2 of body surface area, followed 3–7 days later by vaginal misoprostol, 800 mcg, is 98% successful in terminating pregnancy at 8 weeks or less. Minor side effects, such as nausea, vomiting, and diarrhea, are common with these regimens. There is a 5–10% incidence of hemorrhage or incomplete abortion requiring curettage. There is a 2005 report of four deaths occurring within 1 week of medical abortion, associated with endometritis and toxic shock caused by *Clostridium sordellii*. To improve diagnosis and treatment of this entity, clinicians should be aware of the constellation of presenting symptoms of tachycardia, hypotension, edema, hemoconcentration, profound leukocytosis, and absence of fever.

ACOG. ACOG practice bulletin: Clinical management guidelines of Obstetrician-Gynecologists. Number 67, October 2005. Medical management of abortion. Obstet Gynecol. 2005 Oct;106(4):871–82. [PMID: 16199653]

Fischer M et al. Fatal toxic shock syndrome associated with *Clostridium sordellii* after medical abortion. N Engl J Med. 2005 Dec 1;353(22):2352–60. [PMID: 16319384]

Lipp A. A review of developments in medical termination of pregnancy. J Clin Nurs. 2008 Jun;17(11):1411–8. [PMID: 18482139]

11. Sterilization

In the United States, sterilization is the most popular method of birth control for couples who want no more children. Although sterilization is reversible in some instances, reversal surgery in both men and women is costly, complicated, and not always successful. Therefore, patients should be counseled carefully before sterilization and should view the procedure as final.

Vasectomy is a safe, simple procedure in which the vas deferens is severed and sealed through a scrotal incision under local anesthesia. Long-term follow-up studies on vasectomized men show no excess risk of cardiovascular disease. Several studies have shown a possible association with prostate cancer, but the evidence is weak and inconsistent.

Female sterilization procedures include laparoscopic bipolar electrocoagulation, or plastic ring application on the uterine tubes, or minilaparotomy with Pomeroy tubal resection. The advantages of laparoscopy are minimal postoperative pain, small incisions, and rapid recovery. The advantages of minilaparotomy are that it can be performed with standard surgical instruments under local or general anesthesia. However, there is more postoperative pain and a longer recovery period. The cumulative 10-year failure rate for all methods combined is 1.85%, varying from 0.75% for postpartum partial salpingectomy and laparoscopic unipolar coagulation to 3.65% for spring clips; this fact should be discussed with women preoperatively. Some studies have found an increased risk of menstrual irregularities as a long-term complication of tubal ligation, but findings in different studies have been inconsistent. A new method of transcervical sterilization, Essure, is approved by the FDA. The method involves the placement of an expanding microcoil of titanium into the proximal uterine tube under hysteroscopic guidance. The efficacy rate at 1 year is 99.8%.

▶ When to Refer

Refer to experienced clinicians for Implanon or other subcutaneous insertion, IUD insertion, tubal occlusion or ligation, vasectomy, or therapeutic abortion.

Ogburn T et al. Transcervical sterilization: past, present, and future. Obstet Gynecol Clin North Am. 2007 Mar;34(1):57–72. [PMID: 17472865]

Peterson HB. Sterilization. Obstet Gynecol. 2008 Jan;111(1):189–203. [PMID: 18165410]

RAPE

 ESSENTIALS OF DIAGNOSIS

▶ Women neither secretly want to be raped nor do they expect, encourage, or enjoy rape.

▶ Rape is always a terrifying experience in which most victims fear for their lives.

▶ The rapist is usually a hostile man who uses sexual intercourse to terrorize and humiliate a woman.

▶ General Considerations

Rape, or sexual assault, is legally defined in different ways in various jurisdictions. Clinicians and emergency department personnel who deal with rape victims should be familiar with the laws pertaining to sexual assault in their own state. From a medical and psychological viewpoint, it is essential that persons treating rape victims recognize the nonconsensual and violent nature of the crime. About 95% of reported rape victims are women. Penetration may be vaginal, anal, or oral and may be by the penis, hand, or a foreign object. The absence of genital injury does not imply consent by the victim. The assailant may be unknown to the victim or, more frequently, may be an acquaintance or even the spouse.

"Unlawful sexual intercourse," or statutory rape, is intercourse with a female before the age of majority even with her consent.

Rape represents an expression of anger, power, and sexuality on the part of the rapist. The rapist is usually a hostile man who uses sexual intercourse to terrorize and humiliate a woman. Women neither secretly want to be raped nor do they expect, encourage, or enjoy rape.

Rape involves severe physical injury in 5–10% of cases and is always a terrifying experience in which most victims fear for their lives. Consequently, all victims suffer some psychological aftermath. Moreover, some rape victims may acquire sexually transmissible disease or become pregnant.

Because rape is a personal crisis, each patient will react differently. The rape trauma syndrome comprises two principal phases. (1) Immediate or acute: Shaking, sobbing, and restless activity may last from a few days to a few weeks. The patient may experience anger, guilt, or shame or may repress these emotions. Reactions vary depending on the victim's personality and the circumstances of the attack. (2) Late or chronic: Problems related to the attack may develop weeks or months later. The lifestyle and work patterns of the individual may change. Sleep disorders or phobias often develop. Loss of self-esteem can rarely lead to suicide.

Clinicians and emergency department personnel who deal with rape victims should work with community rape crisis centers whenever possible to provide ongoing support and counseling.

▶ General Office Procedures

The clinician who first sees the alleged rape victim should be empathetic. Begin with a statement such as, "This is a terrible thing that has happened to you. I want to help."

1. Secure written consent from the patient, guardian, or next of kin for gynecologic examination and for photographs if they are likely to be useful as evidence. If police are to be notified, do so, and obtain advice on the preservation and transfer of evidence.

2. Obtain and record the history in the patient's own words. The sequence of events, ie, the time, place, and circumstances, must be included. Note the date of the LMP, whether or not the woman is pregnant, and the time of the most recent coitus prior to the sexual assault. Note the details of the assault such as body cavities penetrated, use of foreign objects, and number of assailants. Note whether the victim is calm, agitated, or confused (drugs or alcohol may be involved). Record whether the patient came directly to the hospital or whether she bathed or changed her clothing. Record findings but do not issue even a tentative diagnosis lest it be erroneous or incomplete.

3. Have the patient disrobe while standing on a white sheet. Hair, dirt, and leaves, underclothing, and any torn or stained clothing should be kept as evidence. Scrape material from beneath fingernails and comb pubic hair for evidence. Place all evidence in separate clean paper bags or envelopes and label carefully.

4. Examine the patient, noting any traumatized areas that should be photographed. Examine the body and genitals with a Wood light to identify semen, which fluoresces; positive areas should be swabbed with a premoistened swab and air-dried in order to identify acid phosphatase. Colposcopy can be used to identify small areas of trauma from forced entry especially at the posterior fourchette.

5. Perform a pelvic examination, explaining all procedures and obtaining the patient's consent before proceeding gently with the examination. Use a narrow speculum lubricated with water only. Collect material with sterile cotton swabs from the vaginal walls and cervix and make two air-dried smears on clean glass slides. Wet and dry swabs of vaginal secretions should be collected and refrigerated for subsequent acid phosphatase and DNA evaluation. Swab the mouth (around molars and cheeks) and anus in the same way, if appropriate. Label all slides carefully. Collect secretions from the vagina, anus, or mouth with a premoistened cotton swab, place at once on a slide with a drop of saline, and cover with a coverslip. Look for motile or nonmotile sperm under high, dry magnification, and record the percentage of motile forms.

6. Perform appropriate laboratory tests as follows. Culture the vagina, anus, or mouth (as appropriate) for *N gonorrhoeae* and *Chlamydia*. Perform a Papanicolaou smear of the cervix, a wet mount for *T vaginalis*, a baseline pregnancy test, and VDRL test. A confidential test for HIV antibody can be obtained if desired by the patient and repeated in 2–4 months if initially negative. Repeat the pregnancy test if the next menses is missed, and repeat the VDRL test in 6 weeks. Obtain blood (10 mL without anticoagulant) and urine (100 mL) specimens if there is a history of forced ingestion or injection of drugs or alcohol.

7. Transfer clearly labeled evidence, eg, laboratory specimens, directly to the clinical pathologist in charge or to the responsible laboratory technician, in the presence of witnesses (never via messenger), so that the rules of evidence will not be breached.

▶ Treatment

Give analgesics or sedatives if indicated. Administer tetanus toxoid if deep lacerations contain soil or dirt particles.

Give ceftriaxone, 125 mg intramuscularly, to prevent gonorrhea. In addition, give metronidazole, 2 g as a single dose, and azithromycin 1 g orally or doxycycline, 100 mg orally twice daily for 7 days to treat chlamydial infection. Incubating syphilis will probably be prevented by these medications, but the VDRL test should be repeated 6 weeks after the assault.

Prevent pregnancy by using one of the methods discussed under Emergency Contraception, if necessary (this chapter).

Vaccinate against hepatitis B. Consider HIV prophylaxis (see Chapter 31).

Make sure the patient and her family and friends have a source of ongoing psychological support.

▶ When to Refer

All women who seek care for sexual assault should be referred to a facility that has expertise in the management of victims of sexual assault and is capable of performing expert forensic examination, if requested.

Martin SL et al. Health-care based interventions for women who have experienced sexual violence: a review of the literature. Trauma Violence Abuse. 2007 Jan;8(1):3–18. [PMID: 17204597]

MENOPAUSAL SYNDROME

 ESSENTIALS OF DIAGNOSIS

▶ Cessation of menses due to aging or to bilateral oophorectomy.

▶ Elevation of FSH and LH levels.

▶ Hot flushes and night sweats (in 80% of women).

▶ Decreased vaginal lubrication; thinned vaginal mucosa with or without dyspareunia.

▶ General Considerations

The term "menopause" denotes the final cessation of menstruation, either as a normal part of aging or as the result of surgical removal of both ovaries. In a broader sense, as the term is commonly used, it denotes a 1- to 3-year period during which a woman adjusts to a diminishing and then absent menstrual flow and the physiologic changes that may be associated—hot flushes, night sweats, and vaginal dryness.

The average age at menopause in Western societies today is 51 years. Premature menopause is defined as ovarian failure and menstrual cessation before age 40; this often has a genetic or autoimmune basis. Surgical menopause due to bilateral oophorectomy is common and can cause more severe symptoms owing to the sudden rapid drop in sex hormone levels.

There is no objective evidence that cessation of ovarian function is associated with severe emotional disturbance or personality changes. However, mood changes toward depression and anxiety can occur at this time. Furthermore, the time of menopause often coincides with other major life changes, such as departure of children from the home, a midlife identity crisis, or divorce. These events, coupled with a sense of the loss of youth, may exacerbate the symptoms of menopause and cause psychological distress.

▶ Clinical Findings

A. Symptoms and Signs

1. Cessation of menstruation—Menstrual cycles generally become irregular as menopause approaches. Anovular cycles occur more often, with irregular cycle length and occasional menorrhagia. Menstrual flow usually diminishes in amount owing to decreased estrogen secretion, resulting in less abundant endometrial growth. Finally, cycles become longer, with missed periods or episodes of spotting only. When no bleeding has occurred for 1 year, the menopausal transition can be said to have occurred. Any bleeding after this time warrants investigation by endometrial curettage or aspiration to rule out endometrial cancer.

2. Hot flushes—Hot flushes (feelings of intense heat over the trunk and face, with flushing of the skin and sweating) occur in 80% of women as a result of the decrease in ovarian hormones. Hot flushes can begin before the cessation of menses. An increase in pulsatile release of GnRH from the hypothalamus is believed to trigger the hot flushes by affecting the adjacent temperature-regulating area of the brain. Hot flushes are more severe in women who undergo surgical menopause. Flushing is more pronounced late in the day, during hot weather, after ingestion of hot foods or drinks, or during periods of tension. Occurring at night, they often cause sweating and insomnia and result in fatigue on the following day.

3. Vaginal atrophy—With decreased estrogen secretion, thinning of the vaginal mucosa and decreased vaginal lubrication occur and may lead to dyspareunia. The introitus decreases in diameter. Pelvic examination reveals pale, smooth vaginal mucosa and a small cervix and uterus. The ovaries are not normally palpable after the menopause. Continued sexual activity will help prevent tissue shrinkage.

4. Osteoporosis—Osteoporosis may occur as a late sequela of menopause.

B. Laboratory Findings

Serum FSH and LH levels are elevated. Vaginal cytologic examination will show a low estrogen effect with predominantly parabasal cells, indicating lack of epithelial maturation due to hypoestrinism.

▶ Treatment

A. Natural Menopause

Education and support from health providers, midlife discussion groups, and reading material will help most women having difficulty adjusting to the menopause. Physiologic symptoms can be treated as follows.

1. Vasomotor symptoms—Oral conjugated estrogens, 0.3 mg or 0.625 mg, estradiol, 0.5 or 1 mg, or estrone sulfate, 0.625 mg; or estradiol can be given transdermally as skin patches that are changed once or twice weekly and secrete 0.05–0.1 mg of hormone daily. When either form of estrogen is used, add a progestin (medroxyprogesterone acetate) to prevent endometrial hyperplasia or cancer. There is also a patch available containing estradiol and the progestin levonorgestrel. The oral hormones can be given in several differing regimens. Give estrogen on days 1–25 of each calendar month, with 5–10 mg of oral medroxy-progesterone acetate added on days 14–25. Withhold hormones from day 26 until the end of the month, when the endometrium will be shed, producing a light, generally painless monthly period. Alternatively, give the estrogen along with 2.5 mg of oral medroxyprogesterone acetate daily, without stopping. This regimen causes some initial bleeding or spotting, but within a few months it produces an atrophic endometrium that will not bleed. If the patient has had a hysterectomy, a progestin need not be used.

Data from the Women's Health Initiative (WHI) study suggest that women should not use combination progestin-estrogen therapy for more than 3 or 4 years. In this study, the increased risk of cardiovascular disease, cerebrovascular disease, and breast cancer with this regimen outweighed the benefits. Women who cannot find relief with alternative approaches may wish to consider continuing use of combination therapy after a thorough discussion of the risks and benefits. Alternatives to hormone therapy for vasomotor symptoms include SSRIs such as paroxetine, 12.5 mg or 25 mg/d orally, or venlafaxine, 75 mg/d orally. Gabapentin, an antiseizure medication, is also effective at 900 mg/d orally. Clonidine given orally or transdermally, 100–150 mcg daily, may also reduce the frequency of hot flushes, but its use is limited by side effects, including dry mouth, drowsiness, and hypotension.

2. Vaginal atrophy—A vaginal ring containing 2 mg of estradiol can be left in place for 3 months and is suitable for long-term use, providing effective relief of vaginal atrophy. There is minimal systemic absorption of estradiol with the ring, and progestin therapy to protect the endometrium is unnecessary. A higher-dose ring with 12.4 mg or 24.8 mg of estradiol acetate delivers a systemic dose and is not appropriate for treatment of vaginal atrophy alone. Short-term use of estrogen vaginal cream will relieve symptoms of atrophy, but because of variable absorption, therapy with either the vaginal ring or systemic hormone replacement is preferable. Testosterone propionate 1–2%, 0.5–1 g, in a vanishing cream base used in the same manner is also effective if estrogen is contraindicated. A bland lubricant such as unscented cold cream or water-soluble gel can be helpful at the time of coitus.

3. Osteoporosis—(See also discussion in Chapter 26.) Women should ingest at least 800 mg of calcium daily throughout life. In addition, 1 g of elemental calcium should be taken as a daily supplement at the time of the menopause and thereafter; calcium supplements should be taken with meals to increase their absorption. Vitamin D, 800 international units/d from food, sunlight, or supplements, is necessary to enhance calcium absorption and maintain bone mass. A daily program of energetic walking and exercise to strengthen the arms and upper body helps maintain bone mass.

Women most at risk for osteoporotic fractures should consider bisphosphonates, raloxifene, or hormone replacement therapy. This includes white and Asian women, especially if they have a family history of osteoporosis; are thin, short, cigarette smokers, and physically inactive; or have had a low calcium intake in adult life.

B. Risks of Hormone Therapy

Double-blinded randomized, controlled trials have shown no overall cardiovascular benefit with estrogen-progestin replacement therapy in a group of postmenopausal women with or without established coronary disease. Both in the WHI trial and the Heart and Estrogen/Progestin Replacement Study (HERS), the overall health risks (increased risk of coronary heart events, strokes, thromboembolic disease, breast cancers, gallstones) exceeded the benefits from the use of combination estrogen and progesterone. Progestins counteract some but not all favorable effects of estrogen. Women who have been receiving long-term estrogen-progestin hormone replacement therapy (HRT), even in the absence of complications should be encouraged to stop, especially if they do not have menopausal symptoms. An ancillary study of the WHI study showed that not only did estrogen-progestin HRT not benefit cognitive function but there was a small increased risk of cognitive decline in that group compared with women in the placebo group. The unopposed estrogen arm of the WHI trial demonstrated a decrease in the risk of hip fracture, a small but nonsignificant decrease in breast cancer, but an increased risk of stroke and no evidence of protection from coronary heart disease. The study also showed a small increase in the combined risk of mild cognitive impairment and dementia with estrogen use compared with placebo, similar to the estrogen-progestin arm. (See also discussions of estrogen and progestin replacement therapy in Chapter 26.)

C. Surgical Menopause

The abrupt hormonal decrease resulting from oophorectomy generally results in severe vasomotor symptoms and rapid onset of dyspareunia and osteoporosis unless treated. Estrogen replacement is generally started immediately after surgery. Conjugated estrogens 1.25 mg orally, estrone sulfate 1.25 mg orally, or estradiol 2 mg orally is given for 25 days of each month. After age 45–50 years, this dose can be tapered to 0.625 mg of conjugated estrogens or equivalent.

Lethaby A et al. Hormone replacement therapy for cognitive function in postmenopausal women. Cochrane Database Syst Rev. 2008 Jan 23;(1):CD003122. [PMID: 18254016]
Nelson HD. Menopause. Lancet. 2008 Mar 1;371(9614):760–70. [PMID: 18313505]

Obstetrics & Obstetric Disorders

Vanessa L. Rogers, MD

Susan Cox, MD

William R. Crombleholme, MD

DIAGNOSIS OF PREGNANCY

It is advantageous to diagnose pregnancy as promptly as possible when a sexually active woman misses a menstrual period or has symptoms suggestive of pregnancy. In the event of a desired pregnancy, prenatal care can begin early, and potentially harmful medications and activities such as drug and alcohol use, smoking, and occupational chemical exposure can be halted. In the event of an unwanted pregnancy, counseling about adoption or termination of the pregnancy can be provided at an early stage.

▶ Pregnancy Tests

All urine or blood pregnancy tests rely on the detection of human chorionic gonadotropin (hCG) produced by the placenta. hCG levels increase shortly after implantation, approximately double every 48 hours, reach a peak at 50–75 days, and fall to lower levels in the second and third trimesters. Laboratory and home pregnancy tests use monoclonal antibodies specific for hCG. These tests are performed on serum or urine and are accurate at the time of the missed period or shortly after it.

Compared with intrauterine pregnancies, ectopic pregnancies may show lower levels of hCG that level off or fall in serial determinations. Quantitative assays of hCG repeated at 48-hour intervals are used in the diagnosis of ectopic pregnancy as well as in cases of molar pregnancy, threatened abortion, and missed abortion. Comparison of hCG levels between laboratories may be misleading in a given patient because different international standards may produce results that vary by as much as twofold. hCG levels can also be problematic because they require a series of measurements. Progesterone levels, however, remain relatively stable in the first trimester and a single measurement can be used to determine whether a pregnancy is viable; a value of less than 5 ng/mL predicts pregnancy failure with a sensitivity of 60%, while a value of 20 ng/mL or higher reflects a viable pregnancy with a sensitivity of 100%.

Mol BW et al. The accuracy of single serum progesterone measurement in the diagnosis of ectopic pregnancy: a meta-analysis. Hum Reprod. 1998;13(11):3220–27. [PMID: 9853884]

▶ Manifestations of Pregnancy

The following symptoms and signs are usually due to pregnancy, but none are diagnostic. A record of the time and frequency of coitus is helpful for diagnosing and dating a pregnancy.

A. Symptoms

Amenorrhea, nausea and vomiting, breast tenderness and tingling, urinary frequency and urgency, "quickening" (perception of first movement noted at about the 18th week), weight gain.

B. Signs (in Weeks from Last Menstrual Period)

Breast changes (enlargement, vascular engorgement, colostrum) start to occur very early in pregnancy and continue until the postpartum period. Cyanosis of vagina and cervical portio and softening of the cervix occur in about the seventh week. Softening of the cervicouterine junction takes place in the eighth week, and generalized enlargement and diffuse softening of the corpus occurs after the eighth week. When a woman's abdomen will start to enlarge depends on her body habitus but typically starts in the sixteenth week.

The uterine fundus is palpable above the pubic symphysis by 12–15 weeks from the last menstrual period and reaches the umbilicus by 20–22 weeks. Fetal heart tones can be heard by Doppler at 10–12 weeks of gestation and at 20 weeks with an ordinary fetoscope.

▶ Differential Diagnosis

The nonpregnant uterus enlarged by myomas can be confused with the gravid uterus, but it is usually very firm and irregular. An ovarian tumor may be found midline, displacing the nonpregnant uterus to the side or posteriorly. Ultrasonography and a pregnancy test will provide accurate diagnosis in these circumstances.

ESSENTIALS OF PRENATAL CARE

The first prenatal visit should occur as early as possible after the diagnosis of pregnancy and should include the

Table 19–1. Common drugs that are teratogenic or fetotoxic.[1]

ACE inhibitors	Lithium
Alcohol	Methotrexate
A-II antagonists	Misoprostol
Androgens	NSAIDs (third trimester)
Anticonvulsants (phenytoin, valproic acid, carbamazepine)	Opioids (prolonged use)
	Progestins
Benzodiazepines	Radioiodine (antithyroid)
Carbarsone (amebicide)	Reserpine
Chloramphenicol (third trimester)	Ribavirin
Cyclophosphamide	Sulfonamides (third trimester)
Diazoxide	SSRIs
Diethylstilbestrol	Tetracycline (third trimester)
Disulfiram	Thalidomide
Ergotamine	Tobacco smoking
Estrogens	Trimethoprim (third trimester)
Griseofulvin	Warfarin and other coumarin
Isotretinoin	anticoagulants

[1]Many other drugs are also contraindicated during pregnancy. Evaluate any drug for its need versus its potential adverse effects. Further information can be obtained from the manufacturer or from any of several teratogenic registries around the country. ACE, angiotensin-converting enzyme; A-II antagonists, angiotensin II receptor blocking agents; NSAIDs, nonsteroidal anti-inflammatory drugs; SSRIs, selective serotonin reuptake inhibitors.

following: history, physical examination, laboratory tests, advice to patients, and tests and procedures.

History

The patient's age, ethnic background, and occupation should be obtained. The onset of the last menstrual period and its normality, possible conception dates, bleeding after the last menstruation, medical history, all prior pregnancies (duration, outcome, and complications), and symptoms of present pregnancy should be documented. The patient's nutritional habits should be discussed with her, as well as any use of caffeine, tobacco, alcohol, or drugs (Table 19–1). Determine whether there is any family history of congenital anomalies and heritable diseases, a personal history of childhood varicella, or prior sexually transmitted diseases (STDs) or risk factors for HIV infection.

Physical Examination

Height, weight, and blood pressure should be measured, and a general physical examination should be done, including a breast examination. Abdominal and pelvic examination should include the following: (1) estimate of uterine size or measure of fundal height; (2) evaluation of bony pelvis for symmetry and adequacy; (3) evaluation of cervix for structural anatomy, infection, effacement, dilation; (4) detection of fetal heart sounds by Doppler device after 10 weeks.

Laboratory Tests

Urinalysis, culture of a clean-voided midstream urine sample, random blood glucose, complete blood count with red cell indices, serologic test for syphilis, rubella antibody titer, varicella immunity, blood group, Rh type, antibody screening, and hepatitis B surface antigen (HBsAg) should be performed. HIV screening should be offered to all pregnant women. Cervical cultures are usually obtained for *Neisseria gonorrhoeae* and *Chlamydia*, along with a Papanicolaou smear of the cervix. All black women should have sickle cell screening. Women of African, Asian, or Mediterranean ancestry with anemia or low mean corpuscular volume (MCV) values should have hemoglobin electrophoresis performed to identify abnormal hemoglobins (Hb S, C, F, α-thalassemia, β-thalassemia). Tuberculosis skin testing is indicated for high-risk populations. Aneuploidy screening is available in the first and second trimester and should be offered to all women, ideally before 20 weeks gestation. Noninvasive first trimester screening for Down syndrome includes ultrasonographic nuchal translucency and serum levels of PAPP-A (pregnancy-associated plasma protein A) and the free β subunit of hCG. In the second trimester, a "quad screen" blood test can be performed; it measures serum alpha-fetoprotein (msAFP), hCG, unconjugated estriol, and inhibin A. First and second trimester tests have similar detection rates. When first and second trimester screening are combined (integrated screening), the detection rates are even higher. Women at increased risk for aneuploidy can then be offered chorionic villus sampling or genetic amniocentesis, depending on gestational age. Blood screening for Tay-Sachs, Canavan disease, and familial dysautonomia is offered to couples who are of Eastern European Jewish (Ashkenazi) descent. Couples of French-Canadian or Cajun ancestry should also be screened as possible Tay-Sachs carriers. Screening for cystic fibrosis is offered to all pregnant women. Hepatitis C antibody screening should be offered to pregnant women who are at high risk for infection.

Pregnant women with high-risk professions and those who are household contacts of a hepatitis B virus carrier or a hemodialysis patient and are HBsAg-negative at prenatal screening are at high risk for acquiring hepatitis B. They should be vaccinated during pregnancy. All women who are pregnant during flu season should receive vaccination for influenza regardless of gestational age.

Advice to Patients

A. Prenatal Visits

Prenatal care should begin early and maintain a schedule of regular prenatal visits: 0–28 weeks, every 4 weeks; 28–36 weeks, every 2 weeks; 36 weeks on, weekly.

B. Diet

Eat a balanced diet containing the major food groups.

1. Take prenatal vitamins with iron and folic acid. Supplements that are not specified for pregnant women should be avoided as they may contain dangerous amounts of certain vitamins.

2. Expect to gain 20–40 lb. Do not diet to lose weight during pregnancy.

3. Decrease caffeine intake to 0–1 cup of coffee, tea, or caffeinated cola daily.

4. Avoid eating raw or rare meat as well as fish known to contain elevated levels of mercury.

5. Eat fresh fruits and vegetables and wash them before eating.

C. Medications

Do not take medications unless prescribed or authorized by your provider.

D. Alcohol and Other Drugs

Abstain from alcohol, tobacco, and all recreational ("street") drugs. No safe level of alcohol intake has been established for pregnancy. Fetal effects are manifest in the **fetal alcohol syndrome**, which includes growth restriction; facial, skeletal, and cardiac abnormalities; and serious central nervous system dysfunction. These effects are thought to result from direct toxicity of ethanol as well as of its metabolites such as acetaldehyde.

Cigarette smoking results in fetal exposure to carbon monoxide and nicotine, and this is thought to eventuate in a number of adverse pregnancy outcomes. An increased risk of abruptio placentae, placenta previa, and premature rupture of the membranes is documented among women who smoke. Premature delivery occurs 20% more frequently among smoking pregnant women, and the birth weights of their infants are on average 200 g lighter than infants of nonsmokers. Women who smoke should quit smoking or at least reduce the number of cigarettes smoked per day to as few as possible. Clinicians should offer smoking cessation counseling during pregnancy, since women are more motivated to change at this time. Pregnant women should also avoid exposure to environmental smoke ("passive smoking").

Sometimes compounding the above effects on pregnancy outcome are the independent adverse effects of illicit drugs. Cocaine use in pregnancy is associated with an increased risk of premature rupture of membranes, preterm delivery, placental abruption, intrauterine growth restriction, neurobehavioral deficits, and sudden infant death syndrome. Similar adverse pregnancy effects are associated with amphetamine use, perhaps reflecting the vasoconstrictive potential of both amphetamines and cocaine. Adverse effects associated with opioid use include intrauterine growth restriction, prematurity, and fetal death.

E. Radiographs and Noxious Exposures

Avoid radiographs unless essential and approved by a physician. Abdominal shielding should be used whenever possible. Inform your dentist and your providers that you are pregnant. Avoid chemical or radiation hazards. Avoid excessive heat in hot tubs or saunas. Avoid handling cat feces or cat litter. Wear gloves when gardening.

F. Rest and Activity

Obtain adequate rest each day. Abstain from strenuous physical work or activities, particularly when heavy lifting or weight bearing is required. Regular exercise can be continued at a mild to moderate level. Avoid exhausting or hazardous exercises or new athletic training programs during pregnancy. Heart rate should be kept below 140 beats/min during exercise.

G. Birth Classes

Enroll with your partner in a childbirth preparation class well before your due date.

▶ Tests & Procedures

A. Each Visit

Weight, blood pressure, fundal height, fetal heart rate are measured, and a urine specimen is obtained and tested for protein and glucose. Review any concerns the patient may have about pregnancy, health, and nutrition.

B. 6–12 Weeks

Confirm uterine size and growth by pelvic examination. Document fetal heart tones (audible at 10–12 weeks of gestation by Doppler). Choices of aneuploidy screening should be discussed at this time (see above). First trimester screening (see Laboratory Tests, above) and transvaginal chorionic villus sampling are performed during this period.

C. 16–20 Weeks

The "quad screen" and amniocentesis are performed as indicated and requested by the patient during this time (see Laboratory Tests, above). Fetal ultrasound examination to determine pregnancy dating and evaluate fetal anatomy is also done. An earlier examination provides the most accurate dating, and a later examination demonstrates fetal anatomy in greatest detail. The best compromise is at 18–20 weeks of gestation.

D. 20–24 Weeks

Instruct patient about symptoms and signs of preterm labor and rupture of membranes. Consider cervical length measurement by ultrasound after 18 weeks with history of prior preterm delivery (> 2.5 cm is normal).

E. 24 Weeks to Delivery

Ultrasound examination is performed as indicated. Typically, fetal size and growth are evaluated when fundal height is 3 cm less than or more than expected for gestational age. In multiple pregnancies, ultrasound should be performed every 4–6 weeks to evaluate for discordant growth.

F. 24–28 Weeks

Screening for gestational diabetes is performed using a 50-g glucose load (Glucola) and a 1-hour post-Glucola blood glucose determination. Abnormal values ($\geq$ 140 mg/dL) should be followed up with a 3-hour glucose tolerance test (see Table 19–4).

G. 28 Weeks

If initial antibody screen is negative, repeat antibody testing for Rh-negative patients is performed, but the result is not required before $Rh_o(D)$ immune globulin is administered.

H. 28–32 Weeks

Repeat the complete blood count to evaluate for anemia of pregnancy. Screening for syphilis is also frequently performed at this time.

I. 28 Weeks to Delivery

Determine fetal position and presentation. Question the patient at each visit for symptoms or signs of preterm labor or rupture of membranes. Assess maternal perception of fetal movement at each visit. Antepartum fetal testing is performed as medically indicated.

J. 36 Weeks to Delivery

Repeat syphilis and HIV testing, cervical cultures for *N gonorrhoeae* and *Chlamydia trachomatis* should be performed in at-risk patients. Discuss with the patient the indicators of onset of labor, admission to hospital, management of labor and delivery, and options for analgesia and anesthesia. Weekly cervical examinations are not necessary unless indicated to assess a specific clinical situation. Elective delivery (whether by induction or cesarean section) prior to 39 weeks of gestation requires confirmation of fetal lung maturity.

The CDC has recommended universal prenatal culture-based screening for group B streptococcal colonization in pregnancy. A single standard culture of the distal vagina and anorectum is collected at 35–37 weeks. No prophylaxis is needed if the screening culture is negative. Patients whose cultures are positive receive intrapartum penicillin prophylaxis during labor. Except when group B streptococci are found in urine, asymptomatic colonization is not to be treated before labor. Patients who have had a previous infant with invasive group B streptococcal disease or who have group B streptococcal bacteriuria during this pregnancy should receive intrapartum prophylaxis regardless, so rectovaginal cultures are not needed. Patients whose cultures at 35–37 weeks were not done or whose results are not known should receive prophylaxis if they have a risk factor for early-onset neonatal disease, including intrapartum temperature greater than 38 °C, membrane rupture greater than 18 hours, or delivery before 37 weeks gestation.

The routine recommended regimen for prophylaxis is penicillin G, 5 million units intravenously as a loading dose and then 2.5 million units intravenously every 4 hours until delivery. In penicillin-allergic patients not at high risk for anaphylaxis, 2 g of cefazolin can be given intravenously as an initial dose and then 1 g intravenously every 8 hours until delivery. In patients at high risk for anaphylaxis, use vancomycin 1 g intravenously every 12 hours until delivery or, after confirmed susceptibility testing of group B streptococcal isolate, clindamycin 900 mg intravenously every 8 hours or erythromycin 500 mg intravenously every 6 hours until delivery.

K. 41 Weeks

Examine the cervix to determine the probability of successful induction of labor. Based on this, induction of labor is undertaken if the cervix is favorable (generally, cervix ≥ 2 cm dilated ≥ 50% effaced, vertex at −1 station, soft cervix, and midposition); if unfavorable, antepartum fetal testing is begun.

ACOG Committee on Genetics. ACOG Committee Opinion No. 298. Prenatal and preconceptional carrier screening for genetic diseases in individuals of Eastern European Jewish descent. Obstet Gynecol. 2004 Aug;104(2):425–28. [PMID: 15292027]

ACOG Committee on Practice Bulletins. ACOG Practice Bulletin No. 77: screening for fetal chromosomal abnormalities. Obstet Gynecol. 2007 Jan;109(1):217–27. [PMID: 17197615]

Kirkham C et al. Evidence-based prenatal care: Part I. General prenatal care and counseling issues. Am Fam Physician. 2005 Apr 1;71(7):1307–16. [PMID: 15832534]

NUTRITION IN PREGNANCY

Nutrition in pregnancy can affect maternal health and infant size and well-being. Pregnant women should have nutrition counseling early in prenatal care and access to supplementary food programs if necessary. Counseling should stress abstention from alcohol, smoking, and recreational drugs. Caffeine and artificial sweeteners should be used only in small amounts. "Empty calories" should be avoided, and the diet should contain the following foods: protein foods of animal and vegetable origin, milk and milk products, whole-grain cereals and breads, and fruits and vegetables—especially green leafy vegetables.

Weight gain in pregnancy should be 20–40 lb, which includes the added weight of the fetus, placenta, and amniotic fluid and of maternal reproductive tissues, fluid, blood, increased fat stores, and increased lean body mass. Maternal fat stores are a caloric reserve for pregnancy and lactation; weight restriction in pregnancy to avoid developing such fat stores may affect the development of other fetal and maternal tissues and is not advisable. Obese women can have normal infants with less weight gain (15–20 lb) but should be encouraged to eat high-quality foods. Normally, a pregnant woman gains 2–5 lb in the first trimester and slightly less than 1 lb/wk thereafter. She needs approximately an extra 200–300 kcal/d (depending on energy output) and 30 g/d of additional protein for a total protein intake of about 75 g/d. Appropriate caloric intake in pregnancy helps prevent the problems associated with low birth weight.

Rigid salt restriction is not necessary. While consumption of highly salted snack foods and prepared foods is not desirable, 2–3 g/d of sodium is permissible. The increased calcium needs of pregnancy (1200 mg/d) can be met with milk, milk products, green vegetables, soybean products, corn tortillas, and calcium carbonate supplements.

The increased need for iron and folic acid should be met from foods as well as vitamin and mineral supplements. (See section on anemia in pregnancy.) Megavitamins should not be taken in pregnancy, as they may result in fetal malformation or disturbed metabolism. However, a balanced prenatal supplement containing 30–60 mg of elemental iron,

0.5–0.8 mg of folate, and the recommended daily allowances of various vitamins and minerals is widely used in the United States and is probably beneficial to many women with marginal diets. There is evidence that periconceptional folic acid supplements can decrease the risk of neural tube defects in the fetus. For this reason, the United States Public Health Service recommends the consumption of 0.4 mg of folic acid per day for all pregnant and reproductive age women. Women with a prior pregnancy complicated by neural tube defect may require higher supplemental doses as determined by their providers. Lactovegetarians and ovolactovegetarians do well in pregnancy; vegetarian women who eat neither eggs nor milk products should have their diets assessed for adequate calories and protein and should take oral vitamin B_{12} supplements during pregnancy and lactation.

Eichholzer M et al. Folic acid: a public-health challenge. Lancet. 2006 Apr 22;367(9519):1352–61. [PMID: 16631914]
Yu CK et al. Obesity in pregnancy. BJOG. 2006 Oct;113(10):1117–25. [PMID: 16903839]

PREVENTION OF HEMOLYTIC DISEASE OF THE NEWBORN (Erythroblastosis Fetalis)

The antibody anti-Rh_o(D) is responsible for most severe instances of hemolytic disease of the newborn (erythroblastosis fetalis). About 15% of whites and much lower proportions of blacks and Asians are Rh_o(D)-negative. If an Rh_o(D)-negative woman carries an Rh_o(D)-positive fetus, antibodies against Rh_o(D) may develop in the mother when fetal red cells enter her circulation during small fetomaternal bleeding episodes in the early third trimester or during delivery, abortion, ectopic pregnancy, abruptio placentae, or other instances of antepartum bleeding. This antibody, once produced, remains in the woman's circulation and poses the threat of hemolytic disease for subsequent Rh-positive fetuses.

Passive immunization against hemolytic disease of the newborn is achieved with Rh_o(D) immune globulin, a purified concentrate of antibodies against Rh_o(D) antigen. The Rh_o(D) immune globulin (one vial of 300 mcg intramuscularly) is given to the mother within 72 hours after delivery (or spontaneous or induced abortion or ectopic pregnancy). The antibodies in the immune globulin destroy fetal Rh-positive cells so that the mother will not produce anti-Rh_o(D). During her next Rh-positive gestation, erythroblastosis will be prevented. An additional safety measure is the routine administration of the immune globulin at the 28th week of pregnancy. The passive antibody titer that results is too low to significantly affect an Rh-positive fetus. The maternal clearance of the globulin is slow enough that protection will continue for 12 weeks.

Hemolytic disease of varying degrees, from mild to serious, continues to occur in association with Rh subgroups (C, c, or E) or Kell, Kidd, and other factors. Therefore, the presence of atypical antibodies should be checked in the third trimester of all pregnancies.

Eder AF. Update on HDFN: new information on long-standing controversies. Immunohematology. 2006;22(4):188–95. [PMID: 17430078]

LACTATION

Breastfeeding should be encouraged by education throughout pregnancy and the puerperium. Mothers should be told the benefits of breastfeeding, including infant immunity, emotional satisfaction, mother-infant bonding, and economic savings. The period of amenorrhea associated with frequent and consistent breastfeeding provides some (although not completely reliable) birth control until menstruation begins at 6–12 months postpartum or the intensity of breastfeeding diminishes. If the mother must return to work, even a brief period of nursing is beneficial. Transfer of immunoglobulins in colostrum and breast milk protects the infant against many systemic and enteric infections. Macrophages and lymphocytes transferred to the infant from breast milk play an immunoprotective role. The intestinal flora of breastfed infants inhibits the growth of pathogens. Breastfed infants have fewer bacterial and viral infections, less severe diarrhea, and fewer allergy problems than bottle-fed infants and are less apt to be obese as children and adults.

Frequent breastfeeding on an infant-demand schedule enhances milk flow and successful breastfeeding. Mothers breastfeeding for the first time need help and encouragement from providers, nurses, and other nursing mothers. Milk supply can be increased by increased suckling and increased rest.

Nursing mothers should have a fluid intake of over 2 L/d. The United States RDA calls for 21 g of extra protein (over the 44 g/d baseline for an adult woman) and 550 extra kcal/d in the first 6 months of nursing. Calcium intake should be 1200 mg/d. Continuation of a prenatal vitamin and mineral supplement is wise. Strict vegetarians who eschew both milk and eggs should always take vitamin B_{12} supplements during pregnancy and lactation.

1. Effects of Drugs in a Nursing Mother

Drugs taken by a nursing mother may accumulate in milk and be transmitted to the infant (Table 19–2). The amount of drug entering the milk depends on the drug's lipid solubility, mechanism of transport, and degree of ionization.

2. Suppression of Lactation

A. Mechanical Suppression

The simplest and safest method of suppressing lactation after it has started is to gradually transfer the baby to a bottle or a cup over a 3-week period. Milk supply will decrease with decreased demand, and minimal discomfort ensues. If nursing must be stopped abruptly, the mother should avoid nipple stimulation, refrain from expressing milk, and use a snug brassiere. Ice packs and analgesics can be helpful. This same technique can be used in cases where suppression is desired before nursing has begun. Engorgement will gradually recede over a 2- to 3-day period.

B. Hormonal Suppression

Oral and long-acting injections of hormonal preparations were used at one time to suppress lactation. Because of

Table 19–2. Drugs and substances that require a careful assessment of risk before they are prescribed for breast-feeding women.[1]

Category	Specific Drugs or Compounds
Analgesic drugs	Meperidine, oxycodone
Antiarthritis drugs	Gold salts, methotrexate, high-dose aspirin
Anticoagulant drugs	Phenindione[2]
Antidepressant drugs and lithium	Fluoxetine, doxepin, lithium[2]
Antiepileptic drugs	Phenobarbital, ethosuximide, primidone
Antimicrobial drugs	Chloramphenicol, tetracycline
Anticancer drugs	All (eg, cyclophosphamide,[2] methotrexate,[2] doxorubicin[2])
Anxiolytic drugs	Diazepam, alprazolam
Cardiovascular and antihypertensive drugs	Acebutolol, amiodarone, atenolol, nadolol, sotalol
Endocrine drugs and hormones	Estrogens, bromocriptine[2]
Immunosuppressive drugs	Cyclosporine,[2] azathioprine
Respiratory drugs	Theophylline
Radioactive compounds	All
Drugs of abuse	All
Nonmedicinal substances	Ethanol, caffeine, nicotine
Miscellaneous compounds	Iodides and iodine, ergotamine,[2] ergonovine

[1]Reproduced with permission from Dershewitz RA, ed. *Ambulatory Pediatric Care*, LWW, 1999. Drugs for which there is no information are not included, although a careful risk assessment is necessary before such drugs are prescribed.
[2]The use of this drug or these drugs by breast-feeding women is contraindicated according to the American Academy of Pediatrics.

their questionable efficacy and particularly because of associated side effects such as thromboembolic episodes and hair growth, their use for this purpose has been abandoned. Similarly, lactation suppression with bromocriptine is to be avoided because of reports of severe hypertension, seizures, strokes, and myocardial infarctions associated with its use.

Britton C et al. Support for breastfeeding mothers. Cochrane Database Syst Rev. 2007 Jan 24;(1):CD001141. [PMID: 17253455]

TRAVEL & IMMUNIZATIONS DURING PREGNANCY

During an otherwise normal low-risk pregnancy, travel can be planned most safely between the 18th and 32nd weeks. Commercial flying in pressurized cabins does not pose a threat to the fetus. An aisle seat will allow frequent walks. Adequate fluids should be taken during the flight.

It is not advisable to travel to endemic areas of yellow fever in Africa or Latin America; similarly, it is inadvisable to travel to areas of Africa or Asia where chloroquine-resistant falciparum malaria is a hazard, since complications of malaria are more common in pregnancy.

Ideally, all immunizations should precede pregnancy. Live virus products are contraindicated during pregnancy (measles, rubella, yellow fever), including smallpox. Inactivated polio vaccine (IPV) should be given subcutaneously instead of the oral live-attenuated vaccine. Vaccines against pneumococcal pneumonia, meningococcal meningitis, and hepatitis A can be used as indicated. Influenza vaccine is indicated in all women who will be pregnant during "flu season." The CDC lists pregnant women as a high-risk group.

Hepatitis A vaccine contains formalin-inactivated virus and can be given in pregnancy when needed. Chloroquine can be used for malaria prophylaxis in pregnancy, and proguanil is also safe. Pooled immune globulin to prevent hepatitis A is safe and does not carry a risk of HIV transmission.

Water should be purified by boiling, since iodine purification may provide more iodine than is safe during pregnancy.

Do not use prophylactic antibiotics or bismuth subsalicylate during pregnancy to prevent diarrhea. Use oral rehydration, and treat bacterial diarrhea with erythromycin or ampicillin if necessary.

▼ OBSTETRIC COMPLICATIONS OF THE FIRST & SECOND TRIMESTER

VOMITING OF PREGNANCY (Morning Sickness) & HYPEREMESIS GRAVIDARUM (Pernicious Vomiting Of Pregnancy)

 ESSENTIALS OF DIAGNOSIS

▶ Morning or evening nausea and vomiting.

▶ Persistent vomiting severe enough to result in weight loss, dehydration, starvation ketosis, hypochloremic alkalosis, hypokalemia.

▶ May have transient elevation of liver enzymes.

▶ Appears related to high or rising serum hCG.

▶ More common with multiple gestation or hydatidiform mole.

▶ General Considerations

Nausea and vomiting begin soon after the first missed period and cease by the fifth month of gestation. Up to three-fourths of women complain of nausea and vomiting during early pregnancy, with the vast majority noting nausea throughout the day. This problem exerts no adverse effects on the pregnancy and does not presage other complications.

Persistent, severe vomiting during pregnancy—hyperemesis gravidarum—can be disabling and require hospitalization. Thyroid dysfunction can be associated with hyperemesis gravidarum, so it is advisable to determine thyroid-stimulating hormone (TSH) and free thyroxine (T_4) values in these patients.

▶ Treatment

A. Mild Nausea and Vomiting of Pregnancy

Reassurance and dietary advice are all that is required in most instances. Because of possible teratogenicity, drugs used during the first half of pregnancy should be restricted to those of major importance to life and health. Antiemetics, antihistamines, and antispasmodics are generally unnecessary to treat nausea of pregnancy. Vitamin B_6 (pyridoxine), 50–100 mg/d orally, is nontoxic and may be helpful in some patients.

B. Hyperemesis Gravidarum

With more severe nausea and vomiting, it may become necessary to hospitalize the patient. In this case, a private room with limited activity is preferred. Give nothing by mouth for 48 hours, and maintain hydration and electrolyte balance by giving appropriate parenteral fluids and vitamin supplements as indicated. Antiemetics such as promethazine (25 mg orally, rectally, or intravenously every 4–6 hours) and metoclopramide (10 mg orally or intravenously every 6 hours) should be started. Antiemetics will likely need to be given intravenously initially. Rarely, total parenteral nutrition may become necessary. As soon as possible, place the patient on a dry diet consisting of six small feedings daily plus clear liquids 1 hour after eating. Antiemetics may be continued orally as needed. After in-patient stabilization, the patient can be maintained at home even if she requires intravenous fluids in addition to her oral intake. There are conflicting studies regarding the use of corticosteroids for the control of hyperemesis gravidarum. Therefore, this treatment should be withheld until more accepted treatments have been exhausted.

▶ When to Refer

- Patient is unable to tolerate any food or water.
- There is concern for other pathology (ie, hydatidiform mole).
- Patient requires hospitalization.

▶ When to Admit

- Patient is unable to tolerate any food or water.
- Condition precludes the patient from ingesting necessary medications.
- Weight loss.
- Presence of a hydatidiform mole.

Bondok RS et al. Pulsed steroid therapy is an effective treatment for intractable hyperemesis gravidarum. Crit Care Med. 2006 Nov;34(11):2781–3. [PMID: 16957638]

Dodds L et al. Outcomes of pregnancies complicated by hyperemesis gravidarum. Obstet Gynecol. 2006 Feb;107(2 Pt 1):285–92. [PMID: 16449113]

SPONTANEOUS ABORTION

 ESSENTIALS OF DIAGNOSIS

- ▶ Intrauterine pregnancy at less than 20 weeks.
- ▶ Low or falling levels of hCG.
- ▶ Bleeding, midline cramping pain.
- ▶ Open cervical os.
- ▶ Complete or partial expulsion of products of conception.

▶ General Considerations

About three-fourths of spontaneous abortions occur before the 16th week; of these, three-fourths occur before the eighth week. Almost 20% of all clinically recognized pregnancies terminate in spontaneous abortion.

More than 60% of spontaneous abortions result from chromosomal defects due to maternal or paternal factors; about 15% appear to be associated with maternal trauma, infections, dietary deficiencies, diabetes mellitus, hypothyroidism, the lupus anticoagulant-anticardiolipin-antiphospholipid antibody syndrome, or anatomic malformations. There is no reliable evidence that abortion may be induced by psychic stimuli such as severe fright, grief, anger, or anxiety. In about one-fourth of cases, the cause of abortion cannot be determined. There is no evidence that video display terminals or associated electromagnetic fields are related to an increased risk of spontaneous abortion.

It is important to distinguish women with a history of incompetent cervix from those with more typical early abortion. Characteristically, incompetent cervix presents as "silent" cervical dilation (ie, with minimal uterine contractions) in the second trimester. Women with incompetent cervix often present with significant cervical dilation (2 cm or more) and minimal symptoms. When the cervix reaches 4 cm or more, active uterine contractions or rupture of the membranes may occur secondary to the degree of cervical dilation. This does not change the primary diagnosis. Factors that predispose to incompetent cervix are a history of incompetent cervix with a previous pregnancy, cervical conization or surgery, cervical injury, diethylstilbestrol (DES) exposure, and anatomic abnormalities of the cervix. Prior to pregnancy or during the first trimester, there are no methods for determining whether the cervix will eventually be incompetent. After 14–16 weeks, ultrasound may be used to evaluate the internal anatomy of the lower uterine segment and cervix for the funneling and shortening abnormalities consistent with cervical incompetence.

▶ Clinical Findings

A. Symptoms and Signs

1. Threatened abortion—Bleeding or cramping occurs, but the pregnancy continues. The cervix is not dilated.

2. Inevitable abortion—The cervix is dilated and the membranes may be ruptured, but passage of the products of conception has not yet occurred. Bleeding and cramping persist, and passage of the products of conception is considered inevitable.

3. Complete abortion—The fetus and placenta are completely expelled. Pain ceases, but spotting may persist.

4. Incomplete abortion—The cervix is dilated. Some portion of the products of conception (usually placental) remain in the uterus. Only mild cramps are reported, but bleeding is persistent and often excessive.

5. Missed abortion—The pregnancy has ceased to develop, but the conceptus has not been expelled. Symptoms of pregnancy disappear. There is a brownish vaginal discharge but no free bleeding. Pain does not develop. The cervix is semifirm and slightly patulous; the uterus becomes smaller and irregularly softened; the adnexa are normal.

B. Laboratory Findings

Pregnancy tests show low or falling levels of hCG. A complete blood count should be obtained if bleeding is heavy. Determine Rh type, and give $Rh_o(D)$ immune globulin if Rh-negative. All tissue recovered should be assessed by a pathologist and may be sent for genetic analysis in selected cases.

C. Ultrasonographic Findings

The gestational sac can be identified at 5–6 weeks from the last menstruation, a fetal pole at 6 weeks, and fetal cardiac activity at 6–7 weeks. Serial observations are often required to evaluate changes in size of the embryo. A small, irregular sac without a fetal pole with accurate dating is diagnostic of an abnormal pregnancy.

▶ Differential Diagnosis

The bleeding that occurs in abortion of a uterine pregnancy must be differentiated from the abnormal bleeding of an ectopic pregnancy and anovular bleeding in a nonpregnant woman. The passage of hydropic villi in the bloody discharge is diagnostic of hydatidiform mole.

▶ Treatment

A. General Measures

1. Threatened abortion—Place the patient on bed rest for 24–48 hours followed by gradual resumption of usual activities, with abstinence from coitus and douching. Hormonal treatment is contraindicated. Antibiotics should be used only if there are signs of infection.

2. Missed abortion—This calls for counseling regarding the fate of the pregnancy and planning for its elective termination at a time chosen by the patient and clinician. Insertion of laminaria to dilate the cervix followed by aspiration is the method of choice for a missed abortion. Prostaglandin vaginal tablets (misoprostol 800 mcg per vagina, repeated 3 days later if products of conception are not expelled) are an effective alternative.

B. Surgical Measures

1. Incomplete or inevitable abortion—Prompt removal of any products of conception remaining within the uterus is required to stop bleeding and prevent infection. Analgesia and a paracervical block are useful, followed by uterine exploration with ovum forceps or uterine aspiration. Regional anesthesia may be required.

2. Cerclage and restriction of activities—A cerclage is the treatment of choice for incompetent cervix, but a viable intrauterine pregnancy should be confirmed prior to placement of the cerclage.

A variety of suture materials including a 5-mm Mersilene band can be used to create a purse-string type of stitch around the cervix, using either the McDonald or Shirodkar method. Cerclage should be undertaken with caution when there is advanced cervical dilation or when the membranes are prolapsed into the vagina. Rupture of the membranes and infection are specific contraindications to cerclage. Cervical cultures for *N gonorrhoeae*, *Chlamydia*, and group B streptococci should be obtained and treated before elective placement of a cerclage.

▶ When to Refer

- Patient with history of two second-trimester losses
- Vaginal bleeding in a pregnant patient that resembles menstruation in a nonpregnant woman.
- Patient with an open cervical os.
- No signs of uterine growth in serial examinations of a pregnant patient.
- Leakage of amniotic fluid.

▶ When to Admit

- Open cervical os.
- Heavy vaginal bleeding.
- Leakage of amniotic fluid.

Maconochie N et al. Risk factors for first trimester miscarriage-results from a UK-population-based case-control study. BJOG. 2007 Feb;114(2):170–86. [PMID: 17305901]

Trinder J et al. Management of miscarriage: expectant, medical, or surgical? Results of randomized controlled trial (miscarriage treatment (MIST) trial). BMJ. 2006 May 27;332(7552):1235–40. [PMID: 16707509]

RECURRENT (Habitual) ABORTION

Recurrent abortion has been defined as the loss of three or more previable (< 500 g) pregnancies in succession. Recurrent abortion occurs in about 0.4–0.8% of all pregnancies. Abnormalities related to recurrent abortion can be identified in approximately half of the couples. If a woman has lost three previous pregnancies without identifiable cause, she still has a 70–80% chance of carrying a fetus to viability. If she has aborted four or five times, the likelihood of a successful pregnancy is 65–70%.

Recurrent abortion is a clinical rather than pathologic diagnosis. The clinical findings are similar to those observed in other types of abortion (see above).

Treatment

A. Preconception Therapy

Preconception therapy is aimed at detection of maternal or paternal defects that may contribute to abortion. A thorough general and gynecologic examination is essential. A random blood glucose test and thyroid function studies (including thyroid antibodies) should be done. Detection of lupus anticoagulant and other hemostatic abnormalities (proteins S and C and antithrombin III deficiency, hyperhomocysteinemia, anticardiolipin antibody, factor V Leiden mutations) and an antinuclear antibody test may be indicated. Endometrial tissue should be examined in the postovulation stage of the cycle to determine the adequacy of the response of the endometrium to hormones. The competency of the cervix must be determined and hysteroscopy or hysterography used to exclude submucosal myomas and congenital anomalies. Chromosomal (karyotype) analysis of both partners can be done to rule out balanced translocations (found in 5% of infertile couples).

Studies have focused on the major histocompatibility complex of chromosome 6, which carries HLA loci and other genes that may influence reproductive success. Some women demonstrate a lack of maternal antibody response to paternal lymphocytes, which is customarily found in normal women after successful childbearing. However, several randomized controlled trials have found no benefit of intravenous immunoglobulin therapy for recurrent spontaneous abortion.

B. Postconception Therapy

Provide early prenatal care and schedule frequent office visits. Bed rest is justified only for bleeding or pain. Empiric sex steroid hormone therapy is contraindicated.

Prognosis

The prognosis is excellent if the cause of abortion can be corrected or treated.

Stephenson M et al. Evaluation and management of recurrent early pregnancy loss. Clin Obstet Gynecol. 2007 Mar;50(1):132–45. [PMID: 17304030]

ECTOPIC PREGNANCY

ESSENTIALS OF DIAGNOSIS

▶ Amenorrhea or irregular bleeding and spotting.

▶ Pelvic pain, usually adnexal.

▶ Adnexal mass by clinical examination or ultrasound.

▶ Failure of serum level of hCG to double every 48 hours.

▶ No intrauterine pregnancy on transvaginal ultrasound with serum β-hCG of > 2000 mU/mL.

General Considerations

Ectopic implantation occurs in about one out of 150 live births. About 98% of ectopic pregnancies are tubal. Other sites of ectopic implantation are the peritoneum or abdominal viscera, the ovary, and the cervix. Any condition that prevents or retards migration of the fertilized ovum to the uterus can predispose to an ectopic pregnancy, including a history of infertility, pelvic inflammatory disease, ruptured appendix, and prior tubal surgery. Combined intrauterine and extrauterine pregnancy (heterotopic) may occur rarely. In the United States, undiagnosed or undetected ectopic pregnancy is currently the most common cause of maternal death during the first trimester.

Clinical Findings

A. Symptoms and Signs

They may be acute or chronic.

1. Acute (40%)—Severe lower quadrant pain occurs in almost every case. It is sudden in onset, lancinating, intermittent, and does not radiate. Backache is present during attacks. Shock occurs in about 10%, often after pelvic examination. At least two-thirds of patients give a history of abnormal menstruation; many have been infertile.

2. Chronic (60%)—Blood leaks from the tubal ampulla over a period of days, and considerable blood may accumulate in the peritoneum. Slight but persistent vaginal spotting is reported, and a pelvic mass can be palpated. Abdominal distention and mild paralytic ileus are often present.

B. Laboratory Findings

Blood studies may show anemia and slight leukocytosis. Quantitative serum pregnancy tests will show levels generally lower than expected for normal pregnancies of the same duration. If pregnancy tests are followed over a few days, there may be a slow rise or a plateau rather than the near doubling every 2 days associated with normal early intrauterine pregnancy or the falling levels that occur with spontaneous abortion. A progesterone level can also be measured to assess the viability of the pregnancy.

C. Imaging

Ultrasonography can reliably demonstrate a gestational sac 6 weeks from the last menstruation and a fetal pole at 7 weeks if located in the uterus. An empty uterine cavity raises a strong suspicion of extrauterine pregnancy, which can occasionally be revealed by transvaginal ultrasound. Specified levels of serum hCG have been reliably correlated with ultrasound findings of an intrauterine pregnancy. For example, an hCG level of 6500 mU/mL with an empty uterine cavity by transabdominal ultrasound is virtually diagnostic of an ectopic pregnancy. Similarly, an hCG value of 2000 mU/mL or more can be indicative of an ectopic pregnancy if no products of conception are detected within the uterine cavity by transvaginal ultrasound.

D. Special Examinations

With the advent of high-resolution transvaginal ultrasound, culdocentesis is rarely used in evaluation of possible ectopic pregnancy. Laparoscopy is the surgical procedure of choice both to confirm an ectopic pregnancy and in most cases to permit removal of the ectopic pregnancy without the need for exploratory laparotomy.

Differential Diagnosis

Clinical and laboratory findings suggestive or diagnostic of pregnancy will distinguish ectopic pregnancy from many acute abdominal illnesses such as acute appendicitis, acute pelvic inflammatory disease, ruptured corpus luteum cyst or ovarian follicle, and urinary calculi. Uterine enlargement with clinical findings similar to those found in ectopic pregnancy is also characteristic of an aborting uterine pregnancy or hydatidiform mole. Ectopic pregnancy should be suspected when postabortal tissue examination fails to reveal chorionic villi. Steps must be taken for immediate diagnosis, including prompt microscopic tissue examination, ultrasonography, and serial hCG titers every 48 hours. Patients must be warned about the complications of an ectopic pregnancy and monitored very closely.

Treatment

In a stable patient, methotrexate (50 mg/m²) intramuscularly—given as single or multiple doses—is acceptable medical therapy for early ectopic pregnancy. Favorable criteria are that the pregnancy should be less than 3.5 cm in largest dimension and unruptured, with no active bleeding and no fetal heart tones.

When a patient with an ectopic pregnancy is unstable or when surgical therapy is planned, the patient is hospitalized. Blood is typed and cross-matched. Ideally, diagnosis and operative treatment should precede frank rupture of the tube and intra-abdominal hemorrhage.

Surgical treatment is definitive. In a stable patient, diagnostic laparoscopy is the initial surgical procedure performed. Depending on the size of the ectopic pregnancy and whether or not it has ruptured, salpingostomy with removal of the ectopic or a partial or complete salpingectomy can usually be performed. Clinical conditions permitting, patency of the contralateral tube can be established by injection of indigo carmine into the uterine cavity and flow through the contralateral tube confirmed visually by the surgeon.

Iron therapy for anemia may be necessary during convalescence. Rh₀(D) immune globulin (300 mcg) should be given to Rh-negative patients.

Prognosis

Repeat tubal pregnancy occurs in about 12% of cases. This should not be regarded as a contraindication to future pregnancy, but the patient requires careful observation and early ultrasound confirmation of an intrauterine pregnancy.

When to Refer

* Severe abdominal pain.

* Palpation of an adnexal mass on pelvic examination.
* Abdominal pain and vaginal bleeding in a pregnant patient.

When to Admit

* Presence of symptoms or signs of a ruptured ectopic pregnancy; methotrexate use is contraindicated.

Alleyassin A et al. Comparison of success rates in the medical management of ectopic pregnancy with single-dose and multiple-dose administration of methotrexate: a prospective, randomized clinical trial. Fertil Steril. 2006 Jun;85(6):1661–6. [PMID: 16650421]

GESTATIONAL TROPHOBLASTIC DISEASE (Hydatidiform Mole & Choriocarcinoma)

 ESSENTIALS OF DIAGNOSIS

Hydatidiform Mole

▶ Amenorrhea.

▶ Irregular uterine bleeding.

▶ Serum hCG β-subunit > 40,000 mU/mL.

▶ Passage of grape-like clusters of enlarged edematous villi per vagina.

▶ Ultrasound of uterus with characteristic heterogeneous echogenic image and no fetus or placenta.

▶ Cytogenetic composition is 46,XX (85%), completely of paternal origin.

Choriocarcinoma

▶ Persistence of detectable hCG after mole evacuation

General Considerations

Gestational trophoblastic disease is a spectrum of disorders that includes hydatidiform mole, invasive mole, and choriocarcinoma. Partial moles generally show evidence of an embryo or gestational sac; are polyploid, slower-growing, and less symptomatic; and often present clinically as a missed abortion. Partial moles tend to follow a benign course, while complete moles have a greater tendency to become choriocarcinomas.

The highest rates of gestational trophoblastic disease occur in some developing countries, with rates of 1:125 pregnancies in certain areas of Asia. In the United States, the frequency is 1:1500 pregnancies. Risk factors include low socioeconomic status, a history of mole, and age younger than 18 or older than 40. Approximately 10% of women require further treatment after evacuation of the mole; 5% develop choriocarcinoma.

Clinical Findings

A. Symptoms and Signs

Excessive nausea and vomiting occur in over one-third of patients with hydatidiform mole. Uterine bleeding, beginning at 6–8 weeks, is observed in virtually all instances. In about one-fifth of cases, the uterus is larger than would be expected in a normal pregnancy of the same duration. Bilaterally enlarged cystic ovaries are sometimes palpable. They are the result of ovarian hyperstimulation due to excess of hCG.

Preeclampsia-eclampsia, frequently of the fulminating type, may develop during the second trimester of pregnancy, but this is unusual.

Choriocarcinoma may be manifested by continued or recurrent uterine bleeding after evacuation of a mole or following delivery, abortion, or ectopic pregnancy. The presence of an ulcerative vaginal tumor, pelvic mass, or evidence of distant metastatic tumor may be the presenting observation. The diagnosis is established by pathologic examination of curettings or by biopsy.

B. Laboratory Findings

Hydatidiform moles are generally characterized by high serum hCG β-subunit values which can range from high normal to the millions. Serum hCG values are more helpful in managing response to treatment than they are for diagnosis.

C. Imaging

Ultrasound has virtually replaced all other means of preoperative diagnosis of hydatidiform mole. Placental vesicles can be easily seen on transvaginal ultrasound. A preoperative chest film is indicated to rule out pulmonary metastases of the trophoblast.

▶ Treatment

A. Specific (Surgical) Measures

The uterus should be emptied as soon as the diagnosis of hydatidiform mole is established, preferably by suction. Ovarian cysts should not be resected nor ovaries removed; spontaneous regression of theca lutein cysts will occur with elimination of the mole.

If malignant tissue is discovered at surgery or during the follow-up examination, chemotherapy is indicated.

Thyrotoxicosis indistinguishable clinically from that of thyroid origin may occur. While hCG usually has minimal TSH-like activity, the very high hCG levels associated with moles result in the release of triidothyronine (T_3) and T_4 and cause hyperthyroidism. Patients who are thyrotoxic on this basis should be stabilized with β-blockers prior to induction of anesthesia. Surgical removal of the mole promptly corrects the thyroid overactivity.

B. Follow-Up Measures

Effective contraception (preferably birth control pills) should be prescribed. Weekly quantitative hCG level measurements are initially required. Following successful surgical evacuation, moles show a progressive decline in hCG. After two negative weekly tests (< 5 mU/mL), the interval may be increased to monthly for 6 months and then to every 2 months for a total of 1 year. If levels plateau or begin to rise, the patient should be evaluated by repeat chest film and dilatation and curettage (D&C) before the initiation of chemotherapy.

C. Antitumor Chemotherapy

For low-risk patients with a good prognosis, methotrexate is considered first-line therapy followed by dactinomycin (see Table 39–10). The side effects—anorexia, nausea and vomiting, stomatitis, rash, diarrhea, and bone marrow depression—usually are reversible in about 3 weeks and can be ameliorated by the administration of leucovorin (0.1 mg/kg) intramuscularly. Repeated courses of methotrexate 2 weeks apart generally are required to destroy the trophoblast and maintain a zero chorionic gonadotropin titer, as indicated by β-hCG determination. Patients with a poor prognosis should be referred to a cancer center, where multiple-agent chemotherapy probably will be given.

D. Supportive Measures

Oral contraceptives (if acceptable) or another reliable birth control method should be prescribed to avoid the hazard and confusion of elevated hCG from a new pregnancy. The hCG levels should be negative for 6 months to 1 year before pregnancy is again attempted. In the pregnancy following a mole, the hCG level should be checked 6 weeks postpartum.

▶ Prognosis

Five year survival after courses of chemotherapy, even when metastases have been demonstrated, can be expected in at least 85% of cases of choriocarcinoma.

▶ When to Refer

- Uterine size exceeds that anticipated for gestational age.
- Vaginal bleeding similar to menstruation.
- Pregnant patient with a history of a molar pregnancy.

▶ When to Admit

- Confirmed molar pregnancy by ultrasound and laboratory studies.
- Heavy vaginal bleeding in a pregnant patient under evaluation.

Golfier F et al. First epidemiological data from the French Trophoblastic Disease Reference Center. Am J Obstet Gynecol. 2007 Feb;196(2):172.e1–5. [PMID: 17306669]

Soper JT. Gestational trophoblastic disease. Obstet Gynecol. 2006 Jul;108(1):176–87. [PMID: 16816073]

▼ OBSTETRIC COMPLICATIONS OF THE SECOND & THIRD TRIMESTER

PREECLAMPSIA-ECLAMPSIA

 ESSENTIALS OF DIAGNOSIS

Preeclampsia

▶ Blood pressure of ≥ 140 mm Hg systolic or ≥ 90 mm Hg diastolic after 20 weeks of gestation.

▶ Proteinuria of ≥ 0.3 g in 24 hours.

Severe Preeclampsia

▶ Blood pressure of ≥ 160 mm Hg systolic or ≥ 110 mm Hg diastolic.

▶ Proteinuria ≥ 5 g in 24 hours or 4+ on dipstick.

▶ Thrombocytopenia.

▶ Hemolysis, elevated liver enzymes, low platelets (HELLP).

▶ Pulmonary edema.

▶ Fetal growth restriction.

Eclampsia

▶ Seizures in a patient with evidence of preeclampsia.

▶ General Considerations

Preeclampsia is defined as the presence of elevated blood pressure and proteinuria during pregnancy. Eclampsia is diagnosed when seizures develop in a patient with evidence of preeclampsia. Historically, the presence of three elements was required for the diagnosis of preeclampsia: hypertension, proteinuria, and edema. Edema was difficult to objectively quantify and is no longer a required element.

Preeclampsia-eclampsia can occur any time after 20 weeks of gestation and up to 6 weeks postpartum. It is a disease unique to pregnancy, with the only cure being delivery of the fetus and placenta. Preeclampsia-eclampsia develops in approximately 7% of pregnant women in the United States. Primiparas are most frequently affected; however, the incidence of preeclampsia-eclampsia is increased with multiple pregnancies, chronic hypertension, diabetes, kidney disease, collagen-vascular and autoimmune disorders, and gestational trophoblastic disease. Five percent of women with preeclampsia progress to eclampsia. Uncontrolled eclampsia is a significant cause of maternal death.

The cause of preeclampsia-eclampsia is not known. Epidemiologic studies suggest an immunologic cause for preeclampsia, since it occurs predominantly in women who have had minimal exposure to sperm (having used barrier methods of contraception) or have new consorts, in primigravidas, and in women both of whose parents have similar HLA antigens. Preeclampsia is an endothelial disorder resulting from poor placental perfusion, which releases a factor that injures the endothelium, causing activation of coagulation and an increased sensitivity to pressors. Before the syndrome becomes clinically manifest in the second half of pregnancy, there has been vasospasm in various small vessel beds, accounting for the pathologic changes in maternal organs and the placenta with consequent adverse effects on the fetus. Investigators have suggested an etiologic role for circulating angiogenic factors in preeclampsia based on studies in an animal model and in women with preeclampsia.

▶ Clinical Findings

Clinically, the severity of preeclampsia-eclampsia can be measured with reference to the six major sites in which it exerts its effects: the central nervous system, the kidneys, the liver, the hematologic and vascular systems, and the fetal-placental unit. By evaluating each of these areas for the presence of mild to severe preeclampsia, the degree of involvement can be assessed, and an appropriate management plan can be formulated that balances the severity of disease and gestational age (Table 19–3).

A. Preeclampsia

1. Mild —With mild preeclampsia, patients usually have few complaints, and the diastolic blood pressure is less than 110 mm Hg. Edema may be present. The platelet count is over 100,000/mcL, antepartum fetal testing is reassuring, central nervous system irritability is minimal, epigastric pain is not present, and liver enzymes are not elevated.

2. Severe—Symptoms are more dramatic and persistent. Patients may complain of headache and vision changes. The blood pressure is often quite high, with readings over 160/110 mm Hg. Thrombocytopenia (platelet counts < 100,000/mcL) may be present and progress to disseminated intravascular coagulation. Severe epigastric pain may be present from hepatic subcapsular hemorrhage with significant stretch or rupture of the liver capsule. HELLP syndrome (hemolysis, elevated liver enzymes, low platelets) is a form of severe preeclampsia.

B. Eclampsia

The occurrence of seizures defines eclampsia. It is a manifestation of severe central nervous system involvement. Other findings of preeclampsia are observed.

▶ Differential Diagnosis

Preeclampsia-eclampsia can mimic and be confused with many other diseases, including chronic hypertension, chronic kidney disease, primary seizure disorders, gallbladder and pancreatic disease, immune or thrombotic thrombocytopenic purpura, and hemolytic-uremic syndrome. It must always be considered a possibility in any pregnant woman beyond 20 weeks of gestation. It is particularly difficult to diagnose when a preexisting disease such as hypertension is present. Uric acid values can be quite helpful in such situations, since hyperuricemia is uncommon in pregnancy except with gout, kidney disease, or preeclampsia-eclampsia.

▶ Treatment

The use of diuretics, dietary restriction or enhancement, sodium restriction, aspirin, and vitamin-mineral supplements such as calcium or vitamin C and E have not been confirmed to be useful in clinical studies. The only cure is termination of the pregnancy at a time as favorable as possible for fetal survival. Magnesium sulfate should be given intravenously, 4- to 6-g load followed by 2–3 g/h maintenance, for seizure prophylaxis in patients with severe preeclampsia.

A. Preeclampsia

Early recognition is the key to treatment. This requires careful attention to the details of prenatal care—especially

Table 19–3. Indicators of mild versus severe preeclampsia-eclampsia.

Site	Indicator	Mild to Moderate	Severe
Central nervous system	Symptoms and signs	Hyperreflexia	Seizures Blurred vision Scotomas Headache Clonus Irritability
Kidney	Proteinuria Uric acid Urinary output	0.3–5 g/24 h ↑ > 4.5 mg/dL > 30 mL/h	> 5 g/24 h or catheterized urine with 4+ protein ↑↑ > 4.5 mg/dL < 30 mL/h
Liver	AST, ALT, LDH	Normal	Elevated LFTs Epigastric pain Ruptured liver
Hematologic	Platelets Hemoglobin	> 100,000/mcL Normal range	< 100,000/mcL Elevated
Vascular	Blood pressure Retina	< 160/110 mm Hg Arteriolar spasm	> 160/110 mm Hg Retinal hemorrhages
Fetal-placental unit	Growth restriction Oligohydramnios Fetal distress	Absent Absent Absent	Present Present Present

AST, aspartate aminotransferase; ALT, alanine aminotransferase; LDH, lactate dehydrogenase; LFTs, liver function tests.

subtle changes in blood pressure and weight. The objectives are to prolong pregnancy if possible, to allow fetal lung maturity while preventing progression to severe disease and eclampsia. The critical factors are the gestational age of the fetus, fetal pulmonary maturity, and the severity of maternal disease. Preeclampsia-eclampsia at term is managed by delivery. Prior to term, severe preeclampsia-eclampsia requires delivery with very few exceptions. Epigastric pain, severe range blood pressures, thrombocytopenia, and visual disturbances are strong indications for delivery of the fetus. Severe disease by protein alone can be managed more conservatively.

For mild preeclampsia, bed rest is the cornerstone of therapy. This increases central blood flow to the kidneys, heart, brain, liver, and placenta and may stabilize or even improve the degree of preeclampsia-eclampsia for a period of time.

Bed rest may be attempted at home or in the hospital. Prior to making this decision, the clinician should evaluate the six sites of involvement listed in Table 19–3 and make an assessment about the severity of disease.

1. Home management—Home management with bed rest may be attempted for patients with mild preeclampsia and a stable home situation. This requires assistance at home, rapid access to the hospital, a reliable patient, and the ability to obtain frequent blood pressure readings. A home health nurse can often provide frequent home visits and assessment.

2. Hospital care—Hospitalization is required for women with severe preeclampsia or those with unreliable home situations. Regular assessment of blood pressure, reflexes, urine protein, and fetal heart tones and activity are required. A complete blood count, platelet count, and electrolyte panel including liver enzymes should be checked every 1 or 2 days. A 24-hour urine collection for creatinine clearance and total protein should be obtained on admission and repeated as indicated. Magnesium sulfate is not used until the diagnosis of severe preeclampsia is made and delivery planned.

Fetal evaluation should be obtained as part of the workup. If the patient is being admitted to the hospital, fetal testing should be performed on the same day to assess fetal wellbeing. This may be done by fetal heart rate testing with nonstress or stress testing or by biophysical profile. A regular schedule of fetal surveillance must then be followed. Daily fetal kick counts can be recorded by the patient herself. Consideration can be given to amniocentesis to evaluate fetal lung maturity if hospitalization occurs at 30–37 weeks of gestation. If immaturity is suspected, corticosteroids (betamethasone 12 mg intramuscularly every 24 h for two doses, or dexamethasone 6 mg intramuscularly every 12 h for four doses) can be administered to the mother. Fetuses between 26 and 30 weeks of gestation can be presumed to be immature, and corticosteroids should be given.

The method of delivery is determined by the maternal and fetal status. A vaginal delivery is preferred because it has less blood loss than a cesarean section and requires less coagulation factors. Cesarean section is reserved for the usual fetal indications.

B. Eclampsia

1. Emergency care—If the patient is convulsing, she is turned on her side to prevent aspiration and to improve blood flow to the placenta. Fluid or food is aspirated from the glottis or trachea. The seizure may be stopped by giving an intravenous bolus of either magnesium sulfate, 4–6 g, or lorazepam, 2–4 mg over 4 minutes or until the seizure stops. Magnesium sulfate is the preferred agent, and alternatives should only be used if magnesium sulfate is unavailable. A continuous intravenous infusion of magnesium sulfate is then started at a rate of 2–3 g/h unless the patient is known to have significantly reduced kidney function. Magnesium blood levels are then checked every 4–6 hours and the infusion rate adjusted to maintain a therapeutic blood level (4–6 mEq/L). Urinary output is checked hourly and the patient assessed for signs of possible magnesium toxicity such as loss of deep tendon reflexes or decrease in respiratory rate and depth, which can be reversed with calcium gluconate, 1 g intravenously over 2 minutes.

2. General care—The occurrence of eclampsia necessitates delivery once the patient is stabilized. It is important, however, that assessment of the status of the patient and fetus take place first. Continuous fetal monitoring must be performed and blood typed and cross-matched quickly. A urinary catheter is inserted to monitor urinary output, and blood is tested for complete blood count, platelets, liver enzymes, uric acid, creatinine, and electrolytes. If hypertension is present with systolic values of ≥ 160 mm Hg or diastolic values ≥ 110 mm Hg, antihypertensive medications should be administered to reduce the blood pressure to 140–150/90–100 mm Hg. Lower blood pressures than this may induce placental insufficiency through reduced perfusion. Hydralazine given in 5- to 10-mg increments intravenously every 20 minutes is frequently used to lower blood pressure. Labetalol, 10–20 mg intravenously, every 20 minutes as needed, can also be used.

3. Delivery—Delivery is mandated once eclampsia has occurred. Vaginal delivery is preferred. The rapidity with which delivery must be achieved depends on the fetal and maternal status following the seizure and the availability of laboratory data on the patient. Oxytocin may be used to induce or augment labor. Regional analgesia or general anesthesia is acceptable. Cesarean section is used for the usual obstetric indications.

4. Postpartum—Magnesium sulfate infusion (2–3 g/h) should be continued until preeclampsia-eclampsia has begun to resolve postpartum (which may take 1–7 days), but in any case for at least 24 hours. The most reliable indicator of this resolution is the onset of diuresis with urinary output of over 100–200 mL/h. When this occurs, magnesium sulfate can be discontinued. Late-onset preeclampsia-eclampsia can occur during the postpartum period. It is usually manifested by either hypertension or seizures. Treatment is the same as prior to delivery—ie, with hydralazine and magnesium sulfate.

► When to Refer

- New onset of hypertension and proteinuria in a pregnant patient > 20 weeks gestation.

- New onset of seizure activity in a pregnant patient.
- Symptoms of severe preeclampsia in a pregnant patient with elevated blood pressure above baseline.

► When to Admit

- Evidence of severe preeclampsia or eclampsia.
- Evaluation for preeclampsia when severe disease is suspected.
- Evaluation for preeclampsia in a patient with an unstable home environment.

Levine R et al; CPEP Study Group. Soluble endoglin and other circulating antiangiogenic factors in preeclampsia. N Engl J Med. 2006 Sep 7;355(10):992–1005. [PMID: 16957146]
Sibai BM. Diagnosis, prevention, and management of eclampsia. Obstet Gynecol. 2005 Feb;105(2):402–10. [PMID: 15684172]

ACUTE FATTY LIVER OF PREGNANCY

Acute fatty liver of pregnancy is a disorder limited to the gravid state. It occurs in the third trimester of pregnancy and involves acute hepatic failure. With improved recognition and immediate delivery, the mortality rate is now 20–30%. The disorder is usually seen after the 35th week of gestation and is more common in primigravidas and those with twins. The incidence is about 1:14,000 deliveries.

The cause of acute fatty liver of pregnancy is not known. However, as many as 20% of cases may be due to a homozygous fetal deficiency of long-chain 3-hydroxyacyl-coenzyme A dehydrogenase (LCHAD) deficiency in a heterozygous mother.

► Clinical Findings

Pathologic findings are unique to the disorder, with fatty engorgement of hepatocytes. Clinical onset is gradual, with flu-like symptoms that progress to the development of abdominal pain, jaundice, encephalopathy, disseminated intravascular coagulation, and death. On examination, the patient shows signs of hepatic failure.

Laboratory findings show marked elevation of alkaline phosphatase but only moderate elevations of alanine aminotransferase (ALT) and aspartate aminotransferase (AST). Prothrombin time and bilirubin are also elevated. The white blood cell count is elevated, and the platelet count is depressed. Hypoglycemia may be extreme.

► Differential Diagnosis

The differential diagnosis is that of fulminant hepatitis. However, liver aminotransferases for fulminant hepatitis are higher (> 1000 units/mL) than those for acute fatty liver of pregnancy (usually 500–1000 units/mL). It is also important to review the appropriate history and perform the appropriate tests for toxins that cause liver failure. Preeclampsia may involve the liver but typically does not cause jaundice. The elevations in liver function tests in patients with preeclampsia usually do not reach the levels seen in patients with acute fatty liver of pregnancy.

Treatment

Diagnosis of acute fatty liver of pregnancy mandates immediate delivery. Supportive care during labor includes administration of glucose, platelets, and fresh frozen plasma as needed. Vaginal delivery is preferred. Resolution of encephalopathy occurs over days, and supportive care with a low-protein diet is needed.

Prognosis

Recurrence rates for this liver disorder are unclear but probably increased in families with proven LCHAD deficiency. Most authorities advise against subsequent pregnancy, but there have been reported cases of successful outcomes in later pregnancies.

Ko H et al. Acute fatty liver of pregnancy. Can J Gastroenterol. 2006 Jan;20(1):25–30. [PMID: 16432556]

PRETERM (Premature) LABOR

ESSENTIALS OF DIAGNOSIS

▶ Regular, rhythmic contractions 5 minutes apart.
▶ Contractions are painful and result in cervical change.
▶ Cervical effacement occurs.

General Considerations

Preterm (premature) labor is labor that begins before the 37th week of gestation; it is responsible for 85% of neonatal morbidity and mortality. Risk factors for preterm labor include a past history of preterm delivery, premature rupture of the membranes, urinary tract infection, exposure to DES, multiple gestation, and abdominal or cervical surgery. In high-risk women (prior preterm birth), ultrasound measurement of cervical length (< 25 mm) in the second trimester may also identify risk. Several prospective randomized controlled trials have failed to demonstrate a benefit of home uterine activity monitoring in preventing preterm birth.

Clinical Findings

Distinguishing true from false labor in patients with a history of previous preterm births can be facilitated by the use of fetal fibronectin measurement in cervicovaginal specimens. Its absence (< 50 ng/mL) in the face of uterine contractions in a patient with a previous preterm birth has a negative predictive value of 93–97% for delivery within 7–14 days.

Treatment

Patients must be educated to identify regular, frequent uterine contractions so they can be evaluated early and treatment initiated if necessary.

Numerous agents have been given in an attempt to stop preterm birth. **Magnesium sulfate** is commonly used. Magnesium sulfate is given intravenously as a 4- to 6-g bolus followed by a continuous infusion of 2–3 g/h. The rate may be increased by 1 g/h every 30 minutes to 2 hours until contractions cease or a maximum blood magnesium concentration of 6–8 mg/dL is reached. Magnesium levels are determined every 4–6 hours to monitor the blood level. After contractions have ceased for 12–24 hours, magnesium can be stopped and the situation reassessed.

β-**Adrenergic drugs** such as terbutaline have also been used. Terbutaline can be given as an intravenous infusion starting at 2.5 mcg/min and increased by 2.5 mcg/min every 20 minutes until contractions cease or until a maximum dose of 20 mcg/min is reached. Terbutaline can also be administered as subcutaneous injections of 250 mcg every 30 minutes up to 1 mg/4 h. Oral terbutaline therapy following parenteral treatment is often elected and consists of giving 2.5–5 mg every 4–6 hours. With terbutaline, a dose-related elevation of heart rate of 20–40 beats/min may occur. An increase of systolic blood pressure up to 10 mm Hg is likely, and the diastolic pressure may fall 10–15 mm Hg during the infusion. Transient elevation of blood glucose, insulin, and fatty acids together with slight reduction of serum potassium have been reported with β-adrenergic drugs. Fetal tachycardia may be slight or absent. No drug-related perinatal deaths have been reported with β-agonists. Maternal side effects requiring dose limitation are tachycardia (≥ 120 beats/min), palpitations, and nervousness. Fluids should be limited to 2500 mL/24 h. Serious side effects (pulmonary edema, chest pain with or without electrocardiographic changes) are often idiosyncratic, not dose-related, and warrant termination of therapy.

Nifedipine, 20 mg orally every 6 h, and indomethacin, 50 mg orally once then 25 mg orally every 6 h up to 48 h, have also been used with limited success. It is recommended that nifedipine not be given in conjunction with magnesium sulfate. Other tocolytics have been given simultaneously in an attempt to stop advanced preterm labor.

Before attempts are made to prevent labor with medication, the patient should be assessed for any conditions that would prompt iatrogenic preterm delivery. Severe preeclampsia, certain fetal anomalies, abruption, and intrauterine infection are all indications for preterm delivery. In these cases, it would be inappropriate to delay delivery with tocolytics.

In pregnancies between 24 and 34 weeks gestation where preterm birth is anticipated, betamethasone, 12 mg intramuscularly repeated once 24 hours later, or dexamethasone, 6 mg intramuscularly, repeated every 12 hours for four doses, is administered to hasten fetal lung maturation. Repeat courses are not recommended.

A prospective randomized controlled study has suggested that weekly injections of 17α-hydroxyprogesterone caproate from 16 to 36 weeks of gestation in women with a history of preterm delivery can reduce the rate of recurrent preterm birth.

When to Refer

- Contractions 5 minutes apart for > 2 hours.
- Rupture of membranes.
- Vaginal bleeding.

When to Admit

- Cervical dilation of ≥ 2 cm prior to 34 weeks gestation.
- Contractions that cause cervical change.
- Rupture of membranes.

Mackenzie R et al. Progesterone for the prevention of preterm birth among women at increased risk: a systematic review and meta-analysis of randomized controlled trials. Am J Obstet Gynecol. 2006 May;194(5):1234–42. [PMID: 16647905]

Spong CY. Prediction and prevention of recurrent spontaneous preterm birth. Obstet Gynecol. 2007 Aug;110(2 Pt 1):405–15. [PMID: 17666618]

THIRD-TRIMESTER BLEEDING

Five to 10 percent of women have vaginal bleeding in late pregnancy. The clinician must distinguish between placental causes (placenta previa, placental abruption, vasa previa) and nonplacental causes (infection, disorders of the lower genital tract, systemic disease). The approach to bleeding in late pregnancy should be conservative and expectant unless fetal distress or excessive maternal hemorrhage occurs.

The patient should be hospitalized and placed on bed rest with continuous fetal monitoring. A complete blood count (including platelets) should be obtained and two to four units of blood typed and cross-matched. Coagulation studies should be ordered as clinically indicated. Ultrasound examination should be performed to determine placental location. Digital pelvic examinations are done only after ultrasound examination has ruled out placenta previa. Continuous electronic fetal monitoring is required to assess for fetal distress. While uterine contractions, pain, or tenderness often indicate placental abruption, an ultrasound examination that is negative for retroplacental clot does not exclude it. In most cases, abruption is an indication for immediate delivery because of the high risk of fetal death. Hypertension is a known risk factor for abruption, and the patient should be assessed with this in mind. Other risk factors include multiparity, cocaine use, smoking, previous abruption, and thrombophilias.

Placenta previa occurs when the placenta grows over the internal cervical os. Its presence at term is an indication for cesarean section. If the patient presents with bleeding at less than 36 weeks of gestation, continued hospitalization and bed rest may be necessary, especially during the initial 7–10 days. If the patient lives in close proximity to the hospital, has immediate access to the hospital, can be on bed rest, and has complete resolution of bleeding and uterine contractions, home management may be considered. She must be well instructed and counseled regarding the risks. Patients with vaginal bleeding at less than 36 weeks of gestation should also be considered for amniocentesis to test for fetal lung maturity. Corticosteroid therapy is indicated if fetal lung maturity is not present.

Usta IM et al. Placenta previa-accreta: risk factors and complications. Am J Obstet Gynecol. 2005 Sep;193(3 Pt 2):1045–9. [PMID: 16157109]

▼ OBSTETRIC COMPLICATIONS OF THE PERIPARTUM PERIOD

PUERPERAL MASTITIS (See Also Chapter 17)

Postpartum mastitis occurs sporadically in nursing mothers shortly after they return home, or it may occur in epidemic form in the hospital. *Staphylococcus aureus* is usually the causative agent. Inflammation is generally unilateral, and women nursing for the first time are more often affected. Rarely, inflammatory carcinoma of the breast can be mistaken for puerperal mastitis.

Mastitis frequently begins within 3 months after delivery and may start with a sore or fissured nipple. There is obvious cellulitis in an area of breast tissue, with redness, tenderness, local warmth, and fever. Treatment consists of antibiotics effective against penicillin-resistant staphylococci (dicloxacillin or a cephalosporin, 500 mg orally every 6 hours for 5–7 days) and regular emptying of the breast by nursing followed by expression of any remaining milk by hand or with a mechanical suction device. Failure to respond to usual antibiotics within 3 days or the presence of an abscess should prompt consideration of resistant staphylococci (methicillin-resistant S aureus [MRSA]).

If the mother begins antibiotic therapy before suppuration begins, infection can usually be controlled in 24 hours. If delay is permitted, breast abscess can result. Incision and drainage are required for abscess formation. Despite puerperal mastitis, the baby usually thrives without prophylactic antimicrobial therapy.

CHORIOAMNIONITIS & ENDOMETRITIS

ESSENTIALS OF DIAGNOSIS

► Fever not attributable to another source.
► Uterine tenderness.
► Foul smelling vaginal discharge.
► Tachycardia in the mother or fetus, or both.

▶ General Considerations

Peripartum infection of the uterus is a common problem encountered during labor and postpartum. Uterine infection when still pregnant is referred to as chorioamnionitis, since the infection involves the chorion. Uterine infection after delivery is called endometritis, endomyometritis, or metritis. It is a polymicrobial infection most commonly attributed to urogential pathogens. Risk factors include cesarean section, prolonged labor, use of internal monitors, many pelvic exams, prolonged rupture of membranes, and lower genital tract infections.

▶ Clinical Findings

Chorioamnionitis and endometritis are diagnosed by the presence of fever (≥ 38 °C) in the absence of any other source and one or more of the following signs: maternal tachycardia, fetal tachycardia, foul-smelling lochia, and uterine tenderness. Cultures of the cervix are not done because of the polymicrobial nature of the infection.

▶ Treatment

Treatment is with broad-spectrum antibiotics that will cover gram-positive organisms and gram-negative organisms if still pregnant and gram-negative organisms and anaerobes if postpartum. A common regimen for chorioamnionitis is ampicillin, 2 g intravenously every 6 hours, and gentamicin, 2 mg/kg intravenous load then 1.5 mg/kg intravenously every 8 hours. A common regimen for metritis is gentamicin, 2 mg/kg intravenous load then 1.5 mg/kg intravenously every 8 hours, and clindamycin, 900 mg intravenously every 8 hours. Antibiotics are stopped when the patient has been afebrile for 24 hours. No oral antibiotics are given. Patients with metritis who do not respond in the first 24–48 hours may have enterococcus and require the addition of ampicillin to the regimen.

▼ MEDICAL CONDITIONS COMPLICATING PREGNANCY

ANEMIA

Plasma volume increases 50% during pregnancy, while red cell volume increases 25%, causing lower hemoglobin and hematocrit values, which are maximally changed around the 24th to 28th weeks. Anemia in pregnancy is often defined as a hemoglobin measurement below 10 g/dL or hematocrit below 30%. Anemia is very common in pregnancy, causing fatigue, anorexia, dyspnea, and edema. Prevention through optimal nutrition and iron and folic acid supplementation is desirable.

A. Iron Deficiency Anemia

Many women enter pregnancy with low iron stores resulting from heavy menstrual periods, previous pregnancies, breastfeeding, or poor nutrition. It is difficult to meet the increased requirement for iron through diet, and anemia often develops unless iron supplements are given. Red cells may not become hypochromic and microcytic until the hematocrit has fallen significantly. When this occurs, a serum iron level below 40 mcg/dL and transferrin saturation less than 10% are consistent with iron deficiency anemia (see Chapter 13). Treatment consists of a diet containing iron-rich foods and 60 mg of oral elemental iron (eg, 300 mg of ferrous sulfate) three times a day with meals. Iron is best absorbed if taken with a source of vitamin C (raw fruits and vegetables, lightly cooked greens). All pregnant women should take daily iron supplements.

B. Folic Acid Deficiency Anemia

Folic acid deficiency anemia is the main cause of macrocytic anemia in pregnancy, since vitamin B_{12} deficiency anemia is rare in the childbearing years. The daily require-

ment of folic acid doubles from 0.4 mg to 0.8 mg in pregnancy. Twin pregnancies, infections, malabsorption, and use of anticonvulsant drugs such as phenytoin can precipitate folic acid deficiency. The anemia may first be seen in the puerperium owing to the increased need for folate during lactation.

The diagnosis is made by finding macrocytic red cells and hypersegmented neutrophils in a blood smear (see Chapter 13). However, blood smears in pregnancy may be difficult to interpret, since they frequently show iron deficiency changes as well. Because the deficiency is hard to diagnose and folate intake is inadequate in some socioeconomic groups, 0.8–1 mg of oral folic acid is given as a supplement in pregnancy; the dose in established deficiency is 1–5 mg/d.

Good sources of folate in food are leafy green vegetables, orange juice, peanuts, and beans. Cooking and storage of food destroy folic acid. Strict vegetarians who eat no eggs or milk products should take vitamin B_{12} supplements during pregnancy and lactation.

C. Sickle Cell Anemia

Women with sickle cell anemia are subject to serious complications in pregnancy. The anemia becomes more severe, and crises may occur more frequently. Complications include infections, bone pain, pulmonary infarction, congestive heart failure, and preeclampsia. There is an increased rate of spontaneous abortion and higher maternal and perinatal mortality rates. Intensive medical treatment may improve the outcome for mother and fetus. Frequent transfusions of packed cells or leukocyte-poor washed red cells to lower the level of hemoglobin S and elevate the level of hemoglobin A is controversial. Management decisions should be made in conjunction with a maternal fetal medicine specialist and a hematologist.

Genetic counseling should be offered to patients with sickle cell disease or sickle trait. They may wish to undergo first-trimester chorionic villus biopsy or second-trimester amniocentesis to determine whether the abnormality has been passed to the fetus. Intrauterine devices and oral contraceptives are relatively contraindicated, but progestin-only contraceptives may be used. Women with sickle cell trait alone usually have an uncomplicated pregnancy except for an increased risk of urinary tract infection. Sickle cell-hemoglobin C disease in pregnancy is similar to sickle cell anemia and is treated similarly.

ACOG Committee on Obstetrics. ACOG Practice Bulletin No. 78: hemoglobinopathies in pregnancy. Obstet Gynecol. 2007 Jan;109(1):229–37. [PMID: 17197616]

LUPUS ANTICOAGULANT-ANTICARDIOLIPIN-ANTIPHOSPHOLIPID ANTIBODY SYNDROME

The presence of antibodies to phospholipids and a variety of clinical symptoms, including vascular thromboses, thrombocytopenia, and recurrent pregnancy loss, characterize the lupus anticoagulant-anticardiolipin-antiphospholipid antibody syndrome. Many of these patients have systemic lupus erythematosus–like symptoms but do not meet specific diagnostic criteria for that disease. The lupus anticoagulant and anticardiolipin antibody may occur in these patients, and both may cause arterial and venous thromboses. Detection of these antiphospholipid antibodies may require a combination of laboratory tests. The lupus anticoagulant will prolong both the partial thromboplastin time and the Russell viper venom time. The latter is a more sensitive predictor of disease. Such patients should also be screened for the presence of the factor V Leiden mutation. Anticardiolipin antibody may be detected with enzyme-linked immunosorbent assay (ELISA) testing. Either antibody may cause false-positive serologic tests for syphilis.

This syndrome may require treatment with anticoagulant medications. In a small number of patients with recurrent pregnancy loss and a diagnosis of lupus anticoagulant syndrome, improved outcomes have been reported following treatment with heparin anticoagulation (8000–20,000 units subcutaneously in two or three doses daily) or low-molecular-weight heparin (1 mg/kg subcutaneously twice daily) and low-dose (81 mg) aspirin begun before or early in pregnancy and continued until the postpartum period. The addition of monthly infusions of intravenous immunoglobulin to this regimen did not improve outcomes in such patients.

Petri M et al. Management of antiphospholipid syndrome in pregnancy. Rheum Dis Clin North Am. 2006 Aug;32(3):591–607. [PMID: 16880086]
Tincani A et al. Pregnancy, lupus and antiphospholipid syndrome (Hughes syndrome). Lupus. 2006;15(3):156–60. [PMID: 16634369]

THYROID DISEASE

Thyrotoxicosis during pregnancy may result in fetal anomalies, late abortion, or preterm labor, and fetal hyperthyroidism with goiter. Thyroid storm in late pregnancy or labor is a life-threatening emergency.

Radioactive isotope therapy must never be given during pregnancy. The thyroid inhibitor of choice is propylthiouracil, which acts to prevent further T_4 formation by blocking iodination of tyrosine. There is a 2- to 3-week delay before the pretreatment hormone level begins to fall. The initial dose of propylthiouracil is 100–150 mg orally three times a day; the dose is lowered as the euthyroid state is approached. It is desirable to keep free T_4 in the high normal range during pregnancy. A maintenance dose of 100 mg/d minimizes the chance of fetal hypothyroidism and goiter. While waiting for the propylthiouracil to take effect, the patient's symptoms can be treated with a β-blocker.

Recurrent postpartum thyroiditis occurs 3–6 months after delivery. A hyperthyroid state of 1–3 months' duration is followed by hypothyroidism, sometimes misdiagnosed as depression. Thyroperoxidase antibodies and thyroglobulin antibodies are present. Recovery is spontaneous in over 90% of cases after 3–6 months.

Maternal hypothyroidism may adversely affect the neuropsychological development of the child. Mothers with known or suspected hypothyroidism should have their TSH and free T_4 level measured at the first prenatal visit. It is not clear if there is a benefit to treating subclinical hypothyroidism. In patients with overt hypothyroidism, replacement therapy with levothyroxine should be adjusted to maintain levels of TSH in the normal range. Levels should be checked every 6-8 weeks. Because of the increased volume of distribution in pregnant women, it is likely that a woman will need a higher dose of levothyroxine than she would when she is not pregnant.

Casey BM et al. Thyroid disease in pregnancy. Obstet Gynecol. 2006 Nov;108(5):1283–92. [PMID: 17077257]

DIABETES MELLITUS

Pregnancy is associated with increased tissue resistance to insulin, resulting in increased levels of blood insulin as well as glucose and triglycerides. These changes are due to placental lactogen and elevated circulating estrogens and progesterone. Although pregnancy does not appear to alter the long-term consequences of diabetes, retinopathy and nephropathy may first appear or become worse during pregnancy. Debate continues over whether gestational diabetics are women whose glucose intolerance is solely a function of their pregnancy compared with their nonpregnant state. Alternatively, pregnancy may merely serve to unmask an underlying propensity for glucose intolerance, which will be evident even in the nonpregnant state at some time in the future if not in the immediate postpartum period. Indeed, 50% of women with gestational diabetes are diagnosed with overt diabetes at some point in their lifetime. The goals for glycemic control during pregnancy are the same whether the diagnosis is made before or during the pregnancy.

Prepregnancy counseling and evaluation of diabetic women should include a complete chemistry panel, HbA_{1c} determination, 24-hour urine collection for total protein and creatinine clearance, funduscopic examination, and an ECG. Any medical problems should be addressed, and HbA_{1c} levels of 6% should be achieved before pregnancy. Euglycemia should be established before conception and maintained during pregnancy with daily home glucose monitoring by the patient. A well-planned dietary program is a key component, with an intake of 1800–2200 kcal/d divided into three meals and three snacks. Insulin is given subcutaneously in a split-dose regimen with frequent dosage adjustments. Patients taking some oral agents prior to pregnancy should be switched to insulin. However, limited information suggests that agents such as glyburide may be safe and effective in pregnancy. The use of continuous insulin pump therapy has been found to be very useful during pregnancy in women with type 1 diabetes mellitus.

Congenital anomalies result from hyperglycemia during the first 4–8 weeks of pregnancy. They occur in 4–10% of diabetic pregnancies (two to three times the rate in nondiabetic pregnancies). Rates are even higher in women with excessive HbA_{1c} levels. Euglycemia in the early weeks of pregnancy, when organogenesis is occurring, reduces the rate of anomalies to near-normal levels. Even so, because few women with diabetes begin a rigorous program to achieve euglycemia until well after they have become pregnant, congenital anomalies are the principal cause of peri-natal fetal deaths in diabetic pregnancies. All women with diabetes should receive counseling about pregnancy and, when the decision has been made to start a family, should receive prepregnancy management by providers experienced in diabetic pregnancies.

Fasting and preprandial glucose values are lower during pregnancy in both diabetic and nondiabetic women. Euglycemia is considered to be 60–90 mg/dL while fasting and 30–45 minutes before meals and < 120 mg/dL 2 hours after meals. This is the target for good diabetic control during pregnancy. Glycated hemoglobin levels help determine the quality of glucose control both before and during pregnancy.

While perinatal problems for mother and baby are decreased by fastidious diabetic control, the incidence of hydramnios, preeclampsia-eclampsia, infections, and prematurity is increased even in carefully managed diabetic pregnancies. Diabetes is an inherently unstable disease characterized by fluctuations of blood glucose levels, particularly late in pregnancy. The risk of fetal demise in the third trimester (stillbirth) and neonatal death increases with the level of hyperglycemia. Consequently, pregnant women with diabetes must receive regular antepartum fetal testing (nonstress testing, contraction stress testing, biophysical profile) during the third trimester. The timing of delivery is dictated by the quality of diabetic control, the presence or absence of medical complications, and fetal status. The goal is to reach 39 weeks (38 completed weeks) and then proceed with delivery. Confirmation of lung maturity is necessary only for delivery prior to 39 weeks. Cesarean sections are performed for obstetric indications.

Because 15% of patients with gestational diabetes require insulin during pregnancy and because the infants of gestational diabetics have some risks similar to those of infants of diabetic mothers (particularly macrosomia), screening of women for glucose intolerance has been recommended between the 24th and 28th weeks of pregnancy (Table 19–4). Patients with gestational diabetes should be evaluated 6–8 weeks postpartum by a 2-hour oral glucose tolerance test (75 g glucose load).

ACOG Committee on Practice Bulletins. ACOG Practice Bulletin. Clinical Management Guidelines for Obstetrician-Gynecologists. Number 60, March 2005. Pregestational diabetes mellitus. Obstet Gynecol. 2005 Mar;105(3):675–85. [PMID: 15738045]

Hollander MH et al. Gestational diabetes: a review of the current literature and guidelines. Obstet Gynecol Surv. 2007 Feb;62(2):125–36. [PMID: 17229329]

Langer O. Oral anti-hyperglycemic agents for the management of gestational diabetes mellitus. Obstet Gynecol Clin North Am. 2007 Jun;34(2):255–74. [PMID: 17572271]

HYPERTENSIVE DISEASE

Hypertensive disease in women of childbearing age is usually essential hypertension, but secondary causes should be considered: coarctation of the aorta, pheochromocytoma, hyperaldosteronism, and renovascular and renal hypertension.

Preeclampsia is superimposed on 20% of pregnancies in hypertensive women and appears earlier, is more severe,

Table 19–4. Screening and diagnostic criteria for gestational diabetes mellitus.

Screening for gestational diabetes mellitus
1. 50-g oral glucose load, administered between the 24th and 28th weeks, without regard to time of day or time of last meal. Universal blood glucose screening is indicated for patients who are of Hispanic, African, Native American, South or East Asian, Pacific Island, or Indigenous Australian ancestry. Other patients who have no known diabetes in first-degree relatives, are under 25 years of age, have normal weight before pregnancy, and have no history of abnormal glucose metabolism or poor obstetric outcome do not require routine screening.
2. Venous plasma glucose measure 1 hour later.
3. Value of 140 mg/dL (7.8 mmol/L) or above in venous plasma indicates the need for a full diagnostic glucose tolerance test.
Diagnosis of gestational diabetes mellitus
1. 100-g oral glucose load, administered in the morning after overnight fast lasting at least 8 hours but not more than 14 hours, and following at least 3 days of unrestricted diet (> 150 g carbohydrate) and physical activity.
2. Venous plasma glucose is measured fasting and at 1, 2, and 3 hours. Subject should remain seated and should not smoke throughout the test.
3. Two or more of the following venous plasma concentrations must be equaled or exceeded for a diagnosis of gestational diabetes: fasting, 95 mg/dL (5.3 mmol/L); 1 hour, 180 mg/dL (10 mmol/L); 2 hours, 155 mg/dL (8.6 mmol/L); 3 hours, 140 mg/dL (7.8 mmol/L).

and is more often associated with intrauterine growth restriction. It may be difficult to determine whether or not hypertension in a pregnant woman precedes or derives from the pregnancy if she is not examined until after the 20th week. Serum uric acid can help differentiate, since it is elevated with preeclampsia and generally normal in chronic hypertension unless the patient is receiving diuretics. If hypertension persists for 6–8 weeks postpartum, essential hypertension is likely.

Pregnant women with chronic hypertension require medication only if the blood pressure is sustained at or above 150/100 mm Hg. For initiation of treatment, methyldopa has the longest record of safety in a starting dosage of 250 mg orally twice daily. Therapy with β-blockers or calcium channel blockers is also acceptable (see Tables 11–7, 11–9). The goal is to keep the blood pressure between 130-150/80-100 mm Hg.

If a hypertensive woman is being managed successfully by medical treatment when she registers for antenatal care, one may generally continue the antihypertensive medication. Diuretics, not usually started in pregnancy, may be continued in patients taking them prior to pregnancy. Angiotensin-converting enzyme inhibitors should be replaced with a drug of another class because of reports of fetal and neonatal kidney failure with these compounds.

Use of antihypertensive medications in preeclampsia remains controversial. This should be attempted only with significant fetal prematurity, absence of fetal compromise, and close supervision of the patient by a maternal fetal medicine specialist.

Therapeutic abortion may be considered in cases of severe hypertension during pregnancy. If pregnancy is allowed to continue, the risk to the fetus must be assessed periodically in anticipation of early delivery. An early first-trimester ultrasound examination will confirm the duration of pregnancy, and follow-up examinations after 26 weeks will evaluate intrauterine growth restriction.

Karthikeyan VJ et al. Hypertension in pregnancy: pathophysiology and management strategies. Curr Pharm Des. 2007;13(25):2567–79. [PMID: 17897001]

HEART DISEASE

Overall, 5% of maternal deaths are due to heart disease. Most heart disease complicating pregnancy in the United States is congenital heart disease. Normal pregnancy causes a faster pulse, an increase of cardiac output of more than 30%, and a rise in plasma volume greater than red cell mass with relative hemodilution. Vital capacity and oxygen consumption rise only slightly.

For practical purposes, the functional capacity of the heart is the best single measurement of cardiopulmonary status (see box, Functional Cardiac Assessment). In general, patients with class I or class II functional disability (80% of pregnant women with heart disease) do well obstetrically, with four-fifths of maternal deaths due to heart disease occurring in women with class III or class IV disability. Congestive failure is the usual cause of death. Most deaths occur in the early puerperium. Pregnancy is contraindicated in Eisenmenger complex, in primary pulmonary hypertension, in severe mitral stenosis with secondary pulmonary hypertension, and in Marfan syndrome, in which the aorta is prone to dissection and rupture. In addition, pregnancy is poorly tolerated in patients with aortic stenosis, aortic coarctation, tetralogy of Fallot, and active rheumatic carditis.

Therapeutic abortion and elective sterilization should be offered to patients with significant cardiac disease. Cesarean section should be performed only for obstetric indications. Women with valvular heart disease, mitral valve prolapse associated with mitral regurgitation, or idiopathic hypertrophic cardiomyopathy should receive appropriate antibiotic prophylaxis against infective endocarditis during labor and delivery or termination of pregnancy.

FUNCTIONAL CARDIAC ASSESSMENT

Class I   Ordinary physical activity causes no discomfort (perinatal mortality rate about 5%).

Class II   Ordinary activity causes discomfort and slight disability (perinatal mortality rate 10–15%).

Class III Less than ordinary activity causes discomfort or disability; patient is barely compensated (perinatal mortality rate about 35%).

Class IV   Patient decompensated; any physical activity causes acute distress (perinatal mortality rate over 50%).

Women intending to carry the pregnancy to term should be monitored in conjunction with a cardiologist. The first 24 hours postpartum, in particular, are a critical time in fluid management, and patients require close observation.

Drenthen W et al. Outcome of pregnancy in women with congenital heart disease: a literature review. J Am Coll Cardiol. 2007 Jun 19;49(24):2303–11. [PMID: 17572244]
Elkayam U et al. Valvular heart disease and pregnancy: part II: prosthetic valves. J Am Coll Cardiol. 2005 Aug 2;46(3):403–10. [PMID: 16053950]

ASTHMA

The effect of pregnancy on asthma is unpredictable. About 50% of patients have no change, 25% improve, and 25% get worse. Management of acute and chronic asthma during pregnancy does not differ significantly from that of nonpregnant women. The goal is to maintain maternal $PO_2 > 80$ mm Hg to sustain normal fetal oxygenation (see Chapter 9).

Namazy JA et al. Current guidelines for the management of asthma during pregnancy. Immunol Allergy Clin North Am. 2006 Feb;26(1):93–102. [PMID: 16443145]

SEIZURE DISORDERS

Epileptic women contemplating pregnancy who have not had a seizure for 5 years should consider a prepregnancy trial of withdrawal from treatment. Those with recurrent epilepsy should use a single drug with blood level monitoring. Commonly used antiepileptics have known teratogenicity. Selecting a medication should be based on the type of seizure disorder and the risks associated with each medication. Phenytoin and levetiracetam are often used. There is promising but limited information available on the safety of newer antiepilepsy drugs (eg, lamotrigine), and they should be used with caution.

Serum levels should be measured as needed, including in cases of ongoing seizure activity or suspected noncompliance. Pregnant women taking phenobarbital and phenytoin should receive vitamin supplements, including folic acid and vitamin D, throughout pregnancy. Oral vitamin K is administered during the last month of pregnancy. Infants should receive an injection of vitamin K_1 subcutaneously immediately after delivery and should have clotting studies 2–4 hours later. Breastfeeding is not contraindicated for infants of mothers taking antiseizure medications.

Tettenborn B et al. Management of epilepsy in women of childbearing age: practical recommendations. CNS Drugs. 2006;20(5):373–87. [PMID: 16696578]

INFECTIOUS CONDITIONS COMPLICATING PREGNANCY

URINARY TRACT INFECTION

The urinary tract is especially vulnerable to infections during pregnancy because the altered secretions of steroid sex hormones and the pressure exerted by the gravid uterus upon the ureters and bladder cause hypotonia and congestion and predispose to urinary stasis. Labor and delivery and urinary retention postpartum also may initiate or aggravate infection. *Escherichia coli* is the offending organism in over two-thirds of cases.

From 2% to 8% of pregnant women have asymptomatic bacteriuria, which some believe to be associated with an increased risk of preterm birth. It is estimated that pyelonephritis will develop in 20–40% of these women if untreated.

An evaluation for asymptomatic bacteriuria at the first prenatal visit is recommended for all pregnant women. If a urine culture is positive, treatment should be initiated. Nitrofurantoin (100 mg orally twice daily), ampicillin (250 mg orally four times daily), and cephalosporins (250 mg orally four times daily) are acceptable medications for 3–7 days. Sulfonamides should be avoided in the third trimester because they may interfere with bilirubin binding and thus impose a risk of neonatal hyperbilirubinemia and kernicterus. Fluoroquinolones are also contraindicated because of their potential teratogenic effects on fetal cartilage and bone. Patients with recurrent bacteriuria should receive suppressive medication (once daily dosing of an appropriate antibiotic) for the remainder of the pregnancy. Acute pyelonephritis requires hospitalization for intravenous administration of antibiotics and crystalloids until the patient is afebrile; this is followed by a full course of oral antibiotics.

Smaill F et al. Antibiotics for asymptomatic bacteriuria in pregnancy. Cochrane Database Syst Rev. 2007 Apr 18;(2):CD000490. [PMID: 17443502]

GROUP B STREPTOCOCCAL INFECTION

Group B streptococci frequently colonize the lower female genital tract, with an asymptomatic carriage rate in pregnancy of 5–30%. This rate depends on maternal age, gravidity, and geographic variation. Vaginal carriage is asymptomatic and intermittent, with spontaneous clearing in approximately 30% and recolonization in about 10% of women. Adverse perinatal outcomes associated with group B streptococcal colonization include urinary tract infection, intrauterine infection, premature rupture of membranes, preterm delivery, and postpartum endometritis.

Women with postpartum endometritis due to infection with group B streptococci, especially after cesarean section, develop fever, tachycardia, and abdominal distention, usually within 24 hours after delivery. Approximately 35% of these women are bacteremic.

Group B streptococcal infection is a common cause of neonatal sepsis. Transmission rates are high, yet the rate of neonatal sepsis is surprisingly low at less than 4:1000 live births. Unfortunately, the mortality rate associated with early-onset disease can be as high as 50% in premature infants and approaches 25% even in those at term. Moreover, these infections can contribute markedly to chronic morbidity, including mental retardation and neurologic disabilities. Late-onset disease develops through contact with hospital nursery personnel. Up to 45% of these health care workers can carry the bacteria on their skin and transmit the infection to newborns.

CDC recommendations for screening and prophylaxis for group B streptococcal colonization are set forth in this chapter in the section on tests and procedures.

Akker-van Marle ME et al. Cost-effectiveness of different treatment strategies with intrapartum antibiotic prophylaxis to prevent early-onset group B streptococcal disease. BJOG. 2005 Jun;112(6):820–6. [PMID: 15924544]

VARICELLA

Commonly known as chickenpox, varicella-zoster virus (VZV) infection has a fairly benign course when incurred during childhood but may result in serious illness in adults, particularly during pregnancy. Infection results in lifelong immunity. Approximately 95% of women born in the United States have VZV antibodies by the time they reach reproductive age. The incidence of VZV infection during pregnancy has been reported as up to 7:10,000.

The incubation period for this infection is 10–20 days. A primary infection follows and is characterized by a flu-like syndrome with malaise, fever, and development of a pruritic maculopapular rash on the trunk which becomes vesicular and then crusts. Pregnant women are prone to the development of VZV pneumonia, often a fulminant infection sometimes requiring respiratory support. After primary infection, the virus becomes latent, ascending to dorsal root ganglia. Subsequent reactivation can occur as zoster, often under circumstances of immunocompromise, although this is rare during pregnancy.

Two types of fetal infection have been documented. The first is congenital VZV syndrome, which typically occurs in 0.4–2% of fetuses exposed to primary VZV infection during the first trimester. Anomalies include limb and digit abnormalities, microphthalmos, and microcephaly.

Infection during the second and third trimesters is less threatening. Maternal IgG crosses the placenta, protecting the fetus. The only infants at risk for severe infection are those born after maternal viremia but before development of maternal protective antibody. Maternal infection manifesting 5 days before or after delivery is the time period believed to be most hazardous for transmission to the fetus.

Diagnosis is commonly made on clinical grounds. Laboratory verification of recent infection is made most often by antibody detection techniques, including ELISA, fluorescent antibody, and hemagglutination inhibition. Serum obtained by cordocentesis may be tested for VZV IgM to document fetal infection.

Varicella-zoster immune globulin (VZIG) has been shown to prevent or modify the symptoms of infection in some women but is no longer readily available. Treatment success depends on identification of susceptible women at or just following exposure. Women with a questionable or negative history of chickenpox should be checked for antibody, since the overwhelming majority will have been previously exposed. If the antibody is negative, VZIG (625 units intramuscularly) should be given within 96 hours after exposure. There are no known adverse effects of

VZIG administration during pregnancy, although the incubation period for disease can be lengthened. Infants born within 5 days after onset of maternal infection should also receive VZIG (125 units).

Infected pregnant women should be closely observed and hospitalized at the earliest signs of pulmonary involvement. Intravenous acyclovir (10 mg/kg intravenously every 8 hours) is recommended in the treatment of VZV pneumonia.

Tan MP et al. Chickenpox in pregnancy: revisited. Reprod Toxicol. 2006 May;21(4):410–20. [PMID: 15979274]

TUBERCULOSIS

The diagnosis of tuberculosis in pregnancy is made by history taking, physical examination, and skin testing, with special attention to women in high-risk groups. Women at high risk include those who are from endemic areas, those infected with HIV, drug users, health care workers, and close contacts of people with tuberculosis. Chest radiographs should not be obtained as a routine screening measure in pregnancy but should be used only in patients with a skin test conversion or with suggestive findings in the history and physical examination. Abdominal shielding must be used if a chest radiograph is obtained.

Decisions on treatment depend on whether the patient has active disease or is at high risk for progression to active disease. Women who are PPD positive but not at high risk for disease progression can receive treatment postpartum, which does not preclude breastfeeding. The concentration of medication in breast milk is neither toxic nor adequate for treatment of the newborn. Treatment is with isoniazid and ethambutol or isoniazid and rifampin (see Chapters 9 and 33). Because isoniazid therapy may result in vitamin B_6 deficiency, a supplement of 50 mg/d of vitamin B_6 should be given simultaneously. Isoniazid, particularly in pregnant women, can cause hepatitis. Liver function tests should be performed regularly in pregnant women who receive treatment. Streptomycin, ethionamide, and most other antituberculous drugs should be avoided in pregnancy. If adequately treated, tuberculosis in pregnancy has an excellent prognosis.

HIV/AIDS DURING PREGNANCY

Heterosexual acquisition and injection drug use are the principal identified modes of HIV infection in women. Asymptomatic infection is associated with a normal pregnancy rate and no increased risk of adverse pregnancy outcomes. There is no evidence that pregnancy causes AIDS progression.

Previously, two-thirds of HIV-positive neonates acquired their infection close to, or during, the time of delivery. Routine HIV screening in pregnancy, including the use of rapid HIV tests in Labor and Delivery units, and the use of highly active antiretroviral therapy (HAART) therapy has markedly reduced this transmission risk. Zidovudine alone (500 mg/d orally) given to the mother antenatally starting at 14 weeks of gestation and during labor (1 mg/kg/h intravenously) and then to the infant (2 mg/kg orally four times daily) for the first 6 weeks of life reduces the transmission rate

from 25% to 8%. HAART reduced the risk even further, to approximately 2%, and has become the standard of care risk. HIV-positive pregnant women should be assessed by CD4 count, plasma RNA levels, resistance testing, and prior or current antiretroviral use. They should also be tested for hepatitis C, toxoplasmosis, and cytomegalovirus.

Pregnant HIV-positive women should be offered HAART with three drugs (commonly two nucleoside analogues and one protease inhibitor, including zidovudine whenever possible) after counseling regarding the potential impact of therapy on both mother and fetus. HAART should be offered regardless of viral load and CD4 count. The majority of drugs used to treat HIV/AIDS have thus far proven to be safe in pregnancy with an acceptable risk/benefit ratio. Efavirenz has been clearly linked with anomalies (myelomeningocele) and should not be used in pregnancy.

The use of prophylactic elective cesarean section before the onset of labor or rupture of the membranes to prevent vertical transmission of HIV infection from mother to fetus has been shown to further reduce the transmission rate. There is limited information on the impact of elective cesarean section on transmission rates in infants of mothers on HAART or with viral loads less than 1000 copies/mL. However, with HAART therapy and undetectable viral loads (< 50 copies/mL), the transmission risk has been estimated to be 1% or less and there may be no additional benefit of cesarean delivery. Women with viral loads less than 1000 copies/mL on HAART can be offered a vaginal delivery. Amniotomy should not be performed and internal monitors, particularly the fetal scalp electrode, should be avoided. HIV-infected women should be advised not to breastfeed their infants.

The Public Health Task Force provides guidelines for the management of HIV/AIDS in pregnancy that are regularly updated and available at http://www.aidsinfo.nih.gov/.

Centers for Disease Control and Prevention (CDC). Achievements in public health. Reduction in perinatal transmission of HIV infection—United States, 1985–2005. MMWR Morb Mortal Wkly Rep. 2006 Jun 2;55(21):592–7. [PMID: 16741495]

Public Health Service Task Force Recommendations for Use of Antiretroviral Drugs in Pregnant HIV-1 Infected Women for Maternal Health and Interventions to Reduce Perinatal HIV-1 Transmission in the United States, October, 2006. http://www.hivatis.org.

MATERNAL HEPATITIS B & C CARRIER STATE

There are an estimated 200 million chronic carriers of hepatitis B virus worldwide. Among these people there is an increased incidence of chronic active hepatitis, cirrhosis, and hepatocellular carcinoma. The frequency of the hepatitis B carrier state varies from 1% in the United States and Western Europe to 35% in parts of Africa and Asia. All pregnant women should be screened for HBsAg. Transmission of the virus to the baby after delivery is likely if both surface antigen and e antigen are positive. Vertical transmission can be blocked by the immediate postdelivery administration to the newborn of 0.5 mL hepatitis B immunoglobulin and hepatitis B vaccine intramuscularly. The vaccine dose is repeated at 1 and 6 months of age.

Successful, but limited, experience has also been reported with lamivudine (150 mg/d) during the last 4 weeks of gestation to prevent vertical transmission of hepatitis B in mothers with high HBV viral loads.

Hepatitis C virus infection is the most common chronic blood-borne infection in the United States. Risk factors for transmission include blood transfusion, injection drug use, employment in patient care or clinical laboratory work, exposure to a sex partner or household member who has had a history of hepatitis, exposure to multiple sex partners, and low socioeconomic level. The average rate of hepatitis C virus (HCV) infection among infants born to HCV-positive, HIV-negative women is 5–6%. However, the average infection rate increases to 14% when mothers are coinfected with HCV and HIV. The principal factor associated with transmission is the presence of HCV RNA in the mother at the time of birth.

Lee C et al. Effect of hepatitis B immunisation in newborn infants of mothers positive for hepatitis B surface antigen: systematic review and meta-analysis. BMJ. 2006 Feb 11;332(7537):328–36. [PMID: 16443611]

HERPES GENITALIS

Infection of the lower genital tract by herpes simplex virus type 2 (HSV-2) (see also Chapter 6) is a common STD of potential seriousness to pregnant women and their newborn infants. Although up to 20% of women in an obstetric practice may have antibodies to HSV-2, a history of the infection is unreliable and the incidence of neonatal infection is low (1:20,000–1:3000 live births). Most infected neonates are born to women with no symptoms, signs, or history of infection.

Women who have had *primary* herpes infection late in pregnancy are at high risk for shedding virus at delivery. Some authors suggest use of prophylactic acyclovir, 400 mg orally twice daily, to decrease the likelihood of active lesions at the time of labor and delivery.

Women with a history of *recurrent* genital herpes have a neonatal attack rate of ≤ 5% and should be monitored by clinical observation and culture of any suspicious lesions. Since asymptomatic viral shedding is not predictable by antepartum cultures, current recommendations do not include routine cultures in individuals with a history of herpes without active disease. However, when labor begins, vulvar and cervical inspection should be performed. Cesarean section is indicated at the time of labor if there are prodromal symptoms, active genital lesions, or a positive cervical culture obtained within the preceding week.

For treatment, see Chapter 32. The use of acyclovir in pregnancy is acceptable, and prophylaxis starting at 36 weeks gestation has been shown to decrease the number of cesarean sections performed for active disease.

Andrews WW et al. Valacyclovir therapy to reduce recurrent genital herpes in pregnant women. Am J Obstet Gynecol. 2006 Mar;194(3):774–81. [PMID: 16522412]

Gardella C et al. Managing genital herpes infections in pregnancy. Cleve Clin J Med. 2007 Mar;74(3):217–24. [PMID: 17375803]

SYPHILIS, GONORRHEA, & *CHLAMYDIA TRACHOMATIS* INFECTION (See Also Chapters 33 and 34)

These STDs have significant consequences for mother and child. Untreated syphilis in pregnancy can cause late abortion, stillbirth, transplacental infection, and congenital syphilis. Gonorrhea can produce large-joint arthritis by hematogenous spread as well as ophthalmia neonatorum. Maternal chlamydial infections are largely asymptomatic but are manifested in the newborn by inclusion conjunctivitis and, at age 2–4 months, by pneumonia. The diagnosis of each can be reliably made by appropriate laboratory tests. All women should be tested for syphilis as part of their routine prenatal care. Women at risk should be tested for gonorrhea and chlamydia. The sexual partners of women with STDs should be identified and treated also if possible; the local health department can assist.

Centers for Disease Control and Prevention. Sexually transmitted disease treatment guidelines 2006. MMWR Recomm Rep. 2006 Aug 4;55(RR-11):1–94. [PMID: 16888612]

SURGICAL COMPLICATIONS DURING PREGNANCY

Elective major surgery should be avoided during pregnancy. Normal uncomplicated pregnancy does not alter operative risk except as it may interfere with the diagnosis of abdominal disorders and increase the technical problems of intra-abdominal surgery. Abortion is not a serious hazard after operation unless peritoneal sepsis or other significant complications occur. During the first trimester, congenital anomalies may theoretically be induced in the developing fetus. Thus, the second trimester is usually the optimal time for operative procedures.

CHOLEDOCHOLITHIASIS, CHOLECYSTITIS, & IDIOPATHIC CHOLESTASIS OF PREGNANCY

Severe choledocholithiasis and cholecystitis are not uncommon during pregnancy. They usually occur in late pregnancy or in the puerperium. About 90% of patients with cholecystitis have gallstones; 90% of stones will be visualized by ultrasonography. Symptomatic relief may be all that is required.

Conventional gallbladder surgery by laparotomy or laparoscopy in pregnant women should be performed when indicated. Traditionally, surgery is considered safest in the second trimester, but it has been successfully performed in all stages of pregnancy. Withholding surgery may result in necrosis and perforation of the gallbladder, pancreatitis, and peritonitis. Cholangitis due to impacted bile duct stone requires surgical removal of gallstones and establishment of biliary drainage. Endoscopic retrograde cholangiopancreatography and endoscopic retrograde sphincterotomy can be performed safely in pregnant women if precautions are taken to minimize exposure to radiation. In the early to mid second trimester, laparoscopic cholecystectomy can be performed with minimal maternal morbidity and fetal mortality.

Idiopathic cholestasis of pregnancy is due to a hereditary metabolic (hepatic) deficiency aggravated by the high estrogen levels of pregnancy. It causes intrahepatic biliary obstruction of varying degrees. The rise in serum bile acids is sufficient in the third trimester to cause severe, intractable, generalized itching and sometimes clinical jaundice. There may be mild elevations in blood bilirubin and alkaline phosphatase levels. The fetus is also threatened by this condition. An increased incidence of preterm delivery has been reported as well as unexplained intrauterine fetal demise. For this reason, antenatal surveillance of the fetus is needed in patients with this diagnosis. Resins such as cholestyramine (4 g orally three times a day) absorb bile acids in the large bowel and relieve pruritus but are difficult to take and may cause constipation. Their use requires vitamin K supplementation. Very encouraging experience has been reported with ursodeoxycholic acid, 8–10 mg/kg/d. The disorder is relieved once the infant has been delivered, but it recurs in subsequent pregnancies and sometimes with the use of oral contraceptives.

APPENDICITIS

Appendicitis occurs in about 1 of 1500 pregnancies. Diagnosis may be difficult, since the appendix is often carried high and to the right, away from McBurney point, as the uterus enlarges, and localization of pain does not always occur. Nausea, vomiting, fever, and leukocytosis occur regularly. Any right-sided abdominal pain associated with these symptoms should arouse suspicion. In at least 20% of obstetric patients, the diagnosis of appendicitis is not made until rupture occurs and peritonitis has become established. Such a delay may lead to premature labor or abortion. With early diagnosis and appendectomy, the prognosis is good for mother and baby.

Parangi S et al. Surgical gastrointestinal disorders during pregnancy. Am J Surg. 2007 Feb;193(2):223–32. [PMID: 17236852]

CARCINOMA OF THE BREAST

Cancer of the breast (see also Chapter 17) is diagnosed approximately once in 3500 pregnancies. Pregnancy may accelerate the growth of cancer of the breast, and delay in diagnosis affects the outcome of treatment. Inflammatory carcinoma is an extremely virulent type of breast cancer that occurs most commonly during lactation. Prepregnancy mammography should be encouraged for women over age 35 who are anticipating a pregnancy.

Breast enlargement during pregnancy obscures parenchymal masses, and breast tissue hyperplasia decreases the accuracy of mammography. Any discrete mass should be evaluated by aspiration to verify its cystic structure, with fine-needle biopsy if it is solid. A definitive diagnosis may require excisional biopsy under local anesthesia. If breast biopsy confirms the diagnosis of cancer, surgery should be done regardless of the stage of the pregnancy. If spread to the regional glands has occurred, irradiation or chemotherapy should be considered. Under these circumstances, the alternatives are termination of an early pregnancy or delay of therapy for fetal maturation.

OVARIAN TUMORS

The most common adnexal mass in early pregnancy is the corpus luteum, which may become cystic and enlarge to 6 cm in diameter. Any persistent mass should be evaluated by ultrasound examination; unilocular cysts are likely to be corpus luteum cysts, whereas septated or semisolid tumors are likely to be neoplasms. The incidence of malignancy in ovarian masses over 6 cm in diameter is 2.5%. Ovarian tumors may undergo torsion and cause abdominal pain and nausea and vomiting and must be differentiated from appendicitis, other bowel disease, and ectopic pregnancy. Patients with suspected ovarian cancer should be referred to a tertiary perinatal center to determine whether the pregnancy can progress to fetal viability or whether treatment should be instituted without delay. There is a paucity of data regarding the removal adnexal masses in pregnancy. It should certainly receive strong consideration in cases where the mass is suspicious for malignancy. If the decision is made to remove the adnexal mass, the second trimester of pregnancy is considered the best time. Removal of a large corpus luteum cyst in the first trimester requires progesterone supplementation and should be avoided.

Giuntoli RL et al. Evaluation and management of adnexal masses during pregnancy. Clin Obstet Gynecol. 2006 Sep;49(3):492–505. [PMID: 16885656]

Musculoskeletal & Immunologic Disorders

David B. Hellmann, MD, MACP

John B. Imboden Jr., MD

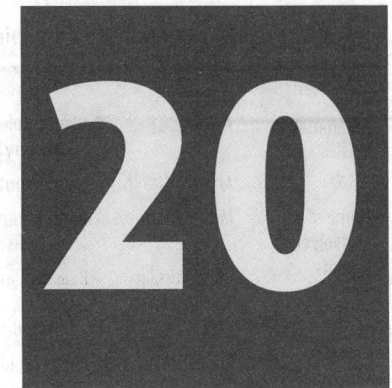

► Diagnosis & Evaluation

A. Examination of the Patient

In the patient with arthritis, the two clinical clues most helpful for diagnosis are the joint pattern and the presence or absence of extra-articular manifestations. The joint pattern is defined by the answers to three questions: (1) Is inflammation present? (2) How many joints are involved? and (3) What joints are affected? Joint inflammation manifests as redness, warmth, swelling, and morning stiffness of at least 30 minutes' duration. Both the number of affected joints and the specific sites of involvement affect the differential diagnosis (Table 20–1). Some diseases—gout, for example—are characteristically monarticular, whereas other diseases, such as rheumatoid arthritis, are usually polyarticular. The location of joint involvement can also be distinctive. Only two diseases frequently cause prominent involvement of the distal interphalangeal (DIP) joint: osteoarthritis and psoriatic arthritis. Extra-articular manifestations such as fever (eg, gout, Still disease, endocarditis), rash (eg, systemic lupus erythematosus, psoriatic arthritis, Still disease), nodules (eg, rheumatoid arthritis, gout), or neuropathy (eg, polyarteritis nodosa, Wegener granulomatosis) narrow the differential diagnosis further.

B. Arthrocentesis and Examination of Joint Fluid

If the diagnosis is uncertain, synovial fluid should be examined whenever possible (Table 20–2). Most large joints are easily aspirated, and contraindications to arthrocentesis are few. The aspirating needle should never be passed through an overlying cellulitis or psoriatic plaque because of the risk of introducing infection. For patients who are receiving long-term anticoagulation therapy with warfarin, joints can be aspirated with a small-gauge needle (eg, 22F) if the international normalized ratio (INR) is less than 3.0.

1. Types of studies

A. Gross examination—Clarity is an approximate guide to the degree of inflammation. Noninflammatory fluid is transparent, mild inflammation produces translucent fluid, and purulent effusions are opaque. Bleeding disorders, trauma, and traumatic taps are the most common causes of bloody effusions.

B. Cell count—The synovial fluid white cell count discriminates between **noninflammatory** (< 2000 white cells/mcL), **inflammatory** (2000–75,000 white cells/mcL), and **purulent** (> 100,000 white cells/mcL) joint effusions. Synovial fluid glucose and protein levels add little information and should not be ordered.

C. Microscopic examination—Compensated polarized light microscopy identifies and distinguishes monosodium urate (gout, negatively birefringent) and calcium pyrophosphate (pseudogout, positive birefringent) crystals. Gram stain has specificity but limited sensitivity (50%) for septic arthritis.

D. Culture—Bacterial cultures as well as special studies for gonococci, tubercle bacilli, or fungi are ordered as appropriate.

2. Interpretation

Synovial fluid analysis is diagnostic in infectious or microcrystalline arthritis. Although the severity of inflammation in synovial fluid can overlap among various conditions, the synovial fluid white cell count is a helpful guide to diagnosis (Table 20–3).

▼ DEGENERATIVE & CRYSTAL-INDUCED ARTHRITIS

DEGENERATIVE JOINT DISEASE (Osteoarthritis)

 ESSENTIALS OF DIAGNOSIS

► A degenerative disorder; no systemic symptoms.

► Commonly secondary to other articular disease.

► Pain relieved by rest; morning stiffness brief; articular inflammation minimal.

► Radiographic findings: narrowed joint space, osteophytes, increased density of subchondral bone, bony cysts.

Table 20–1. Diagnostic value of the joint pattern.

Characteristic	Status	Representative Disease
Inflammation	Present	Rheumatoid arthritis, systemic lupus erythematosus, gout
	Absent	Osteoarthritis
Number of involved joints	Monarticular	Gout, trauma, septic arthritis, Lyme disease, osteoarthritis
	Oligoarticular (2–4 joints)	Reactive arthritis, psoriatic arthritis, inflammatory bowel disease
	Polyarticular (≥ 5 joints)	Rheumatoid arthritis, systemic lupus erythematosus
Site of joint involvement	Distal interphalangeal	Osteoarthritis, psoriatic arthritis (not rheumatoid arthritis)
	Metacarpophalangeal, wrists	Rheumatoid arthritis, systemic lupus erythematosus (not osteoarthritis)
	First metatarsal phalangeal	Gout, osteoarthritis

General Considerations

Osteoarthritis, the most common form of joint disease, is chiefly a disease of aging. Ninety percent of all people have radiographic features of osteoarthritis in weight-bearing joints by age 40. Symptomatic disease also increases with age.

This arthropathy is characterized by degeneration of cartilage and by hypertrophy of bone at the articular margins. Inflammation is usually minimal. Hereditary and mechanical factors may be involved in the pathogenesis.

Obesity is a risk factor for osteoarthritis of the knee and probably of the hip. Recreational running does not increase the incidence of osteoarthritis, but participation in competitive contact sports does. Jobs requiring frequent bending and carrying increase the risk of knee osteoarthritis.

Clinical Findings

A. Symptoms and Signs

Degenerative joint disease is divided into two types: (1) primary, which most commonly affects some or all of the following: the DIP and the proximal interphalangeal (PIP) joints of the fingers, the carpometacarpal joint of the thumb, the hip, the knee, the metatarsophalangeal (MTP) joint of the big toe, and the cervical and lumbar spine; and (2) secondary, which may occur in any joint as a sequela to articular injury resulting from either intra-articular (including rheumatoid arthritis) or extra-articular causes. The injury may be acute, as in a fracture; or chronic, as that due to occupational overuse of a joint, metabolic disease (eg, hyperparathyroidism, hemochromatosis, ochronosis), or neurologic disorders (tabes dorsalis; see below).

The onset is insidious. Initially, there is articular stiffness, seldom lasting more than 15 minutes; this develops later into pain on motion of the affected joint and is made worse by activity or weight bearing and relieved by rest. Bony enlargement of the DIP (Heberden nodes) and PIP (Bouchard nodes) joints are occasionally prominent, and flexion contracture or varus deformity of the knee is not unusual (Plate 79). There is no ankylosis, but limitation of motion of the affected joint or joints is common. Crepitus may often be felt in the joint. Joint effusion and other articular signs of inflammation are mild. There are no systemic manifestations.

B. Laboratory Findings

Osteoarthritis does not cause elevation of the erythrocyte sedimentation rate (ESR) or other laboratory signs of inflammation.

C. Imaging

Radiographs may reveal narrowing of the joint space; osteophyte formation and lipping of marginal bone; and thickened, dense subchondral bone. Bone cysts may also be present.

Table 20–2. Examination of joint fluid.

Measure	(Normal)	Group I (Noninflammatory)	Group II (Inflammatory)	Group III (Purulent)
Volume (mL) (knee)	< 3.5	Often > 3.5	Often > 3.5	Often > 3.5
Clarity	Transparent	Transparent	Translucent to opaque	Opaque
Color	Clear	Yellow	Yellow to opalescent	Yellow to green
WBC (per mcL)	< 200	200–300	2000–75,000[1]	> 100,000[2]
Polymorphonuclear leukocytes	< 25%	< 25%	50% or more	75% or more
Culture	Negative	Negative	Negative	Usually positive[2]

[1]Gout, rheumatoid arthritis, and other inflammatory conditions occasionally have synovial fluid WBC counts > 75,000/mcL but rarely > 100,000/mcL.

[2]Most purulent effusions are due to septic arthritis. Septic arthritis, however, can present with group II synovial fluid, particularly if infection is caused by organisms of low virulence (eg, *Neisseria gonorrhoeae*) or if antibiotic therapy has been started.
WBC, white blood cell count.

Table 20–3. Differential diagnosis by joint fluid groups.

Group I (Noninflammatory) (< 2000 white cells/mcL)	Group II (Inflammatory) (2000–75,000 white cells/mcL)	Group III (Purulent) (> 100,000 white cells/mcL)	Hemorrhagic
Degenerative joint disease	Rheumatoid arthritis	Pyogenic bacterial infections	Hemophilia or other hemorrhagic diathesis
Trauma[1]	Acute crystal-induced synovitis (gout and pseudogout)		Trauma with or without fracture
Osteochondritis dissecans	Reactive arthritis		Neuropathic arthropathy
Osteochondromatosis	Ankylosing spondylitis		Pigmented villonodular synovitis
Neuropathic arthropathy[1]	Rheumatic fever[2]		Synovioma
Subsiding or early inflammation	Tuberculosis		Hemangioma and other benign neoplasms
Hypertrophic osteoarthropathy[2]			
Pigmented villonodular synovitis[1]			

[1]May be hemorrhagic.
[2]Noninflammatory or inflammatory group.
Reproduced, with permission, from Rodnan GP (editor). Primer on the rheumatic diseases, 7th ed. JAMA 1973;224(Suppl):662.

Differential Diagnosis

Because articular inflammation is minimal and systemic manifestations are absent, degenerative joint disease should seldom be confused with other arthritides. The distribution of joint involvement in the hands also helps distinguish osteoarthritis from rheumatoid arthritis. Osteoarthritis chiefly affects the DIP and PIP joints and spares the wrist and metacarpophalangeal (MCP) joints; rheumatoid arthritis involves the wrists and MCP joints and spares the DIP joints. Furthermore, the joint enlargement is bony-hard and cool in osteoarthritis but spongy and warm in rheumatoid arthritis. Skeletal symptoms due to degenerative changes in joints—especially in the spine—may cause coexistent metastatic neoplasia, osteoporosis, multiple myeloma, or other bone disease to be overlooked.

Prevention

Weight reduction reduces the risk of developing symptomatic knee osteoarthritis. Maintaining normal vitamin D levels may reduce the occurrence and progression of osteoarthritis, in addition to being important for bone health.

Treatment

A. General Measures

For patients with mild to moderate osteoarthritis of weight-bearing joints, moderate physical activity (eg, a supervised walking program, hydrotherapy classes, or Tai Chi classes) may result in clinical improvement of functional status without aggravating the joint pain. Weight loss can also improve the symptoms.

B. Analgesic and Anti-inflammatory Drugs

Nonsteroidal anti-inflammatory drugs (NSAIDs) (see Table 5–3) are more effective (and more toxic) than acetaminophen for osteoarthritis of the knee or hip. Their superiority is most convincing in persons with severe disease. Patients with mild disease should start with acetaminophen (2.6–4 g/d). NSAIDs should be considered for patients who do not respond to acetaminophen. (See discussion of NSAID toxicity in the section on treatment of rheumatoid arthritis.) High doses of NSAIDs, as used in the inflammatory arthritides, are unnecessary. Chondroitin sulfate and glucosamine, alone or in combination, are no better than placebo in reducing pain in patients with knee or hip osteoarthritis.

For many patients, it is possible eventually to reduce the dosage or limit use of drugs to periods of exacerbation. For patients with knee osteoarthritis and effusion, intra-articular injection of triamcinolone (20–40 mg) may obviate the need for analgesics or NSAIDs. Corticosteroid injections up to four times a year appear to be safe. Intra-articular injections of sodium hyaluronate reduce symptoms moderately in some patients. Capsaicin cream 0.025–0.075% applied three or four times a day can also reduce knee pain without NSAIDs. Doxycycline, though not approved by the US Food and Drug Administration (FDA) for treating osteoarthritis, has shown promise in slowing the progression of knee osteoarthritis.

C. Surgical Measures

Total hip and knee replacements provide excellent symptomatic and functional improvement when involvement of that joint severely restricts walking or causes pain at rest, particularly at night. Arthroscopic surgery for knee osteoarthritis is ineffective.

Prognosis

Marked disability is less common in patients with osteoarthritis than in those with rheumatoid arthritis, but symptoms may be quite severe and limit activity considerably (especially with involvement of the hips, knees, and cervical spine).

When to Refer

Refer patients to an orthopedic surgeon when recalcitrant symptoms or functional impairment, or both, warrant consideration of joint replacement surgery of the hip or knee.

Kirkley A et al. A randomized trial of arthroscopic surgery for osteoarthritis of the knee. N Engl J Med. 2008 Sep 11;359(11):1097–107. [PMID: 18784099]

Scanzello CR et al. The post-NSAID era: what to use now for the pharmacologic treatment of pain and inflammation in osteoarthritis. Curr Rheumatol Rep. 2008 Jan;10(1):49–56. [PMID: 18457612]

CRYSTAL DEPOSITION ARTHRITIS

1. Gouty Arthritis

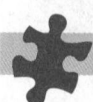 ESSENTIALS OF DIAGNOSIS

▸ Acute onset, typically nocturnal and usually monarticular, often involving the first MTP joint.

▸ Polyarticular involvement more common in patients with long-standing disease.

▸ Identification of urate crystals in joint fluid or tophi is diagnostic.

▸ Dramatic therapeutic response to NSAIDs.

▸ With chronicity, urate deposits in subcutaneous tissue, bone, cartilage, joints, and other tissues.

General Considerations

Gout is a metabolic disease of a heterogeneous nature, often familial, associated with abnormal amounts of urates in the body and characterized early by a recurring acute arthritis, usually monarticular, and later by chronic deforming arthritis. The associated hyperuricemia is due to overproduction or underexcretion of uric acid—sometimes both. The disease is especially common in Pacific islanders, eg, Filipinos and Samoans. Primary gout has a heritable component, and genome-wide surveys have linked risk of gout to several genes whose products regulate urate handling by the kidney. Secondary gout, which may have a heritable component, is related to acquired causes of hyperuricemia, eg, medication use (especially diuretics, low-dose aspirin, cyclosporine, and niacin), myeloproliferative disorders, multiple myeloma, hemoglobinopathies, chronic kidney disease, hypothyroidism, psoriasis, sarcoidosis, and lead poisoning (Table 20–4). Alcohol ingestion promotes hyperuricemia by increasing urate production and decreasing the renal excretion of uric acid. Finally, hospitalized patients frequently suffer attacks of gout because of changes in diet, fluid intake, or medications that lead either to rapid reductions or increases in the serum urate level.

About 90% of patients with primary gout are men, usually over 30 years of age. In women, the onset is typically postmenopausal. The characteristic lesion is the tophus, a nodular deposit of monosodium urate monohydrate crystals with an associated foreign body reaction. Tophi are found in cartilage, subcutaneous and periarticular tissues, tendon, bone, the kidneys, and elsewhere. Urates have been demonstrated in the synovial tissues (and fluid) during acute arthritis; indeed, the acute inflammation of gout is believed to be activated by the phagocytosis by polymorphonuclear cells of urate crystals with the ensuing release from the neutrophils of chemotactic and other substances capable of mediating inflammation. The precise relationship of hyperuricemia to gouty arthritis is still obscure, since chronic hyperuricemia is found in people who never develop gout or uric acid stones. Rapid fluctuations in serum urate levels, either increasing or decreasing, are important factors in precipitating acute gout. The mechanism of the late, chronic stage of gouty arthritis is better understood. This is characterized pathologically by tophaceous invasion of the articular and periarticular tissues, with structural derangement and secondary degeneration (osteoarthritis).

Uric acid kidney stones are present in 5–10% of patients with gouty arthritis. Hyperuricemia correlates highly with the likelihood of developing stones, with the risk of stone formation reaching 50% in patients with a serum urate level above 13 mg/dL. Chronic urate nephropathy is caused by the deposition of monosodium urate crystals in the renal medulla and pyramids. Although progressive chronic kidney disease occurs in a substantial percentage of patients with chronic gout, the role of hyperuricemia in causing this outcome is controversial, because many patients with gout have numerous confounding risk factors for chronic kidney disease (eg, hypertension, alcohol use, lead exposure, and other risk factors for vascular disease).

Table 20–4. Origin of hyperuricemia.

Primary hyperuricemia
A. Increased production of purine
1. Idiopathic
2. Specific enzyme defects (eg, Lesch-Nyhan syndrome, glycogen storage diseases)
B. Decreased renal clearance of uric acid (idiopathic)
Secondary hyperuricemia
A. Increased catabolism and turnover of purine
1. Myeloproliferative disorders
2. Lymphoproliferative disorders
3. Carcinoma and sarcoma (disseminated)
4. Chronic hemolytic anemias
5. Cytotoxic drugs
6. Psoriasis
B. Decreased renal clearance of uric acid
1. Intrinsic kidney disease
2. Functional impairment of tubular transport
a. Drug-induced (eg, thiazides, low-dose aspirin)
b. Hyperlacticacidemia (eg, lactic acidosis, alcoholism)
c. Hyperketoacidemia (eg, diabetic ketoacidosis, starvation)
d. Diabetes insipidus (vasopressin-resistant)
e. Bartter syndrome

Modified, with permission, from Rodnan GP. Gout and other crystalline forms of arthritis. Postgrad Med. 1975 Oct;58(5):6–14.

▶ Clinical Findings

A. Symptoms and Signs

Acute gouty arthritis is sudden in onset and frequently nocturnal. It may develop without apparent precipitating cause or may follow rapid increases or decreases in serum urate levels. Common precipitants are alcohol excess (particularly beer), changes in medications that affect urate metabolism, and, in the hospitalized patient, fasting before medical procedures. The MTP joint of the great toe is the most susceptible joint ("podagra"), although others, especially those of the feet, ankles, and knees, are commonly affected. Gouty attacks may develop in periarticular soft tissues such as the arch of the foot. Hips and shoulders are rarely affected. More than one joint may occasionally be affected during the same attack; in such cases, the distribution of the arthritis is usually asymmetric. As the attack progresses, the pain becomes intense. The involved joints are swollen and exquisitely tender and the overlying skin tense, warm, and dusky red. Fever is common and may reach 39 °C. Local desquamation and pruritus during recovery from the acute arthritis are characteristic of gout but are not always present. Tophi may be found in the external ears, hands, feet, and olecranon and prepatellar bursae (Plate 80). They usually develop years after the initial attack of gout.

Asymptomatic periods of months or years commonly follow the initial acute attack. After years of recurrent severe monarthritis attacks of the lower extremities and untreated hyperuricemia, gout can evolve into a chronic, deforming polyarthritis of upper and lower extremities that mimics rheumatoid arthritis.

B. Laboratory Findings

The serum uric acid is elevated (> 7.5 mg/dL) in 95% of patients who have serial measurements during the course of an attack. However, a single uric acid determination is normal in up to 25% of cases, so it does not exclude gout, especially in patients taking urate-lowering drugs. During an acute attack, the ESR and white cell count are frequently elevated. Identification of sodium urate crystals in joint fluid or material aspirated from a tophus establishes the diagnosis. The crystals, which may be extracellular or found within neutrophils, are needle-like and negatively birefringent when examined by polarized light microscopy.

C. Imaging

Early in the disease, radiographs show no changes. Later, punched-out erosions with an overhanging rim of cortical bone ("rat bite") develop. When these are adjacent to a soft tissue tophus, they are diagnostic of gout.

▶ Differential Diagnosis

Acute gout is often confused with cellulitis. Bacteriologic studies usually exclude acute pyogenic arthritis. Pseudogout is distinguished by the identification of calcium pyrophosphate crystals (positive birefringence) in the joint fluid, usually normal serum uric acid, and the radiographic appearance of chondrocalcinosis.

Chronic tophaceous arthritis may resemble chronic rheumatoid arthritis; gout is suggested by an earlier history of monarthritis and is established by the demonstration of urate crystals in a suspected tophus. Likewise, hips and shoulders are generally spared in tophaceous gout. Biopsy may be necessary to distinguish tophi from rheumatoid nodules. A radiographic appearance similar to that of gout may be found in rheumatoid arthritis, sarcoidosis, multiple myeloma, hyperparathyroidism, or Hand-Schüller-Christian disease. Chronic lead intoxication may result in attacks of gouty arthritis (saturnine gout); abdominal pain, peripheral neuropathy, chronic kidney disease, and basophilic stippling of red cells are clues to the diagnosis.

▶ Treatment

A. Asymptomatic Hyperuricemia

Asymptomatic hyperuricemia should not be treated; uric acid–lowering drugs need not be instituted until arthritis, renal calculi, or tophi become apparent.

B. Acute Attack

Arthritis is treated first and hyperuricemia weeks or months later, if at all. Sudden reduction of serum uric acid often precipitates further episodes of gouty arthritis.

1. NSAIDs—These drugs (see Table 5–3) are the treatment of choice for acute gout. Traditionally, indomethacin has been the most frequently used agent, but all of the other newer NSAIDs are probably equally effective. Indomethacin is initiated at a dosage of 25–50 mg orally every 8 hours and continued until the symptoms have resolved (usually 5–10 days). Active peptic ulcer disease, impaired kidney function, and a history of allergic reaction to NSAIDs are contraindications. For patients at high risk for upper gastrointestinal bleeding, a cyclooxygenase type 2 (COX-2) inhibitor may be an appropriate first choice for management of an acute gout attack. Long-term use of COX-2 inhibitors is not advised because of the association with increased risk of cardiovascular events, which has led to the removal of some drugs from the US market (eg, rofecoxib and valdecoxib).

2. Colchicine—Neither oral nor intravenous colchicine should be used for the treatment of acute gout flares. The use of oral colchicine during the intercritical period to prevent gout attacks is discussed below.

3. Corticosteroids—Corticosteroids often give dramatic symptomatic relief in acute episodes of gout and will control most attacks. They are most useful in patients with contraindications to the use of NSAIDs. If the patient's gout is monarticular, intra-articular administration (eg, triamcinolone, 10–40 mg depending on the size of the joint) is most effective. For polyarticular gout, corticosteroids may be given intravenously (eg, methylprednisolone, 40 mg/d tapered over 7 days) or orally (eg, prednisone, 40–60 mg/d tapered over 7 days). Gouty and septic arthritis can coexist, albeit rarely. Therefore, joint aspiration and Gram stain with culture of synovial fluid should be performed before corticosteroids are given.

C. Management between Attacks

Treatment during symptom-free periods is intended to minimize urate deposition in tissues, which causes chronic tophaceous arthritis, and to reduce the frequency and severity of recurrences.

1. Diet—Potentially reversible causes of hyperuricemia are a high-purine diet, obesity, alcohol consumption, and use of certain medications (see below). Beer consumption appears to confer a higher risk of gout than does whiskey or wine. Higher levels of meat and seafood consumption are associated with increased risks of gout, whereas a higher level of dairy products consumption is associated with a decreased risk. Although dietary purines usually contribute only 1 mg/dL to the serum uric acid level, moderation in eating foods with high purine content is advisable (Table 20–5). A high liquid intake and, more importantly, a daily urinary output of 2 L or more will aid urate excretion and minimize urate precipitation in the urinary tract.

2. Avoidance of hyperuricemic medications—Thiazide and loop diuretics inhibit renal excretion of uric acid and should be avoided in patients with gout. Similarly, low doses of aspirin aggravate hyperuricemia, as does niacin.

3. Colchicine—Patients with a single episode of gout who are willing to lose weight and stop drinking alcohol are at low risk for another attack and unlikely to benefit from chronic medical therapy. In contrast, older individuals with mild chronic kidney disease who require diuretic use and have a history of multiple attacks of gout are more likely to benefit from pharmacologic treatment. In general, the higher the

Table 20–5. The purine content of foods.[1]

Low-purine foods
Refined cereals and cereal products, cornflakes, white bread, pasta, flour, arrowroot, sago, tapioca, cakes
Milk, milk products, and eggs
Sugar, sweets, and gelatin
Butter, polyunsaturated margarine, and all other fats
Fruit, nuts, and peanut butter
Lettuce, tomatoes, and green vegetables (except those listed below)
Cream soups made with low-purine vegetables but without meat or meat stock
Water, fruit juice, cordials, and carbonated drinks
High-purine foods
All meats, including organ meats, and seafood
Meat extracts and gravies
Yeast and yeast extracts, beer, and other alcoholic beverages
Beans, peas, lentils, oatmeal, spinach, asparagus, cauliflower, and mushrooms

[1]The purine content of a food reflects its nucleoprotein content and turnover. Foods containing many nuclei (eg, liver) have many purines, as do rapidly growing foods such as asparagus. The consumption of large amounts of a food containing a small concentration of purines may provide a greater purine load than consumption of a small amount of a food containing a large concentration of purines.
Reproduced, with permission, from Emmerson BT. The management of gout. N Engl J Med. 1996 Feb 15;334(7):445–51.

uric acid level and the more frequent the attacks, the more likely that chronic medical therapy will be beneficial.

There are two indications for daily colchicine administration. First, colchicine can be used to prevent future attacks. For the person who has mild hyperuricemia and occasional attacks of gouty arthritis, chronic colchicine prophylaxis may be all that is needed. The usual dose is 0.6 mg either once or twice a day. Patients who have coexisting moderate chronic kidney disease or heart failure should take colchicine only once a day in order to avoid the peripheral neuromyopathy that can complicate the use of higher doses. Second, colchicine can also be used when uricosuric drugs or allopurinol (see below) are started, to suppress attacks precipitated by abrupt changes in the serum uric acid level.

4. Reduction of serum uric acid—Indications for a urate lowering intervention include frequent acute arthritis not controlled by colchicine prophylaxis, tophaceous deposits, or kidney damage. Hyperuricemia with infrequent attacks of arthritis may not require treatment. If instituted, the goal of medical treatment is to maintain the serum uric acid at or below 5 mg/dL, which should prevent crystallization of urate.

Two classes of agents may be used to lower the serum uric acid—the uricosuric drugs and allopurinol (neither is of value in the treatment of acute gout). The choice of one or the other depends on the result of a 24-hour urine uric acid determination. A value under 800 mg/d indicates undersecretion of uric acid, which is amenable to uricosuric agents if kidney function is preserved or to allopurinol if kidney function is limited. Patients with more than 800 mg of uric acid in a 24-hour urine collection are overproducers and require allopurinol.

A. URICOSURIC DRUGS—Uricosuric drugs, which block the tubular reabsorption of filtered urate thereby reducing the metabolic urate pool, prevent the formation of new tophi and reduce the size of those already present. When administered concomitantly with colchicine, they may lessen the frequency of recurrences of acute gout. The indication for uricosuric treatment is the increasing frequency or severity of acute attacks. Uricosuric agents are ineffective in patients with chronic kidney disease, with a serum creatinine of more than 2 mg/dL.

The following uricosuric drugs may be used: (1) Probenecid, 0.5 g orally daily initially, with gradual increase to 1–2 g daily; or (2) sulfinpyrazone, 50–100 mg orally twice daily initially, with gradual increase to 200–400 mg twice daily. Hypersensitivity to either with fever and rash occurs in 5% of cases; gastrointestinal complaints are observed in 10%. Probenecid also inhibits the excretion of penicillin, indomethacin, dapsone, and acetazolamide.

Precautions with uricosuric drugs include maintaining a daily urinary output of 2000 mL or more in order to minimize the precipitation of uric acid in the urinary tract. This can be further prevented by giving alkalinizing agents (eg, potassium citrate, 30–80 mEq/d orally) to maintain a urine pH of above 6.0. Uricosuric drugs should not be used in patients with a history of uric acid nephrolithiasis. Aspirin in moderate doses antagonizes the action of uricosuric agents, but low doses (325 mg or less per day) do not; doses of aspirin greater than 3 g daily are themselves uricosuric.

B. ALLOPURINOL—The xanthine oxidase inhibitor allopurinol promptly lowers plasma urate and urinary uric acid concentrations and facilitates tophus mobilization. The drug is of special value in uric acid overproducers; in tophaceous gout; in patients unresponsive to the uricosuric regimen; and in gouty patients with uric acid renal calculi. It should be used in low doses in patients with chronic kidney disease and is not indicated in asymptomatic hyperuricemia. The most frequent adverse effect is the precipitation of an acute gouty attack. Hypersensitivity to allopurinol occurs in 2% of cases and can be life-threatening. The most common sign of hypersensitivity is a pruritic rash that may progress to toxic epidermal necrolysis, particularly if allopurinol is continued; vasculitis and hepatitis are other manifestations.

The initial daily dose of allopurinol is 300 mg/d for patients who have normal kidney function and who are taking prophylactic colchicine. In the absence of prophylactic colchicine, the initial dose should be 100 mg/d orally. The dose of allopurinol can be increased in a week if needed to achieve the desired serum uric acid level of ≤ 5.0 mg/dL. Successful treatment usually requires a dose of 300–400 mg of allopurinol daily. The maximum daily dose is 800 mg. Allopurinol can be used in chronic kidney disease, but the dose must be reduced to decrease the chance of side effects.

Allopurinol interacts with other drugs. The combined use of allopurinol and ampicillin causes a drug rash in 20% of patients. Allopurinol can increase the half-life of probenecid, while probenecid increases the excretion of allopurinol. Thus, a patient taking both drugs may need to use slightly higher than usual doses of allopurinol and lower doses of probenecid.

D. Chronic Tophaceous Arthritis

With rigorous medical compliance, allopurinol shrinks tophi and in time can lead to their disappearance. Resorption of extensive tophi requires maintaining a serum uric acid below 5 mg/dL, which may be achievable only with concomitant use of allopurinol and a uricosuric agent. Surgical excision of large tophi offers mechanical improvement in selected deformities.

E. Gout in the Transplant Patient

Hyperuricemia and gout commonly develop in many transplant patients because they have decreased kidney function and require drugs that inhibit uric acid excretion (especially cyclosporine and diuretics). Treating these patients is challenging: NSAIDs are usually contraindicated because of underlying chronic kidney disease; intravenous colchicine should not be used because of its narrow therapeutic index (particularly in kidney dysfunction); and corticosteroids are already being used. Often the best approach for monarticular gout—after excluding infection—is injecting corticosteroids into the joint (see above). For polyarticular gout, increasing the dose of systemic corticosteroid may be the only alternative. Since transplant patients often have multiple attacks of gout, long-term relief requires lowering the serum uric acid with allopurinol. (Kidney dysfunction seen in many transplant patients makes uricosuric agents ineffective.) Allopurinol should be started at a low dose in patients with kidney dysfunction and then adjusted according to its effect on the serum uric acid level. Allopurinol potentiates the effect of azathioprine. If allopurinol cannot be avoided, the dose of azathioprine should be reduced by 75% before allopurinol is started.

► Prognosis

Without treatment, the acute attack may last from a few days to several weeks. The intervals between acute attacks vary up to years, but the asymptomatic periods often become shorter if the disease progresses. Chronic gouty arthritis occurs after repeated attacks of acute gout, but only after inadequate treatment. The younger the patient at the onset of disease, the greater the tendency to a progressive course. Destructive arthropathy is rarely seen in patients whose first attack is after age 50.

Patients with gout are anecdotally thought to have an increased incidence of hypertension, kidney disease (eg, nephrosclerosis, interstitial nephritis, pyelonephritis), diabetes mellitus, hypertriglyceridemia, and atherosclerosis.

Dehghan A et al. Association of three genetic loci with uric acid concentration and risk of gout: a genome-wide association study. Lancet. 2008 Dec 6;372(9654):1953–61. [PMID: 18834626]

Janssens HJ et al. Use of oral prednisolone or naproxen for the treatment of gout arthritis: a double-blind, randomised equivalence trial. Lancet. 2008 May 31;371(9627):1854–60. [PMID: 18514729]

2. Chondrocalcinosis & Pseudogout

Chondrocalcinosis is the presence of calcium-containing salts in articular cartilage. Diagnosed radiologically, it may be familial and is commonly associated with a wide variety of metabolic disorders, eg, hemochromatosis, hyperparathyroidism, ochronosis, diabetes mellitus, hypothyroidism, Wilson disease, and gout. Pseudogout (also called calcium pyrophosphate dihydrate [CPPD] deposition disease) is most often seen in persons age 60 or older, is characterized by acute, recurrent and rarely chronic arthritis involving large joints (most commonly the knees and the wrists) and is almost always accompanied by chondrocalcinosis of the affected joints. Other joints frequently affected are the MCPs, hips, shoulders, elbows, and ankles. Involvement of the DIP and PIP joints is no more common in CPPD deposition disease than in other age-matched controls. Pseudogout, like gout, frequently develops 24–48 hours after major surgery. Identification of calcium pyrophosphate crystals in joint aspirates is diagnostic of pseudogout. With light microscopy, the rhomboid-shaped crystals differ from the needle-shaped gout crystals. A red compensator is used for positive identification, since pseudogout crystals are blue when parallel and yellow when perpendicular to the axis of the compensator. Urate crystals give the opposite pattern. X-ray examination shows not only calcification (usually symmetric) of cartilaginous structures but also signs of degenerative joint disease (osteoarthritis). Unlike gout, pseudogout is usually associated with normal serum urate levels.

Treatment of chondrocalcinosis is directed at the primary disease, if present. NSAIDs (salicylates, indomethacin, naproxen, and other drugs) are helpful in the treatment of acute episodes. Patients at increased risk for upper gastrointestinal bleeding may use a COX-2 inhibitor to treat acute attacks of pseudogout. Long-term use of COX-2 inhibitors is not advised because of the association with increased risk of cardiovascular events. Colchicine, 0.6 mg orally twice daily, is more effective for prophylaxis than for acute attacks. Aspiration of the inflamed joint and intra-articular injection of triamcinolone, 10–40 mg, depending on the size of the joint, are also of value in resistant cases.

Announ N et al. Treating difficult crystal pyrophosphate dihydrate deposition disease. Curr Rheumatol Rep. 2008 Jul;10(3):228–34. [PMID: 18638432]

PAIN SYNDROMES

NECK PAIN

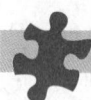 ESSENTIALS OF DIAGNOSIS

► Most chronic neck pain is caused by degenerative joint disease and responds to conservative approaches.

► Whiplash is the most common type of traumatic injury to the neck.

► Serious erosive disease of joints in the neck that may lead to neurologic complications sometimes occurs in rheumatoid arthritis and occasionally in ankylosing spondylitis; the usual joint involved in these disorders is the atlantoaxial joint (C1–2).

General Considerations

At any point in time, about 15% of adults are experiencing neck pain. The prevalence of neck pain peaks at age 50 and develops more commonly in women than in men. A large group of articular and extra-articular disorders are characterized by pain that may involve simultaneously the neck, shoulder girdle, and upper extremity. Diagnostic differentiation may be difficult. Some represent primary disorders of the cervicobrachial region; others are local manifestations of systemic disease. It is frequently not possible to make a specific diagnosis.

Clinical Findings

A. Symptoms and Signs

Neck pain may be limited to the posterior region or, depending on the level of the symptomatic joint, may radiate segmentally to the occiput, anterior chest, shoulder girdle, arm, forearm, and hand. It may be intensified by active or passive neck motions. The general distribution of pain and paresthesias corresponds roughly to the involved dermatome in the upper extremity. Radiating pain in the upper extremity is often intensified by hyperextension of the neck and deviation of the head to the involved side. Limitation of cervical movements is the most common objective finding. Neurologic signs depend on the extent of compression of nerve roots or the spinal cord. Compression of the spinal cord may cause paraparesis or paraplegia.

B. Imaging

The radiographic findings depend on the cause of the pain; many plain radiographs are completely normal in patients who have suffered an acute cervical strain. Loss of cervical lordosis is often seen but is nonspecific. In osteoarthritis, comparative reduction in height of the involved disk space is a frequent finding. The most common late radiographic finding is osteophyte formation anteriorly, adjacent to the disk; other chronic abnormalities occur around the apophysial joint clefts, chiefly in the lower cervical spine.

Use of advanced imaging techniques is indicated in the patient who has severe pain of unknown cause that fails to respond to conservative therapy or in the patient who has evidence of myelopathy. MRI is more sensitive than CT in detecting disk disease, extradural compression, and intramedullary cord disease. CT is preferable for demonstration of fractures.

Differential Diagnosis & Treatment

The causes of neck pain include acute and chronic cervical strain or sprains, herniated nucleus pulposus, osteoarthritis, ankylosing spondylitis, rheumatoid arthritis, fibromyalgia, osteomyelitis, neoplasms, polymyalgia rheumatica, compression fractures, pain referred from visceral structures (eg, angina), and functional disorders.

A. Nonspecific Neck Pain

In the absence of trauma or evidence of infection, malignancy, neurologic findings, or systemic inflammation, the patient can be treated conservatively. Conservative therapy can include rest, analgesics, or physical therapy.

B. Acute Cervical Musculotendinous Strain

Cervical strain is generally caused by mechanical postural disorders, overexertion, or injury (eg, whiplash). Acute episodes are associated with pain, decreased cervical spine motion, and paraspinal muscle spasm, resulting in stiffness of the neck and loss of motion. Muscle trigger points can often be localized. After whiplash injury, patients often experience not only neck pain but also shoulder girdle discomfort and headache. Management includes administration of analgesics. Soft cervical collars are commonly recommended, but evidence suggests they may delay recovery. Acupuncture, manipulation, or physical therapy can help some patients, but the precise role of these treatments is not well established. Corticosteroid injection into cervical facet joints is ineffective. Gradual return to full activity is encouraged.

C. Herniated Nucleus Pulposus

Rupture or prolapse of the nucleus pulposus of the cervical disks into the spinal canal causes pain radiating at a C6–7 level. When intra-abdominal pressure is increased by coughing, sneezing, or other movements, symptoms are aggravated, and cervical muscle spasm may occur. Neurologic abnormalities include decreased reflexes of the deep tendons of the biceps and triceps and decreased sensation and muscle atrophy or weakness in the forearm or hand. Cervical traction, bed rest, and other conservative measures are usually successful. Radicular symptoms usually respond to conservative therapy, including NSAIDs, activity modification, intermittent cervical traction, and neck immobilization. Cervical epidural corticosteroid injections may help those who fail conservative therapy. Surgery is indicated for unremitting pain and progressive weakness despite a full trial of conservative therapy and if a surgically correctable abnormality is identified by MRI or CT myelography. Surgical decompression achieves excellent results in 70–80% of such patients.

D. Arthritic Disorders

Cervical spondylosis (degenerative arthritis) is a collective term describing degenerative changes that occur in the apophysial joints and intervertebral disk joints, with or without neurologic signs. Osteoarthritis of the articular facets is characterized by progressive thinning of the cartilage, subchondral osteoporosis, and osteophytic proliferation around the joint margins. Degeneration of cervical disks and joints may occur in adolescents but is more common after age 40. Degeneration is progressive and is marked by gradual narrowing of the disk space, as demonstrated by radiography. Osteocartilaginous proliferation occurs around the margin of the vertebral body and gives rise to osteophytic ridges that may encroach upon the intervertebral foramina and spinal canal, causing compression of the neurovascular contents.

Osteoarthritis of the cervical spine is often asymptomatic but may cause diffuse neck pain. A minority of patients with neck pain also suffer from radicular pain or myelopathy. Myelopathy develops insidiously and is manifested by sensory dysfunction and clumsy hands. Some patients also complain of unsteady walking, urinary frequency and urgency, or electrical shock sensations with neck flexion or extension (Lhermitte sign). Weakness, sensory loss, and spasticity with exaggerated reflexes develop below the level of spinal cord compression. Amyotrophic lateral sclerosis, multiple sclerosis, syringomyelia, spinal cord tumors, and tropical spastic paresis from HTLV-1 infection can mimic myelopathy from cervical arthritis. The mainstay of conservative therapy is immobilizing the cervical spine with a collar. With moderate to severe neurologic symptoms, surgical treatment is indicated.

Atlantoaxial subluxation may occur in patients with either rheumatoid arthritis or ankylosing spondylitis. Inflammation of the synovial structures resulting from erosion and laxity of the transverse ligament can lead to neurologic signs of spinal cord compression. Treatment may vary from use of a cervical collar or more rigid bracing

to operative treatment, depending on the degree of subluxation and neurologic progression. Surgical treatment for stabilization of the cervical spine is a last resort.

E. Other Disorders

Osteomyelitis and neoplasms are discussed below. Osteoporosis is discussed in Chapter 26.

Gross AR et al. Conservative management of mechanical neck disorders: a systematic review. J Rheumatol. 2007 May;34(5):1083–102. [PMID: 17295434]

THORACIC OUTLET SYNDROMES

Thoracic outlet syndromes result from compression of the neurovascular structures supplying the upper extremity. Symptoms and signs arise from intermittent or continuous pressure on elements of the brachial plexus (> 90% of cases) or the subclavian or axillary vessels (veins or arteries) by a variety of anatomic structures of the shoulder girdle region. The neurovascular bundle can be compressed between the anterior or middle scalene muscles and a normal first thoracic rib or a cervical rib. Most commonly thoracic outlet obstruction is caused by scarred scalene neck muscle secondary to neck trauma or sagging of the shoulder girdle resulting from aging, obesity, or pendulous breasts. Faulty posture, occupation, or thoracic muscle hypertrophy from physical activity (eg, weight-lifting, baseball pitching) may be other predisposing factors.

Thoracic outlet obstruction presents in most patients with some combination of four symptoms involving the upper extremity, namely pain, numbness, weakness, and swelling. The predominant symptoms depend on whether the obstruction chiefly affects neural or vascular structures. The onset of symptoms is usually gradual but can be sudden. Some patients spontaneously notice aggravation of symptoms with specific positioning of the arm. Pain radiates from the point of compression to the base of the neck, the axilla, the shoulder girdle region, arm, forearm, and hand. Paresthesias are common and distributed to the volar aspect of the fourth and fifth digits. Sensory symptoms may be aggravated at night or by prolonged use of the extremities. Weakness and muscle atrophy are the principal motor abnormalities. Vascular symptoms consist of arterial ischemia characterized by pallor of the fingers on elevation of the extremity, sensitivity to cold, and, rarely, gangrene of the digits or venous obstruction marked by edema, cyanosis, and engorgement.

The symptoms of thoracic outlet obstruction can be provoked within 60 seconds over 90% of the time by having a patient elevate the arms in a "stick-em-up" position (ie, abducted 90 degrees in external rotation). Reflexes are usually not altered. Obliteration of the radial pulse with certain maneuvers of the arm or neck, once considered a highly sensitive sign of thoracic outlet obstruction, does not occur in most cases.

Chest radiography will identify patients with cervical rib (although most patients with cervical ribs are asymptomatic). MRI with the arms held in different positions is useful in identifying sites of impaired blood flow. Intra-arterial or venous obstruction is confirmed by angiography. Determination of conduction velocities of the ulnar and other peripheral nerves of the upper extremity may help localize the site of their compression.

Thoracic outlet syndrome must be differentiated from osteoarthritis of the cervical spine, tumors of the superior pulmonary sulcus, cervical spinal cord, or nerve roots, and periarthritis of the shoulder.

Treatment is directed toward relief of compression of the neurovascular bundle. Greater than 95% of patients can be treated successfully with conservative therapy consisting of physical therapy and avoiding postures or activities that compress the neurovascular bundle. Some women will benefit from a support bra. Operative treatment, required by less than 5% of patients, is more likely to relieve the neurologic rather than the vascular component that causes symptoms.

Sadat U et al. Thoracic outlet syndrome: an overview. Br J Hosp Med (Lond). 2008 May;69(5):260–3. [PMID: 18557546]

LOW BACK PAIN

Up to 80% of the population experience low back pain at some time. The differential diagnosis is broad and includes muscular strain, primary spine disease (eg, disk herniation, degenerative arthritis), systemic diseases (eg, metastatic cancer), and regional diseases (eg, aortic aneurysm). A precise diagnosis cannot be made in the majority of cases. Even when anatomic defects—such as vertebral osteophytes or a narrowed disk space—are present, causality cannot be assumed since such defects are common in asymptomatic patients. Most patients will improve in 1–4 weeks and need no evaluation beyond the initial history and physical examination. The diagnostic challenge is to identify those patients who require more extensive or urgent evaluation. In practice, this means identifying those patients with pain caused by (1) infection, (2) cancer, (3) inflammatory back disease such as ankylosing spondylitis, or (4) pain referred from abdominal or pelvic processes, such as penetrating peptic ulcer or expanding aortic aneurysm. Significant or progressive neurologic deficits also require identification. If there is no evidence of these problems, conservative therapy is called for.

1. Clinical Approach to Diagnosis

General History & Physical Examination

Low back pain is a final common pathway of many processes; the pain of vertebral osteomyelitis, for example, is not very different in quality and intensity from that due to back strain of the weekend gardener. Historical factors of importance include smoking, weight loss, age over 50, and cancer, all of which are risk factors for vertebral body metastasis. Osteomyelitis most frequently occurs in adults with a history of recurrent urinary tract infections and is especially common in diabetics and injection drug users. A history of a cardiac murmur should raise concern about endocarditis, since back pain is not an uncommon manifestation. A background of renal calculi might indicate another cause of referred back pain.

History of the Back Pain

Certain qualities of a patient's pain can indicate a specific diagnosis. Low back pain radiating down the buttock and below the knee suggests a herniated disk causing nerve root irritation. Other conditions—including sacroiliitis, facet joint degenerative arthritis, spinal stenosis, or irritation of the sciatic nerve from a wallet—also cause this pattern.

The diagnosis of disk herniation is further suggested by physical examination (see below) and confirmed by imaging techniques. Disk herniation can be asymptomatic, so its presence does not invariably link it to the symptom.

Low back pain at night, unrelieved by rest or the supine position, suggests the possibility of malignancy, either vertebral body metastasis (chiefly from prostate, breast, lung, multiple myeloma, or lymphoma) or a cauda equina tumor. Similar pain can also be caused by compression fractures (from osteoporosis or myeloma).

Symptoms of large or rapidly evolving neurologic deficits identify patients who need urgent evaluation for possible cauda equina tumor, epidural abscess or, rarely, massive disk herniation. When a herniated disk impinges a nerve root, pain is the most prominent symptom; numbness and weakness are less common and, when present, are of the magnitude consistent with compression of a single nerve root. Symptoms of bilateral leg weakness (from multiple lumbar nerve root compressions) or of saddle area anesthesia, bowel or bladder incontinence, or impotence (indicating multiple sacral nerve root compressions) indicate a cauda equina process.

Low back pain that worsens with rest and improves with activity is characteristic of ankylosing spondylitis or other seronegative spondyloarthropathies, especially when the onset is insidious and begins before age 40. Most degenerative back diseases produce precisely the opposite pattern, with rest alleviating and activity aggravating the pain. Low back pain causing the patient to writhe occurs in renal colic but can also indicate a leaking aneurysm. The pain associated with pseudoclaudication from lumbar spinal stenosis is discussed below.

Physical Examination of the Back

Several physical findings should be sought because they help identify those few patients who need more than conservative management.

Neurologic examination of the lower extremities will detect the small deficits produced by disk disease and the large deficits complicating such problems as cauda equina tumors. A positive straight leg raising test indicates nerve root irritation. The examiner performs the test on the supine patient by passively raising the patient's ipsilateral leg. The test is positive if radicular pain is produced with the leg raised 60 degrees or less. It has a specificity of 40% but is 95% sensitive in patients with herniation at the L4–5 or L5–S1 level (the sites of 95% of disk herniations). It can be falsely negative, especially in patients with herniation above the L4–5 level. The crossed straight leg sign is positive when raising the contralateral leg reproduces the sciatica. It has a sensitivity of 25% but is 90% specific for disk herniation.

Table 20–6. Neurologic testing of lumbosacral nerve disorders.

Nerve Root	Motor	Reflex	Sensory Area
L4	Dorsiflexion of foot	Knee jerk	Medial calf
L5	Dorsiflexion of great toe	None	Medial forefoot
S1	Eversion of foot	Ankle jerk	Lateral foot

Detailed examination of the sacral and lumbar nerve roots, especially L5 and S1, is essential for detecting neurologic deficits associated with back pain. Disk herniation produces deficits predictable for the site involved (Table 20–6). Deficits of multiple nerve roots suggest a cauda equina tumor or an epidural abscess, both requiring urgent evaluation and treatment.

Measurement of spinal motion in the patient with acute pain is rarely of diagnostic utility and usually simply confirms that pain limits motion. An exception is the decreased range of motion in multiple regions of the spine (cervical, thoracic, and lumbar) in a diffuse spinal disease such as ankylosing spondylitis. By the time the patient has such limits, however, the diagnosis is usually straightforward.

If back pain is not severe and does not itself limit motion, the modified Schober test of lumbar motion is helpful in early diagnosis of ankylosing spondylitis. To perform this test, two marks are made with the patient upright: one 10 cm above the sacral dimples and another 5 cm below. The patient then bends forward as far as possible, and the distance between the points is measured. Normally, the distance increases from 15 cm to at least 20 cm. Anything less indicates reduced lumbar motion.

Palpation of the spine usually does not yield diagnostic information. Point tenderness over a vertebral body is reported to suggest osteomyelitis, but this association is uncommon. A step-off noted between the spinous process of adjacent vertebral bodies may indicate spondylolisthesis, but the sensitivity of this finding is extremely low. Tenderness of the soft tissues overlying the greater trochanter of the hip is a manifestation of trochanteric bursitis.

Inspection of the spine is not often of value in identifying serious causes of low back pain. The classic posture of ankylosing spondylitis is a late finding. Scoliosis of mild degree is not associated with an increased risk of clinical back disease. Cutaneous neurofibromas can identify the rare patient with nerve root encasement.

Examination of the hips should be part of the complete examination. While hip arthritis usually produces pain chiefly in the groin area, some patients have buttock or low back symptoms.

Further Examination

If the history and physical examination do not suggest the presence of infection, cancer, inflammatory back disease, major neurologic deficits, or pain referred from abdominal or pelvic disease, further evaluation can be eliminated or deferred while conservative therapy is tried. The great majority of patients will improve with conservative care over 1–4 weeks.

Regular radiographs of the lumbosacral spine give 20 times the radiation dose of a chest radiograph and provide limited, albeit important, information. Oblique films double the radiation dose and are not routinely needed. Radiographs can provide evidence of vertebral body osteomyelitis, cancer, fractures, or ankylosing spondylitis. Degenerative changes in the lumbar spine are ubiquitous in patients over 40 and do not prove clinical disease. Plain radiographs have very low sensitivity or specificity for disk disease. Thus, plain radiographs are warranted promptly for patients suspected of having infection, cancer, or fractures; selected other patients who do not improve after 2–4 weeks of conservative therapy are also candidates. The Agency for Healthcare Research and Quality guidelines for obtaining lumbar radiographs are summarized in Table 20–7.

MRI provides exquisite anatomic detail but is reserved for patients who are considering surgery or have evidence of a systemic disease. For example, MRI is needed urgently for any patient in whom an epidural mass or cauda equina tumor is suspected but not for a patient believed to have a routine disk herniation, since most will improve over 4–6 weeks of conservative therapy. Noncontrast CT does not image cauda equina tumors or other intradural lesions, and if used instead of MRI it must include intrathecal contrast.

Radionuclide bone scanning has limited usefulness. It is most useful for early detection of vertebral body osteomyelitis or osteoblastic metastases. The bone scan is normal in multiple myeloma because lytic lesions do not take up isotope.

2. Management

While any management plan must be individualized, key elements of most conservative treatments for back pain include analgesia and education. Analgesia can usually be provided with NSAIDs (see Table 5–3), but severe pain

Table 20–7. AHRQ criteria for lumbar radiographs in patients with acute low back pain.

Possible fracture
Major trauma
Minor trauma in patients > 50 years
Long-term corticosteroid use
Osteoporosis
> 70 years
Possible tumor or infection
> 50 years
< 20 years
History of cancer
Constitutional symptoms
Recent bacterial infection
Injection drug use
Immunosuppression
Supine pain
Nocturnal pain

AHRQ, Agency for Healthcare Research and Quality. Reproduced, with permission, from Suarez-Almazor et al. JAMA 1997;277:1782–6.

may require opioids (see Table 5–4). Rarely does the need for opioids extend beyond 1–2 weeks.

Diazepam, cyclobenzaprine, carisoprodol, and methocarbamol have been prescribed as muscle relaxants, though their sedative effects may limit their use. They should be reserved for patients who do not respond to NSAIDs and usually are needed only for 1–2 weeks, which reduces the chance of dependence. Their use should be avoided in older patients, who are at risk for falling. All patients should be taught how to protect the back in daily activities—ie, not to lift heavy objects, to use the legs rather than the back when lifting, to use a chair with arm rests, and to rise from bed by first rolling to one side and then using the arms to push to an upright position. Back manipulation for benign, mechanical low back pain appears safe and as effective as therapies provided by clinicians.

Rest and back exercises, once thought to be cornerstones of conservative therapy, are now known to be ineffective for acute back pain. Advice to rest in bed is less effective than advice to remain active. No bed rest with continuation of ordinary activities as tolerated is superior to 2 days of bed rest, 7 days of bed rest, and back mobilizing exercises. Similarly, for acute back pain, exercise therapy is not effective. The value of corsets or traction is dubious. Epidural corticosteroid injections can provide short-term relief of sciatica but do not improve functional status or reduce the need for surgery. In double-blind studies, repeated injections have been no more effective than a single injection. For chronic low back pain, yoga is as effective as a back exercise program and more effective than a self-care book. Corticosteroid injections into facet joints are ineffective for chronic low back pain.

Surgical consultation is needed urgently for any patient with a major or evolving neurologic deficit. Randomized controlled trials have shown that for sciatica caused by disk herniation, conservative treatment and surgery achieve similar 1-year outcomes; however, pain relief and perceived recovery were obtained more quickly with surgery. Surgery tends to ameliorate leg pain more quickly and fully than back pain.

Complaints without objective findings suggest a psychological role in symptom formation. Treatment includes reassurance and nonopioid analgesics.

When to Refer

• Suspected malignancy.
• Inflammatory low back pain.

When to Admit

• Neurologic signs indicative of cauda equina syndrome.
• Vertebral osteomyelitis.

Don AS et al. A brief overview of evidence-informed management of chronic low back pain with surgery. Spine J. 2008 Jan–Feb;8(1):258–65. [PMID: 18164474]

Peul WC et al. Surgery versus prolonged conservative treatment for sciatica. N Engl J Med. 2007 May 31;356(22):2245–56. [PMID: 17538084]

Pradhan BB. Evidence-informed management of chronic low back pain with watchful waiting. Spine J. 2008 Jan–Feb;8(1):253–7. [PMID: 18164473]

LUMBAR SPINAL STENOSIS

 ESSENTIALS OF DIAGNOSIS

▶ Most patients are older than 60 years.

▶ Presenting symptom is often back pain radiating to the buttocks and thighs.

▶ Pain often interferes with walking, worsens with lumbar extension, and improves with lumbar flexion.

▶ Back and leg pain often associated with numbness and paresthesias.

▶ Preservation of pedal pulses helps exclude vascular claudication.

▶ Diagnosis best confirmed by MRI.

General Considerations

Lumbar spinal stenosis, defined as narrowing of the spinal canal with compression of the nerve roots, may be congenital or (more commonly) acquired. It most frequently results from enlarging osteophytes at the facet joints, hypertrophy of the ligamentum flavum, and protrusion or bulging of intervertebral disks. Lumbar spinal stenosis may produce symptoms by directly compressing nerve roots or by compressing nutrient arterioles that supply the nerve roots.

Clinical Findings

A. Symptoms and Signs

Since age is the greatest risk factor for spinal degenerative changes, most patients with lumbar spinal stenosis are over 60 years old. Patients typically complain of either leg pain or trouble walking. The pain may originate in the low back but will extend below the buttock into the thigh in nearly 90% of patients. In approximately 50% of patients, the pain will extend below the knee. The pain is often a combination of aching and numbness, which characteristically worsens with walking. The pain can also be brought on by prolonged standing. Not infrequently the symptoms are bilateral. Many patients are more troubled by poor balance, unsteadiness of gait, or leg weakness that develops as they walk. Some describe these neuroclaudication symptoms as developing "spaghetti legs" or "walking like a drunk sailor." Because the lumbar spinal canal volume increases with back flexion and decreases with extension, some patients observe that they have fewer symptoms walking uphill than down. The back and lower extremity examination in patients with lumbar spinal stenosis is often unimpressive. Less than 10% have a positive straight leg raise sign, 25% have diminished deep tendon reflexes, and 60% have slight proximal weakness. Walking with the patient may reveal unsteadiness, although usually the patient's perception of gait disturbance is greater than that of an observer.

B. Imaging

The diagnosis of spinal stenosis in a patient with symptoms is best confirmed by MRI.

Differential Diagnosis

The onset of symptoms with standing, the location of the maximal discomfort to the thighs, and the preservation of pedal pulses help distinguish the "pseudoclaudication" of spinal stenosis from true claudication caused by vascular insufficiency. Distinguishing spinal stenosis from disk herniation can be challenging since both conditions can produce pain radiating down the back of the leg. Features that favor spinal stenosis are the gradual onset of symptoms, the marked exacerbation with walking, and the amelioration of symptoms with sitting or lumbar flexion. Complaints of bilateral aching in the buttocks associated with stiffness may make some practitioners consider the diagnosis of polymyalgia rheumatica. However, patients with lumbar spinal stenosis do not have the shoulder or neck symptoms characteristic of polymyalgia rheumatica.

Treatment

Weight loss and exercises aimed at reducing lumbar lordosis, which aggravates symptoms of spinal stenosis, can help. Lumbar epidural corticosteroid injections provide some immediate relief for about 50% of patients and more sustained relief for approximately 25%. When disabling symptoms persist, surgery will reduce pain and improve function substantially in approximately 75% of patients at 1 and 2 years; only about 25% of patients treated conservatively will experience a similar improvement.

Weinstein JN et al. Surgical versus nonsurgical treatment for lumbar degenerative spondylolisthesis. N Engl J Med. 2007 May 31;356(22):2257–70. [PMID: 17538085]

FIBROMYALGIA

ESSENTIALS OF DIAGNOSIS

▶ Most frequent in women aged 20–50.
▶ Chronic widespread musculoskeletal pain syndrome with multiple tender points.
▶ Fatigue, headaches, numbness common.
▶ Objective signs of inflammation absent; laboratory studies normal.
▶ Partially responsive to exercise, tricyclic antidepressants.

General Considerations

Fibromyalgia is one of the most common rheumatic syndromes in ambulatory general medicine affecting 3–10% of the general population. It shares many features with the chronic fatigue syndrome, namely, an increased frequency among women aged 20–50, absence of objective findings, and absence of diagnostic laboratory test results. While many of the clinical features of the two conditions overlap, musculoskeletal pain predominates in fibromyalgia whereas lassitude dominates the chronic fatigue syndrome.

The cause is unknown, but aberrant perception of painful stimuli, sleep disorders, depression, and viral infections have all been proposed. Fibromyalgia can be a rare complication of hypothyroidism, rheumatoid arthritis or, in men, sleep apnea.

Clinical Findings

The patient complains of chronic aching pain and stiffness, frequently involving the entire body but with prominence of pain around the neck, shoulders, low back, and hips. Fatigue, sleep disorders, subjective numbness, chronic headaches, and irritable bowel symptoms are common. Even minor exertion aggravates pain and increases fatigue. Physical examination is normal except for "trigger points" of pain produced by palpation of various areas such as the trapezius, the medial fat pad of the knee, and the lateral epicondyle of the elbow.

Differential Diagnosis

Fibromyalgia is a diagnosis of exclusion. A detailed history and repeated physical examination can obviate the need for extensive laboratory testing. Rheumatoid arthritis and systemic lupus erythematosus (SLE) present with objective physical findings or abnormalities on routine testing, including the ESR and C-reactive protein. Thyroid function tests are useful, since hypothyroidism can produce a secondary fibromyalgia syndrome. Polymyositis produces weakness rather than pain. The diagnosis of fibromyalgia probably should be made hesitantly in a patient over age 50 and should never be invoked to explain fever, weight loss, or any other objective signs. Polymyalgia rheumatica produces shoulder and pelvic girdle pain, is associated with anemia and an elevated ESR, and occurs after age 50. Hypophosphatemic states, such as oncogenic osteomalacia, should also be included in the differential diagnosis of musculoskeletal pain unassociated with physical findings. In contrast to fibromyalgia, oncogenic osteomalacia usually produces pain in only a few areas and is associated with a low serum phosphate level.

Treatment

Patient education is essential. Patients can be comforted that they have a diagnosable syndrome treatable by specific though imperfect therapies and that the course is not progressive. There is modest efficacy of amitriptyline, fluoxetine, chlorpromazine, cyclobenzaprine, pregabalin, or gabapentin. Amitriptyline is initiated at a dosage of 10 mg orally at bedtime and gradually increased to 40–50 mg depending on efficacy and toxicity. Less than 50% of the patients experience a sustained improvement. Exercise programs are also beneficial. NSAIDs are generally ineffective. Tramadol and acetaminophen combinations have ameliorated symptoms modestly in short-term trials. Opioids and corticosteroids are ineffective and should not be used to treat fibromyalgia. Acupuncture is also ineffective.

Prognosis

All patients have chronic symptoms. With treatment, however, many do eventually resume increased activities. Progressive or objective findings do not develop.

Abeles M et al. Update on fibromyalgia therapy. Am J Med. 2008 Jul;121(7):555–61. [PMID: 18589048]
Carville SF et al. EULAR evidence-based recommendations for the management of fibromyalgia syndrome. Ann Rheum Dis. 2008 Apr;67(4):536–41. [PMID: 17644548]

CARPAL TUNNEL SYNDROME

ESSENTIALS OF DIAGNOSIS

▶ Begins as pain, burning, and tingling in the distribution of the median nerve.

▶ Symptoms initially most bothersome at night.

▶ Weakness or atrophy, especially of the thenar eminence, appears later.

▶ Common in occupations that require repetitive wrist motion and in pregnancy, diabetes, and rheumatoid arthritis.

General Considerations

An entrapment neuropathy, carpal tunnel syndrome is a painful disorder caused by compression of the median nerve between the carpal ligament and other structures within the carpal tunnel. The contents of the tunnel can be compressed by synovitis of the tendon sheaths or carpal joints, recent or malhealed fractures, tumors, and occasionally congenital anomalies. Even though no anatomic lesion is apparent, flattening or even circumferential constriction of the median nerve may be observed during operative section of the ligament. The disorder may occur in pregnancy, is seen in individuals with a history of repetitive use of the hands, and may follow injuries of the wrists. There is a familial type of carpal tunnel syndrome in which no etiologic factor can be identified.

Carpal tunnel syndrome can also be a feature of many systemic diseases: rheumatoid arthritis and other rheumatic disorders (inflammatory tenosynovitis); myxedema, localized amyloidosis in chronic kidney disease, sarcoidosis, and leukemia (tissue infiltration); acromegaly; and hyperparathyroidism.

Clinical Findings

The initial symptoms are pain, burning, and tingling in the distribution of the median nerve (the palmar surfaces of the thumb, the index and long fingers, and the radial half of the ring finger). Aching pain may radiate proximally into the forearm and occasionally proximally to the shoulder and over the neck and chest. Pain is exacerbated by manual activity, particularly by extremes of volar flexion or dorsiflexion of the wrist. It is most bothersome at night. Impairment of sensation in the median nerve distribution may or may not be demonstrable. Subtle disparity between the affected and opposite sides can be shown by testing for two-point discrimination or by requiring the patient to identify different textures of cloth by rubbing them between the tips of the thumb and the index finger. Tinel or Phalen sign may be positive. (Tinel sign is tingling or shock-like pain on volar wrist percussion; Phalen sign is pain or paresthesia in the distribution of the median nerve when the patient flexes both wrists to 90 degrees for 60 seconds.) The carpal compression test, in which numbness and tingling are induced by the direct application of pressure over the carpal tunnel, may be more sensitive and specific than the Tinel and Phalen tests. Muscle weakness or atrophy, especially of the thenar eminence, appears later than sensory disturbances. Specific examinations include electromyography and determinations of segmental sensory and motor conduction delay. Sensory conduction delay is evident before motor delay.

Differential Diagnosis

This syndrome should be differentiated from other cervicobrachial pain syndromes, from compression syndromes of the median nerve in the forearm or arm, and from mononeuritis multiplex. When left-sided, it may be confused with angina pectoris.

Treatment

Treatment is directed toward relief of pressure on the median nerve. When a causative lesion is discovered, it is treated appropriately. Otherwise, patients in whom carpal tunnel syndrome is suspected should modify their hand activities and have the affected wrist splinted for 2–6 weeks. NSAIDs can also be added. Patients should be referred to a specialist for injection of corticosteroid into the carpal tunnel or for operation when they do not improve or when thenar muscle atrophy or weakness develops. Muscle strength returns gradually, but complete recovery cannot be expected when atrophy is pronounced.

When to Refer

• Refer to an orthopedic hand surgeon if symptoms persist despite the use of wrist splints.

• Refer to an orthopedic hand surgeon if weakness or thenar atrophy develops.

Scholten RJ et al. Surgical treatment options for carpal tunnel syndrome. Cochrane Database Syst Rev. 2007 Oct 17;(4):CD003905. [PMID: 17943805]

DUPUYTREN CONTRACTURE

This relatively common disorder is characterized by hyperplasia of the palmar fascia and related structures, with nodule formation and contracture of the palmar fascia. The cause is unknown, but the condition has a genetic predisposition and occurs primarily in white men over 50 years of age. The incidence is higher among alcoholic patients and those with chronic systemic disorders (especially cirrhosis). It is also associated with systemic fibrosing syndrome, which includes Peyronie disease, mediastinal and retroperitoneal fibrosis, and Riedel struma. The onset may be acute, but slowly progressive chronic disease is more common.

Dupuytren contracture manifests itself by nodular or cord-like thickening of one or both hands, with the fourth and fifth fingers most commonly affected. The patient may complain of tightness of the involved digits, with inability to satisfactorily extend the fingers, and on occasion there is tenderness. The resulting cosmetic problems may be unappealing, but in general the contracture is well tolerated since it exaggerates the normal position of function of the hand. Fasciitis involving other areas of the body may lead to plantar fibromatosis (10% of patients) or Peyronie disease (1–2%).

If the palmar nodule is growing rapidly, injections of triamcinolone into the nodule may be of benefit. Surgical intervention is indicated in patients with significant flexion contractures, depending on the location, but recurrence is not uncommon.

Townley WA et al. Dupuytren's contracture unfolded. BMJ. 2006 Feb 18;332(7538):397–400. [PMID: 16484265]

COMPLEX REGIONAL PAIN SYNDROME (Reflex Sympathetic Dystrophy)

Complex regional pain syndrome is a rare disorder of the extremities characterized by autonomic and vasomotor instability. The cardinal symptoms and signs are diffuse pain (characteristically localized to an arm or hand, leg or foot), swelling of the involved extremity, disturbances of color and temperature in the affected limb, dystrophic changes in the overlying skin and nails, and limited range of motion. Use of the former name of this entity, reflex sympathetic dystrophy, is now discouraged because the precise role of the sympathetic nervous system is unclear and dystrophy is not an inevitable sequela of the syndrome. Most cases are preceded by direct physical trauma, often of relatively minor nature, to the soft tissues, bone, or nerve. Early mobilization after injury or surgery reduces the likelihood of developing the syndrome. Any extremity can be involved, but the syndrome most commonly occurs in the hand and is associated with ipsilateral restriction of shoulder motion (shoulder-hand syndrome). The syndrome proceeds through phases: pain, swelling, and skin color and temperature changes develop early and, if untreated, lead to atrophy and dystrophy. The swelling in complex regional pain syndrome is diffuse ("catcher's mitt hand") and not restricted to joints. Pain is often burning in quality, intense, and often greatly worsened by minimal stimuli such as light touch. The shoulder-hand variant of this disorder sometimes complicates myocardial infarction or injuries to the neck or shoulder. Complex regional pain syndrome may occur after a knee injury or after arthroscopic knee surgery. There are no systemic symptoms. In the early phases of the syndrome, bone scans are sensitive,

showing diffuse increased uptake in the affected extremity. Radiographs eventually reveal severe generalized osteopenia. In the posttraumatic variant, this is known as Sudeck atrophy. Symptoms and findings are bilateral in some. This syndrome should be differentiated from other cervicobrachial pain syndromes, rheumatoid arthritis, thoracic outlet obstruction, and scleroderma, among others.

Early treatment offers the best prognosis for recovery. In the acute phase when edema is present, prednisone, 30–60 mg/d orally for 2 weeks and then tapered over 2 weeks, can be effective. Pain management is important and facilitates physical therapy, which plays a critical role in efforts to restore function. Some patients will also benefit from antidepressant agents (eg, nortriptyline initiated at a dosage of 10 mg orally at bedtime and gradually increased to 40–75 mg at bedtime). Regional nerve blocks and dorsal-column stimulation have also been demonstrated to be helpful. Patients who have restricted shoulder motion may benefit from the treatment described for scapulohumeral periarthritis. The prognosis partly depends on the stage in which the lesions are encountered and the extent and severity of associated organic disease.

Albazaz R et al. Complex regional pain syndrome: a review. Ann Vasc Surg. 2008 Mar;22(2):297–306. [PMID: 18346583]

BURSITIS

Inflammation of bursae—the synovium-like cellular membranes overlying bony prominences—may be secondary to trauma, infection, or arthritic conditions such as gout, rheumatoid arthritis, or osteoarthritis. The most common locations are the subdeltoid, olecranon, ischial, trochanteric, semimembranous-gastrocnemius (Baker cyst), and prepatellar bursae.

There are several ways to distinguish bursitis from arthritis. Bursitis is more likely than arthritis to cause focal tenderness and swelling and less likely to affect range of motion of the adjacent joint. Olecranon bursitis, for example, causes an oval (or, if chronic, bulbous) swelling at the tip of the elbow and does not affect elbow motion, whereas an elbow joint inflammation produces more diffuse swelling and reduces range of motion. Similarly, a patient with prepatellar bursitis has a small focus of swelling over the kneecap but no distention of the knee joint itself and preserved knee motion. A patient with trochanteric bursitis will have tenderness over the greater trochanter and normal internal rotation of the hip; a patient with hip arthritis usually will have reduced internal rotation. Bursitis caused by trauma responds to local heat, rest, NSAIDs, and local corticosteroid injections.

Bursitis can result from infection. The two most common sites are the olecranon and prepatellar bursae. Acute swelling and redness at either of these two sites calls for aspiration to rule out infection. The absence of fever does not exclude infection; one-third of those with septic olecranon bursitis are afebrile. A bursal fluid white blood cell count of greater than 1000/mcL indicates inflammation from infection, rheumatoid arthritis, or gout. In septic bursitis, the white cell count averages over 50,000/mcL.

Most cases are caused by *Staphylococcus aureus;* the Gram stain is positive in two-thirds. Treatment involves antibiotics and repeated aspiration for tense effusions.

Chronic, stable olecranon bursa swelling unaccompanied by erythema or other signs of inflammation does not suggest infection and does not require aspiration (Plate 81). Aspiration of the olecranon bursa in rheumatoid arthritis and in gout runs the risk of creating a chronic drainage site, which can be reduced by using a "zig-zag" approach with a small needle (25-gauge if possible) and pulling the skin over the bursa before introducing it. Applying a pressure bandage may also help prevent chronic drainage. Surgical removal of the bursa is indicated only for cases in which repeated infections occur. Repetitive minor trauma to the olecranon bursa should be eliminated by avoiding resting the elbow on a hard surface or by wearing an elbow pad.

A bursa can also become symptomatic when it ruptures. This is particularly true for Baker cyst, whose rupture can cause calf pain and swelling that mimic thrombophlebitis. Ruptured Baker cysts are imaged easily by sonography or MRI. In most cases, imaging is unnecessary because the cyst and an associated knee effusion are detectable on physical examination. It may be important to exclude a deep venous thrombosis, which can be mimicked by a ruptured Baker cyst. Treatment of a ruptured cyst includes rest, leg elevation, and injection of triamcinolone, 20–40 mg into the knee anteriorly (the knee compartment communicates with the cyst). Rarely, Baker cyst can compress vascular structures and cause leg edema and true thrombophlebitis.

Segal NA et al. Greater trochanteric pain syndrome: epidemiology and associated factors. Arch Phys Med Rehabil. 2007 Aug;88(8):988–92. [PMID: 17678660]

SPORTS MEDICINE INJURIES

Musculoskeletal problems commonly occur as a result of both serious athletic pursuits and activities of daily living. For most such disorders, the diagnosis is made easily. Physical therapy is an increasingly important adjunct to the management of these disorders.

1. Rotator Cuff Disorders

Disorders of the rotator cuff, such as tendinitis, subacromial bursitis, and partial and complete tears, account for a substantial majority of shoulder problems. The tendons of the rotator cuff form a musculotendinous unit near their insertions into the proximal humerus. Years of cumulative irritation can lead to attenuation of these tendons, particularly the supraspinatus tendon. Distinguishing between the various soft tissue disorders that cause shoulder pain is difficult because these frequently cause similar symptoms and often occur together. Precise distinction is frequently unimportant for purposes of therapy.

► Clinical Findings

Patients usually present with nonspecific pain localized to the shoulder, often noticed more at night when lying on the affected side. Locking sensations occur with motion of the shoulder, particularly through abduction. Because of the shared innervation, symptoms are frequently referred down the proximal lateral arm. With rotator cuff tears, the patient may be unable to abduct or flex the shoulder, depending on the site of the tear.

The rotator cuff may be palpated just lateral to the head of the acromion. Maximum tenderness is usually noted over the supraspinatus insertion. The acromioclavicular joint may also be tender if there is accompanying degenerative arthritis in that joint. There may be prominent crepitus. Pain with range of motion is most pronounced between 60 and 120 degrees of abduction, the site of greatest impingement of the rotator cuff tissues between the humerus and coracoacromial arch.

For patients with partial rotator cuff tendon ruptures, the findings are identical to those of chronic tendinitis and bursitis. Patients with partial ruptures often demonstrate mild abduction weakness. With complete ruptures, weakness of abduction (and, to a lesser extent, flexion) is substantial, even though full range of motion may be maintained by the shoulder's accessory rotator muscles. Patients with complete tears usually have positive "drop arm" signs: inability to sustain passive abduction of the arm to 90 degrees.

► Treatment

For most rotator cuff disorders, rest and abstention from inciting activities are helpful. NSAIDs and moist heat afford some relief. Injections of a corticosteroid preparation (eg, 1 mL of triamcinolone, 40 mg/mL) mixed with 2–3 mL of lidocaine hydrochloride (1–2%) may be useful. Tears or partial tears of the rotator cuff tendons that are believed to be chronic do not preclude a corticosteroid injection. Most patients obtain significant relief with one injection, but the procedure—along with continued rest—may be repeated after 2–3 weeks. Physical therapy is valuable for refractory cases—if the patient does not maintain the shoulder's normal range of motion, stiffness and impaired function from a "frozen shoulder" may ensue.

Aside from patients with complete rotator cuff tears, only those who do not improve after months of conservative therapy are candidates for operation. Persistent symptoms may be a sign of complete tear, which may be diagnosed by MRI. Patients with symptoms that continue in the absence of a complete tear, however, sometimes require surgery to excise the inferolateral portion of the acromion, release obstructed soft tissue, and repair partial tendon tears. Depending on the patient's symptoms and functional status, complete tears may not always require surgical repair. Patients over 75 years of age rarely have symptoms or limitations that necessitate surgery. Moreover, surgical repairs are frequently less successful because of the attrition of the rotator cuff that occurs with aging.

Burbank KM et al. Chronic shoulder pain: part I. Evaluation and diagnosis. Am Fam Physician. 2008 Feb 15;77(4):453–60. [PMID: 18326164]
Burbank KM et al. Chronic shoulder pain: part II. Treatment. Am Fam Physician. 2008 Feb 15;77(4):493–7. [PMID: 18326169]

2. Lateral & Medial Epicondylitis

These disorders are better known by their sports associations: "tennis elbow" and "golf elbow," respectively. Lateral epicondylitis is the more common of the two. The conditions are caused by overuse, and the pain results from minor tears in the tendons of the forearm's extensor and flexor muscles.

▶ Clinical Findings

The patient complains of pain at the site of tendon insertion. Tasks that require grasping and squeezing, such as shaking hands or opening jars, cause pain.

The diagnoses are easily confirmed on physical examination by elicitation of point tenderness over the involved site. The characteristic pain may also be reproduced by extension or flexion of the wrist against pressure. Clenching the fist and extending the wrist against the pressure of the examiner's palm is a useful maneuver for localizing lateral epicondylitis. Medial epicondylitis may be demonstrated by performing the same maneuver in flexion.

▶ Treatment

NSAIDs and rest are effective in mild cases. Symptoms that persist after 2 weeks of conservative therapy usually respond either to infiltration of triamcinolone, 10–20 mg mixed with 1–2 mL of 1% lidocaine, around the involved epicondyle—or to physiotherapy. Results are quicker with corticosteroid injections but longer-lasting with physiotherapy. Only experienced clinicians should inject the medial epicondyle because of the risk of injury to the ulnar nerve. After the pain and tenderness have subsided, patients may begin a physical therapy program involving daily stretching of the flexor and extensor tendons.

Calfee RP et al. Management of lateral epicondylitis: current concepts. J Am Acad Orthop Surg. 2008 Jan;16(1):19–29. [PMID: 18180389]

3. Patellofemoral Syndrome

Patellofemoral syndrome is among the most common causes of knee complaints in primary care medicine, particularly among adolescent and young adult patients. The syndrome frequently gives rise to the chief complaint of anterior knee pain. A variety of injuries or anatomic abnormalities predispose patients to irregular patellar movements, leading to the patellofemoral syndrome. Such predisposing conditions include imbalance of quadriceps strength, patella alta, recurrent patellar subluxation, direct trauma to the patella, and meniscal injuries. For most of these causes, the therapeutic approach is similar.

▶ Clinical Findings

Patients frequently have difficulty localizing the source of their complaint but generally confirm that the pain is in the front of the knee, around or underneath the patella. Questions regarding specific precipitants of the pain may be useful in establishing the diagnosis. For example,

because of the flexion load, patients have difficulty going up or down staircases (down is usually associated with greater symptoms). Another characteristic symptom is the positive "theater" sign: after remaining seated for a prolonged period, patients describe extreme discomfort with their first few steps after rising. The symptoms improve with further walking. Finally, patients with patellofemoral syndrome often complain of crepitus, joint locking, or sensations of joint instability, all of which lack readily confirmed anatomic explanations.

The physical examination is less useful than the history in establishing the diagnosis, but a significant number of patients have characteristic physical findings. In particular, when the knee is held in slight flexion, gentle pressure against the patella as the patient contracts the quadriceps muscles may reproduce the symptoms. In some cases, with the knee extended and the quadriceps relaxed, the typical pain may be reproduced by digital pressure under the medial or lateral border of the patella, with side-to-side movement of the bone. Inflammatory findings on examination are incompatible with the diagnosis of patellofemoral syndrome and suggest other disorders.

▶ Treatment

Therapy includes avoidance of flexion loads and strengthening of the quadriceps. Referral to a physical therapist is helpful in educating the patient about home exercises. Many patients learn that the most effective therapy is bicycling, with the seat high enough to permit nearly full knee extension with each cycle. Although most cases respond to these interventions and even resolve altogether, some persist for years. Even in the latter, conservative therapy remains the rule; operation is rarely indicated. There is only limited evidence for the effectiveness of NSAIDs in short-term pain reduction associated with the patellofemoral pain syndrome. The evidence supporting the use of glycosaminoglycan polysulfate is conflicting. Bracing is no more effective than a home exercise program.

Fredericson M et al. Physical examination and patellofemoral pain syndrome. Am J Phys Med Rehabil. 2006 Mar;85(3):234–43. [PMID: 16505640]

4. Overuse Syndromes of the Knee

Runners—particularly those who overtrain or do not attain the proper level of conditioning before starting a running program—may develop a variety of painful overuse syndromes of the knee. Most of these conditions are forms of tendinitis or bursitis that can be diagnosed on examination. The most common conditions include anserine bursitis, the iliotibial band syndrome, and popliteal and patellar tendinitis.

▶ Clinical Findings

Symptoms resulting from all of these conditions worsen as the patient continues to run and often require cessation of the activity. Anserine bursitis results in pain medial and inferior to the knee joint over the medial tibia. The iliotibial band syndrome and popliteal tenosynovitis may be difficult to differentiate, because the popliteus tendon inserts into the lateral femoral condyle underneath the iliotibial band. Both conditions result in pain on the lateral side of the knee. Patellar tendinitis, a cause of anterior knee discomfort, typically occurs at the tendon's insertion into the patella rather than at its more inferior insertion.

All of these diagnoses are confirmed by palpation at the relevant sites around the knee. None is associated with joint effusions or other signs of synovitis.

► Treatment

Rest and abstention from the associated physical activities for a period of days to weeks are essential. Once pain has subsided, a program of gentle stretching (particularly prior to resuming exercise) may prevent recurrence. Corticosteroid injections with lidocaine may be useful when intense discomfort is present, but caution must be used when injecting corticosteroids into the region of a tendon to avoid rupture.

Brushøj C et al. Prevention of overuse injuries by a concurrent exercise program in subjects exposed to an increase in training load: a randomized controlled trial of 1020 army recruits. Am J Sports Med. 2008 Apr;36(4):663–70. [PMID: 18337359]

5. Medial Meniscus Injuries

Tears of the medial meniscus are the most common knee injuries encountered in primary care. Because the medial meniscus is tethered firmly to the underlying tibia, injuries to the medial meniscus occur ten times more commonly than injuries to the lateral meniscus. Both result from a twisting action exerted on the knee joint while the foot is in a weight-bearing position.

► Clinical Findings

The injury is heralded by a tearing or popping sensation followed by severe pain. Occasionally, meniscal tears result from seemingly minor trauma. In contrast to ligamentous injuries, in which hemorrhage causes immediate swelling, effusions associated with meniscal injuries accumulate over hours and are typically worse the day after the injury. Several days after resolution (full or partial), the patient may experience the sensation of joint locking or instability, recurrent swelling with activity, and pain. "Pseudolocking" caused by muscle spasm and swelling is more common than mechanical blockage caused by a fragment of torn meniscus.

A knee effusion is usually present. Tenderness may be localized to the medial joint line, and range of motion in the knee may be restricted. In patients without an acutely painful, swollen knee, McMurray test may suggest the diagnosis. This test is performed with the patient supine and the hip and knee in full flexion. The examiner has one hand on the involved knee and the other on the ipsilateral foot. As the foot is externally rotated, the examiner extends the patient's knee. The presence of a "snap" (palpable or audible) suggests a medial meniscus lesion. MRI is the optimal test for confirming the diagnosis if plain films exclude other conditions.

► Treatment

Initial management is conservative, with elevation of the joint and application of a compression dressing and ice. Weight bearing should be minimized for the first few days after the injury but may be resumed slowly thereafter. The patient should perform quadriceps-strengthening exercises under the instruction of a physical therapist. Surgery is reserved for patients with symptoms that recur upon resumption of normal activities or for patients with irreducible locking caused by mechanical problems.

6. Ankle Sprains

Ankle sprains are among the most common of all sports injuries. Most sprains involve the lateral ligament complex, particularly the anterior talofibular ligament. In more severe injuries, the calcaneofibular ligament may also be involved. If both of these ligaments are ruptured, the injury results in significant joint instability and is classified as a grade III (severe) sprain. (Grades I and II correspond to mild and moderate injuries, respectively.) This section reviews only the type of ankle sprain resulting from inversion (varus) injuries, which account for 85% of all sprains.

► Clinical Findings

Varus sprains include a spectrum of severity, ranging from slight loss of function to injuries in which the swelling is prompt, the pain prominent, and weight bearing impossible. A history of hearing a "pop" at the time of injury is frequently associated with the latter.

Hemorrhage resulting from torn ligaments and damaged peroneal muscle tendons may cause substantial ecchymosis. Tenderness is typically present at the site of injury, and the associated swelling may be considerable. Stability of the anterior talofibular and calcaneofibular ligaments should be assessed with the "anterior drawer" sign: With the foot held in slight plantar flexion, the examiner cups the patient's heel with one hand and the patient's shin with the other. The examiner then applies gentle anterior force in the plane of the patient's foot. Excessive anterior motion of the foot constitutes a positive test (grade III sprain). Plain radiographs exclude associated bony injury.

► Treatment

Most ankle sprains—even grade III—are treated identically. The acronym "RICE" (rest, ice, compression, elevation) applies more accurately to ankle sprains than to any other injury. Early application of a compression dressing is essential to control swelling and provide stability to the traumatized joint. An Aircast ankle brace may be more effective than an elastic support bandage. Weight bearing should be minimal, with liberal use of crutches. Elevation of the ankle for several days hastens functional recovery by diminishing pain and swelling, and ice is also helpful (alternating 30 minutes on, 30 minutes off). The ice should be applied on top of the compression dressing and not against the skin both because close apposition of the dressing to the skin is critical to control swelling and because direct application of ice is uncomfortable and even deleterious to the skin. Referral to a physical therapist may expedite recovery. Patients should be informed that symptoms from lateral ankle sprains may take weeks or months to resolve, and that this period will be prolonged by premature attempts to bear weight on the injured ankle. Surgical repairs of ruptured lateral ligaments provide excellent outcomes but are usually necessary only in cases of chronically unstable joints.

van Rijn RM et al. What is the clinical course of acute ankle sprains? A systematic literature review. Am J Med. 2008 Apr;121(4):324–31. [PMID: 18374692]

7. Plantar Fasciitis

The most common cause of foot pain in outpatient medicine is plantar fasciitis, which results from constant strain on the plantar fascia at its insertion into the medial tubercle of the calcaneus. Although certain inflammatory disorders such as the seronegative spondyloarthropathies predispose patients to enthesopathies, the majority of cases occur in patients with no associated disease. Most occur as the result of excessive standing and improper footwear.

▶ Clinical Findings

Patients with plantar fasciitis report severe pain on the bottoms of their feet in the morning—the first steps out of bed in particular—but the pain subsides after a few minutes of ambulation.

The diagnosis may be confirmed by palpation over the plantar fascia's insertion on the medial heel. Radiographs have no role in the diagnosis of this condition—heel spurs frequently exist in patients without plantar fasciitis, and most symptomatic patients do not have heel spurs.

▶ Treatment

Treatment consists of restriction of prolonged standing for days and the use of arch supports. Arch supports give relief by requiring the arches to bear more of the patient's weight, thus unloading the plantar enthesis. NSAIDs may provide some relief. In severe cases, a corticosteroid with lidocaine injection (small volume—no more than a total of 1.5 mL) directly into the most tender area on the sole of the foot is helpful. Rare patients require release of the plantar fascia from its attachment site at the os calcis.

Neufeld SK et al. Plantar fasciitis: evaluation and treatment. J Am Acad Orthop Surg. 2008 Jun;16(6):338–46. [PMID: 18524985]

▼ AUTOIMMUNE DISEASES

RHEUMATOID ARTHRITIS

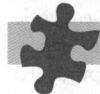

ESSENTIALS OF DIAGNOSIS

▶ Usually insidious onset with morning stiffness and pain in affected joints.

▶ Symmetric polyarthritis with predilection for small joints of the hands and feet; deformities common with progressive disease.

▶ Radiographic findings: juxta-articular osteoporosis, joint erosions, and joint space narrowing.

▶ Rheumatoid factor and antibodies to cyclic citrullinated peptides (anti-CCP) are present in 70–80%.

▶ Extra-articular manifestations: subcutaneous nodules, pleural effusion, pericarditis, lymphadenopathy, splenomegaly with leukopenia, and vasculitis.

▶ General Considerations

Rheumatoid arthritis is a chronic systemic inflammatory disease whose major manifestation is synovitis of multiple joints. It has a prevalence of 1% and is more common in women than men (female:male ratio of 3:1). Rheumatoid arthritis can begin at any age, but the peak onset is in the fourth or fifth decade for women and the sixth to eighth decades for men. The cause is not known. Susceptibility to rheumatoid arthritis is genetically determined with multiple genes contributing. Inheritance of class II HLA molecules with a distinctive five-amino-acid sequence known as the "shared epitope" is the best characterized genetic risk factor. Untreated, rheumatoid arthritis causes joint destruction with consequent disability and shortens life expectancy. Early, aggressive treatment is the standard of care.

The pathologic findings in the joint include chronic synovitis with formation of a pannus, which erodes cartilage, bone, ligaments, and tendons. In the acute phase, effusion and other manifestations of inflammation are common. In the late stage, organization may result in fibrous ankylosis; true bony ankylosis is rare.

▶ Clinical Findings

A. Symptoms and Signs

1. Joint symptoms—The clinical manifestations of rheumatoid disease are highly variable, but joint symptoms usually predominate. Although acute presentations may occur, the onset of articular signs of inflammation is usually insidious, with prodromal symptoms of vague periarticular pain or stiffness. Symmetric swelling of multiple joints with tenderness and pain is characteristic. Monarticular disease is occasionally seen initially. Stiffness persisting for more than 30 minutes (and usually many hours) is prominent in the morning. Stiffness may recur after daytime inactivity and be much more severe after strenuous activity. Although any diarthrodial joint may be affected, PIP joints of the fingers, MCP joints, wrists, knees, ankles, and MTP joints are most often involved (Plate 82). Synovial cysts and rupture of tendons may occur. Entrapment syndromes are not unusual—particularly of the median nerve at the carpal tunnel of the wrist. Rheumatoid arthritis can affect the neck but spares the other components of the spine and does not involve the sacroiliac joints.

2. Rheumatoid nodules—Twenty percent of patients have subcutaneous rheumatoid nodules, most commonly situated over bony prominences but also observed in the bursae and tendon sheaths (Plate 83). Nodules are occasionally seen in the lungs, the sclerae, and other tissues. Nodules correlate with the presence of rheumatoid factor in serum ("seropositivity"), as do most other extra-articular manifestations.

3. Ocular symptoms—Dryness of the eyes, mouth, and other mucous membranes is found especially in advanced disease (see Sjögren syndrome). Other ocular manifestations include episcleritis, scleritis, and scleromalacia due to scleral nodules.

4. Other symptoms—Palmar erythema is common. Occasionally, a small vessel vasculitis develops and manifests as tiny hemorrhagic infarcts in the nail folds or finger pulps. Although necrotizing arteritis is well reported, it is rare. Pericarditis and pleural disease, when present, are usually silent clinically. Additional extra-articular manifestations of rheumatoid arthritis include pulmonary fibrosis, mononuclear cell infiltration of skeletal muscle and perineurium, and hyperplasia of lymph nodes. A small subset of patients with rheumatoid arthritis have Felty syndrome, the occurrence of splenomegaly and neutropenia, usually in the setting of severe, destructive arthritis. Felty syndrome must be distinguished from the large granular lymphocyte syndrome, with which it shares many features.

Aortitis is a rare late complication that can result in aortic regurgitation or rupture and is usually associated with evidence of rheumatoid vasculitis elsewhere in the body.

B. Laboratory Findings

Anti-CCP antibodies and rheumatoid factor, an IgM antibody directed against the Fc fragment of IgG, are present in 70–80% of patients with established rheumatoid arthritis but have sensitivities of only 50% in early disease. Anti-CCP antibodies are the most specific blood test for rheumatoid arthritis (specificity ~95%). Rheumatoid factor can occur in other autoimmune disease and in chronic infections, including hepatitis C, syphilis, subacute bacterial endocarditis, and tuberculosis. The prevalence of rheumatoid factor positivity also rises with age in healthy individuals. Approximately 20% of rheumatoid patients have antinuclear antibodies.

The ESR and levels of C-reactive protein are typically elevated in proportion to disease activity. A moderate hypochromic normocytic anemia is common. The white cell count is normal or slightly elevated, but leukopenia may occur, often in the presence of splenomegaly (eg, Felty syndrome). The platelet count is often elevated, roughly in proportion to the severity of overall joint inflammation. Initial joint fluid examination confirms the inflammatory nature of the arthritis. (See Table 20–2.) Arthrocentesis is needed to diagnose superimposed septic arthritis, which is a common complication of rheumatoid arthritis and should be considered whenever a patient with rheumatoid arthritis has one joint inflamed out of proportion to the rest.

C. Imaging

Of all the laboratory tests, radiographic changes are the most specific for rheumatoid arthritis. Radiographs obtained during the first 6 months of symptoms, however, are usually normal. The earliest changes occur in the wrists or feet and consist of soft tissue swelling and juxta-articular demineralization. Later, diagnostic changes of uniform joint space narrowing and erosions develop. The erosions are often first evident at the ulnar styloid and at the juxta-articular margin, where the bony surface is not protected by cartilage. Diagnostic changes also occur in the cervical spine, with C1–2 subluxation, but these changes usually take many years to develop. Although both MRI and ultrasonography are more sensitive than radiographs in detecting bony and soft tissue changes in rheumatoid arthritis, their value in early diagnosis relative to that of plain radiographs has not been established.

▶ Differential Diagnosis

The differentiation of rheumatoid arthritis from other joint conditions and immune-mediated disorders can be difficult. In contrast to rheumatoid arthritis, osteoarthritis spares the wrist and the MCP joints. Osteoarthritis is not associated with constitutional manifestations, and the joint pain is characteristically relieved by rest, unlike the morning stiffness of rheumatoid arthritis. Signs of articular inflammation, prominent in rheumatoid arthritis, are usually minimal in degenerative joint disease. Although gouty arthritis is almost always intermittent and monarticular in the early years, it may evolve with time into a chronic polyarticular process that mimics rheumatoid arthritis. Gouty tophi resemble rheumatoid nodules both in typical location and appearance. The early history of intermittent monarthritis and the presence of synovial urate crystals are distinctive features of gout. Chronic Lyme arthritis typically involves only one joint, most commonly the knee, and is associated with positive serologic tests (see Chapter 34). Human parvovirus B19 infection in adults can mimic early rheumatoid arthritis. However, arthralgias are more prominent than arthritis, rash—on the cheeks, torso, or extremities—is common, IgM antibodies to parvovirus B19 are present, and the arthritis usually resolves within weeks. Infection with hepatitis C can cause a chronic nonerosive polyarthritis associated with rheumatoid factor; tests for anti-CCP antibodies are negative.

Malar rash, photosensitivity, discoid skin lesions, alopecia, high titer antibodies to double-stranded DNA, glomerulonephritis, and central nervous system abnormalities point to the diagnosis of SLE. Polymyalgia rheumatica occasionally causes polyarthralgias in patients over age 50, but these patients remain rheumatoid factor–negative and have chiefly proximal muscle pain and stiffness, centered on the shoulder and hip girdles. Rheumatic fever is characterized by the migratory nature of the arthritis, an elevated antistreptolysin titer, and a more dramatic and prompt response to aspirin; carditis and erythema marginatum may occur in adults, but chorea and subcutaneous nodules virtually never do. Finally, a variety of cancers produce paraneoplastic syndromes, including polyarthritis. One form is hypertrophic pulmonary osteoarthropathy most often produced by lung and gastrointestinal carcinomas, characterized by a rheumatoid-like arthritis associated with clubbing, periosteal new bone formation, and a negative rheumatoid factor. Diffuse swelling of the hands with palmar fasciitis occurs in a variety of cancers, especially ovarian carcinoma.

► Treatment

The primary objectives in treating rheumatoid arthritis are reduction of inflammation and pain, preservation of function, and prevention of deformity. Success requires early, effective pharmacologic intervention. Disease-modifying antirheumatic drugs (DMARDs) should be started as soon as the diagnosis of rheumatoid disease is certain and then adjusted with the aim of suppressing disease activity. The American College of Rheumatology recommends using standardized assessments, such as the Disease Activity Score 28 Joints (DAS28), to gauge therapeutic responses, with the target of mild disease activity or remission by these measures. In advanced disease, surgical intervention may help improve function of damaged joints and to relieve pain.

A. Nonsteroidal Anti-inflammatory Drugs

NSAIDs provide some symptomatic relief in rheumatoid arthritis but do not prevent erosions or alter disease progression. They are not appropriate for monotherapy and should only be used in conjunction with DMARDs. A large number of NSAIDs are available; all appear equivalent in terms of efficacy (see Table 5–3).

Celecoxib, a selective COX-2 inhibitor, is FDA-approved for the treatment of osteoarthritis and rheumatoid arthritis. Compared with traditional NSAIDs, COX-2 inhibitors are as effective for treating rheumatoid arthritis but less likely in some circumstances to cause upper gastrointestinal tract adverse events (eg, obstruction, perforation, hemorrhage, or ulceration). Long-term use of COX-2 inhibitors, particularly in the absence of concomitant aspirin use, has been associated with an increased risk of cardiovascular events, leading to the removal of some COX-2 inhibitors from the US market and intense scrutiny of all drugs in that class.

1. Gastrointestinal side effects—For traditional NSAIDs that inhibit both COX-1 and COX-2, gastrointestinal side effects, such as gastric ulceration, perforation, and gastrointestinal hemorrhage, are the most common serious side effects. The overall rate of bleeding with NSAID use in the general population is low (1:6000 users or less) but is increased by long-term use, higher NSAID dose, concomitant corticosteroids or anticoagulants, the presence of rheumatoid arthritis, history of peptic ulcer disease or alcoholism, and age over 70. Twenty-five percent of all hospitalizations and deaths from peptic ulcer disease result from traditional NSAID therapy. Each year, 1:1000 patients with rheumatoid arthritis will require hospitalization for NSAID-related gastrointestinal bleeding or perforation. Although all traditional NSAIDs can cause massive gastrointestinal bleeding, the risk may be higher with indomethacin and piroxicam, probably because these drugs preferentially inhibit COX-1 in the stomach.

One approach to reducing the gastrointestinal toxicity of traditional NSAIDs is to add a proton pump inhibitor (eg, omeprazole 20 mg orally daily). Sucralfate, antacids,

and H_2-blockers (such as ranitidine) either do not work or do not work as well as proton pump inhibitors. The expense of proton pump inhibitors and misoprostol dictates that their use should be reserved for patients with risk factors for NSAID-induced gastrointestinal toxicity (noted above). Patients who have recently recovered from an NSAID-induced bleeding gastric ulcer appear to be at high risk for rebleeding (about 5% in 6 months) when an NSAID is reintroduced, even if prophylactic measures such as proton pump inhibitors are used. NSAIDs can also affect the lower intestinal tract, causing perforation or aggravating inflammatory bowel disease.

Acute liver injury from NSAIDs is rare, occurring in about 1 of every 25,000 patients using these agents. Having rheumatoid arthritis or taking sulindac may increase the risk.

2. Renal side effects—All of the NSAIDs, including aspirin and the COX-2 inhibitors, can produce renal toxicity, including interstitial nephritis, nephrotic syndrome, prerenal azotemia, and aggravation of hypertension. Hyperkalemia due to hyporeninemic hypoaldosteronism may also be seen rarely. The risk of renal toxicity is low but is increased by age over 60, a history of kidney disease, congestive heart failure, ascites, and diuretic use. COX-2 inhibitors appear to cause as much nephrotoxicity as traditional NSAIDs.

3. Platelet effects—All NSAIDs except the nonacetylated salicylates and the COX-2 inhibitors interfere with platelet function and prolong bleeding time. For all older NSAIDs except aspirin, the effect on bleeding time resolves as the drug is cleared. Aspirin irreversibly inhibits platelet function, so the bleeding time effect resolves only as new platelets are made. COX-2 inhibitors, which differ from other NSAIDs in not inhibiting platelet function, do not increase the risk of bleeding with surgical procedures as most NSAIDs do. Unfortunately, this failure to inhibit platelets is now known to lead to increased risks of myocardial infarction and stroke, particularly when the medications are used in high doses for prolonged periods of time. Patients requiring low-dose aspirin who are not compliant have a greater risk of developing a thrombotic event while taking a COX-2 inhibitor than while taking a traditional NSAID. Whether combination therapy with low-dose aspirin and a COX-2 inhibitor maintains the gastrointestinal advantage of selective COX-2 inhibitors is not yet known.

Although groups of patients with rheumatoid arthritis respond similarly to NSAIDs, individuals may respond differently—an NSAID that works for one patient may not work for another. Thus, if the first NSAID chosen is not effective after 2–3 weeks of use, another should be tried.

B. Corticosteroids

Low-dose corticosteroids (eg, oral prednisone 5–10 mg daily) produce a prompt anti-inflammatory effect in rheumatoid arthritis and slow the rate of bony destruction. However, their multiple side effects limit their long-term use.

Low-dose corticosteroids often are used as a "bridge" to reduce disease activity until the slower acting DMARDs take effect or as adjunctive therapy for active disease that persists despite treatment with DMARDs. No more than 10 mg of prednisone or equivalent per day is appropriate for articular disease. Many patients do reasonably well on 5–7.5 mg daily. (The use of 1 mg tablets, to facilitate doses of < 5 mg/d, is encouraged.) Higher doses are used to manage serious extra-articular manifestations (eg, pericarditis, necrotizing scleritis). When the corticosteroids are to be discontinued, they should be tapered gradually on a planned schedule appropriate to the duration of treatment. All patients receiving long-term corticosteroid therapy should take measures to prevent osteoporosis.

Intra-articular corticosteroids may be helpful if one or two joints are the chief source of difficulty. Intra-articular triamcinolone, 10–40 mg depending on the size of the joint to be injected, may be given for symptomatic relief but not more than four times a year.

C. Synthetic DMARDs

1. Methotrexate—Methotrexate is usually the initial synthetic DMARD of choice for patients with rheumatoid arthritis. It is generally well tolerated and often produces a beneficial effect in 2–6 weeks. The usual initial dose is 7.5 mg of methotrexate orally once weekly. If the patient has tolerated methotrexate but has not responded in 1 month, the dose can be increased to 15 mg orally once per week. The maximal dose is usually 20–25 mg/wk. The most frequent side effects are gastric irritation and stomatitis. Cytopenia, most commonly leukopenia or thrombocytopenia but rarely pancytopenia, due to bone marrow suppression is another important potential problem. The risk of developing pancytopenia is much higher in patients with elevation of the serum creatinine ($\geq$ 2 mg/dL). Hepatotoxicity with fibrosis and cirrhosis is an important toxic effect that correlates with cumulative dose and is uncommon with appropriate monitoring of liver function tests. Methotrexate is contraindicated in a patient with any form of chronic hepatitis. Heavy alcohol use increases the hepatotoxicity, so patients should be advised to drink alcohol in extreme moderation, if at all. Diabetes, obesity, and kidney disease also increase the risk of hepatotoxicity. Liver function tests should be monitored at least every 12 weeks, along with a complete blood count. The dose of methotrexate should be reduced if aminotransferase levels are elevated, and the drug should be discontinued if abnormalities persist despite dosage reduction. Gastric irritation, stomatitis, cytopenias, and hepatotoxicity are reduced by prescribing either daily folate (1 mg) or weekly leucovorin calcium (2.5–5 mg taken 24 hours after the dose of methotrexate). Hypersensitivity to methotrexate can cause an acute or subacute interstitial pneumonitis that can be life-threatening but which usually responds to cessation of the drug and institution of corticosteroids. Methotrexate is associated with an increased risk of B cell lymphomas, some of which resolve following the discontinuation of the medication. The combination of methotrexate and other folate antagonists, such as trimethoprim-sulfamethoxazole, should be used cautiously, since pancytopenia can result. Probenecid should also be avoided since it increases methotrexate drug levels and toxicity.

2. Sulfasalazine—This drug is a second-line agent for rheumatoid arthritis. It is usually introduced at a dosage of 0.5 g orally twice daily and then increased each week by 0.5 g until the patient improves or the daily dose reaches 3 g. Side effects, particularly neutropenia and thrombocytopenia, occur in 10–25% and are serious in 2–5%. Sulfasalazine also causes hemolysis in patients with glucose-6-phosphate dehydrogenase (G6PD) deficiency, so a G6PD level should be checked before initiating sulfasalazine. Patients taking sulfasalazine should have complete blood counts monitored every 2–4 weeks for the first 3 months, then every 3 months.

3. Leflunomide—Leflunomide, a pyrimidine synthesis inhibitor, is also FDA-approved for treatment of rheumatoid arthritis and is administered as a single daily dose of 20 mg. The most frequent side effects are diarrhea, rash, reversible alopecia, and hepatotoxicity. Some patients experience dramatic unexplained weight loss. The drug is carcinogenic, teratogenic, and has a half-life of 2 weeks. Thus, it is contraindicated in premenopausal women or in men who wish to father children.

4. Antimalarials—Hydroxychloroquine sulfate is the antimalarial agent most often used against rheumatoid arthritis. Monotherapy with hydroxychloroquine should be reserved for patients with mild disease because only a small percentage will respond and in some of those cases only after 3–6 months of therapy. Hydroxychloroquine is often used in combination with other conventional DMARDs, particularly methotrexate and sulfasalazine. The advantage of hydroxychloroquine is its comparatively low toxicity, especially at a dosage of 200–400 mg/d orally (not to exceed 6.5 mg/kg/d). The most important reaction, pigmentary retinitis causing visual loss, is rare at this dose. Ophthalmologic examinations every 12 months are required when this drug is used for long-term therapy. Other reactions include neuropathies and myopathies of both skeletal and cardiac muscle, which usually improve when the drug is withdrawn.

5. Minocycline—Minocycline is more effective than placebo for rheumatoid arthritis. It is reserved for early, mild cases, since its efficacy is modest, and it works better during the first year of rheumatoid arthritis. The mechanism of action is not clear, but tetracyclines do have anti-inflammatory properties, including the ability to inhibit destructive enzymes such as collagenase. The dosage of minocycline is 200 mg orally daily. Adverse effects are uncommon except for dizziness, which occurs in about 10%.

D. Biologic DMARDs

1. Tumor necrosis factor inhibitors—Inhibitors of tumor necrosis factor-α (TNF-α)—a pro-inflammatory cytokine—are fulfilling the aim of targeted therapy for rheumatoid arthritis. These medications are frequently added to the treatment of patients who have not responded adequately to methotrexate and are increasingly used as initial therapy in combination with methotrexate for patients with poor prognostic factors.

Three inhibitors are in use: etanercept, infliximab, and adalimumab. Etanercept, a soluble recombinant TNF receptor:Fc fusion protein, is usually administered at a dosage of 50 mg subcutaneously once per week. Infliximab, a chimeric monoclonal antibody, is administered at a dosage of 3–10 mg/kg intravenously; infusions are repeated after 2, 6, 10, and 14 weeks and then are administered every 8 weeks. Adalimumab, a human monoclonal antibody that binds to TNF, is given at a dosage of 40 mg subcutaneously every other week. Each drug produces substantial improvement in more than 60% of patients. Each is usually very well tolerated. Minor irritation at injection sites is the most common side effect of etanercept and adalimumab. Rarely, nonrecurrent leukopenia develops in patients.

TNF plays a physiologic role in combating many types of infection; TNF inhibitors have been associated with a several-fold increased risk of serious bacterial infections and a striking increase in granulomatous infections, particularly reactivation of tuberculosis. Screening for latent tuberculosis (see Chapter 9) is mandatory before the initiation of TNF blockers. It is prudent to suspend TNF blockers when a fever or other manifestations of a clinically important infection develops in a patient. Demyelinating neurologic complications that resemble multiple sclerosis have been reported rarely in patients taking etanercept, but the true magnitude of this risk—likely quite small—has not been determined with precision. There are conflicting data with respect to increased risk of malignancy. Contrary to expectation, TNF inhibitors were not effective in the treatment of congestive heart failure. The use of infliximab, in fact, was associated with increased morbidity in a congestive heart failure trial. Consequently, TNF inhibitors should be used with extreme caution in patients with congestive heart failure. Infliximab can rarely cause anaphylaxis and induce anti-DNA antibodies (but rarely clinically evident SLE). A final concern about TNF inhibitors is the expense, which is more than $10,000 per year.

2. Abatacept—Abatacept, a recombinant protein made by fusing a fragment of the Fc domain of human IgG with the extracellular domain of a T cell inhibitory receptor (CTLA4), blocks T-cell costimulation. It is approved by the FDA for use in rheumatoid arthritis and produces clinically meaningful responses in approximately 50% of individuals whose disease is active despite the combination of methotrexate and a TNF inhibitor.

3. Rituximab—Rituximab is a humanized mouse monoclonal antibody that depletes B cells. It is approved by the FDA to be used in combination with methotrexate for patients whose disease has been refractory to treatment with a TNF inhibitor.

E. DMARD Combinations

As a general rule, DMARDs have greater efficacy when administered in combination than when used individually. Currently, the most commonly used combination is that of methotrexate with one of the TNF inhibitors, which clearly is superior to methotrexate alone. The urge to use combination therapies with TNF inhibitors as the initial treatment

for rheumatoid arthritis, however, has been tempered by concerns about their safety and cost. The American College of Rheumatology recently published detailed recommendations on the initiation of DMARD combinations.

▶ **Course & Prognosis**

After months or years, deformities may occur; the most common are ulnar deviation of the fingers, boutonnière deformity (hyperextension of the DIP joint with flexion of the PIP joint), "swan-neck" deformity (flexion of the DIP joint with extension of the PIP joint), valgus deformity of the knee, and volar subluxation of the MTP joints. The excess mortality associated with rheumatoid arthritis is largely due to cardiovascular disease that is unexplained by traditional risk factors and that appears to be a result of deleterious effects of chronic systemic inflammation on the vascular system.

▶ **When to Refer**

Early referral to a rheumatologist is essential for appropriate diagnosis and the timely introduction of effective pharmacologic and nonpharmacologic (physical and occupational) therapy.

Donahue KE et al. Systematic review: comparative effectiveness and harms of disease-modifying medications for rheumatoid arthritis. Ann Intern Med. 2008 Jan 15;148(2):124–34. [PMID: 18025440]

Emery P et al. Comparison of methotrexate monotherapy with a combination of methotrexate and etanercept in active, early, moderate to severe rheumatoid arthritis (COMET): a randomised, double-blind, parallel treatment trial. Lancet. 2008 Aug 2;372(9636):375–82. [PMID: 18635256]

Saag KG et al. American College of Rheumatology 2008 recommendations for the use of nonbiologic and biologic disease-modifying antirheumatic drugs in rheumatoid arthritis. Arthritis Rheum. 2008 Jun 15;59(6):762–84. [PMID: 18512708]

ADULT STILL DISEASE

Still disease is a systemic form of juvenile chronic arthritis in which high spiking fevers are much more prominent, especially at the outset, than arthritis. This syndrome also occurs in adults. Most adults are in their 20s or 30s; onset after age 60 is rare. The fever is dramatic, often spiking to 40 °C, associated with sweats and chills, and then plunging to several degrees below normal in the absence of antipyretics. Many patients initially complain of sore throat. An evanescent salmon-colored nonpruritic rash, chiefly on the chest and abdomen, is a characteristic feature. The rash can easily be missed since it often appears only with the fever spike. Many patients also have lymphadenopathy and pericardial effusions. Joint symptoms are mild or absent in the beginning, but a destructive arthritis, especially of the wrists, may develop months later. Anemia and leukocytosis, with white blood counts sometimes exceeding 40,000/mcL, are the rule. Ferritin levels are exceptionally high (> 3000 mg/mL) in more than 70% of cases of adult Still disease—for reasons that are not clear. A low percentage (< 20%) of serum ferritin that is glycosylated may be even more specific for adult Still disease. Although there must be exclusion of other causes of fever, the diagnosis of adult Still disease is strongly suggested by the fever pattern, sore throat, and the classic rash. About half of the patients respond to high-dose aspirin (eg, 1 g three times orally daily) or other NSAIDs, and half require prednisone, sometimes in doses greater than 60 mg/d orally. TNF inhibitors may be helpful for some patients with refractory adult Still disease, but most patients treated with these agents achieve only partial remissions. More complete and dramatic responses have been achieved with the IL-1 receptor antagonist anakinra.

Allantaz F et al. Blood leukocyte microarrays to diagnose systemic onset juvenile idiopathic arthritis and follow the response to IL-1 blockade. J Exp Med. 2007 Sep 3;204(9):2131–44. [PMID: 17724127]

SYSTEMIC LUPUS ERYTHEMATOSUS

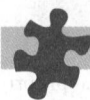

ESSENTIALS OF DIAGNOSIS

▶ Occurs mainly in young women.

▶ Rash over areas exposed to sunlight.

▶ Joint symptoms in 90% of patients. Multiple system involvement.

▶ Anemia, leukopenia, thrombocytopenia.

▶ Glomerulonephritis, central nervous system disease, and complications of antiphospholipid antibodies are major sources of disease morbidity.

▶ Serologic findings: antinuclear antibodies (100%), anti-native DNA antibodies (approximately two-thirds), and low serum complement levels (particularly during disease flares).

▶ General Considerations

SLE is an inflammatory autoimmune disorder characterized by autoantibodies to nuclear antigens. It can affect multiple organ systems. Many of its clinical manifestations are secondary to the trapping of antigen-antibody complexes in capillaries of visceral structures or to autoantibody-mediated destruction of host cells (eg, thrombocytopenia). The clinical course is marked by spontaneous remission and relapses. The severity may vary from a mild episodic disorder to a rapidly fulminant, life-threatening illness.

The incidence of SLE is influenced by many factors, including gender, race, and genetic inheritance. About 85% of patients are women. Sex hormones appear to play some role; most cases develop after menarche and before menopause. Among older individuals, the gender distribution is more equal. Race is also a factor, as SLE occurs in 1:1000 white women but in 1:250 black women. Familial occurrence of SLE has been repeatedly documented, and the disorder is concordant in 25–70% of identical twins. If a mother has SLE, her daughters' risks of developing the disease are 1:40 and her sons' risks are 1:250. Aggregation of serologic abnormalities (positive antinuclear antibody) is seen in asymptomatic family members, and the prevalence

of other rheumatic diseases is increased among close relatives of patients. The importance of specific genes in SLE is emphasized by the high frequency of certain HLA haplotypes, especially DR2 and DR3, and null complement alleles.

Before making a diagnosis of SLE, it is imperative to ascertain that the condition has not been induced by a drug (Table 20–8). Procainamide, hydralazine, and isoniazid are the best-studied drugs. While antinuclear antibody tests and other serologic findings become positive in many persons receiving these agents, clinical manifestations occur in only a few.

Four features of drug-induced lupus separate it from SLE: (1) the sex ratio is nearly equal; (2) nephritis and central nervous system features are not ordinarily present; (3) hypocomplementemia and antibodies to native DNA are absent; and (4) the clinical features and most laboratory abnormalities usually revert toward normal when the offending drug is withdrawn.

The diagnosis of SLE should be suspected in patients having a multisystem disease with serologic positivity (eg, antinuclear antibody, false-positive serologic test for syphilis). Differential diagnosis includes rheumatoid arthritis, systemic vasculitis, scleroderma, inflammatory myopathies, viral hepatitis, sarcoidosis, acute drug reactions, and drug-induced lupus.

The diagnosis of SLE can be made with reasonable probability if 4 of the 11 criteria set forth in Table 20–9 are met. These criteria, developed as guidelines for the inclusion of patients in research studies, do not supplant clinical judgment in the diagnosis of SLE.

▶ Clinical Findings

A. Symptoms and Signs

The systemic features include fever, anorexia, malaise, and weight loss. Most patients have skin lesions at some time; the

Table 20–8. Drugs associated with lupus erythematosus.

Definite association	
Chlorpromazine	Methyldopa
Hydralazine	Procainamide
Isoniazid	Quinidine
Possible association	
β-Blockers	Nitrofurantoin
Captopril	Penicillamine
Carbamazepine	Phenytoin
Cimetidine	Propylthiouracil
Ethosuximide	Sulfasalazine
Levodopa	Sulfonamides
Lithium	Trimethadione
Methimazole	
Unlikely association	
Allopurinol	Penicillin
Chlorthalidone	Phenylbutazone
Gold salts	Reserpine
Griseofulvin	Streptomycin
Methysergide	Tetracyclines
Oral contraceptives	

Modified and reproduced, with permission, from Hess EV et al. Drug-related lupus. Bull Rheum Dis. 1991;40(4):1–8.

Table 20–9. Criteria for the classification of SLE. (A patient is classified as having SLE if any 4 or more of 11 criteria are met.)

1. Malar rash
2. Discoid rash
3. Photosensitivity
4. Oral ulcers
5. Arthritis
6. Serositis
7. Kidney disease
   a. > 0.5 g/d proteinuria, or
   b. ≥ 3+ dipstick proteinuria, or
   c. Cellular casts
8. Neurologic disease
   a. Seizures, or
   b. Psychosis (without other cause)
9. Hematologic disorders
   a. Hemolytic anemia, or
   b. Leukopenia (< 4000/mcL), or
   c. Lymphopenia (< 1500/mcL), or
   d. Thrombocytopenia (< 100,000/mcL)
10. Immunologic abnormalities
    a. Positive LE cell preparation, or
    b. Antibody to native DNA, or
    c. Antibody to Sm, or
    d. False-positive serologic test for syphilis
11. Positive ANA

ANA, antinuclear antibody; SLE, systemic lupus erythematosus. Modified and reproduced, with permission, from Tan EM et al. The 1982 revised criteria for the classification of systemic lupus erythematosus. Arthritis Rheum. 1982 Nov;25(11):1271-7.

characteristic "butterfly" (malar) rash affects less than half of patients. Other cutaneous manifestations are discoid lupus, typical fingertip lesions, periungual erythema, nail fold infarcts, and splinter hemorrhages. Alopecia is common. Mucous membrane lesions tend to occur during periods of exacerbation. Raynaud phenomenon, present in about 20% of patients, often antedates other features of the disease.

Joint symptoms, with or without active synovitis, occur in over 90% of patients and are often the earliest manifestation. The arthritis is seldom deforming; erosive changes are almost never noted on radiographs. Subcutaneous nodules are rare.

Ocular manifestations include conjunctivitis, photophobia, transient or permanent monocular blindness, and blurring of vision. Cotton-wool spots on the retina (cytoid bodies) represent degeneration of nerve fibers due to occlusion of retinal blood vessels.

Pleurisy, pleural effusion, bronchopneumonia, and pneumonitis are frequent. Restrictive lung disease can develop. Alveolar hemorrhage is rare but life-threatening.

The pericardium is affected in the majority of patients. Cardiac failure may result from myocarditis and hypertension. Cardiac arrhythmias are common. Atypical verrucous endocarditis of Libman-Sacks is usually clinically silent but occasionally can produce acute or chronic valvular incompetence—most commonly mitral regurgitation—and can serve as a source of emboli.

Mesenteric vasculitis occasionally occurs in SLE and may closely resemble polyarteritis nodosa, including the presence of aneurysms in medium-sized blood vessels. Abdominal pain (particularly postprandial), ileus, peritonitis, and perforation may result.

Neurologic complications of SLE include psychosis, cognitive impairment, seizures, peripheral and cranial neuropathies, transverse myelitis, and strokes. Severe depression and psychosis are sometimes exacerbated by the administration of large doses of corticosteroids.

Several forms of glomerulonephritis may occur, including mesangial, focal proliferative, diffuse proliferative, and membranous (see Chapter 22). Some patients may also have interstitial nephritis. With appropriate therapy, the survival rate even for patients with serious chronic kidney disease (proliferative glomerulonephritis) is favorable, albeit a substantial portion of patients with severe lupus nephritis still eventually require renal replacement therapy.

B. Laboratory Findings

(Tables 20–10 and 20–11.) SLE is characterized by the production of many different autoantibodies. Antinuclear antibody tests are sensitive but not specific for SLE—ie, they are positive in virtually all patients with lupus but are positive also in many patients with nonlupus conditions such as rheumatoid arthritis, autoimmune thyroid disease, scleroderma, and Sjögren syndrome. Antibodies to double-stranded DNA and to Sm are specific for SLE but not sensitive, since they are present in only 60% and 30% of patients, respectively. Depressed serum complement—a finding suggestive of disease activity—often returns toward normal in remission. Anti-double-stranded DNA antibody levels also correlate with disease activity in some patients; anti-Sm levels do not.

Three types of antiphospholipid antibodies occur (Table 20–11). The first causes the biologic false-positive tests for syphilis; the second is the lupus anticoagulant, which despite its name is a risk factor for venous and arterial thrombosis and for miscarriage. It is most commonly identified by prolongation of the activated partial thromboplastin time, an in vitro phenomenon related to antibody reacting to phospholipid in the test materials. Anticardiolipin antibodies are the third type of antiphospholipid antibodies. In many cases, the "antiphospholipid antibody" appears to be directed at a serum cofactor (β_2-glycoprotein-I) rather than at phospholipid itself. Abnormality of urinary sediment is almost always found in association with renal lesions. Showers of red blood cells, with or without casts, and proteinuria (varying from mild to nephrotic range) are frequent during exacerbation of the disease; these usually abate with remission.

► Treatment

Patient education and emotional support are especially important for patients with lupus. Since the various manifestations of SLE affect prognosis differently and since SLE activity often waxes and wanes, drug therapy—both the choice of agents and the intensity of their use—must be tailored to match disease severity. Patients with photosensitivity should be cautioned against sun exposure and should apply a protective lotion to the skin while out of

Table 20–10. Frequency (%) of autoantibodies in rheumatic diseases.[1]

	ANA	Anti-Native DNA	Rheumatoid Factor	Anti-Sm	Anti-SS-A	Anti-SS-B	Anti-SCL-70	Anti-Centromere	Anti-Jo-1	ANCA
Rheumatoid arthritis	30–60	0–5	80	0	0–5	0–2	0	0	0	0
Systemic lupus erythematosus	95–100	60	20	10–25	15–20	5–20	0	0	0	0–1
Sjögren syndrome	95	0	75	0	65	65	0	0	0	0
Diffuse scleroderma	80–95	0	30	0	0	0	33	1	0	0
Limited scleroderma (CREST syndrome)	80–95	0	30	0	0	0	20	50	0	0
Polymyositis/dermatomyositis	80–95	0	33	0	0	0	0	0	20–30	0
Wegener granulomatosis	0–15	0	50	0	0	0	0	0	0	93–96[1]

[1]Frequency for generalized, active disease.

ANA, antinuclear antibodies; Anti-Sm, anti-Smith antibody; anti-SCL-70, anti-scleroderma antibody; ANCA, antineutrophil cytoplasmic antibody; CREST, calcinosis cutis, Raynaud phenomenon, esophageal motility disorder, sclerodactyly, and telangiectasia.

doors. Skin lesions often respond to the local administration of corticosteroids. Minor joint symptoms can usually be alleviated by rest and NSAIDs.

Antimalarials (hydroxychloroquine) may be helpful in treating lupus rashes or joint symptoms and appear to reduce the incidence of severe disease flares. The dose of hydroxychloroquine is 200 or 400 mg/d orally and should not exceed 6.5 mg/kg/d; annual monitoring for retinal

Table 20–11. Frequency (%) of laboratory abnormalities in systemic lupus erythematosus.

Anemia	60%
Leukopenia	45%
Thrombocytopenia	30%
Biologic false-positive tests for syphilis	25%
Antiphospholipid antibodies	
Lupus anticoagulant	7%
Anti-cardiolipin antibody	25%
Direct Coombs-positive	30%
Proteinuria	30%
Hematuria	30%
Hypocomplementemia	60%
ANA	95–100%
Anti-native DNA	50%
Anti-Sm	20%

ANA, antinuclear antibody; Anti-Sm, anti-Smith antibody.
Modified and reproduced, with permission, from Hochberg MC et al. Systemic lupus erythematosus: a review of clinicolaboratory features and immunologic matches in 150 patients with emphasis on demographic subsets. Medicine (Baltimore). 1985 Sep;64(5):285–95.

changes is recommended. Drug-induced neuropathy and myopathy may be erroneously ascribed to the underlying disease. The androgenic corticosteroid danazol may be effective therapy for thrombocytopenia not responsive to corticosteroids. Dehydroepiandrosterone (DHEA) has a therapeutic role comparable to that of the antimalarial agents in the treatment of SLE, but its side effects (particularly acne) are troubling to some patients.

Corticosteroids are required for the control of certain complications. (Systemic corticosteroids are not usually given for minor arthritis, skin rash, leukopenia, or the anemia associated with chronic disease.) Glomerulonephritis, hemolytic anemia, pericarditis or myocarditis, alveolar hemorrhage, central nervous system involvement, and thrombotic thrombocytopenic purpura all require corticosteroid treatment and often other interventions as well. Forty to 60 mg of oral prednisone is often needed initially; however, the lowest dose of corticosteroid that controls the condition should be used. Central nervous system lupus may require higher doses of corticosteroids than are usually given; however, corticosteroid psychosis may mimic lupus cerebritis, in which case reduced doses are appropriate. Immunosuppressive agents such as cyclophosphamide, mycophenolate mofetil, and azathioprine are used in cases resistant to corticosteroids. Treatment of severe lupus nephritis includes an induction phase and a maintenance phase. Cyclophosphamide, which improves renal survival but not patient survival, has been for many years the standard treatment for both phases of lupus nephritis. Mycophenolate mofetil appears to be an effective alternative treatment for many patients with lupus nephritis. Very close follow-up is needed to watch for potential side effects when immunosuppressants are given; these agents should be administered by clinicians experienced in their use. When cyclophosphamide is required, gonadotropin-releasing hormone analogs can be given to protect a woman against the risk of premature ovarian failure. For patients with the **antiphospholipid syndrome**—the presence of antiphospholipid antibodies and compatible clinical events—anticoagulation is the treatment of choice (see Antiphospholipid Antibody Syndrome, below). Moderate intensive anticoagulation with warfarin to achieve an INR of 2.0–3.0 is as effective as more intensive regimens. Pregnant patients with recurrent fetal loss associated with antiphospholipid antibodies should be treated with low-molecular-weight heparin plus aspirin.

Course & Prognosis

The prognosis for patients with systemic lupus appears to be considerably better than older reports implied. From both community settings and university centers, 10-year survival rates exceeding 85% are routine. In most patients, the illness pursues a relapsing and remitting course. Prednisone, often needed in doses of 40 mg/d orally or more during severe flares, can usually be tapered to low doses (5–10 mg/d) when the disease is inactive. However, there are some in whom the disease pursues a virulent course, leading to serious impairment of vital structures such as lung, heart, brain, or kidneys, and the disease may lead to death. With improved control of lupus activity and with increasing use of corticosteroids and immunosuppressive drugs, the mortality and morbidity patterns in lupus have changed. Mortality in SLE shows a bimodal pattern. In the early years after diagnosis, infections—especially with opportunistic organisms—are the leading cause of death, followed by active SLE, chiefly due to kidney or central nervous system disease. In later years, accelerated atherosclerosis, linked to chronic inflammation, becomes a major cause of death. Indeed, the incidence of myocardial infarction is five times higher in persons with SLE than in the general population. Therefore, it is especially important for SLE patients to avoid smoking and to minimize other conventional risk factors for atherosclerosis (eg, hypercholesterolemia, hypertension, obesity, and inactivity). Patients with SLE should receive influenza vaccination every year and pneumococcal vaccination every 5 years. Since some reports indicate that SLE patients have a higher risk of developing malignancy, preventive cancer screening recommendations should be followed assiduously. With more patients living longer, it has become evident that avascular necrosis of bone, affecting most commonly the hips and knees, is responsible for substantial morbidity. Still, the outlook for most patients with SLE has become increasingly favorable.

When to Refer

- Appropriate management of SLE requires the active participation of a rheumatologist.
- The severity of organ involvement dictates referral to other subspecialists, such as nephrologists and pulmonologists.

When to Admit

- Rapidly progressive glomerulonephritis, pulmonary hemorrhage, transverse myelitis, and other severe organ-

threatening manifestations of lupus usually require inpatient assessment and management.
- Severe infections, particularly in the setting of immunosuppressant therapy, should prompt admission.

Bertsias G et al. Clinical trials in systemic lupus erythematosus (SLE): lessons from the past as we proceed to the future—the EULAR recommendations for the management of SLE and the use of end-points in clinical trials. Lupus. 2008;17(5):437–42. [PMID: 18490423]
Frostegård J. Systemic lupus erythematosus and cardiovascular disease. Lupus. 2008;17(5):364–7. [PMID: 18490408]

ANTIPHOSPHOLIPID ANTIBODY SYNDROME

 ESSENTIALS OF DIAGNOSIS

▶ Hypercoagulability, with recurrent thromboses in either the venous or arterial circulation.

▶ Thrombocytopenia is common.

▶ Pregnancy complications, specifically pregnancy losses after the first trimester.

▶ Lifelong anticoagulation with warfarin is recommended currently for patients with serious complications of this syndrome, as recurrent events are common.

General Considerations

A primary **antiphospholipid antibody syndrome** (APS) is diagnosed in patients who have recurrent venous or arterial occlusions, recurrent fetal loss, or thrombocytopenia in the presence of antiphospholipid antibodies but not other features of SLE. In less than 1% of patients with antiphospholipid antibodies, a potentially devastating syndrome known as the "catastrophic antiphospholipid syndrome" occurs, leading to diffuse thromboses, thrombotic microangiopathy, and multiorgan system failure.

Clinical Findings

A. Symptoms and Signs

Patients are often asymptomatic until suffering a thrombotic complication of this syndrome. Thrombotic events may occur in either the arterial or venous circulations. Thus, deep venous thromboses, pulmonary emboli, cerebrovascular accidents are typical clinical events among patients with the APS. Budd-Chiari syndrome, cerebral sinus vein thrombosis, myocardial or digital infarctions, and other thrombotic events also occur. A variety of other symptoms and signs are often attributed to the APS, including mental status changes, livedo reticularis, skin ulcers, microangiopathic nephropathy, and cardiac valvular dysfunction—typically mitral regurgitation that may mimic Libman-Sacks endocarditis. Livedo reticularis is strongly associated with the subset of patients with APS in whom arterial ischemic events develop.

B. Laboratory Findings

As noted in the discussion of SLE, three types of antiphospholipid antibody are believed to contribute to this syndrome: (1) anti-cardiolipin antibodies; (2) a "lupus anticoagulant" that prolongs certain coagulation tests (see below); and (3) an antibody associated with a biologic false-positive test for syphilis. Anti-cardiolipin antibodies are typically measured with enzyme immunoassays for either IgG or IgM. In general, IgG anti-cardiolipin antibodies are believed to be more pathologic than IgM. A clue to the presence of a lupus anticoagulant, which may occur in individuals who do not have SLE, may be detected by a prolongation of the partial thromboplastin time (which, paradoxically, is associated with a thrombotic tendency rather than a bleeding risk). A finding more sensitive for a lupus anticoagulant, however, is prolongation of a specialized coagulation assay known as the Russell viper venom time (RVVT). In the presence of a lupus anticoagulant, the RVVT is prolonged and does not correct with mixing studies. With the last type of antiphospholipid antibody, the patient has a positive rapid plasma reagin (RPR), but negative specific anti-treponemal assays.

Differential Diagnosis

The exclusion of other autoimmune disorders, particularly those in the SLE spectrum, is essential, as such disorders may be associated with additional complications requiring alternative treatments. Other genetic or acquired conditions associated with hypercoagulability such as protein C, protein S, factor V Leiden, and antithrombin III deficiency should be excluded. The thrombocytopenia associated with APS must be distinguished from immune thrombocytopenic purpura. Catastrophic APS has a broad differential, including sepsis, pulmonary-renal syndromes, systemic vasculitis, disseminated intravascular coagulation, and thrombotic thrombocytopenic purpura.

Treatment

Present recommendations for anticoagulation are to treat patients with warfarin to maintain an INR of 2.0–3.0. Patients who have recurrent thrombotic events on this level of anticoagulation may require higher INRs (> 3.0), but the bleeding risk increases substantially with this degree of anticoagulation. Guidelines indicate that patients with APS should be treated with anticoagulation for life. Because of the teratogenic effects of warfarin, subcutaneous heparin and baby aspirin is the usual approach to prevent pregnancy complications in women with APS. In patients with catastrophic APS, a three-pronged approach is taken in the acute setting: intravenous heparin, high doses of corticosteroids, and either intravenous immune globulin or plasmapheresis.

Bick RL et al. Treatment options for patients who have antiphospholipid syndromes. Hematol Oncol Clin North Am. 2008 Feb;22(1):145–53. [PMID: 18207072]

Lockshin MD et al. New developments in lupus-associated antiphospholipid syndrome. Lupus. 2008;17(5):443–6. [PMID: 18490424]

RAYNAUD PHENOMENON

ESSENTIALS OF DIAGNOSIS

▶ Paroxysmal bilateral symmetric pallor and cyanosis followed by rubor of the skin of the digits.

▶ Precipitated by cold or emotional stress; relieved by warmth.

▶ Primarily affects young women.

▶ Primary form benign; secondary form can cause digital ulceration or gangrene.

General Considerations

Raynaud phenomenon (RP) is a syndrome of paroxysmal digital ischemia, most commonly caused by an exaggerated response of digital arterioles to cold or emotional stress. The initial phase of RP, mediated by excessive vasoconstriction, consists of well-demarcated digital pallor or cyanosis; the subsequent (recovery) phase of RP, caused by vasodilation, leads to intense hyperemia and rubor. Although RP chiefly affects fingers, it can also affect toes and other acral areas such as the nose and ears. RP is classified as primary (idiopathic or Raynaud disease) or secondary. Nearly one-third of the population reports being "sensitive to the cold" but does not experience the paroxysms of digital pallor, cyanosis, and erythema characteristic of RP. Primary RP occurs in 2–6% of adults, is especially common in young women, and poses more a nuisance than a threat to good health. In contrast, secondary RP is less common, is chiefly associated with rheumatic diseases (especially scleroderma), and is frequently severe enough to cause digital ulceration or gangrene.

Clinical Findings

In early attacks of RP, only one or two fingertips may be affected; as it progresses, all fingers down to the distal palm may be involved. The thumbs are rarely affected. During recovery there may be intense rubor, throbbing, paresthesia, pain, and slight swelling. Attacks usually terminate spontaneously or upon returning to a warm room or putting the extremity in warm water. The patient is usually asymptomatic between attacks. Sensory changes that often accompany vasomotor manifestations include numbness, stiffness, diminished sensation, and aching pain.

Primary RP appears first between ages 15 and 30, almost always in women. It tends to be mildly progressive and, unlike secondary RP (which may be unilateral and may involve only one or two fingers), symmetric involvement of the fingers of both hands is the rule. Spasm becomes more frequent and prolonged. Unlike secondary RP, primary RP does not cause digital pitting, ulceration, or gangrene.

Nailfold capillary abnormalities are among the earliest clues that a person has secondary rather than primary RP. The nailfold capillary pattern can be visualized by placing a drop of grade B immersion oil at the patient's cuticle and

Table 20–12. Causes of secondary Raynaud phenomenon.

Rheumatic diseases
Scleroderma
Systemic lupus erythematosus
Dermatomyositis/polymyositis
Sjögren syndrome
Vasculitis (polyarteritis nodosa, Takayasu disease, Buerger disease)
Neurovascular compression and occupational
Carpal tunnel syndrome
Thoracic outlet obstruction
Vibration injury
Medications
Serotonin agonists (sumatriptan)
Sympathomimetic drugs (decongestants)
Chemotherapy (bleomycin, vinblastine)
Ergotamine
Caffeine
Nicotine
Hematologic disorders
Cryoglobulinemia
Polycythemia vera
Paraproteinemia
Cold agglutinins
Endocrine disorders
Hypothyroidism
Pheochromocytoma
Miscellaneous
Atherosclerosis
Embolic disease
Migraine

then viewing the area with an ophthalmoscope set to 20–40 diopters. Dilation or dropout of the capillary loops indicates the patient has a secondary form of RP, most commonly scleroderma (Table 20–12). While highly specific for secondary RP, nailfold capillary changes have a low sensitivity. Digital pitting or ulceration or other abnormal physical findings (eg, skin tightening, loss of extremity pulse, rash, swollen joints) can also provide evidence of secondary RP.

▶ Differential Diagnosis

Primary RP must be differentiated from the numerous causes of secondary RP (Table 20–12). The history and examination may suggest the diagnosis of systemic sclerosis (including its CREST variant), SLE, and mixed connective tissue disease; RP is occasionally the first manifestation of these disorders. The diagnosis of many of these rheumatic diseases can be confirmed with specific serologic tests (see Table 20–10).

The differentiation from Buerger disease (thromboangiitis obliterans) is usually not difficult, since thromboangiitis obliterans is generally a disease of men, particularly smokers; peripheral pulses are often diminished or absent; and, when RP occurs in association with thromboangiitis obliterans, it is usually in only one or two digits.

RP may occur in patients with the thoracic outlet syndromes. In these disorders, involvement is generally unilateral, and symptoms referable to brachial plexus compression tend to dominate the clinical picture. Carpal

tunnel syndrome should also be considered, and nerve conduction tests are appropriate in selected cases.

In acrocyanosis, cyanosis of the hands is permanent and diffuse; the sharp and paroxysmal line of demarcation with pallor does not occur with acrocyanosis. Frostbite may lead to chronic RP. Ergot poisoning, particularly due to prolonged or excessive use of ergotamine, must also be considered but is unusual.

A particularly severe form of RP occurs in up to one-third of patients receiving bleomycin and vincristine in combination, often for testicular cancer. Treatment is unsuccessful, and the problem persists even with discontinuation of the drugs.

Finally, RP may be mimicked by type I cryoglobulinemia, in which a monoclonal antibody cryoprecipitates in the cooler distal circulation. Type I cryoglobulinemia is usually associated with multiple myeloma or with lymphoproliferative disorders.

▶ Treatment

A. General Measures

Keeping the body warm is the cornerstone of initial therapy. Wearing warms shirts, coats, and hats will help prevent the exaggerated vasospasm that causes RP and that is not prevented by warming only the hands. The hands should be protected from injury at all times; wounds heal slowly, and infections are consequently hard to control. Softening and lubricating lotion to control the fissured dry skin should be applied to the hands frequently. Smoking should be stopped. For most patients with primary RP, general measures alone are sufficient to control symptoms. Medical or surgical therapy should be considered in patients who have severe symptoms or are experiencing tissue injury from digital ischemia.

B. Medications

Calcium channel blockers are first-line therapy for RP. Calcium channel blockers produce a modest benefit and are more effective in primary RP than secondary RP. Slow release nifedipine (30–180 mg/d orally), amlodipine (5–20 mg/d orally), felodipine, or nisoldipine are popular and more effective than verapamil and diltiazem. Other medications that are sometimes effective in treating RP include angiotensin-converting enzyme inhibitors, sympatholytic agents (eg, prazosin), topical nitrates, phosphodiesterase inhibitors (eg, sildenafil, tadalafil, and vardenafil), selective serotonin reuptake inhibitors (fluoxetine), and endothelin-receptor inhibitors (ie, bosentan).

C. Surgical Measures

Sympathectomy may be indicated when attacks have become frequent and severe, when they interfere with work and well being, and particularly when trophic changes have developed and medical measures have failed. Cervical sympathectomy is modestly effective for primary but not secondary RP. Digital sympathectomy may improve secondary RP.

Prognosis

Primary PR is benign and largely a nuisance for affected individuals who are exposed to cold winters or excessive air conditioning. The prognosis of secondary RP depends on the severity of the underlying disease. Unfortunately, severe pain from ulceration and gangrene are not rare with scleroderma, especially the CREST variant.

Vinjar B et al. Oral vasodilators for primary Raynaud's phenomenon. Cochrane Database Syst Rev. 2008 Apr 16;(2):CD006687. [PMID: 18425964]

SCLERODERMA (Systemic Sclerosis)

ESSENTIALS OF DIAGNOSIS

▶ Limited disease (80% of patients): thickening of skin confined to the face, neck, and distal extremities.

▶ Diffuse disease (20%): widespread thickening of skin, including truncal involvement, with areas of increased pigmentation and depigmentation.

▶ Raynaud phenomenon and antinuclear antibodies are present in virtually all patients.

▶ Systemic features of gastroesophageal reflux, hypomotility of gastrointestinal tract, pulmonary fibrosis, pulmonary hypertension, and renal involvement.

General Considerations

Scleroderma (systemic sclerosis) is a rare chronic disorder characterized by diffuse fibrosis of the skin and internal organs. Symptoms usually appear in the third to fifth decades, and women are affected two to three times as frequently as men.

Two forms of scleroderma are generally recognized: limited (80% of patients) and diffuse (20%). In limited scleroderma, which is also known as the CREST syndrome (representing calcinosis cutis, Raynaud phenomenon, esophageal motility disorder, sclerodactyly, and telangiectasia), the hardening of the skin (scleroderma) is limited to the face and hands. In contrast, in diffuse scleroderma, the skin changes also involve the trunk and proximal extremities. Tendon friction rubs over the forearms and shins occur uniquely (but not universally) in diffuse scleroderma. In general, patients with limited scleroderma have better outcomes than those with diffuse disease, largely because kidney disease or interstitial lung disease rarely develops in patients with limited disease. Cardiac disease is also more characteristic of diffuse scleroderma. Patients with limited disease, however, are more susceptible to digital ischemia, leading to finger loss, and to life-threatening pulmonary hypertension. Small and large bowel hypomotility, which may occur in either form of scleroderma, can cause constipation alternating with diarrhea, malabsorption due to bacterial overgrowth, pseudoobstruction, and severe bowel distension with rupture.

Clinical Findings

A. Symptoms and Signs

Raynaud phenomenon is usually the initial manifestation and can precede other signs and symptoms by years in cases of limited scleroderma. Polyarthralgia, weight loss, and malaise are common early features of diffuse scleroderma but are infrequent in limited scleroderma. Cutaneous disease usually, but not always, develops before visceral involvement and can manifest initially as non-pitting subcutaneous edema associated with pruritus. With time the skin becomes thickened and hidebound, with loss of normal folds. Telangiectasia, pigmentation, and depigmentation are characteristic. Ulceration about the fingertips and subcutaneous calcification are seen. Dysphagia and symptoms of reflux due to esophageal dysfunction are common and result from abnormalities in motility and later from fibrosis. Fibrosis and atrophy of the gastrointestinal tract cause hypomotility. Large-mouthed diverticuli occur in the jejunum, ileum, and colon. Diffuse pulmonary fibrosis and pulmonary vascular disease are reflected in restrictive lung physiology and low diffusing capacities. Cardiac abnormalities include pericarditis, heart block, myocardial fibrosis, and right heart failure secondary to pulmonary hypertension. Scleroderma renal crisis, resulting from intimal proliferation of smaller renal arteries and usually associated with hypertension, is a marker for a poor outcome even though many cases can be treated effectively with angiotensin-converting enzyme inhibitors.

B. Laboratory Findings

Mild anemia is often present. In scleroderma renal crisis, the peripheral blood smear shows findings consistent with a microangiopathic hemolytic anemia (due to mechanical damage to red cells from diseased small vessels). Elevation of the ESR is unusual. Proteinuria and cylindruria appear in association with renal involvement. Antinuclear antibody tests are nearly always positive, frequently in high titers (Table 20–10). The scleroderma antibody (anti-SCL-70), directed against topoisomerase III, is found in one-third of patients with diffuse systemic sclerosis and in 20% of those with CREST syndrome. Although present in only a small number of patients with diffuse scleroderma, anti-SCL-70 antibodies may portend a poor prognosis, with a high likelihood of serious internal organ involvement (eg, interstitial lung disease). Anticentromere antibodies are seen in 50% of those with CREST syndrome and in 1% of individuals with diffuse scleroderma (Table 20–10). Anticentromere antibodies are highly specific for limited scleroderma, but they also occur occasionally in overlap syndromes.

Differential Diagnosis

Early in its course, scleroderma can cause diagnostic confusion with other causes of Raynaud phenomenon, particularly SLE, mixed connective tissue disease, and the inflammatory myopathies. Scleroderma can be mistaken for other disorders characterized by skin hardening. Eosinophilic fasciitis is a rare disorder presenting with skin changes that resemble diffuse scleroderma. The inflammatory abnormalities, however, are limited to the fascia rather than the dermis and epidermis. Moreover, patients with eosinophilic fasciitis are distinguished from those with scleroderma by the presence of peripheral blood eosinophilia, the absence of Raynaud phenomenon, the good response to prednisone, and an association (in some cases) with paraproteinemias. Diffuse skin thickening and visceral involvement are features of scleromyxedema; the presence of a paraprotein, the absence of Raynaud phenomenon, and distinct skin histology point to scleromyxedema. Diabetic cheiropathy typically develops in long-standing, poorly controlled diabetes and can mimic sclerodactyly. Nephrogenic fibrosing dermopathy produces thickening and hardening of the skin of the trunk and extremities in patients with chronic kidney disease; exposure to gadolinium may play a pathogenic role. Morphea and linear scleroderma cause sclerodermatous changes limited to circumscribed areas of the skin and usually have excellent outcomes.

▶ **Treatment**

Treatment of scleroderma is symptomatic and supportive and focuses on the organ systems involved. There is no effective therapy for the underlying disease process. However, interventions for management of specific organ manifestations of this disease have improved substantially. Severe Raynaud syndrome may respond to calcium channel blockers, eg, long-acting nifedipine, 30–120 mg/d orally, or to losartan, 50 mg/d orally, or to sildenafil 50 mg orally twice daily. Patients with esophageal disease should take medications in liquid or crushed form. Esophageal reflux can be reduced and the risk of scarring diminished by avoidance of late-night meals and by the use of proton pump inhibitors (eg, omeprazole, 20–40 mg/d orally), the only drugs that achieve near-complete inhibition of gastric acid production, are remarkably effective for refractory esophagitis. Patients with delayed gastric emptying maintain their weight better if they eat small, frequent meals and remain upright for at least 2 hours after eating. Long-term octreotide (0.1 mg subcutaneously twice daily), a somatostatin analog, helps some patients with bacterial overgrowth and pseudoobstruction. Malabsorption due to bacterial overgrowth also responds to antibiotics, eg, tetracycline, 500 mg four times orally daily, often prescribed cyclically. The hypertensive crises associated with systemic sclerosis renal crisis must be treated early and aggressively (in the hospital) with angiotensin-converting enzyme inhibitors, eg, captopril, initiated at 25 mg orally every 6 hours and titrated up as needed to a maximum of 100 mg every 6 hours. Apart from the patient with myositis, prednisone has little or no role in the treatment of scleroderma; high doses (> 15 mg daily) have been associated with scleroderma renal crisis. Cyclophosphamide improves dyspnea and pulmonary function tests modestly in patients with severe interstitial lung disease; this highly toxic drug should only be administered by physicians familiar with its use. Bosentan, an endothelin receptor antagonist, improves exercise capacity and cardiopulmonary hemodynamics in patients with pulmonary hypertension and helps prevent digital ulceration. Sildenafil or prostaglandins (delivered by continuous intravenous infusion or intermittent inhalation) may also be useful in treating pulmonary hypertension. At an experimental level, immunoablative therapy with or without stem cell rescue has achieved promising results for some patients with severe, rapidly progressive diffuse scleroderma.

The 9-year survival rate in scleroderma averages approximately 40%. The prognosis tends to be worse in those with diffuse scleroderma, in blacks, in males, and in older patients. Lung disease is now the number one cause of mortality. Death from advanced chronic kidney disease or heart failure is also common. Those persons in whom severe internal organ involvement does not develop in the first 3 years have a substantially better prognosis, with 72% surviving at least 9 years. Breast and lung cancer may be more common in patients with scleroderma.

▶ **When to Refer**

• Appropriate management of scleroderma requires frequent consultations with a rheumatologist.

• Severity of organ involvement dictates referral to other subspecialists, such as pulmonologists or gastroenterologists.

Baroni SS et al. Stimulatory autoantibodies to the PDGF receptor in systemic sclerosis. N Engl J Med. 2006 Jun 22;354(25):2667–76. [PMID: 16790699]

Goldin JG et al; Scleroderma Lung Study Research Group. High-resolution CT scan findings in patients with symptomatic scleroderma-related interstitial lung disease. Chest. 2008 Aug;134(2):358–67. [PMID: 18641099]

Herrick AL. Systemic sclerosis: an update for clinicians. Br J Hosp Med (Lond). 2008 Aug;69(8):464–70. [PMID: 18783099]

Ingegnoli F et al. Prognostic model based on nailfold capillaroscopy for identifying Raynaud's phenomenon patients at high risk for the development of a scleroderma spectrum disorder: PRINCE (prognostic index for nailfold capillaroscopic examination). Arthritis Rheum. 2008 Jul;58(7):2174–82. [PMID: 18576359]

Tashkin DP et al; Scleroderma Lung Study Research Group. Cyclophosphamide versus placebo in scleroderma lung disease. N Engl J Med. 2006 Jun 22;354(25):2655–66. [PMID: 16790692]

Tehlirian CV et al. High-dose cyclophosphamide without stem cell rescue in scleroderma. Ann Rheum Dis. 2008 Jun;67(6):775–81. [PMID: 17974598]

Verrecchia F et al. Skin involvement in scleroderma—where histological and clinical scores meet. Rheumatology (Oxford). 2007 May;46(5):833–41. [PMID: 17255134]

Walker UA et al. Clinical risk assessment of organ manifestations in systemic sclerosis: a report from the EULAR Scleroderma Trials And Research group database. Ann Rheum Dis. 2007 Jun;66(6):754–63. [PMID: 17234652]

IDIOPATHIC INFLAMMATORY MYOPATHIES (Polymyositis & Dermatomyositis)

ESSENTIALS OF DIAGNOSIS

▶ Bilateral proximal muscle weakness.

- Characteristic cutaneous manifestations in dermato-myositis (Gottron papules, heliotrope rash).
- Diagnostic tests: elevated creatine kinase, muscle biopsy, electromyography, MRI.
- Increased risk of malignancy, particularly in dermato-myositis.
- Inclusion body myositis can mimic polymyositis but is less responsive to treatment.

General Considerations

Polymyositis and dermatomyositis are systemic disorders of unknown cause whose principal manifestation is muscle weakness. Although their clinical presentations (aside from the presence of certain skin findings in dermatomyositis, some of which are pathognomonic) and treatments are similar, the two diseases are pathologically quite distinct. They affect persons of any age group, but the peak incidence is in the fifth and sixth decades of life. Women are affected twice as commonly as men, and the diseases (particularly polymyositis) also occur more often among blacks than whites. There is an increased risk of malignancy in adult patients with dermatomyositis. Indeed, up to one patient in four with dermatomyositis has an occult malignancy. Malignancies may be evident at the time of presentation with the muscle disease but may not be detected until months afterward in some cases. Rare patients with dermatomyositis have skin disease without overt muscle involvement, a condition termed "dermatomyositis sine myositis." Myositis may also be associated with other connective tissue diseases, especially scleroderma, lupus, mixed connective tissue disease, and Sjögren syndrome.

Clinical Findings

A. Symptoms and Signs

Polymyositis may begin abruptly, but the usual presentation is one of gradual and progressive muscle weakness. The weakness chiefly involves proximal muscle groups of the upper and lower extremities as well as the neck. Leg weakness (eg, difficulty in rising from a chair or climbing stairs) typically precedes arm symptoms. In contrast to myasthenia gravis, polymyositis and dermatomyositis do not cause facial or ocular muscle weakness. Pain and tenderness of affected muscles occur in one-fourth of cases, but these are rarely the chief complaints. About one-fourth of patients have dysphagia. In contrast to scleroderma, which affects the smooth muscle of the lower esophagus and can cause a "sticking" sensation below the sternum, polymyositis or dermatomyositis involves the striated muscles of the upper pharynx and can make initiation of swallowing difficult. Muscle atrophy and contractures occur as late complications of advanced disease. Clinically significant myocarditis is uncommon even though there is often creatine kinase-MB elevation. Patients who are bed-bound from myositis should be screened for respiratory muscle weakness that can be severe enough to cause CO_2 retention and can progress to require mechanical ventilation.

In **dermatomyositis,** the characteristic rash is dusky red and may appear in a malar distribution mimicking the classic rash of SLE. Facial erythema beyond the malar distribution is also characteristic of dermatomyositis. Erythema also occurs over other areas of the face, neck, shoulders, and upper chest and back ("shawl sign"). Periorbital edema and a purplish (heliotrope) suffusion over the eyelids are typical signs (Plate 84). Periungual erythema, dilations of nailbed capillaries, and scaly patches over the dorsum of PIP and MCP joints (Gottron sign) are highly suggestive. Scalp involvement by dermatomyositis may mimic psoriasis. Infrequently, the cutaneous findings of this disease precede the muscle inflammation by weeks or months. Diagnosing polymyositis in patients over age 70 years can be difficult because weakness may be overlooked or attributed erroneously to idiopathic frailty. Polymyositis can remain undiagnosed or will be misdiagnosed as hepatitis because of elevations in alanine aminotransferase (ALT) and aspartate aminotransferase (AST) levels. A subset of patients with polymyositis and dermatomyositis develop the "antisynthetase syndrome," a group of findings including inflammatory arthritis, Raynaud phenomenon, interstitial lung disease, and often severe muscle disease associated with certain autoantibodies (eg, anti-Jo1 antibodies).

B. Laboratory Findings

Measurement of serum levels of muscle enzymes, especially creatine kinase and aldolase, is most useful in diagnosis and in assessment of disease activity. Anemia is uncommon. The ESR and C-reactive protein are often normal and are not reliable indicators of disease activity. Rheumatoid factor is found in a minority of patients. Antinuclear antibodies are present in many patients, especially those who have an associated connective tissue disease (Table 20-10). Three autoantibodies are seen exclusively in patients with myositis. The most common myositis-specific antibody, anti-Jo-1 antibody, is seen in the subset of patients who have associated interstitial lung disease (Table 20–10). The other myositis-specific autoantibodies are anti-Mi-2, associated with dermatomyositis, and anti-SRP (anti-signal recognition particle), associated with rapidly progressive, severe polymyositis. In the absence of the anti-synthetase syndrome, chest radiographs are usually normal. Electromyographic abnormalities consisting of polyphasic potentials, fibrillations, and high-frequency action potentials are helpful in establishing the diagnosis. None of the studies are specific. MRI can detect early and patchy muscle involvement, can guide biopsies, and may prove to be more useful than electromyography. The malignancies most commonly associated with dermatomyositis in descending order of frequency are ovarian, lung, pancreatic, stomach, colorectal, and non-Hodgkins lymphoma. The search for an occult malignancy should begin with a history and physical examination, supplemented with a complete blood count, comprehensive biochemical panel, serum protein electrophoresis, and urinalysis, and should include age- and risk-appropriate cancer screening tests. Given the especially strong association of ovarian carcinoma and dermatomyositis, pelvic ultrasonography and CT scanning and CA-125 levels may be useful in women. No matter how extensive the initial screening, some malignancies will not become evident for months after the initial presentation.

C. Muscle Biopsy

Biopsy of clinically involved muscle is the only specific diagnostic test. The pathology findings in polymyositis and dermatomyositis are distinct. Although both include lymphoid inflammatory infiltrates, the findings in dermatomyositis are localized to perivascular regions and there is evidence of humoral and complement-mediated destruction of microvasculature associated with the muscle. In addition to its vascular orientation, the inflammatory infiltrate in dermatomyositis centers on the interfascicular septa and is located around, rather than in, muscle fascicles. A pathologic hallmark of dermatomyositis is perifascicular atrophy. In contrast, the pathology of polymyositis characteristically includes endomysial infiltration of the inflammatory infiltrate. Owing to the sometimes patchy distribution of pathologic abnormalities, however, false-negative biopsies sometimes occur in both disorders.

Differential Diagnosis

Muscle inflammation may occur as a component of SLE, scleroderma, Sjögren syndrome, and overlap syndromes. In those cases, associated findings usually permit the precise diagnosis of the primary condition.

Inclusion body myositis, because of its tendency to mimic polymyositis, is a common cause of "treatment-resistant polymyositis." In contrast to the epidemiologic features of polymyositis, however, the typical inclusion body myositis patient is white, male, and over the age of 50. The onset of inclusion body myositis is even more insidious than that of polymyositis or dermatomyositis (eg, occurring over years rather than months), and asymmetric distal motor weakness is common in inclusion body myositis. Creatine kinase levels in inclusion body myositis are often minimally elevated and are normal in 25%. Muscle biopsy shows characteristic intracellular vacuoles by light microscopy either tubular or filamentous inclusions in the nucleus or cytoplasm by electron microscopy. Inclusion body myositis is less likely to respond to therapy.

Hyperthyroidism and hypothyroidism may both be associated with proximal muscle weakness. Hypothyroidism is associated also with elevations of creatine kinase. Patients with polymyalgia rheumatica are over the age of 50 and—in contrast to patients with polymyositis—have pain but no objective weakness; creatine kinase levels are normal. Disorders of the peripheral and central nervous systems (eg, chronic inflammatory polyneuropathy, multiple sclerosis, myasthenia gravis, Eaton-Lambert disease, and amyotrophic lateral sclerosis) can produce weakness but are distinguished by characteristic symptoms and neurologic signs and often by distinctive electromyographic abnormalities. A number of systemic vasculitides (polyarteritis nodosa, microscopic polyangiitis, the Churg-Strauss syndrome, Wegener granulomatosis, and mixed cryoglobulinemia) can produce profound weakness through vasculitic neuropathy. The muscle weakness associated with

these disorders, however, is typically distal and asymmetric, at least in the early stages.

Many drugs, including corticosteroids, alcohol, clofibrate, penicillamine, tryptophan, and hydroxychloroquine, can produce proximal muscle weakness. Chronic use of colchicine at doses as low as 0.6 mg twice a day in patients with moderate chronic kidney disease can produce a mixed neuropathy-myopathy that mimics polymyositis. The weakness and muscle enzyme elevation reverse with cessation of the drug. HMG-CoA reductase inhibitors, which are frequently used to treat hypercholesterolemia, can cause myopathy and rhabdomyolysis. Although only about 0.1% of patients taking a statin drug alone develop myopathy, concomitant administration of other drugs (especially gemfibrozil, cyclosporine, niacin, macrolide antibiotics, azole antifungals, and protease inhibitors) increases the risk. Statin-induced muscle inflammation resolves after cessation of these medications. Polymyositis can occur as a complication of HIV or HTLV-I infection and with zidovudine therapy as well.

Treatment

Most patients respond to corticosteroids. Often a daily dose of 40–60 mg or more of oral prednisone is required initially. The dose is then adjusted downward while monitoring muscle strength and serum levels of muscle enzymes. Long-term use of corticosteroids is often needed, and the disease may recur or reemerge when they are withdrawn. Patients with an associated neoplasm have a poor prognosis, although remission may follow treatment of the tumor; corticosteroids may or may not be effective in these patients. In patients resistant or intolerant to corticosteroids, therapy with methotrexate or azathioprine may be helpful. Intravenous immune globulin is effective for dermatomyositis resistant to prednisone. Mycophenolate mofetil (1.0–1.5 g orally twice daily) may be useful as a steroid-sparing agent. Since the rash of dermatomyositis is often photosensitive, patients should limit sun exposure. Hydroxychloroquine (200–400 mg/d orally not to exceed 6.5 mg/kg) can also help ameliorate the skin disease.

When to Refer

- Appropriate management of myositis usually requires frequent consultations with a rheumatologist or neurologist.
- Severe lung disease may require consultation with a pulmonologist.

When to Admit

- Signs of rhabdomyolysis.
- Respiratory insufficiency with hypoxia or carbon dioxide retention.

Klopstock T. Drug-induced myopathies. Curr Opin Neurol. 2008 Oct;21(5):590–5. [PMID: 18769254]

Suber TL et al. Mechanisms of disease: autoantigens as clues to the pathogenesis of myositis. Nat Clin Pract Rheumatol. 2008 Apr;4(4):201–9. [PMID: 18319710]

Tomasova Studynkova J et al. The role of MRI in the assessment of polymyositis and dermatomyositis. Rheumatology (Oxford). 2007 Jul;46(7):1174–9. [PMID: 17500079]

Ytterberg SR. Treatment of refractory polymyositis and dermatomyositis. Curr Rheumatol Rep. 2006 Jun;8(3):167–73. [PMID: 16901073]

MIXED CONNECTIVE TISSUE DISEASE & OVERLAP SYNDROMES

Many patients with symptoms and signs compatible with a connective tissue disease have features consistent with more than one type of rheumatic disease. Special attention has been drawn to antinuclear antibody–positive patients who have overlapping features of SLE, scleroderma, and inflammatory myopathy together with autoantibodies to ribonuclear protein (RNP). Some consider these patients to have a distinct entity ("mixed connective tissue disease"), and others view this as a subset of SLE characterized by a higher prevalence of Raynaud phenomenon, polyarthritis, myositis, and pulmonary hypertension and a lower incidence of renal involvement. Other patients have features of more than one connective tissue disease (eg, rheumatoid arthritis and SLE, SLE and scleroderma) in the absence of anti-RNP antibodies and are referred to as having an "overlap syndrome." Treatments are guided more by the distribution and severity of patients' organ system involvement than by therapies specific to these overlap syndromes.

Vegh J et al. Clinical and immunoserological characteristics of mixed connective tissue disease associated with pulmonary arterial hypertension. Scand J Immunol. 2006 Jul;64(1):69–76. [PMID: 16784493]

SJÖGREN SYNDROME

ESSENTIALS OF DIAGNOSIS

▶ Women are 90% of patients; the average age is 50 years.

▶ Dryness of eyes and dry mouth (sicca components) are the most common features; they occur alone or in association with rheumatoid arthritis or other connective tissue disease.

▶ Rheumatoid factor and other autoantibodies common.

▶ Increased incidence of lymphoma.

General Considerations

Sjögren syndrome is a systemic autoimmune disorder whose clinical presentation is usually dominated by dryness of the eyes and mouth due to immune-mediated dysfunction of the lacrimal and salivary glands. The disorder is predominantly seen in women, with a ratio of 9:1; most cases develop between the ages of 40 and 60 years. Sjögren syndrome can occur in isolation ("primary" Sjögren syndrome) or in association with another rheumatic disease. Sjögren syndrome is most frequently associated with rheumatoid arthritis but also occurs with SLE, primary biliary cirrhosis, scleroderma, polymyositis, Hashimoto thyroiditis, polyarteritis, and interstitial pulmonary fibrosis.

▶ Clinical Findings

A. Symptoms and Signs

Keratoconjunctivitis sicca results from inadequate tear production caused by lymphocyte and plasma cell infiltration of the lacrimal glands. Ocular symptoms are usually mild. Burning, itching, and the sensation of having a foreign body or a grain of sand in the eye occur commonly. For some patients, the initial manifestation is the inability to tolerate wearing contact lenses. Many patients with more severe ocular dryness notice ropy secretions across their eyes, especially in the morning. Photophobia may signal corneal ulceration resulting from severe dryness. For most patients, symptoms of dryness of the mouth (xerostomia) dominate those of dry eyes. Patients frequently complain of a "cotton mouth" sensation and difficulty swallowing foods, especially dry foods like crackers, unless they are washed down with liquids. The persistent oral dryness causes most patients to carry water bottles or other liquid dispensers from which they sip constantly. A few patients have such severe xerostomia that they have difficulty speaking. Persistent xerostomia results often in rampant dental caries; caries at the gum line strongly suggest Sjögren syndrome. Some patients are most troubled by loss of taste and smell. Parotid enlargement, which may be chronic or relapsing, develops in one-third of patients. Desiccation may involve the nose, throat, larynx, bronchi, vagina, and skin.

Systemic manifestations include dysphagia, vasculitis, pleuritis, obstructive lung disease (in the absence of smoking), neuropsychiatric dysfunction (most commonly peripheral neuropathies), and pancreatitis; they may be related to the associated diseases noted above. Renal tubular acidosis (type I, distal) occurs in 20% of patients. Chronic interstitial nephritis, which may result in impaired kidney function, may be seen. A glomerular lesion is rarely observed but may occur secondary to associated cryoglobulinemia.

B. Laboratory Findings

Laboratory findings include mild anemia, leukopenia, and eosinophilia. Polyclonal hypergammaglobulinemia, rheumatoid factor positivity (70%), and antinuclear antibodies (95%) are all common findings. Antibodies against the cytoplasmic antigens SS-A and SS-B (also called Ro and La, respectively) are often present in primary Sjögren syndrome and tend to correlate with the presence of extraglandular manifestations (Table 20–10). Thyroid-associated autoimmunity is a common finding among patients with Sjögren syndrome.

Useful ocular diagnostic tests include the Schirmer test, which measures the quantity of tears secreted. Lip biopsy, a simple procedure, reveals characteristic lymphoid foci in accessory salivary glands. Biopsy of the parotid gland should be reserved for patients with atypical presentations such as unilateral gland enlargement that suggest a neoplastic process.

Differential Diagnosis

Isolated complaints of dry mouth are most commonly due to medication side effects. Chronic hepatic C can cause sicca symptoms. Minor salivary gland biopsies reveal lymphocytic infiltrates but not to the extent of Sjögren syndrome, and tests for anti-SS-A and anti-SS-B are negative. Diffuse infiltration of CD8 T cells producing parotid gland enlargement can develop in HIV-infected individuals. Involvement of the lacrimal or salivary glands, or both in sarcoidosis can mimic Sjögren syndrome; biopsies reveal noncaseating granulomas. Rarely, amyloid deposits in the lacrimal and salivary glands produce sicca symptoms.

Treatment & Prognosis

Treatment of sicca symptoms is symptomatic and supportive. Artificial tears applied frequently will relieve ocular symptoms and avert further desiccation. The mouth should be kept well lubricated. Sipping water frequently or using sugar-free gums and hard candies usually relieves dry mouth symptoms. Pilocarpine (5 mg orally four times daily) and the acetylcholine derivative cevimeline (30 mg orally three times daily) may improve xerostomia symptoms. Atropinic drugs and decongestants decrease salivary secretions and should be avoided. A program of oral hygiene, including fluoride treatment, is essential in order to preserve dentition. If there is an associated rheumatic disease, its systemic treatment is not altered by the presence of Sjögren syndrome.

Although Sjögren syndrome may compromise patients' quality of life significantly, the disease is usually consistent with a normal life span. Poor prognoses are influenced mainly by the presence of systemic features associated with underlying disorders, the development in some patients of lymphocytic vasculitis, the occurrence of a painful peripheral neuropathy, and the complication (in a minority of patients) of lymphoma. The patients (3–10% of the total Sjögren population) at greatest risk for developing lymphoma are those with severe exocrine dysfunction, marked parotid gland enlargement, splenomegaly, vasculitis, peripheral neuropathy, anemia, and mixed monoclonal cryoglobulinemia.

When to Refer

- Presence of systemic symptoms or signs.
- Symptoms or signs of ocular dryness not responsive to artificial tears.

When to Admit

Presence of severe systemic signs such as vasculitis unresponsive to outpatient management.

Goransson LG et al. Peripheral neuropathy in primary Sjögren syndrome: a population-based study. Arch Neurol. 2006 Nov;63(11):1612–5. [PMID: 17101831]

Ramos-Casals M et al. Atypical autoantibodies in patients with primary Sjögren syndrome: clinical characteristics and follow-up of 82 cases. Semin Arthritis Rheum. 2006 Apr;35(5):312–21. [PMID: 16616154]

Ramos-Casals M et al. The overlap of Sjögren's syndrome with other systemic autoimmune diseases. Semin Arthritis Rheum. 2007 Feb;36(4):246–55. [PMID: 16996579]

Thanou-Stavraki A et al. Primary Sjögren's syndrome: current and prospective therapies. Semin Arthritis Rheum. 2008 Apr;37(5):273–92. [PMID: 17714766]

RHABDOMYOLYSIS

 ESSENTIALS OF DIAGNOSIS

- ▶ Associated with crush injuries to muscle, prolonged immobility, drug toxicities, hypothermia, and other causes.
- ▶ Massive acute elevations of muscle enzymes that peak quickly and usually resolve within days once the inciting injury has been identified and removed.

General Considerations

Defined strictly, rhabdomyolysis is necrosis of skeletal muscle and may be encountered in a wide variety of clinical settings, alone or in concert with other disorders of muscle. When the term "rhabdomyolysis" is used without being otherwise defined, healthcare providers ordinarily think of the syndrome of crush injury to muscle, associated with myoglobinuria, acute kidney injury, markedly elevated creatine kinase levels and, frequently, multiorgan failure as a consequence of other complications of the trauma. Acute kidney injury in myoglobinuria is caused by tubular injury resulting from excessive quantities of filtered myoglobin (See Acute Tubular Necrosis in Chapter 22). This complication is nearly always associated with hypovolemia. Experimental models of severe rhabdomyolysis in which blood volume and pressure are maintained ordinarily are not associated with acute tubular necrosis. From a practical point of view, however, many patients who suffer crush injuries are indeed volume-contracted, and oliguric renal failure is encountered routinely.

In addition to crush injuries, prolonged immobility, particularly after drug overdose or intoxication and commonly associated with exposure hypothermia, may be associated with rhabdomyolysis. Often there is little evidence for muscle injury on external examination of these patients—and specifically, neither myalgia nor myopathy presents. The clue to muscle necrosis in such individuals may be a urinary dipstick testing positive for blood in the absence of red cells in the sediment. This false-positive finding is due to myoglobinuria, which results in a positive reading for blood. Such an abnormality is investigated by serum creatine kinase determination. Other studies elevated in rhabdomyolysis include ALT and lactate dehydrogenase (LDH)—and once again, these studies may be obtained for other reasons, such as suspected liver disease or hemolysis. When disproportionately elevated, it is prudent to establish that they are not of muscle origin by confirming them with creatine kinase determination.

A number of other causes of rhabdomyolysis are encountered. Statins, agents used commonly to treat hyperlipidemia, are common offenders (see above). The presence of compromised kidney and liver function, diabetes, and hypothyroidism as well as concomitant use of other medications all increase the risk of rhabdomyolysis in those patients taking statins. Both acute alcohol intoxication and even intramuscular injections may cause some elevation of creatine kinase.

▶ Treatment

Vigorous fluid resuscitation (4–6 L/d, with careful monitoring for fluid overload), mannitol (100 mg/d), and urine alkalinization are suggested early in the course, but definitive evidence for the efficacy of these measures is lacking. On occasion, oliguric tubular necrosis may be converted to a nonoliguric variety, and—though the prognosis for recovery of kidney function and mortality is the same—many clinicians believe it is easier to care for nonoliguric disease because hyperkalemia and pulmonary edema are less important concerns. Myopathic complications of statins usually resolve within several weeks of discontinuing the drug.

Armitage J. The safety of statins in clinical practice. Lancet. 2007 Nov 24;370(9601):1781–90. [PMID: 17559928]
Kashani A et al. Risks associated with statin therapy: a systematic overview of randomized clinical trials. Circulation. 2006 Dec 19;114(25):2788–97. [PMID: 17159064]

▼ VASCULITIS SYNDROMES

"Vasculitis" is a heterogeneous group of disorders characterized by inflammation within the walls of affected blood

Table 20–13. Classification scheme of primary vasculitides according to size of predominant blood vessels involved.

Predominantly large-vessel vasculitides
Takayasu arteritis
Giant cell arteritis (temporal arteritis)
Behçet disease[1]
Predominantly medium-vessel vasculitides
Polyarteritis nodosa
Buerger disease
Predominantly small-vessel vasculitides
Immune-complex mediated
Cutaneous leukocytoclastic angiitis ("hypersensitivity vasculitis")
Henoch-Schönlein purpura
Essential cryoglobulinemia[2]
"ANCA-associated" disorders[3]
Wegener granulomatosis[2]
Microscopic polyangiitis[2]
Churg-Strauss syndrome[2]

[1]May involve small, medium, and large-sized blood vessels.
[2]Frequent overlap of small and medium-sized blood vessel involvement.
[3]Not all forms of these disorders are always associated with ANCA. ANCA, antineutrophil cytoplasmic antibodies.

Table 20–14. Typical clinical manifestations of large-, medium-, and small-vessel involvement by vasculitis.

Large	Medium	Small
Constitutional symptoms: fever, weight loss, malaise, arthralgias/arthritis		
Limb claudication	Cutaneous	Purpura
Asymmetric blood	nodules	Vesiculobullous lesions
pressures	Ulcers	Urticaria
Absence of pulses	Livedo reticularis	Glomerulonephritis
Bruits	Digital gangrene	Alveolar hemorrhage
Aortic dilation	Mononeuritis	Cutaneous extravascular
	multiplex	necrotizing granulomas
	Microaneurysms	Splinter hemorrhages
		Uveitis
		Episcleritis
		Scleritis

vessels. The major forms of primary systemic vasculitis are listed in Table 20–13. The first consideration in classifying cases of vasculitis is the size of the major vessels involved: large, medium, or small. The presence of the clinical signs and symptoms shown in Table 20–14 help distinguish among these three groups. After determining the size of the major vessels involved, other issues that contribute to the classification include the following:

- Does the process involve arteries, veins, or both?
- What are the patient's demographic characteristics (age, gender, ethnicity, smoking status)?
- Which organs are involved?
- Is there evidence of immune complex deposition?
- Is there granulomatous inflammation on tissue biopsy?
- Are antineutrophil cytoplasmic antibodies (ANCA) present?

In addition to the disorders considered to be primary vasculitides, there are also multiple forms of vasculitis that are associated with other known underlying conditions. These "secondary" forms of vasculitis occur in the setting of chronic infections (eg, hepatitis B or C, subacute bacterial endocarditis), connective tissue disorders, inflammatory bowel disease, malignancies, and reactions to medications. Only the major primary forms of vasculitis are discussed here.

POLYARTERITIS NODOSA

ESSENTIALS OF DIAGNOSIS

- ▶ Medium-sized arteries are always affected; smaller arterioles are sometimes involved; lung is spared but kidney often affected, causing renin-mediated hypertension.
- ▶ Clinical findings depend on the arteries involved.
- ▶ Common features include fever, abdominal pain, livedo reticularis, mononeuritis multiplex, anemia, and ele-

vated acute phase reactants (ESR or C-reactive protein or both).

▶ Associated with hepatitis B (10% of cases).

General Considerations

Polyarteritis nodosa, described in 1866, is acknowledged widely as the first form of vasculitis reported in the medical literature. For many years, all forms of inflammatory vascular disease were termed "polyarteritis nodosa." In recent decades, numerous subtypes of vasculitis have been recognized, greatly narrowing the spectrum of vasculitis called polyarteritis nodosa. Although the term is reserved currently for necrotizing arteritis of medium-sized vessels that has a predilection for involving the skin, peripheral nerves, mesenteric vessels (including renal arteries), heart, and brain, the disease can involve most organs. Polyarteritis nodosa is relatively rare, with a prevalence of about 30 per 1 million people. Approximately 10% of cases of polyarteritis nodosa are caused by hepatitis B. Most cases of hepatitis B–associated disease occur within 6 months of hepatitis B infection.

Stone JH. Vasculitis: a collection of pearls and myths. Rheum Dis Clin North Am. 2007 Nov;33(4):691–739. [PMID: 18037113]

Clinical Findings

A. Symptoms and Signs

The clinical onset is usually insidious, with fever, malaise, weight loss, and other symptoms developing over weeks to months. Pain in the extremities is often a prominent early feature caused by arthralgia, myalgia (particularly affecting the calves), or neuropathy. The combination of mononeuritis multiplex (with the most common finding being footdrop) and features of a systemic illness is one of the earliest specific clues to the presence of an underlying vasculitis. Polyarteritis nodosa is among the forms of vasculitis most commonly associated with vasculitic neuropathy.

In polyarteritis nodosa, the typical skin findings—livedo reticularis, subcutaneous nodules, and skin ulcers—reflect the involvement of deeper, medium-sized blood vessels. Digital gangrene is not an unusual occurrence. The most common cutaneous presentation is lower extremity ulcerations, usually occurring near the malleoli. Involvement of the renal arteries leads to a renin-mediated hypertension (much less characteristic of vasculitides involving smaller blood vessels). For unclear reasons, classic polyarteritis nodosa seldom (if ever) involves the lung, with the occasional exception of the bronchial arteries.

Abdominal pain—particularly diffuse periumbilical pain precipitated by eating—is common but often difficult to attribute to mesenteric vasculitis in the early stages. Nausea and vomiting are common symptoms. Infarction compromises the function of major viscera and may lead to acalculous cholecystitis or appendicitis. Some patients present dramatically with an acute abdomen caused by mesenteric vasculitis and gut perforation or with hypotension resulting from rupture of a microaneurysm in the liver, kidney, or bowel.

Subclinical cardiac involvement is common in polyarteritis nodosa, and overt cardiac dysfunction occasionally occurs (eg, myocardial infarction secondary to coronary vasculitis, or myocarditis).

B. Laboratory Findings

Most patients with polyarteritis nodosa have a slight anemia, and leukocytosis is common. Acute phase reactants are often (but not always) strikingly elevated. A major challenge in making the diagnosis of polyarteritis nodosa, however, is the absence of a disease-specific serologic test (eg, an autoantibody). Patients with classic polyarteritis nodosa are ANCA-negative and may have low titers of rheumatoid factor or antinuclear antibodies, both of which are nonspecific findings. In patients with polyarteritis nodosa, appropriate serologic tests for active hepatitis B infection must be performed.

C. Biopsy and Angiography

The diagnosis of polyarteritis nodosa requires confirmation with either a tissue biopsy or an angiogram. Biopsies of symptomatic sites such as skin (from the edge of an ulcer or the center of a nodule), nerve, or muscle have sensitivities of approximately 70%. The least invasive tests should usually be obtained first, but biopsy of an involved organ is essential. If performed by experienced physicians, tissue biopsies normally have high benefit-risk ratios because of the importance of establishing the diagnosis. Patients in whom polyarteritis nodosa is suspected—eg, on the basis of mesenteric ischemia or new-onset hypertension occurring in the setting of a systemic illness—may be diagnosed by the angiographic finding of aneurysmal dilations in the renal, mesenteric, or hepatic arteries. Angiography must be performed cautiously in patients with baseline renal dysfunction.

Treatment

For polyarteritis nodosa, corticosteroids in high doses (up to 60 mg of oral prednisone daily) may control fever and constitutional symptoms and heal vascular lesions. Pulse methylprednisolone (eg, 1 g intravenously daily for 3 days) may be necessary for patients who are critically ill at presentation. Immunosuppressive agents, especially cyclophosphamide, lower the risk of disease-related death and morbidity among patients who have severe disease. For patients with polyarteritis nodosa associated with hepatitis B, the preferred treatment regimen is a short course of prednisone accompanied by antiviral therapy and plasmapheresis (three times a week for up to 6 weeks).

Prognosis

Without treatment, the 5-year survival rate in these disorders is poor—on the order of 10%. With appropriate therapy, remissions are possible in many cases and the 5-year survival rate has improved to 60–90%. Poor prognostic factors are chronic kidney disease with serum creatinine > 1.6 mg/dL, proteinuria > 1 g/d, gastrointestinal ischemia, central nervous system disease, and cardiac involvement. In the absence of any of these five factors, 5-year survival is nearly 90%. Survival at 5 years drops to 75% with one poor prognostic factor present and to about 50% with two or more factors. Substantial morbidity and even death may result from adverse effects of cyclophosphamide and corticosteroids. Consequently, these therapies require careful monitoring and expert management. In contrast to many other forms of systemic vasculitis, disease relapses in polyarteritis following the successful induction of remission are the exception rather than the rule, occurring in only about 10% of cases.

Bourgarit A et al; French Vasculitis Study Group. Deaths occurring during the first year after treatment onset for polyarteritis nodosa, microscopic polyangiitis, and Churg-Strauss syndrome: a retrospective analysis of causes and factors predictive of mortality based on 595 patients. Medicine (Baltimore). 2005 Sep;84(5):323–30. [PMID: 16148732]

Ebert EC et al. Gastrointestinal involvement in polyarteritis nodosa. Clin Gastroenterol Hepatol. 2008 Sep;6(9):960–6. [PMID: 18585977]

Guillevin L et al; French Vasculitis Study Group. Hepatitis B virus-associated polyarteritis nodosa: clinical characteristics, outcome, and impact of treatment in 115 patients. Medicine (Baltimore). 2005 Sep;84(5):313–22. [PMID: 16148731]

Segelmark M et al. The challenge of managing patients with polyarteritis nodosa. Curr Opin Rheumatol. 2007 Jan;19(1):33–8. [PMID: 17143093]

POLYMYALGIA RHEUMATICA & GIANT CELL ARTERITIS

ESSENTIALS OF DIAGNOSIS

▶ Giant cell (temporal) arteritis is characterized by headache, jaw claudication, polymyalgia rheumatica, visual abnormalities, and a markedly elevated ESR.

▶ The hallmark of polymyalgia rheumatica is pain and stiffness in shoulders and hips lasting for several weeks without other explanation.

▶ General Considerations

Polymyalgia rheumatica and giant cell arteritis probably represent a spectrum of one disease: Both affect the same population (patients over the age of 50), show preference for the same HLA haplotypes, and show similar patterns of cytokines in blood and arteries. Polymyalgia rheumatica and giant cell arteritis also frequently coexist. The important differences between the two conditions are that polymyalgia rheumatica alone does not cause blindness and responds to low-dose (10–20 mg/d orally) prednisone therapy, whereas giant cell arteritis can cause blindness and large artery complications and requires high-dose (40–60 mg/d) prednisone.

▶ Clinical Findings

A. Polymyalgia Rheumatica

Polymyalgia rheumatica is a clinical diagnosis based on pain and stiffness of the shoulder and pelvic girdle areas, fre-

quently in association with fever, malaise, and weight loss. In approximately two-thirds of cases, polymyalgia occurs in the absence of giant cell arteritis. Because of the stiffness and pain in the shoulders, hips, and lower back, patients have trouble combing their hair, putting on a coat, or rising from a chair. In contrast to polymyositis and polyarteritis nodosa, polymyalgia rheumatica does not cause muscular weakness either through primary muscle inflammation or secondary to nerve infarction. A few patients have joint swelling, particularly of the knees, wrists, and sternoclavicular joints. Anemia and elevated acute phase reactants (often markedly elevated ESRs, for example) are present in the most cases, but cases of polymyalgia rheumatica occurring with normal acute phase reactants are well documented. The differential diagnosis of malaise, anemia, and striking acute phase reactant elevations includes rheumatic diseases such as rheumatoid arthritis, other systemic vasculitides, multiple myeloma and other malignant disorders, and chronic infections such as bacterial endocarditis and osteomyelitis.

B. Giant Cell Arteritis

Giant cell arteritis is a systemic panarteritis affecting medium-sized and large vessels in patients over the age of 50. The incidence of this disease increases with each decade of life. The mean age at onset is approximately 72 years. Giant cell arteritis is also called temporal arteritis because that artery is frequently involved, as are other extracranial branches of the carotid artery. About 50% of patients with giant cell arteritis also have polymyalgia rheumatica. The classic symptoms suggesting that a patient has arteritis are headache, scalp tenderness, visual symptoms (particularly amaurosis fugax or diplopia), jaw claudication, or throat pain. Of these symptoms, jaw claudication has the highest positive predictive value. The temporal artery is usually normal on physical examination but may be nodular, enlarged, tender, or pulseless. Blindness usually results from the syndrome of anterior ischemic optic neuropathy, caused by occlusive arteritis of the posterior ciliary branch of the ophthalmic artery. The ischemic optic neuropathy of giant cell arteritis may produce no funduscopic findings for the first 24–48 hours after the onset of blindness.

Asymmetry of pulses in the arms, a murmur of aortic regurgitation, or bruits heard near the clavicle resulting from subclavian artery stenoses identify patients in whom giant cell arteritis has affected the aorta or its major branches. Clinically evident large vessel involvement—characterized chiefly by aneurysm of the thoracic aorta or stenosis of the subclavian, vertebral, carotid, and basilar arteries—occurs in approximately 25% of patients with giant cell arteritis, sometimes years after the diagnosis. Subclinical large artery disease is the rule: positron emission tomography scans reveal inflammation in the aorta and its major branches in nearly 85% of untreated patients. Forty percent of patients with giant cell arteritis have nonclassic symptoms at presentation, chiefly respiratory tract problems (most frequently dry cough), mononeuritis multiplex (most frequently with painful paralysis of a shoulder), or fever of unknown origin. Giant cell arteritis accounts for 15% of all cases of fever of unknown origin in patients over the age of

65. The fever can be as high as 40 °C and is frequently associated with rigors and sweats. In contrast to patients with infection, patients with giant cell arteritis and fever usually have normal white blood cell counts (before prednisone is started). Thus, in an older patient with fever of unknown origin, marked elevations of acute phase reactants, and a normal white blood count, giant cell arteritis must be considered even in the absence of specific features such as headache or jaw claudication. In some cases, instead of having the well-known symptom of jaw claudication, patients complain of vague pain affecting other locations, including the tongue, nose, or ears. Indeed, unexplained head or neck pain in an older patient may signal the presence of giant cell arteritis.

C. Laboratory Findings

Nearly 90% of patients with giant cell arteritis have ESRs > 50 mm/h. The ESR in this disorder is often > 100 mm/h, but cases in which the ESR is low or even normal do occur. In one series, 5% of patients with biopsy-proven giant cell arteritis had ESRs < 40 mm/h. Although the C-reactive protein is slightly more sensitive, patients with biopsy-proven giant cell arteritis with normal C-reactive proteins have also been described. Most patients also have a mild normochromic, normocytic anemia and thrombocytosis. The alkaline phosphatase (liver source) is elevated in 20% of patients with giant cell arteritis.

▶ Treatment

A. Polymyalgia Rheumatica

Patients with isolated polymyalgia rheumatica (ie, those not having "above the neck" symptoms of headache, jaw claudication, scalp tenderness, or visual symptoms) are treated with prednisone, 10–20 mg/d orally. If the patient does not experience a dramatic improvement within 72 hours, the diagnosis should be revisited. Usually after 2–4 weeks of treatment, slow tapering of the prednisone can be attempted. Most patients require some dose of prednisone for a minimum of approximately 1 year; 6 months is too short in most cases. Disease flares are common (50% or more) as prednisone is tapered. The addition of weekly methotrexate may increase the chance of successfully tapering prednisone in some patients.

B. Giant Cell Arteritis

The urgency of early diagnosis and treatment in giant cell arteritis relates to the prevention of blindness. Once blindness develops, it is usually permanent. Therefore, when a patient has symptoms and findings suggestive of temporal arteritis, therapy with prednisone (60 mg/d orally) should be initiated immediately and a temporal artery biopsy performed promptly. For patients who seek medical attention for visual loss, intravenous pulse methylprednisolone (eg, 1 g daily for 3 days) has been advocated; unfortunately, few patients recover vision no matter what the initial treatment. One study—too small and too preliminary to change the standard therapy recommendations mentioned above—suggested that initiating treatment with intravenous pulse

methylprednisolone may increase the chance that a patient with giant cell arteritis will achieve remission and be able to taper off of prednisone. Retrospective studies suggest that low-dose aspirin (~81 mg/d orally) may reduce the chance of visual loss or stroke in patients with giant cell arteritis and should be added to prednisone in the initial treatment. Although it is prudent to obtain a temporal artery biopsy as soon as possible after instituting treatment, diagnostic findings of giant cell arteritis may still be present 2 weeks (or even considerably longer) after starting corticosteroids. Typically, a positive biopsy shows inflammatory infiltrate in the media and adventitia with lymphocytes, histiocytes, plasma cells, and giant cells. An adequate biopsy specimen is essential (at least 2 cm in length is ideal), because the disease may be segmental. Unilateral temporal artery biopsies are positive in approximately 80–85% of patients, but bilateral biopsies add incrementally to the yield (10–15% in some studies, less in others). Prednisone should be continued in a dosage of 60 mg/d orally for about 1 month before tapering. When only the symptoms of polymyalgia rheumatica are present, temporal artery biopsy is not necessary.

After 1 month of high-dose prednisone, almost all patients will have a normal ESR. When tapering and adjusting the dosage of prednisone, the ESR (or C-reactive protein) is a useful but not absolute guide to disease activity. A common error is treating the ESR rather than the patient. The ESR often rises slightly as the prednisone is tapered, even as the disease remains quiescent. Because elderly individuals often have baseline ESRs that are above the normal range, mild ESR elevations should not be an occasion for renewed treatment with prednisone in patients who are asymptomatic. Unfortunately, no highly effective prednisone-sparing therapy has been identified. Methotrexate was modestly effective in one double-blind, placebo-controlled treatment trial but ineffective in another. Anti-TNF therapies do not work in giant cell arteritis. Thoracic aortic aneurysms occur 17 times more frequently in patients with giant cell arteritis than in normal individuals and can result in aortic regurgitation, dissection, or rupture. The aneurysms can develop at any time but typically occur 7 years after the diagnosis of giant cell arteritis is made.

Blockmans D et al. Repetitive 18F-fluorodeoxyglucose positron emission tomography in giant cell arteritis: a prospective study of 35 patients. Arthritis Rheum. 2006 Feb 15;55(1):131–7. [PMID: 16463425]

Gonzalez-Gay MA et al. Giant cell arteritis: disease patterns of clinical presentation in a series of 240 patients. Medicine (Baltimore). 2005 Sep;84(5):269–76. [PMID: 16148727]

Lee MS et al. Antiplatelet and anticoagulant therapy in patients with giant cell arteritis. Arthritis Rheum. 2006 Oct;54(10):3306–9. [PMID: 17009265]

Mazlumzadeh M et al. Treatment of giant cell arteritis using induction therapy with high-dose glucocorticoids: a double-blind, placebo-controlled, randomized prospective clinical trial. Arthritis Rheum. 2006 Oct;54(10):3310–8. [PMID: 17009270]

Parikh M et al. Prevalence of a normal C-reactive protein with an elevated erythrocyte sedimentation rate in biopsy-proven giant cell arteritis. Ophthalmology. 2006 Oct;113(10):1842–5. [PMID: 16884778]

Salvarani C et al. Polymyalgia rheumatica and giant-cell arteritis. Lancet. 2008 Jul 19;372(9634):234–45. [PMID: 18640460]

WEGENER GRANULOMATOSIS

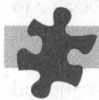

► Classic triad of upper and lower respiratory tract disease and glomerulonephritis.

► Suspect if mild respiratory symptoms (eg, nasal congestion, sinusitis) are refractory to usual treatment.

► Pathology defined by the triad of small vessel vasculitis, granulomatous inflammation, and necrosis.

► ANCAs, usually directed against proteinase-3 (less commonly against myeloperoxidase present in severe, active disease) (90% of patients).

► Kidney disease often rapidly progressive without treatment.

General Considerations

Wegener granulomatosis, which has an estimated incidence of approximately 12 cases per million individuals per year, is the prototype of diseases associated with antineutrophil cytoplasmic antibodies (ANCA). (Other "ANCA-associated vasculitides" include microscopic polyangiitis and the Churg-Strauss syndrome.) Wegener granulomatosis is characterized in its full expression by vasculitis of small arteries, arterioles, and capillaries, necrotizing granulomatous lesions of both upper and lower respiratory tract, glomerulonephritis, and other organ manifestations. Without treatment, generalized disease is invariably fatal, with most patients surviving less than 1 year after diagnosis. It occurs most commonly in the fourth and fifth decades of life and affects men and women with equal frequency.

Clinical Findings

A. Symptoms and Signs

The disorder usually develops over 4–12 months, with 90% of patients presenting with upper or lower respiratory tract symptoms or both. Upper respiratory tract symptoms can include nasal congestion, sinusitis, otitis media, mastoiditis, inflammation of the gums, or stridor due to subglottic stenosis. Since many of these symptoms are common, the underlying disease is not often suspected until the patient develops systemic symptoms or the original problem is refractory to treatment. The lungs are affected initially in 40% and eventually in 80%, with symptoms including cough, dyspnea, and hemoptysis. Other early symptoms can include a migratory oligoarthritis with a predilection for large joints; a variety of symptoms related to ocular disease (unilateral proptosis from orbital pseudotumor; red eye from scleritis, episcleritis, anterior uveitis, or peripheral ulcerative keratitis); purpura or other skin lesions; and dysesthesia due to neuropathy (Plate 85). Renal involvement, which develops in three-fourths of the cases, may be subclinical until chronic kidney disease is advanced. Fever, malaise, and weight loss are common.

Physical examination can be remarkable for congestion, crusting, ulceration, bleeding, and even perforation of the nasal septum. Destruction of the nasal cartilage with "saddle nose" deformity occurs late. Otitis media, proptosis, scleritis, episcleritis, and conjunctivitis are other common findings. Newly acquired hypertension, a frequent feature of polyarteritis nodosa, is rare in Wegener granulomatosis. Venous thrombotic events (eg, deep venous thrombosis and pulmonary embolism) are a common occurrence in Wegener granulomatosis, at least in part because of the tendency of the disease to involve veins as well as arteries. Although limited forms of Wegener granulomatosis have been described in which the kidney is spared initially, kidney disease will develop in the majority of untreated patients.

B. Laboratory Findings

1. Serum tests and urinalysis—Most patients have slight anemia, mild leukocytosis, and elevated acute phase reactants. If there is renal involvement, the urinary sediment invariably contains red cells, with or without white cells, and often has red cell casts.

Serum tests for ANCA help in the diagnosis of Wegener granulomatosis and related forms of vasculitis (Table 20–10). Several different types of ANCA are recognized, but the two subtypes relevant to systemic vasculitis are those directed against proteinase-3 (PR3) and myeloperoxidase (MPO). Antibodies to these two antigens are termed "PR3-ANCA" and "MPO-ANCA," respectively. The cytoplasmic pattern of immunofluorescence (C-ANCA) caused by PR3-ANCA has a high specificity (> 90%) for either Wegener granulomatosis or a closely related disease, microscopic polyangiitis (or, less commonly, the Churg-Strauss syndrome). In the setting of active disease, particularly cases in which the disease is severe and generalized to multiple organ systems, the sensitivity of PR3-ANCA is > 95%. A substantial percentage of patients with "limited" Wegener granulomatosis—disease that does not pose an immediate threat to life and is often confined to the respiratory tract—are ANCA-negative. Although ANCA testing may be very helpful when used properly, it does not eliminate the need in most cases for confirmation of the diagnosis by tissue biopsy. Furthermore, ANCA levels correlate erratically with disease activity, and changes in titer should not dictate changes in therapy in the absence of supporting clinical data. The perinuclear (P-ANCA) pattern, caused by MPO-ANCA, is more likely to occur in microscopic polyangiitis or Churg-Strauss but may also be found in Wegener granulomatosis. Approximately 10–25% of patients with classic Wegener granulomatosis have MPO-ANCA. All positive immunofluorescence assays for ANCA should be confirmed by enzyme immunoassays for the specific autoantibodies directed against PR3 or MPO.

2. Histologic findings—Histologic features of Wegener granulomatosis include vasculitis, granulomatous inflammation, geographic necrosis, and acute and chronic inflammation. The full range of pathologic changes is usually evident only on thoracoscopic lung biopsy. Granulomas, observed only rarely in renal biopsy specimens, are found much more commonly on lung biopsy specimens. Nasal biopsies often do not show vasculitis but may show chronic inflammation and other changes which, interpreted by an experienced pathologist, can serve as convincing evidence of the diagnosis. Renal biopsy discloses a segmental necrotizing glomerulonephritis with multiple crescents; this is characteristic but not diagnostic. Pathologists characterize the renal lesion of Wegener granulomatosis (and other forms of "ANCA-associated vasculitis") as a pauci-immune glomerulonephritis because of the relative absence (compared with immune complex–mediated disorders) of immunoreactants—IgG, IgM, IgA, and complement proteins—within glomeruli.

C. Imaging

Chest CT is more sensitive than chest radiography; lesions include infiltrates, nodules, masses, and cavities. Often the radiographs prompt concern about lung cancer. Hilar adenopathy is unusual in Wegener granulomatosis; if present, sarcoidosis, tumor, or infection is more likely. Other common radiographic abnormalities include extensive sinusitis and even bony sinus erosions.

▶ Differential Diagnosis

In most patients with Wegener granulomatosis, refractory sinusitis or otitis media is initially suspected. When upper respiratory tract inflammation persists and is accompanied by additional systemic inflammatory signs (eg, red eye from scleritis, joint pain and swelling), the diagnosis of Wegener granulomatosis should be considered. Rheumatoid arthritis will wrongly be suspected in a substantial minority of patients who chiefly complain of joint pain. Arriving at the correct diagnosis is aided by awareness that rheumatoid arthritis typically involves small joints of the hand, whereas Wegener granulomatosis favors large joints, such as the hip, knee, elbow, and shoulder. Lung cancer may be the first diagnostic consideration for some middle-aged patients in whom cough, hemoptysis, and lung masses are presenting symptoms and signs; typically, evidence of glomerulonephritis, a positive ANCA or, ultimately, the lung biopsy findings will point to the proper diagnosis. Wegener granulomatosis shares with SLE, Goodpasture syndrome, and microscopic polyangiitis the ability to cause an acute pulmonary-renal syndrome. Approximately 10–25% of patients with classic Wegener granulomatosis have MPO-ANCA. Owing to involvement of the same types of blood vessels, similar patterns of organ involvement, and the possibility of failing to identify granulomatous pathology on tissue biopsies because of sampling error, Wegener granulomatosis is often difficult to differentiate from microscopic polyangiitis. The crucial distinctions between the two disorders are the tendencies for Wegener granulomatosis to involve the upper respiratory tract (including the ears) and to cause granulomatous inflammation.

▶ Treatment

Early treatment is crucial in preventing the devastating end-organ complications of this disease, and often in preserving life. While Wegener granulomatosis may involve the sinuses or lung for months, once proteinuria or hematuria develops, progression to advanced chronic kidney disease can be rapid (over several weeks). Remissions of at least a temporary nature have been induced in more than 90% of patients treated with prednisone (1 mg/kg daily) and cyclophosphamide. Unfortunately, the traditional therapy of oral cyclophosphamide continued for 12 months after the patient achieves remission has resulted in severe toxicity, including a 2.4 times increased risk of all malignancies, a 33-fold increase in bladder cancer, and a 60% chance of ovarian failure. Moreover, disease relapses occur in a substantial proportion of those patients who achieve remission. Still, for patients with severe Wegener granulomatosis, cyclophosphamide and prednisone remain the standard of care for remission induction. Consequently, the current approach to remission induction in severe cases is to use cyclophosphamide for 3–6 months, followed by a switch to a regimen more likely to be tolerated well. Cyclophosphamide is best given daily by mouth; intermittent high-dose intravenous cyclophosphamide is less effective. In patients with remission induced by 3–6 months of cyclophosphamide and corticosteroids, azathioprine (up to 2 mg/kg/d orally) has been shown to be as effective as cyclophosphamide in maintaining disease remissions (at least for up to 12–15 months). Before the institution of azathioprine, patients should be tested (through a commercially available blood test) for deficiencies in the level of thiopurine methyltransferase, an enzyme essential to the metabolism of azathioprine. Another current option for remission maintenance is methotrexate, 20–25 mg/wk (administered either orally or intramuscularly). Because of its superior side-effect profile, methotrexate is viewed as an appropriate substitute for cyclophosphamide in patients who do not have significant renal dysfunction (of any cause) or immediately life-threatening disease. Treatment with TNF inhibitors, particularly etanercept, is not effective. Several small, uncontrolled studies suggest that rituximab, a B-cell-depleting monoclonal antibody, may have efficacy.

Finkielman JD et al; WGET Research Group. Antiproteinase 3 antineutrophil cytoplasmic antibodies and disease activity in Wegener granulomatosis. Ann Intern Med. 2007 Nov 6;147(9):611–9. [PMID: 17975183]

Seo P. Wegener's granulomatosis: managing more than inflammation. Curr Opin Rheumatol. 2008 Jan;20(1):10–6. [PMID: 18281851]

Wegener's Granulomatosis Etanercept Trial (WGET) Research Group. Etanercept plus standard therapy for Wegener's granulomatosis. N Engl J Med. 2005 Jan 27;352(4):351–61. [PMID: 15673801]

Wung PK et al. Therapeutics of Wegener's granulomatosis. Nat Clin Pract Rheumatol. 2006 Apr;2(4):192–200. [PMID: 16932685]

MICROSCOPIC POLYANGIITIS

 ESSENTIALS OF DIAGNOSIS

▶ Necrotizing vasculitis of small- and medium-sized arteries and veins.

▶ Pulmonary alveolar hemorrhage and glomerulonephritis.

▶ Associated with ANCA in 75% of cases, usually antimyeloperoxidase antibodies (MPO-ANCA) that cause a P-ANCA pattern on immunofluorescence testing. ANCA directed against proteinase-3 (PR3-ANCA) can also be observed.

General Considerations

Microscopic polyangiitis is a pauci-immune nongranulomatous necrotizing vasculitis that (1) affects small blood vessels (capillaries, venules, or arterioles), (2) often causes glomerulonephritis and pulmonary capillaritis, and (3) is often associated with ANCA on immunofluorescence testing (directed against MPO, a constituent of neutrophil granules). Because microscopic polyangiitis may involve medium-sized as well as small blood vessels and because it tends to affect capillaries within the lungs and kidneys, its spectrum overlaps those of both polyarteritis nodosa and Wegener granulomatosis.

In a minority of cases, microscopic polyangiitis appears to be induced by reactions to medications, particularly propylthiouracil, hydralazine, allopurinol, penicillamine, minocycline, and sulfasalazine. In rare instances, these drugs induce a systemic vasculitis associated with MPO-ANCA. Such syndromes usually resolve with discontinuation of the offending drug.

Clinical Findings

A. Symptoms and Signs

A wide variety of findings suggesting vasculitis of small blood vessels may develop in microscopic polyangiitis. These include "palpable" (or "raised") purpura and other signs of cutaneous vasculitis (ulcers, splinter hemorrhages, vesiculobullous lesions).

Microscopic polyangiitis is the most common cause of pulmonary-renal syndromes, being several times more common than Goodpasture (antiglomerular basement membrane) syndrome. Interstitial lung fibrosis that mimics usual interstitial pneumonitis is the presenting condition. Pulmonary hemorrhage may occur. The pathologic findings in the lung are typically those of capillaritis.

Hematuria, proteinuria, and red blood cell casts in the urine may occur. The renal lesion is a segmental, necrotizing glomerulonephritis, often with localized intravascular coagulation and the observation of intraglomerular thrombi upon renal biopsy.

Vasculitic neuropathy (mononeuritis multiplex) is also common in microscopic polyangiitis.

B. Laboratory Findings

As noted, three-fourths of patients with microscopic polyangiitis are ANCA-positive. Elevated acute phase reactants are also typical of active disease. Careful scrutiny of the urine sediment is essential to excluding active kidney disease.

Differential Diagnosis

Distinguishing this disease from Wegener granulomatosis may be challenging in some cases. Microscopic polyangiitis is not associated with the chronic destructive upper respiratory tract disease often found in Wegener granulomatosis. Moreover, as noted, a critical difference between the two diseases is the absence of granulomatous inflammation in microscopic polyangiitis. Because their treatments may differ, microscopic polyangiitis must also be differentiated from polyarteritis nodosa.

Treatment

In microscopic polyangiitis, patients are likely to require prednisone and cyclophosphamide because of the urgency in treating pulmonary hemorrhage and glomerulonephritis. Cyclophosphamide may be administered either in an oral daily regimen or via intermittent (usually monthly) intravenous pulses. Whenever cyclophosphamide is used, *Pneumocystis jiroveci* prophylaxis with either single-strength oral trimethoprim-sulfamethoxazole or dapsone 100 mg/d is essential. Following the induction of remission, azathioprine is a reasonable choice to replace cyclophosphamide.

Prognosis

The key to effecting good outcomes is early diagnosis. Compared with patients who have Wegener granulomatosis, those who have microscopic polyangiitis are more likely to have significant fibrosis on renal biopsy because of later diagnosis. The likelihood of disease recurrence following remission in microscopic polyangiitis is about 33%.

Bonaci-Nikolic B et al. Antineutrophil cytoplasmic antibody (ANCA)-associated autoimmune diseases induced by antithyroid drugs: comparison with idiopathic ANCA vasculitides. Arthritis Res Ther. 2005;7(5):R1072–81. [PMID: 16207324]

Haubitz M. ANCA-associated vasculitis: diagnosis, clinical characteristics and treatment. Vasa. 2007 May;36(2):81–9. [PMID: 17708098]

Jayne D. Challenges in the management of microscopic polyangiitis: past, present and future. Curr Opin Rheumatol. 2008 Jan;20(1):3–9. [PMID: 18281850]

Mukhtyar C et al. Outcomes from studies of antineutrophil cytoplasm antibody associated vasculitis: a systematic review by the European League Against Rheumatism Systemic Vasculitis Task Force. Ann Rheum Dis. 2008 Jul;67(7):1004–10. [PMID: 17911225]

CRYOGLOBULINEMIA

Cryoglobulinemia can be associated with an immune-complex mediated, small-vessel vasculitis. Chronic infection with hepatitis C is the most common underlying condition; cryoglobulinemic vasculitis also can occur in the setting of other chronic infections, such as subacute bacterial endocarditis and osteomyelitis, and with connective tissues diseases, especially Sjögren syndrome. The cryoglobulins associated with vasculitis are cold-precipitable immune complexes consisting of rheumatoid factor and IgG (rheumatoid factor is an autoantibody to the constant region of IgG). The rheumatoid factor component can be monoclonal (type II cryoglobulins) or polyclonal (type III cryoglobulins). (Type I cryoglobulins are cryoprecipitable monoclonal proteins that lack rheumatoid factor activity; these cause cold-induced hyperviscosity syndromes, not vasculitis, and are associated with lymphoproliferative disease.) Cryoglobulinemic vasculitis typically manifests as recurrent palpable purpura and peripheral neuropathy. A proliferative glomerulonephritis can develop and can manifest as rapidly progressive glomerulonephritis. Abnormal liver function tests, abdominal pain, and pulmonary disease may also occur. The diagnosis is based on a compatible clinical picture and a positive serum test for cryoglobulins. The presence of a disproportionately low C4 level can be a diagnostic clue to the presence of cryoglobulinemia. The optimal approach to treatment of hepatitis C–associated cryoglobulinemic vasculitis is viral suppression with pegylated forms of interferon-α, with or without ribavirin. Because immunosuppressive agents may facilitate viral replication, corticosteroids, cyclophosphamide, and other interventions (including plasmapheresis) should be reserved for organ-threatening complications. B cell depletion using rituximab appears to be a promising avenue of therapy. Asymptomatic cryoglobulinemia is common in hepatitis C–infected individuals and does not in itself warrant treatment.

Antonelli A et al. HCV infection: pathogenesis, clinical manifestations and therapy. Clin Exp Rheumatol. 2008 Jan–Feb;26(1 Suppl 48):S39–47. [PMID: 18570753]

Kamar N et al. Treatment of hepatitis C-virus-related glomerulonephritis. Kidney Int. 2006 Feb;69(3):436–9. [PMID: 16514428]

Quartuccio L et al. Rituximab treatment for glomerulonephritis in HCV-associated mixed cryoglobulinaemia: efficacy and safety in the absence of steroids. Rheumatology (Oxford). 2006 Jul;45(7):842–6. [PMID: 16418196]

Saadoun D et al. Treatment of hepatitis C-associated mixed cryoglobulinemia vasculitis. Curr Opin Rheumatol. 2008 Jan;20(1):23–8. [PMID: 18281853]

HENOCH-SCHÖNLEIN PURPURA

Henoch-Schönlein purpura, the most common systemic vasculitis in children, occurs in adults as well. Typical features are palpable purpura, abdominal pain, arthritis, and hematuria (Plate 86). Pathologic features include leukocytoclastic vasculitis with IgA deposition. The cause is not known.

The purpuric skin lesions are typically located on the lower extremities but may also be seen on the hands, arms, trunk, and buttocks. Joint symptoms are present in the majority of patients, the knees and ankles being most commonly involved. Abdominal pain secondary to vasculitis of the intestinal tract is often associated with gastrointestinal bleeding. Hematuria signals the presence of a renal lesion that is usually reversible, although it occasionally may progress to chronic kidney disease. Children tend to have more frequent and more serious gastrointestinal vasculitis, whereas adults more often suffer from chronic kidney disease. Biopsy of the kidney reveals segmental glomerulonephritis with crescents and mesangial deposition of IgA.

Chronic courses with persistent or intermittent skin disease are more likely to occur in adults than in children.

The value of corticosteroids has been controversial. In children, prednisone (1 mg/kg/d orally) may benefit those with severe extrarenal manifestations and with evidence of kidney disease. The incremental efficacy of steroid-sparing drugs such as azathioprine and mycophenolate mofetil—often used in the setting of kidney disease—is not known.

Dillon MJ. Henoch-Schönlein purpura: recent advances. Clin Exp Rheumatol. 2007 Jan–Feb;25(1 Suppl 44):S66–8. [PMID: 17428373]

Weiss PF et al. Effects of corticosteroid on Henoch-Schönlein purpura: a systematic review. Pediatrics. 2007 Nov;120(5):1079–87. [PMID: 17974746]

RELAPSING POLYCHONDRITIS

This disease is characterized by inflammatory destructive lesions of cartilaginous structures, principally the ears, nose, trachea, and larynx. Nearly 40% of cases are associated with another disease, especially either other immunologic disorders (such as SLE, rheumatoid arthritis, or Hashimoto thyroiditis) or cancers (such as multiple myeloma) or hematologic disorders (such as myelodysplastic syndrome). The disease, which is usually episodic, affects males and females equally. The cartilage is painful, swollen, and tender during an attack and subsequently becomes atrophic, resulting in permanent deformity. Biopsy of the involved cartilage shows inflammation and chondrolysis. Noncartilaginous manifestations of the disease include fever, episcleritis, uveitis, deafness, aortic insufficiency, and rarely glomerulonephritis. In 85% of patients, a migratory, asymmetric, and seronegative arthropathy occurs, affecting both large and small joints and the costochondral junctions. Diagnosing this uncommon disease is especially difficult since the signs of cartilage inflammation (such as red ears or nasal pain) may be more subtle than the fever, arthritis, rash, or other systemic manifestations.

Prednisone, 0.5–1 mg/kg/d orally, is often effective. Dapsone (100–200 mg/d orally) or methotrexate (7.5–20 mg orally per week) may also have efficacy, sparing the need for long-term high-dose corticosteroid treatment. Involvement of the tracheobronchial tree, leading to tracheomalacia, may lead to difficult management issues.

Dib C et al. Surgical treatment of the cardiac manifestations of relapsing polychondritis: overview of 33 patients identified through literature review and the Mayo Clinic records. Mayo Clin Proc. 2006 Jun;81(6):772–6. [PMID: 16770977]

BEHÇET SYNDROME

 ESSENTIALS OF DIAGNOSIS

▶ Most commonly occurs among persons of Asian, Turkish, or Middle Eastern background, but may affect persons of any demographic profile.

▶ Recurrent, painful aphthous ulcers of the mouth and genitals.

▶ Additional cutaneous findings include erythema nodosum–like lesions, a follicular rash, and the "pathergy" phenomenon (formation of a sterile pustule at the site of a needle stick).

▶ Either anterior or posterior uveitis. Posterior uveitis may be asymptomatic until significant damage to the retina has occurred.

▶ Variety of neurologic lesions that can mimic multiple sclerosis, particularly through involvement of the white matter of the brainstem.

General Considerations

Named after the Turkish dermatologist who first described it, this disease is of unknown cause. Essentially all of its protean manifestations, however, are believed to result from vasculitis that may involve all types of blood vessels: small, medium, and large, on both the arterial and venous side of the circulation.

Clinical Findings

A. Symptoms and Signs

The hallmark of Behçet disease is painful aphthous ulceration in the mouth (Plate 63). These lesions, which usually occur multiply, may be found on the tongue, gums, and inner surfaces of the oral cavity. Genital lesions, similar in appearance, are also common but do not occur in all patients. Other cutaneous lesions of Behçet disease include tender, erythematous, papular lesions that resemble erythema nodosum. (On biopsy, however, many of these lesions are shown to be secondary to vasculitis rather than septal panniculitis.) These erythema nodosum–like lesions have a tendency to ulcerate, a major difference between the lesions of Behçet disease and the erythema nodosum seen in cases of sarcoidosis and inflammatory bowel disease. An erythematous follicular rash that occurs frequently on the upper extremities may be a subtle feature of the disease. The pathergy phenomenon is frequently underappreciated (unless the patient is asked); in this phenomenon, sterile pustules develop at sites where needles have been inserted into the skin (eg, for phlebotomy) in some patients.

A nonerosive arthritis occurs in about two-thirds of patients, most commonly affecting the knees and ankles. Eye involvement may be one of the most devastating complications of Behçet disease. Posterior uveitis, in essence a retinal venulitis, may lead to the insidious destruction of large areas of the retina before the patient becomes aware of visual problems. Anterior uveitis, associated with photophobia and a red eye, is intensely symptomatic. This complication may lead to a hypopyon, the accumulation of pus in the anterior chamber. If not treated properly with mydriatic agents to dilate the pupil and corticosteroid eyedrops to diminish inflammation, the anterior uveitis of Behçet may lead to synechial formation between the iris and lens, resulting in permanent pupillary distortion.

Central nervous system involvement is another cause of major potential morbidity in Behçet disease. The central nervous system lesions that may mimic multiple sclerosis radiologically often result in serious disability or death. Findings include sterile meningitis (recurrent meningeal headaches associated with a lymphocytic pleocytosis), cranial nerve palsies, seizures, encephalitis, mental disturbances, and spinal cord lesions. Finally, patients with Behçet disease have a hypercoagulable tendency that may lead to complicated venous thrombotic events, particularly multiple deep venous thrombosis, pulmonary emboli, cerebral sinus thrombosis, and other problems associated with clotting.

The clinical course may be chronic but is often characterized by remissions and exacerbations.

B. Laboratory Findings

There are no pathognomonic laboratory features of Behçet disease. Although patients with Behçet disease often have elevated acute phase reactants, there is no autoantibody or other assay that is distinctive. No markers of hypercoagulability specific to Behçet have been identified.

Treatment

Corticosteroids (1 mg/kg/d of oral prednisone) are a mainstay of therapy for severe disease manifestations. Azathioprine (2 mg/kg/d orally) may be an effective steroid-sparing agent. Cyclophosphamide (2 mg/kg/d orally) or chlorambucil (0.1–0.2 mg/kg/d orally) is indicated for severe ocular and central nervous system complications of Behçet disease. Both colchicine (0.6 mg once to three times daily orally) and thalidomide (100 mg/d orally) help ameliorate the mucocutaneous findings. TNF inhibition and interferon alfa-2a demonstrates some promise as a therapeutic approach, but large studies are lacking to date.

Alpagut U et al. Major arterial involvement and review of Behcet's disease. Ann Vasc Surg. 2007 Mar;21(2):232–9. [PMID: 17349371]

Calamia KT et al. Behçet's disease: recent advances in early diagnosis and effective treatment. Curr Rheumatol Rep. 2008 Oct;10(5):349–55. [PMID: 18817637]

PRIMARY ANGIITIS OF THE CENTRAL NERVOUS SYSTEM

Primary angiitis of the central nervous system is a syndrome with several possible causes that produces small and medium-sized vasculitis limited to the brain and spinal cord. Biopsy-proved cases have predominated in men who have a history of weeks to months of headaches, encephalopathy, and multifocal strokes. Systemic signs and symptoms are absent, and routine laboratory tests are usually normal. MRI of the brain is almost always abnormal, and the spinal fluid often reveals a mild lymphocytosis and a modest increase in protein level. Angiograms classically reveal a "string of beads" pattern produced by alternating segments of arterial narrowing and dilation. However, neither the MRI nor the angiogram appearance is specific for vasculitis. Indeed, in one study, none of the patients who had biopsy-proved central nervous system vasculitis had an angiogram showing "the string of beads," and none of the patients with the classic angiographic findings had a positive brain biopsy for vasculitis. Many conditions, including vasospasm, can produce the same angiographic pattern as vasculitis. Definitive diagnosis requires a compatible clinical picture; exclusion of infection, neoplasm, or metabolic disorder or drug exposure (eg, cocaine) that can mimic primary angiitis of the central nervous system; and a positive brain biopsy. In contrast to biopsy-proved cases, patients with angiographically defined central nervous system vasculopathy are chiefly women who have had an abrupt onset of headaches and stroke (often in the absence of encephalopathy) with normal spinal fluid findings. Many patients who fit this clinical profile may have reversible cerebral vasoconstriction rather than true vasculitis. Such cases may best be treated with calcium channel blockers (such as nimodipine or verapamil) and possibly short course of corticosteroids. Biopsy-proved cases usually improve with prednisone therapy and often require cyclophosphamide. In recent years, cases of central nervous system vasculitis associated with cerebral amyloid angiopathy have been reported. These cases often respond well to corticosteroids, albeit the long-term natural history remains poorly defined.

Calabrese LH et al. Narrative review: reversible cerebral vasoconstriction syndromes. Ann Intern Med. 2007 Jan 2;146(1):34–44. [PMID: 17200220]

LIVEDO RETICULARIS

Livedo reticularis produces a mottled, purplish discoloration of the skin with reticulated cyanotic areas surrounding paler central cores. This distinctive "fishnet" pattern is caused by spasm or obstruction of perpendicular arterioles, combined with pooling of blood in surrounding venous plexuses. Livedo reticularis can be idiopathic or a manifestation of a serious underlying condition.

Idiopathic livedo reticularis is a benign condition that worsens with cold exposure, improves with warming, and primarily affects the extremities. Apart from cosmetic concerns, it is usually asymptomatic. The presence of systemic symptoms or the development of cutaneous ulcerations points to the presence of an underlying disease.

Secondary livedo reticularis occurs in association with a variety of diseases that cause vascular obstruction or inflammation. Of particular importance is the link with antiphospholipid antibody syndrome. Livedo reticularis is the presenting manifestation of 25% of patients with antiphospholipid antibody syndrome and is strongly associated with the subgroup that has arterial thromboses, including those with Sneddon syndrome (livedo reticularis and cerebrovascular events). Other underlying causes of livedo reticularis include the vasculitides (particularly polyarteritis nodosa), cholesterol emboli syndrome, thrombocythemia, cryoglobulinemia, cold agglutinin disease, primary hyperoxaluria (due to vascular deposits of calcium oxalate), and disseminated intravascular coagulation.

Weinstein S et al. Cutaneous manifestations of antiphospholipid antibody syndrome. Hematol Oncol Clin North Am. 2008 Feb;22(1):67-77. [PMID: 18207066]

SERONEGATIVE SPONDYLOARTHROPATHIES

The seronegative spondyloarthropathies are ankylosing spondylitis, psoriatic arthritis, reactive arthritis (also called Reiter syndrome), the arthritis associated with inflammatory bowel disease, and undifferentiated spondyloarthropathy. These disorders are noted for male predominance, onset usually before age 40, inflammatory arthritis of the spine or the large peripheral joints (or both), enthesopathy (inflammation of where ligaments, tendons, and joint capsule insert into bone), uveitis in a significant minority, the absence of autoantibodies in the serum, and a striking association with HLA-B27. Present in only 8% of normal whites and 4% of normal blacks, HLA-B27 is positive in 90% of patients with ankylosing spondylitis and 75% with reactive arthritis. HLA-B27 also occurs in 50% of the psoriatic and inflammatory bowel disease patients who have sacroiliitis. Patients with only peripheral arthritis in these latter two syndromes do not show an increase in HLA-B27.

ANKYLOSING SPONDYLITIS

 ESSENTIALS OF DIAGNOSIS

▶ Chronic low backache in young adults, generally worst in the morning.

▶ Progressive limitation of back motion and of chest expansion.

▶ Transient (50%) or persistent (25%) peripheral arthritis.

▶ Anterior uveitis in 20–25%.

▶ Diagnostic radiographic changes in sacroiliac joints.

▶ Negative serologic tests for rheumatoid factor.

▶ HLA-B27 testing is most helpful when there is an indeterminate probability of disease.

▶ General Considerations

Ankylosing spondylitis is a chronic inflammatory disease of the joints of the axial skeleton, manifested clinically by pain and progressive stiffening of the spine. The age at onset is usually in the late teens or early 20s. The incidence is greater in males than in females, and symptoms are more prominent in men, with ascending involvement of the spine more likely to occur.

▶ Clinical Findings

A. Symptoms and Signs

The onset is usually gradual, with intermittent bouts of back pain that may radiate into the buttocks. The back pain is worse in the morning and usually associated with stiffness that lasts hours. The pain and stiffness improve with activity, in contrast to back pain due to mechanical causes and degenerative disease, which improves with rest and worsens with activity. As the disease advances, symptoms progress in a cephalad direction and back motion becomes limited, with the normal lumbar curve flattened and the thoracic curvature exaggerated. Chest expansion is often limited as a consequence of costovertebral joint involvement. In advanced cases, the entire spine becomes fused, allowing no motion in any direction. Transient acute arthritis of the peripheral joints occurs in about 50% of cases, and permanent changes in the peripheral joints—most commonly the hips, shoulders, and knees—are seen in about 25%. Enthesopathy, a hallmark of the spondyloarthropathies, can manifest as swelling of the Achilles tendon at its insertion, plantar fasciitis (producing heel pain), or "sausage" swelling of a finger or toe (less common in ankylosing spondylitis than in psoriatic arthritis).

Anterior uveitis is associated in as many as 25% of cases and may be a presenting feature. Spondylitic heart disease, characterized chiefly by atrioventricular conduction defects and aortic insufficiency, occurs in 3–5% of patients with long-standing severe disease. Pulmonary fibrosis of the upper lobes, with progression to cavitation and bronchiectasis mimicking tuberculosis, may rarely occur, characteristically long after the onset of skeletal symptoms. Radicular symptoms due to cauda equina fibrosis may develop years after onset of the disease. Constitutional symptoms similar to those of rheumatoid arthritis are absent in most patients.

B. Laboratory Findings

The ESR is elevated in 85% of cases, but serologic tests for rheumatoid factor are characteristically negative. Anemia may be present but is often mild. HLA-B27 is found in 90% of white patients and 50% of black patients with ankylosing spondylitis. Because this antigen occurs in 8% of the healthy white population (and 2% of healthy blacks), it is not a specific diagnostic test.

C. Imaging

The earliest radiographic changes are usually in the sacroiliac joints. In the first 2 years of the disease process, the sacroiliac changes may be detectable only by MRI. Later, erosion and sclerosis of these joints are evident on plain radiographs; the sacroiliitis of ankylosing spondylitis is bilateral and symmetric. Inflammation where the annulus fibrosus attaches to the vertebral bodies initially causes sclerosis ("the shiny corner sign") and then characteristic squaring of the vertebral bodies. The term "bamboo spine" describes the late radiographic appearance of the spinal column in which the vertebral bodies are fused by vertically oriented, bridging syndesmophytes formed by the ossification of the annulus fibrosus and calcification of the anterior and lateral spinal ligaments. Fusion of the posterior facet joints of the spine is also common.

Additional radiographic findings include periosteal new bone formation on the iliac crest, ischial tuberosities and calcanei, and alterations of the pubic symphysis and sternomanubrial joint similar to those of the sacroiliacs. Radiologic changes in peripheral joints, when present, tend to be asymmetric and lack the demineralization and erosions seen in rheumatoid arthritis.

▶ Differential Diagnosis

Low back pain due to mechanical causes, disk disease, and degenerative arthritis is very common. Onset of back pain prior to age 30 and an "inflammatory" quality of the back pain (ie, morning stiffness and pain that improve with activity) should raise the possibility of ankylosing spondylitis. In contrast to ankylosing spondylitis, rheumatoid arthritis predominantly affects multiple, small, peripheral joints of the hands and feet. Rheumatoid arthritis spares the sacroiliac joints and only affects the cervical component of the spine. Bilateral sacroiliitis indistinguishable from ankylosing spondylitis is seen with the spondylitis associated with inflammatory bowel disease. Sacroiliitis associated with reactive arthritis and psoriasis, on the other hand, is often asymmetric or even unilateral. Osteitis condensans ilii (sclerosis on the iliac side of the sacroiliac joint) is an asymptomatic, postpartum radiographic finding that is occasionally mistaken for sacroiliitis. Diffuse idiopathic skeletal hyperostosis (DISH) causes exuberant osteophytes of the spine that occasionally are difficult to distinguish from the syndesmophytes of ankylosing spondylitis. The osteophytes of DISH are thicker and more anterior than the syndesmophytes of ankylosing spondylitis, and the sacroiliac joints are normal in DISH.

▶ Treatment

A. Basic Program

The general principles of managing chronic arthritis (see above) apply equally well to ankylosing spondylitis. The importance of postural and breathing exercises should be stressed.

B. Drug Therapy

NSAIDs remain first-line treatment of ankylosing spondylitis and may slow radiographic progression of spinal disease. Because individual patients differ in their response to particular NSAIDs, empiric trials of several different NSAIDs are warranted if the response to any given NSAID is not satisfactory. TNF inhibitors have established efficacy for NSAID-resistant axial disease; responses are often substantial and durable. Etanercept (50 mg subcutaneously once a week), adalimumab (40 mg subcutaneously every other week), or infliximab (5 mg/kg every other month by IV infusion) is reasonable for patients whose symptoms are refractory to NSAIDs. Sulfasalazine (1000 mg orally twice daily) is sometimes useful for peripheral arthritis but lacks effectiveness for spinal and sacroiliac joint disease. Corticosteroids have minimal impact on the arthritis—particularly the spondylitis—of ankylosing spondylitis and can worsen osteopenia.

▶ Prognosis

Almost all patients have persistent symptoms over decades; rare individuals experience long-term remissions. The severity of disease varies greatly, with about 10% of patients having work disability after 10 years. Developing hip disease within the first 2 years of disease onset presages a worse prognosis. The availability of TNF inhibitors has improved the outlook dramatically for many patients with ankylosing spondylitis, and the early use of these therapies may attenuate many of the long-term disabilities otherwise characteristic of this disease.

Braun J et al. Efficacy and safety of infliximab in patients with ankylosing spondylitis over a two-year period. Arthritis Rheum. 2008 Sep 15;59(9):1270–8. [PMID: 18759257]

Song IH et al. Benefits and risks of ankylosing spondylitis treatment with nonsteroidal antiinflammatory drugs. Arthritis Rheum. 2008 Apr;58(4):929–38. [PMID: 18383378]

van der Heijde D et al; Ankylosing Spondylitis Study for the Evaluation of Recombinant Infliximab Therapy Study Group. Radiographic findings following two years of infliximab therapy in patients with ankylosing spondylitis. Arthritis Rheum. 2008 Oct;58(10):3063–70. [PMID: 18821688]

Wanders A et al. Nonsteroidal antiinflammatory drugs reduce radiographic progression in patients with ankylosing spondylitis: a randomized clinical trial. Arthritis Rheum. 2005 Jun; 52(6):1756–65. [PMID: 15934081]

PSORIATIC ARTHRITIS

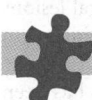 ESSENTIALS OF DIAGNOSIS

► Psoriasis precedes onset of arthritis in 80% of cases.
► Arthritis usually asymmetric, with "sausage" appearance of fingers and toes but a polyarthritis that resembles rheumatoid arthritis also occurs.
► Sacroiliac joint involvement common; ankylosis of the sacroiliac joints may occur.
► Radiographic findings: osteolysis; pencil-in-cup deformity; relative lack of osteoporosis; bony ankylosis; asymmetric sacroiliitis and atypical syndesmophytes.

► General Considerations

Arthritis occurs in 15–20% of patients with psoriasis.

► Clinical Findings

A. Symptoms and Signs

The patterns or subsets of psoriatic arthritis include the following:

1. A symmetric polyarthritis that resembles rheumatoid arthritis. Usually, fewer joints are involved than in rheumatoid arthritis.

2. An oligoarticular form that may lead to considerable destruction of the affected joints.

3. A pattern of disease in which the DIP joints are primarily affected. Early, this may be monarticular, and often the joint involvement is asymmetric. Pitting of the nails and onycholysis frequently accompany DIP involvement.

4. A severe deforming arthritis (arthritis mutilans) in which osteolysis is marked.

5. A spondylitic form in which sacroiliitis and spinal involvement predominate; 50% of these patients are HLA-B27-positive.

Although psoriasis usually precedes the onset of arthritis, arthritis precedes (by up to 2 years) or occurs simultaneously with the skin disease in approximately 20% of cases. Arthritis is at least five times more common in patients with severe skin disease than in those with only mild skin findings. Occasionally, however, patients may have a single patch of psoriasis (typically hidden in the scalp, gluteal cleft, or umbilicus) and are unaware of its connection to the arthritis. Thus, a detailed search for cutaneous lesions is essential in patients with arthritis of new onset. Also, the psoriatic lesions may have cleared when arthritis appears—in such cases, the history is most useful in diagnosing previously unexplained cases of mono- or oligoarthritis. Nail pitting is sometimes a clue. "Sausage" swelling of one or more digits is a common manifestation of enthesopathy in psoriatic arthritis.

B. Laboratory Findings

Laboratory studies show an elevation of the ESR, but rheumatoid factor is not present. Uric acid levels may be high, reflecting the active turnover of skin affected by psoriasis. There is a correlation between the extent of psoriatic involvement and the level of uric acid, but gout is no more common than in patients without psoriasis. Desquamation of the skin may also reduce iron stores.

C. Imaging

Radiographic findings are most helpful in distinguishing the disease from other forms of arthritis. There are marginal erosions of bone and irregular destruction of joint and bone, which, in the phalanx, may give the appearance of a sharpened pencil. Fluffy periosteal new bone may be marked, especially at the insertion of muscles and ligaments into bone. Such changes will also be seen along the shafts of metacarpals, metatarsals, and phalanges. Psoriatic spondylitis causes asymmetric sacroiliitis and syndesmophytes, which are coarser than those seen in ankylosing spondylitis.

► Treatment

NSAIDs are usually sufficient for mild cases. Methotrexate (7.5–20 mg orally once a week) is generally considered the drug of choice for patients who have not responded to NSAIDs; methotrexate can improve both the cutaneous and arthritic manifestations. For cases with disease that is refractory to methotrexate, the addition of TNF inhibitors is usually effective for both arthritis and psoriatic skin disease. Alefacept, a biologic agent that is administered by subcutaneous injection, blocks the activation and proliferation of memory effector T cells by binding to CD2; this drug also appears to be effective in the treatment of psoriatic arthritis as well as cutaneous disease. Corticosteroids are less effective in psoriatic arthritis than in other forms of inflammatory arthritis and may precipitate pustular psoriasis during tapers. Antimalarials may also exacerbate psoriasis. Successful treatment directed at the skin lesions alone (eg, by PUVA therapy) occasionally is accompanied by an improvement in peripheral articular symptoms.

Gottlieb A et al. Guidelines of care for the management of psoriasis and psoriatic arthritis: Section 2. Psoriatic arthritis: overview and guidelines of care for treatment with an emphasis on the biologics. J Am Acad Dermatol. 2008 May;58(5):851–64. [PMID: 18423261]
Griffiths CE et al. Pathogenesis and clinical features of psoriasis. Lancet. 2007 Jul 21;370(9583):263–71. [PMID: 17658397]

REACTIVE ARTHRITIS

 ESSENTIALS OF DIAGNOSIS

▶ Fifty to 80 percent of patients are HLA-B27-positive.

▶ Oligoarthritis, conjunctivitis, urethritis, and mouth ulcers most common features.

▶ Usually follows dysentery or a sexually transmitted infection.

General Considerations

Reactive arthritis (formerly called Reiter syndrome) is precipitated by antecedent gastrointestinal and genitourinary infections and manifests as an asymmetric sterile oligoarthritis, typically of the lower extremities. It is frequently associated with enthesitis. Extra-articular manifestations are common and include urethritis, conjunctivitis, uveitis, and mucocutaneous lesions. Reactive arthritis occurs most commonly in young men and is associated with HLA-B27 in 80% of white patients and 50–60% of blacks.

Clinical Findings

A. Symptoms and Signs

Most cases of reactive arthritis develop within 1–4 weeks after either a gastrointestinal infection (with *Shigella*, *Salmonella*, *Yersinia*, *Campylobacter*) or a sexually transmitted infection (with *Chlamydia trachomatis* or perhaps *Ureaplasma urealyticum*). Whether the inciting infection is sexually transmitted or dysenteric does not affect the subsequent manifestations but does influence the gender ratio: The ratio is 1:1 after enteric infections but 9:1 with male predominance after sexually transmitted infections. Synovial fluid from affected joints is culture-negative. A clinically indistinguishable syndrome can occur without an apparent antecedent infection, suggesting that subclinical infection can precipitate reactive arthritis or that there are other, as yet unrecognized, triggers.

The arthritis is most commonly asymmetric and frequently involves the large weight-bearing joints (chiefly the knee and ankle); sacroiliitis or ankylosing spondylitis is observed in at least 20% of patients, especially after frequent recurrences. Systemic symptoms including fever and weight loss are common at the onset of disease. The mucocutaneous lesions may include balanitis, stomatitis, and keratoderma blennorrhagicum, indistinguishable from pustular

psoriasis (Plates 87 and 88). Involvement of the fingernails in reactive arthritis also mimics psoriatic changes. Carditis and aortic regurgitation may occur. While most signs of the disease disappear within days or weeks, the arthritis may persist for several months or become chronic. Recurrences involving any combination of the clinical manifestations are common and are sometimes followed by permanent sequelae, especially in the joints.

B. Imaging

Radiographic signs of permanent or progressive joint disease may be seen in the sacroiliac as well as the peripheral joints.

▶ Differential Diagnosis

Gonococcal arthritis can initially mimic reactive arthritis, but the marked improvement after 24–48 hours of antibiotic administration and the culture results distinguish the two disorders. Rheumatoid arthritis, ankylosing spondylitis, and psoriatic arthritis must also be considered. By causing similar oral, ocular, and joint lesions, Behçet disease may also mimic reactive arthritis. The oral lesions of reactive arthritis, however, are typically painless, in contrast to those of Behçet disease.

The association of reactive arthritis and HIV has been debated, but evidence now indicates that it is equally common in sexually active men regardless of HIV status.

▶ Treatment

NSAIDs have been the mainstay of therapy. Antibiotics given at the time of a nongonococcal sexually transmitted infection reduce the chance that the individual will develop this disorder. Unfortunately, once reactive arthritis has developed, antibiotics do not alleviate symptoms. Patients who do not respond to NSAIDs may respond to sulfasalazine, 1000 mg orally twice daily, or to methotrexate, 7.5–20 mg orally per week. There are very limited data on the efficacy of the anti-TNF agents, which are effective in the other spondyloarthropathies.

Pope JE et al. *Campylobacter* reactive arthritis: a systematic review. Semin Arthritis Rheum. 2007 Aug;37(1):48–55. [PMID: 17360026]
Rihl M et al. Infection and musculoskeletal conditions: reactive arthritis. Best Pract Res Clin Rheumatol. 2006 Dec;20(6):1119–37. [PMID: 17127200]

ARTHRITIS & INFLAMMATORY INTESTINAL DISEASES

One-fifth of patients with inflammatory bowel disease have arthritis, which complicates Crohn disease somewhat more frequently than it does ulcerative colitis. In both diseases, two distinct forms of arthritis occur. The first is peripheral arthritis—usually a nondeforming asymmetric oligoarthritis of large joints—in which the activity of the joint disease parallels that of the bowel disease. The arthritis usually begins months to years after the bowel disease, but occasionally the joint symptoms develop earlier and may be prominent enough to cause the patient to overlook intestinal symptoms. The second form of arthritis is a spondylitis that is indistinguishable by symptoms or radiographs from ankylosing spondylitis and follows a course independent of the bowel disease. About 50% of these patients are HLA-B27-positive.

Controlling the intestinal inflammation usually eliminates the peripheral arthritis. The spondylitis often requires NSAIDs, which need to be used cautiously since these agents may activate the bowel disease in a few patients. Range-of-motion exercises as prescribed for ankylosing spondylitis can be helpful.

About two-thirds of patients with Whipple disease experience arthralgia or arthritis, most often an episodic, large-joint polyarthritis. The arthritis usually precedes the gastrointestinal manifestations by years. In fact, the arthritis resolves as the diarrhea develops. Thus, Whipple disease should be considered in the differential diagnosis of unexplained episodic arthritis.

Juillerat P et al. Extraintestinal manifestations of Crohn's disease. Digestion. 2007;76(2):141–8. [PMID: 18239406]

▼ INFECTIOUS ARTHRITIS*

NONGONOCOCCAL ACUTE BACTERIAL (Septic) ARTHRITIS

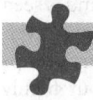 ESSENTIALS OF DIAGNOSIS

- ▶ Acute onset of inflammatory monoarticular arthritis, most often in large weight-bearing joints and wrists.
- ▶ Previous joint damage or injection drug abuse common risk factors.
- ▶ Infection with causative organisms commonly found elsewhere in body.
- ▶ Joint effusions are usually large, with white blood counts commonly > 50,000/mcL.

▶ General Considerations

Nongonococcal acute bacterial arthritis is often a disease that occurs when there is an underlying abnormality. The key risk factors are bacteremia (eg, injection drug use, endocarditis, infection at other sites), damaged or prosthetic joints (eg, rheumatoid arthritis), compromised immunity (eg, diabetes, advanced chronic kidney disease, alcoholism, cirrhosis, and immunosuppressive therapy), and loss of skin integrity (eg, cutaneous ulcer or psoriasis). *Staphylococcus aureus* is the most common cause of nongonococcal septic arthritis, accounting for about 50% of all cases. Methicillin-resistant *S aureus* (MRSA) and group B streptococcus have become increasing frequent and

*Lyme disease is discussed in Chapter 34.

important causes of septic arthritis. Gram-negative septic arthritis causes about 10% of cases and is especially common in injection drug users and in immunocompromised persons. *Escherichia coli* and *Pseudomonas aeruginosa* are the most common gram-negative isolates in adults. Pathologic changes include varying degrees of acute inflammation, with synovitis, effusion, abscess formation in synovial or subchondral tissues, and, if treatment is not adequate, articular destruction.

▶ Clinical Findings

A. Symptoms and Signs

The onset is usually acute, with pain, swelling, and heat of the affected joint worsening over hours. The knee is most frequently involved; other commonly affected sites are the hip, wrist, shoulder, and ankle. Unusual sites, such as the sternoclavicular or sacroiliac joint, can be involved in injection drug users. Chills and fever are common but are absent in up to 20% of patients. Infection of the hip usually does not produce apparent swelling but results in groin pain greatly aggravated by walking. More than one joint is involved in 15% of cases of septic arthritis; risk factors for multiple joint involvement include rheumatoid arthritis, associated endocarditis, and infection with group B streptococci.

B. Laboratory Findings

Synovial fluid analysis is critical for diagnosis. The leukocyte count of the synovial fluid usually exceeds 50,000/mcL and often is greater than 100,000/mcL, with 90% or more polymorphonuclear cells (Table 20–2). Gram stain of the synovial fluid is positive in 75% of staphylococcal infections and in 50% of gram-negative infections. Synovial fluid cultures are positive in 70–90% of cases; administration of antibiotics prior to arthrocentesis reduces the likelihood of a positive culture result. Blood cultures are positive in approximately 50% of patients.

C. Imaging

Imaging tests generally add little to the diagnosis of septic arthritis. Indeed, other than demonstrating joint effusion, radiographs are usually normal early in the disease; evidence of demineralization may develop within days of onset. MRI and CT are more sensitive in detecting fluid in joints that are not accessible to physical examination (eg, the hip). Bony erosions and narrowing of the joint space followed by osteomyelitis and periostitis may be seen within 2 weeks.

▶ Differential Diagnosis

Gout and pseudogout can cause acute, very inflammatory monoarticular arthritis and high-grade fever; the failure to find crystals on synovial fluid analysis excludes these diagnoses. A well-recognized but uncommon initial presentation of rheumatoid arthritis is an acute inflammatory monoarthritis ("pseudoseptic"). Acute rheumatic fever commonly involves many joints; Still disease may mimic septic arthritis, but laboratory evidence of infection is absent. Pyogenic arthritis may be superimposed on other types of joint disease, notably rheumatoid arthritis. Indeed, septic arthritis must be excluded (by joint fluid examination) in any patient with rheumatoid arthritis who has a joint strikingly more inflamed than the other joints.

▶ Treatment

The effective treatment of septic arthritis requires appropriate antibiotic therapy together with drainage of the infected joint. Hospitalization is always necessary. If the likely causative organism cannot be determined clinically or from the synovial fluid Gram stain, treatment should be started with broad-spectrum antibiotic coverage effective against staphylococci, streptococci, and gram-negative organisms. Vancomycin should be used whenever MRSA is reasonably likely. Antibiotic therapy should be adjusted when culture results become available; the duration of antibiotic therapy is usually 6 weeks.

Early orthopedic consultation is essential. Effective drainage is usually achieved through early arthroscopic lavage and debridement together with drain placement. Open surgical drainage should be performed when conservative treatment fails, when there is concomitant osteomyelitis requiring debridement, or when the involved joint (eg, hip, shoulder, sacroiliac joint) cannot be drained by more conservative means. Immobilization with a splint and elevation are used at the onset of treatment. Early active motion exercises within the limits of tolerance will hasten recovery.

▶ Prognosis

The outcome of septic arthritis depends largely on the antecedent health of the patient, the causative organism (eg, *S aureus* bacterial arthritis is associated with a poor functional outcome in about 40% of cases), and the promptness of treatment. Five to 10 percent of patients with an infected joint die of respiratory complications of sepsis. The mortality rate is 30% for patients with polyarticular sepsis. Bony ankylosis and articular destruction commonly also occur if treatment is delayed or inadequate.

Margaretten ME et al. Does this adult patient have septic arthritis? JAMA. 2007 Apr 4;297(13):1478–88. [PMID: 17405973]

Mathews CJ et al. Septic arthritis: current diagnostic and therapeutic algorithm. Curr Opin Rheumatol. 2008 Jul;20(4):457–62. [PMID: 18525361]

GONOCOCCAL ARTHRITIS

ESSENTIALS OF DIAGNOSIS

▶ Prodromal migratory polyarthralgias.

▶ Tenosynovitis most common sign.

▶ Purulent monarthritis in 50%.

▶ Characteristic skin lesions.

▶ Most common in young women during menses or pregnancy.

▶ Symptoms of urethritis frequently absent.

▶ Dramatic response to antibiotics.

▶ General Considerations

In contrast to nongonococcal bacterial arthritis, gonococcal arthritis usually occurs in otherwise healthy individuals. Host factors, however, influence the expression of the disease: Gonococcal arthritis is two to three times more common in women than in men, is especially common during menses and pregnancy, and is rare after age 40. Gonococcal arthritis is also common in male homosexuals, whose high incidence of asymptomatic gonococcal pharyngitis and proctitis predisposes them to disseminated gonococcal infection. Recurrent disseminated gonococcal infection should prompt testing of the patient's CH50 level to evaluate for a congenital deficiency of the terminal complement components C7 and C8.

▶ Clinical Findings

A. Symptoms and Signs

One to 4 days of migratory polyarthralgias involving the wrist, knee, ankle, or elbow are common at the outset. Thereafter, two patterns emerge. The first pattern is characterized by tenosynovitis that most often affects wrists, fingers, ankles, or toes and is seen in 60% of patients. The second pattern is purulent monarthritis that most frequently involves the knee, wrist, ankle, or elbow and is seen in 40% of patients. Less than half of patients have fever, and less than one-fourth have any genitourinary symptoms. Most patients will have asymptomatic but highly characteristic skin lesions that usually consist of two to ten small necrotic pustules distributed over the extremities, especially the palms and soles.

B. Laboratory Findings

The peripheral blood leukocyte count averages about 10,000 cells/mcL and is elevated in less than one-third of patients. The synovial fluid white blood cell count usually ranges from 30,000 to 60,000 cells/mcL. The synovial fluid Gram stain is positive in one-fourth of cases and culture in less than half. Positive blood cultures are seen in 40% of patients with tenosynovitis and virtually never in patients with suppurative arthritis. Urethral, throat, and rectal cultures should be done in all patients, since they are often positive in the absence of local symptoms.

C. Imaging

Radiographs are usually normal or show only soft tissue swelling.

▶ Differential Diagnosis

Reactive arthritis can produce acute monarthritis in a young person but is distinguished by negative cultures, sacroiliitis, and failure to respond to antibiotics. Lyme disease involving the knee is less acute, does not show positive cultures, and may be preceded by known tick exposure and characteristic rash. The synovial fluid analysis will exclude gout, pseudogout, and nongonococcal bacterial arthritis. Rheumatic fever and sarcoidosis can produce migratory tenosynovitis but have other distinguishing features. Infective endocarditis with septic arthritis can mimic disseminated gonococcal infection. Meningococcemia occasionally presents with a clinical picture that resembles disseminated gonococcal infection; blood cultures establish the correct diagnosis.

▶ Treatment

In most cases, patients in whom gonococcal arthritis is suspected should be admitted to the hospital to confirm the diagnosis, to exclude endocarditis, and to start treatment. While outpatient treatment has been recommended in the past, the rapid rise in gonococci resistant to penicillin makes initial inpatient treatment advisable. Approximately 4–5% of all gonococcal isolates produce a β-lactamase that confers penicillin resistance. An additional 15–20% of gonococcal species have chromosomal mutations that result in relative resistance to penicillin. The recommendation for initial treatment is to give a third-generation cephalosporin: ceftriaxone, 1 g intravenously daily (or every 12 hours if concomitant meningitis or endocarditis is suspected); or cefotaxime, 1 g intravenously every 8 hours; or ceftizoxime, 1 g intravenously every 8 hours. Because fluoroquinolone resistance is now found in more than 6% of infected heterosexual men, fluoroquinolone antibiotics are no longer recommended for treatment of gonococcal infections in the United States. Fluoroquinolone antibiotics can be used if antimicrobial sensitivity has been established through culture results. Once improvement from parenteral antibiotics has been achieved for 24–48 hours, patients can be switched to cefixime, 400 mg orally twice daily, or cefpodoxime, 400 mg orally twice daily, to complete a 7- to 10-day course.

▶ Prognosis

Generally, gonococcal arthritis responds dramatically in 24–48 hours after initiation of antibiotics, and drainage of the infected joint(s) is required infrequently. Complete recovery is the rule.

Rice PA. Gonococcal arthritis (disseminated gonococcal infection). Infect Dis Clin North Am. 2005 Dec;19(4):853–61. [PMID: 16297736]

RHEUMATIC MANIFESTATIONS OF HIV INFECTION

Infection with HIV has been associated with various rheumatic disorders, most commonly arthralgias and arthritis. HIV painful articular syndrome causes severe arthralgias in an oligoarticular, asymmetric pattern that resolve within 24 hours; the joint examination is normal. HIV-associated arthritis is an asymmetric oligoarticular process with objective findings of arthritis and a self-limited course that ranges from weeks to months. Psoriatic arthritis and reactive arthritis occur in HIV-infected individuals and can be severe; it remains uncertain whether the incidence of these disorders is increased in HIV-infected populations. These spondyloarthropathies can respond to NSAIDs, though many cases are unresponsive. In the era of highly active antiretroviral therapies, immunosuppressive medications can be used if necessary in HIV patients, though with reluctance and great caution. Muscle weakness associated with an elevated creatine kinase can be due to nucleoside reverse transcriptase inhibitor-associated myopathy or HIV-associated myopathy; the clinical presentations of each resemble idiopathic polymyositis but the muscle biopsies show minimal inflammation. Less commonly, an inflammatory myositis indistinguishable from idiopathic polymyositis occurs.

Louthrenoo W. Rheumatic manifestations of human immunodeficiency virus infection. Curr Opin Rheumatol. 2008 Jan;20(1):92–9. [PMID: 18281864]

VIRAL ARTHRITIS

Arthralgias occur frequently in the course of acute infections with many viruses, but frank arthritis is uncommon. A notable exception is acute parvovirus B19 infection, which leads to acute polyarthritis in 50-60% of adult cases (infected children develop the febrile exanthem known as "slapped cheek fever"). The arthritis can mimic rheumatoid arthritis but is almost always self-limited and resolves within several weeks. The diagnosis is established by the presence of IgM antibodies specific for parvovirus B19. Self-limited polyarthritis is also common in acute hepatitis B infection and typically occurs before the onset of jaundice. Urticaria or other types of skin rash may be present. Indeed, the clinical picture resembles that of serum sickness (see Atopic Disease below). Serum transaminase levels are elevated, and tests for hepatitis B surface antigen are positive. Serum complement levels are often low during active arthritis and become normal after remission of arthritis. The incidence of hepatitis B–associated polyarthritis has fallen substantially with the introduction of hepatitis B vaccination. Effective vaccination programs in the United States have eliminated acute rubella infections, formerly a common cause of virally induced polyarthritis. Changes in the rubella vaccine (an attenuated live vaccine) have greatly reduced the incidence of rubella vaccine–induced polyarthritis as well.

Chronic infection with hepatitis C is associated with chronic polyarthralgia in up to 20% of cases and with chronic polyarthritis in 3-5%. Both can mimic rheumatoid arthritis, and the presence of rheumatoid factor in most hepatitis C–infected individuals leads to further diagnostic confusion. Indeed, hepatitis C–associated arthritis is frequently misdiagnosed as rheumatoid arthritis. Distinguishing viral arthritis/arthralgias from true rheumatoid arthritis can be difficult in hepatitis C–infected individuals. Rheumatoid arthritis always causes objective arthritis (not just arthralgias) and can be erosive (hepatitis C–associated arthritis is nonerosive). The presence of anti-CCP antibodies points to the diagnosis of rheumatoid arthritis.

Franssila R et al. Infection and musculoskeletal conditions: viral causes of arthritis. Best Pract Res Clin Rheumatol. 2006 Dec;20(6):1139–57. [PMID: 17127201]

INFECTIONS OF BONES

ACUTE PYOGENIC OSTEOMYELITIS

 ESSENTIALS OF DIAGNOSIS

► Fever and chills associated with pain and tenderness of involved bone.

► Diagnosis usually requires culture of bone biopsy.

► ESR often extremely high (eg, > 100 mm/h).

► Radiographs early in the course are typically negative.

► General Considerations

Osteomyelitis is a serious infection that is often difficult to diagnose and treat. Infection of bone occurs as a consequence of (1) hematogenous dissemination of bacteria, (2) invasion from a contiguous focus of infection, and (3) skin breakdown in the setting of vascular insufficiency.

► Clinical Findings

A. Symptoms and Signs

1. Hematogenous osteomyelitis—Osteomyelitis resulting from bacteremia is a disease associated with sickle cell disease, injection drug users, or the elderly. Patients with this form of osteomyelitis often present with sudden onset of high fever, chills, and pain and tenderness of the involved bone. The site of osteomyelitis and the causative organism depend on the host. Among patients with hemoglobinopathies such as sickle cell anemia, osteomyelitis is caused by salmonellae ten times as often as by other bacteria. Osteomyelitis in injection drug users develops most commonly in the spine. Although in this setting *S aureus* is most common, gram-negative infections, especially *P aeruginosa* and *Serratia* species, are also frequent pathogens. Rapid progression to epidural abscess causing fever, pain, and sensory and motor loss is not uncommon. In older patients with hematogenous osteomyelitis, the most common sites are the thoracic and lumbar vertebral bodies. Risk factors for these patients include diabetes, intravenous catheters, and indwelling urinary catheters. These patients often have more subtle presentations, with low-grade fever and gradually increasing bone pain.

2. Osteomyelitis from a contiguous focus of infection—Prosthetic joint replacement, decubitus ulcer, neurosurgery, and trauma most frequently cause soft tissue infections that can spread to bone. *S aureus* and *Staphylococcus epidermidis* are the most common organisms. Localized signs of inflammation are usually evident, but high fever and other signs of toxicity are usually absent.

Septic arthritis and cellulitis can also spread to contiguous bone.

3. Osteomyelitis associated with vascular insufficiency—Patients with diabetes and vascular insufficiency are susceptible to developing a very challenging form of osteomyelitis. The foot and ankle are the most commonly affected sites. Infection originates from an ulcer or other break in the skin that is usually still present when the patient presents but may appear disarmingly unimpressive. Bone pain is often absent or muted by the associated neuropathy. Fever is also commonly absent. Two of the best bedside clues that the patient has osteomyelitis are the ability to easily advance a sterile probe through a skin ulcer to bone and an ulcer area greater than 2 cm^2.

B. Imaging and Laboratory Findings

The plain film is the most readily available imaging procedure to establish the diagnosis of osteomyelitis, but it can be falsely negative early. Early radiographic findings may include soft tissue swelling, loss of tissue planes, and periarticular demineralization of bone. About 2 weeks after onset of symptoms, erosion of bone and alteration of cancellous bone appear, followed by periostitis.

MRI, CT, and nuclear medicine bone scanning are more sensitive than conventional radiography. MRI is the most sensitive and is particularly helpful in demonstrating the extent of soft tissue involvement. Radionuclide bone scanning is most valuable when osteomyelitis is suspected but no site is obvious. Nuclear medicine studies may also detect multifocal sites of infection. Ultrasound is useful in diagnosing the presence of effusions within joints and extra-articular soft tissue fluid collections but not in detecting bone infections.

Identifying the offending organism is a crucial step in selection of antibiotic therapy. Bone biopsy for culture is required except in those with hematogenous osteomyelitis, who have positive blood cultures. Cultures from overlying ulcers, wounds, or fistulas are unreliable.

► Differential Diagnosis

Acute hematogenous osteomyelitis should be distinguished from suppurative arthritis, rheumatic fever, and cellulitis. More subacute forms must be differentiated from tuberculosis or mycotic infections of bone and Ewing sarcoma or, in the case of vertebral osteomyelitis, from metastatic tumor. When osteomyelitis involves the vertebrae, it commonly traverses the disk—a finding not observed in tumor.

► Complications

Inadequate treatment of bone infections results in chronicity of infection, and this possibility is increased by delaying diagnosis and treatment. Extension to adjacent bone or joints may complicate acute osteomyelitis. Recurrence of bone infections often results in anemia, a markedly elevated ESR, weight loss, weakness and, rarely, amyloidosis or nephrotic syndrome. Pseudoepitheliomatous hyperplasia, squamous cell carcinoma, or fibrosarcoma may occasionally arise in persistently infected tissues.

Treatment

Most patients require both debridement of necrotic bone and prolonged administration of antibiotics. Patients with vertebral body osteomyelitis and epidural abscess may require urgent neurosurgical decompression. Depending on the site and extent of debridement, surgical procedures to stabilize, fill in, cover, or revascularize may be needed. Traditionally, antibiotics have been administered parenterally for at least 6 weeks. Oral therapy with quinolones (eg, ciprofloxacin, 750 mg twice daily) for 6–8 weeks has been shown to be as effective as standard parenteral antibiotic therapy for chronic osteomyelitis with susceptible organisms. When treating osteomyelitis caused by *S aureus*, quinolones are usually combined with rifampin, 300 mg orally twice daily.

Prognosis

If sterility of the lesion is achieved within 2–4 days, a good result can be expected in most cases if there is no compromise of the patient's immune system. However, progression of the disease to a chronic form may occur. It is especially common in the lower extremities and in patients in whom circulation is impaired (eg, diabetics).

Butalia S et al. Does this patient with diabetes have osteomyelitis of the lower extremity? JAMA. 2008 Feb 20;299(7):806–13. [PMID: 18285592]

Karamanis EM et al. Fluoroquinolones versus beta-lactam based regimens for the treatment of osteomyelitis: a meta-analysis of randomized controlled trials. Spine. 2008 May 1;33(10):E297–304. [PMID: 18449029]

MYCOTIC INFECTIONS OF BONES & JOINTS

Fungal infections of the skeletal system are usually secondary to a primary infection in another organ, frequently the lungs (see Chapter 36). Although skeletal lesions have a predilection for the cancellous portions of long bones and vertebral bodies, the predominant lesion—a granuloma with varying degrees of necrosis and abscess formation—does not produce a characteristic clinical picture.

Differentiation from other chronic focal infections depends on culture studies of synovial fluid or tissue obtained from the local lesion. Serologic tests provide presumptive support of the diagnosis.

1. Candidiasis

Candidal osteomyelitis most commonly develops in debilitated, malnourished patients undergoing prolonged hospitalization for cancer, neutropenia, trauma, complicated abdominal surgical procedures, or injection drug use. Infected intravenous catheters frequently serve as a hematogenous source. Prosthetic joints can also be infected by *Candida*.

For susceptible *Candida* species, fluconazole, 200 mg orally twice daily, is probably as effective as amphotericin B (see Chapter 36).

Richardson M et al. Changing epidemiology of systemic fungal infections. Clin Microbiol Infect. 2008 May;14(Suppl 4):5–24. [PMID: 18430126]

2. Coccidioidomycosis

Coccidioidomycosis of bones and joints is usually secondary to primary pulmonary infection. Arthralgia with periarticular swelling, especially in the knees and ankles, occurring as a nonspecific manifestation of systemic coccidioidomycosis, should be distinguished from actual bone or joint infection. Osseous lesions commonly occur in cancellous bone of the vertebrae or near the ends of long bones at tendinous insertions. These lesions are initially osteolytic and thus may mimic metastatic tumor or myeloma.

The precise diagnosis depends on recovery of *Coccidioides immitis* from the lesion or histologic examination of tissue obtained by open biopsy. Rising titers of complement-fixing antibodies also provide evidence of the disseminated nature of the disease.

Oral azole antifungal agents (fluconazole 200–400 mg daily, or itraconazole 200 mg twice daily) have become the treatment of choice for bone and joint coccidioidomycosis. Chronic infection is rarely cured with antifungal agents and may require operative excision of infected bone and soft tissue; amputation may be the only solution for stubbornly progressive infections. Immobilization of joints by plaster casts and avoidance of weight bearing provide benefit. Synovectomy, joint debridement, and arthrodesis are reserved for more advanced joint infections.

Blair JE. State-of-the-art treatment of coccidioidomycosis skeletal infections. Ann N Y Acad Sci. 2007 Sep;1111:422–33. [PMID: 17395727]

3. Histoplasmosis

Focal skeletal or joint involvement in histoplasmosis is rare and generally represents dissemination from a primary focus in the lungs. Skeletal lesions may be single or multiple and are not characteristic.

Sen D et al. Articular presentation of disseminated histoplasmosis. Clin Rheumatol. 2007 May;26(5):823–4. [PMID: 16724167]

TUBERCULOSIS OF BONES & JOINTS

SPINAL TUBERCULOSIS (Pott Disease)

ESSENTIALS OF DIAGNOSIS

▶ Seen primarily in immigrants from developing countries or immunocompromised patients.

▶ Back pain and gibbus deformity.

▶ Radiographic evidence of vertebral involvement.

▶ Evidence of *Mycobacterium tuberculosis* in aspirates or biopsies of spinal lesions.

General Considerations

In the developing world, children primarily bear the burden of musculoskeletal tuberculosis. In the United States, however, musculoskeletal infection is more often seen in adult immigrants from countries where tuberculosis is prevalent, or it develops in the setting of immunosuppression (eg, HIV infection, therapy with TNF inhibitors). Spinal tuberculosis (Pott disease) accounts for about 50% of musculoskeletal infection due to *M tuberculosis* (see Chapter 9). Seeding of the vertebrae may occur through hematogenous spread from the respiratory tract at the time of primary infection, with clinical disease developing years later as a consequence of reactivation. The thoracic and lumbar vertebrae are the most common sites of spinal involvement; vertebral infection is associated with paravertebral cold abscesses in 75% of cases.

► Clinical Findings

A. Symptoms and Signs

Patients complain of back pain, often present for months and sometimes associated with radicular pain and lower extremity weakness. Constitutional symptoms are usually absent, and less than 20% have active pulmonary disease. Destruction of the anterior aspect of the vertebral body can produce the characteristic gibbus deformity.

B. Laboratory Findings

Most patients have a positive reaction to purified protein derivative (PPD). Cultures of paravertebral abscesses and biopsies of vertebral lesions are positive in up to 70–90%. Biopsies reveal characteristic caseating granulomas in most cases. Isolation of *M tuberculosis* from an extraspinal site is sufficient to establish the diagnosis in the proper clinical setting.

C. Imaging

Radiographs can reveal lytic and sclerotic lesions and bony destruction of vertebrae but are normal early in the disease course. CT scanning can demonstrate paraspinal soft tissue extensions of the infection; MRI is the imaging technique of choice to detect compression of the spinal cord or cauda equina.

► Differential Diagnosis

Spinal tuberculosis must be differentiated from subacute and chronic spinal infections due to pyogenic organisms, *Brucella*, and fungi as well as from malignancy.

► Complications

Paraplegia due to compression of the spinal cord or cauda equina is the most serious complication of spinal tuberculosis.

► Treatment

Antimicrobial therapy should be administered for 6–9 months, usually in the form of isoniazid, rifampin, pyrazinamide, and ethambutol for 2 months followed by isoniazid and rifampin for an additional 4–7 months (see also Chapter 9). Medical management alone is often sufficient. Surgical intervention, however, may be indi-

cated when there is neurologic compromise or severe spinal instability.

Kourbeti IS et al. Spinal infections: evolving concepts. Curr Opin Rheumatol. 2008 Jul;20(4):471–9. [PMID: 18525363]

TUBERCULOUS ARTHRITIS

Infection of peripheral joints by *M tuberculosis* usually presents as a monoarticular arthritis lasting for weeks to months (or longer), but less often, it can have an acute presentation that mimics septic arthritis. Any joint can be involved; the hip and knee are most commonly affected. Constitutional symptoms and fever are present in only a small number of cases. Tuberculosis also can cause a chronic tenosynovitis of the hand and wrist. Joint destruction occurs far more slowly than in septic arthritis due to pyogenic organisms. Synovial fluid is inflammatory but not to the degree seen in pyogenic infections, with synovial white cell counts in the range of 10,000–20,000 cells/mcL. Smears of synovial fluid are positive for acid-fast bacilli in a minority of cases; synovial fluid cultures, however, are positive in 80% of cases. Because culture results may take weeks, the diagnostic procedure of choice usually is synovial biopsy, which yields characteristic pathologic findings and positive cultures in greater than 90%. Antimicrobial therapy is the mainstay of treatment. Rarely, a reactive, sterile polyarthritis associated with erythema nodosum (Poncet disease) develops in patients with active pulmonary tuberculosis.

Gardam M et al. Mycobacterial osteomyelitis and arthritis. Infect Dis Clin North Am. 2005 Dec;19(4):819–30. [PMID: 16297734]

Kroot EJ et al. Poncet's disease: reactive arthritis accompanying tuberculosis. Two case reports and a review of the literature. Rheumatology (Oxford). 2007 Mar;46(3):484–9. [PMID: 16935915]

ARTHRITIS IN SARCOIDOSIS

The frequency of arthritis among patients with sarcoidosis is variously reported between 10% and 35%. It is usually acute in onset, but articular symptoms may appear insidiously and often antedate other manifestations of the disease. Knees and ankles are most commonly involved, but any joint may be affected. Distribution of joint involvement is usually polyarticular and symmetric. The arthritis is commonly self-limited, resolving after several weeks or months and rarely resulting in chronic arthritis, joint destruction, or significant deformity. Sarcoid arthropathy is often associated with erythema nodosum, but the diagnosis is contingent on the demonstration of other extra-articular manifestations of sarcoidosis and, notably, biopsy evidence of noncaseating granulomas. In chronic arthritis, radiographs show typical changes in the bones of the extremities with intact cortex and cystic changes.

Treatment of arthritis in sarcoidosis is usually symptomatic and supportive. Colchicine may be of value. A short course of corticosteroids may be effective in patients with severe and progressive joint disease.

OTHER RHEUMATIC DISORDERS

RHEUMATIC MANIFESTATIONS OF CANCER

Rheumatologic syndromes may be the presenting manifestations for a variety of cancers (see Table 39–13). Dermatomyositis in adults, for example, is often associated with cancer. Hypertrophic pulmonary osteoarthropathy is characterized by the triad of polyarthritis, new onset of clubbing, and periosteal new bone formation. It is associated with both malignant diseases (eg, lung and intrathoracic cancers) and nonmalignant ones (eg, cyanotic heart disease, cirrhosis, and lung abscess). Cancer-associated polyarthritis is rare, has both oligoarticular and polyarticular forms, and should be considered when "seronegative rheumatoid arthritis" develops abruptly in an elderly patient. Palmar fasciitis manifests as bilateral palmar swelling with finger contractures and may be the first indication of cancer, particularly ovarian carcinoma. Remitting seronegative synovitis with non-pitting edema ("RS3PE") presents with a symmetric small joint polyarthritis associated with non-pitting edema of the hands; it can be idiopathic or associated with malignancy. Palpable purpura due to leukocytoclastic vasculitis may be the presenting complaint in myeloproliferative disorders. Hairy cell leukemia can be associated with medium-sized vessel vasculitis such as polyarteritis nodosa. Acute leukemia can produce joint pains that are disproportionately severe in comparison to the minimal swelling and heat that are present. Leukemic arthritis complicates approximately 5% of cases. Rheumatic manifestations of myelodysplastic syndromes include cutaneous vasculitis, lupus-like syndromes, neuropathy, and episodic intense arthritis. Erythromelalgia, a painful warmth and redness of the extremities that (unlike Raynaud) improves with cold exposure or with elevation of the extremity, is often associated with myeloproliferative diseases, particularly essential thrombocythemia.

Naschitz JE et al. Musculoskeletal syndromes associated with malignancy (excluding hypertrophic osteoarthropathy). Curr Opin Rheumatol. 2008 Jan;20(1):100–5. [PMID: 18281865]

Racanelli V et al. Rheumatic disorders as paraneoplastic syndromes. Autoimmun Rev. 2008 May;7(5):352–8. [PMID: 18486921]

NEUROGENIC ARTHROPATHY (Charcot Joint)

Neurogenic arthropathy is joint destruction resulting from loss or diminution of proprioception, pain, and temperature perception. Although traditionally associated with tabes dorsalis, it is more frequently seen in diabetic neuropathy, syringomyelia, spinal cord injury, pernicious anemia, leprosy, and peripheral nerve injury. As normal muscle tone and protective reflexes are lost, secondary degenerative joint disease ensues, resulting in an enlarged, boggy, relatively painless joint with extensive cartilage erosion, osteophyte formation, and multiple loose joint bodies. Radiographic changes may be degenerative or hypertrophic in the same patient.

Treatment is directed toward the primary disease; mechanical devices are used to assist in weight bearing and prevention of further trauma. In some instances, amputation becomes unavoidable.

Wrobel M et al. Charcot's joint of the wrist in type 2 diabetes mellitus. Exp Clin Endocrinol Diabetes. 2007 Jan;115(1):55–7. [PMID: 17286237]

PALINDROMIC RHEUMATISM

Palindromic rheumatism is a disease of unknown cause characterized by frequent recurring attacks (at irregular intervals) of acutely inflamed joints. Periarticular pain with swelling and transient subcutaneous nodules may also occur. The attacks cease within several hours to several days. The knee and finger joints are most commonly affected, but any peripheral joint may be involved. Systemic manifestations other than fever do not occur. Although hundreds of attacks may take place over a period of years, there is no permanent articular damage. Laboratory findings are usually normal. Palindromic rheumatism must be distinguished from acute gouty arthritis and an atypical acute onset of rheumatoid arthritis. In some patients, palindromic rheumatism is a prodrome of rheumatoid arthritis.

Symptomatic treatment with NSAIDs is usually all that is required during the attacks. Hydroxychloroquine may be of value in preventing recurrences.

OSTEONECROSIS (Avascular Necrosis of Bone)

Osteonecrosis is a complication of corticosteroid use, alcoholism, trauma, SLE, pancreatitis, gout, sickle cell disease, dysbaric syndromes (eg, "the bends"), and infiltrative diseases (eg, Gaucher disease). The most commonly affected sites are the proximal and distal femoral heads, leading to hip or knee pain. Other commonly affected sites include the ankle, shoulder, and elbow. Osteonecrosis of the jaw has been rarely associated with use of bisphosphonate therapy, almost always when the bisphosphonate is used for treating metastatic cancer or multiple myeloma rather than osteoporosis. Initially, radiographs are often normal; MRI, CT scan, and bone scan are all more sensitive techniques. Treatment involves avoidance of weight bearing on the affected joint for at least several weeks. The value of surgical core decompression is controversial. For osteonecrosis of the hip, a variety of procedures designed to preserve the femoral head have been developed for early disease, including vascularized and nonvascularized bone grafting procedures. These procedures are most effective in avoiding or forestalling the need for total hip arthroplasty in young patients who do not have advanced disease. Without a successful intervention of this nature, the natural history of avascular necrosis is usually progression of the bony infarction to cortical collapse, resulting in significant joint dysfunction. Total hip replacement is the usual outcome for all patients who are candidates for that procedure.

Petrigliano FA et al. Osteonecrosis of the hip: novel approaches to evaluation and treatment. Clin Ortho Relat Res. 2007 Dec;465:53–62. [PMID: 17906590]

Rizzoli R et al. Osteonecrosis of the jaw and bisphosphonate treatment of osteoporosis. Bone. 2008 May;42(5):841–7. [PMID: 18314405]

ALLERGIC DISEASES

Allergy is an immunologically mediated hypersensitivity reaction to a foreign antigen manifested by tissue inflammation and organ dysfunction. These responses have a genetic basis, but the clinical expression of disease depends on both immunologic responsiveness and antigen exposure. Allergic disorders may be local or systemic. Because the allergen is foreign (ie, environmental), the skin and respiratory tract are the organs most frequently involved in allergic disease. Allergic reactions may also localize to the vasculature, gastrointestinal tract, or other visceral organs. Anaphylaxis is the most extreme form of systemic allergy.

► Immunologic Classification

An immunologic classification for hypersensitivity reactions serves as a rational basis for diagnosis and treatment. The classification follows.

A. Type I—IgE-Mediated (Immediate) Hypersensitivity

IgE antibodies occupy receptor sites on mast cells. Within minutes after exposure to the allergen, a multivalent antigen links adjacent IgE molecules, activating and degranulating mast cells. Clinical manifestations depend on the effects of released mediators on target end organs. Both preformed and newly generated mediators cause vasodilation, visceral smooth muscle contraction, mucus secretory gland stimulation, vascular permeability, and tissue inflammation. Arachidonic acid metabolites, cytokines, and other mediators induce a late-phase inflammatory response that appears several hours later. There are two clinical subgroups of IgE-mediated allergy: atopy and anaphylaxis.

1. Atopy—The term "atopy" is applied to a group of diseases (allergic rhinitis, allergic asthma, atopic dermatitis, and allergic gastroenteropathy) occurring in persons with an inherited tendency to develop antigen-specific IgE reaction to environmental allergens or food antigens. Aeroallergens such as pollens, mold spores, animal danders, and house dust mite antigen are common triggers for allergic conjunctivitis, allergic rhinitis, and allergic asthma. The allergic origin of atopic dermatitis is less well understood, but some patients' symptoms can be triggered by exposure to dust mite antigen and ingestion of certain foods. There is a strong familial tendency toward the development of atopy.

2. Anaphylaxis—Certain allergens—especially drugs, insect venoms, latex, and foods—may induce an IgE antibody response, causing a generalized release of mediators from mast cells and resulting in systemic anaphylaxis. This is characterized by (1) hypotension or shock from widespread vasodilation, (2) bronchospasm, (3) gastrointestinal and uterine muscle contraction, and (4) urticaria or angioedema. The condition is potentially fatal and can affect both nonatopic and atopic persons. Isolated urticaria and angioedema are cutaneous forms of anaphylaxis, are much more common, and have a better prognosis.

B. Type II—Antibody-Mediated (Cytotoxic) Hypersensitivity

Cytotoxic reactions involve the specific reaction of either IgG or IgM antibody to cell-bound antigens. This results in activation of the complement cascade and the destruction of the cell to which the antigen is bound. Examples include immune hemolytic anemia and Rh hemolytic disease in the newborn.

C. Type III—Immune Complex-Mediated Hypersensitivity

Immune complex-mediated reactions occur when antigen and IgG or IgM antibodies form circulating immune complexes. Deposition of these complexes in tissues or in vascular endothelium can produce immune complex-mediated tissue injury through activation of the complement cascade, anaphylatoxin generation, and chemotaxis of polymorphonuclear leukocytes. Serum sickness is the classic example of type III hypersensitivity. Immune complex disease also can develop in the setting of chronic infections such as subacute bacterial endocarditis and hepatitis B.

D. Type IV—T Cell–Mediated Hypersensitivity (Delayed Hypersensitivity, Cell-Mediated Hypersensitivity)

Type IV delayed hypersensitivity is mediated by activated T cells, which accumulate in areas of antigen deposition. The most common expression of delayed hypersensitivity is allergic contact dermatitis, which develops when a low-molecular-weight sensitizing substance haptenates with dermal proteins, becoming a complete antigen. Sensitized T cells release cytokines, activating macrophages and promoting the subsequent dermal inflammation; this occurs 1–2 days after the time of contact. Common topical agents associated with allergic contact dermatitis include nickel, formaldehyde, potassium dichromate, thiurams, mercaptos, parabens, quaternium-15, and ethylenediamine. Rhus (poison oak and ivy) contact dermatitis is caused by cutaneous exposure to oils from the toxicodendron plants. Acute contact dermatitis is characterized by erythema and induration with vesicle formation, often with pruritus, with exudation and crusting in more severe cases. Chronic allergic contact dermatitis may be associated with fissuring, lichenification, or dyspigmentation and may be mistaken for other forms of dermatitis. To diagnose allergic contact dermatitis, patch testing can be performed.

ATOPIC DISEASE

Clinical manifestations resembling allergic hypersensitivity can also occur in the absence of an immunologic mechanism. Therefore, the diagnosis of allergy requires answers to the following questions: (1) What is the nature of the disease? (2) Is the disease caused by an IgE-mediated mechanism? (3) What specific allergens are responsible?

The relevant history includes a survey of allergen exposure associated with home, work, hobbies, and habits as well as medications. Physical examination is most useful if performed during exposure. Demonstration of allergic hypersensitivity by in vivo or in vitro testing confirms clinical suspicions of allergic disease.

▶ Specific IgE Antibody Tests

To maximize the positive predictive value of allergy testing, a positive test result must be correlated with the history. Patients selected for testing include those with moderate to severe disease, those who are potential candidates for allergen immunotherapy, and those with strong predisposing factors for atopic diatheses, eg, a strong family history of atopy or ongoing exposure to potential sources of allergen. Since the development of rhinitis precedes the presentation of asthma in over half of cases, early intervention may decrease the risk of more severe clinical allergic disease. The type of immune response must be consistent with the nature of the disease. IgE antibody causes allergic rhinitis but not allergic contact dermatitis. IgE antibodies are detected by in vivo (skin tests) or in vitro methods.

Akdis CA et al. Diagnosis and treatment of atopic dermatitis in children and adults: European Academy of Allergology and Clinical Immunology/American Academy of Allergy, Asthma and Immunology/PRACTALL Consensus Report. J Allergy Clin Immunol. 2006 Jul;118(1):152–69. [PMID: 16815151]

Antunez C et al. Immediate allergic reactions to cephalosporins: evaluation of cross-reactivity with a panel of penicillins and cephalosporins. J Allergy Clin Immunol. 2006 Feb;117(2):404–10. [PMID: 16461141]

Apter AJ et al. Is there cross-reactivity between penicillins and cephalosporins? Am J Med. 2006 Apr;119(4):354.e11–9. [PMID: 16564780]

Chan LS. Atopic dermatitis in 2008. Curr Dir Autoimmun. 2008;10:76–118. [PMID: 18460882]

Lack G. Clinical practice. Food allergy. N Engl J Med. 2008 Sep 18;359(12):1252–60. [PMID: 18799559]

SERUM SICKNESS

ESSENTIALS OF DIAGNOSIS

▶ Fever, pruritic rash, arthralgias, and arthritis; nephritis in severe cases.

▶ Occurs 7–10 days following administration of an exogenous antigen (eg, heterologous gamma globulin) when specific IgG antibodies develop against the antigen.

▶ Immune-complex mediated small vessel vasculitis and tissue injury.

▶ General Considerations

Serum sickness occurs when an antibody response to exogenously administered antigens results in the formation of immune complexes. Deposition of these complexes in vascular endothelium and tissues produces immune complex–mediated small vessel vasculitis and tissue injury through activation of complement, generation of anaphylatoxins, and chemoattraction of polymorphonuclear leukocytes. The skin, joints, and kidneys are commonly affected. It is self-limited and resolves after the antigen is cleared. First observed in the preantibiotic era when heterologous serum preparations were used for passive immunization, serum sickness is now less common but still occurs with the use of heterologous anti-thymocyte globulin for transplant rejection and, infrequently, after the administration of murine monoclonal antibodies or even non-protein drugs.

▶ Clinical Findings

A. Symptoms and Signs

Sustained high fever (> 101 °F) is typical. The earliest manifestation is often a maculopapular or urticarial pruritic rash. Angioedema can occur. Polyarthralgias, frank polyarthritis, and lymphadenopathy are common. Nephritis is usually mild but can progress to acute renal failure.

B. Laboratory Findings

The ESR is increased, and leukocytosis is common. Other nonspecific laboratory findings include elevated hepatic aminotransferases. When nephritis is present, the urinalysis reveals proteinuria, hematuria, and red cell casts. Hypocomplementemia is usually present in cases due to administration of heterologous gamma globulin but not in milder cases precipitated by non-protein drugs. Circulating immune complexes may be found, but current assays are limited in sensitivity.

▶ Treatment

This disease is self-limited, and treatment is usually conservative for mild cases. NSAIDs help relieve the arthralgias, and antihistamines and topical corticosteroids can be of benefit for the skin manifestation. A high-dose course of corticosteroids is administered for serious reactions, especially those complicated by glomerulonephritis and other manifestations of vasculitis. Plasma exchange may be of benefit for cases refractory to corticosteroids.

Lundquist AL et al. Serum sickness following rabbit antithymocyte globulin induction in a liver transplant recipient: case report and literature review. Liver Transpl. 2007 May;13(5):647–650. [PMID: 17377915]

PSEUDOALLERGIC REACTIONS*

These reactions resemble immediate hypersensitivity reactions but are not mediated by allergen-IgE interaction. Instead, direct mast cell activation occurs. Examples of pseudoallergic or "anaphylactoid" reactions include the now rare "red man syndrome" from rapid infusion of

---

*The contribution of Jeffrey L. Kishiyama, MD and Daniel C. Adelman, MD, is gratefully acknowledged.

vancomycin, direct mast cell activation by opioids, and radiocontrast reactions. In contrast to IgE-mediated reactions, these can often be prevented by prophylactic medical regimens.

Radiocontrast Media Reactions

Reactions to radiocontrast media do not appear to be mediated by IgE antibodies, yet clinically they are similar to anaphylaxis. If a patient has had an anaphylactoid reaction to conventional radiocontrast media, the risk for a second reaction upon reexposure may be as high as 30%. Patients with asthma or those being treated with β-adrenergic blocking medications may be at increased risk. The management of patients at risk for radiocontrast medium reactions includes use of the low-osmolality contrast preparations and prophylactic administration of prednisone (50 mg orally every 6 hours beginning 18 hours before the procedure) and diphenhydramine (25–50 mg intramuscularly 60 minutes before the procedure). The use of the lower-osmolality radiocontrast media in combination with the pretreatment regimen decreases the incidence of reactions to less than 1%.

Liccardi G et al; Cardarelli Hospital Radiocontrast Media and Anesthetic-Induced Anaphylaxis Prevention Working Group. Strategies for the prevention of asthmatic, anaphylactic and anaphylactoid reactions during the administration of anesthetics and/or contrast media. J Investig Allergol Clin Immunol. 2008;18(1):1–11. [PMID: 18361095]

Tramer MR et al. Pharmacological prevention of serious anaphylactic reactions due to iodinated contrast media: systemic review. BMJ. 2006 Sep 30;333(7570):675. [PMID: 16880193]

PRIMARY IMMUNODEFICIENCY DISORDERS

The primary immunologic deficiency diseases include congenital and acquired disorders of humoral immunity (B cell function) or cell-mediated immunity (T cell function). Most of these diseases are rare and, because they are genetically determined, usually present in childhood. Nonetheless, several immunodeficiency disorders can present in adulthood, most notably selective IgA deficiency and common variable immunodeficiency.

Bonilla FA et al. Update on primary immunodeficiency diseases. J Allergy Clin Immunol. 2006 Feb;117(2 Suppl Mini-Primer):S435–41. [PMID: 16455342]

Buckley RH. Primary immunodeficiency or not? Making the correct diagnosis. J Allergy Clin Immunol. 2006 Apr;117(4):756–8. [PMID: 16630930]

Rudd CE. Disabled receptor signaling and new primary immunodeficiency disorders. N Engl J Med. 2006 May 4;354(18):1874–7. [PMID: 16672698]

SELECTIVE IMMUNOGLOBULIN A DEFICIENCY

Selective IgA deficiency is the most common primary immunodeficiency disorder and is characterized by serum IgA levels less than 15 mg/dL with normal levels of IgG and IgM; its prevalence is about 1:500 individuals. Most persons

are asymptomatic because of compensatory increases in secreted IgG and IgM. Some affected patients have frequent and recurrent infections, such as sinusitis, otitis, and bronchitis. Some cases of IgA deficiency may spontaneously remit. When IgG_2 subclass deficiency occurs in combination with IgA deficiency, affected patients are more susceptible to encapsulated bacteria and the degree of immune impairment can be more severe. Patients with a combined IgA and IgG subclass deficiency should be assessed for functional antibody responses to glycoprotein antigen immunization.

Atopic disease and autoimmune disorders can be associated with IgA deficiency. Occasionally, a sprue-like syndrome with steatorrhea has been associated with an isolated IgA deficit. Treatment with commercial immune globulin is ineffective, since IgA and IgM are present only in trace quantities in these preparations.

Individuals with selective IgA deficiency may have high titers of anti-IgA antibodies and are at risk for anaphylactic reactions following exposure to IgA through infusions of plasma (or blood transfusions). These anti-IgA antibodies develop in the absence of prior exposure to human plasma or blood, possibly due to crossreactivity to bovine IgA in cow's milk or prior sensitization to maternal IgA in breast milk.

Woof JM et al. The function of immunoglobulin A in immunity. J Pathol. 2006 Jan;208(2):270–82. [PMID: 16362985]

COMMON VARIABLE IMMUNODEFICIENCY

 ESSENTIALS OF DIAGNOSIS

▸ Defect in terminal differentiation of B cells, with absent plasma cells and deficient synthesis of secreted antibody.

▸ Frequent sinopulmonary infections secondary to humoral immune deficiency.

▸ Confirmation by evaluation of serum immunoglobulin levels and deficient functional antibody responses.

General Considerations

The most common cause of panhypogammaglobulinemia in adults is common variable immunodeficiency, a heterogeneous immunodeficiency disorder clinically characterized by an increased incidence of recurrent infections, autoimmune phenomena, and neoplastic diseases. The onset generally is during adolescence or early adulthood but can occur at any age. The prevalence of common variable immunodeficiency is about 1:80,000 in the United States. Most cases are sporadic; 10–20% are familial.

Clinical Findings

A. Symptoms and Signs

The pattern of immunoglobulin isotype deficiency is variable. Most patients present with significantly depressed IgG levels, but over time all antibody classes (IgG, IgA, and

IgM) may be affected. Increased susceptibility to pyogenic infections is the hallmark of the disease. Virtually all patients suffer from recurrent sinusitis, with bronchitis, otitis, pharyngitis, and pneumonia also being common infections. Infections may be prolonged or associated with unusual complications such as meningitis or sepsis.

Gastrointestinal disorders are commonly associated with common variable immunodeficiency, and a sprue-like syndrome, with diarrhea, steatorrhea, malabsorption, protein-losing enteropathy, and hepatosplenomegaly, may develop in patients. Paradoxically, there is an increased incidence of autoimmune disease (20%), although patients may not display the usual serologic markers. Autoimmune cytopenias are most common, but autoimmune endocrinopathies, seronegative rheumatic disease, and gastrointestinal disorders are also commonly seen. Lymph nodes may be enlarged in these patients, yet biopsies show marked reduction in plasma cells. Noncaseating granulomas are frequently found in the spleen, liver, lungs, or skin. There is an increased propensity for the development of B cell neoplasms (50- to 400-fold increase risk of lymphoma), gastric carcinomas, and skin cancers.

B. Laboratory Findings

Diagnosis is confirmed in patients with recurrent infections by demonstration of functional or quantitative defects in antibody production. Serum IgG levels are usually less than 250 mg/dL; serum IgA and IgM levels are also subnormal. Decreased to absent functional antibody responses to protein antigen immunizations establish the diagnosis.

The causes of the panhypogammaglobulinemia in common variable immunodeficiency patients include intrinsic B cell defects that prevent terminal maturation into antibody-secreting plasma cells. The absolute B cell count in the peripheral blood in most patients, despite the underlying cellular defect, is normal. A subset of these patients have concomitant T cell immunodeficiency with increased numbers of activated CD8 cells, splenomegaly, and decreased delayed-type hypersensitivity.

▶ Treatment

Patients may be treated aggressively with antibiotics at the first sign of infection. Since antibody deficiency predisposes patients to high-risk pyogenic infections, antibiotic coverage should be sure to cover encapsulated bacteria. Only after the development of bronchiectasis or after sinus surgery do patients become significantly affected by more virulent organisms such as S aureus or P aeruginosa. Maintenance intravenous immune globulin therapy is indicated, with infusions of 300–500 mg/kg of intravenous immune globulin given at about monthly intervals. Adjustment of dosage or of the infusion interval is made on the basis of clinical responses and steady-state trough serum IgG levels. Such therapy is effective in decreasing the incidence of potentially life-threatening infections and increasing quality of life. The yearly cost of monthly infusions can be in excess of $20,000–$30,000.

Bacchelli C et al. Translational mini-review series on immunodeficiency: molecular defects in common variable immunodeficiency. Clin Exp Immunol. 2007 Sep;149(3):401–409. [PMID: 17697196]

Park MA et al. Common variable immunodeficiency: a new look at an old disease. Lancet. 2008 Aug 9;372(9637):489–502. [PMID: 18692715]

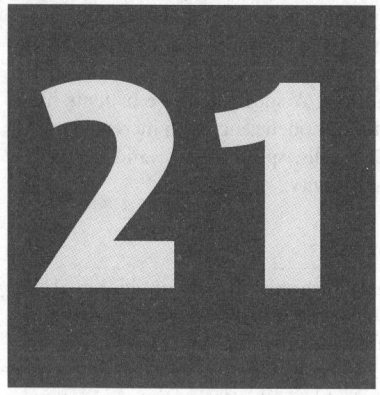

Fluid & Electrolyte Disorders

Kerry C. Cho, MD

ASSESSMENT OF THE PATIENT

The diagnosis and treatment of fluid and electrolyte disorders are based on (1) careful history, (2) physical examination and assessment of total body water and its distribution, (3) serum electrolyte concentrations, (4) urine electrolyte concentrations, and (5) serum osmolality. The pathophysiology of electrolyte disorders is rooted in basic principles of total body water and its distribution across fluid compartments.

A. Body Water and Fluid Distribution

Total body water is different in men than in women, and it decreases with aging (Table 21–1). Approximately 50-60% of total body weight is water; two-thirds (40% of body weight) is intracellular, while one-third (20% of body weight) is extracellular. One-fourth of extracellular fluid (5% of body weight) is intravascular. Water may be lost from either or both compartments (intracellular and extracellular). Changes in total body water content are best evaluated by documenting changes in body weight. Effective circulating volume may be assessed by physical examination (eg, blood pressure, pulse, jugular venous distention). Quantitative measurements of effective circulating volume and intravascular volume may be invasive (ie, central venous pressure or pulmonary wedge pressure) or noninvasive (ie, inferior vena cava diameter and right atrial pressure by echocardiography) but still require careful interpretation.

B. Serum Electrolytes

The cause of electrolyte disorders may be determined by reviewing the history, underlying diseases, and medications.

C. Evaluation of Urine

The urine concentration of an electrolyte indicates renal handling of the electrolyte and whether the kidney is appropriately excreting or retaining the electrolyte. A 24-hour urine collection for daily electrolyte excretion is the gold standard for renal electrolyte handling, but it is slow and onerous. A more convenient method is the fractional

excretion (FE) of an electrolyte X (FE$_X$) calculated from a spot urine sample:

$$F_{E_X}(\%) = \frac{\text{Urine X/Serum X}}{\text{Urine Cr/Serum Cr}} \times 100$$

A low fractional excretion indicates renal reabsorption (high avidity or electrolyte retention), while a high fractional excretion indicates renal wasting (low avidity or electrolyte excretion). Thus, the fractional excretion helps the clinician determine whether the kidney's response is appropriate for a specific electrolyte disorder.

D. Serum Osmolality

Solute concentration is measured by osmolality. Osmoles per kilogram of water is *osmolality*; osmoles per liter of solution is *osmolarity*. At physiological solute concentrations (normally 285–295 mosm/kg), the two measurements are clinically interchangeable. Tonicity refers to osmolytes that are impermeable to cell membranes. Differences in osmolyte concentration across cell membranes lead to osmosis and fluid shifts, stimulation of thirst, and secretion of antidiuretic hormone (ADH). Substances that easily permeate cell membranes (eg, urea, ethanol) are ineffective osmolytes that do not cause fluid shifts across fluid compartments.

Serum osmolality can be estimated from the following formula:

Osmolality =

$$2(\text{Na}^+ \text{mEq/L}) + \frac{\text{Glucose mg/dL}}{18} + \frac{\text{BUN mg/dL}}{2.8}$$

(1 mosm/L of glucose equals 180 mg/L and 1 mosm/L of urea nitrogen equals 28 mg/L). Sodium is the major extracellular cation; doubling the serum sodium in the formula for estimated osmolality accounts for the counterbalancing anions. A discrepancy between measured and estimated osmolality of more than 10 mosm/kg suggests an osmolal gap, which is the presence of other unmeasured osmoles such as ethanol, methanol, isopropanol, and ethylene glycol.

Table 21-1. Total body water (as percentage of body weight) in relation to age and sex.

Age	Male	Female
18-40	60%	50%
41-60	60-50%	50-40%
Over 60	50%	40%

DISORDERS OF SODIUM CONCENTRATION

HYPONATREMIA

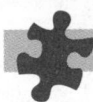

ESSENTIALS OF DIAGNOSIS

► The patient's volume status and serum osmolality are essential to determine etiology.

► Hyponatremia usually reflects excess water retention relative to sodium rather than sodium deficiency.

► Hypotonic fluids commonly cause hyponatremia in hospitalized patients.

► General Considerations

Defined as a serum sodium concentration less than 135 mEq/L, hyponatremia is the most common electrolyte abnormality in hospitalized patients. The clinician should be wary about hyponatremia since mismanagement can result in catastrophic neurologic consequences due to cerebral osmotic demyelination. Indeed, iatrogenic complications from aggressive or inappropriate therapy can be more harmful than hyponatremia itself.

A common misperception is that the sodium concentration is a reflection of total body sodium or total body water. In fact, total body water and total body sodium can be low, normal, or high in hyponatremia since the kidney can regulate sodium and water homeostasis independently. Most cases of hyponatremia reflect water imbalance and abnormal water handling, not sodium imbalance, indicating the primary role of ADH in the pathophysiology of many cases of hyponatremia. A diagnostic algorithm using serum osmolality and volume status separates the causes of hyponatremia into therapeutically useful categories (Figure 21–1).

► Etiology

A. Isotonic & Hypertonic Hyponatremia

Serum osmolality identifies isotonic and hypertonic hyponatremia, although these cases can often be identified by careful history or previous laboratory tests.

Isotonic hyponatremia is seen with severe hyperlipidemia and hyperproteinemia. Lipids (including chylomicrons, triglycerides, and cholesterol) and proteins (> 10 g/dL, eg, paraproteinemias and intravenous immunoglobu-

lin therapy) interfere with the measurement of serum sodium, causing an artifactual pseudohyponatremia. Serum osmolality is isotonic because lipids and proteins do not affect osmolality measurement. Newer sodium measurements using ion-specific electrodes will not produce pseudohyponatremia.

Hypertonic hyponatremia occurs with hyperglycemia and mannitol administration for increased intracranial pressure. Glucose and mannitol osmotically pull intracellular water into the extracellular space. The translocation of water lowers the serum sodium concentration. Translocational hyponatremia is not pseudohyponatremia or an artifact of sodium measurement. The sodium concentration falls 2 mEq/L for every 100 mg/dL rise in glucose when the glucose concentration is between 200 and 400 mg/dL. If the glucose concentration is above 400 mg/dL, the sodium concentration falls 4 mEq/L for every 100 mg/dL rise in glucose. An overall sodium correction factor of 2.4 mEq/L for every 100 mg/dL increase in glucose concentration is more accurate than the 1.6 mg/dL that has been used previously.

B. Hypotonic Hyponatremia

Most cases of hyponatremia are hypotonic, highlighting sodium's role as the predominant extracellular osmole. The next step is classifying hypotonic cases by the patient's volume status.

1. Hypovolemic hypotonic hyponatremia—Hypovolemic hyponatremia occurs with renal or extrarenal volume loss and hypotonic fluid replacement (Figure 21–1). Total body sodium and total body water are decreased. To maintain intravascular volume, the pituitary increases ADH secretion, causing free water retention from hypotonic fluid replacement. The body sacrifices serum osmolality to preserve intravascular volume. In short, losses of water and salt are replaced by water alone. Without ongoing hypotonic fluid intake, the renal or extrarenal volume loss would produce hypovolemic hypernatremia.

Cerebral salt wasting is a distinct and rare subset of hypovolemic hyponatremia seen in patients with intracranial disease (eg, infections, cerebrovascular accidents, tumors, and neurosurgery). Clinical features include refractory hypovolemia and hypotension, often requiring continuous infusion of isotonic or hypertonic saline and ICU monitoring. The exact pathophysiology is unclear but includes renal sodium wasting possibly through brain natriuretic peptide, ADH release, and decreased aldosterone secretion.

2. Euvolemic hypotonic hyponatremia—Euvolemic hyponatremia causes the most anxiety for clinicians because of the broad differential diagnosis. Most processes are mediated directly or indirectly through ADH, including hypothyroidism, adrenal insufficiency, medications, and the syndrome of inappropriate ADH (SIADH). The exceptions are primary polydipsia, beer potomania, and reset osmostat.

A. HORMONAL ABNORMALITIES—Hypothyroidism and adrenal insufficiency can cause hyponatremia. Exactly how hypothyroidism induces hyponatremia is unclear but may be related to ADH. Adrenal insufficiency may be associated

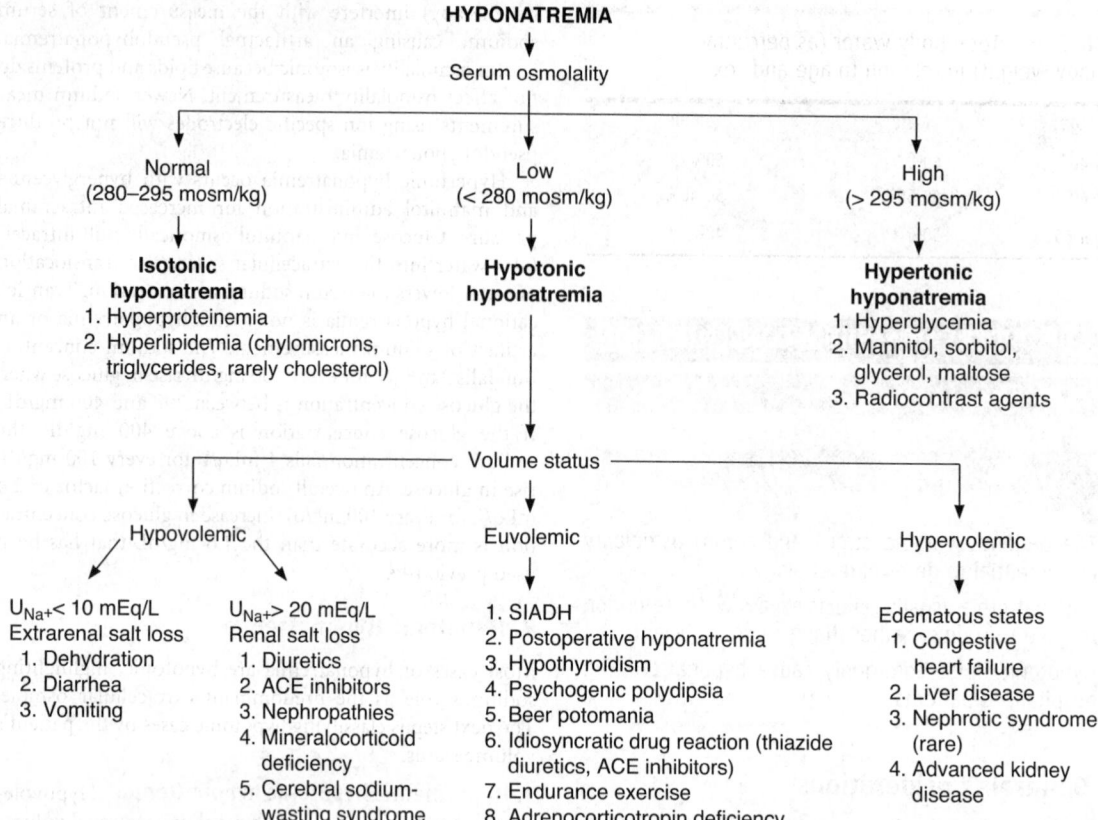

HYPONATREMIA

Serum osmolality

Normal
(280–295 mosm/kg)

Isotonic hyponatremia
1. Hyperproteinemia
2. Hyperlipidemia (chylomicrons, triglycerides, rarely cholesterol)

Low
(< 280 mosm/kg)

Hypotonic hyponatremia

High
(> 295 mosm/kg)

Hypertonic hyponatremia
1. Hyperglycemia
2. Mannitol, sorbitol, glycerol, maltose
3. Radiocontrast agents

Volume status

Hypovolemic

$U_{Na+} < 10$ mEq/L
Extrarenal salt loss
1. Dehydration
2. Diarrhea
3. Vomiting

$U_{Na+} > 20$ mEq/L
Renal salt loss
1. Diuretics
2. ACE inhibitors
3. Nephropathies
4. Mineralocorticoid deficiency
5. Cerebral sodium-wasting syndrome

Euvolemic
1. SIADH
2. Postoperative hyponatremia
3. Hypothyroidism
4. Psychogenic polydipsia
5. Beer potomania
6. Idiosyncratic drug reaction (thiazide diuretics, ACE inhibitors)
7. Endurance exercise
8. Adrenocorticotropin deficiency

Hypervolemic

Edematous states
1. Congestive heart failure
2. Liver disease
3. Nephrotic syndrome (rare)
4. Advanced kidney disease

▲ **Figure 21–1.** Evaluation of hyponatremia using serum osmolality and extracellular fluid volume status. ACE, angiotensin-converting enzyme; SIADH, syndrome of inappropriate antidiuretic hormone. (Adapted, with permission, from Narins RG et al. Diagnostic strategies in disorders of fluid, electrolyte and acid-base homeostasis. Am J Med. 1982 Mar;72(3):496–520.)

with the hyperkalemia and metabolic acidosis of hypoaldosteronism. Cortisol provides feedback inhibition for ADH release.

B. Thiazide diuretics and other medications—Thiazides induce hyponatremia typically in older female patients within days of initiating therapy. The mechanism appears to be a combination of mild diuretic-induced volume contraction, ADH effect, and intact urinary concentrating ability resulting in water retention and hyponatremia. Loop diuretics do not cause hyponatremia as frequently because of disrupted medullary concentrating gradient and impaired urine concentration.

Nonsteroidal anti-inflammatory drugs (NSAIDs) increase ADH by inhibiting prostaglandin formation. Prostaglandins, selective serotonin reuptake inhibitors (eg, fluoxetine, paroxetine, and citalopram) can cause hyponatremia, especially in geriatric patients. Enhanced secretion or action of ADH may result from increased serotonergic tone. Angiotensin-converting enzyme (ACE) inhibitors do not block the conversion of angiotensin I to angiotensin II in the brain. Angiotensin II stimulates thirst and ADH secretion. Hyponatremia during amiodarone-loading has been reported; it usually improves with dose reduction.

Abuse of 3,4-methylenedioxymethylamphetamine (MDMA, also known as Ecstasy) can lead to hyponatremia and severe neurologic symptoms, including seizures, cerebral edema, and brainstem herniation. MDMA and its metabolites increase ADH release from the hypothalamus. There may be a component of primary polydipsia since MDMA users typically increase fluid intake in an attempt to prevent hyperthermia.

C. Nausea, pain, surgery, and medical procedures—Nausea and pain are potent stimulators of ADH release. Severe hyponatremia can develop after elective surgery in healthy patients, especially premenopausal women. Hypotonic fluids in the setting of elevated ADH levels can produce severe and life-threatening hyponatremia. Other medical procedures, such as colonoscopy, have also been associated with hyponatremia.

D. HIV infection—Hyponatremia is seen in up to 50% of hospitalized HIV patients and 20% of ambulatory HIV patients. The differential diagnosis is broad: medication effect, adrenal insufficiency, hypoaldosteronism, central nervous system or pulmonary disease, SIADH, malignancy, and volume depletion.

E. ENDURANCE EXERCISE HYPONATREMIA—Hyponatremia after endurance exercise (eg, triathlon events and marathons) may be caused by a combination of excessive hypotonic fluid intake and continued ADH secretion. Reperfusion of the exercise-induced ischemic splanchnic bed causes delayed absorption of excessive quantities of hypotonic fluid ingested during exercise. Sustained elevation of ADH prevents water excretion in this setting. New guidelines encourage runners to drink between 400 mL/h and 800 mL/h as opposed to the previous "as much as possible" advice. However, the clinical relevance of this new recommendation remains to be determined.

F. SYNDROME OF INAPPROPRIATE ANTIDIURETIC HORMONE SECRETION—Under normal circumstances, hypovolemia and hyperosmolality stimulate ADH secretion. ADH release is inappropriate without these physiological cues. Normal regulation of ADH release occurs from both the central nervous system and the chest via baroreceptors and neural input. The major causes of SIADH (Table 21–2) are disorders affecting the central nervous system (structural, metabolic, psychiatric, or pharmacologic processes) or the lungs (infectious, mechanical, oncologic). Medications commonly cause SIADH by increasing ADH or its action. Some carcinomas, especially small cell lung carcinoma, can autonomously secrete ADH.

G. PSYCHOGENIC POLYDIPSIA AND BEER POTOMANIA—Marked free water intake (generally > 10 L/d) may produce hyponatremia. Euvolemia is maintained through renal excretion of sodium. Urine sodium is therefore generally elevated (> 20 mEq/L), and ADH levels are appropriately suppressed. As the increased free water is excreted, the urine osmolality approaches the minimum urine osmolality of 50 mosm/kg. Psychogenic polydipsia occurs in patients with psychiatric disease. Psychiatric medications may interfere with water excretion or increase thirst through anticholinergic side effects, further increasing water intake. The hyponatremia of beer potomania occurs in patients who consume large amounts of beer. Free water excretion is decreased in these patients because of decreased solute consumption and production; muscle wasting and malnutrition are contributing factors. Without enough solute, these patients have decreased free water excretory capacity even if they can maximally dilute the urine.

H. RESET OSMOSTAT—Reset osmostat is a rare cause of hyponatremia characterized by appropriate ADH regulation in response to water deprivation and fluid challenges. Patients with reset osmostat regulate serum sodium and serum osmolality around a lower set point, concentrating or diluting urine in response to hyperosmolality and hypoosmolality. The mild hypo-osmolality of pregnancy is a form of reset osmostat.

3. Hypervolemic hypotonic hyponatremia—Hypervolemic hyponatremia occurs in the edematous states of cirrhosis, heart failure, nephrotic syndrome, and advanced kidney disease (Figure 21–1). In cirrhosis and heart failure, effective circulating volume is decreased due to peripheral vasodilation or decreased cardiac output. Increased renin-angiotensin-aldosterone system activity and ADH secre-

Table 21–2. Causes of syndrome of inappropriate ADH secretion (SIADH).

Central nervous system disorders
  Head trauma
  Stroke
  Subarachnoid hemorrhage
  Hydrocephalus
  Brain tumor
  Encephalitis
  Guillain-Barré syndrome
  Meningitis
  Acute psychosis
  Acute intermittent porphyria
Pulmonary lesions
  Tuberculosis
  Bacterial pneumonia
  Aspergillosis
  Bronchiectasis
  Neoplasms
  Positive pressure ventilation
Malignancies
  Bronchogenic carcinoma
  Pancreatic carcinoma
  Prostatic carcinoma
  Renal cell carcinoma
  Adenocarcinoma of colon
  Thymoma
  Osteosarcoma
  Malignant lymphoma
  Leukemia
Drugs
  Increased ADH production
    Antidepressants: tricyclics, monoamine oxidase inhibitors, SSRIs
    Antineoplastics: cyclophosphamide, vincristine
    Carbamazepine
    Methylenedioxymethylamphetamine (MDMA; Ecstasy)
    Clofibrate
    Neuroleptics: thiothixene, thioridazine, fluphenazine, haloperidol, trifluoperazine
  Potentiated ADH action
    Carbamazepine
    Chlorpropamide, tolbutamide
    Cyclophosphamide
    NSAIDs
    Somatostatin and analogs
    Amiodarone
Others
  Postoperative
  Pain
  Stress
  AIDS
  Pregnancy (physiologic)
  Hypokalemia

ADH, antidiuretic hormone; NSAIDs, nonsteroidal anti-inflammatory drugs; SSRIs, selective serotonin reuptake inhibitors.

tion result in water retention. Notice the pathophysiological similarity to hypovolemic hyponatremia—the body sacrifices osmolality in an attempt to restore effective circulating volume.

The pathophysiology of hyponatremia in nephrotic syndrome in not completely understood, but the primary disturbance may be renal sodium retention, resulting in overfilling of the intravascular space and secondary edema formation as fluid seeped into the interstitial space. Previously, it was believed that the decreased oncotic pressure of hypoalbuminemia meant that the intravascular space lost fluid to the interstitial compartment. This intravascular underfilling led to secondary renal sodium retention. However, from a clinical standpoint, patients receiving therapy for glomerular disease and nephrotic syndrome often have edema resolution prior to improvements in the serum albumin.

Patients with advanced kidney disease typically have sodium retention with decreased free water excretory capacity, resulting in hypervolemic hyponatremia.

▶ Clinical Findings

A. Symptoms and Signs

Whether hyponatremia is symptomatic depends on its severity and acuity. Chronic disease can be severe (sodium concentration less than 110 mEq/L), yet remarkably asymptomatic because the brain has adapted by decreasing its tonicity over weeks to months. Acute disease that has developed over hours to days can be severely symptomatic with relatively moderate hyponatremia. Mild hyponatremia (sodium concentrations of 130–135 mEq/L) is usually asymptomatic.

Mild symptoms of nausea and malaise progress to headache, lethargy, and disorientation as the sodium concentration drops. The most serious symptoms are respiratory arrest, seizure, coma, permanent brain damage, brainstem herniation, and death. Premenopausal women are much more likely than menopausal women to die or suffer permanent brain injury from hyponatremic encephalopathy, suggesting a hormonal role in the pathophysiology.

Evaluation starts with a careful history for new medications, changes in fluid intake (polydipsia, anorexia, intravenous fluid rates and composition), fluid output (nausea and vomiting, diarrhea, ostomy output, polyuria, oliguria, insensible losses). The physical examination should help categorize the patient's volume status into hypovolemia, euvolemia, or hypervolemia.

B. Laboratory Findings

Laboratory assessment should include serum electrolytes, serum creatinine, serum osmolality, and urine sodium. The etiology of most cases of hyponatremia will be apparent from the history, physical, and these basic laboratory tests. Additional tests of thyroid and adrenal function will occasionally be necessary.

SIADH is a clinical diagnosis characterized by (1) hyponatremia; (2) decreased osmolality (< 280 mosm/kg); (3) absence of heart, kidney, or liver disease; (4) normal thyroid and adrenal function (see Chapter 26); and (5) urine sodium usually over 20 mEq/L. In clinical practice, ADH levels are not measured in these patients. Patients with SIADH may have low blood urea nitrogen (BUN) (< 10 mg/dL) and hypouricemia (< 4 mg/dL), which are not only dilutional but result from increased urea and uric acid clearances in response to the volume-expanded state. An elevated BUN (azotemia) may reflect volume contraction, ruling out SIADH, which is seen in euvolemic patients.

▶ Complications

The most serious complication of hyponatremia is iatrogenic cerebral osmotic demyelination from overly rapid or inappropriate sodium correction.

▶ Treatment

Regardless of the patient's volume status, another common feature is to restrict free water and hypotonic fluid intake, since these solutions can only exacerbate hyponatremia. Free water intake from oral intake and intravenous fluids should generally be less than 1–1.5 L/d.

Hypovolemic patients require adequate fluid resuscitation from isotonic fluids (either normal saline or lactated Ringer solution) to suppress the hypovolemic stimulus for ADH release. Patients with **cerebral salt wasting** may require hypertonic saline or normal saline to prevent circulatory collapse; some may respond to fludrocortisone. **Hypervolemic** patients may require loop diuretics or dialysis, or both, (or other extracorporeal ultrafiltration) to correct the increased total body water and sodium. Euvolemic patients may respond to free water restriction alone.

Pseudohyponatremia from hypertriglyceridemia or hyperproteinemia requires no therapy except perhaps confirmation with the clinical laboratory. **Translocational hyponatremia** from glucose or mannitol can be managed with glucose correction or mannitol discontinuation (if possible). No specific therapy is necessary in patients with **reset osmostat** since they can successfully regulate their serum sodium with fluid challenges and water deprivation.

Symptomatic and/or severe hyponatremia generally requires hospitalization for observation, careful monitoring of fluid balance and weights, and frequent sodium checks. Any inciting medications should be discontinued if possible.

There is no consensus about the optimal rate of sodium correction in symptomatic hyponatremic patients. A reasonable rate is 10–12 mEq/L/d in mildly to moderately symptomatic patients. A more aggressive rate of 1–1.5 mEq/L/h (to a maximum correction of 10–12 mEq/L) has been used in severely symptomatic patients. Sodium concentration should be monitored as frequently as every 1–2 hours. As the symptoms improve or resolve, the correction rate should be reduced to roughly 0.5 mEq/L/h. To avoid overcorrection, the physician should stabilize the sodium in the range of 125 to 130 mEq/L.

Also called central pontine myelinolysis, cerebral osmotic demyelination may occur outside the brainstem. Demyelination may occur days after sodium correction or initial neurologic recovery from hyponatremia. Hypoxic episodes during hyponatremia may contribute to demyelination. Unfortunately, the neurologic effects are generally disastrous and irreversible.

In severely symptomatic patients, the physician should calculate the patient's sodium deficit and deliver **hypertonic saline** (ie, 3% saline) at the appropriate rate. In general the saline infusion rate should be approximately 0.5 mL/kg body weight/h; rates of 1 mL/kg/h or greater may represent a miscalculation of the sodium deficit or mathematical error. Hypertonic saline in hypervolemic patients can be hazardous, resulting in worsening volume overload, pulmonary edema, and ascites.

Demeclocycline (300–600 mg orally twice daily) is used for patients who cannot adequately restrict water restriction or have an inadequate response to conservative measures. It inhibits the effect of ADH on the distal tubule. Onset of action may require 1 week, and urinary concentrating ability may be permanently impaired, resulting in nephrogenic diabetes insipidus and even hypernatremia. Demeclocycline may be more nephrotoxic in patients with cirrhosis.

Vasopressin antagonists may revolutionize the treatment of euvolemic and hypervolemic hyponatremia, especially in persons with heart failure. Unfortunately, oral versions are not available in the United States; these include lixivaptan, tolvaptan, and satavaptan, which are selective vasopressin-2 receptor antagonists. V_2 receptors primarily mediate the diuretic effect of ADH. For hospitalized patients with euvolemic SIADH, conivaptan is given as an intravenous loading dose of 20 mg delivered over 30 minutes, then as 20 mg continuously over 24 hours. Subsequent infusions may be administered every 1–3 days at 20–40 mg/d by continuous infusion.

When to Refer

- Nephrology or endocrinology consultation should be considered in severe, symptomatic, refractory, or complicated cases of hyponatremia.
- Aggressive therapies such as hypertonic saline, demeclocycline, vasopressin antagonists, and dialysis mandate specialist consultation.
- Consultation may be necessary for patients with end-stage liver or heart disease.

When to Admit

Hospital admission is necessary for symptomatic patients or those requiring aggressive therapies for close monitoring and frequent laboratory testing.

Ellison DH et al. Clinical practice. The syndrome of inappropriate antidiuresis. N Engl J Med. 2007 May 17;356(20):2064–72. [PMID: 17507705]

Liamis G et al. A review of drug-induced hyponatremia. Am J Kidney Dis. 2008 Jul;52(1):144–53. [PMID: 18468754]

Lien YH et al. Hyponatremia: clinical diagnosis and management. Am J Med. 2007 Aug;120(8):653–8. [PMID: 17679119]

Schrier RW et al; SALT Investigators. Tolvaptan, a selective oral vasopressin V2-receptor antagonist, for hyponatremia. N Engl J Med. 2006 Nov 16;355(20):2099–112. [PMID: 17105757]

Upadhyay A et al. Incidence and prevalence of hyponatremia. Am J Med. 2006 Jul;119(7 Suppl 1):S30–5. [PMID: 16843082]

Verbalis JG et al. Hyponatremia treatment guidelines 2007: expert panel recommendations. Am J Med. 2007;11(Suppl 1):S1–S21. [PMID: 17981159]

HYPERNATREMIA

ESSENTIALS OF DIAGNOSIS

- Increased thirst and water intake is the first defense against hypernatremia.
- Urine osmolality helps differentiate renal from nonrenal water loss.

General Considerations

Hypernatremia is defined as a sodium concentration > 145 mEq/L. All patients with hypernatremia have hyperosmolality, unlike hyponatremic patients who can have a low, normal, or high serum osmolality. The hypernatremic patient is typically hypovolemic due to free water losses, although hypervolemic hypernatremia is frequently seen, often an iatrogenic complication in hospitalized patients with impaired access to free water. Rarely, excessive sodium intake may cause hypernatremia. Hypernatremia in primary aldosteronism is mild and usually does not cause symptoms.

An intact thirst mechanism and access to water are the primary defense against hypernatremia. The hypothalamus can sense minimal changes in serum osmolality, triggering the thirst mechanism and increased water intake. Thus, whatever the underlying disorder (eg, dehydration, lactulose or mannitol therapy, central and nephrogenic diabetes insipidus), excess water loss can cause hypernatremia only when adequate water intake is not possible, as with unconscious patients.

Clinical Findings

A. Symptoms and Signs

When the patient is dehydrated, orthostatic hypotension and oliguria are typical findings. Because water shifts from the cells to the intravascular space to protect volume status, these symptoms may be delayed. Lethargy, irritability, and weakness are early signs. Hyperthermia, delirium, seizures, and coma may be seen with severe hypernatremia (ie, sodium > 158 mEq/L). Symptoms in the elderly may not be specific; a recent change in consciousness is associated with a poor prognosis. Osmotic demyelination is an uncommon but reported consequence of severe hypernatremia.

B. Laboratory Findings

1. Urine osmolality > 400 mosm/kg—Renal water-conserving ability is functioning.

A. NONRENAL LOSSES—Hypernatremia will develop if water intake falls behind hypotonic fluid losses from excessive sweating, the respiratory tract, or bowel movements. Lactulose causes an osmotic diarrhea with loss of free water.

B. RENAL LOSSES—While severe hyperglycemia can cause translocational hyponatremia (see above), progressive volume depletion from osmotic glucosuria can result in hypernatremia. Osmotic diuresis can occur with the use of mannitol or urea.

2. Urine osmolality < 250 mosm/kg—A dilute urine with osmolality less than 250 mosm/kg with hypernatremia is characteristic of central and nephrogenic diabetes insipidus. Nephrogenic diabetes insipidus results from renal insensitivity to ADH; common causes include lithium, demeclocycline, relief of urinary obstruction, interstitial nephritis, hypercalcemia, and hypokalemia.

▶ Treatment

Treatment of hypernatremia includes correcting the cause of the fluid loss, replacing water, and replacing electrolytes (as needed). In response to increases in plasma osmolality, brain cells synthesize solutes—or idiogenic osmoles—which increase osmotic flow of water back into the brain cells to regulate their volume. This begins 4–6 hours after dehydration and takes several days to reach a steady state. If hypernatremia is too rapidly corrected, the osmotic imbalance may cause water to preferentially enter brain cells, causing cerebral edema and potentially severe neurologic impairment. Fluid therapy should be administered over a 48-hour period, aiming for a decrease in serum sodium of approximately 1 mEq/L/h (1 mmol/L/h). Unfortunately, there is no consensus about the optimal rates of sodium correction in hypernatremia and hyponatremia.

A. Choice of Type of Fluid for Replacement

1. Hypernatremia with hypovolemia—Hypovolemic patients should receive isotonic (0.9%) saline to restore the volume deficit and to treat the hyperosmolality, since the osmolality of isotonic saline (308 mosm/kg) is often lower than that of the plasma. After adequate volume resuscitation with normal saline, 0.45% saline or 5% dextrose (or both) can be used to replace any remaining free water deficit. Milder volume deficits may be treated with 0.45% saline and 5% dextrose.

2. Hypernatremia with euvolemia—Water ingestion or intravenous 5% dextrose will result in the excretion of excess sodium in the urine. If the glomerular filtration rate (GFR) is decreased, diuretics will increase urinary sodium excretion but may impair renal concentrating ability, increasing the quantity of water that needs to be replaced.

3. Hypernatremia with hypervolemia—Treatment includes 5% dextrose solution to reduce hyperosmolality. Loop diuretics may be necessary to promote natriuresis and lower the total body sodium. In severe rare cases with kidney disease, hemodialysis may be necessary to correct the excess total body sodium and water.

B. Calculation of Water Deficit

Fluid replacement should include the free water deficit as well as the maintenance fluid to replace ongoing and anticipated fluid losses.

1. Acute hypernatremia—In acute dehydration without much solute loss, free water loss is similar to the weight loss. Initially, a 5% dextrose solution may be used. As correction of water deficit progresses, therapy should continue with 0.45% saline with dextrose.

2. Chronic hypernatremia—The water deficit is calculated to restore normal sodium concentration, typically 140 mEq/L. Total body water (TBW) (Table 21–1) correlates with muscle mass and therefore decreases with advancing

age, cachexia, and dehydration and is lower in women than in men. Current TBW equals 40–60% current body weight.

$$\text{Volume (in L) to be replaced} = \text{Current TBW} \times \frac{[\text{Na}^+] - 140}{140}$$

▶ When to Refer

Patients with refractory or unexplained hypernatremia should be referred for subspecialist consultation.

▶ When to Admit

- Patients with symptomatic hypernatremia require hospitalization for evaluation and treatment.
- Significant comorbidities or concomitant acute illnesses, especially if contributing to hypernatremia, may necessitate hospitalization.

Adrogue HJ et al. Hypernatremia. N Engl J Med. 2000 May 18;342(20):1493–9. [PMID: 10816188]

Chassagne P et al. Clinical presentation of hypernatremia in elderly patients: a case control study. J Am Geriatr Soc. 2006 Aug;54(8):1225–30. [PMID: 16913989]

Lin M et al. Disorders of water imbalance. Emerg Med Clin North Am. 2005 Aug;23(3):749–70. [PMID: 15982544]

Reynolds RM et al. Disorders of sodium balance. BMJ. 2006 Mar 25;332(7543):702–5. [PMID: 16565125]

VOLUME OVERLOAD

ESSENTIALS OF DIAGNOSIS

▶ Disorder of excessive sodium retention in the setting of low arterial underfilling (eg, congestive heart failure or cirrhosis).

▶ Hyponatremia from water retention in edematous states is associated with sodium retention.

The hallmark of a volume overloaded state is sodium retention. Abnormally low arterial filling, such as from congestive heart failure or cirrhosis, activates the neurohumoral axis, which stimulates the renin-angiotensin-aldosterone system, the sympathetic nervous system, and ADH (vasopressin) release. Sodium retention with edema results. The stimulus for the release of vasopressin is nonosmotic. Instead, vasopressin is released in response to activation of baroreceptors because of a decrease in arterial baroreceptor stretch. Vasopressin stimulates renal V_2 receptors, which increase water reabsorption; hyponatremia may develop in the edematous state.

Adler SM et al. Disorders of body water homeostasis in critical illness. Endocrinol Metab Clin North Am. 2006 Dec;35(4):873–94. [PMID: 17127152]

Chen HH et al. Pathophysiology of volume overload in acute heart failure syndromes. Am J Med. 2006 Dec;119(12 Suppl 1):S11–6. [PMID: 17113395]

Ellis DH. Disorders of sodium and water. Am J Kidney Dis. 2005 Aug;46(2):356–61. [PMID: 16112057]

Sala C et al. Central role of vasopressin in sodium/water retention in hypo- and hypervolemic nephrotic patients: a unifying hypothesis. J Nephrol. 2004 Sep–Oct;17(5):653–7. [PMID: 15593031]

Schrier RW. Water and sodium retention in edematous disorders: role of vasopressin and aldosterone. Am J Med. 2006 Jul;119(7 Suppl 1):S47–53. [PMID: 16843085]

HYPEROSMOLAR DISORDERS & OSMOLAR GAPS

HYPEROSMOLALITY WITH TRANSIENT OR NO SIGNIFICANT SHIFT IN WATER

Urea and alcohol readily cross cell membranes and can produce hyperosmolality. Urea is an ineffective osmole with little effect on osmotic water movement across cell membranes. Alcohol quickly equilibrates between the intracellular and extracellular compartments, adding 22 mosm/L for every 1000 mg/L of ethanol. Ethanol intoxication should be considered in any case of stupor or coma with an elevated osmolal gap (measured osmolality – calculated osmolality > 10 mosm/kg). Other toxic alcohols such as methanol and ethylene glycol cause an osmolal gap and a metabolic acidosis with an increased anion gap (see Chapter 39). The combination of an increased anion gap metabolic acidosis and an osmolal gap exceeding 10 mosm/kg is not specific for toxic alcohol ingestion and may occur with alcoholic ketoacidosis or lactic acidosis (see Metabolic Acidosis).

HYPEROSMOLALITY ASSOCIATED WITH SIGNIFICANT SHIFTS IN WATER

Increased concentrations of solutes that do not readily enter cells cause a shift of water from the intracellular compartment to the extracellular compartment. Hyperosmolality of effective osmoles such as sodium and glucose causes symptoms, primarily in the central nervous system. The severity of symptoms depends on the degree of hyperosmolality and rapidity of development. In acute hyperosmolality, somnolence and confusion can appear when the osmolality exceeds 320–330 mosm/kg; coma, respiratory arrest, and death can result when osmolality exceeds 340–350 mosm/kg.

Stoner GD. Hyperosmolar hyperglycemic state. Am Fam Physician. 2005 May 1;71(9):1723–30. [PMID: 15887451]

Trachtenbarg DE. Diabetic ketoacidosis. Am Fam Physician. 2005 May 1;71(9):1705–14. [PMID: 15887449]

DISORDERS OF POTASSIUM CONCENTRATION

HYPOKALEMIA

 ESSENTIALS OF DIAGNOSIS

► Severe hypokalemia may induce dangerous arrhythmias and rhabdomyolysis.

► Transtubular potassium concentration gradient (TTKG) can distinguish renal from nonrenal loss of potassium.

General Considerations

Hypokalemia can result from insufficient dietary potassium intake, intracellular shifting of potassium from the extracellular space, extrarenal potassium loss, or renal potassium loss (Table 21–3). Cellular uptake of potassium is increased by insulin and β-adrenergic stimulation and blocked by α-adrenergic stimulation. Aldosterone is an important regulator of total body potassium, increasing potassium secretion in the distal renal tubule. The most common cause of hypokalemia, especially in developing countries, is gastrointestinal loss due to infectious diarrhea. The potassium concentration in intestinal secretion is ten times higher (80 mEq/L) than in gastric secretions. Hypokalemia in the presence of acidosis suggests profound potassium depletion and requires urgent treatment. Self-limited hypokalemia occurs in 50–60% of trauma patients, perhaps related to enhanced release of epinephrine.

Table 21–3. Causes of hypokalemia.

Decreased potassium intake
Potassium shift into the cell
Increased postprandial secretion of insulin
Alkalosis
Trauma (via β-adrenergic stimulation?)
Periodic paralysis (hypokalemic)
Barium intoxication
Renal potassium loss
Increased aldosterone (mineralocorticoid) effects
Primary hyperaldosteronism
Secondary aldosteronism (dehydration, heart failure)
Renovascular hypertension
Malignant hypertension
Ectopic ACTH-producing tumor
Gitelman syndrome
Bartter syndrome
Cushing syndrome
Licorice (European)
Renin-producing tumor
Congenital abnormality of steroid metabolism (eg, adrenogenital syndrome, 17α-hydroxylase defect, apparent mineralocorticoid excess, 11β-hydroxylase deficiency)
Increased flow of distal nephron
Diuretics (furosemide, thiazides)
Salt-losing nephropathy
Hypomagnesemia
Unreabsorbable anion
Carbenicillin, penicillin
Renal tubular acidosis (type I or II)
Fanconi syndrome
Interstitial nephritis
Metabolic alkalosis (bicarbonaturia)
Congenital defect of distal nephron
Liddle syndrome
Extrarenal potassium loss
Vomiting, diarrhea, laxative abuse
Villous adenoma, Zollinger-Ellison syndrome

Hypokalemia increases the likelihood of digitalis toxicity. In patients with heart disease, hypokalemia induced by β_2-adrenergic agonists and diuretics may impose a substantial risk. Numerous genetic mutations affect fluid and electrolyte metabolism, including disorders of potassium metabolism (Table 21–4).

Magnesium is an important cofactor for potassium uptake and for maintenance of intracellular potassium levels. Loop diuretics (eg, furosemide) cause substantial renal potassium and magnesium losses. Magnesium depletion should be suspected in refractory hypokalemia.

▶ Clinical Findings

A. Symptoms and Signs

Muscular weakness, fatigue, and muscle cramps are frequent complaints in mild to moderate hypokalemia. Gastrointestinal smooth muscle involvement may result in constipation or ileus. Flaccid paralysis, hyporeflexia, hypercapnia, tetany, and rhabdomyolysis may be seen with severe hypokalemia (< 2.5 mEq/L). The presence of hypertension may be a clue to the diagnosis of hypokalemia from aldosterone or mineralocorticoid excess (Table 21–4). Renal manifestations include nephrogenic diabetes insipidus and interstitial nephritis.

B. Laboratory Findings

Urinary potassium concentration is low (< 20 mEq/L) as a result of extrarenal fluid loss (eg, diarrhea, vomiting) and inappropriately high (> 40 mEq/L) with urinary losses (eg, mineralocorticoid excess, Bartter syndrome, Liddle syndrome) (Table 21–3).

The transtubular $[K^+]$ gradient (TTKG) is a simple and rapid evaluation of net potassium secretion. TTKG is calculated as follows:

$$TTKG = \frac{Urine\ K^+/Plasma\ K^+}{Urine\ osm/Plasma\ osm}$$

Hypokalemia with a TTKG > 4 suggests renal potassium loss with increased distal K^+ secretion. In such cases, plasma renin and aldosterone levels are helpful in differential diagnosis. The presence of nonabsorbed anions, such as bicarbonate, increases TTKG.

C. Electrocardiogram

The electrocardiogram (ECG) shows decreased amplitude and broadening of T waves, prominent U waves, premature ventricular contractions, and depressed ST segments.

▶ Treatment

Oral potassium supplementation is the safest and easiest treatment for mild to moderate deficiency. Dietary potassium is almost entirely coupled to phosphate—rather than chloride—and is therefore not effective in correcting potassium loss associated with chloride depletion from diuretics or vomiting. In the setting of abnormal kidney function and mild to moderate diuretic dosage, 20 mEq/d of oral potassium is generally sufficient to prevent hypokalemia, but 40–

Table 21–4. Genetic disorders associated with electrolyte metabolism disturbances.

Disease	Site of Mutation
Potassium	
Hypokalemia	
Hypokalemic periodic paralysis	Dihydropyridine-sensitive skeletal muscle voltage-gated calcium channel
Bartter syndrome	Na^+-K^+-$2Cl^-$ cotransporter, K^+ channel (ROMK), or Cl^- channel of thick ascending limb of Henle (hypofunction), barttin
Gitelman syndrome	Thiazide-sensitive Na^+-Cl^- cotransporter
Liddle syndrome	β or γ subunit of amiloride-sensitive Na^+ channel (hyperfunction)
Apparent mineralocorticoid excess	11β-hydroxysteroid dehydrogenase (failure to inactivate cortisol)
Glucocorticoid-remediable hyperaldosteronism	Regulatory sequence of 11β-hydroxylase controls aldosterone synthase inappropriately
Hyperkalemia	
Hyperkalemic periodic paralysis	α subunit of calcium channel
Pseudohypoaldosteronism type I	β or γ subunit of amiloride-sensitive Na^+ channel (hypofunction)
Pseudohypoaldosteronism type II (Gordon syndrome)	HNK2, HNK4
Calcium	
Familial hypocalciuric hypercalcemia	Ca^{2+}-sensing protein (hypofunction)
Familial hypocalcemia	Ca^{2+}-sensing protein (hyperfunction)
Phosphate	
Hypophosphatemic rickets	*PEX* gene, FGF23
Magnesium	
Hypomagnesemia-hypercalciuria syndrome	Paracellin-1
Water	
Nephrogenic diabetes insipidus	Vasopressin receptor-2 (Type 1), aquaporin-2
Acid-base	
Proximal RTA	Na^+ HCO_3^- cotransporter
Distal RTA	Cl^- HCO_3^- exchanger H^+-ATPase
Proximal and distal RTA	Carbonic anhydrase II

FGF23, fibroblast growth factor 23; RTA, renal tubular acidosis.

100 mEq/d over a period of days to weeks is needed to treat hypokalemia and fully replete potassium stores.

Intravenous potassium is indicated for patients with severe hypokalemia and for those who cannot take oral supplementation. For severe deficiency, potassium may be given through a peripheral intravenous line in a concentration up to 40 mEq/L and at rates up to 10 mEq/h. A rate of 20 mEq/h may be given through a central venous catheter. Continuous ECG monitoring is indicated, and the serum potassium level should be checked every 3–6 hours. For the initial administration, avoid glucose-containing fluid to prevent further shifts of potassium into the cells. Magnesium deficiency also needs to be corrected at the same time, particularly in refractory hypokalemia.

▶ When to Refer

Patients with unexplained hypokalemia, refractory hyperkalemia, or clinical features suggesting alternative diagnoses (eg, aldosteronism or hypokalemic periodic paralysis) should be referred for endocrinology or nephrology consultation.

▶ When to Admit

Patients with symptomatic or severe hypokalemia, especially with cardiac manifestations, require hospital admission for cardiac monitoring, frequent laboratory testing, and potassium supplementation.

Coca SG et al. The cardiovascular implications of hypokalemia. Am J Kidney Dis. 2005 Feb;45(2):233–47. [PMID: 15685500]

Groeneveld JH et al. An approach to the patient with severe hypokalemia: the potassium quiz. QJM. 2005 Apr;98(4):305–16. [PMID: 15760922]

Schaefer TJ et al. Disorders of potassium. Emerg Med Clin North Am. 2005 Aug;23(3):723–47. [PMID: 15982543]

Wiseman AC et al. Disorders of potassium and acid-base balance. Am J Kidney Dis. 2005 May;45(5):941–9. [PMID: 15861362]

HYPERKALEMIA

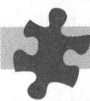

ESSENTIALS OF DIAGNOSIS

▶ Hyperkalemia may develop in patients taking ACE inhibitors, ARBs, potassium-sparing diuretics, or their combination, even with no or only mild kidney dysfunction.

▶ The ECG may show peaked T waves, widened QRS and biphasic QRS–T complexes, or may be normal despite life-threatening hyperkalemia.

▶ Measurement of plasma potassium level differentiates potassium leak from blood cells in cases of clotting, leukocytosis, and thrombocytosis from elevated serum potassium.

▶ Rule out extracellular potassium shift from the cells in acidosis and assess renal potassium excretion.

▶ General Considerations

Hyperkalemia usually occurs in patients with advanced kidney disease but can also develop with no or only mild kidney dysfunction (Table 21–5). Intracellular potassium

Table 21–5. Causes of hyperkalemia.

Spurious
  Leakage from erythrocytes when separation of serum from clot is delayed (plasma K^+ normal)
  Marked thrombocytosis or leukocytosis with release of intracellular K^+ (plasma K^+ normal)
  Repeated fist clenching during phlebotomy, with release of K^+ from forearm muscles
  Specimen drawn from arm with intravenous K^+ infusion

Decreased excretion
  Kidney disease, acute and chronic
  Renal secretory defects (may or may not have frank kidney disease): kidney transplant, interstitial nephritis, systemic lupus erythematosus, sickle cell disease, amyloidosis, obstructive nephropathy
  Hyporeninemic hypoaldosteronism (often in diabetic patients with mild to moderate nephropathy) or selective hypoaldosteronism (some patients with AIDS)
  Drugs that inhibit potassium excretion: spironolactone, eplerenone, drospirenone, NSAIDs, ACE inhibitors, angiotensin II receptor blockers, triamterene, amiloride, trimethoprim, pentamidine, cyclosporine, tacrolimus)

Shift of K^+ from within the cell
  Massive release of intracellular K^+ in burns, rhabdomyolysis, hemolysis, severe infection, internal bleeding, vigorous exercise
  Metabolic acidosis (in the case of organic acid accumulation—eg, lactic acidosis—a shift of K^+ does not occur since organic acid can easily move across the cell membrane)
  Hypertonicity (solvent drag)
  Insulin deficiency (metabolic acidosis may not be apparent)
  Hyperkalemic periodic paralysis
  Drugs: succinylcholine, arginine, digitalis toxicity, β-adrenergic antagonists
  α-Adrenergic stimulation?

Excessive intake of K^+
  Especially in patients taking medications that decrease potassium secretion (see above)

ACE, angiotensin-converting enzyme; NSAIDs, nonsteroidal anti-inflammatory drugs.

shifts to the ECF in hyperkalemia associated with acidosis. Serum potassium concentration rises about 0.7 mEq/L for every decrease of 0.1 pH unit during acidosis. Fist clenching during venipuncture may raise the potassium concentration by 1–2 mEq/L by causing acidosis and potassium shift from cells. In the absence of acidosis, serum potassium concentration rises about 1 mEq/L when there is a total body potassium excess of 1–4 mEq/kg. However, the higher the serum potassium concentration, the smaller the excess necessary to raise the potassium levels further.

Mineralocorticoid deficiency from Addison disease or chronic kidney disease (CKD) is another cause of hyperkalemia with decreased renal excretion of potassium. Mineralocorticoid resistance due to genetic disorders, interstitial kidney disease, or urinary tract obstruction also leads to hyperkalemia.

ACE inhibitors or angiotensin-receptor blockers (ARBs), commonly used in patients with congestive heart failure or CKD, may cause hyperkalemia. The concomitant use of spironolactone, eplerenone, or β-blockers further increases the risk of hyperkalemia. Thiazide or loop diuretics and sodium bicarbonate may minimize hyperkalemia.

Persistent mild hyperkalemia in the absence of ACE inhibitor or ARB therapy is usually due to type IV renal tubular acidosis (RTA). Heparin inhibits aldosterone production in the adrenal glands, causing hyperkalemia.

Trimethoprim is structurally similar to amiloride and triamterene, and all three drugs inhibit renal potassium excretion through suppression of sodium channels in the distal nephron.

Immunosuppressive drugs such as cyclosporine and tacrolimus can induce hyperkalemia in organ transplant recipients, especially kidney transplant patients, partly due to suppression of the basolateral Na^+-K^+-ATPase in principal cells. Hyperkalemia is commonly seen in HIV-infected patients and has been attributed to impaired renal excretion of potassium due to the use of pentamidine or trimethoprim-sulfamethoxazole or to hyporeninemic hypoaldosteronism.

► Clinical Findings

Hyperkalemia impairs neuromuscular transmission, causing muscle weakness, flaccid paralysis, and ileus. Electrocardiography is not a sensitive method for detecting hyperkalemia, since nearly half of patients with a serum potassium level greater than 6.5 mEq/L will not manifest ECG changes. ECG changes in hyperkalemia include bradycardia, PR interval prolongation, peaked T waves, QRS widening, and biphasic QRS–T complexes. Conduction disturbances, such as bundle branch block and atrioventricular block, may occur. Ventricular fibrillation and cardiac arrest are terminal events.

► Prevention

Inhibitors of the renin-angiotensin-aldosterone axis (ie, ACE inhibitors, ARBs, and spironolactone) and potassium-sparing diuretics should be used cautiously in patients with heart failure, liver failure, and kidney disease. Laboratory monitoring should be performed within 1 week of drug initiation or dosage increase.

► Treatment

The diagnosis should be confirmed by repeat laboratory testing to rule out spurious hyperkalemia, especially in the absence of medications that cause hyperkalemia or in patients without kidney disease or a previous history of hyperkalemia. Plasma potassium concentration can be measured to avoid hyperkalemia due to potassium leakage out of red cells, white cells, and platelets. Kidney dysfunction should be ruled out at the initial assessment.

Treatment consists of withholding exogenous potassium, identifying the cause, reviewing the patient's medications and dietary potassium intake, and correcting the hyperkalemia. Emergent treatment of hyperkalemia is indicated when cardiac toxicity or muscular paralysis or severe hyperkalemia (potassium > 6.5 mEq/L) is present, even in the absence of ECG changes. Insulin, bicarbonate, and β-agonists shift potassium intracellularly within minutes of administration (Table 21–6). Intravenous calcium may be given to antagonize the cell membrane effects of potassium, but its use should be restricted to life-threaten-

ing hyperkalemia in patients taking digitalis because hypercalcemia may cause digitalis toxicity. Hemodialysis may be required to remove potassium in patients with acute or chronic kidney injury.

► When to Refer

- Patients with hyperkalemia from kidney disease and reduced renal potassium excretion should see a nephrologist.
- Transplant patients may need adjustment of their immunosuppression regimen by transplant specialists.

► When to Admit

Patients with severe hyperkalemia greater than 6 mEq/L, any degree of hyperkalemia associated with ECG changes, or concomitant illness (eg, tumor lysis, rhabdomyolysis, metabolic acidosis) should be sent to the emergency department or admitted to the hospital for urgent treatment.

de Denus S et al. Quantification of the risk and predictors of hyperkalemia in patients with left ventricular dysfunction: a retrospective analysis of the Studies of Left Ventricular Dysfunction (SOLVD) trials. Am Heart J. 2006 Oct;152(4):705–12. [PMID: 16996842]

Hollander-Rodriguez JC et al. Hyperkalemia. Am Fam Physician. 2006 Jan 15;73(2):283–90. [PMID: 16445274]

Palmer BF. Managing hyperkalemia caused by inhibitors of the renin-angiotensin-aldosterone system. N Engl J Med. 2004 Aug 5;351(6):585–92. [PMID: 15295051]

Weisberg LS. Management of severe hyperkalemia. Crit Care Med. 2008 Dec;36(12):3246–51. [PMID: 18936701]

▼ DISORDERS OF CALCIUM CONCENTRATION

The normal total plasma (or serum) calcium concentration is 9–10.3 mg/dL. Ionized calcium (normal: 4.7–5.3 mg/dL or 1.1–1.3 mmol/L) is physiologically active and necessary for muscle contraction and nerve function.

The calcium-sensing receptor, a transmembrane protein that detects the extracellular calcium concentration, has been identified in the parathyroid gland and the kidney. Functional defects in this protein are associated with diseases of abnormal calcium metabolism such as familial hypocalcemia and familial hypocalciuric hypercalcemia (Table 21–4).

HYPOCALCEMIA

ESSENTIALS OF DIAGNOSIS

- ► Often mistaken as a neurologic disorder.
- ► Check for decreased parathyroid hormone (PTH), vitamin D, or magnesium depletion.
- ► If the ionized calcium level is normal despite a low total serum calcium, calcium metabolism is usually normal.

Table 21–6. Treatment of hyperkalemia.

EMERGENCY					
Modality	Mechanism of Action	Onset	Duration	Prescription	K⁺ Removed from Body
Calcium	Antagonizes cardiac conduction abnormalities	0–5 minutes	1 hour	Calcium gluconate 10%, 5–30 mL intravenously; or calcium chloride 5%, 5–30 mL intravenously	0
Bicarbonate	Distributes K⁺ into cells	15–30 minutes	1–2 hours	NaHCO₃, 44–88 mEq (1–2 ampules) intravenously Note: Sodium bicarbonate may not be effective in end-stage renal disease patients; dialysis is more expedient and effective. Some patients may not tolerate the additional sodium load of bicarbonate therapy.	0
Insulin	Distributes K⁺ into cells	15–60 minutes	4–6 hours	Regular insulin, 5–10 units intravenously, plus glucose 50%, 25 g (1 ampule) intravenously	0
Albuterol	Distributes K⁺ into cells	15–30 minutes	2–4 hours	Nebulized albuterol, 10–20 mg in 4 mL normal saline, inhaled over 10 minutes Note: Much higher doses are necessary for hyperkalemia therapy (10–20 mg) than for airway disease (2.5 mg).	0

NONEMERGENCY				
Modality	Mechanism of Action	Duration of Treatment	Prescription	K⁺ Removed from Body
Loop diuretic	↑ Renal K⁺ excretion	0.5–2 hours	Furosemide, 40–160 mg intravenously or orally with or without NaHCO₃, 0.5–3 mEq/kg daily Note: Diuretics may not be effective in patients with acute and chronic kidney diseases.	Variable
Sodium polystyrene sulfonate (Kayexalate)	Ion-exchange resin binds K⁺	1–3 hours	Oral: 15–30 g in 20% sorbitol (50–100 mL) Rectal: 50 g in 20% sorbitol Note: Resins with sorbitol may cause bowel necrosis and intestinal perforation.	0.5–1 mEq/g
Hemodialysis[1]	Extracorporeal K⁺ removal	48 hours	Blood flow ≥ 200–300 mL/min Dialysate [K⁺] ~ 0 Note: A fast and effective therapy for hyperkalemia, hemodialysis can be delayed by vascular access placement and equipment and staffing availability.	200–300 mEq
Peritoneal dialysis	Peritoneal K⁺ removal	48 hours	Fast exchange, 3–4 L/h	200–300 mEq

[1]Can be both emergency and nonemergency treatment of hyperkalemia.
Modified and reproduced, with permission, from Cogan MG. *Fluid and Electrolytes: Physiology and Pathophysiology*. McGraw-Hill, 1991.

▶ General Considerations

The most common cause of low total serum calcium is hypoalbuminemia. When serum albumin concentration is lower than 4 g/dL, serum Ca^{2+} concentration is reduced by 0.8–1 mg/dL for every 1 g/dL of albumin. Thus,

$$\text{Corrected calcium}^{2+} \text{ (mg/dL)} =$$
$$Ca^{2+} \text{ (mg/dL)} + 0.8 \text{ (4 – albumin [g/dL])}$$

The most accurate measurement of serum calcium is the ionized calcium concentration. True hypocalcemia (decreased ionized calcium) implies insufficient action of PTH or active vitamin D. Important causes of hypocalcemia are listed in Table 21–7.

The most common cause of hypocalcemia is advanced CKD, in which decreased production of active vitamin D_3

(1,25 dihydroxyvitamin D_3) and hyperphosphatemia both play a role (see Chapter 22). Some cases of primary hypoparathyroidism are due to mutations of the calcium-sensing receptor in which inappropriate suppression of PTH release leads to hypocalcemia (see Chapter 26). Magnesium depletion reduces both PTH release and tissue responsiveness to PTH, causing hypocalcemia. Hypocalcemia in pancreatitis is a marker for severe disease. Elderly hospitalized patients with hypocalcemia and hypophosphatemia, with or without an elevated PTH level, are likely vitamin D deficient.

▶ Clinical Findings

A. Symptoms and Signs

Hypocalcemia increases excitation of nerve and muscle cells, primarily affecting the neuromuscular and cardiovascular

Table 21–7. Causes of hypocalcemia.

Decreased intake or absorption
  Malabsorption
  Small bowel bypass, short bowel
  Vitamin D deficit (decreased absorption, decreased production of
    25-hydroxyvitamin D or 1,25-dihydroxyvitamin D)
Increased loss
  Alcoholism
  Chronic kidney disease (CKD)
  Diuretic therapy
Endocrine disease
  Hypoparathyroidism (genetic, acquired; including hypomagnes-
    emia and hypermagnesemia)
  Post-parathyroidectomy (hungry bone syndrome)
  Pseudohypoparathyroidism
  Calcitonin secretion with medullary carcinoma of the thyroid
  Familial hypocalcemia
Associated Diseases
  Pancreatitis
  Rhabdomyolysis
  Septic shock
Physiologic causes
  Associated with decreased serum albumin[1]
  Decreased end-organ response to vitamin D
  Hyperphosphatemia
  Induced by aminoglycoside antibiotics, plicamycin, loop diuretics,
    foscarnet

[1]Ionized calcium concentration is normal.

systems. Spasm of skeletal muscle causes cramps and tetany. Laryngospasm with stridor can obstruct the airway. Convulsions, perioral and peripheral paresthesias, and abdominal pain can develop. Classic physical findings include Chvostek sign (contraction of the facial muscle in response to tapping the facial nerve) and Trousseau sign (carpal spasm occurring with occlusion of the brachial artery by a blood pressure cuff). QT prolongation predisposes to ventricular arrhythmias. In chronic hypoparathyroidism, cataracts and calcification of basal ganglia may appear (see Chapter 26).

B. Laboratory Findings

Serum calcium concentration is low (< 9 mg/dL). In true hypocalcemia, the ionized serum calcium concentration is also low (< 4.7 mg/dL or 1.1 mmol/L). Serum phosphate is usually elevated in hypoparathyroidism or in advanced CKD, whereas it is suppressed in early CKD or vitamin D deficiency.

Serum magnesium concentration is commonly low. In respiratory alkalosis, total serum calcium is normal but ionized calcium is low. The ECG shows a prolonged QT interval.

▶ Treatment*

A. Severe, Symptomatic Hypocalcemia

In the presence of tetany, arrhythmias, or seizures, intravenous calcium gluconate is indicated. Because of the short

*See also Chapter 26 for discussion of the treatment of hypoparathyroidism.

duration of action, continuous calcium infusion is usually required. Ten to 15 milligrams of calcium per kilogram body weight, or six to eight 10-mL vials of 10% calcium gluconate (558–744 mg of calcium), is added to 1 L of D_5W and infused over 4–6 hours. By monitoring the serum calcium level frequently (every 4–6 hours), the infusion rate is adjusted to maintain the serum calcium level at 7–8.5 mg/dL.

B. Asymptomatic Hypocalcemia

Oral calcium (1–2 g) and vitamin D preparations, including active vitamin D sterols, are used. Calcium carbonate is well tolerated and less expensive than many other calcium tablets. A check of urinary calcium excretion is recommended after the initiation of therapy because hypercalciuria (urine calcium excretion > 200 mg/d or urine calcium/urine creatinine ratio > 0.3) may impair kidney function in these patients. The low serum calcium associated with hypoalbuminemia does not require replacement therapy. If serum Mg^{2+} is low, therapy must include magnesium replacement, which by itself will usually correct hypocalcemia.

▶ When to Refer

Patients with complicated hypocalcemia from hypoparathyroidism, familial hypocalcemia, or CKD require referral from an endocrinologist or nephrologist.

▶ When to Admit

Patients with tetany, arrhythmias, seizures, or other symptoms of hypocalcemia require immediate evaluation and therapy in the emergency department or hospital.

Bushinsky DA et al. Electrolyte quintet: calcium. Lancet. 1998 Jul 25;352(9124):306–11. [PMID: 9690425]

Lyman D. Undiagnosed vitamin D deficiency in the hospitalized patient. Am Fam Physician. 2005 Jan 15;71(2):299–304. [PMID: 15686300]

Murphy E et al. Disorders of calcium metabolism. Practitioner. 2006 Sep;250(1686):4–6, 8. [PMID: 17036912]

HYPERCALCEMIA

 ESSENTIALS OF DIAGNOSIS

▶ Primary hyperparathyroidism and malignancy-associated hypercalcemia are the most common causes.

▶ Hypercalciuria usually precedes hypercalcemia.

▶ Most often, asymptomatic, mild hypercalcemia (≤ 11 mg/dL) is due to primary hyperparathyroidism, whereas the symptomatic, severe hypercalcemia (≥ 14 mg/dL) is due to hypercalcemia of malignancy.

▶ General Considerations

Important causes of hypercalcemia are listed in Table 21–8. Primary hyperparathyroidism and malignancy account for 90% of cases. Primary hyperparathyroidism is the most com-

Table 21–8. Causes of hypercalcemia.

Increased intake or absorption
Milk-alkali syndrome
Vitamin D or vitamin A excess
Endocrine disorders
Primary hyperparathyroidism
Secondary or tertiary hyperparathyroidism (usually associated with hypocalcemia)
Acromegaly
Adrenal insufficiency
Pheochromocytoma
Thyrotoxicosis
Neoplastic diseases
Tumors producing PTH-related proteins (ovary, kidney, lung)
Multiple myeloma (elaboration of osteoclast-activating factor)
Lymphoma (occasionally from production of calcitriol)
Miscellaneous causes
Thiazide diuretic use
Granulomatous diseases (production of calcitriol)
Paget disease of bone
Hypophosphatasia
Immobilization
Familial hypocalciuric hypercalcemia
Complications of kidney transplantation
Lithium intake

PTH, parathyroid hormone.

mon cause of hypercalcemia (usually mild) in ambulatory patients. Chronic hypercalcemia (over 6 months) or some manifestation such as nephrolithiasis also suggests a benign cause. Tumor production of PTH-related proteins (PTHrP) is the most common paraneoplastic endocrine syndrome, accounting for most cases of hypercalcemia in inpatients (see Table 39–13). The neoplasm is clinically apparent in nearly all cases when the hypercalcemia is detected, and the prognosis is poor. Granulomatous diseases, such as sarcoidosis and tuberculosis, cause hypercalcemia from production of active vitamin D_3 (1,25 dihydroxyvitamin D_3).

Milk-alkali syndrome has had a resurgence related to calcium ingestion for prevention of osteoporosis. In the milk-alkali syndrome, massive calcium and vitamin D ingestion can cause hypercalcemic nephropathy. Because of the decreased GFR, retention of the alkali in the calcium antacid occurs and causes metabolic alkalosis, which can be worsened by the vomiting associated with this disorder.

Hypercalcemia also causes nephrogenic diabetes insipidus. Development of polyuria is mediated through activation of calcium-sensing receptors in collecting ducts. Volume depletion further worsens hypercalcemia.

Clinical Findings

A. Symptoms and Signs

Hypercalcemia may affect gastrointestinal, kidney, and neurologic function. The history and physical examination should focus on the duration of hypercalcemia and evidence for a neoplasm. Mild hypercalcemia is often asymptomatic. Symptoms usually occur if the serum calcium is above 12 mg/dL and tend to be more severe if hypercalcemia develops acutely. Irrespective of cause, symptoms include constipation and polyuria, except in hypocalciuric hypercalcemia, in which polyuria is absent. Other abdominal symptoms include nausea, vomiting, anorexia, peptic ulcer disease, renal colic, and hematuria from nephrolithiasis. Polyuria from hypercalciuria-induced nephrogenic diabetes insipidus can result in volume depletion and acute kidney injury. Neurologic manifestations may range from mild drowsiness to weakness, depression, lethargy, stupor, and coma in severe hypercalcemia. Ventricular ectopy and idioventricular rhythm occur and can be accentuated by digitalis.

B. Laboratory Findings

The ionized calcium exceeds 1.32 mmol/L. A high serum chloride concentration and a low serum phosphate concentration in a ratio > 33 to 1 suggest primary hyperparathyroidism where PTH decreases proximal tubular phosphate reabsorption. A low serum chloride concentration with a high serum bicarbonate concentration, along with elevated BUN and creatinine, suggests milk-alkali syndrome. The highest serum calcium levels (> 15 mg/dL) generally occur in malignancy. More than 200 mg/d of urinary calcium excretion suggests hypercalciuria; less than 100 mg/d suggests hypocalciuria. Hypercalciuric patients—such as those with malignancy or those receiving oral active vitamin D therapy—may easily develop hypercalcemia in case of volume depletion. Serum phosphate may or may not be low, depending on the cause. Hypocalciuric hypercalcemia occurs in milk-alkali syndrome, thiazide diuretic use, and familial hypocalciuric hypercalcemia.

The chest radiograph may reveal malignancy or granulomatous disease. The ECG shows a shortened QT interval. Measurements of PTH and PTHrP help distinguish between malignancy-associated hypercalcemia (suppressed PTH, elevated PTHrP) and hyperparathyroidism (elevated PTH).

Treatment

Until the primary disease can be brought under control, renal excretion of calcium with resultant decrease in serum calcium concentration is promoted. Excretion of Na^+ is accompanied by excretion of Ca^{2+}. The tendency in hypercalcemia is toward volume depletion from nephrogenic diabetes insipidus. Therefore, intravenous saline for aggressive hydration and forced calciuresis is the mainstay of treatment. In dehydrated patients with normal cardiac and kidney function, 0.45% saline or 0.9% saline can be given rapidly (250–500 mL/h). A recent meta-analysis questioned the efficacy and safety profile of intravenous furosemide for hypercalcemia. Thiazides can worsen hypercalcemia.

Bisphosphonates are the treatment of choice for hypercalcemia of malignancy. Although they are safe, effective, and normalize calcium in more than 70% of patients, bisphosphonates may require up to 48–72 hours before reaching full therapeutic effect. Calcitonin may be helpful to treat hypercalcemia before the onset of action of bisphosphonates. In emergency cases, dialysis with low calcium dialysate may be needed. The calcimimetic agent cinacalcet hydrochloride suppresses PTH secretion and decreases serum calcium concentration and holds promise as a treatment option. See Chapter 39 for a discussion of the treatment of hypercalcemia of malignancy and Chapter 26 for a discussion of the treatment of hypercalcemia of hyperparathyroidism.

Typically, if dialysis patients do not receive proper supplementation of calcium and active vitamin D, hypocalcemia and hyperphosphatemia develop. On the other hand, hypercalcemia can sometimes develop, particularly in the setting of severe secondary hyperparathyroidism, characterized by high levels of PTH and subsequent release of calcium from bone. Therapy may include intravenous vitamin D, which further increases the serum calcium concentration. Another type of hypercalcemia occurs when the PTH levels are low. In this setting, bone turnover is decreased, which results in a low buffering capacity for calcium. When calcium is administered in calcium-containing phosphate binders or in the dialysate, or when vitamin D is administered, hypercalcemia results. Hypercalcemia in dialysis patients usually occurs in the presence of hyperphosphatemia, and metastatic calcification may occur. Malignancy should be considered as a cause of the hypercalcemia.

► When to Refer

- Patients with malignancy-related hypercalcemia should be referred to an oncologist.
- Patients with endocrine disorders should be referred to an endocrinologist.
- Patients with granulomatous diseases (eg, tuberculosis and other chronic infections, Wegener granulomatosis, sarcoidosis) may require assistance from infectious disease specialists, rheumatologists, or pulmonologists.

► When to Admit

- Patients with symptomatic or severe hypercalcemia require immediate treatment.
- Unexplained hypercalcemia with associated conditions, such as acute kidney injury or suspected malignancy, may also require hospitalization for treatment and expedited evaluation.

Jacobs TP et al. Clinical review: rare causes of hypercalcemia. J Clin Endocrinol Metab. 2005 Nov;90(11):6316–22. [PMID: 16131579]

LeGrand SB et al. Narrative review: furosemide for hypercalcemia: an unproven yet common practice. Ann Intern Med. 2008 Aug 19;149(4):259–63. [PMID: 18711156]

Lee CT et al. Hypercalcemia in the emergency department. Am J Med Sci. 2006 Mar;331(3):119–23. [PMID: 16538071]

Stewart AF. Clinical practice. Hypercalcemia associated with cancer. N Engl J Med. 2005 Jan 27;352(4):373–9. [PMID: 15673803]

DISORDERS OF PHOSPHORUS CONCENTRATION

In plasma, phosphate is mainly present as inorganic phosphate, and this fraction is very small (< 0.2% of total phosphate). However, body phosphate metabolism is regulated through plasma inorganic phosphate.

Important determinants of plasma inorganic phosphate concentration are renal excretion, intestinal absorption, and shift between the intracellular and extracellular spaces. The kidney is the most important regulator of the serum phosphate level. PTH decreases the absorption of phosphate in the proximal tubule while 1,25-dihydroxyvitamin D_3 increases tubular phosphate reabsorption. Renal proximal tubular reabsorption of phosphate is decreased by volume expansion, corticosteroids, and proximal tubular dysfunction (as in Fanconi syndrome). Fibroblast growth factor 23 (FGF23) is another potent phosphaturic hormone. Intestinal absorption of phosphate is facilitated by active vitamin D. PTH stimulates phosphate release from bone and renal phosphate excretion; it can lead to hypophosphatemia and depletion of bone phosphate store if hypersecretion continues. By contrast, growth hormone augments proximal tubular reabsorption of phosphate. Cellular phosphate uptake is stimulated by various factors and conditions, including alkalemia, insulin, epinephrine, feeding, hungry bone syndrome, and accelerated cell proliferation.

Phosphorus metabolism and homeostasis are intimately related to calcium metabolism. See sections on metabolic bone disease in Chapter 26.

HYPOPHOSPHATEMIA

ESSENTIALS OF DIAGNOSIS

► Severe hypophosphatemia may cause tissue hypoxia and rhabdomyolysis.

► Renal loss of phosphate can be diagnosed by measuring urinary phosphate excretion and by calculating maximal tubular phosphate reabsorption rate (TmP/GFR).

► PTH and FGF23 are the major factors that decrease TmP/GFR, leading to renal loss of phosphate.

► General Considerations

The leading causes of hypophosphatemia are listed in Table 21–9. Hypophosphatemia may occur in the presence of normal phosphate stores. Serious depletion of body phosphate stores may exist with low, normal, or high serum phosphate concentrations.

Serum phosphate levels decrease transiently after food intake, thus fasting samples are recommended for accuracy. **Moderate** hypophosphatemia (1.0–2.5 mg/dL) occurs commonly in hospitalized patients and may not reflect decreased phosphate stores.

In **severe** hypophosphatemia (1 mg/dL or less), the affinity of hemoglobin for oxygen increases through a decrease in the erythrocyte 2,3-diphosphoglycerate concentration. This impairs tissue oxygenation and thus cell metabolism, which underlies the effects of hypophosphatemia such as muscle weakness or even rhabdomyolysis. **Severe** hypophosphatemia is common and multifactorial in alcoholic patients. In acute alcohol withdrawal, increased plasma insu-

Table 21–9. Causes of hypophosphatemia.

Diminished supply or absorption
  Starvation
  Parenteral alimentation with inadequate phosphate content
  Malabsorption syndrome, small bowel bypass
  Absorption blocked by oral antacids with aluminum or magnesium
  Vitamin D-deficient and vitamin D-resistant osteomalacia
Increased loss
  Phosphaturic drugs: theophylline, diuretics, bronchodilators, corticosteroids
  Hyperparathyroidism (primary or secondary)
  Hyperthyroidism
  Renal tubular defects with excessive phosphaturia (congenital, induced by monoclonal gammopathy, heavy metal poisoning), alcoholism
  Hypokalemic nephropathy
  Inadequately controlled diabetes mellitus
  Hypophosphatemic rickets
  Phosphatonins of oncogenic osteomalacia (eg, FGF23 production)
Intracellular shift of phosphorus
  Administration of glucose
  Anabolic steroids, estrogen, oral contraceptives, β-adrenergic agonists, xanthine derivatives
  Hungry bone syndrome
  Respiratory alkalosis
  Salicylate poisoning
Electrolyte abnormalities
  Hypercalcemia
  Hypomagnesemia
  Metabolic alkalosis
Abnormal losses followed by inadequate repletion
  Diabetes mellitus with acidosis, particularly during aggressive therapy
  Recovery from starvation or prolonged catabolic state
  Chronic alcoholism, particularly during restoration of nutrition; associated with hypomagnesemia
  Recovery from severe burns

FGF23, fibroblast growth factor 23.

lin and epinephrine along with respiratory alkalosis promote intracellular shift of phosphate. Vomiting, diarrhea, and poor dietary intake contribute to hypophosphatemia. Chronic alcohol use results in a decrease in the renal threshold of phosphate excretion. This renal tubular dysfunction reverses after a month of abstinence. Patients with chronic obstructive pulmonary disease and asthma commonly have hypophosphatemia, attributed to xanthine derivatives causing shifts of phosphate intracellularly and the phosphaturic effects of β-adrenergic agonists, loop diuretics, xanthine derivatives, and corticosteroids. The metabolic syndrome, a major contributor to coronary heart disease risk, is associated with low phosphate (and magnesium) levels but the clinical significance of these disturbances is unclear. Refeeding or glucose administration to phosphate-depleted patients may cause fatal hypophosphatemia.

Clinical Findings

A. Symptoms and Signs

Acute, severe hypophosphatemia (< 1.0 mg/dL) can lead to rhabdomyolysis, paresthesias, and encephalopathy (irritabil-

ity, confusion, dysarthria, seizures, and coma). Respiratory failure or failure to wean from mechanical ventilation may occur as a result of diaphragmatic weakness. Arrhythmias and heart failure are uncommon but serious manifestations. Hematologic manifestations include acute hemolytic anemia from increased erythrocyte fragility, platelet dysfunction with petechial hemorrhages, and impaired chemotaxis of leukocytes (leading to increased susceptibility to gram-negative sepsis).

Chronic severe depletion may cause anorexia, pain in muscles and bones, and fractures.

B. Laboratory Findings

Evaluation of urinary phosphate excretion is a useful clue to the diagnosis of hypophosphatemia. A spot urine with > 20 mg/dL of phosphate suggests inappropriate renal phosphate loss. Tubular phosphate reabsorption can be assessed by TmP/GFR:

$$\frac{TmP}{GFR} = \frac{Serum\ Pi - (UPi \times UV)}{GFR}$$

where serum Pi = serum phosphate concentration
UPi = urine phosphate concentration
UV = urine volume
The normal range of TmP/GFR is 2.5–4.5 mg/dL; lower values indicate urinary phosphate loss. The main factors regulating TmP/GFR are PTH and phosphate intake. Increase of PTH or phosphate intake decreases TmP/GFR, so that more phosphate is excreted into the urine.

Measurement of plasma PTH or PTHrP levels may be helpful. The clinical utility of serum FGF levels is underdetermined except in uncommon diseases.

Other clinical features may be suggestive of specific causes of hypophosphatemia. Evidence of hemolytic anemia may be present (eg, elevated serum lactate dehydrogenase). Rhabdomyolysis results in elevated serum creatine kinase, myoglobinuria, and often acute kidney injury. Fanconi syndrome may present with any combination of uricosuria, aminoaciduria, glucosuria (with normoglycemia), normal anion gap metabolic acidosis, and phosphaturia. In chronic depletion, radiographs and bone biopsies show changes resembling osteomalacia.

Treatment

Hypophosphatemia can be prevented by including phosphate in repletion and maintenance fluids. A rapid decline in calcium levels can occur with parenteral administration of phosphate; oral replacement of phosphate is preferable. Moderate hypophosphatemia (1.0–2.5 mg/dL) is usually asymptomatic and does not require treatment. The hypophosphatemia in patients with diabetic ketoacidosis will usually correct with normal dietary intake. Chronic hypophosphatemia can be treated with oral phosphate repletion. Mixtures of sodium and potassium phosphate salts may be given to provide 0.5–1 g (18–32 mmol) of phosphate per day. For severe, symptomatic hypophosphatemia (< 1 mg/dL), an infusion should provide 279–310 mg (9–10 mmol)/12 h until the serum phosphorus exceeds 1 mg/dL and the patient can be switched to oral therapy. The infusion rate should be decreased if hypotension occurs. Monitoring of plasma phosphate, calcium, and potassium every 6 hours is necessary because the response to phosphate supplementation is not predictable. Magnesium deficiency often coexists and should be treated simultaneously.

Contraindications to therapy with phosphate salts include hypoparathyroidism, advanced CKD, tissue damage and necrosis, and hypercalcemia. When an associated hyperglycemia is treated, phosphate accompanies glucose into cells, and hypophosphatemia may ensue.

► When to Refer

- Patients with refractory hypophosphatemia with increased urinary phosphate excretion may require evaluation by an endocrinologist (for such conditions as hyperparathyroidism and vitamin D disorders) or by a nephrologist (for such conditions such as renal tubular defects).
- Patients with decreased gastrointestinal absorption may require referral to a gastroenterologist.

► When to Admit

Patients with severe or refractory hypophosphatemia will require hospitalization for intravenous phosphate.

Amanzadeh J et al. Hypophosphatemia: an evidence-based approach to its clinical consequences and management. Nat Clin Pract Nephrol. 2006 Mar;2(3):136–48. [PMID: 16932412]

Berman E et al. Altered bone and mineral metabolism in patients receiving imatinib mesylate. N Engl J Med. 2006 May 11;354(19):2006–13. [PMID: 16687713]

Brunelli SM et al. Hypophosphatemia: clinical consequences and management. J Am Soc Nephrol. 2007 Jul;18(7):1999–2003. [PMID: 17568018]

Gaasbeek A et al. Hypophosphatemia: an update on its etiology and treatment. Am J Med. 2005 Oct;118(10):1094–101. [PMID: 16194637]

HYPERPHOSPHATEMIA

ESSENTIALS OF DIAGNOSIS

- ▶ Advanced CKD is the most common cause.
- ▶ Hyperphosphatemia in the presence of hypercalcemia imposes a high risk of metastatic calcification.

► General Considerations

Advanced CKD with decreased urinary excretion of phosphate is the most common cause of hyperphosphatemia. Other causes are listed in Table 21–10.

► Clinical Findings

A. Symptoms and Signs

The clinical manifestations are those of the underlying disorder or associated condition.

Table 21–10. Causes of hyperphosphatemia.

Massive load of phosphate into the extracellular fluid
Exogenous sources
Hypervitaminosis D
Laxatives or enemas containing phosphate
Intravenous phosphate supplement
Endogenous sources
Rhabdomyolysis (especially if chronic kidney disease coexists)
Cell lysis by chemotherapy of malignancy, particularly lymphoproliferative diseases
Metabolic acidosis (lactic acidosis, ketoacidosis)
Respiratory acidosis (phosphate incorporation into cells is disturbed)
Decreased excretion into urine
Chronic kidney disease
Acute kidney injury
Hypoparathyroidism
Pseudohypoparathyroidism
Acromegaly
Pseudohyperphosphatemia
Multiple myeloma
Hyperbilirubinemia
Hypertriglyceridemia
Hemolysis in vitro

B. Laboratory Findings

In addition to elevated phosphate, blood chemistry abnormalities are those of the underlying disease.

► Treatment

Treatment is directed at the underlying cause. Exogenous sources of phosphate, including enteral or parenteral nutrition and medications, should be reduced or eliminated. Absorption of dietary phosphate can be reduced by oral phosphate binders, such as calcium carbonate, calcium acetate, sevelamer hydrochloride, lanthanum carbonate, and aluminum hydroxide. Sevelamer, lanthanum, and aluminum may be used in patients with concomitant hypercalcemia, although aluminum should not be used for more than a few days due to the risk of aluminum accumulation and neurotoxicity. In acute kidney injury and advanced CKD, dialysis will reduce serum phosphate.

► When to Admit

Patients with acute severe hyperphosphatemia require hospitalization for emergent therapy, possibly including dialysis. Concomitant illnesses, such as acute kidney injury or cell lysis, may necessitate admission.

Hruska KA et al. Hyperphosphatemia of chronic kidney disease. Kidney Int. 2008 Jul;74(2):148–57. [PMID: 18449174]

Moe SM. Disorders of calcium, phosphorous, and magnesium. Am J Kidney Dis. 2005 Jan;45(1):213–8. [PMID: 18486714]

Tonelli M et al; Cholesterol And Recurrent Events Trial Investigators. Relation between serum phosphate level and cardiovascular event rate in people with coronary disease. Circulation. 2005 Oct 25;112(17):2627–33. [PMID: 16246962]

DISORDERS OF MAGNESIUM CONCENTRATION

Normal plasma magnesium concentration is 1.5–2.5 mEq/L, with about one-third bound to protein and two-thirds existing as free cation. Magnesium excretion is via the kidney. Magnesium's physiologic effects on the nervous system resemble those of calcium.

Altered magnesium concentration usually provokes an associated alteration of Ca^{2+}. Both hypomagnesemia and hypermagnesemia can decrease PTH secretion or action. Severe hypermagnesemia (> 5 mEq/L) suppresses PTH secretion with consequent hypocalcemia; this disorder is typically seen only in patients receiving magnesium therapy for preeclampsia. Severe hypomagnesemia causes PTH resistance in end-organs and eventually decreased PTH secretion in severe cases.

HYPOMAGNESEMIA

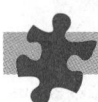

ESSENTIALS OF DIAGNOSIS

▶ Serum concentration of magnesium may not be decreased even in the presence of magnesium depletion. Check urinary magnesium excretion if renal magnesium wasting is suspected.

▶ Causes neurologic symptoms and arrhythmias.

▶ Impairs release of PTH.

▶ General Considerations

Causes of hypomagnesemia are listed in Table 21–11. Normomagnesemia does not exclude magnesium depletion because only 1% of total body magnesium is in the ECF. Hypomagnesemia and hypokalemia share many etiologies, including diuretics, diarrhea, alcoholism, aminoglycosides, and amphotericin. Renal potassium wasting also occurs from hypomagnesemia, and is refractory to potassium replacement until magnesium is repleted. Hypomagnesemia also suppresses PTH release and causes end-organ resistance to PTH and low 1,25-dihydroxyvitamin D_3 levels. This form of hypocalcemia is refractory to calcium replacement until the magnesium is normalized. Molecular mechanisms of magnesium wasting have been revealed in some hereditary disorders.

▶ Clinical Findings

A. Symptoms and Signs

Common symptoms are those of hypokalemia and hypocalcemia, with weakness and muscle cramps. Marked neuromuscular and central nervous system hyperirritability may produce tremors, athetoid movements, jerking, nystagmus, a positive Babinski response, confusion, and disorientation. Cardiovascular manifestations include hypertension, tachycardia, and ventricular arrhythmias.

Table 21–11. Causes of hypomagnesemia.

Diminished absorption or intake
Malabsorption, chronic diarrhea, laxative abuse
Prolonged gastrointestinal suction
Small bowel bypass
Malnutrition
Alcoholism
Total parenteral alimentation with inadequate Mg^{2+} content
Increased renal loss
Diuretic therapy (loop diuretics, thiazide diuretics)
Hyperaldosteronism, Gitelman syndrome (a variant of Bartter syndrome)
Hyperparathyroidism, hyperthyroidism
Hypercalcemia
Volume expansion
Tubulointerstitial diseases
Transplant kidney
Drugs (aminoglycoside, cetuximab, cisplatin, amphotericin B, pentamidine)
Others
Diabetes mellitus
Post-parathyroidectomy (hungry bone syndrome)
Respiratory alkalosis
Pregnancy

B. Laboratory Findings

Urinary excretion of magnesium exceeding 10–30 mg/d or a fractional excretion more than 2% indicates renal magnesium wasting. Hypocalcemia and hypokalemia are often present. The ECG shows a prolonged QT interval, due to lengthening of the ST segment. PTH secretion is often suppressed (see Hypocalcemia, above).

▶ Treatment

Magnesium oxide, 250–500 mg orally once or twice daily, is useful for treating chronic hypomagnesemia. Treatment of symptomatic hypomagnesemia should include infusion of 1–2 g of magnesium sulfate, followed by an infusion of 6 g magnesium sulfate in at least 1 L of fluids over 24 hours, repeated for up to 7 days to replete magnesium stores. Magnesium sulfate may also be given intramuscularly in a dosage of 200–800 mg/d (8–33 mmol/d) in four divided doses. Serum levels must be monitored daily and dosage adjusted to keep the concentration from rising above 2.5 mmol/L. Tendon reflexes may also be checked for hyporeflexia of hypermagnesemia. K^+ and Ca^{2+} replacement may be required as well, but patients with hypokalemia and hypocalcemia of hypomagnesemia do not recover without magnesium supplementation.

Patients with normal kidney function can excrete excess magnesium; hypermagnesemia should not develop with replacement dosages. In patients with CKD, magnesium replacement should be done cautiously to avoid hypermagnesemia. Reduced doses (50–75% dose reduction) and more frequent monitoring (at least twice daily) are indicated.

Mouw DR et al. Clinical inquiries. What are the causes of hypomagnesemia? J Fam Pract. 2005 Feb;54(2):174–6. [PMID: 15689296]

Naderi AS et al. Hereditary etiologies of hypomagnesemia. Nat Clin Pract Nephrol. 2008 Feb;4(2):80–9. [PMID: 18227801]

Pham PC et al. Hypomagnesemia in patients with type 2 diabetes. Clin J Am Soc Nephrol. 2007 Mar;2(2):366–73. [PMID: 17699436]

Tong GM et al. Magnesium deficiency in critical illness. J Intensive Care Med. 2005 Jan–Feb;20(1):3–17. [PMID: 15665255]

HYPERMAGNESEMIA

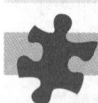 ESSENTIALS OF DIAGNOSIS

▶ Often associated with advanced CKD and chronic intake of magnesium-containing drugs.

▶ General Considerations

Hypermagnesemia is almost always the result of advanced CKD and the inability to excrete excess magnesium. Antacids and laxatives are underrecognized sources of exogenous magnesium. Pregnant patients may have severe hypermagnesemia from intravenous magnesium therapy for preeclampsia and eclampsia. Magnesium replacement should be done cautiously in patients with CKD, and dose reductions up to 75% may be necessary to avoid hypermagnesemia.

▶ Clinical Findings

A. Symptoms and Signs

Muscle weakness, decreased deep tendon reflexes, mental obtundation, and confusion are characteristic manifestations. Weakness, flaccid paralysis, ileus, urinary retention, and hypotension are noted. Serious findings include respiratory muscle paralysis and cardiac arrest.

B. Laboratory Findings

Serum Mg^{2+} is elevated. In the common setting of CKD, BUN, creatinine, potassium, phosphate, and uric acid may all be elevated. Serum Ca^{2+} is often low. The ECG shows increased PR interval, broadened QRS complexes, and peaked T waves, probably related to associated hyperkalemia.

▶ Treatment

Exogenous sources of magnesium should be discontinued. Calcium antagonizes Mg^{2+} and may be given intravenously as calcium chloride, 500 mg or more at a rate of 100 mg (4.5 mmol)/min. Hemodialysis or peritoneal dialysis may be necessary to remove the magnesium, particularly with severe kidney disease.

Long-term use of magnesium-containing drugs, such as magnesium hydroxylate and magnesium sulfate, should be avoided in patients with advanced stages of CKD.

Topf JM et al. Hypomagnesemia and hypermagnesemia. Rev Endocr Metab Disord. 2003 May;4(2):195–206. [PMID: 12766548]

ACID–BASE DISORDERS

Assessment of a patient's acid–base status requires measurement of arterial pH, Pco_2, and plasma bicarbonate (HCO_3^-). Blood gas analyzers directly measure pH and Pco_2. The HCO_3^- value is calculated from the Henderson–Hasselbalch equation:

$$pH = 6.1 + \log \frac{HCO_3^-}{0.3 \times Pco_2}$$

The total venous CO_2 measurement is a more direct determination of HCO_3^-. Because of the dissociation characteristics of carbonic acid (H_2CO_3) at body pH, dissolved CO_2 is almost exclusively in the form of HCO_3^-, and for clinical purposes the total carbon dioxide content is equivalent ($\pm$ 3 mEq/L) to the HCO_3^- concentration:

$$H^+ + HCO_3^- \leftrightarrow H_2CO_3 \leftrightarrow CO_2 + H_2O$$

Venous blood gases can provide useful information for acid–base assessment since the arteriovenous differences in pH and Pco_2 are small and relatively constant. Venous blood pH is usually 0.03–0.04 units lower than arterial blood pH, and venous blood Pco_2 is 7 or 8 mm Hg higher than arterial blood Pco_2. Calculated HCO_3^- concentration in venous blood is at most 2 mEq/L higher than arterial blood HCO_3^-. Arterial and venous blood gases will not be equivalent during a cardiopulmonary arrest; arterial samples should be obtained for the most accurate measurements of pH and Pco_2.

TYPES OF ACID–BASE DISORDERS

There are two types of acid–base disorders: acidoses and alkaloses. These disorders can be either metabolic (decreased or increased HCO_3^-) or respiratory (decreased or increased Pco_2). Primary respiratory disorders affect blood acidity by changes in Pco_2, and primary metabolic disorders are disturbances in the HCO_3^- concentration. A primary disturbance is usually accompanied by a compensatory response, but the compensation does not fully correct the pH disturbance of the primary disorder. If the pH is less than 7.40, the primary process is acidosis, either respiratory ($Pco_2 > 40$ mm Hg) or metabolic ($HCO_3^- < 24$ mEq/L). If the pH is higher than 7.40, the primary process is alkalosis, either respiratory ($Pco_2 < 40$ mm Hg) or metabolic ($HCO_3^- > 24$ mEq/L). One respiratory or metabolic disorder with its appropriate compensatory response is a simple acid-base disorder.

MIXED ACID–BASE DISORDERS

Two or three simultaneous disorders can be present in a mixed acid-base disorder, but there can never be two primary respiratory disorders. Uncovering a mixed acid-base disorder is clinically important, but challenging without a methodical approach to acid–base analysis (see box,

Table 21–12. Primary acid-base disorders and expected compensation.

Disorder	Primary Defect	Compensatory Response	Magnitude of Compensation
Respiratory acidosis			
Acute	$\uparrow P_{CO_2}$	$\uparrow HCO_3^-$	$\uparrow HCO_3^-$ 1 mEq/L per 10 mm Hg $\uparrow P_{CO_2}$
Chronic	$\uparrow P_{CO_2}$	$\uparrow HCO_3^-$	$\uparrow HCO_3^-$ 3.5 mEq/L per 10 mm Hg $\uparrow P_{CO_2}$
Respiratory alkalosis			
Acute	$\downarrow P_{CO_2}$	$\downarrow HCO_3^-$	$\downarrow HCO_3^-$ 2 mEq/L per 10 mm Hg $\downarrow P_{CO_2}$
Chronic	$\downarrow P_{CO_2}$	$\downarrow HCO_3^-$	$\downarrow HCO_3^-$ 5 mEq/L per 10 mm Hg $\downarrow P_{CO_2}$
Metabolic acidosis	$\downarrow HCO_3^-$	$\downarrow P_{CO_2}$	$\downarrow P_{CO_2}$ 1.3 mm Hg per 1 mEq/L $\downarrow HCO_3^-$
Metabolic alkalosis	$\uparrow HCO_3^-$	$\uparrow P_{CO_2}$	$\uparrow P_{CO_2}$ 0.7 mm Hg per 1 mEq/L $\uparrow HCO_3^-$

Step-by-Step Analysis of Acid-Base Status). Once the primary disturbance has been determined, the clinician should assess whether the compensatory response is appropriate (Table 21–12). An inadequate or an exaggerated response indicates the presence of another primary acid-base disturbance.

The anion gap should always be calculated for two reasons. First, it is possible to have an abnormal anion gap even if the sodium, chloride, and bicarbonate levels are normal. Second, a large anion gap (> 20) suggests a primary metabolic acid-base disturbance regardless of the pH or serum bicarbonate level because a markedly abnormal anion gap is never a compensatory response to a respiratory disorder. In patients with an increased anion gap metabolic acidosis, clinicians should calculate the corrected bicarbonate. In increased anion gap acidoses, there should be a mole for mole decrease in HCO_3^- as the anion gap increases. A corrected HCO_3^- value higher or lower than normal (24 mEq/L) indicates the concomitant presence of metabolic alkalosis or normal anion gap metabolic acidosis, respectively.

Herd AM. An approach to complex acid-base problems: keeping it simple. Can Fam Physician. 2005 Feb;51:226–32. [PMID: 15751566]
Kellum JA. Disorders of acid-base balance. Crit Care Med. 2008 Nov;35(11):2630–6. [PMID: 17893626]
Whittier WL et al. Primer on clinical acid-base problem solving. Dis Mon. 2004 Mar;50(3):122–62. [PMID: 15069420]

METABOLIC ACIDOSIS

ESSENTIALS OF DIAGNOSIS

▶ Decreased HCO_3^- with acidemia.

▶ Classified into increased anion gap acidosis and normal anion gap acidosis.

▶ Lactic acidosis, ketoacidosis, and toxins produce metabolic acidoses with the largest anion gaps.

▶ Normal anion gap acidosis is mainly caused by gastrointestinal HCO_3^- loss or RTA. Urinary anion gap may help distinguish between these causes.

▶ General Considerations

The hallmark of metabolic acidosis is decreased HCO_3^-. Metabolic acidoses are classified by the anion gap, either normal or increased (Table 21–13). The anion gap represents the difference between readily measured anions and cations.

In plasma,

$$Na^+ + \underset{\text{cations}}{\text{Unmeasured}} = HCO_3^- + Cl^- + \underset{\text{anions}}{\text{Unmeasured}}$$

$$\text{Anion gap} = Na^+ - (HCO_3^- + Cl^-)$$

Major unmeasured cations are calcium (1 mEq/L), magnesium (2 mEq/L), γ-globulins, and potassium (4 mEq/L). Major unmeasured anions are albumin (2 mEq/L per g/dL), phosphate (2 mEq/L), sulfate (1 mEq/L), lactate (1–2 mEq/L), and other organic anions (3–4 mEq/L). Traditionally, the normal anion gap has been 12 ± 4 mEq/L. With current autoanalyzers, the reference range may be lower (6 ± 1 mEq/L), primarily from an increase in Cl^- values. Despite its usefulness, the anion gap can be misleading. Non-acid–base disorders may cause errors in anion gap interpretation; these disorders include hypoalbuminemia, hypernatremia, or

STEP-BY-STEP ANALYSIS OF ACID-BASE STATUS

Step 1: Determine the primary (or main) disorder—whether it is metabolic or respiratory—from blood, pH, HCO_3^-, and P_{CO_2} values.

Step 2: Determine the presence of mixed acid-base disorders by calculating the range of compensatory responses (Table 21–12).

Step 3: Calculate the anion gap (Table 21–13).

Step 4: Calculate the corrected HCO_3^- concentration if the anion gap is increased (see above).

Step 5: Examine the patient to determine whether the clinical signs are compatible with the acid-base analysis thus obtained.

Table 21–13. Anion gap in metabolic acidosis.[1]

Decreased (< 6 mEq)
  Hypoalbuminemia (decreased unmeasured anion)
  Plasma cell dyscrasias
    Monoclonal protein (cationic paraprotein) (accompanied by
    chloride and bicarbonate)
  Bromide intoxication
Increased (> 12 mEq)
  Metabolic anion
    Diabetic ketoacidosis
    Alcoholic ketoacidosis
    Lactic acidosis
    Chronic kidney disease (advanced stages) (PO_4^{3-}, SO_4^{2-})
    Starvation
    Metabolic alkalosis (increased number of negative charges on
    protein)
  Drug or chemical anion
    Salicylate intoxication
    Sodium carbenicillin therapy
    Methanol (formic acid)
    Ethylene glycol (oxalic acid)
Normal (6–12 mEq)
  Loss of HCO_3^-
    Diarrhea
    Recovery from diabetic ketoacidosis
    Pancreatic fluid loss ileostomy (unadapted)
    Carbonic anhydrase inhibitors
  Chloride retention
    Renal tubular acidosis
    Ileal loop bladder
  Administration of HCl equivalent or NH_4Cl
    Arginine and lysine in parenteral nutrition

[1]Reference ranges for anion gap may vary based on differing laboratory methods.

hyponatremia; antibiotics (eg, carbenicillin is an unmeasured anion; polymyxin is an unmeasured cation) may also cause errors in anion gap interpretation. Although not usually associated with metabolic acidosis, a decreased anion gap can occur because of a reduction in unmeasured anions or an increase in unmeasured cations. In hypoalbuminemia, a 2 mEq/L decrease in anion gap will occur for every 1 g/dL decline in serum albumin.

INCREASED ANION GAP ACIDOSIS (Increased Unmeasured Anions)

Normochloremic metabolic acidosis generally results from addition of organic acids such as lactate, acetoacetate, β-hydroxybutyrate, and exogenous toxins. Other anions such as isocitrate, alpha-ketoglutarate, malate and D-lactate, may contribute to the anion gap of lactic acidosis, diabetic ketoacidosis, and acidosis of unknown etiology. Uremia produces an increased anion gap metabolic acidosis via unexcreted organic acids and anions.

A. Lactic Acidosis

Lactic acid is formed from pyruvate in anaerobic glycolysis, typically in tissues with high rates of glycolysis, such as gut (responsible for over 50% of lactate production), skeletal

muscle, brain, skin, and erythrocytes. Normally, lactate levels remain low (1 mEq/L) because of metabolism of lactate principally by the liver through gluconeogenesis or oxidation via the Krebs cycle. Furthermore, the kidneys metabolize about 30% of lactate.

In lactic acidosis, lactate levels are at least 4–5 mEq/L but commonly 10–30 mEq/L. There are two basic types of lactic acidosis. Type A is characterized by hypoxia or decreased tissue perfusion. Type B has no clinical evidence of hypoxia.

Type A (hypoxic) lactic acidosis is more common, resulting from decreased tissue perfusion; cardiogenic, septic, or hemorrhagic shock; and carbon monoxide or cyanide poisoning. These conditions increase peripheral lactic acid production and decrease hepatic metabolism of lactate as liver perfusion declines.

Type B lactic acidosis may be due to metabolic causes (eg, diabetes, ketoacidosis, liver disease, kidney disease, infection, leukemia, or lymphoma) or toxins (eg, ethanol, methanol, salicylates, isoniazid, or metformin). Propylene glycol can cause lactic acidosis from decreased liver metabolism; it is used as a vehicle for intravenous agents, such as nitroglycerin, etomidate, and diazepam. Parenteral nutrition without thiamine causes severe refractory lactic acidosis from the deranged metabolism of pyruvate. Patients with short bowel syndrome may develop D-lactic acidosis with encephalopathy due to carbohydrate malabsorption and subsequent fermentation by colonic bacteria.

AIDS without AIDS-related lymphoma is associated with type B lactic acidosis. Nucleoside analog reverse transcriptase inhibitors can cause lactic acidosis due to mitochondrial toxicity.

Idiopathic lactic acidosis, usually in debilitated patients, has an extremely high mortality rate. (For treatment of lactic acidosis, see below and Chapter 27.)

B. Diabetic Ketoacidosis

This metabolic abnormality is characterized by hyperglycemia and metabolic acidosis (pH < 7.25 or plasma bicarbonate < 16 mEq/L). Anion gap metabolic acidosis is the acid–base disturbance generally ascribed to diabetic ketoacidosis:

$$H^+ + B^- + NaHCO_3 \leftrightarrow CO_2 + NaB + H_2O$$

where B^- is β-hydroxybutyrate or acetoacetate, the ketones responsible for the increased anion gap. The anion gap should be calculated from the serum electrolytes as measured; correction of the serum sodium for the dilutional effect of hyperglycemia will exaggerate the anion gap. Diabetics with ketoacidosis may have lactic acidosis from tissue hypoperfusion and increased anaerobic metabolism.

During the recovery phase of diabetic ketoacidosis, a hyperchloremic non-anion gap acidosis can develop because saline resuscitation results in chloride retention, restoration of GFR, and ketoaciduria. Ketone salts (NaB) are formed as bicarbonate is consumed:

$$HB + NaHCO_3 \rightarrow NaB + H_2CO_3$$

The kidney reabsorbs ketone anions poorly but can compensate for the loss of anions by increasing the reabsorption of Cl^-.

Patients with diabetic ketoacidosis and normal kidney function may have marked ketonuria and severe metabolic acidosis but only a mildly increased anion gap. Thus, the size of the anion gap correlates poorly with the severity of the diabetic ketoacidosis; the urinary loss of Na^+ or K^+ salts of β-hydroxybutyrate will lower the anion gap without altering the H^+ excretion or the severity of the acidosis. Urine dipsticks for ketones test primarily for acetoacetate and, to a lesser degree, acetone but do not detect the predominant ketoacid, β-hydroxybutyrate. Dipstick tests for ketones may become more positive even as the patient improves due to the metabolism of hydroxybutyrate. Thus, the patient's clinical status and pH are better markers of improvement than the anion gap or ketone levels.

C. Alcoholic Ketoacidosis

This is a common disorder of chronically malnourished patients who consume large quantities of alcohol daily. Most of these patients have mixed acid–base disorders (10% have a triple acid–base disorder). Although decreased HCO_3^- is usual, 50% of the patients may have normal or alkalemic pH. Three types of metabolic acidosis are seen in alcoholic ketoacidosis: (1) Ketoacidosis is due to β-hydroxybutyrate and acetoacetate excess. (2) Lactic acidosis: Alcohol metabolism increases the NADH:NAD ratio, causing increased production and decreased utilization of lactate. Accompanying thiamine deficiency, which inhibits pyruvate carboxylase, further enhances lactic acid production in many cases. Moderate to severe elevations of lactate (> 6 mmol/L) are seen with concomitant disorders such as sepsis, pancreatitis, or hypoglycemia. (3) Hyperchloremic acidosis from bicarbonate loss in the urine is associated with ketonuria (see above). Metabolic alkalosis occurs from volume contraction and vomiting. Respiratory alkalosis results from alcohol withdrawal, pain, or associated disorders such

as sepsis or liver disease. Half of the patients have either hypoglycemia or hyperglycemia. When serum glucose levels are greater than 250 mg/dL, the distinction from diabetic ketoacidosis is difficult. The absence of a diabetic history and normoglycemia after initial therapy support the diagnosis of alcoholic ketoacidosis.

D. Toxins

(See also Chapter 38.) Multiple toxins and drugs increase the anion gap by increasing endogenous acid production. Common examples include methanol (metabolized to formic acid), ethylene glycol (glycolic and oxalic acid), and salicylates (salicylic acid and lactic acid). The latter can cause a mixed disorder of metabolic acidosis with respiratory alkalosis. In toluene poisoning, a metabolite hippurate is rapidly excreted by the kidney and may present as a normal anion gap acidosis. Isopropyl alcohol, which is metabolized to acetone, increases the osmolar gap, but not the anion gap.

E. Uremic Acidosis

As the GFR drops below 15–30 mL/min, the kidneys are increasingly unable to excrete H+ and organic acids, such phosphate and sulfate, resulting in an increased anion gap acidosis. Hyperchloremic normal anion gap acidosis develops in earlier stages of CKD.

NORMAL ANION GAP ACIDOSIS (Table 21–14)

The most common causes are gastrointestinal HCO_3^- loss and defects in renal acidification (renal tubular acidoses). The urinary anion gap can differentiate between these causes (see below).

A. Gastrointestinal HCO_3^- Loss

Bicarbonate is secreted at multiple sites in the gastrointestinal tract. Small bowel and pancreatic secretions contain

Table 21–14. Hyperchloremic, normal anion gap metabolic acidoses.

| | | | Distal H⁺ Secretion | | | |
	Renal Defect	Serum [K^+]	Urinary NH_4^+ Plus Minimal Urine pH	Titratable Acid	Urinary Anion Gap	Treatment
Gastrointestinal HCO_3^- loss	None	↓	< 5.5	↑↑	Negative	Na^+, K^+, and HCO_3^- as required
Renal tubular acidosis						
I. Classic distal	Distal H⁺ secretion	↓	> 5.5	↓	Positive	$NaHCO_3$ (1–3 mEq/kg/d)
II. Proximal secretion	Proximal H⁺	↓	< 5.5	Normal	Positive	$NaHCO_3$ or $KHCO_3$ (10–15 mEq/kg/d), thiazide
IV. Hyporeninemic hypoaldosteronism	Distal Na^+ reabsorption, K^+ secretion, and H⁺ secretion	↑	< 5.5	↓	Positive	Fludrocortisone (0.1–0.5 mg/d), dietary K^+ restriction, furosemide (40–160 mg/d), $NaHCO_3$ (1–3 mEq/kg/d)

Modified and reproduced, with permission, from Cogan MG. *Fluid and Electrolytes: Physiology and Pathophysiology.* McGraw-Hill, 1991.

large amounts of HCO_3^-; massive diarrhea or pancreatic drainage can result in HCO_3^- loss. Hyperchloremia occurs because the ileum and colon secrete HCO_3^- in exchange for Cl^- by countertransport. The resultant volume contraction causes increased Cl^- retention by the kidney in the setting of decreased HCO_3^-. Patients with ureterosigmoidostomies can develop hyperchloremic metabolic acidosis because the colon secretes HCO_3^- in the urine in exchange for Cl^-.

B. Renal Tubular Acidosis (RTA)

Hyperchloremic acidosis with a normal anion gap and normal (or near normal) GFR, and in the absence of diarrhea, defines RTA. The defect is either inability to excrete H^+ (inadequate generation of new HCO_3^-) or inappropriate reabsorption of HCO_3^-. Three major types can be differentiated by the clinical setting, urinary pH, urinary anion gap (see below), and serum K^+ level. Recently, the pathophysiologic mechanisms of RTA have been elucidated by identifying the responsible molecules and their gene mutations.

1. Classic distal RTA (type I)—This disorder is characterized by hypokalemic hyperchloremic metabolic acidosis due to selective deficiency in H^+ secretion in α intercalated cells in the collecting tubule. Despite acidosis, urinary pH cannot be acidified and is above 5.5, which retards the binding of H^+ to phosphate ($H^+ + HPO_4^{2-} \rightarrow H_2PO_4$) and inhibits titratable acid excretion. Furthermore, urinary excretion of $NH_4^+Cl^-$ is decreased, and the urinary anion gap is positive (see below). Enhanced K^+ excretion occurs probably because there is less competition from H^+ in the distal nephron transport system. Furthermore, hyperaldosteronism occurs in response to renal salt wasting, which will increase potassium excretion. Nephrocalcinosis and nephrolithiasis are often seen in patients with distal RTA since chronic acidosis decreases tubular calcium reabsorption. Hypercalciuria, alkaline urine, and lowered level of urinary citrate cause calcium phosphate stones and nephrocalcinosis.

Distal RTA develops as a consequence of dysproteinemic syndromes, autoimmune disease, and drugs and toxins such as amphotericin.

2. Proximal RTA (type II)—Proximal RTA is a hypokalemic hyperchloremic metabolic acidosis due to a selective defect in the proximal tubule's ability to reabsorb filtered HCO_3^-. Carbonic anhydrase inhibitors (acetazolamide) can cause proximal RTA. About 90% of filtered HCO_3^- is absorbed by the proximal tubule. A proximal defect in HCO_3^- reabsorption will overwhelm the limited capacity of the distal tubule to reabsorb HCO_3^-, resulting in bicarbonaturia and metabolic acidosis. Distal delivery of HCO_3^- declines as the plasma HCO_3^- level decreases. When the plasma HCO_3^- level drops to 15–18 mEq/L, the distal nephron can reabsorb the diminished filtered load of HCO_3^-. Bicarbonaturia disappears, and urinary pH can be acidic. Thiazide-induced volume contraction can be used to enhance proximal HCO_3^- reabsorption, leading to the decrease in distal HCO_3^- delivery and improvement of bicarbonaturia and renal acidification. The increased delivery of HCO_3^- to the distal nephron also increases K^+ secretion, and hypokalemia results if a patient is loaded

with excess HCO_3^- and K^+ is not adequately supplemented. Proximal RTA often exists with other defects of absorption in the proximal tubule, resulting in glucosuria, aminoaciduria, phosphaturia, and uricaciduria. Causes include multiple myeloma with Fanconi syndrome and nephrotoxic drugs.

3. Hyporeninemic hypoaldosteronemic RTA (type IV)—Type IV is the most common RTA in clinical practice. The defect is aldosterone deficiency or antagonism, which impairs distal nephron Na^+ reabsorption and K^+ and H^+ excretion. Renal salt wasting and hyperkalemia are frequently present. Common causes are diabetic nephropathy, tubulointerstitial renal diseases, hypertensive nephrosclerosis, and AIDS. In patients with these disorders, caution must be taken when prescribing drugs that can exacerbate the hyperkalemia, such as ACE inhibitors (which will further reduce aldosterone levels), aldosterone receptor blockers such as spironolactone, and NSAIDs.

C. Dilutional Acidosis

Rapid dilution of plasma volume by 0.9% NaCl may cause a mild hyperchloremic acidosis.

D. Recovery from Diabetic Ketoacidosis

See earlier section, Increased Anion Gap Acidosis (Increased Unmeasured Anion).

E. Posthypocapnia

In prolonged respiratory alkalosis, HCO_3^- decreases and Cl^- increases from decreased renal $NH_4^+Cl^-$ excretion. If the respiratory alkalosis is corrected quickly, PCO_2 will increase acutely but HCO_3^- will remain low until the kidneys can generate new HCO_3^-, which generally takes several days. In the meantime, the increased PCO_2 with low HCO_3^- causes metabolic acidosis.

F. Hyperalimentation

Hyperalimentation fluids may contain amino acid solutions that acidify when metabolized, such as arginine hydrochloride and lysine hydrochloride.

▶ Assessment of Hyperchloremic Metabolic Acidosis by Urinary Anion Gap

Increased renal $NH_4^+Cl^-$ excretion to enhance H^+ removal is a normal physiologic response to metabolic acidosis. NH_3 reacts with H^+ to form NH_4^+, which is accompanied by the anion Cl^- for excretion. The normal daily urinary excretion of NH_4Cl of about 30 mEq can be increased up to 200 mEq in response to acid load.

Urinary anion gap from a random urine sample ($[Na^+ + K^+] - Cl^-$) reflects the ability of the kidney to excrete NH_4Cl as in the following equation:

$$Na^+ + K^+ + NH^{4+} = Cl^- + 80$$

where 80 is the average value for the difference in the urinary anions and cations other than Na^+, K^+, NH_4^+, and

Cl. Therefore, urinary anion gap is equal to $(80 - NH_4^+)$, and thus aids in the distinction between gastrointestinal and renal causes of hyperchloremic acidosis. If the cause of the metabolic acidosis is gastrointestinal HCO_3^- loss (diarrhea), the renal acidification ability remains normal and NH_4Cl excretion increases in response to the acidosis. The urinary anion gap is negative (eg, –30 mEq/L). If the cause is distal RTA, the urinary anion gap is positive (eg, +25 mEq/L), since the basic lesion in the disorder is the inability of the kidney to excrete H^+ and thus the inability to increase NH_4Cl excretion. In proximal (type II) RTA, the kidney has defective HCO_3^- reabsorption, leading to increased HCO_3^- excretion rather than decreased NH_4Cl excretion. Thus, the urinary anion gap is often negative in proximal (type II) RTA.

Urinary pH may not as readily differentiate between the two causes. Despite acidosis, if volume depletion from diarrhea causes inadequate Na^+ delivery to the distal nephron and therefore decreased exchange with H^+, urinary pH may not be lower than 5.3. In the presence of this relatively high urine pH, however, H^+ excretion continues due to buffering of NH_3 to NH_4^+, since the pK of this reaction is as high as 9.1. Potassium depletion, which can accompany diarrhea (and surreptitious laxative abuse), may also impair renal acidification. Thus, when volume depletion is present, the urinary anion gap is a better measurement of ability to acidify the urine than urinary pH.

When large amounts of other anions are present in the urine, the urinary anion gap may not be reliable. In such a situation, NH_4^+ excretion can be estimated using the urinary osmolar gap.

$$NH_4^+ \text{ excretion (mmol/L)} =$$
$$0.5 \times \text{Urinary osmolar gap} =$$
$$0.5 [U \text{ osm} - 2(U Na^+ + U K^+) + U \text{ urea} + U \text{ glucose}]$$

where urinary (U) concentrations and osmolality are in millimoles per liter.

▶ Clinical Findings

A. Symptoms and Signs

Symptoms of metabolic acidosis are mainly those of the underlying disorder. Compensatory hyperventilation is an important clinical sign and may be misinterpreted as a primary respiratory disorder; when severe, Kussmaul respirations (deep, regular, sighing respirations) are seen.

B. Laboratory Findings

Blood pH, serum HCO_3^-, and P_{CO_2} are decreased. Anion gap may be normal (hyperchloremic) or increased (normochloremic). Hyperkalemia may be seen (see above).

▶ Treatment

A. Increased Anion Gap Acidosis

Treatment is aimed at the underlying disorder, such as insulin and fluid therapy for diabetes and appropriate volume resuscitation to restore tissue perfusion. The metabolism of lactate will produce HCO_3^- and increase pH. The use of supplemental HCO_3^- is indicated for treatment of hyperkalemia (Table 21–6) and some forms of normal anion gap acidosis but has been controversial for treatment of increased anion gap metabolic acidosis.

Controversy remains about the efficacy and safety of alkali therapy for severe metabolic acidosis. Administration of large amounts of HCO_3^- may have deleterious effects, including hypernatremia, hyperosmolality, volume overload, and worsening of intracellular acidosis.

In addition, alkali administration is known to stimulate phosphofructokinase activity, thus exacerbating lactic acidosis via enhanced lactate production. Ketogenesis is also augmented by alkali therapy.

In salicylate intoxication, alkali therapy must be started unless blood pH is already alkalinized by respiratory alkalosis, since the increment in pH converts salicylate to more impermeable salicylic acid, decreasing central nervous system damage. In alcoholic ketoacidosis, thiamine should be given with glucose to avoid the development of Wernicke encephalopathy. The amount of HCO_3^- deficit can be calculated as follows:

$$\text{Amount of HCO}_3^- \text{ deficit} =$$
$$0.5 \times \text{body weight} \times (24 - HCO_3^-)$$

Half of the calculated deficit should be administered within the first 3–4 hours to avoid overcorrection and volume overload. In methanol intoxication, ethanol had been used as a competitive substrate for alcohol dehydrogenase, which metabolizes methanol to formaldehyde. Inhibition of alcohol dehydrogenase by fomepizole is the standard of care.

B. Normal Anion Gap Acidosis

Treatment of RTA is mainly achieved by administration of alkali (either as bicarbonate or citrate) to correct metabolic abnormalities and prevent nephrocalcinosis and chronic kidney disease.

Large amounts of alkali (10–15 mEq/kg/d) may be required to treat proximal RTA because most of the alkali is excreted into the urine, which exacerbates hypokalemia. Thus, a mixture of sodium and potassium salts is preferred. The addition of thiazides may reduce the amount of alkali required, but hypokalemia may develop. Correction of type 1 distal RTA requires a smaller amount of alkali (1–3 mEq/kg/d) and potassium supplementation as needed.

For the treatment of type IV RTA, dietary potassium restriction may be needed and potassium-retaining drugs should be withdrawn. Fludrocortisone may be effective in cases with hypoaldosteronism, but should be used with care, preferably in combination with loop diuretics. In some cases, alkali supplementation (1–3 mEq/kg/d) may be required.

▶ When to Refer

Most clinicians will refer patients with renal tubular acidoses to a nephrologist for evaluation and possible alkali therapy.

When to Admit

Patients will require emergency department evaluation or hospital admission depending on the severity of the acidosis and underlying conditions.

Adrogue HJ. Metabolic acidosis: pathophysiology, diagnosis and management. J Nephrol. 2006 Mar–Apr;19(Suppl 9):S62–9. [PMID: 16736443]

Casaletto JJ. Differential diagnosis of metabolic acidosis. Emerg Med Clin North Am 2005 Aug;23(3):771–87. [PMID: 15982545]

Eledrisi MS et al. Overview of the diagnosis and management of diabetic ketoacidosis. Am J Med Sci. 2006 May;331(5):243–51. [PMID: 16702793]

Kraut JA et al. Serum anion gap. Clin J Am Soc Nephrol. 2007 Jan;2(1):162–74. [PMID: 17699401]

Morris CG et al. Metabolic acidosis in the critically ill: part 1. Classification and pathophysiology. Anesthesia. 2008 Mar; 63(3):294–301. [PMID: 18289237]

Morris CG et al. Metabolic acidosis in the critically ill: part 2. Causes and treatment. Anesthesia. 2008 Apr;63(4):396–411. [PMID: 18336491]

Rosival V. Metabolic acidosis. Crit Care Med. 2004 Dec;32(12): 2563–4. [PMID: 15599180]

METABOLIC ALKALOSIS

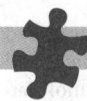

ESSENTIALS OF DIAGNOSIS

▶ High HCO_3^- with alkalemia.

▶ Evaluate effective circulating volume by physical examination and check urinary chloride concentration to differentiate saline-responsive metabolic alkalosis from saline-unresponsive alkalosis.

Classification

Metabolic alkalosis is characterized by high HCO_3^-. Abnormalities that generate HCO_3^- within the body are called "initiation factors" of metabolic alkalosis, whereas abnormalities that promote renal conservation of HCO_3^- are called "maintenance factors." Metabolic alkalosis may remain even after the initiation factors have disappeared.

It is useful to classify the causes of metabolic alkalosis into two groups based on "saline responsiveness" or urinary Cl^-, which are markers for volume status (Table 21–15). Saline-responsive metabolic alkalosis is a sign of extracellular volume contraction, and saline-unresponsive alkalosis implies a volume-expanded state. It is rare for a compensatory increase in P_{CO_2} to exceed 55 mm Hg. Higher P_{CO_2} values imply a superimposed respiratory acidosis.

A. Saline-Responsive Metabolic Alkalosis

Much more common than saline-unresponsive alkalosis, saline-responsive alkalosis is characterized by normotensive extracellular volume contraction and hypokalemia. Less frequently, hypotension or orthostatic hypotension may be seen. In vomiting or nasogastric suction, for example, loss of acid (HCl) initiates the alkalosis, but volume contraction from loss of Cl^- sustains the alkalosis because the decline in GFR causes avid renal Na^+ and HCO_3^- reabsorption. Because there is Cl^- depletion from loss of HCl, NaCl, and KCl from the stomach, the available anion is HCO_3^-, whose reabsorption is increased proximally, and urine pH may remain acidic despite alkalemia (paradoxic aciduria). Renal Cl^- reabsorption (as well as Na^+ reabsorption) is high, and the urinary Cl^- is therefore low (< 10–20 mEq/L). In alkalosis, bicarbonaturia may force Na^+ excretion as the accompanying cation even if volume depletion is present. Therefore, urinary Cl^- is preferred to urinary Na^+ as a

Table 21–15. Metabolic alkalosis.

Saline-Responsive (U_{Cl} < 25 mEq/L)	Saline-Unresponsive (U_{Cl} > 40 mEq/L)
Excessive body bicarbonate content	**Excessive body bicarbonate content**
Renal alkalosis	Renal alkalosis
Diuretic therapy	Normotensive
Poorly reabsorbable anion therapy: carbenicillin, penicillin, sulfate, phosphate	Bartter syndrome (renal salt wasting and secondary hyperaldosteronism)
Posthypercapnia	Severe potassium depletion
Gastrointestinal alkalosis	Refeeding alkalosis
Loss of HCl from vomiting or nasogastric suction	Hypercalcemia and hypoparathyroidism
Intestinal alkalosis: chloride diarrhea	Hypertensive
NaHCO₃ (baking soda)	Endogenous mineralocorticoids
Sodium citrate, lactate, gluconate, acetate	Primary aldosteronism
Transfusions	Hyperreninism
Antacids	Adrenal enzyme deficiency: 11- and 17-hydroxylase
Normal body bicarbonate content	Liddle syndrome
"Contraction alkalosis"	Exogenous alkali
	Exogenous mineralocorticoids
	Licorice

Modified and reproduced, with permission, from Narins RG et al. Diagnostic strategies in disorders of fluid, electrolyte and acid-base homeostasis. Am J Med. 1982 Mar;72(3):496–520.

measure of extracellular volume. An exception to the usefulness of urinary Cl⁻ is in patients who have recently received diuretics. Their urine may contain high Na^+ and Cl^- despite extracellular volume contraction. If diuretics are discontinued, the urinary Cl^- will decrease.

Metabolic alkalosis is generally associated with hypokalemia. This is due partly to the direct effect of alkalosis per se on renal potassium excretion and partly to secondary hyperaldosteronism from volume depletion. Hypokalemia induced in this fashion further worsens the metabolic alkalosis by increasing bicarbonate reabsorption in the proximal tubule and hydrogen ion secretion in the distal tubule. Administration of KCl will correct the disorder. Repletion of KCl is important to reverse the disorder.

1. Contraction alkalosis—Diuretics can quickly decrease extracellular volume from urinary loss of NaCl and water. There is no associated bicarbonaturia, so total body HCO_3^- remains normal. The plasma HCO_3^- concentration increases because the extracellular fluid volume contracts around a stable total body bicarbonate. This process is the reverse of a dilutional acidosis.

2. Posthypercapnia alkalosis—In chronic respiratory acidosis, compensatory increases in HCO_3^- occur (Table 21–12). Hypercapnia also directly affects the proximal tubule to decrease NaCl reabsorption, which can cause extracellular volume depletion. If P_{CO_2} is corrected rapidly, metabolic alkalosis will exist until adequate renal bicarbonate excretion occurs. Hypovolemia will inhibit bicarbonaturia until Cl^- is repleted. Many patients with chronic respiratory acidosis receive diuretics, which further exacerbates the metabolic alkalosis.

B. Saline-Unresponsive Alkalosis

1. Hyperaldosteronism—Primary hyperaldosteronism causes expansion of extracellular volume with hypertension. Metabolic alkalosis with hypokalemia results from the renal mineralocorticoid effect. In an attempt to decrease extracellular volume, high levels of NaCl are excreted, and for that reason the urinary Cl^- is high (> 20 mEq/L, often higher). Therapy with NaCl will only increase volume expansion and hypertension and will not treat the underlying problem of mineralocorticoid excess.

2. Alkali administration with decreased GFR—Despite large ingestions of HCO_3^-, enhanced bicarbonaturia almost always prevents a patient with normal kidney function from developing metabolic alkalosis. However, urinary excretion of bicarbonate is inadequate with CKD. If large amounts of HCO_3^- or metabolizable salts of organic acids such as sodium lactate, sodium citrate, or sodium gluconate are consumed, as with intensive antacid therapy, metabolic alkalosis will occur. In milk-alkali syndrome, large and sustained ingestion of absorbable antacids and milk causes CKD from hypercalcemia. Decreased GFR prevents appropriate bicarbonaturia from the ingested alkali, and metabolic alkalosis occurs. Volume contraction from renal hypercalcemic effects further exacerbates the alkalosis.

► **Clinical Findings**

A. Symptoms and Signs

There are no characteristic symptoms or signs. Orthostatic hypotension may be encountered. Weakness and hyporeflexia occur if serum K^+ is markedly low. Tetany and neuromuscular irritability occur rarely.

B. Laboratory Findings

The arterial blood pH and bicarbonate are elevated. The arterial P_{CO_2} is increased. Serum potassium and chloride are decreased. There may be an increased anion gap. The spot urinary chloride can differentiate between a saline-responsive (< 25 mEq/L) and unresponsive (> 40 mEq/L) disorder.

► **Treatment**

Mild alkalosis is generally well tolerated. Severe or symptomatic alkalosis (pH > 7.60) requires urgent treatment.

A. Saline-Responsive Metabolic Alkalosis

Therapy for saline-responsive metabolic alkalosis is correction of the extracellular volume deficit with isotonic saline. Diuretics should be discontinued. H_2-blockers or proton pump inhibitors may be helpful in patients with alkalosis from nasogastric suctioning. If pulmonary or cardiovascular disease prohibits adequate resuscitation, intravenous acetazolamide will increase renal bicarbonate excretion and improve the metabolic alkalosis. Hypokalemia may develop because bicarbonate excretion may induce kaliuresis. Severe cases, especially those with impaired kidney function, may require dialysis with low-bicarbonate dialysate.

B. Saline-Unresponsive Metabolic Alkalosis

Therapy for saline-unresponsive metabolic alkalosis includes surgical removal of a mineralocorticoid-producing tumor and blockage of aldosterone effect with an ACE inhibitor or with spironolactone. Metabolic alkalosis in primary aldosteronism can be treated only with potassium repletion.

Khanna A et al. Metabolic alkalosis. J Nephrol. 2006 Mar–Apr;19(Suppl 9):S86–96. [PMID: 16736446]

RESPIRATORY ACIDOSIS (HYPERCAPNIA)

Respiratory acidosis results from hypoventilation and subsequent hypercapnia. Pulmonary and extrapulmonary disorders can cause hypoventilation. The clinician should identify readily reversible causes of respiratory acidosis, such as opioid-induced respiratory depression.

Acute respiratory failure is associated with severe acidosis and only a small increase in the plasma bicarbonate. After 6–12 hours, the primary increase in P_{CO_2} evokes a renal compensatory response to excrete more acid and to generate more HCO_3^-, which buffers the respiratory acidosis; complete metabolic compensation by the kidney usually takes several days.

Chronic respiratory acidosis is generally seen in patients with underlying lung disease, such as chronic obstructive pulmonary disease. Urinary excretion of acid in the form of NH_4^+ and Cl^- ions results in the characteristic hypochloremia of chronic respiratory acidosis. When chronic respiratory acidosis is corrected suddenly, there is a 2- to 3-day lag in renal bicarbonate excretion, resulting in posthypercapnic metabolic alkalosis.

▶ Clinical Findings

A. Symptoms and Signs

With acute onset, somnolence, confusion, mental status changes, asterixis, and myoclonus may develop. Severe hypercapnia increases cerebral blood flow, cerebrospinal fluid pressure, and intracranial pressure; papilledema and pseudotumor cerebri may be seen.

B. Laboratory Findings

Arterial pH is low and P_{CO_2} is increased. Serum HCO_3^- is elevated but does not compensate for the hypercapnia or correct the pH. If the disorder is chronic, hypochloremia is seen.

▶ Treatment

If opioid overdose is a possible diagnosis or there is no other obvious cause for hypoventilation, the clinician should consider a diagnostic and therapeutic trial of intravenous naloxone (see Chapter 38). In all forms of respiratory acidosis, treatment is directed at the underlying disorder to improve ventilation.

Epstein SK et al. Respiratory acidosis. Respir Care. 2001 Apr;46 (4):366–83. [PMID: 11262556]
Madias NE et al. Cross-talk between two organs: how the kidney responds to disruption of acid–base balance by the lung. Nephron Physiol. 2003;93(3):61–6. [PMID: 12660492]

RESPIRATORY ALKALOSIS (HYPOCAPNIA)

Respiratory alkalosis occurs when hyperventilation reduces the P_{CO_2}, increasing serum pH. The most common cause of respiratory alkalosis is hyperventilation syndrome (Table 21–16), but bacterial septicemia and cirrhosis are other common causes. Symptoms in acute respiratory alkalosis are related to decreased cerebral blood flow induced by the disorder. Pregnancy is another cause of chronic respiratory alkalosis, probably from progesterone stimulation of the respiratory center, producing an average P_{CO_2} of 30 mm Hg.

Determination of appropriate metabolic compensation in the serum HCO_3^- may reveal an associated metabolic disorder (see above under Mixed Acid–Base Disorders).

As in respiratory acidosis, the changes in HCO_3^- values are greater if the respiratory alkalosis is chronic (Table 21–12). Although serum HCO_3^- is frequently below 15 mEq/L in metabolic acidosis, it is unusual to see such a low level in respiratory alkalosis, and its presence would imply a superimposed (noncompensatory) metabolic acidosis.

Table 21–16. Causes of respiratory alkalosis.

Hypoxia
    Decreased inspired oxygen tension
    High altitude
    Ventilation/perfusion inequality
    Hypotension
    Severe anemia
CNS-mediated disorders
    Voluntary hyperventilation
    Anxiety-hyperventilation syndrome
    Neurologic disease
    Cerebrovascular accident (infarction, hemorrhage)
    Infection
    Trauma
    Tumor
    Pharmacologic and hormonal stimulation
        Salicylates
        Nicotine
        Xanthines
        Pregnancy (progesterone)
    Hepatic failure
    Gram-negative septicemia
    Recovery from metabolic acidosis
    Heat exposure
Pulmonary disease
    Interstitial lung disease
    Pneumonia
    Pulmonary embolism
    Pulmonary edema
Mechanical overventilation

Adapted, with permission, from Gennari FJ. Respiratory acidosis and alkalosis. In: *Maxwell and Kleeman's Clinical Disorders of Fluid and Electrolyte Metabolism*, 5th ed. Narins RG (editor). McGraw-Hill, 1994.

▶ Clinical Findings

A. Symptoms and Signs

In acute cases (hyperventilation), there is light-headedness, anxiety, perioral numbness, and paresthesias. Tetany occurs in more severe alkalosis from a fall in ionized calcium.

B. Laboratory Findings

Arterial blood pH is elevated, and P_{CO_2} is low. Serum bicarbonate is decreased in chronic respiratory alkalosis.

▶ Treatment

Treatment is directed toward the underlying cause. In acute hyperventilation syndrome from anxiety, the traditional treatment of breathing into a paper bag should be discouraged because it does not correct the P_{CO_2} and may decrease the P_{O_2}. Reassurance may be sufficient for the anxious patient, but sedation may be necessary if the process persists. Hyperventilation is usually self-limited since muscle weakness caused by the respiratory alkalemia will suppress ventilation. Rapid correction of chronic respiratory alkalosis may result in metabolic acidosis as P_{CO_2} is increased in the setting of a previous compensatory decrease in HCO_3^-.

Table 21–17. Replacement guidelines for sweat and gastrointestinal fluid losses.

	Average Electrolyte Composition				Replacement Guidelines per Liter Lost				
	Na^+ (mEq/L)	K^+ (mEq/L)	Cl^- (mEq/L)	HCO_3^- (mEq/L)	0.9% Saline (mL)	0.45% Saline (mL)	D_5W (mL)	KCl (mEq/L)	7.5% $NaHCO_3$ (45 mEq HCO_3^-/amp)
Sweat	30–50	5	50			500	500	5	
Gastric secretions	20	10	10			300	700	20	
Pancreatic juice	130	5	35	115		400	600	5	2 amps
Bile	145	5	100	25	600		400	5	0.5 amp
Duodenal fluid	60	15	100	10		1000		15	0.25 amp
Ileal fluid	100	10	60	60		600	400	10	1 amp
Colonic diarrhea	140[1]	10	85	60		1000		10	1 amp

[1]In the absence of diarrhea, colonic fluid Na^+ levels are low (40 mEq/L).

Foster GT et al. Respiratory alkalosis. Respir Care. 2001 Apr; 46(4):384–91. [PMID: 11262557]

Laffey JG et al. Hypocapnia. N Engl J Med. 2002 Jul 4;347(1):43–53. [PMID: 12097540]

FLUID MANAGEMENT

Daily parenteral maintenance fluids and electrolytes for an average adult would include 2500–3000 mL of 5% dextrose in 0.2% saline solution (34 mEq Na^+ plus 34 mEq Cl^-/L) with 30 mEq/L of KCl. Guidelines for gastrointestinal fluid losses are shown in Table 21–17.

Weight loss or gain is the best indication of water balance. Insensible water loss should be considered in febrile patients. Water loss increases by 100–150 mL/d for each degree of body temperature over 37 °C.

In patients requiring maintenance and possibly replacement of fluid and electrolytes by parenteral infusion, the total daily ration should be administered continuously over 24 hours to ensure optimal utilization.

If intravenous fluids are the only source of water, electrolytes, and calories for longer than a week, parenteral nutrition containing amino acids, lipids, trace metals, and vitamins may be indicated. (See Chapter 29.)

For parenteral alimentation, 620 mg (20 mmol) of phosphorus is required for every 1000 nonprotein kcal to maintain phosphate balance and to ensure anabolic function. For prolonged parenteral fluid maintenance, a daily ration is 620–1240 mg (20–40 mmol) of phosphorus.

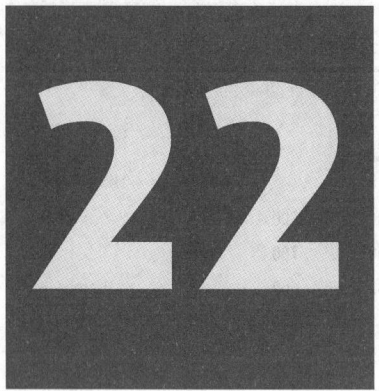

Kidney Disease

Suzanne Watnick, MD
Gail Morrison, MD

Kidney disease presents in one of two ways: discovered incidentally during a routine medical evaluation or with evidence of renal dysfunction, such as hypertension, edema, nausea, and hematuria. The initial approach in both situations should be to assess the cause and severity of renal abnormalities. In all cases this evaluation includes (1) an estimation of disease duration, (2) a careful urinalysis, and (3) an assessment of the glomerular filtration rate (GFR). The history and physical examination, though equally important, are variable among renal syndromes—thus, specific symptoms and signs are discussed under each disease entity.

ASSESSMENT OF KIDNEY DISEASE

▶ Disease Duration

Kidney disease may be acute or chronic. Acute kidney injury, also known as acute renal failure, is worsening of kidney function over hours to days, resulting in the retention of nitrogenous wastes (such as urea nitrogen) and creatinine in the blood. Retention of these substances is called azotemia. Chronic kidney disease results from an abnormal loss of kidney function over months to years. Differentiating between the two is important for diagnosis, treatment, and outcome. Oliguria is unusual in chronic kidney disease. Anemia (from low kidney erythropoietin production) is rare in the initial period of acute kidney disease. Small kidneys are most consistent with chronic kidney disease, whereas normal to large-size kidneys can be seen with both chronic and acute disease.

▶ Urinalysis

A urinalysis has been likened to "a poor man's renal biopsy." The urine is collected in midstream or, if that is not feasible, by bladder catheterization. The urine should be examined within 1 hour after collection to avoid destruction of formed elements. Urinalysis includes a dipstick examination followed by microscopic assessment if the dipstick has positive findings. The dipstick examination measures urinary pH, protein, hemoglobin, glucose, ketones, bilirubin, nitrites, and leukocyte esterase. Urinary specific gravity is often reported, too. Microscopy searches for all formed elements—crystals, cells, casts, and infecting organisms.

Various findings on the urinalysis are indicative of certain patterns of kidney disease. A bland urinary sediment is common, especially in chronic kidney disease and prerenal and postrenal disorders. Casts are composed of Tamm-Horsfall urinary mucoprotein in the shape of the nephron segment where they were formed. Heavy proteinuria and lipiduria are consistent with the nephrotic syndrome. The presence of hematuria with dysmorphic red blood cells, red blood cell casts, and proteinuria is indicative of glomerulonephritis. Dysmorphic red blood cells are misshapen during abnormal passage from the capillary through the glomerular basement membrane (GBM) into the urinary space of Bowman capsule. Pigmented granular casts and renal tubular epithelial cells alone or in casts suggest acute tubular necrosis. White blood cells, including neutrophils and eosinophils, white blood cell casts, red blood cells, and small amounts of protein can be found in interstitial nephritis and pyelonephritis (Table 22–1); Wright and Hansel stains can detect eosinophiluria. Pyuria alone can indicate a urinary tract infection. Hematuria and proteinuria are discussed more thoroughly below.

A. Proteinuria

Proteinuria is defined as excessive protein excretion in the urine, generally greater than 150–160 mg/24 h in adults. Significant proteinuria is a sign of an underlying renal abnormality, usually glomerular in origin when greater than 1 g/d. It can be accompanied by other clinical abnormalities—elevated blood urea nitrogen (BUN) and serum creatinine levels, abnormal urinary sediment, or evidence of systemic illness (eg, fever, rash, vasculitis).

There are four primary reasons for development of proteinuria: (1) Functional proteinuria is a benign process stemming from stressors such as acute illness, exercise, and "orthostatic proteinuria." The latter condition, generally found in people under age 30 years, usually results in urinary protein excretion of less than 1 g/d. The orthostatic nature of the proteinuria is confirmed by measuring an 8-hour overnight supine urinary protein excretion, which

Table 22–1. Significance of specific urinary casts.

Type	Significance
Hyaline casts	Concentrated urine, febrile disease, after strenuous exercise, in the course of diuretic therapy (not indicative of renal disease)
Red cell casts	Glomerulonephritis
White cell casts	Pyelonephritis, interstitial nephritis (indicative of infection or inflammation)
Renal tubular cell casts	Acute tubular necrosis, interstitial nephritis
Coarse, granular casts	Nonspecific; can represent acute tubular necrosis
Broad, waxy casts	Chronic kidney disease (indicative of stasis in enlarged collecting tubules)

should be less than 50 mg. (2) Overload proteinuria can result from overproduction of circulating, filterable plasma proteins (monoclonal gammopathies), such as Bence Jones proteins associated with multiple myeloma. Urinary protein electrophoresis will exhibit a discrete protein peak. Other examples of overload proteinuria include myoglobinuria in rhabdomyolysis and hemoglobinuria in hemolysis. (3) Glomerular proteinuria results from effacement of epithelial cell foot processes and altered glomerular permeability with an increased filtration fraction of normal plasma proteins. Glomerular diseases exhibit some degree of proteinuria. The urinary protein electrophoresis will have a pattern exhibiting a large albumin spike indicative of increased permeability of albumin across a damaged GBM. (4) Tubular proteinuria occurs as a result of faulty reabsorption of normally filtered proteins in the proximal tubule, such as β_2-microglobulin and immunoglobulin light chains. Causes include acute tubular necrosis, toxic injury (lead, aminoglycosides), drug-induced interstitial nephritis, and hereditary metabolic disorders (Wilson disease and Fanconi syndrome).

Evaluation of proteinuria by urinary dipstick primarily detects albumin and intact globulins, while overlooking positively charged light chains of immunoglobulins. These proteins can be detected by the addition of sulfosalicylic acid to the urine specimen. Precipitation indicates the presence of paraproteins.

The next step is a 24-hour urine collection. A finding of greater than 150–160 mg/24 h is abnormal, and greater than 3.5 g/24 h is consistent with nephrotic-range proteinuria. A simpler method is to collect a random urine sample. The ratio of urinary protein concentration to urinary creatinine concentration ($U_{protein}/U_{creatinine}$) correlates with 24-hour urine protein collection (< 0.2 is normal and corresponds to excretion of less than 200 mg/24 h). The benefit of a urine protein-to-creatinine ratio is the ease of collection and the lack of error from overcollection or undercollection of urine. If a patient has proteinuria with or without loss of kidney function, kidney biopsy may be indicated, particularly if the kidney disease is acute in

onset. The clinical consequences of proteinuria are discussed in the section on the nephrotic syndrome.

B. Hematuria

Hematuria is significant if there are more than three red cells per high-power field on at least two occasions. It is usually detected incidentally by the urine dipstick examination or clinically following an episode of macroscopic hematuria. The diagnosis must be confirmed via microscopic examination, as false-positive dipstick tests can be caused by myoglobin, oxidizing agents, beets and rhubarb, hydrochloric acid, and bacteria. Transient hematuria is common, but in patients younger than 40 years, it is less often of clinical significance due to lower concern for malignancy.

Hematuria may be due to renal or extrarenal causes. Extrarenal causes are addressed in Chapters 23 and 39; most worrisome are urologic malignancies. Renal causes account for approximately 10% of cases and are best considered anatomically as glomerular or nonglomerular. The most common extraglomerular sources include cysts, calculi, interstitial nephritis, and renal neoplasia. Glomerular causes include immunoglobulin A (IgA) nephropathy, thin GBM disease, membranoproliferative glomerulonephritis, and systemic nephritic syndromes.

Currently, the United States Health Preventive Services Task Force does not recommend screening for hematuria. See Chapter 23 for evaluation of hematuria.

▶ **Estimation of GFR**

The GFR provides a useful index of overall kidney function; however, patients with kidney disease can actually have a normal or increased GFR. The GFR measures the amount of plasma ultrafiltered across the glomerular capillaries and correlates with the ability of the kidneys to filter fluids and various substances. Daily GFR in normal individuals is variable, with a range of 150–250 L/24 h or 100–120 mL/min/1.73 m^2 of body surface area. GFR can be measured indirectly by determining the renal clearance of plasma substances that are not bound to plasma proteins, are freely filterable across the glomerulus, and are neither secreted nor reabsorbed along the renal tubules. The formula used to determine the renal clearance of a substance is

$$C = \frac{U \times \dot{V}}{P}$$

where C is the clearance, U and P are the urine and plasma concentrations of the substance (mg/dL), and $\dot{V}$ is the urine flow rate (mL/min). In clinical practice, the clearance rate of endogenous creatinine, the creatinine clearance, is one way of estimating GFR. Creatinine is a product of muscle metabolism produced at a relatively constant rate and cleared by renal excretion. It is freely filterable by the glomerulus and not reabsorbed by the renal tubules at steady state. With stable kidney function, creatinine production and excretion are equal; thus, plasma creatinine concentrations remain constant. However, it is not a perfect indicator of GFR for the following reasons: (1) A small amount is normally eliminated by tubular secretion, and

Table 22–2. Conditions affecting serum creatinine independently of glomerular filtration rate.

Condition	Mechanism
Conditions elevating creatinine	
Ketoacidosis, cephalothin, cefoxitin, flucytosine	Noncreatinine chromogen
Other drugs: aspirin, cimetidine, probenecid, trimethoprim	Inhibition of tubular creatinine secretion
Conditions decreasing creatinine	
Advanced age	Physiologic decrease in muscle mass
Cachexia	Pathologic decrease in muscle mass
Liver disease	Decreased hepatic creatine synthesis and cachexia

Table 22–3. Conditions affecting BUN independently of GFR.

Increased BUN
  Reduced effective circulating blood volume (prerenal azotemia)
  Catabolic states (gastrointestinal bleeding, corticosteroid use)
  High-protein diets
  Tetracycline
Decreased BUN
  Liver disease
  Malnutrition
  Sickle cell anemia
  SIADH

BUN, blood urea nitrogen; GFR, glomerular filtration rate; SIADH, syndrome of inappropriate antidiuretic hormone.

the fraction secreted progressively increases as GFR declines (overestimating GFR); (2) with severe kidney failure, gut microorganisms degrade creatinine; (3) an individual's meat intake and muscle mass affect baseline plasma creatinine levels; (4) commonly used drugs such as aspirin, cimetidine, probenecid, and trimethoprim reduce tubular secretion of creatinine, increasing the plasma creatinine concentration and falsely indicating kidney dysfunction; and (5) the accuracy of the measurement necessitates a stable plasma creatinine concentration over a 24-hour period, so that during the development of and recovery from acute kidney injury, the creatinine clearance is of questionable value (Table 22–2).

To measure creatinine clearance, collect a 24-hour urine sample and determine the plasma creatinine level on the same day. An incomplete or prolonged urine collection is a common source of error. One way of estimating the completeness of the collection is to calculate a 24-hour creatinine excretion; the amount should be constant:

$$U_{cr} \times V = 15\text{–}20 \text{ mg/kg for healthy young women}$$

$$U_{cr} \times V = 20\text{–}25 \text{ mg/kg for healthy young men}$$

The creatinine clearance (C_{cr}) is approximately 100 mL/min/1.73 m^2 in healthy young women and 120 mL/min/1.73 m^2 in healthy young men. The C_{cr} declines by an average of 0.8 mL/min/yr after age 40 years as part of the aging process, but 35% of subjects in one study had no decline in kidney function over 10 years.

C_{cr} can be estimated from the formula of Cockcroft and Gault, which incorporates age, sex, and weight to estimate C_{cr} from plasma creatinine levels without any urinary measurements:

$$C_{cr} = \frac{(140 - Age) \times Weight \text{ (kg)}}{P_{cr} \times 72}$$

For women, the creatinine clearance is multiplied by 0.85 because muscle mass is less. This formula overestimates GFR in patients who are obese or edematous and

is most accurate when normalized for body surface area of 1.73 m^2.

Urea is another index helpful in assessing kidney function. It is synthesized mainly in the liver and is the end product of protein catabolism. Urea is freely filtered by the glomerulus, and about 30–70% is reabsorbed in the nephron. Unlike creatinine clearance, which overestimates GFR, urea clearance underestimates GFR. Urea reabsorption may be decreased in volume replete patients, whereas volume depletion causes increased urea reabsorption from the kidney, increasing BUN. A normal BUN:creatinine ratio is 10:1. With volume depletion, the ratio can increase to 20:1 or higher. Other causes of increased BUN include increased catabolism (gastrointestinal bleeding, cell lysis, and corticosteroid usage), increased dietary protein, and decreased renal perfusion (congestive heart failure, renal artery stenosis) (Table 22–3). Reduced BUN is seen in liver disease and in the syndrome of inappropriate antidiuretic hormone (SIADH) secretion.

As patients approach end-stage renal disease (ESRD), a more accurate measure of GFR than creatinine clearance is the average of the creatinine and urea clearances. The creatinine clearance overestimates GFR, as mentioned above, while the urea clearance underestimates GFR. Therefore, an average of the two more accurately approximates the true GFR.

The estimated GFR (eGFR) is a complex four-variable equation, including serum creatinine, age, weight, and race, that is often reported alongside serum creatinine measurements and more accurate than creatinine or urea clearance. This was derived from data collected for the Modification of Diet and Renal Disease study and has been validated in several other populations. Several computer programs exist that will calculate this; one location for this is www.nephron.com.

RENAL BIOPSY

Indications for percutaneous needle biopsy include (1) unexplained acute kidney injury or chronic kidney disease; (2) acute nephritic syndromes; (3) unexplained proteinuria and hematuria; (4) previously identified and treated lesions to plan future therapy; (5) systemic diseases associated with kidney dysfunction, such as systemic lupus erythematosus, Goodpasture syndrome, and Wegener granulomatosis, to confirm the extent of renal involvement and to guide management; (6) suspected transplant rejection, to differentiate it from other causes of acute kidney injury; and (7) to guide treatment. If a patient is unwilling to accept therapy based on biopsy findings, the risk of biopsy may outweigh its benefit. Relative contraindications include a solitary or ectopic kidney (exception: transplant allografts), horseshoe kidney, uncorrected bleeding disorder, severe uncontrolled hypertension, renal infection, renal neoplasm, hydronephrosis, ESRD, congenital anomalies, multiple cysts, or an uncooperative patient.

Prior to biopsy, patients should have well-controlled blood pressure; blood work should include a hemoglobin, platelet count, prothrombin time, and partial thromboplastin time. After biopsy, hematuria occurs in nearly all patients. Fewer than 10% will have macroscopic hematuria. Patients should remain supine for 4–6 hours postbiopsy. A patient with a 6-hour postbiopsy hematocrit more than 3% lower than baseline should be closely monitored.

Percutaneous kidney biopsies are generally safe. Approximately 1% of patients will experience significant bleeding requiring blood transfusions. More than half of patients will have at least a small hematoma. Risk of major bleeding persists up to 72 hours after the biopsy. Any type of anticoagulation therapy should be held for 5–7 days postbiopsy if possible. The risks of nephrectomy and mortality are about 0.06–0.08%. When a percutaneous needle biopsy is technically not feasible and renal tissue is deemed clinically essential, a closed renal biopsy via interventional radiologic techniques or open renal biopsy under general anesthesia can be done.

Bairy M et al. Safety of outpatient kidney biopsy: one center's experience with 178 native kidney biopsies. Am J Kidney Dis. 2008 Sep;52(3):631–2. [PMID: 18725027]

Barnett AH et al; Diabetics Exposed to Telmisartan and Enalapril Study Group. Angiotensin-receptor blockade versus converting-enzyme inhibition in type 2 diabetes and nephropathy. N Engl J Med. 2004 Nov 4;351(19):1952–61. [PMID: 15516696]

Campbell KH et al. Kidney disease in the elderly: update on recent literature. Curr Opin Nephrol Hypertens. 2008 May;17(3):298–303. [PMID: 18408482]

Johnson CA et al. Clinical practice guidelines for chronic kidney disease in adults: Part II. Glomerular filtration rate, proteinuria, and other markers. Am Fam Physician. 2004 Sep 15;70(6):1091–7. [PMID: 15456118]

Patel JV et al. Hematuria: etiology and evaluation for the primary care physician. Can J Urol. 2008 Aug;15 (Suppl 1):54–61. [PMID: 18700066]

Wyatt C et al. Reporting of estimated GFR in the primary care clinic. Am J Kidney Dis. 2007 May;49(5):634–41. [PMID: 17472845]

ACUTE KIDNEY INJURY (ACUTE RENAL FAILURE)

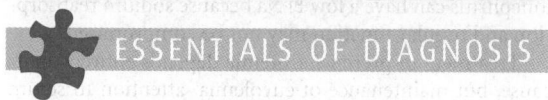

ESSENTIALS OF DIAGNOSIS

► Sudden increase in BUN or serum creatinine.

► Oliguria often associated.

► Symptoms and signs depend on cause.

General Considerations

Acute kidney injury, also known as acute renal failure, is defined as a sudden decrease in kidney function, resulting in an inability to maintain fluid and electrolyte balance and to excrete nitrogenous wastes. Serum creatinine is a convenient marker. In the absence of functioning kidneys, serum creatinine concentration will typically increase by 1–1.5 mg/dL daily—although with certain conditions, such as rhabdomyolysis, serum creatinine can increase more rapidly. Five percent of hospital admissions and 30% of intensive care unit (ICU) admissions carry a diagnosis of acute kidney injury, and it will develop in 25% of hospitalized patients.

Clinical Findings

A. Symptoms and Signs

The uremic milieu of acute kidney injury can cause nonspecific symptoms. When present, they are often due to azotemia or its underlying cause. Azotemia can cause nausea, vomiting, malaise, and altered sensorium. Hypertension is rare, but fluid homeostasis is often altered. Hypovolemia can cause prerenal disease, whereas hypervolemia can result from intrinsic or postrenal disease. Pericardial effusions can occur with azotemia, and a pericardial friction rub can be present. Effusions may result in cardiac tamponade. Arrhythmias occur especially with hyperkalemia. The lung examination may show rales in the presence of hypervolemia. Acute kidney failure can cause nonspecific diffuse abdominal pain and ileus as well as platelet dysfunction; thus, bleeding and clotting disorders are more common in these patients. The neurologic examination reveals encephalopathic changes with asterixis and confusion; seizures may ensue.

B. Laboratory Findings

Elevated BUN and creatinine are present, though these elevations do not in themselves distinguish acute from chronic kidney disease. Hyperkalemia often occurs from impaired renal potassium excretion. The ECG can reveal peaked T waves, PR prolongation, and QRS widening. A long QT segment can occur with hypocalcemia. Anion gap metabolic acidosis (due to decreased organic acid clearance) is often noted. Hyperphosphatemia occurs when phosphorus cannot be secreted by damaged tubules either with or without increased cell catabolism. Hypocalcemia with metastatic calcium phosphate deposition may be observed when the product of calcium and phosphorus exceeds 70 mg^2/dL^2. Anemia can occur as a result of decreased erythropoietin production over weeks, and associated platelet dysfunction is typical.

Classification & Etiology

Acute kidney injury can be divided into three categories: prerenal azotemia, intrinsic renal disease, and postrenal azotemia. Identifying the cause is the first step toward treating the patient (Table 22–4).

Table 22–4. Classification and differential diagnosis of acute kidney injury.

	Prerenal Azotemia	Postrenal Azotemia	Intrinsic Renal Disease		
			Acute Tubular Necrosis (Oliguric or Polyuric)	Acute Glomerulonephritis	Acute Interstitial Nephritis
Etiology	Poor renal perfusion	Obstruction of the urinary tract	Ischemia, nephrotoxins	Immune complex-mediated, pauci-immune, anti-GBM related	Allergic reaction; drug reaction; infection, collagen vascular disease
Serum BUN:Cr ratio	> 20:1	> 20:1	< 20:1	> 20:1	< 20:1
Urinary indices					
U_{Na} (mEq/L)	< 20	Variable	> 20	< 20	Variable
FeNa (%)	< 1	Variable	> 1 (when oliguric)	< 1	< 1; > 1
Urine osmolality (mosm/kg)	> 500	< 400	250–300	Variable	Variable
Urinary sediment	Benign or hyaline casts	Normal or red cells, white cells, or crystals	Granular (muddy brown) casts, renal tubular casts	Red cells, dysmorphic red cells and red cell casts	White cells, white cell casts, with or without eosinophils

BUN:Cr, blood urea nitrogen:creatinine ratio; FeNa, fractional excretion of sodium; U_{Na}, urinary concentration of sodium.

A. Prerenal Azotemia

Prerenal azotemia is the most common cause of acute kidney injury, accounting for 40–80% of cases, depending on the population studied. It is due to renal hypoperfusion. This is an appropriate physiologic change. If it can be immediately reversed with restoration of renal blood flow, renal parenchymal damage often does not occur. If hypoperfusion persists, ischemia can result, causing intrinsic kidney injury.

Decreased renal perfusion can occur in one of three ways: a decrease in intravascular volume, a change in vascular resistance, or low cardiac output. Causes of volume depletion include hemorrhage, gastrointestinal losses, dehydration, excessive diuresis, extravascular space sequestration, pancreatitis, burns, trauma, and peritonitis.

Changes in vascular resistance can occur systemically with sepsis, anaphylaxis, anesthesia, and afterload-reducing drugs. Angiotensin-converting enzyme (ACE) inhibitors prevent efferent renal arteriolar constriction out of proportion to the afferent arteriolar constriction; thus, GFR will decrease. Nonsteroidal anti-inflammatory drugs (NSAIDs) prevent afferent arteriolar vasodilation by inhibiting prostaglandin-mediated signals. Thus, in cirrhosis and congestive heart failure, when prostaglandins are recruited to increase renal blood flow, NSAIDs will have particularly deleterious effects. Epinephrine, norepinephrine, high-dose dopamine, anesthetic agents, and cyclosporine also can cause renal vasoconstriction. Renal artery stenosis causes increased resistance and decreased renal perfusion.

Low cardiac output is a state of low effective renal arterial blood flow. This occurs in states of cardiogenic shock, congestive heart failure, pulmonary embolism, and pericardial tamponade. Arrhythmias and valvular disorders can also reduce cardiac output. In the ICU setting, positive pressure ventilation will decrease venous return, also decreasing cardiac output.

When GFR falls acutely, it is important to determine whether acute kidney injury is due to prerenal or intrinsic renal causes. The history and physical examination are important, and urinalysis can be helpful. The BUN:creatinine ratio will typically exceed 20:1 due to increased urea reabsorption. In an oliguric patient, another useful index is the fractional excretion of sodium (FeNa). With decreased GFR, the kidney will reabsorb salt and water avidly if there is no intrinsic tubular dysfunction. Thus, patients with prerenal failure should have a low fractional excretion percent of sodium (< 1%). Oliguric patients with intrinsic kidney dysfunction will have a high fractional excretion of sodium (> 1%). The FeNa is calculated as follows: FeNa = clearance of Na^+/GFR = clearance of Na^+/creatinine clearance:

$$F_E Na = \frac{Urine_{sodium}/Plasma_{sodium}}{Urine_{creatinine}/Plasma_{creatinine}} \times 100\%$$

Oliguric states are more accurately assessed with this formula than nonoliguric states because the FeNa could be relatively low in nonoliguric acute tubular necrosis if sodium intake and excretion are relatively low. (Oliguria is defined as urinary output < 400–500 mL/d, or < 20 mL/h.) Diuretics can cause increased sodium excretion. Thus, if the FeNa is high within 12–24 hours after diuretic administration, the cause of acute kidney injury may not be accurately predicted. Acute kidney injury due to glomerulonephritis can have a low FeNa because sodium reabsorption and tubular function may not be compromised.

Treatment of prerenal azotemia depends entirely on its cause, but maintenance of euvolemia, attention to serum potassium, and avoidance of nephrotoxic drugs are benchmarks of therapy. This involves careful assessment of volume status, cardiac function, and drug usage.

B. Postrenal Azotemia

Postrenal azotemia is the least common cause of acute kidney injury, accounting for approximately 5–10% of cases, but is important to detect because of its reversibility. It occurs when urinary flow from both kidneys, or a single functioning kidney, is obstructed. Obstruction leads to elevated intraluminal pressure, causing kidney parenchymal damage, with marked effects on renal blood flow and tubular function, and a decrease in GFR.

Causes include urethral obstruction, bladder dysfunction or obstruction, and obstruction of both ureters or renal pelvises. In men, benign prostatic hyperplasia is the most common cause. Patients taking anticholinergic drugs are particularly at risk. Obstruction can also be caused by bladder, prostate, and cervical cancers; retroperitoneal processes; and neurogenic bladder. Less common causes are blood clots, bilateral ureteral stones, urethral stones or stricture, and bilateral papillary necrosis. In patients with a single functioning kidney, obstruction of a solitary ureter can cause postrenal azotemia.

Patients may be anuric or polyuric and may complain of lower abdominal pain. Obstruction can be constant or intermittent and partial or complete. On examination, the patient may have an enlarged prostate, distended bladder, or mass detected on pelvic examination.

Laboratory examination may initially reveal high urine osmolality, low urine sodium, high BUN:creatinine ratio, and low FENa. These indices are similar to a prerenal picture because extensive intrinsic renal damage has not occurred. After several days, the urine sodium increases as the kidneys fail and are unable to concentrate the urine—thus, isosthenuria is present. The urine sediment is generally benign.

Patients with acute kidney injury and suspected postrenal azotemia should undergo bladder catheterization and bladder ultrasonography to assess for hydroureter and hydronephrosis. These patients often undergo a postobstructive saliuresis and diuresis, and care should be taken to avoid volume depletion. Rarely, obstruction is not diagnosed by ultrasonography. For example, patients with retroperitoneal fibrosis from tumor or radiation may not show dilation of the urinary tract. If suspicion does exist, a CT scan or MRI can establish the diagnosis. Prompt treatment of obstruction within days by catheters, stents, or other surgical procedures can result in partial or complete reversal of the acute process.

C. Intrinsic Renal Failure

Intrinsic renal disorders account for up to 50% of all cases of acute kidney injury. Intrinsic (or parenchymal) dysfunction is considered after prerenal and postrenal causes have been excluded. The sites of injury are the tubules, interstitium, vasculature, and glomeruli.

▶ When to Refer

- If a patient has signs of acute kidney injury that have not reversed over 1–2 weeks, but no signs of acute uremia,

the patient can usually be referred to a nephrologist rather than admitted.
- If a patient has signs of urinary tract obstruction, the patient can be referred to a urologist.

▶ When to Admit

The patient should be admitted if he or she has sudden loss of kidney function resulting in abnormalities that cannot be handled expeditiously in an outpatient setting (eg, hyperkalemia, volume overload, uremia) or other requirements for acute dialysis.

ACUTE TUBULAR NECROSIS

ESSENTIALS OF DIAGNOSIS

- ▶ Acute kidney injury.
- ▶ Ischemic or toxic insult.
- ▶ Urine sediment with pigmented granular casts and renal tubular epithelial cells is pathognomonic but not essential.

▶ General Considerations

Acute kidney injury due to tubular damage is termed acute tubular necrosis and accounts for 85% of intrinsic acute kidney injury. The two major causes of acute tubular necrosis are ischemia and nephrotoxin exposure. Ischemia causes tubular damage from states of low perfusion and is often preceded by a state of prerenal azotemia. Ischemic acute kidney injury is characterized not only by inadequate GFR but also by renal blood flow inadequate to maintain parenchymal cellular formation. This occurs in the setting of prolonged hypotension or hypoxemia, such as volume depletion, shock, and sepsis. Major surgical procedures can involve prolonged periods of hypoperfusion, which are exacerbated by vasodilating anesthetic agents.

Exogenous nephrotoxins more commonly cause damage than endogenous nephrotoxins.

A. Exogenous Nephrotoxins

Up to 25% of hospitalized patients receiving therapeutic levels of aminoglycosides sustain some degree of acute tubular necrosis. Nonoliguric kidney injury typically occurs after 5–10 days of exposure. Predisposing factors include underlying kidney damage, volume depletion, and advanced age. Aminoglycosides can remain in renal tissues for up to a month, so kidney function may not recover for some time after stopping the medication. Monitoring of peak and trough levels is important, but trough levels are more helpful in predicting renal toxicity. Gentamicin is as nephrotoxic as tobramycin; streptomycin is the least nephrotoxic of the aminoglycosides, likely due to the number of cationic amino side chains present on each molecule. Amphotericin B is typically nephrotoxic after a dose of 2–3 g. This causes severe vasoconstriction with distal tubular damage and can lead to distal renal tubular acidosis with hypokalemia and nephrogenic diabetes insipidus. Vancomycin, intravenous acyclovir, and several cephalosporins have been known to cause acute tubular necrosis.

Radiographic contrast media can be directly nephrotoxic. Contrast nephropathy is the third leading cause of new acute kidney injury in hospitalized patients. It probably results from the synergistic combination of direct renal tubular epithelial cell toxicity and renal medullary ischemia. Predisposing factors include advanced age, preexisting kidney disease (serum creatinine > 2 mg/dL), volume depletion, diabetic nephropathy, congestive heart failure, multiple myeloma, repeated doses of contrast, and recent exposure to other nephrotoxic agents, including NSAIDs and ACE inhibitors. The combination of diabetes mellitus and kidney dysfunction poses the greatest risk (15–50%) for contrast nephropathy. Lower volumes of contrast with lower osmolality are recommended in high-risk patients. Toxicity usually occurs within 24–48 hours after the radiocontrast study. Nonionic contrast media may be less toxic, but this has not been well proven. Prevention should be the goal when using these agents. The mainstay of therapy is a liter of 0.9% saline over 10–12 hours both before and after the contrast administration—cautiously in patients with preexisting cardiac dysfunction. Neither mannitol nor furosemide offers benefit over normal saline administration. In fact, furosemide may lead to increased rates of renal dysfunction in this setting. In some but not all studies, N-acetylcysteine given before and after contrast decreased the incidence of dye-induced nephrotoxicity. Acetylcysteine is a thiol-containing antioxidant with little toxicity whose mechanism of action is unclear. Its benefit seems more pronounced in subjects with a lower GFR. With little harm and possible benefit, administering acetylcysteine 600 mg orally every 12 hours twice, before and after a dye load, for patients at risk for acute kidney injury, is a reasonable strategy. Intravenous N-acetylcysteine, 1200 mg prior to an emergent procedure, has shown benefit compared with placebo and may be a good option if a patient needs contrast dye urgently. Some investigators have shown a benefit using sodium bicarbonate (154 mEq/L, intravenously at 3 mL/kg/h for 1 hour before the procedure, then 1 mL/kg/h for 6 hours after the procedure) over a more conventional regimen of normal saline as the isotonic volume expander. However, others have shown sodium bicarbonate was not superior to sodium chloride when using similar administration regimens. Other nephrotoxic agents should be avoided during the day before and after dye administration.

Cyclosporine toxicity is usually dose dependent. It causes distal tubular dysfunction from severe vasoconstriction. Regular blood level monitoring is important to prevent nephrotoxicity. With patients who are taking cyclosporine for renal transplant rejection, kidney biopsy is often necessary to distinguish transplant rejection from cyclosporine toxicity. Renal function usually improves after reducing the dose or stopping the drug.

Other exogenous nephrotoxins include antineoplastics, such as cisplatin and organic solvents, and heavy metals such as mercury, cadmium, and arsenic.

B. Endogenous Nephrotoxins

Endogenous nephrotoxins include heme-containing products, uric acid, and paraproteins. **Myoglobinuria** as a consequence of rhabdomyolysis leads to acute tubular necrosis. Necrotic muscle releases large amounts of myoglobin, which is freely filtered across the glomerulus. The myoglobin is reabsorbed by the renal tubules, and direct damage can occur. Distal tubular obstruction from pigmented casts and intrarenal vasoconstriction can also cause damage. This type of kidney injury occurs in the setting of crush injury, or muscle necrosis from prolonged unconsciousness, seizures, cocaine, and alcohol abuse. Dehydration and acidosis predispose to the development of myoglobinuric acute kidney injury. Patients may complain of muscular pain and often have signs of muscle injury. Rhabdomyolysis of clinical importance commonly occurs with a serum creatine kinase (CK) greater than 20,000–50,000 international units/L. One study showed that 58% of patients with acute kidney injury from rhabdomyolysis had CK levels greater than 16,000 international units/L. Only 11% of patients without kidney injury had CK values greater than 16,000 international units/L. The globin moiety of myoglobin will cause the urine dipstick to read falsely positive for hemoglobin: the urine appears dark brown, but no red cells are present. With lysis of muscle cells, patients also become hyperkalemic, hyperphosphatemic, and hyperuricemic. Hypocalcemia may ensue due to phosphorus and calcium precipitation. The mainstay of treatment is volume repletion. Other adjunctive treatments include mannitol for free radical clearance and diuresis as well as alkalinization of the urine. These modalities have not been proved to change outcomes in human trials. Hypocalcemia should not be treated unless the patient is symptomatic; as the patient recovers, calcium can move back from tissues to plasma, so early exogenous calcium administration could result in hypercalcemia.

Hemoglobin can cause a similar form of acute tubular necrosis. Massive intravascular hemolysis is seen in transfusion reactions and in certain hemolytic anemias. Reversal of the underlying disorder and hydration are the mainstays of treatment.

Hyperuricemia can occur in the setting of rapid cell turnover and lysis. Chemotherapy for germ cell neoplasms and leukemia and lymphoma are the primary causes. Acute kidney injury occurs with intratubular deposition of uric acid crystals; serum uric acid levels are often greater than 15–20 mg/dL and urine uric acid levels greater than 600 mg/24 h. A urine uric acid to urine creatinine ratio greater than 1.0 indicates risk of acute kidney injury.

Bence Jones protein seen in conjunction with multiple myeloma can cause direct tubular toxicity and tubular obstruction. Other renal complications from multiple myeloma include hypercalcemia and renal tubular dysfunction, including proximal renal tubular acidosis (see Multiple Myeloma, below).

► Clinical Findings

A. Symptoms and Signs

See Acute Kidney Injury.

B. Laboratory Findings

Hyperkalemia and hyperphosphatemia are commonly encountered. Urinalysis may show evidence of acute tubular damage. The urine may be brown. On microscopic examination, an active sediment may show pigmented granular casts or "muddy brown" casts. Renal tubular epithelial cells and epithelial cell casts can be present (see Table 22–1).

► Treatment

Treatment is aimed at hastening recovery and avoiding complications. Preventive measures should be taken to avoid volume overload and hyperkalemia. Loop diuretics have been used in large doses (eg, furosemide in doses ranging from 20 mg to 160 mg orally or intravenously twice daily, or as a continuous infusion) to affect adequate diuresis and may help convert oliguric to nonoliguric renal failure. Such a conversion has never been shown to affect outcomes such as mortality, though. One retrospective study has shown potentially worse outcomes in patients who receive doses of furosemide, including nonrecovery of renal function and an increased risk of death. A prospective randomized controlled trial has shown no difference between the administration of large doses of diuretics versus placebo on either recovery from acute kidney injury or death. Widespread use of diuretics in critically ill patients with acute kidney injury should be discouraged. Side effects of supranormal dosing include deafness. This is mainly due to peak furosemide levels and can be avoided by the use of a furosemide drip. A starting dose of 0.1–0.3 mg/kg/h is appropriate, increasing to a maximum of 0.5–1 mg/kg/h. A bolus of 1–1.5 mg/kg should be administered at the beginning of each dose escalation. Intravenous thiazide diuretics can be used to augment urinary output; chlorothiazide, 250–500 mg intravenously every 8–12 hours, is a reasonable choice. Short-term effects also include activation of the renin–angiotensin system. One prospective randomized trial showed the long-term benefits of plasma ultrafiltration over the use of intravenous diuretics in patients with decompensated heart failure. This intervention can be considered in ICU patients with acute kidney injury in need of volume removal who are nonresponsive to diuretics. Nutritional support should maintain adequate intake while preventing excessive catabolism. Dietary protein restriction of 0.6 g/kg/d helps prevent metabolic acidosis. Hypocalcemia and hyperphosphatemia can be improved with diet and phosphate-binding agents, such as aluminum hydroxide (500 mg orally with meals) over the short term, calcium carbonate (500–1500 mg orally three times daily), calcium acetate (667 mg, two or three tablets, orally before meals), or sevelamer (800–1600 mg orally three times daily). Lanthanum carbonate (1000 mg orally with meals) is a less well-studied option. Hypocalcemia should not be treated in patients with rhabdomyolysis unless they are symptomatic. Hypermagnesemia can occur because of reduced magnesium excretion by the renal tubules, so magnesium-containing antacids and laxatives should be avoided in these patients. Dosages of all medications must be adjusted according to the estimated degree of renal impairment for drugs eliminated by the kidney.

Indications for dialysis in acute kidney injury from acute tubular necrosis or other intrinsic disorders include life-threatening electrolyte disturbances (such as hyperkalemia), volume overload unresponsive to diuresis, worsening acidosis, and uremic complications (eg, encephalopathy, pericarditis, and seizures). In gravely ill patients, less severe but worsening abnormalities may also be indications for dialytic support. A prospective randomized control trial of 1124 patients showed that an intensive dialysis dose was not superior to a more conventional dose.

► Course & Prognosis

The clinical course of acute tubular necrosis is often divided into three phases: initial injury, maintenance, and recovery. The maintenance phase is expressed as either oliguric (urinary output < 500 mL/d) or nonoliguric. Nonoliguric acute tubular necrosis has a better outcome. Conversion from oliguric to nonoliguric states may be attempted but has not been shown to change the prognosis. Drugs such as dopamine and diuretics are sometimes used for this purpose but have not been shown to improve outcomes. In numerous studies, dopamine use in this setting has been shown to have no benefit. Average duration of the maintenance phase is 1–3 weeks but may be several months. Cellular repair and removal of tubular debris occur during this period. The recovery phase is heralded by diuresis. GFR begins to rise; BUN and serum creatinine fall.

The mortality rate associated with acute kidney injury is 20–50% in medical illness and up to 70% in a surgical setting. Increased mortality is associated with advanced age, severe underlying disease, and multisystem organ failure. Leading causes of death are infections, fluid and electrolyte disturbances, and worsening of underlying disease. Mortality rates may be starting to improve slightly according to two recent retrospective cohort studies.

► When to Refer

- A patient with acute tubular necrosis should be referred to a nephrologist when the etiology is unclear or renal function continues to worsen despite intervention.
- Also, referral is appropriate if fluid, electrolyte, and acid-base abnormalities are recalcitrant to interventions.
- Studies have shown that nephrology referral improves outcome in acute kidney injury.

► When to Admit

Admission is appropriate when a patient has signs or symptoms of acute kidney injury that require immediate intervention, such as intravenous fluids, dialytic therapy, or a team approach that cannot be coordinated as an outpatient.

INTERSTITIAL NEPHRITIS

ESSENTIALS OF DIAGNOSIS

► Fever.
► Transient maculopapular rash.

- ▶ Acute or chronic kidney injury.
- ▶ Pyuria (including eosinophiluria), white blood cell casts, and hematuria.

General Considerations

Acute interstitial nephritis accounts for 10–15% of cases of intrinsic renal failure. An interstitial inflammatory response with edema and possible tubular cell damage is the typical pathologic finding. Cell-mediated immune reactions prevail over humoral responses. T lymphocytes can cause direct cytotoxicity or release lymphokines that recruit monocytes and inflammatory cells.

Although drugs account for over 70% of cases, acute interstitial nephritis also occurs in infectious diseases, immunologic disorders, or as an idiopathic condition. The most common drugs are penicillins and cephalosporins, sulfonamides and sulfonamide-containing diuretics, NSAIDs, rifampin, phenytoin, and allopurinol. Proton pump inhibitors have also been recognized as a cause of acute interstitial nephritis. Infectious causes include streptococcal infections, leptospirosis, cytomegalovirus, histoplasmosis, and Rocky Mountain spotted fever. Immunologic entities are more commonly associated with glomerulonephritis, but systemic lupus erythematosus, Sjögren syndrome, sarcoidosis, and cryoglobulinemia can cause interstitial nephritis.

Clinical Findings

Clinical features can include fever (> 80%), rash (25–50%), arthralgias, and peripheral blood eosinophilia (80%). The urine often contains red cells (95%), white cells, and white cell casts. Proteinuria can be a feature, particularly in NSAID-induced interstitial nephritis, but is usually modest. Eosinophiluria can be detected by Wright or Hansel stain.

Treatment & Prognosis

Acute interstitial nephritis often carries a good prognosis. Recovery occurs over weeks to months, but urgent dialytic therapy may be necessary in up to one-third of all referred patients before resolution. Patients rarely progress to ESRD. Those with prolonged courses of oliguric failure and advanced age have a worse prognosis. Treatment consists of supportive measures and removal of the inciting agent. If kidney injury persists after these steps, a short course of corticosteroids can be given, although the data to support use of corticosteroids are not substantial. Short-term, high-dose methylprednisolone (0.5–1 g/d intravenously for 1–4 days) or prednisone (60 mg/d orally for 1–2 weeks) followed by a prednisone taper can be used in these more severe cases of drug-induced interstitial nephritis.

GLOMERULONEPHRITIS

ESSENTIALS OF DIAGNOSIS

- ▶ Hematuria, dysmorphic red cells, red cell casts, and mild proteinuria.

- ▶ Dependent edema and hypertension.
- ▶ Acute renal insufficiency.

General Considerations

Acute glomerulonephritis is a relatively uncommon cause of acute kidney injury, accounting for about 5% of cases. Pathologically, inflammatory glomerular lesions are seen. These include mesangioproliferative, focal and diffuse proliferative, and crescentic lesions. The larger the percentage of glomeruli involved and the more severe the lesion, the more likely it is that the patient will have a poor clinical outcome.

Categorization of acute glomerulonephritis can be done by serologic analysis. Markers include antineutrophil cytoplasmic antibodies (ANCA), anti-GBM antibodies, and other immune markers of disease.

Immune complex deposition usually occurs when moderate antigen excess over antibody production occurs. Complexes formed with marked antigen excess tend to remain in the circulation. Antibody excess with large antigen–antibody aggregates usually results in phagocytosis and clearance of the precipitates by the mononuclear phagocytic system in the liver and spleen. Causes include IgA nephropathy (Berger disease), peri-infectious or postinfectious glomerulonephritis, endocarditis, lupus nephritis, cryoglobulinemic glomerulonephritis (often associated with hepatitis C virus), and membranoproliferative glomerulonephritis.

Anti-GBM–associated acute glomerulonephritis is either confined to the kidney or associated with pulmonary hemorrhage. The latter is termed "Goodpasture syndrome." Injury is related to autoantibodies aimed against type IV collagen in the GBM rather than to immune complex deposition.

Pauci-immune acute glomerulonephritis is a form of small-vessel vasculitis associated with anti-neutrophil cytoplasmic antibodies (ANCAs), causing primary and secondary kidney diseases that do not have direct immune complex deposition or antibody binding. Tissue injury is believed to be due to cell-mediated immune processes. An example is Wegener granulomatosis, a systemic necrotizing vasculitis of small arteries and veins associated with intravascular and extravascular granuloma formation. In addition to glomerulonephritis, these patients can have upper airway, pulmonary, and skin manifestations of disease. Cytoplasmic ANCA (C-ANCA) is a common pattern. Microscopic polyangiitis is another pauci-immune vasculitis causing acute glomerulonephritis. Perinuclear staining (P-ANCA) is the common pattern. ANCA-associated and anti-GBM-associated acute glomerulonephritis can evolve to crescentic glomerulonephritis and often have poor outcomes unless treatment is started early. Both are described more fully below.

Other vascular causes of acute glomerulonephritis include hypertensive emergencies and the thrombotic microangiopathies such as hemolytic-uremic syndrome and thrombotic thrombocytopenic purpura (see Chapter 14).

Clinical Findings

A. Symptoms and Signs

Patients with acute glomerulonephritis are often hypertensive and edematous, and have an abnormal urinary sediment. The edema is found first in body parts with low tissue tension, such as the periorbital and scrotal regions.

B. Laboratory Findings

Dipstick and microscopic evaluation will reveal evidence of hematuria, moderate proteinuria (usually < 3 g/d), and cellular elements such as red cells, red cell casts, and white cells. Red cell casts are specific for glomerulonephritis, and a detailed search is warranted. Either spot urinary protein-creatinine ratios or twenty-four hour urine collections can quantify protein excretion, the latter can quantify creatinine clearance when renal function is stable. However, in cases of rapidly changing serum creatinine values, the urinary creatinine clearance is an unreliable marker of GFR. The FeNa is usually low unless the renal tubulo-interstitial space is affected, and renal dysfunction is marked.

Further tests include complement levels (C3, C4, CH50), ASO titer, anti-GBM antibody levels, ANCAs, antinuclear antibody titers, cryoglobulins, hepatitis serologies, blood cultures, renal ultrasound, and occasionally renal biopsy.

Treatment

Depending on the nature and severity of disease, treatment can consist of high-dose corticosteroids and cytotoxic agents such as cyclophosphamide. Plasma exchange can be used in Goodpasture disease and pauci-immune glomerulonephritis as a temporizing measure until chemotherapy can take effect. Treatment and prognosis for specific diseases are discussed more fully below.

Bagshaw SM et al. Loop diuretics in the management of acute renal failure: a systematic review and meta-analysis. Crit Care Resusc. 2007 Mar;9(1):60–8. [PMID: 17352669]

Costanzo MR et al. Ultrafiltration versus intravenous diuretics for patients hospitalized for acute decompensated heart failure. J Am Coll Cardiol. 2007 Feb 13;49(6):675–83. [PMID: 17291932]
Cruz DN et al. Acute kidney injury in the intensive care unit: current trends in incidence and outcome. Crit Care. 2007 Jul 24;11(4):149. [PMID: 17666115]
Warnock DG. Towards a definition and classification of acute kidney injury. J Am Soc Nephrol. 2005 Nov;16(11):3149–50. [PMID: 16207828]
Weisbord S et al. Radiocontrast-induced acute renal failure. J Intensive Care Med. 2005 Mar–Apr;20(2):63–75. [PMID: 15855219]

CHRONIC KIDNEY DISEASE

ESSENTIALS OF DIAGNOSIS

► Progressive azotemia over months to years.

► Symptoms and signs of uremia when nearing end-stage disease.

► Hypertension in the majority.

► Isosthenuria and broad casts in urinary sediment are common.

► Bilateral small kidneys on ultrasound are diagnostic.

General Considerations

Chronic kidney disease affects up to 20 million Americans, or one in nine adults. Most are unaware of the condition because they remain asymptomatic until the disease has significantly progressed. The National Kidney Foundation's staging system helps clinicians formulate practice plans (Table 22–5). Over 70% of cases of late-stage (stage 5) chronic kidney disease are due to diabetes mellitus or hypertension. Glomerulonephritis, cystic diseases, and other urologic diseases account for another 12%, and 15% of patients have other or unknown causes. The major causes of chronic kidney disease are listed in Table 22–6.

Table 22–5. Stages of chronic kidney disease: A clinical action plan.[1,2]

Stage	Description	GFR (mL/min/1.73 m^2)	Action[3]
1	Kidney damage with normal or ↑ GFR	≥ 90	Diagnosis and treatment. Treatment of comorbid conditions. Slowing of progression. Cardiovascular disease risk reduction.
2	Kidney damage with mildly ↓	60–89	Estimating progression.
3	Moderately ↓	30–59	Evaluating and treating complications.
4	Severely ↓	15–29	Preparation for kidney replacement therapy.
5	Kidney failure	< 15 (or dialysis)	Replacement (if uremia is present).

[1]From National Kidney Foundation, KDOQI, chronic kidney disease guidelines.
[2]Chronic kidney disease is defined as either kidney damage or GFR < 60 mL/min/1.73 m^2 for 3 or more months. Kidney damage is defined as pathologic abnormalities or markers of damage, including abnormalities in blood or urine tests or imaging studies.
[3]Includes actions from preceding stages.
GFR, glomerular filtration rate.

Table 22–6. Major causes of chronic kidney disease.

Glomerulopathies
Primary glomerular diseases
Focal and segmental glomerulosclerosis
Membranoproliferative glomerulonephritis
IgA nephropathy
Membranous nephropathy
Secondary glomerular diseases
Diabetic nephropathy
Amyloidosis
Postinfectious glomerulonephritis
HIV-associated nephropathy
Collagen-vascular diseases
Sickle cell nephropathy
HIV-associated membranoproliferative glomerulonephritis
Tubulointerstitial nephritis
Drug hypersensitivity
Heavy metals
Analgesic nephropathy
Reflux/chronic pyelonephritis
Idiopathic
Hereditary diseases
Polycystic kidney disease
Medullary cystic disease
Alport syndrome
Obstructive nephropathies
Prostatic disease
Nephrolithiasis
Retroperitoneal fibrosis/tumor
Congenital
Vascular diseases
Hypertensive nephrosclerosis
Renal artery stenosis

Table 22–7. Symptoms and signs of uremia.

Organ System	Symptoms	Signs
General	Fatigue, weakness	Sallow-appearing, chronically ill
Skin	Pruritus, easy bruisability	Pallor, ecchymoses, excoriations, edema, xerosis
ENT	Metallic taste in mouth, epistaxis	Urinous breath
Eye		Pale conjunctiva
Pulmonary	Shortness of breath	Rales, pleural effusion
Cardiovascular	Dyspnea on exertion, retrosternal pain on inspiration (pericarditis)	Hypertension, cardiomegaly, friction rub
Gastrointestinal	Anorexia, nausea, vomiting, hiccups	
Genitourinary	Nocturia, impotence	Isosthenuria
Neuromuscular	Restless legs, numbness and cramps in legs	
Neurologic	Generalized irritability and inability to concentrate, decreased libido	Stupor, asterixis, myoclonus, peripheral neuropathy

Chronic kidney disease is rarely reversible and leads to a progressive decline in kidney function. This occurs even after the inciting event has been removed. Reduction in renal mass leads to hypertrophy of the remaining nephrons with hyperfiltration. The GFR in these nephrons is transiently at supranormal levels. These adaptations place a burden on the remaining nephrons and lead to progressive glomerular sclerosis and interstitial fibrosis, suggesting that hyperfiltration may worsen kidney function. However, decreased renal mass in kidney donors is not associated with chronic kidney disease.

▶ **Clinical Findings**

A. Symptoms and Signs

The symptoms of chronic kidney disease often develop slowly and are nonspecific (Table 22–7). Individuals can remain asymptomatic until kidney disease is far advanced (GFR < 10–15 mL/min). Manifestations include fatigue, weakness, and malaise. Gastrointestinal complaints, such as anorexia, nausea, vomiting, a metallic taste in the mouth, and hiccups, are common. Neurologic problems include irritability, difficulty in concentrating, insomnia, subtle memory defects, restless legs, and twitching. Pruritus is common and difficult to treat. As uremia progresses,

decreased libido, menstrual irregularities, chest pain from pericarditis, and paresthesias can develop. Symptoms of drug toxicity—especially for drugs eliminated by the kidney—increase as renal clearance worsens.

On physical examination, the patient appears chronically ill. Hypertension is common. The skin may be yellow, with signs of easy bruisability. Rarely seen in the current era is uremic frost, a cutaneous reflection of ESRD. Uremic fetor is the characteristic fishy odor of the breath. Cardiopulmonary signs may include rales, cardiomegaly, edema, and a pericardial friction rub. Mental status can vary from decreased concentration to confusion, stupor, and coma. Myoclonus and asterixis are additional signs of uremic effects on the central nervous system.

The term "uremia" is used for this clinical syndrome, but the exact cause remains unknown. BUN and serum creatinine are considered markers for unknown toxins.

In any patient with kidney disease, it is important to identify and correct all possibly reversible causes. Urinary tract infections, obstruction, extracellular fluid volume depletion, nephrotoxins, hypertension, and congestive heart failure should be excluded (Table 22–8). Any of the above can worsen underlying chronic kidney disease.

B. Laboratory Findings

The diagnosis is made by documenting elevations of the BUN and serum creatinine concentrations. Further evaluation is needed to differentiate between acute and chronic

Table 22–8. Reversible causes of kidney injury.

Reversible Factors	Diagnostic Clues
Infection	Urine culture and sensitivity tests
Obstruction	Bladder catheterization, then renal ultrasound
Extracellular fluid volume depletion	Orthostatic blood pressure and pulse: ↓ blood pressure and ↑ pulse upon sitting up from a supine position
Hypokalemia, hypercalcemia, and hyperuricemia (usually > 15 mg/dL)	Serum electrolytes, calcium, phosphate, uric acid
Nephrotoxic agents	Drug history
Hypertension	Blood pressure, chest radiograph
Congestive heart failure	Physical examination, chest radiograph

disease. Evidence of previously elevated BUN and creatinine, abnormal prior urinalyses, and stable but abnormal serum creatinine on successive days is most consistent with a chronic process. It is helpful to plot the inverse of serum creatinine ($1/S_{Cr}$) versus time if three or more prior measurements are available; this can estimate time to ESRD (Figure 22–1). If the slope of the line acutely declines, new causes of kidney disease should be excluded as outlined above. Anemia, metabolic acidosis, hyperphosphatemia, hypocalcemia, and hyperkalemia can occur with both acute and chronic kidney disease. The urinalysis shows isosthenuria if tubular concentrating and diluting ability are impaired. The urinary sediment can show broad waxy casts as a result of dilated, hypertrophic nephrons.

C. Imaging

The finding of small echogenic kidneys bilaterally (< 10 cm) by ultrasonography supports a diagnosis of chronic kidney disease, though normal or even large kidneys can be seen with adult polycystic kidney disease, diabetic nephropathy, HIV-associated nephropathy, multiple myeloma, amyloidosis, and obstructive uropathy. Radiologic evidence of renal osteodystrophy is another helpful finding, since radiographic changes of secondary hyperparathyroidism do not appear unless parathyroid levels have been elevated for at least 1 year. Evidence of subperiosteal reabsorption along the radial sides of the digital bones of the hand confirms hyperparathyroidism.

▶ Complications

A. Hyperkalemia

Potassium balance generally remains intact in chronic kidney disease until the GFR is less than 10–20 mL/min. However, certain states pose an increased risk of hyperkalemia at higher GFRs. Endogenous causes include any type of cellular destruction such as hemolysis and trauma, hyporeninemic hypoaldosteronism (type IV renal tubular acidosis, seen particularly in diabetes mellitus), and acidemic states (0.6 mEq/L elevation in K^+ for each 0.1 unit

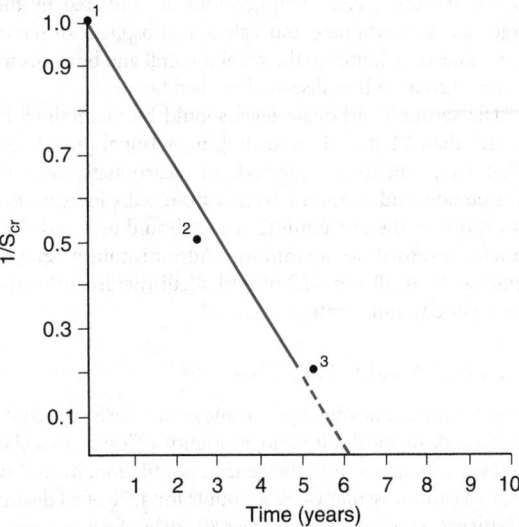

^{1} Value of serum creatinine level = 1.0 mg/dL
^{2} Value of serum creatinine level = 2.0 mg/dL
^{3} Value of serum creatinine level = 5.0 mg/dL

▲ **Figure 22–1.** Decline in kidney function plotted against time to end-stage renal disease (ESRD). The solid line indicates the linear decline in kidney function over time. The dotted line indicates the approximate time to ESRD.

decrease in pH). Exogenous causes include diet (eg, citrus fruits and salt substitutes containing potassium) and drugs that decrease K^+ secretion (amiloride, triamterene, spironolactone, NSAIDs, ACE inhibitors) or block cellular uptake (β-blockers).

Treatment of acute hyperkalemia is discussed in Chapter 21 (Table 21–7). Cardiac monitoring is indicated for any ECG changes seen with hyperkalemia, or a serum potassium level greater than 6.0–6.5 mEq/L. The ion exchange resin, sodium polystyrene sulfonate, exchanges sodium for potassium and can administer a significant sodium load to a patient, although it can cause voluminous diarrhea, which may volume deplete the patient. Chronic hyperkalemia is best treated with dietary potassium restriction (2 g/d) and sodium polystyrene sulfonate when necessary. The usual dose is 15–30 g once a day in juice or sorbitol.

B. Acid–Base Disorders

Damaged kidneys are unable to excrete the 1 mEq/kg/d of acid generated by metabolism of dietary proteins. The resultant metabolic acidosis is primarily due to loss of renal mass. This limits production of ammonia (NH_3) and limits buffering of H^+ in the urine. (Other causes include decreased filtration of titratable acids such as sulfates and phosphates, decreased proximal tubular bicarbonate resorption, and decreased renal tubular hydrogen ion secretion.) Although patients with chronic kidney disease are in positive hydrogen ion balance, the arterial blood pH is maintained at 7.33–7.37 and serum bicarbonate concentration rarely falls below

15 mEq/L. The excess hydrogen ions are buffered by the large calcium carbonate and calcium phosphate stores in bone. This contributes to the renal mineral and bone disorders of chronic kidney disease described below.

The serum bicarbonate level should be maintained at greater than 21 mEq/L according to national guidelines. Alkali supplements include sodium bicarbonate, calcium bicarbonate, and sodium citrate. Citrate salts increase the absorption of dietary aluminum and should be avoided in patients exposed to aluminum. Administration should begin with 20–30 mmol/d of oral alkali divided into two doses per day and titrated as needed.

C. Cardiovascular Complications

Long-term complications of chronic kidney disease include a high risk of morbidity and mortality of cardiovascular disease in comparison to the general population. Mortality due to a cardiovascular cause accounts for 45% of all deaths of patients receiving dialysis. Over 80–90% of patients with chronic kidney disease die, primarily of cardiovascular disease, before reaching the need for dialysis. The precise biologic mechanisms for this are unclear but may have to do with the uremic milieu, underlying coexistent comorbidities, and a hesitancy to perform investigative procedures in patients with chronic kidney disease.

1. Hypertension—As kidney disease progresses, hypertension due to salt and water retention usually develops. Hyperreninemic states and exogenous erythropoietin administration can also exacerbate hypertension. Hypertension is the most common complication of ESRD and must be meticulously controlled. Failure to do so can accelerate the progression of cardiovascular and kidney damage.

Control of hypertension can be achieved with salt and water restriction, weight loss if indicated, and pharmacologic therapy. The ability of the kidney to adjust to variations in sodium and water intake becomes limited as kidney disease progresses. An elevated sodium chloride intake leads to congestive heart failure, edema, and hypertension, whereas low salt intake leads to volume contraction and hypotension. A mildly decreased salt diet (4 g/d) can be started, and salt intake should be reduced to 2 g/d if hypertension persists. Initial drug therapy can include ACE inhibitors or angiotensin II receptor blockers as recommended by national guidelines (if serum potassium and GFR permit), calcium channel-blocking agents, diuretics, and β-blocking agents. The adjunctive drugs that are often needed (eg, α-blocking agents, clonidine, hydralazine, minoxidil) reflect the difficulty of achieving and maintaining hypertensive control in these patients. Goal blood pressure for patients with chronic kidney disease is less than 130/80 mm Hg.

2. Pericarditis—With uremia, pericarditis may develop but is uncommon. The cause is believed to be retention of metabolic toxins. Symptoms include chest pain and fever. Pulsus paradoxus can be present. A friction rub may be auscultated, but the lack of a rub does not rule out a significant pericardial effusion. Chest radiography can show an enlarged cardiac silhouette, and an ECG will show

characteristic findings as explained in Chapter 10. Cardiac tamponade can occur; these patients have signs of poor cardiac output, with jugular venous distention and lungs clear to auscultation. Uremic pericarditis is an absolute indication for initiation of hemodialysis.

3. Congestive heart failure—Patients with ESRD tend toward a high cardiac output. They often have extracellular fluid overload, shunting of blood through an arteriovenous fistula for dialysis, and anemia. In addition to hypertension, these abnormalities cause increased myocardial work and oxygen demand. Patients with chronic kidney disease may also have accelerated rates of atherosclerosis. All of these factors contribute to left ventricular hypertrophy and dilation, present in 75% of patients starting dialysis. Elevated parathyroid hormone (PTH) levels may also play a role in the pathogenesis of the cardiomyopathy of chronic kidney disease.

Water and salt intake should be controlled in patients who are oliguric or anuric. Diuretics are of value, although thiazides are ineffective by themselves when the GFR is less than 20–30 mL/min. Loop diuretics are commonly used, potentially in combination with thiazide diuretics, and higher doses are required as renal function declines. Digoxin should be used with caution since it is excreted by the kidney. The proved efficacy of ACE inhibitors in congestive heart failure holds true for patients with chronic kidney disease. Despite the risks of hyperkalemia and worsening renal function, ACE inhibitors can be used for patients with a serum creatinine greater than 3 mg/dL with close supervision. Along with angiotensin II receptor blockers, ACE inhibitors have been shown to slow the progression to ESRD, even for patients with advanced chronic kidney disease. (See Nephrotic Syndrome section below regarding treatment of proteinuria.) Once a patient is receiving dialysis, these risks become less relevant. When an ACE inhibitor or an angiotensin-receptor blocker (ARB) drug is initiated or uptitrated, patients should have serum creatinine and potassium checked within 5–14 days.

D. Hematologic Complications

1. Anemia—The anemia of chronic kidney disease is characteristically normochromic and normocytic. It is due primarily to decreased erythropoietin production, which becomes clinically significant when GFR falls below 20–40 mL/min. Many patients are iron deficient as well. Low-grade hemolysis and blood loss from platelet dysfunction or hemodialysis play an additional role.

Recombinant erythropoietin-stimulating agents (eg, erythropoietin and darbepoetin) are used in patients whose hemoglobins are less than 11 g/dL if no other causes are present. The effective dose can vary; the starting dose of erythropoietin is 50 units/kg (3000–4000 units/dose) once or twice a week. Darbepoetin is started at 0.45 mcg/kg and can be administered every 2–4 weeks. These agents can be given intravenously (eg, in the hemodialysis patient) or subcutaneously (eg, in any predialysis or dialysis patient). According to national guidelines, both medications should be titrated to a hemoglobin of 11–12 g/dL for optimal safety. Subcutaneous administration is preferable to intravenous administration because it requires a 33% lower dose for the same effect. Hypertension is a complication of erythropoietin therapy in about 20% of patients. It develops more abruptly in the patients with the lowest hemoglobin values at initiation of therapy, and in those with the greatest rate of rise in hemoglobin. The dosage may require adjustment, or antihypertensive drugs may need to given. Hemoglobin levels should rise no more than 1 g/dL every 3–4 weeks.

Iron stores must be adequate to ensure response. Hemodialysis patients typically require 50–200 mg intravenous iron each month due to expected blood loss at dialysis. Other patients with serum ferritin less than 100 ng/mL or iron saturation less than 20% should also receive iron supplementation. Depending on the clinical situation, iron therapy should be withheld if the serum ferritin is greater than 500–800 ng/mL. Oral therapy with ferrous sulfate, 325 mg once daily to three times daily, is adequate but not always well tolerated, and gut absorption of iron is impaired in uremic patients. Ferrous gluconate and fumarate can be better tolerated orally. Intravenous iron may need to be used whether or not a patient is receiving dialysis.

2. Coagulopathy—The coagulopathy of chronic kidney disease is mainly caused by platelet dysfunction. Platelet counts are only mildly decreased, but the bleeding time is prolonged. Platelets show abnormal adhesiveness and aggregation. Clinically, patients can have petechiae, purpura, and an increased tendency for bleeding during surgery.

Treatment is required only in patients who are symptomatic. Raising the hematocrit to 30% can reduce bleeding time in patients with very low hemoglobins (< 10 g/dL) due to the rheologic properties of red blood cells in plasma. Desmopressin (25 mcg intravenously every 8–12 hours for two doses) is effective and often used in preparation for surgery. It causes release of factor VIII bound to von Willebrand factor from endothelial cells. Conjugated estrogens, 0.6 mg/kg diluted in 50 mL of 0.9% sodium chloride infused over 30–40 minutes daily, or 2.5–5 mg orally for 5–7 days, have an effect for several weeks. Dialysis improves the bleeding time but does not normalize it. Cryoprecipitate (10–15 bags) is rarely used and lasts less than 24 hours.

E. Neurologic Complications

Uremic encephalopathy does not occur until GFR falls below 5–15 mL/min. Encephalopathy may be due to the aggregation of uremic toxins. Rarely, hypercalcemia, can be the culprit. Symptoms begin with difficulty in concentrating and can progress to lethargy, confusion, and coma. Physical findings include nystagmus, weakness, asterixis, and hyperreflexia. These symptoms and signs may improve after initiation of dialysis.

Neuropathy is found in 65% of patients who receive dialysis or who will need it soon. Rarely is neuropathy present if the GFR is greater than 10% of normal. Peripheral neuropathies manifest themselves as sensorimotor polyneuropathies (stocking and glove distribution) and isolated or multiple isolated mononeuropathies. Patients can have restless leg syndrome, loss of deep tendon reflexes, and distal pain. The earlier initiation of dialysis may prevent peripheral neuropathies, and the response to dialysis is variable. Other neuropathies result in impotence and autonomic dysfunction.

F. Disorders of Mineral Metabolism

The disorders of calcium, phosphorus, and bone are referred to as **mineral bone disorders of chronic kidney disease**. The most common disorder detected by bone biopsy is osteitis fibrosa cystica—the bony changes of secondary hyperparathyroidism. This affects ~50% of patients nearing ESRD. As GFR decreases below 25% of normal, phosphorus excretion is impaired. Hyperphosphatemia leads to hypocalcemia, stimulating secretion of PTH, which has a phosphaturic effect and normalizes serum phosphorus. This continuous process leads to markedly elevated PTH levels and high bone turnover with osteoclastic bone resorption and subperiosteal lesions. Metastatic calcifications, such as tumoral calcinosis, can occur. Radiographically, lesions are most prominent in the phalanges and lateral ends of the clavicles.

Osteomalacia is a form of renal osteodystrophy with low bone turnover (affecting ~10% of patients nearing ESRD). With worsening kidney function, there is decreased renal conversion of 25-hydroxycholecalciferol to the 1,25-dihydroxy form. Gut absorption of calcium is diminished, leading to hypocalcemia and abnormal bone mineralization. Deposition of aluminum in bone can also lead to osteomalacia. Elevated aluminum levels are seen in patients after years of chronic aluminum hydroxide administration for phosphorus binding. This entity is seen with decreasing frequency because aluminum-based binders are used less in the chronic setting and water used for hemodialysis is now cleared of aluminum.

Adynamic bone disease is a disorder of low bone turnover. More than 25% of patients nearing ESRD show evidence of minimal osteoid and decreased or absent bone remodeling. Its frequency is increasing because of increased use of active vitamin D analogs, which suppress PTH production.

All of the above entities can cause bony pain and proximal muscle weakness. Spontaneous bone fractures can occur that are slow to heal. Patients with advanced chronic kidney disease are also at higher risk for bony fractures. When the calcium-phosphorus product (serum calcium [mg/dL] × serum phosphate [mg/dL]) is above 60–70, metastatic calcifications are commonly seen in blood vessels, soft tissues, lungs, and myocardium. Treatment should begin with dietary phosphorus restriction to 1000 mg/d.

Oral phosphorus-binding agents, such as calcium carbonate (650 mg orally) or calcium acetate (667 mg orally), act in the gut and are given in divided doses three or four times daily with the beginning of meals. These should be titrated to a serum calcium of less than 10 mg/dL (preventing hypercalcemia) and serum phosphorus of 2.7–4.6 mg/dL in patients with a GFR of 15–59 mL/min/1.73 m^2 and serum phosphorus of 3.5–5.5 mg/dL in patients with a GFR of less than 15 mL/min/1.73 m^2. National guidelines recommend maximal elemental calcium doses of 1500 mg/d (eg, nine tablets of calcium acetate).

Phosphorus-binding agents that do not contain calcium are sevelamer and lanthanum. Sevelamer, 800 mg orally, and lanthanum carbonate, 1000 mg orally, are given at the beginning of meals and are particularly useful in patients with hypercalcemia, although long-term effects are unknown. Aluminum hydroxide is an effective phosphorus binder but can cause osteomalacia and neurologic complications. It can be used in the acute setting for serum phosphorus greater than 7 mg/dL or for short periods (eg, 3 weeks) in chronic kidney disease patients, but long-term use should be avoided. If aluminum levels are high, chelation with deferoxamine can be effective. Vitamin D or vitamin D analogs can be given with secondary hyperparathyroidism in stage 3–5 chronic kidney disease (iPTH more than two to three times normal depending on GFR) if phosphorus levels are less than 5.5 mg/dL and calcium less than 10 mg/dL. However, one meta-analysis showed no clear benefit of vitamin D or its analogs in stage 3 and 4 chronic kidney disease. Vitamin D suppresses PTH and increases serum calcium and phosphorus levels; both need to be monitored closely to prevent hypercalcemia and hyperphosphatemia. If calcitriol is used, the dosage should be 0.25–0.5 mcg orally daily or every other day initially. Cinacalcet, 30–90 mg orally once a day, can be used if elevated serum phosphorus or calcium levels prohibit the use of vitamin D analogs. Cinacalcet is a calcimimetic agent that targets the calcium-sensing receptor on the chief cells of the parathyroid gland.

G. Endocrine Disorders

Circulating insulin levels are higher because of decreased renal insulin clearance. Glucose intolerance can occur in chronic renal failure when GFR is less than 10–20 mL/min. Primarily, this is due to peripheral insulin resistance. Fasting glucose levels are usually normal or only slightly elevated. Therefore, patients can be either hyperglycemic or hypoglycemic depending on the predominant disturbance. Most commonly, diabetic patients require decreased doses of hypoglycemic agents.

Decreased libido and impotence are common in chronic kidney disease. Men have decreased testosterone levels; women are often anovulatory. Despite a high degree of infertility, pregnancy can occur—particularly in women who are well dialyzed and well nourished. Fetal mortality approaches 50%. Therefore, contraception is advisable for women who do not wish to become pregnant. Renal transplantation with a stable functioning allograft affords the best chances for a successful pregnancy.

▶ Treatment

A. Dietary Management

Every patient with chronic kidney disease should be evaluated by a renal nutritionist. Specific recommendations should be made concerning protein, salt, water, potassium, and phosphorus intake.

1. Protein restriction—Experimental models have shown that protein restriction slows the progression to ESRD; however, this has not been consistently proved in clinical trials. The Modification of Diet in Renal Disease Study was meant to clarify the issue, but the results were inconclusive. A subsequent meta-analysis of five clinical trials did show a significant benefit but did not control for certain effects such as ACE inhibitor therapy. The benefits of protein restriction in slowing the rate of decline of GFR must be weighed against the risk of cachexia upon the initiation of dialysis. Low serum albumin at the start of dialysis is one of the strongest predictors of mortality in this population. In general, protein intake should not exceed 1 g/kg/d, and if protein restriction proves to be beneficial, the level of restriction may be decreased to 0.6–0.8 g/kg/d.

2. Salt and water restriction—In advanced chronic kidney disease, the kidney is unable to adapt to large changes in sodium intake. Intake greater than 3–4 g/d can lead to edema, hypertension, and congestive heart failure, whereas intake of less than 1 g/d can lead to volume depletion and hypotension. For the nondialysis patient approaching ESRD, 2 g/d of sodium is an initial recommendation. A daily intake of 1–2 L of fluid maintains water balance.

3. Potassium restriction—Restriction is needed once the GFR has fallen below 10–20 mL/min. Patients should receive detailed lists concerning potassium content of foods and should limit their intake to less than 50–60 mEq/d (2 g). Normal intake is about 100 mEq/d.

4. Phosphorus restriction—The phosphorus level should be kept in the 'normal' range (below 4.6 mg/dL) predialysis and between 3.5 and 5.5 mg/dL when on dialysis, with a dietary restriction of 800–1000 mg/d. Foods rich in phosphorus such as cola beverages, eggs, dairy products, nuts, and meat should be limited. Below a GFR of 20–30 mL/min, phosphorus binders are usually required. The treatment of hyperphosphatemia is discussed in the section on disorders of mineral metabolism.

5. Magnesium restriction—Magnesium is excreted primarily by the kidneys. Dangerous hypermagnesemia is rare unless the patient ingests medications high in magnesium or receives it parenterally. All magnesium-containing laxatives and antacids are relatively contraindicated in chronic kidney disease.

B. Dialysis

When conservative management of ESRD is inadequate, hemodialysis, peritoneal dialysis, and kidney transplantation are alternatives (see below). According to the Kidney Disease Outcomes Quality Initiative (KDOQI) guidelines, dialysis should be started when a patient has a GFR of 10 mL/min or serum creatinine of 8 mg/dL. A diabetic patient should start when the GFR reaches 15 mL/min or serum creatinine is 6 mg/dL. Other indications for dialysis include (1) uremic symptoms, such as pericarditis, encephalopathy, or coagulopathy; (2) fluid overload unresponsive to diuresis; (3) refractory hyperkalemia; (4) severe metabolic acidosis (pH < 7.20); and (5) neurologic symptoms, such as seizures or neuropathy. Preparation for dialysis requires a team approach. Dietitians, social workers, and psychiatrists should be involved as well as primary care physicians and nephrologists. The patient and family need early counseling regarding the risks and benefits of therapy. Whether the patient should undergo a 90-day trial period, not start dialysis, or withdraw from dialysis should be discussed openly. Kidney transplantation should be considered prior to initiation of dialysis. This expedites the detailed and time-consuming work-up for transplantation for eligible patients.

1. Hemodialysis—Hemodialysis requires a constant flow of blood along one side of a semipermeable membrane with a cleansing solution, or dialysate, along the other. Diffusion and convection allow the dialysate to remove unwanted substances from the blood while adding back needed components. Vascular access for hemodialysis can be accomplished by an arteriovenous fistula (the preferred method) or prosthetic graft. Indwelling catheters should be considered temporary measures. Native fistulas typically last longer than prosthetic shunts but require a longer time (6–8 weeks or more after surgical construction) for maturation. Infection, thrombosis, and aneurysm formation are complications seen more often in grafts than fistulas. *Staphylococcus* species are the most common infecting agents.

Patients typically require hemodialysis three times a week. Sessions last 3–5 hours depending on patient size, type of dialyzer used, and other factors. More recently, daily dialysis and nocturnal dialysis programs have expanded, improving medical and psychosocial parameters for patients receiving hemodialysis, such as blood pressure control, mineral metabolism, and quality of life. Periodic measurement of dialysis adequacy should determine the duration of treatment. Home hemodialysis is an option but requires a trained helper, large equipment, and hidden costs. Unfamiliarity with home hemodialysis and the financial impact with most current reimbursement schemes can limit the availability of these modalities.

2. Peritoneal dialysis—With peritoneal dialysis, the peritoneal membrane is the "dialyzer." Fluids and solutes move across the capillary bed that lies between the visceral and parietal layers of the membrane into the dialysate. Dialysate enters the peritoneal cavity through a catheter. The most common kind of peritoneal dialysis is continuous ambulatory peritoneal dialysis (CAPD). Patients exchange the dialysate four to six times a day. Continuous cyclic peritoneal dialysis (CCPD) utilizes a cycler machine to automatically perform exchanges at night. The dialysate remains in the peritoneal cavity between exchanges. As with hemodialysis, actual peritoneal dialysis prescriptions are guided by adequacy measurements.

Peritoneal dialysis permits greater patient autonomy; its continuous nature minimizes the symptomatic swings observed in hemodialysis patients; and poorly dialyzable compounds such as phosphates are better cleared, which permits less dietary restriction. The dialysate removes large amounts of albumin, and nutritional status must be closely watched.

The percentage of dialysis patients using peritoneal dialysis has been decreasing over the past several years but is starting to stabilize. The most common complication of peritoneal dialysis is peritonitis. Rates are improving, at less than 0.5 episodes per patient-year. The patient can experience nausea and vomiting, abdominal pain, diarrhea or constipation, and fever. The dialysate can be cloudy with diagnostic criteria being greater than 100 white cells/mcL of which over 50% are polymorphonuclear neutrophils. *Staphylococcus aureus* is the most common infecting organism, but streptococci and gram-negative species are common.

The total costs of peritoneal dialysis and hemodialysis are approximately the same. Equipment expenses are less for peritoneal dialysis, but the costs of peritonitis are high. Patients treated with both modalities more often prefer peritoneal dialysis to hemodialysis.

Survival rates on dialysis depend on the underlying disease process. Five-year Kaplan-Meier survival rates vary from 21% for patients with diabetes to 47% for patients with glomerulonephritis. Overall 5-year survival is currently estimated at 36%. Patients undergoing dialysis have an average life expectancy of 3–5 years, but survival for as long as 25 years is seen depending on the disease entity. Studies are conflicting regarding the survival advantage associated with either peritoneal dialysis or hemodialysis.

C. Kidney Transplantation

Up to 50% of all patients with ESRD are suitable for transplantation. Age is becoming less of a barrier. Two-thirds of kidney transplants come from deceased donors, with the remainder from living related or unrelated donors. Immunosuppressive drugs include corticosteroids, azathioprine, mycophenolate mofetil, tacrolimus, cyclosporine, and sirolimus. A patient with a deceased-donor renal transplant typically requires stronger immunosuppression than a patient with a living related kidney donor transplant. However, this depends to a great extent on the degree of HLA-type matching. The 1- and 3-year kidney graft survival rates are approximately 95% and 88%, respectively, for living donor transplants and 90% and 78%, respectively, for deceased donor transplants. Factors that determine outcome include antigenic disparity (ABO blood groups and major histocompatibility or HLA) between donor and recipient, the type of immunologic response mounted by the host, and the immunosuppressive regimen used to prevent graft rejection. Nonimmunologic factors that affect the risk of chronic rejection include age and race of recipient; donor age; length of time on dialysis; and coexisting hyperlipidemia, hypertension, or cytomegalovirus infection. Kidneys from living related donors who are HLA-identical and also red cell ABO-matched grafts have better survival at 1 year than unrelated donors ABO mismatch. Antigens are matched for HLA-A, -B, and -DR loci, with -DR compatibility most important for long-term graft survival. Grafts from deceased donors with zero HLA mismatches have a half-life of 11 years. Those with six mismatches have a half-life of 7 years, compared with those from HLA-identical siblings, which have a half-life of 24 years.

The average wait for a deceased-donor transplant is 2–6 years depending on geographic location; this is becoming progressively longer as more people are going onto waiting lists while the deceased donor pool is not expanding. Some donors are highly sensitized to HLA antigens from previous transfusions or transplants, ie, possess high panel reactive antibody levels. It may be difficult to find a suitable donor, since a positive cross-match by cytotoxicity testing is likely and would be a contraindication to transplant. Donor screening is performed in all cases to assess suitability, rule out hypertension or anatomic anomalies, and avoid transmission of hepatitis viruses, HIV, and other infectious agents.

Maintenance immunosuppressive regimens are characterized by lower doses of immunosuppressive agents than at the time of transplant, with the aim of preventing recurrent rejection and chronic allograft nephropathy, prolonging graft survival, and minimizing potentially serious medication side effects. Aside from medication use, the life of a transplanted patient can return to nearly normal.

Prognosis

Mortality is higher for patients undergoing dialysis than for age-matched controls. Yearly mortality is 21.2 deaths per 100 patient-years. The expected remaining lifetime for the age group 55–64 is 22 years, whereas that of the ESRD population is 5 years. The most common cause of death is cardiac dysfunction (45%). Other causes include infection (14%), cerebrovascular disease (6%), and malignancy (4%). Diabetes, age, a low serum albumin, lower socioeconomic status, and inadequate dialysis are all significant predictors of mortality.

For those who require dialysis to sustain life but elect not to undergo dialysis, death ensues within days to weeks. In general, uremia develops and patients lose consciousness prior to death. Arrhythmias can occur as a result of electrolyte imbalance. Volume overload and dyspnea can be managed by volume restriction and opioids as described in Chapter 5. Meticulous efforts at palliative care are essential.

When to Refer

- A patient with stage 3–5 chronic kidney disease should be referred to a nephrologist for management of chronic kidney disease in conjunction with the primary care provider.

- A patient with other forms of chronic kidney disease should have an initial visit with a nephrologist to discuss future comanagement needs.

When to Admit

- Admission should be considered for patients with decompensation of problems related to chronic kidney disease, such as worsening of acid-base status, electrolyte abnormalities, volume status that cannot be appropriately treated in the outpatient setting.

- Admission is appropriate when a patient needs to start renal replacement therapy, and is not stable for outpatient initiation.

Coresh J et al. Prevalence of chronic kidney disease in the United States. JAMA. 2007 Nov 7;298(17):2038–47. [PMID: 17986697]

Fox CH et al. A quick guide to evidence-based chronic kidney disease care for the primary care physician. Postgrad Med. 2008 Jul 31;120(2):E01–6. [PMID: 18654062]

Go AS et al. Chronic kidney disease and the risks of death, cardiovascular events, and hospitalization. N Engl J Med. 2004 Sep 23;351(13):1296–305. [PMID: 15385656]

Levey AS et al; National Kidney Foundation. National Kidney Foundation practice guidelines for chronic kidney disease: evaluation, classification, and stratification. Ann Intern Med. 2003 Jul 15;139(2):137–47. [PMID: 12859163]

Meyer TW et al. Uremia. N Engl J Med. 2007 Sep 27;357(13):1316–25. [PMID: 17898101]

Palmer S et al. Meta-analysis: vitamin D compounds in chronic kidney disease. Ann Intern Med. 2007 18 Dec;147(12):841–853. [PMID: 18087055]

Schiffrin EL et al. Chronic kidney disease: effects on the cardiovascular system. Circulation. 2007 Jul 3;116(1):85–97. [PMID: 17606856]

RENAL ARTERY STENOSIS

 ESSENTIALS OF DIAGNOSIS

- ► Produced by atherosclerotic occlusive disease (80–90% of patients) or fibromuscular dysplasia (10–15%).
- ► Hypertension.
- ► Acute kidney injury in patients starting therapy with an ACE inhibitor.

General Considerations

Atherosclerotic ischemic renal disease accounts for nearly all cases of renal artery stenosis. Fibromuscular dysplasia can also cause renal artery stenosis. Approximately 5% of Americans with hypertension suffer from renal artery stenosis. It occurs most commonly in those over 45 years of age with a history of atherosclerotic disease. Other risk factors include chronic kidney disease, diabetes mellitus, tobacco use, and hypertension.

Clinical Findings

A. Symptoms and Signs

Patients with atherosclerotic ischemic renal disease may have refractory hypertension, new-onset hypertension (in an older patient), pulmonary edema with poorly controlled blood pressure, and acute kidney injury upon starting an ACE inhibitor. In addition to hypertension, physical examination may reveal an audible abdominal bruit on the affected side. Fibromuscular dysplasia primarily affects young women. Unexplained hypertension in a young woman is reason to screen for this disorder.

B. Laboratory Findings

Laboratory values can show elevated BUN and serum creatinine levels in the setting of significant renal ischemia.

C. Imaging

Abdominal ultrasound can reveal asymmetric kidney size when one renal artery is affected out of proportion to the other.

Three prevailing methods used for screening are Doppler ultrasonography, CT angiography, and magnetic resonance angiography (MRA). **Doppler ultrasonography** is highly sensitive and specific (> 90% with an experienced ultrasonographer) and relatively inexpensive. However, this method is extremely operator and patient dependent. Measurements of blood flow must be made at the aorta and along each third of the renal artery in order to assess the disease. This test is a poor choice for patients who are obese, unable to lie supine, or have interfering bowel gas patterns.

CT angiography consists of intravenous digital subtraction angiography with arteriography and is a noninvasive procedure. The procedure uses a spiral (helical) CT scan with intravenous contrast injection. The sensitivities from various studies range from 77% to 98%, with less varying specificities in a range of 90–94%.

MRA is an excellent but expensive way to screen for renal artery stenosis, particularly in those with atherosclerotic disease. Sensitivity is 77–100%, although one study with particular flaws showed a sensitivity of only 62%. Specificity ranges from 71% to 96%. Turbulent blood flow can cause false-positive results. The imaging agent for MRA (gadolinium) has been associated with an entity known as nephrogenic systemic fibrosis, which occurs primarily in patients with GFR < 30 mL/min/1.73 m^2, acute kidney injury, and kidney transplant.

Renal angiography is the gold standard for diagnosis. CO_2 subtraction angiography can be used in place of dye when the risk of dye nephropathy exists—eg, in diabetic patients with kidney injury. Lesions are most commonly found in the proximal third or ostial region of the renal artery. The risk of atheroembolic phenomena after angiography is not trivial in this population, ranging from 5% to 10%. Fibromuscular dysplasia has a characteristic "beads-on-a-string" appearance on angiography.

Treatment

Treatment of atherosclerotic ischemic renal disease is controversial. Options include medical management, angioplasty with or without stenting, and surgical bypass. Angioplasty might reduce the number of antihypertensive medications but does not significantly change outcome in comparison to patients medically managed. Stenting produces significantly better angioplastic results. However, blood pressure is equally improved, and serum creatinines are similar at 6 months of observation compared with both angioplasty and stents. Angioplasty is equally as effective as, and safer than, surgical revision. Treatment of **fibromuscular dysplasia** with percutaneous transluminal angioplasty is often curative.

Balk E et al. Effectiveness of management strategies for renal artery stenosis: a systematic review. Ann Intern Med. 2006 Dec 19;145(12):901–12. [PMID: 17062633]

Guo H et al. Atherosclerotic renovascular disease in older US patients starting dialysis, 1996 to 2001. Circulation. 2007 Jan 2;115(1):50–8. [PMID: 17179020]

Kalra PA et al. Atherosclerotic renovascular disease in United States patients aged 67 years or older: risk factors, revascularization, and prognosis. Kidney Int. 2005 Jul;68(1):293–301. [PMID: 15954920]

GLOMERULONEPHROPATHIES

Abnormalities of glomerular function can be caused by damage to the major components of the glomerulus: the epithelium (podocytes), basement membrane, capillary endothelium, or mesangium. The damage is often manifested as an inflammatory process. A specific histologic pattern of glomerular injury can be seen on renal biopsy, one of the most helpful techniques available for defining the cause of glomerular disease. Clinically, hematuria, proteinuria, hypertension, and a reduced GFR are typical findings of glomerular diseases presenting as *nephritic* syndromes; heavy proteinuria (> 3.5 g/24 h), hypoalbuminemia, hyperlipidemia, and edema are typical findings of glomerular diseases presenting as *nephrotic* syndromes.

Classification

Glomerular diseases generally can be classified into one of three major syndromes: nephritic syndrome, nephrotic syndrome, and asymptomatic renal disease. Specific glomerular diseases usually exhibit characteristics of one of the above syndromes, though some can have varying components of all three.

Glomerular diseases can also be classified according to whether they cause only renal abnormalities (primary renal disease) or whether the renal abnormalities result from a systemic disease (secondary renal disease).

NEPHRITIC SYNDROME

 ESSENTIALS OF DIAGNOSIS

► Edema.
► Hypertension.
► Hematuria (with or without dysmorphic red cells, red blood cell casts).

General Considerations

Acute glomerulonephritis usually signifies an inflammatory process causing renal dysfunction over days to weeks that may or may not resolve. If the inflammatory process is severe, the glomerulonephritis may lead to a greater than 50% loss of nephron function over the course of days to weeks to months. Such a process, called rapidly progressive glomerulonephritis, can cause permanent damage to glomeruli if not identified and treated rapidly. Prolonged inflammatory changes can result in chronic glomerulonephritis with persistent renal abnormalities that progress to ESRD.

Clinical Findings

A. Symptoms and Signs

Edema is first seen in regions of low tissue pressure such as the periorbital and scrotal areas. Hypertension, if present, is due to volume overload rather than vasoactive substances such as angiotensin II, whose levels are low.

B. Laboratory Findings

1. Serum chemistries—There are no serum chemistries characteristic of nephritic syndrome, but certain special tests are often performed depending on the history and the results of the preliminary evaluation. These include complement levels, antinuclear antibodies (ANA), cryoglobulins, hepatitis serologies, ANCA, anti-GBM antibodies, antistreptolysin O (ASO) titers, and C3 nephritic factor (Figure 22–2).

2. Urinalysis—The urinalysis shows red blood cells. These may be misshapen from traversing a damaged capillary membrane—so-called dysmorphic red blood cells. Red blood cell casts and moderate degrees of proteinuria are also characteristic of the urinary sediment. Placing the patient in a lordotic position for an hour increases sensitivity for finding red cell casts in the next urine specimen.

3. Biopsy—Renal biopsy should be considered if there are no other contraindications to biopsy (eg, bleeding disorders, thrombocytopenia, uncontrolled hypertension). Rapidly progressive glomerulonephritis is likely when over 50% of glomeruli contain crescents. The type of disease can be categorized according to the immunofluorescent pattern and appearance on electron microscopy (Table 22–9).

► Treatment

Treatment includes aggressive reduction of hypertension and fluid overload and specific therapeutic maneuvers aimed at the underlying cause. Salt and water restriction, diuretic therapy, and possibly dialysis are needed. The inflammatory glomerular injury may require corticosteroids and cytotoxic agents. (See specific diseases discussed below.)

► When to Refer

Any patient in whom a glomerulonephritis is suspected should be referred to a nephrologist immediately.

Vinen CS et al. Acute glomerulonephritis. Postgrad Med J. 2003 Apr;79(930):206–13. [PMID: 12743337]

POSTINFECTIOUS GLOMERULONEPHRITIS

ESSENTIALS OF DIAGNOSIS

► Proteinuria.
► Glomerular hematuria.
► Symptoms 1–3 weeks after infection.

► General Considerations

Postinfectious glomerulonephritis is most often due to infection with nephritogenic group A β-hemolytic streptococci, especially type 12. It can occur sporadically or in clusters and during epidemics can account for up to 10% of known streptococcal infections. It commonly appears after pharyngitis or impetigo. Onset occurs within 1–3 weeks after infection (average, 7–10 days).

Other causes of postinfectious glomerulonephritis include bacteremic states such as systemic *S aureus* infection. Infective endocarditis and shunt infections cause similar lesions.

Viral, fungal, and parasitic causes, including hepatitis B or C, cytomegalovirus infection, infectious mononucleosis, coccidioidomycosis, malaria, and toxoplasmosis, are periinfectious glomerulonephritides.

► Clinical Findings

A. Symptoms and Signs

The patient is oliguric, edematous, and variably hypertensive.

B. Laboratory Findings

Serum complement levels are low; in postinfectious glomerulonephritis due to group A streptococcal infection, ASO titers can be high unless the immune response has been blunted with previous antibiotic treatment. Classically, the urine is described as cola-colored. Urinary red blood cells, red cell casts, and proteinuria under 3.5 g/d are present. On microscopy, this entity appears as a diffuse proliferative glomerulonephritis. Immunofluorescence shows IgG and C3 in a granular pattern in the mesangium and along the capillary basement membrane. Electron microscopy shows large, dense subepithelial deposits or "humps."

► Treatment

Treatment for this entity is supportive. Appropriate antibiotics should be used. Antihypertensives, salt restriction, and diuretics should be used if needed. Corticosteroids have not been shown to improve outcome. Prognosis in children is very favorable, but adults are more prone to crescent formation and chronic kidney disease. A rapidly progressive glomerulonephritis will develop in less than 5% of adults, and a smaller percentage of adults will progress to ESRD.

IGA NEPHROPATHY

ESSENTIALS OF DIAGNOSIS

► Can present with hematuria or proteinuria.
► Proteinuria: minimal to nephrotic range.
► Glomerular hematuria: microscopic is common; macroscopic (gross) after infection.
► Increased serum IgA in 50% of cases.
► Positive IgA staining on renal biopsy, if performed.

► General Considerations

IgA nephropathy (Berger disease) is a primary renal disease of IgA deposition in the glomerular mesangium. The

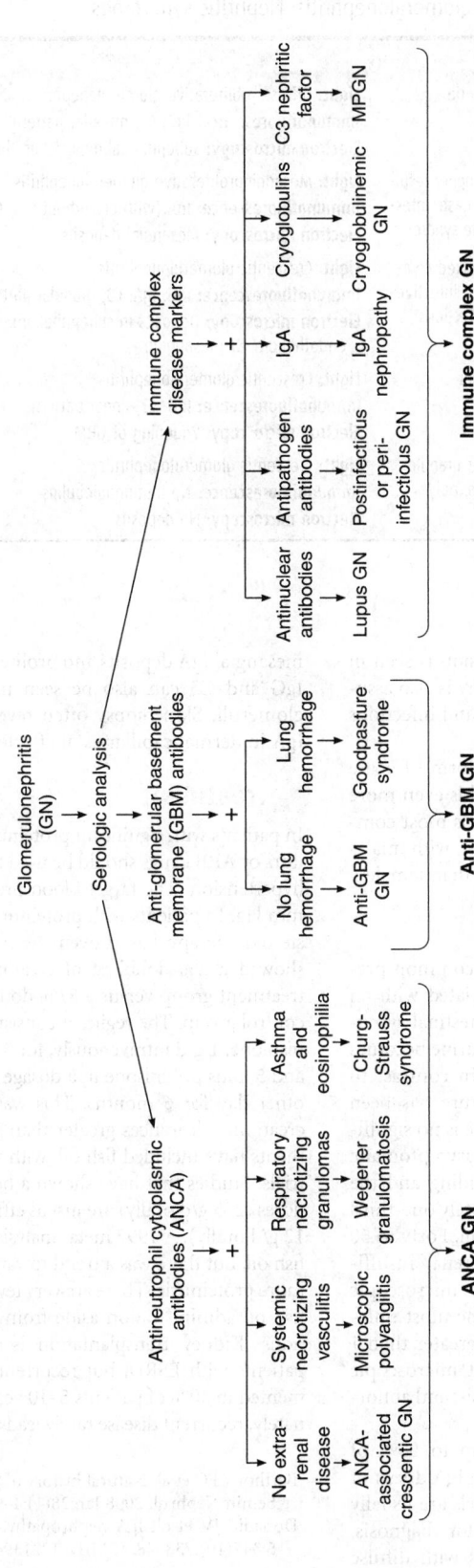

▲ **Figure 22–2.** Serologic analysis of patients with glomerulonephritis. MPGN, membranoproliferative glomerulonephritis. (Reproduced, with permission, from Jennette JC et al. *Primer on Kidney Diseases.* Academic Press, 1994 and Jennette JC, Falk RJ. Diagnosis and management of glomerulonephritis and vasculitis presenting as acute renal failure. Med Clin North Am. 1990;74(4):893–908. © Elsevier.)

Table 22–9. Classification and findings in glomerulonephritis: Nephritic syndromes.

	Etiology	Histopathology	Pathogenesis
Acute (postinfectious) glomerulonephritis	Streptococci, other bacteria	**Light:** Diffuse proliferative glomerulonephritis **Immunofluorescence:** IgG; C3, granular pattern **Electron microscopy:** Subepithelial deposits or "humps"	Trapped immune complexes
IgA nephropathy (Berger disease and Henoch-Schönlein purpura)	In association with viral upper respiratory tract infections; gastrointestinal infection or flu-like syndrome	**Light:** Mesangioproliferative glomerulonephritis **Immunofluorescence:** IgA (with or without IgG, C3) **Electron microscopy:** Mesangial deposits	Unknown
Rapidly progressive glomerulonephritis	Lupus erythematosus, mixed cryoglobulinemia, subacute infective endocarditis, shunt infections	**Light:** Crescentic glomerulonephritis **Immunofluorescence:** IgG, IgA; C3, granular pattern **Electron microscopy:** Deposits in subepithelium, subendothelium, or mesangium	Trapped immune complexes
	Goodpasture syndrome or idiopathic	**Light:** Crescentic glomerulonephritis **Immunofluorescence:** IgG; C3, linear pattern **Electron microscopy:** Widening of GBM	Anti-GBM antibodies
	Pauci-immune (Wegener granulomatosis, Churg-Strauss, polyarteritis, idiopathic)	**Light:** Crescentic glomerulonephritis **Immunofluorescence:** No immunoglobulins **Electron microscopy:** No deposits	Unclear role of ANCAs

GBM, glomerular basement membrane.

inciting cause is unknown, but the same lesion is seen in Henoch-Schönlein purpura. IgA nephropathy is also associated with hepatic cirrhosis, celiac disease, and infections such as HIV and cytomegalovirus.

IgA nephropathy is the most common form of acute glomerulonephritis in the United States and is even more prevalent worldwide, particularly in Asia. It is most commonly seen in children and young adults, with males affected two to three times more commonly than females.

Clinical Findings

An episode of gross hematuria is the most common presenting complaint. Frequently, this is associated with an upper respiratory infection (50%), gastrointestinal symptoms (10%), or a flu-like illness (15%). The urine becomes red or cola-colored 1–2 days after onset. In contrast to postinfectious glomerulonephritis, this feature has been called "synpharyngitic hematuria" since there is no significant latent period. Other findings include asymptomatic microscopic hematuria as an incidental finding and the nephrotic syndrome (see below). Approximately one-third of patients will experience a clinical remission. Forty to 50 percent of patients will have progressive renal insufficiency. The remainder will show chronic microscopic hematuria and a stable serum creatinine. The most unfavorable prognostic indicator is proteinuria greater than 1 g/d; others include hypertension, persistent microscopic hematuria and proteinuria, glomerulosclerosis, and abnormal kidney function.

The serum IgA level is increased in up to 50% of patients, and for that reason a normal serum IgA does not rule out the disease. Serum complement levels are usually normal, and renal biopsy is the standard for diagnosis. Glomeruli show a focal glomerulonephritis with diffuse mesangial IgA deposits and proliferation of mesangial cells. IgG and C3 can also be seen in the mesangium of all glomeruli. Skin biopsy often reveals granular deposits of IgA in dermal capillaries of affected patients.

Treatment

In patients with significant proteinuria (> 1 g/d), ACE inhibitors or ARB drugs should be used to reduce proteinuria and hypertension. The target blood pressure is less than 130/80 mm Hg. In patients with proteinuria of 1.0–3.5 g/d, corticosteroid therapy has proven beneficial. One such regimen showed a 2% doubling of creatinine after 6 years in the treatment group versus a 21% doubling of creatinine in the control group. The regimen consisted of giving methylprednisolone, 1 g/d intravenously, for 3 days during months 1, 3, and 5, plus prednisone in a dosage of 0.5 mg/kg orally every other day for 6 months. This was aimed at patients with creatinine clearances greater than 70 mL/min. Other treatments have included fish oil, with variable results in clinical trials. Studies that have shown a benefit also show that low doses (2–5 g/d orally) are just as efficacious as high doses (9–12 g/d orally). A 1997 meta-analysis showed no benefit from fish oil, but there was a trend toward benefit in patients with more proteinuria. There are very few side effects of long-term fish oil administration aside from fishy breath and eructations. Kidney transplantation is an excellent option for patients with ESRD, but recurrent disease has been documented in 30% of patients 5–10 years posttransplant. Fortunately, recurrent disease rarely leads to failure of the allograft.

Berthoux FC et al. Natural history of primary IgA nephropathy. Semin Nephrol. 2008 Jan;28(1):4–9. [PMID: 18222341]

Donadio JV et al. IgA nephropathy. N Engl J Med. 2002 Sep 5;347(10):738–48. [PMID: 12213946]

HENOCH-SCHÖNLEIN PURPURA

This disease is a leukocytoclastic vasculitis of unknown cause. It is most common in children and has a male predominance. It classically presents with palpable purpura, arthralgias, and abdominal symptoms such as nausea, colic, and melena. Purpuric skin lesions are most often found on the lower extremities. A decrease in GFR is common with a nephritic presentation. The renal lesions are identical to those found in IgA nephropathy. Most patients will recover fully over several weeks.

Further details about Henoch-Schönlein purpura are provided in Chapter 20.

Sanders JT et al. IgA nephropathy and Henoch-Schönlein purpura nephritis. Curr Opin Pediatr. 2008 Apr;20(2):163–70. [PMID: 18332712]

PAUCI-IMMUNE GLOMERULONEPHRITIS (ANCA-Associated)

Pauci-immune glomerular lesions are seen with Wegener granulomatosis, Churg-Strauss disease, and microscopic polyangiitis. All are small-vessel vasculitides. Wegener granulomatosis also involves granulomatous inflammation of the respiratory tract with a necrotizing vasculitis of small and medium-sized vessels. Microscopic polyangiitis (polyarteritis) is similar to Wegener granulomatosis without granulomatous inflammation, but both commonly exhibit a necrotizing glomerulonephritis. ANCA-associated glomerulonephritis can also present as a primary renal lesion. The pathogenesis of these entities is unknown, but more than 95% of pauci-immune glomerulonephritis is associated with antineutrophil cytoplasmic antibodies.

▶ Clinical Findings

A. Symptoms and Signs

Symptoms of a systemic inflammatory disease, including fever, malaise, and weight loss, may be present. In addition to hematuria and proteinuria from glomerular inflammation, some patients exhibit purpura from dermal capillary involvement and mononeuritis multiplex from nerve arteriolar involvement. Ninety percent of patients with Wegener granulomatosis will have upper or lower respiratory tract symptoms with nodular lesions that can cavitate and bleed.

B. Laboratory Findings

Serologically, ANCA subtype analysis can be done. A cytoplasmic pattern (C-ANCA) is specific for antiproteinase-3 antibodies, while a perinuclear pattern (P-ANCA) is specific for antimyeloperoxidase antibodies. Over 90% of patients with Wegener syndrome will have C-ANCA; the remainder can have a P-ANCA pattern. Microscopic angiitis will have either a P-ANCA or C-ANCA pattern about 80% of the time. Pathologically, the small vessels and glomeruli will lack immune deposits (pauci-immune); however, a cell-mediated immune response is often seen. Necrotizing lesions and crescents signify a rapidly progressive glomerulonephritis.

▶ Treatment

Treatment should be instituted early if aggressive disease is suspected. High doses of corticosteroids (methylprednisolone, 1–2 g/d intravenously for 3 days, followed by prednisone, 1 mg/kg orally for 1 month, with a slow taper over the next 6 months) and cytotoxic agents (cyclophosphamide, 0.5–1.0 g/m^2 intravenously per month or 1.5–2 mg/kg orally for 3–6 months with potential conversion to less toxic agents such as azathioprine or mycophenolate mofetil for 12–18 months) are recommended for controlling end-organ damage. Intravenous cyclophosphamide is likely associated with fewer side effects and is just as efficacious as oral cyclophosphamide. Without treatment, prognosis is extremely poor, but with the above regimen, complete remission can be achieved in about 75% of patients. One trial randomized 137 patients with ANCA-associated glomerulonephritis to corticosteroids and cytotoxic medications versus a similar regimen with the addition of plasmapheresis. Those receiving plasmapheresis had improved kidney function and mortality versus those not receiving it. Prognosis also depends on the extent of glomerular involvement before treatment is started. ANCA levels can be monitored to help determine the efficacy of treatment.

Harper L et al. ANCA-associated renal vasculitis at the end of the twentieth century—a disease of older patients. Rheumatology (Oxford). 2005 Apr;44(4):495–501. [PMID: 15613403]

ANTI-GLOMERULAR BASEMENT MEMBRANE GLOMERULONEPHRITIS & GOODPASTURE SYNDROME

Goodpasture syndrome is defined by the clinical constellation of glomerulonephritis and pulmonary hemorrhage; injury to both is mediated by anti-GBM antibodies. Up to one-third of patients with anti-GBM glomerulonephritis have no evidence of lung injury. Anti-GBM-associated glomerulonephritis accounts for about 10% of patients with rapidly progressive acute glomerulonephritis. The incidence in males is approximately six times that in females, and the disease occurs most commonly in the second and third decades but has a wide range. It has been associated with influenza A infection, hydrocarbon solvent exposure, and HLA-DR2 and -B7 antigens.

▶ Clinical Findings

A. Symptoms and Signs

The onset of disease is preceded by an upper respiratory tract infection in 20–60% of cases. Patients experience hemoptysis, dyspnea, and possible respiratory failure. Hypertension and edema are seen as components of the nephritic syndrome.

B. Laboratory Findings

Laboratory evaluation can show iron deficiency anemia, and complement levels are normal. Sputum contains hemosiderin-laden macrophages. Chest radiographs can show shifting pulmonary infiltrates due to pulmonary hemorrhage. The diffusion capacity of carbon monoxide is markedly increased. Diagnosis is confirmed by finding circulating anti-GBM antibodies, which are positive in over 90% of patients. About 15% of patients will have positive serum for ANCAs, too, showing the importance of performing a renal biopsy in such patients.

▶ Treatment

The treatment of choice is a combination of plasma exchange therapy to remove circulating antibodies and administration of immunosuppressive drugs to prevent formation of new antibodies and control the inflammatory response. Corticosteroids are typically given initially in pulse doses of methylprednisolone, 1–2 g/d for 3 days, then prednisone orally 1 mg/kg/d. Cyclophosphamide is administered intravenously at a dose of 0.5–1.0 g/m^2 per month or orally at a dosage of 2–3 mg/kg/d. Daily plasmapheresis is performed for up to 2 weeks. A poorer prognosis exists in patients with oliguria and a serum creatinine greater than 6–7 mg/dL, or requiring dialysis upon presentation. Anti-GBM antibody levels should decrease as the clinical course improves.

Hudson BG et al. Alport's syndrome, Goodpasture's syndrome, and type IV collagen. N Engl J Med. 2003 Jun 19;348(25):2543–56. [PMID: 12815141]

Levy JB et al. Long-term outcome of anti-glomerular basement membrane antibody disease treated with plasma exchange and immunosuppression. Ann Intern Med. 2001 Jun 5;134(11):1033–42. [PMID: 11388816]

CRYOGLOBULIN-ASSOCIATED GLOMERULONEPHRITIS

Essential (mixed) cryoglobulinemia is a disorder associated with cold-precipitable immunoglobulins (cryoglobulins). Glomerular disease results from the precipitation of cryoglobulins in glomerular capillaries. The cause is typically an underlying infection, such as hepatitis B; hepatitis C; or other occult viral, bacterial, and fungal infections.

Patients exhibit necrotizing skin lesions in dependent areas, arthralgias, fever, and hepatosplenomegaly. Serum complement levels are depressed. Rheumatoid factor is often elevated when cryoglobulins are present. Rapidly progressive glomerulonephritis is seen on pathologic examination with the presence of crescents.

Treatment consists of aggressively treating the underlying infection. Pulse corticosteroids, plasma exchange, and cytotoxic agents can be used. Interferon-α (IFN-α) has been shown to benefit patients with hepatitis C–related cryoglobulinemia.

NEPHROTIC SYNDROME

 ESSENTIALS OF DIAGNOSIS

- ▶ Urine protein excretion > 3.5 g/1.73 m^2 per 24 hours.
- ▶ Hypoalbuminemia (albumin < 3 g/dL).
- ▶ Peripheral edema.

▶ General Considerations

In adults, about one-third of patients with nephrotic syndrome have a systemic renal disease such as diabetes mellitus, amyloidosis, or systemic lupus erythematosus. With the current epidemic of type 2 diabetes mellitus, this proportion is slowly increasing. The remainder have idiopathic nephrotic syndrome. The four most common are minimal change disease, focal glomerular sclerosis, membranous nephropathy, and membranoproliferative glomerulonephritis.

▶ Clinical Findings

A. Symptoms and Signs

Peripheral edema is a hallmark of the nephrotic syndrome, occurring when the serum albumin concentration is less than 3 g/dL. Edema is most likely due to sodium retention (from renal disease) rather than arterial underfilling from low plasma oncotic pressure. Initially this presents in the dependent areas of the body such as the lower extremities; however, such edema can become generalized. Patients can experience dyspnea due to pulmonary edema, pleural effusions, and diaphragmatic compromise with ascites. Complaints of abdominal fullness may also be present in patients with ascites.

Patients may show symptoms and signs of infection more frequently than the general population owing to loss of immunoglobulins and certain complement moieties in the urine.

B. Laboratory Findings

1. Urinalysis—Proteinuria occurs as a result of effacement of epithelial cell foot processes and an alteration of the negative charge in the GBM. The screening test for proteinuria is the urinary dipstick analysis; however, this test indicates albumin only. The addition of sulfosalicylic acid to the urine sediment allows abnormal paraproteins to be detected. Urine dipstick testing can detect as little as 15 mg/dL of protein, but the results must be interpreted along with the urine specific gravity. Trace protein seen on highly concentrated specimens may be insignificant, while trace protein on dilute specimens may indicate true renal disease. A spot urine protein to urine creatinine ratio gives a reasonable approximation of grams of protein excreted per day.

Microscopically, the urinary sediment has relatively few cellular elements or casts. However, if marked hyperlipidemia is present, patients can have oval fat bodies in the urine. These represent lipid deposits in sloughed renal tubular epithelial cells. They appear as "grape clusters" under light microscopy and "Maltese crosses" under polarized light.

2. Blood chemistries—Characteristic blood chemistries include a decreased serum albumin (< 3 g/dL) and total serum protein less than 6 g/dL. Hyperlipidemia occurs in over 50% of those with early nephrotic syndrome. As patients excrete larger amounts of protein per day, the frequency and degree of hyperlipidemia increases. There is increased hepatic production of lipids (cholesterol and apolipoprotein B), owing to a fall in oncotic pressure. There is also decreased clearance of very low-density lipoproteins, causing hypertriglyceridemia. Patients can also have an elevated erythrocyte

Table 22–10. Classification and findings in glomerulonephritis: Nephrotic syndromes.

	Etiology	Histopathology	Pathogenesis
Minimal change disease (nil disease; lipoid nephrosis)	Associated with allergy, Hodgkin disease, NSAIDs	**Light:** Normal (with or without mesangial proliferation) **Immunofluorescence:** No immunoglobulins **Electron microscopy:** Fusion foot processes	Unknown
Focal and segmental glomerulosclerosis	Associated with heroin abuse, HIV infection, reflux nephropathy, obesity	**Light:** Focal segmental sclerosis **Immunofluorescence:** IgM and C3 in sclerotic segments **Electron microscopy:** Fusion foot processes	Unknown
Membranous nephropathy	Associated with non-Hodgkin lymphoma, carcinoma (gastrointestinal, renal, bronchogenic, thyroid), gold therapy, penicillamine, lupus erythematosus	**Light:** Thickened GBM and spikes **Immunofluorescence:** Granular IgG and C3 along capillary loops **Electron microscopy:** Dense deposits in subepithelial area	In situ immune complex formation
Membranoproliferative glomerulonephropathy	Type I associated with upper respiratory infection	**Light:** Increased mesangial cells and matrix with splitting of GBM **Immunofluorescence:** Granular C3, C1q, C4 with IgG and IgM **Electron microscopy:** Dense deposits in subendothelium	Unknown
	Type II	**Light:** Same as type I **Immunofluorescence:** C3 only **Electron microscopy:** Dense material in GBM	Unknown

GBM, glomerular basement membrane; NSAIDs, nonsteroidal anti-inflammatory drugs.

sedimentation rate as a result of alterations in some plasma components such as increased levels of fibrinogen.

Other less common tests may be necessary depending on the patient's clinical presentation, including complement levels, serum and urine protein electrophoresis, ANA, and serologic tests for hepatitis. Patients may become deficient in vitamin D, zinc, and copper from loss of binding proteins in the urine; they are prone to infection, in part from urinary losses of immunoglobulins.

3. Renal biopsy—Specific classification and findings are shown in Table 22–10. Specimens are examined by light microscopy, with immunofluorescent stains, and by electron microscopy. Renal biopsy is often performed in adults with new-onset idiopathic nephrotic syndrome if a primary renal disease that may require drug therapy (eg, corticosteroids, cytotoxic agents) is suspected. Significantly elevated creatinine levels may indicate irreversible kidney disease mitigating the usefulness of kidney biopsy. Disease due to amyloidosis or diabetes mellitus often does not need to be biopsied, since nephrotic range proteinuria in these diseases represents irreversible damage, although bone marrow transplant with high-dose chemotherapy can be considered in some patients with amyloidosis. The role of biopsy for other systemic kidney diseases is debated. However, it can be useful for prognosis and treatment. An occasional unexpected diagnosis is made, such as membranous nephropathy due to lupus erythematosus without serologic evidence of that illness.

▶ **Treatment**

A. Protein Loss

The daily total dietary protein intake should replace the daily urinary protein losses so as to avoid negative nitrogen balance. Protein malnutrition often occurs with urinary protein losses greater than 10 g/d. In the past, protein restriction was suggested for patients with kidney disease because experimental animal models had demonstrated a decrease in glomerulosclerosis among those animals fed low-protein diets. The largest human trial to date (the MDRD Study) did not show a significant benefit, but two recent meta-analyses have shown a mild renal benefit. For this reason, the KDOQI recommends protein restriction to 0.6–0.8 g/kg/d in patients with a GFR less than 25 mL/min prior to starting dialysis. However, great care must be taken to avoid malnutrition in these patients.

In both diabetic and nondiabetic patients, therapy that is aimed at reducing proteinuria may also reduce progression of renal disease. ACE inhibitors are effective by lowering efferent arteriolar resistance out of proportion to afferent arteriolar resistance, thereby reducing glomerular capillary pressure, reducing kidney damage, and lowering urinary protein excretion. Other effects include alterations of glomerular mesangial proliferation. ACE inhibitors can be used in patients despite compromised GFR as long as significant hyperkalemia (K^+ > 5.2–5.5 mEq/L) does not occur and serum creatinine rises less than 30%, stabilizing over 2 months. Large randomized controlled trials (ie, the RENAAL and IDNT studies) have also proved the benefit of angiotensin II-receptor blockers in reducing proteinuria and preventing progression of renal disease in diabetic nephropathy. "Head-to-head" comparisons of an ACE-I and an ARB have shown the ARB to be no better than the ACE-I in preventing progression of renal disease in diabetic persons with proteinuria. The combination of ACE-I and ARB versus ARB alone for slowing the progression of diabetic nephropathy is believed to have additional benefits and is being tested in a multi-center, prospective randomized study.

B. Edema

Dietary salt restriction is essential for managing edema; most patients also require diuretic therapy. Commonly used diuretics include thiazide and loop diuretics. Both are highly protein bound. With hypoalbuminemia and poor kidney function, diuretic delivery to the kidney is reduced, and patients often require large doses. The combination of loop and thiazide diuretics can potentiate the diuretic effect. This may be needed for patients with refractory fluid retention associated with pleural effusions and ascites.

C. Hyperlipidemia

Hypercholesterolemia and hypertriglyceridemia occur as outlined above. Dietary management in patients with nephrotic syndrome is of little value; however, dietary modification and exercise should be advocated. Aggressive pharmacologic treatment should be pursued. This is discussed in Chapter 28.

D. Hypercoagulable State

Patients with serum albumin less than 2 g/dL can become hypercoagulable. Nephrotic patients have urinary losses of antithrombin III, protein C, and protein S and increased platelet activation. Patients are prone to renal vein thrombosis and other venous thromboemboli, particularly with membranous glomerulopathy. Anticoagulation therapy is warranted for at least 3–6 months in patients with evidence of thrombosis. Patients with renal vein thrombosis and recurrent thromboemboli require indefinite anticoagulation.

► When to Refer

Any patient noted to have nephritic syndrome should be referred immediately to a nephrologist.

► When to Admit

Patients with edema refractory to outpatient therapy or rapidly worsening kidney function that may require inpatient interventions should be admitted.

Glassock RJ. Prophylactic anticoagulation in nephrotic syndrome: a clinical conundrum. J Am Soc Nephrol. 2007 Aug;18(8):2221–5. [PMID: 17599972]

NEPHROTIC DISEASE IN PRIMARY RENAL DISORDERS

MINIMAL CHANGE DISEASE

ESSENTIALS OF DIAGNOSIS

▶ Nephrotic range proteinuria.

▶ Kidney biopsy shows no changes on light microscopy.

▶ There are characteristic foot-process effacement on electron microscopy.

► General Considerations

Minimal change disease is most commonly seen in children but is occasionally present in adults. In patients over 40 years with primary nephrotic syndrome, the incidence of minimal change disease is 20–25%, with equal distribution between men and women. In younger patients, there is a male predominance. Minimal change disease can be idiopathic but also occurs following viral upper respiratory infections, in association with tumors such as Hodgkin disease, with drugs (gold and lithium), and with hypersensitivity reactions (especially to NSAIDs and bee stings).

► Clinical Findings

A. Symptoms and Signs

Patients can exhibit the manifestations of nephrotic syndrome. They are more susceptible to infection, especially with gram-positive organisms, have a tendency toward thromboembolic events, develop severe hyperlipidemia, and experience protein malnutrition. Minimal change disease can rarely cause acute kidney injury due to tubular changes and interstitial edema.

B. Histologic Findings

Glomeruli show no changes on light microscopy or immunofluorescence. On electron microscopy, there is a characteristic fusion of epithelial foot processes. A subgroup of patients also shows mesangial cell proliferation. These people have more hematuria and hypertension and respond poorly to corticosteroid treatment.

► Treatment

Treatment is with prednisone, 1 mg/kg/d orally. Unlike children, adults often require longer therapy. It can take up to 16 weeks to achieve a response to corticosteroids. Treatment should be continued for several weeks after complete remission of proteinuria. A significant number of patients will relapse and require further corticosteroid treatment. Patients with frequent relapses and corticosteroid resistance may need cyclophosphamide or chlorambucil to induce subsequent remissions. Progression to ESRD is rare. Complications most often arise from prolonged corticosteroid use.

Palmer SC et al. Interventions for minimal change disease in adults with nephrotic syndrome. Cochrane Database Syst Rev. 2008 Jan 23;(1):CD001537. [PMID: 18253993]

MEMBRANOUS NEPHROPATHY

ESSENTIALS OF DIAGNOSIS

▶ Nephrotic range proteinuria.

▶ Associated with coagulopathy, eg, renal vein thrombosis.

- "Spike and dome" pattern on kidney biopsy represents subepithelial deposits.
- Immunofluorescence on kidney biopsy shows IgG and C3 deposits along capillary loops.

General Considerations

Membranous nephropathy is the most common cause of primary nephrotic syndrome in adults. It is an immune-mediated disease characterized by immune complex deposition in the subepithelial portion of glomerular capillary walls. The antigens in primary disease are not known. Secondary disease is associated with infections, such as hepatitis B, endocarditis, and syphilis; autoimmune disease, such as systemic lupus erythematosus, mixed connective tissue disease, and thyroiditis; carcinomas; and certain drugs, such as gold, penicillamine, and captopril. Membranous nephropathy occurs most commonly in adults in their fifth and sixth decades and almost always after age 30 years.

Clinical Findings

A. Symptoms and Signs

Patients exhibit the signs of nephrotic syndrome and have a higher incidence of renal vein thrombosis than most nephrotic patients. A higher incidence of occult neoplasms of lung, stomach, and colon is found in people over 50 years of age. The course of disease is variable, with about 50% of patients progressing to ESRD over 3–10 years. Poorer outcome is associated with concomitant tubulointerstitial fibrosis, male gender, elevated serum creatinine, hypertension, and heavy proteinuria (> 10 g/d).

B. Laboratory Findings

By light microscopy, capillary wall thickness is increased without inflammatory changes or cellular proliferation. When stained with silver methenamine, a "spike and dome" pattern may be observed owing to projections of excess GBM between the subepithelial deposits. Immunofluorescence shows IgG and C3 uniformly along capillary loops. Electron microscopy shows a discontinuous pattern of dense deposits along the subepithelial surface of the basement membrane.

Treatment

Treatment is controversial. After underlying causes are excluded, treatment depends on the risk of renal disease progression. One algorithm is based on the degree of proteinuria. In patients with proteinuria less than 3.5 g/d, the risk of progression is low. These individuals should be closely monitored with a low-salt diet, strict blood pressure control, and an ACE inhibitor for reduction of proteinuria. Patients with proteinuria of 3.5–8 g/d but normal renal function are at medium risk. They should follow the above suggestions and can elect immunosuppressive regimens with corticosteroids and chlorambucil or cyclophosphamide for 6 months, although 65% of these patients experience partial or complete remission within 3–4 years. Cyclo-

sporine is a second choice. The highest-risk patients—those with greater than 8 g/d of proteinuria and possible renal dysfunction—might receive corticosteroids with a cytotoxic agent as first-line immunosuppressant therapy, though the choice of cyclosporine is also reasonable. These treatments should be carefully chosen in consultation with a nephrologist. Patients with membranous nephropathy are excellent candidates for transplant.

Deegens JK et al. Membranous nephropathy in the older adult: epidemiology, diagnosis and management. Drugs Aging. 2007;24(9):717–32. [PMID: 17727303]

FOCAL SEGMENTAL GLOMERULAR SCLEROSIS

This lesion can present as idiopathic disease or secondary to such conditions as heroin use, morbid obesity, and HIV infection. Clinically, patients show evidence of nephrotic syndrome, but they also have more nephritic features than membranous nephropathy or minimal change disease. Eighty percent of patients have microscopic hematuria at presentation, and many are hypertensive. Decreased kidney function is present in 25–50% at time of diagnosis. Patients with focal segmental glomerular sclerosis and nephrotic syndrome typically progress to ESRD in 6–8 years.

Diagnosis requires renal biopsy. Light microscopy shows the lesions of focal segmental glomerular sclerosis. It is thought that these lesions occur first in the juxtamedullary glomeruli and are then seen in the superficial renal cortex. IgM and C3 are seen in the sclerotic lesions on immunofluorescence. Electron microscopy shows fusion of epithelial foot processes as seen in minimal change disease (Table 22–10).

Treatment is controversial, though supportive care for nephrotic patients is indicated. Longer courses of corticosteroids are now being used because a higher percentage of patients enter remission. High-dose oral prednisone (1–1.5 mg/kg/d) for 2–3 months followed by a slow taper can induce remission in over half of patients. Most patients achieve remission within 5–9 months. Other cytotoxic drug therapy can be considered but is disappointing (< 20% remission in most series).

Chun MJ et al. Focal segmental glomerulosclerosis in nephrotic adults: presentation, prognosis, and response to therapy of the histologic variants. J Am Soc Nephrol. 2004 Aug;15(8):2169–77. [PMID: 15284302]

▼ NEPHROTIC DISEASE FROM SYSTEMIC DISORDERS

AMYLOIDOSIS

Amyloidosis consists of extracellular deposition of the fibrous protein amyloid in one or more sites in the body. The amyloid fibrils are composed of proteins that have formed β-pleated sheets, a definitive characteristic. Primary renal amyloidosis (AL amyloidosis) may occur in the absence of systemic disease or associated with multiple myeloma; indeed, both are plasma cell dyscrasias. Secondary amyloidosis (AA amyloidosis) is due to a chronic inflammatory disease, such as rheumatoid arthritis, inflammatory bowel disease, or chronic infection. The acute phase reactant serum amyloid A is synthesized in the liver and deposited in the tissues. Primary amyloidosis usually occurs in older age groups and displays a benign urinary sediment; the amyloid is derived from immunoglobulin light chain. The degree of proteinuria is not associated with the extent of renal lesions. Kidneys can be enlarged as a result of amyloid deposition. Pathologically, glomeruli are filled with amorphous deposits that stain positive with Congo red and show green birefringence.

Treatment options are few. Remissions can occur in secondary amyloidosis if the inciting agent is removed. Primary amyloidosis of the kidney progresses to ESRD in an average of 2–3 years. Five-year overall survival is less than 20%, with death occurring from ESRD and heart disease. The use of alkylating agents and corticosteroids—eg, melphalan and prednisone—can reduce proteinuria and improve renal function in a small percentage of patients. Melphalan and stem cell transplantation are associated with high toxicity (45% mortality) but induce remission in 80% of the remaining patients. Renal transplant is an option in patients with secondary amyloid.

Bergesio F et al; Immunopathology Group, Italian Society of Nephrology. Renal involvement in systemic amyloidosis—an Italian retrospective study on epidemiological and clinical data at diagnosis. Nephrol Dial Transplant. 2007 Jun;22(6):1608–18. [PMID: 17395661]

DIABETIC NEPHROPATHY

ESSENTIALS OF DIAGNOSIS

▸ Prior evidence of diabetes mellitus over years, at minimum.

▸ Albuminuria (microscopic or macroscopic) not due to another kidney disorder.

▸ Signs of diabetic nephropathy on renal biopsy, if done.

▸ Other end-organ damage common, such as diabetic retinopathy, but not required.

▸ General Considerations

Diabetic nephropathy is the most common cause of ESRD in the United States (about 4000 cases a year). Type 1 diabetes mellitus carries a 30–40% chance of nephropathy after 20 years, whereas type 2 has a 15–20% chance after 20 years. ESRD is much more likely to develop in persons with type 1 diabetes mellitus, in part due to fewer comorbidities and deaths before ESRD ensues. With the current epidemic of type 2 diabetes mellitus, rates of diabetic nephropathy are projected to continue to increase over at least the next 2 decades. Patients at higher risk include males, African Americans, and Native Americans.

The most common lesion in diabetic nephropathy is diffuse glomerulosclerosis, but nodular glomerulosclerosis (Kimmelstiel-Wilson nodules) is pathognomonic. The kidneys in these patients are usually enlarged as a result of cellular hypertrophy and proliferation. At the onset of diabetic nephropathy, glomerular disease will cause an increase in GFR. As the nephropathy progresses, with the development of macroalbuminuria, the GFR returns to normal and continues to decrease.

Patients with diabetes are prone to other renal disease. These include papillary necrosis, chronic interstitial nephritis, and type IV (hyporeninemic hypoaldosteronemic) renal tubular acidosis. Patients are more susceptible to acute kidney injury from contrast material and have a poor prognosis once dialysis is begun.

▸ Clinical Findings

The nephrotic syndrome develops in patients at risk for nephropathy. Diabetic retinopathy is often present in these patients. Initial screening of diabetics should always include urine examination for microalbuminuria. Dipstick examination may not be sensitive enough; a 24-hour urine collection is the accepted standard measure. (An albumin excretion of > 30 mg/d is abnormal.) However, an early morning spot urine albumin or albumin-creatinine ratio is adequate. (More than 30 mg of albumin per gram of creatinine is considered abnormal.) In patients prone to nephropathy, microalbuminuria will develop within 10–15 years after onset of diabetes and progress over the next 3–7 years to overt proteinuria.

▸ Treatment

During the onset of microalbuminuria but before clinical proteinuria, aggressive treatment is necessary. Strict glycemic control and treatment of hypertension have been proven to slow progression of disease. In particular, ACE inhibitors and ARBs lower the rate of progression to clinical proteinuria and slow progression to ESRD (see Treatment section under Nephrotic Syndrome, above). They may reduce intraglomerular pressure as well as treat hypertension. Even in the subset of patients with markedly diminished renal function, these agents seem to provide renal benefit if patients can tolerate the medication from the perspective of hyperkalemia and the acute decrease in GFR.

Araki S et al. Reduction in microalbuminuria as an integrated indicator for renal and cardiovascular risk reduction in patients with type 2 diabetes. Diabetes. 2007 Jun;56(6):1727–30. [PMID: 17360976]

Finne P et al. Incidence of end-stage renal disease in patients with type 1 diabetes. JAMA. 2005 Oct 12;294(14):1782–7. [PMID: 16219881]

Gaede P et al. Effect of a multifactorial intervention on mortality in type 2 diabetes. N Engl J Med. 2008 Feb 7;358(6):580–91. [PMID: 18256393]

Strippoli GF et al. Effects of angiotensin converting enzyme inhibitors and angiotensin II receptor antagonists on mortality and renal outcomes in diabetic nephropathy: systematic review. BMJ. 2004 Oct 9;329(7470):828. [PMID: 15459003]

HIV-ASSOCIATED NEPHROPATHY

HIV-associated nephropathy can present as the nephrotic syndrome in patients with HIV infection. Decline in GFR can progress rapidly. Most patients are African American, possibly because of a genetic predisposition (eg, *MYH9* gene). The more common mode of acquisition of HIV in these patients is through injection drug use. Often, patients have low CD4 counts, and have advanced HIV disease, but HIV-associated nephropathy can also be the initial presentation of disease.

Patients can have a nephrotic picture with normal complement levels. Light microscopy shows focal segmental glomerulosclerosis as described above. Lesions are often of the collapsing variety, and renal biopsy specimens exhibit severe tubulointerstitial damage.

Small, uncontrolled studies have shown that highly active antiretroviral therapy (HAART) for a prolonged course can slow progression of disease. Despite this minimal evidence, HAART has been recommended for use in these patients given the therapy's other beneficial effects and reasonable toxicity profile. Either ACE inhibitors or angiotensin II receptor binders augments therapy. Corticosteroid treatment has been used with variable success at a dosage of 1 mg/kg/d, along with cyclosporine.

Atta MG et al. HIV-associated nephropathy: epidemiology, pathogenesis, diagnosis and management. Expert Rev Anti Infect Ther. 2008 Jun;6(3):365–71. [PMID: 18588500]
Szczech LA et al. The clinical epidemiology and course of the spectrum of renal diseases associated with HIV infection. Kidney Int. 2004 Sep;66(3):1145–52. [PMID: 15327410]

DISEASES DEMONSTRATING NEPHRITIC & NEPHROTIC COMPONENTS

SYSTEMIC LUPUS ERYTHEMATOSUS

Systemic lupus erythematosus is a systemic autoimmune disease in which renal involvement is common. In various series, clinical renal involvement ranges from 35% to 90% (see Chapter 20).

Patients present with glomerular syndromes such as nephritic or nephrotic syndromes and asymptomatic kidney disease. Nonglomerular syndromes include tubulointerstitial nephritis and vasculitis. All patients with systemic lupus erythematosus should have routine urinalyses to monitor for the appearance of hematuria or proteinuria. If urinary abnormalities are detected, renal biopsy is often performed. The type of glomerular injury depends on the site of immune complex deposition. The World Health Organization (WHO) classification of renal glomerular lesions follows: type I, normal; type II, mesangial proliferative; type III, focal and segmental proliferative; type IV, diffuse proliferative; and type V, membranous nephropathy. These are further classified as acute or chronic and global or segmental, both of which seem to have prognostic value.

▶ Treatment

Individuals with type I and type II patterns require no treatment. Transformation of these types to a more active lesion is usually accompanied by an increase in lupus serologic activity and evidence of deteriorating renal function (eg, rising serum creatinine, increasing proteinuria). Repeat biopsy to confirm the transformation in these patients is standard. Patients with extensive type III lesions and all type IV lesions should receive aggressive immunosuppressive therapy. Poorest prognostic features in patients with type IV lesions are an elevated serum creatinine, hematocrit less than 26%, and African American race. Indications for treatment of type V disease are unclear; however, if superimposed proliferative lesions exist, aggressive therapy should be instituted. Two different trials have used corticosteroids in conjunction with mycophenolate mofetil.

Corticosteroids are the mainstay of treatment (methylprednisolone 1 g intravenously daily for 3 days followed by prednisone, 1 mg/kg orally daily with subsequent taper for 4–6 weeks) but are associated with many side effects and may not prevent progression of chronic lesions. Higher dose alternating day therapy can be considered in conjunction with a nephrologist or rheumatologist to reduce side effects. Cytotoxic agents, such as cyclophosphamide, are necessary adjuncts because they improve long-term renal survival in patients with aggressive type III and type IV nephritis. However, studies have shown the potential benefit of mycophenolate mofetil as an alternative form of induction therapy. In one randomized noninferiority study, patients using mycophenolate mofetil had similar rates of full remission at 24 weeks in comparison to those using cyclophosphamide. These agents are typically used for 18–24 months (eg, cyclophosphamide intravenously every month for six doses and then every 3 months for six doses or switching to mycophenolate mofetil after induction). Studies suggest that mycophenolate mofetil is less toxic than cyclophosphamide, does not cause ovarian failure, and may be more acceptable to patients, although long-term follow-up needs to be examined. Ongoing trials of other therapies include cyclosporine and azathioprine as longer-term options. The return of serologic measurements to normal can be useful in monitoring treatment. Markers include double-stranded DNA (dsDNA) antibodies, C3, C4, CH50, and serum creatinine. Urinary protein and sediment are also helpful markers. Patients with systemic lupus erythematosus who undergo dialysis have a favorable prospect for long-term survival. Patients with kidney transplants have recurrent renal disease in 8% of cases.

Contreras G et al. Sequential therapies for proliferative lupus nephritis. N Engl J Med. 2004 Mar 4;350(10):971–80. [PMID: 14999109]
Fine DM. Pharmacological therapy of lupus nephritis. JAMA. 2005 Jun 22;293(24):3053–60. [PMID: 15972568]
Ginzler EM et al. Mycophenolate mofetil or intravenous cyclophosphamide for lupus nephritis. N Engl J Med. 2005 Nov 24;353(21):2219–28. [PMID: 16306519]

HEPATITIS C VIRUS INFECTION

Renal disease in the setting of hepatitis C viral infection was not well-recognized until 1993. Now it accounts for approximately 8% of patients with ESRD. Three clinicopathologic glomerular syndromes associated with hepatitis C are secondary membranoproliferative glomerulonephritis, cryoglobulinemic glomerulonephritis, and membranous nephropathy. A type I membranoproliferative glomerulonephritis (MPGN) (see Idiopathic Membranoproliferative Glomerulonephritis, below) is the most common lesion in patients requiring kidney biopsy. These patients typically have hematuria and proteinuria, hypertension, and anemia. Occasionally, they exhibit the nephrotic syndrome. Many have elevated serum transaminases and an elevated rheumatoid factor. Of patients studied in one series, 50% had hepatomegaly. Hypocomplementemia is very common, with C4 typically more reduced than C3. Cryoglobulinemic disease is discussed above. Membranous glomerulopathy is the least common of the three and presents with a typical nephrotic picture. Neither cryoglobulins nor rheumatoid factor is present.

▶ **Treatment**

In patients with MPGN not receiving treatment for liver disease, the question arises whether to initiate therapy for kidney disease. The main indications for therapy are poor renal function, nephrotic syndrome, new or worsening hypertension, fibrosis or tubulointerstitial disease on biopsy, and progressive disease. IFN-α may result in suppression of viremia and improvement in hepatic function. Renal function rarely improves unless viral suppression occurs; however, renal function often worsens when therapy is abated. Ribavirin is relatively contraindicated in kidney disease because of the dose-related hemolysis that occurs with renal dysfunction. Despite this, some case series have shown benefit with combined IFN-α and ribavirin in closely monitored settings.

IDIOPATHIC MEMBRANOPROLIFERATIVE GLOMERULONEPHRITIS

MPGN in its primary form is an idiopathic syndrome that can present with nephritic or nephrotic features. (The secondary form can be seen in the immune complex, paraprotein deposition, and thrombotic microangiopathic glomerulonephritides discussed above.) Most patients are under 30 years of age. At least two major subgroups are recognized: type I and type II.

Patients with **type I MPGN** have a history of recent upper respiratory tract infection about a third of the time. Patients typically have a nephrotic picture, and complement levels are low. Histologically, the GBM is thickened because of immune complex deposition and abnormal mesangial cell proliferation between the GBM and the endothelial cells. This gives a characteristic "splitting" appearance to the capillary wall. Immunofluorescence shows IgG, IgM, and granular deposits of C3, C1q, and C4 (Table 22–10).

Type II MPGN often presents with a nephritic picture and is less common than type I. Light microscopy is similar to type I. Serologically, type II is associated with C3 nephritic factor, which is a circulating IgG antibody. Electron microscopy shows a characteristic dense deposit of homogeneous material that replaces part of the GBM.

Treatment of this disorder is controversial. After ruling out secondary causes, it consists of corticosteroid therapy (there is no standard dosage for adults) and antiplatelet drugs (aspirin, 500–975 mg/d orally, plus dipyridamole 225 mg/d orally). The rationale for antiplatelet therapy is that platelet consumption is increased in MPGN and may play a role in glomerular injury. Fifty percent of patients used to progress to ESRD in 10 years; these rates may now be slightly lower with the introduction of more aggressive therapy. Less favorable prognostic findings include type II disease, early renal insufficiency, hypertension, and persistent nephrotic syndrome. Both types of MPGN will recur after renal transplantation; however, type II recurs more commonly.

Ahmed MS et al. Rapidly deteriorating renal function with membranoproliferative glomerulonephritis type 1 associated with hepatitis C treated successfully with steroids and antiviral therapy: a case report and review of literature. Clin Nephrol. 2008 Apr;69(4):298–301. [PMID: 18397706]

▼ TUBULOINTERSTITIAL DISEASES

Tubulointerstitial disease may be acute or chronic. Acute disease is most commonly associated with toxins and ischemia. Interstitial edema, infiltration with polymorphonuclear neutrophils, and tubular cell necrosis can be seen. (See Acute Kidney Injury, above, and Table 22–11.) Chronic disease is associated with insults from an acute factor or progressive insult without any obvious acute cause. Interstitial fibrosis and tubular atrophy are present, with a mononuclear cell predominance. The chronic disorders are described below.

CHRONIC TUBULOINTERSTITIAL DISEASES

 ESSENTIALS OF DIAGNOSIS

▶ Kidney size is small and contracted.

▶ Decreased urinary concentrating ability.

▶ Hyperchloremic metabolic acidosis.

▶ Reduced GFR.

▶ **General Considerations**

There are four main causes of chronic tubulointerstitial disease. These are discussed below. Other causes include multiple myeloma and gout, which are discussed in the section on multisystem disease with variable kidney involvement.

Table 22–11. Causes of acute tubulointerstitial nephritis (abbreviated list).

Drug reactions
Antibiotics
β-Lactam antibiotics: methicillin, penicillin, ampicillin, cephalosporins
Ciprofloxacin
Erythromycin
Sulfonamides
Tetracycline
Vancomycin
Trimethoprim-sulfamethoxazole
Ethambutol
Rifampin
Nonsteroidal anti-inflammatory drugs
Diuretics
Thiazides
Furosemide
Miscellaneous
Allopurinol
Cimetidine
Phenytoin
Systemic infections
Bacteria
Streptococcus
Corynebacterium diphtheriae
Legionella
Viruses
Epstein-Barr
Others
Mycoplasma
Rickettsia rickettsii
Leptospira icterohaemorrhagiae
Toxoplasma
Idiopathic
Tubulointerstitial nephritis-uveitis (TIN-U)

A. Obstructive Uropathy

The most common cause of chronic tubulointerstitial disease is prolonged obstruction of the urinary tract. In partial obstruction, urinary output alternates between polyuria (due to vasopressin insensitivity) and oliguria (due to decreased GFR). Azotemia and hypertension (due to increased renin-angiotensin production) are usually present. The major causes are prostatic disease in men; ureteral calculus in a single functioning kidney; bilateral ureteral calculi; carcinoma of the cervix, colon, and bladder; and retroperitoneal tumors or fibrosis.

Abdominal, rectal, and genitourinary examinations are helpful. Urinalysis can show hematuria, pyuria, and bacteriuria but is often benign. Abdominal ultrasound may detect mass lesions, hydroureter, and hydronephrosis. CT scanning and MRI provide more detailed information.

B. Vesicoureteral Reflux

Reflux nephropathy is primarily a disorder of childhood and occurs when urine passes retrograde from the bladder to the kidneys during voiding. It is the second most common cause of chronic tubulointerstitial disease. It occurs as a result of an incompetent vesicoureteral sphinc-

ter. Urine can extravasate into the interstitium; an inflammatory response develops, and fibrosis occurs. The inflammatory response is due to either bacteria or normal urinary components.

Patients are adolescents or young adults with hypertension, renal insufficiency, and a history of urinary tract infections as a child. Focal glomerulosclerosis is often seen. This is a cause of substantial proteinuria, unusual in most tubular diseases. Renal ultrasound or IVP can show renal scarring and hydronephrosis. Although most damage occurs before age 5 years, progressive renal deterioration to ESRD continues as a result of the early insults.

C. Analgesics

Analgesic nephropathy is most commonly seen in patients who ingest large quantities of analgesic combinations. The drugs of concern are phenacetin, paracetamol, aspirin, and NSAIDs, with acetaminophen a possible but less certain culprit. Ingestion of 1 g/d for 3 years is the typical amount needed for kidney dysfunction. This disorder occurs most frequently in individuals who are using analgesics for chronic headaches, muscular pains, and arthritis. Most patients grossly underestimate their analgesic use.

Tubulointerstitial inflammation and papillary necrosis are seen on pathologic examination. Papillary tip and inner medullary concentrations of some analgesics are tenfold higher than in the renal cortex. Phenacetin—once a common cause of this disorder and now rarely available—is metabolized in the papillae by the prostaglandin hydroperoxidase pathway to reactive intermediates that bind covalently to interstitial cell macromolecules, causing necrosis. Aspirin and other NSAIDs may worsen the damage by decreasing medullary blood flow (via inhibition of prostaglandin synthesis) and decreasing glutathione levels (which are necessary for detoxification).

Patients can exhibit hematuria, mild proteinuria, polyuria (from tubular damage), anemia (from gastrointestinal bleeding), and sterile pyuria. As a result of papillary necrosis, sloughed papillae can be found in the urine. An IVP may be helpful for detecting these—contrast will fill the area of the sloughed papillae, leaving a "ring shadow" sign at the papillary tip. However, IVP is rarely used in patients with significant kidney dysfunction, given the need for dye and associated acute kidney injury.

D. Heavy Metals

Environmental exposure to heavy metals—such as lead and cadmium—is seen infrequently now in the United States. Chronic lead exposure can lead to tubulointerstitial disease. Individuals at risk are those with occupational exposure (eg, welders who work with lead-based paint) and drinkers of alcohol distilled in automobile radiators (moonshine users). Lead is filtered by the glomerulus and is transported across the proximal convoluted tubules, where it accumulates and causes cell damage. Fibrosed arterioles and cortical scarring also lead to damaged kidneys. Proximal tubular damage leads to decreased secretion of uric acid, resulting in hyperuricemia and saturnine gout. Patients commonly are hypertensive. Diagnosis is most reliably performed with a calcium disodium edetate (EDTA) chelation test. Urinary excretion of more than 600 mg of lead in 24 hours following 1 g of EDTA indicates excessive lead exposure.

Occupational exposure to cadmium also causes proximal tubular dysfunction. Hypercalciuria and nephrolithiasis can be seen. Other heavy metals that can cause tubulointerstitial disease include mercury and bismuth.

▶ Clinical Findings

A. Symptoms and Signs

Polyuria is common because tubular damage leads to inability to concentrate the urine. Dehydration can also occur as a result of a salt-wasting defect in some individuals.

B. Laboratory Findings

Patients are hyperkalemic because the distal tubules become aldosterone resistant. A hyperchloremic renal tubular acidosis is characteristic. The cause of the renal tubular acidosis is threefold: (1) reduced ammonia production, (2) inability to acidify the distal tubules, and (3) proximal tubular bicarbonate wasting. The urinalysis is nonspecific, as opposed to that seen in acute interstitial nephritis. Proteinuria is typically less than 2 g/d (owing to inability of the proximal tubule to reabsorb freely filterable proteins); a few cells may be seen; and broad waxy casts are often present.

▶ Treatment

Treatment depends first upon identifying the disorder responsible for renal dysfunction. The degree of interstitial fibrosis that has developed can help predict recovery of renal function. Once there is evidence for loss of parenchyma (small shrunken kidneys or interstitial fibrosis on biopsy), little can prevent the progression toward ESRD. Treatment is then directed at medical management. Tubular dysfunction may require potassium and phosphorus restriction and sodium, calcium, or bicarbonate supplements.

If hydronephrosis is present, relief of obstruction should be accomplished promptly. Prolonged obstruction leads to further tubular damage—particularly in the distal nephron—which may be irreversible despite relief of obstruction. Neither surgical correction of reflux nor medical therapy with antibiotics can prevent deterioration toward ESRD once renal scarring has occurred.

Patients in whom lead nephropathy is suspected should continue chelation therapy with EDTA if there is no evidence of irreversible renal damage (eg, renal scarring or small kidneys). Continued exposure should be avoided.

Treatment of analgesic nephropathy requires withdrawal of all analgesics. Stabilization or improvement of renal function may occur if significant interstitial fibrosis is not present. Hydration during exposure to analgesics may also have some beneficial effects.

▶ When to Refer

- Patients with stage 3–5 chronic kidney disease should be referred to a nephrologist when tubulointerstitial diseases are suspected. Other select cases of stage 1–2 chronic kidney disease should also be referred.

- Patients with urologic abnormalities should be referred to a urologist.

Gooch K et al. NSAID use and progression of chronic kidney disease. Am J Med. 2007 Mar;120(3):280.e1–7. [PMID: 17349452]

Huerta C et al. Nonsteroidal anti-inflammatory drugs and risk of ARF in the general population. Am J Kidney Dis. 2005 Mar;45(3):531–9. [PMID: 15754275]

▼ CYSTIC DISEASES OF THE KIDNEY

Renal cysts are epithelium-lined cavities filled with fluid or semisolid material. They develop primarily from renal tubular elements. One or more simple cysts are found in 50% of individuals over the age of 50 years. They are rarely symptomatic and have little clinical significance. In contrast, generalized cystic diseases are associated with cysts scattered throughout the cortex and medulla of both kidneys and can progress to ESRD (Table 22–12).

SIMPLE OR SOLITARY CYSTS

Simple cysts account for 65–70% of all renal masses. They are generally found at the outer cortex and contain fluid that is consistent with an ultrafiltrate of plasma. Most are found incidentally on ultrasonographic examination. Simple cysts are typically asymptomatic but can become infected.

The main concern with simple cysts is to differentiate them from malignancy, abscess, or polycystic kidney disease. Renal cystic disease can develop in dialysis patients. These cysts have a potential for progression to malignancy. Ultrasound and CT scanning are the recommended procedures for evaluating these masses. Simple cysts must meet three sonographic criteria to be considered benign: (1) echo free, (2) sharply demarcated mass with smooth walls, and (3) an enhanced back wall (indicating good transmission through the cyst). Complex cysts can have thick walls, calcifications, solid components, and mixed echogenicity. On CT scan, the simple cyst should have a smooth thin wall that is sharply demarcated. It should not enhance with contrast media. A renal cell carcinoma will enhance but typically is of lower density than the rest of the parenchyma. Arteriography can also be used to evaluate a mass preoperatively. A renal cell carcinoma is hypervascular in 80%, hypovascular in 15%, and avascular in 5% of cases.

If a cyst meets the criteria for being benign, periodic reevaluation is the standard of care. If the lesion is not consistent with a simple cyst, surgical exploration is recommended.

Terada N et al. Risk factors for renal cysts. BJU Int. 2004 Jun; 93(9):1300–2. [PMID: 15180627]

Table 22–12. Clinical features of renal cystic disease.

	Simple Renal Cysts	Acquired Renal Cysts	Autosomal Dominant Polycystic Kidney Disease	Medullary Sponge Kidney	Medullary Cystic Kidney
Prevalence	Common	Dialysis patients	1:1000	1:5000	Rare
Inheritance	None	None	Autosomal dominant	None	Autosomal dominant
Age at onset	. . .	. . .	20–40	40–60	Adulthood
Kidney size	Normal	Small	Large	Normal	Small
Cyst location	Cortex and medulla	Cortex and medulla	Cortex and medulla	Collecting ducts	Corticomedullary junction
Hematuria	Occasional	Occasional	Common	Rare	Rare
Hypertension	None	Variable	Common	None	None
Associated complications	None	Adenocarcinoma in cysts	Urinary tract infections, renal calculi, cerebral aneurysms 10–15%, hepatic cysts 40–60%	Renal calculi, urinary tract infections	Polyuria, salt wasting
Kidney failure	Never	Always	Frequently	Never	Always

AUTOSOMAL DOMINANT POLYCYSTIC KIDNEY DISEASE

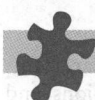 ESSENTIALS OF DIAGNOSIS

▶ Multiple cysts in bilateral kidneys; total number depends on age.

▶ Large, palpable kidneys on examination.

▶ Combination of hypertension and abdominal mass suggestive of disease.

▶ Family history is compelling but not necessary.

▶ Chromosomal abnormalities present in some patients.

▶ General Considerations

This disorder is among the most common hereditary diseases in the United States, affecting 500,000 individuals, or 1 in 800 live births. Fifty percent of patients will have ESRD by age 60 years. The disease has variable penetrance but accounts for 10% of dialysis patients in the United States. At least two genes account for this disorder: *ADPKD1* on the short arm of chromosome 16 (85–90% of patients) and *ADPKD2* on chromosome 4 (10–15%). Patients with the *PKD2* mutation have slower progression of disease and longer life expectancy than those with *PKD1*. Other sporadic cases without these mutations have also been recognized.

▶ Clinical Findings

Abdominal or flank pain and microscopic or gross hematuria are present in most patients. A history of urinary tract infections and nephrolithiasis is common. A family history is positive in 75% of cases, and more than 50% of patients have hypertension (see below) that may antedate the clinical manifestations of the disease. Patients have large kid-

neys that may be palpable on abdominal examination. The combination of hypertension and an abdominal mass should suggest the disease. Forty to 50 percent have concurrent hepatic cysts. Pancreatic and splenic cysts occur also. Hemoglobin and hematocrit tend to be maintained as a result of erythropoietin production by the cysts. The urinalysis may show hematuria and mild proteinuria. In patients with *PKD1*, ultrasonography confirms the diagnosis—two or more cysts in patients under age 30 years (sensitivity of 88.5%), two or more cysts in each kidney in patients age 30–59 years (sensitivity of 100%), and four or more cysts in each kidney in patients age 60 years or older are diagnostic for autosomal dominant polycystic kidney disease. If sonographic results are unclear, CT scan is recommended and highly sensitive.

▶ Complications & Treatment

A. Pain

Abdominal or flank pain is caused by infection, bleeding into cysts, and nephrolithiasis. Bed rest and analgesics are recommended. Cyst decompression can help with chronic pain.

B. Hematuria

Gross hematuria is most commonly due to rupture of a cyst into the renal pelvis, but it can also be caused by a kidney stone or urinary tract infection. Hematuria typically resolves within 7 days with bed rest and hydration. Recurrent bleeding should suggest the possibility of underlying renal cell carcinoma, particularly in men over age 50 years.

C. Renal Infection

An infected renal cyst should be suspected in patients who have flank pain, fever, and leukocytosis. Blood cultures may be positive, and urinalysis may be normal because the cyst does not communicate directly with the urinary tract. CT scans can be helpful because an infected cyst may have an increased wall thickness. Bacterial cyst infections are difficult to treat. Antibiotics with cystic penetration should be used, eg, fluoroquinolones, trimethoprim-sulfamethoxazole, and chloramphenicol. Treatment may require 2 weeks of parenteral therapy followed by long-term oral therapy.

D. Nephrolithiasis

Up to 20% of patients have kidney stones, primarily calcium oxalate. Hydration (2–3 L/d) is recommended.

E. Hypertension

Fifty percent of patients have hypertension at time of presentation, and it will develop in most patients during the course of the disease. Cyst-induced ischemia appears to cause activation of the renin–angiotensin system, and cyst decompression can lower blood pressure temporarily. Hypertension should be treated aggressively, as this may prolong the time to ESRD. (Diuretics should be used cautiously since the effect on renal cyst formation is unknown.)

F. Cerebral Aneurysms

About 10–15% of these patients have arterial aneurysms in the circle of Willis. Screening arteriography is not recommended unless the patient has a family history of aneurysms or is undergoing elective surgery with a high risk of developing hypertension.

G. Other Complications

Vascular problems include mitral valve prolapse in up to 25% of patients, aortic aneurysms, and aortic valve abnormalities. Colonic diverticula are more common in patients with polycystic kidneys.

▶ Prognosis

Significant research is ongoing regarding therapy. Vasopressin receptor antagonists have been successful in animal models but are not yet well-tested in humans. These agents lower renal epithelial cell intracellular cyclic AMP (cAMP) levels, and in vitro evidence suggests that intracellular cAMP plays a significant role in cystogenesis in polycystic kidney disease. Avoidance of caffeine may prevent cyst formation due to effects on G-coupled proteins. Treatment of hypertension and a low-protein diet may slow the progression of disease, although this is not well proven.

Grantham JJ. Clinical practice. Autosomal dominant polycystic kidney disease. N Engl J Med. 2008 Oct 2;359(14):1477–85. [PMID: 18832246]

Pei Y. Diagnostic approach in autosomal dominant polycystic kidney disease. Clin J Am Soc Nephrol. 2006 Sep;1(5):1108–14. [PMID: 17699332]

Torres VE et al. Autosomal dominant polycystic kidney disease. Lancet. 2007 Apr 14;369(9569):1287–301. [PMID: 17434405]

MEDULLARY SPONGE KIDNEY

This disease is a relatively common and benign disorder that is present at birth and not usually diagnosed until the fourth or fifth decade. It is caused by autosomal dominant muta-

tions in the *MCKD1* or *MCKD2* genes on chromosomes 1 and 16, respectively. Kidneys have a marked irregular enlargement of the medullary and interpapillary collecting ducts. This is associated with medullary cysts that are diffuse, giving a "Swiss cheese" appearance in these regions.

▶ Clinical Findings

Medullary sponge kidney presents with gross or microscopic hematuria, recurrent urinary tract infections, or nephrolithiasis. Common abnormalities are a decreased urinary concentrating ability and nephrocalcinosis; less common is incomplete type I distal renal tubular acidosis. The diagnosis is confirmed with IVP, which shows striations in the papillary portions of the kidney produced by the accumulation of contrast in dilated collecting ducts.

▶ Treatment

There is no known therapy. Adequate fluid intake (2 L/d) helps prevent stone formation. If hypercalciuria is present, thiazide diuretics are recommended because they decrease calcium excretion. Alkali therapy is recommended if renal tubular acidosis is present.

▶ Prognosis

Renal function is well maintained unless there are complications from recurrent urinary tract infections and nephrolithiasis.

▼ MULTISYSTEM DISEASES WITH VARIABLE KIDNEY INVOLVEMENT*

MULTIPLE MYELOMA

Multiple myeloma is a malignancy of plasma cells (see Chapter 13). Renal involvement occurs in about 25% of all patients. "Myeloma kidney" is the presence of light chain immunoglobulins (Bence Jones protein) in the urine causing renal toxicity. Bence Jones protein causes direct renal tubular toxicity and results in tubular obstruction by precipitating in the tubules. The earliest tubular damage results in Fanconi syndrome (a type II proximal renal tubular acidosis). The proteinuria seen with multiple myeloma is primarily due to light chains that are not detected on urine dipstick, which mainly detects albumin. Glomerular amyloidosis can develop in patients with multiple myeloma; in these patients, dipstick protein determinations are positive. Hypercalcemia and hyperuricemia are frequently seen. Other conditions resulting in renal dysfunction include plasma cell infiltration of the renal parenchyma and a hyperviscosity syndrome compromising renal blood flow. Therapy for acute kidney injury attributed to multiple myeloma includes correction of hypercalcemia,

---

*Other diseases with variable involvement described elsewhere in this chapter include systemic lupus erythematosus, diabetes mellitus, and the vasculitides such as Wegener granulomatosis and Goodpasture disease.

volume repletion, and chemotherapy for the underlying malignancy. Previously, plasmapheresis had been considered appropriate to decrease the burden of existing monoclonal proteins while awaiting chemotherapeutic regimens to take effect. However, in the largest randomized prospective trial to date, plasmapheresis did not provide any renal benefit to these patients.

Clark WF et al; Canadian Apheresis Group. Plasma exchange when myeloma presents as acute renal failure: a randomized, controlled trial. Ann Intern Med. 2005 Dec 6;143(11):777–84. [PMID: 16330788]
Korbet SM et al. Multiple myeloma. J Am Soc Nephrol. 2006 Sep;17(9):2533–45. [PMID: 16885408]

SICKLE CELL DISEASE

Renal dysfunction associated with sickle cell disease is most commonly due to sickling of red blood cells in the renal medulla because of low oxygen tension and hypertonicity. Congestion and stasis lead to hemorrhage, interstitial inflammation, and papillary infarcts. Clinically, hematuria is common. Damage to renal capillaries also leads to diminished concentrating ability. Isosthenuria (urine osmolality equal to that of serum) is routine, and patients can easily become dehydrated. Papillary necrosis occurs as well. These abnormalities are commonly encountered in sickle cell trait. Sickle cell glomerulopathy is less common but will inexorably progress to ESRD. Its primary clinical manifestation is proteinuria. Optimal treatment requires adequate hydration and control of the sickle cell disease.

Davenport A et al. Sickle cell kidney. J Nephrol. 2008 Mar–Apr;21(2):253–5. [PMID: 18446721]

TUBERCULOSIS

The classic renal manifestation of tuberculosis is the presence of microscopic pyuria with a sterile urine culture—or "sterile pyuria." More often, other bacteria are present in addition. Microscopic hematuria is often present with pyuria. Urine cultures are the gold standard for diagnosis. Three to six first morning midstream specimens should be performed to improve sensitivity. Papillary necrosis and cavitation of the renal parenchyma occur less frequently, as do ureteral strictures and calcifications. Adequate drug therapy can result in resolution of renal involvement.

Figueiredo AA et al. Epidemiology of urogenital tuberculosis worldwide. Int J Urol. 2008 Sep;15(9):827–32. [PMID: 18637157]

GOUT & THE KIDNEY

The kidney is the primary organ for excretion of uric acid. Patients with proximal tubular dysfunction have decreased excretion of uric acid and are more prone to gouty attacks. Depending on the pH and uric acid concentration, deposition can occur in the tubules, the interstitium, or the urinary tract. The more alkaline pH of the interstitium causes urate salt deposition, whereas the acidic environment of the tubules and urinary tract causes uric acid crystal deposition at high concentrations.

Three disorders are commonly seen: (1) uric acid nephrolithiasis, (2) acute uric acid nephropathy, and (3) chronic urate nephropathy. Kidney dysfunction with uric acid nephrolithiasis stems from obstructive nephropathy. Acute uric acid nephropathy presents similarly to acute tubulointerstitial nephritis with direct toxicity from uric acid crystals. Chronic urate nephropathy is caused by deposition of urate crystals in the alkaline medium of the interstitium; this can lead to fibrosis and atrophy. Epidemiologically, hyperuricemia and gout have been associated with worsening cardiovascular outcomes.

Treatment between gouty attacks involves avoidance of food and drugs causing hyperuricemia, aggressive hydration, and pharmacotherapy aimed at reducing serum uric acid levels. These disorders are seen in both "overproducers" and "underexcretors" of uric acid. The latter situation may seem counterintuitive; however, these patients have hyperacidic urine, which explains the deposition of relatively insoluble uric acid crystals.

Edwards NL. The role of hyperuricemia and gout in kidney and cardiovascular disease. Cleve Clin J Med. 2008 Jul;75 (Suppl 5):S13–6. [PMID: 18822470]

NEPHROGENIC SYSTEMIC FIBROSIS

Nephrogenic systemic fibrosis (NSF) is a multi-system disorder seen only in patients with kidney disease. NSF affects several organ systems, including skin, muscles, lungs, and cardiovascular system. The most common manifestation is a debilitating fibrosing skin disorder that can range from skin-colored to erythematous papules, which coalesce to brawny patches. The skin can be thick and woody in areas and is painful out-of-proportion to findings on examination. Histopathologically, there is an increase in dermal spindle cells positive for CD34 and procollagen I. Collagen bundles with mucin and elastic fibers are also noted. This has been reported in cases of chronic kidney disease, primarily with GFR < 30 mL/min/1.73 m^2, acute kidney injury, and after kidney transplantation. It was first recognized in hemodialysis patients in 1997 and has been strongly linked to use of contrast agents containing gadolinium. Incidence is projected to be 1–4% in the highest risk (ESRD) population that has received gadolinium, and lower in patients with less severe kidney dysfunction. The FDA has issued a warning regarding avoidance of exposure to this agent for patients with GFR < 30 mL/min/1.73 m^2, acute kidney injury, and posttransplant, with the caveat that hemodialysis may be beneficial. Despite the latter recommendation, no studies have proven that removal of gadolinium with hemodialysis prevents this disorder. Several case reports and series have described benefit for patients after treatment with corticosteroids, photopheresis, plasmapheresis, and sodium thiosulfate. The true effectiveness of these interventions is still unclear. Alternative imaging agents need to be used for patients requiring MR with contrast at risk for NSF.

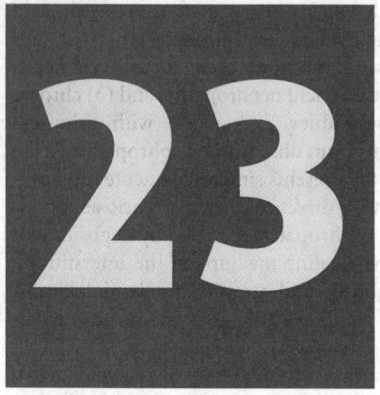

Urologic Disorders

Maxwell V. Meng, MD, FACS
Marshall L. Stoller, MD
Thomas Walsh, MD

HEMATURIA

 ESSENTIALS OF DIAGNOSIS

▶ Both grossly visible and microscopic hematuria require evaluation.

▶ The upper urinary tract should be imaged, and cystoscopy should be performed if there is hematuria in the absence of infection.

▶ General Considerations

In patients with gross or microscopic hematuria, an **upper tract source** (kidneys and ureters) can be identified in 10% of cases. For upper tract sources, stone disease accounts for 40%, medical kidney disease (medullary sponge kidney, glomerulonephritis, papillary necrosis) for 20%, renal cell carcinoma for 10%, and urothelial cell carcinoma of the ureter or renal pelvis for 5%. Drug ingestion and associated medical problems may provide diagnostic clues. Analgesic use (papillary necrosis), cyclophosphamide (chemical cystitis), antibiotics (interstitial nephritis), diabetes mellitus, sickle cell trait or disease (papillary necrosis), a history of stone disease, or malignancy should all be investigated. In the absence of infection, gross hematuria from a **lower tract source** is most commonly from urothelial cell carcinoma of the bladder. Microscopic hematuria in the male is most commonly from benign prostatic hyperplasia. The presence of hematuria in patients receiving anticoagulation therapy cannot be ascribed to the anticoagulation; a complete evaluation is warranted consisting of upper tract imaging, cystoscopy, and urine cytology. **See Chapter 39 for Bladder Cancer, Cancers of the Ureter and Renal Pelvis, Renal Cell Carcinoma, and Kidney and Testis Tumors.**

▶ Clinical Findings

A. Symptoms and Signs

If gross hematuria occurs, a description of the timing (initial, terminal, total) may provide a clue to the localization of disease. Associated symptoms (ie, renal colic, irritative voiding symptoms, constitutional symptoms) should be investigated. Physical examination should emphasize signs of systemic disease (fever, rash, lymphadenopathy, abdominal or pelvic masses) as well as signs of medical kidney disease (hypertension, volume overload). Urologic evaluation may demonstrate an enlarged prostate, flank mass, or urethral disease.

B. Laboratory Findings

Initial laboratory investigations include a urinalysis and urine culture. Proteinuria and casts suggest renal origin. Irritative voiding symptoms, bacteriuria, and a positive urine culture in the female suggest urinary tract infection, but follow-up urinalysis is important after treatment to ensure resolution of the hematuria.

Further evaluation includes urinary cytology to assist in the diagnosis of bladder neoplasm.

C. Imaging

Upper tract imaging (usually abdominal and pelvic CT scanning without and with contrast) may identify neoplasms of the kidney or ureter as well as identifying benign conditions such as urolithiasis, obstructive uropathy, papillary necrosis, medullary sponge kidney, or polycystic kidney disease. CT urography and MRI have replaced intravenous urography (IVU) when imaging the upper tracts for sources of hematuria. The role of ultrasonographic evaluation of the urinary tract for hematuria is unclear. Although it may provide adequate information for the kidney, its sensitivity in detecting ureteral disease is lower. In addition, its higher degree of operator dependence may further confound the issue.

D. Cystoscopy

Cystoscopy can be used to assess for bladder or urethral neoplasm, benign prostatic enlargement, and radiation or chemical cystitis. For gross hematuria, cystoscopy is ideally performed while the patient is actively bleeding to allow better localization (ie, lateralize to one side of the upper tracts, bladder, or urethra).

Follow-up

In patients with negative evaluations, repeat evaluations may be warranted to avoid a missed malignancy; however, the ideal frequency of such evaluations is not defined. Urinary cytology can be repeated in 3–6 months, and cystoscopy and upper tract imaging after a year.

When to Refer

In the absence of infection, hematuria (either gross or microscopic) requires evaluation.

Chow KM et al. Asymptomatic isolated microscopic haematuria: long-term follow-up. QJM. 2004 Nov;97(11):739–45. [PMID: 15496530]

Grossfeld G et al. Evaluation of asymptomatic microscopic hematuria in adults: the American Urological Association best practice policy—part I: definition, detection, prevalence, and etiology. Urology. 2001 Apr;57(4):599–603. [PMID: 11306356]

Ripley TL et al. Early evaluation of hematuria in a patient receiving anticoagulant therapy and detection of malignancy. Pharmacotherapy. 2004 Nov;24(11):1638–40. [PMID: 15537566]

Rodgers MA et al. Diagnostic tests used in the investigation of adult haematuria: A systematic review. BJU Int. 2006 Dec;98(6):1154–60. [PMID: 16879444]

Yun EJ et al. Evaluation of the patient with hematuria. Med Clin North Am. 2004 Mar;88(2):329–43. [PMID: 15049581]

GENITOURINARY TRACT INFECTIONS

1. Acute Cystitis

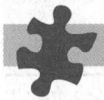

ESSENTIALS OF DIAGNOSIS

- ▶ Irritative voiding symptoms.
- ▶ Patient usually afebrile.
- ▶ Positive urine culture; blood cultures may also be positive.

General Considerations

Acute cystitis is an infection of the bladder most commonly due to the coliform bacteria (especially *Escherichia coli*) and occasionally gram-positive bacteria (enterococci). The route of infection is typically ascending from the urethra. Viral cystitis due to adenovirus is sometimes seen in children but is rare in adults. Cystitis in men is rare and implies a pathologic process such as infected stones, prostatitis, or chronic urinary retention requiring further investigation.

Clinical Findings

A. Symptoms and Signs

Irritative voiding symptoms (frequency, urgency, dysuria) and suprapubic discomfort are common. Women may experience gross hematuria, and symptoms may often appear following sexual intercourse. Physical examination may elicit suprapubic tenderness, but examination is often unremarkable. Systemic toxicity is absent.

B. Laboratory Findings

Urinalysis shows pyuria and bacteriuria and varying degrees of hematuria. The degree of pyuria and bacteriuria does not necessarily correlate with the severity of symptoms. Urine culture is positive for the offending organism, but colony counts exceeding 10^5/mL are not essential for the diagnosis.

C. Imaging

Because uncomplicated cystitis is rare in men, elucidation of the underlying problem with appropriate investigations, such as abdominal ultrasonography or cystoscopy (or both), is warranted. Follow-up imaging using CT scanning is warranted if pyelonephritis, recurrent infections, or anatomic abnormalities are suspected.

Differential Diagnosis

In women, infectious processes such as vulvovaginitis and pelvic inflammatory disease can usually be distinguished by pelvic examination and urinalysis. In men, urethritis and prostatitis may be distinguished by physical examination (urethral discharge or prostatic tenderness).

Noninfectious causes of cystitis-like symptoms include pelvic irradiation, chemotherapy (cyclophosphamide), bladder carcinoma, interstitial cystitis, voiding dysfunction disorders, and psychosomatic disorders.

Prevention

Women who have more than three episodes of cystitis per year are considered candidates for prophylactic antibiotic therapy to prevent recurrence after treatment of urinary tract infection. Prior to institution of therapy, a thorough urologic evaluation is warranted to exclude any anatomic abnormality (eg, stones, reflux, fistula). The three most commonly used oral agents for prophylaxis are trimethoprim-sulfamethoxazole (40 mg/200 mg), nitrofurantoin (100 mg), and cephalexin (250 mg). Single dosing at bedtime or at the time of intercourse is the recommended schedule.

Treatment

Uncomplicated cystitis in women can be treated with short-term antimicrobial therapy, which consists of single-dose therapy or 1–3 days of therapy. Fluoroquinolones and nitrofurantoin are the drugs of choice for uncomplicated cystitis (Table 23–1). Trimethoprim-sulfamethoxazole can be ineffective because of the emergence of resistant organisms. In men, uncomplicated urinary tract infection is rare, and thus, the duration of antibiotic therapy depends on the underlying etiology. Hot sitz baths or urinary analgesics (phenazopyridine, 200 mg orally three times daily) may provide symptomatic relief.

Prognosis

Infections typically respond rapidly to therapy, and failure to respond suggests resistance to the selected drug or anatomic abnormalities requiring further investigation.

Table 23–1. Empiric therapy for urinary tract infections.

Diagnosis	Antibiotic	Route	Duration	Cost per Duration Noted[1]
Acute pyelonephritis	Ampicillin, 1 g every 6 hours, and gentamicin, 1 mg/kg every 8 hours	Intravenous	21 days	$870.00 not including intravenous supplies
	Ciprofloxacin, 750 mg every 12 hours	Oral	21 days	$237.00
	Ofloxacin, 200–300 mg every 12 hours	Oral	21 days	$239.00 (300 mg)
	Trimethoprim-sulfamethoxazole, 160/800 mg every 12 hours[2]	Oral	21 days	$46.00
Chronic pyelonephritis	Same as for acute pyelonephritis, but duration of therapy is 3–6 months			
Acute cystitis	Cephalexin, 250–500 mg every 6 hours	Oral	1–3 days	$16.80/3 days (500 mg)
	Ciprofloxacin, 250–500 mg every 12 hours	Oral	1–3 days	$32.00/3 days (500 mg)
	Nitrofurantoin (macrocrystals), 100 mg every 12 hours	Oral	7 days	$25.90
	Norfloxacin, 400 mg every 12 hours	Oral	1–3 days	$23.00/3 days
	Ofloxacin, 200 mg every 12 hours	Oral	1–3 days	$28.70/3 days
	Trimethoprim-sulfamethoxazole, 160/800 mg, two tablets[2]	Oral	Single dose	$2.20
Acute bacterial prostatitis	Same as for acute pyelonephritis		21 days	
Chronic bacterial prostatitis	Ciprofloxacin, 250–500 mg every 12 hours	Oral	1–3 months	$322.00/1 month (500 mg)
	Ofloxacin, 200–400 mg every 12 hours	Oral	1–3 months	$360.00/1 month (400 mg)
	Trimethoprim-sulfamethoxazole, 160/800 mg every 12 hours[2]	Oral	1–3 months	$69.00/1 month
Acute epididymitis				
Sexually transmitted	Ceftriaxone, 250 mg as single dose, plus:	Intramuscular	Once	$16.00/250 mg
	Doxycycline, 100 mg every 12 hours	Oral	10 days	$12.50
Non-sexually transmitted	Same as for chronic bacterial prostatitis	Oral	3 weeks	

[1]Average wholesale price, (AWP, for AB-rated generic when available) for quantity listed. Source: *Red Book Update,* Vol. 28, No. 3, March 2009. AWP may not accurately represent the actual pharmacy cost because wide contractual variations exist among institutions.
[2]Increasing resistance noted (up to 20%).

▶ **When to Refer**

- Suspicion or radiographic evidence of anatomic abnormality.
- Evidence of urolithiasis.
- Recurrent cystitis due to bacterial persistence.

Fihn SD. Clinical practice. Acute uncomplicated urinary tract infection in women. N Engl J Med. 2003 Jul 17;349(3):259–66. [PMID: 12867610]

Hooton TM et al. Acute uncomplicated cystitis in an era of increasing antibiotic resistance: a proposed approach to empirical therapy. Clin Infect Dis. 2004 Jul 1;39(1):75–80. [PMID: 15206056]

Norris DL 2nd et al. Urinary tract infections: diagnosis and management in the emergency department. 2008 May; 26(2):413–30. [PMID: 18406981]

2. Acute Pyelonephritis

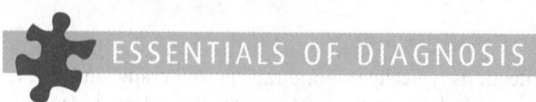

ESSENTIALS OF DIAGNOSIS

▶ Fever.

▶ Flank pain.

▶ Irritative voiding symptoms.

▶ Positive urine culture.

▶ **General Considerations**

Acute pyelonephritis is an infectious inflammatory disease involving the kidney parenchyma and renal pelvis. Gram-negative bacteria are the most common causative agents including *E coli, Proteus, Klebsiella, Enterobacter,* and *Pseudomonas.* Gram-positive bacteria are less commonly seen but include *Enterococcus faecalis* and *Staphylococcus aureus.* The infection usually ascends from the lower urinary tract—with the exception of *S aureus,* which usually is spread by a hematogenous route.

▶ **Clinical Findings**

A. Symptoms and Signs

Symptoms include fever, flank pain, shaking chills, and irritative voiding symptoms (urgency, frequency, dysuria).

Associated nausea and vomiting, and diarrhea are common. Signs include fever and tachycardia. Costovertebral angle tenderness is usually pronounced.

B. Laboratory Findings

Complete blood count shows leukocytosis and a left shift. Urinalysis shows pyuria, bacteriuria, and varying degrees of hematuria. White cell casts may be seen. Urine culture demonstrates heavy growth of the offending agent, and blood culture may also be positive.

C. Imaging

In complicated pyelonephritis, renal ultrasound may show hydronephrosis from a stone or other source of obstruction.

Differential Diagnosis

Acute intra-abdominal disease such as appendicitis, cholecystitis, pancreatitis, or diverticulitis must be distinguished from pyelonephritis. A normal urinalysis is usually seen in gastrointestinal disorders; however, on occasion, inflammation from adjacent bowel (appendicitis or diverticulitis) may result in hematuria or sterile pyuria. Abnormal liver function tests or elevated amylase levels may assist in the differentiation. Lower lobe pneumonia is distinguishable by the abnormal chest radiograph.

In males, the main differential diagnosis for acute pyelonephritis includes acute epididymitis, acute prostatitis, and acute cystitis. Physical examination and the location of the pain should permit this distinction.

Complications

Sepsis with shock can occur with acute pyelonephritis. In diabetic patients, emphysematous pyelonephritis resulting from gas-producing organisms may be life-threatening if not adequately treated. Healthy adults usually recover complete kidney function, yet if coexistent kidney disease is present, scarring or chronic pyelonephritis may result. Inadequate therapy could result in abscess formation.

Treatment

Severe infections or complicating factors require hospital admission. Urine and blood cultures are obtained to identify the causative agent and to determine antimicrobial sensitivity. Intravenous ampicillin and an aminoglycoside are initiated prior to obtaining sensitivity results (Table 23–1). In the outpatient setting, quinolones or nitrofurantoin may be initiated (Table 23–1). Antibiotics are adjusted according to sensitivities. Fevers may persist for up to 72 hours; failure to respond warrants imaging (CT or ultrasound) to exclude complicating factors that may require intervention. Catheter drainage may be necessary in the face of urinary retention and nephrostomy drainage if there is ureteral obstruction. In inpatients, intravenous antibiotics are continued for 24 hours after the fever resolves, and oral antibiotics are then given to complete a 14-day course of therapy. Follow-up urine cultures are mandatory following the completion of treatment.

Prognosis

With prompt diagnosis and appropriate treatment, acute pyelonephritis carries a good prognosis. Complicating factors, underlying kidney disease, and increasing patient age may lead to a less favorable outcome.

When to Refer

- Evidence of complicating factors (urolithiasis, obstruction).
- Absence of clinical improvement in 48 hours.

When to Admit

- Evidence of sepsis and need for parenteral antibiotics.
- Need for radiographic imaging or drainage of urinary tract obstruction.

Meng MV et al. Infections of the upper urinary tract. In: *Urologic Emergencies*, Humana Press, 2005.

3. Acute Bacterial Prostatitis

 ESSENTIALS OF DIAGNOSIS

- ▶ Fever.
- ▶ Irritative voiding symptoms.
- ▶ Perineal or suprapubic pain; exquisite tenderness common on rectal examination.
- ▶ Positive urine culture.

General Considerations

Acute bacterial prostatitis is usually caused by gram-negative rods, especially *E coli* and *Pseudomonas* species and less commonly by gram-positive organisms (eg, enterococci). The most likely routes of infection include ascent up the urethra and reflux of infected urine into the prostatic ducts. Lymphatic and hematogenous routes are probably rare.

Clinical Findings

A. Symptoms and Signs

Perineal, sacral, or suprapubic pain, fever, and irritative voiding complaints are common. Varying degrees of obstructive symptoms may occur as the acutely inflamed prostate swells, which may lead to urinary retention. High fevers and a warm and often exquisitely tender prostate are detected on examination. Care should be taken in performing a gentle rectal examination, as vigorous manipulations may result in septicemia. Prostatic massage is contraindicated.

B. Laboratory Findings

Complete blood count shows leukocytosis and a left shift. Urinalysis shows pyuria, bacteriuria, and varying degrees of hematuria. Urine cultures will demonstrate the offending pathogen.

Differential Diagnosis

Acute pyelonephritis or acute epididymitis should be distinguishable by the location of pain as well as by physical examination. Acute diverticulitis is occasionally confused with acute prostatitis; however, the history and urinalysis should permit clear distinction. Urinary retention from benign or malignant prostatic enlargement is distinguishable by initial or follow-up rectal examination.

Treatment

Hospitalization may be required, and parenteral antibiotics (ampicillin and aminoglycoside) should be initiated until organism sensitivities are available (Table 23–1). After the patient is afebrile for 24–48 hours, oral antibiotics (eg, quinolones) are used to complete 4–6 weeks of therapy. If urinary retention develops, urethral catheterization or instrumentation is contraindicated, and a percutaneous suprapubic tube is required. Follow-up urine culture and examination of prostatic secretions should be performed after the completion of therapy to ensure eradication.

Prognosis

With effective treatment, chronic bacterial prostatitis is rare.

When to Refer

- Evidence of urinary retention.
- Evidence of chronic prostatitis.

When to Admit

- Signs of sepsis.
- Need for surgical drainage of bladder or prostatic abscess.

Hua VN et al. Acute and chronic prostatitis. Med Clin North Am. 2004 Mar;88(2):483–94. [PMID: 15049589]

4. Chronic Bacterial Prostatitis

ESSENTIALS OF DIAGNOSIS

▸ Irritative voiding symptoms.
▸ Perineal or suprapubic discomfort, often dull and poorly localized.
▸ Positive expressed prostatic secretions and culture.

General Considerations

Although chronic bacterial prostatitis may evolve from acute bacterial prostatitis, many men have no history of acute infection. Gram-negative rods are the most common etiologic agents, but only one gram-positive organism (*Enterococcus*) is associated with chronic infection. Routes of infection are the same as discussed for acute infection.

Clinical Findings

A. Symptoms and Signs

Clinical manifestations are variable. Some patients are asymptomatic, but most have varying degrees of irritative voiding symptoms. Low back and perineal pain are not uncommon. Many patients report a history of urinary tract infections. Physical examination is often unremarkable, though the prostate may feel normal, boggy, or indurated.

B. Laboratory Findings

Urinalysis is normal unless a secondary cystitis is present. Expressed prostatic secretions demonstrate increased numbers of leukocytes (> 10 per high-power field), especially lipid-laden macrophages. However, this finding is consistent with inflammation and is not diagnostic of bacterial prostatitis. Leukocyte and bacterial counts from expressed prostatic secretions do not correlate with severity of symptoms. Culture of the secretions or the postprostatic massage urine specimen is necessary to make the diagnosis.

C. Imaging

Imaging tests are not necessary, though pelvic radiographs or transrectal ultrasound may demonstrate prostatic calculi.

Differential Diagnosis

Chronic urethritis may mimic chronic prostatitis, though cultures of the fractionated urine may localize the source of infection to the initial specimen. Cystitis may be secondary to prostatitis, but urine samples after prostatic massage may localize the infection to the prostate. Anal disease may share some of the symptoms of prostatitis, but physical examination should permit a distinction between the two.

Treatment

Few antimicrobial agents attain therapeutic intraprostatic levels in the absence of acute inflammation. Trimethoprim does diffuse into the prostate, and trimethoprim-sulfamethoxazole is associated with the best cure rates (Table 23–1). Other effective agents include carbenicillin, erythromycin, cephalexin, and the quinolones. The optimal duration of therapy remains controversial, ranging from 6 to 12 weeks. Symptomatic relief may be provided by anti-inflammatory agents (indomethacin, ibuprofen) and hot sitz baths.

Prognosis

Chronic bacterial prostatitis is difficult to cure, but its symptoms and tendency to cause recurrent urinary tract infections can be controlled by suppressive antibiotic therapy.

When to Refer

- Persistent symptoms.
- Consideration of enrollment in clinical trials.

5. Nonbacterial Prostatitis

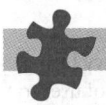

ESSENTIALS OF DIAGNOSIS

▶ Irritative voiding symptoms.

▶ Perineal or suprapubic discomfort, similar to that of chronic bacterial prostatitis.

▶ Positive expressed prostatic secretions, but culture is negative.

▶ General Considerations

Nonbacterial prostatitis is the most common of the prostatitis syndromes, and its cause is unknown. Speculation implicates chlamydiae, mycoplasmas, ureaplasmas, and viruses, but no substantial proof exists. In some cases, nonbacterial prostatitis may represent a noninfectious inflammatory or autoimmune disorder. Because the cause of nonbacterial prostatitis remains unknown, the diagnosis is usually one of exclusion.

▶ Clinical Findings

A. Symptoms and Signs

The clinical presentation is identical to that of chronic bacterial prostatitis; however, no history of urinary tract infections is present. The National Institutes of Health Chronic Prostatitis Symptom Index (NIH-CPSI) (http://www2.niddk.nih.gov/NR/rdonlyres/93B6388F-B429-4603-9C3C-6765BDEB49A1/0/NIHCPSIEnglish.pdf) has been validated to quantify symptoms of chronic nonbacterial prostatitis or chronic pelvic pain syndrome.

B. Laboratory Findings

Increased numbers of leukocytes are seen on expressed prostatic secretions, but all cultures are negative.

▶ Differential Diagnosis

The major distinction is from chronic bacterial prostatitis. The absence of a history of urinary tract infection and of positive cultures makes the distinction (Table 23–2). In older men with irritative voiding symptoms and negative cultures, the possibility of bladder cancer must be excluded. Urinary cytologic examination and cystoscopy are warranted.

▶ Treatment

Because of the uncertainty regarding the etiology of nonbacterial prostatitis, a trial of antimicrobial therapy directed against *Ureaplasma*, *Mycoplasma*, or *Chlamydia* is warranted. Erythromycin (250 mg orally four times daily) can be initiated for 14 days yet should be continued (for 3–6 weeks) only if a favorable clinical response ensues. Some symptomatic relief may be obtained with anti-inflammatory agents or sitz baths. Dietary restrictions are not necessary unless the patient relates a history of symptom exacerbation by certain substances such as alcohol, caffeine, and perhaps certain foods.

▶ Prognosis

Annoying, recurrent symptoms are common, but serious sequelae have not been identified.

Nickel JC. The three As of chronic prostatitis therapy: antibiotics, alpha-blockers and anti-inflammatories. What is the evidence? BJU Int. 2004 Dec;94(9):1230–3. [PMID: 15610095]

Nickel JC et al. Prevalence, diagnosis, characterization, and treatment of prostatitis, interstitial cystitis, and epididymitis in outpatient urological practice: the Canadian PIE Study. Urology. 2005 Nov;66(5):935–40. [PMID: 16286098]

6. Prostatodynia

Prostatodynia is a noninflammatory disorder that affects young and middle-aged men and has variable causes, including voiding dysfunction and pelvic floor musculature dysfunction. The term "prostatodynia" is a misnomer, as the prostate is actually normal.

▶ Clinical Findings

A. Symptoms and Signs

Symptoms are the same as those seen with chronic prostatitis, yet there is no history of urinary tract infection. Additional symptoms may include hesitancy and interruption of flow. Patients may relate a lifelong history of voiding difficulty. Physical examination is unremarkable, but increased anal sphincter tone and periprostatic tenderness may be observed.

Table 23–2. Clinical characteristics of prostatitis and prostatodynia syndromes.

Findings	Acute Bacterial Prostatitis	Chronic Bacterial Prostatitis	Nonbacterial Prostatitis	Prostatodynia
Fever	+	–	–	–
Urinalysis	+	–	–	–
Expressed prostate secretions	Contraindicated	+	+	–
Bacterial culture	+	+	–	–

B. Laboratory Findings

Urinalysis is normal. Expressed prostatic secretions show normal numbers of leukocytes. Urodynamic testing may show signs of dysfunctional voiding (detrusor contraction without urethral relaxation, high urethral pressures, spasms of the urinary sphincter) and is indicated in patients failing empiric trials of α-blockers or anticholinergics.

Differential Diagnosis

Normal urinalysis will distinguish it from acute infectious processes. Examination of expressed prostatic secretions will distinguish this entity from prostatitis syndromes (Table 23–2).

Treatment

Bladder neck and urethral spasms can be treated by α-blocking agents (terazosin, 1–10 mg orally once a day, or doxazosin, 1–8 mg orally once a day). Pelvic floor muscle dysfunction may respond to diazepam and biofeedback techniques. Sitz baths may contribute to symptomatic relief.

Prognosis

Prognosis is variable depending on the specific cause.

Krieger JN. The problem with prostatitis. What do we know? What do we need to know? J Urol. 2004 Aug;172(2):432–3. [PMID: 15247696]
Schaeffer A et al. Chronic prostatitis. Clin Evid. 2003 Dec;(10): 994–1002. [PMID: 15555133]
Zvara P et al. Minimally invasive therapies for prostatitis. Curr Urol Rep. 2004 Aug;5(4):320–6. [PMID: 15260937]

7. Acute Epididymitis

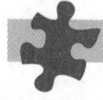

ESSENTIALS OF DIAGNOSIS

- ► Fever.
- ► Irritative voiding symptoms.
- ► Painful enlargement of epididymis.

General Considerations

Most cases of acute epididymitis are infectious and can be divided into one of two categories that have different age distributions and etiologic agents. Sexually transmitted forms typically occur in men under age 40 years, are associated with urethritis, and result from *Chlamydia trachomatis* or *Neisseria gonorrhoeae*. Non-sexually transmitted forms typically occur in older men, are associated with urinary tract infections and prostatitis, and are caused by gram-negative rods. The route of infection is probably via the urethra to the ejaculatory duct and then down the vas deferens to the epididymis. Amiodarone has been associated with self-limited epididymitis, which is a dose-dependent phenomenon.

Clinical Findings

A. Symptoms and Signs

Symptoms may follow acute physical strain (heavy lifting), trauma, or sexual activity. Associated symptoms of urethritis (pain at the tip of the penis and urethral discharge) or cystitis (irritative voiding symptoms) may occur. Pain develops in the scrotum and may radiate along the spermatic cord or to the flank. Fever and scrotal swelling are usually apparent. Early in the course, the epididymis may be distinguishable from the testis; however, later the two may appear as one enlarged, tender mass. The prostate may be tender on rectal examination.

B. Laboratory Findings

Complete blood count shows leukocytosis and a left shift. In the sexually transmitted variety, Gram staining of a smear of urethral discharge may be diagnostic of gram-negative intracellular diplococci (*N gonorrhoeae*). White cells without visible organisms on urethral smear represent nongonococcal urethritis, and *C trachomatis* is the most likely pathogen. In the non-sexually transmitted variety, urinalysis shows pyuria, bacteriuria, and varying degrees of hematuria. Urine cultures will demonstrate the offending pathogen.

C. Imaging

Scrotal ultrasound may aid in the diagnosis if examination is difficult because of the presence of a large hydrocele or because questions exist regarding the diagnosis.

Differential Diagnosis

Tumors generally cause painless enlargement of the testis. Urinalysis is negative, and examination reveals a normal epididymis. Scrotal ultrasound is helpful to define the pathology. Testicular torsion usually occurs in prepubertal males but is occasionally seen in young adults. Acute onset of symptoms and a negative urinalysis favor testicular torsion or torsion of one of the testicular or epididymal appendages. Prehn sign (elevation of the scrotum above the pubic symphysis improves pain from epididymitis) may be helpful but is not reliable.

Treatment

Bed rest with scrotal elevation is important in the acute phase. Treatment is directed toward the identified pathogen (Table 23–1). The sexually transmitted variety is treated with 10–21 days of antibiotics, and the sexual partner must be treated as well. Non-sexually transmitted forms are treated for 21–28 days with appropriate antibiotics, at which time evaluation of the urinary tract is warranted to identify underlying disease.

Prognosis

Prompt treatment usually results in a favorable outcome. Delayed or inadequate treatment may result in epididymo-orchitis, decreased fertility, or abscess formation.

When to Refer

- Persistent symptoms and infection despite antibiotic therapy.
- Signs of sepsis or abscess formation.

Tracy CR et al. Diagnosis and management of epididymitis. Urol Clin North Am. 2008 Feb;35(1):101–8. [PMID: 18061028]

URINARY STONE DISEASE

ESSENTIALS OF DIAGNOSIS

▸ Flank pain.

▸ Nausea and vomiting.

▸ Identification on noncontrast CT.

General Considerations

Urinary stone disease is exceeded in frequency as a urinary tract disorder only by infections and prostatic disease and is estimated to afflict 240,000–720,000 Americans per year. Men are more frequently affected by urolithiasis than women, with a ratio of 3:1. Initial presentation predominates in the third and fourth decades. The ratio of men to women approaches parity in the sixth and seventh decades.

Urinary calculi are polycrystalline aggregates composed of varying amounts of crystalloid and a small amount of organic matrix. Stone formation requires saturated urine that is dependent upon pH, ionic strength, solute concentration, and complexation. There are five major types of urinary stones: calcium oxalate, calcium phosphate, struvite, uric acid, and cystine. The most common types are composed of calcium, and for that reason most urinary stones (85%) are radiopaque. Uric acid stones can be radiolucent yet frequently are composed of a combination of uric acid and calcium oxalate and thus are radiopaque. Cystine stones frequently have a smooth-edged ground-glass appearance.

Geographic factors contribute to the development of stones. Areas of high humidity and elevated temperatures appear to be contributing factors, and the incidence of symptomatic ureteral stones is greatest during hot summer months.

Diet and fluid intake may be important factors in the development of urinary stones. Those afflicted with recurrent urinary stone disease are encouraged to maintain a diet restricted in sodium and protein intake. Sodium should be restricted to 100 mEq/d. Increased sodium intake will increase sodium and calcium excretion, increase monosodium urate saturation (that can act as a nidus for stone growth), increase the relative saturation of calcium phosphate, and decrease urinary citrate excretion. All of these factors encourage stone growth. Protein intake should be limited to 1 g/kg/d. An increased protein load can also increase calcium, oxalate, and uric acid excretion and decrease urinary citrate excretion.

Carbohydrates and fats have not been proved to have any impact on urinary stone disease. Bran can significantly decrease urinary calcium by increasing bowel transit time and mechanically binding to calcium. Excess intake of oxalate and purines can increase the incidence of stones in predisposed individuals. Although a reduction in dietary calcium results in reduced urinary calcium, the concurrent increase in urinary oxalate may promote stone formation. Only type II absorptive hypercalciuric patients (see below) benefit from a low-calcium diet. Persons in sedentary occupations have a higher incidence of stones than manual laborers.

Genetic factors may contribute to urinary stone formation. Cystinuria is an autosomal recessive disorder. Homozygous individuals have markedly increased excretion of cystine and frequently have numerous recurrent episodes of urinary stones despite attempts to optimize medical treatment. Distal renal tubular acidosis may be transmitted as a hereditary trait, and urolithiasis occurs in up to 75% of patients affected with this disorder.

Clinical Findings

A. Symptoms and Signs

Obstructing urinary stones usually present with colic. Pain usually occurs suddenly and may awaken patients from sleep. It is localized to the flank, is usually severe, and may be associated with nausea and vomiting. Patients are constantly moving—in sharp contrast to those with an acute abdomen. The pain may occur episodically and may radiate anteriorly over the abdomen. As the stone progresses down the ureter, the pain may be referred into the ipsilateral testis or labium. If the stone becomes lodged at the ureterovesicular junction, patients will complain of marked urinary urgency and frequency. Stone size does not correlate with the severity of the symptoms.

B. Metabolic Evaluation

Stone analysis should be performed on recovered stones. Controversy exists in deciding which patients need a thorough metabolic evaluation for stone disease. Uncomplicated first-time stone-formers should probably undergo blood screening for abnormalities of serum calcium, phosphate, electrolytes, and uric acid as a baseline.

More extensive evaluation is required in recurrent stone-formers or patients with a family history of stone disease. A 24-hour urine collection on a random diet should ascertain volume, urinary pH, and calcium, uric acid, oxalate, phosphate, sodium, and citrate excretion. A second collection on a restricted calcium (400 mg/d) and sodium (100 mEq/d) diet is undertaken to subcategorize patients, if necessary. Serum parathyroid hormone (PTH) and calcium load tests can be performed at a third visit. A calcium load test is performed as follows: After a patient has been on a restricted calcium diet for at least 1 week, the patient is told to fast from 9 PM. The patient discards the early morning voided specimen (7 AM). While still fasting, the patient voids at 9 AM, which is the fasting sample. The patient then ingests 1 g of calcium gluconate, and all urine is collected from 9 AM to 1 PM, the calcium load sample. Table 23–3 demonstrates the diagnostic criteria for the hypercalciuric states. (See discussion below.)

Table 23-3. Diagnostic criteria of different types of hypercalciuria.

	Absorptive Type I	Absorptive Type II	Absorptive Type III	Resorptive	Renal
Serum					
Calcium	N	N	N	↑	N
Phosphorus	N	N	↓	↓	N
PTH	N	N	N	↑	↑
Vitamin D	N	N	↑	↑	↑
Urinary calcium					
Fasting	N	N	↑	↑	↑
Restricted	↑	N	↑	↑	↑
After calcium load	↑	↑	↑	↑	↑

PTH, parathyroid hormone; ↑, elevated; ↓, low; N, normal.

C. Laboratory Findings

Urinalysis usually reveals microscopic or gross hematuria (~90%). However, the absence of microhematuria does not exclude urinary stones. Infection must be excluded, because the combination of infection and urinary tract obstruction requires prompt intervention as described below. Urinary pH is a valuable clue to the cause of the possible stone. Normal urine pH is 5.9. There is a normal postprandial urinary alkaline tide. Numerous dipstick measurements are valuable in the complete workup of a stone patient. Persistent urinary pH below 5.5 is suggestive of uric acid or cystine stones, both relatively radiolucent as seen on plain films of the abdomen. In contrast, a persistent pH above 7.2 is suggestive of a struvite infection stone, radiopaque on plain films.

D. Imaging

A plain film of the abdomen and renal ultrasound examination will diagnose most stones. Spiral CT has emerged as a first-line tool in evaluating flank pain. All stones whether radiopaque or radiolucent on plain abdominal radiographs will be visible on noncontrast CT except the rare calculi due to the protease inhibitor indinavir. Stones suspected of being located at the ureterovesicular junction can be imaged with abdominal ultrasonography with the aid of the acoustic window of a full bladder. Alternatively, transvaginal or transrectal ultrasonography will help identify calculi near the ureterovesicular junction.

▶ Medical Treatment & Prevention

To reduce the recurrence rate of urinary stones, one must attempt to achieve a stone-free status. Small stone fragments may serve as a nidus for future stone development. Selected patients must be thoroughly evaluated to reduce stone recurrence rates. Uric acid stone-formers may have recurrences within months if appropriate therapy is not initiated. If no medical treatment is provided after surgical stone removal, stones will generally recur in 50% of patients within 5 years. Of greatest importance in reducing stone recurrence is an increased fluid intake. Absolute volumes are

not established, but doubling previous fluid intake is recommended. Patients are encouraged to ingest fluids during meals, 2 hours after each meal (when the body is most dehydrated), and prior to going to sleep in the evening—enough to awaken the patient to void—and to ingest additional fluids during the night. Increasing fluids only during daylight hours may not dilute a supersaturated urine overnight and thus initiate a new stone.

A. Calcium Nephrolithiasis

1. Hypercalciuric—Hypercalciuric calcium nephrolithiasis (> 200 mg/24 h; > 4 mg/kg/24 h) can be caused by absorptive, resorptive, and renal disorders.

Absorptive hypercalciuria is secondary to increased absorption of calcium at the level of the small bowel, predominantly in the jejunum, and can be further subdivided into types I, II, and III. Type I absorptive hypercalciuria is independent of calcium intake. There is increased urinary calcium on a regular or even a calcium-restricted diet. Treatment is centered upon decreasing bowel absorption of calcium. Cellulose phosphate, a chelating agent, is an effective form of therapy. An average dose is 10–15 g in three divided doses. It binds to the calcium and impedes small bowel absorption due to its increased bulk. Cellulose phosphate does not change the intestinal transport mechanism. It should be given with meals so it will be available to bind to the calcium. Taking this chelating agent prior to bedtime is ineffective. Postmenopausal women should be treated with caution. It is interesting, however, that there is no enhanced decline in bone density after long-term use. Inappropriate use without an initial metabolic evaluation (see above) may result in a negative calcium balance and a secondary parathyroid stimulation. Long-term use without follow-up metabolic surveillance may result in hypomagnesuria and secondary hyperoxaluria and recurrent calculi. Routine follow-up every 6–8 months will help encourage medical compliance and permit adjustments in medical therapy based upon repeat metabolic studies.

Thiazide therapy is an alternative to cellulose phosphate in the treatment of type I absorptive hypercalciuria. Thiazides decrease renal calcium excretion but have no impact on intestinal absorption. This therapy results in increased bone density of approximately 1% per year. Thiazides have limited long-term utility ($<$ 5 years) since they may lose their hypocalciuric effect with continued therapy.

Type II absorptive hypercalciuria is diet dependent. Decreasing calcium intake by 50% (approximately 400 mg/d) will decrease the hypercalciuria to normal values (150–200 mg/24 h). There is no specific medical therapy.

Type III absorptive hypercalciuria is secondary to a renal phosphate leak. This results in increased vitamin D synthesis and secondarily increased small bowel absorption of calcium. This can be readily reversed by orthophosphates (250 mg three to four times per day). Orthophosphates do not change intestinal absorption but rather inhibit vitamin D synthesis.

Resorptive hypercalciuria is secondary to hyperparathyroidism. Hypercalcemia, hypophosphatemia, hypercalciuria, and an elevated PTH value are found. Appropriate surgical resection of the parathyroid adenoma cures the disease and the urinary stones. Medical management is invariably a failure.

Renal hypercalciuria occurs when the renal tubules are unable to efficiently reabsorb filtered calcium, and hypercalciuria results. Spilling calcium in the urine results in secondary hyperparathyroidism. Serum calcium typically is normal. Thiazides are effective long-term therapy in patients with this disorder.

2. Hyperuricosuric—Hyperuricosuric calcium nephrolithiasis is secondary to dietary excesses or uric acid metabolic defects. Both disorders can be treated with purine dietary restrictions or allopurinol therapy (or both). In contrast to uric acid nephrolithiasis, patients with hyperuricosuric calcium stones typically maintain a urinary pH greater than 5.5. Monosodium urates absorb and adsorb inhibitors and promote heterogeneous nucleation. Hyperuricosuric calcium nephrolithiasis is probably secondary to epitaxy, or heterogeneous nucleation. In such situations, similar crystal structures (ie, uric acid and calcium oxalate) can grow together with the aid of a protein matrix infrastructure.

3. Hyperoxaluric—Hyperoxaluric calcium nephrolithiasis is usually due to primary intestinal disorders. Patients usually present with a history of chronic diarrhea frequently associated with inflammatory bowel disease or steatorrhea. Increased bowel fat combines with intraluminal calcium to form a soap-like product. Calcium is therefore unavailable to bind to oxalate, which is then freely and rapidly absorbed. A small increase in oxalate absorption will significantly increase stone formation. If the diarrhea or steatorrhea cannot be effectively curtailed, oral calcium supplements should be given with meals. More than 2 g/d of ascorbic acid will increase urinary oxalate levels. Emphasis on encouraging increased fluid intake is required for these patients as for all stone-formers.

4. Hypocitraturic—Hypocitraturic calcium nephrolithiasis may be secondary to chronic diarrhea, type I (distal) renal tubular acidosis, chronic hydrochlorothiazide treatment, and, in rare cases, is idiopathic. Any condition that results in metabolic acidosis (including prolonged fasting, hypomagnesemia, and hypokalemia) will decrease urinary citrate excretion, since it will be consumed by the citric acid cycle within the mitochondria of proximal tubular cells. Hypocitraturia is frequently associated with other forms of calcium stone formation. Citrate appears to bind to calcium in solution, thereby decreasing available calcium for stone formation. Potassium citrate supplements are usually effective. Urinary citrate is decreased in acidosis and is increased during alkalosis. The potassium will supplement the frequently associated hypokalemic states, and citrate will help to correct the acidosis. A typical dose is 20 mEq three times a day (available in solution and in 10-mEq waxed tablets), or 30 mEq of crystal formulations twice a day.

B. Uric Acid Calculi

The average urinary pH is 5.9. Uric acid stone-formers typically have urinary pH values less than 5.5. The pK of uric acid is 5.75, at which point half of the uric acid is ionized as a urate salt and is soluble, while the other half is insoluble. Increasing the pH above 6.5 dramatically increases solubility and can effectively dissolve large calculi. Potassium citrate is the most frequently used medication to increase urinary pH. It can be given in liquid preparation, as crystals that need to be taken with fluids, or as tablets (10 mEq), two by mouth three or four times daily. Compliant urinary alkalinization may dissolve uric acid calculi at a rate of 1 cm (as measured on plain abdominal radiograph) of stone per month. Patients with uric acid calculi should be given Nitrazine pH paper with which to monitor the effectiveness of their urinary alkalinization. Other contributing factors include hyperuricemia, myeloproliferative disorders, malignancy with increased uric acid production, abrupt and dramatic weight loss, and uricosuric medications. If hyperuricemia is present, allopurinol (300 mg/d) may be given. Although pure uric acid stones are relatively radiolucent, most have some calcium components and can be visualized on plain abdominal radiographs. Renal ultrasonography is a helpful adjunct for appropriate diagnosis and long-term management.

C. Struvite Calculi

Struvite stones are synonymous with magnesium-ammonium-phosphate stones. They are commonly seen in women with recurrent urinary tract infections recalcitrant to appropriate antibiotics. They rarely form as ureteral stones without prior upper tract endourologic intervention. Frequently, a struvite stone is discovered as a large staghorn calculus forming a cast of the renal collecting system. Struvite stones are radiodense. Urinary pH is high, usually above 7.2. These stones are formed secondary to urease-producing organisms, including *Proteus*, *Pseudomonas*, *Providencia*, and, less commonly, *Klebsiella*, *Staphylococcus*, and *Mycoplasma*. An *E coli* urinary tract infection is not consistent with an infectious reservoir originating from a struvite calculus. These frequently large stones are relatively soft and amenable to percutaneous nephrolithotomy. Appropriate perioperative antibiotics are required. They can recur rapidly, and efforts should be taken to render the patient stone-free. Postoperative irrigation through nephrostomy tubes can eliminate small fragments. Acetohydroxamic acid is an effective urease inhibitor, but it is poorly tolerated by most patients because of its gastrointestinal toxicity.

D. Cystine Calculi

Cystine stones are a result of abnormal excretion of cystine, ornithine, lysine, and arginine. Cystine is the only amino acid that becomes insoluble in urine. These stones are particularly difficult to manage medically. Prevention is centered around increased fluid intake, alkalinization of the urine above pH 7.5 (monitored with Nitrazine pH paper), and a variety of medications including penicillamine and tiopronin (α-mercaptoproprionylglycine). There are no known inhibitors of cystine calculi.

► Surgical Treatment

Forced intravenous fluids will not push stones down the ureter. Effective peristalsis directing a bolus of urine down the ureter requires opposing ureteral walls to approach each other and touch, which large dilated systems cannot do. In fact, diuresis is counterproductive and will exacerbate the pain. Associated fever may represent infection, a medical emergency requiring prompt drainage by a ureteral catheter or a percutaneous nephrostomy tube. Antibiotics alone are inadequate unless obstruction is drained.

A. Ureteral Stones

Impediment to urine flow by ureteral stones usually occurs at three sites: (1) at the ureteropelvic junction, (2) at the crossing of the ureter over the iliac vessels, and finally (3) as the ureter enters the bladder at the ureterovesicular junction. Prediction of spontaneous stone passage is difficult. Stones less than 6 mm in diameter as seen on a plain abdominal radiograph will usually pass spontaneously. Conservative observation with appropriate pain medications is appropriate for the first 6 weeks. There is evidence that oral corticosteroids, α-blockers, and calcium channel blockers may enhance stone passage of observed ureteral stones. α-Blockers are safe and well tolerated. Typical agents and dosages are tamsulosin, 0.4 mg orally once daily; terazosin, 5 mg orally once daily; or doxazosin, 4 mg orally once daily. If spontaneous stone passage has failed, either because of lack of progression of the stone or intolerance of the pain, therapeutic intervention is required. Distal ureteral stones are best managed either with ureteroscopic stone extraction or in situ extracorporeal shock wave lithotripsy (SWL). Ureteroscopic stone extraction involves placement of a small endoscope through the urethra and into the ureter. Under direct vision, basket extraction or fragmentation followed by extraction is performed. Complications during endoscopic retrieval increase as the duration of conservative observation increases beyond 6 weeks. Indications for earlier intervention include severe pain unresponsive to medications, fever, persistent nausea and vomiting requiring intravenous hydration, social requirements requiring return to work, or anticipated travel. Most upper tract stones that enter the bladder can exit the urethra with minimal discomfort.

In situ SWL, an alternative, utilizes an external energy source that is focused upon the stone. This focused energy is additive, resulting in minimal tissue insult except at the focus where the stone is positioned with the aid of fluoroscopy or ultrasonography. This can be performed under anesthesia as an outpatient procedure and usually results in stone fragmentation. Most stone fragments will pass uneventfully within 2 weeks, but those that have not passed within 3 months are unlikely to pass without intervention. Women of childbearing age are best not treated with SWL for a stone in the lower ureter, as the impact upon the ovary is unknown.

Proximal and midureteral stones—those above the inferior margin of the sacroiliac joint—can be treated with SWL or ureteroscopy. SWL is delivered directly to the stone (in situ) without the need to push the stone back into the renal pelvis. To help ensure adequate drainage after SWL, a double J ureteral stent is frequently placed, but it does not ensure passage of stone fragments. Occasionally, stone fragments will obstruct the ureter after SWL. Conservative management will usually result in spontaneous resolution with eventual passage of the stone fragments. If this is unsuccessful, adequate proximal drainage through a percutaneous nephrostomy tube will facilitate passage. In rare instances, ureteroscopic extraction will be required.

B. Renal Calculi

Patients with renal calculi presenting without pain, urinary tract infections, or obstruction need not be treated. They should be followed with serial abdominal radiographs or renal ultrasonographic examinations. If calculi are growing or become symptomatic, intervention should be undertaken. Renal calculi less than 2 cm in diameter are best treated with SWL. Calculi located in the inferior calix frequently result in suboptimal stone-free rates as measured at 3 months by x-ray. Such calculi and others of larger diameter are best treated via percutaneous nephrolithotomy. Perioperative antibiotic coverage should be given on the basis of preoperative urine cultures.

► When to Refer

- Evidence of urinary obstruction.
- Anatomic abnormalities or solitary kidney.
- Concomitant pyelonephritis.

► When to Admit

- Intractable nausea/vomiting or pain.
- Fever.

Dellabella M et al. Randomized trial of the efficacy of tamsulosin, nifedipine and phloroglucinol in medical expulsive therapy for distal ureteral calculi. J Urol. 2005 Jul;174(1):167–72. [PMID: 15947613]

Pak CY. Medical management of urinary stone disease. Nephron Clin Pract. 2004;98(2):c49–53. [PMID: 15499203]

Pak CY et al. Predictive value of kidney stone composition in the detection of metabolic abnormalities. Am J Med. 2003 Jul;115(1):26–32. [PMID: 12867231]

Stoller ML et al. The primary stone event: a new hypothesis involving a vascular etiology. J Urol. 2004 May;171(5):1920–4. [PMID: 15076312]

INTERSTITIAL CYSTITIS

ESSENTIALS OF DIAGNOSIS

▶ Pain with a full bladder or urinary urgency.
▶ Submucosal petechiae or ulcers on cystoscopic examination.
▶ Diagnosis of exclusion.

General Considerations

Interstitial cystitis is characterized by pain with bladder filling that is relieved by emptying and is often associated with urgency and frequency. This is a diagnosis of exclusion, and patients must have a negative urine culture and cytology and no other obvious cause such as radiation cystitis, chemical cystitis (cyclophosphamide), vaginitis, urethral diverticulum, or genital herpes. Up to 40% of patients referred to urologists for interstitial cystitis may actually be found to have a different diagnosis after careful evaluation.

Population-based studies have demonstrated a prevalence of between 18 and 40 per 100,000 people. Both sexes are involved, but most patients are women, with a mean age of 40 years at onset. Patients with interstitial cystitis are more likely to report bladder problems in childhood, and there appears to be a higher prevalence in white and Jewish women. Up to 50% of patients may experience spontaneous remission of symptoms, with a mean duration of 8 months without treatment.

The etiology of interstitial cystitis is unknown, and it is most likely not a single disease but rather several diseases with similar symptoms. Associated diseases include severe allergies, irritable bowel syndrome, or inflammatory bowel disease. Theories regarding the cause of interstitial cystitis include increased epithelial permeability, neurogenic causes (sensory nervous system abnormalities), and autoimmunity.

Clinical Findings

A. Symptoms and Signs

Pain with bladder filling that is relieved with urination or urgency, frequency, and nocturia are the most common symptoms. Exposures such as pelvic radiation or prior cyclophosphamide should be inquired about. Examination should exclude genital herpes, vaginitis, or a urethral diverticulum.

B. Laboratory Findings

Urinalysis and urine culture are obtained to exclude infectious causes. Urinary cytology is obtained to exclude bladder malignancy. Urodynamic testing assesses bladder sensation and compliance and excludes detrusor instability.

C. Cystoscopy

The bladder is distended with fluid (hydrodistention) to detect glomerulations (submucosal hemorrhage), which

may or may not be present. Biopsy should be performed to exclude other causes such as carcinoma, eosinophilic cystitis, and tuberculous cystitis. The presence of submucosal mast cells is not needed to make the diagnosis of interstitial cystitis.

Differential Diagnosis

Exposures to radiation or cyclophosphamide are obtained by the history. Bacterial cystitis, genital herpes, or vaginitis can be excluded by urinalysis, culture, and physical examination. A urethral diverticulum may be suspected if palpation of the urethra demonstrates an indurated mass that results in the expression of pus from the urethral meatus. Urethral carcinoma presents as a firm mass on palpation.

Treatment

There is no cure for interstitial cystitis, but most patients achieve symptomatic relief from one of several approaches, including hydrodistention, which is usually done as part of the diagnostic evaluation. Approximately 20–30% of patients will notice symptomatic improvement following this maneuver. Also of importance is the measurement of bladder capacity during hydrodistention, since patients with very small bladder capacities (< 200 mL) are unlikely to respond to medical therapy.

Amitriptyline is often used as first-line medical therapy in patients with interstitial cystitis. Both central and peripheral mechanisms may contribute to its activity. Nifedipine and other calcium channel blockers have also demonstrated some activity in patients with interstitial cystitis. Pentosan polysulfate sodium (Elmiron) is an oral synthetic sulfated polysaccharide that helps restore integrity to the epithelium of the bladder in a subset of patients and has been evaluated in a placebo-controlled trial. Other options include intravesical instillation of dimethyl sulfoxide (DMSO), heparin, or bacillus Calmette-Guérin (BCG). A group of investigators and the Interstitial Cystitis Clinical Trials Group performed a randomized controlled trial that showed no statistically significant improvement with intravesical BCG over placebo.

Other treatment modalities include transcutaneous electric nerve stimulation (TENS) and acupuncture. Surgical therapy for interstitial cystitis should be considered only as a last resort and may require cystourethrectomy with urinary diversion.

When to Refer

Persistent and bothersome symptoms in the absence of identifiable cause.

Bogart LM et al. Symptoms of interstitial cystitis, painful bladder syndrome and similar disease in women: a systematic review. J Urol. 2007 Feb;177(2):450–6. [PMID: 17222607]

Dawson TE et al. Intravesical treatment for painful bladder syndrome/interstitial cystitis. Cochrane Database Syst Rev. 2007 Oct;17(4):CD006113. [PMID: 17943887]

Fall M et al. Treatment of bladder pain syndrome/interstitial cystitis 2008: can we make evidence-based decisions? Eur Urol. 2008 Jul;54(1):65–75. [PMID: 18403099]

Irwin P et al. Reinvestigation of patients with a diagnosis of interstitial cystitis: common things are sometimes common. J Urol. 2005 Aug;174(2):584–7. [PMID: 16006903]

Theoharides TC et al. Interstitial cystitis: bladder pain and beyond. Expert Opin Pharmacother. 2008 Dec;9(17):2979–94. [PMID: 19006474]

MALE ERECTILE DYSFUNCTION & SEXUAL DYSFUNCTION

ESSENTIALS OF DIAGNOSIS

▸ Erectile dysfunction can have organic and psychogenic etiologies.

▸ Organic erectile dysfunction may be an early sign of cardiovascular disease and requires evaluation.

▸ Incidence increases with age.

▸ Multiple treatments are effective, and range from oral agents to injectable agents to mechanical devices.

▸ General Considerations

Erectile dysfunction is defined as the consistent inability to attain or maintain a sufficiently rigid penile erection for sexual performance. This condition affects nearly 30 million American men, and its incidence is age related and rising. Approximately 52% of men aged 40–70 years experience this disorder. Most cases of male erectile disorders have an organic rather than a psychogenic cause. Normal male erection is a neurovascular phenomenon relying on an intact autonomic and somatic nerve supply to the penis, smooth and striated musculature of the corpora cavernosa and pelvic floor, and arterial inflow supplied by the paired pudendal arteries. Erection is precipitated and maintained by an increase in arterial flow, active relaxation of the smooth muscle elements of the sinusoids within the corporal bodies of the penis, and an increase in venous resistance. Contraction of the bulbocavernosus and ischiocavernosus muscles results in further rigidity of the penis. Nitric oxide appears to be the pivotal neurotransmitter that initiates and sustains erections; however, other molecules likely contribute, including acetylcholine, prostaglandins, and vasoactive intestinal peptide.

Male sexual dysfunction may be manifested in a variety of ways, and patient history is critical to the proper classification and treatment. Androgens have a strong influence on the sexual desire of men. A **loss of libido** may indicate androgen deficiency on the basis of either hypothalamic, pituitary, or testicular disease. **Loss of erections** may result from arterial, venous, neurogenic, or psychogenic causes. Concurrent medical problems may damage one or more of the mechanisms. Of particular concern is endothelial dysfunction, defined as the decreased bioavailability of nitric oxide with subsequent impairment of arterial vasodilation. Erectile dysfunction may be an early manifestation of endothelial dysfunction, which precedes more severe, systemic atherosclerotic, cardiovascular disease. In addition, many medications, especially antihypertensive and antidepressant agents, are associated with erectile dysfunction. It is impor-

tant to determine whether the patient has any normal erections in the early morning or during sleep. If normal erections occur, an organic cause is less likely. The gradual loss of erections over time is more suggestive of an organic cause. The ability to attain but not maintain an erection may be the first sign of endothelial dysfunction. The **loss of seminal emission** or anejaculation, may result from androgen deficiency by decreasing prostate and seminal vesicle secretions as well as sympathetic denervation as a result of diabetes mellitus or pelvic or retroperitoneal surgery. **Retrograde ejaculation** may occur as a result of mechanical disruption of the bladder neck, especially following transurethral resection of the prostate, treatment with α-blockers, or due to sympathetic denervation. If libido and erection are intact, the **loss of orgasm** is usually of psychological origin. **Premature ejaculation,** the persistent or recurrent ejaculation with minimal stimulation before a person wishes (associated with distress), is usually an anxiety-related disorder and rarely has an organic cause. The history may elucidate the presence of a new partner, unreasonable expectations about performance, or emotional disorders.

▸ Clinical Findings

A. Symptoms and Signs

Erectile dysfunction should be distinguished from problems of ejaculation, libido, and orgasm. The severity of the dysfunction (maintaining vs attaining; chronic, occasional, or situational) as well as its timing should be noted. The history should include inquiries about hyperlipidemia, hypertension, depression, neurologic disease, diabetes mellitus, chronic kidney disease, and endocrine disorders as well as known cardiac or peripheral vascular disease. Pelvic trauma, surgery, or irradiation identifies patients at increased risk for erectile dysfunction. Medication use should be noted, since 25% of all cases of sexual dysfunction may be drug related. The use of alcohol, tobacco, and recreational drugs should be recorded, since each is associated with an increased risk of sexual dysfunction.

During the physical examination, secondary sexual characteristics should be assessed. Motor and sensory examination should be performed as well as palpation and quantification of lower extremity vascular pulsations. The genitalia should be examined, noting the presence of penile scarring or plaque formation (Peyronie disease) and any abnormalities in size or consistency of either testicle.

B. Laboratory Findings

Laboratory evaluation should consist of a complete blood count, fasting lipid profile and glucose, testosterone, and prolactin. Patients with abnormalities of testosterone or prolactin require further evaluation with measurement of serum follicle-stimulating hormone (FSH) and luteinizing hormone (LH) to distinguish hypothalamic-pituitary dysfunction from testes failure.

C. Special Tests

Further testing is based on the patient's goals and history and is performed when etiology is unclear. Organic and psychogenic impotence can be differentiated by use of nocturnal penile tumescence testing, where the frequency and rigidity of erections are recorded by a simple tension meter attached to the penis before sleep. Patients with psychogenic impotence will have nocturnal erections of adequate frequency and rigidity.

Patients with inadequate response to oral medications may undergo further evaluation with direct injection of vasoactive substances into the penis. Such substances (prostaglandin E$_1$, papaverine, phentolamine or a combination of drugs) will induce erections in men with intact vascular systems. Patients who respond with a rigid erection require no further vascular evaluation.

Additional vascular testing is indicated in select patients who do not achieve an erection with injection of vasoactive substances and who are candidates for vascular reconstructive surgery. Diagnostic tests, such as duplex ultrasound, penile cavernosography, and pudendal arteriography, can distinguish arterial from venous erectile dysfunction and help predict which patients may benefit from vascular surgery.

▶ Treatment

Most men suffering from erectile dysfunction can be treated successfully with one of the approaches outlined below. Men who do not suffer from organic dysfunction will probably benefit from behaviorally oriented sex therapy.

A. Hormonal Replacement

Testosterone replacement therapy is offered to men with documented hypogonadism who have undergone endocrinologic evaluation and in whom prostate cancer has been assessed by prostate-specific antigen (PSA) screening and DRE. Although testosterone replacement does not induce the development of prostate cancer, PSA levels do increase and should be monitored at least once a year in addition to DRE.

B. Vasoactive Therapy

Sexual stimulation with subsequent nitric oxide release from the parasympathetic nerves and endothelium initiates penile erection. Nitric oxide enters smooth muscles cells, increases cyclic guanosine monophosphate (cGMP) production, which mediates calcium sequestration and cellular hyperpolarization. Phosphodiesterase 5 (PDE-5) degrades cGMP and fosters penile detumescence.

1. Oral agents—Sildenafil, vardenafil, and tadalafil inhibit PDE-5, allowing cGMP to function unopposed, thereby sustaining inflow of blood into the erect penis. All drugs are similarly effective but have variable half-lives, receptor binding affinity, and side effects. Each drug should be initiated at the lowest dose and titrated to effect. There is no effect on libido, and priapism is exceedingly rare. The additive effect on nitrates may lead to exaggerated cardiac preload reduction and hypotension; therefore, the drug is contraindicated in patients taking nitroglycerin or nitrates. All patients being evaluated for acute chest pain should be asked if they are taking a PDE-5 inhibitor before administering nitroglycerin. Fixed atherosclerotic disease in the aortoiliac system is associated with diminished efficacy. Some patients who do not respond to one PDE-5 inhibitor may respond to one of the other agents.

2. Injectable agents—Direct injection of vasoactive prostaglandins into the penis is an acceptable form of treatment for many men with erectile dysfunction. Injections are performed using a tuberculin syringe or a metered-dose injection device. The base and lateral aspect of the penis is used as the injection site to avoid injury to the superficial blood supply located anteriorly. Complications are rare and include bruising, dizziness, local pain, fibrosis, priapism, and infection. Vasoactive prostaglandins (alprostadil) can also be delivered via a urethral suppository with slightly less effectiveness.

The presence of a prolonged erection requires prompt medical attention to prevent erectile dysfunction and fibrosis of the cavernosal tissues. Initial management may include aspiration of blood from the penis or injection of sympathomimetic drugs (epinephrine or phenylephrine); if these maneuvers fail, surgical shunts may need to be performed to drain blood from the corpora cavernosa.

C. Vacuum Constriction Device

The vacuum constriction device induces erection by creating a vacuum chamber around the penis, whereby blood is drawn into the corpora cavernosa. Once adequate tumescence has been achieved, an elastic constriction band is placed around the proximal penile shaft to prevent loss of erection, and the vacuum cylinder is removed. Such devices are suitable for patients with venous disorders of the penis and those who do not achieve an adequate erection with injection of vasoactive substances. Complications are rare and the device is highly effective, but cumbersome with a high rate of discontinued use.

D. Penile Prostheses

Prosthetic devices may be implanted directly into the paired corporal bodies. Such prostheses may be semi-rigid and malleable or inflatable. Each is manufactured in a variety of sizes and diameters. Inflatable models may result in a more cosmetic appearance and better functionality. Complications are rare but include mechanical failure, infection, and injury to adjacent anatomic structures during surgery.

E. Vascular Reconstruction

Patients with disorders of the arterial system are candidates for various forms of arterial reconstruction, including endarterectomy and balloon dilation for proximal arterial occlusion and arterial bypass procedures utilizing arterial (epigastric) or venous (deep dorsal vein) segments for distal occlusion. Patients with venous disorders may be managed with ligation of certain veins (deep dorsal or emissary veins) or the crura of the corpora cavernosa. Experience with vascular reconstructive procedures is still limited, and many patients so treated still fail to achieve a rigid erection.

When to Refer

- Patients with inadequate response to oral medications.
- Patients with Peyronie disease (penile curvature) or other penile deformity.
- Patients with a history of pelvic or perineal trauma or surgery.
- Young patients or those with lifelong erectile dysfunction.

Basson R et al. Sexual sequelae of general medical disorders. Lancet. 2007 Feb 3;369(9559):409–24. [PMID: 17276781]

Carson CC et al; Patient Response with Vardenafil in Sildenafil Non-Responders (PROVEN) Study Group. Erectile response with vardenafil in sildenafil nonresponders: a multicentre, double-blind, 12-week, flexible-dose, placebo-controlled erectile dysfunction clinical trial. BJU Int. 2004 Dec;94(9):1301–9. [PMID: 15610110]

Jackson G et al. The second Princeton consensus on sexual dysfunction and cardiac risk: new guidelines for sexual medicine. J Sex Med. 2006 Jan;3(1):28–36. [PMID: 16409215]

Kostis JB et al. Sexual dysfunction and cardiac risk (the Second Princeton Consensus Conference). Am J Cardiol. 2005 Dec 26;96(12B):85M-93M. [PMID: 16387575]

Lue TF et al. Summary of recommendations on sexual dysfunctions in men. J Sex Med. 2004 Jul;1(1):6–23. [PMID: 16422979]

McVary KT. Clinical practice. Erectile dysfunction. N Engl J Med. 2007 Dec 13;357(24):2472–81. [PMID: 18077811]

MALE INFERTILITY

 ESSENTIALS OF DIAGNOSIS

- Couple infertility is related to the male partner in 50% of cases.
- Causes include decreased or absent sperm production or function, or obstruction of the male genital tract.
- Detailed history, physical examination, and repeated semen analysis are the cornerstones of diagnosis and treatment.

General Considerations

Infertility, the inability of a couple to conceive a child after 1 year of sexual intercourse without contraceptive use, affects 15–20% of US couples. Approximately one-third of cases result from male factors, one-third from female factors, and one-third from combined factors; therefore, evaluation of both partners is critical. Clinical evaluation is warranted following 6 months of unprotected intercourse in select couples. Following a detailed history and physical examination, a semen analysis is essential for diagnosis and should be performed at least twice, on two separate occasions (Figure 23–1). As spermatogenesis takes approximately 74 days, it is thus important to review events from the past 3 months.

Clinical Findings

A. Symptoms and Signs

The history should include prior testicular insults (torsion, cryptorchidism, trauma), infections (mumps orchitis, epi-

didymitis), environmental factors (excessive heat, radiation, chemotherapy, prolonged pesticide exposure), medications (anabolic steroids, cimetidine, and spironolactone may affect spermatogenesis; phenytoin may lower FSH; sulfasalazine and nitrofurantoin affect sperm motility), and drugs (alcohol, tobacco, marijuana). Sexual habits, frequency and timing of intercourse, use of lubricants, and each partner's previous fertility experiences are important. Loss of libido and headaches, visual disturbances, or galactorrhea may indicate a pituitary tumor. The past medical or surgical history may reveal thyroid or liver disease (abnormalities of spermatogenesis), diabetic neuropathy (retrograde or anejaculation), radical pelvic or retroperitoneal surgery (absent seminal emission secondary to sympathetic nerve injury), or hernia repair (damage to the vas deferens or testicular blood supply).

Physical examination should pay particular attention to features of hypogonadism: underdeveloped secondary sexual characteristics, diminished male pattern hair distribution (axillary, body, facial, pubic), body habitus, and gynecomastia. The scrotal contents should be carefully evaluated. Testicular size should be noted (normal size approximately 4.5 × 2.5 cm, volume 18 mL). Varicoceles are abnormally dilated and refluxing veins of the pampiniform plexus that can be identified in the standing position by gentle palpation of the spermatic cord and, on occasion, may only be appreciated with the Valsalva maneuver. The vas deferens, epididymis, and prostate should be palpated (absence of all or part of the vas deferens may indicate the presence a cystic fibrosis variant, congenital bilateral or unilateral absence of the vas deferens).

B. Laboratory Findings

Semen analysis should be performed after 48–72 hours of abstinence. The specimen should be analyzed within 1 hour after collection. Abnormal sperm concentrations are less than 20 million/mL (**oligospermia** is the presence of less than 20 million sperm/mL in the ejaculate; **azoospermia** is the absence of sperm). Normal semen volumes range between 1.5 and 5 mL (volumes < 1.5 mL may result in inadequate buffering of the vaginal acidity and may be due to retrograde ejaculation or androgen insufficiency). Normal sperm motility and morphology demonstrate 50–60% motile cells and more than 30% or 4% normal (World Health Organization and Krueger guidelines, respectively) morphology. Abnormal motility may result from varicocele, antisperm antibodies, infection, abnormalities of the sperm flagella, or partial ejaculatory duct obstruction. Abnormal morphology may result from a varicocele, infection, or exposure history.

Endocrinologic evaluation is warranted if sperm counts are low or if there is a basis from the history and physical examination for suspecting an endocrinologic origin. Initial testing should include serum FSH and testosterone. Specific abnormalities in these hormones should prompt additional testing, including LH and prolactin. Elevated FSH and LH levels and low testosterone levels (hypergonadotropic hypogonadism) are associated with primary testicular failure. Low FSH and LH associated with low testosterone

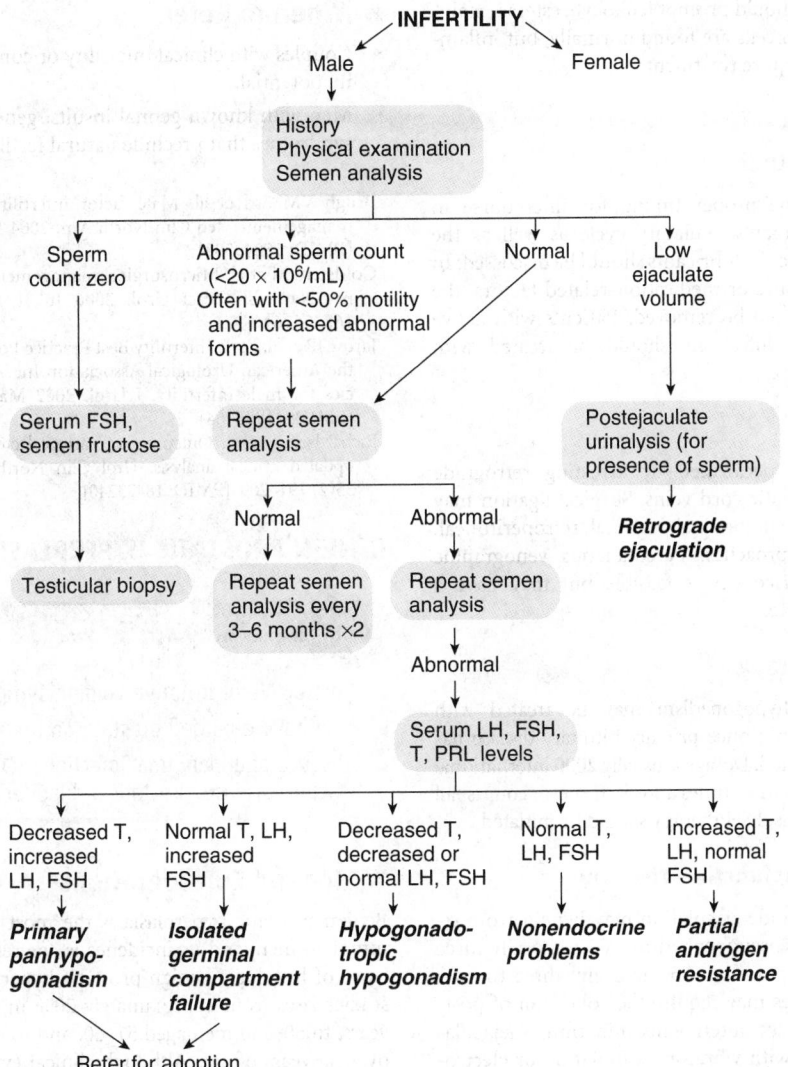

▲ **Figure 23–1.** Male infertility: evaluation of male factor infertility. FSH, follicle-stimulating hormone; LH, luteinizing hormone; PRL, prolactin; T, testosterone. (From Nicoll D et al [editors]: *Pocket Guide to Diagnostic Tests*. McGraw-Hill, 2004. Adapted, with permission, from Swerdloff RS et al. Evaluation of the male partner of an infertile couple. An algorithmic approach. JAMA. 1982 May 7;247(17):2418–22. Copyright © 1982 by The American Medical Association.)

occur in secondary testicular failure (hypogonadotropic hypogonadism) and may be of hypothalamic or pituitary origin. Elevation of serum prolactin may indicate the presence of pituitary prolactinoma.

C. Genetic Testing

Men with sperm concentrations less than 10 million/mL should undergo testing for Y chromosome microdeletions and a karyotyping. Gene deletions from the long arm of the Y chromosome may cause azoospermia or oligospermia with age-related decline in spermatogenesis that is transmissible to male offspring. Karyotyping may reveal Klinefelter syndrome. Partial or complete absence of the vas deferens should prompt testing for cystic fibrosis mutations.

D. Imaging

Scrotal ultrasound may detect a subclinical varicocele. Vasography may be required in patients with suspected genital duct obstruction. Men with low ejaculate volume and no evidence of retrograde ejaculation should undergo transrectal ultrasound to evaluate the prostate and seminal vesicles.

E. Special Tests

Azoospermic patients should have post-ejaculation urine samples centrifuged and analyzed for sperm to evaluate for retrograde ejaculation. In cases of disproportionately low motility, sperm vitality and the presence of autoantibodies should be assessed. Rounds cells in concentrations greater than 1 million/mL should prompt leukocyte esterase staining (immature germ cells are found normally, but inflammatory cells may require treatment).

Treatment

A. General Measures

Education about the proper timing for intercourse in relation to the woman's ovulatory cycle as well as the avoidance of spermicidal lubricants should be discussed. In cases of toxic exposure or medication-related factors, the offending agent should be removed. Patients with active genitourinary tract infections should be treated with appropriate antibiotics.

B. Varicocele

Varicocelectomy is performed by arresting retrograde blood flow in spermatic cord veins. Surgical ligation may be accomplished via subinguinal, inguinal, retroperitoneal, or laparoscopic approaches. Percutaneous venographic embolization of varicoceles is feasible but may have a higher recurrence rate.

C. Endocrine Therapy

Hypogonadotropic hypogonadism may be treated with chorionic gonadotropin once primary pituitary disease has been excluded or treated. Dosage is usually 2000 international units intramuscularly three times a week. If sperm counts fail to rise after 12 months, FSH therapy should be initiated.

D. Ejaculatory Dysfunction Therapy

Patients with retrograde ejaculation may benefit from α-adrenergic agonists (pseudoephedrine, 60 mg orally three times a day) or imipramine (25 mg orally three times a day). Medical failures may require the collection of post-ejaculation urine for intrauterine insemination. Anejaculation can be treated with vibratory stimulation or electroejaculation in select cases.

E. Ductal Obstruction

Obstruction of the ejaculatory ducts may be corrected by transurethral resection of the ducts in the prostatic urethra. If obstruction of the vas deferens or epididymis is suspected, the level of obstruction must be determined via a vasogram prior to operative treatment, with the exception of prior vasectomy. Obstruction of the vas deferens is best managed by a microsurgical approach, and a vasovasostomy or vasoepididymostomy may be required.

F. Assisted Reproductive Techniques

Intrauterine insemination, in vitro fertilization, and intracytoplasmic sperm injection (ICSI) are alternatives to patients in whom other means of treating reduced sperm concentration, motility, or functionality has failed. With the use of ICSI, even azoospermic men can father their genetic progeny by surgical retrieval of sperm from the testicle, epididymis, or vas deferens.

When to Refer

- Couples with clinical infertility or concern about fertility potential.
- Men with known genital insults, genetic diagnoses, or syndromes that preclude natural fertility.

Brugh VM 3rd et al. Male factor infertility: evaluation and management. Med Clin North Am. 2004 Mar;88(2):367–85. [PMID: 15049583]

Goldstein M et al. Microsurgical management of male infertility. Nat Clin Pract Urol. 2006 Jul;3(7):381–91. [PMID: 16835626]

Jarow JP et al; Male Infertility Best Practice Policy Committee of the American Urological Association Inc. Best practice policies for male infertility. J Urol. 2002 May;167(5):2138–44. [PMID: 11956464]

Richardson I et al. Outcomes of varicocelectomy treatment: an updated critical analysis. Urol Clin North Am. 2008 May; 35(2):191–209. [PMID: 18423240]

BENIGN PROSTATIC HYPERPLASIA

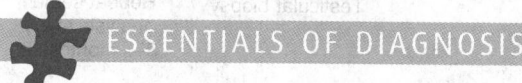

ESSENTIALS OF DIAGNOSIS

- ▸ Obstructive or irritative voiding symptoms.
- ▸ May have enlarged prostate on rectal examination.
- ▸ Absence of urinary tract infection, neurologic disorder, stricture disease, prostatic or bladder malignancy.

General Considerations

Benign prostatic hyperplasia is the most common benign tumor in men, and its incidence is age related. The prevalence of histologic benign prostatic hyperplasia in autopsy studies rises from approximately 20% in men aged 41–50 years, to 50% in men aged 51–60, and to over 90% in men over 80 years of age. Although clinical evidence of disease occurs less commonly, symptoms of prostatic obstruction are also age related. At age 55 years, approximately 25% of men report obstructive voiding symptoms. At age 75 years, 50% of men report a decrease in the force and caliber of the urinary stream.

Risk factors for the development of benign prostatic hyperplasia are poorly understood. Some studies have suggested a genetic predisposition and some have noted racial differences. Approximately 50% of men under age 60 years who undergo surgery for benign prostatic hyperplasia may have a heritable form of the disease. This form is most likely an autosomal dominant trait, and first-degree male relatives of such patients carry an increased relative risk of approximately fourfold.

Clinical Findings

A. Symptoms

The symptoms of benign prostatic hyperplasia can be divided into obstructive and irritative complaints. Obstructive symptoms include hesitancy, decreased force

Table 23–4. American Urological Association symptom index for benign prostatic hyperplasia.[1]

Questions to Be Answered	Not at All	Less Than One Time in Five	Less Than Half the Time	About Half the Time	More Than Half the Time	Almost Always
1. Over the past month, how often have you had a sensation of not emptying your bladder completely after you finish urinating?	0	1	2	3	4	5
2. Over the past month, how often have you had to urinate again less than 2 hours after you finished urinating?	0	1	2	3	4	5
3. Over the past month, how often have you found you stopped and started again several times when you urinated?	0	1	2	3	4	5
4. Over the past month, how often have you found it difficult to postpone urination?	0	1	2	3	4	5
5. Over the past month, how often have you had a weak urinary stream?	0	1	2	3	4	5
6. Over the past month, how often have you had to push or strain to begin urination?	0	1	2	3	4	5
7. Over the past month, how many times did you most typically get up to urinate from the time you went to bed at night until the time you got up in the morning?	0	1	2	3	4	5

[1]Sum of seven circled numbers equals the symptom score. See text for explanation.
Reproduced, with permission, from Barry MJ et al. The American Urological Association symptom index for benign prostatic hyperplasia. J Urol. 1992 Nov;148(5):1549–57.

and caliber of the stream, sensation of incomplete bladder emptying, double voiding (urinating a second time within 2 hours), straining to urinate, and postvoid dribbling. Irritative symptoms include urgency, frequency, and nocturia.

The American Urological Association (AUA) symptom index (Table 23–4) is perhaps the single most important tool used in the evaluation of patients with this disorder and should be calculated for all patients before starting therapy. The answers to seven questions quantitate the severity of obstructive or irritative complaints on a scale of 0–5. Thus, the score can range from 0 to 35, in increasing severity of symptoms.

A detailed history focusing on the urinary tract should be obtained to exclude other possible causes of symptoms such as prostate cancer or disorders unrelated to the prostate such as urinary tract infection, neurogenic bladder, or urethral stricture.

B. Signs

A physical examination, DRE, and a focused neurologic examination should be performed on all patients. The size and consistency of the prostate should be noted, but prostate size does not correlate with the severity of symptoms or the degree of obstruction. Benign prostatic hyperplasia usually results in a smooth, firm, elastic enlargement of the prostate. Induration, if detected, must alert the clinician to the possibility of cancer, and further evaluation is needed (ie, PSA, transrectal ultrasound, and biopsy). Examination of the lower abdomen should be performed to assess for a distended bladder.

C. Laboratory Findings

Urinalysis should be performed to exclude infection or hematuria. A serum PSA is considered optional, yet most clinicians will include it in the initial evaluation, particularly if life expectancy is more than 10 years. PSA certainly increases the ability to detect prostate cancer over DRE alone; however, because there is much overlap between levels seen in benign prostatic hyperplasia and prostate cancer, its use remains controversial (see below in the section on screening for prostate cancer).

D. Imaging

Upper tract imaging (IVU, CT, or renal ultrasound) is recommended only in the presence of concomitant urinary tract disease or complications from benign prostatic hyperplasia (ie, hematuria, urinary tract infection, chronic kidney disease, history of stone disease).

E. Cystoscopy

Cystoscopy is not recommended to determine the need for treatment but may assist in determining the surgical approach in patients opting for invasive therapy.

F. Additional Tests

Cystometrograms and urodynamic profiles should be reserved for patients with suspected neurologic disease or those who have failed prostate surgery. Flow rates, postvoid residual urine determination, and pressure-flow studies are considered optional.

Differential Diagnosis

A history of prior urethral instrumentation, urethritis, or trauma should be elucidated to exclude urethral stricture or bladder neck contracture. Hematuria and pain are commonly associated with bladder stones. Carcinoma of the prostate may be detected by abnormalities on the DRE or an elevated PSA (**see Chapter 39 for Prostate Cancer**). A urinary tract infection can mimic the irritative symptoms of benign prostatic hyperplasia and can be readily identified by urinalysis and culture; however, a urinary tract infection can also be a complication of benign prostatic hyperplasia. Carcinoma of the bladder, especially carcinoma in situ, may also present with irritative voiding complaints; however, urinalysis usually shows evidence of hematuria (**see Chapter 39 for Bladder Cancer**). Patients with a neurogenic bladder may also have many of the same symptoms and signs as those with benign prostatic hyperplasia; however, a history of neurologic disease, stroke, diabetes mellitus, or back injury may be obtained, and diminished perineal or lower extremity sensation or alterations in rectal sphincter tone or the bulbocavernosus reflex might be observed on examination. Simultaneous alterations in bowel function (constipation) might also suggest the possibility of a neurologic disorder.

Treatment

Clinical practice guidelines exist for the evaluation and treatment of patients with benign prostatic hyperplasia (Figure 23–2). Following evaluation as outlined above, patients should be offered various forms of therapy for benign prostatic hyperplasia. Patients are advised to consult with their primary care clinicians and make an educated decision on the basis of the relative efficacy and side effects of the treatment options (Table 23–5).

Patients with mild symptoms (AUA scores 0–7) should be managed by watchful waiting only. Absolute surgical indications are refractory urinary retention (failing at least one attempt at catheter removal), large bladder diverticula, or any of the following sequelae of benign prostatic hyperplasia: recurrent urinary tract infection, recurrent gross hematuria, bladder stones, or chronic kidney disease.

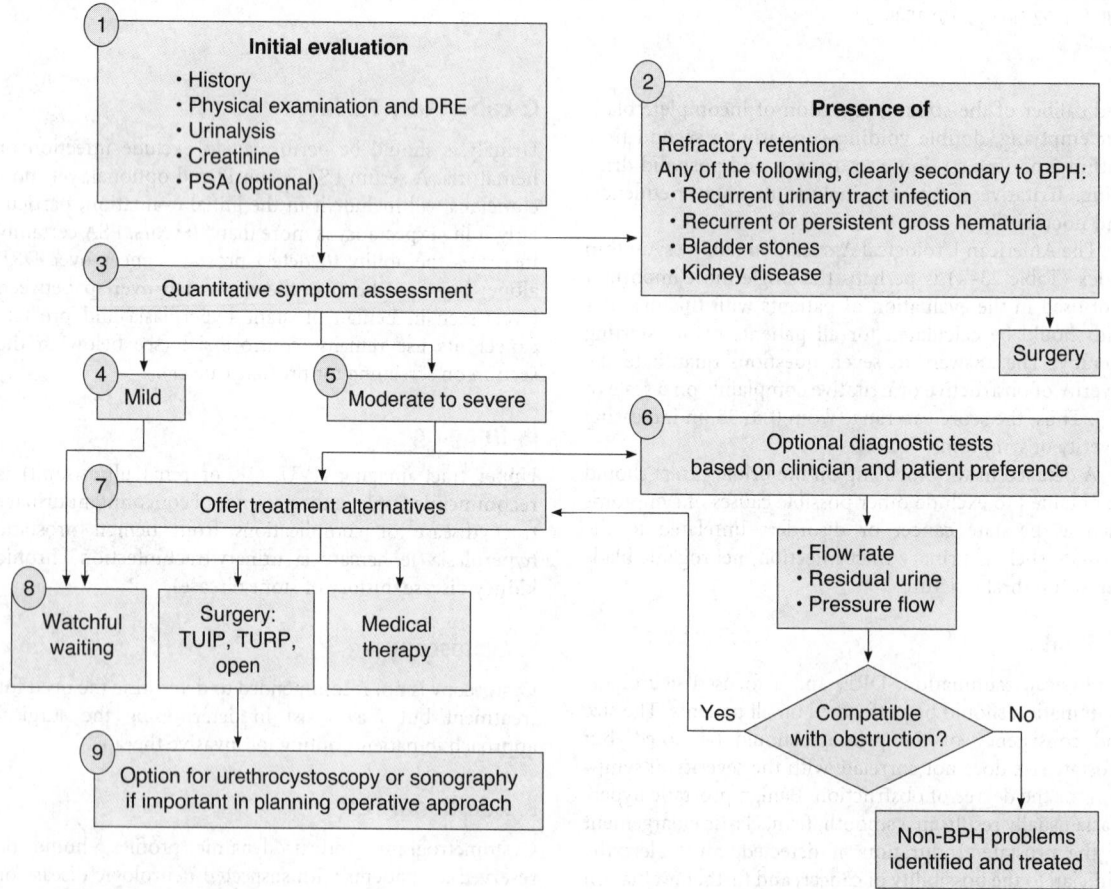

▲ **Figure 23–2.** Benign prostatic hyperplasia decision diagram. DRE, digital rectal examination; PSA, prostate-specific antigen; BPH, benign prostatic hyperplasia; TUIP, transurethral incision of the prostate; TURP, transurethral resection of the prostate.

Table 23–5. Balance sheet for benign prostatic hyperplasia treatment outcomes.[1]

Outcome	TUIP	Open Surgery	TURP	Watchful Waiting	α-Blockers	Finasteride[2]
Chance for improvement[1]	78–83%	94–99.8%	75–96%	31–55%	59–86%	54–78%
Degree of symptom improvement (% reduction in symptom score)	73%	79%	85%	Unknown	51%	31%
Morbidity and complications[1]	2.2–33.3%	7–42.7%	5.2–30.7%	1–5%	2.9–43.3%	13.6–8.8%
Death within 30–90 days[1]	0.2–1.5%	1–4.6%	0.5–3.3%	0.8%	0.8%	0.8%
Total incontinence[1]	0.1–1.1%	0.3–0.7%	0.7–1.4%	2%	2%	2%
Need for operative treatment for surgical complications[1]	1.3–2.7%	0.6–14.1%	0.7–10.1%	0	0	0
Impotence[1]	3.9–24.5%	4.7–39.2%	3.3–34.8%	3%	3%	2.5–5.3%
Retrograde ejaculation	6–55%	36–95%	25–99%	0	4–11%	0
Loss of work in days	7–21	21–28	7–21	1	3.5	1.5
Hospital stay in days	1–3	5–10	3–5	0	0	0

[1] 90% confidence interval.
[2] Most of the data reviewed for finasteride are derived from three trials that have required an enlarged prostate for entry. The chance of improvement in men with symptoms yet minimally enlarged prostates may be much less, as noted from the VA Cooperative Trial.
TUIP, transurethral incision of the prostate; TURP, transurethral resection of the prostate.

A. Watchful Waiting

The risk of progression or complications is uncertain. However, in men with symptomatic disease, it is clear that progression is not inevitable and that some men undergo spontaneous improvement or resolution of their symptoms.

Retrospective studies on the natural history of benign prostatic hyperplasia are inherently subject to bias, relating in part to patient selection and also to the type and extent of follow-up. Very few prospective studies addressing the natural history have been reported. One small series demonstrated that approximately 10% of symptomatic men may progress to urinary retention while 50% of patients demonstrate marked improvement or resolution of symptoms. A large randomized study compared finasteride with placebo in men with moderate to severely symptomatic disease and enlarged prostates on DRE. Patients in the placebo arm demonstrated a 7% risk of developing urinary retention over 4 years.

Men with moderate or severe symptoms can also be observed if they so choose. The optimal interval for follow-up is not defined, nor are the specific end points for intervention.

B. Medical Therapy

1. α-Blockers—α-Blockers can be classified according to their receptor selectivity as well as their half-life (Table 23–6).

Prazosin is effective; however, it requires dose titration and twice daily dosing. Typical side effects include orthostatic hypotension, dizziness, tiredness, retrograde ejaculation, rhinitis, and headache.

Long-acting α-blockers allow for once-a-day dosing, but dose titration is still necessary. Terazosin improves symptoms and in numerous studies is superior to placebo or finasteride. Terazosin is started at a dosage of 1 mg orally daily for 3 days, increased to 2 mg orally daily for 11 days, then 5 mg orally daily. Additional dose escalation to 10 mg orally daily can be performed if necessary. Doxazosin is started at a dosage of 1 mg orally daily for 7 days, increased to 2 mg orally daily for 7 days, then 4 mg orally daily. Additional dose escalation to 8 mg orally daily can be performed if necessary. Side effects are similar to those described above for prazosin. Alfuzosin is a long-acting α-blocker; its dose is 10 mg orally once daily and does not require titration.

α_{1a}-Receptors are localized to the prostate and bladder neck. Selective blockade of these receptors results in fewer systemic side effects than α-blocker therapy (orthostatic hypotension, dizziness, tiredness, rhinitis, and headache), thus obviating the need for dose titration. The typical dose of tamsulosin is 0.4 mg orally daily taken 30 minutes after a meal. Several randomized, double-blind, placebo-controlled trials have been performed comparing terazosin, doxazosin, tamsulosin, and alfuzosin with placebo. All agents have demonstrated safety and efficacy.

Table 23–6. α-Blockade for benign prostatic hyperplasia.

Agent	Action	Oral Dose
Phenoxybenzamine	α_1- and α_2-Blockade	5–10 mg twice daily
Prazosin	α_1-Blockade	1–5 mg twice daily
Terazosin	α_1-Blockade	1–10 mg daily
Doxazosin	α_1-Blockade	1–8 mg daily
Alfuzosin	α_1-Blockade	10 mg daily
Tamsulosin	α_{1a}-Blockade	0.4 or 0.8 mg daily

2. 5α-Reductase inhibitors—Finasteride is a 5α-reductase inhibitor that blocks the conversion of testosterone to dihydrotestosterone. This drug impacts upon the epithelial component of the prostate, resulting in reduction in size of the gland and improvement in symptoms. Six months of therapy is required for maximum effects on prostate size (20% reduction) and symptomatic improvement.

Several randomized, double-blind, placebo-controlled trials have been performed comparing finasteride with placebo. Efficacy, safety, and durability are well established. However, symptomatic improvement is seen only in men with enlarged prostates (> 40 mL by ultrasonographic examination). Side effects include decreased libido, decrease in volume of ejaculate, and impotence. Serum PSA is reduced by approximately 50% in patients receiving finasteride therapy. Therefore, in order to compare with pre-finasteride levels, the serum PSA of a patient taking finasteride should be doubled.

A report suggests that finasteride therapy may decrease the incidence of urinary retention and the need for operative treatment in men with enlarged prostates and moderate to severe symptoms. The larger the prostate over 40 mL, the greater the relative-risk reduction. However, optimal identification of appropriate patients for prophylactic therapy remains to be determined. Dutasteride is a dual 5α-reductase inhibitor that appears to be similar to finasteride in its effectiveness; its dose is 0.5 mg orally daily.

3. Combination therapy—The four-arm Veterans Administration Cooperative Trial compared placebo, finasteride alone, terazosin alone, and combination of finasteride and terazosin. Over 1200 patients participated, and significant decreases in symptom scores and increases in urinary flow rates were seen only in the arms containing terazosin. However, enlarged prostates were not an entry criterion; in fact, prostate size in this study was much smaller than in previous controlled trials using finasteride (32 versus 52 mL). Other randomized, placebo-controlled trials comparing finasteride with placebo in men with lower urinary tract symptoms and large prostates showed finasteride to be beneficial for reducing symptoms, increasing urinary flow rate, and reducing the risk of complications due to benign prostatic hyperplasia as well as reducing the number of men who required surgery for benign prostatic hyperplasia. The Medical Therapy of Prostatic Symptoms (MTOPs) trial is a large, randomized, placebo-controlled trial comparing finasteride, doxazosin, the combination of the two, and placebo in 3047 men observed for a mean of 4.5 years. Long-term combination therapy with doxazosin and finasteride was safe and reduced the risk of overall clinical progression of benign prostatic hyperplasia significantly more than did treatment with either drug alone. Combination therapy and finasteride alone reduced the long-term risk of acute urinary retention and the need for invasive therapy. Combination therapy had the risks of additional side effects and the cost of two medications.

4. Phytotherapy—Phytotherapy is the use of plants or plant extracts for medicinal purposes. Its use in benign prostatic hyperplasia has been popular in Europe for years, and its use in the United States is growing as a result of patient-driven enthusiasm. Several plant extracts have been popularized, including the saw palmetto berry, the bark of *Pygeum africanum*, the roots of *Echinacea purpurea* and *Hypoxis rooperi*, pollen extract, and the leaves of the trembling poplar. The mechanisms of action of these agents are unknown. A 2006 prospective, randomized, double-blind, placebo-controlled trial revealed no improvement in symptoms, urinary flow rate, or quality of life for men with benign prostatic hyperplasia with saw palmetto treatment compared with placebo.

C. Conventional Surgical Therapy

1. Transurethral resection of the prostate (TURP)—Ninety-five percent of simple prostatectomies can be performed endoscopically. Most of these procedures are performed under a spinal anesthetic and require a 1- to 2-day hospital stay. Symptom scores and flow rate improvement are superior following TURP relative to any minimally invasive therapy; however, the length of the hospital stay is greater. Much controversy revolves around possible higher rates of morbidity and mortality associated with TURP in comparison with open surgery, but the higher rates observed in one study probably related to more significant comorbidities in the TURP patients compared with the patients who received open surgical treatment. Several other studies could not confirm the difference in mortality when controlling for age and comorbidities. The risks of TURP include retrograde ejaculation (75%), impotence (5–10%), and urinary incontinence (< 1%). Complications include bleeding, urethral stricture or bladder neck contracture, perforation of the prostate capsule with extravasation, and, if severe, transurethral resection syndrome, a hypervolemic, hyponatremic state resulting from absorption of the hypotonic irrigating solution. Clinical manifestations of the syndrome include nausea, vomiting, confusion, hypertension, bradycardia, and visual disturbances. The risk of transurethral resection syndrome increases with resection times over 90 minutes. Treatment includes diuresis and, in severe cases, hypertonic saline administration.

2. Transurethral incision of the prostate (TUIP)—Men with moderate to severe symptoms and small prostates often have posterior commissure hyperplasia or an "elevated bladder neck." These patients will often benefit from incision of the prostate. The procedure is more rapid and less morbid than TURP. Outcomes in well-selected patients are comparable, though a lower rate of retrograde ejaculation has been reported (25%).

3. Open simple prostatectomy—When the prostate is too large to remove endoscopically, open enucleation is necessary. What size is "too large" depends upon the surgeon's experience with TURP. Glands over 100 g are usually considered for open enucleation. In addition to size, other relative indications for open prostatectomy include concomitant bladder diverticulum or bladder stone and whether dorsal lithotomy positioning is or is not possible.

Open prostatectomies can be performed with either a suprapubic or retropubic approach. Simple suprapubic prostatectomy is performed transvesically and is the operation of choice if there is concomitant bladder pathology. After the adenoma is removed, both a urethral and a suprapubic catheter are inserted prior to closure.

In simple retropubic prostatectomy, the bladder is not entered but rather a transverse incision is made in the surgical capsule of the prostate and the adenoma is enucleated as described above; only a urethral catheter is needed at the end of the case.

D. Minimally Invasive Therapy

1. Laser therapy—Several different coagulation necrosis techniques have been utilized. Transurethral laser-induced prostatectomy (TULIP) is performed under transrectal ultrasound guidance. The instrument is placed in the urethra and transrectal ultrasound is used to direct the device as it is slowly pulled from the bladder neck to the apex. The depth of treatment is monitored with ultrasound.

Most urologists prefer to use visually directed laser techniques. Visual coagulative necrosis is performed under cystoscopic control, and the laser fiber is pulled through the prostate at several designated areas depending upon the size and configuration of the gland. Four-quadrant and sextant approaches have been described for lateral lobes, with additional treatments directed at enlarged median lobes. Coagulative techniques do not create an immediate visual defect in the prostatic urethra—tissue is sloughed over the course of several weeks up to 3 months following the procedure.

Visual contact ablative techniques take longer in the operating room because the fiber is placed in direct contact with the prostate tissue, which is vaporized. Photovaporization of the prostate (PVP), an alternative laser technique, uses a high-power KTP laser. An immediate defect is obtained in the prostatic urethra, similar to that seen during TURP.

Interstitial laser therapy places fibers directly into the prostate, usually under cystoscopic control. Irritative voiding symptoms may be less in these patients as the urethral mucosa is spared and prostate tissue is resorbed by the body rather than sloughed.

Advantages to laser surgery include minimal blood loss, rare occurrence of transurethral resection syndrome, the ability to treat patients while on anticoagulation therapy, and outpatient surgery. Disadvantages are the lack of tissue for pathologic examination, the longer postoperative catheterization time, the more frequent irritative voiding complaints, and the expense of laser fibers and generators.

Large multicenter, randomized studies with long-term follow-up are needed in comparing laser prostate surgery with TURP and other forms of minimally invasive surgery.

2. Transurethral needle ablation of the prostate (TUNA)—This procedure uses a specially designed urethral catheter that is passed into the urethra. Interstitial radiofrequency needles are then deployed from the tip of the catheter, piercing the mucosa of the prostatic urethra. Radiofrequencies are then used to heat the tissue, resulting in coagulative necrosis. Bladder neck and median lobe enlargement are not well treated by TUNA. Subjective and objective improvement in voiding occurs. In randomized trials comparing TUNA to TURP, similar improvement was seen when comparing life scores, peak urinary flow rates, and postvoid residual urine.

3. Transurethral electrovaporization of the prostate—This technique uses the standard resectoscope. High current densities result in heat vaporization of tissue, creating a cavity in the prostatic urethra. Because the device requires slower sweeping speeds over the prostatic urethra and the depth of vaporization is approximately one-third of a standard loop, this procedure usually takes longer than a standard TURP. Long-term comparative data are needed.

4. Hyperthermia—Microwave hyperthermia is most commonly delivered with a transurethral catheter. Some devices cool the urethral mucosa to decrease the risk of injury. However, if temperatures do not go above 45 °C, cooling is unnecessary. Symptom score and flow rate improvement are obtained, but (as with laser surgery) large randomized studies with long-term follow-up are needed to assess durability and cost-effectiveness.

▶ When to Refer

- Progression to urinary retention.
- Patient dissatisfaction with medical therapy.
- Need for surgical intervention or further evaluation (cystoscopy).

AUA Practice Guidelines Committee. AUA guideline on management of benign prostatic hyperplasia (2003). Chapter 1: Diagnosis and treatment recommendations. J Urol. 2003 Aug;170(2 Pt 1):530–47. [PMID: 12853821]

Bent S et al. Saw palmetto for benign prostatic hyperplasia. N Engl J Med. 2006 Feb 9;354(6):557–66. [PMID: 16467543]

Kaplan SA. Use of alpha-adrenergic inhibitors in treatment of benign prostatic hyperplasia and implications on sexual function. Urology. 2004 Mar;63(3):428–34. [PMID: 15028431]

McConnell JD et al; Medical Therapy of Prostatic Symptoms (MTOPS) Research Group. The long-term effect of doxazosin, finasteride, and combination therapy on the clinical progression of benign prostatic hyperplasia. N Engl J Med. 2003 Dec 18;349(25):2387–98. [PMID: 14681504]

Roehrborn CG. BPH progression: concept and key learning from MTOPS, ALTESS, COMBAT, and ALF-ONCE. BJU Int. 2008 Mar;101(Suppl 3):17–21. [PMID: 18307681]

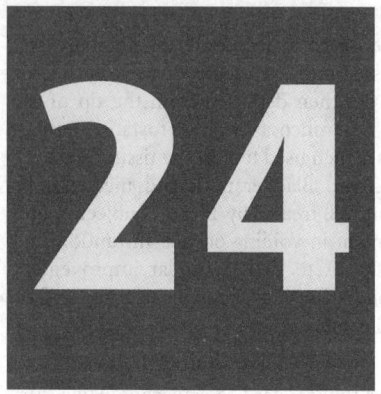

Nervous System Disorders

Michael J. Aminoff, MD, DSc, FRCP

HEADACHE

Headache is such a common complaint and can occur for so many different reasons that its proper evaluation may be difficult. Headaches of acute onset are discussed in Chapter 2. Chronic headaches are commonly due to migraine, tension, or depression, but they may be related to intracranial lesions, head injury, cervical spondylosis, dental or ocular disease, temporomandibular joint dysfunction, sinusitis, hypertension, and a wide variety of general medical disorders. Although underlying structural lesions are not present in most patients presenting with headache, it is nevertheless important to bear this possibility in mind. About one-third of patients with brain tumors, for example, present with a primary complaint of headache.

The intensity, quality, and site of pain—and especially the duration of the headache and the presence of associated neurologic symptoms—may provide clues to the underlying cause. Migraine headaches are often described as pulsating or throbbing; a sense of tightness or pressure is common with tension headache. Sharp lancinating pain suggests a neuritic cause; ocular or periorbital icepick-like pains occur with migraine or cluster headache; and a dull or steady headache is typical of an intracranial mass lesion. Ocular or periocular pain suggests an ophthalmologic disorder; band-like pain is common with tension headaches; and lateralized headache is common with migraine or cluster headache. In patients with sinusitis, there may be tenderness of overlying skin and bone. With intracranial mass lesions, headache may be focal or generalized; in patients with trigeminal or glossopharyngeal neuralgia, the pain is localized to one of the divisions of the trigeminal nerve or to the pharynx and external auditory meatus, respectively.

Inquiry should be made of precipitating factors. Recent sinusitis, dental surgery, head injury, or symptoms suggestive of a systemic viral infection may suggest the underlying cause. Migraine may be exacerbated by emotional stress, fatigue, foods containing nitrite or tyramine, or the menstrual period. Alcohol may precipitate cluster headache. Temporomandibular joint dysfunction causes headache or facial pain that comes on with chewing; trigeminal or glossopharyngeal neuralgia may also be precipitated by chewing, and masticatory claudication sometimes occurs

with giant cell arteritis. Cough-induced headache occurs with structural lesions of the posterior fossa, but in many instances no specific cause can be found.

The timing of symptoms is important. Headaches are typically worse on awakening in patients with an intracranial mass or sleep apnea. Cluster headaches tend to occur at the same time each day or night. Tension headaches are worse with stress or at the end of the day.

The onset of severe headache in a previously well patient is more likely than chronic headache to relate to an intracranial disorder such as subarachnoid hemorrhage or meningitis. The need for further investigation is determined by the initial clinical impression.

A progressive headache disorder, new onset of headache in middle or later life, headaches that disturb sleep or are related to exertion, and headaches that are associated with neurologic symptoms or a focal neurologic deficit usually require cranial MRI or CT scan to exclude an intracranial mass lesion. Signs of meningeal irritation and impairment of consciousness also indicate the need for further investigation (cranial CT scan or MRI and examination of the cerebrospinal fluid) to exclude subarachnoid hemorrhage or meningeal infection. The diagnosis and treatment of primary neurologic disorders associated with headache are considered separately under these disorders.

1. Tension-type Headache

Although this is the most common type of primary headache disorder, many patients do not seek medical attention. Patients frequently complain of pericranial tenderness, poor concentration, and other vague nonspecific symptoms, in addition to constant daily headaches that are often vise-like or tight in quality but are not pulsatile. Headaches may be exacerbated by emotional stress, fatigue, noise, or glare. The headaches are usually generalized, may be most intense about the neck or back of the head, and are not associated with focal neurologic symptoms.

When treatment with simple analgesics is not effective, a trial of antimigrainous agents (see Migraine, below) is worthwhile. Techniques to induce relaxation are also useful and include massage, hot baths, and biofeedback. Exploration of underlying causes of chronic anxiety is often rewarding. Local injection of botulinum toxin type A is sometimes helpful, has few systemic adverse effects, and requires only infrequent administration.

2. Depression Headache

Depression headaches are frequently worse on arising in the morning and may be accompanied by other symptoms of depression. Headaches are occasionally the focus of a somatic delusional system. Antidepressant drugs are often helpful, as may be psychiatric consultation.

3. Migraine

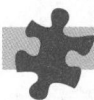

ESSENTIALS OF DIAGNOSIS

▶ Headache, usually pulsatile.

▶ Pain is typically, but not always, unilateral.

▶ Nausea, vomiting, photophobia, and phonophobia are common accompaniments.

▶ May be transient neurologic symptoms (commonly visual) preceding headache of classic migraine.

▶ No preceding aura is common.

▶ General Considerations

The pathophysiology of migraine probably relates to neurovascular dysfunction. Headache results from the dilatation of blood vessels innervated by the trigeminal nerve caused by release of neuropeptides from parasympathetic nerve fibers approximating these vessels. The probable underlying mechanism is activation of the trigeminal nucleus caudalis, nucleus tractus solitarius, and dorsal raphe nucleus. Imaging studies have revealed changes in brainstem regions involved in sensory modulation, suggesting that migraine relates to a failure of normal sensory processing. Before or simultaneous with symptom onset, regional cerebral blood flow is decreased in the cortex corresponding to the clinically affected area; after one to several hours, hyperemia occurs in this same region. Cortical spreading depression of Leão has been implicated.

▶ Clinical Findings

Classic migrainous headache is a lateralized throbbing headache that occurs episodically following its onset in adolescence or early adult life. In many cases, however, the headaches do not conform to this pattern, although their associated features and response to antimigrainous preparations nevertheless suggest that they have a similar basis. In this broader sense, migrainous headaches may be lateralized or generalized, may be dull or throbbing, and are sometimes associated with anorexia, nausea, vomiting, photophobia, phonophobia, osmophobia, cognitive impairment, and blurring of vision. They usually build up gradually and may last for several hours or longer. Focal disturbances of neurologic function may precede or accompany the headaches and have been attributed to constriction of branches of the internal carotid artery. Visual disturbances occur commonly and may consist of field defects; of luminous visual hallucinations such as stars, sparks, unformed light flashes (photopsia), geometric patterns, or zigzags of light; or of some combination of field defects and luminous hallucinations (scintillating scotomas). Other focal disturbances such as aphasia or numbness, paresthesias, clumsiness, dysarthria, disequilibrium, or weakness in a circumscribed distribution may also occur.

In rare instances, the neurologic or somatic disturbance accompanying typical migrainous headaches becomes the sole manifestation of an attack ("migraine equivalent"). Very rarely, the patient may be left with a permanent neurologic deficit following a migrainous attack.

Patients often give a family history of migraine. Attacks may be triggered by emotional or physical stress, lack or excess of sleep, missed meals, specific foods (eg, chocolate), alcoholic beverages, bright lights, loud noise, menstruation, or use of oral contraceptives.

An uncommon variant is **basilar artery migraine**, in which blindness or visual disturbances throughout both visual fields are initially accompanied or followed by dysarthria, disequilibrium, tinnitus, and perioral and distal paresthesias and are sometimes followed by transient loss or impairment of consciousness or by a confusional state. This, in turn, is followed by a throbbing (usually occipital) headache, often with nausea and vomiting.

In **ophthalmoplegic migraine**, lateralized pain—often about the eye—is accompanied by nausea, vomiting, and diplopia due to transient external ophthalmoplegia. The ophthalmoplegia is due to third nerve palsy, sometimes with accompanying sixth nerve involvement, and may outlast the orbital pain by several days or even weeks. The ophthalmic division of the fifth nerve has also been affected in some patients. Ophthalmoplegic migraine is rare; more common causes of a painful ophthalmoplegia are internal carotid artery aneurysms and diabetes.

Familial hemiplegic migraine (FHM) designates the occurrence of migraine with aura including weakness when at least one first- or second-degree relative has a similar disorder. Specific genetic subtypes are recognized: in FHM1, mutations occur in the *CACN1A* gene on chromosome 19, and in FHM2, mutations occur in the *ATP1A2* gene on chromosome 1. In **sporadic hemiplegic migraine**, no other family members are affected.

▶ Treatment

Management of migraine consists of avoidance of any precipitating factors, together with prophylactic or symptomatic pharmacologic treatment if necessary.

A. Symptomatic Therapy

During acute attacks, many patients find it helpful to rest in a quiet, darkened room until symptoms subside. A simple analgesic (eg, aspirin, acetaminophen, ibuprofen, or naproxen) taken right away often provides relief, but treatment with prescription therapy is sometimes necessary. To prevent medication overuse, use of simple analgesics should be limited to 15 days or less per month, and combination analgesics should be limited to less than 10 days per month.

Cafergot, a combination of ergotamine tartrate (1 mg) and caffeine (100 mg), is often particularly helpful; one or two tablets are taken at the onset of headache or warning symptoms, followed by one tablet every 30 minutes, if necessary, up to six tablets per attack and no more than 10 days per month. Because of impaired absorption or vomiting during acute attacks, oral medication sometimes fails to help. Cafergot given rectally as suppositories (one-half to one suppository containing 2 mg of ergotamine) or dihydroergotamine mesylate (0.5–1 mg intravenously or 1–2 mg subcutaneously or intramuscularly) may be useful in such cases. Alternatively, prochlorperazine administered rectally (25 mg suppository) or intravenously (10 mg) may be prescribed. Ergotamine-containing preparations may affect the gravid uterus and thus should be avoided during pregnancy.

Sumatriptan, which has a high affinity for serotonin$_1$ receptors, is a rapidly effective agent for aborting attacks when given subcutaneously by an autoinjection device. It can also be taken in a nasal form, but absorption is limited, and an oral preparation is available. Zolmitriptan, another selective serotonin$_1$ receptor agonist, has high bioavailability after oral administration and is also effective for the acute treatment of migraine. The optimal initial dose is 5 mg, and relief usually occurs within 1 hour. It is also available in a nasal formulation, which has a rapid onset of action. A number of other triptans are available, including rizatriptan, naratriptan, almotriptan, frovatriptan, and eletriptan. Eletriptan (up to 80 mg over 24 hours) is useful for acute therapy and frovatriptan, which has a longer half-life, may be worthwhile for patients with prolonged attacks (up to 7.5 mg over 24 hours). Triptans may cause nausea and vomiting. They should probably be avoided in women who are pregnant, in patients with hemiplegic or basilar migraine, and in patients with risk factors for stroke (such as hypertension, prior stroke or transient ischemic attack, diabetes mellitus, hypercholesterolemia, obesity). Triptans are contraindicated in patients with coronary or peripheral vascular disease. Patients often experience greater benefit when the triptan is combined with naproxen (500 mg).

The neuroleptic droperidol is also helpful in aborting acute attacks. Metoclopramide given intravenously may be helpful and is being studied. Opioid analgesics are needed in rare instances, as when patients are unable to use vasoactive agents or nonsteroidal medications; options include meperidine (100 mg intramuscularly) or butorphanol tartrate by nasal spray (1 mg/spray in one nostril, repeated after 3 or 4 hours if necessary). Intravenous propofol in subanesthetic doses may help in intractable cases.

B. Preventive Therapy

Preventive treatment may be necessary if migrainous headaches occur more frequently than two or three times a month or significant disability is associated with attacks. Some of the more common drugs used for this purpose are listed in Table 24–1. Their mode of action is unclear but may involve alteration of central neurotransmission. Several drugs may have to be tried in turn before the headaches are brought under control. Once a drug has been found to help, it should be continued for several months. If the patient remains headache-free, the dose can then be tapered and the drug eventually withdrawn. Botulinum toxin type A may be effective for migraine prevention in some patients; it has few systemic side effects and need only be given at intervals of several months. However, no statistically significant between-group differences were found in frequency of migraine episodes per 30-day period in a randomized, double-blind, placebo-controlled exploratory study. Although acupuncture has been widely used in the prophylaxis of migraine, a randomized controlled trial failed to show any difference between it and sham acupuncture.

Table 24–1. Prophylactic treatment of migraine.

Drug	Usual Adult Daily Dose	Common Side Effects
Propranolol[1]	80–240 mg	Fatigue, lassitude, depression, insomnia, nausea, vomiting, constipation.
Amitriptyline	10–150 mg	Sedation, dry mouth, constipation, weight gain, blurred vision, edema, hypotension, urinary retention.
Imipramine	10–150 mg	Similar to those of amitriptyline (above).
Sertraline	50–200 mg	Anxiety, insomnia, sweating, tremor, gastrointestinal disturbances.
Fluoxetine	20–60 mg	Similar to those of sertraline (above).
Cyproheptadine	12–20 mg	Sedation, dry mouth, epigastric discomfort, gastrointestinal disturbances.
Clonidine	0.2–0.6 mg	Dry mouth, drowsiness, sedation, headache, constipation.
Verapamil[2]	80–160 mg	Headache, hypotension, flushing, edema, constipation. May aggravate atrioventricular nodal heart block and congestive heart failure.

[1]Other β-blockers (eg, timolol and metoprolol) have also been used.
[2]Other calcium channel antagonists (eg, nimodipine, nicardipine, and diltiazem) have also been used.
Botulinum toxin type A injected locally into the scalp is effective for prophylaxis in some patients. The antiseizure agents valproic acid (500–1500 mg), gabapentin (900–2400 mg), and topiramate (50–200 mg) are also effective and are detailed in Table 24–3. Valproic acid should be avoided during pregnancy.

Calcium channel antagonist drugs may decrease the frequency of attacks after an interval of several weeks, but the severity and duration of attacks are not influenced. They should not be used with β-blockers. The angiotensin-converting enzyme receptor blocker, candesartan, may also be effective and is undergoing evaluation.

4. Cluster Headache

Cluster headache affects predominantly middle-aged men. The pathophysiology is unclear but may relate to activation of cells in the ipsilateral hypothalamus, triggering the trigeminal autonomic vascular system. There is often no family history of headache or migraine. Episodes of severe unilateral periorbital pain occur daily for several weeks and are often accompanied by one or more of the following: ipsilateral nasal congestion, rhinorrhea, lacrimation, redness of the eye, and Horner syndrome. During attacks, patients are often restless and agitated. Episodes often occur at night, awaken the patient, and last for between 15 minutes and 3 hours. Spontaneous remission then occurs, and the patient remains well for weeks or months before another bout of closely spaced attacks occurs. Bouts may last for 4 to 8 weeks and may occur up to several times per year. During a bout, many patients report that alcohol triggers an attack; others report that stress, glare, or ingestion of specific foods occasionally precipitates attacks. In occasional patients, typical attacks of pain and associated symptoms recur at intervals without remission. This variant has been referred to as chronic cluster headache.

Examination reveals no abnormality apart from Horner syndrome that either occurs transiently during an attack or, in longstanding cases, remains as a residual deficit between attacks.

Treatment of an individual attack with oral drugs is generally unsatisfactory, but subcutaneous (6 mg dose) or intranasal (20-mg/spray) sumatriptan or inhalation of 100% oxygen (12–15 L/min for 15 minutes via a non-rebreather mask) may be effective. Zolmitriptan (5- and 10-mg nasal spray) is also effective. Dihydroergotamine (0.5–1 mg intramuscularly or intravenously) is sometimes used. Viscous lidocaine (1 mg of 4–6% solution) intranasally is sometimes effective.

Various prophylactic agents that have been found to be effective in individual patients are cyproheptadine, lithium carbonate (monitored by plasma lithium determination), verapamil (240–960 mg daily), topiramate (100–400 mg daily), valproate (750–1500 mg daily), and methysergide (2–12 mg daily). As there is often a delay before these medications are effective, transitional therapy is often used. Ergotamine tartrate is effective and can be given as rectal suppositories (0.5–1 mg at night or twice daily), by mouth (2 mg daily), or by subcutaneous injection (0.25 mg three times daily for 5 days per week). Other options include prednisone (60 mg daily for 5 days followed by gradual withdrawal), dihydroergotamine (9.25 mg intravenously over several days or 0.5 mg intramuscularly twice daily), or greater occipital nerve injection with lidocaine and corticosteroid.

5. Posttraumatic Headache

A variety of nonspecific symptoms may follow closed head injury, regardless of whether consciousness is lost. Headache is often a conspicuous feature.

The headache itself usually appears within a day or so following injury, may worsen over the ensuing weeks, and then gradually subsides. It is usually a constant dull ache, with superimposed throbbing that may be localized, lateralized, or generalized. It is sometimes accompanied by nausea, vomiting, or scintillating scotomas. Headaches occurring more than 1–2 weeks after the inciting event are probably not directly attributable to the head injury.

Disequilibrium, sometimes with a rotatory component, may also occur and is often enhanced by postural change or head movement. Impaired memory, poor concentration, emotional instability, and increased irritability are other common complaints and occasionally are the sole manifestations of the syndrome. The duration of symptoms relates in part to the severity of the original injury, but even trivial injuries are sometimes followed by symptoms that persist for months.

Special investigations are usually not helpful. The electroencephalogram may show minor nonspecific changes, while the electronystagmogram sometimes suggests either peripheral or central vestibulopathy. CT scans or MRI of the head usually show no abnormal findings.

Treatment is difficult, but optimistic encouragement and graduated rehabilitation, depending on the occupational circumstances, are advised as symptoms often resolve spontaneously within several months. Headaches often respond to simple analgesics, but severe headaches may necessitate treatment with amitriptyline, antiseizure medication, propranolol, or ergot derivatives.

6. Cough Headache

Severe head pain may be produced by coughing (and by straining, sneezing, and laughing) but, fortunately, usually lasts for only a few minutes or less. The pathophysiologic basis of the complaint is not known, and often there is no underlying structural lesion. However, intracranial lesions, usually in the posterior fossa (eg, Arnold-Chiari malformation), are present in about 10% of cases, and brain tumors or other space-occupying lesions may certainly present in this way. Accordingly, CT scanning or MRI should be undertaken in all patients and repeated annually for several years, since a small structural lesion may not show up initially.

The disorder is usually self-limited, although it may persist for several years. For unknown reasons, symptoms sometimes clear completely after lumbar puncture. Indomethacin (75–150 mg daily) may provide relief.

7. Headache Due to Giant Cell (Temporal or Cranial) Arteritis

The superficial temporal, vertebral, ophthalmic, and posterior ciliary arteries are often the most severely affected pathologically. Most patients are elderly. The major symptom is headache, often associated with or preceded by myalgia, malaise, anorexia, weight loss, and other nonspecific complaints. Loss of vision is the most feared manifestation and occurs quite commonly. Clinical examination often reveals tenderness of the scalp and over the temporal arteries. Further details, including approaches to treatment, are given in Chapter 20.

8. Headache Due to Intracranial Mass Lesions

Intracranial mass lesions of all types may cause headache owing to displacement of vascular structures and other pain-sensitive tissues. Posterior fossa tumors often cause occipital pain, and supratentorial lesions lead to bifrontal headache, but such findings are too inconsistent to be of value in attempts at localizing a pathologic process. The headaches are nonspecific in character and may vary in severity from mild to severe. They may be worsened by exertion or postural change and may be associated with nausea and vomiting, but this is true of migraine also. Headaches are also a feature of pseudotumor cerebri (see below). Signs of focal or diffuse cerebral dysfunction or of increased intracranial pressure will indicate the need for further investigation. Similarly, a progressive headache disorder or the new onset of headaches in middle or later life merits investigation if no cause is apparent.

9. Medication Overuse (Analgesic Rebound) Headache

In approximately half of all patients with chronic daily headaches, medication overuse is responsible. They present with chronic pain or with complaints of severe headache unresponsive to medication. Diagnosis is important as patients rarely respond to treatment until the offending medications are discontinued. Withdrawal of analgesics leads to relief of headache within several months.

10. Headache Due to Other Neurologic Causes

Cerebrovascular disease may be associated with headache, but the mechanism is unclear. Headache may occur with internal carotid artery occlusion or carotid dissection and after carotid endarterectomy. Diagnosis is facilitated by the clinical accompaniments and the circumstances in which the headache developed.

Acute severe headache accompanies subarachnoid hemorrhage and meningeal infections; accompanying signs of meningeal irritation and impairment of consciousness indicate the need for further investigations.

Dull or throbbing headache is a frequent sequela of lumbar puncture and may last for several days. It is aggravated by the erect posture and alleviated by recumbency. The exact mechanism is unclear, but it is commonly attributed to leakage of cerebrospinal fluid through the dural puncture site. Its incidence may be reduced if a small-diameter needle is used for the spinal tap, and perhaps also if the patient lies prone or supine after the procedure.

▶ When to Refer

- Acute onset of "worst headache in my life."

- Increasing headache unresponsive to simple measures.
- History of trauma, hypertension, fever, visual changes.
- Presence of neurologic signs or of scalp tenderness.

▶ When to Admit

- Suspected subarachnoid hemorrhage or structural intracranial lesion.
- Depends on underlying cause.

Aurora SK et al. Botulinum toxin type A prophylactic treatment of episodic migraine: a randomized, double-blind, placebo-controlled exploratory study. Headache. 2007 Apr;47(4):486–99. [PMID: 17445098]

Brandes JL et al. Sumatriptan-naproxen for acute treatment of migraine: a randomized trial. JAMA. 2007 Apr 4;297(13):1443–54. [PMID: 17405970]

Capobianco DJ et al. Diagnosis and treatment of cluster headache. Semin Neurol. 2006 Apr;26(2):242–59. [PMID: 16628535]

Goadsby PJ. Recent advances in understanding migraine mechanisms, molecules and therapeutics. Trends Mol Med. 2007 Jan;13(1):39–44. [PMID: 17141570]

Mett A et al. Acute migraine therapy: recent evidence from randomized comparative trials. Curr Opin Neurol. 2008 Jun;21(3):331–7. [PMID: 18451718]

Parmet S et al. JAMA patient page. Headaches. JAMA. 2006 May 17;295(19):2320. [PMID: 16705112]

Rapoport AM. Acute treatment of headache. J Headache Pain. 2006 Oct;7(5):355–9. [PMID: 17058043]

Rapoport AM et al. Zolmitriptan nasal spray in the acute treatment of cluster headache: a double-blind study. Neurology. 2007 Aug 28;69(9):821–6. [PMID: 17724283]

Silberstein SD et al. Efficacy and safety of topiramate for the treatment of chronic migraine: a randomized, double-blind, placebo-controlled trial. Headache. 2007 Feb;47(2):170–80. [PMID: 17300356]

FACIAL PAIN

1. Trigeminal Neuralgia

 ESSENTIALS OF DIAGNOSIS

- ▶ Brief episodes of stabbing facial pain.
- ▶ Pain is in the territory of the second and third division of the trigeminal nerve.
- ▶ Pain exacerbated by touch.

▶ General Considerations

Trigeminal neuralgia ("tic douloureux") is most common in middle and later life. It affects women more frequently than men.

▶ Clinical Findings

Momentary episodes of sudden lancinating facial pain occur and commonly arise near one side of the mouth and shoot toward the ear, eye, or nostril on that side. The pain may be triggered or precipitated by such factors as touch, movement, drafts, and eating. Indeed, in order to lessen the likelihood of triggering further attacks, many patients

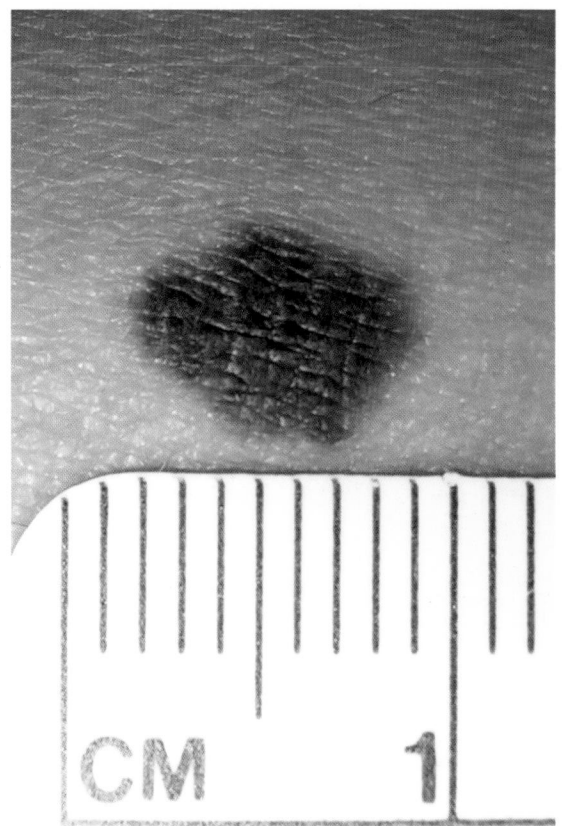

▲ **Plate 1.** Benign, flat and macular compound nevus on the arm. (Courtesy of Richard P. Usatine, MD; used, with permission, from Usatine RP, Smith MA, Mayeaux EJ Jr, Chumley H, Tysinger J. *The Color Atlas of Family Medicine.* McGraw-Hill, 2009.)

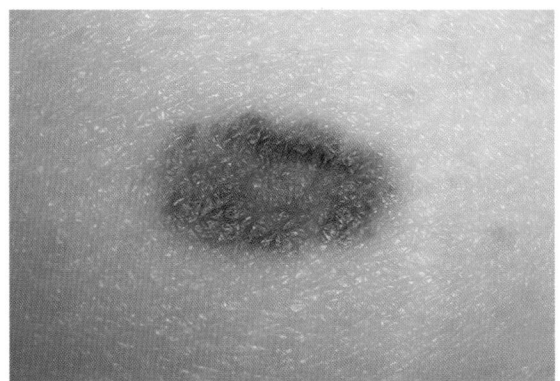

▲ **Plate 2.** Atypical (dysplastic) nevus on the chest. (Courtesy of Richard P. Usatine, MD; used, with permission, from Usatine RP, Smith MA, Mayeaux EJ Jr, Chumley H, Tysinger J. *The Color Atlas of Family Medicine.* McGraw-Hill, 2009.)

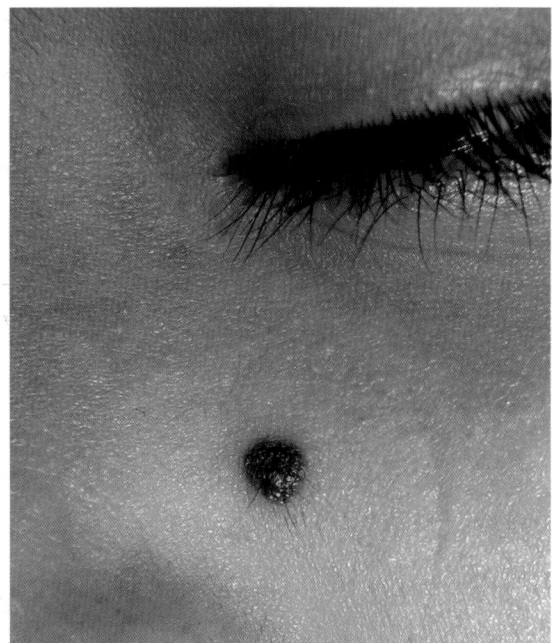

▲ **Plate 3.** Blue nevus on the left cheek, with some resemblance to a melanoma. (Courtesy of Richard P. Usatine, MD; used, with permission, from Usatine RP, Smith MA, Mayeaux EJ Jr, Chumley H, Tysinger J. *The Color Atlas of Family Medicine.* McGraw-Hill, 2009.)

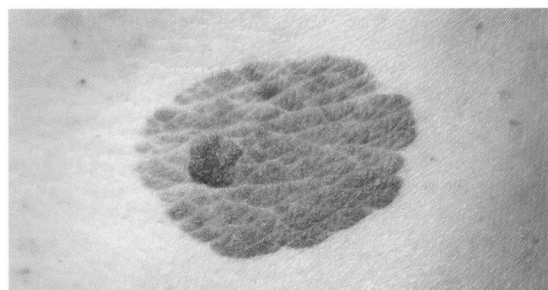

▲ **Plate 4.** Seborrheic keratosis with "stuck on appearance" but irregular borders and color variation suspicious for possible melanoma. (Courtesy of Richard P. Usatine, MD; used, with permission, from Usatine RP, Smith MA, Mayeaux EJ Jr, Chumley H, Tysinger J. *The Color Atlas of Family Medicine.* McGraw-Hill, 2009.)

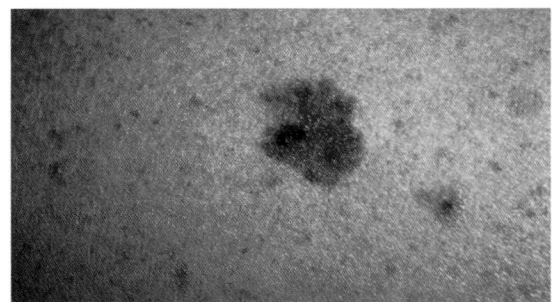

▲ **Plate 5.** Malignant melanoma, with multiple colors and classic "ABCDE" features. (Used, with permission, from Berger TG, Dept Dermatology, UCSF.)

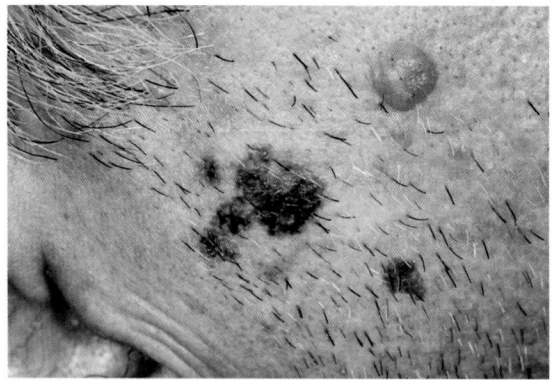

▲ Plate 6. Melanoma resembling a seborrheic keratosis on the lateral face of a man. (Courtesy of Richard P. Usatine, MD; used, with permission, from Usatine RP, Smith MA, Mayeaux EJ Jr, Chumley H, Tysinger J. *The Color Atlas of Family Medicine*. McGraw-Hill, 2009.)

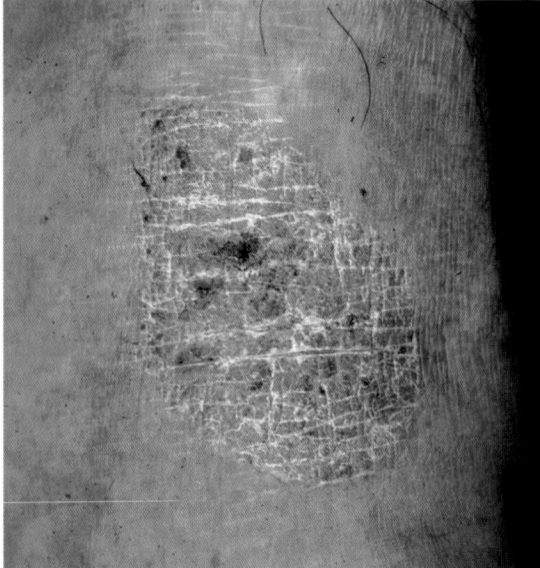

▲ Plate 7. Lichen simplex chronicus. (Used, with permission, from Berger TG, Dept Dermatology, UCSF.)

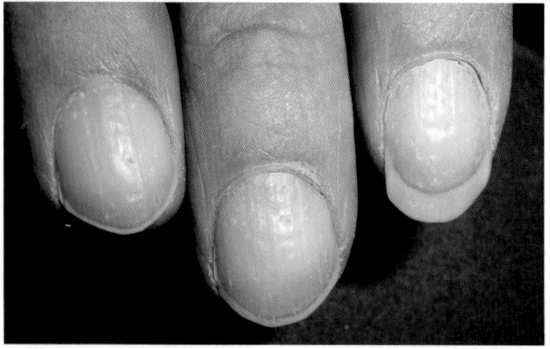

▲ Plate 8. Nail pitting due to psoriasis. (Courtesy of Richard P. Usatine, MD; used, with permission, from Usatine RP, Smith MA, Mayeaux EJ Jr, Chumley H, Tysinger J. *The Color Atlas of Family Medicine*. McGraw-Hill, 2009.)

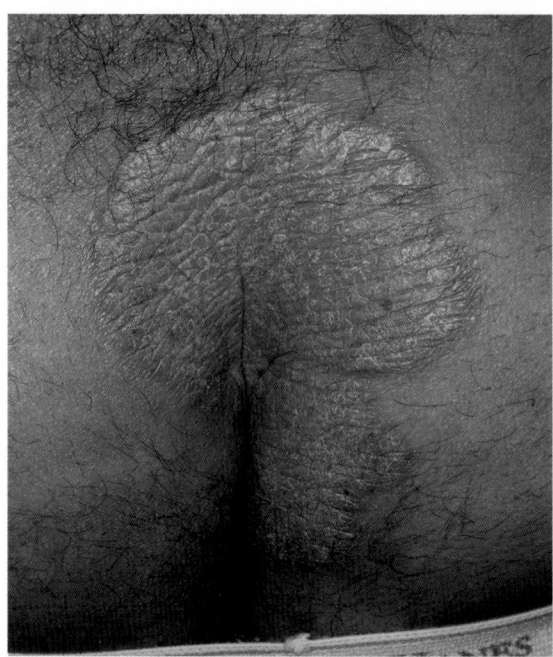

▲ Plate 9. Plaque psoriasis in the sacral region and intergluteal fold. (Courtesy of Richard P. Usatine, MD; used, with permission, from Usatine RP, Smith MA, Mayeaux EJ Jr, Chumley H, Tysinger J. *The Color Atlas of Family Medicine*. McGraw-Hill, 2009.)

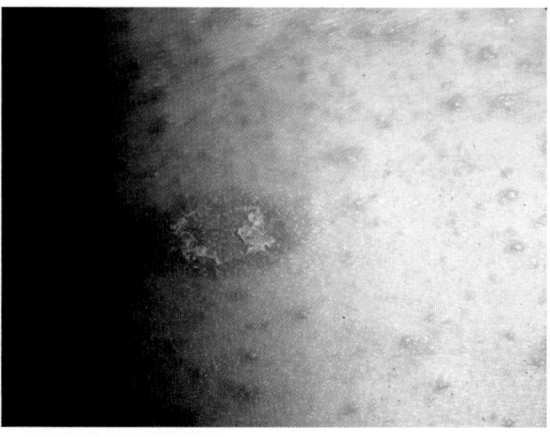

▲ Plate 10. Pityriasis rosea. (Used, with permission, from Berger TG, Dept Dermatology, UCSF.)

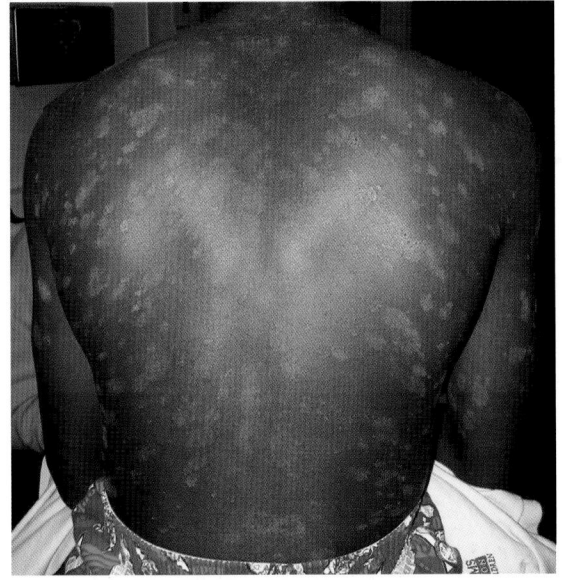

▲ Plate 11. Pityriasis rosea with scaling lesions following skin lines and resembling a Christmas tree. (Courtesy of EJ Mayeaux, MD; used, with permission, from Usatine RP, Smith MA, Mayeaux EJ Jr, Chumley H, Tysinger J. *The Color Atlas of Family Medicine.* McGraw-Hill, 2009.)

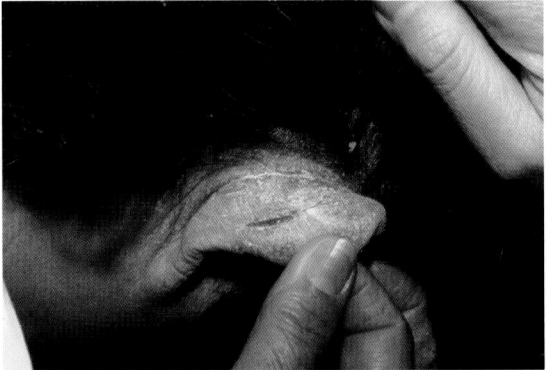

▲ Plate 12. Seborrheic dermatitis. (Used, with permission, from Berger TG, Dept Dermatology, UCSF.)

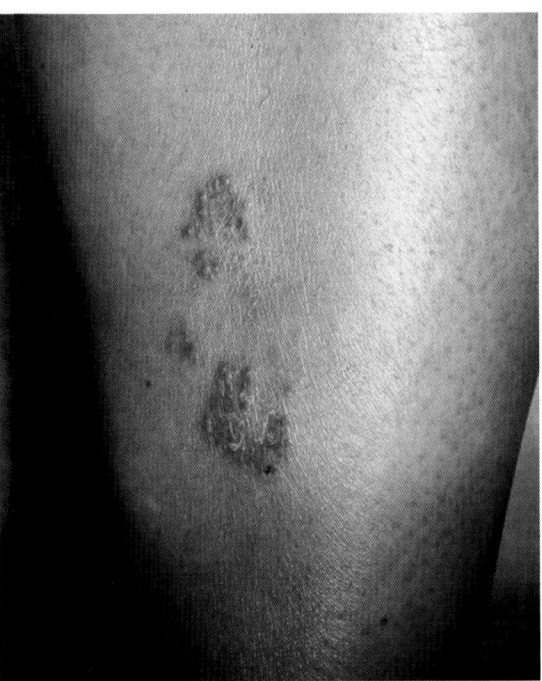

▲ Plate 14. Tinea corporis. (Used, with permission, from Berger TG, Dept Dermatology, UCSF.)

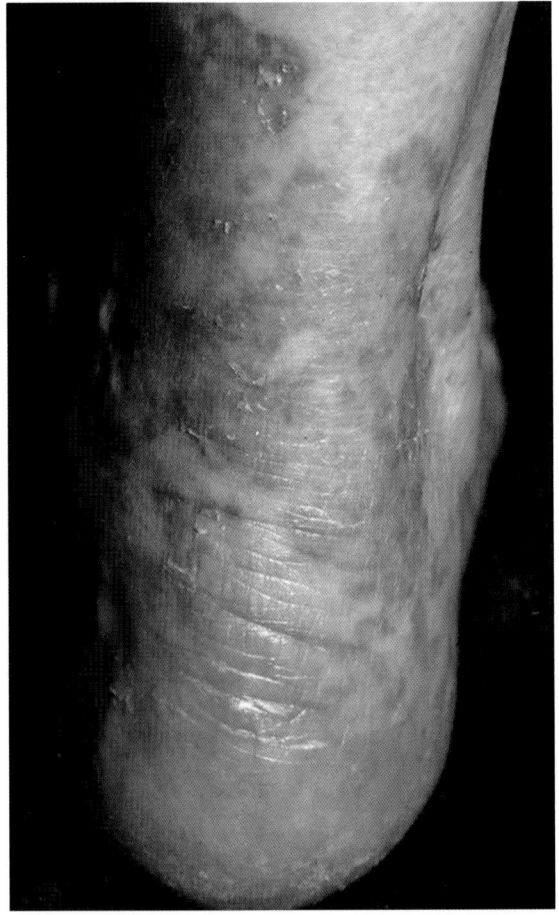

▲ Plate 13. Tinea pedis and corporis. (Used, with permission, from Berger TG, Dept Dermatology, UCSF.)

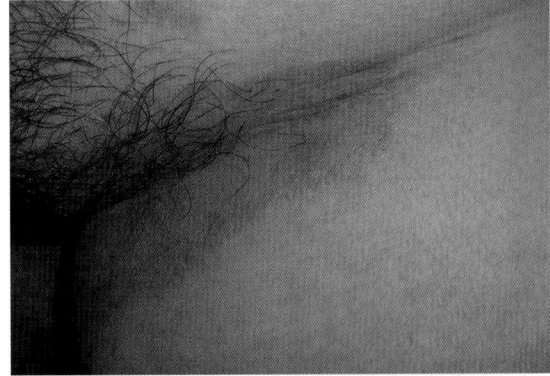

▲ Plate 15. Tinea cruris. (Courtesy of Richard P. Usatine, MD; used, with permission, from Usatine RP, Smith MA, Mayeaux EJ Jr, Chumley H, Tysinger J. *The Color Atlas of Family Medicine.* McGraw-Hill, 2009.)

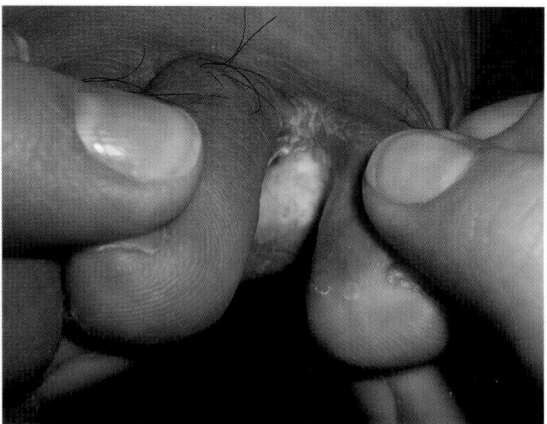

▲ Plate 16. Tinea pedis in the interdigital space between fourth and fifth digits. (Courtesy of Richard P. Usatine, MD; used, with permission, from Usatine RP, Smith MA, Mayeaux EJ Jr, Chumley H, Tysinger J. *The Color Atlas of Family Medicine*. McGraw-Hill, 2009.)

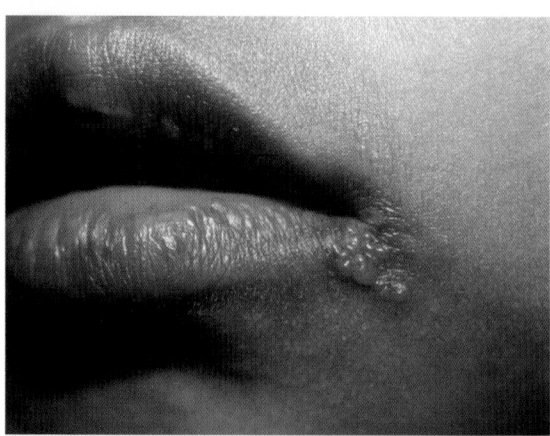

▲ Plate 19. Herpes simplex type 1 vesicles at the vermillion border of the lip. (Courtesy of Richard P. Usatine, MD; used, with permission, from Usatine RP, Smith MA, Mayeaux EJ Jr, Chumley H, Tysinger J. *The Color Atlas of Family Medicine*. McGraw-Hill, 2009.)

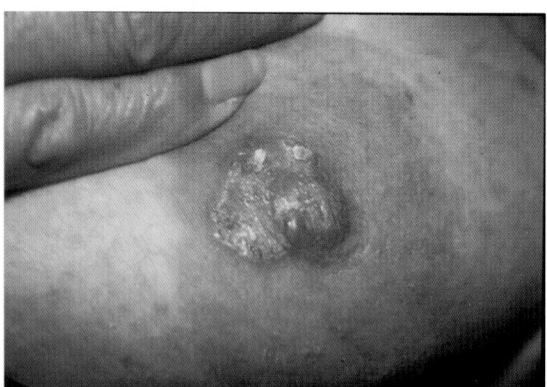

▲ Plate 17. Paget's disease of the breast surrounding the nipple. (Courtesy of the University of Texas Health Sciences Center, Division of Dermatology; used, with permission, from Usatine RP, Smith MA, Mayeaux EJ Jr, Chumley H, Tysinger J. *The Color Atlas of Family Medicine*. McGraw-Hill, 2009.)

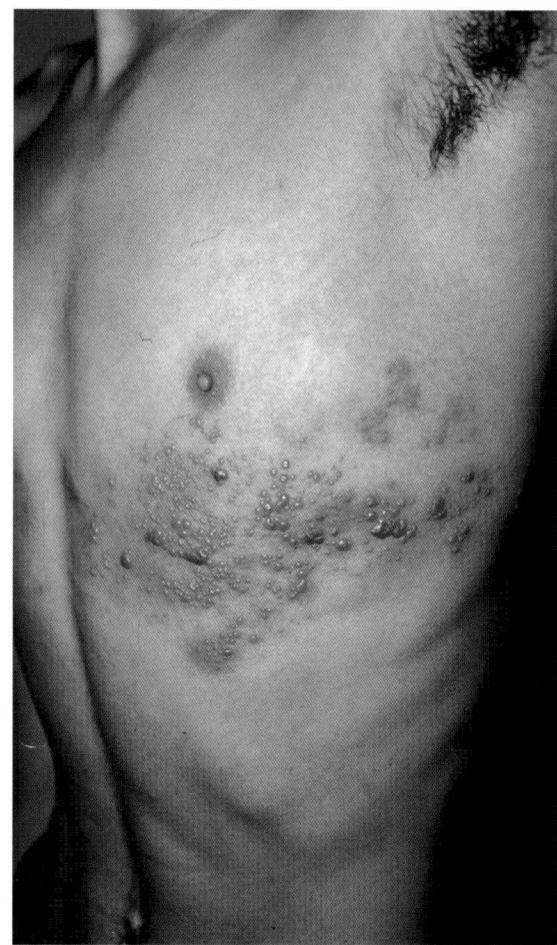

▲ Plate 20. Herpes zoster. (Used, with permission, from Berger TG, Dept Dermatology, UCSF.)

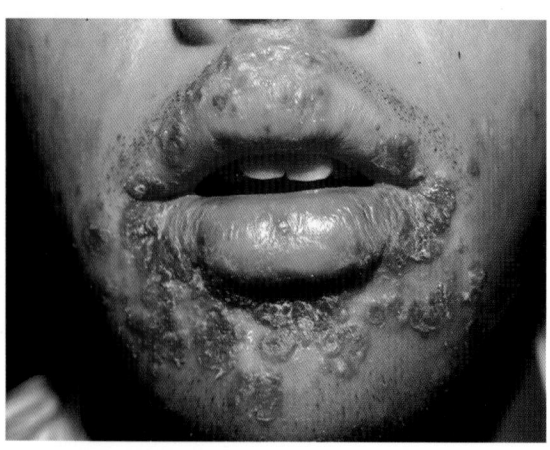

▲ Plate 18. Herpes simplex. (Used, with permission, from Berger TG, Dept Dermatology, UCSF.)

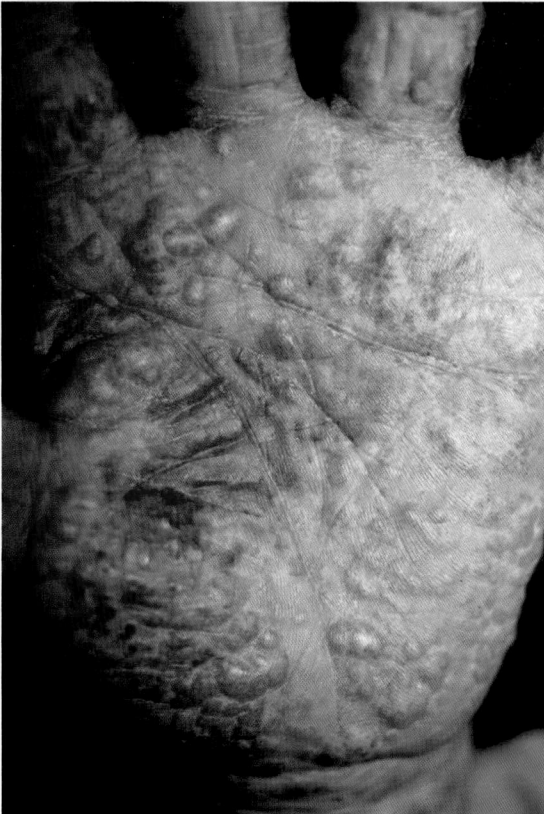

▲ Plate 21. Pompholyx (acute vesiculobullous hand eczema). (Used, with permission, from Berger TG, Dept Dermatology, UCSF.)

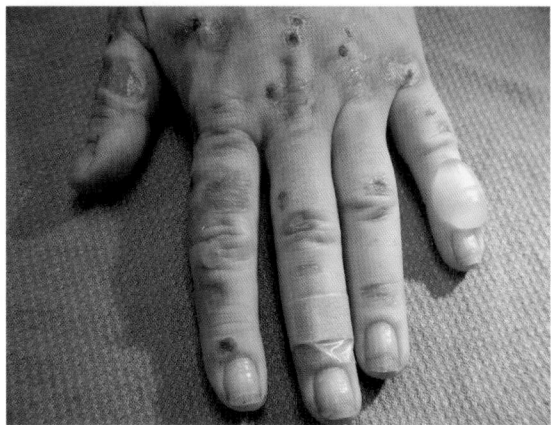

▲ Plate 22. Porphyria cutanea tarda. (Courtesy of Lewis Rose, MD; used, with permission, from Usatine RP, Smith MA, Mayeaux EJ Jr, Chumley H, Tysinger J. *The Color Atlas of Family Medicine.* McGraw-Hill, 2009.)

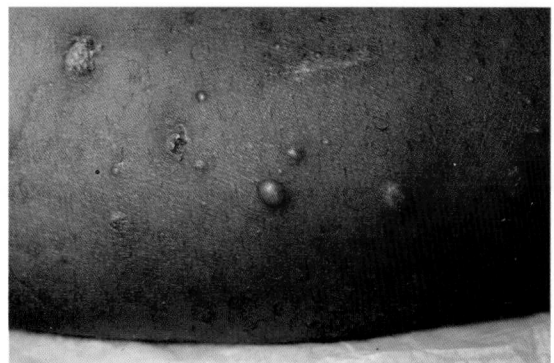

▲ Plate 23. Bullous impetigo. (Used, with permission, from Berger TG, Dept Dermatology, UCSF.)

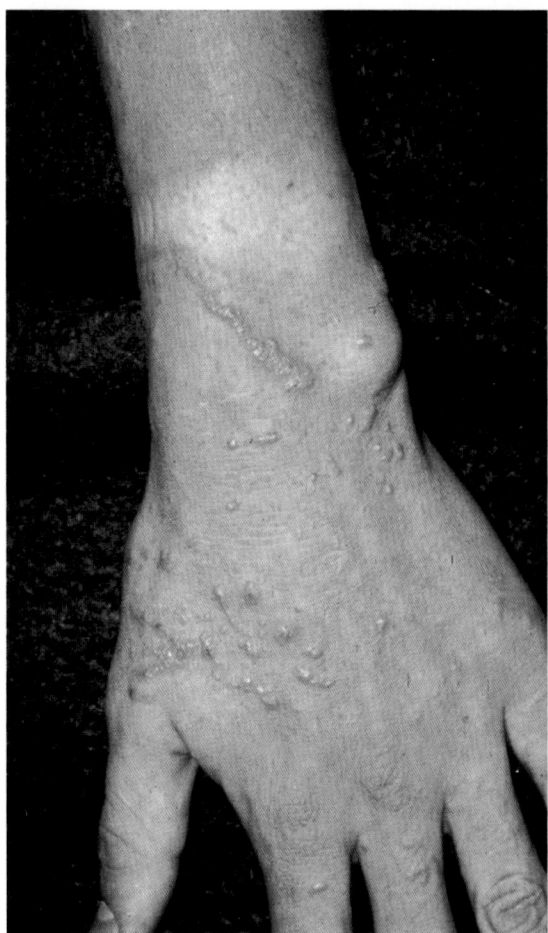

▲ Plate 24. Contact dermatitis with linear pattern due to poison ivy. (Used, with permission, from Berger TG, Dept Dermatology, UCSF.)

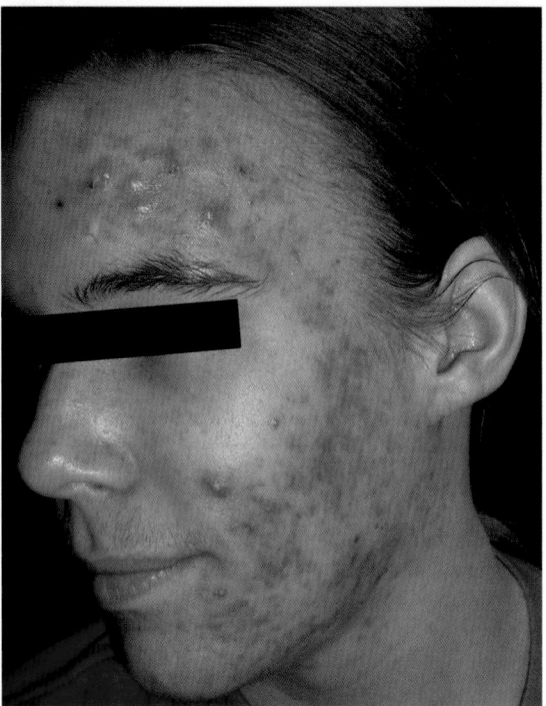

▲ **Plate 25.** Acne vulgaris, severe nodular cystic form with scarring. (Courtesy of Richard P. Usatine, MD; used, with permission, from Usatine RP, Smith MA, Mayeaux EJ Jr, Chumley H, Tysinger J. *The Color Atlas of Family Medicine.* McGraw-Hill, 2009.)

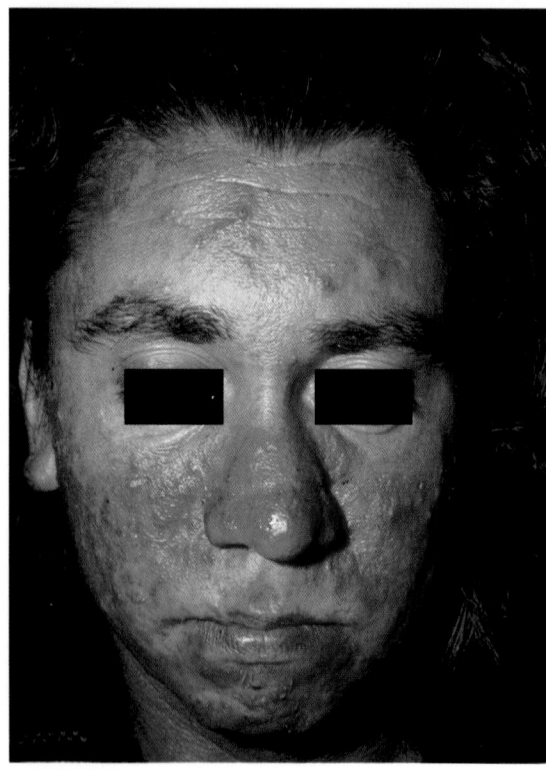

▲ **Plate 26.** Rosacea. (Used, with permission, from Berger TG, Dept Dermatology, UCSF.)

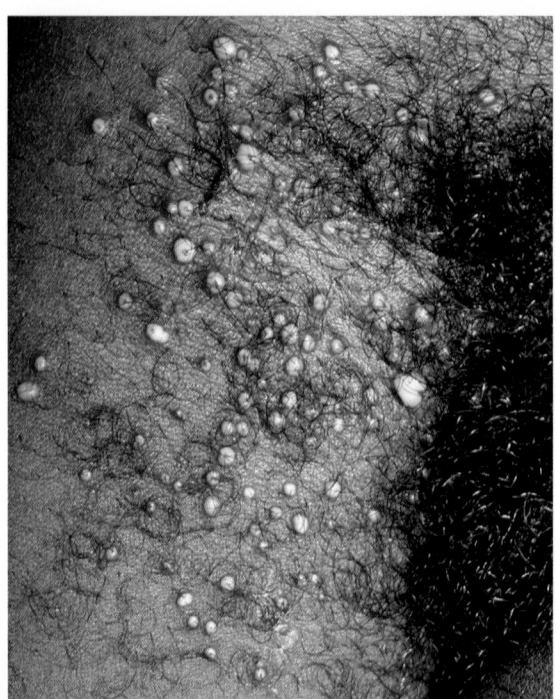

▲ **Plate 27.** Bacterial folliculitis. (Used, with permission, from Berger TG, Dept Dermatology, UCSF.)

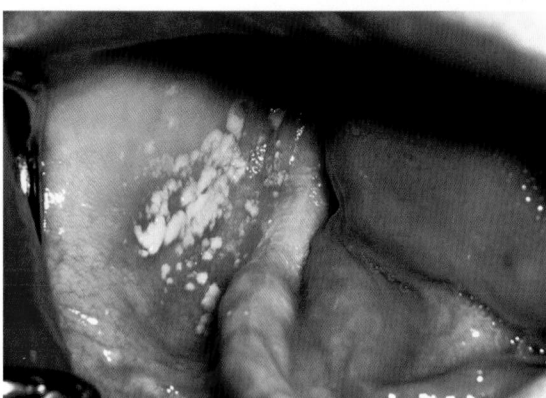

▲ **Plate 28.** Oral mucosal candidiasis. (Courtesy of Sol Silverman, Jr., DDS, Public Health Image Library, CDC.)

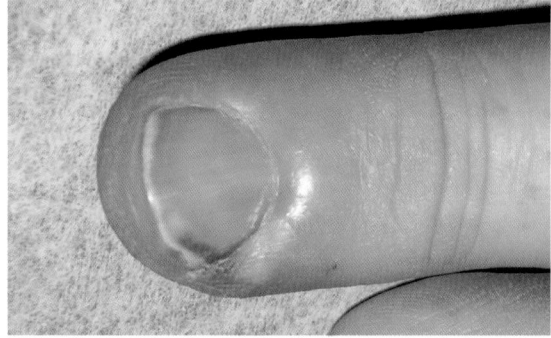

▲ **Plate 29.** Acute paronychia. (Courtesy of EJ Mayeaux, MD; used, with permission, from Usatine RP, Smith MA, Mayeaux EJ Jr, Chumley H, Tysinger J. *The Color Atlas of Family Medicine.* McGraw-Hill, 2009.)

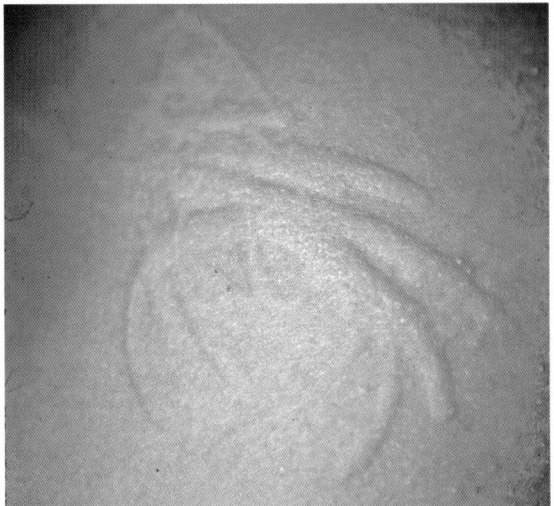

▲ Plate 30. Urticaria. (Used, with permission, from Berger TG, Dept Dermatology, UCSF.)

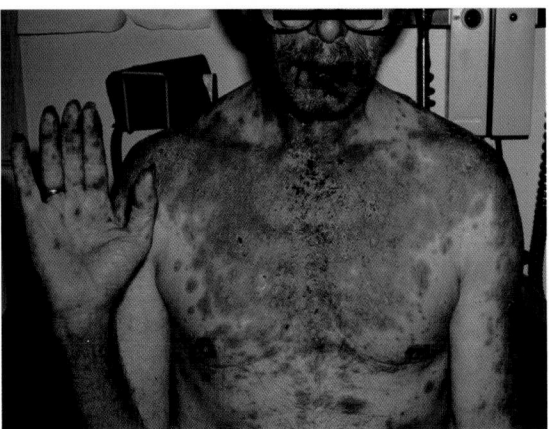

▲ Plate 31. Erythema multiforme. (Used, with permission, from Berger TG, Dept Dermatology, UCSF.)

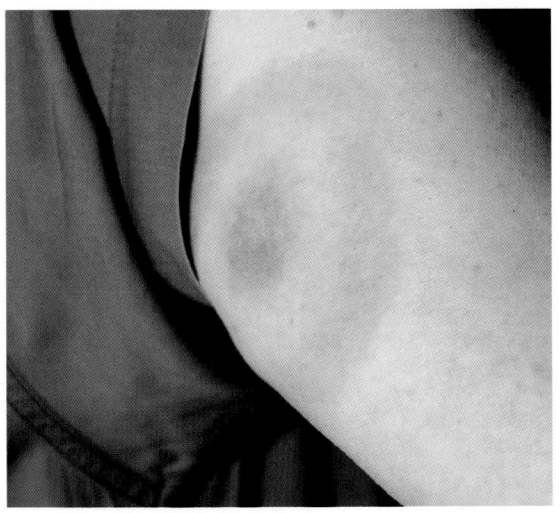

▲ Plate 32. Erythema migrans due to *Borrelia burgdorferi* (Lyme disease). (Courtesy of James Gathany, Public Health Image Library, CDC.)

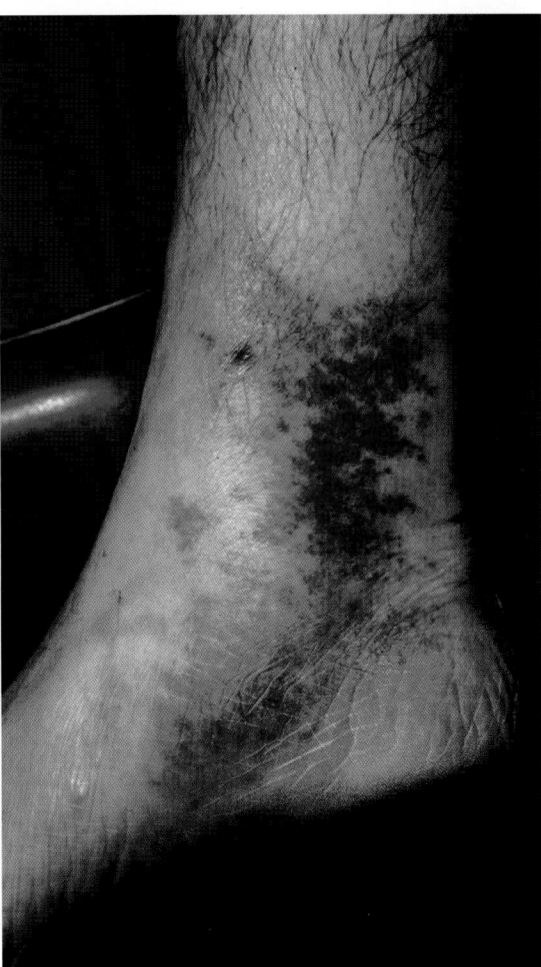

▲ Plate 33. Erysipelas (cellulitis). (Used, with permission, from Berger TG, Dept Dermatology, UCSF.)

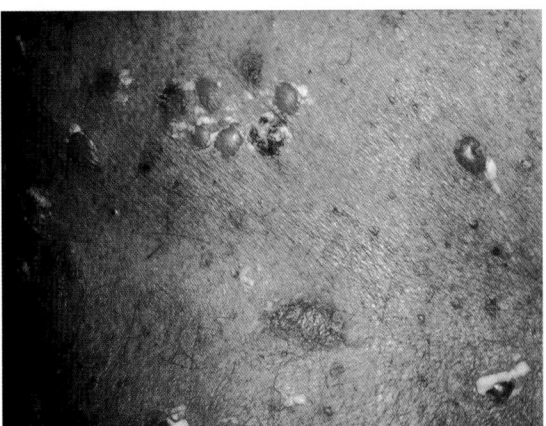

▲ Plate 34. Pemphigus. (Used, with permission, from Berger TG, Dept Dermatology, UCSF.)

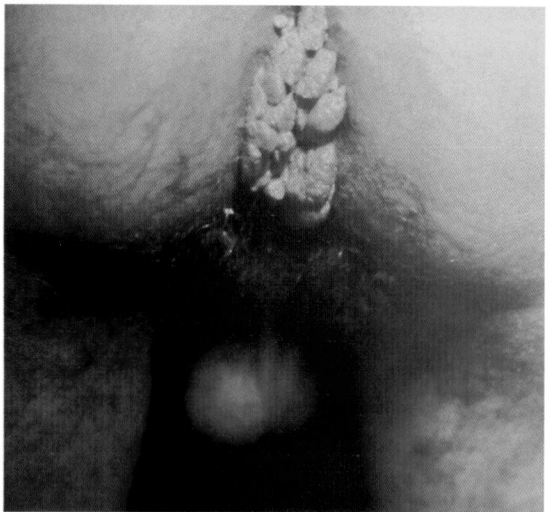

▲ **Plate 35.** Condylomata acuminata, or genital warts, of the anal region due to human papillomavirus. (Public Health Image Library, CDC.)

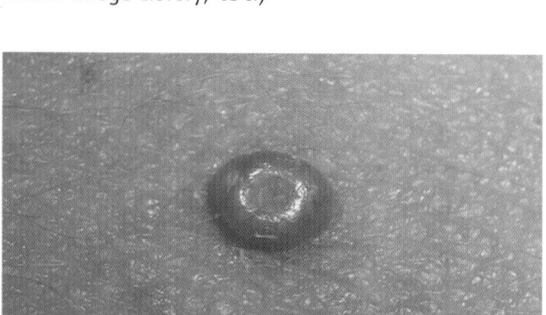

▲ **Plate 36.** Molluscum contagiosum legion on the back. (Courtesy of Richard P. Usatine, MD; used, with permission, from Usatine RP, Smith MA, Mayeaux EJ Jr, Chumley H, Tysinger J. *The Color Atlas of Family Medicine.* McGraw-Hill, 2009.)

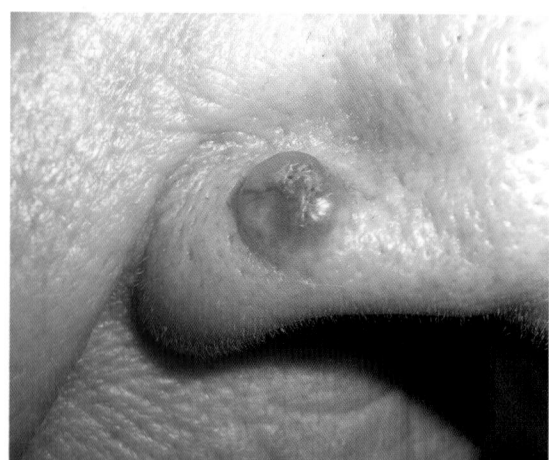

▲ **Plate 37.** Nodular basal cell carcinoma of the nose. (Courtesy of Richard P. Usatine, MD; used, with permission, from Usatine RP, Smith MA, Mayeaux EJ Jr, Chumley H, Tysinger J. *The Color Atlas of Family Medicine.* McGraw-Hill, 2009.)

▲ **Plate 38.** Basal cell carcinoma on the forehead with irregular distribution of the telangiectasias and lack of typical doughnut shape. (Courtesy of Richard P. Usatine, MD; used, with permission, from Usatine RP, Smith MA, Mayeaux EJ Jr, Chumley H, Tysinger J. *The Color Atlas of Family Medicine.* McGraw-Hill, 2009.)

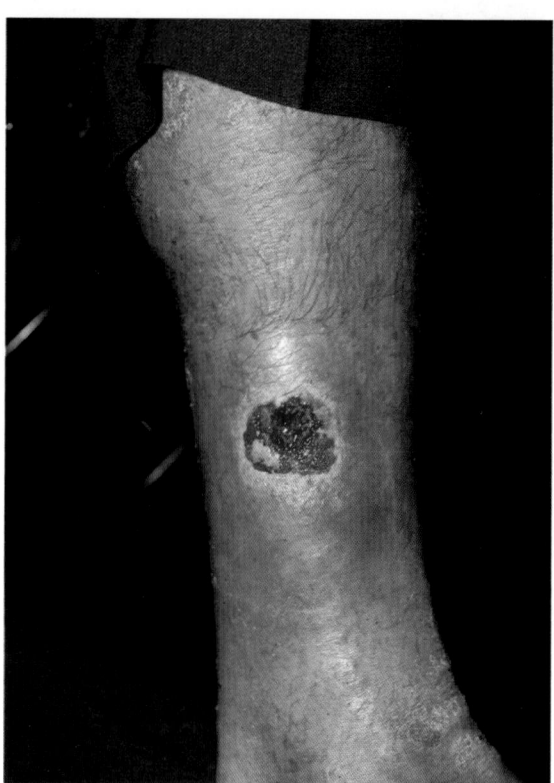

▲ **Plate 39.** Squamous cell carcinoma. (Used, with permission, from Berger TG, Dept Dermatology, UCSF.)

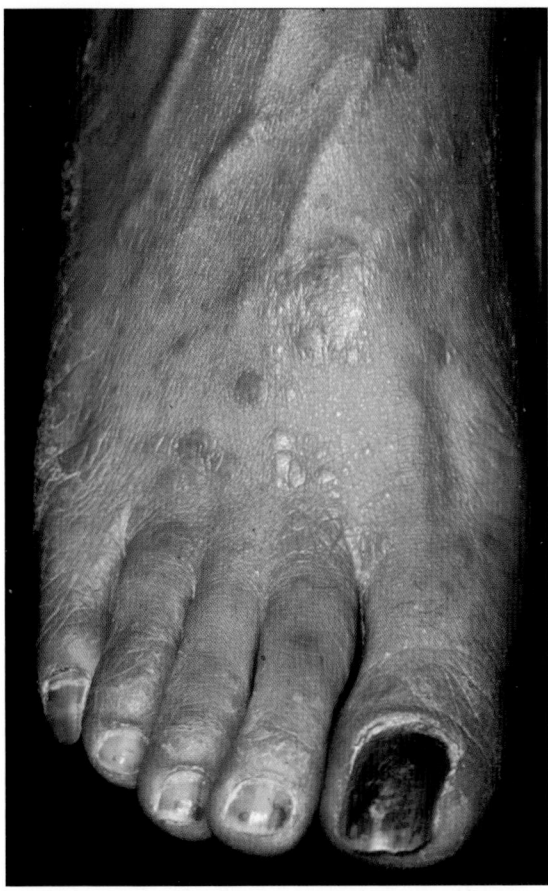

▲ Plate 40. Lichen planus. (Used, with permission, from Berger TG, Dept Dermatology, UCSF.)

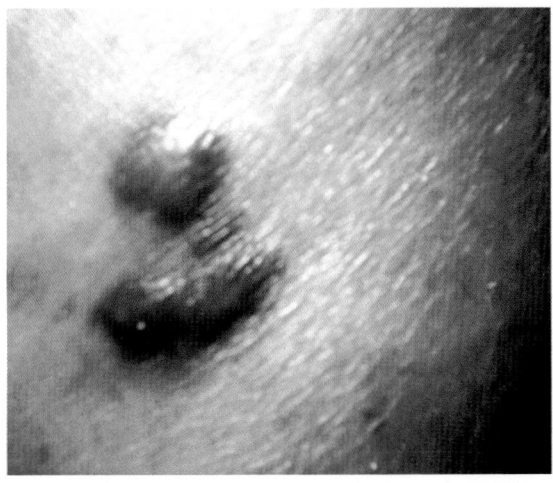

▲ Plate 41. Cutaneous nodule of Kaposi sarcoma in AIDS. (Courtesy of Dr. Steve Kraus, Public Health Image Library, CDC.)

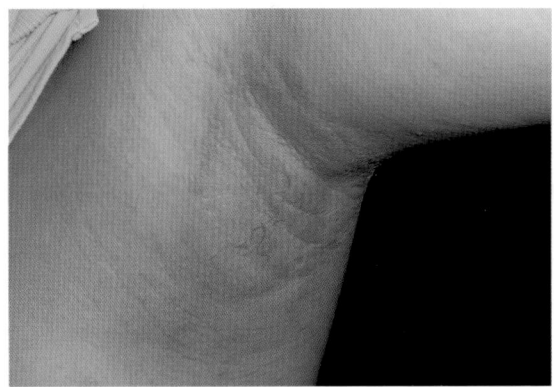

▲ Plate 42. Erythrasma of the axilla. (Courtesy of Richard P. Usatine, MD; used, with permission, from Usatine RP, Smith MA, Mayeaux EJ Jr, Chumley H, Tysinger J. *The Color Atlas of Family Medicine*. McGraw-Hill, 2009.)

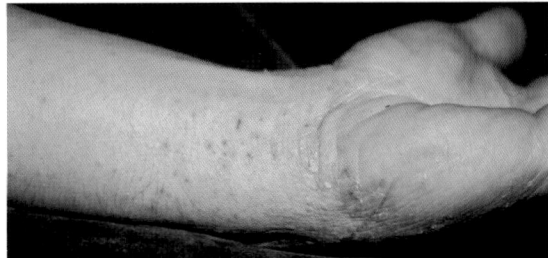

▲ Plate 43. Scabies. (Used, with permission, from Berger TG, Dept Dermatology, UCSF.)

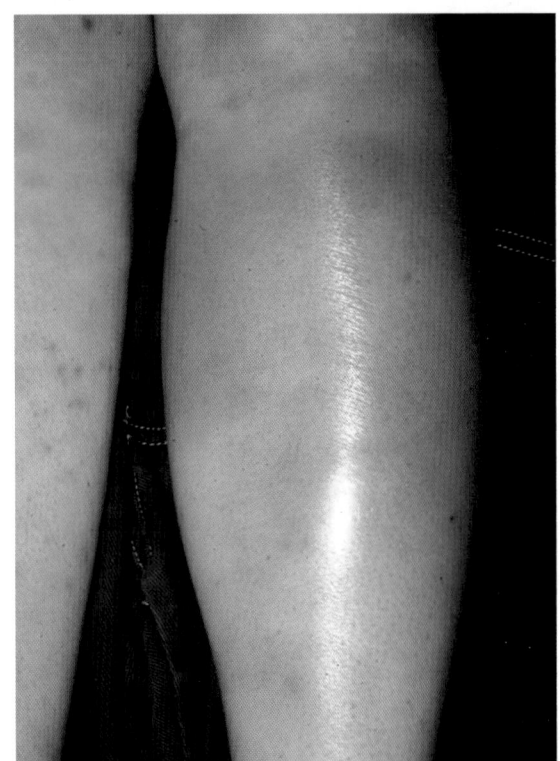

▲ Plate 44. Erythema nodosum. (Used, with permission, from Berger TG, Dept Dermatology, UCSF.)

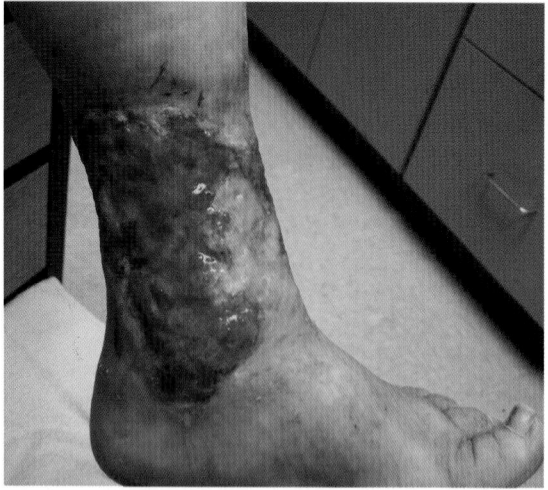

▲ Plate 45. Venous stasis ulcer near the medial malleolus. (Courtesy of Maureen Sheehan, MD; used, with permission, from Usatine RP, Smith MA, Mayeaux EJ Jr, Chumley H, Tysinger J. *The Color Atlas of Family Medicine*. McGraw-Hill, 2009.)

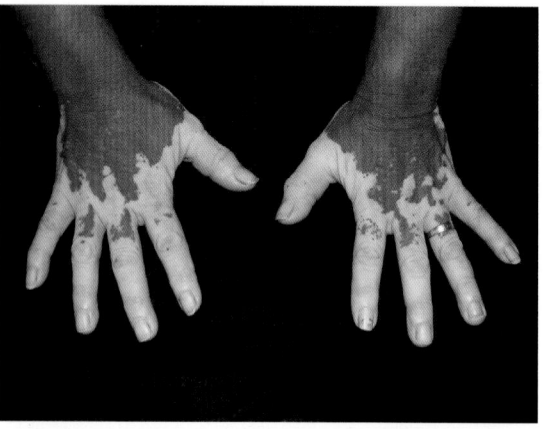

▲ Plate 46. Vitiligo of the hands. (Courtesy of Richard P. Usatine, MD; used, with permission, from Usatine RP, Smith MA, Mayeaux EJ Jr, Chumley H, Tysinger J. *The Color Atlas of Family Medicine*. McGraw-Hill, 2009.)

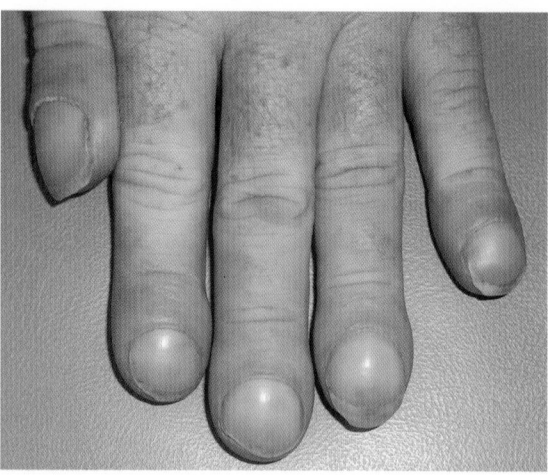

▲ Plate 47. Clubbing of the fingers in congenital heart disease. (Courtesy of Richard P. Usatine, MD; used, with permission, from Usatine RP, Smith MA, Mayeaux EJ Jr, Chumley H, Tysinger J. *The Color Atlas of Family Medicine*. McGraw-Hill, 2009.)

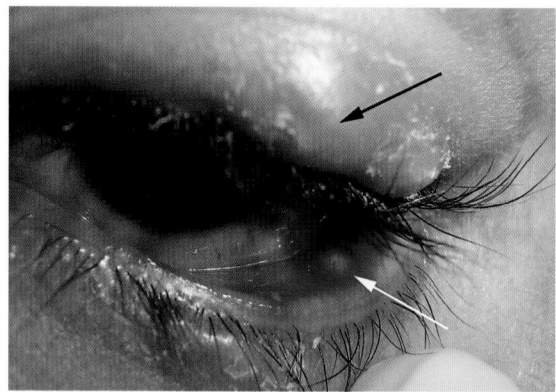

▲ Plate 48. External hordeolum (black arrow) and chalazion (white arrow), which developed from an internal hordeolum. (Courtesy of Richard P. Usatine, MD; used, with permission, from Usatine RP, Smith MA, Mayeaux EJ Jr, Chumley H, Tysinger J. *The Color Atlas of Family Medicine*. McGraw-Hill, 2009.)

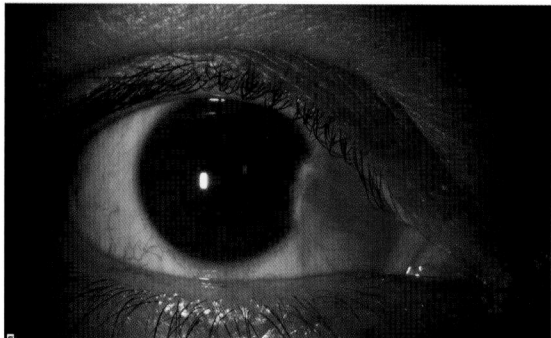

▲ Plate 49. A medial pterygium extending to the cornea. (Courtesy of Paul D. Corneau; used, with permission, from Usatine RP, Smith MA, Mayeaux EJ Jr, Chumley H, Tysinger J. *The Color Atlas of Family Medicine*. McGraw-Hill, 2009.)

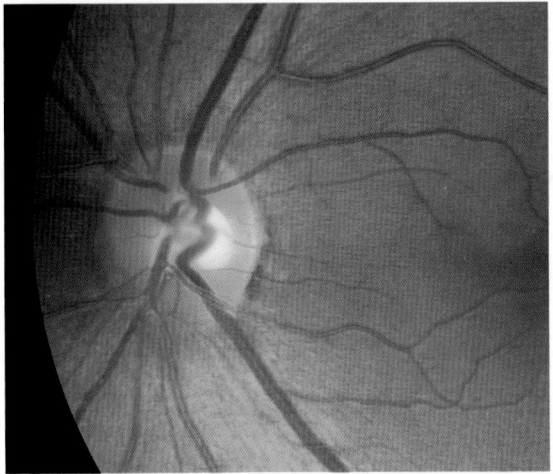

▲ **Plate 50.** Normal eye with a normal optic cup-to-disk ration of 0.4. (Courtesy of Paul D. Corneau; used, with permission, from Usatine RP, Smith MA, Mayeaux EJ Jr, Chumley H, Tysinger J. *The Color Atlas of Family Medicine.* McGraw-Hill, 2009.)

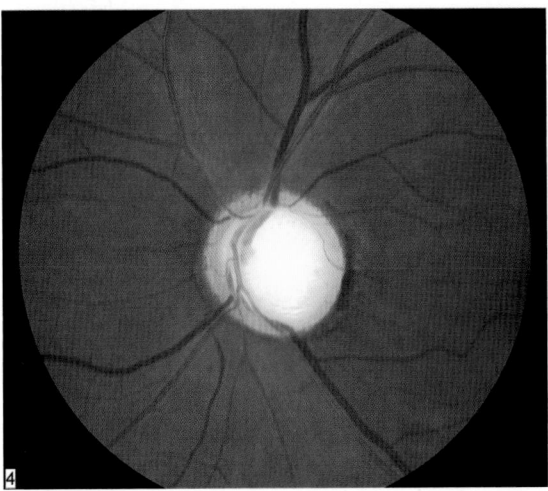

▲ **Plate 51.** Glaucoma with an increased optic cup-to-disk ratio of 0.8. (Courtesy of Paul D. Corneau; used, with permission, from Usatine RP, Smith MA, Mayeaux EJ Jr, Chumley H, Tysinger J. *The Color Atlas of Family Medicine.* McGraw-Hill, 2009.)

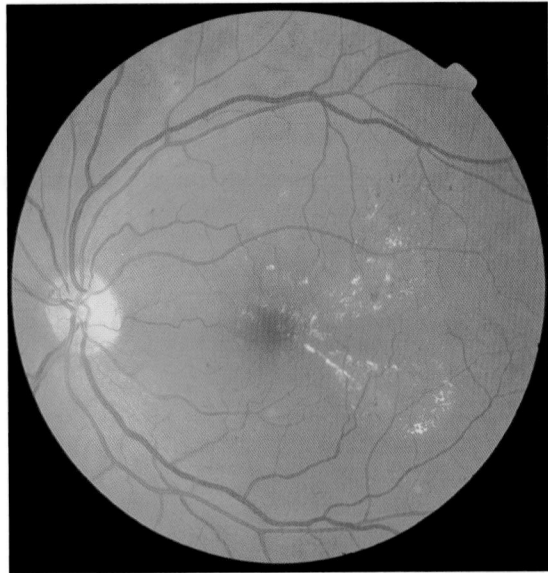

▲ **Plate 52.** Diabetic exudative maculopathy. (Courtesy of Victor Chong; Reproduced with permission from Riordan-Eva, P and Whitcher, JP: *Vaughan & Asbury's General Ophthalmology,* 17th edition, McGraw-Hill, 2008.)

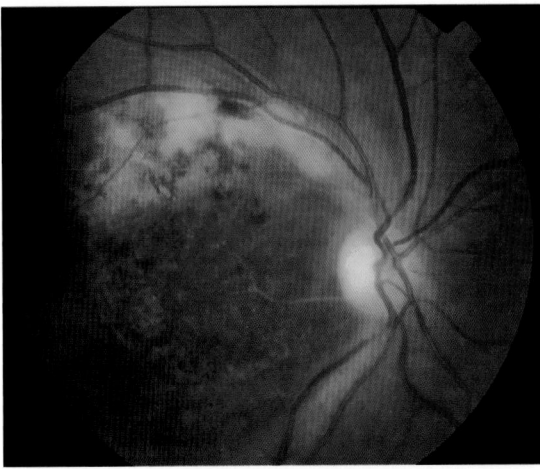

▲ **Plate 53.** Retinal changes in HIV infection: cytomegalovirus retinitis. (Courtesy of Elizabeth Graham; Reproduced with permission from Riordan-Eva, P and Whitcher, JP: *Vaughan & Asbury's General Ophthalmology,* 17th edition, McGraw-Hill, 2008.)

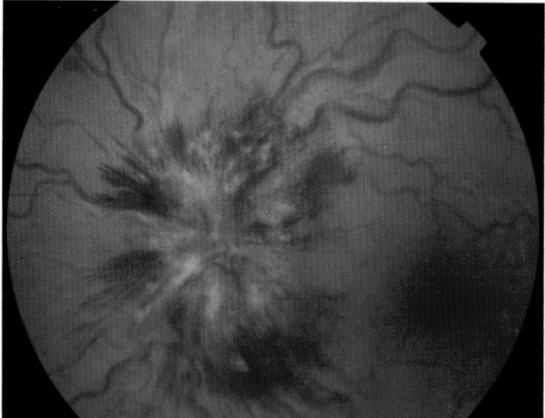

▲ **Plate 54.** Severe acute papilledema. (Used, with permission, from Riordan-Eva, P.)

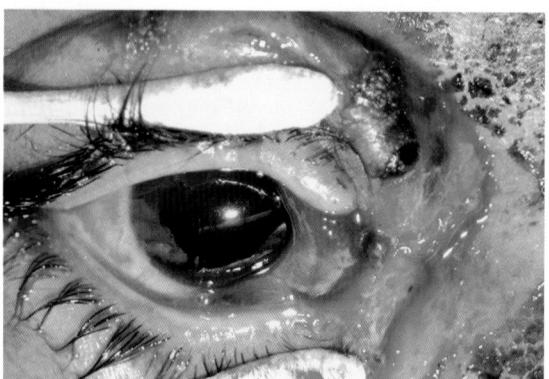

▲ **Plate 55.** Severe ocular injury. (Courtesy of James Augsburger; Reproduced with permission from Riordan-Eva, P and Whitcher, JP: *Vaughan & Asbury's General Ophthalmology*, 17th edition, McGraw-Hill, 2008.)

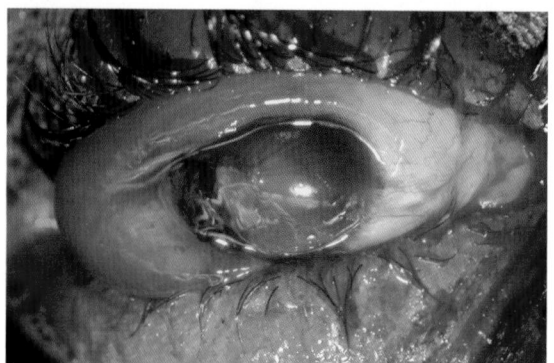

▲ **Plate 56.** Corneal laceration with extrusion of iris. (Courtesy of James Augsburger; Reproduced with permission from Riordan-Eva, P and Whitcher, JP: *Vaughan & Asbury's General Ophthalmology*, 17th edition, McGraw-Hill, 2008.)

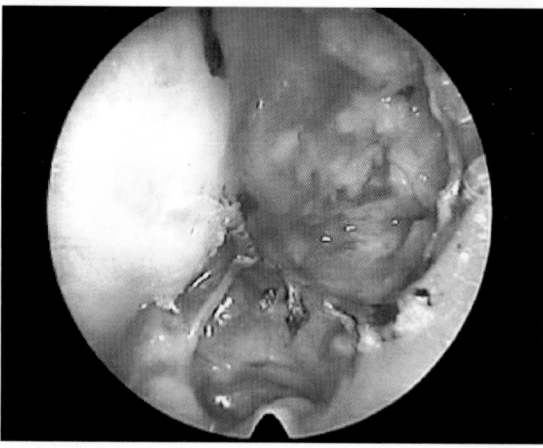

▲ **Plate 57.** Cholesteatoma. (Courtesy of Vladimir Zlinsky, MD in Rory F. Sullivan, PhD: Audiology Forum: Video Otoscopy, www.RCSullivan.com; used, with permission, from Usatine RP, Smith MA, Mayeaux EJ Jr, Chumley H, Tysinger J. *The Color Atlas of Family Medicine.* McGraw-Hill, 2009.)

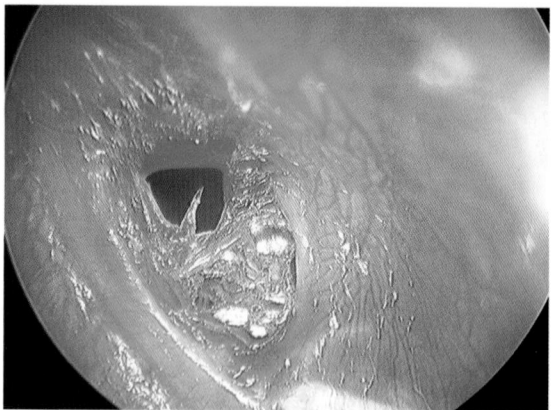

▲ **Plate 58.** Traumatic perforation of the left tympanic membrane. (Courtesy of William Clark, MD; used, with permission, from Usatine RP, Smith MA, Mayeaux EJ Jr, Chumley H, Tysinger J. *The Color Atlas of Family Medicine.* McGraw-Hill, 2009.)

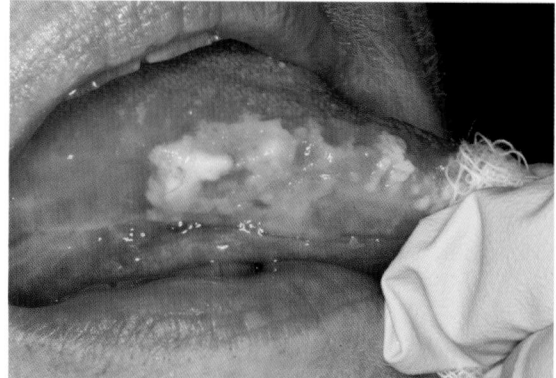

▲ **Plate 59.** Leukoplakia with moderate dysplasia on the lateral border of the tongue. (Courtesy of Ellen Eisenberg, DMD; used, with permission, from Usatine RP, Smith MA, Mayeaux EJ Jr, Chumley H, Tysinger J. *The Color Atlas of Family Medicine.* McGraw-Hill, 2009.)

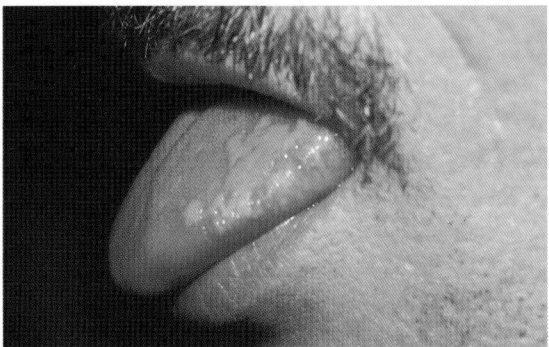

▲ **Plate 60.** Oral hairy leukoplakia on the side of the tongue in AIDS. (Courtesy of Richard P. Usatine, MD; used, with permission, from Usatine RP, Smith MA, Mayeaux EJ Jr, Chumley H, Tysinger J. *The Color Atlas of Family Medicine.* McGraw-Hill, 2009.)

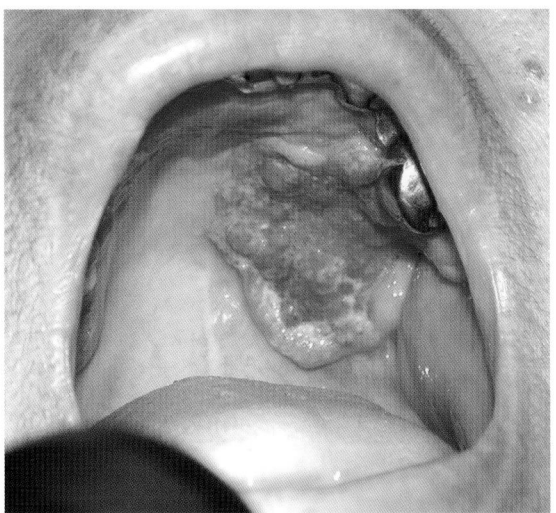

▲ **Plate 61.** Squamous cell carcinoma of the palate. (Courtesy of Frank Miller, MD; used, with permission, from Usatine RP, Smith MA, Mayeaux EJ Jr, Chumley H, Tysinger J. *The Color Atlas of Family Medicine.* McGraw-Hill, 2009.)

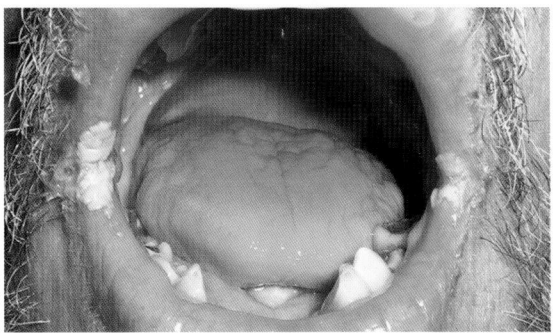

▲ **Plate 62.** Severe angular cheilitis in HIV-positive man with oral thrush. (Courtesy of Richard P. Usatine, MD; used, with permission, from Usatine RP, Smith MA, Mayeaux EJ Jr, Chumley H, Tysinger J. *The Color Atlas of Family Medicine.* McGraw-Hill, 2009.)

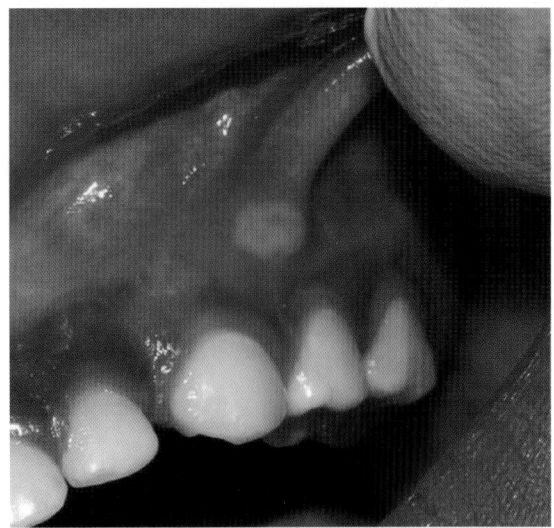

▲ **Plate 63.** Aphthous stomatitis. (Courtesy of Ellen Eisenberg, DMD; used, with permission, from Usatine RP, Smith MA, Mayeaux EJ Jr, Chumley H, Tysinger J. *The Color Atlas of Family Medicine.* McGraw-Hill, 2009.)

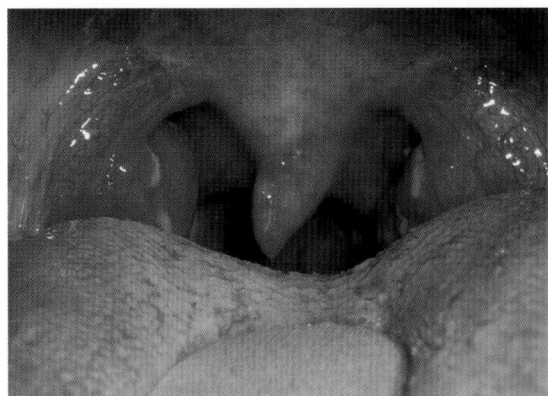

▲ **Plate 64.** Streptococcal pharyngitis showing tonsillar exudate and erythema. (Courtesy of Michael Nguyen, MD; used, with permission, from Usatine RP, Smith MA, Mayeaux EJ Jr, Chumley H, Tysinger J. *The Color Atlas of Family Medicine.* McGraw-Hill, 2009.)

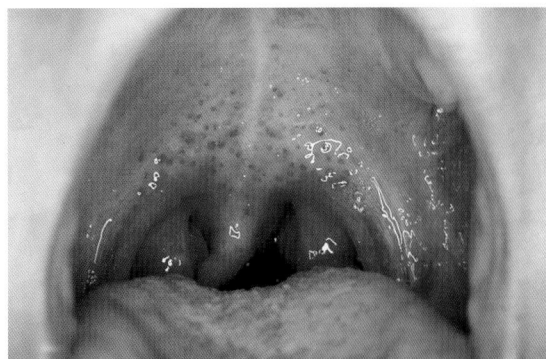

▲ **Plate 65.** Pharyngeal inflammation and petechiae of the soft palate caused by group A *Streptococcus.* (Courtesy of Dr. Heinz F. Eichenwald, Public Health Image Library, CDC.)

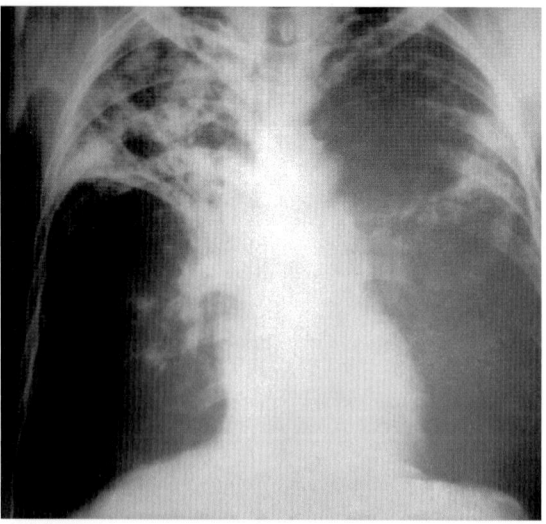

▲ Plate 66. Advanced bilateral pulmonary tuberculosis. (Public Health Image Library, CDC.)

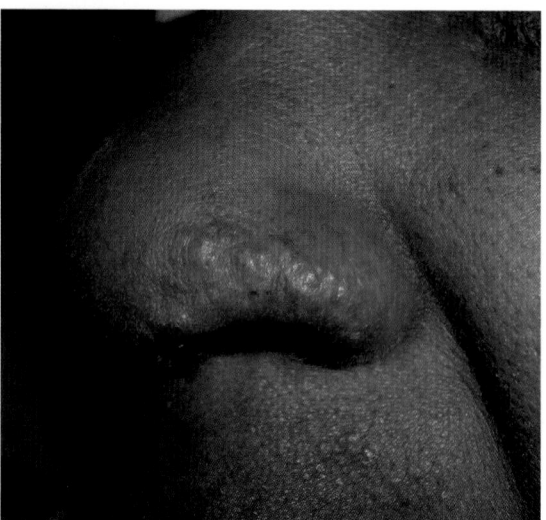

▲ Plate 67. Skin involvement in sarcoidosis (lupus pernio), here involving the nasal rim. (Courtesy of Richard P. Usatine, MD; used, with permission, from Usatine RP, Smith MA, Mayeaux EJ Jr, Chumley H, Tysinger J. *The Color Atlas of Family Medicine.* McGraw-Hill, 2009.)

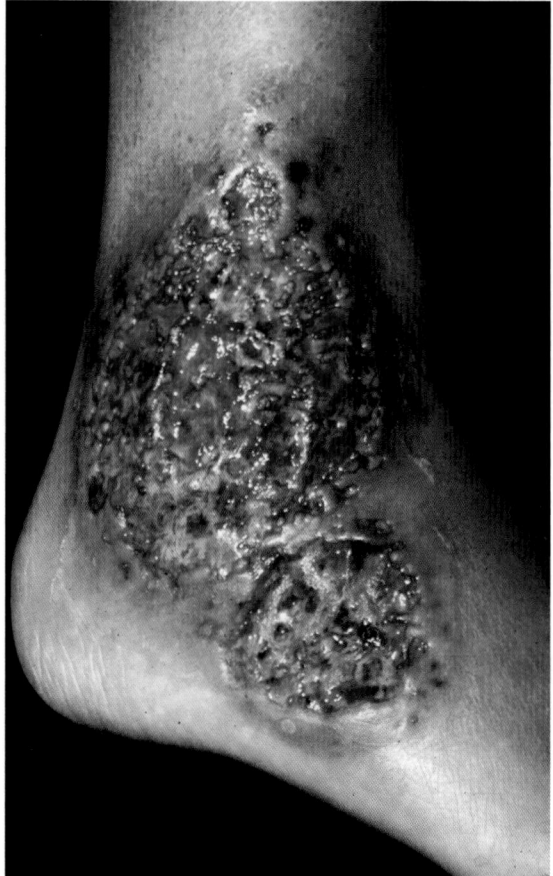

▲ Plate 68. Pyoderma gangrenosum on the leg of the patient with Crohn disease. (Courtesy of Jack Resneck, Sr, MD; used, with permission, from Usatine RP, Smith MA, Mayeaux EJ Jr, Chumley H, Tysinger J. *The Color Atlas of Family Medicine.* McGraw-Hill, 2009.)

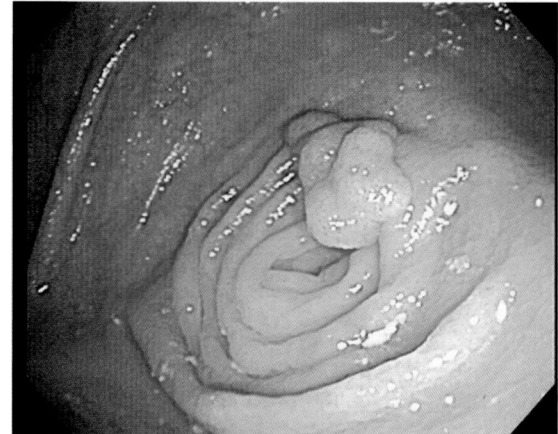

▲ Plate 69. Cecal polyp on colonoscopy. (Courtesy of Marvin Derezin, MD; used, with permission, from Usatine RP, Smith MA, Mayeaux EJ Jr, Chumley H, Tysinger J. *The Color Atlas of Family Medicine.* McGraw-Hill, 2009.)

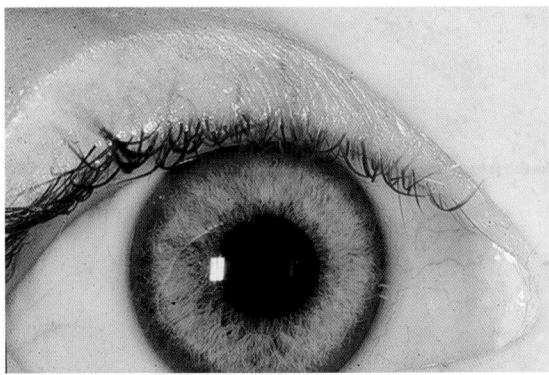

▲ Plate 70. Brownish Kaiser-Fleischer ring at the rim of the cornea in a patient with Wilson disease. (Courtesy of Marc Solioz, University of Berne; used, with permission, from Usatine RP, Smith MA, Mayeaux EJ Jr, Chumley H, Tysinger J. *The Color Atlas of Family Medicine.* McGraw-Hill, 2009.)

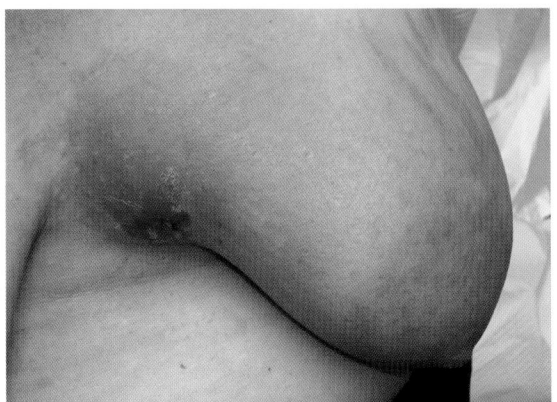

▲ Plate 71. Breast abscess and cellulitis. (Courtesy of Richard P. Usatine, MD; used, with permission, from Usatine RP, Smith MA, Mayeaux EJ Jr, Chumley H, Tysinger J. *The Color Atlas of Family Medicine.* McGraw-Hill, 2009.)

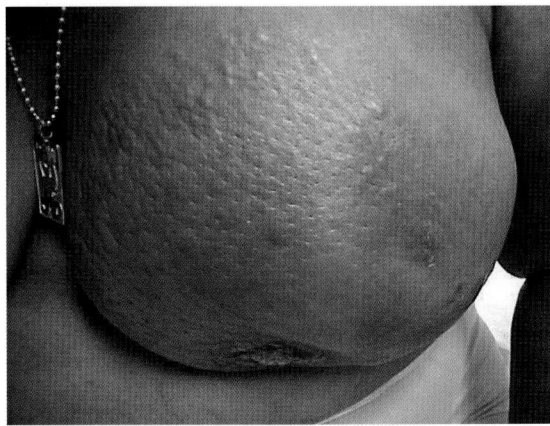

▲ Plate 72. Peau d'orange sign (resemblance to the skin of an orange due to lymphedema) in advanced breast cancer. (Courtesy of Richard P. Usatine, MD; used, with permission, from Usatine RP, Smith MA, Mayeaux EJ Jr, Chumley H, Tysinger J. *The Color Atlas of Family Medicine.* McGraw-Hill, 2009.)

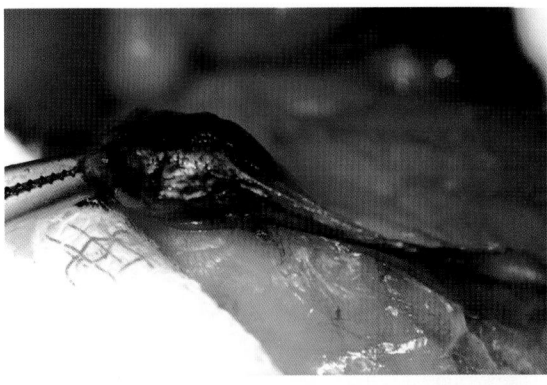

▲ Plate 73. Sentinel node. (Courtesy of Guilano, AE.)

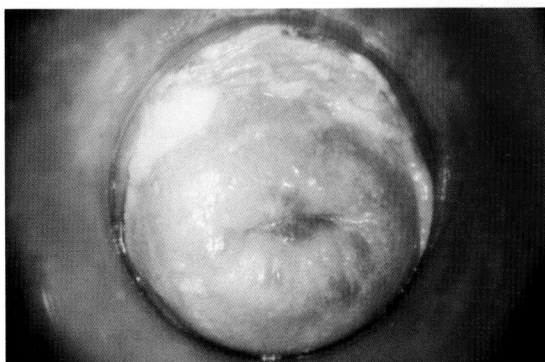

▲ Plate 74. Cervical candidiasis. (Public Health Image Library, CDC.)

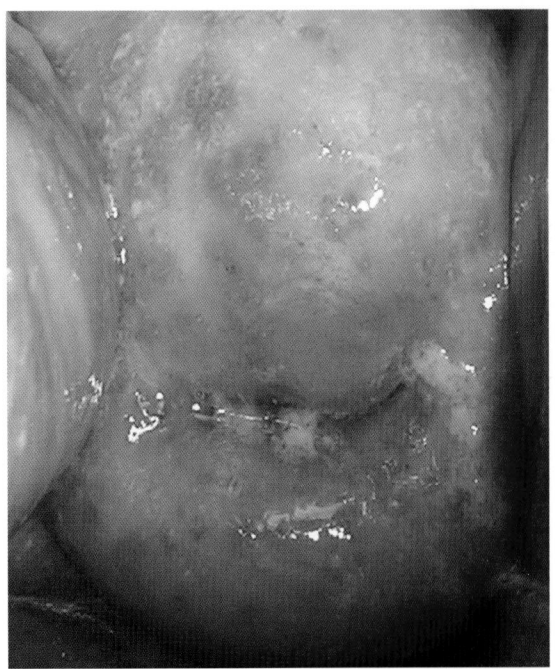

▲ Plate 75. Strawberry cervix in *Trichomonas vaginalis* infection, with inflammation and punctate hemorrhages. (Courtesy of Richard P. Usatine, MD; used, with permission, from Usatine RP, Smith MA, Mayeaux EJ Jr, Chumley H, Tysinger J. *The Color Atlas of Family Medicine.* McGraw-Hill, 2009.)

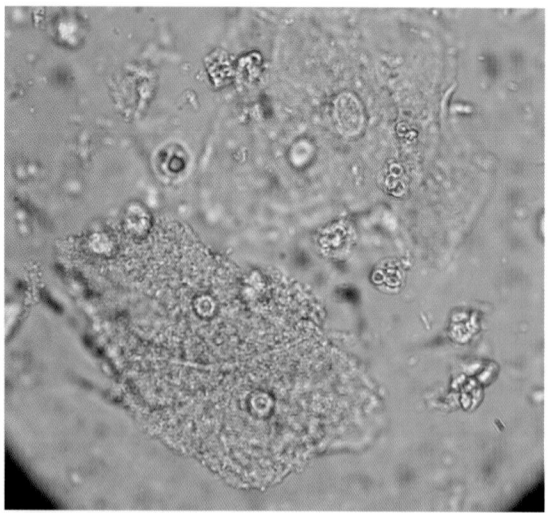

▲ Plate 76. Clue cells seen in bacterial vaginosis due to *Gardnerella* vaginalis. (Courtesy of Richard P. Usatine, MD; used, with permission, from Usatine RP, Smith MA, Mayeaux EJ Jr, Chumley H, Tysinger J. *The Color Atlas of Family Medicine*. McGraw-Hill, 2009.)

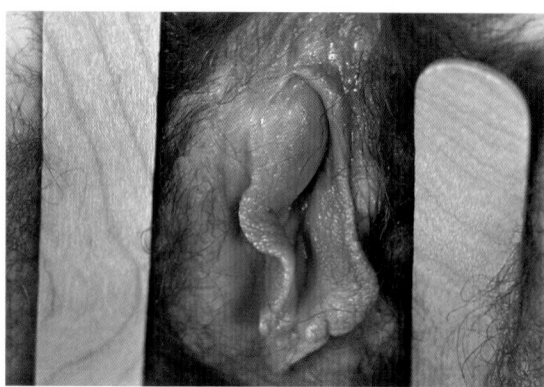

▲ Plate 77. Right-sided Bartholin cyst (abscess). (Courtesy of Susan Lindsley, Public Health Image Library, CDC.)

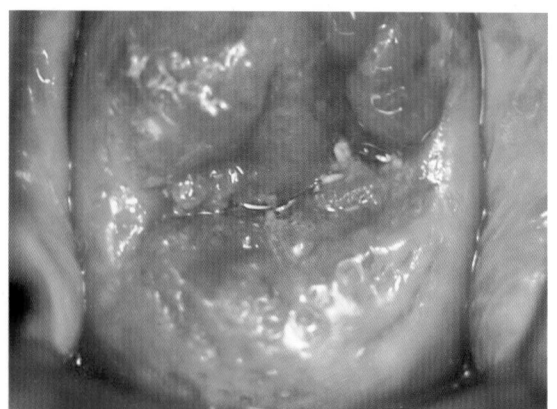

▲ Plate 78. Erosion of the cervix due to cervical intraepithelial neoplasia (CIN), a precursor lesion to cervical cancer. (Public Health Image Library, CDC.)

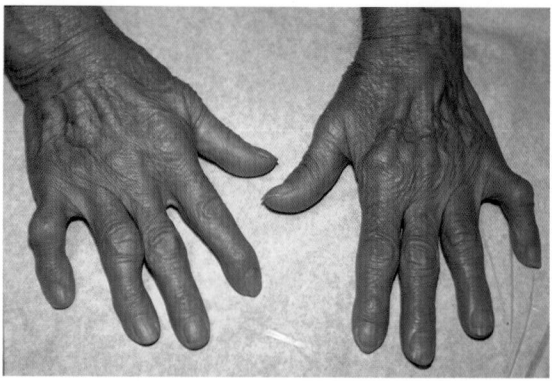

▲ Plate 79. Osteoarthritis with bony enlargement of the distal interphalangeal (DIP) joints (Heberden's nodes) and proximal interphalangeal (PIP) joints (Bouchard's nodes). (Courtesy of Richard P. Usatine, MD; used, with permission, from Usatine RP, Smith MA, Mayeaux EJ Jr, Chumley H, Tysinger J. *The Color Atlas of Family Medicine*. McGraw-Hill, 2009.)

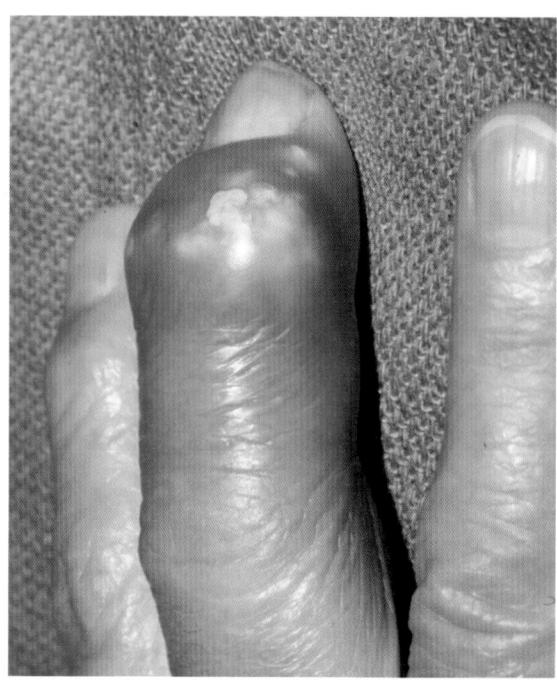

▲ Plate 80. Acute gouty arthritis superimposed on tophaceous gout. (Courtesy of the Western Journal of Medicine and JM Geiderman, MD; used, with permission, from Usatine RP, Smith MA, Mayeaux EJ Jr, Chumley H, Tysinger J. *The Color Atlas of Family Medicine*. McGraw-Hill, 2009.)

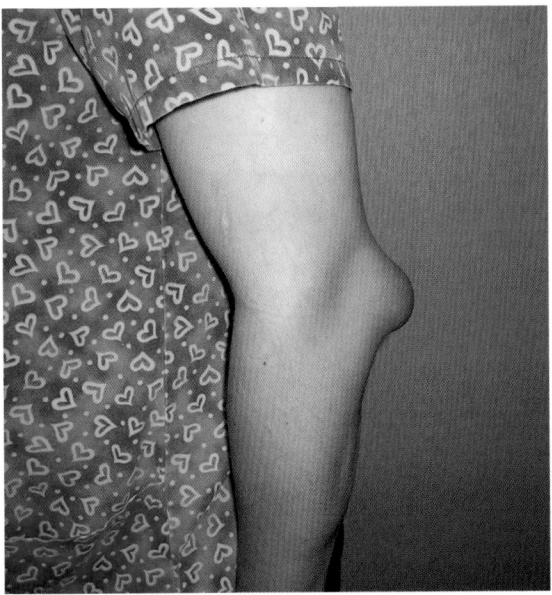

▲ Plate 81. Aseptic olecranon bursitis secondary to repetitive trauma. (Courtesy of Richard P. Usatine, MD; used, with permission, from Usatine RP, Smith MA, Mayeaux EJ Jr, Chumley H, Tysinger J. *The Color Atlas of Family Medicine*. McGraw-Hill, 2009.)

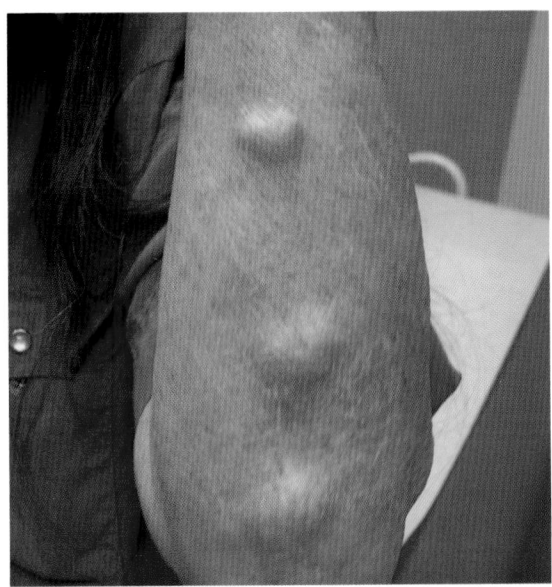

▲ Plate 83. Rheumatoid nodules over the extensive surface of the forearm. (Courtesy of Richard P. Usatine, MD; used, with permission, from Usatine RP, Smith MA, Mayeaux EJ Jr, Chumley H, Tysinger J. *The Color Atlas of Family Medicine*. McGraw-Hill, 2009.)

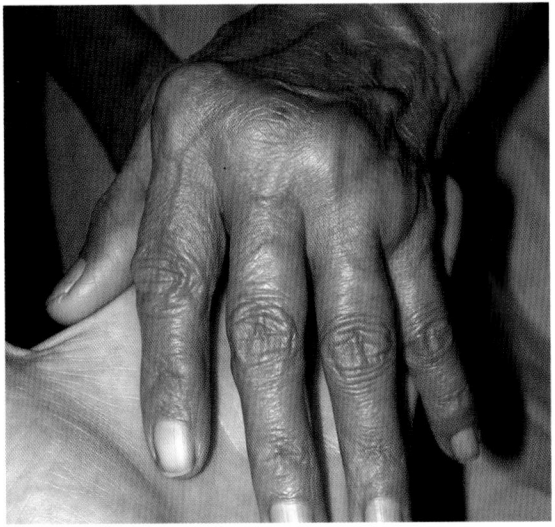

▲ Plate 82. Rheumatoid arthritis with ulnar deviation at the metacarpophalangeal (MCP) joints. (Courtesy of Richard P. Usatine, MD; used, with permission, from Usatine RP, Smith MA, Mayeaux EJ Jr, Chumley H, Tysinger J. *The Color Atlas of Family Medicine*. McGraw-Hill, 2009.)

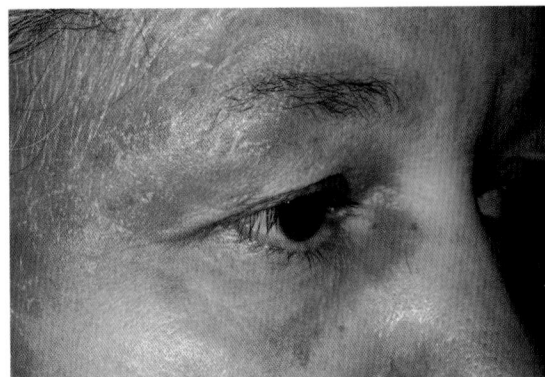

▲ Plate 84. Heliotrope (violaceous) rash around the eyes in a patient with dermatomyositis. (Courtesy of Richard P. Usatine, MD; used, with permission, from Usatine RP, Smith MA, Mayeaux EJ Jr, Chumley H, Tysinger J. *The Color Atlas of Family Medicine*. McGraw-Hill, 2009.)

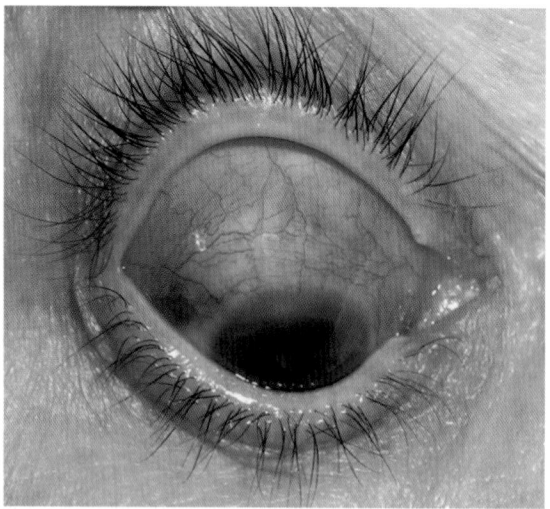

▲ **Plate 85.** Scleritis in a patient with Wegener's granulomatosis. (Courtesy of Everett Allen, MD; used, with permission, from Usatine RP, Smith MA, Mayeaux EJ Jr, Chumley H, Tysinger J. *The Color Atlas of Family Medicine.* McGraw-Hill, 2009.)

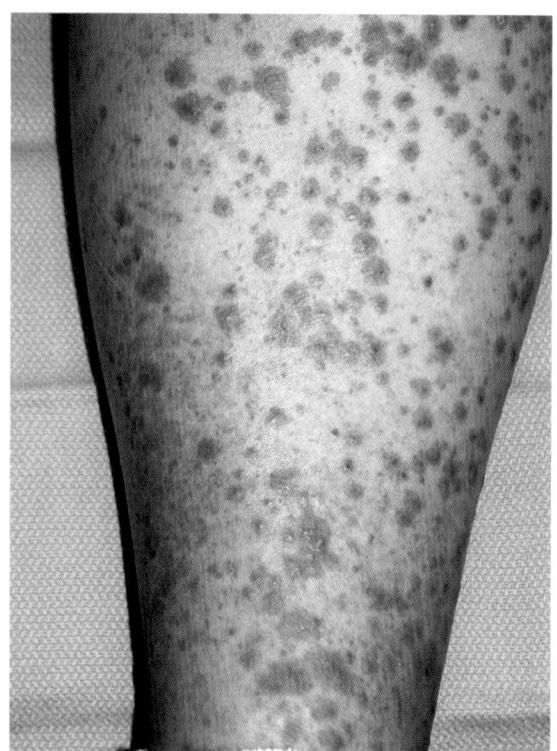

▲ **Plate 86.** Palpable purpura in a woman with leukocytoclastic vasculitis. (Courtesy of Eric Kraus, MD; used, with permission, from Usatine RP, Smith MA, Mayeaux EJ Jr, Chumley H, Tysinger J. *The Color Atlas of Family Medicine.* McGraw-Hill, 2009.)

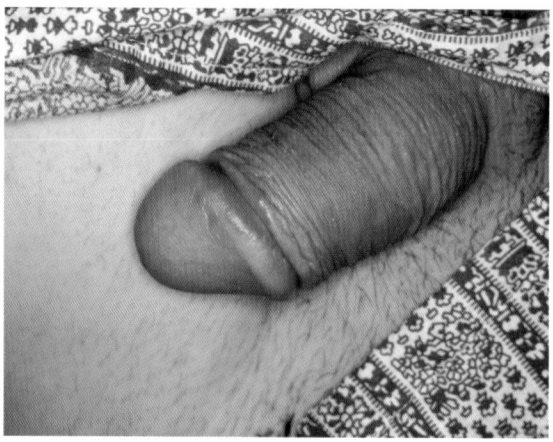

▲ **Plate 87.** Circinate balanitis due to reactive arthritis (Reiter syndrome). (Courtesy of Susan Lindsley, Dr. M. F. Rein, Public Health Image Library, CDC.)

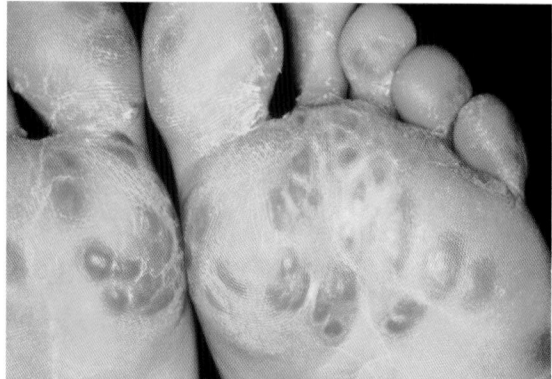

▲ **Plate 88.** Keratoderma blennorrhagica of the soles due to reactive arthritis (Reiter syndrome). (Courtesy of Susan Lindsley, Public Health Image Library, CDC.)

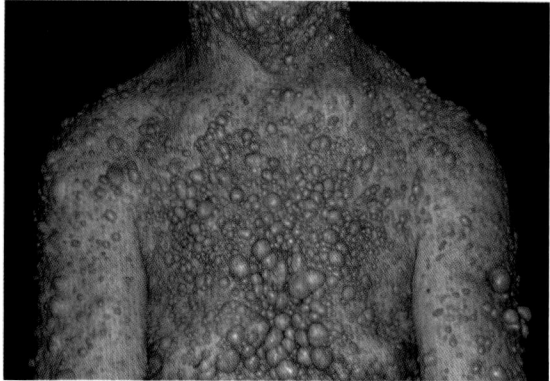

▲ **Plate 89.** Neurofibromatosis. (Courtesy of Jack Resneck, Sr, MD; used, with permission, from Usatine RP, Smith MA, Mayeaux EJ Jr, Chumley H, Tysinger J. *The Color Atlas of Family Medicine.* McGraw-Hill, 2009.)

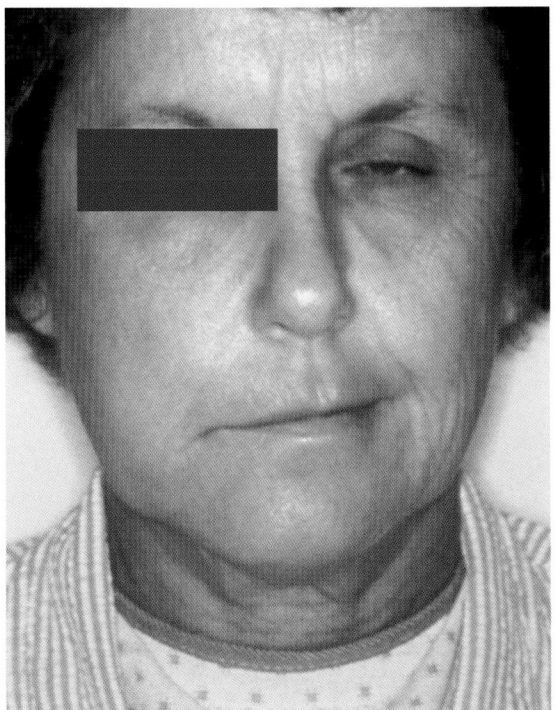

▲ Plate 90. Facial palsy caused by an infection with *Borrelia burgdorferi* (Lyme disease). (Public Health Image Library, CDC.)

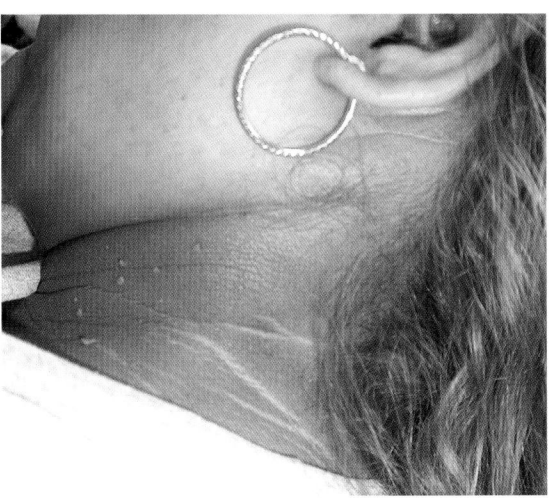

▲ Plate 91. Acanthosis nigricans on the neck of a patient with type 2 diabetes mellitus. (Courtesy of Richard P. Usatine, MD; used, with permission, from Usatine RP, Smith MA, Mayeaux EJ Jr, Chumley H, Tysinger J. *The Color Atlas of Family Medicine*. McGraw-Hill, 2009.)

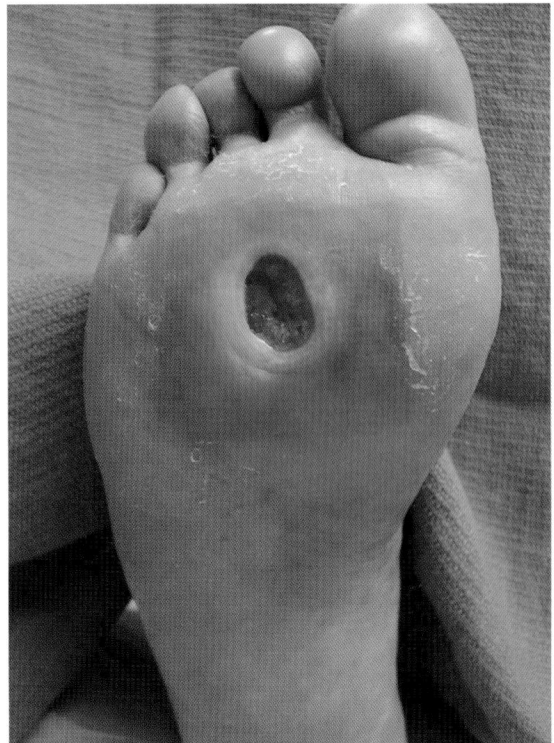

▲ Plate 92. Neuropathic ulcer under the head of the third metatarsal on the foot of a diabetic patient. (Courtesy of Javier La Fontaine, DPM; used, with permission, from Usatine RP, Smith MA, Mayeaux EJ Jr, Chumley H, Tysinger J. *The Color Atlas of Family Medicine*. McGraw-Hill, 2009.)

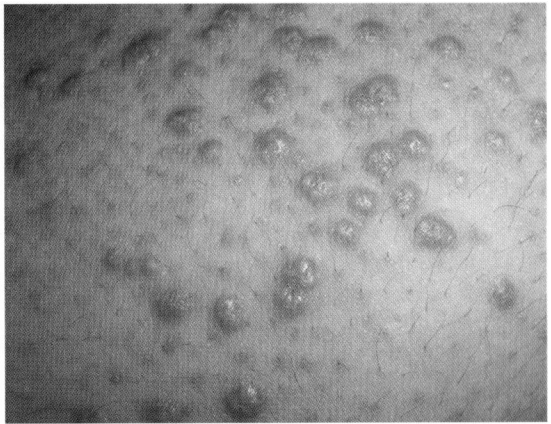

▲ Plate 93. Eruptive xanthoma on the arm of a man with untreated hyperlipidemia and diabetes mellitus. (Courtesy of Richard P. Usatine, MD; used, with permission, from Usatine RP, Smith MA, Mayeaux EJ Jr, Chumley H, Tysinger J. *The Color Atlas of Family Medicine*. McGraw-Hill, 2009.)

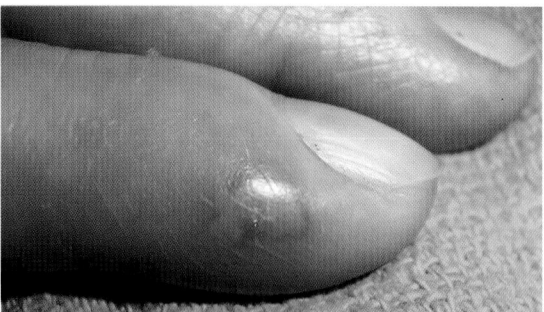

▲ Plate 94. Herpetic whitlow. (Used, with permission, from Usatine RP, Smith MA, Mayeaux EJ Jr, Chumley H, Tysinger J. *The Color Atlas of Family Medicine*. McGraw-Hill, 2009.)

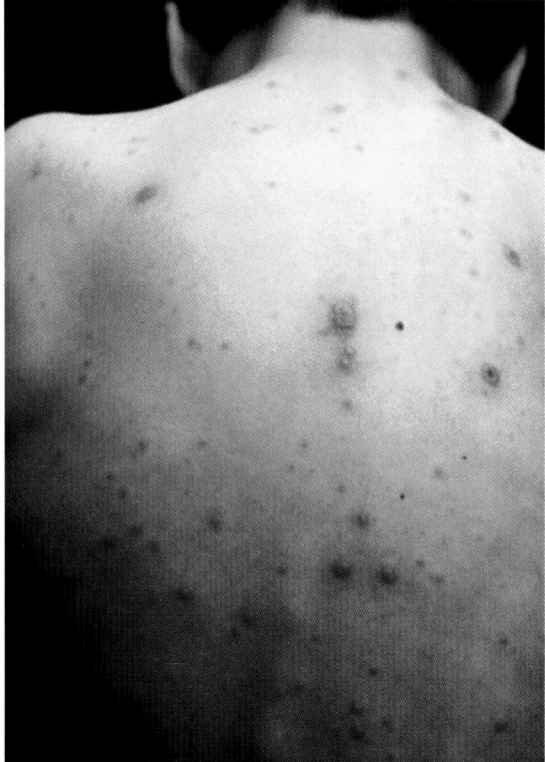

▲ Plate 95. Primary varicella (chickenpox) skin lesions. (Public Health Image Library, CDC.)

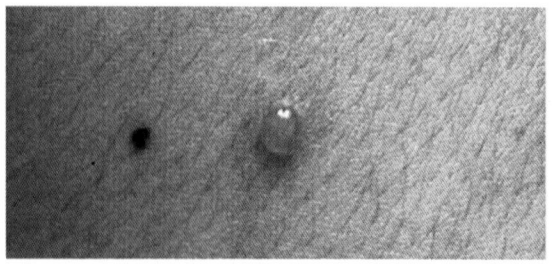

▲ Plate 96. Chickenpox (varicella) with classic "dewdrop on rose petal" appearance. (Courtesy of Richard P. Usatine, MD; used, with permission, from Usatine RP, Smith MA, Mayeaux EJ Jr, Chumley H, Tysinger J. *The Color Atlas of Family Medicine*. McGraw-Hill, 2009.)

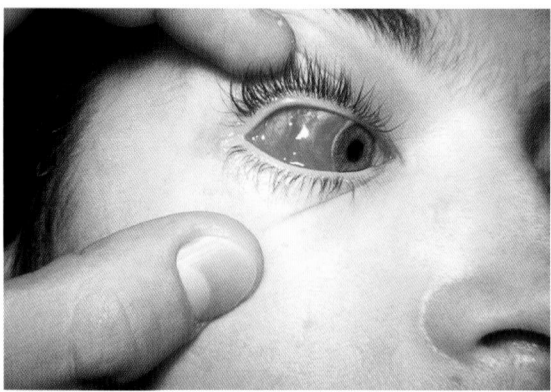

▲ Plate 97. Conjunctival hemorrhage of the eye due to infectious mononucleosis. (Courtesy of Dr. Thomas F. Sellers, Emory University, Public Health Image Library, CDC.)

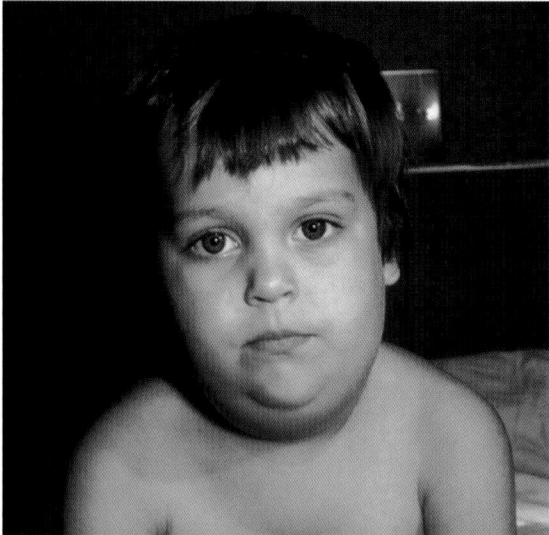

▲ Plate 98. Mumps. (Public Health Image Library, CDC.)

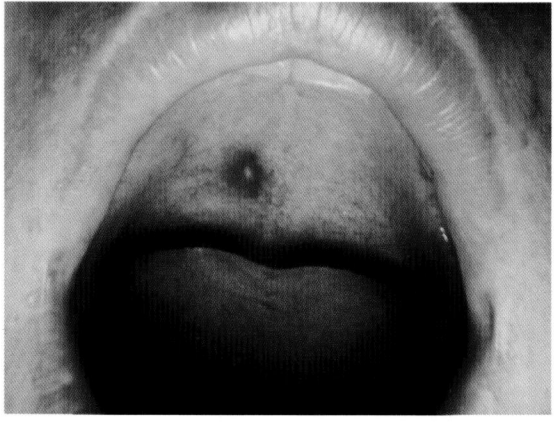

▲ Plate 99. Hard palate lesion caused by Rocky Mountain spotted fever. (Public Health Image Library, CDC.)

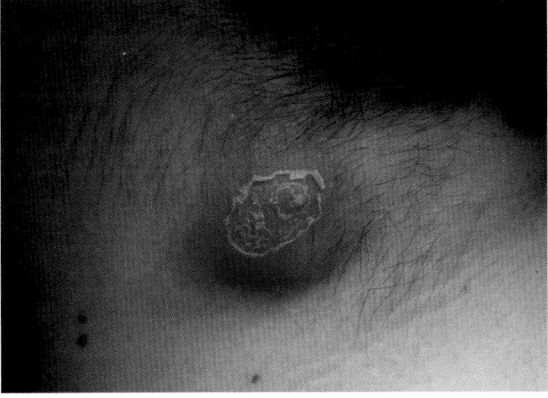

▲ **Plate 100.** Methicillin-resistant *Staphylococcus aureus* (MRSA) abscess of the neck. (Courtesy of Edward Wright, MD; used, with permission, from Usatine RP, Smith MA, Mayeaux EJ Jr, Chumley H, Tysinger J. *The Color Atlas of Family Medicine.* McGraw-Hill, 2009.)

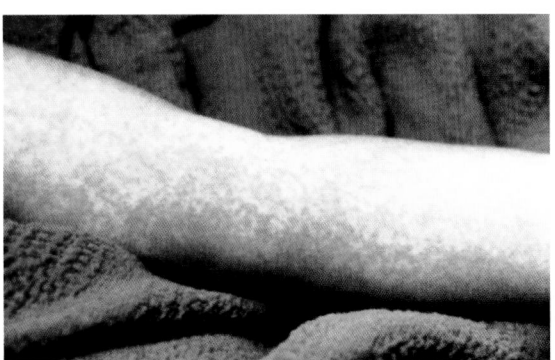

▲ **Plate 101.** Morbilliform rash in toxic shock syndrome caused by *Staphylococcus aureus*. (Public Health Image Library, CDC.)

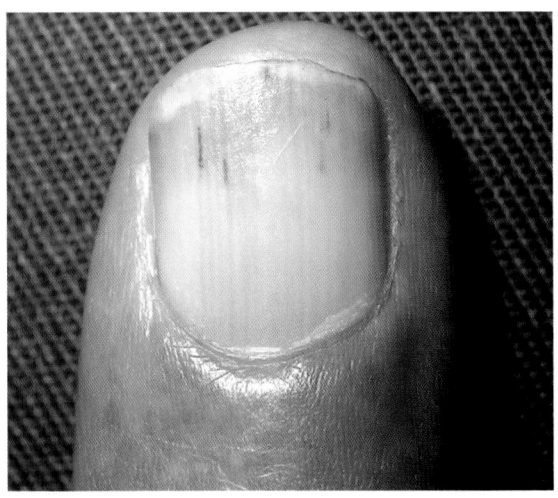

▲ **Plate 102.** Splinter hemorrhages appearing as red lineal streaks under the nail plate and within the nail bed, in endocarditis, psoriasis, and trauma. (Courtesy of Richard P. Usatine, MD; used, with permission, from Usatine RP, Smith MA, Mayeaux EJ Jr, Chumley H, Tysinger J. *The Color Atlas of Family Medicine.* McGraw-Hill, 2009.)

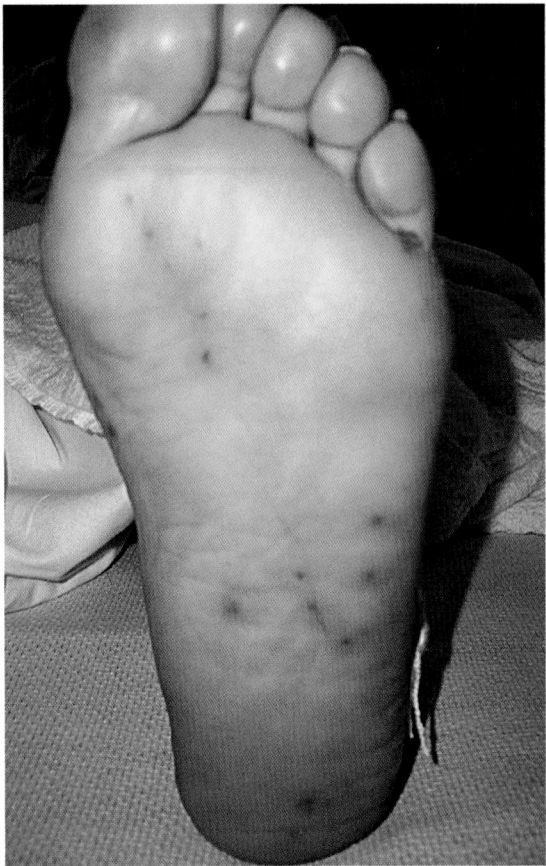

▲ **Plate 103.** Osler's node causing pain within the pulp of the big toe and multiple painless flat Janeway lesions over the sole of the foot. (Courtesy of David A. Kasper, D.O., MBA; used, with permission, from Usatine RP, Smith MA, Mayeaux EJ Jr, Chumley H, Tysinger J. *The Color Atlas of Family Medicine.* McGraw-Hill, 2009.)

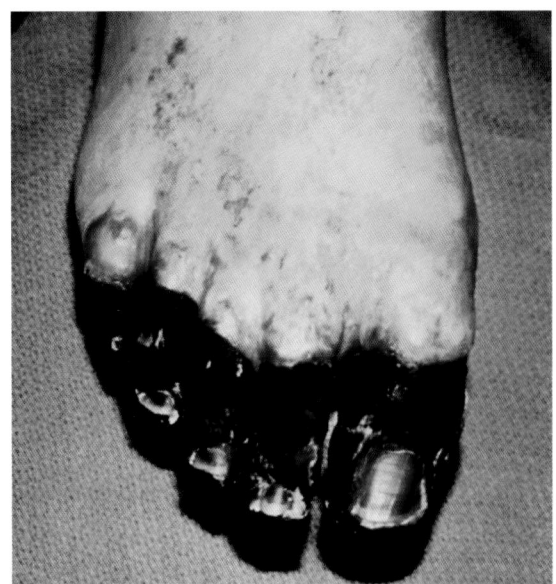

▲ **Plate 104.** Gangrene of the right foot causing necrosis of the toes. (Courtesy of William Archibald, Public Health Image Library, CDC.)

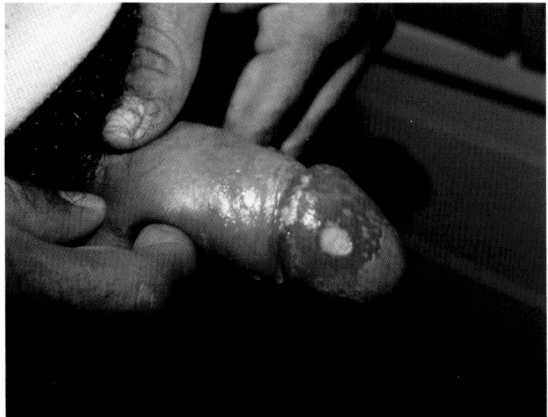

▲ Plate 105. Primary syphilis with a large chancre on the glans of the penis. (Courtesy of Richard P. Usatine, MD; used, with permission, from Usatine RP, Smith MA, Mayeaux EJ Jr, Chumley H, Tysinger J. *The Color Atlas of Family Medicine.* McGraw-Hill, 2009.)

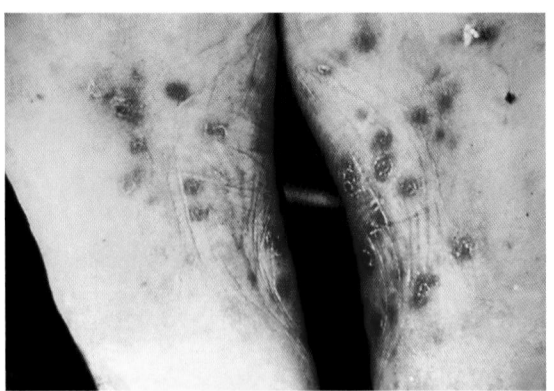

▲ Plate 106. Secondary syphilis lesions on the soles of the feet. (Courtesy of Dr. Gavin Hart, Public Health Image Library, CDC.)

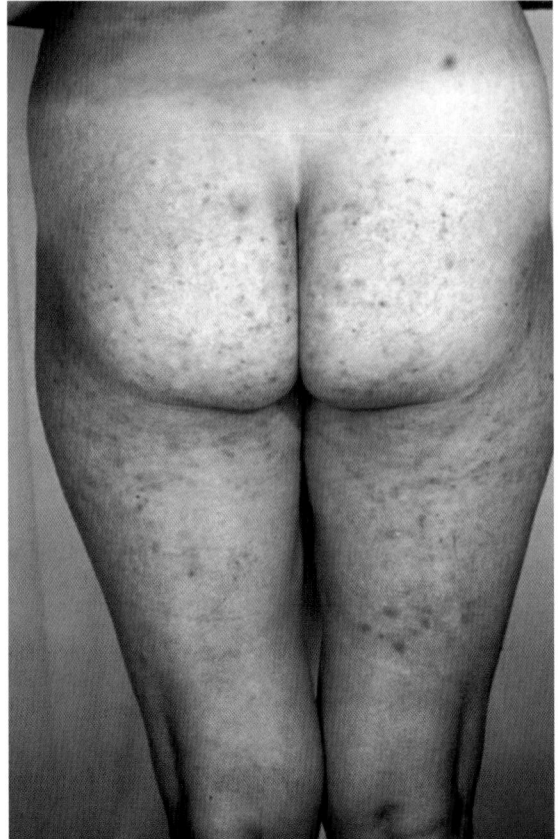

▲ Plate 107. Secondary syphilis rash of the buttocks and legs. (Courtesy of J. Pledger, BSS/VD, Public Health Image Library, CDC.)

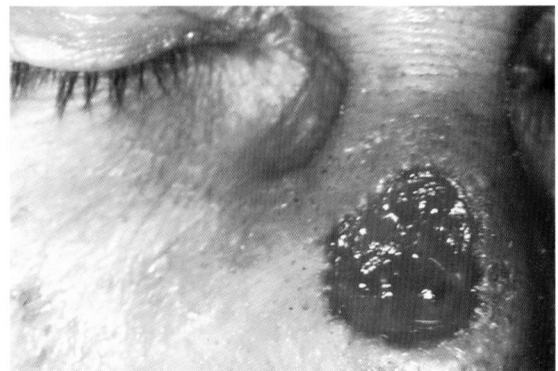

▲ Plate 108. Gumma of the nose due to long-standing tertiary syphilis. (Courtesy of J. Pledger, Public Health Image Library, CDC.)

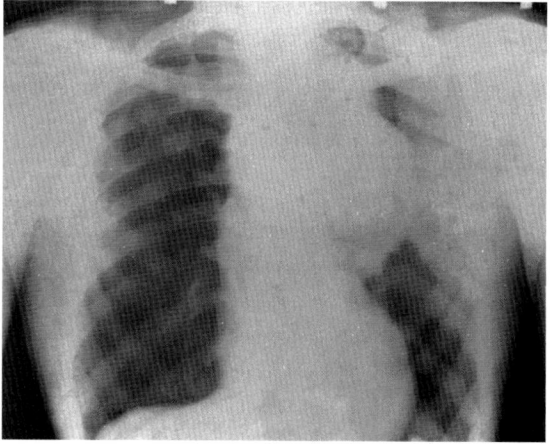

▲ Plate 109. Ascending saccular aneurysm of the thoracic aorta in tertiary syphilis. (Public Health Image Library, CDC.)

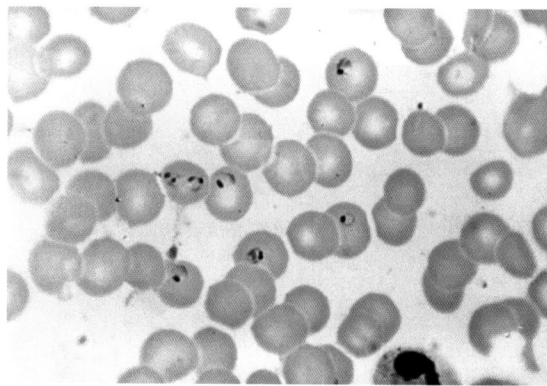

▲ Plate 112. Thin film Giemsa-stained micrograph with *Plasmodium falciparum* trophozoite. (Courtesy of Steven Glenn, Laboratory & Consultation Division, Public Health Image Library, CDC.)

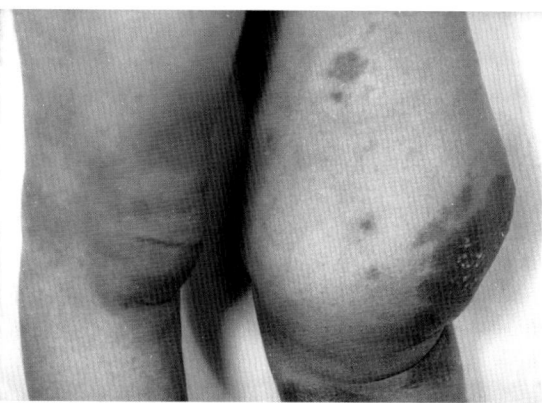

▲ Plate 110. Neuropathic arthropathy (Charcot joint) from tertiary syphilis. (Courtesy of Susan Lindsley, Public Health Image Library, CDC.)

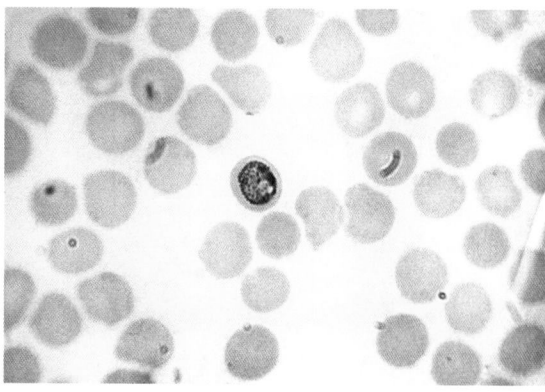

▲ Plate 113. Thin film Giemsa-stained micrograph with *Plasmodium malariae* trophozoite. (Courtesy of Steven Glenn, Laboratory & Consultation Division, Public Health Image Library, CDC.)

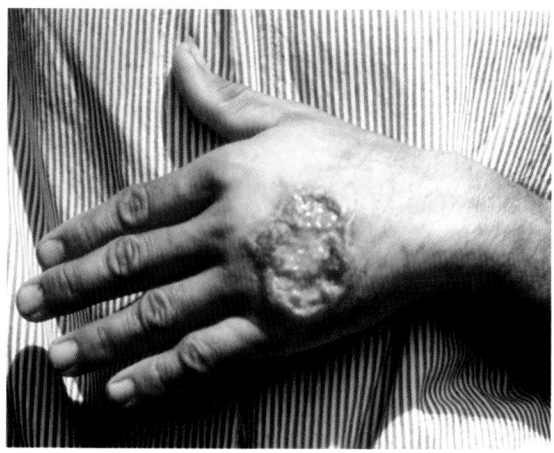

▲ Plate 111. Skin ulcer due to leishmaniasis. (Courtesy of D. S. Martin, Public Health Image Library, CDC.)

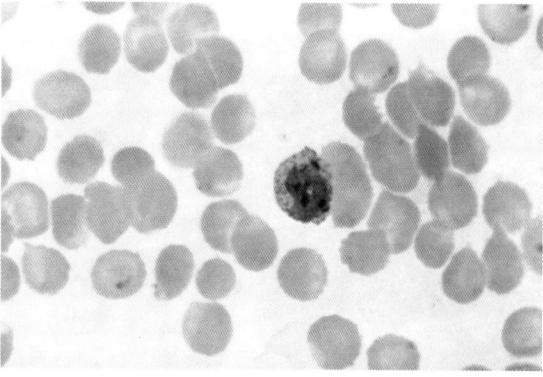

▲ Plate 114. Thin film Giemsa-stained micrograph with *Plasmodium vivax* schizonts. (Courtesy of Steven Glenn, Laboratory & Consultation Division, Public Health Image Library, CDC.)

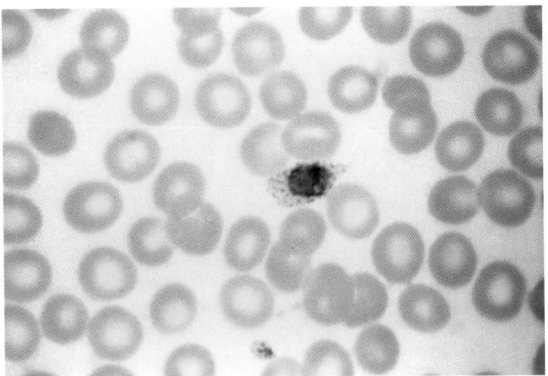

▲ **Plate 115.** Thin film Giemsa-stained micrograph with *Plasmodium ovale* trophozoite. (Courtesy of Steven Glenn, Laboratory & Consultation Division, Public Health Image Library, CDC.)

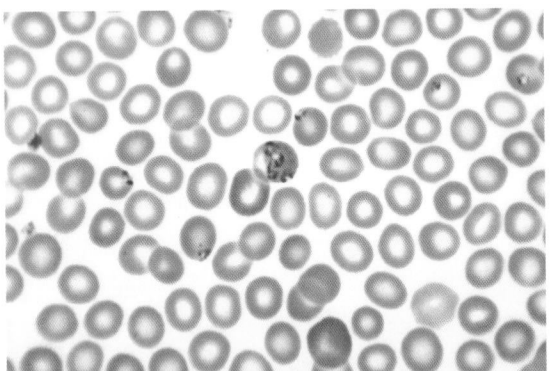

▲ **Plate 116.** Blood smear showing *Babesia* spp. rings with basophilic stippling. (Courtesy of Dr. Mae Melvin, Public Health Image Library, CDC.)

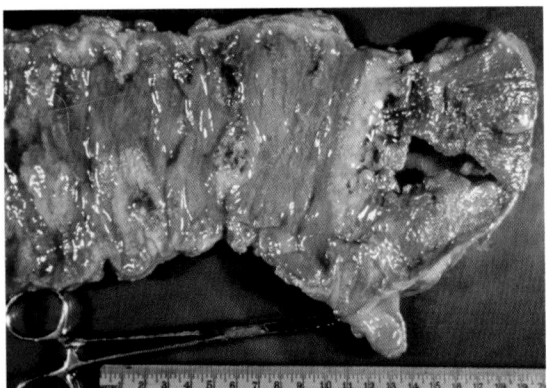

▲ **Plate 117.** Gross pathology showing intestinal ulcers due to amebiasis. (Courtesy of Dr. Mae Melvin, Public Health Image Library, CDC.)

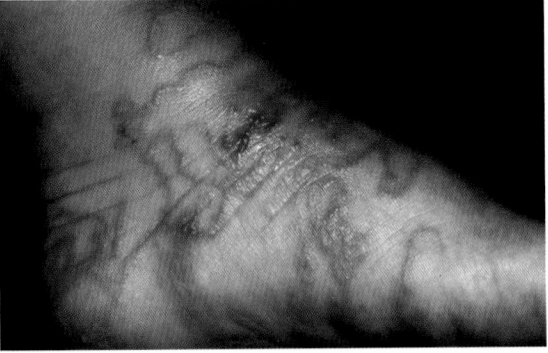

▲ **Plate 118.** Cutaneous larva migrans on the foot. (Courtesy of Richard P. Usatine, MD from Usatine RP: A rash on the feet and buttocks. Western Journal of Medicine 1999;170(6):344; used, with permission, from Usatine RP, Smith MA, Mayeux EJ Jr, Chumley H, Tysinger J. *The Color Atlas of Family Medicine*. McGraw-Hill, 2009.)

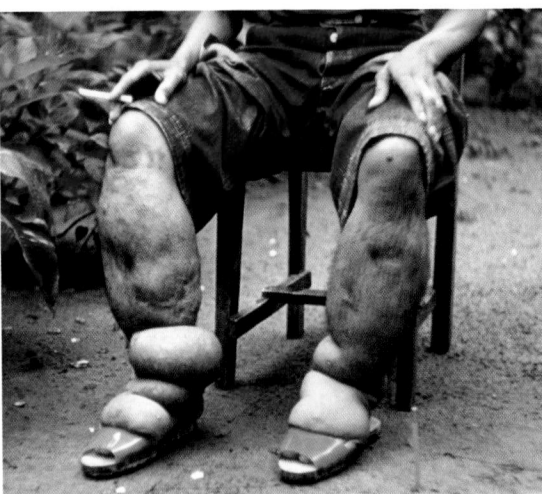

▲ **Plate 119.** Elephantiasis of legs due to filariasis. (Public Health Image Library, CDC.)

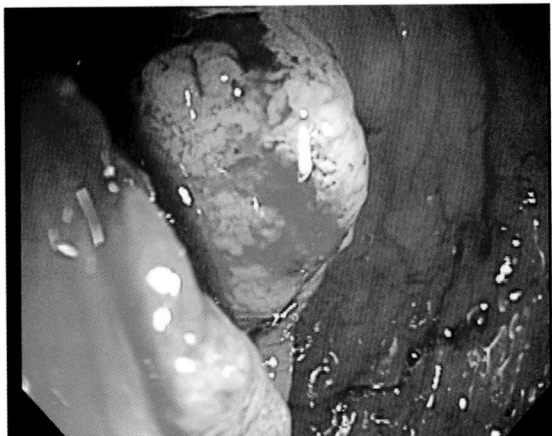

▲ **Plate 120.** Cecal adenocarcinoma on colonoscopy. (Courtesy of Marvin Derezin, MD; used, with permission, from Usatine RP, Smith MA, Mayeaux EJ Jr, Chumley H, Tysinger J. *The Color Atlas of Family Medicine*. McGraw-Hill, 2009.)

try to hold the face still while talking. Spontaneous remissions for several months or longer may occur. As the disorder progresses, however, the episodes of pain become more frequent, remissions become shorter and less common, and a dull ache may persist between the episodes of stabbing pain. Symptoms remain confined to the distribution of the trigeminal nerve (usually the second or third division) on one side only.

▶ Differential Diagnosis

The characteristic features of the pain in trigeminal neuralgia usually distinguish it from other causes of facial pain. Neurologic examination shows no abnormality except in a few patients in whom trigeminal neuralgia is symptomatic of some underlying lesion, such as multiple sclerosis or a brainstem neoplasm, in which case the finding will depend on the nature and site of the lesion. Similarly, CT scans and radiologic contrast studies are often normal in patients with classic trigeminal neuralgia.

In a young patient presenting with trigeminal neuralgia, multiple sclerosis must be suspected even if there are no other neurologic signs. In such circumstances, findings on evoked potential testing and examination of cerebrospinal fluid may be corroborative. When the facial pain is due to a posterior fossa tumor, CT scanning and MRI generally reveal the lesion.

▶ Treatment

The drugs most helpful for treatment are oxcarbazepine (although not approved by the US Food and Drug Administration [FDA] for this indication) or carbamazepine, with monitoring by serial blood counts and liver function tests. If these medications are ineffective or cannot be tolerated, phenytoin should be tried. (Doses and side effects of these drugs are shown in Table 24–3). Baclofen (10–20 mg three or four times daily) or lamotrigine (400 mg orally daily) may also be helpful, either alone or in combination with one of these other agents. Gabapentin may also relieve pain, especially in patients who do not respond to conventional medical therapy and those with multiple sclerosis. Depending on response and tolerance, up to 2400 mg/d is given in divided doses.

In the past, alcohol injection of the affected nerve, rhizotomy, or tractotomy was recommended if pharmacologic treatment was unsuccessful. More recently, however, posterior fossa exploration has frequently revealed some structural cause for the neuralgia (despite normal findings on CT scans, MRI, or arteriograms), such as an anomalous artery or vein impinging on the trigeminal nerve root. In such cases, simple decompression and separation of the anomalous vessel from the nerve root produce lasting relief of symptoms. In elderly patients with a limited life expectancy, radiofrequency rhizotomy is sometimes preferred because it is easy to perform, has few complications, and provides symptomatic relief for a period of time. Gamma radiosurgery to the trigeminal root is another noninvasive approach that appears to be successful in 80% of patients, with essentially no side effects other than facial paresthesias in a few instances. Surgical exploration generally reveals no

abnormality and is inappropriate in patients with trigeminal neuralgia due to multiple sclerosis.

Bennetto L et al. Trigeminal neuralgia and its management. BMJ. 2007 Jan 27;334(7586):201–5. [PMID: 17255614]
Gronseth G et al. Practice Parameter: the diagnostic evaluation and treatment of trigeminal neuralgia (an evidence-based review). Report of the Quality Standards Subcommittee of the American Academy of Neurology and the European Federation of Neurological Societies. Neurology. 2008 Oct 7;71(15):1183–90. [PMID: 18716236]

2. Atypical Facial Pain

Facial pain without the typical features of trigeminal neuralgia is generally a constant, often burning pain that may have a restricted distribution at its onset but soon spreads to the rest of the face on the affected side and sometimes involves the other side, the neck, or the back of the head as well. The disorder is especially common in middle-aged women, many of them depressed, but it is not clear whether depression is the cause of or a reaction to the pain. Simple analgesics should be given a trial, as should tricyclic antidepressants, carbamazepine, oxcarbazepine, and phenytoin; the response is often disappointing. Opioid analgesics pose a danger of addiction in patients with this disorder. Attempts at surgical treatment are not indicated.

3. Glossopharyngeal Neuralgia

Glossopharyngeal neuralgia is an uncommon disorder in which pain similar in quality to that in trigeminal neuralgia occurs in the throat, about the tonsillar fossa, and sometimes deep in the ear and at the back of the tongue. The pain may be precipitated by swallowing, chewing, talking, or yawning and is sometimes accompanied by syncope. In most instances, no underlying structural abnormality is present; multiple sclerosis is sometimes responsible. Oxcarbazepine and carbamazepine (see Table 24–3) are the treatments of choice and should be tried before any surgical procedures are considered. Microvascular decompression is generally preferred over destructive surgical procedures such as partial rhizotomy in medically refractory cases and is often effective without causing severe complications.

4. Postherpetic Neuralgia

Herpes zoster (shingles) is due to infection of the nervous system by varicella-zoster virus. About 15% of patients who develop shingles suffer from postherpetic neuralgia. This complication seems especially likely to occur in the elderly, when the rash is severe, and when the first division of the trigeminal nerve is affected. It also relates to the duration of the rash before medical consultation. A history of shingles and the presence of cutaneous scarring resulting from shingles aid in the diagnosis. Severe pain with shingles correlates with the intensity of postherpetic symptoms.

The incidence of postherpetic neuralgia may be reduced by the treatment of shingles with oral acyclovir or famciclovir, but this is disputed; systemic corticosteroids do not help. Zoster vaccine markedly reduces morbidity from herpes zoster and postherpetic neuralgia among older adults. Management of the established complication is essentially medical. If simple analgesics fail to help, a trial of a tricyclic antidepressant (eg, amitriptyline, up to 100–150 mg/d) in conjunction with a phenothiazine (eg, perphenazine, 2–8 mg/d) is often effective. Other patients respond to carbamazepine (up to 1200 mg/d), phenytoin (300 mg/d), gabapentin (up to 3600 mg/d), or pregabalin (up to 300 mg/d). A combination of gabapentin and morphine taken orally may provide better analgesia at lower doses of each agent than either taken alone. Topical application of capsaicin cream (eg, Zostrix, 0.025%) is sometimes helpful, perhaps because of depletion of pain-mediating peptides from peripheral sensory neurons, and topical lidocaine (5%) is also worthy of trial. The administration of live-attenuated zoster vaccine to patients over the age of 60 years is important in preventing the occurrence of herpes zoster and thus of postherpetic neuralgia.

He L et al. Corticosteroids for preventing postherpetic neuralgia. Cochrane Database Syst Rev. 2008 Jan 23;(1):CD005582. [PMID: 18254083]

Johnson RW et al. Postherpetic neuralgia: epidemiology, pathophysiology and management. Expert Rev Neurother. 2007 Nov;7(11):1581–95. [PMID: 17997705]

Oxman MN et al. Vaccination against herpes zoster and postherpetic neuralgia. J Infect Dis. 2008 Mar 1;197(Suppl 2):S228–36. [PMID: 18419402]

5. Facial Pain Due to Other Causes

Facial pain may be caused by temporomandibular joint dysfunction in patients with malocclusion, abnormal bite, or faulty dentures. There may be tenderness of the masticatory muscles, and an association between pain onset and jaw movement is sometimes noted. This pattern differs from that of jaw (masticatory) claudication, a symptom of giant cell arteritis, in which pain develops progressively with mastication. Treatment of the underlying joint dysfunction relieves symptoms.

A relationship of facial pain to chewing or temperature changes may suggest a dental disturbance. The cause is sometimes not obvious, and diagnosis requires careful dental examination and radiographs. Sinusitis and ear infections causing facial pain are usually recognized by the history of respiratory tract infection, fever, and, in some instances, aural discharge. There may be localized tenderness. Radiologic evidence of sinus infection or mastoiditis is confirmatory.

Glaucoma is an important ocular cause of facial pain, usually localized to the periorbital region.

On occasion, pain in the jaw may be the principal manifestation of angina pectoris. Precipitation by exertion and radiation to more typical areas establish the cardiac origin.

▶ When to Refer

- Worsening pain unresponsive to simple measures.
- Continuing pain of uncertain cause.
- For consideration of surgical treatment (trigeminal or glossopharyngeal neuralgia).

EPILEPSY

 ESSENTIALS OF DIAGNOSIS

▶ Recurrent seizures.

▶ Characteristic electroencephalographic changes accompany seizures.

▶ Mental status abnormalities or focal neurologic symptoms may persist for hours postictally.

▶ General Considerations

The term "epilepsy" denotes any disorder characterized by recurrent unprovoked seizures. A seizure is a transient disturbance of cerebral function due to an abnormal paroxysmal neuronal discharge in the brain. Epilepsy is common, affecting approximately 0.5% of the population in the United States.

▶ Etiology

Epilepsy has several causes. Its most likely cause in individual patients relates to the age at onset.

A. Idiopathic or Constitutional Epilepsy

Seizures usually begin between 5 and 20 years of age but may start later in life. No specific cause can be identified, and there is no other neurologic abnormality.

B. Symptomatic Epilepsy

There are many causes for recurrent seizures.

1. Pediatric age groups—Congenital abnormalities and perinatal injuries may result in seizures presenting in infancy or childhood.

2. Metabolic disorders—Withdrawal from alcohol or drugs is a common cause of recurrent seizures, and other metabolic disorders such as uremia and hypoglycemia or hyperglycemia may also be responsible. Since these seizures are provoked by a readily reversible cause, this would not be considered as epilepsy.

3. Trauma—Trauma is an important cause of seizures at any age, but especially in young adults. Posttraumatic epilepsy is more likely to develop if the dura mater was penetrated and generally becomes manifest within 2 years following the injury. However, seizures developing in the first week after head injury do not necessarily imply that future attacks will occur. There is no clear evidence that prophylactic anticonvulsant drug treatment reduces the incidence of posttraumatic epilepsy.

4. Tumors and other space-occupying lesions—Neoplasms may lead to seizures at any age, but they are an especially important cause of seizures in middle and later life, when the incidence of neoplastic disease increases. The seizures are commonly the initial symptoms of the tumor and often are partial (focal) in character. They are most likely to occur with structural lesions involving the frontal, parietal, or temporal regions. Tumors must be excluded by appropriate imaging studies in all patients with onset of seizures after 30 years of age, focal seizures or signs, or a progressive seizure disorder.

5. Vascular diseases—Vascular diseases become increasingly frequent causes of seizures with advancing age and are the most common cause of seizures with onset at age 60 years or older.

6. Degenerative disorders—Alzheimer disease and other degenerative disorders are a cause of seizures in later life.

7. Infectious diseases—Infectious diseases must be considered in all age groups as potentially reversible causes of seizures. Seizures may occur with an acute infective or inflammatory illness, such as bacterial meningitis or herpes encephalitis, or in patients with more longstanding or chronic disorders such as neurosyphilis or cerebral cysticercosis. In patients with AIDS, they may result from central nervous system toxoplasmosis, cryptococcal meningitis, secondary viral encephalitis, or other infective complications. Seizures are a common sequela of supratentorial brain abscess, developing most frequently in the first year after treatment.

▶ Classification of Seizures

Seizures can be categorized in various ways, but the descriptive classification proposed by the International League Against Epilepsy is clinically the most useful. Seizures are divided into those that are generalized and those affecting only part of the brain (partial seizures) (Table 24–2).

A. Partial Seizures

The initial clinical and electroencephalographic manifestations of partial seizures indicate that only a restricted part of one cerebral hemisphere has been activated. The ictal manifestations depend on the area of the brain involved. Partial seizures are subdivided into simple seizures, in which consciousness is preserved, and complex seizures, in which it is impaired. Partial seizures of either type sometimes become secondarily generalized, leading to a tonic, clonic, or tonic-clonic attack.

1. Simple partial seizures—Simple seizures may be manifested by focal motor symptoms (convulsive jerking) or somatosensory symptoms (eg, paresthesias or tingling) that spread (or "march") to different parts of the limb or body depending on their cortical representation. In other instances, special sensory symptoms (eg, light flashes or buzzing) indicate involvement of visual, auditory, olfactory, or gustatory regions of the brain, or there may be autonomic symptoms or signs (eg, abnormal epigastric sensations, sweating, flushing, pupillary dilation). The sole manifestations of some seizures are phenomena such as dysphasia, dysmnesic symptoms (eg, déjà vu, jamais vu), affective disturbances, illusions, or structured hallucinations, but such symptoms are usually accompanied by impairment of consciousness.

2. Complex partial seizures—Impaired consciousness may be preceded, accompanied, or followed by the psychic symptoms mentioned above, and automatisms may occur. Such seizures may also begin with some of the other simple symptoms mentioned above.

Table 24–2. Seizure classification.

Seizure Type	Key Features	Other Associated Features
Partial seizures	Involvement of only restricted part of brain; may become secondarily generalized	
Simple partial	Consciousness preserved	May be manifested by focal motor, sensory, or autonomic symptoms
Complex partial	Consciousness impaired	Above symptoms may precede, accompany, or follow
Generalized seizures	Diffuse involvement of brain at onset	
Absence (petit mal)	Consciousness impaired briefly; patient often unaware of attacks	May be clonic, tonic, or atonic components (ie, loss of postural tone); autonomic components (eg, enuresis); or accompanying automatisms Almost always begin in childhood and frequently cease by age 20
Atypical absences	May be more gradual in onset and termination than typical absence	More marked changes in tone may occur
Myoclonic	Single or multiple myoclonic jerks	
Tonic-clonic (grand mal)	Tonic phase: Sudden loss of consciousness, with rigidity and arrest of respiration, lasting < 1 minute Clonic phase: Jerking occurs, usually for < 2–3 minutes Flaccid coma: Variable duration	May be accompanied by tongue biting, incontinence, or aspiration; commonly followed by postictal confusion variable in duration
Status epilepticus	Repeated seizures without recovery between them; a fixed and enduring epileptic condition lasting 30 minutes	

B. Generalized Seizures

There are several different varieties of generalized seizures, as outlined below. In some circumstances, seizures cannot be classified because of incomplete information or because they do not fit into any category.

1. Absence (petit mal) seizures—These are characterized by impairment of consciousness, sometimes with mild clonic, tonic, or atonic components (ie, reduction or loss of postural tone), autonomic components (eg, enuresis), or accompanying automatisms. Onset and termination of attacks are abrupt. If attacks occur during conversation, the patient may miss a few words or may break off in mid sentence for a few seconds. The impairment of external awareness is so brief that the patient is unaware of it. Absence seizures almost always begin in childhood and frequently cease by the age of 20 years, although occasionally they are then replaced by other forms of generalized seizure. Electroencephalographically, such attacks are associated with bursts of bilaterally synchronous and symmetric 3-Hz spike-and-wave activity. A normal background in the electroencephalogram and normal or above-normal intelligence imply a good prognosis for the ultimate cessation of these seizures.

2. Atypical absences—There may be more marked changes in tone, or attacks may have a more gradual onset and termination than in typical absences. They commonly occur in patients with multiple seizure types, may be accompanied by developmental delay or mental retardation, and are associated with slower spike-wave discharges than those in typical absence attacks.

3. Myoclonic seizures—Myoclonic seizures consist of single or multiple myoclonic jerks.

4. Tonic-clonic (grand mal) seizures—In these seizures, which are characterized by sudden loss of consciousness, the patient becomes rigid and falls to the ground, and respiration is arrested. This tonic phase, which usually lasts for less than a minute, is followed by a clonic phase in which there is jerking of the body musculature that may last for 2 or 3 minutes and is then followed by a stage of flaccid coma. During the seizure, the tongue or lips may be bitten, urinary or fecal incontinence may occur, and the patient may be injured. Immediately after the seizure, the patient may either recover consciousness, drift into sleep, have a further convulsion without recovery of consciousness between the attacks (**status epilepticus**), or after recovering consciousness have a further convulsion (**serial seizures**). In other cases, patients will behave in an abnormal fashion in the immediate postictal period, without subsequent awareness or memory of events (**postepileptic automatism**). Headache, disorientation, confusion, drowsiness, nausea, soreness of the muscles, or some combination of these symptoms commonly occurs postictally.

5. Tonic, clonic, or atonic seizures—Loss of consciousness may occur with either the tonic or clonic accompaniments described above, especially in children. Atonic seizures (**epileptic drop attacks**) have also been described.

▶ Clinical Findings

A. Symptoms and Signs

Nonspecific changes such as headache, mood alterations, lethargy, and myoclonic jerking alert some patients to an impending seizure hours before it occurs. These prodromal symptoms are distinct from the aura which may precede a generalized seizure by a few seconds or minutes and which is itself a part of the attack, arising locally from a restricted region of the brain.

In most patients, seizures occur unpredictably at any time and without any relationship to posture or ongoing activities. Occasionally, however, they occur at a particular time (eg, during sleep) or in relation to external precipitants such as lack of sleep, missed meals, emotional stress, menstruation, alcohol ingestion (or alcohol withdrawal; see below), or use of certain drugs. Fever and nonspecific infections may also precipitate seizures in known epileptics. In a few patients, seizures are provoked by specific stimuli such as flashing lights or a flickering television set (**photosensitive epilepsy**), music, or reading.

Clinical examination between seizures shows no abnormality in patients with idiopathic epilepsy, but in the immediate postictal period, extensor plantar responses may be seen. The presence of lateralized or focal signs postictally suggests that seizures may have a focal origin. In patients with symptomatic epilepsy, the findings on examination will reflect the underlying cause.

B. Imaging

MRI is indicated for patients with focal neurologic symptoms or signs, focal seizures, or electroencephalographic findings of a focal disturbance; some clinicians routinely order imaging studies for all patients with new-onset seizure disorders. Such studies should certainly be performed in patients with clinical evidence of a progressive disorder and in those presenting with new onset of seizures after the age of 20 years, because of the possibility of an underlying neoplasm. A chest radiograph should also be obtained in such patients, since the lungs are a common site for primary or secondary neoplasms.

C. Laboratory and Other Studies

Initial investigations should always include a full blood count, blood glucose determination, liver and kidney function tests, and serologic tests for syphilis. The hematologic and biochemical screening tests are important both in excluding various causes of seizures and in providing a baseline for subsequent monitoring of long-term effects of treatment.

Electroencephalography may support the clinical diagnosis of epilepsy (by demonstrating paroxysmal abnormalities containing spikes or sharp waves), may provide a guide to prognosis, and may help classify the seizure disorder. Classification of the disorder is important for determining the most appropriate anticonvulsant drug with which to start treatment. For example, absence (petit mal) and complex partial seizures may be difficult to distinguish clinically, but the electroencephalographic findings and treatment of choice differ in these two conditions. Finally, by localizing the epileptogenic source, the electroencephalographic findings are important in evaluating candidates for surgical treatment.

▶ Differential Diagnosis

The distinction between the various disorders likely to be confused with generalized seizures is usually made on the basis of the history. The importance of obtaining an eyewitness account of the attacks cannot be overemphasized.

A. Differential Diagnosis of Partial Seizures

1. Transient ischemic attacks—These attacks are distinguished from seizures by their longer duration, lack of spread, and symptoms. Level of consciousness, which is unaltered, does not distinguish them. There is a loss of motor or sensory function (eg, weakness or numbness) with transient ischemic attacks, whereas positive symptoms (eg, convulsive jerking or paresthesias) characterize seizures.

2. Rage attacks—Rage attacks are usually situational and lead to goal-directed aggressive behavior.

3. Panic attacks—These may be hard to distinguish from simple or complex partial seizures unless there is evidence of psychopathologic disturbances between attacks and the attacks have a clear relationship to external circumstances.

B. Differential Diagnosis of Generalized Seizures

1. Syncope—Syncopal episodes usually occur in relation to postural change, emotional stress, instrumentation, pain, or straining. They are typically preceded by pallor, sweating, nausea, and malaise and lead to loss of consciousness accompanied by flaccidity; recovery occurs rapidly with recumbency, and there is no postictal headache or confusion. In some instances, however, motor accompaniments may simulate a seizure. Serum creatine kinase measured about 3 hours after the event is generally normal after syncopal episodes but markedly elevated after tonic-clonic seizures.

2. Cardiac dysrhythmias—Cerebral hypoperfusion due to a disturbance of cardiac rhythm should be suspected in patients with known cardiac or vascular disease or in elderly patients who present with episodic loss of consciousness. Prodromal symptoms are typically absent. A relationship of attacks to physical activity and the finding of a systolic murmur is suggestive of aortic stenosis. Repeated Holter monitoring may be necessary to establish the diagnosis; monitoring initiated by the patient ("event monitor") may be valuable if the disturbances of consciousness are rare.

3. Brainstem ischemia—Loss of consciousness is preceded or accompanied by other brainstem signs. Basilar artery migraine and vertebrobasilar vascular disease are discussed elsewhere in this chapter.

4. Pseudoseizures—The term "pseudoseizures" is used to denote both hysterical conversion reactions and attacks due to malingering when these simulate epileptic seizures.

Many patients with pseudoseizures also have true seizures or a family history of epilepsy. Although pseudoseizures tend to occur at times of emotional stress, this may also be the case with true seizures.

Clinically, the attacks superficially resemble tonic-clonic seizures, but there may be obvious preparation before pseudoseizures occur. Moreover, there is usually no tonic phase; instead, there is an asynchronous thrashing of the limbs, which increases if restraints are imposed and which rarely leads to injury. Consciousness may be normal or "lost," but in the latter context the occurrence of goal-directed behavior or of shouting, swearing, etc, indicates that it is feigned. Postictally, there are no changes in behavior or neurologic findings.

Laboratory studies may aid in recognition of pseudoseizures. There are no electrocerebral changes, whereas the electroencephalogram changes during organic seizures accompanied by loss of consciousness. The serum level of prolactin has been found to increase dramatically between 15 and 30 minutes after a tonic-clonic convulsion in most patients, whereas it is unchanged after a pseudoseizure. Serum creatine kinase levels also increase after convulsions but not pseudoseizures.

▶ Treatment

A. General Measures

For patients with epilepsy, drug treatment is prescribed with the goal of preventing further attacks and is usually continued until there have been no seizures for at least 3 years. Epileptic patients should be advised to avoid situations that could be dangerous or life-threatening if further seizures should occur. State legislation may require clinicians to report to the state department of public health any patients with seizures or other episodic disturbances of consciousness.

1. Choice of medication—The drug with which treatment is best initiated depends on the type of seizures to be treated (Table 24–3). The dose of the selected drug is gradually increased until seizures are controlled or side effects prevent further increases. If seizures continue despite treatment at the maximal tolerated dose, a second drug is added and the dose increased depending on tolerance; the first drug is then gradually withdrawn. In treatment of partial and secondarily generalized tonic-clonic seizures, the success rate is higher with carbamazepine, phenytoin, or valproic acid than with phenobarbital or primidone. Gabapentin, topiramate, lamotrigine, oxcarbazepine, levetiracetam, and zonisamide are newer antiepileptic drugs that are effective for partial or secondarily generalized seizures. Felbamate is also effective for such seizures but, because it may cause aplastic anemia or fulminant hepatic failure, should be used only in selected patients unresponsive to other measures. Tiagabine is another adjunctive agent for partial seizures. Valproate is better tolerated than topiramate and more efficacious than lamotrigine and is thus preferred for many patients with generalized or unclassified seizures, but its teratogenic potential makes its use undesirable in women of childbearing age.

Table 24–3. Drug treatment for seizures in adults.

Drug	Usual Adult Daily Dose	Minimum No. of Daily Doses	Time to Steady State Drug Levels	Optimal Drug Level	Selected Side Effects and Idiosyncratic Reactions
Generalized tonic-clonic (grand mal) or partial (focal) seizures					
Phenytoin	200–400 mg	1	5–10 days	10–20 mcg/mL	Nystagmus, ataxia, dysarthria, sedation, confusion, gingival hyperplasia, hirsutism, megaloblastic anemia, blood dyscrasias, skin rashes, fever, systemic lupus erythematosus, lymphadenopathy, peripheral neuropathy, dyskinesias.
Carbamazepine (extended-release formulation)	600–1200 mg	2–3 (2)	3–4 days	4–8 mcg/mL	Nystagmus, dysarthria, diplopia, ataxia, drowsiness, nausea, blood dyscrasias, hepatotoxicity, hyponatremia. May exacerbate myoclonic seizures.
Valproic acid	1500–2000 mg	2–3	2–4 days	50–100 mcg/mL	Nausea, vomiting, diarrhea, drowsiness, alopecia, weight gain, hepatotoxicity, thrombocytopenia, tremor, pancreatitis.
Phenobarbital	100–200 mg	1	14–21 days	10–40 mcg/mL	Drowsiness, nystagmus, ataxia, skin rashes, learning difficulties, hyperactivity.
Primidone	750–1500 mg	3	4–7 days	5–15 mcg/mL	Sedation, nystagmus, ataxia, vertigo, nausea, skin rashes, megaloblastic anemia, irritability.
Lamotrigine[1,2,5]	100–500 mg	2	4–5 days	?	Sedation, skin rash, visual disturbances, dyspepsia, ataxia.
Topiramate[1-4]	200–400 mg	2	4 days	?	Somnolence, nausea, dyspepsia, irritability, dizziness, ataxia, nystagmus, diplopia, glaucoma, renal calculi, weight loss, hypohidrosis, hyperthermia.
Oxcarbazepine[1,3]	900–1800 mg	2	2–3 days	?	As for carbamazepine.
Levetiracetam[1,2]	1000–3000 mg	2	2 days	?	Somnolence, ataxia, headache, behavioral changes.
Zonisamide[1]	200–600 mg	1	10 days	?	Somnolence, ataxia, anorexia, nausea, vomiting, rash, confusion, renal calculi. Do not use in patients with sulfonamide allergy.
Tiagabine[1]	32–56 mg	2	2 days	?	Somnolence, anxiety, dizziness, poor concentration, tremor, diarrhea.
Pregabalin[1]	150–300 mg	2	2–4 days	?	Somnolence, dizziness, poor concentration, weight gain, thrombocytopenia, skin rashes, anaphylactoid reactions.
Gabapentin[1]	900–3600 mg	3	1 day	?	Sedation, fatigue, ataxia, nystagmus, weight loss.
Felbamate[1,3,6]	1200–3600 mg	3	4–5 days	?	Anorexia, nausea, vomiting, headache, insomnia, weight loss, dizziness, hepatotoxicity, aplastic anemia.
Absence (petit mal) seizures					
Ethosuximide	100–1500 mg	2	5–10 days	40–100 mcg/mL	Nausea, vomiting, anorexia, headache, lethargy, unsteadiness, blood dyscrasias, systemic lupus erythematosus, urticaria, pruritus.
Valproic acid	1500–2000 mg	3	2–4 days	50–100 mcg/mL	See above.
Clonazepam	0.04–0.2 mg/kg	2	?	20–80 ng/mL	Drowsiness, ataxia, irritability, behavioral changes, exacerbation of tonic-clonic seizures.
Myoclonic seizures					
Valproic acid	1500–2000 mg	3	2–4 days	50–100 mcg/mL	See above.
Clonazepam	0.04–0.2 mg/kg	2	?	20–80 ng/mL	See above.

[1]Approved as adjunctive therapy for partial-onset seizures.
[2]Approved as adjunctive therapy for primary generalized tonic-clonic seizures.
[3]Approved as initial monotherapy for partial-onset seizures.
[4]Approved as initial monotherapy for primary generalized tonic-clonic seizures.
[5]Approved as monotherapy (after conversion from another drug) in partial-onset seizures.
[6]Not to be used as a first-line drug; when used, blood counts should be performed regularly (every 2–4 weeks). Should be used only in selected patients because of risk of aplastic anemia and hepatic failure. It is advisable to obtain written informed consent before use.

Phenytoin, phenobarbital, and carbamazepine are also potentially teratogenic. The teratogenicity of the newer antiseizure medications is less clear, although there is evidence that lamotrigine, oxcarbazepine, and topiramate may be teratogenic. In most patients with seizures of a single type, satisfactory control can be achieved with a single anticonvulsant drug. Treatment with two drugs may further reduce seizure frequency or severity, but usually only at the cost of greater toxicity. Treatment with more than two drugs is almost always unhelpful unless the patient is having seizures of different types.

2. Monitoring—Monitoring serum drug levels has led to major advances in the management of seizure disorders. The same daily dose of a particular drug leads to markedly different blood concentrations in different patients, and this will affect the therapeutic response. In general, the dose of an antiepileptic agent is increased depending on the clinical response regardless of the serum drug level. The trough drug level is then measured to provide a reference point for the maximum tolerated dose. Dosing should not be based simply on serum levels because many patients require levels that exceed the therapeutic range ("toxic levels") but tolerate these without ill effect. Steady-state drug levels in the blood should be measured after treatment is initiated, dosage is changed, or another drug is added to the therapeutic regimen and when seizures are poorly controlled. Dose adjustments are then guided by the laboratory findings. The most common cause of a lower concentration of drug than expected for the prescribed dose is poor patient compliance. Compliance can be improved by limiting to a minimum the number of daily doses. Recurrent seizures or status epilepticus may result if drugs are taken erratically, and in some circumstances noncompliant patients may be better off without any medication.

All anticonvulsant drugs have side effects, and some of these are shown in Table 24–3.

In most patients, a complete blood count should be performed at least annually because of the risk of anemia or blood dyscrasia. Treatment with certain drugs may require more frequent monitoring or use of additional screening tests. For example, periodic tests of hepatic function are necessary if valproic acid, carbamazepine, or felbamate is used, and serial blood counts are important with carbamazepine, ethosuximide, or felbamate.

3. Discontinuance of medication—Only when adult patients have been seizure-free for 2 years should withdrawal of medication be considered. Unfortunately, there is no way of predicting which patients can be managed successfully without treatment, although seizure recurrence is more likely in patients who initially failed to respond to therapy, those with seizures having focal features or of multiple types, and those with continuing electroencephalographic abnormalities. Dose reduction should be gradual over a period of weeks or months, and drugs should be withdrawn one at a time. If seizures recur, treatment is reinstituted with the same drugs used previously. Seizures are no more difficult to control after a recurrence than before.

4. Surgical treatment—Patients with surgically remediable epilepsy or seizures refractory to pharmacologic management may be candidates for operative treatment, which is best undertaken in specialized centers.

5. Vagal nerve stimulation—Treatment by chronic vagal nerve stimulation for adults and adolescents with medically refractory partial-onset seizures is approved in the United States and provides an alternative approach for patients who are not optimal candidates for surgical treatment. The mechanism of therapeutic action is unknown. Adverse effects consist mainly of transient hoarseness during stimulus delivery.

B. Special Circumstances

1. Solitary seizures—In patients who have had only one seizure, investigation as outlined above should exclude an underlying cause requiring specific treatment. An EEG should also be performed, preferably within 24 hours after the seizure, because the findings may influence management—especially when focal abnormalities are present. Prophylactic anticonvulsant drug treatment is generally not required unless further attacks occur or investigations reveal some underlying pathology that itself is untreatable. The risk of seizure recurrence varies in different series between about 30% and 70%. Epilepsy should not be diagnosed on the basis of a solitary seizure. If seizures occur in the context of transient, nonrecurrent systemic disorders such as acute cerebral anoxia, the diagnosis of epilepsy is inaccurate, and long-term prophylactic anticonvulsant drug treatment is unnecessary.

2. Alcohol withdrawal seizures—One or more generalized tonic-clonic seizures may occur within 48 hours or so of withdrawal from alcohol after a period of high or chronic intake. Patients should be hospitalized for at least 24 hours for observation and to follow the severity of withdrawal symptoms. If the seizures have consistently focal features, the possibility of an associated structural abnormality, often traumatic in origin, must be considered. Head CT scan or MRI should be performed in patients with new onset of generalized seizures and whenever there are focal features associated with any seizures. Treatment with anticonvulsant drugs is generally not required for alcohol withdrawal seizures, since they are self-limited. Benzodiazepines (diazepam or lorazepam) are effective and safe for preventing further seizures. Status epilepticus may rarely follow alcohol withdrawal and is managed along conventional lines (see below). Further attacks will not occur if the patient abstains from alcohol.

3. Tonic-clonic status epilepticus—Poor compliance with the anticonvulsant drug regimen is the most common cause; others include alcohol withdrawal, intracranial infection or neoplasms, metabolic disorders, and drug overdose. The mortality rate may be as high as 20%, and among survivors the incidence of neurologic and mental sequelae may be high. The prognosis relates to the length of time between onset of status epilepticus and the start of effective treatment.

Status epilepticus is a medical emergency. Initial management includes maintenance of the airway and 50% dextrose (25–50 mL) intravenously in case hypoglycemia is responsible. If seizures continue, an intravenous bolus of lorazepam, 4 mg, is given and repeated once after 10 minutes if necessary; alternatively, 10 mg of diazepam is given intravenously over the course of 2 minutes, and the dose is repeated after 10 minutes if necessary. This is usually effective in halting seizures for a brief period but occasionally causes respiratory depression.

Regardless of the response to lorazepam or diazepam, phenytoin (18–20 mg/kg) is given intravenously at a rate of 50 mg/min; this provides initiation of long-term seizure control. The drug is best injected directly but can also be given in saline; it precipitates, however, if injected into glucose-containing solutions. Because arrhythmias may develop during rapid administration of phenytoin, electrocardiographic monitoring is prudent. Hypotension may complicate phenytoin administration, especially if diazepam has also been given. In many countries, injectable phenytoin has been replaced by fosphenytoin, which is rapidly and completely converted to phenytoin following intravenous administration. No dosing adjustments are necessary because fosphenytoin is expressed in terms of phenytoin equivalents (PE); fosphenytoin is less likely to cause reactions at the infusion site, can be given with all common intravenous solutions, and may be administered at a faster rate (150 mg PE/min). It is also more expensive.

If seizures continue, phenobarbital is then given in a loading dose of 10–20 mg/kg intravenously by slow or intermittent injection (50 mg/min). Respiratory depression and hypotension are common complications and should be anticipated; they may occur also with diazepam alone, although less commonly. If these measures fail, general anesthesia with ventilatory assistance and neuromuscular junction blockade may be required. Alternatively, intravenous midazolam may provide control of refractory status epilepticus; the suggested loading dose is 0.2 mg/kg, followed by 0.05–0.2 mg/kg/h.

After status epilepticus is controlled, an oral drug program for the long-term management of seizures is started, and investigations into the cause of the disorder are pursued.

4. Nonconvulsive status epilepticus—Absence (petit mal) and complex partial status epilepticus are characterized by fluctuating abnormal mental status, confusion, impaired responsiveness, and automatism. Electroencephalography is helpful both in establishing the diagnosis and in distinguishing the two varieties. Initial treatment with intravenous diazepam or lorazepam is usually helpful regardless of the type of status epilepticus, but phenytoin, phenobarbital, carbamazepine, and other drugs may also be needed to obtain and maintain control in complex partial status epilepticus.

▶ When to Refer

- Behavioral episodes are of uncertain nature.
- Seizures are difficult to control or have focal features.

- There are accompanying neurologic signs.
- There is a progressive neurologic disorder.

▶ When to Admit

- Status epilepticus.
- For monitoring, when pseudoseizures are suspected.
- If surgery is contemplated.

Adams SM et al. Evaluation of a first seizure. Am Fam Physician. 2007 May 1;75(9):1342–7. [PMID: 17508528]

Chen JW et al. Status epilepticus: pathophysiology and management in adults. Lancet Neurol. 2006 Mar;5(3):246–56. [PMID: 16488380]

Hitiris N et al. Modern antiepileptic drugs: guidelines and beyond. Curr Opin Neurol. 2006 Apr;19(2):175–80. [PMID: 16538093]

French JA et al. Clinical Practice. Initial management of epilepsy. N Engl J Med. 2008 Jul 10; 359(2):166–76. [PMID: 18614784]

Marson AG et al. The SANAD study of effectiveness of valproate, lamotrigine, or topiramate for generalised and unclassifiable epilepsy: an unblinded randomised controlled trial. Lancet. 2007 Mar 24;369(9566):1016–26. [PMID: 17382828]

Meierkord H et al. Non-convulsive status epilepticus in adults: clinical forms and treatment. Lancet Neurol. 2007 Apr;6(4):329–39. [PMID: 17362837]

Spencer S et al. Outcomes of epilepsy surgery in adults and children. Lancet Neurol. 2008 Jun;7(6):525–37. [PMID: 18485316]

DYSAUTONOMIA

 ESSENTIALS OF DIAGNOSIS

▶ Abnormalities of blood pressure or heart rate regulation, sweating, intestinal motility, sphincter control, sexual function, respiration, or ocular function, occurring in isolation or any combination.

▶ General Considerations

Dysautonomia may occur as a result of central or peripheral pathologic processes. It is manifested by a variety of symptoms that may occur in isolation or in various combinations and relate to abnormalities of blood pressure regulation, thermoregulatory sweating, gastrointestinal function, sphincter control, sexual function, respiration, and ocular function. Syncope, a symptom of dysautonomia, is characterized by a transient loss of consciousness, usually accompanied by hypotension and bradycardia. It may occur in response to emotional stress, postural hypotension, vigorous exercise in a hot environment, obstructed venous return to the heart, acute pain or its anticipation, fluid loss, and a variety of other circumstances.

A. Central Neurologic Causes

Disease at certain sites in the central nervous system, regardless of its nature, may lead to dysautonomic symptoms. Postural hypotension, which is usually the most troublesome and disabling symptom, may result from spinal cord transection and other myelopathies (eg, due to tumor or syringomyelia) above the T6 level or from brainstem lesions such as syringobulbia and posterior fossa tumors. Sphincter or sexual disturbances may result from cord lesions below T6. Certain primary degenerative disorders are responsible for dysautonomia occurring in isolation (**pure autonomic failure**) or in association with more widespread abnormalities (**multisystem atrophy** or **Shy-Drager syndrome**) that may include parkinsonian, pyramidal symptoms, and cerebellar deficits.

B. Peripheral Neurologic Causes

A pure autonomic neuropathy may occur acutely or subacutely after a viral infection or as a paraneoplastic disorder related usually to small cell lung cancer, particularly in association with certain antibodies, such as anti-Hu or those directed at neuronal nicotinic acetylcholine receptors. Typically, presenting symptoms include postural hypotension, impaired thermoregulatory sweating, xerostomia or xerophthalmia, abnormal gastrointestinal motility, dilated pupils, or acute urinary retention. Dysautonomia is often conspicuous in patients with Guillain-Barré syndrome, manifesting with marked hypotension or hypertension or cardiac arrhythmias that may have a fatal outcome. It may also occur with diabetic, uremic, amyloidotic, and various other metabolic or toxic neuropathies; in association with leprosy or Chagas disease; and as a feature of certain hereditary neuropathies with autosomal dominant or recessive inheritance or an X-linked pattern. Autonomic symptoms are prominent in the crises of hepatic porphyria. Patients with botulism or the Lambert-Eaton myasthenic syndrome may have constipation, urinary retention, and a sicca syndrome as a result of impaired cholinergic function.

▶ Clinical Findings

A. Symptoms and Signs

Dysautonomic symptoms include syncope, postural hypotension, paroxysmal hypertension, persistent tachycardia without other cause, facial flushing, hypohidrosis or hyperhidrosis, vomiting, constipation, diarrhea, dysphagia, abdominal distention, disturbances of micturition or defecation, apneic episodes, and declining night vision. In syncope, prodromal malaise, nausea, headache, diaphoresis, pallor, visual disturbance, loss of postural tone, and a sense of weakness and impending loss of consciousness are followed by actual loss of consciousness. Although the patient is usually flaccid, some motor activity is not uncommon, and urinary (and rarely fecal) incontinence may also occur, thereby simulating a seizure. Recovery is rapid once the patient becomes recumbent, but headache, nausea, and fatigue are common postictally.

B. Evaluation of the Patient

Clinical evaluation is important to exclude reversible, non-neurologic causes of symptoms. Postural hypotension and syncope, for example, may relate to a reduced cardiac output (eg, from aortic stenosis or cardiomyopathy), paroxysmal cardiac dysrhythmias, volume depletion, various medications, and endocrine and metabolic disorders such as Addi-

son disease, hypothyroidism or hyperthyroidism, pheochromocytoma, and carcinoid syndrome. Testing of autonomic function helps establish the diagnosis of dysautonomia, to exclude other causes of symptoms, to assess the severity of involvement, and to guide prognostication. Such testing includes evaluating the cardiovascular response to the Valsalva maneuver, startle, mental stress, postural change, and deep respiration, and the sudomotor (sweating) responses to warming or a deep inspiratory gasp. Tilt-table testing may reproduce syncopal or presyncopal symptoms. Pharmacologic studies to evaluate the pupillary responses, radiologic studies of the bladder or gastrointestinal tract, uroflowmetry and urethral pressure profiles, and recording of nocturnal penile tumescence may also be necessary in selected cases. Further investigation depends on the presence of other associated neurologic abnormalities. In patients with a peripheral cause, work-up for peripheral neuropathy may be required as discussed below and should include testing for ganglionic acetylcholine receptor antibody. For those with evidence of a central lesion, imaging studies will exclude a treatable structural cause.

▶ Treatment

The most disabling symptom of dysautonomia is usually postural hypotension and syncope. Abrupt postural change, prolonged recumbency, and other precipitants should be avoided. Medications associated with postural hypotension should be discontinued or reduced in dose. Treatment may include wearing waist-high elastic hosiery, salt supplementation, sleeping in a semierect position (which minimizes the natriuresis and diuresis that occur during recumbency), and fludrocortisone (0.1–0.2 mg daily). Vasoconstrictor agents may be helpful and include midodrine (2.5–10 mg three times daily) and ephedrine (15–30 mg three times daily). Other agents that have been used occasionally or experimentally are dihydroergotamine, yohimbine, pyridostigmine, and clonidine; refractory cases may respond to erythropoietin (epoetin alfa) or desmopressin. Patients must be monitored for recumbent hypertension. Postprandial hypotension is helped by caffeine. There is no satisfactory treatment for disturbances of sweating, but an air-conditioned environment is helpful in avoiding extreme swings in body temperature.

▶ When to Refer

- When the diagnosis is uncertain.
- When symptoms persist despite conventional treatment.

Klein CM. Evaluation and management of autonomic nervous system disorders. Semin Neurol. 2008 Apr;28(2):195–204. [PMID: 18351521]

Medow MS et al. Pathophysiology, diagnosis, and treatment of orthostatic hypotension and vasovagal syncope. Cardiol Rev. 2008 Jan–Feb;16(1):4–20. [PMID: 18091397]

SENSORY DISTURBANCES

Patients may complain of either lost or abnormal sensations. The term "numbness" is often used by patients to denote loss of feeling, but the word also has other meanings and the patient's intention must be clarified. Abnormal spontaneous sensations are generally called paresthesias, and unpleasant or painful sensations produced by a stimulus that is usually painless are called dysesthesias.

Sensory symptoms may be due to disease located anywhere along the peripheral or central sensory pathways. The character, site, mode of onset, spread, and temporal profile of sensory symptoms must be established and any precipitating or relieving factors identified. These features—and the presence of any associated symptoms—help identify the origin of sensory disturbances, as do the physical signs as well. Sensory symptoms or signs may conform to the territory of individual peripheral nerves or nerve roots. Involvement of one side of the body—or of one limb in its entirety—suggests a central lesion. Distal involvement of all four extremities suggests polyneuropathy, a cervical cord or brainstem lesion, or—when symptoms are transient—a metabolic disturbance such as hyperventilation syndrome. Short-lived sensory complaints may be indicative of sensory seizures or cerebral ischemic phenomena as well as metabolic disturbances. In patients with cord lesions, there may be a transverse sensory level. "Dissociated sensory loss" is characterized by loss of some sensory modalities with preservation of others. Such findings may be encountered in patients with either peripheral or central disease and must therefore be interpreted in the clinical context in which they are found.

The absence of sensory signs in patients with sensory symptoms does not mean that symptoms have a nonorganic basis. Symptoms are often troublesome before signs of sensory dysfunction have had time to develop.

WEAKNESS & PARALYSIS

Loss of muscle power may result from central disease involving the upper or lower motor neurons; from peripheral disease involving the roots, plexus, or peripheral nerves; from disorders of neuromuscular transmission; or from primary disorders of muscle. The clinical findings help localize the lesion and thus reduce the number of diagnostic possibilities.

Weakness due to upper motor neuron lesions is characterized by selective involvement of certain muscle groups and is associated with spasticity, increased tendon reflexes, and extensor plantar responses. The site of upper motor neuron (pyramidal) involvement may be indicated by the presence of other clinical signs or by the distribution of the motor deficit. Lower motor neuron lesions lead to muscle wasting as well as weakness, with flaccidity and loss of tendon reflexes, but no change in the plantar responses unless the neurons subserving them are directly involved. Fasciculations may be evident over affected muscles. In distinguishing between a root, plexus, or peripheral nerve lesion, the distribution of the motor deficit and of any sensory changes is of particular importance. In patients with disturbances of neuromuscular transmission, weakness is patchy in distribution, often fluctuates over short periods of time, and is not associated with sensory changes. In myopathic disorders, weakness is usually most marked proximally in the limbs, is not associated with sensory loss

or sphincter disturbance, and is not accompanied by muscle wasting or loss of tendon reflexes—at least not until an advanced stage.

TRANSIENT ISCHEMIC ATTACKS

ESSENTIALS OF DIAGNOSIS

▶ Focal neurologic deficit of acute onset.
▶ Clinical deficit resolves completely within 24 hours.
▶ Risk factors for vascular disease often present.

General Considerations

Transient ischemic attacks are characterized by focal ischemic cerebral neurologic deficits that last for less than 24 hours (usually less than 1–2 hours). About 30% of patients with stroke have a history of transient ischemic attacks, and proper treatment of the attacks is an important means of prevention. The incidence of stroke does not relate to either the number or the duration of individual attacks but is increased in patients with hypertension or diabetes. The risk of stroke is highest in the month after a transient ischemic attack (particularly in the first 48 hours) and progressively declines thereafter.

Etiology

An important cause of transient cerebral ischemia is embolization. In many patients with these attacks, a source is readily apparent in the heart or a major extracranial artery to the head, and emboli sometimes are visible in the retinal arteries. Moreover, an embolic phenomenon explains why separate attacks may affect different parts of the territory supplied by the same major vessel. Cardiac causes of embolic ischemic attacks include atrial fibrillation, rheumatic heart disease, mitral valve disease, infective endocarditis, atrial myxoma, and mural thrombi complicating myocardial infarction. Atrial septal defects and patent foramen ovale may permit emboli from the veins to reach the brain ("paradoxical emboli"). An ulcerated plaque on a major artery to the brain may serve as a source of emboli. In the anterior circulation, atherosclerotic changes occur most commonly in the region of the carotid bifurcation extracranially, and these changes may cause a bruit. In some patients with transient ischemic attacks or strokes, an acute or recent hemorrhage is found to have occurred into this atherosclerotic plaque, and this finding may have pathologic significance. Patients with AIDS have an increased risk of developing transient ischemic deficits or strokes.

Less common abnormalities of blood vessels that may cause transient ischemic attacks include fibromuscular dysplasia, which affects particularly the cervical internal carotid artery; atherosclerosis of the aortic arch; inflammatory arterial disorders such as giant cell arteritis, systemic lupus erythematosus, polyarteritis, and granulomatous angiitis; and meningovascular syphilis. Hypotension may cause a reduction of cerebral blood flow if a major extracranial artery to the brain is markedly stenosed, but this is a rare cause of transient ischemic attack.

Hematologic causes of ischemic attacks include polycythemia, sickle cell disease, and hyperviscosity syndromes. Severe anemia may also lead to transient focal neurologic deficits in patients with preexisting cerebral arterial disease.

The **subclavian steal syndrome** may lead to transient vertebrobasilar ischemia. Symptoms develop when there is localized stenosis or occlusion of one subclavian artery proximal to the source of the vertebral artery, so that blood is "stolen" from this artery. A bruit in the supraclavicular fossa, unequal radial pulses, and a difference of 20 mm Hg or more between the systolic blood pressures in the arms should suggest the diagnosis in patients with vertebrobasilar transient ischemic attacks.

► Clinical Findings

A. Symptoms and Signs

The symptoms of transient ischemic attacks vary markedly among patients; however, the symptoms in a given individual tend to be constant in type. Onset is abrupt and without warning, and recovery usually occurs rapidly, often within a few minutes.

If the ischemia is in the carotid territory, common symptoms are weakness and heaviness of the contralateral arm, leg, or face, singly or in any combination. Numbness or paresthesias may also occur either as the sole manifestation of the attack or in combination with the motor deficit. There may be slowness of movement, dysphasia, or monocular visual loss in the eye contralateral to affected limbs. During an attack, examination may reveal flaccid weakness with pyramidal distribution, sensory changes, hyperreflexia or an extensor plantar response on the affected side, dysphasia, or any combination of these findings. Subsequently, examination reveals no neurologic abnormality, but the presence of a carotid bruit or cardiac abnormality may provide a clue to the cause of symptoms.

Vertebrobasilar ischemic attacks may be characterized by vertigo, ataxia, diplopia, dysarthria, dimness or blurring of vision, perioral numbness and paresthesias, and weakness or sensory complaints on one, both, or alternating sides of the body. These symptoms may occur singly or in any combination. Drop attacks due to bilateral leg weakness, without headache or loss of consciousness, may occur, sometimes in relation to head movements.

The natural history of attacks is variable. Some patients will have a major stroke after only a few attacks, whereas others may have frequent attacks for weeks or months without having a stroke. The risk of stroke is high in the first 3 months after an attack, particularly in the first month and especially within the first 48 hours. Attacks may occur intermittently over a long period of time, or they may stop spontaneously. In general, carotid ischemic attacks are more liable than vertebrobasilar ischemic attacks to be followed by stroke. The stroke risk is greater in patients older than 60 years, in diabetics, or after transient ischemic attacks that last longer than 10 minutes and with symptoms or signs of weakness, speech impairment, or gait disturbance.

B. Imaging

CT or MRI scan of the head will exclude the possibility of a small cerebral hemorrhage or a cerebral tumor masquerading as a transient ischemic attack. A number of noninvasive techniques, such as ultrasonography, have been developed for studying the cerebral circulation and imaging the major vessels to the head. Carotid duplex ultrasonography is useful for detecting significant stenosis of the internal carotid artery, but arteriography remains important for demonstrating the status of the cerebrovascular system. MR or CT angiography may reveal stenotic lesions of large vessels but is less sensitive than conventional arteriography. Accordingly, if the findings on CT scan or MRI are normal, if there is no cardiac source of embolization, and if age and general condition indicate that the patient is a good operative risk, bilateral carotid arteriography should be considered in the further evaluation of carotid ischemic attacks, although the ultrasound findings may help in selecting patients for study.

C. Laboratory and Other Studies

Clinical and laboratory evaluation must include assessment for hypertension, heart disease, hematologic disorders, diabetes mellitus, hyperlipidemia, and peripheral vascular disease. It should include complete blood count, fasting blood glucose and serum cholesterol and homocysteine determinations, serologic tests for syphilis, and an ECG and chest radiograph. Echocardiography with bubble contrast is performed if a cardiac source is likely, and blood cultures are obtained if endocarditis is suspected. Holter monitoring is indicated if a transient, paroxysmal disturbance of cardiac rhythm is suspected.

► Differential Diagnosis

Focal seizures usually cause abnormal motor or sensory phenomena such as clonic limb movements, paresthesias, or tingling, rather than weakness or loss of feeling. Symptoms generally spread ("march") up the limb and may lead to a generalized tonic-clonic seizure.

Classic migraine is easily recognized by the visual premonitory symptoms, followed by nausea, headache, and photophobia, but less typical cases may be hard to distinguish. The patient's age and medical history (including family history) may be helpful in this regard. Patients with migraine commonly have a history of episodes since adolescence and report that other family members have a similar disorder.

Focal neurologic deficits may occur during periods of hypoglycemia in diabetic patients receiving insulin or oral hypoglycemic agent therapy.

► Treatment

Hospitalization should be considered for patients seen within 48 hours of their first attack or with crescendo attacks, symptoms lasting for more than 1 hour, symptomatic carotid stenosis, or a known cardiac source of emboli or hypercoagulable state; such hospitalization facilitates early intervention for any recurrence and rapid institution of secondary prevention measures. When arteriography reveals a surgically accessible high-grade stenosis (70–99% in luminal diameter) on the side appropriate to carotid ischemic attacks and there is relatively little atherosclerosis elsewhere in the cerebrovascular system, operative treatment (carotid thromboendarterectomy) reduces the risk of ipsilateral carotid stroke, especially when transient ischemic attacks are of recent onset (< 1 month). Surgery is not indicated for mild stenosis (< 30%); its benefits are unclear with severe stenosis plus diffuse intracranial atherosclerotic disease. See Chapter 12 for additional discussion.

In patients with carotid ischemic attacks who are poor operative candidates (and thus have not undergone arteriography) or who are found to have extensive vascular disease, medical treatment should be instituted. Similarly, patients with vertebrobasilar ischemic attacks are treated medically and are not subjected to arteriography unless there is clinical evidence of stenosis or occlusion in the carotid or subclavian arteries.

Medical treatment is aimed at preventing further attacks and stroke. Cigarette smoking should be stopped, and cardiac sources of embolization, hypertension, diabetes mellitus, hyperlipidemia, arteritis, or hematologic disorders should be treated appropriately. Weight reduction and regular physical activity should be encouraged when appropriate.

A. Embolization from the Heart

If anticoagulants are indicated for the treatment of embolism from the heart, they should be started immediately, provided there is no contraindication to their use. There is no advantage in delay, and the common fear of causing hemorrhage into a previously infarcted area is misplaced, since there is a far greater risk of further embolism to the cerebral circulation if treatment is withheld. Treatment with warfarin sodium is introduced in a daily dose of 5–15 mg orally, depending on the international normalized ratio (INR). Warfarin is more effective than aspirin in reducing the incidence of cardioembolic events, but when its use is contraindicated, aspirin (325 mg daily) may be used in patients with nonrheumatic atrial fibrillation to reduce the risk of stroke.

B. Non-cardioembolic Attacks

In patients with presumed or angiographically verified atherosclerotic changes in the extracranial or intracranial cerebrovascular circulation, antithrombotic medication is prescribed. Platelets adhere to and aggregate around an atherosclerotic plaque and release various substances including thromboxane A_2. Treatment with aspirin significantly reduces the frequency of transient ischemic attacks and the incidence of stroke or myocardial infarcts in high-risk patients. A daily dose of 325 mg is adequate. Aspirin can be combined with sustained-release dipyridamole (200 mg twice daily) for optimal stroke prevention. In patients

intolerant of aspirin, clopidogrel (75 mg) can be used; the combination of clopidogrel and aspirin appears to offer no greater benefit than aspirin alone. Anticoagulant drugs (eg, warfarin, with temporary heparinization until the dose of warfarin is adequate) are not recommended; there is no benefit over antiplatelet therapy and the risk of serious hemorrhagic adverse effects is greater.

Surgical extracranial-intracranial arterial anastomosis is generally not helpful in patients with transient ischemic attacks associated with stenotic lesions of the distal internal carotid or the proximal middle cerebral arteries.

▶ When to Refer

All patients should be referred for urgent investigation and treatment to prevent stroke.

▶ When to Admit

All patients with acute or crescendo transient ischemic attacks should be admitted for urgent investigation and treatment to prevent recurrence or stroke.

Giles MF et al. Risk of stroke early after transient ischaemic attack: a systematic review and meta-analysis. Lancet Neurol. 2007 Dec;6(12):1063–72. [PMID: 17993293]

Hankey GJ. Antiplatelet therapy for the prevention of recurrent stroke and other serious vascular events: a review of the clinical trial data and guidelines. Curr Med Res Opin. 2007 May;23(6):1453–62. [PMID: 17559741]

Johnston SC et al. National Stroke Association guidelines for the management of transient ischemic attacks. Ann Neurol. 2006 Sep;60(3):301–13. [PMID: 16912978]

Kennedy J et al. Fast assessment of stroke and transient ischaemic attack to prevent early recurrence (FASTER): a randomised controlled pilot trial. Lancet Neurol. 2007 Nov;6(11):961–9. [PMID: 17931979]

Rothwell PM et al. Recent advances in management of transient ischaemic attacks and minor ischaemic strokes. Lancet Neurol. 2006 Apr;5(4):323–31. [PMID: 16545749]

STROKE

 ESSENTIALS OF DIAGNOSIS

- ▶ Sudden onset of characteristic neurologic deficit.
- ▶ Patient often has history of hypertension, diabetes mellitus, valvular heart disease, or atherosclerosis.
- ▶ Distinctive neurologic signs reflect the region of the brain involved.

▶ General Considerations

In the United States, stroke remains the third leading cause of death, despite a general decline in the incidence of stroke in the last 30 years. The precise reasons for this decline are uncertain, but increased awareness of risk factors (hypertension, diabetes, hyperlipidemia, cigarette smoking, cardiac disease, AIDS, recreational drug abuse, heavy alcohol consumption, family history of stroke) and improved prophylactic measures and surveillance of those at increased risk have been contributory. Elevation of the blood homo-cysteine level is also a risk factor for stroke, but it is unclear whether this risk is reduced by treatment to lower the level. A previous stroke makes individual patients more suscepti-ble to additional strokes.

For years, strokes have been subdivided pathologically into infarcts (thrombotic or embolic) and hemorrhages, and clinical criteria for distinguishing between these possi-bilities have been emphasized. However, it is often difficult to determine on clinical grounds the pathologic basis for stroke (Table 24–4).

1. Lacunar Infarction

Lacunar infarcts are small lesions (usually < 5 mm in diameter) that occur in the distribution of short penetrat-ing arterioles in the basal ganglia, pons, cerebellum, ante-rior limb of the internal capsule, and, less commonly, the deep cerebral white matter. Lacunar infarcts are associated with poorly controlled hypertension or diabetes and have been found in several clinical syndromes, including con-tralateral pure motor or pure sensory deficit, ipsilateral ataxia with crural paresis, and dysarthria with clumsiness of the hand. The neurologic deficit may progress over 24–36 hours before stabilizing.

Lacunar infarcts are sometimes visible on CT scans as small, punched-out, hypodense areas, but in other patients no abnormality is seen. In some instances, patients with a clinical syndrome suggestive of lacunar infarction are found on CT scanning to have a severe hemispheric infarct.

Early mortality and risk of stroke recurrence is higher for patients with nonlacunar than lacunar infarcts. The prognosis for recovery from the deficit produced by a lacunar infarct is usually good, with partial or complete resolution occurring over the following 4–6 weeks in many instances.

Donnan GA et al. Lacunes and lacunar syndromes. Handb Clin Neurol. 2008;93:559–75. [PMID: 18804668]

2. Cerebral Infarction

Thrombotic or embolic occlusion of a major vessel leads to cerebral infarction. Causes include the disorders predis-posing to transient ischemic attacks (see above) and ath-erosclerosis of cerebral arteries. The resulting deficit depends on the particular vessel involved and the extent of any collateral circulation. Cerebral ischemia leads to release of excitatory and other neuropeptides that may augment calcium flux into neurons, thereby leading to cell death and increasing the neurologic deficit.

▶ **Clinical Findings**

A. Symptoms and Signs

Onset is usually abrupt, and there may then be very little progression except that due to brain swelling. Clinical evaluation should always include examination of the heart and auscultation over the subclavian and carotid vessels to determine whether there are any bruits.

1. Obstruction of carotid circulation—Occlusion of the ophthalmic artery is probably symptomless in most cases because of the rich orbital collaterals, but its transient embolic obstruction can lead to amaurosis fugax—sudden and brief loss of vision in one eye.

Occlusion of the anterior cerebral artery distal to its junction with the **anterior communicating artery** causes weakness and cortical sensory loss in the contralateral leg and sometimes mild weakness of the arm, especially proxi-mally. There may be a contralateral grasp reflex, paratonic rigidity, and abulia (lack of initiative) or frank confusion. Urinary incontinence is not uncommon, particularly if behavioral disturbances are conspicuous. Bilateral anterior cerebral infarction is especially likely to cause marked behavioral changes and memory disturbances. Unilateral anterior cerebral artery occlusion proximal to the junction with the anterior communicating artery is generally well tolerated because of the collateral supply from the other side.

Middle cerebral artery occlusion leads to contralateral hemiplegia, hemisensory loss, and homonymous hemian-opia (ie, bilaterally symmetric loss of vision in half of the visual fields), with the eyes deviated to the side of the lesion. If the dominant hemisphere is involved, global aphasia is also present. It may be impossible to distinguish this clinically from occlusion of the internal carotid artery. With occlusion of either of these arteries, there may also be considerable swelling of the hemisphere, leading to drows-iness, stupor, and coma in extreme cases. Occlusions of different branches of the middle cerebral artery cause more limited findings. For example, involvement of the anterior main division leads to a predominantly expressive dyspha-sia and to contralateral paralysis and loss of sensations in the arm, the face, and, to a lesser extent, the leg. Posterior branch occlusion produces a receptive (Wernicke) aphasia and a homonymous visual field defect. With involvement of the nondominant hemisphere, speech and comprehen-sion are preserved, but there may be a confusional state, dressing apraxia, and constructional and spatial deficits.

2. Obstruction of vertebrobasilar circulation—Occlu-sion of the **posterior cerebral artery** may lead to a thalamic syndrome in which contralateral hemisensory disturbance occurs, followed by the development of spontaneous pain and hyperpathia. There is often a macular-sparing homony-mous hemianopia and sometimes a mild, usually tempo-rary, hemiparesis. Depending on the site of the lesion and the collateral circulation, the severity of these deficits varies and other deficits may also occur, including involuntary movements and alexia. Occlusion of the main artery beyond the origin of its penetrating branches may lead solely to a macular-sparing hemianopia.

Vertebral artery occlusion distally, below the origin of the anterior spinal and posterior inferior cerebellar arteries, may be clinically silent because the circulation is main-tained by the other vertebral artery. If the remaining verte-bral artery is congenitally small or severely atherosclerotic, however, a deficit similar to that of basilar artery occlusion is seen unless there is good collateral circulation from the anterior circulation through the circle of Willis. When the small paramedian arteries arising from the vertebral artery

Table 24–4. Features of the major stroke subtypes.

Stroke Type and Subtype	Clinical Features	Diagnosis	Treatment
Ischemic stroke			
Lacunar infarct	Small (< 5 mm) lesions in the basal ganglia, pons, cerebellum, or internal capsule; less often in deep cerebral white matter; prognosis generally good; clinical features depend on location, but may worsen over first 24-36 hours.	CT may reveal small hypodensity but is often normal.	Aspirin; long-term management is to control risk factors (hypertension and diabetes mellitus).
Carotid circulation obstruction	See text—signs vary depending on occluded vessel.	Noncontrast CT to exclude hemorrhage but findings may be normal during first 6–24 hours of an ischemic stroke; when available, diffusion-weighted MRI plus gradient-echo sequences and FLAIR may also be used; electrocardiography, blood glucose, complete blood count, and tests for hypercoagulable states, hyperlipidemia are indicated; echocardiography or Holter monitoring in selected instances; carotid duplex studies, MR angiography and conventional angiography in selected cases.	Select patients for intravenous thrombolytics or intra-arterial mechanical thrombolysis; aspirin (325 mg/d orally) combined with sustained-release dipyridamole (200 mg twice daily) is first-line therapy; anticoagulation with heparin for cardioembolic strokes when no contraindications exist.
Vertebrobasilar occlusion	See text—signs vary based on location of occluded vessel.	As for carotid circulation obstruction.	As for carotid circulation obstruction.
Hemorrhagic stroke			
Spontaneous intracerebral hemorrhage	Commonly associated with hypertension; also with bleeding disorders, amyloid angiopathy. Hypertensive hemorrhage is located commonly in the basal ganglia and less commonly in the pons, thalamus, cerebellum, or cerebral white matter.	Noncontrast CT is superior to MRI for detecting bleeds of < 48 hours duration; laboratory tests to identify bleeding disorder: angiography may be indicated to exclude aneurysm or AVM. Do not perform lumbar puncture.	Most managed supportively, but cerebellar bleeds or hematomas with gross mass effect may require urgent surgical evacuation.
Subarachnoid hemorrhage	Present with sudden onset of worst headache of life, may lead rapidly to loss of consciousness; signs of meningeal irritation often present; etiology usually aneurysm or AVM, but 20% have no source identified.	CT to confirm diagnosis, but may be normal in rare instances; if CT negative and suspicion high, perform lumbar puncture to look for red blood cells or xanthochromia; angiography to determine source of bleed in candidates for treatment.	See sections on AVM and aneurysm.
Intracranial aneurysm	Most located in the anterior circle of Willis and are typically asymptomatic until subarachnoid bleed occurs; 20% rebleed in first 2 weeks.	CT indicates subarachnoid hemorrhage, and angiography then demonstrates aneurysms; angiography may not reveal aneurysm if vasospasm present.	Prevent further bleeding by clipping aneurysm or coil embolization; nimodipine helps prevent vasospasm; reverse vasospasm by intravenous fluids and induced hypertension after aneurysm has been obliterated, if no other aneurysms are present; angioplasty may also reverse symptomatic vasospasm.
AVMs	Focal deficit from hematoma or AVM itself.	CT reveals bleed, and may reveal the AVM; may be seen by MRI. Angiography demonstrates feeding vessels and vascular anatomy.	Surgery indicated if AVM has bled or to prevent further progression of neurologic deficit; other modalities to treat nonoperable AVMs are available at specialized centers.

AVMs, arteriovenous malformations.

are occluded, contralateral hemiplegia and sensory deficit occur in association with an ipsilateral cranial nerve palsy at the level of the lesion. An obstruction of the **posterior inferior cerebellar artery** or an obstruction of the vertebral artery just before it branches to this vessel leads ipsilaterally to spinothalamic sensory loss involving the face, ninth and tenth cranial nerve lesions, limb ataxia and numbness, and Horner syndrome, combined with contralateral spinothalamic sensory loss involving the limbs.

Occlusion of both **vertebral arteries** or the **basilar artery** leads to coma with pinpoint pupils, flaccid quadriplegia and sensory loss, and variable cranial nerve abnormalities. With partial basilar artery occlusion, there may be diplopia, visual loss, vertigo, dysarthria, ataxia, weakness or sensory disturbances in some or all of the limbs, and discrete cranial nerve palsies. In patients with hemiplegia of pontine origin, the eyes are often deviated to the paralyzed side, whereas in patients with a hemispheric lesion, the eyes commonly deviate from the hemiplegic side.

Occlusion of any of the major **cerebellar arteries** produces vertigo, nausea, vomiting, nystagmus, ipsilateral limb ataxia, and contralateral spinothalamic sensory loss in the limbs. If the superior cerebellar artery is involved, the contralateral spinothalamic loss also involves the face; with occlusion of the anterior inferior cerebellar artery, there is ipsilateral spinothalamic sensory loss involving the face, usually in conjunction with ipsilateral facial weakness and deafness. Massive cerebellar infarction may lead to coma, tonsillar herniation, and death.

3. Coma—Infarction in either the carotid or vertebrobasilar territory may lead to loss of consciousness. For example, an infarct involving one cerebral hemisphere may lead to such swelling that the function of the other hemisphere or the rostral brainstem is disturbed and coma results. Similarly, coma occurs with bilateral brainstem infarction when this involves the reticular formation, and it occurs with brainstem compression after cerebellar infarction.

B. Imaging

Radiography of the chest may reveal cardiomegaly or valvular calcification; the presence of a neoplasm would suggest that the neurologic deficit is due to metastasis rather than stroke, or rarely to nonbacterial thrombotic endocarditis. A CT scan of the head (without contrast) is important in excluding cerebral hemorrhage, but it may not permit distinction between a cerebral infarct and tumor. CT scanning is preferable to MRI in the acute stage because it is quicker and because intracranial hemorrhage is not easily detected by MRI within the first 48 hours after a bleeding episode. In selected patients, carotid duplex studies, MRI and MR angiography, and conventional angiography may also be necessary. Diffusion-weighted MRI is more sensitive than standard MRI in detecting cerebral ischemia.

C. Laboratory and Other Studies

Investigations should include a complete blood count, sedimentation rate, blood glucose determination, and serologic tests for syphilis. Antiphospholipid antibodies (lupus anticoagulants and anticardiolipin antibodies) promote thrombosis and are associated with an increased incidence of stroke. Similarly, elevated serum cholesterol and lipids and serum homocysteine may indicate an increased risk of thrombotic stroke. Electrocardiography will help exclude a cardiac arrhythmia or recent myocardial infarction that might be serving as a source of embolization. Blood cultures should be performed if endocarditis is suspected, echocardiography if heart disease is suspected, and Holter monitoring if paroxysmal cardiac arrhythmia requires exclusion. Examination of the cerebrospinal fluid is not always necessary but may be helpful if there is diagnostic uncertainty; it should be delayed until after CT scanning.

▶ Treatment

Prophylactic measures were considered earlier in discussing transient ischemic attacks. The management of acute stroke should be in a stroke care unit, when feasible. Intravenous thrombolytic therapy with recombinant tissue plasminogen activator (0.9 mg/kg to a maximum of 90 mg, with 10% given as a bolus over 1 minute and the remainder over 1 hour) is effective in reducing the neurologic deficit in selected patients without CT evidence of intracranial hemorrhage when administered within 3 hours after onset of ischemic stroke, but later administration has not been proved effective or safe. Recent hemorrhage, increased risk of hemorrhage (eg, treatment with anticoagulants), arterial puncture at a noncompressible site, and systolic pressure above 185 mm Hg or diastolic pressure above 110 mm Hg are among the contraindications to this treatment. Another approach involves the mechanical removal of an embolus or clot from an occluded cerebral artery using an intra-arterial mechanical thrombolytic device.

Early management of a completed stroke otherwise requires general supportive measures. During the acute stage, there may be marked brain swelling and edema, with symptoms and signs of increasing intracranial pressure, an increasing neurologic deficit, or herniation syndrome. Prednisone (up to 100 mg/d) or dexamethasone (16 mg/d) has been used to reduce vasogenic cerebral edema, but evidence of benefit is conflicting; dehydrating hyperosmolar agents are also of uncertain benefit. Decompressive surgery, however, may be worthwhile for major supratentorial hemispheric stroke. Neither hypercapnia nor hypocapnia has any benefit. Attempts to lower the blood pressure of hypertensive patients during the acute phase (ie, within 2 weeks) of a stroke should generally be avoided, as there is loss of cerebral autoregulation and lowering the blood pressure may further compromise ischemic areas. However, if the systolic pressure exceeds 220 mm Hg, it can be lowered using intravenous labetalol or nicardipine with continuous monitoring to 170–200 mm Hg and then, after 2 weeks, it can be reduced further to less than 140/90 mm Hg.

Anticoagulant drugs should be started when there is a cardiac source of embolization. Treatment is with warfarin. The target is an INR of 2.0–3.0 for the prothrombin time. If the CT scan shows no evidence of hemorrhage and the cerebrospinal fluid is clear, anticoagulant treatment may be started without delay. Physical therapy has an important role in the management of patients with impaired motor function. Passive movements at an early stage will help prevent contractures. As cooperation increases and some recovery begins, active movements will improve strength and coordination. In all cases, early mobilization and active rehabilitation are important. Occupational therapy may improve morale and motor skills, while speech therapy may be beneficial in patients with expressive dysphasia or dysarthria. When there is a severe and persisting motor deficit, a device such as a leg brace, toe spring, frame, or cane may help the patient move about, and the provision of other aids to daily living may improve the quality of life.

Prognosis

The prognosis for survival after cerebral infarction is better than after cerebral or subarachnoid hemorrhage. The only proved effective therapy for acute stroke requires initiation within 3 hours after stroke onset, and the prognosis therefore depends on the time that elapses before arrival at the hospital. Patients receiving such treatment with tissue plasminogen activator are at least 30% more likely to have minimal or no disability at 3 months than those not treated by this means. Loss of consciousness after a cerebral infarct implies a poorer prognosis than otherwise. The extent of the infarct governs the potential for rehabilitation. Patients who have had a cerebral infarct are at risk for additional strokes and for myocardial infarcts. Statin therapy to lower serum lipid levels may reduce this risk. Antiplatelet therapy reduces the recurrence rate by 30% among patients without a cardiac cause for the stroke who are not candidates for carotid endarterectomy. Nevertheless, the cumulative risk of recurrence of noncardioembolic stroke is still 3–7% annually. Treatment with aspirin (325 mg) plus extended-release dipyridamole (200 mg) orally twice daily is as effective as clopidogrel (75 mg) orally once daily in reducing the risk of recurrence.

Patients with massive strokes from which meaningful recovery is unlikely should receive palliative care (see Chapter 5).

When to Refer

All patients should be referred.

When to Admit

All patients should be hospitalized, preferably in a stroke care unit.

Amarenco P et al; Stroke Prevention by Aggressive Reduction in Cholesterol Levels (SPARCL) Investigators. High-dose atorvastatin after stroke or transient ischemic attack. N Engl J Med. 2006 Aug 10;355(6):549–59. [PMID: 16899775]

Donnan GA et al. Stroke. Lancet. 2008 May 10;371(9624):1612–23. [PMID: 18468545]

Edgell R et al. Acute endovascular stroke therapy. Curr Neurol Neurosci Rep. 2006 Nov;6(6):531–8. [PMID: 17074290]

Hankey GJ. Antiplatelet therapy for the prevention of recurrent stroke and other serious vascular events: a review of the clinical trial data and guidelines. Curr Med Res Opin. 2007 May;23(6):1453–62. [PMID: 17559741]

Sacco RL et al. Aspirin and extended-release dipyridamole versus clopidogrel for recurrent stroke. N Engl J Med. 2008 Sep 18;359(12):1238–51. [PMID: 18753638]

van der Worp HB et al. Clinical practice. Acute ischemic stroke. N Engl J Med. 2007 Aug 9;357(6):572–9. [PMID: 17687132]

3. Intracerebral Hemorrhage

Spontaneous intracerebral hemorrhage in patients with no angiographic evidence of an associated vascular anomaly (eg, aneurysm or angioma) is usually due to hypertension. The pathologic basis for hemorrhage is probably the presence of microaneurysms that develop on perforating vessels in hypertensive patients. Hypertensive intracerebral hemorrhage occurs most frequently in the basal ganglia and less commonly in the pons, thalamus, cerebellum, and cerebral white matter. Hemorrhage may extend into the ventricular system or subarachnoid space, and signs of meningeal irritation are then found. Hemorrhages usually occur suddenly and without warning, often during activity.

In addition to its association with hypertension, nontraumatic intracerebral hemorrhage may occur with hematologic and bleeding disorders (eg, leukemia, thrombocytopenia, hemophilia, or disseminated intravascular coagulation), anticoagulant therapy, liver disease, cerebral amyloid angiopathy, high alcohol intake, and primary or secondary brain tumors. There is also an association with advancing age and male sex. Bleeding is primarily into the subarachnoid space when it occurs from an intracranial aneurysm or arteriovenous malformation (see below), but it may be partly intraparenchymal as well. In some cases, no specific cause for cerebral hemorrhage can be identified.

Clinical Findings

A. Symptoms and Signs

With hemorrhage into the cerebral hemisphere, consciousness is initially lost or impaired in about one-half of patients. Vomiting occurs very frequently at the onset of bleeding, and headache is sometimes present. Focal symptoms and signs then develop, depending on the site of the hemorrhage. With hypertensive hemorrhage, there is generally a rapidly evolving neurologic deficit with hemiplegia or hemiparesis. A hemisensory disturbance is also present with more deeply placed lesions. With lesions of the putamen, loss of conjugate lateral gaze may be conspicuous. With thalamic hemorrhage, there may be a loss of upward gaze, downward or skew deviation of the eyes, lateral gaze palsies, and pupillary inequalities.

Cerebellar hemorrhage may present with sudden onset of nausea and vomiting, disequilibrium, headache, and loss of consciousness that may terminate fatally within 48 hours. Less commonly, the onset is gradual and the course episodic or slowly progressive—clinical features suggesting an expanding cerebellar lesion. In yet other cases, however, the onset and course are intermediate, and examination shows lateral conjugate gaze palsies to the side of the lesion; small reactive pupils; contralateral hemiplegia; peripheral facial weakness; ataxia of gait, limbs, or trunk; periodic respiration; or some combination of these findings.

B. Imaging

CT scanning (without contrast) is important not only in confirming that hemorrhage has occurred but also in determining the size and site of the hematoma. It is superior to MRI for detecting intracranial hemorrhage of less than 48 hours duration. If the patient's condition permits further intervention, cerebral angiography may be undertaken thereafter to determine whether an aneurysm or arteriovenous malformation is present (see below).

C. Laboratory and Other Studies

A complete blood count, platelet count, bleeding time, prothrombin and partial thromboplastin times, and liver and kidney function tests may reveal a predisposing cause for the hemorrhage. Lumbar puncture is contraindicated because it may precipitate a herniation syndrome in patients with a large hematoma, and CT scanning is superior in detecting intracerebral hemorrhage.

► Treatment

Neurologic management is generally conservative and supportive, regardless of whether the patient has a profound deficit with associated brainstem compression, in which case the prognosis is grim, or a more localized deficit not causing increased intracranial pressure or brainstem involvement. Such therapy may include ventilatory support, blood pressure regulation, seizure prophylaxis, control of fever, osmotherapy, and nutritional supplementation. Intracranial pressure may require monitoring. Ventricular drainage may be required in patients with intraventricular hemorrhage and acute hydrocephalus. Decompression may be helpful when a superficial hematoma in cerebral white matter is exerting a mass effect and causing incipient herniation. In patients with cerebellar hemorrhage, prompt surgical evacuation of the hematoma is appropriate, because spontaneous unpredictable deterioration may otherwise lead to a fatal outcome and because operative treatment may lead to complete resolution of the clinical deficit. The treatment of underlying structural lesions or bleeding disorders depends on their nature. Hemostatic therapy with recombinant activated factor VII given within a few hours of onset reduces hematoma growth but does not appear to improve survival or functional outcome.

► When to Refer

All patients should be referred.

► When to Admit

All patients should be hospitalized.

Broderick J et al. Guidelines for the management of spontaneous intracerebral hemorrhage in adults: 2007 update: a guideline from the American Heart Association/American Stroke Association Stroke Council, High Blood Pressure Research Council, and the Quality of Care and Outcomes in Research Interdisciplinary Working Group. Circulation. 2007 Oct 16;116(16):e391–413. [PMID: 17938297]

Gurol ME et al. Management of intracerebral hemorrhage. Curr Atheroscler Rep. 2008 Aug;10(4):324–31. [PMID: 18606103]

Mayer SA et al. Efficacy and safety of recombinant activated factor VII for acute intracerebral hemorrhage. N Engl J Med. 2008 May 15;358(20):2127–37. [PMID: 18480205]

4. Subarachnoid Hemorrhage

 ESSENTIALS OF DIAGNOSIS

► Sudden severe headache.
► Signs of meningeal irritation usually present.
► Obtundation is common.
► Focal deficits frequently absent.

► General Considerations

Between 5% and 10% of strokes are due to subarachnoid hemorrhage. Although hemorrhage is usually from rupture of an aneurysm or arteriovenous malformation, no specific cause can be found in 20% of cases.

► Clinical Findings

A. Symptoms and Signs

Subarachnoid hemorrhage has a characteristic clinical picture. Its onset is with sudden headache of a severity never experienced previously by the patient. This may be followed by nausea and vomiting and by a loss or impairment of consciousness that can either be transient or progress inexorably to deepening coma and death. If consciousness is regained, the patient is often confused and irritable and may show other symptoms of an altered mental status. Neurologic examination generally reveals nuchal rigidity and other signs of meningeal irritation, except in deeply comatose patients. A focal neurologic deficit is occasionally present and may suggest the site of the underlying lesion.

B. Imaging

A CT scan (preferably a CT angiogram) should be performed immediately to confirm that hemorrhage has occurred and to search for clues regarding its source. It is preferable to MRI because it is faster and more sensitive in detecting hemorrhage in the first 24 hours. CT findings sometimes are normal in patients with suspected hemorrhage, and the cerebrospinal fluid must then be examined for the presence of blood or xanthochromia before the possibility of subarachnoid hemorrhage is discounted.

Cerebral arteriography may be undertaken to determine the source of bleeding; it is not performed unless or until the patient's condition has stabilized and is good enough so that operative treatment is feasible. In general, bilateral carotid and vertebral arteriography are necessary because aneurysms are often multiple, while arteriovenous malformations may be supplied from several sources. MR angiography may also permit these vascular anomalies to be visualized but is less sensitive than conventional arteriography.

Treatment

All patients should be admitted to hospital and seen by a neurologist. The measures outlined below in the section on stupor and coma are applied to comatose patients. Conscious patients are confined to bed, advised against any exertion or straining, treated symptomatically for headache and anxiety, and given laxatives or stool softeners. If there is severe hypertension, the blood pressure can be lowered gradually, but not below a diastolic level of 100 mm Hg. Phenytoin is generally prescribed routinely to prevent seizures. Further comment concerning the specific operative management of arteriovenous malformations and aneurysms follows.

5. Intracranial Aneurysm

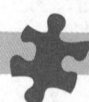

ESSENTIALS OF DIAGNOSIS

▶ Subarachnoid hemorrhage or focal deficit.
▶ Abnormal imaging studies.

General Considerations

Saccular aneurysms ("berry" aneurysms) tend to occur at arterial bifurcations, are frequently multiple (20% of cases), and are usually asymptomatic. They may be associated with polycystic kidney disease and coarctation of the aorta. Risk factors for aneurysm formation include smoking, hypertension, and hypercholesterolemia. Most aneurysms are located on the anterior part of the circle of Willis—particularly on the anterior or posterior communicating arteries, at the bifurcation of the middle cerebral artery, and at the bifurcation of the internal carotid artery.

Clinical Findings

A. Symptoms and Signs

Aneurysms may cause a focal neurologic deficit by compressing adjacent structures. However, most are asymptomatic or produce only nonspecific symptoms until they rupture, at which time subarachnoid hemorrhage results. A higher risk of subarachnoid hemorrhage is associated with older age, female sex, "non-white" ethnicity, hypertension, tobacco smoking, high alcohol consumption (exceeding 150 g per week), previous symptoms, posterior circulation aneurysms, and larger aneurysms. There is often a paucity of focal neurologic signs in patients with subarachnoid hemorrhage, but when present, such signs may relate either to a focal hematoma or to ischemia in the territory of the vessel with the ruptured aneurysm. Hemiplegia or other focal deficit sometimes occurs after a delay of 4–14 days and is due to focal arterial spasm in the vicinity of the ruptured aneurysm. This spasm is of uncertain, probably multifactorial, cause, but it sometimes leads to significant cerebral ischemia or infarction, and it may further aggravate any existing increase in intracranial pressure. Subacute hydrocephalus due to interference with the

flow of cerebrospinal fluid may occur after 2 or more weeks, and this leads to a delayed clinical deterioration that is relieved by shunting.

In some patients, "warning leaks" of a small amount of blood from the aneurysm precede the major hemorrhage by a few hours or days. They lead to headaches, sometimes accompanied by nausea and neck stiffness, but the true cause of these symptoms is often not appreciated until massive hemorrhage occurs.

B. Imaging

The CT scan generally confirms that subarachnoid hemorrhage has occurred, but occasionally it is normal. Angiography (bilateral carotid and vertebral studies) generally indicates the size and site of the lesion, sometimes reveals multiple aneurysms, and may show arterial spasm. CT angiography is becoming increasingly important as a means of evaluating aneurysmal hemorrhage. If subarachnoid hemorrhage is confirmed by lumbar puncture or CT scanning but arteriograms show no abnormality, the examination should be repeated after 2 weeks, because vasospasm may have prevented detection of an aneurysm during the initial study.

C. Laboratory and Other Studies

The cerebrospinal fluid is bloodstained. The electroencephalogram sometimes indicates the side or site of hemorrhage but frequently shows only a diffuse abnormality. Electrocardiographic evidence of arrhythmias or myocardial ischemia has been well described and probably relates to excessive sympathetic activity. Peripheral leukocytosis and transient glycosuria are also common findings.

Treatment

The major aim of treatment is to prevent further hemorrhages. Definitive treatment requires surgical clipping of the aneurysm base or endovascular treatment by interventional radiologists; the latter is sometimes feasible even for inoperable aneurysms. Otherwise, medical management as outlined above for subarachnoid hemorrhage is continued for about 6 weeks and is followed by gradual mobilization.

The risk of further hemorrhage is greatest within a few days of the first hemorrhage; approximately 20% of patients will have further bleeding within 2 weeks and 40% within 6 months. Attempts have been made to reduce this risk pharmacologically. Treatment with an antifibrinolytic agent such as aminocaproic acid during the first 14 days reduces the risk of recurrent hemorrhage but is associated with such an increase in cerebral ischemic complications that the mortality rate and the degree of disability among survivors are unchanged. Thus, early operation (ie, within about 2 days of hemorrhage) is preferred for good operative candidates.

Calcium channel-blocking agents have helped reduce or reverse experimental vasospasm, and nimodipine has been shown to reduce, in neurologically normal patients, the incidence of ischemic deficits from arterial spasm without producing any side effects. The dose of nimodipine is 60 mg every 4 hours orally for 21 days. After surgical obliteration of any aneurysms, symptomatic vasospasm may also be treated by intravascular volume expansion, induced hypertension, or transluminal balloon angioplasty of involved intracranial vessels; aspirin provides no benefit.

With regard to unruptured aneurysms, those that are symptomatic merit prompt treatment, either surgically or by endovascular techniques, whereas small asymptomatic ones discovered incidentally are often monitored arteriographically and corrected only if they increase in size to over 10 mm.

▶ When to Refer

All patients should be referred.

▶ When to Admit

- All patients with a subarachnoid hemorrhage.
- All patients for detailed imaging.
- All patients undergoing surgical or endovascular treatment.

Clarke M. Systematic review of reviews of risk factors for intracranial aneurysms. Neuroradiology. 2008 Aug;50(8):653–64. [PMID: 18560819]

Qureshi AI et al. Comparison of endovascular and surgical treatments for intracranial aneurysms: an evidence-based review. Lancet Neurol. 2007 Sep;6(9):816–25. [PMID: 17706565]

Raja PV et al. Microsurgical clipping and endovascular coiling of intracranial aneurysms: a critical review of the literature. Neurosurgery. 2008 Jun;62(6):1187–202. [PMID: 18824986]

6. Arteriovenous Malformations

ESSENTIALS OF DIAGNOSIS

- ▶ Sudden onset of subarachnoid and intracerebral hemorrhage.
- ▶ Distinctive neurologic signs reflect the region of the brain involved.
- ▶ Signs of meningeal irritation in patients presenting with subarachnoid hemorrhage.
- ▶ Seizures or focal deficits may occur.

▶ General Considerations

Arteriovenous malformations are congenital vascular malformations that result from a localized maldevelopment of part of the primitive vascular plexus and consist of abnormal arteriovenous communications without intervening capillaries. They vary in size, ranging from massive lesions that are fed by multiple vessels and involve a large part of the brain to lesions so small that they are hard to identify at arteriography, surgery, or autopsy. In approximately 10% of cases, there is an associated arterial aneurysm, while 1–2% of patients presenting with aneurysms have associated arteriovenous malformations. Clinical presentation may relate to hemorrhage from the malformation or an associated aneurysm or may relate to cerebral ischemia due to diversion of

blood by the anomalous arteriovenous shunt or due to venous stagnation. Regional maldevelopment of the brain, compression or distortion of adjacent cerebral tissue by enlarged anomalous vessels, and progressive gliosis due to mechanical and ischemic factors may also be contributory. In addition, communicating or obstructive hydrocephalus may occur and lead to symptoms.

▶ Clinical Findings

A. Symptoms and Signs

1. Supratentorial lesions—Most cerebral arteriovenous malformations are supratentorial, usually lying in the territory of the middle cerebral artery. Initial symptoms consist of hemorrhage in 30–60% of cases, recurrent seizures in 20–40%, headache in 5–25%, and miscellaneous complaints (including focal deficits) in 10–15%. Up to 70% of arteriovenous malformations bleed at some point in their natural history, most commonly before the patient reaches the age of 40 years. This tendency to bleed is unrelated to the lesion site or to the patient's sex, but small arteriovenous malformations are more likely to bleed than large ones. Arteriovenous malformations that have bled once are more likely to bleed again. Hemorrhage is commonly intracerebral as well as into the subarachnoid space, and it has a fatal outcome in about 10% of cases. Focal or generalized seizures may accompany or follow hemorrhage, or they may be the initial presentation, especially with frontal or parietal arteriovenous malformations. Headaches are especially likely when the external carotid arteries are involved in the malformation. These sometimes simulate migraine but more commonly are nonspecific in character, with nothing about them to suggest an underlying structural lesion.

In patients presenting with subarachnoid hemorrhage, examination may reveal an abnormal mental status and signs of meningeal irritation. Additional findings may help localize the lesion and sometimes indicate that intracranial pressure is increased. A cranial bruit always suggests the possibility of a cerebral arteriovenous malformation, but bruits may also be found with aneurysms, meningiomas, acquired arteriovenous fistulas, and arteriovenous malformations involving the scalp, calvarium, or orbit. Bruits are best heard over the ipsilateral eye or mastoid region and are of some help in lateralization but of no help in localization. Absence of a bruit in no way excludes the possibility of arteriovenous malformation.

2. Infratentorial lesions—Brainstem arteriovenous malformations are often clinically silent, but they may hemorrhage, cause obstructive hydrocephalus, or lead to progressive or relapsing brainstem deficits. Cerebellar arteriovenous malformations may also be clinically inconspicuous but sometimes lead to cerebellar hemorrhage.

B. Imaging

In patients presenting with suspected hemorrhage, CT scanning indicates whether subarachnoid or intracerebral bleeding has recently occurred, helps localize its source, and may reveal the arteriovenous malformation. If the CT scan shows no evidence of bleeding but subarachnoid hemorrhage is diagnosed clinically, the cerebrospinal fluid should be examined.

When intracranial hemorrhage is confirmed but the source of hemorrhage is not evident on the CT scan, arteriography is necessary to exclude aneurysm or arteriovenous malformation. MR angiography is not sensitive enough for this purpose. Even if the findings on CT scan suggest arteriovenous malformation, arteriography is required to establish the nature of the lesion with certainty and to determine its anatomic features so that treatment can be planned. The examination must generally include bilateral opacification of the internal and external carotid arteries and the vertebral arteries. Arteriovenous malformations typically appear as a tangled vascular mass with distended tortuous afferent and efferent vessels, a rapid circulation time, and arteriovenous shunting. Findings on plain radiographs of the skull are often normal unless an intracerebral hematoma is present, in which case there may be changes suggestive of raised intracranial pressure and displacement of a calcified pineal gland.

In patients presenting without hemorrhage, CT scan or MRI usually reveals the underlying abnormality, and MRI frequently also shows evidence of old or recent hemorrhage that may have been asymptomatic. The nature and detailed anatomy of any focal lesion identified by these means are delineated by angiography, especially if operative treatment is under consideration.

C. Laboratory and Other Studies

Electroencephalography is usually indicated in patients presenting with seizures and may show consistently focal or lateralized abnormalities resulting from the underlying cerebral arteriovenous malformation. This should be followed by CT scanning.

▶ Treatment

Surgical treatment to prevent further hemorrhage is justified in patients with arteriovenous malformations that have bled, provided that the lesion is accessible and the patient has a reasonable life expectancy. Surgical treatment is also appropriate if intracranial pressure is increased and to prevent further progression of a focal neurologic deficit. In patients presenting solely with seizures, anticonvulsant drug treatment is usually sufficient, and operative treatment is unnecessary unless there are further developments.

Definitive operative treatment consists of excision of the arteriovenous malformation if it is surgically accessible. Arteriovenous malformations that are inoperable because of their location are sometimes treated solely by embolization; although the risk of hemorrhage is not reduced, neurologic deficits may be stabilized or even reversed by this procedure. Two other techniques for the treatment of intracerebral arteriovenous malformations are injection of a vascular occlusive polymer through a flow-guided microcatheter and permanent occlusion of feeding vessels by positioning detachable balloon catheters in the desired sites and then inflating them with quickly solidifying contrast material. Stereotactic radiosurgery with the gamma knife or related approaches is also useful in the management of inoperable cerebral arteriovenous malformations.

▶ When to Refer

All patients should be referred.

▶ When to Admit

- All patients with a subarachnoid or cerebral hemorrhage.
- All patients for detailed imaging.
- All patients undergoing surgical or endovascular treatment.

Friedlander RM. Clinical practice. Arteriovenous malformations of the brain. N Engl J Med. 2007 Jun 28;356(26):2704–12. [PMID: 17596605]

Hartmann A et al. Treatment of arteriovenous malformations of the brain. Curr Neurol Neurosci Rep. 2007 Jan;7(1):28–34. [PMID: 17217851]

7. Intracranial Venous Thrombosis

Intracranial venous thrombosis may occur in association with intracranial or maxillofacial infections, hypercoagulable states, polycythemia, sickle cell disease, and cyanotic congenital heart disease and in pregnancy or during the puerperium. It is characterized by headache, focal or generalized convulsions, drowsiness, confusion, increased intracranial pressure, and focal neurologic deficits—and sometimes by evidence of meningeal irritation. The diagnosis is confirmed by CT scanning, MRI, MR venography, or angiography.

Treatment includes anticonvulsant drugs if seizures have occurred and antiedema agents (eg, dexamethasone, 4 mg four times daily and continued as necessary) or other measures to reduce intracranial pressure. Anticoagulation with dose-adjusted intravenous heparin or weight-adjusted subcutaneous low-molecular-weight heparin, followed by oral warfarin anticoagulation for 6 months reduces morbidity and mortality of venous sinus thrombosis. Concomitant intracranial hemorrhage related to the venous thrombosis does not contraindicate heparin therapy. In cases refractory to heparin, endovascular techniques including catheter-directed thrombolytic therapy (urokinase) and thrombectomy, are sometimes helpful.

Masuhr F et al. Treatment of cerebral venous and sinus thrombosis. Front Neurol Neurosci. 2008;23:132–43. [PMID: 18004059]

▶ When to Refer

All patients should be referred.

▶ When to Admit

All patients should be hospitalized.

8. Spinal Cord Vascular Diseases

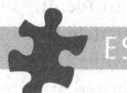

ESSENTIALS OF DIAGNOSIS

- ▶ Sudden onset of back or limb pain and neurologic deficit in limbs.

▶ Motor, sensory, or reflex changes in limbs depending on level of lesion.

▶ Imaging studies distinguish between infarct and hematoma.

Infarction of the Spinal Cord

Infarction of the spinal cord is rare. It typically occurs in the territory of the anterior spinal artery because this vessel, which supplies the anterior two-thirds of the cord, is itself supplied by only a limited number of feeders. Infarction usually results from interrupted flow in one or more of these feeders, eg, with aortic dissection, aortography, polyarteritis, or severe hypotension, or after surgical resection of the thoracic aorta. The paired posterior spinal arteries, by contrast, are supplied by numerous arteries at different levels of the cord. Spinal cord hypoperfusion may lead to a central cord syndrome with distal weakness of lower motor neuron type and loss of pain and temperature appreciation, with preserved posterior column function.

Since the anterior spinal artery receives numerous feeders in the cervical region, infarcts almost always occur caudally. Clinical presentation is characterized by acute onset of flaccid, areflexive paraplegia that evolves after a few days or weeks into a spastic paraplegia with extensor plantar responses. There is an accompanying dissociated sensory loss, with impairment of appreciation of pain and temperature but preservation of sensations of vibration and position. Treatment is symptomatic.

Novy J et al. Spinal cord ischemia: clinical and imaging patterns, pathogenesis, and outcomes in 27 patients. Arch Neurol. 2006 Aug;63(8):1113–20. [PMID: 16908737]

Epidural or Subdural Hemorrhage

Epidural or subdural hemorrhage may lead to sudden severe back pain followed by an acute compressive myelopathy necessitating urgent spinal MRI or myelography and surgical evacuation. It may occur in patients with bleeding disorders or those who are taking anticoagulant drugs, sometimes following trauma or lumbar puncture. Epidural hemorrhage may also be related to a vascular malformation or tumor deposit.

Spinal Dural Arteriovenous Fistulae

Spinal dural arteriovenous fistulae are congenital lesions that present with spinal subarachnoid hemorrhage or myeloradiculopathy. Since most of these malformations are located in the thoracolumbar region, they lead to motor and sensory disturbances in the legs and to sphincter disorders. Pain in the legs or back is often severe. Examination reveals an upper, lower, or mixed motor deficit in the legs; sensory deficits are also present and are usually extensive, although occasionally they are confined to radicular distribution. Cervical spinal dural arteriovenous fistulae lead also to symptoms and signs in the arms. Spinal MRI may not detect the spinal dural arteriovenous fistulae, and negative findings do not exclude the diagno-

sis. Myelography (performed with the patient prone and supine) detects serpiginous filling defects due to enlarged vessels. Selective spinal arteriography confirms the diagnosis. Most lesions are extramedullary, are posterior to the cord (lying either intra- or extradurally), and can easily be treated by ligation of feeding vessels and excision of the fistulous anomaly or by embolization procedures. Delay in treatment may lead to increased and irreversible disability or to death from recurrent subarachnoid hemorrhage.

▶ When to Refer

All patients should be referred.

▶ When to Admit

All patients should be hospitalized.

Narvid J et al. Spinal dural arteriovenous fistulae: clinical features and long-term results. Neurosurgery. 2008 Jan;62(1):159–67. [PMID: 18300903]

INTRACRANIAL & SPINAL TUMORS

1. Primary Intracranial Tumors

ESSENTIALS OF DIAGNOSIS

▶ Generalized or focal disturbance of cerebral function, or both.

▶ Increased intracranial pressure in some patients.

▶ Neuroradiologic evidence of space-occupying lesion.

▶ General Considerations

Half of all primary intracranial neoplasms (Table 24–5) are gliomas and the remainder meningiomas, pituitary adenomas, neurofibromas, and other tumors. Certain tumors, especially neurofibromas, hemangioblastomas, and retinoblastomas, may have a familial basis, and congenital factors bear on the development of craniopharyngiomas. Tumors may occur at any age, but certain gliomas show particular age predilections (Table 24–5).

▶ Clinical Findings

A. Symptoms and Signs

Intracranial tumors may lead to a generalized disturbance of cerebral function and to symptoms and signs of increased intracranial pressure. In consequence, there may be personality changes, intellectual decline, emotional lability, seizures, headaches, nausea, and malaise. If the pressure is increased in a particular cranial compartment, brain tissue may herniate into a compartment with lower pressure. The most familiar syndrome is herniation of the temporal lobe uncus through the tentorial hiatus, which causes compression of the third cranial nerve, midbrain, and posterior cerebral artery. The earliest sign of this is ipsilateral pupillary dilation, followed by stupor, coma, decerebrate postur-

Table 24–5. Primary intracranial tumors.

Tumor	Clinical Features	Treatment and Prognosis
Glioblastoma multiforme	Presents commonly with nonspecific complaints and increased intracranial pressure. As it grows, focal deficits develop.	Course is rapidly progressive, with poor prognosis. Total surgical removal is usually not possible. Radiation therapy and chemotherapy may prolong survival.
Astrocytoma	Presentation similar to glioblastoma multiforme but course more protracted, often over several years. Cerebellar astrocytoma may have a more benign course.	Prognosis is variable. By the time of diagnosis, total excision is usually impossible; tumor may be radiosensitive and chemotherapy may also be helpful. In cerebellar astrocytoma, total surgical removal is often possible.
Medulloblastoma	Seen most frequently in children. Generally arises from roof of fourth ventricle and leads to increased intracranial pressure accompanied by brainstem and cerebellar signs. May seed subarachnoid space.	Treatment consists of surgery combined with radiation therapy and chemotherapy.
Ependymoma	Glioma arising from the ependyma of a ventricle, especially the fourth ventricle; leads to early signs of increased intracranial pressure. Arises also from central canal of cord.	Tumor is best treated surgically if possible. Radiation therapy may be used for residual tumor.
Oligodendroglioma	Slow-growing. Usually arises in cerebral hemisphere in adults. Calcification may be visible on skull radiograph.	Treatment is surgical and usually successful. Radiation and chemotherapy may be used if tumor has malignant features.
Brainstem glioma	Presents during childhood with cranial nerve palsies and then with long tract signs in the limbs. Signs of increased intracranial pressure occur late.	Tumor is inoperable; treatment is by irradiation and shunt for increased intracranial pressure.
Cerebellar hemangioblastoma	Presents with disequilibrium, ataxia of trunk or limbs, and signs of increased intracranial pressure. Sometimes familial. May be associated with retinal and spinal vascular lesions, polycythemia, and renal cell carcinoma.	Treatment is surgical. Radiation is used for residual tumor.
Pineal tumor	Presents with increased intracranial pressure, sometimes associated with impaired upward gaze (Parinaud syndrome) and other deficits indicative of midbrain lesion.	Ventricular decompression by shunting is followed by surgical approach to tumor; irradiation is indicated if tumor is malignant. Prognosis depends on histopathologic findings and extent of tumor.
Craniopharyngioma	Originates from remnants of Rathke pouch above the sella, depressing the optic chiasm. May present at any age but usually in childhood, with endocrine dysfunction and bitemporal field defects.	Treatment is surgical, but total removal may not be possible. Radiation may be used for residual tumor.
Acoustic neurinoma	Ipsilateral hearing loss is most common initial symptom. Subsequent symptoms may include tinnitus, headache, vertigo, facial weakness or numbness, and long tract signs. (May be familial and bilateral when related to neurofibromatosis.) Most sensitive screening tests are MRI and brainstem auditory evoked potential.	Treatment is excision by translabyrinthine surgery, craniectomy, or a combined approach. Outcome is usually good.
Meningioma	Originates from the dura mater or arachnoid; compresses rather than invades adjacent neural structures. Increasingly common with advancing age. Tumor size varies greatly. Symptoms vary with tumor site—eg, unilateral proptosis (sphenoidal ridge); anosmia and optic nerve compression (olfactory groove). Tumor is usually benign and readily detected by CT scanning; may lead to calcification and bone erosion visible on plain radiographs of skull.	Treatment is surgical. Tumor may recur if removal is incomplete.
Primary cerebral lymphoma	Associated with AIDS and other immunodeficient states. Presentation may be with focal deficits or with disturbances of cognition and consciousness. May be indistinguishable from cerebral toxoplasmosis.	Treatment is high-dose methotrexate followed by radiation therapy. Prognosis depends on CD4 count at diagnosis.

ing, and respiratory arrest. Another important herniation syndrome consists of displacement of the cerebellar tonsils through the foramen magnum, which causes medullary compression leading to apnea, circulatory collapse, and death. Other herniation syndromes are less common and of less clear clinical importance.

Intracranial tumors also lead to focal deficits depending on their location.

1. Frontal lobe lesions—Tumors of the frontal lobe often lead to progressive intellectual decline, slowing of mental activity, personality changes, and contralateral grasp reflexes.

They may lead to expressive aphasia if the posterior part of the left inferior frontal gyrus is involved. Anosmia may also occur as a consequence of pressure on the olfactory nerve. Precentral lesions may cause focal motor seizures or contralateral pyramidal deficits.

2. Temporal lobe lesions—Tumors of the uncinate region may be manifested by seizures with olfactory or gustatory hallucinations, motor phenomena such as licking or smacking of the lips, and some impairment of external awareness without actual loss of consciousness. Temporal lobe lesions also lead to depersonalization, emotional changes, behavioral disturbances, sensations of déjà vu or jamais vu, micropsia or macropsia (objects appear smaller or larger than they are), visual field defects (crossed upper quadrantanopia), and auditory illusions or hallucinations. Left-sided lesions may lead to dysnomia and receptive aphasia, while right-sided involvement sometimes disturbs the perception of musical notes and melodies.

3. Parietal lobe lesions—Tumors in this location characteristically cause contralateral disturbances of sensation and may cause sensory seizures, sensory loss or inattention, or some combination of these symptoms. The sensory loss is cortical in type and involves postural sensibility and tactile discrimination, so that the appreciation of shape, size, weight, and texture is impaired. Objects placed in the hand may not be recognized (astereognosis). Extensive parietal lobe lesions may produce contralateral hyperpathia and spontaneous pain (thalamic syndrome). Involvement of the optic radiation leads to a contralateral homonymous field defect that sometimes consists solely of lower quadrantanopia. Lesions of the left angular gyrus cause Gerstmann syndrome (a combination of alexia, agraphia, acalculia, right-left confusion, and finger agnosia), whereas involvement of the left submarginal gyrus causes ideational apraxia. Anosognosia (the denial, neglect, or rejection of a paralyzed limb) is seen in patients with lesions of the nondominant (right) hemisphere. Constructional apraxia and dressing apraxia may also occur with right-sided lesions.

4. Occipital lobe lesions—Tumors of the occipital lobe characteristically produce crossed homonymous hemianopia or a partial field defect. With left-sided or bilateral lesions, there may be visual agnosia both for objects and for colors, while irritative lesions on either side can cause unformed visual hallucinations. Bilateral occipital lobe involvement causes cortical blindness in which there is preservation of pupillary responses to light and lack of awareness of the defect by the patient. There may also be loss of color perception, prosopagnosia (inability to identify a familiar face), simultagnosia (inability to integrate and interpret a composite scene as opposed to its individual elements), and Balint syndrome (failure to turn the eyes to a particular point in space, despite preservation of spontaneous and reflex eye movements). The denial of blindness or a field defect constitutes Anton syndrome.

5. Brainstem and cerebellar lesions—Brainstem lesions lead to cranial nerve palsies, ataxia, incoordination, nystagmus, and pyramidal and sensory deficits in the limbs on one or both sides. Intrinsic brainstem tumors, such as

gliomas, tend to produce an increase in intracranial pressure only late in their course. Cerebellar tumors produce marked ataxia of the trunk if the vermis cerebelli is involved and ipsilateral appendicular deficits (ataxia, incoordination and hypotonia of the limbs) if the cerebellar hemispheres are affected.

6. False localizing signs—Tumors may lead to neurologic signs other than by direct compression or infiltration, thereby leading to errors of clinical localization. These false localizing signs include third or sixth nerve palsy and bilateral extensor plantar responses produced by herniation syndromes, and an extensor plantar response occurring ipsilateral to a hemispheric tumor as a result of compression of the opposite cerebral peduncle against the tentorium.

B. Imaging

CT scanning or MRI with gadolinium enhancement may detect the lesion and may also define its location, shape, and size; the extent to which normal anatomy is distorted; and the degree of any associated cerebral edema or mass effect. CT scanning is less helpful with tumors in the posterior fossa, but MRI is of particular value there. The characteristic appearance of meningiomas on CT scanning is virtually diagnostic, ie, a lesion in a typical site (parasagittal and sylvian regions, olfactory groove, sphenoidal ridge, tuberculum sellae) that appears as a homogeneous area of increased density in noncontrast CT scans and enhances uniformly with contrast. Newer neuroimaging techniques may help identify brain tumors by increased blood perfusion (perfusion-weighted MRI, single photon-emitted computed tomography, positron-emission tomography) and high metabolism or cell turnover (magnetic resonance spectroscopy, positron-emission tomography), but non-neoplastic diseases, such as stroke and inflammatory or infectious diseases, are sometimes associated with hyperperfusion and hypermetabolism. Diffusion-weighted MRI may also be helpful. Arteriography may show stretching or displacement of normal cerebral vessels by the tumor and the presence of tumor vascularity. The presence of an avascular mass is a nonspecific finding that could be due to tumor, hematoma, abscess, or any space-occupying lesion. In patients with normal hormone levels and an intrasellar mass, angiography is necessary to distinguish with confidence between a pituitary adenoma and an arterial aneurysm.

C. Laboratory and Other Studies

The electroencephalogram provides supporting information concerning cerebral function and may show either a focal disturbance due to the neoplasm or a more diffuse change reflecting altered mental status. Lumbar puncture is rarely necessary; the findings are seldom diagnostic, and the procedure carries the risk of causing a herniation syndrome.

► Treatment

Treatment depends on the type and site of the tumor (Table 24–5) and the condition of the patient. Complete surgical removal may be possible if the tumor is extra-axial (eg, meningioma, acoustic neuroma) or is not in a critical or inaccessible region of the brain (eg, cerebellar hemangioblastoma). Surgery also permits the diagnosis to be verified and may be beneficial in reducing intracranial pressure and relieving symptoms even if the neoplasm cannot be completely removed. Clinical deficits are sometimes due in part to obstructive hydrocephalus, in which case simple surgical shunting procedures often produce dramatic benefit. In patients with malignant gliomas, radiation therapy increases median survival rates regardless of any preceding surgery, and its combination with chemotherapy provides additional benefit. Indications for irradiation in the treatment of patients with other primary intracranial neoplasms depend on tumor type and accessibility and the feasibility of complete surgical removal. Corticosteroids help reduce cerebral edema and are usually started before surgery. Herniation is treated with intravenous dexamethasone (10–20 mg as a bolus, followed by 4 mg every 6 hours) and intravenous mannitol (20% solution given in a dose of 1.5 g/kg over about 30 minutes). Anticonvulsants are also commonly administered in standard doses (see Table 24–3) but are not indicated for prophylaxis in patients who have no history of seizures. Long-term neurocognitive deficits may complicate radiation therapy. For those patients whose disease deteriorates despite treatment, palliative care is important (see Chapter 5).

▶ When to Refer

All patients should be referred.

▶ When to Admit

- All patients with increased intracranial pressure.
- All patients requiring biopsy, surgical treatment, or shunting procedures.

Berger MS et al. Surgery of intrinsic cerebral tumors. Neurosurgery. 2007 Jul;61(1 Suppl):279–304. [PMID: 18813160]

Buckner JC et al. Central nervous system tumors. Mayo Clin Proc. 2007 Oct;82(10):1271–86. [PMID: 17908533]

Colman H et al. Molecular predictors in glioblastoma. Arch Neurol. 2008 July; 65(7):877–83. [PMID: 18625854]

Daly FN et al. Supportive management of patients with brain tumors. Expert Rev Neurother. 2007 Oct;7(10):1327–36. [PMID: 17939770]

Omuro AM et al. Pitfalls in the diagnosis of brain tumours. Lancet Neurol. 2006 Nov;5(11):937–48. [PMID: 17052661]

Soffietti R et al. New developments in the treatment of malignant gliomas. Expert Rev Neurother. 2007 Oct;7(10):1313–26. [PMID: 17939769]

Tam Truong M. Current role of radiation therapy in the management of malignant brain tumors. Hematol Oncol Clin North Am. 2006 Apr;20(2):431–53. [PMID: 16730301]

2. Metastatic Intracranial Tumors

Cerebral Metastases

Metastatic brain tumors present in the same way as other cerebral neoplasms, ie, with increased intracranial pressure, with focal or diffuse disturbance of cerebral function, or with both of these manifestations. Indeed, in patients with a single cerebral lesion, the metastatic nature of the lesion may only become evident on histopathologic examination. In other patients, there is evidence of widespread metastatic disease, or an isolated cerebral metastasis develops during treatment of the primary neoplasm.

The most common source of intracranial metastasis is carcinoma of the lung; other primary sites are the breast, kidney, and gastrointestinal tract. Most cerebral metastases are located supratentorially. Laboratory and radiologic studies used to evaluate patients with metastases are those described for primary neoplasms. They include MRI and CT scanning performed both with and without contrast material. Lumbar puncture is necessary only in patients with suspected carcinomatous meningitis (see below). In patients with verified cerebral metastasis from an unknown primary, investigation is guided by symptoms and signs. In women, mammography is indicated; in men under 50, germ cell origin is sought since both have therapeutic implications.

In patients with only a single, surgically accessible cerebral metastasis who are otherwise well (ie, a high level of functioning and little or no evidence of extracranial disease), it may be possible to remove the lesion and then treat with irradiation; the latter may also be selected as the sole treatment. In patients with multiple metastases or widespread systemic disease, the prognosis is poor; stereotactic radiosurgery, whole-brain radiotherapy, or both, may help in some instances, but in others treatment is palliative only.

Eichler AF et al. Brain metastases. Curr Treat Options Neurol. 2008 Jul;10(4):308–14. [PMID: 18579017]

Kanner AA et al. Surgical therapies in brain metastasis. Semin Oncol. 2007 Jun;34(3):197–205. [PMID: 17560981]

Mintz A et al. Management of single brain metastasis: a practice guideline. Curr Oncol. 2007 Aug;14(4):131–43. [PMID: 17710205]

Smith ML et al. Stereotactic radiosurgery in the management of brain metastasis. Neurosurg Focus. 2007 Mar 15;22(3):E5. [PMID: 17608358]

Leptomeningeal Metastases (Carcinomatous Meningitis)

The neoplasms metastasizing most commonly to the leptomeninges are carcinoma of the breast, lymphomas, and leukemia. Leptomeningeal metastases lead to multifocal neurologic deficits, which may be associated with infiltration of cranial and spinal nerve roots, direct invasion of the brain or spinal cord, obstructive hydrocephalus, or some combination of these factors.

The diagnosis is confirmed by examination of the cerebrospinal fluid. Findings may include elevated cerebrospinal fluid pressure, pleocytosis, increased protein concentration, and decreased glucose concentration. Cytologic studies may indicate that malignant cells are present; if not, spinal tap should be repeated at least twice to obtain further samples for analysis.

CT scans showing contrast enhancement in the basal cisterns or showing hydrocephalus without any evidence of a mass lesion support the diagnosis. Gadolinium-enhanced MRI frequently shows enhancing foci in the leptomeninges. Myelography may show deposits on multiple nerve roots.

Treatment is by irradiation to symptomatic areas, combined with intrathecal methotrexate. The long-term prognosis is poor—only about 10% of patients survive for 1 year—and palliative care is therefore important (see Chapter 5).

3. Intracranial Mass Lesions in AIDS Patients

Primary cerebral lymphoma is a common complication in patients with AIDS. This leads to disturbances in cognition or consciousness, focal motor or sensory deficits, aphasia, seizures, and cranial neuropathies. Similar clinical disturbances may result from **cerebral toxoplasmosis**, which is also a common complication in patients with AIDS (see Chapters 31 and 35). Neither CT nor MRI findings distinguish these two disorders, and serologic tests for toxoplasmosis are unreliable in AIDS patients. Accordingly, for neurologically stable patients, a trial of treatment for toxoplasmosis with sulfadiazine (100 mg/kg/d up to 8 g/d in four divided doses) and pyrimethamine (75 mg/d for 3 days, then 25 mg/d) is recommended for 3 weeks; the imaging studies are then repeated, and if any lesion has improved, the regimen is continued indefinitely. If any lesion does not improve, cerebral biopsy is necessary. Primary cerebral lymphoma is treated with whole-brain irradiation.

Cryptococcal meningitis is a common opportunistic infection in AIDS patients. Clinically, it may resemble cerebral toxoplasmosis or lymphoma, but cranial CT scans are usually normal. The diagnosis is made on the basis of cerebrospinal fluid studies, with positive India ink staining in 75–80% and cryptococcal antigen tests in 95% of cases. Treatment is with amphotericin B plus flucytosine, as set forth in Table 36–1, followed by fluconazole.

4. Primary & Metastatic Spinal Tumors

Approximately 10% of spinal tumors are intramedullary. Ependymoma is the most common type of intramedullary tumor; the remainder are other types of glioma. Extramedullary tumors may be extradural or intradural in location. Among the primary extramedullary tumors, neurofibromas and meningiomas are relatively common, are benign, and may be intradural or extradural. Carcinomatous metastases, lymphomatous or leukemic deposits, and myeloma are usually extradural; in the case of metastases, the prostate, breast, lung, and kidney are common primary sites.

Tumors may lead to spinal cord dysfunction by direct compression, by ischemia secondary to arterial or venous obstruction, and, in the case of intramedullary lesions, by invasive infiltration.

▶ Clinical Findings

A. Symptoms and Signs

Symptoms usually develop insidiously. Pain is often conspicuous with extradural lesions; is characteristically aggravated by coughing or straining; may be radicular, localized to the back, or felt diffusely in an extremity; and may be accompanied by motor deficits, paresthesias, or numbness, especially in the legs. When sphincter disturbances occur, they are usually particularly disabling. Pain, however, often precedes specific neurologic symptoms from epidural metastases.

Examination may reveal localized spinal tenderness. A segmental lower motor neuron deficit or dermatomal sensory changes (or both) are sometimes found at the level of the lesion, while an upper motor neuron deficit and sensory disturbance are found below it.

B. Imaging

Findings on plain radiography of the spine may be normal but are commonly abnormal when there are metastatic deposits. CT myelography or MRI may be necessary to identify and localize the site of cord compression. The combination of known tumor elsewhere in the body, back pain, and either abnormal plain films of the spine or neurologic signs of cord compression is an indication to perform these studies on an urgent basis. Some clinicians proceed to myelography based solely on new back pain in a cancer patient. If a complete block is present at lumbar myelography, a cisternal myelogram is performed to determine the upper level of the block and to investigate the possibility of block higher in the cord.

C. Laboratory Findings

The cerebrospinal fluid removed at myelography is often xanthochromic and contains a greatly increased protein concentration with normal cell content and glucose concentration.

▶ Treatment

Intramedullary tumors are treated by decompression and surgical excision (when feasible) and by irradiation. The prognosis depends on the cause and severity of cord compression before it is relieved.

Treatment of epidural spinal metastases consists of irradiation, irrespective of cell type. Dexamethasone is also given in a high dosage (eg, 25 mg four times daily for 3 days, followed by rapid tapering of the dosage, depending on response) to reduce cord swelling and relieve pain. Surgical decompression is reserved for patients with tumors that are unresponsive to irradiation or have previously been irradiated and for cases in which there is some uncertainty about the diagnosis. The long-term outlook is poor, but radiation treatment may at least delay the onset of major disability.

Cole JS et al. Metastatic epidural spinal cord compression. Lancet Neurol. 2008 May;7(5):459–66. [PMID: 18420159]

5. Brain Abscess

ESSENTIALS OF DIAGNOSIS

▶ Symptoms and signs of expanding intracranial mass.

▶ Signs of primary infection or congenital heart disease are sometimes present.

▶ Fever may be absent.

General Considerations

Brain abscess presents as an intracranial space-occupying lesion and arises as a sequela of disease of the ear or nose, may be a complication of infection elsewhere in the body, or may result from infection introduced intracranially by trauma or surgical procedures. The most common infective organisms are streptococci, staphylococci, and anaerobes; mixed infections are not uncommon.

Clinical Findings

A. Symptoms and Signs

Headache, drowsiness, inattention, confusion, and seizures are early symptoms, followed by signs of increasing intracranial pressure and then a focal neurologic deficit. There may be little or no systemic evidence of infection.

B. Imaging and Other Investigations

A CT scan of the head characteristically shows an area of contrast enhancement surrounding a low-density core. Similar abnormalities may be found in patients with metastatic neoplasms. MRI findings often permit earlier recognition of focal cerebritis or an abscess. Arteriography indicates the presence of a space-occupying lesion, which appears as an avascular mass with displacement of normal cerebral vessels, but this procedure provides no clue to the nature of the lesion. Stereotactic needle aspiration may enable a specific etiologic organism to be identified. Examination of the cerebrospinal fluid does not help in diagnosis and may precipitate a herniation syndrome. Peripheral leukocytosis is sometimes present.

Treatment

Treatment consists of intravenous antibiotics, combined with surgical drainage (aspiration or excision) if necessary to reduce the mass effect, or sometimes to establish the diagnosis. Abscesses smaller than 2 cm can often be cured medically. Broad-spectrum antibiotics, selected based on risk factors and likely organisms, are used if the infecting organism is unknown (see Chapter 33). A common regimen is with penicillin G plus a third-generation cephalosporin plus metronidazole. Nafcillin is added if *Staphylococcus aureus* infection is suspected. The regimen is altered once culture and sensitivity data are available. Antimicrobial treatment is usually continued parenterally for 6–8 weeks, followed by orally for 2–3 months. The patient should be monitored by serial CT scans or MRI every 2 weeks and at deterioration. Dexamethasone (4–25 mg four times daily, depending on severity, followed by tapering of dose, depending on response) may reduce any associated edema, but intravenous mannitol is sometimes required.

Carpenter J et al. Retrospective analysis of 49 cases of brain abscess and review of the literature. Eur J Clin Microbiol Infect Dis. 2007 Jan;26(1):1–11. [PMID: 17180609]

NONMETASTATIC NEUROLOGIC COMPLICATIONS OF MALIGNANT DISEASE

A variety of nonmetastatic neurologic complications of malignant disease (see Table 39–13) can be recognized. Metabolic encephalopathy due to electrolyte abnormalities, infections, drug overdose, or the failure of some vital organ may be reflected by drowsiness, lethargy, restlessness, insomnia, agitation, confusion, stupor, or coma. The mental changes are usually associated with tremor, asterixis, and multifocal myoclonus. The electroencephalogram is generally diffusely slowed. Laboratory studies are necessary to detect the cause of the encephalopathy, which must then be treated appropriately.

Immune suppression resulting from either the malignant disease or its treatment (eg, by chemotherapy) predisposes patients to brain abscess, progressive multifocal leukoencephalopathy, meningitis, herpes zoster infection, and other opportunistic infectious diseases. Moreover, an overt or occult cerebrospinal fluid fistula, as occurs with some tumors, may also increase the risk of infection. CT scanning aids in the early recognition of a brain abscess, but metastatic brain tumors may have a similar appearance. Examination of the cerebrospinal fluid is essential in the evaluation of patients with meningitis but is of no help in the diagnosis of brain abscess.

Cerebrovascular disorders that cause neurologic complications in patients with systemic cancer include nonbacterial thrombotic endocarditis and septic embolization. Cerebral, subarachnoid, or subdural hemorrhages may occur in patients with myelogenous leukemia and may be found in association with metastatic tumors, especially malignant melanoma. Spinal subdural hemorrhage sometimes occurs after lumbar puncture in patients with marked thrombocytopenia.

Disseminated intravascular coagulation occurs most commonly in patients with acute promyelocytic leukemia or with some adenocarcinomas and is characterized by a fluctuating encephalopathy, often with associated seizures, that frequently progresses to coma or death. There may be few accompanying neurologic signs. Venous sinus thrombosis, which usually presents with convulsions and headaches, may also occur in patients with leukemia or lymphoma. Examination commonly reveals papilledema and focal or diffuse neurologic signs. Anticonvulsants, anticoagulants, and drugs to lower the intracranial pressure may be of value.

Paraneoplastic cerebellar degeneration occurs most commonly in association with carcinoma of the lung. Symptoms may precede those due to the neoplasm itself, which may be undetected for several months or even longer. Typically, there is a pancerebellar syndrome causing dysarthria, nystagmus, and ataxia of the trunk and limbs. The disorder probably has an autoimmune basis. Treatment is of the underlying malignant disease.

Encephalopathy, characterized by impaired recent memory, disturbed affect, hallucinations, and seizures, occurs in some patients with carcinomas. The cerebrospinal fluid is often abnormal. EEGs may show diffuse slow-wave activity, especially over the temporal regions. Pathologic changes are most marked in the inferomedian portions of the temporal lobes. There is no specific treatment.

Malignant disease may be associated with sensorimotor polyneuropathy and less commonly with pure sensory neuropathy (ie, dorsal root ganglionitis) or autonomic neuropathy. A subacute motor neuronopathy may be associated with lymphomas.

Dermatomyositis or a myasthenic syndrome may be seen in patients with underlying carcinoma (see Chapter

20). The myasthenic syndrome may have an autoimmune basis and differs clinically from myasthenia gravis.

Dalmau J et al. Paraneoplastic syndromes of the CNS. Lancet Neurol. 2008 Apr;7(4):327–40. [PMID: 18339348]

PSEUDOTUMOR CEREBRI (Benign Intracranial Hypertension)

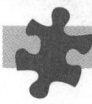 **ESSENTIALS OF DIAGNOSIS**

► Headache, worse on straining.
► Visual obscurations or diplopia may occur.
► Examination reveals papilledema.
► Abducens palsy is commonly present.

General Considerations

There are many causes of pseudotumor cerebri. Thrombosis of the transverse venous sinus as a noninfectious complication of otitis media or chronic mastoiditis is one cause, and sagittal sinus thrombosis may lead to a clinically similar picture. Other causes include chronic pulmonary disease, endocrine disturbances such as hypoparathyroidism or Addison disease, vitamin A toxicity, and the use of tetracycline or oral contraceptives. Cases have also followed withdrawal of corticosteroids after long-term use. In many instances, however, no specific cause can be found, and the disorder remits spontaneously after several months.

Clinical Findings

A. Symptoms and Signs

Symptoms of pseudotumor cerebri consist of headache, diplopia, and other visual disturbances due to papilledema and abducens nerve dysfunction. Pulse-synchronous tinnitus may also occur. Examination reveals the papilledema and some enlargement of the blind spots, but patients otherwise look well.

B. Imaging

Investigations reveal no evidence of a space-occupying lesion, and the CT scan shows small or normal ventricles. MR venography is helpful in screening for thrombosis of the intracranial venous sinuses.

C. Laboratory Findings

Lumbar puncture confirms the presence of intracranial hypertension, but the cerebrospinal fluid is normal. Laboratory studies help exclude some of the other causes mentioned earlier.

Treatment

Untreated pseudotumor cerebri leads to secondary optic atrophy and permanent visual loss. Acetazolamide (250 mg orally three times daily) reduces formation of cerebrospinal fluid and can be used to start treatment. Oral corticosteroids (eg, prednisone, 60–80 mg daily) may also be necessary. Obese patients should be advised to lose weight. Repeated lumbar puncture to lower the intracranial pressure by removal of cerebrospinal fluid is effective, but pharmacologic approaches to treatment are now more satisfactory. Treatment is monitored by checking visual acuity and visual fields, funduscopic appearance, and pressure of the cerebrospinal fluid. The disorder may worsen after a period of stability, indicating the need for long-term follow-up.

If medical treatment fails to control the intracranial pressure, surgical placement of a lumboperitoneal or other shunt or optic nerve sheath fenestration should be undertaken to preserve vision.

In addition to the above measures, any specific cause of pseudotumor cerebri requires appropriate treatment. Thus, hormone therapy should be initiated if there is an underlying endocrine disturbance. Discontinuing the use of tetracycline, oral contraceptives, or vitamin A will allow for resolution of pseudotumor cerebri due to these agents. If corticosteroid withdrawal is responsible, the medication should be reintroduced and then tapered more gradually.

When to Refer

All patients should be referred.

When to Admit

All patients requiring shunt placement or optic nerve sheath fenestration should be hospitalized.

Shah VA et al. Long-term follow-up of idiopathic intracranial hypertension: the Iowa experience. Neurology. 2008 Feb 19;70(8):634–40. [PMID: 18285538]
Wall M. Idiopathic intracranial hypertension (pseudotumor cerebri). Curr Neurol Neurosci Rep. 2008 Mar;8(2):87–93. [PMID: 18460275]

SELECTED NEUROCUTANEOUS DISEASES

1. Tuberous Sclerosis

Tuberous sclerosis may occur sporadically or on a familial basis with autosomal dominant inheritance. There is genetic heterogeneity; mutations involving 9q34 and 16p13 are well described. Neurologic presentation is with seizures and progressive psychomotor retardation beginning in early childhood. The cutaneous abnormality, adenoma sebaceum, becomes manifest usually between 5 and 10 years of age and typically consists of reddened nodules on the face (cheeks, nasolabial folds, sides of the nose, and chin) and sometimes on the forehead and neck. Other typical cutaneous lesions include subungual fibromas, shagreen patches (leathery plaques of subepidermal fibrosis, situated usually on the trunk), and leaf-shaped hypopigmented spots. Associated abnormalities include retinal lesions and tumors, benign rhabdomyomas of the heart, lung cysts, benign tumors in the viscera, and bone cysts.

The disease is slowly progressive and leads to increasing mental deterioration. There is no specific treatment, but anticonvulsant drugs may help in controlling seizures.

Curatolo P et al. Tuberous sclerosis. Lancet. 2008 Aug 23;372(9639):657–68. [PMID: 18722871]

2. Neurofibromatosis

Neurofibromatosis may occur either sporadically or on a familial basis with autosomal dominant inheritance. Two distinct forms are recognized: Type 1 (**Recklinghausen disease**) is characterized by multiple hyperpigmented macules and neurofibromas and type 2 by **eighth nerve tumors**, often accompanied by other intracranial or intraspinal tumors. Among familial cases, the gene for type 1 is located on chromosome 17 and that for type 2 on chromosome 22.

Neurologic presentation is usually with symptoms and signs of tumor. Multiple neurofibromas characteristically are present and may involve spinal or cranial nerves, especially the eighth nerve (Plate 89). Examination of the superficial cutaneous nerves usually reveals palpable mobile nodules. In some cases, there is an associated marked overgrowth of subcutaneous tissues (plexiform neuromas), sometimes with an underlying bony abnormality. Associated cutaneous lesions include axillary freckling and patches of cutaneous pigmentation (café au lait spots). Malignant degeneration of neurofibromas occasionally occurs and may lead to peripheral sarcomas. Meningiomas, gliomas (especially optic nerve gliomas), bone cysts, pheochromocytomas, scoliosis, and obstructive hydrocephalus may also occur.

Yohay K. Neurofibromatosis types 1 and 2. Neurologist. 2006 Mar;12(2):86–93. [PMID: 16534445]

3. Sturge-Weber Syndrome

Sturge-Weber syndrome consists of a congenital, usually unilateral, cutaneous capillary angioma involving the upper face, leptomeningeal angiomatosis, and, in many patients, choroidal angioma. It has no sex predilection and usually occurs sporadically. The cutaneous angioma sometimes has a more extensive distribution over the head and neck and is often quite disfiguring, especially if there is associated overgrowth of connective tissue. Focal or generalized seizures are the usual neurologic presentation and may commence at any age. There may be contralateral homonymous hemianopia, hemiparesis and hemisensory disturbance, ipsilateral glaucoma, and mental subnormality. Skull radiographs taken after the first 2 years of life usually reveal gyriform ("tramline") intracranial calcification, especially in the parieto-occipital region, due to mineral deposition in the cortex beneath the intracranial angioma.

Treatment is aimed at controlling seizures pharmacologically, but surgical treatment may be necessary. Ophthalmologic advice should be sought concerning the management of choroidal angioma and of increased intraocular pressure.

Pascual-Castroviejo I et al. Sturge-Weber syndrome: study of 55 patients. Canad J Neurol Sci. 2008 Jul;35(3):301–7. [PMID: 18714797]

MOVEMENT DISORDERS

1. Benign Essential (Familial) Tremor

ESSENTIALS OF DIAGNOSIS

▶ Postural tremor of hands, head, or voice.

▶ Family history common.

▶ May improve temporarily with alcohol.

▶ No abnormal findings other than tremor.

General Considerations

The cause of benign essential tremor is uncertain, but it is sometimes inherited in an autosomal dominant manner. Responsible genes have been identified at 3q13, 2p22-p25, and 6p23.

Clinical Findings

Tremor may begin at any age and is enhanced by emotional stress. The tremor usually involves one or both hands, the head, or the hands and head, while the legs tend to be spared. Examination reveals no other abnormalities. Ingestion of a small quantity of alcohol commonly provides remarkable but short-lived relief by an unknown mechanism.

Although the tremor may become more conspicuous with time, it generally leads to little disability. Occasionally, it interferes with manual skills and leads to impairment of handwriting. Speech may also be affected if the laryngeal muscles are involved.

Treatment

Treatment is often unnecessary. When it is required because of disability, propranolol may be helpful but will need to be continued indefinitely in daily doses of 60–240 mg. However, intermittent therapy is sometimes useful in patients whose tremor becomes exacerbated in specific predictable situations. Primidone may be helpful when propranolol is ineffective, but patients with essential tremor are often very sensitive to it. Therefore, the starting dose is 50 mg daily, and the daily dose is increased by 50 mg every 2 weeks depending on the patient's response; a maintenance dose of 125 mg three times daily is commonly effective. Occasional patients do not respond to these measures but are helped by alprazolam (up to 3 mg daily in divided doses), clozapine (30–50 mg twice daily), topiramate (titrated up to a dose of 400 mg daily in divided doses over about 8 weeks), gabapentin (1800 mg daily in divided doses), or mirtazapine (15 or 30 mg at night). Other antiepileptic agents including levetiracetam and zonisamide are reportedly sometimes effective. Botulinum toxin A may reduce tremor, but adverse effects include dose-dependent weakness of the injected muscles.

Disabling tremor unresponsive to medical treatment may be helped by contralateral thalamotomy. Unilateral high-frequency thalamic stimulation is an alternative approach that is equally effective, is associated with only mild and transient side effects, and is therefore preferred. Bilateral thalamotomy has significant morbidity, whereas the risks of bilateral stimulation are appreciably lower.

When to Refer

All patients should be referred.

When to Admit

Patients requiring surgical treatment (deep brain stimulator placement) should be hospitalized.

Deng H et al. Genetics of essential tremor. Brain. 2007 Jun;130(Pt 6):1456–64. [PMID: 17353225]

Lorenz D et al. Update on pathogenesis and treatment of essential tremor. Curr Opin Neurol. 2007 Aug;20(4):447–52. [PMID: 17620881]

Ondo WG. Essential tremor: treatment options. Curr Treat Options Neurol. 2006 May;8(3):256–67. [PMID: 16569384]

2. Parkinsonism

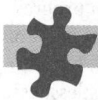
ESSENTIALS OF DIAGNOSIS

► Any combination of tremor, rigidity, bradykinesia, progressive postural instability.

► Cognitive impairment is sometimes prominent.

General Considerations

Parkinsonism is a relatively common disorder that occurs in all ethnic groups, with an approximately equal sex distribution. The most common variety, idiopathic Parkinson disease (paralysis agitans), begins most often between 45 and 65 years of age and is a progressive disease.

Etiology

Parkinsonism may rarely occur on a familial basis, and the parkinsonian phenotype may result from mutations of several different genes (alpha-synuclein, parkin, *LRRK2*, *DJ1*, and *PINK1*). Postencephalitic parkinsonism is becoming increasingly rare. Exposure to certain toxins (eg, manganese dust, carbon disulfide) and severe carbon monoxide poisoning may lead to parkinsonism. Typical parkinsonism has occurred in individuals who have taken 1-methyl-4-phenyl-1,2,5,6-tetrahydropyridine (MPTP) for recreational purposes. This compound is converted in the body to a neurotoxin that selectively destroys dopaminergic neurons in the substantia nigra. Reversible parkinsonism may develop in patients receiving neuroleptic drugs (see Chapter 25), reserpine, or metoclopramide. Only rarely is hemiparkinsonism the presenting feature of a progressive space-occupying lesion.

In idiopathic parkinsonism, dopamine depletion due to degeneration of the dopaminergic nigrostriatal system leads to an imbalance of dopamine and acetylcholine, which are neurotransmitters normally present in the corpus striatum. Treatment is directed at redressing this imbalance by blocking the effect of acetylcholine with anticholinergic drugs or by the administration of levodopa, the precursor of dopamine. The serum urate level may be a prognostic indicator—the rate of progression declines as the urate level increases.

Clinical Findings

Tremor, rigidity, bradykinesia, and postural instability are the cardinal features of parkinsonism and may be present in any combination. There may also be a mild decline in intellectual function. The tremor of about four to six cycles per second is most conspicuous at rest, is enhanced by emotional stress, and is often less severe during voluntary activity. Although it may ultimately be present in all limbs, the tremor is commonly confined to one limb or to the limbs on one side for months or years before it becomes more generalized. In some patients, tremor is absent.

Rigidity (an increase in resistance to passive movement) is responsible for the characteristically flexed posture seen in many patients, but the most disabling symptoms of parkinsonism are due to bradykinesia, manifested as a slowness of voluntary movement and a reduction in automatic movements such as swinging of the arms while walking. Curiously, however, effective voluntary activity may briefly be regained during an emergency (eg, the patient is able to leap aside to avoid an oncoming motor vehicle).

Clinical diagnosis of the well-developed syndrome is usually simple. The patient has a relatively immobile face with widened palpebral fissures, infrequent blinking, and a certain fixity of facial expression. Seborrhea of the scalp and face is common. There is often mild blepharoclonus, and a tremor may be present about the mouth and lips. Repetitive tapping (about twice per second) over the bridge of the nose produces a sustained blink response (Myerson sign). Other findings may include saliva drooling from the mouth, perhaps due to impairment of swallowing; soft and poorly modulated voice; a variable rest tremor and rigidity in some or all of the limbs; slowness of voluntary movements; impairment of fine or rapidly alternating movements; and micrographia. There is typically no muscle weakness (provided that sufficient time is allowed for power to be developed) and no alteration in the tendon reflexes or plantar responses. It is difficult for the patient to arise from a sitting position and begin walking. The gait itself is characterized by small shuffling steps and a loss of the normal automatic arm swing; there may be unsteadiness on turning, difficulty in stopping, and a tendency to fall.

Differential Diagnosis

Diagnostic problems may occur in mild cases, especially if tremor is minimal or absent. For example, mild hypokinesia or slight tremor is commonly attributed to old age. Depression, with its associated expressionless face, poorly modulated voice, and reduction in voluntary activity, can be difficult to distinguish from mild parkinsonism, especially since the two disorders may coexist; in some cases, a trial of antidepressant drug therapy is necessary. The family history, the character of the tremor, and lack of other neurologic signs should distinguish essential tremor from parkinsonism. Wilson disease can be distinguished by its early age at onset, the presence of other abnormal movements, Kayser-Fleischer rings, and chronic hepatitis, and by increased concentrations of copper in the tissues. Huntington disease presenting with rigidity and bradykinesia may be mistaken for parkinsonism unless the family history and accompanying dementia are recognized. In Shy-Drager syndrome (also called multisystem atrophy), the clinical features of parkinsonism are accompanied by autonomic insufficiency (leading to postural hypotension, anhidrosis, disturbances of sphincter control, impotence, etc) and more widespread neurologic deficits (pyramidal, lower motor neuron, or cerebellar signs). In progressive supranuclear palsy, bradykinesia and rigidity are accompanied by a supranuclear disorder of eye movements, pseudobulbar palsy, pseudo-emotional lability (pseudobulbar affect), and axial dystonia. Creutzfeldt-Jakob disease may be accompanied by features of parkinsonism, but dementia is usual, myoclonic jerking is common, ataxia and pyramidal signs may be conspicuous, and the electroencephalographic findings are usually characteristic. In cortical-basal ganglionic degeneration, parkinsonism is accompanied by conspicuous signs of cortical dysfunction (eg, apraxia, sensory inattention, dementia, aphasia).

▶ Treatment

Treatment is symptomatic. Recent studies, however, suggest that rasagiline, 1 mg daily, slows progression of Parkinson disease (see Selective monoamine oxidase inhibitors below), and trials of several other putative neuroprotective agents are in progress, as are various trials of gene therapy.

A. Medical Measures

Drug treatment is not required early in the course of Parkinson disease, but the nature of the disorder and the availability of medical treatment for use when necessary should be discussed with the patient.

1. Amantadine—Patients with mild symptoms but no disability may be helped by amantadine. This drug improves all of the clinical features of parkinsonism, but its mode of action is unclear. Side effects include restlessness, confusion, depression, skin rashes, edema, nausea, constipation, anorexia, postural hypotension, and disturbances of cardiac rhythm. However, these are relatively uncommon with the usual dose (100 mg twice daily).

2. Anticholinergic drugs—Anticholinergics are more helpful in alleviating tremor and rigidity than bradykinesia. Treatment is started with a small dose (Table 24–6) and gradually increased until benefit occurs or side effects limit further increments. If treatment is ineffective, the drug is gradually withdrawn and another preparation then tried.

Common side effects include dryness of the mouth, nausea, constipation, palpitations, cardiac arrhythmias, urinary retention, confusion, agitation, restlessness, drowsiness, mydriasis, increased intraocular pressure, and defective accommodation.

Table 24–6. Some anticholinergic antiparkinsonian drugs.

Drug	Usual Daily Dose
Benztropine mesylate (Cogentin)	1–6 mg
Biperiden (Akineton)	2–12 mg
Orphenadrine (Disipal, Norflex)	150–400 mg
Procyclidine (Kemadrin)	7.5–30 mg
Trihexyphenidyl (Artane)	6–20 mg

Modified, with permission, from Aminoff MJ: Pharmacologic management of parkinsonism and other movement disorders. In: *Basic & Clinical Pharmacology*, 10th ed. Katzung BG (editor). McGraw-Hill, 2007.

Anticholinergic drugs are contraindicated in patients with prostatic hyperplasia, narrow-angle glaucoma, or obstructive gastrointestinal disease and are often tolerated poorly by the elderly.

3. Levodopa—Levodopa, which is converted in the body to dopamine, improves all of the major features of parkinsonism, including bradykinesia, but does not stop progression of the disorder. The most common early side effects of levodopa are nausea, vomiting, and hypotension, but cardiac arrhythmias may also occur. Dyskinesias, restlessness, confusion, and other behavioral changes tend to occur somewhat later and become more common with time. Levodopa-induced dyskinesias may take any conceivable form, including chorea, athetosis, dystonia, tremor, tics, and myoclonus. An even later complication is the "on-off phenomenon," in which abrupt but transient fluctuations in the severity of parkinsonism occur unpredictably but frequently during the day. The "off" period of marked bradykinesia has been shown to relate in some instances to falling plasma levels of levodopa. During the "on" phase, dyskinesias are often conspicuous but mobility is increased.

Carbidopa, which inhibits the enzyme responsible for the breakdown of levodopa to dopamine, does not cross the blood-brain barrier. When levodopa is given in combination with carbidopa, the extracerebral breakdown of levodopa is diminished. This reduces the amount of levodopa required daily for beneficial effects, and it lowers the incidence of nausea, vomiting, hypotension, and cardiac irregularities. Such a combination does not prevent the development of the "on-off phenomenon," and the incidence of other side effects (dyskinesias or psychiatric complications) may actually be increased.

Sinemet, a commercially available preparation that contains carbidopa and levodopa in a fixed ratio (1:10 or 1:4), is generally used. Treatment is started with a small dose— eg, one tablet of Sinemet 25/100 (containing 25 mg of carbidopa and 100 mg of levodopa) three times daily—and gradually increased depending on the response. Sinemet CR is a controlled-release formulation (containing 25 or 50 mg of carbidopa and 100 or 200 mg of levodopa). It is sometimes helpful in reducing fluctuations in clinical response to treatment and in reducing the frequency with which medication must be taken. The commercially available combination of levodopa with both carbidopa and entacapone (Stalevo) may also be helpful in this context and is discussed in the following section on COMT inhibitors. Response fluctuations are also reduced by keeping the daily intake of protein at the recommended minimum and taking the main protein meal as the last meal of the day.

The dyskinesias and behavioral side effects of levodopa are dose-related, but reduction in dose may eliminate any therapeutic benefit. Levodopa-induced dyskinesias may also respond to amantadine.

Levodopa therapy is contraindicated in patients with psychotic illness or narrow-angle glaucoma. It should not be given to patients taking monoamine oxidase A inhibitors or within 2 weeks of their withdrawal, because hypertensive crises may result. Levodopa should be used with care in patients with suspected malignant melanomas or with active peptic ulcers because of concerns that it may exacerbate these disorders.

4. Dopamine agonists—Dopamine agonists act directly on dopamine receptors, and their use in parkinsonism is associated with a lower incidence of the response fluctuations and dyskinesias that occur with long-term levodopa therapy. They were previously reserved for patients who had either become refractory to levodopa or developed the "on-off phenomenon." However, they are now best given either before the introduction of levodopa or with a low dose of Sinemet 25/100 (carbidopa 25 mg and levodopa 100 mg), one tablet three times daily when dopaminergic therapy is first introduced; the dose of Sinemet is kept constant, while the dose of the agonist is gradually increased. Bromocriptine, an ergot derivative is not widely used in the United States because of side effects, including anorexia; nausea; vomiting; constipation; postural hypotension; digital vasospasm; cardiac arrhythmias; various dyskinesias and mental disturbances; headache; nasal congestion; erythromelalgia; pulmonary infiltrates; and pericardial, pleural, or pulmonary fibrosis. In 2007, the manufacturer of pergolide, another ergot derivative and dopamine agonist, withdrew the drug from the US market after two studies showed that serious cardiac valvular abnormalities developed in some patients while taking the drug.

Pramipexole and ropinirole are two newer dopamine agonists that are not ergot derivatives. They are effective in early Parkinson disease as well as in advanced stages of the disease. In each case, the daily dose is built up gradually. Pramipexole is started at a dosage of 0.125 mg three times daily, and the dose is doubled after 1 week and again after another week; the daily dose is then increased by 0.75 mg at weekly intervals depending on response and tolerance. Most patients require between 0.5 and 1.5 mg three times daily. Ropinirole is begun in a dosage of 0.25 mg three times daily, and the total daily dose is increased at weekly intervals by 0.75 mg until the fourth week and by 1.5 mg thereafter. Most patients require between 2 and 8 mg three times daily for benefit. Adverse effects include fatigue, somnolence, nausea, peripheral edema, dyskinesias, confusion, and postural hypotension. Less commonly, an irresistible urge to sleep may occur, sometimes in inappropriate and hazardous circumstances. Impulse control disorders involving gambling, shopping, or sexual activity have also been related to use of dopamine agonists.

5. Selective monoamine oxidase inhibitors—Rasagiline, a selective monoamine oxidase B inhibitor, has a clear symptomatic benefit in a daily oral dose of 1 mg, taken in the morning; it may also be used for adjunctive therapy in patients with response fluctuations to levodopa. Selegiline (5 mg orally with breakfast and lunch) is another monoamine oxidase B inhibitor that is sometimes used as adjunctive treatment for parkinsonism; by inhibiting the metabolic breakdown of dopamine, it may improve fluctuations or declining response to levodopa. Tyramine-rich foods are best avoided when either of these agents is taken because of the theoretical possibility of a hypertensive ("cheese") effect.

Recent studies suggest that rasagiline slows the progression of Parkinson disease and this remains an important consideration for patients who are young or have mild disease.

6. COMT inhibitors—Catecholamine-O-methyltransferase inhibitors reduce the metabolism of levodopa to 3-O-methyldopa and thereby alter the plasma pharmacokinetics of levodopa, leading to more sustained plasma levels and more constant dopaminergic stimulation of the brain. Two such agents, tolcapone and entacapone, are currently available and may be used as an adjunct to levodopa-carbidopa in patients with response fluctuations or an otherwise inadequate response and who either have failed with other adjunctive therapies or are not candidates for such therapies. Treatment results in reduced response fluctuations, with a greater period of responsiveness to administered levodopa. Tolcapone is given in a dosage of 100 mg or 200 mg three times daily, and entacapone is given as 200 mg with each dose of Sinemet (levodopa-carbidopa). With either preparation, the dose of Sinemet taken concurrently may have to be reduced by up to one-third to avoid side effects such as dyskinesias, confusion, hypotension, and syncope. Diarrhea is sometimes troublesome. Because rare cases of fulminant hepatic failure have followed its use, tolcapone should be avoided in patients with preexisting liver disease. Serial liver function tests should be performed at 2-week intervals for the first year and at longer intervals thereafter in patients receiving the drug—as recommended by the manufacturer. Hepatotoxicity has not been reported with entacapone, which is therefore the preferred agent, and serial liver function tests are not required.

Stalevo is the commercial preparation of levodopa combined with both carbidopa and entacapone. It is best used in patients already stabilized on equivalent doses of carbidopa/ levodopa and entacapone. It is priced at or below the price of the individual ingredients (ie, carbidopa/levodopa and entacapone) and has the added convenience of requiring fewer tablets to be taken daily. It is available in three strengths: Stalevo 50 (12.5 mg of carbidopa, 50 mg of levodopa, and 200 mg of entacapone), Stalevo 100 (25 mg of carbidopa, 100 mg of levodopa, and 200 mg of entacapone), and Stalevo 150 (37.5 mg of carbidopa, 150 mg of levodopa, and 200 mg of entacapone).

7. Atypical antipsychotics—Confusion and psychotic symptoms, which may be iatrogenic, often respond to atypical antipsychotic agents, which have few extrapyramidal side effects and do not block the effects of dopaminergic medication. Olanzapine, quetiapine, and risperidone may be tried, but the most effective of these agents is clozapine, a dibenzodiazepine derivative. Clozapine may rarely cause marrow suppression, and weekly blood counts are therefore necessary for patients taking it. The patient is started on 6.25 mg at bedtime and the dosage increased to 25–100 mg/d as needed. In low doses, it may also improve iatrogenic dyskinesias.

B. General Measures

Physical therapy or speech therapy helps many patients. Cognitive impairment and psychiatric symptoms may be helped by rivastigmine (3–12 mg daily). The quality of life can often be improved by the provision of simple aids to daily living, eg, rails or banisters placed strategically about the home, special table cutlery with large handles, nonslip rubber table mats, and devices to amplify the voice.

C. Surgical Measures

Thalamotomy or pallidotomy may be helpful for patients who become unresponsive to medical treatment or have intolerable side effects from antiparkinsonian agents, especially if they have no evidence of diffuse vascular disease or significant cognitive decline. Ablative surgery should generally be confined to one side because the morbidity is considerably greater after bilateral procedures. Because of their morbidity, ablative procedures have generally been supplanted by deep brain stimulation, discussed in the following section.

D. Brain Stimulation

High-frequency thalamic stimulation is effective in suppressing the rest tremor of Parkinson disease, and chronic bilateral stimulation of the subthalamic nuclei or globus pallidus internus may benefit all the major features of the disease. Electrical stimulation of the brain has the advantage over ablative procedures of being reversible and of causing minimal or no damage to the brain, and is therefore the preferred surgical approach to treatment. There is no evidence that the natural history of Parkinson disease is affected.

▶ When to Refer

All patients should be referred.

▶ When to Admit

Patients requiring surgical treatment should be admitted.

Esper CD et al. Failure of recognition of drug-induced parkinsonism in the elderly. Mov Disord. 2008 Feb 15;23(3):401–4. [PMID: 18067180]

Gottwald MD, Aminoff MJ. New frontiers in the pharmacological management of Parkinson's disease. Drugs Today (Barc). 2008 Jul;44(7):531–45. [PMID: 18806903]

Kazantsev AG et al. Central role of alpha-synuclein oligomers in neurodegeneration in Parkinson disease. Arch Neurol. 2008 Dec;65(12):1577–1581. [PMID: 19064744]

Limousin P et al. Deep brain stimulation for Parkinson's disease. Neurotherapeutics. 2008 Apr;5(2):309–19. [PMID: 18394572]

Oertel W et al. Effects of rivastigmine on tremor and other motor symptoms in patients with Parkinson's disease dementia: a retrospective analysis of a double-blind trial and an open-label extension. Drug Saf. 2008;31(1):79–94. [PMID: 18095748]

Pahwa R et al. Practice parameter: Treatment of Parkinson disease with motor fluctuations and dyskinesia (an evidence-based review). Report of the Quality Standards Subcommittee of the American Academy of Neurology. Neurology. 2006 Apr 11;66(7):983–95. [PMID: 16606909]

Schwarzschild MA et al. Serum urate as a predictor of clinical and radiographic progression in Parkinson disease. Arch Neurol. 2008 Jun;65(6):716–23. [PMID: 18413464]

Suchowersky O et al. Practice parameter: Neuroprotective strategies and alternative therapies for Parkinson disease (an evidence-based review). Report of the Quality Standards Subcommittee of the American Academy of Neurology. Neurology. 2006 Apr 11;66(7):976–82. [PMID: 16606908]

Tolosa E et al. The diagnosis of Parkinson's disease. Lancet Neurol. 2006 Jan;5(1):75–86. [PMID: 16361025]

3. Huntington Disease

 ESSENTIALS OF DIAGNOSIS

▶ Gradual onset and progression of chorea and dementia or behavioral change.

▶ Family history of the disorder.

▶ Responsible gene identified on chromosome 4.

▶ General Considerations

Huntington disease is characterized by chorea and dementia. It is inherited in an autosomal dominant manner and occurs throughout the world, in all ethnic groups, with a prevalence rate of about 5 per 100,000. There is an expanded and unstable CAG trinucleotide repeat in the huntingtin gene at 4p16.3; repeat length may affect rate of progression.

▶ Clinical Findings

A. Symptoms and Signs

Clinical onset is usually between 30 and 50 years of age. The disease is progressive and usually leads to a fatal outcome within 15–20 years. The initial symptoms may consist of either abnormal movements or intellectual changes, but ultimately both occur. The earliest mental changes are often behavioral, with irritability, moodiness, antisocial behavior, or a psychiatric disturbance, but a more obvious dementia subsequently develops. The dyskinesia may initially be no more than an apparent fidgetiness or restlessness, but eventually choreiform movements and some dystonic posturing occur. Progressive rigidity and akinesia (rather than chorea) sometimes occur in association with dementia, especially in cases with childhood onset.

B. Imaging

CT scanning or MRI usually demonstrates cerebral atrophy and atrophy of the caudate nucleus in established

occurs on a hereditary or sporadic basis as an isolated phenomenon in otherwise healthy subjects.

Segmental myoclonus is a rare manifestation of a focal spinal cord lesion. It may also be the clinical expression of **epilepsia partialis continua,** a disorder in which a repetitive focal epileptic discharge arises in the contralateral sensorimotor cortex, sometimes from an underlying structural lesion. An electroencephalogram is often helpful in clarifying the epileptic nature of the disorder, and CT or MRI scan may reveal the causal lesion.

Myoclonus may respond to certain anticonvulsant drugs, especially valproic acid, or to one of the benzodiazepines, particularly clonazepam (see Table 24–3). It may also respond to piracetam (up to 16.8 g daily). Myoclonus following anoxic brain damage is often responsive to oxitriptan (5-hydroxytryptophan), an investigational agent that is the precursor of serotonin, and sometimes to clonazepam. Oxitriptan is given in gradually increasing doses up to 1–1.5 mg daily. In patients with segmental myoclonus, a localized lesion should be searched for and treated appropriately.

Chang VC et al. Myoclonus. Curr Treat Options Neurol. 2008 May;10(3):222–9. [PMID: 18579026]

7. Wilson Disease

In this metabolic disorder, abnormal movement and posture may occur with or without coexisting signs of liver involvement. It is discussed in Chapter 16.

8. Drug-Induced Abnormal Movements

Phenothiazines, butyrophenones, and metoclopramide may produce a wide variety of abnormal movements, including parkinsonism, akathisia (ie, motor restlessness), acute dystonia, chorea, and tardive dyskinesias or dystonia; several of these are also produced by aripiprazole. These complications are discussed in Chapter 25. Chorea may also develop in patients receiving levodopa, bromocriptine, anticholinergic drugs, phenytoin, carbamazepine, lithium, amphetamines, or oral contraceptives, and it resolves with withdrawal of the offending substance. Similarly, dystonia may be produced by levodopa, bromocriptine, lithium, or carbamazepine; and parkinsonism by reserpine and tetrabenazine. Postural tremor may occur with a variety of drugs, including epinephrine, isoproterenol, theophylline, caffeine, lithium, thyroid hormone, tricyclic antidepressants, and valproic acid.

9. Restless Legs Syndrome

This disorder may occur as a primary (idiopathic) disorder or in relation to pregnancy, iron deficiency anemia, peripheral neuropathy (especially uremic or diabetic), or periodic leg movements of sleep. It may have a hereditary basis and several genetic loci have been associated with the disorder (12q12-q21, 14q13-q31, 9p24-p22, 2q33, and 20p13). Restlessness and curious sensory disturbances lead to an irresistible urge to move the limbs, especially during periods of relaxation. Disturbed nocturnal sleep and excessive daytime somnolences may result. Therapy is with nonergot dopamine agonists, such as pramipexole (0.125–0.5 mg once

daily or ropinirole (0.25–4.0 mg once daily) 2 to 3 hours before bedtime, or with benzodiazepines, such as clonazepam. Gabapentin may also provide symptom relief and is taken once or twice daily (in the evening and before sleep), starting with 300 mg daily; the dose is built up depending on response and tolerance (to approximately 1800 mg daily). Levodopa is helpful but may lead to an augmentation of symptoms, so that its use is generally reserved for those who do not respond to other measures. In some instances, opioids are required to control symptoms.

Kushida CA. Clinical presentation, diagnosis, and quality of life issues in restless legs syndrome. Am J Med. 2007 Jan;120(1 Suppl 1):S4–S12. [PMID: 17198769]
Trenkwalder C. Treatment of restless legs syndrome: an evidence-based review and implications for clinical practice. Mov Disord. 2008 Dec 15;23(16):2267–302. [PMID: 18925578]
Winkelman JW et al. Efficacy and safety of pramipexole in restless legs syndrome. Neurology. 2006 Sep 26;67(6):1034–9. [PMID: 16931507]

10. Gilles de la Tourette Syndrome

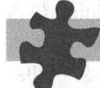

ESSENTIALS OF DIAGNOSIS

▸ Multiple motor and phonic tics.
▸ Symptoms begin before age 21 years.
▸ Tics occur frequently for at least 1 year.
▸ Tics vary in number, frequency, and nature over time.

▸ Clinical Findings

Motor tics are the initial manifestation in 80% of cases and most commonly involve the face, whereas in the remaining 20%, the initial symptoms are phonic tics; ultimately a combination of different motor and phonic tics develop in all patients. These are noted first in childhood, generally between the ages of 2 and 15. Motor tics occur especially about the face, head, and shoulders (eg, sniffing, blinking, frowning, shoulder shrugging, head thrusting, etc). Phonic tics commonly consist of grunts, barks, hisses, throat-clearing, coughs, etc, but sometimes also of verbal utterances including coprolalia (obscene speech). There may also be echolalia (repetition of the speech of others), echopraxia (imitation of others' movements), and palilalia (repetition of words or phrases). Some tics may be self-mutilating in nature, such as nail-biting, hair-pulling, or biting of the lips or tongue. The disorder is chronic, but the course may be punctuated by relapses and remissions. Obsessive-compulsive behaviors are commonly associated and may be more disabling than the tics themselves. A family history is sometimes obtained and inheritance has been attributed to an autosomal dominant gene with variable penetrance. In some instances, mutations in the *SLITRK1* gene on chromosome 13q have been incriminated.

Examination usually reveals no abnormalities other than the tics. In addition to obsessive-compulsive behavior disorders, psychiatric disturbances may occur because of the associated cosmetic and social embarrassment. Electroencephalography may show minor nonspecific abnormalities of no diagnostic relevance.

The diagnosis of the disorder is often delayed for years, the tics being interpreted as psychiatric illness or some other form of abnormal movement. Patients are thus often subjected to unnecessary treatment before the disorder is recognized. The tic-like character of the abnormal movements and the absence of other neurologic signs should differentiate this disorder from other movement disorders presenting in childhood. Wilson disease, however, can simulate the condition and should be excluded.

► **Treatment**

Treatment is symptomatic and may need to be continued indefinitely. Haloperidol is generally regarded as the drug of choice. It is started in a low daily dose (0.25 mg) that is gradually increased (by 0.25 mg every 4 or 5 days) until there is maximum benefit with a minimum of side effects or until side effects limit further increments. A total daily dose of between 2 and 8 mg is usually optimal, but higher doses are sometimes necessary. Treatment with clonazepam (in a dose that depends on response and tolerance) or clonidine (2–5 mcg/kg/d) may also be helpful, and it seems sensible to begin with one of these drugs in order to avoid some of the long-term extrapyramidal side effects of haloperidol. Phenothiazines, such as fluphenazine (2–15 mg daily), have been used, but patients unresponsive to haloperidol are usually unresponsive to these as well.

Pimozide, an oral dopamine-blocking drug related to haloperidol, may be helpful in patients who cannot tolerate or have not responded to haloperidol. Treatment is started with 1 mg daily and the daily dose increased by 1–2 mg every 10 days; the average dose is between 7 and 16 mg daily. Injection of botulinum toxin type A at the site of the most distressing tics is sometimes worthwhile.

Treatment with risperidone, calcium channel blockers, tetrabenazine, clomipramine, or metoclopramide has yielded mixed results or encouraging findings in preliminary studies that require confirmation. Bilateral high-frequency deep brain stimulation at various sites has been helpful in some, otherwise intractable, cases.

► **When to Refer**

All patients with Gilles de la Tourette syndrome should be referred.

► **When to Admit**

Patients undergoing surgical (deep brain stimulation) treatment should be admitted.

Welter ML et al. Internal pallidal and thalamic stimulation in patients with Tourette syndrome. Arch Neurol. 2008 Jul;65(7):952–7. [PMID: 18625864]

DEMENTIA

Dementia, the symptom complex of progressive global impairment of intellectual function, is a major medical, social, and economic problem that is worsening as the num-

ber of elderly people in the general population increases. It is discussed in Chapter 4, and the only point to be reiterated here is the importance of recognizing early any treatable or reversible causes of dementia, such as normal-pressure hydrocephalus, intracranial mass lesions, vascular disease, hypothyroidism, thiamine or vitamin B_{12} deficiency, Wilson disease, liver or kidney failure, neurosyphilis, and the chronic meningitides.

MULTIPLE SCLEROSIS

ESSENTIALS OF DIAGNOSIS

► Episodic neurologic symptoms.
► Patient usually under 55 years of age at onset.
► Single pathologic lesion cannot explain clinical findings.
► Multiple foci best visualized by MRI.

► **General Considerations**

This common neurologic disorder, which probably has an autoimmune basis, has its greatest incidence in young adults. Epidemiologic studies indicate that multiple sclerosis is much more common in persons of western European lineage who live in temperate zones. No population with a high risk for multiple sclerosis exists between latitudes 40° N and 40° S. A genetic susceptibility to the disease is present, based on twin studies, familial cases, and an association with specific HLA antigens (HLA-DR2) and alleles of *IL2RA* (the interleukin-2 receptor α gene) and *IL7RA* (the interleukin-7 receptor α gene). Pathologically, focal—often perivenular—areas of demyelination with reactive gliosis are found scattered in the white matter of brain and spinal cord and in the optic nerves. Axonal damage also occurs.

► **Clinical Findings**

A. Symptoms and Signs

The common initial presentation is weakness, numbness, tingling, or unsteadiness in a limb; spastic paraparesis; retrobulbar neuritis; diplopia; disequilibrium; or a sphincter disturbance such as urinary urgency or hesitancy. Symptoms may disappear after a few days or weeks, although examination often reveals a residual deficit.

Several forms of the disease are recognized. In most patients, there is an interval of months or years after the initial episode before new symptoms develop or the original ones recur (**relapsing-remitting disease**). Eventually, however, relapses and usually incomplete remissions lead to increasing disability, with weakness, spasticity, and ataxia of the limbs, impaired vision, and urinary incontinence. The findings on examination at this stage commonly include optic atrophy, nystagmus, dysarthria, and pyramidal, sensory, or cerebellar deficits in some or all of the limbs. In some of these patients, the clinical course changes so that a steady deterioration occurs, unrelated to acute relapses (**secondary progressive disease**).

Less commonly, symptoms are steadily progressive from their onset, and disability develops at a relatively early stage (**primary progressive disease**). The diagnosis cannot be made with confidence unless the total clinical picture indicates involvement of different parts of the central nervous system at different times.

A number of factors (eg, infection) may precipitate or trigger exacerbations. Relapses are reduced in pregnancy but are more likely during the 2 or 3 months following pregnancy, possibly because of the increased demands and stresses that occur in the postpartum period.

B. Imaging

MRI of the brain or cervical cord has a major role in demonstrating the presence of multiple lesions. In T1-weighted images, hypointense "black holes" probably represent areas of permanent axonal damage; hyperintense lesions are also found. Gadolinium-enhanced T1-weighted images may highlight areas of inflammation with breakdown of the blood-brain barrier. T2-weighted images provide information about disease burden or total number of lesions, which typically appear as areas of high signal intensity. CT scans are less helpful than MRI.

In patients presenting with myelopathy alone and in whom there is no clinical or laboratory evidence of more widespread disease, myelography or MRI may be necessary to exclude a congenital or acquired surgically treatable lesion. The foramen magnum region must be visualized to exclude the possibility of Arnold-Chiari malformation, in which parts of the cerebellum and the lower brainstem are displaced into the cervical canal and produce mixed pyramidal and cerebellar deficits in the limbs.

C. Laboratory and Other Studies

A definitive diagnosis can never be based solely on the laboratory findings. If there is clinical evidence of only a single lesion in the central nervous system, multiple sclerosis cannot properly be diagnosed unless it can be shown that other regions are affected subclinically. The electrocerebral responses evoked by monocular visual stimulation with a checkerboard pattern stimulus, by monaural click stimulation, and by electrical stimulation of a sensory or mixed peripheral nerve have been used to detect subclinical involvement of the visual, brainstem auditory, and somatosensory pathways, respectively. Other disorders may also be characterized by multifocal electrophysiologic abnormalities.

There may be mild lymphocytosis or a slightly increased protein concentration in the cerebrospinal fluid, especially soon after an acute relapse. Elevated IgG in cerebrospinal fluid and discrete bands of IgG (oligoclonal bands) are present in many patients. The presence of such bands is not specific, however, since they have been found in a variety of inflammatory neurologic disorders and occasionally in patients with vascular or neoplastic disorders of the nervous system.

D. Diagnosis

Multiple sclerosis should not be diagnosed unless there is evidence that two or more different regions of the central white matter have been affected at different times. A diagnosis of clinically definite disease can be made in patients with a relapsing-remitting course and evidence on examination of at least two lesions involving different regions of the central white matter. The diagnosis is probable in patients with multifocal white matter disease but only one clinical attack, or with a history of at least two clinical attacks but signs of only a single lesion. Imaging may reveal involvement of the nervous system at different times if a gadolinium-enhancing lesion is present at least 3 months after an initial clinical event at a different site than one corresponding to that event or if a new T2 lesion is found at any time compared with a baseline scan obtained at least 30 days after the initial clinical event. Dissemination in space requires three of the following: (1) at least one gadolinium-enhancing lesion or nine T2 hyperintense lesions if there is no enhancing lesion; (2) one or more infratentorial (or spinal cord) lesions; (3) one or more juxtacortical lesions; and (4) at least three periventricular lesions.

▶ Treatment

At least partial recovery from acute exacerbations can reasonably be expected, but further relapses may occur without warning, and there is no means of preventing progression of the disorder. Some disability is likely to result eventually, but about half of all patients are without significant disability even 10 years after onset of symptoms.

Recovery from acute relapses may be hastened by treatment with corticosteroids, but the extent of recovery is unchanged. A high dose (eg, prednisone, 60 or 80 mg) is given daily for 1 week, after which medication is tapered over the following 2 or 3 weeks. Such a regimen is often preceded by methylprednisolone, 1 g intravenously for 3 days. Long-term treatment with corticosteroids provides no benefit and does not prevent further relapses.

In patients with relapsing-remitting or secondary progressive disease, indefinite treatment with β-interferon (dosing regimen depends on the formulation) or with daily subcutaneous administration of glatiramer acetate reduces the frequency of exacerbations with equal efficacy. Natalizumab, an alpha4 integrin antagonist that reduces the development of brain lesions in experimental models, reduces the relapse rate. However, it can only be prescribed under a risk management plan because of rare reports of progressive multifocal leukoencephalopathy developing in patients while receiving treatment. Natalizumab is sometimes used in patients having lesions with very high disease activity on MRI and in those with progressive or poorly controlled disease despite treatment with β-interferon or glatiramer acetate. Several studies have suggested that immunosuppressive therapy with cyclophosphamide, azathioprine, methotrexate, cladribine, or mitoxantrone may help arrest the course of secondary progressive multiple sclerosis. The evidence of benefit is incomplete, however. Plasmapheresis is sometimes helpful in patients with severe relapses unresponsive to corticosteroids. Intravenous immunoglobulins (IVIGs) may reduce the clinical attack rate in relapsing-remitting disease, but the available studies are inadequate to permit treatment recommendations. Statins may have immunomodulatory effects, and their possible role in the treatment of multiple sclerosis is being studied.

Treatment for spasticity (see below) and for neurogenic bladder may be needed in advanced cases. Excessive fatigue must be avoided, and patients should rest during periods of acute relapse.

► When to Refer

All patients, but especially those with progressive disease despite standard therapy, should be referred.

► When to Admit

- Patients requiring plasma exchange.
- During severe relapses.
- Patient unable to manage at home.

Fox EJ. Management of worsening multiple sclerosis with mitoxantrone: a review. Clin Ther. 2006 Apr;28(4):461–74. [PMID: 16750460]

Goodin DS et al. The use of natalizumab (Tysabri) for the treatment of multiple sclerosis (an evidence-based review): report of the Therapeutics and Technology Assessment Subcommittee of the American Academy of Neurology. Neurology. 2008 Sep 2;71(10):766–73. [PMID: 18765653]

Hemmer B et al. Toward the development of rational therapies in multiple sclerosis: what is on the horizon? Ann Neurol. 2007 Oct;62(4):314–26. [PMID: 17969020]

Miller DH et al. Primary-progressive multiple sclerosis. Lancet Neurol. 2007 Oct;6(10):903–12. [PMID: 17884680]

NEUROMYELITIS OPTICA

This disorder is characterized by optic neuritis and acute myelitis with MRI changes that extend over at least three segments of the spinal cord. An isolated myelitis or optic neuritis may also occur. Previously known as Devic disease and once regarded as a variant of multiple sclerosis, neuromyelitis optica is associated with a specific antibody marker (NMO-IgG) targeting the water channel aquaporin-4. MRI of the brain typically does not show widespread white matter involvement but such changes do not exclude the diagnosis. Treatment is by long-term immunosuppression. Rituximab may help in reducing the risk of relapses and is undergoing clinical trials.

Cree B. Neuromyelitis optica: diagnosis, pathogenesis, and treatment. Curr Neurol Neurosci Rep. 2008 Sep;8(5):427–33. [PMID: 18713580]

VITAMIN E DEFICIENCY

Vitamin E deficiency may produce a disorder somewhat similar to Friedreich ataxia (see below). There is spinocerebellar degeneration involving particularly the posterior columns of the spinal cord and leading to limb ataxia, sensory loss, absent tendon reflexes, slurring of speech, and, in some cases, pigmentary retinal degeneration. The disorder may occur as a consequence of malabsorption or on a hereditary basis. Treatment is with α-tocopheryl acetate (eg, Aquasol E capsules or drops) as discussed in Chapter 29.

SPASTICITY

The term "spasticity" is commonly used for an upper motor neuron deficit, but it properly refers to a velocity-dependent increase in resistance to passive movement that affects different muscles to a different extent, is not uniform in degree throughout the range of a particular movement, and is commonly associated with other features of pyramidal deficit. It is often a major complication of stroke, cerebral or spinal injury, static perinatal encephalopathy, and multiple sclerosis.

Physical therapy with appropriate stretching programs is important during rehabilitation after the development of an upper motor neuron lesion and in subsequent management of the patient. The aim is to prevent joint and muscle contractures and perhaps to modulate spasticity.

Drug management is important also, but treatment may increase functional disability when increased extensor tone is providing additional support for patients with weak legs. Dantrolene weakens muscle contraction by interfering with the role of calcium. It is best avoided in patients with poor respiratory function or severe myocardial disease. Treatment is begun with 25 mg once daily, and the daily dose is built up by 25 mg increments every 3 days, depending on tolerance, to a maximum of 100 mg four times daily. Side effects include diarrhea, nausea, weakness, hepatic dysfunction (that may rarely be fatal, especially in women older than 35), drowsiness, light-headedness, and hallucinations.

Lioresal is an effective drug for treating spasticity of spinal origin and painful flexor (or extensor) spasms. The maximum recommended daily dose is 80 mg; treatment is started with a dose of 5 or 10 mg twice daily and then built up gradually. Side effects include gastrointestinal disturbances, lassitude, fatigue, sedation, unsteadiness, confusion, and hallucinations. Diazepam may modify spasticity by its action on spinal interneurons and perhaps also by influencing supraspinal centers, but effective doses often cause intolerable drowsiness and vary with different patients. Tizanidine, a centrally acting α_2-adrenergic agonist, is as effective as these other agents but is probably better tolerated. The daily dose is built up gradually, usually to 8 mg taken three times daily. Side effects include sedation, lassitude, hypotension, and dryness of the mouth.

Motor-point blocks by intramuscular phenol have been used to reduce spasticity selectively in one or a few important muscles and may permit return of function in patients with incomplete myelopathies. Intramuscular administration of botulinum toxin may also be helpful. Intrathecal injection of phenol or absolute alcohol may be helpful in more severe cases, but greater selectivity can be achieved by nerve root or peripheral nerve neurolysis. These procedures should not be undertaken until the spasticity syndrome is fully evolved, ie, only after about 1 year or so, and only if long-term drug treatment either has been unhelpful or carries a significant risk to the patient.

In patients with severe spasticity and limited use of the legs, a surgically implanted lioresal pump may provide significant relief and improve hygiene. Repeated transcutaneous electrical nerve stimulation may supplement medical treatment. A number of surgical procedures, eg, adductor or heel cord tenotomy, may also help in the management of spasticity and facilitate patient management. For example, obturator neurectomy is helpful in patients with marked adductor spasms that interfere with personal hygiene or cause gait disturbances. Posterior rhizotomy reduces spasticity, but its effect may be short-lived, whereas anterior rhizotomy produces permanent wasting and weakness in the muscles that are denervated.

Spasticity may be exacerbated by decubitus ulcers, urinary or other infections, and nociceptive stimuli.

Simpson DM et al. Botulinum neurotoxin for the treatment of spasticity (an evidence-based review): report of the Therapeutics and Technology Assessment Subcommittee of the American Academy of Neurology. Neurology. 2008 May 6;70(19):1691–8. [PMID: 18458229]

MYELOPATHIES IN AIDS

A variety of myelopathies may occur in patients with AIDS. These are discussed in Chapter 31.

MYELOPATHY OF HUMAN T CELL LEUKEMIA VIRUS INFECTION

Human T cell leukemia virus (HTLV-1), a human retrovirus, is transmitted by breast-feeding, sexual contact, blood transfusion, and contaminated needles. Most patients are asymptomatic, but after a variable latent period (which may be as long as several years) a myelopathy develops in some instances. The MRI, electrophysiologic, and cerebrospinal fluid findings are similar to those of multiple sclerosis, but HTLV-1 antibodies are present in serum and spinal fluid. There is no specific treatment, but intravenous or oral corticosteroids may help in the initial inflammatory phase of the disease. Prophylactic measures are important. Needles or syringes should not be shared; infected patients should not breastfeed their infants or donate blood, semen, or other tissue. Infected patients should use condoms to prevent sexual transmission.

SUBACUTE COMBINED DEGENERATION OF THE SPINAL CORD

Subacute combined degeneration of the spinal cord is due to vitamin B_{12} deficiency, such as occurs in pernicious anemia. It is characterized by myelopathy with predominant pyramidal and posterior column deficits, sometimes in association with polyneuropathy, mental changes, or optic neuropathy. Megaloblastic anemia may also occur, but this does not parallel the neurologic disorder, and the former may be obscured if folic acid supplements have been taken. Treatment is with vitamin B_{12}. For pernicious anemia, a convenient therapeutic regimen is 100 mg cyanocobalamin intramuscularly daily for 1 week, then weekly for 1 month, and then monthly for the remainder of the patient's life.

WERNICKE ENCEPHALOPATHY

Wernicke encephalopathy is characterized by confusion, ataxia, and nystagmus leading to ophthalmoplegia (lateral rectus muscle weakness, conjugate gaze palsies); peripheral neuropathy may also be present. It is due to thiamine deficiency and in the United States occurs most commonly in alcoholics. It may also occur in patients with AIDS or hyperemesis gravidarum, and after surgery for obesity. In suspected cases, thiamine (50 mg) is given intravenously immediately and then intramuscularly on a daily basis until a satisfactory diet can be ensured. Intravenous glucose given before thiamine may precipitate the syndrome or worsen the symptoms. The diagnosis is confirmed by the response in 1 or 2 days to treatment, which must not be delayed while laboratory confirmation is obtained.

Sechi G et al. Wernicke's encephalopathy: new clinical settings and recent advances in diagnosis and management. Lancet Neurol. 2007 May;6(5):442–55. [PMID: 17434099]

STUPOR & COMA

 ESSENTIALS OF DIAGNOSIS

▶ Level of consciousness is depressed.
▶ Stuporous patients respond only to repeated vigorous stimuli.
▶ Comatose patients are unarousable and unresponsive.

General Considerations

The patient who is stuporous is unresponsive except when subjected to repeated vigorous stimuli, while the comatose patient is unarousable and unable to respond to external events or inner needs, although reflex movements and posturing may be present.

Coma is a major complication of serious central nervous system disorders. It can result from seizures, hypothermia, metabolic disturbances, or structural lesions causing bilateral cerebral hemispheric dysfunction or a disturbance of the brainstem reticular activating system. A mass lesion involving one cerebral hemisphere may cause coma by compression of the brainstem. All comatose patients should be admitted to hospital and referred to a neurologist or neurosurgeon.

Assessment & Emergency Measures

The diagnostic workup of the comatose patient must proceed concomitantly with management. Supportive therapy for respiration or blood pressure is initiated; in hypothermia, all vital signs may be absent and all such patients should be rewarmed before the prognosis is assessed.

The patient can be positioned on one side with the neck partly extended, dentures removed, and secretions cleared by suction; if necessary, the patency of the airways is maintained with an oropharyngeal airway. Blood is drawn for serum glucose, electrolyte, and calcium levels; arterial blood gases; liver and kidney function tests; and toxicologic studies as indicated. Dextrose 50% (25 g), naloxone (0.4–1.2 mg), and thiamine (50 mg) are given intravenously.

Further details are then obtained from attendants of the patient's medical history, the circumstances surrounding the onset of coma, and the time course of subsequent events. Abrupt onset of coma suggests subarachnoid hemorrhage, brainstem stroke, or intracerebral hemorrhage, whereas a slower onset and progression occur with other structural or mass lesions. A metabolic cause is likely with a preceding intoxicated state or agitated delirium. On examination, attention is paid to the behavioral response to painful stimuli, the pupils and their response to light, the position of the eyes and their movement in response to passive movement of the head and ice-water caloric stimulation, and the respiratory pattern.

A. Response to Painful Stimuli

Purposive limb withdrawal from painful stimuli implies that sensory pathways from and motor pathways to the stimulated limb are functionally intact. Unilateral absence of responses despite application of stimuli to both sides of the body in turn implies a corticospinal lesion; bilateral absence of responsiveness suggests brainstem involvement, bilateral pyramidal tract lesions, or psychogenic unresponsiveness. Inappropriate responses may also occur. Decorticate posturing may occur with lesions of the internal capsule and rostral cerebral peduncle, decerebrate posturing with dysfunction or destruction of the midbrain and rostral pons, and decerebrate posturing in the arms accompanied by flaccidity or slight flexor responses in the legs in patients with extensive brainstem damage extending down to the pons at the trigeminal level.

B. Ocular Findings

1. Pupils—Hypothalamic disease processes may lead to unilateral Horner syndrome, while bilateral diencephalic involvement or destructive pontine lesions may lead to small but reactive pupils. Ipsilateral pupillary dilation with no direct or consensual response to light occurs with compression of the third cranial nerve, eg, with uncal herniation. The pupils are slightly smaller than normal but responsive to light in many metabolic encephalopathies; however, they may be fixed and dilated following overdosage with atropine, scopolamine, or glutethimide, and pinpoint (but responsive) with opioids. Pupillary dilation for several hours following cardiopulmonary arrest implies a poor prognosis.

2. Eye movements—Conjugate deviation of the eyes to the side suggests the presence of an ipsilateral hemispheric lesion or a contralateral pontine lesion. A mesencephalic lesion leads to downward conjugate deviation. Dysconjugate ocular deviation in coma implies a structural brainstem lesion unless there was preexisting strabismus.

The oculomotor responses to passive head turning and to caloric stimulation relate to each other and provide complementary information. In response to brisk rotation of the head from side to side and to flexion and extension of the head, normally conscious patients with open eyes do not exhibit contraversive conjugate eye deviation (doll's-head eye response) unless there is voluntary visual fixation or bilateral frontal pathology. With cortical depression in lightly comatose patients, a brisk doll's-head eye response is seen. With brainstem lesions, this oculocephalic reflex becomes impaired or lost, depending on the site of the lesion.

The oculovestibular reflex is tested by caloric stimulation using irrigation with ice water. In normal subjects, jerk nystagmus is elicited for about 2 or 3 minutes, with the slow component toward the irrigated ear. In unconscious patients with an intact brainstem, the fast component of the nystagmus disappears, so that the eyes tonically deviate toward the irrigated side for 2–3 minutes before returning to their original position. With impairment of brainstem function, the response becomes perverted and finally disappears. In metabolic coma, oculocephalic and oculovestibular reflex responses are preserved, at least initially.

C. Respiratory Patterns

Diseases causing coma may lead to respiratory abnormalities. Cheyne-Stokes respiration may occur with bihemispheric or diencephalic disease or in metabolic disorders. Central neurogenic hyperventilation occurs with lesions of the brainstem tegmentum; apneustic breathing (in which there are prominent end-inspiratory pauses) suggests damage at the pontine level (eg, due to basilar artery occlusion); and atactic breathing (a completely irregular pattern of breathing with deep and shallow breaths occurring randomly) is associated with lesions of the lower pontine tegmentum and medulla.

1. Stupor & Coma Due to Structural Lesions

Supratentorial mass lesions tend to affect brain function in an orderly way. There may initially be signs of hemispheric dysfunction, such as hemiparesis. As coma develops and deepens, cerebral function becomes progressively disturbed, producing a predictable progression of neurologic signs that suggest rostrocaudal deterioration.

Thus, as a supratentorial mass lesion begins to impair the diencephalon, the patient becomes drowsy, then stuporous, and finally comatose. There may be Cheyne-Stokes respiration; small but reactive pupils; doll's-head eye responses with side-to-side head movements but sometimes an impairment of reflex upward gaze with brisk flexion of the head; tonic ipsilateral deviation of the eyes in response to vestibular stimulation with cold water; and initially a positive response to pain but subsequently only decorticate posturing. With further progression, midbrain failure occurs. Motor dysfunction progresses from decorticate to bilateral decerebrate posturing in response to painful stimuli; Cheyne-Stokes respiration is gradually replaced by sustained central hyperventilation; the pupils become middle-sized and fixed; and the oculocephalic and oculovestibular reflex responses become impaired, perverted, or lost. As the pons and then the medulla fail, the pupils remain unresponsive; oculovestibular responses are unobtainable; respiration is rapid and shallow; and painful stimuli may lead only to flexor responses in the legs. Finally, respiration becomes irregular and stops, the pupils often then dilating widely.

In contrast, a subtentorial (ie, brainstem) lesion may lead to an early, sometimes abrupt disturbance of consciousness without any orderly rostrocaudal progression of neurologic signs. Compressive lesions of the brainstem, especially cerebellar hemorrhage, may be clinically indistinguishable from intraparenchymal processes.

A structural lesion is suspected if the findings suggest focality. In such circumstances, a CT scan should be performed before, or instead of, a lumbar puncture in order to avoid any risk of cerebral herniation. Further management is of the causal lesion and is considered separately under the individual disorders.

2. Stupor & Coma Due to Metabolic Disturbances

Patients with a metabolic cause of coma generally have signs of patchy, diffuse, and symmetric neurologic involvement that cannot be explained by loss of function at any single level or in a sequential manner, although focal or lateralized deficits may occur in hypoglycemia. Moreover, pupillary reactivity is usually preserved, while other brainstem functions are often grossly impaired. Comatose patients with meningitis, encephalitis, or subarachnoid hemorrhage may also exhibit little in the way of focal neurologic signs, however, and clinical evidence of meningeal irritation is sometimes very subtle in comatose patients. Examination of the cerebrospinal fluid in such patients is essential to establish the correct diagnosis.

In patients with coma due to cerebral ischemia and hypoxia, the absence of pupillary light reflexes at the time of initial examination indicates that there is little chance of regaining independence; by contrast, preserved pupillary light responses, the development of spontaneous eye movements (roving, conjugate, or better), and extensor, flexor, or withdrawal responses to pain at this early stage imply a relatively good prognosis.

Treatment of metabolic encephalopathy is of the underlying disturbance and is considered in other chapters. If the cause of the encephalopathy is obscure, all drugs except essential ones may have to be withdrawn in case they are responsible for the altered mental status.

Stevens RD et al. Approach to the comatose patient. Crit Care Med. 2006 Jan;34(1):31–41. [PMID: 16374153]
Wijdicks EF et al. Practice parameter: Prediction of outcome in comatose survivors after cardiopulmonary resuscitation (an evidence-based review): Report of the Quality Standards Subcommittee of the American Academy of Neurology. Neurology. 2006 Jul 25;67(2):203–10. [PMID: 16864809]

3. Brain Death

The definition of brain death is controversial, and diagnostic criteria have been published by many different professional organizations. In order to establish brain death, the irreversibly comatose patient must be shown to have lost all brainstem reflex responses, including the pupillary, corneal, oculovestibular, oculocephalic, oropharyngeal, and respiratory reflexes, and should have been in this condition for at least 6 hours. Spinal reflex movements do not exclude the diagnosis, but ongoing seizure activity or decerebrate or decorticate posturing is not consistent with brain death. The apnea test (presence or absence of spontaneous respiratory activity at a $Paco_2$ of at least 60 mm Hg) serves to determine whether the patient is capable of respiratory activity.

Reversible coma simulating brain death may be seen with hypothermia (temperature < 32 °C) and overdosage with central nervous system depressant drugs, and these conditions must be excluded. Certain ancillary tests may assist the determination of brain death but are not essential. An isoelectric electroencephalogram, when the recording is made according to the recommendations of the American Electroencephalographic Society, may help in confirming the diagnosis. Alternatively, the demonstration of an absent cerebral circulation by intravenous radioisotope cerebral angiography or by four-vessel contrast cerebral angiography is confirmatory.

Wijdicks EF et al. Pronouncing brain death: contemporary practice and safety of the apnea test. Neurology. 2008 Oct 14;71(16):1240–4. [PMID: 18852438]

4. Persistent Vegetative State

Patients with severe bilateral hemispheric disease may show some improvement from an initially comatose state, so that, after a variable interval, they appear to be awake but lie motionless and without evidence of awareness or higher mental activity. This persistent vegetative state has been variously referred to as akinetic mutism, apallic state, or coma vigil. Most patients in this persistent vegetative state will die in months or years, but partial recovery has occasionally occurred and in rare instances has been sufficient to permit communication or even independent living.

5. Minimally Conscious State

In this state, patients exhibit inconsistent evidence of consciousness. There is some degree of functional recovery of behaviors suggesting self- or environmental awareness, such as basic verbalization or context-appropriate gestures, emotional responses (eg, smiling) to emotional but not neutral stimuli, or purposive responses to environmental stimuli (eg, a finger movement or eye blink apparently to command). Further improvement is manifest by the restoration of communication with the patient. The minimally conscious state may be temporary or permanent. Little information is available about its natural history or long-term outlook, which reflect the underlying cause. The likelihood of useful functional recovery diminishes with time; after 12 months, patients are likely to remain severely disabled and without a reliable means of communication. Prognostication is difficult.

6. Locked-In Syndrome (De-efferented State)

Acute destructive lesions (eg, infarction, hemorrhage, demyelination, encephalitis) involving the ventral pons and sparing the tegmentum may lead to a mute, quadriparetic but conscious state in which the patient is capable of blinking and of voluntary eye movement in the vertical plane, with preserved pupillary responses to light. Such a patient can mistakenly be regarded as comatose. Physicians should recognize that "locked-in" individuals are fully aware of their surroundings. The prognosis is variable, but recovery has occasionally been reported—in some cases including resumption of independent daily life, though this may take up to 2 or 3 years.

HEAD INJURY

Trauma is the most common cause of death in young people, and head injury accounts for almost half of these trauma-related deaths. The prognosis following head injury depends on the site and severity of brain damage. Some guide to prognosis is provided by the mental status, since loss of consciousness implies a worse prognosis than otherwise. Similarly, the degree of retrograde and posttraumatic amnesia provides an indication of the severity of injury and thus of the prognosis. Absence of skull fracture does not exclude the possibility of severe head injury. During the physical examination, special attention should be given to the level of consciousness and extent of any brainstem dysfunction.

Note: Patients (especially elderly, >65 years) who are intoxicated with drugs or alcohol or have evidence of soft-tissue injury above the clavicles following head injury should be admitted to the hospital for observation, as should patients with recurrent vomiting, persistent anterograde amnesia, retrograde amnesia for more than 30 minutes, focal neurologic deficits, lethargy, or skull fractures. If admission is declined, responsible family members should be given clear instructions about the need for, and manner of, checking on them at regular (hourly) intervals and for obtaining additional medical help if necessary.

Skull radiographs or CT scans may provide evidence of fractures. Because injury to the spine may have accompanied head trauma, cervical spine radiographs (especially in the lateral projection) should always be obtained in comatose patients and in patients with severe neck pain or a deficit possibly related to cord compression.

CT scanning has an important role in demonstrating intracranial hemorrhage and may also provide evidence of cerebral edema and displacement of midline structures.

1. Cerebral Injuries

These are summarized in Table 24–7 along with comments about treatment. Increased intracranial pressure may result from ventilatory obstruction, abnormal neck position, seizures, dilutional hyponatremia, or cerebral edema; an intracranial hematoma requiring surgical evacuation may also be responsible. Other measures that may be necessary to reduce intracranial pressure include induced hyperventilation, intravenous mannitol infusion, and intravenous furosemide; corticosteroids provide no benefit in this context.

2. Scalp Injuries & Skull Fractures

Scalp lacerations and depressed or compound depressed skull fractures should be treated surgically as appropriate. Simple skull fractures require no specific treatment.

The clinical signs of basilar skull fracture include bruising about the orbit (raccoon sign), blood in the external auditory meatus (Battle sign), and leakage of cerebrospinal fluid (which can be identified by its glucose content) from the ear or nose. Cranial nerve palsies (involving especially the first, second, third, fourth, fifth, seventh, and eighth nerves in any combination) may also occur. If there is any leakage of cerebrospinal fluid, conservative treatment, with elevation of the head, restriction of fluids, and administration of acetazolamide (250 mg four times daily), is often helpful; but if the leak continues for more than a few days, lumbar subarachnoid drainage may be necessary. Antibiotics are given if infection occurs, based on culture and sensitivity studies. Only very occasional patients require intracranial repair of the dural defect because of persistence of the leak or recurrent meningitis.

3. Late Complications of Head Injury

The relationship of chronic subdural hemorrhage to head injury is not always clear. In many elderly persons there is no

Table 24–7. Acute cerebral sequelae of head injury.

Sequelae	Clinical Features	Pathology
Concussion	Transient loss of consciousness with bradycardia, hypotension, and respiratory arrest for a few seconds followed by retrograde and posttraumatic amnesia. Occasionally followed by transient neurologic deficit.	Bruising on side of impact (coup injury) or contralaterally (contrecoup injury).
Cerebral contusion or laceration	Loss of consciousness longer than with concussion. May lead to death or severe residual neurologic deficit.	Cerebral contusion, edema, hemorrhage, and necrosis. May have subarachnoid bleeding.
Acute epidural hemorrhage	Headache, confusion, somnolence, seizures, and focal deficits occur several hours after injury and lead to coma, respiratory depression, and death unless treated by surgical evacuation.	Tear in meningeal artery, vein, or dural sinus, leading to hematoma visible on CT scan.
Acute subdural hemorrhage	Similar to epidural hemorrhage, but interval before onset of symptoms is longer. Treatment is by surgical evacuation.	Hematoma from tear in veins from cortex to superior sagittal sinus or from cerebral laceration, visible on CT scan.
Cerebral hemorrhage	Generally develops immediately after injury. Clinically resembles hypertensive hemorrhage. Surgical evacuation is sometimes helpful.	Hematoma, visible on CT scan.

history of trauma, but in other cases a head injury, often trivial, precedes the onset of symptoms by several weeks. The clinical presentation is usually with mental changes such as slowness, drowsiness, headache, confusion, memory disturbances, personality change, or even dementia. Focal neurologic deficits such as hemiparesis or hemisensory disturbance may also occur but are less common. CT scan is an important means of detecting the hematoma, which is sometimes bilateral. Treatment is by surgical evacuation to prevent cerebral compression and tentorial herniation. There is no clear evidence that prophylactic anticonvulsant therapy reduces the incidence of posttraumatic seizures.

Normal-pressure hydrocephalus may follow head injury, subarachnoid hemorrhage, or meningoencephalitis.

Other late complications of head injury include posttraumatic seizure disorder and posttraumatic headache.

▶ When to Refer

- Patients with focal neurologic deficits, altered consciousness, or skull fracture.
- Patients with late complications of head injury, eg, posttraumatic seizure disorder or normal pressure hydrocephalus.

▶ When to Admit

- Patients (especially elderly, >65 years) who are intoxicated with drugs or alcohol or have evidence of soft-tissue injury above the clavicles should be admitted for observation.
- Patients with recurrent vomiting, focal neurologic deficits, persistent anterograde amnesia, retrograde amnesia for more than 30 minutes, altered consciousness, or skull fracture.
- Patients with acute epidural, subdural, or cerebral hematoma.
- Patients requiring shunt placement for normal pressure hydrocephalus.

Maas AI et al. Moderate and severe traumatic brain injury in adults. Lancet Neurol. 2008 Aug;7(8):728–41. [PMID: 18635021]
Ropper AH et al. Clinical practice. Concussion. N Engl J Med. 2007 Jan 11;356(2):166–72. [PMID: 17215534]

SPINAL TRAUMA

ESSENTIALS OF DIAGNOSIS

- ▶ History of preceding trauma.
- ▶ Development of acute neurologic deficit.
- ▶ Signs of myelopathy on examination.

▶ General Considerations

While spinal cord damage may result from whiplash injury, severe injury usually relates to fracture-dislocation causing compression or angular deformity of the cord either cervically or in the lower thoracic and upper lumbar regions. Extreme hypotension following injury may also lead to cord infarction.

▶ Clinical Findings

Total cord transection results in immediate flaccid paralysis and loss of sensation below the level of the lesion. Reflex activity is lost for a variable period, and there is urinary and fecal retention. As reflex function returns over the following days and weeks, spastic paraplegia or quadriplegia develops, with hyperreflexia and extensor plantar responses, but a flaccid atrophic (lower motor neuron) paralysis may be found depending on the segments of the cord that are affected. The bladder and bowels also regain some reflex function, permitting urine and feces to be expelled at intervals. As spasticity increases, flexor or extensor spasms (or both) of the legs become troublesome, especially if the patient develops bed sores or a urinary tract infection. Paraplegia with the legs in flexion or extension may eventually result.

With lesser degrees of injury, patients may be left with mild limb weakness, distal sensory disturbance, or both. Sphincter function may also be impaired, urinary urgency and urgency incontinence being especially common. More particularly, a unilateral cord lesion leads to an ipsilateral motor disturbance with accompanying impairment of proprioception and contralateral loss of pain and temperature appreciation below the lesion (Brown-Séquard syndrome). A central cord syndrome may lead to a lower motor neuron deficit and loss of pain and temperature appreciation, with sparing of posterior column functions. A radicular deficit may occur at the level of the injury—or, if the cauda equina is involved, there may be evidence of disturbed function in several lumbosacral roots.

▶ Treatment

Treatment of the injury consists of immobilization and—if there is cord compression—decompressive laminectomy and fusion. Early treatment with high doses of corticosteroids (eg, methylprednisolone, 30 mg/kg by intravenous bolus, followed by 5.4 mg/kg/h for 23 hours) may improve neurologic recovery if commenced within 8 hours after injury; the findings from various studies are conflicting, however, and evaluation of the published evidence suggest that significant benefit is unlikely. Various other therapies are being investigated. Anatomic realignment of the spinal cord by traction and other orthopedic procedures is important. Subsequent care of the residual neurologic deficit—paraplegia or quadriplegia—requires treatment of spasticity and care of the skin, bladder, and bowels.

▶ When to Refer

All patients with focal neurologic deficits should be referred.

▶ When to Admit

- Patients with neurologic deficits.

- Patients with spinal cord injury, compression, or acute epidural or subdural hematoma.
- Patients with vertebral fracture-dislocation likely to compress the cord.

Tator CH. Review of treatment trials in human spinal cord injury: issues, difficulties, and recommendations. Neurosurgery. 2006 Nov;59(5):957–82. [PMID: 17143232]
Thuret S et al. Therapeutic interventions after spinal cord injury. Nat Rev Neurosci. 2006 Aug;7(8):628–43. [PMID: 16858391]

SYRINGOMYELIA

Destruction or degeneration of gray and white matter adjacent to the central canal of the cervical spinal cord leads to cavitation and accumulation of fluid within the spinal cord. The precise pathogenesis is unclear, but many cases are associated with Arnold-Chiari malformation, in which there is displacement of the cerebellar tonsils, medulla, and fourth ventricle into the spinal canal, sometimes with accompanying meningomyelocele. In such circumstances, the cord cavity connects with and may merely represent a dilated central canal. In other cases, the cause of cavitation is less clear. There is a characteristic clinical picture, with segmental atrophy and areflexia and loss of pain and temperature appreciation in a "cape" distribution owing to the destruction of fibers crossing in front of the central canal. Thoracic kyphoscoliosis is usually present. With progression, involvement of the long motor and sensory tracts occurs as well, so that a pyramidal and sensory deficit develops in the legs. Upward extension of the cavitation (syringobulbia) leads to dysfunction of the lower brainstem and thus to bulbar palsy, nystagmus, and sensory impairment over one or both sides of the face.

Syringomyelia, ie, cord cavitation, may also occur in association with an intramedullary tumor or following severe cord injury, and the cavity then does not communicate with the central canal.

In patients with Arnold-Chiari malformation, there are commonly skeletal abnormalities on plain radiographs of the skull and cervical spine. CT scans show caudal displacement of the fourth ventricle. MRI or positive contrast myelography may demonstrate the malformation itself. Focal cord enlargement is found at myelography or by MRI in patients with cavitation related to past injury or intramedullary neoplasms.

Treatment of Arnold-Chiari malformation with associated syringomyelia is by suboccipital craniectomy and upper cervical laminectomy, with the aim of decompressing the malformation at the foramen magnum. The cord cavity should be drained, and if necessary an outlet for the fourth ventricle can be made. In cavitation associated with intramedullary tumor, treatment is surgical, but radiation therapy may be necessary if complete removal is not possible. Posttraumatic syringomyelia is also treated surgically if it leads to increasing neurologic deficits or to intolerable pain.

Greitz D. Unraveling the riddle of syringomyelia. Neurosurg Rev. 2006 Oct;29(4):251–63. [PMID: 16752160]

DEGENERATIVE MOTOR NEURON DISEASES

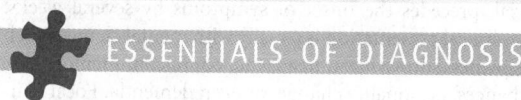
ESSENTIALS OF DIAGNOSIS

▶ Weakness.

▶ No sensory loss or sphincter disturbance.

▶ Progressive course.

▶ No identifiable underlying cause other than genetic basis in familial cases.

▶ General Considerations

This group of degenerative disorders is characterized clinically by weakness and variable wasting of affected muscles, without accompanying sensory changes.

Motor neuron disease in adults generally commences between 30 and 60 years of age. There is degeneration of the anterior horn cells in the spinal cord, the motor nuclei of the lower cranial nerves, and the corticospinal and corticobulbar pathways. The disorder is usually sporadic, but familial cases may occur and several genetic mutations or loci have been identified.

▶ Classification

Five varieties have been distinguished on clinical grounds.

A. Progressive Bulbar Palsy

Bulbar involvement predominates owing to disease processes affecting primarily the motor nuclei of the cranial nerves.

B. Pseudobulbar Palsy

Bulbar involvement predominates in this variety also, but it is due to bilateral corticobulbar disease and thus reflects upper motor neuron dysfunction. There may be a "pseudobulbar affect," with uncontrollable episodes of laughing or crying to stimuli that would not normally have elicited such marked reactions.

C. Progressive Spinal Muscular Atrophy

This is characterized primarily by a lower motor neuron deficit in the limbs due to degeneration of the anterior horn cells in the spinal cord.

D. Primary Lateral Sclerosis

There is a purely upper motor neuron deficit in the limbs.

E. Amyotrophic Lateral Sclerosis

A mixed upper and lower motor neuron deficit is found in the limbs. This disorder is sometimes associated with cognitive decline (in a pattern consistent with frontotemporal dementia), a pseudobulbar affect, or parkinsonism.

▶ Clinical Findings

A. Symptoms and Signs

Difficulty in swallowing, chewing, coughing, breathing, and talking (dysarthria) occur with bulbar involvement. In progressive bulbar palsy, there is drooping of the palate; a depressed gag reflex; pooling of saliva in the pharynx; a weak cough; and a wasted, fasciculating tongue. In pseudobulbar palsy, the tongue is contracted and spastic and cannot be moved rapidly from side to side. Limb involvement is characterized by motor disturbances (weakness, stiffness, wasting, fasciculations) reflecting lower or upper motor neuron dysfunction; there are no objective changes on sensory examination, although there may be vague sensory complaints. The sphincters are generally spared. Cognitive changes or pseudobulbar affect may be present. The disorder is progressive, and amyotrophic lateral sclerosis is usually fatal within 3–5 years; death usually results from pulmonary infections. Patients with bulbar involvement generally have the poorest prognosis.

B. Laboratory and Other Studies

Electromyography may show changes of chronic partial denervation, with abnormal spontaneous activity in the resting muscle and a reduction in the number of motor units under voluntary control. In patients with suspected spinal muscular atrophy or amyotrophic lateral sclerosis, the diagnosis should not be made with confidence unless such changes are found in at least three spinal regions (cervical, thoracic, lumbosacral) or two spinal regions and the bulbar musculature. Motor conduction velocity is usually normal but may be slightly reduced, and sensory conduction studies are also normal. Biopsy of a wasted muscle shows the histologic changes of denervation. The serum creatine kinase may be slightly elevated but never reaches the extremely high values seen in some of the muscular dystrophies. The cerebrospinal fluid is normal.

A familial form of amyotrophic lateral sclerosis has been described with autosomal dominant inheritance, related to mutations in the copper-zinc superoxide dismutase gene on the long arm of chromosome 21. Other familial forms with dominant or recessive inheritance have also been identified and mapped to other genetic loci. X-linked bulbospinal neuronopathy is associated with an expanded trinucleotide repeat sequence on the androgen receptor gene and carries a more benign prognosis than other forms of motor neuron disease. There have been recent reports of juvenile spinal muscular atrophy due to hexosaminidase deficiency, with abnormal findings on rectal biopsy and reduced hexosaminidase A in serum and leukocytes. Pure motor syndromes resembling motor neuron disease may also occur in association with monoclonal gammopathy or multifocal motor neuropathies with conduction block. A motor neuronopathy may also develop in Hodgkin disease and has a relatively benign prognosis. Infective anterior horn cell diseases (polio virus or West Nile virus infection) can generally be distinguished by the acute onset and monophasic course of the illness, as discussed elsewhere in this book.

▶ Treatment

Riluzole, 50 mg orally twice daily, which reduces the presynaptic release of glutamate, may slow progression of amyotrophic lateral sclerosis. There is otherwise no specific treatment except in patients with gammopathy, in whom plasmapheresis and immunosuppression may lead to improvement. Therapeutic trials of various neurotrophic factors to slow disease progression have yielded generally disappointing results as have trials of celecoxib, a cyclooxygenase-2 (COX-2) inhibitor, and pentoxifylline. Symptomatic and supportive measures may include prescription of anticholinergic drugs (such as trihexyphenidyl, amitriptyline, or atropine) or use of a portable suction machine if drooling is troublesome, braces or a walker to improve mobility, and physical therapy to prevent contractures. Behavioral modification (eg, exercising facial muscles and encouraging frequent swallowing) or over-the-counter decongestants may also help mild drooling. Spasticity may be helped by baclofen or diazepam. A semiliquid diet or nasogastric tube feeding may be needed if dysphagia is severe. Gastrostomy or cricopharyngomyotomy is sometimes resorted to in extreme cases of predominant bulbar involvement, and tracheostomy may be necessary if respiratory muscles are severely affected; however, in the terminal stages of these disorders, the aim of treatment should be to keep patients as comfortable as possible. Information on palliative care is provided in Chapter 5.

▶ When to Refer

All patients (to exclude other treatable causes of symptoms and signs) should be referred.

▶ When to Admit

Patients should be admitted during the terminal stages of the disorders for palliative care.

Lomen-Hoerth C. Amyotrophic lateral sclerosis from bench to bedside. Semin Neurol. 2008 Apr;28(2):205–11. [PMID: 18351522]
Mitchell JD et al. Amyotrophic lateral sclerosis. Lancet. 2007 Jun 16;369(9578):2031–41. [PMID: 17574095]
Mitsumoto H et al. Palliative care for patients with amyotrophic lateral sclerosis: "Prepare for the worst and hope for the best". JAMA. 2007 Jul 11;298(2):207–16. [PMID: 17622602]
Phukan J et al. Cognitive impairment in amyotrophic lateral sclerosis. Lancet Neurol. 2007 Nov;6(11):994–1003. [PMID: 17945153]

PERIPHERAL NEUROPATHIES

Peripheral neuropathies can be categorized on the basis of the structure primarily affected. The predominant pathologic feature may be axonal degeneration (axonal or neuronal neuropathies) or paranodal or segmental demyelination. The distinction may be possible on the basis of neurophysiologic findings. Motor and sensory conduction velocity can be measured in accessible segments of peripheral nerves. In axonal neuropathies, conduction velocity is normal or reduced only mildly and needle electromyography provides evidence of denervation in affected muscles. In demyelinating neuropathies, conduction may be slowed considerably in affected fibers, and in more severe cases, conduction is blocked completely, without accompanying electromyographic signs of denervation.

Nerves may be injured or compressed by neighboring anatomic structures at any point along their course. Common **mononeuropathies** of this sort are considered below. They lead to a sensory, motor, or mixed deficit that is restricted to the territory of the affected nerve. A similar clinical disturbance is produced by peripheral nerve tumors, but these are rare except in patients with Recklinghausen disease. Multiple mononeuropathies suggest a patchy multifocal disease process such as vasculopathy (eg, diabetes, arteritis), an infiltrative process (eg, leprosy, sarcoidosis), radiation damage, or an immunologic disorder (eg, brachial plexopathy). Diffuse **polyneuropathies** lead to a symmetric sensory, motor, or mixed deficit, often most marked distally. They include the hereditary, metabolic, and toxic disorders; idiopathic inflammatory polyneuropathy (Guillain-Barré syndrome); and the peripheral neuropathies that may occur as a nonmetastatic complication of malignant diseases. Involvement of motor fibers leads to flaccid weakness that is most marked distally; dysfunction of sensory fibers causes impaired sensory perception. Tendon reflexes are depressed or absent. Paresthesias, pain, and muscle tenderness may also occur.

POLYNEUROPATHIES & MONONEURITIS MULTIPLEX

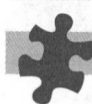 ### ESSENTIALS OF DIAGNOSIS

- ▶ Weakness, sensory disturbances, or both in the extremities.
- ▶ Pain sometimes common.
- ▶ Depressed or absent tendon reflexes.
- ▶ May be family history of neuropathy.
- ▶ May be history of systemic illness or toxic exposure.

The cause of polyneuropathy or mononeuritis multiplex is suggested by the history, mode of onset, and predominant clinical manifestations. Laboratory workup includes a complete blood count and sedimentation rate, serum protein electrophoresis, and immunophoresis, determination of plasma urea and electrolytes, liver and thyroid function tests, tests for rheumatoid factor and antinuclear antibody, HBsAg determination, a serologic test for syphilis, fasting blood glucose level, urinary heavy metal levels, cerebrospinal fluid examination, and chest radiography. These tests should be ordered selectively, as guided by symptoms and signs. Measurement of nerve conduction velocity is important in confirming the peripheral nerve origin of symptoms and providing a means of following clinical changes, as well as indicating the likely disease process (ie, axonal or demyelinating neuropathy). Cutaneous nerve biopsy may help establish a precise diagnosis (eg, polyarteritis, amyloidosis). In about half of cases, no specific cause can be established; of these, slightly less than half are subsequently found to be heredofamilial.

Treatment is of the underlying cause, when feasible, and is discussed below under the individual disorders. Physical therapy helps prevent contractures, and splints can maintain a weak extremity in a position of useful function. Anesthetic extremities must be protected from injury. To guard against burns, patients should check the temperature of water and hot surfaces with a portion of skin having normal sensation, measure water temperature with a thermometer, and use cold water for washing or lower the temperature setting of their hot-water heaters. Shoes should be examined frequently during the day for grit or foreign objects in order to prevent pressure lesions.

Patients with polyneuropathies or mononeuritis multiplex are subject to additional nerve injury at pressure points and should therefore avoid such behavior as leaning on elbows or sitting with crossed legs for lengthy periods.

Neuropathic, burning pain is sometimes troublesome and may respond to simple analgesics, such as aspirin or nonsteroidal anti-inflammatory agents, and to gabapentin. Duloxetine or venlafaxine may be helpful, especially in painful diabetic neuropathy. Opioids may be necessary for severe hyperpathia or pain induced by minimal stimuli, but their use should be avoided as much as possible. The use of a frame or cradle to reduce contact with bedclothes may be helpful. Many patients experience episodic stabbing pains, which may respond to gabapentin, pregabalin, phenytoin, carbamazepine, or tricyclic antidepressants.

Symptoms of autonomic dysfunction are occasionally troublesome. Postural hypotension is often helped by wearing waist-high elastic stockings and sleeping in a semierect position at night. Fludrocortisone reduces postural hypotension, but doses as high as 1 mg/d are sometimes necessary in diabetics and may lead to recumbent hypertension. Midodrine, an α-agonist, is sometimes helpful in a dose of 2.5–10 mg three times daily. Impotence and diarrhea are difficult to treat; a flaccid neuropathic bladder may respond to parasympathomimetic drugs such as bethanechol chloride, 10–50 mg three or four times daily.

1. Inherited Neuropathies

A. Charcot-Marie-Tooth Disease (HMSN Type I, II)

Several distinct varieties of Charcot-Marie-Tooth disease can be recognized. There is usually an autosomal dominant mode of inheritance, but occasional cases occur on a sporadic, recessive, or X-linked basis. The responsible gene is commonly located on the short arm of chromosome 17 and less often shows linkage to chromosome 1 or the X chromosome. It has also been linked to several other chromosomes, emphasizing the genetic heterogeneity of the disorder. Clinical presentation may be with foot deformities or gait disturbances in childhood or early adult life. Slow progression leads to the typical features of polyneuropathy, with distal weakness and wasting that begin in the legs, a variable amount of distal sensory loss, and depressed or absent tendon reflexes. Tremor is a conspicuous feature in some instances. Electrodiagnostic studies show a marked reduction in motor and sensory conduction velocity (hereditary motor and sensory neuropathy [HMSN] type I).

In other instances (HMSN type II), motor conduction velocity is normal or only slightly reduced, sensory nerve action potentials may be absent, and signs of chronic partial denervation are found in affected muscles electromyographically. The predominant pathologic change is axonal loss rather than segmental demyelination.

A similar disorder may occur in patients with progressive distal spinal muscular atrophy, but there is no sensory loss; electrophysiologic investigation reveals that motor conduction velocity is normal or only slightly reduced, and nerve action potentials are normal.

B. Dejerine-Sottas Disease (HMSN Type III)

The disorder may occur on a sporadic, autosomal dominant or, less commonly, autosomal recessive basis. Onset in infancy or childhood leads to a progressive motor and sensory polyneuropathy with weakness, ataxia, sensory loss, and depressed or absent tendon reflexes. The peripheral nerves may be palpably enlarged and are characterized pathologically by segmental demyelination, Schwann cell hyperplasia, and thin myelin sheaths. Electrophysiologically, there is slowing of conduction, and sensory action potentials may be unrecordable.

C. Friedreich Ataxia

Patients generally present in childhood or early adult life with this autosomal recessive disorder, which has been related to an unstable mutation of the *X25* gene on chromosome 9q13–q21.1. The gait becomes atactic, the hands become clumsy, and other signs of cerebellar dysfunction develop accompanied by weakness of the legs and extensor plantar responses. Involvement of peripheral sensory fibers leads to sensory disturbances in the limbs and depressed tendon reflexes. There is bilateral pes cavus. Pathologically, there is a marked loss of cells in the posterior root ganglia and degeneration of peripheral sensory fibers. In the central nervous system, changes are conspicuous in the posterior and lateral columns of the cord. Electrophysiologically, conduction velocity in motor fibers is normal or only mildly reduced, but sensory action potentials are small or absent.

D. Refsum Disease (HMSN Type IV)

This autosomal recessive disorder is due to a disturbance in phytanic acid metabolism. Clinically, pigmentary retinal degeneration is accompanied by progressive sensorimotor polyneuropathy and cerebellar signs. Auditory dysfunction, cardiomyopathy, and cutaneous manifestations may also occur. Motor and sensory conduction velocity are reduced, often markedly, and there may be electromyographic evidence of denervation in affected muscles. Dietary restriction of phytanic acid and its precursors may be helpful therapeutically. Plasmapheresis to reduce stored phytanic acid may help at the initiation of treatment.

E. Porphyria

Peripheral nerve involvement may occur during acute attacks in both variegate porphyria and acute intermittent porphyria. Motor symptoms usually occur first, and weakness is often most marked proximally and in the upper limbs rather than the lower. Sensory symptoms and signs may be proximal or distal in distribution. Autonomic involvement is sometimes pronounced. The electrophysiologic findings are in keeping with the results of neuropathologic studies suggesting that the neuropathy is axonal in type. Hematin (4 mg/kg intravenously over 15 minutes once or twice daily) may lead to rapid improvement. A high-carbohydrate diet and, in severe cases, intravenous glucose or levulose may also be helpful. Propranolol (up to 100 mg every 4 hours) may control tachycardia and hypertension in acute attacks.

2. Neuropathies Associated with Systemic & Metabolic Disorders

A. Diabetes Mellitus

In this disorder, involvement of the peripheral nervous system may lead to symmetric sensory or mixed polyneuropathy, asymmetric motor radiculoneuropathy or plexopathy (diabetic amyotrophy), thoracoabdominal radiculopathy, autonomic neuropathy, or isolated lesions of individual nerves. These may occur singly or in any combination and are discussed in Chapter 27.

B. Uremia

Uremia may lead to a symmetric sensorimotor polyneuropathy that tends to affect the lower limbs more than the upper limbs and is more marked distally than proximally (see Chapter 22). The diagnosis can be confirmed electrophysiologically, for motor and sensory conduction velocity is moderately reduced. The neuropathy improves both clinically and electrophysiologically with kidney transplantation and to a lesser extent with chronic dialysis.

C. Alcoholism and Nutritional Deficiency

Many alcoholics have an axonal distal sensorimotor polyneuropathy that is frequently accompanied by painful cramps, muscle tenderness, and painful paresthesias and is often more marked in the legs than in the arms. Symptoms of autonomic dysfunction may also be conspicuous. Motor and sensory conduction velocity may be slightly reduced, even in subclinical cases, but gross slowing of conduction is uncommon. A similar distal sensorimotor polyneuropathy is a well-recognized feature of beriberi (thiamine deficiency). In vitamin B_{12} deficiency, distal sensory polyneuropathy may develop but is usually overshadowed by central nervous system manifestations (eg, myelopathy, optic neuropathy, or intellectual changes).

D. Paraproteinemias

A symmetric sensorimotor polyneuropathy that is gradual in onset, progressive in course, and often accompanied by pain and dysesthesias in the limbs may occur in patients (especially men) with multiple myeloma. The neuropathy is of the axonal type in classic lytic myeloma, but segmental demyelination (primary or secondary) and axonal loss may occur in sclerotic myeloma and lead to predominantly motor clinical manifestations. Both demyelinating and axonal neuropathies are also observed in patients with paraproteinemias without myeloma. A small fraction will develop myeloma if serially followed. The demyelinating neuropathy in these patients may be due to the monoclonal protein's reacting to a component of the nerve myelin. The neuropathy of classic multiple myeloma is poorly responsive to therapy. The polyneuropathy of benign monoclonal gammopathy may respond to immunosuppressant drugs and plasmapheresis.

Polyneuropathy may also occur in association with macroglobulinemia and cryoglobulinemia and sometimes responds to plasmapheresis. Entrapment neuropathy, such as carpal tunnel syndrome, is more common than polyneuropathy in patients with (nonhereditary) generalized amyloidosis. With polyneuropathy due to amyloidosis, sensory and autonomic symptoms are especially conspicuous, whereas distal wasting and weakness occur later; there is no specific treatment.

3. Neuropathies Associated with Infectious & Inflammatory Diseases

A. Leprosy

Leprosy is an important cause of peripheral neuropathy in certain parts of the world. Sensory disturbances are mainly due to involvement of intracutaneous nerves. In tuberculoid leprosy, they develop at the same time and in the same distribution as the skin lesion but may be more extensive if nerve trunks lying beneath the lesion are also involved. In lepromatous leprosy, there is more extensive sensory loss, and this develops earlier and to a greater extent in the coolest regions of the body, such as the dorsal surfaces of the hands and feet, where the bacilli proliferate most actively. Motor deficits result from involvement of superficial nerves where their temperature is lowest, eg, the ulnar nerve in the region proximal to the olecranon groove, the median nerve as it emerges from beneath the forearm flexor muscle to run toward the carpal tunnel, the peroneal nerve at the head of the fibula, and the posterior tibial nerve in the lower part of the leg; patchy facial muscular weakness may also occur owing to involvement of the superficial branches of the seventh cranial nerve.

Motor disturbances in leprosy are suggestive of multiple mononeuropathy, whereas sensory changes resemble those of distal polyneuropathy. Examination, however, relates the distribution of sensory deficits to the temperature of the tissues; in the legs, for example, sparing frequently occurs between the toes and in the popliteal fossae, where the temperature is higher. Treatment is with antileprotic agents (see Chapter 33).

B. AIDS

A variety of neuropathies occur in HIV-infected patients (see Chapter 31). Patients with AIDS may develop a chronic symmetric sensorimotor axonal **polyneuropathy** associated usually with no abnormal cerebrospinal fluid findings. Treatment is symptomatic. AIDS patients may also develop progressive **polyradiculopathy** or radiculomyelopathy that leads to leg weakness and urinary reten-

tion; sensory loss is less conspicuous than in polyneuropathy. The cerebrospinal fluid may show mononuclear pleocytosis and increased protein and low glucose concentrations. Cytomegalovirus is responsible in at least some cases. The prognosis is generally poor, but some patients respond to intravenous ganciclovir (2.5 mg/kg every 8 hours for 10 days, then 7.5 mg/kg daily 5 days per week).

An inflammatory **demyelinating polyradiculoneuropathy** sometimes occurs in HIV-seropositive patients without AIDS and may follow an acute, subacute, or chronic course. Weakness is usually more conspicuous distally than proximally and tends to overshadow sensory symptoms. Tendon reflexes are depressed or absent. The cerebrospinal fluid shows an increased cell count and protein concentration. Treatment with plasmapheresis has helped some patients. Spontaneous improvement may also occur. Seropositive patients without AIDS may also develop a **mononeuropathy multiplex** that sometimes responds to treatment with plasmapheresis.

C. Lyme Borreliosis

The neurologic manifestations of Lyme disease include meningitis, meningoencephalitis, polyradiculoneuropathy, mononeuropathy multiplex, and cranial neuropathy. Serologic tests establish the underlying disorder. Treatment is described in Chapter 34.

D. Sarcoidosis

Cranial nerve palsies (especially facial palsy), multiple mononeuropathy and, less commonly, symmetric polyneuropathy may all occur, the latter sometimes preferentially affecting either motor or sensory fibers. Improvement may occur with use of corticosteroids.

E. Polyarteritis

Involvement of the vasa nervorum by the vasculitic process may result in infarction of the nerve. Clinically, one encounters an asymmetric sensorimotor polyneuropathy (mononeuritis multiplex) that pursues a waxing and waning course. Corticosteroids and cytotoxic agents—especially cyclophosphamide—may be of benefit in severe cases.

F. Rheumatoid Arthritis

Compressive or entrapment neuropathies, ischemic neuropathies, mild distal sensory polyneuropathy, and severe progressive sensorimotor polyneuropathy can occur in rheumatoid arthritis.

4. Neuropathy Associated with Critical Illness

Patients in intensive care units with sepsis and multiorgan failure sometimes develop polyneuropathies. This may be manifested initially by unexpected difficulty in weaning patients from a mechanical ventilator and in more advanced cases by wasting and weakness of the extremities and loss of tendon reflexes. Sensory abnormalities are relatively inconspicuous. The neuropathy is axonal in type. Its pathogenesis is obscure, and treatment is supportive. The prognosis is good provided patients recover from the underlying critical illness.

5. Toxic Neuropathies

Axonal polyneuropathy may follow exposure to industrial agents or pesticides such as acrylamide, organophosphorus compounds, hexacarbon solvents, methyl bromide, and carbon disulfide; metals such as arsenic, thallium, mercury, and lead; and drugs such as phenytoin, perhexiline, isoniazid, nitrofurantoin, vincristine, and pyridoxine in high doses. Detailed occupational, environmental, and medical histories and recognition of clusters of cases are important in suggesting the diagnosis. Treatment is by preventing further exposure to the causal agent. Isoniazid neuropathy is prevented by pyridoxine supplementation.

Diphtheritic neuropathy results from a neurotoxin released by the causative organism and is common in many areas. Palatal weakness may develop 2–4 weeks after infection of the throat, and infection of the skin may similarly be followed by focal weakness of neighboring muscles. Disturbances of accommodation may occur about 4–5 weeks after infection and distal sensorimotor demyelinating polyneuropathy after 1–3 months.

6. Neuropathies Associated with Malignant Diseases

Both a sensorimotor and a purely sensory polyneuropathy may occur as a nonmetastatic complication of malignant diseases (see Table 39–13), and have been associated with circulating anti-MAG or anti-Hu antibodies that can be detected by a paraneoplastic antibody panel that is available commercially. The sensorimotor polyneuropathy may be mild and occur in the course of known malignant disease, or it may have an acute or subacute onset, lead to severe disability, and occur before there is any clinical evidence of the cancer, occasionally following a remitting course. An autonomic neuropathy may also occur as a paraneoplastic disorder related to the presence of anti-Hu antibodies or to an antibody against ganglionic acetylcholine receptors (anti-nAChR).

7. Acute Idiopathic Polyneuropathy (Guillain-Barré Syndrome)

ESSENTIALS OF DIAGNOSIS

▶ Acute or subacute progressive polyradiculoneuropathy.
▶ Weakness is more severe than sensory disturbances.
▶ Acute dysautonomia may be life-threatening.

General Considerations

This acute or subacute polyradiculoneuropathy sometimes follows infective illness, inoculations, or surgical procedures. There is an association with preceding *Campylo-*

bacter jejuni enteritis. The disorder probably has an immunologic basis, but the precise mechanism is unclear.

▶ Clinical Findings

A. Symptoms and Signs

The main complaint is of weakness that varies widely in severity in different patients and often has a proximal emphasis and symmetric distribution. It usually begins in the legs, spreading to a variable extent but frequently involving the arms and often one or both sides of the face. The muscles of respiration or deglutition may also be affected. Sensory symptoms are usually less conspicuous than motor ones, but distal paresthesias and dysesthesias are common, and neuropathic or radicular pain is present in many patients. Autonomic disturbances are also common, may be severe, and are sometimes life-threatening; they include tachycardia, cardiac irregularities, hypotension or hypertension, facial flushing, abnormalities of sweating, pulmonary dysfunction, and impaired sphincter control. The axonal subtypes of the syndrome (acute motor axonal neuropathy [AMAN] and acute motor and sensory axonal neuropathy [AMSAN]) are caused by antibodies to gangliosides on the axon membrane and especially by antibodies to GM1, GM1b, and GD1a (and GalNac-GD1a to AMAN).

B. Laboratory Findings

The cerebrospinal fluid characteristically contains a high protein concentration with a normal cell content, but these changes may take 2 or 3 weeks to develop. Electrophysiologic studies may reveal marked abnormalities, which do not necessarily parallel the clinical disorder in their temporal course. Pathologic examination shows primary demyelination or, less commonly, axonal degeneration.

▶ Differential Diagnosis

When the diagnosis is made, the history and appropriate laboratory studies should exclude the possibility of porphyric, diphtheritic, or toxic (heavy metal, hexacarbon, organophosphate) neuropathies. The temporal course excludes other peripheral neuropathies. Poliomyelitis, botulism, and tick paralysis must also be considered as they cause weakness of acute onset. The presence of pyramidal signs, a markedly asymmetric motor deficit, a sharp sensory level, or early sphincter involvement should suggest a focal cord lesion.

▶ Treatment

Treatment with prednisone is ineffective and may prolong recovery time. Plasmapheresis is of value; it is best performed within the first few days of illness and is particularly useful for clinically severe or rapidly progressive cases or those with ventilatory impairment. IVIG (400 mg/kg/d for 5 days) is equally helpful and imposes less stress on the cardiovascular system than plasmapheresis. Patients should be admitted to intensive care units if their forced vital capacity is declining, and intubation is considered if the forced vital capacity reaches 15 mL/kg, dyspnea becomes evident, or the oxygen saturation declines. Respiratory toilet and chest physical therapy help prevent atelectasis. Marked hypotension may respond to volume replacement or pressor agents. Low-dose heparin to prevent pulmonary embolism should be considered.

Approximately 3% of patients with acute idiopathic polyneuropathy have one or more clinically similar relapses, sometimes several years after the initial illness. Plasma exchange therapy may produce improvement in chronic and relapsing inflammatory polyneuropathy.

▶ Prognosis

Most patients eventually make a good recovery, but this may take many months, and about 20% of patients are left with persisting disability.

▶ When to Refer

All patients should be referred.

▶ When to Admit

All patients should be hospitalized until their condition is stable and there is no respiratory compromise.

8. Chronic Inflammatory Polyneuropathy

Chronic inflammatory demyelinating polyneuropathy, an acquired immunologically mediated disorder, is clinically similar to Guillain-Barré syndrome except that it has a relapsing or steadily progressive course over months or years and that autonomic dysfunction is generally less common. It may present as an exclusively motor disorder or with a mixed sensorimotor disturbance. In the relapsing form, partial recovery may occur after some relapses, but in other instances there is no recovery between exacerbations. Although remission may occur spontaneously with time, the disorder frequently follows a progressive downhill course leading to severe functional disability.

Electrodiagnostic studies show marked slowing of motor and sensory conduction, and focal conduction block. Signs of partial denervation may also be present owing to secondary axonal degeneration. Nerve biopsy may show chronic perivascular inflammatory infiltrates in the endoneurium and epineurium, without accompanying evidence of vasculitis. However, a normal nerve biopsy result or the presence of nonspecific abnormalities does not exclude the diagnosis.

Corticosteroids may arrest or reverse the downhill course. Treatment is usually begun with prednisone, 60–80 mg daily, continued for 2–3 months or until a definite response has occurred. If no response has occurred despite 3 months of treatment, a higher dose may be tried. In responsive cases, the dose is gradually tapered, but most patients become corticosteroid-dependent, often requiring prednisone, 20 mg daily on alternate days, on a long-term basis. IVIG can be used in place of—or in addition to—corticosteroids and is best used as the initial treatment in pure motor syndromes. When both IVIG and corticosteroids are ineffective, plasma exchange may be worthwhile. Immunosuppressant or immunomodulatory drugs (such

as azathioprine) may be added when the response to other measures is unsatisfactory or to enable maintenance doses of corticosteroids to be lowered. Symptomatic treatment is also important.

Freeman R. Autonomic peripheral neuropathy. Neurol Clin. 2007 Feb;25(1):277–301. [PMID: 17324728]

Hughes RA et al. Corticosteroids for Guillain-Barré syndrome. Cochrane Database Syst Rev. 2006 Apr 19;(2):CD001446. [PMID: 16625544]

Hughes RA et al. Immunotherapy for Guillain-Barré syndrome: a systematic review. Brain. 2007 Sep;130(Pt 9):2245–57. [PMID: 17337484]

Krishnan AV et al. Uremic neuropathy: clinical features and new pathophysiological insights. Muscle Nerve. 2007 Mar;35(3): 273–90. [PMID: 17195171]

Lo YL. Clinical and immunological spectrum of the Miller Fisher syndrome. Muscle Nerve. 2007 Nov;36(5):615–27. [PMID: 17657801]

Stamboulis E et al. Clinical and subclinical autonomic dysfunction in chronic inflammatory demyelinating polyradiculoneuropathy. Muscle Nerve. 2006 Jan;33(1):78–84. [PMID: 16184605]

van Doorn PA et al. Clinical features, pathogenesis, and treatment of Guillain-Barré syndrome. Lancet Neurol. 2008 Oct;7(10):939–50. [PMID: 18848313]

Vernino S et al. Antibody testing in peripheral neuropathies. Neurol Clin. 2007 Feb;25(1):29–46. [PMID: 17324719]

Yuki N. Ganglioside mimicry and peripheral nerve disease. Muscle Nerve. 2007 Jun;35(6):691–711. [PMID: 17373701]

Zochodne DW. Diabetic polyneuropathy: an update. Curr Opin Neurol. 2008 Oct;21(5):527–33. [PMID: 18769245]

MONONEUROPATHIES

 ESSENTIALS OF DIAGNOSIS

▶ Focal motor or sensory deficit.

▶ Deficit is in territory of an individual peripheral nerve.

An individual nerve may be injured along its course or may be compressed, angulated, or stretched by neighboring anatomic structures, especially at a point where it passes through a narrow space (entrapment neuropathy). The relative contributions of mechanical factors and ischemia to the local damage are not clear. With involvement of a sensory or mixed nerve, pain is commonly felt distal to the lesion. Symptoms never develop with some entrapment neuropathies, resolve rapidly and spontaneously in others, and become progressively more disabling and distressing in yet other cases. The precise neurologic deficit depends on the nerve involved. Percussion of the nerve at the site of the lesion may lead to paresthesias in its distal distribution.

Entrapment neuropathy may be the sole manifestation of subclinical polyneuropathy, and this must be borne in mind and excluded by nerve conduction studies. Such studies are also indispensable for the accurate localization of the focal lesion.

In patients with acute compression neuropathy such as may occur in intoxicated individuals ("Saturday night palsy"), no treatment is necessary. Complete recovery generally occurs, usually within 2 months, presumably because the underlying pathology is demyelination. However, axonal degeneration can occur in severe cases, and recovery then takes longer and may never be complete.

In chronic compressive or entrapment neuropathies, avoidance of aggravating factors and correction of any underlying systemic conditions are important. Local infiltration of the region about the nerve with corticosteroids may be of value; in addition, surgical decompression may help if there is a progressively increasing neurologic deficit or if electrodiagnostic studies show evidence of partial denervation in weak muscles.

Peripheral nerve tumors are uncommon, except in Recklinghausen disease, but also give rise to mononeuropathy. This may be distinguishable from entrapment neuropathy only by noting the presence of a mass along the course of the nerve and by demonstrating the precise site of the lesion with appropriate electrophysiologic studies. Treatment of symptomatic lesions is by surgical removal if possible.

1. Carpal Tunnel Syndrome

See Chapter 20.

2. Pronator Teres or Anterior Interosseous Syndrome

The median nerve gives off its motor branch, the anterior interosseous nerve, below the elbow as it descends between the two heads of the pronator teres muscle. A lesion of either nerve may occur in this region, sometimes after trauma or owing to compression from, for example, a fibrous band. With anterior interosseous nerve involvement, there is no sensory loss, and weakness is confined to the pronator quadratus, flexor pollicis longus, and the flexor digitorum profundus to the second and third digits. Weakness is more widespread and sensory changes occur in an appropriate distribution when the median nerve itself is affected. The prognosis is variable. If improvement does not occur spontaneously, decompressive surgery may be helpful.

3. Ulnar Nerve Lesions

Ulnar nerve lesions are likely to occur in the elbow region as the nerve runs behind the medial epicondyle and descends into the cubital tunnel. In the condylar groove, the ulnar nerve is exposed to pressure or trauma. Moreover, any increase in the carrying angle of the elbow, whether congenital, degenerative, or traumatic, may cause excessive stretching of the nerve when the elbow is flexed. Ulnar nerve lesions may also result from thickening or distortion of the anatomic structures forming the cubital tunnel, and the resulting symptoms may also be aggravated by flexion of the elbow, because the tunnel is then narrowed by tightening of its roof or inward bulging of its floor. A severe lesion at either site causes sensory changes in the medial $1^1/2$ digits and along the medial border of the hand. There is weakness of the ulnar-innervated muscles in the forearm and hand. With a cubital tunnel lesion, however, there may be relative sparing of the flexor carpi ulnaris muscle. Electrophysiologic evaluation using nerve stimulation techniques allows more precise localization of the lesion.

If conservative measures are unsuccessful in relieving symptoms and preventing further progression, surgical treatment may be necessary. This consists of nerve transposition if the lesion is in the condylar groove, or a release procedure if it is in the cubital tunnel.

Ulnar nerve lesions may also develop at the wrist or in the palm of the hand, usually owing to repetitive trauma or to compression from ganglia or benign tumors. They can be subdivided depending on their presumed site. Compressive lesions are treated surgically. If repetitive mechanical trauma is responsible, this is avoided by occupational adjustment or job retraining.

4. Radial Nerve Lesions

The radial nerve is particularly liable to compression or injury in the axilla (eg, by crutches or by pressure when the arm hangs over the back of a chair). This leads to weakness or paralysis of all the muscles supplied by the nerve, including the triceps. Sensory changes may also occur but are often surprisingly inconspicuous, being marked only in a small area on the back of the hand between the thumb and index finger. Injuries to the radial nerve in the spiral groove occur characteristically during deep sleep, as in intoxicated individuals (Saturday night palsy), and there is then sparing of the triceps muscle, which is supplied more proximally. The nerve may also be injured at or above the elbow; its purely motor posterior interosseous branch, supplying the extensors of the wrist and fingers, may be involved immediately below the elbow, but then there is sparing of the extensor carpi radialis longus, so that the wrist can still be extended. The superficial radial nerve may be compressed by handcuffs or a tight watch strap.

5. Femoral Neuropathy

The clinical features of femoral nerve palsy consist of weakness and wasting of the quadriceps muscle, with sensory impairment over the anteromedian aspect of the thigh and sometimes also of the leg to the medial malleolus, and a depressed or absent knee jerk. Isolated femoral neuropathy may occur in diabetics or from compression by retroperitoneal neoplasms or hematomas (eg, expanding aortic aneurysm). Femoral neuropathy may also result from pressure from the inguinal ligament when the thighs are markedly flexed and abducted, as in the lithotomy position.

6. Meralgia Paresthetica

The lateral femoral cutaneous nerve, a sensory nerve arising from the L2 and L3 roots, may be compressed or stretched in obese or diabetic patients and during pregnancy. The nerve usually runs under the outer portion of the inguinal ligament to reach the thigh, but the ligament sometimes splits to enclose it. Hyperextension of the hip or increased lumbar lordosis—such as occurs during pregnancy—leads to nerve compression by the posterior fascicle of the ligament. However, entrapment of the nerve at any point along its course may cause similar symptoms, and several other anatomic variations predispose the nerve to damage when it is stretched. Pain, paresthesia, or numbness occurs about the outer aspect of the thigh, usually unilaterally, and is sometimes relieved by sitting. Examination shows no abnormalities except in severe cases when cutaneous sensation is impaired in the affected area. Symptoms are usually mild and commonly settle spontaneously. Hydrocortisone injections medial to the anterosuperior iliac spine often relieve symptoms temporarily, while nerve decompression by transposition may provide more lasting relief.

7. Sciatic & Common Peroneal Nerve Palsies

Misplaced deep intramuscular injections are probably still the most common cause of sciatic nerve palsy. Trauma to the buttock, hip, or thigh may also be responsible. The resulting clinical deficit depends on whether the whole nerve has been affected or only certain fibers. In general, the peroneal fibers of the sciatic nerve are more susceptible to damage than those destined for the tibial nerve. A sciatic nerve lesion may therefore be difficult to distinguish from peroneal neuropathy unless there is electromyographic evidence of involvement of the short head of the biceps femoris muscle. The common peroneal nerve itself may be compressed or injured in the region of the head and neck of the fibula, eg, by sitting with crossed legs or wearing high boots. There is weakness of dorsiflexion and eversion of the foot, accompanied by numbness or blunted sensation of the anterolateral aspect of the calf and dorsum of the foot.

8. Tarsal Tunnel Syndrome

The tibial nerve, the other branch of the sciatic, supplies several muscles in the lower extremity, gives origin to the sural nerve, and then continues as the posterior tibial nerve to supply the plantar flexors of the foot and toes. It passes through the tarsal tunnel behind and below the medial malleolus, giving off calcaneal branches and the medial and lateral plantar nerves that supply small muscles of the foot and the skin on the plantar aspect of the foot and toes. Compression of the posterior tibial nerve or its branches between the bony floor and ligamentous roof of the tarsal tunnel leads to pain, paresthesias, and numbness over the bottom of the foot, especially at night, with sparing of the heel. Muscle weakness may be hard to recognize clinically. Compressive lesions of the individual plantar nerves may also occur more distally, with clinical features similar to those of the tarsal tunnel syndrome. Treatment is surgical decompression.

9. Facial Neuropathy

An isolated facial palsy may occur in patients with HIV seropositivity, sarcoidosis, or Lyme disease (Plate 90; also see Chapter 34), but most often it is idiopathic (Bell palsy).

▶ When to Refer

• If there is uncertainty about the diagnosis.

• Symptoms or signs are progressing despite treatment.

▶ When to Admit

When a patient should be hospitalized depends on the cause and treatment.

BELL PALSY

ESSENTIALS OF DIAGNOSIS

▶ Sudden onset of lower motor neuron facial palsy.

▶ Hyperacusis or impaired taste may occur.

▶ No other neurologic abnormalities

▶ General Considerations

Bell palsy is an idiopathic facial paresis of lower motor neuron type that has been attributed to an inflammatory reaction involving the facial nerve near the stylomastoid foramen or in the bony facial canal. Increasing evidence incriminates reactivation of herpes simplex virus infection in the geniculate ganglion at least in some instances. The disorder is more common in pregnant women or in persons with diabetes.

▶ Clinical Findings

The facial paresis generally comes on abruptly, but it may worsen over the following day or so. Pain about the ear precedes or accompanies the weakness in many cases but usually lasts for only a few days. The face itself feels stiff and pulled to one side. There may be ipsilateral restriction of eye closure and difficulty with eating and fine facial movements. A disturbance of taste is common, owing to involvement of chorda tympani fibers, and hyperacusis due to involvement of fibers to the stapedius occurs occasionally.

▶ Treatment

Other disorders that can produce a facial palsy and require specific treatment, such as tumors, Lyme disease, AIDS, sarcoidosis, and herpes zoster infection of the geniculate ganglion, must be excluded. The management of Bell palsy is controversial. Approximately 60% of cases recover completely without treatment, presumably because the lesion is so mild that it leads merely to conduction block. Considerable improvement occurs in most other cases, and only about 10% of all patients have permanent disfigurement or other long-term sequelae. Treatment is unnecessary in most cases but is indicated for patients in whom an unsatisfactory outcome can be predicted. The best clinical guide to progress is the severity of the palsy during the first few days after presentation. Patients with clinically complete palsy when first seen are less likely to make a full recovery than those with an incomplete one. A poor prognosis for recovery is also associated with advanced age, hyperacusis, and severe initial pain. Electromyography and nerve excitability or conduction studies provide a guide to prognosis but not early enough to aid in the selection of patients for treatment.

The only medical treatment that may influence the outcome is administration of corticosteroids, but this must be commenced within 5 days of onset. Treatment with prednisone, 60 or 80 mg daily in divided doses for 4 or 5 days, followed by tapering of the dose over the next 7–10 days, is a satisfactory regimen. It is helpful to protect the eye with lubricating drops (or lubricating ointment at night) and a patch if eye closure is not possible. Acyclovir does not confer any additional benefit. There is no evidence that surgical procedures to decompress the facial nerve are of benefit.

Sullivan FM et al. Early treatment with prednisolone or acyclovir in Bell's palsy. N Engl J Med. 2007 Oct 18;357(16):1598–607. [PMID: 17942873]

DISCOGENIC NECK PAIN

ESSENTIALS OF DIAGNOSIS

- ▶ Neck pain, sometimes radiating to arms.
- ▶ Restricted neck movements.
- ▶ Motor, sensory, or reflex changes in arms with root involvement.
- ▶ Neurologic deficit in legs, gait disorder, or sphincter disturbance with cord involvement.

General Considerations

A variety of congenital abnormalities may involve the cervical spine and lead to neck pain; these include hemivertebrae, fused vertebrae, basilar impression, and instability of the atlantoaxial joint. Traumatic, degenerative, infective, and neoplastic disorders may also lead to pain in the neck. When rheumatoid arthritis involves the spine, it tends to affect especially the cervical region, leading to pain, stiffness, and reduced mobility; displacement of vertebrae or atlantoaxial subluxation may lead to cord compression that can be life-threatening if not treated by fixation. Further details are given in Chapter 20 (including a discussion on low back pain), and discussion here is restricted to disk disease.

1. Acute Cervical Disk Protrusion

Acute cervical disk protrusion leads to pain in the neck and radicular pain in the arm, exacerbated by head movement. With lateral herniation of the disk, motor, sensory, or reflex changes may be found in a radicular (usually C6 or C7) distribution on the affected side (Figure 24–1); with more centrally directed herniations, the spinal cord may also be involved, leading to spastic paraparesis and sensory disturbances in the legs, sometimes accompanied by impaired sphincter function. The diagnosis is confirmed by MRI or CT myelography. In mild cases, bed rest or intermittent neck traction may help, followed by immobilization of the neck in a collar for several weeks. If these measures are unsuccessful or the patient has a significant neurologic deficit, surgical removal of the protruding disk may be necessary.

2. Cervical Spondylosis

Cervical spondylosis results from chronic cervical disk degeneration, with herniation of disk material, secondary calcification, and associated osteophytic outgrowths. One or more of the cervical nerve roots may be compressed, stretched, or angulated; and myelopathy may also develop as a result of compression, vascular insufficiency, or recurrent minor trauma to the cord. Patients present with neck pain and restricted head movement, occipital headaches, radicular pain and other sensory disturbances in the arms, weakness of the arms or legs, or some combination of these symptoms. Examination generally reveals that lateral flexion and rotation of the neck are limited. A segmental pattern of weakness or dermatomal sensory loss (or both) may be found unilaterally or bilaterally in the upper limbs, and tendon reflexes mediated by the affected root or roots are depressed. The C5 and C6 nerve roots are most commonly involved, and examination frequently then reveals weakness of muscles supplied by these roots (eg, deltoids, supraspinatus and infraspinatus, biceps, brachioradialis), pain or sensory loss about the shoulder and outer border of the arm and forearm, and depressed biceps and brachioradialis reflexes. Spastic paraparesis may also be present if there is an associated myelopathy, sometimes accompanied by posterior column or spinothalamic sensory deficits in the legs.

Plain radiographs of the cervical spine show osteophyte formation, narrowing of disk spaces, and encroachment on the intervertebral foramina, but such changes are common in middle-aged persons and may be unrelated to the presenting complaint. CT or MRI helps confirm the diagnosis and exclude other structural causes of the myelopathy.

Restriction of neck movements by a cervical collar may relieve pain. Operative treatment may be necessary to prevent further progression if there is a significant neurologic deficit or if root pain is severe, persistent, and unresponsive to conservative measures.

When to Refer

- Pain unresponsive to simple measures.
- Patients with neurologic deficits.
- Patients in whom surgical treatment is under consideration.

When to Admit

- Patients with progressive or significant neurologic deficit.
- Patients with sphincter involvement (from cord compression).
- Patients requiring surgical treatment.

BRACHIAL & LUMBAR PLEXUS LESIONS

1. Brachial Plexus Neuropathy

Brachial plexus neuropathy may be idiopathic, sometimes occurring in relationship to a number of different nonspecific illnesses or factors. In other instances, brachial plexus

Peripheral nerve

Nerve root

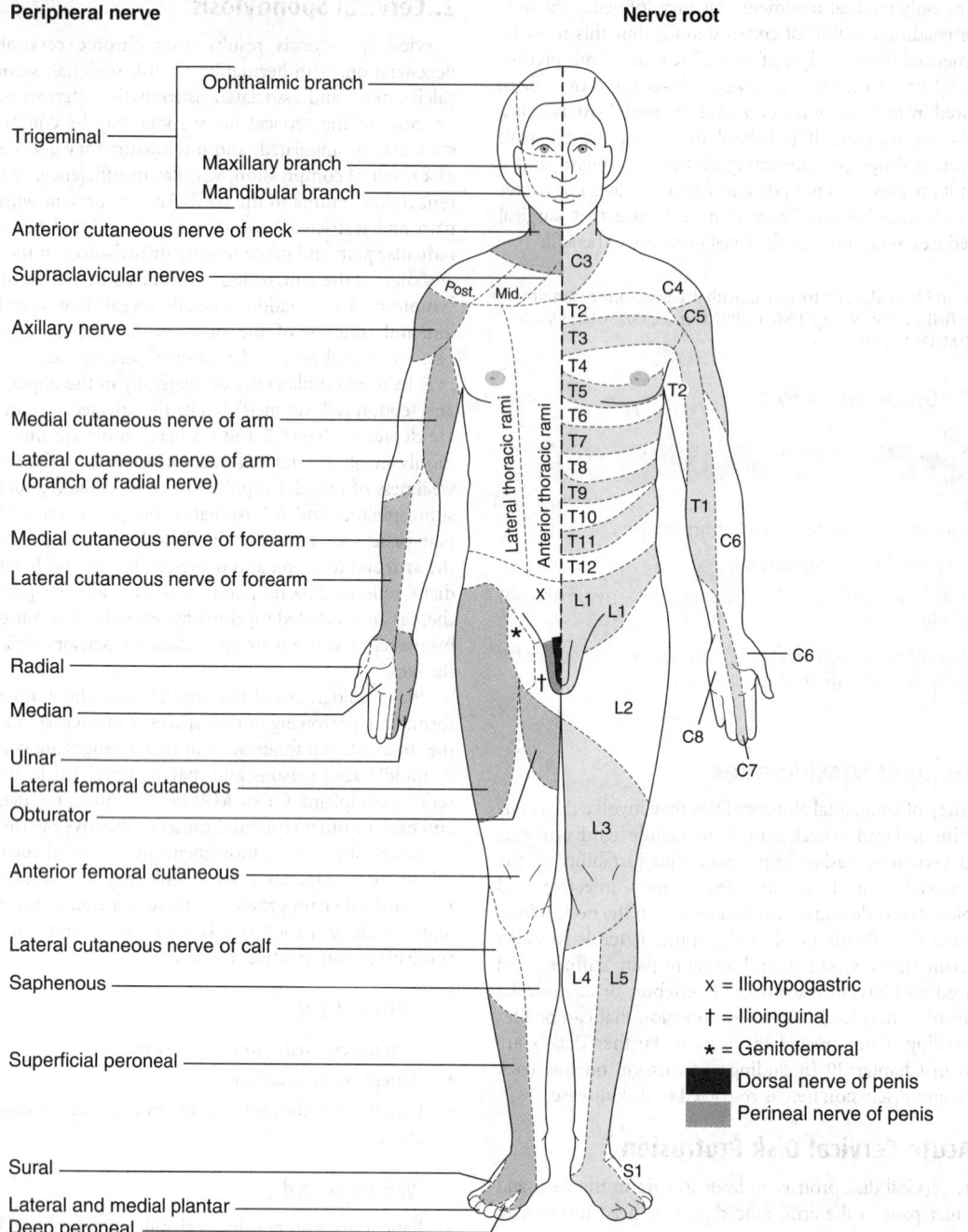

Trigeminal
- Ophthalmic branch
- Maxillary branch
- Mandibular branch

Anterior cutaneous nerve of neck

Supraclavicular nerves

Axillary nerve

Medial cutaneous nerve of arm

Lateral cutaneous nerve of arm (branch of radial nerve)

Medial cutaneous nerve of forearm

Lateral cutaneous nerve of forearm

Radial

Median

Ulnar

Lateral femoral cutaneous

Obturator

Anterior femoral cutaneous

Lateral cutaneous nerve of calf

Saphenous

Superficial peroneal

Sural

Lateral and medial plantar

Deep peroneal

Post. Mid.

C3
C4
C5
T2
T3
T4
T5
T6
T7
T8
T9
T10
T11
T12
L1
L2
L3
L4 L5
S1

Lateral thoracic rami
Anterior thoracic rami

T2
T1
C6
C6
C8
C7

x = Iliohypogastric
† = Ilioinguinal
★ = Genitofemoral
■ Dorsal nerve of penis
▨ Perineal nerve of penis

▲ **Figure 24–1.** Cutaneous innervation. The segmental or radicular (root) distribution is shown on the left side of the body and the peripheral nerve distribution on the right side. Above: anterior view; facing page: posterior view. (Reproduced, with permission, from Simon RP et al. *Clinical Neurology*, 4th ed. McGraw-Hill, 1999.) (*Continued*)

lesions follow trauma or result from congenital anomalies, neoplastic involvement, or injury by various physical agents. In rare instances, the disorder occurs on a familial basis.

Idiopathic brachial plexus neuropathy (neuralgic amyotrophy) characteristically begins with severe pain about the shoulder, followed within a few days by weakness, reflex changes, and sensory disturbances involving especially the C5 and C6 segments but affecting any nerve in the brachial plexus. Symptoms and signs are usually unilateral but may be bilateral. Wasting of affected muscles is sometimes pro-

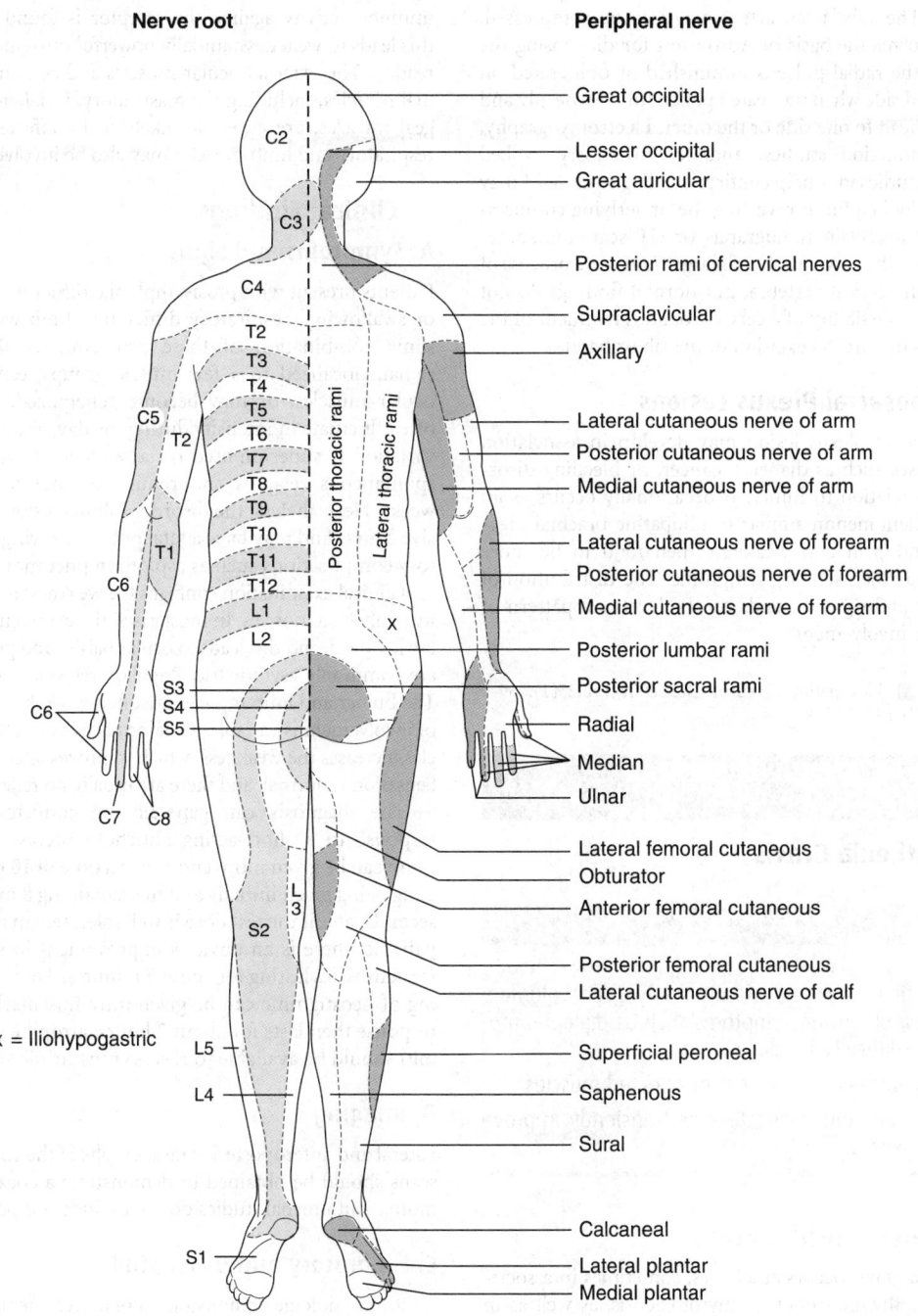

Nerve root

C2
C3
C4
T2
T3
T4
T5
T6
T7
T8
T9
T10
T11
T12
L1
L2
C5
T2
T1
C6
S3
S4
S5
C6
C7 C8

Posterior thoracic rami
Lateral thoracic rami
L3
S2
x

x = Iliohypogastric

L5
L4
S1

Peripheral nerve

Great occipital
Lesser occipital
Great auricular
Posterior rami of cervical nerves
Supraclavicular
Axillary
Lateral cutaneous nerve of arm
Posterior cutaneous nerve of arm
Medial cutaneous nerve of arm
Lateral cutaneous nerve of forearm
Posterior cutaneous nerve of forearm
Medial cutaneous nerve of forearm
Posterior lumbar rami
Posterior sacral rami
Radial
Median
Ulnar
Lateral femoral cutaneous
Obturator
Anterior femoral cutaneous
Posterior femoral cutaneous
Lateral cutaneous nerve of calf
Superficial peroneal
Saphenous
Sural
Calcaneal
Lateral plantar
Medial plantar

▲ **Figure 24–1.** (*Continued*)

found. The disorder relates to disturbed function of cervical roots or part of the brachial plexus, but its precise cause is unknown. Recovery occurs over the ensuing months but may be incomplete. Treatment is purely symptomatic.

van Alfen N et al. The clinical spectrum of neuralgic amyotrophy in 246 cases. Brain. 2006 Feb;129(Pt 2):438–50. [PMID: 16371410]

2. Cervical Rib Syndrome

Compression of the C8 and T1 roots or the lower trunk of the brachial plexus by a cervical rib or band arising from the seventh cervical vertebra leads to weakness and wasting of intrinsic hand muscles, especially those in the thenar eminence, accompanied by pain and numbness in the medial two fingers and the ulnar border of the hand and forearm. The subclavian artery may also be compressed, and this forms the basis of Adson test for diagnosing the disorder; the radial pulse is diminished or obliterated on the affected side when the seated patient inhales deeply and turns the head to one side or the other. Electromyography, nerve conduction studies, and somatosensory evoked potential studies may help confirm the diagnosis. MRI may be especially helpful in revealing the underlying compressive structure. Plain radiographs or CT scanning sometimes shows the cervical rib or a large transverse process of the seventh cervical vertebra, but normal findings do not exclude the possibility of a cervical band. Treatment of the disorder is by surgical excision of the rib or band.

3. Lumbosacral Plexus Lesions

A lumbosacral plexus lesion may develop in association with diseases such as diabetes, cancer, or bleeding disorders or in relation to injury. It occasionally occurs as an isolated phenomenon similar to idiopathic brachial plexopathy, and pain and weakness then tend to be more conspicuous than sensory symptoms. The distribution of symptoms and signs depends on the level and pattern of neurologic involvement.

Wilbourn AJ. Plexopathies. Neurol Clin. 2007 Feb;25(1):139–71. [PMID: 17324724]

DISORDERS OF NEUROMUSCULAR TRANSMISSION

1. Myasthenia Gravis

ESSENTIALS OF DIAGNOSIS

▶ Fluctuating weakness of commonly used voluntary muscles, producing symptoms such as diplopia, ptosis, and difficulty in swallowing.

▶ Activity increases weakness of affected muscles.

▶ Short-acting anticholinesterases transiently improve the weakness.

General Considerations

Myasthenia gravis occurs at all ages, sometimes in association with a thymic tumor or thyrotoxicosis, as well as in rheumatoid arthritis and lupus erythematosus. It is most common in young women with HLA-DR3; if thymoma is associated, older men are more commonly affected. Onset is usually insidious, but the disorder is sometimes unmasked by a coincidental infection that leads to exacerbation of symptoms. Exacerbations may also occur before the menstrual period and during or shortly after pregnancy. Symptoms are due to a variable degree of block of neuromuscular transmission caused by autoantibodies binding to acetylcholine receptors; these are found in most patients with the disease and have a primary role in reducing the number of functioning acetylcholine receptors. Additionally, cellular

immune activity against the receptor is found. Clinically, this leads to weakness; initially powerful movements fatigue readily. The external ocular muscles and certain other cranial muscles, including the masticatory, facial, and pharyngeal muscles, are especially likely to be affected, and the respiratory and limb muscles may also be involved.

Clinical Findings

A. Symptoms and Signs

Patients present with ptosis, diplopia, difficulty in chewing or swallowing, respiratory difficulties, limb weakness, or some combination of these problems. Weakness may remain localized to a few muscle groups, especially the ocular muscles, or may become generalized. Symptoms often fluctuate in intensity during the day, and this diurnal variation is superimposed on a tendency to longer-term spontaneous relapses and remissions that may last for weeks. Nevertheless, the disorder follows a slowly progressive course and may have a fatal outcome owing to respiratory complications such as aspiration pneumonia.

Clinical examination confirms the weakness and fatigability of affected muscles. In most cases, the extraocular muscles are involved, and this leads to ocular palsies and ptosis, which are commonly asymmetric. Pupillary responses are normal. The bulbar and limb muscles are often weak, but the pattern of involvement is variable. Sustained activity of affected muscles increases the weakness, which improves after a brief rest. Sensation is normal, and there are usually no reflex changes.

The diagnosis can generally be confirmed by the response to a short-acting anticholinesterase. Edrophonium can be given intravenously in a dose of 10 mg (1 mL), 2 mg being given initially and the remaining 8 mg about 30 seconds later if the test dose is well tolerated; in myasthenic patients, there is an obvious improvement in strength of weak muscles lasting for about 5 minutes. Alternatively, 1.5 mg of neostigmine can be given intramuscularly, and the response then lasts for about 2 hours; atropine sulfate (0.6 mg) should be available to reverse muscarinic side effects.

B. Imaging

Lateral and anteroposterior radiographs of the chest and CT scans should be obtained to demonstrate a coexisting thymoma, but normal studies do not exclude this possibility.

C. Laboratory and Other Studies

Electrophysiologic demonstration of a decrementing muscle response to repetitive 2- or 3-Hz stimulation of motor nerves indicates a disturbance of neuromuscular transmission. Such an abnormality may even be detected in clinically strong muscles with certain provocative procedures. Needle electromyography of affected muscles shows a marked variation in configuration and size of individual motor unit potentials, and single-fiber electromyography reveals an increased jitter, or variability, in the time interval between two muscle fiber action potentials from the same motor unit.

Assay of serum for elevated levels of circulating acetylcholine receptor antibodies is useful because it has a sensitivity of 80–90% for the diagnosis of myasthenia gravis. Certain patients without antibodies to acetylcholine receptors have serum antibodies to muscle-specific tyrosine kinase (MuSK), which should therefore be determined; these patients are more likely to have facial, respiratory, and proximal muscle weakness than those with antibodies to acetylcholine receptors.

Treatment

Medication such as aminoglycosides that may exacerbate myasthenia gravis should be avoided. Anticholinesterase drugs provide symptomatic benefit without influencing the course of the disease. Neostigmine, pyridostigmine, or both can be used, the dose being determined on an individual basis. The usual dose of neostigmine is 7.5–30 mg (average, 15 mg) taken four times daily; of pyridostigmine, 30–180 mg (average, 60 mg) four times daily. Overmedication may temporarily increase weakness, which is then unaffected or enhanced by intravenous edrophonium.

Thymectomy usually leads to symptomatic benefit or remission and should be considered in all patients younger than age 60, unless weakness is restricted to the extraocular muscles. If the disease is of recent onset and only slowly progressive, operation is sometimes delayed for a year or so, in the hope that spontaneous remission will occur.

Treatment with corticosteroids is indicated for patients who have responded poorly to anticholinesterase drugs and have already undergone thymectomy. It is often introduced with the patient in the hospital, since weakness may initially be aggravated. Once weakness has stabilized after 2–3 weeks or any improvement is sustained, further management can be on an outpatient basis. Alternate-day treatment is usually well tolerated, but if weakness is enhanced on the nontreatment day it may be necessary for medication to be taken daily. The dose of corticosteroids is determined on an individual basis, but an initial high daily dose (eg, prednisone, 60–100 mg) can gradually be tapered to a relatively low maintenance level as improvement occurs; total withdrawal is difficult, however. Treatment with azathioprine may also be effective. The usual dose is 2–3 mg/kg orally daily after a lower initial dose.

In patients with major disability, plasmapheresis or IVIG therapy may be beneficial. It is also useful for stabilizing patients before thymectomy and for managing acute crisis. Mycophenolate mofetil, an immunosuppressant, may provide symptomatic benefit and allow the corticosteroid dose to be reduced.

When to Refer

All patients should be referred.

When to Admit

- Patients with acute exacerbation or bulbar involvement.
- Patients requiring plasmapheresis.
- Patients who are starting corticosteroid therapy.
- For thymectomy.

Benatar M et al. Evidence report: the medical treatment of ocular myasthenia (an evidence-based review). Report of the Quality Standards Subcommittee of the American Academy of Neurology. Neurology. 2007 Jun 12;68(24):2144–9. [PMID: 17460154]

Jani-Acsadi A et al. Myasthenic crisis: guidelines for prevention and treatment. J Neurol Sci. 2007 Oct 15;261(1–2):127–33. [PMID: 17544450]

Mahadeva B et al. Autoimmune disorders of neuromuscular transmission. Semin Neurol. 2008 Apr;28(2):212–27. [PMID: 18351523]

2. Myasthenic Syndrome (Lambert-Eaton Syndrome)

 ESSENTIALS OF DIAGNOSIS

- ▶ Variable weakness, typically improving with activity.
- ▶ Dysautonomic symptoms may also be present.
- ▶ A history of malignant disease may be obtained.

General Considerations

Myasthenic syndrome (see Table 39–13) may be associated with small-cell carcinoma, sometimes developing before the tumor is diagnosed, and occasionally occurs with certain autoimmune diseases. There is defective release of acetylcholine in response to a nerve impulse, caused by P/Q-type voltage-gated calcium-channel antibody, and this leads to weakness, especially of the proximal muscles of the limbs. Unlike myasthenia gravis, however, power steadily increases with sustained contraction. The diagnosis can be confirmed electrophysiologically, because the muscle response to stimulation of its motor nerve increases remarkably if the nerve is stimulated repetitively at high rates, even in muscles that are not clinically weak.

Treatment with plasmapheresis and immunosuppressive drug therapy (prednisone and azathioprine) may lead to clinical and electrophysiologic improvement, in addition to therapy aimed at tumor when present. Prednisone is usually initiated in a daily dose of 60–80 mg and azathioprine in a daily dose of 2 mg/kg. Guanidine hydrochloride (25–50 mg/kg/d in divided doses) is occasionally helpful in seriously disabled patients, but adverse effects of the drug include marrow suppression. The response to treatment with anticholinesterase drugs such as pyridostigmine or neostigmine, either alone or in combination with guanidine, is variable.

3. Botulism

The toxin of *Clostridium botulinum* prevents the release of acetylcholine at neuromuscular junctions and autonomic synapses. Botulism occurs most commonly following the ingestion of contaminated home-canned food and should be suggested by the development of sudden, fluctuating, severe weakness in a previously healthy person. Symptoms begin within 72 hours following ingestion of the toxin and may progress for several days. Typically, there is diplopia, ptosis, facial weakness, dysphagia, and nasal speech, followed by respiratory difficulty and finally by weakness that appears last in the limbs. Blurring of vision (with unreactive dilated pupils) is characteristic, and there may be dryness of the mouth, constipation (paralytic ileus), and postural hypotension. Sensation is preserved, and the tendon reflexes are not affected unless the involved muscles are very weak. If the diagnosis is suspected, the local health authority should be notified and a sample of serum and contaminated food (if available) sent to be assayed for toxin. Support for the diagnosis may be obtained by electrophysiologic studies; with repetitive stimulation of motor nerves at fast rates, the muscle response increases in size progressively.

Patients should be hospitalized in case respiratory assistance becomes necessary. Treatment is with trivalent antitoxin, once it is established that the patient is not allergic to horse serum. Guanidine hydrochloride (25–50 mg/kg/d in divided doses) to facilitate release of acetylcholine from nerve endings sometimes helps to increase muscle strength. Anticholinesterase drugs are of no value. Respiratory assistance and other supportive measures should be provided as necessary. Further details are provided in Chapter 33.

4. Disorders Associated with Use of Aminoglycosides

Aminoglycoside antibiotics, eg, gentamicin, may produce a clinical disturbance similar to botulism by preventing the release of acetylcholine from nerve endings, but symptoms subside rapidly as the responsible drug is eliminated from the body. These antibiotics are particularly dangerous in patients with preexisting disturbances of neuromuscular

transmission and are therefore best avoided in patients with myasthenia gravis.

MYOPATHIC DISORDERS

1. Muscular Dystrophies

ESSENTIALS OF DIAGNOSIS

► Muscle weakness, often in a characteristic distribution.
► Age at onset and inheritance pattern depend on the specific dystrophy.

► General Considerations

These inherited myopathic disorders are characterized by progressive muscle weakness and wasting. They are subdivided by mode of inheritance, age at onset, and clinical features, as shown in Table 24–8. In the Duchenne type, pseudohypertrophy of muscles frequently occurs at some stage; intellectual retardation is common; and there may be skeletal deformities, muscle contractures, and cardiac involvement. The serum creatine kinase level is increased, especially in the Duchenne and Becker varieties, and mildly increased also in limb-girdle dystrophy. Electromyography may help confirm that weakness

Table 24–8. The muscular dystrophies.[1]

Disorder	Inheritance	Age at Onset (years)	Distribution	Prognosis	Genetic Locus
Duchenne type	X-linked recessive	1–5	Pelvic, then shoulder girdle; later, limb and respiratory muscles.	Rapid progression. Death within about 15 years after onset.	Xp21
Becker	X-linked recessive	5–25	Pelvic, then shoulder girdle.	Slow progression. May have normal life span.	Xp21
Limb-girdle (Erb)	Autosomal recessive, dominant or sporadic	10–30	Pelvic or shoulder girdle initially, with later spread to the other.	Variable severity and rate of progression. Possible severe disability in middle life.	Multiple
Facioscapulo-humeral	Autosomal dominant	Any age	Face and shoulder girdle initially; later, pelvic girdle and legs.	Slow progression. Minor disability. Usually normal life span.	4q35
Emery-Dreifuss	X-linked recessive or autosomal dominant	5–10	Humeroperoneal or scapulo-peroneal.	Variable.	Xq28, 1q21.2
Distal	Autosomal dominant or recessive	40–60	Onset distally in extremities; proximal involvement later.	Slow progression.	2p13, 14q12
Ocular	Autosomal dominant (may be recessive)	Any age (usually 5–30)	External ocular muscles; may also be mild weakness of face, neck, and arms.		
Oculopharyngeal	Autosomal dominant	Any age	As in the ocular form but with dysphagia.		14q11.2–q13
Myotonic dystrophy	Autosomal dominant	Any age (usually 20–40)	Face, neck, distal limbs.	Slow progression.	19q13.2-q13.3; 3q13.3-q24

[1]Not all possible genetic loci are shown.

is myopathic rather than neurogenic. Similarly, histopathologic examination of a muscle biopsy specimen may help confirm that weakness is due to a primary disorder of muscle and to distinguish between various muscle diseases.

A genetic defect on the short arm of the X chromosome has been identified in Duchenne dystrophy. The affected gene codes for the protein dystrophin, which is markedly reduced or absent from the muscle of patients with the disease. Dystrophin levels are generally normal in the Becker variety, but the protein is qualitatively altered.

Duchenne muscular dystrophy can now be recognized early in pregnancy in about 95% of women by genetic studies; in late pregnancy, DNA probes can be used on fetal tissue obtained for this purpose by amniocentesis. The genes causing some of the other muscular dystrophies are listed in Table 24–8.

There is no specific treatment for the muscular dystrophies, but it is important to encourage patients to lead as normal lives as possible. Prednisone (0.75 mg/kg daily) improves muscle strength and function in boys with Duchenne dystrophy, but side effects need to be monitored. Prolonged bed rest must be avoided, as inactivity often leads to worsening of the underlying muscle disease. Physical therapy and orthopedic procedures may help counteract deformities or contractures.

Angelini C. The role of corticosteroids in muscular dystrophy: a critical appraisal. Muscle Nerve. 2007 Oct;36(4):424–35. [PMID: 17541998]

Guglieri M et al. Limb-girdle muscular dystrophies. Curr Opin Neurol. 2008 Oct;21(5):576–84. [PMID: 18769252]

Rodino-Klapac LR et al. Gene therapy for Duchenne muscular dystrophy: expectations and challenges. Arch Neurol. 2007 Sep;64(9):1236–41. [PMID: 17846262]

Tawil R et al. Facioscapulohumeral muscular dystrophy. Muscle Nerve. 2006 Jul;34(1):1–15. [PMID: 16508966]

2. Myotonic Dystrophy

Myotonic dystrophy, a slowly progressive, dominantly inherited disorder, usually manifests itself in the third or fourth decade but occasionally appears early in childhood. The genetic defect has been localized to the long arm of chromosome 19 in the type 1 disorder. Myotonia leads to complaints of muscle stiffness and is evidenced by the marked delay that occurs before affected muscles can relax after a contraction. This can often be demonstrated clinically by delayed relaxation of the hand after sustained grip or by percussion of the belly of a muscle. In addition, there is weakness and wasting of the facial, sternocleidomastoid, and distal limb muscles. Associated clinical features include cataracts, frontal baldness, testicular atrophy, diabetes mellitus, cardiac abnormalities, and intellectual changes. In myotonic dystrophy type 2, the clinical features are similar but a different gene is involved (3q21.3). Electromyographic sampling of affected muscles reveals myotonic discharges in addition to changes suggestive of myopathy.

It is difficult to determine whether drug therapy for myotonia is safe or effective. Myotonia is widely treated with phenytoin (100 mg three times daily), quinine sulfate (300–400 mg three times daily), or procainamide (0.5–1 g four times daily). More recently, tocainide and mexiletine have been used. Phenytoin is preferred, since the other drugs may have undesirable effects on cardiac conduction. Neither the weakness nor the course of the disorder is influenced by treatment.

Miller TM. Differential diagnosis of myotonic disorders. Muscle Nerve. 2008 Mar;37(3):293–9. [PMID: 18067134]

Trip J et al. Drug treatment for myotonia. Cochrane Database Syst Rev. 2006 Jan 25;(1):CD004762. [PMID: 16437496]

3. Myotonia Congenita

Myotonia congenita is commonly inherited as a dominant trait. The responsible gene may be on the long arm of chromosome 7. Generalized myotonia without weakness is usually present from birth, but symptoms may not appear until early childhood. Patients complain of muscle stiffness that is enhanced by cold and inactivity and relieved by exercise. Muscle hypertrophy, at times pronounced, is also a feature. A recessive form with later onset is associated with slight weakness and atrophy of distal muscles. Treatment with quinine sulfate, procainamide, tocainide, mexiletine, or phenytoin may help the myotonia, as in myotonic dystrophy.

4. Polymyositis & Dermatomyositis

See Chapter 20.

5. Inclusion Body Myositis

This disorder, of unknown cause, begins insidiously, usually after middle age, with progressive proximal weakness of first the lower and then the upper extremities, and affecting facial and pharyngeal muscles. Weakness often begins in the quadriceps femoris in the lower limbs and the forearm flexors in the upper limbs. Distal weakness is usually mild. Serum creatine kinase levels may be normal or increased. The diagnosis is confirmed by muscle biopsy. Corticosteroid and immunosuppressive therapy is usually ineffective, but IVIG therapy is occasionally of mild benefit.

Griggs RC. The current status of treatment for inclusion-body myositis. Neurology. 2006 Jan 24;66(2 Suppl 1):S30–2. [PMID: 16432142]

6. Mitochondrial Myopathies

The mitochondrial myopathies are a clinically diverse group of disorders that on pathologic examination of skeletal muscle with the modified Gomori stain show characteristic "ragged red fibers" containing accumulations of abnormal mitochondria. Patients may present with progressive external ophthalmoplegia or with limb weakness that is exacerbated or induced by activity. Other patients present with central neurologic dysfunction, eg, myoclonic epilepsy (myoclonic epilepsy, ragged red fiber syndrome, or MERRF), or the combination of myopathy, encephalopathy, lactic acidosis, and stroke-like episodes (MELAS). These disorders result from separate abnormalities of mitochondrial DNA. (See also Chapter 20.) Treatment is symptomatic and palliative, but various experimental approaches are being explored.

A mitochondrial myopathy may develop in patients receiving zidovudine for treatment of AIDS, and patients receiving highly active antiretroviral therapy (HAART) for HIV-1 infection may develop a **lipodystrophy**, with fat accumulating in muscle.

DiMauro S et al. Approaches to the treatment of mitochondrial diseases. Muscle Nerve. 2006 Sep;34(3):265–83. [PMID: 16810684]

7. Myopathies Associated with Other Disorders

Myopathy may occur in association with chronic hypokalemia, any endocrinopathy, and in patients taking corticosteroids, chloroquine, colchicine, clofibrate, emetine, aminocaproic acid, lovastatin, bretylium tosylate, or drugs causing potassium depletion. Weakness is mainly proximal, and serum creatine kinase is typically normal, except in hypothyroidism and some of the toxic myopathies. Treatment is of the underlying cause. Myopathy also occurs with chronic alcoholism, whereas acute reversible muscle necrosis may occur shortly after acute alcohol intoxication. Inflammatory myopathy may occur in patients taking penicillamine; myotonia may be induced by clofibrate, and preexisting myotonia may be exacerbated or unmasked by depolarizing muscle relaxants (eg, suxamethonium), β-blockers (eg, propranolol), fenoterol, ritodrine and, possibly, certain diuretics.

▶ **When to Refer**

All patients should be referred (to establish the diagnosis and underlying cause).

▶ **When to Admit**

- For respiratory assistance.
- For rhabdomyolysis.

PERIODIC PARALYSIS SYNDROMES

Periodic paralysis may have a familial (dominant inheritance) basis. The syndromes to be described are channelopathies that manifest as abnormal, often potassium-sensitive, muscle-membrane excitability and lead clinically to episodes of flaccid weakness or paralysis, sometimes in association with abnormalities of the plasma potassium level. Strength is normal between attacks. Mutations in genes encoding three ion channels [*CACNA1S (1q32), SCN4A (17q23.1-q25.3),* and *KCNJ2 (17q23.1-q24.2)*] account for most cases. **Hypokalemic periodic paralysis** has been related to mutations in the *CACNL1A3, SCN4A,* or *KCNE3 (11q13-q14)* gene and is characterized by attacks that tend to occur on awakening, after exercise, or after a heavy meal and may last for several days. Patients should avoid excessive exertion. A low-carbohydrate and low-salt diet may help prevent attacks, as may acetazolamide, 250–750 mg/d. Nonselective β-adrenergic blockers may also prevent recurrent paralytic attacks. An ongoing attack may be aborted by potassium chloride given orally or by intravenous drip, provided the ECG can be monitored and kidney function is satisfactory. In young Asian men, it is commonly associated with hyperthyroidism and has been related to polymorphism in the *CACNA1S* gene; treatment of the endocrine disorder prevents recurrences. In **hyperkalemic periodic paralysis**, which is mostly associated with mutations in the *SCN4A* gene, attacks also tend to occur after exercise but usually last for less than an hour. They may be terminated by intravenous calcium gluconate (1–2 g) or by intravenous diuretics (furosemide, 20–40 mg), glucose, or glucose and insulin; daily acetazolamide or chlorothiazide may prevent recurrences. **Normokalemic periodic paralysis** is similar clinically to the hyperkalemic variety, but the plasma potassium level remains normal during attacks; treatment is with acetazolamide.

▶ **When to Refer**

All patients should be referred.

Venance SL et al. The primary periodic paralyses: diagnosis, pathogenesis and treatment. Brain. 2006 Jan;129(Pt 1):8–17. [PMID: 16195244]

Psychiatric Disorders

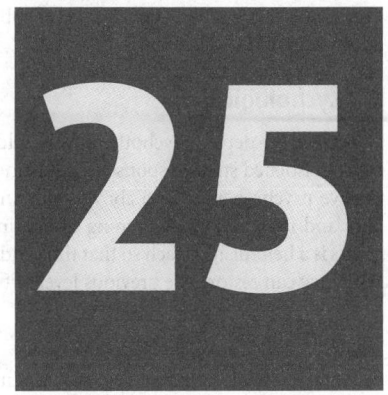

Stuart J. Eisendrath, MD
Jonathan E. Lichtmacher, MD

STRESS & ADJUSTMENT DISORDERS (Situational Disorders)

 ESSENTIALS OF DIAGNOSIS

▶ Anxiety or depression clearly secondary to an identifiable stress.

▶ Subsequent symptoms of anxiety or depression commonly elicited by similar stress of lesser magnitude.

▶ Alcohol and other drugs are commonly used in self-treatment.

▶ General Considerations

Stress exists when the adaptive capacity of the individual is overwhelmed by events. The event may be an insignificant one objectively considered, and even favorable changes (eg, promotion and transfer) requiring adaptive behavior can produce stress. For each individual, stress is subjectively defined, and the response to stress is a function of each person's personality and physiologic endowment.

Opinion differs about what events are most apt to produce stress reactions. The causes of stress are different at different ages—eg, in young adulthood, the sources of stress are found in the marriage or parent-child relationship, the employment relationship, and the struggle to achieve financial stability; in the middle years, the focus shifts to changing spousal relationships, problems with aging parents, and problems associated with having young adult offspring who themselves are encountering stressful situations; in old age, the principal concerns are apt to be retirement, loss of physical capacity, major personal losses, and thoughts of death.

▶ Clinical Findings

An individual may react to stress by becoming anxious or depressed, by developing a physical symptom, by running away, having a drink, starting an affair, or in limitless other ways. Common subjective responses are fear (of repetition of the stress-inducing event), rage (at frustration), guilt (over aggressive impulses), and shame (over helplessness). Acute and reactivated stress may be manifested by restlessness, irritability, fatigue, increased startle reaction, and a feeling of tension. Inability to concentrate, sleep disturbances (insomnia, bad dreams), and somatic preoccupations often lead to self-medication, most commonly with alcohol or other central nervous system depressants. Maladaptive behavior in response to stress is called adjustment disorder, with the major symptom specified (eg, "adjustment disorder with depressed mood").

▶ Differential Diagnosis

Adjustment disorders must be distinguished from anxiety disorders, affective disorders, and personality disorders exacerbated by stress and from somatic disorders with psychic overlay.

▶ Treatment

A. Behavioral

Stress reduction techniques include immediate symptom reduction (eg, rebreathing in a bag for hyperventilation) or early recognition and removal from a stress source before full-blown symptoms appear. It is often helpful for the patient to keep a daily log of stress precipitators, responses, and alleviators. Relaxation and exercise techniques are also helpful in reducing the reaction to stressful events.

B. Social

The stress reactions of life crisis problems are a function of psychosocial upheaval, and patients frequently present with somatic symptoms. While it is not easy for the patient to make necessary changes (or they would have been made long ago), it is important for the therapist to establish the framework of the problem, since the patient's denial system may obscure the issues. Clarifying the problem allows the patient to begin viewing it within the proper context and facilitates the sometimes difficult decisions the patient eventually must make (eg, change of job or relocation of adult-dependent offspring).

C. Psychological

Prolonged in-depth psychotherapy is seldom necessary in cases of isolated stress response or adjustment disorder. Supportive psychotherapy (see above) with an emphasis on the here and now and strengthening of existing coping mechanisms is a helpful approach so that time and the patient's own resiliency can restore the previous level of function.

D. Medical

Judicious use of sedatives (eg, lorazepam, 1–2 mg orally daily) for a limited time and as part of an overall treatment plan can provide relief from acute anxiety symptoms. Problems arise when the situation becomes chronic through inappropriate treatment or when the treatment approach supports the development of chronicity.

▶ Prognosis

Return to satisfactory function after a short period is part of the clinical picture of this syndrome. Resolution may be delayed if others' responses to the patient's difficulties are thoughtlessly harmful or if the secondary gains outweigh the advantages of recovery. The longer the symptoms persist, the worse the prognosis.

Alim TN et al. Trauma, resilience and recovery in a high-risk African-American population. Am J Psychiatry. 2008 Dec; 165(12):1566–75. [PMID: 19015233]

Ehlers A et al. Early psychological interventions for survivors of trauma: a review. Biol Psychiatry. 2003 May 1;53(9):817–26. [PMID: 12725974]

Katon WJ et al. Dissemination of evidence-based mental health interventions: importance to the trauma field. J Trauma Stress. 2006 Oct;19(5):611–23. [PMID: 17075915]

POSTTRAUMATIC STRESS DISORDER

ESSENTIALS OF DIAGNOSIS

▶ Exposure to traumatic (life-threatening) event.

▶ Symptoms, such as flashbacks, intrusive images, and nightmares, often represent reexperiencing the event.

▶ Avoidance symptoms, including numbing, social withdrawal, and avoidance of stimuli associated with the event.

▶ Increased vigilance, such as startle reactions and difficulty falling asleep.

▶ Symptoms impair functioning.

▶ General Considerations

Posttraumatic stress disorder (PTSD)—included among the anxiety disorders in *DSM-IV*—is a syndrome characterized by "reexperiencing" a traumatic event (eg, rape, severe burns, military combat) and decreased responsiveness and avoidance of current events associated with the trauma. The 2005 National Comorbidity Survey Report estimated the lifetime prevalence of PTSD among adult Americans at 6.8% with women having rates twice as high as men. These rates indicate that traumas are not invariably associated with producing PTSD since approximately 60% of men and 50% of women report having experienced at least one lifetime trauma. The National Veterans Vietnam Readjustment Survey indicated that 53.4% of male and 48.1% of female Vietnam war veterans experienced some symptoms of PTSD, with approximately 60% of these affected veterans experiencing the full syndrome. Of the male veterans, 44.7% experienced a lifetime prevalence of alcohol or drug abuse, with 13% experiencing current abuse or dependence. Data indicate that 13% of veterans who served in Iraq and 6% of those who served in Afghanistan have experienced PTSD. In the US population, recent estimates indicate a lifetime prevalence of 7% with a current prevalence of 3.6%. PTSD is more common when the event is associated with physical injury than when it is not. Many individuals with PTSD (20–40%) have experienced other associated problems, including divorce, parenting problems, difficulties with the law, and substance abuse. Since the terrorist attacks in the United States on September 11, 2001, estimates of PTSD have ranged from 4.7% to 10.2% and have been associated with functional impairment as well as increased rates of substance use.

▶ Clinical Findings

Patients with PTSD experience physiologic hyperarousal, including startle reactions, intrusive thoughts, illusions, overgeneralized associations, sleep problems, nightmares, dreams about the precipitating event, impulsivity, difficulties in concentration, and hyperalertness. The symptoms may be precipitated or exacerbated by events that are a reminder of the original stress. Symptoms frequently arise after a long latency period (eg, child abuse can result in later-onset posttraumatic stress disorder).

▶ Differential Diagnosis

In 75% of cases, PTSD occurs with comorbid depression or panic disorder, and there is considerable overlap in the symptom complexes of all three conditions. The key to establishing the PTSD diagnosis lies in the history of exposure to a life-threatening event followed by intrusive (eg, flashbacks, nightmares) or avoidance (eg, withdrawal) symptoms. Acute stress disorder occurs during or shortly after a traumatic event and has many of the same symptoms as PTSD but lasts between 2 and 28 days. Some individuals with dissociative features, such as borderline personality disorders, may mimic some of the symptoms of PTSD, but those disorders are typically more related to chronic childhood maltreatment not a specific traumatic event.

▶ Treatment

A. Psychotherapy

Psychotherapy should be initiated as soon as possible after the traumatic event, and it should be brief and simple (once in a safe environment). Psychological debriefing in a single session, once a mainstay in prevention of PTSD, is now considered to be ineffective and possibly harmful. Posttraumatic stress syndromes respond to interventions that help patients integrate the event in an adaptive way with some sense of mastery in having survived the trauma. Early cognitive behavioral therapy has been shown to speed recovery. Marital problems are a major area of concern, and it is important that the clinician have available a dependable referral source when marriage counseling is indicated.

Treatment initiated later, when symptoms have crystallized, includes programs for cessation of alcohol and other drug abuse, group and individual psychotherapy, and improved social support systems. The therapeutic approach is to facilitate the normal recovery that was blocked at the time of the trauma.

B. Medication

Early treatment of anxious arousal with β-blockers (eg, propranolol, 80–160 mg orally daily) may lessen the peripheral symptoms of anxiety (eg, tremors, palpitations) and help prevent development of PTSD; however, research in this area is preliminary. Antidepressant drugs—particularly selective serotonin reuptake inhibitors (SSRIs)—in full dosage are helpful in ameliorating depression, panic attacks, sleep disruption, and startle responses in chronic PTSD. Sertraline and paroxetine are approved by the US Food and Drug Administration (FDA) for this purpose. Antiseizure medications such as carbamazepine (400–800 mg orally daily) will often mitigate impulsivity and difficulty with anger management. Benzodiazepines, such as clonazepam (1–4 mg orally daily), will reduce anxiety and panic attacks when used in adequate dosage, but dependency problems are a concern, particularly when the patient has had such problems in the past. The α-adrenergic blocking agent prazosin (2–10 mg orally at bedtime) has been successfully used to decrease nightmares and improve quality of sleep in PTSD.

▶ Prognosis

The sooner therapy is initiated after the trauma, the better the prognosis. Treatment reduces the duration of symptoms significantly from an average of 64 months to 36 months. Approximately half of patients experience chronic symptoms. Prognosis is best in those with good premorbid psychiatric functioning. Individuals experiencing an acute stress disorder typically do better than those experiencing a delayed posttraumatic disorder. Individuals who experience trauma resulting from a natural disaster (eg, earthquake or hurricane) tend to do better than those who experience a traumatic interpersonal encounter (eg, rape or combat).

Mellman T et al. Posttraumatic stress disorder: characteristics and treatment. J Clin Psychiatry. 2008 Jan;69(1):e2. [PMID: 18312029]

Sijbrandij M et al. Treatment of acute posttraumatic stress disorder with brief cognitive behavioral therapy: a randomized controlled trial. Am J Psychiatry. 2007 Jan;164(1):82–90. [PMID: 17202548]

Stevens LM et al. JAMA patient page. Posttraumatic stress disorder. JAMA. 2006 Aug 2;296(5):614. [PMID: 16882969]

Taylor FB et al. Prazosin effects on objective sleep measures and clinical symptoms in civilian trauma posttraumatic stress disorder: a placebo-controlled study. Biol Psychiatry. 2008 Mar 15;63(6):629–32. [PMID: 17868655]

Zhang W, Davidson JR. Post-traumatic stress disorder: an evaluation of existing pharmacotherapies and new strategies. Expert Opin Pharmacother. 2007;8(12):1861–70. [PMID: 17696789]

ANXIETY DISORDERS & DISSOCIATIVE DISORDERS

 ESSENTIALS OF DIAGNOSIS

▶ Overt anxiety or an overt manifestation of a coping mechanism (such as a phobia), or both.

▶ Not limited to an adjustment disorder.

▶ Somatic symptoms referable to the autonomic nervous system or to a specific organ system (eg, dyspnea, palpitations, paresthesias).

▶ Not a result of physical disorders, psychiatric conditions (eg, schizophrenia), or drug abuse (eg, cocaine).

▶ General Considerations

Stress, fear, and anxiety all tend to be interactive. The principal components of anxiety are **psychological** (tension, fears, difficulty in concentration, apprehension) and **somatic** (tachycardia, hyperventilation, palpitations, tremor, sweating). Other organ systems (eg, gastrointestinal) may be involved in multiple-system complaints. Fatigue and sleep disturbances are common. Sympathomimetic symptoms of anxiety are both a response to a central nervous system state and a reinforcement of further anxiety. Anxiety can become self-generating, since the symptoms reinforce the reaction, causing it to spiral. This is often the case when the anxiety is an epiphenomenon of other medical or psychiatric disorders.

Anxiety may be free-floating, resulting in acute anxiety attacks, occasionally becoming chronic. When one or several coping mechanisms (see above) are functioning, the consequences are well-known problems such as phobias, conversion reactions, dissociative states, obsessions, and compulsions. Lack of structure is frequently a contributing factor, as noted in those people who have "Sunday neuroses." They do well during the week with a planned work schedule but cannot tolerate the unstructured weekend. Planned-time activities tend to bind anxiety, and many people have increased difficulties when this is lost, as in retirement.

Some believe that various manifestations of anxiety are not a result of unconscious conflicts but are "habits"— persistent patterns of nonadaptive behavior acquired by learning. The "habits," being nonadaptive, are unsatisfactory ways of dealing with life's problems—hence the resultant anxiety. Help is sought only when the anxiety becomes too painful. Exogenous factors such as stimulants (eg, caffeine, cocaine) must be considered as a contributing factor.

▶ Clinical Findings

A. Generalized Anxiety Disorder

This is the most common of the clinically significant anxiety disorders. Initial manifestations appear at age 20–35 years, and there is a slight predominance in women. The anxiety symptoms of apprehension, worry, irritability, difficulty in concentrating, insomnia, and somatic complaints are present more days than not for at least 6 months. Manifestations can include cardiac (eg, tachycardia, increased blood pressure), gastrointestinal (eg, increased acidity, nausea, epigastric pain), and neurologic (eg, headache, near-syncope) systems. The focus of the anxiety may be a number of everyday activities.

B. Panic Disorder

This is characterized by short-lived, recurrent, unpredictable episodes of intense anxiety accompanied by marked physiologic manifestations. **Agoraphobia**, fear of being in places where escape is difficult, such as open spaces or public places, may be present and may lead the individual to confine his or her life to the home environment. Distressing symptoms and signs such as dyspnea, tachycardia, palpitations, headaches, dizziness, paresthesias, choking, smothering feelings, nausea, and bloating are associated with feelings of impending doom (alarm response). Recurrent **sleep panic attacks** (not nightmares) occur in about 30% of panic disorders. Anticipatory anxiety develops in all these patients and further constricts their daily lives. Panic disorder tends to be familial, with onset usually under age 25; it affects 3–5% of the population, and the female-to-male ratio is 2:1. The premenstrual period is one of heightened vulnerability. Patients frequently undergo emergency medical evaluations (eg, for "heart attacks" or "hypoglycemia") before the correct diagnosis is made. Gastrointestinal symptoms are especially common, occurring in about one-third of cases. Myocardial infarction, pheochromocytoma, hyperthyroidism, and various recreational drug reactions can mimic panic disorder. Mitral valve prolapse may be present but is not usually a significant factor. Patients who have recurrent panic disorder often become **demoralized, hypochondriacal, agoraphobic,** and **depressed**. These individuals are at increased risk for major depression and the suicide attempts associated with that disorder. Alcohol abuse (about 20%) results from self-treatment and is not infrequently combined with dependence on sedatives. Some patients have atypical panic attacks associated with seizure-like symptoms that often include psychosensory phenomena (a history of stimulant abuse often emerges). About 25% of panic disorder patients also have obsessive-compulsive disorder (OCD).

C. Obsessive-Compulsive Disorder

In the obsessive-compulsive reaction, the irrational idea or the impulse persistently intrudes into awareness. Obsessions (constantly recurring thoughts such as fears of exposure to germs) and compulsions (repetitive actions such as washing the hands many times) are recognized by the individual as absurd and are resisted, but anxiety is alleviated only by ritualistic performance of the action or by deliberate contemplation of the intruding idea or emotion. Many patients do not mention the symptoms and must be asked about them. These patients are usually predictable, orderly, conscientious, and intelligent—traits that are seen in many compulsive behaviors such as food binging and purging and compulsive exercise. There is an overlapping of OCD and other behaviors ("OCD spectrum"), including tics, trichotillomania (hair pulling), onychophagia (nail biting), hypochondriasis, Tourette syndrome, and eating disorders (see Chapter 29). The 2–3% incidence of OCD in the general population is much higher than was previously recognized. In addition, there is a high comorbidity of OCD and major depression; two-thirds of OCD patients will develop major depression during their lifetime. Male to female ratios are similar, with the highest rates occurring in the young, divorced, separated, and unemployed (all high-stress categories). Neurologic abnormalities of fine motor coordination and involuntary movements are common. Under extreme stress, these patients sometimes exhibit paranoid and delusional behaviors, often associated with depression, and can mimic schizophrenia.

D. Phobic Disorder

Phobic ideation can be considered a form of "displacement" in which patients transfer feelings of anxiety from their true object to one that can be avoided. However, since phobias are ineffective coping mechanisms, there tends to be an increase in their scope, intensity, and number. Social phobias are global or specific; in the former, all social situations are poorly tolerated, while the latter group includes performance anxiety or well-delineated phobias (eg, fear of bridges). Agoraphobia (fear of open places and public areas) is frequently associated with severe panic attacks, and it often develops in early adult life, making a normal lifestyle difficult.

E. Dissociative Disorder

Fugue (the sudden, unexpected travel away from one's home with inability to recall one's past), amnesia, somnambulism, dissociative identity disorder (multiple personality disorder), and depersonalization are all dissociative states. The reaction is precipitated by emotional crisis. The symptom produces anxiety reduction and a temporary solution of the crisis. Mechanisms include repression and isolation as well as particularly limited scope of attention as seen in hypnotic states. Dissociative symptoms are similar in many ways to symptoms seen in patients with temporal lobe dysfunction.

▶ Treatment

In all cases, underlying medical disorders must be ruled out (eg, cardiovascular, endocrine, respiratory, and neurologic disorders and substance-related syndromes, both intoxication and withdrawal states). These and other disorders can coexist with panic disorder.

Table 25-1. Commonly used antianxiety and hypnotic agents.

Drug	Usual Daily Oral Doses	Usual Daily Maximum Doses	Cost for 30 Days Treatment Based on Maximum Dosage[1]
Benzodiazepines (used for anxiety)			
Alprazolam (Xanax)[2]	0.5 mg	4 mg	$117.87
Chlordiazepoxide (Librium)[3]	10–20 mg	100 mg	$40.82
Clonazepam (Klonopin)[3]	1–2 mg	10 mg	$177.68
Clorazepate (Tranxene)[3]	15–30 mg	60 mg	$260.94
Diazepam (Valium)[3]	5–15 mg	30 mg	$28.13
Lorazepam (Ativan)[2]	2–4 mg	4 mg	$76.80
Oxazepam (Serax)[2]	10–30 mg	60 mg	$98.40
Benzodiazepines (used for sleep)			
Estazolam (Prosom)[2]	1 mg	2 mg	$29.70
Flurazepam (Dalmane)[3]	15 mg	30 mg	$10.50
Midazolam (Versed IV)[4]	5 mg IV		$3.58/dose
Quazepam (Doral)[3]	7.5 mg	15 mg	$138.00
Temazepam (Restoril)[2]	15 mg	30 mg	$26.40
Triazolam (Halcion)[5]	0.125 mg	0.25 mg	$20.25
Miscellaneous (used for anxiety)			
Buspirone (Buspar)[2]	10–30 mg	60 mg	$218.10
Phenobarbital[3]	15–30 mg	90 mg	$3.15
Miscellaneous (used for sleep)			
Chloral hydrate (Noctec)[2]	500 mg	1000 mg	$9.41
Eszopiclone (Lunesta)[5]	2–3 mg	3 mg	$151.92
Hydroxyzine (Vistaril)[2]	50 mg	100 mg	$19.20
Zolpidem (Ambien)[5]	5–10 mg	10 mg	$138.59
Zaleplon (Sonata)[6]	5–10 mg	10 mg	$121.20
Ramelteon (Rozerem)	8 mg	8 mg	$126.70

[1]Average wholesale price (AWP, for AB-rated generic when available) for quantity listed. Source: *Red Book Update*, Vol. 28, No. 3, March 2009. AWP may not accurately represent the actual pharmacy cost because wide contractual variations exist among institutions.
[2]Intermediate physical half-life (10–20 hours).
[3]Long physical half-life (> 20 hours).
[4]Intravenously for procedures.
[5]Short physical half-life (1–6 hours).
[6]Short physical half-life (about 1 hour).

A. Medical

1. Generalized anxiety—Benzodiazepines are the anxiolytics of choice in the acute management of generalized anxiety (Table 25–1). They are almost immediately effective. Antidepressants can be efficacious for the long-term treatment of generalized anxiety disorder, panic disorder, social phobia, and OCD.

All of the benzodiazepines may be given orally, and several are available in parenteral formulations. Benzodiazepines such as lorazepam are absorbed rapidly when given intramuscularly. In psychiatric disorders, the benzodiazepines are usually given orally; in controlled medical environments (eg, the ICU), where the rapid onset of respiratory depression can be assessed, they are often given

intravenously. Onset of action is a function of the rate of absorption (related to lipophilic property) and varies, with diazepam and clorazepate being the most rapidly absorbed orally. This characteristic, along with high lipid solubility, may explain the popularity of diazepam. In the average case of anxiety, diazepam, 5–10 mg orally twice daily as needed, is a reasonable starting regimen.

The duration of action of the benzodiazepines varies as a function of the active metabolites they produce. Benzodiazepines such as lorazepam do not produce active metabolites and have intermediate half-lives of 10–20 hours, characteristics useful in treating elderly patients. Ultrashort-acting agents such as triazolam have half-lives of 1–3 hours and may lead to rebound withdrawal anxiety. Longer-acting benzodiazepines such as flurazepam and diazepam produce active metabolites, have half-lives of 20–120 hours, and should be avoided in the elderly. Since people vary widely in their response and since the drugs are long-lasting, the dosage must be individualized. Once this is established, an adequate dose early in the course of symptom development will obviate the need for "pill popping," which contributes to dependency problems. Panic disorder does not usually respond to benzodiazepines other than clonazepam and alprazolam. Those high-potency benzodiazepines and the antidepressants are most commonly used for panic disorder. Notably, alprazolam has a relatively short half-life and over time can lead to interdose rebound anxiety, although the extended release form is available and obviates some of this difficulty.

Whether the indications for benzodiazepines are anxiety or insomnia, the drugs should be used judiciously. The longer-acting benzodiazepines are used for the treatment of alcohol withdrawal and anxiety symptoms; the intermediate drugs are useful as sedatives for insomnia (eg, lorazepam), while short-acting agents (eg, midazolam) are used for medical procedures such as endoscopy.

The side effects of all the benzodiazepine antianxiety agents are patient and dose dependent. As the dosage exceeds the levels necessary for sedation, the side effects include disinhibition, ataxia, dysarthria, nystagmus, and delirium. (The patient should be told not to operate machinery until he or she is well stabilized without side effects.)

Paradoxical agitation, anxiety, psychosis, confusion, mood lability, and anterograde amnesia have been reported, particularly with the shorter-acting benzodiazepines. These agents produce cumulative clinical effects with repeated dosage (especially if the patient has not had time to metabolize the previous dose), additive effects when given with other classes of sedatives or alcohol (many apparently "accidental" deaths are the result of concomitant use of sedatives and alcohol), and residual effects after termination of treatment (particularly in the case of drugs that undergo slow biotransformation).

Overdosage results in respiratory depression, hypotension, shock syndrome, coma, and death. Flumazenil, a benzodiazepine antagonist, is effective in overdosage. Overdosage (see Chapter 38) and withdrawal states are medical emergencies. Serious side effects of chronic excessive dosage are development of tolerance, resulting in increasing dose requirements, and physiologic dependence, resulting in withdrawal symptoms similar in appearance to alcohol and barbiturate withdrawal (withdrawal effects must be distinguished from reemergent anxiety). Abrupt withdrawal of sedative drugs may cause serious and even fatal convulsive seizures. Psychosis, delirium, and autonomic dysfunction have also been described. Both duration of action and duration of exposure are major factors related to likelihood of withdrawal.

Common withdrawal symptoms after low to moderate daily use of benzodiazepines are classified as somatic (disturbed sleep, tremor, nausea, muscle aches), psychological (anxiety, poor concentration, irritability, mild depression), or perceptual (poor coordination, mild paranoia, mild confusion). The presentation of symptoms will vary depending

Table 25–2. Benzodiazepine interactions with other drugs.

Drug	Effects
Antacids	Decreased absorption of benzodiazepines
Cimetidine	Increased half-life of diazepam and triazolam
Contraceptives	Increased levels of diazepam and triazolam
Digoxin	Alprazolam and diazepam raise digoxin level
Disulfiram	Increased duration of action of sedatives
Isoniazid	Increased plasma diazepam
Levodopa	Inhibition of antiparkinsonism effect
Propoxyphene	Impaired clearance of diazepam
Rifampin	Decreased plasma diazepam
Warfarin	Decreased prothrombin time

on the half-life of the drug. There are no significant side effects on organ systems other than the brain, and the drugs are safe in most medical conditions. Benzodiazepine interactions with other drugs are listed in Table 25–2.

Antidepressants are the first-line medications for sustained treatment of generalized anxiety disorder, having the advantage of not causing serious physiologic dependency problems. At initiation of treatment, antidepressants can themselves be anxiogenic—thus, an initial dose, in conjunction with short-term treatment with a benzodiazepine, is often indicated. Venlafaxine and duloxetine (serotonin and norepinephrine reuptake inhibitors) are FDA-approved for the treatment of generalized anxiety disorder in usual antidepressant doses. Initial daily dosing should start low (37.5–75 mg for venlafaxine and 30 mg for duloxetine) and be titrated upward as needed. SSRIs, such as paroxetine, are also used. Similarly, buspirone, sometimes used as an augmenting agent in the treatment of depression and compulsive behaviors, is also effective for generalized anxiety. Buspirone is usually given in a total dosage of 15–60 mg/d in three divided doses. Higher doses tend to be counterproductive and produce gastrointestinal symptoms and dizziness. There is a 2- to 4-week delay before antidepressants and buspirone take effect, and patients require education regarding this lag. Sleep is sometimes negatively affected. β-Blockers such as propranolol may help reduce peripheral somatic symptoms. Alcohol is the most frequently self-administered drug and should be interdicted. The highly addicting drugs with a narrow margin of safety such as glutethimide, ethchlorvynol, methprylon, meprobamate, and the barbiturates (with the exception of phenobarbital) should be avoided. Phenobarbital, in addition to its anticonvulsant properties, is a reasonably safe and very inexpensive sedative but has the disadvantage of causing hepatic microsomal enzyme stimulation (not the case with benzodiazepines), which may affect the metabolism of other medications.

2. Panic attacks—Panic attacks may be treated in several ways. A sublingual dose of lorazepam (0.5–2 mg) or alprazolam (0.5–1 mg) is often effective for urgent treatment.

For sustained treatment, SSRIs are the initial drugs of choice (adequate blood levels will require dosages similar to those used in the treatment of depression). For example, sertraline starting at 25 mg/d and increased after 1 week to 50 mg/d may be effective. Because of initial agitation in response to antidepressants, doses should start low and be very gradually increased. High-potency benzodiazepines may be used for symptomatic treatment as the antidepressant dose is titrated upward. Clonazepam (1–6 mg/d orally) and alprazolam (0.5–6 mg/d orally) are effective alternatives to antidepressants. Both drugs may produce marked withdrawal if stopped abruptly and should always be tapered. Because of chronicity of the disorders and the problem of dependency with benzodiazepine drugs, it is generally desirable to use antidepressant drugs as the principal pharmacologic approach. Antidepressants have been used in conjunction with β-blockers in resistant cases. Propranolol (40–160 mg/d orally) can mute the peripheral symptoms of anxiety without significantly affecting motor and cognitive performance. They block symptoms mediated by sympathetic stimulation (eg, palpitations, tremulousness) but not nonadrenergic symptoms (eg, diarrhea, muscle tension). Contrary to current belief, they usually do not cause depression as a side effect and can be used cautiously in patients with depression. Valproate has been found to be as effective in panic disorder as the antidepressants and is another useful alternative.

3. Phobic disorder—Phobic disorder may be part of the panic disorder and is treated within that framework. Global social phobias may be treated with SSRIs, such as paroxetine, sertraline, and fluvoxamine, or monoamine oxidase (MAO) inhibitors in the same dosage as used for depression. Gabapentin, an anticonvulsant with anxiolytic properties, may be an alternative to antidepressants in the treatment of social phobia in a dosage of 300–3600 mg/d, depending on response versus sedation. Specific phobias such as performance anxiety may respond to moderate doses of β-blockers, such as propranolol, 20–40 mg 1 hour prior to exposure. D-cycloserine (DCS), an antituberculosis drug, has recently been investigated as an augmenting agent in exposure treatment. As a partial agonist at the NMDA receptor in the amygdala, DCS may be useful in reducing fear responses. Importantly, such medications must be used in combination with cognitive behavioral exposure strategies.

4. Obsessive-compulsive disorder—OCD responds to serotonergic drugs in about 60% of cases and usually requires a longer response time than for depression (up to 12 weeks). Clomipramine has proved effective in doses equivalent to those used for depression. Fluoxetine (an SSRI drug) has been widely used in this disorder but in doses higher than those used in depression (up to 60–80 mg/d). The other SSRI drugs such as sertraline, paroxetine, and fluvoxamine are being used with comparable efficacy, each with its own side-effect profile. Buspirone in doses of 15–60 mg/d appears to be effective primarily as an antiobsessional augmenting agent for the SSRI drugs. There is some evidence that antipsychotics may be helpful as adjuncts to the SSRIs in treatment-resistant cases. Psycho-

surgery has a limited place in selected cases of severe unremitting OCD. The stereotactic techniques now being used, including modified cingulotomy, are great improvements over the crude methods of the past. Recently, experimental work has suggested a role for deep brain stimulation in OCD.

B. Behavioral

Behavioral approaches are widely used in various anxiety disorders, often in conjunction with medication. Any of the behavioral techniques can be used beneficially in altering the contingencies (precipitating factors or rewards) supporting any anxiety-provoking behavior. Relaxation techniques can sometimes be helpful in reducing anxiety. Desensitization, by exposing the patient to graded doses of a phobic object or situation, is an effective technique and one that the patient can practice outside the therapy session. Emotive imagery, wherein the patient imagines the anxiety-provoking situation while at the same time learning to relax, helps decrease the anxiety when the patient faces the real-life situation. Physiologic symptoms in panic attacks respond well to relaxation training. Exposure techniques with response prevention are useful for OCD.

C. Psychological

Cognitive behavioral approaches have been effective in treatment of panic disorders, phobias, and OCD when erroneous beliefs need correction. These approaches share a common technique of exposing the individual to the feared object or situation. The combination of medical and cognitive behavioral therapy is more effective than either alone. Group therapy is the treatment of choice when the anxiety is clearly a function of the patient's difficulties in dealing with social settings.

D. Social

Peer support groups for panic disorder and agoraphobia have been particularly helpful. Social modification may require measures such as family counseling to aid acceptance of the patient's symptoms and avoid counterproductive behavior in behavioral training. Any help in maintaining the social structure is anxiety-alleviating, and work, school, and social activities should be maintained. School and vocational counseling may be provided by professionals, who often need help from the clinician in defining the patient's limitations.

▶ Prognosis

Anxiety disorders are usually of longstanding and may be quite difficult to treat. All can be relieved to varying degrees with medications and behavioral techniques. The prognosis is much better if the commonly observed anxiety-panic-phobia-depression cycle can be broken with a combination of the therapeutic interventions discussed above.

Bergstrom J et al. An open label study of the effectiveness of Internet treatment for panic disorder delivered in a psychiatric setting. Nord J Psychiatry. 2009;63(1):44–50. [PMID: 18985514]

Kopell BH et al. Anatomy and physiology of the basal ganglia: implications for DBS in psychiatry. Neurosci Biobehav Rev. 2008;32(3):408–22. [PMID: 17854894]

Kushner MG et al. D-cycloserine augmented exposure therapy for obsessive-compulsive disorder. Biol Psychiatry. 2007 Oct 15;62(8):835–8. [PMID: 17588545]

SOMATOFORM DISORDERS
(Abnormal Illness Behaviors)

 ESSENTIALS OF DIAGNOSIS

▸ Physical symptoms may involve one or more organ systems and are not intentional.

▸ Subjective complaints exceed objective findings.

▸ Correlations of symptom development and psychosocial stresses.

▸ Combination of biogenetic and developmental patterns.

▸ General Considerations

Somatoform disorders can occur focused on any organ system. Vulnerability in one or more organ systems and exposure to family members with somatization problems play a major role in the development of particular symptoms, and the "functional" versus "organic" dichotomy is a hindrance to good treatment. Clinicians should suspect psychiatric disorders in a number of conditions. For example, 45% of patients complaining of palpitations had lifetime psychiatric diagnoses including generalized anxiety, depression, panic, and somatization disorders. Similarly, 33–44% of patients who undergo coronary angiography for chest pain but have negative results have been found to have panic disorder.

In any patient presenting with a condition judged to be somatoform, depression must be considered in the diagnosis.

▸ Clinical Findings

A. Conversion Disorder

"Conversion" (formerly "hysterical conversion") of psychic conflict into physical symptoms in parts of the body innervated by the sensorimotor system (eg, paralysis, aphonia) is a disorder that is more common in individuals from lower socioeconomic classes and certain cultures. The coping mechanisms used in this condition are repression (a barring from consciousness) and isolation (a splitting of the affect from the idea). The somatic manifestation that takes the place of anxiety is typically paralysis, and in some instances the organ dysfunction may have symbolic meaning (eg, arm paralysis in marked anger). Pseudoepileptic ("hysterical") seizures are often difficult to differentiate from intoxication states or panic attacks. Retention of consciousness, random flailing with asynchronous movements of the right and left sides, and resistance to having the nose and mouth pinched closed during the attack, all point toward a pseudoepileptic event. Electroencephalography, particularly in a video-EEG assessment unit, during the attack is the most helpful diag-

nostic aid in excluding genuine seizure states. Serum prolactin levels rise abruptly in the postictal state only in true epilepsy. La belle indifférence (an unconcerned affect) is not a significant identifying characteristic, as commonly believed, since individuals even with genuine medical illness, may exhibit a high level of denial. Important conversion disorder criteria include a history of conversion or somatization disorder, modeling the symptom after someone else who had a similar presentation, a serious precipitating emotional event, associated psychopathology (eg, depression, schizophrenia, personality disorders), a temporal correlation between the precipitating event and the symptom, and a temporary "solving of the problem" by the conversion. It is important to identify physical disorders with unusual presentations (eg, multiple sclerosis, systemic lupus erythematosus).

B. Somatization Disorder (Briquet Syndrome, Hysteria)

This is characterized by multiple physical complaints referable to several organ systems. Anxiety, panic disorder, and depression are often present, and **major depression** is an important consideration in the differential diagnosis. There is a significant relationship (20%) to a lifetime history of panic-agoraphobia-depression. It usually occurs before age 30 and is ten times more common in women. Polysurgery is often a feature of the history. Preoccupation with medical and surgical therapy becomes a lifestyle that excludes most other activities. The symptoms are a reflection of maladaptive coping techniques and reactivity of the particular organ system. There is often evidence of longstanding somatic symptoms (particularly dysmenorrhea, a lump in the throat, vomiting, shortness of breath, burning in the sex organs, painful extremities, and amnesia), often with a history of similar organ system involvement in other family members. Multiple symptoms that constantly change and inability of more than three doctors to make a diagnosis are strong clues to the problem.

C. Pain Disorder Associated with Psychological Factors (Formerly Somatoform Pain Disorder)

This involves a long history of complaints of severe pain not consonant with anatomic and clinical signs. This diagnosis must not be one of exclusion and should be made only after extended evaluation has established a clear correlation of psychogenic factors with exacerbations and remissions of complaints.

D. Hypochondriasis

This is a fear of disease and preoccupation with the body, with perceptual amplification and heightened responsiveness. A process of social learning is usually involved, frequently with a role model who was a member of the family and may be a part of the underlying psychodynamic causation. It is common in panic disorders.

E. Factitious Disorders

These disorders, in which symptom production is intentional, are not somatoform conditions in that symptoms are produced consciously, in contrast to the unconscious process of the above conditions. They are characterized by self-induced symptoms or false physical and laboratory findings for the purpose of deceiving clinicians or other hospital personnel. The deceptions may involve self-mutilation, fever, hemorrhage, hypoglycemia, seizures, and an almost endless variety of manifestations—often presented in an exaggerated and dramatic fashion (Munchausen syndrome). "Munchausen by proxy" is the term used when a parent creates an illness in a child so the adult (usually the mother) can maintain a relationship with clinicians. The duplicity may be either simple or extremely complex and difficult to recognize. The patients are frequently connected in some way with the health professions; they are often migratory; and there is no apparent external motivation other than achieving the patient role.

Complications

A poor doctor-patient relationship, with iatrogenic disorders and "doctor shopping," tends to exacerbate the problem. Sedative and analgesic dependency is the most common iatrogenic complication.

Treatment

A. Medical

Medical support with careful attention to building a therapeutic practitioner-patient relationship is the mainstay of treatment. It must be accepted that the patient's distress is real. Every problem not found to have an organic basis is not necessarily a mental disease. Diligent attempts should be made to relate symptoms to adverse developments in the patient's life. It may be useful to have the patient keep a meticulous diary, paying particular attention to various pertinent factors evident in the history. Regular, frequent, short appointments that are not symptom-contingent may be helpful. Drugs (frequently abused) should not be prescribed to replace appointments. One person should be the primary clinician, and consultants should be used mainly for evaluation. An empathic, realistic, optimistic approach must be maintained in the face of the expected ups and downs. Ongoing reevaluation is necessary, since somatization can coexist with a concurrent physical illness.

B. Psychological

Psychological approaches can be used by the primary clinician when it is clear that the patient is ready to make some changes in lifestyle in order to achieve symptomatic relief. This is often best approached on a here-and-now basis and oriented toward pragmatic changes rather than an exploration of early experiences that the patient frequently fails to relate to current distress. Group therapy with other individuals who have similar problems is sometimes of value to improve coping, allow ventilation, and focus on interpersonal adjustment. Hypnosis or lorazepam interviews used early are helpful in resolving conversion disorders. If the primary clinician has been working with the patient on psychological problems

related to the physical illness, the groundwork is often laid for successful psychiatric referral.

For patients who have been identified as having a factitious disorder, early psychiatric consultation is indicated. There are two main treatment strategies for these patients. One consists of a conjoint confrontation of the patient by both the primary clinician and the psychiatrist. The patient's disorder is portrayed as a cry for help, and psychiatric treatment is recommended. The second approach avoids direct confrontation and attempts to provide a face-saving way to relinquish the symptom without overt disclosure of the disorder's origin. Techniques such as biofeedback and self-hypnosis may foster recovery using this strategy. Another face-saving approach is to use a double bind with the patient. For example, the patient is told there are two possible diagnoses: (1) an organic disease that should respond to the next medical intervention (usually modest and noninvasive), or (2) factitious disorder for which the patient will need psychiatric treatment. Given these options, many patients will choose to recover and not have to admit the origin of their problem.

C. Behavioral

Behavioral therapy is probably best exemplified by biofeedback techniques. In biofeedback, the particular abnormality (eg, increased peristalsis) must be recognized and monitored by the patient and therapist (eg, by an electronic stethoscope to amplify the sounds). This is immediate feedback, and after learning to recognize it, the patient can then learn to identify any change thus produced (eg, a decrease in bowel sounds) and so become a conscious originator of the feedback instead of a passive recipient. Relief of the symptom operantly conditions the patient to utilize the maneuver that relieves symptoms (eg, relaxation causing a decrease in bowel sounds). With emphasis on this type of learning, the patient is able to identify symptoms early and initiate the countermaneuvers, thus decreasing the symptomatic problem. Migrainoid and tension headaches have been particularly responsive to biofeedback methods.

D. Social

Social endeavors include family, work, and other interpersonal activity. Family members should come for some appointments with the patient so they can learn how best to live with the patient. This is particularly important in treatment of somatization and pain disorders. Peer support groups provide a climate for encouraging the patient to accept and live with the problem. Ongoing communication with the employer may be necessary to encourage long-term continued interest in the employee. Employers can become just as discouraged as clinicians in dealing with employees who have chronic problems.

Prognosis

The prognosis is much better if the primary clinician is able to intervene early before the situation has deteriorated. After the problem has crystallized into chronicity, it is very difficult to effect change.

Krahn LE et al. Patients who strive to be ill: factitious disorder with physical symptoms. Am J Psychiatry. 2003 Jun;160(6):1163–8. [PMID: 12777276]

Kroenke K et al. Efficacy of treatment for somatoform disorders: a review of randomized controlled trials. Psychosom Med. 2007 Dec;69(9):881–8. [PMID: 18040099]

CHRONIC PAIN DISORDERS

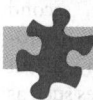 ESSENTIALS OF DIAGNOSIS

▶ Chronic complaints of pain.

▶ Symptoms frequently exceed signs.

▶ Minimal relief with standard treatment.

▶ History of having seen many clinicians.

▶ Frequent use of several nonspecific medications.

▶ General Considerations

A problem in the management of pain is the lack of distinction between acute and chronic pain syndromes. Most clinicians are adept at dealing with acute pain problems but have difficulty handling the patient with a chronic pain disorder. This type of patient frequently takes too many medications, stays in bed a great deal, has seen many clinicians, has lost skills, and experiences little joy in either work or play. All relationships suffer (including those with clinicians), and life becomes a constant search for succor. The search results in complex clinician-patient relationships that usually include many drug trials, particularly sedatives, with adverse consequences (eg, irritability, depressed mood) related to long-term use. Treatment failures provoke angry responses and depression from both the patient and the clinician, and the pain syndrome is exacerbated. When frustration becomes too great, a new clinician is found, and the cycle is repeated. The longer the existence of the pain disorder, the more important become the psychological factors of anxiety and depression. As with all other conditions, it is counterproductive to speculate about whether the pain is "real." It is real to the patient, and acceptance of the problem must precede a mutual endeavor to alleviate the disturbance.

▶ Clinical Findings

Components of the chronic pain syndrome consist of anatomic changes, chronic anxiety and depression, anger, and changed lifestyle. Usually, the anatomic problem is irreversible, since it has already been subjected to many interventions with increasingly unsatisfactory results. An algorithm for assessing chronic pain and differentiating it from other psychiatric conditions is illustrated in Figure 25–1.

Chronic anxiety and depression produce heightened irritability and overreaction to stimuli. A marked decrease in pain threshold is apparent. This pattern develops into a hypochondriacal preoccupation with the body and a constant need for reassurance. The pressure on the clinician becomes wearing and often leads to covert rejection of the patient, such as not being available or making referrals to other clinicians.

This is perceived by the patient, who then intensifies the effort to find help, and the typical cycle is repeated. Anxiety and depression are seldom discussed, almost as if there is a tacit agreement not to deal with these issues.

Changes in lifestyle involve some of the pain behaviors. These usually take the form of a family script in which the patient accepts the role of being sick, and this role then becomes the focus of most family interactions and may become important in maintaining the family, so that neither the patient nor the family wants the patient's role to change. Demands for attention and efforts to control the behavior of others revolve around the central issue of control of other people (including clinicians). Cultural factors frequently play a role in the behavior of the patient and how the significant people around the patient cope with the problem. Some cultures encourage demonstrative behavior, while others value the stoic role.

Another secondary gain that frequently maintains the patient in the sick role is financial compensation or other benefits. Frequently, such systems are structured so that they reinforce the maintenance of sickness and discourage any attempts to give up the role. Clinicians unwittingly reinforce this role because of the very nature of the practice of medicine, which is to respond to complaints of illness. Helpful suggestions from the clinician are often met with responses like, "Yes, but…." Medications then become the principal approach, and drug dependency problems may develop.

▶ Treatment

A. Behavioral

The cornerstone of a unified approach to chronic pain syndromes is a comprehensive behavioral program. This is necessary to identify and eliminate pain reinforcers, to decrease drug use, and to use effectively those positive reinforcers that shift the focus from the pain. It is critical that the patient be made a partner in the effort to alleviate pain. The clinician must shift from the idea of biomedical cure to ongoing care of the patient. The patient should agree to discuss the pain only with the clinician and not with family members; this tends to stabilize the patient's personal life, since the family is usually tired of the subject. At the beginning of treatment, the patient should be assigned self-help tasks graded up to maximal activity as a means of positive reinforcement. The tasks should not exceed capability. The patient can also be asked to keep a self-rating chart to log accomplishments, so that progress can be measured and remembered. Instruct the patient to record degrees of pain on a self-rating scale in relation to various situations and mental attitudes so that similar circumstances can be avoided or modified.

Avoid positive reinforcers for pain such as marked sympathy and attention to pain. Emphasize a positive response to productive activities, which remove the focus of attention from the pain. Activity is also desensitizing, since the patient learns to tolerate increasing activity levels.

Biofeedback techniques (see Somatoform Disorders, above) and hypnosis have been successful in ameliorating some pain syndromes. Hypnosis tends to be most effective

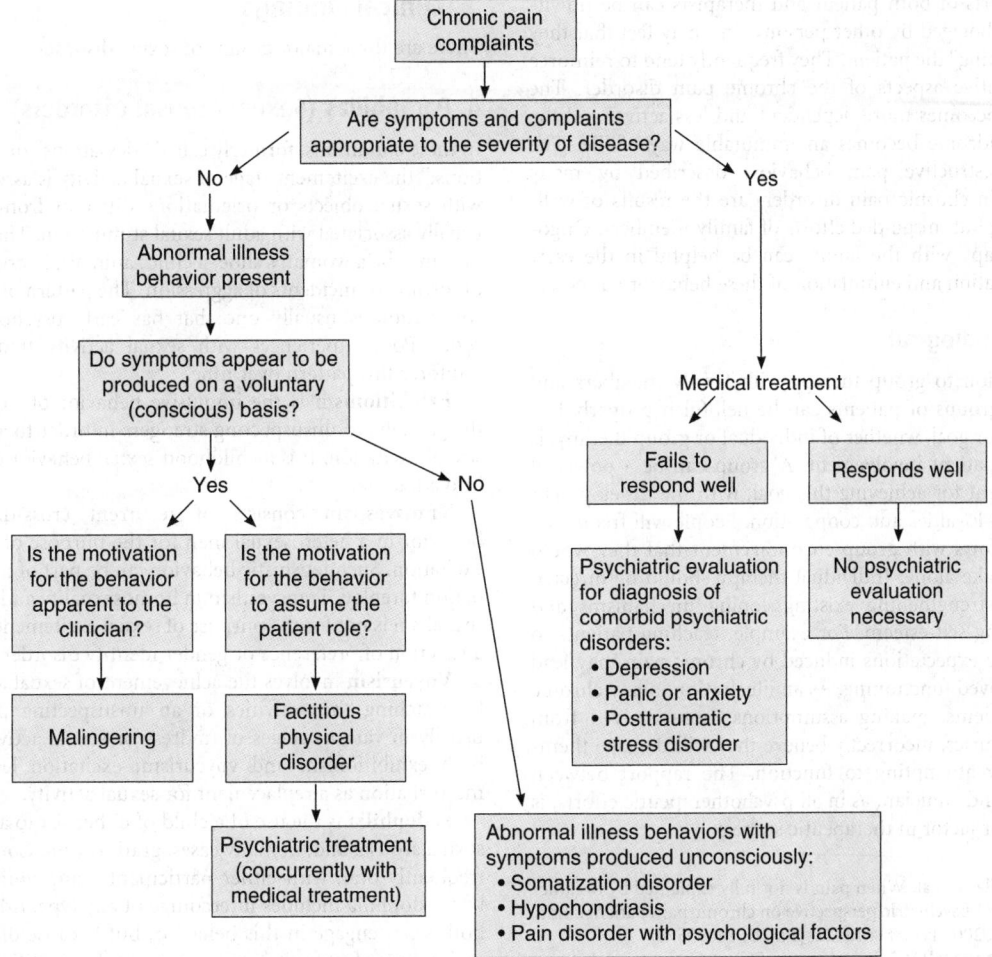

▲ **Figure 25–1.** Algorithm for assessing psychiatric component of chronic pain. (Adapted and reproduced, with permission, from Eisendrath SJ. Psychiatric aspects of chronic pain. Neurology. 1995 Dec;45(12 Suppl 9):S26–34.)

in patients with a high level of denial, who are more responsive to suggestion. Hypnosis can be used to lessen anxiety, alter perception of the length of time that pain is experienced, and encourage relaxation. Mindfulness-based stress reduction programs have been useful in helping individuals develop an enhanced capacity to live a higher quality life with persistent pain (see Chapter 41).

B. Medical

A *single clinician* in charge of the comprehensive treatment approach is the highest priority. Consultations as indicated and technical procedures done by others are appropriate, but the care of the patient should remain in the hands of the primary clinician. Referrals should not be allowed to raise the patient's hopes unrealistically or to become a way for the clinician to reject the case. The attitude of the doctor should be one of honesty, interest, and hopefulness—not for a cure but for control of pain and improved function. If the patient manifests opioid addiction, detoxification may be an early treatment goal.

Nonsteroidal anti-inflammatory drugs are often the first-line of treatment for pain. If opioid analgesics or sedatives are prescribed, they should not be given on an "as-needed" schedule (see Chapter 5). A fixed schedule lessens the conditioning effects of these drugs. Tricyclic antidepressants (TCAs) (eg, nortriptyline), venlafaxine, and duloxetine in doses up to those used in depression may be helpful, particularly in neuropathic pain syndromes. In other conditions, their effects on pain may be less clear, but ameliorating depression is usually important nonetheless. Gabapentin, an anticonvulsant with possible applications in the treatment of anxiety disorders, has been shown to be useful in postherpetic and diabetic neuropathy and somatoform disorders.

In addition to medications, a variety of alternative strategies may be offered, including physical therapy and acupuncture.

C. Social

Involvement of family members and other significant persons in the patient's life should be an early priority. The best efforts of both patient and therapists can be unwittingly sabotaged by other persons who may feel that they are "helping" the patient. They frequently tend to reinforce the negative aspects of the chronic pain disorder. The patient becomes more dependent and less active, and the pain syndrome becomes an immutable way of life. The more destructive pain behaviors described by many experts in chronic pain disorders are the results of well-meaning but misguided efforts of family members. Ongoing therapy with the family can be helpful in the early identification and elimination of these behavior patterns.

D. Psychological

In addition to group therapy with family members and others, groups of patients can be helpful if properly led. The major goal, whether of individual or group therapy, is to gain patient involvement. A group can be a powerful instrument for achieving this goal, with the development of group loyalties and cooperation. People will frequently make efforts with group encouragement that they would never make alone. Individual therapy should be directed toward strengthening existing coping mechanisms and improving self-esteem. For example, teaching patients to challenge expectations induced by chronic pain may lead to improved functioning. As an illustration, many chronic pain patients, making assumptions more derived from acute injuries, incorrectly believe they will damage themselves by attempting to function. The rapport between patient and clinician, as in all psychotherapeutic efforts, is the major factor in therapeutic success.

Ciaramella A et al. When pain is not fully explained by organic lesion: a psychiatric perspective on chronic pain patients. Eur J Pain. 2004 Feb;8(1):13–22. [PMID: 14690670]

Lin EH et al; IMPACT Investigators. Effect of improving depression care on pain and functional outcomes among older adults with arthritis: a randomized controlled trial. JAMA. 2003 Nov 12;290(18):2428–9. [PMID: 14612479]

Thielke SM et al. Pain limits the effectiveness of collaborative care for depression. Am J Geriatr Psychiatry. 2007 Aug;15(8):699–707. [PMID: 17670998]

Verdu B et al. Antidepressants for the treatment of chronic pain. Drugs. 2008;68(18):2611–32. [PMID: 19093703]

PSYCHOSEXUAL DISORDERS

The stages of sexual activity include **excitement** (arousal), **orgasm**, and **resolution**. The precipitating excitement or arousal is psychologically determined. Arousal response leading to plateau is a physiologic and psychological phenomenon of vasocongestion, a parasympathetic reaction causing erection in men and labial-clitoral congestion in women. The orgasmic response includes emission in men and clonic contractions of the analogous striated perineal muscles of both men and women. Resolution is a gradual return to normal physiologic status.

While the arousal stimuli—vasocongestive and orgasmic responses—constitute a single response in a well-adjusted person, they can be considered as separate stages that can produce different syndromes responding to different treatment procedures.

▶ Clinical Findings

There are three major groups of sexual disorders.

A. Paraphilias (Sexual Arousal Disorders)

In these conditions, formerly called "deviations" or "variations," the excitement stage of sexual activity is associated with sexual objects or orientations different from those usually associated with adult sexual stimulation. The stimulus may be a woman's shoe, a child, animals, instruments of torture, or incidents of aggression. The pattern of sexual stimulation is usually one that has early psychological roots. Poor experiences with sexual activity frequently reinforce this pattern over time.

Exhibitionism is the impulsive behavior of exposing the genitalia to unsuspecting strangers in order to achieve sexual excitation. It is a childhood sexual behavior carried into adult life.

Transvestism consists of recurrent cross-dressing behavior in a heterosexual man for the purpose of sexual excitation. Such fetishistic behavior can be part of masturbation foreplay. Transvestism in homosexuality and transsexualism is not for the purpose of sexual excitement but is a function of preference or gender identity disorder.

Voyeurism involves the achievement of sexual arousal by watching the activities of an unsuspecting person, usually in various stages of undress or sexual activity. In both exhibitionism and voyeurism, excitation leads to masturbation as a replacement for sexual activity.

Pedophilia is the use of a child of either sex to achieve sexual arousal and, in many cases, gratification. Contact is frequently oral, with either participant being dominant, but pedophilia includes intercourse of any type. Adults of both sexes engage in this behavior, but because of social and cultural factors it is more commonly identified with men. The pedophile has difficulty in adult sexual relationships, and men who perform this act are frequently impotent.

Incest involves a sexual relationship with a person in the immediate family, most frequently a child. In many ways it is similar to pedophilia (intrafamilial pedophilia). Incestuous feelings are fairly common, but cultural mores are usually sufficiently strong to act as a barrier to the expression of sexual feelings.

Sexual sadism is the attainment of sexual arousal by inflicting pain upon the sexual object. Much sexual activity has aggressive components (eg, biting, scratching). However, forced sexual acquiescence (eg, rape) is considered to be primarily an act of aggression.

Sexual masochism is the achievement of erotic pleasure by being humiliated, enslaved, physically bound, and restrained. It may be life-threatening, since neck binding or partial asphyxiation usually forms part of the ritual. The practice is much more common in men than in women.

B. Gender Identity Disorder

Core gender identity reflects a biologic self-image—the conviction that "I am a boy" or "I am a girl" that is usually well developed by age 3 or 4. Gender dysphoria refers to the development of a sexual identity that is the opposite of the biologic one.

Transsexualism is an attempt to deny and reverse biologic sex by maintaining sexual identity with the opposite gender. Transsexuals do not alternate between gender roles; rather, they assume a fixed role of attitudes, feelings, fantasies, and choices consonant with those of the opposite sex, all of which clearly date back to early development. For example, male to female transsexuals in early childhood behave, talk, and fantasize as if they were girls. They do not grow out of feminine patterns; they do not work in professions traditionally considered to be masculine; and they have no interest in their own penises either as evidence of maleness or as organs for erotic behavior. The desire for sex change starts early and may culminate in assumption of a feminine lifestyle, hormonal treatment, and use of surgical procedures, eg, castration and vaginoplasty.

C. Psychosexual Dysfunction

This category includes a large group of vasocongestive and orgasmic disorders. Often, they involve problems of sexual adaptation, education, and technique that are often initially discussed with, diagnosed by, and treated by the primary care provider.

There are two conditions common in men: erectile dysfunction and ejaculation disturbances.

Erectile dysfunction (impotence) is inability to achieve or maintain an erection firm enough for satisfactory intercourse; patients sometimes use the term to mean premature ejaculation. Careful questioning is necessary, since causes of this vasocongestive disorder can be psychological, physiologic, or both. The majority are pathophysiologic and, to varying degrees, treatable. After onset of the problem, a history of occasional erections—especially nocturnal penile tumescence, which may be evaluated by a simple monitoring device, or a sleep study in the sleep laboratory—is usually evidence that the dysfunction is psychological in origin, with the caveat that decreased nocturnal penile tumescence occurs in some depressed patients. **Psychological erectile dysfunction** is caused by interpersonal or intrapsychic factors (eg, marital disharmony, depression). **Organic factors** are discussed in Chapter 23.

Ejaculation disturbances include premature ejaculation, inability to ejaculate, and retrograde ejaculation. (One may ejaculate even though impotent.) Ejaculation is usually connected with orgasm, and ejaculatory control is an acquired behavior that is minimal in adolescence and increases with experience. Pathogenic factors are those that interfere with learning control, most frequently sexual ignorance. Intrapsychic factors (anxiety, guilt, depression) and interpersonal maladaptation (marital problems, unresponsiveness of mate, power struggles) are also common. Organic causes include interference with sympathetic nerve distribution (often due to surgery or trauma) and the effects of pharmacologic agents (eg, SSRIs or sympatholytics).

In women, the two most common forms of sexual dysfunction are vaginismus and frigidity.

Vaginismus is a conditioned response in which a spasm of the perineal muscles occurs if there is any stimulation of the area. The desire is to avoid penetration. Sexual responsiveness and vasocongestion may be present, and orgasm can result from clitoral stimulation.

Frigidity is a complex condition in which there is a general lack of sexual responsiveness. The woman has difficulty in experiencing erotic sensation and does not have the vasocongestive response. Sexual activity varies from active avoidance of sex to an occasional orgasm. Orgasmic dysfunction—in which a woman has a vasocongestive response but varying degrees of difficulty in reaching orgasm—is sometimes differentiated from frigidity. Causes for the dysfunctions include poor sexual techniques, early traumatic sexual experiences, interpersonal disharmony (marital struggles, use of sex as a means of control), and intrapsychic problems (anxiety, fear, guilt). Organic causes include any conditions that might cause pain in intercourse, pelvic pathology, mechanical obstruction, and neurologic deficits.

Disorders of sexual desire consist of diminished or absent libido in either sex and may be a function of organic or psychological difficulties (eg, anxiety, phobic avoidance). Any chronic illness can reduce desire. Hormonal disorders, including hypogonadism or use of antiandrogen compounds such as cyproterone acetate, and chronic kidney disease contribute to deterioration in sexual activity. Although menopause may lead to diminution of sexual desire in some women, the relationship between menopause and libido is complicated and may be influenced by sociocultural factors. Alcohol, sedatives, opioids, marijuana, and some medications may affect sexual drive and performance.

► Treatment

A. Paraphilias and Gender Identity Disorders

1. Psychological—Sexual arousal disorders involving variant sexual activity (paraphilia), particularly those of a more superficial nature (eg, voyeurism) and those of recent onset, are responsive to psychotherapy in a moderate percentage of cases. The prognosis is much better if the motivation comes from the individual rather than the legal system; unfortunately, however, judicial intervention is frequently the only stimulus to treatment, because the condition persists and is reinforced until conflict with the law occurs. Therapies frequently focus on barriers to normal arousal response; the expectation is that the variant behavior will decrease as normal behavior increases.

2. Behavioral—Aversive and operant conditioning techniques have been tried frequently in gender role disorders but have only occasionally been successful. In some cases, the sexual arousal disorders improve with modeling, role-playing, and conditioning procedures. Emotive imagery is occasionally helpful in lessening anxiety in fetish problems.

3. Social—Although they do not produce a change in sexual arousal patterns or gender role, self-help groups have facilitated adjustment to an often hostile society. Attention to the family is particularly important in helping persons in such groups to accept their situation and alleviate their guilt about the role they think they had in creating the problem.

4. Medical—Medroxyprogesterone acetate, a suppressor of libidinal drive, is used to mute disruptive sexual behavior in men of all ages. Onset of action is usually within 3 weeks, and the effects are generally reversible. Fluoxetine or other SSRIs at depression doses (see Table 25–8) may reduce some of the compulsive sexual behaviors including the paraphilias. A focus of study in the treatment of severe paraphilia has been agonists of luteinizing hormone–releasing hormone. Although some transsexuals are treated with genital reconstructive surgery, many others are screened out by trial periods of living as the other sex prior to operation.

B. Psychosexual Dysfunction

1. Medical—Identification of a contributory reversible cause is most important. Even if the condition is not reversible, identification of the specific cause helps the patient to accept the condition. Marital disharmony, with its exacerbating effects, may thus be avoided. Of all the sexual dysfunctions, erectile dysfunction is the condition most likely to have an organic basis. Sildenafil, tadalafil, and vardenafil are phosphodiesterase type 5 inhibitors that are effective oral agents for the treatment of penile erectile dysfunction (eg, sildenafil 25–100 mg orally 1 hour prior to intercourse). These agents are effective for SSRI-induced erectile dysfunction in men and in some cases for SSRI-associated sexual dysfunction in women. Use of the medications in conjunction with any nitrates, particularly in individuals with coronary artery disease, can have significant hypotensive effects leading to death in some cases. The medication, which does not appear to impact sexual desire, should be used only once a day. Because of their common effect in delaying ejaculation, the SSRIs have been effective in premature ejaculation.

2. Behavioral—Syndromes resulting from conditioned responses have been treated by conditioning techniques, with excellent results. Vaginismus responds well to desensitization with graduated Hegar dilators along with relaxation techniques. Masters and Johnson have used behavioral approaches in all of the sexual dysfunctions, with concomitant supportive psychotherapy and with improvement of the communication patterns of the couple.

3. Psychological—The use of psychotherapy by itself is best suited for those cases in which interpersonal difficulties or intrapsychic problems predominate. Anxiety and guilt about parental injunctions against sex may contribute to sexual dysfunction. Even in these cases, however, a combined behavioral-psychological approach usually produces results most quickly.

4. Social—The proximity of other people (eg, a mother-in-law) in a household is frequently an inhibiting factor in sexual relationships. In such cases, some social engineering may alleviate the problem.

Kostis JB et al. Sexual dysfunction and cardiac risk (The Second Princeton Consensus Conference). Am J Cardiol. 2005 Jul 15;96(2):313–21. [PMID: 16018863]

Nurnburg HG et al. Sildenafil treatment of women with antidepressant-associated sexual dysfunction: a randomized controlled trial. JAMA. 2008 Jul 23;300(4):395–404. [PMID: 18647982]

Sivalingam S et al. An overview of the diagnosis and treatment of erectile dysfunction. Drugs. 2006;66(18):2339–55. [PMID: 17181376]

PERSONALITY DISORDERS

 ESSENTIALS OF DIAGNOSIS

- ▸ Long history dating back to childhood.
- ▸ Recurrent maladaptive behavior.
- ▸ Low self-esteem and lack of confidence.
- ▸ Minimal introspective ability with a tendency to blame others for all problems.
- ▸ Major difficulties with interpersonal relationships or society.
- ▸ Depression with anxiety when maladaptive behavior fails.

▸ General Considerations

An individual's personality structure, or character, is an integral part of self-image. It reflects genetics, interpersonal influences, and recurring patterns of behavior adopted in order to cope with the environment. The classification of subtypes of personality disorders depends on the predominant symptoms and their severity. The most severe disorders—those that bring the patient into greatest conflict with society—tend to be classified as antisocial (psychopathic) or borderline.

Personality disorders can be considered a matrix for some of the more severe psychiatric problems (eg, schizotypal, relating to schizophrenia, and avoidance types, relating to some anxiety disorders).

▸ Classification & Clinical Findings

See Table 25–3.

▸ Differential Diagnosis

Patients with personality disorders tend to show anxiety and depression when pathologic coping mechanisms fail, and their symptoms can be similar to those disorders. Occasionally, the more severe cases may decompensate into psychosis under stress and mimic other psychotic disorders.

▸ Treatment

A. Social

Social and therapeutic environments such as day hospitals, halfway houses, and self-help communities utilize peer pressures to modify the self-destructive behavior. The patient with a personality disorder often has failed to profit from experience, and difficulties with authority impair the learning experience. The use of peer relationships and the repetition possible in a structured setting of a helpful community enhance the behavioral treatment opportunities and increase learning. When problems are detected

Table 25-3. Personality disorders: Classification and clinical findings.

Personality Disorder	Clinical Findings
Paranoid	Defensive, oversensitive, secretive, suspicious, hyperalert, with limited emotional response.
Schizoid	Shy, introverted, withdrawn, avoids close relationships.
Obsessive compulsive	Perfectionist, egocentric, indecisive, with rigid thought patterns and need for control.
Histrionic (hysterical)	Dependent, immature, seductive, egocentric, vain, emotionally labile.
Schizotypal	Superstitious, socially isolated, suspicious, with limited interpersonal ability, eccentric behaviors, and odd speech.
Narcissistic	Exhibitionist, grandiose, preoccupied with power, lacks interest in others, with excessive demands for attention.
Avoidant	Fears rejection, hyperreacts to rejection and failure, with poor social endeavors and low self-esteem.
Dependent	Passive, overaccepting, unable to make decisions, lacks confidence, with poor self-esteem.
Antisocial	Selfish, callous, promiscuous, impulsive, unable to learn from experience, has legal problems.
Borderline	Impulsive; has unstable and intense interpersonal relationships; is suffused with anger, fear, and guilt; lacks self-control and self-fulfillment; has identity problems and affective instability; is suicidal (a serious problem—up to 80% of hospitalized borderline patients make an attempt at some time during treatment, and the incidence of completed suicide is as high as 5%); aggressive behavior, feelings of emptiness, and occasional psychotic decompensation. This group has a high drug abuse rate, which plays a role in symptoms. There is extensive overlap with other diagnostic categories, particularly mood disorders and posttraumatic stress disorder.

early, both the school and the home can serve as foci of intensified social pressure to change the behavior, particularly with the use of behavioral techniques.

B. Behavioral

The behavioral techniques used are principally operant conditioning and aversive conditioning. The former simply emphasizes the recognition of acceptable behavior and its reinforcement with praise or other tangible rewards. Aversive responses usually mean punishment, although this can range from a mild rebuke to some specific punitive responses such as deprivation of privileges. Extinction plays a role in that an attempt is made not to respond to inappropriate behavior, and the lack of response eventually causes the person to abandon that type of behavior. Pouting and tantrums, for example, diminish quickly when such behavior elicits no reaction. Dialectical behavioral therapy is a program of individual and group therapy specifically designed for patients with chronic suicidality and borderline personality disorder. It blends mindfulness and a cognitive-behavioral model to address self-awareness, interpersonal functioning, affective lability, and reactions to stress.

C. Psychological

Psychological intervention is best conducted in group settings. Group therapy is helpful when specific interpersonal behavior needs to be improved. This mode of treatment also has a place with so-called acting-out patients, ie, those who frequently act in an impulsive and inappropriate way. The peer pressure in the group tends to impose restraints on rash behavior. The group also quickly identifies the patient's types of behavior and helps improve the validity of the patient's self-assessment, so that the antecedents of the unacceptable behavior can be effectively handled, thus decreasing its frequency. Individual therapy

should initially be supportive, ie, helping the patient to restabilize and mobilize coping mechanisms. If the individual has the ability to observe his or her own behavior, a longer-term and more introspective therapy may be warranted. The therapist must be able to handle countertransference feelings (which are frequently negative), maintain appropriate boundaries in the relationship (no physical contacts, however well-meaning), and refrain from premature confrontations and interpretations.

D. Medical

Hospitalization is indicated in the case of serious suicidal or homicidal danger. In most cases, treatment can be accomplished in the day treatment center or self-help community. Antipsychotics may be required for short periods in conditions that have temporarily decompensated into transient psychoses (eg, haloperidol, 2–5 mg orally every 3–4 hours until the patient has quieted down and is regaining contact with reality). Olanzapine (2.5–10 mg/d orally) or risperidone (0.5–2 mg/d orally) may be given with lorazepam (1–2 mg orally every 4 hours as needed). In some cases, these drugs are required only for several days and can be discontinued after the patient has regained a previously established level of adjustment; they can also provide ongoing support. Carbamazepine, 400–800 mg orally daily in divided doses, decreases the severity of behavioral dyscontrol. Antidepressants have improved anxiety, depression, and sensitivity to rejection in some borderline patients. SSRIs may have a role in reducing aggressive behavior in impulsive aggressive patients.

► Prognosis

Antisocial and borderline categories generally have a guarded prognosis. Those patients with a history of parental abuse and a family history of mood disorder tend to have the most challenging treatments.

Binks CA et al. Pharmacological interventions for people with borderline personality disorder. Cochrane Database Syst Rev. 2006 Jan 25;(1):CD005653. [PMID: 16437535]

Linehann MM et al. Two-year randomized controlled trial and follow-up of dialectical behavior therapy vs therapy by experts for suicidal behaviors and borderline personality disorder. Arch Gen Psychiatry. 2006 Jul;63(7):757–66. [PMID: 16818865]

SCHIZOPHRENIC & OTHER PSYCHOTIC DISORDERS

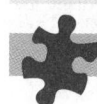

ESSENTIALS OF DIAGNOSIS

▶ Social withdrawal, usually slowly progressive, often with deterioration in personal care.

▶ Loss of ego boundaries, with inability to perceive oneself as a separate entity.

▶ Loose thought associations, often with slowed thinking or overinclusive and rapid shifting from topic to topic.

▶ Autistic absorption in inner thoughts and frequent sexual or religious preoccupations.

▶ Auditory hallucinations, often of a derogatory nature.

▶ Delusions, frequently of a grandiose or persecutory nature.

▶ Symptoms of at least 6 months' duration.

Frequent additional signs:

▶ Flat affect and rapidly alternating mood shifts irrespective of circumstances.

▶ Hypersensitivity to environmental stimuli, with a feeling of enhanced sensory awareness.

▶ Variability or changeable behavior incongruent with the external environment.

▶ Concrete thinking with inability to abstract; inappropriate symbolism.

▶ Impaired concentration worsened by hallucinations and delusions.

▶ Depersonalization, wherein one behaves like a detached observer of one's own actions.

▶ General Considerations

The schizophrenic disorders are a group of syndromes manifested by massive disruption of thinking, mood, and overall behavior as well as poor filtering of stimuli. The characterization and nomenclature of the disorders are quite arbitrary and are influenced by sociocultural factors and schools of psychiatric thought.

It is currently believed that the schizophrenic disorders are of multifactorial cause, with genetic, environmental, and neurotransmitter pathophysiologic components. At present, there is no laboratory method for confirming the diagnosis of schizophrenia. There may or may not be a history of a major disruption in the individual's life (failure, loss, physical illness) before gross psychotic deterioration is evident.

Schizophrenic symptoms have been classified into positive and negative categories. Positive symptoms include hallucinations, delusions, and formal thought disorders; these symptoms appear to be related to increased dopaminergic (D_2) activity in the mesolimbic region. Negative symptoms include diminished sociability, restricted affect, and poverty of speech; these symptoms appear to be related to decreased D_2 activity in the mesocortical system.

"Other psychotic disorders" are conditions that are similar to schizophrenic disorders in their acute symptoms but have a less pervasive influence over the long term. The patient usually attains higher levels of functioning. The acute psychotic episodes tend to be less disruptive of the person's lifestyle, with a fairly quick return to previous levels of functioning.

▶ Classification

A. Schizophrenic Disorders

Schizophrenic disorders are subdivided on the basis of certain prominent phenomena that are frequently present. **Disorganized (hebephrenic) schizophrenia** is characterized by marked incoherence and an incongruous or silly affect. **Catatonic schizophrenia** is distinguished by a marked psychomotor disturbance of either excitement (purposeless and stereotyped) or rigidity with mutism. Infrequently, there may be rapid alternation between excitement and stupor (see under catatonic syndrome, below). **Paranoid schizophrenia** includes marked persecutory or grandiose delusions often consonant with hallucinations of similar content and with less marked disorganization of speech and behavior. **Undifferentiated schizophrenia** denotes a category in which symptoms are not specific enough to warrant inclusion of the illness in the other subtypes. **Residual schizophrenia** is a classification that includes persons who have clearly had an episode warranting a diagnosis of schizophrenia but who at present have no overt psychotic symptoms, although they show milder signs such as social withdrawal, flat affect, and eccentric behaviors.

B. Delusional Disorders

Delusional disorders are psychoses in which the predominant symptoms are persistent, nonbizarre delusions with minimal impairment of daily functioning. (The schizophrenic disorders show significant impairment.) Intellectual and occupational activities are little affected, whereas social and marital functioning tend to be markedly involved. Hallucinations are not usually present. Common delusional themes include paranoid delusions of persecution, delusions of being related to or loved by a well-known person, and delusions that one's partner is unfaithful.

C. Schizoaffective Disorders

Schizoaffective disorders are those cases that fail to fit comfortably either in the schizophrenic or in the affective categories. They are usually cases with affective symptoms that precede or develop concurrently with psychotic manifestations. There has been increasing interest in studying prodromal schizophrenia with a goal of prevention or early treatment.

D. Schizophreniform Disorders

Schizophreniform disorders are similar in their symptoms to schizophrenic disorders except that the duration of prodromal, acute, and residual symptoms is more than 1 week but less than 6 months.

E. Brief Psychotic Disorders

These disorders last less than 1 week. They are the result of psychological stress. The shorter duration is significant and correlates with a more acute onset and resolution as well as a much better prognosis.

F. Late Life Psychosis

Brain abnormalities occur in 40% of patients who develop psychotic symptoms after age 60. The psychotic symptoms are typical, and there are other findings such as low IQ scores and diminished cognitive function.

G. Atypical Psychoses

This group includes a wide range of conditions with psychotic symptoms. The cause is often not clear, but later events (eg, new symptoms) may clarify the diagnosis. The most common example is chronic psychosis developing either during periods of heavy abuse of drugs or at some time after the drug use has ceased. Other conditions include temporal lobe dysfunction, HIV infection, and a number of the conditions noted in the differential diagnosis (see below). They often have a good premorbid history, a precipitous onset, and an episodic course with symptom-free intervals.

▶ Clinical Findings

A. Symptoms and Signs

The symptoms and signs of schizophrenia vary markedly among individuals as well as in the same person at different times. The patient's **appearance** may be bizarre, although the usual finding is a mild to moderate unkempt blandness. **Motor activity** is generally reduced, although extremes ranging from catatonic stupor to frenzied excitement occur. **Social behavior** is characterized by marked withdrawal coupled with disturbed interpersonal relationships and a reduced ability to experience pleasure. Dependency and a poor self-image are common. **Verbal utterances** are variable, the language being concrete yet symbolic, with unassociated rambling statements (at times interspersed with mutism) during an acute episode. Neologisms (made-up words or phrases), echolalia (repetition of words spoken by others), and verbigeration (repetition of senseless words or phrases) are occasionally present. **Affect** is usually flattened, with occasional inappropriateness. **Depression** is present in almost all cases but may be less apparent during the acute psychotic episode and more obvious during recovery. Depression is sometimes confused with akinetic side effects of antipsychotic drugs. It is also related to **boredom**, which increases symptoms and decreases the response to treatment. Work is generally unavailable and time unfilled, providing opportunities for counterproductive activities

such as drug abuse, withdrawal, and increased psychotic symptoms.

Thought content may vary from a paucity of ideas to a rich complex of delusional fantasy with archaic thinking. One frequently notes after a period of conversation that little if any information has actually been conveyed. Incoming stimuli produce varied responses. In some cases a simple question may trigger explosive outbursts, whereas at other times there may be no overt response whatsoever (catatonia). When paranoid ideation is present, the patient is often irritable and less cooperative. **Delusions** (false beliefs) are characteristic of paranoid thinking, and they usually take the form of a preoccupation with the supposedly threatening behavior exhibited by other individuals. This ideation may cause the patient to adopt active countermeasures such as locking doors and windows, taking up weapons, covering the ceiling with aluminum foil to counteract radar waves, and other bizarre efforts. Somatic delusions revolve around issues of bodily decay or infestation. **Perceptual distortions** usually include auditory hallucinations—visual hallucinations are more commonly associated with organic mental states—and may include illusions (distortions of reality) such as figures changing in size or lights varying in intensity. Cenesthetic hallucinations (eg, a burning sensation in the brain, feeling blood flowing in blood vessels) occasionally occur. Lack of humor, feelings of dread, depersonalization (a feeling of being apart from the self), and fears of annihilation may be present. Any of the above symptoms generate higher anxiety levels, with heightened arousal and occasional panic and suicidal ideation, as the individual fails to cope.

The development of the acute episode in schizophrenia frequently is the end product of a gradual decompensation. Frustration and anxiety appear early, followed by depression and alienation, along with progressive ineffectiveness in day-to-day coping. This often leads to feelings of panic and increasing disorganization, with loss of the ability to test and evaluate the reality of perceptions. The stage of so-called psychotic resolution includes delusions, autistic preoccupations, and psychotic insight, with acceptance of the decompensated state. The process is frequently complicated by the use of caffeine, alcohol, and other recreational drugs. Life expectancy of schizophrenic patients is as much as 20% shorter than that of cohorts in the general population and is often associated with comorbid conditions such as the metabolic syndrome.

Polydipsia may produce water intoxication with hyponatremia—characterized by symptoms of confusion, lethargy, psychosis, seizures, and occasionally death—in any psychiatric disorder, but most commonly in schizophrenia. These problems exacerbate the schizophrenic symptoms and can be confused with them. Possible pathogenetic factors in polydipsia include a hypothalamic defect, inappropriate antidiuretic hormone (ADH) secretion, neuroleptic medications (anticholinergic effects, stimulation of hypothalamic thirst center, effect on ADH), smoking (nicotine and syndrome of inappropriate antidiuretic hormone [SIADH]), psychotic thought processes (delusions), and other medications (eg, diuretics, antidepressants, lithium, alcohol). Other causes of polydipsia must be ruled out (eg, diabetes mellitus, diabetes insipidus, kidney disease).

B. Imaging

Ventricular enlargement and cortical atrophy, as seen on CT scan, have been correlated with chronic course, severe cognitive impairment, and nonresponsiveness to neuroleptic medications. Decreased frontal lobe activity seen on PET scan has been associated with negative symptoms.

▶ Differential Diagnosis

One should not hesitate to reconsider the diagnosis of schizophrenia in any person who has received that diagnosis in the past, particularly when the clinical course has been atypical. A number of these patients have been found to actually have atypical episodic affective disorders that have responded well to lithium. Manic episodes often mimic schizophrenia. Furthermore, schizophrenia has been diagnosed in many individuals because of inadequacies in psychiatric nomenclature. Thus, schizophrenia was often inappropriately diagnosed in persons with brief reactive psychoses, OCD, paranoid disorders, and schizophreniform disorders.

Psychotic depressions, psychotic organic mental states, and any illness with psychotic ideation tend to be confused with schizophrenia, partly because of the regrettable tendency to use the terms interchangeably. Adolescent phases of growth and counterculture behaviors constitute another area of diagnostic confusion. It is particularly important to avoid a misdiagnosis in these groups, because of the long-term implications arising from having such a serious diagnosis made in a formative stage of life.

Medical disorders such as thyroid dysfunction, adrenal and pituitary disorders, reactions to toxic materials (eg, mercury, PCBs), and almost all of the organic mental states in the early stages must be ruled out. Postpartum psychosis is discussed under Mood Disorders. **Complex partial seizures,** especially when psychosensory phenomena are present, are an important differential consideration. Toxic drug states arising from prescription, over-the-counter, herbal and street drugs may mimic all of the psychotic disorders. The chronic use of amphetamines, cocaine, and other stimulants frequently produces a psychosis that is almost identical to the acute paranoid schizophrenic episode. The presence of formication and stereotypy suggests the possibility of stimulant abuse. Phencyclidine (see below), a very common street drug, may cause a reaction that is difficult to distinguish from other psychotic disorders. Cerebellar signs, excessive salivation, dilated pupils, and increased deep tendon reflexes should alert the clinician to the possibility of a toxic psychosis. Industrial chemical toxicity (both organic and metallic), degenerative disorders, and metabolic deficiencies must be considered in the differential diagnosis.

Catatonic syndrome, frequently assumed to exist solely as a component of schizophrenic disorders, is actually the end product of a number of illnesses, including various organic conditions. Neoplasms, viral and bacterial encephalopathies, central nervous system hemorrhage, metabolic derangements such as diabetic ketoacidosis, sedative withdrawal, and hepatic and renal malfunction have all been implicated. It is particularly important to realize that drug toxicity (eg, overdoses of antipsychotic medications such as fluphenazine or haloperidol) can cause catatonic syndrome, which may be misdiagnosed as a catatonic schizophrenic disorder and inappropriately treated with more antipsychotic medication.

▶ Treatment

A. Medical

Hospitalization is often necessary, particularly when the patient's behavior shows gross disorganization. The presence of competent family members lessens the need for hospitalization, and each case should be judged individually. The major considerations are to prevent self-inflicted harm or harm to others and to provide the patient's basic needs. A full medical evaluation and CT scan or MRI should be considered in first episodes of schizophreniform disorder and other psychotic episodes of unknown cause.

Antipsychotic medications (see below) are the treatment of choice. They block the response to stimulation. The relapse rate can be reduced by 50% with proper maintenance neuroleptic therapy. Long-acting, injectable depot neuroleptics are used in noncompliant patients or nonresponders to oral medication.

Antipsychotic drugs include the "typical" neuroleptics **phenothiazines, thioxanthenes** (both similar in structure), **butyrophenones, dihydroindolones, dibenzoxazepines,** and **benzisoxazoles,** and the newer "atypical" neuroleptics clozapine, risperidone, olanzapine, quetiapine, aripiprazole, and ziprasidone (Table 25–4). Generally, increasing milligram potency of the typical neuroleptics is associated with decreasing anticholinergic and adrenergic side effects and increasing extrapyramidal symptoms (Table 25–5). For example, chlorpromazine has lower potency and more severe anticholinergic and adrenergic side effects. The increased anticholinergic effect of chlorpromazine, however, lowers the risk of extrapyramidal symptoms.

The Clinical Antipsychotic Trials of Intervention Effectiveness (CATIE) study was a complex investigation that compared "atypical" and "typical" neuroleptic drugs. Although it was not definitive, it suggested similar antipsychotic efficacy for both classes and a tendency for the atypicals, particularly olanzapine, to be better tolerated leading to enhanced compliance. It also highlighted lack of patient adherence as a major factor in treatments.

The phenothiazines comprise the bulk of the currently used "typical" neuroleptic drugs. The only butyrophenone commonly used in psychiatry is haloperidol, which is different in structure but similar in action and side effects to the piperazine phenothiazines such as fluphenazine, perphenazine, and trifluoperazine. These drugs and haloperidol (dopamine [D_2] receptor blockers) have high potency and a paucity of autonomic side effects and act to markedly lower arousal levels. Molindone and loxapine, while less potent, are similar in action, side effects, and safety to the piperazine phenothiazines.

Table 25–4. Commonly used antipsychotics.

Drug	Usual Daily Oral Dose	Usual Daily Maximum Dose[1]	Cost per Unit	Cost for 30 Days Treatment Based on Maximum Dosage[2]
Phenothiazines				
Chlorpromazine (Thorazine; others)	100–400 mg	1 g	$1.05/200 mg	$157.50
Thioridazine (Mellaril)	100–400 mg	600 mg	$.67/100 mg	$120.60
Mesoridazine (Serentil)	50–200 mg	400 mg		Not available in United States
Perphenazine (Trilafon)[3]	16–32 mg	64 mg	$1.85/16 mg	$222.00
Trifluoperazine (Stelazine)	5–15 mg	60 mg	$1.63/10 mg	$293.60
Fluphenazine (Permitil, Prolixin)[3]	2–10 mg	60 mg	$1.25/10 mg	$225.00
Thioxanthenes				
Thiothixene (Navane)[3]	5–10 mg	80 mg	$0.65/10 mg	$156.00
Dihydroindolone				
Molindone (Moban)	30–100 mg	225 mg	$4.03/50 mg	$544.05
Dibenzoxazepine				
Loxapine (Loxitane)	20–60 mg	200 mg	$2.57/50 mg	$308.40
Dibenzodiazepine				
Clozapine (Clozaril)	300–450 mg	900 mg	$3.42/100 mg	$923.40
Butyrophenone				
Haloperidol (Haldol)	2–5 mg	60 mg	$2.76/20 mg	$248.40
Benzisoxazole				
Risperidone[4] (Risperdal)	2–6 mg	10 mg	$7.59/2 mg	$946.16
Thienobenzodiazepine				
Olanzapine (Zyprexa)	5–10 mg	10 mg	$14.64/10 mg	$439.20
Dibenzothiazepine				
Quetiapine (Seroquel)	200–400 mg	800 mg	$8.18/200 mg	$755.92
Benzisothiazolyl piperazine				
Ziprasidone (Geodon)	40–160 mg	160 mg	$7.66/80 mg	$459.37
Dipiperazine				
Aripiprazole (Abilify)	10–15 mg	30 mg	$21.57/30 mg	$646.97

[1]Can be higher in some cases.
[2]Average wholesale price (AWP, for AB-rated generic when available) for quantity listed. Source: *Red Book Update*, Vol. 28, No. 3, March 2009. AWP may not accurately represent the actual pharmacy cost because wide contractual variations exist among institutions.
[3]Indicates piperazine structure.
[4]For risperidone, daily doses above 6 mg increase the risk of extrapyramidal syndrome. Risperidone 6 mg is approximately equivalent to haloperidol 20 mg.

The first "atypical" (novel) antipsychotic drug developed, clozapine, a dibenzodiazepine derivative, has dopamine (D_4) receptor-blocking activity as well as central serotonergic, histaminergic, and α-noradrenergic receptor-blocking activity. It is effective in the treatment of about 30% of psychoses resistant to other neuroleptic drugs. Research suggests that clozapine may have specific efficacy in decreasing suicidality in patients with schizophrenia. It is associated with a 1% risk of agranulocytosis, which requires weekly white blood cell count monitoring for the first 6 months followed by monitoring every other week. Weekly monitoring for 1 month after discontinuation of the medication is recommended. Because of an association between clozapine and myocarditis, the drug is contraindicated in patients with severe heart disease.

Risperidone is an antipsychotic that blocks some serotonin receptors ($5\text{-}HT_2$) and dopamine receptors (D_2). Risperidone causes fewer extrapyramidal side effects than the typical antipsychotics at doses less than 6 mg. It appears to be as effective as haloperidol and possibly as effective as clozapine in treatment-resistant patients without requiring weekly white cell counts. Risperidone-induced hyperprolactinemia, even on low doses, has been reported, and that effect is thought to be more common with risperidone than with other atypical antipsychotics. Risperidone is available in a long-acting injectable preparation.

Table 25–5. Relative potency and side effects of antipsychotics.

Drug	Chlorpromazine: Drug Potency Ratio	Anticholinergic Effects[1]	Extrapyramidal Effect[1]
Phenothiazines			
Chlorpromazine	1:1	4	1
Thioridazine	1:1	4	1
Mesoridazine	1:2	3	2
Perphenazine	1:10	2	3
Trifluoperazine	1:20	1	4
Fluphenazine	1:50	1	4
Thioxanthene			
Thiothixene	1:20	1	4
Dihydroindolone			
Molindone	1:10	2	3
Dibenzoxazepine			
Loxapine	1:10	2	3
Butyrophenone			
Haloperidol	1:50	1	4
Dibenzodiazepine			
Clozapine	1:1	4	—
Benzisoxazole			
Risperidone	1:50	1	1
Thienobenzodiazepine			
Olanzapine	1:20	1	1
Dibenzothiazepine			
Quetiapine	1:1	1	—
Benzisothiazolyl piperazine			
Ziprasidone	1:1	1	1
Dipiperazine			
Aripiprazole	1:20	1	0

[1]4, strong effect; 1, weak effect.

Olanzapine is a potent blocker of muscarinic, anticholinergic, 5-HT$_2$, and dopamine D$_1$, D$_2$, and D$_4$ receptors. High doses of olanzapine (12.5–17.5 mg daily) appear to be more effective than lower doses. The drug appears to be more effective than haloperidol in the treatment of negative symptoms, such as withdrawal, psychomotor retardation, and poor interpersonal relationships. It is available in an orally disintegrating form for patients who are unable to tolerate standard oral dosing and in an injectable form for the management of acute agitation associated with schizophrenia and bipolar disorder. Serum alanine aminotransferase is more elevated in patients taking olanzapine than in those taking haloperidol. Olanzapine is associated with a much lower incidence of dystonic reaction than haloperidol and is perhaps less likely to induce tardive dyskinesia. Its most common side effects include somnolence, agitation, nervousness, headache, insomnia, dizziness, and significant weight gain. Multiple case reports have linked olanzapine

and clozapine to new-onset type 2 diabetes and other atypical drugs should be monitored for this adverse effect as well. Further investigation is ongoing to clarify the risk, risk factors, and pathophysiology. The manufacturer has alerted physicians to an association between olanzapine and a significantly higher risk of stroke and death in elderly patients, which has also been noted with other atypical agents.

Quetiapine is a neuroleptic with greater 5-HT$_2$ relative to D$_2$ receptor blockade as well as a relatively high affinity for α_1- and α_2-adrenergic receptors. It appears to be as efficacious as haloperidol in treating positive and negative symptoms of schizophrenia, with less extrapyramidal side effects even at high doses. More common side effects include somnolence, dizziness, and postural hypotension. Because of an association with lens changes seen in patients on long-term treatment, an eye examination to detect cataract formation is recommended at initiation of treatment and then at 6-month intervals during treatment.

Ziprasidone has both anti-dopamine receptor and anti-serotonin receptor effects, with good efficacy for both positive and negative symptoms of schizophrenia. Ziprasidone is not associated with significant weight gain, hyperlipidemia, or new-onset diabetes and offers a good alternative for some patients. It has been implicated in QTc interval delay of > 500 ms in some patients, although in several cases of overdose there were no incidents of torsades de pointes or sudden death. Patients taking ziprasidone should be screened for cardiac risk factors. A pretreatment ECG is indicated for patients at risk for cardiac sequelae (including patients taking other medications that might prolong the QTc interval).

Aripiprazole is the first neuroleptic that is a dopamine stabilizer. A partial agonist at the dopamine D_2 and serotonin 5-HT$_1$ receptors and an antagonist at 5-HT$_2$ receptors, it is effective against positive and negative symptoms of schizophrenia. It functions as an antagonist or agonist, depending on the dopaminergic activity at the dopamine receptors. This may help decrease side effects. More activating than sedating, aripiprazole is thought to impose a low risk of extrapyramidal symptoms, weight gain, hyperprolactinemia, and delayed QT interval. Aripiprazole has been approved as an augmentation agent for treatment-resistant depression even when psychosis is not present.

None of the antipsychotics produce true physical dependency. All decrease adrenergic responses. Despite higher costs, atypical neuroleptics are often considered preferable to traditional antipsychotics because they are thought to be associated with reduced extrapyramidal symptoms and a lesser risk of tardive dyskinesia.

Clinical Indications

The antipsychotics are used to treat all forms of the schizophrenias as well as psychotic ideation in organic brain psychoses, delirium and dementia, drug-induced psychoses, psychotic depression, and mania. They are also effective in Tourette disorder. They quickly lower the arousal (activity) level and, perhaps indirectly, gradually improve socialization and thinking. The improvement rate is about 80%. Patients whose behavioral symptoms worsen with use of antipsychotic drugs may have an undiagnosed organic condition such as anticholinergic toxicity.

Symptoms that are ameliorated by these drugs include hyperactivity, hostility, aggression, delusions, hallucinations, irritability, and poor sleep. Individuals with acute psychosis and good premorbid function respond quite well. The most common cause of failure in the treatment of acute psychosis is inadequate dosage, and the most common cause of relapse is noncompliance.

Although typical antipsychotics are efficacious in the treatment of so-called positive symptoms of schizophrenia, such as hallucinations and delusions, atypical antipsychotics are thought to have efficacy in reducing both positive and negative symptoms. Antidepressant drugs may be used in conjunction with neuroleptics if significant depression is present. Resistant cases may require concomitant use of lithium, carbamazepine, or valproic acid. The addition of a benzodiazepine drug to the neuroleptic regimen may prove helpful in treating the agitated or catatonic psychotic patient who has not responded to neuroleptics alone—lorazepam, 1–2 mg orally, can produce a rapid resolution of catatonic symptoms and may allow maintenance with a lower neuroleptic dose. Electroconvulsive therapy (ECT) has also been effective in treating catatonia.

Dosage Forms & Patterns

The dosage range is quite broad. For example, risperidone, 0.25–1 mg orally at bedtime, may be sufficient for the elderly person with mild dementia with psychosis (especially in view of the increased risk of stroke and death in the elderly), whereas up to 6 mg/d may be used in a young patient with acute schizophrenia. For quick response, an atypical antipsychotic may be started in combination with a benzodiazepine (eg, risperidone oral solution, 2 mg, or olanzapine, 10 mg orally, and lorazepam, 2 mg orally, every 2–4 hours as needed). In an acutely distressed, psychotic patient one might use haloperidol, 10 mg intramuscularly, which is absorbed rapidly and achieves an initial tenfold plasma level advantage over equal oral doses. Psychomotor agitation, racing thoughts, and general arousal are quickly reduced. The dose can be repeated every 3–4 hours; when the patient is less symptomatic, oral doses can replace parenteral administration in most cases. In the elderly, both atypical (eg, risperidone 0.25 mg–0.5 mg daily or olanzapine 1.25 mg daily) and conventional (eg haloperidol 0.5 mg daily or perphenazine 2 mg daily) antipsychotics, often used effectively in small doses for behavioral control, have been linked to premature death in some cases.

Various factors play a role in the absorption of oral medications. Of particular importance are previous gastrointestinal surgery and concomitant administration of other drugs. There are racial differences in metabolizing the neuroleptic drugs—eg, many Asians require only about half the usual dosage. Bioavailability is influenced by other factors such as smoking or hepatic microsomal enzyme stimulation with alcohol or barbiturates and enzyme-altering drugs such as carbamazepine or methylphenidate. Neuroleptic plasma drug level determinations are not currently of major clinical assistance.

Divided daily doses are not necessary after a maintenance dose has been established, and most patients can then be maintained on a single daily dose, usually taken at bedtime. This is particularly appropriate in a case where the sedative effect of the drug is desired for nighttime sleep, and undesirable sedative effects can be avoided during the day. Risperidone is an exception, being given twice daily. First-episode patients especially should be tapered off medications after about 6 months of stability and carefully monitored; their rate of relapse is lower than that of multiple-episode patients.

Psychiatric patients—particularly paranoid individuals—often neglect to take their medication. In these cases and in nonresponders to oral medication, the enanthate and decanoate (the latter is slightly longer-lasting and has fewer extrapyramidal side effects) forms of fluphenazine or the decanoate form of haloperidol may be given by deep subcutaneous injection or intramuscularly to achieve an effect that will usually last 7–28 days. A patient who cannot be depended on to take oral medication (or who overdoses on minimal provocation) will generally agree to come to the clinician's office for a "shot." The usual dose of the fluphenazine long-acting preparations is 25 mg every 2 weeks. Dosage and frequency of administration vary from about 100 mg weekly to 12.5 mg monthly. Use the smallest effective amount as infrequently as possible. A monthly injection of 25 mg of fluphenazine decanoate is equivalent to about 15–20 mg of oral fluphenazine daily. Risperidone is the first atypical neuroleptic available in a long-acting injectable form (25–50 mg intramuscularly every 2 weeks). Concomitant use of a benzodiazepine (eg, lorazepam, 2 mg orally twice daily) may permit reduction of the required dosage of oral or parenteral antipsychotic drug.

Intravenous haloperidol, the neuroleptic most commonly used by this route, is often used in critical care units in the management of agitated, delirious patients. Intravenous haloperidol should be given no faster than 1 mg/min to reduce cardiovascular side effects, such as torsades de pointes. Current practice indicates that ECG monitoring should be used whenever haloperidol is being administered intravenously.

▶ Side Effects

For both typical and atypical neuroleptic agents, a range of side effects has been reported. The most common anticholinergic side effects include dry mouth (which can lead to ingestion of caloric liquids and weight gain or hyponatremia), blurred near vision, urinary retention (particularly in elderly men with enlarged prostates), delayed gastric emptying, esophageal reflux, ileus, delirium, and precipitation of acute glaucoma in patients with narrow anterior chamber angles. Other autonomic effects include orthostatic hypotension and sexual dysfunction—problems in achieving erection, ejaculation (including retrograde ejaculation), and orgasm in men (approximately 50% of cases) and women (approximately 30%). Delay in achieving orgasm is often a factor in medication noncompliance. Electrocardiographic changes occur frequently, but clinically significant arrhythmias are much less common. Elderly patients and those with preexisting cardiac disease are at greater risk. The most frequently seen electrocardiographic changes include diminution of the T wave amplitude, appearance of prominent U waves, depression of the ST segment, and prolongation of the QT interval. Thioridazine has been given an FDA warning for dose-related QTc delay and risk of fatal cardiac arrhythmias. As noted above, ziprasidone can produce QTc prolongation. An ECG prior to treatment in some patients may be indicated. In some critical care patients, torsades de pointes has been associated with the use of high-dose intravenous haloperidol (usually > 30 mg/24 h).

Associations have been suggested between the atypical neuroleptics and new-onset diabetes, hyperlipidemia, QTc prolongation, and weight gain (Table 25–6). The FDA has particularly noted the risk of hyperglycemia and new-onset diabetes in this class of medication that is not related to weight gain. Monitoring of weight, fasting blood sugar and lipids prior to initiation of treatment and at regular intervals thereafter is an important part of medication monitoring. Early research suggests that the addition of metformin to olanzapine may improve drug-induced weight gain in patients with drug-naïve, first-episode schizophrenia. Neuroleptic medications in general may have metabolic and endocrine effects, including weight gain, hyperglycemia, impaired temperature regulation in hot weather, and water intoxication, that may be due to inappropriate ADH secretion. Lactation and menstrual irregularities are common (antipsychotic drugs should be avoided, if possible, in breast cancer patients because of potential trophic effects of elevated prolactin levels on the breast). Both antipsychotic and antidepressant drugs inhibit sperm motility. Bone marrow depression and cholestatic jaundice occur rarely; these are hypersensitivity reactions, and they usually appear in the first 2 months of treatment. They subside on discontinuance of the drug. There is cross-sensitivity among all of the phenothiazines, and a drug from a different group should be used when allergic reactions occur.

Clozapine is associated with a 1.6% risk of **agranulocytosis** (higher in persons of Ashkenazi Jewish ancestry), and its use must be strictly monitored with weekly blood counts during the first 6 months of treatment, with monitoring every other week thereafter. Discontinuation of the medication requires weekly monitoring of the white blood cell count for 1 month. Clozapine has been associated with fatal

Table 25–6. Adverse factors associated with atypical antipsychotics.

	Weight Gain	Hyperlipidemia	New-Onset Diabetes	QTc Prolongation[1]
Clozapine	+++	+	+	+/–
Olanzapine	+++	+	+	+/–
Risperidone	++	Unclear data	Unclear data	+
Quetiapine	++	Unclear data	Unclear data	++
Ziprasidone	+/–	–	–	+++

[1]QTc prolongation is a side effect of many medications and suggests a possible risk for arrhythmia. Among atypical neuroleptics, only ziprasidone carries a special warning regarding the risk of QTc prolongation.

Adapted, with permission, from American Diabetes Association: Consensus Development Conference on Antipsychotic Drugs and Obesity and Diabetes. Diabetes Care. 2004 Feb;27(2):596–601.

myocarditis and is contraindicated in patients with severe heart disease. In addition, clozapine lowers the seizure threshold and has many side effects, including sedation, hypotension, increased liver enzyme levels, hypersalivation, respiratory arrest, weight gain, and changes in both the ECG and the EEG.

Photosensitivity, retinopathy, and hyperpigmentation are associated with use of fairly high dosages of chlorpromazine and thioridazine. The appearance of particulate melanin deposits in the lens of the eye is related to the total dose given, and patients on long-term medication should have periodic eye examinations. Teratogenicity has not been causally related to these drugs, but prudence is indicated particularly in the first trimester of pregnancy. The seizure threshold is lowered, but it is safe to use these medications in epileptics who take anticonvulsants.

The **neuroleptic malignant syndrome (NMS)** is a catatonia-like state manifested by extrapyramidal signs, blood pressure changes, altered consciousness, and hyperpyrexia; it is an uncommon but serious complication of neuroleptic treatment. Muscle rigidity, involuntary movements, confusion, dysarthria, and dysphagia are accompanied by pallor, cardiovascular instability, fever, pulmonary congestion, and diaphoresis and may result in stupor, coma, and death. The cause may be related to a number of factors, including poor dosage control of neuroleptic medication, affective illness, decreased serum iron, dehydration, and increased sensitivity of dopamine receptor sites. Lithium in combination with a neuroleptic drug may increase vulnerability, which is already increased in patients with an affective disorder. In most cases, the symptoms develop within the first 2 weeks of antipsychotic drug treatment. The syndrome may occur with small doses of the drugs. Intramuscular administration is a risk factor. Elevated creatine kinase and leukocytosis with a shift to the left are present early in about half of cases. Treatment includes controlling fever and providing fluid support. Dopamine agonists such as bromocriptine, 2.5–10 mg orally three times a day, and amantadine, 100–200 mg orally twice a day, have also been useful. Dantrolene, 50 mg intravenously as needed, is used to alleviate rigidity (do not exceed 10 mg/kg/d due to hepatotoxicity risk). There is ongoing controversy about the efficacy of these three agents as well as the use of calcium channel blockers and benzodiazepines. ECT has been used effectively in resistant cases. Clozapine has been used with relative safety and fair success as an antipsychotic drug for patients who have had NMS. The syndrome must be differentiated from acute lethal catatonia, malignant hyperthermia, neurotoxic syndromes (including AIDS), and a variety of other conditions such as viral encephalitis, Wilson disease, central anticholinergic syndrome, and hypertonic states (eg, tetany, strychnine poisoning).

Akathisia is the most common (about 20%) so-called **extrapyramidal symptom**. It usually occurs early in treatment (but may persist after neuroleptics are discontinued) and is frequently mistaken for anxiety or exacerbation of psychosis. It is characterized by a subjective desire to be in constant motion followed by an inability to sit or stand still and consequent pacing. It may induce suicidality or feelings of fright, rage, terror, or sexual torment. Insomnia is often

present. It is crucial to educate patients in advance about these potential side effects so that the patients do not misinterpret them as signs of increased illness. In all cases, reevaluate the dosage requirement or the type of neuroleptic drug. One should inquire also about cigarette smoking, which in women has been associated with an increased incidence of akathisia. Antiparkinsonism drugs (such as trihexyphenidyl, 2–5 mg orally three times daily) may be helpful, but first-line treatment often includes a benzodiazepine (such as clonazepam 0.5–1.0 mg orally three times daily). In resistant cases, symptoms may be alleviated by propranolol, 30–80 mg/d orally, diazepam, 5 mg orally three times daily, or amantadine, 100 mg orally three times daily.

Acute dystonias usually occur early, although a late (tardive) occurrence is reported in patients (mostly men after several years of therapy) who previously had early severe dystonic reactions and a mood disorder (see below). Younger patients are at higher risk for acute dystonias. The most common signs are bizarre muscle spasms of the head, neck, and tongue. Frequently present are torticollis, oculogyric crises, swallowing or chewing difficulties, and masseter spasms. Laryngospasm is particularly dangerous. Back, arm, or leg muscle spasms are occasionally reported. Diphenhydramine, 50 mg intramuscularly, is effective for the acute crisis; one should then give benztropine mesylate, 2 mg orally twice daily, for several weeks, and then discontinue gradually, since few of the extrapyramidal symptoms require long-term use of the antiparkinsonism drugs (all of which are about equally efficacious—though trihexyphenidyl tends to be mildly stimulating and benztropine mildly sedating).

Drug-induced parkinsonism is indistinguishable from idiopathic parkinsonism, but it is reversible, occurs later in treatment than the preceding extrapyramidal symptoms, and in some cases appears after neuroleptic withdrawal. The condition includes the typical signs of apathy and reduction of facial and arm movements (akinesia, which can mimic depression), festinating gait, rigidity, loss of postural reflexes, and pill-rolling tremor. AIDS patients seem particularly vulnerable to extrapyramidal side effects. High-potency neuroleptics often require antiparkinsonism drugs (see Table 24–6). The neuroleptic dosage should be reduced, and immediate relief can be achieved with antiparkinsonism drugs in the same dosages as above. After 4–6 weeks, these antiparkinsonism drugs can often be discontinued with no recurrent symptoms. In any of the extrapyramidal symptoms, amantadine, 100–400 mg orally daily, may be used instead of the antiparkinsonism drugs. Neuroleptic-induced catatonia is similar to catatonic stupor with rigidity, drooling, urinary incontinence, and cogwheeling. It usually responds slowly to withdrawal of the offending medication and use of antiparkinsonism agents.

Tardive dyskinesia is a syndrome of abnormal involuntary stereotyped movements of the face, mouth, tongue, trunk, and limbs that may occur after months or (usually) years of treatment with neuroleptic agents. The syndrome affects 20–35% of patients who have undergone long-term neuroleptic therapy. Predisposing factors include older age, many years of treatment, cigarette smoking, and diabetes mellitus. Pineal calcification is higher in this condition by a margin of 3:1. There are no known differences among any of the antipsychotic drugs in the development of this syndrome. Although the atypical antipsychotics appear to offer lower risk, the CATIE study did not address the long-term effects of these drugs.

Early manifestations include fine worm-like movements of the tongue at rest, difficulty in sticking out the tongue, facial tics, increased blink frequency, or jaw movements of recent onset. Later manifestations may include bucco-linguo-masticatory movements, lip smacking, chewing motions, mouth opening and closing, disturbed gag reflex, puffing of the cheeks, disrupted speech, respiratory distress, or choreoathetoid movements of the extremities (the last being more prevalent in younger patients). The symptoms do not necessarily worsen and in rare cases may lessen even though neuroleptic drugs are continued. The dyskinesias do not occur during sleep and can be voluntarily suppressed for short periods. Stress and movements in other parts of the body will often aggravate the condition.

Early signs of dyskinesia must be differentiated from those reversible signs produced by ill-fitting dentures or nonneuroleptic drugs such as levodopa, TCAs, antiparkinsonism agents, anticonvulsants, and antihistamines. Other neurologic conditions such as Huntington chorea can be differentiated by history and examination.

The emphasis should be on prevention. Use the least amount of neuroleptic drug necessary to mute the psychotic symptoms; atypical drugs appear to offer less risk as first line agents. Detect early manifestations of dyskinesias. When these occur, stop anticholinergic drugs and gradually discontinue neuroleptic drugs, if clinically feasible. Weight loss and cachexia sometimes appear on withdrawal of neuroleptics. In an indeterminate number of cases, the dyskinesias will remit. Keep the patient off the drugs until reemergent psychotic symptoms dictate their resumption, at which point they are restarted in low doses and gradually increased until there is clinical improvement. If neuroleptic drugs are restarted, clozapine and olanzapine appear to offer less risk of recurrence. The use of adjunctive agents such as benzodiazepines or lithium may help directly or indirectly by allowing control of psychotic symptoms with a low dosage of neuroleptics. If the dyskinesic syndrome recurs and it is necessary to continue neuroleptic drugs to control psychotic symptoms, informed consent should be obtained. Benzodiazepines, buspirone (in doses of 15–60 mg/d orally), phosphatidylcholine, clonidine, calcium channel blockers, vitamin E, omega-3 fatty acids, and propranolol all have had limited usefulness in treating the dyskinetic side effects.

B. Social

Environmental considerations are most important in the individual with a chronic illness, who usually has a history of repeated hospitalizations, a continued low level of functioning, and symptoms that never completely remit. Family rejection and work failure are common. In these cases, board and care homes staffed by personnel experienced in caring for psychiatric patients are most important. There is frequently an inverse relationship between stability of the living situation and the amounts of required antipsychotic drugs, since the most salutary environment is one that reduces stimuli. Nonresidential self-help groups such as Recovery, Inc., should be utilized whenever possible. They provide a setting for sharing, learning, and mutual support and are frequently the only social involvement with which this type of patient is comfortable. Vocational rehabilitation and work agencies (eg, Goodwill Industries, Inc.) provide assessment, training, and job opportunities at a level commensurate with the person's clinical condition.

C. Psychological

The need for psychotherapy varies markedly depending on the patient's current status and history. In a person with a single psychotic episode and a previously good level of adjustment, supportive psychotherapy may help the patient reintegrate the experience, gain some insight into antecedent problems, and become a more self-observant individual who can recognize early signs of stress. Insight-oriented psychotherapy is often counterproductive in this type of disorder. Research suggests that cognitive behavioral therapy—in conjunction with medication management—may have some efficacy in the treatment of symptoms of schizophrenia. Cognitive behavioral therapy for schizophrenia involves helping the individual challenge psychotic thinking and alters response to hallucinations. Similarly, a new form of psychotherapy called acceptance and commitment therapy has shown value in helping prevent hospitalizations in schizophrenia. Cognitive remediation therapy is another new approach to treatment that shows promise in helping schizophrenics become better able to focus their disorganized thinking. Family therapy may also help alleviate the patient's stress and to assist relatives in coping with the patient.

D. Behavioral

Behavioral techniques (see above) are most frequently used in therapeutic settings such as day treatment centers, but there is no reason why they cannot be incorporated into family situations or any therapeutic setting. Many behavioral techniques (eg, positive reinforcement—whether it be a word of praise or an approving nod—after some positive behavior), can be a powerful instrument for helping a person learn behaviors that will facilitate social acceptance. Music from portable digital players with earphones is one of many ways to divert the patient's attention from auditory hallucinations.

▶ Prognosis

In any psychosis, in the large majority of patients the prognosis is excellent for alleviation of positive symptoms such as hallucinations or delusions treated with medication. Negative symptoms such as diminished affect and sociability are much more difficult to treat but appear responsive to atypical antipsychotics. Unavailability of structured work situations and lack of family therapy are two other reasons why the prognosis is so guarded in such a large percentage of schizophrenic patients. Psychosis connected with a history of serious drug abuse has a guarded prognosis because of the central nervous system damage, usually from the drugs themselves and associated medical illnesses.

Freedman R. Schizophrenia. N Engl J Med. 2003 Oct 30;349(18): 1738–49. [PMID: 14585943]

Newcomer JW. Second-generation (atypical) antipsychotics and metabolic effects: a comprehensive literature review. CNS Drugs. 2005;19 Suppl 1:1–93. [PMID: 15998156]

Swartz et al. What CATIE found: results from the schizophrenia trial. Psychiatr Serv. 2008 May;59(5):500–6. [PMID: 18451005]

Wang PS et al. Risk of death in elderly users of conventional vs. atypical antipsychotic medications. N Engl J Med. 2005 Dec 1;353(22):2335–41. [PMID: 16319382]

Wu R-R et al. Metformin addition attenuates olanzapine-induced weight gain in drug-naïve first-episode schizophrenia patients: a double-blind, placebo-controlled study. Am J Psychiatry. 2008 Mar;165(3):352–8. [PMID: 18245179]

MOOD DISORDERS (Depression & Mania)

ESSENTIALS OF DIAGNOSIS

Present in most depressions:

► Mood varies from mild sadness to intense feelings of guilt, worthlessness, and hopelessness.

► Difficulty in thinking, including inability to concentrate, ruminations, and lack of decisiveness.

► Loss of interest, with diminished involvement in work and recreation.

► Somatic complaints such as headache; disrupted, lessened, or excessive sleep; loss of energy; change in appetite; decreased sexual drive.

► Anxiety.

Present in some severe depressions:

► Psychomotor retardation or agitation.

► Delusions of a hypochondriacal or persecutory nature.

► Withdrawal from activities.

► Physical symptoms of major severity, eg, anorexia, insomnia, reduced sexual drive, weight loss, and various somatic complaints.

► Suicidal ideation.

Present in mania:

► Mood ranging from euphoria to irritability.

► Sleep disruption.

► Hyperactivity.

► Racing thoughts.

► Grandiosity.

► Variable psychotic symptoms.

► General Considerations

Depression is extremely common, with up to 30% of primary care patients having depressive symptoms. Depression may be the final expression of (1) genetic factors (neu-

rotransmitter dysfunction), (2) developmental problems (personality problems, childhood events), or (3) psychosocial stresses (divorce, unemployment). It frequently presents in the form of somatic complaints with negative medical workups. Although sadness and grief are normal responses to loss, depression is not. Patients experiencing normal grief tend to produce sympathy and sadness in the clinician caregiver; depression often produces frustration and irritation in the clinician. Grief is usually accompanied by intact self-esteem, whereas depression is marked by a sense of guilt and worthlessness.

Mania is often combined with depression and may occur alone, together with mania in a mixed episode, or in cyclic fashion with depression.

► Clinical Findings

In general, there are four major types of depressions, with similar symptoms in each group.

A. Adjustment Disorder with Depressed Mood

Depression may occur in reaction to some identifiable stressor or adverse life situation, usually loss of a person by death (grief reaction), divorce, etc; financial reversal (crisis); or loss of an established role, such as being needed. Anger is frequently associated with the loss, and this in turn often produces a feeling of guilt. The disorder occurs within 3 months of the stressor and causes significant impairment in social or occupational functioning. The symptoms range from mild sadness, anxiety, irritability, worry, lack of concentration, discouragement, and somatic complaints to the more severe symptoms of the next group.

B. Depressive Disorders

The subclassifications include major depressive disorder and dysthymia.

1. Major depressive disorder—A major depressive disorder (eg, "endogenous" unipolar disorder, melancholia) consists of at least one episode of serious mood depression that occurs at any time of life. Many consider a physiologic or metabolic aberration to be causative. Complaints vary widely but most frequently include a loss of interest and pleasure (anhedonia), withdrawal from activities, and feelings of guilt. Also included are inability to concentrate, some cognitive dysfunction, anxiety, chronic fatigue, feelings of worthlessness, somatic complaints (unidentifiable somatic complaints frequently indicate depression), loss of sexual drive, and thoughts of death. Diurnal variation with improvement as the day progresses is common. Vegetative signs that frequently occur are insomnia, anorexia with weight loss, and constipation. Occasionally, severe agitation and psychotic ideation (paranoid thinking, somatic delusions) are present. These symptoms are more common in depressed persons who are older than 50 years. Paranoid symptoms may range from general suspiciousness to ideas of reference with delusions. The somatic delusions frequently revolve around feelings of impending annihilation or hypochondriacal beliefs (eg, that the body is rotting away with cancer). Hallucinations are uncommon.

Subcategories include **major depression with atypical features** characterized by hypersomnia, overeating, lethargy, and rejection sensitivity. **Major depression with a seasonal onset (seasonal affective disorder)** is a dysfunction of circadian rhythms that occurs more commonly in the winter months and is believed to be due to decreased exposure to full-spectrum light. Common symptoms include carbohydrate craving, lethargy, hyperphagia, and hypersomnia. **Major depression with postpartum onset** usually occurs 2 weeks to 6 months postpartum.

Most women (up to 80%) experience some mild letdown of mood in the postpartum period. For some of these (10–15%), the symptoms are more severe and similar to those usually seen in serious depression, with an increased emphasis on concerns related to the baby (obsessive thoughts about harming it or inability to care for it). When psychotic symptoms occur, there is frequently associated sleep deprivation, volatility of behavior, and manic-like symptoms. Postpartum psychosis is much less common (< 2%), often occurs within the first 2 weeks, and requires early and aggressive management. Biologic vulnerability with hormonal changes and psychosocial stressors all play a role. The chances of a second episode are about 25% and may be reduced with prophylactic treatment.

2. Dysthymia—Dysthymia is a chronic depressive disturbance. Sadness, loss of interest, and withdrawal from activities over a period of 2 or more years with a relatively persistent course is necessary for this diagnosis. Generally, the symptoms are milder but longer-lasting than those in a major depressive episode.

3. Premenstrual dysphoric disorder—Depressive symptoms occur during the late luteal phase (last 2 weeks) of the menstrual cycle.

C. Bipolar Disorders

Bipolar disorders consist of episodic mood shifts into mania, major depression, hypomania, and mixed mood states. The ability of bipolar disorder to mimic aspects of many other Axis I disorders and a high comorbidity with substance abuse can make the initial diagnosis of bipolar disorder difficult.

1. Mania—A manic episode is a mood change characterized by elation with hyperactivity, over involvement in life activities, increased irritability, flight of ideas, easy distractibility, and little need for sleep. The overenthusiastic quality of the mood and the expansive behavior initially attract others, but the irritability, mood lability with swings into depression, aggressive behavior, and grandiosity usually lead to marked interpersonal difficulties. Activities may occur that are later regretted, eg, excessive spending, resignation from a job, a hasty marriage, sexual acting out, and exhibitionistic behavior, with alienation of friends and family. Atypical manic episodes can include gross delusions, paranoid ideation of severe proportions, and auditory hallucinations usually related to some grandiose perception. The episodes begin abruptly (sometimes precipitated by life stresses) and may last from several days to months. Spring and summer tend to be the peak periods. Generally, the manic episodes are of shorter duration than the depressive episodes. In almost all cases, the manic episode is part of a broader bipolar (manic-depressive) disorder. Patients with four or more discrete episodes of a mood disturbance in 1 year are called "rapid cyclers." (Substance abuse, particularly cocaine, can mimic rapid cycling.) These patients have a higher incidence of hypothyroidism. Manic patients differ from patients with schizophrenia in that the former use more effective interpersonal maneuvers, are more sensitive to the social maneuvers of others, and are more able to utilize weakness and vulnerability in others to their own advantage. Creativity has been positively correlated with mood disorders, but the best work done is between episodes of mania and depression.

2. Cyclothymic disorders—These are chronic mood disturbances with episodes of depression and hypomania. The symptoms must have at least a 2-year duration and are milder than those that occur in depressive or manic episodes. Occasionally, the symptoms will escalate into a full-blown manic or depressive episode, in which case reclassification as bipolar I or bipolar II disorder would be warranted.

D. Mood Disorders Secondary to Illness and Drugs

Any illness, severe or mild, can cause significant depression. Conditions such as rheumatoid arthritis, multiple sclerosis, and chronic heart disease are particularly likely to be associated with depression, as are other chronic illnesses. Hormonal variations clearly play a role in some depressions. Varying degrees of depression occur at various times in schizophrenic disorders, central nervous system disease, and organic mental states. **Alcohol dependency** frequently coexists with serious depression.

The classic model of drug-induced depression occurs with the use of reserpine, both in a clinical and a neurochemical sense. Corticosteroids and oral contraceptives are commonly associated with affective changes. Antihypertensive medications such as methyldopa, guanethidine, and clonidine have been associated with the development of depressive syndromes, as have digitalis and antiparkinsonism drugs (eg, levodopa). It is unusual for β-blockers to produce depression when given for short periods, such as in the treatment of performance anxiety. Sustained use of β-blockers for medical conditions such as hypertension may produce depression in some patients, although most individuals do not suffer this adverse effect. Infrequently, disulfiram and anticholinesterase drugs may be associated with symptoms of depression. All stimulant use results in a depressive syndrome when the drug is withdrawn. Alcohol, sedatives, opiates, and most of the psychedelic drugs are depressants and, paradoxically, are often used in self-treatment of depression.

▶ Differential Diagnosis

Since depression may be a part of any illness—either reactively or as a secondary symptom—careful attention must be given to personal life adjustment problems and the role of medications (eg, reserpine, corticosteroids, levodopa).

Schizophrenia, partial complex seizures, organic brain syndromes, panic disorders, and anxiety disorders must be differentiated. Subtle thyroid dysfunction must be ruled out.

▶ **Complications**

The most important complication is suicide, which often includes some elements of aggression. Suicide rates in the general population vary from 9 per 100,000 in Spain to 20 per 100,000 in the United States to 58 per 100,000 in Hungary. In individuals with depression, the lifetime risk rises to 10–15%. Men tend toward successful suicide, particularly in older age groups, whereas women make more attempts with lower mortality rates. An increased suicide rate is being observed in the younger population, ages 15–35. Patients with cancer, respiratory illnesses, AIDS, and those being maintained on hemodialysis have higher suicide rates. Alcohol is a significant factor in many suicide attempts.

There are several groups of people who make suicide attempts. One group includes those individuals with acute **situational problems.** These individuals may be acutely distressed by a recent breakup in a relationship or another type of disappointment. This group also includes those who may not be diagnosed as having depression but who are overwhelmed by a stressful situation often with an aspect of public humiliation (eg, the man charged with child molestation who hangs himself in his cell). A suicide attempt in such cases may be an impulsive or aggressive act not associated with significant depression. In such cases, a suicide attempt is clearly a stratagem for **controlling or hurting others or an attempted escape**.

Another high-risk group includes individuals with severe depression. **Severe depression** may be due to conditions such as medical illness (eg, AIDS, whose victims have a suicide rate over 30 times that of the general population) or comorbid psychiatric disorders (eg, panic disorders). Anxiety, panic, and fear are major findings in suicidal behavior. A patient may seem to make a dramatic improvement, but the lifting of depression may be due to the patient's decision to commit suicide. Another high-risk group are individuals with **psychotic illness** who tend not to verbalize their concerns, are unpredictable, and are often successful in their suicide attempt, although they make up only a small percentage of the total.

Finally, suicide is ten times more prevalent in patients with schizophrenia than in the general population, and jumping from bridges is a more common means of attempted suicide by schizophrenics than by others. In one study of 100 jumpers, 47% had schizophrenia.

The immediate goal of psychiatric evaluation is to assess the current suicidal risk and the need for hospitalization versus outpatient management. The intent is less likely to be truly suicidal, for example, if small amounts of poison or drugs were ingested or scratching of wrists was superficial, if the act was performed in the vicinity of others or with early notification of others, or if the attempt was arranged so that early detection would be anticipated. Alcohol, hopelessness, delusional thoughts, and complete or nearly complete loss of interest in life or ability to experience pleasure

are all positively correlated with suicide attempts. Other risk factors are previous attempts, a family history of suicide, medical or psychiatric illness (eg, anxiety, depression, psychosis), male sex, older age, contemplation of violent methods, a humiliating social stressor, and drug use (including long-term sedative or alcohol use), which contributes to impulsiveness or mood swings. Successful treatment of the patient at risk for suicide cannot be achieved if the patient continues to abuse drugs.

The patient's current mood status is best evaluated by direct evaluation of plans and concerns about the future, personal reactions to the attempt, and thoughts about the reactions of others. The patient's immediate resources should be assessed—people who can be significantly involved (most important), family support, job situation, financial resources, etc.

If hospitalization is not indicated (eg, gestures, impulsive attempts; see above), the clinician must formulate and institute a treatment plan or make an adequate referral. Medication should be dispensed in small amounts to at-risk patients. Although TCAs and SSRIs are associated with an equal incidence of suicide attempts, the risk of successful suicide is higher with TCA overdose. Guns and drugs should be removed from the patient's household. Driving should be interdicted until the patient improves. The problem is often worsened by the long-term complications of the suicide attempt, eg, brain damage due to hypoxia, peripheral neuropathies caused by staying for long periods in one position causing nerve compressions, and medical or surgical problems such as esophageal strictures and tendon dysfunctions.

The reasons for self-mutilation, most commonly wrist cutting (but also autocastration, autoamputation, and autoenucleation, which are associated with psychoses), may be very different from the reasons for a suicide attempt. The initial treatment plan, however, should presume suicidal ideation, and conservative treatment should be initiated.

Sleep disturbances in the depressions are discussed below.

▶ **Treatment of Depression**

A. Medical

Depression associated with reactive disorders usually does not call for drug therapy and can be managed by psychotherapy and the passage of time. In severe cases—particularly when vegetative signs are significant and symptoms have persisted for more than a few weeks—antidepressant drug therapy is often effective. Drug therapy is also suggested by a family history of major depression in first-degree relatives or a past history of prior episodes.

The antidepressant drugs may be conveniently classified into three groups: (1) the newer antidepressants, including the SSRIs and bupropion, duloxetine, venlafaxine, nefazodone, and mirtazapine, (2) the TCAs and clinically similar drugs, and (3) the MAO inhibitors (see Table 25–8). These groups are described in greater detail below. ECT is effective in all types of depression and will also rapidly resolve a manic episode. It is also very effective for postpartum depression. Megavitamin treatment, acupuncture, and electrosleep are of unproved usefulness for any psychiatric condition.

Hospitalization is necessary if suicide is a major consideration or if complex treatment modalities are required.

Drug selection is influenced by the history of previous responses if that information is available. If a relative has responded to a particular drug, this suggests that the patient may respond similarly. If no background information is available, a drug such as sertraline, 25 mg orally daily and increasing gradually up to 200 mg orally, or desipramine, starting with 50 mg orally and gradually increasing to 150 mg daily, can be selected and a *full trial* instituted. The medication trial should be monitored for worsening mood or suicidal ideation with patient assessments every 1–2 weeks until week 6. If successful, the medication should be continued for 6–12 months at the full therapeutic dose before tapering is considered. Antidepressants should usually be continued indefinitely at full dosage in individuals with more than two episodes after age 40 or one episode after age 50. If the response is inadequate the best alternatives are to switch to a second agent or to try augmenting the first agent according to the STAR*D study. The latter course is often taken when there has been at least a partial response to the initial drug. If a second drug is tried, it does not appear to matter whether that drug is from the same or different class. If the second drug fails or augmentation was selected as the second step, the choices include lithium (eg, 600–900 mg/d orally), buspirone (eg, 30–60 mg/d orally), or thyroid medication (eg, liothyronine, 25 mcg/d orally). Dysthymia is also treated in this way. The Agency for Health Care Policy and Research has produced clinical practice guidelines that outline one algorithm of treatment decisions (Figure 25–2).

Psychotic depression should be treated with a combination of an antipsychotic such as olanzapine and an antidepressant such as an SSRI at their usual doses. Mifepristone may have specific and early activity against psychotic depression.

Major depression with atypical features or seasonal onset can be treated with an MAO inhibitor or an SSRI with good results.

Stimulants such as dextroamphetamine (5–30 mg/d orally) and methylphenidate (10–45 mg/d orally) have enjoyed a resurgence of interest for the short-term treatment of depression in medically ill and geriatric patients. Their 50–60% efficacy rate is slightly below that of other agents. The stimulants are notable for rapid onset of action (hours) and a paucity of side effects (tachycardia, agitation) in most patients. They are usually given in two divided doses early in the day (eg, 7 am and noon) so as to avoid interfering with sleep. These agents may also be useful as adjunctive agents in refractory depression.

Caution: Depressed patients may have suicidal thoughts, and the amount of drug dispensed should be appropriately controlled. It appears that in children and adolescent populations, antidepressants may be associated with some slightly increased risk of suicidality, but this diminishes by age 25. After that, antidepressants have neutral or possibly protective effects until age 65 years or older when they have

protective effects. The older TCAs have a narrow therapeutic index, and one advantage of the newer drugs is their wider margin of safety. Nonetheless, even with newer agents, because of the possibility of suicidality early in antidepressant treatment, close follow-up is indicated. In all cases of pharmacologic management of depressed states, caution is indicated until the risk of suicide is considered minimal.

1. SSRIs and atypical antidepressants—The chief advantages of these agents are that they do not generally cause significant cardiovascular or anticholinergic side effects, and they have much lower lethality in overdose compared to TCAs. The SSRIs include fluoxetine, sertraline, paroxetine, fluvoxamine, citalopram and its enantiomer escitalopram. The atypical antidepressants are bupropion, which appears to exert its effect through the dopamine neurotransmitter system; venlafaxine and duloxetine, both of which inhibit the reuptake of both serotonin and norepinephrine; nefazodone, which blocks the reuptake of serotonin but also inhibits the 5-HT$_2$ postsynaptic receptors; and mirtazapine, which selectively blocks presynaptic α_2-adrenergic receptors and enhances both noradrenergic and serotonergic transmission. All of these antidepressants are effective in the treatment of depression, both typical and atypical. The SSRI drugs have been effective in the treatment of panic attacks, bulimia, generalized anxiety disorder, OCD, and PTSD. They do not seem to be as clearly effective in some pain syndromes as the TCAs, although venlafaxine may have some efficacy in the treatment of neuropathic pain, and duloxetine is FDA-approved for the treatment of diabetic peripheral neuropathy.

Most of the drugs in this group tend to be activating and are given in the morning so as not to interfere with sleep. Some patients, however, may have sedation, requiring that the drug be given at bedtime. This reaction occurs most commonly with paroxetine, fluvoxamine, and mirtazapine. The SSRIs can be given in once-daily dosage. Nefazodone and venlafaxine are usually given twice daily. Bupropion and venlafaxine are available in extended-release formulations and can be given once daily. There is usually some delay in response; fluoxetine, for example, requires 2–6 weeks to act in depression, 4–8 weeks to be effective in panic disorder, and 6–12 weeks in treatment of OCD. The starting dose (10 mg) is given for 1 week before increasing to the average daily oral dose of 20 mg for depression, while OCD may require up to 80 mg daily. Some patients, particularly the elderly, may tolerate and benefit from as little as 10 mg/d or every other day. The other SSRIs have shorter half-lives and a lesser effect on hepatic enzymes, which reduces their impact on the metabolism of other drugs (thus not increasing significantly the serum concentrations of other drugs as much as fluoxetine). The shorter half-lives also allow for more rapid clearing if adverse side effects appear. Venlafaxine appears to be more effective with doses greater than 200 mg/d, although some individuals respond to doses as low as 75 mg/d.

The side effects common to all of these drugs are headache, nausea, tinnitus, insomnia, and nervousness. Akathisia has been common with the SSRIs; other extrapyramidal symptoms (eg, dystonias) have occurred infrequently but

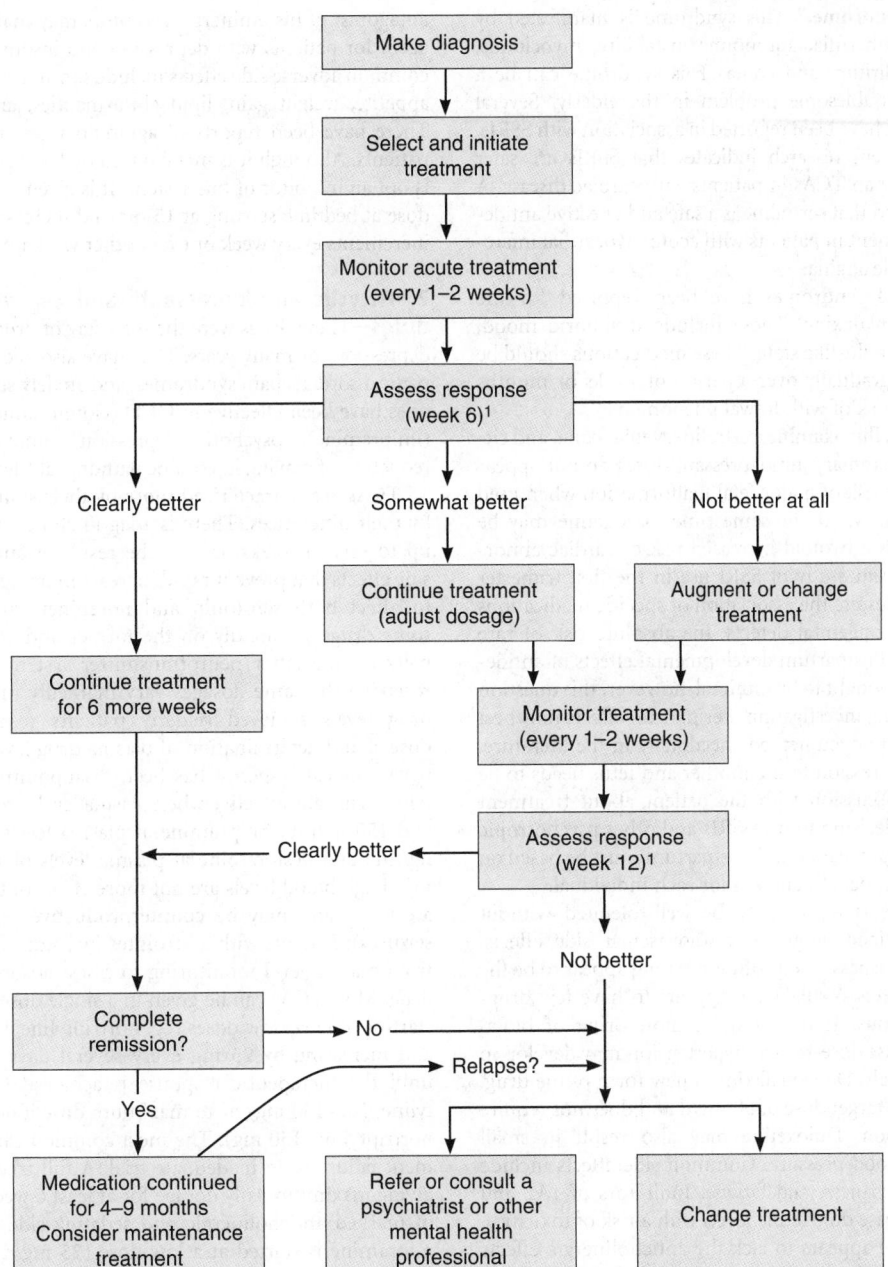

▲ **Figure 25–2.** Overview of treatment for depression. (Reproduced from Agency for Health Care Policy and Research: *Depression in Primary Care. Vol. 2: Treatment of Major Depression.* United States Department of Health and Human Services, 1993.)

particularly in withdrawal states. Sexual side effects of erectile dysfunction, retrograde ejaculation, and dysorgasmia are very common with the SSRIs. Antidotes to SSRI-induced sexual dysfunction are occasionally helpful. Sildenafil, 25–50 mg orally 1 hour prior to sexual activity, can improve erectile dysfunction in some patients. Cyproheptadine, 4 mg

orally prior to sexual activity, may be helpful in countering drug-induced anorgasmia. Adjunctive bupropion (75–150 mg orally daily) may also help with restoring erectile function. The SSRIs are strong serotonin uptake blockers and may in high dosage or in combination with MAO inhibitors, including the antiparkinsonian drug selegiline, cause a "serotonin syndrome." This syndrome is manifested by rigidity, hyperthermia, autonomic instability, myoclonus, confusion, delirium, and coma. This syndrome can be a particularly troublesome problem in the elderly. Several cases of angina have been reported in association with SSRIs. However, current research indicates that SSRIs are safer agents to use than TCAs in patients with cardiac disease. A study has found that sertraline is a safe and effective antidepressant treatment in patients with acute myocardial infarction or unstable angina.

Withdrawal syndromes have been reported for the SSRIs and venlafaxine. These include dysphoric mood, agitation, and a flu-like state. These medications should be discontinued gradually over a period of weeks or months to reduce the risk of withdrawal phenomena.

Fluoxetine, fluvoxamine, sertraline, venlafaxine, and citalopram in customary antidepressant doses do not appear to increase the risk of major fetal malformation when used during pregnancy. At the same time, paroxetine may be associated with a twofold increased risk of cardiac abnormalities. A recent study of SSRI use in the first trimester suggests that despite the association of specific medications with specific congenital defects, the absolute risk of rare defects is low. Postpartum developmental effects of antidepressants are thought to be minimal, however, this question calls for ongoing investigation. Peripartum effects may be a concern and are documented anecdotally in the literature. The risk of depression to the mother and fetus needs to be part of the discussion with the patient about treatment options. The decision to use SSRIs and other psychotropic agents during pregnancy and postpartum must be based on a thorough risk-benefit analysis for each individual.

Venlafaxine is reported to be well-tolerated without significant anticholinergic or cardiovascular side effects. Nausea, nervousness, and profuse sweating appear to be the major side effects. Venlafaxine appears to have few drug-drug interactions. It does require monitoring of blood pressure because dose-related hypertension may develop in some individuals. Desvenlafaxine, a new form of the drug, is started at its target dose of 50 mg/d and does not require upward titration. Duloxetine may also result in small increases in blood pressure. Common side effects include dry mouth, dizziness, and fatigue. Inhibitors of 1A2 and 2D6 may increase duloxetine levels with a risk of toxicity.

Nefazodone appears to lack the anticholinergic effects of the TCAs and the agitation sometimes induced by SSRIs. Nefazodone should not be given with terfenadine, astemizole, or cisapride. (Terfenadine and astemizole are not commercially available in the United States.) Because nefazodone inhibits the liver's cytochrome P450 3A4 isoenzymes, concurrent use of these medications can lead to serious QT prolongation, ventricular tachycardia, or death. Through the same mechanism of enzyme inhibition, nefazodone can elevate cyclosporine levels sixfold to tenfold. Nefazodone has been given an FDA warning because it has been implicated in liver failure in rare cases. Pretreatment and ongoing monitoring of liver enzymes are indicated.

Mirtazapine is thought to enhance central noradrenergic and serotonergic activity with minimal sexual side effects compared with the SSRIs. Its action as a potent antagonist of histaminergic receptors may make it a useful agent for patients with depression and insomnia. Its most common adverse side effects include somnolence, increased appetite, weight gain, lipid abnormalities, and dizziness. There have been reports of agranulocytosis in 2 of 2796 patients. Although it is metabolized by P450 isoenzymes, it is not an inhibitor of this system. It is given in a single oral dose at bedtime starting at 15 mg and increasing in 15-mg increments every week or every other week up to 45 mg.

2. Tricyclic antidepressants and clinically similar drugs—These drugs were the mainstay of drug therapy for depression for many years. They have also been effective in panic disorders, pain syndromes, and anxiety states. Specific ones have been effective in OCD (clomipramine), enuresis (imipramine), psychotic depression (amoxapine), and reduction of craving in cocaine withdrawal (desipramine).

TCAs are characterized more by their similarities than by their differences. There is a lag in clinical response for up to several weeks, largely the result of anticholinergic side effects that prevent rapid increase in dosage. They tend to affect both serotonin and norepinephrine reuptake; some drugs act mainly on the former and others principally on the latter neurotransmitter system. Individuals receiving the same dosages vary markedly in therapeutic drug levels achieved (elderly patients require smaller doses), and determination of plasma drug levels is helpful when clinical response has been disappointing. Nortriptyline is usually effective when plasma levels are between 50 and 150 ng/mL; imipramine at plasma levels of 200–250 ng/mL; and desipramine at plasma levels of 100–250 ng/mL. High blood levels are not more effective than moderate levels and may be counterproductive (eg, delirium, seizures). Patients with gastrointestinal side effects benefit from plasma level monitoring to assess absorption of the drug. Most TCAs can be given in a single dose at bedtime, starting at fairly low doses (eg, nortriptyline 25 mg orally) and increasing by 25 mg every several days as tolerated until the therapeutic response is achieved (eg, nortriptyline, 100–150 mg) or to maximum dose if necessary (eg, nortriptyline, 150 mg). The most common cause of treatment failure is an inadequate trial. A full trial consists of giving maximum daily dosage for at least 6 weeks. Because of marked anticholinergic and sedating side effects, clomipramine is started at a low dose (25 mg/d orally) and increased slowly in divided doses up to 100 mg/d, held at that level for several days, and then gradually increased as necessary up to 250 mg/d. Any of the TCA-like drugs should be started at very low doses (eg, 10–25 mg/d) and increased slowly in the treatment of panic disorder.

The TCAs have anticholinergic side effects to varying degrees (amitriptyline 100 mg is equivalent to atropine 5 mg). One must be particularly wary of the effect in elderly men with prostatic hyperplasia. The anticholinergic effects also predispose to other medical problems such as constipation, heat stroke, or dental problems from xerostomia. Orthostatic hypotension is fairly common, is not dose-dependent and may not remit with time on medication; this may predispose to falls and hip fractures in the elderly. Cardiac effects of the TCAs are functions of the anticholinergic effect, direct myocardial depression (quinidine-like effect), and interference with adrenergic neurons. These factors may produce altered rate, rhythm, and contractility, particularly in patients with preexisting cardiac disease, such as bundle-branch or bifascicular block. Electrocardiographic changes range from benign ST segment and T wave changes and sinus tachycardia to a variety of complex and serious arrhythmias, the latter requiring a change in medication. Because TCAs have class I antiarrhythmic effects, they should be used with caution in patients with ischemic heart disease, arrhythmias, or conduction disturbances. SSRIs or the atypical antidepressants are better initial choices for this population. TCAs lower the seizure threshold so this is of particular concern in patients with a propensity for seizures (eg, previous head injury, alcohol withdrawal). Loss of libido and erectile, ejaculatory, and orgasmic dysfunction are fairly common and can compromise compliance. Trazodone rarely causes priapism, which requires treatment within 12 hours (epinephrine 1:1000 injected into the corpus cavernosum). Delirium, agitation, and mania are infrequent complications. Sudden discontinuation of some of these drugs can produce "cholinergic rebound," manifested by headaches and nausea with abdominal cramps. Overdoses of TCAs are often serious because of the narrow therapeutic index and quinidine-like effects (see Chapter 38).

3. Monoamine oxidase inhibitors—The MAO inhibitors are generally used as third-line drugs for depression (after a failure of SSRIs, TCAs, or the atypical antidepressants) because of the dietary and other restrictions required (see below and Table 25–7). They should be considered third-line drugs for refractory panic disorder and depression; however, this has changed since MAO inhibitor skin patches (selegilene) have become available. They deliver the MAO inhibitor to the bloodstream bypassing the gastrointestinal tract so that dietary restrictions are not necessary in the lowest dosage strength (6 mg/24h).

Oral MAO inhibitors are administered in gradual stepwise dosage and may be given in the morning or evening, depending upon their effect on sleep. They tend to take effect in a fairly low dosage range (Table 25–8). Blood levels are not congruent with therapeutic response.

The MAO inhibitors commonly cause symptoms of orthostatic hypotension (which may persist) and sympathomimetic effects of tachycardia, sweating, and tremor. Nausea, insomnia (often associated with intense afternoon drowsiness), and sexual dysfunction are common. Trazo-

Table 25–7. Principal dietary restrictions in MAOI use.

1. Cheese, except cream cheese and cottage cheese and fresh yogurt
2. Fermented or aged meats such as bologna, salami
3. Broad bean pods such as Chinese bean pods
4. Liver of all types
5. Meat and yeast extracts
6. Red wine, sherry, vermouth, cognac, beer, ale
7. Soy sauce, shrimp paste, sauerkraut

MAOI, monoamine oxidase inhibitor.

done, 25–75 mg orally at bedtime, may ameliorate the MAO-induced insomnia. Central nervous system effects include agitation and toxic psychoses. Dietary limitations (see Table 25–7) and abstinence from drug products containing phenylpropanolamine, phenylephrine, meperidine, dextromethorphan, and pseudoephedrine are mandatory for MAO-A type inhibitors (those marketed for treatment of depression), since the reduction of available MAO leaves the patient vulnerable to exogenous amines (eg, tyramine in foodstuffs).

Treatment for a resultant hypertensive crisis has been the same as for pheochromocytoma (see Chapter 26), but there have been reports of success with nifedipine, 10 mg chewed and placed under the tongue, normalizing blood pressure in 1–5 minutes. The restrictions on the proscribed foodstuffs and sympathomimetic drugs are in effect during treatment and for 2–3 weeks after cessation of therapy. Termination of therapy with MAO inhibitors may be associated with anxiety, agitation, cognitive slowing, and headache. Very gradual withdrawal and short-term benzodiazepine therapy will ameliorate symptoms.

4. Switching and combination therapy—If the therapeutic response has been poor after an adequate trial with the chosen drug, the diagnosis should be reassessed. Assuming that the trial has been adequate and the diagnosis is correct, a trial with a second drug is appropriate. In switching from one group to another, an adequate "washout time" must be allowed. This is critical in certain situations—eg, in switching from an MAO inhibitor to a TCA, allow 2–3 weeks between stopping one drug and starting another; in switching from an SSRI to an MAO inhibitor, allow 4–5 weeks. In switching within groups—eg, from one TCA to another (amitriptyline to desipramine, etc)—no washout time is needed, and one can rapidly decrease the dosage of one drug while increasing the other. The adjunctive use of low-dose atypical antipsychotics such as aripiprazole and risperidone in the treatment of patients with refractory depression is supported by recent research, although the side effect risk is the same as when treating psychosis. The FDA recently approved aripiprazole for this purpose. Combining two antidepressants, or adding an antipsychotic to an antidepressant, requires caution and is usually reserved for clinicians who feel comfortable managing this or after psychiatric consultation.

5. Maintenance and tapering—When clinical relief of symptoms is obtained, medication is continued for 12 months in the effective maintenance dosage, which is the dosage required in the acute stage. The full dosage should be continued indefinitely when the individual has a first episode before age 20 or after age 50, is over age 40 with two episodes, or has had three episodes at any age. Major depression should often be considered as a chronic disease. If the medication is being tapered, it should be done gradually over several months, monitoring closely for relapse.

6. Drug interactions—Interactions with other drugs are listed in Table 25–9.

7. Electroconvulsive therapy—ECT causes a generalized central nervous system seizure (peripheral convulsion is not

Table 25–8. Commonly used antidepressants.

Drug	Usual Daily Oral Dose (mg)	Usual Daily Maximum Dose (mg)	Sedative Effects[1]	Anticholinergic Effects[1]	Cost per Unit	Cost for 30 Days Treatment Based on Maximum Dosage[2]
SSRIs						
Fluoxetine (Prozac, Sarafem)	5–40	80	< 1	< 1	$2.67/20 mg	$320.40
Fluvoxamine (Luvox)	100–300	300	1	< 1	$2.64/100 mg	$237.60
Nefazodone (Serzone)	300–600	600	2	< 1	$1.60/200 mg	$144.00
Paroxetine (Paxil)	20–30	50	1	1	$2.73/20 mg	$163.80
Sertraline (Zoloft)	50–150	200	< 1	< 1	$2.72/100 mg	$163.20
Citalopram (Celexa)	20	40	< 1	1	$2.53/40 mg	$75.78
Escitalopram (Lexapro)	10	20	< 1	1	$3.38/20 mg	$101.40
Tricyclic and clinically similar compounds						
Amitriptyline (Elavil)	150–250	300	4	4	$1.16/150 mg	$69.60
Amoxapine (Asendin)	150–200	400	2	2	$1.67/100 mg	$200.40
Clomipramine (Anafranil)	100	250	3	3	$1.48/75 mg	$158.92
Desipramine (Norpramin)	100–250	300	1	1	$1.50/100 mg	$135.00
Doxepin (Sinequan)	150–200	300	4	3	$1.00/100 mg	$90.00
Imipramine (Tofranil)	150–200	300	3	3	$1.22/50 mg	$219.60
Maprotiline (Ludiomil)	100–200	300	4	2	$1.14/75 mg	$136.50
Nortriptyline (Aventyl, Pamelor)	100–150	150	2	2	$1.46/50 mg	$131.40
Protriptyline (Vivactil)	15–40	60	1	3	$3.10/10 mg	$558.00
Monoamine oxidase inhibitors						
Phenelzine (Nardil)	45–60	90	…	…	$0.80/15 mg	$144.00
Tranylcypromine (Parnate)	20–30	50	…	…	$1.03/10 mg	$154.50
Selegiline transdermal (Emsam)	6 (skin patch)	12			$17.56/6 mg patch	$526.67
Other compounds						
Desvenlafaxine	50	100	1	< 1		
Venlafaxine XR (Effexor)	150–225	225	1	< 1	$4.45/75 mg	$400.50
Duloxetine (Cymbalta)	40	60	2	3	$4.49/60 mg	$134.78
Mirtazapine (Remeron)	15–45	45	4	2	$2.80/30 mg	$85.50
Bupropion XL (Wellbutrin XL)	300[3]	450[3]		< 1	$4.00/300 mg	$178.05
Bupropion SR (Wellbutrin SR)	300	400[4]		< 1	$3.77/200 mg	$226.12
Trazodone (Desyrel)	100–300	400	4	< 1	$0.73/100 mg	$87.60
Trimipramine (Surmontil)	75–200	200	4	4	$4.03/100 mg	$241.80

[1]4, strong effect; 1, weak effect.
[2]Average wholesale price (AWP, for AB-rated generic when available) for quantity listed. Source: *Red Book Update*, Vol. 28, No. 3, March 2009. AWP may not accurately represent the actual pharmacy cost because wide contractual variations exist among institutions.
[3]Wellbutrin XL is a once-daily form of bupropion. Bupropion is still available as immediate release, and, if used, no single dose should exceed 150 mg.
[4]200 mg twice daily.
SSRIs, serotonin selective reuptake inhibitors.

necessary) by means of electric current. The key objective is to exceed the seizure threshold, which can be accomplished by a variety of means. The mechanism of action is not known, but it is thought to involve major neurotransmitter responses at the cell membrane. Electrical current insufficient to cause a seizure produces no therapeutic benefit.

ECT is the most effective (about 70–85%) treatment of severe depression—particularly the delusions and agitation commonly seen with depression in the elderly. It is indicated when medical conditions preclude the use of antidepressants, nonresponsiveness to these medications, and extreme suicidality. Comparative controlled studies of ECT in severe

Table 25–9. Antidepressant drug interactions with other drugs.

Drug	Effects
Tricyclic and other non-MAOI antidepressants	
Antacids	Decreased absorption of antidepressants
Anticoagulants	Increased hypoprothrombinemic effect
Cimetidine	Increased antidepressant blood levels and psychosis
Clonidine	Decreased antihypertensive effect
Digitalis	Increased incidence of heart block
Disulfiram	Increased antidepressant blood levels
Guanethidine	Decreased antihypertensive effect
Haloperidol	Increased clomipramine levels
Insulin	Decreased blood sugar
Lithium	Increased lithium levels with fluoxetine
Methyldopa	Decreased antihypertensive effect
Other anticholinergic drugs	Marked anticholinergic responses
Phenytoin	Increased blood levels
Procainamide	Decreased ventricular conduction
Procarbazine	Hypertensive crisis
Propranolol	Increased hypotension
Quinidine	Decreased ventricular conduction
Rauwolfia derivatives	Increased stimulation
Sedatives	Increased sedation
Sympathomimetic drugs	Increased pressor effect
Terfenadine,[1] astemizole,[1] cisapride[1]	Torsades de pointes
MAOIs	
Antihistamines	Increased sedation
Belladonna-like drugs	Increased blood pressure
Dextromethorphan	Same as meperidine
Guanethidine	Decreased blood pressure
Insulin	Decreased blood sugar
Levodopa	Increased blood pressure
Meperidine	Increased agitation, seizures, coma, death
Methyldopa	Decreased blood pressure
Pseudoephedrine	Hypertensive crisis (increased blood pressure)
Reserpine	Increased blood pressure and temperature
Succinylcholine	Increased neuromuscular blockade
Sulfonylureas	Decreased blood sugar
Sympathomimetic drugs	Increased blood pressure

[1]Terfenadine, astemizole, and cisapride are not commercially available in the United States.
MAOIs, monoamine oxidase inhibitors.

depression show that it is more effective than chemotherapy. It is also effective in the manic disorders and psychoses during pregnancy (when drugs may be contraindicated). It has not been shown to be helpful in chronic schizophrenic disorders, and it is generally not used in acute schizophrenic episodes unless drugs are not effective and it is urgent that the psychosis be controlled (eg, a catatonic stupor complicating an acute medical condition).

The most common side effects are memory disturbance and headache. Memory loss or confusion is usually related to the number and frequency of ECT treatments and proper oxygenation during treatment. Unilateral ECT is associated with less memory loss than bilateral ECT. Some memory loss is occasionally permanent, but most memory faculties return to full capacity within several weeks. There have been reports that lithium administration concurrent with ECT resulted in greater memory loss.

Increased intracranial pressure is a serious contraindication. Other problems such as cardiac disorders, aortic aneurysms, bronchopulmonary disease, and venous thrombosis are relative contraindications and must be evaluated in light of the severity of the medical problem versus the need for ECT. Serious complications arising from ECT occur in less than 1 in 1000 cases. Most of these problems are cardiovascular or respiratory in nature (eg, aspiration of gastric contents). Poor patient understanding and lack of acceptance of the technique by the public are the biggest obstacles to the use of ECT.

8. Phototherapy—Phototherapy is used in major depression with seasonal onset. It consists of exposure (at a 3-foot distance) to a light source of 2500 lux for 2 hours daily. Light visors are an adaptation that provides greater mobility and an adjustable light intensity. The dosage varies, with some patients requiring morning and night exposure. One effect is alteration of biorhythm through melatonin mechanisms.

9. Experimental treatments—In preliminary studies, transcranial magnetic stimulation appears to be effective in nonpsychotic depression. Its use in this condition has been approved by the FDA for individuals who have not responded to an antidepressant. It is usually delivered in a course of 16–20 sessions over 1 month. Vagal nerve stimulation has shown some promise in extremely refractory cases and is approved by the FDA but has not been approved by many insurers.

B. Psychological

It is seldom possible to engage an individual in penetrating psychotherapeutic endeavors during the acute stage of a severe depression. While medications may be taking effect, a supportive approach to strengthen existing coping mechanisms and appropriate consideration of the patient's continuing need to function at work, to engage in recreational activities, etc, are necessary as the severity of the depression lessens. If the patient is not seriously depressed, it is often quite appropriate to initiate intensive psychotherapeutic efforts, since flux periods are a good time to effect change. A catharsis of repressed anger and guilt may be beneficial.

Therapy during or just after the acute stage may focus on coping techniques, with some practice of alternative choices. Depression-specific psychotherapies help improve self-esteem, increase assertiveness, and lessen dependency. Interpersonal psychotherapy for depression has shown efficacy in the treatment of acute depression, helping patients master interpersonal stresses and develop new coping strategies. Cognitive behavioral therapy for depression addresses patients' patterns of negative thoughts, called cognitive distortions, that lead to feelings of depression and anxiety. Treatment usually includes homework assignments such as keeping a journal of cognitive distortions and of positive responses to them. As previously noted, numerous studies have shown that the combination of drug therapy plus interpersonal psychotherapy or cognitive behavioral therapy is more effective than either modality alone. It is usually helpful to involve the spouse or other significant family members early in treatment. Mindfulness-based cognitive therapy is a new form of therapy that has reduced relapse rates in several randomized controlled trials. In one study, it was as effective as maintenance medication in preventing relapse. This therapy incorporates meditation and teaches patients to distance themselves from depressive thinking.

C. Social

Flexible use of appropriate social services can be of major importance in the treatment of depression. Since alcohol is often associated with depression, early involvement in alcohol treatment programs such as Alcoholics Anonymous can be important to future success (see Alcohol Dependency and Abuse, below). The structuring of daily activities during severe depression is often quite difficult for the patient, and loneliness is often a major factor. The help of family, employer, or friends is often necessary to mobilize the patient who experiences no joy in daily activities and tends to remain uninvolved and to deteriorate. Insistence on sharing activities will help involve the patient in simple but important daily functions. In some severe cases, the use of day treatment centers or support groups of a specific type (eg, mastectomy groups) is indicated. It is not unusual for a patient to have multiple legal, financial, and vocational problems requiring legal and vocational assistance.

D. Behavioral

When depression is a function of self-defeating coping techniques such as passivity, the role-playing approach can be useful. Behavioral techniques, including desensitization, may be used in problems such as phobias where depression is a by-product. When depression is a regularly used interpersonal style, behavioral counseling to family members or others can help in extinguishing the behavior in the patient.

▶ Treatment of Mania

Acute manic or hypomanic symptoms will respond to lithium or valproic acid after several days of treatment, but it is increasingly common to use atypical neuroleptics as adjunctive treatment or monotherapy. High-potency benzodiazepines (eg, clonazepam) may also be useful adjuncts

in managing acute cases. Some schizoaffective disorders and some cases of so-called schizophrenia are probably atypical bipolar affective disorder, for which lithium treatment may be effective.

A. Neuroleptics

Acute manic symptoms of agitation and psychosis may be treated initially with the atypical antipsychotic olanzapine, (eg, 5–20 mg orally), risperidone (2–3 mg orally), or aripiprazole (15–30 mg) in conjunction with a benzodiazepine if indicated. Alternatively, when behavioral control is immediately necessary, olanzapine in an injectable form (2.5–10 mg intramuscularly) or haloperidol, 5–10 mg orally or intramuscularly repeated as needed until symptoms subside, may be used. The dosage of the neuroleptic may be gradually reduced after lithium or another mood stabilizer is started (see below). Olanzapine is approved as a maintenance treatment for bipolar disorder.

B. Clonazepam

Clonazepam can be an alternative or adjunct to a neuroleptic in controlling acute behavioral symptoms. Clonazepam has the advantage of causing no extrapyramidal side effects. Although 1–2 mg orally every 4–6 hours may be effective, up to 16 mg/d may be necessary.

C. Lithium

As a prophylactic drug for bipolar affective disorder, lithium significantly decreases the frequency and severity of both manic and depressive attacks in about 70% of patients. A positive response is more predictable if the patient has a low frequency of episodes (no more than two per year with intervals free of psychopathology). A positive response occurs more frequently in individuals who have blood relatives with a diagnosis of manic or hypomanic attacks. Patients who swing rapidly back and forth between manic and depressive attacks (at least four cycles per year) usually respond poorly to lithium prophylaxis initially, but some improve with continued long-term treatment. Carbamazepine (see below) has been used with success in this group.

In addition to its use in manic states, lithium is sometimes useful in the prophylaxis of recurrent unipolar depressions (perhaps undiagnosed bipolar disorder). Lithium may ameliorate nonspecific aggressive behaviors and dyscontrol syndromes. The dosages are the same as used in bipolar disorder. Most patients with bipolar disease can be managed long-term with lithium alone, although some will require continued or intermittent use of a neuroleptic, antidepressant, or carbamazepine. An excellent resource for information is the Lithium Information Center, Madison Institute of Medicine, 7617 Mineral Point Road, Suite 300, Madison, WI 53717-1914, http://www.miminc.org/aboutlithinfoctr.html.

Before treatment, the clinical workup should include a medical history and physical examination; complete blood count; T4, thyroid-stimulating hormone, blood urea nitrogen (BUN), serum creatinine, and serum electrolyte determinations; urinalysis; and electrocardiography in patients over age 45 or with a history of cardiac disease.

1. Dosage—The common starting dosage of lithium carbonate is 300 mg two or three times daily, with trough blood levels measured after 5 days of treatment. In a small minority of patients, a slow release form or units of different dosage may be required. Lithium citrate is available as a syrup. The dosage is that required to maintain blood levels in the therapeutic range. For acute attacks, this ranges from 1 to 1.5 mEq/L. Although there is controversy about the optimal long-term maintenance dose, many clinicians reduce the acute level to 0.6–1 mEq/L in order to reduce side effects. The dose required to meet this need will vary in different individuals. For acute mania, doses of 1200–1800 mg/d are generally recommended. Augmentation of antidepressants is usually achieved with half of these doses. Once-a-day dosage is acceptable, but most patients have less nausea when they take the drug in divided doses with meals.

Lithium is readily absorbed, with peak serum levels occurring within 1–3 hours and complete absorption in 8 hours. Half of the total body lithium is excreted in 18–24 hours (95% in the urine). Blood for lithium levels should be drawn 12 hours after the last dose. Serum levels should be measured 5–7 days after initiation of treatment and changes in dose. For maintenance treatment, lithium levels should be monitored initially every 1–2 months but may be measured every 6–12 months in stable, long-term patients. Levels should be monitored more closely when there is any condition that causes volume depletion (eg, diarrhea, dehydration, use of diuretics).

2. Side effects—Mild gastrointestinal symptoms (take lithium with food and in divided doses), fine tremors (treat with propranolol, 20–60 mg/d orally, only if persistent), slight muscle weakness, and some degree of somnolence are early side effects that are usually transient. Moderate polyuria (reduced renal responsiveness to ADH) and polydipsia (associated with increased plasma renin concentration) are often present. Potassium administration can blunt this effect, as may once-daily dosing of lithium. Weight gain (often a result of calories in fluids taken for polydipsia) and leukocytosis not due to infection are fairly common.

Other side effects include goiter (3%; often euthyroid), hypothyroidism (10%; concomitant administration of lithium and iodide or lithium and carbamazepine enhances the hypothyroid and goitrogenic effect of either drug), changes in the glucose tolerance test toward a diabetes-like curve, nephrogenic diabetes insipidus (usually resolving about 8 weeks after cessation of lithium therapy), nephrotic syndrome, edema, folate deficiency, and pseudotumor cerebri (ophthalmoscopy is indicated if there are complaints of headache or blurred vision). A metallic taste, hair loss, and Raynaud phenomenon have been reported in a few cases. Thyroid and kidney function should be checked at 3- to 4-month intervals. Most of these side effects subside when lithium is discontinued; when residual side effects exist, they are usually not serious. Most clinicians treat lithium-induced hypothyroidism (more common in women) with thyroid hormone while continuing lithium therapy. Hypercalcemia and elevated parathyroid hormone levels occur in some patients. Electrocardiographic abnormalities (principally T wave flattening or inversion) may occur during lithium administration but are not of major clinical significance. Sinoatrial block may occur, particularly in the elderly. Other drugs that prolong intraventricular conduction, such as TCAs, must be used cautiously in conjunction with lithium. Lithium impairs ventilatory function in patients with airway obstruction. Lithium alone does not have a significant effect on sexual function, but when combined with benzodiazepines (clonazepam in most symptomatic patients) it causes sexual dysfunction in about 50% of men. Lithium may precipitate or exacerbate psoriasis in some patients.

Patients receiving long-term lithium therapy may have cogwheel rigidity and, occasionally, other extrapyramidal signs. Lithium potentiates the parkinsonian effects of haloperidol. Long-term lithium therapy has also been associated with a relative lowering of the level of memory and perceptual processing (affecting compliance in some cases). Some impairment of attention and emotional reactivity has also been noted. Lithium-induced delirium with therapeutic lithium levels is an infrequent complication usually occurring in the elderly and may persist for several days after serum levels have become negligible. Encephalopathy has occurred in patients receiving combined lithium and neuroleptic therapy and in those who have cerebrovascular disease, thus requiring careful evaluation of patients who develop neurotoxic signs at subtoxic blood levels.

Some reports have suggested that the long-term use of lithium may have adverse effects on kidney function (with interstitial fibrosis or tubular atrophy). A rise in serum creatinine levels is an indication for in-depth evaluation of kidney function and consideration of alternative treatments if the individual can tolerate a change. Incontinence has been reported in women, apparently related to changes in bladder cholinergic-adrenergic balance.

Prospective studies suggest that the overall risk imposed by lithium in pregnancy may be overemphasized. However, lithium exposure in early pregnancy does increase the frequency of congenital anomalies, especially Ebstein and other major cardiovascular anomalies. For women who take psychotropic medications who become pregnant, the decision to make a change in medication is complex and requires informed consent regarding the relative risks to the patient and fetus. Indeed, the risk of untreated bipolar disorder carries its own risks for pregnancy. Formula feeding should be considered in mothers taking lithium, since concentration in breast milk is one-third to half that in serum.

Frank toxicity usually occurs at blood lithium levels above 2 mEq/L. Because sodium and lithium are reabsorbed at the same loci in the proximal renal tubules, any sodium loss (diarrhea, use of diuretics, or excessive perspiration) results in increased lithium levels. Symptoms and signs include vomiting and diarrhea, the latter exacerbating the problem since more sodium is lost and more lithium is absorbed. Other symptoms and signs, some of which may not be reversible, include tremors, marked muscle weakness, confusion, dysarthria, vertigo, choreoathetosis, ataxia, hyperreflexia, rigidity, lack of coordination, myoclonus, seizures, opisthotonos, and coma. Toxicity is more severe in the elderly, who should be maintained on slightly lower serum levels. Lithium overdosage may be accidental or intentional or may occur as a result of poor monitoring.

Patients with massive ingestions of lithium or blood lithium levels above 2.5 mEq/L should be treated with induced emesis and gastric lavage. If kidney function is normal, osmotic and saline diuresis increases renal lithium clearance. Urinary alkalinization is also helpful, since sodium bicarbonate decreases lithium reabsorption in the proximal tubule, as does acetazolamide as well. Aminophylline potentiates the diuretic effect by increasing the clearance of lithium. Drugs affecting the distal loop have no effect on lithium reabsorption. Blood lithium levels above 2.5 mEq/L (confirmed by cerebrospinal fluid lithium levels) should be considered an indication for hemodialysis.

Compliance with lithium therapy is adversely affected by the loss of some hypomanic experiences valued by the patient. These include social extroversion and a sense of heightened enjoyment in many activities such as sex and business dealings, often with increased productivity in the latter.

3. Drug interactions—Patients receiving lithium should use diuretics with caution and only under close medical supervision. The thiazide diuretics cause increased lithium reabsorption from the proximal renal tubules, resulting in increased serum lithium levels (Table 25–10), and adjustment of lithium intake must be made to compensate for this. Reduce lithium dosage by 25–40% when the patient is receiving 50 mg of hydrochlorothiazide daily. Potassium-sparing diuretics (spironolactone, amiloride, triamterene) may also increase serum lithium levels and require careful monitoring of lithium levels. Loop diuretics (furosemide, ethacrynic acid, bumetanide) do not appear to alter serum

Table 25–10. Lithium interactions with other drugs.

Drug	Effects
ACE inhibitors	↑ Lithium levels
Fluoxetine	↑ Lithium levels
Ibuprofen	↑ Lithium levels
Indomethacin	↑ Lithium levels
Methyldopa	Rigidity, mutism, fascicular twitching
Osmotic diuretics (urea, mannitol)	↑ Lithium excretion
Phenylbutazone	↑ Lithium levels
Potassium-sparing diuretics (spironolactone, amiloride, triamterene)	↑ Lithium levels
Sodium bicarbonate	↑ Lithium excretion
Succinylcholine	↑ Duration of action of succinylcholine
Theophylline, aminophylline	↑ Lithium excretion
Thiazide diuretics	↑ Lithium levels
Valproic acid	↓ Lithium levels
COX-2 inhibitors	↑ Lithium levels

ACE, angiotensin-converting enzyme; COX-2, cyclooxygenase-2.

lithium levels. Concurrent use of lithium and angiotensin-converting enzyme inhibitors requires a 50–75% reduction in lithium intake to achieve therapeutic lithium levels.

D. Valproic Acid

Valproic acid (divalproex) is an antiseizure drug whose activity is at least partially related to GABA neurotransmission. It is a first-line treatment for mania because it has a broader index of safety than lithium. This issue is particularly important in AIDS or other medically ill patients prone to dehydration or malabsorption with wide swings in serum lithium levels. Valproic acid has also been used effectively in panic disorder and migraine headache. Treatment is often started at a dose of 750 mg/d orally in divided doses, and dosage is then titrated to achieve therapeutic serum levels. Oral loading in acutely manic bipolar patients in an inpatient setting (initiated at a dosage of 20 mg/kg/d) can safely achieve serum therapeutic levels in 2–3 days. Concomitant use of aspirin, carbamazepine, warfarin, or phenytoin may affect serum levels. Gastrointestinal symptoms and weight gain are the main side effects. Liver function tests, complete blood counts, glucose levels, and weight should be monitored, and significant teratogenic effects are a concern so pregnancy should be ruled out prior to initiation.

E. Carbamazepine

Carbamazepine, an antiseizure drug that stabilizes the activity of cell membranes, has been used with increasing frequency in the treatment of bipolar patients who cannot be satisfactorily treated with lithium (nonresponsive, excessive side effects, or rapid cycling). It is often effective at 800–1600 mg/d orally. It has also been used in the treatment of resistant depressions, alcohol withdrawal, and hallucinations (in conjunction with neuroleptics) and in patients with behavioral dyscontrol or panic attacks. It suppresses some phases of kindling (see Stimulants) and has been used to treat residual symptoms in previous stimulant abusers (eg, PTSD with impulse control problems). Dose-related side effects include sedation and ataxia. Dosages start at 400–600 mg orally daily and are increased slowly to therapeutic levels. Skin rashes and a mild reduction in white count are common. SIADH occurs rarely. Nonsteroidal anti-inflammatory drugs (except aspirin), the antibiotics erythromycin and isoniazid, the calcium channel blockers verapamil and diltiazem (but not nifedipine), fluoxetine, propoxyphene, and cimetidine all increase carbamazepine levels. Carbamazepine can be effective in conjunction with lithium, although there have been reports of reversible neurotoxicity with the combination. Carbamazepine stimulates hepatic microsomal enzymes and so tends to decrease levels of haloperidol and oral contraceptives. It also lowers T_4, free T_4, and T_3 levels. Cases of fetal malformation (particularly spina bifida) have been reported along with growth deficiency and developmental delay. Liver tests and complete blood counts should be monitored in patients taking carbamazepine. **Oxcarbazepine**, a derivative of carbamazepine, does not appear to induce its own metabolism and is associated with fewer drug interactions, although it may impose a higher risk of hyponatremia. FDA-approved for partial seizures, oxcarbazepine may have efficacy in acute mania. It appears to be a safer alternative to carbamazepine due to its lower risk of hepatotoxicity.

F. Lamotrigine

Lamotrigine is thought to inhibit neuronal sodium channels and the release of the excitatory amino acids, glutamate and aspartate. It is FDA approved for long-term maintenance of bipolar disorder. Two double-blind studies support its efficacy in the treatment of acute bipolar depression as adjunctive therapy or as monotherapy. Its metabolism is inhibited by coadministration of valproic acid—doubling its half-life—and accelerated by hepatic enzyme-inducing agents such as carbamazepine. More frequent mild side effects include headache, dizziness, nausea, and diplopia. Rash occurring in 10% of patients is an indication for immediate cessation of dosing, since lamotrigine has been associated with Stevens-Johnson syndrome (1:1000) and, rarely, toxic epidermal necrolysis. Dosing starts at 25–50 mg/d orally and is titrated upward slowly to decrease the likelihood of rash. Slower titration and a lower total dose are indicated for patients taking valproic acid.

G. Calcium Channel Blockers

Calcium channel blockers (eg, verapamil) have been used in bipolar states that have failed to respond to lithium, carbamazepine, or valproic acid. This has come about with the realization that a number of drugs used in psychiatry (eg, lithium, antidepressants, neuroleptics, and carbamazepine) have calcium channel–blocking activity. Verapamil may be safer than lithium or carbamazepine during pregnancy, although it decreases uterine contractility and must be discontinued before delivery.

▶ Prognosis

Reactive depressions are usually time-limited, and the prognosis with treatment is good if a pathologic pattern of adjustment does not intervene. Major affective disorders frequently respond well to a full trial of drug treatment.

Mania and bipolar disorder have a good prognosis with adequate treatment, although patient adherence to treatment is often quite challenging.

ACOG Committee on Practice Bulletins—Obstetrics. ACOG Practice Bulletin: Clinical management guidelines for obstetrician-gynecologists number 92, April 2008 (replaces practice bulletin number 87, November 2007). Use of psychiatric medications during pregnancy and lactation. Obstet Gynecol. 2008 Apr;111(4):1001–20. [PMID: 18378767]

Belmaker RH et al. Major depressive disorder. N Engl J Med. 2008 Jan 3;358(1):55–68. [PMID: 18172175]

Cohen LS et al. Relapse of major depression during pregnancy in women who maintain or discontinue antidepressant treatment. JAMA. 2006 Feb 1;295(5):499–507. [PMID: 16449615]

Fava M et al. Efficacy and safety of sildenafil in men with serotonergic antidepressant-associated erectile dysfunction: results from a randomized, double-blind, placebo-controlled trial. J Clin Psychiatry. 2006 Feb;67(2):240–6. [PMID: 16566619]

Kuyken W et al. Mindfulness-based cognitive therapy to prevent relapse in recurrent depression. J Consult Clin Psychol. 2008 Dec;76(6):966–78. [PMID: 19045965]

Oberlander TF et al. Effects of timing and duration of gestational exposure to serotonin reuptake inhibitor antidepressants: population-based study. Br J Psychiatry. 2008 May;192(5):338–43. [PMID: 18450656]

Papakostas GI et al. Augmentation of antidepressants with atypical antipsychotic medications for treatment-resistant major depressive disorder: a meta-analysis. J Clin Psychiatry. 2007 Jun;68(6):826–31. [PMID: 17592905]

Rush AJ et al. Acute and longer-term outcomes in depressed outpatients requiring one or several treatment steps: a STAR*D report. Am J Psychiatry. 2006 Nov;163(11):1905–17. [PMID: 17074942]

Weissman MM et al. Remissions in maternal depression and child psychopathology: STAR*D-child report. JAMA. 2006 Mar 22;295(12):1389–98. [PMID: 16551710]

Williams M et al. Paroxetine (Paxil) and congenital malformations. CMAJ. 2005 Nov 22;173(11):1320–1. [PMID: 16272192]

SLEEP DISORDERS

Sleep consists of two distinct states as shown by electroencephalographic studies: (1) REM (rapid eye movement) sleep, also called dream sleep, D state sleep, paradoxic sleep, and (2) NREM (non-REM) sleep, also called S stage sleep, which is divided into stages 1, 2, 3, and 4 and is recognizable by different electroencephalographic patterns. Stages 3 and 4 are "delta" sleep. Dreaming occurs mostly in REM and to a lesser extent in NREM sleep.

Sleep is a cyclic phenomenon, with four or five REM periods during the night accounting for about one-fourth of the total night's sleep (1.5–2 hours). The first REM period occurs about 80–120 minutes after onset of sleep and lasts about 10 minutes. Later REM periods are longer (15–40 minutes) and occur mostly in the last several hours of sleep. Most stage 4 (deepest) sleep occurs in the first several hours.

Age-related changes in normal sleep include an unchanging percentage of REM sleep and a marked decrease in stage 3 and stage 4 sleep, with an increase in wakeful periods during the night. These normal changes, early bedtimes, and daytime naps play a role in the increased complaints of insomnia in older people. Variations in sleep patterns may be due to circumstances (eg, "jet lag") or to idiosyncratic patterns ("night owls") in persons who perhaps because of different "biologic rhythms" habitually go to bed late and sleep late in the morning. Creativity and rapidity of response to unfamiliar situations are impaired by loss of sleep. There are also rare individuals who have chronic difficulty in adapting to a 24-hour sleep-wake cycle (desynchronization sleep disorder), which can be resynchronized by altering exposure to light.

The three major sleep disorders are discussed below.

1. Dyssomnias (Insomnia)

▶ Classification & Clinical Findings

Patients may complain of difficulty getting to sleep or staying asleep, intermittent wakefulness during the night, early morning awakening, or combinations of any of these. Transient episodes are usually of little significance. Stress, caffeine, physical discomfort, daytime napping, and early bedtimes are common factors.

Psychiatric disorders are often associated with persistent insomnia. **Depression** is usually associated with fragmented sleep, decreased total sleep time, earlier onset of REM sleep, a shift of REM activity to the first half of the night, and a loss of slow wave sleep—all of which are nonspecific findings. In **manic disorders,** sleeplessness is a cardinal feature and an important early sign of impending mania in bipolar cases. Total sleep time is decreased, with shortened REM latency and increased REM activity. Sleep-related panic attacks occur in the transition from stage 2 to stage 3 sleep in some patients with a longer REM latency in the sleep pattern preceding the attacks.

Abuse of alcohol may cause or be secondary to the sleep disturbance. There is a tendency to use alcohol as a means of getting to sleep without realizing that it disrupts the normal sleep cycle. Acute alcohol intake produces a decreased sleep latency with reduced REM sleep during the first half of the night. REM sleep is increased in the second half of the night, with an increase in total amount of slow wave sleep (stages 3 and 4). Vivid dreams and frequent awakenings are common. Chronic alcohol abuse increases stage 1 and decreases REM sleep (most drugs delay or block REM sleep), with symptoms persisting for many months after the individual has stopped drinking. Acute alcohol or other sedative withdrawal causes delayed onset of sleep and REM rebound with intermittent awakening during the night.

Heavy smoking (more than a pack a day) causes difficulty falling asleep—apparently independently of the often associated increase in coffee drinking. Excess intake near bedtime of caffeine, cocaine, and other stimulants (eg, over-the-counter cold remedies) causes decreased total sleep time—mostly NREM sleep—with some increased sleep latency.

Sedative-hypnotics—specifically, the benzodiazepines, which are the most commonly prescribed drugs to promote sleep—tend to increase total sleep time, decrease sleep latency, and decrease nocturnal awakening, with variable effects on NREM sleep. Withdrawal causes just the opposite effects and results in continued use of the drug for the purpose of preventing withdrawal symptoms. Antidepressants decrease REM sleep (with marked rebound on withdrawal in the form of nightmares) and have varying effects on NREM sleep. The effect on REM sleep correlates with reports that REM sleep deprivation produces improvement in some depressions.

Persistent insomnias are also related to a wide variety of medical conditions, particularly delirium, pain, respiratory distress syndromes, uremia, asthma, and thyroid disorders. Adequate analgesia and proper treatment of medical disorders will reduce symptoms and decrease the need for sedatives.

▶ **Treatment**

In general, there are two broad classes of treatment for insomnia, and the two may be combined: psychological (cognitive-behavioral) and pharmacologic. In situations of acute distress, such as a grief reaction, pharmacologic measures may be most appropriate. With primary insomnia, however, initial efforts should be psychologically based. This is particularly true in the elderly to avoid the potential adverse reactions of medications. The elderly population is at risk for complaints of insomnia because sleep becomes lighter and more easily disrupted with aging. Medical disorders that become more common with age may also predispose to insomnia.

A. Psychological

Psychological strategies should include educating the patient regarding good sleep hygiene: (1) Go to bed only when sleepy. (2) Use the bed and bedroom only for sleeping and sex. (3) If still awake after 20 minutes, leave the bedroom and only return when sleepy. (4) Get up at the same time every morning regardless of the amount of sleep during the night. (5) Discontinue caffeine and nicotine, at least in the evening if not completely. (6) Establish a daily exercise regimen. (7) Avoid alcohol as it may disrupt continuity of sleep. (8) Limit fluids in the evening. (9) Learn and practice relaxation techniques. A recent study suggests that cognitive behavioral therapy for insomnia was as effective as zolpidem with benefits sustained 1 year after treatment.

B. Medical

When the above measures are insufficient, medications may be useful. Pharmacologic measures currently rely primarily on safe hypnotic medications that are difficult to overdose with. Lorazepam (0.5 mg orally nightly), temazepam (7.5–15 mg orally nightly) and the nonbenzodiazepine hypnotics, zolpidem (5–10 mg orally nightly), and zaleplon (5–10 mg orally nightly), are often effective for the elderly population and can be given in larger doses—twice what is prescribed for the elderly—in younger patients. A nonbenzodiazepine hypnotic, eszopiclone (2–3 mg), is similar in action to zolpidem and zaleplon but dissimilar in that it is not restricted to short-term use. A lower dose of 1 mg is indicated in the elderly or those with hepatic impairment. It is important to note that short-acting agents like triazolam or zolpidem may lead to amnestic episodes if used on a daily ongoing basis. Longer-acting agents such as flurazepam (half-life of > 48 hours) may accumulate in the elderly and lead to cognitive slowing, ataxia, falls, and somnolence. In general, it is appropriate to use medications for short courses of 1–2 weeks. The medications described above have largely replaced barbiturates as hypnotic agents because of their greater safety in overdose and their lesser hepatic enzyme induction effects. Antihistamines such as diphenhydramine (25 mg nightly) or hydroxyzine (25 mg nightly) may also be useful for sleep, as they produce no pharmacologic dependency; their anticholinergic effects may, however, produce confusion or urinary symptoms in the elderly. Trazodone, an atypical antidepressant, is a non–habit-forming, effective sleep medication in lower than antidepressant doses (25–150 mg at bedtime). Priapism is a rare side effect requiring emergent treatment. Ramelteon, 8 mg orally at bedtime, is a melatonin receptor agonist that helps with sleep onset and does not appear to have abuse potential. It appears to be safe for ongoing use without the development of tolerance.

Triazolam has achieved popularity as a hypnotic drug because of its very short duration of action. However, because it has been associated with dependency, transient psychotic reactions, anterograde amnesia, and rebound anxiety, it has been removed from the market in several European countries. If used, it must be prescribed only for short periods of time.

2. Hypersomnias (Disorders of Excessive Sleepiness)

The hypersomnias are a more severe problem than insomnia.

▶ Classification & Clinical Findings

A. Sleep Apnea

This disorder is characterized by cessation of breathing for at least 30 episodes (each lasting about 10 seconds) during the night. There are two types: obstructive and central. (See Chapter 9.)

B. Narcolepsy

Narcolepsy consists of a tetrad of symptoms: (1) Sudden, brief (about 15 minutes) sleep attacks that may occur during any type of activity; (2) cataplexy—sudden loss of muscle tone involving specific small muscle groups or generalized muscle weakness that may cause the person to slump to the floor, unable to move, often associated with emotional reactions and sometimes confused with seizure disorder; (3) sleep paralysis—a generalized flaccidity of muscles with full consciousness in the transition zone between sleep and waking; and (4) hypnagogic hallucinations, visual or auditory, which may precede sleep or occur during the sleep attack. The attacks are characterized by an abrupt transition into REM sleep—a necessary criterion for diagnosis. The disorder begins in early adult life, affects both sexes equally, and usually levels off in severity at about 30 years of age.

REM sleep behavior disorder, characterized by motor dyscontrol and often violent dreams during REM sleep, may be related to narcolepsy.

C. Kleine-Levin Syndrome

This syndrome, which occurs mostly in young men, is characterized by hypersomnic attacks three or four times a year lasting up to 2 days, with hyperphagia, hypersexuality, irritability, and confusion on awakening. It has often been associated with antecedent neurologic insults. It usually remits after age 40.

D. Nocturnal Myoclonus

Periodic lower leg movements occur during sleep with subsequent daytime sleepiness, anxiety, depression, and cognitive impairment.

▶ Treatment

Narcolepsy can be managed by daily administration of a stimulant such as dextroamphetamine sulfate, 10 mg orally in the morning, with increased dosage as necessary. Modafinil is a schedule IV medication FDA-approved for treating the excessive daytime fatigue of narcolepsy. Usual dosing is 200 mg orally each morning. Its mechanism of action is unknown, yet it is thought to be less of an abuse risk than stimulants that are primarily dopaminergic. Common side effects include headache and anxiety; however, modafinil appears to be generally well tolerated. Modafinil may reduce the efficacy of cyclosporine, oral contraceptives, and other medications by inducing their hepatic metabolism. Imipramine, 75–100 mg orally daily, has been effective in treatment of cataplexy but not narcolepsy.

Nocturnal myoclonus and REM sleep behavior disorder can be treated with clonazepam with variable results. There is no treatment for Kleine-Levin syndrome.

Treatment of sleep apnea is discussed in Chapter 9.

3. Parasomnias (Abnormal Behaviors during Sleep)

These disorders are fairly common in children and less so in adults.

▶ Classification & Clinical Findings

A. Sleep Terror

Sleep terror (pavor nocturnus) is an abrupt, terrifying arousal from sleep, usually in preadolescent boys although it may occur in adults as well. It is distinct from sleep panic attacks. Symptoms are fear, sweating, tachycardia, and confusion for several minutes, with amnesia for the event.

B. Nightmares

Nightmares occur during REM sleep; sleep terrors in stage 3 or stage 4 sleep.

C. Sleepwalking

Sleepwalking (somnambulism) includes ambulation or other intricate behaviors while still asleep, with amnesia for the event. It affects mostly children aged 6–12 years, and episodes occur during stage 3 or stage 4 sleep in the first third of the night and in REM sleep in the later sleep hours. Sleepwalking in elderly people may be a feature of dementia. Idiosyncratic reactions to drugs (eg, marijuana, alcohol) and medical conditions (eg, partial complex seizures) may be causative factors in adults.

D. Enuresis

Enuresis is involuntary micturition during sleep in a person who usually has voluntary control. Like other parasomnias, it is more common in children, usually in the 3–4 hours after bedtime, but is not limited to a specific stage of sleep. Confusion during the episode and amnesia for the event are common.

▶ Treatment

Treatment for sleep terrors is with benzodiazepines (eg, diazepam, 5–20 orally mg at bedtime), since it will suppress stage 3 and stage 4 sleep. Somnambulism responds to the same treatment for the same reason, but simple safety measures should not be neglected. Enuresis may respond to imipramine, 50–100 mg orally at bedtime, although desmopressin nasal spray (an ADH preparation) has increasingly become the treatment of choice for nocturnal enuresis. Behavioral approaches (eg, bells that ring when the pad gets wet) have also been successful.

Johnson MW et al. Ramelteon: a novel hypnotic lacking abuse liability and sedative adverse affects. Arch Gen Psychiatry. 2006 Oct;63(10):1149–57. [PMID: 17015817]

Parmet S et al. JAMA patient page. Insomnia. JAMA. 2006 Jun 28;295(24):2952. [PMID: 16804158]

Siversten B et al. Cognitive behavioral therapy vs zopiclone for treatment of chronic primary insomnia in older adults: a randomized controlled trial. JAMA. 2006 Jun 28;295(24):2851–8. [PMID: 16804151]

DISORDERS OF AGGRESSION

Aggression and violence are symptoms rather than diseases, and most frequently they are not associated with an underlying medical condition. Clinicians are unable to predict dangerous behavior with greater than chance accuracy. Depression, schizophrenia, personality disorders, mania, paranoia, temporal lobe dysfunction, and organic mental states may be associated with acts of aggression. Impulse control disorders are characterized by physical abuse (usually of the aggressor's domestic partner or children), by pathologic intoxication, by impulsive sexual activities, and by reckless driving. Anabolic steroid usage by athletes has been associated with increased tendencies toward violent behavior.

In the United States, a significant proportion of all violent deaths are alcohol-related. The ingestion of even small amounts of alcohol can result in pathologic intoxication that resembles an acute organic mental condition. Amphetamines, crack cocaine, and other stimulants are frequently associated with aggressive behavior. Phencyclidine is a drug commonly associated with violent behavior that is occasionally of a bizarre nature, partly due to lowering of the pain threshold. Domestic violence and rape are much more widespread than previously recognized. Awareness of the problem is to some degree due to increasing recognition of the rights of women and the understanding by women that they do not have to accept abuse. Acceptance of this kind of aggressive behavior inevitably leads to more, with the ultimate aggression being murder— 20–50% of murders in the United States occur within the family. Police are called in more domestic disputes than all other criminal incidents combined. Children living in such family situations frequently become victims of abuse.

Features of individuals who have been subjected to long-term physical or sexual abuse are as follows: trouble expressing anger, staying angry longer, general passivity in relationships, feeling "marked for life" with an accompanying feeling of deserving to be victimized, lack of trust, and dissociation of affect from experiences. They are prone to express their psychological distress with somatization symptoms, often pain complaints. They may also have symptoms related to posttraumatic stress, as discussed above. The clinician should be suspicious about the origin of any injuries not fully explained, particularly if such incidents recur.

▶ Treatment

A. Psychological

Management of any violent individual includes appropriate psychological maneuvers. Move slowly, talk slowly, with clarity and reassurance, and evaluate the situation. Strive to create a setting that is minimally disturbing, and eliminate people or things threatening to the violent individual. Do not threaten or abuse, and do not touch or crowd the person. Allow no weapons in the area (an increasing problem in hospital emergency departments). Proximity to a door is comforting to both the patient and the examiner. Use a negotiator the violent person can relate to comfortably. Food and drink are helpful in defusing the situation (as are cigarettes for those who smoke). Honesty is important. Make no false promises, bolster the patient's self-esteem, and continue to engage the subject verbally until the situation is under control. This type of individual does better with strong external controls to replace the lack of inner controls over the long term. Close probationary supervision and judicially mandated restrictions can be most helpful. There should be a major effort to help the individual avoid drug use (eg, Alcoholics Anonymous). Victims of abuse are essentially treated as any victim of trauma and, not infrequently, have evidence of PTSD.

B. Pharmacologic

Pharmacologic means are often necessary whether or not psychological approaches have been successful. This is particularly true in the agitated or psychotic patient. The drug of choice in psychotic aggressive states is haloperidol, 5–10 mg intramuscularly every hour until symptoms are alleviated. Benzodiazepine sedatives (eg, diazepam, 5 mg orally or intravenously every several hours) can be used for mild to moderate agitation, but an antipsychotic drug is preferred for management of the seriously violent and psychotic patient. Chronic aggressive states, particularly in retardation and brain damage (rule out causative organic conditions and medications such as anticholinergic drugs in amounts sufficient to cause confusion), have been ameliorated with risperidone, 0.5–2 mg/d orally, propranolol, 40–240 mg/d orally, or pindolol, 5 mg twice daily orally (pindolol causes less bradycardia and hypotension). Carbamazepine and valproic acid are effective in the treatment of aggression and explosive disorders, particularly when associated with known or suspected brain lesions. Lithium and SSRIs are also effective for some intermittent explosive outbursts. Buspirone (10–45 mg/d orally) is helpful for aggression, particularly in mentally retarded patients.

C. Physical

Physical management is necessary if psychological and pharmacologic means are not sufficient. It requires the active and visible presence of an adequate number of personnel (five or six) to reinforce the idea that the situation is under control despite the patient's lack of inner controls. Such an approach often precludes the need for actual physical restraint. When adequate personnel are not available, however, two people shielded by a mattress (single-bed size) can usually corner and subdue the patient without injury to anyone. Seclusion rooms and restraints should be used only when necessary (ambulatory restraints are an alternative), and the patient must then be observed at frequent intervals. Design of corridors and seclusion rooms is important. Narrow corridors, small spaces, and crowded areas exacerbate the potential for violence in an anxious patient.

D. Other Interventions

The treatment of victims (eg, battered women) is challenging and often complicated by their reluctance to leave the situation. Reasons for staying vary, but common themes include the fear of more violence because of leaving, the hope that the situation may ameliorate (in spite of steady worsening), and the financial aspects of the situation, which are seldom to the woman's advantage. Concerns for the children often finally compel the woman to seek help. An early step is to get the woman into a therapeutic situation that provides the support of others in similar straits. Al-Anon is frequently a valuable asset and quite appropriate when alcohol is a factor. The group can support the victim while she gathers strength to consider alternatives without being paralyzed by fear. Many cities now offer temporary emergency centers and counseling. Use the available resources, attend to any medical or psychiatric problems, and maintain a compassionate interest. Some states now require physicians to report injuries caused by abuse to police authorities.

Ellsberg M et al. Intimate partner violence and women's physical and mental health in the WHO multi-country study on women's health and domestic violence: an observational study. Lancet. 2008 Apr 5;371(9619):1165–72. [PMID: 18395577]

Hassouneh D et al. The influence of gender role stereotyping on women's experiences of female same-sex intimate partner violence. Violence Against Women. 2008 Mar;14(3):310–25. [PMID: 18292372]

Siever LJ. Neurobiology of aggression and violence. Am J Psychiatry. 2008 Apr;165(4):429–42. [PMID: 18346997]

▼ SUBSTANCE USE DISORDERS (DRUG DEPENDENCY, DRUG ABUSE)

The term "drug dependency" is used in a broad sense here to include both addictions and habituations. It involves the triad of compulsive drug use referred to as drug addiction, which includes: (1) a **psychological dependence** or craving and the behavior involved in procurement of the drug; (2) **physiologic dependence**, with withdrawal symptoms on discontinuance of the drug; and (3) **tolerance**, ie, the need to increase the dose to obtain the desired effects. Drug dependency is a function of the amount of drug used and the duration of usage. The amount needed to produce dependency varies with the nature of the drug and the idiosyncratic nature of the user. The frequency of use is usually daily, and the duration is inevitably greater than 2–3 weeks. Polydrug abuse is very common. Transgenerational continuity of drug abuse is also common.

There is accumulating evidence that an impairment syndrome exists in many former (and current) drug users. It is believed that drug use produces damaged neurotransmitter receptor sites and that the consequent imbalance produces symptoms that may mimic other psychiatric illnesses. "Kindling"—repeated stimulation of the brain—renders the individual more susceptible to focal brain activity with minimal stimulation. Stimulants and depressants can produce kindling, leading to relatively spontaneous effects no longer dependent on the original stimulus. These effects may be manifested as mood swings, panic, psychosis, and occasionally overt seizure activity. The imbalance also results in frequent job changes, marital problems, and generally erratic behavior. Patients with PTSD frequently have treated themselves with a variety of drugs. Chronic abusers of a wide variety of drugs exhibit cerebral atrophy on CT scans, a finding that may relate to the above symptoms. Early recognition is important, mainly to establish realistic treatment programs that are chiefly symptom-directed.

The clinician faces three problems with substance abuse: (1) the prescribing of substances such as sedatives, stimulants, or opioids that might produce dependency; (2) the treatment of individuals who have already abused drugs, most commonly alcohol; and (3) the detection of illicit drug use in patients presenting with psychiatric symptoms. The usefulness of urinalysis for detection of drugs varies markedly with different drugs and under different circumstances (pharmacokinetics is a major factor). Water-soluble drugs (eg, alcohol, stimulants, opioids) are eliminated in a day or so. Lipophilic substances (eg, barbiturates, tetrahydrocannabinol) appear in the urine over longer periods of time: several days in most cases, 1–2 months in chronic marijuana users. Sedative drug determinations are quite variable, amount of drug and duration of use being important determinants. False-positives can be a problem related to ingestion of some legitimate drugs (eg, phenytoin for barbiturates, phenylpropanolamine for amphetamines, chlorpromazine for opioids) and some foods (eg, poppy seeds for opioids, coca leaf tea for cocaine). Manipulations can alter the legitimacy of the testing. Dilution, either in vivo or in vitro, can be detected by checking urine specific gravity. Addition of ammonia, vinegar, or salt may invalidate the test, but odor and pH determinations are simple. Hair analysis can determine drug use over longer periods, particularly sequential drug-taking patterns. The sensitivity and reliability of such tests are considered good, and the method may be complementary to urinalysis.

Kosten TR et al. Management of drug and alcohol withdrawal. N Engl J Med. 2003 May 1;348(18):1786–95. [PMID: 12724485]

Prochaska JJ et al. Addressing nicotine dependence in psychodynamic psychotherapy: perspectives from residency training. Acad Psychiatry. 2007 Jan–Feb;31(1):8–14. [PMID: 17242046]

Thom B. From alcoholism treatment to the alcohol harm reduction strategy for England: an overview of alcohol policy since 1950. Am J Addict. 2005 Oct–Dec;14(5):416–25. [PMID: 16257879]

ALCOHOL DEPENDENCY & ABUSE (Alcoholism)

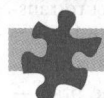 ESSENTIALS OF DIAGNOSIS

Major criteria:

▶ Physiologic dependence as manifested by evidence of withdrawal when intake is interrupted.

▶ Tolerance to the effects of alcohol.

▶ Evidence of alcohol-associated illnesses, such as alcoholic liver disease, cerebellar degeneration.

▶ Continued drinking despite strong medical and social contraindications and life disruptions.

▶ Impairment in social and occupational functioning.

▶ Depression.

▶ Blackouts.

Other signs:

▶ Alcohol stigmas: alcohol odor on breath, alcoholic facies, flushed face, scleral injection, tremor, ecchymoses, peripheral neuropathy.

▶ Surreptitious drinking.

▶ Unexplained work absences.

▶ Frequent accidents, falls, or injuries of vague origin; in smokers, cigarette burns on hands or chest.

▶ Laboratory tests: elevated values of liver function tests, mean corpuscular volume, serum uric acid, and triglycerides.

General Considerations

Alcoholism is a syndrome consisting of two phases: problem drinking and alcohol addiction. Problem drinking is the repetitive use of alcohol, often to alleviate anxiety or solve other emotional problems. Alcohol addiction is a true addiction similar to that which occurs following the repeated use of other sedative-hypnotics. Alcohol and other drug abuse patients have a much higher prevalence of lifetime psychiatric disorders. While male-to-female ratios in alcoholic treatment agencies remain at 4:1, there is evidence that the rates are converging. Women delay seeking help, and when they do they tend to seek it in medical or mental health settings. Adoption and twin studies indicate some genetic influence. Ethnic distinctions are important—eg, 40% of Japanese have aldehyde dehydrogenase deficiency and are more susceptible to the effects of alcohol. Depression is often present and should be evaluated carefully. The majority of suicides and intrafamily homicides involve alcohol. Alcohol is a major factor in rapes and other assaults.

There are several screening instruments that may help identify alcoholism. One of the most useful is the CAGE questionnaire (see Table 1–10).

Clinical Findings

A. Acute Intoxication

The signs of alcoholic intoxication are the same as those of overdosage with any other central nervous system depressant: drowsiness, errors of commission, psychomotor dysfunction, disinhibition, dysarthria, ataxia, and nystagmus. For a 70-kg person, an ounce of whiskey, a 4- to 6-oz glass of wine, or a 12-oz bottle of beer (roughly 15, 11, and 13 grams of alcohol, respectively) may raise the level of alcohol in the blood by 25 mg/dL. For a 50-kg person, the blood alcohol level would rise even higher (35 mg/dL) with the same consumption. Blood alcohol levels below 50 mg/dL rarely cause significant motor dysfunction (the legal limit for driving under the influence is commonly 80 mg/dL). Intoxication as manifested by ataxia, dysarthria, and nausea and vomiting indicates a blood level above 150 mg/dL, and lethal blood levels range from 350 to 900 mg/dL. In severe cases, overdosage is marked by respiratory depression, stupor, seizures, shock syndrome, coma, and death. Serious overdoses are frequently due to a combination of alcohol with other sedatives.

B. Withdrawal

There is a wide spectrum of manifestations of alcoholic withdrawal, ranging from anxiety, decreased cognition, and tremulousness through increasing irritability and hyperreactivity to full-blown delirium tremens. Symptoms of mild withdrawal, including tremor, elevated vital signs, and anxiety, begin within about 8 hours after the last drink and usually have passed by day 3. Generalized seizures occur within the first 24–38 hours and are more prevalent in persons who have a history of withdrawal syndromes. Delirium tremens is an acute organic psychosis that is usually manifest within 24–72 hours after the last drink (but may occur up to 7–10 days later). It is characterized by mental confusion, tremor, sensory hyperacuity, visual hallucinations (often of snakes, bugs, etc), autonomic hyperactivity, diaphoresis, dehydration, electrolyte disturbances (hypokalemia, hypomagnesemia), seizures, and cardiovascular abnormalities. The acute withdrawal syndrome is often completely unexpected and occurs when the patient has been hospitalized for some unrelated problem and presents as a diagnostic problem. Suspect alcohol withdrawal in every unexplained delirium. The mortality rate from delirium tremens has steadily decreased with early diagnosis and improved treatment.

In addition to the immediate withdrawal symptoms, there is evidence of persistent longer-term ones, including sleep disturbances, anxiety, depression, excitability, fatigue, and emotional volatility. These symptoms may persist for 3–12 months, and in some cases they become chronic.

C. Alcoholic (Organic) Hallucinosis

This syndrome occurs either during heavy drinking or on withdrawal and is characterized by a paranoid psychosis without the tremulousness, confusion, and clouded sensorium seen in withdrawal syndromes. The patient appears normal except for the auditory hallucinations, which are frequently persecutory and may cause the patient to behave aggressively and in a paranoid fashion.

D. Chronic Alcoholic Brain Syndromes

These encephalopathies are characterized by increasing erratic behavior, memory and recall problems, and emotional instability—the usual signs of organic brain injury due to any cause. Wernicke-Korsakoff syndrome due to thiamine deficiency may develop with a series of episodes. Wernicke encephalopathy consists of the triad of confusion, ataxia, and ophthalmoplegia (typically sixth nerve). Early recognition and treatment with thiamine can minimize damage. One of the possible sequelae is Korsakoff psychosis, characterized by both anterograde and retrograde amnesia, with confabulation early in the course. Early recognition and treatment of the alcoholic with intravenous thiamine and B complex vitamins can minimize damage.

E. Laboratory Findings

Ethanol may contribute to the presence of an otherwise unexplained osmolar gap. There may also be elevated liver function tests, increased serum uric acid and triglycerides, and decreased serum potassium and magnesium. The most definitive biologic marker for chronic alcoholism is carbohydrate deficient transferrin, which can detect heavy use (60 mg/d over 7–10 days) with high specificity. Two other tests that may provide clues to an alcohol problem are γ-glutamyl transpeptidase measurement (levels above 30 units/L are suggestive of heavy drinking) and mean corpuscular volume (> 95 fL in men and > 100 fL in women). If both are elevated, a serious drinking problem is likely. Use of other recreational drugs with alcohol skews and negates the significance of these tests. High-density lipoprotein cholesterol elevations combined with elevated γ-glutamyl transpeptidase concentrations also can help identify heavy drinkers.

▶ Differential Diagnosis

The differential diagnosis of problem drinking is essentially between primary alcoholism (when no other major psychiatric diagnosis exists) and secondary alcoholism, when alcohol is used as self-medication for major underlying psychiatric problems such as schizophrenia or affective disorder. The differentiation is important, since the latter group requires treatment for the specific psychiatric problem.

The differential diagnosis of alcohol withdrawal includes other sedative withdrawals and other causes of delirium. Acute alcoholic hallucinosis must be differentiated from other acute paranoid states such as amphetamine psychosis or paranoid schizophrenia. The history and laboratory test results are the most important features in differentiating chronic organic brain syndromes due to alcohol from those due to other causes. The form of the brain syndrome is of

little help—eg, chronic brain syndromes from lupus erythematosus may be associated with confabulation similar to that resulting from longstanding alcoholism.

▶ Complications

The medical, economic, and psychosocial problems of alcoholism are staggering. The central and peripheral nervous system complications include chronic brain syndromes, cerebellar degeneration, cardiomyopathy, and peripheral neuropathies. Direct effects on the liver include cirrhosis, esophageal varices, and eventual hepatic failure. Indirect effects include protein abnormalities, coagulation defects, hormone deficiencies, and an increased incidence of liver neoplasms.

Fetal alcohol syndrome includes one or more of the following developmental defects in the offspring of alcoholic women: (1) low birth weight and small size with failure to catch up in size or weight, (2) mental retardation, with an average IQ in the 60s, and (3) a variety of birth defects, with a large percentage of facial and cardiac abnormalities. The fetuses are very quiet in utero, and there is an increased frequency of breech presentations. There is a higher incidence of delayed postnatal growth and behavior development. The risk is appreciably higher the more alcohol ingested by the mother each day. Cigarette and marijuana smoking as well as cocaine use can produce similar effects on the fetus.

▶ Treatment of Problem Drinking

A. Psychological

The most important consideration for the clinician is to suspect the problem early and take a nonjudgmental attitude, although this does not mean a passive one. The problem of **denial** must be faced, preferably with significant family members at the first meeting. This means dealing from the beginning with any enabling behavior of the spouse or other significant people. Enabling behavior allows the alcoholic to avoid facing the consequences of his or her behavior.

There must be an emphasis on the things that can be done. This approach emphasizes the fact that the clinician cares and strikes a positive and hopeful note early in treatment. Valuable time should not be wasted trying to find out why the patient drinks; come to grips early with the immediate problem of how to stop the drinking. Although total abstinence should be the ultimate goal, a harm reduction model indicates that gradual progress toward abstinence can be a useful treatment stratagem.

B. Social

Get the patient into Alcoholics Anonymous and the spouse into Al-Anon. Success is usually proportionate to the utilization of Alcoholics Anonymous, religious counseling, and other resources. The patient should be seen frequently for short periods and charged an appropriate fee.

Do not underestimate the importance of religion, particularly since the alcoholic is often a dependent person who needs a great deal of support. Early enlistment of the help of a concerned religious adviser can often provide the turning point for a personal conversion to sobriety.

One of the most important considerations is the patient's job—fear of losing a job is one of the most powerful motivations for giving up drink. The business community has become painfully aware of the problem, with the result that about 70% of the Fortune 500 companies offer programs to their employees to help with the problem of alcoholism. In the latter case, some specific recommendations to employers can be offered: (1) Avoid placement in jobs where the alcoholic must be alone, eg, as a traveling buyer or sales executive. (2) Use supervision but not surveillance. (3) Keep competition with others to a minimum. (4) Avoid positions that require quick decision making on important matters (high-stress situations). In general, commitment to abstinence and avoidance of situations that might be conducive to drinking are most predictive of a good outcome.

C. Medical

Hospitalization is not usually necessary. It is sometimes used to dramatize a situation and force the patient to face the problem of alcoholism, but generally it should be used for medical indications.

Because of the many medical complications of alcoholism, a complete physical examination with appropriate laboratory tests is mandatory, with special attention to the liver and nervous system. Use of sedatives as a replacement for alcohol is not desirable. The usual result is concomitant use of sedatives and alcohol and worsening of the problem. Lithium is not helpful in the treatment of alcoholism.

Disulfiram (250–500 mg/d orally) has been used for many years as an aversive drug to discourage alcohol use. Disulfiram inhibits alcohol dehydrogenase, causing toxic reactions when alcohol is consumed. The results have generally been of limited effectiveness and depend on the motivation of the individual to be compliant.

Naltrexone, an opiate antagonist, in a dosage of 50 mg orally daily, has been helpful in lowering relapse rates over the 3–6 months after cessation of drinking, apparently by lessening the pleasurable effects of alcohol. One study suggests that naltrexone is most effective when given during periods of drinking in combination with therapy that supports abstinence but accepts the fact that relapses occur. Naltrexone is FDA-approved for maintenance therapy. Studies indicate that it reduces alcohol craving when used as part of a comprehensive treatment program. Acamprosate (333–666 mg orally three times daily) helps reduce craving and maintain abstinence, and can be continued even during periods of relapse.

D. Behavioral

Conditioning approaches historically have been used in some settings in the treatment of alcoholism, most commonly as a type of aversion therapy. For example, the patient is given a drink of whiskey and then a shot of apomorphine, and proceeds to vomit. In this way a strong association is built up between the drinking and vomiting. Although this kind of treatment has been successful in some cases, after appropriate informed consent, many people do not sustain the learned aversive response.

▶ Treatment of Hallucinosis & Withdrawal

A. Medical

1. Alcoholic hallucinosis—Alcoholic hallucinosis, which can occur either during or on cessation of a prolonged drinking period, is not a typical withdrawal syndrome and is handled differently. Since the symptoms are primarily those of a psychosis in the presence of a clear sensorium, they are handled like any other psychosis: hospitalization (when indicated) and adequate amounts of antipsychotic drugs. Haloperidol, 5 mg orally twice a day for the first day or so, usually ameliorates symptoms quickly, and the drug can be decreased and discontinued over several days as the patient improves. It then becomes necessary to deal with the chronic alcohol abuse, which has been discussed.

2. Withdrawal symptoms—The onset of withdrawal symptoms is usually 8–12 hours and the peak intensity of symptoms is 48–72 hours after alcohol consumption is stopped. Providing adequate central nervous system depressants (eg, benzodiazepines) is important to counteract the excitability resulting from sudden cessation of alcohol intake. The choice of a specific sedative is less important than using adequate doses to bring the patient to a level of moderate sedation, and this will vary from person to person. Mild dependency requires "drying out." In some instances for outpatients, a short course of tapering benzodiazepines—eg, diazepam, 20 mg orally daily initially, decreasing by 5 mg daily—may be a useful adjunct. In moderate to severe withdrawal, hospitalize the patient and use diazepam orally in a dosage of 5–10 mg hourly depending on the clinical need as judged by withdrawal symptoms, including nausea, tremor, autonomic hyperactivity, agitation; tactile, visual, and auditory hallucinations; and disorientation. This type of symptom-driven medication regimen for withdrawal appears to reduce total benzodiazepine usage over fixed-dose schedules. Antipsychotic drugs should not be used. Monitoring of vital signs and fluid and electrolyte levels is essential for the severely ill patient.

In very severe withdrawal, intravenous administration is necessary. After stabilization, the amount of diazepam required to maintain a sedated state may be given orally every 8–12 hours. If restlessness, tremulousness, and other signs of withdrawal persist, the dosage is increased until moderate sedation occurs. The dosage is then gradually reduced by 20% every 24 hours until withdrawal is complete. This usually requires a week or so of treatment. Clonidine, 5 mcg/kg orally every 2 hours, or the patch formulation of appropriate dosage strength, suppresses cardiovascular signs of withdrawal and has some anxiolytic effect. Carbamazepine, 400–800 mg daily orally, compares favorably with benzodiazepines for alcohol withdrawal.

Atenolol, as an adjunct to benzodiazepines, can reduce symptoms of alcohol withdrawal. The daily oral atenolol dose is 100 mg when the heart rate is above 80 beats per minute and 50 mg for a heart rate between 50 and 80 beats per minute. Atenolol should not be used when bradycardia is present.

Meticulous examination for other medical problems is necessary. Alcoholic hypoglycemia can occur with low blood alcohol levels (see Chapter 27). Alcoholics commonly have liver disease and associated clotting problems and are also prone to injury—and the combination all too frequently leads to undiagnosed subdural hematoma.

Phenytoin does not appear to be useful in managing alcohol withdrawal seizures per se. Sedating doses of benzodiazepines are effective in treating alcohol withdrawal seizures. Thus, other anticonvulsants are not usually needed unless there is a preexisting seizure disorder.

A general diet should be given, and vitamins in high doses: thiamine, 50 mg intravenously initially, then intramuscularly on a daily basis; pyridoxine, 100 mg/d; folic acid, 1 mg/d; and ascorbic acid, 100 mg twice a day. Intravenous glucose solutions should not be given prior to thiamine for fear of precipitating Wernicke syndrome. Thiamine is necessary as a ketolase enzyme cofactor. Concurrent administration is satisfactory, and hydration should be meticulously assessed on an ongoing basis.

Chronic brain syndromes secondary to a long history of alcohol intake are not clearly responsive to thiamine and vitamin replenishment. Attention to the social and environmental care of this type of patient is paramount.

B. Psychological and Behavioral

The comments in the section on problem drinking apply here also; these methods of treatment become the primary consideration after successful treatment of withdrawal or alcoholic hallucinosis. Psychological and social measures should be initiated in the hospital prior to discharge. This increases the possibility of continued post-hospitalization treatment.

Anton RF et al; COMBINE Study Research Group. Combined pharmacotherapies and behavioral interventions for alcohol dependence: the COMBINE study: a randomized controlled trial. JAMA. 2006 May 3;295(17):2003–17. [PMID: 16670409]

Dongier M. What are the treatment options for comorbid alcohol abuse and depressive disorders? J Psychiatry Neurosci. 2005 May;30(3):224. [PMID: 15944746]

Mayo-Smith MF et al. Management of alcohol withdrawal delirium. An evidence-based practice guideline. Arch Intern Med. 2004 Jul 12;164(13):1405–12. Erratum in: Arch Intern Med. 2004 Oct 11;164(18):2068. dosage error in text. [PMID: 15249349]

Ringold S et al. JAMA patient page. Alcohol abuse and alcoholism. JAMA. 2006 May 3;295(17):2100. [PMID: 16670424]

Williams SH. Medications for treating alcohol dependence. Am Fam Physician. 2005 Nov 1;72(9):1775–80. [PMID: 16300039]

OTHER DRUG & SUBSTANCE DEPENDENCIES

1. Opioids

The terms "opioids" and "narcotics" are used interchangeably and include a group of drugs with actions that mimic those of morphine. The group includes natural derivatives of opium (opiates), synthetic surrogates (opioids), and a number of polypeptides, some of which have been discovered to be natural neurotransmitters. The principal narcotic of abuse is heroin (metabolized to morphine), which is not used as a legitimate medication. The other common opioids are prescription drugs that differ in milligram potency, duration of action, and agonist and antagonist capabilities (see Chapter 1). All of the opioid analgesics can be reversed by the opioid antagonist naloxone.

The clinical symptoms and signs of mild narcotic intoxication include changes in mood, with feelings of euphoria; drowsiness; nausea with occasional emesis; needle tracks; and miosis. The incidence of snorting and inhaling heroin ("smoking") is increasing, particularly among cocaine users. This coincides with a decrease in the availability of methaqualone (no longer marketed) and other sedatives used to temper the cocaine "high" (see discussion of cocaine under Stimulants, below). Overdosage causes respiratory depression, peripheral vasodilation, pinpoint pupils, pulmonary edema, coma, and death.

Dependency is a major concern when continued use of narcotics occurs, although withdrawal causes only moderate morbidity (similar in severity to a bout of "flu"). Addicted patients sometimes consider themselves more addicted than they really are and may not require a withdrawal program. Grades of withdrawal are categorized from 0 to 4: grade 0 includes craving and anxiety; grade 1, yawning, lacrimation, rhinorrhea, and perspiration; grade 2, previous symptoms plus mydriasis, piloerection, anorexia, tremors, and hot and cold flashes with generalized aching; grades 3 and 4, increased intensity of previous symptoms and signs, with increased temperature, blood pressure, pulse, and respiratory rate and depth. In withdrawal from the most severe addiction, vomiting, diarrhea, weight loss, hemoconcentration, and spontaneous ejaculation or orgasm commonly occur. Complications of heroin administration include infections (eg, pneumonia, septic emboli, hepatitis, and HIV infection from using nonsterile needles), traumatic insults (eg, arterial spasm due to drug injection, gangrene), and pulmonary edema.

Treatment for overdosage (or suspected overdosage) is naloxone, 2 mg intravenously. If an overdose has been taken, the results are dramatic and occur within 2 minutes. Since the duration of action of naloxone is much shorter than that of the narcotics, the patient must be under close observation. Hospitalization, supportive care, repeated naloxone administration, and observation for withdrawal from other drugs should be maintained for as long as necessary.

Treatment for withdrawal begins if grade 2 signs develop. If a withdrawal program is necessary, use methadone, 10 mg orally (use parenteral administration if the patient is vomiting), and observe. If signs (piloerection, mydriasis, cardiovascular changes) persist for more than 4–6 hours, give another 10 mg; continue to administer methadone at 4- to 6-hour intervals until signs are not present (rarely more than 40 mg of methadone in 24 hours). Divide the total amount of drug required over the first 24-hour period by 2 and give that amount every 12 hours. Each day, reduce the total 24-hour dose by 5–10 mg. Thus, a moderately addicted patient initially requiring 30–

40 mg of methadone could be withdrawn over a 4- to 8-day period. Clonidine, 0.1 mg orally several times daily over a 10- to 14-day period, is both an alternative and an adjunct to methadone detoxification; it is not necessary to taper the dose. Clonidine is helpful in alleviating cardiovascular symptoms but does not significantly relieve anxiety, insomnia, or generalized aching. There is a protracted abstinence syndrome of metabolic, respiratory, and blood pressure changes over a period of 3–6 months.

Narcotic antagonists (eg, naltrexone) can also be used successfully for treatment of the patient who has been free of opioids for 7–10 days. Naltrexone blocks the narcotic "high" of heroin when 50 mg is given orally every 24 hours initially for several days and then 100 mg is given every 48–72 hours. Liver disorders are a major contraindication. Compliance tends to be poor, partly because of the dysphoria that can persist long after opioid discontinuance. Buprenorphine, a partial agonist, is a mainstay of office-based treatment of opiate dependency. Its use requires special training.

Alternative strategies for the treatment of opioid withdrawal have included rapid and ultrarapid detoxification techniques. However, recent data do not support the use of either method. Methadone maintenance programs are of some value in chronic recidivism. Under carefully controlled supervision, the narcotic addict is maintained on fairly high doses of methadone (40–120 mg/d) that satisfy craving and block the effects of heroin to a great degree.

2. Sedatives (Anxiolytics)

See Anxiety Disorders, this chapter.

3. Psychedelics

About 6000 species of plants have psychoactive properties. All of the common psychedelics (LSD, mescaline, psilocybin, dimethyltryptamine, and other derivatives of phenylalanine and tryptophan) can produce similar behavioral and physiologic effects. An initial feeling of tension is followed by emotional release such as crying or laughing (1–2 hours). Later, perceptual distortions occur, with visual illusions and hallucinations, and occasionally there is fear of ego disintegration (2–3 hours). Major changes in time sense and mood lability then occur (3–4 hours). A feeling of detachment and a sense of destiny and control occur (4–6 hours). Of course, reactions vary among individuals, and some of the drugs produce markedly different time frames. Occasionally, the acute episode is terrifying (a "bad trip"), which may include panic, depression, confusion, or psychotic symptoms. Preexisting emotional problems, the attitude of the user, and the setting where the drug is used affect the experience.

Treatment of the acute episode primarily involves protection of the individual from erratic behavior that may lead to injury or death. A structured environment is usually sufficient until the drug is metabolized. In severe cases, antipsychotic drugs with minimal side effects (eg, haloperidol, 5 mg intramuscularly) may be given every several hours until the individual has regained control. In cases where "flashbacks" occur (mental imagery from a "bad trip" that

is later triggered by mild stimuli such as marijuana, alcohol, or psychic trauma), a short course of an antipsychotic drug—eg, olanzapine, 5–10 mg/d, or risperidone, 2 mg/d, initially, and up to 20 mg/d and 6 mg/d, respectively—is usually sufficient. Lorazepam, 1–2 mg orally or intramuscularly every 2 hours as needed for acute agitation, may be a useful adjunct. An occasional patient may have "flashbacks" for much longer periods and require small doses of neuroleptic drugs over the longer term.

4. Phencyclidine

Phencyclidine (PCP, angel dust, peace pill, hog), developed as an anesthetic agent, first appeared as a street drug deceptively sold as tetrahydrocannabinol (THC). Because it is simple to produce and mimics to some degree the traditional psychedelic drugs, PCP has become a common deceptive substitute for LSD, THC, and mescaline. It is available in crystals, capsules, and tablets to be inhaled, injected, swallowed, or smoked (it is commonly sprinkled on marijuana).

Absorption after smoking is rapid, with onset of symptoms in several minutes and peak symptoms in 15–30 minutes. Mild intoxication produces euphoria accompanied by a feeling of numbness. Moderate intoxication (5–10 mg) results in disorientation, detachment from surroundings, distortion of body image, combativeness, unusual feats of strength (partly due to its anesthetic activity), and loss of ability to integrate sensory input, especially touch and proprioception. Physical symptoms include dizziness, ataxia, dysarthria, nystagmus, retracted upper eyelid with blank stare, hyperreflexia, and tachycardia. There are increases in blood pressure, respiration, muscle tone, and urine production. Usage in the first trimester of pregnancy is associated with an increase in spontaneous abortion and congenital defects. Severe intoxication (20 mg or more) produces an increase in degree of moderate symptoms, with the addition of seizures, deepening coma, hypertensive crisis, and severe psychotic ideation. The drug is particularly long-lasting (several days to several weeks) owing to high lipid solubility, gastroenteric recycling, and the production of active metabolites. Overdosage may be fatal, with the major causes of death being hypertensive crisis, respiratory arrest, and convulsions. Acute rhabdomyolysis has been reported and can result in myoglobinuric kidney failure.

Differential diagnosis involves the whole spectrum of street drugs, since in some ways phencyclidine mimics sedatives, psychedelics, and marijuana in its effects. Blood and urine testing can detect the acute problem.

Treatment is discussed in Chapter 38.

5. Marijuana

Cannabis sativa, a hemp plant, is the source of marijuana. The parts of the plant vary in potency. The resinous exudate of the flowering tops of the female plant (hashish, charas) is the most potent, followed by the dried leaves and flowering shoots of the female plant (bhang) and the resinous mass from small leaves of inflorescence (ganja). The least potent parts are the lower branches and the leaves of the female plant and all parts of the male plant. Mercury may be a contaminant in marijuana grown in volcanic soil. The drug is usually inhaled by smoking. Effects occur in 10–20 minutes and last 2–3 hours. "Joints" of good quality contain about 500 mg of marijuana (which contains approximately 5–15 mg of tetrahydrocannabinol with a half-life of 7 days). Marijuana soaked in formaldehyde and dried ("AMP") has produced unusual effects, including autonomic discharge and severe though transient cognitive impairment.

With moderate dosage, marijuana produces two phases: mild euphoria followed by sleepiness. In the acute state, the user has an altered time perception, less inhibited emotions, psychomotor problems, impaired immediate memory, and conjunctival injection. High doses produce transient psychotomimetic effects. No specific treatment is necessary except in the case of the occasional "bad trip," in which case the person is treated in the same way as for psychedelic usage. Marijuana frequently aggravates existing mental illness and adversely affects motor performance.

Studies of long-term effects have conclusively shown abnormalities in the pulmonary tree. Laryngitis and rhinitis are related to prolonged use, along with chronic obstructive pulmonary disease. Electrocardiographic abnormalities are common, but no chronic cardiac disease has been linked to marijuana use. Long-term usage has resulted in depression of plasma testosterone levels and reduced sperm counts. Abnormal menstruation and failure to ovulate have occurred in some women. Cognitive impairments are common. Health care utilization for a variety of health problems is increased in long-term marijuana smokers. Sudden withdrawal produces insomnia, nausea, myalgia, and irritability. Psychological effects of long-term marijuana usage are still unclear. Urine testing is reliable if samples are carefully collected and tested. Detection periods span 4–6 days in short-term users and 20–50 days in long-term users.

6. Stimulants: Amphetamines & Cocaine

Stimulant abuse is quite common, either alone or in combination with abuse of other drugs. The **amphetamines**, including Methedrine ("speed")—one variant is a smokable form called "ice," which gives an intense and fairly long-lasting high—methylphenidate, and phenmetrazine, are under prescription control, but street availability remains high. Moderate usage of any of the stimulants produces hyperactivity, a sense of enhanced physical and mental capacity, and sympathomimetic effects. The clinical picture of acute stimulant intoxication includes sweating, tachycardia, elevated blood pressure, mydriasis, hyperactivity, and an acute brain syndrome with confusion and disorientation. Tolerance develops quickly, and, as the dosage is increased, hypervigilance, paranoid ideation (with delusions of parasitosis), stereotypy, bruxism, tactile hallucinations of insect infestation, and full-blown psychoses occur, often with persecutory ideation and aggressive responses. Stimulant withdrawal is characterized by depression with symptoms of hyperphagia and hypersomnia.

People who have used stimulants chronically (eg, anorexigenics) occasionally become sensitized ("**kindling**") to future use of stimulants. In these individuals, even small amounts of mild stimulants such as caffeine can cause symptoms of paranoia and auditory hallucinations.

Cocaine is a stimulant. It is a product of the coca plant. The derivatives include seeds, leaves, coca paste, cocaine hydrochloride, and the free base of cocaine. Cocaine hydrochloride is the salt and the most commonly used form. Free base, a purer (and stronger) derivative called "crack," is prepared by simple extraction from cocaine hydrochloride.

There are various modes of use. Coca leaf chewing involves toasting the leaves and chewing with alkaline material (eg, the ash of other burned leaves) to enhance buccal absorption. One achieves a mild high, with onset in 5–10 minutes and lasting for about an hour. Intranasal use is simply snorting cocaine through a straw. Absorption is slowed somewhat by vasoconstriction (which may eventually cause tissue necrosis and septal perforation); the onset of action is in 2–3 minutes, with a moderate high (euphoria, excitement, increased energy) lasting about 30 minutes. The purity of the cocaine is a major determinant of the high. Intravenous use of cocaine hydrochloride or "freebase" is effective in 30 seconds and produces a short-lasting, fairly intense high of about 15 minutes' duration. The combined use of cocaine and ethanol results in the metabolic production of cocaethylene by the liver. This substance produces more intense and long-lasting cocaine-like effects. Smoking freebase (volatilized cocaine because of the lower boiling point) acts in seconds and results in an intense high lasting several minutes. The intensity of the reaction is related to the marked lipid solubility of the freebase form and produces by far the most severe medical and psychiatric symptoms.

Cardiovascular collapse, arrhythmias, myocardial infarction, and transient ischemic attacks have been reported. Seizures, strokes, migraine symptoms, hyperthermia, and lung damage may occur, and there are several obstetric complications, including spontaneous abortion, abruptio placentae, teratogenic effects, delayed fetal growth, and prematurity. Cocaine can cause anxiety, mood swings, and delirium, and chronic use can cause the same problems as other stimulants (see above).

Clinicians should be alert to cocaine use in patients presenting with unexplained nasal bleeding, headaches, fatigue, insomnia, anxiety, depression, and chronic hoarseness. Sudden withdrawal of the drug is not life-threatening but usually produces craving, sleep disturbances, hyperphagia, lassitude, and severe depression (sometimes with suicidal ideation) lasting days to weeks.

Treatment is imprecise and difficult. Since the high is related to blockage of dopamine reuptake, the dopamine agonist bromocriptine, 1.5 mg orally three times a day, alleviates some of the symptoms of craving associated with acute cocaine withdrawal. Other dopamine agonists such as apomorphine, levodopa, and amantadine are under study for this purpose. Carbamazepine may be a useful adjunct in treating symptoms of alcohol withdrawal, and desipramine in moderate doses has been useful in helping maintain abstinence in the early stages of treatment. Treatment of psychosis is the same as that of any psychosis: antipsychotic drugs in dosages sufficient to alleviate the symptoms. Any medical symptoms (eg, hyperthermia, seizures, hypertension) are treated specifically. These approaches should be used in conjunction with a structured program, most often based on the Alcoholics Anonymous model. Hospitalization may be required if self-harm or violence toward others is a perceived threat (usually indicated by paranoid delusions).

7. Caffeine

Caffeine, along with nicotine and alcohol, is one of the most commonly used drugs worldwide. About 10 billion pounds of coffee (the richest source of caffeine) are consumed yearly throughout the world. Tea, cocoa, and cola drinks also contribute to an intake of caffeine that is often astoundingly high in a large number of people. Low to moderate doses (30–200 mg/d) tend to improve some aspects of performance (eg, vigilance). The approximate content of caffeine in a (180-mL) cup of beverage is as follows: brewed coffee, 80–140 mg; instant coffee, 60–100 mg; decaffeinated coffee, 1–6 mg; black leaf tea, 30–80 mg; tea bags, 25–75 mg; instant tea, 30–60 mg; cocoa, 10–50 mg; and 12-oz cola drinks, 30–65 mg. A 2-oz chocolate candy bar has about 20 mg. Some herbal teas (eg, "morning thunder") contain caffeine. Caffeine-containing analgesics usually contain approximately 30 mg per unit. Symptoms of caffeinism (usually associated with ingestion of over 500 mg/d) include anxiety, agitation, restlessness, insomnia, a feeling of being "wired," and somatic symptoms referable to the heart and gastrointestinal tract. It is common for a case of caffeinism to present as an anxiety disorder. It is also common for caffeine and other stimulants to precipitate severe symptoms in compensated schizophrenic and manic-depressive patients. Chronically depressed patients often use caffeine drinks as self-medication. This diagnostic clue may help distinguish some major affective disorders. Withdrawal from caffeine (> 250 mg/d) can produce headaches, irritability, lethargy, and occasional nausea.

8. Miscellaneous Drugs, Solvents

The principal over-the-counter drugs of concern have been phenylpropanolamine and an assortment of antihistaminic agents, frequently in combination with a mild analgesic promoted as cold remedies. Medications containing phenylpropanolamine have been removed from sale in the United States due to an FDA ban. The major problem in use of phenylpropanolamine relates to its side effects as a stimulant, including precipitation of anxiety states, increased pressure effects, auditory and visual hallucinations, paranoid ideation, and occasionally delirium. Aggressiveness and some loss of impulse control were reported as well as sleep disturbances even with small doses.

Antihistamines usually produce some central nervous system depression—thus their use as over-the-counter sedatives. Practically all of the so-called sleep aids are antihistamines. The mixture of antihistamines with alcohol usually exacerbates the central nervous system effects. Scopolamine and bromides have generally been removed from over-the-counter products.

The abuse of laxatives sometimes can lead to electrolyte disturbances that may contribute to the manifestations of a delirium. The greatest use of laxatives tends to be in the elderly and in those with eating disorders, both of whom are the most vulnerable to physiologic changes.

Anabolic steroids are being abused by people who wish to increase muscle mass for cosmetic reasons or for greater strength. In addition to the medical problems, the practice is associated with significant mood swings, aggressiveness, and paranoid delusions. Alcohol and stimulant use is higher in these individuals. Withdrawal symptoms of steroid dependency include fatigue, depressed mood, restlessness, and insomnia.

Amyl nitrite has been used as an "orgasm expander." The changes in time perception, "rush," and mild euphoria caused by the drug prompted its nonmedical use, and popular lore concerning the effects of inhalation just prior to orgasm has led to increased use. Subjective effects last from 5 seconds to 15 minutes. Tolerance develops readily, but there are no known withdrawal symptoms. Abstinence for several days reestablishes the previous level of responsiveness. Long-term effects may include damage to the immune system and respiratory difficulties.

Sniffing of solvents and inhaling of gases (including aerosols) produce a form of inebriation similar to that of the volatile anesthetics. Agents include gasoline, toluene, petroleum ether, lighter fluids, cleaning fluids, paint thinners, and solvents that are present in many household products (eg, nail polish, typewriter correction fluid). Typical intoxication states include euphoria, slurred speech, hallucinations, and confusion, and with high doses, acute manifestations are unconsciousness and cardiorespiratory depression or failure; chronic exposure produces a variety of symptoms related to the liver, kidney, bone marrow, or heart. Lead encephalopathy can be associated with sniffing leaded gasoline. In addition, studies of workers chronically exposed to jet fuel showed significant increases in neurasthenic symptoms, including fatigue, anxiety, mood changes, memory difficulties, and somatic complaints. These same problems have been noted in long-term solvent abuse.

The so-called designer drugs are synthetic substitutes for commonly used recreational drugs and are produced in small, clandestine laboratories. The most common designer drugs have been methyl analogues of fentanyl and have been used as heroin substitutes. MDMA (methylenedioxymethamphetamine), an amphetamine derivative sometimes called "ecstasy," is also a designer drug with high abuse potential and neurotoxicity. Often not detected by standard toxicology screens, these substances can present a vexing problem for clinicians faced with symptoms from a totally unknown cause.

Collins ED et al. Anesthesia-assisted vs buprenorphine- or clonidine-assisted heroin detoxification and naltrexone induction: a randomized trial. JAMA. 2005 Aug 24;294(8):903–13. [PMID: 16118380]

Donaher PA et al. Managing opioid addiction with buprenorphine. Am Fam Physician. 2007 May 1;73(9):1573–8. [PMID: 16719249]

Lundqvist T. Cognitive consequences of cannabis use: comparison with abuse of stimulants and heroin with regard to attention, memory and executive functions. Pharmacol Biochem Behav. 2005 Jun;81(2):319–30. [PMID: 15925403]

Moore BA et al. Primary care office-based buprenorphine treatment: comparison of heroin and prescription opioid dependent patients. J Gen Intern Med. 2007 Apr;22(4):527–30. [PMID: 17372805]

DELIRIUM, DEMENTIA, & OTHER COGNITIVE DISORDERS (FORMERLY: ORGANIC BRAIN SYNDROME)

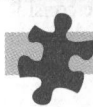

ESSENTIALS OF DIAGNOSIS

▶ Transient or permanent brain dysfunction.

▶ Cognitive impairment to varying degrees.

▶ Impaired recall and recent memory, inability to focus attention, random psychomotor activity such as stereotypy, and problems in perceptual processing, often with psychotic ideation.

▶ Emotional disorders frequently present: depression, anxiety, irritability.

▶ Behavioral disturbances: impulse control, sexual acting-out, attention deficits, aggression, and exhibitionism.

▶ General Considerations

The organic problem may be a primary brain disease or a secondary manifestation of some general disorder. All of the cognitive disorders show some degree of impaired thinking depending on the site of involvement, the rate of onset and progression, and the duration of the underlying brain lesion. Emotional disturbances (eg, depression) are often present as significant comorbidities. The behavioral disturbances tend to be more common with chronicity, more directly related to the underlying personality or central nervous system vulnerability to drug side effects, and not necessarily correlated with cognitive dysfunction.

The causes of cognitive disorders are listed in Table 25–11.

▶ Clinical Findings

The manifestations are many and varied and include problems with orientation, short or fluctuating attention span, loss of recent memory and recall, impaired judgment, emotional lability, lack of initiative, impaired impulse control, inability to reason through problems, depression (worse in

Table 25–11. Etiology of delirium and other cognitive disorders.

Disorder	Possible Causes
Intoxication	Alcohol, sedatives, bromides, analgesics (eg, pentazocine), psychedelic drugs, stimulants, and household solvents.
Drug withdrawal	Withdrawal from alcohol, sedative-hypnotics, corticosteroids.
Long-term effects of alcohol	Wernicke-Korsakoff syndrome.
Infections	Septicemia; meningitis and encephalitis due to bacterial, viral, fungal, parasitic, or tuberculous organisms or to central nervous system syphilis; acute and chronic infections due to the entire range of microbiologic pathogens.
Endocrine disorders	Thyrotoxicosis, hypothyroidism, adrenocortical dysfunction (including Addison disease and Cushing syndrome), pheochromocytoma, insulinoma, hypoglycemia, hyperparathyroidism, hypoparathyroidism, panhypopituitarism, diabetic ketoacidosis.
Respiratory disorders	Hypoxia, hypercapnia.
Metabolic disturbances	Fluid and electrolyte disturbances (especially hyponatremia, hypomagnesemia, and hypercalcemia), acid-base disorders, hepatic disease (hepatic encephalopathy), kidney failure, porphyria.
Nutritional deficiencies	Deficiency of vitamin B_1 (beriberi), vitamin B_{12} (pernicious anemia), folic acid, nicotinic acid (pellagra); protein-calorie malnutrition.
Trauma	Subdural hematoma, subarachnoid hemorrhage, intracerebral bleeding, concussion syndrome.
Cardiovascular disorders	Myocardial infarctions, cardiac arrhythmias, cerebrovascular spasms, hypertensive encephalopathy, hemorrhages, embolisms, and occlusions indirectly cause decreased cognitive function.
Neoplasms	Primary or metastatic lesions of the central nervous system, cancer-induced hypercalcemia.
Seizure disorders	Ictal, interictal, and postictal dysfunction.
Collagen-vascular and immunologic disorders	Autoimmune disorders, including systemic lupus erythematosus, Sjögren syndrome, and AIDS.
Degenerative diseases	Alzheimer disease, Pick disease, multiple sclerosis, parkinsonism, Huntington chorea, normal pressure hydrocephalus.
Medications	Anticholinergic drugs, antidepressants, H_2-blocking agents, digoxin, salicylates (long-term use), and a wide variety of other over-the-counter and prescribed drugs.

mild to moderate types), confabulation (not limited to alcohol organic brain syndrome), constriction of intellectual functions, visual and auditory hallucinations, and delusions. Physical findings will naturally vary according to the cause. The EEG usually shows generalized slowing in delirium.

A. Delirium

Delirium (acute confusional state) is a transient global disorder of attention, with clouding of consciousness, usually a result of systemic problems (eg, drugs, hypoxemia). Onset is usually rapid. The mental status fluctuates (impairment is usually least in the morning), with varying inability to concentrate, maintain attention, and sustain purposeful behavior. ("Sundowning"—mild to moderate delirium at night—is more common in patients with preexisting dementia and may be precipitated by hospitalization, drugs, and sensory deprivation.) There is a marked deficit of short-term memory and recall. Anxiety and irritability are common. Amnesia is retrograde (impaired recall of past memories) and anterograde (inability to recall events after the onset of the delirium). Orientation problems follow the inability to retain information. Perceptual disturbances (often visual hallucinations) and psychomotor restlessness with insomnia are common. Autonomic changes include tachycardia, dilated pupils, and sweating. The average duration is about 1 week, with full recovery in most cases. Delirium can coexist with dementia.

B. Dementia

(See also Chapter 4.) Dementia is characterized by chronicity and deterioration of selective mental functions. Onset is insidious over months to years in most cases. Formal cognitive screens can quantify impairments and point to the need for further evaluation. The Mini-Mental State Examination produces a numerical score with up to 30 points given for correct answers to questions (likely organic < 27 points) (see Figure 4–3). Specific cognitive assessment must be performed, since many patients are able to cover a deficit in routine conversation.

Dementia is usually progressive, more common in the elderly, and rarely reversible even if underlying disease can be corrected. Dementia can be classified as cortical or subcortical.

There are three types of cortical dementia: (1) primary degenerative dementia (eg, Alzheimer dementia), accounting for about 50–60% of cases; (2) atherosclerotic (multi-infarct) dementia, 15–20% of cases (this figure is probably low because of the tendency to overuse the diagnosis of Alzheimer dementia); and (3) mixtures of the first two types or dementia due to miscellaneous causes, 15–20% of cases (see also Chapter 4). Examples of primary degenerative dementia are Alzheimer dementia (most common) and Pick, Creutzfeldt-Jakob, and Huntington dementias (less common).

In all types, loss of impulse control (sexual and language) is common. The tenuous level of functioning makes the individual most susceptible to minor physical and psychological stresses. The course depends on the underlying cause, and the general trend is steady deterioration.

HIV infection can produce a primary neurogenic disorder (partially due to neuronal loss) and secondary effects due to opportunistic infections, neoplasias, or the effects of drug therapy. At present there has been a reduction in dementia symptoms in both early and late stages, perhaps due to earlier use of zidovudine. The general trend is variable, and patients require ongoing monitoring of neuropsychiatric status.

Pseudodementia is a term applied to depressed patients who appear to be demented. These patients are often identifiable by their tendency to complain about memory problems vociferously rather than try to cover them up. They usually say they can't complete cognitive tasks but with encouragement can often do so. They can be considered to have depression-induced reversible dementia that remits when the depression resolves.

C. Amnestic Syndrome

This is a memory disturbance without delirium or dementia. It is usually associated with thiamine deficiency and chronic alcohol use (eg, Korsakoff syndrome). There is an impairment in the ability to learn new information or recall previously learned information.

D. Substance-Induced Hallucinosis

This condition is characterized by persistent or recurrent hallucinations (usually auditory) without the other symptoms usually found in delirium or dementia. Alcohol or hallucinogens are often the cause. There does not have to be any other mental disorder, and there may be complete spontaneous resolution.

E. Personality Changes Due to a General Medical Condition (Formerly Organic Personality Syndrome)

This syndrome is characterized by emotional lability and loss of impulse control along with a general change in personality. Cognitive functions are preserved. Social inappropriateness is common. Loss of interest and lack of concern with the consequences of one's actions are often present. The course depends on the underlying cause (eg, frontal lobe contusion may resolve completely).

▶ Differential Diagnosis

The differential diagnosis consists mainly of schizophrenia and the other psychoses, which are sometimes confused with cognitive disorders and are often accompanied by psychotic symptoms.

▶ Complications

Chronicity may result from delayed correction of the defect, eg, subdural hematoma, low-pressure hydrocephalus. Accidents secondary to impulsive behavior and poor judgment are a major consideration. Secondary depression and impulsive behavior not infrequently lead to suicide attempts. Drugs—particularly sedatives—may worsen thinking abilities and contribute to the overall problems.

Treatment

(See also Chapter 4.)

A. Medical

Delirium should be considered a syndrome of acute brain dysfunction analogous to acute kidney failure. The first aim of treatment is to identify and correct the etiologic medical problem. Evaluation should consist of a comprehensive physical examination including a search for neurologic abnormalities, infection, or hypoxia. Routine laboratory tests may include serum electrolytes, serum glucose, BUN, serum creatinine, liver function tests, thyroid function tests, arterial blood gases, complete blood count, serum calcium, phosphorus, magnesium, vitamin B_{12}, folate, blood cultures, urinalysis, and cerebrospinal fluid analysis. Discontinue drugs that may be contributing to the problem (eg, analgesics, corticosteroids, cimetidine, lidocaine, anticholinergic drugs, central nervous system depressants, mefloquine). Do not overlook any possibility of reversible organic disease. Electroencephalography, CT, and MRI evaluations may be helpful in diagnosis. Ideally, the patient should be monitored without further medications while the evaluation is carried out. There are, however, two indications for medication in delirious states: behavioral control (eg, pulling out lines) and subjective distress (eg, pronounced fear due to hallucinations). If these indications are present, medications may be used. If there is any hint of alcohol or substance withdrawal (the most common cause of delirium in the general hospital), a benzodiazepine such as lorazepam (1–2 mg every hour) can be given parenterally. If there is little likelihood of withdrawal syndrome, haloperidol is often used in doses of 1–10 mg every hour. Given intravenously under ECG monitoring, it appears to impose slight risk of extrapyramidal side effects. In addition to the medication, a pleasant, comfortable, nonthreatening, and physically safe environment with adequate nursing or attendant services should be provided. Once the underlying condition has been identified and treated, adjunctive medications can be tapered.

Treatment of dementia syndrome usually involves symptomatic management with one exception. Since there is a cholinergic deficiency in Alzheimer disease, research has focused on drugs to increase cholinergic activity by inhibiting cholinesterase. Tacrine was the first reversible cholinesterase inhibitor approved by the FDA. Three better-tolerated FDA-approved cholinesterase inhibitors are donepezil (5–10 mg at night), rivastigmine (3–6 mg orally twice daily), and galantamine (8–12 mg orally twice daily). Donepezil and galantamine doses need adjustment for liver disease, and the galantamine dose should be adjusted for kidney failure. They are thought to be efficacious in the short-term preservation of cognitive function and activities of daily living in mild to moderate dementia and, unlike tacrine, are not thought to be hepatotoxic. Gastrointestinal side effects are common but may be least frequent with donepezil. Further research continues to clarify the long-term efficacy of these medications on cognition and behavior. None of the cholinesterase inhibitors to date are thought to slow disease progression. An N-methyl-D-aspartate (NMDA) receptor antagonist, memantine 20 mg orally daily (begin at 5 mg daily and titrate upwards by 5 mg weekly) is the first medication approved by the FDA for the treatment of moderate to severe Alzheimer disease. Memantine may improve performance and cognition in some patients and has been used as an augmenting agent with the cholinesterase inhibitors. Although not yet FDA approved, preliminary research suggests that the nonselective antihistamine dimebon may also improve cognition and function in patients with mild to moderate Alzheimer disease.

Aggressiveness and rage states in central nervous system disease can be reduced with lipophilic β-blockers (eg, propranolol, metoprolol) in moderate doses. Since the serotonergic system has been implicated in arousal conditions, drugs that affect serotonin have been found to be of some benefit in aggression and agitation. Included in this group are lithium, trazodone, buspirone, and clonazepam. Dopamine blockers (eg, the neuroleptic drugs such as haloperidol) have been used for many years to attenuate aggression. Atypical neuroleptics may have a role in selected geriatric patients; however, there are reports of increased mortality in some studies related to the use of atypical neuroleptics in this population. There are also reports of reduced agitation in Alzheimer disease from carbamazepine, 100–400 mg/d orally (with slow increase as needed). Emotional lability in some cases responds to small doses of imipramine (25 mg orally one to three times per day) or fluoxetine (5–20 mg/d orally); depression, which often occurs early in the course of Alzheimer dementia, responds to the usual doses of antidepressant drugs, preferably those with the least anticholinergic side effects (eg, SSRIs and MAO inhibitors).

Cerebral vasodilators were originally used on the assumption that cerebral arteriosclerosis and ischemia were the principal causes of the dementias. Although there is a slight reduction of blood flow in primary degenerative dementia (probably as a result of the basic disorder), there is no evidence that this is a major factor in this group of disorders or that vasodilators are of value. Ergotoxine alkaloids (ergoloid mesylates: Hydergine, others) have been studied with mixed results; improvement in ambulatory self-care and depressed mood has been noted, but there has been no improvement of cognitive functioning on any standardized tests. Hyperbaric oxygen treatment has not produced significant improvement. Stimulant drugs (eg, methylphenidate) do not change cognitive function but can improve affect and mood, which helps the caretakers cope with the problem.

Failing sensory functions should be supported as necessary, with hearing aids, cataract surgery, etc.

B. Social

Substitute home care, board and care, or convalescent home care may be most useful when the family is unable to care for the patient. The setting should include familiar people and objects, lights at night, and a simple schedule. Counseling may help the family to cope with problems and may help keep the patient at home as long as possible. Information about local groups can be obtained from the Alzheimer's Disease and Related Disorders Association, 70

East Lake Street, Suite 600, Chicago, IL 60601. Volunteer services, including homemakers, visiting nurses, and adult protective services, may be helpful in maintaining the patient at home.

C. Behavioral

Behavioral techniques include operant responses that can be used to induce positive behaviors, eg, paying attention to the patient who is trying to communicate appropriately, and extinction by ignoring inappropriate responses. Patients with Alzheimer disease can learn skills and retain them but do not recall the circumstances in which they were learned.

D. Psychological

Formal psychological therapies are not usually helpful and may make things worse by taxing the patient's limited cognitive resources.

▶ Prognosis

The prognosis is good for recovery of mental functioning in delirium when the underlying condition is reversible. For most dementia syndromes, the prognosis is for gradual deterioration, although new drug treatments may prove helpful.

Doody R et al. Effect of dimebon on cognition, activities of daily living, behavior, and global function in patients with mild-to-moderate Alzheimer's disease: a randomized, double-blind, placebo-controlled study. Lancet. 2008 Jul 19;372(9634):207–15. [PMID: 18640457]

McShane R et al. Memantine for dementia. Cochrane Database Syst Rev. 2006 Apr 19;(2):CD003154. [PMID: 16625572]

Schneider LS et al. Risk of death with atypical antipsychotic drug treatment for dementia: meta-analysis of randomized placebo-controlled trials. JAMA. 2005 Oct 19;294(15):1934–43. [PMID: 16234500]

PSYCHIATRIC PROBLEMS ASSOCIATED WITH HOSPITALIZATION & ILLNESS

▶ Diagnostic Categories

A. Acute Problems

1. Delirium with psychotic features secondary to the medical or surgical problem, or compounded by effect of treatment.
2. Acute anxiety, often related to ignorance and fear of the immediate problem as well as uncertainty about the future.
3. Anxiety as an intrinsic aspect of the medical problem (eg, hyperthyroidism).
4. Denial of illness, which may present during acute or intermediate phases of illness.

B. Intermediate Problems

1. Depression as a function of the illness or acceptance of the illness, often associated with realistic or fantasied hopelessness about the future.

2. Behavioral problems, often related to denial of illness and, in extreme cases, causing the patient to leave the hospital against medical advice.

C. Recuperative Problems

1. Decreasing cooperation as the patient sees improvement and compliance are not compelled.
2. Readjustment problems with family, job, and society.

▶ General Considerations

A. Acute Problems

1. "Intensive care unit psychosis"—The stressful ICU environment may be a cause of delirium. Critical care unit factors include sleep deprivation, increased arousal, mechanical ventilation, and social isolation. Other causes include those common to delirium and require vigorous investigation (see Delirium, above).

2. Pre- and postsurgical anxiety states—Such problems are common and commonly ignored. Presurgical anxiety is very common and is principally a fear of death (many surgical patients make out their wills). Patients may be fearful of anesthesia (improved by the preoperative anesthesia interview), the mysterious operating room, and the disease processes that might be uncovered by the surgeon. Such fears frequently cause people to delay examinations that might result in earlier surgery and a greater chance of cure.

The opposite of this is **surgery proneness**, the quest for surgery to escape from overwhelming life stresses. Polysurgery patients may be classified as having factitious disorders. Dynamic motivations include the need to get medical care as a way of getting dependency needs met, the desire to outwit authority figures, unconscious guilt, or a masochistic need to suffer. Frequent surgery may also be related to a somatoform disorder, particularly body dysmorphic disorder (an obsession that a body part is disfigured). More apparent reasons may include an attempt to get relief from pain and a lifestyle that has become almost exclusively medically oriented, with all of the risks entailed in such an endeavor.

Postsurgical anxiety states are usually related to pain, procedures, and loss of body image. Acute pain problems are quite different from chronic pain disorders (see Chronic Pain Disorders, this chapter); the former are readily handled with adequate analgesic medication (see Chapter 5). Alterations in body image, as with amputations, ostomies, and mastectomies, often raise concerns about relationships with others.

3. Iatrogenic problems—These usually pertain to medications, complications of diagnostic and treatment procedures, and impersonal and unsympathetic staff behavior. Polypharmacy is often a factor. Patients with unsolved diagnostic problems are at higher risk. They are desirous of relief, and the quest engenders more diagnostic procedures with a higher incidence of complications. The upset patient and family may be very demanding. Excessive demands usually result from anxiety. Such behavior is best handled with calm and measured responses.

B. Intermediate Problems

1. Prolonged hospitalization—Prolonged hospitalization presents unique problems in certain hospital services, eg, burn units, orthopedic services, and tuberculosis wards. The acute problems of the severely burned patient are discussed in Chapter 37. The problems often are behavioral difficulties related to length of hospitalization and necessary procedures. For example, in burn units, pain is a major problem in addition to anxiety about procedures. Disputes with staff are common and often concern pain medication or ward privileges. Some patients regress to infantile behavior and dependency. Staff members must agree about their approach to the patient in order to ensure the smooth functioning of the unit.

Denial of illness may present in some patients. Intervention by an authority figure (eg, immediate work supervisor) may help the patient accept treatment and eventually abandon the coping mechanism of denial.

2. Depression—Depression frequently occurs during this period. Therapeutic drugs (eg, corticosteroids) may be a factor. Depression can contribute to irritability and overt anger. Severe depression can lead to anorexia, which further complicates healing and metabolic balance. It is during this period that the issue of disfigurement arises—relief at survival gives way to concern about future function and appearance.

C. Recuperative Problems

1. Anxiety—Anxiety about return to the posthospital environment can cause regression to a dependent position. Complications increase, and staff forbearance again is tested. Anxiety occurring at this stage usually is handled more easily than previous behavior problems.

2. Posthospital adjustment—Adjustment difficulties after discharge are related to the severity of the deficits and the use of outpatient facilities (eg, physical therapy, rehabilitation programs, psychiatric outpatient treatment). Some patients may experience posttraumatic stress symptoms (eg, from traumatic injuries or even from necessary medical treatments). Lack of appropriate follow-up can contribute to depression in the patient, who may feel that he or she is making poor progress and may have thoughts of "giving up." Reintegration into work, educational, and social endeavors may be slow. Life is simply much more difficult when one is disfigured, disabled, or disenfranchised.

▶ Clinical Findings

The symptoms that occur in these patients are similar to those discussed in previous sections of this chapter, eg, delirium, stress and adjustment disorders, anxiety, and depression. Behavior problems may include lack of cooperation, increased complaints, demands for medication, sexual approaches to nurses, threats to leave the hospital, and actual signing out against medical recommendations. The underlying personality structure of the individual is a major factor in coping styles (eg, the compulsive individual increases indecision, the hysterical individual increases dramatic behavior).

▶ Differential Diagnosis

Delirium and dementia (including cases associated with HIV infection and drug abuse) must always be ruled out, since they often present with symptoms resembling anxiety, depression, or psychosis. Personality disorders existing prior to hospitalization often underlie the various behavior problems, but particularly the management problems.

▶ Complications

Prolongation of hospitalization causes increased expense, deterioration of patient-staff relationships, and increased probabilities of iatrogenic and legal problems. The possibility of increasing posthospital treatment problems is enhanced.

▶ Treatment

A. Medical

The most important consideration by far is to have one clinician in charge, a clinician whom the patient trusts and who is able to oversee multiple treatment approaches (see Somatoform Disorders, above). In acute problems, attention must be paid to metabolic imbalance, alcohol withdrawal, and previous drug use—prescribed, recreational, or over-the-counter. Adequate sleep and analgesia are important in the prevention of delirium. When absolute behavioral control is urgently needed, agents such as propofol, dexmedetomidine, opioids, and midazolam have been used.

Many clinicians are attuned to the early detection of the surgery-prone patient. Plastic and orthopedic surgeons are at particular risk. Appropriate consultations may help detect some problems and mitigate future ones.

Postsurgical anxiety states can be alleviated by personal attention from the surgeon. Anxiety is not so effectively lessened by ancillary medical personnel, whom the patient perceives as lesser authorities, until after the physician has reassured the patient. Inappropriate use of "as needed" analgesia places an unfair burden on the nurse. "Patient-controlled analgesia" can improve pain control, decrease anxiety, and minimize side effects.

Depression should be recognized early. If severe, it may be treated by antidepressant medications (see Antidepressant Drugs, above). High levels of anxiety can be lowered with judicious use of anxiolytic agents. Unnecessary medications tend to reinforce the patient's impression that there must be a serious illness or medication would not be required.

B. Psychological

Prepare the patient and family for what is to come. This includes the types of units where the patient will be quartered, the procedures that will be performed, and any disfigurements that will result from surgery. Repetition improves understanding. The nursing staff can be helpful, since patients frequently confide a lack of understanding to a nurse but are reluctant to do so to the physician.

Denial of illness is frequently a block to acceptance of treatment. This too should be handled with family members present (to help the patient face the reality of the situation) in a series of short interviews (for reinforcement). Dependency problems resulting from long hospitalization are best handled by focusing on the changes to come as the patient makes the transition to the outside world. Key figures are teachers, vocational counselors, and physical therapists. Challenges should be realistic and practical and handled in small steps.

Depression is usually related to the loss of familiar hospital supports, and the outpatient therapists and counselors help to lessen the impact of the loss. Some of the impact can be alleviated by anticipating, with the patient and family, the signal features of the common depression to help prevent the patient from assuming a permanent sick role (invalidism).

Suicide is always a concern when a patient is faced with despair. An honest, compassionate, and supportive approach will help sustain the patient during this trying period.

C. Behavioral

Prior desensitization can significantly allay anxiety about medical procedures. A "dry run" can be done to reinforce the oral description. Cooperation during acute problem periods can be enhanced by the use of appropriate reinforcers such as a favorite nurse or helpful family member. People who are positive reinforcers are even more helpful during the intermediate phases when the patient becomes resistant to the seemingly endless procedures (eg, debridement of burned areas).

Specific situations (eg, psychological dependency on the respirator) can be corrected by weaning with appropriate reinforcers (eg, watching a favorite movie on a video recorder when disconnected from the ventilator). Behavioral approaches should be used in a positive and optimistic way for maximal reinforcement.

Relaxation techniques and attentional distraction can be used to block side effects of a necessary treatment (eg, nausea in cancer chemotherapy).

D. Social

A change in environment requires adaptation. Because of the illness, admission and hospitalization may be more easily handled than discharge. Reintegration into society can be difficult. In some cases, the family is a negative influence. A predischarge evaluation must be made to determine whether the family will be able to cope with the physical or mental changes in the patient. Working with the family while the patient is in the acute stage may presage a successful transition later on.

Development of a new social life can be facilitated by various self-help organizations (eg, the stoma club). Sharing problems with others in similar circumstances eases the return to a social life, which may be quite different from that prior to the illness.

► Prognosis

The prognosis is good in all patients who have reversible medical and surgical conditions. It is guarded when there is serious functional loss that impairs vocational, educational, or societal possibilities—especially in the case of progressive and ultimately life-threatening illness.

Hogarth DK et al. Management of sedation in mechanically ventilated patients. Curr Opin Crit Care. 2004 Feb;10(1):40–6. [PMID: 15166848]

Katon W et al. Depression and diabetes: a potentially lethal combination. J Gen Intern Med. 2008 Oct;23(10):1571–5. [PMID: 18649108]

Whooley MA. Depression and cardiovascular disease: healing the broken hearted. JAMA. 2006 Jun 28;295(24):2874–81. [PMID: 16804154]

Endocrine Disorders

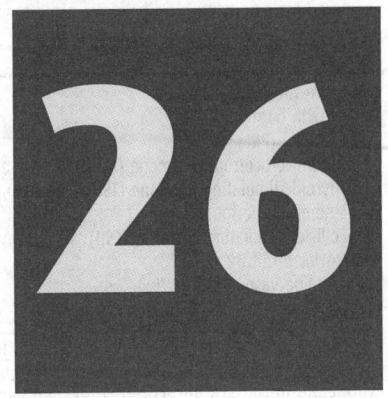

Paul A. Fitzgerald, MD

26

ANTERIOR HYPOPITUITARISM

ESSENTIALS OF DIAGNOSIS

▶ Loss of one, all, or any combination of anterior pituitary hormones.

▶ Adrenocorticotropic hormone deficiency reduces adrenal secretion of cortisol, testosterone, and epinephrine; aldosterone secretion remains intact.

▶ Growth hormone (GH) deficiency in children causes short stature; GH deficiency in adults causes asthenia, obesity, and increased cardiac mortality.

▶ Prolactin deficiency inhibits postpartum lactation.

▶ Thyroid-stimulating hormone deficiency causes secondary hypothyroidism.

▶ Luteinizing hormone and follicle-stimulating hormone deficiency cause hypogonadism and infertility in men and women.

▶ General Considerations

Hypopituitarism can be caused by either hypothalamic or pituitary dysfunction. Patients with hypopituitarism may have single or multiple hormonal deficiencies (Table 26–1). When one hormonal deficiency is discovered, others may be present.

Mass lesions causing hypopituitarism are commonly pituitary adenomas, which are usually sporadic but are sometimes part of multiple endocrine neoplasia type 1 (MEN 1). Pituitary tumors that arise in MEN 1 usually secrete prolactin (63%), GH (9%), or both (10%) and are more aggressive than sporadic adenomas. Other types of mass lesions include granulomas, Rathke cleft cysts, apoplexy, metastatic carcinomas, aneurysms, and brain tumors (craniopharyngioma, meningioma, germinoma, glioma, chondrosarcoma, chordoma of the clivus). Langerhans cell histiocytosis usually presents in youth with diabetes insipidus or hypopituitarism. Osteolytic bone lesions are noted on radiographs. Autoimmune hypophysitis, postpartum pituitary necrosis (Sheehan syndrome), eclampsia–preeclampsia, sickle cell disease, and African trypanosomiasis are rare causes.

Hypopituitarism without mass lesions may be congenital malformations in syndromes such as septo-optic dysplasia (de Morsier syndrome). Hypopituitarism may also be caused by trauma, cranial radiation, surgery, encephalitis, hemochromatosis, autoimmunity, or stroke. It may also occur after coronary artery bypass grafting. At least one pituitary hormone deficiency develops in about 25–30% of survivors of moderate to severe traumatic brain injury (Glasgow Coma Scale ≤ 13/15) and in about 55% of survivors of aneurysmal subarachnoid hemorrhage.

Kallmann syndrome is the most common cause of congenital isolated gonadotropin deficiency. It is usually sporadic but may be familial. Three different genetic inheritance patterns can occur: X-linked recessive (Kal 1), autosomal dominant (Kal 2), or autosomal recessive (Kal 3). Kallmann syndrome has an incidence of 1:10,000 males and 1:50,000 females. It is associated with hyposmia caused by hypoplasia of the olfactory bulbs. Another cause of congenital gonadotropin deficiency is congenital adrenal hypoplasia that can be caused by *DAX 1* gene mutations. Congenital hypopituitarism also develops in patients with *PROP 1* gene mutations.

▶ Clinical Findings

Manifestations of hypopituitarism vary depending on which specific hormones are lacking and whether their deficiency is partial or complete.

A. Symptoms and Signs

Gonadotropin deficiency includes loss of luteinizing hormone (LH) and follicle-stimulating hormone (FSH), which causes hypogonadism and infertility. This condition is also known as hypogonadotropic hypogonadism and may be associated with anosmia (Kallmann syndrome) or normal olfaction. In Kallmann syndrome, about 50% of patients have unilateral renal agenesis; some patients may

Table 26–1. Pituitary hormones.

Anterior pituitary
Growth hormone (GH)[1]
Prolactin (PRL)
Adrenocorticotropic hormone (ACTH)
Thyroid-stimulating hormone (TSH)
Luteinizing hormone (LH)[2]
Follicle-stimulating hormone (FSH)
Posterior pituitary
Arginine vasopressin (AVP)[3]
Oxytocin

[1]GH closely resembles human placental lactogen (hPL).
[2]LH closely resembles human chorionic gonadotropin (hCG).
[3]AVP is identical with antidiuretic hormone (ADH).

also exhibit cryptorchidism, sensorineural deafness, cerebellar dysfunction, bilateral synkinesis, nystagmus, cleft lip, or high-arched palate. Patients with isolated gonadotropin deficiency may seek medical attention for delayed adolescence. (See also discussion of primary amenorrhea.) Congenital gonadotropin deficiency in males may be associated with congenital micropenis or cryptorchidism.

Hypogonadotropic hypogonadism is also seen in patients with *congenital adrenal hypoplasia*, a rare autosomal recessive or X-linked disorder; the X-linked form is caused by a mutation in the *DAX 1* gene. Adrenal insufficiency, caused by failure to form the permanent zone of the adrenal cortex, can present during infancy or childhood in boys with *DAX 1* gene mutations. Boys who survive beyond childhood usually do not enter puberty as a result of hypogonadotropic hypogonadism. However, hypogonadotropic hypogonadism and subtle signs of adrenal failure can present in adulthood in males with partial loss-of-function mutations in *DAX 1*.

In *acquired* gonadotropin deficiency, both men and women lose axillary, pubic, and body hair gradually, particularly if they are also hypoadrenal. Men may note diminished beard growth. Libido is diminished. Women have amenorrhea; men note decreased erections. Most patients are infertile. Androgen deficiency predisposes patients to osteopenia and muscle atrophy. (See section on secondary amenorrhea.)

Thyroid-stimulating hormone (TSH) deficiency causes hypothyroidism with manifestations such as fatigue, weakness, weight change, and hyperlipidemia. (See Hypothyroidism and Myxedema.)

Adrenocorticotropic hormone (ACTH) deficiency results in diminished cortisol secretion (see Adrenocortical Hypofunction). Symptoms may include weakness, fatigue, weight loss, and hypotension. Patients with partial ACTH deficiency continue to have some cortisol secretion and may not have symptoms until stressed by illness or surgery. Adrenal mineralocorticoid secretion continues, so manifestations of adrenal insufficiency in hypopituitarism are usually less striking than in bilateral adrenal gland destruction (Addison disease); hyponatremia may occur, especially when ACTH and TSH deficiencies are both present.

GH deficiency in adulthood tends to cause mild to moderate central obesity, increased systolic blood pressure,

increased low-density lipoprotein (LDL) cholesterol, and reduced cardiac output. Affected patients may also have reduced muscle and bone mass, reduced physical and mental energy, impaired concentration and memory, and depression. Laron syndrome is an autosomal recessive disorder that is mainly associated with mutations in GH receptor gene. This causes resistance to GH and severe IGF-I deficiency, resulting in short stature (dwarfism). Affected individuals have a prominent forehead, depressed nasal bridge, small mandible, and central obesity. They may have recurrent hypoglycemic seizures. Partial resistance to GH may cause some cases of idiopathic short stature without features of Laron syndrome.

Panhypopituitarism is the absence of all anterior pituitary hormones. Combined pituitary hormone deficiency (CPHD) refers to a deficiency of several anterior pituitary hormones. CPHD gradually develops in patients with *PROP 1* gene mutations, usually presenting with short stature and growth failure due to GH and TSH deficiency; lack of pubertal development occurs due to deficiencies in FSH and LH. ACTH-cortisol deficiency gradually develops in patients with *PROP 1* gene mutations; these patients typically require corticosteroid replacement therapy by age 18 years. In addition to the manifestations noted above, patients with long-standing hypopituitarism tend to have dry, pale, finely textured skin. The face has fine wrinkles and an apathetic countenance.

B. Laboratory Findings

The fasting blood glucose may be low. Hyponatremia is often present due to hypothyroidism or hypoadrenalism. Hyperkalemia usually does not occur, since aldosterone production is not affected.

For men, an accurate serum total testosterone measurement must be obtained with an assay that uses extraction and chromatography, followed by mass spectrometry or immunoassay. For older men, free testosterone is best measured by calculation, using accurate assays for testosterone and sex hormone binding globulin (SHBG). Serum gonadotropins (FSH and LH) are obtained if the serum testosterone is low in order to distinguish primary hypogonadism from pituitary dysfunction.

The free thyroxine (FT$_4$) level is low, and TSH is not elevated. Plasma levels of sex steroids (testosterone and estradiol) are low or low normal, as are the serum gonadotropins as well. Elevated prolactin (PRL) levels are found in patients with prolactinomas, acromegaly, and hypothalamic disease.

ACTH deficiency causes functional atrophy of the adrenal cortex within 2 weeks of pituitary damage. Therefore, the diagnosis of secondary hypoadrenalism may be confirmed by holding any corticosteroid medication on the day of the test and by administering cosyntropin (synthetic ACTH$_{1-24}$), 0.25 mg (intramuscularly or intravenously); blood is drawn 30–60 minutes after the injection. A serum cortisol of ≥ 20 mcg/dL (550 nmol/mL), random or stimulated, rules out the diagnosis. A baseline ACTH level is low or normal in secondary hypoadrenalism, distinguishing it from primary adrenal disease. Serum dehydroepiandrosterone (DHEA) levels are low in patients with ACTH deficiency, helping confirm the diagnosis. Metyrapone testing is unnecessary.

Deficiency of epinephrine occurs with secondary adrenal insufficiency, since high local concentrations of cortisol are required to induce the production of the enzyme phenylethanolamine *N*-methyltransferase (PNMT) that catalyzes the conversion of norepinephrine to epinephrine in the adrenal medulla.

The diagnosis of GH deficiency is difficult since normal GH secretion is pulsatile and serum GH levels are nearly undetectable for most of the day. Also, adults normally tend to produce less GH as they age. Therefore, GH deficiency is often inferred by symptoms of GH deficiency in the presence of pituitary destruction or other pituitary hormone deficiencies. GH deficiency is present in 96% of patients with three or more other pituitary hormone deficiencies. GH stimulates the production of insulin-like growth factor-I (IGF-I). Unfortunately, serum IGF-I is not sensitive for GH deficiency since IGF-I levels are in the normal range in about 50% of adults with GH deficiency. Low serum IGF-I levels are not specific for GH deficiency. However, very low levels of IGF-I (< 84 mcg/L) are indicative of GH deficiency, except in conditions that naturally suppress serum IGF-I (eg, malnutrition, prolonged fasting, oral estrogen, hypothyroidism, uncontrolled diabetes mellitus, liver failure). In GH deficiency, exercise-stimulated serum GH levels remain at < 5 ng/mL and usually fail to rise; however, by age 40 years, most normal adults have lost their GH response to exercise.

Provocative GH-stimulation tests are commonly used but are poor tests for GH deficiency. The insulin hypoglycemia test, long considered the "gold standard," is insensitive; it is contraindicated in the elderly, in patients with cardiovascular or cerebrovascular disease, and in patients with any history of seizures, an abnormal electroencephalogram (EEG), or recent brain surgery. Other GH stimulation tests require the administration of intravenous arginine and growth hormone–releasing hormone (GHRH) and oral clonidine or carbidopa/levodopa (combination) in patients pretreated with propranolol or estrogen. However, these tests do not discriminate well between normal individuals and patients with presumed GH deficiency (patients with three or more other pituitary hormone deficiencies). Also, normal overweight adults (body mass index [BMI] ≥ 25 kg/m^2) typically have blunted peak GH levels (below 20 ng/mL) after arginine-GHRH administration.

Despite the limitations of intravenous GHRH/arginine sulfhydryl stimulation testing, some insurance companies insist that patients have an abnormal test before covering the costs of GH replacement therapy. However, the latter test has a sensitivity of only 66% for GH deficiency. Therefore, when patients have a serum insulin-like growth factor (IGF-I) < 84 mcg/L or three other pituitary hormone deficiencies, the likelihood of GH deficiency is so high that symptomatic patients should have a therapeutic trial of GH therapy, even with a "normal" stimulation test.

The differential diagnosis of GH deficiency is congenital GH resistance with deficiency of IGF-I; at its worst, IGF-I deficiency results in Laron dwarfism that is resistant to GH therapy.

Because hemochromatosis can cause hypopituitarism, in patients with hypopituitarism without an established etiology, it is prudent to screen for hemochromatosis with a serum iron and transferrin saturation or ferritin.

C. Imaging

MRI provides the best visualization of pituitary tumors. Thickening of the pituitary stalk can be caused by sarcoidosis or hypophysitis.

▶ Differential Diagnosis

Reversible hypogonadotropic hypogonadism may occur with serious illness, malnutrition, or anorexia nervosa. The clinical situation and the presence of normal adrenal and thyroid function allow ready distinction from hypopituitarism. Profound hypogonadotropic hypogonadism develops in men who receive gonadotropin-releasing hormone (GnRH) therapy for prostate cancer; it usually persists following cessation of therapy. Hypogonadotropic hypogonadism usually develops in patients receiving high-dose methadone or chronic intrathecal infusion of opioids; both GH deficiency and secondary adrenal insufficiency occur in 15% of such patients. Secondary adrenal insufficiency may persist for many months following high-dose corticosteroid therapy.

Severe illness causes functional suppression of TSH and T$_4$. Hyperthyroxinemia reversibly suppresses TSH. Administration of triiodothyronine (Cytomel) suppresses TSH and T$_4$. Bexarotene, used to treat cutaneous T cell lymphoma, suppresses TSH secretion, resulting in temporary central hypothyroidism. Corticosteroids or megestrol treatment reversibly suppresses endogenous ACTH and cortisol secretion.

▶ Complications

Among patients with craniopharyngiomas, diabetes insipidus is found in 16% preoperatively and in 60% postoperatively. Hyponatremia often presents abruptly during the first 2 weeks following pituitary surgery. Visual field impairment may occur. Hypothalamic damage may result in morbid obesity as well as cognitive and emotional problems. Conventional radiation therapy results in an increased incidence of small vessel ischemic strokes and second tumors.

Patients with untreated hypoadrenalism and a stressful illness may become febrile and die in shock and coma.

Adults with GH deficiency have experienced an increased cardiovascular morbidity. Rarely, acute hemorrhage may occur in large pituitary tumors, manifested by rapid loss of vision, headache, and evidence of acute pituitary failure (pituitary apoplexy) requiring emergency decompression of the sella.

▶ Treatment

Transsphenoidal removal of pituitary tumors will sometimes reverse hypopituitarism. Postoperative hyponatremia often occurs; serum sodium must be checked frequently for 2 weeks after pituitary surgery. Hypogonadism due to PRL excess usually resolves during treatment with dopamine agonists. Endocrine substitution therapy must be given before, during, and, often, permanently after such procedures.

GH-secreting tumors may respond to octreotide (see section on acromegaly). Radiation therapy with x-ray, gamma knife, or heavy particles may be necessary but increases the likelihood of hypopituitarism.

The mainstay of substitution therapy for pituitary insufficiency remains lifetime hormone replacement.

A. Corticosteroids

Hydrocortisone tablets, 15–35 mg/d orally in divided doses, should be given. Most patients do well with 10-20 mg in the morning and 5–15 mg in the late afternoon. Patients with partial ACTH deficiency (basal morning serum cortisol above 8 mg/dL [220 mmol/L]) require hydrocortisone replacement in lower doses of about 5 mg orally twice daily. Some patients feel better taking prednisone, 3–7.5 mg/d orally. A mineralocorticoid is rarely needed. To determine the optimal corticosteroid replacement dosage, it is necessary to monitor patients carefully for manifestations of overreplacement (Cushing syndrome) or underreplacement. A serum white blood cell count (WBC) with a relative differential can be useful, since a relative neutrophilia and lymphopenia can indicate overreplacement with corticosteroid, and vice versa. Additional corticosteroids must be given during states of stress, eg, during infection, trauma, or surgical procedures. For mild illness, corticosteroid doses are doubled or tripled. For trauma or surgical stress, hydrocortisone is given in doses of 50 mg intramuscularly or intravenously every 6 hours and then reduced to normal doses as the stress subsides. Patients with adrenal insufficiency are advised to wear a medical alert bracelet describing their condition and treatment.

Patients with secondary adrenal insufficiency due to treatment with corticosteroids at supraphysiologic doses require their usual daily dose of corticosteroid during surgery and acute illness; supplemental hydrocortisone is not usually required.

B. Thyroid

Levothyroxine is given to correct hypothyroidism only after the patient is assessed for cortisol deficiency or is already receiving corticosteroids. (See Hypothyroidism.) The typical maintenance dose is about 1.6 mcg/kg body weight. However, dosage requirements vary widely, averaging 125 mcg daily with a range of 25–300 mcg daily. The optimal replacement dose of thyroxine for each patient must be carefully assessed clinically on an individual basis. Serum FT_4 levels usually need to be in the high-normal range for adequate replacement. Assessment of serum TSH is useless for monitoring patients, since levels are always low with TSH deficiency.

C. Sex Hormones

Hypogonadotropic hypogonadism often develops in patients with hyperprolactinemia; it may be reversed with treatment of the hyperprolactinemia. (See Hyperprolactinemia.)

Androgen replacement is discussed in the section on male hypogonadism. Estrogen replacement is discussed in the section on female hypogonadism. Patients with idiopathic hypogonadotropic hypogonadism, who have received several years of hormone replacement therapy, may have a trial off hormonal therapy to assess whether spontaneous sexual maturation may have occurred.

Women with hypopituitarism and androgen deficiency may be treated with compounded DHEA in doses of about 50 mg/d orally. DHEA therapy tends to increase pubic and axillary hair and may modestly improve libido, alertness, stamina, and overall psychological well-being after 6 months of therapy.

To improve spermatogenesis, human chorionic gonadotropin (hCG) (equivalent to LH) may be given at a dosage of 2000–3000 units intramuscularly three times weekly and testosterone replacement is discontinued. The dose of hCG is adjusted to normalize serum testosterone levels. After 6–12 months of hCG treatment, if the sperm count remains low, hCG injections are continued along with injections of FSH: follitropin-β (synthetic recombinant FSH) or urofollitropins (urine-derived FSH). An alternative for patients with an intact pituitary (eg, Kallmann syndrome) is the use of leuprolide (GnRH analog) by intermittent subcutaneous infusion. With either treatment, testicular volumes double within 5–12 months, and spermatogenesis occurs in most cases. With persistent treatment and the help of intracytoplasmic sperm injection for some cases, the total pregnancy success rate is about 70%. Clomiphene, 25–50 mg orally daily, can sometimes stimulate a man's own pituitary gonadotropins (when his pituitary is intact), thereby increasing testosterone and sperm production.

For fertility induction in females, ovulation may be induced with clomiphene, 50 mg daily for 5 days every 2 months. Follitropins and hCG can induce multiple births and should be used only by those experienced with their administration. (See Hypogonadism.)

D. Human Growth Hormone (hGH)

Symptomatic adults with severe GH deficiency (serum IGF-I below 85 mcg/L) may be treated with a subcutaneous recombinant human growth hormone (rhGH) injection starting at a dosage of about 0.2 mg (0.6 international units)/day, administered three or four times weekly. The dosage of rhGH is increased every 2–4 weeks by increments of 0.1 mg (0.3 international units) until side effects occur or a sufficient salutary response and a normal serum IGF-I level are achieved. A sustained-release injectable suspension of depot GH is available (Nutropin Depot). It can be given twice monthly and is therefore more convenient than standard rhGH preparations. In a study of 20 Brazilian GH-deficient adults, depot GH, given in doses of 13.5 mg subcutaneously twice monthly over 6 months, improved body morphology and lipid profiles but was associated with an increase in carotid plaque. Therefore, more long-term studies are required to determine the safety and optimal dosing and method for administering GH to adults. If the desired effects (eg, improved energy and mentation, reduction in visceral adiposity) are not seen within 3–6 months at maximum tolerated dosage, rhGH therapy is discontinued.

During pregnancy, rhGH may be safely administered to women with hypopituitarism at their usual pregestational dose during the first trimester, tapering the dose during the second trimester, and discontinuing rhGH during the third trimester.

Oral estrogen replacement reduces hepatic IGF-I production. Therefore, prior to commencing rhGH therapy, oral estrogen is changed to a transdermal or transvaginal estradiol.

Side effects of rhGH therapy may include peripheral edema, hand stiffness, arthralgias, myalgias, headache, pseudotumor cerebri, gynecomastia, carpal tunnel syndrome, tarsal tunnel syndrome, hypertension, and proliferative retinopathy. Side effects are more common in older patients, those with greater weight and higher BMI, and those with adult-onset GH deficiency. Such symptoms usually remit promptly after a sufficient reduction in dosage. Excessive doses of rhGH could cause acromegaly; patients receiving long-term therapy require careful clinical monitoring. Serum IGF-I levels should be kept in the normal range and periodic determinations of serum IGF-I levels are helpful in guiding therapeutic dosing.

GH should not be administered during critical illness since, in one study, administration of very high doses of rhGH to patients in an intensive care unit was shown to increase overall mortality. There is no role for GH replacement in the somatopause of aging.

IGF-I (mecasermin) is available to treat patients with Laron syndrome.

E. Other Treatment

Selective transsphenoidal resection of pituitary adenomas can often restore normal pituitary function. Cabergoline, bromocriptine, or quinagolide may reverse the hypogonadism seen in hyperprolactinomas. (See Disorders of Prolactin Secretion.) Disseminated Langerhans cell histiocytosis may be treated with bisphosphonates to improve bone pain; treatment with 2-chlorodeoxyadenosine (cladribine) has been reported to produce remissions.

▶ Prognosis

The prognosis depends on the primary cause. Hypopituitarism resulting from a pituitary tumor may be reversible with dopamine agonists or with careful selective resection of the tumor. Spontaneous recovery from hypopituitarism associated with pituitary stalk thickening has been reported. Patients can also recover from functional hypopituitarism, eg, hypogonadism due to starvation or severe illness, suppression of ACTH by corticosteroids, or suppression of TSH by hyperthyroidism. Spontaneous reversal of isolated idiopathic hypogonadotropic hypogonadism occurs in about 10% of patients after several years of hormone replacement therapy.

Functionally, most patients with hypopituitarism do very well with hormone replacement. Men with infertility who are treated with hCG/FSH or GnRH are likely to resume spermatogenesis if they have a history of sexual maturation, descended testicles, and a baseline serum inhibin level over 60 pg/mL. Women under age 40 years, with infertility due to hypogonadotropic hypogonadism, can usually have successful induction of ovulation.

Abrams P et al. Growth hormone replacement in hypopituitarism improves lipid profile and quality of life independently of changes in obesity variables. Eur J Endocrinol. 2008 Dec;159(6):825–32. [PMID: 18713841]

Agha A et al. The long-term predictive accuracy of the short synacthen (corticotropin) stimulation test for assessment of the hypothalamic-pituitary-adrenal axis. J Clin Endocrinol Metab. 2006 Jan;91(1):43–7. [PMID: 16249286]

Brooke AM et al. Dehydroepiandrosterone improves psychological well-being in male and female hypopituitary patients on maintenance growth hormone replacement. J Clin Endocrinol Metab. 2006 Oct;91(10):3773–9. [PMID: 16849414]

Raivio T et al. Reversal of idiopathic hypogonadotropic hypogonadism. N Engl J Med. 2007 Aug 30;357(9):863–73. [PMID: 17761590]

Schneider HJ et al. Hypopituitarism. Lancet. 2007 Apr 28;369 (9571):1461–70. [PMID: 17467517]

Schneider HJ et al. Hypothalamopituitary dysfunction following traumatic brain injury and aneurysmal subarachnoid hemorrhage: a systematic review. JAMA. 2007 Sep 26;298(12):1429–38. [PMID: 17895459]

DIABETES INSIPIDUS

 ESSENTIALS OF DIAGNOSIS

▶ Antidiuretic hormone (ADH) deficiency causes central diabetes insipidus with polyuria (2–20 L/d) and polydipsia.

▶ Hypernatremia occurs if fluid intake is inadequate.

▶ General Considerations

Diabetes insipidus is an uncommon disease characterized by an increase in thirst and the passage of large quantities of urine of low specific gravity (usually < 1.006 with ad libitum fluid intake). The urine is otherwise normal. It is caused by a deficiency of vasopressin or resistance to vasopressin.

Primary central diabetes insipidus (without an identifiable lesion noted on MRI of the pituitary and hypothalamus) accounts for about one-third of all cases of diabetes insipidus. Many such cases appear to be due to autoimmunity against hypothalamic arginine vasopressin (AVP)-secreting cells; pituitary stalk thickening can often be detected on pituitary MRI scanning. The cause may also be genetic. Familial diabetes insipidus occurs as a dominant genetic trait with symptoms developing at about 2 years of age. Diabetes insipidus also occurs in Wolfram syndrome, a rare autosomal recessive disorder that is also known by the acronym DIDMOAD (diabetes insipidus, type 1 diabetes mellitus, optic atrophy, and deafness). DIDMOAD manifestations usually present in childhood but may not occur until adulthood, along with depression and cognitive problems. **Secondary central diabetes insipidus** is due to damage to the hypothalamus or pituitary stalk by tumor, hypophysitis, anoxic encephalopathy, surgical or accidental trauma, infection (eg, encephalitis, tuberculosis, syphilis), sarcoidosis, or multifocal Langerhans cell (eosinophilic) granulomatosis ("histiocytosis X"). Metastases to the pituitary are more likely to cause diabetes insipidus (33%) than are pituitary adenomas (1%).

Vasopressinase-induced diabetes insipidus may be seen in the last trimester of pregnancy and in the puerperium; it is often associated with oligohydramnios, preeclampsia, or hepatic dysfunction. A circulating enzyme destroys native vasopressin; however, synthetic desmopressin is unaffected. The condition usually responds to desmopressin therapy (see below) and subsides spontaneously.

Nephrogenic diabetes insipidus is a disorder caused by a defect in the kidney tubules that interferes with water reabsorption. These patients have normal secretion of vasopressin, and the polyuria is unresponsive to it. Congenital nephrogenic diabetes insipidus is present from birth and is due to defective expression of renal vasopressin V2 receptors or vasopressin-sensitive water channels. It occurs as a familial X-linked trait; adults often have hyperuricemia as well.

Acquired forms of vasopressin-resistant diabetes insipidus are usually less severe and are seen in pyelonephritis, renal amyloidosis, myeloma, potassium depletion, Sjögren syndrome, sickle cell anemia, or chronic hypercalcemia. The disorder may occur also as a corticosteroid effect or as an acute side effect of diuretics. Certain drugs (eg, demeclocycline, lithium, foscarnet, or methicillin) may induce nephrogenic diabetes insipidus. The recovery from acute tubular necrosis may also be associated with transient nephrogenic diabetes insipidus. (See Kidney Disorders.)

Clinical Findings

A. Symptoms and Signs

The symptoms of the disease are intense thirst, especially with a craving for ice water, and polyuria, the volume of ingested fluid varying from 2 L to 20 L daily, with correspondingly large urine volumes. Partial diabetes insipidus presents with less intense symptoms and should be suspected in patients with unremitting enuresis. Most patients with diabetes insipidus are able to maintain fluid balance by continuing to ingest large volumes of water. However, diabetes insipidus may present with hypernatremia and dehydration in patients without free access to water, or with a damaged hypothalamic thirst center and altered thirst sensation. Diabetes insipidus is aggravated by administration of high-dose corticosteroids, which increases renal free water clearance.

B. Laboratory Findings

The diagnosis of diabetes insipidus as a cause of polyuria or hypernatremia requires clinical judgment. There is no single diagnostic laboratory test. Evaluation for diabetes insipidus should include an accurate 24-hour urine collection that is measured for volume and creatinine. A urine volume of < 2 L/24 h (in the absence of hypernatremia) essentially rules out diabetes insipidus. Serum is assayed for glucose, urea nitrogen, calcium, potassium, sodium, and uric acid. Hyperuricemia occurs in many patients with diabetes insipidus, since reduced vasopressin stimulation of the renal V1 receptor causes a reduction in the renal tubular clearance of urate.

A supervised "vasopressin challenge test" may be given: Desmopressin acetate is given in an initial dose of 0.05–0.1 mL (5–10 mcg) intranasally (or 1 mcg subcutaneously or intravenously), with measurement of urine volume for 12 hours before and 12 hours after administration. Serum sodium must be obtained immediately in the event of symptoms of hyponatremia. The dosage of desmopressin is doubled if the response is marginal. Patients with central diabetes insipidus notice a distinct reduction in thirst and polyuria; serum sodium stays normal except in some salt-losing conditions.

In **nonfamilial central diabetes insipidus**, MRI of the pituitary and hypothalamus and of the skull is done to look for mass lesions. The pituitary stalk may be thickened, which may be a manifestation of Langerhans cell histiocytosis, sarcoidosis, or lymphocytic hypophysitis. When **nephrogenic diabetes insipidus** is a diagnostic consideration, measurement of serum vasopressin is done during modest fluid restriction; typically, the vasopressin level is high.

Differential Diagnosis

Central diabetes insipidus must be distinguished from polyuria caused by diabetes mellitus, Cushing syndrome or corticosteroid treatment, lithium, hypercalcemia, hypokalemia, and the nocturnal polyuria of Parkinson disease. It must also be distinguished from nephrogenic diabetes insipidus (see above), psychogenic polydipsia, central nervous system sarcoidosis, and intravenous fluid administration.

Complications

If water is not readily available, the excessive output of urine will lead to severe dehydration. Patients with an impaired thirst mechanism are very prone to hypernatremia, particularly since they usually also have impaired mentation and forget to take their desmopressin. All the complications of the primary disease may eventually become evident. In patients who are receiving desmopressin acetate therapy, there is a danger of induced water intoxication.

Treatment

Mild cases of diabetes insipidus require no treatment other than adequate fluid intake. Reduction of aggravating factors (eg, corticosteroids, which directly increase renal free water clearance) will improve polyuria.

Desmopressin acetate is the treatment of choice for central diabetes insipidus. It is also useful in diabetes insipidus associated with pregnancy or the puerperium, since desmopressin is resistant to degradation by the circulating vasopressinase.

Desmopressin is available as an oral preparation (0.1 or 0.2 mg tablets) that is given in a starting dose of 0.05 mg twice daily and increased to a maximum of 0.4 mg every 8 hours, if required. Oral desmopressin is particularly useful for patients with sinusitis from the nasal preparation.

Gastrointestinal symptoms, asthenia, and mild increases in hepatic enzymes can occur with the oral preparation.

The nasal preparation (100 mcg/mL solution) is given every 12–24 hours as needed for thirst and polyuria. It may be administered via metered-dose nasal inhaler containing 0.1 mL/spray or via a plastic calibrated tube. The starting dose is 0.05–0.1 mL every 12–24 hours, and the dose is then individualized according to response. Nasal desmopressin may cause nasal irritation.

Desmopressin is also available as a parenteral preparation containing 4 mcg/mL. For central diabetes insipidus, it is given intravenously, intramuscularly, or subcutaneously in doses of 1–4 mcg every 12–24 hours as needed to treat thirst or hypernatremia.

All desmopressin preparations may cause hyponatremia, which is uncommon if minimum effective doses are used and the patient allows thirst to occur periodically. All preparations of desmopression can sometimes cause emotional changes, such as depression or agitation; erythromelalgia occurs rarely. All desmopression preparations, including tablets, are subject to heat degradation and should be refrigerated.

Both central and nephrogenic diabetes insipidus respond partially to hydrochlorothiazide, 50–100 mg/d orally (with potassium supplement or amiloride). Nephrogenic diabetes insipidus may respond to combined treatments of indomethacin-hydrochlorothiazide, indomethacin-desmopressin, or indomethacin-amiloride. Indomethacin, 50 mg orally every 8 hours, is effective in acute cases.

Psychotherapy is required for most patients with psychogenic polydipsia. Thioridazine and lithium are best avoided if psychiatric drug therapy is needed, since they cause polyuria.

Prognosis

Central diabetes insipidus appearing after pituitary surgery usually remits after days to weeks but may be permanent if the upper pituitary stalk is cut.

Chronic central diabetes insipidus is ordinarily more an inconvenience than a dire medical condition. Treatment with desmopressin allows normal sleep and activity. Hypernatremia can occur, especially when the thirst center is damaged, but diabetes insipidus does not otherwise reduce life expectancy, and the prognosis is that of the underlying disorder.

Loh JA et al. Disorders of water and salt metabolism associated with pituitary disease. Endocrinol Metab Clin North Am. 2008 Mar;37(1):213–234. [PMID: 18226738]

Makaryus AN et al. Diabetes insipidus: diagnosis and treatment of a complex disease. Cleve Clin J Med. 2006 Jan;73(1):65–71. [PMID: 16444918]

ACROMEGALY & GIGANTISM

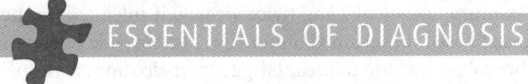

ESSENTIALS OF DIAGNOSIS

▶ Excessive growth of hands, feet, jaw, and internal organs; or gigantism before closure of epiphyses.

▶ Amenorrhea, headaches, visual field loss, weakness.

▶ Soft, doughy, sweaty handshake.

▶ Elevated IGF-I.

▶ Serum GH not suppressed following oral glucose.

General Considerations

GH exerts much of its growth-promoting effects by stimulating the release of IGF-I from the liver and other tissues.

Acromegaly is nearly always caused by a pituitary adenoma. These tumors may be locally invasive, particularly into the cavernous sinus. Less than 1% are malignant. Most are macroadenomas (over 1 cm in diameter). Acromegaly is usually sporadic but may rarely be familial. The disease may also be associated with endocrine tumors of the parathyroids or pancreas (MEN 1). Acromegaly may also be seen in McCune–Albright syndrome and as part of Carney syndrome (atrial myxoma, acoustic neuroma, lentigines, adrenal hypercortisolism). Acromegaly is rarely caused by ectopic secretion of GHRH or GH secreted by a lymphoma, hypothalamic tumor, bronchial carcinoid, or pancreatic tumor.

Clinical Findings

A. Symptoms and Signs

Excessive GH causes tall stature and gigantism if it occurs in youth, before closure of epiphyses. Afterward, acromegaly develops. The term "acromegaly," meaning extremity enlargement, seriously understates the manifestations. The hands enlarge and a doughy, moist handshake is characteristic. The fingers widen, causing patients to enlarge their rings. Carpal tunnel syndrome is common. The feet also grow, particularly in shoe width. Facial features coarsen since the bones and sinuses of the skull enlarge; hat size increases. The mandible becomes more prominent, causing prognathism and malocclusion. Tooth spacing widens.

Macroglossia occurs, as does hypertrophy of pharyngeal and laryngeal tissue; this causes a deep, coarse voice and sometimes makes intubation difficult. Obstructive sleep apnea may occur. A goiter may be noted. Hypertension (50%) and cardiomegaly are common. At diagnosis, about 10% of acromegalic patients have overt heart failure, with a dilated left ventricle and a reduced ejection fraction. Weight gain is typical, particularly of muscle and bone. Insulin resistance is usually present and frequently causes diabetes mellitus (30%). Arthralgias and degenerative arthritis occur. Overgrowth of vertebral bone can cause spinal stenosis. Colon polyps are common, especially in patients with skin papillomas. The skin may also manifest hyperhidrosis, thickening, cystic acne, skin tags, and areas of acanthosis nigricans.

GH-secreting pituitary tumors usually cause some degree of hypogonadism, either by cosecretion of PRL or by direct pressure upon normal pituitary tissue. Decreased libido and impotence are common, as are irregular menses or amenorrhea. Secondary hypothyroidism sometimes occurs; hypoadrenalism is unusual. Headaches are frequent.

Temporal hemianopia may occur as a result of the optic chiasm being impinged by a suprasellar growth of the tumor.

B. Laboratory Findings

For screening purposes, a random serum IGF-I can be obtained. If it is normal for age, acromegaly is ruled out. For further evaluation, the patient should be fasting for at least 8 hours (except for water), not acutely ill, and should not have exercised on the day of testing. Assay for the following: IGF-I (increased to over five times normal in most acromegalic patients), PRL (cosecreted by many GH-secreting tumors), glucose (diabetes is common in acromegaly), liver enzymes and blood urea nitrogen (BUN) (liver failure or kidney disease can misleadingly elevate GH), serum calcium (to screen for hyperparathyroidism), serum inorganic phosphorus (frequently elevated), serum free T_4, and TSH (secondary hypothyroidism is common in acromegaly; primary hypothyroidism may increase PRL; hyperthyroidism may occur as a result of excess TSH).

Glucose syrup (75 g) is then administered orally, and serum GH is measured 60 minutes afterward; acromegaly is excluded if the serum GH is less than 1 ng/mL (immunoradiometric assay [IRMA] or chemiluminescent assays). For ultrasensitive GH assays, GH should be suppressed to less than 0.3 ng/mL to exclude acromegaly.

C. Imaging

MRI shows a pituitary tumor in 90% of acromegalic patients. These tumors ordinarily involve the sella and cavernous sinus; rare ectopic tumors may arise in the sphenoid bone. MRI is generally superior to CT scanning, especially in the postoperative setting. Radiographs of the skull may show an enlarged sella and thickened skull. Radiographs may also show tufting of the terminal phalanges of the fingers and toes. A lateral view of the foot shows increased thickness of the heel pad.

▶ Differential Diagnosis

Active acromegaly must be distinguished from familial coarse features, large hands and feet, and isolated prognathism and from inactive ("burned-out") acromegaly in which there has been a spontaneous remission due to infarction of the pituitary adenoma. GH-induced gigantism must be differentiated from familial tall stature and from aromatase deficiency. (See Osteoporosis.)

Misleadingly high serum GH levels can be caused by exercise or eating just prior to the test; acute illness or agitation; liver failure or kidney disease; malnourishment; diabetes mellitus; or concurrent treatment with estrogens, β-blockers, or clonidine. During normal adolescence, serum IGF-I is usually elevated and GH may fail to be suppressed.

▶ Complications

Complications include hypopituitarism, hypertension, glucose intolerance or frank diabetes mellitus, cardiac enlargement, and cardiac failure. Carpal tunnel syndrome may cause thumb weakness and thenar atrophy. Arthritis of hips, knees, and spine can be troublesome. Cord compression may be seen. Visual field defects may be severe and progressive. Acute loss of vision or cranial nerve palsy may occur if the tumor undergoes spontaneous hemorrhage and necrosis (pituitary apoplexy). Colon polyps are more likely to develop in patients with acromegaly.

▶ Treatment

Pituitary microsurgery is the treatment of choice for patients with acromegaly. Many patients have an apparent surgical cure and a remission in all clinical symptoms but continue to have a mildly elevated serum GH or IGF-I postoperatively. If no residual tumor is apparent on MRI, the patient may elect to be monitored closely, rather than embark on adjuvant medical therapy that is expensive and carries its own risks (see below).

A. Pituitary Microsurgery

Endoscopic transnasal, transsphenoidal pituitary microsurgery removes the adenoma while preserving anterior pituitary function in most patients. Surgical remission is achieved in about 70% of patients followed over 3 years. GH levels fall immediately; diaphoresis and carpal tunnel syndrome often improve within a day after surgery. Transsphenoidal surgery is usually well tolerated, but complications occur in about 10% of patients, including infection, cerebrospinal fluid leak, and hypopituitarism. Transsphenoidal pituitary surgery may be difficult in patients with McCune–Albright syndrome because of fibrous dysplasia of the skull base. Hyponatremia can occur 4–13 days postoperatively and is manifested by nausea, vomiting, headache, malaise, or seizure. It is prudent to monitor serum sodium levels postoperatively. Dietary salt supplements for 2 weeks postoperatively may prevent this complication. Corticosteroids are administered perioperatively and tapered to replacement doses over 1 week; hydrocortisone is discontinued and cosyntropin stimulation test is performed about 6 weeks after surgery. At that time, a serum T_4 can be checked (to screen for secondary hypothyroidism) and the patient is screened for secondary hypogonadism (see above).

B. Medications

Patients who do not have a clinical or biochemical remission after surgery are treated with a dopamine agonist (eg, cabergoline), somatostatin analogs, pegvisomant, or a combination of these medications. **Cabergoline** may be used first, since it is an oral medication. Cabergoline therapy is most successful for tumors that secrete both PRL and GH but can also be effective for patients with normal serum PRL levels. Therapy with cabergoline will shrink one-third of such tumors by more than 50%. The initial dose is 0.25 mg orally twice weekly, which is gradually increased to a maximum dosage of 1 mg twice weekly, if tolerated by the patient based on serum GH and IGF-I levels. Side effects of cabergoline include nausea, fatigue, constipation, abdominal pain, and dizziness. Cabergoline is expensive. Long-term, high-dose therapy with the dopamine agonists cabergoline, bromocriptine, and pergolide for Parkinson disease has caused some cases of serious cardiac valve regurgitation, similar to that seen with other ergot alkaloids such as methysergide. In such cases of valvulopathy, cabergoline or pergolide had been given in doses of > 2.8 mg/d for over 6 months. Doses such as these are seldom used for patients with pituitary tumors. In a study of 78 patients who had taken cabergoline for a mean of 8 years, there was no increased risk of significant valvular insufficiency, but there was an increased risk of aortic valve calcification and mild tricuspid regurgitation compared with controls. Therefore, it is prudent to minimize cabergoline doses and to obtain baseline and periodic echocardiograms in patients receiving long-term cabergoline therapy.

Octreotide and **lanreotide** are somatostatin analogs that are given by subcutaneous injection. Octreotide (Sandostatin LAR depot) is given at a dose of 20–40 mg intragluteally monthly. Lanreotide acetate (Somatuline Depot) is given by subcutaneous intragluteal injection at a dosage of 60–120 mg monthly. Whichever preparation is used, the dosage can be adjusted to achieve serum GH levels under 2 ng/mL. Such long-acting somatostatin analogs can achieve serum GH levels under 2 ng/mL in 79% of patients and normal serum IGF-I levels in 53% of patients. Headaches often improve, and tumor shrinkage of about 30% may be expected. Acromegalic patients with pretreatment serum GH levels exceeding 20 ng/mL are less likely to respond to octreotide or lanreotide therapy. Side effects are experienced by about one-third of patients and include injection site pain, loose acholic stools, abdominal discomfort, or cholelithiasis. All somatostatin analogs are expensive and must be continued indefinitely or until other treatment has been effective.

Pegvisomant is a GH receptor antagonist that blocks hepatic IGF-I production. Pegvisomant therapy produces symptomatic relief and normalizes serum IGF-I levels in over 90% of patients. The starting dosage is 10 mg subcutaneously daily. The maintenance dosage can be increased by 5–10 mg every 4–6 weeks, based on serum IGF-I levels and liver transaminase levels; the maximum dosage is 40 mg subcutaneously daily. Pegvisomant does not shrink GH-secreting tumors. Patients need to be monitored carefully with visual field examinations, GH levels, and MRI scanning of the pituitary. Side effects of pegvisomant can include hepatitis, edema, flu-like syndrome, nausea, and hypertension. Lipohypertrophy can occur at injection sites, so injection sites must be diligently rotated and inspected. In acromegalic diabetics, hypoglycemic drugs are reduced to avoid hypoglycemia during pegvisomant therapy. The effectiveness of pegvisomant is reduced by coadministration of opioids or propoxyphene. Pegvisomant is detected in some GH assays, which could overestimate serum GH levels. Pegvisomant is extremely expensive.

C. Stereotactic Radiosurgery

Acromegalic patients who have not had a complete remission with transsphenoidal surgery or medical therapy may be treated with **stereotactic radiosurgery** administered by gamma knife, heavy particle radiation, or adapted linear accelerator. Some medical centers are using pituitary gamma knife radiosurgery as the initial treatment with reported success rates of 20–90%. Radiosurgery precisely radiates the pituitary tumor in a single session and reduces radiation to the normal brain. However, it cannot be used for pituitary tumors with suprasellar extension due to the risk of damaging the optic chiasm. Radiosurgery can be used for pituitary tumors invading the cavernous sinus, since cranial nerves III, IV, V, and VI are less susceptible to radiation damage. Radiosurgery can also be used for patients who have not responded to conventional radiation therapy.

▶ Prognosis

Patients with acromegaly have increased morbidity and mortality from cardiovascular disorders and progressive acromegalic symptoms; those who are treated and have a glucose-suppressed serum GH level less than 2.5 ng/mL (radioimmunoassay) or under 1 ng/mL (immunofluorometric assay) and normal age-adjusted serum IGF-I levels have reduced morbidity and mortality. Transsphenoidal pituitary surgery is successful in 80–90% of patients with tumors less than 2 cm in diameter and GH levels less than 50 ng/mL. Extrasellar extension of the pituitary tumor, particularly cavernous sinus invasion, reduces the likelihood of surgical cure.

Adjuvant medical therapy has been quite successful in treating patients who are not cured by pituitary surgery. Postoperatively, normal pituitary function is usually preserved. Soft tissue swelling regresses but bone enlargement is permanent. Hypertension frequently persists despite successful surgery. Conventional radiation therapy (alone) produces a remission in about 40% of patients by 2 years and 75% of patients by 5 years after treatment. Gamma knife or cyberknife radiosurgery reduces GH levels an average of 77%, with 20% of patients having a full remission after 12 months. Patients with pituitary adenomas that abut the optic chiasm can be treated with cyberknife radiosurgery, controlling tumor growth and preserving vision in most patients. Heavy particle pituitary radiation produces a remission in about 70% of patients by 2 years and 80% of patients by 5 years. Radiation therapy eventually produces some degree of hypopituitarism in most patients. Conventional radiation therapy may cause some degree of organic brain syndrome and predisposes to small strokes. Patients must receive lifelong follow-up, with regular monitoring of serum GH and IGF-I levels. Serum GH levels over 5 ng/mL and rising IGF-I levels usually indicate a recurrent tumor.

Hypopituitarism may occur, due to the tumor itself, pituitary surgery, or radiation therapy. Hypopituitarism may develop years following radiation therapy, so patients must have regular clinical monitoring of their pituitary function.

Ben-Shlomo A et al. Acromegaly. Endocrinol Metab Clin North Am. 2008 Mar;37(1):101–22. [PMID: 18226732]

Galland F et al. McCune-Albright syndrome and acromegaly: Effects of hypothalamopituitary radiotherapy and/or pegvisomant in somatostatin analog-resistant patients. J Clin Endocrinol Metab. 2006 Dec;91(12):4957–61. [PMID: 16984995]

Jagannathan J et al. Gamma knife radiosurgery for acromegaly: outcomes after failed transsphenoidal surgery. Neurosurgery. 2008 Jun;62(6):1262–9. [PMID: 18824992]

Kars M et al. Aortic valve calcification and mild tricuspid regurgitation but no clinical heart disease after 8 years of dopamine agonist therapy for prolactinoma. J Clin Endocrinol Metab. 2008 Sep;93(9):3348–56. [PMID: 18559921]

Kobayashi T. Long-term results of stereotactic gamma knife radiosurgery for pituitary adenomas. Prog Neurol Surg. 2009;22:77–95. [PMID: 18948721]

HYPERPROLACTINEMIA

 ESSENTIALS OF DIAGNOSIS

▶ Women: Oligomenorrhea, amenorrhea; galactorrhea; infertility.

▶ Prolactin normally elevated during pregnancy.

▶ Men: Hypogonadism; decreased libido and erectile dysfunction; infertility.

▶ Elevated serum PRL.

▶ CT scan or MRI often demonstrates pituitary adenoma.

▶ General Considerations

Non-gestational elevations in serum PRL can be caused by numerous conditions (Table 26–2). PRL-secreting pituitary tumors are more common in women than in men and are usually sporadic but may rarely be familial as part of MEN 1. Most are microadenomas (< 1 cm in diameter) that do not grow even with pregnancy or oral contraceptives. However, some giant prolactinomas (over 3 cm in diameter) can spread into the cavernous sinuses and suprasellar areas; rarely, they may erode the floor of the sella to invade the sinuses.

▶ Clinical Findings

A. Symptoms and Signs

Hyperprolactinemia may result in hypogonadotropic hypogonadism and reduced fertility. Men usually have erectile dysfunction and diminished libido; gynecomastia sometimes occurs but rarely with galactorrhea. Women may note oligomenorrhea or amenorrhea, although some women continue to menstruate normally. Galactorrhea, defined as lactation in the absence of nursing, is common. Of women with secondary amenorrhea and galactorrhea, about 70% have hyperprolactinemia. Untreated hypogonadism ultimately increases the risk of developing osteoporosis.

Pituitary prolactinomas may cosecrete GH and cause acromegaly (see above). Large tumors may cause headaches, visual symptoms, and pituitary insufficiency.

Aside from pituitary tumors, some women secrete an abnormal form of prolactin that appears to cause peripartum cardiomyopathy (see Chapter 10). Suppression of prolactin secretion with dopamine agonists has reversed the cardiomyopathy.

Table 26–2. Causes of hyperprolactinemia.

Physiologic Causes	Pharmacologic Causes	Pathologic Causes
Exercise	Amoxapine	Acromegaly
Idiopathic	Amphetamines	Chronic chest wall
Macroprolactin-	Anesthetic agents	stimulation (post-
emia ("big	Antipsychotics (con-	thoracotomy, post-
prolactin")	ventional and	mastectomy, herpes
Pregnancy	atypical)	zoster, breast prob-
Puerperium	Butyrophenones	lems, chest acu-
Sleep (REM	Cimetidine and raniti-	puncture, nipple
phase)	dine (not famoti-	rings, etc)
Stress (trauma,	dine or nizatidine)	Cirrhosis
surgery)	Estrogens	Hypothalamic disease
Suckling	Hydroxyzine	Hypothyroidism
	Methyldopa	Kidney disease (espe-
	Metoclopramide	cially with zinc
	Opioids	deficiency)
	Nicotine	Multiple sclerosis
	Phenothiazines	Optic neuromyelitis
	Protease inhibitors	Pituitary stalk section
	Progestins	Prolactin-secreting
	Reserpine	tumors
	Risperidone	Pseudocyesis (false
	Selective serotonin	pregnancy)
	reuptake inhibitors	Spinal cord lesions
	Testosterone	Systemic lupus ery-
	Tricyclic antidepres-	thematosus
	sants	
	Verapamil	

B. Laboratory Findings

Evaluate for conditions known to cause hyperprolactinemia, particularly pregnancy (serum hCG), hypothyroidism (serum FT_4 and TSH), kidney disease (BUN and serum creatinine), cirrhosis (clinical evaluation and serum bilirubin and liver enzymes) and hyperparathyroidism (serum calcium). Men are evaluated for hypogonadism with determinations of serum total and free testosterone, LH, and FSH. Women who have amenorrhea are assessed for hypogonadism with determinations of serum estradiol, LH, and FSH. An assay for macroprolactinemia should be considered for patients with hyperprolactinemia who are relatively asymptomatic and have no apparent cause for hyperprolactinemia. Patients with pituitary macroadenomas (> 3 cm in diameter) should have PRL measured on serial dilutions of serum, since IRMA assays may otherwise report falsely low titers, the "high-dose hook effect." Patients with macroprolactinomas or manifestations of possible hypopituitarism should be evaluated for hypopituitarism as described above.

C. Imaging

When hyperprolactinemia persists without obvious cause, MRI of the pituitary and hypothalamus is indicated. Small prolactinomas may thus be demonstrated, but clear differentiation from normal variants is not always possible.

Differential Diagnosis

The causes of hyperprolactinemia are shown in Table 26–2. Chronic nipple stimulation, nipple piercing, augmentation or reduction mammoplasty, and mastectomy may stimulate PRL secretion. The pituitary tumor of acromegaly can cosecrete GH and PRL. Hyperprolactinemia may also be idiopathic. Increased pituitary size is a normal variant in young women. About 10% of hyperprolactinemic patients are found to be secreting macroprolactin, a relatively inactive "big prolactin"; pituitary MRI is normal in 78% of cases.

The differential diagnosis for galactorrhea includes the small amount of breast milk that can be expressed from the nipple in many parous women that is not cause for concern. Nipple stimulation from nipple rings, chest surgery, or acupuncture can cause galactorrhea; serum PRL levels may be normal or minimally elevated. Some women can have galactorrhea with normal serum PRL levels and no discernible cause (idiopathic). Normal breast milk may be various colors besides white. Bloody galactorrhea requires an evaluation for breast malignancy.

Treatment

Medications known to increase PRL should be stopped if possible. Hyperprolactinemia due to hypothyroidism is corrected by thyroxine. Patients with hyperprolactinemia not induced by drugs, hypothyroidism, or pregnancy should be examined by pituitary MRI.

Women with microprolactinomas who have amenorrhea or are desirous of contraception may safely take oral contraceptives or estrogen replacement—there is minimal risk of stimulating enlargement of the microadenoma. Patients with infertility and hyperprolactinemia may be treated with a dopamine agonist in an effort to improve fertility. Women with amenorrhea who elect to receive no treatment have an increased risk of developing osteoporosis; such women require periodic bone densitometry.

Pituitary macroprolactinomas (> 10 mm in diameter) have a higher risk of progressive growth, particularly during treatment with estrogen or testosterone replacement therapy or during pregnancy. Therefore, patients with macroprolactinomas should not be treated with sex hormone replacement therapy (HRT) unless they are in remission with dopamine agonist medication or surgery. Pregnant women with macroprolactinomas should continue to receive treatment with dopamine agonists throughout the pregnancy to prevent tumor growth.

A. Dopamine Agonists

Dopamine agonists are the initial treatment of choice for patients with giant prolactinomas and those with hyperprolactinemia desiring restoration of normal sexual function and fertility. Of the ergot-derived dopamine agonists, cabergoline is usually the best tolerated. The beginning dosage is 0.25 mg orally once weekly for 1 week, then 0.25 mg twice weekly for the next week, then 0.5 mg twice weekly. Further dosage increases may be required monthly, based on serum PRL levels, up to a maximum of 1.5 mg twice weekly. Alternative drugs include bromocriptine (1.25–20 mg/d orally). Women who experience nausea with oral preparations may find relief with deep vaginal insertion of cabergoline or bromocriptine tablets; vaginal irritation sometimes occurs. Quinagolide (Norprolac; not available in the United States) is a non-ergot-derived dopamine agonist for patients intolerant or resistant to ergot-derived medications; the starting dosage is 0.075 mg/d orally, increasing as needed and tolerated to a maximum of 0.6 mg/d. Patients whose tumor is resistant to one dopamine agonist may be switched to another in an effort to induce a tolerable remission.

Dopamine agonists are given at bedtime to minimize side effects of fatigue, nausea, dizziness, and orthostatic hypotension. These symptoms usually improve with dosage reduction and continued use. Erythromelalgia is rare. Dopamine agonists can cause a variety of psychiatric side effects that are not dose related and may take weeks to resolve once the dopamine agonist is discontinued. Therefore, dopamine agonists should be used judiciously in psychiatric patients whose antipsychotic medications have caused hyperprolactinemia. Cabergoline has caused cardiac valve insufficiency in patients with Parkinson disease after prolonged administration at doses greater than 3 mg/d, but such doses are not used for suppression of pituitary prolactinomas.

With dopamine agonist treatment, 90% of patients with prolactinomas experience a fall in serum PRL to 10% or less of pretreatment levels; about 80% of treated patients achieve a normal serum PRL level. Shrinkage of a pituitary adenoma occurs early, but the maximum effect may take up to a year. Nearly half of prolactinomas—even massive tumors—shrink more than 50%. Such shrinkage of giant prolactinomas can result in spinal fluid rhinorrhea. Discontinuing therapy after months or years usually results in the reappearance of hyperprolactinemia and galactorrhea-amenorrhea, but some patients with microadenomas remain in remission.

Because dopamine agonists usually restore fertility promptly, many pregnancies have resulted; no teratogenicity has been noted with any of the dopamine agonists. However, women with microadenomas may have treatment withdrawn during pregnancy. Macroadenomas may enlarge significantly during pregnancy; if therapy is withdrawn, such patients must be monitored clinically with serum PRL determinations and with computer-assisted visual field perimetry. Women with macroprolactinomas who have responded to dopamine agonists may safely receive oral contraceptive agents as long as they continue receiving therapy.

The initial dose is 0.25 mg orally twice weekly, which is gradually increased to a maximum dosage of 1 mg twice weekly according to serum prolactin levels. Side effects of cabergoline include nausea, fatigue, constipation, abdominal pain, and dizziness. Cabergoline is expensive. Long-term high-dose therapy for patients with Parkinson disease with the dopamine agonists cabergoline, bromocriptine, and pergolide has caused some cases of serious cardiac valve regurgitation, similar to that seen with other ergot alkaloids such as methysergide. In such cases of valvulopathy, cabergoline or pergolide had been given in doses of > 2 mg/d for over 6 months. Doses such as these are seldom used for patients with pituitary tumors. In a study of 78 patients who had taken cabergoline for a mean of 8 years, there was no increased risk of significant valvular insufficiency, but there was an increased risk of aortic valve calcification and mild tricuspid regurgitation compared with controls. Therefore, it is prudent to minimize cabergoline doses and to obtain baseline and periodic echocardiograms in patients receiving long-term cabergoline therapy.

B. Surgical Treatment

Transsphenoidal pituitary surgery may be urgently required for large tumors undergoing apoplexy or those severely compromising visual fields. It is also used electively for patients who do not tolerate or respond to dopamine agonists. Pituitary transsphenoidal surgery is generally well-tolerated, with a surgical mortality rate of less than 0.5%. Complications, such as cerebrospinal fluid leakage, meningitis, stroke, or visual loss, occur in about 3% of cases; sinusitis, nasal septal perforation, or infection complicates about 6.5% of surgeries. Postoperative hyponatremia occurs quite commonly, and it is advisable to monitor serum sodium levels for the first 2 weeks postoperatively. For pituitary microprolactinomas, skilled neurosurgeons are successful in normalizing prolactin in 87% of patients; the 10-year recurrence rate is 13%. Pituitary function can be preserved in over 95% of cases. However, the surgical success rate for macroprolactinomas is much lower, and the complication rates are higher. Craniotomy is rarely indicated, since even large tumors can usually be decompressed via the transsphenoidal approach.

C. Radiation Therapy

Radiation therapy is reserved for patients with macroadenomas that are growing despite treatment with dopamine agonists. A single gamma knife or cyberknife treatment is preferable for certain patients whose optic chiasm is clear of tumor, since it is generally safer and more convenient than conventional radiation therapy. Conventional radiation therapy must be given over 5 weeks and carries a high risk of eventual hypopituitarism. Other possible side effects include some degree of memory impairment and an increased long-term risk of second tumors and small vessel ischemic strokes. After radiation therapy, patients are advised to take low-dose aspirin daily for life to reduce their stroke risk.

Hilfiker-Kleiner D et al. A cathepsin D-cleaved 16 kDa form of prolactin mediates postpartum cardiomyopathy. Cell. 2007 Feb 9;128(3):589–600. [PMID: 17289576]

Hilfiker-Kleiner D et al. Recovery from postpartum cardiomyopathy in 2 patients by blocking prolactin release with bromocriptine. J Am Coll Cardiol. 2007 Dec 11;50(24):2354–5. [PMID: 1806804]

Kars M et al. Aortic valve calcification and mild tricuspid regurgitation but no clinical heart disease after 8 years of dopamine agonist therapy for prolactinoma. J Clin Endocrinol Metab. 2008 Sep;93(9):3348–56. [PMID: 18559921]

Schlechte JA. Long-term management of prolactinomas. J Clin Endocrinol Metab. 2007 Aug;92(8):2861–5. [PMID: 17682084]

▼ DISEASES OF THE THYROID GLAND

THYROID TESTING

Assays for FT_4, total triiodothyronine (T_3), and free triiodothyronine (FT_3) have largely supplanted measurements of total T_4, resin T_3 uptake (RT_3U), and free thyroxine index (FT_4I). It is particularly important to determine "free" serum levels (FT_4 and FT_3) in conditions associated with high circulating levels of thyroxine-binding globulin, such as during pregnancy or therapy with oral estrogen. Ultrasensitive assays for serum TSH have largely replaced older TSH assays. Table 26–3 shows the appropriate use of thyroid tests.

▶ Effects of Nonthyroidal Illness & Drugs on Thyroid Function Tests

Many factors affect thyroid function tests, causing misleading laboratory evidence of hypothyroidism (Table 26–4) or hyperthyroidism (Table 26–5) in patients who are clinically euthyroid.

Serum T_4 is frequently low in patients with severe illness, caloric deprivation, or major surgery who have accelerated peripheral metabolism of serum T_4 to reverse T_3 (rT_3). Furthermore, in most patients who are critically ill, there is a circulating inhibitor of thyroid hormone binding to serum thyroxine-binding proteins (TBPs). This causes the RT_3U to be misleadingly low, causing the computed FT_4I to be very low. The presence of a very low serum T_4 in severe nonthyroidal illness indicates a poor prognosis.

Direct assays of FT_4 often show low levels of FT_4 in severe illness. Because studies of giving replacement T_4 to such patients have shown no improvement in survival, they are considered **"euthyroid sick."** Serum TSH tends to be suppressed in severe nonthyroidal illness, making the diagnosis of concurrent primary hypothyroidism quite difficult, although the presence of a goiter suggests the diagnosis.

The clinician must decide whether such severely ill patients (with a low serum T_4 but nonelevated TSH) might have hypothyroidism due to pituitary insufficiency. Patients without symptoms of prior brain lesion or hypopituitarism are very unlikely to suddenly develop hypopituitarism during an unrelated illness. Patients with diabetes insipidus, hypopituitarism, or other signs of a central nervous system lesion may have T_4 given empirically. True secondary hypothyroidism due to direct dopamine suppression of TSH-secreting cells may develop in patients receiving prolonged dopamine infusions.

Certain antiseizure medications cause low serum FT_4 levels by accelerating hepatic conversion of T_4 to T_3; serum TSH levels are normal.

Adler SM et al. The nonthyroidal illness syndrome. Endocrinol Metab Clin North Am. 2008 Sep;36(3):657–72. [PMID: 17673123]

Beltran S et al. Subclinical hypothyroidism in HIV-infected patients is not an autoimmune disease. Horm Res. 2006;66(1):21–6. [PMID: 16685132]

Table 26–3. Appropriate use of thyroid tests.

	Test	Comment
Screening	Serum thyroid-stimulating hormone (TSH) (sensitive assay)	Most sensitive test for primary hypothyroidism and hyperthyroidism
	Free thyroxine (FT_4)	Excellent test
For hypothyroidism	Serum TSH	High in primary and low in secondary hypothyroidism
	Antithyroglobulin and antithyroperoxidase antibodies	Elevated in Hashimoto thyroiditis
For hyperthyroidism	Serum TSH (sensitive assay)	Suppressed except in TSH-secreting pituitary tumor or pituitary hyperplasia (rare)
	Triiodothyronine (T_3) or free triiodothyronine (FT_3)	Elevated
	^{123}I uptake and scan	Increased uptake; diffuse versus "hot" areas on scan
	Antithyroglobulin and antimicrosomal antibodies	Elevated in Graves disease
	Thyroid-stimulating immunoglobulin (TSI); TSH receptor antibody (TSH-R Ab [stim])	Usually (65%) positive in Graves disease
For thyroid nodules	Fine-needle aspiration (FNA) biopsy	Best diagnostic method for thyroid cancer
	^{123}I uptake and scan	Cancer is usually "cold"; less reliable than FNA biopsy
	^{99m}Tc scan	Vascular versus avascular
	Ultrasonography	Useful to assist FNA biopsy. Useful in assessing the risk of malignancy (multinodular goiter or pure cysts are less likely to be malignant). Useful to monitor nodules and patients after thyroid surgery for carcinoma.

Koenig RJ. Modeling the nonthyroidal illness syndrome. Curr Opin Endocrinol Diabetes Obes. 2008 Oct;15(5):466–9. [PMID: 18769221]

HYPOTHYROIDISM & MYXEDEMA

ESSENTIALS OF DIAGNOSIS

► Weakness, fatigue, cold intolerance, constipation, weight change, depression, menorrhagia, hoarseness.

► Dry skin, bradycardia, delayed return of deep tendon reflexes.

► Anemia, hyponatremia, hyperlipidemia.

► FT_4 level is usually low.

► TSH elevated in primary hypothyroidism.

► General Considerations

Hypothyroidism is common, affecting over 1% of the general population and about 5% of individuals over age 60 years. Thyroid hormone deficiency affects almost all body functions. The degree of severity ranges from mild and unrecognized hypothyroid states to striking myxedema. The fluid retention seen in myxedema is caused by the interstitial accumulation of hydrophilic mucopolysaccharides, which leads to lymphedema. Hyponatremia is the result of impaired renal tubular sodium reabsorption due to reductions in Na^+–K^+-ATPase.

Hypothyroidism may be due to failure or resection of the thyroid gland itself or deficiency of pituitary TSH (see Hypopituitarism, above). The condition must be distinguished from the functional hypothyroidism that occurs in severe nonthyroidal illness, which does not require treatment with thyroxine (see Euthyroid Sick, above).

Maternal hypothyroidism during pregnancy results in offspring with IQ scores that are an average 7 points lower than those of euthyroid mothers.

Goiter may be present with thyroiditis, iodide deficiency, genetic thyroid enzyme defects, drug goitrogens (lithium, iodide, propylthiouracil or methimazole, phenylbutazone, sulfonamides, amiodarone, interferon-α, interferon-β, interleukin-2), food goitrogens in iodide-deficient areas (eg, turnips, cassavas) or, rarely, peripheral resistance to thyroid hormone or infiltrating diseases (eg, cancer, sarcoidosis). A hypothyroid phase occurs in subacute (de Quervain) viral thyroiditis following initial hyperthyroidism. Hashimoto thyroiditis is the most common cause of hypothyroidism (see Thyroiditis section).

Goiter is usually absent when hypothyroidism is due to destruction of the gland by surgery, radiation therapy (to the head, neck, chest, and shoulder region), or ^{131}I. Chemotherapy can reduce thyroid function, causing hypothyroidism. Sunitinib, a protein-tyrosine kinase inhibitor used to treat gastrointestinal stromal malignancies, causes transient primary hypothyroidism in about 50% of treated patients.

Amiodarone, because of its high iodine content, causes clinically significant hypothyroidism in about 8% of patients who receive it. The T_4 level is normal or low, and the TSH is elevated, usually over 20 ng/dL. Another 17% of

Table 26–4. Factors that may cause aberrations in laboratory tests that may be mistaken for primary hypothyroidism.[1]

Low Serum T$_4$ or T$_3$	High Serum TSH
Laboratory error	Laboratory error
Acute psychiatric problems	Autoimmune disease (assay
Cirrhosis	interference)
Nephrotic syndrome	Heterophile antibodies
Familial thyroid-binding globulin	Anti-mouse antibodies
deficiency	Strenuous exercise (acute)
Severe illness	Sleep deprivation (acute)
Drugs	Recovery from nonthyroidal
Androgens	illness (transient)
Asparaginase	Acute psychiatric admissions
Carbamazepine	(14% transient)
Chloral hydrate	Elderly—especially women
Corticosteroids	(10%, mild elevations)
Diclofenac (T$_3$)	
Didanosine	
Fenclofenac	
Fluoracil	
Halofenate	
Mitotane	
Naproxen (T$_3$)	
Nicotinic acid	
Oxcarbazepine	
Phenobarbital	
Phenytoin (total T$_4$ may be as	
low as 2 mcg/dL)	
Salicylates—large doses (T$_3$ and T$_4$)	
Sertraline	
Stavudine	
T$_3$ therapy	

[1]True primary hypothyroidism may coexist.

T$_4$, levothyroxine; T$_3$, triiodothyronine; TSH, thyroid-stimulating hormone.

Table 26–5. Factors that can cause aberrations in laboratory tests that may be mistaken for spontaneous clinical primary hyperthyroidism.[1]

High Serum T$_4$ or T$_3$	Low Serum TSH
Laboratory error	Laboratory error
Collecting serum in vial with gel	Autonomous thyroid or
barrier for T$_3$	thyroid nodule
Acute psychiatric problems (30%)	Acute corticosteroid
Acute medical illness (eg, acute inter-	administration
mittent porphyria	Elderly euthyroid
AIDS (increased thyroid-binding globulin)	Nonthyroidal illness
Autoimmunity	(severe)
Hepatitis: acute or chronic active	Pregnancy (especially
Primary biliary cirrhosis	with morning sickness)
Pregnancy (especially with morning	hCG-secreting tropho-
sickness)	blastic tumors
Hyperemesis gravidarum	Drugs
Familial thyroid-binding abnormalities	Thyroid hormone
Familial generalized resistance to thy-	Amphetamines
roid (Refetoff syndrome)	Dopamine
Drugs	Dopamine agonists
Amiodarone	Calcium channel
Amphetamines	blockers (nifedi-
Clofibrate	pine, verapamil)
Estrogens (oral)	
Heparin (dialysis method)	
Heroin	
Thyroid hormone therapy	
Methadone	
Perphenazine	
Tamoxifen	

[1]True clinical hyperthyroidism may coexist.

hCG, human chorionic gonadotropin; NSAIDs, nonsteroidal anti-inflammatory drugs; T$_4$, levothyroxine; T$_3$, triiodothyronine; TSH, thyroid-stimulating hormone.

patients develop milder elevations of TSH and are asymptomatic. Low-dose amiodarone is less likely to cause hypothyroidism. Cardiac patients with amiodarone-induced symptomatic hypothyroidism are treated with just enough thyroxine to relieve symptoms. Hypothyroidism usually resolves over several months if amiodarone is discontinued. Hypothyroidism may also develop in patients with a high iodine intake from other sources, especially if they have underlying lymphocytic thyroiditis.

Hepatitis C is associated with an increased risk of autoimmune thyroiditis, with 21% of affected patients having antithyroid antibodies and 13% having hypothyroidism. The risk of thyroid dysfunction is even higher when patients are treated with interferon. Interferon-α and interferon-β treatment can induce thyroid dysfunction (usually hypothyroidism, sometimes hyperthyroidism) in 6% of patients. Spontaneous resolution occurs in over 50% of cases once interferon is discontinued.

▶ **Clinical Findings**

These may vary from the rather rare full-blown myxedema to mild states of hypothyroidism, which are far more

common. Mild hypothyroidism often escapes detection without screening (ie, serum TSH). Hypothyroidism is a common disorder; therefore, a clinician should request thyroid function tests for any patient with the nonspecific symptoms or signs of hypothyroidism.

A. Symptoms and Signs

1. Common manifestations—Common symptoms of hypothyroidism include weight gain, fatigue, lethargy, depression, weakness, dyspnea on exertion, arthralgias or myalgias, muscle cramps, paresthesias, cold intolerance, constipation, dry skin, headache, carpal tunnel syndrome, and menorrhagia. Physical findings can include bradycardia; diastolic hypertension; thin, brittle nails; thinning of hair; peripheral edema; puffy face and eyelids; and skin pallor or yellowing (carotenemia). Delayed relaxation of deep tendon reflexes may be present. Patients often have a palpably enlarged thyroid (goiter) that arises due to elevated serum TSH levels or the underlying thyroid pathology, such as Hashimoto thyroiditis.

2. Less common manifestations—Less common symptoms of hypothyroidism include diminished appetite and weight loss, hoarseness, decreased sense of taste and smell, and diminished auditory acuity. Some patients may complain of dysphagia or neck discomfort. Although most menstruating women have menorrhagia, some women have scant menses or amenorrhea. Physical findings may include thinning of the outer halves of the eyebrows; thickening of the tongue; hard pitting edema; and effusions into the pleural and peritoneal cavities as well as into joints. Galactorrhea may also be present. Cardiac enlargement ("myxedema heart") and pericardial effusions may occur. Psychosis may occur and is termed "myxedema madness." Hypothermia and stupor or myxedema coma, which is often associated with infection (especially pneumonia), may develop in patients with severe hypothyroidism. Pituitary enlargement due to hyperplasia of TSH-secreting cells, which is reversible following thyroid therapy, may be seen in long-standing hypothyroidism.

B. Laboratory Findings

The single best screening test for hypothyroidism is the serum TSH (Table 26-3). Serum TSH is increased with primary hypothyroidism but is low or normal with pituitary insufficiency. The FT_4 may be low or low-normal. Other laboratory abnormalities may often be seen: increased serum LDL cholesterol, triglycerides, lipoprotein (a), liver enzymes, and creatine kinase; increased serum PRL; and hyponatremia, hypoglycemia, and anemia (with normal or increased mean corpuscular volume). Semen analysis shows an increase in abnormal sperm morphology. In patients with autoimmune thyroiditis, titers of antibodies against thyroperoxidase and thyroglobulin are high; serum antinuclear antibodies (ANA) are usually present and are not indicative of lupus.

The normal range for ultrasensitive TSH levels is generally stated to be 0.4–4.0 mU/L. However, the normal range of TSH varies with age such that newborns have a much higher normal range; children and elderly patients have a mildly higher normal range. Over 95% of normal adults have serum TSH concentrations under 3.0 mU/L. There is a high risk of finding antithyroid antibodies in patients with serum TSH in the upper range of normal, but most such patients are asymptomatic. TSH may be mildly elevated in some euthyroid individuals, especially elderly women (10% incidence). Such patients with normal FT_4 levels must be evaluated carefully for subtle signs of hypothyroidism (eg, fatigue, depression, hyperlipidemia). About 18% later become definitely hypothyroid.

C. Imaging

Radiologic imaging is usually not necessary for patients with hypothyroidism. However, on CT or MRI, a goiter may be noted in the neck or in the mediastinum (retrosternal goiter). An enlarged thymus is frequently seen in the mediastinum in cases of autoimmune thyroiditis. In primary hypothyroidism with elevated serum TSH levels, MRI of the head will frequently show an enlargement of the pituitary gland from thyrotrophe hyperplasia; such enlargement can be mistaken for a pituitary tumor.

Differential Diagnosis

Many clinical manifestations of hypothyroidism (see above) are common in the general population without thyroid illness. The differential diagnoses are the conditions and drugs that can cause aberrations in laboratory tests, resulting in a low serum T_4 or T_3 or high serum TSH in the absence of hypothyroidism (see Table 26–4). The pituitary is often quite enlarged in primary hypothyroidism due to reversible hyperplasia of TSH-secreting cells; the concomitant hyperprolactinemia seen in hypothyroidism can lead to the mistaken diagnosis of a TSH-secreting or PRL-secreting pituitary adenoma.

Complications

Complications are mostly cardiac in nature, occurring as a result of advanced coronary artery disease and congestive heart failure, which may be precipitated by overly vigorous thyroid therapy. There is an increased susceptibility to infection. Megacolon has been described in long-standing hypothyroidism. Organic psychoses with paranoid delusions may occur ("myxedema madness"). Rarely, adrenal crisis may be precipitated by thyroid therapy. Hypothyroidism is a rare cause of infertility, which may respond to thyroid medication. Pregnancy in a woman with untreated hypothyroidism often results in miscarriage. Sellar enlargement and even well-defined TSH-secreting tumors may develop in untreated cases. These tumors decrease in size after replacement therapy is instituted.

Myxedema crisis refers to severe, life-threatening hypothyroidism. The manifestations of hypothyroidism are present and more severe. Affected patients have impaired cognition, ranging from confusion to somnolence to coma (myxedema coma). Convulsions and abnormal central nervous system signs may occur. Patients have severe hypothermia, hypoventilation, hyponatremia, hypoglycemia, and hypotension. Rhabdomyolysis and acute kidney injury may occur. Myxedema coma is often induced by an underlying infection; cardiac, respiratory, or central nervous system illness; cold exposure; or drug use. It is most often seen in elderly women who have had a stroke or who have stopped taking their thyroxine medication. The mortality rate from myxedema coma is high. Myxedematous patients are unusually sensitive to opioids and may die from average doses. Patients with severe myxedema may have hyponatremia that is severe and refractory to treatment.

Treatment

Levothyroxine (thyroxine; T_4) is the treatment of choice. It is partially converted in the body to T_3, the active thyroid hormone. Hypothyroid patients who are taking thyroxine replacement typically have serum T_3 levels that are lower than normal, owing to their lack of thyroidal T_3 secretion. Oral administration of T_3 or T_4/T_3 combination preparations causes abnormal peaks in serum T_3 and the usefulness of T_3 for hypothyroidism is controversial; a sustained-release T_3 preparation is not commercially available.

In patients taking levothyroxine daily, significant increases in serum T_4 levels are seen within 1–2 weeks, and near-peak levels are seen within 3–4 weeks. Thyroxine is best taken in the morning with water, avoiding concomitant intake of foods and drugs that may interfere with its absorption (see below).

Before therapy with thyroid hormone is commenced, the hypothyroid patient requires at least a clinical assessment for adrenal insufficiency, for which the patient would require evaluation and concurrent treatment.

A. Beginning Treatment for Hypothyroidism

Otherwise healthy young and middle-age adults with hypothyroidism may be treated initially with levothyroxine in doses of 25–75 mcg daily. The lower doses are used for very mild hypothyroidism, while higher doses are given for more symptomatic hypothyroidism. The average daily thyroxine requirement averages 1.7 mcg/kg for this group of patients. The thyroxine dosage may be increased according to clinical response and serum TSH measurements, trying to keep the serum TSH level between 0.4 mU/L and 2.0 mU/L. The ultimate levothyroxine dosage requirement varies considerably.

Women who are pregnant with significant hypothyroidism may begin therapy with levothyroxine at higher doses of 100–150 mcg orally daily.

Patients with coronary disease or those who are over age 60 years are treated with smaller initial doses of levothyroxine, 25–50 mcg daily; higher initial doses may be used if such patients are severely hypothyroid. The dose can be increased by 25 mcg every 1–3 weeks until the patient is euthyroid. The average daily requirement for elderly patients averages 1 mcg/kg. Patients with hypothyroidism and known ischemic heart disease may begin thyroxine therapy following restoration of coronary perfusion by coronary artery angioplasty or bypass.

Myxedema crisis requires larger initial doses of levothyroxine intravenously, since myxedema itself can interfere with levothyroxine's intestinal absorption. Levothyroxine sodium 400 mcg is given intravenously as a loading dose, followed by 50–100 mcg intravenously daily; the lower dose is given to patients with suspected coronary insufficiency. In patients with myxedema coma, liothyronine (T_3, Triostat) can be given intravenously in doses of 5–10 mcg every 8 hours for the first 48 hours. The hypothermic patient is warmed only with blankets, since faster warming can precipitate cardiovascular collapse. Patients with hypercapnia require intubation and assisted mechanical ventilation. Infections must be detected and treated aggressively. Patients in whom concomitant adrenal insufficiency is suspected are treated with hydrocortisone, 100 mg intravenously, followed by 25–50 mg every 8 hours.

B. Monitoring & Optimizing Treatment of Hypothyroidism

It is important to stress to the patient that levothyroxine therapy must be continued long-term (usually in doses 50–250 mcg orally daily) and that regular clinical reassessments will be required for life.

For most patients with hypothyroidism, a stable maintenance dose can usually be found. However, the dosage requirement can rise due to increased hepatic metabolism of thyroxine induced by certain medications: carbamazepine, phenobarbitol, primidone, phenytoin, rifabutin, rifampin, and the antitumor drug imatinib (Gleevec). Amiodarone can cause changes in thyroxine dose requirements, making it necessary to closely monitor serum TSH and adjust the thyroxine dosage accordingly in these patients. Malabsorption of thyroxine can be caused by coadministration of binding substances, particularly iron preparations (including iron found in multivitamins), raloxifene, sucralfate, aluminum hydroxide antacids, calcium and magnesium supplements, and soy milk or soy protein supplements. Bile acid-binding resins such as cholestyramine can bind T_4 and impair its absorption even when administered 5 hours before the T_4. Proton pump inhibitors interfere slightly with the absorption of levothyroxine. Compared with Synthyroid brand of T_4 (100%), there are varying bioavailabilities of different thyroxine preparations: Lannet generic T_4 (Unithyroid), 103%; Mylar generic T_4, 109%; Sandoz generic T_4, 109%; and Levoxyl brand T_4, 114%. Such differences in bioavailability of different T_4 formulations may have a subtle but significant clinical impact. It is therefore recommended that patients always continue to take the same brand name of thyroxine or the same manufacturer's generic thyroxine.

Women with hypothyroidism typically require increased doses of T_4 during pregnancy and during therapy with oral estrogen. Conversely, T_4 dosage requirements for women often decrease with delivery, cessation of oral estrogen, and menopause.

There is no standardized optimal dose of levothyroxine, so each patient's dose must be based on careful clinical assessment. Although serum TSH levels can be helpful in determining optimal dosing, it is important not to rely entirely on this test alone.

During pregnancy, it is critical to administer adequate levothyroxine to a hypothyroid woman. Although the fetal thyroid begins secreting thyroid hormone at about 18 weeks of gestation, fetal thyroid development is not complete until term. The fetus is at least partially dependent upon maternal T_4 for central nervous system development—particularly in the second trimester. Maternal hypothyroidism after the first trimester appears to cause some developmental delay in offspring. It is therefore important to carefully monitor women with hypothyroidism during their pregnancies with serum TSH (FT_4 concentrations in hypopituitarism) determinations every 4–6 weeks and to increase T_4 replacement progressively as required (see Chapter 19, Obstetrics & Obstetric Disorders).

There is considerable individual variation in the requirement for additional T_4 replacement during pregnancy. An increase in thyroxine requirement has been noted as early as the fifth week of pregnancy. Therefore, for women receiving replacement thyroxine, it is prudent to increase thyroxine dosages by approximately 30% as soon as pregnancy is confirmed. By mid pregnancy, women require an average of 47% increase in their thyroxine dosage.

The increased T_4 dosage requirements during pregnancy are believed to be due to several factors: (1) Rising estrogen levels during pregnancy increase thyroxine binding globulin

(TBG) serum concentrations, reducing FT_4 levels. (2) Placental deiodinase promotes the turnover of T_4. (3) Supplemental iron and prenatal multivitamins containing iron can bind to oral T_4 and reduce its intestinal absorption. Similarly, supplemental calcium can also reduce T_4 absorption. Therefore, it is important that patients take their T_4 replacement at least 4 hours before or after such dietary supplements. Postpartum, T_4 replacement requirements ordinarily return to prepregnancy levels.

Elevated serum TSH levels usually indicate underreplacement with levothyroxine. However, before increasing the T_4 dosage, confirm compliance and ask the patient about the presence of angina. It is also important to consider the following: A high TSH in a patient receiving standard replacement doses of T_4 may indicate malabsorption of levothyroxine due to concurrent administration with binding substances (see above). Malabsorption of T_4 can also occur in short bowel syndrome; therapy with medium chain triglyceride oil may improve absorption. Impaired absorption of T_4 can also be caused by diarrhea of any cause or malabsorption due to sprue, regional enteritis, liver disease, or pancreatic exocrine insufficiency. Serum TSH may be elevated transiently in acute psychiatric illness and during recovery from nonthyroidal illness. Autoimmune disease can cause false elevations of TSH by interfering with the assay. A high TSH can also be caused by thyrotropin-secreting pituitary tumors. TSH may be increased by phenothiazines and atypical antipsychotics.

Suppressed serum TSH levels < 0.1 mU/L (using a sensitive assay) may indicate overreplacement with levothyroxine; if such a patient has manifestations of hyperthyroidism, the dosage of levothyroxine is reduced. However, some patients with suppressed serum TSH levels exhibit no symptoms of hyperthyroidism. For such patients, it is important to determine whether hypopituitarism or severe nonthyroidal illness is present, which can result in low serum TSH levels without hyperthyroidism. TSH can also be suppressed by certain medications, such as nonsteroidal anti-inflammatory drugs, opioids, nifedipine, verapamil, and urgent administration of corticosteroids. Absent such conditions, a clinically euthyroid patient with a low serum TSH should be given a lower dosage of levothyroxine. Patients who exhibit hypothyroid symptoms on the reduced dosage of levothyroxine may have their higher dosage resumed, unless they have coronary insufficiency.

Some hypothyroid patients treated with levothyroxine complain of hypothyroid-type symptoms, particularly fatigue, despite having normal or suppressed levels of TSH and normal levels of FT_4. Such patients require careful assessment for other concurrent illnesses such as adrenal insufficiency, hypogonadism, anemia, or depression. If such conditions are treated and hypothyroid-type symptoms persist despite normal or low TSH levels, a serum T_3 level (FT_3 in pregnancy and women receiving oral estrogens) may help make the difficult decision about whether to increase the levothyroxine dose. If the serum T_3 level is low or low normal, such a patient may benefit from a careful increase in T_4 dosage; if a definite clinical benefit is achieved, the higher dose is continued. However, long-term monitoring for atrial arrhythmias and for osteoporosis is recommended for such patients, though such complications are uncommon in those who are clinically euthyroid. The malaise felt by some hypothyroid patients despite apparent optimal replacement therapy with T_4 may be caused by a low concentration of T_3 in certain tissues. Studies adding T_3 to T_4 therapy have not typically shown objective improvement, but patients tend to lose weight and to subjectively prefer combined T_4/T_3 mixtures to T_4 alone. A Dutch double-blind study of 141 hypothyroid patients found that most patients subjectively preferred not T_4 but a combined T_4/T_3 preparation in 5:1 or 10:1 ratios, such that TSH was often suppressed; satisfaction correlated with weight loss.

► **Prognosis**

Hypothyroidism caused by interferon-α resolves within 17 months of stopping the drug in 50% of patients. Patients with mild hypothyroidism caused by Hashimoto thyroiditis have a remission rate of 11%. With early treatment of hypothyroidism, striking transformations take place both in appearance and mental function. Return to a normal state is usually the rule, but relapses will occur if treatment is interrupted. On the whole, response to thyroid treatment is most satisfactory. However, untreated hypothyroid patients with myxedema crisis have a mortality rate approaching 100%. Even with optimal treatment, patients with myxedema crisis have a mortality rate of 20–50%.

Abalovich M et al. Management of thyroid dysfunction during pregnancy and postpartum: an Endocrine Society Clinical Practice Guideline. J Clin Endocrinol Metab. 2007 Aug;92(8 Suppl):S1–47. [PMID: 17948378]

Dutta P et al. Predictors of outcome in myxoedema coma: a study from a tertiary care centre. Crit Care. 2008;12(1):R1. [PMID: 18173846]

Fitzgerald PA. Hypothyroidism. https://knol.google.com/k/paul-fitzgerald/hypothyroidism/muAutpdJ/nreXcw?path_author=paul-fitzgerald&path_title=hypothyroidism#

Hennessey JV. Levothyroxine dosage and the limitations of current bioequivalence standards. Nat Clin Pract Endocrinol Metab. 2006 Sep;2(9):474–5. [PMID: 16957756]

Krassas GE et al. Hypothyroidism has an adverse effect on hyman spermatogenesis: a prospective, controlled study. Thyroid. 2008 Dec;18(12):1255–9. [PMID: 19012472]

Wong E et al. Sunitinib induces hypothyroidism in advanced cancer patients and may inhibit thyroid peroxidase activity. Thyroid. 2007 Apr;17(4):351–5. [PMID: 17465866]

HYPERTHYROIDISM (Thyrotoxicosis)

 ESSENTIALS OF DIAGNOSIS

► Sweating, weight loss or gain, anxiety, palpitations, loose stools, heat intolerance, irritability, fatigue, weakness, menstrual irregularity.

► Tachycardia; warm, moist skin; stare; tremor.

► In Graves disease: goiter (often with bruit); ophthalmopathy.

► Suppressed TSH in primary hyperthyroidism; increased T_4, FT_4, T_3, FT_3.

General Considerations

The term "thyrotoxicosis" refers to the clinical manifestations associated with serum levels of T_4 or T_3 that are excessive for the individual (hyperthyroidism). Serum TSH levels are suppressed in primary hyperthyroidism. However, laboratory tests can be affected by certain conditions and drugs that may lead to the erroneous diagnosis of hyperthyroidism in euthyroid individuals (Table 26–5). The causes of hyperthyroidism are many and diverse, as described below.

A. Graves Disease

Graves disease (known as Basedow disease in Europe) is the most common cause of thyrotoxicosis. It is an autoimmune disorder affecting the thyroid gland, characterized by an increase in synthesis and release of thyroid hormones; the thyroid gland is typically enlarged. Graves disease is much more common in women than in men (8:1), and its onset is usually between the ages of 20 and 40 years. It may be accompanied by infiltrative ophthalmopathy (Graves exophthalmos) and, less commonly, by infiltrative dermopathy (pretibial myxedema). The thymus gland is typically hyperplastic and enlarged. Graves disease may also be associated with other systemic autoimmune disorders such as pernicious anemia, myasthenia gravis, and diabetes mellitus. It has a familial tendency, and histocompatibility studies have shown an association with group HLA-B8 and HLA-DR3. The pathogenesis of the hyperthyroidism of Graves disease involves the formation of autoantibodies that bind to the TSH receptor in thyroid cell membranes and stimulate the gland to hyperfunction. Antibodies increased in most patients include thyrotropin receptor antibody (TRAb), ANA, and thyroperoxidase (TPO) or thyroglobulin (Tg) antibodies.

Patients with Graves disease have an increased risk of developing Sjögren syndrome, Addison disease, alopecia areata, vitiligo, celiac disease, autoimmune diabetes mellitus type 1, hypoparathyroidism, myasthenia gravis, and cardiomyopathy.

B. Toxic Multinodular Goiter and Thyroid Adenomas

Autonomous toxic adenomas of the thyroid may be single (Plummer disease) or multiple (toxic multinodular goiter). **Jodbasedow disease**, or iodine-induced hyperthyroidism, may occur in patients with multinodular goiters after intake of large amounts of iodine in the diet or in the form of radiographic contrast materials or drugs, especially amiodarone. This condition is not associated with infiltrative ophthalmopathy or dermopathy. Antithyroid antibodies are usually not present in the plasma, and tests for TRAb are negative.

C. Subacute (de Quervain) Thyroiditis

Subacute thyroiditis typically presents with a moderately enlarged, tender thyroid, and hyperthyroidism. It is thought to be due to a viral infection. If the gland is nontender, the disorder is called "silent thyroiditis." Hyperthyroidism is followed by hypothyroidism. During thyrotoxicosis, thyroid radioactive iodine (RAI) uptake is low. A similar problem of low RAI is seen with interleukin-2 therapy and after neck surgery for hyperparathyroidism. Patients taking lithium may rarely experience thyrotoxicosis due to silent thyroiditis. Symptoms mimic a manic episode such that the diagnosis is often missed.

D. Thyrotoxicosis Factitia

Thyrotoxicosis factitia is due to ingestion of excessive amounts of exogenous thyroid hormone. Isolated epidemics of thyrotoxicosis have been caused by consumption of ground beef contaminated with bovine thyroid gland.

E. Struma Ovarii

Thyroid tissue is contained in about 3% of ovarian dermoid tumors and teratomas. This thyroid tissue may autonomously secrete thyroid hormone due to a toxic nodule or in concert with the woman's thyroid gland in Graves disease or toxic multinodular goiter.

F. Pituitary Tumor

TSH hypersecretion by the pituitary may be caused by a tumor or thyrotroph cell hyperplasia and is a rare cause of hyperthyroidism. Serum TSH is elevated or normal in the presence of true thyrotoxicosis. Pituitary hyperplasia may be detected on MRI scan as pituitary enlargement without a discrete adenoma being visible. This condition appears to be due to a diminished feedback effect of T_4 upon the pituitary. It may be familial, but it can also be caused by prolonged untreated hypothyroidism, especially in youth.

G. Hashimoto Thyroiditis

Hashimoto thyroiditis may cause transient hyperthyroidism during the initial destructive phase. This is also seen in some patients receiving interferon-α, interferon-β, and interleukin-2. Postpartum thyroiditis refers to Hashimoto thyroiditis that occurs in the first 6 months after delivery. It is common, occurring postpartum in 5–10% of women in the United States. Hyperthyroidism results from the release of stored thyroid hormone following damage to the thyroid (see Thyroiditis, below).

H. Pregnancy and Trophoblastic Tumors

The prevalence of hyperthyroidism in pregnancy—most commonly due to Graves disease—is about 0.2%. Struma ovarii is rare. Newborns have an increased risk of intrauterine growth retardation, prematurity, and transient thyrotoxicosis from transplacental transfer of TRAb.

Although hCG generally has a low affinity for the thyroid's TSH receptors, very high serum levels of hCG may cause sufficient receptor activation to cause thyrotoxicosis. Mild gestational hyperthyroidism may occur during the first 4 months of pregnancy, when hCG levels are very high. Pregnant women are more likely to have thyrotoxicosis and hyperemesis gravidarum if they have high serum levels of asialo-hCG, a subfraction of hCG with greater affinity for TSH receptors.

Thyrotoxicosis may also be caused by the high serum levels of hCG seen in molar pregnancy, choriocarcinoma, and testicular malignancies.

I. Thyroid Carcinoma

Metastatic functioning thyroid carcinoma is a rare cause of thyrotoxicosis. (See Thyroid Cancer section.)

J. Amiodarone-Induced Thyrotoxicosis

Amiodarone is 38% iodine by weight; its elimination half-life can be as long as 100 days. Among patients in the United States taking amiodarone, hyperthyroidism develops in about 3%; the incidence of hyperthyroidism is higher in Europe and in iodine-deficient geographic areas. Hyperthyroidism can occur 4 months to 3 years after initiation of amiodarone and may develop many months after amiodarone has been discontinued.

Type I amiodarone-induced thyrotoxicosis is caused by active elaboration of excessive thyroid hormone and may occur by either of two mechanisms: (1) Free iodine may cause toxic multinodular goiter in iodine-deficient patients with preexisting autonomous thyroid nodules (jodbasedow phenomenon). This is infrequently encountered in iodine-sufficient countries such as the United States. Thyroid RAI uptake ranges from low to high. (2) Excessive free iodine can trigger an immunologic attack on the thyroid; this may cause Graves disease, commonly with diffuse thyroid enlargement and antithyroid peroxidase antibodies (70%). Type II amiodarone-induced thyrotoxicosis is caused by destructive thyroiditis, which releases stored thyroid hormone from damaged cells; hyperthyroidism can last 1–3 months and may be followed by hypothyroidism.

▶ Clinical Findings

A. Symptoms and Signs

Thyrotoxicosis due to any cause produces many different manifestations of variable intensity among different individuals. Patients may complain of nervousness, restlessness, heat intolerance, increased sweating, pruritus, fatigue, weakness, muscle cramps, frequent bowel movements, or weight change (usually loss). There may be palpitations or angina pectoris. Women frequently report menstrual irregularities.

Signs of thyrotoxicosis may include stare and lid lag, fine resting finger tremors, moist warm skin, hyperreflexia, fine hair, and onycholysis. Certain eye findings—such as upper eyelid retraction (Dalrymple sign), lid lag with downward gaze (von Graefe sign), and a staring appearance (Kocher sign)—can occur with hyperthyroidism of any etiology. Chronic thyrotoxicosis may cause osteoporosis. Clubbing and swelling of the fingers (acropachy) develop in a small number of patients. Graves disease usually presents with additional findings of goiter (often with a bruit), but some patients have no palpable thyroid enlargement.

Cardiac manifestations of thyrotoxicosis commonly include a forceful heart beat, premature atrial contractions, and sinus tachycardia. Atrial fibrillation or atrial tachycardia occurs in about 8% of patients with thyrotoxicosis, more commonly in men, the elderly, and those with ischemic or valvular heart disease. The ventricular response from the atrial fibrillation may be difficult to control. Thyrotoxicosis itself can cause a thyrotoxic cardiomyopathy, and the onset of atrial fibrillation can precipitate congestive heart failure.

Ophthalmopathy is clinically apparent in 20–40% of patients with Graves disease and type I amiodarone-induced thyrotoxicosis, but in no other conditions causing hyperthyroidism. It usually consists of conjunctival edema (chemosis), conjunctivitis, and mild exophthalmos (proptosis). More severe lymphocytic infiltration of the eye muscles occurs in 5–10%, pushing the eye forward, producing clinical exophthalmos and sometimes diplopia due to extraocular muscle entrapment. There may be weakness of upward gaze (Stellwag sign). The optic nerve may be compressed in severe cases, causing progressive loss of color vision, visual fields, and visual acuity. Corneal drying may occur with inadequate lid closure. Eye changes may sometimes be asymmetric or unilateral. The severity of the eye disease is not closely correlated with the severity of the thyrotoxicosis. Some patients with Graves ophthalmopathy are clinically euthyroid.

Exophthalmometry should be performed on all patients with Graves disease to document their degree of exophthalmos and detect progression of orbitopathy. The protrusion of the eye beyond the orbital rim is measured with a prism instrument (Hertel exophthalmometer). Maximum normal eye protrusion varies between kindreds and races, being about 22 mm for blacks, 20 mm for whites, and 18 mm for Asians.

Diplopia can be caused by exophthalmus or by coexistent **ocular myasthenia gravis,** which is more common in Graves disease and is usually mild, often with selective eye involvement. Acetylcholinesterase receptor antibody (AChR Ab) levels are elevated in only 36% of such patients, and a thymoma is present in 9%.

Graves dermopathy (pretibial myxedema) occurs in about 3% of patients with Graves disease, usually in the pretibial region. Glycosaminoglycan accumulation and lymphoid infiltration occur in affected skin, which becomes erythematous with a thickened, rough texture.

Thyroid acropachy is an extreme and unusual manifestation of Graves disease. It presents with digital clubbing, swelling of fingers and toes, and a periosteal reaction of extremity bones. It is ordinarily associated with ophthalmopathy and thyroid dermopathy. Most patients are smokers. The presence of thyroid acropachy is an indication of the severity of the autoimmunity; most patients have high serum titers of thyroid-stimulating immunoglobulin. Patients with thyroid acropachy are at greater risk for having concurrent Graves dermopathy and severe ophthalmopathy. However, acropachy itself does not usually cause clinical complaints.

Hyperthyroidism during pregnancy shares many of the features of normal pregnancy: tachycardia, warm skin, heat intolerance, increased sweating, and a palpable thyroid. Pregnancy can have a beneficial effect on the thyrotoxicosis of Graves disease. However, there is an increased risk of thyroid storm, preeclampsia–eclampsia, congestive heart failure, premature delivery, and abruptio placentae.

Hypokalemic periodic paralysis occurs in about 15% of Asian or Native American men with thyrotoxicosis. It usually presents abruptly with symmetric flaccid paralysis (and few thyrotoxic symptoms), often after intravenous dextrose, oral carbohydrate, or vigorous exercise. Attacks last 7–72 hours.

B. Laboratory Findings

Serum T_3, T_4, thyroid resin uptake, and FT_4 are usually all increased. Sometimes the T_4 level may be normal but the serum T_3 is elevated. Serum T_3 can be misleadingly elevated when blood is collected in tubes using a gel barrier, which causes certain immunoassays (eg, Immulite but not Axsym analyzers) to report serum total T_3 levels that are falsely elevated in 24% of normal patients. Serum T_4 or T_3 can be elevated in other nonthyroidal conditions (Table 26–5).

Serum TSH is suppressed in hyperthyroidism, except in the very rare cases of pituitary inappropriate secretion of thyrotropin. Serum TSH may be misleadingly low in other nonthyroidal conditions. Hyperthyroidism can cause other laboratory abnormalities, including hypercalcemia, increased alkaline phosphatase, anemia, and decreased granulocytes. Hypokalemia and hypophosphatemia occur in thyrotoxic periodic paralysis.

Problems of diagnosis occur in patients with acute psychiatric disorders; about 30% of these patients have hyperthyroxinemia without thyrotoxicosis. The TSH is not usually suppressed, distinguishing psychiatric disorder from true hyperthyroidism. T_4 levels return to normal gradually.

In **Graves disease**, TSH receptor antibody (TRAb) levels are usually detectable (65%). Antithyroglobulin or antithyroperoxidase antibodies are usually elevated but are nonspecific. Serum ANA and anti-double-stranded DNA antibodies are also usually elevated without any evidence of lupus erythematosus or other collagen-vascular disease.

With **subacute thyroiditis,** patients often have an increased erythrocyte sedimentation rate (ESR).

With **hyperthyroidism during pregnancy,** women have an elevated FT_4 while the TSH is suppressed. However, apparent lack of full TSH suppression can be seen due to misidentification of hCG as TSH in certain assays. Although the total T_4 is elevated in most pregnant women, values over 20 mcg/dL are encountered only in hyperthyroidism. The T_3 resin uptake, which is low in normal pregnancy because of high TBG concentration, is normal or high in thyrotoxic persons. Pregnancy can have a beneficial effect on the thyrotoxicosis of Graves disease, with decreasing antibody titers and decreasing FT_4 levels as the pregnancy advances.

Since high levels of T_4 and FT_4 are normally seen in patients taking **amiodarone,** suppressed TSH (sensitive assay) must be present along with a greatly elevated T_4 (> 20 mcg/dL) or T_3 (> 200 ng/dL) in order to diagnose hyperthyroidism. (**Note:** *Hypo*thyroidism occurs in an additional 6% of patients receiving amiodarone after 2–39 weeks of therapy.) In **type I amiodarone-induced thyrotoxicosis,** the presence of proptosis, TSH-R Ab[stim], or thyrotropin-binding inhibitory immunoglobulin (TBII) is diagnostic. In **type II amiodarone-induced thyrotoxicosis,** serum levels of interleukin-6 (IL-6) are usually quite elevated.

C. Imaging

Patients with an established diagnosis of thyrotoxicosis usually undergo thyroid RAI uptake and scan. Women with hyperthyroidism due to Graves disease should ideally have the RAI scan extended to include the pelvis in order to screen for concomitant struma ovarii (rare). A high RAI uptake is seen in **Graves disease** and **toxic nodular goiter** but can be seen in other conditions as well. A low RAI uptake is characteristic of subacute thyroiditis but can also be seen after an iodine load and in other conditions. In the United States, thyroid RAI uptake is usually negligible in patients with **type I amiodarone-induced thyrotoxicosis;** however, in Europe, up to 80% of such patients have detectable or normal RAI uptake. In **type II amiodarone-induced thyrotoxicosis,** thyroid RAI uptake is very low.

MRI of the orbits is the imaging method of choice to visualize Graves ophthalmopathy affecting the extraocular muscles. CT scanning and ultrasonography can also be used. Imaging is required only in severe or unilateral cases or in euthyroid exophthalmos that must be distinguished from orbital pseudotumor, tumors, and other lesions.

▶ Differential Diagnosis

True thyrotoxicosis must be distinguished from those conditions elevating serum T_4 and T_3 or suppressing serum TSH without affecting clinical status.

Some states of hypermetabolism without thyrotoxicosis—notably severe anemia, leukemia, polycythemia, and cancer—rarely cause confusion. Pheochromocytoma is often associated with hypermetabolism, tachycardia, weight loss, and profuse sweating. Acromegaly may also produce tachycardia, sweating, and thyroid enlargement. Appropriate laboratory tests will easily distinguish these entities.

Cardiac disease (eg, atrial fibrillation, angina) refractory to treatment suggests the possibility of underlying ("apathetic") hyperthyroidism. Other causes of ophthalmoplegia (eg, myasthenia gravis) and exophthalmos (eg, orbital tumor, pseudotumor) must be considered. Thyrotoxicosis must also be considered in the differential diagnosis of muscle weakness and osteoporosis. Diabetes mellitus and Addison disease may coexist with thyrotoxicosis.

▶ Complications

Hypercalcemia, osteoporosis, and nephrocalcinosis may occur. Decreased libido, impotence, diminished sperm motility, and gynecomastia may be noted in men with hyperthyroidism. Other complications include cardiac arrhythmias and heart failure, thyroid crisis, ophthalmopathy, dermopathy, and thyrotoxic hypokalemic periodic paralysis (see below.)

▶ Treatment

A. Graves Disease

The treatment of Graves disease involves a choice of methods rather than a method of choice.

1. Propranolol—Propranolol is generally used for symptomatic relief until the hyperthyroidism is resolved. It effectively relieves the tachycardia, tremor, diaphoresis, and anxiety that occur with hyperthyroidism due to any cause. It is the initial treatment of choice for thyroid storm. The periodic paralysis seen in association with thyrotoxicosis is also effectively treated with β-blockade. It has no effect on thyroid hormone secretion. Treatment is usually begun with propranolol ER 60 mg orally twice daily, with dosage increases every 2 days. The available doses of propranolol ER are 60, 80, 120, and 160 mg. Propranolol ER is initially given every 12 hours for patients with severe hyperthyroidism, due to accelerated metabolism of the propranolol; it may be given once daily as hyperthyroidism improves.

2. Thiourea drugs—Methimazole or propylthiouracil is generally used for young adults or patients with mild thyrotoxicosis, small goiters, or fear of isotopes. Carbimazole is another thiourea that is converted to methimazole in vivo and is available outside the United States. Elderly patients usually respond particularly well. These drugs are also useful for preparing hyperthyroid patients for surgery and elderly patients for RAI treatment. The drugs do not permanently damage the thyroid and are associated with a lower chance of posttreatment hypothyroidism (compared with RAI or surgery). When thiourea therapy is discontinued, there is a high recurrence rate for hyperthyroidism (about 50%). A better likelihood of long-term remission is seen in patients with small goiters or mild hyperthyroidism and those requiring small doses of thiourea. Patients whose thyroperoxidase and thyroglobulin antibodies remain high after 2 years of therapy have been reported to have only a 10% rate of relapse. Thiourea therapy may be continued long-term for patients who are tolerating it well.

Agranulocytosis occurs in about 0.3% of patients taking methimazole and about 0.4% of patients taking propylthiouracil. Agranulocytosis usually occurs in the first 60 days of therapy, and it develops in a few patients after 5 months of therapy. There is a genetic tendency to develop agranulocytosis with thiourea therapy; if a close relative has had this adverse reaction, other therapies should be considered for the patient. Patients are warned that if a sore throat or febrile illness develops, they should stop the drug while a WBC is rechecked. The agranulocytosis is generally reversible; recovery is not improved by filgrastim (granulocyte colony-stimulating factor [G-CSF]). Periodic surveillance of the WBC during treatment has been advocated, but the onset of agranulocytosis is generally abrupt.

Other side effects common to thiourea drugs include pruritus, allergic dermatitis, nausea, and dyspepsia. Antihistamines may control mild pruritus without discontinuation of the drug. Since the two thiourea drugs are similar, patients who have had a major allergic reaction from one should not be given the other.

Primary hypothyroidism may occur. The patient may become clinically hypothyroid for 2 weeks or more before TSH levels rise, having been suppressed by the preceding hyperthyroidism. Therefore, the patient's changing thyroid status is best monitored clinically and with serum levels of FT_4. Rapid growth of the goiter usually occurs if prolonged hypothyroidism is allowed to develop; the goiter may some-times become massive but usually regresses rapidly with thyroid hormone replacement.

A. Methimazole—Methimazole is generally preferred over propylthiouracil since the methimazole is more convenient to use and is less likely to cause fulminant hepatic necrosis. Methimazole therapy is also less likely to cause ^{131}I treatment failure. Rare complications peculiar to methimazole include serum sickness, cholestatic jaundice, loss of taste, alopecia, nephrotic syndrome, and hypoglycemia. Methimazole is given orally in initial doses of 30–60 mg once daily. Some patients with very mild hyperthyroidism may respond well to smaller initial doses of methimazole (10–20 mg daily). Methimazole may also be administered twice daily to reduce the likelihood of gastrointestinal upset. Methimazole use in pregnancy has been associated with a possibly increased risk of fetal anomalies such as aplasia cutis, esophageal atresia, and coanal atresia. However, methimazole may be used if the patient cannot tolerate propylthiouracil (see below). If methimazole is used during pregnancy or breastfeeding, the dose should not exceed 20 mg daily. The dosage is reduced as manifestations of hyperthyroidism resolve and as the FT_4 level falls toward normal. For patients who have elected to receive ^{131}I therapy, methimazole is discontinued 4 days prior to receiving the ^{131}I and is resumed at a lower dose 3 days afterwards to avoid recurrence of hyperthyroidism. About 4 weeks after ^{131}I therapy, methimazole may be discontinued if the patient is euthyroid.

B. Propylthiouracil—Propylthiouracil has been the drug of choice during breastfeeding since it is not concentrated in the milk as much as methimazole. Propylthiouracil is also favored during pregnancy, possibly causing fewer problems in the newborn. Rare complications peculiar to propylthiouracil include arthritis, lupus erythematosus, aplastic anemia, thrombocytopenia, and hypoprothrombinemia. Acute hepatitis occurs rarely and is treated with prednisone but may progress to liver failure. Propylthiouracil is given orally in initial doses of 300–600 mg daily in four divided doses. The dosage and frequency of administration are reduced as symptoms of hyperthyroidism resolve and the FT_4 level approaches normal. During pregnancy, the dose of propylthiouracil is kept below 200 mg/d to avoid goitrous hypothyroidism in the infant.

3. Iodinated contrast agents—These agents provide effective temporary treatment for thyrotoxicosis of any cause. Iopanoic acid (Telepaque) or ipodate sodium (Bilivist, Oragrafin) is given orally in a dosage of 500 mg twice daily for 3 days, then 500 mg once daily. These agents inhibit peripheral 5'-monodeiodination of T_4, thereby blocking its conversion to active T_3. Within 24 hours, serum T_3 levels fall an average of 62%. For patients with Graves disease, methimazole is begun first to block iodine organification; the next day, ipodate sodium or iopanoic acid may be added. The iodinated contrast agents are particularly useful for patients who are very symptomatically thyrotoxic (see Thyroid Storm, below). They offer a therapeutic option for patients with T_4 overdosage, subacute thyroiditis, and amiodarone-induced thyrotoxicosis and for those intolerant to thioureas and for newborns with thyrotoxicosis (due to maternal Graves disease). Treatment periods of 8 months or more are possible, but efficacy tends to wane with time. In Graves disease, thyroid RAI uptake may be suppressed during treatment but typically returns to pretreatment uptake by 7 days after discontinuation of the drug, allowing ^{131}I treatment.

4. Radioactive iodine (^{131}I, RAI)—The administration of ^{131}I is an excellent method of destroying overactive thyroid tissue (either diffuse or toxic nodular goiter). There are ample data to conclude that patients who are treated with RAI in adulthood do not have an increased risk of subsequent thyroid cancer, leukemia, or other malignancies. Similarly, individuals who were treated with RAI as teenagers have not shown any increased risk of malignancy in a 36-year retrospective study. Children born to parents previously treated with ^{131}I show normal rates of congenital abnormalities.

Because fetal radiation is harmful, *RAI should not be given to pregnant women.* It is prudent to obtain a sensitive pregnancy test (serum β-hCG) on all women of reproductive age prior to ^{131}I therapy.

Most patients may receive ^{131}I while being symptomatically treated with just propranolol LA, which is then reduced in dosage as hyperthyroxinemia resolves. However, some patients (those with coronary diseases, the elderly, or those with severe hyperthyroidism) are usually rendered euthyroid with a thiouracil drug (see above) while the dosage of propranolol is reduced. A higher rate of ^{131}I treatment failure has been reported in patients with Graves disease who have been receiving methimazole or propylthiouracil. However, therapy with ^{131}I will usually be effective if the methimazole is discontinued at least 4 days before RAI therapy and if the therapeutic dosage of ^{131}I is adjusted (upward) according to RAI uptake on the pretherapy scan. Prior to ^{131}I therapy, patients are instructed against receiving intravenous iodinated contrast or ingesting large quantities of dietary iodine, but severe restriction of dietary iodine is not usually necessary.

Following ^{131}I treatment for hyperthyroidism, Graves ophthalmopathy appears or worsens in 15% of patients (23% in smokers and 6% in nonsmokers) and improves in none, whereas during treatment with methimazole, ophthalmopathy worsens in 3% and improves in 2% of patients. Among patients receiving 3 months of prednisone following ^{131}I treatment, preexistent ophthalmopathy worsens in none and improves in 67%.

Smoking increases the risk of having a flare in ophthalmopathy following ^{131}I treatment and also reduces the effectiveness of prednisone treatment. Therefore, patients who smoke are strongly encouraged to quit prior to ^{131}I treatment.

FT$_4$ levels may sometimes drop within 2 months after ^{131}I treatment, but then rise again to thyrotoxic levels, at which time thyroid RAI uptake is low. This phenomenon is caused by a release of stored thyroid hormone from injured thyroid cells and does not indicate a treatment failure. In fact, serum FT$_4$ then falls abruptly to hypothyroid levels.

There is a high incidence of hypothyroidism in the months to years after ^{131}I, even when small doses are given. However, hypothyroidism also occurs quite frequently years after surgical or medical treatment of Graves disease, and eventual hypothyroidism may be part of the natural history of this condition. Lifelong clinical follow-up is mandatory, with measurements of FT$_4$ and TSH when indicated.

5. Thyroid surgery—Thyroid surgery for Graves disease and toxic nodular goiter has been performed less frequently since the increased use of RAI treatment. Thyroidectomy may be performed for pregnant women whose thyrotoxicosis is not controlled with low doses of thioureas, and for women who desire to become pregnant in the very near future. Surgery is also an option for nodular goiters, when there is a suspicion for malignancy. The Hartley–Dunhill operation is the surgical procedure of choice for patients with Graves disease; this operation consists of a total resection of one lobe and a subtotal resection of the other lobe, leaving about 4 g of thyroid tissue. Subtotal thyroidectomy of both lobes is often used, but ultimately results in a 9% recurrence rate for hyperthyroidism. Total thyroidectomy of both lobes poses an increased risk for hypoparathyroidism and damage to the recurrent laryngeal nerve.

Patients are ordinarily rendered euthyroid preoperatively with a thiourea drug. Ipodate sodium or iopanoic acid (500 mg orally twice daily) may be used in addition to a thiourea to accelerate the decline in serum T$_3$. Propranolol is given until the serum T$_3$ (or free T$_3$) is normal preoperatively. Thyroid vascularity is reduced by preoperative treatment with either ipodate sodium or iopanoic acid (500 mg twice daily for 3 days) or iodine (eg, Lugol solution, two or three drops orally daily for several days). If a patient undergoes surgery while thyrotoxic, larger doses of propranolol are given perioperatively to reduce the likelihood of thyroid crisis.

Morbidity includes possible damage to the recurrent laryngeal nerve, with resultant vocal cord paralysis. Hypoparathyroidism also occurs, which means that calcium levels must be checked postoperatively. When a thyroidectomy is performed by a competent, experienced neck surgeon, surgical complications are uncommon. Thyroid surgery should be performed as an inpatient, with at least an overnight observational period.

B. Toxic Solitary Thyroid Nodules

Toxic solitary thyroid nodules are usually benign but may rarely be malignant. If a nonsurgical therapy is elected, the nodule should be evaluated with a fine-needle aspiration biopsy (FNA). Hyperthyroidism caused by a single hyperfunctioning thyroid nodule may be treated symptomatically with propranolol ER and methimazole or propylthiouracil, as in Graves disease (see above). Patients who tolerate methimazole well may elect to continue it for long-term therapy. When using methimazole, the serum TSH should be monitored and the dose of methimazole adjusted to be kept slightly suppressed, so the risk of TSH-stimulated growth of the nodule is reduced. For patients under age 40 years and for healthy older patients, surgery is usually recommended; patients are made euthyroid with a thiourea preoperatively and given several days of iodine, ipodate sodium, or iopanoic acid before surgery as in Graves disease (see above). Transient postoperative hypothyroidism resolves spontaneously. Permanent hypothyroidism occurs in about 14% of patients by 6 years after surgery. Patients with a toxic solitary nodule who are over age 40 years or in poor health may be offered ^{131}I therapy. If the patient has been receiving methimazole preparatory to ^{131}I, the TSH should be kept slightly suppressed in order to reduce the uptake of ^{131}I by the normal thyroid. Nevertheless, permanent hypothyroidism occurs in about one-third of patients after 8 years of ^{131}I therapy. The nodule remains palpable in 50% and may grow in 10% of patients after [131]I.

C. Toxic Multinodular Goiter

Hyperthyroidism caused by a toxic multinodular goiter may also be treated with propranolol ER and methimazole, as in Graves disease. Methimazole does reverse hyperthyroidism, but there is a 95% recurrence rate if it is stopped. Definitive treatment for large multinodular goiters is surgery, prior to which patients are rendered euthyroid. Surgery is particularly indicated to relieve pressure symptoms or for cosmetic indications. Patients with toxic multinodular goiter are prepared for surgery the same as those with Graves disease (see above). Patients who are to receive ^{131}I treatment are rendered nearly euthyroid with methimazole, which is stopped at least 4 days before RAI treatment. Meanwhile, the patient follows a low-iodine diet; this is done to enhance the thyroid gland's uptake of RAI, which may be relatively low in this condition (compared to Graves disease). Relatively high doses of ^{131}I are usually required; recurrent thyrotoxicosis and hypothyroidism are common, so patients must be monitored closely. Peculiarly, in about 5% of patients with diffusely nodular toxic goiter, the administration of ^{131}I therapy may induce Graves disease. Also, Graves' eye disease has occurred rarely following ^{131}I therapy for multinodular goiter.

D. Subacute (de Quervain) Thyroiditis

Patients with hyperthyroidism due to subacute thyroiditis are treated symptomatically with propranolol ER. Ipodate sodium or iopanoic acid, 500 mg orally daily, promptly corrects elevated T_3 levels and is continued for 15–60 days until the serum FT_4 level normalizes. The condition subsides spontaneously within weeks to months. Thioureas are ineffective, since thyroid hormone production is actually low in this condition. RAI is ineffective, since the thyroid's iodine uptake is low. Since periods of hypothyroidism may occur following the initial inflammatory episode, patients should have close clinical follow-up, with serum FT_4 measurement when necessary. Prompt treatment of the transient hypothyroidism may reduce the incidence of recurrent thyroiditis. Pain can usually be managed with non-aspirin nonsteroidal anti-inflammatory drugs.

E. Hashimoto Thyroiditis (Hashitoxicosis)

Rarely, hyperthyroidism develops as a result of release of stored thyroid hormone during severe Hashimoto thyroiditis. The thyroperoxidase or thyroglobulin antibodies are usually high, but RAI uptake is low, thus distinguishing it from Graves disease. This is especially common in postpartum women, in whom it may be transient. Treatment is with propranolol ER. Ipodate sodium or iopanoic acid may also be used as described above. Patients are monitored carefully for the development of hypothyroidism and treated.

F. Hyperthyroidism during Pregnancy and Lactation

Pregnant women with hyperthyroidism are treated with propylthiouracil, which is generally preferred over methimazole on the basis of uncontrolled reports of fetal anomalies in the offspring of women taking methimazole during pregnancy. Whichever thiourea is used, it should be given in the smallest dose possible, permitting mild hyperthyroidism to occur since it is usually well tolerated. Both propylthiouracil and methimazole cross the placenta and can induce hypothyroidism, with fetal TSH hypersecretion and goiter. Thyroid hormone administration to the mother does not prevent hypothyroidism in the fetus, since T_4 and T_3 do not freely cross the placenta. Fetal hypothyroidism is rare if the mother's hyperthyroidism is controlled with small daily doses of propylthiouracil (50–150 mg/d orally) or methimazole (5–15 mg/d orally). Thyroidectomy is reserved for women who are allergic or resistant to antithyroid drugs (usually due to noncompliance) or who have very large goiters. Fetal ultrasound at 32 weeks gestation can visualize any fetal goiter, so fetal thyroid dysfunction can be diagnosed and treated.

During lactation, women treated with propylthiouracil secrete very little of it into breast milk. Methimazole is secreted in somewhat higher concentrations in breast milk. However, the use of either propylthiouracil or methimazole during breast-feeding does not significantly affect the infant's thyroid hormone levels, and both drugs are approved for nursing mothers by the American Academy of Pediatrics. No adverse reactions to these drugs (eg, rash, hepatic dysfunction, leukopenia) have been reported in breast-fed infants. Recommended doses are 20 mg orally daily or less for methimazole and 450 mg orally daily or less for propylthiouracil. It is recommended that the medication be taken just after breast-feeding.

G. Other Causes of Hyperthyroidism

Patients with thyrotoxicosis from **thyrotrophe pituitary hyperplasia** are treated with propranolol LA as described above. Definitive treatment is with RAI or thyroid surgery. Patients with thyrotoxicosis caused by a **thyrotrophe pituitary adenoma** are treated with propranolol LA and methimazole, followed by transsphenoidal resection of the pituitary tumor, when possible. Treatment of patients with **type I amiodarone-induced thyrotoxicosis** usually requires propranolol ER and a prolonged course of methimazole. After two doses of methimazole, iopanoic acid or sodium ipodate may be added to the regimen to further block conversion of T_4 to T_3; the recommended dosage for each is 500 mg orally twice daily for 3 days, followed by 500 mg once daily until thyrotoxicosis is resolved. β-Blockers may be required. Withdrawal of amiodarone does not have a significant therapeutic effect for several months. Therapy with ^{131}I may be successful in some patients with adequate RAI uptake. Thyroidectomy is reserved for resistant cases. Treatment of patients with **type II amiodarone-induced thyrotoxicosis** consists of propranolol ER and prednisone plus either iopanoic acid or ipodate sodium (see above). Withdrawal of amiodarone is not usually necessary. Because the condition is transient, thyroidectomy is rarely required.

H. Treatment of Complications

1. Graves ophthalmopathy—The risk of having a "flare" of ophthalmopathy following ^{131}I treatment for hyperthyroidism is about 6% for nonsmokers and 23% for smokers. Graves ophthalmopathy can also be aggravated by thiazolidinediones (eg, pioglitazone, rosiglitazone); these oral diabetic agents should be avoided or withdrawn in patients with Graves disease. For acute, progressive exophthalmos, intravenous methylprednisolone, begun promptly, is superior to oral prednisone, possibly due to improved compliance. Methylprednisolone is given intravenously, 500 mg weekly for 6 weeks, then 250 mg weekly for 6 weeks. If oral prednisone is chosen for treatment, it must be given promptly in daily doses of 40–60 mg/d orally, with dosage reduction over several weeks. Higher initial prednisone doses of 80–120 mg/d are used when there is optic nerve compression. Prednisone alleviates eye symptoms in 64% of nonsmokers, but only 14% of smokers respond well.

Progressive active exophthalmos may be treated with retrobulbar radiation therapy using a supervoltage linear accelerator (4–6 MeV) to deliver 20 Gy over 2 weeks to the extraocular muscles, avoiding the cornea and lens. Prednisone in high doses is given concurrently. Patients who respond well to orbital radiation include those with signs of acute inflammation, recent exophthalmos (< 6 months), or optic nerve compression. Patients with chronic proptosis and orbital muscle restriction respond less well. Retrobulbar radiation does not cause cataracts or tumors; however, it can cause radiation-induced retinopathy (usually subclinical) in about 5% of patients overall, mostly in diabetics.

For severe cases, orbital decompression surgery may save vision, though diplopia often persists postoperatively. General eye protective measures include wearing glasses to protect the protruding eye and taping the lids shut during sleep if corneal drying is a problem. Methylcellulose drops and gels ("artificial tears") may also help. Tarsorrhaphy or canthoplasty can frequently help protect the cornea and provide improved appearance. Hypothyroidism and hyperthyroidism must be treated promptly.

2. Cardiac complications

A. Sinus tachycardia—Treatment consists of treating the thyrotoxicosis. A β-blocker (as described above) such as propranolol is used in the interim unless there is an associated cardiomyopathy.

B. Atrial fibrillation—Electrical cardioversion is unlikely to convert atrial fibrillation to normal sinus rhythm while the patient is thyrotoxic. Spontaneous conversion to normal sinus rhythm tends to occur in about 56% of patients with achievement of euthyroidism, but that likelihood decreases with age. Elective cardioversion may be used for those patients in whom atrial fibrillation persists for 4 months after resolution of hyperthyroidism. Hyperthyroidism must be treated immediately (see above). Other drugs, including digoxin, β-blockers, anticoagulants, may be required.

(1) Digoxin—Digoxin is used to slow a fast ventricular response to thyrotoxic atrial fibrillation; it must be used in larger than normal doses because of increased clearance and an increased number of cardiac cellular sodium pumps requiring inhibition. Digoxin doses are reduced as hyperthyroidism is corrected.

(2) β-Blockers—β-Blockers may also reduce the ventricular rate, but they must be used with caution—particularly in patients with cardiomegaly or signs of heart failure—since their negative inotropic effect may precipitate congestive heart failure. Therefore, an initial trial of a short-duration β-blocker should be considered, such as esmolol intravenously. If a β-blocker is used, doses of digoxin must be reduced.

(3) Anticoagulants—Anticoagulation is indicated in the following situations: left atrial enlargement on echocardiogram, global left ventricular dysfunction, recent congestive heart failure, hypertension, recurrent atrial fibrillation, or a history of previous thromboembolism. The doses of warfarin required in thyrotoxicosis are smaller than normal because of an accelerated plasma clearance of vitamin K–dependent clotting factors. Higher warfarin doses are usually required as hyperthyroidism subsides.

C. Heart failure—Heart failure due to thyrotoxicosis may be caused by extreme tachycardia, cardiomyopathy, or both. Very aggressive treatment of the hyperthyroidism is required in either case (see Thyroid Crisis, below). The tachycardia from atrial fibrillation is treated with digoxin as above. Intravenous furosemide is typically required. Oral spironolactone or eplerenone may be helpful. If tachycardia appears to be the main cause of the failure, β-blockers are administered cautiously as described above.

Congestive heart failure may occur as a result of low-output dilated cardiomyopathy in the setting of hyperthyroidism. It is uncommon and may be caused by an idiosyncratic severe toxic effect of hyperthyroidism upon certain hearts. Cardiomyopathy may occur at any age and without preexisting cardiac disease. β-Blockers and calcium channel blockers are avoided. Emergency treatment may include afterload reduction, diuretics, digoxin, and other inotropic agents while the patient is being rendered euthyroid. Heart failure usually persists despite correction of hyperthyroidism.

D. Apathetic hyperthyroidism—Apathetic hyperthyroidism may present with angina pectoris. Treatment is directed at reversing the hyperthyroidism as well as providing standard antianginal therapy. Coronary angioplasty or bypass grafting can often be avoided by prompt diagnosis and treatment.

3. Thyroid crisis or "storm"—This disorder, rarely seen today, is an extreme form of thyrotoxicosis that may be triggered by stressful illness, thyroid surgery, or RAI administration and is manifested by marked delirium, severe tachycardia, vomiting, diarrhea, dehydration and, in many cases, very high fever. The mortality rate is high.

A thiourea drug is given (eg, methimazole, 15–25 mg orally every 6 hours or propylthiouracil, 150–250 mg orally every 6 hours). Ipodate sodium (500 mg/d orally) can be helpful if begun 1 hour after the first dose of thiourea. Iodide is given 1 hour later as Lugol solution (10 drops three times daily orally) or as sodium iodide (1 g intravenously slowly). Propranolol is given (cautiously in the presence of heart failure; see above) in a dosage of 0.5–2 mg intravenously every 4 hours or 20–120 mg orally every 6 hours. Hydrocortisone is usually given in doses of 50 mg orally every 6 hours, with rapid dosage reduction as the clinical situation improves. Aspirin is avoided since it displaces T_4 from TBG, raising FT_4 serum levels. Definitive treatment with ^{131}I or surgery is delayed until the patient is euthyroid.

4. Hyperthyroidism from postpartum thyroiditis—Propranolol ER is given during the hyperthyroid phase followed by levothyroxine during the hypothyroidism phase (see Thyroiditis, below).

5. Graves dermopathy—Treatment involves application of a topical corticosteroid (eg, fluocinolone) with nocturnal plastic occlusive dressings.

6. Thyrotoxic hypokalemic periodic paralysis—Sudden symmetric flaccid paralysis, along with hypokalemia and hypophosphatemia and few signs of thyrotoxicosis, may develop in Asian and Native American men with hyperthyroidism. Therapy with oral propranolol, 3 mg/kg, normalizes the serum potassium and phosphate levels and reverses the paralysis within 2–3 hours. No intravenous potassium or phosphate is ordinarily required. Intravenous dextrose and oral carbohydrate aggravate the condition and are to be avoided. Therapy is continued with propranolol, 60–80 mg every 8 hours (or sustained-action propranolol ER daily at equivalent daily dosage), along with a thiourea drug such as methimazole to treat the hyperthyroidism.

▶ **Prognosis**

Graves disease may rarely subside spontaneously, particularly when it is mild or subclinical. However, it usually persists. The ocular, cardiac, and psychological complications can become very serious and persistent even after treatment. Permanent hypoparathyroidism and vocal cord palsy are risks of surgical thyroidectomy. Recurrences are common following thiourea therapy but also occur after low-dose ^{131}I therapy or subtotal thyroidectomy. With adequate treatment and long-term follow-up, the results

are usually good. However, despite treatment for their hyperthyroidism, women experience an increased long-term risk of death from thyroid disease, cardiovascular disease, stroke, and fracture of the femur. Posttreatment hypothyroidism is common. It may occur within a few months or up to several years after RAI therapy or subtotal thyroidectomy. Malignant exophthalmos has a poor prognosis unless treated aggressively.

Subclinical hyperthyroidism refers to a condition in which asymptomatic individuals have a low serum TSH and normal FT_4 and T_3. Most such patients do well without treatment. In one series, clinical hyperthyroidism developed in only one of seven patients after 2 years. However, most patients do not progress to overt thyrotoxicosis, and the serum TSH may revert to normal within 2 years. Most such patients do not have accelerated bone loss. However, if a baseline bone density shows significant osteopenia, bone densitometry may be performed periodically. In persons over age 60 years, serum TSH is very low (< 0.1 mU/L) in 3% and mildly low (0.1–0.4 mU/L) in 9%. The chance of developing atrial fibrillation is 2.8% yearly in elderly patients with very low TSH and 1.1% yearly in those with mildly low TSH. Asymptomatic persons with very low TSH are monitored closely but are not treated unless atrial fibrillation or other manifestations of hyperthyroidism develop.

Laurberg P et al. Management of Graves' hyperthyroidism in pregnancy: focus on both maternal and foetal thyroid function, and caution against surgical thyroidectomy in pregnancy. Eur J Endocrinol. 2009 Jan;160(1):1–8. [PMID: 18849306]

Meller J et al. Incidence of radioiodine induced Graves' disease in patients with multinodular toxic goiter. Exp Clin Endocrinol Diabetes. 2006 May;114(5):235–9. [PMID: 16804797]

Porterfield JR Jr et al. Evidence-based management of toxic multinodular goiter (Plummer's disease). World J Surg. 2008 Jul;32(7):1278–84. [PMID: 18357484]

Tahrani AA et al. Graves' eye disease developing following radioiodine treatment for toxic nodular goitre. Exp Clin Endocrinol Diabetes. 2007 Jul;115(7):471–3. [PMID: 17647147]

THYROIDITIS

ESSENTIALS OF DIAGNOSIS

▶ Swelling of thyroid gland, sometimes causing pressure symptoms in acute and subacute forms; painless enlargement and rubbery firmness in chronic form.

▶ Thyroid function tests variable.

▶ Serum antithyroperoxidase and antithyroglobulin antibody levels usually elevated in Hashimoto thyroiditis.

▶ **General Considerations**

Thyroiditis may be classified as follows: (1) chronic lymphocytic thyroiditis due to autoimmunity (also called Hashimoto thyroiditis), (2) subacute thyroiditis, (3) suppurative thyroiditis, and (4) Riedel thyroiditis.

Hashimoto thyroiditis is an autoimmune condition and the most common thyroid disorder in the United States. B-lymphocytes invade the thyroid gland, such that the condition is also known as *chronic lymphocytic thyroiditis*. Detectable levels of antithyroid antibodies are usually present: antithyroperoxidase (antimitochondrial) antibodies or antithyroglobulin antibodies, or both. However, only a small subset of individuals with elevated antithyroid antibody levels ever develops thyroid dysfunction. Elevated serum levels of antithyroid antibodies are found in 3% of men and 13% of women. Women over the age of 60 years have a 25% incidence of elevated serum levels of antithyroid antibodies. The incidence of Hashimoto thyroiditis varies by kindred and by race; in persons older than 12 years of age in the United States, elevated levels of antithyroid antibodies are found in 14.3% of whites, 10.9% of Mexican-Americans, and 5.3% of blacks. Subclinical thyroiditis is extremely common, as evidenced in autopsy series that have found focal thyroiditis in about 40% of women and 20% of men. However, only 1% of the population has serum antithyroid antibody titers greater than 1:6400.

Hashimoto thyroiditis tends to be familial and is six times more common in women than in men. Its frequency is increased by dietary iodine supplementation. Certain drugs (amiodarone, interferon-α, interferon-β, interleukin-2, G-CSF) frequently induce thyroid autoantibodies. Childhood or occupational exposure to head–neck external beam radiation increases the lifetime risk of Hashimoto thyroiditis.

Hashimoto thyroiditis often progresses to hypothyroidism. The development of hypothyroidism may be linked to thyrotropin receptor–blocking antibodies, which are detected in 10% of patients with Hashimoto thyroiditis. Among patients with Hashimoto thyroiditis, hypothyroidism is more likely to develop in smokers than in nonsmokers, possibly due to the thiocyanates found in cigarette smoke. High serum levels of thyroid peroxidase antibody also predict progression from subclinical hypothyroidism to symptomatic hypothyroidism. Although the hypothyroidism is usually permanent, up to 11% of patients experience a remission after several years. There are two possible causes for such remissions: (1) the Hashimoto thyroiditis may improve spontaneously; and (2) thyroid-stimulating immunoglobulin (TSI) is produced in sufficient quantities to overwhelm the destructive effects of concurrent Hashimoto thyroiditis, causing the thyroid to produce more thyroid hormone. Rarely, if the thyroid gland goes on to produce *excessive* thyroid hormone, the result is an autoimmune hyperthyroidism (see Graves disease).

Hashimoto thyroiditis is sometimes associated with other endocrine deficiencies as part of polyglandular autoimmunity (PGA). Adults with type 2 PGA are prone to autoimmune thyroiditis, diabetes mellitus type 1, autoimmune gonadal failure, hypoparathyroidism, and adrenal insufficiency (see Adrenal Insufficiency). Thyroiditis is associated with other autoimmune conditions, such as pernicious anemia, Sjögren syndrome, vitiligo, inflammatory bowel disease, and celiac disease. The incidence of celiac disease in patients with Hashimoto thyroiditis is about 5%. Hashimoto thyroiditis is very rarely associated with other autoimmune conditions such as myocarditis, hypophysitis, alopecia areata, encephalitis, primary pulmonary hypertension, or membranous nephropathy. Women with gonadal dysgenesis (Turner syndrome) have a 15% incidence of significant thyroid dysfunction by age 40 years. Thyroiditis is also commonly seen in patients with hepatitis C.

Painless postpartum thyroiditis refers to autoimmune thyroiditis that occurs soon after delivery in 7.2% of women. Women in whom postpartum thyroiditis develops have a 70% chance of recurrence after subsequent pregnancies. It occurs most commonly in women who have high levels of thyroid peroxidase antibody in the first trimester of pregnancy or immediately after delivery. It is also more common in women with other autoimmunity or a family history of Hashimoto thyroiditis. There is some evidence that the autoimmunity may be triggered by the accumulation of fetal cells in the maternal thyroid during pregnancy, a condition known as microchimerism.

Painless sporadic thyroiditis is thought to be a subacute form of Hashimoto thyroiditis that is similar to painless postpartum thyroiditis (see above), except that it is not related to pregnancy. It accounts for about 1% of cases of thyrotoxicosis.

Subacute thyroiditis—also called de Quervain thyroiditis, granulomatous thyroiditis, and giant cell thyroiditis—is relatively common and is believed to be caused by a viral infection. It accounts for up to 5% of clinical thyroid disease.

Suppurative thyroiditis refers to a nonviral infection of the thyroid gland. It is usually bacterial. However, mycobacterial, fungal, and parasitic infections can occur, particularly in immunosuppressed individuals. Suppurative thyroiditis is quite rare, since the thyroid is resistant to infection, largely due to its high iodine content. Congenital pyriform sinus fistulas are a cause for recurrent suppurative thyroiditis in otherwise normal individuals.

Riedel thyroiditis is also called invasive fibrous thyroiditis, Riedel struma, woody thyroiditis, ligneous thyroiditis, and invasive thyroiditis. It is usually a manifestation of a multifocal systemic fibrosis syndrome.

▶ **Clinical Findings**

A. Symptoms and Signs

In **Hashimoto thyroiditis,** the thyroid gland is usually diffusely enlarged, firm, and finely nodular. One thyroid lobe may be asymmetrically enlarged, raising concerns about neoplasm. Although patients may complain of neck tightness, pain and tenderness are not usually present. About 10% of cases are atrophic, the gland being fibrotic, particularly in elderly women.

Systemic manifestations are mostly related to ambient levels of thyroid hormone. However, depression and chronic fatigue are more common in such patients, even after correction of hypothyroidism. About one-third of patients have mild dry mouth (xerostomia) or dry eyes (keratoconjunctivitis sicca) of an autoimmune nature related to Sjögren syndrome. It may be associated with myasthenia gravis, which is usually of mild severity, mainly affecting the extraocular muscles and having a relatively low incidence of detectable AChR Ab or thymic disease.

Postpartum thyroiditis is typically accompanied by hyperthyroidism that begins 1–6 months after delivery and persists for only 1–2 months. Then, hypothyroidism tends to develop in affected women beginning 4–8 months after delivery. Although 80% of affected women subsequently recover normal thyroid function, permanent hypothyroidism eventually develops in about 50% within 7 years. Permanent hypothyroidism is more common in women who are multiparous or who have had a spontaneous abortion.

Thyrotoxic symptoms in **painless sporadic thyroiditis** are usually mild; a small, nontender goiter may be palpated in about 50% of such patients. High serum thyroid peroxidase antibody concentrations are found in only 50% of such patients. The course is similar to painless postpartum thyroiditis.

Subacute thyroiditis usually presents with an acute, usually painful enlargement of the thyroid gland, often with dysphagia. The pain may radiate to the ears. Patients usually have a low-grade fever and fatigue. The manifestations may persist for weeks or months and may be associated with malaise. In patients who experience pain, it is called **painful subacute thyroiditis.** If there is no pain, it is called **silent thyroiditis.** Subacute thyroiditis often follows an upper respiratory infection and its incidence peaks in the summer. A viral etiology has been proposed but not firmly established. Thyrotoxicosis develops in 50% of affected patients and tends to last for several weeks. Subsequently, hypothyroidism develops that lasts 4–6 months. Normal thyroid function typically returns within 12 months, but persistent hypothyroidism develops in 5% of patients. Young and middle-aged women are most commonly affected.

Patients with **suppurative thyroiditis** usually are febrile and have severe pain, tenderness, redness, and fluctuation in the region of the thyroid gland. It tends to affect patients with preexistent thyroid disease. It is also more likely to affect patients who are immunosuppressed or infirm.

Riedel thyroiditis usually causes hypothyroidism and may cause hypoparathyroidism as well. It is the rarest form of thyroiditis and is found most frequently in middle-aged or elderly women. Thyroid enlargement is often asymmetric; the gland is stony hard and adherent to the neck structures, causing signs of compression and invasion, including dysphagia, dyspnea, pain, and hoarseness. Related conditions include retroperitoneal fibrosis, fibrosing mediastinitis, sclerosing cervicitis, subretinal fibrosis, and biliary tract sclerosis. It may respond to therapy with tamoxifen (see Treatment, below).

B. Laboratory Findings

With hyperthyroidism due to Hashimoto thyroiditis or subacute thyroiditis, serum FT_4 levels tend to be proportionally higher than T_3 levels, since the hyperthyroidism is due to the passive release of stored thyroid hormone, which is predominantly T_4; this is in contrast to Graves disease and toxic nodular goiter, where T_3 is relatively more elevated. Because T_4 is less active than T_3, the hyperthyroidism seen in thyroiditis is usually less severe. Serum levels of TSH are suppressed in hyperthyroidism due to thyroiditis.

Thyroid autoantibodies are most commonly demonstrable in Hashimoto thyroiditis but may also be present in the other types of thyroiditis. Patients with Hashimoto thyroiditis and clinically evident disease usually have increased circulating levels of antithyroid peroxidase (90%) or antithyroglobulin (40%) antibodies. Antithyroid antibodies decline during pregnancy and are often undetectable in the third trimester. Once Hashimoto thyroiditis has been diagnosed, monitoring of these antibody levels is not necessary. The serum TSH level is elevated if thyroid hormone is not elaborated in adequate amounts by the thyroid gland. In subacute thyroiditis, the ESR is markedly elevated while antithyroid antibody titers are low, distinguishing it from autoimmune thyroiditis. In **suppurative thyroiditis, both** the leukocyte count and ESR are usually elevated.

C. Imaging

Ultrasound in cases of Hashimoto thyroiditis typically shows a gland with characteristic diffuse heterogeneous density and hypoechogenicity. Ultrasonography of the thyroid helps distinguish thyroiditis from multinodular goiter or thyroid nodules that are suspicious for malignancy. It is also helpful in guiding FNA biopsy of small suspicious thyroid nodules. Color-flow Doppler ultrasonography can help distinguish thyroiditis from Graves disease, since patients with Graves disease have a hypervascular thyroid gland, whereas in thyroiditis there is normal or reduced vascularity.

RAI uptake and scan may be helpful in determining the cause of hyperthyroidism, distinguishing thyroiditis from Graves disease, since patients with subacute thyroiditis exhibit a very low RAI uptake. In patients with chronic Hashimoto thyroiditis (euthyroid or hypothyroid), RAI uptake may be normal or high with uneven uptake on the scan; scanning is not useful in making the diagnosis.

D. Fine-Needle Aspiration Biopsy

Patients with **Hashimoto thyroiditis** who have a thyroid nodule should have an ultrasound-guided FNA biopsy, since the risk of papillary thyroid cancer is about 8% in such nodules. When **suppurative thyroiditis** is suspected, an FNA biopsy with Gram stain and culture is required. FNA biopsy is usually not required for subacute thyroiditis but shows characteristic giant multinucleated cells.

► Complications

In the suppurative forms of thyroiditis, any of the complications of infection may occur; the subacute and chronic forms of the disease are complicated by the effects of pressure on the neck structures: dyspnea and, in Riedel struma, vocal cord palsy. Hashimoto thyroiditis may lead to hypothyroidism or transient thyrotoxicosis. Perimenopausal women with high serum levels of antithyroperoxidase antibodies have a higher relative risk of depression independently of ambient thyroid hormone levels.

Pregnant women with Hashimoto thyroiditis have an increased risk of spontaneous miscarriage in the first trimester of pregnancy. Hyperthyroidism may develop in patients with Hashimoto thyroiditis, either due to the emergence of Graves disease or due to the release of stored hormone by the thyroid, which is caused by inflammation. The latter condition has variably been termed "hashitoxicosis" or "painless sporadic thyroiditis;" it is known as postpartum painless thyroiditis when it occurs in women after delivery.

Papillary thyroid carcinoma or thyroid lymphoma may rarely be associated with chronic thyroiditis and must be considered in the diagnosis of uneven painless enlargements that continue in spite of treatment; such patients require FNA biopsy. Hashimoto thyroiditis may be associated with Addison disease, hypoparathyroidism, diabetes, pernicious anemia, biliary cirrhosis, vitiligo, and other autoimmune conditions.

▶ Differential Diagnosis

Thyroiditis must be considered in the differential diagnosis of all types of goiters, especially if enlargement is rapid. The very low RAI uptake in subacute thyroiditis with elevated T_4 and T_3 is helpful. Chronic thyroiditis, especially if the enlargement is uneven and if there is pressure on surrounding structures, may resemble carcinoma, and both disorders may be present in the same gland. The subacute and suppurative forms of thyroiditis may resemble any infectious process in or near the neck structures. Thyroid autoantibody tests have been of help in the diagnosis of Hashimoto thyroiditis, but the tests are not specific and may also be positive in patients with multinodular goiters, malignancy (eg, thyroid carcinoma, lymphoma), and concurrent Graves disease.

▶ Treatment

A. Hashimoto Thyroiditis

If hypothyroidism is present, levothyroxine should be given in the usual replacement doses (0.05–0.2 mg orally daily). In patients with a large goiter and normal or elevated serum TSH, T_4 may be given in doses sufficient to suppress serum TSH in an effort to shrink the thyroid. Suppressive doses of T_4 tend to shrink the goiter an average of 30% over 6 months. If the goiter does not regress, lower replacement doses of T_4 may be given. If the thyroid gland is only minimally enlarged and the patient is euthyroid (with normal TSH levels), regular observation is in order, since hypothyroidism may develop subsequently—often years later. (See Hypothyroidism section.)

In one study involving 21 patients with Hashimoto thyroiditis and subclinical hypothyroidism, simvastatin (20 mg orally daily) improved thyroid function over 8 weeks, possibly by stimulating apoptosis of certain types of lymphocytes. In another study, selenium selenite (200 mcg daily orally for 3 months) reduced the serum levels of antithyroperoxidase antibodies by 49% versus a 10% reduction in the placebo arm. The long-term effectiveness of statins or selenium therapy on the course of Hashimoto thyroiditis is unknown.

B. Subacute Thyroiditis

All treatment is empiric and must be continued for several weeks. Recurrence is common. The drug of choice is aspirin, which relieves pain and inflammation. Thyrotoxic symptoms are treated with propranolol, 10–40 mg orally every 6 hours. Iodinated contrast agents cause a prompt fall in serum T_3 levels and a dramatic improvement in thyrotoxic symptoms. Sodium ipodate (Oragrafin, Bilivist) or iopanoic acid (Telepaque) is given orally in doses of 500 mg orally daily until serum FT_4 levels return to normal. Transient hypothyroidism is treated with T_4 (0.05–0.1 mg orally daily) if symptomatic.

C. Suppurative Thyroiditis

Treatment is with antibiotics and with surgical drainage when fluctuation is marked.

D. Riedel Struma

The treatment of choice for invasive fibrous thyroiditis, like that of its related conditions, is tamoxifen, 20 mg orally twice daily, which must be continued for years. Tamoxifen can induce partial to complete remissions in most patients within 3–6 months. Its mode of action appears to be unrelated to its antiestrogen activity. Short-term corticosteroid treatment may be added for partial alleviation of pain and compression symptoms. Surgical decompression usually fails to permanently alleviate compression symptoms; such surgery is difficult due to dense fibrous adhesions, making surgical complications more likely.

▶ Prognosis

In subacute thyroiditis, spontaneous remissions and exacerbations are common, and therapy is supportive; the disease process may smolder for months. Hashimoto thyroiditis is occasionally associated with other autoimmune disorders (diabetes mellitus, Addison disease, pernicious anemia, etc). In general, however, patients with Hashimoto thyroiditis have an excellent prognosis, since the condition either remains stable for years or progresses slowly to hypothyroidism, which is easily treated. Women with postpartum thyroiditis usually regain normal thyroid function. Papillary thyroid carcinoma carries a relatively good prognosis when it occurs in patients with Hashimoto thyroiditis.

Ch'ng CL et al. Celiac disease and autoimmune thyroid disease. Clin Med Res. 2007 Oct;5(3):184–92. [PMID: 18056028]

Duntas LH. Environmental factors and autoimmune thyroiditis. Nat Clin Pract Endocrinol Metab. 2008 Aug;4(8):454–60. [PMID: 18607401]

Ladenson PW. Thyroiditis. https://knol.google.com/k/paul-w-ladenson-md/thyroiditis/Jk6Nt39x/pQbtmw#

Moinuddin S et al. Acute blastomycosis thyroiditis. Thyroid. 2008 Jun;18(6):659–61. [PMID: 18578618]

Tamagno G et al. Clinical and diagnostic aspects of encephalopathy associated with autoimmune thyroid disease (or Hashimoto's encephalopathy). Intern Emerg Med. 2006;1(1):15–23. [PMID: 16941808]

Tomer Y et al. Interferon alpha treatment and thyroid dysfunction. Endocrinol Metab Clin North Am. 2007 Dec;36(4):1051–66. [PMID: 17983936]

THYROID NODULES & MULTINODULAR GOITER

ESSENTIALS OF DIAGNOSIS

▶ Single or multiple thyroid nodules are commonly found with careful thyroid examinations.

▶ Thyroid function tests mandatory.

▶ Thyroid biopsy for single or dominant nodules or for a history of prior head–neck or chest–shoulder radiation.

▶ Ultrasound examination useful for biopsy and follow-up.

▶ Clinical follow-up required.

General Considerations

Nodular enlargement of the thyroid is detectable by palpation in 4–7% of the adult population in areas of the world with sufficient intake of iodine. Each year in the United States, about 275,000 thyroid nodules are detected by palpation. Palpable thyroid nodules are even more common in iodine-deficient geographic areas (see Iodine Deficiency Disorder & Endemic Goiter, below). Palpable thyroid nodules are increasingly prevalent with age. A thyroid nodule is four times more likely to develop in women than men. On thyroid ultrasound, about 50% palpable "solitary nodules" are found to be just one nodule in a multinodular goiter.

About 95% of thyroid nodules are benign, but the presence of a thyroid nodule warrants follow-up and further testing for function and malignancy. Most patients with a thyroid nodule are euthyroid, but there is a high incidence of hypothyroidism or hyperthyroidism. Goiter may be caused by numerous conditions, including multinodular goiter, iodine deficiency, pregnancy (in areas of iodine deficiency), Graves disease, Hashimoto thyroiditis, subacute thyroiditis, or infections. About 95% of thyroid nodules are benign adenoma, colloid nodule, or cyst but may sometimes be a primary thyroid malignancy or (less frequently) a metastatic neoplasm. Patients with multiple thyroid nodules have the same overall risk of thyroid cancer as patients with solitary nodules. The risk of a thyroid nodule being malignant is higher among patients with a history of head–neck radiation, a family history of thyroid cancer, or a personal history of another malignancy. The risk of malignancy is also higher if a thyroid nodule is large, adherent to the trachea or strap muscles, or associated with lymphadenopathy. The presence of Hashimoto thyroiditis does not reduce the risk of malignancy; a nodule of ≥ 1 cm in a gland with thyroiditis carries an 8% chance of malignancy.

▶ Clinical Findings

Table 26–6 illustrates the approach to the evaluation of thyroid nodules based on the index of suspicion for malignancy.

A. Symptoms and Signs

Most small thyroid nodules cause no symptoms. They may sometimes be detected only by having the patient swallow during careful inspection and palpation of the thyroid.

A thyroid nodule or multinodular goiter can grow to become visible and of concern to the patient. Particularly large nodular goiters can become a cosmetic embarrassment. Nodules can grow large enough to cause discomfort, hoarseness, or dysphagia. Retrosternal large multinodular goiters can cause dyspnea due to tracheal compression. Large substernal goiters may cause superior vena cava syndrome, manifested by facial erythema and jugular vein distention that progress to cyanosis and facial edema when both arms are kept raised over the head (Pemberton sign).

Depending on their cause, goiters and thyroid nodules may be associated with hypothyroidism (Hashimoto thy-

Table 26–6. Clinical evaluation of thyroid nodules.[1]

Clinical Evidence	Low Index of Suspicion	High Index of Suspicion
History	Family history of goiter; residence in area of endemic goiter	Previous therapeutic radiation of head, neck, or chest; hoarseness
Physical characteristics	Older women; soft nodule; multinodular goiter	Young adults, men; solitary, firm nodule; vocal cord paralysis; enlarged lymph nodes; distant metastatic lesions
Serum factors	High titer of antithyroid antibody; hypothyroidism; hyperthyroidism	Elevated serum calcitonin
Fine-needle aspiration biopsy	Colloid nodule or adenoma	Papillary carcinoma, follicular lesion, medullary or anaplastic carcinoma
Scanning techniques		
Uptake of ^{123}I	"Hot" nodule	"Cold" nodule
Ultrasonogram	Cystic lesion	Solid lesion
Roentgenogram	Shell-like calcification	Punctate calcification
Thyroxine therapy	Regression after 0.05–0.1 mg/d for 6 months or more	Increase in size

[1]Clinically suspicious nodules should be evaluated with fine-needle aspiration biopsy.

roiditis, endemic goiter) or hyperthyroidism (Graves disease, toxic nodular goiter, subacute thyroiditis, and thyroid cancer with metastases).

B. Laboratory Findings

Thyroid nodules are an indication for thyroid function testing. Serum determinations for TSH (sensitive assay) and FT_4 are preferred. Tests for antithyroperoxidase antibodies and antithyroglobulin antibodies may also be helpful. Very high antibody levels are found in Hashimoto thyroiditis. However, thyroiditis frequently coexists with malignancy, so suspicious nodules should always be biopsied. Serum calcitonin is obtained if a medullary thyroid carcinoma is suspected in a family member with a history of familial medullary thyroid carcinoma or MEN type 2.

C. Imaging

Neck ultrasonography should be performed to measure the size of a nodule and to determine whether a palpable nodule is part of a multinodular goiter. The following ultrasound characteristics of thyroid nodules increase the likelihood of malignancy: irregular or indistinct margins, heterogenous nodule echogenicity, intranodular vascular images, microcalcifications, complex cyst, or diameter over 1 cm. Ultrasound is also useful for long-term surveillance of thyroid nodules and multinodular goiter. Ultrasonography is generally preferred over CT and MRI because of its accuracy, ease of use, and lower cost.

RAI (^{123}I or ^{131}I) scans have limited usefulness in the evaluation of thyroid nodules. Hypofunctioning (cold) nodules have a somewhat increased risk of being malignant but most are benign. Hyperfunctioning (hot) nodules are ordinarily benign but may sometimes be malignant. RAI uptake and scanning is helpful if a patient is found to have evidence of hyperthyroidism. (See Hyperthyroidism, above.)

CT scanning is helpful for larger thyroid nodules and multinodular goiter; it can determine the degree of tracheal compression and the degree of extension into the mediastinum.

D. Incidentally Discovered Thyroid Nodules

Thyroid nodules are frequently discovered as an incidental finding, with an incidence that depends on the imaging modality: MRI, 50%; CT, 13%; and [^{18}F]fluorodeoxyglucose positron emission tomography (^{18}FDG-PET), 2%. When such scanning detects a thyroid nodule, an ultrasound is performed to better determine the nodule's risk for malignancy and the need for FNA biopsy (see above), and to establish a baseline for ultrasound follow-up. The malignancy risk is about 17% for nodules discovered incidentally on CT or MRI, and 25–50% for nodules discovered incidentally by ^{18}FDG-PET. For incidentally discovered thyroid nodules of borderline concern, follow-up thyroid ultrasound in 3–6 months may be helpful; growing lesions may be biopsied or resected.

E. Fine-Needle Aspiration Biopsy

FNA biopsy is the best method to assess a thyroid nodule for malignancy. FNA biopsy can be done while patients con-

tinue taking anticoagulants or aspirin. For multinodular goiters, the four largest nodules ($\geq$ 1 cm diameter) should be biopsied to minimize the risk of missing a malignancy. Smaller thyroid nodules (8–10 mm) with a suspicious appearance on ultrasound should also be considered for ultrasound-guided FNA biopsy. Using ultrasound guidance for FNA biopsy improves the diagnostic accuracy for both palpable and nonpalpable thyroid nodules. The chance of an optimal tissue sampling is also improved by having an experienced clinician perform the FNA biopsy and by having the aspirate interpreted by a skilled cytopathologist.

In one review of thyroid FNA biopsies, about 70% were benign, 5% were malignant, 15% were nondiagnostic, and 10% were indeterminate or "suspicious."

When FNA cytology is "suspicious" for papillary thyroid carcinoma, the risk of malignancy is 57%. When FNA cytology yields a "suspicious" follicular lesion, the overall risk of the lesion being malignant is about 20–25%. However, the risk is lower in patients aged 50 years. The risk that a follicular lesion is malignant increases for patients who are much younger or older than age 50. Most patients with suspicious FNA cytology undergo thyroid surgery.

Cystic nodules yielding serous fluid are usually benign, but fluid should be submitted for cytologic testing. Cystic nodules yielding bloody fluid have a higher chance of being malignant. Repeat FNA biopsy is done with ultrasound guidance if the cytologic test results are nondiagnostic (eg, diluted with blood or hypocellular) and the lesion remains palpable.

False-positive thyroid FNA biopsy results occur at a rate of about 4%. False-negative thyroid FNA biopsy results also occur at an overall rate of about 4%, less commonly when performed under ultrasound guidance and interpreted by cytopathologists. False-negative results delay surgical excision and lead to an increased risk of vascular and capsular invasion by the malignancy. Some false-negative FNA biopsy results may not have actually been inaccurate, since truly benign thyroid nodules can later become malignant. Patients who have a negative thyroid FNA should have observational follow-up, ideally with both palpation and ultrasound; nodules that continue to grow should be rebiopsied or excised.

▶ Treatment

All thyroid nodules, including those that are benign, need to be monitored by regular periodic palpation and ultrasound and rebiopsied if growth occurs. A toxic multinodular goiter and hyperthyroidism, associated with the ingestion or intravenous administration of large amounts of iodine, may develop in patients with multinodular goiters. It is therefore prudent to minimize excessive dietary iodine intake and intravenous iodinated contrast. Patients found to have hyperthyroidism may have a RAI uptake and scan for additional evaluation, especially if ^{131}I is a therapeutic consideration. Patients with toxic multinodular goiters may also be treated with methimazole, propranolol, or surgery (see Hyperthyroidism section).

A. Levothyroxine Suppression Therapy

Patients with elevated levels of serum TSH are treated with levothyroxine replacement. Otherwise, for small benign thyroid nodules, levothyroxine suppression therapy is not required. For larger nodules (> 2 cm), if TSH levels are elevated or normal, "suppression" with levothyroxine (starting doses of 50 mcg daily) can be considered. Levothyroxine should not be administered if the baseline TSH is low, since that is an indication of autonomous thyroid secretion, such that levothyroxine therapy will be ineffective and liable to cause clinical thyrotoxicosis. Long-term levothyroxine suppression of TSH tends to keep nodules from enlarging, but only a few will actually shrink. In one 5-year study, thyroid nodule size increased in 29% of patients treated with levothyroxine, compared to growth in 56% of nodules in patients not receiving levothyroxine. Levothyroxine suppression also reduces the emergency of new nodules: 8% with levothyroxine and 29% without levothyroxine.

Levothyroxine suppression needs to be carefully monitored, since it carries a 17% risk of inducing symptoms of hyperthyroidism. This can occur due to excessive levothyroxine dosing, the emergence of an autonomous or toxic nodule or Graves disease, or a reduction in thyroid binding globulin seen in early menopause or with discontinuing oral estrogen therapy. Therefore, levothyroxine suppression therapy is most suitable for younger patients. All patients require regular careful clinical evaluation and thyroid palpation or ultrasound examinations. Levothyroxine suppression therapy is not usually given to patients with cardiac disease, since it increases the risk for angina and atrial fibrillation. Levothyroxine suppression causes a small loss of bone density, particularly in postmenopausal women. Patients at risk for osteoporosis are advised to have periodic bone density testing. Bisphosphonate or other therapy for osteoporosis may be indicated.

B. Surgery

Total thyroidectomy is required for thyroid nodules that are malignant on FNA biopsy (see Thyroid Cancer section). More limited thyroid surgery is indicated for benign nodules with indeterminate or suspicious cytologic test results, compression symptoms, discomfort, or cosmetic embarrassment. Surgery may also be used to remove hyperfunctioning "hot" thyroid adenomas or toxic multinodular goiter causing hyperthyroidism (see Hyperthyroidism section).

C. Ethanol Injection

Percutaneous ethanol injection has been used to shrink benign (biopsy proven) thyroid nodules, both solid and cystic. Most nodules undergo partial shrinkage after percutaneous ethanol injection. The complication rate is about 9%, although serious or permanent complications are rare.

D. Radioiodine (^{131}I) Therapy

Radioactive ^{131}I is a treatment option for hyperthyroid patients with toxic thyroid adenomas, multinodular goiter, or Graves disease (see Hyperthyroidism section). It may also be used to shrink benign nontoxic thyroid nodules. Thyroid nodules shrink an average of 40% by 1 year and 59% by 2 years after ^{131}I therapy. Nodules that shrink after ^{131}I therapy generally remain palpable and become firmer;

they may develop unusual cytologic characteristics on FNA biopsy. Hypothyroidism is a risk and may occur years after ^{131}I therapy, so thyroid function testing must be performed regularly.

Prognosis

The great majority of thyroid nodules are benign. Benign thyroid nodules may involute but usually persist or grow slowly. About 90% of thyroid nodules will increase their volume by ≥ 15% over 5 years; cystic nodules are less likely to grow. Cytologically benign nodules that grow are unlikely to be malignant; in one series, only 1 of 78 rebiopsied nodules was found to be malignant. The prognosis for patients with thyroid nodules that prove to be malignant is determined by the histologic type and other factors (see below). Multinodular goiters tend to persist or grow slowly, even in iodine-deficient areas where iodine repletion usually does not shrink established goiters. Patients with very small, incidentally discovered, nonpalpable thyroid nodules do require follow-up with thyroid ultrasound but are at low risk for malignancy. Nodules that are malignant have a minor effect on morbidity and mortality.

Alexander EK. Approach to the patient with a cytologically indeterminate thyroid nodule. J Clin Endocrinol Metab. 2008 Nov;93(11):4175–82. [PMID: 18987277]

Banks ND et al. A diagnostic predictor model for indeterminate or suspicious thyroid FNA samples. Thyroid. 2008 Sep;18(9): 933–41. [PMID: 18788917]

Bogsrud TV et al. The value of quantifying 18F-FDG uptake in thyroid nodules found incidentally on whole-body PET-CT. Nucl Med Commun. 2007 May;28(5):373–381. [PMID: 17414887]

Gharib H et al. Thyroid nodules: clinical importance, assessment, and treatment. Endocrinol Metab Clin North Am. 2007 Sep;36(3):707–735. [PMID: 17673125]

Kim DW et al. Ultrasound-guided fine-needle aspiration biopsy of thyroid nodules: comparison in efficacy according to nodule size. Thyroid. 2009 Jan;19(1):27–31. [PMID: 19021460]

Mihai R et al. One in four patients with follicular thyroid cytology (THY3) has a thyroid carcinoma. Thyroid. 2009 Jan;19(1):33–7. [PMID: 18976164]

THYROID CANCER

ESSENTIALS OF DIAGNOSIS

► Painless swelling in region of thyroid.

► Thyroid function tests usually normal.

► Past history of irradiation to head and neck region may be present.

► Positive thyroid needle aspiration.

General Considerations

The incidence of papillary and follicular (differentiated) thyroid carcinomas increases with age. The overall female:male ratio is 3:1. The yearly incidence of thyroid cancer has been increasing in the United States, with the

Table 26–7. Some characteristics of thyroid cancer.

	Papillary	Follicular	Medullary	Undifferentiated
Incidence	Most common	Common	Uncommon	Uncommon
Average age	42	50	50	57
Females	70%	72%	56%	56%
Invasion				
Juxtanodal	+++++	+	++++++	+++
Blood vessels	+	+++	+++	+++++
Distant sites	+	+++	++	++++
^{123}I uptake	+	++++	0	0
Mortality	+	++ to +++	+ to ++++	+++++++

number of cases diagnosed annually reaching 33,500, probably as a result of the wider use of CT, MRI, PET, and ultrasound that incidentally find small thyroid malignancies. Thyroid cancer mortality has been stable, accounting for about 1500 deaths in the United States annually. At autopsy, microscopic thyroid cancer is found with surprising frequency. Clearly, most thyroid cancers remain microscopic and indolent. However, larger thyroid cancers (palpable or ≥ 1 cm in diameter) are more malignant and require treatment.

Papillary thyroid carcinoma is the most common thyroid malignancy (Table 26–7).

Pure papillary and mixed papillary-follicular carcinoma represent about 80% of all thyroid cancers. It usually presents as a single thyroid nodule, but it can arise out of a multinodular goiter. Papillary thyroid carcinoma is commonly multifocal within the gland, with other foci usually arising de novo rather than representing intraglandular metastases. About 10% of cases present with palpable cervical lymph node metastases from a small thyroid cancer. Papillary thyroid carcinomas tend to grow slowly and often remain confined to the thyroid and regional lymph nodes for years. However, they may become more aggressive, especially in patients over age 45 years, and most particularly in the elderly. The cancer may invade the trachea and local muscles and may spread to the lungs.

Papillary thyroid carcinoma is caused by certain genetic mutations or translocations. Activating mutations of the *ras* oncogene can cause benign thyroid adenomas or nodular goiter. Additional activating mutations in *BRAF* or *TRK* genes can lead to papillary carcinoma. About 45% of papillary thyroid carcinomas are caused by over expression of the *ret* oncogene by the translocation of certain gene promoters to it, producing *retPTC-1*, *retPTC-2*, or *retPTC-3*. Radiation treatments to the head and neck region tend to cause *retPTC-1*. Nuclear fallout exposure tends to cause *retPTC-3*, resulting in more aggressive papillary thyroid carcinomas. Additional loss of the *p53* tumor suppressor gene can cause progression of papillary thyroid carcinoma to anaplastic thyroid carcinoma.

Exposure to radiation therapy to the head and neck poses a particular threat to children who then have an

increased lifetime risk of developing thyroid pathology, including papillary thyroid carcinoma; thyroid malignancy may emerge between 10 and 40 years after exposure, with a peak occurrence 20–25 years later. After an explosion at the Chernobyl Nuclear Plant in the Ukraine in 1986, the risk of developing papillary thyroid carcinoma was highest among children who were under age 5 at the time of exposure to radiation; emergence of more aggressive papillary thyroid carcinoma occurred within 6–7 years after exposure.

Papillary thyroid carcinoma can occur in familial syndromes as an autosomal dominant trait, caused by loss of various tumor suppressor genes. Such syndromes (with associated features) include familial papillary carcinoma (with papillary renal carcinoma); familial nonmedullary thyroid carcinoma; familial polyposis (with large intestine polyps and gastrointestinal tumors); Gardner syndrome (with small and large intestine polyps, fibromas, lipomas, osteomas); and Turcot syndrome (with large intestine polyps and brain tumors). Older patients with multinodular goiter may rarely develop a papillary thyroid carcinoma. Papillary carcinoma can sometimes undergo a late anaplastic transformation into an aggressive carcinoma.

Generally speaking, papillary carcinoma is the least aggressive thyroid malignancy. However, the tumor spreads via lymphatics within the thyroid, appearing to be multifocal in 60% of patients and involving both lobes in 30% of patients. About 80% of patients have microscopic metastases to cervical lymph nodes. Unlike other forms of cancer, patients with papillary thyroid carcinoma who have palpable lymph node metastases do not have a particularly increased mortality rate; however, their risk of local recurrence is increased.

Occult metastases to the lung occur in 10–15% of differentiated thyroid cancer. About 70% of small lung metastases resolve following ^{131}I therapy; however, larger pulmonary metastases have only a 10% remission rate.

Microscopic "micropapillary" carcinoma (≤ 1 mm and invisible even on thyroid ultrasound) is a variant of normal, being found in 24% of thyroidectomies performed for benign thyroid disease when 2-mm sections were carefully examined. It thus appears that the overwhelming majority of these microscopic foci never become clinically significant. The surgical pathology report of such a tiny papillary carcinoma that is otherwise benign does not justify aggressive follow-up or treatment because a cancer diagnosis is unwarranted and harmful. All that may be required is yearly follow-up with palpation of the neck and mild TSH suppression by thyroxine.

Follicular thyroid carcinoma and its variants (eg, Hürthle cell carcinoma) account for about 14% of thyroid malignancies; follicular thyroid carcinoma is generally more aggressive than papillary carcinoma. Rarely, some follicular carcinomas secrete enough T_4 to cause thyrotoxicosis if the tumor load becomes significant. Metastases commonly are found in neck nodes, bones, and lungs. Most follicular thyroid carcinomas avidly absorb iodine, making possible diagnostic scanning and treatment with ^{131}I after total thyroidectomy. Certain follicular histopathologic features are associated with a high risk of metastasis and recurrence: poorly differentiated and Hürthle cell (oncocytic) variants. The latter variants do not take up RAI.

Follicular carcinoma results from certain gene mutations or translocations. Aberrant DNA methylation, activation of the *ras* oncogene, and mutations of the *MEN1* gene can result in benign follicular adenomas. Loss of function of PPARγ or the *3P* tumor suppressor gene can lead to follicular carcinoma, and additional loss of the *p53* tumor suppressor gene can produce anaplastic carcinoma.

Follicular thyroid carcinoma and adenomas develop in patients with Cowden disease, a rare autosomal dominant familial syndrome caused by loss of a tumor suppressor gene; such patients tend to have macrocephaly, multiple hamartomas, early-onset breast cancer, intestinal polyps, facial papules, and other skin and mucosal lesions.

Medullary thyroid carcinoma represents about 3% of thyroid cancers. About one-third of cases are sporadic, one-third are familial, and one-third are associated with MEN type 2. Medullary thyroid carcinoma is often caused by an activating mutation of the *ret* oncogene on chromosome 10. Mutation analysis of the *ret* oncogene's exons 10, 11, 13, and 14 detects 95% of the mutations causing MEN 2A and 90% of the mutations causing familial medullary thyroid carcinoma. Patients with MEN 2B have activating mutations in exon 16 of the *ret* oncogene. These germline mutations can be detected by DNA analysis of peripheral WBCs. Therefore, discovery of a medullary thyroid carcinoma makes genetic analysis mandatory. If a gene defect is discovered, related family members must have genetic screening for that specific gene defect. When a family member with MEN 2A or familial medullary thyroid carcinoma does not have an identifiable *ret* oncogene mutation, gene carriers may still be identified using family linkage analysis. Even when no gene defect is detectable, family members should have regular thyroid surveillance. Somatic mutations of the *ret* oncogene can be identified in the tumors of 30% of patients with sporadic (nonfamilial) medullary thyroid carcinoma. (See Multiple Endocrine Neoplasia.)

Medullary thyroid carcinoma arises from parafollicular thyroid cells that can secrete calcitonin, prostaglandins, serotonin, ACTH, corticotropin-releasing hormone (CRH), and other peptides. These peptides can cause symptoms and can be used as tumor markers. Early local metastases are usually present, usually to adjacent muscle and trachea as well as to local and mediastinal lymph nodes. Eventually, late metastases may appear in the bones, lungs, adrenals, or liver. Medullary thyroid carcinoma does not concentrate iodine.

Anaplastic thyroid carcinoma represents about 2% of thyroid cancers. It usually presents in an older patient as a rapidly enlarging mass in a multinodular goiter. It is the most aggressive thyroid carcinoma and metastasizes early to surrounding nodes and distant sites. Local pressure symptoms include dysphagia or vocal cord paralysis. This tumor does not concentrate iodine.

Anaplastic thyroid carcinoma is caused by certain gene mutations, including inactivating mutations of the *p53* tumor suppressor gene, as described above for papillary and follicular thyroid carcinomas.

Other thyroid malignancies together represent about 3% of thyroid cancers. **Lymphoma** of the thyroid is more common in older women. Thyroid lymphomas are most commonly B cell lymphomas (50%) or mucosa-associated lymphoid tissue (MALT; 23%); other types include follicular, small lymphocytic, and Burkitt lymphoma and Hodgkin disease. Thyroidectomy is rarely required. **Other cancers** may sometimes metastasize to the thyroid, particularly bronchogenic, breast, and renal carcinomas and malignant melanoma.

▶ **Clinical Findings**

A. Symptoms and Signs

Thyroid carcinoma usually presents as a palpable, firm, nontender nodule in the thyroid. Most thyroid carcinomas are asymptomatic, but large thyroid cancers can cause neck discomfort, dysphagia, or hoarseness (due to pressure on the recurrent laryngeal nerve). About 3% of thyroid malignancies present with a metastasis, usually to local lymph nodes but sometimes to distant sites such as bone or lung. Palpable lymph node involvement is present in 15% of adults and 60% of youths. Metastatic functioning differentiated thyroid carcinoma can sometimes secrete enough thyroid hormone to produce thyrotoxicosis. **Anaplastic thyroid carcinoma** is more apt to be advanced at the time of diagnosis, presenting with dysphagia, hoarseness, dyspnea, and metastases to the lungs. Occasionally, such carcinomas may be discovered while they are still relatively small and localized.

Medullary thyroid carcinoma frequently causes flushing and persistent diarrhea (30%), which may be the initial clinical feature. Patients with metastases often experience fatigue as well as other symptoms. Cushing syndrome develops in about 5% of patients from secretion of ACTH or CRH. Signs of pressure or invasion of surrounding tissues are present in anaplastic or large tumors; recurrent laryngeal nerve palsy can occur.

Lymphoma usually presents as a rapidly enlarging, painful mass arising out of a multinodular or diffuse goiter affected by autoimmune thyroiditis, with which it may be confused microscopically. About 20% of cases have concomitant hypothyroidism.

B. Laboratory Findings

(FNA biopsy is discussed above in the section on nodular thyroid.) Thyroid function tests are generally normal unless there is concomitant thyroiditis. Follicular carcinoma may secrete enough T_4 to suppress TSH and cause clinical hyperthyroidism.

Serum thyroglobulin is high in most metastatic papillary and follicular tumors, making this a useful marker for recurrent or metastatic disease. Caution must be exercised for the following reasons: (1) Circulating antithyroglobulin antibodies can cause erroneous thyroglobulin determinations. (2) Thyroglobulin levels may be misleadingly elevated in thyroiditis, which often coexists with carcinoma. (3) Certain thyroglobulin assays falsely report the continued presence of thyroglobulin after total thyroidectomy and tumor resection, causing undue concern about possible metastases. Therefore, unexpected thyroglobulin levels should prompt a repeat assay in another reference laboratory.

Serum calcitonin levels are usually elevated in medullary thyroid carcinoma, making this a marker for metastatic disease. However, serum calcitonin may be elevated in many other conditions, such as thyroiditis; pregnancy; azotemia; hypercalcemia; and other malignancies, including pheochromocytomas, carcinoid tumors, and carcinomas of the lung, pancreas, breast, and colon.

Serum calcitonin and carcinoembryonic antigen (CEA) determinations should be obtained before surgery for medullary carcinoma, then regularly in postoperative follow-up: every 4 months for 5 years, then every 6 months for life. Calcitonin levels remain elevated in patients with persistent tumor but also in some patients with apparent cure or indolent disease. Therefore, rising levels of calcitonin (or CEA) are the best indication for recurrence. Serum calcitonin levels > 250 pg/mL are also an indication for recurrent or metastatic medullary thyroid carcinoma. Serum CEA levels are usually elevated with medullary carcinoma, making this a useful second marker; however, it is not specific for this carcinoma.

C. Imaging

1. Ultrasound of the neck—Ultrasound of the neck should be performed routinely on all patients with thyroid cancer for the initial diagnosis and for follow-up. Ultrasound is useful in determining the size and location of the malignancy as well as the location of any neck metastases.

2. Radioactive iodine scanning—RAI (^{131}I or ^{123}I) thyroid and whole-body scanning is used after thyroidectomy for surveillance as described below, supplanting its previous use to determine whether a nodule was "cold" as a sign of malignancy.

3. CT scanning—CT scanning may demonstrate metastases and is particularly useful for localizing and monitoring lung metastases. However, CT scanning is less sensitive than ultrasound for detecting metastases within the neck. Iodinated contrast should never be given prior to RAI scanning or RAI therapy, since the large amounts of iodine in contrast media competitively inhibit the uptake of RAI

by the thyroid, greatly reducing the effectiveness of subsequent RAI scanning and therapy. Medullary carcinoma in the thyroid, nodes, and liver may calcify, but lung metastases rarely do so.

4. MRI—MRI is particularly useful for imaging bone metastases.

5. PET scanning—PET scanning is particularly useful for detecting thyroid cancer metastases that do not have sufficient iodine uptake to be visible on RAI scans. Metastases are best detected using ^{18}FDG-PET whole-body scanning. The sensitivity of ^{18}FDG-PET scanning for differentiated thyroid cancer is enhanced if the patient is hypothyroid or receiving thyrotropin, which increases the metabolic activity of differentiated thyroid cancer. Disadvantages of PET scanning include its lack of specificity for thyroid cancer as well as its expense and lack of availability in many locations. ^{18}FDG-PET scanning has prognostic implications, since differentiated thyroid cancer metastases with low standard uptake value scores are associated with a better prognosis.

▶ Differential Diagnosis

Neuroendocrine carcinomas may metastasize to the thyroid and be confused with medullary thyroid carcinoma.

False-positive ^{131}I scans are common with normal residual thyroid tissue and have been reported with Zenker diverticulum, struma ovarii, pleuropericardial cyst, gastric pull-up, and ^{131}I-contaminated bodily secretions. False-negative ^{131}I scans are common in early metastatic differentiated thyroid carcinoma but occur also in more advanced disease, including 14% of bone metastases.

▶ Complications

The complications vary with the type of carcinoma. Differentiated thyroid carcinomas may have local or distant metastases. One-third of medullary carcinomas may secrete serotonin and prostaglandins, producing flushing and diarrhea, and may be complicated by the coexistence of pheochromocytomas or hyperparathyroidism. The risks of radical neck surgery include permanent hypoparathyroidism and vocal cord palsy due to recurrent laryngeal nerve damage; permanent hypothyroidism is expected after thyroidectomy and should always be treated adequately.

▶ Treatment of Differentiated Thyroid Carcinoma

A. Surgical Treatment

Surgical removal is the treatment of choice for thyroid carcinomas. For differentiated papillary and follicular carcinoma, thyroidectomy with limited removal of cervical lymph nodes is adequate. The advantage of near-total thyroidectomy for differentiated thyroid carcinoma is that multicentric foci of carcinoma are more apt to be resected and there is then less normal thyroid tissue to compete with cancer for ^{131}I administered later for scans or treatment. Subtotal thyroidectomy is acceptable for adults under age 45 years who have a single small tumor (≤ 1 cm in diameter). Patients with bulky metastases in the neck region also benefit from surgery. Neck muscle resections are usually avoided for differentiated thyroid carcinoma. However, patients with the Hürthle cell variant of follicular carcinoma may benefit from a modified radical neck dissection. Metastases to the brain are best treated surgically, since treatment with radiation or RAI is ineffective. Levothyroxine is prescribed in doses of 0.05–0.1 mg/d immediately postoperatively (see Thyroxine Suppression and Chemotherapy, below). About 2–4 months after surgery, patients require reevaluation and often require therapy with [131]I (see below).

Highly skilled surgeons can perform near-total thyroidectomies with a less than 1% rate of serious complications (hypoparathyroidism or recurrent laryngeal nerve damage). Other series have reported up to an 11% incidence of permanent hypoparathyroidism after total thyroidectomy. The incidence of hypoparathyroidism may be reduced if accidentally resected parathyroids are immediately autotransplanted into the neck muscles.

Thyroidectomy requires at least an overnight hospital admission, since late bleeding, airway problems, and tetany can occur. Ambulatory thyroidectomy is potentially dangerous and should not be done.

B. Thyroxine Suppression and Chemotherapy

Patients who have had a thyroidectomy for differentiated thyroid cancer must take thyroxine replacement for life. Oral thyroxine should be given in doses that suppress serum TSH without causing clinical thyrotoxicosis. An ultrasensitive TSH assay should be used; serum TSH should be suppressed below 0.1 mU/L for patients with stage II disease and below 0.05 mU/L for patients with stage III–IV disease. (See Table 26–8.) Patients receiving thyroxine suppression therapy have been reported, as a group, to have slightly lower bone density than age-matched controls. However, for patients who are clinically euthyroid, thyroxine suppression therapy has a minimal effect upon bone and fracture risk. Nevertheless, patients receiving thyroxine suppression therapy are advised to have periodic bone densitometry.

Thyroid carcinomas are extraordinarily resistant to chemotherapy. Zoledronic acid, an intravenous bisphosphonate, has proven useful for osteolytic metastases from other solid tumors and has been used for patients with thyroid bone metastases, but its effectiveness is unknown.

C. Radioactive Iodine Therapy

Differentiated thyroid cancers variably retain the normal thyroid's ability to respond to TSH, secrete thyroglobulin, and concentrate iodine. Patients with stage II–IV cancer are usually treated with adjuvant ^{131}I therapy, when possible. The use of postoperative RAI therapy for patients with stage I differentiated thyroid cancer is controversial; there has been no demonstrable improvement in survival in this group of patients following RAI therapy. Most clinicians give RAI therapy to patients with stage I cancer only if the primary tumor was greater than 1–2 cm in diameter or of histologic higher risk.

About 2–4 months after thyroidectomy, patients follow a low iodine diet for at least 2 weeks before RAI therapy. **The low iodine diet** consists of avoiding the following: iodized table salt, sea salt, fish, shellfish, seaweed, commercial bread, dairy products, processed meats, canned or dried fruit, canned fruit juices, highly salted soups and snack foods, black tea, instant coffee, food coloring with Red Dye #3, egg yolks, multivitamins with iodine, or topical iodine. Patients must not be given intravenous radiologic contrast dyes containing iodine.

In order to stimulate radioiodine uptake by residual cancer tissue, patients are given recombinant human thyroid stimulating hormone (rhTSH, Thyrogen) as described below. Thyroxine withdrawal (2 weeks before ^{131}I therapy) is an alternative to Thyrogen, allowing the body's TSH levels to rise naturally and increasing the body's retention of administered [131]I. This technique avoids the high costs of Thyrogen. Also, whether Thyrogen-stimulated ^{131}I therapy is adequate to treat patients with stage III–IV cancer remains controversial. However, hypothyroidism is uncomfortable for most patients.

Just before ^{131}I therapy, serum is obtained for measurement of TSH (to make certain it is > 30 mcU/mL), thyro-

Table 26–8. Pathologic tumor-node-metastasis (pTNM) staging and tumor-related approximate survival rates for adults with appropriately treated differentiated (papillary) thyroid carcinoma based upon patient age, primary tumor size and invasiveness (T), lymph node involvement (N), and distant metastases (M).[1]

Stage	Description	Five-Year Survival	Ten-Year Survival
1	Under 45: any T, any N, no M Over 45: T ≤ 1 cm, no N, no M	99%	98%
2	Under 45: any T, any N, any M Over 45: T > 1 cm limited to thyroid, no N, no M	99%	90%
3	Over 45: T beyond thyroid capsule, no N, no M; or any T, regional N, no M	95%	75%
4	Over 45: any T, any N, any M	85%	65%

[1]Patients having a relatively worse prognosis include those with follicular thyroid carcinoma and those with familial differentiated thyroid carcinoma.

globulin, and hCG (in all reproductive-age women). Pregnant women may not receive RAI therapy. Women are advised to avoid pregnancy for at least 4 months following ^{131}I therapy. Men have been found to have abnormal spermatozoa for up to 6 months following ^{131}I therapy and are advised to use contraceptive methods during that time.

^{131}I is administered orally. The dose of ^{131}I for thyroid "remnant ablation" in those with no nodal involvement is 30 mCi (1110 MBq). Higher doses (50–100 mCi) of ^{131}I may be given to patients with large primary tumors or tumors at the surgical margin. Patients with local lymph node involvement typically receive 100 mCi of ^{131}I; patients with more extensive neck node involvement or distant metastases receive ^{131}I at a dose of 125–200 mCi (4625–7400 MBq). A post-therapy whole-body scan, performed about 1 week after ^{131}I treatment, will often detect metastases that were not visible on pretreatment scans. Unfortunately, about 35% of patients with differentiated thyroid carcinoma have poor uptake of ^{131}I into metastases.

Patients who have been withdrawn from thyroid hormone may resume thyroxine at the full replacement dose 4 days following ^{131}I therapy. They may also cease their low iodine diet. To accelerate the return to euthyroidism, Cytomel may be added to thyroxine for 2 weeks at a dose of 25 mcg orally twice daily for 1 week, reduced to 12.5 mcg twice daily for the next week.

^{131}I therapy in doses over 100 mCi (3800 MBq) can cause gastritis, temporary oligospermia, sialadenitis, and xerostomia. RAI therapy can cause neurologic decompensation in patients with brain metastases; it is advisable to treat such patients with prednisone 30–40 mg orally daily for several days before and after ^{131}I therapy. Cumulative doses of ^{131}I over 500 mCi can cause infertility, pancytopenia (4%), and leukemia (0.3%). The kidneys excrete RAI. Patients receiving dialysis for kidney disease require a dosage reduction to only 20% of the usual dose of ^{131}I.

National Cancer Institute surveillance data for 30,278 patients with thyroid cancer has indicated that patients with differentiated thyroid cancer, treated with only surgery, had a 5% increased risk of developing a second nonthyroid malignancy (especially breast cancer). Patients with thyroid cancer who received ^{131}I therapy had a 20% increased risk of developing a second non-thyroid malignancy (especially leukemia and lymphoma). The greatest risk of second cancers appeared within 5 years of ^{131}I therapy and was most significant for younger patients.

D. Treatment of Other Thyroid Malignancies

Patients with anaplastic thyroid carcinoma are treated with local resection and radiation. Lovastatin, an HMG-CoA inhibitor, has been demonstrated to cause differentiation and apoptosis of anaplastic thyroid carcinoma cells in vitro; however, clinical studies have not been performed. Anaplastic thyroid carcinoma does not respond to ^{131}I therapy and is resistant to chemotherapy.

Patients with thyroid MALT lymphomas have a low risk of recurrence after simple thyroidectomy. Patients with other thyroid lymphomas are best treated with external radiation therapy; chemotherapy is added for extensive lymphoma. Patients with systemic lymphomas involving the thyroid are usually treated with chemotherapy.

Patients with a *ret* protooncogene mutation should have a prophylactic total thyroidectomy, ideally by age 6 years (MEN 2A) or at age 6 months (MEN 2B). Patients with medullary thyroid carcinoma are treated surgically; repeated neck dissections are often required over time. Medullary thyroid carcinomas do not respond to ^{131}I therapy and are generally resistant to chemotherapy.

E. External Radiation Therapy

External radiation may be delivered to bone metastases. Brain metastases do not usually respond to ^{131}I and are best resected or treated with gamma knife radiosurgery.

F. Surveillance

Patients with differentiated thyroid carcinoma must be observed long-term for recurrent or metastatic disease. Follow-up must include physical examinations and laboratory testing to ensure that patients remain clinically euthyroid with a suppressed TSH. To achieve suppression of serum TSH, the required dose of thyroxine may be such that serum FT_4 levels may be slightly elevated; in that case, measurement of serum T_3 or free T_3 (women who are pregnant or receiving oral estrogens) can be useful to ensure the patient is not frankly hyperthyroid. Thyrotoxicosis can be caused by overreplacement with thyroxine or by the growth of functioning metastases.

Neck palpation has a sensitivity of only 16% for detecting cervical lymph node metastases. For surveillance, neck ultrasound and serum thyroglobulin determinations (baseline and rhTSH-stimulated) have largely repeated whole-body radioiodine scanning, which has a false-negative rate of about 80%. Follow-up intervals of 4–6 months are usually satisfactory.

1. Neck ultrasound—Neck ultrasound should be used in all patients with thyroid carcinoma to supplement neck palpation. It is prudent to perform a thyroid/neck ultrasound in all patients with thyroid cancer preoperatively, 3 months postoperatively, and regularly thereafter. Ultrasound is more sensitive for lymph node metastases than either CT or MRI scanning. Small inflammatory nodes may be detected postoperatively and do not necessarily indicate metastatic disease, but follow-up is necessary. Ultrasound-guided FNA biopsy should be performed on suspicious lesions.

2. Serum thyroglobulin (Tg)—Thyroglobulin is produced by normal thyroid tissue and by most differentiated thyroid carcinomas. It is only after a total or near-total thyroidectomy and ^{131}I remnant ablation that Tg becomes a useful tumor marker for patients with differentiated papillary or follicular thyroid cancer, particularly for patients who do not have serum anti-Tg antibodies. Anti-Tg antibodies mainly interfere with immunometric assays and interfere less with radioimmunoassays for Tg. Anti-Tg antibodies tend to persist but may become less evident several years after total thyroidectomy and during the last trimester of pregnancy.

Detectable levels of thyroglobulin are commonly encountered in patients who have had incomplete thyroidectomies and ^{131}I remnant ablations. Detectable thyroglobulin levels do not necessarily indicate the presence of residual or metastatic thyroid cancer. However, baseline or stimulated serum Tg levels ≥ 2 ng/mL indicate the need for a repeat neck ultrasound and further scanning with RAI or ^{18}FDG-PET. If serum Tg levels remain ≥ 2 ng/mL in the presence of normal scanning, it is prudent to repeat the serum Tg in a national reference laboratory. Rising serum levels of thyroglobulin are particularly worrisome.

In one series of patients with differentiated thyroid cancer following thyroidectomy, there was a 21% incidence of metastases in patients with serum Tg < 1 ng/mL (while receiving thyroxine for TSH suppression). Therefore, baseline serum Tg levels are inadequately sensitive and *stimulated* serum Tg measurements should be used and *always* with neck ultrasound. The usefulness of routinely doing a radioiodine scan (see below) in low-risk patients is controversial but continues to be done in many centers during stimulation following either rhTSH or thyroid hormone withdrawal, according to the protocols described below.

3. Radioactive iodine (RAI: ^{131}I or ^{123}I) whole-body scanning—Despite its limitations, RAI has traditionally been used to detect metastatic differentiated thyroid cancer and to determine whether the cancer is amenable to treatment with ^{131}I. RAI scanning is particularly useful for high-risk patients and those with persistent anti-thyroglobulin antibodies that make serum thyroglobulin determinations unreliable.

The ^{131}I isotope may be used in scanning doses of < 3 mCi (111 MBq) or given within 2 weeks of RAI treatment to avoid "stunning" metastases such that they take up less of the RAI therapy dose. The radioisotope ^{123}I may be used in scanning doses of 5 mCi (185 MBq), does not stun tumors, and allows single-photon emission computed tomography (SPECT) to better localize metastases. Initial RAI scanning is typically performed about 2–4 months following surgery for differentiated thyroid carcinoma. Whole-body scanning should be performed for at least 30 minutes for at least 140,000 counts and spot views of the neck should be obtained for at least 35,000 counts.

About 65% of metastases are detectable by RAI scanning, but only after optimal preparation: Patients should ideally have a total or near-total thyroidectomy, since any residual normal thyroid competes for RAI with metastases, which are less avid for iodine. To avoid nonradioactive iodine competitive inhibition of RAI uptake, intravenous iodinated contrast must be avoided for at least 2 months before scanning; patients must follow a low-iodine diet for at least 2 weeks before scanning and continue to limit iodine consumption until the scan is complete or until after ^{131}I therapy. In addition, patients must have high levels of TSH to stimulate metastases to take up more RAI, making them visible on scanning. This can be accomplished by administering synthetic rhTSH or by allowing the patient to become hypothyroid. The use of rhTSH has become more widespread for surveillance scanning and

stimulated thyroglobulin determinations following thyroidectomy for differentiated thyroid carcinoma, due to its convenience for the patient. For stage I–II patients, it is reasonable to perform a rhTSH-stimulated scan and thyroglobulin level 2–3 months after the initial neck surgery; if the scan is negative and the serum thyroglobulin is < 2 ng/mL, the patient may be monitored with yearly neck ultrasound and serum thyroglobulin levels. For higher-risk patients, the rhTSH-stimulated thyroglobulin and RAI scan may be repeated about 1 year after surgery and then again if warranted.

A. Thyrotropin-stimulated serum Tg and radioiodine scanning—For surveillance, recombinant human thyrotropin-α (Thyrogen; rhTSH) is given in order to increase the sensitivity of serum thyroglobulin and RAI scanning. The use of rhTSH is particularly suited to "low-risk" patients: those with a small papillary thyroid carcinoma who have had a total or near-total thyroidectomy and have no known local or distal metastases and a serum thyroglobulin < 1 mcg/L during thyroxine suppression of serum TSH. In about 21% of such low-risk patients, rhTSH stimulates serum thyroglobulin to above 2 mcg/L; such patients have a 23% risk of local neck metastases and a 13% risk of distant metastases. Stimulated radioiodine neck and whole-body scanning can detect only about half of these metastases because they are small or not avid for iodine.

Thyrotropin must be kept refrigerated and may be administered according to the following protocol: Thyroxine replacement is held for 2 days before rhTSH and for 3 days afterward. On Monday and Tuesday, thyrotropin 0.9 mg is administered intragluteally (not intravenously). On Wednesday, serum is drawn for TSH and thyroglobulin determinations. Immediately thereafter, RAI is administered in a scanning dose (see above). On Friday, serum is drawn for thyroglobulin and the whole-body scan is performed.

Side effects of thyrotropin injections include nausea (11%) and headache (7%). Hyperthyroidism can occur in patients with significant metastases or residual normal thyroid. Thyrotropin has caused neurologic deterioration in 7% of patients with central nervous system metastases.

The combination of thyrotropin-stimulated scanning and thyroglobulin levels detects a thyroid remnant or cancer with a sensitivity of 84%. However, the presence of anti-thyroglobulin antibodies renders the serum thyroglobulin determination uninterpretable. Thyrotropin stimulation does not prepare patients for ^{131}I treatment; they must be prepared for treatment by becoming hypothyroid as described below.

B. Thyroid withdrawal-stimulated serum Tg and radioiodine scanning—Recombinant human TSH (rhTSH, Thyrogen) has largely replaced thyroid withdrawal, as noted above. But thyroid hormone withdrawal is still used, allowing the patient to become hypothyroid; high levels of endogenous TSH stimulate the uptake of RAI and production of thyroglobulin by thyroid cancer or residual thyroid. Serum thyroxine is held for 14 days. Prior to scanning, serum TSH is assayed to confirm that it is > 30 mcU/mL; serum hCG is assayed to screen for pregnancy; serum thyroglobulin titers are also determined.

Following radioisotope scanning, or 4 days after ^{131}I therapy (see above), thyroxine therapy may be resumed at full replacement dose.

Patients with **differentiated thyroid carcinoma** have traditionally required at least two annual consecutively negative stimulated serum thyroglobulin determinations < 1 mcg/L and normal RAI scans (if done) and neck ultrasound before they are considered to be in remission. Patients with persistent RAI uptake restricted to the thyroid bed need not have repeated ^{131}I therapies if neck ultrasound appears benign and serum thyroglobulin is < 5 ng/mL. Further radioiodine or other scans may be required for patients with more aggressive papillary-follicular, follicular, or medullary thyroid carcinomas, prior metastases, rising serum thyroglobulin levels, or other evidence of metastases.

Patients often have a negative whole-body radioiodine scan but have serum thyroglobulin levels that are > 2 ng/mL. In such cases, another thyroglobulin assay should be sent to a different reference laboratory to confirm the accuracy of the thyroglobulin determination. Patients with serum Tg levels > 2 ng/mL require close continued monitoring. Those with progressively rising Tg levels are at high risk for occult thyroid cancer metastases. Other scanning methods may be used in an effort to detect such metastases.

4. Positron emission tomography scanning—PET whole-body scanning using ^{18}FDG-PET is a relatively sensitive method for detecting thyroid cancer metastases—particularly those that are not revealed on RAI scanning. PET scanning is particularly useful for detecting thyroid cancer metastases in patients with a detectable serum thyroglobulin (especially serum thyroglobulin levels > 10 ng/mL and rising) who have a normal whole-body RAI scan and an unrevealing neck ultrasound. PET scanning can be combined with a CT scan; the resultant PET/CT fusion scan is 60% sensitive for detecting metastases that are not visible by other methods. This scan is less sensitive for small brain metastases. ^{18}FDG-PET scanning detects the metabolic activity of tumor tissue; for differentiated thyroid carcinoma, this scan is more sensitive when the patient is pretreated with thyrotropin as described above. One problem with ^{18}FDG-PET scanning is its lack of specificity. For example, false-positives can occur with benign hepatic tumors, sarcoidosis, radiation therapy, suture granulomas, reactive lymph nodes, or inflammation at surgical sites that can persist for months. False-positive uptake can also occur in muscles and brown fat in the neck and shoulders, axillae, mediastinum, perinephric regions, intercostal paravertebral spaces, and paravertebral muscles. A fusion ^{18}FDG-PET/CT (noniodine contrast) scan improves specificity but cannot distinguish thyroid carcinoma from other unrelated malignancies that may be present concurrently. Smaller metastases are often present on PET scanning before becoming visible on CT or MRI scanning.

^{18}FDG-PET scanning is particularly sensitive for detecting medullary thyroid carcinoma metastases, and prescan thyrotropin does not improve the PET scan sensitivity for medullary thyroid carcinoma.

5. Other scanning—Thallium-201 (^{201}Tl) scans may be useful for detecting metastatic differentiated thyroid carcinoma when the ^{131}I scan is normal but serum thyroglobulin is elevated. MRI scanning is particularly useful for imaging metastases in the brain, mediastinum, or bones. CT scanning is useful for imaging and monitoring pulmonary metastases.

► Staging & Prognosis

Staging and survival for **papillary thyroid cancer** is shown on Table 26–8. Papillary thyroid cancer carries a generally good prognosis, particularly for adults under age 45 years, despite the fact that about 15% of these patients are subsequently found to have metastases. The following characteristics imply a worse prognosis: older age, male sex, bone or brain metastases, large pulmonary metastases, and lack of ^{131}I uptake into metastases. Younger patients with pulmonary metastases tend to respond better to ^{131}I therapy than do older adults. Certain papillary histologic types are associated with a higher risk of recurrence: tall cell, columnar cell, and diffuse sclerosing types. Brain metastases are detected in 1%; they reduce median survival to 12 months, but the patient's prognosis is improved by surgical resection. Patients with a **follicular variant of papillary carcinoma** have a prognosis somewhere between that of papillary and follicular thyroid carcinoma.

Patients with **follicular carcinoma** have a cancer mortality rate that is 3.4 times higher than patients with papillary carcinoma. The Hürthle cell variant of follicular carcinoma is even more aggressive. Patients with primary tumors over 1 cm in diameter who undergo limited thyroid surgery (subtotal thyroidectomy or lobectomy) have a 2.2-fold increased mortality over those having total or near-total thyroidectomies. Patients who have not received ^{131}I ablation have mortality rates that are increased twofold by 10 years and threefold by 25 years (over those who have received ablation). The risk of cancer recurrence is twofold higher in men than in women and 1.7-fold higher in multifocal than in unifocal tumors.

Medullary thyroid carcinoma is more aggressive than differentiated thyroid cancer but is typically fairly indolent. The overall 10-year survival rate is 90% when the tumor is confined to the thyroid, 70% for those with metastases to cervical lymph nodes, and 20% for those with distant metastases. Patients with sporadic disease usually have lymph node involvement noted at the time of diagnosis, whereas distal metastases may not be noted for years. For patients with medullary thyroid carcinoma who have metastases to lymph nodes, modified radical neck dissection is recommended. Familial cases or those associated with MEN 2A tend to be less aggressive; the 10-year survival rate is higher, in part due to earlier detection. Medullary thyroid carcinoma that is seen in MEN 2B is more aggressive, arises earlier in life, and carries a worse overall prognosis. Women with medullary thyroid carcinoma who are under age 40 years have a better prognosis. A better prognosis is also obtained in patients undergoing total thyroidectomy and neck dissection; radiation therapy reduces recurrence in patients with metastases to neck nodes. The mortality rate is increased 4.5-fold when primary or metastatic tumor tissue stains heavily for myelomonocytic antigen M-1. Conversely, tumors with heavy immunoperoxidase staining for calcitonin are associated with prolonged survival even in the presence of significant metastases.

Anaplastic thyroid carcinoma carries a 1-year survival rate of about 10% and a 5-year survival rate of about 5%. Patients with fully localized tumors on MRI have a better prognosis.

Localized lymphoma carries a 5-year survival of nearly 100%. Those with disease outside the thyroid have a 63% 5-year survival. However, the prognosis is better for those with the MALT type. Patients presenting with stridor, pain, laryngeal nerve palsy, or mediastinal extension tend to fare worse.

Brown AP et al. The risk of second primary malignancies up to three decades after the treatment of differentiated thyroid cancer. J Clin Endocrinol Metab. 2008 Feb;93(2):504–15. [PMID: 18029468]

McCarthy RP et al. Molecular evidence for the same clonal origin of multifocal papillary thyroid carcinoma. Clin Cancer Res. 2006 Apr;12(8):2414–8. [PMID: 1663846]

Pilli T et al. A comparison of 1850 (50 mCi) and 3700 MBq (100 mCi) 131-iodine administered doses for recombinant thyrotropin-stimulated postoperative thyroid remnant ablation in differentiated thyroid cancer. J Clin Endocrinol Metab. 2007 Sep;92(9):3542–6. [PMID: 17609306]

Robbins RJ et al. Real-time prognosis for metastatic thyroid carcinoma based on 2-[18F]fluoro-2-deoxy-D-glucose-positron emission tomography scanning. J Clin Endocrinol Metab. 2006 Feb;91(2):498–505. [PMID: 16303836]

IODINE DEFICIENCY DISORDER & ENDEMIC GOITER

ESSENTIALS OF DIAGNOSIS

▶ Common in regions of the world with low-iodine diets.

▶ High rate of congenital hypothyroidism and cretinism.

▶ Goiters may become multinodular and grow to great size.

▶ Most adults with endemic goiter are found to be euthyroid; however, some are hypothyroid or hyperthyroid.

▶ Impaired cognition and hearing may be subtle or severe in congenital hypothyroidism.

General Considerations

About 1 billion people are iodine deficient, having no access to iodized salt and living in areas with iodine-depleted soil. Severe iodine deficiency increases the risk of miscarriage and stillbirth. About 0.5% of live births in iodine-deficient areas have full-blown cretinism. Moderate iodine deficiency during gestation and infancy cause other manifestations of congenital hypothyroidism, such as deafness and short stature and permanently lowers a child's IQ by 10–15 points. Such children belong to the most isolated and impoverished families whose affected children serve to perpetuate the cycle of poverty in these areas.

Populations in areas of iodine deficiency have a high incidence of goiter. One such area is Pescopagano, Italy, where 60% of adults have goiters. Hyperthyroidism (present or past) occurred in 2.9%; hypothyroidism was overt in 0.2% and subclinical in 3.8%.

Although iodine deficiency is the most common cause of endemic goiter, certain foods (eg, sorghum, millet, maize, cassava), mineral deficiencies (selenium, iron), and water pollutants can themselves cause goiter or aggravate a goiter proclivity caused by iodine deficiency. In iodine-deficient patients, smoking can induce goiter growth. Pregnancy aggravates iodine deficiency and is associated with an increase in size of thyroid nodules and the emergence of new nodules. Some individuals are particularly susceptible to goiter owing to congenital partial defects in thyroid enzyme activity.

Clinical Findings

A. Symptoms and Signs

Endemic goiters may become multinodular and very large. Growth often occurs during pregnancy and may cause compressive symptoms.

Substernal goiters are usually asymptomatic but can cause tracheal compression, respiratory distress and failure, dysphagia, superior vena cava syndrome, gastrointestinal bleeding from esophageal varices, palsies of the phrenic or recurrent laryngeal nerves, or Horner syndrome. Cerebral ischemia and stroke can result from arterial compression or thyrocervical steal syndrome. Substernal goiters can rarely cause pleural or pericardial effusions. The incidence of significant malignancy is less than 1%.

Some patients with endemic goiter may become hypothyroid. Others may become thyrotoxic as the goiter grows and becomes more autonomous, especially if iodine is added to the diet.

B. Laboratory Findings

The serum T_4 is usually normal. Serum TSH is generally normal. TSH falls in the presence of hyperthyroidism if a multinodular goiter has become autonomous in the presence of sufficient amounts of iodine for thyroid hormone synthesis. TSH rises with hypothyroidism. Thyroid RAI uptake is usually elevated, but it may be normal if iodine intake has improved. Serum levels of antithyroid antibodies are usually either undetectable or in low titers. Serum thyroglobulin is often elevated.

Differential Diagnosis

Endemic goiter must be distinguished from all other forms of nodular goiter that may coexist in an endemic region (see above).

Prevention

Iodine deficiency is prevented by adding iodine to commercial salt. In the United States, potassium iodide is used. Some tropical countries use potassium iodate, since it is more stable than potassium iodide in hot and humid climates. Iodized salt contains iodine at about 20 mg per kg salt. The minimum dietary requirement for iodine is about 50 mcg daily, with optimal iodine intake being 150–300 mcg daily. Iodine sufficiency is assessed by measurement of urinary iodide excretion, the target being more than 10 mcg/dL. Initiating iodine supplementation in an iodine-deficient area greatly reduces the emergence of new goiters but causes an increased frequency of hyperthyroidism during the first year.

▶ Treatment

The addition of potassium iodide to table salt greatly reduces the prevalence of endemic goiter and cretinism but is less effective in shrinking established goiter. Concurrent deficiencies in both vitamin A and iodine increase the risk of endemic goiter and concurrent repletion of both iodide and vitamin A reduces goiter in endemic goiter regions.

Adults with large multinodular goiter may require thyroidectomy for cosmesis, compressive symptoms, or thyrotoxicosis. Following partial thyroidectomy in iodine-deficient geographic areas, there is a high goiter recurrence rate, so near-total thyroidectomy is preferred when surgery is indicated. Certain patients may be treated with ^{131}I for large compressive goiters.

▶ Complications

Dietary iodine supplementation increases the risk of autoimmune thyroid dysfunction, which may cause hypothyroidism or hyperthyroidism. Excessive iodine supplementation increases the risk of goiter. Thyroxine suppression carries the risk of inducing hyperthyroidism, particularly in patients with autonomous multinodular goiters; therefore, thyroxine suppression should not be started in patients with a low TSH level. Rarely, Graves disease can develop 3–10 months after ^{131}I treatment in patients with large multinodular goiters.

Pearce EN. National trends in iodine nutrition: is everyone getting enough? Thyroid. 2007 Sep;17(9):823–7. [PMID: 17956156]
Zimmerman MB. Iodine requirements and the risks and benefits of correcting iodine deficiency in populations. J Trace Elem Biol. 2008 May;22(2):81–92. [PMID: 18565420]

▼ THE PARATHYROIDS

Parathyroid hormone (PTH) increases osteoclastic activity in bone, increases the renal tubular reabsorption of calcium, and stimulates the synthesis of 1,25-dihydroxycholecalciferol by the kidney. Meanwhile, PTH inhibits the absorption of phosphate and bicarbonate by the renal tubule. All of these actions cause a net increase in serum calcium.

HYPOPARATHYROIDISM & PSEUDOHYPOPARATHYROIDISM

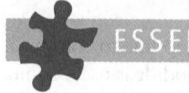

ESSENTIALS OF DIAGNOSIS

▶ Tetany, carpopedal spasms, tingling of lips and hands, muscle and abdominal cramps, psychological changes.

▶ Positive Chvostek sign and Trousseau phenomenon.

▶ Serum calcium low; serum phosphate high; alkaline phosphatase normal; urine calcium excretion reduced.

▶ Low or low-normal serum PTH in presence of hypocalcemia.

▶ Serum magnesium may be low.

▶ General Considerations

Acquired hypoparathyroidism is most commonly seen following thyroidectomy, when it is usually transient but may be permanent. It may also occur after multiple parathyroidectomies. Hypoparathyroidism may occur transiently after surgical removal of a parathyroid adenoma for primary hyperparathyroidism due to suppression of the remaining normal parathyroids and accelerated remineralization of the skeleton (hungry bone syndrome). Neck irradiation may rarely cause hypoparathyroidism.

Parathyroid deficiency may also be the result of damage from heavy metals such as copper (Wilson disease) or iron (hemochromatosis, transfusion hemosiderosis), granulomas, sporadic autoimmunity, Riedel thyroiditis, tumors, or infection.

Functional hypoparathyroidism may also occur as a result of magnesium deficiency (malabsorption, chronic alcoholism), which prevents the secretion of PTH. Correction of hypomagnesemia results in rapid disappearance of the condition.

PGA type I (PGA-1) is also known as autoimmune polyendocrinopathy-candidiasis-ectodermal dystrophy (APECED). PGA-1 presents in childhood with at least two of the following manifestations: candidiasis, hypoparathyroidism, or Addison disease. Cataracts, uveitis, alopecia, vitiligo, or autoimmune thyroid disease may also develop.

Fat malabsorption occurs in 20% of patients with PGA-1 and may present as weight loss, diarrhea, or malabsorption of vitamin D, a fat-soluble vitamin used to treat the hypoparathyroidism. The fat malabsorption may be due to a deficiency in the jejunal enteroendocrine cells that produce cholecystokinin, causing a reduction in bile acid secretion.

In **congenital hypoparathyroidism,** parathyroid cells have calcium-sensing receptors (CaSR) that sense the serum calcium concentration and suppress PTH secretion by way of G-protein-coupled mechanisms. Gain-of-function mutations (constitutive activation) of the *CaSR* gene suppress the parathyroid glands, resulting in hypocalcemia without elevations in serum PTH levels. Such mutations cause "autosomal dominant hypocalcemia with hypercalciuria" (ADHH) from deficient secretion of PTH. The prevalence of ADHH in the population is about 1 in 70,000, and it typically presents in infancy with hypocalcemic seizures.

Hypoparathyroidism, deafness, and renal dysplasia (HDR or Barakat) syndrome is an autosomal dominant condition caused by haploinsufficiency or mutations of the gene *GATA3*. The hypocalcemia is present from birth but may not be detected until the occurrence of mental retardation or hypocalcemic tetany. The mostly high-frequency deafness is present at birth. Various renal and vesicoureteral anomalies occur.

Hypoparathyroidism may also be seen in DiGeorge syndrome, along with congenital cardiac and facial anomalies; hypocalcemia usually presents with tetany in infancy, but some cases are not detected until adulthood.

▶ Clinical Findings

A. Symptoms and Signs

Acute hypoparathyroidism causes tetany, with muscle cramps, irritability, carpopedal spasm, and convulsions; tingling of the circumoral area, hands, and feet is almost always present. Symptoms of the chronic disease are lethargy, personality changes, anxiety state, blurring of vision due to cataracts, parkinsonism, and mental retardation.

Chvostek sign (facial muscle contraction on tapping the facial nerve in front of the ear) is positive, and Trousseau phenomenon (carpal spasm after application of a sphygmomanometer cuff) is present. Cataracts may occur; the nails may be thin and brittle; the skin is dry and scaly, at times with fungus infection (candidiasis), and there may be loss of hair (eyebrows); and deep tendon reflexes may be hyperactive. Papilledema and elevated cerebrospinal fluid pressure are occasionally seen. Teeth may be defective if the onset of the disease occurs in childhood.

B. Laboratory Findings

Serum calcium is low, serum phosphate high, urinary calcium low, and alkaline phosphatase normal. Serum calcium is largely bound to albumin. In hypoalbuminemia, the serum ionized calcium may be determined, but it has had surprisingly poor clinical utility. Alternatively, the serum calcium level can be corrected for serum albumin level as follows:

$$\text{"Corrected" serum } Ca^{2+} = \text{Serum } Ca^{2+} \text{ mg/dL} + (0.8 \times [4.0 - \text{Albumin g/dL}])$$

PTH levels are low. Serum magnesium should be determined since hypomagnesemia frequently accompanies hypocalcemia and may exacerbate symptoms and decrease parathyroid function.

C. Imaging

Radiographs or CT scans of the skull may show basal ganglia calcifications; the bones may be denser than normal. Cutaneous calcification may occur.

D. Other Examinations

Slit-lamp examination may show early posterior lenticular cataract formation. The electrocardiogram (ECG) shows prolonged QT intervals and T wave abnormalities. Patients with chronic hypoparathyroidism tend to have increased bone mineral density, particularly in the lumbar spine.

▶ Complications

Acute tetany with stridor, especially if associated with vocal cord palsy, may lead to respiratory obstruction requiring tracheostomy. The complications of chronic hypoparathyroidism largely depend on the duration of the disease. There may be associated autoimmunity causing sprue syndrome, pernicious anemia, or Addison disease. In long-standing cases, cataract formation and calcification of the basal ganglia are seen. Occasionally, parkinsonian symptoms or choreoathetosis develop. Ossification of the paravertebral ligaments may occur with nerve root compression; surgical decompression may be required. Seizures are common in untreated patients. Overtreatment with vitamin D and calcium may produce nephrocalcinosis and impairment of kidney function. Chronic hypocalcemia can cause heart failure.

▶ Differential Diagnosis

Paresthesias, muscle cramps, or tetany due to respiratory alkalosis, in which the serum calcium is normal, can be confused with hypocalcemia. In fact, hyperventilation tends to accentuate hypocalcemic symptoms.

At times hypoparathyroidism is misdiagnosed as idiopathic epilepsy, choreoathetosis, or brain tumor (on the basis of brain calcifications, convulsions, choked disks) or, more rarely, as "asthma" (on the basis of stridor and dyspnea). In patients with hypoalbuminemia, serum levels of ionized calcium are normal.

Hypocalcemia may also be due to malabsorption of calcium, magnesium, or vitamin D; patients do not always have diarrhea. Hypocalcemia may also be caused by certain drugs: loop diuretics, plicamycin, phenytoin, alendronate, and foscarnet. In addition, hypocalcemia may be seen in cases of rapid intravascular volume expansion or due to chelation from transfusions of large volumes of citrated blood. It is also observed in patients with acute pancreatitis. Hypocalcemia may develop in some patients with certain osteoblastic metastatic carcinomas (especially breast, prostate) instead of the expected hypercalcemia. Hypocalcemia with hyperphosphatemia (simulating hypoparathyroidism) is seen in azotemia but may also be caused by large doses of intravenous, oral, or rectal phosphate preparations and by chemotherapy of responsive lymphomas or leukemias.

Hypocalcemia with hypercalciuria may be due to a familial syndrome involving a mutation in the calcium-sensing receptor; such patients have levels of serum PTH that are in the normal range, distinguishing it from hypoparathyroidism. It is transmitted as an autosomal dominant disorder. Such patients are hypercalciuric; treatment with calcium and vitamin D may cause nephrocalcinosis.

Congenital pseudohypoparathyroidism is a group of disorders characterized by resistance to PTH. There are several subtypes caused by different mutations involving the PTH receptor or its G protein or adenylyl cyclase. Renal tubular resistance to PTH causes hypercalciuria with resultant hypocalcemia. PTH levels are high and the PTH receptors in bone are typically not involved, such that bony changes of hyperparathyroidism may be evident. Various phenotypic abnormalities—classically, short stature, round face, obesity, short fourth metacarpals, ectopic bone formation, and mental retardation—may be associated with congenital pseudohypoparathyroidism. Patients without hypo-

Table 26–9. Vitamin D preparations used in the treatment of hypoparathyroidism.

	Available Preparations	Daily Dose	Duration of Action
Ergocalciferol ergosterol, (vitamin D₂, Calciferol)	Capsules of 50,000 international units; 8000 international units/mL oral solution	2000–200,000 units	1–2 weeks
Cholecalciferol (vitamin D₃)	Capsules of 50,000 international units not available commercially in United States; may be compounded	10,000–50,000 units	4–8 weeks
Calcitriol (Rocaltrol)	Capsules of 0.25 and 0.5 mcg; 1 mcg/mL oral solution; 1 mcg/mL for injection	0.25–4 mcg	¹/₂–2 weeks

calcemia but sharing the phenotypic abnormalities are said to have "pseudopseudohypoparathyroidism."

▶ **Treatment**

A. Emergency Treatment for Acute Attack (Hypoparathyroid Tetany)

This usually occurs after surgery and requires immediate treatment.

1. Airway—Be sure an adequate airway is present.

2. Intravenous calcium gluconate—Calcium gluconate, 10–20 mL of 10% solution intravenously, may be given *slowly* until tetany ceases. Ten to 50 mL of 10% calcium gluconate may be added to 1 L of 5% glucose in water or saline and administered by slow intravenous drip. The rate should be adjusted so that the serum calcium is maintained between 8 mg/dL and 9 mg/dL.

3. Oral calcium—Calcium salts should be given orally as soon as possible to supply 1–2 g of calcium daily. Liquid calcium carbonate, 500 mg/5 mL, may be especially useful. The dosage is 1–3 g calcium daily. Calcium citrate contains 21% calcium, but a higher proportion is absorbed with less gastrointestinal intolerance.

4. Vitamin D preparations—(Table 26–9.) Therapy should be started as soon as oral calcium is begun. The active metabolite of vitamin D, 1,25-dihydroxycholecalciferol (calcitriol), has a very rapid onset of action and is not long-lasting if hypercalcemia occurs. It is of great use in the treatment of acute hypocalcemia. Therapy is commenced at a dosage of 0.25 mcg orally each morning with upward dosage titration to near normocalcemia. Ultimately, doses of 0.5–2 mcg/d are usually required.

Calcifediol (25-hydroxyvitamin D₃), another option for treatment, has an intermediate onset and duration of action; the usual starting dose is 20 mcg/d orally.

5. Magnesium—If hypomagnesemia is present (chronic alcoholism, malnutrition, renal loss, drugs such as cisplatin, etc), it must be corrected to treat the resulting hypocalcemia. Acutely, magnesium sulfate is given intravenously, 1–2 g every 6 hours. Long-term magnesium replacement may be given as magnesium oxide tablets (600 mg), one or two per day, or as a combined magnesium and calcium preparation (CalMag, others).

6. Transplantation of cryopreserved parathyroid tissue removed during prior surgery—Transplantation restores normocalcemia in about 23% of cases.

B. Maintenance Treatment

The goal should be to maintain the serum calcium in a slightly low but asymptomatic range (8–8.6 mg/dL). This will minimize the hypercalciuria that would otherwise occur and provides a margin of safety against overdosage and hypercalcemia, which may produce permanent damage to kidney function. Calcium supplementation (1–2 g/d) is given, along with a vitamin D preparation.

Patients with chronic hypoparathyroidism must usually be treated with some type of vitamin D (Table 26–9). Vitamin D₂ (ergocalciferol) is derived from plants and is commercially available. The usual dose ranges from 25,000 to 150,000 units/d. Vitamin D₃ (cholecalciferol), the form of vitamin D that is naturally produced in unprotected human skin with UV sunlight exposure, is not generally commercially available in the United States in large doses but may be compounded. Vitamin D₃ is at least three times more bioavailable than vitamin D₂, so that appropriate dosing adjustments must be made when changing from one type of vitamin D to another. Both forms of vitamin D are slow-acting preparation, and if toxicity develops, hypercalcemia—treatable with hydration and prednisone—may persist for weeks after it is discontinued. Ergocalciferol and cholecalciferol usually produce a more stable serum calcium level than do the shorter-acting preparations.

Despite its high cost, calcitriol is being used with increasing frequency for the treatment of chronic hypoparathyroidism; the maintenance dosage of calcitriol ranges from 0.25 mcg/d to 2.0 mcg/d. Monitoring of serum calcium at regular intervals (at least every 3 months) is mandatory.

PTH acts upon the kidney to increase tubular reabsorption of calcium. Therefore, patients with hypoparathyroidism are prone to hypercalciuria and calcium nephrolithiasis during treatment. Target serum calcium levels should be 8–8.6 mg/dL, keeping it mildly low to avoid hypercalciuria. It is prudent to monitor urine calcium with "spot" urine determinations and keep the level below 30 mg/dL if possible. Hypercalciuria may respond to oral hydrochlorothiazide, usually given with a potassium supplement.

Caution: Phenothiazine drugs should be administered with caution, since they may precipitate extrapyramidal symptoms in hypocalcemic patients. Furosemide should be avoided, since it may worsen hypocalcemia.

Prognosis

The outlook is good if the diagnosis is made promptly and treatment instituted. Any dental changes, cataracts, and brain calcifications are permanent. Periodic blood chemical evaluation is required, since changes in calcium levels may call for modification of the treatment schedule. Hypercalcemia that develops in patients with seemingly stable, treated hypoparathyroidism may be a presenting sign of Addison disease.

Shalitin S et al. Clinical heterogeneity of pseudohypoparathyroidism: from hyper- to hypocalcemia. Horm Res. 2008;70(3):137–44. [PMID: 18663313]
Shoback D. Clinical practice. Hypoparathyroidism. N Engl J Med. 2008 Jul;359(4):391–403. [PMID: 18650515]

HYPERPARATHYROIDISM

ESSENTIALS OF DIAGNOSIS

- ▶ Frequently detected incidentally by screening.
- ▶ Renal calculi, polyuria, hypertension, constipation, fatigue, mental changes.
- ▶ Bone pain; rarely, cystic lesions and pathologic fractures.
- ▶ Serum and urine calcium elevated; urine phosphate high with low to normal serum phosphate; alkaline phosphatase normal to elevated.
- ▶ Elevated PTH.

General Considerations

Primary hyperparathyroidism is characterized by chronic poorly regulated excessive secretion of PTH by one or more parathyroid glands that results in hypercalcemia. It is an increasingly recognized disorder, present in up to 0.1% of adult patients examined. It can be seen at any age but is more frequent in persons over the age of 50 years and is three times more common in women than in men.

The disease is caused by hypersecretion of PTH, usually by a single parathyroid adenoma (80%), and less commonly by hyperplasia by two or more parathyroid glands (20%), or carcinoma (≤ 1%). However, when hyperparathyroidism presents before age 30 years, there is a higher incidence of multiglandular disease (36%) and carcinoma (5%). The size of the parathyroid adenoma correlates with the serum PTH level.

Hyperparathyroidism is familial in about 10% of cases. Parathyroid hyperplasia may arise in MEN types 1, 2A, and 2B. In MEN 1, multiglandular hyperparathyroidism is usually the initial manifestation and ultimately occurs in 90% of affected individuals. Hyperparathyroidism in MEN 2A is less frequent that in MEN 1 and is usually milder. Familial hyperparathyroidism can also occur in the hyperparathyroidism-jaw tumor syndrome, a rare autosomal

dominant familial condition in which parathyroid cystic adenomas or carcinomas are associated with ossifying fibromas of the mandible and maxilla as well as renal lesions (cysts, hamartomas, Wilms tumors). Affected individuals usually present with severe hypercalcemia as teenagers or young adults; the pathology is usually a single parathyroid adenoma. (See Table 26–16.)

Hyperparathyroidism results in the excessive excretion of calcium and phosphate by the kidneys. PTH stimulates renal tubular reabsorption of calcium; however, hyperparathyroidism causes hypercalcemia and an increase in calcium in the glomerular filtrate that overwhelms tubular reabsorption capacity, resulting in hypercalciuria. At least 5% of renal calculi are associated with this disease. Diffuse parenchymal calcification (nephrocalcinosis) is seen less commonly. Chronic bone resorption induced by excessive PTH in the circulation may produce diffuse demineralization, pathologic fractures, or cystic bone lesions throughout the skeleton ("osteitis fibrosa cystica").

In chronic kidney disease, hyperphosphatemia and decreased renal production of 1,25-dihydroxycholecalciferol ($1,25[OH]_2D_3$) initially produce a decrease in ionized calcium. The parathyroid glands are stimulated (secondary hyperparathyroidism) and may enlarge, becoming autonomous (tertiary hyperparathyroidism). The bone disease seen in this setting is known as "renal osteodystrophy." Parathyroid hyperplasia in uremia can result in extremely high serum PTH levels that are associated with uremic vascular calcification. Hypercalcemia often occurs after kidney transplant.

Parathyroid carcinoma is a rare cause of hyperparathyroidism but is more common in patients with severe hypercalcemia. About 50% of parathyroid carcinomas are palpable.

Clinical Findings

A. Symptoms and Signs

Hypercalcemia of hyperparathyroidism is typically discovered accidentally by routine chemistry panels. Many patients are asymptomatic or have mild symptoms that may be elicited only upon questioning. Parathyroid adenomas are usually so small and deeply located in the neck that they are almost never palpable; when a mass is palpated, it usually turns out to be an incidental thyroid nodule.

Symptomatic patients are said to have problems with "bones, stones, abdominal groans, psychic moans, with fatigue overtones." The manifestations are categorized as skeletal, urinary tract, and those associated with hypercalcemia.

1. Skeletal manifestations—Hyperparathyroidism causes a loss of cortical bone and a gain of trabecular bone. Significant bone demineralization is uncommon in mild hyperparathyroidism, but osteitis fibrosa cystica may present as pathologic fractures or as "brown tumors" or cysts of the jaw. More commonly, patients have bone pain and arthralgias.

2. Manifestations of hypercalcemia—Mild hypercalcemia may be asymptomatic. However, hypercalcemia has a variety of manifestations that become progressively worse with more severe hypercalcemia. Paresthesias, muscular weakness, and diminished deep tendon reflexes are examples of **neuromuscular manifestations. Central nervous system** manifestations include malaise, fatigue, intellectual weariness, depression, increased sleep requirement, progressing to cognitive impairment, disorientation, psychosis, or stupor. **Cardiovascular symptoms** that can indicate hypercalcemia are hypertension, prolonged P-R interval, shortened Q-T interval, sensitivity to arrhythmic effects of digitalis, bradyarrhythmias, heart block, asystole. **Renal** manifestations include polyuria and polydipsia, caused by hypercalcemia-induced nephrogenic diabetes insipidus. Calcium-containing kidney stones are reported in about 18% of those with newly discovered primary hyperparathyroidism. Nephrocalcinosis and kidney disease can occur. Gastrointestinal symptoms include anorexia, nausea, vomiting, abdominal pain, weight loss, constipation, and obstipation. Pancreatitis occurs in 3%. **Pruritus** may be present. **Calcium** may precipitate in the corneas ("band keratopathy"). Calcium may also precipitate in extravascular tissues as well as in small arteries, causing small vessel thrombosis and skin necrosis (calciphylaxis).

3. Hyperparathyroidism during pregnancy—About 67% of women with primary hyperparathyroidism during pregnancy experience complications such as nephrolithiasis, hyperemesis, pancreatitis, muscle weakness, cognitive changes, and hypercalcemic crisis. About 80% of fetuses experience complications of maternal hyperparathyroidism, including fetal demise, preterm delivery, low birth weight, postpartum neonatal tetany, and permanent hypoparathyroidism.

B. Laboratory Findings

The hallmark of primary hyperparathyroidism is the serum calcium > 10.5 mg/dL (Figure 26–1). In hyperproteinemic states, the total serum calcium may be elevated but the ionized fraction is normal, whereas in primary hyperparathyroidism, the ionized calcium is almost always over 5.4 mg/dL (1.4 mmol/L). In practice, serum ionized calcium determinations have not proved to be very helpful clinically. The serum phosphate is often low (< 2.5 mg/dL). The urine calcium excretion may be high or normal (averaging 250 mg/g creatinine) but it is usually low for the degree of hypercalcemia. There is an excessive loss of phosphate in the urine in the presence of hypophosphatemia (25% of cases). (In secondary hyperparathyroidism due to kidney disease, the serum phosphate is high.) The alkaline phosphatase is elevated only if bone disease is present. The plasma chloride and uric acid levels may be elevated. Vitamin D deficiency is common in patients with hyperparathyroidism, and it is prudent to screen for vitamin D deficiency with a serum 25-OH vitamin D determination. Low serum 25-OH vitamin D levels (< 20 mcg/L; < 50 nmol/L) can aggravate hyperparathyroidism and its bone manifestations; vitamin D replacement may be helpful in treating patients with hyperparathyroidism. (See below.)

Elevated serum levels of intact PTH (IRMA assay) confirm the diagnosis of hyperparathyroidism. Patients with apparent hyperparathyroidism should be screened for familial benign hypocalciuric hypercalcemia with a 24-hour urine for calcium and creatinine.

Patients should discontinue thiazide diuretics prior to this test. Calcium excretion of < 50 mg/24 hours (or < 5 mg/dL on a random urine) is not typical for primary

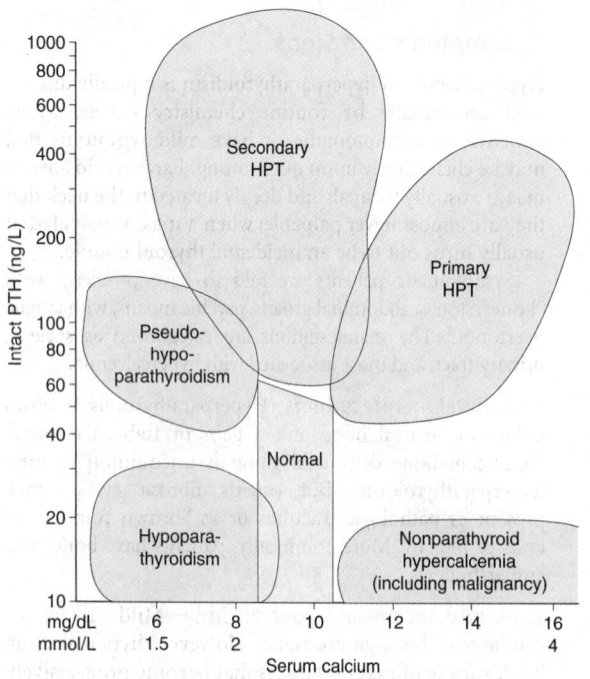

▲ **Figure 26–1.** Parathyroid hormone and calcium nomogram. Relationship between serum intact parathyroid hormone (PTH) and serum calcium levels in patients with hypoparathyroidism, pseudohypoparathyroidism, nonparathyroid hypercalcemia, primary hyperparathyroidism (HPT), and secondary hyperparathyroidism. (Courtesy of GJ Strewler.)

hyperparathyroidism and indicates possible familial benign hypocalciuric hypercalcemia. (See below.)

C. Imaging

Preoperative sestamibi-iodine subtraction scanning and neck ultrasonography have been used to locate parathyroid adenomas in patients with hyperparathyroidism, in an effort to improve the outcome and limit the invasiveness of neck surgery. Parathyroid imaging is crucial for patients who have had prior neck surgery. However, the usefulness of preoperative parathyroid localizing imaging studies for first neck explorations remains controversial. Imaging is not useful for the diagnosis of hyperparathyroidism, which must be made by serum calcium and PTH determinations. Preoperative scanning does not improve the outcome of initial bilateral neck explorations performed by a surgeon with special expertise in parathyroid surgery. Therefore, preoperative imaging has been used mainly to improve the outcome for limited neck exploration, with only modest success. (See Surgery, below.) Small benign thyroid nodules are discovered incidentally in nearly 50% of patients with hyperparathyroidism who have imaging with ultrasound or MRI.

CT and MRI scanning are not ordinarily required or useful for initial preoperative parathyroid localizing studies, since these scanning techniques are less sensitive for identifying tiny parathyroid adenomas. However, for repeat neck operations and when ectopic parathyroids are suspected, MRI is preferred since it offers better soft tissue contrast than CT scanning and is less adversely affected by postoperative changes in the neck. Three-dimensional technetium-99m sestamibi scanning can also help localize ectopic parathyroid glands.

Bone density measurements by dual energy x-ray absorptiometry (DXA) is helpful in determining the amount of bone loss in patients with hyperparathyroidism. Bone loss occurs mostly in long bones, and DXA should ideally include three areas: lumbar spine, hip, and distal radius.

Bone radiographs are usually normal and are not required to make the diagnosis of hyperparathyroidism. There may be demineralization, subperiosteal resorption of bone (especially in the radial aspects of the fingers), or loss of the lamina dura of the teeth. There may be cysts throughout the skeleton, mottling of the skull ("salt-and-pepper appearance"), or pathologic fractures. Articular cartilage calcification (chondrocalcinosis) is sometimes found.

Patients with renal osteodystrophy may have ectopic calcifications around joints or in soft tissue. Such patients may exhibit radiographic changes of osteopenia, osteitis fibrosa, or osteosclerosis, alone or in combination. Osteosclerosis of the vertebral bodies is known as "rugger jersey spine."

▶ Complications

Pathologic long bone fractures are more common in patients with hyperparathyroidism than in the general population. Urinary tract infection due to stone and obstruction may lead to kidney disease and uremia. If the serum calcium level rises rapidly, clouding of sensorium, kidney disease, and rapid precipitation of calcium throughout the soft tissues may occur. Peptic ulcer and pancreatitis may be intractable before surgery. Insulinomas or gastrinomas may be associated, as well as pituitary tumors (MEN type 1). Pseudogout may complicate hyperparathyroidism both before and after surgical removal of tumors. Hypercalcemia during gestation produces neonatal hypocalcemia.

In tertiary hyperparathyroidism due to chronic kidney disease, high serum calcium and phosphate levels may cause disseminated calcification in the skin, soft tissues, and arteries (calciphylaxis); this can result in painful ischemic necrosis of skin and gangrene, cardiac arrhythmias, and respiratory failure. The actual serum levels of calcium and phosphate have not correlated well with calciphylaxis, but a calcium (mg/dL) × phosphate (mg/dL) product over 70 is usually present.

▶ Differential Diagnosis

A. Artifact

A report of hypercalcemia may be due to laboratory error or excess tourniquet time and should always be repeated. Hypercalcemia may be due to high serum protein concentrations; in the presence of high or low serum albumin concentrations, a serum ionized calcium is more dependable than the total serum calcium concentration. Hypercalcemia may also be seen with dehydration; spurious elevations in serum calcium have been reported with severe hypertriglyceridemia, when the calcium assay uses spectrophotometry.

B. Vitamin D Deficiency

Secondary hyperparathyroidism predictably develops in patients with a deficiency in vitamin D. Serum calcium levels are typically in the normal range, but may rise to become borderline elevated with time, due to parathyroid glandular hyperplasia. (See Osteomalacia section.)

C. Hypercalcemia of Malignancy

Many malignant tumors (breast, lung, pancreas, uterus, hypernephroma, paraganglioma, etc) can produce hypercalcemia. In some cases (breast carcinoma especially), bony metastases are present. In others, no metastases to bone can be demonstrated. Most of these tumors secrete PTH-related protein (PTHrP), which has tertiary structural homologies to PTH and causes bone resorption and hypercalcemia similar to those of PTH. The clinical features of the hypercalcemia of cancer can closely simulate hyperparathyroidism. Serum phosphate is often low, but the plasma level of PTH by IRMA is *low*. Serum PTHrP may be elevated.

Multiple myeloma is a common cause of hypercalcemia in the older population. Many other hematologic cancers, such as monocytic leukemia, T cell leukemia and lymphoma, and Burkitt lymphoma, have also been associated with hypercalcemia. Multiple myeloma causes kidney dysfunction; resultant increased levels of carboxyl terminal PTH may cause it to be confused with hyperparathyroidism if a carboxyl terminal PTH assay is used.

D. Sarcoidosis and Other Granulomatous Disorders

Macrophages and perhaps other cells present in granulomatous tissue have the ability to synthesize $1,25(OH)_2D_3$. Hypercalcemia has been reported in patients with sarcoidosis, tuberculosis, berylliosis, histoplasmosis, coccidioidomycosis, leprosy, and even foreign-body granuloma. Increased intestinal calcium absorption and hypercalciuria are more common than hypercalcemia. Serum levels of $1,25(OH)_2D_3$ are elevated.

E. Calcium or Vitamin D Ingestion

Ingestion of large amounts of calcium or vitamin D can cause hypercalcemia, especially in patients who concurrently take thiazide diuretics, which reduce urinary calcium loss. Hypercalcemia is reversible following withdrawal of calcium and vitamin D supplements. If hypercalcemia persists, the possibility of associated hyperparathyroidism should be strongly considered.

In vitamin D intoxication, patients may be taking large amounts of vitamin D for unclear reasons, so a thorough review of all medications is important. Hypercalcemia may persist for several weeks. Serum levels of 25-hydroxycholecalciferol $(25[OH]D_3)$ are helpful to confirm the diagnosis. A brief course of corticosteroid therapy may be necessary if hypercalcemia is severe.

F. Familial Benign Hypocalciuric Hypercalcemia

Familial benign hypocalciuric hypercalcemia can be easily mistaken for mild hyperparathyroidism. It is a common autosomal dominant inherited disorder (prevalence: 1 in 16,000) caused by a loss-of-function mutation in the gene encoding the CaSR. CaSRs are found on the surface of the parathyroid glands and allow the parathyroid glands to vary PTH secretion according to serum calcium levels. Reduced function of the CaSR causes the parathyroid glands to falsely "sense" hypocalcemia and inappropriately release slightly excessive amounts of PTH. At the same time, the renal tubule CaSRs are also affected, causing hypocalciuria. Familial benign hypocalciuric hypercalcemia is characterized by hypercalcemia, hypocalciuria (usually < 50 mg/24 h), variable hypermagnesemia, and normal or minimally elevated levels of PTH. These patients do not normalize their hypercalcemia after subtotal parathyroid removal and should not be subjected to surgery. The condition has an excellent prognosis and is easily diagnosed with a family history and urinary calcium clearance determination.

G. Adrenal Insufficiency

Hypercalcemia is common in untreated Addison disease. This is partly due to disinhibition of calcium uptake by the renal tubule and gut. Additionally, Addison disease can cause dehydration and hyperproteinemia, resulting in higher levels of nonionized calcium.

H. Hyperthyroidism

Increased bone turnover is a feature of thyrotoxicosis. Mild hypercalcemia may also be present.

I. Other Causes

Other causes of hypercalcemia are shown in Table 21–8. Modest hypercalcemia is also occasionally seen in patients taking thiazide diuretics or lithium; such patients may have an inappropriately nonsuppressed PTH level with hypercalcemia. Prolonged immobilization at bed rest may also cause hypercalcemia, especially in adolescents and patients with extensive Paget disease of bone. Hypercalcemia is noted in up to one-third of acutely ill patients being treated in intensive care units, particularly patients with acute renal injury. Serum PTH levels are usually slightly elevated, consistent with mild hyperparathyroidism. Bisphosphonates can increase serum calcium in 20% and serum PTH becomes high in 10%, mimicking hyperparathyroidism.

▶ Treatment

A. Surgical Parathyroidectomy

Parathyroidectomy is recommended for patients with symptomatic hyperparathyroidism, kidney stones, bone disease, and pregnancy.

Some patients with seemingly asymptomatic hyperparathyroidism may be surgical candidates for other reasons such as (1) serum calcium 1 mg/dL above the upper limit of normal with urine calcium excretion > 50 mg/24 h (off thiazide diuretics), (2) urine calcium excretion over 400 mg/24 h, (3) cortical bone density (wrist, hip) ≥ 2 SD below normal, (4) relative youth (under age 50–60 years), (5) difficulty ensuring medical follow-up, or (6) pregnancy. During pregnancy, parathyroidectomy is performed in the second trimester.

Patients who undergo surgery for "asymptomatic" hyperparathyroidism have been reported to have modest benefits in social and emotional function, with improvements in anxiety and phobias being reported in comparison to similar patients who are monitored without surgery.

Preoperative parathyroid imaging has been used in an attempt to allow unilateral minimally invasive neck surgery. The usefulness of preoperative parathyroid imaging was evaluated in a series of 350 patients with sporadic primary hyperparathyroidism. A single gland was predicted by sestamibi in 83%, by ultrasound in 85%, and by concordance of both in 59% of patients. Unilateral neck exploration, directed by these studies, resulted in success rate of only 73%, 77%, and 82%, respectively, despite the intraoperative quick PTH assay predicting success. Even in patients with concordant sestamibi and ultrasound scans, and an intraoperative PTH drop of > 50%, at least one additional abnormal parathyroid gland is left behind in the contralateral neck in 15% of patients.

Bilateral neck exploration is usually advisable for all patients without preoperative localization studies for the following: (1) patients with a family history of hyperparathyroidism, (2) patients with a personal or family history of MEN, and (3) patients wanting an optimal chance of success with a single surgery. Patients undergoing unilateral neck exploration can have the incision widened for bilateral neck exploration if two abnormal glands are found or if the serum quick PTH falls by < 50%. Parathyroid glands are not uncommonly supernumerary (five or more) or ectopic (eg, intrathyroidal, carotid sheath, mediastinum).

Parathyroid hyperplasia is commonly seen with uremic calciphylaxis. When surgery is performed, a subtotal parathyroidectomy is optimally treated surgically; three and one-half glands are usually removed, and a metal clip is left to mark the location of residual parathyroid tissue.

Parathyroid carcinoma can cause severe hypercalcemia associated with very high serum levels of PTH. Preoperative localizing studies usually detect a large invasive tumor. Therapy consists of en bloc resection of the tumor and the ipsilateral thyroid lobe. Metastases to local and to distant sites occur in about 50% of patients. Reoperation for neck recurrence is usually necessary. Adjuvant treatment includes radiation therapy. Intravenous bisphosphonate (zoledronic acid) and calcimimetic agents (NPS R-568) are used for treatment of hypercalcemia.

Complications: Serum PTH levels fall below normal in 70% of patients within hours after successful surgery, commonly causing hypocalcemic paresthesias or even tetany. Hypocalcemia tends to occur the evening after surgery or on the next day. Therefore, frequent postoperative monitoring of serum ionized calcium (or serum calcium plus albumin) is advisable beginning the evening after surgery. Once hypercalcemia has resolved, liquid or chewable calcium carbonate is given orally to reduce the likelihood of hypocalcemia. Symptomatic hypocalcemia is treated with larger doses of calcium; calcitriol (0.25–1 mcg daily orally) may be added, with the dosage depending on symptom severity. Magnesium salts are sometimes required postoperatively, since adequate magnesium is required for functional recovery of the remaining suppressed parathyroid glands.

In about 12% of patients having successful parathyroid surgery, PTH levels rise above normal (while serum calcium is normal or low) by 1 week postoperatively. This secondary hyperparathyroidism is probably due to "hungry bones" and is treated with calcium and vitamin D preparations. Such therapy is usually needed only for 3–6 months but is required long-term by some patients.

Hyperthyroidism commonly occurs immediately following parathyroid surgery. It is caused by release of stored thyroid hormone during surgical manipulation of the thyroid. Short-term treatment with propranolol may be required for several days.

B. Medical Measures

1. Fluids—Hypercalcemia is treated with a large fluid intake unless contraindicated. Severe hypercalcemia requires hospitalization and intensive hydration with intravenous saline. (See Chapter 21.)

2. Bisphosphonates—Intravenous bisphosphonates are potent inhibitors of bone resorption and can temporarily treat the hypercalcemia of hyperparathyroidism, malignancy, or immobilization. They may relieve bone pain as with patients with metastatic breast or prostate cancer. Pamidronate in doses of 30–90 mg (in 0.9% saline) is administered intravenously over 2–4 hours. Zoledronic acid 2–4 mg is administered intravenously over 15 to 20 minutes; it is quite effective but also very expensive. These drugs cause a gradual decline in serum calcium over several days that may last for weeks to months. Such intravenous bisphosphonates are used generally for patients with severe hyperparathyroidism in preparation for surgery. Oral bisphosphonates, such as alendronate, are not effective for treating the hypercalcemia or hypercalciuria of hyperparathyroidism. However, oral alendronate has been shown to improve bone mineral density in the lumbar spine and hip (not distal radius) and may be used for asymptomatic patients with hyperparathyroidism who have a low bone mineral density.

3. Cinacalcet—Cinacalcet hydrochloride is a calcimimetic agent that binds to sites of the parathyroid glands' extracellular CaSRs to increase their affinity for extracellular calcium, thereby decreasing PTH secretion. Cinacalcet may be administered orally in doses of 30–250 mg daily. Patients with primary hyperparathyroidism have also been treated successfully with cinacalcet in oral doses of 30–50 mg twice daily, with 73% of patients achieving normocalcemia. Administering cinacalcet for secondary parathyroidism of kidney disease causes a drop of serum PTH levels to < 250 pg/mL in 41% of patients receiving dialysis. Cinacalcet is given to patients with severe hypercalcemia due to parathyroid carcinoma at initial doses of 30 mg orally twice daily and increased progressively to 60 mg twice daily, then 90 mg twice daily to a maximum of 90 mg every 6–8 hours. Cinacalcet is usually well tolerated but may cause nausea and vomiting, which are usually transient. It is very expensive.

4. Vitamin D and vitamin D analogs

A. Primary hyperparathyroidism—For patients with vitamin D deficiency, careful vitamin D replacement may be beneficial to patients with hyperparathyroidism. Aggravation of hypercalcemia does not ordinarily occur. Serum PTH levels may fall with vitamin D replacement in doses of 800–2000 units daily. Occasionally, larger doses are required to achieve normal 25-OH vitamin D levels.

B. Secondary and tertiary hyperparathyroidism associated with kidney disease—Calcitriol, given orally or intravenously after dialysis, suppresses parathyroid hyperplasia of kidney disease. Certain vitamin D analogs suppress PTH secretion but cause less hypercalcemia than calcitriol. Doxercalciferol (Hectorol) is administered three times weekly orally with hemodialysis to patients with azotemic secondary hyperparathyroidism in the following doses according to serum immunoradiometric PTH (iPTH) levels: give 10 mcg three times weekly for iPTH > 400 pg/mL and increase the dose by 2.5 mcg every 8 weeks if iPTH remains > 300 pg/mL, to a maximum dose of 20 mcg three times weekly. If iPTH drops to < 100 pg/mL, doxercalciferol is held for 1 week and the dose is reduced by at least 2.5 mcg. Paricalcitol (Zemplar) is administered intravenously during dialysis three times weekly in starting doses of 0.04–0.1 mcg/kg body weight; the dosage is increased for iPTH levels > 300 pg/mL to a maximum of 0.24 mcg/ kg three times weekly; paricalcitol is held if iPTH levels drop to < 100 pg/mL.

5. Other measures—Patients with mild, asymptomatic hyperparathyroidism may be monitored closely medically.

Such patients are advised to keep active, avoid immobilization, and drink adequate fluids. They need to avoid thiazide diuretics, large doses of vitamins A, and calcium-containing antacids or supplements. Serum calcium and albumin are checked about twice yearly, kidney function and urine calcium once yearly, and three-site bone density (distal radius, hip, and spine) every 2 years.

Estrogen replacement, given to postmenopausal women, reduces hypercalcemia slightly. Similarly, raloxifene also reduces the hypercalcemia of hyperparathyroidism, reducing serum calcium levels an average of 0.4 mg/dL. Propranolol may be useful for preventing the adverse cardiac effects of hypercalcemia.

Renal osteodystrophy is caused by secondary or tertiary hyperparathyroidism during kidney disease. It can be prevented or delayed by reducing hyperphosphatemia with phosphate binding medication and dietary phosphate restriction.

C. Monitoring Patients with Asymptomatic Primary Hyperparathyroidism

Patients with mild asymptomatic hyperparathyroidism may not need therapy. However, they should be monitored closely for the development of symptoms of hypercalcemia and worsening hypercalcemia. Patients should be evaluated every 6 months with determination of blood pressure and serum calcium. Rising serum calcium should prompt further evaluation and determination of PTH levels. Serum creatinine should be measured yearly. A bone density should ideally be determined every 1 to 2 years at 3 points: wrist, hip, and vertebrae.

▶ Prognosis

Completely asymptomatic patients with mild hypercalcemia may be observed and treated medically without compromising survival. There can be unexplained exacerbations and partial remissions. Surgical removal of sporadic parathyroid adenomas generally results in a permanent cure. Patients with MEN 1 undergoing subtotal parathyroidectomy may experience long remissions, but hyperparathyroidism usually recurs.

Spontaneous cure due to necrosis of the tumor has been reported but is exceedingly rare. The bones, in spite of severe cyst formation, deformity, and fracture, will heal if a parathyroid tumor is successfully removed. The presence of pancreatitis increases the mortality rate. Acute pancreatitis usually resolves with correction of hypercalcemia, whereas subacute or chronic pancreatitis tends to persist. Significant renal damage may progress even after removal of an adenoma. Parathyroid carcinoma tends to invade local structures and may sometimes metastasize; repeat surgical resections and radiation therapy can prolong life. Aggressive surgical and medical management of parathyroid carcinoma can result in an 85% 5-year survival rate and a 57% 10-year survival rate.

Carlson AL et al. Primary hyperparathyroidism and jaw tumor syndrome: a novel mutation of the HRPT2 gene. Endocr Pract. 2008 Sep;14(6):743–7. [PMID: 18996796]

DeLellis RA et al. Primary hyperparathyroidism: a current perspective. Arch Pathol Lab Med. 2008 Aug;132(8):1251–62. [PMID: 18684024]

Silverberg SJ et al. Cinacalcet hydrochloride reduces the serum calcium concentration in inoperable parathyroid carcinoma. J Clin Endocrinol Metab. 2007 Oct;92(10):3803–8. [PMID: 17666472]

Vanderwalde LH et al. Effect of bone mineral density and parathyroidectomy on fracture risk in primary hyperparathyroidism. World J Surg. 2009 Mar;33(3):406–11. [PMID: 18763015]

▼ METABOLIC BONE DISEASE

The term "metabolic bone disease" denotes those conditions producing diffusely decreased bone density and diminished bone strength. It is categorized by histologic appearance: osteoporosis (bone matrix and mineral both decreased) and osteomalacia (bone matrix intact, mineral decreased). Osteoporosis and osteomalacia often coexist in the same patient.

OSTEOPOROSIS

ESSENTIALS OF DIAGNOSIS

▶ Asymptomatic to severe backache from vertebral fractures.

▶ Spontaneous fractures often discovered incidentally on radiography; loss of height.

▶ Serum PTH, calcium, phosphorus, and alkaline phosphatase usually normal.

▶ Serum 25-hydroxyvitamin D levels often low as a comorbid condition.

▶ Demineralization, especially of spine, hip, pelvis, and wrist.

▶ General Considerations

Osteoporosis is estimated to cause 1.5 million fractures annually in the United States—mainly of the spine and hip. The morbidity and indirect mortality rates are very high. Since the usual form of the disease is clinically evident in middle life and beyond and since women are more frequently affected than men, it is often referred to as "postmenopausal" osteoporosis. It is characterized by a decrease in the amount of bone present to a level below which it is capable of maintaining the structural integrity of the skeleton. The rate of bone formation is often normal, whereas the rate of bone resorption is increased.

Osteoporosis can be caused by a variety of factors. The long-term use of a selective serotonin reuptake inhibitor (SSRI) has been associated with reduced hip density, increased falls, and increased fracture risk, particularly in the elderly. Rosiglitazone appears to decrease bone mineral density in men with type 2 diabetes mellitus. The causes of osteoporosis are listed in Table 26–10.

Table 26–10. Causes of osteoporosis.[1]

Hormone deficiency	Genetic disorders
Estrogen (women)	Aromatase deficiency
Androgen (men)	Type I collagen mutations
Hormone excess	Osteogenesis imperfecta
Cushing syndrome or cortico-	Idiopathic juvenile and
steroid administration	adult osteoporosis
Thyrotoxicosis	Ehlers-Danlos syndrome
Hyperparathyroidism	Marfan syndrome
Immobilization and microgravity	Homocystinuria
Tobacco	Miscellaneous
Alcoholism	Celiac disease
Malignancy, especially	Anorexia nervosa
multiple myeloma	Hyponatremia (chronic)
Medications	Protein-calorie malnutrition
Excessive vitamin D intake	Vitamin C deficiency
Excessive vitamin A intake	Copper deficiency
Heparin therapy	Liver disease
Selective serotonin reuptake	Rheumatoid arthritis
inhibitors	Uncontrolled diabetes
Rosiglitazone	mellitus
	Systemic mastocytosis

[1]See Table 26–11 for causes of osteomalacia.

Osteoporosis is caused by a reduction and disarray of bone's microarchitectural organic collagenous matrix, which normally accounts for about 40% of bone mass and provides bone's tensile strength. Inorganic calcium and phosphate compounds, largely calcium hydroxyapetite, mineralize the available collagenous bone matrix and normally provide about 60% of bone mass and most of bone's compressive strength.

Osteogenesis imperfecta is caused by a major mutation in the gene encoding for type I collagen, the major collagen constituent of bone. This causes severe osteoporosis; spontaneous fractures occur in utero or during childhood. Blue sclerae may be present. Certain polymorphisms in the genes encoding type I collagen are common, particularly in whites, resulting in collagen disarray and predisposing to hypogonadal (eg, menopausal) or idiopathic osteoporosis.

► Clinical Findings

A. Symptoms and Signs

Osteoporosis is usually asymptomatic until fractures occur. It may present as backache of varying degrees of severity or as a spontaneous fracture or collapse of a vertebra. Loss of height is common. Once osteoporosis is identified, a carefully directed history and physical examination must be performed to determine its cause (Table 26–10).

B. Laboratory Findings

Serum calcium, phosphate, and PTH are normal. The alkaline phosphatase is usually normal but may be slightly elevated, especially following a fracture. Vitamin D deficiency is very common and serum determination of 25-hydroxyvitamin D should be obtained for every individual with low bone density. Serum 25-hydroxyvitamin D levels below 20 ng/mL are considered frank vitamin D deficiency.

Lesser degrees of vitamin D deficiency (serum 25-hydroxyvitamin D levels between 20 ng/mL and 30 ng/mL) may also increase the risk for hip fracture. (See Osteomalacia, below.) Testing for thyrotoxicosis and hypogonadism may be required. Celiac disease may be screened for with serum immunoglobulin A (IgA) endomysial antibody and tissue transglutaminase antibody determinations.

C. Bone Densitometry

DXA is used to determine the bone density of the lumbar spine and hip. Bone densitometry should be performed on all patients who are at risk for osteoporosis or osteomalacia or have pathologic fractures or radiographic evidence of diminished bone density. This test delivers negligible radiation, and the measurements are quite accurate. However, bone densitometry cannot distinguish osteoporosis from osteomalacia; in fact, both are often present. Also, the bone mineral density does not directly measure bone quality and is only fairly successful at predicting fractures. Vertebral bone mineral density may be misleadingly high in compressed vertebrae and in patients with extensive arthritis. DXA also overestimates the bone mineral density of taller persons and underestimates the bone mineral density of smaller persons. Quantitative CT delivers more radiation but is more accurate in the latter situations.

Bone mineral density in typically expressed in g/cm^2, for which there are different normal ranges for each bone and for each type of DXA-measuring machine. The "T score" is a simplified way of reporting bone density in which the patient's bone mineral density is compared to the young normal mean and expressed as a standard deviation score. The World Health Organization has established criteria for defining osteoporosis in postmenopausal white women, based on T score:

T score ≥ -1.0: Normal.

T score -1.0 to -2.5: Osteopenia ("low bone density").

T score < -2.5: Osteoporosis.

T score < -2.5 with a fracture: Severe osteoporosis.

This classification is somewhat arbitrary and there really is no bone mineral density fracture threshold; instead, the fracture risk increases about twofold for each standard deviation drop in bone mineral density. In fact, most women with fragility fractures have bone densities above -2.5. Surveillance DXA bone densitometry is recommended for postmenopausal women with a frequency according to their T scores: obtain DXA every 5 years for T scores -1.0 to -1.5, every 3–5 years for scores -1.5 to -2.0, and every 1–2 years for scores under -2.0.

The "Z score" is used to express bone density in premenopausal women, younger men, and children, The Z score is a statistical term that is used for expressing an individual's bone density as standard deviation from age-matched, race-matched, and sex-matched means.

► Differential Diagnosis

Osteoporosis has many causes (see Table 26–10). Additionally, osteopenia and fractures can be caused by osteomalacia (see below) and bone marrow neoplasia such as myeloma or metastatic bone disease. These conditions coexist in many patients.

▶ **Treatment**

A. Specific Measures

Several treatment options are available, so a regimen is tailored to each patient. Generally, treatment is indicated for all women with osteoporosis (T scores below –2.5) and for all patients who have had fragility fractures. Prophylactic treatment should also be considered for patients with advanced osteopenia (T scores between –2.0 and –2.5).

1. Vitamin D and calcium—Osteoporosis and osteomalacia often coexist (see Osteomalacia section). Sun exposure and vitamin D supplementation are useful in preventing and treating osteomalacia. Vitamin D supplementation reduces the incidence of vertebral fractures by 37% and may slightly reduce the incidence of nonvertebral fractures. Oral vitamin D is given in doses of 800-2000 international units daily. Higher doses of vitamin D may be required during winter months and for patients having prolonged hospitalization or nursing home care, for patients with serum levels of 25-hydroxyvitamin D below 20 ng/mL, and those with intestinal malabsorption.

Calcium supplementation has not reduced the fracture risk in otherwise healthy postmenopausal women. Therefore, calcium supplementation is indicated principally for those with diets low in calcium. More important is the assurance of adequate vitamin D through sun exposure or oral vitamin D supplementation, and calcium supplementation should include vitamin D. Calcium supplementation may be given as calcium citrate (0.4–0.7 g elemental calcium per day) or calcium carbonate (1–1.5 g elemental calcium per day).

2. Bisphosphonates—Bisphosphonates work similarly, inhibiting osteoclast-induced bone resorption. They increase bone density significantly and reduce the incidence of both vertebral and nonvertebral fractures. Bisphosphonates have also been effective in preventing corticosteroid-induced osteoporosis. To ensure intestinal absorption, oral bisphosphonates must be taken in the morning with at least 8 oz of plain water at least 40 minutes before consumption of anything else. The patient must remain upright after taking bisphosphonates to reduce the risk of esophagitis. These medications are excreted in the urine. However, no dosage adjustments are required for patients with creatinine clearances above 35 mL/min. There has been little experience giving bisphosphonates to patients with severe kidney disease; if given, the dose would need to be greatly reduced and serum phosphate levels monitored.

Bisphosphonates may be given orally once monthly or weekly; which is more convenient than daily therapy and equally effective. Available oral preparations include **alendronate**, 70 mg orally once weekly (tablet or solution), and **risedronate**, 35 mg orally once weekly. Both these medications reduce the risk of both vertebral and nonvertebral fractures. Studies sponsored by the manufacturer of alen-

dronate found that alendronate was significantly more potent than risedronate and equally well tolerated. Another bisphosphonate, **ibandronate sodium,** is taken once monthly in a dose of 150 mg orally. Once-monthly ibandronate is convenient and reduces the risk of vertebral fractures but not nonvertebral fractures; its effectiveness has not been directly compared with other bisphosphonates. Oral bisphosphonates can cause esophagitis, especially in patients with hiatal hernia and gastroesophageal reflux.

For patients who cannot tolerate oral bisphosphonates or for whom oral bisphosphonates are contraindicated, intravenous bisphosphonates are available. **Zoledronic acid** is a third-generation bisphosphonate and a potent osteoclast inhibitor. It can be given every 12 months in doses of 2–4 mg intravenously over 15–30 minutes. **Pamidronate** is an older parenteral bisphosphonate that can be given in doses of 30–60 mg by slow intravenous infusion in normal saline solution every 3–6 months. Transient postinfusion fever occurs fairly commonly (26%).

Both oral and parenteral bisphosphonates can cause bone, joint, or muscle pains as well as fatigue, particularly after the first dose. The onset of pain may occur from 1 day to 1 year after therapy is initiated, with a mean of 14 days. The pain can be transient, lasting several days and usually resolving spontaneously but typically recurring with subsequent doses. When the bisphosphonate is discontinued, most patients experience gradual relief of pain. Some patients taking alendronate or risedronate for osteoporosis have experienced bone osteonecrosis: painful, necrotic, nonhealing lesions of the jaw, particularly after tooth extraction. The incidence of osteonecrosis is very low. In a prospective 3-year trial of 7714 women who received intravenous zoledronic acid 5 mg/y or placebo, there were no cases of osteonecrosis. For such patients with painful exposed bone, treatment is 90% effective (without resolution of the exposed bone) using antibiotics along with 0.12% chlorohexidine antiseptic mouth wash. Patients receiving bisphosphonates must receive regular dental care and try to avoid dental extraction. Osteonecrosis of the jaw has also been reported in patients receiving intravenous zoledronic acid and pamidronate for treatment of hypercalcemia and bone metastases, for which the drugs had been administered more frequently than for osteoporosis. Another adverse effect reported with bisphosphonates is ocular inflammation, manifested by blurred vision, eye pain, uveitis, conjunctivitis, and scleritis, which remits after discontinuation of the drug. Other side effects can include nausea, anemia, dyspnea, and leg edema. In patients taking bisphosphonates, hypercalcemia is seen in 20% and serum PTH levels increase above normal in 10%, mimicking primary hyperparathyroidism.

The half-life of alendronate in bone is 10 years. Therefore, patients with mild osteoporosis may discontinue bisphosphonates after a 5-year course of therapy. Bone density falls in 18% of patients during their first year of treatment with bisphosphonates, but 80% of such patients have gain in bone density with continued bisphosphonate treatment.

3. Sex hormones—Hypogonadal women who take estrogen replacement therapy (ERT) have a lower risk of developing osteoporosis. Postmenopausal estrogen replacement is valuable as an osteoporosis prevention measure and this should be one factor in the complex decision about whether to take ERT. Low doses of estrogen appear to be adequate to prevent postmenopausal osteoporosis (see Estrogen Replacement Therapy). Once osteoporosis has developed, estrogen replacement is not an effective treatment. Although ERT does increase bone mineral density in postmenopausal women with osteoporosis, it has not been demonstrated to significantly reduce fracture rates. Men with hypogonadism may be treated with testosterone (see Male Hypogonadism).

4. Selective estrogen receptor modulators—Raloxifene, 60 mg/d orally, can be used by postmenopausal women in place of estrogen for prevention of osteoporosis. Bone density increases about 1% over 2 years in postmenopausal women versus 2% increases with estrogen replacement. It reduces the risk of vertebral fractures by about 40% but does not appear to reduce the risk of nonvertebral fractures. Raloxifene produces a reduction in LDL cholesterol but not the rise in high-density lipoprotein (HDL) cholesterol seen with estrogen. It has no direct effect on coronary plaque. Unlike estrogen, raloxifene does not reduce hot flushes; in fact, it often intensifies them. It does not relieve vaginal dryness. Unlike estrogen, raloxifene does not cause endometrial hyperplasia, uterine bleeding, or cancer, nor does it cause breast soreness. The risk of breast cancer is reduced 76% in women taking raloxifene for 3 years. Since it is a potential teratogen, it is relatively contraindicated in women capable of pregnancy.

Raloxifene increases the risk for thromboembolism and should not be used by women with such a history. Leg cramps can also occur.

5. Teriparatide—Teriparatide (Forteo, Parathar) is an analog of PTH. Teriparatide stimulates the production of new collagenous bone matrix that must be mineralized. Patients receiving teriparatide must have sufficient intake of vitamin D and calcium. When administered to patients with osteoporosis in doses of 20 mcg/d subcutaneously for 2 years, teriparatide dramatically improves bone density in most bones except the distal radius. The recommended dose should not be exceeded, since teriparatide has caused osteosarcoma in rats when administered in very high doses. Patients with Paget disease of bone or patients with open epiphyses or hypercalcemia should not use the drug. Patients with a past history of osteosarcoma or chondrosarcoma should not use this medication. Side effects may include dizziness and leg cramps. Teriparatide is approved only for a 2-year course of treatment.

Precautions: Hypercalcemia may develop in patients who are taking teriparatide if they also take corticosteroids and thiazide diuretics along with oral calcium supplementation.

Following a course of teriparatide, a course of bisphosphonates should be considered in order to retain the improved bone density.

6. Calcitonin—A nasal spray of calcitonin-salmon (Miacalcin) is available that contains 2200 units/mL in 2-mL metered-dose bottles. The usual dose is one puff (0.09 mL, 200 international units) once daily, alternating nostrils. Nasal administration causes significantly less nausea and flushing than the parenteral route. However, nasal symptoms such as rhinitis and epistaxis occur commonly; other less common adverse reactions include flu-like symptoms, allergy, arthralgias, back pain, and headache. Five years of therapy increases bone 2–3% and reduces the number of new vertebral fractures. Both nasal and parenteral calcitonin have analgesic effects on bone pain; reduction of pain may be noted within 2–4 weeks after commencing therapy. Calcitonin reduces the incidence of vertebral fractures, but its effect upon nonvertebral fractures has not been established.

7. Denosumab—Denosumab is a promising treatment for osteoporosis that is in clinical trials. It is a monoclonal antibody that inhibits osteoclast activation by binding to the osteoclasts' receptor activator of nuclear factor-kappa B ligand (RANKL). Denosumab is effective at doses of 60 mg subcutaneously every 6 months. It has been relatively well tolerated, with an 8% incidence of flu-like symptoms.

B. General Measures

For prevention and treatment of osteoporosis, the diet should be adequate in protein, total calories, calcium, and vitamin D. Pharmacologic corticosteroid doses should be reduced or discontinued if possible. Thiazides may be useful if hypercalciuria is present. High-impact physical activity (eg, jogging) significantly increases bone density in men and women. Stair-climbing increases bone density in women. Patients who cannot exercise vigorously should be encouraged to engage in other exercise regularly, thereby increasing strength and reducing the risk of falling. Weight training is helpful to increase muscle strength as well as bone density. Measures should be taken to avoid falls at home (eg, adequate lighting, handrails on stairs, handholds in bathrooms). Patients who have weakness or balance problems must use a cane or a walker; rolling walkers should have a brake mechanism. Balance exercises can reduce the risk of falls. Patients should be kept active; bedridden patients should be given active or passive exercises. The spine may be adequately supported (though braces or corsets are usually not well tolerated), but rigid or excessive immobilization must be avoided. Alcohol and smoking should be avoided.

▶ Prognosis

Bone mineral density densitometries can detect whether progressive osteopenia or frank osteoporosis is developing. Hypogonadal women, especially those not receiving HRT, must ensure sufficient intake of vitamin D to prevent osteomalacia. Bisphosphonates and raloxifene can reverse progressive osteopenia and osteoporosis and decrease fracture risk.

Hypogonadal men are also at risk for developing osteoporosis. Testosterone administration can prevent osteoporosis. Men with prostate cancer may not receive testosterone replacement and should be monitored with bone densitometries. Bisphosphonate therapy can reverse progressive osteopenia and osteoporosis in men.

Black DM et al. Effects of continuing or stopping alendronate after 5 years of treatment: The Fracture Intervention Trial Long-term Extension (FLEX): a randomized trial. JAMA. 2006 Dec 27;296(24):2927–38. [PMID: 17190893]

Black DM et al. HORIZON Pivotal Fracture Trial. Once-yearly zoledronic acid for treatment of postmenopausal osteoporosis. N Engl J Med. 2007 May 3;356(18):1809–22. [PMID: 17476007]

Brown JP et al. Comparison of the effect of denosumab and alendronate on bone mineral density and biochemical markers of bone turnover in postmenopausal women with low bone mass: a randomized, blinded, phase 3 trial. J Bone Miner Res. 2009 Jan;24(1):153–61. [PMID: 18767928]

Grbic JT et al. Incidence of osteonecrosis of the jaw in women with postmenopausal osteoporosis in the health outcomes and reduced incidence with zoledronic acid once yearly pivotal fracture trial. J Am Dent Assoc. 2008 Jan;13991):32–40. [PMID: 18167382]

Jackson RD et al; Women's Health Initiative Investigators. Calcium plus vitamin D supplementation and the risk of fractures. N Engl J Med. 2006 Feb 16;354(7):669–83. [PMID: 16481635]

McClung MR et al. Denosumab in postmenopausal women with low bone mineral density. N Engl J Med. 2006 Feb 23;354(8):821–31. [PMID: 16495394]

Richards JB et al. Effect of selective serotonin reuptake inhibitors on the risk of fracture. Arch Intern Med. 2007 Jan 22;167(2):188–94. [PMID: 17242321]

Shoback D. Update in osteoporosis and metabolic bone disorders. J Clin Endocrinol Metab. 2007 Mar;92(3):747–53. [PMID: 17341572]

OSTEOMALACIA

 ESSENTIALS OF DIAGNOSIS

▶ Painful proximal muscle weakness (especially pelvic girdle); bone pain and tenderness.

▶ Decreased bone density from defective mineralization.

▶ Laboratory abnormalities may include increases in alkaline phosphatase, decreased 25-hydroxyvitamin D, or hypocalcemia, hypocalciuria, hypophosphatemia, secondary hyperparathyroidism.

▶ Classic radiologic features may be present.

▶ General Considerations

Defective mineralization of the growing skeleton in childhood causes permanent bone deformities (rickets). Defective skeletal mineralization in adults is known as osteomalacia. It is caused by any condition that results in inadequate calcium or phosphate mineralization of bone osteoid.

▶ Etiology (Table 26–11)

A. Vitamin D Deficiency and Resistance

Vitamin D deficiency decreases the intestinal absorption of calcium and is the most common cause of osteomalacia. Significant vitamin D deficiency (serum 25[OH]D < 50 nmol/L or < 20 ng/mL) was found in 24.3% of postmenopausal women from 25 countries in the MORE study. The incidence varied: < 1% in Southeast Asia, 29% in the

Table 26–11. Causes of osteomalacia.[1]

Vitamin disorders
Decreased availability of vitamin D
Insufficient sunlight exposure
Nutritional deficiency of vitamin D
Malabsorption; aging, excess wheat bran, bariatric surgery, pancreatic enzyme deficiency
Nephrotic syndrome
Vitamin D–dependent rickets type I
Liver disease
Chronic kidney disease
Kidney transplantation
Phenytoin, carbamazepine, or barbiturate therapy
Dietary calcium deficiency
Phosphate deficiency
Decreased intestinal absorption
Nutritional deficiency of phosphorus
Malabsorption
Phosphate-binding antacid therapy
Increased renal loss
X-linked hypophosphatemic rickets
Tumoral hypophosphatemic osteomalacia
Association with other disorders, including paraproteinemias, glycogen storage diseases, neurofibromatosis, Wilson disease, Fanconi syndrome, renal tubular acidosis, and alcoholism
Disorders of bone matrix
Hypophosphatasia
Fibrogenesis imperfecta
Axial osteomalacia
Inhibitors of mineralization
Aluminum
Bisphosphonates

[1]See Table 26–10 for causes of osteoporosis.

United States, and 36% in Italy. Severe vitamin D deficiency (serum 25[OH]D < 25 nmol/L or < 10 ng/mL) was found in 4% of these women; 3.5% in the United States and 12.5% in Italy. Vitamin D deficiency is particularly common in the institutionalized elderly, with the incidence exceeding 60% in some groups not receiving vitamin D supplementation. Deficiency of vitamin D may arise from insufficient sun exposure, malnutrition, or malabsorption (due to pancreatic insufficiency, cholestatic liver disease, sprue, inflammatory bowel disease, jejunoileal bypass, Billroth type II gastrectomy, etc). Cholestyramine binds bile acids necessary for vitamin D absorption. Patients with severe nephrotic syndrome lose large amounts of vitamin D–binding protein in the urine, and osteomalacia may also develop.

Anticonvulsants (eg, phenytoin, carbamazepine, valproate, phenobarbital) inhibit the hepatic production of 25(OH)D and sometimes cause osteomalacia. Phenytoin can also directly inhibit bone mineralization. Serum levels of 1,25(OH)$_2$D are usually normal.

Vitamin D–dependent rickets type I is caused by a rare autosomal recessive disorder with a defect in the renal enzyme 1-α-hydroxylase leading to defective synthesis of 1,25(OH)$_2$D. It presents in childhood with rickets and alopecia; osteomalacia develops in adults with this condition unless treated with oral calcitriol in doses of 0.5–1 mcg daily.

Vitamin D–dependent rickets type II (better known as hereditary 1,25[OH]$_2$D-resistant rickets) is caused by a genetic defect in the 1,25(OH)$_2$D receptor. Patients have hypocalcemia with childhood rickets and adult osteomalacia. Alopecia is common. These patients respond variably to oral calcitriol in very large doses (2–6 mcg daily).

B. Deficient Calcium Intake

Rickets and osteomalacia continue to be common problems in many tropical countries despite adequate exposure to sunlight. A nutritional deficiency of calcium can occur in any severely malnourished patient. Some degree of calcium deficiency is common in the elderly, since intestinal calcium absorption declines with age. Ingestion of excessive wheat bran also causes calcium malabsorption.

C. Phosphate Deficiency

Phosphatonin is a circulating peptide that inhibits sodium-dependent phosphate transport in the renal tubule; high levels of this peptide cause excessive phosphaturia, resulting in hypophosphatemia. X-linked hypophosphatemic rickets is associated with high levels of phosphatonin, probably caused by familial or sporadic mutations in PHEX endopeptidase, which fails to cleave phosphatonin.

Oncogenic osteomalacia is caused by excessive production of phosphatonin by a wide variety of soft tissue tumors (87% benign). Such tumors may be hard to find. OctreoScan has been reported to detect many of these small tumors. The condition is characterized by hypophosphatemia, excessive phosphaturia, reduced or normal serum 1,25(OH)$_2$D concentrations, and osteomalacia. Excessive renal phosphate losses are also seen in proximal renal tubular acidosis and Fanconi syndrome. Some cases of hyperphosphaturia are idiopathic.

Other causes of hypophosphatemic osteomalacia include poor nutrition, alcoholism, or chelation of phosphate in the gut by aluminum hydroxide antacids, calcium acetate (Phos-Lo), or sevelamer hydrochloride (Renagel).

D. Aluminum Toxicity

Bone mineralization is inhibited by aluminum. Osteomalacia may occur in patients receiving long-term renal hemodialysis with tap water dialysate or from aluminum-containing antacids used to reduce phosphate levels. Osteomalacia may develop in patients being maintained on long-term total parenteral nutrition if the casein hydrolysate used for amino acids contains high levels of aluminum.

E. Hypophosphatasia

Hypophosphatasia, a deficiency of bone alkaline phosphatase effect, is a rare genetic cause of osteomalacia that is commonly misdiagnosed as osteoporosis. The incidence in the United States is about 1 in 100,000 live births; about 1 in 300 adults is a carrier. Many different mutations in the gene (designated *ALPL*) encoding bone alkaline phosphatase have been described, and transmission can be either autosomal recessive or autosomal dominant. The phenotypic presentation of hypophosphatasia is extremely vari-

able. At its worst extreme, it can present as a stillborn without dentition or calcified bones. At its mildest, hypophosphatasia can present in middle age with premature loss of teeth, foot pain (due to metatarsal stress fractures), thigh pain (due to femoral pseudofractures), or arthritis (due to chondrocalcinosis). Serum alkaline phosphatase (collected in a non-EDTA tube) is low for age in patients with hypophosphatasia. To confirm the diagnosis, a 24-hour urine should be assayed for phosphoethanolamine, a substrate for tissue-nonspecific alkaline phosphatase, whose excretion is always elevated in patients with hypophosphatasia. Prenatal genetic testing, by way of chorionic villus biopsy, is available for the infantile form of hypophosphatasia. There is no proven therapy for hypophosphatasia, except for supportive care. Teriparatide, a useful therapy for osteoporosis, has been administered to some patients with hypophosphatasia, but its long-term efficacy is unknown.

F. Fibrogenesis Imperfecta Ossium

This rare condition sporadically affects middle-aged patients, who present with progressive bone pain and pathologic fractures. Bones have a dense "fishnet" appearance on radiographs. Serum alkaline phosphatase levels are elevated. Some patients have a monoclonal gammopathy, indicating a possible plasma cell dyscrasia causing an impairment in osteoblast function and collagen disarray. Remission has been reported after repeated courses of melphalan, corticosteroids, and vitamin D analog over 3 years.

► Clinical Findings

The clinical manifestations of defective bone mineralization depend on the age at onset and the severity. In adults, osteomalacia is typically asymptomatic at first. Eventually, bone pain occurs, along with muscle weakness due to calcium deficiency. Pathologic fractures may occur with little or no trauma. Vitamin D deficiency has also been associated with a possible increased risk of multiple sclerosis, rheumatoid arthritis, and diabetes mellitus (types 1 and 2).

► Diagnostic Tests

Serum is obtained for calcium, albumin, phosphate, alkaline phosphatase, PTH, and 25[OH]D$_3$ determinations. Bone densitometry helps document the degree of osteopenia. Radiographs may show diagnostic features.

In one series of biopsy-proved osteomalacia, alkaline phosphatase was elevated in 94% of patients; the calcium or phosphorus was low in 47% of patients; 25(OH)D$_3$ was low in 29% of patients; pseudofractures were seen in 18% of patients; and urinary calcium was low in 18% of patients. 1,25(OH)$_2$D$_3$ may be low even when 25(OH)D$_2$ levels are normal.

Bone biopsy is not usually necessary but is diagnostic of osteomalacia if there is significant unmineralized osteoid.

► Differential Diagnosis

Osteomalacia is often seen together with osteoporosis, and its presence can be inferred by finding low serum levels of 25(OH) vitamin D, low serum calcium, or low serum phosphate. A high serum alkaline phosphatase may be present in severe osteomalacia but not osteoporosis. The relative contribution of the two entities to diminished bone density may not be apparent until treatment, since a dramatic rise in bone density is often seen with therapy for osteomalacia. Phosphate deficiency must be distinguished from hypophosphatemia seen in hyperparathyroidism.

Prevention & Treatment

To obtain adequate sunshine vitamin D, the face, arms, hands, or back must have sun exposure without sunscreen for 15 minutes at least twice weekly. The main natural food source of vitamin D is fish, particularly, salmon, mackerel, cod liver oil, and sardines or tuna canned in oil. Most commercial cow's milk is fortified with vitamin D at about 400 international units per quart; however, skim milk and other dairy products contain much less vitamin D. Vitamin supplements containing vitamin D are widely available, but contain plant-derived vitamin D_2, which has less biologic availability than once believed. In sunlight-deprived individuals (eg, veiled women, confined patients, or residents of higher latitudes during winter), the recommended daily allowance should be 1000 international units daily. In such individuals, vitamin D supplements should be given prophylactically. Patients receiving long-term phenytoin therapy may be treated prophylactically with vitamin D, 50,000 international units orally every 2–4 weeks.

Frank vitamin D deficiency is treated with ergocalciferol (D_2), 50,000 international units orally once or twice weekly for 6–12 months, followed by 1000–2000 international units daily. Some patients require long-term supplementation with ergocalciferol of up to 50,000 international units weekly. In patients with intestinal malabsorption, oral doses of 25,000–100,000 international units of vitamin D_2 daily may be required. Some patients with steatorrhea respond better to oral 25(OH)D_3 (calcifediol), 50–100 mcg/d.

Beyond increasing the intestinal absorption of calcium, vitamin D supplementation may have additional effects. Vitamin D supplementation has been associated with improved muscle strength and a reduced fall risk, factors that reduce the risk of bone fracture.

The addition of calcium supplements to vitamin D is probably not necessary for the prevention of osteomalacia in the majority of otherwise well-nourished patients. However, patients with malabsorption or poor nutrition should receive calcium supplementation. Recommended doses of calcium are as follows: calcium citrate (eg, Citracal), 0.4–0.6 g elemental calcium per day, or calcium carbonate (eg, OsCal, Tums), 1–1.5 g elemental calcium per day. Calcium supplements are best administered with meals.

In hypophosphatemic osteomalacia, nutritional deficiencies are corrected, aluminum-containing antacids are discontinued, and patients with renal tubular acidosis are given bicarbonate therapy. In patients with sporadic adult-onset hypophosphatemia, hyperphosphaturia, and low serum 1,25(OH)$_2$D levels, a search is conducted for occult tumors that may be resected; whole-body MRI scanning may be required.

For those with X-linked or idiopathic hypophosphatemia and hyperphosphaturia, oral phosphate supplements must be given long-term; calcitriol, 0.25–0.5 mcg/d, is given also to improve the impaired calcium absorption caused by the oral phosphate. Human recombinant growth hormone reduces phosphaturia and may be added to the above regimen.

Ceglia L. Vitamin D and skeletal muscle tissue and function. Mol Aspects Med. 2008 Dec;29(6):407–14. [PMID: 18727936]

Prentice A. Vitamin D deficiency: a global perspective. Nutr Rev. 2008 Oct;66(10 Suppl 2):S153–64. [PMID: 18844843]

Whyte MP et al. Adult hypophosphatasia treated with teriparatide. J Clin Endocrinol Metab. 2007 Apr;92(4):1203–8. [PMID: 17213282]

Woznowski M et al. Oncogenic osteomalacia, a rare paraneoplastic syndrome due to phosphate wasting–a case report and review of the literature. Clin Nephrol. 2008 Nov;70(5):431–8. [PMID: 19000546]

PAGET DISEASE OF BONE (Osteitis Deformans)

 ESSENTIALS OF DIAGNOSIS

▶ Often asymptomatic.

▶ Bone pain may be the first symptom.

▶ Kyphosis, bowed tibias, large head, deafness, and frequent fractures.

▶ Serum calcium and phosphate normal; alkaline phosphatase elevated; urinary hydroxyproline elevated.

▶ Dense, expanded bones on radiographs.

General Considerations

Paget disease of bone is a common condition manifested by one or more bony lesions having high bone turnover and disorganized osteoid formation. Involved bones become vascular, weak, and deformed. Paget disease is most common in the United Kingdom but is also common in other areas of the world, particularly in those with British ancestry. It is uncommon in Africa, Asia, and Scandinavia. Paget disease is present in 1–2% of the population of the United States and affects men more commonly than women. It is usually diagnosed in patients over age 40 years and its prevalence doubles with each decade thereafter, reaching an incidence of about 10% after age 80. It is usually discovered incidentally during radiology imaging or because of incidentally discovered elevations in serum alkaline phosphatase. The cause of Paget disease is unknown. However, there is often a genetic component since about 15% of affected patients have a first-degree relative with the disease. Similar familial disorders occur at an earlier age and their genetics has been established (see Differential Diagnosis).

Clinical Findings

A. Symptoms and Signs

Paget disease is often mild and asymptomatic. Only 27% of affected individuals are symptomatic at the time of diagnosis. It can involve just one bone (monostotic) or multiple bones (polyostotic), particularly the skull, femur, tibia, pelvis, and humerus. The affected bones are typically involved right away and the disease tends not to involve additional bones during its course. Pain is the usual first symptom. It may occur in the involved bone or in an adjacent joint, which can be involved with degenerative arthritis. The bones can become soft, leading to bowed tibias, kyphosis, and frequent "chalkstick" fractures with slight trauma. If the skull is involved, the patient may report headaches and an increased hat size. Deafness may occur. Increased vascularity over the involved bones causes increased warmth and can cause vascular "steal" syndromes (see Complications).

B. Laboratory Findings

Serum alkaline phosphatase is usually markedly elevated. However, some patients with limited monostotic involvement may have serum alkaline phosphatase levels within the normal range. A serum bone-specific alkaline phosphatase determination can be useful for patients with a normal serum total alkaline phosphatase level and to distinguish the source of an elevated serum alkaline phosphatase as being from bone (rather than liver). Other markers of bone turnover may be elevated. Serum C-telopeptide (CTx) is usually high. Urinary hydroxyproline is also elevated in active disease. Serum calcium may be elevated, particularly if the patient is at bed rest. A serum 25-OH vitamin D determination should be obtained to screen for vitamin D deficiency, which can also present with an increased alkaline phosphatase and bone pain. Also, any vitamin D deficiency should be corrected before prescribing a bisphosphonate.

C. Imaging

On radiographs, the initial lesions are typically osteolytic, with focal radiolucencies ("osteoporosis circumscripta") in the skull or advancing flame-shaped lytic lesions in long bones. Bone lesions may subsequently become sclerotic and have a mixed lytic and sclerotic appearance. The affected bones eventually become thickened and deformed. Technetium pyrophosphate bone scans are helpful in delineating activity of bone lesions even before any radiologic changes are apparent.

▶ Differential Diagnosis

Certain rare familial osteoclastic bone disorders share phenotypic homologies with Paget disease of bone. Familial expansile osteolysis, familial early-onset Paget disease, and familial skeletal hyperphosphatasia are autosomal dominant disorders caused by different tandem duplications of the gene encoding RANK, resulting in its constitutive activation. Juvenile Paget disease is an autosomal recessive disorder caused by an inactivating mutation in the gene encoding osteoprotegerin. The syndrome of Paget disease, inclusion body myopathy, and frontotemporal dementia is caused by a mutation in the gene that encodes valosin-containing protein.

Paget disease must be differentiated from primary bone lesions such as osteogenic sarcoma, multiple myeloma, and

fibrous dysplasia and from secondary bone lesions such as metastatic carcinoma and osteitis fibrosa cystica. Fibrogenesis imperfecta ossium is a rare symmetric disorder that can mimic the features of Paget disease; alkaline phosphatase is likewise elevated. If serum calcium is elevated, hyperparathyroidism may be present in some patients as well.

▶ Complications

If immobilization occurs, hypercalcemia and renal calculi may develop. Vertebral collapse may lead to spinal cord compression. The increased vascularity may give rise to high-output cardiac failure. Arthritis frequently develops in joints adjacent to involved bone.

Extensive skull involvement may cause cranial nerve palsies from impingement of the neural foramina. Involvement of the petrous temporal bone frequently causes hearing loss (mixed sensorineural and conductive) and occasionally tinnitus or vertigo. Vertebral involvement can cause compression of spinal nerves, resulting in radiculopathy or paralysis. The affected bones have a high blood flow and can thereby cause a vascular "steal" syndrome. Skull involvement can cause a vascular steal syndrome with somnolence or ischemic neurologic events; the optic nerve may be affected, resulting in loss of vision. Vertebral involvement can cause a vascular steal syndrome with paralysis. Jaw involvement can cause the teeth to spread intraorally and become misaligned.

Osteosarcoma may develop in long-standing lesions but is rare (< 1%). Sarcomatous change is suggested by a marked increase in bone pain, sudden rise in alkaline phosphatase, and appearance of a new lytic lesion.

▶ Treatment

Asymptomatic patients may require only clinical surveillance and no treatment. However, treatment should be considered for asymptomatic patients who have extensive involvement of the skull, long bones, or vertebrae. Patients must be monitored carefully before, during, and after treatment with clinical examinations and serial serum alkaline phosphatase determinations.

A. Bisphosphonates

Bisphosphonates are the treatment of choice for Paget disease. Bisphosphonates are usually given cyclically. Therapy is given until a therapeutic response occurs, as evidenced by normalization of the serum alkaline phosphatase. After a course of therapy, patients are given a break for about 3 months or until the serum alkaline phosphatase begins rising again; another cycle is then commenced.

Patients frequently experience a paradoxical increase in pain soon after commencing bisphosphonate therapy; this is the "first dose effect" and the pain usually subsides with further treatment. Flu-like symptoms occur fairly frequently. Osteonecrosis, particularly of the jaw, is rare but can occur spontaneously or after tooth extraction.

The oral bisphosphonates should all be taken with 8 oz of plain water only; they are relatively contraindicated in patients with a history of esophagitis, esophageal stricture, dysphagia, hiatal hernia, or achalasia. **Alendronate**, 40 mg orally daily for 3–6 month cycles, must be taken in the morning with water only, at least 30-40 minutes before any other food, liquids, or medications. Patients should not lie down for at least 30 minutes after taking alendronate to reduce the risk of esophagitis. **Tiludronate**, 400 mg orally daily for 3-month cycles, should not be taken within 2 hours of meals, aspirin, indomethacin, calcium, magnesium, or aluminum-containing antacids. Esophagitis is uncommon, but it is still advisable to avoid recumbency for 30 minutes after dosing; but the drug may be taken in the evening as well as during the day. The most common side effects have been gastrointestinal, including abdominal pain in 13% and nausea in 9%. **Risedronate**, 30 mg orally daily for 2-month cycles, must be taken in the morning with water only, at least 30–40 minutes before any other food, liquids, or medications. Patients should not lie down for at least 30 minutes after taking risedronate to reduce the risk of esophagitis.

Parenteral bisphosphonates are particularly useful for patients who cannot tolerate oral bisphosphonates. Intravenous bisphosphonates can produce clinical improvements that last several months. Serum alkaline phosphatase levels may continue to drop for 6 months after treatment. They appear to be more effective than oral bisphosphonates but have more systemic side effects. Postinfusion fever, fatigue, myalgia, bone pain, and ocular problems occur commonly and may sometimes be severe. Serious side effects are rare but include uveitis and acute kidney disease. Hypocalcemia is common and may be severe, especially if intravenous bisphosphonates are given along with loop diuretics. It is advisable to administer calcium and vitamin D supplements, especially during the first 2 weeks following treatment. Asthma may occur in aspirin-sensitive patients. **Pamidronate**, 30–60 mg is infused intravenously over 2–4 hours. Depending on the disease severity, one to three additional doses may be given days or weeks apart. **Zoledronic acid** can be given every 6–12 months in doses of 2–5 mg intravenously over 20 minutes. Six months following a single infusion of zoledronic acid, patients had a clinical response rate of 96%, compared with 74% in patients receiving daily oral risedronate. Intravenous zoledronic acid has been demonstrated to be significantly more effective than daily risedronate.

B. Nasal Calcitonin-Salmon

Miacalcin, 200 international units/unit dose spray, is administered as one spray daily, alternating nostrils. It is just as effective as the parenteral preparation and is associated with fewer side effects. Nasal irritation may occur, as may occasional epistaxis. Calcitonin has been used for many years to treat Paget disease. However, its use has declined dramatically with the introduction of more potent bisphosphonates.

▶ Prognosis

The prognosis in general is good, but sarcomatous changes (in 1–3%) can alter it unfavorably. In general, the prognosis is worse the earlier in life the disease starts. Fractures usually heal well. In the severe forms, marked deformity, intractable pain, and cardiac failure are found. These complications should become rare with prompt bisphosphonate treatment.

Colina M et al. Paget's disease of bone: a review. Rheumatol Int. 2008 Sep;28(11):1069–75. [PMID: 18592244]

Ralston SH. Juvenile Paget's disease, familial expansile osteolysis and other genetic osteolytic disorders. Best Pract Res Clin Rheumatol. 2008 Mar;22(1):101–11. [PMID: 18328984]

Watts GD et al. Novel VCP mutations in inclusion body myopathy associated with Paget disease of bone and frontotemporal dementia. Clin Genet. 2007 Nov;72(5):420–6. [PMID: 17935506]

Whyte MP. Clinical practice: Paget's disease of bone. N Engl J Med. 2006 Aug 10;355(6):593–600. [PMID: 16899779]

DISEASES OF THE ADRENAL CORTEX

ACUTE ADRENOCORTICAL INSUFFICIENCY (Adrenal Crisis)

 ESSENTIALS OF DIAGNOSIS

▶ Weakness, abdominal pain, fever, confusion, nausea, vomiting, and diarrhea.

▶ Low blood pressure, dehydration; skin pigmentation may be increased.

▶ Serum potassium high, sodium low, BUN high.

▶ Cosyntropin (ACTH$_{1-24}$) unable to stimulate an increase in serum cortisol to $\geq$ 20 mcg/dL.

▶ General Considerations

Acute adrenal insufficiency is an emergency caused by insufficient cortisol. Crisis may occur in the course of treatment of chronic insufficiency, or it may be the presenting manifestation of adrenal insufficiency. Acute adrenal crisis is more commonly seen in primary adrenal insufficiency (Addison disease) than in disorders of the pituitary gland causing secondary adrenocortical hypofunction.

Adrenal crisis may occur in the following situations: (1) during stress, (eg, trauma, surgery, infection, hyperthyroidism, or prolonged fasting) in a patient with latent or treated adrenal insufficiency; (2) following sudden withdrawal of adrenocortical hormone in a patient with chronic insufficiency or in a patient with temporary insufficiency due to suppression by exogenous corticosteroids or megestrol; (3) following bilateral adrenalectomy or removal of a functioning adrenal tumor that had suppressed the other adrenal; (4) following sudden destruction of the pituitary gland (pituitary necrosis), or when thyroid hormone is given to a patient with hypoadrenalism; and (5) following injury to both adrenals by trauma, hemorrhage, anticoagulant therapy, thrombosis, infection or, rarely, metastatic carcinoma; (6) following administration of etomidate, which is used intravenously for rapid anesthesia induction or intubation.

Clinical Findings

A. Symptoms and Signs

The patient complains of headache, lassitude, nausea and vomiting, abdominal pain, and often diarrhea. Confusion or coma may be present. Fever may be 40.6 °C or more. The blood pressure is low. Recurrent hypoglycemia and reduced insulin requirements may present in patients with preexisting type 1 diabetes mellitus. Other signs may include cyanosis, dehydration, skin hyperpigmentation, and sparse axillary hair (if hypogonadism is also present). Meningococcemia may be associated with purpura and adrenal insufficiency secondary to adrenal infarction (Waterhouse–Friderichsen syndrome).

B. Laboratory Findings

The eosinophil count may be high. Hyponatremia or hyperkalemia (or both) are usually present. Hypoglycemia is frequent. Hypercalcemia may be present. Blood, sputum, or urine culture may be positive if bacterial infection is the precipitating cause of the crisis.

The diagnosis is made by a simplified cosyntropin stimulation test, which is performed as follows: (1) Synthetic $ACTH_{1-24}$ (cosyntropin), 0.25 mg, is given parenterally. (2) Serum is obtained for cortisol between 30 and 60 minutes after cosyntropin is administered. Normally, serum cortisol rises to at least 20 mcg/dL. For patients receiving corticosteroid treatment, hydrocortisone must not be given for at least 8 hours before the test. Other corticosteroids (eg, prednisone, dexamethasone) do not interfere with specific assays for cortisol.

Plasma ACTH is markedly elevated if the patient has primary adrenal disease (generally > 200 pg/mL).

Differential Diagnosis

Acute adrenal insufficiency must be distinguished from other causes of shock (eg, septic, hemorrhagic, cardiogenic). Hyperkalemia is also seen with gastrointestinal bleeding, rhabdomyolysis, hyperkalemic paralysis, and certain drugs (eg, angiotensin-converting enzyme [ACE] inhibitors, spironolactone). Hyponatremia is seen in many other conditions (eg, hypothyroidism, diuretic use, heart failure, cirrhosis, vomiting, diarrhea, severe illness, or major surgery). Acute adrenal insufficiency must be distinguished from an acute abdomen in which neutrophilia is the rule, whereas adrenal insufficiency is characterized by a relative lymphocytosis and eosinophilia.

More than 90% of serum cortisol is protein bound and low serum levels of binding proteins result in misleadingly low serum cortisol determinations by most assays. Nearly 40% of critically ill patients, with serum albumin < 2.5 g/dL, have low serum total cortisol levels but normal serum free cortisol or salivary cortisol levels and normal adrenal function.

Treatment

A. Acute Phase

If the diagnosis is suspected, draw a blood sample for cortisol determination and treat with hydrocortisone, 100–300 mg intravenously, and saline *immediately*, without waiting for the results. Thereafter, give hydrocortisone phosphate or hydrocortisone sodium succinate, 100 mg intravenously immediately, and continue intravenous infusions of 50–100 mg every 6 hours for the first day. Give the same amount every 8 hours on the second day and then adjust the dosage in view of the clinical picture.

Since bacterial infection frequently precipitates acute adrenal crisis, broad-spectrum antibiotics should be administered empirically while waiting for the results of initial cultures. Hypoglycemia should be vigorously treated while serum electrolytes, BUN, and creatinine are monitored.

B. Convalescent Phase

When the patient is able to take food by mouth, give oral hydrocortisone, 10–20 mg every 6 hours, and reduce dosage to maintenance levels as needed. Most patients ultimately require hydrocortisone twice daily (am, 10–20 mg; pm, 5–10 mg). Mineralocorticoid therapy is not needed when large amounts of hydrocortisone are being given, but as the dose is reduced it is usually necessary to add fludrocortisone acetate, 0.05–0.2 mg daily. Some patients never require fludrocortisone or become edematous at doses of more than 0.05 mg once or twice weekly. Once the crisis has passed, the patient must be evaluated to assess the degree of permanent adrenal insufficiency and to establish the cause if possible.

Prognosis

Rapid treatment will usually be life-saving. However, acute adrenal insufficiency is frequently unrecognized and untreated since its manifestations mimic more common conditions; lack of treatment leads to shock that is unresponsive to volume replacement and vasopressors, resulting in death.

Lewandowsi KC et al. New onset Graves' disease as a cause of an adrenal crisis in an individual with panhypituitaris: brief report. Thyroid Res. 2008 Nov 19;1(1):7. [PMID: 19019235]
Lundy JB et al. Acute adrenal insufficiency after a single dose of etomidate. J Intensive Care Med. 2007 Mar–Apr;22(2):111–7. [PMID: 17456730]

CHRONIC ADRENOCORTICAL INSUFFICIENCY (Addison Disease)

ESSENTIALS OF DIAGNOSIS

▶ Weakness, fatigability, anorexia, weight loss; nausea and vomiting, diarrhea; abdominal pain, muscle and joint pains; amenorrhea.

▶ Sparse axillary hair; increased skin pigmentation, especially of creases, pressure areas, and nipples.

▶ Hypotension, small heart.

▶ Serum sodium may be low; potassium, calcium, and BUN may be elevated; neutropenia, mild anemia, eosinophilia, and relative lymphocytosis may be present.

- Plasma cortisol levels are low or fail to rise after administration of corticotropin.
- Plasma ACTH level is elevated.

General Considerations

Addison disease is an uncommon disorder caused by destruction or dysfunction of the adrenal cortices. It is characterized by chronic deficiency of cortisol, aldosterone, and adrenal androgens and causes skin pigmentation that can be subtle or strikingly dark. Volume and sodium depletion and potassium excess eventually occur in primary adrenal failure. In contrast, if chronic adrenal insufficiency is secondary to pituitary failure (atrophy, necrosis, tumor), mineralocorticoid production (controlled by the renin–angiotensin system) persists and hyperkalemia is not present. Furthermore, if ACTH is not elevated, skin pigmentary changes are not encountered.

Etiology

Autoimmune destruction of the adrenals is the most common cause of Addison disease in the United States (accounting for about 80% of spontaneous cases). With such autoimmunity, adrenal function decreases over several years as it progresses to overt adrenal insufficiency. It may occur alone or as part of a **polyglandular autoimmune (PGA) syndrome.** *Type 1 PGA* is also known as autoimmune polyendocrinopathy-candidiasis-ectodermal dystrophy (APCED) syndrome and is caused by a defect in T cell-mediated immunity inherited as an autosomal recessive trait. Type 1 PGA usually presents in early childhood with mucocutaneous candidiasis, followed by hypoparathyroidism and dystrophy of the teeth and nails; Addison disease usually appears by age 15 years. Partial or late expression of the syndrome is common. A varied spectrum of associated diseases may be seen in adulthood, including hypogonadism, hypothyroidism, pernicious anemia, alopecia, vitiligo, hepatitis, malabsorption, and Sjögren syndrome.

Type 2 PGA usually presents in young adults age 20–40 years, usually women (female:male ration is 3:1). The following conditions may be presentations of type 2 PGA: autoimmune adrenal insufficiency, type 1 diabetes mellitus, or autoimmune thyroid disease (usually hypothyroidism, sometimes hyperthyroidism). The combination of Addison disease and hypothyroidism is known as Schmidt syndrome. Patients may also have vitiligo, alopecia areata, Sjögren syndrome, or celiac sprue. Type 2 PGA is also associated with autoimmune primary ovarian failure; testicular failure (5%); pernicious anemia (4%); and, rarely, autoimmune hypophysitis, encephalitis, or hypoparathyroidism (late-onset).

Tuberculosis as a leading cause of Addison disease is relatively rare in the United States but common where tuberculosis is more prevalent.

Bilateral **adrenal hemorrhage** may occur during sepsis, heparin-associated thrombocytopenia or anticoagulation, or with antiphospholipid antibody syndrome. It may occur in association with major surgery or trauma, presenting about 1 week later with pain, fever, and shock. It may also occur spontaneously.

Adrenoleukodystrophy is an X-linked peroxisomal disorder causing accumulation of very long-chain fatty acids in the adrenal cortex, testes, brain, and spinal cord. It may present at any age and accounts for one-third of cases of Addison disease in boys. Aldosterone deficiency occurs in 9%. Hypogonadism is common. Psychiatric symptoms often include mania, psychosis, or cognitive impairment. Neurologic deterioration may be severe or mild (particularly in heterozygote women), mimics symptoms of multiple sclerosis, and can occur years after the onset of adrenal insufficiency.

Rare causes of adrenal insufficiency include lymphoma, metastatic carcinoma, coccidioidomycosis, histoplasmosis, cytomegalovirus infection (more frequent in patients with AIDS), syphilitic gummas, scleroderma, amyloid disease, and hemochromatosis.

Congenital adrenal insufficiency occurs in several conditions. **Familial glucocorticoid deficiency** is caused by a mutation in the gene encoding the adrenal ACTH receptor. **Triple A (Allgrove) syndrome** is characterized by variable expression of the following: adrenal ACTH resistance with cortisol deficiency, achalasia, alacrima, nasal voice, and neuromuscular disease of varying severity (hyperreflexia to spastic paraplegia). Cortisol deficiency usually presents in infancy but may not occur until the third decade of life. **Congenital adrenal hypoplasia** causes adrenal insufficiency due to absence of the adrenal cortex; patients may also have hypogonadotropic hypogonadism, myopathy, and high-frequency hearing loss. Patients with hereditary defects in adrenal enzymes for cortisol synthesis develop **congenital adrenal hyperplasia** due to ACTH stimulation. The most common enzyme defect is P450c21 (21-hydroxylase). Patients with severely defective P450c21 enzymes manifest deficiency of mineralocorticoids (salt wasting) in addition to deficient cortisol and excessive androgens. Women with milder enzyme defects have adequate cortisol but develop hirsutism in adolescence or adulthood and are said to have "late-onset" congenital adrenal hyperplasia. (See Hirsutism section.)

Clinical Findings

A. Symptoms and Signs

The symptoms may include weakness and fatigability, weight loss, myalgias, arthralgias, fever, anorexia, nausea and vomiting, anxiety, and mental irritability. Some of these symptoms may be due to high serum levels of IL-6. Pigmentary changes consist of diffuse tanning over nonexposed as well as exposed parts or multiple freckles; hyperpigmentation is especially prominent over the knuckles, elbows, knees, and posterior neck and in palmar creases. Nail beds may develop longitudinal pigmented bands. Nipples and areolas tend to darken. The skin in pressure areas such as the belt or brassiere lines and the buttocks also darkens. New scars are pigmented. Some patients have associated vitiligo (10%). Emotional changes are common. Hypoglycemia, when present, may worsen the patient's weakness and mental functioning, rarely leading to coma.

Manifestations of other autoimmune disease (see above) may be present. Patients tend to be hypotensive and orthostatic; about 90% have systolic blood pressures under 110 mm Hg; blood pressure over 130 mm Hg is rare. Other findings may include a small heart, hyperplasia of lymphoid tissues, and scant axillary and pubic hair (especially in women).

Patients with adult-onset adrenoleukodystrophy may present with neuropsychiatric symptoms, sometimes without adrenal insufficiency.

B. Laboratory Findings

The WBC count usually shows moderate neutropenia, lymphocytosis, and a total eosinophil count over 300/mcL. Among patients with *chronic* Addison disease, the serum sodium is usually low (90%) while the potassium is elevated (65%). Patients with diarrhea may not be hyperkalemic. Fasting blood glucose may be low. Hypercalcemia may be present. Young men with idiopathic Addison disease are screened for adrenoleukodystrophy by determining plasma very long-chain fatty acid levels; affected patients have high levels.

Low plasma cortisol (< 3 mcg/dL) at 8 am is diagnostic, especially if accompanied by simultaneous elevation of the plasma ACTH level (usually > 200 pg/mL). The diagnosis is made by a simplified cosyntropin stimulation test, which is performed as follows: (1) Synthetic $ACTH_{1-24}$ (cosyntropin), 0.25 mg, is given parenterally. (2) Serum is obtained for cortisol between 30 and 60 minutes after cosyntropin is administered. Normally, serum cortisol rises to at least 20 mcg/dL. For patients receiving corticosteroid treatment, hydrocortisone must not be given for at least 8 hours before the test. Other corticosteroids (eg, prednisone, dexamethasone) do not interfere with specific assays for cortisol.

Serum DHEA levels are under 1000 ng/mL in 100% of patients with Addison disease and a serum DHEA above 1000 ng/mL excludes the diagnosis. However, serum DHEA levels below 1000 ng/mL are not helpful, since about 15% of the general population have such low DHEA levels, particularly children and elderly individuals. Antiadrenal antibodies are found in the serum in about 50% of cases of autoimmune Addison disease. Antibodies to thyroid (45%) and other tissues may be present.

Elevated plasma renin activity (PRA) indicates the presence of depleted intravascular volume and the need for higher doses of fludrocortisone replacement. Serum epinephrine levels are low in patients with adrenal insufficiency, since these patients do not have the high local concentrations of cortisol that are required to induce the enzyme PNMT in adrenal medulla for the synthesis of epinephrine from norepinephrine.

C. Imaging

When Addison disease is not clearly autoimmune, a chest radiograph is obtained to look for tuberculosis, fungal infection, or cancer as possible causes. CT scan of the abdomen will show small noncalcified adrenals in autoimmune Addison disease. The adrenals are enlarged in about 85% of cases due to metastatic or granulomatous disease.

Calcification is noted in about 50% of cases of tuberculous Addison disease but is also seen with hemorrhage, fungal infection, pheochromocytoma, and melanoma.

▶ Differential Diagnosis

Addison disease should be considered in any patient with unexplained hypotension, but shock is usually caused by more common conditions such as gastrointestinal bleeding or sepsis. Hyponatremia or hyperkalemia may be seen in numerous other conditions (see Chapter 21). Drospirenone, the progestin component in certain oral contraceptives, may cause hyperkalemia.

Unexplained weight loss, weakness, and anorexia may be mistaken for occult cancer. Nausea, vomiting, diarrhea, and abdominal pain may be misdiagnosed as intrinsic gastrointestinal disease. The hyperpigmentation may be confused with that due to ethnic or racial factors. Weight loss may simulate anorexia nervosa. The neurologic manifestations of Allgrove syndrome and adrenoleukodystrophy (especially in women) may mimic multiple sclerosis. Hemochromatosis also enters the differential diagnosis of skin hyperpigmentation, but it should be remembered that it may truly be a cause of Addison disease as well as diabetes mellitus and hypoparathyroidism. Serum ferritin is increased in most cases of hemochromatosis and is a useful screening test. About 17% of patients with AIDS have symptoms of cortisol resistance. AIDS can also cause frank adrenal insufficiency.

Hyperkalemia can be caused by isolated hypoaldosteronism and is seen in various conditions. Hyporeninemic hypoaldosteronism can be caused by renal tubular acidosis type IV and is commonly seen with diabetic nephropathy, hypertensive nephrosclerosis, tubulointerstitial diseases, and AIDS; hyperkalemia, hyperchloremia, and metabolic acidosis (see Chapter 21) are presenting signs. Hyperreninemic hypoaldosteronism can be seen in patients with myotonic dystrophy, aldosterone synthase deficiency, and congenital adrenal hyperplasia. Hyperkalemia, hypertension, and hypogonadism may present as delayed adolescence or in adulthood in some patients with congenital adrenal hyperplasia (CYP17 deficiency); cortisol deficiency is also usually present but may not be clinically evident.

▶ Complications

Any of the complications of the underlying disease (eg, tuberculosis) are more likely to occur, and the patient is susceptible to intercurrent infections that may precipitate crisis. Associated autoimmune diseases are common (see above).

▶ Treatment

A. Specific Therapy

Replacement therapy should include a combination of corticosteroids and mineralocorticoids. In mild cases, hydrocortisone alone may be adequate.

Hydrocortisone is the drug of choice. Most addisonian patients are well maintained on 15–30 mg of hydrocortisone orally daily in two divided doses, two-thirds in the morning and one-third in the late afternoon or early evening. Some patients respond better to prednisone in a dosage of about 2–4 mg in the morning and 1–2 mg in the evening. Adjustments in dosage are made according to the clinical response. A proper dose usually results in a normal differential WBC count.

Fludrocortisone acetate has a potent sodium-retaining effect. The dosage is 0.05–0.3 mg orally daily or every other day. In the presence of postural hypotension, hyponatremia, or hyperkalemia, the dosage is increased. Similarly, in patients with fatigue, elevated PRA indicates the need for a higher replacement dose of fludrocortisone. If edema, hypokalemia, or hypertension ensues, the dose is decreased.

DHEA is given to some patients with adrenal insufficiency. In a double-blind clinical trial, patients taking DHEA 50 mg orally each morning have experienced an improvement in their overall sense of well-being, an increase in muscle mass, and a reversal in bone loss at the femoral neck. DHEA replacement did not improve fatigue or sexual dysfunction; however, its placebo effect may be significant in that regard. Older women who receive DHEA should be monitored for androgenic effects. Because over-the-counter preparations of DHEA have variable potencies, it is best to have the pharmacy formulate this with pharmaceutical-grade micronized DHEA.

B. General Measures

Patients with Addison disease must be thoroughly informed about their condition. All infections should be treated immediately and vigorously, with the dose of hydrocortisone increased appropriately. The dose of corticosteroid should also be raised in case of trauma, surgery, stressful diagnostic procedures, or other forms of stress. The maximum hydrocortisone dose for severe stress is 50 mg intravenously or intramuscularly every 6 hours. Lower doses, oral or parenteral, are used for less severe stress. The dose is reduced back to normal as the stress subsides. Patients are advised to wear a medical alert bracelet or medal reading, "Adrenal insufficiency—takes hydrocortisone."

▶ Prognosis

The life expectancy of patients with Addison disease has been considered reasonably normal, as long as they are very compliant with taking their medications and are knowledgeable about their condition. However, a retrospective Swedish study of 1675 patients with Addison disease found an unexpected increase in all-cause mortality, mostly from cardiovascular disease, malignancy, and infectious causes. Associated conditions can pose additional health risks. For example, patients with adrenoleukodystrophy or Allgrove syndrome may suffer from neurologic disease. Patients with adrenal tuberculosis may have a serious systemic infection that requires treatment. Adrenal crisis can occur in patients who stop their medication or who experience stress such as infection, trauma, or surgery without appropriately higher doses of corticosteroids. Patients who take excessive doses of corticosteroid replacement can develop Cushing syndrome, which imposes its own risks.

Many patients with treated Addison disease complain of chronic low-grade fatigue.

Many patients with Addison disease do not feel entirely normal, despite glucocorticoid and mineralocorticoid replacement. This may be due, in part, to the inadequacy of oral replacement to duplicate cortisol's normal circadian rhythm. Also, patients with Addison disease are deficient in epinephrine, but replacement epinephrine is not available. Fatigue may also be an indication of suboptimal dosing of medication, electrolyte imbalance, or concurrent problems such as hypothyroidism or diabetes mellitus. However, most patients with Addison disease are able to live fully active lives.

Ferraz-de-Souza B et al. Disorders of adrenal development. Endocr Dev. 2008;13:19–32. [PMID: 18493131]

Gurnell EM et al. Long-term DHEA replacement in primary adrenal insufficiency: a randomized, controlled trial. J Clin Endocrinol Metab. 2008 Feb;93(2):400–9. [PMID: 18000094]

Kyriazopoulou V. Glucocorticoid replacement therapy in patients with Addison's disease. Expert Opin Pharmacother. 2007 Apr;8(6):725–9. [PMID: 17425469]

Lovas K et al. Continuous subcutaneous hydrocortisone infusion in Addison's disease. Eur J Endocrinol. 2007 Jul;157(1):109–12. [PMID: 17609409]

CUSHING SYNDROME (Hypercortisolism)

ESSENTIALS OF DIAGNOSIS

▶ Central obesity, muscle wasting, thin skin, hirsutism, purple striae.

▶ Psychological changes.

▶ Osteoporosis, hypertension, poor wound healing.

▶ Hyperglycemia, glycosuria, leukocytosis, lymphocytopenia, hypokalemia.

▶ Elevated serum cortisol and urinary free cortisol. Lack of normal suppression by dexamethasone.

▶ General Considerations

The term Cushing "syndrome" refers to the manifestations of excessive corticosteroids, commonly due to supraphysiologic doses of corticosteroid drugs and rarely due to spontaneous production of excessive corticosteroids by the adrenal cortex. Cases of spontaneous Cushing syndrome are rare (2.6 new cases yearly per million population) and have several possible causes.

About 40% of cases are due to Cushing "disease," by which is meant the manifestations of hypercortisolism due to ACTH hypersecretion by the pituitary. Cushing disease is caused by a benign pituitary adenoma that is typically very small (< 5 mm) and usually located in the anterior pituitary (98%) or in the posterior pituitary (2%). It is at least three times more frequent in women than men.

About 10% of cases are due to nonpituitary ACTH-secreting neoplasms (eg, small cell lung carcinoma), which produce excessive amounts of ectopic ACTH. Hypokalemia and hyperpigmentation are commonly found in this group.

About 15% of cases are due to ACTH from a source that cannot be initially located.

About 30% of cases are due to excessive autonomous secretion of cortisol by the adrenals—independently of ACTH, serum levels of which are usually low. Most such cases are due to a unilateral adrenal tumor: Benign adrenal adenomas are generally small and produce mostly cortisol; adrenal carcinomas are usually large when discovered and can produce excessive cortisol as well as androgens, with resultant hirsutism and virilization. ACTH-independent macronodular adrenal hyperplasia can also produce hypercortisolism due to the adrenal cortex cells' abnormal stimulation by hormones such as catecholamines, arginine vasopressin, serotonin, hCG/LH, or gastric inhibitory polypeptide; in the latter case, hypercortisolism may be intermittent and food dependent and serum ACTH may not be completely suppressed. Pigmented bilateral adrenal macronodular adrenal hyperplasia is a rare cause of Cushing syndrome in children and young adults; it may be an isolated condition or part of the Carney complex.

▶ Clinical Findings

A. Symptoms and Signs

Patients with Cushing syndrome usually have central obesity with a plethoric "moon face," "buffalo hump," supraclavicular fat pads, protuberant abdomen, and thin extremities; oligomenorrhea or amenorrhea (or impotence in the male); weakness, backache, and headache; hypertension; osteoporosis; avascular bone necrosis; and acne and superficial skin infections. Patients may have thirst and polyuria (with or without glycosuria), renal calculi, glaucoma, purple striae (especially around the thighs, breasts, and abdomen), and easy bruisability. Wound healing is impaired. Mental symptoms may range from diminished ability to concentrate to increased lability of mood to frank psychosis. Patients are susceptible to opportunistic infections.

B. Laboratory Findings

Glucose tolerance is impaired as a result of insulin resistance. Polyuria is present as a result of increased free water clearance; diabetes mellitus with glycosuria may worsen it. Patients with Cushing syndrome often have leukocytosis with relative granulocytosis and lymphopenia. Hypokalemia may be present, particularly in cases of ectopic ACTH secretion.

▶ Tests for Hypercortisolism

The easiest screening test for Cushing syndrome is the dexamethasone suppression test: dexamethasone 1 mg is given orally at 11 pm and serum is collected for cortisol determination at about 8 am the next morning; a cortisol level under 5 mcg/dL (< 135 nmol/L, fluorometric assay) or under 2 mcg/dL (< 54 nmol/L, high-performance liquid chromatography [HPLC] assay) excludes Cushing syndrome with some certainty. However, 8% of established

patients with pituitary Cushing disease have dexamethasone-suppressed cortisol levels < 2 mcg/dL. Therefore, when other clinical criteria suggest hypercortisolism, further evaluation is warranted even in the face of normal dexamethasone-suppressed serum cortisol. Antiseizure drugs (eg, phenytoin, phenobarbital, primidone) and rifampin accelerate the metabolism of dexamethasone, in that way causing a lack of cortisol suppression by dexamethasone. Estrogens—during pregnancy or as oral contraceptives or ERT—may also cause lack of dexamethasone suppressibility.

Patients with an abnormal dexamethasone suppression test require further investigation, which includes a 24-hour urine collection for free cortisol and creatinine. An abnormally high 24-hour urine free cortisol (or free cortisol to creatinine ratio of > 95 mcg cortisol/g creatinine) helps confirm hypercortisolism. A misleadingly high urine free cortisol excretion occurs with high fluid intake. In pregnancy, urine free cortisol is increased, while 17-hydroxycorticosteroids remain normal and diurnal variability of serum cortisol is normal. Carbamazepine and fenofibrate cause false elevations of urine free cortisol when determined by HPLC.

A midnight serum cortisol level > 7.5 mcg/dL is indicative of Cushing syndrome and distinguishes it from other conditions associated with a high urine free cortisol (pseudo-Cushing states; see Differential Diagnosis, below). Requirements for this test include being in the same time zone for at least 3 days, being without food for at least 3 hours, and having an indwelling intravenous line established in advance for the blood draw.

Due to the inconvenience of obtaining a midnight blood specimen for serum cortisol, late-night salivary cortisol assays have proved useful. Salivary cortisol kits can be ordered at www.acllaboratories.com. A standardized enzyme-linked immunosorbent assay (ELISA) is used by reliable laboratories. Using ELISA, midnight salivary cortisol levels are normally < 0.15 mcg/dL (4.0 nmol/L). Midnight salivary cortisol levels that are consistently > 0.25 mcg/dL (7.0 nmol/L) are considered very abnormal. The late-night salivary cortisol test has a high sensitivity and specificity for Cushing syndrome, but false-positive and false-negative tests have occurred.

Interestingly, hypercortisolism without Cushing syndrome can occur in several conditions, such as severe depression, anorexia nervosa, alcoholism, and familial cortisol resistance. (See Differential Diagnosis, below.)

▶ Finding the Cause of Hypercortisolism

Once hypercortisolism is confirmed, a plasma or serum ACTH is obtained. It must be collected properly in a plastic tube on ice and processed quickly by a laboratory with a reliable, sensitive assay. A level of ACTH below about 20 pg/mL indicates a probable adrenal tumor, whereas higher levels are produced by pituitary or ectopic ACTH-secreting tumors.

▶ Localizing Techniques

In ACTH-dependent Cushing syndrome, MRI of the pituitary demonstrates a pituitary lesion in about 50% of cases.

Premature cerebral atrophy is often noted. When the pituitary MRI is normal or shows a tiny (< 5 mm diameter) irregularity that may be incidental, selective catheterization of the inferior petrosal sinus veins draining the pituitary is performed. ACTH levels in the inferior petrosal sinus that are more than twice the simultaneous peripheral venous ACTH levels are indicative of pituitary Cushing disease. Inferior petrosal sinus sampling is also done during CRH administration, which ordinarily causes the ACTH levels in the inferior petrosal sinus to be over three times the peripheral ACTH level when the pituitary is the source of ACTH.

When inferior petrosal sinus ACTH concentrations are not above the requisite levels, a search for an ectopic source of ACTH is undertaken. Location of ectopic sources of ACTH commences with CT scanning of the chest and abdomen, with special attention to the lungs (for carcinoid or small cell carcinomas), the thymus, the pancreas, and the adrenals. In patients with ACTH-dependent Cushing syndrome, chest masses should not be assumed to be the source of ACTH, since opportunistic infections are common, so it is prudent to biopsy a chest mass to confirm the pathologic diagnosis prior to resection.

CT scanning fails to detect the source of ACTH in about 40% of patients with ectopic ACTH secretion. ^{111}In-octreotide (OCT, somatostatin receptor scintigraphy) scanning is also useful in detecting occult tumors. A low-dose scan with 6 mCi OCT is used first; a high-dose scan with 12 mCi OCT may be used if the low-dose scan gives equivocal results. [18]FDG-PET scanning is not usually helpful. Some ectopic ACTH-secreting tumors elude discovery, necessitating bilateral adrenalectomy. The ectopic source of ACTH should continue to be sought, since they may become detectable by OCT or CT scanning at a later date.

In non-ACTH-dependent Cushing syndrome, a CT scan of the adrenals can localize the adrenal tumor in most cases.

Differential Diagnosis

Alcoholic patients can have hypercortisolism and many clinical manifestations of Cushing syndrome. Regular use of the "party drug" gamma hydroxybutyrate (GHB, sodium oxybate) has been reported to cause reversible ACTH-dependent Cushing syndrome. Depressed patients also have hypercortisolism that can be nearly impossible to distinguish biochemically from Cushing syndrome but without clinical signs of Cushing syndrome. Some adolescents develop violaceous striae on the abdomen, back, and breasts; these are known as "striae distensae" and are not indicative of Cushing syndrome. Cushing syndrome can be misdiagnosed as anorexia nervosa (and vice versa) owing to the muscle wasting and extraordinarily high urine free cortisol levels found in anorexia. Patients with severe obesity frequently have an abnormal dexamethasone suppression test, but the urine free cortisol is usually normal, as is diurnal variation of serum cortisol. Patients with familial cortisol resistance have hyperandrogenism, hypertension, and hypercortisolism without actual Cushing syndrome. In patients with familial partial lipodystrophy type I, central obesity and a moon facies develop, along with thin extremities due to atrophy of subcutaneous fat. However, these patients' muscles are strong and may be hypertrophic, distinguishing this condition from Cushing syndrome. Patients receiving antiretroviral therapy for HIV-1 infection frequently develop partial lipodystrophy with thin extremities and central obesity with a dorsocervical fat pad ("buffalo hump") that may mimic Cushing syndrome.

Complications

Cushing syndrome, if untreated, produces serious morbidity and even death. The patient may suffer from any of the complications of hypertension or of diabetes. Susceptibility to infections is increased. Compression fractures of the osteoporotic spine and aseptic necrosis of the femoral head may cause marked disability. Nephrolithiasis and psychosis may occur. Following bilateral adrenalectomy for Cushing disease, a pituitary adenoma may enlarge progressively, causing local destruction (eg, visual field impairment) and hyperpigmentation; this complication is known as Nelson syndrome.

Treatment

Cushing disease is best treated by transsphenoidal selective resection of the pituitary adenoma. After pituitary surgery, the rest of the pituitary usually returns to normal function; however, the pituitary corticotrophs remain suppressed and require 6–36 months to recover normal function. Hydrocortisone or prednisone replacement therapy is necessary in the meantime. Patients who do not have a remission (or who have a recurrence) should be treated by bilateral laparoscopic adrenalectomy. Another treatment option for patients with ACTH-secreting pituitary tumors is stereotactic pituitary radiosurgery (gamma knife or cyberknife), which normalizes urine free cortisol in two-thirds of patients within 12 months. Conventional radiation therapy results in a 23% cure rate.

Pituitary radiosurgery can also be used to treat Nelson syndrome, the progressive enlargement of ACTH-secreting pituitary tumors following bilateral adrenalectomy. Patients who are not surgical candidates may be given a trial of ketoconazole in doses of about 200 mg every 6 hours; liver enzymes must be monitored for progressive elevation.

Adrenal neoplasms secreting cortisol are resected laparoscopically. The contralateral adrenal is suppressed, so postoperative hydrocortisone replacement is required until recovery occurs. Metastatic adrenal carcinoma may be treated with mitotane; ketoconazole or metyrapone can help suppress hypercortisolism in unresectable adrenal carcinoma. The thiazolidinedione rosiglitazone has slowed the growth of adrenal carcinomas in-vitro, but clinical trials are lacking.

Ectopic ACTH-secreting tumors should be located, when possible, and surgically resected. If that cannot be done, laparoscopic bilateral adrenalectomy is recommended. Medical treatment with ketoconazole or metyrapone (or both) may partially suppress the hypercortisolism; however, metyrapone may exacerbate female virilization. The somatostatin analog octreotide, given parenterally, suppresses ACTH secretion in about one-third of such cases.

Patients who are successfully treated for Cushing syndrome typically develop "cortisol withdrawal syndrome," even when given replacement corticosteroids for adrenal insufficiency. Manifestations can include hypotension, nausea, fatigue, arthralgias, myalgias, pruritus, and flaking skin. Increasing the hydrocortisone replacement to 30 mg twice daily can improve these symptoms; the dosage is then reduced as tolerated.

Prognosis

Patients with Cushing syndrome from a benign adrenal adenoma experience a 5-year survival of 95% and a 10-year survival of 90%, following a successful adrenalectomy. Patients with Cushing disease from a pituitary adenoma experience a similar survival if their pituitary surgery is successful. However, transsphenoidal surgery incurs a failure rate of about 10–20%, often due to the adenoma's ectopic position or invasion of the cavernous sinus. Those patients who have a complete remission after transsphenoidal surgery have about a 15–20% chance of recurrence over the next 10 years. Patients with failed pituitary surgery may require pituitary radiation therapy, which has its own morbidity. Bilateral adrenalectomy is often complicated by infection; recurrence of hypercortisolism may occur as a result of growth of an adrenal remnant stimulated by high levels of ACTH. The prognosis for patients with ectopic ACTH-producing tumors depends on the aggressiveness and stage of the particular tumor. Patients with ACTH of unknown source have a 5-year survival rate of 65% and a 10-year survival rate of 55%. Patients with adrenal carcinoma have a median survival of 7 months.

Carroll T et al. Late-night salivary cortisol measurement in the diagnosis of Cushing's syndrome. Nat Clin Pract Endocrinol Metab. 2008 Jun;4(6):344–50. [PMID: 18446140]

Kidambi S et al. Limitations of nocturnal salivary cortisol and urine free cortisol in the diagnosis of mild Cushing's syndrome. Eur J Endocrinol. 2007 Dec;157(6):725–31. [PMID: 18057379]

Razenberg AJ et al. A 'smart' type of Cushing's syndrome. Eur J Endocrinol. 2007 Dec;157(6):779–81. [PMID: 18057386]

HIRSUTISM & VIRILIZATION

ESSENTIALS OF DIAGNOSIS

- ▶ Hirsutism, acne, menstrual disorders.
- ▶ Virilization: increased muscularity, androgenic alopecia, deepening of the voice, clitoromegaly.
- ▶ Rarely, a palpable pelvic tumor.
- ▶ Urinary 17-ketosteroids and serum DHEAS and androstenedione elevated in adrenal disorders; variable in others.
- ▶ Serum testosterone is often elevated.

General Considerations

Hirsutism is defined as excessive terminal hair growth that appears in a male pattern in women. Hirsutism is frequently quantitated according to the Ferriman-Gallwey scale, which grades the presence of androgen sensitive hair from 0 (no hair) to 4 (virile) in 9 areas of the body (maximum score = 36). About 5% of reproductive age women are hirsute, with Ferriman-Gallwey scores 8.

Etiology

Hirsutism may be idiopathic or familial or be caused by the following disorders: polycystic ovary syndrome (PCOS), steroidogenic enzyme defects, neoplastic disorders or rarely by medications, acromegaly, or ACTH-induced Cushing disease.

A. Idiopathic or Familial

Most women with hirsutism or androgenic alopecia have no detectable hyperandrogenism. Patients often have a strong familial predisposition to hirsutism that may be considered normal in the context of their genetic background. Such patients may have elevated serum levels of androstenediol glucuronide, a metabolite of dihydrotestosterone that is produced by skin in cosmetically unacceptable amounts.

B. Polycystic Ovary Syndrome (Hyperthecosis, Stein–Leventhal Syndrome)

PCOS is a common functional disorder of the ovaries, affecting about 4–6% of premenopausal women in the United States and accounting for at least 50% of all cases of hirsutism associated with elevated testosterone levels. It is familial and transmitted as a modified autosomal dominant trait. Affected women have elevated serum testosterone or free testosterone levels. Affected women have signs of androgen excess, including hirsutism, acne, and male-pattern thinning of scalp hair. About 50% of affected women have oligomenorrhea or amenorrhea with anovulation. Despite the syndrome's name, the presence of ovarian cysts is not helpful diagnostically, since about 30% of women with PCOS do *not* have cystic ovaries and 25–30% of normal menstruating women *have* cystic ovaries. Obesity and high serum insulin levels (due to insulin resistance) contribute to the syndrome in 70% of women. The serum LH:FSH ratio is often greater than 2.0. Both adrenal and ovarian androgen hypersecretion are commonly present. Women with PCOS have a 35% risk of depression, compared with 11% in age-matched controls. Diabetes mellitus is present in about 13% of cases. Untreated women with amenorrhea have a slightly increased risk of endometrial carcinoma. Hypertension and hyperlipidemia are often present, increasing the risk of cardiovascular disease. Women frequently regain normal menstrual cycles with aging.

C. Steroidogenic Enzyme Defects

Baby girls with "classic" 21-hydroxylase deficiency have ambiguous genitalia and may become virilized unless treated with corticosteroid replacement; about 50% of such patients have clinically evident mineralocorticoid deficiency (salt-wasting) as well.

About 2% of patients with adult-onset hirsutism have been found to have a partial defect in adrenal 21-hydroxylase, whose phenotypic expression is delayed until adolescence or adulthood; such patients do not have salt-wasting. Polycystic ovaries and adrenal adenomas are more likely to develop in these women.

Some rare patients with hyperandrogenism and hypertension have 11-hydroxylase deficiency. This is distinguished from cortisol resistance by high cortisol serum levels in the latter and by high serum 11-deoxycortisol levels in the former.

Patients with an XY karyotype and a deficiency in 17β-hydroxysteroid dehydrogenase-3 or a deficiency in 5α-reductase-2 may present as phenotypic girls in whom virilization develops at puberty.

D. Neoplastic Disorders

Ovarian tumors are very uncommon causes of hirsutism (0.8%) and include arrhenoblastomas, Sertoli-Leydig cell tumors, dysgerminomas, and hilar cell tumors. Adrenal carcinoma is a rare cause of Cushing syndrome and hyperandrogenism that can be quite virilizing. Pure androgen-secreting adrenal tumors occur very rarely; about 50% are malignant.

E. Rare Causes of Hirsutism

Acromegaly and ACTH-induced Cushing syndrome can cause hirsutism. Maternal virilization during pregnancy may occur as a result of a luteoma of pregnancy, hyperreactio luteinalis, or polycystic ovaries. In postmenopausal women, diffuse stromal Leydig cell hyperplasia is a rare cause of hyperandrogenism. Acquired hypertrichosis lanuginosa is manifested by the appearance of diffuse fine lanugo hair growth on the face and body along with stomatologic symptoms; the disorder is usually associated with an internal malignancy, especially colorectal cancer, and may regress after tumor removal. Pharmacologic causes include minoxidil, cyclosporine, phenytoin, anabolic steroids, diazoxide, and certain progestins.

▶ Clinical Findings

A. Symptoms and Signs

Modest androgen excess from any source increases sexual hair (chin, upper lip, abdomen, and chest) and increases sebaceous gland activity, producing acne. Menstrual irregularities, anovulation, and amenorrhea are common. If androgen excess is pronounced, defeminization (decrease in breast size, loss of feminine adipose tissue) and virilization (frontal balding, muscularity, clitoromegaly, and deepening of the voice) occur. Virilization implicates the presence of an androgen-producing neoplasm.

Hypertension may be seen in rare patients with Cushing syndrome, adrenal 11-hydroxylase deficiency, or cortisol resistance syndrome.

A pelvic examination may disclose clitoromegaly or ovarian enlargement that may be cystic or neoplastic.

B. Laboratory Testing and Imaging

Serum androgen testing is mainly useful to screen for rare occult adrenal or ovarian neoplasms. Some general guidelines are presented here, though exceptions are common.

Serum is assayed for total testosterone and free testosterone. A serum testosterone level > 200 ng/dL or free testosterone > 40 ng/dL indicates the need for pelvic examination and ultrasound. If that is negative, an adrenal CT scan is performed.

Most radioimmunoassays and ELISA for testosterone are inaccurate below serum testosterone levels of 300 ng/dL. The more accurate testosterone assays rely upon extraction and chromatography, followed by mass spectrometry or immunoassay. Free testosterone is best measured by calculation, using accurate assays for testosterone and SHBG.

A serum androstenedione level > 1000 ng/dL also implicates an ovarian or adrenal neoplasm.

Patients with milder elevations of serum testosterone or androstenedione usually are treated with an oral contraceptive.

Patients with very elevated serum DHEAS (> 700 mcg/dL) have an adrenal source of androgen. This usually is due to adrenal hyperplasia and rarely to adrenal carcinoma. An adrenal CT scan is performed.

No firm guidelines exist as to which patients (if any) with hyperandrogenism should be screened for "late-onset" 21-hydroxylase deficiency. The evaluation requires levels of serum 17-hydroxyprogesterone to be drawn at baseline and at 30–60 minutes after the intramuscular injection of 0.25 mg of cosyntropin ($ACTH_{1-24}$). This test should ideally be done during the follicular phase of a woman's menstrual cycle. Patients with congenital adrenal hyperplasia will usually have a baseline 17-hydroxyprogesterone level over 300 ng/dL or a stimulated level over 1000 ng/dL. The diagnosis, once made, is interesting academically but not helpful to the patient since corticosteroid treatment is not particularly more effective in this condition than are other treatment modalities (see below).

Patients with any clinical signs of Cushing syndrome should receive a screening test. (See Cushing Syndrome.)

Serum levels of FSH and LH are elevated if amenorrhea is due to ovarian failure. An LH:FSH ratio greater than 2.0 is common in patients with PCOS. On abdominal ultrasound, about 25–30% of normal young women have polycystic ovaries, so the appearance of ovarian cysts on ultrasound is not helpful. So, the "polycystic" ovary syndrome is actually a misnomer and the diagnostic criteria for PCOS does not include imaging evidence of polycystic ovaries.

Virilizing tumors of the ovary can usually be detected by pelvic ultrasound or MRI. However, small virilizing ovarian tumors may not be detectable on imaging studies; selective venous sampling for testosterone may be used for diagnosis in such patients.

▶ Treatment

Postmenopausal women with severe hyperandrogenism should undergo laparoscopic bilateral oophorectomy (if CT scan of the adrenals and ovaries is normal), since small hilar cell tumors of the ovary may not be visible on scans. Girls with hyperandrogenism due to classic salt-wasting congenital adrenal hyperplasia may be treated with laparoscopic bilateral adrenalectomy. Any drugs causing hirsutism are stopped.

Spironolactone may be taken in doses of 50–100 mg orally twice daily on days 5–25 of the menstrual cycle or daily if used concomitantly with an oral contraceptive. Hyperkalemia or hyponatremia is uncommon.

Cyproterone acetate is a potent antiandrogen with progestational activity. A dose of 2 mg orally is effective. An oral contraceptive is usually prescribed also. Cyproterone is not available in the United States but is available elsewhere as the progestin element in an oral contraceptive (Diane-35: ethinyl estradiol 35 mcg with cyproterone acetate 2 mg). Side effects may include fatigue, nausea, depression, or hyperlipidemia.

Finasteride inhibits 5α-reductase, the enzyme that converts testosterone to active dihydrotestosterone in the skin. Given as 2.5-mg doses orally daily, it provides modest reduction in hirsutism over 6 months—somewhat less than that achieved with spironolactone. Finasteride is ineffective for androgenic alopecia in women. Side effects are rare.

Flutamide inhibits androgen reception uptake and also suppresses serum androgen. It is given orally in a dosage of 250 mg/d for the first year and then 125 mg/d for maintenance. Used with an oral contraceptive, it appears to be more effective than spironolactone in improving hirsutism, acne, and male pattern baldness. Women with congenital adrenal hyperplasia who take replacement hydrocortisone experience decreased renal cortisol clearance when treated with flutamide, resulting in lower hydrocortisone dosage requirements; corticosteroid replacement doses should be reduced when flutamide is added for treatment of hirsutism. Hepatotoxicity has been reported but is rare.

Oral contraceptives stimulate menses (if that is desired) and reduce acne vulgaris, but are less effective for hirsutism. Contraceptives containing antiandrogen progestins (either desogestrel 0.15 mg or levonorgestrel 0.15 mg) may be more effective for treating hirsutism but are associated with an increased risk of deep venous thrombosis. Simvastatin, when added to oral contraceptive therapy, has been reported to further decrease serum free testosterone by 16%, besides improving patients' serum lipid profiles.

Metformin may improve menstrual function in women with PCOS and amenorrhea or oligomenorrhea, but is less effective than oral contraceptives. Metformin is not effective in promoting fertility or in improving hirsutism in women with PCOS. Metformin therapy is usually given with meals and is started at a dose of 500 mg/d with breakfast for 1 week, then 500 mg with breakfast and dinner for 1 week, then 500 mg with breakfast and 1000 mg with dinner for 1 week, then 1000 mg with breakfast and dinner. The most common side effects are dose-related gastrointestinal upset and diarrhea. Patients are advised to take the highest tolerated dosage. Metformin appears to be nonteratogenic. Although metformin reduces insulin resistance, it does not cause hypoglycemia in nondiabetics. Metformin is contraindicated in renal and hepatic disease.

Clomiphene is the treatment of choice for women with PCOS and infertility. Over 6 months, clomiphene therapy resulted in a 22.5% rate of conception with live births. The rate of pregnancy with multiple fetuses is 6%.

Women with classic congenital adrenal hyperplasia (21-hydroxylase deficiency) have hirsutism and adrenal insufficiency that requires glucocorticoid and mineralocorticoid replacement. However, women with partial "late onset" 21-hydroxylase deficiency do not require hormone replacement. Treating such women with dexamethasone risks iatrogenic Cushing syndrome and is not particularly more effective than the other treatments for hirsutism listed in this section.

Local treatment by shaving or depilatories, waxing, electrolysis, or bleaching should be encouraged. Eflornithine (Vaniqua 13.9%) topical cream retards hair growth when applied twice daily to unwanted facial hair; improvement is noted within 4–8 weeks. However, local skin irritation may occur. Hirsutism returns with discontinuation. Laser therapy (photoepilation) is an effective treatment for facial hirsutism, particularly for women with dark hair and light skin; complications include skin hypopigmentation (rare) and hyperpigmentation, which occurs in 20% but usually resolves.

Women with androgenic alopecia may be effectively treated with topical minoxidil 2% solution applied twice daily to a dry scalp. Hypertrichosis is an unwanted side effect of topical minoxidil, occurring in 3–5% of treated women; it may affect the forehead, cheeks, upper lip, or chin. Hypertrichosis resolves within 1–6 months after the drug is stopped.

Note: Antiandrogen treatments must be given only to nonpregnant women. Women must be counseled to take oral contraceptives, when indicated, and avoid pregnancy, since use during pregnancy causes malformations and pseudohermaphroditism in male infants.

Banaszewska B et al. Effects of simvastatin and oral contraceptive agent on polycystic ovary syndrome: prospective, randomized, crossover trial. J Clin Endocrinol Metab. 2007 Feb;92(2):456–61. [PMID: 17105841]

Nestler JE. Metformin for the treatment of the polycystic ovary syndrome. N Engl J Med. 2008 Jan;358(1):47–54. [PMID: 18172174]

Norman RJ et al. Polycystic ovary syndrome. Lancet. 2007 Aug 25;370(9588):685–97. [PMID: 17720020]

Nouri K et al. Photoepilation: a growing trend in laser-assisted cosmetic dermatology. J Cosmet Dermatol. 2008 Mar;7(1):61–7. [PMID: 18254814]

Somani N et al. The clinical evaluation of hirsutism. Dermatol Ther. 2008 Sep–Oct;21(5):376–91. [PMID: 18844715]

PRIMARY ALDOSTERONISM

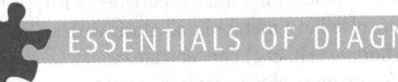
ESSENTIALS OF DIAGNOSIS

► Hypertension that may be severe or drug-resistant.
► Hypokalemia (in minority of patients) may cause polyuria, polydipsia, muscle weakness.
► Elevated plasma and urine aldosterone levels and low plasma renin level.

General Considerations

Primary aldosteronism (hyperaldosteronism) is common, accounting for 5–10% of all cases of hypertension. Patients of all ages may be affected, but the peak incidence is between 30–60 years. Excessive aldosterone production increases sodium retention and suppresses plasma renin. It increases renal potassium excretion that can lead to hypokalemia. Cardiovascular events are more prevalent in patients with aldosteronism (35%) than in those with essential hypertension (11%). Primary aldosteronism is most commonly caused by an adrenal adenoma (Conn syndrome), and unilateral or bilateral adrenal hyperplasia. Bilateral aldosteronism may be corticosteroid suppressible, due to an autosomal-dominant genetic defect allowing ACTH stimulation of aldosterone production.

▶ Clinical Findings

A. Symptoms and Signs

Patients have hypertension that is typically moderate. Some patients have only diastolic hypertension, without other symptoms and signs. Malignant hypertension is rare. Edema is rarely seen in primary aldosteronism. About 37% of patients have hypokalemia and may consequently have symptoms of muscular weakness (at times with paralysis simulating periodic paralysis), paresthesias with frank tetany, headache, polyuria, and polydipsia.

B. Laboratory Findings

Ideally, all hypertensive patients should be screened for hyperaldosteronism prior to treatment. Such screening can include PRA. About 20% of hypertensive patients have a low PRA, and a significant portion of these patients have primary aldosteronism. Initial screening can also include both PRA and aldosterone to determine a renin:aldosterone ratio (see below).

Plasma potassium should also be determined in all hypertensive individuals. However, hypokalemia, once thought to be the hallmark of hyperaldosteronism, is present in only 37% of affected patients: 50% of those with an adrenal adenoma and 17% of those with adrenal hyperplasia. Proper phlebotomy technique is important to avoid spurious increases in potassium. The blood should be drawn slowly with a syringe and needle (rather than a vacutainer) at least 5 seconds after tourniquet release and without fist-clenching. Plasma potassium should be measured, with the separation of plasma from cells within 30 minutes of collection. Besides hypokalemia, many patients with primary aldosteronism also have metabolic alkalosis with an elevated serum bicarbonate (HCO_3^-) concentration.

Testing for primary aldosteronism should be done for all hypertensive patients with hypokalemia, whether spontaneous or diuretic induced. But since only a minority of patients have hypokalemia, testing should also be considered for normokalemic hypertensive patients with (1) treatment-resistant hypertension (despite three drugs); (2) severe hypertension: > 160 mm Hg systolic or > 100 mm Hg diastolic; (3) early-onset hypertension; (4) low-renin hypertension; (5) hypertension with an adrenal mass; and (6) family history of aldosteronism.

For a patient to be properly tested for primary aldosteronism, certain antihypertensive medications should

ideally be held. Diuretics should be discontinued for 3 weeks. Dihydropyridine calcium channel blockers can normalize aldosterone secretion, thus interfering with the diagnosis. β-Blockers suppress PRA in patients with essential hypertension. ACE inhibitors and α-blockers are less likely to affect testing. Antihypertensive medications that have minimal effects on the plasma aldosterone:renin ratio include verapamil, hydralazine, prazosin, doxazosin, and terazosin. However, it may be impractical to hold or change antihypertensive medicines; in such cases, testing should proceed.

During the testing period, the patient should have an unrestricted high sodium intake. The patient should be out of bed for at least 2 hours and seated for 5–15 minutes before the blood draw, which should preferably be obtained between 8 am and 10 am. Renin is measured as either PRA or direct renin concentration. Serum aldosterone should ideally be measured with a tandem mass spectrometry assay.

For patients who have not been receiving diuretics for at least 3 weeks, a plasma renin that is normal or elevated makes primary aldosteronism very unlikely. However, a low plasma renin is insufficient to establish the presence of primary aldosteronism, since many patients with essential hypertension have low plasma renin activity. A plasma aldosterone:renin ratio is a sensitive screening test. Plasma aldosterone (ng/dL):PRA (ng/mL/h) ratios < 24 exclude primary aldosteronism, whereas ratios between 24 and 67 are suspicious and ratios > 67 are very suggestive of primary aldosteronism. Such elevated ratios are not diagnostic; rather, they indicate the need to document increased aldosterone secretion with a 24-hour urine collection. Another problem with the aldosterone:renin ratio is the use of different units and measurements. For aldosterone, 1 ng/dL converts to 27.7 pmol/L. For renin, a PRA of 1 ng/mL/h (12.8 pmol/L/min) converts to a direct renin concentration of 5.2 ng/L (8.2 mU/L).

When the aldosterone:renin ratio is high, a 24-hour urine collection is assayed for aldosterone, free cortisol, and creatinine. A low PRA (< 5 mcg/L/h) with a urine aldosterone over 20 mcg/24 h indicates primary aldosteronism.

Once primary aldosteronism is diagnosed, unilateral adrenal aldosteronism may be distinguished from bilateral adrenal aldosteronism by adrenal vein sampling (see below) and by further biochemical testing. Plasma may be assayed for 18-hydroxycorticosterone; a level > 100 ng/dL is seen with adrenal neoplasms, whereas levels < 100 ng/dL are nondiagnostic. In addition, a posture stimulation test may be performed, but this requires overnight hospitalization. The test is performed by drawing blood for aldosterone at 8 am while the patient is supine after overnight recumbency and again after the patient is upright for 4 hours. Patients with a unilateral adrenal adenoma usually have a baseline plasma aldosterone level > 20 ng/dL that does not rise. Patients with bilateral adrenal hyperplasia typically have a baseline plasma aldosterone level < 20 ng/dL that rises during upright posture. The accuracy of the posture stimulation test is about 85%.

C. Imaging

All patients with biochemically confirmed primary aldosteronism require a thin-section CT scan of the adrenals to screen for a rare adrenal carcinoma. In the absence of a large adrenal carcinoma, adrenal CT scanning cannot reliably distinguish unilateral from bilateral aldosterone excess, having a sensitivity of 78% and a specificity of 78% for unilateral aldosteronism. Therefore, the decision to perform a unilateral adrenalectomy should not be based solely on an adrenal CT scan. Instead, patients with primary aldosteronism should be considered for a trial of medical therapy with spironolactone or eplerenone (see below). If medical therapy is ineffective or if surgery is desired for an apparent adrenal adenoma, further evaluation for surgical candidacy should be done with laboratory testing (see above). However, since CT scanning and laboratory testing is often inconclusive, adrenal vein sampling is often required.

D. Adrenal Vein Sampling

Bilateral selective adrenal vein sampling is the most accurate way to determine whether primary aldosteronism is due to unilateral aldosterone excess, which can be treated by adrenalectomy. It is indicated only to direct the surgeon to the correct adrenal and should be performed only if surgery is contemplated. It is particularly useful for patients who are not hypokalemic, who are over age 40 years, or who have an adrenal adenoma < 1 cm diameter. It is particularly difficult to catheterize the right adrenal vein. Therefore, the venous samples are assayed for both aldosterone and cortisol during a cosyntropin ($ACTH_{1-24}$) infusion to be sure that the sampling has included both adrenal veins. The procedure has a sensitivity of 95% and a specificity of 100% but only when performed by an experienced radiologist. The complication rate is 2.5%. Risks can be minimized if the radiologist avoids adrenal venography and limits the use of contrast.

► Differential Diagnosis

The differential diagnosis of primary aldosteronism includes other causes of hypokalemia (see Chapter 21) in patients with essential hypertension, especially diuretic therapy. Chronic depletion of intravascular volume stimulates renin secretion and secondary hyperaldosteronism. Thus, it is important to discontinue diuretics and ensure adequate hydration and sodium intake when assessing a patient for primary hyperaldosteronism (see above).

Excessive ingestion of real licorice (black and derived from anise) can cause hypertension and hypokalemia. Licorice contains glycrrhizinic acid, which has a metabolite that inhibits the adrenal enzyme 11β-hydroxysteroid dehydrogenase, thereby blocking the production of cortisol and causing accumulation of the precursor mineralocorticoid deoxycorticosterone. Oral contraceptives may increase aldosterone secretion in some patients. Renal vascular disease can cause severe hypertension with hypokalemia; PRA is high, distinguishing it from primary aldosteronism.

Excessive adrenal secretion of other corticosteroids (besides aldosterone) may also cause hypertension with hypokalemia. This occurs with certain congenital adrenal enzyme disorders such as P450c11 deficiency (increased deoxycorticosterone with virilization and deficient cortisol) or P450c17 deficiency (increased deoxycorticosterone, corticosterone, and progesterone but deficient estradiol and testosterone). P450c17 deficiency results from a defect in the 17-hydroxylase enzyme in both the adrenal and ovarian steroidogenic pathways. Presenting signs include hypertension and ambiguous genitalia or primary amenorrhea. Urinary aldosterone secretion is less than 20 mcg/24 h and plasma renin is low in both P450c11 and P450c17 deficiencies. Primary cortisol resistance can cause hypertension and hypokalemia; renin and aldosterone are suppressed, while plasma levels of cortisol, ACTH, and deoxycorticosterone are high. Liddle syndrome is an autosomal dominant cause of hypertension and hypokalemia resulting from excessive sodium absorption from the renal tubule; renin and aldosterone levels are low. Thyrotoxicosis and familial periodic paralysis may also present with hypokalemia. Hyperaldosteronism may rarely be due to a malignant ovarian tumor.

► Complications

The incidence of cardiovascular complications from hypertension are higher in primary aldosteronism than in idiopathic hypertension. Following unilateral adrenalectomy for Conn syndrome, suppression of the contralateral adrenal may result in temporary postoperative hypoaldosteronism, characterized by hyperkalemia and hypotension.

► Treatment

Conn syndrome (unilateral aldosterone-secreting adrenal adenoma) is treated by laparoscopic adrenalectomy, though long-term therapy with spironolactone or eplerenone is an option. Bilateral adrenal hyperplasia is best treated with spironolactone or eplerenone. Spironolactone also has anti-androgen activity and frequently causes breast tenderness, gynecomastia, or reduced libido; it is given at initial doses of 12.5–25 mg once daily. Eplerenone is becoming favored for men since it does not have anti-androgen effects; it is usually given at an initial dose of 25 mg twice daily. Eplerenone is metabolized by hepatic CYP 3A4 and drugs that inhibit or compete for this enzyme may increase serum eplerenone levels excessively. Blood pressure must be monitored daily when beginning these anti-mineralocorticoid medications; significant drops in blood pressure have occurred when these drugs are added to other antihypertensives. Other antihypertensive drugs may also be required. Glucocorticoid-remediable aldosteronism is very rare but may respond well to suppression with low-dose dexamethasone.

► Prognosis

The hypertension is reversible in about two-thirds of cases but persists or returns in spite of surgery in the remainder. The prognosis is much improved by early diagnosis and treatment. Only 2% of aldosterone-secreting adrenal tumors are malignant.

Funder JW et al. Case detection, diagnosis, and treatment of patients with primary aldosteronism: an Endocrine Society clinical practice guideline. J Clin Endocrinol Metab. 2008 Sep;93(9):3266–81. [PMID: 18552288]

White ML et al. The role of radiologic studies in the evaluation and management of primary hyperaldosteronism. Surgery. 2008 Dec;144(6):926–33. [PMID: 19040999]

PHEOCHROMOCYTOMA & PARAGANGLIOMA

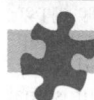 ESSENTIALS OF DIAGNOSIS

► "Attacks" of headache, perspiration, palpitations, anxiety.

► Hypertension, frequently sustained but often paroxysmal, especially during surgery or delivery.

► Elevated urinary catecholamines or their metabolites. Normal serum T_4 and TSH.

► General Considerations

Both pheochromocytomas and non–head-neck paragangliomas are tumors of the sympathetic nervous system. Pheochromocytomas arise from the adrenal medulla and usually secrete both epinephrine and norepinephrine. Paragangliomas ("extra-adrenal pheochromocytomas") arise from sympathetic paraganglia, often metastasize, and secrete norepinephrine or are nonsecretory. Excessive levels of norepinephrine or neuropeptide Y cause hypertension, while epinephrine causes tachyarrhythmias. These tumors may be located in either or both adrenals or anywhere along the sympathetic nervous chain, and rarely in such aberrant locations as the mediastinum, heart, or bladder.

These rare tumors are deceptive and deadly. They are a rare cause of hypertension, being found in less than 0.3% of hypertensive individuals. The incidence is higher in patients with moderate to severe hypertension. About two to three new cases per million population are diagnosed annually. However, in autopsy cases, the incidence of pheochromocytoma is 250–1300 cases per million, indicating that most cases are not diagnosed during life.

About 25% of patients with pheochromocytomas/paragangliomas harbor germline mutations making them prone to develop the tumor. The chance of harboring a germline mutation is nearly 100% in patients with a family history of pheochromocytomas/paragangliomas and 17% in patients without any known family history of pheochromocytomas/paragangliomas.

Pheochromocytomas develop in about 20% of patients with type 2 von Hippel–Lindau (VHL) disease (hemangiomas of the retina, cerebellum, brainstem, and spinal cord; hyperparathyroidism; pancreatic cysts; endolymphatic sac tumors; cystadenomas of the adnexa or epididymis; renal cysts, adenomas, and carcinomas); inheritance is autosomal dominant. Patients with VHL develop pheochromocytomas that are less likely to be malignant or extra-adrenal,

more likely to be bilateral, and more likely to present at an early age. Pheochromocytomas that arise in patients with VHL secrete exclusively norepinephrine and its metabolite normetanephrine. Therefore, individuals who carry type 2 VHL mutations should be screened for pheochromocytoma with plasma normetanephrine levels.

MEN 2A is associated with pheochromocytomas and medullary thyroid carcinoma. *MEN 2B* is associated with pheochromocytomas, aggressive medullary thyroid carcinoma, mucosal neuromas, and marfinoid habitus. *von Recklinghausen neurofibromatosis type 1 (NF-1)* is associated with an increased risk of pheochromocytomas/paragangliomas as well as cutaneous neurofibromas, optic gliomas, vascular anomalies, hamartomas, malignant nerve sheath tumors, and smooth-bordered café au lait spots. *Familial paraganglioma* can be caused by mutations in the genes encoding succinate dehydrogenase (SDH) subunits B, C, or D. Patients with such germline mutations are more apt to have bilateral pheochromocytomas or multicentric paragangliomas.

► Clinical Findings

A. Symptoms and Signs

Pheochromocytomas can be lethal unless they are diagnosed and treated appropriately. They typically cause attacks or "paroxysms" that can be spontaneous or triggered by exercise, bending, lifting, emotional stress, surgery, or minor procedures. Certain drugs can precipitate attacks: monoamine oxidase (MAO) inhibitors, caffeine, nicotine, decongestants, amphetamines, cocaine, ionic intravenous contrast, and epinephrine. Bladder paragangliomas may present with paroxysms during micturation. Paroxysms typically produce hypertension and symptoms such as severe headache (80%), perspiration (70%), and palpitations (60%); other symptoms may include anxiety (50%), a sense of impending doom, or tremor (40%). Vasomotor changes during an attack cause mottled cyanosis and facial pallor; as the attack subsides, facial flushing may occur as a result of reflex vasodilation. Epinephrine secretion by an adrenal pheochromocytoma may cause episodic tachyarrhythmias, hypotension, or even syncope. Acute coronary syndrome can be caused by coronary vasoconstriction. Confusion, psychosis, seizures, transient ischemic attacks, or stroke may occur with cerebrovascular vasoconstriction or hemorrhagic stroke. Aortic aneurysms may dissect and rupture. Abdominal pain, nausea, vomiting, and even ischemic bowel can be due to splanchnic vasoconstriction. Large or hemorrhagic abdominal tumors can also cause abdominal pain. Peripheral vasoconstriction can cause Raynaud phenomenon or even gangrene. Patients may experience nervousness and irritability, increased appetite, and loss of weight. Other patients have pulmonary edema and heart failure due to cardiomyopathy. Cytokine release can cause nephrotic syndrome or acute respiratory distress syndrome (ARDS). Other manifestations can include hyperglycemia, bradycardia, constipation, and paresthesias.

Physical findings usually include hypertension (90% of patients), which may be sustained (20% of patients), sustained with paroxysms (50% of patients), or paroxysmal only (25% of patients). Postural changes in blood pressure and pulse are often encountered, with blood pressure decreasing and pulse increasing (change of > 20 beats/min) after arising from a supine to a standing position. There may be cardiac enlargement and cardiomyopathy. Fever and elevation of basal body temperature can occur. Retinal hemorrhage or cerebrovascular hemorrhage occurs occasionally. Although most patients are symptomatic, some patients are normotensive and asymptomatic, particularly when the tumor is nonsecretory or discovered at an early stage.

Catastrophic hypertensive crisis and fatal cardiac arrhythmias can occur spontaneously or may be triggered by intravenous contrast dye or glucagon injection, needle biopsy of the mass, anesthesia, and surgical procedures.

In addition to catecholamines and their metabolites, pheochromocytomas secrete a wide range of other peptides that can sometimes cause symptoms of Cushing syndrome (ACTH), erythrocytosis (erythropoietin), or hypercalcemia (PTHrP).

B. Laboratory Findings

Plasma fractionated free metanephrines is the single most sensitive test for secretory pheochromocytomas and paragangliomas. Normal levels rule out pheochromocytoma and paraganglioma with some certainty and the work-up can usually end there. However, misleading elevations in metanephrines or normetanephrines can be caused by factors such as physical or emotional stress, sleep apnea, and MAO inhibitors. Therefore, patients with elevated plasma metanephrines or normetanephrines levels require further evaluation.

Assay of urinary fractionated metanephrines and creatinine effectively confirms most pheochromocytomas that were detected by elevated plasma fractionated metanephrines. A 24-hour urine specimen is usually obtained, although an overnight or shorter collection may be used; patients with pheochromocytomas generally have more that 2.2 mcg of total metanephrine per milligram of creatinine, and more than 135 mcg total catecholamines per gram creatinine. Urinary assay for total metanephrines is about 97% sensitive for detecting functioning pheochromocytomas. Urinary assay for vanillylmandelic acid (VMA) is about 89% sensitive and is not usually required.

Some drugs and foods can interfere with certain assays for catecholamines, and stresses can also cause misleading elevations in catecholamine excretion (Table 26–12). About 10% of hypertensive patients have a misleadingly elevated level of one or more tests.

Direct assay of epinephrine and norepinephrine in blood and urine during or following an attack is a sensitive test for pheochromocytoma associated with paroxysmal hypertension. Plasma free metanephrine concentrations may also be used. Proper, quiet collection of plasma specimens is essential.

Serum chromogranin A is elevated in 90% of patients with pheochromocytoma and the levels correlate with tumor size, being higher in patients with metastatic disease. Serum chromogranin A levels can be misleadingly elevated in patients with azotemia or hypergastrinemia, and in those treated with corticosteroids or proton pump

Table 26–12. Factors potentially causing misleading catecholamine results: High-performance liquid chromatography with electrochemical detection (HPLC-ECD).

Drugs	Foods	Conditions
Acetaminophen[2]	Bananas[1]	Amyotrophic lateral sclerosis[1]
Aldomet[2]	Caffeine[1]	Brain lesions[1]
Amphetamines[1]	Coffee[2]	Carcinoid[1]
Bronchodilators[1]	Peppers[2]	Eclampsia[1]
Buspirone[2]		Emotion, severe[1]
Captopril[2]		Exercise, vigorous[1]
Cocaine[1]		Guillain-Barré syndrome[1]
Cimetidine[2]		Hypoglycemia[1]
Codeine[2]		Kidney disease[3]
Decongestants[1]		Lead poisoning[1]
Ephedrine[1]		Myocardial infarct, acute[1]
Fenfluramine[3]		Pain, severe[1]
Isoproterenol[1]		Porphyria, acute[1]
Levodopa[2]		Psychosis, acute[1]
Labetalol[1,2]		Quadriplegia[1]
Mandelamine[2]		Sleep apnea
Metoclopramide[2]		
Nitroglycerin[1]		
Phenoxybenzamine		
Tricyclic anti-depressants		
Viloxazine[2]		

[1]Increases catecholamine excretion.
[2]May cause confounding peaks on HPLC chromatograms.
[3]Decreases catecholamine excretion.

inhibitors. Serum may also be assayed for neuron-specific enolase; high levels implicate a malignant pheochromocytoma, while normal levels are nonspecific.

Pharmacologic provocative and suppressive tests that evaluate the rise or fall in blood pressure are usually not required or recommended.

Hyperglycemia is present in about 35% of patients but is usually mild. Leukocytosis is common. The ESR is sometimes elevated. PRA may be increased by catecholamines.

Genetic testing should ideally be performed on all patients with pheochromocytoma or paraganglioma. Testing for VHL, *ret* protooncogene, and SDHB/SDHD mutations is advisable. Family members may then be screened for the specific gene mutation.

C. Imaging

1. CT and MRI scanning—Imaging should not usually replace biochemical testing, since incidental adrenal adenomas are common (2–4% of scans) and can be misleading. When a pheochromocytoma is suspected because of biochemical testing or a genetic condition predisposing to pheochromocytoma, a CT scan of the abdomen is performed, with thin sections through the adrenals. *A noncontrast CT should be followed by a CT scan using nonionic contrast, which reduces the risk of catecholamine release from a pheochromocytoma and a hypertensive crisis.* Glucagon should not be used during scanning, since it can provoke hypertensive crisis; similarly, intravenous contrast can precipitate hypertensive crisis, particularly in patients whose hypertension is uncontrolled.

MRI scanning has the advantage of not requiring intravenous contrast dye; its lack of radiation makes it the imaging of choice during pregnancy and childhood. Both CT and MRI scanning have a sensitivity of about 90% for adrenal pheochromocytoma and a sensitivity of 95% for adrenal tumors over 0.5 cm in diameter. However, both CT and MRI are less sensitive for detecting recurrent tumors, metastases, and extra-adrenal paragangliomas. If no adrenal tumor is found, the scan is extended to include the entire abdomen, pelvis, and chest.

2. Nuclear imaging—A whole-body [^{123}I]m-Iodobenzylguanidine (^{123}I-MIBG) scan can localize tumors with a sensitivity of 85% and a specificity of 99%. It is less sensitive for MEN 2A- or MEN 2B-related pheochromocytomas. Preoperative ^{123}I-MIBG scanning is not usually required to confirm that a unilateral adrenal mass is a pheochromocytoma in a patient with classic clinical and biochemical presentation. Preoperative whole-body ^{123}I-MIBG scanning can be useful when the CT scan cannot locate a suspected pheochromocytoma, making a paraganglioma more likely; it can also be useful when the CT scan is ambiguous for pheochromocytoma. It is prudent to perform a whole-body ^{123}I-MIBG scan about 3 months postoperatively to determine if metastatic or recurrent tumor is present. Drugs that reduce ^{123}I-MIBG uptake should be avoided, including tricyclic antidepressants and cyclobenzaprine (6 weeks), amphetamines, nasal decongestants, phenothiazines, haloperidol, diet pills, labetalol, and cocaine (2 weeks).

Somatostatin receptor imaging using ^{111}In-labeled octreotide is only 25% sensitive for detecting an adrenal pheochromocytoma. However, ^{111}In-labeled octreotide scanning is quite sensitive for detecting extra-adrenal pheochromocytomas (paragangliomas) and metastatic pheochromocytomas, sometimes locating tumors that were missed by ^{123}I-MIBG scanning.

PET scanning usually detects tumors using ^{18}F-labeled deoxyglucose (^{18}FDG-PET) or ^{18}F-labeled dopamine (^{18}FDA-PET), and may demonstrate tumors that are not visible on ^{123}I-MIBG scanning. Combining PET scan with noncontrast CT produces a PET/CT fusion scan with exceptional sensitivity.

Differential Diagnosis

Pheochromocytoma may be misdiagnosed as thyrotoxicosis, essential hypertension, myocarditis, glomerulonephritis or other renal lesions, toxemia of pregnancy, eclampsia, and psychoneurosis (anxiety attack). It can sometimes be mistaken for an acute abdomen.

Conditions that have manifestations similar to those of pheochromocytoma include the following: essential labile hypertension, renal hypertension, anxiety attacks, thyrotoxicosis, toxemia of pregnancy, acute intermittent porphyria, hypogonadal vascular instability (hot flushes), cocaine or amphetamine use, and clonidine withdrawal. Patients taking nonselective MAO inhibitor antidepressants can have hypertensive crisis after eating foods that contain tyramine (eg, fermented cheeses, aged wines, certain beers, fava beans, vegemite, marmite). Patients with erythromelalgia can have hypertensive crises; their episodic painful flushing and leg swelling are relieved by cold, distinguishing this condition from pheochromocytoma. Pheochromocytomas can cause chest pain and ECG changes that mimic acute cardiac ischemia. Renal artery stenosis can cause severe hypertension and may coexist with pheochromocytoma.

False-positive testing for catecholamines and metabolites occurs in about 10% of hypertensives, but levels are usually less than 50% above normal and typically normalize with repeat testing.

▶ Complications

All of the complications of severe hypertension may be encountered. In addition, a catecholamine-induced cardiomyopathy may develop. Severe heart failure and cardiovascular collapse may develop in patients during a paroxysm. Sudden death may occur due to cardiac arrhythmia. ARDS has been reported. Hypertensive crises with sudden blindness or cerebrovascular accidents are not uncommon. Paroxysms may be precipitated by sudden movement, by manipulation during or after pregnancy, by emotional stress or trauma, or during surgical removal of the tumor. Decongestant medications, fluoxetine, and other selective serotonin reuptake inhibitors may induce hypertensive paroxysms and death. Occasionally, the initial manifestation of pheochromocytoma may be hypotension or even shock.

After removal of the tumor, a state of severe hypotension and shock (resistant to epinephrine and norepinephrine) may ensue with precipitation of kidney disease or myocardial infarction. Hypotension and shock may occur from spontaneous infarction or hemorrhage of the tumor.

On rare occasions, a patient dies as a result of the complications of diagnostic tests or during surgery. During surgery, pheochromocytoma cells may be seeded within the peritoneum, resulting in multifocal recurrent tumors.

▶ Medical Treatment

Patients must receive adequate treatment for hypertension and tachyarrhythmias prior to surgery for pheochromocytoma/paraganglioma. Patients are advised to use a portable sphyngomanometer and measure their blood pressures daily and immediately during paroxysms.

α-Blockers (prazocin or phenoxybenzamine) are typically administered preparatory to surgery. Many surgeons insist upon α-blockade preoperatively. Phenoxybenzamine is given initially in a dosage of 10 mg orally every 12 hours, increasing gradually—about every 3 days—until hypertension is controlled. Maintenance doses range from 10 mg/d to 120 mg/d. Optimal α-blockade is achieved when supine arterial pressure is below 140/90 mm Hg or as low as possible for the patient to have a standing arterial pressure above 80/45 mm Hg.

Calcium channel blockers (nifedipine ER or nicardipine ER) are very effective and may be used with or without α-blockers. They are superior to phenoxybenzamine for long-term use, since they cause less fatigue, nasal congestion, and orthostatic hypotension. For acute hypertensive crisis (systolic blood pressure > 170 mm Hg) a nifedipine 10-mg capsule may be chewed and swallowed. Nifedipine is quite successful for treating acute hypertension in patients with pheochromocytoma/paraganglioma, even at home; it is reasonably safe as long as the blood pressure is monitored.

β-**Blockers** (eg, metoprolol XL) are required by most patients after institution of α-blockade or calcium channel blockade. The use of a β-blocker as initial antihypertensive therapy has resulted in "unopposed alpha" that causes paradoxical worsening of hypertension. Labetalol has combined α- and β-blocking activity and is an effective agent but can cause paradoxical hypertension if used as the initial antihypertensive agent. Labetalol can also interfere with catecholamine determinations in some laboratories and reduces the tumor's uptake-1, such that it must be discontinued for at least 4–7 days before diagnostic scanning with ^{123}I-MIBG or [18]FDA-PET or ^{131}I-MIBG therapy.

Surgical Treatment

Surgical removal of pheochromocytomas or abdominal paragangliomas is the treatment of choice. For surgery, a team approach—endocrinologist, anesthesiologist, and surgeon—is critically important. Laparoscopic surgery is preferred, but large and invasive tumors require open laparotomy. Patients with small familial or bilateral pheochromocytomas may undergo selective resection of the tumors, sparing the adrenal cortex; however, there is a recurrence rate of 10% over 10 years.

Prior to surgery, blood pressure control should be maintained for a minimum of 4–7 days or until optimal cardiac status is established. The ECG should be monitored until it becomes stable. (It may take a week or even months to correct ECG changes in patients with catecholamine myocarditis, and it may be prudent to defer surgery until then in such cases.) Patients must be very closely monitored during surgery to promptly detect sudden changes in blood pressure or cardiac arrhythmias.

Intraoperative severe hypertension is managed with continuous intravenous nicardipine (a short-acting calcium channel blocker), 2–6 mcg/kg/min, or nitroprusside, 0.5–10 mcg/kg/min. Prolonged nitroprusside administration can cause cyanide toxicity. Tachyarrhythmia is treated with intravenous atenolol (1 mg boluses), esmolol, or lidocaine.

Autotransfusion of 1–2 units of blood at 12 hours preoperatively plus generous intraoperative volume replacement reduces the risk of postresection hypotension caused by desensitization of the vascular $α_1$-receptors. Shock may therefore occur following removal of the pheochromocytoma. It is treated with intravenous saline or colloid and high doses of intravenous norepinephrine. Intravenous 5% dextrose is infused postoperatively to prevent hypoglycemia.

Surgical histopathology for pheochromocytoma/paraganglioma cannot reliably determine whether a tumor is malignant. Therefore, all pheochromocytomas and paragangliomas must be approached as possibly malignant. Even if no metastases are visible at the time of surgery, patients require lifetime follow-up. Therefore, it is essential to recheck plasma fractionated metanephrine levels postoperatively, at least 2–4 weeks after surgery and when the patient has minimal residual pain. It is also prudent to perform a whole-body [123]I mIBG scan about 3 months postoperatively, since previously undetected metastases may become visible. Thereafter, blood pressure and symptoms must be rechecked regularly for life; plasma fractionated metanephrines are also rechecked regularly, at least every 6 months for 5 years, and immediately if hypertension or symptoms recur or if metastases become evident.

For inoperable or metastatic tumors, metyrosine reduces catecholamine synthesis; the initial dosage is 250 mg four times daily, increased daily by increments of 250–500 mg to a maximum of 4 g/d. Metyrosine causes central nervous system side effects and crystalluria; hydration must be ensured. Metastatic pheochromocytomas may be treated with combination chemotherapy (eg, cyclophosphamide, vincristine, and dacarbazine) or with high doses of ^{131}I-MIBG.

Prognosis

The malignancy of a pheochromocytoma cannot be determined by histologic examination. A tumor is considered malignant if metastases are present; this may take many years to become clinically evident. Therefore, lifetime surveillance is required. Malignancy is more likely for paragangliomas and for large pheochromocytomas (> 7 cm in diameter). The prognosis is good for patients with smaller, benign pheochromocytomas that are resected before causing cardiovascular damage. Hypertension usually resolves after successful surgery but may persist or return in 25% of patients despite successful surgery. Although this may be essential hypertension, biochemical reevaluation is then required, looking for a second or metastatic pheochromocytoma.

Before the advent of blocking agents, the surgical mortality rate was as high as 30%, but this has rapidly decreased. With optimal management, the surgical mortality rate is less than 3%.

Patients with metastatic pheochromocytoma and paraganglioma have a 5-year survival rate of 44% after surgery; patients who have their primary tumor resected and subsequently receive high-dose [131]I mIBG therapy have been reported to have a 5-year survival rate of 75%. Patients with a heavy and increasing tumor burden and distant metastases have a worse prognosis; patients with multiple pulmonary metastases have limited survival. Those with metastases limited to the abdomen have a better prognosis. Some patients have an indolent malignancy and experience a prolonged survival.

Amar L et al. Succinate dehydrogenase B gene mutations predict survival in patients with malignant pheochromocytomas or paragangliomas. J Clin Endocrinol Metab. 2007 Oct;92(10):3822–8. [PMID: 17652212]

Fitzgerald PA et al. Malignant pheochromocytomas and paragangliomas: a phase II study of therapy with high-dose ^{131}I-metaiodobenzylguanidine (^{131}I-MIBG). Ann N Y Acad Sci. 2006 Aug;1073:465–90. [PMID: 17102115]

Lee JA et al. Adrenal incidentaloma, borderline elevations of urine or plasma metanephrine levels, and the "subclinical" pheochromocytoma. Arch Surg. 2007 Sep;142(9):870–3. [PMID: 17875842]

Pacak K. Preoperative management of the pheochromocytoma patient. J Clin Endocrinol Metab. 2007 Nov;92(11):4069–79. [PMID: 17989126]

PANCREATIC & DUODENAL NEUROENDOCRINE TUMORS*

ISLET CELL TUMORS

 ESSENTIALS OF DIAGNOSIS

▸ Half the tumors are nonsecretory; weight loss, abdominal pain, or jaundice may be presenting signs.

▸ Secretory tumors cause a variety of manifestations depending on the hormones secreted.

General Considerations

The pancreatic islets are composed of several types of cells, each with distinct chemical and microscopic features: the A cells (20%) secrete glucagon, the B cells (70%) secrete insulin, and the D cells (5%) secrete somatostatin or gastrin. F cells secrete "pancreatic polypeptide." Although most pancreatic and duodenal neuroendocrine tumors arise spontaneously, they may occur as part four different inherited disorders: multiple endocrine neoplasia type 1 (MEN 1), von Hippel-Lindau disease (VHL), neurofibromatosis 1 (NF-1) and the rare tuberous sclerosis complex (TSC).

Insulinomas are usually (about 82%) benign and secrete excessive amounts of insulin (as well as proinsulin and C-peptide), which causes hypoglycemia. The tumors may be multiple, especially in familial MEN 1—about 12% of cases (see Chapter 27).

Gastrinomas secrete excessive quantities of the hormone gastrin (as well as "big" gastrin), which stimulates the stomach to hypersecrete acid, thereby causing hyperplastic gastric rugae and peptic ulceration (Zollinger–Ellison syndrome). Most gastrinomas are benign, but some are malignant and metastasize to the liver. Gastrinomas are typically found in the duodenum (49%), pancreas (24%), or lymph nodes (11%). Sporadic Zollinger–Ellison syndrome is rarely suspected at the onset of symptoms; typically, there is a 5-year delay in diagnosis. About 22% of patients have MEN 1. MEN 1 usually presents in patients who are younger; hyperparathyroidism may occur from 14 years preceding the Zollinger–Ellison diagnosis to 38 years afterward. (See Multiple Endocrine Neoplasia, below.)

Glucagonomas are usually malignant; liver metastases are ordinarily present by the time of diagnosis. They usually secrete other hormones besides glucagon, often gastrin.

Somatostatinomas are very rare and are associated with weight loss, diabetes mellitus, malabsorption, and hypochlorhydria.

Other rare tumors secrete excessive amounts of **vasoactive intestinal polypeptide (VIP)**, a substance that causes profuse watery diarrhea (Verner–Morrison syndrome).

Clinical Findings

A. Symptoms and Signs

Presenting symptoms and signs of **gastrinomas** include abdominal pain (75%), diarrhea (73%), heartburn (44%), bleeding (25%), or weight loss (17%). Endoscopy usually discovers prominent gastric folds (94%).

The 5-, 10-, and 20-year survival rates with MEN 1 are 94%, 75%, and 58%, respectively, while the survival rates for sporadic Zollinger–Ellison syndrome are 62%, 50%, and 31%, respectively. (See Chapter 15.)

Initial symptoms of **glucagonoma** often include weight loss, diarrhea, nausea, peptic ulcer, or necrolytic migratory erythema. About 35% of patients ultimately develop diabetes. The median survival is 2.8 years after diagnosis.

Islet cell tumors can secrete ectopic hormones in addition to native hormones, often in combinations producing a variety of clinical syndromes. They may secrete ACTH, producing Cushing syndrome. Secretion of serotonin can produce an atypical carcinoid syndrome manifested by pain, diarrhea, and weight loss; skin flushing occurs in only 39% of patients. Pancreatic carcinoid tumors grow slowly but usually metastasize to local and distant sites, particularly to other endocrine organs.

Islet cell tumors may be part of the syndrome of multiple endocrine adenomatosis type I (with pituitary and parathyroid adenomas).

B. Imaging

Localization of noninsulinoma pancreatic islet cell tumors and their metastases is best done with somatostatin receptor scintigraphy (SRS); SRS detects about 75% of noninsulinomas. CT and MRI are also useful. Insulinomas can usually be located preoperatively by endoscopic ultrasonography. For insulinomas, preoperative localization studies are less successful and have the following sensitivities: ultrasonography 25%, CT 25%, endoscopic ultrasonography 27%, transhepatic portal vein sampling 40%, arteriography 45%, intraoperative palpation 55%, and intraoperative pancreatic ultrasound 75%. Nearly all insulinomas can be successfully located at surgery by intraoperative palpation and ultrasound. An abdominal CT scan is usually obtained, but extensive preoperative localization procedures, especially with invasive methods, are not required. Tumors may be located in the pancreatic head or neck (57%), body (15%), or tail (19%) or in the duodenum (9%).

Treatment

Direct resection of the tumor (or tumors), which often spreads locally, is the primary form of therapy for all types of islet cell neoplasm except Zollinger–Ellison syndrome, where use of high doses of a proton pump inhibitor is the therapy of choice (quadruple the usual doses). Note that serum gastrin levels tend to be high in any patient who is taking a proton pump inhibitor; hypercalcemia also stimulates gastrin release. Insulinomas are resected. However, in MEN 1, insulinomas are rarely cured, so surgery is reserved for dominant masses in such cases. Palliation of

---

*Diabetes mellitus and hyperglycemia are discussed in Chapter 27.

functioning malignant disease often requires both antihormonal and anticancer chemotherapy. The use of streptozocin, doxorubicin, and asparaginase, especially for malignant insulinoma, has produced some encouraging results, though these drugs are quite toxic (see Table 39–11). The hypoglycemia of insulinoma may be counteracted by verapamil or diazoxide. Octreotide LAR is useful in the therapy of islet cell tumors with the exception of insulinoma; monthly subcutaneous injections of 20–30 mg are required. Treatment with octreotide improves the symptoms of **VIP** but does not halt tumor growth. Symptomatic improvement with calcitonin treatment has also been reported.

The prognosis in these neoplasms is variable. The surgical complication rate is about 40%, with patients commonly developing fistulas and infections. Extensive pancreatic resection may cause diabetes mellitus. The overall 5-year survival is higher with functional tumors (77%) than with nonfunctional ones (55%) and higher with benign tumors (91%) than with malignant ones (55%).

Baldelli R et al. Malignant insulinoma presenting as metastatic liver tumor. Case report and review of the literature. J Exp Clin Cancer Res. 2007 Dec;26(4):603–7. [PMID: 18365560]

Cisco RM et al. Surgery for gastrinoma. Adv Surg. 2007;41:165–76. [PMID: 17972563]

Jani N et al. Pancreatic endocrine tumors. Gastroenterol Clin North Am. 2007 Jun;36(2):431–9. [PMID: 17533088]

Jensen RT et al. Inherited pancreatic endocrine tumor syndromes: advances in molecular pathogenesis, diagnosis, management, and controversies. Cancer. 2008 Oct;113(7 Suppl):1807–43. [PMID: 18798544]

DISEASES OF THE TESTES & MALE BREAST

MALE HYPOGONADISM

 ESSENTIALS OF DIAGNOSIS

▶ Diminished libido and erections.

▶ Decreased growth of body hair.

▶ Testes may be small or normal in size. Serum testosterone is usually decreased.

▶ Serum gonadotropins (LH and FSH) are decreased in hypogonadotropic hypogonadism; they are increased in testicular failure (hypergonadotropic hypogonadism).

▶ General Considerations

Male hypogonadism is caused by deficient testosterone secretion by the testes. It may be classified according to whether it is due to (1) insufficient gonadotropin secretion by the pituitary (hypogonadotropic) or (2) pathology in the testes themselves (hypergonadotropic) (Table 26–13).

Table 26–13. Causes of male hypogonadism.

Hypogonadotropic (Low or Normal LH)	Hypergonadotropic (High LH)
Alcohol	Antitumor chemotherapy
Chronic illness	Bilateral anorchia
Congenital syndromes	Idiopathic
Constitutional delay	Klinefelter syndrome
Cushing syndrome	Leprosy
Drugs	Lymphoma
Estrogen-secreting tumors (testicular, adrenal)	Male climacteric
GnRH agonist (leuprolide)	Mumps
Hemochromatosis	Myotonic dystrophy
Hypopituitarism	Noonan syndrome
Hypothyroidism	Orchitis
Idiopathic	Radiation therapy
Kallmann syndrome	Sertoli cell-only syndrome
Ketoconazole	Testicular trauma
17-Ketosteroid reductase deficiency	Tuberculosis
Malnourishment	Uremia
Marijuana	
Obesity (BMI > 40)	
Prader-Willi syndrome	
Prior androgens	
Spironolactone	

BMI, body mass index; GnRH, gonadotropin-releasing hormone; LH, luteinizing hormone.

▶ Etiology

A. Hypogonadotropic Hypogonadism

A deficiency in FSH and LH may be isolated or associated with other pituitary hormonal abnormalities. (See Hypopituitarism.) Patients must be evaluated for signs of Cushing syndrome or adrenal insufficiency, growth hormone excess or deficiency, and thyroid hormone excess or deficiency.

Acquired hypogonadotropic hypogonadism may be due to pituitary or hypothalamic factors but may be idiopathic. Hyperprolactinemia (see Table 26–2) may also induce hypogonadism.

Hypogonadotropic hypogonadism can develop in men receiving GnRH agonist therapy for prostate cancer and can persist following cessation of therapy.

B. Hypergonadotropic Hypogonadism

A failure in testicular secretion of testosterone causes a rise in LH. If testicular Sertoli cell function is deficient, FSH will be elevated. Conditions that can cause testicular failure include viral infection (eg, mumps), irradiation, cancer chemotherapy, autoimmunity, myotonic dystrophy, uremia, XY gonadal dysgenesis, partial 17-ketosteroid reductase deficiency, Klinefelter syndrome, and male climacteric.

Klinefelter syndrome (47,XXY and its variants) is the most common chromosomal abnormality among males, with an incidence of about 1:500. It is caused by the expression of an abnormal karyotype, classically 47,XXY. Other forms are common, eg, 46,XY/47,XXY mosaicism, 48,XXYY, 48,XXXY, or 46,XX males.

The manifestations of Klinefelter syndrome are variable. Testes feel normal during childhood, but during adolescence they usually become firm, fibrotic, small, and nontender to palpation. Although puberty occurs at the normal time, the degree of virilization is variable. About 85% of patients have some gynecomastia at puberty.

Other common findings include tall stature and abnormal body proportions that are unusual for hypogonadal men (height greater than arm span; crown-pubis length greater than pubis-floor). Patients with multiple X or Y chromosomes are more apt to have mental deficiency and other abnormalities such as clinodactyly or synostosis. They may also exhibit problems with coordination and social skills. Other problems include a higher incidence of breast cancer, chronic pulmonary disease, varicosities of the legs, and diabetes mellitus (8% of patients); impaired glucose tolerance occurs in an additional 19% of patients.

On semen analysis, most men (about 95%) with classic Klinfelter syndrome have azoospermia, but men with 46,XY/47,XXY mosaicism may have spontaneous fertility. Also, testicular biopsy reveals sperm in up to 50% of affected patients, allowing some of them to be fertile with the use of in vitro fertilization using intracytoplasmic sperm injection (ICSI). The diagnosis is confirmed by karyotyping or by determining the presence of RNA for X-inactive-specific transcriptase (XIST) in peripheral blood leukocytes by polymerase chain reaction.

All causes of gynecomastia (see Table 26–14) must be differentiated from Klinefelter syndrome.

C. Androgen Insensitivity

Partial resistance to testosterone is a rare condition in which phenotypic males have variable degrees of apparent hypogonadism, hypospadias, cryptorchism, and gynecomastia. Serum testosterone levels are normal.

▶ Clinical Findings

A. Symptoms and Signs

Hypogonadism that is congenital or acquired during childhood presents as delayed puberty. Men with acquired hypogonadism have variable manifestations. Most men experience decreased libido. Others complain of erectile dysfunction, hot sweats, fatigue, or depression. Their presenting complaint may also be infertility, gynecomastia, headache, fracture, or other symptoms related to the cause or result of the hypogonadism. The patient's history often gives a clue to the cause (Table 26–13).

Physical signs associated with hypogonadism may include decreased body, axillary, beard, or pubic hair; such diminished sexual hair growth is not reliably present except after years of severe hypogonadism. Men in whom hypogonadism develops tend to lose muscle mass and gain weight due to an increase in subcutaneous fat. Examination should include measurements of arm span and height. Testicular size should be assessed with an orchidometer (normal volume is about 10–25 mL; normal length is usually over 6 cm). Testicular size may decrease but usually remains within the normal range in men with postpubertal

Table 26–14. Causes of gynecomastia.

Idiopathic	Busulfan
	Chorionic gonadotropin
Physiologic causes	Cimetidine
Neonatal period	Clomiphene
Puberty	Cyclophosphamide
Aging	Diazepam
Obesity	Diethylstilbestrol
	Digitalis preparations
Endocrine diseases	Estrogens (oral or topical)
Androgen resistance	Ethionamide
syndromes	Finasteride
Aromatase excess syndrome	Flutamide
(sporadic or familial)	Goserelin
Diabetic lymphocytic mastitis	HAART (highly active antiret-
Hyperprolactinemia	roviral therapy)
Hyperthyroidism	Haloperidol
Klinefelter syndrome	Hydroxyzine
Male hypogonadism	Isoniazid
Partial 17-ketosteroid reduc-	Ketoconazole
tase deficiency	Leuprolide
	Marijuana
Systemic diseases	Meprobamate
Chronic liver disease	Methadone
Chronic kidney disease	Methyldopa
Neurologic disorders	Metoclopramide
Refeeding after starvation	Mirtazapine
Spinal cord injury	Molindone
	Nilutamide
Neoplasms	Omeprazole
Adrenal tumors	Opioids
Bronchogenic carcinoma	Penicillamine
Carcinoma of the breast	Phenothiazines
Hepatocellular carcinoma (rare)	Progestins
Testicular tumors	Protease inhibitors
	Reserpine
Drugs (partial list)	Risperidone
Alcohol	Somatropin (growth hormone)
Alkylating agents	Soy ingestion
Amiodarone	Spironolactone
Anabolic steroids	Testosterone
Androgens	Thioridazine
Bicalutamide	Tricyclic antidepressants

hypogonadotropic hypogonadism, but it may be diminished with testicular injury or Klinefelter syndrome. The testes must also be carefully palpated for masses, since Leydig cell tumors may secrete estrogen and present with hypogonadism. The testicles must be carefully examined for evidence of trauma, infiltrative lesions (eg, lymphoma), or ongoing infection (eg, leprosy, tuberculosis).

B. Laboratory Findings

The evaluation for hypogonadism begins with a morning serum testosterone or free testosterone measurement. Normal ranges for serum testosterone have been derived from nonfasting morning blood specimens, which tend to be the highest of the day. Later in the day, serum testosterone levels can be 25–50% lower. Therefore, a serum testosterone drawn fasting or late in the day may be misleadingly below the "normal range." Serum testosterone levels in men are highest at age 20–30 years and slightly lower at age 30–40 years; testosterone falls gradually but progressively after age 40 years. Testing for serum free testosterone is especially important for detecting hypogonadism in elderly men, who generally have high levels of SHBG. A low serum testosterone is evaluated with serum LH and FSH levels. LH and FSH tend to be high in patients with hypergonadotropic hypogonadism but low or inappropriately normal in men with hypogonadotropic hypogonadism. Patients with low gonadotropins are further evaluated for other pituitary abnormalities, including hyperprolactinemia.

Testosterone stimulates erythropoiesis in men, causing the normal red blood count range to be higher in men than in women; mild anemia is common in men with hypogonadism, with red blood counts below the normal male range. For men with long-standing male hypogonadism, bone densitometry is recommended. Men with severe osteoporosis may require treatment with bisphosphonates and vitamin D, in addition to testosterone replacement therapy. (See Osteoporosis section.)

Most radioimmunoassays and ELISA for testosterone are inaccurate below serum testosterone levels of 300 ng/dL. The more accurate testosterone assays rely upon extraction and chromatography, followed by mass spectrometry or immunoassay. Free testosterone is best measured by calculation, using accurate assays for testosterone and SHBG.

1. Hypogonadotropic hypogonadism—A serum PRL determination is obtained but may be elevated for many reasons (see Table 26–2). Men with gynecomastia may be screened for partial 17-ketosteroid reductase deficiency with serum determinations for androstenedione and estrone, which are elevated in this condition. X-linked congenital adrenal hypoplasia is a rare condition in which a *DAX-1* gene mutation causes hypogonadotropic hypogonadism and azoospermia, which usually presents in adolescence; the associated primary adrenal insufficiency usually presents in childhood, but it may remain undiagnosed into adulthood. The serum estradiol level may be elevated in patients with cirrhosis and in rare cases of estrogen-secreting tumors (testicular Leydig cell tumor or adrenal carcinoma). Men with no discernible definite cause for hypogonadotropic hypogonadism should be screened for hemochromatosis and have an MRI of the pituitary and hypothalamic region to look for a tumor or other lesion. (See Hypopituitarism.)

2. Hypergonadotropic hypogonadism—Men with hypergonadotropic hypogonadism have low serum testosterone levels with a compensatory increase in FSH and LH. Klinefelter syndrome can be confirmed by karyotyping or by measurement of leukocyte XIST. Testicular biopsy is usually reserved for younger patients in whom the reason for primary hypogonadism is unclear.

► **Treatment**

Testosterone replacement is the usual treatment for hypogonadism. It is prudent to screen older men for prostate cancer before testosterone therapy is begun. Testosterone helps reverse sexual dysfunction and muscle atrophy. Men with Klinefelter syndrome have a reduced risk of developing verbal fluency problems if testosterone therapy is begun at the time of normal puberty.

Topical testosterone gel is the preferred method for administering testosterone. Topical 1% testosterone gel is commercially available as Androgel or Testim (2.5-g and 5-g packets); Androgel is odorless, while Testim has a musky odor. The starting dose is 5 g (50 mg testosterone) applied once daily to clean, dry skin of the shoulders, upper arms, or abdomen. The skin serves as a reservoir that slowly releases about 10% of the testosterone into the blood; serum testosterone levels reach a steady state in 1–3 days. The gel should not be applied to the genitals. The entire contents of a packet are squeezed onto the palm and then immediately applied. After the application of testosterone gel, the hands should be washed. The application site should be allowed to dry for 5–10 minutes before donning a shirt to prevent the gel from rubbing off the skin. A shirt must be worn during contact with women or children to prevent transfer of testosterone to them. The serum testosterone level should be determined about 14 days after starting therapy; if the level remains below normal or the clinical response is inadequate, the daily dose may be increased to 7.5 g or 10 g.

Testosterone transdermal systems (skin patches) are available in two formulations for application to nongenital skin. Testoderm II, 5 mg/d leaves a sticky residue but causes little skin irritation. Androderm adheres more tightly to the skin but may cause more skin irritation. Both produce reliable serum levels of testosterone that are somewhat lower that those achieved with injections. The patch systems also suffer from being rather inconvenient and expensive.

Hypogonadism may also be treated with parenteral testosterone (enanthate or cypionate). The usual dose is about 300 mg intramuscularly in the gluteal area every 3 weeks or 200 mg every 2 weeks. The preparation is oil based and is usually given in the gluteal area. The dose is adjusted according to the patient's response.

Oral androgen preparations include methyltestosterone and fluoxymesterone. These oral preparations have rarely caused liver tumors or peliosis hepatis with long-term use. Cholestatic jaundice occurs in 1–2% of patients but usually remits after the medication is discontinued. The oral androgens are not as effective as parenteral testosterone.

Men with mosaic Klinefelter syndrome (eg, 46,XY/47,XXY) may be fertile. However, men with nonmosaic Klinefelter syndrome (eg, 47,XXY) are usually azoospermic; fertility may be achieved by testicular sperm retrieval and in vitro intracytoplasmic sperm injection (ICSI) into an ovum.

Testosterone replacement therapy may cause a minimal reduction in serum HDL levels and has no effect on LDL levels; testosterone therapy has never been demonstrated to increase the incidence of cardiovascular disease, myocardial infarction, or stroke.

Testosterone therapy can aggravate benign prostatic hypertrophy (BPH). However, aggravation of voiding problems is uncommon. In men with BPH, finasteride may be coadministered with testosterone to reduce prostate size. The incidence of prostate cancer does not appear to be increased by testosterone therapy. However, testosterone therapy is contraindicated in the presence of active prostate cancer. In men over age 50 years, serum prostate-specific antigen (PSA) levels should be monitored before testosterone therapy as well as each year during therapy. Hypogonadal men who have had a prostatectomy for low-grade prostate cancer, and who have remained in complete remission for several years, may have testosterone therapy given cautiously while monitoring sensitive serum PSA levels.

Erythrocytosis develops in some men who are treated with testosterone. Erythrocytosis is more common with intramuscular injections of testosterone enanthate than with transcutaneous testosterone. It is particularly common in men receiving intramuscular testosterone enanthate in doses of 200 mg intramuscularly every 2 weeks. However, no increase in the incidence of thromboembolic events has been reported.

Testosterone therapy tends to aggravate sleep apnea in older men, likely through central nervous system effects. Surveillance for sleep apnea is recommended during testosterone therapy and a formal evaluation with nocturnal pulse oximetry recording is recommended for all high-risk patients. A man's risk for sleep apnea may be approximated by determining an "adjusted neck circumference" with the following algorithm: Measure the neck circumference in centimeters; add 4 cm if the patient is hypertensive; add 3 cm if the patient snores; add 3 cm if the patient chokes or gasps most nights. Adjusted neck circumference: < 43 = low risk; 43–48 = moderate risk; > 48 = high risk.

Men who are treated with testosterone frequently experience some increase in acne, which is usually mild and tolerated; topical antiacne therapy or a reduction in testosterone replacement dosage may be required. Increases in intraocular pressure have occurred during testosterone therapy. During the initiation of testosterone replacement therapy, gynecomastia develops in some men, which usually is mild and tends to resolve spontaneously; switching from testosterone injections to testosterone transdermal gel may help this condition.

▶ Prognosis of Male Hypogonadism

If hypogonadism is due to a pituitary lesion, the prognosis is that of the primary disease (eg, tumor, necrosis). The prognosis for restoration of virility is good if testosterone is given.

Kalyani RR et al. Male hypogonadism in systemic disease. Endocrinol Metab Clin North Am. 2007 Jun;36(2):333–48. [PMID: 17543722]

Paduch DA et al. New concepts in Klinefelter syndrome. Curr Opin Urol. 2008 Nov;18(6):621–7. [PMID: 18832949]

Rosner W et al. Position statement: utility, limitations, and pitfalls in measuring testosterone: an Endocrine Society position statement. J Clin Endocrinol Metab. 2007 Feb;92(2):405–13. [PMID: 17090633]

TESTICULAR TUMORS IN ADULTS
(See Also Chapter 39)

About 95% of testicular tumors are germ cell tumors (seminomas or nonseminomas). Seminomas do not pro-duce α-fetoprotein, but about 5–10% produce some hCG. Nonseminomas, on the other hand, produce increased serum levels of one or both of these markers in about 90% of cases. Men with liver disease may have misleadingly high levels of α-fetoprotein. Most germ cell tumors are sensitive to cisplatin-based combined chemotherapy. Sperm banking is advised.

About 5% of testicular tumors are Leydig or Sertoli cell tumors. Leydig cell tumors tend to produce estrogen (75%) and cause gynecomastia and impotence on that basis; they may sometimes produce androgens that can cause pseudoprecocious puberty in boys. Sertoli cell tumors may also produce estrogen (30%) with feminization; gynecomastia may be due to hCG secretion (25%).

Some testicular tumors may be small and nonpalpable yet may secrete sufficient amounts of hCG or estrogen to cause gynecomastia or impotence. Testicular ultrasound may help reveal small tumors.

After unilateral orchiectomy for testicular cancer, an elevated FSH level prior to further treatment indicates a patient at higher risk for cancer in the remaining testis.

CRYPTORCHISM

One or both testes may be absent from the scrotum at birth in about 20% of premature or low-birth-weight male infants and in 3–6% at full term infants. Cryptorchism is found in 1–2% of males after 1 year of age but must be distinguished from retractile testes, which require no treatment. Cryptorchism should be corrected before age 12–24 months in an attempt to reduce the risk of infertility, which occurs in up to 75% of men with bilateral cryptorchism and in 50% of men with unilateral cryptorchism. It is not clear, however, whether such early orchiopexy improves ultimate fertility. Some patients have underlying hypogonadism.

The ultimate incidence of significant testicular neoplasia is about 0.002% in normal males, 0.06% in cryptorchid males, and up to 5% in patients with intra-abdominal testes.

If the testes are not palpable, ultrasound or MRI can be used to locate them. Alternatively, hCG, 1500 units intramuscularly daily for 3 days, causes a significant rise in testosterone if the testes are present. Therapy with hCG results in a testicular descent rate of about 25%.

Orchiopexy decreases the risk of neoplasia when performed before 10 years of age. Orchiectomy after puberty is an option for intra-abdominal testes.

Thorsson AV et al. Efficacy and safety of hormonal treatment of cryptorchidism: current state of the art. Acta Paediatr. 2007 May;96(5):628–30. [PMID: 17462056]

Thorup J et al. Surgical treatment of undescended testes. Acta Paediatr. 2007 May;96(5):631–7. [PMID: 1738147]

GYNECOMASTIA

ESSENTIALS OF DIAGNOSIS

▶ Enlargement of the male breast, often asymmetric or unilateral.

- Glandular gynecomastia characterized by tenderness.
- Fatty gynecomastia typically nontender.
- Must be distinguished from tumors or mastitis.

General Considerations

Gynecomastia refers to a female-appearing male breast. Pubertal gynecomastia is common and the swelling usually subsides spontaneously within a year. Gynecomastia is particularly common in teenagers who are very tall or overweight. Gynecomastia develops in about 50% of athletes who abuse androgens and anabolic steroids. It is seen in Klinefelter syndrome, which affects 1:500 men. (See section on Klinefelter syndrome.) Gynecomastia can develop in HIV-infected patients treated with highly active antiretroviral therapy (HAART), especially in men receiving efavirenz or didanosine; breast enlargement resolves spontaneously in 73% of patients within 9 months. Gynecomastia is common among elderly men, particularly when there is associated weight gain. However, it can be the first sign of a serious disorder. Patients with Peutz–Jeghers syndrome are prone to development of gynecomastia caused by testicular tumors.

The causes of gynecomastia are multiple and diverse (Table 26–14).

Clinical Findings

A. Symptoms and Signs

Gynecomastia is graded according to severity: I, mild; II, moderate; III, severe. Fatty gynecomastia is usually diffuse and nontender. Glandular enlargement beneath the areola may be tender. Pubertal gynecomastia is characterized by tender discoid enlargement of breast tissue 2–3 cm in diameter beneath the areola.

B. Laboratory Findings

Laboratory measurements of plasma levels of PRL (see Hyperprolactinemia) and the β-subunit of hCG (β-hCG). Detectable levels of β-hCG implicate a testicular tumor (germ cell or Sertoli cell) or other malignancy (usually lung or liver). Detectable low levels of serum β-hCG (< 5 mU/mL) may be reported in men with primary hypogonadism and high serum LH levels if the assay for β-hCG cross-reacts with LH. Measurements of plasma testosterone and LH are valuable in the diagnosis of primary or secondary hypogonadism. A low testosterone and high LH are seen in primary hypogonadism. High testosterone levels plus high LH levels characterize partial androgen resistance. Serum estradiol is determined but is usually normal; increased levels may result from testicular tumors, increased β-hCG, liver disease, obesity, adrenal tumors (rare), true hermaphroditism (rare), or gain of function mutations affecting the aromatase gene (rare). Many estrogens and substances with estrogenic activity are not detected by estradiol assays. Serum TSH (sensitive) and FT_4 levels are also determined. A karyotype (for Klinefelter syndrome) is obtained in men with persistent gynecomastia without obvious cause.

Investigation of unclear cases should include a chest radiograph to search for metastatic or bronchogenic carcinoma. Needle biopsy with cytologic examination may be performed on suspicious areas of male breast enlargement (especially when unilateral or asymmetric) to distinguish gynecomastia from tumor or mastitis.

Treatment

Pubertal gynecomastia often resolves spontaneously within 1–2 years. Drug-induced gynecomastia resolves after the offending drug is removed. Spironolactone can be stopped, with substitution of a selective aldosterone antagonist such as eplerenone. Patients with painful or persistent (> 12 months) gynecomastia may be treated with a 3- to 9-month course of a SERM (eg, raloxifene or tamoxifen). SERM therapy is much more effective for glandular ("lumpy") gynecomastia than for diffuse fatty gynecomastia. There is some evidence that raloxifene, taken orally in a dose of 60 mg daily, may be the more effective drug. Aromatase inhibitors (eg, letrozole, anastrozole, or exemestane) are marginally effective and should not ordinarily be used for adolescent boys, since long-term therapy may prevent epiphyseal fusion. Surgical correction is reserved for patients with persistent or severe gynecomastia, since results are often disappointing. Endoscopically assisted transaxillary liposuction and subcutaneous mastectomy may produce acceptable results. Generally, it is prudent to treat patients for gynecomastia only when it becomes a troubling and continuing problem for them.

Braunstein GD. Clinical practice. Gynecomastia. N Engl J Med. 2007 Sep 20;357(12):1229–37. [PMID: 17881754]

Martinez J et al. An unusual case of gynecomastia associated with soy product consumption. Endocr Pract. 2008 May–Jun;14(4):415–8. [PMID: 18558591]

▼ AMENORRHEA & MENOPAUSE (SEE ALSO CHAPTER 18)

PRIMARY AMENORRHEA

Menarche ordinarily occurs between ages 11 and 15 years (average in the United States: 12.7 years). The failure of any menses to appear is termed "primary amenorrhea," and evaluation is commenced (1) at age 14 years if neither menarche nor breast development has occurred or if height is in the lowest 3%, or (2) at age 16 years if menarche has not occurred.

Etiology of Primary Amenorrhea

The causes of primary amenorrhea include hypothalamic-pituitary causes, hyperandrogenism, ovarian causes, pseudohermaphroditism, uterine causes, and pregnancy.

A. Hypothalamic-Pituitary Causes (with Low or Normal FSH)

A genetic deficiency of GnRH and gonadotropins may be isolated or associated with other pituitary deficiencies or diminished olfaction (Kallmann syndrome). Hypothalamic lesions, particularly craniopharyngioma, may be present. Pituitary tumors may be nonsecreting or may secrete PRL or GH. Cushing syndrome may be caused by corticosteroid treatment, a cortisol-secreting adrenal tumor, or an ACTH-secreting pituitary tumor. Hypothyroidism can delay adolescence. Head trauma or encephalitis can cause gonadotropin deficiency. Primary amenorrhea may also be caused by constitutional delay of adolescence, organic illness, vigorous exercise (eg, ballet dancing, running), stressful life events, dieting, or anorexia nervosa; however, these conditions should not be assumed to account for amenorrhea without a full physical and endocrinologic evaluation. (See section on Hypopituitarism.)

B. Hyperandrogenism (with Low or Normal FSH)

Excess testosterone may be secreted by adrenal tumors or by adrenal hyperplasia caused by steroidogenic enzyme defects such as P450c21 deficiency (salt-wasting) or P450c11 deficiency (hypertension). Ovarian tumors or polycystic ovaries may also secrete excess testosterone. Androgenic steroids may also cause this syndrome.

C. Ovarian Causes (with High FSH)

Gonadal dysgenesis (Turner syndrome and variants; see below) is a frequent cause of primary amenorrhea. Ovarian failure due to autoimmunity is a common cause. Rare deficiencies in certain ovarian steroidogenic enzymes are causes of primary hypogonadism without virilization: 3β-hydroxysteroid dehydrogenase deficiency (adrenal insufficiency with low serum 17-hydroxyprogesterone) and P450c17 deficiency (hypertension and hypokalemia with high serum 17-hydroxyprogesterone). A whole-body deficiency in P450 aromatose (P450arom) activity produces female hypogonadism associated with polycystic ovaries, tall stature, osteoporosis, and virilization.

D. Pseudohermaphroditism (with High LH)

An enzymatic defect in testosterone synthesis may present as a sexually immature phenotypic girl with primary amenorrhea. Complete androgen resistance (testicular feminization) presents as a phenotypic young woman without sexual hair but with normal breast development and primary amenorrhea. In both cases, the uterus is absent and testes are intra-abdominal or cryptorchid. Intra-abdominal testes are surgically resected. Such patients are treated as normal but infertile, hypogonadal women.

E. Uterine Causes (with Normal FSH)

Congenital absence or malformation of the uterus may be responsible for primary amenorrhea, as may an unresponsive or atrophic endometrium. An imperforate hymen is occasionally the reason for the absence of visible menses.

F. Pregnancy (with High hCG)

Pregnancy may be the cause of primary amenorrhea even when the patient denies ever having had sexual intercourse.

▶ Clinical Findings

A. Symptoms and Signs

Patients with primary amenorrhea require a thorough history and physical examination to look for signs of the conditions noted above. Headaches or visual field abnormalities implicate a hypothalamic or pituitary tumor. Signs of pregnancy may be present. Blood pressure abnormalities, acne, and hirsutism should be noted. Short stature may be seen with an associated GH or thyroid hormone deficiency. Short stature with manifestations of gonadal dysgenesis indicates Turner syndrome (see below). Olfaction testing screens for Kallmann syndrome. Obesity and short stature may be signs of Cushing syndrome. Tall stature may be due to eunuchoidism or gigantism. Hirsutism or virilization suggests excessive testosterone.

An external pelvic examination plus a rectal examination should be performed to assess hymenal patency and the presence of a uterus.

B. Laboratory Findings

The initial endocrine evaluation should include serum determinations of FSH, LH, PRL, testosterone, TSH, FT_4, and hCG (pregnancy test). Patients who are virilized or hypertensive require serum electrolyte determinations and further hormonal evaluation. Girls with low-normal FSH and LH—especially those with high PRL levels—are evaluated by MRI of the hypothalamus and pituitary. Girls who have a normal uterus and high FSH without the classic features of Turner syndrome may require a karyotype to diagnose X chromosome mosaicism.

▶ Treatment

Treatment of primary amenorrhea is directed at the underlying cause. Girls with permanent hypogonadism are treated with ERT (see below).

Torstveit MK et al. Participation in leanness sports but not training volume is associated with menstrual dysfunction: a national survey of 1276 elite athletes and controls. Br J Sports Med. 2005 Mar;39(3):141–7. [PMID: 15728691]

SECONDARY AMENORRHEA & MENOPAUSE

Secondary amenorrhea is defined as the absence of menses for 3 consecutive months in women who have passed menarche. Menopause is defined as the terminal episode of naturally occurring menses; it is a retrospective diagnosis, usually made after 6 months of amenorrhea.

▶ Etiology

The causes of secondary amenorrhea include pregnancy, hypothalamic-pituitary causes, hyperandrogenism, uterine causes, premature ovarian failure, and menopause.

A. Pregnancy (High hCG)

Pregnancy is the most common cause for secondary amenorrhea in women of childbearing age. The differential diagnosis includes rare ectopic secretion of hCG by a choriocarcinoma or bronchogenic carcinoma.

B. Hypothalamic-Pituitary Causes (with Low or Normal FSH)

The hypothalamus must release GnRH in a pulsatile manner for the pituitary to secrete gonadotropins. GnRH pulses occurring more than once per hour favor LH secretion, while less frequent pulses favor FSH secretion. In normal ovulatory cycles, GnRH pulses in the follicular phase are rapid and favor LH synthesis and ovulation; ovarian luteal progesterone is then secreted that slows GnRH pulses, causing FSH secretion during the luteal phase. Most women with hypothalamic amenorrhea have a persistently low frequency of GnRH pulses.

Secondary "hypothalamic" amenorrhea may be caused by stressful life events such as school examinations or leaving home. Such women usually have a history of normal sexual development and irregular menses since menarche. Amenorrhea may also be the result of strict dieting, vigorous exercise, organic illness, or anorexia nervosa. Intrathecal infusion of opioids causes amenorrhea in most women. These conditions should not be assumed to account for amenorrhea without a full physical and endocrinologic evaluation. Young women in whom the results of evaluation and progestin withdrawal test are normal have noncyclic secretion of gonadotropins resulting in anovulation. Such women typically recover spontaneously but should have regular evaluations and a progestin withdrawal test about every 3 months to detect loss of estrogen effect.

PRL elevation due to any cause (see section on hyperprolactinemia) may cause amenorrhea. Pituitary tumors or other lesions may cause hypopituitarism. Corticosteroid excess of any cause suppresses gonadotropins.

C. Hyperandrogenism (with Low-Normal FSH)

Elevated serum levels of testosterone can cause hirsutism, virilization, and amenorrhea. In PCOS, GnRH pulses are persistently rapid, favoring LH synthesis with excessive androgen secretion; reduced FSH secretion impairs follicular maturation. Progesterone administration can slow the GnRH pulses, thus favoring FSH secretion that induces follicular maturation. Rare causes include adrenal P450c21 deficiency, ovarian or adrenal malignancies, ectopic ACTH secretion by a malignancy, and Cushing disease. Anabolic steroids also cause amenorrhea.

D. Uterine Causes (with Normal FSH)

Infection of the uterus commonly occurs following delivery or D&C but may occur spontaneously. Endometritis due to tuberculosis or schistosomiasis should be suspected in endemic areas. Endometrial scarring may result, causing amenorrhea (Asherman syndrome). Such women typically continue to have monthly premenstrual symptoms. The vaginal estrogen effect is normal.

E. Premature Ovarian Failure (with High FSH)

This refers to primary hypogonadism that occurs before age 40 years. It affects about 1% of women. About 30% of such cases are due to autoimmunity against the ovary. About 8% of cases are due to X chromosome mosaicism. Other causes include surgical bilateral oophorectomy, radiation therapy for pelvic malignancy, and chemotherapy. Women who have undergone hysterectomy are prone to premature ovarian failure even though the ovaries were left intact. Myotonic dystrophy, galactosemia, and mumps oophoritis are additional causes. Other cases may be familial or idiopathic. Ovarian failure is usually irreversible.

F. Menopause (with High FSH)

"Climacteric" is defined as the period of natural physiologic decline in ovarian function, generally occurring over about 10 years. By about age 40 years, the remaining ovarian follicles are those that are the least sensitive to gonadotropins. Increasing titers of FSH are required to stimulate estradiol secretion. Estradiol levels may actually rise during early climacteric.

The normal age for menopause in the United States ranges between 48 and 55 years, with an average of about 51.5 years. Serum estradiol levels fall and the remaining estrogen after menopause is estrone, derived mainly from peripheral aromatization of adrenal androstenedione. Such peripheral production of estrone is enhanced by obesity and liver disease. Individual differences in estrone levels partly explain why the symptoms noted above may be minimal in some women but severe in others.

► Clinical Findings

A. Symptoms and Signs

All women with amenorrhea require a complete history and physical examination. Nausea and breast engorgement are typical signs of early pregnancy. Headache or visual field abnormalities are seen with pituitary or hypothalamic tumors. Complaints of thirst and polyuria require evaluation; diabetes insipidus implicates a hypothalamic lesion. Goiter may be due to hyperthyroidism. Weight loss, diarrhea, or skin darkening may indicate adrenal insufficiency. Weight loss with a distorted body image implicates anorexia nervosa. The breasts are examined carefully for galactorrhea, a common sign of hyperprolactinemia. Hirsutism or virilization may be a sign of hyperandrogenism. Manifestations of hypercortisolism (eg, weakness, psychiatric changes, hypertension, central obesity, hirsutism, thin skin, ecchymoses) may indicate alcoholism or Cushing syndrome. Signs of acromegaly or gigantism may also indicate a pituitary tumor. Signs of systemic illness (eg, cirrhosis, kidney disease) should be appreciated. Various drugs may elevate PRL and cause amenorrhea (see section on Hyperprolactinemia). Needle tracks may indicate heroin or amphetamine abuse.

Psychological symptoms of "climacteric" may include depression and irritability. Women may experience fatigue, insomnia, headache, diminished libido, or rheumatologic symptoms. Vasomotor instability (hot flushes) is experienced by 80% of women, lasting seconds to many minutes. Hot flushes with drenching sweats may be most severe at night or may be triggered by emotional stress. Some women continue to menstruate for many months despite symptoms of estrogen deficiency. The acute symptoms of estrogen deficiency noted above tend to decline in severity within several years after menopause. However, about 35% of women have symptoms for more than 5 years. The late manifestations of estrogen deficiency include urogenital atrophy with vaginal dryness and dyspareunia; dysuria, frequency, and incontinence may occur. Increased bone osteoclastic activity increases the risk for osteoporosis and fractures. The skin becomes more wrinkled. Increases in the LDL:HDL cholesterol ratio cause an increased risk for arteriosclerosis.

A careful pelvic examination is always required to check for uterine or adnexal enlargement and to obtain a Papanicolaou smear and a vaginal smear for assessment of estrogen effect. Various life stresses, vigorous exercise, and "crash" dieting all predispose to amenorrhea; however, such factors should not be assumed to account for amenorrhea without a complete workup to screen for other causes.

B. Laboratory Findings

Since pregnancy is the most common cause of amenorrhea, women of childbearing age are immediately screened with a serum or urine hCG (pregnancy test). An elevated hCG overwhelmingly indicates pregnancy; false-positive testing may occur very rarely with ectopic hCG secretion (eg, choriocarcinoma or bronchogenic carcinoma). Women without an elevated hCG receive further laboratory evaluation including serum PRL, FSH, LH, TSH, and plasma potassium. Hyperprolactinemia or hypopituitarism (without obvious cause; see section on Hypopituitarism) should prompt an MRI study of the pituitary region. Routine testing for kidney and liver function (eg, BUN, serum creatinine, bilirubin, alkaline phosphatase, and alanine aminotransferase) is also performed. A serum testosterone level is obtained in hirsute or virilized women. Patients with manifestations of hypercortisolism receive a 1-mg overnight dexamethasone suppression test for initial screening (see section on Cushing syndrome). Nonpregnant women without any laboratory abnormality may receive a 10-day course of a progestin (eg, medroxyprogesterone acetate, 10 mg/d); absence of withdrawal menses typically indicates a lack of estrogen or a uterine abnormality.

▶ Treatment

Therapy of symptomatic hypogonadism generally consists of ERT (see below). Slow, deep breathing can ameliorate hot flushes. For women with severe hot flushes who cannot take estrogen, gabapentin is quite effective in oral doses titrated up to 800 mg every 8 hours; gabapentin is frequently associated with side effects such as fatigue, headache, dizziness, and cognitive impairment. Tamoxifen and raloxifene offer bone protection but aggravate hot flushes. Treatment or prevention of postmenopausal osteoporosis with bisphosphonates such as alendronate, risedronate, or intravenous zoledronic acid (see section on Osteoporosis) is another therapeutic option. Women with low serum testosterone levels may experience hypoactive sexual desire disorder (HSDD) that may respond to low-dose testosterone replacement.

▶ Estrogen Replacement Therapy

The Women's Health Initiative (WHI) monitored 16,606 postmenopausal women in the United States in a prospective, double-blinded, placebo-controlled study of postmenopausal HRT. A control group of women taking a daily placebo was compared with (1) women receiving daily conventional-dose oral combined HRT (conjugated equine estrogens [CEE] 0.625 mg/d with medroxyprogesterone acetate [MPA] 2.5 mg/d) and (2) women, having had a hysterectomy, receiving only CEE 0.625 mg/d.

The WHI risk–benefit findings (described below) have dramatically changed postmenopausal HRT. To reduce the risks of HRT, lower-dose estrogen regimens are preferred over conventional-dose therapy. Estrogen preparations other than CEE are increasingly favored. Transdermal and vaginal estrogen preparations are widely preferred over oral estrogen replacement. Also, the potential adverse effects of progestins are now recognized, such that women taking very low-dose estrogen replacement may receive progestin therapy only periodically, if at all. For moderate to high-dose estrogen therapy, progestins are being used in lower doses. Also, clinicians are now tending to prescribe progestins other than MPA or progesterone-eluting intrauterine devices. **Oral estrogen preparations** include CEEs (0.3, 0.45, 0.625, 0.9, and 1.25 mg), ethinyl estradiol (20 and 50 mcg), estradiol (0.5, 1, 1.5, and 2 mg), estropipate (0.75, 1.5, 3, and 6 mg), plant-derived esterified estrogens (eg, Menest, Estratab, 0.3, 0.625, and 2.5 mg), and synthetic estrogens (eg, Cenestin, 0.3, 0.625, 0.9, and 1.25 mg).

Oral estrogen plus progestin preparations include CEE with MPA (Prempro 0.3/1.5, 0.45/1.5, 0.625/2.5, and 0.625/5), CEE for 14 days cycled with CEE plus MPA for 14 days (Premphase 0.625, 0.625/5), estradiol with norethindrone acetate (Activella 1/0.5), ethinyl estradiol with norethindrone acetate (Femhrt 1/5, 5 mcg/1 mg/tablet), and estradiol with norgestimate (Ortho-Prefest, sequences of estradiol 1 mg/d for 3 days, alternating with a combination of 1 mg estradiol/0.09 mg norgestimate daily for 3 days). Oral contraceptives can also be used for combined HRT.

Transdermal estradiol: Estradiol can be delivered systemically with different transdermal systems. Because transdermal absorption of estradiol is somewhat variable, this delivery method will not work for all women.

1. Transdermal systems with estradiol mixed with adhesive: These systems tend to cause minimal skin irritation. Of the following preparations, the Vivelle-Dot patches are the smallest and least obtrusive. Available preparations include Esclim, Vivelle, and Vivelle-Dot (0.025, 0.0375, 0.05, 0.075, or 0.1 mg/d), replaced twice weekly; Alora (0.025, 0.05, 0.075, or 0.1 mg/d), replaced twice weekly; Climara (0.025, 0.0375, 0.05, 0.06, 0.075, or 0.1 mg/d), replaced weekly; FemPatch (0.025 mg/d), replaced weekly; and Menostar (0.014 mg/d), replaced weekly. This type of estradiol skin patch can be cut in half and applied to the skin without proportionately greater loss of potency.

2. Transdermal systems with estradiol in a drug reservoir: These systems cause significant skin irritation in some women. Available preparations include Estraderm (0.05 or 0.1 mg/d), replaced twice weekly.

3. Transdermal systems with estradiol (E) and norethindrone acetate (NA) mixed with adhesive: Available preparations include Combipatch (0.05 mg/d E and 0.14 mg/d NA or 0.05 mg/d E and 0.25 mg/d NA), replaced twice weekly. The addition of a progestin increases the likelihood of side effects compared with therapy with estrogen alone.

4. Transdermal estradiol gel (EstroGel, 0.6%) is available in a metered-dose dispenser that delivers 1.25 g estradiol per actuation. The gel is applied to one arm from the wrist to the shoulder daily after bathing. To avoid spreading the estradiol to others, the hands should be washed and precautions taken to avoid prolonged skin contact with children. Application of sunscreen prior to estradiol gel has been reported to *increase* the transdermal absorption of estradiol.

Vaginal estrogen: Urogenital atrophy commonly develops in postmenopausal women and can cause dryness of the vagina, genital itching, burning, and dyspareunia. Urinary symptoms can include urgency and dysuria. Vaginal estrogen is intended to deliver estrogen directly to local tissues in an effort to reduce these symptoms, while minimizing systemic estrogen exposure. Some estrogen is absorbed systemically and can relieve menopausal symptoms. Systemically absorbed estrogen avoids first-pass liver metabolism, causing less hypertriglyceridemia and prothrombotic effects than oral estrogen. Manufacturers recommend that these preparations be used for only 3–6 months in women with an intact uterus, since vaginal estrogen can cause endometrial proliferation. However, most clinicians use them for longer periods. Vaginal estrogen can be administered in three different ways:

1. Estrogen vaginal creams: These creams are administered intravaginally with a measured-dose applicator daily for 2 weeks for atrophic vaginitis, then administered one to three times weekly. Available preparations include CEEs (Premarin, 0.626 mg/g cream), 0.25–0.5 g cream vaginally; dienestrol (Ortho Dienestrol, 10 mg/g cream), 0.25–0.5 g cream vaginally; estradiol (Estrace, 0.1 mg/g cream), 1 g cream vaginally; and estropipate (Ogen, 1.5 mg/g cream), 0.25–0.5 g vaginally.

2. Estradiol vaginal tablets: These tablets are sold prepackaged in a disposable applicator and can be administered deep intravaginally daily for 2 weeks for atrophic vaginitis, then twice weekly. The tablets dissolve into a gel that gradually releases estradiol. Available preparations include vaginal estradiol tablets (Vagifem, 25 mcg/tablet).

3. Estradiol vaginal rings: These rings are inserted manually into the upper third of the vagina, worn continuously, and replaced every 90 days. Only a small amount of the released estradiol enters the systemic circulation. Vaginal rings do not usually interfere with sexual intercourse. If a ring is removed or descends into the introitus, it may be washed in warm water and reinserted. Available preparations include Estring (2 mg estradiol/ring, releasing 0.0075 mg/d) and Femring (12.4 mg estradiol/ring, releasing 0.05 mg/d, or 24.8 mg estradiol/ring, releasing 0.10 mg/d).

Oral progestins: For a woman with an intact uterus, long-term conventional-dose unopposed systemic estrogen therapy can cause endometrial hyperplasia, which typically results in dysfunctional uterine bleeding (DUB)

and can rarely lead to endometrial cancer. Progestin therapy transforms proliferative into secretory endometrium, causing a menses when given intermittently or no bleeding when given continuously.

The type of progestin preparation, its dosage, and the timing of administration may be tailored to the given situation. Progestins may be given daily, monthly, or at longer intervals. When given episodically, progestins are usually administered for 7–14 day periods. Progestins are available in different formulations: Micronized progesterone (Prometrium, 100 mg/capsule), medroxyprogesterone acetate (Provera, Amen, Cycrin; 2.5, 5.0, and 10 mg/scored tablet), norethindrone acetate (Aygestin, 5 mg/tablet), and norethindrone (Micronor, Nor-QD; 0.35 mg/tablet).

Topical progesterone (20–50 mg/d) may reduce hot flushes in women who are intolerant to oral HRT. It may be applied to the upper arms, thighs, or inner wrists daily. It may be compounded as micronized progesterone 250 mg/mL in a transdermal gel. Its effects upon the breast and endometrium are unknown.

Progesterone-releasing intrauterine devices: Progesterone-releasing intrauterine devices can be useful for women receiving ERT, since they can reduce the incidence of DUB and endometrial carcinoma without exposing women to the significant risks of systemic progestins.

Benefits of ERT: Estrogen replacement without progestin (unopposed): Surprisingly, the WHI study found that postmenopausal women who received conventional-dose estrogen-only therapy had a reduced risk for breast cancer (seven fewer cases/year per 10,000 women) compared with a placebo group. The WHI study also found that women who received estrogen therapy experienced a reduced number of hip fractures (six fewer fractures/year per 10,000 women) compared with placebo. In the WHI study, unopposed estrogen therapy had no discernible effect upon the risk for heart attacks, colorectal cancer, or overall mortality. A 20-year study of 8801 women living in a retirement community found that estrogen use was associated with improved survival. Age-adjusted mortality rates were 56.4 (per 1000 person-years) among nonusers and 50.4 among women who had used estrogen for 15 years or longer.

Women receiving unopposed conventional-dose daily conjugated estrogen and medroxyprogesterone acetate (0.625 mg and 2.5 mg, respectively) for an average of 5.6 years, experienced a lower risk of developing diabetes (3.5%) versus those taking a placebo (4.2%).

Serum levels of atherogenic lipoprotein(a) are reduced by estrogen replacement with or without daily or cycled progestins. Improvement in serum HDL cholesterol is greatest with unopposed estrogen but is also seen with the addition of a progestin.

Estrogen replacement improves or eliminates postmenopausal hot flushes and diaphoretic episodes. Vaginal moisture is improved. Libido is enhanced in some women. Sleep disturbances are common in menopause and can be reversed with estrogen replacement. Sex hormone replacement may also improve the body pain and reduced physical function experienced by some women at the time of menopause.

Perimenopause-related depression is improved by unopposed estrogen replacement; the addition of a progestin may negate this effect. Estrogen replacement, when initiated at the time of menopause or oophorectomy, has been reported to help protect cognitive function, particularly verbal memory, whereas estrogen replacement that is begun many years after menopause confers little or no benefit on cognition. Estrogen therapy does not appear to reduce the risk of Alzheimer dementia.

Unopposed estrogen replacement improves glycemic control in women with type 2 diabetes mellitus. Estrogen replacement does not prevent facial skin wrinkling; however, it may improve facial skin moisture and thickness, reducing seborrhea and atrophy.

Risks of ERT: The risks of estrogen replacement depend on the dose. Conventional doses (eg, oral conjugated estrogens ≥ 0.625 mg/d or transdermal estradiol ≥ 0.05 mg/d) carry higher risks than lower doses (eg, oral conjugated estrogens, ≤ 0.3 mg/d or transdermal estradiol ≤ 0.025 mg/d). Route of administration also affects risks, since oral estrogens pass through the liver and increase hepatic production of clotting factors (thereby increasing the risks of thrombotic stroke), whereas transdermal or vaginal administration of estrogen does not significantly increase clotting proclivity. The risks for HRT also depend on whether estrogen is administered alone (unopposed HRT) or with a progestin (combined HRT).

Estrogen replacement without progestin (unopposed HRT): Conventional-dose unopposed estrogen replacement increases the risk of endometrial hyperplasia and DUB, which often prompts patients to stop the estrogen. Lower-dose unopposed estrogen has a much lower risk of DUB. Recurrent dysfunctional bleeding necessitates a pelvic examination and possibly an endometrial biopsy.

Unopposed estrogen in conventional doses may increase the risk for endometrial carcinoma, although the absolute risk remains low. A Cochrane Database Review found no increased risk of endometrial carcinoma in a review of 30 randomized controlled trials. Therefore, lower-dose unopposed estrogen replacement confers a negligible risk for endometrial cancer.

Long-term conventional-dose unopposed estrogen increases the mortality risk from ovarian cancer, although the absolute risk is small. The annual age-adjusted ovarian cancer death rates for women taking estrogen replacement for ≥ 10 years are 64:100,000 for current users, 38:100,000 for former users, and 26:100,000 for women who had never taken estrogen. Lower-dose estrogen replacement is believed to confer a negligible increased risk for ovarian cancer.

The WHI study has reported that conventional doses of unopposed oral estrogen do not increase the risk of breast cancer; in fact, somewhat fewer breast cancers were found in women taking estrogen alone, compared with placebo. However, the WHI trial was stopped in 2002 because of an increased risk of stroke among women taking conjugated oral estrogens in doses of 0.625 mg daily; the risk was about 44 strokes per 10,000 person-years versus about 32 per 10,000 person-years in women taking placebo. Transdermal or transvaginal estrogen is not expected to increase the risk of stroke.

Conventional-dose oral estrogen replacement increases the risk of deep venous thrombosis. It can cause hypertri-

glyceridemia, particularly in women with preexistent hyperlipidemia, rarely resulting in pancreatitis. Postmenopausal estrogen therapy also slightly increases the risk of gallstones and cholecystitis. Oral estrogens reduce the effectiveness of growth hormone replacement. These side effects can be reduced or avoided by using nonoral estrogen replacement.

Elderly women, receiving long-term conventional-dose estrogen replacement, experience an increased risk of urinary incontinence. Some women complain of estrogen-induced edema or mastalgia. Estrogen replacement has been reported to lower the seizure threshold in some women with epilepsy. Untreated large pituitary prolactinomas may enlarge if exposed to estrogen.

Estrogen replacement with a progestin (combined HRT): The WHI study found that women who received long-term conventional oral doses of combined HRT (conjugated estrogens 0.625 mg/d plus medroxyprogesterone acetate 2.5 mg/d) had an increased risk of deep venous thrombosis (3.5 per 1000 person-years) compared with women receiving placebo (1.7 per 1000 person-years).

Conventional-dose oral combined HRT results in an increased risk for myocardial infarction (24% or six additional heart attacks per 10,000 women), mostly in women with high-risk LDL levels or preexistent coronary disease. Most of the risk for myocardial infarction occurs in the first year of therapy. This increased risk is attributable to the progestin component, since the estrogen-only arm of the WHI study found no increased risk of myocardial infarction.

Long-term conventional-dose oral combined HRT increases breast density and increases the risk for abnormal mammograms (9.4% versus 5.4% for placebo). There is also a higher risk for breast cancer (8 cases per 10,000 women/year versus 6.5 cases per 10,000 women/year for placebo); no increased risk of breast cancer has been found with estrogen-only HRT. This increased risk for breast cancer appears to mostly affect relatively thin women with a BMI < 24.4. The Iowa Women's Health Study reported an increase in breast cancer with HRT only in women consuming more than 1 oz of alcohol weekly. No accelerated risk of breast cancer has been seen in users of HRT who have benign breast disease or a family history of breast cancer.

The Women's Health Initiative Mental Study (WHIMS) followed the effect of combined conventional-dose oral HRT on cognitive function in women 65–79 years old. HRT did not protect these older women from cognitive decline. In fact, they experienced an increased risk for severe dementia at a rate of 23 more cases/year for every 10,000 women over age 65 years.

In the WHI study, women receiving conventional-dose combined oral HRT experienced an increased risk of stroke (31 strokes per 10,000 women/year versus 26 strokes per 10,000 women/year for placebo). Stroke risk was also increased by hypertension, diabetes, and smoking.

Women taking combined estrogen–progestin replacement do not experience an increased risk of ovarian cancer. They do experience an increased risk of developing asthma.

Progestins may cause moodiness, particularly in women with a history of premenstrual dysphoric disorder. Cycled progestins may trigger migraines in certain women. Many other adverse reactions have been reported, including breast tenderness, alopecia, and fluid retention. Contraindications to the use of progestins include thromboembolic disorders, liver disease, breast cancer, and pregnancy.

SERMs (eg, raloxifene; Evista) are an alternative to estrogen replacement for hypogonadal women at risk for osteoporosis who prefer not to take estrogens because of their contraindications (eg, breast or uterine cancer) or side effects. Raloxifene does not reduce hot flushes, vaginal dryness, skin wrinkling, or breast atrophy; it does not improve cognition. However, in doses of 60 mg/d orally, it inhibits bone loss without stimulating effects upon the breasts or endometrium. Because raloxifene may slightly increase the risk of venous thromboembolism, it should not be used by women at prolonged bed rest or by those prone to thrombosis. In contrast with the use of ERT, concomitant progesterone therapy is not needed, and raloxifene does not increase the risk of development of breast cancer. Tibolone (Livial) is an SERM whose metabolites have mixed estrogenic, progestogenic, and weak androgenic activity. It is comparable to HRT for the treatment of climacteric-related complaints. It does not appear to significantly stimulate proliferation of breast or endometrial tissue. It depresses both serum triglycerides and HDL cholesterol. Long-term studies are lacking. It is not available in the United States.

Phytoestrogens are substances found in plants that bind to estrogen receptors. Phytoestrogens, found in soy and red clover extracts, do not appear to significantly improve menopausal hot flushes, cognitive function, bone density, or plasma lipids.

Testosterone replacement therapy in women: In premenopausal women, serum testosterone levels decline with age. Between 25 and 45 years of age, women's testosterone levels fall 50%. After natural menopause, the ovaries remain a significant source for testosterone. In fact, following natural menopause, serum testosterone levels do not fall abruptly and serum free testosterone levels may actually rise. In contrast, very low serum testosterone levels are found in women after bilateral oophorectomy, autoimmune ovarian failure, adrenalectomy, and hypopituitarism. Testosterone deficiency contributes to hot flushes, loss of sexual hair, muscle atrophy, osteoporosis, and diminished libido, also known as hypoactive sexual desire disorder (HSDD).

In women, diminished libido is common and multifactorial. Although low serum testosterone levels may contribute to HSDD, hysterectomy and sexual isolation are major causes. Low serum testosterone levels may also cause fatigue, a diminished sense of well-being, and a dulled enthusiasm for life. Androgen replacement may improve these problems.

Testosterone therapy is often effective, while DHEA therapy is not. Selected women may be treated with low-dose testosterone. Methyltestosterone can be taken orally in doses of 1.25–2.5 mg daily. Testosterone can also be compounded as a cream containing 1 mg/mL, with 1 mL applied to the low abdomen daily. Methyltestosterone is also available in combination with conjugated estrogens (eg, Estrat-

est). This formulation is convenient but carries the same disadvantage as oral estrogen—increased risk of thromboembolism. Tablets contain either 1.25 mg conjugated estrogens with 2.5 mg methyltestosterone or 0.625 mg conjugated estrogens with 1.25 mg methyltestosterone. Estratest is usually started at the lowest strength. It should be given cyclically at the lowest dose that controls symptoms.

Women receiving testosterone therapy must be monitored for the appearance of any acne or hirsutism, and serum testosterone levels are determined periodically if women feel that they are benefitting and long-term testosterone therapy is instituted. Side effects of low-dose testosterone therapy are usually minimal but may include polycythemia, emotional changes hirsutism, acne, an adverse effect on lipids, and potentiation of warfarin anticoagulation therapy. Testosterone replacement tends to reduce both triglyceride and HDL cholesterol levels. Hepatocellular neoplasms and peliosis hepatis, rare complications of oral androgens at higher doses, have not been reported with methyltestosterone at lower doses of 2.5 mg orally daily. Androgens should not be given to women with liver disease or during pregnancy or breast-feeding. Testosterone replacement therapy for women should be used judiciously, since long-term prospective clinical trials are lacking. An analysis of the Nurses' Health Study found that women who had been taking CEEs plus methyltestosterone experienced an increased risk of breast cancer. Yearly mammography is recommended for all women over 40 years of age.

Basaria S et al. Clinical review: controversies regarding transdermal androgen therapy in postmenopausal women. J Clin Endocrinol Metab. 2006 Dec;91(12):4743–52. [PMID: 16984993]

Goswami D et al. Premature ovarian failure. Horm Res. 2007;68(4):196–202. [PMID: 17495481]

Maddalozzo GF et al. The effects of hormone replacement therapy and resistance training on spine bone mineral density in early postmenopausal women. Bone. 2007 May;40(5):1244–51. [PMID: 17291843]

Nair KS et al. DHEA in elderly women and DHEA or testosterone in elderly men. N Engl J Med. 2006 Oct 19;355(16):1647–59. [PMID: 17050889]

Paganini-Hill A et al. Increased longevity in older users of postmenopausal estrogen therapy: the Leisure World Cohort Study. Menopause. 2006 Jan–Feb;13(1):12–8. [PMID: 16607094]

Reddy SY et al. Gabapentin, estrogen, and placebo for treating hot flushes: a randomized controlled trial. Obstet Gynecol. 2006 Jul;108(1):41–8. [PMID: 16816054]

Shulman LLP. Transdermal hormone therapy and bone health. Clin Interv Aging. 2008;3(1):51–4. [PMID: 18488878]

Tamimi RM et al. Combined estrogen and testosterone use and risk of breast cancer in postmenopausal women. Arch Intern Med. 2006 Jul 24;166(14):1483–9. [PMID: 16864758]

Warren MP et al. Exercise-induced amenorrhea and bone health in the adolescent athlete. Ann N Y Acad Sci. 2008;1135:244–52. [PMID: 18574231]

TURNER SYNDROME (Gonadal Dysgenesis)

 ESSENTIALS OF DIAGNOSIS

► Short stature with normal growth hormone levels.

► Primary amenorrhea or early ovarian failure.

▶ Epicanthal folds, webbed neck, short fourth metacarpals.

▶ Renal and cardiovascular anomalies.

Turner syndrome comprises a group of X chromosome disorders that are associated with spontaneous abortion, primary hypogonadism, short stature, and other phenotypic anomalies. It affects 1–2% of fetuses, of which about 97% abort, accounting for about 10% of all spontaneous abortions. Nevertheless, it affects about 1 in every 2500 live female births. Patients with the classic syndrome (about 50% of cases) lack one of the two chromosomes (45,XO karyotype). Other patients with Turner syndrome have X chromosome abnormalities, such as ring X or Xq (X/abnormal X) or X chromosome deletions affecting all or some somatic cells (mosaicism, XX/XO).

1. Classic Turner Syndrome (Table 26–15) (45,XO Gonadal Dysgenesis)

Features of Turner syndrome are variable and may be subtle in girls with mosaicism. Typical manifestations in adulthood include short stature, hypogonadism, webbed neck, high-arched palate, wide-spaced nipples, hypertension, and renal abnormalities. Emotional disorders are common.

Girls with Turner syndrome may be diagnosed at birth, since they tend to be small and may exhibit severe lymphedema. Evaluation for childhood short stature often leads to the diagnosis. Growth hormone and IGF-1 levels are normal. Hypogonadism presents as "delayed adolescence" (primary amenorrhea, 80%) or early ovarian failure (20%); girls with 45,XO Turner (blood karyotyping) who enter puberty are typically found to have mosaicism if other tissues are karyotyped. Hypogonadism is confirmed in girls who have high serum levels of FSH and LH. A blood karyotype showing 45,XO (or X chromosome abnormalities or mosaicism) establishes the diagnosis.

Treatment of short stature with daily injections of GH (0.1 unit/kg/d) plus an androgen (eg, oxandrolone) for at least 4 years before epiphysial fusion increases final height by a mean of about 10.3 cm over the mean predicted height of 144.2 cm. Such GH treatment rarely causes pseudotumor cerebri. After age 12 years, estrogen therapy is begun with low doses of conjugated estrogens (0.3 mg) or ethinyl estradiol (5 mcg) given on days 1–21 per month. When growth stops, HRT is begun with estrogen and progestin; transdermal estrogen may be used to initiate pubertal development.

Girls and women with Turner syndrome have an increased risk of aortic coarctation (11%) and bicuspid aortic valves (16%); these cardiac abnormalities are more common in patients with webbed necks. Bicuspid aortic valves are associated with an increased risk for infective endocarditis, aortic valvular stenosis or insufficiency, and ascending aortic aneurysm and dissection. Partial anomalous pulmonary vein connections occur in 13% and can lead to left-to-right shunting of blood. Adults with Turner syndrome have a high incidence of ECG abnormalities.

Women with Turner syndrome have a reduced life expectancy due in part to their increased risk for diabetes mellitus (types 1 and 2), hypertension, dyslipidemia, and osteoporosis.

Table 26–15. Manifestations of Turner syndrome.

Short stature
Distinctive facial features
  Ptosis
  Micrognathia
  Low-set ears
  Epicanthal folds
Sexual infantilism due to gonadal dysgenesis with primary amenorrhea (80%)
Early ovarian failure with secondary amenorrhea (20%)
Webbed neck (40%)
Low hairline
High-arched palate
Cubitus valgus
Short fourth metacarpals (50%)
Lymphedema of hands and feet (30%)
Hypoplastic widely spaced nipples
Hyperconvex nails
Pigmented nevi
Keloid formation (eg, surgical scars or after ear piercing)
Recurrent otitis media
Renal abnormalities (60%)
  Horseshoe kidney
  Hydronephrosis
Hypertension (idiopathic or due to coarctation or kidney disease)
Gastrointestinal disorders
  Telangiectasis with bleeding
  Celiac disease
  Inflammatory bowel disease
  Colon carcinoma
  Liver disease
Impaired space-form recognition, direction sense, and mathematical reasoning
Cardiovascular anomalies
  Coarctation of the aorta (10–20%)
  Partial anomalous pulmonary venous connection
  Bicuspid aortic valve (with aortic stenosis or insufficiency)
  Aortic dissection due to coarctation and cystic medial necrosis of the aorta
Associated conditions
  Obesity
  Diabetes mellitus (types 1 and 2)
  Dyslipidemia
  Hyperuricemia
  Hashimoto thyroiditis
  Achlorhydria
  Cataracts, corneal opacities
  Neuroblastoma (1%)
  Rheumatoid arthritis
  Inflammatory bowel disease

Diagnostic vigilance and aggressive treatment of these conditions reduce the risk of aortic aneurysm dissection, ischemic heart disease, stroke, and fracture. Patients are prone to keloid formation after surgery or ear piercing. Yearly ocular examinations and periodic thyroid evaluations are recommended. It is advisable to evaluate all patients with Turner syndrome with an ultrasound, along with MRI examination of the chest and abdomen, looking for cardiac, aortic, and renal abnormalities. Repeat cardiovascular evaluations should be done every 3–4 years. Patients with the classic 45,XO karyotype have a high risk of renal structural abnormalities, whereas those with 46 X/abnormal X are more prone to malformations of the urinary collecting system. The risk of aortic dissection is increased more than 100-fold in women with Turner syndrome, particularly those with pronounced neck webbing and shield chest. Patients with aortic root enlargement are usually treated with β-blockade and serial imaging. Women with Turner syndrome who are able to become pregnant are strongly advised to deliver via cesarean section due to the risk of aortic aneurysm rupture during vaginal delivery.

2. Turner Syndrome Variants

A. 46,X (Abnormal X) Karyotype

Patients with small distal short arm deletions of the X chromosome (Xp-) that include the SHOX gene often have short stature and skeletal abnormalities but have a low risk of ovarian failure. Transmission of Turner syndrome from mother to daughter can occur. There may be an increased risk of trisomy 21 in the conceptuses of women with Turner syndrome. Patients with deletions of the long arm of the X chromosome (distal to Xq24) often have amenorrhea without short stature or other features of Turner syndrome. Abnormalities or deletions of other genes located on both the long and short arms of the X chromosome can produce gonadal dysgenesis with few other somatic features.

B. 45,XO/46,XX Mosaicism

This karyotype results in a modified form of Turner syndrome. Such girls tend to be taller and may have more gonadal function and fewer other manifestations of Turner syndrome.

C. Other Variants

45,XO/46,XY mosaicism can produce some manifestations of Turner syndrome. Patients may have ambiguous genitalia or male infertility with an otherwise normal phenotype. Germ cell tumors, such as gonadoblastomas and seminomas, develop in about 10% of patients with 45,XO/46,XY mosaicism; most such tumors are benign.

Baxter L et al. Recombinant growth hormone for children and adolescents with Turner syndrome. Cochrane Database Syst Rev. 2007 Jan 24;(1):CD003887. [PMID: 17253498]

Bondy CA. Aortic dissection in Turner syndrome. Curr Opin Cardiol. 2008 Nov;23(6):519–26. [PMID: 18839441]

Bondy CA et al. Care of girls and women with Turner syndrome: a guideline of the Turner Syndrome Study Group. J Endocrinol Metab. 2007 Jan;92(1):10–25. [PMID: 17047017]

Matura LA et al. Aortic dilatation and dissection in Turner syndrome. Circulation. 2007 Oct 9;116(15):1663–70. [PMID: 17875973]

MULTIPLE ENDOCRINE NEOPLASIA

 ESSENTIALS OF DIAGNOSIS

► MEN 1: tumors of the parathyroid glands, endocrine pancreas and duodenum, pituitary, adrenal, thyroid; lipomas and facial angiofibromas.

► MEN 2A: medullary thyroid cancers, pheochromocytomas, Hirschsprung disease.

► MEN 2B: medullary thyroid cancers, pheochromocytomas, Marfan-like habitus, mucosal neuromas, intestinal ganglioneuroma, delayed puberty.

Syndromes of MEN are inherited as autosomal dominant traits and cause a predisposition to the development of tumors in different tissues, particularly involving endocrine glands (Table 26–16).

1. MEN 1 (Wermer Syndrome)

MEN 1 is a familial multiglandular endocrine tumor syndrome, with a prevalence of 2–10 per 100,000 people. The presentation of MEN 1 is quite variable, even in the same kindred. Parathyroid, enteropancreatic, and pituitary tumors can be present in one individual, though not necessarily at the same time. Nonendocrine tumors also occur, such as subcutaneous lipomas, facial angiofibromas, and collagenomas. In some affected individuals, tumors may start developing in childhood, whereas in others, tumors develop late in adult life.

About 90% of patients with MEN 1 have germline mutations that are inherited as an autosomal dominant trait. Patients with MEN 1 usually have detectable mutations in the *menin* gene, located on the long arm of chromosome 11 (11q13). MEN 1 gene testing is available at a few centers and is able to detect the specific mutation in 60–95% of cases. If no mutation is detected, genetic linkage analysis can be done if there are several affected members in the kindred. Gene testing permits the rest of the kindred to be tested for the specific gene defect and allows informed genetic counseling.

With close endocrine surveillance of affected individuals, the initial biochemical manifestations (usually hypercalcemia) can often be detected as early as age 14–18 years in patients with a MEN 1 gene mutation, although clinical manifestations do not usually present until the third or fourth decade.

Hyperparathyroidism is the first clinical manifestation of MEN 1 in two-thirds of affected patients, but it may present at any time of life. Patients with the MEN 1 mutation have a > 90% lifetime risk of developing hyperparathyroidism. The hyperparathyroidism of MEN 1 is notoriously difficult to treat surgically, due to multiple gland involvement and the frequency of supernumerary glands and ectopic parathyroid tissue. Typically, three and one-half glands are resected, leaving one-half of the most normal-appearing gland intact. Also, during neck surgery, a thymectomy is performed to resect any intrathymic parathyroid glands or occult thymic carcinoid tumors. Nevertheless, the surgical failure rate is about 38%, and there is a recurrence rate of about 16%, with hypercalcemia often recurring many years after neck surgery. Aggressive parathyroid resection can cause permanent hypoparathyroidism. Patients with persistent or recurrent hyperparathyroidism should avoid oral calcium supplements and thiazide diuretics; oral therapy with calcimimetic drug, such as cinacalcet, is effective but expensive. The diagnosis

Table 26–16. Multiple endocrine neoplasia (MEN) syndromes: Incidence of tumor types.

Tumor Type	MEN 1 (Wermer Syndrome)	MEN 2A (Sipple Syndrome)	MEN 2B
Parathyroid	95%	20–50%	Rare
Pancreatic	54%		
Pituitary	42%		
Medullary thyroid carcinoma		> 90%	80%
Pheochromocytoma	Rare	20–35%	60%
Mucosal and gastrointestinal ganglioneuromas		Rare	> 90%
Subcutaneous lipoma	30%		
Adrenocortical adenoma	30%		
Thoracic carcinoid	15%		
Thyroid adenoma	55%		
Facial angiofibromas and collagenomas	85%		

and treatment of hyperparathyroidism is described earlier in this chapter.

Enteropancreatic tumors occur in about 75% of patients with MEN 1. **Nonsecretory neuroendocrine tumors** occur and do not secrete hormones; they tend to be large and very aggressive. **Gastrinomas** occur in about 35% of patients with MEN 1; they secrete gastrin, thereby causing severe gastric hyperacidity (Zollinger–Ellison syndrome) with peptic ulcer disease or diarrhea. Concurrent hypercalcemia, due to hyperparathyroidism (see above), stimulates gastrin and gastric acid secretion; control of the hypercalcemia often reduces gastric acid secretion and serum gastrin levels. These gastrinomas tend to be small, multiple, and ectopic; they are frequently found outside the pancreas, usually in the duodenum. Gastrinomas of MEN 1 can metastasize to the liver; but in patients with MEN 1, depending upon the kindred, hepatic metastases tend to be less aggressive than those from sporadic gastrinomas. Treatment of patients with gastrinomas in MEN 1 is usually conservative, utilizing long-term high-dose proton pump inhibitor therapy and control of hypercalcemia; surgery is palliative and usually reserved for aggressive gastrinomas and those tumors arising in the duodenum. Zollinger–Ellison syndrome is also discussed in Chapter 15.

Insulinomas cause hyperinsulinism and fasting hypoglycemia. They occur in about 15% of patients with MEN 1. Surgery is usually attempted, but the tumors can be small, multiple, and difficult to detect. The diagnosis and treatment of insulinomas are described in Chapter 27. Glucagonomas (1.6%) secrete glucagon and cause diabetes and migratory necrolytic erythema. VIPomas (1%) secrete VIP and cause profuse watery diarrhea, hypokalemia, and achlorhydria (WDHA, Verner–Morrison syndrome). Somatostatinomas (0.7%) can cause diabetes mellitus, steatorrhea, and cholelithiasis.

Pituitary adenomas occur in about 42% of patients with MEN 1. They are more common in women (50%) than men (31%) and are the presenting tumor in 17% of patients with MEN 1. These tumors tend to be more aggressive macroadenomas (> 1 cm diameter, 85%) com-

pared to sporadic pituitary tumors (42%). Of MEN 1–associated pituitary tumors, about 62% secrete PRL, 8% secrete GH, 13% secrete both PRL and GH, and 13% are nonsecretory; only 4% secrete ACTH and cause Cushing disease. The diagnosis and treatment of pituitary tumors and Cushing disease were described earlier in this chapter. These pituitary tumors can produce local pressure effects and hypopituitarism.

Adrenal adenomas or **hyperplasia** occurs in about 37% of patients with MEN 1 and 50% are bilateral. They are generally benign and nonfunctional. In one series, one out of 12 of these patients developed a feminizing adrenal carcinoma. These adrenal lesions are pituitary independent.

Nonendocrine tumors occur commonly in MEN 1. Small facial angiofibromas and subcutaneous lipomas are common. Collagenomas can present as firm dermal nodules. Malignant melanomas have been reported.

The differential diagnosis of MEN 1 includes sporadic or familial tumors of the pituitary, parathyroids, or pancreatic islets. Hypercalcemia (from any cause) may cause gastrointestinal symptoms and increased gastrin levels, simulating a gastrinoma. Routine suppression of gastric acid secretion with H_2-blockers or proton pump inhibitors causes a physiologic increase in serum gastrin that can be mistaken for a gastrinoma. H_2-blockers and metoclopramide cause hyperprolactinemia, simulating a pituitary prolactinoma.

Variants of MEN 1 also occur. Kindreds with MEN 1 Burin variant have a high prevalence of prolactinomas, late-onset hyperparathyroidism, and carcinoid tumors, but rarely enteropancreatic tumors.

2. MEN 2A (Sipple Syndrome)

MEN 2A is a rare familial multiglandular syndrome that is inherited as an autosomal dominant trait. Patients with MEN 2A should have genetic testing for a *ret* protooncogene (RET) mutation. Their first-degree relatives may then be tested for the specific RET mutation. Patients with MEN 2A may have **medullary thyroid carcinoma** (> 90%); hyperparathyroidism (20–50%), due to hyperplasia or multiple adenomas in over 70% of cases; **pheochromocytomas** (20–35%), which are often bilateral; or **Hirschsprung disease**. The medullary thyroid carcinoma is of mild to moderate aggressiveness. Children harboring an MEN 2A RET gene mutation are advised to have a prophylactic total thyroidectomy by age 6 years.

Siblings or children of patients with MEN 2A should have genetic testing to determine if they have a mutation of the *ret* protooncogene (RET) on chromosome 10cen-10q11.2; this identifies about 95% of affected individuals. Each kindred has a certain *ret* codon mutation that correlates with the particular variation in the MEN 2 syndrome, such as the age of onset and aggressiveness of medullary thyroid cancer. The specific mutation as well as case histories of family members should guide the timing for prophylactic thyroidectomy. Before any surgical procedure, MEN 2 carriers should be screened for pheochromocytoma. There is incomplete penetrance, and about 30% of those with such mutations never manifest endocrine tumors.

Patients may be screened for medullary thyroid carcinoma with a serum calcitonin drawn after 3 days of omeprazole, 20 mg orally twice daily; calcitonin levels rise in the presence of medullary thyroid carcinoma to above 80 pg/mL in women or above 190 pg/mL in men.

3. MEN 2B

MEN 2B is a familial, autosomal dominant multiglandular syndrome that is caused by a mutation of the *ret* protooncogene (RET) on chromosome 10. MEN 2B is characterized by mucosal neuromas (> 90%) with bumpy and enlarged lips and tongue, Marfan-like habitus (75%), adrenal pheochromocytomas (60%) that are rarely malignant and often bilateral, and medullary thyroid carcinoma (80%). Patients also have intestinal abnormalities (75%) such as intestinal ganglioneuromas, skeletal abnormalities (87%), and delayed puberty (43%). Medullary thyroid carcinoma is aggressive and presents early in life. Therefore, infants having a parent with MEN 2B receive genetic screening; those carrying the RET mutation undergo a prophylactic total thyroidectomy by age 6 months.

OTHER SYNDROMES OF MULTIPLE ENDOCRINE NEOPLASIA

Patients with *Carney complex* develop tumors in the adrenal cortex, pituitary, thyroid, and gonads as well as cardiac myxomas and hyperpigmentation. Patients with *Cowden disease* develop thyroid abnormalities (66%) such as benign adenomas and follicular adenocarcinomas, along with breast cancer (20–36% in women), and multiple hamartomas that affect the skin and multiple other organs. Patients with McCune-Albright syndrome may develop precocious puberty (particularly girls) due to gonadal hypersecretion, Cushing syndrome caused by multiple adrenal nodules, hyperthyroidism from hypersecretory thyroid nodules, and acromegaly caused by GH-secreting pituitary tumors. Patients have fibrous dysplasia of bones and hypophosphatemia, with bone fractures being common. Sudden death has been reported. It is caused by a postzygotic

somatic mutatin in the gene coding for the stimulatory G_s protein, resulting in constitutive activation of affected cells.

Callender GG et al. Multiple endocrine neoplasia syndromes. Surg Clin North Am. 2008 Aug;88(4):863–95. [PMID: 18672144]

Kann PH et al. Natural course of small, asymptomatic neuroendocrine pancreatic tumours in multiple endocrine neoplasia type 1: an endoscopic ultrasound imaging study. Endocr Relat Cancer. 2006 Dec;13(4):1195–202. [PMID: 17158764]

Waldmann J et al. Adrenal involvement in multiple endocrine neoplasia type 1: results of 7 years of prospective screening. Langenbecks Arch Surg. 2007 Aug;392(4):437–43. [PMID: 17235589]

▼ CLINICAL USE OF CORTICOSTEROIDS

▶ Mechanisms of Action

Cortisol is a steroid hormone that is normally secreted by the adrenal cortex in response to ACTH. It exerts its action by binding to nuclear receptors, which then act upon chromatin to regulate gene expression, producing effects throughout the body.

▶ Relative Potencies (Table 26-17)

Hydrocortisone and cortisone acetate, like cortisol, have mineralocorticoid effects that become excessive at higher doses. Other synthetic corticosteroids such as prednisone, dexamethasone, and deflazacort (an oxazoline derivative of prednisolone) have minimal mineralocorticoid activity. Anticonvulsant drugs (eg, phenytoin, carbamazepine, phenobarbital) accelerate the metabolism of corticosteroids other than hydrocortisone, making them significantly less potent. Megestrol, a synthetic progestin, has slight corticosteroid activity that becomes significant when administered in high doses for appetite stimulation.

Table 26–17. Systemic versus topical activity of corticosteroids.[1]

	Systemic Activity	Topical Activity
Prednisone	4–5	1–2
Fluprednisolone	8–10	10
Triamcinolone	5	1
Triamcinolone acetonide	5	40
Dexamethasone	30–120	10
Betamethasone	30	5–10
Betamethasone valerate	—	50–150
Methylprednisolone	5	5
Fluocinolone acetonide	—	40–100
Flurandrenolone acetonide	—	20–50
Fluorometholone	1–2	40
Deflazacort	3–4	—

[1]Hydrocortisone = 1 in potency.

Table 26–18. Management of patients receiving systemic corticosteroids.

Recommendations for prescribing
- Do not administer corticosteroids unless absolutely indicated or more conservative measures have failed.
- Keep dosage and duration of administration to the minimum required for adequate treatment.

Monitoring recommendations
- Screen for tuberculosis with a purified protein derivative (PPD) test or chest radiograph before commencing long-term corticosteroid therapy.
- Screen for diabetes mellitus before treatment and at each physician visit.
  - Have patient test urine weekly for glucose.
  - Teach patient about the symptoms of hyperglycemia.
- Screen for hypertension before treatment and at each clinician visit.
- Screen for glaucoma and cataracts before treatment, 3 months after treatment inception, and then at least yearly.
- Monitor plasma potassium for hypokalemia and treat as indicated.
- Obtain bone densitometry before treatment and then periodically. Treat osteoporosis.
- Weigh daily. Use dietary measures to avoid obesity and optimize nutrition.
- Measure height frequently to document the degree of axial spine demineralization and compression.
- Watch for fungal or yeast infections of skin, nails, mouth, vagina, and rectum, and treat appropriately.
- With dosage reduction, watch for signs of adrenal insufficiency or corticosteroid withdrawal syndrome.

Patient information
- Prepare the patient and family for possible adverse effects on mood, memory, and cognitive function.
- Inform the patient about other possible side effects, particularly weight gain, osteoporosis, and aseptic necrosis of bone.
- Counsel to avoid smoking and excessive ethanol consumption.

Prophylactic measures
- Institute a vigorous physical exercise and isometric regimen tailored to each patient's disabilities.
- Administer calcium (1 g elemental calcium) and vitamin D_3, 400–800 international units orally daily.
  - Check spot morning urines, and alter dosage to keep urine calcium concentration below 30 mg/dL.
  - If the patient is receiving thiazide diuretics, check for hypercalcemia, and administer only 500 mg elemental calcium daily.
  - Consider a bisphosphonate such as alendronate (70 mg orally weekly) or periodic intravenous infusions of pamidronate or zoledronic acid.
- Avoid prolonged bed rest that will accelerate muscle weakness and bone mineral loss. Ambulate early after fractures.
- Avoid elective surgery, if possible. Vitamin A in a daily dose of 20,000 units orally for 1 week may improve wound healing, but it is not prescribed in pregnancy.
- Avoid activities that could cause falls or other trauma.
- For ulcer prophylaxis, if administering corticosteroids with nonsteroidals, prescribe a proton pump inhibitor (not required for corticosteroids alone). Avoid large doses of antacids containing aluminum hydroxide (many popular brands) because aluminum hydroxide binds phosphate and may cause a hypophosphatemic osteomalacia that can compound corticosteroid osteoporosis.
- Treat hypogonadism.
- Treat infections aggressively. Consider unusual pathogens.
- Treat edema as indicated.

▶ Adverse Effects

Prolonged treatment with systemic corticosteroids causes a variety of adverse effects that can be life-threatening. Patients should be thoroughly informed of the major possible side effects of treatment such as insomnia, personality change, weight gain, muscle weakness, polyuria, kidney stones, diabetes mellitus, sex hormone suppression, occasional amenorrhea in women, candidiasis and opportunistic infections, osteoporosis with fractures, or aseptic necrosis of bones (particularly of the hips), which may become manifest many months after even brief treatment (see section on Cushing syndrome). Patients who receive intermittent high-dose corticosteroids (eg, prednisone ≥ 15 mg daily and cumulative dose > 1 g) are at increased risk for osteoporotic fractures. Avascular necrosis of bone develops in about 15% of patients who receive corticosteroids at high doses (eg, prednisone ≥ 15 mg daily) for more than 1 month with cumulative prednisone doses of ≥ 10 g.

Bisphosphonates (eg, alendronate, 70 mg orally weekly) prevent the development of osteoporosis among patients receiving prolonged courses of corticosteroids. For patients who are unable to tolerate oral bisphosphonates (due to esophagitis, hiatal hernia, or gastritis), periodic intravenous infusions of pamidronate, 60–90 mg, or zoledronic acid, 2–4 mg, should also be effective. Teriparatide, 20 mcg subcutaneously daily for up to 2 years, is also effective against corticosteroid-induced osteoporosis. (See further discussion in Osteoporosis section.) It is wise to follow an organized treatment plan such as the one outlined in Table 26–18.

Ce P et al. Avascular necrosis of the bones: an overlooked complication of pulse steroid treatment of multiple sclerosis. Eur J Neurol. 2006 Aug; 13(8):857–61. [PMID: 16879296]

De Vries F et al. Fracture risk with intermittent high-dose oral glucocorticoid therapy. Arthritis Rheum. 2007 Jan;56(1):208–14. [PMID: 17195223]

Saag KG et al. Teriparatide or alendronate in glucocorticoid-induced osteoporosis. N Engl J Med. 2007 Nov;357(20):2028–39. [PMID: 18003959]

Diabetes Mellitus & Hypoglycemia

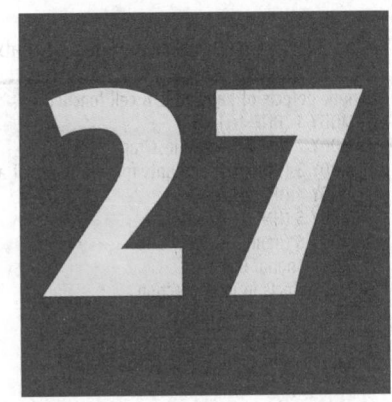

Umesh Masharani, MB, BS, MRCP(UK)

▼ DIABETES MELLITUS

ESSENTIALS OF DIAGNOSIS

Type 1 diabetes:

▶ Polyuria, polydipsia, and weight loss associated with random plasma glucose ≥ 200 mg/dL.

▶ Plasma glucose of 126 mg/dL or higher after an overnight fast, documented on more than one occasion.

▶ Ketonemia, ketonuria, or both.

▶ Islet autoantibodies are frequently present.

Type 2 diabetes:

▶ Most patients are over 40 years of age and obese.

▶ Polyuria and polydipsia. Ketonuria and weight loss generally are uncommon at time of diagnosis. Candidal vaginitis in women may be an initial manifestation. Many patients have few or no symptoms.

▶ Plasma glucose of 126 mg/dL or higher after an overnight fast on more than one occasion. After 75 g oral glucose, diagnostic values are 200 mg/dL or more 2 hours after the oral glucose.

▶ Hypertension, dyslipidemia, and atherosclerosis are often associated.

▶ Epidemiologic Considerations

In 2007, an estimated 23.6 million people in the United States had diabetes mellitus, of which approximately 1 million have type 1 diabetes and the rest mostly have type 2 diabetes. A third group that was designated as "other specific types" by the American Diabetes Association (ADA) (Table 27–1) number only in the thousands. Among these are the rare monogenic defects of either B cell function or of insulin action, primary diseases of the exocrine pancreas, endocrinopathies, and drug-induced diabetes. Updated information about the prevalence of diabetes in the United States is available from the Centers for Disease Control and Prevention (http://www.cdc.gov/diabetes/pubs/estimates. htm#prev).

▶ Classification & Pathogenesis

Diabetes mellitus is a syndrome with disordered metabolism and inappropriate hyperglycemia due to either a deficiency of insulin secretion or to a combination of insulin resistance and inadequate insulin secretion to compensate. Type 1 diabetes is due to pancreatic islet B cell destruction predominantly by an autoimmune process, and these patients are prone to ketoacidosis. Type 2 diabetes is the more prevalent form and results from insulin resistance with a defect in compensatory insulin secretion (Table 27–2).

A. Type 1 Diabetes Mellitus

This form of diabetes is immune-mediated in over 90% of cases and idiopathic in less than 10%. The rate of pancreatic B cell destruction is quite variable, being rapid in some individuals and slow in others. Type 1 diabetes is usually associated with ketosis in its untreated state. It occurs at any age but most commonly arises in children and young adults with a peak incidence before school age and again at around puberty. It is a catabolic disorder in which circulating insulin is virtually absent, plasma glucagon is elevated, and the pancreatic B cells fail to respond to all insulinogenic stimuli. Exogenous insulin is therefore required to reverse the catabolic state, prevent ketosis, reduce the hyperglucagonemia, and reduce blood glucose.

1. Immune-mediated type 1 diabetes mellitus (type 1A)—The highest incidence of immune-mediated type 1 diabetes mellitus is in Scandinavia and northern Europe, where the annual incidence is as high as 37 per 100,000 children aged 14 years or younger in Finland, 27 per 100,000 in Sweden, 22 per 100,000 in Norway, and 19 per 100,000 in the United Kingdom. The annual incidence of type 1 diabetes decreases across the rest of Europe to 10 per 100,000 in Greece and 8 per 100,000 in France. Surprisingly, the island of Sardinia has as high an annual incidence as Finland (37 per 100,000) even though in the rest of Italy, including the island of Sicily, it is only 10 per 100,000 per year. In the United States, the annual incidence of type 1 diabetes averages 15 per 100,000, with higher rates in states more densely populated with persons of Scandinavian descent such as Minnesota. Worldwide, the lowest incidence of type 1 diabe-

Table 27–1. Other specific types of diabetes mellitus.

Genetic defects of pancreatic B cell function
    MODY 1 (HNF-4α); rare
    MODY 2 (glucokinase); less rare
    MODY 3 (HNF-1α); accounts for two-thirds of all MODY
    MODY 4 (IPF-1); very rare
    MODY 5 (HNF-1β); very rare
    MODY 6 (neuroD1); very rare
    Mitochondrial DNA
Genetic defects in insulin action
    Type A insulin resistance
    Leprechaunism
    Rabson-Mendenhall syndrome
    Lipoatrophic diabetes
Diseases of the exocrine pancreas
Endocrinopathies
Drug- or chemical-induced diabetes
Other genetic syndromes (Down, Klinefelter, Turner, others) sometimes associated with diabetes

MODY, maturity-onset diabetes of the young.

Table 27–3. Diagnostic sensitivity and specificity of autoimmune markers in patients with newly diagnosed type 1 diabetes mellitus.

	Sensitivity	Specificity
Glutamic acid decarboxylase (GAD65)	70–90%	99%
Insulin (IAA)	40–70%	99%
Tyrosine phosphatase (IA-2)	50–70%	99%

Most patients with type 1 diabetes mellitus have circulating antibodies to islet cells (ICA), insulin (IAA), glutamic acid decarboxylase (GAD65), and tyrosine phosphatases (IA-2 and IA2-β) at the time the diagnosis is made. These antibodies facilitate screening for an autoimmune cause of diabetes, particularly screening siblings of affected children, as well as adults with atypical features of type 2 diabetes (Table 27–3). An additional autoantibody to a zinc transporter ZnT8 (Slc30A8) was recently found to be present in about 28% of type 1 diabetes patients who were negative for the other antibodies. Screening with zinc transporter, GAD65, IA2 and IAA autoantibodies may identify about 98% of people who have an autoimmune basis for their beta cell loss. Antibody levels decline with increasing duration of disease. Also, low levels of anti-insulin antibodies develop in almost all patients once they are treated with insulin.

Family members of diabetic probands are at increased lifetime risk for developing type 1 diabetes. A child whose mother has type 1 diabetes has a 3% risk of developing the disease and a 6% risk if the child's father has it. The risk in siblings is related to the number of HLA haplotypes that the sibling shares with the diabetic proband. If one haplotype is shared, the risk is 6% and if two haplotypes are shared, the risk increases to 12–25%. The highest risk is for identical twins, where the concordance rate is 25–50%.

Some patients with a milder expression of type 1 diabetes mellitus initially retain enough B cell function to avoid ketosis, but as their B cell mass diminishes later in life, dependence on insulin therapy develops. Islet cell antibody surveys among northern Europeans indicate that up to 15% of "type 2" diabetic patients may actually have this mild

tes (< 1 case per 100,000 per year) is in China and parts of South America. The global incidence of type 1 diabetes is increasing (approximately 3% each year).

Approximately one-third of the disease susceptibility is due to genes and two-thirds to environmental factors. Genes that are related to the HLA locus contribute about 40% of the genetic risk. About 95% of patients with type 1 diabetes possess either HLA-DR3 or HLA-DR4, compared with 45–50% of white controls. *HLA-DQ* genes are even more specific markers of type 1 susceptibility, since a particular variety *(HLA-DQB1*0302)* is found in the DR4 patients with type 1, while a "protective" gene *(HLA-DQB1*0602)* is often present in the DR4 controls. The other important gene that contributes to about 10% of the genetic risk is found at the 5′ polymorphic region of the insulin gene. This polymorphic region affects the expression of the insulin gene in the thymus and results in depletion of insulin-specific T lymphocytes. In linkage studies, 16 other genetic regions of the human genome have been identified as being important to pathogenesis but less is known about them.

Table 27–2. Clinical classification of common diabetes mellitus syndromes.

Type	Ketosis	Islet Cell Antibodies	HLA Association	Treatment
Type 1				
(A) Immune-mediated	Present	Present at onset	Positive	Eucaloric healthy diet and preprandial rapidly acting insulin, plus basal
(B) Idiopathic	Present	Absent	Absent	insulin replacement with intermediate-acting or long-acting insulin
Type 2				
(A) Nonobese	Absent	Absent	Negative	(1) Eucaloric diet alone
				(2) Diet plus insulin or oral agents
(B) Obese	Absent	Absent	Negative	(1) Weight reduction
				(2) Hypocaloric diet, plus oral agents or insulin

form of type 1 diabetes (latent autoimmune diabetes of adulthood; LADA). Evidence for environmental factors playing a role in the development of type 1 diabetes include the observation that the disease is more common in Scandinavian countries and becomes progressively less frequent in countries nearer and nearer to the equator. Also, the risk for type 1 diabetes increases when individuals who normally have a low risk emigrate to the Northern Hemisphere. For example, it was recently shown that Pakistani children born and raised in Bradford, England have a higher risk for developing type 1 diabetes compared with children who lived in Pakistan all their lives.

Which environmental factor is responsible for the increased risk is not known. There have been a number of different hypotheses including infections with certain viruses (rubella, Coxsackie B4) and consumption of cow's milk. Also, in developed countries, childhood infections have become less frequent and so perhaps the immune system becomes dysregulated with development of autoimmunity and conditions such as asthma and diabetes. This theory is referred to as the hygiene hypothesis. None of these factors has so far been confirmed as the culprit. Part of the difficulty is that autoimmune injury undoubtedly starts many years before clinical diabetes mellitus develops.

2. Idiopathic type 1 diabetes mellitus (type 1B)—

Less than 10% of subjects have no evidence of pancreatic B cell autoimmunity to explain their insulinopenia and ketoacidosis. This subgroup has been classified as "idiopathic type 1 diabetes" and designated as "type 1B." Although only a minority of patients with type 1 diabetes fall into this group, most of these are of Asian or African origin. It was recently reported that about 4% of the West Africans with ketosis-prone diabetes are homozygous for a mutation in *PAX-4* (*Arg133Trp*)—a gene that is essential for the development of pancreatic islets.

B. Type 2 Diabetes Mellitus

This represents a heterogeneous group of conditions that used to occur predominantly in adults, but it is now more frequently encountered in children and adolescents. More than 90% of all diabetic persons in the United States are included under this classification. Circulating endogenous insulin is sufficient to prevent ketoacidosis but is inadequate to prevent hyperglycemia in the face of increased needs owing to tissue insensitivity (insulin resistance).

Genetic and environmental factors combine to cause both the insulin resistance and the beta cell loss. Most epidemiologic data indicate strong genetic influences, since in monozygotic twins over 40 years of age, concordance develops in over 70% of cases within a year whenever type 2 diabetes develops in one twin. Genome-wide association studies have made considerable progress in identifying the at-risk genes. So far, 18 different genetic loci have been associated with an increased risk of type 2 diabetes. A significant number of the identified loci appear to code for proteins that have a role in beta cell function or development. One of the genetic loci with the largest risk effect is *TCF7L2*. This gene codes for a transcription factor involved in the WNT signaling pathway that is required for normal pancreatic development. Alleles at other genetic loci (*CDKAL1*, *SLC30A8*, *HHEX-IDE*, *CDKN2A/B*, *KCNJ11*, and *IGF2BP2*) are thought to affect insulin secretion. Two loci (*FTO* and *MC4R*) affect fat mass and obesity risk. The *PPARG* locus has been implicated in insulin resistance. The loci identified to date still explain only some of the heritable risk for diabetes; clearly, other loci remain to be discovered.

Early in the disease process, hyperplasia of pancreatic B cells occurs and probably accounts for the fasting hyperinsulinism and exaggerated insulin and proinsulin responses to glucose and other stimuli. With time, chronic deposition of amyloid in the islets may combine with inherited genetic defects progressively to impair B cell function.

Obesity is the most important environmental factor causing insulin resistance. The degree and prevalence of obesity varies among different racial groups with type 2 diabetes. While obesity is apparent in no more than 30% of Chinese and Japanese patients with type 2, it is found in 60–70% of North Americans, Europeans, or Africans with type 2 and approaches 100% of patients with type 2 among Pima Indians or Pacific Islanders from Nauru or Samoa.

Visceral obesity, due to accumulation of fat in the omental and mesenteric regions, correlates with insulin resistance; subcutaneous abdominal fat seems to have less of an association with insulin insensitivity. There are many patients with type 2 diabetes who, while not overtly obese, have increased visceral fat; they are termed the "metabolically obese." Exercise may affect the deposition of visceral fat as suggested by CT scans of Japanese wrestlers, whose extreme obesity is predominantly subcutaneous. Their daily vigorous exercise program prevents accumulation of visceral fat, and they have normal serum lipids and euglycemia despite daily intakes of 5000–7000 kcal and development of massive subcutaneous obesity. Several **adipokines**, secreted by fat cells, can affect insulin action in obesity. Two of these, **leptin** and **adiponectin**, seem to increase sensitivity to insulin, presumably by increasing hepatic responsiveness. Two others—**tumor necrosis factor**-α, which inactivates insulin receptors, and **resistin,** which interferes with insulin action on glucose metabolism—have been reported to be elevated in obese animal models. Abnormal levels of these adipokines may contribute to the development of insulin resistance in human obesity.

Hyperglycemia per se can impair insulin action by causing accumulation of hexosamines in muscle and fat tissue and by inhibiting glucose transport (acquired glucose toxicity). Correction of hyperglycemia reverses this acquired insulin resistance.

C. Other Specific Types of Diabetes Mellitus

1. Maturity-onset diabetes of the young (MODY)—

This subgroup is a relatively rare monogenic disorder characterized by non–insulin-dependent diabetes with autosomal dominant inheritance and an age at onset of 25 years or younger. Patients are nonobese, and their hyperglycemia is due to impaired glucose-induced secretion of insulin. Six types of MODY have been described. Except for MODY 2, in which a glucokinase gene is defective, all other types involve mutations of a nuclear transcription factor that regulates islet gene expression.

MODY 2 is quite mild, associated with only slight fasting hyperglycemia and few if any microvascular diabetic complications. It generally responds well to hygienic measures or low doses of oral hypoglycemic agents. MODY 3—the most common form—accounts for two-thirds of all MODY cases. The clinical course is similar to that of idiopathic type 2 diabetes in terms of microangiopathy and failure to respond to oral agents with time.

2. Diabetes due to mutant insulins—This is a very rare subtype of nonobese type 2 diabetes, with no more than ten families having been described. Since affected individuals were heterozygous and possessed one normal insulin gene, diabetes was mild, did not appear until middle age, and showed autosomal dominant genetic transmission. There is generally no evidence of clinical insulin resistance, and these patients respond well to standard therapy.

3. Diabetes due to mutant insulin receptors—Defects in one of their insulin receptor genes have been found in more than 40 people with diabetes, and most have extreme insulin resistance associated with acanthosis nigricans (Plate 91). In very rare instances when both insulin receptor genes are abnormal, newborns present with a leprechaun-like phenotype and seldom live through infancy.

4. Diabetes mellitus associated with a mutation of mitochondrial DNA—Since sperm do not contain mitochondria, only the mother transmits mitochondrial genes to her offspring. Diabetes due to mutations of mitochondrial DNA occurs in less than 2% of patients with diabetes. The most common cause is the A3243G mutation in the gene coding for the tRNA (Leu,UUR). Diabetes occurs even when a small percentage of the mitochondria in the cell carry the mutation; the heteroplasmy levels in the leukocytes range from 1% to 40%. Diabetes usually develops in these patients in their late 30s, and characteristically, they also have hearing loss (maternally inherited diabetes and deafness [MIDD]). In some patients, the beta cell failure can be rapidly progressive and patients require insulin soon after diagnosis. Other patients can be managed by diet or oral agents for a while but most eventually require insulin. MIDD patients are not usually overweight; they resemble patients with type 1 diabetes mellitus but without evidence for autoimmunity.

5. Wolfram syndrome—Wolfram syndrome is an autosomal recessive neurodegenerative disorder first evident in childhood. It consists of diabetes insipidus, diabetes mellitus, optic atrophy, and deafness, hence the acronym DIDMOAD. It is due to mutations in a gene named *WFS1*, which encodes a 100.3 KDa transmembrane protein localized in the endoplasmic reticulum. Diabetes develops in mice with mutated form of this protein; and isolated islets from these mice show impairment in insulin secretion to glucose stimulus and increased apoptosis. The diabetes mellitus usually presents in the first decade together with the optic atrophy. Cranial diabetes insipidus and sensorineural deafness develop during the second decade in 60–75% of patients. Ureterohydronephrosis, neurogenic bladder, cerebellar ataxia, peripheral neuropathy, and psychiatric illness develop later in many patients.

Insulin Resistance Syndrome (Syndrome X; Metabolic Syndrome)

Twenty-five percent of the general nonobese nondiabetic population has insulin resistance of a magnitude similar to that seen in type 2 diabetes. These insulin-resistant nondiabetic individuals are at much higher risk for developing type 2 diabetes than insulin-sensitive persons. In addition to diabetes, these individuals have increased risk for elevated plasma triglycerides, lower high-density lipoproteins (HDLs), and higher blood pressure—a cluster of abnormalities termed syndrome X. These associations have now been expanded to include small, dense, low-density lipoprotein (LDL), hyperuricemia, abdominal obesity, prothrombotic state with increased levels of plasminogen activator inhibitor type 1 (PAI-1), and proinflammatory state. These clusters of abnormalities significantly increase the risk of atherosclerotic disease.

It has been postulated that hyperinsulinemia and insulin resistance play a direct role in these metabolic abnormalities, but supportive evidence is inconclusive. Although hyperinsulinism and hypertension often coexist in whites, that is not the case in blacks or Pima Indians. Moreover, patients with hyperinsulinism due to insulinoma are not hypertensive, and there is no fall in blood pressure after surgical removal of the insulinoma restores normal insulin levels. The main value of grouping these disorders as a syndrome, however, is to remind clinicians that the therapeutic goals are not only to correct hyperglycemia but also to manage the elevated blood pressure and dyslipidemia that result in increased cerebrovascular and cardiac morbidity and mortality in these patients.

Clinical Findings

The principal clinical features of the two major types of diabetes mellitus are listed for comparison in Table 27–4.

Patients with type 1 diabetes have a characteristic symptom complex.

An absolute deficiency of insulin results in accumulation of circulating glucose and fatty acids, with consequent hyperosmolality and hyperketonemia.

Patients with type 2 diabetes may or may not have characteristic features. The presence of obesity or a strongly

Table 27–4. Clinical features of diabetes at diagnosis.

	Type 1 Diabetes	Type 2 Diabetes
Polyuria and thirst	++	+
Weakness or fatigue	++	+
Polyphagia with weight loss	++	–
Recurrent blurred vision	+	++
Vulvovaginitis or pruritus	+	++
Peripheral neuropathy	+	++
Nocturnal enuresis	++	–
Often asymptomatic	–	++

positive family history for mild diabetes suggests a high risk for the development of type 2 diabetes.

A. Symptoms and Signs

1. Type 1 diabetes—Increased urination is a consequence of osmotic diuresis secondary to sustained hyperglycemia. This results in a loss of glucose as well as free water and electrolytes in the urine. Thirst is a consequence of the hyperosmolar state, as is blurred vision, which often develops as the lenses are exposed to hyperosmolar fluids.

Weight loss despite normal or increased appetite is a common feature of type 1 when it develops subacutely. The weight loss is initially due to depletion of water, glycogen, and triglycerides; thereafter, reduced muscle mass occurs as amino acids are diverted to form glucose and ketone bodies.

Lowered plasma volume produces symptoms of postural hypotension. Total body potassium loss and the general catabolism of muscle protein contribute to the weakness.

Paresthesias may be present at the time of diagnosis, particularly when the onset is subacute. They reflect a temporary dysfunction of peripheral sensory nerves, which clears as insulin replacement restores glycemic levels closer to normal, suggesting neurotoxicity from sustained hyperglycemia.

When absolute insulin deficiency is of acute onset, the above symptoms develop abruptly. Ketoacidosis exacerbates the dehydration and hyperosmolality by producing anorexia and nausea and vomiting, interfering with oral fluid replacement.

The patient's level of consciousness can vary depending on the degree of hyperosmolality. When insulin deficiency develops relatively slowly and sufficient water intake is maintained, patients remain relatively alert and physical findings may be minimal. When vomiting occurs in response to worsening ketoacidosis, dehydration progresses and compensatory mechanisms become inadequate to keep serum osmolality below 320–330 mosm/L. Under these circumstances, stupor or even coma may occur. The fruity breath odor of acetone further suggests the diagnosis of diabetic ketoacidosis.

Hypotension in the recumbent position is a serious prognostic sign. Loss of subcutaneous fat and muscle wasting are features of more slowly developing insulin deficiency. In occasional patients with slow, insidious onset of insulin deficiency, subcutaneous fat may be considerably depleted.

2. Type 2 diabetes—While many patients with type 2 diabetes present with increased urination and thirst, many others have an insidious onset of hyperglycemia and are asymptomatic initially. This is particularly true in obese patients, whose diabetes may be detected only after glycosuria or hyperglycemia is noted during routine laboratory studies. Occasionally, type 2 patients may present with evidence of neuropathic or cardiovascular complications because of occult disease present for some time prior to diagnosis. Chronic skin infections are common. Generalized pruritus and symptoms of vaginitis are frequently the initial complaints of women. Diabetes should be suspected in women with chronic candidal vulvovaginitis as well as in those who have delivered large babies (> 9 lb, or 4.1 kg) or

have had polyhydramnios, preeclampsia, or unexplained fetal losses.

Obese diabetics may have any variety of fat distribution; however, diabetes seems to be more often associated in both men and women with localization of fat deposits on the upper segment of the body (particularly the abdomen, chest, neck, and face) and relatively less fat on the appendages, which may be quite muscular. Standardized tables of waist-to-hip ratio indicate that ratios of "greater than 0.9" in men and "greater than 0.8" in women are associated with an increased risk of diabetes in obese subjects. Mild hypertension is often present in obese diabetics. Eruptive xanthomas on the flexor surface of the limbs and on the buttocks and lipemia retinalis due to hyperchylomicronemia can occur in patients with uncontrolled type 2 diabetes who also have a familial form of hypertriglyceridemia.

B. Laboratory Findings

1. Urinalysis

A. GLUCOSURIA—A specific and convenient method to detect glucosuria is the paper strip impregnated with glucose oxidase and a chromogen system (Clinistix, Diastix), which is sensitive to as little as 0.1% glucose in urine. Diastix can be directly applied to the urinary stream, and differing color responses of the indicator strip reflect glucose concentration.

A normal renal threshold for glucose as well as reliable bladder emptying is essential for interpretation.

B. KETONURIA—Qualitative detection of ketone bodies can be accomplished by nitroprusside tests (Acetest or Ketostix). Although these tests do not detect β-hydroxybutyric acid, which lacks a ketone group, the semiquantitative estimation of ketonuria thus obtained is nonetheless usually adequate for clinical purposes. Many laboratories now measure β-hydroxybutyric acid, and there is now a meter available (Precision Xtra, Abbott Diabetes Care) for patient use that measures β-hydroxybutyric acid levels in capillary glucose samples.

2. Blood testing procedures

A. GLUCOSE TOLERANCE TEST

(1) Methodology and normal fasting glucose—Plasma or serum from venous blood samples has the advantage over whole blood of providing values for glucose that are independent of hematocrit and that reflect the glucose concentration to which body tissues are exposed. For these reasons, and because plasma and serum are more readily measured on automated equipment, they are used in most laboratories. If serum is used or if plasma is collected from tubes that lack an agent to block glucose metabolism (such as fluoride), samples should be refrigerated and separated within 1 hour after collection. The glucose concentration is 10–15% higher in plasma or serum than in whole blood because structural components of blood cells are absent.

(2) Criteria for laboratory confirmation of diabetes mellitus—If the fasting plasma glucose level is 126 mg/dL or higher on more than one occasion, further evaluation of the patient with a glucose challenge is unnecessary. How-

Table 27–5. The Diabetes Expert Committee criteria for evaluating the standard oral glucose tolerance test.[1]

	Normal Glucose Tolerance	Impaired Glucose Tolerance	Diabetes Mellitus[2]
Fasting plasma glucose (mg/dL)	< 100	100–125	≥ 126
Two hours after glucose load (mg/dL)	< 140	≥ 140–199	≥ 200

[1]Give 75 g of glucose dissolved in 300 mL of water after an overnight fast in persons who have been receiving at least 150–200 g of carbohydrate daily for 3 days before the test.
[2]A fasting plasma glucose ≥ 126 mg/dL is diagnostic of diabetes if confirmed on a subsequent day.

ever, when fasting plasma glucose is less than 126 mg/dL in suspected cases, a standardized oral glucose tolerance test may be done (Table 27–5).

For proper evaluation of the test, the subjects should be normally active and free from acute illness. Medications that may impair glucose tolerance include diuretics, contraceptive drugs, glucocorticoids, niacin, and phenytoin.

Because of difficulties in interpreting oral glucose tolerance tests and the lack of standards related to aging, these tests are being replaced by documentation of fasting hyperglycemia.

B. GLYCATED HEMOGLOBIN (HEMOGLOBIN A₁) MEASUREMENTS—Hemoglobin becomes glycated by ketoamine reactions between glucose and other sugars and the free amino groups on the α and β chains. Only glycation of the N-terminal valine of the beta chain imparts sufficient negative charge to the hemoglobin molecule to allow separation by charge dependent techniques. These charge separated hemoglobins are collectively referred to as hemoglobin A₁ (HbA₁). The major form of HbA₁ is hemoglobin A₁c (HbA₁c) where glucose is the carbohydrate. HbA₁c comprises 4–6% of total hemoglobin A₁. The remaining HbA₁ species contain fructose-1,6 diphosphate (HbA₁a₁); glucose-6-phosphate (HbA₁a₂); and unknown carbohydrate moiety (HbA₁b). The hemoglobin A₁c fraction is abnormally elevated in diabetic persons with chronic hyperglycemia. Methods for measuring HbA₁c include electrophoresis, cation-exchange chromatography, boronate affinity chromatography, and immunoassays. Office-based immunoassays using capillary blood give a result in about 9 minutes and this allows for immediate feedback to the patients regarding their glycemic control.

Since glycohemoglobins circulate within red blood cells whose life span lasts up to 120 days, they generally reflect the state of glycemia over the preceding 8–12 weeks, thereby providing an improved method of assessing diabetic control. The HbA₁c value, however, is weighted to more recent glucose levels (previous month) and this explains why significant changes in HbA₁c are observed with short-term (1 month) changes in mean plasma glucose levels. Measurements should be made in patients with either type of diabetes mellitus at 3- to 4-month intervals so that adjust-

ments in therapy can be made if HbA₁c is either subnormal or if it is more than 2% above the upper limits of normal for a particular laboratory. In patients monitoring their own blood glucose levels, HbA₁c values provide a valuable check on the accuracy of monitoring. In patients who do not monitor their own blood glucose levels, HbA₁c values are essential for adjusting therapy. There is a linear relationship between the HbA₁c and the average glucose levels in the previous 3 months as determined from continuous glucose monitoring data and from seven-point capillary blood glucose profiles (preprandial, postprandial, and bedtime). Table 27–6 gives the mean capillary glucose values for HbA₁c values ranging from 5% to 12%. Use of HbA₁c for screening is controversial. Sensitivity in detecting known diabetes cases by HbA₁c measurements is only 85%, indicating that diabetes cannot be excluded by a normal value. On the other hand, elevated HbA₁c assays are fairly specific (91%) in identifying the presence of diabetes.

The accuracy of HbA₁c values can be affected by hemoglobin variants or derivatives; the effect depends on the specific hemoglobin variant or derivative and the specific assay used. Immunoassays that use an antibody to the glycated amino terminus of β globin do not recognize the terminus of the γ globin of hemoglobin F. Thus, in patients with high levels of hemoglobin F, immunoassays give falsely low values of HbA₁c. Cation-exchange chromatography separates hemoglobin species by charge differences. Hemoglobin variants that co-elute with HbA₁c can lead to an overestimation of the HbA₁c value. Chemically modified derivatives of hemoglobin such as carbamoylation (in end-stage chronic kidney disease) or acetylation (high-dose aspirin therapy) can similarly co-elute with HbA₁c by some assay methods.

Any condition that shortens erythrocyte survival or decreases mean erythrocyte age (eg, recovery from acute blood loss, hemolytic anemia) will falsely lower HbA₁c irrespective of the assay method used. Alternative methods such as fructosamine (see below) should be considered for these

Table 27–6. Correlations of HbA₁c levels with average of capillary glucose measurements (preprandial, postprandial and bedtime) in the previous 3 months.

HbA₁c Value (%) Determined Using DCCT Aligned Assays	Mean Capillary Blood Glucose Levels (mg/dL)
5	97
6	126
7	154
8	183
9	212
10	240
11	269
12	298

Adapted, with permission, from Nathan et al. Translating the A₁c assay into estimated average glucose values. Diabetes Care 2008 Aug;31(8):1473–8.

patients. Vitamins C and E are reported to falsely lower test results possibly by inhibiting glycation of hemoglobin.

C. Serum fructosamine—Serum fructosamine is formed by nonenzymatic glycosylation of serum proteins (predominantly albumin). Since serum albumin has a much shorter half-life than hemoglobin, serum fructosamine generally reflects the state of glycemic control for only the preceding 1–2 weeks. Reductions in serum albumin (eg, nephrotic state or hepatic disease) will lower the serum fructosamine value. When abnormal hemoglobins or hemolytic states affect the interpretation of glycohemoglobin or when a narrower time frame is required, such as for ascertaining glycemic control at the time of conception in a diabetic woman who has recently become pregnant, serum fructosamine assays offer some advantage. Normal values vary in relation to the serum albumin concentration and are 1.5–2.4 mmol/L when the serum albumin level is 5 g/dL.

D. Self-monitoring of blood glucose—Capillary blood glucose measurements performed by patients themselves, as outpatients, are extremely useful. In type 1 patients in whom "tight" metabolic control is attempted, they are indispensable. There are several paper strip (glucose oxidase, glucose dehydrogenase, or hexokinase) methods for measuring glucose on capillary blood samples. A reflectance photometer or an amperometric system is then used to measure the reaction that takes place on the reagent strip. A large number of blood glucose meters are now available. All are accurate, but they vary with regard to speed, convenience, size of blood samples required, and cost. Popular models include those manufactured by LifeScan (One Touch), Bayer Corporation (Ascencia), Roche Diagnostics (Accu-Chek), Abbott Laboratories (Precision, FreeStyle), and Home Diagnostics (Prestige). These blood glucose meters are relatively inexpensive, ranging from $50 to $100 each. Test strips remain a major expense, costing $.50 to $.75 apiece. Each glucose meter comes with a lancet device and disposable 26- to 33-gauge lancets. For some meters, there is a code associated with every batch of test strips, and this code needs to be entered into the meter before the strips can be used. Failure to properly code the meter can result in inaccurate readings. Patients not infrequently forget to change the code and it is preferable to give patients meters that do not require coding. The accuracy of data obtained by home glucose monitoring does require education of the patient in sampling and measuring procedures as well as in properly calibrating the instruments.

The clinician should be aware of the limitations of the self-monitoring glucose systems. First, a few of the older meters (such as the One Touch Profile) are calibrated against whole blood glucose concentrations even though the test strip measures the glucose in the plasma fraction. This means the displayed values are 10% to 15% *lower* than the laboratory glucose result. Second, increases or decreases in hematocrit can decrease or increase the measured glucose values. The mechanism underlying this effect is not known but presumably it is due to the impact of red cells on the diffusion of plasma into the reagent layer. Third, the meters and the test strips are calibrated over the glucose concentrations ranging from 60 mg/dL to 160 mg/dL, and

the accuracy is not as good for higher and lower glucose levels. When the glucose is less than 60 mg/dL, the difference between the meter and the laboratory value may be as much as 20%. Fourth, glucose oxidase–based amperometric systems underestimate glucose levels in the presence of high oxygen tension. This may be important in the critically ill who are receiving supplemental oxygen; under these circumstances, a glucose dehydrogenase–based system may be preferable. Fifth, some meters have been approved for measuring glucose in blood samples obtained at alternative sites such as the forearm and thigh. There is, however, a 5- to 20-minute lag in the glucose response on the arm with respect to the glucose response on the finger. Forearm blood glucose measurements could therefore result in a delay in detection of rapidly developing hypoglycemia.

E. Continuous glucose monitoring systems—Three continuous glucose monitoring systems are currently available for clinical use. The MiniMed Medtronic, Navigator, and DexCom systems involve inserting a subcutaneous sensor (rather like an insulin pump cannula) that measures glucose concentrations in the interstitial fluid for 3, 5, or 7 days, respectively. The data are transmitted to a separate pager-like device with a screen. The MiniMed system also has the option to wirelessly transmit the data to the screen of their insulin pump. The systems allow the patient to set "alerts" for low and high glucose values and rate of change of glucose levels. Patients still have to calibrate the devices with periodic fingerstick glucose levels, and since there are concerns regarding reliability, it is still necessary to confirm the displayed glucose level with a fingerstick glucose before making interventions such as injecting extra insulin or eating extra carbohydrates. A 6-month randomized controlled study of type 1 patients showed that adults (25 years and older) using these systems had improved glycemic control without an increase in the incidence of hypoglycemia. A randomized controlled study of continuous glucose monitoring during pregnancy showed improved glycemic control in the third trimester, lower birth weight, and reduced risk of macrosomia. The individual glucose values are not that critical—what matters is the direction and the rate at which the glucose is changing, allowing the user to take corrective action. The wearer also gains insight into the way particular foods and activities affect their glucose levels. The other main benefit is the low glucose alert warning. These systems are not covered by insurance and the initial cost is about $800 to $1000, and the sensor, which has to be changed every 3 to 7 days, costs $35 to $60. This adds up to an out-of-pocket expense of about $4000 annually.

3. Lipoprotein abnormalities in diabetes—Circulating lipoproteins are just as dependent on insulin as is the plasma glucose. In type 1 diabetes, moderately deficient control of hyperglycemia is associated with only a slight elevation of LDL cholesterol and serum triglycerides and little if any change in HDL cholesterol. Once the hyperglycemia is corrected, lipoprotein levels are generally normal. However, in patients with type 2 diabetes, a distinct "diabetic dyslipidemia" is characteristic of the insulin resistance syndrome. Its features are a high serum triglyceride level (300–400 mg/dL), a low HDL cholesterol (less than 30 mg/dL), and a qualitative change in LDL particles, producing a smaller dense particle whose membrane carries supranormal amounts of free cholesterol. These smaller dense LDL particles are more susceptible to oxidation, which renders them more atherogenic. Since a low HDL cholesterol is a major feature predisposing to macrovascular disease, the term "dyslipidemia" has preempted the term "hyperlipidemia," which mainly denoted the elevated triglycerides. Measures designed to correct the obesity and hyperglycemia, such as exercise, diet, and hypoglycemic therapy, are the treatment of choice for diabetic dyslipidemia, and in occasional patients in whom normal weight was achieved, all features of the lipoprotein abnormalities cleared. Since primary disorders of lipid metabolism may coexist with diabetes, persistence of lipid abnormalities after restoration of normal weight and blood glucose should prompt a diagnostic workup and possible pharmacotherapy of the lipid disorder. Chapter 28 discusses these matters in detail.

▶ Differential Diagnosis

A. Hyperglycemia Secondary to Other Causes

Secondary hyperglycemia has been associated with various disorders of insulin target tissues (liver, muscle, and adipose tissue) (Table 27–7). Other secondary causes of carbohydrate intolerance include endocrine disorders—often specific endocrine tumors—associated with excess production of growth hormone, glucocorticoids, catecholamines, glucagon, or somatostatin. In the first four situations, peripheral responsiveness to insulin is impaired. With excess of glucocorticoids, catecholamines, or glucagon, increased hepatic output of glucose is a contributory factor; in the case of catecholamines, decreased insulin release is an additional factor in producing carbohydrate intolerance, and with excess somatostatin production it is the major factor.

A rare syndrome of extreme insulin resistance associated with acanthosis nigricans afflicts either young women with androgenic features as well as insulin receptor mutations or older people, mostly women, in whom a circulating immunoglobulin binds to insulin receptors and reduces their affinity to insulin.

Table 27–7. Secondary causes of hyperglycemia.

Hyperglycemia due to tissue insensitivity to insulin
Hormonal tumors (acromegaly, Cushing syndrome, glucagonoma, pheochromocytoma)
Pharmacologic agents (corticosteroids, sympathomimetic drugs, niacin)
Liver disease (cirrhosis, hemochromatosis)
Muscle disorders (myotonic dystrophy)
Adipose tissue disorders (lipodystrophy, truncal obesity)
Insulin receptor disorders (acanthosis nigricans syndromes, leprechaunism)
Hyperglycemia due to reduced insulin secretion
Hormonal tumors (somatostatinoma, pheochromocytoma)
Pancreatic disorders (pancreatitis, hemosiderosis, hemochromatosis)
Pharmacologic agents (thiazide diuretics, phenytoin, pentamidine)

Medications such as diuretics, phenytoin, niacin, and high-dose corticosteroids can produce hyperglycemia that is reversible once the drugs are discontinued or when diuretic-induced hypokalemia is corrected. Chronic pancreatitis or subtotal pancreatectomy reduces the number of functioning B cells and can result in a metabolic derangement very similar to that of genetic type 1 diabetes except that a concomitant reduction in pancreatic A cells may reduce glucagon secretion so that relatively lower doses of insulin replacement are needed. Insulin-dependent diabetes is occasionally associated with Addison disease and autoimmune thyroiditis (**Schmidt syndrome**, or **polyglandular failure syndrome**). This occurs more commonly in women and represents an autoimmune disorder in which there are circulating antibodies to adrenocortical and thyroid tissue, thyroglobulin, and gastric parietal cells.

B. Nondiabetic Glycosuria

Nondiabetic glycosuria (renal glycosuria) is a benign asymptomatic condition wherein glucose appears in the urine despite a normal amount of glucose in the blood, either basally or during a glucose tolerance test. Its cause may vary from an autosomally transmitted genetic disorder to one associated with dysfunction of the proximal renal tubule (Fanconi syndrome, chronic kidney disease), or it may merely be a consequence of the increased load of glucose presented to the tubules by the elevated glomerular filtration rate during pregnancy. As many as 50% of pregnant women normally have demonstrable sugar in the urine, especially during the third and fourth months. This sugar is practically always glucose except during the late weeks of pregnancy, when lactose may be present.

▶ Clinical Trials in Diabetes

Findings of the Diabetes Complications and Control Trial (DCCT) and of the United Kingdom Prospective Diabetes Study (UKPDS), have confirmed the beneficial effects of improved glycemic control in both type 1 and type 2 diabetes, respectively (see below). In addition, with increased understanding of the pathophysiology of both type 1 and type 2 diabetes, large prospective studies—Diabetes Prevention Trial 1 (DPT-1) and the Diabetes Prevention Program (DPP)—have been performed in attempts to prevent onset of these disorders (see below).

A. Clinical Trials in Type 1 Diabetes

1. Diabetes Prevention Trial-1—This multicenter study sponsored by the National Institutes of Health was designed to determine whether the development of type 1 diabetes mellitus could be prevented or delayed by immune intervention therapy. Daily low-dose insulin injections were administered for up to 8 years in first-degree relatives of type 1 diabetic patients who were selected as being at high risk for development of type 1 diabetes because of detectable islet cell antibodies and reduced early-insulin release. Unfortunately, this immune intervention failed to affect the onset of type 1 diabetes compared with a randomized untreated group. A related study using oral insulin in lower risk first-degree relatives who have islet cell antibodies but whose early insulin release remains intact also failed to show an effect on the onset of type 1 diabetes. After an average of 4.3 years of observation, type 1 diabetes developed in about 35% of persons in both the oral insulin and the placebo groups.

2. The Diabetes Control and Complications Trial—

A long-term therapeutic study involving 1441 patients with type 1 diabetes mellitus reported that "near" normalization of blood glucose resulted in a delay in the onset and a major slowing of the progression of established microvascular and neuropathic complications of diabetes during a follow-up period of up to 10 years. Multiple insulin injections (66%) or insulin pumps (34%) were used in the intensively treated group, who were trained to modify their therapy in response to frequent glucose monitoring. The conventionally treated groups used no more than two insulin injections, and clinical well-being was the goal with no attempt to modify management based on HbA_{1c} determinations or the glucose results.

In half of the patients, a mean hemoglobin A_{1c} of 7.2% (normal: < 6%) and a mean blood glucose of 155 mg/dL were achieved using intensive therapy, while in the conventionally treated group HbA_{1c} averaged 8.9% with an average blood glucose of 225 mg/dL. Over the study period, which averaged 7 years, there was an approximately 60% reduction in risk between the two groups in regard to diabetic retinopathy, nephropathy, and neuropathy. The intensively treated group also had a nonsignificant reduction in the risk of macrovascular disease of 41% (95% CI, −10 to 68). Intensively treated patients had a threefold greater risk of serious hypoglycemia as well as a greater tendency toward weight gain. However, there were no deaths definitely attributable to hypoglycemia in any persons in the DCCT study, and no evidence of posthypoglycemic cognitive damage was detected.

Subjects participating in the DCCT study were subsequently enrolled in a follow-up observational study, the Epidemiology of Diabetes Interventions and Complications (EDIC) study. Even though the between-group differences in mean HbA_{1c} narrowed over 4 years, the group assigned to intensive therapy had a lower risk of retinopathy at 4 years and microalbuminuria at 7 to 8 years of continued study follow-up. Moreover, by the end of the 11-year follow-up period, the intensive therapy group had significantly reduced their risk of any cardiovascular disease events by 42% (95% CI, 9% to 23%; $P = 0.02$). Thus, it seems that the benefits of good glucose control persist even if control deteriorates at a later date.

The general consensus of the ADA is that intensive insulin therapy associated with comprehensive self-management training should become standard therapy in patients with type 1 diabetes mellitus after the age of puberty. Exceptions include those with advanced chronic kidney disease and the elderly, since in these groups the detrimental risks of hypoglycemia outweigh the benefits of tight glycemic control.

3. Immune intervention trials in new-onset type 1 diabetes—

At the time of diagnosis of type 1 diabetes, patients still have significant B cell function. This explains why soon after diagnosis patients go into a partial clinical remission ("honeymoon") requiring little or no insulin. This clinical remission is short-lived, however, and eventually patients lose all B cell function and have more labile glucose control. Attempts have been made to prolong this partial clinical remission using drugs such as cyclosporine, azathioprine, prednisone, and antithymocyte globulin. These drugs have had limited efficacy, and there are concerns about toxicity and the need for continuous treatment.

Newer agents that may induce immune tolerance and appear to have few side effects have been used in new-onset type 1 patients. Two studies with anti-CD3 antibodies have demonstrated that these agents can preserve endogenous insulin production. Larger phase 2 clinical trials are currently in progress.

B. Clinical Trials in Type 2 Diabetes

1. The Diabetes Prevention Program—

This study was aimed at discovering whether treatment with either diet and exercise or metformin could prevent the onset of type 2 diabetes in people with impaired glucose tolerance; 3234 overweight men and women aged 25–85 years with impaired glucose tolerance participated in the study. Intervention with a low-fat diet and 150 minutes of moderate exercise (equivalent to a brisk walk) per week reduced the risk of progression to type 2 diabetes by 71% compared with a matched control group. Participants taking 80 mg of metformin twice a day reduced their risk of developing type 2 diabetes by 31%, but this intervention was relatively ineffective in those who were either less obese or in the older age group.

With the demonstration that intervention can be successful in preventing progression to diabetes in these subjects, a recommendation has been made to change the terminology from the less comprehensible "impaired glucose tolerance" to "prediabetes." The latter is a term that the public can better understand and thus respond to by implementing healthier diet and exercise habits.

2. Kumamoto study—

The Kumamoto study involved a relatively small number of patients with type 2 diabetes (n = 110) who were nonobese and only slightly insulin-resistant, requiring less than 30 units of insulin per day for intensive therapy. Over a 6-year period, it was shown that intensive insulin therapy, achieving a mean HbA_{1c} of 7.1%, significantly reduced microvascular end points compared with conventional insulin therapy achieving a mean HbA_{1c} of 9.4%. Cardiovascular events were neither worsened nor improved by intensive therapy, and weight changes were likewise not influenced by either form of treatment.

3. The United Kingdom Prospective Diabetes Study—

This multicenter study was designed to establish, in type 2 diabetic patients, whether the risk of macrovascular or microvascular complications could be reduced by intensive blood glucose control with oral hypoglycemic agents or insulin and whether any particular therapy was of advantage. A total of 3867 patients aged 25–65 years with newly diagnosed diabetes were recruited between 1977 and 1991, and studied over 10 years. The median age at baseline was 54 years; 44% were overweight (> 120% over ideal weight); and baseline HbA_{1c} was 9.1%. Therapies were randomized to include a control group on diet alone and separate groups intensively treated with either insulin or sulfonylurea (chlorpropamide, glyburide, or glipizide). Metformin was included as a randomization option in a subgroup of 342 overweight or obese patients, and much later in the study an additional subgroup of both normal-weight and overweight patients who were responding unsatisfactorily to sulfonylurea therapy were randomized to either continue on their sulfonylurea therapy alone or to have metformin combined with it.

A. HYPERTENSION CONTROL SUBSTUDY—In 1987, an additional modification was made to evaluate whether tight control of blood pressure with stepwise antihypertensive therapy would prevent macrovascular and microvascular complications in 758 hypertensive patients among this UKPDS population compared with 390 of them whose blood pressure was treated less intensively. The tight control group was randomly assigned to treatment with either an angiotensin-converting enzyme (ACE) inhibitor (captopril) or a β-blocker (atenolol). Both drugs were stepped up to maximum dosages of 100 mg/d and then, if blood pressure remained higher than the target level of < 150/85 mm Hg, more drugs were added in the following stepwise sequence: a diuretic, slow-release nifedipine, methyldopa, and prazosin—until the target level of tight control was achieved. In the control group, hypertension was conventionally treated to achieve target levels < 180/105 mm Hg, but these patients were not prescribed either ACE inhibitors or β-blockers.

B. RESULTS OF THE UKPDS—Intensive treatment with either sulfonylureas, metformin, combinations of those two, or insulin achieved mean HbA_{1c} levels of 7%. This level of glycemic control decreases the risk of microvascular complications (retinopathy and nephropathy) in comparison with conventional therapy (mostly diet alone), which achieved mean levels of HbA_{1c} of 7.9%. Weight gain occurred in intensively treated patients except when metformin was used as monotherapy. No cardiovascular benefit and no adverse cardiovascular outcomes were noted regardless of the therapeutic agent. Hypoglycemic reactions occurred in the intensive treatment groups, but only one death from hypoglycemia was documented during 27,000 patient-years of intensive therapy.

When therapeutic subgroups were analyzed, some unexpected and paradoxical results were noted. Among the obese patients, intensive treatment with insulin or sulfonylureas did not reduce microvascular complications compared with diet therapy alone. This was in contrast to the significant benefit of intensive therapy with these drugs in the total group. Furthermore, intensive therapy with metformin was more beneficial in the overweight or obese persons than diet alone with regard to fewer myocardial infarctions, strokes, and diabetes-related deaths, but there was no significant reduction by metformin of diabetic microvascular complications as compared with the diet group. Moreover, in the subgroup of obese and nonobese patients in whom metformin was added to sulfonylurea failures, rather than showing a benefit, there was a 96% *increase* in diabetes-related deaths compared with the matched cohort of patients with unsatisfactory glycemic

control on sulfonylureas who remained on their sulfonylurea therapy. Chlorpropamide also came out poorly on subgroup analysis in that those receiving it as intensive therapy did less well regarding progression to retinopathy than those conventionally treated with diet.

Intensive antihypertensive therapy to a mean of 144/82 mm Hg had beneficial effects on microvascular disease as well as on all diabetes-related end points, including virtually all cardiovascular outcomes, in comparison with looser control at a mean of 154/87 mm Hg. In fact, the advantage of reducing hypertension by this amount was substantially more impressive than the benefit achieved by improving the degree of glycemic control from a mean HbA_{1c} of 7.9% to 7%. More than half of the patients needed two or more drugs for adequate therapy of their hypertension, and there was no demonstrable advantage of ACE inhibitor therapy over therapy with β-blockers with regard to diabetes end points. Use of a calcium channel blocker added to both treatment groups appeared to be safe over the long term in this diabetic population despite some controversy in the recent literature about its safety in diabetics.

Like the DCCT trialists, the UKPDS researchers performed post-trial monitoring to determine whether there were long-term benefits of having been in the intensively treated glucose and blood pressure arms of the study. The between-group differences in HbA1c were lost within the first year of follow-up, but the reduced risk (24%, $P = 0.001$) of development or progression of microvascular complications in the intensively treated group persisted for 10 years. The intensively treated group also had significantly reduced risk of myocardial infarction (15%, $P = 0.01$) and death from any cause (13%, $P = 0.007$) during the follow-up period. The subgroup of overweight or obese subjects who were initially randomized to metformin therapy showed sustained reduction in risk of myocardial infarction and death from any cause in the follow-up period. The between-group blood pressure differences disappeared within 2 years of the end of the trial. Unlike the sustained benefits seen with glucose control, there were no sustained benefits from having been in the more tightly controlled blood pressure group. Both blood pressure groups were at similar risk for microvascular events and diabetes-related end points during the follow-up period.

Thus, the follow-up of the UKPDS type 2 diabetes cohort showed that, as in type 1 diabetes, the benefits of good glucose control persist even if control deteriorates at a later date. Blood pressure benefits, however, last only as long as the blood pressure is well controlled.

4. The Steno-2 study—The Steno-2 study was designed in 1990 to validate the efficacy of targeting multiple concomitant risk factors for both microvascular and macrovascular disorders in type 2 diabetes. A prospective, randomized, open, blinded end point design was used where 160 patients with type 2 diabetes and microalbuminuria were assigned to conventional therapy with their general practitioner or to intensive care at the Steno Diabetes Center. The intensively treated group had step-wise introduction of lifestyle and pharmacologic interventions aimed at keeping glycated hemoglobin less than 6.5%, blood pressure less than 130/80 mm Hg; total cholesterol < 175 mg/dL, and triglycerides < 150 mg/dL. All the intensively treated group received ACE inhibitors and if intolerant, an angiotensin II-receptor blocker. The lifestyle component of intensive intervention included reduction in dietary fat intake to less than 30% of total calories; smoking cessation program; light to moderate exercise; daily vitamin-mineral supplement of vitamin C, E, and chromium picolinate. Initially, aspirin was only given as secondary prevention to patients with a history of ischemic cardiovascular disease; later, all patients received aspirin. After a mean follow-up of 7.8 years, cardiovascular events (eg, myocardial infarction, angioplasties, coronary bypass grafts, strokes, amputations, vascular surgical interventions) developed in 44% of patients in the conventional arm and only in 24% in the intensive multifactorial arm—about a 50% reduction. Rates of nephropathy, retinopathy, and autonomic neuropathy were also lower in the multifactorial intervention arm by 62% and 63%, respectively.

The data from the UKPDS and this study provide support for guidelines recommending vigorous treatment of concomitant microvascular and cardiovascular risk factors in patients with type 2 diabetes.

5. ACCORD and ADVANCE studies—The ACCORD study was a randomized controlled study designed to determine whether normal HbA$_{1c}$ levels would reduce the risk of cardiovascular events in middle-aged or older individuals with type 2 diabetes. About 35% of the 10,251 recruited subjects had established cardiovascular disease at study entry. The intensive arm of the study was discontinued after 3.5 years of follow-up because of more unexplained deaths in the intensive arm when compared with the control arm (22%, P = 0.020). Analysis of the data at time of discontinuation showed that the intensively treated group (mean HbA$_{1c}$ 6.4%) had a 10% reduction in cardiovascular event rate compared with the standard treated group (mean HbA$_{1c}$ 7.5%), but this difference was not statistically significant.

The ADVANCE trial randomly assigned 11,140 patients with type 2 diabetes to standard or intensive glucose control. The primary outcomes were major macrovascular cardiovascular events (nonfatal myocardial infarction or stroke or death from cardiovascular causes) or microvascular events. Overall, one-third (32%) of the subjects had established cardiovascular disease at study entry. After a median follow-up of 5 years, there was a nonsignificant reduction (6%) in major macrovascular event rate in the intensively treated group (mean HbA$_{1c}$ 6.5%) compared with the standard therapy group (HbA$_{1c}$ 7.3%).

Thus, the ACCORD and ADVANCE results do not provide support for the hypothesis that near-normal glucose control in patients with type 2 diabetes will reduce cardiovascular events. It is, however, important not to over-interpret the results of these two studies. The results do not exclude the possibility that cardiovascular benefits might accrue with longer duration of near-normal glucose control. In the UKPDS, risk reductions for myocardial infarction and death from any cause were only observed during 10 years of post-trial follow-up. Specific subgroups of type 2 diabetic patients may also have different outcomes. The ACCORD and ADVANCE studies recruited patients who had diabetes

for 8–10 years and one-third of them already had established cardiovascular disease. Patients in the UKPDS, in contrast, had newly diagnosed diabetes and only 7.5% had a history of macrovascular disease. It is possible that the benefits of tight glycemic control on macrovascular events are attenuated in patients with longer duration of diabetes or with established vascular disease. Specific therapies used to lower glucose may also affect cardiovascular event rate or mortality. Severe hypoglycemia occurred more frequently in the intensively treated groups of the ACCORD and ADVANCE studies; the ACCORD investigators were not able to exclude undiagnosed hypoglycemia as a potential cause for the increased death rate in the intensive treatment group.

▶ Treatment Regimens

A. Diet

A well-balanced, nutritious diet remains a fundamental element of therapy. The American Diabetes Association (ADA) recommends about 45–65% of total daily calories in the form of carbohydrates; 25–35% in the form of fat (of which less than 7% are from saturated fat), and 10–35% in the form of protein. In patients with type 2 diabetes, limiting the carbohydrate intake and substituting some of the calories with monounsaturated fats, such as olive oil, rapeseed (canola) oil, or the oils in nuts and avocados, can lower triglycerides and increase HDL cholesterol. Patients with type 1 diabetes or type 2 diabetes who take insulin should be taught "carbohydrate counting," so they can administer their insulin bolus for each meal based on its carbohydrate content. In obese individuals with diabetes, an additional goal is weight reduction by caloric restriction (see Chapter 29).

The current recommendations for both types of diabetes continue to limit cholesterol to 300 mg daily, and individuals with LDL cholesterol more than 100 mg/dL should limit dietary cholesterol to 200 mg daily. High protein intake may cause progression of kidney disease in patients with diabetic nephropathy; for these individuals, a reduction in protein intake to 0.8 kg/day (or about 10% of total calories daily) is recommended.

Exchange lists for meal planning can be obtained from the American Diabetes Association and its affiliate associations or from the American Dietetic Association, 216 W. Jackson Blvd., Chicago, IL 60606 (312-899-0040). Their Internet address is http://www.eatright.org.

1. Dietary fiber—Plant components such as cellulose, gum, and pectin are indigestible by humans and are termed dietary "fiber." Insoluble fibers such as cellulose or hemicellulose, as found in bran, tend to increase intestinal transit and may have beneficial effects on colonic function. In contrast, soluble fibers such as gums and pectins, as found in beans, oatmeal, or apple skin, tend to retard nutrient absorption rates so that glucose absorption is slower and hyperglycemia may be slightly diminished. Although its recommendations do not include insoluble fiber supplements such as added bran, the ADA recommends food such as oatmeal, cereals, and beans with relatively high soluble fiber content as staple components of the diet in diabetics. High soluble fiber content in the diet may also have a favorable effect on blood cholesterol levels.

2. Artificial and other sweeteners—Aspartame (Nutra Sweet) consists of two major amino acids, aspartic acid and phenylalanine, which combine to produce a sweetener 180 times as sweet as sucrose. A major limitation is that it is not heat stable, so it cannot be used in cooking. Saccharin (Sweet 'N Low), Sucralose (Splenda), and Acesulfame potassium (Sweet One) are other "artificial" sweeteners that can be used in cooking and baking.

Fructose represents a "natural" sugar substance that is a highly effective sweetener, induces only slight increases in plasma glucose levels, and does not require insulin for its metabolism. However, because of potential adverse effects of large amounts of fructose on raising serum cholesterol, triglycerides, and LDL cholesterol, it does not have any advantage as a sweetening agent in the diabetic diet. This does not preclude, however, ingestion of fructose-containing fruits and vegetables or fructose-sweetened foods in moderation.

Sugar alcohols, also known as polyols or polyalcohol, are commonly used as sweeteners and bulking agents. They occur naturally in a variety of fruits and vegetables but are also commercially made from sucrose, glucose, and starch. Examples are sorbitol, xylitol, mannitol, lactitol, isomalt, maltitol, and hydrogenated starch hydrolysates (HSH). They are not as easily absorbed as sugar, so they do not raise blood glucose levels as much. Therefore, sugar alcohols are often used in food products that are labeled as "sugar free," such as chewing gum, lozenges, hard candy, and sugar-free ice cream. However, if consumed in large quantities, they will raise blood glucose and can cause bloating and diarrhea.

B. Drugs for Treating Hyperglycemia

(Table 27–8.) The drugs for treating type 2 diabetes fall into several categories: (1) Drugs that primarily stimulate insulin secretion by binding to the sulfonylurea receptor. Sulfonylureas remain the most widely prescribed drugs for treating hyperglycemia. The meglitinide analog repaglinide and the D-phenylalanine derivative nateglinide also bind the sulfonylurea receptor and stimulate insulin secretion. (2) Drugs that alter insulin action: Metformin works in the liver. The thiazolidinediones appear to have their main effect on skeletal muscle and adipose tissue. (3) Drugs that principally affect absorption of glucose: The α-glucosidase inhibitors acarbose and miglitol are such currently available drugs. (4) Drugs that mimic incretin effect or prolong incretin action: Exenatide and DPP 1V inhibitors fall into this category. (5) Other: Pramlintide lowers glucose by suppressing glucagon and slowing gastric emptying.

1. Drugs that primarily stimulate insulin secretion by binding to the sulfonylurea receptor on the beta cell

A. SULFONYLUREAS—The primary mechanism of action of the sulfonylureas is to stimulate insulin release from pancreatic B cells. Specific receptors on the surface of pancreatic B cells bind sulfonylureas in the rank order of their insulinotropic potency (glyburide with the greatest affinity and tolbutamide with the least affinity). It has been shown

that activation of these receptors closes potassium channels, resulting in depolarization of the B cell. This depolarized state permits calcium to enter the cell and actively promote insulin release.

Sulfonylureas are not indicated for use in type 1 diabetes patients since these drugs require functioning pancreatic B cells to produce their effect on blood glucose. These drugs are used in patients with type 2 diabetes, in whom acute administration improves the early phase of insulin release that is refractory to acute glucose stimulation. Sulfonylureas are metabolized by the liver and apart from acetohexamide, whose metabolite is more active than the parent compound, the metabolites of all the other sulfonylureas are weakly active or inactive. The metabolites are excreted by the kidney and, in the case of the second-generation sulfonylureas, partly excreted in the bile. Sulfonylureas are generally contraindicated in patients with severe liver or kidney impairment. Idiosyncratic reactions are rare, with skin rashes or hematologic toxicity (leukopenia, thrombocytopenia) occurring in less than 0.1% of users.

(1) First-generation sulfonylureas (tolbutamide, tolazamide, acetohexamide, chlorpropamide)—**Tolbutamide** is supplied as 500-mg tablets. It is rapidly oxidized in the liver to inactive metabolites, and its approximate duration of effect is relatively short (6–10 hours). Tolbutamide is probably best administered in divided doses (eg, 500 mg before each meal and at bedtime); however, some patients require only one or two tablets daily with a maximum dose of 3000 mg/d. Because of its short duration of action, which is independent of kidney function, tolbutamide is probably the safest sulfonylurea to use if liver function is normal. Prolonged hypoglycemia has been reported rarely with tolbutamide, mostly in patients receiving certain antibacterial sulfonamides (sulfisoxazole), phenylbutazone for arthralgias, or the oral azole antifungal drugs to treat candidiasis. These drugs apparently compete with tolbutamide for oxidative enzyme systems in the liver, resulting in maintenance of high levels of unmetabolized, active sulfonylurea in the circulation.

Tolazamide, acetohexamide, and chlorpropamide are rarely used. Chlorpropamide has a prolonged biologic effect, and severe hypoglycemia can occur especially in the elderly as their renal clearance declines with aging. Its other side effects include alcohol-induced flushing and hyponatremia due to its effect on vasopressin secretion and action.

(2) Second-generation sulfonylureas (glyburide, glipizide, gliclazide, glimepiride)—Glyburide, glipizide, gliclazide, and glimepiride are 100–200 times more potent than tolbutamide. These drugs should be used with caution in patients with cardiovascular disease or in elderly patients, in whom prolonged hypoglycemia would be especially dangerous.

Glyburide is available in 1.25-mg, 2.5-mg, and 5-mg tablets. The usual starting dose is 2.5 mg/d, and the average maintenance dose is 5–10 mg/d given as a single morning dose; maintenance doses higher than 20 mg/d are not recommended. Some reports suggest that 10 mg is a maximum daily therapeutic dose, with 15–20 mg having no additional benefit in poor responders and doses over 20 mg actually worsening hyperglycemia. Glyburide is metabolized

Table 27–8. Drugs for treatment of type 2 diabetes mellitus.

Drug	Tablet Size	Daily Dose	Duration of Action
Sulfonylureas			
Tolbutamide (Orinase)	500 mg	0.5–2 g in two or three divided doses	6–12 hours
Tolazamide (Tolinase)	100, 250, and 500 mg	0.1–1 g as single dose or in two divided doses	Up to 24 hours
Acetohexamide (Dymelor)	250 and 500 mg	0.25–1.5 g as single dose or in two divided doses	8–24 hours
Chlorpropamide (Diabinese)	100 and 250 mg	0.1–0.5 g as single dose	24–72 hours
Glyburide			
(Diaβeta, Micronase)	1.25, 2.5, and 5 mg	1.25–20 mg as single dose or in two divided doses	Up to 24 hours
(Glynase)	1.5, 3, and 6 mg	1.5–12 mg as single dose or in two divided doses	Up to 24 hours
Glipizide			
(Glucotrol)	5 and 10 mg	2.5–20 mg twice a day 30 minutes before meals	6–12 hours
(Glucotrol XL)	2.5, 5, and 10 mg	2.5 to 10 mg once a day is usual dose; 20 mg once a day is maximal dose	Up to 24 hours
Gliclazide (not available in US)	80 mg	40–80 mg as single dose; 160–320 mg as divided dose	12 hours
Glimepiride (Amaryl)	1, 2, and 4 mg	1–4 mg once a day is usual dose; 8 mg once a day is maximal dose	Up to 24 hours
Meglitinide analogs			
Repaglinide (Prandin)	0.5, 1, and 2 mg	0.5 to 4 mg three times a day before meals	3 hours
ᴅ-Phenylalanine derivative			
Nateglinide (Starlix)	60 and 120 mg	60 or 120 mg three times a day before meals	1.5 hours
Biguanides			
Metformin (Glucophage)	500, 850, and 1000 mg	1–2.5 g; 1 tablet with meals two or three times daily	7–12 hours
Extended-release metformin (Glucophage XR)	500 mg	500–2000 mg once a day	Up to 24 hours
Thiazolidinediones			
Rosiglitazone (Avandia)	2, 4, and 8 mg	4–8 mg daily (can be divided)	Up to 24 hours
Pioglitazone (Actos)	15, 30, and 45 mg	15–45 mg daily	Up to 24 hours
α-Glucosidase inhibitors			
Acarbose (Precose)	50 and 100 mg	25 to 100 mg three times a day just before meals	4 hours
Miglitol (Glyset)	25, 50, and 100 mg	25–100 mg three times a day just before meals	4 hours
Incretins			
Exenatide (Byetta)	1.2 mL and 2.4 mL pre-filled pens containing 5 mcg and 10 mcg (subcutaneous injection)	5 mcg subcutaneously twice a day within 1 hour of breakfast and dinner. Increase to 10 mcg subcutaneously twice a day after about a month. Do not use if calculated creatinine clearance is less than 30 mL/min.	6 hours
Sitagliptin (Januvia)	25, 50, and 100 mg	100 mg once daily is usual dose; dose is 50 mg once daily if calculated creatinine clearance is 30 to 50 mL/min and 25 mg once daily if clearance is less than 30 mL/min.	24 hours
Others			
Pramlintide (Symlin)	5 mL vial containing 0.6 mg/mL; also available as prefilled pens. Symlin pen 60 or Symlin pen 120 (subcutaneous injection)	For insulin-treated type 2 patients, start at 60 mcg dose three times a day (10 units on U100 insulin syringe). Increase to 120 mcg three times a day (20 units on U100 insulin syringe) if no nausea for 3–7 days. Give immediately before meal.	
		For type 1 patients, start at 15 mcg three times a day (2.5 units on U100 insulin syringe) and increase by increments of 15 mcg to a maximum of 60 mcg three times a day, as tolerated.	
		To avoid hypoglycemia, lower insulin dose by 50% on initiation of therapy.	

in the liver into products with hypoglycemic activity, which probably explains why assays specific for the unmetabolized compound suggest a plasma half-life of only 1–2 hours, yet the biologic effects of glyburide are clearly persistent 24 hours after a single morning dose in diabetic patients. Glyburide is unique among sulfonylureas in that it not only binds to the pancreatic B cell membrane sulfonylurea receptor but also becomes sequestered within the B cell. This may also contribute to its prolonged biologic effect despite its relatively short circulating half-life. A "Press Tab" formulation of "micronized" glyburide—easy to divide in half with slight pressure if necessary—is available in tablet sizes of 1.5 mg, 3 mg, and 6 mg.

Glyburide has few adverse effects other than its potential for causing hypoglycemia, which at times can be prolonged. Flushing has rarely been reported after ethanol ingestion. It does not cause water retention, as chlorpropamide does, but rather slightly enhances free water clearance. Glyburide is absolutely contraindicated in the presence of hepatic impairment and should not be used in patients with chronic kidney disease, in elderly patients, or in those who would be put at serious risk from an episode of hypoglycemia.

Glipizide is available in 5-mg and 10-mg tablets. For maximum effect in reducing postprandial hyperglycemia, this agent should be ingested 30 minutes before meals, since rapid absorption is delayed when the drug is taken with food. The recommended starting dose is 5 mg/d, with up to 15 mg/d given as a single daily dose before breakfast. When higher daily doses are required, they should be divided and given before meals. The maximum dose recommended by the manufacturer is 40 mg/d, although doses above 10–15 mg probably provide little additional benefit in poor responders and may even be *less* effective than smaller doses.

At least 90% of glipizide is metabolized in the liver to inactive products, and 10% is excreted unchanged in the urine. Glipizide therapy is therefore contraindicated in patients with liver or kidney impairment, who would be at high risk for hypoglycemia; but because of its lower potency and shorter duration of action, it is preferable to glyburide in elderly patients. Glipizide has also been marketed as Glucotrol-XL in 5-mg and 10-mg tablets. It provides extended release during transit through the gastrointestinal tract with greater effectiveness in lowering prebreakfast hyperglycemia than the shorter-duration immediate-release standard glipizide tablets. However, this formulation appears to have sacrificed its lower propensity for severe hypoglycemia compared with longer-acting glyburide without showing any demonstrable therapeutic advantages over glyburide.

Gliclazide (not available in the United States) is another intermediate duration sulfonylurea with a duration of action of about 12 hours. It is available as 80 mg tablets. The recommended starting dose is 40–80 mg/d with a maximum dose of 320 mg. Doses of 160 mg and above are given as divided doses before breakfast and dinner. The drug is metabolized by the liver; the metabolites and conjugates have no hypoglycemic effect. An extended release preparation is available.

Glimepiride is given once daily as monotherapy or in combination with insulin to lower blood glucose in diabetes patients who cannot control their glucose level through diet and exercise. Glimepiride achieves blood glucose lowering with the lowest dose of any sulfonylurea compound, and this tends to increase its cost-effectiveness. A single daily dose of 1 mg/d has been shown to be effective, and the maximal recommended dose is 8 mg. It has a long duration of action with a pharmacodynamic half-life of 5 hours, allowing once-daily administration, which improves compliance. It is completely metabolized by the liver to relatively inactive metabolic products.

B. Meglitinide analogs—**Repaglinide** is structurally similar to glyburide but lacks the sulfonic acid-urea moiety. It acts by binding to the sulfonylurea receptor and closing the ATP-sensitive potassium channel. It is rapidly absorbed from the intestine and then undergoes complete metabolism in the liver to inactive biliary products, giving it a plasma half-life of less than 1 hour. The drug therefore causes a brief but rapid pulse of insulin. The starting dose is 0.5 mg three times a day 15 minutes before each meal. The dose can be titrated to a maximal daily dose of 16 mg. Like the sulfonylureas, repaglinide can be used in combination with metformin. Hypoglycemia is the main side effect. In clinical trials, when the drug was compared with a long-duration sulfonylurea (glyburide), there was a trend toward less hypoglycemia. Like the sulfonylureas also, repaglinide causes weight gain. Metabolism is by cytochrome P450 3A4 isoenzyme, and other drugs that induce or inhibit this isoenzyme may increase or inhibit (respectively) the metabolism of repaglinide. The drug may be useful in patients with kidney impairment or in the elderly.

C. D-Phenylalanine derivative—**Nateglinide** stimulates insulin secretion by binding to the sulfonylurea receptor and closing the ATP-sensitive potassium channel. This compound is rapidly absorbed from the intestine, reaching peak plasma levels within 1 hour. It is metabolized in the liver and has a plasma half-life of about 1.5 hours. Like repaglinide, it causes a brief rapid pulse of insulin, and when given before a meal it reduces the postprandial rise in blood glucose. The drug is available as 60-mg and 120-mg tablets. The 60-mg dose is used in patients who have mild elevations in HbA_{1c}. For most patients, the recommended starting and maintenance dose is 120 mg three times a day before meals. Like the other insulin secretagogues, its main side effects are hypoglycemia and weight gain.

2. Drugs that alter insulin action

A. Metformin—Metformin (1,1-dimethylbiguanide hydrochloride) is used, either alone or in conjunction with other oral agents or insulin, in the treatment of patients with type 2 diabetes.

Metformin's primary action is on the liver, reducing hepatic gluconeogenesis by activating adenosine monophosphate-activated protein kinase (AMPK), which acts as an intracellular energy sensor, and has a critical role regulating gluconeogenesis. LKB1 is a protein threonine kinase that phosphorylates and activates AMPK; it was recently reported that in mice the deletion of LKB1 function in the liver results in hyperglycemia with increased gluconeogenic and lipogenic gene expression. The deletion of LKB1 also eliminated the glucose lowering effect of metformin, providing genetic proof for the hypothesis that metformin lowers glucose levels by AMP kinase activation.

Metformin has a half-life of 1.5–3 hours, is not bound to plasma proteins, and is not metabolized in humans, being excreted unchanged by the kidneys.

Metformin may be used as an adjunct to diet for the control of hyperglycemia and its associated symptoms in patients with type 2 diabetes, particularly those who are obese or are not responding optimally to maximal doses of sulfonylureas. A side benefit of metformin therapy is its tendency to improve both fasting and postprandial hyperglycemia and hypertriglyceridemia in obese diabetics without the weight gain associated with insulin or sulfonylurea therapy. Metformin is not indicated for patients with type 1 diabetes and is contraindicated in diabetics with serum creatinine levels of 1.5 mg/dL or higher, hepatic insufficiency, alcoholism, or a propensity to develop tissue hypoxia.

Metformin is dispensed as 500 mg, 850 mg, and 1000 mg tablets. A 500 mg extended-release preparation is also available. Although the maximal dosage is 2.55 g, little benefit is seen above a total dose of 2000 mg. It is important to begin with a low dose and increase the dosage very gradually in divided doses—taken with meals—to reduce minor gastrointestinal upsets. A common schedule would be one 500 mg tablet three times a day with meals or one 850 mg or 1000 mg tablet twice daily at breakfast and dinner. One to four tablets of the extended-release preparation can be given once a day.

The most frequent side effects of metformin are gastrointestinal symptoms (anorexia, nausea, vomiting, abdominal discomfort, diarrhea), which occur in up to 20% of patients. These effects are dose-related, tend to occur at onset of therapy, and often are transient. However, in 3–5% of patients, therapy may have to be discontinued because of persistent diarrheal discomfort. In a retrospective analysis, it has been reported that patients switched from immediate-release metformin to comparable dose of extended-release metformin experienced fewer gastrointestinal side effects.

Hypoglycemia does not occur with therapeutic doses of metformin, which permits its description as a "euglycemic" or "antihyperglycemic" drug rather than an oral hypoglycemic agent. Dermatologic or hematologic toxicity is rare.

Lactic acidosis has been reported as a side effect but is uncommon with metformin in contrast to phenformin. While therapeutic doses of metformin reduce lactate uptake by the liver, serum lactate levels rise only minimally if at all, since other organs such as the kidney can remove the slight excess. However, if tissue hypoxia occurs, the metformin-treated patient is at higher risk for lactic acidosis due to compromised lactate removal. Similarly, when kidney function deteriorates, affecting not only lactate removal by the kidney but also metformin excretion, plasma levels of metformin rise far above the therapeutic range and block hepatic uptake enough to provoke lactic acidosis without associated increases in lactic acid production. Almost all reported cases have involved subjects with associated risk factors that should have contraindicated its use (kidney, liver, or cardiorespiratory insufficiency, alcoholism, advanced age). Acute kidney failure can occur rarely in certain patients receiving radiocontrast agents. Metformin therapy should therefore be temporarily halted on the day of the test and for 2 days following injection of radiocontrast agents to avoid potential lactic acidosis if end-stage chronic kidney failure occurs.

B. THIAZOLIDINEDIONES—Drugs of this class of antihyperglycemic agents sensitize peripheral tissues to insulin. They bind a nuclear receptor called peroxisome proliferator-activated receptor gamma (PPAR-γ) and affect the expression of a number of genes and regulate the release of the adipokines—resistin and adiponectin—from adipocytes. Adiponectin secretion is stimulated, which sensitizes tissues to the effects of insulin, and resistin secretion is inhibited, which reduces insulin resistance. Observed effects of thiazolidinediones include increased glucose transporter expression (GLUT 1 and GLUT 4), decreased free fatty acid levels, decreased hepatic glucose output, and increased differentiation of preadipocytes into adipocytes. Like the biguanides, this class of drugs does not cause hypoglycemia.

Two drugs of this class, rosiglitazone and pioglitazone, are available for clinical use. Both are effective as monotherapy and in combination with sulfonylureas or metformin or insulin. When used as monotherapy, these drugs lower HbA_{1c} by about 1 or 2 percentage points. When used in combination with insulin, they can result in a 30–50% reduction in insulin dosage, and some patients can come off insulin completely. The dosage of rosiglitazone is 4–8 mg daily and of pioglitazone, 15–45 mg daily, and the drugs do not have to be taken with food. Rosiglitazone is primarily metabolized by the CYP 2C8 isoenzyme and pioglitazone is metabolized by CYP 2C8 and CYP 3A4.

The combination of a thiazolidinedione and metformin has the advantage of not causing hypoglycemia. Patients inadequately managed on sulfonylureas can do well on a combination of sulfonylurea and rosiglitazone or pioglitazone. About 25% of patients in clinical trials fail to respond to these drugs, presumably because they are significantly insulinopenic.

These drugs have some additional effects apart from glucose lowering. Rosiglitazone therapy is associated with increases in total cholesterol, LDL-cholesterol (15%), and HDL-cholesterol (10%). There is a reduction in free fatty acids of about 8–15%. The changes in triglycerides were generally not different from placebo. Pioglitazone in clinical trials lowered triglycerides (9%) and increased HDL-cholesterol (15%), but did not cause a consistent change in total cholesterol and LDL-cholesterol levels. A prospective randomized comparison of the metabolic effects of pioglitazone and rosiglitazone on patients who had previously taken troglitazone (now withdrawn from the US market) showed similar effects on HbA_{1c} and weight gain. Pioglitazone-treated persons, however, had lower total cholesterol, LDL-cholesterol, and triglycerides when compared with rosiglitazone-treated persons. The thiazolidinediones have also been demonstrated to decrease levels of plasminogen activator inhibitor type 1, matrix metalloproteinase 9, C-reactive protein, and interleukin 6. Small prospective studies have demonstrated that treatment with these drugs leads to improvements in the biochemical and histologic features of nonalcoholic fatty liver disease. The thiazolidinediones also may limit vascular smooth muscle proliferation after injury, and there are reports that pioglitazone and troglitazone (subsequently withdrawn from the US market) reduced neointimal proliferation after coronary stent placement. Finally, in one double-blind, placebo-controlled study, rosiglitazone was shown to be associated with a decrease in the ratio of urinary albumin to creatinine excretion.

Safety concerns and some troublesome side effects have emerged about this class of drugs that potentially limit their use.

A meta-analysis of 42 randomized clinical trials with rosiglitazone suggested that this drug increases the risk of angina pectoris or myocardial infarction. Even though definitive evidence is lacking, the FDA has required the manufacturer to include a boxed warning about the potential risk of heart attacks on the drug label. A meta-analysis of clinical trials with pioglitazone did not show a similar finding. Many physicians, because of these findings, have stopped prescribing rosiglitazone and instead use pioglitazone, if indicated.

Edema occurs in about 3–4% of patients receiving monotherapy with rosiglitazone or pioglitazone. The edema occurs more frequently (10–15%) in patients receiving concomitant insulin therapy and may result in congestive heart failure. The drugs are contraindicated in diabetic individuals with New York Heart Association class III and IV cardiac status. Thiazolidinediones have also been reported as being associated with new onset or worsening macular edema. Apparently, this is a rare side effect, and most of these patients also had peripheral edema. The macular edema resolved or improved once the drug was discontinued.

In experimental animals, rosiglitazone stimulates bone marrow adipogenesis at the expense of osteoblastogenesis resulting in a decrease in bone density. An increase in fracture risk in women (but not men) has been reported with both rosiglitazone and pioglitazone. The fracture risk is in the range of 1.9 per 100 patient-years with the thiazolidinedione compared to 1.1 per 100 patient years on comparison treatment. In at least one study of rosiglitazone, the fracture risk was increased in premenopausal as well as postmenopausal women.

Other side effects include anemia, which occurs in 4% of patients treated with these drugs; it may be due to a dilutional effect of increased plasma volume rather than a reduction in red cell mass. Weight gain occurs, especially when the drug is combined with a sulfonylurea or insulin. Some of the weight gain is fluid retention, but there is also an increase in total fat mass.

Troglitazone, the first drug in this class to go into widespread clinical use, was withdrawn from clinical use because of drug-associated fatal liver failure. The two currently available agents, rosiglitazone and pioglitazone, have thus far not caused hepatotoxicity. The FDA has, however, recommended that patients should not initiate drug therapy if there is clinical evidence of active liver disease or pre-treatment elevation of the alanine aminotransferase (ALT) level that is 2.5 times greater than the upper limit of normal. Obviously, caution should be used in initiation of therapy in patients with even mild ALT elevations. Liver biochemical tests should be performed prior to initiation of treatment and periodically thereafter.

3. Drugs that affect absorption of glucose—α-Glucosidase inhibitors competitively inhibit the α-glucosidase enzymes in the gut that digest dietary starch and sucrose. Two of these drugs—acarbose and miglitol—are available for clinical use. Both are potent inhibitors of glucoamylase, α-amylase, and sucrase but have less effect on isomaltase and hardly any on trehalase and lactase. Acarbose binds 1000 times more avidly to the intestinal disaccharidases than do products of carbohydrate digestion or sucrose. A fundamental difference between acarbose and miglitol is in their absorption. Acarbose has the molecular mass and structural features of a tetrasaccharide, and very little (about 2%) crosses the microvillar membrane. Miglitol, however, has a structural similarity with glucose and is absorbable. Both drugs delay the absorption of carbohydrate and lower postprandial glycemic excursion.

A. ACARBOSE—Acarbose is available as 50-mg and 100-mg tablets. The recommended starting dose of acarbose is 50 mg twice daily, gradually increasing to 100 mg three times daily. For maximal benefit on postprandial hyperglycemia, acarbose should be given with the first mouthful of food ingested. In diabetic patients, it reduces postprandial hyperglycemia by 30–50%, and its overall effect is to lower the HbA_{1c} by 0.5–1%.

The principal adverse effect, seen in 20–30% of patients, is flatulence. This is caused by undigested carbohydrate reaching the lower bowel, where gases are produced by bacterial flora. In 3% of cases, troublesome diarrhea occurs. This gastrointestinal discomfort tends to discourage excessive carbohydrate consumption and promotes improved compliance of type 2 patients with their diet prescriptions. When acarbose is given alone, there is no risk of hypoglycemia. However, if combined with insulin or sulfonylureas, it might increase the risk of hypoglycemia from these agents. A slight rise in hepatic aminotransferases has been noted in clinical trials with acarbose (5% versus 2% in placebo controls, and particularly with doses > 300 mg/d). The levels generally return to normal on stopping the drug.

In the UKPDS, approximately 2000 patients on diet, sulfonylurea, metformin, or insulin therapy were randomized to acarbose or placebo therapy. By 3 years, 60% of the patients had discontinued the drug, mostly because of gastrointestinal symptoms. If one looked only at the 40% who remained on the drug, they had an 0.5% lower HbA_{1c} compared with placebo.

B. MIGLITOL—Miglitol is similar to acarbose in terms of its clinical effects. It is indicated for use in diet- or sulfonylurea-treated patients with type 2 diabetes. Therapy is initiated at the lowest effective dosage of 25 mg three times a day. The usual maintenance dose is 50 mg three times a day, although some patients may benefit from increasing the dose to 100 mg three times a day. Gastrointestinal side effects occur as with acarbose. The drug is not metabolized and is excreted unchanged by the kidney. Theoretically, absorbable α-glucosidase inhibitors could induce a deficiency of one or more of the α-glucosidases involved in cellular glycogen metabolism and biosynthesis of glycoproteins. This does not occur in practice because, unlike the intestinal mucosa, which sees a high concentration of the drug, the blood level is 200-fold to 1000-fold lower than the concentration needed to inhibit intracellular α-glucosidases. Miglitol should not be used in end-stage chronic kidney disease, when its clearance would be impaired.

4. Incretins—Oral glucose provokes a threefold to fourfold higher insulin response than an equivalent dose of glucose given intravenously. This is because the oral glucose causes a release of gut hormones, principally glucagon-like peptide 1 (GLP-1) and glucose-dependent insulinotropic polypeptide (GIP1), that amplify the glucose-induced insulin release. This "incretin effect" is reduced in patients with type 2 diabetes. GLP-1 secretion (but not GIP1 secretion) is impaired in patients with type 2 diabetes and when GLP-1 is infused in patients with type 2 diabetes, it stimulates insulin secretion and lowers glucose levels. GLP-1, unlike the sulfonylureas, has only a modest insulin stimulatory effect at normoglycemic concentrations. This means that GLP-1 has a lower risk for hypoglycemia than the sulfonylureas.

In addition to its insulin stimulatory effect, GLP-1 also has a number of other pancreatic and extrapancreatic effects. It suppresses glucagon secretion and so may ameliorate the hyperglucagonemia that is present in people with diabetes and improve postprandial hyperglycemia. GLP-1 preserves islet integrity and reduces apoptotic cell death of human islet cells in culture. In mice, streptozotocin-induced apoptosis is significantly reduced by coadministration of exendin-4 or exenatide, a GLP-1 receptor agonist. GLP-1 acts on the stomach delaying gastric emptying; the importance of this effect on glucose lowering is illustrated by the observation that antagonizing the deceleration of gastric emptying markedly reduces the glucose lowering effect of GLP-1. GLP-1 receptors are present in the central nervous system, and intracerebroventricular administration of GLP-1 in wild type mice, but not in GLP-1 receptor knockout mice, inhibits feeding. Type 2 diabetic patients undergoing GLP-1 infusion are less hungry; it is unclear whether this is mainly due to a deceleration of gastric emptying or whether there is a central nervous system effect as well.

A. Exenatide—GLP-1 is rapidly proteolyzed by dipeptidyl peptidase 4 (DPP-4), and therefore for clinical effect would need to be administered as a continuous infusion. Exendin 4 or exenatide is a GLP-1 receptor agonist isolated from the saliva of the Gila Monster (a venomous lizard) that is more resistant to DPP-4 action and so its half-life is 2.4 hours and its glucose lowering effect is about 6 hours. When this drug is given to patients with type 2 diabetes by subcutaneous injection twice daily, it lowers blood glucose and HbA$_{1c}$ levels. Exenatide appears to have the same effects as GLP-1 on glucagon suppression and gastric emptying. In clinical trials, adding exenatide therapy to patients with type 2 diabetes already taking metformin or a sulfonylurea, or both, further lowered the HbA$_{1c}$ value by 0.4% to 0.6% over a 30-week period. These patients also experienced a weight loss of 3–6 pounds. In an open label extension study up to 80 weeks, the HbA$_{1c}$ reduction was sustained and there was further weight loss (to a total loss of about 10 pounds). The

main side effect was nausea, affecting over 40% of the patients. The nausea was dose-dependent and declined with time. The risk of hypoglycemia was higher in persons taking sulfonylureas. The FDA has received 30 post-marketing reports of acute pancreatitis in patients taking exenatide. Many of these patients had other risk factors for pancreatitis, but the possibility remains that the drug was causally responsible for some cases. Patients taking exenatide should be advised to seek immediate medical care if they experience unexplained persistent severe abdominal pain. The delay in gastric emptying may affect the absorption of some other drugs; therefore, antibiotics and oral contraceptives should be taken 1 hour before exenatide doses. Low-titer antibodies against exenatide develop in over one-third (38%) of patients, but the clinical effects are not attenuated. High-titer antibodies develop in a subset of patients (~6%), and in about half of these cases, an attenuation of glycemic response has been seen.

Exenatide is dispensed as two fixed-dose pens (5 mcg and 10 mcg). It is injected 60 minutes before breakfast and before dinner. Patients should be prescribed the 5 mcg pen for the first month and, if tolerated, the dose can then be increased to 10 mcg twice a day. The drug is not recommended in patients with glomerular filtration rate less than 30 mL/min.

B. Sitagliptin—The oral DPP-4 inhibitors prolong the action of endogenously released GLP-1 and GIP. A number of neuropeptides, growth factors, cytokines, and chemokines are potential DPP-4 substrates; DPP-4 inhibitors prolong the actions of neuropeptide Y and substance P. Sitagliptin in clinical trials was shown to be effective in lowering glucose when used alone and in combination with metformin and pioglitazone. In various clinical trials, improvements in HbA$_{1c}$ ranged from 0.5% to 1.4%. The usual dose of sitagliptin is 100 mg once daily, but the dose is reduced to 50 mg daily if the calculated creatinine clearance is 30–50 mL/min and to 25 mg for clearances less than 30 mL/min. Unlike exenatide, sitagliptin does not cause nausea or vomiting. It also does not result in weight loss. The main adverse effect appears to be a predisposition to nasopharyngitis or upper respiratory tract infection. A small increase in neutrophil count of ~200 cells/mcL has also occurred. Since its FDA approval and clinical use, there have been reports of serious allergic reactions to sitagliptin, including anaphylaxis, angioedema, and exfoliative skin conditions including Stevens-Johnson syndrome. The frequency of these events is unclear.

5. Others—**Pramlintide** is a synthetic analog of islet amyloid polypeptide (IAPP or amylin). When given subcutaneously, it delays gastric emptying, suppresses glucagon secretion, and decreases appetite. It is approved for use both in type 1 diabetes and in insulin-treated type 2 diabetes. In 6-month clinical studies with type 1 and insulin-treated type 2 patients, those on the drug had an approximately 0.4% reduction in HbA$_{1c}$ and about 1.7 kg weight loss compared with placebo. The HbA$_{1c}$ reduction was sustained for 2 years but some of the weight was regained. The drug is given by injection immediately before the meal. Hypoglycemia can occur, and it is recommended that the short-acting or premixed insulin doses be reduced by 50% when the drug is started. Nausea was the other main side effect, affecting 30–50% of persons but tended to improve with time. In patients with type 1 diabetes, the initial dose of pramlintide is 15 mcg before each meal and titrated up by 15 mcg increments to a maintenance dose of 30 mcg or 60 mcg before each meal. In patients with type 2 diabetes, the starting dose is 60 mcg premeals increased to 120 mcg in 3 to 7 days if no significant nausea occurs.

6. Drug combinations—Several drug combinations are available in different dose sizes, including glyburide and metformin (Glucovance); glipizide and metformin (Metaglip); rosiglitazone and metformin (Avandamet); pioglitazone and metformin (ACTOplus Met); rosiglitazone and glimepiride (Avandaryl); pioglitazone and glimepiride (Duetact); and sitagliptin and metformin (Janumet). These drug combinations, however, limit the clinician's ability to optimally adjust dosage of the individual drugs and for that reason are not recommended.

C. Insulin

Insulin is indicated for type 1 diabetes as well as for type 2 diabetic patients with insulinopenia whose hyperglycemia does not respond to diet therapy either alone or combined with other hypoglycemic drugs.

With the development of highly purified human insulin preparations, immunogenicity has been markedly reduced, thereby decreasing the incidence of therapeutic complications such as insulin allergy, immune insulin resistance, and localized lipoatrophy at the injection site. However, the problem of achieving optimal insulin delivery remains unsolved with the present state of technology. It has not been possible to reproduce the physiologic patterns of intraportal insulin secretion with subcutaneous injections of short-acting or longer-acting insulin preparations. Even so, with the help of appropriate modifications of diet and exercise and careful monitoring of capillary blood glucose levels at home, it has often been possible to achieve acceptable control of blood glucose by using various mixtures of short- and longer-acting insulins injected at least twice daily or portable insulin infusion pumps.

1. Characteristics of available insulin preparations—Commercial insulin preparations differ with respect to the time of onset and duration of their biologic action (Table 27–9).

A. SPECIES OF INSULIN—Human insulin is produced by recombinant DNA techniques (biosynthetic human insulin) as Humulin (Eli Lilly) and as Novolin (Novo Nordisk). It is dispensed as either regular (R) or NPH (N) formulations. Five analogs of human insulin—three rapidly acting (insulin lispro, insulin aspart, insulin glulisine) and two long-acting (insulin glargine and insulin detemir)—have been approved by the FDA for clinical use (see below) (Table 27–10). Animal insulins are no longer available in the United States.

B. PURITY OF INSULIN—"Purified" insulin is defined by FDA regulations as the degree of purity wherein proinsulin contamination is less than 10 ppm. All insulins presently

Table 27–9. Summary of bioavailability characteristics of the insulins.

Insulin Preparations	Onset of Action	Peak Action	Effective Duration
Insulins lispro, aspart, glulisine	5–15 minutes	1–1.5 hours	3–4 hours
Human regular	30–60 minutes	2 hours	6–8 hours
Human NPH	2–4 hours	6–7 hours	10–20 hours
Insulin glargine	1.5 hours	Flat	~24 hours
Insulin detemir	1 hour	Flat	17 hours

available contain less than 10 ppm of proinsulin and are labeled as "purified." These purified insulins seem to preserve their potency quite well, so that refrigeration is recommended but not crucial. During travel, reserve supplies of insulin can thus be readily transported for weeks without losing potency if protected from extremes of heat or cold.

C. CONCENTRATION OF INSULIN—At present, insulins in the United States are available in a concentration of 100 units/mL (U100), and all are dispensed in 10-mL vials. With the popularity of "low-dose" (0.5- or 0.3-mL) disposable insulin syringes, U100 can be measured with acceptable accuracy in doses as low as 1–2 units. For use in rare cases of severe insulin resistance in which large quantities of insulin are required, U500 regular human insulin (Humulin R) is available from Eli Lilly.

2. Insulin preparations—Insulins are classified into short-acting and long-acting insulin preparations. The short-act-

Table 27–10. Insulin preparations available in the United States.[1]

Rapidly acting human insulin analogs
  Insulin lispro (Humalog, Lilly)
  Insulin aspart (Novolog, Novo Nordisk)
  Insulin glulisine (Apidra, Sanofi Aventis)
Short-acting regular insulin
  Regular insulin (Lilly, Novo Nordisk)
Intermediate-acting insulins
  NPH insulin (Lilly, Novo Nordisk)
Premixed insulins
  70% NPH/30% regular (70/30 insulin—Lilly, Novo Nordisk)
  50% NPH/50% regular (50/50 insulin—Lilly)
  70% NPL/25% insulin lispro (Humalog Mix 75/25—Lilly)
  50% NPL/50% insulin lispro (Humalog Mix 50/50—Lilly)
  70% insulin aspart protamine/30% insulin aspart (Novolog Mix 70/30—Novo Nordisk)
Long-acting human insulin analogs
  Insulin glargine (Lantus, Sanofi Aventis)
  Insulin detemir (Levemir, Novo Nordisk)

[1]All insulins available in the United States are recombinant human or human insulin analog origin. All the insulins are dispensed at U100 concentration. There is an additional U500 preparation of regular insulin.
NPH, neutral protamine Hagedorn.

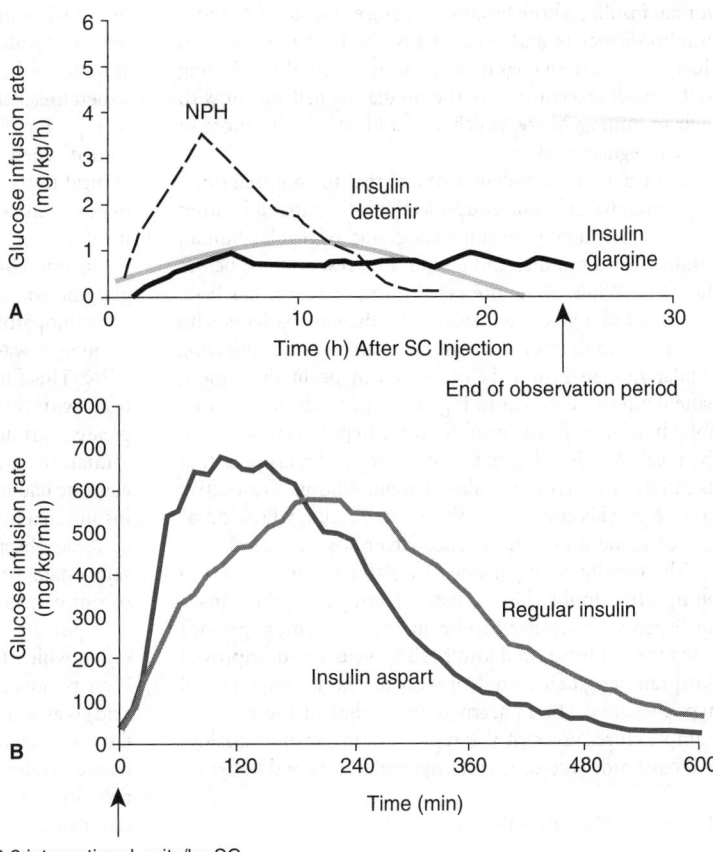

▲ **Figure 27–1.** Extent and duration of action of various types of insulin–euglycemic hyperinsulinemic clamps in normal volunteers. **A.** Intermediate neutral protamine Hagedorn (NPH) insulin and long-acting insulin analogs. **B.** Regular insulin and rapidly acting insulin analogs.

ing preparations are regular insulin and the rapidly acting insulin analogs (Figure 27–1). They are dispensed as clear solutions at neutral pH and contain small amounts of zinc to improve their stability and shelf life. The long-acting preparations are NPH insulin and the long-acting insulin analogs. NPH insulin is dispensed as a turbid suspension at neutral pH with protamine in phosphate buffer. The long-acting insulin analogs are also dispensed as clear solutions; insulin glargine is at acidic pH and insulin detemir is at neutral pH. The Lente series of insulin (ultralente and lente) are no longer available in the United States. The rapidly acting insulin analogs and the long-acting insulins are designed for subcutaneous administration, while regular insulin can also be given intravenously. While insulin aspart has been approved for intravenous use (eg, in hyperglycemic emergencies), there is no advantage in using insulin aspart over regular insulin by this route.

A. SHORT-ACTING INSULIN PREPARATIONS

(1) Regular insulin—Regular insulin is a short-acting soluble crystalline zinc insulin whose effect appears within 30 minutes after subcutaneous injection and lasts 5–7 hours when usual quantities are administered. Intravenous infusions of regular insulin are particularly useful in the treatment of diabetic ketoacidosis and during the perioperative management of insulin-requiring diabetics. Regular insulin

is indicated when the subcutaneous insulin requirement is changing rapidly, such as after surgery or during acute infections—although the rapidly acting insulin analogs may be preferable in these situations.

For markedly insulin-resistant persons who would otherwise require large volumes of insulin solution, a U500 preparation of human regular insulin is available. Since a U500 syringe is not available, a U100 insulin syringe or tuberculin syringe is used to measure doses. The physician should carefully note dosages in both units and volume to avoid overdosage.

(2) Rapidly acting insulin analogs—Insulin lispro (Humalog) is an insulin analog produced by recombinant technology, wherein two amino acids near the carboxyl terminal of the B chain have been reversed in position: Proline at position B28 has been moved to B29 and lysine has been moved from B29 to B28. Insulin aspart (Novolog) is a single substitution of proline by aspartic acid at position B28. Insulin glulisine (Apidra) differs from human insulin in that the amino acid asparagine at position B3 is replaced by lysine and the lysine in position B29 by glutamic acid. These changes result in these three analogs having less tendency to form hexamers, in contrast to human insulin. When injected subcutaneously, the analogs quickly dissociate into monomers and are absorbed very rapidly, reaching peak serum values in as soon as 1 hour—in contrast to regular

human insulin, whose hexamers require considerably more time to dissociate and become absorbed. The amino acid changes in these analogs do not interfere with their binding to the insulin receptor, with the circulating half-life, or with their immunogenicity, which are all identical with those of human regular insulin.

Clinical trials have demonstrated that the optimal times of preprandial subcutaneous injection of comparable doses of the rapidly acting insulin analogs and of regular human insulin are 20 minutes and 60 minutes, respectively, before the meal. While this more rapid onset of action has been welcomed as a great convenience by diabetic patients who object to waiting as long as 60 minutes after injecting regular human insulin before they can begin their meal, patients must be taught to ingest adequate absorbable carbohydrate early in the meal to avoid hypoglycemia during the meal. Another desirable feature of insulin lispro is that its duration of action remains at about 4 hours irrespective of dosage. This contrasts with regular insulin, whose duration of action is prolonged when larger doses are used.

The rapidly acting analogs are also commonly used in pumps. In a double-blind crossover study comparing insulin lispro with regular insulin in insulin pumps, persons using insulin lispro had lower HbA_{1c} values and improved postprandial glucose control with the same frequency of hypoglycemia. The concern remains that in the event of pump failure, users of the rapidly acting insulin analogs will have more rapid onset of hyperglycemia and ketosis.

B. Long-acting Insulin Preparations

(1) NPH (neutral protamine Hagedorn or isophane) insulin—NPH is an intermediate-acting insulin whose onset of action is delayed by combining 2 parts soluble crystalline zinc insulin with 1 part protamine zinc insulin. This produces equivalent amounts of insulin and protamine, so that neither is present in an uncomplexed form ("isophane").

Its onset of action is delayed to 2–4 hours, and its peak response is generally reached in about 8–10 hours. Because its duration of action is often less than 24 hours (with a range of 10–20 hours), most patients require at least two injections daily to maintain a sustained insulin effect. Occasional vials of NPH insulin have tended to show unusual clumping of their contents or "frosting" of the container, with considerable loss of bioactivity. This instability is rare and occurs less frequently if NPH human insulin is refrigerated when not in use and if bottles are discarded after 1 month of use.

(2) Insulin glargine—Insulin glargine is an insulin analog in which the asparagine at position 21 of the A chain of the human insulin molecule is replaced by glycine and two arginines are added to the carboxyl terminal of the B chain. The arginines raise the isoelectric point of the molecule closer to neutral, making it more soluble in an acidic environment. In contrast, human insulin has an isoelectric point of pH 5.4. Insulin glargine is a clear insulin which, when injected into the neutral pH environment of the subcutaneous tissue, forms microprecipitates that slowly release the insulin into the circulation. It lasts for about 24

hours without any pronounced peaks and is given once a day to provide basal coverage. This insulin cannot be mixed with the other human insulins because of its acidic pH. When this insulin was given as a single injection at bedtime to type 1 patients, fasting hyperglycemia was better controlled when compared with bedtime NPH insulin. The clinical trials also suggest that there may be less nocturnal hypoglycemia with this insulin when compared with NPH insulin.

In one clinical trial involving type 2 patients, insulin glargine was associated with a slightly higher progression of retinopathy when compared with NPH insulin. The frequency was 7.5% with the analog and 2.7% with the NPH. This finding, however, was not seen in other clinical trials with this analog. Insulin glargine does have a sixfold greater affinity for IGF-1 receptor compared with the human insulin. There has also been a report that insulin glargine had increased mitogenicity compared with human insulin in a human osteosarcoma cell line. The significance of these observations is not yet clear. Because of lack of safety data, use of insulin glargine during pregnancy is not recommended.

(3) Insulin detemir—Insulin detemir is an insulin analog in which the tyrosine at position 30 of the β chain has been removed and a 14-C fatty acid chain (tetradecanoic acid) is attached to the lysine at position 29 by acylation. The fatty acid chain makes the molecule more lipophilic than native insulin and the addition of zinc stabilizes the molecule and leads to formation of hexamers. After injection, self-association at the injection site and albumin binding in the circulation via the fatty acid side chain, leads to slower distribution to peripheral target tissues and prolonged duration of action. The affinity of insulin detemir is fourfold to fivefold lower than that of human soluble insulin and therefore the U100 formulation of insulin detemir has an insulin concentration of 2400 nmol/mL compared with 600 nmol/mL for NPH. The duration of action for insulin detemir is about 17 hours at therapeutically relevant doses. It is recommended that the insulin be injected once or twice a day to achieve a stable basal coverage. This insulin has been reported to have lower within-subject pharmacodynamic variability compared with NPH insulin and insulin glargine. In vitro studies do not suggest any clinically relevant albumin binding interactions between insulin detemir and fatty acids or protein-bound drugs. Since there is a vast excess (~400,000) of albumin binding sites available in plasma per insulin detemir molecule, it is unlikely that hypoalbuminemic disease states will affect the ratio of bound to free insulin detemir.

C. Mixed Insulin Preparations

Since intermediate insulins require several hours to reach adequate therapeutic levels, their use in patients with type 1 diabetes requires supplements of regular or rapidly acting insulin analogs preprandially. For convenience, regular or rapidly acting insulin analogs and NPH insulin may be mixed together in the same syringe and injected subcutaneously in split dosage before breakfast and supper. It is recommended that the regular insulin or rapidly acting insulin analog be withdrawn first, then the NPH insulin and that the injection be given immediately after loading the syringe. Stable premixed insulins (70% NPH and 30% regular or 50% of each) are available as a convenience to patients who have difficulty mixing insulin because of visual problems or impairment of manual dexterity. Premixed preparations of insulin lispro and NPH insulins are unstable because of exchange of insulin lispro with the human insulin in the protamine complex. Consequently, the soluble component becomes over time a mixture of regular and insulin lispro at varying ratios. In an attempt to remedy this, an intermediate insulin composed of isophane complexes of protamine with insulin lispro was developed called NPL (neutral protamine lispro). This insulin has the same duration of action as NPH insulin. Premixed combinations of NPL and insulin lispro (eg, 75:25, 50:50, and 25:75 of NPL:insulin lispro) have been tested. Both 75% NPL/25% insulin lispro mixture (Humalog Mix 75/25) and 50% NPL/50% insulin lispro mixture (Humalog Mix 50/50) are available for clinical use. Similarly, a 70% insulin aspart protamine/ 30% insulin aspart (NovoLog Mix 70/30) is available. The main advantages of these mixtures are that they can be given within 15 minutes of starting a meal and they are superior in controlling the postprandial glucose rise after a carbohydrate rich meal. These benefits have not translated into improvements in HbA$_{1c}$ levels when compared with the usual 70% NPH/30% regular mixture.

The longer-acting insulin analogs cannot be mixed with either regular insulin or the rapidly acting insulin analogs.

3. Methods of insulin administration

A. INSULIN SYRINGES AND NEEDLES—Plastic disposable syringes are available in 1-mL, 0.5-mL, and 0.3-mL sizes. The "low-dose" 0.3-mL syringes have become increasingly popular, because many diabetics do not take more than 30 units of insulin in a single injection except in rare instances of extreme insulin resistance. Two lengths of needles are available: short (8 mm) and long (12.7 mm). Long needles are preferable in obese patients to reduce variability of insulin absorption. Ultrafine needles as small as 31 gauge reduce the pain of injections. "Disposable" syringes may be reused until blunting of the needle occurs (usually after three to five injections). Sterility adequate to avoid infection with reuse appears to be maintained by recapping syringes between uses. Cleansing the needle with alcohol may not be desirable since it can dissolve the silicone coating and can increase the pain of skin puncturing.

Any part of the body covered by loose skin can be used, such as the abdomen, thighs, upper arms, flanks, and upper buttocks. Preparation with alcohol is no longer required prior to injection as long as the skin is clean. Rotation of sites continues to be recommended to avoid delayed absorption when fibrosis or lipohypertrophy occurs from repeated use of a single site. However, considerable variability of absorption rates from different sites, particularly with exercise, may contribute to the instability of glycemic control in certain type 1 patients if injection sites are rotated too frequently in different areas of the body. Consequently, it is best to limit injection sites to a single region of the body and rotate sites within that region. The abdomen is recommended for subcutaneous injections, since regular insulin has been shown to absorb more rapidly from there than from other subcutaneous sites. The effect of anatomic regions appears to be much less pronounced with the analog insulins.

B. INSULIN PEN INJECTOR DEVICES—Insulin pens eliminate the need for carrying insulin vials and syringes. Cartridges of insulin lispro, insulin aspart, insulin glargine, regular insulin, NPH insulin, and 70% NPH/30% regular insulin are available for reusable pens (Novo Nordisk, Becton Dickinson, and Sanofi Aventis pens). Disposable prefilled pens are also available for insulin lispro, insulin aspart, insulin detemir, insulin glargine, NPH, 70% NPH/ 30% regular, 75% NPL/25% insulin lispro, 50% NPL/50% insulin lispro, and 70% insulin aspart protamine/30% insulin aspart. Thirty-one gauge needles (5, 6, and 8 mm long) for these pens make injections almost painless.

C. INSULIN PUMPS—In the United States, Medtronic MiniMed, Animas, Deltec. Insulet, and Roche make insulin infusion pumps for subcutaneous delivery of insulin. These pumps are small (about the size of a pager) and very easy to program. They offer many features, including the ability to set a number of different basal rates throughout the 24 hours and to adjust the time over which bolus doses are given. They also are able to detect pressure build-up if the catheter is kinked. Improvements have also been made in the infusion sets. The catheter connecting the insulin reservoir to the subcutaneous cannula can be disconnected, allowing the patient to remove the pump temporarily (eg, for bathing). The great advantage of continuous subcutaneous insulin infusion (CSII) is that it allows for establishment of a basal profile tailored to the patient. The patient therefore is able to eat with less regard to timing because the basal insulin infusion should maintain constant blood glucose between meals. Also the ability to adjust the basal insulin infusion makes it easier for the patient to manage glycemic excursions that occur with exercise.

CSII therapy is appropriate for patients who are motivated, mechanically inclined, educated about diabetes (diet, insulin action, treatment of hypoglycemia and hyperglycemia), and willing to monitor their blood glucose four to six times a day. Known complications of CSII include ketoacidosis, which can occur when insulin delivery is interrupted, and skin infections. Another disadvantage is its cost and the time demanded of physicians and staff in initiating therapy.

D. INHALED INSULIN—Exubera, the first inhaled insulin preparation approved by the FDA is no longer available; the manufacturer stopped marketing it because of lack of demand. In clinical trials, Exubera was as effective as subcutaneous regular insulin in controlling postprandial glucose excursions. Physicians, however, were reluctant to prescribe Exubera for a number of reasons, including a lack of longterm safety data on pulmonary function, awkward dosing schedule, availability of other insulin delivery systems, and cost and lack of insurance coverage.

D. Transplantation

Pancreas transplantation at the time of kidney transplantation is becoming more widely accepted. Patients undergoing simultaneous pancreas and kidney transplantation have an 85% chance of pancreatic graft survival and a 92% chance of kidney graft survival after 1 year. Solitary pancreatic transplantation in the absence of a need for kidney transplantation should be considered only in those rare patients who fail all other insulin therapeutic approaches and who have frequent severe hypoglycemia or who have life-threatening complications related to their lack of metabolic control.

Islet cell transplantation is a minimally invasive procedure, and investigators in Edmonton, Canada, have reported initial insulin independence in a small number of patients with type 1 diabetes who underwent this procedure. Using islets from multiple donors and corticosteroid-free immunosuppression, percutaneous transhepatic portal vein transplantation of islets was achieved in over 20 subjects. Although all of the initial cohort was able to achieve insulin independence posttransplantation (some for more than 2 years of follow-up), a decline in insulin secretion has occurred over time and the subjects have again required supplemental insulin. All patients had complete correction of severe hypoglycemic reactions, leading to a marked improvement in overall quality of life. Even if long-term insulin independence is demonstrated, wide application of this procedure for the treatment of type 1 diabetes is limited by the dependence on multiple donors and the requirement for potent long-term immunotherapy.

General Considerations in Treatment of Diabetes

Insulin-treated patients with diabetes can have a full and satisfying life. However, "free" diets and unrestricted activity are still not advised. Until new methods of insulin replacement are developed that provide more normal patterns of insulin delivery in response to metabolic demands, multiple feedings with carbohydrate counting will continue to be recommended, and certain occupations potentially hazardous to the patient or others will continue to be prohibited because of risks due to hypoglycemia. The American Diabetic Association can act as a patient advocate in case of employment questions.

Exercise increases the effectiveness of insulin, and moderate exercise is an excellent means of improving utilization of fat and carbohydrate in diabetic patients. A judicious balance of the size and frequency of meals with moderate regular exercise can often stabilize the insulin dosage in diabetics who tend to slip out of control easily. Strenuous exercise can precipitate hypoglycemia in an unprepared patient, and diabetics must therefore be taught to reduce their insulin dosage in anticipation of strenuous activity or to take supplemental carbohydrate. Injection of insulin into a site farthest away from the muscles most involved in exercise may help ameliorate exercise-induced hypoglycemia, since insulin injected in the proximity of exercising muscle may be more rapidly mobilized.

All diabetic patients must receive adequate instruction on personal hygiene, especially with regard to care of the feet, skin, and teeth. All infections (especially pyogenic ones) provoke the release of high levels of insulin antagonists such as catecholamines or glucagon and thus bring about a marked increase in insulin requirements. Supplemental regular insulin is often required to correct hyperglycemia during infection.

Steps in the Management of the Diabetic Patient

A. Diagnostic Examination

Any features of the clinical picture that suggest end-organ insensitivity to insulin, such as visceral obesity, must be identified. The family history should document not only the incidence of diabetes in other members of the family but also the age at onset, whether it was associated with obesity, and whether insulin was required. An attempt should be made to characterize the diabetes as type 1 or type 2, based on the clinical features present and on whether or not ketonuria accompanies the glycosuria. For the occasional patient, measurement of ICA, GAD65, IAA, and ICA 512 antibodies can help distinguish between type 1 and type 2 diabetes. Many patients in whom type 1 diabetes is newly diagnosed still have significant endogenous insulin production, and C peptide levels do not reliably distinguish between type 1 and type 2 diabetes. Other factors that increase cardiac risk, such as smoking history, presence of hypertension or hyperlipidemia, or oral contraceptive pill use, should be recorded.

Laboratory diagnosis should document fasting plasma glucose levels above 126 mg/dL or postprandial values consistently above 200 mg/dL and whether ketonuria accompanies the glycosuria. A glycohemoglobin measurement is useful for assessing the effectiveness of future therapy. Some flexibility of clinical judgment is appropriate when diagnosing diabetes mellitus in the elderly patient with borderline hyperglycemia.

Baseline values include fasting plasma triglycerides, total cholesterol and HDL-cholesterol, electrocardiography, kidney function studies, peripheral pulses, and neurologic, podiatric, and ophthalmologic examinations to help guide future assessments.

B. Patient Education (Self-Management Training)

Since diabetes is a lifelong disorder, education of the patient and the family is probably the most important obligation of the clinician who provides initial care. The best persons to manage a disease that is affected so markedly by daily fluctuations in environmental stress, exercise, diet, and infections are the patients themselves and their families. The "teaching curriculum" should include explanations by the physician or nurse of the nature of diabetes and its potential acute and chronic hazards and how they can be recognized early and prevented or treated. Self-monitoring of blood glucose should be emphasized, especially in insulin-requiring diabetic patients, and instructions must be given on proper testing and recording of data. Patients should be provided with algorithms they can use to adjust the timing and quantity of their insulin dose, food, and exercise in response to measured blood glucose values. The targets for blood glucose control should be elevated appropriately in elderly patients since they have the greatest risk if subjected to hypoglycemia and the least long-term benefit from more rigid glycemic control. Advice on personal hygiene, including detailed instructions on foot care as well as individual instruction on diet and specific hypoglycemic therapy, should be provided. Patients should be told about community agencies, such as Diabetes Association chapters, that can serve as a continuing source of instruction. Finally, vigorous efforts should be made to persuade new diabetics who smoke to give up the habit, since large vessel peripheral vascular disease and debilitating retinopathy are less common in nonsmoking diabetic patients.

C. Therapy

Treatment must be individualized on the basis of the type of diabetes and specific needs of each patient. However, certain general principles of management can be outlined for hyperglycemic states of different types.

1. Type 2 diabetes

A. THE OBESE PATIENT WITH TYPE 2 DIABETES—The most common type of diabetic patient is obese, is non–insulin-dependent, and has hyperglycemia because of a combination of insulin resistance and beta cell failure.

(1) Weight reduction—Treatment is directed toward achieving weight reduction, and prescribing a diet is only one means to this end. Behavior modification to achieve adherence to the diet—as well as increased physical activity to expend energy—is also required. Cure can be achieved by reducing adipose stores, with consequent restoration of tissue sensitivity to insulin, but weight reduction is hard to achieve and even more difficult to maintain with our current therapies. The presence of diabetes with its added risk factors may motivate the obese diabetic to greater efforts to lose weight. (See also Chapter 29.)

(2) Hypoglycemic agents—If the patient is not able to achieve target glycemic control with weight management and exercise, then pharmacologic therapy is indicated. The choice of initial agent depends on a number of factors, including comorbid conditions, adverse reactions to the medications, ability of the patient to monitor for hypoglycemia, drug cost, and patient and physician preferences. **Metformin** is advantageous because apart from lowering glucose without the risk of hypoglycemia, it also lowers triglycerides and promotes some modest weight loss. The drug, however, cannot be used in patients with end-stage chronic kidney disease, and gastrointestinal side effects develop in some patients at even the lowest doses. **Thiazolidinediones** improve peripheral insulin resistance and lower glucose without causing hypoglycemia. Both of the available thiazolidinediones, however, can cause fluid retention and are contraindicated in patients with heart failure. They also very commonly increase weight, which patients find distressing, affecting adherence. The drugs increase fracture risk in women further limiting their use. Pioglitazone is the preferred choice until there is more definitive data regarding rosiglitazone and the risk of ischemic heart disease. Both drugs are contraindicated in patients with active liver disease and in patients with liver enzymes ≥ 2.5 times the upper limit of normal. **Sulfonylureas** have been

available for many years and their use in combination with metformin is well established. They do, however, have the propensity of causing hypoglycemia and weight gain. The α-**glucosidase inhibitors** have modest glucose lowering effects and have gastrointestinal side effects. **Exenatide** has a lower risk of hypoglycemia than the sulfonylureas and promotes weight loss. However, it needs to be given by injection, causes nausea, may cause pancreatitis, and is contraindicated in patients with gastroparesis. **Sitagliptin** also has a low risk of hypoglycemia, and it does not cause nausea or vomiting. It can also be used in patients with kidney impairment. There are, however, reports of serious allergic reactions, including anaphylaxis, angioedema, and Stevens-Johnson syndrome.

For most obese patients with mild type 2 diabetes, metformin is the first-line agent. If it proves to be inadequate, then a second agent should be added. In those patients where the problem is hyperglycemia after a carbohydrate rich meal (such as dinner), then a short-acting secretagogue before meals may suffice to get the glucose levels into the target range. Patients with severe insulin resistance may be candidates for pioglitazone. Subjects who are very concerned about weight gain may benefit from a trial of exenatide. If two agents are inadequate, then a third agent is added, although data regarding efficacy of such combined therapy are limited. Experienced clinicians have found that instead of maximizing the dose of each agent before adding another agent, some patients are more tolerant of submaximal combinations of drugs. Insulin therapy should be instituted if combination of oral agents (and exenatide) fail to restore euglycemia or if there are concerns about side effects. Weight-reducing interventions should continue and may allow for simplification of this regimen in the future.

When the combination of oral agents (and exenatide) fail to achieve euglycemia in patients with type 2 diabetes, various insulin regimens may be effective. One proposed regimen is to continue the oral combination therapy and then simply add a bedtime dose of NPH or long-acting insulin analog (insulin glargine or insulin detemir) to reduce excessive nocturnal hepatic glucose output and improve fasting glucose levels. If the patient does not achieve target glucose levels during the day, then daytime insulin treatment can be initiated. A convenient insulin regimen under these circumstances is a split dose of 70/30 NPH/regular mixture (or Humalog Mix 75/25 or NovoLogMix 70/30) before breakfast and before dinner. If this regimen fails to achieve satisfactory glycemic goals or is associated with unacceptable frequency of hypoglycemic episodes, then a more intensive regimen of multiple insulin injections can be instituted as in patients with type 1 diabetes. Metformin principally reduces hepatic glucose output and pioglitazone improves peripheral insulin resistance, so it is a reasonable option to continue these drugs when insulin therapy is instituted. The sulfonylureas also have been shown to be of continued benefit. Thus, the continued use of the oral drugs may permit the use of lower doses of insulin and simpler regimens. There is no data on the continued administration of exenatide under these circumstances.

B. THE NONOBESE PATIENT WITH TYPE 2 DIABETES—Nonobese patients with type 2 diabetes frequently have increased visceral adiposity—the so-called metabolically obese normal weight patient—and the treatment algorithm is much the same as in the obese patient except there is not as much emphasis on weight loss. However, exercise remains an important aspect of treatment. Persons who do not have central obesity or insulin resistance should be evaluated for other types of diabetes such as LADA or MODY. Patients with LADA can initially be treated with oral agents but require insulin within a few years, so experienced clinicians often prescribe insulin for these patients when the diagnosis is made.

2. Type 1 diabetes—Traditional once- or twice-daily insulin regimens are usually ineffective in type 1 patients without residual endogenous insulin. In these patients, information and counseling based on the findings of the DCCT (see above) should be provided about the advantages of taking multiple injections of insulin in conjunction with self-blood glucose monitoring. If near-normalization of blood glucose is attempted, at least four measurements of capillary blood glucose and three or four insulin injections are necessary.

A combination of rapidly acting insulin analogs and long-acting insulin analogs allows for more physiologic insulin replacement. The rapidly acting insulin analogs have been advocated as a safer and much more convenient alternative to regular human insulin for preprandial use. In a study comparing regular insulin with insulin lispro, daily insulin doses and HbA_{1c} levels were similar, but insulin lispro improved postprandial control, reduced hypoglycemic episodes, and improved patient convenience compared with regular insulin. However, because of their relatively short duration (no more than 3–4 hours), the rapidly acting insulin analogs need to be combined with longer-acting insulins to provide basal coverage and avoid hyperglycemia prior to the next meal. In addition to carbohydrate content of the meal, the effect of simultaneous fat ingestion must also be considered a factor in determining the rapidly acting insulin analog dosage required to control the glycemic increment during and just after the meal. With low-carbohydrate content and high-fat intake, there is an increased risk of hypoglycemia from insulin lispro within 2 hours after the meal. Table 27–11 illustrates a regimen with a rapidly acting insulin analog and insulin detemir or insulin glargine that might be appropriate for a 70-kg person with type 1 diabetes eating meals providing standard carbohydrate intake and moderate to low fat content.

Insulin glargine is usually given once in the evening to provide 24-hour coverage. This insulin *cannot be mixed* with any of the other insulins and must be given as a separate injection. There are occasional patients in whom insulin glargine does not seem to last for 24 hours, and in such cases it needs to be given twice a day. As shown, insulin detemir may also need to be given twice a day to get adequate 24-hour basal coverage. Alternatively, small doses of NPH (~ 3 to 4 units) can be given with each meal to provide daytime basal coverage with a larger dose at night. Unlike the long-acting insulin analogs, NPH can be mixed in the same syringe as the insulin lispro, insulin aspart, and insulin glulisine.

Continuous subcutaneous insulin infusion (CSII) by portable battery-operated "open loop" devices currently

Table 27–11. Examples of intensive insulin regimens using rapidly acting insulin analogs (insulin lispro, aspart, or glulisine) and insulin detemir, or insulin glargine in a 70-kg man with type 1 diabetes.[1-3]

	Pre-Breakfast	Pre-Lunch	Pre-Dinner	At Bedtime
Rapidly acting insulin analog	5 units	4 units	6 units	—
Insulin detemir	6–7 units			8–9 units
OR				
Rapidly acting insulin analog	5 units	4 units	6 units	—
Insulin glargine	—	—	—	15–16 units

[1]Assumes that patient is consuming approximately 75 g carbohydrate at breakfast, 60 g at lunch, and 90 g at dinner.
[2]The dose of rapidly acting insulin can be raised by 1 or 2 units if extra carbohydrate (15–30 g) is ingested or if premeal blood glucose is > 170 mg/dL.
[3]Insulin glargine or insulin detemir must be given as a separate injection.

provides the most flexible approach, allowing the setting of different basal rates throughout the 24 hours and permitting patients to delay or skip meals and vary meal size and composition. The dosage is usually based on providing 50% of the estimated insulin dose as basal and the remainder as intermittent boluses prior to meals. For example, a 70-kg man requiring 35 units of insulin per day may require a basal rate of 0.7 units per hour throughout the 24 hours with the exception of 3 AM to 8 AM, when 0.8 units per hour might be appropriate (for the dawn phenomenon). The meal bolus would depend on the carbohydrate content of the meal and the premeal blood glucose value. One unit per 15 g of carbohydrate plus 1 unit for 50 mg/dL of blood glucose above a target value (eg, 120 mg/dL) is a common starting point. Further adjustments to basal and bolus dosages would depend on the results of blood glucose monitoring. The majority of patients use the rapidly acting insulin analogs in the pumps. One of the more difficult therapeutic problems in managing patients with type 1 diabetes is determining the proper adjustment of insulin dose when the prebreakfast blood glucose level is high. Occasionally, the prebreakfast hyperglycemia is due to the Somogyi effect, in which nocturnal hypoglycemia leads to a surge of counterregulatory hormones to produce high blood glucose levels by 7 AM. However, a more common cause for prebreakfast hyperglycemia is the waning of circulating insulin levels by the morning. Also, the "dawn phenomenon"—reduced tissue sensitivity to insulin between 5 AM and 8 AM—is present in as many as 75% of type 1 patients and can aggravate the hyperglycemia.

Table 27–12 shows that diagnosis of the cause of prebreakfast hyperglycemia can be facilitated by self-monitoring of blood glucose at 3 AM in addition to the usual bedtime and 7 AM measurements. This is required for only a few

Table 27–12. Prebreakfast hyperglycemia: Classification by blood glucose and insulin levels.

	Blood Glucose (mg/dL)			Free Immunoreactive Insulin (microunit/mL)		
	10:00 PM	3:00 AM	7:00 AM	10:00 PM	3:00 AM	7:00 AM
Somogyi effect	90	40	200	High	Slightly high	Normal
Dawn phenomenon	110	110	150	Normal	Normal	Normal
Waning of insulin dose plus dawn phenomenon	110	190	220	Normal	Low	Low
Waning of insulin dose plus dawn phenomenon plus Somogyi effect	110	40	380	High	Normal	Low

nights, and when a particular pattern emerges from monitoring blood glucose levels overnight, appropriate therapeutic measures can be taken. The Somogyi effect can be treated by eliminating the dose of intermediate insulin at dinnertime and giving it at a lower dosage at bedtime or by supplying more food at bedtime. When a waning insulin level is the cause, then either increasing the evening dose or shifting it from dinnertime to bedtime (or both) can be effective. A bedtime dose either of insulin glargine or insulin detemir provides more sustained overnight insulin levels than human NPH and may be effective in managing refractory prebreakfast hyperglycemia. If this fails, insulin pump therapy may be required. When the dawn phenomenon alone is present, the dosage of intermediate insulin can be divided between dinnertime and bedtime; when insulin pumps are used, the basal infusion rate can be increased (eg, from 0.8 unit/h to 0.9 unit/h from 6 AM until breakfast).

▶ Acceptable Levels of Glycemic Control

A reasonable aim of therapy is to approach normal glycemic excursions without provoking severe or frequent hypoglycemia. What has been considered "acceptable" control includes blood glucose levels of 90–130 mg/dL before meals and after an overnight fast, and levels no higher than 180 mg/dL 1 hour after meals and 150 mg/dL 2 hours after meals. Glycohemoglobin levels should be no higher than 1% above the upper limit of the normal range for any particular laboratory. It should be emphasized that the value of blood pressure control was as great as or greater than glycemic control in type 2 patients as regards microvascular as well as macrovascular complications.

▶ Complications of Insulin Therapy

A. Hypoglycemia

When the blood glucose falls to around 54 mg/dL, the patient starts to experience both sympathetic (tachycardia, palpitations, sweating, tremulousness) and parasympathetic (nausea, hunger) nervous system symptoms. If these autonomic symptoms are ignored and the glucose levels fall further (to around 50 mg/dL), then neuroglycopenic symptoms appear, including irritability, confusion, blurred vision, tiredness, headache, and difficulty speaking. A further decline in glucose can then lead to loss of consciousness or even a seizure. With repeated episodes of hypoglycemia,

there is adaptation, and autonomic symptoms do not occur until the blood glucose levels are much lower and so the first symptoms are often due to neuroglycopenia. This condition is referred to as "hypoglycemic unawareness." It has been shown that hypoglycemic unawareness can be reversed by keeping glucose levels high for a period of several weeks. Except for sweating, most of the sympathetic symptoms of hypoglycemia are blunted in patients receiving β-blocking agents for angina pectoris or hypertension. Though not absolutely contraindicated, these drugs must be used with caution in insulin-requiring diabetics, and β₁-selective blocking agents are preferred.

Hypoglycemia in insulin-treated patients with diabetes occurs as a consequence of three factors: behavioral issues, impaired counterregulatory systems, and complications of diabetes.

Behavioral issues include injecting too much insulin for the amount of carbohydrates ingested. Drinking alcohol in excess, especially on an empty stomach, can also cause hypoglycemia. In patients with type 1 diabetes, hypoglycemia can occur during or even several hours after exercise, and so glucose levels need to be monitored and food and insulin adjusted. Some patients do not like their glucose levels to be high, and they treat every high glucose level aggressively. These individuals who "stack" their insulin—that is, give another dose of insulin before the first injection has had its full action—can develop hypoglycemia.

Counterregulatory issues resulting in hypoglycemia include impaired glucagon response, sympatho-adrenal responses, and cortisol deficiency. Patients with diabetes of greater than 5 years duration lose their glucagon response to hypoglycemia. As a result, they are at a significant disadvantage in protecting themselves against falling glucose levels. Once the glucagon response is lost, their sympatho-adrenal responses take on added importance. Unfortunately, aging, autonomic neuropathy, or hypoglycemic unawareness due to repeated low glucose levels further blunts the sympatho-adrenal responses. Occasionally, Addison disease develops in persons with type 1 diabetes mellitus; when this happens, insulin requirements fall significantly, and unless insulin dose is reduced, recurrent hypoglycemia will develop.

Complications of diabetes that increase the risk for hypoglycemia include autonomic neuropathy, gastroparesis, and end-stage chronic kidney disease. The sympathetic nervous system is an important system alerting the individual that the glucose level is falling by causing symptoms of tachycardia, palpitations, sweating, and tremulousness. Failure of the sympatho-adrenal responses increases the risk of hypoglycemia. In addition, in patients with gastroparesis, if insulin is given before a meal, the peak of insulin action may occur before the food is absorbed causing the glucose levels to fall. Finally, in end-stage chronic kidney disease, hypoglycemia can occur presumably because of decreased insulin clearance as well as loss of renal contribution to gluconeogenesis in the postabsorptive state.

To prevent and treat insulin-induced hypoglycemia, the diabetic patient should carry glucose tablets or juice at all times. For most episodes, ingestion of 15 grams of carbohydrate is sufficient to reverse the hypoglycemia. The patient should be instructed to check the blood glucose in 15 minutes and treat again if the glucose level is still low. A parenteral glucagon emergency kit (1 mg) should be provided to every patient with diabetes who is receiving insulin therapy. Family or friends should be instructed how to inject it subcutaneously or intramuscularly into the buttock, arm, or thigh in the event that the patient is unconscious or refuses food. The drug can occasionally cause vomiting, and the unconscious patient should be turned on his or her side to protect the airway. The glucagon mobilizes glycogen from the liver, raising the blood glucose by about 36 mg/dL in about 15 minutes. After the patient recovers consciousness, additional oral carbohydrate should be given. People with diabetes receiving hypoglycemic drug therapy should also wear an identification MedicAlert bracelet or necklace or carry a card in his or her wallet. The telephone number for the MedicAlert Foundation International in Turlock, California, is 1-800-ID-ALERT and the Internet address is www.medicalert.org.

Medical personnel treating severe hypoglycemia can give 50 mL of 50% glucose solution by rapid intravenous infusion. If intravenous therapy is not available, 1 mg of glucagon can be injected intramuscularly. If the patient is stuporous and glucagon is not available, small amounts of honey or syrup or glucose gel (15 g) can be inserted within the buccal pouch, but, in general, oral feeding is contraindicated in unconscious patients. Rectal administration of syrup or honey (30 mL per 500 mL of warm water) has been effective.

B. Immunopathology of Insulin Therapy

At least five molecular classes of insulin antibodies are produced during the course of insulin therapy in diabetes, including IgA, IgD, IgE, IgG, and IgM. With the increased therapeutic use of purified pork and especially human insulin, the various immunopathologic syndromes such as insulin allergy, immune insulin resistance, and lipoatrophy have become quite rare since the titers and avidity of these induced antibodies are generally quite low.

1. Insulin allergy—Insulin allergy, or immediate-type hypersensitivity, is a rare condition in which local or systemic urticaria is due to histamine release from tissue mast cells sensitized by adherence of anti-insulin IgE antibodies. In severe cases, anaphylaxis results. When only human insulin has been used from the onset of insulin therapy, insulin allergy is exceedingly rare. Antihistamines, corticosteroids, and even desensitization may be required, especially for systemic hypersensitivity. There have been case reports of successful use of insulin lispro in those rare patients who have a generalized allergy to human insulin or insulin resistance due to a high titer of insulin antibodies.

2. Immune insulin resistance—Most insulin-treated patients develop a low titer of circulating IgG anti-insulin antibodies that neutralize to a small extent the action of insulin. With the old animal insulins, a high titer of circulating antibodies sometimes developed, resulting in extremely high insulin requirements—often more than 200 units daily. This is now rarely seen with the switch to highly purified pork or human insulins and has not been reported with the analogs.

C. Lipodystrophy at Injection Sites

Atrophy of subcutaneous fatty tissue leading to disfiguring excavations and depressed areas may rarely occur at the site of injection. This complication results from an immune reaction, and it has become rarer with the development of pure and human insulin preparations. Lipohypertrophy, on the other hand, is a consequence of the pharmacologic effects of insulin being deposited in the same location repeatedly. It can occur with purified insulins as well. Rotation of injection sites will prevent lipohypertrophy. There is a case report of a patient who had intractable lipohypertrophy with human insulin but no longer had the problem when he switched to insulin lispro.

▶ Chronic Complications of Diabetes

Late clinical manifestations of diabetes mellitus include a number of pathologic changes that involve small and large blood vessels, cranial and peripheral nerves, the skin, and the lens of the eye. These lesions lead to hypertension, end-stage chronic kidney disease, blindness, autonomic and peripheral neuropathy, amputations of the lower extremities, myocardial infarction, and cerebrovascular accidents. These late manifestations correlate with the duration of the diabetic state subsequent to the onset of puberty. In type 1 diabetes, end-stage chronic kidney disease develops in up to 40% of patients, compared with less than 20% of patients with type 2 diabetes. As regards proliferative retinopathy, it ultimately develops in both types of diabetes but has a slightly higher prevalence in type 1 patients (25% after 15 years' duration). In patients with type 1 diabetes, complications from end-stage chronic kidney disease are a major cause of death, whereas patients with type 2 diabetes are more likely to have macrovascular diseases leading to myocardial infarction and stroke as the main causes of death. Cigarette use adds significantly to the risk of both microvascular and macrovascular complications in diabetic patients.

A. Ocular Complications

1. Diabetic cataracts—Premature cataracts occur in diabetic patients and seem to correlate with both the duration of diabetes and the severity of chronic hyperglycemia. Nonenzymatic glycosylation of lens protein is twice as high in diabetic patients as in age-matched nondiabetic persons and may contribute to the premature occurrence of cataracts.

2. Diabetic retinopathy—Three main categories exist: background, or "simple," retinopathy, consisting of microaneurysms, hemorrhages, exudates, and retinal edema; preproliferative retinopathy with arteriolar ischemia manifested as cotton-wool spots (small infarcted areas of retina); and proliferative, or "malignant," retinopathy, consisting of newly formed vessels. Proliferative retinopathy is a leading cause of blindness in the United States, particularly since it increases the risk of retinal detachment. Vision-threatening retinopathy virtually never appears in type 1 patients in the first 3–5 years of diabetes or before puberty. Up to 20% of patients with type 2 diabetes have retinopathy at the time of diagnosis. Annual consultation with an ophthalmologist should be arranged for patients who have had type 1 diabetes for more than 3–5 years and for all patients with type 2 diabetes, because many were probably diabetic for an extensive period of time before diagnosis. Patients with any macular edema, severe nonproliferative retinopathy, or any proliferative retinopathy require the care of an ophthalmologist. Extensive "scatter" xenon or argon photocoagulation and focal treatment of new vessels reduce severe visual loss in those cases in which proliferative retinopathy is associated with recent vitreous hemorrhages or in which extensive new vessels are located on or near the optic disk. Macular edema, which is more common than proliferative retinopathy in patients with type 2 diabetes (up to 20% prevalence), has a guarded prognosis, but it has also responded to scatter therapy with improvement in visual acuity if detected early. Injection of bevacizumab (Avastin), an anti-vascular endothelial growth factor (anti-VEGF), into the eye has been shown to stop the growth of the new blood vessels in diabetic eye disease. Avoiding tobacco use and correction of associated hypertension are important therapeutic measures in the management of diabetic retinopathy. There is no contraindication to using aspirin in patients with proliferative retinopathy.

3. Glaucoma—Glaucoma occurs in approximately 6% of persons with diabetes. It is responsive to the usual therapy for open-angle disease. Neovascularization of the iris in diabetics can predispose to closed-angle glaucoma, but this is relatively uncommon except after cataract extraction, when growth of new vessels has been known to progress rapidly, involving the angle of the iris and obstructing outflow.

B. Diabetic Nephropathy

As many as 4000 cases of end-stage chronic kidney disease occur each year among diabetic people in the United States. This is about one-third of all patients being treated for end-stage chronic kidney disease and represents a considerable national health expense.

The cumulative incidence of nephropathy differs between the two major types of diabetes. Patients with type 1 diabetes have a 30–40% chance of having nephropathy after 20 years—in contrast to the much lower frequency in type 2 diabetes patients, in whom only about 15–20% develop clinical kidney disease. However, since there are many more individuals affected with type 2 diabetes, end-stage chronic kidney disease is much more prevalent in type 2 than in type 1 diabetes in the United States and especially

throughout the rest of the world. Improved glycemic control and more effective therapeutic measures to correct hypertension—and with the beneficial effects of ACE inhibitors—can reduce the development of end-stage chronic kidney disease among diabetics.

Diabetic nephropathy is initially manifested by proteinuria; subsequently, as kidney function declines, urea and creatinine accumulate in the blood.

1. Microalbuminuria—Sensitive radioimmunoassay methods of detecting small amounts of urinary albumin have permitted detection of microgram concentrations—in contrast to the less sensitive dipstick strips, whose minimal detection limit is 0.3–0.5%. Conventional 24-hour urine collections, in addition to being inconvenient for patients, also show wide variability of albumin excretion, since several factors such as sustained erect posture, dietary protein, and exercise tend to increase albumin excretion rates. For these reasons, a timed overnight urine collection or albumin-creatinine ratio in an early morning spot urine collected upon awakening is preferable. Normal subjects excrete less than 15 mcg/min during overnight urine collections; values of 20 mcg/min or higher are considered to represent abnormal microalbuminuria. In the early morning spot urine, a ratio of albumin (mcg/L) to creatinine (mg/L) of < 30 mcg/mg creatinine is normal, and a ratio of 30–300 mcg/mg creatinine suggests abnormal microalbuminuria. At least two of three timed overnight or early morning spot urine collections over a 3- to 6-month period should be abnormal before a diagnosis of microalbuminuria is justified.

Subsequent end-stage chronic kidney disease can be predicted by persistent urinary albumin excretion rates exceeding 30 mcg/min. Increased microalbuminuria correlates with increased levels of blood pressure and increased LDL cholesterol, and this may explain why increased proteinuria in diabetic patients is associated with an increase in cardiovascular deaths even in the absence of end-stage chronic kidney disease. Glycemic control as well as a low-protein diet (0.8 g/kg/d) may reduce both the hyperfiltration and the elevated microalbuminuria in patients in the early stages of diabetes and those with incipient diabetic nephropathy. Antihypertensive therapy also decreases microalbuminuria. Evidence from some studies—but not the UKPDS—supports a specific role for ACE inhibitors in reducing intraglomerular pressure in addition to their lowering of systemic hypertension. An ACE inhibitor (captopril, 50 mg twice daily) in normotensive diabetics impedes progression to proteinuria and prevents the increase in albumin excretion rate. Since microalbuminuria has been shown to correlate with elevated *nocturnal* systolic blood pressure, it is possible that "normotensive" diabetic patients with microalbuminuria have slightly elevated systolic blood pressure during sleep, which is lowered during antihypertensive therapy. This action may contribute to the reported efficacy of ACE inhibitor drugs in reducing microalbuminuria in "normotensive" patients.

2. Progressive diabetic nephropathy—Progressive diabetic nephropathy consists of proteinuria of varying severity occasionally leading to nephrotic syndrome with hypoalbuminemia, edema, and an increase in circulating LDL cholesterol as well as progressive azotemia. In contrast to all other kidney disorders, the proteinuria associated with diabetic nephropathy does not diminish with progressive end-stage chronic kidney disease (patients continue to excrete 10–11 g daily as creatinine clearance diminishes). As end-stage chronic kidney disease progresses, there is an elevation in the renal threshold at which glycosuria appears.

Hypertension develops with progressive kidney involvement, and coronary and cerebral atherosclerosis seems to be accelerated. Approximately two-thirds of adult patients with diabetes have hypertension. Once diabetic nephropathy has progressed to the stage of hypertension, proteinuria, or early chronic kidney disease, glycemic control is not beneficial in influencing its course. In this circumstance, antihypertensive medications, including ACE inhibitors, and restriction of dietary protein to 0.8 g/kg body weight per day are recommended. ACE inhibitors have been shown to protect against deterioration in kidney function in type 1 diabetic patients with clinical nephropathy. This beneficial effect appears to be due to improved glomerular hemodynamics that cannot be explained only by the antihypertensive action of these drugs. Captopril (25 mg three times daily) has shown a 50% reduction in the risk of the combined end points of death, dialysis, and transplantation in type 1 subjects with diabetic nephropathy and clinical proteinuria. During initiation of ACE inhibitor therapy, an increment in serum creatinine greater than 2 mg/dL due to a rapid fall in intraglomerular pressure—or the occurrence of persistent hyperkalemia (above 6 mEq/L) due to hyporeninemic hypoaldosteronism—is an indication to stop this medication.

Dialysis has been of limited value in the long-term treatment of chronic kidney disease due to diabetic nephropathy. At present, experience in kidney transplantation—especially from related donors—is more promising and is the treatment of choice in cases where there are no contraindications such as severe cardiovascular disease.

C. Diabetic Neuropathy

Diabetic neuropathies are the most common complications of diabetes affecting up to 50% of older patients with type 2 diabetes.

1. Peripheral neuropathy

A. Distal symmetric polyneuropathy—This is the most common form of diabetic peripheral neuropathy where loss of function appears in a stocking-glove pattern and is due to an axonal neuropathic process. Longer nerves are especially vulnerable, hence the impact on the foot. Both motor and sensory nerve conduction is delayed in the peripheral nerves, and ankle jerks may be absent.

Sensory involvement usually occurs first and is generally bilateral, symmetric, and associated with dulled perception of vibration, pain, and temperature. The pain can range from mild discomfort to severe incapacitating symptoms (see below). The sensory deficit may eventually be of sufficient degree to prevent patients from feeling pain. Patients who have a sensory neuropathy should therefore be examined with a 5.07 Semmes Weinstein filament and

those who cannot feel the filament must be considered at risk for unperceived neuropathic injury.

The denervation of the small muscles of the foot result in clawing of the toes and displacement of the submetatarsal fat pads anteriorly. These changes, together with the joint and connective tissue changes, alter the biomechanics of the foot and increase plantar pressures. This combination of decreased pain threshold, abnormally high foot pressures, and repetitive stress (such as from walking) can lead to calluses and ulcerations in the high-pressure areas such as over the metatarsal heads (Plate 92). Peripheral neuropathy, autonomic neuropathy, and trauma also predisposes to the development of Charcot arthropathy. An acute case of Charcot foot arthropathy presents with pain and swelling, and if left untreated, leads to a "rocker bottom" deformity and ulceration. The early radiologic changes show joint subluxation and periarticular fractures. As the process progresses, there is frank osteoclastic destruction leading to deranged and unstable joints particularly in the midfoot. Not surprisingly, the key issue for the healing of neuropathic ulcers in a foot with good vascular supply is mechanical unloading. In addition, any infection should be treated with debridement and appropriate antibiotics; healing duration of 8–10 weeks is typical. Occasionally, when healing appears refractory, **platelet-derived growth factor** (becaplermin [Regranex]) should be considered for local application. A post-marketing epidemiologic study showed increased cancer deaths in patients who had used three or more tubes of becaplermin on their leg or feet ulcers, and there is now a "black box" warning on the drug label. Once ulcers are healed, therapeutic footwear is key to preventing recurrences. Custom molded shoes are reserved for patients with significant foot deformities. Other patients with neuropathy may require accommodative insoles that distribute the load over as wide an area as possible. Patients with foot deformities and loss of their protective threshold should get regular care from a podiatrist. Patients should be educated on appropriate footwear and those with loss of their protective threshold should be instructed to inspect their feet daily for reddened areas, blisters, abrasions, or lacerations.

B. Isolated peripheral neuropathy—Involvement of the distribution of only one nerve ("mononeuropathy") or of several nerves ("mononeuropathy multiplex") is characterized by sudden onset with subsequent recovery of all or most of the function. This neuropathology has been attributed to vascular ischemia or traumatic damage. Cranial and femoral nerves are commonly involved, and motor abnormalities predominate. The patient with cranial nerve involvement usually has diplopia and single third, fourth, or sixth nerve weakness on examination but the pupil is spared. A full recovery of function occurs in 6–12 weeks. Diabetic amyotrophy presents with onset of severe pain in the front of the thigh. Within a few days or weeks of the onset of pain, weakness and wasting of the quadriceps develops. As the weakness appears, the pain tends to improve. Management includes analgesia and improved diabetes control. The symptoms improve over 6–18 months.

C. Painful diabetic neuropathy—Hypersensitivity to light touch and occasionally severe "burning" pain, particularly at night, can become physically and emotionally disabling. Amitriptyline, 25–75 mg at bedtime, has been recommended for pain associated with diabetic neuropathy. Dramatic relief has often resulted within 48–72 hours. This rapid response is in contrast to the 2 or 3 weeks required for an antidepressive effect. Patients often attribute the benefit to having a full night's sleep. Mild to moderate morning drowsiness is a side effect that generally improves with time or can be lessened by giving the medication several hours before bedtime. This drug should not be continued if improvement has not occurred after 5 days of therapy. If amitriptyline's anticholinergic effects are too troublesome, then nortriptyline can be used. Desipramine in doses of 25–150 mg/d seems to have the same efficacy as amitriptyline. Tricyclic antidepressants, in combination with the phenothiazine, fluphenazine, have been shown in two studies to be efficacious in painful neuropathy, with benefits unrelated to relief of depression. Gabapentin (900–1800 mg/d in three divided doses) has also been shown to be effective in the treatment of painful neuropathy and should be tried if the tricyclic drugs prove ineffective. Pregabalin, a congener of gabapentin, has been shown in an 8-week study to be more effective than placebo in treating painful diabetic peripheral neuropathy. However, this drug was not compared with an active control. Also, because of its abuse potential, it has been categorized as a schedule V controlled substance. Duloxetine, a serotonin and norepinephrine reuptake inhibitor, has been approved for the treatment of painful diabetic neuropathy. In clinical trials, this drug reduced the pain sensitivity score by 40–50%. Capsaicin, a topical irritant, has been found to be effective in reducing local nerve pain; it is dispensed as a cream (Zostrix 0.025%, Zostrix-HP 0.075%) to be rubbed into the skin over the painful region two to four times daily. Gloves should be used for application since hand contamination could result in discomfort if the cream comes in contact with eyes or sensitive areas such as the genitalia.

Diabetic neuropathic cachexia is a syndrome characterized by a symmetric peripheral neuropathy associated with profound weight loss (up to 60% of total body weight) and painful dysesthesias affecting the proximal lower limbs, the hands, or the lower trunk. Treatment is usually with insulin and analgesics. The prognosis is generally good, and patients typically recover their baseline weight with resolution of the painful sensory symptoms within 1 year.

2. Autonomic neuropathy—With autonomic neuropathy, there is evidence of postural hypotension, decreased cardiovascular response to the Valsalva maneuver, gastroparesis, alternating bouts of diarrhea (particularly nocturnal) and constipation, inability to empty the bladder, and impotence. Gastroparesis should be considered in type 1 diabetic patients in whom unexpected fluctuations and variability in their blood glucose levels develops after meals. Impotence due to neuropathy differs from psychogenic impotence in that the latter may be intermittent (erections occur under special circumstances), whereas diabetic impotence is usually persistent; aortoiliac occlusive disease may contribute to this problem.

A. MANAGEMENT OF AUTONOMIC NEUROPATHY—There is no consistently effective treatment for diabetic autonomic neuropathy. Metoclopramide has been of some help in treating diabetic gastroparesis over the short term, but its effectiveness seems to diminish over time. It is a dopamine antagonist that has central antiemetic effects as well as a cholinergic action to facilitate gastric emptying. It is given in a dose of 10 mg orally three or four times a day, 30 minutes before meals and at bedtime. Drowsiness, restlessness, fatigue, and lassitude are common adverse effects. Tardive dyskinesia and extrapyramidal effects also occur. Erythromycin appears to bind to motilin receptors in the stomach and has been found to improve gastric emptying in doses of 250 mg three times daily. Tegaserod (Zelnorm), the partial 5-HT4 agonist, has been withdrawn from the US market by the FDA, so it is no longer used for this indication. In selected patients, injections of botulinum toxin into the pylorus can reduce pylorus sphincter resistance and enhance gastric emptying. Gastric electrical stimulation has been reported to improve symptoms and quality of life indices in patients with gastroparesis refractory to pharmacologic therapy. Diarrhea associated with autonomic neuropathy has occasionally responded to broad-spectrum antibiotic therapy, although it often undergoes spontaneous remission. Refractory diabetic diarrhea is often associated with impaired sphincter control and fecal incontinence. Therapy with loperamide, 4–8 mg daily, or diphenoxylate with atropine, two tablets up to four times a day, may provide relief. In more severe cases, tincture of paregoric or codeine (60-mg tablets) may be required to reduce the frequency of diarrhea and improve the consistency of the stools. Clonidine has been reported to lessen diabetic diarrhea; however, its usefulness is limited by its tendency to lower blood pressure in these patients who already have autonomic neuropathy, resulting in orthostatic hypotension. Constipation usually responds to stimulant laxatives such as senna. Bethanechol in doses of 10–50 mg three times a day has occasionally improved emptying of the atonic urinary bladder. Catheter decompression of the distended bladder has been reported to improve its function, and considerable benefit has been reported after surgical severing of the internal vesicle sphincter. Mineralocorticoid therapy with fludrocortisone, 0.2–0.3 mg/d, and elastic stockings or pressure suits have reportedly been of some help in patients with orthostatic hypotension occurring as a result of loss of postural reflexes.

B. MANAGEMENT OF ERECTILE DYSFUNCTION—There are medical, mechanical, and surgical treatments available for treatment of erectile dysfunction. Penile erection depends on relaxation of the smooth muscle in the arteries of the corpus cavernosum, and this is mediated by nitric oxide-induced cyclic 3′,5′-guanosine monophosphate (cGMP) formation. cGMP-specific phosphodiesterase type 5 (PDE5) inhibitors impair the breakdown of cGMP and improve the ability to attain and maintain an erection. Sildenafil (Viagra), vardenafil (Levitra), and tadalafil (Cialis) have been shown in placebo-controlled clinical trials to improve erections in response to sexual stimulation. The recommended dose of sildenafil for most patients is one 50-mg tablet taken approximately 1 hour before sexual activity. The peak effect is at 1.5–2 hours, with some effect persisting for 4 hours.

Patients with diabetes mellitus using sildenafil reported 50–60% improvement in erectile function. The maximum recommended dose is 100 mg. The recommended dose of both vardenafil and tadalafil is 10 mg. The doses may be increased to 20 mg or decreased to 5 mg based on efficacy and side effects. Tadalafil has been shown to improve erectile function for up to 36 hours after dosing. In clinical trials, only a few adverse effects have been reported—transient mild headache, flushing, dyspepsia, and some altered color vision. Priapism can occur with these drugs and patients should be advised to seek immediate medical attention if an erection persists for longer than 4 hours. The PDE5 inhibitors potentiate the hypotensive effects of nitrates and their use is contraindicated in patients who are concurrently using organic nitrates in any form. Caution is advised for men who have suffered a heart attack, stroke, or life-threatening arrhythmia within the previous 6 months; men who have resting hypotension or hypertension; and men who have a history of cardiac failure or have unstable angina. Rarely, a decrease in vision or permanent visual loss has been reported after PDE5 inhibitor use.

Intracorporeal injection of vasoactive drugs causes penile engorgement and erection. Drugs most commonly used include papaverine alone, papaverine with phentolamine, and alprostadil (prostaglandin E_1). Alprostadil injections are relatively painless, but careful instruction is essential to prevent local trauma, priapism, and fibrosis. Intraurethral pellets of alprostadil avoid the problem of injection of the drug.

External vacuum therapy (Erec-Aid System) is a nonsurgical treatment consisting of a suction chamber operated by a hand pump that creates a vacuum around the penis. This draws blood into the penis to produce an erection which is maintained by a specially designed tension ring inserted around the base of the penis and which can be kept in place for up to 20–30 minutes. While this method is generally effective, its cumbersome nature limits its appeal.

In view of the recent development of nonsurgical approaches to therapy of erectile dysfunction, resort to surgical implants of penile prostheses is becoming less common.

D. Cardiovascular Complications

1. Heart disease—Microangiopathy occurs in the heart and may explain the etiology of congestive cardiomyopathies in diabetic patients who do not have demonstrable coronary artery disease. More commonly, however, heart disease in patients with diabetes is due to coronary atherosclerosis. Myocardial infarction is three to five times more common in diabetic patients and is the leading cause of death in patients with type 2 diabetes. Cardiovascular disease risk is increased in patients with type 1 diabetes as well, although the absolute risk is lower than in patients with type 2 diabetes. Premenopausal women who normally have lower rates of coronary artery disease lose this protection once diabetes develops. The increased risk in patients with type 2 diabetes reflects the combination of hyperglycemia, hyperlipidemia, abnormalities of platelet adhesiveness, coagulation factors, hypertension, oxidative stress, and inflammation. Large intervention studies of risk factor reduction in diabetes are lacking, but it

is reasonable to assume that reducing these risk factors would have a beneficial effect. Lowering LDL cholesterol reduces first events in patients without known coronary disease and secondary events in patients with known coronary disease. These intervention studies included some patients with diabetes, and the benefits of LDL cholesterol lowering was apparent in this group. The National Cholesterol Education Program clinical practice guidelines have designated diabetes as a coronary risk equivalent and have recommended that patients with diabetes should have an LDL cholesterol goal of < 100 mg/dL.

The ADA also recommends lowering blood pressure to 130/80 mm Hg or less. The Heart Outcomes Prevention Evaluation (HOPE) study randomized 9297 high-risk patients who had evidence of vascular disease or diabetes plus one other cardiovascular risk factor to receive ramipril or placebo for a mean of 5 years. Treatment with ramipril resulted in a 25% reduction of the risk of myocardial infarction, stroke, or death from cardiovascular disease. The mean difference between the placebo and ramipril group was 2.2 mm Hg systolic and 1.4 mm Hg diastolic blood pressure. The reduction in cardiovascular event rate remained significant after adjustment for this small difference in blood pressure. The mechanism underlying this protective effect of ramipril is unknown. Patients with type 2 diabetes who already have cardiovascular disease or microalbuminuria should therefore be considered for treatment with an ACE inhibitor. More clinical studies are needed to address the question of whether patients with type 2 diabetes who do not have cardiovascular disease or microalbuminuria would specifically benefit from ACE inhibitor treatment.

Aspirin at a dose of 81–325 mg daily has been shown to effectively inhibit thromboxane synthesis by platelets and reduce the risk of diabetic atherothrombosis without increasing risks of gastrointestinal hemorrhage. Use of low-dose enteric-coated aspirin is recommended in diabetic adults with evident macrovascular disease or in those with increased cardiovascular risk factors or those older than 30 years. Contraindications for aspirin therapy are patients with aspirin allergy, bleeding tendency, recent gastrointestinal bleeding, or active hepatic disease. The Early Treatment Diabetic Retinopathy Study (ETDRS) showed that aspirin does not influence the course of proliferative retinopathy. There was no statistically significant difference in the severity of vitreous/preretinal hemorrhages or their rate of resolution between the aspirin and placebo groups. Thus, it appears that there is no contraindication to aspirin use to achieve cardiovascular benefit in diabetic patients who have proliferative retinopathy.

2. Peripheral vascular disease—Atherosclerosis is markedly accelerated in the larger arteries. It is often diffuse, with localized enhancement in certain areas of turbulent blood flow, such as at the bifurcation of the aorta or other large vessels. Clinical manifestations of peripheral vascular disease include ischemia of the lower extremities, impotence, and intestinal angina.

The incidence of **gangrene of the feet** in diabetics is 30 times that in age-matched controls. The factors responsible for its development, in addition to peripheral vascular disease, are small vessel disease, peripheral neuropathy with loss of both pain sensation and neurogenic inflammatory responses, and secondary infection. In two-thirds of patients with ischemic gangrene, pedal pulses are not palpable. In the remaining one-third who have palpable pulses, reduced blood flow through these vessels can be demonstrated by plethysmographic or Doppler ultrasound examination. Prevention of foot injury is imperative. Agents that reduce peripheral blood flow such as tobacco and propranolol should be avoided. Control of other risk factors such as hypertension is essential. Cholesterol-lowering agents are useful as adjunctive therapy when early ischemic signs are detected and when dyslipidemia is present. Patients should be advised to seek immediate medical care if a diabetic foot ulcer develops. Improvement in peripheral blood flow with endarterectomy and bypass operations is possible in certain patients.

E. Skin and Mucous Membrane Complications

Chronic pyogenic infections of the skin may occur, especially in poorly controlled diabetic patients. Eruptive xanthomas can result from hypertriglyceridemia, associated with poor glycemic control. An unusual lesion termed **necrobiosis lipoidica diabeticorum** is usually located over the anterior surfaces of the legs or the dorsal surfaces of the ankles. They are oval or irregularly shaped plaques with demarcated borders and a glistening yellow surface and occur in women two to four times more frequently than in men.

"Shin spots" are not uncommon in adult diabetics. They are brownish, rounded, painless atrophic lesions of the skin in the pretibial area. Candidal infection can produce erythema and edema of intertriginous areas below the breasts, in the axillas, and between the fingers. It causes vulvovaginitis in most chronically uncontrolled diabetic women with persistent glucosuria and is a frequent cause of pruritus.

While antifungal creams containing miconazole or clotrimazole offer immediate relief of vulvovaginitis, recurrence is frequent unless glucosuria is reduced.

F. Special Situations

1. Insulin replacement during surgery—A number of studies have observed that hospitalized patients with diabetes and those with new-onset hyperglycemia (ie, those without a preadmission diagnosis of diabetes) have higher inpatient morbidity and mortality. These observations have led to the question of whether tight glycemic control in the hospital improves outcomes.

A prospective trial in surgical ICU patients (Leuven 1 study) reported that aggressive treatment of hyperglycemia (blood glucose > 110 mg/dL) reduced mortality and morbidity. Only a small number of persons in this study (204 of 1548) had a diagnosis of diabetes preoperatively, and so this study suggests that controlling hyperglycemia per se (independent of a diagnosis of diabetes) was beneficial. The benefits, however, were principally seen in patients who were in the ICU for longer than 5 days, and it is unclear whether the benefits also apply to most surgical patients who stay in the ICU for only 1 to 2 days.

The same investigators performed a similar prospective trial among 1200 medical ICU patients (Leuven 2 study) and reported that aggressive treatment of hyperglycemia reduced morbidity (decreased acquired kidney injury and increased early weaning from mechanical ventilation) but not mortality. Again, as in the surgical ICU study, only a small number of persons (16.9%) had a diagnosis of diabetes at admission. One of the inclusion criteria for the study was that patients would only be enrolled if they were likely to stay in the ICU for 3 days or longer. Some patients stayed in the ICU less than 3 days, and in that subgroup, intensive insulin therapy was associated with *increased* mortality. On the other hand, patients who stayed in the ICU for 3 days or longer had *reduced* mortality (and morbidity).

The findings of the Leuven studies have not been independently confirmed. Two other ICU-based studies (Glucontrol and VISEP) that attempted to confirm the findings were unable to do so. These two studies, however, were stopped prematurely for the following reasons: an interim analysis (falsely) suggested increased mortality in the test group in the Glucontrol study and hypoglycemic events increased sevenfold in the intensive treatment group in the VISEP study.

A study on tight intraoperative glycemic control during cardiac surgery also failed to show any benefit; if anything, the intensively treated group had more events. The United Kingdom Glucose Insulin in Stroke Trial (GIST-UK) failed to show beneficial effect of tight glycemic control in stroke patients; however, the investigators acknowledged that, because of slow recruitment, the study was underpowered. A large multicenter, multinational study (NICE-SUGAR) is currently reenrolling patients and the results of this study will hopefully resolve the question of how tightly to control glucose levels in the ICU.

Thus, based on the evidence available so far, keeping blood glucose values close to 100 mg/dL should be considered in the surgical and medical ICUs. When patients leave the ICU, target glucose values between 100 mg/dL and 180 mg/dL may be appropriate, although this view is based on clinical observations rather than conclusive evidence.

During major surgery and in the immediate recovery period in patients with type 1 diabetes—and in most patients with type 2 diabetes—regular insulin (25 units insulin in 250 mL 0.9% saline) is infused at a rate of 1-3 units/h. The insulin infusion is "piggy backed" onto a 5% dextrose in physiologic saline containing 20 mEq of potassium chloride, which is infused intravenously at a rate of ~100 mL/h. The patient's blood glucose should be monitored every 30 minutes to 2 hours and the insulin dose adjusted to maintain target blood glucose levels. Type 2 patients facing minor surgical procedures not requiring general anesthesia who have previously been controlled on oral agents or diet alone do not generally require insulin infusions. Glucose-containing solutions should be avoided during surgery in these patients, and blood glucose levels should be monitored every 4 hours. Regular human insulin or one of the rapidly acting insulin analogs should be administered subcutaneously if needed to maintain blood glucose below 200 mg/dL (see Chapter 3).

2. Pregnancy and the diabetic patient—Tight glycemic control with normal HbA$_{1c}$ levels is very important during pregnancy. Early in pregnancy, poor control increases the risk of spontaneous abortion and congenital malformations. Late in pregnancy, poor control can result in polyhydramnios, preterm labor, stillbirth, and fetal macrosomia with its associated problems. Diabetes complications can impact both maternal and fetal health. Diabetic retinopathy can first develop during pregnancy or retinopathy that is already present can worsen. Diabetic women with microalbuminuria can have worsening albuminuria during pregnancy and are at higher risk for preeclampsia. Patients who have preexisting kidney failure (prepregnancy creatinine clearance less than 80 mL/min) are at high risk for further decline in kidney function during the pregnancy, and this may not reverse after delivery. Diabetic gastroparesis can severely exacerbate the nausea and vomiting of pregnancy and some patients may require fluid and nutritional support.

Although there is evidence that glyburide is safe during pregnancy, the current practice is to control diabetes with insulin therapy. Every effort should be made, utilizing multiple injections of insulin or a continuous infusion of insulin by pump, to maintain near-normalization of fasting and preprandial blood glucose values while avoiding hypoglycemia. The fast-acting insulin analogs insulin aspart and insulin lispro can be used, but data on using the long-acting insulin analogs are limited. A small study using insulin glargine in 32 pregnancies did not reveal any problems. There are no data on insulin detemir use in pregnancy. NPH is currently the preferred intermediate insulin for basal coverage during pregnancy.

Unless there are fetal or maternal complications, diabetic women should be able to carry the pregnancy to full-term, delivering at 38 to 41 weeks. Induction of labor before 39 weeks may be considered if there is concern about increasing fetal weight. See Chapter 19 for further details.

▶ **Prognosis**

The DCCT showed that the previously poor prognosis for as many as 40% of patients with type 1 diabetes is markedly improved by optimal care. DCCT participants were generally young and highly motivated and were cared for in academic centers by skilled diabetes educators and endocrinologists who were able to provide more attention and services than are usually available. Improved training of primary care providers may be beneficial.

For type 2 diabetes, the UKPDS documented a reduction in microvascular disease with glycemic control, although this was not apparent in the obese subgroup. Cardiovascular outcomes were not improved by glycemic control, although antihypertensive therapy showed benefit in reducing the number of adverse cardiovascular complications as well as in reducing the occurrence of microvascular disease among hypertensive patients. In patients with visceral obesity, successful management of type 2 diabetes remains a major challenge in the attempt to achieve appropriate control of hyperglycemia, hypertension, and dyslipidemia. Once safe and effective methods are devised to prevent or manage

obesity, the prognosis of type 2 diabetes with its high cardiovascular risks should improve considerably.

In addition to poorly understood genetic factors relating to differences in individual susceptibility to development of long-term complications of hyperglycemia, it is clear that in both types of diabetes, the diabetic patient's intelligence, motivation, and awareness of the potential complications of the disease contribute significantly to the ultimate outcome.

ADVANCE Collaborative Group; Patel A et al. Intensive blood glucose control and vascular outcomes in patients with type 2 diabetes. N Engl J Med. 2008 Jun 12;358(24):2560–72. [PMID: 18539916]

American Association of Diabetes Educators http://www.aadenet.org/

American Diabetes Association http://www.diabetes.org/home

American Diabetes Association. Standards of Medical Care in Diabetes–2008. Diabetes Care. 2008 Jan;31(Suppl 1):S1–110. [PMID: 18165335]

American Dietetic Association http://www.eatright.org

ACCORD Study Group; Gerstein HC et al. Effects of intensive glucose lowering in type 2 diabetes. N Engl J Med. 2008 Jun 12;358(24):2545–59. [PMID: 18539917]

Brunkhorst FM et al. German Competence Network Sepsis (SepNet). Intensive insulin therapy and pentastarch resuscitation in severe sepsis. N Engl J Med. 2008 Jan 10;358(2):125–39. [PMID: 18184958]

Cryer PE et al. Hypoglycemia in diabetes. Diabetes Care. 2003 Jun;26(6):1902–12. [PMID: 12766131]

Daneman D. Type 1 diabetes. Lancet. 2006 Mar 11;367(9513):847–58. [PMID: 16530579]

DeFronzo RA et al. Effects of exenatide (exendin-4) on glycemic control and weight over 30 weeks in metformin-treated patients with type 2 diabetes. Diabetes Care. 2005 May;28(5):1092–100. [PMID: 15855572]

Dey J et al. Evaluation and treatment of erectile dysfunction in men with diabetes mellitus. Mayo Clin Proc. 2002 Mar; 77(3):276–82. [PMID: 11888032]

Diabetes Prevention Trial—Type 1 Diabetes Study Group. Effects of insulin in relatives of patients with type 1 diabetes mellitus. N Engl J Med. 2002 May 30;346(22):1685–91. [PMID: 12037147]

Drucker DJ et al. The incretin system: glucagon-like peptide-1 receptor agonists and dipeptidyl peptidase-4 inhibitors in type 2 diabetes. Lancet. 2006 Nov 11;368(9548):1696–705. [PMID: 17098089]

Effect of intensive blood-glucose control with metformin on complications in overweight patients with type 2 diabetes (UKPDS 34). UK Prospective Diabetes Study (UKPDS) Group. Lancet. 1998 Sep 12;352(9131):854–65. [PMID: 9742977]

Efficacy of atenolol and captopril in reducing risk of macrovascular and microvascular complications in type 2 diabetes: UKPDS 39. UK Prospective Diabetes Study Group. BMJ. 1998 Sep 12;317(7160):713–20. [PMID: 9732338]

Gaede P et al. Multifactorial intervention and cardiovascular disease in patients with type 2 diabetes. N Engl J Med. 2003 Jan 30;348(5):383–93. [PMID: 12556541]

Gandhi GY et al. Intensive intraoperative insulin therapy versus conventional glucose management during cardiac surgery: a randomized trial. Ann Intern Med. 2007 Feb 20;146(4):233–43. [PMID: 17310047]

Genuth S et al; Expert Committee on the Diagnosis and Classification of Diabetes Mellitus. Follow-up report on the diagnosis of diabetes mellitus. Diabetes Care. 2003 Nov;26(11):3160–7. [PMID: 14578255]

Gray CS et al. Glucose-potassium-insulin infusions in the management of post-stroke hyperglycaemia: the UK Glucose Insulin in Stroke Trial (GIST-UK). Lancet Neurol. 2007 May;6(5):397–406. [PMID: 17434094]

Grundy SM. Metabolic syndrome: a multiplex cardiovascular risk factor. J Clin Endocrinol Metab. 2007 Feb;92(2):399–404. [PMID: 17284640]

Harris R et al. Screening adults for type 2 diabetes: a review of the evidence for the U.S. Preventive Services Task Force. Ann Intern Med. 2003 Feb 4;138(3):215–29. [PMID: 12558362]

Intensive blood-glucose control with sulphonylureas or insulin compared with conventional treatment and risk of complications in patients with type 2 diabetes (UKPDS 33). UK Prospective Diabetes Study (UKPDS) Group. Lancet. 1998 Sep 12;352(9131):837–53. [PMID: 9742976]

Juvenile Diabetes Foundation http://www.jdf.org/index.html

Kahn SE et al. Mechanisms linking obesity to insulin resistance and type 2 diabetes. Nature. 2006 Dec 14;444(7121):840–6. [PMID: 17167471]

Knowler WC et al; Diabetes Prevention Program Research Group. Reduction in the incidence of type 2 diabetes with lifestyle intervention or metformin. N Engl J Med. 2002 Feb 7;346(6):393–403. [PMID: 11832527]

Marso SP et al. Peripheral arterial disease in patients with diabetes. J Am Coll Cardiol. 2006 Mar 7;47(5):921–9. [PMID: 16516072]

Mayfield JA et al; American Diabetes Association. Preventive foot care in diabetes. Diabetes Care. 2004 Jan;27(Suppl 1):S63–4. [PMID: 14693928]

Mohamed Q et al. Management of diabetic retinopathy: a systematic review. JAMA. 2007 Aug 22;298(8):902–16. [PMID: 17712074]

Molitch ME et al; American Diabetes Association. Nephropathy in diabetes. Diabetes Care. 2004 Jan;27(Suppl 1):S79–83. [PMID: 14693934]

Mooradian AD et al. Narrative review: a rational approach to starting insulin therapy. Ann Intern Med. 2006 Jul 18;145(2):125–34. [PMID: 16847295]

Murphy HR et al. Effectiveness of continuous glucose monitoring in pregnant women with diabetes: randomised clinical trial. BMJ. 2008 Sep 25;337:a1680. [PMID: 18818254]

Nathan DM et al. Management of hyperglycemia in type 2 diabetes: a consensus algorithm for the initiation and adjustment of therapy: update regarding thiazolidinediones: a consensus statement from the American Diabetes Association and the European Association for the Study of Diabetes. Diabetes Care. 2008 Jan;31(1):173–5. [PMID: 18165348]

Nathan DM et al; A_{1c}-Derived Average Glucose Study Group. Translating the A_{1c} assay into estimated average glucose values. Diabetes Care. 2008 Aug;31(8):1473–8. [PMID: 18540046]

Ohkubo Y et al. Intensive insulin therapy prevents the progression of diabetic microvascular complications in Japanese patients with non-insulin-dependent diabetes mellitus: a randomized prospective 6-year study. Diabetes Res Clin Pract. 1995 May;28(2):103–17. [PMID: 7587918]

Robertson RP et al; American Diabetes Association. Pancreas and islet transplantation in type 1 diabetes. Diabetes Care. 2006 Apr;29(4):935. [PMID: 16567844]

Rosenstock J et al. Inhaled insulin improves glycemic control when substituted for or added to oral combination therapy in type 2 diabetes: a randomized, controlled trial. Ann Intern Med. 2005 Oct 18;143(8):549–58. Summary for patients in: Ann Intern Med. 2005 Oct 18;143(8):I28 [PMID: 16230721]

Screening for type 2 diabetes mellitus in adults: U.S. Preventive Services Task Force recommendation statement. Ann Intern Med. 2008 Jun 3;148(11):846–54. [PMID: 18519930]

Snow V et al; Clinical Efficacy Assessment Subcommittee of the American College of Physicians. The evidence base for tight blood pressure control in the management of type 2 diabetes mellitus. Ann Intern Med. 2003 Apr 1;138(7):587–92. [PMID: 12667031]

Tamborlane WV et al; Juvenile Diabetes Research Foundation Continuous Glucose Monitoring Study Group. Continuous glucose monitoring and intensive treatment of type 1 diabetes. N Engl J Med. 2008 Oct 2;359(14):1464–76. [PMID: 18779236]

Tight blood pressure control and risk of macrovascular and microvascular complications in type 2 diabetes: UKPDS 38. UK Prospective Diabetes Study Group. BMJ. 1998 Sep 12;317(7160):703–13. [PMID: 9732337]

Van den Berghe G et al. Intensive insulin therapy in the critically ill patient. N Engl J Med. 2001 Nov 8;345(19):1359–67. [PMID: 11794168]

Van den Berghe G et al. Intensive insulin therapy in the medical ICU. N Engl J Med. 2006 Feb 2;354(5):449–61. [PMID: 16452557]

Vardi M et al. Phosphodiesterase inhibitors for erectile dysfunction in patients with diabetes mellitus. Cochrane Database Syst Rev. 2007 Jan 24;(1):CD002187. [PMID: 17253475]

Vijan S et al. Treatment of hypertension in type 2 diabetes mellitus: blood pressure goals, choice of agents, and setting priorities in diabetes care. Ann Intern Med. 2003 Apr 1;138(7):593–602. [PMID: 12667032]

Wajchenberg BL. Subcutaneous and visceral adipose tissue: their relation to the metabolic syndrome. Endocr Rev. 2000 Dec;21(6):697–738. [PMID: 11133069]

Weissberg-Benchell J et al. Insulin pump therapy: a meta-analysis. Diabetes Care. 2003 Apr;26(4):1079–87. [PMID: 12663577]

Yki-Jarvinen H. Thiazolidinediones. N Engl J Med. 2004 Sep 9;351(11):1106–18. [PMID: 15356308]

Yusuf S et al. Effects of an angiotensin-converting-enzyme inhibitor, ramipril, on cardiovascular events in high-risk patients. The Heart Outcomes Prevention Evaluation Study Investigators. N Engl J Med. 2000 Jan 20;342(3):145–53. [PMID: 10639539]

Zinman B et al; American Diabetes Association. Physical activity/exercise and diabetes. Diabetes Care. 2004 Jan;27(Suppl 1):S58–62. [PMID: 14693927]

DIABETIC COMA

Coma may be due to a variety of causes not directly related to diabetes. Certain causes directly related to diabetes require differentiation: (1) Hypoglycemic coma resulting from excessive doses of insulin or oral hypoglycemic agents. (2) Hyperglycemic coma associated with either severe insulin deficiency (diabetic ketoacidosis) or mild to moderate insulin deficiency (hyperglycemic hyperosmolar state). (3) Lactic acidosis associated with diabetes, particularly in diabetics stricken with severe infections or with cardiovascular collapse.

DIABETIC KETOACIDOSIS

 ESSENTIALS OF DIAGNOSIS

- ▶ Hyperglycemia > 250 mg/dL.
- ▶ Acidosis with blood pH < 7.3.
- ▶ Serum bicarbonate < 15 mEq/L.
- ▶ Serum positive for ketones.

▶ General Considerations

Diabetic ketoacidosis may be the initial manifestation of type 1 diabetes or may result from increased insulin requirements in type 1 diabetes patients during the course of infection, trauma, myocardial infarction, or surgery. It is a life-threatening medical emergency with a mortality rate just under 5% in individuals under 40 years of age, but with a more serious prognosis in the elderly, who have mortality rates over 20%. The National Data Group report an annual incidence of five to eight episodes of diabetic ketoacidosis per 1000 diabetic persons. Ketoacidosis may develop in patients with type 2 diabetes when severe stress such as sepsis or trauma is present. Diabetic ketoacidosis has been found to be one of the more common serious complications of insulin pump therapy, occurring in approximately 1 per 80 patient-months of treatment. Many patients who monitor capillary blood glucose regularly ignore urine ketone measurements, which would signal the possibility of insulin leakage or pump failure before serious illness develops. Poor compliance is one of the most common causes of diabetic ketoacidosis, particularly when episodes are recurrent.

▶ Clinical Findings

A. Symptoms and Signs

The appearance of diabetic ketoacidotic coma is usually preceded by a day or more of polyuria and polydipsia associated with marked fatigue, nausea and vomiting, and, finally, mental stupor that can progress to coma. On physical examination, evidence of dehydration in a stuporous patient with rapid deep breathing and a "fruity" breath odor of acetone would strongly suggest the diagnosis. Hypotension with tachycardia indicates profound fluid and electrolyte depletion, and mild hypothermia is usually present. Abdominal pain and even tenderness may be present in the absence of abdominal disease. Conversely, cholecystitis or pancreatitis may occur with minimal symptoms and signs.

B. Laboratory Findings

(Table 27–13.) Glycosuria of 4+ and strong ketonuria with hyperglycemia, ketonemia, low arterial blood pH, and low plasma bicarbonate are typical of diabetic ketoacidosis. Serum potassium is often elevated despite total body potassium depletion resulting from protracted polyuria or vomiting. Elevation of serum amylase is common but often

represents salivary as well as pancreatic amylase. Thus, in this setting, an elevated serum amylase is not specific for acute pancreatitis. Serum lipase may be useful if the diagnosis of acute pancreatitis is being seriously considered. Azotemia may be a better indicator of renal status than serum creatinine, since multichannel chemical analysis of serum creatinine (SMA-6) is falsely elevated by nonspecific chromogenicity of keto acids and glucose. Most laboratories, however, now routinely eliminate this interference. Leukocytosis as high as 25,000/mcL with a left shift may occur with or without associated infection. The presence of an elevated or even a normal temperature would suggest the presence of an infection, since patients with diabetic ketoacidosis are generally hypothermic if uninfected.

▶ Complications

Hyperglycemia and ketoacidemia are due to insulin lack, hyperglucagonemia, and elevated levels of the stress hormones catecholamines, cortisol, and growth hormone.

A. Hyperglycemia

Hyperglycemia results from increased hepatic production of glucose as well as diminished glucose uptake by peripheral tissues. Hepatic glucose output is a consequence of increased gluconeogenesis resulting from insulinopenia as well as from an associated hyperglucagonemia.

B. Ketoacidemia

Ketoacidemia represents the effect of insulin lack at multiple enzyme loci. Insulin lack associated with elevated levels of growth hormone, catecholamines, and glucagon contributes to an increase in lipolysis from adipose tissue and in hepatic ketogenesis. In addition, there is evidence that reduced ketolysis by insulin-deficient peripheral tissues contributes to the ketoacidemia. The only true "keto" acid present is acetoacetic acid, which, along with its by-product acetone, is measured by nitroprusside reagents (Acetest and Ketostix). The sensitivity for acetone, however, is poor, requiring over 10 mmol, which is seldom reached in the plasma of ketoacidotic subjects—

Table 27–13. Laboratory diagnosis of coma in diabetic patients.

	Urine Glucose	Acetone	Plasma Glucose	Bicarbonate	Acetone
Related to diabetes					
Hypoglycemia	0[1]	0 or +	Low	Normal	0
Diabetic ketoacidosis	++++	++++	High	Low	++++
Hyperglycemic hyperosmolar state coma	++++	0	High	Normal or slightly low	0
Lactic acidosis	0 or +	0 or +	Normal or low or high	Low	0 or +
Unrelated to diabetes					
Alcohol or other toxic drugs	0 or +	0 or +	May be low	Normal or low[2]	0 or +
Cerebrovascular accident or head trauma	+ or 0	0	Often high	Normal	0
Uremia	0 or +	0	High or normal	Low	0 or +

[1]Leftover urine in bladder might still contain glucose from earlier hyperglycemia.
[2]Alcohol can elevate plasma lactate as well as keto acids to reduce pH.

although this detectable concentration is readily achieved in urine. Thus, in the plasma of ketotic patients, only acetoacetate is measured by these reagents. The more prevalent β-hydroxybutyric acid has no ketone group and is therefore not detected by conventional nitroprusside tests. This takes on special importance in the presence of circulatory collapse during diabetic ketoacidosis, wherein an increase in lactic acid can shift the redox state to increase β-hydroxybutyric acid at the expense of the readily detectable acetoacetic acid. Bedside diagnostic reagents would then be unreliable, suggesting no ketonemia in cases where β-hydroxybutyric acid is a major factor in producing the acidosis. A combined glucose and ketone meter (Precision Xtra, Abbott Diabetes Care) that is able to measure blood β-hydroxybutyrate concentration on capillary blood is available. Many clinical laboratories now offer β-hydroxybutyrate measurement.

C. Fluid and Electrolyte Depletion

Hyperglycemia results in an osmotic diuresis and dehydration and secondary loss of electrolytes. Ketonuria similarly causes loss of water and electrolytes. Balance studies during withdrawal of insulin and treatment in patients with type 1 diabetes show that on average the water depletion is about 5 L; sodium, 300–500 mmol; potassium, 270–400 mmol; chloride, 100–400 mmol.

Drowsiness is fairly common but frank coma only occurs in about 10% of patients. There is a correlation between the degree of depression of the sensorium and extracellular osmolarity. When serum hyperosmolality exceeds 320–330 mosm/L, central nervous system depression or coma may ensue. Coma in a diabetic patient with a lower osmolality should prompt a search for cause of coma other than hyperosmolality.

▶ Treatment

A. Prevention

Education of diabetic patients to recognize the early symptoms and signs of ketoacidosis has done a great deal to prevent severe acidosis. Urine ketones or capillary blood β-hydroxybutyrate should be measured in patients with signs of infection or in insulin pump-treated patients when capillary blood glucose is unexpectedly and persistently high. When heavy ketonuria and glycosuria persist on several successive examinations, supplemental regular insulin should be administered and liquid foods such as lightly salted tomato juice and broth should be ingested to replenish fluids and electrolytes. The patient should be instructed to contact the physician if ketonuria persists, and especially if vomiting develops or if appropriate adjustment of the infusion rate on an insulin pump does not correct the hyperglycemia and ketonuria. In juvenile-onset diabetics, particularly in the teen years, recurrent episodes of severe ketoacidosis often indicate poor compliance with the insulin regimen, and these patients will require intensive family counseling.

B. Emergency Measures

If ketosis is severe, the patient should be placed in the hospital for correction of the hyperosmolality as well as the ketoacidemia. An ICU or, at the least, a step-down unit is preferable for more severe cases.

1. Therapeutic flow sheet—One of the most important steps in initiating therapy is to start a flow sheet listing vital signs and the time sequence of diagnostic laboratory values in relation to therapeutic maneuvers. Indices of the metabolic defects include urine glucose and ketones as well as arterial pH, plasma glucose, acetone, bicarbonate, serum urea nitrogen, and electrolytes. Serum osmolality should be measured or estimated and tabulated during the course of therapy.

A convenient method of estimating effective serum osmolality is as follows (normal values in humans are 280–300 mosm/kg):

$$\text{mosm/kg} = 2[\text{Na}^+] + \frac{\text{Glucose (mg/dL)}}{18}$$

These calculated estimates are usually 10–20 mosm/kg lower than values measured by standard cryoscopic techniques in patients with diabetic coma. Urea is freely permeable across cell membranes and therefore not included in calculations of effective serum osmolality. One physician should be responsible for maintaining this therapeutic flow sheet and prescribing therapy. An indwelling urinary catheter is required in all comatose patients but should be avoided if possible in a fully cooperative diabetic because of the risk of introducing bladder infection. Fluid intake and output should be recorded. Gastric intubation is recommended in the comatose patient to correct the commonly associated gastric dilatation that may lead to vomiting and aspiration. The patient should not receive sedatives or opioids.

2. Insulin replacement—Only regular insulin should be used initially in all cases of severe ketoacidosis, and it should be given immediately after the diagnosis is established. Regular insulin can be given in a loading dose of 0.15 unit/kg as an intravenous bolus to prime the tissue insulin receptors. Following the initial bolus, doses of insulin as low as 0.1 unit/kg/h are continuously infused or given hourly as an intramuscular injection; this is sufficient to replace the insulin deficit in most patients. Replacement of insulin deficiency helps correct the acidosis by reducing the flux of fatty acids to the liver, reducing ketone production by the liver, and also improving removal of ketones from the blood. Insulin treatment reduces the hyperosmolality by reducing the hyperglycemia. It accomplishes this by increasing removal of glucose through peripheral utilization as well as by decreasing production of glucose by the liver. This latter effect is accomplished by direct inhibition of gluconeogenesis and glycogenolysis, as well as by lowered amino acid flux from muscle to liver and reduced hyperglucagonemia.

The insulin dose should be "piggy-backed" into the fluid line so the rate of fluid replacement can be changed without altering the insulin delivery rate. If the plasma glucose level fails to fall at least 10% in the first hour, a repeat loading dose is recommended. The availability of bedside glucometers and of laboratory instruments for rapid and accurate glucose analysis (Beckman or Yellow Springs glucose analyzer) has contributed much to achieving optimal insulin replacement. Rarely, a patient with immune insulin resistance is encountered, and this requires doubling the insulin dose every 2–4 hours if hyperglycemia does not improve after the first two doses of insulin.

3. Fluid replacement—In most patients, the fluid deficit is 4–5 L. Initially, 0.9% saline solution is the solution of choice to help reexpand the contracted vascular volume and should be started in the emergency department as soon as the diagnosis is established. The saline should be infused rapidly to provide 1 L/h over the first 1–2 hours. After the first 2 L of fluid have been given, the intravenous infusion should be at the rate of 300–400 mL/h. Use 0.9% ("normal") saline unless the serum sodium is greater than 150 mEq/L, when 0.45% ("half normal") saline solution should be used. The volume status should be very carefully monitored. Failure to give enough volume replacement (at least 3–4 L in 8 hours) to restore normal perfusion is one of the most serious therapeutic shortcomings adversely influencing satisfactory recovery. Excessive fluid replacement (more than 5 L in 8 hours) may contribute to acute respiratory distress syndrome or cerebral edema. When blood glucose falls to approximately 250 mg/dL, the fluids should be changed to a 5% glucose-containing solution to maintain serum glucose in the range of 250–300 mg/dL. This will prevent the development of hypoglycemia and will also reduce the likelihood of cerebral edema, which could result from too rapid decline of blood glucose. Intensive insulin therapy should be continued until the ketoacidosis is corrected.

4. Sodium bicarbonate—The use of sodium bicarbonate in management of diabetic ketoacidosis has been questioned since clinical benefit was not demonstrated in one prospective randomized trial and because of the following potentially harmful consequences: (1) development of hypokalemia from rapid shift of potassium into cells if the acidosis is overcorrected, (2) tissue anoxia from reduced dissociation of oxygen from hemoglobin when acidosis is rapidly reversed (leftward shift of the oxygen dissociation curve), and (3) cerebral acidosis resulting from lowering of cerebrospinal fluid pH. It must be emphasized, however, that these considerations are less important when severe acidosis exists. It is therefore recommended that bicarbonate be administered to diabetic patients in ketoacidosis if the arterial blood pH is 7.0 or less, with careful monitoring to prevent overcorrection. One or two ampules of sodium bicarbonate (one ampule contains 44 mEq/50 mL) should be added to 1 L of 0.45% saline. (**Note:** Addition of sodium bicarbonate to 0.9% saline would produce a markedly hypertonic solution that could aggravate the hyperosmolar state already present.) This should be administered rapidly (over the first hour). It can be repeated until the arterial pH reaches 7.1, but *it should not be given if the pH is 7.1 or greater* since additional bicarbonate would increase the risk of rebound metabolic alkalosis as ketones are metabolized. Alkalosis shifts potassium from serum into cells, which could precipitate a fatal cardiac arrhythmia.

5. Potassium—Total body potassium loss from polyuria and vomiting may be as high as 200 mEq. However, because of shifts of potassium from cells into the extracellular space as a consequence of acidosis, serum potassium is usually normal to slightly elevated prior to institution of treatment. As the acidosis is corrected, potassium flows back into the cells, and hypokalemia can develop if potassium replacement is not instituted. If the patient is not uremic and has an adequate urinary output, potassium chloride in doses of 10–30 mEq/h should be infused during the second and third hours after beginning therapy as soon as the acidosis starts to resolve. Replacement should be started sooner if the initial serum potassium is inappropriately normal or low and should be delayed if serum potassium fails to respond to initial therapy and remains above 5 mEq/L, as in cases of chronic kidney disease. An ECG can be of help in monitoring the patient's potassium status: High peaked T waves are a sign of hyperkalemia, and flattened T waves with U waves are a sign of hypokalemia. Foods high in potassium content should be prescribed when the patient has recovered sufficiently to take food orally. Tomato juice has 14 mEq of potassium per 240 mL, and a medium-sized banana provides about 10 mEq.

6. Phosphate—Phosphate replacement is seldom required in treating diabetic ketoacidosis. However, if severe hypophosphatemia of less than 1 mg/dL (< 0.32 mmol/L) develops during insulin therapy, a small amount of phosphate can be replaced per hour as the potassium salt. Correction of hypophosphatemia helps restore the buffering capacity of the plasma, thereby facilitating renal excretion of hydrogen. It also corrects the impaired oxygen dissociation from hemoglobin by regenerating 2,3-diphosphoglycerate. However, three randomized studies in which phosphate was replaced in only half of a group of patients with diabetic ketoacidosis did not show any apparent clinical benefit from phosphate administration. Moreover, attempts to use the phosphate salt of potassium as the sole means of replacing potassium have led to a number of reported cases of severe hypocalcemia with tetany. To minimize the risk of inducing tetany from too-rapid replacement of phosphate, the average deficit of 40–50 mmol of phosphate should be replaced intravenously at a rate *no greater than 3–4 mmol/h* in a 60–70-kg person. A stock solution (Abbott) provides a mixture of 1.12 g KH_2PO_4 and 1.18 g K_2HPO_4 in a 5-mL single-dose vial (this equals 22 mmol of potassium and 15 mmol of phosphate). One-half of this vial (2.5 mL) should be added to 1 L of either 0.45% saline or 5% dextrose in water. Two liters of this solution, infused at a rate of 400 mL/h, will correct the phosphate deficit at the optimal rate of 3 mmol/h while providing 4.4 mEq of potassium per hour. (Additional potassium should be administered as potassium chloride to provide a total of 10–30 mEq of potassium per hour, as noted above.) If the serum phosphate remains below 2.5 mg/dL after this infusion, a repeat 5-hour infusion can be given.

7. Hyperchloremic acidosis during therapy—Because of the considerable loss of keto acids in the urine during the initial phase of therapy, substrate for subsequent regeneration of bicarbonate is lost and correction of the total bicarbonate deficit is hampered. A portion of the bicarbonate deficit is replaced with chloride ions infused in large amounts as saline to correct the dehydration. In most patients, as the ketoacidosis clears during insulin replacement, a hyperchloremic, low-bicarbonate pattern emerges with a normal anion gap. This is a relatively benign condition that reverses itself over the subsequent 12–24 hours once intravenous saline is no longer being administered.

8. Treatment of associated infection—Antibiotics are prescribed as indicated. Cholecystitis and pyelonephritis may be particularly severe in these patients.

Prognosis

The frequency of deaths due to diabetic ketoacidosis has been dramatically reduced by improved therapy of young diabetics, but this complication remains a significant risk in the aged and in patients in profound coma in whom treatment has been delayed. Acute myocardial infarction and infarction of the bowel following prolonged hypotension worsen the outlook. A serious prognostic sign is end-stage chronic kidney disease, and prior kidney dysfunction worsens the prognosis considerably because the kidney plays a key role in compensating for massive pH and electrolyte abnormalities. Cerebral edema has been reported to occur rarely as metabolic deficits return to normal. This is best prevented by avoiding sudden reversal of marked hyperglycemia. Maintaining glycemic levels of 200–300 mg/dL for the initial 24 hours after correction of severe hyperglycemia reduces this risk.

Kitabchi AE et al. Management of hyperglycemic crises in patients with diabetes. Diabetes Care. 2001 Jan;24(1):131–53. [PMID: 11194218]

HYPERGLYCEMIC HYPEROSMOLAR STATE

 ESSENTIALS OF DIAGNOSIS

▶ Hyperglycemia > 600 mg/dL.

▶ Serum osmolality > 310 mosm/kg.

▶ No acidosis; blood pH above 7.3.

▶ Serum bicarbonate > 15 mEq/L.

▶ Normal anion gap (< 14 mEq/L).

General Considerations

This second most common form of hyperglycemic coma is characterized by severe hyperglycemia in the absence of significant ketosis, with hyperosmolality and dehydration. It occurs in patients with mild or occult diabetes, and most patients are at least middle-aged to elderly. Accurate figures are not available as to its true incidence, but from data on hospital discharges it is rarer than diabetic ketoacidosis even in older age groups. Lethargy and confusion develop as serum osmolality exceeds 310 mosm/kg, and coma can occur if osmolality exceeds 320–330 mosm/kg. A committee of the ADA has recommended replacing the previous name of this disorder (hyperglycemic, hyperosmolar, nonketotic coma) with the consensus term "hyperglycemic hyperosmolar state." Underlying chronic kidney disease or

congestive heart failure is common, and the presence of either worsens the prognosis. A precipitating event such as infection, myocardial infarction, stroke, or recent operation is often present. Certain drugs such as phenytoin, diazoxide, corticosteroids, and diuretics have been implicated in its pathogenesis, as have procedures associated with glucose loading such as peritoneal dialysis.

Pathogenesis

A partial or relative insulin deficiency may initiate the syndrome by reducing glucose utilization of muscle, fat, and liver while inducing hyperglucagonemia and increasing hepatic glucose output. With massive glycosuria, obligatory water loss ensues. If a patient is unable to maintain adequate fluid intake because of an associated acute or chronic illness or has suffered excessive fluid loss, marked dehydration results. As plasma volume contracts, chronic kidney disease develops, and the resultant limitation of renal glucose loss leads to increasingly higher blood glucose concentrations. Severe hyperosmolality develops that causes mental confusion and finally coma. It is not clear why ketosis is virtually absent under these conditions of insulin insufficiency, although reduced levels of growth hormone may be a factor, along with portal vein insulin concentrations sufficient to restrain ketogenesis.

Clinical Findings

A. Symptoms and Signs

Onset may be insidious over a period of days or weeks, with weakness, polyuria, and polydipsia. The lack of features of ketoacidosis may retard recognition of the syndrome and delay therapy until dehydration becomes more profound than in ketoacidosis. Reduced intake of fluid is not an uncommon historical feature, due to either inappropriate lack of thirst, nausea, or inaccessibility of fluids to elderly, bedridden patients. Lethargy and confusion develop, progressing to convulsions and deep coma. Physical examination confirms the presence of profound dehydration in a lethargic or comatose patient without Kussmaul respirations.

B. Laboratory Findings

(Table 27–13.) Severe hyperglycemia is present, with blood glucose values ranging from 600 mg/dL to 2400 mg/dL. In mild cases, where dehydration is less severe, dilutional hyponatremia as well as urinary sodium losses may reduce serum sodium to 120–125 mEq/L, which protects to some extent against extreme hyperosmolality. However, as dehydration progresses, serum sodium can exceed 140 mEq/L, producing serum osmolality readings of 330–440 mosm/kg. Ketosis and acidosis are usually absent or mild. Prerenal azotemia is the rule, with serum urea nitrogen elevations over 100 mg/dL being typical.

Treatment

A. Saline

Fluid replacement is of paramount importance in treating nonketotic hyperglycemic coma. The onset of hyperosmolarity is more insidious in elderly people without ketosis than in younger individuals with high serum ketone levels, which provide earlier indicators of severe illness (vomiting, rapid deep breathing, acetone odor, etc). Consequently, diagnosis and treatment are often delayed until fluid deficit has reached levels of 6–10 L.

If hypovolemia is present as evidenced by hypotension and oliguria, fluid therapy should be initiated with 0.9% saline. In all other cases, 0.45% saline appears to be preferable as the initial replacement solution because the body fluids of these patients are markedly hyperosmolar. As much as 4–6 L of fluid may be required in the first 8–10 hours. Careful monitoring of the patient is required for proper sodium and water replacement. Once blood glucose reaches 250 mg/dL, fluid replacement should include 5% dextrose in either water, 0.45% saline solution, or 0.9% saline solution. The rate of dextrose infusion should be adjusted to maintain glycemic levels of 250–300 mg/dL in order to reduce the risk of cerebral edema. An important end point of fluid therapy is to restore urinary output to 50 mL/h or more.

B. Insulin

Less insulin may be required to reduce the hyperglycemia in nonketotic patients as compared to those with diabetic ketoacidotic coma. In fact, fluid replacement alone can reduce hyperglycemia considerably by correcting the hypovolemia, which then increases both glomerular filtration and renal excretion of glucose. An initial dose of 0.15 unit/kg is followed by an insulin infusion of 1–2 units/h, which is titrated to lower blood glucose levels by 50–70 mg/dL per hour.

C. Potassium

With the absence of acidosis, there may be no initial hyperkalemia unless associated end-stage chronic kidney disease is present. This results in less severe total potassium depletion than in diabetic ketoacidosis, and less potassium replacement is therefore needed. However, because initial serum potassium is usually not elevated and because it declines rapidly as a result of insulin's effect on driving potassium intracellularly, it has been recommended that potassium replacement be initiated earlier than in ketotic patients, assuming that no chronic kidney disease or oliguria is present. Potassium chloride (10 mEq/L) can be added to the initial bottle of fluids administered if the patient's serum potassium is not elevated.

D. Phosphate

If severe hypophosphatemia (serum phosphate < 1 mg/dL [< 0.32 mmol/L]) develops during insulin therapy, phosphate replacement can be given as described for ketoacidotic patients (at 3 mmol/h).

▶ Prognosis

The overall mortality rate of hyperglycemic hyperosmolar state coma is more than ten times that of diabetic ketoacidosis, chiefly because of its higher incidence in older patients, who may have compromised cardiovascular systems or associated major illnesses and whose dehydration

is often excessive because of delays in recognition and treatment. (When patients are matched for age, the prognoses of these two hyperglycemic emergencies are reasonably comparable.) When prompt therapy is instituted, the mortality rate can be reduced from nearly 50% to that related to the severity of coexistent disorders.

American Diabetes Association. Hyperglycemic crises in patients with diabetes mellitus. Diabetes Care. 2001 Jan;24(1):154–61. [PMID: 11221603]

LACTIC ACIDOSIS

 ESSENTIALS OF DIAGNOSIS

- ▶ Severe acidosis with hyperventilation.
- ▶ Blood pH below 7.30.
- ▶ Serum bicarbonate < 15 mEq/L.
- ▶ Anion gap > 15 mEq/L.
- ▶ Absent serum ketones.
- ▶ Serum lactate > 5 mmol/L.

▶ General Considerations

Lactic acidosis is characterized by accumulation of excess lactic acid in the blood. Normally, the principal sources of this acid are the erythrocytes (which lack enzymes for aerobic oxidation), skeletal muscle, skin, and brain. Conversion of lactic acid to glucose and its oxidation principally by the liver but also by the kidneys represent the chief pathways for its removal. Overproduction of lactic acid (tissue hypoxia), deficient removal (hepatic failure), or both (circulatory collapse) can cause accumulation. Lactic acidosis is not uncommon in any severely ill patient suffering from cardiac decompensation, respiratory or hepatic failure, septicemia, or infarction of bowel or extremities. With the discontinuance of phenformin therapy in the United States, lactic acidosis in patients with diabetes mellitus has become uncommon but occasionally occurs in metformin-treated patients (see above) and it still must be considered in the acidotic diabetic, especially if the patient is seriously ill.

▶ Clinical Findings

A. Symptoms and Signs

The main clinical feature of lactic acidosis is marked hyperventilation. When lactic acidosis is secondary to tissue hypoxia or vascular collapse, the clinical presentation is variable, being that of the prevailing catastrophic illness. However, in the idiopathic, or spontaneous, variety, the onset is rapid (usually over a few hours), blood pressure is normal, peripheral circulation is good, and there is no cyanosis.

B. Laboratory Findings

Plasma bicarbonate and blood pH are quite low, indicating the presence of severe metabolic acidosis. Ketones are usually absent from plasma and urine or at least not prominent. The first clue may be a high anion gap (serum sodium minus the sum of chloride and bicarbonate anions [in mEq/L] should be no greater than 15). A higher value indicates the existence of an abnormal compartment of anions. If this cannot be clinically explained by an excess of keto acids (diabetes), inorganic acids (uremia), or anions from drug overdosage (salicylates, methyl alcohol, ethylene glycol), then lactic acidosis is probably the correct diagnosis. (See also Chapter 21.) In the absence of azotemia, hyperphosphatemia may be a clue to the presence of lactic acidosis for reasons that are not clear. The diagnosis is confirmed by demonstrating, in a sample of blood that is promptly chilled and separated, a plasma lactic acid concentration of 5 mmol/L or higher (values as high as 30 mmol/L have been reported). Normal plasma values average 1 mmol/L, with a normal lactate/pyruvate ratio of 10:1. This ratio is greatly exceeded in lactic acidosis.*

▶ Treatment

Aggressive treatment of the precipitating cause of lactic acidosis is the main component of therapy, such as ensuring adequate oxygenation and vascular perfusion of tissues. Empiric antibiotic coverage for sepsis should be given after culture samples are obtained in any patient in whom the cause of the lactic acidosis is not apparent.

Alkalinization with intravenous sodium bicarbonate to keep the pH above 7.2 has been recommended by some in the emergency treatment of lactic acidosis; as much as 2000 mEq in 24 hours has been used. However, there is no evidence that the mortality rate is favorably affected by administering bicarbonate, and its use remains controversial. Hemodialysis may be useful in cases where large sodium loads are poorly tolerated.

▶ Prognosis

The mortality rate of spontaneous lactic acidosis is high. The prognosis in most cases is that of the primary disorder that produced the lactic acidosis.

Forsythe SM et al. Sodium bicarbonate for the treatment of lactic acidosis. Chest. 2000 Jan;117(1):260–7. [PMID: 10631227]
Salpeter S et al. Risk of fatal and nonfatal lactic acidosis with metformin use in type 2 diabetes mellitus. Cochrane Database Syst Rev. 2006 Jan 25;(1):CD002967. [PMID: 16437448]

▼ THE HYPOGLYCEMIC STATES

Spontaneous hypoglycemia in adults is of two principal types: fasting and postprandial. Symptoms begin at plasma glucose levels in the range of 60 mg/dL and impairment of brain function at approximately 50 mg/dL. Fasting hypoglycemia is often subacute or chronic and usually presents with

---

*In collecting samples, it is essential to rapidly chill and separate the blood in order to remove red cells, whose continued glycolysis at room temperature is a common source of error in reports of high plasma lactate. Frozen plasma remains stable for subsequent assay.

Table 27–14. Common causes of hypoglycemia in adults.[1]

Fasting hypoglycemia
Hyperinsulinism
Pancreatic B cell tumor
Surreptitious administration of insulin or sulfonylureas
Extrapancreatic tumors
Postprandial (reactive) hypoglycemia
Early hypoglycemia (alimentary)
Postgastrectomy
Functional (increased vagal tone)
Late hypoglycemia (occult diabetes mellitus)
Delayed insulin release due to B cell dysfunction
Counterregulatory hormone and neurogenic autonomic response deficiency
Idiopathic
Alcohol-related hypoglycemia
Immunopathologic hypoglycemia
Idiopathic anti-insulin antibodies (which release their bound insulin)
Antibodies to insulin receptors (which act as agonists)
Drug-induced hypoglycemia

[1]In the absence of clinically obvious endocrine, renal, or hepatic disorders and exclusive of diabetes mellitus treated with hypoglycemic agents.

neuroglycopenia as its principal manifestation; postprandial hypoglycemia is relatively acute and is often heralded by symptoms of neurogenic autonomic discharge (sweating, palpitations, anxiety, tremulousness).

▶ Differential Diagnosis (Table 27–14)

Fasting hypoglycemia may occur in certain endocrine disorders, such as hypopituitarism, Addison disease, or myxedema; in disorders related to liver malfunction, such as acute alcoholism or liver failure; and in instances of end-stage chronic kidney disease, particularly in patients requiring dialysis. These conditions are usually obvious, with hypoglycemia being only a secondary feature. When fasting hypoglycemia is a primary manifestation developing in adults without apparent endocrine disorders or inborn metabolic diseases from childhood, the principal diagnostic possibilities include: (1) hyperinsulinism, due to either pancreatic B cell tumors or islet hyperplasia or surreptitious administration of insulin (or sulfonylureas), and (2) hypoglycemia due to non–insulin-producing extrapancreatic tumors.

Postprandial (reactive) hypoglycemia may be classified as early (within 2–3 hours after a meal) or late (3–5 hours after eating). Early, or alimentary, hypoglycemia occurs when there is a rapid discharge of ingested carbohydrate into the small bowel followed by rapid glucose absorption and hyperinsulinism. It may be seen after gastrointestinal surgery and is particularly associated with the dumping syndrome after gastrectomy and Roux-en-Y gastric bypass surgery. In some cases, it is functional and may represent overactivity of the parasympathetic nervous system mediated via the vagus nerve. Rarely, it results from defective counterregulatory responses such as deficiencies of growth hormone, glucagon, cortisol, or autonomic responses.

Alcohol-related hypoglycemia is due to hepatic glycogen depletion combined with alcohol-mediated inhibition of gluconeogenesis. It is most common in malnourished alcohol abusers but can occur in anyone who is unable to ingest food after an acute alcoholic episode followed by gastritis and vomiting.

Immunopathologic hypoglycemia is an extremely rare condition in which anti-insulin antibodies or antibodies to insulin receptors develop spontaneously. In the former case, the mechanism appears to relate to increasing dissociation of insulin from circulating pools of bound insulin. When antibodies to insulin receptors are found, most patients do not have hypoglycemia but rather severe insulin-resistant diabetes and acanthosis nigricans. However, during the course of the disease in these patients, certain anti-insulin receptor antibodies with agonist activity mimicking insulin action may develop, producing severe hypoglycemia.

Factitious hypoglycemia is self-induced hypoglycemia due to surreptitious administration of insulin or sulfonylureas.

HYPOGLYCEMIA DUE TO PANCREATIC B CELL TUMORS

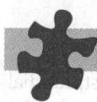

ESSENTIALS OF DIAGNOSIS

▶ Hypoglycemic symptoms—frequently neuroglyco-penic (confusion, blurred vision, diplopia, anxiety, convulsions).

▶ Immediate recovery upon administration of glucose.

▶ Blood glucose < 40 mg/dL with a serum insulin level of 6 microunit/mL or more.

▶ General Considerations

Fasting hypoglycemia in an otherwise healthy, well-nourished adult is rare and is most commonly due to an adenoma of the islets of Langerhans. Ninety percent of such tumors are single and benign, but multiple adenomas can occur as well as malignant tumors with functional metastases. Adenomas may be familial, and multiple adenomas have been found in conjunction with tumors of the parathyroids and pituitary (multiple endocrine neoplasia type 1 [MEN 1]).

▶ Clinical Findings

A. Symptoms and Signs

The most important prerequisite to diagnosing an insulinoma is simply to consider it, particularly in relatively healthy-appearing persons who have fasting hypoglycemia associated with some degree of central nervous system dysfunction such as confusion or abnormal behavior. A delay in diagnosis can result in unnecessary treatment for psychomotor epilepsy or psychiatric disorders and may cause irreversible brain damage. In longstanding cases, obesity can result as a consequence of overeating to relieve symptoms.

The so-called Whipple triad is characteristic of hypoglycemia regardless of the cause. It consists of: (1) a history of hypoglycemic symptoms; (2) an associated fasting blood glucose of 40 mg/dL or less; and (3) immediate recovery upon administration of glucose. The hypoglycemic symptoms in insulinoma often develop in the early morning or after missing a meal. Occasionally, they occur after exercise. They typically begin with evidence of central nervous system glucose lack and can include blurred vision or diplopia, headache, feelings of detachment, slurred speech, and weakness. Personality and mental changes vary from anxiety to psychotic behavior, and neurologic deterioration can result in convulsions or coma. Sweating and palpitations may not occur.

Hypoglycemic unawareness is very common in patients with insulinoma. They adapt to chronic hypoglycemia by increasing their efficiency in transporting glucose across the blood-brain barrier, which masks awareness that their blood glucose is approaching critically low levels. Counterregulatory hormonal responses as well as neurogenic symptoms such as tremor, sweating, and palpitations are therefore blunted during hypoglycemia. If lack of these warning symptoms prevents recognition of the need to eat to correct the problem, patients can lapse into severe hypoglycemic coma. However, symptoms and normal hormone responses during experimental insulin-induced hypoglycemia have been shown to be restored after successful surgical removal of the insulinoma. Presumably with return of euglycemia, adaptive effects on glucose transport into the brain are corrected, and thresholds of counterregulatory responses and neurogenic autonomic symptoms are therefore restored to normal.

B. Laboratory Findings

B cell adenomas do not reduce secretion in the presence of hypoglycemia, and the critical diagnostic test is to demonstrate inappropriately elevated serum insulin levels at a time when hypoglycemia is present. A reliable serum insulin level (radioimmunoassay) of 6 microunit/mL or more in the presence of blood glucose values below 40 mg/dL is diagnostic of inappropriate hyperinsulinism. Immunochemiluminometric assays (ICMA) have sensitivities of less than 1 microunit/mL, and with these assays, the cutoffs for insulinomas is insulin level of 3 microunit/mL or higher. Other causes of hyperinsulinemic hypoglycemia must be considered, including factitious administration of insulin or sulfonylureas. Factitious use of insulin will result in suppression of endogenous insulin secretion and a low C-peptide levels. An elevated circulating proinsulin level in the presence of fasting hypoglycemia is characteristic of most B cell adenomas and does not occur in factitious hyperinsulinism. Thus, C-peptide and proinsulin levels (by ICMA) of > 200 pmol/L and > 5 pmol/L, respectively, are characteristic of insulinomas.

In patients with epigastric distress, a history of renal calculi, or menstrual or erectile dysfunction, a serum calcium, gastrin, or prolactin level may be useful in screening for MEN 1 associated with insulinoma.

C. Diagnostic Tests

1. Prolonged fasting—Prolonged fasting under hospital supervision until hypoglycemia is documented is probably the most dependable means of establishing the diagnosis, especially in men. In 30% of patients with insulinoma, the blood glucose levels often drop below 40 mg/dL after an overnight fast, but some patients require up to 72 hours to develop symptomatic hypoglycemia. However, the term "72-hour fast" is actually a misnomer in most cases since the fast should be immediately terminated as soon as symptoms appear and laboratory confirmation of hypoglycemia is available. In normal male subjects, the blood glucose does not fall below 55–60 mg/dL during a 3-day fast. In contrast, in normal premenopausal women who have fasted for only 24 hours, the plasma glucose may fall normally to such an extent that it can reach values as low as 35 mg/dL. In these cases, however, the women are not symptomatic, presumably owing to the development of sufficient ketonemia to supply energy needs to the brain. Insulinoma patients, on the other hand, become symptomatic when plasma glucose drops to subnormal levels, since inappropriate insulin secretion restricts ketone formation. Moreover, the demonstration of a nonsuppressed insulin level ≥ 6 microunit/mL using a RIA assay (> 3 microunit/mL using an ICMA assay) in the presence of hypoglycemia suggests the diagnosis of insulinoma. If hypoglycemia does not develop in a male patient after fasting for up to 72 hours—and particularly when this prolonged fast is terminated with a period of moderate exercise—insulinoma must be considered an unlikely diagnosis. A suggested protocol for the supervised fast is shown in Table 27–15.

2. Stimulation tests—Stimulation with pancreatic B cell secretagogues such as tolbutamide, glucagon, or leucine is generally not needed in most cases if basal insulin is found

---

Table 27–15. Suggested hospital protocol for supervised fast in diagnosis of insulinoma.

(1) Obtain baseline serum glucose, insulin, proinsulin, and C-peptide measurements at onset of fast and place intravenous cannula.

(2) Permit only calorie-free and caffeine-free fluids and encourage supervised activity (such as walking).

(3) Measure urine for ketones at the beginning and every 12 hours and at end of fast.

(4) Obtain capillary glucose measurements with a reflectance meter every 4 hours until values < 60 mg/dL are obtained. Then increase the frequency of fingersticks to each hour, and when capillary glucose value is < 49 mg/dL send a venous blood sample to the laboratory for serum glucose, insulin, proinsulin, and C-peptide measurements. Check frequently for manifestations of neuroglycopenia.

(5) If symptoms of hypoglycemia occur or if a laboratory value of serum glucose is < 45 mg/dL, or if 72 hours have elapsed then conclude the fast with a final blood sample for serum glucose, insulin, proinsulin, C-peptide, β-hydroxybutyrate or acetone and sulfonylurea measurements. Then give oral fast-acting carbohydrate followed by a meal. If the patient is confused or unable to take oral agents, then administer 50 mL of 50% dextrose intravenously over 3 to 5 minutes. Do not conclude a fast based simply on a capillary blood glucose measurement—wait for the laboratory glucose value—unless the patient is very symptomatic and it would be dangerous to wait.

---

to be nonsuppressible and therefore inappropriately elevated during fasting hypoglycemia.

Intravenous glucagon (1 mg over 1 minute) can be useful in patients with "borderline" fasting inappropriate hyperinsulinism. A serum insulin rise above baseline of 200 microunit/mL or more at 5 and 10 minutes strongly suggests insulinoma, although poorly differentiated tumors may not respond. Glucagon has the advantage over tolbutamide of correcting rather than provoking hypoglycemia during stimulation testing and is diagnostic in 60–70% of patients with insulinoma. False-negative results can occur if the tumor is poorly differentiated and agranular.

D. Preoperative Localization of B Cell Tumors

After the diagnosis of insulinoma has been unequivocally made by clinical and laboratory findings, studies to localize the tumor should be initiated. The focus of attention should be directed to the pancreas since that is where virtually all insulinomas originate.

A spiral CT angiography of the pancreas should be performed to rule out a large tumor of the pancreas or hepatic metastases from a malignant islet cell tumor. Endoscopic ultrasonographic examination of the pancreas can also be helpful in identifying the pancreatic lesions. Because of the small size of these tumors (averaging 1.5 cm in diameter in one large series), imaging studies do not necessarily identify all the tumors. Patients who do not have an obvious tumor on imaging (but have a definite biochemical diagnosis) should undergo selective calcium-stimulated angiography. In this test, angiography is combined with injections of calcium gluconate into the gastroduodenal, splenic, and superior mesenteric arteries and insulin levels are measured in the hepatic vein effluent. Calcium stimulates insulin release from insulinomas but not normal islets, and so a step-up of insulin levels regionalizes the hyperinsulinism to the head of the pancreas for the gastroduodenal artery, to the uncinate process for the superior mesenteric artery, and to the body and tail of the pancreas for the splenic artery. This technique may also provide data that are particularly helpful when multiple insulinomas are suspected (MEN 1) and it has become a major tool in confirming the diagnosis of diffuse islet hyperplasia in the recently described noninsulinoma pancreatogenous hypoglycemia syndrome (NIPHS) (see below). Since diazoxide might interfere with this test, it should be discontinued for at least 48–72 hours before sampling. An infusion of dextrose may be required, therefore, and patients should be closely monitored during the procedure to avoid hypoglycemia (as well as hyperglycemia, which could affect insulin gradients). These studies combined with careful intraoperative ultrasonography and palpation by a surgeon experienced in insulinoma surgery identifies up to 98% of tumors.

▶ Treatment

A. Surgical Measures

It is imperative that the surgeon be convinced that the diagnosis of insulinoma has been unequivocally made by clinical and laboratory findings. Only then should surgery be considered, as there is no justification for exploratory operation—just as there is none for the use of current localization techniques as a preoperative diagnostic tool. Resection by a surgeon with previous experience in removing pancreatic B cell tumors is the treatment of choice. In patients with a single benign adenoma, 90–95% have a successful cure at the first surgical attempt when intraoperative ultrasound is used by a skilled surgeon. Blood glucose should be monitored throughout surgery, and 10% dextrose in water should be infused at a rate of 100 mL/h or faster. In cases where the diagnosis has been established but no adenoma is located after careful palpation and use of intraoperative ultrasound, it is no longer advisable to blindly resect the body and tail of the pancreas, since a nonpalpable tumor missed by ultrasound is most likely embedded within the fleshy head of the pancreas that is left behind with subtotal resections. Most surgeons prefer to close the incision and schedule a selective arterial calcium stimulation with hepatic venous sampling to locate the tumor site prior to a repeat operation. Laparoscopy using ultrasound and enucleation has been successful with a single tumor of the body or tail of the pancreas, but open surgery remains necessary for tumors in the head of the pancreas.

B. Diet and Medical Therapy

In patients with inoperable functioning islet cell carcinoma and in approximately 5–10% of MEN 1 cases when subtotal removal of the pancreas has failed to produce cure, reliance on frequent feedings is necessary. Since most tumors are not responsive to glucose, carbohydrate feedings every 2–3 hours are usually effective in preventing hypoglycemia, although obesity may become a problem. Diazoxide, 300–600 mg (or 3 mg to 8 mg/kg; 50 mg/mL oral suspension) daily orally in two or three divided doses, is the treatment of choice. Hydrochlorothiazide, 25–50 mg daily, should also be prescribed to counteract the sodium retention and edema secondary to diazoxide therapy as well as to potentiate its hyperglycemic effect. If patients are unable to tolerate diazoxide because of gastrointestinal upset, hirsutism, or edema, the calcium channel blocker verapamil may be beneficial in view of its inhibitory effect on insulin release from insulinoma cells. Octreotide, a potent long-acting synthetic octapeptide analog of somatostatin, has been used to inhibit release of hormones from a number of endocrine tumors. A dose of 50 mcg of octreotide injected subcutaneously twice daily has been tried in cases where surgery failed to remove the source of hyperinsulinism. However, its effectiveness is limited since its affinity for somatostatin receptors of the pancreatic B cell is very much less than for those of the anterior pituitary somatotrophs for which it was originally designed as treatment for acromegaly. When hypoglycemia persists after attempted surgical removal of the insulinoma and if diazoxide or verapamil is poorly tolerated or ineffective, multiple small feedings may be the only recourse until more selective somatostatin receptor agonists are available. Streptozocin can decrease insulin secretion in islet cell carcinomas, and effective doses have been delivered via selective arterial catheter so that the undue renal toxicity that characterized early experience is less of a problem.

► Prognosis

When insulinoma is diagnosed early and cured surgically, complete recovery is likely, although brain damage following prolonged severe hypoglycemia is not reversible. A significant increase in survival rate has been shown in streptozocin-treated patients with islet cell carcinoma, with reduction in tumor mass as well as decreased hyperinsulinism.

Griffiths MJ et al. Adult spontaneous hypoglycaemia. Hosp Med. 2005 May;66(5):277–83. [PMID: 15920857]

Hirshberg B et al. Forty-eight-hour fast: the diagnostic test for insulinoma. J Clin Endocrinol Metab. 2000 Sep;85(9):3222–6. [PMID: 10999812]

Koch B. Selected topics of hypoglycemia care. Can Fam Physician. 2006 Apr;52:466–71. [PMID: 16639972]

Service FJ. Diagnostic approach to adults with hypoglycemic disorders. Endocrinol Metab Clin North Am. 1999 Sep; 28(3):519–32. [PMID: 10500929]

Tucker ON et al. The management of insulinoma. Br J Surg. 2006 Mar;93(3):264–75. [PMID: 16498592]

PERSISTENT ISLET HYPERPLASIA (Noninsulinoma Pancreatogenous Hypoglycemia Syndrome)

In a very small number of patients with organic hyperinsulinism, islet hyperplasia rather than an adenoma is present. These patients typically have documented hyperinsulinemic hypoglycemia after meals but not with fasting up to 72 hours. The patients have a positive response to calcium-stimulated angiography. A gradient-guided partial pancreatectomy leads to clinical remission, and the pathology of the pancreas shows evidence of islet hyperplasia and nesidioblastosis. These patients do not have mutations in the *Kir 6.2* and *SUR1* genes, which has been reported in children with familial hyperinsulinemic hypoglycemia.

HYPOGLYCEMIA DUE TO EXTRAPANCREATIC TUMORS

These rare causes of hypoglycemia include mesenchymal tumors such as retroperitoneal sarcomas, hepatocellular carcinomas, adrenocortical carcinomas, and miscellaneous epithelial-type tumors. The tumors are frequently large and readily palpated or visualized on CT scans or MRI.

The expression and release of an incompletely processed insulin-like growth factor-2 (IGF-2) has provided the best explanation for the clinical manifestations of hypoglycemia in these cases. A larger immature form of the IGF-2 molecule is released which binds to a carrier protein but not to an acid-labile component of serum which inactivates normal IGF-2. This immature IGF-2 complex therefore remains active and binds to insulin receptors in muscle to promote glucose transport and to insulin receptors in liver and kidney to reduce glucose output. It also binds to receptors for IGF-1 in the pancreatic B cell to inhibit insulin secretion. Serum levels of IGF-2 may be increased but often are "normal" in quantity, despite the presence of the immature, higher-molecular-weight form of IGF-2, which can only be detected by special laboratory techniques. Laboratory diagnosis depends on documenting fasting hypoglycemia associated with undetectable serum insulin levels.

The prognosis for these tumors is generally poor, and surgical removal should be attempted when feasible. Dietary management of the hypoglycemia is the mainstay of medical treatment, since diazoxide is usually ineffective.

Escobar GA et al. Severe paraneoplastic hypoglycemia in a patient with a gastrointestinal stromal tumor with an exon 9 mutation: a case report. BMC Cancer. 2007 Jan 17;7:13. [PMID: 17229322]

Le Roith D. Tumor-induced hypoglycemia. N Engl J Med. 1999 Sep 2;341(10):757–8. [PMID: 10471466]

POSTPRANDIAL HYPOGLYCEMIA (Reactive Hypoglycemia)

1. Postgastrectomy Alimentary Hypoglycemia

Reactive hypoglycemia following gastrectomy is a consequence of hyperinsulinism resulting from rapid gastric emptying of ingested food. Symptoms result from adrenergic hyperactivity in response to the hypoglycemia. Treatment consists of more frequent feedings with smaller portions of less rapidly assimilated carbohydrate combined with more slowly absorbed fat and protein. Cases of hypoglycemia have been reported in patients who have undergone Roux-en-Y gastric bypass surgery for the treatment of obesity. The hypoglycemia occurs after meals and can be severe. There have been case reports of islet hyperplasia but this is probably uncommon; other studies report normal islet pathology.

2. Functional Alimentary Hypoglycemia

This syndrome is classified as functional when no postsurgical explanation exists for the presence of early alimentary type reactive hypoglycemia. It is most often associated with chronic fatigue, anxiety, irritability, weakness, poor concentration, decreased libido, headaches, hunger after meals, and tremulousness. However, most patients with these symptoms do not have hypoglycemia after a mixed meal. (See Chronic Fatigue Syndrome in Chapter 2.)

Indiscriminate use and overinterpretation of glucose tolerance tests have led to an unfortunate tendency to overdiagnose functional hypoglycemia. As many as one-third or more of normal subjects have blood glucose levels as low as 40–50 mg/dL with or without symptoms during a 4-hour glucose tolerance test. Accordingly, to increase diagnostic reliability, hypoglycemia should preferably be documented during a spontaneous symptomatic episode accompanying routine daily activity, with clinical improvement following feeding. Oral glucose tolerance tests are overly sensitive and mixed meals are relatively insensitive in detecting postprandial reactive hypoglycemia. It has been shown that a high-carbohydrate breakfast has proved useful in differentiating persons with postprandial reactive hypoglycemia from normal controls. The test resulted in reactive hypoglycemia to levels below 59 mg/dL in 47% of 38 subjects, in contrast to only 2.2% of the 43 controls. This test was found to be much more sensitive than a standard mixed meal, which was also given to these two groups.

In patients with documented postprandial hypoglycemia on a functional basis, there is no harm and occasional benefit in reducing the proportion of carbohydrate in the diet while increasing the frequency and reducing the size of meals. Acarbose has also been reported to provide symptomatic relief and can be tried if dietary manipulations alone are ineffective.

3. Late Hypoglycemia (Occult Diabetes)

This condition is characterized by a delay in early insulin release from pancreatic B cells, resulting in initial exaggeration of hyperglycemia during a glucose tolerance test. In response to this hyperglycemia, an exaggerated insulin release produces a late hypoglycemia 4–5 hours after ingestion of glucose. These patients are usually quite different from those with early hypoglycemia occurring 2–3 hours after glucose ingestion, often being obese and frequently having a family history of diabetes mellitus.

In obese patients, treatment is directed at weight reduction to achieve ideal weight. Like all patients with postprandial hypoglycemia, regardless of cause, these patients often respond to reduced carbohydrate intake with multiple, spaced, small feedings. They should be considered potential diabetics and advised to have periodic medical evaluations.

Service GJ et al. Hyperinsulinemic hypoglycemia with nesidioblastosis after gastric-bypass surgery. N Engl J Med. 2005 Jul 21;353(3):249–54. [PMID: 16034010]

ALCOHOL-RELATED HYPOGLYCEMIA

1. Fasting Hypoglycemia after Ethanol

During the postabsorptive state, normal plasma glucose is maintained by hepatic glucose output derived from both glycogenolysis and gluconeogenesis. With prolonged starvation, glycogen reserves become depleted within 18–24 hours and hepatic glucose output becomes totally dependent on gluconeogenesis. Under these circumstances, a blood concentration of ethanol as low as 45 mg/dL can induce profound hypoglycemia by blocking gluconeogenesis. Neuroglycopenia in a patient whose breath smells of alcohol may be mistaken for alcoholic stupor. Prevention consists of adequate food intake during ethanol ingestion. Therapy consists of glucose administration to replenish glycogen stores until gluconeogenesis resumes.

▶ Postethanol Reactive Hypoglycemia

When sugar-containing soft drinks are used as mixers to dilute alcohol in beverages (gin and tonic, rum and cola), there seems to be a greater insulin release than when the soft drink alone is ingested and a tendency for more of a late hypoglycemic overswing to occur 3–4 hours later. Prevention would consist of avoiding sugar mixers while ingesting alcohol and ensuring supplementary food intake to provide sustained absorption.

van de Wiel A. Diabetes mellitus and alcohol. Diabetes Metab Res Rev. 2004 Jul–Aug;20(4):263–7. [PMID: 15250029]

FACTITIOUS HYPOGLYCEMIA

Factitious hypoglycemia may be difficult to document. A suspicion of self-induced hypoglycemia is supported when the patient is associated with the health professions or has access to insulin or sulfonylurea drugs taken by a diabetic member of the family. The triad of hypoglycemia, high immunoreactive insulin, and suppressed plasma C peptide immunoreactivity is pathognomonic of exogenous insulin administration. Demonstration of circulating insulin antibodies supports this diagnosis in suspected cases. When sulfonylureas, repaglinide and nateglinide are suspected as a cause of factitious hypoglycemia, a plasma level of these drugs to detect their presence may be required to distinguish laboratory findings from those of insulinoma.

Charlton R et al. Munchausen's syndrome manifesting as factitious hypoglycaemia. Diabetologia. 2001 Jun;44(6):784–5. [PMID: 11440375]

Hirshberg B et al. Repaglinide-induced factitious hypoglycemia. J Clin Endocrinol Metab. 2001 Feb;86(2):475–7. [PMID: 11157993]

Trenque T et al. Prevalence of factitious hypoglycaemia associated with sulphonylurea drugs in France in the year 2000. Br J Clin Pharmacol. 2002 Nov;54(5):548. [PMID: 12445037]

IMMUNOPATHOLOGIC HYPOGLYCEMIA

This rare cause of hypoglycemia, documented in isolated case reports, may occur as two distinct disorders: one associated with spontaneous development of circulating anti-insulin antibodies and another associated with antibodies to insulin receptors, in which the antibodies apparently have agonist capabilities. This latter disorder is extremely rare, having been documented in no more than five cases. However, development of anti-insulin antibodies has been reported in over 200 patients most of whom were being treated with methimazole for thyrotoxicosis. In Western countries, 23 cases have been reported and include patients with a lupus-like syndrome or with various paraproteinemias. The hypoglycemia occurs 3–4 hours after meals following an initial postprandial hyperglycemic phase that is due to the antibodies interfering with the exit of insulin from the plasma to reach its target tissues. Later, after most of the meal is absorbed, inappropriate high levels of insulin dissociate from this antibody-bound compartment, resulting in hypoglycemia. Insulin levels in excess of 1000 pmol/L are observed at time of hypoglycemia, and these persons have high titers of insulin autoantibodies.

Basu A et al. Insulin autoimmunity and hypoglycemia in seven white patients. Endocr Pract. 2005 Mar–Apr;11(2):97–103. [PMID: 15901524]

Kim CH et al. Autoimmune hypoglycemia in a type 2 diabetic patient with anti-insulin and insulin receptor antibodies. Diabetes Care. 2004 Jan;27(1):288–9. [PMID: 14694017]

Sahin M et al. Autoimmune hypoglycemia in a type 2 diabetic patient with anti-insulin and insulin receptor antibodies. Diabetes Care. 2004 May;27(5):1246–7. [PMID: 15111569]

Yaturu S et al. Severe autoimmune hypoglycemia with insulin antibodies necessitating plasmapheresis. Endocr Pract. 2004 Jan–Feb;10(1):49–54. [PMID: 15251622]

DRUG-INDUCED HYPOGLYCEMIA

A number of drugs apart from the sulfonylureas can occasionally cause hypoglycemia, especially when ingested in large amounts. These include quinine, quinidine, disopyramide, and salicylates. ACE inhibitors, when taken with antidiabetic drugs, can cause hypoglycemia possibly by improving insulin sensitivity. Recently, it has been reported that the use of gatifloxacin (an antibiotic that is no longer available in the United States) in diabetic patients is associated with serious hypoglycemic and hyperglycemic reactions.

Ten to 20 percent of patients receiving pentamidine for *Pneumocystis jiroveci* pneumonia develop symptomatic hypoglycemia, particularly when the drug is administered intravenously. This apparently is due to lytic destruction of pancreatic B cells, causing acute hyperinsulinemia and hypoglycemia. It is later followed by insulinopenia and hyperglycemia, which occasionally is persistent. Since other drugs have been found to be as effective in treating *Pneumocystis* pneumonia, pentamidine administration and its hypoglycemic sequelae are less frequently encountered.

Lipid Disorders

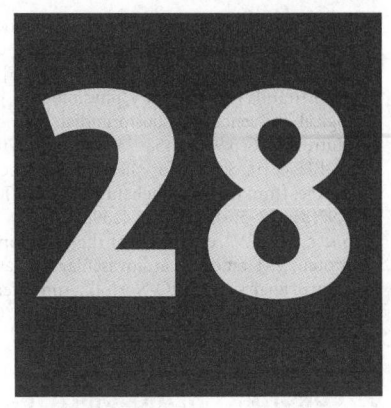

Robert B. Baron, MD, MS

For patients with known cardiovascular disease (secondary prevention), cholesterol lowering leads to a consistent reduction in total mortality and recurrent cardiovascular events in men and women and in middle-aged and older patients. Among patients without cardiovascular disease (primary prevention), the data are less conclusive, with rates of cardiovascular events, heart disease mortality, and all-cause mortality differing among studies. Nonetheless, treatment algorithms have been designed to assist clinicians in selecting patients for cholesterol-lowering therapy based on their lipid levels and their overall risk of developing cardiovascular disease.

LIPOPROTEINS & ATHEROGENESIS

The plaques in the arterial walls of patients with atherosclerosis contain large amounts of cholesterol. The higher the level of low-density lipoproteins (LDL) cholesterol, the greater the risk of atherosclerotic heart disease; conversely, the higher the high-density lipoproteins (HDL) cholesterol, the lower the risk of coronary heart disease (CHD). This is true in men and women, in different racial and ethnic groups, and at all ages up to age 75 years. Because most cholesterol in serum is LDL, high total cholesterol levels are also associated with an increased risk of CHD. Middle-aged men whose serum cholesterol levels are in the highest quintile for age (above about 230 mg/dL) have a risk of coronary death before age 65 years of about 10%; men in the lowest quintile (below about 170 mg/dL) have a 3% risk. Death from CHD before age 65 years is less common in women, with equivalent risks one-third those of men. In men, each 10-mg/dL increase in cholesterol (or LDL cholesterol) increases the risk of CHD by about 10%; each 5-mg/dL increase in HDL reduces the risk by about 10%. The effect of HDL cholesterol is greater in women, whereas the effects of total and LDL cholesterol are smaller.

There are several genetic disorders that provide insight into the pathogenesis of lipid-related diseases. **Familial hypercholesterolemia**, rare in the homozygous state (about one per million) is a condition in which the cell-surface receptors for the LDL molecule are absent or defective, resulting in unregulated synthesis of LDL. Patients with two abnormal genes (homozygotes) have extremely high levels—up to eight times normal—and present with atherosclerotic disease in childhood. Homozygotes may require liver transplantation to correct their severe lipid abnormalities. Those with one defective gene (heterozygotes) have LDL concentrations twice normal; persons with this condition may develop CHD in their 30s or 40s.

Another rare condition is caused by an abnormality of lipoprotein lipase, the enzyme that enables peripheral tissues to take up triglyceride from chylomicrons and very-low-density lipoproteins (VLDL) particles. Patients with this condition, one cause of **familial hyperchylomicronemia**, have marked hypertriglyceridemia with recurrent pancreatitis and hepatosplenomegaly in childhood.

Numerous other genetic abnormalities of lipid metabolism are named for the abnormality noted when serum is electrophoresed (eg, dysbetalipoproteinemia) or from combinations of lipid abnormalities in families (eg, familial combined hyperlipidemia). Thus, family members of patients with severe lipid disorders are appropriately studied. Other patients have abnormalities in the production of apoproteins, such as increased apoprotein B and its affiliated lipoproteins, LDL and VLDL; reduced apoprotein AII and its affiliated particle; or excess lipoprotein(a). Other mutations occur in lipoprotein lipase and in the gene encoding for cholesterol efflux regulatory protein.

▶ When to Refer

- Known genetic lipid disorders.
- Striking family history of hyperlipidemia or premature atherosclerosis.
- Extremely high serum LDL cholesterol or triglyceride, or extremely low serum HDL cholesterol.

Amarenco P et al. High-density lipoprotein-cholesterol and risk of stroke and carotid atherosclerosis: a systematic review. Atherosclerosis. 2008 Feb;196(2):489–96. [PMID: 17923134]

Bennet AM et al. Association of apolipoprotein E genotypes with lipid levels and coronary risk. JAMA. 2007 Sep 19;298(11):1300–11. [PMID: 17878422]

Brener SJ et al. The relation between extent of coronary artery disease measured by quantitative coronary angiography and changes in lipid profile: insights from trials of atherosclerosis regression. J Invasive Cardiol. 2008 Jun;20(6):261–5. [PMID: 18523316]

Grundy SM. Atherogenic dyslipidemia associated with metabolic syndrome and insulin resistance. Clin Cornerstone. 2006;8(Suppl 1):S21–7. [PMID: 16903166]

Lopez-Miranda J et al. Dietary, physiological, genetic and pathological influences on postprandial lipid metabolism. Br J Nutr. 2007 Sep;98(3):458–73. [PMID: 17705891]

Nam BH et al. Search for the optimal atherogenic lipid risk profile: from the Framingham study. Am J Cardiol. 2006 Feb 1;97(3):372–5. [PMID: 16442398]

Van der Steeg WA et al. Role of the apolipoprotein B-apolipoprotein A-I ratio in cardiovascular risk assessment: a case-control analysis in EPIC-Norfolk. Ann Intern Med. 2007 May 1;146(9):640–8. [PMID: 17470832]

LIPID FRACTIONS & THE RISK OF CORONARY HEART DISEASE

In fasting serum, cholesterol is carried primarily on three different lipoproteins—the VLDL, LDL, and HDL molecules. Total cholesterol equals the sum of these three components:

$$\text{Total cholesterol} = \text{HDL cholesterol} +$$
$$\text{VLDL cholesterol} + \text{LDL cholesterol}$$

Most clinical laboratories measure the total cholesterol, the total triglycerides, and the amount of cholesterol found in the HDL fraction, which is easily precipitated from serum. Most triglyceride is found in VLDL particles, which contain five times as much triglyceride by weight as cholesterol. The amount of cholesterol found in the VLDL fraction can be estimated by dividing the triglyceride by 5:

$$\text{VLDL cholesterol} = \frac{\text{Triglycerides}}{5}$$

Because the triglyceride level is used as a proxy for the amount of VLDL, this formula works only in fasting samples and when the triglyceride level is less than 400 mg/dL. At higher triglyceride levels, LDL and VLDL cholesterol levels can be determined after ultracentrifugation or by direct chemical measurement.

The total cholesterol is reasonably stable over time; however, measurements of HDL and especially triglycerides may vary considerably because of analytic error in the laboratory and biologic variation in a patient's lipid level. Thus, the LDL should always be estimated as the mean of at least two determinations; if those two estimates differ by more than 10%, a third lipid profile is obtained. The LDL is estimated as follows:

$$\underset{\text{terol}}{\overset{\text{LDL}}{\text{choles-}}} = \underset{\text{(mg/dL)}}{\overset{\text{Total}}{\text{cholesterol}}} - \underset{\text{(mg/dL)}}{\overset{\text{HDL}}{\text{cholesterol}}} - \frac{\overset{\text{Triglycerides}}{\text{(mg/dL)}}}{5}$$

When using SI units, the formula becomes

$$\underset{\text{terol}}{\overset{\text{LDL}}{\text{choles-}}} = \underset{\text{(mmol/L)}}{\overset{\text{Total}}{\text{cholesterol}}} - \underset{\text{(mmol/L)}}{\overset{\text{HDL}}{\text{cholesterol}}} - \frac{\overset{\text{Triglycerides}}{\text{(mmol/L)}}}{2.2}$$

Understanding the relationships of the different lipid fractions leads to a more accurate understanding of a patient's lipid-related coronary risk than the total choles-terol. Two persons with the same total cholesterol of 275 mg/dL may have very different lipid profiles. One may have an HDL cholesterol of 110 mg/dL with a triglyceride of 150 mg/dL, giving an estimated LDL cholesterol of 135 mg/dL; the other may have an HDL cholesterol of 25 mg/dL with a triglyceride of 200 mg/dL and an LDL cholesterol of 210 mg/dL. The second would have more than a tenfold higher CHD risk than the first, assuming no differences in other factors. Because of high HDL cholesterol levels in women, many with apparently high total cholesterol levels have favorable lipid profiles. Thus, evaluation of the lipid fractions is essential before therapy is initiated.

Some authorities use the ratio of the total to HDL cholesterol as an indicator of lipid-related coronary risk: the lower this ratio is, the better. (In the example above, the first person would have a ratio of 275 ÷ 110 = 2.5, while the second would have a much less favorable ratio of 275 ÷ 25 = 11.) Although ratios are useful predictors within populations of patients, they may obscure important information in individual patients. (A total cholesterol of 300 mg/dL and an HDL of 60 mg/dL result in the same ratio of 5 as a total cholesterol of 150 mg/dL with an HDL of 30 mg/dL.) Moreover, the total cholesterol-to-HDL cholesterol ratio will magnify the importance of variations in HDL measurement.

There is no true "normal" range for serum lipids. In Western populations, cholesterol values are about 20% higher than in Asian populations and exceed 300 mg/dL in nearly 5% of adults. About 10% of adults have LDL cholesterol levels above 200 mg/dL. Total and LDL cholesterol levels tend to rise with age in persons who are otherwise in good health.

Declines are seen in acute illness, and lipid studies in such patients are of little value with the exception of the serum triglyceride level in a patient with pancreatitis. Cholesterol levels (even when expressed as an age-matched percentile rank, such as the highest 20%) do not remain constant over time, especially from childhood through adolescence and young adulthood. Thus, children and young adults with relatively high cholesterol may have lower levels later in life, whereas those with low cholesterol may show increases.

THERAPEUTIC EFFECTS OF LOWERING CHOLESTEROL

Reducing cholesterol levels in healthy middle-aged men without CHD (primary prevention) reduces their risk in proportion to the reduction in LDL cholesterol and the increase in HDL cholesterol. Treated patients have statistically significant and clinically important reductions in the rates of myocardial infarctions, new cases of angina, and need for coronary artery bypass procedures. The West of Scotland Study showed a 31% decrease in myocardial infarctions in middle-aged men treated with pravastatin compared with placebo. The Air Force/Texas Coronary Atherosclerosis Prevention Study (AFCAPS/TexCAPS) study showed similar results with lovastatin. As with any primary prevention interventions, large numbers of healthy patients need to be treated to prevent a single event. The numbers of patients needed to treat (NNT) to prevent a nonfatal myocardial infarction or a coronary artery disease death in these two studies were 46 and 50, respectively. The Anglo-Scandinavian Cardiac Outcomes Trial (ASCOT) study of atorvastatin in subjects with hypertension and other risk factors but without CHD also demonstrated a convincing 36% reduction in CHD events. The Justification for the Use of Statins in Prevention: an Intervention Trial Evaluating Rosuvastatin (JUPITER) showed a 44% reduction in a combined end point of myocardial infarction, stroke, revascularization, hospitalization for unstable angina, or death from cardiovascular causes. The NNT for 1 year to prevent one event was 169.

Primary prevention studies have found a less consistent effect on total mortality. The West of Scotland study found a 20% decrease in total mortality, tending toward statistical significance. The AFCAPS/TexCAPS study with lovastatin showed no difference in total mortality. The Antihypertensive and Lipid-Lowering Treatment to Prevent Heart Attack Trial (ALLHAT-LLT) also showed no reduction either in all-cause mortality or in CHD events when pravastatin was compared with usual care. Subjects treated with atorvastatin in the ASCOT study had a 13% reduction in mortality, but the result was not statistically significant. This study, however, was stopped early due to the marked reduction in CHD events. The JUPITER trial demonstrated a statistically significant 20% reduction in death from any cause. The NNT for 1 year was 400.

In patients with CHD, the benefits of cholesterol lowering are clearer. Major studies with statins have shown significant reductions in cardiovascular events, cardiovascular deaths, and all-cause mortality in men and women with coronary artery disease. The NNT to prevent a nonfatal myocardial infarction or a coronary artery disease death in these three studies were between 12 and 34. Aggressive cholesterol lowering with these agents causes regression of atherosclerotic plaques in some patients, reduces the progression of atherosclerosis in saphenous vein grafts, and can slow or reverse carotid artery atherosclerosis. Meta-analysis suggests that this latter effect results in a significant decrease in strokes. Results with other classes of medications have been less consistent. For example, gemfibrozil treatment subjects had fewer cardiovascular events, but there was no benefit in all-cause mortality when compared with placebo.

The disparities in results between primary and secondary prevention studies highlight several important points. The benefits and adverse effects of cholesterol lowering may be specific to each type of drug; the clinician cannot assume that the effects will generalize to other classes of medication. Second, the net benefits from cholesterol lowering depend on the underlying risk of CHD and of other disease. In patients with atherosclerosis, morbidity and mortality rates associated with CHD are high, and measures that reduce it are more likely to be beneficial even if they have no effect—or even slightly harmful effects—on other diseases.

Baigent C et al. Efficacy and safety of cholesterol-lowering treatment: prospective meta-analysis of data from 90,056 participants in 14 randomised trials. Lancet. 2005 Oct 8;366(9493):1267–78. [PMID: 16214597]

Barter P et al. HDL cholesterol, very low levels of LDL cholesterol, and cardiovascular events. N Engl J Med. 2007 Sept 27:357(13):1301–1310. [PMID: 17898099]

Cholesterol Treatment Trialists (CTT) Collaborators; Kearney PM et al. Efficacy of cholesterol-lowering therapy in 18,686 people with diabetes in 14 randomised trials of statins: a meta-analysis. Lancet. 2008 Jan 12;371(9607):117–25. [PMID: 18191683]

Ford ES et al. Explaining the decrease in U.S. deaths from coronary disease, 1980–2000. N Engl J Med. 2007 Jun 7;356(23):2388–98. [PMID: 17554120]

Ford I et al. Long-term follow-up of the West of Scotland Coronary Prevention Study. N Engl J Med. 2007 Oct 11;357(15):1477–86. [PMID: 17928595]

Grundy SM. Cardiovascular and metabolic risk factors: how can we improve outcomes in the high-risk patient? Am J Med. 2007 Sep;120(9 Suppl 1):S3–8. [PMID: 17720359]

Ingelsson E et al. Clinical utility of different lipid measures for prediction of coronary heart disease in men and women. JAMA. 2007 Aug 15;298(7):776–85. [PMID: 17699011]

Nicholls SJ et al. Statins, high-density lipoprotein cholesterol, and regression of coronary atherosclerosis. JAMA. 2007 Feb 7;297:499–508. [PMID: 17284700]

Ridker PM et al. Development and validation of improved algorithms for the assessment of global cardiovascular risk in women: the Reynolds Risk Score. JAMA. 2007 Feb 14;297(6):611–9. [PMID: 17299196]

Ridker PM et al; JUPITER Study Group. Rosuvastatin to prevent vascular events in men and women with elevated C-reactive protein. N Engl J Med. 2008 Nov 20;359(21):2195–207. [PMID: 18997196]

SECONDARY CONDITIONS THAT AFFECT LIPID METABOLISM

Several factors, including drugs, can influence serum lipids (Table 28–1). These are important for two reasons: Abnormal lipid levels (or changes in lipid levels) may be the presenting sign of some of these conditions, and correction of the underlying condition may obviate the need to treat an apparent lipid disorder. Diabetes and alcohol use, in particular, are commonly associated with high triglyceride levels that decline with improvements in glycemic control or reduction in alcohol use, respectively. Thus, secondary causes of high blood lipids should be considered in each patient with a lipid disorder before lipid-lowering therapy is started. In most instances, special testing is not needed: a history and physical examination are sufficient. However, screening for hypothyroidism in patients with hyperlipidemia is cost effective.

CLINICAL PRESENTATIONS

Most patients with high cholesterol levels have no specific symptoms or signs. The vast majority of patients with lipid abnormalities are detected by the laboratory, either as part of the workup of a patient with cardiovascular disease or as part of a preventive screening strategy. Extremely high levels of chylomicrons or VLDL particles (triglyceride level above 1000 mg/dL) result in the formation of **eruptive xanthomas** (Plate 93) (red-yellow papules, especially on the buttocks). High LDL concentrations result in **tendinous xanthomas** on certain tendons (Achilles, patella, back of the hand). Such xanthomas usually indicate one of the underlying genetic hyperlipidemias. **Lipemia retinalis**

Table 28-1. Secondary causes of lipid abnormalities.

Cause	Associated Lipid Abnormality
Obesity	Increased triglycerides, decreased HDL cholesterol
Sedentary lifestyle	Decreased HDL cholesterol
Diabetes mellitus	Increased triglycerides, increased total cholesterol
Alcohol use	Increased triglycerides, increased HDL cholesterol
Hypothyroidism	Increased total cholesterol
Hyperthyroidism	Decreased total cholesterol
Nephrotic syndrome	Increased total cholesterol
Chronic kidney disease	Increased total cholesterol, increased triglycerides
Liver disease (cirrhosis)	Decreased total cholesterol
Obstructive liver disease	Increased total cholesterol
Malignancy	Decreased total cholesterol
Cushing disease (or corticosteroid use)	Increased total cholesterol
Oral contraceptives	Increased triglycerides, increased total cholesterol
Diuretics[1]	Increased total cholesterol, increased triglycerides
β-Blockers[1,2]	Increased total cholesterol, decreased HDL

[1]Short-term effects only.
[2]β-Blockers with intrinsic sympathomimetic activity, such as pindolol and acebutolol, do not affect lipid levels.

(cream-colored blood vessels in the fundus) is seen with extremely high triglyceride levels (above 2000 mg/dL).

SCREENING FOR HIGH BLOOD CHOLESTEROL

All patients with CHD or CHD risk equivalents (other clinical forms of atherosclerosis such as peripheral artery disease, abdominal aortic aneurysm, and symptomatic carotid artery disease; patients with diabetes mellitus; and patients with multiple risk factors that confer a greater than 20% 10-year risk for developing CHD) should be screened for elevated lipids. The only exceptions are patients in whom lipid lowering is not indicated or desirable for other reasons. Patients who already have evidence of atherosclerosis are the group at highest risk of suffering additional manifestations in the near term and thus have the most to gain from reduction of blood lipids. Additional risk reduction measures for atherosclerosis are discussed in Chapter 10; lipid lowering should be just one aspect of a program to reduce the progression and effects of the disease.

In patients with cardiovascular disease, a complete lipid profile (total cholesterol, HDL cholesterol, and triglyceride levels) after an overnight fast should be obtained as a screening test. Those whose estimated LDL cholesterol level is high should have at least one repeat measurement.

Specific treatments for high LDL cholesterol levels are discussed below. The goal of therapy should be to reduce the LDL cholesterol to below 100 mg/dL or optimally to below 70 mg/dL. Evidence suggests that treatment with a statin is effective even if the starting LDL cholesterol is below 100 mg/dL. These data suggest that most patients with CHD or CHD risk equivalents should be treated with statin therapy.

The best screening and treatment strategy for adults who do not have atherosclerotic cardiovascular disease is less clear. Several algorithms have been developed to guide the clinician in treatment decisions, but management decisions are individualized based on the patient's risk.

Although the National Cholesterol Education Program (NCEP) recommends screening of all adults aged 20 years or older for high blood cholesterol, the United States Preventive Services Task Force (USPSTF) suggests beginning at age 35 years in men and age 45 years in women unless there are other risk factors for CHD. For men and women with an increased risk for CHD, however, screening should begin at age 20. Although there is no established interval for screening, screening can be repeated every 5 years for those with average or low risk and more often for those whose levels are close to therapeutic thresholds. This strategy focuses cholesterol screening on those at the greatest risk of coronary artery disease and increases the cost effectiveness of cholesterol screening.

Individuals without cardiovascular disease can then be stratified according to risk factors as defined by the NCEP. Those with two or more risk factors are considered to be at intermediate risk of coronary artery disease, and those with less than two are at low risk. These include age and gender (men aged 45 years or older, women aged 55 years or older), a family history of premature CHD (myocardial infarction or sudden cardiac death before age 55 years in a first-degree male relative or before age 65 years in a first-degree female relative), hypertension (whether treated or not), current cigarette smoking (10 or more cigarettes per day), and low HDL cholesterol (< 40 mg/dL). Because HDL cholesterol is protective against CHD, a risk factor is subtracted if the level is greater than 60 mg/dL. Patients with two or more risk factors are then further stratified by evaluating their 10-year risk of developing CHD using Framingham projections of 10-year risk (Table 28–2). Because risk factors alone are an imprecise measure of CHD risk, estimating the 10-year risk using Framingham data is helpful even in patients with one or no risk factors. Other measures may also be useful to further refine risk in selected patients. For example, high-sensitivity C-reactive protein (hs-CRP) may be useful in intermediate-risk patients if the decision to initiate medications might change based on the hs-CRP level.

Several strategies for obtaining the initial cholesterol measurement have been proposed, including: (1) measuring total cholesterol alone, (2) measuring total cholesterol and HDL cholesterol, or (3) measuring LDL and HDL cholesterol. Each is acceptable, but treatment decisions are based on the LDL and HDL cholesterol levels. Measurement of the total cholesterol alone is the least expensive strategy and is adequate for low-risk individuals; those with total cholesterol greater than 200 mg/dL should then be reevaluated

Table 28–2. Framingham 10-year coronary heart disease risk projections. Calculate the number of points for each risk factor. Sum the total risk score and estimate the 10-year risk.

MEN

Age	Points
20–34	–9
35–39	–4
40–44	0
45–49	3
50–54	6
55–59	8
60–64	10
65–69	11
70–74	12
75–79	13

WOMEN

Age	Points
20–34	–7
35–39	–3
40–44	0
45–49	3
50–54	6
55–59	8
60–64	10
65–69	12
70–74	14
75–79	16

MEN

Total Cholesterol	Points				
	Age 20–39	Age 40–49	Age 50–59	Age 60–69	Age 70–79
< 160	0	0	0	0	0
160–199	4	3	2	1	0
200–239	7	5	3	1	0
240–279	9	6	4	2	1
≥ 280	11	8	5	3	1

WOMEN

Total Cholesterol	Points				
	Age 20–39	Age 40–49	Age 50–59	Age 60–69	Age 70–79
< 160	0	0	0	0	0
160–199	4	3	2	1	1
200–239	8	6	4	2	1
240–279	11	8	5	3	2
≥ 280	13	10	7	4	2

MEN

Age	Points				
	20–39	40–49	50–59	60–69	70–79
Nonsmoker	0	0	0	0	0
Smoker	8	5	3	1	1

WOMEN

Age	Points				
	20–39	40–49	50–59	60–69	70–79
Nonsmoker	0	0	0	0	0
Smoker	9	7	4	2	1

MEN

HDL (mg/dL)	Points
≥ 60	–1
50–59	0
40–49	1
< 40	2

WOMEN

HDL (mg/dL)	Points
≥ 60	–1
50–59	0
40–49	1
< 40	2

MEN

Systolic BP (mm Hg)	Points if Untreated	Points if Treated
< 120	0	0
120–129	0	1
130–139	1	2
140–159	1	2
≥ 160	2	3

WOMEN

Systolic BP (mm Hg)	Points if Untreated	Points if Treated
< 120	0	0
120–129	1	3
130–139	2	4
140–159	3	5
≥ 160	4	6

(continued)

Table 28–2. Framingham 10-year coronary heart disease risk projections. Calculate the number of points for each risk factor. Sum the total risk score and estimate the 10-year risk. (continued)

MEN			WOMEN		
Point Total	10-Year Risk %		Point Total	10-Year Risk %	
< 0	< 1		< 9	< 1	
0	1		9	1	
1	1		10	1	
2	1		11	1	
3	1		12	1	
4	1		13	2	
5	2		14	2	
6	2		15	3	
7	3		16	4	
8	4		17	5	
9	5		18	6	
10	6		19	8	
11	8		20	11	
12	10		21	14	
13	12	Ten-Year Risk	22	17	Ten-Year Risk
14	16		23	22	
15	20		24	27	
16	25		≥ 25	≥ 30	
≥ 17	≥ 30	%			%

with a fasting LDL and HDL cholesterol measurement. Measurement of the total cholesterol and HDL cholesterol allows for better characterization of the risk factor profile but also requires reevaluation if the total cholesterol is greater than 200 mg/dL as recommended by the USPSTF. Initial measurement of the LDL and HDL cholesterol is least likely to lead to patient misinformation and misclassification and is the strategy recommended by the NCEP.

Treatment decisions are based on the LDL cholesterol, and the patient's risk factor profile (including the HDL cholesterol level) and estimated 10-year risk. Patients in the intermediate-risk group (two or more risk factors) are selected for diet therapy (therapeutic lifestyle changes) if LDL cholesterol is greater than 130 mg/dL. If the 10-year risk of CHD is < 10%, drug treatment is recommended if LDL is > 160 mg/dL; if the 10-year CHD risk is between 10% and 20%, drug treatment is recommended if LDL is > 130 mg/dL. Low-risk individuals with one or no risk factors and estimated 10-year CHD risk less than 10% are selected for diet therapy if LDL cholesterol is greater than 160 mg/dL and for drug therapy if it is greater than 190 mg/dL (Table 28–3).

Screening in Women

The foregoing screening and treatment guidelines, based largely on LDL cholesterol levels, are designed for both men and women. Yet several observational studies suggest that a low HDL cholesterol is a more important risk factor for CHD in women than a high LDL cholesterol. Meta-analysis of studies including women with known heart disease, however, has found that medications that primarily lower LDL cholesterol do prevent recurrent myocardial infarctions in women. There is insufficient evidence to be certain of a similar effect from LDL-lowering therapy in women without evidence of CHD. Although most experts recommend application of the same primary prevention guidelines for women as for men, clinicians should be aware of the uncertainty in this area. Using estimates of 10-year CHD risk may be particularly helpful in women since a larger percentage of women than men will have estimated 10-year CHD risks below 10% per year and thus women are less likely to benefit from therapy unless their LDL cholesterol is extremely high (greater than 190 mg/dL).

Screening in Older Patients

Meta-analysis of evidence relating cholesterol to CHD in the elderly suggests that cholesterol is not a risk factor for CHD for persons over age 75 years. Clinical trials have rarely included such individuals. One exception is the Prospective Study of Pravastatin in the Elderly at Risk (PROSPER). In this study, elderly patients with cardiovascular disease (sec-

Table 28–3. LDL goals and treatment cutpoints: Recommendations of the NCEP Adult Treatment Panel III.

Risk Category	LDL Goal (mg/dL)	LDL Level at Which to Initiate Lifestyle Changes (mg/dL)	LDL Level at Which to Consider Drug Therapy[1] (mg/dL)
High risk: CHD[2] or CHD risk equivalents[3] (10-year risk > 20%)	< 100 (optional goal: < 70 mg/dL)[4]	≥ 100[5]	≥ 100[6] (< 100: consider drug options)[1]
Moderately high risk: 2+ risk factors[7] (10-year risk 10% to 20%)[8]	< 130[9]	≥ 130[5]	≥ 130 (100–129; consider drug options)[10]
Moderate risk: 2+ risk factors[7] (10-year risk < 10%)[8]	< 130	≥ 130	≥ 160
Low risk: 0–1 risk factors[11]	< 160	≥ 160	≥ 190 (160–189: LDL-lowering drug optional)

[1]When LDL-lowering drug therapy is used, it is advised that intensity of therapy be sufficient to achieve at least a 30–40% reduction in LDL cholesterol levels.

[2]CHD includes history of myocardial infarction, unstable angina, coronary artery procedures (angioplasty or bypass surgery), or evidence of clinically significant myocardial ischemia.

[3]CHD risk equivalents include clinical manifestations of noncoronary forms of atherosclerotic disease (peripheral arterial disease, abdominal aortic aneurysm, and carotid artery disease [transient ischemic attacks or stroke of carotid origin with > 50% obstruction of a carotid artery]), diabetes mellitus, and ≥ 2 risk factors with 10-year risk for CHD > 20%.

[4]Very high risk favors the optional LDL cholesterol goal of < 70 mg/dL, or in patients with high triglycerides, non-high density lipoprotein (HDL) cholesterol < 100 mg/dL.

[5]Any person at high risk or moderately high risk who has lifestyle-related risk factors (eg, obesity, physical inactivity, elevated triglyceride, low HDL cholesterol, or metabolic syndrome) is a candidate for therapeutic lifestyle changes to modify these risk factors regardless of LDL cholesterol.

[6]If baseline LDL cholesterol is < 100 mg/dL, institution of an LDL-lowering drug is a therapeutic option on the basis of available clinical trial results. If a high-risk person has high triglycerides or low HDL cholesterol, combining a fibrate or nicotinic acid with an LDL-lowering drug can be considered.

[7]Risk factors include cigarette smoking, hypertension (blood pressure ≥ 140/90 mm Hg or on antihypertensive medication), low HDL cholesterol (< 40 mg/dL), family history of premature CHD (CHD in male first-degree relative < 55 years of age; CHD in female first-degree relative < 65 years of age), and age (men ≥ 45 years; women ≥ 55 years).

[8]Electronic 10-year risk calculators are available at www.nhlbi.nih.gov/guidelines/cholesterol.

[9]Optional LDL cholesterol goal < 100 mg/dL.

[10]For moderately high-risk persons, when the LDL cholesterol level is 100–129 mg/dL at baseline or on lifestyle therapy, initiation of an LDL-lowering drug to achieve an LDL cholesterol level < 100 mg/dL is a therapeutic option on the basis of available clinical trial results.

[11]Almost all people with zero or one risk factor have a 10-year CHD risk < 10%, and 10-year risk assessment in these people is thus not necessary.

LDL, low-density lipoprotein; NCEP, National Cholesterol Education Program; CHD, coronary heart disease.

Reproduced, with permission, from Grundy SM et al. Implications of recent clinical trials for the National Cholesterol Education Program Adult Treatment Panel III guidelines. Circulation. 2004 Jul 13;110(2):227–39.

ondary prevention) benefited from statin therapy, whereas those without cardiovascular disease (primary prevention) did not. Although the NCEP recommends continuing treatment in the elderly, many clinicians will prefer to stop screening and treatment in patients age 75 years or older who do not have CHD. In patients age 75 years or older who have CHD, LDL-lowering therapy can be continued as recommended for younger patients with the disease. Decisions to discontinue therapy should be based on overall functional status and life expectancy, comorbidities, and patient preference and should be made in context with overall therapeutic goals and end-of-life decisions.

Greenland P et al. ACCF/AHA 2007 clinical expert consensus document on coronary artery calcium scoring by computed tomography in global cardiovascular risk assessment and in evaluation of patients with chest pain: a report of the ACCF Clinical Expert Consensus Task Force. J Am Coll Cardiol. 2007 Jan 23;49(3):378–402. [PMID: 17239724]

Lakaski SG. Coronary artery calcium scores and risk for cardiovascular events in women classified as "low risk" based on Framingham risk score: the multi-ethnic study of atherosclerosis (MESA). Arch Intern Med. 2007 Dec 10;167(22):2437–42. [PMID: 18071165]

McCrindle BW et al. Drug therapy of high-risk lipid abnormalities in children and adolescents: a scientific statement from the American Heart Association Atherosclerosis, Hypertension, and Obesity in Youth Committee, Council of Cardiovascular Disease in the Young, with the Council on Cardiovascular Nursing. Circulation. 2007 Apr 10;115(14):1948–67. [PMID: 17377073]

Mora S et al. Fasting compared with nonfasting lipids and apolipoproteins for predicting incident cardiovascular events. Circulation. 2008 Sep 2;118(10):993–1001. [PMID: 18711012]

Mosca L et al. Evidence-based guidelines for cardiovascular disease prevention in women: 2007 update. J Am Coll Cardiol. 2007 Mar 20;49(11):1230–50. [PMID: 17367675]

Wald DS et al. Child-parent screening for familial hypercholesterolaemia: screening strategy based on a meta-analysis. BMJ. 2007 Sep 22;335(7620):599. [PMID: 17855284]

TREATMENT OF HIGH LOW-DENSITY LIPOPROTEIN CHOLESTEROL

Reduction of LDL cholesterol is just one part of a program to reduce the risk of cardiovascular disease. Other measures—including smoking cessation, hypertension control, and aspirin—are also of central importance. Less well studied but of potential value is raising the HDL cholesterol level. Quitting smoking reduces the effect of other cardiovascular risk factors (such as a high cholesterol level); it may also increase the HDL cholesterol level. Exercise (and weight loss) may reduce the LDL cholesterol and increase the HDL. Modest alcohol use (1–2 ounces a day) also raises HDL levels and appears to have a salutary effect on CHD rates.

Several new classes of medications are being actively tested to raise HDL cholesterol levels. One such class of these medications, the cholesteryl ester transfer protein inhibitors, raises HDL cholesterol levels. However, studies to date of one agent in this class, torcetrapib, have shown adverse effects on cardiovascular outcomes. The effects of reconstituted HDL infusions have also been studied but have shown only modest effects on indirect measures of atherosclerosis.

▶ Diet Therapy

Studies of nonhospitalized adults have reported only modest cholesterol-lowering benefits of dietary therapy, typically in the range of a 5–10% decrease in LDL cholesterol, with even less in the long term. The effect of diet therapy, however, varies considerably among individuals, as some patients will have striking reductions in LDL cholesterol—up to a 25–30% decrease—whereas others will have clinically important increases. Thus, the results of diet therapy should be assessed about 4 weeks after initiation.

Cholesterol-lowering diets may also have a variable effect on lipid fractions. Diets very low in total fat or in saturated fat may lower HDL cholesterol as much as LDL cholesterol. It is not known how these diet-induced changes affect coronary risk.

Several nutritional approaches to diet therapy are available. Most Americans currently eat over 35% of calories as fat, of which 15% is saturated fat. Dietary cholesterol intake averages 400 mg/d. A cholesterol-lowering diet recommends reducing total fat to 25–30% and saturated fat to less than 7% of calories. Dietary cholesterol should be limited to less than 200 mg/d. These diets replace fat, particularly saturated fat, with carbohydrate. In most instances, this approach will also result in fewer total calories consumed and will facilitate weight loss in overweight patients. Other diet plans, including the Dean Ornish Diet, the Pritikin Diet, and most vegetarian diets, restrict fat even further. Low-fat, high-carbohydrate diets may, however, result in reductions in HDL cholesterol.

An alternative strategy is the "Mediterranean diet," which maintains total fat at approximately 35–40% of total calories but replaces saturated fat with monounsaturated fat such as that found in canola oil and in olives, peanuts, avocados, and their oils. This diet is equally effective at lowering LDL cholesterol but is less likely to lead to reductions in HDL cholesterol. Recent studies have demonstrated that this approach may also be associated with reductions in endothelial dysfunction, insulin resistance, and markers of vascular inflammation and may result in better resolution of the metabolic syndrome than traditional cholesterol-lowering diets.

Other dietary changes may also result in beneficial changes in blood lipids. Soluble fiber, such as that found in oat bran or psyllium, may reduce LDL cholesterol by 5–10%. Garlic, soy protein, vitamin C, pecans, and plant sterols may also result in reduction of LDL cholesterol. Because oxidation of LDL cholesterol is a potential initiating event in atherogenesis, diets rich in antioxidants, found primarily in fruits and vegetables, may be helpful (see Chapter 29). Studies have suggested that when all of these elements are combined into a single dietary prescription, the impact of diet on LDL cholesterol may approach that of statin medications, lowering LDL cholesterol by close to 30%.

Brunner E et al. Dietary advice for reducing cardiovascular risk. Cochrane Database Syst Rev. 2005 Oct 19;(4):CD002128. [PMID: 16235299]

Coodley GO et al. Lowering LDL cholesterol in adults: a prospective, community-based practice initiative. Am J Med. 2008 Jul;121(7):604–10. [PMID: 18538295]

Estruch R et al. Effects of a Mediterranean-style diet on cardiovascular risk factors: a randomized trial. Ann Intern Med. 2006 Jul 4;145(1):1–11. [PMID: 16818923]

Jenkins DJ et al. Effect of plant sterols in combination with other cholesterol-lowering foods. Metabolism. 2008 Jan;57(1):130–139. [PMID: 18078870]

Krauss RM et al. Separate effects of reduced carbohydrate intake and weight loss on atherogenic dyslipidemia. Am J Clin Nutr. 2006 May;83(5):1025–31. [PMID: 16685042]

Sacks FM et al. Soy protein, isoflavones, and cardiovascular health. An American Heart Association Science Advisory for professionals from the Nutrition Committee. Circulation. 2006 Feb 21;113(7):1034–44. [PMID: 16418439]

Tall AR. CETP inhibitors to increase HDL cholesterol levels. N Engl J Med. 2007 Mar 29;356(13):1364–6. [PMID: 17387130]

Tardif JC et al. Effects of reconstituted high-density lipoprotein infusions on coronary atherosclerosis: a randomized controlled trial. JAMA. 2007 Apr 18;297(15):1675–82. [PMID: 17387133]

▶ Pharmacologic Therapy

All patients whose risk from CHD is considered high enough to warrant pharmacologic therapy of an elevated LDL cholesterol should be given aspirin prophylaxis at a dose of 81 mg/d unless there are contraindications such as aspirin sensitivity, bleeding diatheses, or active peptic ulcer disease. The benefit of aspirin in reducing the risk of CHD is equivalent to that of cholesterol lowering. Other CHD risk factors, such as hypertension and smoking, should also be controlled.

If the decision to treat a patient with an LDL-lowering drug is made, a goal for treatment is set. The National Cholesterol Education Program's Adult Treatment Panel III (NCEP ATP III) published revised, more intensive LDL treatment goals in 2004, and these guidelines remain the mainstay of clinical practice. For patients with CHD or CHD risk equivalents, the goal is LDL < 100 mg/dL, but for patients with very high risk, a goal of LDL < 70 mg/dL is a therapeutic option (see Table 28–3). This goal may also be appropriate for patients with very high risk who have a baseline LDL < 100 mg/dL. For patients with two or more risk factors and a 10-year CHD risk of 10–20%, the recommended goal is LDL < 130 mg/dL, but a goal of < 100 mg/dL is optional. For those with two or more risk factors and a 10-year CHD risk of < 10%, the goal is < 130 mg/dL. For those with zero or one risk factor, the goal is LDL < 160 mg/dL (see Table 28–3). In most instances, intensity of therapy should be sufficient to achieve a 30–40% reduction in LDL cholesterol. Combinations of drugs may be necessary. Once the goal is reached, the lipid profile should be monitored periodically (every 6–12 months), with consideration given to periodic reductions in drug dose. Most lipid-lowering agents are expensive and may need to be given for decades. Thus, their cost effectiveness is low for some groups of patients, especially in primary prevention.

A. Niacin (Nicotinic Acid)

Niacin was the first lipid-lowering agent that was associated with a reduction in total mortality. Long-term follow-up of a secondary prevention trial of middle-aged men with previous myocardial infarction disclosed that about half of those who had been previously treated with niacin had died, compared with nearly 60% of the placebo group. This favorable effect on mortality was not seen during the trial itself, though there was a reduction in the incidence of recurrent coronary events.

Niacin reduces the production of VLDL particles, with secondary reduction in LDL and increases in HDL cholesterol levels. The average effect of full-dose niacin therapy, 3–4.5 g/d, is a 15–25% reduction in LDL cholesterol and a 25–35% increase in HDL cholesterol. Full doses are required to obtain the LDL effect, but the HDL effect is observed at lower doses, eg, 1 g/d. Niacin will also reduce triglycerides by half and will lower lipoprotein(a) (Lp[a]) levels and will increase plasma homocysteine levels. Thus, its effect on blood lipids and CHD risk is nearly optimal. Intolerance to niacin is common; only 50–60% of patients can take full doses. Niacin causes a prostaglandin-mediated flushing that patients may describe as "hot flashes" or pruritus and that can be decreased with aspirin (81–325 mg/d) or other nonsteroidal anti-inflammatory agents taken during the same day. Flushing may also be decreased by initiating niacin therapy with a very small dose, eg, 100 mg with the evening meal. The dose can be doubled each week until 1.5 g/d is tolerated. After rechecking blood lipids, the dose is increased and divided over three meals until the goal of 3–4.5 g/d is reached (eg, 1 g with each meal). Extended-release niacin is also available and is better tolerated by most patients. It is not known whether routine monitoring of liver enzymes results in early detection and thus reduced severity of this side effect. Niacin can also exacerbate gout and peptic ulcer disease. Although niacin may increase blood sugar in some patients, clinical trials have shown that niacin can be safely used in diabetics.

B. Bile Acid–Binding Resins

The bile acid–binding resins include cholestyramine, colesevelam, and colestipol. Treatment with these agents reduces the incidence of coronary events in middle-aged men by about 20%, with no significant effect on total mortality. The resins work by binding bile acids in the intestine. The resultant reduction in the enterohepatic circulation causes the liver to increase its production of bile acids, using hepatic cholesterol to do so. Thus, hepatic LDL receptor activity increases, with a decline in plasma LDL levels. The triglyceride level tends to increase slightly in some patients treated with bile acid–binding resins; they should be used with caution in those with elevated triglycerides and probably not at all in patients who have triglyceride levels above 500 mg/dL. The clinician can anticipate a reduction of 15–25% in the LDL cholesterol level, with insignificant effects on the HDL level.

The usual dose of cholestyramine is 12–36 g of resin per day in divided doses with meals, mixed in water or, more palatably, juice. Doses of colestipol are 20% higher (each packet contains 5 g of resin). The dose of colesevelam is 625 mg, 6–7 tablets per day.

These agents often cause gastrointestinal symptoms, such as constipation and gas. They may interfere with the absorption of fat-soluble vitamins (thereby complicating the management of patients receiving warfarin) and may bind other drugs in the intestine. Concurrent use of psyllium may ameliorate the gastrointestinal side effects.

C. Hydroxymethylglutaryl-Coenzyme A (HMG-CoA) Reductase Inhibitors (Statins)

The HMG-CoA reductase inhibitors include atorvastatin, fluvastatin, lovastatin, pravastatin, rosuvastatin, and simvastatin. These agents work by inhibiting the rate-limiting enzyme in the formation of cholesterol. They reduce myocardial infarctions and total mortality in secondary prevention, as well as in older middle-aged men free of CHD. A meta-analysis has demonstrated significant reduction in risk of stroke. Cholesterol synthesis in the liver is reduced, with a compensatory increase in hepatic LDL receptors (presumably so that the liver can take more of the cholesterol that it needs from the blood) and a reduction in the circulating LDL cholesterol level by up to 35%. There are also modest increases in HDL levels and decreases in triglyceride levels.

Oral doses are as follows: atorvastatin, 10–80 mg/d; fluvastatin, 20–40 mg/d; lovastatin, 10–80 mg/d; pravastatin, 10–40 mg/d; rosuvastatin, 5–40 mg/d; and simvastatin, 5–40 mg/d. These agents are usually given once a day in the evening (most cholesterol synthesis takes place overnight); at the high end of the dose ranges, twice-a-day dosing may be used. Side effects include myositis, whose incidence may be higher in patients concurrently taking fibrates or niacin. Manufacturers recommend monitoring liver and muscle enzymes. Several agents (notably erythromycin, cyclosporine, and azole antifungals) reduce the metabolism of these agents.

D. Fibric Acid Derivatives

The fibric acid derivatives or fibrates approved for use in the United States are gemfibrozil and fenofibrate. Ciprofibrate and bezafibrate are also available for use internationally. Gemfibrozil reduced CHD rates in hypercholesterolemic middle-aged men free of coronary disease in the Helsinki

Heart Study. The effect was observed only among those who also had lower HDL cholesterol levels and high triglyceride levels. In a VA study, gemfibrozil was also shown to reduce cardiovascular events in men with existing CHD whose primary lipid abnormality was a low HDL cholesterol. There was no effect on all-cause mortality.

The fibrates are peroxisome proliferative-activated receptor-alpha (PPAR-alpha) agonists that result in potent reductions of plasma triglycerides and increases in HDL cholesterol. They reduce LDL levels by about 10–15%, although the result is quite variable, and triglyceride levels by about 40% and raise HDL levels by about 15–20%. The usual dose of gemfibrozil is 600 mg once or twice a day. Side effects include cholelithiasis, hepatitis, and myositis. The incidence of the latter two conditions may be higher among patients also taking other lipid-lowering agents. In the largest clinical trial that used clofibrate, there were significantly more deaths—especially due to cancer—in the treatment group; it should not be used.

E. Ezetimibe

Ezetimibe is a lipid-lowering drug that inhibits the intestinal absorption of dietary and biliary cholesterol by blocking passage across the intestinal wall by inhibiting a cholesterol transporter. The usual dose of ezetimibe is 10 mg/d orally. Ezetimibe reduces LDL cholesterol between 15% and 20% when used as monotherapy and can further reduce LDL in patients taking statins who are not yet at therapeutic goal.

However, the effects of ezetimide on CHD and its long-term safety are not yet known. Results from one small clinical trial, ENHANCE (a study of 720 persons with heterozygous familial hypercholesterolemia), showed no significant difference of intimal media thickness with ezetimibe plus an HMG-CoA reductase inhibitor compared with an HMG-CoA reductase inhibitor alone. Concern has also been raised about a greater risk of cancer with ezetimibe. A meta-analysis of three trials of ezetimibe showed no increase in cancer incidence but did find a nonsignificant increase in deaths from cancer.

► Initial Selection of Medication

At present there are no absolute guidelines for selection of available lipid-modifying medications in particular patients. Nonetheless, clinical trials provide guidance (Table 28–4). For most patients who require a lipid-modifying medication, an HMG-CoA reductase inhibitor is preferred. Although niacin will also have beneficial effects on lipids in both men and women with CHD, there is less evidence demonstrating the desired effects on CHD and all-cause mortality. Resins are the only lipid-modifying medication considered safe in pregnancy.

Combination therapy may be used to meet lipid targets in some patients or to achieve other therapeutic goals. For example, ezetimibe plus an HMG-CoA reductase inhibitor will typically lower the LDL cholesterol more than either medication alone. Similarly, low-dose niacin (0.5–1 g/d),

Table 28–4. Effects of selected lipid-modifying drugs.

Drug	Lipid-Modifying Effects			Initial Daily Dose	Maximum Daily Dose	Cost for 30 Days Treatment with Dose Listed[1]
	LDL	HDL	Triglyceride			
Atorvastatin (Lipitor)	−25 to −40%	+5 to 10%	↓↓	10 mg once	80 mg once	$130.87 (20 mg once)
Cholestyramine (Questran, others)	−15 to −25%	+5%	±	4 g twice a day	24 g divided	$126.65 (8 g divided)
Colesevelam (WelChol)	−10 to −20%	+10%	±	625 mg, 6–7 tablets once	625 mg, 6–7 tablets once	$222.48 (6 tablets once)
Colestipol (Colestid)	−15 to −25%	+5%	±	5 g twice a day	30 g divided	$120.00 (10 g divided)
Ezetimibe (Zetia)	−20%	+5%	±	10 mg once	10 mg once	$108.66 (10 mg once)
Fenofibrate (Tricor, others)	−10 to −15%	+15 to 25%	↓↓	48 mg once	145 mg once	$130.06 (145 mg once)
Fenofibric Acid (Trilpix)	−10 to −15%	+15 to 25%	↓↓	45 mg once	135 mg once	$124.00 (135 mg once)
Fluvastatin (Lescol)	−20 to −30%	+5 to 10%	↓	20 mg once	40 mg once	$90.40 (20 mg once)
Gemfibrozil (Lopid)	−10 to −15%	+15 to 20%	↓↓	600 mg once	1200 mg divided	$74.80 (600 mg twice a day)
Lovastatin (Mevacor)	−25 to −40%	+5 to 10%	↓	10 mg once	80 mg divided	$71.19 (20 mg once)
Niacin (OTC, Niaspan)	−15 to −25%	+25 to 35%	↓↓	100 mg once	3–4.5 g divided	$15.28 (1.5 g twice a day, OTC) $254.00 (2 g Niaspan)
Pravastatin (Pravachol)	−25 to −40%	+5 to 10%	↓	20 mg once	40 mg once	$98.01 (20 mg once)
Rosuvastatin (Crestor)	−40 to −50%	+10 to 15%	↓↓	10 mg once	40 mg once	$114.37 (20 mg once)
Simvastatin (Zocor)	−25 to −40%	+5 to 10%	↓↓	5 mg once	80 mg once	$84.60 (10 mg once)

[1]Average wholesale price (AWP, for AB-rated generic when available) for quantity listed. Source: *Red Book Update*, Vol. 28, No. 3, March 2009. AWP may not accurately represent the actual pharmacy cost because wide contractual variations exist among institutions. LDL, low-density lipoprotein; HDL, high-density lipoprotein; ± variable, if any; OTC, over the counter.

will substantially increase the HDL cholesterol when added to an HMG-CoA reductase inhibitor. Despite improvements in the lipid profile, however, there are few data demonstrating improved clinical outcomes of combination therapy when compared with HMG-CoA reductase inhibitors alone. Combinations may also increase the risk of complications of drug therapy. The combination of gemfibrozil and HMG-CoA reductase inhibitors increases the risk of myopathy more than either drug alone.

Dale KM et al. Statins and cancer risk: a meta-analysis. JAMA. 2006 Jan 4;295(1):74–80. [PMID: 16391219]

Kastelein JJ et al; ENHANCE Investigators. Simvastatin with or without ezetimibe in familial hypercholesterolemia. N Engl J Med. 2008 Apr 3;358(14):1431–43. [PMID: 18376000]

Keating GM et al. Fenofibrate: a review of its use in primary dyslipidaemia, the metabolic syndrome and type 2 diabetes mellitus. Drugs. 2007;67(1):121–53. [PMID: 17209672]

Khush KK et al. Effect of high-dose atorvastatin on hospitalizations for heart failure: subgroup analysis of the Treating to New Targets (TNT) study. Circulation. 2007 Feb 6;115(5):576–83. [PMID: 17261662]

Maroo BP et al. Efficacy and safety of intensive statin therapy in the elderly. Am J Geriatr Cardiol. 2008 Mar–Apr;17(2):92–100. [PMID: 18326948]

Nicholls SJ et al. Statins, high-density lipoprotein cholesterol, and regression of coronary atherosclerosis. JAMA. 2007 Feb 7;297(5):499–508. [PMID: 17284700]

Peto R et al. Analyses of cancer data from three ezetimibe trials. N Engl J Med. 2008 Sep 25;359(13):1357–66. [PMID: 18765432]

Pignone M et al. Aspirin, statins, or both drugs for the primary prevention of coronary heart disease events in men: a cost-utility analysis. Ann Intern Med. 2006 Mar 7;144(5):326–36. [PMID: 16520473]

Singh U et al. Comparison effect of atorvastatin (10 versus 80 mg) on biomarkers of inflammation and oxidative stress in subjects with metabolic syndrome. Am J Cardiol. 2008 Aug 1;102(3):321–5. [PMID: 18638594]

HIGH BLOOD TRIGLYCERIDES

Patients with very high levels of serum triglycerides are at risk for pancreatitis. The pathophysiology is not certain, since pancreatitis never develops in some patients with very high triglyceride levels. Most patients with congenital abnormalities in triglyceride metabolism present in childhood; hypertriglyceridemia-induced pancreatitis first presenting in adults is more commonly due to an acquired problem in lipid metabolism.

Although there are no clear triglyceride levels that predict pancreatitis, most clinicians treat fasting levels above 500 mg/dL. The risk of pancreatitis may be more related to the triglyceride level following consumption of a fatty meal. Because postprandial increases in triglyceride are inevitable if fat-containing foods are eaten, fasting triglyceride levels in persons prone to pancreatitis should be kept well below that level.

The primary therapy for high triglyceride levels is dietary, avoiding alcohol, simple sugars, refined starches, saturated and trans fatty acids, and restricting total calories. Control of secondary causes of high triglyceride levels (see Table 28–1) may also be helpful. In patients with fasting triglycerides ≥ 500 mg/dL despite adequate dietary compliance—and certainly in those with a previous episode of pancreatitis—therapy with a triglyceride-lowering drug (eg, niacin, a fibric acid derivative, or an HMG-CoA reductase inhibitor) is indicated.

Whether patients with elevated triglycerides (> 150 mg/dL) should be treated to prevent CHD is not known. Meta-analysis of 17 observational studies suggests that after adjustment for other risk factors, elevated triglycerides increased CHD risk in men by 14% and in women by 37%. Triglyceride-rich lipoproteins (partially degraded VLDL, commonly called remnant lipoproteins) have been found in human atheromas, and elevated triglycerides are associated with small dense LDL in most instances. Elevated triglycerides are also an important feature of the metabolic syndrome, found in an estimated 25% of Americans—defined by three or more of the following five abnormalities: waist circumference > 102 cm in men or > 88 cm in women, serum triglyceride level of at least 150 mg/dL, HDL level of < 40 mg/dL in men or < 50 mg/dL in women, blood pressure of at least 130/85 mm Hg, and serum glucose level of at least 110 mg/dL. Other data, however, suggest that triglyceride measurements do not improve discrimination between those with and without CHD events, and clinical trial data are not available to support the routine treatment of high triglycerides in all patients.

The NCEP ATP III guidelines, however, recommend an aggressive approach to triglyceride management. For those with borderline levels (150–199 mg/dL), emphasis is placed on calorie restriction and exercise. For patients with high triglycerides (> 200 mg/dL), the non-HDL cholesterol should be measured (total cholesterol – HDL cholesterol). The ATP III report recommends that non-HDL cholesterol should be treated with diet and medications to result in levels 30 mg/dL higher than the LDL goal. The ATP III report does not differentiate between primary and secondary prevention. It is reasonable to use this approach for patients with CHD and risk equivalents for that disease but not for lower-risk patients.

Bersot T et al. Hypertriglyceridemia: management of atherogenic dyslipidemia. J Fam Pract. 2006 Jul;55(7):S1–8. [PMID: 16822443]

Brunzell JD. Clinical practice. Hypertriglyceridemia. N Engl J Med. 2007 Sep 6;357(10):1009–17. [PMID: 17804845]

Oh RC et al. Management of hypertriglyceridemia. Am Fam Physician. 2007 May 1;75(9):1365–71. [PMID: 17508532]

Yuan G et al. Hypertriglyceridemia: its etiology, effects and treatment. CMAJ. 2007 Apr 10;176(8):1113–20. [PMID: 17420495]

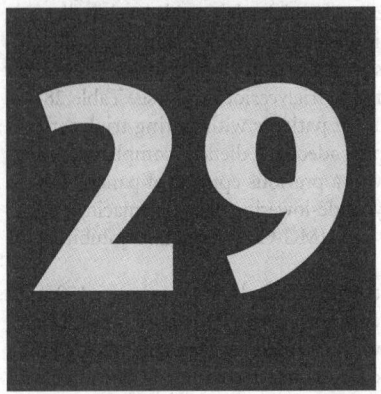

Nutritional Disorders

Robert B. Baron, MD, MS

PROTEIN–ENERGY MALNUTRITION

ESSENTIALS OF DIAGNOSIS

▶ History of decreased intake of energy or protein, increased nutrient losses, or increased nutrient requirements.

▶ Manifestations range from weight loss and growth failure to distinct syndromes, kwashiorkor, and marasmus.

▶ In severe cases, virtually all organ systems are affected.

▶ Protein loss correlates with weight loss: 35–40% total body weight loss is usually fatal.

General Considerations

Protein–energy malnutrition occurs as a result of a relative or absolute deficiency of energy and protein. It may be primary, due to inadequate food intake, or secondary, as a result of other illness. For most developing nations, primary protein–energy malnutrition remains among the most significant health problems. Protein–energy malnutrition has been described as two distinct syndromes. **Kwashiorkor**, caused by a deficiency of protein in the presence of adequate energy, is typically seen in weaning infants at the birth of a sibling in areas where foods containing protein are insufficiently abundant. **Marasmus**, caused by combined protein and energy deficiency, is most commonly seen where adequate quantities of food are not available.

In industrialized societies, protein–energy malnutrition is most often secondary to other diseases. **Kwashiorkor-like secondary protein–energy malnutrition** occurs primarily in association with hypermetabolic acute illnesses such as trauma, burns, and sepsis. **Marasmus-like secondary protein–energy malnutrition** typically results from chronic diseases such as chronic obstructive pulmonary disease (COPD), congestive heart failure, cancer, or AIDS. These syndromes have been estimated to be present in at least 20% of hospitalized patients. A substantially greater number of patients have risk factors that could result in these syndromes. In both syndromes, protein–energy malnutrition is caused either by decreased intake of energy and protein, increased nutrient losses, or increased nutrient requirements dictated by the underlying illness. For example, diminished oral intake may result from poor dentition or various gastrointestinal disorders. Loss of nutrients results from malabsorption and diarrhea as well as from glycosuria. Nutrient requirements are increased by fever, surgery, neoplasia, and burns.

▶ Pathophysiology

Protein–energy malnutrition affects every organ system. The most obvious results are loss of body weight, adipose stores, and skeletal muscle mass. Weight losses of 5–10% are usually tolerated without loss of physiologic function; losses of 35–40% of body weight usually result in death. Loss of protein from skeletal muscle and internal organs is usually proportionate to weight loss. Protein mass is lost from the liver, gastrointestinal tract, kidneys, and heart.

As protein–energy malnutrition progresses, organ dysfunction develops. Hepatic synthesis of serum proteins decreases, and depressed levels of circulating proteins are observed. Cardiac output and contractility are decreased, and the electrocardiogram (ECG) may show decreased voltage and a rightward axis shift. Autopsies of patients who die with severe undernutrition show myofibrillar atrophy and interstitial edema of the heart.

Respiratory function is affected primarily by weakness and atrophy of the muscles of respiration. Vital capacity and tidal volume are depressed, and mucociliary clearance is abnormal. The gastrointestinal tract is affected by mucosal atrophy and loss of villi of small intestine, resulting in malabsorption. Intestinal disaccharidase deficiency and mild pancreatic insufficiency also occur.

Changes in immunologic function are among the most important changes seen in protein–calorie undernutrition. T lymphocyte number and function are depressed. Changes in B cell function are more variable. Impaired complement activity, granulocyte function, and anatomic barriers to infection are noted, and wound healing is poor.

Clinical Findings

The clinical manifestations of protein–energy malnutrition range from mild growth retardation and weight loss to a number of distinct clinical syndromes. Children in the developing world manifest marasmus and kwashiorkor. In secondary protein–energy malnutrition as seen in industrialized nations, clinical manifestations are affected by the degree of protein and energy deficiency, the underlying illness that resulted in the deficiency, and the patient's nutritional status prior to illness.

Progressive wasting that begins with weight loss and proceeds to more severe cachexia typically develops in most patients with marasmus-like secondary protein–energy malnutrition. In the most severe form of this disorder, most body fat stores disappear and muscle mass decreases, most noticeably in the temporalis and interosseous muscles. Laboratory studies may be unremarkable—serum albumin, for example, may be normal or slightly decreased, rarely decreasing to < 2.8 g/dL. In contrast, owing to its rapidity of onset, kwashiorkor-like secondary protein–energy malnutrition may develop in patients with normal subcutaneous fat and muscle mass or, if the patient is obese, in patients with excess fat and muscle. The serum protein level, however, typically declines and the serum albumin is often < 2.8 g/dL. Dependent edema, ascites, or anasarca may develop. As with primary protein–energy malnutrition, combinations of the marasmus-like and kwashiorkor-like syndromes can occur simultaneously, typically in patients with progressive chronic disease in whom a superimposed acute illness develops.

Treatment

The treatment of severe protein–energy malnutrition is a slow process requiring great care. Initial efforts should be directed at correcting fluid and electrolyte abnormalities and infections. Of particular concern are depletion of potassium, magnesium, and calcium and acid–base abnormalities. The second phase of treatment is directed at repletion of protein, energy, and micronutrients. Treatment is started with modest quantities of protein and calories calculated according to the patient's actual body weight. Adult patients are given 1 g of protein and 30 kcal/kg. Concomitant administration of vitamins and minerals is obligatory. Either the enteral or parenteral route can be used, although the former is preferable. Enteral fat and lactose are withheld initially. Patients with less severe protein–calorie undernutrition can be given calories and protein simultaneously with the correction of fluid and electrolyte abnormalities. Similar quantities of protein and calories are recommended for initial treatment.

Patients treated for protein–energy malnutrition require close follow-up. In adults, both calories and protein are advanced as tolerated, adults to 1.5 g/kg/d of protein and 40 kcal/kg/d of calories.

Patients who are re-fed too rapidly may develop a number of untoward clinical sequelae. During refeeding, circulating potassium, magnesium, phosphorus, and glucose move intracellularly and can result in low serum levels of each. The administration of water and sodium with carbohydrate refeeding can overload hearts with depressed cardiac function and result in congestive heart failure. Enteral refeeding can lead to malabsorption and diarrhea due to abnormalities in the gastrointestinal tract.

Refeeding edema is a benign condition to be differentiated from congestive heart failure. Changes in renal sodium reabsorption and poor skin and blood vessel integrity result in the development of dependent edema without other signs of heart disease. Treatment includes reassurance, elevation of the dependent area, and modest sodium restriction. Diuretics are usually ineffective, may aggravate electrolyte deficiencies, and should not be used.

The prevention and early detection of protein–energy malnutrition in hospitalized patients require awareness of its risk factors and early symptoms and signs. Patients at risk require formal assessment of nutritional status and close observation of dietary intake, body weight, and nutritional requirements during the hospital stay.

Bejon P et al. Fraction of all hospital admissions and deaths attributable to malnutrition among children in rural Kenya. Am J Clin Nutr. 2008 Dec;88(6):1626–31. [PMID: 19064524]

Brewster DR. Critical appraisal of the management of severe malnutrition: 2. Dietary management. J Paediatr Child Health. 2006 Oct;42(10):575–82. [PMID: 16972962]

Delano MJ et al. The origins of cachexia in acute and chronic inflammatory diseases. Nutr Clin Pract. 2006 Feb;21(1):68–81. [PMID: 16439772]

Franfenfield D. Energy expenditure and protein requirements after traumatic injury. Nutr Clin Pract. 2006 Oct;21(5):430–7. [PMID: 16998142]

Furman EF. Undernutrition in older adults across the continuum of care: nutritional assessment, barriers, and interventions. J Gerontol Nurs. 2006 Jan;32(1):22–7. [PMID: 16475461]

Huhmann MB et al. Review of American Society for Parenteral and Enteral Nutrition (ASPEN) Clinical Guidelines for Nutrition Support in Cancer Patients: nutrition screening and assessment. Nutr Clin Pract. 2008 Apr–May;23(2):182–8. [PMID: 18390787]

Thomas DR. Loss of skeletal muscle mass in aging: examining the relationship of starvation, sarcopenia and cachexia. Clin Nutr. 2007 Aug;26(4):389–99. [PMID: 17499396]

OBESITY

 ESSENTIALS OF DIAGNOSIS

▶ Excess adipose tissue, resulting in BMI > 30.

▶ Upper body obesity (abdomen and flank) of greater health consequence than lower body obesity (buttocks and thighs).

▶ Associated with multiple metabolic and structural disorders, including diabetes mellitus, hypertension, and hyperlipidemia.

General Considerations

Obesity is one of the most common disorders in medical practice and among the most frustrating and difficult to manage. Little progress has been made in prevention or treatment, yet major changes have occurred in our understanding of its causes and its implications for health.

▶ Definition & Measurement

Obesity is defined as an excess of adipose tissue. Accurate quantification of body fat requires sophisticated techniques not usually available in clinical practice. Physical examination is usually sufficient to detect excess body fat. More quantitative evaluation is performed by calculating the BMI.

The **BMI** closely correlates with excess adipose tissue. It is calculated by dividing measured body weight in kilograms by the height in meters squared.

The National Institutes of Health (NIH) define a normal BMI as 18.5–24.9. Overweight is defined as BMI = 25–29.9. Class I obesity is 30–34.9, class II obesity is 35–39.9, and class III (extreme) obesity is BMI > 40. Factors other than total weight, however, are also important. Upper body obesity (excess fat around the waist and flank) is a greater health hazard than lower body obesity (fat in the thighs and buttocks). Obese patients with increased abdominal circumference (> 102 cm in men and 88 cm in women) or with high waist–hip ratios (> 1.0 in men and > 0.85 in women) have a greater risk of diabetes mellitus, stroke, coronary artery disease, and early death than equally obese patients with lower ratios. Further differentiation of the location of excess fat suggests that visceral fat within the abdominal cavity is more hazardous to health than subcutaneous fat around the abdomen.

Current U.S. survey data demonstrate that 65% of Americans are overweight and 30.4% are obese. Women in the United States are more apt to be obese than men, and African-American and Mexican-American women are more obese than whites. The poor are more obese than the rich regardless of race.

▶ Health Consequences of Obesity

Obesity is associated with significant increases in both morbidity and mortality. A great many disorders occur with greater frequency in obese people. The most important and common of these are hypertension, type 2 diabetes mellitus, hyperlipidemia, coronary artery disease, degenerative joint disease, and psychosocial disability. Approximately 60% of individuals with obesity in the United States have the metabolic syndrome (including three or more of the following factors: elevated abdominal circumference, blood pressure, blood triglycerides, and fasting blood sugar, and low high-density lipoprotein [HDL] cholesterol). Certain cancers (colon, ovary, and breast), thromboembolic disorders, digestive tract diseases (gallbladder disease, gastroesophageal reflux disease), and skin disorders are also more prevalent in the obese. Surgical and obstetric risks are greater. Obese patients also have a greater risk of pulmonary functional impairment including sleep apnea, endocrine abnormalities, proteinuria, and increased hemoglobin concentration. Patients with obesity have increased rates of major depression and binge eating disorder. Several studies have documented that obese individuals are also subject to various forms of social discrimination.

In young and middle-aged adults, mortality from all causes and mortality from cardiovascular disease increase in proportion to the degree of obesity. The relative risk associated with obesity, however, decreases with age, and weight is no longer a risk factor in adults over age 75 years. Recent analysis of data from the National Health and Nutrition Examination Survey (NHANES) has suggested that lesser amounts of excess weight (BMI between 25 and 29.9) may not be associated with excess mortality.

▶ Etiology

Until recently, obesity was considered to be the direct result of a sedentary lifestyle plus chronic ingestion of excess calories. Although these factors are undoubtedly the principal cause in many cases, there is evidence for strong genetic influences on the development of obesity. Adopted children demonstrate a close relationship between their body mass index and that of their biologic parents. No such relationship is found between the children and their adoptive parents. Twin studies also demonstrate substantial genetic influences on BMI with little influence from the childhood environment. As much as 40–70% of obesity may be explained by genetic influences.

Genetic determinants of some types of obesity have now been established. Five genes affecting control of appetite have been identified in mice. Mutations of each gene result in obesity, and each has a human homolog. One gene codes for a protein expressed by adipose tissue—leptin—and another for the leptin receptor in the brain. The other three genes affect brain pathways downstream from the leptin receptor. Numerous other candidate genes for human obesity have been identified. Only a small percentage (4–6%) of human obesity is thought to be due to single gene mutations. Most human obesity undoubtedly develops from the interactions of multiple genes, environmental factors, and behavior. The rapid increase in obesity in the last several decades clearly points to a major role of environmental factors in the development of obesity.

▶ Medical Evaluation of the Obese Patient

Historical information should be obtained about age at onset, recent weight changes, family history of obesity, occupational history, eating and exercise behavior, cigarette and alcohol use, previous weight loss experience, and psychosocial factors including assessment for depression and eating disorders. Particular attention should be directed at use of laxatives, diuretics, hormones, nutritional supplements, and over-the-counter medications.

Physical examination should assess the degree and distribution of body fat, overall nutritional status, and signs of secondary causes of obesity.

Less than 1% of obese patients have an identifiable secondary, nonpsychiatric, cause of obesity. Hypothyroidism and Cushing syndrome are important examples that can usually be diagnosed by physical examination in patients with unexplained recent weight gain. Such patients require further endocrinologic evaluation, including serum thyroid-stimulating hormone (TSH) determination and dexamethasone suppression testing (see Chapter 26).

All obese patients should be assessed for medical consequences of their obesity by screening for the metabolic syndrome. Blood pressure, waist circumference, fasting glucose, low-density lipoprotein (LDL) and HDL cholesterol, and triglycerides should be measured.

▶ Treatment

Using conventional dietary techniques, only 20% of patients will lose 20 lb and maintain the loss for over 2 years; 5% will maintain a 40-lb loss. Average weight loss is approximately 7% of baseline weight. Continued close provider–patient contact appears to be more important for success of treatment than the specific features of any given treatment regimen. Careful patient selection will improve success rates and decrease frustration of both patients and therapists. Only sufficiently motivated patients should enter active treatment programs. Specific attempts to identify motivated patients—eg, requesting a 3-day diet record— are often useful.

Most successful programs employ a multidisciplinary approach to weight loss, with hypocaloric diets, behavior modification to change eating behavior, aerobic exercise, and social support. Emphasis must be on *maintenance* of weight loss.

Dietary instructions for most patients incorporate the same principles that apply to healthy people who are not obese. This is achieved by emphasizing intake of a wide variety of predominantly "unprocessed" foods. Special attention is usually paid to limiting foods that provide large amounts of calories without other nutrients, ie, fat, sucrose, and alcohol. There is no physiologic advantage to diets that restrict carbohydrates, advocate relatively larger amounts of protein or fats, or recommend ingestion of foods one at a time. Diets that are restricted in carbohydrates, however, can be effective in achieving a lower total calorie intake. Several studies have demonstrated that low-carbohydrate diets can be used safely for weight loss without adverse effects on lipids or other metabolic parameters. Meal replacement diets can also be used effectively and safely to achieve weight loss.

Long-term changes in eating behavior are required to maintain weight loss. Although formal **behavior modification** programs are available to which patients can be referred, the clinician caring for obese patients can teach a number of useful behavioral techniques. The most important technique is to emphasize planning and record keeping. Patients can be taught to plan menus and exercise sessions and to record their actual behavior. Record keeping not only aids in behavioral change, but also helps the provider to make specific suggestions for problem solving. Patients can be taught to recognize "eating cues" (emotional, situational, etc) and how to avoid or control them. Regular self-monitoring of weight is also associated with improved long-term weight maintenance.

Exercise offers a number of advantages to patients trying to lose weight and keep it off. Aerobic exercise directly increases the daily energy expenditure and is particularly useful for long-term weight maintenance. Exercise will also preserve lean body mass and partially prevent the decrease in basal energy expenditure (BEE) seen with semi-starvation. When compared with no treatment, exercise alone results in small amounts of weight loss. Exercise plus diet results in greater weight loss than diet alone. A greater intensity of exercise is associated with a greater amount of weight loss. Up to 1 hour of moderate exercise per day is associated with long-term weight maintenance in individuals who have successfully lost weight. **Social support** is essential for a successful weight loss program. Continued close contact with clinicians and involvement of the family and peer group are useful techniques for reinforcing behavioral change and preventing social isolation.

Patients with severe obesity may require more aggressive treatment regimens. Very-low-calorie diets ($\leq$ 800 kcal/d) result in rapid weight loss and marked initial improvement in obesity-related metabolic complications. Patients are commonly maintained on such programs for 4–6 months and lose an average of 2 lb per week. Average weight loss is approximately 15% of initial weight. Most programs use meal replacement diets to achieve the very-low-calorie intake. Long-term weight maintenance is less predictable and requires concurrent behavior modification, long-term use of low-calorie diets, careful self-monitoring, and regular exercise. Side effects such as fatigue, orthostatic hypotension, cold intolerance, and fluid and electrolyte disorders are observed in proportion to the degree of calorie reduction and require regular supervision by a physician. Other less common complications include gout, gallbladder disease, and cardiac arrhythmias. Although weight loss is more rapidly achieved with very-low-calorie diets as compared with traditional diets, long-term outcomes are equivalent.

Medications for the treatment of obesity are available both over the counter and by prescription. Considerable controversy exists as to the appropriate use of medications for obesity. NIH clinical obesity guidelines state that obesity drugs may be used as part of a comprehensive weight loss program for patients with BMI > 30 or those with BMI > 27 with obesity-related risk factors. There are few data, however, to suggest that medications can improve long-term outcomes associated with obesity.

Several medications are approved by the US Food and Drug Administration (FDA) for treatment of obesity. Catecholaminergic medications (eg, phentermine, diethylpropion, mazindol) are approved for short-term use only and have limited utility. Two additional medications are approved for weight loss: sibutramine and orlistat. Sibutramine blocks uptake of both serotonin and norepinephrine in the central nervous system. Orlistat reduces fat absorption in the gastrointestinal tract.

Sibutramine, typically at doses of 10 mg/d, results in average weight losses of 3–5 kg more than placebo in studies extending over 6–12 months. Sibutramine also appears to improve 1-year outcomes in patients on very-low-calorie diets. Side effects include dry mouth, anorexia, constipation, insomnia, and dizziness. In some patients (< 5%), sibutramine may substantially increase blood pressure.

Orlistat is the first approved medication for obesity that works in the gastrointestinal tract rather than the central nervous system. By inhibiting intestinal lipase, orlistat reduces fat absorption. As expected, orlistat may result in diarrhea, gas, and cramping and perhaps also reduced absorption of fat-soluble vitamins. In randomized trials with up to 2 years of follow-up, orlistat has resulted in 2–4 kg greater weight loss than placebo. The recommended dose of orlistat is 120 mg three times daily with meals. A 60-mg dose is available over-the-counter in the United States. Despite FDA approval of sibutramine and orlistat and NIH guidelines supporting their use, long-term clinical benefits have not been demonstrated. Although these medications result in some additional weight loss at the end of 1- and 2-year clinical trials and, in some studies, improved obesity-related metabolic parameters, a beneficial impact of these medications on obesity-related clinical outcomes has not been established. Another class of medications under investigation is selective cannabinoid-1 receptor antagonists (eg, rimonabant). In four initial year-long studies of rimonabant, a 20-mg dose resulted in 5 kg greater weight loss than placebo. Rimonabant, however, caused more adverse affects than placebo, including nervous system, psychiatric, and gastrointestinal symptoms, and attrition rates at 1 year were approximately 40%. Because of concerns related to depression and suicidality, the FDA did not approve rimonabant for use in the United States.

Bariatric surgery is an increasingly prevalent treatment option for patients with severe obesity. In the United States, gastric operations are considered the procedures of choice. Most popular is the Roux-en-Y gastric bypass (RYGB). In most centers, the operation can be done laparoscopically. RYGB typically results in substantial amounts of weight loss—close to 50% of initial body weight in some studies. Complications occur in up to 40% of persons undergoing RYGB surgery and include peritonitis due to anastomotic leak, abdominal wall hernias, staple line disruption, gallstones, neuropathy, marginal ulcers, stomal stenosis, wound infections, thromboembolic disease, gastrointestinal symptoms, and nutritional deficiencies including iron, vitamin B_{12}, folate, calcium, and vitamin D. Operative mortality rates within 30 days are nil to 1% in low-risk populations but have been reported to be substantially higher in Medicare beneficiaries. One-year mortality rates have been reported as high as 7.5% in men with Medicare. The surgical volume (the number of cases performed by the surgeon or hospital) has been demonstrated to be an important predictor of outcome. Gastric banding (GB) surgeries are increasing as an alternative procedure. GB results in less dramatic weight loss than RYGB but with fewer short-term complications. Frequent follow-up is required to adjust the gastric band. Longer-term follow-up suggests that both procedures are associated with significant regaining of weight. NIH consensus panel recommendations are to limit obesity surgery to patients with BMIs over 40, or over 35 if obesity-related comorbidities are present. The procedure is cost-effective for patients with severe obesity and most third-party payers now cover the procedure in selected patients. Recent outcomes studies have suggested that bariatric surgery is associated with a significant reduction in deaths at 11-year follow-up. In one prospective study, the number needed to treat to prevent one death in 11 years was 77 operations.

When to Refer

Patients with BMI over 40 (or over 35 with obesity-related morbidities) who are interested in considering weight loss surgery.

Adams TD et al. Long-term mortality after gastric bypass surgery. N Engl J Med. 2007 Aug 23;357(8):753–761. [PMID: 17715409]

Bravata DM et al. Using pedometers to increase physical activity and improve health: a systematic review. JAMA. 2007 Nov 21;298(19):2296–304. [PMID: 18029834]

Christakis NA et al. The spread of obesity in a large social network over 32 years. N Engl J Med. 2007 Jul 26;357(4):370–9. [PMID: 17652652]

Davis MM et al. Recommendations for prevention of childhood obesity. Pediatrics. 2007 Dec;120(Suppl 4):S229-53. [PMID: 18055653]

DeMaria EJ. Bariatric surgery for morbid obesity. N Engl J Med. 2007 May 24;356(21):2176-83. [PMID: 17522401]

Fabricatore AN. Behavior therapy and cognitive-behavioral therapy of obesity: is there a difference? J Am Diet Assoc. 2007 Jan;107(1):92–9. [PMID: 17197276]

Flegal KM et al. Cause-specific excess deaths associated with underweight, overweight, and obesity. JAMA. 2007;298(17):2028–2037. [PMID: 17986696]

Flum DR et al. Toward the rational and equitable use of bariatric surgery. JAMA. 2007 Sep 26;298(12):1442–4. [PMID: 17895461]

Franz MJ et al. Weight-loss outcomes: a systematic review and meta-analysis of weight-loss clinical trials with a minimum 1-year follow-up. J Am Diet Assoc. 2007 Oct;107(10):1755–67. [PMID: 17904936]

Gardner CD et al. Comparison of the Atkins, Zone, Ornish, and LEARN diets for change in weight and related risk factors among overweight premenopausal women: the A TO Z Weight Loss Study: a randomized trial. JAMA. 2007 Mar 7;297(9):969–77. [PMID: 17341711]

Ogden CL et al. The epidemiology of obesity. Gastroenterology. 2007 May;132(6):2087–102. [PMID: 17498505]

Poitou Bernert C et al. Nutritional deficiency after gastric bypass: diagnosis, prevention and treatment. Diabetes Metab. 2007 Feb;33(1):13–24. [PMID: 17258928]

Puhl MR et al. The stigma of obesity: A review and update. Obesity (Silver Spring). 2009 Jan 22. 2009 May;17(5):941–64. [PMID: 19165161]

Santry HP et al. Predictors of patient selection in bariatric surgery. Ann Surg. 2007 Jan;245(1):59–67. [PMID: 17197966]

Sharma B et al. Sibutramine: current status as an anti-obesity drug and its future perspectives. Expert Opin Pharmacother. 2008 Aug;9(12):2161–73. [PMID: 18671470]

Sjöström L et al. Effects of bariatric surgery on mortality in Swedish obese subjects. N Engl J Med. 2007 Aug 23;357(8):741–752. [PMID: 17715408]

Sui X et al. Cardiorespiratory fitness and adiposity as mortality predictors in older adults. JAMA. 2007 Dec 5;298(21):2507-16. [PMID: 18056904]

EATING DISORDERS

ANOREXIA NERVOSA

 ESSENTIALS OF DIAGNOSIS

▶ Disturbance of body image and intense fear of becoming fat.

▶ Weight loss leading to body weight 15% below expected.

▶ In females, absence of three consecutive menstrual cycles.

General Considerations

Anorexia nervosa typically begins in the years between adolescence and young adulthood. Ninety percent of patients are females, most from the middle and upper socioeconomic strata. The diagnosis is based on weight loss leading to body weight 15% below expected, a distorted body image, fear of weight gain or of loss of control over food intake and, in females, the absence of at least three consecutive menstrual cycles. Other medical or psychiatric illnesses that can account for anorexia and weight loss must be excluded.

The prevalence of anorexia nervosa is greater than previously suggested. In Rochester, Minnesota, for example, the prevalence per 100,000 population is estimated to be 270 for females and 22 for males. Many other adolescent girls have features of the disorder without the severe weight loss.

The cause of anorexia nervosa is not known. Although multiple endocrinologic abnormalities exist in these patients, most authorities believe they are secondary to malnutrition and not primary disorders. Most experts favor a primary psychiatric origin, but no hypothesis explains all cases. The patient characteristically comes from a family whose members are highly goal and achievement oriented. Interpersonal relationships may be inadequate or destructive. The parents are usually overly directive and concerned with slimness and physical fitness, and much of the family conversation centers around dietary matters. One theory holds that the patient's refusal to eat is an attempt to regain control of her body in defiance of parental control. The patient's unwillingness to inhabit an "adult body" may also represent a rejection of adult responsibilities and the implications of adult interpersonal relationships. Patients are commonly perfectionistic in behavior and exhibit obsessional personality characteristics. Marked depression or anxiety may be present.

Clinical Findings

A. Symptoms and Signs

Patients with anorexia nervosa may exhibit severe emaciation and may complain of cold intolerance or constipation. Amenorrhea is almost always present. Bradycardia, hypotension, and hypothermia may be present in severe cases. Examination demonstrates loss of body fat, dry and scaly skin, and increased lanugo body hair. Parotid enlargement and edema may also occur.

B. Laboratory Findings

Laboratory findings are variable but may include anemia, leukopenia, electrolyte abnormalities, and elevations of blood urea nitrogen (BUN) and serum creatinine. Serum cholesterol levels are often increased. Endocrine abnormal-ities include depressed levels of luteinizing and follicle-stimulating hormones and impaired response of luteinizing hormone to luteinizing hormone-releasing hormone.

Diagnosis & Differential Diagnosis

The diagnosis can be difficult, since many common social and cultural factors promote and maintain anorexic behavior. The diagnosis depends on identification of the common behavioral features and exclusion of medical disorders that would account for weight loss.

Behavioral features required for the diagnosis include intense fear of becoming obese, disturbance of body image, weight loss of at least 15%, and refusal to exceed a minimal normal weight.

The differential diagnosis includes endocrine and metabolic disorders, such as panhypopituitarism, Addison disease, hyperthyroidism, and diabetes mellitus; gastrointestinal disorders, such as Crohn disease and celiac sprue; chronic infections and cancers, such as tuberculosis and lymphoma; and rare central nervous system disorders, such as hypothalamic tumors.

Treatment

The goal of treatment is restoration of normal body weight and resolution of psychological difficulties. Hospitalization may be necessary. Treatment programs conducted by experienced teams are successful in about two-thirds of cases, restoring normal weight and menstruation. One-half continue to experience difficulties with eating behavior and psychiatric problems. Occasional patients with anorexia develop obesity after treatment. Two to 6% of patients die of the complications of the disorder or commit suicide.

Various treatment methods have been used without clear evidence of superiority of one over another. Supportive care by physicians and nurses is probably the most important feature of therapy. Structured behavioral therapy, intensive psychotherapy, and family therapy may be tried. A variety of medications including tricyclic antidepressants, SSRIs, and lithium carbonate are effective in some cases; overall, however, clinical trial results have been disappointing. Patients with severe malnutrition must be hemodynamically stabilized and may require enteral or parenteral feeding. Forced feedings should be reserved for life-threatening situations, since the goal of treatment is to reestablish normal eating behavior.

When to Refer

• Adolescents and young adults with otherwise unexplained weight loss should be evaluated by a psychiatrist.

• All patients with diagnosed anorexia nervosa should be co-managed with a psychiatrist.

When to Admit

• Signs of hypovolemia, major electrolyte disorders, and severe protein-energy malnutrition.

• Failure to improve with outpatient management.

American Dietetic Association. Position of the American Dietetic Association: Nutrition intervention in the treatment of anorexia nervosa, bulimia nervosa, and other eating disorders. J Am Diet Assoc. 2006 Dec;106(12):2073–82. [PMID: 17186637]

Court A et al. What is the scientific evidence for the use of antipsychotic medication in anorexia nervosa? Eat Disord. 2008 May–Jun;16(3):217–23. [PMID: 18443980]

Mayer LE et al. Does percent body fat predict outcome in anorexia nervosa? Am J Psychiatry. 2007 Jun;164(6):970–2. [PMID: 17541059]

Taylor CB et al. Prevention of eating disorders in at-risk college-age women. Arch Gen Psychiatry. 2006 Aug;63(8):881–8. [PMID: 16894064]

Walsh BT et al. Fluoxetine after weight restoration in anorexia nervosa: a randomized controlled trial. JAMA. 2006 Jun 14;295(22):2605–12. [PMID: 16772623]

Yager J et al. Clinical practice. Anorexia nervosa. N Engl J Med. 2005 Oct 6;353(14):1481–8. [PMID: 16207850]

BULIMIA NERVOSA

 ESSENTIALS OF DIAGNOSIS

► Uncontrolled episodes of binge eating at least twice weekly for 3 months.

► Recurrent inappropriate compensation to prevent weight gain such as self-induced vomiting, laxatives, diuretics, fasting, or excessive exercise.

► Overconcern with weight and body shape.

General Considerations

Bulimia nervosa is the episodic uncontrolled ingestion of large quantities of food followed by recurrent inappropriate compensatory behavior to prevent weight gain such as self-induced vomiting, diuretic or cathartic use, or strict dieting or vigorous exercise.

Like anorexia nervosa, bulimia nervosa is predominantly a disorder of young, white, middle- and upper-class women. It is more difficult to detect than anorexia, and some studies have estimated that the prevalence may be as high as 19% in college-aged women.

Clinical Findings

Patients with bulimia nervosa typically consume large quantities of easily ingested high-calorie foods, usually in secrecy. Some patients may have several such episodes a day for a few days; others report regular and persistent patterns of binge eating. Binging is usually followed by vomiting, cathartics, or diuretics and is usually accompanied by feelings of guilt or depression. Periods of binging may be followed by intervals of self-imposed starvation. Body weights may fluctuate but generally are within 20% of desirable weights.

Some patients with bulimia nervosa also have a cryptic form of anorexia nervosa with significant weight loss and amenorrhea. Family and psychological issues are generally similar to those encountered among patients with anorexia nervosa. Bulimics, however, have a higher incidence of premorbid obesity, greater use of cathartics and diuretics, and more impulsive or antisocial behavior. Menstruation is usually preserved.

Medical complications are numerous. Gastric dilatation and pancreatitis have been reported after binges. Vomiting can result in poor dentition, pharyngitis, esophagitis, aspiration, and electrolyte abnormalities. Cathartic and diuretic abuse also cause electrolyte abnormalities or dehydration. Constipation and hemorrhoids are common.

► Treatment

Treatment of bulimia nervosa and bulimarexia requires supportive care and psychotherapy. Individual, group, family, and behavioral therapy have all been utilized. Antidepressant medications may be helpful. The best results have been with fluoxetine hydrochloride and other SSRIs. Although death from bulimia is rare, the long-term psychiatric prognosis in severe bulimia is worse than that in anorexia nervosa.

► When to Refer

All patients with diagnosed bulimia should be co-managed with a psychiatrist.

American Dietetic Association. Position of the American Dietetic Association: Nutrition intervention in the treatment of anorexia nervosa, bulimia nervosa, and other eating disorders. J Am Diet Assoc. 2006 Dec;106(12):2073–82. [PMID: 17186637]

Krysanki VL et al. Review of controlled psychotherapy treatment trials for binge eating disorder. Psychol Rep. 2008 Apr;102(2):339–68. [PMID: 18567205]

le Grange D et al. A randomized controlled comparison of family-based treatment and supportive psychotherapy for adolescent bulimia nervosa. Arch Gen Psychiatry. 2007 Sep;64(9):1049–56. [PMID: 17768270]

Schmidt U et al. A randomized controlled trial of family therapy and cognitive behavior therapy guided self-care for adolescents with bulimia nervosa and related disorders. Am J Psychiatry. 2007 Apr;164(4):591–8. [PMID: 17403972]

▼ **DISORDERS OF VITAMIN METABOLISM**

THIAMINE (B₁) DEFICIENCY

 ESSENTIALS OF DIAGNOSIS

► Most common in patients with chronic alcoholism.

► Early symptoms of anorexia, muscle cramps, paresthesias, irritability.

► Advanced syndromes of high output heart failure ("wet beriberi"), peripheral nerve disorders, and Wernicke-Korsakoff syndrome ("dry beriberi").

► Clinical Findings

Most thiamine deficiency in the United States is due to alcoholism. Patients with chronic alcoholism may have poor dietary intakes of thiamine and impaired thiamine absorption, metabolism, and storage. Thiamine deficiency is also associated with malabsorption, dialysis, and other causes of chronic protein–calorie undernutrition. Thiamine deficiency can be precipitated in patients with marginal thiamine status with intravenous dextrose solutions.

Early manifestations of thiamine deficiency include anorexia, muscle cramps, paresthesias, and irritability. Advanced deficiency primarily affects the cardiovascular system ("wet beriberi") or the nervous system ("dry beriberi"). Wet beriberi occurs in thiamine deficiency accompanied by severe physical exertion and high carbohydrate intakes. Dry beriberi occurs in thiamine deficiency accompanied by inactivity and low calorie intake.

Wet beriberi is characterized by marked peripheral vasodilation resulting in high-output heart failure with dyspnea, tachycardia, cardiomegaly, and pulmonary and peripheral edema, with warm extremities mimicking cellulitis.

Dry beriberi involves both the peripheral and the central nervous systems. Peripheral nerve involvement is typically a symmetric motor and sensory neuropathy with pain, paresthesias, and loss of reflexes. The legs are affected more than the arms. Central nervous system involvement results in Wernicke–Korsakoff syndrome. Wernicke encephalopathy consists of nystagmus progressing to ophthalmoplegia, truncal ataxia, and confusion. Korsakoff syndrome includes amnesia, confabulation, and impaired learning.

► Diagnosis

A variety of biochemical tests are available to assess thiamine deficiency. In most instances, however, the clinical response to empiric thiamine therapy is used to support a diagnosis of thiamine deficiency. The most commonly used and widely available biochemical tests are measurement of erythrocyte transketolase activity and urinary thiamine excretion. A transketolase activity coefficient greater than 15–20% suggests thiamine deficiency.

► Treatment

Thiamine deficiency is treated with large parenteral doses of thiamine. Fifty to 100 mg/d is administered intravenously for the first few days, followed by daily oral doses of 5–10 mg/d. All patients should simultaneously receive therapeutic doses of other water-soluble vitamins. Although treatment results in complete resolution in half of patients (one-fourth immediately and another one-fourth over days), the other half obtain only partial resolution or no benefit.

► When to Refer

Patients with signs of beriberi or Wernicke-Korsakoff syndrome should be referred to a neurologist.

THIAMINE TOXICITY

There is no known toxicity of thiamine.

Clements RH et al. Incidence of vitamin deficiency after laparoscopic Roux-en-Y gastric bypass in a university hospital setting. Am Surg. 2006 Dec;72(12):1196–202. [PMID: 17216818]

Francini-Pesenti F et al. Wernicke's encephalopathy during parenteral nutrition. J Parenter Enteral Nutr. 2007 Jan–Feb; 31(1):69–71. [PMID: 17202444]

Harper C. Thiamine (vitamin B₁) deficiency and associated brain damage is still common throughout the world and prevention is simple and safe! Eur J Neurol. 2006 Oct; 13(10):1078–82. [PMID: 16987159]

Singh S et al. Wernicke encephalopathy after obesity surgery: a systematic review. Neurology. 2007 Mar 13;68(11):807–11. [PMID: 17353468]

Zuccoli G et al. Wernicke encephalopathy: MR findings at clinical presentation in twenty-six alcoholic and nonalcoholic patients. AJNR Am J Neuroradiol. 2007 Aug;28(7):1328–31. [PMID: 17698536]

RIBOFLAVIN (B₂) DEFICIENCY

► Clinical Findings

Riboflavin deficiency almost always occurs in combination with deficiencies of other vitamins. Dietary inadequacy, interactions with a variety of medications, alcoholism, and other causes of protein–calorie undernutrition are the most common causes of riboflavin deficiency.

Manifestations of riboflavin deficiency include cheilosis, angular stomatitis, glossitis, seborrheic dermatitis, weakness, corneal vascularization, and anemia.

► Diagnosis

Riboflavin deficiency can be confirmed by measuring the riboflavin-dependent enzyme erythrocyte glutathione reductase. Activity coefficients greater than 1.2–1.3 are suggestive of riboflavin deficiency. Urinary riboflavin excretion and serum levels of plasma and red cell flavins can also be measured.

► Treatment

Riboflavin deficiency is usually treated empirically when the diagnosis is suspected. It is easily treated with foods such as meat, fish, and dairy products or with oral preparations of the vitamin. Administration of 5–15 mg/d until clinical findings are resolved is usually adequate. Riboflavin can also be given parenterally, but it is poorly soluble in aqueous solutions.

RIBOFLAVIN TOXICITY

There is no known toxicity of riboflavin.

Chuang CZ et al. Effects of riboflavin and folic acid supplementation on plasma homocysteine levels in healthy subjects. Am J Med Sci. 2006 Feb;331(2):65–71. [PMID: 16479177]

Dainty JR et al. Quantification of the bioavailability of riboflavin from foods by use of stable-isotope labels and kinetic modeling. Am J Clin Nutr. 2007 Jun;85(6):1557–64. [PMID: 17556693]

McNulty H et al. Intake and status of folate and related B-vitamins: considerations and challenges in achieving optimal status. Br J Nutr. 2008 Jun;99(Suppl 3):S48–54. [PMID: 18598588]

Said HM et al. Intestinal absorption of water-soluble vitamins: an update. Curr Opin Gastroenterol. 2006 Mar;22(2):140–6. [PMID: 16462170]

NIACIN DEFICIENCY

▶ General Considerations

Niacin is a generic term for nicotinic acid and other derivatives with similar nutritional activity. Unlike most other vitamins, niacin can be synthesized from the amino acid tryptophan. Niacin is an essential component of the coenzymes nicotinamide adenine dinucleotide (NAD) and nicotinamide adenine dinucleotide phosphate (NADP), which are involved in many oxidation-reduction reactions. The major food sources of niacin are protein foods containing tryptophan and numerous cereals, vegetables, and dairy products.

Niacin in the form of nicotinic acid is used therapeutically for the treatment of hypercholesterolemia and hypertriglyceridemia. Daily doses of 3–6 g can result in significant reductions in levels of LDL and very-low-density lipoproteins (VLDL) and in elevation of HDL. Niacinamide (the form of niacin usually used to treat niacin deficiency) does not exhibit the lipid-lowering effects of nicotinic acid. Historically, niacin deficiency occurred when corn, which is relatively deficient in both tryptophan and niacin, was the major source of calories. Currently, niacin deficiency is more commonly due to alcoholism and nutrient–drug interactions. Niacin deficiency can also occur in inborn errors of metabolism.

▶ Clinical Findings

As with other B vitamins, the early manifestations of niacin deficiency are nonspecific. Common complaints include anorexia, weakness, irritability, mouth soreness, glossitis, stomatitis, and weight loss. More advanced deficiency results in the classic triad of pellagra: dermatitis, diarrhea, and dementia. The dermatitis is symmetric, involving sun-exposed areas. Skin lesions are dark, dry, and scaling. The dementia begins with insomnia, irritability, and apathy and progresses to confusion, memory loss, hallucinations, and psychosis. The diarrhea can be severe and may result in malabsorption due to atrophy of the intestinal villi. Advanced pellagra can result in death.

▶ Diagnosis

In early deficiency, diagnosis requires a high index of suspicion and attempts at confirmation of niacin deficiency. Niacin metabolites, particularly N-methylnicotinamide, can be measured in the urine. Low levels suggest niacin deficiency but may also be found in patients with generalized undernutrition. Serum and red cell levels of NAD and NADP are also low but are similarly nonspecific. In advanced cases, the diagnosis of pellagra can be made on clinical grounds.

▶ Treatment

Niacin deficiency can be effectively treated with oral niacin, usually given as nicotinamide. Doses ranging from 10 mg/d to 150 mg/d have been used without difficulty.

NIACIN TOXICITY

At the high doses of niacin used to treat hyperlipidemia, side effects are common. These include cutaneous flushing (partially prevented by pretreatment with aspirin, 325 mg/d, and use of extended-release preparations) and gastric irritation. Elevation of liver enzymes, hyperglycemia, and gout are less common untoward effects.

Alsheikh-Ali AA et al. Safety of lovastatin/extended release niacin compared with lovastatin alone, atorvastatin alone, pravastatin alone, and simvastatin alone (from the United States Food and Drug Administration Adverse Event Reporting System). Am J Cardiol. 2007 Feb 1;99(3):379–81. [PMID: 17261402]

Canner PL et al. Benefits of niacin in patients with versus without the metabolic syndrome and healed myocardial infarction (from the Coronary Drug Project). Am J Cardiol. 2006 Feb 15;97(4):477–9. [PMID: 16461040]

Guyton JR. Niacin in cardiovascular prevention: mechanisms, efficacy, and safety. Curr Opin Lipidol. 2007 Aug;18(4):415–20. [PMID: 17620858]

McKenney JM et al. Comparative effects on lipid levels of combination therapy with a statin and extended-release niacin or ezetimibe versus a statin alone (the COMPELL study). Atherosclerosis. 2007 Jun;192(2):432–7. [PMID: 17239888]

VITAMIN B$_6$ DEFICIENCY

Vitamin B$_6$ deficiency most commonly occurs as a result of interactions with medications—especially isoniazid, cycloserine, penicillamine, and oral contraceptives—or of alcoholism. A number of inborn errors of metabolism and other pyridoxine-responsive syndromes, particularly pyridoxine-responsive anemia, are not clearly due to vitamin deficiency but commonly respond to high doses of the vitamin.

▶ Clinical Findings

Vitamin B$_6$ deficiency results in a clinical syndrome similar to that seen with deficiencies of other B vitamins, including mouth soreness, glossitis, cheilosis, weakness, and irritability. Severe deficiency can result in peripheral neuropathy, anemia, and seizures. Recent studies have suggested a potential relationship of low vitamin B$_6$ levels and a variety of clinical conditions including cardiovascular diseases, inflammatory diseases, and certain cancers.

▶ Diagnosis

The diagnosis of vitamin B$_6$ deficiency can be confirmed by measurement of pyridoxal phosphate in blood. Normal levels are greater than 50 ng/mL.

▶ Treatment

Vitamin B$_6$ deficiency can be effectively treated with oral vitamin B$_6$ supplements. Doses of 10–20 mg/d are usually adequate, though some patients taking medications that interfere with pyridoxine metabolism may need doses as high as 100 mg/d. Inborn errors of metabolism and the pyridoxine-responsive syndromes often require doses up to 600 mg/d.

Vitamin B$_6$ should be routinely prescribed for patients receiving medications (such as isoniazid) that interfere with pyridoxine metabolism to prevent vitamin B$_6$ deficiency. This is particularly true for elderly patients, the urban poor, and alcoholics, who are more likely to have diets marginally adequate in vitamin B_6. Recent clinical trials have shown that vitamin B_6 supplementation, combined with other B vitamins, has no benefit on cardiovascular disease outcomes.

VITAMIN B_6 TOXICITY

A sensory neuropathy, at times irreversible, occurs in patients receiving large doses of vitamin B_6. Although most patients have taken 2 g or more per day, some patients have taken only 200 mg/d.

Biewirth J et al. Association of common variable immunodeficiency with vitamin B6 deficiency. Eur J Clin Nutr. 2008 Mar;62(3):332–5. [PMID: 17311052]

Kumar N. Nutritional neuropathies. Neurol Clin. 2007 Feb; 25(1):209–55. [PMID: 17324726]

Lonn E et al. Homocysteine lowering with folic acid and B vitamins in vascular disease. N Engl J Med. 2006 Apr 13;354(15):1567–77. [PMID: 16531613]

Peeters AC et al. Low vitamin B_6, and not plasma homocysteine concentration, as risk factor for abdominal aortic aneurysm: a retrospective case-control study. J Vasc Surg. 2007 Apr;45(4):701–5. [PMID: 17398378]

Raman G et al. Heterogeneity and lack of good quality studies limit association between folate, vitamins B-6 and B-12, and cognitive function. J Nutr. 2007 Jul;137(7):1789–94. [PMID: 17585032]

Spinneker A et al. Vitamin B_6 status, deficiency and its consequences–an overview. Nutr Hosp. 2007 Jan–Feb;22(1):7–24. [PMID: 17260529]

VITAMIN B_{12} & FOLATE

Vitamin B_{12} (cobalamin) and folate are discussed in Chapter 13.

VITAMIN C (Ascorbic Acid) DEFICIENCY

Most cases of vitamin C deficiency seen in the United States are due to dietary inadequacy in the urban poor, the elderly, and chronic alcoholics. Patients with chronic illnesses such as cancer and chronic kidney disease and individuals who smoke cigarettes are also at risk.

▶ Clinical Findings

Early manifestations of vitamin C deficiency are nonspecific and include malaise and weakness. In more advanced stages, the typical features of scurvy develop. Manifestations include perifollicular hemorrhages, perifollicular hyperkeratotic papules, petechiae and purpura, splinter hemorrhages, bleeding gums, hemarthroses, and subperiosteal hemorrhages. Periodontal signs do not occur in edentulous patients. Anemia is common, and wound healing is impaired. The late stages of scurvy are characterized by edema, oliguria, neuropathy, intracerebral hemorrhage, and death.

▶ Diagnosis

The diagnosis of advanced scurvy can be made clinically on the basis of the skin lesions in the proper clinical situation. Atraumatic hemarthrosis is also highly suggestive. The diagnosis can be confirmed with decreased plasma ascorbic acid levels, typically below 0.1 mg/dL.

▶ Treatment

Adult scurvy can be treated orally with 300–1000 mg of ascorbic acid per day. Improvement typically occurs within days. Clinical trials have shown that supplemental vitamin C has no benefit on cardiovascular disease or cancer outcomes.

VITAMIN C TOXICITY

Very large doses of vitamin C can cause gastric irritation, flatulence, or diarrhea. Oxalate kidney stones are of theoretic concern because ascorbic acid is metabolized to oxalate, but stone formation has not been frequently reported. Vitamin C can also confound common diagnostic tests by causing false-negative tests for fecal occult blood and both false-negative and false-positive tests for urine glucose.

Bjelakovic G et al. Mortality in randomized trials of antioxidant supplements for primary and secondary prevention: systematic review and meta-analysis. JAMA. 2007 Feb 28;297(8):842–57. [PMID: 17327526]

Douglas RM et al. Vitamin C for preventing and treating the common cold. Cochrane Database Syst Rev. 2007 Jul 18;(3):CD000980. [PMID: 17636648]

Huang HY et al. The efficacy and safety of multivitamin and mineral supplement use to prevent cancer and chronic disease in adults: a systematic review for a National Institutes of Health state-of-the-science conference. Ann Intern Med. 2006 Sep 5;145(5):372–85. [PMID: 16880453]

Li Y et al. New developments and novel therapeutic perspectives for vitamin C. J Nutr. 2007 Oct;137(10):2171–84. [PMID: 17884994]

Olmedo JM et al. Scurvy: a disease almost forgotten. Int J Dermatol. 2006 Aug;45(8):909–13. [PMID: 16911372]

Rohrmann S et al. Fruit and vegetable consumption, intake of micronutrients, and benign prostatic hyperplasia in US men. Am J Clin Nutr. 2007 Feb;85(2):523–9. [PMID: 17284753]

VITAMIN A DEFICIENCY

▶ Clinical Findings

Vitamin A deficiency is one of the most common vitamin deficiency syndromes, particularly in developing countries. In many such regions, it is the most common cause of blindness. In the United States, vitamin A deficiency is usually due to fat malabsorption syndromes or mineral oil laxative abuse and occurs most commonly in the elderly and urban poor.

Night blindness is the earliest symptom. Dryness of the conjunctiva (xerosis) and the development of small white patches on the conjunctiva (Bitot spots) are early signs. Ulceration and necrosis of the cornea (keratomalacia), perforation, endophthalmitis, and blindness are late manifestations. Xerosis and hyperkeratinization of the skin and loss of taste may also occur.

▶ Diagnosis

Abnormalities of dark adaptation are strongly suggestive of vitamin A deficiency. Serum levels below the normal range of 30–65 mg/dL are commonly seen in advanced deficiency.

Treatment

Night blindness, poor wound healing, and other signs of early deficiency can be effectively treated orally with 30,000 international units of vitamin A daily for 1 week. Advanced deficiency with corneal damage calls for administration of 20,000 international units/kg orally for at least 5 days. The potential antioxidant effects of β-carotene can be achieved with supplements of 25,000–50,000 international units of β-carotene.

VITAMIN A TOXICITY

Excess intake of β-carotenes (hypercarotenosis) results in staining of the skin a yellow-orange color but is otherwise benign. Skin changes are most marked on the palms and soles, while the scleras remain white, clearly distinguishing hypercarotenosis from jaundice.

Excessive vitamin A (hypervitaminosis A), on the other hand, can be quite toxic. Chronic toxicity usually occurs after ingestion of daily doses of over 50,000 international units/d for more than 3 months. Early manifestations include dry, scaly skin, hair loss, mouth sores, painful hyperostoses, anorexia, and vomiting. More serious findings include hypercalcemia; increased intracranial pressure, with papilledema, headaches, and decreased cognition; and hepatomegaly, occasionally progressing to cirrhosis. Excessive vitamin A has also recently been related to increased risk of hip fracture. Acute toxicity can result from ingestion of massive doses of vitamin A, such as in drug overdoses or consumption of polar bear liver. Manifestations include nausea, vomiting, abdominal pain, headache, papilledema, and lethargy.

The diagnosis can be confirmed by elevations of serum vitamin A levels. The only treatment is withdrawal of vitamin A from the diet. Most symptoms and signs improve rapidly.

Age-Related Eye Disease Study Research Group; SanGiovanni JP et al. The relationship of dietary carotenoid and vitamin A, E, and C intake with age-related macular degeneration in a case-control study: AREDS Report No. 22. Arch Ophthalmol. 2007 Sep;125(9):1225–32. [PMID: 17846363]

Canter PH et al. The antioxidant vitamins A, C, E and selenium in the treatment of arthritis: a systematic review of randomized clinical trials. Rheumatology (Oxford). 2007 Aug;46(8):1223–33. [PMID: 17522095]

Darlow BA et al. Vitamin A supplementation to prevent mortality and short and long-term morbidity in very low birthweight infants. Cochrane Database Syst Rev. 2007 Oct 17;(4):CD000501. [PMID: 17943744]

Penniston KL et al. The acute and chronic toxic effects of vitamin A. Am J Clin Nutr. 2006 Feb;83(2):191–201. [PMID: 16469975]

Swami HM et al. Impact of mass supplementation of vitamin A. Indian J Pediatr. 2007 May;74(5):443–7. [PMID: 17526954]

VITAMIN D

Vitamin D is discussed in Chapter 26. The major food source of vitamin D is fortified milk, but sunlight on the skin is a prime resource as well.

VITAMIN E DEFICIENCY

Clinical Findings

Clinical deficiency of vitamin E is most commonly due to severe malabsorption, the genetic disorder abetalipoproteinemia, or, in children with chronic cholestatic liver disease, biliary atresia or cystic fibrosis. Manifestations of deficiency include areflexia, disturbances of gait, decreased proprioception and vibration, and ophthalmoplegia.

Diagnosis

Plasma vitamin E levels can be measured; normal levels are 0.5–0.7 mg/dL or higher. Since vitamin E is normally transported in lipoproteins, the serum level should be interpreted in relation to circulating lipids.

Treatment

The optimum therapeutic dose of vitamin E has not been clearly defined. Large doses, often administered parenterally, can be used to improve the neurologic complications seen in abetalipoproteinemia and cholestatic liver disease. The potential antioxidant benefits of vitamin E can be achieved with supplements of 100–400 international units/d. Clinical trials of supplemental vitamin E to prevent cardiovascular disease, however, have shown no beneficial effects.

VITAMIN E TOXICITY

Vitamin E has been thought to be the least toxic of the fat-soluble vitamins. Large doses—many times the recommended daily requirement—have been taken for extended periods of time without apparent harm, though nausea, flatulence, and diarrhea have been reported. Clinical trials, however, have suggested an increase in all-cause mortality with high dose (≥ 400 international units/d) vitamin E supplements. Large doses of vitamin E can also increase the vitamin K requirement and can result in bleeding in patients taking oral anticoagulants.

Cook NR et al. A randomized factorial trial of vitamins C and E and beta carotene in the secondary prevention of cardiovascular events in women: results from the Women's Antioxidant Cardiovascular Study. Arch Intern Med. 2007 Aug 13–27;167(15):1610–8. [PMID: 17698683]

Glynn RJ et al. Effects of random allocation to vitamin E supplementation on the occurrence of venous thromboembolism: report from the Women's Health Study. Circulation. 2007 Sep 25;116(13):1497–503. [PMID: 17846285]

Lee IM et al. Vitamin E in the primary prevention of cardiovascular disease and cancer: the Women's Health Study: a randomized controlled trial. JAMA. 2005 Jul 6;294(1):56–65. [PMID: 15998891]

Miller ER 3rd et al. Meta-analysis: high-dosage vitamin E supplementation may increase all-cause mortality. Ann Intern Med. 2005 Jan 4;142(1):37–46. [PMID: 15537682]

Traber MG et al. Vitamin E revisited: do new data validate benefits for chronic disease prevention? Curr Opin Lipidol. 2008 Feb;19(1):30–8. [PMID: 18196984]

VITAMIN K

Vitamin K is discussed in Chapter 13. Vitamin K is synthesized by intestinal bacteria.

▼ DIET THERAPY

Specific therapeutic diets can be designed to facilitate the medical management of most common illnesses. In most cases, consultation with a registered dietitian is necessary in order to design and implement major dietary changes. Clinicians should be familiar with the indications for special diets and their basic composition to facilitate patient referrals and to maximize patient compliance. Diet therapy is a difficult process, and not all patients are able to cooperate fully. Requesting the patient to record dietary intake for 3–5 days may provide useful insight into the patient's motivation as well as providing nutrient information about the current diet.

Therapeutic diets can be divided into three groups: (1) diets that alter the consistency of food, (2) diets that restrict or otherwise modify dietary components, and (3) diets that supplement dietary components.

DIETS THAT ALTER CONSISTENCY

▶ Clear Liquid Diet

This diet provides adequate water, 500–1000 kcal as simple sugar, and some electrolytes. It is fiber free and requires minimal digestion or intestinal motility.

A clear liquid diet is useful for patients with resolving postoperative ileus, acute gastroenteritis, partial intestinal obstruction, and as preparation for diagnostic gastrointestinal procedures. It is commonly used as the first diet for patients who have been taking nothing by mouth for long periods. Because of the low calorie and minimal protein content of the clear liquid diet, it is used only for short periods.

▶ Full Liquid Diet

The full liquid diet provides adequate water and can be designed to provide adequate calories and protein. Vitamins and minerals—especially folic acid, iron, and vitamin B_6—may be inadequate and should be provided in the form of supplements. Dairy products, soups, eggs, and soft cereals are used to supplement clear liquids. Commercial oral supplements can also be incorporated into the diet or used alone.

This diet is low in residue and can be used in many instances instead of the clear liquid diet described above—especially in patients with difficulty in chewing or swallowing, with partial obstructions, or in preparation for some diagnostic procedures. Full liquid diets are commonly used following clear liquid diets to advance diets in patients who have been taking nothing by mouth for long periods.

▶ Soft Diets

Soft diets are designed for patients unable to chew or swallow hard or coarse food. Tender foods are used, and most raw fruits and vegetables and coarse breads and cereals are eliminated. Soft diets are commonly used to assist in progression from full liquid diets to regular diets in postoperative patients, in patients who are too weak or those whose dentition is too poor to handle a general diet, in head and neck surgical patients, in patients with esophageal strictures, and in other patients who have difficulty with chewing or swallowing.

The soft diet can be designed to meet all nutritional requirements.

DIETS THAT RESTRICT NUTRIENTS

Diets can be designed to restrict (or eliminate) virtually any nutrient or food component. The most commonly used restricted diets are those that limit sodium, fat, and protein. Other restrictive diets include gluten restriction in sprue, potassium and phosphate reduction in chronic kidney disease, and various elimination diets for food allergies.

▶ Sodium-Restricted Diets

Low-sodium diets are useful in the management of hypertension and in conditions in which sodium retention and edema are prominent features, particularly congestive heart failure, chronic liver disease, and chronic kidney disease. Sodium restriction is beneficial with or without diuretic therapy. When used in conjunction with diuretics, sodium restriction allows lower dosage of the diuretic medication and may prevent side effects. Potassium excretion, in particular, is directly related to distal renal tubule sodium delivery, and sodium restriction will decrease diuretic-related potassium losses.

Typical American diets contain a minimum of 4–6 g (175–260 mEq) of sodium per day. A no-added-salt diet contains approximately 3 g (132 mEq) of sodium per day. Further restriction can be achieved with sodium diets of 2 or 1 g/d. Diets with more severe restriction are poorly accepted by patients and are rarely used.

Dietary sodium includes sodium naturally occurring in foods, sodium added during food processing, and sodium added by the consumer during cooking and at the table. About a third of current dietary intake is derived from each. Diets that allow 2000 mg of sodium daily are easiest to design and implement. Such diets generally eliminate added salt, most processed foods, and selected foods with particularly high sodium content. Patients who follow such diets for 2–3 months lose their craving for salty foods and can often continue to restrict their sodium intake indefinitely. Many patients with mild hypertension will achieve significant reductions in blood pressure (approximately 5 mm Hg diastolic) with this degree of sodium restriction. Other patients require more severe sodium restriction (approximately 1000 mg of sodium per day) for reduction in blood pressure.

Diets allowing 1000 mg of sodium require further restriction of commonly eaten foods. Special "low-sodium" products are now available to facilitate such diets. These diets are difficult for most people to follow and are generally reserved for hospitalized patients and highly motivated outpatients—most commonly those with severe liver disease and ascites.

Fat-Restricted Diets

Traditional fat-restricted diets are useful in the treatment of fat malabsorption syndromes. Such diets will improve the symptoms of diarrhea with steatorrhea independently of the primary physiologic abnormality by limiting the quantity of fatty acids that reach the colon. The degree of fat restriction necessary to control symptoms must be individualized. Patients with severe malabsorption can be limited to 40–60 g of fat per day. Diets containing 60–80 g of fat per day can be designed for patients with less severe abnormalities.

In general, fat-restricted diets require broiling, baking, or boiling meat and fish; discarding the skin of poultry and fish and using those foods as the main protein source; using nonfat dairy products; and avoiding desserts, sauces, and gravies.

Low-Cholesterol, Low-Saturated-Fat Diets

Fat-restricted diets that specifically restrict saturated fats and dietary cholesterol are the mainstay of dietary treatment of hyperlipidemia (see Chapter 28). Similar diets are recommended also for diabetes mellitus (see Chapter 27) and for the prevention of coronary artery disease (see Chapter 10). Current recommendations for the prevention of cancer by dietary modification also include fat restriction. The large Women's Health Initiative Dietary Modification Trial, however, did not show any significant benefit of a low-fat diet on weight control or prevention of cardiovascular disease or cancer.

The aim of these diets is to restrict total fat to less than 30% of calories and to achieve a normal body weight by caloric restriction and increased physical activity. Saturated fat is restricted to 7% of calories and dietary cholesterol to 200 mg/d. Saturated fat can be replaced either with complex carbohydrates or, if energy balance permits, with monounsaturated fats. Saturated fat, total fat, and dietary cholesterol can be restricted further, but studies suggest that more extreme restriction offers little further advantage in overall modification of serum lipids. Cholesterol-lowering diets can be further augmented with the addition of plant stanols and sterols and with soluble dietary fiber.

Protein-Restricted Diets

Protein-restricted diets are most commonly used in patients with hepatic encephalopathy due to chronic liver disease and in patients with advanced chronic kidney disease to slow the progression of early disease and to decrease symptoms of uremia in more severe disease. Patients with selected inborn errors of amino acid metabolism and other abnormalities resulting in hyperammonemia also require restriction of protein or of specific amino acids.

Protein restriction is intended to limit the production of nitrogenous waste products. Energy intake must be adequate to facilitate the efficient use of dietary protein. Proteins must be of high biologic value and be provided in sufficient quantity to meet minimal requirements. For most patients, the diet should contain at least 0.6 g/kg/d of protein. Patients with encephalopathy who do not respond to this degree of restriction are unlikely to respond to more severe restriction.

DIETS THAT SUPPLEMENT NUTRIENTS

High-Fiber Diet

Dietary fiber is a diverse group of plant constituents that is resistant to digestion by the human digestive tract. Typical American diets contain about 5–10 g of dietary fiber per day. Epidemiologic evidence has suggested that populations consuming greater quantities of fiber have a lower incidence of certain gastrointestinal disorders, including diverticulitis and colon cancer. Most authorities currently recommend higher intakes of dietary fiber for health maintenance.

Diets high in dietary fiber (20–35 g/d) are also commonly used in the management of a variety of gastrointestinal disorders, particularly irritable bowel syndrome and recurrent diverticulitis. Diets high in fiber may also be useful to reduce blood sugar in patients with diabetes and to reduce cholesterol levels in patients with hypercholesterolemia. Such diets include greater intakes of fresh fruits and vegetables, whole grains, legumes and seeds, and bran products. For some patients, the addition of psyllium seed (2 tsp per day) or natural bran (one-half cup per day) may be preferable.

High-Potassium Diets

Potassium-supplemented diets are used most commonly to compensate for potassium losses caused by diuretics. Although potassium losses can be partially prevented by using lower doses of diuretics, concurrent sodium restriction, and potassium-sparing diuretics, some patients require additional potassium to prevent hypokalemia. High-potassium diets may also have a direct antihypertensive effect. Typical American diets contain about 3 g (80 mEq) of potassium per day. High-potassium diets commonly contain 4.5–7 g (120–180 mEq) of potassium per day.

Most fruits, vegetables, and their juices contain high concentrations of potassium. Supplemental potassium can also be provided with potassium-containing salt substitutes (up to 20 mEq in one-quarter tsp) or as potassium chloride in solution or capsules, but this is rarely necessary if the above measures are followed to prevent potassium losses and supplement dietary potassium.

High-Calcium Diets

Additional intakes of dietary calcium have been recommended for the prevention of postmenopausal osteoporosis, the prevention and treatment of hypertension, and the prevention of colon cancer. The recent Women's Health Initiative, however, suggested that calcium and vitamin D supplementation did not prevent fractures or colon cancer. Nonetheless, many authorities recommend intakes of 1 g of calcium per day for most adults and 1.5 g/d for postmenopausal women. Average American daily intakes are approximately 700 mg/d.

Dairy products are the primary dietary sources of calcium in the United States. Patients with lactose intolerance who cannot tolerate liquid dairy products may be able to tolerate nonliquid products such as cheese and yogurt. Leafy green vegetables and canned fish with bones also contain high concentrations of calcium, although the latter is also high in sodium.

Dansinger ML et al. Meta-analysis: the effect of dietary counseling for weight loss. Ann Intern Med. 2007 Jul 3;147(1):41–50. [PMID: 17606960]

Delahanty LM et al. Implications of the diabetes prevention program and Look AHEAD clinical trials for lifestyle interventions. J Am Diet Assoc. 2008 Apr;108(4 Suppl 1):S66–72. [PMID: 18358260]

Ebbeling CB et al. Effects of a low-glycemic load vs low-fat diet in obese young adults: a randomized trial. JAMA. 2007 May 16;297(19):2092–102. [PMID: 17507345]

Helsel DL et al. Comparison of techniques for self-monitoring eating and exercise behaviors on weight loss in a correspondence-based intervention. J Am Diet Assoc. 2007 Oct; 107(10):1807–10. [PMID: 17904942]

Howard BV et al. Low-fat dietary pattern and weight change over 7 years: the Women's Health Initiative Dietary Modification Trial. JAMA. 2006 Jan 4;295(1):39–49. [PMID: 16391215]

Pan Y et al. Low-protein diet for diabetic nephropathy: a meta-analysis of randomized controlled trials. Am J Clin Nutr. 2008 Sep;88(3):660–6. [PMID: 18779281]

Pedersen SD et al. Portion control plate for weight loss in obese patients with type 2 diabetes mellitus: a controlled clinical trial. Arch Intern Med. 2007 Jun 25;167(12):1277–83. [PMID: 17592101]

Westman EC et al. Low-carbohydrate nutrition and metabolism. Am J Clin Nutr. 2007 Aug;86(2):276–84. [PMID: 17684196]

Zivkovic AM et al. Comparative review of diets for the metabolic syndrome: implications for nonalcoholic fatty liver disease. Am J Clin Nutr. 2007 Aug;86(2):285–300. [PMID: 17684197]

▼ NUTRITIONAL SUPPORT

Nutritional support is the provision of nutrients to patients who cannot meet their nutritional requirements by eating standard diets. Nutrients may be delivered enterally, using oral nutritional supplements, nasogastric and nasoduodenal feeding tubes, and tube enterostomies, or parenterally, using lines or catheters placed in peripheral or central veins, respectively. Current nutritional support techniques permit adequate nutrient delivery to most patients. Nutrition support should be utilized, however, only if it is likely to improve the patient's clinical outcome. The financial costs and risks of side effects must be balanced against the potential advantages of improved nutritional status in each clinical situation.

INDICATIONS FOR NUTRITIONAL SUPPORT

The precise indications for nutritional support remain controversial. Most authorities agree that nutritional support is indicated for at least four groups of adult patients: (1) those with inadequate bowel syndromes, (2) those with severe prolonged hypercatabolic states (eg, due to extensive burns, multiple trauma, mechanical ventilation), (3) those requir-

ing prolonged therapeutic bowel rest, and (4) those with severe protein–calorie undernutrition with a treatable disease who have sustained a loss of over 25% of body weight.

It has been difficult to prove the efficacy of nutritional support in the treatment of most other conditions. In most cases it has not been possible to show a clear advantage of treatment by means of nutritional support over treatment without such support.

The American Society for Parenteral and Enteral Nutrition (ASPEN) has published recommendations for the rational use of nutritional support. The recommendations emphasize the need to individualize the decision to begin nutritional support, weighing the risks and costs against the benefits to each patient. They also reinforce the need to identify high-risk malnourished patients by nutritional assessment.

NUTRITIONAL SUPPORT METHODS

Selection of the most appropriate nutritional support method involves consideration of gastrointestinal function, the anticipated duration of nutritional support, and the ability of each method to meet the patient's nutritional requirements. The method chosen should meet the patient's nutritional needs with the lowest risk and lowest cost possible. For most patients, enteral feeding is safer and cheaper and offers significant physiologic advantages. An algorithm for selection of the most appropriate nutritional support method is presented in Figure 29–1.

Prior to initiating specialized enteral nutritional support, efforts should be made to supplement food intake. Attention to patient preferences, timing of meals and diagnostic procedures and use of medications, and the use of foods brought to the hospital by family and friends can often increase oral intake. Patients unable to eat enough at regular mealtimes to meet nutritional requirements can be given **oral supplements** as snacks or to replace low-calorie beverages. Oral supplements of differing nutritional composition are available for the purpose of individualizing the diet in accordance with specific clinical requirements (see below). Fiber and lactose content, caloric density, protein level, and amino acid profiles can all be modified as necessary.

Patients unable to take adequate oral nutrients who have functioning gastrointestinal tracts and who meet the criteria for nutritional support are candidates for **tube feedings**. Small-bore feeding tubes are placed via the nose into the stomach or duodenum. Patients able to sit up in bed who can protect their airways can be fed into the stomach. Because of the increased risk of aspiration, patients who cannot adequately protect their airways should be fed nasoduodenally. Feeding tubes can usually be passed into the duodenum by leaving an extra length of tubing in the stomach and placing the patient in the right decubitus position. Metoclopramide, 10 mg intravenously, can be given 20 minutes prior to insertion and continued every 6 hours thereafter to facilitate passage through the pylorus. Occasionally patients will require fluoroscopic or endoscopic guidance to insert the tube distal to the pylorus. Placement of nasogastric and, particularly, nasoduodenal tubes should be confirmed radiographically before delivery of feeding solutions.

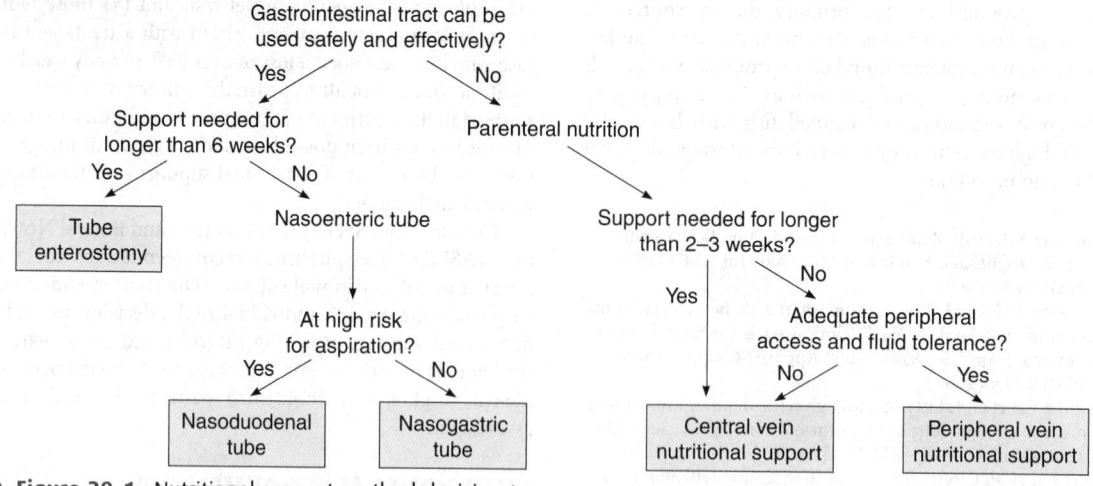

▲ **Figure 29–1.** Nutritional support method decision tree.

Feeding tubes can also be placed directly into the gastrointestinal tract using **tube enterostomies**. Most tube enterostomies are placed in patients who require long-term enteral nutritional support. Gastrostomies have the advantage of allowing bolus feedings, while jejunostomies require continuous infusions. Gastrostomies—like nasogastric feeding—should be used only in patients at low risk for aspiration. Gastrostomies can also be placed percutaneously with the aid of endoscopy. These tubes can then be advanced to jejunostomies. Tube enterostomies can also be placed surgically.

Patients who require nutritional support but whose gastrointestinal tracts are nonfunctional should receive **parenteral nutritional support**. Most patients receive parenteral feedings via a central vein—most commonly the subclavian vein. Peripheral veins can be used in some patients, but because of the high osmolality of parenteral solutions this is rarely tolerated for more than a few weeks.

Peripheral vein nutritional support is most commonly used in patients with nonfunctioning gastrointestinal tracts who require immediate support but whose clinical status is expected to improve within 1–2 weeks, allowing enteral feeding. Peripheral vein nutritional support is administered via standard intravenous lines. Solutions should always include lipid and dextrose in combination with amino acids to provide adequate nonprotein calories. Serious side effects are infrequent, but there is a high incidence of phlebitis and infiltration of intravenous lines.

Central vein nutritional support is delivered via intravenous catheters placed percutaneously using aseptic technique. Proper placement in the superior vena cava is documented radiographically before the solution is infused. Catheters must be carefully maintained by experienced nursing personnel and used solely for nutritional support to prevent infection and other catheter-related complications.

NUTRITIONAL REQUIREMENTS

Each patient's nutritional requirements should be determined independently of the method of nutritional sup-

port. In most situations, solutions of equal nutrient value can be designed for delivery via enteral and parenteral routes, but differences in absorption must be considered. A complete nutritional support solution must contain water, energy, amino acids, electrolytes, vitamins, minerals, and essential fatty acids.

▶ Water

For most patients, water requirements can be calculated by allowing 1500 mL for the first 20 kg of body weight plus 20 mL for every kilogram over 20. Additional losses should be replaced as they occur. For average-sized adult patients, fluid needs are about 30–35 mL/kg, or approximately 1 mL/kcal of energy required (see below).

▶ Energy

Energy requirements can be estimated by one of three methods: (1) by using standard equations to calculate BEE plus additional calories for activity and illness, (2) by applying a simple calculation based on calories per kilogram of body weight, or (3) by measuring energy expenditure with indirect calorimetry.

BEE can be estimated by the **Harris–Benedict equation:** for men, BEE = 666 + (13.7 × weight in kg) + (5 × height in cm) − (6.8 × age in years). For women, BEE = 655 + (9.5 × weight in kg) + (1.8 × height in cm) − (4.7 × age in years). For undernourished patients, actual body weight should be used; for obese patients, ideal body weight should be used. For most patients, an additional 20–50% of BEE is administered as nonprotein calories to accommodate energy expenditures during activity or relating to the illness. Occasional patients are noted to have energy expenditures greater than 150% of BEE.

Energy requirements can be estimated also by multiplying actual body weight in kilograms (for obese patients, ideal body weight) by 30–35 kcal.

Both of these methods provide imprecise estimates of actual energy expenditures, especially for the markedly underweight, overweight, and critically ill patient. Studies using indirect calorimetry have demonstrated that as many as 30–40% of patients will have measured expenditures 10% above or below estimated values. For accurate determination of energy expenditure, indirect calorimetry should be used.

Protein

Protein and energy requirements are closely related. If adequate calories are provided, most patients can be given 0.8–1.2 g of protein per kilogram per day. Patients undergoing moderate to severe stress should receive up to 1.5 g/kg/d. As in the case of energy requirements, actual weights should be used for normal and underweight patients and ideal weights for patients with significant obesity.

Patients who are receiving protein without adequate calories will catabolize protein for energy rather than utilizing it for protein synthesis. Thus, when energy intake is low, excess protein is needed for nitrogen balance. If both energy and protein intakes are low, extra energy will have a more significant positive effect on nitrogen balance than extra protein.

Electrolytes & Minerals

Requirements for sodium, potassium, and chloride vary widely. Most patients require 45–145 mEq/d of each. The actual requirement in individual patients will depend on the patient's cardiovascular, renal, endocrine, and gastrointestinal status as well as measurements of serum concentration.

Patients receiving enteral nutritional support should receive adequate vitamins and minerals according to the recommended daily allowances. Most premixed enteral solutions provide adequate vitamins and minerals as long as adequate calories are administered.

Patients receiving parenteral nutritional support require smaller amounts of minerals: calcium, 10–15 mEq/d; phosphorus, 15–20 mEq per 1000 nonprotein calories; and magnesium, 16–24 mEq/d. Most patients receiving nutritional support do not require supplemental iron because body stores are adequate. Iron nutrition should be monitored closely by following the hemoglobin concentration, mean corpuscular volume, and iron studies. Parenteral administration of iron is associated with a number of adverse effects and should be reserved for iron-deficient patients unable to take oral iron.

Patients receiving parenteral nutritional support should be given the trace elements zinc (about 5 mg/d) and copper (about 2 mg/d). Patients with diarrhea will require additional zinc to replace fecal losses. Additional trace elements—especially chromium, manganese, and selenium—are provided to patients receiving long-term parenteral nutrition.

Parenteral vitamins are provided daily. Standardized multivitamin solutions are currently available to provide adequate quantities of vitamins A, B_{12}, C, D, E, thiamine, riboflavin, niacin, pantothenic acid, pyridoxine, folic acid, and biotin. Vitamin K is not given routinely but administered when the prothrombin time becomes abnormal.

Essential Fatty Acids

Patients receiving nutritional support should be given 2–4% of their total calories as linoleic acid to prevent essential fatty acid deficiency. Most prepared enteral solutions contain adequate linoleic acid. Patients receiving parenteral nutrition should be given at least 250 mL of a 20% intravenous fat (emulsified soybean or safflower oil) about two or three times a week. Intravenous fat can also be used as an energy source in place of dextrose.

ENTERAL NUTRITIONAL SUPPORT SOLUTIONS

Most patients who require enteral nutritional support can be given commercially prepared enteral solutions (Table 29–1). Nutritionally complete solutions have been designed to provide adequate proportions of water, energy, protein, and micronutrients. Nutritionally incomplete solutions are also available to provide specific macronutrients (eg, protein, carbohydrate, and fat) to supplement complete solutions for patients with unusual requirements or to design solutions that are not available commercially.

Nutritionally complete solutions are characterized as follows: (1) by osmolality (isotonic or hypertonic), (2) by

Table 29–1. Enteral solutions.

Complete
  Blenderized (eg, Compleat Regular, Compleat Modified,[1] Vitaneed[1])
  Whole protein, lactose-containing (eg, Mentene, Carnation and Delmark Instant Breakfast, Forta Shake)
  Whole protein, lactose-free, low-residue:
    1 kcal/mL (eg, Ensure, Isocal, Osmolite, Nutren 1.0,[1] Nutrilan, Isolan,[1] Sustacal, Resource)
    1.5 kcal/mL (eg, Ensure Plus, Sustacal HC, Comply, Nutren 1.5, Resource Plus)
    2 kcal/mL (eg, Isocal HCN, Magnacal, TwoCal HN)
    High-nitrogen: > 15% total calories from protein (eg, Ensure HN, Attain,[1] Osmolite HN,[1] Replete, Entrition HN,[1] Isolan,[1] Isocal HN,[1] Sustacal HC, Isosource HN,[1] Ultralan)
  Whole protein, lactose-free, high-residue:
    1 kcal/mL (eg, Jevity,[1] Profiber,[1] Nutren 1.0 with fiber,[1] Fiberian,[1] Sustacal with fiber, Ultracal,[1] Ensure with fiber, Fibersource)
    Chemically defined peptide- or amino acid-based (eg, Accu-pep HPF, Criticare HN, Peptamen,[1] Reabfin, Vital HN, AlitraQ, Tolerex, Vivonex TEN)
"Disease-specific" formulas
  Advanced chronic kidney disease: with essential amino acids (eg, Amin-Aid, Travasorb Renal, Aminess)
  Malabsorption: with medium-chain triglycerides (eg, Portagen,[1] Travasorb MCT)
  Respiratory failure: with > 50% calories from fat (eg, Pulmocare, NutriVent)
  Hepatic encephalopathy: with high amounts of branched-chain amino acids (eg, Hepatic-Acid II, Travasorb Hepatic)
Incomplete (modular)
  Protein (eg, Nutrisource Protein, Promed, Propac)
  Carbohydrate (eg, Nutrisource Carbohydrate, Polycose, Sumacal)
  Fat (eg, MCT Oil, Microlipid, Nutrisource Lipid)
  Vitamins (eg, Nutrisource Vitamins)
  Minerals (eg, Nutrisource Minerals)

[1]Isotonic.

lactose content (present or absent), (3) by the molecular form of the protein component (intact proteins; peptides or amino acids), (4) by the quantity of protein and calories provided, and (5) by fiber content (present or absent). For most patients, isotonic solutions containing no lactose or fiber are preferable. Such solutions generally contain moderate amounts of fat and intact protein. Most commercial isotonic solutions contain 1000 kcal and about 37–45 g of protein per liter.

Solutions containing hydrolyzed proteins or crystalline amino acids and with no significant fat content are called elemental solutions, since macronutrients are provided in their most "elemental" form. These solutions have been designed for patients with malabsorption, particularly pancreatic insufficiency and limited fat absorption. Elemental diets are extremely hypertonic and often result in more severe diarrhea. Their use should be limited to patients who cannot tolerate isotonic solutions.

Although formulas have been designed for specific clinical situations—solutions containing primarily essential amino acids (for advanced chronic kidney disease), medium-chain triglycerides (for fat malabsorption), more fat (for respiratory failure and CO_2 retention), and more branched-chain amino acids (for hepatic encephalopathy and severe trauma)—they have not been shown to be superior to standard formulas for most patients.

Enteral solutions should be administered via continuous infusion, preferably with an infusion pump. Isotonic feedings should be started at full strength at about 25–33% of the estimated final infusion rate. Feedings can be advanced by similar amounts every 12 hours as tolerated. Hypertonic feedings should be started at half strength. The strength and the rate can then be advanced every 6 hours as tolerated.

COMPLICATIONS OF ENTERAL NUTRITIONAL SUPPORT

Minor complications of tube feedings occur in 10–15% of patients. Gastrointestinal complications include diarrhea (most common), inadequate gastric emptying, emesis, esophagitis, and occasionally gastrointestinal bleeding. Diarrhea associated with tube feeding may be due to intolerance to the osmotic load or to one of the macronutrients (eg, fat, lactose) in the solution. Patients being fed in this way may also have diarrhea from other causes (as side effects of antibiotics or other drugs, associated with infection, etc), and these possibilities should always be investigated in appropriate circumstances.

Mechanical complications of tube feedings are potentially the most serious. Of particular importance is aspiration. All patients receiving nasogastric tube feedings are at risk for this life-threatening complication. Limiting nasogastric feedings to those patients who can adequately protect their airway and careful monitoring of patients being fed by tube should limit these serious complications to 1–2% of cases. Minor mechanical complications are common and include tube obstruction and dislodgment.

Metabolic complications during enteral nutritional support are common but in most cases are easily managed.

The most important problem is hypernatremic dehydration, most commonly seen in elderly patients given excessive protein intake who are unable to respond to thirst. Abnormalities of potassium, glucose, and acid–base balance may also occur.

PARENTERAL NUTRITIONAL SUPPORT SOLUTIONS

Parenteral nutritional support solutions can be designed to deliver adequate nutrients to most patients. The basic parenteral solution is composed of dextrose, amino acids, and water. Electrolytes, minerals, trace elements, vitamins, and medications can also be added. Most commercial solutions contain the monohydrate form of dextrose that provides 3.4 kcal/g. Crystalline amino acids are available in a variety of concentrations, so that a broad range of solutions can be made up that will contain specific amounts of dextrose and amino acids as required.

Typical solutions for central vein nutritional support contain 25–35% dextrose and 2.75–6% amino acids depending upon the patient's estimated nutrient and water requirements. These solutions typically have osmolalities in excess of 1800 mosm/L and require infusion into a central vein. A typical formula for patients without organ failure is shown in Table 29–2.

Solutions with lower osmolalities can also be designed for infusion into peripheral veins. Typical solutions for peripheral infusion contain 5–10% dextrose and 2.75–4.25% amino acids. These solutions have osmolalities between 800 and 1200 mosm/L and result in a high inci-

Table 29–2. Typical parenteral nutrition solution (for stable patients without organ failure).

Dextrose (3.4 kcal/g)	25%
Amino acids (4 kcal/g)	6%
Na^+	50 mEq/L
K^+	40 mEq/L
Ca^{2+}	5 mEq/L
Mg^{2+}	8 mEq/L
Cl^-	60 mEq/L
P	12 mEq/L
Acetate	Balance
MVI-12 (vitamins)	10 mL/d
MTE (trace elements)	5 mL/d
Fat emulsion 20%	250 mL five times a week
Typical rate	Day 1: 30 mL/h
	Day 2: 60 mL/h
By day 2, solution provides:	Calories: 1925 kcal total
	Protein: 86 g
	Fat: 19% of total kcal
	Fluid: 1690 mL

dence of thrombophlebitis and line infiltration. These solutions will provide adequate protein for most patients but inadequate energy. Additional energy must be provided in the form of emulsified soybean or safflower oil. Such intravenous fat solutions are currently available in 10% and 25% solutions providing 1.1 and 2.2 kcal/mL, respectively. Intravenous fat solutions are isosmotic and well tolerated by peripheral veins.

Typical patients are given 200–500 mL of a 20% solution each day. As much as 60% of total calories can be administered in this manner.

Intravenous fat can also be provided to patients receiving central vein nutritional support. In this instance, dextrose concentrations should be decreased to provide a fixed concentration of energy. Intravenous fat has been shown to be equivalent to intravenous dextrose in providing energy to spare protein. Intravenous fat is associated with less glucose intolerance, less production of carbon dioxide, and less fatty infiltration of the liver and has been increasingly utilized in patients with hyperglycemia, respiratory failure, and liver disease. Intravenous fat has also been increasingly used in patients with large estimated energy requirements. Recent studies suggest that the maximum glucose utilization rate is approximately 5–7 mg/min/kg. Patients who require additional calories can be given them as fat to prevent excess administration of dextrose. Intravenous fat can also be used to prevent essential fatty acid deficiency. The optimal ratio of carbohydrate and fat in parenteral nutritional support has not been determined.

Infusion of parenteral solutions should be started slowly to prevent hyperglycemia and other metabolic complications. Typical solutions are given initially at a rate of 50 mL/h and advanced by about the same amount every 24 hours until the desired final rate is reached.

COMPLICATIONS OF PARENTERAL NUTRITIONAL SUPPORT

Complications of central vein nutritional support occur in up to 50% of patients. Although most are minor and easily managed, significant complications will develop in about 5% of patients. Complications of central vein nutritional support can be divided into catheter-related complications and metabolic complications.

Catheter-related complications can occur during insertion or while the catheter is in place. Pneumothorax, hemothorax, arterial laceration, air emboli, and brachial plexus injury can occur during catheter placement. The incidence of these complications is inversely related to the experience of the physician performing the procedure but will occur in at least 1–2% of cases even in major medical centers. Each catheter placement should be documented by chest radiograph prior to initiation of nutritional support.

Catheter thrombosis and catheter-related sepsis are the most important complications of indwelling catheters. Patients with indwelling central vein catheters in whom fever develops without an apparent source should have their lines changed over a wire or removed immediately, the tip quantitatively cultured, and antibiotics begun empirically. Quantitative tip cultures and blood cultures will help guide further antibiotic therapy. Catheter-related sepsis occurs in 2–3% of patients even if maximal efforts are made to prevent infection.

Metabolic complications of central vein nutritional support occur in over 50% of patients (Table 29–3). Most are minor and easily managed, and termination of support is seldom necessary.

PATIENT MONITORING DURING NUTRITIONAL SUPPORT

Every patient receiving enteral or parenteral nutritional support should be monitored closely. Formal nutritional support teams composed of a physician, a nurse, a dietitian, and a pharmacist have been shown to decrease the rate of complications.

Patients should be monitored both for the adequacy of treatment and to prevent complications or detect them early when they occur. Because estimates of nutritional requirements are imprecise, frequent reassessment is necessary. Daily intakes should be recorded and compared with estimated requirements. Body weight, hydration status, and

Table 29–3. Metabolic complications of parenteral nutritional support.

Complication	Common Causes	Possible Solutions
Hyperglycemia	Too rapid infusion of dextrose, "stress," corticosteroids	Decrease glucose infusion; insulin; replacement of dextrose with fat
Hyperosmolar nonketotic dehydration	Severe, undetected hyperglycemia	Insulin, hydration, potassium
Hyperchloremic metabolic acidosis	High chloride administration	Decrease chloride
Azotemia	Excessive protein administration	Decrease amino acid concentration
Hyperphosphatemia, hypokalemia, hypomagnesemia	Extracellular to intracellular shifting with refeeding	Increase solution concentration
Liver enzyme abnormalities	Lipid trapping in hepatocytes, fatty liver	Decrease dextrose
Acalculous cholecystitis	Biliary stasis	Oral fat
Zinc deficiency	Diarrhea, small bowel fistulas	Increase concentration
Copper deficiency	Biliary fistulas	Increase concentration

overall clinical status should be followed. Patients who do not appear to be responding as anticipated can be evaluated for nitrogen balance by means of the following equation:

$$\text{Nitrogen balance} = \frac{\text{24-hour protein intake (g)}}{6.25} - \left(\text{25-hour urinary nitrogen (g)} + 4 \right)$$

Patients with positive nitrogen balances can be continued on their current regimens; patients with negative balances should receive moderate increases in calorie and protein intake and then be reassessed. Monitoring for metabolic complications includes daily measurements of electrolytes; serum glucose, phosphorus, magnesium, calcium, and creatinine; and BUN until the patient is stabilized. Once the patient is stabilized, electrolytes, phosphorus, calcium, magnesium, and glucose should be obtained at least twice weekly. Red blood cell folate, zinc, and copper should be checked at least once a month.

Curtis CS et al. Nutrition support in pancreatitis. Surg Clin North Am. 2007 Dec;87(6):1403–15, viii. [PMID: 18053838]

Forbes A. Parenteral nutrition. Curr Opin Gastroenterol. 2006 Mar;22(2):160–4. [PMID: 16462173]

Gariballa S et al. A randomized, double-blind, placebo-controlled trial of nutritional supplementation during acute illness. Am J Med. 2006 Aug;119(8):693–9. [PMID: 16887416]

Grau T et al; Working Group on Nutrition and Metabolism of the Spanish Society of Critical Care. Liver dysfunction associated with artificial nutrition in critically ill patients. Crit Care. 2007;11(1):R10. [PMID: 17254321]

Han-Geurts IJ et al. Randomized clinical trial of the impact of early enteral feeding on postoperative ileus and recovery. Br J Surg. 2007 May;94(5):555–61. [PMID: 17443854]

Heidegger CP et al. Enteral vs. parenteral nutrition for the critically ill patient: a combined support should be preferred. Curr Opin Crit Care. 2008 Aug;14(4):408–14. [PMID: 18614904]

Howard L. Home parenteral nutrition: survival, cost, and quality of life. Gastroenterology. 2006 Feb;130(2 Suppl 1):S52–9. [PMID: 16473073]

Koretz RL. Do data support nutrition support? Part I: intravenous nutrition. J Am Diet Assoc. 2007 Jun;107(6):988–98. [PMID: 17524720]

Koretz RL. Do data support nutrition support? Part II: enteral artificial nutrition. J Am Diet Assoc. 2007 Aug;107(8):1374–80. [PMID: 17659905]

Murray SM et al. Nutrition support for bone marrow transplant patients. Cochrane Database Syst Rev. 2009 Jan 21;(1): CD002920. [PMID: 19160213]

Sayers GM et al. Parenteral nutrition: ethical and legal considerations. Postgrad Med J. 2006 Feb;82(964):79–83. [PMID: 16461468]

Stapleton RD et al. Feeding critically ill patients: what is the optimal amount of energy? Crit Care Med. 2007 Sep;35(9 Suppl):S535–40. [PMID: 17713405]

Thomson A. The enteral vs parenteral nutrition debate revisited. JPEN J Parenter Enteral Nutr. 2008;Jul–Aug;32(4):474–81. [PMID: 18596321]

Common Problems in Infectious Diseases & Antimicrobial Therapy

Peter V. Chin-Hong, MD

B. Joseph Guglielmo, PharmD

Richard A. Jacobs, MD, PhD

COMMON PROBLEMS IN INFECTIOUS DISEASES

FEVER OF UNKNOWN ORIGIN (FUO)

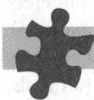 ESSENTIALS OF DIAGNOSIS

▶ Illness of at least 3 weeks duration.

▶ Fever over 38.3 °C on several occasions.

▶ Diagnosis has not been made after three outpatient visits or 3 days of hospitalization.

General Considerations

The intervals specified in the criteria for the diagnosis of FUO are arbitrary ones intended to exclude patients with protracted but self-limited viral illnesses and to allow time for the usual radiographic, serologic, and cultural studies to be performed. Because of costs of hospitalization and the availability of most screening tests on an outpatient basis, the original criterion requiring 1 week of hospitalization has been modified to accept patients in whom a diagnosis has not been made after three outpatient visits or 3 days of hospitalization.

Several additional categories of FUO have been added: (1) Hospital-associated FUO refers to the hospitalized patient with fever of 38.3 °C or higher on several occasions, due to a process not present or incubating at the time of admission, in whom initial cultures are negative and the diagnosis remains unknown after 3 days of investigation (see Hospital-Associated Infections, below). (2) Neutropenic FUO includes patients with fever of 38.3 °C or higher on several occasions with less than 500 neutrophils per microliter in whom initial cultures are negative and the diagnosis remains uncertain after 3 days (see Chapter 2 and Infections in the Immunocompromised Patient, below). (3) HIV-associated FUO pertains to HIV-positive patients with fever of 38.3 °C or higher who have been febrile for 4 weeks or more as an outpatient or 3 days as an inpatient, in whom the diagnosis remains uncertain after 3 days of

investigation with at least 2 days for cultures to incubate (see Chapter 31). Although not usually considered separately, FUO in solid organ transplant recipients is a common scenario with a unique differential diagnosis and is discussed below.

For a general discussion of fever, see the section on fever and hyperthermia in Chapter 2.

A. Common Causes

Most cases represent unusual manifestations of common diseases and not rare or exotic diseases—eg, tuberculosis, endocarditis, gallbladder disease, and HIV (primary infection or opportunistic infection) are more common causes of FUO than Whipple disease or familial Mediterranean fever.

B. Age of Patient

In adults, infections (25–40% of cases) and cancer (25–40% of cases) account for the majority of FUOs. In children, infections are the most common cause of FUO (30–50% of cases) and cancer a rare cause (5–10% of cases). Autoimmune disorders occur with equal frequency in adults and children (10–20% of cases), but the diseases differ. Juvenile rheumatoid arthritis is particularly common in children, whereas systemic lupus erythematosus, Wegener granulomatosis, and polyarteritis nodosa are more common in adults. Still disease, giant cell arteritis, and polymyalgia rheumatica occur exclusively in adults. In the elderly (over 65 years of age), multisystem immune-mediated diseases such as temporal arteritis, polymyalgia rheumatica, sarcoidosis, rheumatoid arthritis, and Wegener granulomatosis account for 25–30% of all FUOs.

C. Duration of Fever

The cause of FUO changes dramatically in patients who have been febrile for 6 months or longer. Infection, cancer, and autoimmune disorders combined account for only 20% of FUOs in these patients. Instead, other entities such as granulomatous diseases (granulomatous hepatitis, Crohn disease, ulcerative colitis) and factitious fever become important causes. One-fourth of patients who say they have been febrile for 6 months or longer actually have no true fever or underlying disease. Instead, the usual normal circadian variation in temperature (temperature 0.5–1 °C higher in the afternoon than in the morning) is interpreted as abnormal. Patients with episodic or recurrent fever (ie, those who meet the criteria for FUO but have fever-free periods of 2 weeks or longer) are similar to those with prolonged fever. Infection, malignancy, and autoimmune disorders account for only 20–25% of such fevers, whereas various miscellaneous diseases (Crohn disease, familial Mediterranean fever, allergic alveolitis) account for another 25%. Approximately 50% of cases remain undiagnosed but have a benign course with eventual resolution of symptoms.

D. Immunologic Status

In the neutropenic patient, fungal infections and occult bacterial infection are important causes of FUO. In the patient taking immunosuppressive medications (particularly organ transplant patients), cytomegalovirus (CMV) infections are a frequent cause of fever, as are fungal infections, nocardiosis, *Pneumocystis jiroveci* (formerly *Pneumocystis carinii*) pneumonia, and mycobacterial infections.

E. Classification of Causes of FUO

Most patients with FUO will fit into one of five categories.

1. Infection—Both systemic and localized infections can cause FUO. Tuberculosis and endocarditis are the most common systemic infections, but mycoses, viral diseases (particularly infection with Epstein-Barr virus and CMV), toxoplasmosis, brucellosis, Q fever, cat-scratch disease, salmonellosis, malaria, and many other less common infections have been implicated. Primary infection with HIV or opportunistic infections associated with AIDS—particularly mycobacterial infections—can also present as FUO. The most common form of localized infection causing FUO is an occult abscess. Liver, spleen, kidney, brain, and bone abscesses may be difficult to detect. A collection of pus may form in the peritoneal cavity or in the subdiaphragmatic, subhepatic, paracolic, or other areas. Cholangitis, osteomyelitis, urinary tract infection, dental abscess, or paranasal sinusitis may cause prolonged fever.

2. Neoplasms—Many cancers can present as FUO. The most common are lymphoma (both Hodgkin and non-Hodgkin) and leukemia. Other diseases of lymph nodes, such as angioimmunoblastic lymphoma and Castleman disease, can also cause FUO. Primary and metastatic tumors of the liver are frequently associated with fever, as are renal cell carcinomas. Atrial myxoma is an often forgotten neoplasm that can result in fever. Chronic lymphocytic leukemia and multiple myeloma are rarely associated with fever, and the presence of fever in patients with these diseases should prompt a search for infection.

3. Autoimmune disorders—Still disease, systemic lupus erythematosus, cryoglobulinemia, and polyarteritis nodosa are the most common causes of autoimmune-associated FUO. Giant cell arteritis and polymyalgia rheumatica are seen almost exclusively in patients over 50 years of age and

are nearly always associated with an elevated erythrocyte sedimentation rate (> 40 mm/h).

4. Miscellaneous causes—Many other conditions have been associated with FUO but less commonly than the foregoing types of illness. Examples include thyroiditis, sarcoidosis, Whipple disease, familial Mediterranean fever, recurrent pulmonary emboli, alcoholic hepatitis, drug fever, and factitious fever.

5. Undiagnosed FUO—Despite extensive evaluation, the diagnosis remains elusive in 15% or more of patients. Of these patients, the fever abates spontaneously in about 75% with no diagnosis; in the remainder, more classic manifestations of the underlying disease appear over time.

▶ Clinical Findings

Because the evaluation of a patient with FUO is costly and time-consuming, it is imperative to first document the presence of fever. This is done by observing the patient while the temperature is being taken to ascertain that fever is not factitious (self-induced). Associated findings that accompany fever include tachycardia, chills, and piloerection. A thorough history—including family, occupational, social (sexual practices, use of injection drugs), dietary (unpasteurized products, raw meat), exposures (animals, chemicals), and travel—may give clues to the diagnosis. Repeated physical examination may reveal subtle, evanescent clinical findings essential to diagnosis.

A. Laboratory Tests

In addition to routine laboratory studies, blood cultures should always be obtained, preferably when the patient has not taken antibiotics for several days, and should be held by the laboratory for 2 weeks to detect slow-growing organisms. Cultures on special media are requested if *Legionella*, *Bartonella*, or nutritionally deficient streptococci are possible pathogens. "Screening tests" with immunologic or microbiologic serologies ("febrile agglutinins") are of low yield and should not be done. If the history or physical examination suggests a specific diagnosis, specific serologic tests with an associated fourfold rise or fall in titer may be useful. Because infection is the most common cause of FUO, other body fluids are usually cultured, ie, urine, sputum, stool, cerebrospinal fluid, and morning gastric aspirates (if one suspects tuberculosis). Direct examination of blood smears may establish a diagnosis of malaria or relapsing fever (*Borrelia*).

B. Imaging

All patients with FUO should have a chest radiograph. Studies such as sinus films, upper gastrointestinal series with small bowel follow-through, barium enema, proctosigmoidoscopy, and evaluation of gallbladder function are reserved for patients who have symptoms, signs, or a history that suggest disease in these body regions. CT scan of the abdomen and pelvis is also frequently performed and is particularly useful for looking at the liver, spleen, and retroperitoneum. When the CT scan is abnormal, the findings often lead to a specific diagnosis. A normal CT scan is not quite as useful; more invasive procedures such as biopsy or exploratory laparotomy may be needed. The role of MRI in the investigation of FUO has not been evaluated. In general, however, MRI is better than CT for detecting lesions of the nervous system and is useful in diagnosing various vasculitides. Ultrasound is sensitive for detecting lesions of the kidney, pancreas, and biliary tree. Echocardiography should be used if one is considering endocarditis or atrial myxoma. Transesophageal echocardiography is more sensitive than surface echocardiography for detecting valvular lesions, but even a negative transesophageal study does not exclude endocarditis (10% false-negative rate). The usefulness of radionuclide studies in diagnosing FUO is variable. Theoretically, a gallium or positron emission tomography (PET) scan would be more helpful than an indium-labeled white blood cell scan, because gallium and fluorodeoxy-glucose may be useful for detecting infection, inflammation, and neoplasm whereas the indium scan is useful only for detecting infection. Indium-labeled immunoglobulin may prove to be useful in detecting infection and neoplasm and can be used in the neutropenic patient. It is not sensitive for lesions of the liver, kidney, and heart because of high background activity. In general, radionuclide scans are plagued by high rates of false-positive and false-negative results that are not useful when used as screening tests and, if done at all, are limited to those patients whose history or examination suggests local inflammation or infection.

C. Biopsy

Invasive procedures are often required for diagnosis. Any abnormal finding should be aggressively evaluated: Headache calls for lumbar puncture to rule out meningitis; skin rash should be biopsied for cutaneous manifestations of collagen vascular disease or infection; and enlarged lymph nodes should be aspirated or biopsied for neoplasm and sent for culture. Bone marrow aspiration with biopsy is a relatively low-yield procedure (except in HIV-positive patients, in whom mycobacterial infection is a common cause of FUO), but the risk is low and the procedure should be done if other less invasive tests have not yielded a diagnosis. Liver biopsy will yield a specific diagnosis in 10–15% of patients with FUO and should be considered in any patient with abnormal liver function tests even if the liver is normal in size. CT scanning and MRI have decreased the need for exploratory laparotomy; however, surgical intervention should be considered with continued deterioration or lack of diagnosis.

▸ Treatment

An empiric course of antimicrobials should be considered if an infectious diagnosis is strongly suspected. However, if there is no clinical response, it is imperative to stop therapy and reevaluate. Once definitive culture results return, streamlining therapy to the most narrow spectrum antimicrobial should take place. Antituberculosis medications (particularly in the elderly or foreign-born) and broad-spectrum antibiotics may be reasonable in this setting.

Empiric administration of corticosteroids should be discouraged because they can suppress fever and exacerbate many infections.

▸ When to Refer

- Any patient with FUO and progressive weight loss and other constitutional signs.
- Any immunocompromised patient (eg, transplant recipients and HIV-infected patients).
- Infectious diseases specialists may also be able to coordinate and interpret specialized testing (eg, Q fever serologies) with outside agencies, such as the US Centers for Disease Control and Prevention.

▸ When to Admit

- Any patient who is rapidly declining with weight loss where hospital admission may expedite work-up.
- If FUO is present in immunocompromised patients, such as those who are neutropenic from recent chemotherapy or those who have undergone transplantation (particularly in the previous 6 months).

Bleeker-Rovers et al. A prospective multicenter study on fever of unknown origin: the yield of a structured diagnostic protocol. Medicine. 2007 Jan;86(1):26–38. [PMID: 17220753]

Cunha BA. Fever of unknown origin: clinical overview of classic and current concepts. Infect Dis Clin North Am. 2007;21(4):867–915. [PMID: 18061081]

Ozaras R et al. Is laparotomy necessary in the diagnosis of fever of unknown origin? Acta Chir Belg. 2005 Feb;105(1):89–92. [PMID: 15790210]

Woolery WA et al. Fever of unknown origin: keys to determining the etiology in older patients. Geriatrics. 2004 Oct;59(10):41–5. [PMID: 15508555]

Zernone T. Fever of unknown origin in adults: evaluation of 144 cases in a non-university hospital. Scand J Infect Dis. 2006;38(8):632–8. [PMID: 16857607]

INFECTIONS IN THE IMMUNOCOMPROMISED PATIENT

 ESSENTIALS OF DIAGNOSIS

- ▸ Fever and other symptoms may be blunted because of immunosuppression.
- ▸ A contaminating organism in an immunocompetent individual may be a pathogen in an immunocompromised one.
- ▸ The interval since transplantation and the degree of immunosuppression can narrow the differential diagnosis.
- ▸ Empiric broad-spectrum antibiotics may be appropriate in high-risk patients whether or not symptoms are localized.

▸ General Considerations

Immunocompromised patients have defects in their natural defense mechanisms resulting in an increased risk for infection. In addition, infection is often severe, rapidly progressive, and life-threatening. Organisms that are not usually problematic in the immunocompetent person may be important pathogens in the compromised patient (eg, *Staphylococcus epidermidis, Corynebacterium jeikeium, Propionibacterium acnes, Bacillus* species). Therefore, culture results must be interpreted with caution, and isolates should not be disregarded as merely contaminants. Although the type of immunodeficiency is associated with specific infectious disease syndromes, any pathogen can cause infection in any immunosuppressed patient at any time. Thus, a systematic evaluation is required to identify a specific organism.

A. Impaired Humoral Immunity

Defects in humoral immunity are often congenital, although hypogammaglobulinemia can occur in multiple myeloma, chronic lymphocytic leukemia, and in patients who have undergone splenectomy. Patients with ineffective humoral immunity lack opsonizing antibodies and are at particular risk for infection with encapsulated organisms, such as *Haemophilus influenzae, Neisseria meningitidis* and *Streptococcus pneumoniae.*

B. Granulocytopenia (Neutropenia)

Granulocytopenia is common following hematopoietic cell transplantation ("stem cell transplantation") and among patients with solid tumors—as a result of myelosuppressive chemotherapy—and in acute leukemias. The risk of infection begins to increase when the absolute granulocyte count falls below 1000/mcL, with a dramatic increase in frequency and severity when the granulocyte count falls below 100/ mcL. The infection risk is also increased with a rapid rate of decline of neutrophils and with a prolonged period of neutropenia. The granulocytopenic patient is particularly susceptible to infections with gram-negative enteric organisms, *Pseudomonas,* gram-positive cocci (particularly *Staphylococcus aureus, S epidermidis,* and viridans streptococci), *Candida, Aspergillus,* and other fungi that have recently emerged as pathogens such as *Trichosporon, Scedosporium, Fusarium,* and the mucormycoses.

C. Impaired Cellular Immunity

Patients with cellular immune deficiency encompass a large and heterogeneous group, including patients with HIV infection (see Chapter 31); patients with lymphoreticular malignancies, such as Hodgkin disease; and patients receiving immunosuppressive medications, such as corticosteroids, cyclosporine, tacrolimus, and other cytotoxic drugs. This latter group—those who are immunosuppressed as a result of medications—includes patients who have undergone solid organ transplantation, many patients receiving therapy for solid tumors, and patients receiving prolonged high-dose corticosteroid treatment (eg, for asthma, temporal arteritis, systemic lupus). Patients taking tumor necrosis factor (TNF)-α inhibitors, such as etanercept and infliximab, for a variety of inflammatory conditions are also included in this category. Patients with cellular immune dysfunction are susceptible to infections by a large number of organisms, particularly ones that replicate intracellularly. Examples include bacteria, such as *Listeria, Legionella, Salmonella,* and

Mycobacterium; viruses, such as herpes simplex, varicella, and CMV; fungi, such as *Cryptococcus, Coccidioides, Histoplasma,* and *Pneumocystis;* and protozoa, such as *Toxoplasma.* Patients taking TNF-α inhibitors have specific defects that increase risk of bacterial, mycobacterial (particularly tuberculosis), and fungal infections (primary and reactivation).

D. Hematopoietic Cell Transplant Recipients

The length of time it takes for complications to occur in hematopoietic cell transplant recipients can be helpful in determining the etiologic agent. In the early (preengraftment) posttransplant period (day 1–21), patients will become severely neutropenic for 7–21 days. Patients are at risk for gram-positive (particularly catheter-related) and gram-negative bacterial infections, as well as herpes simplex virus, respiratory syncytial virus, and fungal infections. In contrast to solid organ transplant recipients, the source of fever is unknown in 60–70% of hematopoietic cell transplant patients. Between 3 weeks and 3 months posttransplant, infections with CMV, adenovirus, *Aspergillus,* and *Candida* are most common. *P jiroveci* pneumonia is possible, particularly in patients in whom graft-versus-host disease has developed resulting in additional immunosuppression. Patients continue to be at risk for infectious complications beyond 3 months following transplantation, particularly those who have received allogeneic transplantation and those who are taking immunosuppressive therapy for chronic graft-versus-host disease. Varicella-zoster is common, and *Aspergillus* and CMV infections are increasingly seen in this period as well.

E. Solid Organ Transplant Recipients

The length of time it takes for infection to occur following solid organ transplantation can also be helpful in determining the infectious origin. Immediate postoperative infections often involve the transplanted organ. Following lung transplantation, pneumonia and mediastinitis are particularly common; following liver transplantation, intraabdominal abscess, cholangitis, and peritonitis may be seen; after kidney transplantation, urinary tract infections, perinephric abscesses, and infected lymphoceles can occur.

Most infections that occur in the first 2–4 weeks posttransplant are related to the operative procedure and to hospitalization itself (wound infection, intravenous catheter infection, urinary tract infection from a Foley catheter) or are related to the transplanted organ. Infections that occur between the first and sixth months are often related to immunosuppression. During this period, reactivation of viruses, such as herpes simplex, varicella-zoster, and CMV is quite common. Opportunistic infections with fungi (eg, *Candida, Aspergillus, Cryptococcus, Pneumocystis), Listeria monocytogenes, Nocardia,* and *Toxoplasma* are also common. After 6 months, if immunosuppression has been reduced to maintenance levels, infections that would be expected in any population occur. Patients with poorly functioning allografts receiving long-term immunosuppression therapy continue to be at risk for opportunistic infections.

F. Other Immunocompromised States

A large group of patients who are not specifically immunodeficient are at increased risk for infection due to debilitating injury (eg, burns or severe trauma), invasive procedures (eg, chronic central intravenous catheters, Foley catheters, dialysis catheters), central nervous system dysfunction (which predisposes patients to aspiration pneumonia and decubitus ulcers), obstructing lesions (eg, pneumonia due to an obstructed bronchus, pyelonephritis due to nephrolithiasis, cholangitis secondary to cholelithiasis), and use of broad-spectrum antibiotics. Patients with diabetes mellitus have alterations in cellular immunity, resulting in mucormycosis, emphysematous pyelonephritis, and foot infections.

Clinical Findings

A. Laboratory Findings

Routine evaluation includes complete blood count with differential, chest radiograph, and blood cultures; urine and respiratory cultures should be obtained if indicated clinically or radiographically. Any focal complaints (localized pain, headache, rash) should prompt imaging and cultures appropriate to the site.

Patients who remain febrile without an obvious source should be evaluated for viral infection (serum CMV antigen test or polymerase chain reaction), abscesses (which usually occur near previous operative sites), candidiasis involving the liver or spleen, or aspergillosis. Serologic evaluation may be helpful if toxoplasmosis, aspergillosis (detected by galactomannan level in serum), or an endemic fungal infection (coccidioidomycosis, histoplasmosis) is a possible cause.

B. Special Diagnostic Procedures

Special diagnostic procedures should also be considered. The cause of pulmonary infiltrates can be easily determined with simple techniques in some situations—eg, induced sputum yields a diagnosis of *Pneumocystis* pneumonia in 50–80% of AIDS patients with this infection. In other situations, more invasive procedures may be required (bronchoalveolar lavage, transbronchial biopsy, open lung biopsy). Skin, liver, or bone marrow biopsy may be helpful in establishing a diagnosis.

Differential Diagnosis

Transplant rejection, organ ischemia and necrosis, thrombophlebitis, and lymphoma (posttransplant lymphoproliferative disease) may all present as fever and must be considered in the differential diagnosis.

Prevention

There is great interest in preventing infection with prophylactic antimicrobial regimens but no uniformity of opinion about optimal drugs or dosage regimens. Hand washing is the simplest and most effective means of decreasing hospital-associated infections, especially in the compromised patient. Invasive devices such as central and peripheral lines and Foley catheters are potential sources of infection. Some centers use laminar airflow isolation or high-efficiency particulate air (HEPA) filtering in hematopoietic cell transplant patients. Rates of infection and episodes of febrile neutropenia, but not mortality, are decreased if colony-stimulating factors are used during chemotherapy or during stem-cell transplantation.

A. *Pneumocystis* & Herpes Simplex Infections

Trimethoprim-sulfamethoxazole (TMP-SMZ), one double-strength tablet orally three times a week, one double-strength tablet twice daily on weekends, or one single-strength tablet daily for 3–6 months, is frequently used to prevent *Pneumocystis* infections in transplant patients. In patients allergic to TMP-SMZ, dapsone, 50 mg orally daily or 100 mg three times weekly, is recommended. Glucose-6-phosphate dehydrogenase (G6PD) levels should be determined before therapy when the latter is instituted. Acyclovir prevents herpes simplex infections in bone marrow and solid organ transplant recipients and is given to seropositive patients who are not receiving acyclovir or ganciclovir for CMV prophylaxis. The usual dose is 200 mg orally three times daily for 4 weeks (hematopoietic cell transplants) to 12 weeks (other solid organ transplants).

B. CMV

No uniformly accepted approach has been adopted for prevention of CMV. Prevention strategies often depend on the serologic status of the donor and recipient and the organ transplanted, which determines the level of immunosuppression after transplant. In solid organ transplants (liver, kidney, heart, lung), the greatest risk of developing CMV disease is in seronegative patients who receive organs from seropositive donors. These high-risk patients usually receive oral valganciclovir, 900 mg daily, or oral ganciclovir, 1 g three times daily for 3 months. Other solid organ transplant recipients (seropositive recipients) are at lower risk for developing CMV disease but still usually receive either oral valganciclovir or oral ganciclovir for 3 months. The lowest risk group for the development of CMV disease is in seronegative patients who receive organs from seronegative donors. Typically, no CMV prophylaxis is used in this group. Ganciclovir and valganciclovir also prevent herpes virus reactivation. Because immunosuppression is increased during periods of rejection, patients treated for rejection usually receive CMV prophylaxis during rejection therapy.

Recipients of hematopoietic cell transplants are more severely immunosuppressed than recipients of solid organ transplants, are at greater risk for developing serious CMV infection (usually CMV reactivation), and thus usually receive more aggressive prophylaxis. Two approaches have been used: universal prophylaxis or preemptive therapy. In the former, all high-risk patients (seropositive patients who receive allogeneic transplants) may receive oral valganciclovir, 900 mg daily to day 100. This method is costly and associated with significant bone marrow toxicity. Alternatively, patients can be monitored without specific prophylaxis and have blood sampled weekly for the presence of CMV. If CMV is detected by an antigenemia assay or by polymerase chain reaction, preemptive therapy is instituted with oral valganciclovir, 900 mg twice daily for a minimum of 2–3 weeks followed by oral valganciclovir at 900 mg daily until day 100. This preemptive approach is effective but does miss a small number of patients in whom CMV disease would have been prevented had prophylaxis been used. Other preventive strategies include use of CMV-negative or leukocyte-depleted blood products for CMV-seronegative recipients.

C. Other Organisms

Routine decontamination of the gastrointestinal tract to prevent bacteremia in the neutropenic patient is not recommended. Prophylactic administration of antibiotics in the afebrile, asymptomatic neutropenic patient is controversial, although many centers have adopted this strategy. Rates of bacteremia are decreased, but overall mortality is not affected and emergence of resistant organisms is a risk. Use of intravenous immunoglobulin is reserved for the small number of patients with severe hypogammaglobulinemia following bone marrow transplantation and should not be routinely administered to all transplant patients.

Prophylaxis with antifungal agents to prevent invasive mold (primarily *Aspergillus*) and yeast (primarily *Candida*) infections is routinely used, but the optimal agent, dose, and duration have not been standardized. Moderate-dose (0.5 mg/kg/d) and low-dose (0.1–0.25 mg/kg/d) intravenous amphotericin, lipid-based preparations of amphotericin B, aerosolized amphotericin B, intravenous and oral voriconazole, and oral posaconazole solution have all been used in the neutropenic patient. Because voriconazole appears to be more effective than amphotericin for documented *Aspergillus* infections and because posaconazole prophylaxis (compared with fluconazole) has been shown to result in fewer cases of invasive aspergillosis among allogeneic stem cell transplant recipients with graft-versus-host disease, one approach to prophylaxis is to use oral fluconazole (400 mg/d) for patients at low risk for developing fungal infections (those who receive autologous bone marrow transplants) and oral voriconazole (200 mg twice daily) or oral posaconazole (200 mg solution three times daily) for those at high risk (allogeneic transplants, graft-versus-host disease) at least until engraftment (usually 30 days). In solid organ transplant recipients, the risk of invasive fungal infection varies considerably (1–2% in liver, pancreas, and kidney transplants and 6–8% in heart and lung transplants). Whether universal prophylaxis or observation with preemptive therapy is the best approach has not been determined. Although fluconazole is effective in preventing yeast infections, emergence of fluconazole-resistant *Candida* and molds (*Fusarium, Aspergillus, Mucor*) has raised concerns about its routine use as a prophylactic agent.

Given the high risk of reactivation of tuberculosis in patients taking TNF-α inhibitors, all patients should be screened for latent tuberculosis infection (LTBI) with a tuberculin skin test or an interferon-gamma release assay prior to the start of therapy. If LTBI is diagnosed, treatment with the TNF-α inhibitors should be delayed until treatment for LTBI is completed.

▶ Treatment

A. General Measures

Because infections in the immunocompromised patient can be rapidly progressive and life-threatening, diagnostic procedures must be performed promptly, and empiric therapy is usually instituted.

While reduction or discontinuation of immunosuppressive medication may jeopardize the viability of the transplanted organ, this measure may be necessary if the infection is life-threatening. Hematopoietic growth factors (granulocyte and granulocyte-macrophage colony-stimulating factors) stimulate proliferation of bone marrow stem cells, resulting in an increase in peripheral leukocytes. These agents shorten the period of neutropenia and have been associated with reduction in infection.

B. Specific Measures

Antimicrobial drug therapy ultimately should be based on culture results. While combinations of antimicrobials may be used to provide synergy or to prevent resistance, the primary reason for empiric combination therapy is broad-spectrum coverage of multiple pathogens (since infections in these patients are often polymicrobial).

Empiric therapy is often instituted at the earliest sign of infection in the immunosuppressed patient because prompt therapy favorably affects outcome. The antibiotic or combination of antibiotics used depends on the type of immunocompromise and the site of infection. For example, in the febrile neutropenic patient, an algorithmic approach to therapy is often used. Febrile neutropenic patients should be empirically treated with broad-spectrum agents active against gram-positive organisms, *Pseudomonas aeruginosa*, and other gram-negative bacilli (such as cefepime 2 g every 8 hours intravenously). The addition of vancomycin, 10–15 mg/kg/dose intravenously every 12 hours, should be considered in those patients with suspected infection due to methicillin-resistant *S aureus* (MRSA), *S epidermidis*, and enterococcus. Continued neutropenic fever necessitates broadening of antibacterial coverage from cefepime to agents such as imipenem 500 mg every 6 hours intravenously with or without tobramycin, 5 mg/kg intravenously every 24 hours. Antifungal agents (such as voriconazole 200 mg intravenously or orally every 12 hours, or caspofungin, 50 mg daily intravenously) should be added if fevers continue after 5–7 days of broad-spectrum antibacterial therapy. Regardless of whether the patient becomes afebrile, therapy is continued until resolution of neutropenia. Failure to continue antibiotics through the period of neutropenia has been associated with increase morbidity and mortality.

Patients with fever and low-risk neutropenia (neutropenia expected to persist for less than 10 days, no comorbid complications requiring hospitalization, and cancer adequately treated) can be treated with oral antibiotic regimens, such as ciprofloxacin, 750 mg every 12 hours, plus amoxicillin-clavulanic acid, 500 mg every 8 hours. Antibiotics are continued as long as the patient is neutropenic even if a source is not identified. In the organ transplant patient with interstitial infiltrates, the main concern is infection with *Pneumocystis* or *Legionella* species, so that empiric treatment with a macrolide (or fluoroquinolone) and TMP-SMZ, 15 mg/kg/d orally or intravenously (based on trimethoprim component) would be reasonable in those patients not receiving TMP-SMZ prophylaxis. If the patient does not respond to empiric treatment, a decision must be made to add more antimicrobial agents or perform invasive procedures (see above) to make a specific diagnosis. By making a specific diagnosis, therapy can be specific and polypharmacy with multiple potentially toxic agents can be avoided.

When to Refer

- Any immunocompromised patient with an opportunistic infection.
- Patients with potential drug toxicities and drug interactions related to antimicrobials where alternative agents are sought.
- Patients with LTBI in whom therapy with TNF-α inhibitors is planned.

When to Admit

Immunocompromised patients who are febrile, or those without fevers in whom an infection is suspected, particularly in the following groups: solid-organ or hematopoietic stem cell transplant recipient (particularly in the first 6 months), neutropenic patients, patients receiving TNF-α inhibitors, transplant recipients who have had recent rejection episodes (including graft-versus-host disease).

Bucaneve G et al. Levofloxacin to prevent bacterial infection in patients with cancer and neutropenia. N Engl J Med. 2005 Sep 8;353(10):977–87. [PMID: 16148283]

Fishman JA. Infection in solid-organ transplant recipients. N Engl J Med. 2007;357(25):2601–14. [PMID: 18094380]

Small LN et al. Preventing post-organ transplantation cytomegalovirus disease with ganciclovir: a meta-analysis comparing prophylactic and preemptive therapies. Clin Infect Dis. 2006 Oct 1;43(7):869–80. [PMID: 16941368]

Ullmann AJ et al. Posaconazole or fluconazole for prophylaxis in severe graft-versus-host disease. N Engl J Med. 2007 Jan 25; 356(4):335–47. [PMID: 17251530]

Walsh TJ et al. Treatment of aspergillosis: clinical practice guidelines of the Infectious Diseases Society of America. Clin Infect Dis. 2008 Feb 1;46(3):327–60. [PMID: 18177225]

Winthrop KL et al. Mycobacterial and other serious infections in patients receiving anti-tumor necrosis factor and other newly approved biologic therapies: case finding through the Emerging Infections Network. Clin Infect Dis. 2008 Jun 1;46(11):1738–40. [PMID: 18419421]

HOSPITAL-ASSOCIATED INFECTIONS

ESSENTIALS OF DIAGNOSIS

- Hospital-associated infections are defined as those not present or incubating at the time of hospital admission and developing 48–72 hours after admission.

- Hand washing is the most effective means of preventing hospital-associated infections and should be done routinely even when gloves are worn.

General Considerations

In the United States, approximately 5% of patients acquire a hospital-associated infection, resulting in prolongation of the hospital stay, increase in cost of care, significant morbidity, and a 5% mortality rate. The most common infections are urinary tract infections, usually associated with Foley catheters or urologic procedures; bloodstream infections, most commonly from indwelling catheters but also from secondary sites, such as surgical wounds, abscesses, pneumonia, the genitourinary tract, and the gastrointestinal tract; pneumonia in intubated patients or those with altered levels of consciousness; surgical wound infections; MRSA infections; and *Clostridium difficile* colitis.

Some general principles are helpful in preventing, diagnosing, and treating hospital-associated infections:

1. Many infections are a direct result of the use of invasive devices for monitoring or therapy, such as intravenous catheters, Foley catheters, shunts, surgical drains, catheters placed by interventional radiology for drainage, nasogastric tubes, and orotracheal or nasotracheal tubes for ventilatory support. Early removal of such devices reduces the possibility of infection.

2. Patients in whom hospital-associated infections develop are often critically ill, have been hospitalized for extended periods, and have received several courses of broad-spectrum antibiotic therapy. As a result, hospital-associated infections are often due to multidrug resistant pathogens and are different from those encountered in community-acquired infections. For example, *S aureus* and *S epidermidis* (a frequent cause of prosthetic device infection) are often resistant to nafcillin and cephalosporins and require vancomycin for therapy; *Enterococcus faecium* resistant to ampicillin and vancomycin; gram-negative infections caused by *Pseudomonas, Citrobacter, Enterobacter, Acinetobacter,* and *Stenotrophomonas,* which may be resistant to most antibacterials. When choosing antibiotics to treat the seriously ill patient with a hospital-associated infection, antimicrobial history and the "local ecology" must be considered. In seriously ill patients, broad-spectrum coverage with vancomycin and a carbapenem with or without an aminoglycoside is recommended. Once a pathogen is isolated and susceptibilities are known, the most narrow spectrum, least toxic, most cost-effective drug should be used.

Widespread use of antimicrobial drugs contributes to the selection of drug-resistant organisms, thus every effort should be made to limit the spectrum of coverage and unnecessary duration. All too often, unreliable or uninterpretable specimens are obtained for culture that result in unnecessary use of antibiotics. The best example of this principle is the diagnosis of line-related or bloodstream infection in the febrile patient (see below). To avoid unnecessary use of antibiotics, thoughtful consideration of culture results is mandatory. A positive wound culture without signs of inflammation or infection, a positive sputum culture without pulmonary infiltrates on chest radiograph, or a positive urine culture in a catheterized patient without symptoms or signs of pyelonephritis are all likely to represent colonization, not infection.

▶ **Clinical Findings**

A. Symptoms and Signs

Catheter-associated infections have a variable presentation, depending on the type of catheter used (peripheral or central venous catheters, nontunneled or tunneled). Local signs of infection may be present at the insertion site, with pain, erythema, and purulence. Fever is often absent in uncomplicated infections and if present, may indicate more disseminated disease such as bacteremia, cellulitis and septic thrombophlebitis. Often signs of infection at the insertion site are absent.

1. Fever in an intensive care unit patient—Fever complicates up to 70% of patients in intensive care units, and the etiology of the fever may be infectious or noninfectious. Common infectious causes include catheter-associated infections, hospital-acquired and ventilator-associated pneumonia (see Chapter 9), surgical site infections, urinary tract infections, and sepsis. Clinically relevant sinusitis is relatively uncommon in the patient in the intensive care unit.

An important noninfectious cause is thromboembolic disease. Fever in conjunction with refractory hypotension and shock may suggest sepsis; however, adrenal insufficiency, thyroid storm, and transfusion reaction may have a similar clinical presentation. Drug fever is difficult to diagnose and is usually a diagnosis of exclusion unless there are other signs of hypersensitivity, such as a typical maculopapular rash.

2. Fever in the postoperative patient—Postoperative fever is very common and in many cases resolves spontaneously. Etiologies are both infectious and noninfectious. Timing of the fever in relation to the surgery and the nature of the surgical procedure may help diagnostically.

A. Immediate fever (in the first few hours after surgery)—Immediate fever can be due to medications that were given perioperatively, to the trauma of surgery itself, or to infections that were present before surgery. Necrotizing fasciitis due to group A streptococci or mixed organisms may present in this period. Malignant hyperthermia is rare and presents 30 minutes to several hours following inhalational anesthesia and is characterized by extreme hyperthermia, muscle rigidity, rhabdomyolysis, electrolyte abnormalities, and hypotension. Aggressive cooling and dantrolene are the mainstays of therapy. Aspiration of acidic gastric contents during surgery can cause a chemical pneumonitis (Mendelson syndrome) that rapidly develops but is transient and does not require intervention. Fever due to the trauma of surgery itself usually resolves in 2–3 days, longer in more complicated operative cases and in patients with head trauma.

B. Acute fever (within 1 week of surgery)—Acute fever is usually due to common causes of hospital-associated infections, such as ventilator-associated pneumonia (including aspiration pneumonia in patients with decreased gag reflex) and line infections. Noninfectious causes include alcohol withdrawal, gout, pulmonary embolism, and pancreatitis. Atelectasis following surgery is commonly invoked as a cause of postoperative fever but there is no good evidence to support a causal association between the presence or degree of atelectasis and fever.

C. Subacute fever (at least 1 week after surgery)—Surgical site infections commonly present at least 1 week after surgery. The type of surgery that was performed predicts specific infectious etiologies. Patients undergoing cardiothoracic surgery may be at higher risk for pneumonia and deep and superficial sternal wound infections. Meningitis without typical signs of meningismus may complicate neurosurgical procedures. Abdominal surgery may result in deep abdominal abscesses that require drainage.

B. Laboratory Findings

Blood cultures are universally recommended, and chest radiographs are frequently obtained. A properly prepared sputum Gram stain and semi-quantitative sputum cultures may be useful in selected patients where there is a high pretest probability of pneumonia but multiple exclusion criteria probably limit generalizability in most patients, such as immunocompromised patients and those with drug resistance. Other diagnostic strategies will be dictated by the clinical context (eg, transesophageal echocardiogram in a patient with *S aureus* bacteremia).

Any fever in a patient with a central venous catheter should prompt the collection of blood. The best method to evaluate bacteremia is to gather at least two peripherally obtained blood cultures. Blood cultures from unidentified sites, a single blood culture from any site, or a blood culture through an existing line will often be positive for *S epidermidis*, resulting in the inappropriate use of vancomycin. Unless two separate venipuncture cultures are obtained—not through catheters—interpretation of results is impossible and unnecessary therapy may be given. Every such "pseudobacteremia" increases laboratory costs, antibiotic use, and length of stay. Microbiologic evaluation of the removed catheter can sometimes be helpful, but only in addition to (not instead of) blood cultures drawn from peripheral sites. The differential time to positivity measures the difference in time that cultures simultaneously drawn through a catheter and a peripheral site become positive. A positive test (about 120 minutes difference in time) supports a catheter-related bloodstream infection, and a negative test may permit catheters to be retained.

▶ **Complications**

Patients who have persistent bacteremia and fever despite removal of the infected catheter may have complications such as septic thrombophlebitis, endocarditis, or metastatic foci of infection (particularly with *S aureus*). Additional studies such as venous Doppler studies, transesophageal echocardiogram, and chest radiographs may be indicated, and 4–6 weeks of antibiotics may be needed. In the case of septic thrombophlebitis, anticoagulation with heparin is also recommended if there are no contraindications.

Differential Diagnosis

Although most fevers are due to infections, about 25% of patients will have fever of noninfectious origin, including drug fever, nonspecific postoperative fevers (tissue damage or necrosis), hematoma, pancreatitis, pulmonary embolism, myocardial infarction, and ischemic bowel disease.

Prevention

The concept of universal precautions emphasizes that all patients are treated as though they have a potential bloodborne transmissible disease, and thus all body secretions are handled with care to prevent spread of disease. Body substance isolation requires use of gloves whenever a health care worker anticipates contact with blood or other body secretions. Even though gloves are worn, health care workers should routinely wash their hands, since it is the easiest and most effective means of preventing hospital-associated infections. Application of a rapid drying, alcohol-based antiseptic is simple, takes less time than traditional hand washing with soap and water, is more effective at reducing hand colonization, and promotes compliance with hand decontamination.

Peripheral intravenous lines should be replaced every 3 days, and arterial lines should be replaced every 4 days. Lines in the central venous circulation (including those placed peripherally) can be left in place indefinitely and are changed or removed when they are clinically suspected of being infected, when they are nonfunctional, or when they are no longer needed. Using sterile barrier precautions (including cap, mask, gown, gloves, and drape) is recommended while inserting central venous catheters. Silver alloy–impregnated Foley catheters reduce the incidence of catheter-associated bacteriuria, and antibiotic-impregnated (minocycline plus rifampin or chlorhexidine plus silver sulfadiazine) venous catheters reduce line infections and bacteremia. Silver-coated endotracheal tubes may reduce the incidence of ventilator-associated pneumonia. Whether the increased cost of these devices justifies their routine use should be determined by individual institutions. Perioperative administration of chlorhexadine intranasal ointment and oropharyngeal rinse has been shown to reduce the incidence of infection following surgery. Daily bathing of ICU patients with chlorhexadine-impregnated washcloths versus soap and water may result in lower risk of catheter-associated bloodstream infections. Selective decontamination of the digestive tract with nonabsorbable or parenteral antibiotics, or both, may prevent hospital-acquired pneumonia and decrease mortality.

Attentive nursing care (positioning to prevent decubitus ulcers, wound care, elevating the head during tube feedings to prevent aspiration) is critical in preventing hospital-associated infections. In addition, monitoring of high-risk areas by hospital epidemiologists is critical in the prevention of infection. Some guidelines advocate rapid screening for MRSA on admission to acute care facilities among certain subpopulations of patients (eg, those recently hospitalized, admission to the intensive care unit, patients undergoing hemodialysis). However, it is not clear whether this strategy decreases the incidence of hospital-associated MRSA infections.

Vaccines, including hepatitis A, hepatitis B, and the varicella, pneumococcal, influenza vaccination are important adjuncts. (See section below on Immunization against Infectious Diseases.)

Treatment

A. Fever in an Intensive Care Unit Patient

Unless the patient has a central neurologic injury with elevated intracranial pressure or has a temperature > 41 °C, there is less physiologic need to maintain euthermia. Empiric broad-spectrum antibiotics (as noted above) are recommended for neutropenic and other immunocompromised patients and in patients who are clinically unstable.

B. Catheter-Associated Infections

Factors that inform treatment decisions include the type of catheter, the causative pathogen, the availability of alternate catheter access sites, the need for ongoing intravascular access, and the severity of disease.

In general, catheters should be removed if there is purulence at the exit site; if the organism is S aureus, gram-negative rods, or Candida species; if there is persistent bacteremia (> 48 hours while receiving antibiotics); or if complications, such as septic thrombophlebitis, endocarditis, or other metastatic disease exist. Central venous catheters may be exchanged over a guidewire provided there is no erythema or purulence at the exit site and the patient does not appear to be septic. Methicillin-resistant, coagulase-negative staphylococci are the most common pathogens; thus, empiric therapy with vancomycin, 15 mg/kg IV twice daily, should be given assuming normal kidney function. Empiric gram-negative coverage may be considered in patients who are immunocompromised or who are critically ill.

Antibiotic treatment duration depends on the pathogen and the extent of disease. For uncomplicated bacteremia, 5–7 days of therapy is usually sufficient for coagulase-negative staphylococci, even if the original catheter is retained. Fourteen days of therapy is generally recommended for uncomplicated bacteremia caused by gram-negative rods, Candida species, and S aureus.

When to Refer

- Any patient with multidrug-resistant infection.
- Any patient with fungemia or persistent bacteremia.
- Patients with multisite infections.
- Patients with impaired or fluctuating kidney function for assistance with dosing of antimicrobials.

Bleasdale SC et al. Effectiveness of chlorhexidine bathing to reduce catheter-associated bloodstream infections in medical intensive care unit patients. Arch Intern Med. 2007;167(19):2073–9. [PMID: 17954801]

Bouza E et al. A randomized and prospective study of 3 procedures for the diagnosis of catheter-related bloodstream infection without catheter withdrawal. Clin Infect Dis. 2007;44(6):820–6. [PMID: 17304454]

Canadian Critical Care Trials Group. A randomized trial of diagnostic techniques for ventilator-associated pneumonia. N Engl J Med. 2006 Dec 21;355(25):2619–30. [PMID: 17182987]

Harbarth S et al. Universal screening for methicillin-resistant *Staphylococcus aureus* at hospital admission and nosocomial infection in surgical patients. JAMA. 2008 Mar 12;299(10):1149–57. [PMID: 18334690]

Kollef MH et al. Silver-coated endotracheal tubes and incidence of ventilator-associated pneumonia: the NASCENT randomized trial. JAMA. 2008 Aug 20;300(7):805–13. [PMID: 18714060]

Pronovost P et al. An intervention to decrease catheter-related bloodstream infections in the ICU. N Engl J Med. 2006 Dec 28;355(26):2725–32. [PMID: 17192537]

Segers P et al. Prevention of nosocomial infection in cardiac surgery by decontamination of the nasopharynx and oropharynx with chlorhexadine gluconate: a randomized controlled trial. JAMA. 2006 Nov 22;296(20):2460–6. [PMID: 17119142]

Yokoe DS et al. A compendium of strategies to prevent healthcare-associated infections in acute care hospitals. Infect Control Hosp Epidemiol. 2008 Oct;29(Suppl 1):S12–21. [PMID: 18840084]

INFECTIONS OF THE CENTRAL NERVOUS SYSTEM

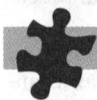 ESSENTIALS OF DIAGNOSIS

- ▶ Central nervous system infection is a medical emergency.
- ▶ Symptoms and signs common to all central nervous system infections include headache, fever, sensorial disturbances, neck and back stiffness, positive Kernig and Brudzinski signs, and cerebrospinal fluid abnormalities.

▶ General Considerations

Infections of the central nervous system can be caused by almost any infectious agent, including bacteria, mycobacteria, fungi, spirochetes, protozoa, helminths, and viruses. The classic triad of fever, stiff neck and altered mental status has a low sensitivity (44%) for bacterial meningitis. However, nearly all patients with bacterial meningitis have at least two of the following symptoms—fever, headache, stiff neck, or altered mental status.

▶ Etiologic Classification

Central nervous system infections can be divided into several categories that usually can be readily distinguished from each other by cerebrospinal fluid examination as the first step toward etiologic diagnosis (Table 30–1).

A. Purulent Meningitis

Patients with bacterial meningitis usually seek medical attention within hours or 1–2 days after onset of symptoms. The organisms responsible depend primarily on the age of the patient as summarized in Table 30–2. The diagnosis is usually based on the Gram-stained smear (positive in 60–90%) or culture (positive in over 90%).

B. Chronic Meningitis

The presentation of chronic meningitis is less acute than purulent meningitis. Patients with chronic meningitis usually have a history of symptoms lasting weeks to months. The most common pathogens are *Mycobacterium tuberculosis*, atypical mycobacteria, fungi (*Cryptococcus, Coccidioides, Histoplasma*), and spirochetes (*Treponema pallidum* and *Borrelia burgdorferi*, the cause of Lyme disease). The diagnosis is made by culture or in some cases by serologic tests (cryptococcosis, coccidioidomycosis, syphilis, Lyme disease).

Table 30–1. Typical cerebrospinal fluid findings in various central nervous system diseases.

Diagnosis	Cells/mcL	Glucose (mg/dL)	Protein (mg/dL)	Opening Pressure
Normal	0–5 lymphocytes	45–85[1]	15–45	70–180 mm H$_2$O
Purulent meningitis (bacterial)[2] community-acquired	200–20,000 polymorphonuclear neutrophils	Low (< 45)	High (> 50)	Markedly elevated
Granulomatous meningitis (mycobacterial, fungal)[3]	100–1000, mostly lymphocytes[3]	Low (< 45)	High (> 50)	Moderately elevated
Spirochetal meningitis	100–1000, mostly lymphocytes[3]	Normal	Moderately high (> 50)	Normal to slightly elevated
Aseptic meningitis, viral or meningoencephalitis[4]	25–2000, mostly lymphocytes[3]	Normal or low	High (> 50)	Slightly elevated
"Neighborhood reaction"[5]	Variably increased	Normal	Normal or high	Variable

[1]Cerebrospinal fluid glucose must be considered in relation to blood glucose level. Normally, cerebrospinal fluid glucose is 20–30 mg/dL lower than blood glucose, or 50–70% of the normal value of blood glucose.
[2]Organisms in smear or culture of cerebrospinal fluid; counterimmunoelectrophoresis or latex agglutination may be diagnostic.
[3]Polymorphonuclear neutrophils may predominate early.
[4]Viral isolation from cerebrospinal fluid early; antibody titer rise in paired specimens of serum; polymerase chain reaction for herpesvirus.
[5]May occur in mastoiditis, brain abscess, epidural abscess, sinusitis, septic thrombus, brain tumor. Cerebrospinal fluid culture results usually negative.

Table 30–2. Initial antimicrobial therapy for purulent meningitis of unknown cause.

Population	Common Microorganisms	Standard Therapy
18–50 years	Streptococcus pneumoniae, Neisseria meningitidis	Vancomycin[1] **plus** cefotaxime or ceftriaxone[2]
Over 50 years	S pneumoniae, N meningitidis, Listeria monocytogenes, gram-negative bacilli	Vancomycin[1] **plus** ampicillin,[3] **plus** cefotaxime or ceftriaxone[2]
Impaired cellular immunity	L monocytogenes, gram-negative bacilli, S pneumoniae	Vancomycin[1] **plus** ampicillin[3] **plus** ceftazidime[4]
Postsurgical or posttraumatic	Staphylococcus aureus, S pneumoniae, gram-negative bacilli	Vancomycin[1] **plus** ceftazidime[4]

[1]The dose of vancomycin is 10–15 mg/kg/dose IV every 6 hours.
[2]The usual dose of cefotaxime is 2 g IV every 6 hours and that of ceftriaxone is 2 g IV every 12 hours. If the organism is sensitive to penicillin, 3–4 million units IV every 4 hours is given.
[3]The dose of ampicillin is usually 2 g IV every 4 hours.
[4]Ceftazidime is given in a dose of 50–100 mg/kg IV every 8 hours.

C. Aseptic Meningitis

Aseptic meningitis—a much more benign and self-limited syndrome than purulent meningitis—is caused principally by viruses, especially herpes simplex virus and the enterovirus group (including coxsackieviruses and echoviruses). Infectious mononucleosis may be accompanied by aseptic meningitis. Leptospiral infection is also usually placed in the aseptic group because of the lymphocytic cellular response and its relatively benign course. This type of meningitis also occurs during secondary syphilis and disseminated Lyme disease. Prior to the routine administration of measles-mumps-rubella (MMR) vaccines, mumps was the most common cause of viral meningitis.

D. Encephalitis

Encephalitis (due to herpesviruses, arboviruses, rabies virus, flaviviruses [West Nile encephalitis, Japanese encephalitis], and many others) produces disturbances of the sensorium, seizures, and many other manifestations. Patients are more ill than those with aseptic meningitis. Cerebrospinal fluid may be entirely normal or may show some lymphocytes and in some instances (eg, herpes simplex) red cells as well.

E. Partially Treated Bacterial Meningitis

Previous effective antibiotic therapy given for 12–24 hours will decrease the rate of positive Gram stain results by 20% and culture by 30–40% but will have little effect on cell count, protein, or glucose. Occasionally, previous antibiotic therapy will change a predominantly polymorphonuclear response to a lymphocytic pleocytosis, and some of the cerebrospinal fluid findings may be similar to those seen in aseptic meningitis.

F. Neighborhood Reaction

As noted in Table 30–1, this term denotes a purulent infectious process in close proximity to the central nervous system that spills some of the products of the inflammatory process—white blood cells or protein—into the cerebrospinal fluid. Such an infection might be a brain abscess, osteomyelitis of the vertebrae, epidural abscess, subdural empyema, or bacterial sinusitis or mastoiditis.

G. Noninfectious Meningeal Irritation

Carcinomatous meningitis, sarcoidosis, systemic lupus erythematosus, chemical meningitis, and certain drugs—nonsteroidal anti-inflammatory drugs, muromonab-CD3 (OKT3), TMP-SMZ, and others—can also produce symptoms and signs of meningeal irritation with associated cerebrospinal fluid pleocytosis, increased protein, and low or normal glucose. Meningismus with normal cerebrospinal fluid findings occurs in the presence of other infections such as pneumonia and shigellosis.

H. Brain Abscess

Brain abscess presents as a space-occupying lesion; symptoms may include vomiting, fever, change of mental status, or focal neurologic manifestations. When brain abscess is suspected, a CT scan should be performed. If positive, lumbar puncture should *not* be performed since results rarely provide clinically useful information and herniation can occur. The bacteriology of brain abscess is usually polymicrobial and includes S aureus, gram-negative bacilli, streptococci, and anaerobes (including anaerobic streptococci and Prevotella species).

I. Amebic Meningoencephalitis

These infections are caused by free-living amebas and present as two distinct syndromes. The diagnosis is confirmed by culture (Acanthamoeba species and Balamuthia mandrillaris) or identification of the organism in a wet mount of cerebrospinal fluid (Naegleria fowleri) or on biopsy specimens. No effective therapy is available.

Primary amebic meningoencephalitis is caused by N fowleri and is an acute fulminant disease, usually seen in children and young adults with recent fresh water exposure, and is characterized by signs of meningeal irritation that rapidly progresses to encephalitis and death. Rare cures have been reported with intravenous and intraventricular administration of amphotericin B.

Granulomatous amebic encephalitis is caused by *Acanthamoeba* species. It is an indolent disease, frequently seen in immunocompromised patients and associated with cutaneous lesions. Central nervous system disease is characterized by headache, nausea, vomiting, cranial neuropathies, seizures, and hemiparesis. Infections with *Balamuthia* are similar to *Acanthamoeba* in that the course is subacute to chronic, but unlike *Acanthamoeba* both immunocompromised and immunocompetent persons can be affected.

▶ Clinical Findings

A. Laboratory Tests

Evaluation of a patient with suspected meningitis includes a history, physical examination, blood count, blood culture, lumbar puncture followed by careful study and culture of the cerebrospinal fluid, and a chest film. The fluid must be examined for cell count, glucose, and protein, and a smear stained for bacteria (and acid-fast organisms when appropriate) and cultured for pyogenic organisms and for mycobacteria and fungi when indicated. Latex agglutination tests can detect antigens of encapsulated organisms (*S pneumoniae, H influenzae, N meningitidis,* and *Cryptococcus neoformans*) but are rarely used except for detection of *Cryptococcus* or in partially treated patients. Polymerase chain reaction (PCR) testing of cerebrospinal fluid has been used to detect bacteria (*S pneumoniae, H influenzae, N meningitidis, M tuberculosis, B burgdorferi,* and *Tropheryma whippelii*) and viruses (herpes simplex, varicella-zoster, CMV, Epstein-Barr virus, and enteroviruses) in patients with meningitis. The greatest experience is with PCR for herpes simplex and varicella-zoster, and the tests are very sensitive (> 95%) and specific. Tests to detect the other organisms may not be any more sensitive than culture, but the real value is the rapidity with which results are available, ie, hours compared with days or weeks. At present, with the exception of PCR for herpes simplex, these tests are performed only in reference laboratories. Although it is difficult to prove with existing clinical data that early antibiotic therapy improves outcome in bacterial meningitis, prompt therapy is still recommended.

B. Lumbar Puncture and Imaging

Since performing a lumbar puncture in the presence of a space-occupying lesion (brain abscess, subdural hematoma, subdural empyema, necrotic temporal lobe from herpes encephalitis) may result in brainstem herniation, a CT scan is performed prior to lumbar puncture if a space-occupying lesion is suspected on the basis of papilledema, seizures, or focal neurologic findings. Other indications for CT scan are an immunocompromised patient or moderate to severely impaired level of consciousness. If delays are encountered in obtaining a CT scan and bacterial meningitis is suspected, blood cultures should be drawn and antibiotics and corticosteroids administered even before cerebrospinal fluid is obtained for culture to avoid delay in treatment (Table 30–1). Antibiotics given within 4 hours

before obtaining cerebrospinal fluid probably do not affect culture results.

▶ Treatment

Increased intracranial pressure due to brain edema often requires therapeutic attention. Hyperventilation, mannitol (25–50 g as a bolus intravenous infusion), and even drainage of cerebrospinal fluid by repeated lumbar punctures or by placement of ventricular catheters have been used to control cerebral edema and increased intracranial pressure. Dexamethasone (4 mg intravenously every 4–6 hours) may also decrease cerebral edema. In purulent meningitis, the identity of the causative microorganism may remain unknown or doubtful for a few days and initial antibiotic treatment as set forth in Table 30–2 should be directed against the microorganisms most common for each age group.

The duration of therapy for bacterial meningitis varies depending on the etiologic agent: *H influenzae,* 7 days; *N meningitidis,* 3–7 days; *S pneumoniae,* 10–14 days; *L monocytogenes,* 14–21 days; and gram-negative bacilli, 21 days.

Dexamethasone therapy is recommended for adults with pneumococcal meningitis. Ten milligrams of dexamethasone administered intravenously 15–20 minutes before or simultaneously with the first dose of antibiotics and continued every 6 hours for 4 days decreases morbidity and mortality. Patients most likely to benefit from corticosteroids are those infected with gram-positive organisms (*Streptococcus pneumoniae* or *Streptococcus suis*), and those who are HIV negative. The number of patients with meningitis due to *N meningitidis* and other bacterial pathogens studied does not support similar conclusions.

Therapy of brain abscess consists of drainage (excision or aspiration) in addition to 3–4 weeks of systemic antibiotics directed against organisms isolated. An empiric regimen often includes metronidazole, 500 mg intravenously or orally every 8 hours, plus ceftriaxone, 2 g intravenously every 12 hours, with or without vancomycin, 10–15 mg/kg/dose intravenously every 12 hours. In cases where abscesses are less than 2 cm in size, where there are multiple abscesses that cannot be drained, or if an abscess is located in an area where significant neurologic sequelae would result from drainage, antibiotics for 6–8 weeks without drainage can be used.

Therapy of other types of meningitis is discussed elsewhere in this book (fungal meningitis, Chapter 36; syphilis and Lyme borreliosis, Chapter 34; tuberculous meningitis, Chapter 33; herpes encephalitis, Chapter 32).

▶ When to Refer

- Patients with acute meningitis, particularly if culture negative or atypical (eg, fungi, syphilis, Lyme disease, *M tuberculosis*), or if the patient is immunosuppressed.
- Patients with chronic meningitis.
- All patients with brain abscesses and encephalitis.
- Patients with suspected hospital-acquired meningitis (eg, in patients who have undergone recent neurosurgery).
- Patients with recurrent meningitis.

When to Admit

- Patients with suspected acute meningitis, encephalitis, and brain abscess should be admitted for urgent evaluation and treatment.

- There is less urgency to admit patients with chronic meningitis; these patients may be admitted to expedite diagnostic procedures and coordinate care, particularly if no diagnosis has been made in the outpatient setting.

Bernardini GL. Diagnosis and management of brain abscess and subdural empyema. Curr Neurol Neurosci. 2004 Nov;4(6):448–56. [PMID: 15509445]

Glaser CA et al. Beyond viruses: Clinical profiles and etiologies associated with encephalitis. Clin Infect Dis. 2006 Dec 15;43(12):1565–77. [PMID: 17109290]

Logan SA et al. Viral meningitis. BMJ. 2008 Jan 5;336(7634):36–40. [PMID: 18174598]

Nguyen TH et al. Dexamethasone in Vietnamese adolescents and adults with bacterial meningitis. N Engl J Med. 2007 Dec 13;357(24):2431–40. [PMID: 18077808]

Tunkel AR et al. Practice guidelines for the management of bacterial meningitis. Clin Infect Dis. 2004 Nov 1;39(9):1267–84. [PMID: 15494903]

van de Beek D et al. Community-acquired bacterial meningitis in adults. N Engl J Med. 2006 Jan 5;354(1):44–53. [PMID: 16394301]

van de Beek D et al. Corticosteroids for acute bacterial meningitis. Cochrane Database Syst Rev. 2007 Jan 24;(1):CD004405. [PMID: 17253505]

ANIMAL & HUMAN BITE WOUNDS

ESSENTIALS OF DIAGNOSIS

- ▶ Cat and human bites have higher rates of infection than dog bites.

- ▶ Hand bites are particularly concerning for the possibility of closed-space infection.

- ▶ Antibiotic prophylaxis indicated for noninfected bites of the hand and hospitalization required for infected hand bites.

- ▶ All infected wounds need to be cultured to direct therapy.

General Considerations

About 1000 dog bite injuries require emergency department attention each day, most often in urban areas. Dog bites occur most commonly in the summer months. Biting animals are usually known by their victims, and most biting incidents are provoked (ie, bites occur while playing with the animal or after surprising the animal or waking it abruptly from sleep). Failure to elicit a history of provocation is important, because an unprovoked attack raises the possibility of rabies. Human bites are usually inflicted by children while playing or fighting; in adults, bites are associated with alcohol use and closed-fist injuries that occur during fights.

The animal inflicting the bite, the location of the bite, and the type of injury inflicted are all important determinants of whether they become infected. Cat bites are more likely to become infected than human bites—between 30% and 50% of all cat bites become infected. Infections following human bites are variable: Those inflicted by children rarely become infected because they are superficial, and bites by adults become infected in 15–30% of cases, with a particularly high rate of infection in closed-fist injuries. "Through and through" bites (eg involving the mucosa and the skin) have an infection rate similar to closed-fist injuries. Dog bites, for unclear reasons, become infected only 5% of the time. Bites of the head, face, and neck are less likely to become infected than bites on the extremities. Puncture wounds become infected more frequently than lacerations, probably because the latter are easier to irrigate and debride.

The bacteriology of bite infections is polymicrobial. Following dog and cat bites, over 50% of infections are caused by aerobes and anaerobes and 36% are due to aerobes alone. Pure anaerobic infections are rare. *Pasteurella* species are the single most common isolate (75% of cat bites and 50% of dog bites). Other common aerobic isolates include streptococci, staphylococci, *Moraxella,* and *Neisseria;* the most common anaerobes are *Fusobacterium, Bacteroides, Porphyromonas,* and *Prevotella.* The median number of isolates following human bites is four (three aerobes and one anaerobe). Like dog and cat bites, most human bites are a mixture of aerobes and anaerobes (54%) or are due to aerobes alone (44%). *Streptococcus, Staphylococcus,* and *Eikenella corrodens* (found in 30% of patients) are the most common aerobes. *Prevotella* and *Fusobacterium* are the most common anaerobes. Although the organisms noted are the most common, innumerable others have been isolated—including *Capnocytophaga* (dog and cats), *Pseudomonas,* and *Haemophilus*—emphasizing the point that all infected bites should be cultured to define the microbiology.

HIV can be transmitted from bites (either from biting or receiving a bite from an HIV-infected patient) but has rarely been reported.

Treatment

A. Local Care

Vigorous cleansing and irrigation of the wound as well as debridement of necrotic material are the most important factors in decreasing the incidence of infections. Radiographs should be obtained to look for fractures and the presence of foreign bodies. Careful examination to assess the extent of the injury (tendon laceration, joint space penetration) is critical to appropriate care.

B. Suturing

If wounds require closure for cosmetic or mechanical reasons, suturing can be done. However, one should never suture an infected wound, and wounds of the hand should generally not be sutured since a closed-space infection of the hand can result in loss of function.

C. Prophylactic Antibiotics

Prophylaxis is indicated in high-risk bites and in high-risk patients. Cat bites in any location and hand bites by any animal, including humans, should receive prophylaxis. Individuals with certain comorbidities (diabetes, liver disease) are at increased risk for severe complications and should receive prophylaxis even for low-risk bites, as should patients without functional spleens who are at increased risk for overwhelming sepsis (primarily with *Capnocytophaga* species). Amoxicillin-clavulanate (Augmentin) 500 mg orally three times daily for 5–7 days is the regimen of choice. For patients with serious allergy to penicillin, a combination of clindamycin 300 mg orally three times daily plus doxycycline 100 mg orally twice daily, or double-strength TMP-SMZ orally twice daily, or a fluoroquinolone (ciprofloxacin 500 mg orally twice daily or levofloxacin 500–750 mg orally once daily) is recommended. Agents such as dicloxacillin, cephalexin, erythromycin, and clindamycin should not be used alone because they lack activity against *Pasteurella* species. Doxycycline and TMP-SMZ have poor activity against anaerobes and should only be used in combination with clindamycin. Moxifloxacin, a fluoroquinolone with good aerobic and anaerobic activity, may be suitable as monotherapy.

Because the risk of HIV transmission is so low following a bite, routine postexposure prophylaxis is not recommended. Each case should be evaluated individually and consideration for prophylaxis should be given to those who present within 72 hours of the incident, the source is known to be HIV infected, and the exposure is high risk.

D. Antibiotics for Documented Infection

For wounds that are infected, antibiotics are clearly indicated. How they are given (orally or intravenously) and the need for hospitalization are individualized clinical decisions. The most commonly encountered pathogens are adequately covered by a combination of a β-lactam plus a β-lactamase inhibitor (ampicillin-sulbactam [Unasyn], 1.5–3.0 g intravenously every 6–8 hours; piperacillin-tazobactam [Zosyn], 3.375 g intravenously every 6–8 hours; or amoxicillin-clavulanate [Augmentin], 500 mg orally three times daily) or carbapenems (ertapenem, 1 g intravenously daily; imipenem, 500 mg intravenously every 6–8 hours; meropenem, 1 g intravenously every 8 hours). For the patient with severe penicillin allergy, a combination of clindamycin 600–900 mg intravenously every 8 hours plus a fluoroquinolone (ciprofloxacin, 400 mg intravenously every 12 hours; levofloxacin, 500–750 mg intravenously once daily) or TMP-SMZ (10 mg/kg of trimethoprim daily in two or three divided doses) is indicated. Duration of therapy is usually 2–3 weeks unless complications such as septic arthritis or osteomyelitis are present; if these complications are present, therapy should be extended to 4 and 6 weeks, respectively.

E. Tetanus and Rabies

All patients must be evaluated for the need for tetanus (see Chapter 33) and rabies (see Chapter 32) prophylaxis.

▶ When to Refer

• If septic arthritis or osteomyelitis is suspected.

• For exposure to bites by dogs, cats, reptiles, amphibians, and rodents.
• When rabies is a possibility.

▶ When to Admit

• Patients with infected hand bites.
• Deep bites, particularly if over joints.

Stevens DL et al; Infectious Diseases Society of America. Practice guidelines for the diagnosis and management of skin and soft-tissue infections. Clin Infect Dis. 2005 Nov 15;41(10):1373–406. [PMID: 16231249]

Taplitz RA. Managing bite wounds. Currently recommended antibiotics for treatment and prophylaxis. Postgrad Med. 2004 Aug;116(2):49–52, 55–6, 59. [PMID: 15323154]

Warrell MJ. Emerging aspects of rabies infection: with a special emphasis on children. Curr Opin Infect Dis. 2008 Jun;21(3):251–7. [PMID: 18448969]

SEXUALLY TRANSMITTED DISEASES

ESSENTIALS OF DIAGNOSIS

▶ All sexually transmitted diseases (STDs) have subclinical or latent periods, and patients may be asymptomatic.

▶ Simultaneous infection with several organisms is common.

▶ All patients who seek STD testing should be offered HIV screening.

▶ Partner notification and treatment are important to prevent further transmission and reinfection in the index case.

▶ General Considerations

The most common STDs are gonorrhea,* syphilis,* human papillomavirus (HPV)-associated condyloma acuminatum, chlamydial genital infections,* herpesvirus genital infections, trichomonas vaginitis, chancroid,* granuloma inguinale, scabies, louse infestation, and bacterial vaginosis (among women who have sex with women). However, shigellosis*; hepatitis A, B, and C*; amebiasis; giardiasis*; cryptosporidiosis*; salmonellosis*; and campylobacteriosis may also be transmitted by sexual (oral-anal) contact, especially in men who have sex with men. Both homosexual and heterosexual contact are risk factors for the transmission of HIV (see Chapter 31). All STDs have subclinical or latent phases that play an important role in long-term persistence of the infection or in its transmission from infected (but largely asymptomatic) persons to other contacts. Simultaneous infection by several different agents is common.

Infections typically present in one of several ways, each of which has a defined differential diagnosis, which should prompt appropriate diagnostic tests.

---

*Reportable to public health authorities.

A. Genital Ulcers

Potential etiologies include herpes simplex virus, primary syphilis, and chancroid most commonly. Other possibilities include lymphogranuloma venerum (see Chapter 33), granuloma inguinale caused by *Klebsiella granulomatis* (see Chapter 33), as well as lesions caused by infection with Epstein-Barr virus and HIV. Noninfectious causes are Behçet disease (see Chapter 20), neoplasm, trauma, drugs, and irritants.

B. Urethritis with or without Urethral Discharge

The most common infections causing urethral discharge are *Neisseria gonorrhoeae* and *Chlamydia trachomatis*. *N gonorrhoeae* and *C trachomatis* are also frequent causes of prostatitis among sexually active men. Other sexually transmitted infections that can cause urethritis include *Mycoplasma genitalium*, *Ureaplasma urealyticum*, and *Trichomonas vaginalis*. Noninfectious causes of urethritis includes reactive arthritis with associated urethritis (Reiter syndrome).

C. Vaginal Discharge

Common causes of vaginitis are bacterial vaginosis (caused by overgrowth of anaerobes such as *Gardnerella vaginalis*), candidiasis, and *T vaginalis* (see Chapter 18). Less common infectious causes of vaginitis include HPV-associated condyloma acuminata and group A streptococcus. Noninfectious causes are physiologic changes related to the menstrual cycle, irritants, and lichen planus. Even though *N gonorrhoeae* and *C trachomatis* are frequent causes of cervicitis, they rarely produce vaginal discharge.

▶ Clinical Findings

Any person with an STD should be tested for syphilis; a repeat study should be performed in 3 months if results are negative, since seroconversion is delayed after primary infection. All persons who seek STD testing should also undergo routine screening for HIV infection, using rapid HIV-testing (if patients may not follow-up for results obtained by standard methods) or nucleic acid amplification followed by confirmatory serology (if primary HIV infection may be a possibility) as indicated. Although it is not recommended to perform tests-of-cure for those in whom STDs have been diagnosed and treated, these patients are at a high risk for reinfection and should be encouraged to be rescreened for STDs at 3 months following the initial STD diagnosis.

▶ Screening & Prevention

Asymptomatic patients often request STD screening at the time of initiating a new sexual relationship. Routine HIV testing and hepatitis B serology testing should be offered to all such patients. In sexually active women who have not been recently screened, cervical Papanicolaou testing and nucleic acid amplification testing of a urine specimen for gonorrhea and chlamydia are recommended. Among men who have sex with men, additional screening is recom-

mended for syphilis; hepatitis A; urethral, pharyngeal, and rectal gonorrhea; as well as urethral and rectal chlamydia. Nucleic acid amplification testing is FDA-cleared for testing urine for gonorrhea or chlamydia. However, the use of nucleic acid amplification testing in the rectum and pharynx has not been validated in many laboratories. The periodicity of screening thereafter depends on sexual risk, but most screening should be offered at least annually to sexually active adults. If not immune, hepatitis B vaccination is recommended for all sexually active adults, and hepatitis A vaccination in men who have sex with men. Girls and women between the ages of 9 and 26 may be offered vaccination against HPV.

The risk of developing an STD following a **sexual assault** has not been established. Victims of assault have a high baseline rate of infection (*N gonorrhoeae*, 6%; *C trachomatis*, 10%; *T vaginalis*, 15%; and bacterial vaginosis, 34%), and the risk of acquiring infection as a result of the assault is significant but is often lower than the preexisting rate (*N gonorrhoeae*, 6–12%; *C trachomatis*, 4–17%; *T vaginalis*, 12%; syphilis, 0.5–3%; and bacterial vaginosis, 19%). Victims should be evaluated within 24 hours after the assault, and cultures or nucleic acid amplification tests for *N gonorrhoeae* and *C trachomatis* should be obtained. Vaginal secretions are cultured and examined for *Trichomonas*. If a discharge is present, if there is itching, or if secretions are malodorous, a wet mount should be examined for *Candida* and bacterial vaginosis. In addition, a blood sample should be obtained for immediate serologic testing for syphilis, hepatitis B, and HIV. Follow-up examination for STD should be repeated within 1–2 weeks, since concentrations of infecting organisms may not have been sufficient to produce a positive test at the time of initial examination. If prophylactic treatment was given (may include postexposure hepatitis B vaccination without hepatitis B immune globulin; treatment for chlamydial, gonorrheal, or trichomonal infection; and emergency contraception), tests should be repeated only if the victim has symptoms. If prophylaxis was not administered, the individual should be seen in 1 week so that any positive tests can be treated. Follow-up serologic testing for syphilis and HIV infection should be performed in 6, 12, and 24 weeks if the initial tests are negative. The usefulness of presumptive therapy is controversial, some feeling that all patients should receive it and others that it should be limited to those in whom follow-up cannot be ensured or to patients who request it.

Although seroconversion to HIV has been reported following sexual assault when this was the only known risk, this risk is believed to be low. The likelihood of HIV transmission from vaginal or anal receptive intercourse when the source is known to be HIV positive is 1 per 1000 and 5 per 1000, respectively. Although prophylactic antiretroviral therapy has not been studied in this setting, the Department of Health and Human Services recommends the prompt institution of postexposure prophylaxis with highly active antiretroviral therapy if the person seeks care within 72 hours of the assault, the source is known to be HIV positive, and the exposure presents a substantial risk of transmission.

In addition to screening asymptomatic patients with STDs, other strategies for preventing further transmission include evaluating sex partners and administering preexposure vaccination of preventable STDs to individuals at risk; other strategies include the consistent use of male and female condoms. For each patient, there are one or more sexual contacts who require diagnosis and treatment. Prompt treatment of contacts by giving antibiotics to the index case to distribute all sexual contacts (patient-delivered therapy) is an important strategy for preventing further transmission and to prevent reinfection in the index case.

Note that vaginal spermicides and condoms containing nonoxynol-9 provide no additional protection against STDs. Male circumcision has been demonstrated to protect against HIV and HPV acquisition in heterosexual men with HIV-infected partners.

▶ When to Refer

- Patients with a new diagnosis of HIV.
- Patients with persistent, refractory or recurrent STDs, particularly when drug resistance is suspected.

Auvert B et al. Effect of male circumcision on the prevalence of high-risk human papillomavirus in young men: results of a randomized controlled trial conducted in Orange Farm, South Africa. J Infect Dis. 2009 Jan 1;199(1):14–9. [PMID: 19086814]

Peterman TA et al. High incidence of new sexually transmitted infections in the year following a sexually transmitted infection: a case for rescreening. Ann Intern Med. 2006 Oct 17;145(8):564–72. [PMID: 17043338]

Screening for chlamydial infection: U.S. Preventive Services Task Force recommendation statement. Ann Intern Med. 2007;147(2):128–34. [PMID: 17576996]

Sexually transmitted diseases treatment guidelines 2006. Centers for Disease Control and Prevention. MMWR Recomm Rep. 2006 Aug 4;55(RR-11):1–94. [PMID: 16888612]

Smith DK et al. Antiretroviral postexposure prophylaxis after sexual, injection-drug use, or other nonoccupational exposure to HIV in the United States: recommendations from the U.S. Department of Health and Human Services. MMWR Recomm Rep. 2005 Jan 21;54(RR-2):1–20. [PMID: 15660015]

INFECTIONS IN DRUG USERS

ESSENTIALS OF DIAGNOSIS

Common infections that occur with greater frequency in drug users include:

- ▶ Skin infections, aspiration pneumonia, tuberculosis.
- ▶ Hepatitis A, B, C, D; STDs; AIDS.
- ▶ Pulmonary septic emboli, infective endocarditis.
- ▶ Osteomyelitis and septic arthritis.
- ▶ Rare infections in the United States include tetanus, malaria, and melioidosis.

▶ General Considerations

The use of parenterally administered recreational drugs has increased enormously in recent years. There are now an estimated 300,000 or more injection drug users in the United States.

1. Common Infections That Occur with Greater Frequency in Drug Users

Skin infections are associated with poor hygiene and use of nonsterile technique when injecting drugs. *S aureus* (including community-acquired methicillin-resistant strains) and oral flora (streptococci, *Eikenella, Fusobacterium, Peptostreptococcus*) are the most common organisms, with enteric gram-negatives generally more likely seen in those who inject into the groin. Cellulitis and subcutaneous abscesses occur most commonly, particularly in association with subcutaneous ("skin-popping") or intramuscular injections and the use of cocaine and heroin mixtures (probably due to ischemia). Myositis, clostridial myonecrosis, and necrotizing fasciitis occur infrequently but are life-threatening. Wound botulism in association with black tar heroin occurs sporadically but often in clusters.

Aspiration pneumonia and its complications (lung abscess, empyema, brain abscess) result from altered consciousness associated with drug use. Mixed aerobic and anaerobic mouth flora are usually involved.

Tuberculosis also occurs in drug users, and infection with HIV has fostered the spread of tuberculosis in this population. Morbidity and mortality rates are increased in HIV-infected individuals with tuberculosis. Classic radiographic findings are often absent; tuberculosis is suspected in any patient with infiltrates who does not respond to antibiotics.

Hepatitis is very common among habitual drug users and is transmissible both by the parenteral (hepatitis B, C, and D) and by the fecal-oral route (hepatitis A). Multiple episodes of hepatitis with different agents can occur.

Pulmonary septic emboli may originate from venous thrombi or right-sided endocarditis.

STDs are not directly related to drug use, but the practice of exchanging sex for drugs has resulted in an increased frequency of STDs. Syphilis, gonorrhea, and chancroid are the most common.

AIDS has a high incidence among injection drug users and their sexual contacts and among the offspring of infected women (see Chapter 31).

Infective endocarditis in persons who use drugs intravenously is most commonly caused by *S aureus, Candida* (usually *C albicans* or *C parapsilosis*), *Enterococcus faecalis*, other streptococci, and gram-negative bacteria (especially *Pseudomonas* and *Serratia marcescens*). See Chapter 33.

Other vascular infections include septic thrombophlebitis and mycotic aneurysms. Mycotic aneurysms resulting from direct trauma to a vessel with secondary infection most commonly occur in femoral arteries and less commonly in arteries of the neck. Aneurysms resulting from hematogenous spread of organisms frequently involve intracerebral vessels and thus are seen in association with endocarditis.

Osteomyelitis and septic arthritis involving vertebral bodies, sternoclavicular joints, the pubic symphysis, the sacroiliac joints, and other sites usually results from hematogenous distribution of injected organisms or septic venous thrombi. Pain and fever precede radiographic changes, sometimes by several weeks. While staphylococci—often methicillin-resistant—are common organisms, *Serratia, Pseudomonas, Candida* (often not *C albicans*), and other pathogens rarely encountered in spontaneous bone or joint disease are found in injection drug users.

2. Infections Rare in United States

A. Tetanus

In the 1950s and 1960s, tetanus was commonly seen in drug users, especially in unimmunized women who injected drugs subcutaneously ("skin-popping"). Increased tetanus immunization among drug users has resulted in a decline in this disease, although cases are still reported.

B. Malaria

Needle transmission occurs from injection drug users who acquired the infection in malaria-endemic areas outside the United States.

C. Melioidosis

This chronic pulmonary infection caused by *Burkholderia pseudomallei* occurs occasionally in debilitated drug users, but most cases are reported in Asia and Australia.

Treatment

A common and difficult clinical problem is management of the parenteral drug user who presents with fever. In general, after obtaining appropriate cultures (blood, urine, and sputum if the chest radiograph is abnormal), empiric therapy is begun. If the chest radiograph is suggestive of a community-acquired pneumonia (consolidation), therapy for outpatient pneumonia is begun with a third-generation cephalosporin, such as ceftriaxone, 1 g intravenously every 24 hours, plus azithromycin, 500 mg orally or intravenously every 24 hours, or doxycycline, 100 mg orally or intravenously twice daily. If the chest radiograph is suggestive of septic emboli (nodular infiltrates), therapy for presumed endocarditis is initiated, usually with a combination of vancomycin 15 mg/kg/dose every 12 hours intravenously (due to the high prevalence of MRSA and the possibility of enterococcus) and gentamicin, 3 mg/kg/d in two to three doses intravenously. If the chest radiograph is normal and no focal site of infection can be found, endocarditis is presumed. While awaiting the results of blood cultures, empiric treatment with vancomycin and gentamicin is started. If blood cultures are positive for organisms that frequently cause endocarditis in drug users (see above), endocarditis is presumed to be present and treated accordingly. If blood cultures are positive for an organism that is an unusual cause of endocarditis, evaluation for an occult source of infection should go forward. In this setting, a transesophageal echocardiogram may be quite helpful since it is 90% sensitive in detecting vegetations and a negative study is strong evidence against endocarditis. If blood cultures are negative and the patient responds

to antibiotics, therapy should be continued for 7–14 days (oral therapy can be given once an initial response has occurred). In every patient, careful examination for an occult source of infection (eg, genitourinary, dental, sinus, gallbladder) should be done.

When to Refer

- Any patient with suspected or proven infective endocarditis.
- Patients with persistent bacteremia.

When to Admit

- Injection drug users with fever.
- Patients with abscesses or progressive skin and soft tissue infection that require debridement.

Gordon RJ et al. Bacterial infections in drug users. N Engl J Med. 2005 Nov 3;353(18):1945–54. [PMID: 16267325]

Infections in injection drug users (entire issue). Infect Dis Clin North Am. 2002 Sep;16(3).

Rajendran PM et al. Randomized, double-blind, placebo-controlled trial of cephalexin for treatment of uncomplicated skin abscesses in a population at risk for community-acquired methicillin-resistant *Staphylococcus aureus* infection. Antimicrob Agents Chemother. 2007;51(11):4044–8. [PMID: 17846141]

Jain V et al. Infective endocarditis in an urban medical center: association of individual drugs with valvular involvement. J Infect. 2008 Aug;57(2):132–8. [PMID: 18597851]

ACUTE INFECTIOUS DIARRHEA

 ESSENTIALS OF DIAGNOSIS

- ▶ Diarrhea is acute if lasts < 2 weeks and chronic if lasts > 2 weeks.
- ▶ Disease is mild if there are three or fewer stools per day, moderate if there are four or more stools in association with local symptoms (abdominal cramps, nausea, tenesmus), and severe if there are four or more stools per day with systemic symptoms (fevers, chills, dehydration).

General Considerations

Acute diarrhea can be caused by a number of different factors, including emotional stress, food intolerance, inorganic agents (eg, sodium nitrite), organic substances (eg, mushrooms, shellfish), drugs, and infectious agents (including viruses, bacteria, and protozoa) (Table 30–3). From a diagnostic and therapeutic standpoint, it is helpful to classify infectious diarrhea into syndromes that produce inflammatory or bloody diarrhea and those that are noninflammatory, nonbloody, or watery. In general, the term "inflammatory diarrhea" suggests colonic involvement by invasive bacteria or parasites or by toxin production. Patients complain of frequent bloody, small-volume stools, often associated with fever, abdominal cramps, tenesmus, and fecal urgency. Common causes of this

Table 30–3. Acute bacterial diarrheas and "food poisoning."

Organism	Incubation Period	Vomiting	Diarrhea	Fever	Associated Foods	Diagnosis	Clinical Features and Treatment
Staphylococcus (preformed toxin)	1–8 hours	+++	±	±	Staphylococci grow in meats, dairy, and bakery products and produce enterotoxin.	Clinical. Food and stool can be tested for toxin.	Abrupt onset, intense nausea and vomiting for up to 24 hours, recovery in 24–48 hours. Supportive care.
Bacillus cereus (preformed toxin)	1–8 hours	+++	±	–	Reheated fried rice causes vomiting or diarrhea.	Clinical. Food and stool can be tested for toxin.	Acute onset, severe nausea and vomiting lasting 24 hours. Supportive care.
B cereus (diarrheal toxin)	10–16 hours	±	+++	–	Toxin in meats, stews, and gravy.	Clinical. Food and stool can be tested for toxin.	Abdominal cramps, watery diarrhea, and nausea lasting 24–48 hours. Supportive care.
Clostridium perfringens	8–16 hours	±	+++	–	Clostridia grow in rewarmed meat and poultry dishes and produce an enterotoxin.	Stools can be tested for enterotoxin or cultured.	Abrupt onset of profuse diarrhea, abdominal cramps, nausea; vomiting occasionally. Recovery usual without treatment in 24–48 hours. Supportive care; antibiotics not needed.
Clostridium botulinum	12–72 hours	±	–	–	Clostridia grow in anaerobic acidic environment eg, canned foods, fermented fish, foods held warm for extended periods.	Stool, serum, and food can be tested for toxin. Stool and food can be cultured.	Diplopia, dysphagia, dysphonia, respiratory embarrassment. Treatment requires clear airway, ventilation, and intravenous polyvalent antitoxin (see text). Symptoms can last for days to months.
Clostridium difficile	Usually occurs after 7–10 days of antibiotics. Can occur after a single dose or several weeks after completion of antibiotics.	–	+++	++	Associated with antimicrobial drugs; clindamycin and cephalosporins most commonly implicated.	Stool tested for toxin.	Abrupt onset of diarrhea that may be bloody; fever. Oral metronidazole first-line therapy. If no response, oral vancomycin can be given.
Enterohemorrhagic *Escherichia coli*, including *E coli* O157:H7 and other Shiga-toxin producing strains (STEC)	1–8 days	+	+++	+	Undercooked beef, especially hamburger; unpasteurized milk and juice; raw fruits and vegetables.	*E coli* O157:H7 can be cultured on special medium. Other toxins can be detected in stool.	Usually abrupt onset of diarrhea, often bloody; abdominal pain. In adults, it is usually self-limited to 5–10 days. In children, it is associated with hemolytic-uremic syndrome (HUS). Antibiotic therapy may increase risk of HUS.
Enterotoxigenic *E coli* (ETEC)	1–3 days	±	+++	+	Water, food contaminated with feces.	Stool culture. Special tests required to identify toxin-producing strains.	Watery diarrhea and abdominal cramps, usually lasting 3–7 days. In travelers, fluoroquinolones shorten disease.
Vibrio parahaemolyticus	2–48 hours	+	+	+	Undercooked or raw seafood.	Stool culture on special medium.	Abrupt onset of watery diarrhea, abdominal cramps, nausea and vomiting. Recovery is usually complete in 2–5 days.

Organism	Incubation Period				Common Food Sources	Diagnosis	Clinical Features
Vibrio cholerae	24–72 hours	+	++		Contaminated water, fish, shellfish, street vendor food.	Stool culture on special medium.	Abrupt onset of liquid diarrhea in endemic area. Needs prompt intravenous or oral replacement of fluids and electrolytes. Tetracyclines shorten excretion of vibrios.
Campylobacter jejuni	2–5 days	±	+++	+	Raw or undercooked poultry, unpasteurized milk, water.	Stool culture on special medium.	Fever, diarrhea that can be bloody, cramps. Usually self-limited in 2–10 days. Early treatment (erythromycin) shortens course. May be associated with Guillain-Barré syndrome.
Shigella species (mild cases)	24–48 hours	±	+	+	Food or water contaminated with human feces. Person to person spread.	Routine stool culture.	Abrupt onset of diarrhea, often with blood and pus in stools, cramps, tenesmus, and lethargy. Stool cultures are positive. Therapy depends on sensitivity testing, but the fluoroquinolones are most effective. Do not give opioids. Often mild and self-limited.
Salmonella species	1–3 days	–	++		Eggs, poultry, unpasteurized milk, cheese, juices, raw fruits and vegetables.	Routine stool culture.	Gradual or abrupt onset of diarrhea and low-grade fever. No antimicrobials unless high risk (see text) or systemic dissemination is suspected, in which case give a fluoroquinolone. Prolonged carriage can occur.
Yersinia enterocolitica	24–48 hours	±	+		Undercooked pork, contaminated water, unpasteurized milk, tofu.	Stool culture on special medium.	Severe abdominal pain, (appendicitis-like symptoms) diarrhea, fever. Polyarthritis, erythema nodosum in children. If severe, give tetracycline or fluoroquinolone. Without treatment, self-limited in 1–3 weeks.
Rotavirus	1–3 days	++	+++		Fecally contaminated foods touched by infected food handlers.	Immunoassay on stool.	Acute onset, vomiting, watery diarrhea that lasts 4–8 days. Supportive care.
Noroviruses and other caliciviruses	12–48 hours	++	+++		Shell fish and fecally contaminated foods touched by infected food handlers.	Clinical diagnosis with negative stool cultures. PCR available on stool.	Nausea, vomiting (more common in children) diarrhea (more common in adults), fever, myalgias, abdominal cramps. Lasts 12–60 hours. Supportive care.

PCR, polymerase chain reaction.

syndrome include *Shigella, Salmonella, Campylobacter, Yersinia,* invasive strains of *Escherichia coli, E coli* O157:H7, *Entamoeba histolytica,* and *C difficile.* Tests for fecal leukocytes or the neutrophil marker lactoferrin are frequently positive, and definitive etiologic diagnosis requires stool culture. Non-inflammatory diarrhea is generally milder and is caused by viruses or toxins that affect the small intestine and interfere with salt and water balance, resulting in large-volume watery diarrhea, often with nausea, vomiting, and cramps. Common causes of this syndrome include viruses (eg, rotavirus, Norwalk virus, enteric adenoviruses, astrovirus, coronavirus), vibriones *(Vibrio cholerae, Vibrio parahaemolyticus),* enterotoxin-producing *E coli, Giardia lamblia,* cryptosporidia, and agents that can cause food-borne gastroenteritis.

The term "food poisoning" denotes diseases caused by toxins present in consumed foods. When the incubation period is short (1–6 hours after consumption), the toxin is usually preformed. Vomiting is usually a major complaint, and fever is usually absent. Examples include intoxication from *S aureus* or *Bacillus cereus,* and toxin can be detected in the food. When the incubation period is longer—between 8 hours and 16 hours—the organism is present in the food and produces toxin after being ingested. Vomiting is less prominent, abdominal cramping is frequent, and fever is often absent. The best example of this disease is that due to *Clostridium perfringens.* Toxin can be detected in food or stool specimens.

The inflammatory and noninflammatory diarrheas discussed above can also be transmitted by food and water and usually have incubation periods between 12 and 72 hours. *Cyclospora,* cryptosporidia, and *Isospora* are protozoans capable of causing disease in both immunocompetent and immunocompromised patients. Characteristics of disease include profuse watery diarrhea that is prolonged but usually self-limited (1–2 weeks) in the immunocompetent patient but can be chronic in the compromised host. Epidemiologic features may be helpful in determining etiology. Recent hospitalization or antibiotic use suggests *C difficile;* recent foreign travel suggests *Salmonella, Shigella, Campylobacter, E coli,* or *V cholerae;* undercooked hamburger suggests *E coli,* especially O157:H7; and fried rice consumption is associated with *B cereus* toxin. Prominent features of some of these causes of diarrhea are listed in Table 30–3.

► Treatment

Treatment usually consists of replacement of fluids and electrolytes and, very rarely, management of hypovolemic shock and respiratory compromise. In mild diarrhea, increasing ingestion of juices and clear soups is adequate. In more severe cases of dehydration (postural lightheadedness, decreased urination), oral glucose-based rehydration solutions can be used (Ceralyte, Pedialyte). In general, most cases of acute gastroenteritis are self-limited and do not require therapy other than supportive measures. When symptoms persist beyond 3–4 days, initial presentation is accompanied by fever or bloody diarrhea, or if the patient is immunocompromised, cultures of stool are usually obtained. Symptoms have often resolved by the time cultures are completed. In this case, even if a pathogen is isolated, therapy is not needed (except for *Shigella,* since the infecting dose is so small that

therapy to eradicate organisms from the stool is indicated for epidemiologic reasons). If symptoms persist and a pathogen is isolated, it is reasonable to institute specific treatment even though therapy has not been conclusively shown to alter the natural history of disease for most pathogens. Exceptions include infection with *Shigella* where antibiotic therapy has been shown to shorten the duration of symptoms by 2–3 days, infections with *E coli* O157:H7 (antibiotic therapy does not ameliorate symptoms and may increase the risk of developing hemolytic-uremic syndrome), and *Campylobacter* infections (early therapy, within 4 days of onset of symptoms, shortens the course of disease). Uncomplicated gastroenteritis due to *Salmonella* does not require therapy because the disease is usually self-limited and therapy may prolong carriage and perhaps increase relapses. Because bacteremia with complications can occur in high-risk patients, some experts have recommended therapy for *Salmonella* in patients over the age of 50, in organ transplant recipients, in those with HIV, in patients taking corticosteroids, in those with lymphoproliferative diseases, and in those with vascular grafts. Ciprofloxacin, 500 mg every 12 hours for 5 days, is effective in shortening the course of illness compared with placebo in patients presenting with diarrhea, whether a pathogen is isolated or not. However, because of concerns about selecting for resistant organisms (especially *Campylobacter,* where increasing resistance to fluoroquinolones has been documented and erythromycin is the drug of choice) coupled with the fact that most infectious diarrhea is self-limited, routine use of antibiotics for all patients with diarrhea is not recommended. Antibiotics should be considered in patients with evidence of invasive disease (white cells in stool, dysentery), with symptoms 3–4 days or more in duration, with multiple stools (eight to ten or more per day), and in those with impaired immune responses. Antimotility drugs are useful in mild cases. Their use should be limited to patients without fever and without dysentery (bloody stools), and they should be used in low doses because of the risk of producing toxic megacolon.

Therapeutic recommendations for specific agents can be found elsewhere in this book.

American Medical Association; American Nurses Association-American Nurses Foundation; Centers for Disease Control and Prevention; Center for Food Safety and Applied Nutrition, Food and Drug Administration; Food Safety and Inspection Service, US Department of Agriculture. Diagnosis and management of foodborne illnesses: a primer for physicians and other health care professionals. MMWR Recomm Rep. 2004 Apr 16;53(RR-4):1–33. [PMID: 15123984]

Musher DM et al. Contagious acute gastrointestinal infections N Engl J Med. 2004 Dec 2;351(23):2417–27. [PMID: 15575058]

Thielman NM et al. Clinical practice. Acute infectious diarrhea. N Engl J Med. 2004 Jan 1;350(1):38–47. [PMID: 14702426]

INFECTIOUS DISEASES IN THE RETURNING TRAVELER

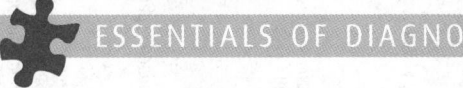

ESSENTIALS OF DIAGNOSIS

► Most infections are common and self-limited.

- ▶ Identify patients with transmissible diseases that require isolation.
- ▶ The incubation period may be helpful in diagnosis.
- ▶ Less than 3 weeks following exposure may suggest dengue, leptospirosis and yellow fever; greater than 3 weeks suggest typhoid fever, malaria, and tuberculosis.

General Considerations

The differential diagnosis of fever in the returning traveler is broad, ranging from self-limited viral infections to life-threatening illness. The evaluation is best done by identifying whether a particular syndrome is present, then refining the differential diagnosis based on an exposure history. The travel history should include directed questions regarding geography (rural versus urban), animal or arthropod contact, unprotected sexual intercourse, ingestion of untreated water or raw foods, historical or pretravel immunizations, and adherence to malaria prophylaxis.

Etiologies

The most common infectious causes of fever—excluding simple causes such as upper respiratory infections, bacterial pneumonia and urinary tract infections—in returning travelers are malaria (see Chapter 35), diarrhea (see next section), and dengue (see Chapter 32). Others include respiratory infections, leptospirosis (see Chapter 34), typhoid fever (see Chapter 33), and rickettsial infections (see Chapter 32). Systemic febrile illnesses without a diagnosis also occurs commonly, particularly in travelers returning from sub-Saharan Africa or Southeast Asia.

A. Fever and Rash

Potential etiologies include dengue, Chikungunya, viral hemorrhagic fever, leptospirosis, meningococcemia, yellow fever, typhus, *Salmonella typhi*, and acute HIV infection.

B. Pulmonary Infiltrates

Tuberculosis, ascaris, *Paragonimus*, and *Strongyloides* can all cause pulmonary infiltrates.

C. Meningoencephalitis

Etiologies include *N meningitidis*, leptospirosis, arboviruses, rabies, and (cerebral) malaria.

D. Jaundice

Consider hepatitis A, yellow fever, hemorrhagic fever, leptospirosis, and malaria.

E. Fever without Localizing Symptoms or Signs

Malaria, typhoid fever, acute HIV infection, rickettsial illness, visceral leishmaniasis, trypanosomiasis, and dengue are possible etiologies.

F. Traveler's Diarrhea

See next section.

Clinical Findings

Fever and rash in the returning traveler should prompt blood cultures and various serologic tests based on the exposure history. The work-up of a pulmonary infiltrate should include the placement of a PPD, examination of sputum for acid-fast bacilli and possibly for ova and parasites. Patients with evidence of meningoencephalitis should receive lumbar puncture, blood cultures, thick/thin smears of peripheral blood, history-guided serologies, and a nape biopsy (if rabies is suspected). Jaundice in a returning traveler should be evaluated for hemolysis, and the following tests should be performed: liver function tests, thick/thin smears of peripheral blood, and directed serologic testing. The work-up of traveler's diarrhea is presented in the following section. Finally, patients with fever but no localizing signs or symptoms should have blood cultures performed. Routine laboratory studies usually include complete blood count with differential, electrolytes, liver function tests, urine analysis, and blood cultures. Thick and thin peripheral blood smears should be done (and repeated in 12–24 hours if clinical suspicion remains high) for malaria if there has been travel to endemic areas. Other studies are directed by the results of history, physical examination, and initial laboratory tests. They may include stool for ova and parasites, chest radiograph, HIV test, and specific serologies (eg, dengue, leptospirosis, rickettsial disease, schistosomiasis, *Strongyloides*). Bone marrow biopsy to diagnose typhoid fever could be helpful in the appropriate patient.

When to Refer

Travelers with fever, particularly if immunocompromised.

When to Admit

Any evidence of hemorrhage, respiratory distress, hemodynamic instability, and neurologic deficits.

Freedman DO et al; GeoSentinel Surveillance Network. Spectrum of disease and relation to place of exposure among ill returned travelers. N Engl J Med. 2006 Jan 12;354(2):119–30. [PMID: 16407507]

Griffith KS et al. Treatment of malaria in the United States: a systematic review. JAMA. 2007 May 23;297(20):2264–77. [PMID: 17519416]

Hochedez P et al. Management of travelers with fever and exanthema, notably dengue and chikungunya infections. Am J Trop Med Hyg. 2008 May;78(5):710–3. [PMID: 18458301]

Luna LK et al. Spectrum of viruses and atypical bacteria in intercontinental air travelers with symptoms of acute respiratory infection. J Infect Dis. 2007 Mar 1;195(5):675–9. [PMID: 17262708]

Monsel G et al. Recent developments in dermatological syndromes in returning travelers. Curr Opin Infect Dis. 2008 Oct;21(5):495–9. [PMID: 18725799]

TRAVELER'S DIARRHEA

 ESSENTIALS OF DIAGNOSIS

- ▶ Usually a benign, self-limited disease occurring about 1 week into travel.

▶ Prophylaxis not recommended unless there is a comorbid disease (inflammatory bowel syndrome, HIV, immunosuppressive medication).

▶ Single-dose therapy of a fluoroquinolone usually effective if significant symptoms develop.

General Considerations

Whenever a person travels from one country to another—particularly if the change involves a marked difference in climate, social conditions, or sanitation standards and facilities—diarrhea may develop within 2–10 days. Bacteria cause 80% of cases of traveler's diarrhea, with enterotoxigenic *E coli*, *Shigella* species, and *Campylobacter jejuni* being the most common pathogens. Less common are *Aeromonas*, *Salmonella*, noncholera vibriones, *E histolytica*, and *G lamblia*. Contributory causes include unusual food and drink, change in living habits, occasional viral infections (adenoviruses or rotaviruses), and change in bowel flora. Chronic watery diarrhea may be due to amebiasis or giardiasis or, rarely, tropical sprue.

Clinical Findings

A. Symptoms and Signs

There may be up to ten or even more loose stools per day, often accompanied by abdominal cramps and nausea, occasionally by vomiting, and rarely by fever. The stools are usually watery and not associated with fever when caused by enterotoxigenic *E coli*. With invasive bacterial pathogens (*Shigella*, *Campylobacter*, *Salmonella*) stools can be bloody and fever may be present. The illness usually subsides spontaneously within 1–5 days, although 10% remain symptomatic for 1 week or longer, and symptoms persist for longer than 1 month in 2%. Traveler's diarrhea is also a significant risk factor for developing irritable bowel syndrome.

B. Laboratory Findings

In patients with fever and bloody diarrhea, stool culture is indicated, but in most cases, cultures are reserved for those who do not respond to antibiotics.

Prevention

A. General Measures

Avoidance of fresh foods and water sources that are likely to be contaminated is recommended for travelers to developing countries, where infectious diarrheal illnesses are endemic.

B. Specific Measures

Prophylaxis is recommended for those with significant underlying disease (inflammatory bowel disease, AIDS, diabetes, heart disease in the elderly, conditions requiring immunosuppressive medications) and for those whose full activity status during the trip is so essential that even short periods of diarrhea would be unacceptable. Prophylaxis is started upon entry into the destination country and is continued for 1 or 2 days after leaving. For stays of more than 3 weeks, prophylaxis is not recommended because of the cost and increased toxicity. For prophylaxis, numerous oral antimicrobial once-daily regimens are effective, such as norfloxacin, 400 mg; ciprofloxacin, 500 mg; or rifaximin, 200 mg. Bismuth subsalicylate is effective but turns the tongue and the stools black and can interfere with doxycycline absorption, which may be needed for malaria prophylaxis; it is rarely used.

Because not all travelers will have diarrhea and because most episodes are brief and self-limited, an alternative approach currently recommended is to provide the traveler with a supply of antimicrobials to be taken if significant diarrhea occurs during the trip. In areas where toxin-producing bacteria are the major cause of diarrhea (Latin America and Africa), loperamide (4 mg oral loading dose, then 2 mg after each loose stool to a maximum of 16 mg/d) with a single oral dose of ciprofloxacin (750 mg), levofloxacin (500 mg), or ofloxacin (200 mg), cures most cases of traveler's diarrhea. If diarrhea is associated with bloody stools or persists despite a single dose of a fluoroquinolone, 1000 mg of azithromycin should be taken. In pregnant women and in areas where invasive bacteria more commonly cause diarrhea (Indian subcontinent, Asia, especially Thailand where fluoroquinolone-resistant *Campylobacter* is prevalent), azithromycin is the drug of choice. Rifaximin, a nonabsorbable agent, is also approved for therapy of traveler's diarrhea at a dose of 200 mg orally three times per day or 400 mg twice a day for 3 days. Because luminal concentrations are high, but tissue levels are insufficient, it should not be used in situations where there is a high likelihood of invasive disease (eg, fever, systemic toxicity, or bloody stools).

Treatment

For most individuals, the affliction is short-lived, and symptomatic therapy with loperamide is all that is required, provided the patient is not systemically ill (fever ≥ 39 °C) and does not have dysentery (bloody stools), in which case antimotility agents should be avoided. Packages of oral rehydration salts to treat dehydration are available over the counter in the United States (Infalyte, Pedialyte, others) and in many foreign countries.

When to Refer

- Cases refractory to treatment.
- Persistent infection.
- Immunocompromised patient.

When to Admit

Patients who are severely dehydrated or hemodynamically unstable should be admitted to the hospital.

DuPont HL. Azithromycin for the self-treatment of traveler's diarrhea. Clin Infect Dis. 2007 Feb 1;44(3):347–9. [PMID: 17205439]

Hill DR et al. The practice of travel medicine: guidelines by the Infectious Disease Society of America. Clin Infect Dis. 2006 Dec 15;43(12):1499–539. [PMID: 17109284]

Thielman NM et al. Clinical practice. Acute infectious diarrhea. N Engl J Med. 2004 Jan 1;350(1):38–47. [PMID: 14702426]

Tuteja AK et al. Development of functional diarrhea, constipation, irritable bowel syndrome, and dyspepsia during and after traveling outside the USA. Dig Dis Sci. 2008 Jan;53(1):271–6. [PMID: 17549631]

▼ ANTIMICROBIAL THERAPY

SELECTED PRINCIPLES OF ANTIMICROBIAL THERAPY

Specific steps (outlined below) are required when considering antibiotic therapy for patients. Drugs within classes, drugs of first choice, and alternative drugs are presented in Tables 30–4, 30–5, 30–6, 30–7, and 30–8.

A. Etiologic Diagnosis

Based on the organ system involved, the organism causing infection can often be predicted. See Tables 30–9 and 30–10.

B. "Best Guess"

Select an empiric regimen that is likely to be effective against the suspected pathogens.

C. Laboratory Control

Specimens for laboratory examination should be obtained before institution of therapy to determine susceptibility.

D. Clinical Response

Based on clinical response and other data, the laboratory reports are evaluated and then the desirability of changing the regimen is considered. If the specimen was obtained from a normally sterile site (eg, blood, cerebrospinal fluid, pleural fluid, joint fluid), the recovery of a microorganism in significant amounts is meaningful even if the organism recovered is different from the clinically suspected agent, and this may force a change in treatment. Isolation of unexpected microorganisms from the respiratory tract, gastrointestinal tract, or surface lesions (sites that have a complex flora) may represent colonization or contamination, and cultures must be critically evaluated before drugs are abandoned that were judiciously selected on a "best guess" basis.

E. Drug Susceptibility Tests

Some microorganisms are predictably inhibited by certain drugs; if such organisms are isolated, they need not be tested for drug susceptibility. For example, all group A hemolytic streptococci are inhibited by penicillin. Other organisms (eg, enteric gram-negative rods) are variably susceptible and generally require susceptibility testing whenever they are isolated. Organisms that once had predictable susceptibility patterns have now become resistant and require testing. Examples include the pneumococci, which may be resistant to multiple drugs (including penicillin, macrolides, and TMP-SMZ); the enterococci, which may be resistant to penicillin, aminoglycosides, and

vancomycin; and extended-spectrum β-lactamase producing–E coli resistant to third-generation cephalosporins and fluoroquinolones.

Over the past 10 years, pharmaceutical companies have shifted away from developing and producing antibacterial medications, particularly those active against gram-negative pathogens. The lack of new drugs and increasing bacterial resistance reinforce the need to use these drugs judiciously.

Antimicrobial drug susceptibility tests may be performed on solid media as disk diffusion tests, in broth in tubes, in wells of microdilution plates, or as E-tests (strips with increasing concentration of antibiotic). The latter three methods yield results expressed as MIC (minimal inhibitory concentration), and the broth and microdilution techniques can be modified to give MBC (minimal bactericidal concentration) results. In most infections, the MIC is the appropriate in vitro test to guide selection of an antibacterial agent. When there appear to be marked discrepancies between susceptibility testing and clinical response, the following possibilities must be considered:

1. Selection of an inappropriate drug, drug dosage, or route of administration.
2. Failure to drain a collection of pus or to remove a foreign body.
3. Failure of a poorly diffusing drug to reach the site of infection (eg, central nervous system) or to reach intracellular phagocytosed bacteria.
4. Superinfection in the course of prolonged chemotherapy.
5. Emergence of drug-resistant organisms.
6. Participation of two or more microorganisms in the infectious process, of which only one was originally detected and used for drug selection.
7. Inadequate host defenses, including immunodeficiencies and diabetes.
8. Noninfectious causes, including drug fever, malignancy, and autoimmune disease.

F. Promptness of Response

Response depends on a number of factors, including the patient (immunocompromised patients respond slower than immunocompetent patients), the site of infection (deep-seated infections such as osteomyelitis and endocarditis respond more slowly than superficial infections such as cystitis or cellulitis), the pathogen (virulent organisms such as S aureus respond more slowly than viridans streptococci; mycobacterial and fungal infections respond slower than bacterial infections), and the duration of illness (in general, the longer the symptoms are present, the longer it takes to respond). Thus, depending on the clinical situation, persistent fever and leukocytosis several days after initiation of therapy may not indicate improper choice of antibiotics but may be due to the natural history of the disease being treated. In most infections, either a bacteriostatic or a bactericidal agent can be used. In some infections (eg, infective endocarditis and meningitis), a bactericidal agent should be used. When potentially toxic drugs (eg, aminoglycosides, flucytosine) are used, serum levels of the drug are measured

Table 30–4. Drugs of choice for suspected or proved microbial pathogens, 2009.[1]

Suspected or Proved Etiologic Agent	Drug(s) of First Choice	Alternative Drug(s)
Gram-negative cocci		
Moraxella catarrhalis	TMP-SMZ,[2] a fluoroquinolone[3]	Cefuroxime, cefotaxime, ceftriaxone, cefuroxime axetil, an erythromycin,[4] a tetracycline,[5] azithromycin, amoxicillin-clavulanic acid, clarithromycin
Neisseria gonorrhoeae (gonococcus)	Cefixime, ceftriaxone	Cefpodoxime proxetil
Neisseria meningitidis (meningococcus)	Penicillin[6]	Cefotaxime, ceftriaxone, ampicillin
Gram-positive cocci		
Streptococcus pneumoniae[8] (pneumococcus)	Penicillin[6]	An erythromycin,[4] a cephalosporin,[7] vancomycin, TMP-SMZ,[2] clindamycin, azithromycin, clarithromycin, a tetracycline,[5] certain fluoroquinolones[3]
Streptococcus, hemolytic, groups A, B, C, G	Penicillin[6]	An erythromycin,[4] a cephalosporin,[7] vancomycin, clindamycin, azithromycin, clarithromycin
Viridans streptococci	Penicillin[6] ± gentamicin	Cephalosporin,[7] vancomycin
Staphylococcus, methicillin-resistant	Vancomycin ± gentamicin	TMP-SMZ,[2] doxycycline, minocycline, a fluoroquinolone,[3] linezolid, daptomycin, quinupristin-dalfopristin
Staphylococcus, non-penicillinase-producing	Penicillin[6]	A cephalosporin,[8] clindamycin
Staphylococcus, penicillinase-producing	Penicillinase-resistant penicillin[9]	Vancomycin, a cephalosporin,[7] clindamycin, amoxicillin-clavulanic acid, ampicillin-sulbactam, piperacillin-tazobactam, TMP-SMZ[2]
Enterococcus faecalis	Ampicillin ± gentamicin[10]	Vancomycin ± gentamicin
Enterococcus faecium	Vancomycin ± gentamicin[10]	Linezolid, quinupristin-dalfopristin, daptomycin
Gram-negative rods		
Acinetobacter	Imipenem, meropenem	Tigecycline, minocycline, doxycycline, aminoglycosides,[11] colistin
Prevotella, oropharyngeal strains	Clindamycin	Metronidazole
Bacteroides, gastrointestinal strains	Metronidazole	Clindamycin, ampicillin-sulbactam, piperacillin-tazobactam
Brucella	Tetracycline + rifampin[5]	TMP-SMZ[2] ± gentamicin; chloramphenicol ± gentamicin; doxycycline ± gentamicin
Campylobacter jejuni	Erythromycin[4] or azithromycin	Tetracycline,[5] a fluoroquinolone[3]
Enterobacter	TMP-SMZ,[2] imipenem, meropenem	Aminoglycoside, a fluoroquinolone,[3] cefepime
Escherichia coli (sepsis)	Cefotaxime, ceftriaxone,	Imipenem or meropenem, aminoglycosides,[11] a fluoroquinolone[3]
Escherichia coli (uncomplicated outpatient urinary infection)	Fluoroquinolones,[3] nitrofurantoin	TMP-SMZ,[2] oral cephalosporin
Haemophilus (meningitis and other serious infections)	Cefotaxime, ceftriaxone	Aztreonam
Haemophilus (respiratory infections, otitis)	TMP-SMZ[2]	Ampicillin, amoxicillin, doxycycline, azithromycin, clarithromycin, cefotaxime, ceftriaxone, cefuroxime, cefuroxime axetil, ampicillin-clavulanate
Helicobacter pylori	Amoxicillin + clarithromycin + proton pump inhibitor (PPI)	Bismuth subsalicylate + tetracycline + metronidazole + PPI
Klebsiella	A cephalosporin	TMP-SMZ,[2] aminoglycoside,[11] imipenem or meropenem, a fluoroquinolone,[3] aztreonam
Legionella species (pneumonia)	Erythromycin[4] or clarithromycin or azithromycin, or fluoroquinolones[3] ± rifampin	Doxycycline ± rifampin
Proteus mirabilis	Ampicillin	An aminoglycoside,[11] TMP-SMZ,[2] a fluoroquinolone,[3] a cephalosporin[7]

(continued)

Table 30–4. Drugs of choice for suspected or proved microbial pathogens, 2009.[1] (continued)

Suspected or Proved Etiologic Agent	Drug(s) of First Choice	Alternative Drug(s)
Proteus vulgaris and other species (*Morganella, Providencia*)	Cefotaxime, ceftriaxone	Aminoglycoside,[11] imipenem, TMP-SMZ,[2] a fluoroquinolone[3]
Pseudomonas aeruginosa	Aminoglycoside[11] + antipseudomonal penicillin[12]	Ceftazidime ± aminoglycoside; imipenem or meropenem ± aminoglycoside; aztreonam ± aminoglycoside; ciprofloxacin (or levofloxacin) ± piperacillin-tazobactam; ciprofloxacin (or levofloxacin) ± ceftazidime; ciprofloxacin (or levofloxacin) ± cefepime
Burkholderia pseudomallei (melioidosis)	Ceftazidime	Tetracycline,[5] TMP-SMZ,[2] amoxicillin-clavulanic acid, imipenem or meropenem
Burkholderia mallei (glanders)	Streptomycin + tetracycline[5]	Chloramphenicol + streptomycin
Salmonella (bacteremia)	Ceftriaxone	A fluoroquinolone[3]
Serratia	Cefotaxime, ceftriaxone	TMP-SMZ,[2] aminoglycosides,[11] imipenem or meropenem, a fluoroquinolone[3]
Shigella	A fluoroquinolone[3]	Ampicillin, TMP-SMZ,[2] ceftriaxone
Vibrio (cholera, sepsis)	A tetracycline[5]	TMP-SMZ,[2] a fluoroquinolone[3]
Yersinia pestis (plague, tularemia)	Streptomycin ± a tetracycline[5]	Chloramphenicol, TMP-SMZ[2]
Gram-positive rods		
Actinomyces	Penicillin[6]	Tetracycline,[5] clindamycin
Bacillus (including anthrax)	Penicillin[6] (ciprofloxacin or doxycycline for anthrax; see Table 33–2)	Erythromycin,[4] a fluoroquinolone[3]
Clostridium (eg, gas gangrene, tetanus)	Penicillin[6]	Metronidazole, clindamycin, imipenem or meropenem
Corynebacterium diphtheriae	Erythromycin[4]	Penicillin[6]
Corynebacterium jeikeium	Vancomycin	A fluoroquinolone
Listeria	Ampicillin ± aminoglycoside[11]	TMP-SMZ[2]
Acid-fast rods		
Mycobacterium tuberculosis[13]	Isoniazid (INH) + rifampin + pyrazinamide ± ethambutol (or streptomycin)	Other antituberculous drugs (see Tables 9–12 and 9–13)
Mycobacterium leprae	Dapsone + rifampin ± clofazimine	Minocycline, ofloxacin, clarithromycin
Mycobacterium kansasii	INH + rifampin ± ethambutol	Ethionamide, cycloserine
Mycobacterium avium complex	Clarithromycin or azithromycin + one or more of the following: ethambutol, rifampin or rifabutin, ciprofloxacin	Amikacin
Mycobacterium fortuitum-chelonei	Amikacin + clarithromycin	Cefoxitin, sulfonamide, doxycycline, linezolid
Nocardia	TMP-SMZ[2]	Minocycline, imipenem or meropenem, linezolid
Spirochetes		
Borrelia burgdorferi (Lyme disease)	Doxycycline, amoxicillin, cefuroxime axetil	Ceftriaxone, cefotaxime, penicillin, azithromycin, clarithromycin
Borrelia recurrentis (relapsing fever)	Doxycycline[5]	Penicillin[6]
Leptospira	Penicillin,[6] ceftriaxone	Doxycycline[5]
Treponema pallidum (syphilis)	Penicillin[6]	Doxycycline, ceftriaxone
Treponema pertenue (yaws)	Penicillin[6]	Doxycycline
Mycoplasmas	**Erythromycin[4] or doxycycline**	**Clarithromycin, azithromycin, a fluoroquinolone[3]**
Chlamydiae		
C psittaci	Doxycycline	Chloramphenicol
C trachomatis (urethritis or pelvic inflammatory disease)	Doxycycline or azithromycin	Ofloxacin

(continued)

Table 30–4. Drugs of choice for suspected or proved microbial pathogens, 2009.[1] (continued)

Suspected or Proved Etiologic Agent	Drug(s) of First Choice	Alternative Drug(s)
C pneumoniae	Doxycycline[5]	Erythromycin,[4] clarithromycin, azithromycin, a fluoroquinolone[3,14]
Rickettsiae	**Doxycycline[5]**	**Chloramphenicol, a fluoroquinolone[3]**

[1]Adapted, with permission, from Treat Guide Med Lett. 2007 May;5(57):33–50.
[2]TMP-SMZ is a mixture of 1 part trimethoprim and 5 parts sulfamethoxazole.
[3]Fluoroquinolones include ciprofloxacin, ofloxacin, levofloxacin, moxifloxacin, and others (see text). Gemifloxacin, levofloxacin, and moxifloxacin have the best activity against gram-positive organisms, including penicillin-resistant S pneumoniae and methicillin-sensitive S aureus. Activity against enterococci and S epidermidis is variable.
[4]Erythromycin estolate is best absorbed orally but carries the highest risk of hepatitis; erythromycin stearate and erythromycin ethylsuccinate are also available.
[5]All tetracyclines have similar activity against most microorganisms. Minocycline and doxycycline have increased activity against S aureus.
[6]Penicillin G is preferred for parenteral injection; penicillin V for oral administration—to be used only in treating infections due to highly sensitive organisms.
[7]Most intravenous cephalosporins (with the exception of ceftazidime) have good activity against gram-positive cocci.
[8]Infections caused by isolates with intermediate resistance may respond to high doses of penicillin, cefotaxime, or ceftriaxone. Infections caused by highly resistant strains should be treated with vancomycin. Many strains of penicillin-resistant pneumococci are resistant to macrolides, cephalosporins, tetracyclines, and TMP-SMZ.
[9]Parenteral nafcillin or oxacillin; oral dicloxacillin, cloxacillin, or oxacillin.
[10]Addition of gentamicin indicated only for severe enterococcal infections (eg, endocarditis, meningitis).
[11]Aminoglycosides—gentamicin, tobramycin, amikacin, netilmicin—should be chosen on the basis of local patterns of susceptibility.
[12]Antipseudomonal penicillins: ticarcillin, piperacillin.
[13]Resistance is common and susceptibility testing should be done.
[14]Ciprofloxacin has inferior antichlamydial activity compared with newer fluoroquinolones.
Key: ±, alone or combined with.

to minimize toxicity and ensure appropriate dosage. In patients with altered renal or hepatic clearance of drugs, the dosage or frequency of administration must be adjusted; it is best to measure levels in the elderly, morbidly obese patients, or those with altered kidney function when possible and adjust therapy accordingly.

In kidney disease or liver failure, the dosage should be adjusted as shown in Table 30–11.

G. Duration of Antimicrobial Therapy

Generally, effective antimicrobial treatment results in reversal of the clinical and laboratory parameters of active infection and marked clinical improvement. However, varying periods of treatment may be required for cure. Key factors include (1) the type of infecting organism (bacterial infections generally can be cured more rapidly than fungal or mycobacterial ones), (2) the location of the process (eg, endocarditis and osteomyelitis require prolonged therapy), and (3) the immunocompetence of the patient. Recommendations about duration of therapy are often given based on clinical experience, not prospective controlled studies of large numbers of patients.

H. Adverse Reactions and Toxicity

These include hypersensitivity reactions, direct toxicity, superinfection by drug-resistant microorganisms, and drug interactions. If the infection is life-threatening and treatment cannot be stopped, the reactions are managed symptomatically or another drug is chosen that does not cross-react with the offending one (Table 30–4). If the infection is less serious, it may be possible to stop all antimicrobials and monitor the patient closely.

I. Route of Administration

Parenteral therapy is preferred for acutely ill patients with serious infections (eg, endocarditis, meningitis, sepsis, severe pneumonia) when dependable levels of antibiotics are required for successful therapy. Certain drugs (eg, fluconazole, voriconazole, rifampin, metronidazole, TMP-SMZ, and fluoroquinolones) are so well absorbed that they generally can be administered orally in seriously ill—but not hemodynamically unstable—patients.

Table 30–5. Major groups of cephalosporins.

First Generation	Second Generation	Third Generation	Fourth Generation
Cephalothin	Cefamandole	Cefotaxime	Cefepime
Cephapirin	Cefuroxime	Ceftizoxime	
Cefazolin	Cefotetan	Ceftriaxone	
Cephalexin[1]	Cefaclor[1]	Ceftazidime	
Cephradine[1]	Cefoxitin	Cefoperazone	
Cefadroxil	Cefprozil[1]	Cefpodoxime proxetil[1]	
	Cefuroxime axetil[1]	Ceftibuten[1]	
		Cefdinir[1]	
		Cefditoren pivoxil[1]	

[1]Oral agents.

Food does not significantly influence the bioavailability of most oral antimicrobial agents. However, the tetracyclines and the quinolones chelate heavy metals resulting in decreased antibacterial absorption. Azithromycin capsules are associated with decreased bioavailability when taken with food and should be given 1 hour before or 2 hours after meals. Posaconazole solution should always be administered with food.

Table 30–6. Pharmacology of the cephalosporins.

Drug	Peak Serum Level (mcg/mL) after 1 g IV	Serum Half-Life (min)	Total Daily Dose (mg/kg)	Dosage Interval (hrs)	Dosage Adjustments in Kidney Disease		
					Moderate (Cl$_{cr}$ 10–50 mL/min)	Severe (Cl$_{cr}$ < 10 mL/min)	Post-hemodialysis Dose
Cephapirin	40–60	40	50–200	4–6	1–2 g q6–12h	1 g q12h	1 g
Cefazolin	90–120	90	25–100	8	0.5–1 g q6–12h	0.5 g daily	0.5 g
Cephalexin, cephradine[1]	15–20	50–60	15–30	6	0.25–0.5 g q8–12h	0.25–0.5 g daily	0.5 g
Cefadroxil[1]	15	75	15–30	12–24	1 g daily	0.5 g daily	0.5 g
Cefamandole	60–80	45	75–200	6–8	1 g q12h	1–2 g daily	0.5 g
Cefditoren pivoxil	2–3	90	6	12	0.2 g q12h	0.2 g q12h	None
Cefepime	60–70	120	50–75	8–12	1 g q12h	1 g q24h	1 g
Ceftibuten[1]	20	120	9	12–24	0.4 g daily	0.1–0.2 g daily	0.7 g
Cefuroxime	80–100	80	50	6–12	1 g q12h	1–2 g daily	0.5 g
Cefuroxime axetil[1]	6–8	75	5–15	12	0.5 g q24h	0.25 g daily	0.25 g
Cefonicid	200–250	240	15–30	24	0.5 g daily	1 g q72h	0.25 g
Ceforanide	125	180	15–30	12	1 g daily	1 g q48h	0.25 g
Cefaclor[1]	15–20	50	10–15	6–8	0.5 g q8–12h	0.25–0.5 g q12–24h	0.25–0.5 g
Cefpodoxime proxetil[1]	2	150	5	12	0.2 g q24h	0.2 g 3 times/wk after dialysis	0.2 g
Cefprozil[1]	10	90	10–15	12	0.5 g q12–24h	0.25–0.5 g q12–24h	0.5 g
Cefotaxime	40–60	60	50–75	6–8	1–2 g q6–8h	1–2 g q24h	1–2 g
Cefoxitin	60–80	60	50–100	6–8	1 g q12h	1–2 g daily	0.5 g
Ceftizoxime	80–100	100	50–75	8–12	0.5–1 g q8–12h	0.25–0.5 g q12–24h	0.5 g
Ceftriaxone	150	480	30–50	12–24	1–2 g daily	1–2 g daily	None
Ceftazidime	100–120	120	50–75	8–12	1 g q12h	0.5–1 g daily	0.5 g
Cefoperazone	150	120	30–200	8–12	1–2 g q12h	1–2 g q12h	None
Loracarbef[1]	10	60	10–15	12	0.2 g q24h	0.2 g 3 times/wk after dialysis	0.2 g

[1]Oral agents. Serum levels based on 0.5 g oral dose.

Table 30–7. Dosing of aminoglycosides.[1]

Drug (IV)	Creatinine Clearance (mL/min)				
	> 80	60–80	40–60	20–40	< 20
Gentamicin, tobramycin, netilmicin	5 mg/kg q24h	1.5–2.5 mg/kg q12h	1.2–1.5 mg/kg q24h	1.2–1.5 mg/kg q12–24h	2 mg/kg as loading dose and then 1–1.5 mg/kg q24–48h
Amikacin	15 mg/kg q24h	4.5–7.5 mg/kg q12h	3.5–4.5 mg/kg q12h	3.5–4.5 mg/kg q12–24h	7.5 mg/kg as loading dose and then 3–4.5 mg/kg q24–48h

[1]Traditional dosing should be guided by serum level measurements (peaks 30 minutes after the end of intravenous infusion and troughs ≤ 30 minutes before the next dose). When a single large daily dose is given, peak levels are not required. Trough levels should be undetectable with high-dose (5 mg/kg) once-daily gentamicin or amikacin. For those patients with creatinine clearances less than 80 mL/min, the dosage ranges in the table are used to treat gram-negative infections and are intended to achieve, for gentamicin, tobramycin, and netilmicin, peak levels of 6–10 mg/L and trough levels of ≤ 2 mg/L; for amikacin, peak levels of 20–30 mg/L and trough levels of ≤ 5 mg/L. (See text.)

Table 30–8. Pharmacology of the quinolones.

Drug	Peak Serum Levels (mcg/mL)	Serum Half-Life (h)	Total Daily Dose	Dosage Adjustments in Kidney Disease			
				Dosage Interval (h)	Moderate (Cl$_{cr}$ 10–50 mL/min)	Severe (Cl$_{cr}$ < 10 mL/min)	Post-hemodialysis Dose
Ciprofloxacin	3–4 (400 mg IV, 500–750 mg PO)	3–6	800–1200 mg (IV), 0.5–1.5 g (PO)	8–12	400 mg q12h	200 mg q12h	None
Gemifloxacin	2–4 (320 mg PO)	7	320 mg PO	Not known	Not known	Not known	Not known
Levofloxacin	5–7 (500 mg PO or IV)	6–8	250–750 mg (PO/IV)	24	250–500 mg q24–48h	250–500 mg q48h	None
Moxifloxacin	3–4 (400 mg PO)	12	400 mg (PO)	24	400 mg q24h	400 mg q24h	Not known
Ofloxacin	5–7 (400 mg PO or IV)	6–8	400–800 mg (PO/IV)	12	200–400 mg q24h	200 mg q24h	None

A major complication of intravenous antibiotic therapy is catheter infections. Peripheral catheters are changed every 48–72 hours to prevent phlebitis, and antimicrobial-coated central venous catheters (minocycline and rifampin, chlorhexidine and sulfadiazine) have been associated with a decreased incidence of catheter-related infections. Most of these infections present with local signs of infection (erythema, tenderness) at the insertion site. In a patient with fever who is receiving intravenous therapy, the catheter must always be considered a potential source. Small-gauge (20–23F) peripherally inserted silicone or polyurethane catheters (Per Q Cath, A-Cath, Ven-A-Cath, and others) are associated with a low infection rate and can be maintained for 3–6 months without replacement. Such catheters are ideal for long-term outpatient antibiotic therapy.

J. Cost of Antibiotics

The cost of these agents can be substantial. In addition to acquisition cost, monitoring costs, (drug levels, liver function tests, electrolytes, etc), the cost of treating adverse reactions, the cost of treatment failure, and the costs associated with drug administration must be considered.

Drusano GL. Antimicrobial pharmacodynamics: critical interactions of 'bug and drug'. Nat Rev Microbiol. 2004 Apr;2(4):289–300. [PMID: 15031728]

Lampiris HW et al. Clinical use of antimicrobial agents. In: *Basic & Clinical Pharmacology*, 9th ed. Katzung BG (editor). McGraw-Hill, 2004.

Spellberg B et al. Trends in antimicrobial drug development: implications for the future. Clin Infec Dis. 2004 May 1;38(9):1279–86. [PMID: 15127341]

HYPERSENSITIVITY TESTS & DESENSITIZATION

▶ Penicillin Allergy

All penicillins are cross-sensitizing and cross-reacting. The responsible antigenic determinants appear to be degradation products of penicillins, particularly penicilloic acid and products of alkaline hydrolysis (minor antigenic determinants) bound to host protein. Skin tests with penicilloyl-polylysine, with minor antigenic determinants, and with undegraded penicillin can identify most individuals with IgE-mediated reactions (hives, bronchospasm). Among positive reactors to skin tests, the incidence of subsequent immediate severe penicillin reactions is high. Although IgG antibodies to antigenic determinants of penicillin develop in many persons, the presence of such antibodies is not correlated with allergic reactivity (except for rare instances of hemolytic anemia), and serologic tests have little predictive value. A history of a penicillin reaction in the past is not reliable. Only 15–20% of patients with a history of penicillin allergy have an adverse reaction when challenged with the drug. The decision to administer penicillin or related drugs (other β-lactams) to patients with an allergic history depends on the severity of the reported reaction, the severity of the infection being treated, and the availability of alternative drugs. For patients with a history of severe reaction (anaphylaxis), alternative drugs should be used. In the rare situations when there is a strong indication for using penicillin (eg, syphilis in pregnancy) in allergic patients, desensitization can be performed. If the reaction is mild (nonurticarial rash), the patient may be rechallenged with penicillin or may be given another β-lactam antibiotic.

Allergic reactions include anaphylaxis, serum sickness (urticaria, fever, joint swelling, angioedema 7–12 days after exposure), skin rashes, fever, interstitial nephritis, eosinophilia, hemolytic anemia, other hematologic disturbances, and vasculitis. The incidence of hypersensitivity to penicillin is estimated to be 1–5% among adults in the United States. Life-threatening anaphylactic reactions are very rare (0.05%). Ampicillin produces maculopapular skin rashes more frequently than other penicillins, but many ampicillin (and other β-lactam) rashes are not allergic in origin. The nonallergic ampicillin rash usually occurs after 3–4 days of therapy, is maculopapular, is more common in patients with coexisting viral illness (especially Epstein-Barr infection), and resolves with continued therapy. The maculopapular rash may or may not reappear with rechallenge. Rarely, penicillins can induce nephritis with primary tubular lesions associated with anti-basement membrane antibodies.

Table 30–9. Examples of initial antimicrobial therapy for acutely ill, hospitalized adults pending identification of causative organism.

Suspected Clinical Diagnosis	Likely Etiologic Diagnosis	Drugs of Choice
(A) Meningitis, bacterial, community-acquired	Pneumococcus,[1] meningococcus	Cefotaxime,[2] 2–3 g IV every 6 hours; **or** ceftriaxone, 2 g IV every 12 hours plus vancomycin, 10 mg/kg IV every 8 hours
(B) Meningitis, bacterial, age > 50, community-acquired	Pneumococcus, meningococcus, *Listeria monocytogenes*,[3] gram-negative bacilli	Ampicillin, 2 g IV every 4 hours, plus cefotaxime **or** ceftriaxone and vancomycin as in (A)
(C) Meningitis, postoperative (or posttraumatic)	*S aureus*, gram-negative bacilli (pneumococcus, in posttraumatic)	Vancomycin, 10 mg/kg IV every 8 hours, plus ceftazidime, 3 g IV every 8 hours
(D) Brain abscess	Mixed anaerobes, pneumococci, streptococci	Penicillin G, 4 million units IV every 4 hours, plus metronidazole, 500 mg orally every 8 hours; **or** cefotaxime or ceftriaxone as in (A) plus metronidazole, 500 mg orally every 8 hours
(E) Pneumonia, acute, community-acquired, severe	Pneumococci, *M pneumoniae*, *Legionella*, *C pneumoniae*	Cefotaxime, 2 g IV every 8 hours (or ceftriaxone, 1 g IV every 24 hours or ampicillin 2 g IV every 6 hours) plus azithromycin 500 mg IV every 24 hours; **or** a fluoroquinolone[5] alone
(F) Pneumonia, postoperative or nosocomial	*S aureus*, mixed anaerobes, gram-negative bacilli	Cefepime, 2 g IV every 8 hours; **or** ceftazidime, 2 g IV every 8 hours; **or** piperacillin-tazobactam, 45 g IV every 6 hours; **or** imipenem, 500 mg IV every 6 hours; **or** meropenem, 1 g IV every 8 hours plus tobramycin, 5 mg/kg IV every 24 hours; **or** ciprofloxacin, 400 mg IV every 12 hours; **or** levofloxacin, 500 mg IV every 24 hours plus vancomycin, 15 mg/kg IV every 12 hours
(G) Endocarditis, acute (including injection drug user)	*S aureus*, *E faecalis*, gram-negative aerobic bacteria, viridans streptococci	Vancomycin, 15 mg/kg IV every 12 hours, plus gentamicin, 1 mg/kg every 8 hours
(H) Septic thrombophlebitis (eg, IV tubing, IV shunts)	*S aureus*, gram-negative aerobic bacteria	Vancomycin, 15 mg/kg IV every 12 hours plus ceftriaxone, 1 g IV every 24 hours
(I) Osteomyelitis	*S aureus*	Nafcillin, 2 g IV every 4 hours; **or** cefazolin, 2 g IV every 8 hours
(J) Septic arthritis	*S aureus*, *N gonorrhoeae*	Ceftriaxone, 1–2 g IV every 24 hours
(K) Pyelonephritis with flank pain and fever (recurrent urinary tract infection)	*E coli*, *Klebsiella*, *Enterobacter*, *Pseudomonas*	Ceftriaxone, 1g IV every 24 hours; **or** ciprofloxacin, 400 mg IV every 12 hours (500 mg orally); **or** levofloxacin, 500 mg once daily (IV/PO)
(L) Fever in neutropenic patient receiving cancer chemotherapy	*S aureus*, *Pseudomonas*, *Klebsiella*, *E coli*	Ceftazidime, 2 g IV every 8 hours; **or** cefepime, 2 g IV every 8 hours
(M) Intra-abdominal sepsis (eg, postoperative, peritonitis, cholecystitis)	Gram-negative bacteria, *Bacteroides*, anaerobic bacteria, streptococci, clostridia	Piperacillin-tazobactam as in (F) **or** ertapenem, 1 g every 24 hours

[1]Some strains may be resistant to penicillin. Vancomycin can be used with or without rifampin.
[2]Cefotaxime, ceftriaxone, ceftazidime, or ceftizoxime can be used. Most studies on meningitis have been with cefotaxime or ceftriaxone (see text).
[3]TMP-SMZ can be used to treat *Listeria monocytogenes* in patients allergic to penicillin in a dosage of 15–20 mg/kg of TMP in three or four divided doses.
[4]Depending on local drug susceptibility pattern, use tobramycin, 5 mg/kg/d, or amikacin, 15 mg/kg/d, in place of gentamicin.
[5]Levofloxacin 750 mg/d, moxifloxacin 400 mg/d.

If the intradermal test described below is negative, desensitization is not necessary, and a full dose of the material may be given. If the test is positive, alternative drugs should be strongly considered. If that is not feasible, desensitization is necessary.

Patients with a history of allergy to penicillin are also at an increased risk for having a reaction to **cephalosporins**. Since the specific immunogens responsible for anaphylaxis are not known for drugs other than penicillin, skin testing with cephalosporins is not recommended. A common approach to these patients is to assess the severity of the reaction. If an IgE-mediated reaction to penicillin can be excluded by history, a cephalosporin can be administered. When the history justifies concern about an immediate-type reaction, penicillin skin testing should be performed. If the test is negative, a cephalosporin can be given. If the test is positive, there is a 5–10% chance of cross reactivity, and the decision whether to use cephalosporins depends on the availability of alternative agents and the severity of the infection.

Table 30–10. Examples of empiric choices of antimicrobials for adult outpatient infections.

Suspected Clinical Diagnosis	Likely Etiologic Agents	Drugs of Choice	Alternative Drugs
Erysipelas, impetigo, cellulitis, ascending lymphangitis	Group A streptococcus	Phenoxymethyl penicillin, 0.5 g orally four times daily for 7–10 days	Cephalexin, 0.5 g orally four times daily for 7–10 days; or azithromycin, 500 mg on day 1 and 250 mg on days 2–5
Furuncle with surrounding cellulitis	Staphylococcus aureus	Dicloxacillin, 0.5 g orally four times daily for 7–10 days (If high-risk for MRSA, clindamycin 0.3 g orally four times daily for 7–10 days)	Cephalexin, 0.5 g orally four times daily for 7–10 days. (If high-risk for MRSA, TMP-SMZ two double strength tablets twice daily for 7–10 days)
Pharyngitis	Group A streptococcus	Phenoxymethyl penicillin, 0.5 g orally four times daily for 10 days	Clindamycin, 300 mg orally four times daily for 10 days; or erythromycin, 0.5 g orally four times daily for 10 days; or azithromycin, 500 mg on day 1 and 250 mg on days 2–5; or clarithromycin, 500 mg twice daily for 10 days
Otitis media	Streptococcus pneumoniae, Haemophilus influenzae, Moraxella catarrhalis	Amoxicillin, 0.5–1.0 g orally three times daily for 10 days	Augmentin,[2] 0.875 g orally twice daily; or cefuroxime, 0.5 g orally twice daily; or cefpodoxime, 0.2–0.4 g daily; or doxycycline, 100 mg twice daily; or TMP-SMZ,[1] one double-strength tablet twice daily (all regimens for 10 days).
Acute sinusitis	S pneumoniae, H influenzae, M catarrhalis	Amoxicillin, 0.5–1.0 g orally three times daily; or TMP-SMZ, one double-strength tablet twice daily for 10 days	Augmentin,[2] 0.875 g orally twice daily; or cefuroxime, 0.5 g orally twice daily; or cefpodoxime, 0.2–0.4 g daily; or doxycycline, 100 mg twice daily (all regimens for 10 days)
Aspiration pneumonia	Mixed oropharyngeal flora, including anaerobes	Clindamycin, 0.3 g orally four times daily for 10–14 days	Phenoxymethyl penicillin, 0.5 g orally four times daily for 10–14 days
Pneumonia	S pneumoniae, Mycoplasma pneumoniae, Legionella pneumophila, Chlamydophila pneumoniae	Doxycycline, 100 mg orally twice daily; or clarithromycin, 0.5 g orally twice daily, for 10–14 days; or azithromycin, 0.5 g orally on day 1 and 0.25 g on days 2–5	Amoxicillin, 0.5–1.0 g orally four times daily; or a fluoroquinolone[5] for 10–14 days
Cystitis	Escherichia coli, Klebsiella pneumoniae, Proteus species, Staphylococcus saprophyticus	Fluoroquinolones,[4] 3 days for uncomplicated cystitis, nitrofurantoin macrocrystals, 100 mg orally four times daily for 7 days; nitrofurantoin monohydrate macrocrystals, 100 mg twice daily for 7 days	TMP-SMZ,[1] one double-strength tablet twice daily for 3 days; or cephalexin, 0.5 g orally four times daily for 7 days
Pyelonephritis	E coli, K pneumoniae, Proteus species, S saprophyticus	Fluoroquinolones[4] for 7–14 days	TMP-SMZ,[1] one double-strength tablet twice daily for 7–14 days
Gastroenteritis	Salmonella, Shigella, Campylobacter, Entamoeba histolytica	See Note 3.	
Urethritis, epididymitis	Neisseria gonorrhoeae, Chlamydia trachomatis	Ceftriaxone, 250 mg IM once or cefpodoxime 200–400 mg orally once, for N gonorrhoeae; plus doxycycline, 100 mg orally twice daily for 10 days, for C trachomatis	Ciprofloxacin, 500 mg orally once, for N gonorrhoeae; plus doxycycline, 100 mg orally twice daily for 10 days, or ofloxacin, 300 mg orally twice daily for 10 days
Pelvic inflammatory disease	N gonorrhoeae, C trachomatis, anaerobes, gram-negative rods	Ofloxacin, 400 mg orally twice daily, for 14 days, plus metronidazole, 500 mg orally twice daily, for 14 days	Cefoxitin, 2 g IM, with probenecid, 1 g orally, followed by doxycycline, 100 mg orally twice daily for 14 days; or ceftriaxone, 250 mg IM once, followed by doxycycline, 100 mg orally twice daily for 14 days

(continued)

Table 30–10. Examples of empiric choices of antimicrobials for adult outpatient infections. (continued)

Suspected Clinical Diagnosis	Likely Etiologic Agents	Drugs of Choice	Alternative Drugs
Syphilis			
Early syphilis (primary, secondary, or latent of < 1 year's duration)	*Treponema pallidum*	Benzathine penicillin G, 2.4 million units IM once	Doxycycline, 100 mg orally twice daily for 2 weeks
Latent syphilis of > 1 year's duration or cardiovascular syphilis	*T pallidum*	Benzathine penicillin G, 2.4 million units IM once a week for 3 weeks (total: 7.2 million units)	Doxycycline, 100 mg orally twice daily, for 4 weeks
Neurosyphilis	*T pallidum*	Aqueous penicillin G, 12–24 million units/d IV for 10–14 days	

[1]TMP-SMZ is a fixed combination of 1 part trimethoprim and 5 parts sulfamethoxazole. Single-strength tablets: 80 mg TMP, 400 mg SMZ; double-strength tablets: 160 mg TMP, 800 mg SMZ.

[2]Augmentin is a combination of amoxicillin, 250 mg, 500 mg, or 875 mg, plus 125 mg of clavulanic acid. Augmentin XR is a combination of amoxicillin 1 g and clavulanic acid 62.5 mg.

[3]The diagnosis should be confirmed by culture before therapy. *Salmonella* gastroenteritis does not require therapy. For susceptible *Shigella* isolates, give TMP-SMZ double-strength tablets twice daily for 5 days; or ampicillin, 0.5 g orally four times daily for 5 days; or ciprofloxacin, 0.5 g orally twice daily for 5 days. For *Campylobacter* infection, give azithromycin, 1 g orally times one dose, or ciprofloxacin, 0.5 g orally twice daily for 5 days. For *E histolytica* infection, give metronidazole, 750 mg orally three times daily for 5–10 days, followed by diiodohydroxyquin, 600 mg orally three times daily for 3 weeks.

[4]Fluoroquinolones and dosages include ciprofloxacin, 500 mg orally twice daily; ofloxacin, 400 mg orally twice daily; levofloxacin, 500 mg orally daily. For others see text.

[5]Fluoroquinolones with activity against *S pneumoniae*, including penicillin-resistant isolates, include levofloxacin (500 mg orally once daily), gemifloxacin (320 mg orally once daily), and moxifloxacin (400 mg orally once daily).

MRSA, methicillin-resistant *Staphylococcus aureus*; TMP-SMZ, trimethoprim-sulfamethoxazole.

▶ Intradermal Test for Hypersensitivity

Penicillin is the drug that most frequently serves as an indication for sensitivity testing and desensitization. A clinical history of penicillin allergy has a positive predictive value of only 15%. In determining whether allergy testing should be performed, its nature should be determined. IgG-mediated delayed reactions such as erythematous or maculopapular skin rash or serum sickness should be distinguished from immediate-type IgE-mediated reactions, such as urticaria, angioedema, and anaphylaxis. Only patients with the latter history who require penicillin or a cephalosporin should undergo hypersensitivity testing. Skin testing requires two preparations: PPL (penicilloyl-polylysine) and a minor determinant mixture. Several points should be emphasized in performing and interpreting these tests. Whenever possible, both PPL and a minor determinant should be used, since 85% of skin test reactors are positive to PPL but 15% react only to the minor determinant mixture. In addition, if penicillin G is used instead of the minor determinant mixture, some allergic patients will be missed. About 25% of individuals who react to minor determinant mixture may not react to penicillin G, and such patients may still have an anaphylactic or accelerated reaction to penicillin. A pinprick test is performed with each solution at different sites by placing a small drop of solution on the skin and making small indentations of the skin with a needle. If there is no reaction within 10 minutes, 0.01–0.02 mL is injected intradermally, raising a small bleb. Development of a wheal greater than 5 mm in diameter is considered a positive test and an indication for desensitization. Even if the test is negative, about 1–2% of patients will have an immediate or accelerated reaction, but an anaphylactic reaction is rare. Thus, if the test is negative, the drug can be administered with relative safety, but the first dose should be medically supervised and the patient observed for 1 hour (serious reactions after 1 hour are rare).

▶ Desensitization

A. Precautions

1. The desensitization procedure is not innocuous—deaths from anaphylaxis have been reported. If extreme hypersensitivity is suspected, it is advisable to use an alternative structurally unrelated drug and to reserve desensitization for situations when treatment cannot be withheld and no alternative drug is available.

2. An antihistaminic drug (25–50 mg of hydroxyzine or diphenhydramine intramuscularly or orally) should be administered before desensitization is begun in order to lessen any reaction that occurs.

3. Desensitization should be conducted in an intensive care unit where cardiac monitoring and emergency endotracheal intubation can be performed.

4. Epinephrine, 1 mL of 1:1000 solution, must be ready for immediate administration.

B. Desensitization Method

Several methods of desensitization have been described for penicillin, including use of both oral and intravenous

Table 30–11. Use of antimicrobials in patients with kidney failure[1] and liver failure.

| Drug | Principal Mode of Excretion or Detoxification | Approximate Half-Life in Serum | | Proposed Dosage Regimen in End-Stage Kidney Disease (all doses IV unless stated otherwise) | | Removal of Drug by Hemodialysis | Dose after Hemodialysis | Dosage in Hepatic Failure |
		Normal	Kidney Disease	Initial Dose[3]	Maintenance Dose			
Acyclovir	Renal	2.5–3.5 hours	20 hours	2.5 mg/kg	2.5 mg/kg q24h	Yes	2.5 mg/kg	No change
Amphotericin B	Unknown	360 hours	360 hours	No change	No change	No	None	No change
Ampicillin	Tubular secretion	0.5–1 hour	8–12 hours	1 g	1 g q8–12h	Yes	1 g	No change
Ampicillin-sulbactam	Renal	0.5–1 hour	8–12 hours	3 g	1.5 g q8–12h	Yes	1.5 g	No change
Azithromycin	Renal 20%; hepatic 35%	3–4 hours	Not known	500 mg	250 mg q24h	No	None	Not known[4]
Aztreonam	Renal	1.7 hours	6 hours	1–2 g	0.5–1 g q6–8h	Yes	0.5–1 g	No change
Caspofungin	Liver	9–10 hours	9–10 hours	70 mg	50 mg q24h	No	None	35 mg q24h
Chloramphenicol	Mainly liver	3 hours	4 hours	0.5 g	0.5 g q6h	Yes	0.5 g	0.25–0.5 g q12h
Clarithromycin	Renal 30%; hepatic > 50%	3–4 hours	15 hours	500 mg PO	250 mg q12h PO	No	None	Not known[4]
Clindamycin	Liver	2–4 hours	2–4 hours	0.6 g IV	0.6 g q8h	No	None	0.3–0.6 g q8h
Daptomycin	Renal	8–12 hours	> 24 hours	4–6 mg/kg	4–6 mg/kg q48h	No	None	No change
Doxycycline	Renal	15–24 hours	15–24 hours	100 mg	100 mg q12h	No	None	Not known[4]
Ertapenem	Renal	4 hours	20 hours	1 g	0.5 g q24h	Yes	0.15 g	No change
Erythromycin	Mainly liver	1.5 hours	1.5 hours	0.5–1 g	0.5–1 g q6h	No	None	0.25–0.5 g q6h
Famciclovir[5]	Renal	2.5 hours	13–20 hours	500 mg PO	500 mg q24h PO	Yes	500 mg	No change
Fluconazole	Renal	30 hours	98 hours	0.2 g	0.1 g q24h	Yes	Give q24h dose	No change
Flucytosine	Renal	3–6 hours	30–250 hours	37.5 mg/kg PO	25 mg/kg q24h PO	Yes	25 mg/kg	No change
Foscarnet	Renal	3–8 hours	Not known	90–120 mg	Not known[6]	No	None	No change
Fosfomycin	Renal	6 hours	11–50 hours	NA	NA	NA	NA	No change
Ganciclovir[7]	Renal	3 hours	11–28 hours	1.25 mg/kg	1.25 mg/kg q24h	Yes	Give q24h dose	No change
Gemifloxacin	Renal and liver	7 hours	Not known	320 mg PO	160 mg q24h PO	Not known	Not known	Not known
Imipenem	Glomerular filtration	1 hour	3 hours	0.5 g	0.25–0.5 g q12h	Yes	0.25–0.5 g	No change
Isoniazid	Renal	1–5 hours	2.5 hours	300 mg PO	300 mg q24h PO	Yes	None	Not known[4]
Itraconazole	Hepatic	21 hours	25 hours	50–200 mg PO	50–200 mg q24h PO	No	None	Not known[4]
Ketoconazole	Hepatic	8 hours	8 hours	200 mg PO	200–400 mg q24h PO	No	None	Not known[4]
Meropenem	Renal	1 hour	5–10 hours	1 g	0.5–1 g q24h	Yes	0.5 g	No change
Metronidazole	Liver	6–10 hours	6–10 hours	0.5 g IV	0.5 g q8h	Yes	0.25 g	0.25 g q12h

Micafungin	Biliary/hepatic	15 hours	15 hours	150 mg	150 mg q24h	No	None	No change
Nafcillin	Liver 80%; kidney 20%	0.75 hour	1.5 hours	1.5 g	1.5 g q4h	No	None	2–3 g q12h
Penicillin G	Tubular secretion	0.5 hour	7–10 hours	1–2 million units	1 million units q8h	Yes	500,000 units	No change
Pentamidine	Not known	6–9 hours	6–9 hours	4 mg/kg	4 mg/kg q24h	No	None needed	No change
Piperacillin and piperacillin + tazobactam	Renal 50–70%; biliary 20–30%	1 hour	3–6 hours	3 g	2 g q6–8h	Yes	1 g	1–2 g q8h
Posaconazole	Hepatic	20–66 hours	20–66 hours	200–400 mg	200 mg q6–8h PO 400 mg q12h PO	No		Not known[4]
Rifampin	Hepatic	2–3 hours	3–5 hours	600 mg PO	600 mg q24h PO	No	None	Not known
Telithromycin	Hepatic	7–10 hours	7–10 hours	800 mg PO	800 mg q24h PO	Not known	Not known	Not known
Tigecycline	Hepatic	25–40 hours	25–40 hours	100 mg	50 mg q12h	No	None	No change
Trimethoprim-sulfamethoxazole	Some liver	TMP 10–12 hours; SMZ 8–10 hours	TMP 24–48 hours; SMZ 18–24 hours	320 mg TMP + 1600 mg SMZ	80 mg TMP + 400 mg SMZ q12h	Yes	80 mg TMP + 400 mg SMZ	No change
Vancomycin	Glomerular filtration	6 hours	6–10 days	1 g	1 g q6–10d based on serum levels[8]	No	None	No change
Voriconazole	Hepatic	6–24 hours; dose-dependent	6–24 hours	200 mg orally; avoid IV in kidney disease	200 mg orally twice daily; avoid IV in kidney disease	No	None	100 mg twice daily

[1] For cephalosporins, see text and Tables 30–5 and 30–6; for aminoglycosides, see Table 30–7.

[2] Considered here to be marked by creatinine clearance of 10 mL/min or less.

[3] For a 70-kg adult with a serious systemic infection.

[4] Dose adjustment in hepatic failure has not been studied, but because clearance of the drug is principally hepatic, dose reduction may be required.

[5] Pharmacokinetics and dosing are in reference to the active agent, penciclovir.

[6] When creatinine clearance is 30 mL/min, a dose of 60 mg/kg is given once daily. For clearances less than 30 mL/min, the dose has not been established.

[7] Oral valganciclovir is same as IV ganciclovir except that the initial dose is 900 mg, maintenance dose is 450 mg twice weekly in patients with creatinine clearance 10–40 mL/min. Post doses not known.

[8] When serum levels reach 10–15 mcg/mL, another dose should be given.

preparations. All methods start with very small doses of drug and gradually increase the dose until therapeutic doses are achieved. For penicillin, 1 unit of drug is given intravenously and the patient observed for 15–30 minutes. If there is no reaction, some recommend doubling the dose while others recommend increasing it tenfold every 15–30 minutes until a dosage of 2 million units is reached; then give the remainder of the desired dose.

For recommendations on skin testing and desensitization for other preparations (eg, botulism antitoxin and diphtheria antitoxin), the manufacturer's package inserts should be consulted.

▶ Treatment of Reactions

A. Mild Reactions

If a mild reaction occurs, drop back to the next lower dose and continue with desensitization. If a severe reaction occurs, administer epinephrine (see below) and discontinue the drug unless treatment is urgently needed. If desensitization is imperative, continue slowly, increasing the dosage of the drug more gradually.

B. Severe Reactions

If bronchospasm occurs, epinephrine, 0.3–0.5 mL of 1:1000 dilution, should be given subcutaneously every 10–20 minutes, followed by corticosteroids (250 mg of hydrocortisone or 50 mg of methylprednisolone intravenously every 6 hours for two to four doses), if needed. Hypotension should be treated with intravenous fluids (saline or colloid), epinephrine (1 mL of 1:1000 dilution in 500 mL of D_5W intravenously at a rate of 0.5–5 mcg/min), and antihistamines (25–50 mg of hydroxyzine or diphenhydramine intramuscularly or orally every 6–8 hours as needed). Cutaneous reactions, manifested as urticaria or angioedema, respond to epinephrine subcutaneously and antihistamines in the doses set forth above.

Arroliga ME et al. Penicillin allergy: consider trying penicillin again. Cleve Clin J Med. 2003 Apr;70(4):313–4, 317–8, 320–1 passim. [PMID: 12701985]
Gruchalla RS et al. Clinical practice. Antibiotic allergy. N Engl J Med. 2006 Feb 9;354(6):601–9. [PMID: 16467547]

▌IMMUNIZATION AGAINST INFECTIOUS DISEASES

RECOMMENDED IMMUNIZATION OF INFANTS, CHILDREN, & ADOLESCENTS

The recommended schedules and dosages of vaccination change often, so the manufacturer's package inserts should always be consulted.

The schedule for active immunizations in children is presented in Table 30–12 (see also www.cdc.gov/vaccines/recs/schedules). All adolescents should see a health care provider to ensure vaccination of those who have not received varicella or hepatitis B vaccine, to make certain that a second dose of MMR has been given, to receive a

booster of tetanus toxoid, reduced diphtheria toxoid and acellular pertussis vaccine (Tdap adolescent preparation), to receive meningococcal vaccine conjugate vaccine, and to receive immunizations (influenza and pneumococcal vaccines) that may be indicated for certain high-risk individuals.

RECOMMENDED IMMUNIZATION OF ADULTS

Several vaccines are recommended for adults depending on the individual's previous vaccination status and the risks of exposure to certain diseases. Recommendations are summarized in Table 30–13.

▶ Hepatitis A

Two inactivated hepatitis A vaccines (Havrix, VAQTA) are approved for use in the United States for individuals 12 months of age or older. Hepatitis A vaccination is recommended as part of the routine childhood vaccination for all those 1 year of age or older. Vaccination is also recommended for adults at increased risk for developing infection, including travelers to areas where hepatitis is endemic (Africa, Asia, Central and South America, Mexico, parts of the Caribbean); certain populations that experience outbreaks (such as indigenous Alaskans, certain American Indian reservations, various religious communities and states where the risk of hepatitis A is high among children); employees of day care centers, caretakers for developmentally impaired institutionalized individuals, and laboratory workers who handle live hepatitis A virus or work closely with nonhuman primates; men who have sex with men; illicit drug users; persons who receive clotting factor concentrates; and those with chronic liver disease. A single intramuscular injection of vaccine in adults elicits antibodies in 55–60% of individuals at 2 weeks and 95% by 1 month, although rates of seroconversion may be lower in immunocompromised individuals. The different formulations come in different strengths, and dosage depends on the age of the vaccine and the preparation used (see package insert). In general, two doses are required, the second 6–18 months after the first. The duration of immunity may be lifelong, and at present, repeat vaccination is not recommended. A single dose of hepatitis A vaccine can be used as postexposure prophylaxis and is recommended for those between the ages of 12 months and 40 years of age. For those older than 40 years of age, 0.02 mL/kg of immunoglobulin is recommended. Preparation of immunoglobulin from plasma involves steps that inactivate HIV, thus making it incapable of transmitting HIV infection.

▶ Hepatitis B

Recombinant hepatitis B vaccine is recommended for all individuals at increased risk for developing hepatitis B, including individuals at risk for acquiring disease by sexual exposure (sex partners of hepatitis B surface antigen (HBsAg)–positive individuals, persons with more than one sex partner in the last 6 months, persons seeking evaluation and treatment for STDs, and men who have sex with men) and those at risk for infection from percutaneous or mucosal exposure to blood (current or recent injection drug users; household contacts of HBsAg–positive individuals; residents and staff of facilities for developmentally disabled individuals; healthcare and public safety workers with likely exposure to infected blood or body fluids; and persons with end-stage renal disease, including predialysis and dialysis patients). Others who are candidates for vaccination include travelers to regions with high rates of endemic disease, those with chronic liver disease or HIV infection, and anyone who wants protection from hepatitis B. In settings where a high proportion of individuals are likely to be at risk for hepatitis B (such as STD and HIV screening and treatment facilities, drug abuse treatment centers, health care settings targeting care for men who have sex with men, and correctional facilities), all patients who seek care at those facilities be vaccinated. In addition, it is recommended that primary and specialty care practices establish standing orders to identify adults at risk for hepatitis B and administer vaccine as part of their routine services. In immunocompromised patients and individuals undergoing hemodialysis, seroresponse to standard doses of vaccine is low, and a special preparation delivering a higher vaccine dose (40 mcg/mL) is recommended. In addition to higher vaccine doses, these patients may require more frequent immunizations, and some authorities recommend annual screening to determine whether booster doses are needed. Although most often used for preexposure prophylaxis, the vaccine is also given as postexposure prophylaxis along with hepatitis B immunoglobulin following needlestick injury or mucous membrane exposure to blood from an individual who is HBsAg-positive. It is also given along with hepatitis B immunoglobulin to infants of mothers who are HBsAg-positive (Table 30–12). Immunity wanes with time, but protection against infection lasts at least 20 years, making periodic serologic monitoring and routine administration of booster doses unnecessary.

Ten micrograms of recombinant hepatitis B vaccine is given intramuscularly in the deltoid (gluteal injection often results in deposition of vaccine in fat rather than muscle with fewer serologic conversions) on three separate occasions: the first two doses 1 month apart and the last dose 5 months after the second one. Seroconversion occurs after the first dose in 30–55% of healthy adults less than 40 years of age, in 75% after two doses, and in greater than 90% after 3 doses. No apparent effect on immunogenicity has been documented if this timing is not strictly adhered to. A number of factors decrease serologic response, including age over 40, kidney disease, HIV infection, diabetes, chronic liver disease, obesity, and smoking. Post-vaccination serologic testing is not routinely performed. It is reserved for those whose clinical management would be influenced by their immune status (eg, health care workers, infants born to HBsAg-positive mothers, dialysis patients), and those who may have an impaired response. Those who do not respond should receive a second three-dose vaccine series with serologic testing 1–2 months after completion. Those who do not respond are unlikely to respond to further vaccination even with a different recombinant

vaccine and should be considered susceptible; if exposed, they should receive hepatitis B immune globulin.

▶ **Herpes Zoster**

Waning cell-mediated immunity that occurs with aging increases the risk of reactivation of latent varicella virus, as does immunosuppression. More than 90% of adults have been exposed to varicella and are at risk for developing herpes zoster. Most cases of herpes zoster occur in those over the age of 60 years, and postherpetic neuralgia (a severe and debilitating sequela that can last months to years) occurs in about 30% of those over age 60 in whom herpes zoster develops.

Zostavax is a live attenuated varicella-zoster vaccine that contains 14 times as much virus as that used for varicella vaccination (see above). Compared with placebo, a single subcutaneous dose of vaccine significantly decreased the incidence of herpes zoster, the incidence of postherpetic neuralgia, and the severity and duration of pain in those in whom postherpetic neuralgia developed.

A single dose of zoster vaccine is recommended for adults 60 years of age or older whether or not they have had a prior episode of herpes zoster. Serologic status should be checked prior to immunization. Individuals lacking immunity should be vaccinated against varicella (see above).

▶ **Human Papillomavirus**

Genital HPV is the most common STD in the United States with more than 6 million new cases annually. There are over 100 different types of virus, about 40 of which cause genital disease. "Low risk" strains are associated with genital warts or benign low-grade cervical cell changes, whereas "high-risk" strains are associated with cervical and other anogenital neoplasms. Although most HPV infections are transient, those that persist can be associated with cervical intraepithelial neoplasia and may progress to cervical cancer. Approximately 70% of cervical cancers are associated with HPV types 16 and 18, and 90% of anogenital warts are associated with types 6 and 11.

A recombinant quadrivalent HPV vaccine (Gardasil) composed of the L1 major capsid protein from "low risk" types 6 and 11 and "high risk" types 16 and 18 has been approved for use in girls and women 9–26 years of age to prevent disease associated with these HPV types. Clinical studies indicated a high efficacy of prevention of vaccine type persistent infections, cervical intraepithelial neoplasia, and genital warts. There was no evidence of protection against nonvaccine strains or protection against strains that were present before vaccination. The Advisory Committee on Immunization Practices (ACIP) recommends routine vaccination of females 11–12 years of age with three intramuscular doses; the second and third doses should be given 2 and 6 months after the first. No changes in cervical cancer screening have been recommended in vaccinated individuals. The vaccine has also been evaluated in boys, heterosexual men, and men who have sex with men. Currently, there are no guidelines for vaccination in these groups pending final analysis and review of the data.

Table 30–12. Recommended childhood and adolescent immunization schedule–United States, 2009.[1]

Recommended Immunization Schedule for Persons Aged 0 Through 6 Years—United States • 2009

For those who fall behind or start late, see the catch-up schedule

Vaccine ▼ Age ▶	Birth	1 month	2 months	4 months	6 months	12 months	15 months	18 months	19–23 months	2–3 years	4–6 years
Hepatitis B[1]	HepB	HepB		see footnote 1		HepB					
Rotavirus[2]			RV	RV	RV[2]						
Diphtheria, Tetanus, Pertussis[3]			DTaP	DTaP	DTaP	see footnote 3	DTaP	DTaP			DTaP
Haemophilus influenzae type b[4]			Hib	Hib	Hib[4]	Hib	Hib				
Pneumococcal[5]			PCV	PCV	PCV	PCV	PCV			PPSV	
Inactivated Poliovirus			IPV	IPV		IPV	IPV				IPV
Influenza[6]						Influenza (Yearly)					
Measles, Mumps, Rubella[7]						MMR	MMR		see footnote 7		MMR
Varicella[8]						Varicella	Varicella		see footnote 8		Varicella
Hepatitis A[9]						HepA (2 doses)	HepA (2 doses)			HepA Series	
Meningococcal[10]										MCV4	MCV4

■ Range of recommended ages

■ Certain high-risk groups

This schedule indicates the recommended ages for routine administration of currently licensed vaccines, as of December 1, 2008, for children aged 0 through 6 years. Any dose not administered at the recommended age should be administered at a subsequent visit, when indicated and feasible. Licensed combination vaccines may be used whenever any component of the combination is indicated and other components are not contraindicated and if approved by the Food and Drug Administration for that dose of the series.

Providers should consult the relevant Advisory Committee on Immunization Practices statement for detailed recommendations, including high-risk conditions: http://www.cdc.gov/vaccines/ pubs/acip-list.htm. Clinically significant adverse events that follow immunization should be reported to the Vaccine Adverse Event Reporting System (VAERS). Guidance about how to obtain and complete a VAERS form is available at http://www.vaers.hhs.gov or by telephone, 800-822-7967.

1. Hepatitis B vaccine (HepB). *(Minimum age: birth)*

At birth:

- Administer monovalent HepB to all newborns before hospital discharge.
- If mother is hepatitis B surface antigen (HBsAg)-positive, administer HepB and 0.5 mL of hepatitis B immune globulin (HBIG) within 12 hours of birth.
- If mother's HBsAg status is unknown, administer HepB within 12 hours of birth. Determine mother's HBsAg status as soon as possible and, ifHBsAg-positive, administer HBIG (no later than age 1 week).

After the birth dose:

- The HepB series should be completed with either monovalent HepB or a combination vaccine containing HepB. The second dose should be administered at age 1 or 2 months. The final dose should be administered no earlier than age 24 weeks.
- Infants born to HBsAg-positive mothers should be tested for HBsAg and antibody to HBsAg (anti-HBs) after completion of at least 3 doses of the HepB series, at age 9 through 18 months (generally at the next well-child visit).

4-month dose:

- Administration of 4 doses of HepB to infants is permissible when combination vaccines containing HepB are administered after the birth dose.

2. Rotavirus vaccine (RV). *(Minimum age: 6 weeks)*

- Administer the first dose at age 6 through 14 weeks (maximum age: 14 weeks 6 days). Vaccination should not be initiated for infants aged 15 weeks or older (i.e., 15 weeks 0 days or older).
- Administer the final dose in the series by age 8 months 0 days.
- If Rotarix® is administered at ages 2 and 4 months, a dose at 6 months is not indicated.

3. Diphtheria and tetanus toxoids and acellular pertussis vaccine (DTaP). *(Minimum age: 6 weeks)*

- The fourth dose may be administered as early as age 12 months, provided at least 6 months have elapsed since the third dose.
- Administer the final dose in the series at age 4 through 6 years.

4. Haemophilus influenzae type b conjugate vaccine (Hib). *(Minimum age: 6 weeks)*

- If PRP-OMP (PedvaxHIB® or Comvax® (HepB-Hib)) is administered at ages 2 and 4 months, a dose at age 6 months is not indicated.
- TriHiBit® (DTaP/Hib) should not be used for doses at ages 2, 4, or 6 months but can be used as the final dose in children aged 12 months or older.

5. Pneumococcal vaccine. *(Minimum age: 6 weeks for pneumococcal conjugate vaccine [PCV]; 2 years for pneumococcal polysaccharide vaccine [PPSV])*

- PCV is recommended for all children aged younger than 5 years. Administer 1 dose of PCV to all healthy children aged 24 through 59 months who are not completely vaccinated for their age.
- Administer PPSV to children aged 2 years or older with certain underlying medical conditions (see MMWR 2000;49[No. RR-9]), including a cochlear implant.

6. Influenza vaccine. *(Minimum age: 6 months for trivalent inactivated influenza vaccine [TIV]; 2 years for live, attenuated influenza vaccine [LAIV])*

- Administer annually to children aged 6 months through 18 years.
- For healthy nonpregnant persons (i.e., those who do not have underlying medical conditions that predispose them to influenza complications) aged 2 through 49 years, either LAIV or TIV may be used.
- Children receiving TIV should receive 0.25 mL if aged 6 through 35 months or 0.5 mL if aged 3 years or older.
- Administer 2 doses (separated by at least 4 weeks) to children aged younger than 9 years who are receiving influenza vaccine for the first time or who were vaccinated for the first time during the previous influenza season but only received 1 dose.

7. Measles, mumps, and rubella vaccine (MMR). *(Minimum age: 12 months)*

- Administer the second dose at age 4 through 6 years. However, the second dose may be administered before age 4, provided at least 28 days have elapsed since the first dose.

8. Varicella vaccine. *(Minimum age: 12 months)*

- Administer the second dose at age 4 through 6 years. However, the second dose may be administered before age 4, provided at least 3 months have elapsed since the first dose.
- For children aged 12 months through 12 years the minimum interval between doses is 3 months. However, if the second dose was administered at least 28 days after the first dose, it can be accepted as valid.

9. Hepatitis A vaccine (HepA). *(Minimum age: 12 months)*

- Administer to all children aged 1 year (i.e., aged 12 through 23 months). Administer 2 doses at least 6 months apart.
- Children not fully vaccinated by age 2 years can be vaccinated at subsequent visits.
- HepA also is recommended for children older than 1 year who live in areas where vaccination programs target older children or who are at increased risk of infection. See MMWR 2006;55(No. RR-7).

10. Meningococcal vaccine. *(Minimum age: 2 years for meningococcal conjugate vaccine [MCV] and for meningococcal polysaccharide vaccine [MPSV])*

- Administer MCV to children aged 2 through 10 years with terminal complement component deficiency, anatomic or functional asplenia, and certain other high-risk groups. See MMWR 2005;54(No. RR-7).
- Persons who received MPSV 3 or more years previously and who remain at increased risk for meningococcal disease should be revaccinated with MCV.

The Recommended Immunization Schedules for Persons Aged 0 Through 18 Years are approved by the Advisory Committee on Immunization Practices (www.cdc.gov/vaccines/recs/acip), the American Academy of Pediatrics (http://www.aap.org), and the American Academy of Family Physicians (http://www.aafp.org).

(continued)

Table 30–12. Recommended childhood and adolescent immunization schedule—United States, 2009. (continued)

Recommended Immunization Schedule for Persons Aged 7 Through 18 Years—United States • 2009

For those who fall behind or start late, see the schedule below and the catch-up schedule

Vaccine ▼ Age ►	7–10 years	11–12 years	13–18 years
Tetanus, Diphtheria, Pertussis[1]	see footnote 1	Tdap	Tdap
Human Papillomavirus[2]	see footnote 2	HPV (3 doses)	HPV Series
Meningococcal[3]	MCV	MCV	MCV
Influenza[4]	Influenza (Yearly)		
Pneumococcal[5]	PPSV		
Hepatitis A[6]	HepA Series		
Hepatitis B[7]	HepB Series		
Inactivated Poliovirus[8]	IPV Series		
Measles, Mumps, Rubella[9]	MMR Series		
Varicella[10]	Varicella Series		

Range of recommended ages

Catch-up immunization

Certain high-risk groups

This schedule indicates the recommended ages for routine administration of currently licensed vaccines, as of December 1, 2008, for children aged 7 through 18 years. Any dose not administered at the recommended age should be administered at a subsequent visit, when indicated and feasible. Licensed combination vaccines may be used whenever any component of the combination is indicated and other components are not contraindicated and if approved by the Food and Drug Administration for that dose of the series. Providers should consult the relevant Advisory Committee on Immunization Practices statement for detailed recommendations, including high-risk conditions: http://www.cdc.gov/vaccines/pubs/acip-list.htm. Clinically significant adverse events that follow immunization should be reported to the Vaccine Adverse Event Reporting System (VAERS). Guidance about how to obtain and complete a VAERS form is available at http://www.vaers.hhs.gov or by telephone, 800-822-7967.

1. Tetanus and diphtheria toxoids and acellular pertussis vaccine (Tdap). *(Minimum age: 10 years for BOOSTRIX® and 11 years for ADACEL®)*
- Administer at age 11 or 12 years for those who have completed the recommended childhood DTP/DTaP vaccination series and have not received a tetanus and diphtheria toxoid (Td) booster dose.
- Persons aged 13 through 18 years who have not received Tdap should receive a dose.
- A 5-year interval from the last Td dose is encouraged when Tdap is used as a booster dose; however, a shorter interval may be used if pertussis immunity is needed.

2. Human papillomavirus vaccine (HPV). *(Minimum age: 9 years)*
- Administer the first dose to females at age 11 or 12 years.
- Administer the second dose 2 months after the first dose and the third dose 6 months after the first dose (at least 24 weeks after the first dose).
- Administer the series to females at age 13 through 18 years if not previously vaccinated.

3. Meningococcal conjugate vaccine (MCV).
- Administer at age 11 or 12 years, or at age 13 through 18 years if not previously vaccinated.
- Administer to previously unvaccinated college freshmen living in a dormitory.
- MCV is recommended for children aged 2 through 10 years with terminal complement component deficiency, anatomic or functional asplenia, and certain other groups at high risk. See MMWR 2005;54(No. RR-7).
- Persons who received MPSV 5 or more years previously and remain at increased risk for meningococcal disease should be revaccinated with MCV.

4. Influenza vaccine.
- Administer annually to children aged 6 months through 18 years.
- For healthy nonpregnant persons (i.e., those who do not have underlying medical conditions that predispose them to influenza complications) aged 2 through 49 years, either LAIV or TIV may be used.
- Administer 2 doses (separated by at least 4 weeks) to children aged younger than 9 years who are receiving influenza vaccine for the first time or who were vaccinated for the first time during the previous influenza season but only received 1 dose.

5. Pneumococcal polysaccharide vaccine (PPSV).
- Administer to children with certain underlying medical conditions (see MMWR 1997;46[No. RR-8]), including a cochlear implant. A single revaccination should be administered to children with functional or anatomic asplenia or other immunocompromising condition after 5 years.

6. Hepatitis A vaccine (HepA).
- Administer 2 doses at least 6 months apart.
- HepA is recommended for children older than 1 year who live in areas where vaccination programs target older children or who are at increased risk of infection. See MMWR 2006;55(No. RR-7).

7. Hepatitis B vaccine (HepB).
- Administer the 3-dose series to those not previously vaccinated.
- A 2-dose series (separated by at least 4 months) of adult formulation Recombivax HB® is licensed for children aged 11 through 15 years.

8. Inactivated poliovirus vaccine (IPV).
- For children who received an all-IPV or all-oral poliovirus (OPV) series, a fourth dose is not necessary if the third dose was administered at age 4 years or older.
- If both OPV and IPV were administered as part of a series, a total of 4 doses should be administered, regardless of the child's current age.

9. Measles, mumps, and rubella vaccine (MMR).
- If not previously vaccinated, administer 2 doses or the second dose for those who have received only 1 dose, with at least 28 days between doses.

10. Varicella vaccine.
- For persons aged 7 through 18 years without evidence of immunity (see MMWR 2007;56[No. RR-4]), administer 2 doses if not previously vaccinated or the second dose if they have received only 1 dose.
- For persons aged 7 through 12 years, the minimum interval between doses is 3 months. However, if the second dose was administered at least 28 days after the first dose, it can be accepted as valid.
- For persons aged 13 years and older, the minimum interval between doses is 28 days.

The Recommended Immunization Schedules for Persons Aged 0 Through 18 Years are approved by the Advisory Committee on Immunization Practices (www.cdc.gov/vaccines/recs/acip), the American Academy of Pediatrics (http://www.aap.org), and the American Academy of Family Physicians (http://www.aafp.org).

(continued)

Table 30–12. Recommended childhood and adolescent immunization schedule—United States, 2009. (continued)

Catch-up Immunization Schedule for Persons Aged 4 Months Through 18 Years Who Start Late or Who Are More Than 1 Month Behind—United States • 2009

The table below provides catch-up schedules and minimum intervals between doses for children whose vaccinations have been delayed. A vaccine series does not need to be restarted, regardless of the time that has elapsed between doses. Use the section appropriate for the child's age.

Vaccine	Minimum Age for Dose 1	Dose 1 to Dose 2	Minimum Interval Between Doses		
			Dose 2 to Dose 3	Dose 3 to Dose 4	Dose 4 to Dose 5
CATCH-UP SCHEDULE FOR PERSONS AGED 4 MONTHS THROUGH 6 YEARS					
Hepatitis B[1]	Birth	4 weeks	8 weeks (and at least 16 weeks after first dose)		
Rotavirus[2]	6 wks	4 weeks	4 weeks[2]		
Diphtheria, Tetanus, Pertussis[3]	6 wks	4 weeks	4 weeks	6 months	6 months[3]
Haemophilus influenzae type b[4]	6 wks	4 weeks if first dose administered at younger than age 12 months / 8 weeks (as final dose) if first dose administered at age 12-14 months / No further doses needed if first dose administered at age 15 months or older	4 weeks[4] if current age is younger than 12 months / 8 weeks (as final dose)[4] if current age is 12 months or older and second dose administered at younger than age 15 months / No further doses needed if previous dose administered at age 15 months or older	8 weeks (as final dose) This dose only necessary for children aged 12 months through 59 months who received 3 doses before age 12 months	
Pneumococcal[5]	6 wks	4 weeks if first dose administered at younger than age 12 months / 8 weeks (as final dose for healthy children) if first dose administered at age 12 months or older or current age 24 through 59 months / No further doses needed for healthy children if first dose administered at age 24 months or older	4 weeks if current age is younger than 12 months / 8 weeks (as final dose for healthy children) if current age is 12 months or older / No further doses needed for healthy children if previous dose administered at age 24 months or older	8 weeks (as final dose) This dose only necessary for children aged 12 months through 59 months who received 3 doses before age 12 months or for high-risk children who received 3 doses at any age	
Inactivated Poliovirus[6]	6 wks	4 weeks	4 weeks	4 weeks[6]	
Measles, Mumps, Rubella[7]	12 mos	4 weeks			
Varicella[8]	12 mos	3 months			
Hepatitis A[9]	12 mos	6 months			
CATCH-UP SCHEDULE FOR PERSONS AGED 7 THROUGH 18 YEARS					
Tetanus, Diphtheria/ Tetanus, Diphtheria, Pertussis[10]	7 yrs[10]	4 weeks	4 weeks if first dose administered at younger than age 12 months / 6 months if first dose administered at age 12 months or older	6 months if first dose administered at younger than age 12 months	
Human Papillomavirus[11]	9 yrs	Routine dosing intervals are recommended[11]			
Hepatitis A[9]	12 mos	6 months			
Hepatitis B[1]	Birth	4 weeks	8 weeks (and at least 16 weeks after first dose)		
Inactivated Poliovirus[6]	6 wks	4 weeks	4 weeks	4 weeks[6]	
Measles, Mumps, Rubella[7]	12 mos	4 weeks			
Varicella[8]	12 mos	3 months if the person is younger than age 13 years / 4 weeks if the person is aged 13 years or older			

1. Hepatitis B vaccine (HepB).

- Administer the 3-dose series to those not previously vaccinated.
- A 2-dose series (separated by at least 4 months) of adult formulation Recombivax HB® is licensed for children aged 11 through 15 years.

2. Rotavirus vaccine (RV).

- The maximum age for the first dose is 14 weeks 6 days. Vaccination should not be initiated for infants aged 15 weeks or older (i.e., 15 weeks 0 days or older).
- Administer the final dose in the series by age 8 months 0 days.
- If Rotarix® was administered for the first and second doses, a third dose is not indicated.

3. Diphtheria and tetanus toxoids and acellular pertussis vaccine (DTaP).

- The fifth dose is not necessary if the fourth dose was administered at age 4 years or older.

4. Haemophilus influenzae type b conjugate vaccine (Hib).

- Hib vaccine is not generally recommended for persons aged 5 years or older. No efficacy data are available on which to base a recommendation concerning use of Hib vaccine for older children and adults. However, studies suggest good immunogenicity in persons who have sickle cell disease, leukemia, or HIV infection, or who have had a splenectomy; administering 1 dose of Hib vaccine to these persons is not contraindicated.
- If the first 2 doses were PRP-OMP (PedvaxHIB® or Comvax®), and administered at age 11 months or younger, the third (and final) dose should be administered at age 12 through 15 months and at least 8 weeks after the second dose.
- If the first dose was administered at age 7 through 11 months, administer 2 doses separated by 4 weeks and a final dose at age 12 through 15 months.

5. Pneumococcal vaccine.

- Administer 1 dose of pneumococcal conjugate vaccine (PCV) to all healthy children aged 24 through 59 months who have not received at least 1 dose of PCV on or after age 12 months.
- For children aged 24 through 59 months with underlying medical conditions, administer 1 dose of PCV if 3 doses were received previously or administer 2 doses of PCV at least 8 weeks apart if fewer than 3 doses were received previously.
- Administer pneumococcal polysaccharide vaccine (PPSV) to children aged 2 years or older with certain underlying medical conditions (see MMWR 2000;49[No. RR-9]), including a cochlear implant, at least 8 weeks after the last dose of PCV.

6. Inactivated poliovirus vaccine (IPV).

- For children who received an all-IPV or all-oral poliovirus (OPV) series, a fourth dose is not necessary if the third dose was administered at age 4 years or older.
- If both OPV and IPV were administered as part of a series, a total of 4 doses should be administered, regardless of the child's current age.

7. Measles, mumps, and rubella vaccine (MMR).

- Administer the second dose at age 4 through 6 years. However, the second dose may be administered before age 4, provided at least 28 days have elapsed since the first dose.
- If not previously vaccinated, administer 2 doses with at least 28 days between doses.

8. Varicella vaccine.

- Administer the second dose at age 4 through 6 years. However, the second dose may be administered before age 4, provided at least 3 months have elapsed since the first dose.
- For persons aged 12 months through 12 years, the minimum interval between doses is 3 months. However, if the second dose was administered at least 28 days after the first dose, it can be accepted as valid.
- For persons aged 13 years and older, the minimum interval between doses is 28 days.

9. Hepatitis A vaccine (HepA).

- HepA is recommended for children older than 1 year who live in areas where vaccination programs target older children or who are at increased risk of infection. See MMWR 2006;55(No. RR-7).

10. Tetanus and diphtheria toxoids vaccine (Td) and tetanus and diphtheria toxoids and acellular pertussis vaccine (Tdap).

- Doses of DTaP are counted as part of the Td/Tdap series
- Tdap should be substituted for a single dose of Td in the catch-up series or as a booster for children aged 10 through 18 years; use Td for other doses.

11. Human papillomavirus vaccine (HPV).

- Administer the series to females at age 13 through 18 years if not previously vaccinated.
- Use recommended routine dosing intervals for series catch-up (i.e., the second and third doses should be administered at 2 and 6 months after the first dose). However, the minimum interval between the first and second doses is 4 weeks. The minimum interval between the second and third doses is 12 weeks, and the third dose should be given at least 24 weeks after the first dose.

Information about reporting reactions after immunization is available online at http://www.vaers.hhs.gov or by telephone, 800-822-7967. Suspected cases of vaccine-preventable diseases should be reported to the state or local health department. Additional information, including precautions and contraindications for immunization, is available from the National Center for Immunization and Respiratory Diseases at http://www.cdc.gov/vaccines or telephone, 800-CDC-INFO (800-232-4636).

Table 30–13. Recommended adult immunization schedule—United States, 2009.

Recommended Adult Immunization Schedule
UNITED STATES · 2009

Note: These recommendations *must* **be read with the footnotes that follow containing number of doses, intervals between doses, and other important information.**

Recommended adult immunization schedule, by vaccine and age group

VACCINE ▼ AGE GROUP ▶	19–26 years	27–49 years	50–59 years	60–64 years	≥65 years
Tetanus, diphtheria, pertussis (Td/Tdap)[1],*	Substitute 1-time dose of Tdap for Td booster; then boost with Td every 10 yrs				Td booster every 10 yrs
Human papillomavirus (HPV)[2],*	3 doses (females)				
Varicella[3],*	2 doses				
Zoster[4]				1 dose	
Measles, mumps, rubella (MMR)[5],*	1 or 2 doses		1 dose		
Influenza[6],*	1 dose annually				
Pneumococcal (polysaccharide)[7,8]	1 or 2 doses				1 dose
Hepatitis A[9],*	2 doses				
Hepatitis B[10],*	3 doses				
Meningococcal[11],*	1 or more doses				

*Covered by the Vaccine Injury Compensation Program.

For all persons in this category who meet the age requirements and who lack evidence of immunity (e.g., lack documentation of vaccination or have no evidence of prior infection)

Recommended if some other risk factor is present (e.g., on the basis of medical, occupational, lifestyle, or other indications)

No recommendation

Report all clinically significant postvaccination reactions to the Vaccine Adverse Event Reporting System (VAERS). Reporting forms and instructions on filing a VAERS report are available at www.vaers.hhs.gov or by telephone, 800-822-7967.

Information on how to file a Vaccine Injury Compensation Program claim is available at www.hrsa.gov/vaccinecompensation or by telephone, 800-338-2382. To file a claim for vaccine injury, contact the U.S. Court of Federal Claims, 717 Madison Place, N.W., Washington, D.C. 20005; telephone, 202-357-6400.

Additional information about the vaccines in this schedule, extent of available data, and contraindications for vaccination is also available at www.cdc.gov/vaccines or from the CDC-INFO Contact Center at 800-CDC-INFO (800-232-4636) in English and Spanish, 24 hours a day, 7 days a week.

Use of trade names and commercial sources is for identification only and does not imply endorsement by the U.S. Department of Health and Human Services.

Vaccines that might be indicated for adults based on medical and other indications

VACCINE ▼ INDICATION ▶	Pregnancy	Immuno-compromising conditions (excluding human immunodeficiency virus [HIV])[1,*]	HIV infection[1,12,13] CD4+ T lymphocyte count <200 cells/μL	HIV infection[1,12,13] CD4+ T lymphocyte count ≥200 cells/μL	Diabetes, heart disease, chronic lung disease, chronic alcoholism	Asplenia[12] (including elective splenectomy and terminal complement component deficiencies)	Chronic liver disease	Kidney failure, end-stage renal disease, receipt of hemodialysis	Health-care personnel
Tetanus, diphtheria, pertussis (Td/Tdap)[1,*]	Td	Substitute 1-time dose of Tdap for Td booster; then boost with Td every 10 yrs →							
Human papillomavirus (HPV)[2,*]		3 doses for females through age 26 yrs →							
Varicella[3,*]	Contraindicated	Contraindicated	Contraindicated		2 doses				
Zoster[4]	Contraindicated	Contraindicated	Contraindicated				1 dose		
Measles, mumps, rubella (MMR)[5,*]	Contraindicated	Contraindicated	Contraindicated				1 or 2 doses		
Influenza[6,*]			1 dose TIV annually →						1 dose TIV or LAIV annually
Pneumococcal (polysaccharide)[7,8]			1 or 2 doses →						
Hepatitis A[9,*]			2 doses →						
Hepatitis B[10,*]			3 doses →						
Meningococcal[11,*]			1 or more doses →						

* Covered by the Vaccine Injury Compensation Program.

■ For all persons in this category who meet the age requirements and who lack evidence of immunity (e.g., lack documentation of vaccination or have no evidence of prior infection)

■ Recommended if some other risk factor is present (e.g., on the basis of medical, occupational, lifestyle, or other indications)

☐ No recommendation

These schedules indicate the recommended age groups and medical indications for which administration of currently licensed vaccines is commonly indicated for adults ages 19 years and older, as of January 1, 2009. Licensed combination vaccines may be used whenever any components of the combination are indicated and when the vaccine's other components are not contraindicated. For detailed recommendations on all vaccines, including those used primarily for travelers or that are issued during the year, consult the manufacturers' package inserts and the complete statements from the Advisory Committee on Immunization Practices (www.cdc.gov/vaccines/pubs/acip-list.htm).

The Recommended Immunization Schedules for Persons Aged 0 Through 18 Years are approved by the Advisory Committee on Immunization Practices (www.cdc.gov/vaccines/recs/acip), the American Academy of Pediatrics (http://www.aap.org), and the American Academy of Family Physicians (http://www.aafp.org).

(continued)

Table 30-13. Recommended adult immunization schedule—United States, 2009. (continued)

Footnotes

Recommended Adult Immunization Schedule—UNITED STATES · 2009

For complete statements by the Advisory Committee on Immunization Practices (ACIP), visit www.cdc.gov/vaccines/pubs/ACIP-list.htm.

1. Tetanus, diphtheria, and acellular pertussis (Td/Tdap) vaccination

Tdap should replace a single dose of Td for adults aged 19 through 64 years who have not received a dose of Tdap previously.

Adults with uncertain or incomplete history of primary vaccination series with tetanus and diphtheria toxoid-containing vaccines should begin or complete a primary vaccination series. A primary series for adults is 3 doses of tetanus and diphtheria toxoid-containing vaccines; administer the first 2 doses at least 4 weeks apart and the third dose 6–12 months after the second. However, Tdap can substitute for any one of the doses of Td in the 3-dose primary series. The booster dose of tetanus and diphtheria toxoid-containing vaccine should be administered to adults who have completed a primary series and if the last vaccination was received 10 or more years previously. Tdap or Td vaccine may be used, as indicated.

If a woman is pregnant and received the last Td vaccination 10 or more years previously, administer Td during the second or third trimester. If the woman received the last Td vaccination less than 10 years previously, administer Tdap during the immediate postpartum period. A dose of Tdap is recommended for postpartum women, close contacts of infants aged less than 12 months, and all health-care personnel with direct patient contact if they have not previously received Tdap. An interval as short as 2 years from the last Td is suggested; shorter intervals can be used. Td may be deferred during pregnancy and Tdap substituted in the immediate postpartum period, or Tdap may be administered instead of Td to a pregnant woman after an informed discussion with the woman.

Consult the ACIP statement for recommendations for administering Td as prophylaxis in wound management.

2. Human papillomavirus (HPV) vaccination

HPV vaccination is recommended for all females aged 11 through 26 years (and may begin at 9 years) who have not completed the vaccine series. History of genital warts, abnormal Papanicolaou test, or positive HPV DNA test is not evidence of prior infection with all vaccine HPV types; HPV vaccination is recommended for persons with such histories.

Ideally, vaccine should be administered before potential exposure to HPV through sexual activity; however, females who are sexually active should still be vaccinated consistent with age-based recommendations. Sexually active females who have not been infected with any of the four HPV vaccine types receive the full benefit of the vaccination. Vaccination is less beneficial for females who have already been infected with one or more of the HPV vaccine types.

A complete series consists of 3 doses. The second dose should be administered 2 months after the first dose; the third dose should be administered 6 months after the first dose.

HPV vaccination is not specifically recommended for females with the medical indications described in Figure 2, "Vaccines that might be indicated for adults based on medical and other indications." Because HPV vaccine is not a live-virus vaccine, it may be administered to persons with the medical indications described in Figure 2. However, the immune response and vaccine efficacy might be less for persons with the medical indications described in Figure 2 than in persons who do not have the medical indications described or who are immunocompetent. Health-care personnel are not at increased risk because of occupational exposure, and should be vaccinated consistent with age-based recommendations.

3. Varicella vaccination

All adults without evidence of immunity to varicella should receive 2 doses of single-antigen varicella vaccine if not previously vaccinated or the second dose if they have received only one dose unless they have a medical contraindication. Special consideration should be given to those who 1) have close contact with persons at high risk for severe disease (e.g., health-care personnel and family contacts of persons with immunocompromising conditions) or 2) are at high risk for exposure or transmission (e.g., teachers; child care employees; residents and staff members of institutional settings, including correctional institutions; college students; military personnel; adolescents and adults living in households with children; nonpregnant women of childbearing age; and international travelers).

Evidence of immunity to varicella in adults includes any of the following: 1) documentation of 2 doses of varicella vaccine at least 4 weeks apart; 2) U.S.-born before 1980 (although for health-care personnel and pregnant women, birth before 1980 should not be considered evidence of immunity); 3) history of varicella based on diagnosis or verification of varicella by a health-care provider (for a patient reporting a history of or presenting with an atypical case, a mild case, or both, health-care providers should seek either an epidemiologic link with a typical varicella case or to a laboratory-confirmed case or evidence of laboratory confirmation, if it was performed at the time of acute disease); 4) history of herpes zoster based on health-care provider diagnosis or verification of herpes zoster by a health-care provider; or 5) laboratory evidence of immunity or laboratory confirmation of disease.

Pregnant women should be assessed for evidence of varicella immunity. Women who do not have evidence of immunity should receive the first dose of varicella vaccine upon completion or termination of pregnancy and before discharge from the health-care facility. The second dose should be administered 4–8 weeks after the first dose.

4. Herpes zoster vaccination

A single dose of zoster vaccine is recommended for adults aged 60 years and older regardless of whether they report a prior episode of herpes zoster. Persons with chronic medical conditions may be vaccinated unless their condition constitutes a contraindication.

5. Measles, mumps, rubella (MMR) vaccination

Measles component: Adults born before 1957 generally are considered immune to measles. Adults born during or after 1957 should receive 1 or more doses of MMR unless they have a medical contraindication, documentation of 1 or more doses, history of measles based on health-care provider diagnosis, or laboratory evidence of immunity.

A second dose of MMR is recommended for adults who 1) have been recently exposed to measles or are in an outbreak setting; 2) have been vaccinated previously with killed measles vaccine; 3) have been vaccinated with an unknown type of measles vaccine during 1963–1967; 4) are students in postsecondary educational institutions; 5) work in a health-care facility; or 6) plan to travel internationally.

Mumps component: Adults born before 1957 generally are considered immune to mumps. Adults born during or after 1957 should receive 1 dose of MMR unless they have a medical contraindication, history of mumps based on health-care provider diagnosis, or laboratory evidence of immunity.

A second dose of MMR is recommended for adults who 1) live in a community experiencing a mumps outbreak and are in an affected age group; 2) are students in postsecondary educational institutions; 3) work in a health-care facility; or 4) plan to travel internationally. For unvaccinated health-care personnel born before 1957 who do not have other evidence of mumps immunity, administering 1 dose on a routine basis should be considered and administering a second dose during an outbreak should be strongly considered.

Rubella component: 1 dose of MMR vaccine is recommended for women whose rubella vaccination history is unreliable or who lack laboratory evidence of immunity. For women of childbearing age, regardless of birth year, rubella immunity should be determined and women should be counseled regarding congenital rubella syndrome. Women who do not have evidence of immunity should receive MMR upon completion or termination of pregnancy and before discharge from the health-care facility.

6. **Influenza vaccination**

Medical indications: Chronic disorders of the cardiovascular or pulmonary systems, including asthma; chronic metabolic diseases, including diabetes mellitus, renal or hepatic dysfunction, hemoglobinopathies, or immunocompromising conditions (including immunocompromising conditions caused by medications or human immunodeficiency virus [HIV]); any condition that compromises respiratory function or the handling of respiratory secretions or that can increase the risk of aspiration (e.g., cognitive dysfunction, spinal cord injury, or seizure disorder or other neuromuscular disorder); and pregnancy during the influenza season. No data exist on the risk for severe or complicated influenza disease among persons with asplenia; however, influenza is a risk factor for secondary bacterial infections that can cause severe disease among persons with asplenia.

Occupational indications: All health-care personnel, including those employed by long-term care and assisted-living facilities, and caregivers of children less than 5 years old.

Other indications: Residents of nursing homes and other long-term care and assisted-living facilities; persons likely to transmit influenza to persons at high risk (e.g., in-home household contacts and caregivers of children aged less than 5 years old, persons 65 years old and older and persons of all ages with high-risk condition[s]); and anyone who would like to decrease their risk of getting influenza. Healthy, nonpregnant adults aged less than 50 years without high-risk medical conditions who are not contacts of severely immunocompromised persons in special care units can receive either intranasally administered live, attenuated influenza vaccine (FluMist®) or inactivated vaccine. Other persons should receive the inactivated vaccine.

7. **Pneumococcal polysaccharide (PPSV) vaccination**

Medical indications: Chronic lung disease (including asthma); chronic cardiovascular diseases; diabetes mellitus; chronic liver diseases, cirrhosis; chronic alcoholism, chronic renal failure or nephrotic syndrome; functional or anatomic asplenia (e.g., sickle cell disease or splenectomy [if elective splenectomy is planned, vaccinate at least 2 weeks before surgery]); immunocompromising conditions; and cochlear implants and cerebrospinal fluid leaks. Vaccinate as close to HIV diagnosis as possible.

Other indications: Residents of nursing homes or long-term care facilities and persons who smoke cigarettes. Routine use of PPSV is not recommended for Alaska Native or American Indian persons younger than 65 years unless they have underlying medical conditions that are PPSV indications. However, public health authorities may consider recommending PPSV for Alaska Natives and American Indians aged 50 through 64 years who are living in areas in which the risk of invasive pneumococcal disease is increased.

8. **Revaccination with PPSV**

One-time revaccination after 5 years for persons with chronic renal failure or nephrotic syndrome; functional or anatomic asplenia (e.g., sickle cell disease or splenectomy); and for persons with immunocompromising conditions. For persons aged 65 years and older, one-time revaccination if they were vaccinated 5 or more years previously and were aged less than 65 years at the time of primary vaccination.

9. **Hepatitis A vaccination**

Medical indications: Persons with chronic liver disease and persons who receive clotting factor concentrates.

Behavioral indications: Men who have sex with men and persons who use illegal drugs.

Occupational indications: Persons working with hepatitis A virus (HAV)-infected primates or with HAV in a research laboratory setting.

Other indications: Persons traveling to or working in countries that have high or intermediate endemicity of hepatitis A (a list of countries is available at wwvw.cdc.gov/travel/contentdiseases.aspx) and any person seeking protection from HAV infection.

Single-antigen vaccine formulations should be administered in a 2-dose schedule at either 0 and 6-12 months (Havrix®), or 0 and 6-18 months (Vaqta®). If the combined hepatitis A and hepatitis B vaccine (Twinrix®) is used, administer 3 doses at 0, 1, and 6 months; alternatively, a 4-dose schedule, administered on days 0, 7 and 21 to 30 followed by a booster dose at month 12 may be used.

10. **Hepatitis B vaccination**

Medical indications: Persons with end-stage renal disease, including patients receiving hemodialysis; persons with HIV infection; and persons with chronic liver disease.

Occupational indications: Health-care personnel and public-safety workers who are exposed to blood or other potentially infectious body fluids.

Behavioral indications: Sexually active persons who are not in a long-term, mutually monogamous relationship (e.g., persons with more than 1 sex partner during the previous 6 months); persons seeking evaluation or treatment for a sexually transmitted disease (STD); current or recent injection-drug users; and men who have sex with men.

Other indications: Household contacts and sex partners of persons with chronic hepatitis B virus (HBV) infection; clients and staff members of institutions for persons with developmental disabilities; international travelers to countries with high or intermediate prevalence of chronic HBV infection (a list of countries is available at wwvm.cdc.gov/travel/contentdiseases.aspx); and any adult seeking protection from HBV infection.

Hepatitis B vaccination is recommended for all adults in the following settings: STD treatment facilities; HIV testing and treatment facilities; facilities providing drug-abuse treatment and prevention services; health-care settings targeting services to injection-drug users or men who have sex with men; correctional facilities; end-stage renal disease programs and facilities for chronic hemodialysis patients; and institutions and nonresidential daycare facilities for persons with developmental disabilities.

If the combined hepatitis A and hepatitis B vaccine (Twinrix®) is used, administer 3 doses at 0, 1, and 6 months; alternatively, a 4-dose schedule, administered on days 0, 7 and 21 to 30 followed by a booster dose at month 12 may be used.

Special formulation indications: For adult patients receiving hemodialysis or with other immunocompromising conditions, 1 dose of 40 µg/mL (Recombivax HB®) administered on a 3-dose schedule or 2 doses of 20 µg/mL (Engerix-B®) administered simultaneously on a 4-dose schedule at 0, 1, 2 and 6 months.

11. **Meningococcal vaccination**

Medical indications: Adults with anatomic or functional asplenia, or terminal complement component deficiencies.

Other indications: First-year college students living in dormitories; microbiologists who are routinely exposed to isolates of Neisseria meningitidis; military recruits; and persons who travel to or live in countries in which meningococcal disease is hyperendemic or epidemic (e.g., the "meningitis belt" of sub-Saharan Africa during the dry season [December–June]), particularly if their contact with local populations will be prolonged. Vaccination is required by the government of Saudi Arabia for all travelers to Mecca during the annual Hajj.

Meningococcal conjugate (MCV) vaccine is preferred for adults with any of the preceding indications who are aged 55 years or younger, although meningococcal polysaccharide vaccine (MPSV) is an acceptable alternative. Revaccination with MCV after 5 years might be indicated for adults previously vaccinated with MPSV who remain at increased risk for infection (e.g., persons residing in areas in which disease is epidemic).

12. **Selected conditions for which Haemophilus influenzae type b (Hib) vaccine may be used**

Hib vaccine generally is not recommended for persons aged 5 years and older. No efficacy data are available on which to base a recommendation concerning use of Hib vaccine for older children and adults. However, studies suggest good immunogenicity in persons who have sickle cell disease, leukemia, or HIV infection or who have had a splenectomy; administering 1 dose of vaccine to these persons is not contraindicated.

13. **Immunocompromising conditions**

Inactivated vaccines generally are acceptable (e.g., pneumococcal, meningococcal, and influenza [trivalent inactivated influenza vaccine]), and live vaccines generally are avoided in persons with immune deficiencies or immunocompromising conditions. Information on specific conditions is available at www.cdc.gov/vaccines/pubs/acip-list.htm.

The vaccine is not advised for pregnant women at this time. Unanswered questions include the need for booster doses to prevent the development of cervical cancer and whether males should also be vaccinated.

▶ Influenza

Influenza vaccination is recommended yearly for all children aged 6 months-18 years and any adult wishing to reduce the likelihood of either becoming infected with or transmitting influenza. However, those at greatest risk for severe complications of influenza should have priority in vaccination programs: (1) Adults and children with chronic cardiopulmonary disease, including asthmatics. (2) Residents, health care workers, and employees of long-term care facilities. (3) Healthy adults 50 years of age or older. (4) Adults and children who have required either regular medical follow-up or hospitalization in the last year for chronic metabolic disorders (including diabetes) or kidney disease, those with hemoglobinopathies, and those receiving immunosuppressive drugs. (5) Children and teenagers (age 6 months to 18 years) who are receiving long-term aspirin therapy and would be at increased risk for developing Reye syndrome following influenza. (6) Women who will become pregnant during the influenza season. (7) Persons who are likely to transmit influenza to persons of high risk as defined above, such as in-home or out-of-home caregivers or household and close contacts of persons at high risk.

Certain high-risk groups of patients (the elderly, persons with AIDS, transplant patients) may have a poor antibody response to vaccine, but they should still be vaccinated. Concern that vaccination of HIV-positive patients may result in a brief (2- to 4-week) period of increased HIV viremia and viral replication has been raised, but the clinical significance is unclear and should not preclude vaccination.

A trivalent, live-attenuated influenza vaccine administered as a single-dose intranasal spray is as effective as inactivated vaccine in preventing disease. It is approved for use in otherwise healthy individuals between the ages of 2 and 49 years. Because the risk of transmission of the live-attenuated vaccine virus to immunocompromised individuals is unknown, it should not be used in household members of immunosuppressed individuals, health care workers, or others with close contact with immunosuppressed persons. Two neuraminidase inhibitors (zanamivir and oseltamivir) are available for prevention and therapy of influenza A and B. The dose of oseltamivir is 75 mg/d for prophylaxis and 75 mg twice daily for 5 days for therapy. Zanamivir is administered by inhaler (10 mg dose) and is given twice daily for therapy and once daily for prophylaxis. The duration of prophylaxis depends on the clinical setting. The 2008-2009 flu season was associated with a very high rate of oseltamivir-resistant virus, particularly in influenza A (H1N1 virus). Current recommendations are that influenza A be treated with zanamivir or a combination of oseltamivir and rimantadine. Influenza B can be treated with either oseltamivir or zanamivir. For chemoprophylaxis against influenza A, zanamivir should be used. If this is contraindicated, patients should be given rimantadine. In an outbreak associated with influenza B, either oseltamivir or zanamivir can be used for prophylaxis.

▶ Measles, Mumps, & Rubella (MMR)

A. Measles

Adults born before 1957 are considered immune to measles. Adults born in 1957 or later who lack documentation of immunization after age 1 or who do not have a provider-documented history or laboratory evidence of previous infection should receive at least one dose of vaccine. Persons born between 1963 and 1967—a period when less effective inactivated measles vaccine was the only product available—and persons vaccinated before their first birthday should receive a single dose of vaccine. Because most adults do not have detailed information about childhood immunization or illnesses, a practical approach is to administer a single dose of MMR to all healthy adults born after 1956. Because outbreaks of measles have occurred in young adults who have received a single dose of measles vaccine, revaccination is recommended, particularly before going to college, entering a health care profession, or embarking on foreign travel to areas where measles is endemic. Even though birth before 1957 implies immunity, unvaccinated health care workers (especially women of childbearing age) who do not have a history of measles or laboratory evidence of immunity should be vaccinated. Entrants to colleges and universities and employees of health care institutions who have not previously been vaccinated should receive two doses of vaccine at least 1 month apart. Revaccination of an immune person is not associated with adverse effects—if the vaccination status is unknown and an indication for vaccination exists, it can be safely done. Vaccination of susceptible adults within 72 hours after exposure to an active case of measles is protective.

B. Mumps

Mumps vaccine is recommended for all adults thought to be susceptible. Persons born before 1957 are considered to be naturally immune. Those born in 1957 or later are believed to be susceptible unless they can document infection, prove vaccination, or have laboratory evidence of immunity. Because of recent outbreaks of mumps, the definition of adequate vaccination is more stringent—it is one dose of vaccine for preschool-aged children and adults not at high risk and two doses for school-aged children (grades kindergarten through high school) and for adults at high risk (health care workers, international travelers, and students at post high school institutions). Thus, all health care workers should have evidence of immunity or should have received two doses of vaccine. Because birth before 1957 is only presumptive evidence of immunity, healthcare workers born before 1957 should receive a single dose of vaccine unless they have laboratory evidence of immunity or have a history of physician diagnosed mumps.

C. Rubella

The purpose of rubella vaccination is to prevent transmission to the fetus. Immunization is recommended for all adults but particularly for women of childbearing age not previously immunized. Although persons born before 1957 are considered immune, this is not an acceptable criterion of immunity for women who could become pregnant. Thus, women of childbearing age, regardless of birth year, should have rubella immunity checked and should be vaccinated if they lack evidence of antibody. They should be counseled not to become pregnant within 4 weeks of immunization. Women who are already pregnant and lack immunity should be vaccinated in the postpartum period. In addition, both male and female hospital workers who may be exposed to patients with rubella or who might have contact with pregnant patients should be immunized. A single immunization is given. MMR trivalent vaccine is recommended, but if immunity to one or more of the components can be demonstrated, monovalent or bivalent vaccines can be used.

Meningococcal Disease

Two vaccines are currently available, a polysaccharide vaccine (MPSV4) and the newer protein conjugated vaccine (MCV4). Both are highly immunogenic to serogroups A, C, Y, and W-135 and well tolerated. Whereas the polysaccharide vaccine requires revaccination of at-risk groups every 3–5 years due to waning immunity, the protein conjugated vaccine likely will provide longer protection, although data on need for revaccination with MCV4 are not available. Both vaccines are approved for individuals 2 years and older.

Vaccination with MCV4 is routinely recommended for adolescents aged 11–12. For those who miss that vaccination, "catch up" is recommended at high school entry (approximately age 15). MCV4 is also recommended for certain high-risk groups, including college freshman living in dormitories (the risk to nonfreshman and freshman not living in dormitories is the same as the general population and vaccination of these groups is elective), microbiologists who are routinely exposed to *N meningitidis*, military recruits, persons who travel to or reside in areas in which *N meningitidis* is hyperendemic or epidemic (see below), those with terminal complement deficiencies, and persons with anatomic or functional asplenia. HIV-infected patients may be at increased risk for meningococcal disease, and vaccination should be considered elective in that group. MCV4 is the preferred preparation, but if availability is an issue, MPSV4 can be substituted. MCV4 is administered as a single 0.5-mL dose intramuscularly and MPSV4 as a single 0.5-mL dose subcutaneously. Both can be administered with other vaccines, but at different sites and both produce an antibody response in 7–10 days. Both are inactivated vaccines and can be administered to immunocompromised patients. MPSV4 is safe in pregnancy, but there are no safety or efficacy data for MCV4 in pregnancy.

Pneumococcal Disease

Pneumococcal vaccine contains purified polysaccharide from 23 of the most common strains of *S pneumoniae*, which cause 90% of bacteremic episodes in the United States. Antibody response following vaccination depends on the patient's immune status and the presence of concomitant disease. Healthy adults have an excellent antibody response, as do patients who are postsplenectomy

and those with sickle cell disease. Elderly individuals and those with chronic diseases (diabetes mellitus, alcoholic cirrhosis, chronic obstructive pulmonary disease, chronic kidney disease, lupus erythematosus, rheumatoid arthritis) have less vigorous response than young healthy adults. Patients with Hodgkin disease respond to vaccination if it is given before splenectomy, radiation, or chemotherapy, whereas patients with leukemia, lymphoma, and HIV infection respond sluggishly.

Although the efficacy of pneumococcal vaccine has been questioned, most authorities believe that vaccination is about 60–70% effective in preventing bacteremic disease in immunocompetent persons, but less effective at preventing pneumonia. Fifty percent efficacy is observed in patients with underlying diseases (not severely immunocompromised), and less in immunocompromised patients (10%), largely because of inability to mount an antibody response in this population. It is presently recommended for patients at increased risk for developing severe pneumococcal disease, especially asplenic patients and those with sickle cell disease. It is also indicated for adults at increased risk for developing pneumococcal disease, including those with chronic illnesses (eg, cardiopulmonary disease, alcoholism, cirrhosis, chronic kidney disease, nephrotic syndrome, cerebrospinal fluid leaks), those with asthma, cigarette smokers, those who are immunocompromised (eg, patients with Hodgkin disease, lymphoma, chronic lymphocytic leukemia, multiple myeloma, congenital immunodeficiency, asymptomatic or symptomatic HIV infection, organ or bone marrow transplant recipients), those receiving immunosuppressive therapy (eg, long-term systemic corticosteroids, alkylating agents, and antimetabolites) and Alaskan Natives. Because of the increased risk of developing pneumococcal meningitis following cochlear implants, patients receiving these implants should be given age-appropriate vaccination. In addition, it is recommended for all individuals over 65 years of age. A single dose of vaccine usually confers lifelong immunity. One-time revaccination 5 years after initial vaccination is recommended for those at highest risk (see list above). In addition, a single revaccination is recommended for those 65 or more years of age who received the vaccine 5 years or more previously and were under age 65 at the time of primary vaccination. Elderly individuals with unknown vaccination status should be immunized once. Revaccination should also be considered for high-risk individuals previously immunized with the older 14-valent vaccine. Since immunocompetent patients respond best to the vaccine, it should be given 2 weeks before splenectomy or before starting chemotherapy if that can be anticipated.

A protein-conjugated heptavalent pneumococcal vaccine used in children under 2 years of age is very effective at preventing meningitis and pneumonia but only modestly effective at preventing otitis media. Unlike the adult polysaccharide vaccine, the pediatric conjugated vaccine decreases nasopharyngeal colonization, which results in less transmission to nonimmunized children and adults (herd immunity). Limited information about use of this vaccine in adults suggests that those with poor antibody response to the 23-valent vaccine (such as kidney transplant recipients) also have poor antibody response to the protein-conjugated vaccine despite its higher immunogenicity.

Tetanus, Diphtheria, & Pertussis

A tetanus toxoid, reduced diphtheria toxoid and acellular pertussis vaccine (Tdap) is approved for use in persons 11–64 years of age. All should receive a primary series of immunizations against tetanus, diphtheria, and pertussis (Table 30–12). Adults who have not previously been immunized should receive a dose of Tdap followed by a dose Td 4 weeks later, and a booster with Td 6–12 months after the second dose.

The ACIP recommends that adults aged 19–64 years should receive a single dose of Tdap to replace tetanus and diphtheria toxoids vaccine (Td) for booster immunization if they received their last dose of Td ≥ 10 years earlier and they have not previously received Tdap. To prevent pertussis among infants less than 12 months of age, a single dose of Tdap is recommended at an interval as short as 2 years from the previous Td vaccination for those adults anticipating close contact with these infants (eg, parents, grandparents aged < 65 years, child-care providers). When possible, women should receive Tdap before becoming pregnant. Women who have not previously received Tdap should receive a dose of Tdap in the immediate postpartum period. Health-care personnel who work in hospitals or ambulatory care settings and have direct patient contact should receive a single dose of Tdap as soon as feasible if they have not previously received Tdap. For wound management, adults between the ages of 19 and 64 should receive Tdap instead of Td if they have not previously received Tdap. Tdap is contraindicated if there is a history of anaphylaxis to vaccine components or if there is a history of unexplained encephalitis within 7 days of administration of a pertussis-containing vaccine.

Varicella

A live attenuated varicella virus vaccine is currently recommended as part of routine childhood immunization (Table 30–12) and its use has been associated with decreased mortality due to varicella across all age ranges. Although only 10% of adults remain susceptible, varicella in adolescents and adults is a more serious disease. Only about 2% of all cases of varicella occur in adults, but almost 50% of all deaths are in adults. Thus, all susceptible adolescents and adults should be immunized, with special emphasis on certain high-risk groups, ie, health care workers; household contacts of immunosuppressed individuals; persons who live or work in environments where transmission can occur, eg, teachers in day care centers or elementary schools, residents and workers in institutional settings such as military and correctional institutions, college students; nonpregnant women of childbearing age; and international travelers. The role of the present vaccine in postexposure prophylaxis has not been widely studied, but it has been suggested that it is 90% effective in preventing varicella in an outbreak, particularly when given within 3–5 days after exposure. The ACIP recommends vaccination in susceptible persons following exposure. The vaccine is very immunogenic. Sero-

conversion occurs in 95% of children after a single dose. In adolescents (older than 12 years of age) and adults, seroconversion is seen in 78% after one dose and 99% after two doses. For this reason, two doses given 4–8 weeks apart are recommended in persons 12 years of age and older. The duration of immunity is not known but is probably 10 years.

RECOMMENDED IMMUNIZATIONS FOR TRAVELERS

Individuals traveling to other countries frequently require immunizations in addition to those listed above and may benefit from chemoprophylaxis against various diseases. These are listed in *Health Information for International Travel*, published by the CDC. An updated version is published yearly and is available from the Superintendent of Documents, United States Government Printing Office, Washington, DC 20402, or on the Internet: http://www.cdc.gov/nip.

Various vaccines can be given simultaneously at different sites. Some, such as cholera, plague, and typhoid vaccine, cause significant discomfort and are best given at different times. In general, live attenuated vaccines (measles, mumps, rubella, yellow fever, and oral typhoid vaccine) should not be given to immunosuppressed individuals or household members of immunosuppressed people or to pregnant women. Immunoglobulin should not be given for 3 months before or at least 2 weeks after live virus vaccines, because it may attenuate the antibody response.

Chemoprophylaxis of malaria is discussed in Chapter 35.

Cholera

Because cholera among travelers is rare and the vaccine marginally effective, the World Health Organization (WHO) does not require immunization for persons traveling to endemic areas. The only cholera vaccine licensed in the United States is no longer manufactured. Two oral vaccines are available in other countries and appear to be slightly more immunogenic than previous vaccines. However, the CDC does not recommend either of these two vaccines, and they are not available in the United States. No country requires vaccination for entry, but some local authorities may require documentation for entry. In such cases, a medical waiver will suffice or a single dose of the oral vaccine is usually sufficient. Information is available at http://www.bernaproducts.com.

Hepatitis B

The risk of hepatitis B infection for most international travelers is low. Hepatitis B vaccination should be considered for those traveling to areas with high (≥ 8%) or intermediate (2–7%) rates of endemic hepatitis B infection if the individual will have contact with blood or secretions, have unprotected sex, or will be using illicit drugs. Examples of high and intermediate risk areas include all of Africa, South Asia (except Sri Lanka), the Middle East (except Cyprus), Eastern Europe (except Hungary), Newly Independent States of the former Soviet Union, Italy, Spain, Portugal, Greenland, Belize, Guatemala, Honduras, Panama, Argentina, Bolivia, Brazil, Ecuador, Venezuela, certain Caribbean Islands. Alaskan natives and indigenous populations of Northern Canada are at intermediate and high risk for hepatitis B infection. Vaccination should begin at least 6 months before travel to allow for completion of the series.

Hepatitis A

Protection is recommended for susceptible persons traveling to areas where sanitation is poor and the risk of exposure to hepatitis A high because of contaminated food and water supplies and contact with infected persons (eg, anywhere except Canada, western Europe, Japan, Australia, and New Zealand). Either hepatitis A vaccine or immunoglobulin can be used, although vaccination is preferred. The first dose of vaccine should be given as soon as travel is considered. In healthy individuals, a single dose of vaccine administered any time prior to travel will provide adequate protection. In older patients, those who are immunocompromised, and those with chronic liver disease or other chronic medical problems who are planning to travel in 2 weeks or less should receive hepatitis A vaccine and immunoglobulin 0.02 mL/kg simultaneously at different anatomic sites. Those who choose not to receive vaccine should receive immunoglobulin.

Meningococcal Meningitis

If travel is contemplated to an area where meningococcal meningitis is epidemic (Nepal, sub-Saharan Africa, the "meningitis belt" from Senegal in the west to Ethiopia in the east, northern India) or highly endemic, vaccination with MCV4 is indicated for those 2–55 years of age, otherwise MPSV should be used. (Saudi Arabia requires immunization for pilgrims to Mecca.)

Plague

The risk of plague is so small to travelers that vaccine is no longer commercially available and vaccination is not required for entry into any country. Travelers at unavoidable high risk of exposure to rodents should consider chemoprophylaxis with doxycycline or TMP-SMZ.

Poliomyelitis

Polio remains endemic in five countries (Afghanistan, India, Pakistan, Nigeria, and Niger), and sporadic outbreaks from reinfection continues to occur in Somalia, Ethiopia, Angola, and Bangladesh. Adults traveling to endemic or epidemic areas who have not previously been immunized against poliomyelitis should receive a primary series of three doses of inactivated enhanced-potency poliovaccine (IPV), as follows: two doses of 0.5 mL subcutaneously 4–8 weeks apart and then a third dose 6–12 months after the second dose. If more than 8 weeks will elapse before travel, three doses of IPV can be given 4 weeks apart. If 4–8 weeks will elapse before travel, two doses are given 4 weeks apart, and if less than 4 weeks will elapse, a single dose is given. Vaccination can be completed upon return if continued or future exposure to polio is anticipated. Travelers who have previously been fully immunized with OPV

or IPV should receive a one-time booster dose with IPV. Data do not indicate the need for more than one adult booster. Live attenuated poliovaccine is no longer recommended because of the risk of vaccine-associated disease and is no longer available in the United States, although it continues to be used in many other countries.

Rabies

For travelers to areas where rabies is common in domestic animals (eg, India, Asia, Mexico, Africa, areas of Central and South America), with extensive outdoor activities or certain professional activities (veterinarians, animal handlers, field biologists), preexposure prophylaxis with human diploid cell vaccine (HDCV), rabies vaccine adsorbed (RVA), or purified chick embryo cell culture (PCEC) vaccine should be considered. It usually consists of two intramuscular (deltoid area) injections of 1 mL given 1 week apart with a booster dose 2–3 weeks later. Alternatively, two intradermal injections of 0.1 mL of HDCV are given 1 week apart, with a booster dose given 2–3 weeks later. Chloroquine can blunt the immunologic response to rabies vaccine. If malaria prophylaxis with chloroquine is required, vaccination should be given intramuscularly (*not* intradermally) to ensure adequate antibody response. Until further studies are done, interaction between mefloquine and rabies vaccine, while not established, makes intramuscular administration prudent if mefloquine is to be given.

Typhoid

Typhoid vaccination is recommended for travelers to developing countries (especially the Indian subcontinent, Asia, Africa, Central and South America, and the Caribbean) who will have prolonged exposure to contaminated food and water. Two preparations of approximately equal efficacy (50–75% effective) are available in the United States: (1) an oral live-attenuated Ty21a vaccine supplied as enteric-coated capsules, and (2) a Vi capsular polysaccharide (Vi CPS) vaccine for parenteral use. The Ty21a vaccine is given as one capsule every other day for four doses. The capsules must be refrigerated and taken with cool liquids (37 °C or less) at least 1 hour before meals. All four doses must be taken for maximum protection and should be completed 1 week before travel. It is not recommended for infants or children younger than 6 years. Adverse effects are minimal and consist primarily of gastrointestinal upset. The Vi CPS vaccine is given as a single intramuscular injection at least 2 weeks prior to travel. It is not recommended for infants younger than 2 years. Adverse effects consist mainly of local irritation at the site of injection, but fever and headache occur. If continued or repeated exposures are anticipated, boosters are recommended every 2 years for the Vi CPS and every 5 years for the Ty21a. The live attenuated vaccine should not be used in immunosuppressed patients, including those with HIV infection.

Yellow Fever

The live attenuated yellow fever virus vaccine is administered once subcutaneously. Although the risk of yellow fever

Table 30–14. Adverse effects and contraindications to vaccinations.

Vaccine	Adverse Effects	Contraindications
Hepatitis A	Minimal Consist mainly of pain at the injection site	
Hepatitis B	Minimal Consist mainly of pain at the injection site	Hypersensitivity to yeast Severe reaction to a previous dose
Human papillomavirus	Minimal Consists mainly of mild to moderate localized pain, erythema, swelling Systemic reactions, mainly fever, seen in 4% of recipients	History of hypersensitivity to yeast or to any vaccine component

Influenza (intramuscular inactivated and intra-nasal live attenuated vaccines)	**Intramuscular, inactivated vaccine:** Local reactions (erythema and tenderness) at the site of injection common, but fevers, chills, and malaise (which last in any case only 2–3 days) rare.
	Either inactivated or live attenuated vaccine: The risk of Guillain-Barré syndrome is not increased following vaccination. Influenza vaccination may be associated with multiple false-positive serologic tests to HIV, HTLV-1, and hepatitis C, but it is self-limited, lasting 2–5 months.
		Intranasal, live attenuated vaccine [FluMist]: Should not be used in:
		  People 50 years of age and over
		  Household members of immunosuppressed individuals
		  Health care workers, or others with close contact with immunosuppressed persons
		  Presence of reactive airway disease; chronic underlying metabolic, pulmonary, or cardiovascular diseases (use intramuscular inactivated vaccine)
		  Long-term aspirin therapy in children or adolescents (because of the risk of Reye syndrome)
		  Pregnancy[1]
		Contraindication to both inactivated and live attenuated vaccine: History of Guillain-Barré syndrome, especially within 6 weeks of receiving a previous influenza vaccine
		History of egg allergy[2]

Measles, mumps, and rubella (MMR)[3]	Fever will develop in about 5–15% of unimmunized individuals, and a mild rash will develop in about 5% 5–12 days after vaccination. Fever and rash are self-limiting, lasting only 2–3 days. Local swelling and induration are particularly common in individuals previously vaccinated with inactivated vaccine.	Pregnancy[4] Immunosuppressed persons should not be vaccinated (with the exception of asymptomatic HIV-infected individuals whose CD4 count is > 200/mcL). History of anaphylaxis to neomycin or to related agents such as streptomycin
Meningococcal	Minor reactions (fever, redness, swelling, erythema, pain) occur slightly more commonly with MCV4. Major reactions are rare. A potential association between Guillain-Barré syndrome and vaccination with MCV4 has been reported, but current recommendations favor continued use of MCV4, since the benefits of preventing the serious consequences of meningococcal infection outweigh the theoretical risk of Guillain-Barré syndrome.	Persons with history of adverse reaction to diphtheria toxoid should not receive MCV4 since the protein conjugate used in MCV4 is diphtheria toxoid
Pneumococcal (polysaccharide)	Mild local reactions (erythema and tenderness) occur in up to 50% of recipients, but systemic reactions are uncommon. Similarly, revaccination at least 5 years after initial vaccination is associated with mild self-limited local but not systemic reactions.	Revaccination is not recommended for those who had a severe reaction (anaphylaxis or Arthus reaction) to the initial vaccination.
Tetanus, diphtheria, and pertussis	Minimal Consist mainly of pain at the injection site	Any history of anaphylaxis to vaccine components or if there is a history of unexplained encephalitis within 7 days of administration of a pertussis-containing vaccine.

(continued)

Table 30–14. Adverse effects and contraindications to vaccinations. (continued)

Vaccine	Adverse Effects	Contraindications
Varicella	Can occur as late as 4–6 weeks after vaccination. Tenderness and erythema at the injection site are seen in 25%, fever in 10–15%, and a localized maculopapular or vesicular rash in 5%; a diffuse rash, usually with five or fewer vesicular lesions, develops in a smaller percentage. Spread of virus from vaccinees to susceptible individuals is possible, but the risk of such transmission even to immunocompromised patients is small and disease, when it develops, is mild and treatable with acyclovir.	Allergy to neomycin Avoid in immunocompromised individuals, including HIV-positive children and adults, or pregnant women. For theoretic reasons, it is recommended that salicylates should be avoided for 6 weeks following vaccination (to prevent Reye syndrome).
Zoster	Mild and limited to local reactions Although it is theoretically possible to transmit the virus to susceptible contacts, no such cases have been reported.	Presence of primary or acquired immunodeficiency state (leukemia, lymphoma, any malignant neoplasm affecting the bone marrow, HIV infection) Therapy with immunosuppressive medications (including high-dose corticosteroids) Pregnancy Persons with an anaphylactic type reaction to gelatin or neomycin should not receive the vaccine.

[1]The inactivated influenza vaccine can be given during any trimester.
[2]The vaccine is prepared using embryonated chicken eggs.
[3]MMR vaccine can be safely given to patients with a history of egg allergy even when severe.
[4]Although vaccination of pregnant women is *not* recommended, with the currently available RA27/3 vaccine strain the congenital rubella syndrome does not occur in the offspring of those inadvertently vaccinated during pregnancy or within 3 months before conception.

is low for most travelers, a number of countries require vaccination for all visitors and others require it for travelers to or from endemic areas (mainly equatorial Africa and parts of South and Central America). The WHO certificate requires registration of the manufacturer and the batch number of the vaccine. Vaccination is available in the United States only at approved centers; the local health department should be contacted for available resources. Reimmunization is recommended at 10-year intervals if continued risk exists.

Because it is a live attenuated vaccine prepared in embryonated eggs, the yellow fever vaccine should not be given to immunosuppressed individuals or those with a history of anaphylaxis to eggs. Pregnancy is a relative contraindication to vaccination.

Two very severe adverse reactions have been associated with yellow fever vaccination. Viscerotropic disease presents with fever, jaundice, and multiple organ system failure within 30 days of yellow fever vaccination. Clinically and histopathologically, the illness is identical to yellow fever and is associated with a high mortality rate. The other adverse reaction is neurotropic disease and presents as encephalitis, encephalomyelitis, and Guillain-Barré syndrome. Because yellow fever is a severe disease and deaths have been reported in travelers, and these serious adverse reactions are rare (3–5 cases of viscerotropic disease and 4–6 cases of neurotropic disease per 1,000,000 doses of vaccine distributed), vaccination is still recommended but limited to those traveling to areas reporting epidemic or endemic yellow fever. (Current information about the vaccine and yellow

fever activity can be found at http://www2.ncid.cdc.gov/travel/yb/utils/ybGet.asp?section=dis&obj=yellowfever.htm.) The risk for serious adverse reactions are age-related (infants < 9 months; age > 60 years) and is greater in those with a history of thymus disease.

▶ **Japanese B Encephalitis**

Japanese B encephalitis is a mosquito-borne viral encephalitis that affects primarily children and older adults (65 years and older) and usually occurs from May to September. It is the leading cause of encephalitis in Asia. Because the risk of infection is low and because adverse effects of the vaccine can be serious, not all travelers to Asia should be vaccinated. Vaccine should be given to travelers to endemic areas who will be staying at least 30 days and who are traveling during the transmission season, particularly if they are visiting rural areas. Travelers who spend less than 30 days in the region should be considered for vaccination if they intend to visit areas of epidemic transmission or if extensive outdoor activities are planned in rural rice-growing areas. The recommended primary immunization schedule is 1 mL of vaccine administered subcutaneously on days 0, 7, and 30. If time constraints are compelling, the last dose can be given on day 14. The last dose should be given at least 10 days before embarkation because urticaria and angioedema have been described, occurring from minutes up to 10 days after vaccination. Following vaccination, patients should be observed for 30 minutes and advised of the possibility of delayed reactions of angioedema and urticaria. In addition, local reactions have been reported in 20% of vaccinees and systemic reactions (fever, chills, malaise, headache) in 10%.

VACCINE SAFETY

Most vaccines are safe to administer. In general, it is recommended that the use of live vaccines be avoided in immunocompromised patients, including pregnant women. Vaccines are generally not contraindicated in the following situations: mild, acute illness with low-grade fevers (<40.5 °C); concurrent antibiotic therapy; soreness or redness at the site; family history of adverse reactions to vaccinations. Absolute contraindications to vaccines are rare (Table 30–14).

Advisory Committee on Immunization Practices. Recommended adult immunization schedule: United States, 2009. Ann Intern Med. 2009 Jan 6;150(1):40–4. [PMID: 19124819]

Advisory Committee on Immunization Practices (ACIP) Centers for Disease Control and Prevention (CDC). Update: Prevention of hepatitis A after exposure to hepatitis A virus and in international travelers. MMWR Morb Mortal Wkly Rep. 2007 Oct 19;56(41):1080–4. [PMID: 17947967]

Bilukha OO et al; National Center for Infectious Diseases, Centers for Disease Control and Prevention (CDC). Prevention and control of meningococcal disease. Recommendations of the Advisory Committee on Immunization Practices (ACIP). MMWR Recomm Rep. 2005 May 27;54(RR-7):1–21. [PMID: 15917737]

Centers for Disease Control and Prevention. Health Information for International Travel 2005–2006. http://www.cdc.gov/travel/yb/

Centers for Disease Control and Prevention (CDC). Notice to readers: updated recommendations of the Advisory Committee on Immunization Practices (ACIP) for the control and elimination of mumps. MMWR Morb Mortal Wkly Rep. 2006 Jun 9;55(22):629–30. [PMID: 16761359]

Centers for Disease Control and Prevention (CDC). Vaccine safety. http://www.cdc.gov/vaccinesafety/

Kimberlin DW et al. Varicella-zoster vaccine for the prevention of herpes zoster. N Engl J Med. 2007 Mar 29;356(13):1338–13. [PMID: 17392303]

Kretsinger K et al. Preventing tetanus, diphtheria, and pertussis among adults: use of tetanus toxoid, reduced diphtheria toxoid and acellular pertussis vaccine recommendations of the Advisory Committee on Immunization Practices (ACIP) and recommendation of ACIP, supported by the Healthcare Infection Control Practices Advisory Committee (HICPAC), for use of Tdap among health-care personnel. MMWR Recomm Rep. 2006 Dec 15;55(RR-17):1–37. [PMID: 17167397]

Markowitz LE et al; Centers for Disease Control and Prevention (CDC); Advisory Committee on Immunization Practices (ACIP). Quadrivalent Human Papillomavirus Vaccine: Recommendations of the Advisory Committee on Immunization Practices (ACIP). MMWR Recomm Rep. 2007 Mar 23;56(RR-2):1–24. [PMID: 17380109]

Mast EE et al; Advisory Committee on Immunization Practices (ACIP) Centers for Disease Control and Prevention (CDC). A comprehensive immunization strategy to eliminate transmission of hepatitis B virus infection in the United States: recommendations of the Advisory Committee on Immunization Practices (ACIP) Part II: immunization of adults. MMWR Recomm Rep. 2006 Dec 8;55(RR-16):1–33. [PMID: 17159833]

Ward JI et al; APERT Study Group. Efficacy of an acellular pertussis vaccine among adolescents and adults. N Engl J Med. 2005 Oct 13;353(15):1555–63. [PMID: 16221778]

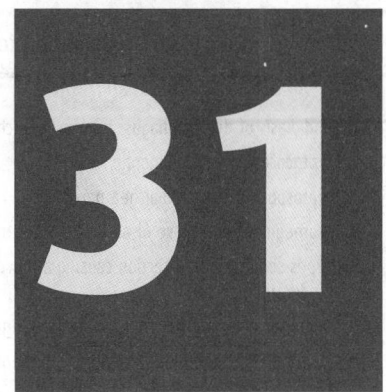

HIV Infection & AIDS

Andrew R. Zolopa, MD
Mitchell H. Katz, MD

ESSENTIALS OF DIAGNOSIS

▶ Risk factors: sexual contact with an infected person, parenteral exposure to infected blood by transfusion or needle sharing, perinatal exposure.

▶ Prominent systemic complaints such as sweats, diarrhea, weight loss, and wasting.

▶ Opportunistic infections due to diminished cellular immunity—often life-threatening.

▶ Aggressive cancers, particularly Kaposi sarcoma and extranodal lymphoma.

▶ Neurologic manifestations, including dementia, aseptic meningitis, and neuropathy.

▶ General Considerations

When AIDS was first recognized in the United States in 1981, cases were identified by finding severe opportunistic infections such as *Pneumocystis* pneumonia that indicated profound defects in cellular immunity in the absence of other causes of immunodeficiency. When the syndrome was found to be caused by HIV, it became obvious that severe opportunistic infections and unusual neoplasms were at one end of a spectrum of disease, while healthy seropositive individuals were at the other end.

The Centers for Disease Control and Prevention (CDC) AIDS case definition (Table 31–1) includes opportunistic infections and malignancies that rarely occur in the absence of severe immunodeficiency (eg, *Pneumocystis* pneumonia, central nervous system lymphoma). It also classifies persons as having AIDS if they have positive HIV serology and certain infections and malignancies that can occur in immunocompetent hosts but that are more common among persons infected with HIV (pulmonary tuberculosis, invasive cervical cancer). Several nonspecific conditions, including dementia and wasting (documented weight loss)—in the presence of a positive HIV serology—are considered AIDS. The definition includes criteria for both definitive and presumptive diagnoses of certain infections and malignancies. Finally, persons with positive HIV serology who have ever had a CD4 lymphocyte count below 200 cells/mcL or a CD4 lymphocyte percentage below 14% are considered to have AIDS. Inclusion of persons with low CD4 counts as AIDS cases reflects the recognition that immunodeficiency is the defining characteristic of AIDS. The choice of a cutoff point at 200 cells/mcL is supported by several cohort studies showing that AIDS will develop within 3 years in over 80% of persons with counts below this level in the absence of effective antiretroviral therapy (ART). The 1993 definition was also expanded to include persons with positive HIV serology and pulmonary tuberculosis (Plate 66), recurrent pneumonia, and invasive cervical cancer. The prognosis of persons with HIV/AIDS has dramatically improved due to the introduction of highly active antiretroviral therapy (HAART) in the mid 1990s. One consequence is that fewer persons with HIV ever develop an infection or malignancy or have a low enough CD4 count to classify them as having AIDS, which means that the CDC definition has become a less useful measure of the impact of HIV/AIDS in the United States. Conversely, persons in whom AIDS had been diagnosed based on a serious opportunistic infection, malignancy, or immunodeficiency may now be markedly healthier, with high CD4 counts, due to the use of HAART. Therefore, the Social Security Administration as well as most social service agencies focus on functional assessment for determining eligibility for benefits rather than the simple presence or absence of an AIDS-defined illness.

▶ Epidemiology

The modes of transmission of HIV are similar to those of hepatitis B, in particular with respect to sexual, parenteral, and vertical transmission. Although certain sexual practices (eg, receptive anal intercourse) are significantly riskier than other sexual practices (eg, oral sex), it is difficult to quantify per-contact risks. The reason is that studies of sexual transmission of HIV show that most people at risk for HIV infection engage in a variety of sexual practices and have sex with multiple persons, only some of whom may actually be HIV infected. Thus, it is difficult to determine which practice with which person actually resulted in HIV transmission.

Table 31–1. CDC AIDS case definition for surveillance of adults and adolescents.

Definitive AIDS diagnoses (with or without laboratory evidence of HIV infection)

1. Candidiasis of the esophagus, trachea, bronchi, or lungs.

2. Cryptococcosis, extrapulmonary.

3. Cryptosporidiosis with diarrhea persisting > 1 month.

4. Cytomegalovirus disease of an organ other than liver, spleen, or lymph nodes.

5. Herpes simplex virus infection causing a mucocutaneous ulcer that persists longer than 1 month; or bronchitis, pneumonitis, or esophagitis of any duration.

6. Kaposi sarcoma in a patient < 60 years of age.

7. Lymphoma of the brain (primary) in a patient < 60 years of age.

8. *Mycobacterium avium* complex or *Mycobacterium kansasii* disease, disseminated (at a site other than or in addition to lungs, skin, or cervical or hilar lymph nodes).

9. *Pneumocystis jiroveci* pneumonia.

10. Progressive multifocal leukoencephalopathy.

11. Toxoplasmosis of the brain.

Definitive AIDS diagnoses (with laboratory evidence of HIV infection)

1. Coccidioidomycosis, disseminated (at a site other than or in addition to lungs or cervical or hilar lymph nodes).

2. HIV encephalopathy.

3. Histoplasmosis, disseminated (at a site other than or in addition to lungs or cervical or hilar lymph nodes).

4. Isosporiasis with diarrhea persisting > 1 month.

5. Kaposi sarcoma at any age.

6. Lymphoma of the brain (primary) at any age.

7. Other non-Hodgkin lymphoma of B cell or unknown immunologic phenotype.

8. Any mycobacterial disease caused by mycobacteria other than *Mycobacterium tuberculosis,* disseminated (at a site other than or in addition to lungs, skin, or cervical or hilar lymph nodes).

9. Disease caused by extrapulmonary *M tuberculosis.*

10. *Salmonella* (nontyphoid) septicemia, recurrent.

11. HIV wasting syndrome.

12. CD4 lymphocyte count below 200 cells/mcL or a CD4 lymphocyte percentage below 14%.

13. Pulmonary tuberculosis.

14. Recurrent pneumonia.

15. Invasive cervical cancer.

Presumptive AIDS diagnoses (with laboratory evidence of HIV infection)

1. Candidiasis of esophagus: (a) recent onset of retrosternal pain on swallowing; and (b) oral candidiasis.

2. Cytomegalovirus retinitis. A characteristic appearance on serial ophthalmoscopic examinations.

3. Mycobacteriosis. Specimen from stool or normally sterile body fluids or tissue from a site other than lungs, skin, or cervical or hilar lymph nodes, showing acid-fast bacilli of a species not identified by culture.

4. Kaposi sarcoma. Erythematous or violaceous plaque-like lesion on skin or mucous membrane.

5. *Pneumocystis jiroveci* pneumonia: (a) a history of dyspnea on exertion or nonproductive cough of recent onset (within the past 3 months); and (b) chest x-ray evidence of diffuse bilateral interstitial infiltrates or gallium scan evidence of diffuse bilateral pulmonary disease; and (c) arterial blood gas analysis showing an arterial oxygen partial pressure of < 70 mm Hg or a low respiratory diffusing capacity of < 80% of predicted values or an increase in the alveolar-arterial oxygen tension gradient; and (d) no evidence of a bacterial pneumonia.

6. Toxoplasmosis of the brain: (a) recent onset of a focal neurologic abnormality consistent with intracranial disease or a reduced level of consciousness; and (b) brain imaging evidence of a lesion having a mass effect or the radiographic appearance of which is enhanced by injection of contrast medium; and (c) serum antibody to toxoplasmosis or successful response to therapy for toxoplasmosis.

7. Recurrent pneumonia: (a) more than one episode in a 1-year period; and (b) acute pneumonia (new symptoms, signs, or radiologic evidence not present earlier) diagnosed on clinical or radiologic grounds by the patient's physician.

8. Pulmonary tuberculosis: (a) apical or miliary infiltrates and (b) radiographic and clinical response to antituberculous therapy.

Nonetheless, the best available estimates indicate that the risk of HIV transmission with receptive anal intercourse is between 1:100 and 1:30, with insertive anal intercourse 1:1000, with receptive vaginal intercourse 1:1000, with insertive vaginal intercourse 1:10,000, and with receptive fellatio with ejaculation 1:1000. The per-contact risk of HIV transmission with other behaviors, including receptive fellatio without ejaculation, insertive fellatio, and cunnilingus, is not known.

All per-contact risk estimates assume that the source is HIV infected. If the HIV status of the source is unknown, the risk of transmission is the risk of transmission multiplied by the probability that the source is HIV infected. This would vary by risk practices, age, and geographic area. A number of cofactors are known to increase the risk of HIV transmission during a given encounter, including the presence of ulcerative or inflammatory sexually transmitted diseases, trauma, menses, and lack of male circumcision.

The risk of acquiring HIV infection from a needlestick with infected blood is approximately 1:300. Factors known to increase the risk of transmission include depth of penetration, hollow bore needles, visible blood on the needle, and advanced stage of disease in the source. The risk of HIV transmission from a mucosal splash with infected blood is unknown but is assumed to be significantly lower.

The risk of acquiring HIV infection from illicit drug use with sharing of needles from an HIV-infected source is estimated to be 1:150. Use of clean needles markedly decreases the chance of HIV transmission but does not eliminate it if other drug paraphernalia are shared (eg, cookers).

When blood transfusion from an HIV-infected donor occurs, the risk of transmission is 95%. Fortunately, since 1985, blood donor screening using the HIV enzyme-linked immunosorbent assay (ELISA) has been universally practiced in the United States. Also, persons who have recently engaged in unsafe behaviors (eg, sex with a person at risk for HIV, injection drug use) are not allowed to donate. This eliminates donations from persons who are HIV infected but have not yet developed antibodies (ie, persons in the "window" period). In recent years, HIV antigen and viral load testing have been added to the screening of blood to further lower the chance of HIV transmission. With these precautions, the chance of HIV transmission with receipt of blood transfusion is about 1:1,000,000.

In the absence of perinatal HIV prophylaxis, between 13% and 40% of children born to HIV-infected mothers contract HIV infection. The risk is higher with vaginal than with cesarean delivery, higher among mothers with high viral loads, and higher among those who breast-feed their children. The risk can be decreased by administering antiretroviral treatment to the mother during pregnancy and to the infant immediately after birth (see below).

HIV has not been shown to be transmitted by respiratory droplet spread, by vectors such as mosquitoes, or by casual nonsexual contact.

Current estimates are that about 950,000 Americans are infected with HIV, and there are about 53,000 new infections each year. At the end of 2006, there were an estimated 448,871 persons in the United States living with AIDS. Of those, 76% are men, of whom 60% were exposed through male-to-male sexual contact, 19% were exposed through injection drug use, 12% were exposed through heterosexual contact, and 8% were exposed through male-to-male sexual contact and injection drug use. Women account for 23% of living persons, of whom 66% were infected through heterosexual contact and 32% were exposed through injection drug use. Children account for less than 1% of living cases. African Americans have been disproportionately hard hit by the epidemic. The estimated rate in 2006 of new AIDS cases in the United States per 100,000 population was 60.3 among African Americans, 20.8 among Latinos, 7.8 among native Americans and native Alaskans, 6.4 among whites, and 4.4 among Asians and Pacific Islanders.

In general, the progression of HIV-related illness is similar in men and women. However, there are some important differences. Women are at risk for gynecologic complications of HIV, including recurrent candidal vaginitis, pelvic inflammatory disease, and cervical dysplasia. Violence directed against women, pregnancy, and frequent occurrence of drug use and poverty all complicate the treatment of HIV-infected women. Although "safer sex" campaigns dramatically decreased the rates of seroconversions among men who have sex with men (MSM) living in metropolitan areas in the United States by the mid 1980s, relapse to unsafe sexual practices among MSM in several large cities in the United States and in western Europe has been observed. The higher rates of unsafe sex appear to be related to decreased concern about acquiring HIV due to the availability of HAART. Decreased interest in following safer sex recommendations and increasing use of crystal methamphetamine among certain risk groups also appears to be playing a role in the increased unsafe sex rates.

Worldwide there are an estimated 33 million persons infected with HIV. In Central and East Africa in some urban areas, as many as one-third of sexually active adults are infected. HIV infection began to spread in Asia in the late 1980s. The most common mode of transmission is bidirectional heterosexual spread. The reason for the greater risk for transmission with heterosexual intercourse in Africa and Asia than in the United States may relate to cofactors such as general health status, the presence of genital ulcers, relative lack of male circumcision, the number of sexual partners, and different HIV serotypes.

Centers for Disease Control and Prevention: HIV/AIDS Surveillance Reports. Available at http://www.cdc.gov/hiv/topics/surveillance/resources/reports/index.htm.

Colfax G et al. The methamphetamine epidemic: implications for HIV prevention and treatment. Curr HIV/AIDS Rep. 2005 Nov;2(4):194–9. [PMID: 16343378]

Fowler MG et al. Reducing the risk of mother-to-child human immunodeficiency virus transmission: past successes, current progress and challenges, and future directions. Am J Obstet Gynecol. 2007 Sep;197(3 Suppl):S3–9. [PMID: 17825648]

Hall HI et al; HIV Incidence Surveillance Group. Estimation of HIV incidence in the United States. JAMA. 2008 Aug 6;300(5):520–9. [PMID: 18677024]

Public Health Service Task Force recommendations for use of antiretroviral drugs in pregnant HIV-1 infected women for maternal health and interventions to reduce perinatal HIV-1 transmission in the United States. October 12, 2006 Guideline. Available at http://aidsinfo.nih.gov/ContentFiles/PerinatalGL.pdf

Santibanez SS et al. Update and overview of practical epidemiologic aspects of HIV/AIDS among injection drug users in the United States. J Urban Health. 2006 Jan;83(1):86–100. [PMID: 16736357]

Stevens LM et al. JAMA patient page. HIV infection: the basics. JAMA. 2006 Aug 16;296(7):892. [PMID: 16905793]

Vittinghoff E et al. Per-contact risk of human immunodeficiency virus transmission between male sexual partners. Am J Epidemiol. 1999 Aug 1;150(3):306–11. [PMID: 10430236]

▶ Etiology

HIV, like other retroviruses, depends on a unique enzyme, reverse transcriptase (RNA-dependent DNA polymerase), to replicate within host cells. The other major pathogenic human retrovirus, human T cell lymphotropic/leukemia virus (HTLV)-I, is associated with lymphoma, while HIV is not known to be directly oncogenic. The HIV genomes contain genes for three basic structural proteins and at least five other regulatory proteins; *gag* codes for group antigen proteins, *pol* codes for polymerase, and *env* codes for the external envelope protein. The greatest variability in strains of HIV occurs in the viral envelope. Since neutralizing activity is found in antibodies directed against the envelope, this variability presents problems for vaccine development.

In addition to the classic AIDS virus (HIV-1), a group of related viruses, HIV-2, has been isolated in West African patients. HIV-2 has the same genetic organization as HIV-1, but there are significant differences in the envelope glycoproteins. Some infected individuals exhibit AIDS-like illnesses, but the rate of progression in individuals infected with HIV-2 appears to be slower than that of HIV-1 infection. HIV-2 remains relatively rare in the United States but has become more common in Western Europe due to immigration from endemic areas. Cases have been documented in which AIDS-like illnesses have occurred in the absence of HIV infection or other known infectious causes of immunodeficiency.

▶ Pathogenesis

The hallmark of symptomatic HIV infection is immunodeficiency caused by continuing viral replication. The virus can infect all cells expressing the T4 (CD4) antigen, which HIV uses to attach to the cell. Chemokine co-receptors (CCR5 and CXCR4) are required for virus entry, and individuals with CCR5 deletions are less likely to become infected and, once infected, the disease is more likely to progress slowly. Once it enters a cell, HIV can replicate and cause cell fusion or death. A latent state is also established, with integration of the HIV genome into the cell's genome. The cell principally infected is the CD4 (helper-inducer) lymphocyte, which directs many other cells in the immune network. With increasing duration of infection, the number of CD4 lymphocytes falls. Some of the immunologic defects, however, are explained not by *quantitative* abnormalities of lymphocyte subsets but by *qualitative* defects in CD4 responsiveness induced by HIV.

Other cells in the immune network that are infected by HIV include B lymphocytes and macrophages. The defect in B cells is partly due to disordered CD4 lymphocyte function. These direct and indirect effects can lead to generalized hypergammaglobulinemia and can also depress B cell responses to new antigen challenges. Because of these defects, the immunodeficiency of HIV is mixed. Elements of humoral and cellular immunodeficiency are present, especially in children. Macrophages act as a reservoir for HIV and serve to disseminate it to other organ systems (eg, the central nervous system).

Apart from the immunologic effects of HIV, the virus can also directly cause a variety of neurologic effects. Neuropathology largely results from the release of cytokines and other neurotoxins by infected macrophages. Perturbations of excitatory neurotransmitters and calcium flux may contribute to neurologic dysfunction. Direct HIV infection of renal tubular cells and gastrointestinal epithelium may contribute to these organ system manifestations of infection.

▶ Pathophysiology

Clinically, the syndromes caused by HIV infection are usually explicable by one of three known mechanisms: immunodeficiency, autoimmunity, and allergic and hypersensitivity reactions.

A. Immunodeficiency

Immunodeficiency is a direct result of the effects of HIV upon immune cells. A spectrum of infections and neoplasms is seen, as in other congenital or acquired immunodeficiency states. Two remarkable features of HIV immunodeficiency are the low incidence of certain infections such as listeriosis and aspergillosis and the frequent occurrence of certain neoplasms such as lymphoma or Kaposi sarcoma. This latter complication has been seen primarily in MSM or in bisexual men, and its incidence has steadily declined through the first 15 years of the epidemic. A herpesvirus (KSHV or HHV-8) is the cause of Kaposi sarcoma.

B. Autoimmunity/Allergic & Hypersensitivity Reactions

Autoimmunity can occur as a result of disordered cellular immune function or B lymphocyte dysfunction. Examples of both lymphocytic infiltration of organs (eg, lymphocytic interstitial pneumonitis) and autoantibody production (eg, immunologic thrombocytopenia) occur. These phenomena may be the only clinically apparent disease or may coexist with obvious immunodeficiency. Moreover, HIV-infected individuals appear to have higher rates of allergic reactions to unknown allergens as seen with eosinophilic pustular folliculitis ("itchy red bump syndrome") as well as increased rates of hypersensitivity reactions to medications (for example, the fever and sunburn-like rash seen with trimethoprim-sulfamethoxazole reactions).

▶ Clinical Findings

The complications of HIV-related infections and neoplasms affect virtually every organ. The general approach to the HIV-infected person with symptoms is to evaluate the organ systems involved, aiming to diagnose treatable conditions rapidly. As can be seen in Figure 31–1, the CD4

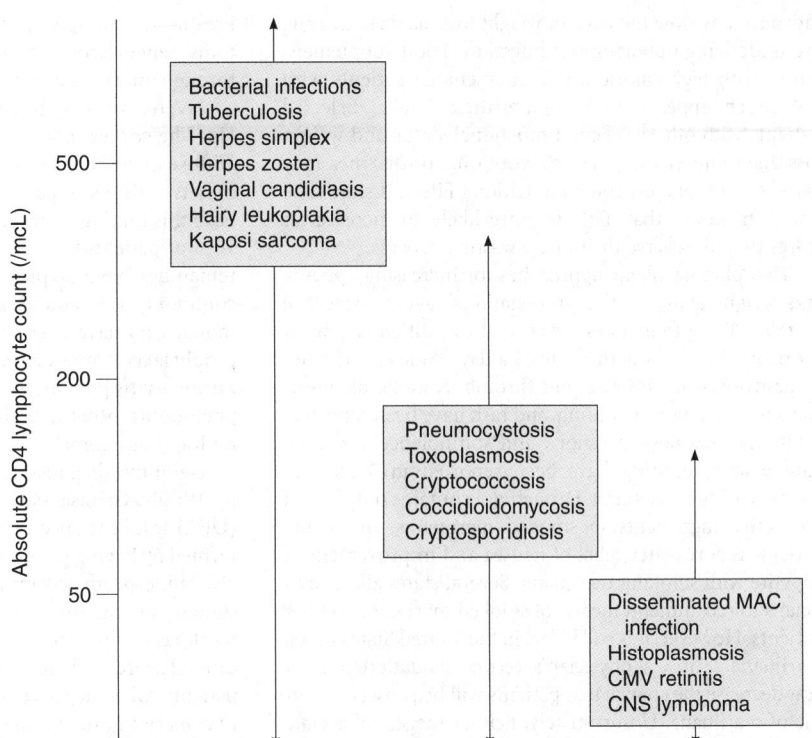

▲ **Figure 31–1.** Relationship of CD4 count to development of opportunistic infections. MAC, *Mycobacterium avium* complex; CMV, cytomegalovirus; CNS, central nervous system.

lymphocyte count provides very important prognostic information. Certain infections may occur at any CD4 count, while others rarely occur unless the CD4 lymphocyte count has dropped below a certain level. For example, a patient with a CD4 count of 600 cells/mcL, cough, and fever may have a bacterial pneumonia but would be very unlikely to have *Pneumocystis* pneumonia.

A. Symptoms and Signs

Many individuals with HIV infection remain asymptomatic for years even without antiretroviral therapy, with a mean time of approximately 10 years between exposure and development of AIDS. When symptoms occur, they may be remarkably protean and nonspecific. Since virtually all the findings may be seen with other diseases, a combination of complaints is more suggestive of HIV infection than any one symptom.

Physical examination may be entirely normal. Abnormal findings range from completely nonspecific to highly specific for HIV infection. Those that are specific for HIV infection include hairy leukoplakia of the tongue, disseminated Kaposi sarcoma, and cutaneous bacillary angiomatosis. Generalized lymphadenopathy is common early in infection.

1. Systemic complaints—Fever, night sweats, and weight loss are common symptoms in HIV-infected patients and may occur without a complicating opportunistic infection. Patients with persistent fever and no localizing symptoms should nonetheless be carefully examined, and evaluated with a chest radiograph (*Pneumocystis* pneumonia can present without respiratory symptoms), bacterial blood cultures if the fever is greater than 38.5 °C, serum cryptococcal antigen, and mycobacterial cultures of the blood. Sinus CT scans or sinus radiographs should be considered to evaluate occult sinusitis. If these studies are normal, patients should be observed closely. Antipyretics are useful to prevent dehydration.

Weight loss is a particularly distressing complication of long-standing HIV infection. Patients typically have disproportionate loss of muscle mass, with maintenance or less substantial loss of fat stores. The mechanism of HIV-related weight loss is not completely understood but appears to be multifactorial.

AIDS patients frequently suffer from anorexia, nausea, and vomiting, all of which contribute to weight loss by decreasing caloric intake. In some cases, these symptoms are secondary to a specific infection, such as viral hepatitis. In other cases, however, evaluation of the symptoms yields no specific pathogen, and it is assumed to be due to a primary effect of HIV. Malabsorption also plays a role in decreased caloric intake. Patients may suffer diarrhea from infections with bacterial, viral, or parasitic agents.

Exacerbating the decrease in caloric intake, many AIDS patients have an increased metabolic rate. This increased rate has been shown to exist even among asymptomatic HIV-infected persons, but it accelerates with disease progression and secondary infection. AIDS patients with secondary infections also have decreased protein synthesis, which makes maintaining muscle mass difficult.

Several strategies have been developed to slow AIDS wasting. Effective fever control decreases the metabolic rate and may slow the pace of weight loss, as does treating the underlying opportunistic infection. Food supplementation with high-calorie drinks may enable patients with not much appetite to maintain their intake. Selected patients with otherwise good functional status and weight loss due to unrelenting nausea, vomiting, or diarrhea may benefit from total parenteral nutrition (TPN). It should be noted, however, that TPN is more likely to increase fat stores than to reverse the muscle wasting process.

Two pharmacologic approaches for increasing appetite and weight gain are the progestational agent megestrol acetate (80 mg four times a day) and the antiemetic agent dronabinol (2.5–5 mg three times a day). Side effects from megestrol acetate are rare, but thromboembolic phenomena, edema, nausea, vomiting, and rash have been reported. Euphoria, dizziness, paranoia, and somnolence and even nausea and vomiting have been reported in 3–10% of patients using dronabinol. Dronabinol contains only one of the active ingredients in smoked marijuana, and many patients report better relief of nausea and improvement of appetite with smoking marijuana. Several states allow physicians to recommend the use of smoked marijuana to their patients. However, it is still illegal in the United States to sell marijuana. Thus, a physician's recommendation may at best decrease the chance that patients will be prosecuted for use of marijuana. Unfortunately, neither megestrol acetate nor dronabinol increases lean body mass.

Two regimens that have resulted in increases in lean body mass are growth hormone and anabolic steroids. Growth hormone at a dose of 0.1 mg/kg/d (up to 6 mg) subcutaneously for 12 weeks has resulted in modest increases in lean body mass. Treatment with growth hormone can cost as much as $10,000 per month. Anabolic steroids also increase lean body mass among HIV-infected patients. They seem to work best for patients who are able to do weight training. The most commonly used regimens are testosterone enanthate or testosterone cypionate (100–200 mg intramuscularly every 2–4 weeks). Testosterone transdermal system (apply 5 mg system each evening) and testosterone gel (1%; apply a 5-g packet [50 mg testosterone] to clean, dry skin daily) are also available. The anabolic steroid oxandrolone (20 mg orally in two divided doses) has also been found to increase lean body mass.

Nausea leading to weight loss is sometimes due to esophageal candidiasis. Patients with oral candidiasis and nausea should be empirically treated with an oral antifungal agent. Patients with weight loss due to nausea of unclear origin may benefit from use of antiemetics prior to meals (prochlorperazine, 10 mg three times daily; metoclopramide, 10 mg three times daily; or ondansetron, 8 mg three times daily). Dronabinol (5 mg three times daily) can also be used to increase appetite. Depression and adrenal insufficiency are two potentially treatable causes of weight loss.

2. Pulmonary disease

A. PNEUMOCYSTIS PNEUMONIA—(See also discussions in Chapter 36.) *Pneumocystis jiroveci* pneumonia is the most common opportunistic infection associated with AIDS. *Pneumocystis* pneumonia may be difficult to diagnose because the symptoms—fever, cough, and shortness of breath—are nonspecific. Furthermore, the severity of symptoms ranges from fever and no respiratory symptoms through mild cough or dyspnea to frank respiratory distress.

Hypoxemia may be severe, with a Po_2 less than 60 mm Hg. The cornerstone of diagnosis is the chest radiograph. Diffuse or perihilar infiltrates are most characteristic, but only two-thirds of patients with *Pneumocystis* pneumonia have this finding. Normal chest radiographs are seen in 5–10% of patients with *Pneumocystis* pneumonia, while the remainder have atypical infiltrates. Apical infiltrates are commonly seen among patients with *Pneumocystis* pneumonia who have been receiving aerosolized pentamidine prophylaxis. Large pleural effusions are uncommon with *Pneumocystis* pneumonia; their presence suggests bacterial pneumonia, other infections such as tuberculosis, or pleural Kaposi sarcoma.

Definitive diagnosis can be obtained in 50–80% of cases by Wright-Giemsa stain or direct fluorescence antibody (DFA) test of induced sputum. Sputum induction is performed by having patients inhale an aerosolized solution of 3% saline produced by an ultrasonic nebulizer. Patients should not eat for at least 8 hours and should not use toothpaste or mouthwash prior to the procedure since they can interfere with test interpretation. The next step for patients with negative sputum examinations in whom *Pneumocystis* pneumonia is still suspected should be bronchoalveolar lavage. This technique establishes the diagnosis in over 95% of cases.

In patients with symptoms suggestive of *Pneumocystis* pneumonia but with negative or atypical chest radiographs and negative sputum examinations, other diagnostic tests may provide additional information in deciding whether to proceed to bronchoalveolar lavage. Elevation of serum lactate dehydrogenase occurs in 95% of cases of *Pneumocystis* pneumonia, but the specificity of this finding is at best 75%. Either a normal diffusing capacity of carbon monoxide (DL_{CO}) or a high-resolution CT scan of the chest that demonstrates no interstitial lung disease makes the diagnosis of *Pneumocystis* pneumonia very unlikely. In addition, a CD4 count above 250 cells/mcL within 2 months prior to evaluation of respiratory symptoms makes a diagnosis of *Pneumocystis* pneumonia unlikely; only 1–5% of cases occur above this CD4 count level (Figure 31–1). This is true even if the patient previously had a CD4 count lower than 200 cells/mcL but has had an increase with antiretroviral therapy. Pneumothoraces can be seen in HIV-infected patients with a history of *Pneumocystis* pneumonia, especially if they have received aerosolized pentamidine treatment.

B. OTHER INFECTIOUS PULMONARY DISEASES—Other infectious causes of pulmonary disease in AIDS patients include bacterial, mycobacterial, and viral pneumonias. Community-acquired pneumonia is the most common cause of pulmonary disease in HIV-infected persons. An increased incidence of pneumococcal pneumonia with septicemia and *Haemophilus influenzae* pneumonia has been reported. *Pseudomonas aeruginosa* is an important respiratory pathogen in advanced disease. The incidence of infection with *Mycobacterium tuberculosis* has markedly increased in metropolitan areas because of HIV infection as well as homelessness. Tuberculosis occurs in an estimated 4% of persons in the United States who have AIDS. Apical infiltrates and disseminated disease occur more commonly than among immunocompetent persons. Although a purified protein derivative (PPD) test should be performed on all HIV-infected persons in whom a diagnosis of tuberculosis is being considered, the lower the CD4 cell count, the greater the likelihood of anergy. Because "anergy" skin test panels do not accurately classify those patients who are infected with tuberculosis but unreactive to the PPD, they are not recommended. Treatment of HIV-infected persons with active tuberculosis is similar to treatment of HIV-uninfected tubercular individuals (see Figure 31–1). However, rifampin should not be given to patients receiving indinavir, nelfinavir, amprenavir, lopinavir, or delavirdine. In these cases, rifabutin may be substituted, but it may require dosing modifications depending on the antiretroviral regimen. Multidrug-resistant tuberculosis is a major problem in several metropolitan areas. Noncompliance with prescribed antituberculous drugs is a major risk factor. Several of the reported outbreaks appear to implicate nosocomial spread. The emergence of drug resistance makes it essential that antibiotic sensitivities be performed on all positive cultures. Drug therapy should be individualized. Patients with multidrug-resistant *M tuberculosis* infection should receive at least three drugs to which their organism is sensitive. Atypical mycobacteria can cause pulmonary disease in AIDS patients with or without preexisting lung disease and responds variably to treatment. Making a distinction between *M tuberculosis* and atypical mycobacteria requires culture of sputum specimens. If culture of the sputum produces acid-fast bacilli, definitive identification may take several weeks using traditional techniques. DNA probes allow for presumptive identification usually within days of a positive culture. While awaiting definitive diagnosis, clinicians should err on the side of treating patients as if they have *M tuberculosis* infection. In cases in which the risk of atypical mycobacteria is very high (eg, a person without risk for tuberculosis exposure with a CD4 count under 50 cells/mcL—see Figure 31–1), clinicians may wait for definitive diagnosis if the person is smear-negative for acid-fast bacilli, clinically stable, and not living in a communal setting. Isolation of cytomegalovirus (CMV) from bronchoalveolar lavage fluid occurs commonly in AIDS patients but does not establish a definitive diagnosis. Diagnosis of CMV pneumonia requires biopsy; response to treatment is poor. Histoplasmosis, coccidioidomycosis, and cryptococcal disease should also be considered in the differential diagnosis of unexplained pulmonary infiltrates.

C. Noninfectious pulmonary diseases—Noninfectious causes of lung disease include Kaposi sarcoma, non-Hodgkin lymphoma, and interstitial pneumonitis. In patients with known Kaposi sarcoma, pulmonary involvement complicates the course in approximately one-third of cases. However, pulmonary involvement is rarely the presenting manifestation of Kaposi sarcoma. Non-Hodgkin lymphoma may involve the lung as the sole site of disease but more commonly involves other organs as well, especially the brain, liver, and gastrointestinal tract. Both of

these processes may show nodular or diffuse parenchymal involvement, pleural effusions, and mediastinal adenopathy on chest radiographs.

Nonspecific interstitial pneumonitis may mimic *Pneumocystis* pneumonia. Lymphocytic interstitial pneumonitis seen in lung biopsies has a variable clinical course. Typically, these patients present with several months of mild cough and dyspnea; chest radiographs show interstitial infiltrates. Many patients with this entity undergo transbronchial biopsies in an attempt to diagnose *Pneumocystis* pneumonia. Instead, the tissue shows interstitial inflammation ranging from an intense lymphocytic infiltration (consistent with lymphoid interstitial pneumonitis) to a mild mononuclear inflammation. Corticosteroids may be helpful in some cases refractory to antiretroviral therapy.

D. Sinusitis—Chronic sinusitis can be a frustrating problem for HIV-infected patients even in those on adequate antiretroviral therapy. Symptoms include sinus congestion and discharge, headache, and fever. Some patients may have radiographic evidence of sinus disease on sinus CT scan or sinus x-ray in the absence of significant symptoms. Nonsmoking patients with purulent drainage should be treated with amoxicillin (500 mg orally three times a day). Patients who smoke should be treated with amoxicillin-potassium clavulanate (500 mg orally three times a day) to cover *H influenzae*. Prolonged treatment (3–6 weeks) with an antibiotic and guaifenesin (600 mg orally twice daily) to decrease sinus congestion may be required. For patients not responding to amoxicillin-potassium clavulanate, levofloxacin should be tried (400 mg orally daily). Some patients may require referral to an otolaryngologist for sinus drainage.

3. Central nervous system disease—Central nervous system disease in HIV-infected patients can be divided into intracerebral space-occupying lesions, encephalopathy, meningitis, and spinal cord processes. Many of these complications have declined markedly in prevalence in the era of HAART.

A. Toxoplasmosis—Toxoplasmosis is the most common space-occupying lesion in HIV-infected patients. Headache, focal neurologic deficits, seizures, or altered mental status may be presenting symptoms. The diagnosis is usually made presumptively based on the characteristic appearance of cerebral imaging studies in an individual known to be seropositive for *Toxoplasma*. Typically, toxoplasmosis appears as multiple contrast-enhancing lesions on CT scan. Lesions tend to be peripheral, with a predilection for the basal ganglia.

Single lesions are atypical of toxoplasmosis. When a single lesion has been detected by CT scanning, MRI scanning may reveal multiple lesions because of its greater sensitivity. If a patient has a single lesion on MRI and is neurologically stable, clinicians may pursue a 2-week empiric trial of toxoplasmosis therapy. A repeat scan should be performed at 2 weeks. If the lesion has not diminished in size, biopsy of the lesion should be performed. Since many HIV-infected patients will have detectable titers, a positive *Toxoplasma* serologic test does not confirm the diagnosis. Conversely, less than 3% of patients with toxoplasmosis have negative titers. Therefore, negative *Toxoplasma* titers in an HIV-infected patient with a space-occupying lesion should be a cause for aggressively pursuing an alternative diagnosis.

B. CENTRAL NERVOUS SYSTEM LYMPHOMA—Primary non-Hodgkin lymphoma is the second most common space-occupying lesion in HIV-infected patients. Symptoms are similar to those with toxoplasmosis. While imaging techniques cannot distinguish these two diseases with certainty, lymphoma more often is solitary. Other less common lesions should be suspected if there is preceding bacteremia, positive tuberculin test, fungemia, or injection drug use. These include bacterial abscesses, cryptococcomas, tuberculomas, and *Nocardia* lesions.

Because techniques for stereotactic brain biopsy have improved, this procedure plays an increasing role in diagnosing cerebral lesions. Biopsy should be strongly considered if lesions are solitary or do not respond to toxoplasmosis treatment, especially if they are easily accessible. Diagnosis of lymphoma is important because many patients benefit from treatment (radiation therapy). In the future, it may be possible to avoid brain biopsy by utilizing polymerase chain reaction (PCR) assay of cerebrospinal fluid for Epstein–Barr virus DNA, which is present in 90% of CNS lymphoma cases.

C. AIDS DEMENTIA COMPLEX—The diagnosis of AIDS dementia complex (HIV-associated cognitive-motor complex) is one of exclusion based on a brain imaging study and on spinal fluid analysis that excludes other pathogens. Neuropsychiatric testing is helpful in distinguishing patients with dementia from those with depression. Patients with AIDS dementia complex typically have difficulty with cognitive tasks and exhibit diminished motor speed. Patients may first notice a deterioration in their handwriting. The manifestations of dementia may wax and wane, with persons exhibiting periods of lucidity and confusion over the course of a day. Many patients improve with effective antiretroviral treatment. Metabolic abnormalities may also cause changes in mental status: hypoglycemia, hyponatremia, hypoxia, and drug overdose are important considerations in this population. Other less common infectious causes of encephalopathy include progressive multifocal leukoencephalopathy (discussed below), CMV, syphilis, and herpes simplex encephalitis.

D. CRYPTOCOCCAL MENINGITIS—Cryptococcal meningitis typically presents with fever and headache. Less than 20% of patients have meningismus. Diagnosis is based on a positive latex agglutination test that detects cryptococcal antigen (or "CRAG") or positive culture of spinal fluid for *Cryptococcus*. Seventy to 90% of patients with cryptococcal meningitis have a positive serum CRAG. Thus, a negative serum CRAG test makes a diagnosis of cryptococcal meningitis unlikely and can be useful in the initial evaluation of a patient with headache, fever, and normal mental status. HIV meningitis, characterized by lymphocytic pleocytosis of the spinal fluid with negative culture, is common early in HIV infection.

E. HIV MYELOPATHY—Spinal cord function may also be impaired in HIV-infected individuals. HIV myelopathy

presents with leg weakness and incontinence. Spastic paraparesis and sensory ataxia are seen on neurologic examination. Myelopathy is usually a late manifestation of HIV disease, and most patients will have concomitant HIV encephalopathy. Pathologic evaluation of the spinal cord reveals vacuolation of white matter. Because HIV myelopathy is a diagnosis of exclusion, symptoms suggestive of myelopathy should be evaluated by lumbar puncture to rule out CMV polyradiculopathy (described below) and an MRI or CT scan to exclude epidural lymphoma.

F. PROGRESSIVE MULTIFOCAL LEUKOENCEPHALOPATHY (PML)—PML is a viral infection of the white matter of the brain seen in patients with very advanced HIV infection. It typically results in focal neurologic deficits such as aphasia, hemiparesis, and cortical blindness. Imaging studies are strongly suggestive of the diagnosis if they show nonenhancing white matter lesions without mass effect. Extensive lesions may be difficult to differentiate from the changes caused by HIV. Several patients have stabilized or improved after the institution of combination antiretroviral therapy or cidofovir.

4. Peripheral nervous system—Peripheral nervous system syndromes include inflammatory polyneuropathies, sensory neuropathies, and mononeuropathies.

An inflammatory demyelinating polyneuropathy similar to Guillain-Barré syndrome occurs in HIV-infected patients, usually prior to frank immunodeficiency. The syndrome in many cases improves with plasmapheresis, supporting an autoimmune basis of the disease. CMV can cause an ascending polyradiculopathy characterized by lower extremity weakness and a neutrophilic pleocytosis on spinal fluid analysis with a negative bacterial culture. Transverse myelitis can be seen with herpes zoster or CMV.

Peripheral neuropathy is common among HIV-infected persons. Patients typically complain of numbness, tingling, and pain in the lower extremities. Symptoms are disproportionate to findings on gross sensory and motor evaluation. Beyond HIV infection itself, the most common cause is prior antiretroviral therapy with stavudine or didanosine. Patients who report these symptoms should be switched to an alternative agent if possible. Caution should be used when administering these agents to patients with a history of peripheral neuropathy. Unfortunately, drug-induced neuropathy is not always reversed when the offending agent is discontinued. Patients with advanced disease may also develop peripheral neuropathy even if they have never taken antiretroviral therapy. Evaluation should rule out other causes of sensory neuropathy such as alcoholism, thyroid disease, vitamin B_{12} deficiency, and syphilis.

Treatment of peripheral neuropathy is aimed at symptomatic relief. Patients should be initially treated with gabapentin (start at 300 mg at bedtime and increase to 300–900 mg orally three times a day).

5. Rheumatologic manifestations—Arthritis, involving single or multiple joints, with or without effusion, has been commonly noted in HIV-infected patients. Involvement of large joints is most common. Although the cause of HIV-related arthritis is unknown, most patients will respond to nonsteroidal anti-inflammatory drugs. Patients with a sizable effusion, especially if the joint is warm or erythematous, should have the joint tapped, followed by culture of the fluid to rule out suppurative arthritis as well as fungal and mycobacterial disease.

Several rheumatologic syndromes, including reactive arthritis (Reiter syndrome), psoriatic arthritis, sicca syndrome, and systemic lupus erythematosus, have been reported in HIV-infected patients (see Chapter 20). However, it is unclear if the prevalence is greater than in the general population. Cases of avascular necrosis of the femoral heads have been reported sporadically, generally in the setting of advanced disease with long-standing infection and in patients receiving long-term antiretroviral therapy. The etiology is not clear but is probably multifactorial in nature.

6. Myopathy—Myopathies are infrequent in the era of effective antiretroviral therapy but can be related to either HIV-infection or antiretroviral therapy, particularly with use of zidovudine (azidothymidine [AZT]). Proximal muscle weakness is typical, and patients may have varying degrees of muscle tenderness. A muscle biopsy can distinguish HIV myopathy from zidovudine myopathy and should be considered in patients for whom continuation of zidovudine is essential.

7. Retinitis—Complaints of visual changes must be evaluated immediately in HIV-infected patients. CMV retinitis, characterized by perivascular hemorrhages and white fluffy exudates, is the most common retinal infection in AIDS patients and can be rapidly progressive. In contrast, cotton wool spots, which are also common in HIV-infected people, are benign, remit spontaneously, and appear as small indistinct white spots without exudation or hemorrhage. This distinction may be difficult at times for the nonspecialist, and patients with visual changes should be seen by an ophthalmologist. Other rare retinal processes include other herpesvirus infections or toxoplasmosis.

8. Oral lesions—The presence of oral candidiasis or hairy leukoplakia is significant for several reasons. First, these lesions are highly suggestive of HIV infection in patients who have no other obvious cause of immunodeficiency. Second, several studies have indicated that patients with candidiasis have a high rate of progression to AIDS even with statistical adjustment for CD4 count.

Hairy leukoplakia is caused by the Epstein-Barr virus. The lesion is not usually troubling to patients and sometimes regresses spontaneously. Hairy leukoplakia is commonly seen as a white lesion on the lateral aspect of the tongue. It may be flat or slightly raised, is usually corrugated, and has vertical parallel lines with fine or thick ("hairy") projections. Oral candidiasis can be bothersome to patients, many of whom report an unpleasant taste or mouth dryness. There are two major types of oral candidiasis: pseudomembranous (removable white plaques) and erythematous (red friable plaques). Treatment is with topical agents such as clotrimazole 10-mg troches (one troche four or five times a day). Patients with candidiasis who do not respond to topical antifungals can be treated

with fluconazole (50–100 mg orally once a day for 3–7 days). Chronic suppression of oral candidiasis with fluconazole has been associated with development of candidiasis resistant to all available azoles and thus should be avoided except in frequently recurring cases.

Angular cheilitis—fissures at the sides of the mouth—is usually due to *Candida* as well and can be treated topically with ketoconazole cream (2%) twice a day.

Gingival disease is common in HIV-infected patients and is thought to be due to an overgrowth of microorganisms. It usually responds to professional dental cleaning and chlorhexidine rinses. A particularly aggressive gingivitis or periodontitis will develop in some HIV-infected patients; these patients should be given antibiotics that cover anaerobic oral flora (eg, metronidazole, 250 mg four times a day for 4 or 5 days) and referred to oral surgeons with experience with these entities.

Aphthous ulcers are painful and may interfere with eating. They can be treated with fluocinonide (0.05% ointment mixed 1:1 with plain Orabase and applied six times a day to the ulcer). For lesions that are difficult to reach, patients should use dexamethasone swishes (0.5 mg in 5 mL elixir three times a day). The pain of the ulcers can be relieved with use of an anesthetic spray (10% lidocaine). For patients with refractory ulcers, thalidomide, starting at a dose of 50 mg orally daily and increasing to 100–200 mg daily, has proved useful. Because it is teratogenic; it should be administered only to patients at zero risk of procreation. The most common side effects are sedation and peripheral neuropathy. Other lesions seen in the mouths of HIV-infected patients include Kaposi sarcoma (usually on the hard palate) and warts.

9. Gastrointestinal manifestations

A. CANDIDAL ESOPHAGITIS—(See also discussion in Chapter 15.) Esophageal candidiasis is a common AIDS complication. In a patient with characteristic symptoms, empiric antifungal treatment is begun with fluconazole (200 mg daily for 10–14 days). Further evaluation to identify other causes of esophagitis (herpes simplex, CMV) is reserved for patients who do not improve with antifungal treatment.

B. HEPATIC DISEASE—Autopsy studies have demonstrated that the liver is a frequent site of infections and neoplasms in HIV-infected patients. However, many of these infections are not clinically symptomatic. Clinicians may note elevations of alkaline phosphatase and aminotransferases on routine chemistry panels. Mycobacterial disease, CMV, hepatitis B virus, hepatitis C virus, and lymphoma cause liver disease and can present with varying degrees of nausea, vomiting, right upper quadrant abdominal pain, and jaundice. Sulfonamides, imidazole drugs, antituberculous medications, pentamidine, clarithromycin, and didanosine have also been associated with hepatitis. HIV-infected patients with chronic hepatitis may have more rapid progression of liver disease because of the concomitant immunodeficiency or hepatotoxicity of antiretroviral therapy. Percutaneous liver biopsy may be helpful in diagnosing liver disease, but some common causes of liver disease (eg, *Mycobacterium avium* complex, lymphoma) can be determined by less invasive measures (eg, blood culture, biopsy of a more accessible site). With patients living longer as a result of advances in antiretroviral therapy, advanced liver disease and hepatic failure due to chronic active hepatitis B and or C are increasing causes of morbidity and mortality. HIV-infected individuals who are coinfected with hepatitis B, should be treated with antiretroviral regimens that include drugs with activity against both viruses (eg, lamivudine [3TC], emtricitabine [FTC], tenofovir [TDF]). Treatment of HIV-infected persons with hepatitis C with peginterferon and ribavirin has been shown to be efficacious, although less so than in HIV-uninfected persons. HIV-infected persons are also more likely to have difficulty tolerating treatment with peginterferon than uninfected persons. Liver transplants have been performed successfully in HIV-infected patients. This strategy is most likely to be successful in persons who have CD4 counts above 100 cells/mcL and nondetectable viral loads.

C. BILIARY DISEASE—Cholecystitis presents with manifestations similar to those seen in immunocompetent hosts but is more likely to be acalculous. Sclerosing cholangitis and papillary stenosis have also been reported in HIV-infected patients. Typically, the syndrome presents with severe nausea, vomiting, and right upper quadrant pain. Liver function tests generally show alkaline phosphatase elevations disproportionate to elevation of the aminotransferases. Although dilated ducts can be seen on ultrasound, the diagnosis is made by endoscopic retrograde cholangiopancreatography, which reveals intraluminal irregularities of the proximal intrahepatic ducts with "pruning" of the terminal ductal branches. Stenosis of the distal common bile duct at the papilla is commonly seen with this syndrome. CMV, *Cryptosporidium*, and microsporidia are thought to play inciting roles in this syndrome.

D. ENTEROCOLITIS—Enterocolitis is a common problem in HIV-infected individuals. Organisms known to cause enterocolitis include bacteria (*Campylobacter, Salmonella, Shigella*), viruses (CMV, adenovirus), and protozoans (*Cryptosporidium, Entamoeba histolytica, Giardia, Isospora*, microsporidia). HIV itself may cause enterocolitis. Several of the organisms causing enterocolitis in HIV-infected individuals also cause diarrhea in immunocompetent persons. However, HIV-infected patients tend to have more severe and more chronic symptoms, including high fevers and severe abdominal pain that can mimic acute abdominal catastrophes. Bacteremia and concomitant biliary involvement are also more common with enterocolitis in HIV-infected patients. Relapses of enterocolitis following adequate therapy have been reported with both *Salmonella* and *Shigella* infections.

Because of the wide range of agents known to cause enterocolitis, a stool culture and multiple stool examinations for ova and parasites (including modified acid-fast staining for *Cryptosporidium*) should be performed. Those patients who have *Cryptosporidium* in one stool with improvement in symptoms in less than 1 month should not be considered to have AIDS, as *Cryptosporidium* is a cause of self-limited diarrhea in HIV-negative persons. More commonly, HIV-infected patients with *Cryptospo-ridium* infection have persistent enterocolitis with profuse watery diarrhea.

To date, no consistently effective treatments have been developed for *Cryptosporidium* infection. The most effective treatment of cryptosporidiosis is to improve immune function through the use of effective antiretroviral treatment. The diarrhea can be treated symptomatically with diphenoxylate with atropine (one or two tablets orally three or four times a day). Those who do not respond may be given paregoric with bismuth (5–10 mL orally three or four times a day). Octreotide in escalating doses (starting at 0.05 mg subcutaneously every 8 hours for 48 hours) has been found to ameliorate symptoms in approximately 40% of patients with cryptosporidia or idiopathic HIV-associated diarrhea.

Patients with a negative stool examination and persistent symptoms should be evaluated with colonoscopy and biopsy. Patients whose symptoms last longer than 1 month with no identified cause of diarrhea are considered to have a presumptive diagnosis of AIDS enteropathy. Patients may respond to institution of effective antiretroviral treatment. Upper endoscopy with small bowel biopsy is not recommended as a routine part of the evaluation.

E. OTHER DISORDERS—Two other important gastrointestinal abnormalities in HIV-infected patients are gastropathy and malabsorption. It has been documented that some HIV-infected patients do not produce normal levels of stomach acid and therefore are unable to absorb drugs that require an acid medium. This decreased acid production may explain, in part, the susceptibility of HIV-infected patients to *Campylobacter, Salmonella*, and *Shigella*, all of which are sensitive to acid concentration. There is no evidence that *Helicobacter pylori* is more common in HIV-infected persons.

A malabsorption syndrome occurs commonly in HIV-infected patients. It can be due to infection of the small bowel with *M avium* complex, *Cryptosporidium*, or microsporidia.

10. Endocrinologic manifestations—Hypogonadism is probably the most common endocrinologic abnormality in HIV-infected men. The adrenal gland is also a commonly afflicted endocrine gland in patients with AIDS. Abnormalities demonstrated on autopsy include infection (especially with CMV and *M avium* complex), infiltration with Kaposi sarcoma, and injury from hemorrhage and presumed autoimmunity. The prevalence of clinically significant adrenal insufficiency is low. Patients with suggestive symptoms should undergo a cosyntropin stimulation test.

Although frank deficiency of cortisol is rare, an isolated defect in mineralocorticoid metabolism may lead to salt-wasting and hyperkalemia. Such patients should be treated with fludrocortisone (0.1–0.2 mg daily).

AIDS patients appear to have abnormalities of thyroid function tests different from those of patients with other chronic diseases. AIDS patients have been shown to have high levels of triiodothyronine (T_3), thyroxine (T_4), and thyroid-binding globulin and low levels of reverse triiodothyronine (rT_3). The causes and clinical significance of these abnormalities are unknown.

11. Skin manifestations—The skin manifestations that commonly develop in HIV-infected patients can be grouped into viral, bacterial, fungal, neoplastic, and nonspecific dermatitides.

Herpes simplex infections occur more frequently, tend to be more severe, and are more likely to disseminate in AIDS patients than in immunocompetent persons. Because of the risk of progressive local disease, all herpes simplex attacks should be treated with acyclovir (400 mg orally three times a day until healed, usually 7 days), famciclovir (500 mg orally twice daily until healed), or valacyclovir (500 mg orally twice daily until healed). To avoid the complications of attacks, many clinicians recommend suppressive therapy for HIV-infected patients with a history of recurrent herpes. Options for suppressive therapy include acyclovir (400 mg orally twice daily), famciclovir (250 mg orally twice daily), and valacyclovir (500 mg orally daily). A randomized trial of women infected with both herpes simplex and HIV showed that suppressive therapy with valacyclovir at a dose of 500 mg orally twice daily decreased genital and plasma HIV-1 RNA levels, suggesting the possibility that suppressive treatment may reduce HIV transmission.

Herpes zoster is a common manifestation of HIV infection. As with herpes simplex infections, patients with zoster should be treated with acyclovir to prevent dissemination (800 mg orally four or five times per day for 7 days). Alternatively, famciclovir (500 mg orally three times a day) or valacyclovir (500 mg three times a day) may be used. Vesicular lesions should be cultured if there is any question about their origin, since herpes simplex responds to much lower doses of acyclovir. Disseminated zoster and cases with ocular involvement should be treated with intravenous (10 mg/kg every 8 hours for 7–10 days) rather than oral acyclovir.

Molluscum contagiosum caused by a pox virus is seen in HIV-infected patients, as in other immunocompromised patients. The characteristic umbilicated fleshy papular lesions have a propensity for spreading widely over the patient's face and neck and should be treated with topical liquid nitrogen.

Staphylococcus is the most common bacterial cause of skin disease in HIV-infected patients; it usually presents as **folliculitis, superficial abscesses (furuncles)**, or **bullous impetigo**. Because dissemination with sepsis has been reported, attempts should be made to treat these lesions aggressively. Folliculitis is initially treated with topical clindamycin or mupirocin, and patients may benefit from regular washing with an antibacterial soap such as chlorhexidine. Intranasal mupirocin has been used successfully for staphylococcal decolonization in other settings. In HIV-infected patients with recurrent staphylococcal infections, weekly intranasal mupirocin should be considered in addition to topical care and systemic antibiotics. Abscesses often require incision and drainage. Patients may need antistaphylococcal antibiotics as well. Due to high frequency of methicillin-resistant *Staphylococcus aureus* (MRSA) skin infections in HIV-infected populations, lesions should be cultured prior to initiating empiric antistaphylococcal therapy. Although there is limited experience treating MRSA with oral antibiotics, current recommendations for empiric

treatment are trimethoprim-sulfamethoxazole (one double-strength tablet orally twice daily) or doxycycline (100 mg orally twice daily) with close follow-up.

Bacillary angiomatosis is a well-described entity in HIV-infected patients. It is caused by two closely related organisms: *Bartonella henselae* and *Bartonella quintana*. The epidemiology of these infections suggests zoonotic transmission from fleas of infected domestic cats. The most common manifestation is raised, reddish, highly vascular skin lesions that can mimic the lesions of Kaposi sarcoma. Fever is a common manifestation of this infection; involvement of bone, lymph nodes, and liver has also been reported. The infection responds to doxycycline, 100 mg orally twice daily, or erythromycin, 250 mg orally four times daily. Therapy is continued for at least 14 days, and patients who are seriously ill with visceral involvement may require months of therapy.

The majority of **fungal rashes** afflicting AIDS patients are due to dermatophytes and *Candida*. These are particularly common in the inguinal region but may occur anywhere on the body. Fungal rashes generally respond well to topical clotrimazole (1% twice a day) or ketoconazole (2% twice a day).

Seborrheic dermatitis is more common in HIV-infected patients. Scrapings of seborrhea have revealed *Malassezia furfur (Pityrosporum ovale)*, implying that the seborrhea is caused by this fungus. Consistent with the isolation of this fungus is the clinical finding that seborrhea responds well to topical clotrimazole (1% cream) as well as hydrocortisone (1% cream).

Xerosis presents in HIV-infected patients with severe pruritus. The patient may have no rash, or nonspecific excoriations from scratching. Treatment is with emollients (eg, absorption base cream) and antipruritic lotions (eg, camphor 9.5% and menthol 0.5%).

Psoriasis can be very severe in HIV-infected patients. Phototherapy and etretinate (0.25–9.75 mg/kg/d orally in divided doses) may be used for recalcitrant cases in consultation with a dermatologist. Because of the underlying immunodeficiency, methotrexate should be avoided.

12. HIV-related malignancies—Four cancers are currently included in the CDC classification of AIDS: Kaposi sarcoma, non-Hodgkin lymphoma, primary lymphoma of the brain, and invasive cervical carcinoma. Epidemiologic studies have shown that between 1973 and 1987 among single men in San Francisco, the risk of Kaposi sarcoma increased more than 5000-fold and the risk of non-Hodgkin lymphoma more than tenfold. The increase in incidence of malignancies is probably a function of impaired cell-mediated immunity.

Kaposi sarcoma lesions may appear anywhere; careful examination of the eyelids, conjunctiva, pinnae, palate, and toe webs is mandatory to locate potentially occult lesions. In light-skinned individuals, Kaposi lesions usually appear as purplish, nonblanching lesions that can be papular or nodular (Plate 41). In dark-skinned individuals, the lesions may appear more brown. In the mouth, lesions are most often palatal papules, though exophytic lesions of the tongue and gingivae may also be seen. Kaposi lesions may be confused with other vascular lesions such as angiomas and pyogenic granulomas. Visceral disease (eg, gastrointestinal, pulmonary) will develop in about 40% of patients with dermatologic Kaposi sarcoma. Rapidly progressive dermatologic or visceral disease is best treated with systemic chemotherapy. Liposomally encapsulated doxorubicin given intravenously every 3 weeks has a response rate of approximately 70%. α-Interferon (10 million units subcutaneously three times a week) also has activity against Kaposi sarcoma. However, symptoms such as malaise and anorexia limit the utility of this therapy. Patients with milder forms of Kaposi sarcoma do not require specific treatment as the lesions usually improve and can completely resolve with antiretroviral therapy. However, it should be noted that the lesions may flare when antiretroviral therapy is first initiated—probably as a result of an immune reconstitution process (see Inflammatory reactions below).

Non-Hodgkin lymphoma in HIV-infected persons tends to be very aggressive. The malignancies are usually of B cell origin and characterized as diffuse large-cell tumors. Over 70% of the malignancies are extranodal.

The prognosis of patients with systemic non-Hodgkin lymphoma depends primarily on the degree of immunodeficiency at the time of diagnosis. Patients with high CD4 counts do markedly better than those diagnosed at a late stage of illness. Patients with primary central nervous system lymphoma are treated with radiation. Response to treatment is good, but prior to the availability of HAART, most patients died within a few months after diagnosis due to their underlying disease. Systemic disease is treated with chemotherapy. Common regimens are CHOP (cyclophosphamide, doxorubicin, vincristine, and prednisone) and modified M-BACOD (methotrexate, bleomycin, doxorubicin, cyclophosphamide, vincristine, and dexamethasone). Granulocyte colony-stimulating factor (G-CSF; filgrastim) is used to maintain white blood counts with this latter regimen. Intrathecal chemotherapy is administered to prevent or treat meningeal involvement.

Although **Hodgkin disease** is not included as part of the CDC definition of AIDS, studies have found that HIV infection is associated with a fivefold increase in the incidence of Hodgkin disease. HIV-infected persons with Hodgkin disease are more likely to have mixed cellularity and lymphocyte depletion subtypes of Hodgkin disease and to seek medical attention at an advanced stage of disease.

Anal dysplasia and squamous cell carcinoma have been noted in HIV-infected men and women. These lesions have been strongly correlated with previous infection by human papillomavirus (HPV). Although many of the infected MSM report a history of anal warts or have visible warts, a significant percentage have silent papillomavirus infection. Cytologic (using Papanicolaou smears) and papillomavirus DNA studies can easily be performed on specimens obtained by anal swab. Because of the risk of progression from dysplasia to cancer in immunocompromised patients, some experts suggest that annual anal swabs for cytologic examination should be done in all HIV-infected persons. An anal Papanicolaou smear is performed by rotating a moistened Dacron swab about 2 cm into the anal canal. The swab is immediately inserted into a cytology bottle.

HPV also appears to play a causative role in **cervical dysplasia and neoplasia**. The incidence and clinical course of cervical disease in HIV-infected women are discussed below.

13. Gynecologic manifestations—Vaginal candidiasis, cervical dysplasia and neoplasia, and pelvic inflammatory disease are more common in HIV-infected women than in uninfected women. These manifestations also tend to be more severe when they occur in association with HIV infection. Therefore, HIV-infected women need frequent gynecologic care. Vaginal candidiasis may be treated with topical agents (see Chapter 36). However, HIV-infected women with recurrent or severe vaginal candidiasis may need systemic therapy.

The incidence of cervical dysplasia in HIV-infected women is 40%. Because of this finding, HIV-infected women should have Papanicolaou smears every 6 months (as opposed to the Agency for Healthcare Research and Quality [AHRQ] Guideline recommendation for every 12 months). Some clinicians recommend routine colposcopy or cervicography because cervical intraepithelial neoplasia has occurred in women with negative Papanicolaou smears. Cone biopsy is indicated in cases of serious cervical dysplasia. For 1 year following treatment of an abnormal Papanicolaou smear, women should have repeat smears every 3 to 4 months.

Cervical neoplasia appears to be more aggressive among HIV-infected women. Most HIV-infected women with cervical cancer die of that disease rather than of AIDS. Because of its frequency and severity, cervical neoplasia was added to the CDC definition of AIDS in 1993.

While pelvic inflammatory disease appears to be more common in HIV-infected women, the bacteriology of this condition appears to be the same as among HIV-uninfected women. At present, HIV-infected women with pelvic inflammatory disease should be treated with the same regimens as uninfected women (see Chapter 18). However, inpatient therapy is generally recommended.

14. Coronary artery disease—HIV-infected persons are at higher risk for coronary artery disease than age- and sex-matched controls. Part of this increase in coronary artery disease is due to changes in lipids caused by antiretroviral agents (see Treatment section on Antiretroviral Therapy below), especially stavudine and most of the protease inhibitors. However, some of the risk appears to be due to HIV infection, independent of its therapy. It is important that clinicians pay close attention to this issue because the first presentation of coronary artery disease in HIV-infected persons may be sudden death. HIV-infected patients with symptoms of coronary artery disease such as chest pain or dyspnea should be rapidly evaluated. Clinicians should aggressively treat conditions that result in increased risk of heart disease, especially smoking, hypertension, hyperlipidemia, obesity, diabetes mellitus, and sedentary lifestyle.

15. Inflammatory reactions (immune reconstitution syndromes)—With initiation of HAART, some patients experience inflammatory reactions that appear to be associated with immune reconstitution as indicated by a rapid increase in CD4 count. These inflammatory reactions may present with generalized signs of fevers, sweats, and malaise with or without more localized manifestations that usually represent unusual presentations of opportunistic infections. For example, vitreitis has developed in patients with CMV retinitis after they have been treated with HAART. *M avium* can present as focal lymphadenitis or granulomatous masses in patients receiving HAART. Tuberculosis may paradoxically worsen with new or evolving pulmonary infiltrates and lymphadenopathy. PML and cryptococcal meningitis may also behave atypically. Clinicians should be alert to these syndromes, which are most often seen in patients who have initiated antiretroviral therapy in the setting of advanced disease and who show rapid increases in CD4 counts with treatment. The diagnosis of IRIS is one of exclusion and can be made only after recurrence or new opportunistic infection has been ruled out as the cause of the clinical deterioration. Management of IRIS is conservative and supportive with use of corticosteroids only for severe reactions. Most authorities recommend that antiretroviral therapy be continued unless the reaction is life-threatening.

B. Laboratory Findings

Specific tests for HIV include antibody and antigen detection (Table 31–2). Conventional HIV antibody testing is done by ELISA. Positive specimens are then confirmed by a different method (eg, Western blot). The sensitivity of screening serologic tests is greater than 99.5%. The specificity of positive results by two different techniques approaches 100% even in low-risk populations. False-positive screening tests may occur as normal biologic variants or in association with recent influenza vaccination or other disease states, such as connective tissue disease. These are usually detected by negative confirmatory tests. Molecular biology techniques (PCR) show a small incidence of individuals (< 1%)

who are infected with HIV for up to 36 months without generating an antibody response. However, antibodies that are detectable by screening serologic tests will develop in 95% of persons within 6 weeks after infection.

Rapid HIV antibody tests are now available. They provide results within 10–20 minutes and can be performed in physician offices, including by personnel without laboratory training and without a Clinical Laboratory Improvement Amendment (CLIA) approved laboratory. Persons who test positive on a rapid test should be told that they may be HIV-infected or their test may be falsely reactive. Standard testing (ELISA with Western blot confirmation) should be performed to distinguish these two possibilities. Rapid testing is particularly helpful in settings where a result is needed immediately (eg, a woman in labor who has not recently been tested for HIV) or when the patient is unlikely to return for a result.

Nonspecific laboratory findings with HIV infection may include anemia, leukopenia (particularly lymphopenia), and thrombocytopenia in any combination, elevation of the erythrocyte sedimentation rate, polyclonal hypergammaglobulinemia, and hypocholesterolemia. Cutaneous anergy is common.

Several laboratory markers are available to provide prognostic information and guide therapy decisions (Table 31–2). The most widely used marker is the absolute CD4 lymphocyte count. As counts decrease, the risk of serious opportunistic infection over the subsequent 3–5 years increases (Figure 31–1).

There are many limitations to using the CD4 count, including diurnal variation, depression with intercurrent illness, and intralaboratory and interlaboratory variability. Therefore, the trend is more important than a single determination. The frequency of performance of counts depends on the patient's health status. Patients whose CD4 counts are substantially above the threshold for initiation of antivi-

Table 31–2. Laboratory findings with HIV infection.

Test	Significance
HIV enzyme-linked immunosorbent assay (ELISA)	Screening test for HIV infection. Of ELISA tests 50% are positive within 22 days after HIV transmission; 95% are positive within 6 weeks after transmission. Sensitivity > 99.9%; to avoid false-positive results, repeatedly reactive results must be confirmed with Western blot.
Western blot	Confirmatory test for HIV. Specificity when combined with ELISA > 99.99%. Indeterminate results with early HIV infection, HIV-2 infection, autoimmune disease, pregnancy, and recent tetanus toxoid administration.
HIV rapid antibody test	Screening test for HIV. Produces results in 10-20 minutes. Can be performed by personnel with limited training. Positive results must be confirmed with standard HIV test (ELISA and Western blot).
Complete blood count	Anemia, neutropenia, and thrombocytopenia common with advanced HIV infection.
Absolute CD4 lymphocyte count	Most widely used predictor of HIV progression. Risk of progression to an AIDS opportunistic infection or malignancy is high with CD4 < 200 cells/mcL in the absence of treatment.
CD4 lymphocyte percentage	Percentage may be more reliable than the CD4 count. Risk of progression to an AIDS opportunistic infection or malignancy is high with percentage < 14% in the absence of treatment.
HIV viral load tests	These tests measure the amount of actively replicating HIV virus. Correlate with disease progression and response to antiretroviral drugs. Best tests available for diagnosis of acute HIV infection (prior to seroconversion); however, caution is warranted when the test result shows low-level viremia (ie, < 500 copies/mL) as this may represent a false-positive test.

ral therapy (350 cells/mcL) should have counts performed every 6 months. Those who have counts near or below 350 cells/mcL should have counts performed every 3 months. This is necessary for evaluating the efficacy of antiviral therapy and for initiating *P jiroveci* prophylactic therapy when the CD4 count drops below 200 cells/mcL. Some studies suggest that the percentage of CD4 lymphocytes is a more reliable indicator of prognosis than the absolute counts because the percentage does not depend on calculating a manual differential. While the CD4 count measures immune dysfunction, it does not provide a measure of how actively HIV is replicating in the body. HIV viral load tests (discussed below) assess the level of viral replication and provide useful prognostic information that is independent of the information provided by CD4 counts.

Dominguez S et al. Efficacy of early treatment of acute hepatitis C infection with pegylated interferon and ribavirin in HIV-infected patients. AIDS. 2006 May 12;20(8):1157–61. [PMID: 16691067]

Fitch KV et al. Effects of a lifestyle modification program in HIV-infected patients with the metabolic syndrome. AIDS. 2006 Sep 11;20(14):1843–50. [PMID: 16954725]

Grubb JR et al. The changing spectrum of pulmonary disease in patients with HIV infection on antiretroviral therapy. AIDS. 2006 May 12;20(8):1095–107. [PMID: 16691060]

Kohli R et al; HER Study Group. Bacterial pneumonia, HIV therapy, and disease progression among HIV-infected women in the HIV epidemiologic research (HER) study. Clin Infect Dis. 2006 Jul 1;43(1):90–8. [PMID: 16758423]

Koziel MJ et al. Viral hepatitis in HIV infection. N Engl J Med. 2007 Apr 5;356(14):1445–54. [PMID: 17409326]

Lima MA et al. New features of progressive multifocal leukoencephalopathy in the era of highly active antiretroviral therapy and natalizumab. J Neurovirol. 2005;11 (Suppl 3):52–7. [PMID: 16540456]

McArthur JC et al. Neurological complications of HIV infection. Lancet Neurol. 2005 Sep;4(9):543–55. [PMID: 16109361]

Manzardo C et al. Central nervous system opportunistic infections in developed countries in the highly active antiretroviral therapy era. J Neurovirol. 2005;11 (Suppl 3):72–82. [PMID: 16540459]

Maurer TA. Dermatologic manifestations of HIV infection. Top HIV Med. 2005 Dec–2006 Jan;13(5):149–54. [PMID: 16377853]

Nagot N et al. Reduction of HIV-1 RNA levels with therapy to suppress herpes simplex virus. N Engl J Med. 2007 Feb 22;356(8):790–9. [PMID: 17314338]

Nath A et al. Influence of highly active antiretroviral therapy on persistence of HIV in the central nervous system. Curr Opin Neurol. 2006 Aug;19(4):358–61. [PMID: 16914973]

Roberts MT. AIDS-associated progressive multifocal leukoencephalopathy: current management strategies. CNS Drugs. 2005;19(8):671–82. [PMID: 16097849]

Skiest DJ et al. Cryptococcal immune reconstitution inflammatory syndrome: report of four cases in three patients and review of the literature. J Infect. 2005 Dec;51(5):e289–97. [PMID: 16321643]

Stevens DL et al. Practice guidelines for the diagnosis and management of skin and soft-tissue infections. Clin Infect Dis. 2005 Nov 15;41(10):1373–406. [PMID: 16231249]

Sullivan PS et al. Effect of hepatitis C infection on progression of HIV disease and early response to initial antiretroviral therapy. AIDS. 2006 May 12;20(8):1171–9. [PMID: 16691069]

Thorne JE et al. Effect of cytomegalovirus retinitis on the risk of visual acuity loss among patients with AIDS. Ophthalmology. 2007 Mar;114(3):591–8. [PMID: 17123624]

Weis N et al. Impact of hepatitis C virus coinfection on response to highly active antiretroviral therapy and outcome in HIV-infected individuals: a nationwide cohort study. Clin Infect Dis. 2006 May 15;42(10):1481–7. [PMID: 16619163]

▶ Differential Diagnosis

HIV infection may mimic a variety of other medical illnesses. Specific differential diagnosis depends on the mode of presentation. In patients presenting with constitutional symptoms such as weight loss and fevers, differential considerations include cancer, chronic infections such as tuberculosis and endocarditis, and endocrinologic diseases such as hyperthyroidism. When pulmonary processes dominate the presentation, acute and chronic lung infections must be considered as well as other causes of diffuse interstitial pulmonary infiltrates. When neurologic disease is the mode of presentation, conditions that cause mental status changes or neuropathy—eg, alcoholism, liver disease, kidney dysfunction, thyroid disease, and vitamin deficiency—should be considered. If a patient presents with headache and a cerebrospinal fluid pleocytosis, other causes of chronic meningitis enter the differential. When diarrhea is a prominent complaint, infectious enterocolitis, antibiotic-associated colitis, inflammatory bowel disease, and malabsorptive symptoms must be considered.

▶ Prevention

A. Primary Prevention

Until vaccination is a reality, prevention of HIV infection will depend on effective precautions regarding sexual practices and injection drug use, use of perinatal HIV prophylaxis, screening of blood products, and infection control practices in the health care setting. Primary care clinicians should routinely obtain a sexual history and provide risk factor assessment of their patients. Because approximately one-fourth of the HIV-infected persons in the United States do not know they are infected, the CDC recommends all adults be routinely tested for HIV. Prior to testing, clinicians should obtain informed consent and review the risk factors for HIV infection with the patient and discuss safer sex and safer needle use as well as the meaning of a positive test. For persons whose test results are positive, information on available medical and mental health services should be provided as well as guidance for contacting sexual or needle-sharing partners. Interventions focused on the importance of HIV-infected persons not putting others at risk have been successful. For patients whose test results are negative, clinicians should review safer sex and needle use practices, including counseling not to exchange bodily fluids unless they are in a long-term mutually monogamous relationship with someone who has tested HIV antibody-negative and has not engaged in unsafe sex, injection drug use, or other HIV risk behaviors for at least 6 months prior to or at any time since the negative test.

Only latex condoms should be used, along with a water-soluble lubricant. Although nonoxynol-9, a spermicide, kills HIV, it is contraindicated because in some patients it may cause genital ulcers that could facilitate HIV transmission. Patients should be counseled that condoms are not 100% effective. They should be made familiar with the use of condoms, including, specifically, the advice that condoms must be used every time, that space should be left at the tip of the condom as a receptacle for semen, that intercourse with a condom should not be attempted if the penis is only partially erect, that men should hold on to the base of the condom when withdrawing the penis to prevent slippage, and that condoms should not be reused. Although anal intercourse remains the sexual practice at highest risk for transmitting HIV, seroconversions have been documented with vaginal and oral intercourse as well. Therefore, condoms should be used when engaging in these activities. Women as well as men should understand how to use condoms so as to be sure that their partners are using them correctly. A randomized trial in Africa demonstrated that male circumcision significantly reduced HIV incidence in men, but there are a number of barriers to performing widespread circumcisions among men in Africa.

Persons using injection drugs should be cautioned never to exchange needles or other drug paraphernalia. When sterile needles are not available, bleach does appear to inactivate HIV and should be used to clean needles.

Current efforts to screen blood and blood products have lowered the risk of HIV transmission with transfusion of a unit of blood to 1:1,000,000.

In the hospital, concerns about nosocomial infection have led to the recommendation for universal body fluid precautions. This involves the rigorous use of gloves when handling any body fluid and the addition of gown, mask, and goggles for procedures that may result in splash or droplet spread as well as the use of specially designed needles with sheath devices to decrease the risk of needle sticks. Reports of transmission of drug-resistant tuberculosis in health care settings also have had infection control implications. All patients with cough in outpatient settings should be encouraged to wear masks. Hospitalized HIV-infected patients with cough should be placed in respiratory isolation until tuberculosis can be excluded by chest radiograph and sputum smear examination.

Primate model data have suggested that development of a protective vaccine may be possible, but clinical trials in humans using gp120 or its precursor gp160 have shown development of neutralizing antibodies to laboratory but not field isolates of HIV and may not be protective of infection. Many scientists have abandoned the quest for a fully protective HIV vaccine and are focusing on developing a vaccine that would reduce the chances of HIV transmission given a particular exposure.

B. Secondary Prevention

In the era prior to the development of highly effective antiretroviral treatment, cohort studies of individuals with documented dates of seroconversion demonstrate that AIDS develops within 10 years in approximately 50% of untreated seropositive persons. With currently available treatment, progression of disease has been markedly decreased. In addition to antiretroviral treatment, prophy-

lactic regimens can prevent opportunistic infections and improve survival. Prophylaxis and early intervention prevent several infectious diseases, including tuberculosis and syphilis, which are transmissible to others. Recommendations for screening tests, vaccinations, and prophylaxis are listed in Table 31–3.

Because of the increased occurrence of tuberculosis among HIV-infected patients, all such individuals should undergo PPD testing. Although anergy is common among AIDS patients, the likelihood of a false-negative result is much lower when the test is done early in infection. Those with positive tests (defined for HIV-infected patients as > 5 mm of induration) need a chest radiograph. Patients with an infiltrate in any location, especially if accompanied by mediastinal adenopathy, should have sputum sent for acid-fast staining. Patients with a positive PPD but negative evaluations for active disease should receive isoniazid (300 mg daily) with pyridoxine (50 mg daily) for 9 months to a year. An alternative regimen of rifampin plus pyrazinamide for 2 months is no longer recommended because of the high associated incidence of hepatotoxicity. Recent analysis suggests also that HIV-infected individuals at high risk for tuberculosis should receive a course of isoniazid

Table 31–3. Health care maintenance of HIV-infected individuals.

For all HIV-infected individuals:
CD4 counts every 3-6 months
Viral load tests every 3-6 months and 1 month following a change in therapy
PPD
INH for those with positive PPD and normal chest radiograph
RPR or VDRL
Toxoplasma IgG serology
Hepatitis serologies: hepatitis A antibody, hepatitis B surface antigen, hepatitis B surface antibody, hepatitis B core antibody, hepatitis C antibody.
Pneumococcal vaccine
Inactivated influenza vaccine in season
Hepatitis A vaccine for those without immunity to hepatitis A.
Hepatitis B vaccine for those who are hepatitis B surface antigen and antibody negative. (Use 40 mcg formulation at 0, 1, and 6 months; repeat if no immunity 1 month after three-shot series.)
Tetanus/diphtheria vaccine
Human papillomavirus vaccine for HIV-infected women age 26 years or less.
Haemophilus influenzae type b vaccination
Papanicolaou smears every 6 months for women
Consider anal swabs for cytologic evaluation.
For HIV-infected individuals with CD4 < 200 cells/mcL:
Pneumocystis jiroveci prophylaxis (see Prophylaxis of Opportunistic Infections section under Treatment and Table 31–4)
For HIV-infected individuals with CD4 < 75 cells/mcL:
Mycobacterium avium complex prophylaxis (see Prophylaxis of Opportunistic Infections section under Treatment)
For HIV-infected individuals with CD4 < 50 cells/mcL:
Consider CMV prophylaxis

PPD, purified protein derivative; INH, isoniazid; RPR, rapid plasma reagin; VDRL, Venereal Disease Research Laboratories; IgG, immunoglobulin G.

prophylaxis regardless of the PPD status. This may include homeless individuals and injection drug users. Although not yet widely available, a blood test (QuantiFERON Gold test) can be used to assess prior tuberculosis exposure. Blood samples are mixed with synthetic antigens representing *M tuberculosis*. Patients infected with *M tuberculosis* produce interferon-gamma in response to contact with the antigens. Unlike the PPD, the patient does not have to return for a second visit. The test is less likely to result in false-positive results than a PPD. Unfortunately, HIV-infected persons may not produce sufficient interferon-gamma, in which case the test may be falsely negative.

Because of recent increases in the number of cases of syphilis among MSM, including those who are HIV infected, all such men should be screened for syphilis by rapid plasma reagin (RPR) or Venereal Disease Research Laboratories (VDRL) test every 6 months. Increases of syphilis cases among HIV-infected persons are of particular concern because these individuals are at increased risk for reactivation of syphilis and progression to tertiary syphilis despite standard treatment. Because the only widely available tests for syphilis are serologic and because HIV-infected individuals are known to have disordered antibody production, there is concern about the interpretation of these titers. This concern has been fueled by a report of an HIV-infected patient with secondary syphilis and negative syphilis serologic testing. Furthermore, HIV-infected individuals may lose fluorescent treponemal antibody absorption (FTA-ABS) reactivity after treatment for syphilis, particularly if they have low CD4 counts. Thus, in this population, a nonreactive treponemal test does not rule out a past history of syphilis. In addition, persistence of treponemes in the spinal fluid after one dose of benzathine penicillin has been demonstrated in HIV-infected patients with primary and secondary syphilis. Therefore, the CDC has recommended an aggressive diagnostic approach to HIV-infected patients with reactive RPR or VDRL tests of greater than 1 year or unknown duration. All such patients should have a lumbar puncture with cerebrospinal fluid cell count and cerebrospinal fluid VDRL. Those with a normal cerebrospinal fluid evaluation are treated as having late latent syphilis (benzathine penicillin G, 2.4 million units intramuscularly weekly for 3 weeks) with follow-up titers. Those with a pleocytosis or a positive cerebrospinal fluid-VDRL test are treated as having neurosyphilis (aqueous penicillin G, 2–4 million units intravenously every 4 hours, or procaine penicillin G, 2.4 million units intramuscularly daily, with probenecid, 500 mg four times daily, for 10 days). Some clinicians take a less aggressive approach to patients who have low titers (less than 1:8), a history of having been treated for syphilis, and a normal neurologic examination. Close follow-up of titers is mandatory if such a course is taken. For a more detailed discussion of this topic, see Chapter 34.

HIV-infected individuals should receive the pneumococcal vaccine and the inactivated influenza vaccine. Patients without immunity to hepatitis A should be vaccinated against it. Patients without evidence of hepatitis B surface antigen or surface antibody should receive hepatitis B vaccination, using the 40 mcg formulation; the higher dose is to increase the chance of developing protective immunity. If the patient does not have immunity 1 month after the three-shot series, then the series should be repeated. HIV-infected persons should also receive the standard inactivated vaccines such as tetanus and diphtheria boosters that would be given to uninfected persons. Live vaccines, such as yellow fever vaccine, should be avoided. Measles vaccination, while a live virus vaccine, appears relatively safe when administered to HIV-infected individuals and should be given if the patient has never had measles or been adequately vaccinated. Herpes zoster vaccine is contraindicated in HIV-infected persons with evidence of immune suppression.

A randomized study found that multivitamin supplementation decreased HIV disease progression and mortality in HIV-infected women in Africa. However, supplementation is unlikely to be as effective in well-nourished populations.

HIV-infected individuals should be counseled with regard to safe sex. Because of the risk of transmission, they should be warned to use condoms with sexual intercourse, including oral intercourse. Partners of HIV-infected women should use latex barriers such as dental dams (available at dental supply stores) to prevent direct oral contact with vaginal secretions. Substance abuse treatment should be recommended for persons who are using recreational drugs. They should be warned to avoid consuming raw meat or eggs to avoid infections with *Toxoplasma*, *Campylobacter*, and *Salmonella*. HIV-infected patients should wash their hands thoroughly after cleaning cat litter or should forgo this household chore to avoid possible exposure to toxoplasmosis. To reduce the likelihood of infection with *Bartonella* species, patients should avoid activities that might result in cat scratches or bites. Although the data are not conclusive, many clinicians recommend that HIV-infected persons—especially those with low CD4 counts—drink bottled water instead of tap water to prevent cryptosporidia infection.

Because of the emotional impact of HIV infection and subsequent illness, many patients will benefit from supportive counseling.

C. HIV Risk for Health Care Professionals

Epidemiologic studies show that needle sticks occur commonly among health care professionals, especially among surgeons performing invasive procedures, inexperienced hospital house staff, and medical students. Efforts to reduce needle sticks should focus on avoiding recapping needles and use of safety needles whenever doing invasive procedures under controlled circumstances. The risk of HIV transmission from a needle stick with blood from an HIV-infected patient is about 1:300. The risk is higher with deep punctures, large inocula, and source patients with high viral loads. The risk from mucous membrane contact is too low to quantitate.

Health care professionals who sustain needle sticks should be counseled and offered HIV testing as soon as possible. HIV testing is done to establish a negative baseline for worker's compensation claims in case there is a subsequent conversion. Follow-up testing is usually performed at 6 weeks, 3 months, and 6 months.

A case-control study by the CDC indicates that administration of zidovudine following a needle stick decreases the rate of HIV seroconversion by 79%. Therefore, providers should be offered therapy with Combivir (zidovudine 300 mg plus lamivudine 150 mg orally twice daily). Providers who have exposures to persons who are likely to have antiretroviral drug resistance (eg, persons receiving therapy who have detectable viral loads) should have their therapy individualized, using at least two drugs to which the source is unlikely to be resistant. Some clinicians recommend triple combination regimens, including a protease inhibitor for all occupational exposures, because of uncertainty about drug resistance. Others save these more aggressive regimens for the higher-risk exposures listed above. Because reports have noted hepatotoxicity due to nevirapine in this setting, this agent should be avoided. Therapy should be started as soon as possible after exposure and continued for 4 weeks. Unfortunately, there have been documented cases of seroconversion following potential parenteral exposure to HIV despite prompt use of zidovudine prophylaxis. Counseling of the provider should include "safer sex" guidelines.

D. Postexposure Prophylaxis for Sexual and Drug Use Exposures to HIV

Following publication of a case-control study indicating that antiretroviral therapy decreased the odds of seroconversion among health care workers who had occupational exposure, some experts have recommended offering antiretroviral therapy following potential exposure to HIV through sexual activity or drug use. Although there are no efficacy data to support this practice, there are similarities between the immune response following transcutaneous and transmucosal exposures. The goal of postexposure prophylaxis is to reduce or prevent local viral replication prior to dissemination such that the infection can be aborted.

The choice of antiretroviral agents and the duration of treatment are the same as those for exposures that occur through the occupational route (see above). In contrast to those with occupational exposures, some individuals may present very late after exposure. Because the likelihood of success declines with length of time from HIV exposure, it is not recommended that treatment be offered after 72 hours. In addition, because the psychosocial issues involved with postexposure prophylaxis for sexual and drug use exposures are complex, it should be offered only in the context of prevention counseling. Counseling should focus on how to prevent future exposures. Clinicians needing more information on postexposure prophylaxis for occupational or nonoccupational exposures should contact the National Clinician's Post-exposure Hotline (1-888-448-4911; www.ucsf.edu/hivcntr/PEPline/).

E. Preventing Perinatal Transmission of HIV

A multicenter trial showed that when zidovudine is administered to women during pregnancy, labor, and delivery and to their newborns, the rate of HIV transmission is decreased by two-thirds. An observational trial demonstrated that zidovudine treatment is almost as effective when begun during labor or when administered only to the infant, as long as treatment is begun within 48 hours after birth. Nonetheless, treatment begun by at least the second trimester is still recommended. Many women are currently being offered combination antiretroviral treatment to further lower the risk of transmission. The availability of treatment makes it essential that all women who are pregnant or considering pregnancy be offered HIV counseling and testing. Many obstetricians recommend combination antiretroviral treatment, especially if zidovudine resistance is suspected. HIV-infected women receiving antiretroviral therapy in whom pregnancy is recognized during the first trimester should be counseled about the benefits and potential risks to the fetus of treatment during the first trimester. Because healthy mothers make healthy babies, continuation of therapy should be strongly considered. Because about half of fetal infections in non–breast-feeding women occur shortly before or during the birth process, antiretroviral therapy should be administered whenever a woman initiates perinatal care even if she did not begin therapy in the second trimester. Breast-feeding is thought to increase the rate of transmission by 10–20% and should be avoided.

Branson BM et al; Centers for Disease Control and Prevention (CDC). Revised recommendations for HIV testing of adults, adolescents, and pregnant women in health-care settings. MMWR Recomm Rep. 2006 Sep 22;55(RR-14):1–17. [PMID: 16988643]

Chiao EY et al. Screening HIV-infected individuals for anal cancer precursor lesions: a systematic review. Clin Infect Dis. 2006 Jul 15;43(2):223–33. [PMID: 16779751]

Gray RH et al. Male circumcision for HIV prevention in men in Rakai, Uganda: a randomized trial. Lancet 2007 Feb 24; 369(9562):657–66. [PMID: 17321311]

Johnson BT et al. Sexual risk reduction for persons living with HIV: research synthesis of randomized controlled trials, 1993 to 2004. J Acquir Immune Defic Syndr. 2006 Apr 15;41(5):642–50. [PMID: 16652039]

Roland ME et al. Seroconversion following nonoccupational postexposure prophylaxis against HIV. Clin Infect Dis. 2005 Nov 15;41(10):1507–13. [PMID: 16231265]

Smith DK. Antiretroviral postexposure prophylaxis after sexual, injection-drug use, or other nonoccupational exposure to HIV in the United States: recommendations from the U.S. Department of Health and Human Services. MMWR Recomm Rep. 2005 Jan 21;54(RR-2):1–20. [PMID: 15660015]

▶ Treatment

Treatment for HIV infection can be broadly divided into the following categories: (1) prophylaxis for opportunistic infections, malignancies, and other complications of HIV infection; (2) treatment of opportunistic infections, malignancies, and other complications of HIV infection; and (3) treatment of the HIV infection itself with combination ART.

Treatment regimens for HIV infection are constantly changing. Clinicians may obtain up-to-date information on new and experimental treatments by calling the AIDS Clinical Trials Information Service (ACTIS), 800-TRIALS-A (English and Spanish), and the National AIDS Hot Line, 800-342-AIDS (English), 800-344-SIDA (Spanish), and 800-AIDS-TTY (hearing-impaired).

A. Prophylactic Treatment of Complications of HIV Infection

In general, decisions about prophylaxis of opportunistic infections are based on the CD4 count, other evidence of severe immunosuppression (eg, oral candidiasis), and a history of having had the infection in the past. In the era prior to HAART, patients who started taking prophylactic regimens were maintained on them indefinitely. However, studies have shown that in patients with robust improvements in immune function—as measured by increases in CD4 counts above the levels that are used to initiate treatment—prophylactic regimens can safely be discontinued.

Because individuals with advanced HIV infection are susceptible to a number of opportunistic pathogens, the use of agents with activity against more than one pathogen is preferable. It has been shown, for example, that trimethoprim-sulfamethoxazole confers some protection against toxoplasmosis in individuals receiving this drug for *Pneumocystis* prophylaxis.

1. Prophylaxis against *Pneumocystis* pneumonia— Patients with CD4 counts below 200 cells/mcL, a CD4 lymphocyte percentage below 14%, or weight loss or oral candidiasis should be offered primary prophylaxis for *Pneumocystis* pneumonia. Patients with a history of *Pneumocystis* pneumonia should receive secondary prophylaxis until they have had a durable virologic response to HAART for at least 3–6 months and maintain a CD4 count of > 250 cells/mcL. Regimens for *Pneumocystis* prophylaxis are given in Table 31–4.

2. Prophylaxis against *M avium* complex infection— Patients whose CD4 counts fall to below 75–100 cells/mcL should be given prophylaxis against *M avium* complex infection. Clarithromycin (500 mg orally twice daily) and azithromycin (1200 mg orally weekly) have both been shown to decrease the incidence of disseminated *M avium* complex infection by approximately 75%, with a low rate of breakthrough of resistant disease. The azithromycin regimen is generally preferred based on high compliance and low cost. Adding rifabutin increases the toxicity of the regimen but does not significantly increase its efficacy and is therefore not recommended. Prophylaxis against *M avium* complex infection may be discontinued in patients whose CD4 counts rise above 100 cells/mcL in response to HAART and whose plasma viral load has been optimally suppressed to < 50–75 copies/mL.

3. Prophylaxis against *M tuberculosis* infection— Isoniazid, 300 mg daily, plus pyridoxine, 50 mg orally daily, for 9-12 months should be given to all HIV-infected patients with positive PPD reactions (defined as > 5 mm of induration for HIV-infected patients).

4. Prophylaxis against toxoplasmosis— Toxoplasmosis prophylaxis is desirable in patients with a positive IgG toxoplasma serology and CD4 counts below 100 cells/mcL. Trimethoprim-sulfamethoxazole (one double-strength tablet daily) offers good protection against toxoplasmosis, as does a combination of pyrimethamine, 25 mg orally once a week, plus dapsone, 50 mg orally daily, plus leucovorin, 25 mg orally once a week. A glucose-6-phosphate dehydrogenase (G6PD) level should be checked prior to dapsone therapy, and a methemoglobin level should be checked at 1 month.

5. Prophylaxis against CMV infection— Oral ganciclovir (1000 mg orally three times daily with food) is approved for CMV prophylaxis among HIV-infected persons with advanced disease (eg, CD4 counts below 50 cells/mcL). However, because the drug causes neutropenia, it is not widely used. Clinicians should consider performing serum CMV IgG antibody testing prior to starting ganciclovir. Persons who are CMV IgG-negative are not at risk for development of CMV disease, although it is important that such patients receive only CMV-negative blood if they require transfusion. Because over 99% of MSM are positive for CMV IgG, it is appropriate to reserve such testing for heterosexuals with HIV.

6. Prophylaxis against cryptococcosis, candidiasis, and endemic fungal diseases— One trial showed a decreased incidence of cryptococcal disease with prophy-

Table 31–4. *Pneumocystis jiroveci* prophylaxis.

Drug	Dose	Side Effects	Limitations
Trimethoprim-sulfamethoxazole	One double-strength tablet three times a week to one tablet daily	Rash, neutropenia, hepatitis, Stevens-Johnson syndrome	Hypersensitivity reaction is common but, if mild, it may be possible to treat through.
Dapsone	50–100 mg daily or 100 mg two or three times per week	Anemia, nausea, methemoglobinemia, hemolytic anemia	Less effective than above. Glucose-6-phosphate dehydrogenase (G6PD) level should be checked prior to therapy. Check methemoglobin level at 1 month.
Atovaquone	1500 mg daily with a meal	Rash, diarrhea, nausea	Less effective than suspension trimethoprim-sulfamethoxazole; equal efficacy to dapsone, but more expensive.
Aerosolized pentamidine	300 mg monthly	Bronchospasm (pretreat with bronchodilators); rare reports of pancreatitis	Apical *Pneumocystis jiroveci* pneumonia, extrapulmonary *P jiroveci* infections, pneumothorax.

laxis using fluconazole, 200 mg orally daily, but the treated group had no benefit in terms of mortality. Fluconazole (200 mg orally once a week) was found to prevent oral and vaginal candidiasis in women with CD4 counts below 300 cells/mcL. In areas of the world where histoplasmosis and coccidioidomycosis are endemic and are frequent complications of HIV infection, prophylactic use of fluconazole or itraconazole may prove to be useful strategies. However, the problem of identifying individuals at highest risk makes appropriate targeting of prophylaxis difficult.

B. Treatment of Complications of HIV Infection

Treatment of common AIDS-related complications is detailed in Table 31–5. In the era prior to the use of HAART, patients required lifelong treatment for many infections, including CMV retinitis, toxoplasmosis, and cryptococcal meningitis. However, among patients who have a good response to HAART, maintenance therapy for some opportunistic infections can be terminated. For example, in consultation with an ophthalmologist, maintenance treatment for CMV infection can be discontinued when persons receiving HAART have durable suppression of viral load (ie, < 50 copies/mL) and a CD4 count > 100–150 cells/mcL. Similar results have been observed in patients with *M avium* complex bacteremia. Prophylaxis for *Pneumocystis* pneumonia is also commonly discontinued in patients who have achieved and maintained a CD4 > 200 cells/mcL with good virologic control.

Treating patients with repeated episodes of the same opportunistic infection can pose difficult therapeutic challenges. For example, patients with second or third episodes of *Pneumocystis* pneumonia may have developed allergic reactions to standard treatments with a prior episode. Fortunately, there are several alternatives available for the treatment of *Pneumocystis* infection. Trimethoprim with dapsone and primaquine with clindamycin are two combinations that often are tolerated in patients with a prior allergic reaction to trimethoprim-sulfamethoxazole and intravenous pentamidine. On the positive side, patients in whom second episodes of *Pneumocystis* pneumonia develop while taking prophylaxis tend to have milder courses.

Well-established alternative regimens now also exist for most AIDS-related opportunistic infections: amphotericin B or fluconazole for cryptococcal meningitis; ganciclovir, cidofovir, or foscarnet for CMV infection; and sulfadiazine or clindamycin with pyrimethamine for toxoplasmosis.

Adjunctive Treatments Although conceptually it would seem that **corticosteroids** should be avoided in HIV-infected patients, corticosteroid therapy has been shown to improve the course of patients with moderate to severe *Pneumocystis jiroveci* pneumonia (oxygen saturation < 90%, Po_2 < 65 mm Hg) when administered within 72 hours after diagnosis. The mechanism of action is presumed to be a decrease in alveolar inflammation.

Corticosteroids have also been used to treat immune reconstitution and inflammatory syndromes (IRIS) that can sometimes complicate the early treatment course when ART is initiated in patients with advanced AIDS (see section Inflammatory reactions [immune reconstitution syndromes]).

Epoetin alfa (erythropoietin) is approved for use in HIV-infected patients with anemia, including those with anemia secondary to zidovudine use. It has been shown to decrease the need for blood transfusions. The drug is expensive, and therefore an erythropoietin level < 500 mU/mL should be demonstrated before starting therapy. The starting dose of epoetin alfa is 8000 units subcutaneously three times a week. The target hematocrit is 35–40%. The dose may be increased by 12,000 units every 4–6 weeks as needed to a maximum dose of 48,000 units per week. Hypertension is the most common side effect.

Human G-CSF (filgrastim) and **granulocyte-macrophage colony-stimulating factor (GM-CSF [sargramostim])** have been shown to increase the neutrophil counts of HIV-infected patients. Because of the high cost of this therapy, the dosage should be closely monitored and minimized, aiming for a neutrophil count of 1000/mcL. When the drug is used for indications other than cytotoxic chemotherapy, one or two doses at 5 mcg/kg per week are usually sufficient.

C. Antiretroviral Therapy

The availability of agents that in combination suppress HIV replication (Table 31–6) has had a profound impact on the natural history of HIV infection. Patients who achieve excellent suppression of HIV generally have stabilization or improvement of their clinical course that results from immunologic reconstitution and a subsequent decrease in AIDS-related complications. The greater potency and the improved side effect profile have led to recommendations to start treatment earlier in the course of HIV disease. Treatment should be initiated for all symptomatic patients, and for asymptomatic persons who (1) have CD4 cell counts below 350 cells/mcL; (2) have rapidly dropping CD4 counts or very high viral loads (> 100,000/mcL); (3) have dual infection with hepatitis B or C (rapid HIV replication is thought to hasten progression of hepatitis B and C); (4) have risk factors for cardiac disease (rapid HIV replication may increase the risk of cardiac disease); or (5) have risk factors for non–AIDS-related cancers (rapid HIV replication may increase such cancers). However, for patients who might have difficulty adhering to such therapy, deferring ART for some time may be a better strategy. In addition, because 5–20% of patients in developed countries who are treatment-naïve have a virus that is resistant to some drugs, resistance testing is recommended for all patients prior to initiating ART.

Once a decision to initiate therapy has been made, several important principles should guide therapy. First, because drug resistance to antiretroviral agents develops in HIV-infected patients, a primary goal of therapy should be complete suppression of viral replication as measured by the serum viral load. Therapy that achieves a plasma viral load of < 40 or < 50 copies/mL (depending on the test used) has been shown to provide a durable response to the therapy. To achieve this and maintain virologic control over time, combination therapy with at least 3 drugs from at least two different classes is necessary, and partially suppressive combinations such as dual nucleoside therapy

Table 31–5. Treatment of AIDS-related opportunistic infections and malignancies.[1]

Infection or Malignancy	Treatment	Complications
Pneumocystis jiroveci infection[2]	Trimethoprim-sulfamethoxazole, 15 mg/kg/d (based on trimethoprim component) orally or intravenously for 14–21 days.	Nausea, neutropenia, anemia, hepatitis, drug rash, Stevens-Johnson syndrome.
	Pentamidine, 3–4 mg/kg/d intravenously for 14–21 days.	Hypotension, hypoglycemia, anemia, neutropenia, pancreatitis, hepatitis.
	Trimethoprim, 15 mg/kg/d orally, with dapsone, 100 mg/d orally, for 14–21 days.[3]	Nausea, rash, hemolytic anemia in G6PD[3]-deficient patients. Methemoglobinemia (weekly levels should be < 10% of total hemoglobin).
	Primaquine, 15–30 mg/d orally, and clindamycin, 600 mg every 8 hours orally, for 14–21 days.	Hemolytic anemia in G6PD-deficient patients. Methemoglobinemia, neutropenia, colitis.
	Atovaquone, 750 mg orally three times daily for 14–21 days.	Rash, elevated aminotransferases, anemia, neutropenia.
	Trimetrexate, 45 mg/m² intravenously for 21 days (given with leucovorin calcium) if intolerant of all other regimens.	Leukopenia, rash, mucositis.
Mycobacterium avium complex infection	Clarithromycin, 500 mg orally twice daily with ethambutol, 15 mg/kg/d orally (maximum, 1 g). May also add:	Clarithromycin: hepatitis, nausea, diarrhea; ethambutol: hepatitis, optic neuritis.
	Rifabutin, 300 mg orally daily.	Rash, hepatitis, uveitis.
Toxoplasmosis	Pyrimethamine, 100–200 mg orally as loading dose, followed by 50–75 mg/d, combined with sulfadiazine, 4–6 g orally daily in four divided doses, and folinic acid, 10 mg daily for 4–8 weeks; then pyrimethamine, 25–50 mg/d, with clindamycin, 2–2.7 g/d in three or four divided doses, and folinic acid, 5 mg/d, until clinical and radiographic resolution is achieved.	Leukopenia, rash.
Lymphoma	Combination chemotherapy (eg, modified CHOP, M-BACOD, with or without G-CSF or GM-CSF). Central nervous system disease: radiation treatment with dexamethasone for edema.	Nausea, vomiting, anemia, leukopenia, cardiac toxicity (with doxorubicin).
Cryptococcal meningitis	Amphotericin B, 0.6 mg/kg/d intravenously, with or without flucytosine, 100 mg/kg/d orally in four divided doses for 2 weeks, followed by:	Fever, anemia, hypokalemia, azotemia.
	Fluconazole, 400 mg orally daily for 6 weeks, then 200 mg orally daily.	Hepatitis.
Cytomegalovirus infection	Valganciclovir, 900 mg orally twice a day for 21 days with food (induction), followed by 900 mg daily with food (maintenance).	Neutropenia, anemia, thrombocytopenia.
	Ganciclovir, 10 mg/kg/d intravenously in two divided doses for 10 days, followed by 6 mg/kg 5 days a week indefinitely. (Decrease dose for kidney disease.) May use ganciclovir as maintenance therapy (1 g orally with fatty foods three times a day).	Neutropenia (especially when used concurrently with zidovudine), anemia, thrombocytopenia.
	Foscarnet, 60 mg/kg intravenously every 8 hours for 10–14 days (induction), followed by 90 mg/kg once daily. (Adjust for changes in kidney function.)	Nausea, hypokalemia, hypocalcemia, hyperphosphatemia, azotemia.
Esophageal candidiasis or recurrent vaginal candidiasis	Fluconazole, 100–200 mg orally daily for 10–14 days.	Hepatitis, development of imidazole resistance.
Herpes simplex infection	Acyclovir, 400 mg orally three times daily until healed; or acyclovir, 5 mg/kg intravenously every 8 hours for severe cases.	Resistant herpes simplex with chronic therapy.
	Famciclovir, 500 mg orally twice daily until healed.	Nausea.
	Valacyclovir, 500 mg orally twice daily until healed.	Nausea.
	Foscarnet, 40 mg/kg intravenously every 8 hours, for acyclovir-resistant cases. (Adjust for changes in kidney function.)	See above.

(continued)

Table 31–5. Treatment of AIDS-related opportunistic infections and malignancies.[1] (continued)

Infection or Malignancy	Treatment	Complications
Herpes zoster	Acyclovir, 800 mg orally four or five times daily for 7 days. Intravenous therapy at 10 mg/kg every 8 hours for ocular involvement, disseminated disease.	See above.
	Famciclovir, 500 mg orally three times daily for 7 days.	Nausea.
	Valacyclovir, 500 mg orally three times daily for 7 days.	Nausea.
	Foscarnet, 40 mg/kg intravenously every 8 hours for acyclovir-resistant cases. (Adjust for changes in kidney function.)	See above.
Kaposi sarcoma		
Limited cutaneous disease	Observation, intralesional vinblastine.	Inflammation, pain at site of injection.
Extensive or aggressive cutaneous disease	Systemic chemotherapy (eg, liposomal doxorubicin). Interferon-α (for patients with CD4 > 200 cells/mcL and no constitutional symptoms). Radiation (amelioration of edema).	Bone marrow suppression, peripheral neuritis, flu-like syndrome.
Visceral disease (eg, pulmonary)	Combination chemotherapy (eg, daunorubicin, bleomycin, vinblastine).	Bone marrow suppression, cardiac toxicity, fever.

[1]For treatment of *Mycobacterium tuberculosis* infection, see Chapter 9.
[2]For moderate to severe *P jiroveci* infection (oxygen saturation < 90%), corticosteroids should be given with specific treatment. The dose of prednisone is 40 mg orally twice daily for 5 days, then 40 mg daily for 5 days, and then 20 mg daily until therapy is complete.
[3]When considering use of dapsone, check glucose-6-phosphate dehydrogenase (G6PD) level in black patients and those of Mediterranean origin.
CHOP, cyclophosphamide, doxorubicin (hydroxydaunomycin), vincristine (Oncovin), and prednisone; G-CSF, granulocyte-colony stimulating factor (filgrastim); GM-CSF, granulocyte-macrophage colony-stimulating factor (sargramostim); modified M-BACOD, methotrexate, bleomycin, doxorubicin (Adriamycin), cyclophosphamide, vincristine (Oncovin), and dexamethasone.

should be avoided. Similarly, if toxicity develops, it is preferable to either interrupt the entire regimen or change the offending drug rather than reduce individual doses.

A recent randomized trial compared early initiation of ART (within 2 weeks of starting treatment for an opportunistic infection) with ART that was deferred until after treatment of the opportunistic infection was completed (6 weeks after its start); results demonstrated that early initiation reduced death or AIDS progression by 50%. The reduced progression rates were related to more rapid improvements in CD4 counts in patients with advanced immunodeficiency. Furthermore, IRIS and other adverse events were no more frequent in the early ART arm. Based on these results, most treatment guidelines recommend that ART be initiated as early as is clinically feasible for patients with an acute AIDS-related opportunistic infection. For hospitalized patients, this recommendation requires close coordination between inpatient and outpatient physicians to ensure that treatment is continued once patients are discharged.

The current standard is to use at least three agents simultaneously usually from at least two different classes. Because the number of drugs and potential combinations is finite and the development of drug resistance may severely compromise the efficacy of treatment, patients must be able to adhere to these regimens. Adherence can be promoted through the use of medication boxes with compartments (eg, Medisets), supportive counseling, or daily supervision of therapy. Therefore, decisions to withhold treatment should not be based on a patient's circumstances (eg, active

drug use or housing status) alone. Often, a trial intervention such as offering *Pneumocystis* pneumonia prophylaxis may be helpful in determining the likelihood of adherence to a more complex antiretroviral regimen.

Monitoring of ART has two goals. Laboratory evaluation for toxicity depends on the specific drugs in the combination but generally should be done approximately every 3 months once a patient is on a stable regimen. Patients who are intolerant of their initial regimen (eg, patients who cannot tolerate the neurologic side effects of efavirenz) should be changed to an alternative drug or regimen. The second aspect of monitoring is to regularly measure objective markers of efficacy. The CD4 cell count and HIV viral load should be repeated 1–2 months after the initiation or change of antiretroviral regimen and every 3–4 months thereafter in clinically stable patients. In a patient who is adherent to an effective regimen, viral loads should be undetectable within 12–24 weeks. For patients in whom viral loads are not suppressed or who have viral rebound after suppression, the major question facing the clinician is whether the patient is nonadherent or has resistance to the regimen, or both. The issue is complicated because many patients report being more compliant than they really are, not because they wish to be untruthful but because they wish to tell the clinician what he or she wants to hear. Patients who are having trouble adhering to their treatment should receive counseling on how to better comply to their treatment. In patients who are adherent or who have missed enough doses to make resistance possible, resistance testing

Table 31–6. Antiretroviral therapy.

Drug	Dose	Common Side Effects	Special Monitoring[1]	Cost[2]	Cost/Month
Nucleoside reverse transcriptase inhibitors					
Zidovudine (AZT) (Retrovir)	600 mg orally daily in two divided doses	Anemia, neutropenia, nausea, malaise, headache, insomnia, myopathy	No special monitoring	$6.08/300 mg	$365.09
Didanosine (ddI) (Videx)	400 mg orally daily (enteric-coated capsule) for persons ≥ 60 kg	Peripheral neuropathy, pancreatitis, dry mouth, hepatitis	Bimonthly neurologic questionnaire for neuropathy, K^+, amylase, bilirubin, triglycerides	$10.70/400 mg	$321.00
Zalcitabine (ddC) (Hivid)	0.375–0.75 mg orally three times daily	Peripheral neuropathy, aphthous ulcers, hepatitis	Monthly neurologic questionnaire for neuropathy	$3.03/0.75 mg	$272.70
Stavudine (d4T) (Zerit)	40 mg orally twice daily for persons ≥ 60 kg	Peripheral neuropathy, hepatitis, pancreatitis	Monthly neurologic questionnaire for neuropathy, amylase	$7.31/40 mg	$438.61
Lamivudine (3TC) (Epivir)	150 mg orally twice daily	Rash, peripheral neuropathy	No special monitoring	$6.80/150 mg	$408.00
Emtricitabine (Emtriva)	200 mg orally once daily	Skin discoloration palms/soles (mild)	No special monitoring	$13.15/200 mg	$394.38
Abacavir (Ziagen)	300 mg orally twice daily	Rash, fever—if occur, rechallenge may be fatal	No special monitoring	$9.14/300 mg	$548.21
Nucleotide reverse transcriptase inhibitors					
Tenofovir (Viread)	300 mg orally once daily	Gastrointestinal distress	Kidney function	$22.09/300 mg	$662.70
Protease inhibitors (PIs)					
Indinavir (Crixivan)	800 mg orally three times daily	Renal calculi	Cholesterol, triglycerides, bilirubin level	$3.05/400 mg	$548.12
Saquinavir hard gel (Invirase)	1000 mg orally twice daily with 100 mg ritonavir orally twice daily	Gastrointestinal distress	Cholesterol, triglycerides	$6.91/500 mg	$829.18 (plus cost of ritonavir)
Ritonavir (Norvir)	600 mg orally twice daily or in lower doses (eg, 100 mg orally once or twice daily) for boosting other PIs	Gastrointestinal distress, peripheral paresthesias	Cholesterol, triglycerides	$10.29/100 mg	$3703.20 ($617.20 in lower doses)
Nelfinavir (Viracept)	750 mg orally three times daily or 1250 mg twice daily	Diarrhea	Cholesterol, triglycerides	$2.52/250 mg $6.30/625 mg	$680.99 $726.40
Fosamprenavir (Lexiva)	For PI-experienced patients: 700 mg orally twice daily and 100 mg of ritonavir 100 orally twice daily. For PI-naïve patients: above or 1400 mg orally twice daily or 1400 mg orally once daily and 200 mg of ritonavir orally once daily	Gastrointestinal rash	Cholesterol, triglycerides	$12.91/700 mg	$774.52–$1549.04 (plus cost of ritonavir for lower dose)
Lopinavir/ ritonavir (Kaletra)	400 mg/100 mg orally twice daily	Diarrhea	Cholesterol, triglycerides	$7.02/200 mg (lopinavir)	$841.90
Atazanavir (Reyataz)	400 mg orally once daily	Hyperbilirubinemia	Bilirubin level; when used with ritonavir: cholesterol and triglycerides	$17.12/200 mg	$1026.90

(continued)

Table 31–6. Antiretroviral therapy. (continued)

Drug	Dose	Common Side Effects	Special Monitoring[1]	Cost[2]	Cost/Month
Tipranavir/ ritonavir (Aptivus/ Norvir)	500 mg of tipranavir and 200 mg of ritonavir orally twice daily	Gastrointestinal, rash	Cholesterol, triglycerides	$8.94/250 mg (tipranavir) $10.29/100 mg (ritonavir)	$2307.20 (for combination)
Darunavir/ ritonavir (Prezista/ Norvir)	600 mg of darunavir and 100 mg of ritonavir orally twice daily	Rash	Cholesterol, triglycerides	$7.80/300 mg (darunavir) $10.29/100 mg (ritonavir)	$1553.40 (for combination)
Nonnucleoside reverse transcriptase inhibitors (NNRTIs)					
Nevirapine (Viramune)	200 mg orally daily for 2 weeks, then 200 mg orally twice daily	Rash	No special monitoring	$8.56/200 mg	$513.80
Delavirdine (Rescriptor)	400 mg orally three times daily	Rash	No special monitoring	$1.69/200 mg	$303.70
Efavirenz (Sustiva)	600 mg orally daily	Neurologic disturbances	No special monitoring	$20.07/600 mg	$602.00
Etravirine (Intelence)	200 mg orally daily	Rash, nausea	No special monitoring		
Entry inhibitors					
Enfuvirtide (Fuzeon)	90 mg subcutaneously twice daily	Injection site pain and allergic reaction	No special monitoring	$42.89/90 mg	$2573.16
Maraviroc (Selzentry)	150–300 mg orally daily	Cough, fever, rash	No special monitoring	$17.40/150 mg or 300 mg	$1044.00
Integrase inhibitor					
Raltegravir (Isentress)	400 mg orally twice daily	Diarrhea, nausea, headache	No special monitoring	$16.20/400 mg	$972.00

[1]Standard monitoring is complete blood count (CBC) and differential, and serum aminotransferases.
[2]Average wholesale price (AWP, for AB-rated generic when available) for quantity listed. Source: *Red Book Update*, Vol. 28, No. 3, March 2009. AWP may not accurately represent the actual pharmacy cost because wide contractual variations exist among institutions.

must be performed. Based on the results of resistance testing, and assessment of the patient's capability to comply with complicated regimens or to tolerate predictable side effects, the clinician should prescribe a combination of three medications to which there is no or only minimal resistance. Some patients whose counts rise dramatically on ART and who are fully suppressed (ie, plasma viral load < 50 copies/mL) may be successfully transitioned from a high potency regimen to a lower potency regimen with fewer side effects; however, this "induction-maintenance" strategy is still being evaluated in clinical trials. Stopping therapy in patients with high CD4 counts will generally result in patients reverting to their pretreatment nadir CD4 count in a matter of months and is therefore not recommended.

Although the ideal combination of drugs has not yet been defined for all possible clinical situations, possible choices can be better understood after a review of the available agents. These drugs can be grouped into five major categories: nucleoside and nucleotide reverse transcriptase inhibitors (NRTI), protease inhibitors (PI), nonnucleoside reverse transcriptase inhibitors (NNRTI), entry inhibitors (including fusion inhibitors and CCR5 antagonists), and integrase inhibitors. Once ART has been initiated in a

patient, it is not advisable to stop the therapy unless there is a compelling reason (eg, toxicity, poor adherence, etc). So-called "drug holidays" or "structured treatment interruptions" have been shown to increase risk of AIDS-related complications, increase CD4 declines, and increase morbidity from non–AIDS-related complications (eg, myocardial infarctions and liver failure) and are not recommended.

1. Nucleoside and nucleotide reverse transcriptase inhibitors—There are currently seven nucleoside or nucleotide agents approved for use. The choice of which agent to use depends primarily on the patient's prior treatment experience, results of resistance testing, drug side effects, other underlying conditions, and convenience of formulation. However, most clinicians use fixed-dose combinations of either tenofovir/emtricitabine (TDF/FTC) or abacavir/lamivudine (ABC/3TC), both of which can be given once a day. Zidovudine/lamivudine (AZT/3TC) is usually reserved for second- or third-line regimens because of toxicity and dosing schedule. Recent studies have raised some concerns about the efficacy of ABC/3TC in patients with high viral loads (eg, > 100,000 copies/mL) as well as concerns about increase risks of myocardial infarction with abacavir. Therefore, TDF/FTC is the preferred fixed-dose combination as part of initial treatment regimens.

Of the available agents, zidovudine is the most likely to cause anemia. Zidovudine and didanosine are the most likely to cause neutropenia. Stavudine is the most likely to cause lipoatrophy (loss of fat in the face, extremities, and buttocks) followed by zidovudine. Zalcitabine and didanosine are the most likely to cause peripheral neuropathy. Lamivudine, emtricitabine, and tenofovir have activity against hepatitis B. Didanosine, lamivudine, emtricitabine, and tenofovir can be administered daily. Generally, didanosine and tenofovir should not be given together due to toxicity of the combination that can result in decreasing CD4 counts. Information specific to each drug is given below, and recommendations on how to combine them appear in the Constructing regimens section below.

A. ZIDOVUDINE—Zidovudine was the first approved antiviral drug for HIV infection and remains an important agent. It is administered at a dose of 300 mg orally twice daily. A combination of zidovudine 300 mg and lamivudine 150 mg (Combivir) allows more convenient dosing of medication for individuals taking both of these agents. Side effects seen with zidovudine are listed in Table 31–6. Approximately 40% of patients experience subjective side effects that usually remit within 6 weeks. The common dose-limiting side effects are anemia and neutropenia, which require ongoing laboratory monitoring. Long-term use has been associated with lipoatrophy.

B. DIDANOSINE—The most convenient formulation of didanosine (ddI) is the enteric-coated capsule. For adults weighing at least 60 kg, the dose is one 400-mg enteric-coated capsule orally daily; for those 30–59 kg, the dose is one 250-mg enteric-coated capsule orally daily. Didanosine should be taken on an empty stomach.

Didanosine does not cause anemia but may cause neutropenia. It has also been associated with pancreatitis. The incidence of pancreatitis with didanosine is 5–10%—of fatal pancreatitis, less than 0.4%. Patients with a history of pancreatitis, as well as those taking other medications associated with pancreatitis (including trimethoprim-sulfamethoxazole and intravenous pentamidine) are at higher risk for this complication. Patients should be warned to use alcohol judiciously while taking didanosine. Other common side effects with didanosine include a dose-related, reversible, painful peripheral neuropathy, which occurs in about 15% of patients, and dry mouth. Fulminant hepatic failure and electrolyte abnormalities, including hypokalemia, hypocalcemia, and hypomagnesemia, have been reported in patients taking didanosine.

C. STAVUDINE—Stavudine (d4T) has shown good activity as an antiretroviral drug. The dose is 40 mg orally twice daily for individuals weighing 60 kg or more. However, because of its side effects including lipoatrophy, lipodystrophy (see below), peripheral neuropathy and, rarely, lactic acidosis and hepatitis, this drug should no longer be used except when there is no alternative. Patients taking stavudine should be routinely changed to abacavir or tenofovir, both of which are less likely to cause lipoatrophy.

D. LAMIVUDINE—Lamivudine (3TC) is a safe and well-tolerated agent. The dosage is 150 mg orally twice daily or 300 mg orally once a day. The dose should be reduced with chronic kidney disease. There are no significant side effects with lamivudine, and it has activity also against hepatitis B.

E. EMTRICITABINE—Emtricitabine is a nucleoside analog that is dosed at 200 mg orally. It was developed primarily as a once a day alternative to lamivudine. However, lamivudine can be dosed daily, eliminating the special indication for emtricitabine. As is true of lamivudine, emtricitabine has activity against hepatitis B and its dosage should be reduced in patients with chronic kidney disease.

F. ABACAVIR—A daily dose of 300 mg orally twice daily results in potent antiretroviral activity. Prior to initiation of abacavir, patients should undergo testing for HLA typing. Those with the B*5701 allele should not be treated with abacavir because the likelihood of a hypersensitivity reaction developing is high; the reaction is characterized by a flu-like syndrome with rash and fever that worsens with successive doses. Unfortunately, the absence of this allele does not guarantee that the patient will avoid the hypersensitivity reaction. Individuals in whom the hypersensitivity reaction develops *should not* be rechallenged with this agent because subsequent hypersensitivity reactions can be fatal. Two studies have reported an apparent increased risk of myocardial infarctions with abacavir use in patients who have underlying risks of cardiovascular disease. Consequently, abacavir should be avoided in such patients if effective alternative nucleoside or nucleotide analog agents exist.

Abacavir is formulated with zidovudine and lamivudine in a single pill (Trizivir, one tablet orally twice daily). Trizivir is not recommended as solo treatment for HIV because it is not as efficacious as combining two nucleoside/nucleotide analogs with a PI/ritonavir or an NNRTI; its use as a sole regimen should be reserved only for exceptional cases. Abacavir is also available as a fixed dose combination pill with lamivudine for use as a once daily pill (Epzicom).

G. ZALCITABINE—Zalcitabine (ddC) is thought to be one of the least effective antiretroviral agents and is therefore not commonly used. Zalcitabine, like didanosine, may cause peripheral neuropathy. It is also associated with aphthous ulcers, rash, and rare cases of pancreatitis.

H. TENOFOVIR—Tenofovir is the only licensed nucleotide analog. It is given as a single daily oral dose of 300 mg and is generally well tolerated. Tenofovir is available in a fixed dose combination pill with emtricitabine (Truvada) for daily dosing and is the only recommended fixed-dose combination for initial regimens. A once-a-day single fixed-dose combination pill that contains tenofovir, emtricitabine, and efavirenz (Atripla) is also available. Tenofovir is active against hepatitis B, including isolates that have resistance to lamivudine.

2. Protease inhibitors—Ten PIs—indinavir, nelfinavir, ritonavir, saquinavir, amprenavir, fosamprenavir, lopinavir (in combination with ritonavir), atazanavir, darunavir, and tipranavir are available. PIs have been shown to potently suppress HIV replication and are administered as part of a combination regimen.

All the PIs—to differing degrees—are metabolized by the cytochrome P450 system, and each can inhibit and induce various P450 isoenzymes. Therefore, drug interactions are common and difficult to predict. Clinicians should consult the product inserts before prescribing PIs with other medications. Drugs such as rifampin that are known to induce the P450 system should be avoided.

The fact that the PIs are dependent on metabolism through the cytochrome P450 system has led to the use of ritonavir to boost the drug levels of saquinavir, lopinavir, indinavir, atazanavir, tipranavir, darunavir and amprenavir, allowing use of lower doses and simpler dosing schedules of these PIs. In fact, current guidelines recommend that all PI-containing regimens use ritonavir boosting if possible. The only PIs that can be safely used without ritonavir boosting are nelfinavir and atazanavir.

When choosing which PI to use, prior patient experience, resistance patterns, side effects, and ease of administration are the major considerations. The first three PIs to be developed—indinavir, saquinavir, and ritonavir (as single agents)—are now rarely used because of the superiority of the second generation of PIs. Amprenavir has been almost entirely replaced by its prodrug, fosamprenavir. Unfortunately, all PIs, with the exception of unboosted atazanavir have been linked to a constellation of metabolic abnormalities, including elevated cholesterol levels, elevated triglyceride levels, insulin resistance, diabetes mellitus, and changes in body fat composition (eg, buffalo hump, abdominal obesity). The lipid abnormalities and body habitus changes are referred to as lipodystrophy. Although lipodystrophy is commonly associated with PIs, it has been seen also in HIV-infected persons who have never been treated with these agents. In particular, the lipoatrophy effects seen in patients receiving ART appears to be more related to the nucleoside toxicity and in particular to the thymidine analogs (stavudine and zidovudine).

Of the different manifestations of lipodystrophy, the dyslipidemias that occur are of particular concern because of the likelihood that increased levels of cholesterol and triglycerides will result in increased prevalence of heart disease. All patients taking PIs or NRTIs should have fasting serum cholesterol, low-density lipoprotein (LDL) cholesterol, and triglyceride levels performed every 3–6 months. Clinicians should calculate the Framingham 10-year coronary heart disease risk (see Chapter 28) and consider initiating dietary or drug therapy (or both) to achieve target LDL levels depending on the individual's risk factors. Patients who are unable to meet their LDL goal based solely on dietary interventions should be given pravastatin (20 mg daily orally) or atorvastatin (10 mg daily orally). Lovastatin and simvastatin should be avoided because of their interactions with PIs. Fish oil (3000 mg daily) combined with exercise and dietary counseling has been found to decrease triglycerides levels by 25%. Patients with persistently elevated fasting serum triglyceride levels of 500 mg/dL or more who do not respond to dietary intervention should be treated with gemfibrozil (600 mg twice daily prior to the morning and evening meals).

A. INDINAVIR—The standard dose of indinavir is 800 mg orally three times a day, although it is usually dosed twice daily in combination with ritonavir. Nausea and headache are common complaints with this drug. Indinavir crystals are present in the urine in approximately 40% of patients; this results in clinically apparent nephrolithiasis in about 15% of patients receiving indinavir. Lower urinary tract symptoms and acute kidney injury also have been reported. Patients taking this drug should be instructed to drink at least 48 ounces of fluid a day to ensure adequate hydration in an attempt to limit these complications. Mild indirect hyperbilirubinemia is also commonly observed in patients taking indinavir but is not an indication for discontinuation of the drug.

B. SAQUINAVIR—Saquinavir is formulated only as a hard-gel capsule (Invirase). It should only be used with ritonavir (1000 mg of hard-gel saquinavir with 100 mg of ritonavir orally twice daily). The soft-gel capsule (Fortovase) has been removed from the market in the United States. The most common side effects with saquinavir are diarrhea, nausea, dyspepsia, and abdominal pain.

C. RITONAVIR—Use of this potent PI at full dose (600 mg orally twice daily) has been limited by its inhibition of the cytochrome P450 pathway causing a large number of drug–drug interactions and by its frequent side effects of fatigue, nausea, and paresthesias. However, it is widely used in lower dose (eg, 100 mg daily to 100 mg twice daily) as a booster of other PIs.

D. NELFINAVIR—Nelfinavir is the only PI for which ritonavir boosting is not recommended. Unboosted nelfinavir is generally not as potent as a boosted PI regimen (eg, lopinavir plus ritonavir). The dose of nelfinavir is 1250 mg orally twice daily. Diarrhea is a side effect in 25% of patients taking nelfinavir, but this symptom may be controlled with over-the-counter antidiarrheal agents in most patients.

E. AMPRENAVIR—Amprenavir has efficacy and side effects similar to those of other PIs. Common side effects are nausea, vomiting, diarrhea, rash, and perioral paresthesia. The dose is 1200 mg orally twice daily. The concentration of amprenavir decreases when coadministered with ethinyl estradiol; therefore, amprenavir should be used with circumspection in the treatment of transgender persons requiring high-dose estrogen.

F. FOSAMPRENAVIR—Fosamprenavir is a prodrug of amprenavir. Its major advantage over using amprenavir is a much lower pill burden. For PI-naïve patients, it can be dosed at 1400 mg orally twice daily (four capsules a day) or at 1400 mg orally daily (two capsules) with ritonavir 200 mg orally daily (two capsules) or at 700 mg orally with ritonavir 100 mg orally twice daily. Patients previously treated with PIs should receive 700 mg orally with ritonavir 100 mg orally twice daily. Side effects are similar to those with amprenavir—most commonly gastrointestinal distress and hyperlipidemia. As with amprenavir, the concentration of fosamprenavir decreases when coadministered with ethinyl estradiol; therefore, fosamprenavir should be used with circumspection in the treatment of transgender persons requiring high-dose estrogen.

G. LOPINAVIR/R—Lopinavir/r is lopinavir (200 mg) coformulated with a low dose of ritonavir (50 mg) to maximize the bioavailability of lopinavir. It has been shown to be more effective than nelfinavir when used in combination with stavudine and lamivudine. The usual dose is 400 mg lopinavir with 100 mg of ritonavir (two tablets) orally twice daily with food. When given along with efavirenz or nevirapine, a higher dose (600 mg/150 mg—three tablets) is usually prescribed. The most common side effect is diarrhea, and lipid abnormalities are frequent.

H. ATAZANAVIR—Atazanavir can be dosed only once daily (two 200-mg capsules with food) or 300 mg in combination with 100 mg of ritonavir once daily). When used without ritonavir, it has only minimal or no impact on cholesterol and triglyceride levels. The most common side effect is mild hyperbilirubinemia that resolves with discontinuation of the drug. Both tenofovir and efavirenz lower the serum concentration of atazanavir. Therefore, when either of these two drugs is used with atazanavir, it should be boosted by administering ritonavir. Proton pump inhibitors are contraindicated in patients taking atazanavir because atazanavir requires an acidic pH to remain in solution.

I. TIPRANAVIR—Tipranavir is the only nonpeptidic PI currently approved by the US Food and Drug Administration (FDA). Because of its unique structure, it is active against some strains of HIV that are resistant to other PIs. It is dosed with ritonavir (two 250 mg capsules of tipranavir with two 100 mg capsules of ritonavir orally twice daily with food). The most common side effects are nausea, vomiting, diarrhea, fatigue, and headache. Tipranavir/ritonavir has been also associated with liver damage and should be used very cautiously in patients with underlying liver disease. Recent reports of intracranial hemorrhage in patients taking tipranavir-containing regimens have raised additional safety concerns about this potent PI. Because it is a sulfa-containing drug, its use should be closely monitored in patients with sulfa allergy.

J. DARUNAVIR—Darunavir is the most recently approved PI with impressive antiviral activity in the setting of significant PI resistance and in treatment-naïve patients. Darunavir has been added to the list of recommended PIs for initial treatment of HIV where it can be dosed daily (darunavir, 800 mg, with ritonavir, 100 mg). Darunavir, 600 mg orally twice daily, with ritonavir, 100 mg orally twice daily, is recommended for patients with prior PI treatment experience or PI resistance. Darunavir appears to be reasonably well tolerated with a safety profile similar to other PIs, such as lopinavir/ritonavir. Like tipranavir, darunavir is a sulfa-containing drug, and its use should be closely monitored in patients with sulfa allergy.

3. Nonnucleoside reverse transcriptase inhibitors—
NNRTIs inhibit reverse transcriptase at a site different from that of the nucleoside and nucleotide agents described above. All four NNRTIs have shown antiviral

activity as measured by HIV viral load and CD4 responses. The major advantage of the NNRTIs is that two of them (nevirapine and efavirenz) have potencies comparable to that of PIs—with lower pill burden and fewer side effects. In particular, they do not appear to cause lipodystrophy; patients with cholesterol and triglyceride elevations who are switched from a PI to an NNRTI may have improvement in their lipids. The resistance patterns of the NNRTIs are distinct from those of the PIs, so their use still leaves open the option for future PI use.

The NNRTIs can be used with PIs in patients who are difficult to suppress on simpler regimens or when it is difficult to identify at least two nucleoside/nucleotide agents to which the patient is not resistant. Because these agents may cause alterations in the clearance of PIs, dose modifications may be necessary when these two classes of medications are administered concomitantly. There is a high degree of cross-resistance between the "first generation" NNRTIs, such that resistance to one drug in this class uniformly predicts resistance to other drugs. However, etravirine has been approved as a "second-generation" NNRTI and appears to have consistent antiviral activity in patients with prior exposure and resistance to the "first generation" drugs of this class. In particular, the K103N mutation, which is associated with a high level of resistance to nevirapine, efavirenz, and delavirdine, does not appear to have an impact on etravirine. There is no therapeutic reason for using more than one NNRTI at the same time.

A. EFAVIRENZ—The major advantage of efavirenz is that it can be given once daily in a single dose (600 mg orally). The side effects are neurologic, with patients reporting symptoms ranging from lack of concentration and strange dreams to delusions and mania. Fortunately, the neurologic side effects of efavirenz subside over time, usually within a month. Administration of efavirenz with food, especially fatty food, may increase its serum levels and consequent neurotoxicity. Due to teratogenicity, efavirenz should be avoided in women who wish to conceive or are already pregnant. A once-daily fixed-dose combination of efavirenz, tenofovir, and emtricitabine in a single pill (Atripla) is available and is probably the best first choice for treatment-naïve patients without significant drug resistance.

B. NEVIRAPINE—The target dose of nevirapine is 200 mg orally twice daily, but it is initiated at a dose of 200 mg once a day to decrease the incidence of rash, which is as high as 40% when full doses are begun immediately. If rash develops while the patient is taking 200 mg a day, liver enzymes should be checked and the dose should not be increased until the rash resolves. Patients with mild rash and no evidence of hepatotoxicity can continue to be treated with nevirapine. Nevirapine should not be used in treatment-naïve women with high CD4 counts (> 250/mcL). Because of potential fatal hepatotoxicity, nevirapine should only be used in patients who cannot tolerate efavirenz.

C. DELAVIRDINE—Of the available "first generation" NNRTIs, delavirdine is used the least largely because of its less convenient dosing and pill burden compared with the other available NNRTIs. Unlike nevirapine and efavirenz, delavirdine inhibits P450 cytochromes rather than inducing these enzymes. This means that delavirdine can act like ritonavir and boost other antiretrovirals, although delavirdine is not as potent as ritonavir in this capacity. The dosage is 400 mg orally three times a day. The major side effect is rash.

D. Etravirine—Etravirine is the most recently approved NNRTI for the treatment of patients with prior NNRTI intolerance or resistance. The DUET trials demonstrated potent and durable antiviral activity in patients with NNRTI resistance to "first-generation" NNRTIs. Etravirine dosage is two 100-mg tablets twice daily. It should be used with a PI and a nucleoside/nucleotide analog and not just with two nucleoside/nucleotide analogs. The most common side effects are rash and nausea. Prior rash due to treatment with one of the other NNRTIs does not make rash more likely with etravirine.

4. Entry inhibitors

A. Enfuvirtide—Enfuvirtide (Fuzeon) is known as a fusion inhibitor; it blocks the entry of HIV into cells by blocking the fusion of the HIV envelope to the cell membrane. The addition of enfuvirtide to an optimized antiretroviral regimen improved CD4 counts and lowered viral loads in heavily pretreated patients with multidrug-resistant HIV. Unfortunately, resistance develops rapidly in patients receiving nonsuppressive treatment. The dose is 90 mg by subcutaneous injection twice daily; unfortunately, painful injection site reactions develop in most patients.

B. Maraviroc—Maraviroc is the first CCR5 co-receptor antagonist to be approved for use. Drugs in this class work by preventing the virus from entering uninfected cells by blocking the CCR5 co-receptor. Unfortunately, this class of entry inhibitors is only active against "CCR5-tropic virus." This form of the HIV-1 virus tends to predominate early in infection, while so-called "dual/mixed tropic virus" (which utilizes either R5 or CXCR4 co-receptors) emerges later as infection progresses. Approximately 50–60% of previously treated HIV-infected patients have circulating CCR5-tropic HIV. The drug has been shown to be effective in HIV-infected persons with ongoing viral replication despite being heavily treated and who have CCR5-tropic virus. Tropism testing should be performed before beginning the medication. The dose of maraviroc is 150–300 mg orally twice daily, based on the other drugs the patient is taking at the time. Common side effects are cough, fever, rash, musculoskeletal problems, abdominal pain, and dizziness.

5. Integrase inhibitors

A. Raltegravir—Raltegravir is the first HIV integrase inhibitor to be approved by the FDA. Integrase inhibitors slow HIV replication by blocking the HIV integrase enzyme needed for the virus to multiply. Raltegravir was impressively effective (when combined with other active drugs) in the treatment of HIV-infected patients with documented resistance to at least one drug in each of the three main classes of antiretroviral medications (nucleoside analogs, PIs, NNRTIs). Clinical trials of integrase inhibitors reveal a consistent pattern of more rapid decline in viral load compared with more standard PI/r or NNRTI-based regimens. The clinical significance of this observation is yet to be defined. Despite the impressive antiviral potency of this new exciting class of antiretroviral drugs, it appears that high-level resistance to integrase inhibitors emerges quickly in the setting of virologic failure (much like with the NNRTIs). Therefore, it is critical that raltegravir be used in combination with other active antiretroviral agents.

Recent studies in treatment-naïve patients have demonstrated that raltegravir in combination with TDF/FTC is as effective as the current first-line choice of EFV/TDF/FTC for daily treatment and has fewer side effects. Furthermore, the CD4 response appeared better in patients treated with the raltegravir combination. These results led to FDA approval for raltegravir in treatment-naïve patients. The dose of raltegravir is 400 mg orally twice daily. Common side effects are diarrhea, nausea, and headache.

B. Elvitegravir—Elvitegravir is another integrase inhibitor that is in phase 3 studies. The dose is 125 mg once daily, given with ritonavir (100 mg) for boosting. Elvitegravir showed impressive short-term virologic responses in phase 2 studies.

6. Constructing regimens—There is now little debate about the necessity for combining drugs to achieve long-term suppression of HIV and its associated clinical benefit. Only combinations of three or more drugs have been able to decrease HIV viral load by 2–3 logs and allow long-term suppression of HIV RNA to below the threshold of detection.

Current evidence supports the use of Truvada (tenofovir and emtricitabine) as the "nucleoside/nucleotide backbone" combined with efavirenz as the initial regimen. This regimen has been shown to be more effective and better tolerated than Combivir (zidovudine and lamivudine) and Epzicom (abacavir/lamivudine). It has the advantages of once daily dosing and is available as a single pill (Atripla). Because 8–10% of newly infected persons in some urban areas of the United States have NNRTI resistance, resistance testing should be performed before initiating efavirenz in this population. Regimens that include only nucleoside and nucleotide analogs without nonnucleoside agents or PIs are clinically inferior and should only be used for patients that cannot adhere to a more complicated regimen.

In the absence of head-to-head comparisons of different regimens in different situations, several general principles should guide the choice of combinations. The most important determinant of treatment efficacy is adherence to the regimen. Therefore, it is vitally important that the regimen chosen be one to which the patient can easily adhere. In general, patients are more compliant with medication regimens that are once or twice a day only, do not require special timing with regard to meals, can be taken at the same time as other medications, do not require refrigeration or special preparation, and do not have bothersome side effects. To the extent possible, agents to which the patient has not been exposed are preferable to drugs for which resistance mutations may have already occurred. Toxicities should ideally be nonoverlapping. An individual's relative contraindications to a given drug or drugs should be considered. The regimen should not include agents that are either virologically antagonistic or incompatible in terms of drug–drug interactions. For example, etravirine should not be used with boosted tipranavir because of drug-drug interactions. Compatible dosing schedules—prescribing medications that can be taken at the same time—improve adherence to treatment. Finally, highly complex therapeutic regimens should be reserved for individuals who are capable of adhering to the rigorous demands of taking multiple medications and having this therapy closely monitored. Conversely, simplified regimens that deliver the lowest number of pills given at the longest possible dosing intervals are desirable for patients who have difficulty taking multiple medications.

Possible ways of incorporating nonnucleoside agents and PIs into combinations are displayed in Figure 31–2.

A number of points about the "nucleoside/nucleotide backbone" of regimens have become clearer. The combination of stavudine plus didanosine should be avoided, since there is increased risk of toxicities, in particular in pregnant women because of the increased risk of lactic acidosis, which can be fatal. Moreover, the nucleoside pair of zidovudine and stavudine should be avoided because of increased toxicity and the potential for antagonism that results from intracellular competition for phosphorylation. Finally, the

combination of didanosine with tenofovir should be avoided due to observed declines in CD4 counts.

In choosing which agents to include in an initial antiretroviral regimen, ease of administration, minimization of side effects, drug resistance pattern, and future treatment options should all be considered. In designing second-line regimens for patients with resistance to initial therapy, the goal is to identify three drugs from at least two different classes to which the virus is not resistant. This can be quite complicated because of the problem of cross-resistance between drugs within a class. For example, the resistance patterns of lopinavir/ritonavir and indinavir are overlapping, and patients with virus resistant to these agents are unlikely to respond to nelfinavir or saquinavir even though they have never received treatment with these agents. Similarly, the resistance patterns of nevirapine and efavirenz are overlapping. With several new classes of drugs and new generations of existing drug classes now available, the ability to provide fully suppressive regimens even to patients with extensive treatment experience and drug resistance has become more realistic. The goal of therapy, therefore, should be to fully suppress viral loads to < 50 copies/mL even for highly treatment-experienced patients.

In addition to taking a careful history of what antiretroviral agents a patient has taken and for how long, genotypic

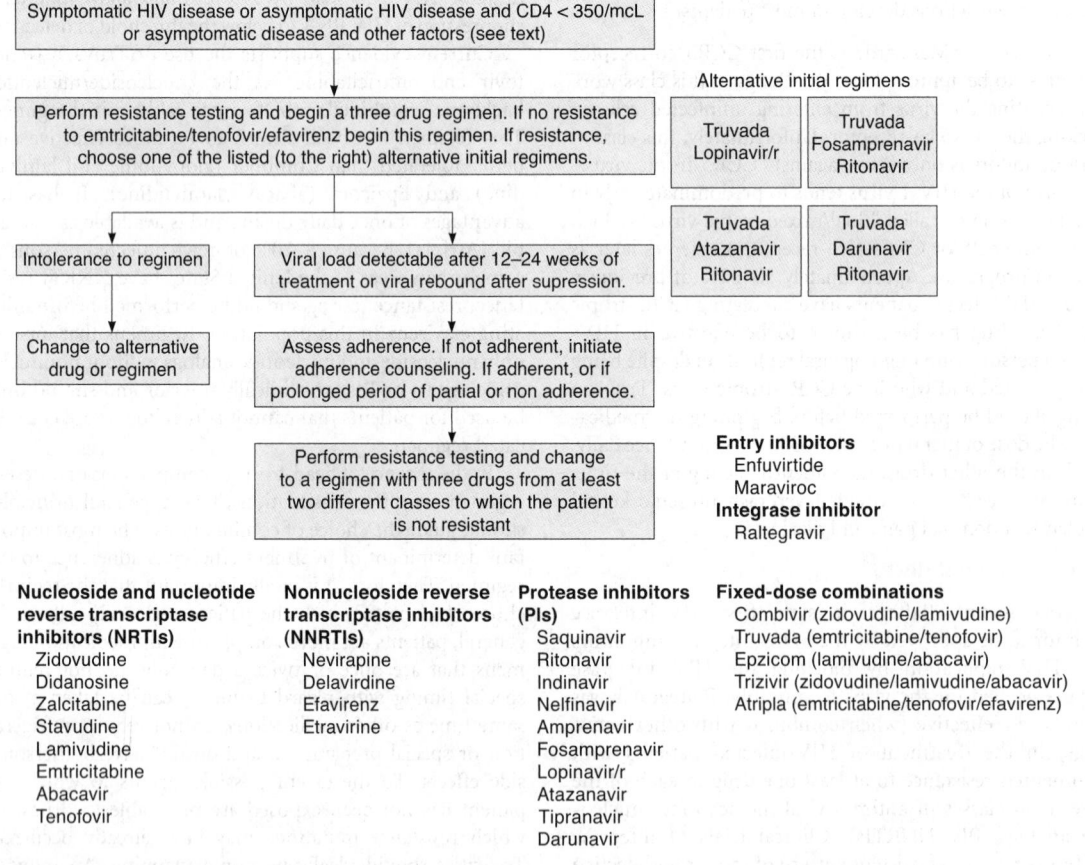

▲ Figure 31–2. Approach to initial and subsequent antiretroviral therapy.

and phenotypic resistance testing can provide useful information in designing second-line regimens (see below).

Whatever regimen is chosen, patients should be coached in ways to improve adherence. For certain populations (eg, unstably housed individuals), specially tailored programs that include drug dispensing are needed.

For some patients, it is impossible to construct a tolerable regimen that fully suppresses HIV. In such cases, clinicians and patients should consider their goals. Patients maintained on effective antiretroviral agents often benefit from these regimens (eg, higher CD4 counts, fewer opportunistic infections) even if their virus is detectable. In some cases, patients may request a drug holiday during which they are taken off all medications. Patients often immediately feel better because of the absence of drug side effects. Unfortunately, structured treatment interruptions generally result in viral rebound and CD4 decline, and patients who interrupt their treatment fare poorly compared with patients who continue their regimens without interruption.

7. The challenge of drug resistance—HIV-1 drug resistance limits the ability to fully control HIV replication and is a leading cause for antiretroviral regimen failure. Resistance has been documented for all currently available antiretrovirals including the new classes of fusion inhibitors, CCR5 inhibitors, and integrase inhibitors. The problem of drug resistance is widespread in HIV-infected patients undergoing treatment in countries where ART is widely available. A cohort study revealed that some degree of resistance developed over the first 30 months of therapy in nearly one-third of patients starting a HAART regimen. Patients who have taken various antiretroviral regimens and who now have resistant HIV-1 represent a major challenge for the treating clinician. Resistance is now also documented in patients who are ART-naive, but who have been infected with a drug resistant strain—"primary resistance." Cohort studies of antiretroviral treatment–naive patients entering care in North America and Western Europe show that roughly 10–12% (and as high as 25%) of recently infected individuals have been infected with a drug-resistant strain of HIV-1.

Current expert guidelines recommend resistance testing as part of standard baseline testing in all patients. Resistance testing is also recommended for patients who are on an antiretroviral regimen and have suboptimal viral suppression (ie, viral loads > 1000 copies/mL). Both genotypic and phenotypic tests are commercially available and in randomized controlled studies their use has been shown to result in improved short-term virologic outcomes compared to making treatment choices without resistance testing. Furthermore, multiple retrospective studies have conclusively demonstrated that resistance tests provide prognostic information about virologic response to newly initiated therapy that cannot be gleaned from standard clinical information (ie, treatment history, examination, CD4 count, and viral load tests).

Because of the complexity of resistance tests, many clinicians require expert interpretation of results. In the case of genotypic assays, results may show that the mutations that are selected for during ART are drug-specific or contribute to broad cross-resistance to multiple drugs within a therapeutic class. An example of a drug-specific mutation for the reverse transcriptase inhibitors would be the M184V mutation that is selected for by lamivudine or emtricitabine therapy—this mutation causes resistance only to those two drugs. Conversely, the thymidine analog mutations ("TAMs") of M41L, D67N, K70R, L210W, T215Y/F, and T219Q/K/E are selected for by either zidovudine or stavudine therapy, but cause resistance to all the drugs in the class and often extend to the nucleotide inhibitor tenofovir when three or more of these TAMs are present. Further complicating the interpretation of genotypic tests is the fact that some mutations that cause resistance to one drug can actually make the virus that contains this mutation more sensitive to another drug. The M184V mutation, for example, is associated with increased sensitivity to zidovudine, stavudine, and tenofovir. The most common mutations associated with drug resistance and cross-resistance patterns for NRTIs, NNRTIs, and PIs can be found at http://hivdb.stanford.edu. Phenotypic tests also require interpretation in that the distinction between a resistant virus and sensitive one is not fully defined for all available drugs.

Both methods of resistance testing are limited by the fact that they may measure resistance in only some of the viral strains present in an individual. Resistance results may also be misleading if a patient is not taking antiretroviral medications at the time of testing. Thus, resistance results must be viewed cumulatively—ie, if resistance is reported to an agent on one test, it should be presumed to be present thereafter even if subsequent tests do not give the same result.

► Course & Prognosis

With improvements in therapy, patients are living longer after the diagnosis of AIDS. A population-based study conducted in Denmark found that HIV-infected persons at age 25 years without hepatitis C had a life expectancy of 39 additional years. Unfortunately, not all HIV-infected persons have access to treatment. Studies consistently show less access to treatment for blacks, the homeless, and injection drug users. In addition to access to treatment, sustaining lower mortality will require developing new treatments for patients in whom resistance to existing agents develops. For patients whose disease progresses even though they are receiving appropriate treatment, meticulous palliative care must be provided (see Chapter 5), with attention to pain control, spiritual needs, and family (biologic and chosen) dynamics.

► When to Refer

- Clinicians with limited experience in HIV/AIDS should refer HIV-infected patients to specialists with experience, given the increasing number and complexity of treatment regimens available.

- Extra efforts should be made to obtain specialty consultation for those patients with detectable viral loads on ART; those intolerant of standard medications; those in need of systemic chemotherapy; and those with complicated opportunistic infections, particularly when invasive procedures or experimental therapies are needed.

▶ **When to Admit**

Patients with opportunistic infections who are acutely ill (eg, who are febrile, who have had rapid change of mental status, or who are in respiratory distress) or who require intravenous medications.

Cooper DA et al; BENCHMRK Study Teams. Subgroup and resistance analyses of raltegravir for resistant HIV-1 infection. N Engl J Med. 2008 Jul 24;359(4):355–65. [PMID: 18650513]

El-Sadr WM et al; Strategies for Management of Antiretroviral Therapy (SMART) Study Group. CD4+ count-guided interruption of antiretroviral treatment. N Engl J Med. 2006 Nov 30;355(22):2283–96. [PMID: 17135583]

Gallant JE et al; Study 934 Group. Tenofovir DF, emtricitabine, and efavirenz vs. zidovudine, lamivudine, and efavirenz for HIV. N Engl J Med. 2006 Jan 19;354(3):251–60. [PMID: 16421366]

Grinspoon S et al. Cardiovascular risk and body-fat abnormalities in HIV-infected adults. N Engl J Med. 2005 Jan 6;352(1):48–62. [PMID: 15635112]

Gulick RM et al; AIDS Clinical Trials Group (ACTG) A5095 Study Team. Three- vs four-drug antiretroviral regimens for the initial treatment of HIV-1 infection: a randomized controlled trial. JAMA. 2006 Aug 16;296(7):769–81. [PMID: 16905783]

Hammer SM et al. Antiretroviral treatment of adult HIV infection: 2008 recommendations of the International AIDS Society-USA panel. JAMA. 2008 Aug 6;300(5):555–70. [PMID: 18677028]

Lohse N et al. Survival of persons with and without HIV infection in Denmark, 1995–2005. Ann Intern Med. 2007 Jan 16;146(2):87–95. [PMID: 17227932]

Viral & Rickettsial Infections

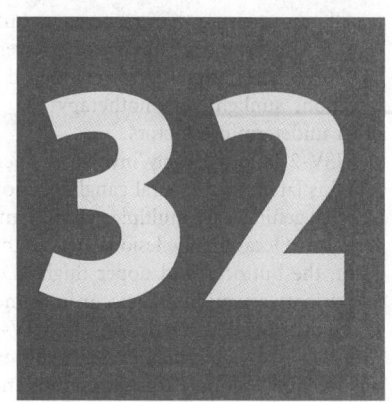

Vicente F. Corrales-Medina, MD

Wayne X. Shandera, MD

VIRAL DISEASES

HUMAN HERPESVIRUSES

Herpesviruses cause a wide spectrum of human disease. Eight identified human herpesviruses (HHV) include herpes simplex virus (HSV) (type 1), HSV (type 2), varicella zoster virus (VZV) (type 3), Epstein–Barr infectious mononucleosis virus (type 4), and cytomegalovirus (CMV) (type 5). A sixth type (HHV-6) has been identified as a causative agent of roseola (exanthema subitum), and a seventh (HHV-7) is serologically associated with several syndromes. Another herpesvirus (HHV-8) is linked with Kaposi sarcoma (see Chapter 31).

Subclinical primary infection with the herpesviruses is more common than clinically manifest illness. Each persists in a latent state for the remainder of the person's life. With HSV and VZV, virus remains latent in sensory ganglia; upon reactivation, lesions appear in the distal sensory nerve distribution. As a result of disease-, drug-, or radiation-induced immunosuppression, virus reactivation may lead to widespread lesions in affected organs such as the viscera or the central nervous system (CNS). Severe or fatal illness may occur in infants and immunodeficient persons. Herpesviruses can transform cells in tissue culture. Associations with malignancies include Epstein–Barr virus (EBV) with Burkitt lymphoma and nasopharyngeal carcinoma and HHV-8 with primary effusion lymphoma and Kaposi sarcoma.

1. Herpesviruses 1 & 2

ESSENTIALS OF DIAGNOSIS

► Spectrum of illness from stomatitis and urogenital lesions to facial nerve paralysis (Bell palsy) and encephalitis.

► Variable intervals between exposure and clinical disease, since HSV causes both primary (which may be subclinical) and reactivation disease.

► Successful management with acyclovir or related acyclic compounds (valacyclovir, famciclovir).

General Considerations

Herpesviruses 1 and 2 affect primarily the oral and genital areas, respectively. Seroprevalence to both viruses increases with age; seroprevalence to HSV-2 increases with sexual activity. Disease is typically a manifestation of reactivation. Although HSV-2 is the most common cause of genital ulcers in the developed world, HSV-1 is increasingly recognized as causing primary urogenital infections. Genital recurrences are much more frequent with HSV-2 and gradually decrease over time, whereas HSV-1 recurrences are rare after the first year. Risk factors for HSV transmission include black race, female gender, a history of sexually transmitted infections (STIs), an increased number of partners, contact with commercial sex workers, lower socioeconomic status, young age of onset of sexual activity, and total duration of sexual activity. Asymptomatic shedding of either virus is common, especially following primary infection or symptomatic recurrences, and may be responsible for transmission. HSV-2 increases the risk of HIV acquisition, and in advanced HIV infection, HSV reactivates more frequently. HIV replication is increased by interaction with HSV proteins; suppression of HSV-2 can decrease genital tract shedding of HIV as well as plasma HIV RNA levels.

Clinical Findings

A. Symptoms and Signs

1. Mucocutaneous disease—HSV-1 mucocutaneous disease largely involves the mouth and oral cavity ("herpes labialis" or "gingivostomatitis;" the latter largely in children). Digital lesions (**whitlows**) are an occupational hazard in medicine, nursing, and dentistry (Plate 94). Certain contact sports (eg, wrestling) are associated with outbreaks of skin infections ("herpes gladiatorum"). Asymptomatic shedding of HSV-1 is frequent, with most infected individuals shedding virus at least once a month.

Vesicles form moist ulcers after several days and epithelialize over 1–2 weeks if untreated. Primary infection is usually more severe than recurrences but may be asymptomatic. Recurrences often involve fewer lesions, tend to be labial, heal faster, and are induced by stress, fever, infection, sunlight, chemotherapy (eg, fludarabine), or other undetermined factors.

HSV-2 lesions largely involve the genital tract. Virus remains latent in presacral ganglia. Lesions arising on the external genitalia are multiple, painful, small, grouped, and vesicular. Occasionally, lesions arise in the perianal region or on the buttocks and upper thighs. Dysuria, cervicitis, and urinary retention may occur in women.

Proctitis and sacral lesions in HIV-infected persons with CD4 cytopenia may present with extensive, ulcerating, weeping lesions. Large ulcerations and atypical lesions suggest drug-resistant isolates (see below).

2. Ocular disease—HSV can cause keratitis, blepharitis, and keratoconjunctivitis. Keratitis is usually unilateral, often with impaired visual acuity. Lesions limited to the epithelium usually heal without affecting vision, whereas stromal involvement can cause uveitis, scarring, and eventually blindness. Recurrences are frequent. HSV is the second most common cause, after VZV, of acute retinal necrosis.

3. Neonatal and congenital infection—Both herpesviruses can infect the fetus and induce congenital malformations (organomegaly, bleeding, and CNS abnormalities). Neonatal transmission during delivery is more common than intrauterine infection. Maternal infection during the third trimester is associated with the highest risk of neonatal transmission; about 70% of these infections are asymptomatic or unrecognized. Invasive fetal monitoring and vacuum or forceps delivery can facilitate the risk of transmitting herpes.

4. Central nervous system disease—HSV-1 predominantly causes herpes simplex encephalitis, while HSV-1 and HSV-2 are both associated with benign recurrent lymphocytic (Mollaret) meningitis. Primary HSV-2 infection in women often presents as aseptic meningitis. HSV-1 and HSV-2 are increasingly recognized as a cause of mild, nonspecific neurologic symptoms.

Herpes simplex encephalitis presents with nonspecific symptoms: a flu-like prodrome, followed by headache, fever, behavioral and speech disturbances, and focal or generalized seizures. The temporal lobe is often involved. Untreated disease and presentation with coma carry a high mortality rate, with many survivors suffering neurologic sequelae. In children, nonspecific symptoms may complicate establishing a diagnosis.

5. Disseminated infection—Disseminated HSV infection occurs in the setting of immunosuppression, either primary or iatrogenic, or rarely with pregnancy. In disseminated disease, skin lesions are not always present. Disseminated skin lesions are a particular complication in patients with atopic eczema (eczema herpeticum) and burns.

6. Bell palsy—An association between HSV-1 and Bell palsy is established.

7. Esophagitis and proctitis—HSV-1 can cause esophagitis in those with AIDS and other immunocompromised patients. CMV esophagitis is distinguished by the size and depth of the lesion (smaller and deeper for HSV). HSV-1 is also postulated to activate mononuclear cells in the pathogenesis of achalasia. Proctitis often occurs mainly in men who have sex with men.

8. Erythema multiforme—Herpes simplex viruses remain, with drugs, the leading association with erythema multiforme and with the more severe, mucosally involved Stevens–Johnson syndrome.

9. Other—Rarely, HSV causes fulminant hepatitis. HSV lower respiratory tract infection is common in mechanically ventilated patients, but its clinical significance is unknown. HSV-1 is associated with *Helicobacter pylori*–negative upper gastrointestinal tract ulcers. An association between HSV-1 and endocardial inflammation in the pathogenesis of atrial myxoma is postulated.

B. Laboratory Findings

1. Mucocutaneous disease—Diagnosis is usually made clinically, but viral cultures of vesicular fluid or direct fluorescent antibody staining of scraped lesions remain the standard of diagnosis. Polymerase chain reaction (PCR) is a more sensitive diagnostic assay. The presence of intranuclear inclusion bodies and multinucleated giant cells on a Tzanck preparation or Calcofluor stain is supportive of a diagnosis of herpetic viral infection. Type-specific serologies are useful for counseling HIV-infected individuals; pregnant women; sexual partners of persons infected with HSV; and those with an uncertain clinical history, high-risk behavior, or increased number of sexual partners.

2. Ocular disease—Keratitis is diagnosed by branching (dendritic) ulcers that stain with fluorescein.

3. Encephalitis and recurrent meningitis—Cerebrospinal fluid pleocytosis is common, with roughly equal numbers of red cells. HSV DNA PCR of the cerebrospinal fluid is a rapid, sensitive, and specific tool for early diagnosis. Antibodies to HSV in cerebrospinal fluid can confirm the diagnosis but appear late in the course of the disease. Viral culture shows a sensitivity of only 10%. MRI scanning is often a useful adjunct showing increased signal in the temporal and frontal lobes. Temporal lobe seizure foci may be demonstrated on electroencephalograms (EEGs).

4. Esophagitis and proctitis—Esophagitis is diagnosed by endoscopic biopsy and cultures. Proctitis may be diagnosed by rectal swab for PCR or culture, or both, although complicated cases may require biopsy.

▶ Prevention

Besides antiviral suppressive therapy, prevention also requires counseling and the use of barrier precautions during sexual activity. Disclosure of partner status is associated with about a 50% reduction in the HSV-2 acquisition. Arguments favoring partner testing include confirming exposure, assistance with management, reducing the risk of transmission, and aiding in public health strategies.

Preventing spread to hospital staff and other patients from cases with mucocutaneous, disseminated, or genital disease requires isolation and the usage of handwashing and gloving–gowning precautions. Staff with active lesions (eg, whitlows) should not have contact with patients. Asymptomatic transmission occurs, especially with HSV-2. An HSV-2 glycoprotein-D vaccine under development appears to prevent infection and disease among women who are seronegative at baseline.

▶ Treatment & Prophylaxis

Drugs that inhibit replication of HSV-1 and HSV-2 include trifluridine and vidarabine (both for keratitis), acyclovir and related compounds, foscarnet, and cidofovir (Table 32–1).

A. Mucocutaneous Disease

While treatment is often not necessary in immunocompetent patients, it can ameliorate and shorten the duration of symptoms if initiated early. For primary genital infection, oral agents are generally used and include acyclovir, 200 mg five times a day or 400 mg three times a day; valacyclovir, 1 g twice daily; or famciclovir, 250 mg three times daily; all given for 7–10 days. Most experience in treating primary herpes labialis is with acyclovir (same doses and duration as for genital infection). Intravenous acyclovir (5–10 mg/kg every 8 hours for 7–14 days) should be considered in immunosuppressed patients.

For recurrent genital disease, acyclovir, 800 mg three times daily for 2 days; valacyclovir, 500 mg twice daily for 3 days; or famciclovir, 1 g twice daily for 1 day all show efficacy in controlled trials. Patient-initiated therapy with short courses of antivirals at first symptoms of recurrence is a frequently used and favorable approach. For the treatment of recurrences of herpes labialis, lesions heal faster with topical penciclovir than with topical acyclovir. Docosanol cream offers modest benefit. Oral acyclovir (same doses as above for 5 days) is more effective than topical agents. Recent data promote short-course therapy with higher doses of antivirals (eg, valacyclovir, 2 g twice daily for 1 day, or famciclovir, 1.5 g single dose).

Atypical isolates, large ulcerations, new lesions, or poor response to therapy suggest acyclovir resistance, which often occurs in immunodeficient patients. Alternatives include high dose acyclovir (4–5 g), which is effective in treating proctitis in the HIV-positive population, or foscarnet (40–60 mg/kg intravenously every 8 hours), adjusting the dose interval in patients with kidney dysfunction. Cidofovir is used in rare cases of infection resistant to both acyclovir and foscarnet.

Patients with frequent recurrent genital infections may be given **secondary prophylaxis** with acyclovir, 400 mg twice a day; valacyclovir, 500–1000 mg once daily; or famciclovir, 250 mg twice a day. For herpes labialis, valacyclovir, 500 mg daily, is the best option. Sunscreen may be useful for recurrences associated with sunlight exposure. Advantages of suppressive therapy include a significant reduction in acquisition of disease among the HSV-2 discordant heterosexual partners. AIDS patients with a history of mucocutaneous disease should continued receiving suppressive therapy unless a sustained improve-

ment of immune status occurs. Among the HIV-infected, the use of highly active antiretroviral therapy (HAART) is associated with fewer days of HSV-1 or -2 lesions.

B. Keratitis

For the treatment of acute epithelial keratitis, topical antivirals (ophthalmic trifluridine, vidarabine, acyclovir, and ganciclovir are all nearly equivalent in efficacy) are recommended. Combination of topical antivirals with interferon or debridement (or both) hastens healing. The usage of topical corticosteroids may exacerbate the infection, although systemic corticosteroids may help with selected cases of stromal infection. Long-term treatment (greater than 1 year) with acyclovir at a dosage of 800 mg/d orally decreases recurrence rates.

C. Neonatal Disease

Acyclovir intravenously is effective for disseminated lesions in neonatal disease. The dosage is 20 mg/kg intravenously every 8 hours for 14–21 days. Counseling with serologic screening should be offered to pregnant mothers. The use of maternal antenatal suppressive therapy with acyclovir (typically, 400 mg three times daily) beginning at 36 weeks gestation decreases the presence of detectable HSV, the rates of recurrence at delivery, and the need for cesarean section. Cesarean section is recommended for pregnant women with active genital lesions or typical prodromal symptoms.

D. Encephalitis

Because of the need for rapid treatment and the difficulties associated with brain biopsy, patients with suspected HSV encephalitis are given intravenous acyclovir (10 mg/kg every 8 hours for 10 days or more, adjusting for kidney dysfunction), starting upon suspicion of diagnosis, and stopping if another diagnosis is established. If the PCR is negative and clinical suspicion remains high in the absence of a biopsy, treatment should be continued for 10 days because the false-negative rate for PCR can be as high as 25% (especially in children) and acyclovir is relatively nontoxic. Long-term neurologic sequelae are common and late pediatric relapse is recognized.

E. Disseminated Disease

Disseminated disease responds best to parenteral acyclovir (see the preceding paragraph for dosages) when treatment is initiated early.

F. Bell Palsy

Prednisolone, 25 mg orally twice daily for 10 days started within 72 h of onset, significantly increases the rate of recovery. Valacyclovir (but not acyclovir), 1 g orally daily for 5 days, may be beneficial if started within 7 days of onset along with corticosteroid therapy.

G. Esophagitis and Proctitis

Patients with esophagitis should receive either intravenous acyclovir at a dosage of 5–10 mg/kg every 8 hours or oral

Table 32–1. Agents for viral infections.[1]

Drug	Dosing	Spectrum	Renal Clearance/ Hemodialysis	CNS/CSF Penetration	Toxicities
Acyclovir	200–800 mg orally five times daily; 250–500 mg/m^2 intravenously every 8 hours for 7 days	HSV, VZV	Yes/Yes	Yes	Neurotoxic reactions, reversible renal dysfunction, local reactions
Adefovir	10 mg daily orally	HBV	Yes/Yes	NA	Gastrointestinal symptoms, transaminitis, lactic acidosis, nephrotoxicity
Cidofovir	5 mg/kg intravenously weekly for 2 weeks, then every other week	CMV	Yes/NA	NA	Neutropenia, renal failure, ocular hypotonia
Entecavir	0.5 mg orally daily, increase to 1 mg orally daily in lamivudine-resistant patients	HBV	Yes/NA	NA	Lactic acidosis, rare exacerbation of HBV infection
Famciclovir	500 mg orally three times daily for 7 days for acute VZV; 250 mg three times daily for 7–10 days for genital or cutaneous HSV-1/HSV-2 infection; 125 mg twice daily for 5 days for recurrences (500 mg twice daily for 7 days if HIV-infected)	HSV, VZV	Yes/NA	NA	NA
Fomivirsen	165 mcg by intravitreal injection once weekly for 3 weeks, then every other week	CMV	NA	NA	Ocular inflammation, retinal detachment
Foscarnet	20 mg/kg intravenous bolus, then 120 mg/kg intravenously every 8 hours for 2 weeks; maintain with 60 mg/kg/d intravenously for 5 days each week	CMV, HSV resistant to acyclovir, VZV, HIV-1	Yes/Yes	Variable	Nephrotoxicity, genital ulcerations, calcium disturbances
Ganciclovir	5 mg/kg intravenous bolus every 12 hours for 14–21 days; maintain with 3.75 mg/kg/d intravenously for 5 days each week	CMV	Yes/Yes	Yes	Neutropenia, thrombocytopenia, CNS side effects
Idoxuridine	Topical, 0.1% every 1–2 hours for 3–5 days	HSV keratitis	—	—	Local reactions
Interferon α-2b	3–5 million international units subcutaneously three times weekly to daily. Intralesionally: 1 million international units per 0.1 mL in up to five warts three times weekly for 3 weeks	HBV, HCV, HPV	Yes/Yes	—	Influenza-like syndrome, myelosuppression, neurotoxicity
Interferon α-n3	0.05 mL/wart biweekly up to 8 weeks	HPV	NA/NA	NA	Local reactions
	3 mU intravenously three times per week	? HCV	NA/NA	NA	Influenza-like syndrome, myelosuppression, neurotoxicity
Lamivudine (3TC)	12 mg/kg/d	HIV-1, ?HIV-2, HBV	Yes/NA	Yes	Skin rash, headache, insomnia
Oseltamivir	75 mg twice daily for 5 days beginning 48 hours after onset of symptoms	Influenza A and B	Yes/NA	NA	Few
Penciclovir	Topical, 1% cream every 2 hours for 4 days	HSV	No/No	No	Local reactions
Palivizumab	15 mg/kg intramuscularly every month in RSV season	RSV	No/No	No	Upper respiratory infection symptoms
Ribavirin	Aerosol: 1.1 g/d as 20 mg/mL dilution over 12–18 hours for 3–7 days (See text for Lassa fever doses.)	RSV, severe influenza A or B, Lassa fever	Yes/No	Yes	Wheezing

(continued)

Table 32–1. Agents for viral infections.[1] (continued)

Drug	Dosing	Spectrum	Renal Clearance/ Hemodialysis	CNS/CSF Penetration	Toxicities
Trifluridine	Topical, 1% drops every 2 hours to 9 drops/d	HSV keratitis	—	—	Local reactions
Valacyclovir	1 g orally three times daily for 7 days for acute VZV; 1 g twice daily for primary genital HSV-1/HSV-2 infection with 500 mg three times daily for recurrences	VZV, HSV	Yes/Poorly	NA	Thrombotic thrombocytopenic purpura or hemolytic-uremic syndrome in AIDS
Valganciclovir	900 mg orally twice daily for 3 weeks; 900 mg daily as maintenance	CMV	Yes/Yes	Yes	See ganciclovir
Vidarabine	15 mg/kg/d intravenously for 10 days	HSV, VZV	Yes/Yes	Yes	Teratogenic, megaloblastosis, neurotoxicity
Zanamivir	2–5 mg inhalations twice daily for 5 days	Influenza A and B	Yes/NA	NA	Few

[1]Agents used exclusively in the management of HIV infection and AIDS are found in Chapter 31.
CNS, central nervous system; CSF, cerebrospinal fluid; HSV, herpes simplex virus; VZV, varicella-zoster virus; HBV, hepatitis B virus; CMV, cytomegalovirus; HPV, human papillomavirus; HCV, hepatitis C virus; RSV, respiratory syncytial virus.

acyclovir, 400 mg five times daily. Maintenance therapy for AIDS patients is acyclovir at a dosage of 400 mg three to five times daily. Proctitis is treated with similar dosages and usually responds within 5 days.

H. Erythema Multiforme

Suppressive therapy with oral acyclovir (400 mg twice a day for 6 months) decreases the recurrence rate of HSV-associated erythema multiforme. Valacyclovir (500 mg twice a day) may be effective in cases unresponsive to acyclovir.

Berger JR et al. Neurological complications of herpes simplex virus type 2 infection. Arch Neurol. 2008 Jun;65(5):596–600. [PMID: 18474734]

Cernik C et al. The treatment of herpes simplex infections: an evidence-based review. Arch Intern Med. 2008 Jun 9;168(11):1137–44. [PMID: 18541820]

Hollier LM et al. Third trimester antiviral prophylaxis for preventing maternal genital herpes simplex virus (HSV) recurrences and neonatal infection. Cochrane Database Syst Rev. 2008 Jan 23;(1):CD004946. [PMID: 18254066]

Koelle DM et al. Herpes simplex: insights on pathogenesis and possible vaccines. Annu Rev Med. 2008;59:381–95. [PMID: 18186706]

2. Varicella (Chickenpox) & Herpes Zoster (Shingles)

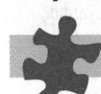

ESSENTIALS OF DIAGNOSIS

▶ Exposure 14–21 days before onset.

▶ Fever and malaise just before or with eruption.

▶ Rash: pruritic, centrifugal, papular, changing to vesicular ("dewdrops on a rose petal"), pustular, and finally crusting.

▶ General Considerations

Varicella zoster virus (VZV) is HHV-3. Disease manifestations include chickenpox (varicella) and shingles (herpes zoster). Chickenpox is generally a disease of the childhood. It has an incubation period of 10–20 days (average 2 weeks) and is highly contagious, spreading by inhalation of infective droplets or contact with lesions.

The incidence and severity of herpes zoster ("shingles") increases with age due to an age-related decline in immunity against VZV. More than half of all patients in whom herpes zoster develops are older than 60 years. The annual incidence of herpes zoster in the United States is at least 1 million cases, which is expected to increase as the mean population age increases.

▶ Clinical Findings

A. Varicella

1. Symptoms and signs—(Table 32–2.) Fever and malaise are mild in children and more marked in adults. The pruritic rash begins prominently on the face, scalp, and trunk, and later involves the extremities. Maculopapules change in a few hours to vesicles that become pustular and eventually form crusts (Plates 95 and 96). New lesions may erupt for 1–5 days, so that different stages of the eruption are usually present simultaneously. The crusts slough in 7–14 days. The vesicles and pustules are superficial and elliptical, with slightly serrated borders. Pitted scars are frequent sequelae.

After the primary infection, the virus remains dormant in cranial nerves sensory ganglia and spinal dorsal root ganglia. Latent VZV will reactivate as herpes zoster in about 10–30% of persons (see below). Varicella is more severe in older patients and immunocompromised persons. In the latter, atypical presentations, including widespread dissemination in the absence of skin lesions, are often described.

Table 32–2. Diagnostic features of some acute exanthems.

Disease	Prodromal Signs and Symptoms	Nature of Eruption	Other Diagnostic Features	Laboratory Tests
Eczema herpeticum	None.	Vesiculopustular lesions in area of eczema.		Herpes simplex virus isolated in cell culture. Multinucleate giant cells in smear of lesion.
Varicella (chicken-pox)	0–1 day of fever, anorexia, head-ache.	Rapid evolution of macules to pap-ules, vesicles, crusts; all stages simultaneously present; lesions superficial, distribution centripetal.	Lesions on scalp and mucous membranes.	Specialized complement fixation and virus neutralization in cell culture. Fluorescent antibody test of smear of lesions.
Infectious mono-nucleosis (EBV)	Fever, adenopa-thy, sore throat.	Maculopapular rash resembling rubella, rarely papulovesicular.	Splenomegaly, tonsillar exudate.	Atypical lymphocytes in blood smears; heterophil agglutina-tion (Monospot test).
Exanthema subi-tum (HHV-6, 7; roseola)	3–4 days of high fever.	As fever falls by crisis, pink macu-lopapules appear on chest and trunk; fade in 1–3 days.		White blood count low.
Measles (rubeola)	3–4 days of fever, coryza, conjunc-tivitis, and cough.	Maculopapular, brick-red; begins on head and neck; spreads down-ward and outward, in 5–6 days rash brownish, desquamating. See atypical measles, below.	Koplik spots on buccal mucosa.	White blood count low. Virus isolation in cell culture. Anti-body tests by hemagglutina-tion inhibition or neutralization.
Atypical measles	Same as measles.	Maculopapular centripetal rash, becoming confluent.	History of measles vaccination.	Measles antibody present in past, with titer rise during illness.
Rubella	Little or no pro-drome.	Maculopapular, pink; begins on head and neck, spreads down-ward, fades in 3 days. No des-quamation.	Lymphadenopathy, post-auricular or occipital.	White blood count normal or low. Serologic tests for immu-nity and definitive diagnosis (hemagglutination inhibition).
Erythema infectio-sum (parvovirus B19)	None. Usually in epidemics.	Red, flushed cheeks; circumoral pallor; maculopapules on extremities.	"Slapped face" appear-ance.	White blood count normal.
Enterovirus infections	1–2 days of fever, malaise.	Maculopapular rash resembling rubella, rarely papulovesicular or petechial.	Aseptic meningitis.	Virus isolation from stool or cerebrospinal fluid; comple-ment fixation titer rise.
Typhus	3–4 days of fever, chills, severe headaches.	Maculopapules, petechiae, initial distribution centrifugal (trunk to extremities).	Endemic area, lice.	Complement fixation.
Rocky Mountain spotted fever	3–4 days of fever, vomiting.	Maculopapules, petechiae, initial distribution centripetal (extremi-ties to trunk, including palms).	History of tick bite.	Indirect fluorescent antibody; complement fixation.
Ehrlichiosis	Headache, malaise.	Rash in one-third, similar to Rocky Mountain spotted fever.	Pancytopenia, elevated liver function tests.	Polymerase chain reaction, immunofluorescent antibody.
Scarlet fever	One-half to 2 days of malaise, sore throat, fever, vomiting.	Generalized, punctate, red; prominent on neck, in axillae, groin, skin folds; circumoral pallor; fine desquama-tion involves hands and feet.	Strawberry tongue, exu-dative tonsillitis.	Group A β-hemolytic strepto-cocci in cultures from throat; antistreptolysin O titer rise.
Meningococcemia	Hours of fever, vomiting.	Maculopapules, petechiae, purpura.	Meningeal signs, toxic-ity, shock.	Cultures of blood, cerebrospinal fluid. High white blood count.
Kawasaki disease	Fever, adenopathy, conjunctivitis.	Cracked lips, strawberry tongue, maculopapular polymorphous rash, peeling skin on fingers and toes.	Edema of extremities. Angiitis of coronary arteries.	Thrombocytosis, electrocardio-graphic changes.
Smallpox (based on prior experience)	Fever, malaise, prostration.	Maculopapules to vesicles to pus-tules to scars (lesions develop at the same pace).	Centrifugal rash; fulmi-nant sepsis in small percentage of patients, gastrointestinal and skin hemorrhages.	Contact CDC[1] for suspicious rash; EM and gel diffusion assays.

[1] http://www.bt.cdc.gov/agent/smallpox/response-plan/.
EBV, Epstein–Barr virus; EM, electron microscopy HHV, human herpesvirus.

2. Laboratory findings—Diagnosis is usually made clinically, with confirmation by direct immunofluorescent antibody (DFA) staining or PCR of scrapings from lesions. Multinucleated giant cells are usually apparent on a Tzanck smear or Calcofluor stain of material from the vesicle bases. Leukopenia and subclinical transaminase elevation are often present and thrombocytopenia occasionally occurs.

B. Herpes Zoster

Herpes zoster ("**shingles**") usually occurs among adults, but cases are reported among infants and children. Skin lesions resemble those of chickenpox. Pain is often severe and commonly precedes the appearance of rash. Lesions follow a dermatomal distribution, with thoracic and lumbar roots being the most common. In most cases, a single unilateral dermatome is involved, but occasionally, neighboring and distant areas are involved. Lesions on the tip of the nose, inner corner of the eye, and root and side of the nose (Hutchinson sign) indicate involvement of the trigeminal nerve (herpes zoster ophthalmicus). Facial palsy, lesions of the external ear with or without tympanic membrane involvement, vertigo and tinnitus, and deafness signify geniculate ganglion involvement (Ramsay Hunt syndrome).

▶ Complications

A. Varicella

Secondary bacterial skin superinfections, particularly with group A β-hemolytic streptococci and *Staphylococcus aureus*, are the most common complications in children. Cellulitis, erysipelas, and scarlet fever are described. Bullous impetigo and necrotizing fasciitis are less often seen. Other associations with varicella include epiglottitis, necrotizing pneumonia, osteomyelitis, septic arthritis, epidural abscess, meningitis, endocarditis, and purpura fulminans. Toxic shock syndrome can also occur.

Interstitial VZV pneumonia is more common in adults (especially smokers, HIV-infected patients, and pregnant women) and may result in acute respiratory distress syndrome (ARDS). After healing, numerous densely calcified lesions are seen throughout the lung fields on chest radiographs.

Cerebellar ataxia occurs among younger people at a frequency of 1:4000. A limited course and complete recovery are the rule. Encephalitis is infrequent (1:1000), occurs mostly in adults, and is characterized by delirium, seizures, and focal neurologic signs. Both mortality and long-term neurologic sequelae rates are about 10%. Ischemic strokes in the wake of acute VZV infection present a mean of 4 months after rashes and may be due to an associated vasculitis. Multifocal encephalitis, ventriculitis, myeloradiculitis, arterial aneurysm formation, and arteritis are also described in immunosuppressed persons.

Clinical hepatitis is uncommon and mostly presents in the immunosuppressed patient but can be fulminant and fatal. Reye syndrome (fatty liver with encephalopathy) also complicates varicella (and other viral infections, especially influenza B), usually in childhood, and is associated with aspirin therapy (see Influenza, below).

When contracted during the first or second trimesters of pregnancy, varicella carries a very small risk of congenital malformations, including cicatricial lesions of an extremity, growth retardation, microphthalmia, cataracts, chorioretinitis, deafness, and cerebrocortical atrophy. If varicella develops around the time of delivery, the newborn is at risk for disseminated disease.

B. Herpes Zoster

Postherpetic neuralgia occurs in 60–70% of patients who have herpes zoster and are older than 60 years. The pain can be prolonged and debilitating. Risk factors for postherpetic neuralgia include age, female sex, prodrome, and severity of rash or pain.

Other less common complications include bacterial skin superinfections; herpes zoster ophthalmicus, which occurs with involvement of the trigeminal nerve and is a sight-threatening complication, especially when it involves the cornea or the iris; involvement of the geniculate ganglion of cranial nerve VII as well as cranial nerves V, VIII, IX, and X; aseptic meningitis; peripheral motor neuropathy; transverse myelitis; encephalitis; vasculopathy; acute retinal necrosis; and progressive outer retinal necrosis (largely among HIV infected persons). VZV is a major cause of Bell palsy in patients who are HSV seronegative. Diagnosis of neurologic complications requires the detection of VZV DNA or anti-VZV IgG in cerebrospinal fluid or the detection of VZV DNA in tissue. Zoster sine herpete (pain without rash) can also be associated with most of the above complications.

▶ Prevention

Health care workers should be screened for varicella and vaccinated if seronegative. Patients with active varicella or herpes zoster are promptly separated from seronegative patients. For those with varicella, airborne and contact isolation is recommended, whereas for those with zoster, contact precautions are sufficient. For immunosuppressed patients with zoster, precautions should be the same as if the patient had varicella. Exposed serosusceptible patients should be placed in isolation and exposed serosusceptible employees should stay away from work between days 10 and 21 after exposure. Health care workers with zoster should receive antivirals during the first 72 hours of disease and withdraw from work until lesions are crusted. Postexposure prophylaxis should be evaluated (see below).

A. Varicella

1. Vaccination—Universal childhood vaccination against varicella is effective. A single antigen live attenuated vaccine (VARIVAX) or a quadrivalent measles, mumps, rubella, and varicella vaccine (ProQuad) are available. The first dose should be administered at 12–15 months of age and the second at 4–6 years. Aspirin should be avoided for at least 6 weeks because of the risk of Reye syndrome. This vaccine is safe, well tolerated, and is not associated with neurologic sequelae. Rashes, when secondary to the varicella vaccine, appear 15–42 days after vaccination.

For serosusceptible individuals older than 13 years, two doses of varicella vaccine (single antigen) administered 4 to 8 weeks apart is recommended. For those who received a single dose in the past, a catch-up second dose is advised. Household contacts of immunocompromised patients should adhere to these recommendations. Susceptible pregnant women need to receive the first dose of vaccine before discharge after delivery and the second dose 4–8 weeks later.

The vaccine, administered 3 months apart, should also be considered for HIV-infected children with age-specific CD4+ T lymphocyte percentages of 15–24% and adolescents and adults with CD4+ T lymphocyte counts ≥ 200 cells/mcL. The vaccine may also be given to patients with impaired humoral immunity or receiving corticosteroids at a dose < 2 mg/kg or a total of < 20 mg/d of prednisone. Persons who are receiving higher doses for over 2 weeks may be vaccinated after the corticosteroid therapy has been discontinued for over 1 month. Patients with leukemia, lymphoma, or other malignancies whose disease is in remission and who have not undergone chemotherapy for at least 3 months may be vaccinated, although the presence of both ancillary antiviral treatment and expert guidance are encouraged.

2. Postexposure—Postexposure vaccination is recommended for unvaccinated persons without other evidence of immunity. Varicella-zoster immune globulin (VZIG) (in short supply with production stopped in 2004) or VariZIG (a lyophilized product available under expanded access since December 2007) should be considered for susceptible exposed patients who cannot receive the vaccine, including immunosuppressed patients, neonates from mothers with varicella around the time of delivery, exposed premature infants born from serosusceptible mothers at > 28 weeks of gestation, neonates born at < 28 weeks of gestation regardless of maternal serostatus, and pregnant women. No controlled studies have evaluated the use of acyclovir in this setting. VZIG is given by intramuscular injection in a dosage of 12.5 units/kg up to a maximum of 625 units, with a repeat identical dose in 3 weeks if a high-risk patient remains exposed. VZIG has no place in therapy of established disease.

Further information may be obtained by calling the Centers for Disease Control and Prevention's Immunization Information Hotline (800-232-2522).

B. Herpes Zoster

A live attenuated VZV vaccine is available and should be offered to persons 60 years and older. In this population, the vaccine reduces the incidence of postherpetic neuralgia and herpes zoster by 67% and 51%, respectively.

Prophylaxis with acyclovir, 800 mg twice daily, can be considered in patients at high risk for reactivation (eg, allogeneic hematopoietic cell transplant patients).

▶ Treatment

A. General Measures

In general, patients with varicella should be isolated until primary crusts have disappeared and kept at bed rest until afebrile. The skin is kept clean. Pruritus can be relieved with antihistamines, calamine lotion, and colloidal oatmeal baths. As an antipyretic, acetaminophen is used. Fingernails can be closely cropped to avoid skin excoriation and infection.

B. Antiviral Therapy

Acyclovir, 20 mg/kg (up to 800 mg per dose) orally four times daily for 5 days, should be given within the first 24 hours after the onset of rash and should be considered for patients older than 12 years, secondary household contacts (secondary cases tend to be more severe disease), patients with chronic cutaneous and cardiopulmonary diseases, and children receiving long-term therapy with salicylates (to decrease the risk of Reye syndrome). Experience with valacyclovir and famciclovir in these settings is scant.

In immunocompromised patients, in pregnant women during the third trimester, and in patients with extracutaneous disease (encephalitis, pneumonitis), antiviral therapy with high-dose acyclovir (30 mg/kg/d in three divided doses intravenously for at least 7 days) should be started once the diagnosis is suspected. Corticosteroids may be useful in the presence of pneumonia.

For uncomplicated herpes zoster, acyclovir (800 mg orally five times daily) or valacyclovir (1 g three times daily) for 7 days is recommended. Therapy should start within the first 72 hours of the onset of the lesions. Intravenous acyclovir is used for extradermatomal complications of zoster, although acyclovir is not fully effective in retinal disease. Foscarnet may be used for acyclovir-resistant VZV infections seen in immunosuppressed patients. The Ramsay Hunt syndrome is less responsive to antiviral therapy.

C. Treatment of Complications

Once established, postherpetic neuralgia may respond to gabapentin or lidocaine patches (FDA approved drugs for neuropathic pain). Tricyclic antidepressants, opioids, and capsaicin cream are also widely used and effective. The epidural injection of corticosteroids and local anesthetics appears to modestly reduce herpetic pain at 1 month but is not effective for prevention of long-term postherpetic neuralgia. Secondary bacterial infections are treated with antibiotics providing coverage for staphylococci.

▶ Prognosis

The total duration of varicella from onset of symptoms to disappearance of crusts rarely exceeds 2 weeks. Fatalities are rare except in immunosuppressed patients.

Herpes zoster resolves in 2–6 weeks. Antibodies persist longer and at higher levels than with primary varicella. Eye involvement with herpes zoster necessitates periodic future examinations.

Macartney K et al. Vaccines for post-exposure prophylaxis against varicella (chickenpox) in children and adults. Cochrane Database Syst Rev. 2008 Jul 16;(3):CD001833. [PMID: 18646079]

Marin M et al. Prevention of varicella: recommendations of the Advisory Committee on Immunization Practices (ACIP). MMWR Recomm Rep.2007 Jun 22;56(RR-4):1–40. [PMID: 17585291]

Nagel MA et al. The varicella zoster viral vasculopathies: clinical, CSF, imaging, and virologic features. Neurology. 2008 Mar 11;70(11):853–60. [PMID: 18332343]

Oxman MN et al; Shingles Prevention Study Group. A vaccine to prevent herpes zoster and postherpetic neuralgia in older adults. N Engl J Med. 2005 Jun 2;352(22):2271–84. [PMID: 15930418]

Uscategui T et al. Corticosteroids as adjuvant to antiviral treatment in Ramsay Hunt syndrome (herpes zoster oticus with facial palsy) in adults. Cochrane Database Syst Rev. 2008 Jul 16;(3):CD006852. [PMID: 18646170]

3. Epstein–Barr Virus & Infectious Mononucleosis

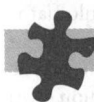 ESSENTIALS OF DIAGNOSIS

▶ Malaise, fever, and sore throat, sometimes with exudates.

▶ Palatal petechiae, lymphadenopathy, splenomegaly, and, occasionally, a maculopapular rash.

▶ Positive heterophil agglutination test (Monospot).

▶ Atypical large lymphocytes in blood smear; lymphocytosis.

▶ Possible complications: hepatitis, myocarditis, neuropathy, encephalitis, airway obstruction secondary to lymph node enlargement, anti-i hemolytic anemia, thrombocytopenia.

▶ General Considerations

Infectious mononucleosis is usually due to the EBV (HHV-4). More than 90% of adults worldwide are seropositive for EBV. Infectious mononucleosis may be seen at any age but usually occurs in the United States in persons between the ages of 10 and 35 years, sporadically or epidemically. In the developing world, infectious mononucleosis occurs at younger ages and tends to be less symptomatic. Rare cases in the elderly occur usually without the full symptomatology. EBV is largely transmitted by saliva but can also be recovered from genital secretions. Saliva may remain infectious during convalescence for 6 months or longer from symptom onset. The incubation period lasts several weeks.

▶ Clinical Findings

A. Symptoms and Signs

The protean manifestations of infectious mononucleosis reflect the dissemination of the virus in the oral cavity and through peripheral blood lymphocytes and cell-free plasma (Plate 97). Fever, sore throat, fatigue, malaise, anorexia, and myalgia typically occur in the early phase of the illness. Physical findings include lymphadenopathy (discrete, non-suppurative, slightly painful, especially along the posterior cervical chain) and splenomegaly (in up to 50% of patients). A maculopapular or occasionally petechial rash occurs in less than 15% of patients unless ampicillin has been given (when rash is seen in > 90%). Exudative pharyngitis, tonsillitis, or gingivitis may occur and soft palatal petechiae may be noted.

Other manifestations include hepatitis, cholestasis, nervous system involvement (mononeuropathies and occasionally aseptic meningitis, encephalitis, optic neuritis, transverse myelitis, or Guillain–Barré syndrome), kidney disease (mostly interstitial nephritis), pneumonia, pleural involvement, and myocarditis. Airway obstruction from lymph node enlargement, pericarditis, life-threatening thrombocytopenia, severe CNS complications, and massive splenomegaly are all considered indications for hospitalization or close observation. Mesenteric adenitis may mimic acute abdomen.

B. Laboratory Findings

Initially infectious mononucleosis is associated with granulocytopenia followed within 1 week by a lymphocytic leukocytosis (> 50% of all leukocytes) with atypical lymphocytes (larger than normal mature lymphocytes, staining more darkly, and showing vacuolated, foamy cytoplasm and dark nuclear chromatin) comprising more than 10% of the leukocyte count. Hemolytic anemia, with anti-i antibodies, occurs occasionally as does thrombocytopenia (at times marked).

Heterophil (sheep cell agglutination) antibody tests and the correlated mononucleosis spot (Monospot) test usually become positive within 4 weeks after onset of illness and are specific but often not sensitive in early illness. During acute illness, there occurs a rise and fall in immunoglobulin M (IgM) antibody to EB virus capsid antigen (VCA) and a rise in IgG antibody to VCA, which persists for life. Antibodies (IgG) to EBV nuclear antigen (EBNA) appear after 4 weeks of onset and also persist. Absence of IgG and IgM VCA or the presence of IgG EBNA should make one reconsider the diagnosis of acute EBV infection. PCR for EBV DNA is useful in the evaluation of malignancies associated with EBV. For instance, detection of EBV DNA in cerebrospinal fluid shows a sensitivity of 90% and specificity of nearly 100% for the diagnosis of primary CNS lymphoma in patients with AIDS. Monitoring of EBV DNA load in blood may be useful in early detection of posttransplant lymphoproliferative disorder in high-risk patients. PCR analysis may also be helpful in detecting primary infection and infectious mononucleosis in children, in narrowing the differential diagnosis of CNS processes, and in monitoring disease and treatment response in primary CNS lymphoma and posttransplant lymphoproliferative disorder. Detection of specific IgA antibodies is also being studied as a marker of primary infection in children. Hepatic aminotransferases and bilirubin are commonly elevated. In aseptic meningitis, the cerebrospinal fluid may show increased opening pressure, lymphocytosis with abnormal morphology, and increased protein concentration.

▶ Differential Diagnosis

CMV infection, toxoplasmosis, acute HIV infection, secondary syphilis, HHV-6, rubella, and drug hypersensitivity reactions may be indistinguishable from infectious mononucleosis due to EBV, but exudative pharyngitis is usually absent and the heterophil antibody tests are negative. With acute HIV infection, rash and mucocutaneous ulceration are common but atypical lymphocytosis is much less common. Heterophil-negative infectious mononucleosis with nonsignificant lymphocytosis (especially if rash or mucocutaneous ulcers are present) should prompt investigation for acute HIV infection. Heterophil-negative infectious mononucleosis with atypical lymphocytosis can be caused by CMV, toxoplasmosis and, on occasion, EBV itself. Mycoplasmal infection may also present as pharyngitis, though lower respiratory symptoms usually predominate. A hypersensitivity syndrome induced by carbamazepine or phenytoin may mimic infectious mononucleosis.

The differential diagnosis of acute exudative pharyngitis includes diphtheria, gonococcal and streptococcal infections, and infections with adenovirus and herpes simplex. Head and neck soft tissue infections (pharyngeal and tonsillar abscesses) may occasionally be mistaken as the lymphadenopathy of mononucleosis.

► Complications

Secondary bacterial pharyngitis can occur and is often streptococcal. Splenic rupture is a rare but dramatic complication, and a history of preceding trauma can be elicited in 50% of the cases. Acalculous cholecystitis, fulminant hepatitis with massive necrosis, pericarditis and myocarditis are also infrequent complications. Neurologic involvement—including transverse myelitis, encephalitis, and Guillain–Barré syndrome—is infrequent.

► Treatment

A. General Measures

Over 95% of patients recover without specific antiviral therapy. Treatment is symptomatic with acetaminophen or other nonsteroidal anti-inflammatory drugs and warm saline throat irrigations or gargles three or four times daily. Acyclovir decreases viral shedding but has no clinical benefit. Corticosteroid therapy, although widespread, is not recommended in uncomplicated cases; its use is reserved for impending airway obstruction from enlarged lymph nodes, hemolytic anemia, and severe thrombocytopenia. The value of corticosteroid therapy in impending splenic rupture, pericarditis, myocarditis, and nervous system involvement is less well defined. If a throat culture grows β-hemolytic streptococci, a 10-day course of penicillin or erythromycin is indicated. Ampicillin and amoxicillin are avoided because of the frequent association with rash.

B. Treatment of Complications

Hepatitis, myocarditis, and encephalitis are treated symptomatically. Rupture of the spleen requires splenectomy and is most often caused by deep palpation of the spleen or vigorous activity. Patients should avoid contact or collision sports for at least 4 weeks to decrease the risk of splenic rupture (even if splenomegaly is not detected by physical examination which can be insensitive).

► Prognosis

In cases without complications, fever disappears in 10 days and lymphadenopathy and splenomegaly in 4 weeks. The debility sometimes lingers for 2–3 months.

Death is uncommon and is usually due to splenic rupture, hypersplenic phenomena (severe hemolytic anemia, thrombocytopenic purpura), or encephalitis.

4. Other Epstein–Barr Virus Syndromes

EBV viral antigens have been found in over 90% of patients with African Burkitt lymphoma or nasopharyngeal carcinoma (among whom quantified EBV DNA can be used to follow disease). A causative role for EBV has been postulated with both neoplasms. Chronic EBV infection is associated with aberrant cellular immunity (a low frequency of EBV-specific CD8 cells), an X-linked lymphoproliferative syndrome (Duncan disease), lymphomatoid granulomatosis, and a fatal T cell lymphoproliferative disorder in children. EBV is an important cause of hemophagocytic lymphohistiocytosis EBV-induced lymphoproliferation gives rise to B-cell lymphomas among immunodeficient patients, such as primary CNS lymphoma in HIV-infected individuals or posttransplant lymphoproliferative disorder in persons who have undergone transplantation. Rituximab (CD20 monoclonal antibody) is effective in treating some cases of posttransplant lymphoproliferative disorder and is often administered in conjunction with monitoring levels of EBV DNA load in the blood and, if indicated, CNS. Infusion of EBV-specific cytotoxic T cell lymphocytes (adoptive cell therapy) is also used but with a less established role.

Age is a major determinant of the type of tumor EBV causes, with T and NK cell tumors in childhood caused by chronic active EBV infections and peripheral T cell lymphomas and diffuse large B cell lymphomas in the elderly due to waning immunity. EBV is also associated with leiomyomas in children with AIDS and with nasal T cell lymphomas. There is no persuasive evidence that chronic fatigue syndrome is caused by EBV infection. Oral hairy leukoplakia and its association with EBV are discussed in Chapter 8.

EBV is also implicated in the pathogenesis of a host of disorders from Hodgkin disease and gastric carcinoma to multiple sclerosis, chronic obstructive pulmonary disease (COPD), and rheumatic diseases.

► When to Admit

- Acute meningitis, encephalitis, or acute Guillain-Barré.
- Severe thrombocytopenia.
- Potential splenic rupture.
- Airway obstruction from severe adenitis.
- Significant hemolysis.
- Pericarditis.
- Abdominal findings mimicking an acute abdomen.

Brady G et al. Epstein-Barr virus and Burkitt lymphoma. J Clin Pathol. 2007 Dec;60(12):1397–402. [PMID: 18042696]

Merlo A et al. Adoptive cell therapy against EBV-related malignancies: a survey of clinical results. Expert Opin Biol Ther. 2008 Sep;8(9):1265–94. [PMID: 18694349]

Rouphael NG et al. Infections associated with haemophagocytic syndrome. Lancet Infect Dis. 2007 Dec;7(12):814–22. [PMID: 18045564]

Shimomaya Y et al. Age-related Epstein-Barr virus-associated B-cell lymphoproliferative disorders: special references to lymphomas surrounding this newly recognized clinicopatholgic disease. Cancer Sci. 2008 Jun;99(6):1085–91. [PMID: 18429953]

5. Cytomegalovirus Disease

ESSENTIALS OF DIAGNOSIS

- ▶ Mononucleosis-like syndrome.
- ▶ Frequent pathogen seen in transplant populations.
- ▶ Diverse clinical syndromes in HIV (retinitis, esophagitis, pneumonia, encephalitis).
- ▶ Major pathogen to consider in neonates in the differential of maternally transmitted agents.

▶ General Considerations

Most CMV infections are asymptomatic. After primary infection, the virus remains latent in different cells including vascular endothelium, monocytes, macrophages, polymorphonuclear neutrophils, and renal and pulmonary epithelial cells. Seroprevalence in adults of Western developed countries is about 60–80% but is higher in developing countries. CMV seroprevalence increases with age, number of sexual partners, history of prior STIs, and low socioeconomic status. The virus can be isolated from a variety of tissues under nonpathogenic conditions. Transmission occurs through sexual contact, breastfeeding, blood products, or transplantation; it may also occur person-to-person (eg, day care centers) or be congenital. Serious disease occurs primarily in immunocompromised persons.

There are three recognizable clinical syndromes: (1) perinatal disease and CMV inclusion disease; (2) diseases in immunocompetent persons; and (3) diseases in immunocompromised persons. **Congenital CMV infection** is the most common congenital infection in developed countries (1% of all neonates). Transmission is much higher from mothers with primary disease than those with reactivation. About 10% of infected newborns will be symptomatic with CMV inclusion disease. In **immunocompetent persons**, acute CMV infection is the most common cause of mononucleosis-like syndrome with negative heterophil antibodies. CMV appears to play a role in critically ill immunocompetent adults wherein it is reactivated and associated with prolonged hospitalization and death. Other syndromes associated with CMV and whose role in pathogenesis requires further elucidation include inflammatory bowel disease, atherosclerosis, cognitive decline, and breast cancer. In **immunocompromised persons**, tissue and bone marrow transplant patients are mainly at risk in the first 100 days after allograft transplantation and in particular when graft-versus-host disease or CMV seropositivity, or both, are present in the donor and recipient. Depending on the serostatus of the donor and recipient, disease may present as primary infection or reactivation. The risk of CMV disease is proportionate to the intensity of immunosuppression. CMV is itself immunosuppressive. CMV may contribute to transplanted organ dysfunction, which often mimics organ rejection. CMV disease in HIV-infected patients (retinitis, serious gastrointestinal disease) occurs most prominently when the CD4 count is < 50 cells/mcL. HAART reduces the frequency of retinitis and may reverse active disease. CMV retinitis may also develop after solid organ or bone marrow transplantation. CMV retinitis associated with intravitreal delivery of corticosteroids (injections or implants) or systemic anti-tumor necrosis factor-α antibodies is also described. Occasionally, CMV retinitis presents in immunocompetent persons. Serious gastrointestinal CMV disease also occurs after organ transplantation, cancer chemotherapy, or corticosteroid therapy. CMV has been identified—often with other pathogens such as *Cryptosporidium*—in up to 15% of patients with AIDS cholangiopathy. CMV pneumonitis occurs in transplant recipients (mainly bone marrow and lung) with a mortality rate up to 60–80%, and less commonly in AIDS patients. CMV pneumonitis in hematologic malignancies (eg, lymphoma) is increasingly reported. Neurologic CMV in patients with advanced AIDS is usually associated with disseminated CMV infection.

▶ Clinical Findings

A. Symptoms and Signs

1. Perinatal disease and CMV inclusion disease—CMV inclusion disease in infected newborns is characterized by jaundice, hepatosplenomegaly, thrombocytopenia, purpura, microcephaly, periventricular CNS calcifications, mental retardation, and motor disability. Hearing loss develops in greater than 50% of infants who are symptomatic at birth. Most infected neonates are asymptomatic, but neurologic deficits may ensue later in life. Perinatal infection acquired through breastfeeding or blood products typically shows a benign clinical course.

2. Disease in immunocompetent persons—Acute acquired CMV infection is characterized by fever, malaise, myalgias and arthralgias, and splenomegaly. Exudative pharyngitis or cervical lymphadenopathies are uncommon, but cutaneous rashes (including the typical maculopapular rash after exposure to ampicillin) are common. The mean duration of symptoms is 7–8 weeks. Notorious complications include mucosal gastrointestinal damage, encephalitis, severe hepatitis, Guillain–Barré syndrome, pericarditis, and myocarditis.

3. Disease in immunocompromised persons

A. CMV RETINITIS—A funduscopic examination reveals neovascular, proliferative lesions ("pizza-pie" retinopathy). Immune restoration with HAART is associated with CMV vitreitis and cystoid macular edema. Infants with CMV retinitis tend to have more macular than peripheral disease.

B. GASTROINTESTINAL AND HEPATOBILIARY CMV—Esophagitis presents with odynophagia. Gastritis can occasionally cause bleeding, and small bowel disease may mimic inflammatory bowel disease or may present as ulceration or perforation. Colonic CMV disease causes diarrhea, hematochezia, abdominal pain, fever, and weight loss. CMV hepatitis commonly complicates liver transplantation.

C. Respiratory CMV—CMV pneumonitis is characterized by cough, dyspnea, and relatively little sputum production.

D. Neurologic CMV—Neurologic syndromes associated with CMV include polyradiculopathy, transverse myelitis, ventriculoencephalitis (suspected with ependymitis), and focal encephalitis. These manifestations are more prominent in patients with advanced AIDS in whom the encephalitis has a subacute onset.

B. Laboratory Findings

PCR assays of dried blood samples from neonates are becoming the easiest method of diagnosing congenital CMV infection and are preferred over serologies or classic throat or urine cultures.

1. Immunocompetent persons—The acute mononucleosis-like syndrome is characterized by initial leukopenia; within 1 week, it is followed by absolute lymphocytosis with atypical lymphocytes. Abnormal liver function tests are common in the first 2 weeks of the disease (often 2 weeks after the fever). Detection of specific IgM or a fourfold increase of specific IgG levels support the diagnosis of acute infection.

2. Immunocompromised persons—CMV retinitis is diagnosed on the basis of the characteristic ophthalmoscopic findings. In HIV-infected patients, negative CMV serologies lower the possibility of the diagnosis but do not eliminate it. Cultures alone are of little use in diagnosing AIDS-related CMV infections, since viral shedding of CMV is common. PCR analysis should be used to diagnose CNS infection since cultures are insensitive.

Detection of pp65 antigen in blood and determination of CMV viral load by PCR are increasingly used in post-transplant patients for guidance on both treatment and prevention and should be interpreted in the context of clinical and pathologic findings. PCR appears to be more useful in predicting clinical disease. Quantitative PCR of bronchoalveolar lavage fluid seems to be useful for diagnosing CMV pneumonia.

Rapid shell-vial cultures for detection of early CMV antigens with fluorescent antibodies have largely replaced the conventional tube culture (for detection of cytopathic changes) since the time to positivity is greatly reduced (24–48 hours compared to weeks).

A variety of false-positive immunologic assays occur in the setting of acute CMV infections, including positive rheumatoid factor, direct Coombs test, cryoglobulins, and speckled antinuclear antibody.

C. Imaging

The chest radiographic findings of CMV pneumonitis are consistent with interstitial pneumonia.

D. Biopsy

Tissue confirmation is especially useful in diagnosing CMV pneumonitis and CMV gastrointestinal disease; the diagnosis of colonic CMV disease is made by mucosal biopsy showing characteristic CMV histopathologic findings of intranuclear ("owl's eye") and intracytoplasmic inclusions.

► Prevention

No vaccine is currently available. HAART is effective in preventing CMV infections in HIV-infected patients. Use of leukocyte-depleted blood products effectively reduces the incidence of CMV disease in patients who have undergone transplantation. Prophylactic and preemptive strategies (eg, antivirals only when antigen detection or PCR assays show evidence of active CMV replication) are effective in preventing disease in the early transplantation period but are associated with a risk of a late-onset form of the disease after the prophylaxis is discontinued. All effective anti-CMV agents can serve as prophylactic agents for CMV-seropositive transplants or for CMV-seronegative recipients of CMV-positive organ transplants. CMV immune globulin may be useful in reducing the incidence of bronchiolitis obliterans in the bone marrow transplant population and is used in some centers as part of the prophylaxis in kidney, liver, and lung transplantation patients.

Withdrawal of infected children from day care centers, reduction of patient contact by health care workers, screening for women of childbearing age, or restrictions to breastfeeding are not recommended because the virus is ubiquitous.

► Treatment

Sight-threatening CMV retinitis (lesions close to the fovea or optic nerve head) is treated with ganciclovir induction therapy (5 mg/kg intravenously every 12 hours for 14–21 days) followed by maintenance therapy at lower doses (5 mg/kg intravenously daily). Sustained-release ganciclovir intraocular implants (always accompanied by systemic valganciclovir) are another option. In less severe retinal disease, valganciclovir (900 mg twice daily for 14–21 days followed by 900 mg/d maintenance) is preferred. Due to potential toxicities, foscarnet, cidofovir, and fomivirsen are usually reserved for CMV infections that are resistant to ganciclovir. Combinations of ganciclovir and foscarnet are shown to be safe and effective in treating clinically resistant CMV retinitis. The role of HAART in reducing the need for CMV antivirals is essential. Other forms of CMV disease in AIDS are managed initially with intravenous ganciclovir and subsequently with oral valganciclovir; alternative agents (listed above) are used when resistance evolves.

Therapy for CMV disease resulting from a transplantation procedure is ganciclovir (at same doses as for retinitis) for 2–3 weeks. Oral valganciclovir (900 mg twice daily for 21 days followed by 900 mg daily for 28 days) is noninferior to intravenous ganciclovir-based therapy in solid organ transplant patients with CMV disease and is associated with less clinical resistance than ganciclovir. Dosage adjustments of all medications are needed for kidney dysfunction. Reduction of immunosuppression should be attempted when possible (especially for muromonab, azathioprine, or mycophenolate mofetil). New agents that may be useful in resistant CMV infections include leflunomide, sirolimus-based therapy, and artenusate.

In pregnant women with primary CMV infection, passive immunization with hyperimmune globulin appears preliminarily to be effective in both treatment and prevention of fetal infection, but controlled clinical trials are lacking.

When to Refer

- Neonatal infections consistent with CMV inclusion disease.
- AIDS patients with retinitis, esophagitis, colitis, hepatobiliary disease, or encephalitis.
- Organ transplants with suspected reactivation CMV.

When to Admit

- Risk of colonic perforation.
- Evaluation of unexplained, advancing encephalopathy.
- Biopsy of tissues in the differential diagnosis of transplant rejection vs infection.
- Initiation of treatment with intravenous anti-CMV agents.

Avery RK. Update in management of ganciclovir-resistant cytomegalovirus infection. Curr Opin Infect Dis. 2008 Aug;21(4):433–7. [PMID: 18594298]

Baroco AL et al. Gastrointestinal cytomegalovirus disease in the immunocompromised patient. Curr Gastroenterol Rep. 2008 Aug;10(4):409–16. [PMID: 18627655]

Kedhar SR et al. Cytomegalovirus retinitis in the era of highly active antiretroviral therapy. Herpes. 2007 Dec;14(3):66–71. [PMID: 18371289]

Limaye AP et al. Cytomegalovirus reactivation in critically ill immunocompetent patients. JAMA. 2008 Jun 23;300(4):413–22. [PMID: 18647984]

6. Human Herpesviruses 6, 7, & 8

HHV-6 is a B cell lymphotropic virus that is the principal cause of exanthema subitum (roseola infantum, sixth disease). Primary HHV-6 infection occurs most commonly in children under 2 years of age and is a major cause of infantile febrile seizures. HHV-6 is also associated with encephalitis and with acute liver failure. Primary infection in immunocompetent adults is rare and can produce a mononucleosis-like illness. Reactivation of HHV-6 in immunocompetent adults is rare and can present as encephalitis. Infection during pregnancy and congenital transmission is recognized. Most cases of reactivation, however, occur in immunocompromised persons. Reactivation is associated with graft rejection and bone marrow suppression in transplant patients and with encephalitis and pneumonitis in AIDS patients and in recipients of hematopoietic cell transplants. HHV-6 is on occasion also associated with drug-induced hypersensitivity syndromes that may evolve into diabetes mellitus. The roles of HHV-6 in multiple sclerosis, chronic fatigue syndrome, certain malignancies, myocarditis and progressive multifocal leukoencephalopathy remain unproven.

Two variants (A and B) of HHV-6 have been identified. HHV-6B is the predominant strain found in both normal and immunocompromised persons. Ganciclovir and foscarnet (but not acyclovir) appear to be clinically active against HHV-6.

HHV-7 is a T cell lymphotropic virus that is associated with roseola (serologically), seizures and, rarely, encephalitis. Pregnant women are often infected. Infection with HHV-7 is synergistic with CMV in kidney transplant recipients. The membrane glycoprotein CD4 is involved in HHV-7 recognition, but a clinical interaction between HHV-7 and HIV is not established.

HHV-8 is associated with Kaposi sarcoma, multicentric Castleman disease and primary effusion (body cavity) lymphoma. See Chapter 31 for pathogenesis and management.

Caserta MT et al. Human herpesvirus (HHV)-6 and HHV-7 infections in pregnant women. J Infect Dis. 2007 Nov 1;196(9):1296–303. [PMID: 17922393]

Gewurz BE et al. Human herpesvirus 6 encephalitis. Curr Infect Dis Rep. 2008 Jul;10(4):292–9. [PMID: 18765102]

MAJOR VACCINE-PREVENTABLE VIRAL INFECTIONS

1. Measles

 ESSENTIALS OF DIAGNOSIS

▶ Exposure 10–14 days before onset in an unvaccinated patient.

▶ Prodrome of fever, coryza, cough, conjunctivitis, malaise, irritability, photophobia, Koplik spots.

▶ Rash: brick-red, irregular, maculopapular; onset 3–4 days after onset of prodrome; begins on the face and proceeds "downward and outward," affecting the palms and soles last.

▶ Leukopenia.

General Considerations

Measles is a reportable acute systemic paramyxoviral infection transmitted by inhalation of infective droplets. It is a major worldwide cause of pediatric morbidity and mortality, with nearly 800,000 estimated deaths annually. Illness confers permanent immunity. It is highly contagious and communicability is greatest during the preeruptive and catarrhal stages but continues as long as the rash remains. The largest recent outbreak in the Americas was in São Paulo, Brazil, in 1997, with over 42,000 cases among largely unvaccinated young adults. This and other sporadic recent outbreaks of the disease in adults, adolescents, and unvaccinated preschool children in dense urban areas and among sporting events participants emphasize the need for specific recommendations concerning prevention (see below).

In the United States, measles was declared eliminated in 2000. The few reported cases since then are largely imported and geographically dispersed, and the associated isolates fail to show a recurrent strain. Although the number of cases reported during the first half of 2008 was significantly higher than that for previous years, most cases were again associated with importation, especially from

Europe. New immigrants and refugees can show serosusceptibility rates to measles in excess of 35%.

▶ Clinical Findings

A. Symptoms and Signs

(Table 32–2.) Fever is often as high as 40–40.6 °C. It persists through the prodrome and early rash (about 5–7 days). Malaise may be marked. Coryza (nasal obstruction, sneezing, and sore throat) resembles that seen with upper respiratory infections. Cough is persistent and nonproductive. Conjunctivitis manifests as redness, swelling, photophobia, and discharge. These symptoms intensify over the 2–4 days before the onset of the rash and peak on the first day of the rash.

Koplik spots (small, irregular, and red with whitish center on the mucous membranes) are pathognomonic of measles. They appear about 2 days before the rash and last 1–4 days as tiny "table salt crystals" in the buccal mucosa opposite the molars and vaginal membranes. The rash usually appears on the face and behind the ears 4 days after the onset of symptoms. The initial lesions are pinhead-sized papules that coalesce to form a brick-red, irregular, blotchy maculopapular rash. In severe cases, the rash coalesces to form a nearly uniform erythema on some body areas. The rash next appears on the trunk, followed by the extremities, including the palms (25–50% of those infected) and soles. The rash lasts for 3–7 days and fades in the same manner it appeared. Hyperpigmentation remains in fair-skinned individuals and severe cases. Slight desquamation may follow.

Other findings in measles include pharyngeal erythema, a tonsillar yellowish exudate, coating of the tongue in the center with a red tip and margins, moderate generalized lymphadenopathy and, at times, splenomegaly.

Atypical measles is a syndrome occurring in adults who received inactivated measles vaccine (1963–1968) or who received live measles vaccine before age 12 months and as a result developed hypersensitivity rather than protective immunity. When persons are infected later with wild measles virus, a potentially fatal illness may develop, with high fever; unusual rashes (papular, hemorrhagic), most prominent on the extremities, without Koplik spots; headache; arthralgias; hepatitis; a high rate of pneumonitis, and sometimes pleural effusions. Measles antibody titers tend to be very high after the appearance of the exanthem.

Measles may be distinctive in HIV-infected individuals, with higher rates of pneumonitis, higher mortality, and prolonged viral shedding. Vaccine failure rates, primary and secondary, are higher in HIV-infected children. The frequent difficulty in establishing a diagnosis suggests that measles may be more prevalent in epidemics than heretofore recognized.

Measles during pregnancy is not known to cause congenital abnormalities of the fetus. It is, however, associated with spontaneous abortion and premature delivery and can cause severe disease in the mother. Although measles does not always develop in the offspring of mothers with the disease, it can be severe when it does. It is therefore recommended that infants born to such mothers be passively immunized with immunoglobulin at birth.

The virologic clearance of measles can take months.

B. Laboratory Findings

Leukopenia is usually present unless secondary bacterial complications exist. A lymphocyte count under 2000/mcL is a poor prognostic sign. Thrombocytopenia is common. Proteinuria is often observed. Although technically difficult, virus can be cultured from nasopharyngeal washings and from blood. Detection of IgM measles antibodies with enzyme-linked immunosorbent assay (ELISA) or a fourfold rise in serum hemagglutination inhibition antibody supports the diagnosis. Fluorescent antibody staining of respiratory or urinary epithelial cells can also confirm the diagnosis. PCR techniques are available in research settings.

▶ Differential Diagnosis

Measles is usually diagnosed clinically but may be mistaken for other exanthematous infections (see Table 32–2).

▶ Complications

A. Central Nervous System

Postinfectious encephalomyelitis occurs in about 0.05–0.1% of cases. Higher rates of encephalitis occur in adolescents and adults than in school-aged children. Its onset is usually 3–7 days after the rash. Vomiting, convulsions, coma, and diverse, severe neurologic symptoms and signs may develop. Treatment is symptomatic and supportive. Virus is usually not found in the CNS, though demyelination is prominent. There is an appreciable mortality rate (10–20%), and 33% of survivors are left with neurologic deficit.

A similar form, "inclusion body encephalitis," occurs months after exposure. This complication is reported to occur after measles vaccination in patients with inadequate cellular immunity but is associated with isolation of the measles virus.

Subacute sclerosing panencephalitis (SSPE) is a very late CNS complication (5–15 years after infection); the measles virus acts as a "slow virus" to produce degenerative CNS disease years after the initial infection. SSPE is rare (1:100,000 cases of measles) and occurs more often when measles develops early in life among males who live in rural environments. SSPE very rarely develops in adults.

Measles virus can opportunistically invade the CNS. An acute progressive encephalitis (subacute measles encephalitis), characterized by seizures, neurologic deficits, and often progressive stupor and death, can occur among immunosuppressed patients. Treatment is supportive, withholding immunosuppressive chemotherapy when feasible. Interferon and ribavirin are variably successful.

B. Respiratory Tract Disease

Early in the course of the disease, bronchopneumonia or bronchiolitis due to the measles virus may occur in up to 5% of patients and result in serious respiratory difficulties.

Bronchiectases may occur in up to a quarter of nonvaccinated children. Pneumonia occurring with or without an evanescent rash is seen in atypical measles.

C. Secondary Bacterial Infections

Immediately following measles, secondary bacterial infection, particularly cervical adenitis, otitis media (the most common complication), and pneumonia, occurs in about 15% of patients.

D. Immune Reactivity

Measles produces temporary anergy to cell-mediated skin tests.

E. Gastroenteritis

Diarrhea and protein-losing enteropathy (prodromal rectal Koplik spots may be seen) are significant complications among malnourished children.

F. Other Complications

Other complications include conjunctivitis, keratitis, and otosclerosis.

▶ Prevention

In the United States, children receive their first vaccine dose at 12–15 months and a second at age 4–6 years prior to entry into school (see Table 32–2). Combination measles-mumps-rubella-varicella vaccines (MMRV) can be used in place of the traditional measles, mumps, and rubella (MMR) vaccine.

American students beyond high school and medical staff starting employment require documentation of the above vaccination schedule or must show serologic evidence of immunity if they were born after 1956. For individuals born before 1957, herd immunity is assumed. Health care workers, immigrants, and refugees should be screened and vaccinated if necessary regardless of date of birth.

In outbreaks occurring in infants under 1 year of age, initial vaccination may be given at 6 months, with repeat at 15 months. When outbreaks take place in day care centers, K–12 institutions, or colleges and universities, revaccination is probably indicated for all, in particular for students and their siblings born after 1956 who do not have documentation of immunity as defined above. Susceptible personnel who have been exposed should be isolated from patient contact between the fifth and the twenty-first day after exposure regardless of whether they were vaccinated or given immune globulin. If measles develop in these persons, they should be isolated from patient contact until 7 days after the rash develops.

When susceptible individuals are exposed to measles, the live virus vaccine can prevent disease if given within 5 days of exposure. In addition, immune globulin (0.25 mL/kg [0.11 mL/lb] body weight) can be injected intramuscularly for prevention or modification of clinical illness if given within 6 days after exposure. This must be followed by active immunization with live measles vaccine 3 months later. Vaccination of all immunocompetent persons born after 1956 who travel to the developing world is important. In the developing world, the use of the second vaccine dose is an important aspect of achieving control of measles in the community-at-large.

Pregnant women and immunosuppressed persons should *not* receive this vaccine. The exception to this contraindication is asymptomatic HIV-infected patients including children, who have not shown adverse effects from measles vaccination. In asymptomatic HIV-infected children, exposure to vaccines improves survival after measles, and HAART therapy is associated with an improved vaccine response. Repeat vaccination may be necessary in HIV-infected children. Immune globulin should be considered for postexposure prophylaxis in any high-risk person exposed to measles. This group includes children with malignant disease and patients with AIDS, in whom severe disease or fatal measles is likely to develop. To be effective, immune globulin should be administered within 6 days after an exposure.

Severe allergic reactions to the MMR vaccine are rare, though fever and rash appear to occur slightly more often among female recipients. An aerosolized measles vaccine shows promising results in small clinical trials with hopes for availability in the near future. Future vaccines for a variety of infectious agents may utilize measles vectors, thereby augmenting immunity to measles.

▶ Treatment

A. General Measures

The patient should be isolated for the week following onset of rash and kept at bed rest until afebrile. Treatment is symptomatic including antipyretics and fluids as needed. Vitamin A, 200,000 units/d orally for 2 days (the benefit being maintenance of gastrointestinal and respiratory epithelial mucosa), reduces pediatric morbidity rates although high-dose vitamin A exposure increases the severity and risk of antibiotic failure in nonmeasles pneumonia. Measles virus is susceptible to ribavirin in vitro and has been used in selected severe cases of pneumonitis (35 mg/kg/d intravenously in three divided doses for 2 days, followed by 20 mg/kg/d intravenously in three divided doses for 5 days).

B. Treatment of Complications

Secondary bacterial infections, including pneumonia, are treated with appropriate antibacterial antibiotics. Post-measles encephalitis, including SSPE, can be managed only symptomatically.

▶ Prognosis

Between 1999 and 2005, measles mortality rate was reduced an estimated 60%. In the last decade, the case-fatality rate in the United States stayed around 3 per 1000 reported cases, with deaths principally due to encephalitis (15% mortality rate) and secondary bacterial pneumonia. Deaths in the developing world are mainly related to diarrhea and protein-losing enteropathy.

When to Refer

- Any suspect cases should be reported to public health authorities.
- HIV infection.
- Pregnancy.

When to Admit

- Meningitis, encephalitis, or myelitis.
- Severe pneumonia.
- Diarrhea that significantly compromises fluid or electrolyte status.

Aurpibul L et al. Response to measles, mumps, and rubella revaccination in HIV-infected children with immune recovery after highly active antiretroviral therapy. Clin Infect Dis. 2007 Sep 1;45(5):637–42. [PMID: 17683001]

Centers for Disease Control and Prevention (CDC). Update: measles—United States, January–July 2008. MMWR Morb Mortal Wkly Rep. 2008 Aug 22;57(33):893–6. [PMID: 18716580]

de Vries RD et al. Measles vaccination: new strategies and formulations. Expert Rev Vaccines. 2008 Oct;7(8):1215–23. [PMID: 18844595]

Kabra SK et al. Antibiotics for preventing complications in children with measles. Cochrane Database Syst Rev. 2008 Jul 16;(3):CD001477. [PMID: 18646073]

Moss WJ et al. Global measles elimination. Nat Rev Microbiol. 2006 Dec;4(12):900–8. [PMID: 17088933]

2. Mumps

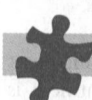

ESSENTIALS OF DIAGNOSIS

- ▶ Exposure 14–21 days before onset.
- ▶ Painful, swollen salivary glands, usually parotid.
- ▶ Frequent involvement of testes, pancreas, and meninges in unvaccinated individuals.

General Considerations

Mumps is a paramyxoviral disease spread by respiratory droplets. While children are the age group most affected, recent outbreaks involved patients in the late second or early third decades of life. The incidence of mumps is highest in spring. The incubation period is 14–21 days (average, 18 days). Infectivity occurs via saliva and urine and precedes the symptoms by about 1 day and is maximal for 3 days, although it may last a week. Up to one-third of affected individuals have subclinical infection. In 2006, an outbreak of mumps in the United States occurred and involved over 6000 persons; 85% of these cases were reported from eight Midwestern states.

Clinical Findings

A. Symptoms and Signs

Mumps is more serious in adults than in children. Parotid tenderness and overlying facial edema are the most common physical findings (Plate 98) and typically develop within 48 hours of the prodromal symptoms. Usually, one parotid gland enlarges before the other, but unilateral parotitis alone occurs in 25% of patients. The orifice of Stensen duct may be red and swollen. Trismus may result from parotitis. The parotid glands return to normal within a week. Involvement of other salivary glands (submaxillary and sublingual) occurs in 10% of cases.

Fever and malaise are variable but often minimal in young children. High fever accompanies meningitis or orchitis. Neck stiffness, headache, and lethargy suggest meningitis. Testicular swelling and tenderness (unilateral in 75% of cases) denote orchitis; the testes are the most common extrasalivary site of disease in adults. Orchitis develops 7–10 days after the onset of parotitis in about 25–40% of postpubertal men, but sterility is rare. Upper abdominal pain, nausea, and vomiting suggest pancreatitis. Mumps is the leading cause of pancreatitis in children. Lower abdominal pain and ovarian enlargement suggest oophoritis (which occurs in 5% of postpubertal women, usually unilateral); it is a difficult diagnosis to establish.

B. Laboratory Findings

Mild leukopenia with relative lymphocytosis may be present. Serum amylasemia usually reflects salivary gland involvement rather than pancreatitis. Lymphocytic pleocytosis (and hypoglychorrhachia) of the cerebrospinal fluid in meningitis may be asymptomatic. Mild kidney function abnormalities are found in up to 60% of patients.

A characteristic clinical picture is usually sufficient for diagnosis. A confirmatory diagnosis of mumps is made by isolating the virus preferably from a swab of the duct of the parotid or other affected salivary gland. The virus can also be isolated from cerebrospinal fluid early in the course of aseptic meningitis. Isolation from urine is no longer advised. Nucleic acid amplification techniques are more sensitive than viral cultures but their availability is limited. An elevated serum IgM is also considered diagnostic and a repeat test 2–3 weeks after the onset of symptoms is recommended if the first assay is negative due to a delay in IgM rise, especially in vaccinated persons. A fourfold rise in complement-fixing antibodies to mumps virus in paired serum IgG also confirms infection.

Differential Diagnosis

Swelling of the parotid gland may be due to calculi in the parotid ducts, tumors, or cysts, or to a reaction to iodides. Other causes include starch ingestion, sarcoidosis, cirrhosis, diabetes, bulimia, pilocarpine usage, and Sjögren syndrome. Parotitis may be produced by pyogenic organisms (eg, S aureus, gram-negative organisms), particularly in debilitated individuals with poor oral intake, drug reaction (phenothiazines, propylthiouracil), and other viruses (influenza A, parainfluenza, EBV infection, coxsackieviruses, adenoviruses, HHV-6). Swelling of the parotid gland must be differentiated from inflammation of the lymph nodes located more posteriorly and inferiorly than the parotid gland.

Complications

Other manifestations of the disease are less common. These usually follow the parotitis but may precede it or occur without salivary gland involvement and include meningitis (30%), orchitis (which on rare occasion leads to priapism or testicular infarction), pancreatitis (usually mild), oophoritis, thyroiditis, neuritis, hepatitis, myocarditis, thrombocytopenia, migratory arthralgias (noted infrequently among adults and rarely in children), and nephritis. Mumps has also been associated with cases of endocardial fibroelastosis.

Rare neurologic complications include encephalitis, Guillain–Barré syndrome, cerebellar ataxia, facial palsy, and transverse myelitis. Encephalitis is associated with cerebral edema, serious neurologic manifestations, and sometimes death. Deafness develops from eighth nerve neuritis, and data from Japan report an incidence of 0.3% among patients.

Prevention

Mumps live virus vaccine is safe and highly effective with long lasting immunity. It is recommended for routine immunization for children over age 1 year, either alone or in combination with other virus vaccines (eg, in the measles-mumps-rubella (MMR) vaccine or as a quadrivalent vaccine with varicella). A second dose is recommended for children (ages 4–6 years) before starting school. Two doses of the vaccine should also be considered for high-risk individuals (eg, health care workers) born before 1957 and without evidence of immunity. There are no known cases of long-term sequelae associated with mumps vaccination and the currently used mumps strain (Jeryl Lynn) shows the lowest associated incidence of postvaccine aseptic meningitis (from 1 in 150,000 to 1 in 1.8 million). This vaccine is less effective in epidemic than in nonepidemic settings. Reactions are reviewed in the measles section. It should not be given to pregnant women or to immunocompromised individuals, though the vaccine has been given to asymptomatic HIV-infected individuals without adverse sequelae especially when the individuals are taking HAART. In the developed world, persons in whom mumps develops are less likely to have received a second vaccine dose. The mumps skin tests are less reliable than serum neutralization titers in determining immunity.

Treatment

A. General Measures

The patient should be isolated until swelling subsides (about 9 days from onset) and kept at bed rest while febrile. Treatment is symptomatic. Topical application of compresses may relieve parotid discomfort.

B. Management of Complications

1. Meningitis—The treatment of aseptic meningitis is symptomatic. The management of encephalitis requires attention to cerebral edema, the airway, and vital functions.

2. Orchitis—The scrotum should be supported with a suspensory or toweling "bridge" and ice bags applied.

Incision of the tunica may be necessary in severe cases. Pain can be relieved with opioids, or by injecting the spermatic cord at the external inguinal ring with 10–20 mL of 1% procaine solution. The merit of hydrocortisone sodium succinate (100 mg intravenously, followed by 20 mg orally every 6 hours for 2 or 3 days) in reducing inflammation is not firmly established.

3. Pancreatitis—Symptomatic treatment should be provided, with emphasis on parenteral hydration.

Prognosis

The entire course of mumps rarely exceeds 2 weeks. Rare fatalities are usually due to encephalitis.

When to Refer

Any suspect cases should be reported to public health authorities.

When to Admit

- Trismus.
- Meningitis, encephalitis.
- Severe abdominal pain or vomiting suggesting pancreatitis.
- Severe testicular pain.
- Priapism.
- Severe thrombocytopenia.
- Myocarditis.

Dayan GH et al. Recent resurgence of mumps in the United States. N Engl J Med. 2008 Apr 10;358(15):1580–9. [PMID: 18403766]

Hviid A et al. Mumps. Lancet. 2008 Mar 15;371(9616):932–44. [PMID: 18342688]

Peltola H et al. Mumps outbreaks in Canada and the United States: time for new thinking on mumps vaccines. Clin Infect Dis. 2007 Aug 15;45(4):459–66. [PMID: 17638194]

3. Poliomyelitis

 ESSENTIALS OF DIAGNOSIS

▶ Incubation period 9–12 days from exposure.

▶ Muscle weakness, headache, stiff neck, fever, nausea and vomiting, sore throat.

▶ Lower motor neuron lesion (flaccid paralysis) with decreased deep tendon reflexes and muscle wasting.

▶ Cerebrospinal fluid shows excess leukocytes, with lymphocytic predominance; count is rarely more than 500/mcL.

General Considerations

Poliomyelitis virus, an enterovirus, is present in throat washings and stools (excretion may last for several weeks after infection). Infection is highly contagious through the fecal–oral route, especially during the first week of the disease. The global poliomyelitis eradication initiative was launched in 1988 and led to the virtual elimination of wild poliovirus from the Western hemisphere (a few cases of vaccine-associated disease were reported in Hispaniola, see below). The Pacific Rim and much of Central Asia also appear to be polio free. Between 1988 and 2007, the number of cases decreased globally from 350,000 to just over 1000. Only four countries had not yet documented interruption of wild poliovirus transmission (Afghanistan, India, Nigeria, and Pakistan). Resurgence in wildtype polio cases and vaccine-derived poliomyelitis still pose problems for elimination of poliomyelitis virus. Recent vaccine-associated cases were reported from Cambodia, Myanmar, and Nigeria, and cases among immunodeficient persons were reported from China, Iran, Syria, and Egypt. The last vaccine-associated case in the United States occurred in 2005; the woman acquired the infection while traveling in Central America.

Three antigenically distinct types of poliomyelitis virus are recognized, with little cross-immunity between them. Disease with type 2 in particular is on the verge of extinction.

Clinical Findings

A. Symptoms and Signs

At least 95% of infections are asymptomatic, but in those who become ill, manifestations include abortive poliomyelitis (minor illness), nonparalytic poliomyelitis, and paralytic poliomyelitis.

1. Abortive poliomyelitis (minor illness)—Such minor illness occurs in 4–8% of infections and the symptoms are fever, headache, vomiting, diarrhea, constipation, and sore throat lasting 2–3 days. This entity is suspected clinically only during an epidemic.

2. Nonparalytic poliomyelitis—In addition to the above symptoms, signs of meningeal irritation and muscle spasm occur in the absence of frank paralysis. This disease is indistinguishable from aseptic meningitis caused by other viruses.

3. Paralytic poliomyelitis—Paralytic poliomyelitis represents 0.1% of all poliomyelitis cases (the incidence is higher when infections are acquired later in life). Paralysis may occur at any time during the febrile period. Tremors, muscle weakness, constipation, and ileus may appear. Paralytic poliomyelitis is divided into two forms, which may coexist: (1) **spinal poliomyelitis**, with involvement of the muscles innervated by the spinal nerves, and (2) **bulbar poliomyelitis**, with weakness of the muscles supplied by the cranial nerves (especially nerves IX and X) and of the respiratory and vasomotor centers.

In spinal poliomyelitis, paralysis of the shoulder girdle often precedes intercostal and diaphragmatic paralysis, which leads to diminished chest expansion and decreased vital capacity. The paralysis occurs over 2–3 days, is flaccid, has an asymmetric distribution, and affects the proximal muscles of the lower extremities more frequently. Sensory loss is very rare.

In bulbar poliomyelitis, symptoms include diplopia (uncommonly), facial weakness, dysphagia, dysphonia, nasal voice, weakness of the sternocleidomastoid and trapezius muscles, difficulty in chewing, inability to swallow or expel saliva, and regurgitation of fluids through the nose. The most life-threatening aspect of bulbar poliomyelitis is respiratory paralysis. Lethargy or coma may be due to hypoxia, most often from hypoventilation. Vasomotor disturbances in blood pressure and heart rate may occur. Convulsions are rare. Bulbar poliomyelitis is more common in adults.

B. Laboratory Findings

The peripheral white blood cell count may be normal or mildly elevated. Cerebrospinal fluid pressure and protein are normal or slightly increased. Glucose is not decreased. White blood cells usually number < 500/mcL and are principally lymphocytes after the first 24 hours. Cerebrospinal fluid is normal in 5% of patients. The virus may be recovered from throat washings (early) and stools (early and late). Neutralizing and complement-fixing antibodies appear during the first or second week of illness. Serologic testing cannot distinguish between wild-type and vaccine-related virus infections.

Differential Diagnosis

Nonparalytic poliomyelitis is similar to other forms of enteroviral meningitis; the distinction is made serologically. Acute flaccid paralysis is the term used in the developing world for the variety of neurologic illnesses that both include and mimic poliomyelitis. Acute flaccid paralysis due to poliomyelitis is distinguished by the greater frequency of fever and asymmetric neurologic signs. Acute inflammatory polyneuritis (Guillain–Barré syndrome), Japanese B virus encephalitis, West Nile virus infection, and tick paralysis may resemble poliomyelitis. In Guillain–Barré syndrome (see Chapter 24), the weakness is more symmetric and ascending in most cases, but the Miller–Fisher variant is quite similar to bulbar polio. Paresthesias are uncommon in poliomyelitis but common in Guillain–Barré syndrome. The cerebrospinal fluid usually has a high protein content but normal cell count in Guillain–Barré syndrome.

Complications

Urinary tract infection, atelectasis, pneumonia, myocarditis, paralytic ileus, gastric dilation, and pulmonary edema may occur. Respiratory failure may be a result of paralysis of respiratory muscles, airway obstruction from involvement of cranial nerve nuclei, or lesions of the respiratory center.

Prevention

Given the epidemiologic distribution of poliomyelitis and the continued concern about vaccine-associated disease (estimated in 1:750,000 recipients) with the trivalent oral live poliovirus vaccine (OPV), the inactive (Salk) parenteral vaccination is currently used in the United States for all four recommended doses (at ages 2 months, 4 months, and 6–18 months and at 4–6 years). Inactivated vaccine is also routinely used elsewhere in the developed world. Oral vaccines are limited to usage for outbreak control, travel to endemic areas within the ensuing month, and protection of children whose parents do not comply with the recommended number of immunizations. The advantages of oral vaccination are the ease of administration, low cost, effective local gastrointestinal and circulating immunity, and herd immunity.

Routine immunization of adults in the United States is no longer recommended because of the low incidence of the disease. Exceptions include adults not vaccinated within the prior decade who are exposed to poliomyelitis or who plan to travel to endemic areas (mentioned above). Vaccination should also be considered for adults engaged in high-risk activities (eg, laboratory workers handling stools). Such adults should be given inactivated poliomyelitis vaccine (Salk) as should immunodeficient or immunosuppressed individuals and members of their households.

In the developing world, three doses of OPV seem sufficient for adequate immunization and the interval between doses should probably be longer than 1 month (because of interference from enteric pathogens). Intramuscular injections should be routinely avoided during the month following oral poliomyelitis vaccination to prevent provocation paralysis. Ancillary useful control measures in polio-endemic countries include national immunization days (mass campaigns in which all children are vaccinated twice, 4–6 weeks apart, regardless of vaccine history); cross-border vaccination activities; surveillance for acute flaccid paralysis, an indicator for poliomyelitis; and aggressive outbreak responses as well as intensified immunization activities in countries recently affected by armed conflicts. Vaccine-associated poliomyelitis with the oral Sabin vaccination is due to mutations leading to neurovirulence. Outbreaks of vaccine-derived poliomyelitis are reported sporadically globally (listed above) with the last major outbreak in the Western Hemisphere occurring in Hispaniola (both Haiti and the Dominican Republic) from 2000 to 2001. Such incidents serve as a reminder of the need to maintain high levels of immunization coverage even in the absence of overt disease. A monovalent type 1 oral vaccine that seems more immunogenic than the three-valent OPV and has the advantage of single administration was successfully used in India, Egypt, and Nigeria. Cost considerations along with effective herd immunity remain major reasons the oral Sabin is still administered.

There is no epidemiologic evidence to implicate poliomyelitis vaccination as a cause for recurrent worsening wheezing or eczema in childhood.

► Treatment

In the acute phase of paralytic poliomyelitis patients should be hospitalized. Strict bed rest in the first few days of illness reduces the rate of paralysis. Cranial nerve involvement must be vigilantly sought. Comfortable but rotating positions should be maintained in a "polio bed": firm mattress, footboard, sponge rubber pads or rolls, sandbags, and light splints. Intensive physiotherapy may help recover some motor function with paralysis. Fecal impaction and urinary retention (especially with paraplegia) are managed appropriately. In cases of respiratory weakness or paralysis, inten-

sive care is needed. The antiviral pleconaril shows no clear benefit in cases of polio meningoencephalitis.

► Prognosis

During the febrile period, paralysis may develop or progress. Mild weakness of small muscles is more likely to regress than is severe weakness of large muscles. Bulbar poliomyelitis carries a mortality rate of up to 50%. New muscle weakness and pain may develop and progress slowly years after recovery from acute paralytic poliomyelitis. This entity is called **postpoliomyelitis syndrome** and presents with signs of chronic and new denervation, is not infectious in origin, and patients do not shed the virus. The syndrome is associated with increasing dysfunction of surviving motor neurons. Different immune modulators such as prednisone, interferon, and intravenous immunoglobulin have been tested for treatment of postpoliomyelitis syndrome but have not shown clear benefits. Series that report increased incidences of multiple sclerosis or other motor neuron diseases among poliomyelitis survivors need to be evaluated in the context of what is known about the postpoliomyelitis syndrome. Although bulbar poliomyelitis causes the greatest threat to life, it is rarely responsible for permanent damage among surviving patients.

► When to Refer

- Neurologic compromise.
- Any suspicious cases should be referred to public health authorities.

► When to Admit

Patients with neurologic compromise should be admitted to the hospital.

Centers for Disease Control and Prevention (CDC). Update on vaccine-derived polioviruses–worldwide, January 2006–August 2007. MMWR Morb Mortal Wkly Rep. 2007 Sept 28;56(38):996–1001. [PMID: 17898693]

El-Sayed N et al. Monovalent type 1 oral poliovirus vaccine in newborns. N Engl J Med. 2008 Oct 16;359(16):1655–65. [PMID: 18923170]

Howard RS. Poliomyelitis and the postpolio syndrome. BMJ. 2005 Jun 4;330(7503):1314–8. [PMID: 15933355]

Jenkins HE et al. Effectiveness of immunization against paralytic poliomyelitis in Nigeria. N Engl J Med. 2008 Oct 16; 359(16):1666–74. [PMID: 18923171]

4. Rubella

ESSENTIALS OF DIAGNOSIS

- ► Exposure 14–21 days before onset.
- ► Arthralgia, particularly in young women.
- ► No prodrome in children, mild prodrome in adults; mild symptoms (fever, malaise, coryza) coinciding with eruption.
- ► Posterior cervical and postauricular lymphadenopathy 5–10 days before rash.

▸ Fine maculopapular rash of 3 days duration; face to trunk to extremities.

▸ Leukopenia, thrombocytopenia.

General Considerations

Rubella is a systemic disease caused by a togavirus transmitted by inhalation of infective droplets. It is only moderately communicable. One attack usually confers permanent immunity but reinfection is possible. The incubation period is 14–21 days (average, 16 days). The disease is transmissible from 1 week before the rash appears until 15 days afterward.

The clinical picture of rubella is difficult to distinguish from other viral illnesses such as infectious mononucleosis, measles, echovirus infections, and coxsackievirus infections; however, arthritis is more prominent in rubella. In the United States, endemic rubella and congenital rubella syndrome are eliminated. Surveillance of female military recruits suggests, however, that serologic protection against rubella, measles, and mumps are inadequate. In 2004, fewer than ten cases were reported to the Centers for Disease Control and Prevention (CDC) with all them likely imported from other countries. In parts of the world (eg, Eastern Europe) where vaccination against rubella was more recently introduced, significant outbreaks still occur. Serosusceptibility to the infection in immigrants to developed countries is still significant.

The principal importance of rubella lies in its devastating effects on the fetus in utero, producing teratogenic effects and a continuing congenital infection. More than 100,000 cases of **congenital rubella syndrome** are reported annually in the developing world.

Clinical Findings

A. Symptoms and Signs

While fetal rubella can be devastating, postnatally acquired rubella is usually innocuous with up to 50% cases asymptomatic. In the postnatally acquired infection, fever and malaise, usually mild, accompanied by tender suboccipital adenitis, may precede the eruption by 1 week. Mild coryza may be present. Polyarticular arthritis occurs in about 25% of adult cases and involves the fingers, wrists, and knees. Rarely does chronic arthritis develop. The polyarthritis usually subsides within 7 days but may persist for weeks. Early posterior cervical and postauricular lymphadenopathy is very common. Erythema of the palate and throat, sometimes patchy, may be noted.

A fine, pink maculopapular rash appears on the face, trunk, and extremities in rapid progression (2–3 days) and fades quickly, usually lasting 1 day in each area (Table 32–2). Rubella without rash may be at least as common as the exanthematous disease. Diagnosis, when suspected because of disease in the community, requires serologic confirmation.

B. Laboratory Findings

Leukopenia may be present early and may be followed by an increase in plasma cells. The definitive diagnosis of acute rubella infection is based on elevated IgM antibody, fourfold or greater rise in IgG antibody titers, or isolation of the virus. False-positive IgM antibodies, however, are associated with Epstein-Barr virus, cytomegalovirus, parvovirus, and rheumatoid factor. Detection of antibodies against rubella in other body fluids, such as urine and saliva, seem promising diagnostic aids. PCR techniques are also available.

Complications

A. Exposure during Pregnancy

When a pregnant woman is exposed to a possible case of rubella, an immediate hemagglutination-inhibiting rubella antibody level should be obtained to document immunity, since fetal infection during the first trimester leads to congenital rubella in at least 80% of fetuses.

Positive tests for IgG antibodies alone indicate past infection or vaccination. If no antibodies are found, clinical observation and serologic follow-up are essential. An isolated IgM-positive test needs to be interpreted with caution because it does not necessarily imply acute infection. Confirmation of rubella in the expectant mother raises the question of therapeutic abortion, an alternative to be considered in light of personal, religious, legal, and other factors.

B. Congenital Rubella

An infant acquiring the infection in utero may be normal at birth but probably—50% in a series of nearly 70 pregnant women with rubella in Mexico—will have a wide variety of manifestations, including early-onset cataracts and glaucoma, microphthalmia, hearing deficits, psychomotor retardation, congenital heart defects, organomegaly, and maculopapular rash. In general, the younger the fetus when infected, the more severe the illness. Deafness is the primary complication in the second trimester. Viral excretion in the throat and urine persists for many months despite high antibody levels. A specific test for IgM rubella antibody is useful for diagnosis in the newborn. A confirmatory diagnosis is made by isolation of the virus or PCR detection of viral RNA in tissues. Treatment is directed toward the many anomalies.

C. Postinfectious Encephalopathy

In 1:6000 cases, postinfectious encephalopathy develops 1–6 days after the rash; the virus cannot always be isolated. The mortality rate is 20%, but residual deficits are rare among the recovered. The mechanism is unknown.

Other unusual complications of rubella include hemorrhagic manifestations due to thrombocytopenia and vascular damage, duodenal stenosis, and mild hepatitis.

Prevention

Live attenuated rubella virus vaccine should be given to all infants and to susceptible girls before the menarche. When women are immunized, they should not be pregnant, and the absence of antibodies should be established. (In the United States, about 80% of 20-year-old women are immune to rubella.) Postpartum administration to susceptible female hospital employees is recommended. It is recommended that women not become pregnant for at least 3 months after vaccine administration. Nonetheless, there are no reports of congenital rubella syndrome after rubella immunization, and inadvertent immunization of a pregnant woman is not considered an indication for therapeutic abortion. Arthritis is more marked after rubella vaccination than in native disease and appears to be immunologically mediated. The association between chronic arthropathies and rubella vaccination is controversial. MMR may be given in conjunction with diphtheria–pertussis–tetanus (DPT) boosters as adequate serologic responses are documented. The administration of two or more doses appears to overcome an immunogenetic risk for vaccine failure in some vaccinees.

Treatment

Acetaminophen provides symptomatic relief. Encephalitis and non–life-threatening thrombocytopenia should be treated symptomatically.

Prognosis

Rubella is a mild illness and rarely lasts more than 3–4 days. Congenital rubella, on the other hand, has a high mortality rate, and the associated congenital defects are largely permanent.

When to Refer

- Pregnancy.
- Meningitis/encephalitis.
- Any suspect cases should be reported to public health authorities.

Centers for Disease Control and Prevention (CDC). Elimination of rubella and congenital rubella syndrome—United States, 1969–2004. MMWR Morb Mortal Wkly Rep. 2005 Mar 25;54(11):279–82. [PMID: 15788995]

Dontigny L et al. Rubella in pregnancy. J Obstet Gynaecol Can. 2008 Feb;30(2):152–68. [PMID: 18254998]

Greenaway C et al. Susceptibility to measles, mumps, and rubella in newly arrived adult immigrants and refugees. Ann Intern Med. 2007 Jan 2;146(1):20–4. [PMID: 17200218]

Weir E et al. A refresher on rubella. CMAJ. 2005 Jun 21;172(13):1680–1. [PMID: 15967968]

OTHER NEUROTROPIC VIRUSES

1. Rabies

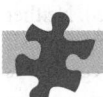

ESSENTIALS OF DIAGNOSIS

- ► History of animal bite.
- ► Paresthesia, hydrophobia, rage alternating with calm.
- ► Convulsions, paralysis, thick tenacious saliva.

General Considerations

Rabies is a viral (rhabdovirus) encephalitis transmitted by infected saliva that gains entry into the body by an animal bite or an open wound. Globally, an estimated 50,000 to 100,000 deaths occur annually from rabies, mostly in rural areas of Africa and Asia. In the United States, domestically acquired rabies cases are rare but probably underreported. One bat-associated human case was reported from Minnesota in 2007. Raccoons, skunks, bats, and foxes are common wildlife reservoirs. Unique geographic biting species that cause rabies in the United States include raccoons in the East, including New England; skunks in the Midwest, Southwest, and in California; and foxes in the Southwest and in Alaska. Bats are the second most reported rabid animal behind raccoons and most cases in the United States from 2000 through 2006 (17 of 24 total) were associated with bat rabies virus variants. Hawaii is the only rabies-free state. Vaccination campaigns are very successful in preventing dog-associated cases. Cats are rarely infected in the United States, although an increase in the number of cases was reported in 2006. Rodents and lagomorphs (eg, rabbits) are unlikely to spread rabies because they cannot survive the disease long enough to transmit it, although woodchucks and groundhogs can become infected and transmit the virus. In developing countries, greater than 90% of human cases are due to infected dog bites. Rabies among travelers to rabies-endemic areas (usually the Middle East and sub-Saharan Africa) is usually associated with animal injuries.

The virus gains entry into the salivary glands of dogs 5–7 days before their death from rabies, thus limiting their period of infectivity. Less common routes of transmission include contamination of mucous membranes with saliva or brain tissue, aerosol transmission, and corneal transplantation. Transmission through solid organ and vascular segment transplantation from donors with unrecognized infection is also reported.

The incubation period may range from 10 days to many years but is usually 3–7 weeks depending in part on the distance of the wound from the CNS. The virus travels in the nerves to the brain, multiplies there, and then migrates along the efferent nerves to the salivary glands.

Rabies is almost uniformly fatal, with only six documented surviving cases to date. Five received either preexposure or postexposure prophylaxis. In 2004, a teenager survived with only naturally acquired immunity, but received intense treatment including antiviral therapy and an intentionally induced drug coma. The most common clinical problem confronting clinicians is the management of a patient bitten by an animal.

Clinical Findings

A. Symptoms and Signs

While there is usually a history of animal bite, bat bites may not be recognized. The prodromal syndrome consists of pain at the site of the bite in association with fever, malaise, headache, nausea, and vomiting. The skin is sensitive to changes of temperature, especially air currents (aerophobia). Percussion myoedema can be present and persist throughout the disease. The CNS stage begins about 10 days after the prodome and may be either encephalitic ("furious") or paralytic ("dumb"). The encephalitic form (about 80% of the cases) produces the classic rabies manifestations of delirium alternating with periods of calm, extremely painful laryngeal spasms on attempting drinking (hydrophobia), autonomic stimulation (hypersalivation), and seizures. In the less common paralytic form, an acute ascending paralysis resembling Guillain–Barré syndrome predominates with relative sparing of higher cortical functions initially. Both forms progress relentlessly to coma, autonomic nervous system dysfunction, and death.

B. Laboratory Findings

Biting animals that appear well should be quarantined and observed for 10 days. Sick or dead animals should be tested for rabies. A wild animal, if captured, should be sacrificed and the head shipped on ice to the nearest laboratory qualified to examine the brain for evidence of rabies virus. When the animal cannot be examined, raccoons, skunks, bats, and foxes should be presumed to be rabid.

Direct fluorescent antibody testing of skin biopsy material from the posterior neck (where hair follicles are highly innervated) has a sensitivity of 60–80%.

Reverse transcriptase PCR (RT-PCR), nucleic acid sequence-based amplification, and viral isolation from the cerebrospinal fluid or saliva are being advocated as definitive diagnostic assays. Antibodies can be detected in the serum and the cerebrospinal fluid. Pathologic specimens often demonstrate round or oval eosinophilic inclusion bodies (Negri bodies) in the cytoplasm of neuronal cells, but the finding is neither sensitive nor specific. MRI signs are diffuse and nonspecific.

▶ Prevention

Immunization of household dogs and cats and active immunization of persons with significant animal exposure (eg, veterinarians) are important. The most important decisions, however, concern animal bites.

In the developing world, education, surveillance, and animal (particularly dog) vaccination programs are preferred over mass destruction of dogs, which is followed typically by invasion of susceptible feral animals into urban areas. In some Western European countries, campaigns of oral vaccination of wild animals led to the elimination of rabies in wildlife.

A. Local Treatment of Animal Bites and Scratches

Thorough cleansing, debridement, and repeated flushing of wounds with soap and water are important. Rabies immune globulin or antiserum should be given as stated below. Wounds caused by animal bites should not be sutured.

B. Postexposure Immunization

The decision to treat should be based on the circumstances of the bite, including the extent and location of the wound, the biting animal, the history of prior vaccination, and the local epidemiology of rabies. Any contact or suspect contact with a bat is usually deemed a sufficient indication to warrant prophylaxis. Consultation with state and local health departments is recommended. Postexposure treatment including

both immune globulin and vaccination should be administered as promptly as possible when indicated.

The optimal form of passive immunization is human rabies immune globulin (HRIG; 20 international units/kg), administered once. As much as possible of the full dose should be infiltrated around the wound, with any remaining injected intramuscularly at a site distant from the wound. Finger spaces can be safely injected without development of a compartment syndrome. If HRIG is not available, equine rabies antiserum (20–40 international units/kg) can be used if available (it was last produced in 2001) after appropriate tests for horse serum sensitivity.

Two vaccines are licensed and available for use in humans in the United States: a human diploid cell vaccine (HDCV) and a purified chick embryo cell vaccine (PCEC). The current vaccines are given as five injections of 1 mL intramuscularly in the deltoid or, in small children, into the anterolateral thigh muscles on days 0, 3, 7, 14, and 28 after exposure. The vaccine should not be given in the gluteal area due to suboptimal response.

Rabies vaccines and HRIG should never be given in the same syringe or at the same site. Allergic reactions to the vaccine are rare, although local reactions (pruritus, erythema, tenderness) occur in about 25% and mild systemic reactions (headaches, myalgias, nausea) in about 20% of recipients. Adverse reactions to HRIG seem to be more frequent in women and rare in young children. The vaccine is commercially available or can be obtained through health departments.

Globally diverse anti-rabies vaccines are used. After Pasteur's research in the 19th century with increasingly virulent strains, the first licensed vaccine (1911) was inactivated and grown on bovine brain tissue. Subsequent vaccines were grown using duck or chick embryo cells but remained allergenic. Recent increasingly purified vaccines were grown on verocells, and a sixth-generation verocell rabies vaccine (VRVg) is under development. In some countries, the full spectrum of vaccines, from human diploid rabies (HDRV) to chromatographically purified rabies vaccine (CPRV) are available, whereas in others, the gamut is smaller and intradermal application of smaller vaccine doses at multiple sites and at different times is commonly practiced in an attempt to lower costs, and is deemed safe and effective by the World Health Organization.

In patients with history of past vaccination, the need for HRIG is eliminated (RIG is in short supply worldwide) but postexposure vaccination is still required. The vaccine should be given 1 mL in the deltoid twice (on days 0 and 3). Neither the passive nor the active form of postexposure prophylaxis is associated with fetal abnormalities and thus pregnancy is not considered a contraindication to vaccination.

C. Preexposure Immunization

Preexposure prophylaxis with three injections of HDCV intramuscularly (1 mL on days 0, 7, and 21 or 28) is recommended for persons at high risk for exposure: veterinarians (who should have rabies antibody titers checked every 2 years and be boosted with 1 mL intramuscularly or 0.1 mL intradermally if seronegative); animal handlers; laboratory workers; Peace Corps workers; and travelers with stays over 1 month to remote areas in endemic countries in Africa, Asia, and Latin America. An intradermal route is also available. Intradermal preexposure prophylaxis (0.1 mL on days 0, 7, and 21 over the deltoid) is not available in the United States. Immunosuppressive illnesses and agents including corticosteroids as well as antimalarials—in particular chloroquine—may diminish the antibody response.

Treatment

Management requires intensive care with attention to the airway, maintenance of oxygenation, and control of seizures. Universal precautions are essential. The induction of coma by ketamine, midazolam, and supplemental barbiturates along with the use of amantadine and ribavirin, was reportedly helpful in one case but has failed to reproduce success in two subsequent cases. Corticosteroids are of no use.

Prognosis

If postexposure prophylaxis is given expediently, before clinical signs develop, it is nearly 100% successful in prevention of disease. Once the symptoms have appeared, death almost inevitably occurs after 7 days, usually from respiratory failure. Most deaths occur in persons with unrecognized disease who do not seek medical care or in individuals who do not receive postexposure prophylaxis.

When to Refer

Suspicion of rabies requires contact with public health personnel to initiate appropriate passive and active prophylaxis and observation of suspect cases.

When to Admit

- Respiratory, neuromuscular, or CNS dysfunction consistent with rabies.
- Patients with suspect rabies require initiation of therapy until the disease is ruled out in suspect animals, and this requires coordination of care based on likelihood of patient compliance, availability of inpatient and outpatient facilities, and response of local public health teams.

Manning SE et al; Advisory Committee on Immunization Practices Centers for Disease Control and Prevention (CDC). Human rabies prevention—United States, 2008: recommendations of the Advisory Committee on Immunization Practices. MMWR Recomm Rep. 2008 May 23;57(RR-3):1–28. [PMID: 18496505]

Rupprecht CE et al. Can rabies be eradicated? Dev Biol (Basel). 2008;131:95–121. [PMID: 18634470]

Wilde H. Failures of post-exposure rabies prophylaxis. Vaccine. 2007 Nov 1;25(44):7605–9. [PMID: 17905484]

2. Arbovirus Encephalitides

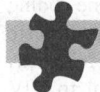

ESSENTIALS OF DIAGNOSIS

- ▸ Fever, malaise, stiff neck, sore throat, and nausea and vomiting, progressing to stupor, coma, and convulsions.

- ▸ Signs of an upper motor neuron lesion (exaggerated deep tendon reflexes, absent superficial reflexes, pathologic reflexes, and spastic paralysis).

- ▸ Cerebrospinal fluid protein and opening pressure often increased, with lymphocytic pleocytosis.

General Considerations

The arboviruses are arthropod-borne pathogens that produce clinical manifestations in humans. The **mosquito-borne pathogens** that cause encephalitis include three togaviruses (causing Western, Eastern, and Venezuelan equine encephalitis), five flaviviruses (causing West Nile fever, St. Louis encephalitis, Japanese B encephalitis, dengue, and Murray Valley encephalitis), and bunyaviruses (the California serogroup of viruses, including the Lacrosse agent of California encephalitis). The **tick-borne** causes of encephalitis include the flavivirus of the Powassan encephalitis (northeastern United States and Canada) and tick-borne encephalitis virus of Europe; and the Colorado tick fever reovirus. Tick-borne encephalitis virus, Colorado tick fever, and the arboviruses associated with viral hemorrhagic fever (including dengue) are discussed below, and only those viruses causing primarily encephalitis in the United States will be discussed here.

Infection with West Nile virus was first identified in the United States in the New York City area in 1999. The virus spread rapidly, and current cases are reported throughout the continental United States. The homeless appear to be at increased risk for infection. In 2008, 1370 cases of WNV infection were reported to the CDC with more than half of them occurring in four states: California (411), Arizona (109), Mississippi (99), and Colorado (95). The highest incidences (> 100 per million population), however, were reported from Midwestern states (North Dakota, South Dakota, Nebraska, and Kansas).

Pathogen-specific reservoirs (typically small mammals or birds) are responsible for maintaining the encephalitis-producing viruses in nature. Birds are the main reservoir for West Nile virus and substantial avian mortality accompanies West Nile fever outbreaks. Outbreaks tend to occur in late summer and early fall. Real-time data at the county-level for sentinel cases (animal and human) of this infection in the United States can be found at http://diseasemaps.usgs.gov/.

Only dengue and Venezuelan equine encephalitis viruses produce viremias high enough to allow continued transmission to other mosquitoes and ticks. Human to human transmission of the other arboviruses are usually related to blood transfusion or organ transplantation. West Nile virus perinatal, transplacental, breast-feeding (rarely), laboratory, and possibly aerosol transmission can also occur. It is estimated that fever develops in 1 of 5 patients infected with West Nile virus, while severe neurologic disease presents in 1 of 150. St. Louis encephalitis and Powassan encephalitis occur among adults; Western equine encephalitis, Venezuelan equine encephalitis, and California encephalitis occur primarily among children, while West Nile fever and Eastern equine encephalitis are diseases of both children and adults.

Clinical Findings

A. Symptoms and Signs

The human incubation period for arboviral encephalitides is 2–14 days. Symptoms include fever, malaise, sore throat, headache, gastrointestinal upset, lethargy, and stupor progressing to coma. A nonpruritic maculopapular rash is variably present. Stiff neck and mental status changes are the most common neurologic signs. About 50% of hospitalized patients with West Nile virus infection in the United States have significant muscle weakness that may be initially confused with the Guillain–Barré syndrome. Acute flaccid (poliomyelitis-like) paralysis is seen in 10% of West Nile virus neuroinvasive disease and less commonly with the other arboviruses. Other signs include tremors, seizures, cranial nerve palsies, and pathologic reflexes. Myocarditis and hearing loss are also reported. The disease manifestations associated with West Nile virus infection are strongly age-dependent: the acute febrile syndrome and mild neurologic symptoms are more common in the young, aseptic meningitis and poliomyelitis-like syndromes are seen in the middle aged, and frank encephalopathy is seen in the elderly.

B. Laboratory Findings

The peripheral white blood cell count is variable. Cerebrospinal fluid protein is elevated; cerebrospinal fluid glucose is normal; there is usually a lymphocytic pleocytosis; and polymorphonuclear cells may predominate early. The diagnosis of arboviral encephalitides depends on serologic tests. Antibodies to arboviruses persist for life and the presence of IgG in the absence of a rising titer of IgM may indicate past exposure rather than acute infection. Documentation of a four-fold increase in acute/convalescence titers IgG or the presence of IgM antibodies is confirmatory. For West Nile virus, an IgM capture ELISA in serum or cerebrospinal fluid is almost always positive by the time the disease is clinically evident, and the presence of IgM in cerebrospinal fluid indicates neuroinvasive disease. These tests are commercially available but also obtainable through local or state health departments. Serologic tests specific for other arboviral encephalitides can be obtained through the CDC (http://www.cdc.gov/ncidod/dvbid/misc/specimen-submission.htm). Cross-reactivity exists among the different flaviviruses, so a plaque reduction assay may be needed to definitively distinguish between West Nile fever and St. Louis encephalitis. PCR assays (also available through the CDC) are less sensitive than serologic tests for the diagnosis of acute infections but are the preferred method for screening blood products and may be particularly useful in immunocompromised patients with abnormal antibody responses. CT scans of the brain usually show no acute disease, but MRI may reveal leptomeningeal, basal ganglia, thalamic, or periventricular enhancement.

Differential Diagnosis

Mild forms of encephalitis must be differentiated from aseptic meningitis, lymphocytic choriomeningitis, and nonparalytic poliomyelitis.

Severe forms of arbovirus encephalitides (Table 32–2) are to be differentiated from other causes of viral encephalitis (HSV, mumps virus, poliovirus or other enteroviruses, HIV), encephalitis accompanying exanthematous diseases of childhood (measles, varicella, infectious mononucleosis, rubella), encephalitis following vaccination (a demyelinating type following rabies, measles, pertussis), toxic encephalitis (from drugs, poisons, or bacterial toxins such as *Shigella dysenteriae* type 1), Reye syndrome, and severe forms of stroke, brain tumors, brain abscess, autoimmune processes such as lupus cerebritis, and intoxications. In the California Encephalitis Project, the cause for most cases of encephalitis was not identified.

Complications

Bronchial pneumonia, urinary retention and infection, prolonged weakness, and decubitus ulcers may occur. St. Louis encephalitis is reportedly associated with a postinfectious encephalomyelitis.

Prevention

No human vaccine is currently available for the arboviruses prevalent in North America, although yellow fever virus-based chimeric vaccines and recombinant vaccines are under development for West Nile virus. Mosquito control (repellents, protective clothing, and insecticides) is effective in prevention. Since 2003, all blood donations in the United States are screened with nucleic acid amplification tests for West Nile virus. Laboratory precautions are indicated for handling all these pathogens, in particular the West Nile virus.

A vaccine against Japanese B encephalitis is recommended for travelers to rural areas of East Asia, though the risk of disease acquisition among the exposed is estimated at only 1:1,000,000. This vaccination appears to provide some protection against West Nile virus (both agents are related flaviviruses).

Treatment

Although specific antiviral therapy is not available for most causative entities, vigorous supportive measures can be helpful. Such measures include reduction of intracranial pressure (mannitol) and monitoring of intraventricular pressure. The efficacy of corticosteroids in these infections is not established. Preliminary evidence that ribavirin was useful in West Nile virus encephalitis is not substantiated. Other therapeutic options such as IVIG or interferon-α await confirmation of effectiveness.

Prognosis

Although most infections are mild or asymptomatic, the prognosis is always guarded, especially at the extremes of age. Homozygosity for a 32bp deletion in the gene coding for the chemokine receptor CCR5, associated with complete loss of function, predisposes to symptomatic West Nile virus infection. People with this mutation are resistant to HIV infection. The case fatality rate for West Nile virus neuroinvasive disease in the United States was 5.8% in 2008. Age older than 50 years is the most important risk factor for severe disease and death. Other risk factors for mortality include black race, chronic kidney disease, hepatitis C virus infection, and immunosuppression. Recovery of persons with severe neurologic compromise may take months. Sequelae of West Nile virus infection include a poliomyelitis-like syndrome, cognitive complaints, movement disorders, epilepsy, and depression; and they may become apparent late in the course of what appears to be a successful recovery. The prognosis is generally better for Western equine than for Eastern equine or St. Louis encephalitis.

Centers for Disease Control and Prevention (CDC). National Center for Infectious Diseases. Division of Vector-Borne Infectious Diseases. http://www.cdc.gov/ncidod/dvbid/misc/adb.htm

Davis LE et al. North American encephalitic arboviruses. Neurol Clin. 2008 Aug;26(3):727–57. [PMID: 18657724]

Murray K et al. Risk factors for encephalitis and death from West Nile virus infection. Epidemiol Infect. 2006 Dec;134(6):1325–32. [PMID: 16672108]

Lim JK et al. Genetic deficiency of chemokine receptor CCR5 is a strong risk factor for symptomatic West Nile virus infection: a meta-analysis of 4 cohorts in the US epidemic. J Infect Dis. 2008 Jan 15;197(2):262–5. [PMID: 18179388]

3. Lymphocytic Choriomeningitis

ESSENTIALS OF DIAGNOSIS

▶ "Influenza-like" prodrome of fever, chills, malaise, and cough, followed by meningitis with associated stiff neck.

▶ Aseptic meningitis with positive Kernig sign, headache, nausea, vomiting, and lethargy.

▶ Cerebrospinal fluid: slight increase of protein, lymphocytic pleocytosis (500–3000/mcL); low glucose in 25% of patients.

▶ Complement-fixing antibodies within 2 weeks.

▶ General Considerations

The lymphocytic choriomeningitis virus is an arenavirus (related to the pathogen causing Lassa fever, discussed below) that causes infection of the CNS. The main reservoir for lymphocytic choriomeningitis virus is the house mouse. Other rodents (such as rats, guinea pigs, and even pet hamsters), monkeys, dogs, and swine are also potential reservoirs. Lymphocytic choriomeningitis virus is shed by the infected animal via nasal secretions, urine, and feces; transmission to humans probably occurs through aerosolized particles, direct contact, or animal bites. Human cases are most common in autumn. The virus is typically not spread person to person, though vertical transmission occurs, and lymphocytic choriomeningitis virus is an underrecognized neuroteratogen. Rare cases related to solid organ transplantation and autopsies of infected individuals are reported. Outbreaks tend to occur among persons with rodent exposure (eg, in the laboratory setting). Complications of clinical disease are rare.

This disease is principally confined to the eastern seaboard and northeastern states of the United States. Serologic evidence of past infection is present in 5% of adults in some urban areas of those regions and is higher in women, the elderly, and members of lower socioeconomic groups.

▶ Clinical Findings

A. Symptoms and Signs

The incubation period is 8–13 days to the appearance of systemic manifestations and 15–21 days to the appearance of meningeal symptoms. Symptoms are biphasic, with a prodromal illness characterized by fever, chills, headache, myalgia, cough, and vomiting, occasionally with lymphadenopathy and maculopapular rash. After 3–5 days, the fever subsides and recurs in 2–4 days with the meningeal phase, characterized by headache, nausea and vomiting, lethargy, and variably present meningeal signs. Obstructive hydrocephalus is a rare complication. Arthralgias can develop late.

Chorioretinitis also appears to be a sequela. Occasionally, a syndrome resembling the viral hemorrhagic fevers (see below) is described in transplant recipients of infected organs and in patients with lymphoma.

B. Laboratory Findings

Leukocytosis or leukopenia and thrombocytopenia may be present. Cerebrospinal fluid lymphocytic pleocytosis (total count is often 500–3000/mcL) may occur, with a slight increase in protein and normal to low glucose in at least 25%. The virus may be recovered from the blood and cerebrospinal fluid by mouse inoculation. Complement-fixing antibodies appear during or after the second week. Detection of specific IgM by ELISA is becoming widely used. Detection of lymphocytic choriomeningitis virus by PCR is available in research settings.

▶ Differential Diagnosis

The influenza-like prodrome and latent period may distinguish this from other aseptic meningitides, and bacterial and granulomatous meningitis. A history of exposure to mice or other potential vectors is an important diagnostic clue.

▶ Prevention

Pregnant women should be advised of the dangers to their unborn children inherent in exposure to rodents.

▶ Treatment

Treatment is supportive. In the survivor of a transplant-associated outbreak, ribavirin (which is effective against other arenaviruses) was used successfully along with decreasing immunosuppression.

▶ Prognosis

Fatalities are rare. The illness usually lasts 1–2 weeks, though convalescence may be prolonged. Congenital infection is more severe with about 30% mortality rate among infected infants, and more than 90% of survivors suffering long-term neurologic abnormalities.

Centers for Disease Control and Prevention (CDC). Brief report: Lymphocytic choriomeningitis virus transmitted through solid organ transplantation—Massachusetts, 2008. MMWR Morb Mortal Wkly Rep. 2008 Jul 25;57(29):799–801. [PMID: 18650788]

Palacios G et al. A new arenavirus in a cluster of fatal transplant-associated diseases. N Engl J Med. 2008 Mar 6;358(10):991–8. [PMID: 18256387]

4. Prion Diseases

ESSENTIALS OF DIAGNOSIS

▶ Rare in humans.

▶ Cognitive decline.

▶ Myoclonic fasciculations, ataxia, visual disturbances, pyramidal and extrapyramidal symptoms.

▶ Variant disease in younger people with prominent psychiatric or sensory symptoms.

▶ Specific EEG patterns.

▶ General Considerations

Several non-treatable neurodegenerative diseases are caused by communicable pathogens that contain protein but apparently lack nucleic acid as they are resistant to most procedures that modify it. They are called "prions" for *proteinaceous infectious particles*. These agents show slow replicative capacity and long latent intervals in the host. They induce the conformational change of a normal brain protein (prion protein; PrP^C) into an abnormal isoform (PrP^{Sc}) that accumulates and causes neuronal vacuolation (spongiosis), reactive proliferation of astrocytes and microglia and, in some cases, amyloid plaques. The term "transmissible spongiform encephalopathies" (TSE) refers to the spongiform appearance of the brain tissue observed in these conditions. A variety of animal diseases exhibit characteristics of TSE but those affecting humans include **classic Creutzfeldt–Jakob disease** (cCJD) and its **variant form** (vCJD), **kuru**, **Gerstmann-Sträussler-Scheinker syndrome** (GSS), and **fatal familial insomnia** (FFI). Infectious transmission of disease has only been described for vCJD, kuru and the iatrogenic form of cCJD (see below), whereas genetically determined mutations of PrP^C are the cause for the remainder. **Kuru** (characterized by cerebellar ataxia, tremors, dysarthria and emotional liability) was once prevalent in central New Guinea but now rare since the abandonment of cannibalism in the late 1950s. **FFI** occurs in kindreds (rarely sporadic) and **GSS** (ataxia and dysarthria, progressing to dementia and spastic paraparesis) is extremely rare. Only cCJD and vCJD will be further discussed here.

There are three forms cCJD: sporadic (80–85%), familial (15%), and iatrogenic (< 1%). There are no definitive risk factors for cCJD, and its annual incidence is about 1 in one million people per year. Familial cases are inherited in an autosomal dominant pattern with variable penetrance.

vCJD probably results from ingestion of beefsteak contaminated with neural tissue (brain, spinal cord) from livestock infected with **bovine spongiform encephalopathy (BSE)** ("mad cow disease"). A genetic variation in codon 129 of the PrP^C is highly prevalent in those patients affected. Since the first documented cases in Great Britain in the mid 1990s, more than 200 cases of vCJD have been reported with most cases reported from the United Kingdom. Only three cases of **vCJD** to date were reported in the United States (the last one in 2005), and all had documented former residence in the United Kingdom or Saudi Arabia. As of January 2009, only three cases of BSE were documented in the United States (from Washington, Texas, and Alabama), the last one in 2006. Canada in turn, has reported 15 cases to date, the last three in 2008. The risk for vCJD associated with the ingestion of beef products in these countries, thus, is very small. There is no animal-to-animal spread of BSE and milk and its derived products are not infected. Transmission through blood transfusions is documented in the United Kingdom.

▶ Clinical Findings

A. Symptoms and Signs

The sporadic and familial cases of **cCJD** usually present in the sixth or seventh decade of life, whereas the iatrogenic form tends to occur in much younger patients. The typical clinical picture is dementia that progresses over several months, myoclonic fasciculations, ataxia, visual disturbances, pyramidal or extrapyramidal symptoms (or both), and akinetic mutism. **vCJD**, in contrast, usually affects younger people, the duration of disease is longer, and the clinical symptoms are unique (prominent psychiatric and sensory symptoms).

B. Laboratory Findings

The diagnosis of **CJD** should be considered in the proper clinical setting and in the absence of alternative diagnoses after routine investigations. Abnormalities in cerebrospinal fluid are subtle and rarely helpful. The detection of 14-3-3 protein in the cerebrospinal fluid is supportive of the diagnosis of **cCJD** but is not helpful in **vCJD**. Cerebrospinal fluid detection of other proteins like tau and neuron-specific enolase do not as yet show clinical utility. EEG typically shows a pattern of paroxysms with high voltages and slow waves in **cCJD**, and the MRI is characteristic for bilateral areas of increased signal intensity, predominantly in the caudate and putamen. **vCJD**, in contrast, shows diffusely abnormal but not diagnostic EEGs; and the MRI characteristically reveals hyperintensity of the posterior thalamus ("pulvinar sign"). The differentiation and definitive diagnosis of these diseases are ultimately established by neuropathologic confirmation.

▶ Treatment & Prevention

There is no specific treatment for CJD and once symptoms appear, the infection invariably leads to death. Flupirtine (an analgesic drug) may slow cognitive decline but does not affect survival.

Iatrogenic cCJD can be prevented by limiting patient exposure to potentially infectious sources, which include human cadaveric growth hormones, gonadotrophins, corneal grafts, and dural grafts, and by restricting unnecessary exposure to stereotactic electroencephalography electrodes. Disinfection of equipment requires autoclaving at 15 psi for 1 hour, and disinfection of contaminated surfaces requires 5% hypochlorite or 0.1 N sodium hydroxide solution. Prevention of vCJD relies on surveillance of potentially infected livestock.

Kovacs GG. Prion diseases: from protein to cell pathology. Am J Pathol. 2008 Mar;172(3):555–65. [PMID: 18245809]
Stewart LA et al. Systematic review of therapeutic interventions in human prion disease. Neurology. 2008 Apr 8;70(15):1272–81. [PMID: 18391159]
United States Department of Health and Human Services, Centers for Disease Control and Prevention. vCJD (Variant Creutzfeldt-Jakob Disease). http://www.cdc.gov/ncidod/dvrd/vcjd/

5. Progressive Multifocal Leukoencephalopathy

Progressive multifocal leukoencephalopathy (PML) is a rare demyelinating CNS disorder caused by the reactivation of JC virus (JCV; a polyomavirus). JCV infects children and has a reported seropositivity in adults of greater than 60%. The virus stays latent in the kidneys and lymphoid organs until reactivation. PML mainly occurs in adults with impaired cell-mediated immunity, especially AIDS patients but also in those with lymphoproliferative and myeloproliferative disorders, granulomatous, inflammatory and rheumatic diseases, solid and hematopoietic cell transplantation. Use of natalizumab, an anti-integrin monoclonal antibody used in multiple sclerosis and inflammatory bowel disease is associated with a reported incidence of PML of 1:1000 after 18 months of therapy. Case reports also implicate rituximab use. JCV causes lytic infection of oligodendrocytes in the white matter and the symptoms presenting subacutely reflect the diverse areas of CNS involvement. Symptoms include altered mental status, aphasia, ataxia, hemiparesis or hemiplegia and visual field disturbances. Seizures occur in about 18%. Involvement of cranial nerves and cervical spine is rare.

PCR for JCV in cerebrospinal fluid is used for diagnosis in patients with compatible clinical and radiologic findings. MRI of the brain shows multifocal areas of white matter demyelination with no mass effect nor contrast enhancement. HAART for HIV improves survival as well as the clinical and radiographic features, although a small number of cases appear to worsen with immune restoration. Immune reconstitution syndromes do not alter mortality but are associated with a distinct form of PML called non-determined leukoencephalopathy associated with a distinct chemokine polymorphism. Significant neurologic sequelae to PML infections are the rule.

Decreasing immunosuppression in non-AIDS patients with PML (eg, transplant patients) is typically beneficial. Cidofovir may be beneficial in non-AIDS related cases;

corticosteroids may be useful with immune reconstitution. Anecdotal responses to risperidone and mirtazapine are reported (The JC virus infects cells through serotonin receptors). Future reports will assess the role of small inhibitory RNAs.

Aksamit AJ. Progressive multifocal leukoencephalopathy. Curr Treat Options Neurol. 2008 May;10(3):178–85. [PMID: 18579021]
Boren EJ et al. The emergence of progressive multifocal leukoencephalopathy (PML) in rheumatic diseases. J Autoimmun. 2008 Feb–Mar;30(1–2):90–8. [PMID: 18191544]
De Luca A et al. Cidofovir in addition to antiretroviral treatment is not effective for AIDS-associated progressive multifocal leukoencephalopathy: a multicohort analysis. AIDS. 2008 Sep 12;22(14):1759–67. [PMID: 18753934]
Falcó V et al. Influence of HAART on the clinical course of HIV-1-infected patients with progressive multifocal leukoencephalopathy: results of an observational multicenter study. J Acquir Immune Defic Syndr. 2008 Sep 1;49(1):26–31. [PMID: 18667930]

6. Human T Cell Lymphotropic Virus (HTLV)

HTLV-1 and -2 are retroviruses. HTLV-1 is endemic to many regions in the world including the Caribbean, southern Japan (where more than 10% of the population is infected), sub-Saharan Africa, Latin America, Eastern Europe, Oceania, and the southeastern United States (where seroprevalence is most common among injection drug users). The virus is transmitted horizontally (sex), vertically (intrauterine, peripartum, and breast-feeding), and parenterally (injection drug use and blood transfusion).

The association of HTLV-1 with adult T cell lymphoma/leukemia (ATL) is well established. The lifetime risk of developing ATL among seropositive persons is estimated to be 3% in women and 7% in men, with an incubation period of at least 15 years. The mean age of diagnosis of ATL is 40–50 years in Central and South America but 60 years in Japan.

ATL clinical syndromes may be classified as chronic, acute (leukemic), smoldering, or lymphomatous. Presentation as a primary cutaneous tumor is also described and has a prognosis worse than the smoldering type. Clinical features of ATL include diffuse lymphadenopathy, maculopapular skin lesions that may evolve into erythroderma, organomegaly, lytic bone lesions, and hypercalcemia. Opportunistic infections, such as *Pneumocystis jiroveci* pneumonia and cryptococcal meningitis, are more common. HTLV seropositivity is associated with an increased risk of tuberculosis. The identification of HTLV-1 antibodies supports the diagnosis. The peripheral smear can show atypical lymphoid cells with basophilic cytoplasm and convoluted nuclei (flower cells) but the diagnostic standard is evidence of clonal integration of the proviral DNA genome into tumor cell. Management of ATL is similar to that for non-Hodgkin lymphoma. The use of interferon-α, zidovudine, monoclonal antibodies or protein inhibitors is under evaluation.

HTLV-1 also causes HTLV-associated myelopathy (HAM; tropical spastic paraparesis). HAM develops in 0.3–4% of seropositive individuals and is more common in women. A chronic inflammation of the spinal cord leads to progressive motor weakness and symmetric spastic parapa- resis or paraplegia with hyperreflexia. Bladder and sexual disorders, sensory disturbances, and constipation are also common.

HTLV-1 provirus load in peripheral blood mononu- clear cells and in cerebrospinal fluid cells, and HTLV-1 mRNA load have all been proposed as markers of HAM risk and progression. HTLV positivity is associated with erythrocytosis and lymphocytosis (HTLV-II) and with thrombocytosis (HTLV-I and –II).

HAM is treated with a variety of immune-modulating agents (including corticosteroids) without consistent results. Combination of antiretrovirals does not show benefit. Inter- feron-a may be of some efficacy.

Patients infected with HTLV-1 show a risk of *Strongy- loides stercoralis* hyperinfection. Other associations are with tuberculosis, crusted scabies, and infective dermatitis. Inflammatory states associated with HTLV-1 infection include arthropathy, polymyositis, uveitis, Sjögren syn- drome, vasculitis, cryoglobulinemia, infiltrative pneumoni- tis, and ichthyosis.

HTLV-2 is no longer considered associated with hairy cell leukemia. HTLV-2 seropositivity is common in injec- tion drug users. HTLV-2 causes a myelopathy that is milder and slower to progress than HAM.

HTLV-1/HIV coinfection is associated both with higher CD4 counts and a higher risk of HAM.

Screening of the blood supply for HTLV-1 is required in the United States. There is significant cross-reactivity between HTLV-1 and HTLV-2 by serologic studies, but PCR can distinguish the two.

Oh U et al. Treatment of HTLV-I-associated myelopathy/tropi- cal spastic paraparesis: toward rational targeted therapy. Neu- rol Clin. 2008 Aug;26(3):781–97. [PMID: 18657726]
Verdonck K et al. Human T-lymphotropic virus 1: recent knowledge about an ancient infection. Lancet Infect Dis. 2007 Apr;7(4):266–81. [PMID: 17376384]

OTHER SYSTEMIC VIRAL DISEASES

1. Hemorrhagic Fevers

This diverse group of illnesses results from infection with one of several single-stranded RNA viruses (members of the families Arenaviridae, Bunyaviridae, Filoviridae, and Fla- viviridae). Flaviviruses, such as the pathogens causing den- gue and yellow fever (both with occasional hemorrhagic complications), are discussed in the following sections.

Modes of transmission are diverse. Lassa fever (an Old World arenavirus) is rodent associated and transmission usually occurs through aerosolized particles (from rodents or infected individuals) although contagion through direct contact with infected biologic fluids or tissues is also documented. Similar modes of transmission are assumed for Junin hemorrhagic fever and other diseases due to New World Arenaviridae. Ebola fever and Marburg fever (out- breaks in the Democratic Republic of Congo from 1998 to 2000 and in Angola from 2004 to 2005) are due to filovi- ruses with unknown vectors. Bats are the suspected reser-

voir for Ebola and Marburg viruses, and infection with the latter is associated with mining in the Congo. The bunyavi- ruses include the tick-borne Crimean-Congo hemorrhagic fever, the mosquito-borne Rift Valley fever (cause of a major outbreak in Saudi Arabia in 2000–2001 involving over 800 persons), and the hantaviruses (associated with rodent exposure and discussed separately below). Hospi- tal-associated transmission of Crimean-Congo hemor- rhagic fever is well documented in Iran.

▶ Clinical Findings

A. Symptoms and Signs

The incubation period can be as short as 2 days for the Rift Valley fever or as long as 21 days for Lassa fever. The clinical symptoms in the early phase of a viral hemorrhagic fever are very similar, irrespective of the causative virus, and resemble a flu-like illness or gastroenteritis. Hepatitis is common.

The late phase is more specific and is characterized by organ failure, persistent leukopenia, altered mental status, and hemorrhage. Exanthemas and mucosal lesions can occur. Adrenal dysfunction is a common sequela and a cause for the development of the late-stage shock associ- ated with these infections. The case-fatality rate ranges from 5% to 30% and may be as high as 90% in Ebola fever. The convalescence period can be long and complicated. There is no evidence of chronic infection among survivors.

B. Laboratory Findings

Laboratory features usually include thrombocytopenia, leu- kopenia, (although with Lassa fever leukocytosis is noted), anemia, increased hematocrit, oftenly elevated liver function tests, and findings consistent with disseminated intravascu- lar coagulation (although less prominently in Lassa fever). Urinalysis can reveal proteinuria and hematuria.

Special care should be taken for handling clinical spec- imens of suspected cases. Laboratory personnel should be warned about the diagnostic suspicion and the CDC must be contacted for guidance (Special Pathogens Branch, 404- 639-1115). Diagnosis may be made by growing the virus from blood obtained early in the disease, antigen detection (by ELISA), nucleic acid amplification (PCR techniques), or by demonstration of a significant specific fourfold or greater rise in antibody titer. Detection of Ebola virus antigen in oral fluid samples by ELISA and RT-PCR may be possible; sample collection in this manner will be useful since certain ethnic customs prohibit blood collection. These tests are generally available only through the CDC.

▶ Differential Diagnosis

The differential diagnosis for hemorrhagic fever includes meningococcemia or other septicemias, Rocky Mountain spotted fever, dengue, typhoid fever, and malaria. The likeli- hood of acquiring hemorrhagic fevers among travelers is low.

▶ Treatment

Patients should be placed in private rooms with standard contact and droplet precautions. Barrier precautions to prevent contamination of skin or mucous membranes should also be adopted by the caring personnel. Airborne precautions should be considered in patients with significant pulmonary involvement or undergoing procedures that stimulate cough.

Certain arenaviruses (the Lassa pathogen, Junin virus in its viscerotropic phase, Machupo virus) and bunyaviruses (the Congo-Crimean hemorrhagic fever and Rift Valley fever pathogens) respond to oral ribavirin if it is started promptly: 30 mg/kg as loading dose, followed by 16 mg/kg every 6 hours for 4 days and then 8 mg/kg every 8 hours for 3 days. The filoviruses and the flaviviruses do not respond to ribavirin. Live attenuated vaccines are available for Junin hemorrhagic fever and the Rift Valley fever, and they are under study for the Crimean-Congo hemorrhagic fever, Ebola, and Marburg viruses. In addition, recombinant vaccines are under development for most of these pathogens (including the Lassa fever virus but not the Junin hemorrhagic fever virus). Therapeutic interventions that target the hematologic system are either ineffective or only marginally effective.

When to Admit

- Persons with symptoms compatible with those of any hemorrhagic fever and who have traveled from a possible endemic area should be isolated for diagnosis and symptomatic treatment.
- Isolation is particularly important because diseases due to some of these agents, such as Ebola virus, are highly transmissible and carry a mortality rate of 50–90%.

Basuch DG et al; International Scientific and Technical Committee for Marburg Hemorrhagic Fever Control in the Democratic Republic of the Congo. Marburg hemorrhagic fever associated with multiple genetic lineages of virus. N Engl J Med. 2006 Aug 31;355(9):909–19. [PMID: 16943403]

Cleri DJ et al. Viral hemorrhagic fevers: current status of endemic disease and strategies for control. Infect Dis Clin North Am. 2006;20(2):359–93. [PMID: 16762743]

Jeffs B. A clinical guide to viral haemorrhagic fevers: Ebola, Marburg and Lassa. Trop Doct. 2006 Jan;36(1):1–4. [PMID: 16483416]

Marty AM et al. Viral hemorrhagic fevers. Clin Lab Med. 2006 Jun;26(2):345–86. [PMID: 16815457]

Mohamadzadeh M et al. How Ebola and Marburg viruses battle the immune system. Nat Rev Immunol. 2007 Jul;7(7):556–67. [PMID: 17589545]

Vorou R et al. Crimean-Congo hemorrhagic fever. Curr Opin Infect Dis. 2007 Oct;20(5):495–500. [PMID: 17762783]

2. Dengue

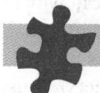

ESSENTIALS OF DIAGNOSIS

- Exposure 7–10 days before onset.
- Sudden onset of high fever, chills, severe myalgias and arthralgias, headache, sore throat, and depression.
- Biphasic fever curve: initial phase, 3–7 days; remission, few hours to 2 days; second phase, 1–2 days.
- Biphasic rash: evanescent, then maculopapular, scarlatiniform, morbilliform, or petechial changes from extremities to torso.
- Leukopenia and thrombocytopenia in the hemorrhagic form.

General Considerations

Dengue is due to a flavivirus transmitted by the bite of the *Aedes* mosquito. It may be caused by one of four serotypes widely distributed globally between the tropics of Capricorn and Cancer. An estimated 50–100 million cases of dengue fever and several hundred thousand cases of dengue hemorrhagic fever occur each year. The incubation period is 3–15 days (usually 7–10 days). When the virus is introduced into susceptible populations, usually by viremic travelers, epidemic attack rates range from 50% to 70%. Dengue is endemic in the lower Rio Grande Valley and adjacent border towns, with 40% of Brownsville, Texas residents showing serologic evidence of past infection and the virus being detected in mosquito larvae among 30% of households.

Severe epidemics of dengue hemorrhagic fever (serotype 3) occurred over the past 20 years in East Africa, Sri Lanka, and Latin America. In general, the more advanced forms of disease (hemorrhagic fever and shock) occur less often in the Americas than in Asia. In 2005, the first outbreak of dengue hemorrhagic fever in the continental United States was documented. The outbreak was binational and involved more than 6000 persons in Brownsville, Texas and Matamoros, Mexico with primarily serotype 2. Dengue is the second most common cause of fever (after malaria) in the traveler returning from developing countries. Nosocomial (via needlesticks or mucocutaneous exposure) and vertical transmission occur rarely.

Clinical Findings

A. Symptoms and Signs

Dengue infection may range from asymptomatic to severe hemorrhagic fever and fatal shock (**dengue shock syndrome**). Dengue fever is usually a nonspecific, self-limited biphasic febrile illness. More than half of infected children are asymptomatic. The illness is more severe and begins more suddenly in adults. After an incubation period of 4–5 days, there is a sudden onset of high fever, chills, and "break bone" aching of the head, back, and extremities accompanied by sore throat, prostration, and malaise. There may be conjunctival redness. Initially, the skin appears flushed or blotched, but 3–4 days after the lysis of the fever, a maculopapular rash, which spares palms and soles, appears in over 50% of cases. As the rash fades, localized clusters of petechiae on the extensor surface of the limbs become apparent. Hepatitis frequently complicates dengue fever.

Dengue hemorrhagic fever usually affects children living in endemic areas and is most likely to occur in secondary infections and in infections with serotype 2. A few days into the illness, signs of hemorrhage such as ecchymoses, gastrointestinal bleeding, and epistaxis appear. Symptoms found more often among the hemorrhagic fever subset of patients include restlessness, epistaxis, and abdominal pain.

A subset of patients, often with secondary infection, may progress to dengue shock syndrome in which acute fever, hemorrhagic manifestations, and marked capillary leak are prominent; the latter manifests as pleural effusions and ascites, and there is a tendency for shock to develop. While the infection is difficult to distinguish from malaria, yellow fever, or influenza, the rash makes dengue far more likely. Continuous abdominal pain with vomiting, bleeding, a decrease in the level of consciousness, and hypothermia should raise concern about dengue shock syndrome. A history of travel to a dengue-endemic area within 14 days of symptom onset is helpful for diagnosis.

B. Laboratory Findings

Leukopenia is characteristic, and elevated transaminases are found frequently in dengue fever. Thrombocytopenia, increased fibrinolysis, and hemoconcentration occur more often in the hemorrhagic form of the disease. Liver function abnormalities are nearly universal. The nonspecific nature of the illness mandates laboratory verification for diagnosis, usually with IgM and IgG ELISAs after the febrile phase. Virus may be recovered from the blood during the acute phase. PCR or detection of the specific viral protein NS1 by ELISA may be diagnostic during the first few days of infection. Immunohistochemistry for antigen detection in tissue samples can also be used. Chest radiographs in dengue hemorrhagic fever show infiltrates and effusions, which follow the course of laboratory abnormalities.

▶ Complications

Usual complications include pneumonia; bone marrow failure; hepatitis; iritis, retinal hemorrhages, and maculopathy; orchitis; and oophoritis. Depression and chronic fatigue, occurring more often in older women, are also reported. Neurologic complications, such as encephalitis, Guillain–Barré syndrome, and transverse myelitis, are less common. Bacterial superinfection occurs more commonly with advanced age, higher fever, gastrointestinal bleeding, kidney disease, and altered consciousness.

▶ Prevention

Available prophylactic measures include control of mosquitoes by screening and insect repellents, particularly during early morning and late afternoon exposures.

Tetravalent live attenuated vaccines and genetically modified chimeric virus vaccines are under study and entering clinical trials.

▶ Treatment

Treatment entails the appropriate use of volume support (with Ringer lactate in moderately severe shock and colloids in more severe cases), blood products, and pressor agents, and acetaminophen rather than nonsteroidal antiinflammatory drugs for analgesia. Activities are gradually

restored during prolonged convalescences. Endoscopic therapy is useful in evaluating and managing gastrointestinal hemorrhage, although injection therapy with sclerosing agents is not beneficial in most dengue hemorrhagic states. Platelet counts do not usefully predict clinically significant bleeding. Platelet transfusions, however, should be considered for severe thrombocytopenia (< 10,000/mL) or when there is evidence of bleeding. Monitoring for hemoconcentration may help in anticipating the complications of dengue hemorrhagic fever or shock syndrome.

▶ Prognosis

Fatalities are rare but do occur, especially during epidemic outbreaks, with occasional patients dying of fulminant hepatitis. Convalescence for most patients is slow.

Centers for Disease Control and Prevention (CDC). Dengue hemorrhagic fever–U.S.-Mexico border, 2005. MMWR Morb Mortal Wkly Rep. 2007 Aug 10;56(31):785–9. [PMID: 17687243]

Edelman R. Dengue vaccines approach the finish line. Clin Infect Dis. 2007;45(Suppl 1):S56–60. [PMID: 17582571]

Halstead SB. Dengue. Lancet. 2007 Nov 10;370(9599):1644–52. [PMID: 17993365]

Morens DM et al. Dengue and hemorrhagic fever: a potential threat to public health in the United States. JAMA. 2008 Jan 9;299(2):214–6. [PMID: 18182605]

Schwartz E et al. Seasonality, annual trends, and characteristics of dengue among ill returned travelers, 1997–2006. Emerg Infect Dis. 2008 Jul;14(7):1081–8. [PMID: 18598629]

3. Hantaviruses

Hantaviruses are rodent-borne enveloped RNA bunyaviruses with several distinct serotypes. These differ in rodent hosts, geographic distribution, and degree of pathogenicity for humans. They cause two major clinical syndromes: **hemorrhagic fever** (discussed above) and the **hantavirus pulmonary syndrome** (HPS). Each year, over 150,000 cases of these two syndromes occur globally, with HPS being far less common. Aerosols of virus-contaminated rodent urine and perhaps feces are thought to be the main vehicle for transmission to humans. The ubiquity of hantaviruses is recognized, with descriptions of infections from North and South America (New World hantaviruses) and additional infections from Europe and Asia (Old World hantaviruses). The Hantaan serotype viruses cause severe hemorrhagic fever with renal syndrome and are found primarily in Korea, China, and eastern Russia. The Seoul viruses produce a less severe form and are found primarily in Korea and China. The Puumala and Dobrava viruses are found in Scandinavia and Europe and are associated with a milder form of the syndrome, nephropathia epidemica, which usually presents with fever, headache, gastrointestinal symptoms, and impaired kidney function.

The Sin Nombre (Muerto Canyon, Four Corners) virus is the most common hantavirus infection in the United States and is the chief North American virus responsible for HPS; it is usually seen in the southwestern United States. Between 1993 and 2006, 438 cases were reported in 32 states in an area roughly coterminous with the distribution of plague. Outbreaks of HPS with other hantavirus types are also reported from Central and South America. HPS (the mean incubation period for which is 18 days) begins as a nonspecific febrile illness followed by a severe increase in pulmonary vascular permeability associated with a CD8 immune response, leading to respiratory failure, and rapid progression to a shock-like state. Laboratory features include thrombocytopenia, hemoconcentration, leukocytosis (with abnormal lymphocytes and immature myeloid cells), and elevated lactate dehydrogenase and transaminases. Clinical similarities, including a propensity toward kidney involvement exist between the New World hantaviruses and their Old World counterparts.

Diagnosis can be made serologically, with most patients having both IgM and IgG antibodies at the time of presentation; by immunohistochemical staining; or by PCR amplification of viral tissue DNA (the agents may be isolated from blood or saliva). A viral load assay correlates with severity of disease among patients with HPS caused by the Sin Nombre virus.

Treatment is mainly supportive. Intravenous ribavirin has been used with some success in hemorrhagic fever with renal syndrome (Hantaan virus), but studies in HPS suggest it is not effective. Cardiorespiratory support with pressors and sometimes extracorporeal membrane oxygenation may be considered. Because infection is thought to occur by inhalation of rodent wastes, prevention is aimed at eradication of rodents in houses and avoidance of exposure to rodent excreta in rural settings, including forest service facilities.

Abel Borges A et al. Mechanisms of shock in hantavirus pulmonary syndrome. Curr Opin Infect Dis. 2008 Jun;21(3):293–7. [PMID: 18448975]

Eisen RJ et al. A spatial model of shared risk for plague and hantavirus pulmonary syndrome in the southwestern United States. Am J Trop Med Hyg. 2007 Dec;77(6):999–1004. [PMID: 18165511]

Ferluga D et al. Hantavirus nephropathy. J Am Soc Nephrol. 2008 Sep;19(9):1653–8. [PMID: 18650483]

Jonsson CB et al. Treatment of hantavirus pulmonary syndrome. Antiviral Res. 2008 Apr;78(1):162–9. [PMID: 18093668]

4. Yellow Fever

ESSENTIALS OF DIAGNOSIS

► Endemic area exposure (tropical South and Central America, Africa, but not Asia).

► Sudden onset of severe headache, aching in legs, and tachycardia.

► Brief (1 day) remission, followed by bradycardia, hypotension, jaundice, hemorrhagic tendency.

► Proteinuria, leukopenia, bilirubinemia, bilirubinuria.

► Rare and potentially fatal reactions to vaccination.

▶ General Considerations

Yellow fever is a zoonotic flavivirus infection transmitted by *Aedes* and jungle mosquitoes. It occurs in an urban and jungle cycle in Africa and in a jungle cycle in South America (where genetic studies suggest it arose through the slave trade 300–400 years ago). Epidemics have extended far into the temperate zone during warm seasons.

The mosquito transmits the infection by first biting an individual having the disease and then biting a susceptible individual after the virus has multiplied within the mosquito's body. The incubation period in humans is 3–6 days. Adults and children are equally susceptible, though attack rates are highest among adult males because of their work habits. Between 5% and 50% of infections are asymptomatic.

▶ Clinical Findings

A. Symptoms and Signs

1. Mild form—Symptoms are malaise, headache, fever, retroorbital pain, nausea, vomiting, and photophobia. Relative bradycardia, conjunctival injection, and facial flushing may be present.

2. Severe form—Severe illness develops in about 15%. Initial symptoms are similar to the mild form, but a brief fever remission lasting hours to a few days is followed by a "period of intoxication" manifested by fever and relative bradycardia (Faget sign), hypotension, jaundice, hemorrhage (gastrointestinal, nasal, oral), and delirium that may progress to coma.

B. Laboratory Findings

Leukopenia occurs, although it may not be present at the onset. Kidney disease with proteinuria is present, sometimes as high as 5–6 g/L, and usually disappears completely with recovery. Levels of liver enzymes and bilirubin can be remarkably abnormal with the levels of aspartate aminotransferase (AST) usually doubling those of alanine aminotransferase (ALT). Prothrombin time may be elevated as well. Serologic diagnosis is primarily by measurement of IgM by capture ELISA during the acute and convalescent phases. Viral culture is possible and has been used in epidemic settings. Rapid test involving PCR protocols and immunoassays of monoclonal antibodies against circulating viral antigens are becoming more widely available.

▶ Differential Diagnosis

It may be difficult to distinguish yellow fever from hepatitis, malaria, leptospirosis, louse-borne relapsing fever, dengue, and other hemorrhagic fevers on clinical evidence alone. Albuminuria is a constant feature in yellow fever patients and its presence helps differentiate yellow fever from other viral hepatitides. Serologic confirmation is often needed.

▶ Prevention

Transmission is prevented through mosquito control. Live virus vaccine is highly effective and should be provided for immunocompetent persons over 9 months of age living in or traveling to endemic areas. Revaccination is recommended every 10 years for persons with continued exposure. Vaccine-induced reactions, including neurotropic (encephalitis-like syndrome) and viscerotropic (resembling yellow fever) diseases are reported (particularly among patients of 60 years or older and patients with thymic dysfunction; the former should probably not be vaccinated and the latter definitely not be vaccinated). The safety of the vaccine in pregnant patients is not verified, and pregnant women should, if possible, defer travel to endemic areas (see Chapter 30). Eradication is difficult because of the sylvatic cycle (mainly maintained by non-human primates).

▶ Treatment

No specific antiviral therapy is available. Treatment is directed toward symptomatic relief and management of complications. If not in an endemic area, the patient should be isolated from mosquitoes to prevent transmission, since blood in the acute phase is potentially infectious.

▶ Prognosis

The mortality rate of the severe form is 20–50%, with death occurring most commonly between the sixth and the tenth days. In survivors, the temperature returns to normal by the seventh or eighth day. The prognosis in any individual case is guarded at the onset, since sudden changes for the worse are common. Intractable hiccups, copious black vomitus, melena, anuria, jaundice, and elevated AST are unfavorable signs. Convalescence is prolonged, including 1–2 weeks of asthenia. Infection confers lifelong immunity to those who recover.

Barnett ED. Yellow fever: epidemiology and prevention. Clin Infect Dis. 2007 Mar 15;44(6):850–6. [PMID: 17304460]
Monath TP. Dengue and yellow fever-challenges for the development and use of vaccines. N Engl J Med. 2007 Nov 29;357(22):2222–5. [PMID: 18046026]

5. Tick-Borne Encephalitis

ESSENTIALS OF DIAGNOSIS

▶ Flaviviral encephalitis found in Eastern, Central, and occasionally Northern Europe and Asia.

▶ Transmitted via ticks or ingestion of unpasteurized milk.

▶ Long-term neurologic sequelae occur in 2–25% of cases.

▶ Therapy is largely supportive.

▶ Prevention is based on avoiding tick exposure, pasteurization of milk, and vaccination.

▶ General Considerations

Tick-borne encephalitis (TBE) is a flaviviral infection caused by TBE virus. This infection is endemic in Russia and in eastern and central Europe, but cases are also well recognized in western Europe, China, and Japan. An estimated 10,000 to 12,000 cases occur each year in parts of Europe and the Baltic, with annual increases thought to be

a function of increased recognition, climatic changes, and personal or social habits. TBE occurs predominantly in the late spring through fall. It is usually a consequence of exposure to infected ticks, although unpasteurized milk from viremic livestock is also a recognized form of transmission. The incubation period is 7–14 days for tick-borne exposures but only 3–4 days for milk ingestion. The principal reservoirs for TBE virus are small rodents; humans are an accidental host. The vectors for most cases are *Ixodes ricinus* (most of Europe, including Turkey, Iran, and the Caucasus) and *Ixodes persulcatus* (in the belt from eastern Europe to China and Japan).

▶ Clinical Findings
A. Symptoms and Signs

Most cases are subclinical and many resemble a flu-like syndrome. There are two variants of clinical presentation: the Western subtype occurs mainly in the fall and is most severe among the elderly, and the Eastern subtype is more severe among children.

Western subtype disease is biphasic in which after 2–10 days of fever (usually with malaise, headache, and myalgias), a 1–21 day symptom-free interval leads to a second phase with resumed fevers followed by neurologic symptoms. Eastern subtype disease is progressive without an asymptomatic interval. The neurologic manifestations range from febrile headache (accounting for up to 50% of Eastern subtype cases) to aseptic meningitis and encephalitis with or without myelitis (preferentially of the cervical anterior horn) and spinal paralysis (usually flaccid). A myeloradiculitic form can also develop but is less common. Double infection with *Borrelia burgdorferi* (the agent if Lyme disease; transmitted by the same tick vector) may result in a more severe disease. Homozygosity for a 32bp deletion in the gene coding for the chemokine receptor CCR5, producing its complete loss of function, predisposes to severe disease. People with this mutation are, however, naturally resistant to HIV infection and CCR5 is the target of blockage by newer antiretroviral medications (eg, maraviroc and vicriviroc). Mortality in TBE is usually a consequence of brain edema or bulbar involvement.

B. Diagnosis

Leukocytosis and neutrophilia are common. Abnormal cerebrospinal fluid findings include a pleocytosis that may persist for up to 4 months. Neuroimaging shows hyperintense lesions in the thalamus, brainstem, and basal ganglia. TBE virus IgM and IgG are detected by ELISA techniques when neurologic symptoms occur. Cross-reactivity with other flaviviruses or a vaccinated state (see below) may require confirmation by detection of TEB virus–specific antibodies in cerebrospinal fluid. RT-PCR of blood (at earlier stages of the disease) or cerebrospinal fluid can sometimes, if available, assist with the diagnosis.

▶ Complications

The main sequela of disease is paresis, which occurs in up to 10% of Western and up to 25% of Eastern subtype disease. Other causes of long-term morbidity include protracted cognitive dysfunction and persistent spinal nerve paralysis. The postencephalitic syndrome, characterized by headache, difficulties concentrating, balance disorders, dysphasia, hearing defects, and chronic fatigue, occurs with both subtypes. A progressive motor neuron disease may occur with the Eastern subtype.

Differential Diagnosis

The differential diagnosis includes other causes of aseptic meningitis such as enteroviral infections, herpes simplex encephalitis, and a variety of tick-borne pathogens including tularemia, the rickettsial diseases, babesiosis, Lyme disease, poliomyelitis (no longer reported from Eastern Europe) and other flaviviral infections.

Prevention

There are two inactivated TBE virus vaccines for adults and two vaccines for children licensed in Europe. Their effectiveness is about 99% when properly administered. The initial vaccination schedule requires 1 year with boosters every 3–5 years. Other prevention recommendations include avoidance of tick exposure and pasteurization of milk.

Treatment

Therapy is largely supportive. Some clinicians believe corticosteroids may be useful, although no controlled clinical trials exist.

Kaiser R. Tick-borne encephalitis. Infect Dis Clin North Am. 2008 Sep;22(3):561–75. [PMID: 18755391]

Kindberg E et al. A deletion in the chemokine receptor 5 (CCR5) gene is associated with tickborne encephalitis. J Infect Dis. 2008 Jan 15;197(2):266–9. [PMID: 18179389]

Lindquist L et al. Tick-borne encephalitis. Lancet. 2008 May 31;371(9627):1861–71. [PMID: 18514730]

6. Colorado Tick Fever

ESSENTIALS OF DIAGNOSIS

▶ Onset 1–19 days (average, 4 days) following tick bite.

▶ Fever, chills, myalgia, headache, prostration.

▶ Leukopenia, thrombocytopenia.

▶ Second attack of fever after remission lasting 2–3 days.

General Considerations

Colorado tick fever is a reportable acute reovirus infection transmitted by *Dermacentor andersoni* bites. The disease is limited to the western United States and Canada and is most prevalent during the tick season (March to November). There is a discrete history of tick bite or exposure in 90% of cases. The virus infects the marrow erythrocyte precursors, leading to viremia lasting the life span of the infected red cells. Blood transfusions can be a vehicle of transmission.

Clinical Findings

A. Symptoms and Signs

The incubation period is 3–6 days. The onset is usually abrupt with fever (to 38.9–40.6 °C), sometimes with chills. Severe myalgia, headache, photophobia, anorexia, nausea and vomiting, and generalized weakness are prominent. Physical findings are limited to an occasional faint rash. The acute symptoms resolve within a week. The remission is followed in 50% of cases by recurrent fever and a full recrudescence lasting 2–4 days. In an occasional case, there may be three bouts of fever.

The differential diagnosis includes influenza, Rocky Mountain spotted fever, numerous other viral infections and, in the right setting, relapsing fevers.

B. Laboratory Findings

Leukopenia (2000–3000/mcL) with a shift to the left and atypical lymphocytes occurs, reaching a nadir 5–6 days after the onset of illness. Thrombocytopenia may occur. Viremia may be demonstrated by inoculation of blood into mice or by fluorescent antibody staining of the patient's red cells (with adsorbed virus). An RT-PCR assay may be used to detect early viremia. Detection of IgM by capture ELISA or plaque reduction neutralization is possible after 2 weeks from symptom onset and is the most frequently used diagnostic tool.

Complications

Aseptic meningitis (particularly in children), encephalitis, and hemorrhagic fever occur rarely. Malaise may last weeks to months. Fatalities are very rare. There is one reported case of spontaneous abortion and multiple congenital anomalies associated with Colorado tick fever infection during pregnancy.

Treatment

No specific treatment is available. Ribavirin has shown efficacy in an animal model. Antipyretics are used, although aspirin should be avoided. Tick-avoidance is the best prevention.

Prognosis

The disease is usually self-limited and benign.

Romero JR et al. Powassan encephalitis and Colorado tick fever. Infect Dis Clin North Am. 2008 Sep;22(3):545–59. [PMID: 18755390]

7. Chikungunya Fever

Chikungunya ("that which bends up" in Bantu) is a flaviviral infection transmitted to humans by *Aedes aegypti* and *Aedes albopictus*. While historically limited to tropical Africa and Asia, a major ongoing outbreak starting in 2004 spread the disease to the Indian subcontinent and to northeastern Italy, with attack rates of around 50% in some regions. Travelers return often viremic from these areas. The endemicity of *A aegypti* in the Americas and the introduction of

A albopictus into Europe and the New World raise the concerns of a global extension of the epidemic.

Clinical Findings

A. Symptoms and Signs

After an incubation period of 1–12 days (average 2–4), there is an abrupt onset of fever; headache; intestinal complaints; myalgias; and arthralgias/arthritis affecting small, large, ans axial joints. The simultaneous involvement of more than 10 joints and the presence of tenosynovitis (especially in the wrist) are characteristic. The stooped posture of patients gives the disease its name. Joint symptoms persists for 4 months in 33% and linger for years in about 10%. A centrally distributed pruritic maculopapular rash is reported in 50% of the patients, but it can be bullous with sloughing in children. Facial edema and localized petechiae are reported. Meningoencephalitis is occasional and hemorrhagic fever-like presentation exceptional. Coinfection with other respiratory viruses is common. Death is rare and usually related to underlying comorbidities.

B. Laboratory Findings

Diagnosis is made epidemiologically and clinically. Mild leukopenia occurs as does thrombocytopenia, which is seldom severe. Elevated inflammatory markers do not correlate with the severity of arthritis. Radiographs of affected joints are normal.

Serologic confirmation requires elevated IgM titers or fourfold increases in convalescent IgG levels. RT-PCR and culture techniques (viral isolation in insect or mammalian cell lines or by inoculation of mosquitoes or mice) are seldom available. Suspected cases in the United States should be promptly reported to public health authorities including the CDC Arboviral Diseases Branch, 970-221-6400. The differential includes other tropical febrile diseases, such as malaria or dengue.

Treatment

Treatment is largely supportive with nonsteroidal anti-inflammatory drugs. Chloroquine may be useful for managing refractory arthritis. No vaccine is available, and prevention relies on avoidance of the mosquito vectors. Vertical transmission is documented, but teratogenicity is not established.

Pialoux G et al. Chikungunya, an epidemic arbovirosis. Lancet Infect Dis. 2007 May;7(5):319–27. [PMID: 17448935]
Simon F et al. Chikungunya: a paradigm of emergence and globalization of vector-borne diseases. Med Clin North Am. 2008 Nov;92(6):1323–43. [PMID: 19061754]

COMMON VIRAL RESPIRATORY INFECTIONS

1. Respiratory Syncytial Virus & Other Paramyxoviruses

General Considerations

Respiratory syncytial virus (RSV) is a paramyxovirus that causes annual outbreaks, in winter and early spring, of pneumonia, bronchiolitis, and tracheobronchitis, with the majority of cases occurring in the very young. Risk factors include prematurity, low birth weight, younger age (especially younger than 6 months), bronchopulmonary dysplasia, congenital heart disease, later birth order, and day care exposure. Reinfections are common but usually milder. In older children and adults, RSV infection is typically manifested as an upper respiratory tract infection and tracheobronchitis. The virus enters through contact with mucosal surfaces, as the eye or nose. The average incubation period is 5 days. RSV infection in children has been associated with persistence of airway reactivity later in life in some studies.

In immunocompromised patients, such as bone marrow transplant recipients, serious pneumonia can occur and outbreaks with a high mortality rate (> 70%) are reported. RSV infection is also an important illness in elderly and other high-risk adults (eg, those with chronic heart or lung diseases).

Other paramyxoviruses important in human disease include human metapneumovirus and parainfluenza virus. **Human metapneumovirus** is less common and less pathogenic than RSV. It appears to cause bronchiolitis; croup; exacerbation of pneumonia; and pneumonia during the winter and spring among slightly older children and is responsible for lower respiratory tract infections among immunocompromised and elderly adults. **Parainfluenza viruses,** the most common cause of croup, also causes respiratory tract infections in the very young, the elderly, the immunocompromised, and those with chronic illnesses. **Bocavirus** infections are discussed under parvoviruses.

Clinical Findings

A. Symptoms and Signs

In RSV bronchiolitis, proliferation and necrosis of bronchiolar epithelium develop, producing obstruction from sloughed epithelium and increased mucus secretion. Signs include low-grade fever, tachypnea, and wheezes. Apnea is a common presenting symptom. Hyperinflated lungs, decreased gas exchange, and increased work of breathing are present. In children, RSV is a common cause of acute and recurrent otitis media. RSV-confirmed bronchiolitis in children under age 13 is associated with the development of asthma. RSV pneumonia is a serious condition in the elderly and debilitated patient as well as in the immunocompromised person.

B. Laboratory Findings

A rapid diagnosis of RSV infection is made by viral antigen identification of nasal washings using an ELISA or immunofluorescent assay. Culture of nasopharyngeal or lower respiratory tract secretions remain the standard of diagnosis, although PCR is increasingly used. Coinfection with bacteria is relatively uncommon in industrialized countries. Coinfection with *B pertussis* and other viruses occurs in a subset of patients hospitalized for RSV infection. Detection of parainfluenza virus usually requires culture, but tests for rapid detection of viral antigens with immunofluorescence or ELISA, and PCR techniques are also available. Human metapneumovirus is best diagnosed by PCR.

Treatment

Treatment of RSV consists of supportive care, including hydration, humidification of inspired air, and ventilatory support as needed. Neither bronchodilating agents nor corticosteroids have demonstrated efficacy in bronchiolitis although individual patients with significant bronchospasm or history of asthma might respond to them. Use of nebulized ribavarin might be considered in some high risk and very sick children (eg, immunosuppressed, those with underlying pulmonary or congenital heart conditions, and those with severe respiratory compromise) but the evidence of its efficacy is not well documented and this therapy is expensive and cumbersome. There is no evidence that macrolides are beneficial to infants or children with lower respiratory tract disease caused by RSV.

Ribavirin can also be considered in high-risk adults, such as those with a history of bone marrow transplantation. Pregnant women, including hospital staff, should avoid ribavirin exposure. Therapy with surfactant lacks evidence to make recommendations on its use. Passive immunotherapy has no role in treating acute infections in children. The combination of hyperimmune RSV immunoglobulin G (RSVIG) and ribavarin appears to be beneficial in uncontrolled studies of infected adult bone marrow transplant patients. In the United States, RSVIG is no longer available and has been replaced with palivizumab, a monoclonal RSV antibody. Administration of palivizumab prophylactically (parenterally at 15 mg/kg monthly during the season of high transmission) to infants with high-risk factors, such as congenital heart disease, is well recommended. Future studies may entail the use of small inhibitory RNA molecules and of newer generation monoclonal antibodies, such as motavizumab.

Live attenuated vaccines fail to show significant clinical protection or immunogenicity in adults and their use in infants raises safety concerns. Prevention in hospitals entails rapid diagnosis, handwashing, contact isolation, and perhaps passive immunization. Therapeutic modalities for human metapneumovirus and parainfluenzavirus infections under investigation include ribavirin administration. The use of conjugated pneumococcal vaccination appears to decrease the incidence of concomitant pneumonia associated with viral infections in children in some countries.

Mohapatra SS et al. Epidemiologic, experimental, and clinical links between respiratory syncytial virus infection and asthma. Clin Microbiol Rev. 2008 Jul;21(3):495–504. [PMID: 18625684]

Panickar J et al. Oral prednisolone for preschool children with acute virus-induced wheezing. N Engl J Med. 2009 Jan 22;360(4):329–38. [PMID: 19164186]

Power UF. Respiratory syncytial virus (RSV) vaccines—two steps back for one leap forward. J Clin Virol. 2008 Jan;41(1):38–44. [PMID: 18340669]

Rossi GA et al. Risk factors for severe RSV-induced lower respiratory tract infection over four consecutive epidemics. Eur J Pediatr. 2007 Dec;166(12):1267–72. [PMID: 17308898]

2. Influenza

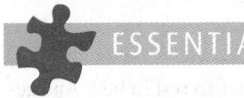

ESSENTIALS OF DIAGNOSIS

▶ Cases usually in epidemic pattern.

▶ Abrupt onset with fever, chills, malaise, cough, coryza, and myalgias.

▶ Aching, fever, and prostration out of proportion to catarrhal symptoms.

▶ Leukopenia.

General Considerations

Influenza (an orthomyxovirus) is a highly contagious disease transmitted by the respiratory route. In contrast to RSV and rhinoviruses, transmission occurs primarily by droplet nuclei rather than fomites or large particle aerosols. There are three types of influenza viruses. While type A can infect a variety of mammals (humans, swine, horses, etc) and birds, types B and C almost exclusively infect humans. Type A viruses are further divided into subtypes based on the hemagglutinin (H) and the neuraminidase (N) expressed in their surface. There are 16 subtypes of hemagglutinin and 9 subtypes of neuraminidase. Annual epidemics usually appear in the fall or winter (although sporadic cases occur as summer outbreaks in northern areas such as Alaska); they affect 10–20% of the global population on average each year and are rarely the result of frequent minor antigenic variations of the virus, or antigenic drift, which are more common in influenza A virus. On the other hand, pandemics—associated with higher mortality—appear at longer (3–5 decades) and varying intervals as a consequence of a major genetic reassortment of the virus (antigenic shift) or the mutation of an animal virus that adapts to the human (as with the avian-origin (H5N1) pandemic virus of 1918). Currently, the main circulating influenza viruses are the human-origin A (H1N1) and (H3N2) subtypes, as well as type B. A novel swine-origin influenza A (H1N1) virus of pandemic potential emerged in Mexico in March of 2009 and quickly spread through North America and elsewhere. In addition, a highly pathogenic avian (H5N1) subtype that caused occasional human infections in Asia and Europe over the last decade is still cause of ongoing global concern. The infections with influenza viruses of human origin will be discussed here, whereas those due to avian- and swine-origin viruses will be covered in the next sections.

Clinical Findings

A. Symptoms and Signs

Human-origin influenza viruses of antigenic types A and B produce clinically indistinguishable infections, whereas type C usually causes a minor illness. Typically, the infection has an incubation period is 1–4 days. In unvaccinated persons, typical uncomplicated influenza often begins abruptly. Symptoms include fever, chills, malaise, myalgias, substernal soreness, headache, nasal stuffiness, and occasionally nausea. Fever lasts 1–7 days (usually 3–5). Coryza, nonproductive cough, and sore throat are present. Elderly patients may present with only lassitude and confusion, often without fever or respiratory symptoms. Signs include mild pharyngeal injection, flushed face, and conjunctival redness. Moderate enlargement of the cervical lymph nodes may be observed. The presence of fever (> to

38.2 °C) and cough during influenza season is highly predictive of influenza infection in those older than 4 years of age.

B. Laboratory Findings

Leukopenia is common, but leukocytosis can occur. Proteinuria may be present. The virus may be isolated from throat swabs or nasal washings by inoculation of embryonated eggs or cell cultures. Rapid immunofluorescence assays and enzyme immunoassays for detection of influenza antigens from nasal or throat swabs are becoming widely available; however, their sensitivity is suboptimal (60–80%) and only a few can distinguish between influenza A and B. Nucleic acid (PCR) techniques still remain less accessible. Complement-fixing and hemagglutination-inhibiting antibodies appear during the second week. Microarrays may be used in the future to monitor the spread of pathogenic viral variants.

▶ Complications

Influenza causes necrosis of the respiratory epithelium, which predisposes to secondary bacterial infections. In turn, bacterial enzymes (eg, proteases, trypsin-like compounds, streptokinase) activate influenza viruses. Frequent complications are acute sinusitis, otitis media, purulent bronchitis, and pneumonia. Children (6–59 months), pregnant women, the elderly (aged 65 years or older), and the chronically ill (including HIV-infected individuals) are at high risk for complications.

Primary viral pneumonia (caused by the influenza virus itself) may occur, particularly in patients with cardiovascular disease and pregnant women and has a high mortality. Secondary bacterial pneumonia due to pneumococci or, less often, staphylococci or *Haemophilus* spp is common. Pericarditis and myocarditis occur infrequently. Rhabdomyolysis is a rare late complication.

Reye syndrome (fatty liver with encephalopathy) is a rare and severe complication of influenza (usually B type) and other viral diseases (eg, varicella), particularly in young children. It consists of rapidly progressive hepatic failure and encephalopathy, and there is a 30% mortality rate. The pathogenesis is unknown, but the syndrome is associated with aspirin use in a variety of viral infections. Hypoglycemia, elevation of serum aminotransferases and blood ammonia, prolonged prothrombin time, and change in mental status all occur within 2–3 weeks after onset of the viral infection. Histologically, the periphery of liver lobules shows striking fatty infiltration and glycogen depletion. Treatment is supportive and directed toward the management of cerebral edema. Other encephalopathic complications of influenza are equally rare and include an acute necrotizing encephalopathy associated with disseminated intravascular coagulation and cytokine storm, with worsening when treated with certain nonsteroidal anti-inflammatory drugs (diclofenac and mefenamic acid), and an acute encephalopathy associated with febrile seizures and the use of theophylline. Influenza infections appear to be an infrequent trigger of Guillain-Barré syndrome.

▶ Prevention

If no contraindication is present, influenza vaccination in October or November each year is recommended for persons over 50 years of age; children (6 months–18 years of age); nursing home residents; patients of any age with chronic medical problems, including lung or heart disease, active malignancy, diabetes, kidney disease, chronic liver disease, immunodeficiencies (such as HIV infection or organ transplant), hemoglobinopathies, or neurologic conditions that impair the clearance of respiratory secretions; pregnant women; and contacts of these high-risk groups, including health care workers, service personnel, and caretakers of children younger than 2 years (see Chapter 30).

The vaccine is contraindicated in persons with well-substantiated hypersensitivity to chicken eggs (based on dietary history) or other components of the vaccine (skin testing can be performed by an allergist), in persons with Guillain–Barré syndrome, or in persons with an acute febrile illness until symptomatic improvement. Concomitant warfarin or corticosteroid therapy is not a contraindication. Side effects are infrequent and include tenderness, redness, or induration at the site for the trivalent inactivated vaccine (intramuscular); and respiratory symptoms for the live attenuated intranasal vaccine.

Chemoprophylaxis can be considered for certain individuals (see Treatment section for definitions) exposed to an infected patient within 2 weeks after vaccination with the trivalent inactivated vaccine; this does not apply for the intranasal live attenuated vaccine since it confers more rapid protection. Chemoprophylaxis may also be considered for those in whom vaccination is contraindicated or not available. Special circumstances that may also warrant consideration of chemoprophylaxis include outbreaks in long-term care facilities, persons living with or in close contact with high risk unvaccinated individuals (eg, health-care providers), persons with immune deficiencies who might not respond to vaccination, unvaccinated staff during response to an outbreak in a closed institutional setting with residents at high risk, and first responders to epidemic situations. Chemoprophylaxis against influenza A and B is traditionally accomplished with the neuraminidase inhibitors oseltamivir (75 mg/d, oral) and zanamivir (10 mg/d, inhaled) but resistance to the former is increasingly prevalent in H1N1 strains. These agents reduce the attack rate among unvaccinated individuals if begun within 48 hours after exposure. In the United States, the M2 inhibitors amantadine and rimantadine are effective against current human H1N1 strains but not the epidemic H1N1 virus of swine origin (see below). In addition, these drugs are not active against other circulating influenza A viruses (H3N2) or B viruses and hence, their use as first-line agents is limited. Occasionally, chemoprophylaxis may need to be continued for the duration of influenza activity in the community, but cost, compliance, and potential adverse effects should be considered as well.

▶ Treatment

Many patients with influenza prefer to rest in bed. Analgesics and a cough mixture may be used. Treatment should be considered for those with a suggestive clinical presentation or with laboratory confirmed influenza and at high risk for developing complications (nursing home residents; patients with chronic pulmonary, cardiovascular, kidney, or liver disease; those with diabetes, active malignancy, immunosuppression, or impairment for managing respiratory secretions), or living with persons at significant risk for them. Maximum benefit is expected with the earliest initiation of therapy. Although the benefit of antiviral therapy after 48 hours of illness is unproven, it should be considered if the patient is hospitalized.

The neuraminidase inhibitors, either inhaled zanamivir (two 5-mg inhalations twice daily for 5 days) or oral oseltamivir (75 mg twice daily for 5 days), are equally effective in the treatment of susceptible strains of influenza. Clinical trials have shown a reduction in the duration of symptoms as well as secondary complications such as otitis, sinusitis, or pneumonia, but not in the rate of hospitalizations or mortality when using these agents. These drugs, when administered early, are effective mainly in high-risk patients over age 12 years. Resistance to neuraminidase inhibitors can occur with prolonged use in immunocompromised patients or in avian (H5N1)-infected patients. High rates (greater than 25%) of oseltamivir resistance in influenza A viruses are reported in surveillance data from several areas of Europe and Africa. In the United States, unfortunately, resistance to oseltamivir is also progressively becoming more prevalent, especially among influenza A (H3N2) strains. No comprehensive data on global emergence of resistance to zanamivir are available. Both oseltamivir and zanamivir appear less effective in treating influenza B than influenza A viruses. Zanamivir is relatively contraindicated among persons with asthma because of the risk of bronchospasm. Transient neuropsychiatric events, occasionally resulting in self-injury and death, have been reported postmarketing for both neuraminidase inhibitors. Patients receiving these drugs should be closely monitored for any unusual behavior, and healthcare professionals should be notified immediately if such signs occur. Ribavirin (unlabeled usage, 1.1 g/d, diluted to 20 mg/mL, delivered as particulate aerosol with oxygen over 12–18 hours a day for 3–7 days [see Table 32–1]) may be effective in severely ill patients with influenza A or B. Amantadine and rimantadine are inactive against influenza A (H3N2) and influenza B, but they can be used for treatment in the United States, in conjunction with neuraminidase inhibitors, when human-origin influenza A (H1N1) is the predominant viral strain in the community.

Antibacterial antibiotics should be reserved for treatment of bacterial complications. Acetaminophen rather than aspirin should be used for fever in children.

Prognosis

The duration of the uncomplicated illness is 1–7 days, and the prognosis is excellent in healthy, nonelderly adults. Purulent bronchitis and bronchiectasis may result in chronic pulmonary disease and fibrosis that persist throughout life. Most fatalities are due to bacterial pneumonia although exacerbations of other diseases processes,

in particular cardiac diseases, occur which contributed to the overall increase in fatalities. Influenza pneumonia has a high mortality rate among pregnant women and persons with a history of rheumatic heart disease. In recent epidemics, the mortality rate has been low except in debilitated individuals.

If the fever persists for more than 4 days with productive cough and white cell count over 10,000/mcL, secondary bacterial infection should be suspected. Pneumococcal pneumonia is the most common such infection, and staphylococcal pneumonia is the most serious.

When to Admit

- Limited availability of supporting services.
- Pneumonia.
- Changes in mental status.

Dharan NJ et al. Infections with oseltamivir-resistant influenza A(H1N1) virus in the United States. JAMA. 2009 Mar 11;301(10):1034–41.

Glezen WP. Clinical practice. Prevention and treatment of seasonal influenza. N Engl J Med. 2008 Dec 11;359(24):2579–85. [PMID: 19073977]

Hayden F. Developing new antiviral agents for influenza treatment: what does the future hold? Clin Infect Dis. 2009 Jan 1;48 Suppl 1:S3–13. [PMID: 19067613]

Jefferson T et al. Antivirals for influenza in healthy adults: systematic review. Lancet. 2006 Jan 28;367(9507):303–13. [PMID: 16443037]

Rothberg MB et al. Complications of viral influenza. Am J Med. 2008 Apr;121(4):258–64. [PMID: 18374680]

Taubenberger JK et al. The pathology of influenza virus infections. Annu Rev Pathol. 2008;3:499–522. [PMID: 18039138]

3. Avian Influenza (H5N1)

ESSENTIALS OF DIAGNOSIS

▶ Cases to date in humans, mostly from Southeast Asia.

▶ Clinically indistinguishable from influenza.

▶ Epidemiologic factors assist in diagnosis.

▶ Rapid antigen assays are the means of confirming diagnosis.

General Considerations

The normal hosts for avian influenza viruses are aquatic waterfowl. Although avian influenza was first recognized in Italy in 1878, the current outbreak of highly pathogenic influenza A subtype (H5N1) in poultry was recognized in 1997 in Hong Kong and was followed by the first documented human cases. A massive slaughter of poultry was attempted to contain the disease. New outbreaks of H5N1 influenza in poultry emerged, however, in 2003 and now involve more than 65 countries of East and Southeast Asia, Eurasia, Western and Eastern Europe, and Northern Africa. The 387 confirmed human cases as of January 2009 include 245 deaths (from Azerbaijan, Bangladesh,

Cambodia, China, Djibouti, Egypt, Indonesia, Iraq, Lao PDR, Myanmar, Nigeria, Pakistan, Thailand, Turkey, and Vietnam).

Although highly contagious among birds, the transmission of this H5N1 strain from human to human is relatively inefficient and not sustained. The result is only rare cases of person-to-person infection. Occasional transmission to other mammals, including domestic cats and dogs, is also documented.

Most human cases occur after exposure to infected poultry or surfaces contaminated with poultry droppings. Because infection in humans is associated with a mortality rate greater than 50% (over 80% [91 of 113] for Indonesian cases) and the avian H5N1 subtype continues to spread among birds (with many parts of Southeast Asia now considered endemic for the virus), there is worldwide concern that the virus may undergo genetic reassortment or mutation (as with the 1918 strain) and develop greater human-human transmissibility with the potential to produce a global pandemic.

▶ Clinical Findings

A. Symptoms and Signs

Distinguishing avian influenza from regular influenza is difficult. History of exposure to dead or ill poultry in the prior 10 days, recent travel to Southeast Asia, or contact with known cases should be investigated. The symptoms and signs include predominantly respiratory symptoms (cough and dyspnea), but a variety of other systems may be involved, producing headaches and gastrointestinal complaints in particular. Subclinical disease is relatively rare. With high levels of cytokines being responsible for much of the pathology, prolonged febrile states and generalized malaise are common. Children are preferentially impacted. Most patients die of respiratory failure.

B. Laboratory Findings

Current commercial rapid antigen tests are not optimally sensitive or specific for detection of H5N1 influenza but are still first-line diagnostic tests because of their widespread availability. Diagnostic yield can be improved by earlier collection of samples. More sensitive RT-PCR assays are usually available through state health departments. An initial negative result in the right clinical setting warrants retesting. Throat or lower respiratory swabs may provide higher yield of detection than nasal swabs. When highly pathogenic strains (eg, H5N1) are suspected, extreme care in the handling of these samples must be observed during preliminary testing. Positive samples must then be forwarded to the appropriate public health authorities for further investigations (eg, culture) in laboratories with the adequate level of biosafety (level 3).

▶ Treatment

Resistance of asian H5N1 influenza strains to amantadine and rimantadine is present in most geographic areas where the virus is found. Reacquisition of sensitivity to

these drugs through genetic reassortment is possible. The current first-line recommendation is to use the neuraminidase inhibitor oseltamivir, 75 mg twice daily for 5 days administered within 48 hours from onset of illness. A higher dose (150 mg twice daily), longer duration, and possible combination therapy with amantadine or rimantadine (in countries where A (H5N1) viruses are likely to be susceptible to adamantanes) may be considered in those patients with pneumonia or progressive disease. Recent evidence of resistance to oseltamivir is reported. Although inhaled zanamivir has proven effective in treating seasonal influenza, no data of its efficacy against H5N1 strains are available. Therapy should still be considered for patients with severe avian influenza disease even after several days of onset. Postexposure prophylaxis with 75 mg of oseltamivir once daily for 7–10 days should be given to household contacts of documented cases. Personnel exposed to those patients should be monitored for symptoms. Careful surveillance of new human cases and prudent stockpiling of medications with establishment of an infrastructure for dissemination are essential modalities of control. Nonpharmacologic means of control include masks; social distancing; quarantine; travel limitations; and infrastructure development, particularly for emergency departments.

One human vaccine against H5N1 influenza is licensed but not yet marketed in the United States. This vaccine does not contain adjuvant and as a result, its immunogenicity is only modest. A vaccine with oil-in-water emulsion-based adjuvant is available in Europe. Several other vaccine candidates are undergoing clinical trials. Conventional tricomponent inactivated influenza vaccines provide only partial protection.

Prevention of exposure to avian influenza strains also includes hygienic practices during handling of poultry products, including handwashing and prevention of cross-contamination, as well as thorough cooking of poultry products (to 70 °C). Nonetheless, the risk of acquiring avian influenza through the consumption of poultry products is still very small.

Ehrlich HJ et al; Baxter H5N1 Pandemic Influenza Vaccine Clinical Study Team. A clinical trial of a whole-virus H5N1 vaccine derived from cell culture. N Engl J Med. 2008 Jun 12;358(24):2573–84. [PMID: 18550874]

Gambotto A et al. Human infection with highly pathogenic H5N1 influenza virus. Lancet. 2008 Apr 26;371(9622):1464–75. [PMID: 18440429]

Keitel WA et al. Preparing for a possible pandemic: influenza A/H5N1 vaccine development. Curr Opin Pharmacol. 2007 Oct;7(5):484–90. [PMID: 17644429]

Writing Committee of the Second World Health Organization Consultation on Clinical Aspects of Human Infection with Avian Influenza A (H5N1) Virus; Abdel-Ghafar AN et al. Update on avian influenza A (H5N1) virus infection in humans. N Engl J Med. 2008 Jan 17;358(3):261–73. [PMID: 18199865]

World Health Organization. Avian Influenza Frequently Asked Questions. http://www.who.int/csr/disease/avian_influenza/avian_faqs/en/print.html

World Organization for Animal Health. Avian influenza data. http://www.oie.int/

4. Swine-origin Influenza (H1N1/A/California/04/2009)

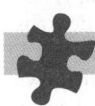

▶ Influenza-like illness with consistent epidemiologic background.

▶ Respiratory swab allows local screen and more specific analysis by state public health laboratories.

General Considerations

Because the human influenza virus of avian, human, and swine sources can grow readily in the respiratory tract of pigs, they are considered a "mixing vessel" for gene reassortment between strains. A current outbreak of pandemic swine-origin (H1N1) influenza virus (S-OIV) emerged in Mexico City in March 2009. In the United States, the first cases occurred in metropolitan San Diego and San Antonio, and the outbreak rapidly spread throughout the United States. As of June 1, 2009, cases were also reported from over 40 nations among the five continents. Although referred in the popular press to as "swine flu," this infection is caused by a new influenza A strain that is a reassortment of swine, avian, and human influenza strains (eg, triple-reassortant); thus, "swine flu" is a misnomer. The WHO guidelines suggest that influenza viruses be named after their viral type (A, B, or C), host (if non-human), place of isolation, isolation number, and year of isolation (separated by slashes). Hence, a more appropriate term to identify this virus is influenza A/California/04/2009, but its utility might be restricted to physicians and scientists.

Clinical Findings

A. Symptoms and Signs

This current strain of S-OIV appears to cause typical influenza symptoms (fever, malaise, myalgias, cough, sore throat, rhinorrhea, shortness of breath) commonly accompanied by gastrointestinal manifestations (especially diarrhea). The disease has an incubation period of 2–9 days and preferentially impacts young adults. This age specificity might reflect previous exposure with related strains in people over the age of 40 years (conferring some degree of cross-protection) but also to some case-ascertainment bias due to more young people being tested as part of outbreaks in schools or the workplace. The infectivity of the new strain appears to be unusually high. Most patients report a relatively mild illness with full recovery. While a number of deaths were reported from early cases in metropolitan Mexico City, S-OIV seems less likely to cause death than other pandemic viruses (ie, 1918 pandemic virus). The mortality rate of S-OIV seems to be similar to seasonal influenza (mortality rate < 0.5%); however, this could change as the pandemic evolves.

B. Laboratory Findings

A respiratory swab for novel S-OIV testing should be taken and placed in a refrigerator (not a freezer). State public health laboratories can then perform a PCR and subtype testing on identified samples. For current case definitions and guidelines on specimen collecting and processing and for confirmation testing, see www.cdc.gov/h1n1flu/ or contact the local public health department. While waiting for confirmatory results, local laboratories can perform rapid immunofluorescence or enzyme immunoassays that can differentiate between influenza viruses types A and B, but their results should be interpreted with caution due to their limited sensitivity (typically about 60%) and inability to differentiate between human- and swine-origin viruses.

Treatment

Treatment entails using neuraminidase inhibitors (oseltamivir or zanamivir) at standard dosages. The virus is usually resistant to the adamantanes (amantadine or rimantadine). Please see the regular influenza section for side effects and concerns with these medications. At the time of this review, the recommendations on which patients should receive specific antiviral therapy for S-OIV infections are similar to those for seasonal influenza. As additional information becomes available, however, specific recommendations may change. Updated advice can be found at http://www.cdc.gov/h1n1flu/recommendations.htm.

Prevention

A polyvalent vaccine is under development, and this vaccine may require that patients at risk take the vaccine (which may be two dosages) plus the standard vaccine (for a total of three dosages). In general, persons with S-OIV infection should be considered potentially infectious from 1 day before to 7 days following illness onset. Children, especially younger ones, may be infectious up to 10 days. Any hospital patient in whom the infection is suspected should be isolated in individual rooms with standard and contact precautions plus eye protection. Strict adherence to hand hygiene with soap and water or an alcohol-based hand sanitizer and immediate removal of gloves and other equipment after contact with respiratory secretions is essential. For procedures likely to generate aerosols (eg, bronchoscopy, elective intubation, suctioning, administering nebulized medications), an airborne infection isolation room (AIIR) can be used, with air exhausted directly outside or recirculated after filtration by a high efficiency particulate air (HEPA) filter. The patient should wear surgical masks to contain secretions when outside a patient room, and healthcare personnel in contact with patients should wear a fit-tested disposable N95 respirator or equivalent (eg, powered air purifying respirator). This latter recommendation differs from that for cases of seasonal influenza because of the undetermined potential transmissibility of this new reassortment virus. Precautions should be maintained until 7 days from symptom onset or until the resolution of symptoms, whichever is longer. Postexposure prophylaxis should be considered for close contacts of patients (confirmed, probable, or suspected) who are at high risk for complications of influenza (see section on seasonal influenza) as well as for healthcare personnel, public health workers, or first responders who have had a recognized, unprotected close contact exposure to a person with novel (H1N1) influenza virus infection (confirmed, probable, or suspected) during that person's infectious period. Despite limited data of the safety of neuraminidase inhibitors, the CDC recommends considering postexposure prophylaxis as well in this population. Healthcare professionals should frequently refer to the CDC guidelines for changes in these recommendations (http://www.cdc.gov/h1n1flu/recommendations.htm). There are no currently documented or substantiated indications for travel restrictions, culling of animals, or widespread school closures. There is concern that in heavily impacted, dense urban areas (major cities of Asia or Africa, for example) the number of cases may significantly increase in the winter of 2009–2010. Concerned professionals should refer to MMWR or the CDC (www.cdc.gov/h1n1flu/) and WHO websites (http://www.who.int/csr/disease/swineflu/en/) for evolving updates about this pandemic.

Fraser C et al; The WHO Rapid Pandemic Assessment Collaboration. Pandemic Potential of a Strain of Influenza A (H1N1): Early Findings. Science. 2009 May 14;[Epub ahead of print]. [PMID: 19433588]

Garten RJ et al. Antigenic and Genetic Characteristics of Swine-Origin 2009 A (H1N1) Influenza Viruses Circulating in Humans. Science. 2009 May 22;[Epub ahead of print]. [PMID: 19465683]

Novel Swine-Origin Influenza A (H1N1) Virus Investigation Team. Emergence of a Novel Swine-Origin Influenza A (H1N1) Virus in Humans.. N Engl J Med. 2009 May 22;[Epub ahead of print]. [PMID: 19423869]

Stein RA. Lessons From Outbreaks of H1N1 Influenza. Ann Intern Med. 2009 May 26;[Epub ahead of print]. [PMID: 19470591]

5. Severe Acute Respiratory Syndrome (SARS)

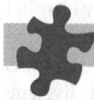

ESSENTIALS OF DIAGNOSIS

▸ Mild, moderate, or severe respiratory illness.

▸ Travel to endemic area within 10 days before symptom onset, including mainland China, Hong Kong, Singapore, Taiwan, Vietnam, and Toronto.

▸ Persistent fever; dry cough, dyspnea in most.

▸ Diagnosis confirmed by antibody testing or isolation of virus.

▸ No specific treatment; mortality as high as 10% in clinically diagnosed cases.

General Considerations

SARS is a respiratory syndrome of varying severity but capable of causing death in as many as 10% of clinically established cases. It is caused by an apparently unique coronavirus. The earliest cases were traced to a health care worker in Guangdong Province in China in late 2002, with rapid spread thereafter to Hong Kong, Singapore, Vietnam, Taiwan, and Toronto. The primary mode of transmission appears to be through direct or indirect contact of mucous membranes (eyes, nose, or mouth) with infectious respiratory droplets or fomites. Epidemiologic data also suggest airborne spread. The use of aerosol-generating procedures (endotracheal intubation, bronchoscopy, nebulization treatments) in hospitals may amplify the transmission of the SARS coronavirus. The virus is shed in stools but the role of fecal–oral transmission is unknown. The natural reservoir appears to be the horseshoe bat (which eats and drops fruits ingested by civets, the earlier presumed reservoir and a likely amplifying host).

The variable distribution of cases throughout Asia and Canada is considered a consequence of spread through travel. The virus is sufficiently virulent that it may be transmitted and acquired by patients during brief stops in airports. As a result, sporadic confirmed and suspected cases have appeared throughout the United States. The 2003 outbreak involved 8096 probable cases in about 28 countries, with 774 fatalities. In 2004, nine cases associated with laboratory and subsequent secondary exposure were reported from Beijing, China. No new cases have been reported since then.

▸ Clinical Findings

A. Symptoms and Signs

SARS is considered an atypical pneumonia that affects persons in all age groups. The CDC recognizes asymptomatic or mild cases, moderate disease, and severe respiratory illness. The incubation period is 2–7 days, and it can be spread to contacts of affected patients for 10 days. The mean time from onset of clinical symptoms to hospital admission is 3–5 days. In all clinical cases, persistent fever is present; chills or rigor (or both), cough, shortness of breath, rales, and rhonchi are the rule. Many patients report headache, myalgias, and sore throat as well. A watery diarrhea occurs in some patients during the course of the illness. Elderly patients may report malaise and delirium, without the typical febrile response. No single symptom or sign is diagnostic or highly suggestive, and the history and physical examination of a patient in whom SARS in suspected are to be interpreted in this context.

B. Laboratory Findings and Imaging

Leukopenia and especially lymphopenia are observed commonly. A low-grade disseminated intravascular coagulation (thrombocytopenia, prolonged activated thromboplastin time, and elevated D-dimer level) is present in many patients. Other abnormalities include modest elevations of ALT and creatine kinase. Arterial oxygen saturation is less than 95% in 80% of affected individuals, and pulmonary infiltrates are noted in all. The roentgenographic pattern is not specific, and severe cases may progress to ARDS, with extensive bilateral consolidation. A high-resolution CT scan is abnormal (ground-glass opacifications or focal consolidation) in 67% of patients with initially normal chest radiographs. Serum serologies, including enzyme immunoassays and fluorescent antibody assays, are available through public health departments at the state level, although seroconversion may not occur until 3 weeks after the onset of symptoms.

The detection rates for the virus using conventional RT-PCR are generally low in the first week of illness. Urine, nasopharyngeal aspirate, and stool specimens are positive in 42%, 68%, and 97%, respectively, on day 14 of illness. Although viral isolation is possible, it is a technically laborious and time-consuming procedure.

Complications

As with any viral pneumonia, pulmonary decompensation is the most feared problem. ARDS occurs in about 16% patients, and about 20–30% of patients require intubation and mechanical ventilation. Sequelae of intensive care include infection with nosocomial pathogens, tension pneumothorax from ventilation at high peak pressures, and noncardiogenic pulmonary edema.

Prevention

Health care workers engaged in procedures that involve activities such as intubation, suctioning, and nebulization are at high risk for acquiring the virus. Transmission may occur shortly after the development of symptoms and perhaps before the appearance of fever, cough, and dyspnea. Thus, an increased level of suspicion is critical, and isolation of high-risk patients is essential. Simple hygienic measures (such as handwashing after touching patients, use of appropriate and well-fitted face masks, and early introduction of infection control measures, including quarantine) may help reduce transmission.

Measures enacted for air travelers have included screening for fever and compatible symptoms and quarantining in the home for high-risk exposed persons. Continual reporting of suspected cases is crucial, as is awareness of restrictions on international travel. The most cautious modalities include monitoring for 10 days after the last potential exposure and confinement of recovering patients for a similar interval. The efficacy of facemasks is established for preventing hospital-acquired infections, although the validity for their usage in the community remains unsubstantiated.

Treatment

Severe cases require intensive support. Although a number of different agents including ribavirin (400–600 mg/d and 4 g/d), lopinavir/ritonavir (400 mg/100 mg), interferon type I, intravenous immunoglobulin, and systemic corticosteroids were used to treat SARS patients during the 2003 epidemic, the treatment efficacy of these therapeutic agents remains inconclusive and further research is needed. Subsequent studies with ribavirin show no activity against the virus in vitro, and a retrospective analysis of the epidemic in Toronto suggests worse outcomes in patients who receive the drug.

Prognosis

The overall mortality rate of identified cases is about 14%. Mortality is age-related, ranging from less than 1% in persons under 24 years of age to greater than 50% in persons over 65 years of age. Poor prognostic factors include advanced age, chronic hepatitis B infection treated with lamivudine, high initial or high peak lactate dehydrogenase concentration, high neutrophil count on presentation, diabetes mellitus, acute kidney disease, and low counts of CD4 and CD8 on presentation. Many subclinical cases probably go undiagnosed. Seasonality, as with influenza, is not established.

Cheng VC et al. Severe acute respiratory syndrome coronavirus as an agent of emerging and reemerging infection. Clin Microbiol Rev. 2007 Oct;20(4):660–94. [PMID: 17934078]
Golda A et al. Recent antiviral strategies against human coronavirus-related respiratory illnesses. Curr Opin Pulm Med. 2008 May;14(3):248–53. [PMID: 18427249]
Hui DS et al. Clinical features, pathogenesis and immunobiology of severe acute respiratory syndrome. Curr Opin Pulm Med. 2008 May;14(3):2417. [PMID: 18427248]
Nishiyama A et al. Risk factors for SARS infection within hospitals in Hanoi, Vietnam. Jpn J Infect Dis. 2008;61(5):388–90. [PMID: 18806349]

ADENOVIRUS INFECTIONS

Adenoviruses (there are over at least 52 serotypes) produce a variety of clinical syndromes. These infections are usually self-limited or clinically inapparent and most common among infants, young children, and military recruits. Adenoviruses, however, may cause significant morbidity and mortality in immunocompromised persons, such as HIV-infected persons and liver, kidney, and lung and hematopoietic stem cell transplant, cancer chemotherapy, and COPD patients. The incubation period is 4–9 days. Adenoviruses, although a common cause of human disease, also receive particular recognition through their role as vectors in gene therapy.

Clinical syndromes of adenovirus infection, often overlapping, include the following. The common cold (see Chapter 8) is characterized by rhinitis, pharyngitis, and mild malaise without fever. Nonstreptococcal exudative pharyngitis is characterized by fever lasting 2–12 days and accompanied by malaise and myalgia. Conjunctivitis is often present. Lower respiratory tract infection may occur, including bronchiolitis, suggested by cough and râles, or pneumonia (types 3, 4, and 7 commonly cause acute respiratory disease and pneumonia). Adenovirus type 14 is increasingly reported as a cause of severe and sometimes fatal pneumonia in those with chronic lung disease, but it is also seen in healthy young adults. Pharyngoconjunctival fever is manifested by fever and malaise, conjunctivitis (often unilateral), mild pharyngitis, and cervical adenitis. Epidemic keratoconjunctivitis (transmissible person to person) occurs in adults and is manifested by bilateral conjunctival redness, pain, tearing, and an enlarged preauricular lymph node (multiple types may be involved in a single outbreak). Keratitis may lead to subepithelial opacities (especially with types 8, 19, or 37). Acute hemorrhagic cystitis is a disorder of children often associated with adenovirus type 11 and 21. Sexually transmitted genitourinary ulcers and urethritis may be caused by types 2, 8, and 37 in particular. Adenoviruses also cause acute gastroenteritis (types 40 and 41), mesenteric adenitis, acute appendicitis, and intussusception. Rarely, they are associated with encephalitis, acute flaccid paralysis, and pericarditis. Adenovirus is commonly identified in endomyocardial tissue of patients with myocarditis and dilated cardiomyopathy. Risk factors associated with severity of infection include youth, chronic underlying infections, recent transplantation, and serotypes 5 or 21.

Hepatitis (type 5 adenovirus), pneumonia, and hemorrhagic cystitis (types 11 and 34) tend to develop in infected liver, lung, or kidney transplant recipients, respectively. Syndromes that may develop in hematopoietic stem cell transplant patients, include hepatitis, pneumonia, hemorrhagic cystitis, tubulointerstitial nephritis, colitis, and encephalitis.

A rapid diagnostic direct fluorescence assay or enzyme immunoassay may assist with diagnosis and a quantitative real-time rapid-cycle PCR is useful in distinguishing disease from colonization, especially in hematologic cell transplant patients. Viral culture remains the gold standard, but cultures delay the diagnosis.

Treatment is symptomatic. Ribavirin and cidofovir are used in immunocompromised individuals with occasional success, although the latter is attendant with significant renal toxicity, in immunocompromised persons among whom reduced immunosuppression is indicated. Adoptive immunotherapy with transfusion of adenovirus-specific T cells is currently being investigated. Typing of isolates is useful epidemiologically and in distinguishing transmission from endogenous reactivation. Complications of adenovirus pneumonia in children include bronchiolitis obliterans.

Vaccines are not available for general use. Live oral vaccines containing attenuated type 4 and type 7 were used in military personnel, but they have been discontinued.

Gray GC et al. Genotype prevalence and risk factors for severe clinical adenovirus infection, United States 2004–2006. Clin Infect Dis. 2007 Nov 1;45(9):1120–31. [PMID: 17918073]
Louie JK et al. Severe pneumonia due to adenovirus serotype 14: a new respiratory threat? Clin Infect Dis. 2008 Feb 1;46(3):421–5. [PMID: 18173356]

OTHER EXANTHEMATOUS VIRAL INFECTIONS

1. Parvovirus Infections

Parvovirus B19 infects human erythroid precursor cells. It is quite widespread (by age 15 years about 50% of children have detectable IgG) and its transmission occurs through respiratory secretions and saliva, through the placenta (vertical transmission), and through administration of blood products. The incubation period is 4–14 days. Chronic forms of the infection can occur. **Bocavirus,** another parvovirus, was recently uncovered as a cause of winter acute respiratory disease in children and adults.

▶ Clinical Findings

A. Symptoms and Signs

Parvovirus B19 causes several syndromes and manifests differently in various populations.

1. Children—In children, an exanthematous illness ("fifth disease," erythema infectiosum) is characterized by a fiery red "slapped cheek" appearance, circumoral pallor, and a subsequent lacy, maculopapular, evanescent rash on the trunk and limbs. Malaise, headache, and pruritus (especially on the palms and soles) occur. Systemic symptoms and fever are mostly abated by the time of rash appearance.

2. Immuncompromised patients—In immunosuppressed patients, including those with HIV infection or transplanted organs, or with hematologic conditions such as sickle cell disease, transient aplastic crisis and pure red blood cell aplasia may occur. Bone marrow aspirates reveal absence of mature erythroid precursors and characteristic giant pronormoblasts.

3. Adults—A limited nonerosive symmetric polyarthritis that mimics lupus erythematosus and rheumatoid arthritis, preferentially involving the metacarpophalangeal joints of the hands and the wrists and knees, can develop in middle-aged persons (especially women) but can also occur in children. Rashes, especially facial, are less common in adults.

Rare reported presentations include myocarditis with infarction, constrictive pericarditis, hepatitis, pneumonitis, neutropenia, thrombocytopenia, a lupus-like syndrome, glomerulopathy, CNS vasculitis, and a chronic fatigue syndrome. Subclinical infection is documented among patients with sickle cell disease.

In pregnancy, fetal loss and hydrops fetalis are reported sequelae. Pregnant women with a recent exposure or with suggestive symptoms should be tested for the disease and carefully monitored if results are positive.

B. Laboratory Findings

The diagnosis is clinical (Table 32–2) but may be confirmed by an elevated titer of IgM anti-parvovirus antibodies in serum or with PCR in serum or bone marrow. Autoimmune antibodies (antiphospholipid and antineutrophil cytoplasmic antibodies) can be present and are thought to be a consequence of molecular mimicry.

▶ Complications

Uncommon complications include encephalitis, chronic hemolytic anemia, thrombotic thrombocytopenic purpuric syndrome, acute postinfectious glomerulonephritis, and hepatitis.

▶ Treatment

Treatment in healthy persons is symptomatic (nonsteroidal anti-inflammatory drugs are used to treat arthralgias, and transfusions are used to treat transient aplastic crises). In immunosuppressed patients, intravenous immunoglobulin can aid in the reduction of anemia. Intrauterine blood transfusion can be considered in severe fetal anemia.

▶ Prevention & Prognosis

Screening of donated blood could potentially prevent transfusion-related infection. Several nosocomial outbreaks have been documented. In these cases, standard containment guidelines, including handwashing after patient exposure and avoiding contact with pregnant women are paramount.

The prognosis is generally excellent in immunocompetent individuals. In immunosuppressed patients, persistent anemia may require prolonged transfusion dependence. Remission of parvovirus infection in AIDS patients may occur with HAART, though the immune restoration syndrome is also reported.

Christensen A et al. Human bocavirus commonly involved in multiple viral airway infections. J Clin Virol. 2008 Jan;41(1):34–7. [PMID: 18069504]

Servey JT et al. Clinical presentations of parvovirus B19 infection. Am Fam Physician. 2007 Feb 1;75(3):373–6. [PMID: 17304869]

2. Poxvirus Infections

Among the nine poxviruses causing disease in humans, the following are clinically important.

1. **Variola/vaccinia:** Smallpox (variola) was a highly contagious disease associated with high mortality and disabling sequelae. Its manifestations included severe headache, acute onset of fever, prostration and a rash characterized by the uniform progression from macules to papules to firm, deep seated vesicles or pustules. The synchronous progression in smallpox readily differentiates lesions from those of varicella (see also Chapter 6).

Complications of smallpox included bacterial superinfections (cellulitis and pneumonia), encephalitis, and keratitis with corneal ulcerations a risk factor for blindness. Effective vaccination led to its global elimination by 1979 and routine vaccination stopped in 1985. Despite the recommendation of destroying remaining samples of this virus, significant concern exists for the potential misuse of these repositories in military or terrorist activities. Smallpox should be considered, in concordance with the CDC's Smallpox Response Plan (www.bt.cdc.gov/agent/smallpox/response-plan/index.asp), in any patient with fever and a characteristic rash (see above) for which other etiologies such as herpes infections, drug reactions, erythema multiforme or other infections are unlikely. Such patients should be placed in airborne and contact isolation and the official agency contacted (CDC Emergency Preparedness and Response Branch; 770-488-7100). The Department of Defense and the US Department of Health and Human Services (DHHS) launched military and civilian vaccination programs by January 2003.

The presence of any of the following in the person being vaccinated or in his or her household contacts is a contraindication to vaccination: any form of immunosuppression, eczema or other forms of dermatitis (active or in remission), or allergy to any component of the vaccine. Infants younger than 1 year and pregnant or breastfeeding women should not receive the vaccine.

Adverse reactions to the vaccine include generalized vaccinia; eczema vaccinatum, which is a more serious local or disseminated vesicular rash in patients with preexisting eczema or atopic dermatitis; and progressive vaccinia occurring in immunocompromised persons associated with significant widespread necrosis and a high mortality even after administration of vaccinia immune globulin (VIG). Other adverse reactions are generalized symptoms (fatigue, headache, muscle aches, and fever, referred as the **acute vaccinia syndrome**), myocarditis, pericarditis, unexpected ischemic cardiac events, postvaccinial encephalitis, and erythema multiforme major. The occurrence of vaccinia-related disease is also described in contacts of vaccinees, including rare cases of sexually transmitted disease. Inoculation of the vaccine in inappropriate sites (eg, eyes) is unfortunately common. Asymptomatic vaccinia viremia can be detected up to 21 days post vaccination and no blood donation should occur during this interval. Cidofovir shows activity against poxviruses and can be considered for treatment of these poxviral conditions.

2. **Molluscum contagiosum** may be transmitted sexually or by other close contact. It is manifested by pearly, raised, umbilicated skin nodules sparing the palms and soles. Keratoconjunctivitis can occur. Marked and persistent lesions in AIDS patients respond readily to combination antiretroviral therapy. Curettage is most effective for limited lesions. Reportedly effective forms of therapy include catharidin (blisters are a side effect), cimetidine and CO_2 laser therapy combined with natural interferon-β gel, salicylic and glycolic acids, and imiquimod cream (5%). Multiple courses of therapy are often needed.

3. **Orf** (contagious pustular dermatitis, or ecthyma contagiosa) and **paravaccinia** (milker's nodules) are occupational diseases acquired by contact with sheep and cattle, respectively. Orf also occurs among children with ruminant exposures. Orf anecdotally responds to imiquimod.

4. **Monkeypox**, first identified in 1970, is enzootic in the rain forests of equatorial Africa and presents in humans as a syndrome similar to smallpox. The incubation period is about 12 days, and limited person-to-person spread occurs. African mortality rates vary from 3% to 11% depending on the immune status of the patient. Secondary attack rates appear to be about 10%. The first community-acquired outbreak in the United States of monkeypox occurred in 2003 in Wisconsin and other states of the upper Midwest. The source appeared to be imported Gambian giant rats via consequent exposure of prairie dogs. Other susceptible animals include nonhuman primates, rabbits, and rodents. Confusion with smallpox and varicella occurs; however, lymphadenopathy is a prominent feature of monkeypox infection (seen in up to 90% of unvaccinated persons), and skin lesions of the palms and soles, frequently seen in these poxviruses, are uncommon in varicella infection. Suspected cases should be placed on standard, contact and droplet precautions; and local and state public health officials, and the CDC should be notified for assistance with the confirmation of the diagnosis (electron microscopy, viral culture, ELISA, PCR). Cidofovir is effective against monkeypox, and IVIG can be used in selected cases.

Other general precautions that should be taken are avoidance of contact with prairie dogs and Gambian giant rats (whose illness is manifested by alopecia, rash, and ocular or nasal discharge), appropriate care and isolation of those exposed within 3 prior weeks to such animals, and veterinary examination and investigation of suspect animals through health departments. Vaccinia immunization is effective against monkeypox and is recommended, if no contraindication exists (outlined above), for those involved in the investigation of the outbreak and for healthcare workers caring for those infected with monkeypox. Post exposure vaccination is also advised for documented contacts of infected persons or animals. US federal agencies currently prohibit the importation of African rodents.

Centers for Disease Control and Prevention (CDC). Laboratory-acquired vaccinia exposures and infections—United States, 2005-2007. MMWR Morb Mortal Wkly Rep. 2008 Apr 18;57(15):401–4. [PMID: 18418346]

CDC. Updated interim CDC guidance for use of smallpox vaccine, cidofovir, and vaccinia immune globulin (VIG) for prevention and treatment in the setting of an outbreak of monkeypox infections. Available at: http://www.cdc.gov/ncidod/monkeypox/treatmentguidelines.htm.

Taub DD et al. Immunity from smallpox vaccine persists for decades: a longitudinal study. Am J Med. 2008 Dec;121 (12):1058–64. [PMID: 19028201]

VIRUSES & GASTROENTERITIS

Viruses are responsible for at least 30–40% of cases of infectious diarrhea in the United States. These agents include rotaviruses; caliciviruses, including noroviruses such as Norwalk virus; astroviruses; enteric adenoviruses; and, less often, toroviruses, coronaviruses, picornaviruses, and pestiviruses.

Rotaviruses are the leading worldwide cause of dehydrating gastroenteritis in young children and are associated with significant morbidity and mortality (nearly 600,000 persons die each year in developing countries). Children aged 6 months to 2 years are the most affected. By age 5, virtually every child has been infected with this pathogen. There are **seven groups of rotaviruses** (A-G), but group A strains cause the vast majority of these infections while group B and C strains are limited to outbreaks in more restricted settings. Rotavirus infections follow an endemic pattern, especially in the tropics, although they peak during the winter in temperate regions. The virus is transmitted by fecal-oral route and can be shed in feces for up to 3 weeks in severe infections. In outbreak settings (eg, daycare centers), the virus is ubiquitously found in the environment, and secondary attack rates are between 16% and 30% (including household contacts). The disease is usually mild and self-limiting. A 2- to 3-day prodrome of fever and vomiting is followed by nonbloody diarrhea (up to 10–20 bowel movements per day) lasting for 1–4 days. The method of choice for diagnosis is PCR of the stool. Treatment is symptomatic, with fluid and electrolyte replacement. Local intestinal immunity gives protection against successive infection. Two oral rotavirus vaccines are available in the United States: pentavalent human-bovine reassortment rotavirus vaccine (PRV, RotaTeq; to be given at 2, 4, and 6 months of age) and attenuated human rotavirus vaccine (HRV, Rotarix; to be given at 2 and 4 months of age). Contraindications include allergy to any of the vaccine ingredients, previous allergic reaction to the vaccine, and immunodeficiency.

Noroviruses, such as **Norwalk virus,** are the major cause of epidemic gastroenteritis. They appear to evolve by antigenic drift (similar to influenza). While 90% of young adults show serologic evidence of past infection, no long-lasting protective immunity develops and reinfections are common. In the United States, noroviruses are responsible for over 90% of reported nonbacterial gastroenteritis outbreaks during cold weather intervals (hence the colloquial name "gastric flu"). Outbreak environments include restaurants, long-term care facilities, hospitals, schools, daycare centers, vacation destinations (including cruise ships), and Middle Eastern military bases deployed abroad. Although transmission is usually fecal–oral, airborne and waterborne transmission are also documented. A short incubation period (24–48 hours), a short symptomatic illness (12–60 hours), a high frequency (> 50%) of vomiting, and absence of bacterial pathogens in stool samples are highly predictive of norovirus gastroenteritis. RT-PCR of stool samples is used for epidemiologic purposes. Treatment is largely symptomatic.

Outbreak control for both rotavirus and noroviurs infections include strict adherence to general hygienic measures, cohorting of sick patients, contact precautions for symptomatic hospitalized patients, exclusion from work of symptomatic staff until symptom resolution (or 48–72 h after this for norovirus disease), and proper decontamination procedures.

The presence of antibodies is not associated with protection against reinfection.

Atmar RL et al. The epidemiologic and clinical importance of norovirus infection. Gastroenterol Clin North Am. 2006 Jun;35(2):275–90. [PMID: 16880066]

Grimwood K. Clinical update: rotavirus gastroenteritis and its prevention. Lancet. 2007 Jul 28;370(9584):302–4. [PMID: 17662867]

Said MA et al. Healthcare epidemiology: gastrointestinal flu: norovirus in health care and long-term care facilities. Clin Infect Dis. 2008 Nov 1;47(9):1202–8. [PMID: 18808354]

Ward RL. Rotarix: a rotavirus vaccine for the world. Clin Infect Dis. 2009 Jan 15;48(2):222–8. [PMID: 19072246]

ENTEROVIRUSES THAT PRODUCE SEVERAL SYNDROMES

1. Coxsackievirus Infections

Coxsackievirus infections cause several clinical syndromes. As with other enteroviruses, infections are most common during the summer. Two groups, A and B, are defined either serologically or by mouse bioassay. There are more than 50 serotypes.

► Clinical Findings

A. Symptoms and Signs

The clinical syndromes associated with coxsackievirus infection may be described briefly as follows.

1. Summer grippe (A and B)—A febrile illness, principally of children, summer grippe usually lasts 1–4 days. Minor symptoms of upper respiratory tract infection are often present.

2. Herpangina (A2–6, 10: B3)—Sudden onset of fever, which may be as high as 40.6 °C, sometimes with febrile convulsions; headache, myalgia, and vomiting; and sore throat, characterized early by petechiae or papules on the soft palate that become shallow ulcers in about 3 days and then heal. Treatment is symptomatic.

3. Epidemic pleurodynia (Bornholm disease) (B1–5)—

Pleuritic pain is prominent, and tenderness, hyperesthesia, and muscle swelling are present over the area of diaphragmatic attachment. Other findings include headache, sore throat, malaise, nausea, and fever. Orchitis and aseptic meningitis occur in less than 10% of patients. Most patients are ill for 4–6 days.

4. Aseptic meningitis (A and B) and other neurologic syndromes—

Fever, headache, nausea, vomiting, stiff neck, drowsiness, and cerebrospinal fluid lymphocytosis without chemical abnormalities may occur, and pediatric clusters of group B (especially B5) meningitis are reported. Focal encephalitis and transverse myelitis are reported with coxsackievirus group A. A disseminated encephalitis occurs after group B infection, and acute flaccid paralysis is reported with both coxsackievirus group A and B. Severe neonatal illnesses are reported including encephalomyocarditis.

5. Acute nonspecific pericarditis (B types)—

Sudden onset of anterior chest pain, often worse with inspiration and in the supine position, is typical. Fever, myalgia, headache, and pericardial friction rub appear early and these symptoms are often transient. Evidence for pericardial effusion on imaging studies is often present, and the occasional patient has a paradoxical pulse. Electrocardiographic evidence of pericarditis is often present. Relapses may occur.

6. Myocarditis (B1–5)—

Heart failure in the neonatal period secondary to in utero myocarditis and over 20% of adult cases of myocarditis and dilated cardiomyopathy are associated with group B (especially B3) infections.

7. Hand, foot, and mouth disease (A5, 10, 16)—

This disease is sometimes epidemic and is characterized by stomatitis and a vesicular rash on hands and feet. Enterovirus 71 is also a causative agent.

8. Epidemic conjunctivitis—

As with enterovirus 70 (see below), the A24 variant of coxsackievirus is associated with acute epidemic hemorrhagic conjunctivitis in tropical areas with recent outbreaks in southern China and Pakistan.

9. Other syndromes associated with coxsackievirus infections—

These include rhabdomyolysis, fulminant neonatal hepatitis (occurs rarely), glomerulopathy (group B infections), and type 1 diabetes mellitus (mainly with group B infections), although definitive causality is not established. A pathogenic role in primary Sjögren syndrome and acute myocardial infarction has also been proposed for group B coxsackievirus infections.

B. Laboratory Findings

Routine laboratory studies show no characteristic abnormalities. Neutralizing antibodies appear during convalescence. The virus may be isolated from throat washings or stools inoculated into suckling mice. Viral culture is expensive, labor demanding, and requires several days for

results. A PCR test for enterovirus RNA is available and, although it cannot identify the serotype, it appears to be useful, particularly in cases of meningitis.

▶ Treatment & Prognosis

Treatment is symptomatic. With the exception of meningitis, myocarditis, pericarditis, perhaps diabetes, and rare illnesses such as pancreatitis or polio-like syndrome, the syndromes caused by coxsackieviruses are benign and self-limited. Two controlled trials showed a potential clinical benefit with pleconaril for patients with enteroviral meningitis although the compassionate use of this drug has stopped. There are anecdotal reports of success with intravenous immunoglobulin in severe disease.

Brunetti L et al. Treatment of viral myocarditis caused by coxsackievirus B. Am J Health Syst Pharm. 2008 Jan 15;65(2):132–7. [PMID: 18192257]
Centers for Disease Control and Prevention (CDC). Increased detections and severe neonatal disease associated with coxsackievirus B1 infection—United States, 2007. MMWR Morb Mortal Wkly Rep. 2008 May 23;57(20):553–6. [PMID: 18496504]

2. Echovirus Infections

Echoviruses are enteroviruses that produce several clinical syndromes, particularly in children. Infection is most common during summer. Among reported specimens, death ensues in about 3%. Males younger than 20 years are more commonly infected than other persons.

Over 30 serotypes have been demonstrated and the most common serotypes for disease are types 6, 9, 11, and 30. Most can cause aseptic meningitis, which may be associated with a rubelliform rash. Types 30 and 13 (the latter also associated with meningitis) outbreaks are increasingly reported globally, including five epidemics of the latter in the United States. Transmission is primarily fecal–oral. Handwashing is an effective control measure in outbreaks of aseptic meningitis. Outbreaks related to fecal contamination of water sources, including drinking water and swimming and bathing pools, were reported in the past.

Besides meningitis, other conditions associated with echoviruses range from common respiratory diseases (bronchiolitis occurs often in children) and epidemic diarrhea to myocarditis, a hemorrhagic obstetric syndrome, keratoconjunctivitis, hepatitis with coagulopathy, leukocytoclastic vasculitis, and neonatal as well as adult cases of encephalitis and sepsis, interstitial pneumonitis, hemophagocytic syndromes (in children with cancer), sudden deafness, encephalitis, optic neuritis, uveitis, and septic shock. Echoviruses, and enteroviruses in general, are also a common cause of nonspecific exanthems.

The role of enteroviruses in the development of type 1 diabetes mellitus and in the chronic fatigue syndrome are under study.

As with other enterovirus infections, diagnosis is best established by correlation of clinical, epidemiologic, and laboratory evidence. Cytopathic effects are produced in tissue culture after recovery of virus from throat washings, blood, or cerebrospinal fluid. An enterovirus PCR of the cerebrospinal fluid can assist in the diagnosis. Fourfold or greater rises in antibody titer signify systemic infection.

Treatment is usually symptomatic, and the prognosis is excellent, though there are reports of mild paralysis after CNS infection. Pleconaril, investigational, appears to be of some use among meningitis patients with more severe disease in shortening the course of illness.

From a public health standpoint, the prevention of fecal-oral contamination and the maintenance of pool hygiene through chlorination and pH control are important.

Jacques J et al. Epidemiological, molecular, and clinical features of enterovirus respiratory infections in French children between 1999 and 2005. J Clin Microbiol. 2008 Jan;46(1):206–13. [PMID: 18003804]

3. Enteroviruses 70 & 71

Several clinical syndromes are being described in association with newer enteroviruses. **Enterovirus 70,** a ubiquitous agent first identified in 1969 and responsible for abrupt bilateral eye discharge and subconjunctival hemorrhage with occasional systemic symptoms, is most commonly associated with **acute hemorrhagic conjunctivitis. Enterovirus 71** is associated with **hand, foot, and mouth disease** (HFMD) as well as a form of **epidemic encephalitis** associated on occasion with pulmonary edema, and **acute flaccid paralysis.** Because of lower herd immunity, HFMD tends to infect the very young (under age 5) in nonendemic areas. Disease is usually more severe and sequelae more common than with other enteroviruses. The sequelae include central hypoventilation, dysphagia, and limb weakness. An outbreak of enterovirus 71 infections occurred in Colorado between 2003 and 2005.

Diagnosis of both entities is facilitated by the clinical and epidemiologic findings with the isolation of the suspect agent from conjunctival scraping for enterovirus 70 or vesicle swabs, body secretions, or cerebrospinal fluid for enterovirus 71. An IgM capture ELISA is being developed for the latter agent.

Treatment of both entities remains largely symptomatic, though pleconaril (see above) may be of some use. The major complication associated with enterovirus 70 is the rare development of an acute neurologic illness with motor paralysis akin to poliomyelitis. Attention-deficit with hyperactivity occurs in about 20% with confirmed infection.

Household contacts, especially children under 6 months of age, are at particular risk for enterovirus 71 acquisition. A commercial disinfectant, Virkon S, at 1–2% application, appears to reduce infectivity titers. A stage-based supportive treatment for enterovirus 71 infections, recognizing the potential for late onset CNS disease and cardiopulmonary failure is important.

Enterovirus 72 is another term for hepatitis A virus (see Chapter 16).

Gau SS et al. Attention-deficit/hyperactivity-related symptoms among children with enterovirus 71 infection of the central nervous system. Pediatrics. 2008 Aug;122(2):e452–8. [PMID: 18606624]

Hamaguchi T et al. Acute encephalitis caused by intrafamilial transmission of enterovirus 71 in adult. Emerg Infect Dis. 2008 May;14(5):828–30. [PMID: 18439374]
Qiu J. Enterovirus 71 infection: a new threat to global public health? Lancet Neurol. 2008 Oct;7(10):868–9. [PMID: 18848307]

4. Human Parechovirus Infection

Four types of parechovirus (a picornavirus first recognized in 2000) were recognized by 2007. They are responsible for otitis, respiratory, and gastrointestinal illness in young children; neonatal sepsis; flaccid paralysis; and cerebral infections, including aseptic meningitis and encephalitis. Severe disease is most often found with the third serotype. Cases are reported from Europe and North America. Disease can also occur in older adults. Treatment at this stage is largely supportive. Reported complications of neonatal cerebral infections include learning disabilities, epilepsy, and cerebral palsy.

Harvala H et al. Epidemiology and clinical associations of human parechovirus respiratory infections. J Clin Microbiol. 2008 Oct;46(10):3446–53. [PMID: 18753351]
Wolthers KC et al. Human parechoviruses as an important viral cause of sepsis-like illness and meningitis in young children. Clin Infect Dis. 2008 Aug 1;47(3):358–63. [PMID: 18558876]

▼ RICKETTSIAL DISEASES

TYPHUS GROUP

1. Epidemic Louse-Borne Typhus

ESSENTIALS OF DIAGNOSIS

▶ Prodrome of headache, then chills and fever.

▶ Severe, intractable headaches, prostration, persisting high fever.

▶ Macular rash appearing on the fourth to seventh days on the trunk and in the axillae, spreading to the rest of the body but sparing the face, palms, and soles.

▶ Diagnosis confirmed by specific antibodies using complement fixation, microagglutination, or immunofluorescence.

▶ General Considerations

Epidemic louse-borne typhus is due to infection with *Rickettsia prowazekii,* a parasite of the body louse (Table 32–3). Transmission is favored by crowded, unsanitary living conditions, famine, war, or any circumstances that predispose to heavy infestation with lice. When the louse sucks the blood of a person infected with *R prowazekii,* the organism becomes established in the gut of the louse and grows there. When the louse is transmitted to another person (through contact or clothing) and has a blood meal,

Table 32–3. Rickettsial diseases.

Disease	Rickettsial Pathogen	Geographic Areas of Prevalence	Insect Vector	Mammalian Reservoir	Travel Association
Typhus group					
Epidemic (louse-borne) typhus	*Rickettsia prowazekii*	South America, Central Africa	Louse	Humans, flying squirrels	Rare
Endemic (murine) typhus	*Rickettsia typhi*	Worldwide; small foci (United States: southeastern gulf coast)	Flea	Rodents	Often
Scrub typhus group					
Scrub typhus	*Orientia tsutsugamushi*	Southeast Asia, Japan, Australia, Western Siberia	Mite[1]	Rodents	Often
Spotted fever group					
Rocky Mountain spotted fever	*Rickettsia rickettsii*	Western Hemisphere; United States (especially mid-Atlantic coast region)	Tick[1]	Rodents, dogs	Rare
California flea rickettsiosis	*Rickettsia felis*	Worldwide?	Flea	Cats, opossums	
Mediterranean spotted fever, Boutonneuse fever, Kenya tick typhus, South African tick fever, Indian tick typhus	*Rickettsia conorii*	Africa, India, Mediterranean regions	Tick[1]	Rodents, dogs	Often
Queensland tick typhus	*Rickettsia australis*	Eastern Australia	Tick[1]	Rodents, marsupials	Rare
Siberian Asian tick typhus	*Rickettsia sibirica*	Siberia, Mongolia	Tick[1]	Rodents	Rare
African tick bite fever	*Rickettsia africae*	Rural sub-Saharan Africa, Eastern Caribbean	Tick[1]	Cattle	Often
Rickettsialpox	*Rickettsia akari*	United States, Korea, former USSR	Mite[1]	Mice	
Other					
Ehrlichiosis and anaplasmosis, human Monocytic	*Ehrlichia chaffeensis, Anaplasma equi, Ehrlichia canis*	Southeastern United States	Tick[1]	Dogs	
Granulocytic	*Anaplasma phagocytophilum, Ehrlichia ewingii*	Northeastern United States	Tick[1]	Rodents, deer, sheep	
Q fever	*Coxiella burnetii*	Worldwide	None[2]	Cattle, sheep, goats	

[1]Also serve as arthropod reservoir by maintaining rickettsiae through transovarian transmission.
[2]Human infection results from inhalation of dust.

it defecates simultaneously, and the infected feces are rubbed into the itching bite wound or mucous membranes. Dry, infectious louse feces may also enter the respiratory tract. Cases can be acquired by travel to pockets of infection (eg, central and northeastern Africa, Central and South America). Recent outbreaks were reported from Peru, Burundi, and Russia. *R prowazekii* is considered a possible bioterrorist agent.

R prowazekii can survive in lymphoid tissues after primary infection, and years later, produce recrudescence of disease (Brill-Zinsser disease) without exposure to infected lice. This phenomenon can serve as a point source for future outbreaks.

An extrahuman reservoir of *R prowazekii* in the United States is flying squirrels. Transmission to humans can occur through their ectoparasites, usually causing atypical mild disease.

▶ Clinical Findings

A. Symptoms and Signs

(Table 32–2.) Prodromal malaise, cough, headache, backache, arthralgia, and chest pain begin after an incubation period of 10–14 days, followed by an abrupt onset of chills, high fever, and prostration, with flu-like symptoms progressing to delirium and stupor. The headache is severe and the fever is prolonged.

Other findings consist of conjunctivitis, hearing loss from neuropathy of the eighth cranial nerve, flushed facies, rales at the lung bases, and often splenomegaly. A macular rash (that may become confluent) appears first in the axillae and then over the trunk, spreading to the extremities but rarely involving the face, palms, or soles. In severely ill patients, the rash becomes hemorrhagic, and hypotension becomes marked. There may be acute kidney injury, stupor, and delirium. In spontaneous recovery, improvement begins 13–16 days after onset with a rapid drop of fever.

B. Laboratory Findings

The white blood cell count is variable. Thrombocytopenia, elevated liver enzymes, proteinuria and hematuria commonly occur. Serum obtained 5–12 days after onset of symptoms usually shows specific antibodies for R prowazekii antigens as demonstrated by complement fixation, microagglutination, or immunofluorescence. In primary rickettsial infection, early antibodies are IgM; in recrudescence (Brill disease), early antibodies are predominantly IgG. A PCR test is developed, but its availability is limited. R prowazekii is differentiated into 7 genotypes.

C. Imaging

Radiographs of the chest may show patchy consolidation.

▶ Differential Diagnosis

The prodromal symptoms and the early febrile stage are not specific enough to permit diagnosis in nonepidemic situations. The rash is usually sufficiently distinctive for diagnosis, but it may be absent in up to 50% of cases or may be difficult to observe in dark-skinned persons. A variety of other acute febrile diseases should be considered, including typhoid fever, meningococcemia, and measles.

Brill-Zinsser disease (recrudescent epidemic typhus) has a more gradual onset than primary R prowazekii infection, fever and rash are of shorter duration, and the disease is milder and rarely fatal.

▶ Complications

Pneumonia, thromboses, vasculitis with major vessel obstruction and gangrene, circulatory collapse, myocarditis, and uremia may occur.

▶ Prevention

Prevention consists of louse control with insecticides, particularly by applying chemicals to clothing or treating it with heat, and frequent bathing. A deloused and bathed typhus patient is not infectious. The disease is not transmitted from person to person. Patients are infectious for the lice during the febrile period and perhaps 2–3 days after the fever returns to normal. Infected lice pass rickettsiae in their feces within 2–6 days after the blood meal and can be infectious earlier if crushed. Rickettsiae remain viable in a dead louse for weeks.

No vaccine is currently available for the prevention of R prowazekii infection. Past use of crude antigen or inactivated Rickettsia provided partial protection but was associated with undesirable toxic reactions and difficulties in standardization. Efforts to identify new candidate antigens through DNA technology are underway.

▶ Treatment

Treatment consists of either doxycycline (100 mg orally twice daily for adults and children weighing > 45 kg, and 2.2 mg/kg twice daily for children weighing < 45 kg) or chloramphenicol (50–100 mg/kg/d in four divided doses, orally or intravenously; it is the drug of choice in pregnant women) for 4–10 days. In epidemic conditions, a single dose of doxycycline can be effective and is less costly.

▶ Prognosis

The prognosis depends greatly on the patient's age and immune status. In children under age 10 years, the disease is usually mild. The mortality rate is 10% in the second and third decades but in the past reached 60% in the sixth decade.

Azad AF et al. Pathogenic rickettsiae as bioterrorism agents. Clin Infect Dis. 2007 Jul 15;45 (Suppl 1):S52–5. [PMID: 17582570]
Bechah Y et al. Epidemic typhus. Lancet Infect Dis. 2008 Jul;8(7):417–26. [PMID: 18582834]
Zhu Y et al. Genotyping *Rickettsia prowazekii* isolates. Emerg Infect Dis. 2008 Aug;14(8):1300–2. [PMID: 18680662]

2. Endemic Flea-Borne Typhus (Murine Typhus)

Rickettsia typhi, a ubiquitous pathogen recognized on all continents, is transmitted from rat to rat through the rat flea (Table 32–3). Humans usually acquire the infection in an urban or suburban setting when bitten by an infected flea, which releases infected feces while sucking blood. Rare human cases in the developed world follow travel, usually to Southeast Asia. Seroprevalence to R typhi among children in South Texas is reported as high as 14% and among the homeless in Houston about 10%.

Endemic typhus resembles recrudescent epidemic typhus in that it has a gradual onset, less severe symptoms, and a shorter duration of illness than epidemic typhus (7–10 days versus 14–21 days). The presentation is nonspecific, including fever, headache, and chills. Maculopapular rash occurs in around 50% of cases; it is concentrated on the trunk and fades fairly rapidly. Peripheral facial paralysis and splenic infarction are reported to occur. Severe disease with mental confusion and signs of hepatic, cardiac, renal, and pulmonary involvement may develop. Fatalities are uncommon but occur especially in the elderly. Jaundice, bradycardia, and the absence of a headache are correlated with a delayed defervescence (in both epidemic and endemic typhus).

The most common entity in the differential diagnosis is Rocky Mountain spotted fever, usually occurring after a rural exposure and with a different rash (centripetal versus centrifugal for endemic typhus). Serologic confirmation may be necessary for differentiation, with complement-fixing or immunofluorescent antibodies detectable within 15 days after onset, with specific R typhi antigens. A fourfold rise in serum antibody titers between the acute and the convalescence phase is diagnostic.

Preventive measures are directed at control of rats and ectoparasites (rat fleas) with insecticides, rat poisons, and rat-proofing of buildings. Antibiotic treatment is the same as for epidemic typhus (see above). Ciprofloxacin (500–

750 mg orally twice a day) is another alternative in pregnant women.

Lai CH et al. Clinical characteristics of acute Q fever, scrub typhus, and murine typhus with delayed defervescence despite doxycycline treatment. Am J Trop Med Hyg. 2008 Sep;79(3):441–6. [PMID: 18784240]

Reeves WK et al. Serological evidence of typhus group rickettsia in a homeless population in Houston, Texas. J Vector Ecol. 2008 Jun;33(1):205–7. [PMID: 18697325]

3. Scrub Typhus (Tsutsugamushi Fever)

ESSENTIALS OF DIAGNOSIS

▶ Exposure to mites in endemic area of Southeast Asia, the western Pacific (including Korea), and Australia.

▶ Black eschar at site of the bite, with regional and generalized lymphadenopathy.

▶ Conjunctivitis and a short-lived macular rash.

▶ Frequent pneumonitis, encephalitis, and cardiac failure.

General Considerations

Scrub typhus is caused by *Orientia tsutsugamushi*, which is principally a parasite of rodents transmitted by mites in the endemic areas listed above (Table 32–3). The mites live on vegetation but complete their maturation cycle by biting humans who come in contact with infested vegetation. Vertical transmission occurs, and blood transfusions may transmit the pathogen as well. Rare occupational transmission via inhalation is documented among laboratory workers. The disease in endemic in Korea; China; Taiwan; Japan; Pakistan; India; Thailand; Malaysia; and Queensland, Australia.

Clinical Findings

A. Symptoms and Signs

After a 1- to 3-week incubation period, malaise, chills, severe headache, and backache develop. At the site of the bite, a papule evolves into a flat black eschar. The regional lymph nodes are enlarged and tender, and there may be generalized adenopathy. Fever rises gradually, and a macular rash appears primarily on the trunk after a week of fever and may be fleeting or may last a week. The patient may become obtunded. During the second or third week, pneumonitis, myocarditis and cardiac failure, encephalitis or meningitis, acute abdominal pain, granulomatous hepatitis, disseminated intravascular coagulation, acute respiratory distress syndrome, or acute kidney disease may develop, although not often. Gastrointestinal symptoms including nausea, vomiting, and diarrhea occur in nearly two-thirds of patients and correspond to the presence of superficial mucosal hemorrhage, multiple erosions, or ulcers in the gastrointestinal tract. An attack confers prolonged immunity against homologous strains and transient immunity against heterologous strains. Heterologous strains produce mild disease if infection occurs within a year after the first episode.

B. Laboratory Findings

Thrombocytopenia and elevation of liver enzymes, bilirubin, and creatinine are common. Serologic testing with immunofluorescence and immunoperoxidase assays or commercial dot-blot ELISA dipstick assays are convenient diagnostic aids, but a conclusive diagnosis requires documentation of a fourfold increase between acute and convalescence titers of antibodies. PCR (from the eschar or blood) may be the most sensitive diagnostic test while culture of the organism (by mouse inoculation) from blood obtained during the first few days of illness is another diagnostic modality. Unfortunately, both tests are of limited availability. A reticulonodular infiltrate is the most common finding on chest radiograph.

Differential Diagnosis

Leptospirosis, typhoid, dengue, malaria, hemorrhagic fevers, and other rickettsial infections should be considered. The headache may mimic trigeminal neuralgia. Scrub typhus is a recognized cause of obscure tropical fevers, especially in children.

Prevention

Repeated application of long-acting miticides can make endemic areas safe. Insect repellents on clothing and skin provide some protection. For short exposure, chemoprophylaxis with doxycycline (200 mg weekly) can prevent the disease but permits infection. No effective vaccines are available.

Treatment & Prognosis

Without treatment, fever subsides spontaneously after 2 weeks, but the mortality rate may be 10–30%. Empiric treatment for 3 days with doxycycline, 100 mg orally twice daily, or for 7 days with chloramphenicol, 25 mg/kg/d orally or intravenously in four divided doses, eliminates most deaths and relapses. Chloramphenicol- and tetracycline-resistant strains have been reported from Southeast Asia, where azithromycin or roxythromycin may become the drug of choice for children, pregnant women, and patients with refractory disease. Rifampin reduces the duration of fever by 1 day when used with doxycycline. HIV infection does not appear to influence the severity of scrub typhus.

Botelho-Nevers E et al. Fever of unknown origin due to rickettsioses. Infect Dis Clin North Am. 2007 Dec;21(4):997–1011. [PMID: 18061086]

Nachega JB. Travel-acquired scrub typhus: emphasis on the differential diagnosis, treatment, and prevention strategies. J Travel Med. 2007 Sep–Oct;14(5):352–5. [PMID: 17883470]

SPOTTED FEVERS

1. Rocky Mountain Spotted Fever

ESSENTIALS OF DIAGNOSIS

▶ Exposure to tick bite in an endemic area.

- An influenza-like prodrome followed by chills, fever, severe headache, myalgias, restlessness, and prostration; occasionally, delirium and coma.

- Red macular rash appears between the second and sixth days of fever, first on the wrists and ankles and then spreading centrally; it may become petechial.

- Serial serologic examinations by indirect fluorescent antibody (IFA) confirm the diagnosis retrospectively.

General Considerations

Despite its name, most cases of Rocky Mountain spotted fever (RMSF) occur outside the Rocky Mountain area. Passive surveillance data from 1997 to 2002 reported cases of RMSF from each of the contiguous states except Vermont and Maine. More than half (56%) of these cases were from only five states: North Carolina, South Carolina, Tennessee, Oklahoma, and Arkansas. The causative agent, *R rickettsii*, is transmitted to humans by the bite of ticks, including the Rocky Mountain wood tick, *D andersoni*, in the western United States, and the American dog tick, *Dermacentor variabilis*, in the eastern United States. The brown dog tick, *Rhipicephalus sanguineus*, is a vector in eastern Arizona. In the United States, the estimated annual incidence of RMSF is 2.2 cases per million persons with cases primarily occurring from April through September, and with a higher incidence among children and men.

Other hard ticks transmit the organism in the southern United States and in Central and South America and are responsible for transmitting it among rodents, dogs, porcupines, and other animals.

Clinical Findings

A. Symptoms and Signs

Two to 14 days (mean, 7 days) after the bite of an infectious tick, symptoms begin with fever, chills, headache, nausea and vomiting, myalgias, restlessness, insomnia, and irritability. Cough and pneumonitis may develop. Delirium, lethargy, seizures, stupor, and coma may appear. The face is flushed and the conjunctiva injected (Plate 99). The rash (faint macules that progress to maculopapules and then petechiae) appears between days 2 and 6 of fever, first on the wrists and ankles, spreading centrally to the arms, legs, and trunk for 2–3 days; involvement of the palms and soles is characteristic. About 10% of cases, however, occur without rash or with minimal rash. In some cases there is splenomegaly, hepatomegaly, jaundice, myocarditis (which may mimic an acute coronary syndrome), or uremia. ARDS and necrotizing vasculitis are of greatest concern.

B. Laboratory Findings

Thrombocytopenia, hyponatremia, elevated aminotransferases, and hyperbilirubinemia are common. Cerebrospinal fluid may show hypoglycorrhachia and mild pleocytosis. Disseminated intravascular coagulation is observed in severe cases. Diagnosis during the acute phase of the illness can be made by immunohistologic demonstration of *R*

rickettsiae in skin biopsy specimens, but this must be performed as soon as skin lesions become apparent and before antibiotics are started to achieve maximum sensitivity. Isolation of the organism using the shell-vial technique is available in some laboratories but is hazardous.

Serologic studies confirm the diagnosis, but most patients do not mount an antibody response until the second week of illness. The indirect fluorescent antibody test is most commonly used. No PCR technique has been validated for clinical use.

Differential Diagnosis

The diagnosis is challenging. Up to 40% of patients do not recall a tick bite, and initial diagnosis is made clinically. Early symptoms may resemble those of many other infections. The rash may be confused with that of measles, typhoid, and ehrlichiosis, or—most importantly—meningococcemia. Blood cultures and examination of cerebrospinal fluid establish the latter.

Prevention

Protective clothing, tick-repellent chemicals, and the removal of ticks at frequent intervals are helpful measures. Prophylactic therapy after a tick bite is not currently recommended.

Treatment & Prognosis

Treatment with doxycycline or, in pregnant women, chloramphenicol at similar doses and duration as for epidemic typhus (see above) is recommended. Patients usually defervesce within 48–72 hours. Therapy should be maintained for at least 3 days after defervescence. Mild cases in low-risk individuals may be observed without treatment.

Although the reported mortality rate in the United States is about 3–5%, it can be as high as 70% in the untreated elderly. Myocarditis is the leading cause of death. Other risk factors for a fatal outcome include very young age, atypical clinical features (absence of headache, no history of tick attachment, gastrointestinal symptoms), underlying chronic diseases, and a delay in initiation of appropriate antibiotic therapy. The usual cause of death is pneumonitis with respiratory or cardiac failure. Sequelae, more common than formerly recognized, may include seizures, encephalopathy, peripheral neuropathy, paraparesis, bowel and bladder incontinence, cerebellar and vestibular dysfunction, hearing loss, and motor deficits.

Chen LF et al. What's new in Rocky Mountain spotted fever? Infect Dis Clin North Am. 2008 Sep;22(3):415–32. [PMID: 18755382]
Cunha BA. Clinical features of Rocky Mountain spotted fever. Lancet Infect Dis. 2008 Mar;8(3):143–4. [PMID: 18291332]

2. Rickettsialpox

Rickettsia akari is a parasite of mice, transmitted by mites *Liponyssoides sanguineus* (Table 32–2). Rickettsialpox occurs in humans when crowded conditions and mouse-infested housing allow transmission of the pathogen to humans. In a free clinic in downtown Los Angeles, California, serologic evidence of infection was detected in 8% of patients. The incubation period is 7–12 days. Onset is sudden, with chills, fever, headache, photophobia, and disseminated aches and pains. The primary lesion is a painless red papule that vesiculates and forms a black eschar. Two to 4 days after onset of symptoms, a widespread papular eruption appears that becomes vesicular and forms crusts that are shed in about 10 days. Early lesions may resemble those of chickenpox (typically vesicular versus papulovesicular in rickettsialpox). Pathologic findings include dermal edema, subepidermal vesicles, and at times a lymphocytic vasculitis.

Transient leukopenia and thrombocytopenia and acute hepatitis can occur. A fourfold rise in serum antibody titers to rickettsial antigen, detected by complement fixation or indirect fluorescent assays, is diagnostic. Conjugated antirickettsial globulin can identify antigen in punch biopsies of skin lesions. PCR detection of rickettsial DNA in fresh tissue also appears of value. *R akari* is also reported to be isolable from eschar biopsy specimens.

Treatment includes doxycycline (200 mg/d) for 7 days. The disease is usually mild and self-limited without treatment, but occasionally severe symptoms may require hospitalization. Control requires the elimination of mice from human habitations and insecticide applications to suppress the mite vectors.

Bennett SG et al. Serologic evidence of a *Rickettsia akari*-like infection among wild-caught rodents in Orange County and humans in Los Angeles County, California. J Vector Ecol. 2007 Dec;32(2):198–201. [PMID: 18260508]

3. Tick Typhus (Rickettsial Fever)

The term "tick typhus" denotes a variety of spotted rickettsial fevers. They are often named by geography, eg, Mediterranean spotted fever, Queensland tick typhus, Oriental spotted fever, African tick bite fever, Siberian tick typhus, North Asian tick typhus, or by morphology, eg, boutonneuse fever. These illnesses are transmitted by tick vectors of the rickettsial organisms *R conorii*, *R australis*, *R japonica*, *R africae*, and *R sibirica* (Table 32–3). Dogs and wild animals, usually rodents but even reptiles, may serve as reservoirs. Travel is a risk factor for disease, particularly among elderly ecotourists. The pathogens usually produce an eschar or black spot (tâche noire) at the site of the tick bite that may be useful in diagnosis, though spotless boutonneuse fever occurs. Symptoms include fever, headache, myalgias, and rash. Rarely, papulovesicular lesions may resemble rickettsialpox. Endothelial injury produces perivascular edema and dermal necrosis. Regional adenopathy, disseminated lesions, kidney disease, splenic rupture, and focal hepatic necrosis may occur. Diabetes, dehydration, and uremia were risk factors for mortality in one series. The disease occurs among travelers, the most common travel-associated rickettsiosis being African tick bite fever. Diagnosis is clinical, with serologic or PCR confirmation. Prevention entails protective clothing, repellents, and inspection for and removal of ticks. Treatment is with the following drugs given for 7–10 days: doxycycline (200 mg/d), chloramphenicol (50–75 mg/kg/d

in four divided doses), or ciprofloxacin (500 mg twice daily). The combination of erythromycin and rifampin is effective and safe in pregnancy. Delayed therapy is the usual cause of morbidity.

Another rickettsial infection, formerly classified as an endemic or murine typhus, is more properly classified as a spotted fever. The causative agent, *R felis*, is an organism that has been linked to the cat flea and opossum exposures. Most cases in the United States occur in the spring and summer, are reported from southern Texas and California; it also appears to be present in Hawaii. Cases are treated as above.

Civen R et al. Murine typhus: an unrecognized suburban vector-borne disease. Clin Infect Dis. 2008 Mar 15;46(6):913–8. [PMID: 18260783]
Lee N et al. Risk factors associated with life-threatening rickettsial infections. Am J Trop Med Hyg. 2008 Jun;78(6):973–8. [PMID: 18541779]
Rovery C et al. Mediterranean spotted fever. Infect Dis Clin North Am. 2008 Sep;22(3):515–30. [PMID: 18755388]

OTHER RICKETTSIAL & RICKETTSIAL-LIKE DISEASES

1. Ehrlichiosis & Anaplasmosis

 ESSENTIALS OF DIAGNOSIS

► Infection of monocyte or granulocyte by tick-borne gram-negative bacteria.

► Nine-day incubation period, with variable clinical illness, ranging from asymptomatic to persistent or life-threatening.

► Common symptoms are malaise, nausea, fever, and headaches.

► Excellent response to therapy with tetracyclines.

► General Considerations

Ehrlichiae and anaplasmae are small tick-borne gram-negative obligate intracellular bacteria that infect monocytes or granulocytes. Human monocytic ehrlichiosis is caused by *Ehrlichia chaffeensis* (Table 32–3). Human granulocytic anaplasmosis is caused by *Anasplasma phagocytophilium*. *Ehrlichia ewingii* (infecting primarily dogs) can rarely cause human granulocytic ehrlichiosis similar to human granulocytic anaplasmosis. Another ehrlichia-like organism, *Neorickettsia sennetsu*, is the etiologic agent of sennetsu fever, which is confined to western Japan.

Human monocytic ehrlichiosis is seen primarily in the Southeast, mid-Atlantic, and South Central states of the United States, though cases are also recognized in Israel, Japan, Mexico, South America, and Europe. Human granulocytic anaplasmosis is more frequent in Northeastern and Midwestern United States; but infections in Europe and China are also well documented. Human infection with *E ewingii* is limited to Missouri, Oklahoma, and Tennessee and occurs mainly among the immunocompromised. In

North America, the major vectors for these pathogens are the Lone Star tick (*Amblyomma americanus* for *E chaffeensis* and *E ewingii*), the western black-legged tick (*Ixodes pacificus*, for *E chaffeensis*), and *Ixodes scapularis* (the same vector for Lyme disease and babesiosis) for *A phagocytophilium*). Reported incidences of both human monocytic and granulocytic ehrlichiosis are about 0.6 and 1.4 per million, respectively, with higher rates in the summer. The highest attack rate is in men over 60 years of age.

The principal reservoirs for human monocytic ehrlichiosis and human granulocytic anaplasmosis are the white tail deer and the white footed mouse, respectively. Other mammals can be implicated as well. A nosocomial outbreak was recently reported from China. Perinatal transmission of human granulocytic anaplasmosis is also documented.

Clinical Findings

A. Symptoms and Signs

Clinical disease of human monocytic ehrlichiosis ranges from mild to life-threatening. Typically, after about a 9-day incubation period and a prodrome consisting of malaise, rigors, and nausea, worsening fever and headache develop. A pleomorphic rash may occur. The presentation in immunosuppressed patients and the elderly tends to be more severe than in immunocompetent and younger patients. Serious sequelae include acute respiratory failure and ARDS, encephalopathy, and acute kidney disease, which may mimic thrombotic thrombocytopenic purpura.

The symptoms of human granulocytic ehrlichiosis and *E ewingii* infection are similar to those seen with human monocytic ehrlichiosis. Rash, however, is infrequent in human granulocytic ehrlichiosis and should prompt the consideration of other infections (eg, Lyme disease). Persistent fever and malaise are reported to occur for 2 or more years. Coinfection with Lyme disease or basesiosis may occur.

B. Laboratory Findings

Diagnosis can be made by the history of tick exposure followed by a characteristic clinical presentation. Leukopenia, absolute lymphopenia, thrombocytopenia, and transaminitis occur often. Thrombocytopenia occurs more often than leukopenia in human granulocytic ehrlichiosis. Examination of peripheral blood with Giemsa stain may reveal characteristic intraleukocytic vacuoles (morulae). An indirect fluorescent antibody assay is available through the CDC and requires acute and convalescent sera. A PCR assay, if available, is a rapid diagnostic tool, especially for early disease.

Treatment

Treatment for both forms of ehrlichiosis is with doxycycline, 100 mg twice daily (orally or intravenously) for at least 10 days or until 3 days of defervescence. Rifampin is an alternative in pregnant women and children. Treatment should not be withheld while awaiting confirmatory serol-

ogy when suspicion is high. Lack of clinical improvement and defervescence 48 hours after doxycycline initiation suggests an alternate diagnosis.

Bakken JS et al. Human granulocytic anaplasmosis. Infect Dis Clin North Am. 2008 Sep;22(3):433–48. [PMID: 18755383]

Dumler JS et al. Ehrlichioses in humans: epidemiology, clinical presentation, diagnosis, and treatment. Clin Infect Dis. 2007 Jul 15;45(Suppl 1):S45–51. [PMID: 17582569]

Hamburg BJ et al. The importance of early treatment with doxycycline in human ehrlichiosis. Medicine (Baltimore). 2008 Mar;87(2):53–60. [PMID: 18344803]

Zhang L et al. Nosocomial transmission of human granulocytic anaplasmosis in China. JAMA. 2008 Nov 19;300(19):2263–70. [PMID: 19017912]

2. Q Fever

 ESSENTIALS OF DIAGNOSIS

▶ Exposure to sheep, goats, cattle, or their products is common; some infections are laboratory acquired.

▶ An acute or chronic febrile illness with severe headache, cough, prostration, and abdominal pain.

▶ Extensive pneumonitis, hepatitis, or encephalopathy; less often, endocarditis, vascular infections, or chronic fatigue syndrome.

▶ A common cause of culture-negative endocarditis.

General Considerations

Q fever (for "query" in view of its formerly unknown cause) is a reportable disease in the United States caused by *Coxiella burnetii*, an organism previously classified as a rickettsia but now considered a proteobacteria. Unlike rickettsiae, *C burnetii* is usually transmitted to humans not by arthropods but by inhalation or ingestion. *Coxiella* infections occur mostly in cattle, sheep, and goats, in which they cause mild or subclinical disease (Table 32–3). In these animals, reactivation of the infection occurs during pregnancy and causes abortions or low birth weight offspring. *Coxiella* is resistant to heat and drying and remains infective in the environment for months. Humans become infected by inhalation of aerosolized bacteria (in dust or droplets) from feces, urine, milk, or products of conception of infected animals. Ingestion and skin penetration are recognized routes of transmission as well. Outbreaks associated with other mammals such as cats and dogs are also described. There is an occupational risk for animal handlers, slaughterhouse workers, veterinarians, laboratory workers, and other workers exposed to animal products. Outbreaks in military personnel returning from Iraq and Afghanistan were recently described. Endocarditis, an uncommon but serious form of *Coxiella* infection, has been linked to preexisting valvular conditions, immunocompromise, urban residence, and raw milk ingestion. Horizontal spread from one human to another does not seem to occur even in the presence of florid pneumonitis, but maternal–fetal infection can occur.

Clinical Findings

A. Symptoms and Signs

Asymptomatic infection is common. For the remaining cases, a febrile illness develops after an incubation period of 1–3 weeks, usually accompanied by headache, prostration, and muscle pains. The clinical course may be acute, chronic (duration ≥ 6 months), or relapsing. Pneumonia and granulomatous hepatitis are the predominant manifestation in the acute form, whereas other less common manifestations include skin rashes (maculopapular or purpuric), fever of unknown origin, myocarditis, pericarditis, aseptic meningitis, encephalitis, hemolytic anemia, orchitis, acute kidney disease, spondylodiscitis, tenosynovitis, and regional (mediastinal) or diffuse lymphadenopathies. The most common presentation of chronic Q fever is culture-negative endocarditis, which occurs in less than 1% of infected individuals. It is found mainly in the setting of preexisting valve disease. Vascular infections, particularly of the aorta (and potentially causing aneurysms) are the second most common form of Q fever and are associated with a high mortality (25%). A Q fever chronic fatigue syndrome is thought by some experts to involve bacteremic shedding from bone marrow reservoirs and to be immunogenetically determined.

Reactivation of Q fever in pregnant women may cause spontaneous abortions, intrauterine growth retardation, intrauterine fetal death, premature delivery, and oligamnios.

B. Laboratory Findings

Laboratory examination during the acute phase may show elevated liver function tests and occasional leukocytosis. Patients with acute Q fever usually produce antibodies to *C burnetii* phase II antigen. A fourfold rise between acute and convalescent sera by indirect immunofluorescence is diagnostic.

The diagnosis of chronic Q fever is established on the basis of serologic tests done at 3- and 6-month intervals. The IgG titer against phase I antigen is usually 1:200 or greater. In some cases, the diagnosis is not made until the time of valve replacement, with PCR of tissue samples. Isolation of *C burnetii* from affected valves is also possible using the shell-vial technique, but the organism is highly transmissible to laboratory workers and culture techniques should be carried out in biosafety level 3 settings.

C. Imaging

Radiographs of the chest show patchy pulmonary infiltrates, often more prominent than the physical signs would suggest.

Differential Diagnosis

Viral, mycoplasmal, and bacterial pneumonias, viral hepatitis, brucellosis, tuberculosis, psittacosis, and other animal-borne diseases must be considered. Q fever should be considered in cases of unexplained fevers with negative blood cultures in association with embolic or cardiac disease.

Prevention

Prevention is based on detection of the infection in livestock, reduction of contact with infected animals or dusts contaminated by them, special care when working with animal tissues, and effective pasteurization of milk. No Q fever vaccine is approved for use in the United States, although a whole-cell vaccine, with a 5-year efficacy of more than 95%, is available in Australia for persons with high-risk exposures.

C burnetii is category B bioterrorism agent. In the setting of a bioterrorist attack, postexposure prophylaxis should be started 8–12 days after exposure, doxycycline (100 mg orally twice daily) should be taken for 5 days, and a pregnant woman should take trimethoprim-sulfamethoxazole (160 mg/800 mg twice daily) for the duration of the pregnancy.

Treatment & Prognosis

For acute infection, treatment with doxycycline (100 mg orally twice daily) for 14 days or at least 3 full days after defervescence is recommended. Even in untreated patients, the mortality rate is usually low, except when endocarditis develops.

For the treatment of endocarditis, most experts recommend a combination of oral doxycycline (200 mg/d) plus oral hydroxychloroquine (600 mg/d) for at least 2 years. Serologic responses can be monitored to determine cessation of therapy. Heart valve replacement may be necessary in refractory disease. Given the difficulty in treating endocarditis, transthoracic echocardiography is recommended for all patients with acute Q fever, and the same aforementioned therapy for 1 year should be offered if a valvulopathy is observed.

Because of the many and serious obstetric complications that occur among pregnant women in whom Q fever develops (listed above), a regimen of long-term trimethoprim-sulfamethoxasole (320/1600 mg for at least 5 weeks) should be given to all infected, pregnant women.

Faix DJ et al. Outbreak of Q fever among US military in western Iraq, June–July 2005. Clin Infect Dis. 2008 Apr 1;46(7):e65–8. [PMID: 18444807]
Scott JW et al. Q fever endocarditis: the Mayo Clinic experience. Am J Med Sci. 2008 Jul;336(1):53–7. [PMID: 18626237]
Tissot-Dupont H et al. Q fever. Infect Dis Clin North Am. 2008 Sep;22(3):505–14. [PMID: 18755387]

KAWASAKI DISEASE

ESSENTIALS OF DIAGNOSIS

▸ Fever, bilateral conjunctivitis, oral mucosal changes, rash, cervical lymphadenopathy, peripheral extremity changes.

▸ Elevated erythrocyte sedimentation rate and C-reactive protein levels.

General Considerations

Kawasaki disease is a worldwide multisystemic disease initially described by Tomisaku Kawasaki in 1967. It is also known as the "mucocutaneous lymph node syndrome." It occurs mainly in children between the ages of 3 months and 5 years but can occur occasionally in adults as well. Kawasaki disease occurs more frequently in Asians or Pacific Islanders but rarely in whites. It is a vasculitis characterized by the infiltration of vessel walls with mononuclear cells and later by IgA secreting plasma cells that can result in the destruction of the media and aneurysm formation. Several infectious agents (New Haven coronavirus, parvovirus, bocavirus, CMV, *Yersinia pseudotuberculosis*), bacterial superantigens, and genetic polymorphisms in components of the immune system have been implicated in its pathogenesis.

Clinical Findings

A clinical diagnosis of "complete" Kawasaki disease requires, in the absence of other processes, explaining the current illness of fever and four of the following criteria for at least 5 days: bilateral nonexudative conjunctivitis, mucous membrane changes of at least one type (injected pharynx, erythema, swelling and fissuring of the lips, strawberry tongue), peripheral extremity changes of at least one type (edema, desquamation, erythema of the palms and soles, induration of the hands and feet, Beau lines [transverse grooves of the nails]), a polymorphous rash, and cervical lymphadenopathy greater than 1.5 cm. An "incomplete" form is diagnosed when only two criteria are met.

A major complication is arteritis of the coronary vessels, occurring in about 25% of untreated patients, on occasion causing myocardial infarction. It is more common among patients over 6 years or below 1 year of age. Noninvasive diagnosis of this complication can be made with magnetic resonance angiography or transthoracic echocardiography. Other factors associated with the development of coronary aneurysms are relentless fever (after the administration of IVIG), high C-reactive protein, anemia, hypoalbuminemia, hyponatremia, thrombocytopenia, and male gender. Pericardial effusions, myocarditis, and mitral regurgitation (usually mild) are also common. Arteritis of extremity vessels, peripheral gangrene, syndrome of inappropriate secretion of antidiuretic hormone (SIADH), and the hemophagocytic syndrome are also reported. Cerebrospinal fluid pleocytosis is found in one-third of cases.

Differentiation from disseminated adenovirus infection is important and can be performed with rapid adenovirus assays.

Treatment

Every patient with a clinical diagnosis of Kawasaki disease (complete or incomplete) should be treated. IVIG (2 g/kg over 10–12 hours) is given within the first 10 days of illness. For those presenting later, but with persistent fever, ongoing systemic inflammation, or aneurysm formation, IVIG should be offered as well. Concomitant aspirin should be started at 80–100 mg/kg/d (divided into four doses and not exceeding 4 g/d) until the patient is afebrile for 48 hours and then reduced to 3–5 mg/kg/d until markers of acute inflammation normalize. Aspirin therapy is continued if coronary aneurysm develops. If fevers persist beyond 36 hours after the initial IVIG infusion, a new dose of 2 g/kg should be given if no other source of fever is found. Methylprednisolone (30 mg/kg/d for a maximum of 3 days) should follow if the disease persists after the second IVIG administration. Further options for refractory cases include TNF-α blockers (eg, infliximab), cyclophosphamide, methotrexate, and plasmapheresis. An echocardiogram is essential in the acute phase of illness and 6–8 weeks after onset. Warfarin is indicated along with low-dose aspirin in patients with aneurysms larger than 8 mm in diameter. If myocardial infarction occurs, therapy with thrombolytics, percutaneous coronary intervention, coronary artery bypass grafts, and even cardiac transplantation should be considered. Manifestation of coronary aneurysms can occur as late as in the third or fourth decade of life and regular follow-up with a cardiologist is recommended for those with coronary complications.

When to Refer

All cases of Kawasaki disease merit referral to specialists.

Ashouri N et al. Risk factors for nonresponse to therapy in Kawasaki disease. J Pediatr. 2008 Sep;153(3):365–8. [PMID: 18534243]

Burns JC. Infliximab treatment of intravenous immunoglobulin-resistant Kawasaki disease. J Pediatr. 2008 Dec;153(6):833–8. [PMID: 18672254]

De Rosa G et al. Current recommendations for the pharmacologic therapy in Kawasaki syndrome and management of its cardiovascular complications. Eur Rev Med Pharmacol Sci. 2007 Sep–Oct;11(5):301–8. [PMID: 18074939]

Furukawa T et al. Effects of steroid pulse therapy on immunoglobulin-resistant Kawasaki disease. Arch Dis Child. 2008 Feb;93(2):142–6. [PMID: 17962370]

Pinna GS et al. Kawasaki disease: an overview. Curr Opin Infect Dis. 2008 Jun;21(3):263–70. [PMID: 18448971]

Bacterial & Chlamydial Infections

Brian S. Schwartz, MD
Henry F. Chambers, MD

INFECTIONS CAUSED BY GRAM-POSITIVE BACTERIA

STREPTOCOCCAL INFECTIONS

1. Pharyngitis

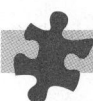

ESSENTIALS OF DIAGNOSIS

- ▶ Abrupt onset of sore throat, fever, malaise, nausea, and headache.
- ▶ Throat red and edematous, with or without exudate; cervical nodes tender.
- ▶ Diagnosis confirmed by culture of throat.

General Considerations

Group A β-hemolytic streptococci (*Streptococcus pyogenes*) are the most common bacterial cause of pharyngitis. Transmission occurs by droplets of infected secretions. Group A streptococci producing erythrogenic toxin may cause scarlet fever in susceptible persons.

Clinical Findings

A. Symptoms and Signs

"Strep throat" is characterized by a sudden onset of fever, sore throat, pain on swallowing, tender cervical adenopathy, malaise, and nausea. The pharynx, soft palate, and tonsils are red and edematous. There may be a purulent exudate. The Centor clinical criteria for the diagnosis of streptococcal pharyngitis are temperature > 38 °C, tender anterior cervical adenopathy, lack of a cough, and pharyngotonsillar exudate.

The rash of scarlet fever is diffusely erythematous, resembling a sunburn, with superimposed fine red papules, and is most intense in the groin and axillas. It blanches on pressure, may become petechial, and fades in 2–5 days, leaving a fine desquamation. The face is flushed, with circumoral pallor, and the tongue is coated with enlarged red papillae (strawberry tongue).

B. Laboratory Findings

Leukocytosis with neutrophil predominance is common. Throat culture onto a single blood agar plate has a sensitivity of 80–90%. Rapid diagnostic tests based on detection of streptococcal antigen are slightly less sensitive than culture.

Complications

Suppurative complications include sinusitis, otitis media, mastoiditis, peritonsillar abscess, and suppuration of cervical lymph nodes.

Nonsuppurative complications are rheumatic fever and glomerulonephritis. Rheumatic fever may follow recurrent episodes of pharyngitis beginning 1–4 weeks after the onset of symptoms. Glomerulonephritis follows a single infection with a nephritogenic strain of streptococcus group A (eg, types 4, 12, 2, 49, and 60), more commonly on the skin than in the throat, and begins 1–3 weeks after the onset of the infection.

Differential Diagnosis

Streptococcal sore throat resembles (and cannot be reliably distinguished clinically from) pharyngitis caused by adenoviruses, Epstein-Barr virus, *Arcanobacterium haemolyticum* (which also may cause a rash), and other agents. Pharyngitis and lymphadenopathy are common findings in primary HIV infection. Generalized lymphadenopathy, splenomegaly, atypical lymphocytosis, and a positive serologic test distinguish mononucleosis from streptococcal pharyngitis. Diphtheria is characterized by a pseudomembrane; candidiasis shows white patches of exudate and less erythema; and necrotizing ulcerative gingivostomatitis (Vincent fusospirochetal gingivitis or stomatitis) presents with shallow ulcers in the mouth. Retropharyngeal abscess or bacterial epiglottitis should be considered when odynophagia and difficulty in handling secretions are present and when the severity of symptoms is disproportionate to findings on examination of the pharynx.

Treatment

Antimicrobial therapy has a modest effect on resolution of symptoms and primarily is administered for prevention of complications. Antibiotic therapy can be safely delayed until the diagnosis is established on the basis of a positive antigen test or culture. Empiric therapy usually is not a cost-effective approach to the management of most adults with pharyngitis because in typical clinical settings, the prevalence of streptococcal pharyngitis is likely to be no more than 10–20% and the positive predictive value of clinical criteria is low. Clinical criteria, such as the Centor criteria, are useful for identifying patients in whom a rapid antigen test or throat culture is indicated. Patients who meet two or more of these criteria merit further testing. When three of the four are present, laboratory sensitivity of rapid antigen testing exceeds 90%. When only one criterion is present, streptococcal pharyngitis is unlikely. In high-prevalence settings or if clinical suspicion for streptococcal pharyngitis is high, a negative antigen test or culture should be confirmed by a follow-up culture.

A. Benzathine Penicillin G

Benzathine penicillin G, 1.2 million units intramuscularly as a single dose, is optimal therapy.

B. Penicillin VK

Penicillin VK, 500 mg orally four times a day (or amoxicillin, 750 mg orally twice daily) for 10 days, is effective, but compliance may be poor after the patient becomes asymptomatic in 2–4 days.

C. Cephalosporins

Cefdinir, 300 mg orally twice daily for 5–10 days or 600 mg orally once daily for 10 days, and cefpodoxime, 100 mg orally twice daily for 5–10 days, are both approved by the US Food and Drug Administration (FDA) for the treatment of streptococcal pharyngitis but should be reserved for penicillin-allergic patients able to tolerate cephalosporins.

D. Macrolides

Erythromycin, 500 mg orally four times a day, or azithromycin, 500 mg orally once daily for 3 days, is an alternative for the penicillin-allergic patient. Macrolides are less effective than penicillins and are considered second-line agents. Macrolide-resistant strains almost always are susceptible to clindamycin, a suitable alternative to penicillins; a 10-day course of 300 mg orally twice daily is effective.

▶ Prevention of Recurrent Rheumatic Fever

Effectively controlling rheumatic fever depends on identification and treatment of primary streptococcal infection and secondary prevention of recurrences. Patients who have had rheumatic fever should be treated with a continuous course of antimicrobial prophylaxis for at least 5 years. Effective regimens are erythromycin, 250 mg orally twice daily, or penicillin G, 500 mg orally daily.

Casey JR et al. The evidence base for cephalosporin superiority over penicillin in streptococcal pharyngitis. Diagn Microbiol Infect Dis. 2007 Mar;57(3 Suppl):39S–45S. [PMID: 17292576]

Falagas ME et al. Effectiveness and safety of short-course vs long-course antibiotic therapy for group A beta hemolytic streptococcal tonsillopharyngitis: a meta-analysis of randomized trials. Mayo Clin Proc. 2008 Aug;83(8):880–9. [PMID: 18674472]

2. Streptococcal Skin Infections

Group A β-hemolytic streptococci are not normal skin flora. Streptococcal skin infections result from colonization of normal skin by contact with other infected individuals or by preceding streptococcal respiratory infection.

▶ Clinical Findings

A. Symptoms and Signs

Impetigo is a focal, vesicular, pustular lesion with a thick, amber-colored crust with a "stuck-on" appearance.

Erysipelas is a painful superficial cellulitis that frequently involves the face. It is well demarcated from the surrounding normal skin. It affects skin with impaired lymphatic drainage, such as edematous lower extremities or wounds.

B. Laboratory Findings

Cultures obtained from a wound or pustule are likely to grow group A streptococci. Blood cultures are occasionally positive.

▶ Treatment

Parenteral antibiotics are indicated for patients with facial erysipelas or evidence of systemic infection. Penicillin, 2 million units intravenously every 4 hours, is the drug of choice. However, staphylococci infections may at times be difficult to differentiate from streptococcal infections. In practice, initial therapy for patients with risk factors for *Staphylococcus aureus* (eg, injection drug use, diabetes, wound infection) should cover this organism. Nafcillin, 1.5 g every 6 hours intravenously, and cefazolin, 1 g intravenously or intramuscularly every 8 hours, are reasonable choices. In the patient at risk for methicillin-resistant *S aureus* infection or with a serious penicillin allergy (ie, anaphylaxis), vancomycin, 1000 mg intravenously every 12 hours, should be used.

Patients who do not require parenteral therapy may be treated with amoxicillin, 750 mg twice daily for 7–10 days. A first-generation oral cephalosporin, eg, cephalexin, 500 mg four times daily, or clindamycin, 300 mg orally three times daily, is an alternative to amoxicillin.

3. Other Group A Streptococcal Infections

Arthritis, pneumonia, empyema, endocarditis, and necrotizing fasciitis are relatively uncommon infections that may be caused by group A streptococci. Toxic shock-like syndrome also occurs.

Arthritis generally occurs in association with cellulitis. In addition to intravenous therapy with penicillin G, 2 million units every 4 hours (or cefazolin or vancomycin in doses recommended above for penicillin-allergic patients), frequent percutaneous needle aspiration should be performed to remove joint effusions. Open surgical drainage may be necessary when the hip or shoulder is infected.

Pneumonia and **empyema** often are characterized by extensive tissue destruction and an aggressive, rapidly progressive clinical course associated with significant morbidity and mortality. High-dose penicillin and chest tube drainage are indicated for treatment of empyema. Vancomycin is an acceptable substitute in penicillin-allergic patients.

Group A streptococci can cause **endocarditis.** Endocarditis should be treated with 4 million units of penicillin G intravenously every 4 hours for 4–6 weeks. Vancomycin, 1 g intravenously every 12 hours, is recommended for persons allergic to penicillin.

Necrotizing fasciitis is a rapidly spreading infection involving the fascia of deep muscle. The clinical findings at presentation may be those of severe cellulitis, but the presence of systemic toxicity and severe pain, which may be followed by anesthesia of the involved area due to destruction of nerves as infection advances through the fascial planes, is a clue to the diagnosis. Surgical exploration is mandatory when the diagnosis is suspected. Early and extensive debridement is essential for survival.

Any streptococcal infection—and necrotizing fasciitis in particular—can be associated with **streptococcal toxic shock syndrome**, typified by invasion of skin or soft tissues, acute respiratory distress syndrome, and kidney failure. The very young, the elderly, and those with underlying medical conditions are at particularly high risk for invasive disease. Bacteremia occurs in most cases. Skin rash and desquamation may not be present. Mortality rates can be up to 80%. The syndrome is due to elaboration of pyrogenic erythrotoxin (which also causes **scarlet fever**), a superantigen that stimulates massive release of inflammatory cytokines believed to mediate the shock. A β-lactam remains the drug of choice for treatment of serious streptococcal infections, but clindamycin, which is a potent inhibitor of toxin production, should also be administered at a dose of 600 mg every 8 hours intravenously for invasive disease, especially in the presence of shock. Intravenous immune globulin has also been recommended for streptococcal toxic shock syndrome for presumed, although unproven, therapeutic benefit from specific antibody to streptococcal exotoxins in immune globulin preparations. Two dosage regimens have been used: 450 mg/kg once daily for 5 days or a single dose of 2 g/kg with a repeat dose at 48 hours if the patient remains unstable.

Outbreaks of invasive disease have been associated with colonization by invasive clones that can be transmitted to close contacts who, though asymptomatic, may be a reservoir for disease. Tracing contacts of patients with invasive disease is controversial.

Anaya DA et al. Necrotizing soft-tissue infection: diagnosis and management. Clin Infect Dis. 2007 Mar 1;44(5):705–10. [PMID: 17278065]

Eisenstein BI. Treatment challenges in the management of complicated skin and soft-tissue infections. Clin Microbiol Infect. 2008 Mar;14(Suppl 2):17–25. [PMID: 18226086]

4. Non-Group A Streptococcal Infections

Non-group A hemolytic streptococci (eg, groups B, C, and G) produce a spectrum of disease similar to that of group A streptococci. The treatment of infections caused by these strains is the same as for group A streptococci.

Group B streptococci are an important cause of sepsis, bacteremia, and meningitis in the neonate. Antepartum screening to identify carriers and peripartum antimicrobial prophylaxis are recommended in pregnancy. This organism, part of the normal vaginal flora, may cause septic abortion, endometritis, or peripartum infections and, less commonly, cellulitis, bacteremia, and endocarditis in adults. Treatment of infections caused by group B streptococci is with either penicillin or vancomycin in doses recommended for group A streptococci. Because of in vitro synergism, some experts recommend the addition of low-dose gentamicin, 1 mg/kg every 8 hours.

Viridans streptococci, which are nonhemolytic or α-hemolytic (ie, producing a green zone of hemolysis on blood agar), are part of the normal oral flora. Although these strains may produce focal pyogenic infection, they are most notable as the leading cause of native valve endocarditis (see below).

Group D streptococci include *Streptococcus bovis* and the enterococci. *S bovis* is a cause of endocarditis in association with bowel neoplasia or cirrhosis and is treated like viridans streptococci.

Larsen JW et al. Group B Streptococcus and pregnancy: a review. Am J Obstet Gynecol. 2008 Apr;198(4):440–8. [PMID: 18201679]

ENTEROCOCCAL INFECTIONS

Two species, *Enterococcus faecalis* and *Enterococcus faecium*, are responsible for most human enterococcal infections. Enterococci cause wound infections, urinary tract infections, bacteremia, and endocarditis. Infections caused by penicillin-susceptible strains should be treated with penicillin 3–4 million units every 4 hours; ampicillin 3 g every 6 hours; or if the patient is penicillin-allergic, vancomycin 15 mg/kg every 12 hours intravenously. If the patient has endocarditis or meningitis, gentamicin 1 mg/kg every 8 hours intravenously should be added to the regimen in order to achieve the bactericidal activity that is required to cure these infections.

Resistance to vancomycin, penicillin, and gentamicin is common among enterococcal isolates, especially *E faecium*; it is essential to determine antimicrobial susceptibility of isolates. Infection control measures that may be indicated to limit their spread include isolation, barrier precautions, and avoidance of overuse of vancomycin and gentamicin. Consultation with an infectious diseases specialist is strongly advised when treating infections caused by resistant strains of enterococci. Quinupristin/dalfopristin and linezolid are approved by the FDA for treatment of infections caused by vancomycin-resistant strains of enterococci. Quinupristin/dalfopristin is not active against strains of *E faecalis* and should be used only for infections caused by *E faecium*. The dose is 7.5 mg/kg intravenously every 8–12 hours. Phlebitis and irritation at the infusion site (often requiring a central line) and an arthralgia-myalgia syndrome are relatively common side effects. Linezolid, an oxazolidinone, is active against both *E faecalis* and *E faecium*. The dose is 600 mg twice daily, and both intravenous and oral preparations are available. Its two principal side effects are thrombocytopenia and bone marrow suppression; however, peripheral neuropathy, optic neuritis, and lactic acidosis have been observed with prolonged use due to mitochondrial toxicity. Emergence of resistance has occurred during therapy with either quinupristin/dalfopristin or linezolid.

Gavaldà J et al. Brief communication: treatment of *Enterococcus faecalis* endocarditis with ampicillin plus ceftriaxone. Ann Intern Med. 2007 Apr 17;146(8):574–9. [PMID: 17438316]
Willems RJ et al. Glycopeptide-resistant enterococci: deciphering virulence, resistance and epidemicity. Curr Opin Infect Dis. 2007 Aug;20(4):384–90. [PMID: 17609597]

PNEUMOCOCCAL INFECTIONS

1. Pneumococcal Pneumonia

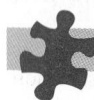 ESSENTIALS OF DIAGNOSIS

▶ Productive cough, fever, rigors, dyspnea, early pleuritic chest pain.

▶ Consolidating lobar pneumonia on chest radiograph.

▶ Gram-positive diplococci on Gram stain of sputum.

General Considerations

The pneumococcus is the most common cause of community-acquired pyogenic bacterial pneumonia. Alcoholism, asthma, HIV infection, sickle cell disease, splenectomy, and hematologic disorders are predisposing factors. The mortality rate remains high in the setting of advanced age, multilobar disease, severe hypoxemia, extrapulmonary complications, and bacteremia.

Clinical Findings

A. Symptoms and Signs

Presenting symptoms and signs include high fever, productive cough, occasionally hemoptysis, and pleuritic chest pain. Rigors occur within the first few hours of infection but are uncommon thereafter. Bronchial breath sounds are an early sign.

B. Laboratory Findings

Pneumococcal pneumonia classically is a lobar pneumonia with radiographic findings of consolidation and occasionally effusion. However, differentiating it from other pneumonias is not possible radiographically or clinically because of significant overlap in presentations. Diagnosis requires isolation of the organism in culture, although the Gram stain appearance of sputum can be suggestive. Sputum and

blood cultures, positive in 60% and 25% of cases of pneumococcal pneumonia, respectively, should be obtained prior to initiation of antimicrobial therapy in patients who are admitted to the hospital. A good-quality sputum sample (less than 10 epithelial cells and more than 25 polymorphonuclear leukocytes per high-power field) shows gram-positive diplococci in 80–90% of cases. A rapid urinary antigen test for *S pneumoniae*, with sensitivity of 70–80% and specificity greater than 95%, can assist with early diagnosis.

Complications

Parapneumonic (sympathetic) effusion is common and may cause recurrence or persistence of fever. These sterile fluid accumulations need no specific therapy. Empyema occurs in 5% or less of cases and is differentiated from sympathetic effusion by the presence of organisms on Gram-stained fluid or positive pleural fluid cultures.

Pneumococcal pericarditis is a rare complication that can cause tamponade. Pneumococcal arthritis also is uncommon. Pneumococcal endocarditis usually involves the aortic valve and often occurs in association with meningitis and pneumonia (sometimes referred to as Austrian or Osler triad). Early heart failure and multiple embolic events are typical.

Treatment

A. Specific Measures

Initial antimicrobial therapy for pneumonia is empiric (see Chapter 9 for specific recommendations) pending isolation and identification of the causative agent. Once the pneumonia is determined to be caused by *Streptococcus pneumoniae*, any of several antimicrobial agents may be used depending on the clinical setting, community patterns of penicillin resistance, and susceptibility of the particular isolate. Uncomplicated pneumococcal pneumonia (ie, arterial P_{O_2} > 60 mm Hg, no coexisting medical problems, and single-lobe disease without signs of extrapulmonary infection) caused by penicillin-susceptible strains of pneumococcus may be treated on an outpatient basis with amoxicillin, 750 mg orally twice daily for 7–10 days. For penicillin-allergic patients, alternatives are azithromycin, one 500-mg dose orally on the first day and 250 mg for the next 4 days; clarithromycin, 500 mg orally twice daily for 10 days; doxycycline, 100 mg orally twice daily for 10 days; levofloxacin, 750 mg orally for 5 days; or moxifloxacin, 400 mg orally for 7–14 days. Patients should be monitored for clinical response (eg, less cough, defervescence within 2–3 days) because pneumococci have become increasingly resistant to penicillin and the second-line agents.

Parenteral therapy is generally recommended for the hospitalized patient at least until there has been clinical improvement. Aqueous penicillin G, 2 million units intravenously every 4 hours, or ceftriaxone, 1 g intravenously every 24 hours, is effective for strains that are not highly penicillin-resistant (ie, strains for which the minimum inhibitory concentration [MIC] of penicillin is ≤ 1 mcg/mL). For serious penicillin allergy or infection caused by a highly penicillin-resistant strain, vancomycin, 1 g intravenously every 12 hours, is effective. Alternatively, a fluoroquinolone (eg, levofloxacin, 500 mg, or a comparable dose of any one of several newer fluoroquinolones now on the market, orally or intravenously) can be used. The total duration of therapy is not well defined but 10–14 days is standard.

B. Treatment of Complications

Pleural effusions developing after initiation of antimicrobial therapy usually are sterile, and thoracentesis need not be performed if the patient is otherwise improving. Thoracentesis is indicated for an effusion present prior to initiation of therapy and in the patient who has not responded to antibiotics after 3–4 days. Chest tube drainage may be required if pneumococci are identified by culture or Gram stain, especially if aspiration of the fluid is difficult.

Echocardiography should be done if pericardial effusion is suspected. Patients with pericardial effusion who are responding to therapy and have no signs of tamponade may be monitored and treated with indomethacin, 50 mg orally three times daily, for pain. In patients with increasing effusion, unsatisfactory clinical response, or evidence of tamponade, pericardiocentesis will determine whether the pericardial space is infected. Infected fluid must be drained either percutaneously (by tube placement or needle aspiration), by placement of a pericardial window, or by pericardiectomy. Pericardiectomy eventually may be required to prevent or treat constrictive pericarditis, a common sequela of bacterial pericarditis.

Endocarditis should be treated for 4 weeks with 3–4 million units of penicillin G every 4 hours intravenously; ceftriaxone, 2 g once daily intravenously; or vancomycin, 15 mg/kg every 12 hours intravenously. Mild heart failure may respond to medical therapy, but moderate to severe heart failure is an indication for prosthetic valve implantation, as are systemic emboli or large friable vegetations as determined by echocardiography.

C. Penicillin-Resistant Pneumococci

Susceptibility breakpoints defining penicillin-resistant pneumococci for isolates causing pneumonia were revised in 2008. Resistance breakpoints for parenterally administered penicillin and high-dose oral amoxicillin (2 g twice daily) are as follows: susceptible, penicillin MIC ≤ 2 mcg/mL; intermediate, MIC = 4 mcg/mL; resistant, MIC ≥ 8 mcg/mL. This change reflected results from studies demonstrating equivalent cure rates when high doses of parenteral penicillin were used for treatment of pneumococcal pneumonia due to isolates with penicillin MIC ≤ 2 mcg/mL. Note, however, that these new breakpoints do not apply to orally administered penicillin, which are the same as for use of penicillin in treatment of meningitis (see below). In cases of pneumococcal pneumonia where the isolate has a penicillin MIC > 2 mcg/mL, cephalosporin cross-resistance is common, and a non–β-lactam antimicrobial, such as vancomycin, 1 g intravenously every 12 hours or a fluoroquinolone with enhanced gram-positive activity (eg, levofloxacin, 750 mg intravenously or orally once daily or moxifloxacin, 400 mg intravenously or orally once daily), is recommended. Penicillin-resistant strains of pneumococci may be resistant to macrolides, trimethoprim-sulfamethoxazole, and chloramphenicol, and susceptibility must be documented prior to their use. All blood and cerebrospinal fluid isolates should still be tested for resistance to penicillin. There has been no change to the penicillin susceptibility breakpoint for pneumococcal isolates causing meningitis, nor any change in treatment recommendations (see below).

Li JZ. Efficacy of short-course antibiotic regimens for community-acquired pneumonia: a meta-analysis. Am J Med. 2007 Sep;120(9):783–90. [PMID: 17765048]
Mandell LA et al. Infectious Diseases Society of America/American Thoracic Society consensus guidelines on the management of community-acquired pneumonia in adults. Clin Infect Dis. 2007 Mar 1;44 (Suppl 2):S27–72. [PMID: 17278083]
Tleyjeh IM et al. The impact of penicillin resistance on short-term mortality in hospitalized adults with pneumococcal pneumonia: a systematic review and meta-analysis. Clin Infect Dis. 2006 Mar 15;42(6):788–97. [PMID: 16477555]

2. Pneumococcal Meningitis

 ESSENTIALS OF DIAGNOSIS

▶ Fever, headache, altered mental status.
▶ Meningismus.
▶ Gram-positive diplococci on Gram stain of cerebrospinal fluid.

▶ General Considerations

S pneumoniae is the most common cause of meningitis in adults. Head trauma, with cerebrospinal fluid leaks, sinusitis, and pneumonia may precede it.

▶ Clinical Findings

A. Symptoms and Signs

The onset is rapid, with fever, headache, meningismus, and altered mentation. Pneumonia may be present. Compared with meningitis caused by the meningococcus, pneumococcal meningitis lacks a rash, and focal neurologic deficits, cranial nerve palsies, and obtundation are more prominent features.

B. Laboratory Findings

The cerebrospinal fluid typically has more than 1000 white blood cells per microliter, over 60% of which are polymorphonuclear leukocytes; the glucose concentration is less than 40 mg/dL, or less than 50% of the simultaneous serum concentration; and the protein usually exceeds 150 mg/dL. Not all cases of meningitis will have these typical findings, and alterations in cerebrospinal fluid cell counts and chemistries may be surprisingly minimal, overlapping with those of aseptic meningitis.

Gram stain of cerebrospinal fluid shows gram-positive cocci in 80–90% of cases, and in untreated cases, blood or cerebrospinal fluid cultures are almost always positive.

Treatment

Antibiotics should be given as soon as the diagnosis is suspected. If lumbar puncture must be delayed (eg, while awaiting results of an imaging study to exclude a mass lesion), the patient should be treated empirically for presumed meningitis with intravenous ceftriaxone, 2 g, plus vancomycin, 15 mg/kg, plus dexamethasone, 0.15 mg/kg administered concomitantly after blood cultures (positive in 50% of cases) have been obtained. Once susceptibility to penicillin has been confirmed, penicillin, 24 million units intravenously daily in six divided doses, or ceftriaxone, 2 g every 12 hours intravenously, is continued for 10–14 days in documented cases.

The best therapy for penicillin-resistant strains is not known. Penicillin-resistant strains (MIC > 0.06 mcg/mL) are often cross-resistant to the third-generation cephalosporins as well as other antibiotics. Susceptibility testing is essential to proper management of this infection. If the MIC of ceftriaxone or cefotaxime is ≤ 0.5 mcg/mL, single-drug therapy with either of these cephalosporins is likely to be effective; when the MIC is ≥ 1 mcg/mL, treatment with a combination of ceftriaxone, 2 g intravenously every 12 hours, plus vancomycin, 30 mg/kg/d intravenously in two or three divided doses, is recommended. If a patient with a penicillin-resistant organism is slow to respond clinically, repeat lumbar puncture may be indicated to assess bacteriologic response.

Dexamethasone administered with antibiotic to adults has been associated with a 60% reduction in mortality and a 50% reduction in unfavorable outcomes, primarily in patients with pneumococcal meningitis. It is recommended that adults with acute bacterial meningitis be given 10 mg of dexamethasone intravenously immediately prior to or concomitantly with the first dose of appropriate antibiotic and continued in those with pneumococcal disease every 6 hours thereafter for a total of 4 days. Patients with pneumococcal meningitis and AIDS who do not have access to resources may not benefit from dexamethasone. The effect of dexamethasone on outcome of meningitis caused by penicillin-resistant organisms is not known.

Scarborough M et al. Corticosteroids for bacterial meningitis in adults in sub-Saharan Africa. N Engl J Med. 2007 Dec 13;357(24):2441–50. [PMID: 18077809]

Van de Beek D et al. Corticosteroids for acute bacterial meningitis. Cochrane Database Syst Rev. 2007 Jan 24;(1):CD004405. [PMID: 17253505]

Weisfelt M et al. Pneumococcal meningitis in adults: new approaches to management and prevention. Lancet Neurol. 2006 Apr;5(4):332–42. [PMID: 16545750]

STAPHYLOCOCCUS AUREUS INFECTIONS

1. Skin & Soft Tissue Infections

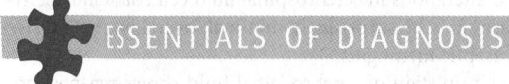

ESSENTIALS OF DIAGNOSIS

- Localized erythema with induration and purulent drainage.
- Abscess formation.
- Folliculitis commonly observed.
- Gram stain of pus with gram-positive cocci in clusters; cultures usually positive.

General Considerations

Approximately one-quarter of people are asymptomatic nasal carriers of *S aureus*, which is spread by direct contact. Carriage often precedes infection, which occurs as a consequence of disruption of the cutaneous barrier or impairment of host defenses. *S aureus* tends to cause more localized skin infections than streptococci, and abscess formation is common. The prevalence of methicillin-resistant strains in community settings is increasing, and these strains have been associated with recurrent and severe skin and soft tissue infections, including necrotizing fasciitis.

Clinical Findings

A. Symptoms and Signs

S aureus skin infections may begin around one or more hair follicles, causing folliculitis; may become localized to form boils (or furuncles); or may spread to adjacent skin and deeper subcutaneous tissue (ie, a carbuncle) (Plate 100). Deep abscesses involving muscle or fascia may occur, often in association with a deep wound or other inoculation or injection. Necrotizing fasciitis, a rare form of *S aureus* skin and soft tissues infection, has been reported with community strains of methicillin-resistant *S aureus*.

B. Laboratory Findings

Cultures of the wound or abscess material will almost always yield the organism. In patients with systemic signs of infection, blood cultures should be obtained because of potential endocarditis, osteomyelitis, or metastatic seeding of other sites. Patients who are bacteremic should have blood cultures taken early during therapy to exclude persistent bacteremia, an indicator of severe or complicated infection.

Treatment

Proper drainage of abscess fluid or other focal infections is the mainstay of therapy. Incision and drainage alone may be sufficient for cutaneous abscess. For uncomplicated skin infections, oral antimicrobial therapy is satisfactory. Before the emergence of community methicillin-resistant strains of *S aureus*, an oral penicillinase-resistant penicillin or cephalosporin, such as dicloxacillin or cephalexin, 500 mg four times a day for 7–10 days, was the drug of choice for empiric therapy. However, increasing prevalence of methicillin-resistant strains of *S aureus* among community isolates may necessitate use of other oral agents to which the isolate is susceptible in vitro, such as clindamycin, 300 mg three times daily; doxycycline or minocycline, 100 mg twice daily; or trimethoprim-sulfamethoxazole, given in two divided doses based on 5–10 mg/kg/d of the trimethoprim component. Unfortunately, the efficacy of these agents is not well defined and not evidence based. Because of the high prevalence of macrolide resistance among *S aureus* strains, these agents should not be used unless susceptibility is documented.

For more complicated infections with extensive cutaneous or deep tissue involvement or fever, parenteral therapy is indicated initially. A penicillinase-resistant penicillin such as nafcillin or oxacillin in a dosage of 1.5 g every 6 hours intravenously or cefazolin 1 g intravenously or intramuscularly is preferred for infections caused by methicillin-susceptible isolates. In patients with a serious allergy to β-lactam antibiotics or if the strain is methicillin-resistant, vancomycin, 1 g intravenously every 12 hours, is a drug of choice. If the local prevalence of methicillin-resistance is high (eg, 10% or more), and particularly if the patient is seriously ill, vancomycin is indicated empirically pending strain isolation and determination of susceptibility.

Linezolid is FDA-approved for treatment of skin and skin-structure infections as well as hospital-acquired pneumonia caused by methicillin-resistant strains of *S aureus* and clinically is as effective as vancomycin. The dose is 600 mg orally (bioavailability of 100%) or intravenously twice a day for 10–14 days. Its considerable cost makes it an unattractive choice for most routine outpatient infections, and its safety in treatment courses lasting longer than 2–3 weeks is not well characterized; nevertheless, it is the only proven effective oral alternative to parenteral vancomycin. Daptomycin, 4 mg/kg once daily (or every other day in the patient with creatinine clearance < 30 mL/min) intravenously for 7–14 days, is also an option for treatment of complicated skin and skin structure infections. Tigecycline, a glycylcycline class antimicrobial, has been approved by the FDA for treatment of complicated skin and skin structure infections due to methicillin-resistant strains of *S aureus* at a dose of 100 mg intravenously once followed by 50 mg intravenously twice a day for 10–14 days.

Hersh AL et al. National trends in ambulatory visits and antibiotic prescribing for skin and soft-tissue infections. Arch Intern Med. 2008 Jul 28;168(14):1585–91. [PMID: 18663172]
Seaton RA. Daptomycin: rationale and role in the management of skin and soft tissue infections. J Antimicrob Chemother. 2008 Nov;62(Suppl 3):iii15–23. [PMID: 18829721]
Stryjewski ME et al. Skin and soft-tissue infections caused by community-acquired methicillin-resistant *Staphylococcus aureus*. Clin Infect Dis. 2008 Jun 1;46(Suppl 5):S368–77. [PMID: 18462092]

2. Osteomyelitis

S aureus causes approximately 60% of all cases of osteomyelitis. Osteomyelitis may be caused by direct inoculation, eg, from an open fracture or as a result of surgery; by extension from a contiguous focus of infection or open wound; or by hematogenous spread. Long bones and vertebrae are the usual sites. Epidural abscess is a common complication of vertebral osteomyelitis and should be suspected if fever and severe back or neck pain are accompanied by radicular pain or symptoms or signs indicative of spinal cord compression (eg, incontinence, extremity weakness, pathologic reflexes).

► **Clinical Findings**

A. Symptoms and Signs

The infection may be acute, with abrupt development of local symptoms and systemic toxicity, or indolent, with insidious onset of vague pain over the site of infection, progressing to local tenderness. Fever is absent in one-third or more of cases. Abscess formation is a late and unusual manifestation. Draining sinus tracts occur in chronic infections or infections of foreign body implants.

B. Laboratory Findings

The diagnosis is established by isolation of *S aureus* from the blood, bone, or a contiguous focus of a patient with signs and symptoms of focal bone infection. Blood culture will be positive in approximately 60% of untreated cases. Bone biopsy and culture are indicated if blood cultures are sterile.

C. Imaging

Bone scan and gallium scan, each with a sensitivity of approximately 95% and a specificity of 60–70%, are useful in identifying or confirming the site of bone infection. Plain bone films early in the course of infection are often normal but will become abnormal in most cases even with effective therapy. Spinal infection (unlike malignancy) traverses the disk space to involve the contiguous vertebral body. CT is more sensitive than plain films and helps localize associated abscesses. MRI is slightly less sensitive than bone scan but has a specificity of 90%. It is indicated when epidural abscess is suspected in association with vertebral osteomyelitis.

► **Treatment**

Prolonged therapy is required to cure staphylococcal osteomyelitis. Durations of 4–6 weeks or longer are recommended. In cases of staphylococcal osteomyelitis with associated epidural abscess and spinal cord compression, other abscesses (psoas, paraspinal) or extensive disease, surgical treatment is often indicated. Although oral regimens can be effective, parenteral therapy is preferred, particularly during the acute phase of the infection for patients with systemic toxicity. Nafcillin or oxacillin, 9–12 g/d in six divided doses, is the drug of choice for infection with methicillin-sensitive isolates. Cefazolin, 2 g every 6–8 hours, also is effective. Patients with infections due to methicillin-resistant strains of *S aureus* or who have severe penicillin allergies should be treated with vancomycin, 30 mg/kg/d intravenously divided in two or three doses. Doses should be adjusted to achieve a vancomycin trough of 15-20 mcg/mL. Oral step-down therapy to a rifampin combination regimen appears to be as effective as parenterally administered regimens. The role of newer agents, daptomycin or linezolid, remains to be defined.

Daver NG et al. Oral step-down therapy is comparable to intravenous therapy for *Staphylococcus aureus* osteomyelitis. J Infect. 2007 Jun;54(60):539–44. [PMID: 17198732]
Lamp KC et al. Clinical experience with daptomycin for the treatment of patients with osteomyelitis. Am J Med. 2007 Oct;120(10 Suppl 1):S13–20. [PMID: 17904946]

3. Staphylococcal Bacteremia

S aureus readily invades the bloodstream and infects sites distant from the primary site of infection, which may be relatively minor or even inapparent. Whenever *S aureus* is recovered from blood cultures, the possibility of endocarditis, osteomyelitis, or other metastatic deep infection must be considered. Bacteremia that persists for more than 48 to 96 hours after initiation of therapy is strongly predictive of worse outcome and complicated infection. The appropriate duration of therapy for uncomplicated bacteremia arising from a removable source (eg, intravenous device) or drainable focus (eg, skin abscess) has not been well defined, but a 10- to 14-day course of therapy appears to be the minimum. However, 5% or more of patients may relapse, usually with endocarditis or osteomyelitis, even if treated for 2 weeks.

Nafcillin or oxacillin, 2 g intravenously every 4 hours or cefazolin, 2 g every 8 hours is recommended for uncomplicated methicillin-susceptible *S aureus* bacteremia. Vancomycin, 30 mg/kg/d intravenously in two or three divided doses, as definitive therapy should be reserved for patients with serious penicillin allergy or with infections caused by methicillin-resistant strains because it is less active than β-lactam antibiotics and treatment failures are more common than with β-lactams. Maintaining a vancomycin trough concentration of 15–20 mcg/mL may improve outcomes and is recommended. Transesophageal echocardiography (TEE) is a sensitive and cost-effective method for excluding underlying endocarditis. It is considered for patients for whom the pretest probability of endocarditis is 5% or higher—and for all patients with unexplained *S aureus* bacteremia.

Vancomycin treatment failures are relatively common, particularly for complicated bacteremia, in foreign body infection, or when the MIC of the isolate is ≥ 2 mcg/mL. Consultation should be sought with an infectious diseases specialist when vancomycin treatment failure is encountered. Daptomycin, 6 mg/kg once daily, is approved by the FDA for treatment of *S aureus* bacteremia and is an alternative to vancomycin, especially if a β-lactam cannot be used or if the patient is not responding to vancomycin. Cases of vancomycin treatment failures in which the staphylococcal isolate exhibits a vancomycin MIC ≥ 4 mcg/mL should be reported to the Centers for Disease Control and Prevention (CDC) to help track this potentially serious and emerging problem of vancomycin resistance.

Empiric therapy of suspected staphylococcal infection, whether of community or hospital onset, depends on the severity of the infection and the likelihood that it is caused by methicillin-resistant strains. If the prevalence exceeds 5–10% for more seriously ill patients, initial therapy should include vancomycin, 30 mg/kg/d intravenously divided in two or three doses, until results of susceptibility tests are known. Resistance to vancomycin fortunately remains rare and should not affect the choice of empiric therapy.

Cosgrove SE et al. Management of methicillin-resistant *Staphylococcus aureus* bacteremia. Clin Infect Dis. 2008 Jun 1;46 Suppl 5:S386–93. [PMID: 18462094]

Hawkins C et al. Persistent *Staphylococcus aureus* bacteremia: an analysis of risk factors and outcomes. Arch Intern Med. 2007 Sep 24;167(17):1861–7. [PMID: 17893307]

Stryjewski ME et al. Use of vancomycin or first-generation cephalosporins for the treatment of hemodialysis-dependent patients with methicillin-susceptible *Staphylococcus aureus* bacteremia. Clin Infect Dis. 2007 Jan 15;44(2):190–6. [PMID: 17173215]

4. Toxic Shock Syndrome

S aureus produces toxins that cause three important entities: "scalded skin syndrome" in children, toxic shock syndrome in adults, and enterotoxin food poisoning. Toxic shock syndrome is characterized by abrupt onset of high fever, vomiting, and watery diarrhea. Sore throat, myalgias, and headache are common. Hypotension with kidney and heart failure is associated with a poor outcome. A diffuse macular erythematous rash (Plate 101) and nonpurulent conjunctivitis are common, and desquamation, especially of palms and soles, is typical during recovery. Fatality rates may be as high as 15%. Although originally associated with tampon use, any focus (eg, nasopharynx, bone, vagina, rectum, abscess, or wound) harboring a toxin-producing *S aureus* strain can cause toxic shock syndrome and nonmenstrual cases of toxic shock syndrome are common. Classically, blood cultures are negative because symptoms are due to the effects of the toxin and not systemic infection.

Important aspects of treatment include rapid rehydration, antistaphylococcal drugs, management of kidney or heart failure, and addressing sources of toxin, eg, removal of tampon or drainage of abscess.

5. Infections Caused by Coagulase-Negative Staphylococci

Coagulase-negative staphylococci are an important cause of infections of intravascular and prosthetic devices and of wound infection following cardiothoracic surgery. These organisms infrequently cause infections such as osteomyelitis and endocarditis in the absence of a prosthesis, but rates may be increasing. Most human infections are caused by *Staphylococcus epidermidis, Staphylococcus haemolyticus, Staphylococcus hominis, Staphylococcus warnerii, Staphylococcus saprophyticus, Staphylococcus saccharolyticus,* and *Staphylococcus cohnii*. These common hospital-acquired pathogens are less virulent than *S aureus*, and infections caused by them tend to be more indolent.

Because coagulase-negative staphylococci are normal inhabitants of human skin, it is difficult to distinguish infection from contamination, the latter perhaps accounting for three-fourths of blood culture isolates. Infection is more likely if the patient has a foreign body (eg, sternal wires, prosthetic joint, prosthetic cardiac valve, pacemaker, intracranial pressure monitor, cerebrospinal fluid shunt, peritoneal dialysis catheter) or an intravascular device in place. Purulent or serosanguineous drainage, erythema, pain, or tenderness at the site of the foreign body or device suggests infection. Instability and pain are signs of prosthetic joint infection. Fever, a new murmur, instability of the prosthesis, or signs of systemic embolization are evidence of prosthetic valve endocarditis. Immunosuppression and recent antimicrobial therapy are risk factors.

Infection is also more likely if the same strain is consistently isolated from two or more blood cultures (particularly if samples were obtained at different times) and from the foreign body site. Contamination is more likely when a single blood culture is positive or if more than one strain is isolated from blood cultures. The antimicrobial susceptibility pattern and speciation are used to determine whether one or more strains have been isolated. More sophisticated typing methods, eg, pulse-field gel electrophoresis of restriction enzyme digested chromosomal DNA, may be required to identify distinct strains.

Whenever possible, the intravascular device or foreign body suspected of being infected by coagulase-negative staphylococci should be removed. However, removal and replacement of some devices (eg, prosthetic joint, prosthetic valve, cerebrospinal fluid shunt) can be a difficult or risky procedure, and it may sometimes be preferable to treat with antibiotics alone with the understanding that the probability of cure is reduced and that surgical management may eventually be necessary.

Coagulase-negative staphylococci are commonly resistant to β-lactams and multiple other antibiotics. For patients with normal kidney function, vancomycin, 1 g intravenously every 12 hours, is the treatment of choice for suspected or confirmed infection caused by these organisms until susceptibility to penicillinase-resistant penicillins or other agents has been confirmed. Duration of therapy has not been established for relatively uncomplicated infections, such as those secondary to intravenous devices, which may be eliminated by simply removing the infected device. Infection involving bone or a prosthetic valve should be treated for 6 weeks. A combination regimen of vancomycin plus rifampin, 300 mg orally twice daily, and gentamicin, 1 mg/kg intravenously every 8 hours, is recommended for treatment of prosthetic valve endocarditis caused by methicillin-resistant strains.

Chu VH et al. Emergence of coagulase-negative staphylococci as a cause of native valve endocarditis. Clin Infect Dis. 2008 Jan 15;46(2):232–42. [PMID: 18171255]

CLOSTRIDIAL DISEASES

1. Clostridial Myonecrosis (Gas Gangrene)

 ESSENTIALS OF DIAGNOSIS

▶ Sudden onset of pain and edema in an area of wound contamination.

▶ Prostration and systemic toxicity.

▶ Brown to blood-tinged watery exudate, with skin discoloration of surrounding area.

▶ Gas in the tissue by palpation or radiograph.

▶ Gram-positive rods in culture or smear of exudate.

▶ General Considerations

Gas gangrene or clostridial myonecrosis is produced by any one of several clostridia (*Clostridium perfringens, Clostridium ramosum, Clostridium bifermentans, Clostridium histolyticum, Clostridium novyi*, etc). Trauma and injection drug use are common predisposing conditions. Toxins produced in devitalized tissues under anaerobic conditions result in shock, hemolysis, and myonecrosis.

▶ Clinical Findings

A. Symptoms and Signs

The onset is usually sudden, with rapidly increasing pain in the affected area, hypotension, and tachycardia. Fever is present but is not proportionate to the severity of the infection. In the last stages of the disease, severe prostration, stupor, delirium, and coma occur.

The wound becomes swollen, and the surrounding skin is pale. There is a foul-smelling brown, blood-tinged serous discharge. As the disease advances, the surrounding tissue changes from pale to dusky and finally becomes deeply discolored, with coalescent, red, fluid-filled vesicles. Gas may be palpable in the tissues.

B. Laboratory Findings

Gas gangrene is a clinical diagnosis, and empiric therapy is indicated if the diagnosis is suspected. Radiographic studies may show gas within the soft tissues, but this finding is not specific. The smear shows absence of neutrophils and the presence of gram-positive rods. Anaerobic culture confirms the diagnosis.

▶ Differential Diagnosis

Other bacteria can produce gas in infected tissue, eg, enteric gram-negative organisms, or anaerobes.

▶ Treatment

Penicillin, 2 million units every 3 hours intravenously, is effective. Other agents (eg, tetracycline, clindamycin, metronidazole, chloramphenicol, cefoxitin) are active against *Clostridium* species in vitro and probably in vivo as well. Adequate surgical debridement and exposure of infected areas are essential, with radical surgical excision often necessary. Hyperbaric oxygen therapy has been used empirically but must be used in conjunction with administration of an appropriate antibiotic and surgical debridement.

2. *Clostridium sordellii* Toxic Shock Syndrome

 ESSENTIALS OF DIAGNOSIS

▶ Sudden onset after medical abortion.

▶ Abdominal pain.

▶ Absence of fever.

▶ Tachycardia, severe hypotension, capillary leak syndrome with edema.

▶ Profound leukocytosis, hemoconcentration.

General Considerations & Clinical Findings

C sordellii is a rare cause of endometritis and toxic shock syndrome following childbirth. Four cases, all fatal, of uterine infection following medically induced abortion with mifepristone were reported in 2005. Onset of illness was within 4–5 days of ingestion of mifepristone and the clinical course fulminant. Infection appeared to be limited to the uterus, which showed necrosis, edema, hemorrhage, and acute inflammatory changes.

Treatment

Early recognition, aggressive resuscitation from shock, immediate surgical debridement with hysterectomy, and administration of an antimicrobial that is active against *C sordellii* are essential to survival. Based on in vitro susceptibility data, any of several agents should be active, including penicillin, ampicillin, a macrolide, clindamycin, a tetracycline, or metronidazole. Whether a protein synthesis inhibitor to block further toxin production offers any advantage over a β-lactam is unknown.

Cohen AL et al. Toxic shock associated with *Clostridium sordellii* and *Clostridium perfringens* after medical and spontaneous abortion. Obstet Gynecol. 2007 Nov;110(5):1027–33. [PMID: 17978116]

3. Tetanus

ESSENTIALS OF DIAGNOSIS

▶ History of wound and possible contamination.

▶ Jaw stiffness followed by spasms of jaw muscles (trismus).

▶ Stiffness of the neck and other muscles, dysphagia, irritability, hyperreflexia.

▶ Finally, painful convulsions precipitated by minimal stimuli.

General Considerations

Tetanus is caused by the neurotoxin tetanospasmin, elaborated by *Clostridium tetani*. Spores of this organism are ubiquitous in soil and may germinate when introduced into a wound. The vegetative bacteria produce tetanospasmin, a zinc metalloprotease that cleaves synaptobrevin, a protein essential for neurotransmitter release. Tetanospasmin interferes with neurotransmission at spinal synapses of inhibitory neurons. As a result, minor stimuli result in uncontrolled spasms, and reflexes are exaggerated. The incubation period 5 days to 15 weeks, with the average being 8–12 days.

Most cases occur in unvaccinated individuals. Persons at are the elderly, migrant workers, newborns, and injec-

tion drug users. While puncture wounds are particularly prone to causing tetanus, any wound, including bites or decubiti, may become colonized and infected by *C tetani*.

Clinical Findings

A. Symptoms and Signs

The first symptom may be pain and tingling at the site of inoculation, followed by spasticity of the muscles nearby. Stiffness of the jaw, neck stiffness, dysphagia, and irritability are other early signs. Hyperreflexia develops later, with spasms of the jaw muscles (trismus) or facial muscles and rigidity and spasm of the muscles of the abdomen, neck, and back. Painful tonic convulsions precipitated by minor stimuli are common. Spasms of the glottis and respiratory muscles may cause acute asphyxia. The patient is awake and alert throughout the illness. The sensory examination is normal. The temperature is normal or only slightly elevated.

B. Laboratory Findings

The diagnosis of tetanus is made clinically.

Differential Diagnosis

Tetanus must be differentiated from various acute central nervous system infections such as meningitis. Trismus may occasionally develop with the use of phenothiazines. Strychnine poisoning should also be considered.

Complications

Airway obstruction is common. Urinary retention and constipation may result from spasm of the sphincters. Respiratory arrest and cardiac failure are late, life-threatening events.

Prevention

Tetanus is completely preventable by active immunization. For primary immunization of adults, Td (tetanus and diphtheria toxoids vaccine) is administered as two doses 4–6 weeks apart, with a third dose 6–12 months later. For one of the doses, Tdap (tetanus toxoid, reduced dose diphtheria toxoid, acellular pertussis vaccine) should be substituted for Td. Booster doses are given every 10 years or at the time of major injury if it occurs more than 5 years after a dose. A single dose of Tdap is preferred to Td for wound prophylaxis if the patient has not been previously vaccinated with Tdap.

Passive immunization should be used in nonimmunized individuals and those whose immunization status is uncertain whenever a wound is contaminated or likely to have devitalized tissue. Tetanus immune globulin, 250 units, is given intramuscularly. Active immunization with tetanus toxoid is started concurrently. Table 33–1 provides a guide to prophylactic management.

Treatment

A. Specific Measures

Human tetanus immune globulin, 500 units, should be administered intramuscularly within the first 24 hours of

Table 33–1. Guide to tetanus prophylaxis in wound management.

History of Absorbed Tetanus Toxoid	Clean, Minor Wounds		All Other Wounds[1]	
	Tdap or Td[2]	TIG[3]	Tdap or Td[2]	TIG[3]
Unknown or < 3 doses	Yes	No	Yes	Yes
3 or more doses	No[4]	No	No[5]	No

[1]Such as, but not limited to, wounds contaminated with dirt, feces, soil, saliva, etc; puncture wounds; avulsions; and wounds resulting from missiles, crushing, burns, and frostbite.
[2]Td indicates tetanus toxoid and diphtheria toxoid, adult form. Tdap indicates tetanous toxoid, reduced diphtheria toxoid, and acellular pertussis vaccine, which may be substituted as a single dose for Td. Unvaccinated individuals should receive a complete series of three doses, one of which is Tdap.
[3]Human tetanus immune globulin, 250 units intramuscularly.
[4]Yes if more than 10 years have elapsed since last dose.
[5]Yes if more than 5 years have elapsed since last dose. (More frequent boosters are not needed and can enhance side effects.) Tdap has been safely administered within 2 years of Td vaccination, although local reactions to the vaccine may be increased.

presentation. Whether intrathecal administration has any additional benefit is controversial. An unblinded, randomized trial comparing intramuscular tetanus immune globulin to intramuscular plus intrathecal tetanus immune globulin found more rapid resolution of spasms, fewer days of ventilatory support, and a shorter hospital stay in the intrathecal group. However, the exact immunoglobulin preparation that was used was not specified and the total dose was 4000 units. Tetanus does not produce natural immunity, and a full course of immunization with tetanus toxoid should be administered once the patient has recovered.

B. General Measures

Minimal stimuli can provoke spasms, so the patient should be placed at bed rest and monitored under the quietest conditions possible. Sedation, paralysis with curare-like agents, and mechanical ventilation are often necessary to control tetanic spasms. Penicillin, 20 million units intravenously daily, is given to all patients—even those with mild illness—to eradicate toxin-producing organisms.

▶ Prognosis

High mortality rates are associated with a short incubation period, early onset of convulsions, and delay in treatment. Contaminated lesions about the head and face are more dangerous than wounds on other parts of the body.

Kretsinger K et al; Centers for Disease Control and Prevention; Advisory Committee on Immunization Practices; Healthcare Infection Control Practices Advisory Committee. Preventing tetanus, diphtheria, and pertussis among adults: use of tetanus toxoid, reduced diphtheria toxoid and acellular pertussis vaccine recommendations of the Advisory Committee on Immunization Practices (ACIP) and recommendation of ACIP, supported by the Healthcare Infection Control Practices Advisory Committee (HICPAC), for use of Tdap among health-care personnel. MMWR Recomm Rep. 2006 Dec 15; 55(RR-17):1–37. [PMID: 17167397]

Thwaites CL et al. Magnesium sulphate for treatment of severe tetanus: a randomised controlled trial. Lancet. 2006 Oct 21; 368(9545):1436–43. [PMID: 17055945]

4. Botulism

ESSENTIALS OF DIAGNOSIS

▶ History of recent ingestion of home-canned or smoked foods or of injection drug use and demonstration of toxin in serum or food.

▶ Sudden onset of diplopia, dry mouth, dysphagia, dysphonia, and muscle weakness progressing to respiratory paralysis.

▶ Pupils are fixed and dilated in most cases.

▶ General Considerations

Botulism is a paralytic disease caused by botulinum toxin, which is produced by *Clostridium botulinum*, a ubiquitous, strictly anaerobic, spore-forming bacillus found in soil. Four toxin types—A, B, E, and F—cause human disease. Botulinum toxin is a zinc metalloprotease that cleaves a specific component of the synaptic vesicle membrane docking and fusion complex at the neuromuscular junction blocking release of the neurotransmitter acetylcholine. Botulinum toxin is extremely potent and is classified by the CDC as a high-priority agent because of its potential for use as an agent of bioterrorism. Naturally occurring botulism occurs in one of three forms: food-borne botulism, infant botulism, or wound botulism. Food-borne botulism is caused by ingestion of preformed toxin present in canned, smoked, or vacuum-packed foods such as home-canned vegetables, smoked meats, and vacuum-packed fish. Commercial foods have also been associated with outbreaks of botulism. Infant botulism (associated with ingestion of honey) and wound botulism (which typically occurs in association with injection drug use) result from organisms present in the gut or wound that elaborate toxin in vivo.

Clinical Findings

A. Symptoms and Signs

Twelve to 36 hours after ingestion of the toxin, visual disturbances appear, particularly diplopia and loss of accommodation. Ptosis, cranial nerve palsies with impairment of extraocular muscles, and fixed dilated pupils are characteristic signs. The sensory examination is normal. Other symptoms are dry mouth, dysphagia, and dysphonia. Nausea and vomiting may be present, particularly with type E toxin. The sensorium remains clear and the temperature normal. Paralysis progressing to respiratory failure and death may occur unless mechanical assistance is provided.

B. Laboratory Findings

Toxin in patients' serum and in suspected foods can be demonstrated by mouse inoculation and identified with specific antiserum.

Differential Diagnosis

Because the clinical presentation of botulism is so distinctive and the differential diagnosis limited, botulism once considered is not easily confused with other diseases. Cranial nerve involvement may be seen with vertebrobasilar insufficiency, the C. Miller Fisher variant of Guillain-Barré syndrome, myasthenia gravis, or any basilar meningitis (infectious or carcinomatous). Intestinal obstruction or other types of food poisoning are considered when nausea and vomiting are present.

Treatment

If botulism is suspected, the practitioner should contact the state health authorities or the CDC for advice and help with procurement of botulinus antitoxin and for assistance in obtaining assays for toxin in serum, stool, or food. Skin testing is recommended to exclude hypersensitivity to the antitoxin preparation. Antitoxin should be administered as early as possible, ideally within 24 hours of the onset of symptoms or signs, to arrest progression of disease; its administration should not be delayed for laboratory confirmation of the diagnosis. Respiratory failure is managed with intubation and mechanical ventilation. Parenteral fluids or alimentation should be given while swallowing difficulty persists. The removal of unabsorbed toxin from the gut may be attempted. Any remnants of suspected foods should be assayed for toxin. Persons who might have eaten the suspected food must be located and observed.

Villar RG et al. Botulism: the many faces of botulinum toxin and its potential for bioterrorism. Infect Dis Clin North Am. 2006 Jun;20(2):313–27. [PMID: 16762741]

Wongtanate M et al. Signs and symptoms predictive of respiratory failure in patients with foodborne botulism in Thailand. Am J Trop Med Hyg. 2007 Aug;77(2):386–9. [PMID: 7690419]

ANTHRAX

ESSENTIALS OF DIAGNOSIS

▶ Appropriate epidemiologic setting, eg, exposure to animals or animal hides, or potential exposure resulting from an act of bioterrorism.

▶ A painless cutaneous black eschar on exposed areas of the skin, with marked surrounding edema and vesicles.

▶ Nonspecific flu-like symptoms that rapidly progress to extreme dyspnea and shock in association with mediastinal widening and pleural effusions on chest radiograph.

General Considerations

The death of a Florida photo editor from inhalational anthrax acquired from a letter deliberately contaminated with spores of *Bacillus anthracis* thrust this extremely rare infection into the public awareness. Between September 18 and November 21 of 2001, there were 13 cases of cutaneous anthrax and 11 cases of inhalational anthrax associated with exposure to anthrax spores in contaminated mail.

Naturally occurring anthrax is a disease of sheep, cattle, horses, goats, and swine. *B anthracis* is a gram-positive spore-forming aerobic rod. Spores—not vegetative bacteria—are the infectious form of the organism. These are transmitted to humans from contact with contaminated animals, animal products, or animal hides, or from soil by inoculation of broken skin or mucous membranes; by inhalation of aerosolized spores; or, rarely, by ingestion resulting in cutaneous, inhalational, or gastrointestinal forms of anthrax, respectively. Spores germinate into vegetative bacteria that multiply locally in cutaneous and gastrointestinal anthrax but may also disseminate to cause systemic infection. Inhaled spores are ingested by pulmonary macrophages and carried via lymphatics to regional lymph nodes, where they germinate. The bacteria rapidly multiply within the lymphatics, causing a hemorrhagic lymphadenitis. Invasion of the bloodstream leads to overwhelming sepsis, killing the host.

Clinical Findings

A. Symptoms and Signs

1. Cutaneous anthrax—This occurs within 2 weeks after exposure to spores; there is no latency period for cutaneous disease. The initial lesion is an erythematous papule, often on an exposed area of skin that vesiculates and then ulcerates and undergoes necrosis, ultimately progressing to a purple to black eschar. The eschar typically is painless; pain indicates secondary staphylococcal or streptococcal infection. The surrounding area is edematous and vesicular but not purulent. Regional adenopathy, fever, malaise, headache, and nausea and vomiting may be present. The infection is self-limited in most cases, but hematogenous spread with sepsis or meningitis may occur.

2. Inhalational anthrax—Illness occurs in two stages, beginning on average 10 days after exposure, but may begin up to 6 weeks after exposure. Nonspecific viral-like symptoms such as fever, malaise, headache, dyspnea, cough, and congestion of the nose, throat, and larynx are characteristic of the initial stage. Anterior chest pain is an early symptom of mediastinitis. Within hours to a few days, progression to the fulminant stage of infection occurs in which symptoms or signs of overwhelming sepsis predominate. Delirium, obtundation, or findings of meningeal irritation suggest an accompanying hemorrhagic meningitis.

3. Gastrointestinal anthrax—This form has not been reported in the United States. Fever, diffuse abdominal pain, rebound abdominal tenderness, vomiting, constipation, and diarrhea occur 2–5 days after ingestion of meat contaminated with anthrax spores. The primary lesion is ulcerative, producing emesis that may be blood-tinged or coffee-grounds and stool that may be blood-tinged or melenic. Bowel perforation can occur. The oropharyngeal form of the disease is characterized by local lymphadenopathy, cervical edema, dysphagia, and upper respiratory tract obstruction.

B. Laboratory Findings

Laboratory findings are nonspecific. The white blood cell count initially may be normal or modestly elevated, with polymorphonuclear predominance and an increase in early forms. Pleural fluid from patients with inhalational anthrax is typically hemorrhagic with few white cells. Cerebrospinal fluid from meningitis cases is also hemorrhagic. Gram stain of pleural fluid, cerebrospinal fluid, unspun blood, blood culture, or fluid from a cutaneous lesion may show the characteristic boxcar-shaped encapsulated rods in chains.

The diagnosis is established by isolation of the organism from culture of the skin lesion (or fluid expressed from it), blood, or pleural fluid—or cerebrospinal fluid in cases of meningitis. In the absence of prior antimicrobial therapy, cultures are invariably positive. Cultures obtained after initiation of antimicrobial therapy may be negative. If anthrax is suspected on clinical or epidemiologic grounds, immunohistochemical tests (eg, to detect capsular antigen), polymerase chain reaction assays, and serologic tests (useful for documenting past cutaneous infection) are available through the CDC and should be used to establish the diagnosis. Any suspected case of anthrax should be immediately reported to the CDC so that a complete investigation can be conducted.

C. Imaging

The chest radiograph is the most sensitive test for inhalational disease, being abnormal (though the findings can be subtle) initially in every case of bioterrorism-associated disease. Mediastinal widening due to hemorrhagic lymphadenitis, a hallmark feature of the disease, has been present in 70% of the bioterrorism-related cases. Pleural effusions were present initially or occurred over the course of illness in all cases, and approximately three-fourths had pulmonary infiltrates or signs of consolidation.

▶ Differential Diagnosis

Cutaneous anthrax, despite its characteristic appearance, can be confused with a variety of other also uncommon or rare conditions such as ecthyma gangrenosum, rat-bite fever, ulceroglandular tularemia, plague, glanders, rickettsialpox, orf (parapoxvirus infection), or cutaneous mycobacterial infection. Inhalational anthrax must be differentiated from mediastinitis due to other bacterial causes, fibrous mediastinitis due to histoplasmosis, coccidioidomycosis, atypical or viral pneumonia, silicosis, sarcoidosis, and other causes of mediastinal widening (eg, superior vena cava syndrome or aortic aneurysm or dissection). Gastrointestinal anthrax shares clinical features with a variety of common intra-abdominal disorders, including bowel obstruction, perforated viscus, peritonitis, gastroenteritis, and peptic ulcer disease.

▶ Treatment

Strains of *B anthracis* (including the strain isolated in the bioterrorism cases) are susceptible in vitro to penicillin, amoxicillin, chloramphenicol, clindamycin, imipenem, doxycycline, ciprofloxacin (as well as other fluoroquinolones), macrolides, rifampin, and vancomycin. Susceptibility to cephalosporins is variable. *B anthracis* may express β-lactamases that confer resistance to cephalosporins and penicillins. For this reason, penicillin or amoxicillin is no longer recommended for use as a single agent in treatment of disseminated disease. Based on results of animal experiments and because of concern for engineered drug resistance in strains of *B anthracis* used in bioterrorism or weaponized, ciprofloxacin is considered the drug of choice (Table 33–2) for treatment and for prophylaxis following exposure to anthrax spores. Other fluoroquinolones with activity against gram-positive bacteria (eg, levofloxacin, moxifloxacin) are likely to be just as effective as ciprofloxacin. Doxycycline is an alternative first-line agent. Combination therapy with at least one additional agent is recommended for inhalational or disseminated disease and in cutaneous infection involving the face, head, and neck or associated with extensive local edema or systemic signs of

---

Table 33–2. Antimicrobial agents for treatment of anthrax or for prophylaxis against anthrax.

First-line agents and recommended doses
Ciprofloxacin, 500 mg twice daily orally or 400 mg every 12 hours intravenously
Doxycycline, 100 mg every 12 hours orally or intravenously
Second-line agents and recommended doses
Amoxicillin, 500 mg three times daily orally
Penicillin G, 2–4 million units every 4 hours intravenously
Alternative agents with in vitro activity and suggested doses
Rifampin, 10 mg/kg/d orally or intravenously
Clindamycin, 450–600 mg every 8 hours orally or intravenously
Clarithromycin, 500 mg orally twice daily
Erythromycin, 500 mg every 6 hours intravenously
Vancomycin, 1 g every 12 hours intravenously
Imipenem, 500 mg every 6 hours intravenously

infection, eg, fever, tachycardia and elevated white blood cell count. Anecdotally, four of the six survivors of the 2001 inhalational cases were treated with combinations that included both a fluoroquinolone and rifampin. Single-drug therapy is recommended for prophylaxis following exposure to spores.

The required duration of therapy is poorly defined. In naturally occurring disease, treatment for 7–10 days for cutaneous disease and for at least 2 weeks following clinical response for disseminated, inhalational, or gastrointestinal infection have been standard recommendations. Because of concern about relapse from latent spores acquired by inhalation of aerosol in bioterrorism-associated cases, the initial recommendation was treatment for 60 days. In 2001, the CDC offered one of two options for postal workers receiving prophylaxis for exposure to contaminated mail: (1) antibiotics for 100 days (fearing that even with 60 days of treatment late relapses might occur) or (2) vaccination with an investigative agent (three doses administered over a 1-month period) in conjunction with 40 days of antibiotic administration to cover the time required for a protective antibody response to develop. Insufficient information exists to favor one recommendation over the other.

There is also an FDA-approved vaccine for persons at high risk for exposure to anthrax spores. The vaccine is cell-free antigen prepared from an attenuated strain of *B anthracis*. Multiple injections over 18 months and an annual booster dose are required to achieve and maintain protection. Existing supplies have been reserved for vaccination of military personnel.

The prognosis in cutaneous infection is excellent. Death is unlikely if the infection has remained localized, and lesions heal without complications in most cases. The reported mortality rate for gastrointestinal and inhalational infections is up to 85%. The experience with bioterrorism-associated inhalational cases in which six of eleven victims survived suggests a somewhat better outcome with modern supportive care and antibiotics provided that treatment is initiated before the patient has progressed to the fulminant stage of disease. No cases of anthrax have occurred among the several thousand individuals receiving antimicrobial prophylaxis following exposure to spores.

Kyriacou DN et al. Discriminating inhalational anthrax from community-acquired pneumonia using chest radiograph findings and a clinical algorithm. Chest. 2007 Feb;131(2):489–96. [PMID: 17296652]

DIPHTHERIA

ESSENTIALS OF DIAGNOSIS

- ...cious gray membrane at portal of entry in pharynx.
- ...roat, nasal discharge, hoarseness, malaise, fever.
- ...tis, neuropathy.
- ...firms the diagnosis.

▶ General Considerations

Diphtheria is an acute infection caused by *Corynebacterium diphtheriae* that usually attacks the respiratory tract but may involve any mucous membrane or skin wound. The organism is spread chiefly by respiratory secretions. Exotoxin produced by the organism is responsible for myocarditis and neuropathy. This exotoxin inhibits elongation factor, which is required for protein synthesis.

▶ Clinical Findings

A. Symptoms and Signs

Nasal, laryngeal, pharyngeal, and cutaneous forms of diphtheria occur. Nasal infection produces few symptoms other than a nasal discharge. Laryngeal infection may lead to upper airway and bronchial obstruction. In pharyngeal diphtheria, the most common form, a tenacious gray membrane covers the tonsils and pharynx. Mild sore throat, fever, and malaise are followed by toxemia and prostration.

Myocarditis and neuropathy are the most common and most serious complications. Myocarditis causes cardiac arrhythmias, heart block, and heart failure. The neuropathy usually involves the cranial nerves first, producing diplopia, slurred speech, and difficulty in swallowing.

B. Laboratory Findings

The diagnosis is made clinically but can be confirmed by culture of the organism.

▶ Differential Diagnosis

Diphtheria must be differentiated from streptococcal pharyngitis, infectious mononucleosis, adenovirus or herpes simplex infection, Vincent angina, pharyngitis due to *Arcanobacterium haemolyticum*, and candidiasis. A presumptive diagnosis of diphtheria should be made on clinical grounds without waiting for laboratory verification, since emergency treatment is needed.

▶ Prevention

Active immunization with diphtheria toxoid is part of routine childhood immunization with appropriate booster injections. The immunization schedule for adults is the same as for tetanus.

Susceptible persons exposed to diphtheria should receive a booster dose of diphtheria toxoid (or a complete series if previously unimmunized), as well as a course of penicillin or erythromycin.

▶ Treatment

Antitoxin, which is prepared from horse serum, must be given in all cases when diphtheria is suspected. For mild early pharyngeal or laryngeal disease, the dose is 20,000–40,000 units; for moderate nasopharyngeal disease, 40,000–60,000 units; for severe, extensive, or late (3 days or more) disease, 80,000–100,000 units. Diphtheria equine antitoxin can be obtained from the CDC.

Removal of membrane by direct laryngoscopy or bronchoscopy may be necessary to prevent or alleviate airway obstruction.

Either penicillin, 250 mg orally four times daily, or erythromycin, 500 mg orally four times daily, for 14 days is effective therapy, although erythromycin is slightly more effective in eliminating the carrier state. Azithromycin or clarithromycin is probably as effective as erythromycin. The patient should be isolated until three consecutive cultures at the completion of therapy have documented elimination of the organism from the oropharynx. Contacts to a case should receive erythromycin, 500 mg orally four times daily for 7 days, to eradicate carriage.

LISTERIOSIS

Listeria monocytogenes is a facultative, motile, gram-positive rod that is capable of invading several cell types and causes intracellular infection. Most cases of infection caused by *L monocytogenes* are sporadic, but outbreaks have been traced to eating contaminated food, including unpasteurized dairy products, hot dogs, and delicatessen meats. Five types of infection are recognized:

(1) **Infection during pregnancy,** usually in the last trimester, is a mild febrile illness without an apparent primary focus. This relatively benign disease for the mother may resolve without specific therapy. However, approximately one in five pregnancies complicated by listeriosis result in spontaneous abortion or stillbirth and surviving infants are at high risk for clinical neonatal listeriosis.

(2) **Granulomatosis infantisepticum** is a neonatal infection acquired in utero, characterized by disseminated abscesses, granulomas, and a high mortality rate.

(3) **Bacteremia** with or without sepsis syndrome is an infection of neonates or immunocompromised adults. The presentation is of a febrile illness without a recognized source.

(4) **Meningitis** caused by *L monocytogenes* affects infants under 2 months of age as well as older adults, ranking third after the meningococcus and pneumococcus among the common causes of bacterial meningitis. Cerebrospinal fluid shows a *neutrophilic* pleocytosis. Adults with meningitis are often immunocompromised, and cases have been associated with HIV infection and therapy with tumor necrosis factor-α (TNF-α) inhibitors such as infliximab.

(5) Finally, **focal infections**, including adenitis, brain abscess, endocarditis, osteomyelitis, and arthritis, occur rarely.

Ampicillin, 8–12 g/d intravenously in four to six divided doses (the higher dose for meningitis) is considered the treatment of choice. It penetrates well into cerebrospinal fluid, and clinical response is better than with penicillin, erythromycin, or chloramphenicol. Gentamicin is synergistic with ampicillin against *Listeria* in vitro and in animal models, and the use of combination therapy may be considered during the first few days of treatment to enhance eradication of organisms. Mortality and morbidity rates still are high, and relapses occur, perhaps related to poor intracellular penetration of ampicillin. Trimethoprim-sulfamethoxazole with its excellent intracellular and cerebrospi-

nal fluid penetration may be more efficacious. The dose is 10–20 mg/kg/d intravenously of the trimethoprim component. Therapy should be administered for at least 2–3 weeks. Longer durations—between 3 and 6 weeks—have been recommended for treatment of meningitis, especially in immunocompromised persons.

Bennion JR et al. Decreasing listeriosis mortality in the United States, 1990–2005. Clin Infect Dis. 2008 Oct 1;47(7):867–74. [PMID: 18752441]

▼ INFECTIVE ENDOCARDITIS

 ESSENTIALS OF DIAGNOSIS

▶ Fever
▶ Preexisting organic heart lesion.
▶ Positive blood cultures.
▶ Evidence of vegetation on echocardiography.
▶ New or changing heart murmur.
▶ Evidence of systemic emboli.

▶ General Considerations

Endocarditis is a bacterial or fungal infection of the valvular or endocardial surface of the heart. The clinical presentation depends on the infecting organism and the valve or valves that are infected. More virulent organisms—*S aureus* in particular—tend to produce a more rapidly progressive and destructive infection. Endocarditis caused by more virulent organisms often presents as an acute febrile illnesses and is complicated by early embolization, acute valvular regurgitation, and myocardial abscess formation. Viridans strains of streptococci, enterococci, other bacteria, yeasts, and fungi tend to cause a more subacute picture.

Underlying valvular disease, less common than in the past, is present in about 50% of cases. Valvular disease alters blood flow and produces jet effects that disrupt the endothelial surface, providing a nidus for attachment and infection of microorganisms that enter the bloodstream. Predisposing valvular abnormalities include rheumatic involvement of any valve, bicuspid aortic valves, calcific or sclerotic aortic valves, hypertrophic subaortic stenosis, mitral valve prolapse, and a variety of congenital disorders such as ventricular septal defect, tetralogy of Fallot, coarctation of the aorta, or patent ductus arteriosus. Rheumatic disease is no longer the major predisposing factor in developed countries. Regurgitation lesions are more susceptible than stenotic ones.

The initiating event in native valve endocarditis is colonization of the valve by bacteria or yeast that gain access to the bloodstream. Transient bacteremia is common during dental, upper respiratory, urologic, and lower gastrointestinal diagnostic and surgical procedures. It is less common during upper gastrointestinal and gynecologic proced

Intravascular devices are increasingly implicated as a portal of access of microorganisms into the bloodstream. A large proportion of cases of *S aureus* endocarditis are attributable to healthcare-associated bacteremia.

Native valve endocarditis is usually caused by viridans streptococci, group D streptococci, *S aureus*, enterococci, or HACEK organisms (an acronym for *Haemophilus aphrophilus, Haemophilus parainfluenzae, Actinobacillus actinomycetemcomitans, Cardiobacterium hominis, Eikenella corrodens,* and *Kingella kingae*). Streptococcal species formerly accounted for the majority of native valve endocarditis cases, but the proportion of cases caused by *S aureus* has been increasing, and this organism is now the leading cause. Gram-negative organisms and fungi account for a small percentage.

In injection drug users, *S aureus* accounts for over 60% of all endocarditis cases and for 80–90% of cases in which the tricuspid valve is infected. Enterococci and streptococci comprise the balance in about equal proportions. Gram-negative aerobic bacilli, fungi, and unusual organisms may cause endocarditis in injection drug users.

The microbiology of prosthetic valve endocarditis also is distinctive. Early infections (ie, those occurring within 2 months after valve implantation) are commonly caused by staphylococci—both coagulase-positive and coagulase-negative—gram-negative organisms, and fungi. In late prosthetic valve endocarditis, streptococci are commonly identified, although coagulase-negative and coagulase-positive staphylococci still cause many cases.

▶ **Clinical Findings**

A. Symptoms and Signs

Virtually all patients have fever at some point in the illness, although it may be very low grade (less than 38 °C) in elderly individuals and in patients with heart failure or kidney failure. Rarely, there may be no fever at all.

The duration of illness typically is a few days to a few weeks. Nonspecific symptoms are common. The initial symptoms and signs of endocarditis may be caused by direct arterial, valvular, or cardiac damage. Although a changing regurgitant murmur is significant diagnostically, it is the exception rather than the rule. Symptoms also may occur as a result of embolization, metastatic infection or immunologically mediated phenomena. These include cough; dyspnea; arthralgias or arthritis; diarrhea; and abdominal, back, or flank pain.

The characteristic peripheral lesions—petechiae (on the palate or conjunctiva or beneath the fingernails), subungual ("splinter") hemorrhages, Osler nodes (painful, violaceous raised lesions of the fingers, toes, or feet), Janeway lesions (painless erythematous lesions of the palms or soles), and Roth spots (exudative lesions in the retina)—occur in about 25% of patients (Plates 102 and ...). Strokes and major systemic embolic events are ... about 25% of patients, and tend to occur before ... first week of antimicrobial therapy. Hematuria may result from emboli or immuno...ed glomerulonephritis, which can cause ...

B. Diagnostic Studies

Blood cultures establish the diagnosis. Three sets of blood cultures at least 1 hour apart before starting antibiotics are recommended to maximize the opportunity for a microbiologic diagnosis. Approximately 5% of cases will be culture-negative, usually attributable to administration of antimicrobials prior to obtaining cultures. If antimicrobial therapy has been administered prior to obtaining cultures and the patient is clinically stable, it is reasonable to withhold further antimicrobial therapy for 2–3 days so that appropriate cultures can be obtained. Culture-negative endocarditis may also be due to a fungus, organisms that require special media for growth (eg, *Legionella, Bartonella, Abiotrophia* species, formerly referred to as nutritionally deficient streptococci), organisms that do not grow on artificial media (*Tropheryma whippelii,* or pathogens of Q fever or psittacosis), or those that are slow-growing and may require prolonged incubation (eg, *Brucella,* anaerobes, HACEK organisms). *Bartonella quintana* has emerged as an important cause of culture-negative endocarditis.

Chest radiograph may show evidence for the underlying cardiac abnormality and, in right-sided endocarditis, pulmonary infiltrates. The electrocardiogram is nondiagnostic, but new conduction abnormalities suggest myocardial abscess formation. Echocardiography is useful in identifying vegetations and other characteristic features suspicious for endocarditis and may provide adjunctive information about the specific valve or valves that are infected. The sensitivity of transthoracic echocardiography is between 55% and 65%; it cannot reliably rule out endocarditis but may confirm a clinical suspicion. TEE is 90% sensitive in detecting vegetations and is particularly useful for identifying valve ring abscesses as well as prosthetic valve endocarditis.

Clinical criteria, referred to as the **Modified Duke criteria,** for the diagnosis of endocarditis have been proposed. Major criteria include: (1) two positive blood cultures for a microorganism that typically causes infective endocarditis or persistent bacteremia; (2) evidence of endocardial involvement documented by echocardiography (eg, definite vegetation, myocardial abscess, or new partial dehiscence of a prosthetic valve); or (3) development of a new regurgitant murmur. Minor criteria include the presence of a predisposing condition; fever ≥ 38 °C; vascular phenomena, such as cutaneous hemorrhages, aneurysm, systemic emboli, pulmonary infarction; immunologic phenomena, such as glomerulonephritis, Osler nodes, Roth spots, rheumatoid factor; and positive blood cultures not meeting the major criteria or serologic evidence of an active infection. A definite diagnosis can be made with 80% accuracy if two major criteria, one major criterion and three minor criteria, or five minor criteria are fulfilled. A possible diagnosis of endocarditis is made if one major and one minor criterion or three minor criteria are met. If fewer criteria are found, or a sound alternative explanation for illness is identified, or the endocarditis syndrome has resolved and the patient has defervesced within 4 days, endocarditis is unlikely.

▶ **Complications**

The course of infective endocarditis is determined by the degree of damage to the heart, by the site of infection (right-

is sensitive to methicillin, either nafcillin or oxacillin or cefazolin can be used in combination with rifampin and gentamicin. Combination therapy with nafcillin or oxacillin (vancomycin for methicillin-resistant strains or patients allergic to β-lactams), rifampin, and gentamicin is also recommended for treatment of *S aureus* prosthetic valve infection.

E. HACEK Organisms

HACEK organisms are slow-growing, fastidious gram-negative coccobacilli or bacilli that are normal oral flora and cause less than 5% of all cases of endocarditis. They may produce β-lactamase, and thus the treatment of choice is ceftriaxone (or some other third-generation cephalosporin), 2 g intravenously once daily for 4 weeks. Prosthetic valve endocarditis should be treated for 6 weeks. In the penicillin-allergic patient, experience is limited, but trimethoprim-sulfamethoxazole, quinolones, and aztreonam have in vitro activity and should be considered; desensitization may be preferable.

F. Role of Surgery

While many cases can be successfully treated medically, operative management is frequently required. Acute heart failure unresponsive to medical therapy is an indication for valve replacement even if active infection is present, especially for aortic valve infection. Infections unresponsive to appropriate antimicrobial therapy after 7–10 days (ie, persistent fevers, positive blood cultures despite therapy) are more likely to be eradicated if the valve is replaced. Surgery is nearly always required for cure of fungal endocarditis and is more often necessary with gram-negative bacilli. It is also indicated when the infection involves the sinus of Valsalva or produces septal abscesses. Recurrent infection with the same organism prompts an operative approach, especially with infected prosthetic valves. Continuing embolization presents a difficult problem when the infection is otherwise responding; surgery may be the proper approach. Particularly challenging is a large and fragile vegetation demonstrated by echo in the absence of embolization. Most clinicians favor an operative approach, vegetectomy with valve repair if the patient is a good candidate. Embolization after bacteriologic cure does not necessarily imply recurrence of endocarditis.

G. Role of Anticoagulation

Anticoagulation is contraindicated in native valve endocarditis because of an increased risk of intracerebral hemorrhage. The role of anticoagulant therapy during active prosthetic valve endocarditis is more controversial. Reversal of anticoagulation may result in thrombosis of the mechanical prosthesis, particularly in the mitral position. On the other hand, anticoagulation during active prosthetic valve endocarditis caused by *S aureus* has been associated with fatal intracerebral hemorrhage. One approach is to discontinue anticoagulation during the septic phase of *S aureus* prosthetic valve endocarditis. In patients with *S aureus* prosthetic valve endocarditis complicated by a central ner-

vous system embolic event, anticoagulation should be discontinued for the first 2 weeks of therapy. Indications for anticoagulation following prosthetic valve implantation for endocarditis are the same as for patients with prosthetic valves without endocarditis (eg, nonporcine mechanical valves and valves in the mitral position).

Response to Therapy

If infection is caused by viridans streptococci, enterococci, or coagulase-negative staphylococci, defervescence occurs in 3–4 days on average; with *S aureus* or *Pseudomonas aeruginosa*, fever commonly persists for 9–12 days. Blood cultures should be obtained to document sterilization of the blood. Other causes of persistent fever are myocardial or metastatic abscess, sterile embolization, superimposed hospital-acquired infection, and drug reaction. Most relapses occur within 1–2 months after completion of therapy. Obtaining one or two blood cultures during this period is prudent.

Baddour LM et al. Infective endocarditis: diagnosis, antimicrobial therapy, and management of complications: a statement for healthcare professionals from the Committee on Rheumatic Fever, Endocarditis, and Kawasaki Disease, Council on Cardiovascular Disease in the Young, and the Councils on Clinical Cardiology, Stroke, and Cardiovascular Surgery and Anesthesia, American Heart Association: endorsed by the Infectious Diseases Society of America. Circulation. 2005 Jun 14;111(23):e394–434. [PMID: 15956145]

Durante-Mangoni E et al. Current features of infective endocarditis in elderly patients: results of the International Collaboration on Endocarditis Prospective Cohort Study. Arch Intern Med. 2008 Oct 27;168(19):2095–103. [PMID: 18955638]

Hill EE et al. Management of prosthetic valve infective endocarditis. Am J Cardiol. 2008 Apr 15;101(8):1174–8. [PMID: 18394454]

Wilson W et al. Prevention of infective endocarditis: guidelines from the American Heart Association: a guideline from the American Heart Association Rheumatic Fever, Endocarditis, and Kawasaki Disease Committee, Council on Cardiovascular Disease in the Young, and the Council on Clinical Cardiology, Council on Cardiovascular Surgery and Anesthesia, and the Quality of Care and Outcomes Research Interdisciplinary Working Group. Circulation. 2007 Oct 9;116(15):1736–54. [PMID: 17446442]

INFECTIONS CAUSED BY GRAM-NEGATIVE BACTERIA

BORDETELLA PERTUSSIS INFECTION (Whooping Cough)

ESSENTIALS OF DIAGNOSIS

► Predominantly in infants under age 2 years. Adolescents and adults are an important reservoir of infection.

► Two-week prodromal catarrhal stage of malaise, cough, coryza, and anorexia.

▶ Paroxysmal cough ending in a high-pitched inspiratory "whoop."

▶ Absolute lymphocytosis, often striking; culture confirms diagnosis.

General Considerations

Pertussis is an acute infection of the respiratory tract caused by *B pertussis* that is transmitted by respiratory droplets. The incubation period is 7–17 days. Half of all cases occur before age 2 years. Neither immunization nor disease confers lasting immunity to pertussis. Consequently, adults are an important reservoir of the disease.

Clinical Findings

The symptoms of classic pertussis last about 6 weeks and are divided into three consecutive stages. The catarrhal stage is characterized by its insidious onset, with lacrimation, sneezing, and coryza, anorexia and malaise, and a hacking night cough that becomes diurnal. The paroxysmal stage is characterized by bursts of rapid, consecutive coughs followed by a deep, high-pitched inspiration (whoop). The convalescent stage begins 4 weeks after onset of the illness with a decrease in the frequency and severity of paroxysms of cough. The diagnosis often is not considered in adults, who may not have a typical presentation. Cough persisting more than 2 weeks is suggestive. Infection may also be asymptomatic.

The white blood cell count is usually 15,000–20,000/mcL (rarely, as high as 50,000/mcL or more), 60–80% of which are lymphocytes. The diagnosis is established by isolating the organism from nasopharyngeal culture. A special medium (eg, Bordet-Gengou agar) must be requested. Polymerase chain reaction assays for diagnosis of pertussis may be available in some clinical or health department laboratories.

Prevention

Acellular pertussis vaccine is recommended for all infants, combined with diphtheria and tetanus toxoids (DTaP). Infants and susceptible adults with significant exposure should receive prophylaxis with an oral macrolide (see below). In recognition of their importance as a reservoir of disease, vaccination of adolescents and adults against pertussis is now recommended. The FDA licensed two tetanus toxoid, reduced diphtheria toxoid and acellular pertussis vaccine (Tdap) products (BOOSTRIX, GlaxoSmithKline and ADACEL, Sanofi Pasteur) in 2005. Adolescents aged 11–18 years who have completed the DTP or DTaP vaccination series should receive a single dose of either Tdap product instead of Td (tetanus and diphtheria toxoids vaccine) for booster immunization against tetanus, diphtheria, and pertussis. Either vaccine may be used in place of Td for prophylaxis of tetanus in wound management. The ADACEL vaccine is indicated as a one-time dose for booster immunization for pertussis in children and adults (ages 11 through 64 years). It may be used as a replacement dose for one of the Td doses when completing a primary immunization series or in place of Td for tetanus wound prophylaxis. Postpartum women and adults who have not been previously vaccinated with Tdap and who have close contact to an infant younger than 12 months should receive a single dose of Tdap. Women of childbearing age are also candidates for one dose of Tdap.

Treatment

Erythromycin, 500 mg four times a day orally for 7 days, shortens the duration of carriage. It also may diminish the severity of coughing paroxysms. Azithromycin, 500 mg orally on day 1 and 250 mg for 4 more days; or clarithromycin, 500 mg orally twice daily for 7 days, is probably as effective as erythromycin and likely to be better tolerated. Trimethoprim-sulfamethoxazole 160 mg–800 mg orally twice a day for 7 days also is effective. These same regimens are indicated for prophylaxis of contacts to an active case of pertussis who are exposed within 3 weeks of the onset of cough in the index case.

Kretsinger K et al; Centers for Disease Control and Prevention; Advisory Committee on Immunization Practices; Healthcare Infection Control Practices Advisory Committee. Preventing tetanus, diphtheria, and pertussis among adults: use of tetanus toxoid, reduced diphtheria toxoid and acellular pertussis vaccine recommendations of the Advisory Committee on Immunization Practices (ACIP) and recommendation of ACIP, supported by the Healthcare Infection Control Practices Advisory Committee (HICPAC), for use of Tdap among health-care personnel. MMWR Recomm Rep. 2006 Dec 15;55(RR-17):1–37. [PMID: 17167397]

Singh M et al. Whooping cough: the current scene. Chest. 2006 Nov;130(5):1547–53. [PMID: 17099036]

OTHER *BORDETELLA* INFECTIONS

Bordetella bronchiseptica is a pleomorphic gram-negative coccobacillus causing kennel cough in dogs. On occasion it causes upper and lower respiratory infection in humans, principally HIV-infected patients. Infection has been associated with contact with dogs and cats, suggesting animal-to-human transmission. Treatment of *B bronchiseptica* infection is guided by results of in vitro susceptibility tests.

MENINGOCOCCAL MENINGITIS

ESSENTIALS OF DIAGNOSIS

▶ Fever, headache, vomiting, confusion, delirium, convulsions.

▶ Petechial rash of skin and mucous membranes in many.

▶ Neck and back stiffness with positive Kernig and Brudzinski signs is characteristic.

▶ Purulent spinal fluid with gram-negative intracellular and extracellular diplococci.

▶ Culture of cerebrospinal fluid, blood, or petechial aspiration confirms the diagnosis.

General Considerations

Meningococcal meningitis is caused by *Neisseria meningitidis* of groups A, B, C, Y, and W-135, among others. Meningitis due to serogroup A is uncommon in the United States. Serogroup B generally causes sporadic cases. The frequency of outbreaks of meningitis caused by group C *meningococcus* has increased, and this serotype is the most common cause of epidemic disease in the United States. Up to 40% of persons are nasopharyngeal carriers of meningococci, but disease develops in relatively few of these persons. Infection is transmitted by droplets. The clinical illness may take the form of meningococcemia (a fulminant form of septicemia without meningitis), meningococcemia with meningitis, or meningitis. Recurrent meningococcemia with fever, rash, and arthritis is seen rarely in patients with certain terminal complement deficiencies.

Clinical Findings

A. Symptoms and Signs

High fever, chills, and headache; back, abdominal, and extremity pains; and nausea and vomiting are typical. Rapidly developing confusion, delirium, seizures, and coma occur in some.

On examination, nuchal and back rigidity are typical, with positive Kernig and Brudzinski signs. (Kernig sign is pain in the hamstrings upon extension of the knee with the hip at 90-degree flexion; Brudzinski sign is flexion of the knee in response to flexion of the neck.) A petechial rash appearing in the lower extremities and at pressure points is found in most cases. Petechiae may vary in size from pinpoint lesions to large ecchymoses or even skin gangrene that may later slough if the patient survives.

B. Laboratory Findings

Lumbar puncture typically reveals a cloudy or purulent cerebrospinal fluid, with elevated pressure, increased protein, and decreased glucose content. The fluid usually contains more than 1000 cells/mcL, with polymorphonuclear cells predominating and containing gram-negative intracellular diplococci. The absence of organisms in a Gram-stained smear of the cerebrospinal fluid sediment does not rule out the diagnosis. The capsular polysaccharide can be demonstrated in cerebrospinal fluid or urine by latex agglutination; this is useful in partially treated patients, though sensitivity is 60–80%. The organism is usually demonstrated by smear and culture of the cerebrospinal fluid, oropharynx, blood, or aspirated petechiae.

Disseminated intravascular coagulation is an important complication of meningococcal infection and is typically present in toxic patients with ecchymotic skin lesions.

Differential Diagnosis

Meningococcal meningitis must be differentiated from other meningitides. In small infants and in the elderly, fever or stiff neck is often missing, and altered mental status may dominate the picture.

Rickettsial, echovirus and, rarely, other bacterial infections (eg, staphylococcal infections, scarlet fever) also cause petechial rash.

Prevention

Two vaccines, meningococcal polysaccharide vaccine (MPSV4, indicated for vaccination of persons over age 55) and a conjugate vaccine (MCV4, indicated for persons aged 2–55 years) are effective for meningococcal groups A, C, Y, and W-135. The Advisory Committee on Immunization Practices recommends immunization with a single dose of MCV4 for preadolescents ages 11–12, and for those not previously vaccinated, upon entry into high school. MCV4 is also recommended for college freshmen—particularly those living in dormitories (see Tables 30–12 and 30–13). Vaccine is also recommended for military recruits, asplenic individuals, those with deficiencies in terminal component of complement, and exposed persons during outbreaks.

Eliminating nasopharyngeal carriage of meningococci is an effective prevention strategy in closed populations and to prevent secondary cases in household or otherwise close contacts. Rifampin, 600 mg orally twice a day for 2 days, ciprofloxacin, 500 mg orally once, or one intramuscular 250-mg dose of ceftriaxone is effective. A cluster of cases of fluoroquinolone-resistant meningococcal infections was recently identified in the United States. However, ciprofloxacin remains a recommended empiric agent for eradication of nasopharyngeal carriage. School and work contacts ordinarily need not be treated. Hospital contacts receive therapy only if intense exposure has occurred (eg, mouth-to-mouth resuscitation). Accidentally discovered carriers without known close contact with meningococcal disease do not require prophylactic antimicrobials.

Treatment

Blood cultures must be obtained and intravenous antimicrobial therapy started immediately. This may be done prior to lumbar puncture in patients in whom the diagnosis is not straightforward and for those in whom MR or CT imaging is indicated to exclude mass lesions. Aqueous penicillin G is the antibiotic of choice (24 million units/24 h intravenously in divided doses every 4 hours). The prevalence of strains of *N meningitidis* with intermediate resistance to penicillin in vitro (MICs 0.1 to 1 mcg/mL) is increasing, particularly in Europe. At what level of resistance penicillin treatment failure can occur is not known. Penicillin-intermediate strains thus far remain fully susceptible to ceftriaxone and other third-generation cephalosporins used to treat meningitis, and these should be effective alternatives to penicillin. In penicillin-allergic patients or those in whom *Haemophilus influenzae* or gram-negative meningitis is a consideration, ceftriaxone, 2 g intravenously every 12 hours, should be used. Treatment should be continued in full doses by the intravenous route until the patient is afebrile for 5 days. Shorter courses—as few as 4 days if ceftriaxone is used—are also effective.

Heckenberg SG et al. Clinical features, outcome, and meningococcal genotype in 258 adults with meningococcal meningitis: a prospective cohort study. Medicine (Baltimore). 2008 Jul;87(4):185–92. [PMID: 18626301]

Stephens DS et al. Epidemic meningitis, meningococcaemia, and *Neisseria meningitidis*. Lancet. 2007 Jun 30;369(9580):2196–210. [PMID: 17604802]

INFECTIONS CAUSED BY *HAEMOPHILUS* SPECIES

H influenzae and other *Haemophilus* species may cause sinusitis, otitis, bronchitis, epiglottitis, pneumonia, cellulitis, arthritis, meningitis, and endocarditis. Nontypeable strains are responsible for most disease in adults. Alcoholism, smoking, chronic lung disease, advanced age, and HIV infection are risk factors. *Haemophilus* species colonize the upper respiratory tract in patients with chronic obstructive pulmonary disease and frequently cause purulent bronchitis.

β-Lactamase-producing strains are less common in adults than in children. For adults with sinusitis, otitis, or respiratory tract infection, oral amoxicillin, 750 mg twice daily for 10–14 days, is adequate. For β-lactamase-producing strains, use of the oral fixed drug combination of amoxicillin, 875 mg, with clavulanate, 125 mg, is indicated. For the penicillin-allergic patient, oral cefuroxime axetil, 250 mg twice daily; trimethoprim-sulfamethoxazole, 800/160 mg orally twice daily; or a fluoroquinolone (ciprofloxacin, 500 mg orally twice daily; levofloxacin, 500 mg orally once daily; or moxifloxacin, 400 mg orally once daily) for 10 days is effective. Azithromycin and clarithromycin are less effective.

In the more seriously ill patient (eg, the toxic patient with multilobar pneumonia), ceftriaxone, 1 g/d intravenously is recommended pending determination of whether the infecting strain is a β-lactamase producer. Trimethoprim-sulfamethoxazole administered intravenously based on a dose of 10 mg/kg/d of trimethoprim or a fluoroquinolone (see above for dosages) can be used for the penicillin-allergic patient. A 10- to 14-day course of therapy is adequate for most cases.

Epiglottitis is characterized by an abrupt onset of high fever, drooling, and inability to handle secretions. An important clue to the diagnosis is complaint of a severe sore throat despite an unimpressive examination of the pharynx. Stridor and respiratory distress result from laryngeal obstruction. The diagnosis is best made by direct visualization of the cherry-red, swollen epiglottis at laryngoscopy. Because laryngoscopy may provoke laryngospasm and obstruction, especially in children, it should be performed in an intensive care unit or similar setting, and only at a time when intubation can be performed promptly. Ceftriaxone, 1 g intravenously every 24 hours for 7–10 days, is the drug of choice. Trimethoprim-sulfamethoxazole or a fluoroquinolone (see above for dosage) may be used in the patient with serious penicillin allergy.

Meningitis, rare in adults, is a consideration in the patient who has meningitis associated with sinusitis or otitis. Initial therapy for suspected *H influenzae* meningitis should be with ceftriaxone, 4 g/d in two divided doses, until the strain is proved not to produce β-lactamase. Meningitis is treated for 10–14 days. Dexamethasone, 0.15 mg/kg intravenously every 6 hours may reduce the incidence of long-term sequelae, principally hearing loss.

Tristam S et al. Antimicrobial resistance in *Haemophilus influenzae*. Clin Microbiol Rev. 2007 Apr;20(2):368–89. [PMID: 17428889]

INFECTIONS CAUSED BY *MORAXELLA CATARRHALIS*

M catarrhalis is a gram-negative aerobic coccus morphologically and biochemically similar to *Neisseria*. It causes sinusitis, bronchitis, and pneumonia. Bacteremia and meningitis have also been reported in immunocompromised patients. The organism frequently colonizes the respiratory tract, making differentiation of colonization from infection difficult. If *M catarrhalis* is the predominant isolate, therapy is directed against it. *M catarrhalis* typically produces β-lactamase and therefore is usually resistant to ampicillin and amoxicillin. It is susceptible to amoxicillin-clavulanate, ampicillin-sulbactam, trimethoprim-sulfamethoxazole, ciprofloxacin, and second- and third-generation cephalosporins.

Heininger N et al. A reservoir of *Moraxella catarrhalis* in human pharyngeal lymphoid tissue. J Infect Dis. 2007 Oct 1;196(7): 1080–7. [PMID: 17763332]

LEGIONNAIRES DISEASE

 ESSENTIALS OF DIAGNOSIS

▶ Patients are often immunocompromised, smokers, or have chronic lung disease.

▶ Scant sputum production, pleuritic chest pain, toxic appearance.

▶ Chest radiograph shows focal patchy infiltrates or consolidation.

▶ Gram stain of sputum shows polymorphonuclear leukocytes and no organisms.

▶ General Considerations

Legionella infection ranks among the three or four most common causes of community-acquired pneumonia and is considered whenever the etiology of a pneumonia is in question. Legionnaires disease is more common in immunocompromised persons, in smokers, and in those with chronic lung disease. Outbreaks have been associated with contaminated water sources, such as showerheads and faucets in patient rooms and air conditioning cooling towers.

▶ Clinical Findings

A. Symptoms and Signs

Legionnaires disease is one of the atypical pneumonias, so called because a Gram-stained smear of sputum does not show organisms. However, many features of Legionnaires disease are more like typical pneumonia, with high fevers, a toxic patient, pleurisy, and grossly purulent sputum. Classically, this pneumonia is caused by *Legionella pneumophila*, though other species can cause identical disease.

B. Laboratory Findings

Several laboratory abnormalities can be associated with Legionnaires disease, which include hyponatremia, elevated liver enzymes, and elevated creatine kinase. Culture of *Legionella* species onto charcoal-yeast extract agar or similar enriched medium is the most sensitive method (80–90% sensitivity) for diagnosis and permits identification of infections caused by species and serotypes other than *L pneumophila* serotype 1. Dieterle silver staining of tissue, pleural fluid, or other infected material is also a reliable method for detecting *Legionella* species. Direct fluorescent antibody stains and serologic testing are less sensitive because these will detect only *L pneumophila* serotype 1. In addition, making a serologic diagnosis requires that the host respond with sufficient specific antibody production. Urinary antigen tests, which are targeted for detection of *L pneumophila* serotype 1, are also less sensitive than culture.

▶ Treatment

Azithromycin (500 mg orally once daily), clarithromycin (500 mg orally twice daily), or a fluoroquinolone (eg, levofloxacin 500 mg orally once daily), and not erythromycin, are the drugs of choice for treatment of legionellosis because of their excellent intracellular penetration and in vitro activity, as well as desirable pharmacokinetic properties that permit oral administration and once or twice daily dosing. Duration of therapy is 10–14 days, although a 21-day course of therapy is recommended for immunocompromised patients.

Bartlett JG. Is activity against "atypical" pathogens necessary in the treatment protocols for community-acquired pneumonia? Issues with combination therapy. Clin Infect Dis. 2008 Dec 1;47(Suppl 3):S232–6. [PMID: 18986295]

Jacobson KL et al. *Legionella* pneumonia in cancer patients. Medicine (Baltimore). 2008 May;87(3):152–9. [PMID: 18520324]

GRAM-NEGATIVE BACTEREMIA & SEPSIS

Gram-negative bacteremia can originate in a number of sites, the most common being the genitourinary system, hepatobiliary tract, gastrointestinal tract, and lungs. Less common sources include intravenous lines, infusion fluids, surgical wounds, drains, and decubitus ulcers.

Patients with potentially fatal underlying conditions in the short term such as neutropenia or immunoparesis have a mortality rate of 40–60%; those with serious underlying diseases likely to be fatal in 5 years, such as solid tumors, cirrhosis, and aplastic anemia, die in 15–20% of cases; and individuals with no underlying diseases have a mortality rate of 5% or less.

▶ Clinical Findings

A. Symptoms and Signs

Most patients have fevers and chills, often with abrupt onset. However, 15% of patients are hypothermic (temperature ≤ 36.4 °C) at presentation, and 5% never develop a temperature above 37.5 °C. Hyperventilation with respiratory alkalosis and changes in mental status are important

early manifestations. Hypotension and shock, which occur in 20–50% of patients, are unfavorable prognostic signs.

B. Laboratory Findings

Neutropenia or neutrophilia, often with increased numbers of immature forms of polymorphonuclear leukocytes, is the most common laboratory abnormality in septic patients. Thrombocytopenia occurs in 50% of patients, laboratory evidence of coagulation abnormalities in 10%, and overt disseminated intravascular coagulation in 2–3%. Both clinical manifestations and the laboratory abnormalities are nonspecific and insensitive, which accounts for the relatively low rate of blood culture positivity (approximately 20–40%). If possible, three blood cultures from separate sites should be obtained in rapid succession before starting antimicrobial therapy. The chance of recovering the organism in at least one of the three blood cultures is greater than 95%. The false-negative rate for a single culture of 5–10 mL of blood is 30%. This may be reduced to 5–10% (albeit with a slight false-positive rate due to isolation of contaminants) if a single volume of 30 mL is inoculated into several blood culture bottles. Because blood cultures may be falsely negative, when a patient with presumed septic shock, negative blood cultures, and inadequate explanation for the clinical course responds to antimicrobials, therapy should be continued for 10–14 days.

▶ Treatment

Several factors are important in the management of patients with sepsis.

A. Removal of Predisposing Factors

This usually means decreasing or stopping immunosuppressive medications and in certain circumstances (eg, positive blood cultures) giving granulocyte colony-stimulating factor (filgrastim; G-CSF) to the neutropenic patient.

B. Identifying the Source of Bacteremia

By simply finding the source of bacteremia and removing it (intravenous line) or draining it (abscess), a fatal disease becomes easily treatable.

C. Supportive Measures

The use of fluids and pressors for maintaining blood pressure is discussed in Chapter 12; management of disseminated intravascular coagulation is discussed in Chapter 13.

D. Antibiotics

Antibiotics should be given as soon as the diagnosis is suspected, since delays in therapy have been associated with increased mortality rates, particularly once hypotension develops. In general, bactericidal antibiotics should be used and given intravenously to ensure therapeutic serum levels. Penetration of antibiotics into the site of primary infection is critical for successful therapy—ie, if the infection originates in the central nervous system, antibiotics that penetrate the blood-brain barrier should be used—eg, penicillin, ampicillin, chloramphenicol, and third-generation cephalosporins—but not first-generation cephalosporins or aminoglycosides, which penetrate poorly. Sepsis caused by gram-positive organisms cannot be differentiated on clinical grounds from that due to gram-negative bacteria. Therefore, initial therapy should include antibiotics active against both types of organisms.

The number of antibiotics necessary remains controversial and depends on the cause. Table 30–9 provides a guide for empiric therapy. Although a combination of antibiotics is often recommended for "synergism," combination therapy has not been shown to be superior to a single-drug regimen with any of several broad-spectrum antibiotics (eg, a third-generation cephalosporin, piperacillin-tazobactam, carbapenem). If multiple drugs are used initially, the regimen should be modified and coverage narrowed based on the results of culture and sensitivity testing.

E. Corticosteroids

The role of corticosteroids in treatment of septic shock is still quite controversial. Clinical data have suggested an association between mortality in patients with septic shock and poor adrenal reserve to cosyntropin (Cortrosyn) stimulation testing. Administration of "stress doses" of hydrocortisone to patients with relative adrenal insufficiency and pressor-dependent septic shock was shown to reduce mortality in earlier studies. However, the CORTICUS trial, the largest randomized control trial to evaluate the effect of stress-dose hydrocortisone on mortality in septic shock, refuted these earlier findings. This study failed to demonstrate a survival benefit from the addition of stress-dose hydrocortisone, 50 mg intravenously four times a day for 5 days followed by a 6-day tapering dose regimen, in subjects with or without a normal cosyntropin stimulation test. The usefulness of cosyntropin stimulation testing and use of stress-dose hydrocortisone in patients with septic shock are therefore not considered to be standard care.

F. Adjunctive Therapy

Expanded knowledge of the pathophysiology of sepsis and septic shock and recognition that cytokines play a critical role suggest novel approaches to therapy. Strategies include blocking the effects of endotoxin with anti-endotoxin monoclonal antibodies; blockade of TNF-α, a potent cytokine mediator of septic shock, with anti-TNF monoclonal antibody or soluble TNF receptor; use of IL-1 receptor antagonists to inhibit the proinflammatory effects of IL-1 binding to its receptor; use of corticosteroids; and blocking platelet or thrombin activation. None of these strategies have been met with improved survival. However, a single randomized placebo-controlled trial showed that recombinant human activated protein C (drotrecogin alfa) reduced mortality of septic patients with APACHE II scores $\geq$ 25, but the benefits of this agent remain controversial. This drug should be used cautiously because of the risk of bleeding. Drotrecogin alfa is not beneficial for patients with severe sepsis and low risk of death (eg, APACHE II score < 25 or single organ failure), and since it is associated with serious bleeding complications, it should not be used in these patients. Patients considered to have an

infectious cause of severe sepsis (defined as three or more signs of systemic inflammation—eg, fever or hypothermia, tachycardia, tachypnea—plus sepsis-induced dysfunction of at least one organ system) of less than 24 hours' duration are the best candidates. Platelet counts less than 30,000/mcL, conditions associated with an increased risk of bleeding (eg, recent trauma, surgery, or bleeding episode; anticoagulation), or hypercoagulable states have not been investigated. These criteria should be followed when selecting candidates for treatment with drotrecogin alfa (activated). The agent is administered intravenously by constant infusion at a dosage of 24 mcg/kg/h for 96 hours.

Dellinger RP et al. Surviving Sepsis Campaign: international guidelines for management of severe sepsis and septic shock: 2008. Crit Care Med. 2008 Jan;36(1):296–327. [PMID: 18158437]

Sprung CL et al. Hydrocortisone therapy for patients with septic shock. N Engl J Med. 2008 Jan 10;358(2):111–24. [PMID: 18184957]

SALMONELLOSIS

Salmonellosis includes infection by any of approximately 2000 serotypes of salmonellae. The taxonomy of *Salmonella* species has been confusing. All *Salmonella* serotypes are members of a single species, *Salmonella enterica*. Human infections are caused almost exclusively by *S enterica* subsp *enterica*, of which three serotypes—*typhi*, *typhimurium*, and *choleraesuis*—are predominantly isolated. Three clinical patterns of infection are recognized: (1) enteric fever, the best example of which is typhoid fever, due to serotype *typhi*; (2) acute enterocolitis, caused by serotype *typhimurium*, among others; and (3) the "septicemic" type, characterized by bacteremia and focal lesions, exemplified by infection with serotype *choleraesuis*. All types are transmitted by ingestion of the organism, usually from contaminated food or drink.

1. Enteric Fever (Typhoid Fever)

 ESSENTIALS OF DIAGNOSIS

► Gradual onset of malaise, headache, nausea, vomiting, abdominal pain.

► Rose spots, relative bradycardia, splenomegaly, and abdominal distention and tenderness.

► Slow (stepladder) rise of fever to maximum and then slow return to normal.

► Leukopenia; blood, stool, and urine culture positive for salmonella.

► General Considerations

Enteric fever is a clinical syndrome characterized by constitutional and gastrointestinal symptoms and by headache. It can be caused by any *Salmonella* species. The term "typhoid fever" applies when serotype *typhi* is the cause. Infection is transmitted by consumption of contaminated food or drink. The incubation period is 5–14 days. *Salmonella* is an intracellular pathogen. Infection begins when organisms breach the mucosal epithelium of the intestines by transcytosis, an organism-mediated transport process through the cell via an endocytic vesicle. Having crossed the epithelial barrier, organisms invade and replicate in macrophages in Peyer patches, mesenteric lymph nodes, and the spleen. Serotypes other than *typhi* usually do not cause invasive disease, presumably because they lack the necessary human-specific virulence factors. Bacteremia occurs, and the infection then localizes principally in the lymphoid tissue of the small intestine (particularly within 60 cm of the ileocecal valve). Peyer patches become inflamed and may ulcerate, with involvement greatest during the third week of disease. The organism may disseminate to the lungs, gallbladder, kidneys, or central nervous system.

Clinical Findings

A. Symptoms and Signs

During the prodromal stage, there is increasing malaise, headache, cough, and sore throat, often with abdominal pain and constipation, while the fever ascends in a stepwise fashion. After about 7–10 days, it reaches a plateau and the patient is much more ill, appearing exhausted and often prostrated. There may be marked constipation, especially early, or "pea soup" diarrhea; marked abdominal distention occurs as well. If there are no complications, the patient's condition will gradually improve over 7–10 days. However, relapse may occur for up to 2 weeks after defervescence.

During the early prodrome, physical findings are few. Later, splenomegaly, abdominal distention and tenderness, relative bradycardia, and occasionally meningismus appear. The rash (rose spots) commonly appears during the second week of disease. The individual spot, found principally on the trunk, is a pink papule 2–3 mm in diameter that fades on pressure. It disappears in 3–4 days.

B. Laboratory Findings

Typhoid fever is best diagnosed by blood culture, which is positive in the first week of illness in 80% of patients who have not taken antimicrobials. The rate of positivity declines thereafter, but one-fourth or more of patients still have positive blood cultures in the third week. Cultures of bone marrow occasionally are positive when blood cultures are not. Stool culture is unreliable because it may be positive in gastroenteritis without typhoid fever. Relative bradycardia and leukopenia are typical.

Differential Diagnosis

Enteric fever must be distinguished from other gastrointestinal illnesses and from other infections that have few localizing findings. Examples include tuberculosis, infective endocarditis, brucellosis, lymphoma, and Q fever. Often there is a history of recent travel to endemic areas, and viral hepatitis, malaria, or amebiasis may be in the differential as well.

Complications

Complications occur in about 30% of untreated cases and account for 75% of deaths. Intestinal hemorrhage, mani-

fested by a sudden drop in temperature and signs of shock followed by dark or fresh blood in the stool, or intestinal perforation, accompanied by abdominal pain and tenderness, is most likely to occur during the third week. Appearance of leukocytosis and tachycardia should suggest these complications. Urinary retention, pneumonia, thrombophlebitis, myocarditis, psychosis, cholecystitis, nephritis, osteomyelitis, and meningitis are less often observed.

Prevention

Immunization is not always effective but should be considered for household contacts of a typhoid carrier, for travelers to endemic areas, and during epidemic outbreaks. A multiple-dose oral vaccine and a single-dose parenteral vaccine are available. Their efficacies are similar, but oral vaccine causes fewer side effects. Boosters, when indicated, should be given every 5 years and 2 years for oral and parenteral preparations, respectively.

Adequate waste disposal and protection of food and water supplies from contamination are important public health measures to prevent salmonellosis. Carriers cannot work as food handlers.

Treatment

A. Specific Measures

Several antibiotics, including ampicillin, azithromycin, chloramphenicol, third-generation cephalosporins, and trimethoprim-sulfamethoxazole all are effective for treatment of enteric fever caused by drug-susceptible strains. These drugs can be given orally or intravenously depending on the patient's condition. Because many salmonella strains are resistant to ampicillin, chloramphenicol, and trimethoprim-sulfamethoxazole, a fluoroquinolone—such as ciprofloxacin 750 mg orally twice daily or levofloxacin 500 mg orally once daily, 5–7 days for uncomplicated enteric fever and 10–14 days for severe infection—is the agent of choice for treatment of salmonella infections. Ceftriaxone, 2 g intravenously for 7 days, is also effective. Although resistance to fluoroquinolones or cephalosporins occurs uncommonly, the prevalence appears to be increasing. When an infection is caused by a multidrug-resistant strain, select an antibiotic to which the isolate is susceptible in vitro. Alternatively, increasing the dose of ceftriaxone to 4 g/d and treating for 10–14 days or using azithromycin 500 mg orally for 7 days in uncomplicated cases may be effective.

B. Treatment of Carriers

Chemotherapy often is unsuccessful in eradicating the carrier state. While treatment of carriage with ampicillin, trimethoprim-sulfamethoxazole, or chloramphenicol may be successful, ciprofloxacin, 750 mg orally twice a day for 4 weeks, has proved to be highly effective. Cholecystectomy may also achieve this goal.

Prognosis

The mortality rate of typhoid fever is about 2% in treated cases. Elderly or debilitated persons are likely to do poorly.

With complications, the prognosis is poor. Relapses occur in up to 15% of cases. A residual carrier state frequently persists in spite of chemotherapy.

Fraser A et al. Vaccines for preventing typhoid fever. Cochrane Database Syst Rev. 2007 Jul 18;(3):CD001261. [PMID: 17636661]

Parry CM et al. A randomised controlled comparison of ofloxacin, azithromycin and an ofloxacin-azithromycin combination for treatment of multidrug-resistant and nalidixic acid resistant typhoid fever. Antimicrob Agents Chemother. 2007 Mar;51(3):819–25. [PMID: 17145784]

2. *Salmonella* Gastroenteritis

By far the most common form of salmonellosis is acute enterocolitis caused by numerous *Salmonella* serotypes. The incubation period is 8–48 hours after ingestion of contaminated food or liquid.

Symptoms and signs consist of fever (often with chills), nausea and vomiting, cramping abdominal pain, and diarrhea, which may be grossly bloody, lasting 3–5 days. Differentiation must be made from viral gastroenteritis, food poisoning, shigellosis, amebic dysentery, and acute ulcerative colitis. The diagnosis is made by culturing the organism from the stool.

The disease is usually self-limited, but bacteremia with localization in joints or bones may occur, especially in patients with sickle cell disease.

Treatment of uncomplicated enterocolitis is symptomatic only. Malnourished or severely ill patients, those with sickle cell disease, and HIV-positive patients should be treated for 3–5 days with trimethoprim-sulfamethoxazole (one double-strength tablet twice a day), ampicillin (100 mg/kg intravenously or orally), or ciprofloxacin (750 mg orally twice a day).

Swanson SJ et al. Multidrug-resistant *Salmonella enterica* serotype *Typhimurium* associated with pet rodents. N Engl J Med. 2007 Jan 4;356(1):21–8. [PMID: 17202452]

3. *Salmonella* Bacteremia

Salmonella infection may be manifested by prolonged or recurrent fevers accompanied by bacteremia and local infection in bone, joints, pleura, pericardium, lungs, or other sites. Mycotic abdominal aortic aneurysms may also occur. Serotypes other than typhi usually are isolated. This complication tends to occur in immunocompromised persons and is seen in HIV-infected individuals, who typically have bacteremia without an obvious source. Treatment is the same as for typhoid fever, plus drainage of any abscesses. In HIV-infected patients, relapse is common, and lifelong suppressive therapy may be needed. Ciprofloxacin, 750 mg orally twice a day, is effective both for therapy of acute infection and for suppression of recurrence. Incidence of infections caused by drug-resistant strains may be on the rise.

SHIGELLOSIS

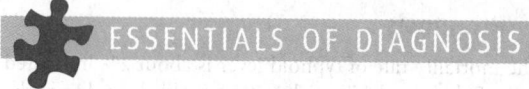

▶ Diarrhea, often with blood and mucus.

▶ Crampy abdominal pain and systemic toxicity.

▶ White blood cells in stools; organism isolated on stool culture.

General Considerations

Shigella dysentery is a common disease, often self-limited and mild but occasionally serious. *Shigella sonnei* is the leading cause in the United States, followed by *Shigella flexneri*. *Shigella dysenteriae* causes the most serious form of the illness. Shigellae are invasive organisms. The infective dose is 10^2–10^3 organisms. There has been a rise in strains resistant to multiple antibiotics.

Clinical Findings

A. Symptoms and Signs

The illness usually starts abruptly, with diarrhea, lower abdominal cramps, and tenesmus. The diarrheal stool often is mixed with blood and mucus. Systemic symptoms are fever, chills, anorexia and malaise, and headache. The abdomen is tender. Sigmoidoscopic examination reveals an inflamed, engorged mucosa with punctate and sometimes large areas of ulceration.

B. Laboratory Findings

The stool shows many leukocytes and red cells. Stool culture is positive for shigellae in most cases, but blood cultures grow the organism in less than 5% of cases.

Differential Diagnosis

Bacillary dysentery must be distinguished from salmonella enterocolitis and from disease due to enterotoxigenic *Escherichia coli*, *Campylobacter*, and *Yersinia enterocolitica*. Amebic dysentery may be similar clinically and is diagnosed by finding amebas in the fresh stool specimen. Ulcerative colitis is also an important cause of bloody diarrhea.

Complications

Temporary disaccharidase deficiency may follow the diarrhea. Reactive arthritis is an uncommon complication, usually occurring in HLA-B27 individuals infected by *Shigella*. Hemolytic-uremic syndrome occurs rarely.

Treatment

Treatment of dehydration and hypotension is lifesaving in severe cases. The antimicrobial treatments of choice are trimethoprim-sulfamethoxazole, one double-strength tablet twice a day for 7–10 days, or a fluoroquinolone (ciprofloxacin 750 mg orally twice daily for 7–10 days, or levofloxacin, 500 mg orally once daily) for 3 days. Fluoroquinolones are contraindicated in pregnancy. Shigellae resistant to ampicillin are common, but if the isolate is susceptible, a dose of 500 mg orally four times a day is also effective. Amoxicillin, which is less effective, should not be used.

Aragón TJ et al. Case-control study of shigellosis in San Francisco: the role of sexual transmission and HIV infection. Clin Infect Dis. 2007 Feb 1;44(3):327–34. [PMID: 17205436]

GASTROENTERITIS CAUSED BY *ESCHERICHIA COLI*

E coli causes gastroenteritis by a variety of mechanisms. Enterotoxigenic *E coli* (ETEC) elaborates either a heat-stable or heat-labile toxin that mediates the disease. ETEC is an important cause of traveler's diarrhea. Enteroinvasive *E coli* (EIEC) differs from other *E coli* bowel pathogens in that these strains invade cells, causing bloody diarrhea and dysentery similar to infection with *Shigella* species. EIEC is uncommon in the United States. Neither ETEC nor EIEC strains are routinely isolated and identified from stool cultures because there is no selective medium. Antimicrobial therapy directed against *Salmonella* and *Shigella* shortens the clinical course, but the disease is self-limited.

Enterohemorrhagic *E coli* (EHEC) produces two shiga-like toxins that mediate the clinical manifestations, which include an asymptomatic carriage stage, nonbloody diarrhea, hemorrhagic colitis, hemolytic-uremic syndrome, and thrombotic thrombocytopenic purpura. Although there are several serotypes of EHEC, O157:H7 is responsible for most cases in the United States. *E coli* O157:H7 has caused several outbreaks of diarrhea and hemolytic-uremic syndrome related to consumption of undercooked hamburger and unpasteurized apple juice. Older individuals and young children are most affected, with hemolytic-uremic syndrome being more common in the latter group. *E coli* O157:H7 is not identified by routine stool cultures. Isolation requires identification of sorbitol-negative colonies of *E coli* on sorbitol-MacConkey agar followed by serologic testing to confirm the serotype. Antimicrobial therapy does not alter the course of the disease, and may increase the risk of hemolytic-uremic syndrome. Treatment is primarily supportive. Hemolytic-uremic syndrome or thrombotic thrombocytopenic purpura occurring in association with a diarrheal illness suggests the diagnosis and should prompt evaluation for EHEC. Confirmed infections should be reported to public health officials.

Riddle MS. Effect of adjunctive loperamide in combination with antibiotics on treatment outcomes in traveler's diarrhea: a systematic review and meta-analysis. Clin Infect Dis. 2008 Oct 15;47(8):1007–14. [PMID: 18781873]

Serna A 4th et al. Pathogenesis and treatment of Shiga toxin-producing *Escherichia coli* infections. Curr Opin Gastroenterol. 2008 Jan;24(1):38–47. [PMID: 18043231]

CHOLERA

ESSENTIALS OF DIAGNOSIS

▶ History of travel in endemic area or contact with infected person.

▶ Voluminous diarrhea.

▶ Stool is liquid, gray, turbid, and without fecal odor, blood, or pus ("rice water stool").

▶ Rapid development of marked dehydration.

▶ Positive stool cultures and agglutination of vibrios with specific sera.

▶ General Considerations

Cholera is an acute diarrheal illness caused by certain serotypes of *Vibrio cholerae*. The disease is toxin-mediated, and fever is unusual. The toxin activates adenylyl cyclase in intestinal epithelial cells of the small intestines, producing hypersecretion of water and chloride ion and a massive diarrhea of up to 15 L/d. Death results from profound hypovolemia.

Cholera occurs in epidemics under conditions of crowding, war, and famine (eg, in refugee camps) and where sanitation is inadequate. Infection is acquired by ingestion of contaminated food or water. Cholera was rarely seen in the United States until 1991, when epidemic cholera returned to the Western Hemisphere, originating as an outbreak in coastal cities of Peru. The epidemic spread to involve several countries in South and Central America as well as Mexico, and cases have been imported into the United States. Cholera should be considered in the differential diagnosis of severe watery diarrhea, especially in those who have traveled to affected countries.

▶ Clinical Findings

Cholera is characterized by a sudden onset of severe, frequent watery diarrhea (up to 1 L/h). The liquid stool is gray; turbid; and without fecal odor, blood, or pus ("rice water stool"). Dehydration and hypotension develop rapidly. Stool cultures are positive, and agglutination of vibrios with specific sera can be demonstrated.

▶ Prevention

A vaccine is available that confers short-lived, limited protection and may be required for entry into or reentry after travel to some countries. It is administered in two doses 1–4 weeks apart. A booster dose every 6 months is recommended for persons remaining in areas where cholera is a hazard.

Vaccination programs are expensive and not particularly effective in managing outbreaks of cholera. When outbreaks occur, efforts should be directed toward establishing clean water and food sources and proper waste disposal.

▶ Treatment

Treatment is by replacement of fluids. In mild or moderate illness, oral rehydration usually is adequate. A simple oral replacement fluid can be made from 1 teaspoon of table salt and 4 heaping teaspoons of sugar added to 1 L of water. Intravenous fluids are indicated for persons with signs of severe hypovolemia and those who cannot take adequate fluids orally. Lactated Ringer infusion is satisfactory.

Antimicrobial therapy will shorten the course of illness. Several antimicrobials are active against *V cholerae*, including tetracycline, ampicillin, chloramphenicol, trimethoprim-sulfamethoxazole, fluoroquinolones, and azithromycin. Multiple drug-resistant strains are increasingly encountered, so susceptibility testing, if available, is advisable. A single 1 g oral dose of azithromycin was effective for severe cholera caused by strains with reduced susceptibility to fluoroquinolones, but resistance is emerging to this drug as well.

Tobin-D'Angelo M et al. Severe diarrhea caused by cholera toxin-producing *Vibrio cholerae* serogroup O75 infections acquired in the southeastern United States. Clin Infect Dis. 2008 Oct 15;47(8):1035–40. [PMID: 18781876]

Zuckerman JN et al. The true burden and risk of cholera: implications for prevention and control. Lancet Infect Dis. 2007 Aug;7(8):521–30. [PMID: 17584531]

INFECTIONS CAUSED BY OTHER *VIBRIO* SPECIES

Vibrios other than *V cholerae* that cause human disease are *Vibrio parahaemolyticus*, *Vibrio vulnificus*, and *Vibrio alginolyticus*. All are halophilic marine organisms. Infection is acquired by exposure to organisms in contaminated, undercooked, or raw crustaceans or shellfish and warm (> 20 °C) ocean waters and estuaries. Infections are more common during the summer months from regions along the Atlantic coast and the Gulf of Mexico in the United States and from tropical waters around the world. Oysters are implicated in up to 90% of food-related cases. *V parahaemolyticus* causes an acute watery diarrhea with crampy abdominal pain and fever, typically occurring within 24 hours after ingestion of contaminated shellfish. The disease is self-limited, and antimicrobial therapy is usually not necessary. *V parahaemolyticus* may also cause cellulitis and sepsis, though these findings are more characteristic of *V vulnificus* infection.

V vulnificus and *V alginolyticus*—neither of which is associated with diarrheal illness—are important causes of cellulitis and primary bacteremia following ingestion of contaminated shellfish or exposure to sea water. Cellulitis with or without sepsis may be accompanied by bulla formation and necrosis with extensive soft tissue destruction, at times requiring debridement and amputation. The infection can be rapidly progressive and is particularly severe in immunocompromised individuals—especially those with cirrhosis—with death rates as high as 50%. Patients with chronic liver disease and those who are immunocompromised should be cautioned to avoid eating raw oysters.

Tetracycline at a dose of 500 mg orally four times a day for 7–10 days is the drug of choice for treatment of suspected or documented primary bacteremia or cellulitis caused by *Vibrio* species. *V vulnificus* is susceptible in vitro to penicillin, ampicillin, cephalosporins, chloramphenicol, aminoglycosides, and fluoroquinolones, and these agents may also be effective. *V parahaemolyticus* and *V alginolyticus* produce β-lactamase and therefore are resistant to penicillin and ampicillin, but susceptibilities otherwise are similar to those listed for *V vulnificus*.

Bross MH et al. *Vibrio vulnificus* infection: diagnosis and treatment. Am Fam Physician. 2007 Aug 15;76(4):539–44. [PMID: 17853628]

Dechet AM. Nonfoodborne *Vibrio* infections: an important cause of morbidity and mortality in the United States, 1997–2006. Clin Infect Dis. 2008 Apr 1;46(7):970–6. [PMID: 18444811]

INFECTIONS CAUSED BY *CAMPYLOBACTER* SPECIES

Campylobacter organisms are microaerophilic, motile, gram-negative rods. Two species infect humans: *Campylo-*bacter jejuni*, an important cause of diarrheal disease, and *Campylobacter fetus* subsp *fetus*, which typically causes systemic infection and not diarrhea. Dairy cattle and poultry are an important reservoir for campylobacters. Outbreaks of enteritis have been associated with consumption of raw milk. Campylobacter gastroenteritis is associated with fever, abdominal pain, and diarrhea characterized by loose, watery, or bloody stools. The differential diagnosis includes shigellosis, *Salmonella* gastroenteritis, and enteritis caused by *Y enterocolitica* or invasive *E coli*. The disease is self-limited, but its duration can be shortened with antimicrobial therapy. Either azithromycin, 1 g orally as a single dose, or ciprofloxacin, 500 mg orally twice daily for 3 days, is effective therapy. However, fluoroquinolone resistance among *C jejuni* isolates has been increasing and susceptibility testing should be routinely performed.

C fetus causes systemic infections that can be fatal, including primary bacteremia, endocarditis, meningitis, and focal abscesses. It infrequently causes gastroenteritis. Patients infected with *C fetus* are often older, debilitated, or immunocompromised. Closely related species, collectively termed "campylobacter-like organisms," cause bacteremia in HIV-infected individuals. Systemic infections respond to therapy with gentamicin, chloramphenicol, ceftriaxone, or ciprofloxacin. Ceftriaxone or chloramphenicol should be used to treat infections of the central nervous system because of their ability to penetrate the blood-brain barrier.

Alfredson DA et al. Antibiotic resistance and resistance mechanisms in *Campylobacter jejuni* and *Campylobacter coli*. FEMS Microbiol Lett. 2007 Dec;277(2):123–32. [PMID: 18031331]

Gazaigne L et al. Campylobacter fetus bloodstream infection: risk factors and clinical features. Eur J Clin Microbiol Infect Dis. 2008 Mar;27(3):185–9. [PMID: 17999095]

BRUCELLOSIS

 ESSENTIALS OF DIAGNOSIS

▶ History of animal exposure, ingestion of unpasteurized milk or cheese.

▶ Insidious onset: easy fatigability, headache, arthralgia, anorexia, sweating, irritability.

▶ Intermittent and persistent fever.

▶ Cervical and axillary lymphadenopathy; hepatosplenomegaly.

▶ Lymphocytosis, positive blood culture, positive serologic test.

▶ General Considerations

The infection is transmitted from animals to humans. *Brucella abortus* (cattle), *Brucella suis* (hogs), and *Brucella melitensis* (goats) are the main agents. Transmission to humans occurs by contact with infected meat (slaughterhouse workers), placentae of infected animals (farmers, veterinarians), or ingestion of infected unpasteurized milk or cheese. The incubation period varies from a few days to several weeks. Brucellosis is a systemic infection that may become chronic. In the United States, brucellosis is very rare. Almost all US cases are imported from countries where brucellosis is endemic (eg, Mexico, Mediterranean Europe, Spain, South American countries).

Clinical Findings

A. Symptoms and Signs

The onset may be acute, with fever, chills, and sweats, but more often is insidious with symptoms of weakness, weight loss, low-grade fevers, sweats, and exhaustion upon minimal activity. Headache, abdominal or back pain with anorexia and constipation, and arthralgias are also common. The chronic form may assume an undulant nature, with periods of normal temperature between acute attacks; symptoms may persist for years, either continuously or intermittently.

Fever, hepatosplenomegaly, and lymphadenopathy are the most common physical findings. Infection may present with or be complicated by specific organ involvement with signs of endocarditis, meningitis, epididymitis, orchitis, arthritis (especially sacroiliitis), spondylitis, or osteomyelitis.

B. Laboratory Findings

The organism can be recovered from cultures of blood, cerebrospinal fluid, urine, bone marrow, or other sites. Modern automated systems have shortened the time to detection of the organism in blood culture. Cultures are more likely to be negative in chronic cases. The diagnosis often is made by serologic testing. Rising serologic titers or an absolute agglutination titer of greater than 1:160 supports the diagnosis.

Differential Diagnosis

Brucellosis must be differentiated from any other acute febrile disease, especially influenza, tularemia, Q fever, mononucleosis, and enteric fever. In its chronic form it resembles Hodgkin disease, tuberculosis, HIV infection, malaria, and disseminated fungal infections such as histoplasmosis and coccidioidomycosis.

Complications

The most frequent complications are bone and joint lesions such as spondylitis and suppurative arthritis (usually of a single joint), endocarditis, and meningoencephalitis. Less common complications are pneumonitis with pleural effusion, hepatitis, and cholecystitis.

Treatment

Single-drug regimens are not recommended because the relapse rate may be as high as 50%. Combination regimens of two or three drugs are most effective. Regimens of doxycycline (200 mg/d orally for 6 weeks) plus rifampin (600 mg/d orally for 6 weeks) or streptomycin (1 g/d intramuscularly for 2 weeks) or gentamicin (240 mg intramuscularly once daily for 7 days) have the lowest recurrence

rates. Longer courses of therapy may be required to prevent relapse of meningitis, osteomyelitis, or endocarditis.

Franco MP et al. Human brucellosis. Lancet Infect Dis. 2007 Dec;7(12):775–86. [PMID: 18045560]

Skalsky K et al. Treatment of human brucellosis: systematic review and meta-analysis of randomised controlled trials. BMJ. 2008 Mar 29;336(7646):701–4. [PMID: 18321957]

TULAREMIA

ESSENTIALS OF DIAGNOSIS

- History of contact with rabbits, other rodents, and biting arthropods (eg, ticks in summer) in endemic area.
- Fever, headache, nausea, and prostration.
- Papule progressing to ulcer at site of inoculation.
- Enlarged regional lymph nodes.
- Serologic tests or culture of ulcer, lymph node aspirate, or blood confirm the diagnosis.

General Considerations

Tularemia is a zoonotic infection of wild rodents and rabbits caused by *Francisella tularensis*. Humans usually acquire the infection by contact with animal tissues (eg, trapping muskrats, skinning rabbits) or from a tick or insect bite. Hamsters and prairie dogs also may carry the organism. An investigation of an outbreak of pneumonic tularemia on Martha's Vineyard in Massachusetts implicated lawn-mowing and brush-cutting as risk factors for infection, underscoring the potential for probable aerosol transmission of the organism. *F tularensis* has been classified as a high-priority agent for potential bioterrorism use because of its virulence and relative ease of dissemination. Infection in humans often produces a local lesion and widespread organ involvement but may be entirely asymptomatic. The incubation period is 2–10 days.

Clinical Findings

A. Symptoms and Signs

Fever, headache, and nausea begin suddenly, and a local lesion—a papule at the site of inoculation—develops and soon ulcerates. Regional lymph nodes may become enlarged and tender and may suppurate. The local lesion may be on the skin of an extremity or in the eye. Pneumonia may develop from hematogenous spread of the organism or may be primary after inhalation of infected aerosols, which are responsible for human-to-human transmission. Following ingestion of infected meat or water, an enteric form may be manifested by gastrointestinal symptoms, stupor, and delirium. In any type of involvement, the spleen may be enlarged and tender and there may be nonspecific rashes, myalgias, and prostration.

B. Laboratory Findings

Culturing the organism from blood or infected tissue requires special media. For this reason and because cultures of *F tularensis* may be hazardous to laboratory personnel, the diagnosis is usually made serologically. A positive agglutination test (> 1:80) develops in the second week after infection and may persist for several years.

Differential Diagnosis

Tularemia must be differentiated from rickettsial and meningococcal infections, cat-scratch disease, infectious mononucleosis, and various bacterial and fungal diseases.

Complications

Hematogenous spread may produce meningitis, perisplenitis, pericarditis, pneumonia, and osteomyelitis.

Treatment

Streptomycin is drug of choice for treatment of tularemia. The recommended dose is 7.5 mg/kg intramuscularly every 12 hours for 7–14 days. Gentamicin, which has good in vitro activity against *F tularensis*, is generally less toxic than streptomycin and probably just as effective. Doxycycline (200 mg/d orally) is also effective but has a higher relapse rate. A variety of other agents (eg, fluoroquinolones) are active in vitro but their clinical effectiveness is less well established.

Hepburn MJ et al. Tularemia: current diagnosis and treatment options. Expert Rev Anti Infect Ther. 2008 Apr;6(2):231–40. [PMID: 18380605]

Nigrovic LE et al. Tularemia. Infect Dis Clin North Am. 2008 Sep;22(3):489–504. [PMID: 18755386]

PLAGUE

ESSENTIALS OF DIAGNOSIS

▶ History of exposure to rodents in endemic area.

▶ Sudden onset of high fever, malaise, muscular pains, and prostration.

▶ Axillary or inguinal lymphadenitis (bubo).

▶ Bacteremia, pneumonitis, and meningitis may occur.

▶ Positive smear and culture from bubo and positive blood culture.

General Considerations

Plague is an infection of wild rodents with *Yersinia pestis*, a small bipolar-staining gram-negative rod. It is endemic in California, Arizona, Nevada, and New Mexico. It is transmitted among rodents and to humans by the bites of fleas or from contact with infected animals. Following a fleabite, the organisms spread through the lymphatics to the lymph nodes, which become greatly enlarged (bubo). They may then reach the bloodstream to involve all organs. When pneumonia or meningitis develops, the outcome is often fatal. The patient with pneumonia can transmit the infection to other individuals by droplets. The incubation

period is 2–10 days. Because of its extreme virulence, its potential for dissemination and person-to-person transmission, and efforts to develop the organism as an agent of biowarfare, plague bacillus is considered a high-priority agent for bioterrorism.

Clinical Findings

A. Symptoms and Signs

The onset is sudden, with high fever, malaise, tachycardia, intense headache, delirium, and severe myalgias. The patient appears profoundly ill. If pneumonia develops, tachypnea, productive cough, blood-tinged sputum, and cyanosis also occur. There may be signs of meningitis. A pustule or ulcer at the site of inoculation and lymphangitis may be observed. Axillary, inguinal, or cervical lymph nodes become enlarged and tender and may suppurate and drain. With hematogenous spread, the patient may rapidly become toxic and comatose, with purpuric spots (black plague) appearing on the skin.

Primary plague pneumonia is a fulminant pneumonitis with bloody, frothy sputum and sepsis. It is usually fatal unless treatment is started within a few hours after onset.

B. Laboratory Findings

The plague bacillus may be found in smears from aspirates of buboes examined with Gram stain. Cultures from bubo aspirate or pus and blood are positive but may grow slowly. In convalescing patients, an antibody titer rise may be demonstrated by agglutination tests.

Differential Diagnosis

The lymphadenitis of plague is most commonly mistaken for the lymphadenitis accompanying staphylococcal or streptococcal infections of an extremity, sexually transmitted diseases such as lymphogranuloma venereum or syphilis, and tularemia. The systemic manifestations resemble those of enteric or rickettsial fevers, malaria, or influenza. The pneumonia resembles other bacterial pneumonias, and the meningitis is similar to those caused by other bacteria.

Prevention

Drug prophylaxis may provide temporary protection for persons exposed to the risk of plague infection, particularly by the respiratory route. Tetracycline hydrochloride, 500 mg orally once or twice daily for 5 days, is effective.

Plague vaccines—both live and killed—have been used for many years, but their efficacy is not clearly established.

Treatment

Therapy should be started immediately once plague is suspected. Either streptomycin (the agent with which there is greatest experience), 1 g every 12 hours intravenously, or gentamicin, administered as a 2-mg/kg loading dose, then 1.7 mg/kg every 8 hours intravenously, is effective. Alternatively, doxycycline, 100 mg orally or intravenously, may be used. The duration of therapy is 10 days. Patients with plague pneumonia are placed in strict respiratory isolation, and prophylactic therapy is given to any person who came in contact with the patient.

Prentice MB et al. Plague. Lancet. 2007 Apr 7;369(9568):1196–207. [PMID: 17416264]
Stenseth NC et al. Plague: past, present, and future. PLoS Med. 2008 Jan 15;5(1):e3. [PMID: 18198939]

GONOCOCCAL INFECTIONS

ESSENTIALS OF DIAGNOSIS

▶ Purulent and profuse urethral discharge, especially in men, with dysuria, yielding positive smear.

▶ Epididymitis, prostatitis, periurethral inflammation, proctitis in men.

▶ Cervicitis in women with purulent discharge, or asymptomatic, yielding positive culture; vaginitis, salpingitis, proctitis also occur.

▶ Fever, rash, tenosynovitis, and arthritis with disseminated disease.

▶ Gram-negative intracellular diplococci seen in a smear or cultured from any site, particularly the urethra, cervix, pharynx, and rectum.

General Considerations

Gonorrhea is caused by *Neisseria gonorrhoeae*, a gram-negative diplococcus typically found inside polymorphonuclear cells. It is transmitted during sexual activity and has its greatest incidence in the 15- to 29-year-old age group. The incubation period is usually 2–8 days.

Classification

A. Urethritis and Cervicitis

In men, there is initially burning on urination and a serous or milky discharge. One to 3 days later, the urethral pain is more pronounced and the discharge becomes yellow, creamy, and profuse, sometimes blood-tinged. The disorder may regress and become chronic or progress to involve the prostate, epididymis, and periurethral glands with painful inflammation. Chronic infection leads to prostatitis and urethral strictures. Rectal infection is common in homosexual men. Atypical sites of primary infection (eg, the pharynx) must always be considered. Asymptomatic infection is common and occurs in both sexes.

Gonococcal infection in women often becomes symptomatic during menses. Women may have dysuria, urinary frequency, and urgency, with a purulent urethral discharge. Vaginitis and cervicitis with inflammation of Bartholin glands are common. Infection may be asymptomatic, with only slightly increased vaginal discharge and moderate cervicitis on examination. Infection may remain as a chronic cervicitis—an important reservoir of gonococci. It can progress to involve the uterus and tubes with acute and chronic salpingitis, with scarring of tubes and sterility. In pelvic inflammatory disease, anaerobes and chlamydiae often accompany gonococci. Rectal infection may result from spread of the organism from the genital tract or from anal coitus.

Gram stain of urethral discharge in men, especially during the first week after onset, shows gram-negative diplococci in polymorphonuclear leukocytes. Gram stain is less often positive in women. Culture has been the gold standard for diagnosis, particularly when the Gram stain is negative. Nucleic acid amplification tests for *N gonorrhoeae* in cervical and urethral swab specimens and urine permit rapid diagnosis, have excellent sensitivity and specificity, and have largely replaced culture. Identification of *N gonorrhoeae* from rectal or pharyngeal sites, blood, and in joint fluid still requires culture.

B. Disseminated Disease

Systemic complications follow the dissemination of gonococci from the primary site via the bloodstream. Gonococcal bacteremia is associated with intermittent fever, arthralgia, and skin lesions ranging from maculopapular to pustular or hemorrhagic, which tend to be few in number and peripherally located. Rarely, gonococcal endocarditis or meningitis develops. Arthritis and tenosynovitis are common complications, particularly involving the knees, ankles, and wrists. One or occasionally a few joints usually are involved. Gonococci are isolated by culture from less than half of patients with gonococcal arthritis.

C. Conjunctivitis

The most common form of eye involvement is direct inoculation of gonococci into the conjunctival sac. In adults, this occurs by autoinoculation of a person with genital infection. The purulent conjunctivitis may rapidly progress to panophthalmitis and loss of the eye unless treated promptly. A single 1-g dose of ceftriaxone is effective.

Differential Diagnosis

Gonococcal urethritis or cervicitis must be differentiated from nongonococcal urethritis; cervicitis or vaginitis due to *Chlamydia trachomatis*, *Gardnerella vaginalis*, *Trichomonas*, *Candida*, and many other pathogens associated with sexually transmitted diseases; and pelvic inflammatory disease, arthritis, proctitis, and skin lesions. Often, several such pathogens coexist in a patient. Reactive arthritis (urethritis, conjunctivitis, arthritis) may mimic gonorrhea or coexist with it.

Prevention

Prevention is based on education and mechanical or chemical prophylaxis. The condom, if properly used, can reduce the risk of infection. Effective drugs taken in therapeutic doses within 24 hours of exposure can abort an infection. Partner notification and referral of contacts for treatment has been the standard method used to control sexually transmitted diseases. Expedited treatment of sex partners by patient-delivered partner therapy is more effective than partner notification in reducing persistence and recurrence rates of gonorrhea and chlamydia. This strategy is being increasingly adopted as a means of disease control.

▶ Treatment

Therapy typically is administered before antimicrobial susceptibilities are known. The choice of which regimen to use should be based on the national prevalences of antibiotic-resistant organisms. Nationwide, strains of gonococci that are resistant to penicillin, tetracycline, or ciprofloxacin have been increasingly observed. Consequently, these drugs can no longer be considered first-line therapy. All sexual partners should be treated and tested for HIV infection and syphilis, as should the patient.

A. Uncomplicated Gonorrhea

For uncomplicated gonococcal infections of the cervix, urethra, and rectum, either ceftriaxone (125 mg intramuscularly) or cefixime (400 mg orally as a single dose) is the treatment of choice. Fluoroquinolones are no longer recommended because of high rates of resistance. Spectinomycin, 1 g intramuscularly once, may be used for the penicillin-allergic patient but is not currently available in the United States. Other single-dose cephalosporin therapies that are considered alternative treatment regimens for uncomplicated urogenital and anorectal gonococcal infections include ceftizoxime, 500 mg intramuscularly once; or cefoxitin, 2 g intramuscularly once, administered with probenecid, 1 g orally; or cefotaxime, 500 mg intramuscularly once. Some evidence indicates that single-dose cefpodoxime, 400 mg and cefuroxime axetil, 1 g might be oral alternatives.

Pharyngeal gonorrhea is treated by ceftriaxone, 125 mg intramuscularly. Since coexistent chlamydial infection is common, doxycycline, 100 mg orally twice daily for 7 days, or azithromycin, given as a single 1-g oral dose, concurrently, should be administered unless chlamydial infection has been ruled out with a negative nucleic acid amplification test for *C trachomatis;* women should have a pregnancy test before a tetracycline (such as doxycycline) is prescribed.

B. Treatment of Other Infections

Disseminated gonococcal infection should be treated with ceftriaxone, 1 g intravenously daily, until 48 hours after improvement begins, at which time therapy may be switched to cefixime, 400 mg orally daily to complete at least 1 week of antimicrobial therapy. An oral fluoroquinolone (ciprofloxacin, 500 mg twice daily, or levofloxacin, 500 mg once daily) for 7 days also is effective, provided the isolate is susceptible. Endocarditis should be treated with ceftriaxone, 2 g every 24 hours intravenously, for at least 3 weeks. Postgonococcal urethritis and cervicitis, which are usually caused by chlamydia, are treated with a regimen of erythromycin, doxycycline, or azithromycin as described above.

Pelvic inflammatory disease requires cefoxitin, 2 g parenterally every 6 hours, or cefotetan, 2 g intravenously every 12 hours. Clindamycin, 900 mg intravenously every 8 hours, plus gentamicin, administered intravenously as a 2-mg/kg loading dose followed by 1.5 mg/kg every 8 hours, is also effective. Cefoxitin, 2 g intramuscularly, plus

probenecid, 1 g orally as a single dose, followed by a 14-day oral regimen of doxycycline, 100 mg twice a day, with or without metronidazole, 500 mg twice daily, is an effective outpatient regimen. Concurrent treatment for chlamydial infection also is indicated.

Centers for Disease Control and Prevention (CDC). Availability of cefixime 400 mg tablets—United States, April 2008. MMWR Morb Mortal Wkly Rep. 2008 Apr 25;57(16):435. [PMID: 18437119]

Workowski KA et al. Emerging antimicrobial resistance in *Neisseria gonorrhoeae*: urgent need to strengthen prevention strategies. Ann Intern Med. 2008 Apr 15;148(8):606–13. [PMID: 18413622]

Workowski KA et al; Centers for Disease Control and Prevention. Sexually transmitted diseases treatment guidelines, 2006. MMWR Recomm Rep. 2006 Aug 4;55(RR-11):1–94. [PMID: 16888612]

CHANCROID

Chancroid is a sexually transmitted disease caused by the short gram-negative bacillus *Haemophilus ducreyi*. The incubation period is 3–5 days. At the site of inoculation, a vesicopustule develops that breaks down to form a painful, soft ulcer with a necrotic base, surrounding erythema, and undermined edges. There may be multiple lesions due to autoinoculation. The adenitis is usually unilateral and consists of tender, matted nodes of moderate size with overlying erythema. These may become fluctuant and rupture spontaneously. With lymph node involvement, fever, chills, and malaise may develop. Balanitis and phimosis are frequent complications in men. Women may have no external signs of infection. The diagnosis is established by culturing a swab of the lesion onto a special medium.

Chancroid must be differentiated from other genital ulcers. The chancre of syphilis is clean and painless, with a hard base. Mixed sexually transmitted disease is very common (including syphilis, herpes simplex, and HIV infection), as is infection of the ulcer with fusiforms, spirochetes, and other organisms.

A single dose of either azithromycin, 1 g orally, or ceftriaxone, 250 mg intramuscularly, is effective treatment. Effective multiple-dose regimens are erythromycin, 500 mg orally four times a day for 7 days, or ciprofloxacin, 500 mg orally twice a day for 3 days.

Mohammed TT et al. Chancroid and human immunodeficiency virus infection–a review. Int J Dermatol. 2008 Jan;47(1):1–8. [PMID: 18173591]

GRANULOMA INGUINALE

Granuloma inguinale is a chronic, relapsing granulomatous anogenital infection due to *Calymmatobacterium (Donovania) granulomatis*. The pathognomonic cell, found in tissue scrapings or secretions, is large (25–90 mcm) and contains intracytoplasmic cysts filled with bodies (Donovan bodies) that stain deeply with Wright stain.

The incubation period is 8 days to 12 weeks. The onset is insidious. The lesions occur on the skin or mucous membranes of the genitalia or perineal area. They are relatively painless infiltrated nodules that soon slough. A shallow, sharply demarcated ulcer forms, with a beefy-red friable base of granulation tissue. The lesion spreads by contiguity. The advancing border has a characteristic rolled edge of granulation tissue. Large ulcerations may advance onto the lower abdomen and thighs. Scar formation and healing occur along one border while the opposite border advances.

Superinfection with spirochete-fusiform organisms is common. The ulcer then becomes purulent, painful, foul-smelling, and extremely difficult to treat.

Several therapies are available. Because of the indolent nature of the disease, duration of therapy is relatively long. The following recommended regimens should be given for 3 weeks or until all lesions have healed: doxycycline, 100 mg orally twice daily; or azithromycin, 1 g orally once weekly; or ciprofloxacin, 750 mg orally twice daily; or erythromycin, 500 mg orally four times a day.

BARTONELLA SPECIES

Bartonella species are responsible for a wide variety of clinical syndromes. **Bacillary angiomatosis**, an important manifestation of bartonellosis, is discussed in Chapter 31. A variety of atypical infections, including retinitis, encephalitis, osteomyelitis, and persistent bacteremia and endocarditis have been described.

Trench fever is a self-limited, louse-borne relapsing febrile disease caused by *B quintana*. The disease has occurred epidemically in louse-infested troops and civilians during wars and endemically in residents of scattered geographic areas (eg, Central America). An urban equivalent of trench fever has been described among the homeless. Humans acquire infection when infected lice feces enter sites of skin breakdown. Onset of symptoms is abrupt and fever lasts 3–5 days, with relapses. The patient complains of weakness and severe pain behind the eyes and typically in the back and legs. Lymphadenopathy, splenomegaly, and a transient maculopapular rash may appear. Subclinical infection is frequent, and a carrier state is recognized. The differential diagnosis includes other febrile, self-limited states such as dengue, leptospirosis, malaria, relapsing fever, and typhus. Recovery occurs regularly even in the absence of treatment.

Cat-scratch disease is an acute infection of children and young adults caused by *Bartonella henselae*. It is transmitted from cats to humans as the result of a scratch or bite. Within a few days, a papule or ulcer will develop at the inoculation site in one-third of patients. One to 3 weeks later, fever, headache, and malaise occur. Regional lymph nodes become enlarged, often tender, and may suppurate. Lymphadenopathy from cat scratches resembles that due to neoplasm, tuberculosis, lymphogranuloma venereum, and bacterial lymphadenitis. The diagnosis is usually made clinically. Special cultures for bartonellae, serology, or excisional biopsy, though rarely necessary, confirm the diagnosis. The biopsy reveals necrotizing lymphadenitis and is itself not specific for cat-scratch disease. Cat-scratch disease is usually self-limited, requiring no specific therapy. Encephalitis occurs rarely.

Disseminated forms of the disease—bacillary angiomatosis, peliosis hepatis, and retinitis—occur in HIV-infected persons. The lesions are vasculoproliferative and histopathologically distinct from those of cat-scratch disease. Unexplained fever in patients with late stages of HIV infection is not uncommonly due to bartonellosis. *B quintana*, the agent of trench fever, can also cause bacillary angiomatosis and persistent bacteremia or endocarditis (which will be "culture-negative" unless specifically sought), the latter two entities being associated with homelessness. Due to the fastidious nature of the organism and its special growth requirements, serologic testing (eg, demonstration of a high antibody titer in an indirect immunofluorescence assay) or nucleic acid amplification tests are often required to establish a diagnosis.

Bacillary angiomatosis responds to treatment with a macrolide or doxycycline administered in standard doses for 4–8 weeks. Bacteremia and endocarditis can be effectively treated with a 6-week course of doxycycline (200 mg orally or intravenously in two divided doses per day) plus gentamicin 3 mg/kg/d intravenously for the first 2 weeks. Relapse may occur.

Eremeeva ME et al. Bacteremia, fever, and splenomegaly caused by a newly recognized bartonella species. N Engl J Med. 2007 Jun 7;356(23):2381–7. [PMID: 17554119]
Florin TA et al. Beyond cat scratch disease: widening spectrum of *Bartonella henselae* infection. Pediatrics. 2008 May;121(5):e1413–25. [PMID: 18443019]
Maman E et al. Musculoskeletal manifestations of cat scratch disease. Clin Infect Dis. 2007 Dec 15;45(12):1535–40. [PMID: 18190312]

ANAEROBIC INFECTIONS

Anaerobic bacteria comprise the majority of normal human flora. Normal microbial flora of the mouth (anaerobic spirochetes, *Prevotella,* fusobacteria), the skin (anaerobic diphtheroids), the large bowel (bacteroides, anaerobic streptococci, clostridia), and the female genitourinary tract (bacteroides, anaerobic streptococci, fusobacteria) produce disease when displaced from their normal sites into tissues or closed body spaces.

Anaerobic infections tend to be polymicrobial and abscesses are common. Pus and infected tissue often are malodorous. Septic thrombophlebitis and metastatic infection are frequent and may require incision and drainage. Diminished blood supply that favors proliferation of anaerobes because of reduced tissue oxygenation may interfere with the delivery of antimicrobials to the site of anaerobic infection. Cultures, unless carefully collected under anaerobic conditions, may yield negative results.

Important types of infections that are most commonly caused by anaerobic organisms are listed below. Treatment of all these infections consists of surgical exploration and judicious excision in conjunction with administration of antimicrobial drugs.

1. Head & Neck Infections

Prevotella melaninogenica (formerly *Bacteroides melaninogenicus*) and anaerobic spirochetes are commonly involved in periodontal infections. These organisms, fusobacteria, and peptostreptococci may cause chronic sinusitis, peritonsillar abscess, chronic otitis media, and mastoiditis. Hygiene, drainage, and surgical debridement are as important in treatment as antimicrobials. Oral anaerobic organisms have been uniformly susceptible to penicillin, but there has been a recent trend of increasing penicillin resistance, usually due to β-lactamase production. Penicillin, 1–2 million units intravenously every 4 hours (if parenteral therapy is required) or 0.5 g orally four times daily for less severe infections, or clindamycin can be used (600 mg intravenously every 8 hours or 300 mg orally every 6 hours). Antimicrobial treatment is continued for a few days after signs and symptoms of infection have resolved. Indolent, established infections (eg, mastoiditis or osteomyelitis) may require prolonged courses of therapy, eg, 4–6 weeks or longer.

2. Chest Infections

Usually in the setting of poor oral hygiene and periodontal disease, aspiration of saliva (which contains 10^8 anaerobic organisms per milliliter in addition to aerobes) may lead to necrotizing pneumonia, lung abscess, and empyema. Polymicrobial infection is the rule and anaerobes—particularly *P melaninogenica,* fusobacteria, and peptostreptococci—are common etiologic agents. Septic internal jugular thrombophlebitis (Lemierre syndrome) may originate from mouth anaerobes, classically *Fusobacterium necrophorum,* and cause septic pulmonary embolization. Severe sore throat is a concomitant symptom. Most pulmonary infections respond to antimicrobial therapy alone. Percutaneous chest tube or surgical drainage is indicated for empyema.

Penicillin-resistant *Bacteroides fragilis* and *P melaninogenica* are commonly isolated and have been associated with clinical failures. Clindamycin, 600 mg intravenously once, followed by 300 mg orally every 6–8 hours, is the treatment of choice for these infections. Metronidazole does not cover facultative streptococci, which often are present, and if used, a second agent that is active against streptococci, such as ceftriaxone 1 g intravenously or intramuscularly daily, should be added. Penicillin, 2 million units intravenously every 4 hours, followed by amoxicillin, 500 mg every 8 hours orally, is an alternative; however, increasing prevalence of β-lactamase producing organisms is a concern. Moxifloxacin, 400 mg orally or intravenously once daily, may be used. Because these infections respond slowly, a prolonged course of therapy (eg, 4–6 weeks) is generally recommended.

Bartlett JG. The role of anaerobic bacteria in lung abscess. Clin Infect Dis. 2005 Apr 1;40(7):923–5. [PMID: 15824980]

3. Central Nervous System

Anaerobes are a common cause of brain abscess, subdural empyema, or septic central nervous system thrombophlebitis. The organisms reach the central nervous system by direct extension from sinusitis, otitis, or mastoiditis or by hematogenous spread from chronic lung infections. Antimicrobial therapy—eg, ceftriaxone, 2 g intravenously every

12 hours, plus metronidazole, 750 mg intravenously every 8 hours—is an important adjunct to surgical drainage. Duration of therapy is 6–8 weeks. Some small multiple brain abscesses can be treated with antibiotics alone without surgical drainage.

Menon S et al. Current epidemiology of intracranial abscesses: a prospective 5 year study. J Med Microbiol. 2008 Oct;57(Pt 10):1259–68. [PMID: 18809555]

4. Intra-abdominal Infections

In the colon there are up to 10^{11} anaerobes per gram of content—predominantly *B fragilis*, clostridia, and peptostreptococci. These organisms play a central role in most intra-abdominal abscesses following trauma to the colon, diverticulitis, appendicitis, or perirectal abscess and may also participate in hepatic abscess and cholecystitis, often in association with aerobic coliform bacteria. The bacteriology includes anaerobes as well as enteric gram-negative rods and on occasion enterococci. Therapy should be directed both against anaerobes and gram-negative aerobes. Agents that are active against *B fragilis* include metronidazole, chloramphenicol, moxifloxacin, tigecycline, ertapenem, imipenem, doripenem, ampicillin-sulbactam, ticarcillin-clavulanic acid, and piperacillin-tazobactam. Resistance to cefoxitin, cefotetan, and clindamycin is increasingly encountered. Most third-generation cephalosporins have poor efficacy. Non-fragilis species of bacteroides may be less susceptible to the cephalosporins.

Table 33–6 summarizes the antibiotic regimens for management of moderate to moderately severe infections (eg, patient hemodynamically stable, good surgical drainage possible or established, low APACHE score, no multiple organ failure) and severe infections (eg, major peritoneal soilage, large or multiple abscesses, patient hemodynamically unstable), particularly if drug-resistant organisms are suspected. An effective oral regimen for patients able to take it is presented also.

Table 33–6. Treatment of anaerobic intra-abdominal infections.

Oral therapy
Moxifloxacin 400 mg every 24 hours
Intravenous therapy
Moderate to moderately severe infections:
Ertapenem 1 g every 24 hours
or—
Ceftriaxone 1 g every 24 hours (or ciprofloxacin 400 mg every 12 hours, if penicillin allergic) plus metronidazole 500 mg every 8 hours
or—
Tigecycline 100 mg once followed by 50 mg every 12 hours
or—
Moxifloxacin 400 mg every 24 hours
Severe infections:
Imipenem, 0.5 g every 6–8 hours; meropenem 1 g every 8 hours; doripenem 0.5 g every 8 hours; piperacillin/tazobactam 3.75 g every 6 hours

Brook I. Treatment of anaerobic infection. Expert Rev Anti Infect Ther. 2007 Dec;5(6):991–1006. [PMID: 18039083]

5. Female Genital Tract & Pelvic Infections

The normal flora of the vagina and cervix includes several species of bacteroides, peptostreptococci, group B streptococci, lactobacilli, coliform bacteria, and, occasionally, spirochetes and clostridia. These organisms commonly cause genital tract infections and may disseminate from there.

While salpingitis is often caused by gonococci and chlamydiae, tubo-ovarian and pelvic abscesses are associated with anaerobes in most cases. Postpartum infections may be caused by aerobic streptococci or staphylococci, but anaerobes are often found, and the worst cases of postpartum or postabortion sepsis are associated with clostridia and bacteroides. These have a high mortality rate, and treatment requires both antimicrobials directed against anaerobes and coliforms (see above) and abscess drainage or early hysterectomy.

Trigg BG et al. Sexually transmitted infections and pelvic inflammatory disease in women. Med Clin North Am. 2008 Sep;92(5):1083–113. [PMID: 18721654]

6. Bacteremia & Endocarditis

Anaerobic bacteremia usually originates from the gastrointestinal tract, the oropharynx, decubitus ulcers, or the female genital tract. Endocarditis due to anaerobic and microaerophilic streptococci and bacteroides originates from the same sites. Most cases of anaerobic or microaerophilic streptococcal endocarditis can be effectively treated with 12–20 million units of penicillin G daily for 4–6 weeks, but optimal therapy of other types of anaerobic bacterial endocarditis must rely on laboratory guidance. Anaerobic corynebacteria (propionibacteria), clostridia, and bacteroides occasionally cause endocarditis.

7. Skin & Soft Tissue Infections

Anaerobic infections in the skin and soft tissue usually follow trauma, inadequate blood supply, or surgery and are most common in areas that are contaminated by oral or fecal flora. These infections also occur in injection drug users and persons sustaining animal to human bites. There may be progressive tissue necrosis (Plate 104) and a putrid odor.

Several terms, such as bacterial synergistic gangrene, synergistic necrotizing cellulitis, necrotizing fasciitis, and nonclostridial crepitant cellulitis, have been used to classify these infections. Although there are some differences in microbiology among them, their differentiation on clinical grounds alone is difficult. All are mixed infections caused by aerobic and anaerobic organisms and require aggressive surgical debridement of necrotic tissue for cure. Surgical consultation is obligatory to assist in diagnosis and treatment.

Broad-spectrum antibiotics active against both anaerobes and gram-positive and gram-negative aerobes (eg, vancomycin plus piperacillin-tazobactam) should be instituted empirically and modified by culture results (see

Table 30–9). They are given for about a week after progressive tissue destruction has been controlled and the margins of the wound remain free of inflammation.

Anaya DA et al. Necrotizing soft-tissue infection: diagnosis and management. Clin Infect Dis. 2007 Mar 1;44(5):705–10. [PMID: 17278065]

ACTINOMYCOSIS

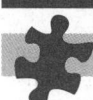

ESSENTIALS OF DIAGNOSIS

▶ History of recent dental infection or abdominal trauma.

▶ Chronic pneumonia or indolent intra-abdominal or cervicofacial abscess.

▶ Sinus tract formation.

General Considerations

Actinomyces israelii and other species of *Actinomyces* occur in the normal flora of the mouth and tonsillar crypts. They are anaerobic, gram-positive, branching filamentous bacteria (1 mcm in diameter) that may fragment into bacillary forms. When introduced into traumatized tissue and associated with other anaerobic bacteria, these actinomycetes become pathogens.

The most common site of infection is the cervicofacial area (about 60% of cases). Infection typically follows extraction of a tooth or other trauma. Lesions may develop in the gastrointestinal tract or lungs following ingestion or aspiration of the organism from its endogenous source in the mouth. Interestingly, *T whippelii*, the causative agent of Whipple disease, is an actinomycete and therefore is related to the species that cause actinomycosis.

Clinical Findings

A. Symptoms and Signs

1. Cervicofacial actinomycosis—Cervicofacial actinomycosis develops slowly. The area becomes markedly indurated, and the overlying skin becomes reddish or cyanotic. Abscesses eventually draining to the surface persist for long periods. Sulfur granules—masses of filamentous organisms—may be found in the pus. There is usually little pain unless there is secondary infection. Trismus indicates that the muscles of mastication are involved. Radiography may reveal bony involvement.

2. Thoracic actinomycosis—Thoracic involvement begins with fever, cough, and sputum production with night sweats and weight loss. Pleuritic pain may be present. Multiple sinuses may extend through the chest wall, to the heart, or into the abdominal cavity. Ribs may be involved. Radiography shows areas of consolidation and in many cases pleural effusion. Cervicofacial or thoracic disease may occasionally involve the central nervous system, most commonly brain abscess or meningitis.

3. Abdominal actinomycosis—Abdominal actinomycosis usually causes pain in the ileocecal region, spiking fever and chills, vomiting, and weight loss; it may be confused with Crohn disease. Irregular abdominal masses may be palpated. Pelvic inflammatory disease caused by actinomycetes has been associated with prolonged use of an intrauterine contraceptive device. Sinuses draining to the exterior may develop. CT scanning reveals an inflammatory mass extended to involve bone.

B. Laboratory Findings

The anaerobic, gram-positive organism may be demonstrated as a granule or as scattered branching gram-positive filaments in the pus. Anaerobic culture is necessary to distinguish actinomycetes from nocardiae because specific therapy differs for the two infections.

▶ **Treatment**

Penicillin G is the drug of choice. Ten to 20 million units are given via a parenteral route for 4–6 weeks, followed by oral penicillin V, 500 mg four times daily. Alternatives include ampicillin, 12 g/d intravenously for 4–6 weeks followed by oral amoxicillin 500 mg three times daily or doxycycline 100 mg twice daily intravenously or orally. Response to therapy is slow. Therapy should be continued for weeks to months after clinical manifestations have disappeared in order to ensure cure. Surgical procedures such as drainage and resection may be beneficial.

With penicillin and surgery, the prognosis is good. The difficulties of diagnosis, however, may permit extensive destruction of tissue before the diagnosis is identified and therapy is started.

Sharkawy AA. Cervicofacial actinomycosis and mandibular osteomyelitis. Infect Dis Clin North Am. 2007 Jun;21(2):543–56. [PMID: 17561082]

▼ **NOCARDIOSIS**

Nocardia asteroides, an aerobic filamentous soil bacterium, causes pulmonary and systemic nocardiosis. Bronchopulmonary abnormalities (eg, alveolar proteinosis) predispose to colonization, but infection is unusual unless the patient is also receiving systemic corticosteroids or is otherwise immunosuppressed.

Pulmonary involvement usually begins with malaise, loss of weight, fever, and night sweats. Cough and production of purulent sputum are the chief complaints. Radiography may show infiltrates accompanied by pleural effusion. The lesions may penetrate to the exterior through the chest wall, invading the ribs.

Dissemination involves any organ. Brain abscesses and subcutaneous nodules are most frequent. This is seen exclusively in immunocompromised patients.

N asteroides is usually found as delicate, branching, gram-positive filaments. It may be weakly acid-fast, occasionally causing diagnostic confusion with tuberculosis. Identification is made by culture.

For cutaneous infections, therapy is initiated with intravenous trimethoprim-sulfamethoxazole administered at a dosage of 5–10 mg/kg/d (based on trimethoprim) and continued with oral trimethoprim-sulfamethoxazole, one double-strength tablet twice a day. Surgical procedures such as drainage and resection may be needed as adjunctive therapy. A higher dose of 15 mg/kg/d (based on trimethoprim) should be used for disseminated or pulmonary infections. Imipenem 500 mg intravenously every 6 hours is an alternative.

Response may be slow, and therapy must be continued for at least 6 months. The prognosis in systemic nocardiosis is poor when diagnosis and therapy are delayed.

Nocardia brasiliensis typically causes a digital lesion—resembling herpetic whitlow—and ascending lymphangitis in normal hosts. Antimicrobial treatment is as for *N asteroides* infection, and the prognosis is excellent.

Martínez R et al. Pulmonary nocardiosis: risk factors, clinical features, diagnosis and prognosis. Curr Opin Pulm Med. 2008 May;14(3):219–27. [PMID: 18427245]
Peleg AY et al. Risk factors, clinical characteristics, and outcome of *Nocardia* infection in organ transplant recipients: a matched case-control study. Clin Infect Dis. 2007 May 15;44(10):1307–14. [PMID: 17443467]

▼ **INFECTIONS CAUSED BY MYCOBACTERIA**

NONTUBERCULOUS ATYPICAL MYCOBACTERIAL DISEASES

About 10% of mycobacterial infections are caused by atypical mycobacteria. Atypical mycobacterial infections are among the most common opportunistic infections in advanced HIV disease. These organisms have distinctive laboratory characteristics, occur ubiquitously in the environment, are not communicable from person to person, and are often resistant to standard antituberculous drugs.

1. Disseminated *Mycobacterium avium* Infection

Mycobacterium avium complex (MAC) produces asymptomatic colonization or a wide spectrum of diseases, including coin lesions, bronchitis in patients with chronic lung disease, and invasive pulmonary disease that is often cavitary and occurs in patients with underlying lung disease. MAC causes disseminated disease in the late stages of HIV infection, when the CD4 cell count is less than 50/mcL. Persistent fever and weight loss are the most common symptoms. The organism can usually be cultured from multiple sites, including blood, liver, lymph node, or bone marrow. Blood culture is the preferred means of establishing the diagnosis and has a sensitivity of 98%.

Agents with proved activity against MAC are rifabutin, azithromycin, clarithromycin, and ethambutol. Amikacin and ciprofloxacin work in vitro, but clinical results are inconsistent. A combination of two or more active agents should be used to prevent rapid emergence of secondary resistance. Clarithromycin, 500 mg orally twice daily, plus ethambutol, 15 mg/kg/d orally as a single dose, with or without rifabutin, 300 mg/d orally, is the treatment of choice. Azithromycin, 500 mg orally once daily, may be used instead of clarithromycin. Insufficient data are available to permit specific recommendations about second-line regimens for patients intolerant of macrolides or those with macrolide-resistant organisms. MAC therapy may be discontinued in patients who have been treated with 12 months of therapy for disseminated MAC, who have no evidence of active disease, and whose CD4 counts exceed 100 cells/mcL while receiving highly active antiretroviral therapy (HAART). Antimicrobial prophylaxis of MAC prevents disseminated disease and prolongs survival. It is the standard of care to offer it to all HIV-infected patients with CD4 counts ≤ 50/mcL. In contrast to active infection, single-drug oral regimens of clarithromycin, 500 mg twice daily, azithromycin, 1200 mg once weekly, or rifabutin, 300 mg once daily, are appropriate. Clarithromycin or azithromycin is more effective and better tolerated than rifabutin, and therefore preferred. Primary prophylaxis for MAC infection can be stopped in patients who have responded to antiretroviral combination therapy with elevation of CD4 counts above 100 cells/mcL for 3 months.

2. Pulmonary Infections

MAC causes a chronic, slowly progressive pulmonary infection resembling tuberculosis in immunocompetent patients, who typically have underlying pulmonary disease.

Treatment of immunocompetent patients with pulmonary infection is empiric and based entirely on anecdotal data. A combination of agents is probably best. Rifampin, 600 mg orally once daily, plus ethambutol, 15–25 mg/kg/d orally, plus streptomycin, 1 g intramuscularly three to five times a week for the first 4–6 months, have been used. The role of rifabutin, fluoroquinolones, and the macrolides is not known, but based on their excellent efficacy in immunocompromised AIDS patients, they may actually be more effective than the relatively weak agents traditionally used in immunocompetent patients. Clarithromycin is a very potent drug in the treatment of MAC in AIDS patients. Based on this, inclusion of clarithromycin in the initial treatment regimen of immunocompetent patients is prudent. Therapy is continued for a total of 18–24 months.

Mycobacterium kansasii can produce clinical disease resembling tuberculosis, but the illness progresses more slowly. Most such infections occur in patients with preexisting lung disease, though 40% of patients have no known pulmonary disease. Microbiologically, *M kansasii* is similar to *Mycobacterium tuberculosis* and is sensitive to the same drugs except pyrazinamide, to which it is resistant. Therapy with isoniazid, ethambutol, and rifampin for 2 years (or 1 year after sputum conversion) has been successful.

Less common causes of pulmonary disease include *Mycobacterium xenopi*, *Mycobacterium szulgai*, and *Mycobacterium gordonae*. These organisms have variable sensitivities, and treatment is based on results of sensitivity tests. The rapid growing mycobacteria, *Mycobacterium abscessus*, *Mycobacterium chelonae*, and *Mycobacterium fortuitum* also can cause pneumonia in the occasional patient.

3. Lymphadenitis

Most cases of lymphadenitis (scrofula) in adults are caused by *M tuberculosis* and can be a manifestation of disseminated disease. In children, the majority of cases are due to nontuberculous mycobacterial species, with MAC being the most common followed by *Mycobacterium scrofulaceum* in the United States and *Mycobacterium malmoense* and *Mycobacterium haemophilum* in Northern Europe. *M kansasii*, *Mycobacterium bovis*, *M chelonae*, and *M fortuitum* are less commonly observed. Unlike disease caused by *M tuberculosis*, which requires systemic therapy for 6 months, infection with nontuberculous mycobacteria can be successfully treated by surgical excision without antituberculous therapy.

4. Skin & Soft Tissue Infections

Skin and soft tissue infections such as abscesses, septic arthritis, and osteomyelitis can result from direct inoculation or hematogenous dissemination or may occur as a complication of surgery.

M abscessus, *M chelonae*, and *M fortuitum* are frequent causes of this type of infection. Most cases occur in the extremities and initially present as nodules. Ulceration with abscess formation often follows. The organisms are resistant to the usual antituberculous drugs but may be sensitive to a variety of antibiotics, including erythromycin, doxycycline, amikacin, cefoxitin, sulfonamides, imipenem, and ciprofloxacin. Therapy includes surgical debridement along with drug therapy. Initially, parenteral drugs are given for several weeks, and this is followed by an oral regimen to which the organism is sensitive. The duration of therapy is variable but usually continues for several months after the soft tissue lesions have healed.

Mycobacterium marinum infection ("swimming pool granuloma") presents as a nodular skin lesion following exposure to nonchlorinated water. The lesions respond to therapy with clarithromycin, doxycycline, minocycline, or trimethoprim-sulfamethoxazole.

Mycobacterium ulcerans infection (Buruli ulcer) is seen mainly in Africa and Australia and produces a large ulcerative lesion. Therapy consists of surgical excision and skin grafting.

Bodle EE et al. Epidemiology of nontuberculous mycobacteria in patients without HIV infection, New York City. Emerg Infect Dis. 2008 Mar;14(3):390–6. [PMID: 18325252]

Glassroth J. Pulmonary disease due to nontuberculous mycobacteria. Chest. 2008 Jan;133(1):243–51. [PMID: 18187749]

Griffith DE et al; ATS Mycobacterial Diseases Subcommittee; American Thoracic Society; Infectious Disease Society of America. An official ATS/IDSA statement: diagnosis, treatment, and prevention of nontuberculous mycobacterial diseases. Am J Respir Crit Care Med. 2007 Feb 15;175(4):367–416. [PMID: 17277290]

MYCOBACTERIUM TUBERCULOSIS INFECTIONS

Tuberculosis is discussed in Chapter 9. Further information and expert consultation can be obtained from the Francis J. Curry National Tuberculosis Center at the Web site http://www.nationaltbcenter.edu or, by phone, 415-502-4600, or fax, 415-502-4620.

TUBERCULOUS MENINGITIS

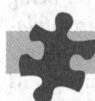

ESSENTIALS OF DIAGNOSIS

▶ Gradual onset of listlessness, irritability, and anorexia.

▶ Headache, vomiting, and seizures common.

▶ Cranial nerve abnormalities typical.

▶ Tuberculosis focus may be evident elsewhere.

▶ Cerebrospinal fluid shows several hundred lymphocytes, low glucose, and high protein.

General Considerations

Tuberculous meningitis is caused by rupture of a meningeal tuberculoma resulting from earlier hematogenous seeding of tubercle bacilli from a pulmonary focus, or it may be a consequence of miliary spread.

Clinical Findings

A. Symptoms and Signs

The onset is usually gradual, with listlessness, irritability, anorexia, and fever, followed by headache, vomiting, convulsions, and coma. In older patients, headache and behavioral changes are prominent early symptoms. Nuchal rigidity and cranial nerve palsies occur as the meningitis progresses. Evidence of active tuberculosis elsewhere or a history of prior tuberculosis is present in up to 75% of patients.

B. Laboratory Findings

The spinal fluid is frequently yellowish, with increased pressure, 100–500 cells/mcL (predominantly lymphocytes, though neutrophils may be present early during infection), increased protein, and decreased glucose. Acid-fast stains of cerebrospinal fluid usually are negative, and cultures also may be negative in 15–25% of cases. Nucleic acid amplification tests for rapid diagnosis of tuberculosis have variable sensitivity and specificity and none are FDA-approved for use in meningitis. Chest x-ray often reveals abnormalities compatible with tuberculosis but may be normal.

Differential Diagnosis

Tuberculous meningitis may be confused with any other type of meningitis, but the gradual onset, the predominantly lymphocytic pleocytosis of the spinal fluid, and evidence of tuberculosis elsewhere often point to the diagnosis. The tuberculin skin test is usually (not always) positive. Fungal and other granulomatous meningitides, syphilis, and carcinomatous meningitis are in the differential diagnosis.

Complications

Complications of tuberculous meningitis include seizure disorders, cranial nerve palsies, stroke, and obstructive hydrocephalus with impaired cognitive function. These result from inflammatory exudate primarily involving the basilar meninges and arteries.

Treatment

Presumptive diagnosis followed by early, empiric antituberculous therapy is essential for survival and to minimize sequelae. Even if cultures are not positive, a full course of therapy is warranted if the clinical setting is suggestive of tuberculous meningitis.

Regimens that are effective for pulmonary tuberculosis are effective also for tuberculous meningitis (see Table 9–13). Rifampin, isoniazid, and pyrazinamide all penetrate into cerebrospinal fluid well. The penetration of ethambutol is more variable, but therapeutic concentrations can be achieved, and the drug has been successfully used for meningitis. Aminoglycosides penetrate less well. Regimens that do not include both isoniazid and rifampin may be effective but are less reliable and generally must be given for longer periods.

Many authorities recommend the addition of corticosteroids for patients with focal deficits or altered mental status. Dexamethasone, 0.15 mg/kg intravenously or orally four times daily for 1–2 weeks, then discontinued in a tapering regimen over 4 weeks, may be used.

Prasad K et al. Corticosteroids for managing tuberculous meningitis. Cochrane Database Syst Rev. 2008 Jan 23;(1):CD002244. [PMID: 18254003]

Török ME et al. Clinical and microbiological features of HIV-associated tuberculous meningitis in Vietnamese adults. PLoS ONE. 2008 Mar 19;3(3):e1772. [PMID: 18350135]

Török ME et al. Validation of a diagnostic algorithm for adult tuberculous meningitis. Am J Trop Med Hyg. 2007 Sep;77(3):555–9. [PMID: 17827378]

LEPROSY (Hansen Disease)

ESSENTIALS OF DIAGNOSIS

▶ Pale, anesthetic macular—or nodular and erythematous—skin lesions.

▶ Superficial nerve thickening with associated anesthesia.

▶ History of residence in endemic area in childhood.

▶ Acid-fast bacilli in skin lesions or nasal scrapings, or characteristic histologic nerve changes.

General Considerations

Leprosy (Hansen disease) is a chronic infectious disease caused by the acid-fast rod *Mycobacterium leprae*. The mode of transmission probably is respiratory and involves prolonged exposure in childhood. The disease is endemic in tropical and subtropical Asia, Africa, Central and South

America, and the Pacific regions, and rarely seen sporadically in the southern United States.

Clinical Findings

A. Symptoms and Signs

The onset is insidious. The lesions involve the cooler body tissues: skin, superficial nerves, nose, pharynx, larynx, eyes, and testicles. Skin lesions may occur as pale, anesthetic macular lesions 1–10 cm in diameter; discrete erythematous, infiltrated nodules 1–5 cm in diameter; or diffuse skin infiltration. Neurologic disturbances are caused by nerve infiltration and thickening, with resultant anesthesia, and motor abnormalities. Bilateral ulnar neuropathy is highly suggestive. In untreated cases, disfigurement due to the skin infiltration and nerve involvement may be extreme, leading to trophic ulcers, bone resorption, and loss of digits.

The disease is divided clinically and by laboratory tests into two distinct types: lepromatous and tuberculoid. The **lepromatous** type (also referred to as multibacillary leprosy) occurs in persons with defective cellular immunity. The course is progressive and malignant, with nodular skin lesions; slow, symmetric nerve involvement; abundant acid-fast bacilli in the skin lesions; and a negative lepromin skin test. In the **tuberculoid** type (paucibacillary leprosy), cellular immunity is intact and the course is more benign and less progressive, with macular skin lesions, severe asymmetric nerve involvement of sudden onset with few bacilli present in the lesions, and a positive lepromin skin test. Intermediate ("borderline") cases are frequent. Eye involvement (keratitis and iridocyclitis), nasal ulcers, epistaxis, anemia, and lymphadenopathy may occur.

B. Laboratory Findings

Laboratory confirmation of leprosy requires the demonstration of acid-fast bacilli in a skin biopsy. Biopsy of skin or of a thickened involved nerve also gives a typical histologic picture. *M leprae* does not grow in artificial media but does grow in the foot pads of armadillos.

Differential Diagnosis

The skin lesions of leprosy often resemble those of lupus erythematosus, sarcoidosis, syphilis, erythema nodosum, erythema multiforme, cutaneous tuberculosis, and vitiligo.

Complications

Kidney failure and hepatomegaly from secondary amyloidosis may occur with long-standing disease.

Treatment

Combination therapy is recommended for treatment of all types of leprosy. Single-drug treatment is accompanied by emergence of resistance, and primary resistance to dapsone also occurs. For borderline and lepromatous cases (ie, multibacillary disease), the World Health Organization recommends a triple drug-regimen of rifampin, 600 mg once a month; dapsone, 100 mg daily; and clofazimine, 300 mg once a month and 50 mg daily for 12 months. For

indeterminate and tuberculoid leprosy (paucibacillary disease), the recommendation is rifampin, 600 mg once a month, plus dapsone, 100 mg daily for 6 months.

Two reactional states—erythema nodosum leprosum and reversal reactions—may occur as a consequence of therapy. The reversal reaction, typical of borderline lepromatous leprosy, probably results from enhanced host immunity. Skin lesions and nerves become swollen and tender, but systemic manifestations are not seen. Erythema nodosum leprosum, typical of lepromatous leprosy, is a consequence of immune injury from antigen-antibody complex deposition in skin and other tissues; in addition to skin and nerve manifestations, fever and systemic involvement may be seen. Prednisone, 60 mg/d orally, or thalidomide, 300 mg/d orally (in the nonpregnant patient only), is effective for erythema nodosum leprosum. Improvement is expected within a few days after initiating prednisone, and thereafter the dose may be tapered over several weeks to avoid recurrence. Thalidomide is also tapered over several weeks to a 100-mg bedtime dose. Erythema nodosum leprosum is usually confined to the first year of therapy, and prednisone or thalidomide can be discontinued. Thalidomide is ineffective for reversal reactions, and prednisone, 60 mg/d, is indicated. Reversal reactions tend to recur, and the dose of prednisone should be slowly tapered over weeks to months. Therapy for leprosy should not be discontinued during treatment of reactional states.

Walker SL et al. Leprosy. Clin Dermatol. 2007 Mar–Apr;25(2):165–72. [PMID: 17350495]

INFECTIONS CAUSED BY CHLAMYDIAE

Chlamydiaceae is a family of obligate intracellular parasites closely related to gram-negative bacteria. They include two important genera of human pathogens—*Chlamydia*, which includes the species *Chlamydia trachomatis*, and *Chlamydophila*, which include the species *Chlamydophila psittaci* (formerly known as *Chlamydia psittaci*) and *Chlamydophila pneumoniae* (formerly known as *Chlamydia pneumoniae*). The differentiation of genera is based on differences in intracellular inclusions, sulfonamide susceptibility, antigenic composition, and disease production. *C trachomatis* causes many different human infections involving the eye (trachoma, inclusion conjunctivitis), the genital tract (lymphogranuloma venereum, nongonococcal urethritis, cervicitis, salpingitis), or the respiratory tract in infants (pneumonitis). *C psittaci* causes psittacosis and *C pneumoniae* is a cause of respiratory tract infections.

CHLAMYDIA TRACHOMATIS INFECTIONS

1. Lymphogranuloma Venereum

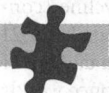

ESSENTIALS OF DIAGNOSIS

► Evanescent primary genital lesion.

▶ Lymph node enlargement, softening, and suppuration, with draining sinuses.

▶ Proctitis and rectal stricture in women or homosexual men.

▶ Positive complement fixation test.

General Considerations

Lymphogranuloma venereum (LGV) is an acute and chronic sexually transmitted disease caused by *C trachomatis* types L1–L3. The disease is acquired during intercourse or through contact with contaminated exudate from active lesions. The incubation period is 5–21 days. After the genital lesion disappears, the infection spreads to lymph channels and lymph nodes of the genital and rectal areas. Inapparent infections and latent disease are not uncommon.

Clinical Findings

A. Symptoms and Signs

In men, the initial vesicular or ulcerative lesion (on the external genitalia) is evanescent and often goes unnoticed. Inguinal buboes appear 1–4 weeks after exposure, are often bilateral, and have a tendency to fuse, soften, and break down to form multiple draining sinuses, with extensive scarring. In women, the genital lymph drainage is to the perirectal glands. Early anorectal manifestations are proctitis with tenesmus and bloody purulent discharge; late manifestations are chronic cicatrizing inflammation of the rectal and perirectal tissue. These changes lead to obstipation and rectal stricture and, occasionally, rectovaginal and perianal fistulas. They are also seen in homosexual men.

B. Laboratory Findings

The complement fixation test may be positive (titers > 1:64), but cross-reaction with other chlamydiae occurs. Although a positive reaction may reflect remote infection, high titers usually indicate active disease. Nucleic acid detection tests are sensitive, but not FDA-approved for rectal specimens and cannot differentiate LGV from non-LGV strains.

Differential Diagnosis

The early lesion of LGV must be differentiated from the lesions of syphilis, genital herpes, and chancroid; lymph node involvement must be distinguished from that due to tularemia, tuberculosis, plague, neoplasm, or pyogenic infection; and rectal stricture must be distinguished from that due to neoplasm and ulcerative colitis.

Treatment

If diagnostic testing for LGV is not available, patients with a clinical presentation suggestive of LGV should be treated empirically. The antibiotic of choice is doxycycline (contraindicated in pregnancy), 100 mg orally twice daily for 21 days. Erythromycin, 500 mg orally four times a day for 21 days, is also effective. Azithromycin, 1 g orally once weekly for 3 weeks, may also be effective.

McLean CA et al. Treatment of lymphogranuloma venereum. Clin Infect Dis. 2007 Apr 1;44 (Suppl 3):S147–52. [PMID: 17342667]

2. Chlamydial Urethritis & Cervicitis

C trachomatis immunotypes D–K are isolated in about 50% of cases of nongonococcal urethritis and cervicitis by appropriate techniques. In other cases, *Ureaplasma urealyticum* or *Mycoplasma genitalium* can be grown as a possible etiologic agent. *C trachomatis* is an important cause of postgonococcal urethritis. Coinfection with gonococci and chlamydiae is common, and postgonococcal (ie, chlamydial) urethritis may persist after successful treatment of the gonococcal component. Occasionally, epididymitis, prostatitis, or proctitis is caused by chlamydial infection.

Females infected with chlamydiae may be asymptomatic or may have symptoms and signs of cervicitis, salpingitis, or pelvic inflammatory disease. Chlamydiae are a leading cause of infertility in females in the United States. Active screening for chlamydial infection is recommended in certain settings: pregnant women; all sexually active women 25 years of age and under; older women with risk factors for sexually transmitted diseases; and men with risk factors for sexually transmitted diseases, such as HIV-positive men or men who have sex with men.

The urethral or cervical discharge due to *C trachomatis* tends to be less painful, less purulent, and watery compared with gonococcal infection. A patient with urethritis or cervicitis and absence of gram-negative diplococci on Gram stain and of *N gonorrhoeae* on culture is assumed to have chlamydial infection until proven otherwise. In the past, the diagnosis of chlamydial infection has been clinical because *C trachomatis* is difficult and expensive to culture; therefore, therapy often was given presumptively. The advent of FDA-approved, highly sensitive nucleic acid amplification tests for use with urine or vaginal swabs has simplified matters, and the diagnosis should be confirmed whenever possible. A negative nucleic acid amplification test for chlamydia reliably excludes the diagnosis of chlamydial urethritis or cervicitis and therapy need not be administered. Presumptively administered therapy still may be indicated in some cases (such as for an individual with gonococcal infection in whom no chlamydial testing was performed or a test other than a nucleic acid amplification test was used to exclude the diagnosis, an individual for whom a test result is pending but is considered unlikely to follow-up, and for sexual contacts of documented cases).

Recommended regimens are a single oral 1-g dose of azithromycin (preferred and safe in pregnancy), 100 mg of doxycycline orally for 7 days (contraindicated in pregnancy), or 500 mg of levofloxacin once daily for 7 days (also contraindicated in pregnancy). As for all sexually transmitted diseases, studies for HIV and syphilis should be performed.

Lusk MJ et al. Cervicitis: a review. Curr Opin Infect Dis. 2008 Feb;21(1):49–55. [PMID: 18192786]

Meyers DS et al. Screening for chlamydial infection: an evidence update for the U.S. Preventive Services Task Force. Ann Intern Med. 2007 Jul 17;147(2):135–42. [PMID: 17576995]

Workowski KA et al; Centers for Disease Control and Prevention. Sexually transmitted diseases treatment guidelines, 2006. MMWR Recomm Rep. 2006 Aug 4;55(RR-11):1–94. [PMID: 16888612]

CHLAMYDOPHILA PSITTACI & PSITTACOSIS (Ornithosis)

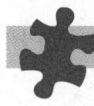 ESSENTIALS OF DIAGNOSIS

► Fever, chills, and cough; headache common.
► Atypical pneumonia with slightly delayed appearance of signs of pneumonitis.
► Contact with infected bird (psittacine, pigeons, many others) 7–15 days previously.
► Isolation of chlamydiae or rising titer of complement-fixing antibodies.

General Considerations

Psittacosis is acquired from contact with birds (parrots, parakeets, pigeons, chickens, ducks, and many others), which may or may not be ill. The history may be difficult to obtain if the patient acquired infection from an illegally imported bird.

Clinical Findings

The onset is usually rapid, with fever, chills, myalgia, dry cough, and headache. Signs include temperature-pulse dissociation, dullness to percussion, and rales. Pulmonary findings may be absent early. Dyspnea and cyanosis may occur later. Endocarditis, which is culture-negative, may occur. The radiographic findings in typical psittacosis are those of atypical pneumonia, which tends to be interstitial and diffuse in appearance, though consolidation can occur. Psittacosis is indistinguishable from other bacterial or viral pneumonias by radiography.

The organism is rarely isolated from cultures. The diagnosis is usually made serologically; antibodies appear during the second week and can be demonstrated by complement fixation or immunofluorescence. Antibody response may be suppressed by early chemotherapy.

Differential Diagnosis

The illness is indistinguishable from viral, mycoplasmal, or other atypical pneumonias except for the history of contact with birds. Psittacosis is in the differential diagnosis of culture-negative endocarditis.

Treatment

Treatment consists of giving tetracycline, 0.5 g orally every 6 hours or 0.5 g intravenously every 12 hours, for 14–21 days. Erythromycin, 500 mg orally every 6 hours, may be effective as well.

CHLAMYDOPHILA PNEUMONIAE INFECTION

C pneumoniae causes pneumonia and bronchitis. The clinical presentation of pneumonia is that of an atypical pneumonia. The organism accounts for approximately 10% of community-acquired pneumonias, ranking second to mycoplasma as an agent of atypical pneumonia. A putative role in coronary artery disease has not held up to close scientific scrutiny.

Like *C psittaci*, strains of *C pneumoniae* are resistant to sulfonamides. Erythromycin or tetracycline, 500 mg orally four times a day for 10–14 days, appears to be effective therapy. Fluoroquinolones, such as levofloxacin (500 mg once daily for 7–14 days) or moxifloxacin (400 mg once daily for 7–14 days), are active in vitro against *C pneumoniae* and probably are effective. It is unclear if empiric coverage for atypical pathogens in hospitalized patients with community-acquired pneumonia provides a survival benefit or improves clinical outcome.

Kumar S et al. Acute respiratory infection due to *Chlamydia pneumoniae*: current status of diagnostic methods. Clin Infect Dis. 2007 Feb 15;44(4):568–76. [PMID: 17243062]

Luna LK et al. Spectrum of viruses and atypical bacteria in intercontinental air travelers with symptoms of acute respiratory infection. J Infect Dis. 2007 Mar 1;195(5):675–9. [PMID: 17262708]

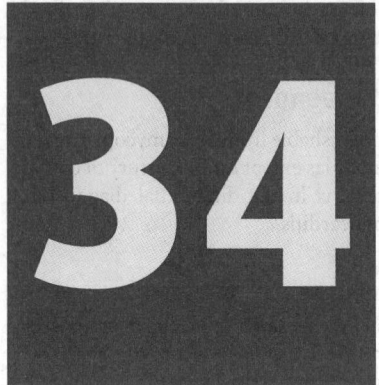

Spirochetal Infections

Susan S. Philip, MD, MPH

▼ SYPHILIS

NATURAL HISTORY & PRINCIPLES OF DIAGNOSIS & TREATMENT

Syphilis is a complex infectious disease caused by *Treponema pallidum*, a spirochete capable of infecting almost any organ or tissue in the body and causing protean clinical manifestations (Table 34–1). Transmission occurs most frequently during sexual contact (including oral sex), through minor skin or mucosal lesions; sites of inoculation are usually genital but may be extragenital. The risk of developing syphilis after unprotected sex with an individual with infectious syphilis is approximately 30–50%. Rarely, it can also be transmitted through nonsexual contact, blood transfusion, or via the placenta from mother to fetus (congenital syphilis).

The natural history of acquired syphilis is generally divided into two major clinical stages: **early (infectious) syphilis** and **late syphilis**. The two stages are separated by a symptom-free latent phase during the first part of which (early latency) infectious lesions are liable to recur. Infectious syphilis includes the primary lesions (chancre and regional lymphadenopathy), the secondary lesions (commonly involving skin and mucous membranes, occasionally bone, central nervous system, or liver), relapsing lesions during early latency, and congenital lesions. The hallmark of these lesions is an abundance of spirochetes; tissue reaction is usually minimal. Late syphilis consists of so-called benign (gummatous) lesions involving skin, bones, and viscera; cardiovascular disease (principally aortitis); and a variety of central nervous system and ocular syndromes. These forms of syphilis are not contagious. The lesions contain few demonstrable spirochetes, but tissue reactivity (vasculitis, necrosis) is severe and suggestive of hypersensitivity phenomena.

COURSE & PROGNOSIS

The lesions associated with primary and secondary syphilis are self-limiting, even without treatment, and resolve with few or no residua. Late syphilis may be highly destructive and permanently disabling and may lead to death. Many experts now believe that while infection is almost never completely eradicated in the absence of treatment, most infections remain latent without sequelae, and only a small number of latent infections progress to further disease.

CLINICAL STAGES OF SYPHILIS

1. Primary Syphilis

ESSENTIALS OF DIAGNOSIS

▶ History of sexual contact (often unreliable).

▶ Painless ulcer on genitalia, perianal area, rectum, pharynx, tongue, lip, or elsewhere 2–6 weeks after exposure.

▶ Nontender enlargement of regional lymph nodes.

▶ Fluid expressed from lesion contains *T pallidum* by immunofluorescence or darkfield microscopy.

▶ Serologic test for syphilis may be positive.

▶ Clinical Findings

A. Symptoms and Signs

This is the stage of invasion and may pass unrecognized. The typical lesion is the chancre at the site or sites of inoculation, most frequently located on the penis, labia, cervix, or anorectal region (Plate 105). Anorectal lesions are especially common among men who have sex with men. Chancres also occur occasionally in the oropharynx (lip, tongue, or tonsil) and rarely on the breast or finger. An initial small erosion 10–90 days (average, 3–4 weeks) after inoculation then rapidly develops into a painless superficial ulcer with a clean base and firm, indurated margins, which is associated with enlargement of regional lymph nodes, which are rubbery, discrete, and nontender. Bacterial infection of the chancre may occur and may lead to pain. Healing occurs without treatment, but a scar may form, especially with secondary bacterial infection. Multiple chancres may be present, particularly in HIV-positive patients. Although the "classic" ulcer of syphilis has been described as nontender, nonpurulent, and indurated, only 31% of patients have this triad.

Table 34–1. Stages of syphilis and common clinical manifestations.

Primary syphilis
    Genital ulcer: painless ulcer with clean base and firm indurated borders
    Regional lymphadenopathy
Secondary syphilis
    Skin and mucous membranes
        Rash: diffuse (including palms and soles), macular, papular, pustular, and combinations
        Condylomata lata
        Mucous patches: painless, silvery ulcerations of mucous membrane with surrounding erythema
    Generalized lymphadenopathy
    Constitutional symptoms
        Fever, usually low-grade
        Malaise
        Anorexia
        Arthralgias and myalgias
    Central nervous system
        Asymptomatic
        Symptomatic
        Headache
        Meningitis
        Cranial neuropathies (II–VIII)
    Ocular
        Iritis
        Iridocyclitis
    Other
        Renal: glomerulonephritis, nephrotic syndrome
        Liver: hepatitis
        Bone and joint: arthritis, periostitis
Late syphilis
    Late benign (gummatous): granulomatous lesion usually involving skin, mucous membranes and bones, but any organ can be involved
    Cardiovascular
        Aortic regurgitation
        Coronary ostial stenosis
        Aortic aneurysm
    Neurosyphilis
        Asymptomatic
        Meningovascular
            Seizures
            Hemiparesis or hemiplegia
        Tabes dorsalis
            Impaired proprioception and vibratory sensation
            Argyll Robertson pupil
            Shooting pains
            Ataxia
            Romberg sign
            Urinary and fecal incontinence
            Charcot joint
            Cranial nerve involvement (II–VIII)
        General paresis
            Personality changes
            Hyperactive reflexes
            Argyll Robertson pupil
            Decreased memory
            Slurred speech
            Optic atrophy

B. Laboratory Findings

1. Microscopic examination—In early (infectious) syphilis, darkfield microscopic examination by a skilled observer

Table 34–2. Percentage of patients with positive serologic tests for syphilis.[1]

Test	Stage		
	Primary	Secondary	Tertiary
VDRL	75–85%	99%	95%
FTA-ABS	85–95%	100%	98%

[1]Based on untreated cases.
FTA-ABS, fluorescent treponemal antibody absorption test; VDRL, Venereal Disease Research Laboratory test.

of fresh exudate from lesions or material aspirated from regional lymph nodes is up to 90% sensitive for diagnosis. The darkfield examination requires considerable experience for proper specimen collection and identification of characteristic features of morphology and motility of pathogenic spirochetes, and repeated examinations may be necessary. Therefore, this testing is usually only available in select sexually transmitted disease clinics. Darkfield examination of oral lesions is not recommended because of the presence of nonpathogenic treponemes in the mouth. Spirochetes usually are not found in late syphilitic lesions by this technique.

An immunofluorescent staining technique for demonstrating *T pallidum* in dried smears of fluid taken from early syphilitic lesions is available. Slides are fixed and treated with fluorescein-labeled antitreponemal antibody that has been preabsorbed with nonpathogenic treponemes. The slides are then examined for fluorescing spirochetes in an ultraviolet microscope. Because of its simplicity and convenience to clinicians (slides can be mailed), this technique has replaced darkfield microscopy in most health departments and medical center laboratories.

2. Serologic tests for syphilis—(Table 34–2.) There are two general categories of serologic tests for syphilis: (1) Nontreponemal tests detect antibodies to lipoidal antigens present in the host after modification by *T pallidum*. (2) Treponemal tests use live or killed *T pallidum* as antigen to detect antibodies specific for pathogenic treponemes.

A. NONTREPONEMAL ANTIGEN TESTS—The most commonly used nontreponemal antigen tests are the Venereal Disease Research Laboratory (VDRL) and rapid plasma reagin (RPR), which measure the ability of heated serum to flocculate a suspension of cardiolipin–cholesterol–lecithin. The flocculation tests are inexpensive, rapid, and easy to perform and are therefore used primarily for routine screening. Quantitative expression of the reactivity of the serum, based on titration of dilutions of serum, is valuable in establishing the diagnosis and in evaluating the efficacy of treatment, since titers usually correlate with disease activity.

Nontreponemal tests generally become positive 4–6 weeks after infection or 1–3 weeks after the appearance of a primary lesion; they are almost invariably positive in the secondary stage, with titers ≥ 1:32. In the late stages, titers tend to be lower (< 1:4). These serologic tests are not highly specific and must be closely correlated with other clinical and laboratory findings. The tests are positive in patients with non–sexually transmitted treponematoses (see below). More important, false-positive serologic reactions are frequently encountered in a wide variety of nontreponemal states, including connective tissue diseases, infectious mononucleosis, malaria, febrile diseases, leprosy, injection drug use, infective endocarditis, old age, hepatitis C viral infection, and pregnancy. False-positive tests also occur more commonly in HIV-seropositive patients (4%) than in HIV-seronegative patients (0.8%). False-positive reactions are usually of low titer and transient and may be distinguished from true positives by specific treponemal antibody tests. False-negative results can be seen when very high antibody titers are present (the prozone phenomenon). If syphilis is strongly suspected and the nontreponemal test is negative, the laboratory should be instructed to dilute the specimen to detect a positive reaction. The RPR and VDRL tests are equally reliable, but titers of RPR tend to be higher than the VDRL. Thus, when these tests are used to follow disease activity, the same testing method should be used and preferably should be performed at the same laboratory.

Nontreponemal antibody titers are used to assess adequacy of therapy. The time required for the VDRL or RPR to become negative depends on the stage of the disease, the level of the initial titer, and whether the infection is an initial or repeat episode. In general, persons with repeat infections, higher initial titers, more advanced stages of disease, or those who are HIV positive at the time of treatment have a slower seroconversion rate and are more likely to remain serofast (ie, titers do not become negative). Data based on currently recommended treatment regimens (see below) suggest that in primary and secondary syphilis it may take 6 months to see a fourfold decrease in titer and 12 months to see an eightfold drop. In patients with early latent syphilis, response is even slower, with a fourfold drop in titer taking 12–24 months. Seronegativity was seen in 72% of patients with primary syphilis and only 56% of those with secondary syphilis after 3 years.

B. TREPONEMAL ANTIBODY TESTS—These tests measure antibodies capable of reacting with *T pallidum* antigens. The *T pallidum* hemagglutination (TPHA) test and the *T pallidum* particle agglutination (TPPA) test are comparable in specificity and sensitivity to the fluorescent treponemal antibody absorption test (FTA-ABS). The TPPA test, because of ease of performance, has supplanted the FTA-ABS test as the means of confirming the diagnosis of syphilis.

The treponemal tests are of value principally in determining whether a positive nontreponemal antigen test is false-positive or is indicative of syphilis. Because of their great sensitivity, particularly in the late stages of the disease, these tests are also of value when there is clinical evidence of syphilis but the nontreponemal serologic test for syphilis is negative. Treponemal tests are positive in most patients with primary syphilis and in almost all patients with secondary syphilis. Like nontreponemal antigen tests, the specific treponemal antibody test may revert to negative with adequate therapy. This is seen almost exclusively in initial infections in persons with primary

syphilis. In one study, 11% of individuals with a first episode of primary syphilis were seronegative by the FTA-ABS test at 1 year posttreatment and 24% were negative by 3 years. Immunologic status may also affect antibody titers. Seven percent of asymptomatic HIV-infected patients became seronegative after treatment, compared with 38% of symptomatic HIV-infected individuals. The long-held belief that a positive treponemal test persists indefinitely is clearly not valid, and this test therefore cannot be used as a reliable marker of previous infection. False-positive test results occur rarely in persons with systemic lupus erythematosus and in other disorders associated with increased levels of γ-globulins, malaria, leprosy, and other spirochetal infections. It is noteworthy that Lyme disease may cause a false-positive treponemal test but rarely causes a false-positive nontreponemal test. Final decisions about the significance of the results of serologic tests for syphilis must be based on a total clinical appraisal.

3. Polymerase chain reaction—There is increasing interest in the use of polymerase chain reaction (PCR) for the diagnosis of genital ulcer disease, including syphilis, but it is not yet widely available in the United States.

4. Cerebrospinal fluid examination—See Neurosyphilis (below).

▶ **Differential Diagnosis**

The syphilitic chancre may be confused with genital herpes, chancroid (usually painful and uncommon in the United states), lymphogranuloma venereum (also uncommon), or neoplasm. Any genital ulcer should be considered a possible primary syphilitic lesion. Simultaneous evaluation for herpes simplex virus types 1 and 2 using PCR or culture should also be done in these cases.

▶ **Prevention & Screening**

Avoidance of sexual contact is the only completely reliable method of prevention but is an impractical public health measure for obvious reasons. The standard latex condom is effective but protects covered areas only. Screening every 6–12 months for syphilis among men who have sex with men has been recommended based on preliminary data suggesting that this may decrease the rate of transmission. High-risk individuals (those who have multiple encounters with anonymous partners or who have sex in conjunction with the use of drugs) should be screened every 3–6 months. Patients treated for other sexually transmitted diseases should also be tested for syphilis, and persons who have known or suspected contact with patients who have syphilis should be evaluated and treated to abort development of infectious syphilis (see Treating Syphilis Contacts below).

▶ **Treatment**

A. Antibiotic Therapy

Penicillin remains the preferred treatment for syphilis, since there have been no documented cases of penicillin resistant *T pallidum* (Table 34–3). Although doxycycline is

Table 34–3. Recommended treatment for syphilis.[1]

Stage of Syphilis	Treatment	Alternative[2]	Comment
Early			
Primary, secondary, or early latent	Benzathine penicillin G 2.4 million units IM once	Doxycycline 100 mg orally twice daily for 14 days or Tetracycline 500 mg orally four times daily for 28 days or Ceftriaxone 1 g IM daily for 8–10 days	
Late			
Late latent or uncertain duration	Benzathine penicillin G 2.4 million units IM weekly for 3 weeks	Doxycycline 100 mg orally twice daily for 28 days or Tetracycline 500 mg orally four times a day for 28 days	
Tertiary without neurosyphilis	Benzathine penicillin G 2.4 million units IM weekly for 3 weeks	Doxycycline 100 mg orally twice daily for 28 days or Tetracycline 500 mg orally four times a day for 28 days	Cerebrospinal fluid evaluation recommended in all patients
Neurosyphilis	Aqueous penicillin G 18–24 million units IV daily, given every 3–4 hours or as continuous infusion for 10–14 days	Procaine penicillin, 2.4 million units IM daily with probenecid 500 mg orally four times a day for 10–14 days or Ceftriaxone 2 g IM daily for 10–14 days	Follow treatment with benzathine penicillin G, 2.4 million units IM weekly for up to 3 weeks

[1]Penicillin is the only documented effective treatment in pregnancy, so pregnant patients with true allergy should be desensitized and treated with penicillin according to stage of disease as above.
[2]Patients treated with alternative therapies require close clinical and serologic monitoring.

an alternative for some patients, pregnant women must be treated with penicillin (see below).

There are limited data for ceftriaxone, although optimum dose and duration are not well defined. Azithromycin is no longer recommended due to increasing resistance. Patients treated for neurosyphilis should receive at least one dose of long-acting penicillin at the completion of therapy. All patients treated with a non-penicillin regimen must have close clinical and serologic follow up, as noted below.

B. Local Measures (Mucocutaneous Lesions)

Local treatment is usually not necessary. No local antiseptics or other chemicals should be applied to a suspected syphilitic lesion until specimens for microscopy have been obtained.

C. Public Health Measures

Patients with infectious syphilis must abstain from sexual activity for 7–10 days after treatment, or until lesions have resolved. All cases of syphilis must be reported to the appropriate local public health agency for assistance in identifying and treating contacts. In addition, all patients with syphilis should have an HIV test at the time of diagnosis. In areas of high HIV prevalence, a repeat HIV test should be performed in 3 months if the initial test result was negative.

D. Treating Syphilis Contacts

Patients who have been sexually exposed to infectious syphilis within the preceding 3 months may be infected but seronegative and thus should be treated as for early syphilis. Persons exposed more than 90 days previously should

be treated based on serologic results. If their partners are unavailable for testing or unreliable for follow-up, empiric therapy is indicated.

Persons at high risk for infection (ie, those with other sexually transmitted diseases and those infected with HIV) and pregnant women should undergo serologic tests for syphilis. Patients with gonorrhea and a known exposure to syphilis should be treated with separate regimens effective against both diseases.

▶ Complications of Specific Therapy

The Jarisch–Herxheimer reaction, manifested by fever and aggravation of the existing clinical picture in the hours following treatment, is ascribed to the sudden massive destruction of spirochetes. It is most common in early syphilis, particularly secondary syphilis where it can occur in 66% of cases. The reaction resolves spontaneously within 24 hours; treatment should not be discontinued unless the symptoms become severe or life-threatening or unless syphilitic laryngitis, auditory neuritis, or labyrinthitis is present, where the reaction may cause irreversible damage. It may prompt preterm labor in pregnant women.

The reaction may be prevented or modified by simultaneous administration of antipyretics, although no proved method of prevention exists. Patients should be reminded it does not represent an allergic reaction to penicillin.

▶ Follow-Up Care

Because treatment failures and reinfection may occur, patients treated for syphilis should be monitored clinically and serologically at 3–6 month intervals. Response to therapy may be difficult to assess, and no definite criteria exist for cure in patients with primary or secondary syphilis. In primary and secondary syphilis, failure of nontreponemal antibody titers to decrease fourfold by 6 months may identify a group at high risk for treatment failure. Optimal management of these patients is unclear, but at a minimum, close clinical and serologic follow-up is indicated. If titers fail to decrease fourfold by 6 months, an HIV test should be repeated (all patients with syphilis should have an HIV test at the time of diagnosis); a lumbar puncture should be considered since unrecognized neurosyphilis can be a cause of treatment failure; and, if careful follow-up cannot be ensured (3-month intervals for HIV-positive individuals and 6-month intervals for HIV-negative patients), treatment should be repeated with 2.4 million units of benzathine penicillin intramuscularly weekly for 3 weeks. If symptoms or signs persist or recur after initial therapy or there is a fourfold or greater increase in nontreponemal titers, therapy has either failed or the patient has been reinfected. In those individuals, an HIV test should be performed, a lumbar puncture done (unless reinfection is a certainty), and re-treatment given as indicated above.

2. Secondary Syphilis

ESSENTIALS OF DIAGNOSIS

- ▶ Generalized maculopapular skin rash.
- ▶ Mucous membrane lesions, including patches and ulcers.
- ▶ Weeping papules (condylomas) in moist skin areas.
- ▶ Generalized nontender lymphadenopathy.
- ▶ Fever.
- ▶ Meningitis, hepatitis, osteitis, arthritis, iritis.
- ▶ Many treponemes in scrapings of mucous membrane or skin lesions by immunofluorescence or darkfield microscopy.
- ▶ Serologic tests for syphilis always positive.

▶ General Considerations & Treatment

The secondary stage of syphilis usually appears a few weeks (or up to 6 months) after development of the chancre, when dissemination of *T pallidum* produces systemic signs (fever, lymphadenopathy) or infectious lesions at sites distant from the site of inoculation. The most common manifestations are skin and mucosal lesions. The skin lesions are nonpruritic, macular, papular, pustular, or follicular (or combinations of any of these types, but *not* vesicular), though the maculopapular rash is the most common. The skin lesions usually are generalized; involvement of the palms and soles occurs in 80% of cases (Plate 106). Annular lesions simulating ringworm may be observed in dark-skinned individuals. Mucous membrane lesions range from ulcers and papules of the lips, mouth,

throat, genitalia, and anus ("mucous patches") to a diffuse redness of the pharynx. Both skin and mucous membrane lesions are highly infectious at this stage. Specific lesions—**condylomata lata**—are fused, weeping papules on the moist areas of the skin and mucous membranes and are sometimes mistaken for genital warts.

Meningeal (aseptic meningitis or acute basilar meningitis), hepatic, renal, bone, and joint invasion may occur, with resulting cranial nerve palsies, jaundice, nephrotic syndrome, and periostitis. Alopecia (moth-eaten appearance) and uveitis may also occur.

The serologic tests for syphilis are positive in almost all cases (see Primary Syphilis, above). The moist cutaneous and mucous membrane lesions often show *T pallidum* on darkfield microscopic examination. A transient cerebrospinal fluid (CSF) pleocytosis is seen in 30–70% of patients with secondary syphilis, though only 5% have positive serologic CSF reactions. There may be evidence of hepatitis or nephritis (immune complex type). Circulating immune complexes exist in the blood and are deposited in blood vessel walls.

Skin lesions may be confused with the infectious exanthems, pityriasis rosea, and drug eruptions (Plate 107). Visceral lesions may suggest nephritis or hepatitis due to other causes. The diffusely red throat may mimic other forms of pharyngitis.

Treatment is as for primary syphilis unless central nervous system or ocular disease is present, in which case a lumbar puncture should be performed and, if positive, treatment is as for neurosyphilis (Table 34–3). Isolation of the patient is important. See Primary Syphilis for follow-up care and treatment of contacts.

3. Early Latent Syphilis

ESSENTIALS OF DIAGNOSIS

- ▶ No physical signs.
- ▶ History of syphilis with inadequate treatment.
- ▶ Positive serologic tests for syphilis.

▶ General Considerations & Treatment

Latent syphilis is the clinically quiescent phase during the interval after the disappearance of secondary lesions and is defined as the first year after primary infection. Early latent syphilis may relapse to secondary syphilis if undiagnosed or inadequately treated (see above). Unlike the usual asymptomatic neurologic involvement of secondary syphilis, neurologic relapses may be fulminating, leading to death. Relapse is almost always accompanied by a rising titer in quantitative serologic tests; indeed, a rising titer may be the first or only evidence of relapse. About 90% of relapses occur during the first year after infection. If untreated, a small proportion of patients progress to tertiary syphilis.

Treatment and follow up is as for primary syphilis unless central nervous system disease is present (Table 34–3).

4. Late Latent ("Hidden") Syphilis

▶ No physical signs.

▶ History of syphilis with inadequate treatment.

▶ Positive serologic tests for syphilis.

General Considerations & Treatment

After the first year of latent syphilis, the patient is said to be in the late latent phase. Transmission to the fetus, however, can probably occur in any phase. There are (by definition) no clinical manifestations during the latent phase, and the only significant laboratory findings are positive serologic tests. A diagnosis of latent syphilis is justified only when the CSF is entirely negative, radiographic studies and physical examination show no evidence of cardiovascular involvement, and false-positive tests for syphilis have been ruled out. The latent phase may last from months to a lifetime.

Treatment of late latent syphilis is shown in Table 34–3. The treatment of this stage of the disease is intended to prevent the late sequelae. If there is evidence of central nervous system involvement, a lumbar puncture should be performed and, if positive, the patient should receive treatment as for neurosyphilis. Titers may not decline as rapidly following treatment as in early syphilis. Nontreponemal serologic tests should be repeated at 6, 12, and 24 months. If titers increase fourfold or if initially high titers (≥ 1:32) fail to decrease fourfold by 12–24 months or if symptoms or signs consistent with syphilis develop, an HIV test and lumbar puncture should be performed and re-treatment given according to the stage of the disease.

5. Late (Tertiary) Syphilis

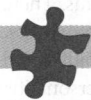

▶ Infiltrative tumors of skin, bones, liver (gummas).

▶ Aortitis, aneurysms, aortic regurgitation.

▶ Central nervous system disorders, including meningovascular and degenerative changes, paresthesias, shooting pains, abnormal reflexes, dementia, or psychosis.

General Considerations

This stage may occur at any time after secondary syphilis, even after years of latency, and is rarely seen in the modern antibiotic era. Late lesions probably represent, at least in part, a delayed hypersensitivity reaction of the tissue to the organism and are usually divided into two types: (1) a localized gummatous reaction, with a relatively rapid onset and generally prompt response to therapy ("benign late syphilis") and (2) diffuse inflammation of a more insidious onset that characteristically involves the central nervous system and large arteries, is often fatal if untreated, and is at best arrested by treatment. Gummas may involve any area or organ of the body but most often affect the skin or long bones. Cardiovascular disease is usually manifested by aortic aneurysm, aortic regurgitation, or aortitis. Various forms of diffuse or localized central nervous system involvement may occur.

Late syphilis must be differentiated from neoplasms of the skin, liver, lung, stomach, or brain; other forms of meningitis; and primary neurologic lesions.

Although almost any tissue and organ may be involved in late syphilis, the following are the most common types of involvement: skin, mucous membranes, skeletal system, eyes, respiratory system, gastrointestinal system, cardiovascular system, and nervous system.

Clinical Findings

A. Symptoms and Signs

1. Skin—Cutaneous lesions of late syphilis are of two varieties: (1) multiple nodular lesions that eventually ulcerate (lues maligna) or resolve by forming atrophic, pigmented scars and (2) solitary gummas that start as painless subcutaneous nodules, then enlarge, attach to the overlying skin, and eventually ulcerate (Plate 108).

2. Mucous membranes—Late lesions of the mucous membranes are nodular gummas or leukoplakia, highly destructive to the involved tissue.

3. Skeletal system—Bone lesions are destructive, causing periostitis, osteitis, and arthritis with little or no associated redness or swelling but often marked myalgia and myositis of the neighboring muscles. The pain is especially severe at night.

4. Eyes—Late ocular lesions are gummatous iritis, chorioretinitis, optic atrophy, and cranial nerve palsies, in addition to the lesions of central nervous system syphilis.

5. Respiratory system—Respiratory involvement by late syphilis is caused by gummatous infiltrates into the larynx, trachea, and pulmonary parenchyma, producing discrete pulmonary densities. There may be hoarseness, respiratory distress, and wheezing secondary to the gummatous lesion itself or to subsequent stenosis occurring with healing.

6. Gastrointestinal system—Gummas involving the liver produce the usually benign, asymptomatic hepar lobatum. A picture resembling Laennec cirrhosis is occasionally produced by liver involvement. Gastric involvement can consist of diffuse infiltration into the stomach wall or focal lesions that endoscopically and microscopically can be confused with lymphoma or carcinoma. Epigastric pain, early satiety, regurgitation, belching, and weight loss are common symptoms.

7. Cardiovascular system—Cardiovascular lesions (10–15% of late syphilitic lesions) are often progressive, disabling, and life-threatening. Central nervous system lesions are often present concomitantly. Involvement usually starts as an arteritis in the supracardiac portion of the aorta and progresses to one or more of the following: (1) narrowing of the coronary ostia, with resulting decreased coronary circulation, angina, and acute myocardial infarction; (2) scarring of the aortic valves, producing aortic regurgitation, and eventually congestive heart failure; and (3) weakness of the wall of the aorta, with saccular aneurysm formation (Plate 109) and associated pressure symptoms of dysphagia, hoarseness, brassy cough, back pain (vertebral erosion), and occasionally rupture of the aneurysm. Recurrent respiratory infections are common as a result of pressure on the trachea and bronchi.

8. Nervous system (neurosyphilis)—See following section.

▶ Treatment

Treatment of tertiary syphilis (excluding neurosyphilis) is the same as late latent syphilis (Table 34–3). Reversal of positive serologic tests does not usually occur. A second course of penicillin therapy may be given, but there is no known method for reliable eradication of the treponeme from humans in the late stages of syphilis. Viable spirochetes are occasionally found in the eyes, in CSF, and elsewhere in patients with "adequately" treated syphilis, but claims for their capacity to cause progressive disease are speculative.

In the presence of definite CSF or neurologic abnormalities, one should treat for neurosyphilis. The pretreatment clinical and laboratory evaluation should include neurologic, ocular, cardiovascular, psychiatric, and CSF examinations.

6. Neurosyphilis

ESSENTIALS OF DIAGNOSIS

▶ Can occur at any stage of disease.

▶ Consider both clinical presentation and laboratory data.

▶ Carefully evaluate HIV-positive patients and consider CSF evaluation for atypical symptoms or lack of decrease in nontreponemal serology titers.

▶ General Considerations

Neurosyphilis can occur at any stage of disease and can be a progressive, disabling, and life-threatening complication. CSF pleocytosis has been reported in 10–20% of patients with primary syphilis. Asymptomatic and meningovascular syphilis occur earlier (months to years after infection, sometimes coexisting with primary and secondary syphilis) than tabes dorsalis and general paresis (2–50 years after infection).

▶ Clinical Findings

A. Classification

There are four clinical types.

1. Asymptomatic neurosyphilis—This form is characterized by spinal fluid abnormalities (positive spinal fluid

serology, increased cell count, occasionally increased protein) without symptoms or signs of neurologic involvement.

2. Meningovascular syphilis—This form is characterized by meningeal involvement or changes in the vascular structures of the brain (or both), producing symptoms of chronic meningitis (headache, irritability); cranial nerve palsies (basilar meningitis); unequal reflexes; irregular pupils with poor light and accommodation reflexes; and when large vessels are involved, cerebrovascular accidents. The CSF shows increased cells (100–1000/mcL), elevated protein, and usually a positive serologic test for syphilis. The symptoms of acute meningitis are rare in late syphilis.

3. Tabes dorsalis—This form is a chronic progressive degeneration of the parenchyma of the posterior columns of the spinal cord and of the posterior sensory ganglia and nerve roots. The symptoms and signs are impairment of proprioception and vibration sense, Argyll Robertson pupils (which react poorly to light but well to accommodation), and muscular hypotonia and hyporeflexia. Impairment of proprioception results in a wide-based gait and inability to walk in the dark. Paresthesias, analgesia, or sharp recurrent pains in the muscles of the leg ("shooting" or "lightning" pains) may occur. Crises are also common in tabes: gastric crises, consisting of sharp abdominal pains with nausea and vomiting (simulating an acute abdomen); laryngeal crises, with paroxysmal cough and dyspnea; urethral crises, with painful bladder spasms; and rectal and anal crises. Crises may begin suddenly, last for hours to days, and cease abruptly. Neurogenic bladder with overflow incontinence is also seen. Painless trophic ulcers may develop over pressure points on the feet. Joint damage may occur as a result of lack of sensory innervation (Charcot joint, Plate 110). The CSF may have a normal or increased cell count (3–200/mcL), elevated protein, and variable results of serologic tests.

4. General paresis—This is generalized involvement of the cerebral cortex with insidious onset of symptoms. There is usually a decrease in concentrating power, memory loss, dysarthria, tremor of the fingers and lips, irritability, and mild headaches. Most striking is the change of personality; the patient becomes slovenly, irresponsible, confused, and psychotic. The CSF findings resemble those of tabes dorsalis. Combinations of the various forms of neurosyphilis (especially tabes and paresis) are not uncommon.

B. Laboratory Findings

See Serologic Tests for Syphilis, above; these tests should also be performed in cases of suspected neurosyphilis.

1. Indications for a lumbar puncture—It is most important to prevent neurosyphilis by prompt diagnosis, adequate treatment, and follow-up of early syphilis. Indications for lumbar puncture vary depending on the stage of the disease and the patient's immune status. In early syphilis (primary and secondary syphilis and early latent syphilis of less than 1 year duration), invasion of the central nervous system by *T pallidum* with CSF abnormalities occurs commonly, but clinical neurosyphilis rarely develops in patients who have received the standard therapy outlined above. Thus, unless clinical symptoms and signs of neurosyphilis or ophthalmologic involvement (uveitis, neuroretinitis, optic neuritis, iritis) are present, a lumbar puncture in early syphilis is not recommended as part of the routine evaluation. In latent syphilis, the decision to perform a lumbar puncture should be individualized. Routine lumbar puncture for all patients is not indicated since the yield is low and findings rarely influence therapeutic decisions. CSF evaluation is recommended, however, in the later stages of syphilis if neurologic or ophthalmologic symptoms and signs are present, if therapy other than with penicillin is to be given, if the patient is HIV positive (see next section), if there is evidence of treatment failure (see earlier discussion), or if there is evidence of active tertiary syphilis (eg, aortitis, iritis, optic atrophy, the presence of a gumma). Some experts also routinely recommend lumbar puncture for all persons with latent syphilis if the serum nontreponemal antibody titer is ≥ 1:32 or the CD4 count is < 350/mcL in HIV-infected persons.

2. Spinal fluid examination—CSF findings in neurosyphilis are variable. In "classic" cases, there is an elevation of total protein, lymphocytic pleocytosis, and a positive CSF reagin test (VDRL). However, CSF may be completely normal in neurosyphilis, and the VDRL may be negative. In one study, 25% of patients with primary or secondary syphilis in whom *T pallidum* was isolated from CSF had normal findings. In later stages of syphilis, normal CSF analysis in the presence of infection can occur, but it is unusual. Because false-positive reagin tests rarely occur in the CSF, a positive test confirms the presence of neurosyphilis. Because the CSF VDRL may be negative in 30–70% of cases of neurosyphilis, *a negative test does not exclude neurosyphilis*. The CSF FTA-ABS is sometimes used; it is a highly sensitive test but lacks specificity, and a high serum titer of FTA-ABS may result in a positive CSF titer in the absence of neurosyphilis.

▶ **Treatment**

Current recommendations for the therapy of neurosyphilis include higher doses of short-acting penicillin to achieve better penetration and higher levels of drug in the CSF than is possible with benzathine penicillin (Table 34–3). Because of concerns about slowly dividing organisms that may persist after only 10–14 days of therapy, many experts recommend subsequent administration of 2.4 million units of benzathine penicillin intramuscularly once weekly for up to 3 weeks as additional therapy. There are some data for using ceftriaxone as well, but because other regimens for neurosyphilis have not been adequately studied, patients with a history of an IgE-mediated reaction to penicillin should be skin tested for allergy to penicillin and, if positive, desensitized.

All patients should have nontreponemal serologic tests done every 3 months. Guidelines established by the Centers for Disease Control and Prevention (CDC) recommend spinal fluid examinations at 6-month intervals until the CSF cell count is normal; however, a recent study suggested that in certain patients normalization of serum titers are an acceptable surrogate for CSF response. In general, CSF white blood cell count and CSF VDRL normalize more quickly (usually in 12 months) than CSF protein concentration, which can remain abnormal for extended periods. If the serum nontreponemal titers do not normalize, the CSF analysis should be repeated. A second course of penicillin therapy may be given if the CSF cell count has not decreased at 6 months or is not normal at 2 years.

7. Syphilis in HIV-Infected Patients

Interpretation of serologic tests should be the same for HIV-positive and HIV-negative persons. Although unusual serologic responses have been reported in HIV-positive patients, including high titers of nontreponemal tests, delayed appearance of positive titers, and false-negative tests, most HIV-positive patients respond serologically in largely the same way as noninfected patients. All HIV-positive patients in care should be screened at least twice a year by RPR or VDRL to identify latent disease because by establishing a serologic history, unnecessary lumbar punctures and prolonged treatment for latent syphilis of uncertain duration can be avoided. If the diagnosis of syphilis is suggested on clinical grounds but reagin tests are negative, alternative tests should be performed. These tests include darkfield examination of lesions and direct fluorescent antibody staining for *T pallidum* of lesion exudate or biopsy specimens.

Treatment of HIV-positive patients with primary and secondary syphilis is the same as for HIV-negative patients. Because of concerns about the adequacy of this therapy, some experts recommend additional therapy with 2.4 million units of benzathine penicillin intramuscularly weekly for 3 weeks instead of single-dose therapy. However, despite occasional reports of neurosyphilis developing in HIV-infected patients despite appropriate therapy for early disease, most HIV-infected patients with primary or secondary syphilis respond appropriately to currently recommended regimens. In all cases, careful clinical and serologic follow-up should be done at 3, 6, 9, 12, and 24 months. HIV-infected patients with late latent syphilis, syphilis of uncertain duration, and neurosyphilis should be treated like HIV-negative individuals, with follow-up at 6, 12, 18, and 24 months. A study among HIV-clinic patients in Baltimore found that the use of antiretroviral therapy was associated with reduced serologic failure rates after syphilis treatment.

The diagnosis of neurosyphilis in HIV-infected patients is complicated by the fact that CSF abnormalities are frequently seen and may be due to neurosyphilis or HIV infection itself. The significance of these abnormalities is unknown, and similar abnormalities are frequently seen in non–HIV-infected patients with primary or secondary syphilis. Thus, although some experts recommend a CSF examination for all HIV-positive patients with syphilis, such testing is probably not needed in those with early disease. In contrast, a lumbar puncture should be performed in HIV-positive patients if they have late latent syphilis or syphilis of uncertain duration, if neurologic signs are present, or if therapy has failed. A recent study found that HIV-positive patients with a nontreponemal antibody titer ≥ 1:32 had a sixfold increased risk of having neurosyphilis, and if the CD4 count was ≤ 350/mcL, there was a threefold increased risk of neurosyphilis, suggesting that these subgroups should also undergo lumbar puncture. Following treatment, CSF white blood cell counts normalize within 12 months regardless of HIV status, while the CSF VDRL is slower to normalize in HIV-infected individuals, especially those with CD4 counts < 200 cells/mcL. As discussed above, the same criteria for failure apply to HIV-positive and HIV-negative patients, and re-treatment regimens are the same.

Because clinical experience in treating HIV-infected patients with syphilis is based on penicillin regimens, few options exist for treating the penicillin-allergic patient. Doxycycline or tetracycline regimens can be used for primary, secondary, and early latent syphilis as well as for late latent syphilis and latent syphilis of unknown duration though with caution and close follow-up. For neurosyphilis, penicillin regimens are optimal even if this requires skin testing and desensitization; limited data exist for ceftriaxone.

8. Syphilis in Pregnancy

All pregnant women should have a nontreponemal serologic test for syphilis at the time of the first prenatal visit. In women who may be at increased risk for syphilis or for populations in which there is a high prevalence of syphilis, additional nontreponemal tests should be performed during the third trimester at 28 weeks and again at delivery. The serologic status of all women who have delivered should be known before discharge from the hospital. Seropositive women should be considered infected and should be treated unless prior treatment with fall in antibody titer is medically documented.

The only acceptable treatment for syphilis in pregnancy is penicillin in dosage schedules appropriate for the stage of disease (see above). Penicillin prevents congenital syphilis in 90% of cases, even when treatment is given late in pregnancy. Tetracycline and doxycycline are contraindicated in pregnancy. Erythromycin should not be used because of failure to eradicate infection in the fetus, and insufficient data are available to justify a recommendation for ceftriaxone or azithromycin. Thus, women with a history of penicillin allergy should be skin tested and desensitized if necessary.

The infant should be evaluated immediately, as noted below, and at 6–8 weeks of age.

9. Congenital Syphilis

Congenital syphilis is a transplacentally transmitted infection that occurs in infants of untreated or inadequately treated mothers. The physical findings at birth are quite variable: The infant may have many or minimal signs or even no signs until 6–8 weeks of life (delayed form). The most common findings are on the mucous membranes and skin—maculopapular rash, condylomas, mucous membrane patches, and serous nasal discharge (snuffles). These lesions are infectious; *T pallidum* can easily be found microscopically, and the infant must be isolated. Other common findings are hepatosplenomegaly, anemia, or osteochondritis. These early active lesions subsequently

heal, and if the disease is left untreated it produces the characteristic stigmas of syphilis—interstitial keratitis, Hutchinson teeth, saddle nose, saber shins, deafness, and central nervous system involvement.

The presence of negative serologic tests at birth in both the mother and the infant usually means that the newborn is free of infection. However, recent infection near the time of delivery may result in negative tests because there has been insufficient time to develop a serologic response. Thus, it is necessary to maintain a high index of suspicion in infants with delayed onset of symptoms despite negative serologic tests at birth, especially in infants born to high-risk mothers (HIV-positive, illicit drug users). All infants born to mothers with positive nontreponemal and treponemal antibody titers should have blood drawn for an RPR or VDRL test and, if positive, be referred to a pediatrician for further evaluation and therapy.

▶ When to Refer

Consultation with the local public health department may help obtain all prior positive syphilis serologic results and may be helpful in complicated or atypical cases.

▶ When to Admit

- Pregnant women with syphilis and true penicillin allergy should be admitted for desensitization and treatment.

- Women in late pregnancy treated for early syphilis should have close outpatient monitoring or be admitted because the Jarisch-Herxheimer reaction can induce premature labor.

- Patients with neurosyphilis usually require admission for treatment with aqueous penicillin.

Fenton KA et al. Infectious syphilis in high-income settings in the 21st century. Lancet Infect Dis. 2008 Apr;8(4):244–53. [PMID: 18353265]

Marra CM et al. Normalization of serum rapid plasma reagin titer predicts normalization of cerebrospinal fluid and clinical abnormalities after treatment of neurosyphilis. Clin Infect Dis. 2008 Oct 1;47(7):893–9. [PMID: 18715154]

O'Donnell JA et al. Neurosyphilis: A current review. Curr Infect Dis Rep. 2005 Jul;7(4):277–284. [PMID: 15963329]

Sexually transmitted diseases treatment guidelines 2006. MMWR Recomm Rep. 2006 Aug 4;55(RR-11):1–94. [PMID: 16888612]

Zetola et al. Syphilis in the United States: an update for clinicians with an emphasis on HIV coinfection. Mayo Clin Proc. 2007 Sep;82(9):1091–102. [PMID: 17803877]

NON–SEXUALLY TRANSMITTED TREPONEMATOSES

A variety of treponemal diseases other than syphilis occur endemically in many tropical areas of the world. They are distinguished from disease caused by *T pallidum* by their nonsexual transmission, their relatively high incidence in certain geographic areas and among children, and their tendency to produce less severe visceral manifestations. As in syphilis, organisms can be demonstrated in infectious lesions with darkfield microscopy or immunofluorescence but cannot be cultured in artificial media; the serologic tests for syphilis are positive; the diseases have primary, secondary, and sometimes tertiary stages; and penicillin is the drug of choice. There is evidence that infection with these agents may provide partial resistance to syphilis and vice versa. Treatment with penicillin in doses appropriate to primary syphilis (eg, 2.4 million units of benzathine penicillin G intramuscularly) is generally curative in any stage of the non–sexually transmitted treponematoses. In cases of penicillin hypersensitivity, tetracycline, 500 mg orally four times a day for 10–14 days, is usually the recommended alternative.

YAWS (Frambesia)

Yaws is a contagious disease largely limited to tropical regions that is caused by *T pallidum* subspecies *pertenue*. It is characterized by granulomatous lesions of the skin, mucous membranes, and bone. Yaws is rarely fatal, though if untreated it may lead to chronic disability and disfigurement. Yaws is acquired by direct nonsexual contact, usually in childhood, although it may occur at any age. The "mother yaw," a painless papule that later ulcerates, appears 3–4 weeks after exposure. There is usually associated regional lymphadenopathy. Six to 12 weeks later, secondary lesions that are raised papillomas and papules that weep highly infectious material appear and last for several months or years. Painful ulcerated lesions on the soles are called "crab yaws" because of the resulting gait. Late gummatous lesions may occur, with associated tissue destruction involving large areas of skin and subcutaneous tissues. The late effects of yaws, with bone change, shortening of digits, and contractions, may be confused with similar changes occurring in leprosy. Central nervous system, cardiac, or other visceral involvement is rare. See above for therapy.

PINTA

Pinta is a non–sexually transmitted spirochetal infection caused by *Treponema carateum*. It occurs endemically in rural areas of Latin America, especially in Mexico, Colombia, and Cuba, and in some areas of the Pacific. A nonulcerative, erythematous primary papule spreads slowly into a papulosquamous plaque showing a variety of color changes (slate, lilac, black). Secondary lesions resemble the primary one and appear within a year after it. These appear successively, new lesions together with older ones; are most common on the extremities; and later show atrophy and depigmentation. Some cases show pigmentary changes and atrophic patches on the soles and palms, with or without hyperkeratosis, that are indistinguishable from "crab yaws." Very rarely, central nervous system or cardiovascular disease is observed late in the course of infection. See above for therapy.

ENDEMIC SYPHILIS

Endemic syphilis is an acute or chronic infection caused by *T pallidum* subspecies *endemicum*. It has been reported in a number of countries, particularly in the eastern Mediterranean area, often with local names: bejel in Syria, Saudi Arabia, and Iraq, and dichuchwa, njovera, and siti in Africa. It also occurs in Southeast Asia. The local forms have distinctive features. Moist ulcerated lesions of the skin or oral or nasopharyngeal mucosa are the most common manifestations. Generalized lymphadenopathy and secondary and tertiary bone and skin lesions are also common. Deep leg pain points to periostitis or osteomyelitis. In the late stages of disease, destructive gummatous lesions similar to those seen in yaws can develop, resulting in loss of cartilage and saber shin deformity. Cardiovascular and central nervous system involvement are rare. See above for therapy.

Farnsworth N et al. Endemic treponematosis: review and update. Clin Dermatol. 2006 May–Jun;24(3):181–90. [PMID: 16714199]
Rinaldi A. Yaws: a second (and maybe last?) chance for eradication. PLoS Negl Trop Dis. 2008;2(8):e275. [PMID: 18846236]

▼ SELECTED SPIROCHETAL DISEASES

RELAPSING FEVER

Relapsing fever is endemic in many parts of the world. The main reservoir is rodents, which serve as the source of infection for ticks (eg, ornithodoros). The distribution and seasonal incidence of the disease are determined by the ecology of the ticks in different areas. In the United States, infected ticks are found throughout the West, especially in mountainous areas, but clinical cases are uncommon in humans.

The infectious organisms are spirochetes of the genus *Borrelia*. The infection has two forms: tick-borne and louse-borne. Tick-borne relapsing fever may be transmitted transovarially from one generation of ticks to the next. Humans can be infected by tick bites or by rubbing crushed tick tissues or feces into the bite wound. Tick-borne relapsing fever is endemic but is not transmitted from person to person. Different species (or strain) names have been given to *Borrelia* in different parts of the world where the organisms are transmitted by different ticks.

The louse-borne form is primarily seen in the developing world. Large epidemics may occur in louse-infested populations, and transmission is favored by crowding, malnutrition, and cold climate.

► Clinical Findings

A. Symptoms and Signs

There is an abrupt onset of fever, chills, tachycardia, nausea and vomiting, arthralgia, and severe headache. Hepatomegaly and splenomegaly may develop, as well as various types of rashes (macular, popular, petechial) that usually occur at the end of a febrile episode. Delirium occurs with high fever, and there may be various neurologic and psychic abnormalities. The attack terminates, usually abruptly, after 3–10 days. After an interval of 1–2 weeks, relapse occurs, but often it is somewhat milder. Three to ten relapses may occur before recovery in tick-borne disease, whereas louse-borne disease is associated with only one or two relapses.

B. Laboratory Findings

During episodes of fever, large spirochetes are seen in blood smears stained with Wright or Giemsa stain. The organisms can be cultured in special media but rapidly lose pathogenicity. The spirochetes can multiply in injected rats or mice and can be seen in their blood.

A variety of anti-borrelia antibodies develop during the illness; sometimes the Weil–Felix test for rickettsioses and nontreponemal serologic tests for syphilis may also be falsely positive. Infection with *B recurrentis* can cause false-positive indirect fluorescent antibody and Western blot tests for *Borrelia burgdorferi*, and some cases may be misdiagnosed as Lyme disease. CSF abnormalities occur in patients with meningeal involvement. Mild anemia and thrombocytopenia are common, but the white blood cell count tends to be normal.

Differential Diagnosis

The manifestations of relapsing fever may be confused with malaria, leptospirosis, meningococcemia, yellow fever, typhus, or rat-bite fever.

Prevention

Prevention of tick bites (as described for rickettsial diseases) and delousing procedures applicable to large groups can prevent illness. Arthropod vectors should be controlled if possible.

Doxycycline 200 mg orally on day 1 and 100 mg daily for 4 days has been shown to prevent recurrent fever following tick bites in highly endemic areas.

Treatment

A single dose of tetracycline or erythromycin, 0.5 g orally, or a single dose of procaine penicillin G, 400,000–600,000 units intramuscularly, probably constitutes adequate treatment for louse-borne relapsing fevers. Because of higher relapse rates, tick-borne disease is treated with 0.5 g of tetracycline or erythromycin given orally four times daily for 5–10 days. Jarisch–Herxheimer reactions occur commonly following treatment and may be life-threatening, so patients should be closely monitored. There is evidence that administration of anti-TNF antibodies prior to antibiotic therapy can be effective in preventing the reaction.

Prognosis

The overall mortality rate is usually about 5%. Fatalities are most common in old, debilitated, or very young patients. With treatment, the initial attack is shortened and relapses are largely prevented.

Dworkin MS et al. Tick-borne relapsing fever. Infect Dis Clin North Am. 2008 Sept 22(3):449–68. [PMID: 18755384]

Hasin T et al. Postexposure treatment with doxycycline for prevention of tick-borne relapsing fever. N Engl J Med. 2006 Jul 13;355(2):148–55. [PMID: 16837678]

RAT-BITE FEVER

Rat-bite fever is an uncommon acute infectious disease caused by the treponeme *Spirillum minus* (Asia), covered in this section, or the bacteria *Streptobacillus moniliformis* (North America). It is transmitted to humans by the bite of a rat. Inhabitants of rat-infested dwellings and laboratory workers are at greatest risk.

▶ Clinical Findings

A. Symptoms and Signs

In Spirillum infections, the original rat bite, unless secondarily infected, heals promptly, but 1 to several weeks later the site becomes swollen, indurated, and painful; assumes a dusky purplish hue; and may ulcerate. Regional lymphangitis and lymphadenitis, fever, chills, malaise, myalgia, arthralgia, and headache are present. Splenomegaly may occur. A sparse, dusky-red maculopapular rash appears on the trunk and extremities in many cases, and there may be frank arthritis.

After a few days, both the local and systemic symptoms subside, only to reappear several days later. This relapsing pattern of fever for 3–4 days alternating with afebrile periods lasting 3–9 days may persist for weeks. The other features, however, usually recur only during the first few relapses. Endocarditis is a rare complication of infection.

B. Laboratory Findings

Leukocytosis is often present, and the nontreponemal test for syphilis is often falsely positive. The organism may be identified in darkfield examination of the ulcer exudate or aspirated lymph node material; more commonly, it is observed after inoculation of a laboratory animal with the patient's exudate or blood. It has not been cultured in artificial media.

▶ Differential Diagnosis

Rat-bite fever must be distinguished from the rat-bite–induced lymphadenitis and rash of streptobacillary fever. Clinically, the severe arthritis and myalgias seen in streptobacillary disease are rarely seen in disease caused by *S minus*. Reliable differentiation requires an increasing titer of agglutinins against *S moniliformis* or isolation of the causative organism. Other diseases in the differential include tularemia, rickettsial disease, *Pasteurella multocida* infections, and relapsing fever.

▶ Treatment

Penicillin is given for 10–14 days. During the acute phase of illness, the intravenous route is used (1–2 million units every 4–6 hours) and once improvement has occurred, therapy is completed with oral medication, penicillin V 500 mg four times daily to complete 10–14 days of therapy. For the penicillin-allergic patient, tetracycline 500 mg orally four times daily or doxycycline 100 mg twice a day can be used.

▶ Prognosis

The reported mortality rate of about 10% should be markedly reduced by prompt diagnosis and antimicrobial treatment.

Elliot SP. Rat bite fever and *Streptobacillus moniliformis*. Clin Microbiol Rev. 2007 Jan;20(1):13–22. [PMID: 17223620]

LEPTOSPIROSIS

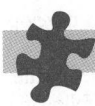

ESSENTIALS OF DIAGNOSIS

▶ Clinical illness can vary from asymptomatic to fatal liver and kidney disease.

▶ Anicteric leptospirosis is the more common and milder form of the disease.

▶ Icteric leptospirosis (Weil syndrome) is characterized by impaired kidney and liver function, abnormal mental status, and hemorrhagic pneumonia and has a 5–40% mortality rate.

General Considerations

Leptospirosis is an acute and often severe treponemal infection that frequently affects the liver or other organs and is caused by multiple species within the genus *Leptospira*. The disease is worldwide in distribution, and it is among the most common zoonotic diseases. The leptospires are often transmitted to humans by the ingestion of food and drink contaminated by the urine of the reservoir animal. The organism may also enter through minor skin lesions and probably via the conjunctiva. Recreational cases have followed swimming or rafting in contaminated water, and occupational cases occur among sewer workers, rice planters, abattoir workers, and farmers. Sporadic urban cases have been seen in the homeless exposed to rat urine. The incubation period is 2–20 days.

Clinical Findings

A. Symptoms and Signs

Anicteric leptospirosis, the more common and milder form of the disease, is often biphasic. The initial or "septicemic" phase begins with abrupt fever to 39–40 °C, chills, abdominal pain, severe headache, and myalgias, especially of the calf muscles. There may be marked conjunctival suffusion. Leptospires can be isolated from blood, CSF, and tissues. Following a 1- to 3-day period of improvement in symptoms and absence of fever, the second or "immune" phase begins. Leptospires are absent from blood and CSF but are still present in the kidney, and specific antibodies appear. A recurrence of symptoms is seen as in the first phase of disease with the onset of meningitis. Uveitis (which can be unilateral or bilateral and usually involves the entire uveal tract), rash, and adenopathy may occur. A rare but severe manifestation is hemorrhagic pneumonia. The illness is usually self-limited, lasting 4–30 days, and complete recovery is the rule.

Icteric leptospirosis (Weil syndrome) is the most severe form of the disease, characterized by impaired kidney and liver function, abnormal mental status, hemorrhagic pneumonia, hypotension, and a 5–40% mortality rate. Symptoms and signs often are continuous and not biphasic.

Leptospirosis with jaundice must be distinguished from hepatitis, yellow fever, and relapsing fever.

B. Laboratory Findings

The leukocyte count may be normal or as high as 50,000/mcL, with neutrophils predominating. The urine may contain bile, protein, casts, and red cells. Oliguria is common, and in severe cases uremia may occur. Elevated bilirubin and aminotransferases are seen in 75%, and elevated creatinine (> 1.5 mg/dL) is seen in 50% of cases. In cases with meningeal involvement, organisms may be found in the CSF during the first 10 days of illness. Early in the disease, the organism may be identified by darkfield examination of the patient's blood (a test requiring expertise since false-positives are frequent in inexperienced hands) or by culture on a semisolid medium (eg, Fletcher EMJH). Cultures take 1–6 weeks to become positive. The organism may also be grown from the urine from the tenth day to the sixth week. Diagnosis is usually made by means of serologic tests, of which several are available. Agglutination tests (microscopic, using live organisms, and macroscopic, using killed antigen) become positive after 7–10 days of illness, peak at 3–4 weeks, and may persist at high levels for many years. Thus, to make a diagnosis, a fourfold or greater rise in titer must be documented. The agglutination tests are cumbersome to perform and require trained personnel. Indirect hemagglutination and enzyme-linked immunosorbent assay (ELISA) tests are also available. The IgM EIA is particularly useful in making an early diagnosis, since it is positive as early as 2 days into illness, a time when the clinical manifestations may be nonspecific, and it is extremely sensitive and specific (93%). PCR methods (presently investigational) appear to be sensitive, specific, positive early in disease, and able to detect leptospiral DNA in blood, urine, CSF, and aqueous humor. Serum creatine kinase (CK) is usually elevated in persons with leptospirosis and normal in persons with hepatitis.

Complications

Myocarditis, aseptic meningitis, acute kidney injury, and pulmonary infiltrates with hemorrhage are not common but are the usual causes of death. Iridocyclitis may occur.

Prevention

The mainstay of prevention is avoidance of potentially contaminated food and water.

Prophylaxis with doxycycline, 200 mg orally once weekly, can be given during periods of possible exposure. Human vaccine is used in some limited settings but is not widely available.

Treatment

Various antimicrobial drugs, including penicillin, ceftriaxone, and tetracyclines, show antileptospiral activity. Penicillin (eg, 1.5 million units every 6 hours intravenously) or ceftriaxone (1 g daily intravenously) is the drug of choice in severe leptospirosis and is especially effective if started within the first 4 days of illness. Jarisch–Herxheimer reactions may occur. Doxycycline, 100 mg orally twice daily for 7 days, is also effective as therapy if started early, but this agent is most often used in mild to moderate disease. Although therapy for mild disease is controversial, most clinicians treat with oral penicillin, 500 mg four times daily, or doxycycline, 100 mg orally twice daily, for 7 days. Azithromycin is also active, but clinical experience is limited.

▶ Prognosis

Without jaundice, the disease is almost never fatal. With jaundice, the mortality rate is 5% for those under age 30 years and 30% for those over age 60 years.

Ahmad SN et al. Laboratory diagnosis of leptospirosis. J Postgrad Med. 2005 Jul–Sep;51(3):195–200. [PMID: 16333192]

Palaniappan RU et al. Leptospirosis: pathogenesis, immunity, and diagnosis. Curr Opin Infect Dis. 2007 Jun;20(3):284–92. [PMID: 17471039]

Pavli A et al. Travel-acquired leptospirosis. J Travel Med. 2008 Nov–Dec;15(6):447–53. [PMID: 19090801]

Ricaldi JN et al. Leptospirosis in the tropics and in travelers. Curr Infect Dis Rep. 2006 Jan;8(1):51–8. [PMID: 16448601]

LYME DISEASE (Lyme Borreliosis)

ESSENTIALS OF DIAGNOSIS

▶ Erythema migrans, a flat or slightly raised red lesion that expands with central clearing.

▶ Headache or stiff neck.

▶ Arthralgias, arthritis, and myalgias; arthritis is often chronic and recurrent.

▶ Wide geographic distribution, with most United States cases in the Northeast, mid-Atlantic, upper Midwest, and Pacific coastal regions.

▶ General Considerations

This illness, named after the town of Old Lyme, Connecticut, is the most common tickborne disease in the United States and Europe. In the United States, the causative organism is the spirochete *B burgdorferi*, whereas in Europe and Asia the predominant organisms are *Borrelia garinii* and *Borrelia afzelii*. Most cases (90%) are reported from the mid-Atlantic, northeastern, and north central regions of the country, whereas far fewer cases are reported from the West Coast. The true incidence of Lyme disease is not known and overreporting continues to be a problem for a number of reasons: (1) serologic tests are not standardized (see below); (2) clinical manifestations are nonspecific; (3) even with reliable testing, serology is insensitive in early disease; and (4) other as yet unidentified organisms may cause illnesses similar to Lyme disease, eg, the Lone Star tick (*Amblyomma americanum*) found in the midwestern and southern regions of the United States can carry a spirochete that produces skin lesions indistinguishable from erythema migrans.

The vector of Lyme disease varies geographically and is *Ixodes scapularis* in the northeastern, north central, and mid-Atlantic regions of the United States; *Ixodes pacificus* on the West Coast; *Ixodes ricinus* in Europe; and *Ixodes persulcatus* in Asia. The disease also occurs in Australia. Mice and deer make up the major animal reservoir of *B burgdorferi*, but other rodents and birds may also be infected. Domestic animals such as dogs, cattle, and horses can also develop clinical illness, usually manifested as arthritis.

Ticks feed once during each of their three stages of life. Larval ticks feed in late summer, nymphs in the following spring and early summer, and adults during the fall. In the northeastern United States and the mid-Atlantic states, the preferred host for the nymphs and larvae is the white-footed mouse (the black-striped mouse in Europe). This animal is tolerant of infection—a fact that is critical in maintaining infection, since the mouse can remain spirochetemic and transmit the agent to the larvae the following spring after being infected by the nymphal form in early summer. Adult ticks prefer the white-tailed deer as host. Although only 20–25% of nymphs harbor spirochetes compared with 50–65% of adults, most infections occur in the spring and summer (when nymphs are active), and fewer cases occur in the cooler months (October to April), when adults feed. This is probably due to the greater abundance of nymphs; greater human outdoor activity in spring and summer, when nymphs feed; and the fact that adult ticks are larger, easier to detect by the human host, and thus can be removed before disease is transmitted. Less than 1% of larvae are infected with spirochetes, and transmission of the disease through contact with larvae is unlikely. In the western United States, the *I pacificus* nymph prefers to feed on lizards, which are not susceptible to infection. It is only the few nymph and larval ticks that feed on wood rats, which can be infected, that are capable of transmitting disease.

Under experimental conditions, ticks must feed for 24–36 hours or longer to transmit infections. Human epidemiologic studies have indicated that the incidence of disease is significantly higher when tick attachment is for longer than 72 hours than if it is less than 72 hours, though rare cases have been documented with attachment of less than 24 hours. In addition, the percentage of ticks infected varies on a regional basis. In the northeastern and midwestern regions, 15–65% of *I scapularis* ticks are infected with the spirochete; in the western United States, only 2% of *I pacificus* are infected. These are important epidemiologic features in assessing the likelihood that tick exposure will result in disease. Exposure to *I pacificus* is unlikely to result in disease, since so few ticks are infected, but this is not true of exposure to *I scapularis*. Eliciting a history of brushing a tick off the skin (ie, the tick was not feeding) or removing a tick on the same day as exposure (ie, the tick did not feed long enough) decreases the likelihood that infection will develop.

Ixodes ticks are smaller than the more common dog ticks (*Dermacentor variabilis*). Larvae are less than 1 mm in size, and the adult female is 2–3 mm in size, with a red body and black legs. After a blood meal, ticks can reach two to three times their unengorged size. Because the tick is so small, the bite is usually painless and goes unnoticed. After feeding, the tick drops off in 2–4 days. If a tick is found, it should be removed immediately. The best way to accomplish this is to use a fine-tipped tweezers to pull firmly and repeatedly on the tick's mouth part—not the tick's body—until the tick releases its hold. Saving the tick in a bottle of alcohol for future identification may be useful, especially if symptoms develop.

Congenital infection has been documented, but the exact frequency and manifestations have not been clearly defined. Similarly, because the organism can be latent, it is not known if women infected prior to becoming pregnant can activate the disease and transmit infection to the fetus. In one retrospective study, 5 of 19 pregnancies complicated by Lyme disease resulted in an adverse outcome, but all of the outcomes were different and could not be conclusively linked to infection. Several serosurveys involving over 2000 pregnant women in endemic areas have not found any association between seropositivity in prospective mothers and the prevalence of congenital malformations, fetal death, and prematurity. Thus, if *B burgdorferi* causes a congenital syndrome like some other spirochetal illnesses, it must be extremely uncommon.

▶ Clinical Findings

The typical clinical description of Lyme disease divides the illness into three stages: stage 1, flu-like symptoms and a typical skin rash (**erythema migrans**, Plate 32); stage 2, weeks to months later, Bell palsy or meningitis; and stage 3, months to years later, arthritis. The problem with this simplified scheme is that there is a great deal of overlap, and the skin, central nervous system, and musculoskeletal system can be involved early or late. A more accurate classification divides disease into early and late manifestations and specifies whether disease is localized or disseminated.

A. Symptoms and Signs

1. Stage 1, early localized infection—Stage 1 infection is characterized by erythema migrans. About 1 week after the tick bite (range, 3–30 days; median 7–10 days), a flat or slightly raised red lesion appears at the site, which is commonly seen in areas of tight clothing such as the groin, thigh, or axilla. This lesion expands over several days. Although originally described as a lesion that progresses with central clearing ("bulls-eye" lesion), often there is a more homogeneous appearance or even central intensification. About 10–20% of patients either do not have typical skin lesions or the lesions go unnoticed. Most patients with erythema migrans will have a concomitant viral-like illness (the "summer flu") characterized by myalgias, arthralgias, headache, and fatigue. Fever may or may not be present. Even without treatment, the symptoms and signs of erythema migrans resolve in 3–4 weeks. Although the classic lesion of erythema migrans is not difficult to recognize, atypical forms can occur that may lead to misdiagnosis. Vesicular, urticarial, and evanescent erythema migrans have all been reported. Similarly, chemical reactions to tick and spider bites (these usually recede in 24–48 hours whereas erythema migrans increases in size in this time period), drug eruptions, urticaria, and staphylococcal and streptococcal cellulitis have been mistaken for erythema migrans.

Completely asymptomatic disease, without erythema migrans or flu-like symptoms, can occur but is very uncommon in the United States. Serosurveys done as part of vaccination trials found asymptomatic seroconversion in 7% or less of the population.

2. Stage 2, early disseminated infection—Up to 50–60% of patients with erythema migrans are bacteremic (especially if multiple lesions are present) leading to dissemination of the spirochete resulting in a wide variety of symptoms and signs. Within days to weeks of the original infection, secondary skin lesions that are not associated with a tick bite develop in about 50% of patients. These lesions are similar in appearance to the primary lesion but are usually smaller. Malaise, fatigue, fever, headache (sometimes severe), neck pain, and generalized achiness are common with the skin lesions. Most symptoms are transient, although fatigue may persist for months. After hematogenous spread, the organism may sequester itself in certain areas and produces focal symptoms. Some patients experience cardiac (4–10% of patients) or neurologic (10–15% of patients) manifestations. Involvement of the heart includes myopericarditis, with atrial or ventricular arrhythmias and heart block. Neurologic manifestations include both the central and peripheral nervous systems. The most common central nervous system manifestation is an aseptic meningitis with mild headache and neck stiffness. The most common peripheral manifestation is a cranial neuropathy, ie, Bell palsy (usually unilateral but can be bilateral, Plate 90). A sensory or motor radiculopathy and mononeuritis multiplex occur less frequently. Conjunctivitis, keratitis and, rarely, panophthalmitis can also occur.

3. Stage 3, late persistent infection—Stage 3 infection occurs months to years after the initial infection and again primarily manifests itself as musculoskeletal, neurologic, and skin disease. In early reports, musculoskeletal complaints developed in up to 60% of patients. With early recognition and treatment of disease, joint complaints develop in less than 10% of patients. The classic manifestation of late disease is a monarticular or oligoarticular arthritis most commonly affecting the knee or other large weight bearing joints. Knees are swollen out of proportion to the pain experienced by the patient. Even if untreated, the arthritis is self-limited, resolving in a few weeks to months. Multiple recurrences are common but are usually less severe than the original disease. Joint fluid reflects an inflammatory arthritis with a mean white blood cell count of 25,000/mcL with a predominance of neutrophils. Chronic arthritis develops in about 10% of patients. The pathogenesis of chronic Lyme arthritis may be an immunologic phenomenon rather than persistence of infection. The observations that persons with chronic arthritis have an increased frequency of HLA-DR4 gene expression, antibodies to OspA and OspB protein in joint fluid (major outer surface proteins of *B burgdorferi*), lack *B burgdorferi* DNA in synovial fluid as detected by PCR, and often do not respond to antibiotics—all support the inference of an immunologic mechanism.

Rarely, the nervous system (both central and peripheral) can be involved in late Lyme disease. In the United States, a subacute encephalopathy, characterized by memory loss, mood changes, and sleep disturbance, is seen. In Europe, a more severe encephalomyelitis caused by *B garinii* is seen and presents with cognitive dysfunction, spastic paraparesis, ataxia, and bladder dysfunction. Peripheral nervous system involvement includes intermittent paresthesias, often in a stocking glove distribution, or radicular pain.

The cutaneous manifestation of late infection, which can occur up to 10 years after infection, is **acrodermatitis chronicum atrophicans**. It has been described mainly in Europe and is due to infection with *B afzelii*, a species that commonly causes disease in Europe but not the United States. There is usually bluish-red discoloration of a distal extremity with associated swelling. These lesions become atrophic and sclerotic with time and eventually resemble localized scleroderma. At least two cases of diffuse fasciitis with eosinophilia, a rare entity that resembles scleroderma, have been associated with infection with *B burgdorferi*.

B. Laboratory Findings

The diagnosis of Lyme disease is based on both clinical manifestations and laboratory findings. The National Surveillance Case Definition specifies a person with exposure to a potential tick habitat (within the 30 days just prior to developing erythema migrans) with (1) erythema migrans diagnosed by a physician or (2) at least one late manifestation of the disease and (3) laboratory confirmation as fulfilling the criteria for Lyme disease.

Laboratory confirmation requires detection of specific antibodies to *B burgdorferi* in serum, either by indirect immunofluorescence assay (IFA) or ELISA; the latter is preferred because it is more sensitive and specific. A Western blot assay that can detect both IgM and IgG antibodies is used as a confirmatory test. IgM antibody appears first 2–4 weeks after onset of erythema migrans, peaks at 6–8 weeks, and then declines to low levels after 4–6 months of illness. The presence of IgM antibody in patients with prolonged symptoms persisting for several months is likely to be a false-positive result. IgG occurs later (6–8 weeks after onset of disease), peaks at 4–6 months, and may remain elevated at low levels indefinitely despite appropriate therapy and resolution of symptoms. A two-test approach is recommended for the diagnosis of active Lyme disease. All specimens positive or equivocal by ELISA or IFA should be tested by Western immunoblot. When Western immunoblot is done during the first 4 weeks of illness, both IgM and IgG should be tested. If a patient with suspected early Lyme disease has negative serologic studies, acute and convalescent titers should be obtained since up to 50% of patients with early disease can be antibody negative in the first several weeks of illness. A fourfold rise in antibody titer would be diagnostic of recent infection. In patients with later stages of disease, almost all are antibody positive. False-positive reactions in the ELISA and IFA have been reported in juvenile rheumatoid arthritis, rheumatoid arthritis, systemic lupus erythematosus, infectious mononucleosis, subacute infective endocarditis, syphilis, relapsing fever, leptospirosis, enteroviral and other viral illnesses, and patients with gingival disease (presumably because of cross-reactivity with oral treponemes). False-negative serologic reactions occur early in

illness, and antibiotic therapy early in disease can abort subsequent seroconversion.

An ELISA test measures antibodies against a peptide in the invariant region of VlsE, an outer surface lipoprotein of *B burgdorferi*. The test is done in a single step (as opposed to the current two-step test recommended by the Centers for Disease Control and Prevention), is easy to standardize, and is less expensive than two-step testing. The ELISA appears to be as sensitive and specific as the current two-step test in the diagnosis of late stage disease and it is more sensitive for early disease.

Caution should be exercised in interpreting serologic tests because they are not subject to national standards, and inter-laboratory variation is a major problem. In addition, some laboratories perform tests that are entirely unreliable and should never be used to support the diagnosis of Lyme disease (eg, the Lyme urinary antigen test, immunofluorescent staining for cell wall-deficient forms of *B burgdorferi*, lymphocyte transformation tests, using PCR on inappropriate specimens such as blood or urine). Finally, testing is often done in patients with nonspecific symptoms such as headache, arthralgia, myalgia, fatigue, and palpitations. Even in endemic areas, the pretest probability of having Lyme disease is low in these patients, and the probability of a false-positive test result is greater than that of a true-positive result. For these reasons, the American College of Physicians has established guidelines for laboratory evaluation of patients with suspected Lyme disease:

1. The diagnosis of early Lyme disease is clinical (ie, exposure in an endemic area, with physician-documented erythema migrans), and does *not* require laboratory confirmation. (Tests are often negative at this stage.)

2. Late disease requires objective evidence of clinical manifestations (recurrent brief attacks of monarticular or oligoarticular arthritis of the large joints; lymphocytic meningitis, cranial neuritis [Bell palsy], peripheral neuropathy or, rarely, encephalomyelitis—but *not* headache, fatigue, paresthesias, or stiff neck alone; atrioventricular conduction defects with or without myocarditis) and laboratory evidence of disease (two-stage testing with ELISA and Western blot, as described above).

3. Patients with nonspecific symptoms without objective signs of Lyme disease should *not* have serologic testing done. It is in this setting that false-positive tests occur more commonly than true-positive tests.

4. The role of serologic testing in neuroborreliosis is unclear, as sensitivity and specificity of CSF serologic tests have not been determined. However, it is rare for a patient with neuroborreliosis to have positive serologic tests on CSF without positive tests on serum (see below).

5. Other tests such as the T cell proliferative assay, PCR testing, and urinary antigen detection have not yet been studied well enough to be routinely used (see discussion below).

Cultures for *B burgdorferi* can be performed but are not routine and are usually reserved for clinical studies. Aspiration of erythema migrans lesions has yielded positive cultures in up to 30% of cases, whereas culture of a 2-mm punch biopsy is positive in 50–70%. PCR of a skin biopsy is even more sensitive, with positivity rates of 80%. In early disease, blood cultures are positive in up to 50% if large volumes (9 mL) are used, but CSF is rarely culture positive. The ability to culture organisms from skin lesions is greatly influenced by antibiotic therapy. Even a brief course of several days will result in negative cultures. Special silver staining of chronically inflamed synovial tissue demonstrates spirochetes in one-third of patients.

PCR is very specific for detecting the presence of *Borrelia* DNA, but sensitivity is variable and depends on which body fluid is tested and the stage of the disease. In general, PCR is more sensitive than culture, especially in chronic disease. Up to 85% of synovial fluid samples are positive in active arthritis. In contrast, 38% of CSF samples in acute neuroborreliosis are PCR positive, and only 25% are positive in chronic neuroborreliosis. The significance of a positive reaction is unclear. Whether a positive PCR indicates persistence of viable organisms that will respond to further treatment or is a marker for residual DNA (not active infection) has not been clarified. In chronic Lyme arthritis, some have suggested that a positive PCR indicates active infection that requires further therapy, while others have found a positive reaction despite months of therapy, suggesting that the presence of DNA is indicative of an autoimmune arthritis.

The diagnosis of late **neuroborreliosis** is often difficult since clinical manifestations, such as subtle memory impairment, may be difficult to document. Most patients with neuroborreliosis have a history of previous erythema migrans or monarticular or polyarticular arthritis, and the vast majority have antibody present in serum. When CSF is sampled from patients with encephalopathy, there may be evidence of inflammation (pleocytosis or elevated protein, or both), and localized antibody production, ie, a ratio of CSF to serum antibody of > 1.0. The role of other tests such as PCR in detection of DNA or ELISA in detecting the presence of outer surface protein A (OspA) antigen is unclear, but in difficult cases these tests can be performed and, if positive, help establish the diagnosis. Patients with late disease and peripheral neuropathy almost always have positive serum antibody tests, usually have abnormal electrophysiology tests, and may have abnormal nerve biopsies showing perivascular collections of lymphocytes. Because disease involves peripheral nerves, the cerebral spinal fluid is usually normal and does not demonstrate local antibody production.

Nonspecific laboratory abnormalities can be seen, particularly in early disease. The most common are an elevated sedimentation rate of > 20 mm/h seen in 50% of cases and mildly abnormal liver function tests present in 30%. The abnormal liver function tests are transient and return to normal within a few weeks of treatment. A mild anemia, leukocytosis (11,000–18,000/mcL), and microscopic hematuria have been reported in 10% or less of patients.

► Prevention

Simple preventive measures such as avoiding tick-infested areas, covering exposed skin with long-sleeved shirts and wearing long trousers tucked into socks, wearing light-colored clothing, using repellents, and inspecting for ticks after exposure will greatly reduce the number of tick bites. Environmental controls directed at limiting ticks on residential property would be helpful, but trying to limit the deer, tick, or white-footed mouse populations over large areas is not feasible.

Prophylactic antibiotics following tick bites is recommended in certain high risk situations if all of the following criteria are met: (1) a tick identified as an adult or nymphal *I scapularis* has been attached for at least 36 hours; (2) prophylaxis can be started within 72 hours of the time the tick was removed; (3) more than 20% of ticks in the area are known to be infected with *B burgdorferi*; and (4) there is no contraindication to the use of doxycycline (not pregnant, age greater than 8 years, not allergic). As noted above, *I scapularis* ticks in the northeastern, mid-Atlantic, and upper midwestern states are infected with *B burgdorferi* at a high rate (> 20%) whereas *I pacificus* ticks on the West Coast are not (about 2%). The drug of choice for prophylaxis is a single 200 mg dose of doxycycline. If doxycycline is contraindicated, no prophylaxis should be given, since short course prophylactic therapy with other agents has not been studied and if early disease does develop appropriate therapy is very effective in preventing long-term sequelae. Individuals who have removed ticks (including those who have had prophylaxis) should be monitored carefully for 30 days. If skin lesions or a viral-like illness develop, they should be evaluated for possible Lyme disease, human granulocytic anaplasmosis, and babesiosis. There is no human vaccine currently available.

► Treatment

Present recommendations for therapy are outlined in Table 34–4. For erythema migrans, antibiotic therapy shortens the duration of rash and prevents late sequelae. Doxycycline is most commonly used and has the advantage of being active against *Anaplasma phagocytophilum* (formerly *Ehrlichia*). Amoxicillin is also effective and is recommended for pregnant or lactating women and for those who cannot tolerate doxycycline. Cefuroxime axetil, is as effective as doxycycline, but because of its cost it should be considered an alternative choice for those who cannot tolerate doxycycline or amoxicillin or for those in whom the drugs are contraindicated. Erythromycin and azithromycin are less effective, associated with higher rates of relapse, and are not recommended as first-line therapy.

Isolated Bell palsy (without meningitis or peripheral neuropathy) can be treated with doxycycline, amoxicillin, or cefuroxime axetil for 2–3 weeks. Although therapy does not affect the rate of resolution of the cranial neuropathy, it does prevent development of late manifestations of disease.

The need for a lumbar puncture in patients with seventh nerve palsy is controversial. Some clinicians perform lumbar puncture on all patients with Bell palsy and others only if there are symptoms or signs of meningitis. If meningitis is present, therapy with a parenteral antibiotic is indicated. Ceftriaxone is most commonly used, but penicillin is equally efficacious. In European countries, doxycycline 400 mg/d for 14 days is frequently used and is comparable in efficacy to ceftriaxone.

Table 34–4. Treatment of Lyme disease.

Manifestations	Drug and Dosage
Tick bite	No treatment in most circumstances (see text); observe
Erythema migrans	Doxycycline, 100 mg orally twice daily, or amoxicillin, 500 mg orally three times daily, or cefuroxime axetil, 500 mg orally twice daily—all for 2-3 weeks
Neurologic disease	
Bell palsy (without meningitis)	Doxycycline, amoxicillin, or cefuroxime axetil as above for 2-3 weeks
Other central nervous system disease	Ceftriaxone, 2 g intravenously once daily, or penicillin G, 18-24 million units daily intravenously in six divided doses, or cefotaxime, 2 g intravenously every 8 hours—all for 2-4 weeks
Cardiac disease	
Atrioventricular block and myopericarditis[1]	An oral or parenteral regimen as described above can be used
	Ceftriaxone or penicillin G as above for 30-60 days (see text)
Arthritis	
Oral dosage	Doxycycline, amoxicillin, or cefuroxime axetil as above for 28 days (see text)
Parenteral dosage	Ceftriaxone, cefotaxime, or penicillin G as above for 2-4 weeks
Acrodermatitis chronicum atrophicans	Doxycycline, amoxicillin, or cefuroxime axetil as above for 3 weeks
"Chronic Lyme disease" or "post-Lyme disease syndrome"	Symptomatic therapy

[1]Symptomatic patients, those with second- or third-degree block and those with first-degree block with a PR interval ≥ 30 milliseconds should be hospitalized for observation.

Patients with atrioventricular block or myopericarditis (or both) can be treated with either oral or parenteral agents for 2–3 weeks. Hospitalization and observation is indicated for symptomatic patients, those with second- or third-degree block, and those with first-degree block with a PR interval ≥ 30 milliseconds. Once stabilized, hospitalized patients can be transitioned to one of the oral regimens to complete therapy.

Therapy of arthritis is difficult because some patients do not respond to any therapy, and those who do respond may do so slowly. Oral agents (doxycycline, amoxicillin, or cefuroxime axetil) are as effective as intravenous regimens (ceftriaxone, cefotaxime, or penicillin). A reasonable approach to the patient with Lyme arthritis is to start with oral therapy for 28 days, and if this fails (persistent or recurrent joint swelling), to re-treat with an oral regimen for 28 days or switch to an intravenous regimen for 2–4 weeks. If some improvement has occurred with initial treatment with an oral regimen, another course of oral therapy is reasonable. If there has been no response or worsening with initial oral therapy, a parenteral regimen should be used. Re-treatment should be delayed for several months because of the slow resolution of joint symptoms. If arthritis persists after re-treatment, symptomatic therapy with nonsteroidal anti-inflammatory drugs is recommended. For severe refractory pain, synovectomy may be required.

Based on the limited published data, therapy of Lyme disease in pregnancy should be the same as therapy in other patients with the exception that doxycycline should not be used.

Clinicians are often confronted with patients with non-specific symptoms (such as fatigue and myalgias) and positive serologic tests for Lyme disease who request (or demand) therapy for their illness. It is important in managing these patients to remember (1) that the diagnosis of Lyme disease is primarily a clinical one, and nonspecific symptoms alone are not diagnostic; (2) that serologic tests are fraught with difficulty (as noted above), and in areas where disease prevalence is low, false-positive serologic tests are much more common than true-positive tests; and (3) that parenteral therapy with ceftriaxone for 2–4 weeks is costly (approximately $5000) and has been associated with significant adverse effects (cholelithiasis). Parenteral therapy should be reserved for those most likely to benefit, ie, those with cutaneous, neurologic, cardiac, or rheumatic manifestations that are characteristic of Lyme disease.

▶ **Coinfections**

Lyme disease, babesiosis (see Chapter 35), and human granulocytic anaplasmosis (formerly human granulocytic ehrlichiosis) (see Chapter 32) are endemic in similar areas of the country and are transmitted by the same tick, *I scapularis*. Coinfection with two or even all three of these organisms can occur, causing a clinical picture that is not "classic" for any of these diseases. The presence of erythema migrans is highly suggestive of Lyme disease, whereas flu-like symptoms without rash are more suggestive of babesiosis or anaplasmosis. The complete blood count is usually normal in Lyme disease, but in patients with Lyme disease and babesiosis, anemia and thrombocytopenia are more common. Patients with Lyme disease and anaplasmosis are more likely to have leukopenia. Coinfection should be considered and excluded in patients who have persistent high fevers 48 hours after starting appropriate therapy for Lyme disease; in patients with persistent symptoms despite resolution of rash; and in those with anemia, leukopenia, or thrombocytopenia.

Even in patients with documented Lyme disease, immunity is not complete. Reinfection, although uncommon, is predominantly seen in patients successfully treated for early disease (erythema migrans) who do not develop antibody titers. Clinical manifestations and serologic response is similar to an initial infection.

▶ **Prognosis**

Most patients respond to appropriate therapy with prompt resolution of symptoms within 4 weeks. True treatment failures are thus uncommon, and in most cases re-treatment or prolonged treatment of Lyme disease is instituted because of misdiagnosis or misinterpretation of serologic results (both IgG and IgM antibodies can persist for prolonged periods despite adequate therapy) rather than inadequate therapy or response. The terms "chronic Lyme disease" or "post-Lyme disease syndrome" have been applied to a heterogeneous group of patients with documented Lyme disease who have been adequately treated but have persistent poorly defined, nonspecific symptoms such as fatigue, arthralgias, myalgias, and neurocognitive complaints. Although some providers treat these patients with multiple or prolonged courses of oral or intravenous antibiotics, there are no data suggesting that this is efficacious, and the prolonged use of antibiotics in this setting is emphatically discouraged.

The long-term outcome of adult patients with Lyme disease is generally favorable, but some patients have chronic complaints. Joint pain, memory impairment, and poor functional status secondary to pain are common subjective complaints in patients with Lyme disease, but physical examination and neurocognitive testing fail to document the presence of these symptoms as objective sequelae. Similarly, in highly endemic areas, patients with a diagnosis of Lyme disease commonly complain of pain, fatigue, and an inability to perform certain physical activities when followed for several years. However, these complaints occur just as commonly in age-matched controls without a history of Lyme disease. Attempts to document chronic cardiac disease in patients treated for Lyme disease also have been unsuccessful. The long-term outcome of treated neuroborreliosis is favorable, with complete recovery in 75% of patients. Of the remaining individuals, only 12% had sequelae that affected their daily activities.

▶ When to Refer

Consultation with an infectious diseases specialist with experience in treating Lyme disease can be helpful in atypical or prolonged cases.

▶ When to Admit

Admission for parenteral antibiotics is indicated for any patient with symptomatic CNS or cardiac disease as well as those with second- or third-degree atrioventricular block, or first-degree block with a PR interval ≥ 30 milliseconds.

Dandache P et al. Erythema migrans. Infect Dis Clin North Am. 2008 Jun;22(2):235–60. [PMID: 18452799]

Feder HM et al. A critical appraisal of "chronic Lyme disease." N Engl J Med. 2007 Oct 4;357(14):1422–1430. [PMID: 17914043]

Halperin JJ. Nervous system Lyme disease. Infect Dis Clin North Am. 2008 Jun;22(2):261–74. [PMID: 18452800]

Nadelman RB et al. Reinfection in patients with Lyme disease. Clin Infect Dis. 2007 Oct 15;45(8):1032–8. [PMID: 17879922]

Wormser GP. Clinical practice. Early Lyme disease. N Engl J Med. 2006 Jun 29;354(26):2794–801. [PMID: 16807416]

Wormser GP et al. The clinical assessment, treatment, and prevention of Lyme disease, human granulocytic anaplasmosis, and babesiosis: clinical practice guidelines by the Infectious Diseases Society of America. Clin Infect Dis. 2006 Nov 1;43(9):1089–134. [PMID: 17029130]

Protozoal & Helminthic Infections

Philip J. Rosenthal, MD

AFRICAN TRYPANOSOMIASIS
(Sleeping Sickness)

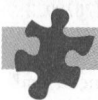 ESSENTIALS OF DIAGNOSIS

▶ Exposure to tsetse flies, with subsequent bite lesion.

▶ Irregular fever, headache, joint pain, rash, edema, lymphadenopathy progressing to somnolence, and neurologic abnormalities.

▶ Trypanosomes in blood or lymph node aspirates; positive serologic tests.

▶ Trypanosomes and increased white cells and protein in cerebrospinal fluid.

▶ General Considerations

African trypanosomiasis is caused by the hemoflagellates *Trypanosoma brucei rhodesiense* and *Trypanosoma brucei gambiense*. The organisms are transmitted by bites of tsetse flies (genus *Glossina*), which inhabit shaded areas along streams and rivers. Trypanosomes ingested in a blood meal develop over 18–35 days in the fly; when the fly feeds again on a mammalian host, the infective stage is injected. Human disease occurs in rural areas of sub-Saharan Africa from south of the Sahara to about 15 degrees south latitude. *T b gambiense* causes West African trypanosomiasis, and is transmitted in the moist sub-Saharan savannas and forests of west and central Africa. *T b rhodesiense* causes East African trypanosomiasis, and is transmitted in the savannas of east and southeast Africa.

T b rhodesiense infection is primarily a zoonosis of game animals and cattle; humans are infected sporadically. Humans are the principal mammalian host for *T b gambiense*, but domestic animals can be infected. African trypanosomiasis is an increasing threat, especially where control has been disrupted by civil strife. The largest number of cases is in the Democratic Republic of the Congo. Annual incidence estimates are about 100,000 cases and 48,000 deaths, mostly due to *T b gambiense*, leading to the loss of 1.5 million disability-adjusted life years. Infections are rare among travelers, including visitors to game parks.

▶ Clinical Findings

A. Symptoms and Signs

1. West African trypanosomiasis—Chancres at the site of the bite are uncommon. After an asymptomatic period that may last for months, hemolymphatic disease presents with fever, headache, myalgias, arthralgias, weight loss, and lymphadenopathy, with discrete, nontender, rubbery nodes, referred to as Winterbottom sign when in a posterior cervical distribution. Other common signs are mild splenomegaly, transient edema, and a pruritic erythematous rash. Febrile episodes may be broken by afebrile periods of up to several weeks. The hemolymphatic stage progresses over months to meningoencephalitic disease, with somnolence, irritability, personality changes, severe headache, and parkinsonian symptoms progressing to coma and death.

2. East African trypanosomiasis—Chancres are more commonly recognized with *T b rhodesiense* infection, with a painful lesion of 3–10 cm and regional lymphadenopathy that appears about 48 hours after the tsetse fly bite and lasts 2–4 weeks. East African disease follows a much more acute course, with the onset of symptoms usually within a few days of the insect bite. The hemolymphatic stage includes intermittent fever and rash, but lymphadenopathy is less common than with West African disease. Myocarditis can cause tachycardia and death due to arrhythmias or heart failure. If untreated, East African trypanosomiasis progresses over weeks to months to meningoencephalitic disease, somnolence, coma, and death.

B. Laboratory Findings

Definitive diagnosis requires identification of trypanosomes. Microscopic examination of fluid expressed from a chancre or lymph node may show motile trypanosomes or, in fixed specimens, parasites stained with Giemsa. During the hemolymphatic stage, detection of parasites in Giemsa-stained blood smears is common in East African disease but difficult in West African disease. Serial specimens should be examined, since parasitemias vary greatly over time. With meningoencephalitic disease, cerebrospinal fluid (CSF) shows increased mononuclear cells and protein as well as trypanosomes. Concentration techniques can aid identification of parasites in blood or CSF. Serologic tests are also available. The simple card agglutination test for trypanosomes (CATT) has excellent sensitivity and specificity and can be performed in the field; however, the diagnosis should be confirmed by identification of the parasites.

Treatment

Detection of trypanosomes is a prerequisite for treatment of African trypanosomiasis because of the significant toxicity of most available therapies. Treatment recommendations depend on the type of trypanosomiasis, which is determined by geography, and stage of disease, which requires examination of CSF (Table 35–1).

A. West African Trypanosomiasis

1. Early stage infection—Pentamidine (4 mg/kg intramuscularly or intravenously every day or every other day for 7 days) is used to treat infection that does not involve the central nervous system (CNS). The side effects of pentamidine include immediate hypotension; tachycardia; gastrointestinal symptoms during administration; sterile abscesses; and pancreatic, liver, and kidney abnormalities. An alternate drug is eflornithine (100 mg/kg/d intravenously every 6 hours for 14 days).

2. Late stage infection—Eflornithine is the drug of choice for infection that involves the CNS; the dosage is the same as that used to treat early disease. Eflornithine has less toxicity than older trypanocidal drugs, but it can cause gastrointestinal symptoms and bone marrow suppression and is limited by lack of availability and the need for frequent infusions. Alternative therapies are melarsoprol (see below) or nifurtimox (5 mg/kg orally three times per day for 14 days), and drug combinations may offer improved efficacy over monotherapies, with simplified regimens and decreased doses of toxic drugs.

B. East African Trypanosomiasis

Pentamidine and eflornithine are not reliably effective, and early disease is treated with suramin. The dosing regimens

Table 35–1. Treatment of African trypanosomiasis.

Disease	Stage	Treatment First Line	Treatment Alternative
West African	Early	Pentamidine	Suramin
			Eflornithine
	CNS involvement	Eflornithine	Melarsoprol
			Eflornithine
			Nifurtimox
East African	Early	Suramin	Pentamidine
	CNS involvement	Melarsoprol	

CNS, central nervous system.

of suramin vary (eg, 100–200 mg test dose, then 20 mg/kg [maximum 1 g] intravenously on days 1, 3, 7, 14, and 21 or weekly for 5 doses). Suramin toxicities include vomiting and, rarely, seizures and shock during infusions as well as subsequent fever, rash, headache, neuropathy, and kidney and bone marrow dysfunction.

Suramin does not enter the CNS, so East African trypanosomiasis involving the CNS is treated with melarsoprol (three series of 3.6 mg/kg/d intravenously for 3 days, with 7-day breaks between the series or a 10-day intravenous course with 0.6 mg/kg on day 1, 1.2 mg/kg on day 2, and 1.8 mg/kg on days 3–10). Although melarsoprol acts against both early West and East African disease, it is very toxic. Immediate side effects of melarsoprol include fever and gastrointestinal symptoms. The most important side effect is a reactive encephalopathy that can progress to seizures, coma, and death. To help avoid this side effect, corticosteroids are coadministered (recommended regimens include dexamethasone 1 mg/kg/d intravenously for 2–3 days or oral prednisolone 1 mg/kg/d for 5 days, and then 0.5 mg/kg/d until treatment completion). In addition, increasing resistance to melarsoprol is a serious concern. Suramin and melarsoprol are available in the United States from the CDC Drug Service, Centers for Disease Control and Prevention, Atlanta, GA 30333; telephone: 404-639-3670.

Prevention & Control

Individual prevention in endemic areas should include long sleeves and pants, insect repellents, and mosquito nets. Control programs focusing on vector elimination and treatment of infected persons and animals have shown good success in many areas but suffer from limited resources.

Bisser S et al. Equivalence trial of melarsoprol and nifurtimox monotherapy and combination therapy for the treatment of second-stage *Trypanosoma brucei gambiense* sleeping sickness. J Inf Dis. 2007 Feb 1;195(3):322–9. [PMID: 17205469]

Croft SL et al. Chemotherapy of trypanosomiases and leishmaniasis. Trends Parasitol. 2005 Nov;21(11):508–12. [PMID: 16150644]

Priotto G et al. Nifurtimox-eflornithine combination therapy for second-stage *Trypanosoma brucei gambiense* sleeping sickness: a randomized clinical trial in Congo. Clin Inf Dis. 2007 Dec 1;45(11):1435–42. [PMID: 17990225]

Priotto G et al. Three drug combinations for late-stage *Trypanosoma brucei gambiense* sleeping sickness: a randomized clinical trial in Uganda. PLoS Clin Trials. 2006 Dec 8;1(8):e39. [PMID: 17160135]

Schmid C et al. Effectiveness of a 10-day melarsoprol schedule for the treatment of late-stage human African trypanosomiasis: confirmation from a multinational study (IMPAMEL II). J Infect Dis. 2005 Jun 1;191:1922–31. [PMID: 15871127]

AMERICAN TRYPANOSOMIASIS (Chagas Disease)

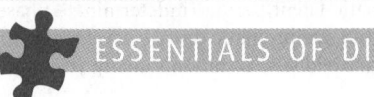
ESSENTIALS OF DIAGNOSIS

Acute stage

► Inflammatory lesion at inoculation site.

► Fever.

▶ Hepatosplenomegaly.

▶ Lymphadenopathy.

▶ Myocarditis.

▶ Parasites in blood is diagnostic.

Chronic stage

▶ Heart failure, cardiac arrhythmias.

▶ Thromboembolism.

▶ Megaesophagus.

▶ Megacolon.

▶ Serologic tests are usually diagnostic.

▶ General Considerations

Chagas disease is caused by *Trypanosoma cruzi*, a protozoan parasite found only in the Americas; it infects wild animals and to a lesser extent humans from southern South America to the southern United States. An estimated 10–12 million people are infected, mostly in rural areas, resulting in about 45,000 deaths annually. The disease is often acquired in childhood. In many countries in South America, Chagas disease is the most important cause of heart disease. In the United States, the vector is found and some animals are infected, but only a few instances of local transmission have been reported.

T cruzi is transmitted by reduviid (triatomine) bugs infected by ingesting blood from animals or humans who have circulating trypanosomes. Multiplication occurs in the digestive tract of the bug and infective forms are eliminated in feces. Infection in humans occurs when the parasite penetrates the skin through the bite wound, mucous membranes, or the conjunctiva. Transmission can also occur by blood transfusion or in utero. From the bloodstream, *T cruzi* invades many cell types but has a predilection for myocardium, smooth muscle, and CNS glial cells. Multiplication causes cellular destruction, inflammation, and fibrosis, with progressive disease over decades.

▶ Clinical Findings

A. Symptoms and Signs

As many as 70% of infected persons remain asymptomatic. The **acute stage** is seen principally in children and lasts 1–2 months. The earliest findings are at the site of inoculation either in the eye—Romaña sign (unilateral edema, conjunctivitis, and lymphadenopathy)—or in the skin—a chagoma (swelling with local lymphadenopathy). Subsequent findings include fever, malaise, headache, mild hepatosplenomegaly, and generalized lymphadenopathy. Acute myocarditis and meningoencephalitis are rare but can be fatal.

An asymptomatic latent period (indeterminate phase) may last for life, but symptomatic disease develops in 10–30% of infected individuals, commonly many years after infection.

Chronic Chagas disease generally manifests as abnormalities in cardiac and smooth muscle. Cardiac disease includes arrhythmias, congestive heart failure, and embolic disease. Smooth muscle abnormalities lead to megaesophagus and megacolon, with dysphagia, regurgitation, aspiration, constipation, and abdominal pain. These findings can be complicated by superinfections. In immunosuppressed persons, including AIDS patients and transplant recipients, latent Chagas disease may reactivate; findings have included brain abscesses.

B. Diagnostic Testing

Diagnosis should be considered in persons with suggestive findings who have resided in an endemic area. Transmission by blood transfusion and congenital transmission should also be considered. The diagnosis is made by detecting parasites. With **acute** infection, evaluation of fresh blood or buffy coats may show motile trypanosomes, and fixed preparations may show Giemsa-stained parasites. Trypanosomes may be identified in lymph nodes, bone marrow, or pericardial or spinal fluid. When initial tests are unrevealing in a suspicious case, xenodiagnosis using laboratory vectors, laboratory culture, or animal inoculation may provide a diagnosis, but these methods are expensive and slow.

Chronic Chagas disease is usually diagnosed serologically. Many different serologic assays are available, but sensitivity and specificity are not ideal, so confirmatory assays are advised after an initial positive test, as is standard for blood bank testing in South America. Polymerase chain reaction (PCR) may offer an important new modality for diagnosis, but sensitivity of PCR assays has been disappointing.

▶ Treatment

Treatment is inadequate because the two drugs used, nifurtimox and benznidazole, often cause severe side effects, must be used for long periods, and are ineffective against chronic infection. In acute and congenital infections, the drugs can reduce the duration and severity of infection, but cure is achieved in only about 70% of patients. During the chronic phase of infection, although parasitemia may disappear in up to 70% of patients, treatment does not clearly alter the progression of the disease. Nevertheless, there is general consensus that treatment should be considered in all *T cruzi*-infected persons regardless of clinical status or time since infection.

Nifurtimox is given orally in daily doses of 8–10 mg/kg in four divided doses after meals for 90–120 days. Side effects include gastrointestinal and neurologic symptoms, which appear to be reversible and to lessen with dosage reduction. Benznidazole is an alternative therapy that is given orally at a dosage of 5 mg/kg/d in divided doses for 60 days. Its side effects include granulocytopenia, rash, and peripheral neuropathy. In the United States, nifurtimox and benznidazole are available only from the CDC Drug Service, Centers for Disease Control and Prevention, Atlanta, GA 30333; telephone: 404-639-3670. Patients with chronic Chagas disease may also benefit from antiarrhythmic therapy, standard therapy for congestive heart failure, and conservative and surgical management of megaesophagus and megacolon.

Prevention & Control

In South America, a major eradication program based on improved housing, use of residual pyrethroid insecticides and pyrethroid-impregnated bed curtains, and screening of blood donors has achieved striking reductions in new infections. In endemic areas and ideally in donors from endemic areas, blood should not be used for transfusion unless at least two serologic tests are negative.

Bern C et al. Evaluation and treatment of Chagas disease in the United States: a systematic review. JAMA. 2007 Nov 14; 298(18):2171–81. [PMID: 18000201]

Reyes PA et al. Trypanocidal drugs for late stage, symptomatic Chagas disease (*Trypanosoma cruzi* infection). Cochrane Database Syst Rev. 2005 Oct 19;(4):CD004102. [PMID: 16235350]

Schofield CJ. The future of Chagas disease control. Trends Parasitol. 2006 Dec;22(12):583–8. [PMID: 17049308]

Yamagata Y et al. Control of Chagas disease. Adv Parasitol. 2006;61:129–65. [PMID: 16735164]

LEISHMANIASIS

ESSENTIALS OF DIAGNOSIS

- ▶ Sand fly bite in an endemic area.
- ▶ Visceral leishmaniasis: irregular fever, progressive hepatosplenomegaly, pancytopenia, wasting.
- ▶ Cutaneous leishmaniasis: chronic, painless, moist ulcers or dry nodules.
- ▶ Mucocutaneous leishmaniasis: destructive nasopharyngeal lesions.
- ▶ Amastigotes in macrophages in aspirates, touch preparations, or biopsies.
- ▶ Positive culture, serologic tests, PCR, or skin test.

General Considerations

Leishmaniasis is a zoonosis transmitted by bites of sand flies of the genus *Lutzomyia* in the Americas and *Phlebotomus* elsewhere. When sand flies feed on an infected host, the parasitized cells are ingested with the blood meal. Leishmaniasis is caused by about 20 species of *Leishmania;* taxonomy is complex. Clinical syndromes are generally dictated by the infecting species, but some species can cause more than one syndrome.

An estimated 350 million persons are at risk for leishmaniasis. The estimated annual incidence of disease is 1–1.5 million new cases of cutaneous and 500,000 cases of visceral disease, leading to an estimated 50,000–60,000 deaths. The incidence of disease is increasing in many areas.

Visceral leishmaniasis (kala azar) is caused mainly by *Leishmania donovani* in the Indian subcontinent and East Africa; *Leishmania infantum* in the Mediterranean, Middle East, China, parts of Asia, and Horn of Africa; and *Leishmania chagasi* in South and Central America. Other species may occasionally cause visceral disease. Over 90% of cases occur in five countries: India, Bangladesh, Nepal, Sudan,

and Brazil. In each locale, the disease has particular clinical and epidemiologic features. The incubation period is usually 4–6 months (range: 10 days to 24 months). Without treatment, the fatality rate reaches 90%. Early diagnosis and treatment reduces mortality to 2–5%.

Old World cutaneous leishmaniasis is caused mainly by *Leishmania tropica, Leishmania major,* and *Leishmania aethiopica* in the Mediterranean, Middle East, Africa, Central Asia, and Indian subcontinent. New World cutaneous leishmaniasis is caused by *Leishmania mexicana* and *Leishmania amazonensis* in Central and South America. Mucocutaneous leishmaniasis (espundia) occurs in lowland forest areas of the Americas and is caused by *Leishmania braziliensis, Leishmania panamensis,* and *Leishmania peruviana.*

Clinical Findings

A. Symptoms and Signs

1. Visceral leishmaniasis (kala azar)—Most infections are subclinical, but a small number progress to full-blown disease. A local nonulcerating nodule at the site of the sand fly bite may precede systemic manifestations but usually is inapparent. The onset of illness may be acute, within 2 weeks of infection, or insidious. Symptoms and signs include fever, chills, sweats, weakness, anorexia, weight loss, cough, and diarrhea. The spleen progressively becomes greatly enlarged, firm, and nontender. The liver is somewhat enlarged, and generalized lymphadenopathy may occur. Hyperpigmentation of skin can be seen, leading to the name kala azar ("black fever"). Other signs include skin lesions, petechiae, gingival bleeding, jaundice, edema, and ascites. As the disease progresses, severe wasting and malnutrition are seen; death eventually occurs often due to secondary infections, within months to a few years. Post-kala azar dermal leishmaniasis may appear after apparent cure in the Indian subcontinent and Sudan. It may simulate leprosy, with hypopigmented macules or nodules developing on preexisting lesions. Viscerotropic leishmaniasis has been reported in small numbers of American military personnel in the Middle East, with mild systemic febrile illnesses after *L tropica* infections.

2. Cutaneous leishmaniasis—Cutaneous swellings appear 2 weeks to several months after sand fly bites and can be single or multiple. Characteristics of lesions and courses of disease vary depending on the leishmanial species and host immune response. Lesions begin as small papules and develop into nonulcerated dry plaques or large encrusted ulcers with well-demarcated raised and indurated margins (Plate 111). Satellite lesions may be present. The lesions are painless unless secondarily infected. Local lymph nodes may be enlarged. Systemic symptoms are uncommon, but fever, constitutional symptoms, and regional lymphadenopathy may be seen. For most species, healing occurs spontaneously in months to a few years, but scarring is commonly seen.

Leishmaniasis recidivans is a relapsing form of *L tropica* infection associated with hypersensitivity, in which the primary lesion heals centrally, but spreads laterally, with extensive scarring. Diffuse cutaneous leishmaniasis involves spread from a central lesion to local dissemination of nodules and a protracted course. Disseminated cutaneous leishmaniasis involves multiple nodular or ulcerated lesions, often with mucosal involvement.

3. Mucocutaneous leishmaniasis (espundia)—In Latin America, mucosal lesions develop in a small percentage of persons infected with *L braziliensis* and some other species, usually months to years after resolution of a cutaneous lesion. Nasal congestion is followed by ulceration of the nasal mucosa and septum, progressing to involvement of the mouth, lips, palate, pharynx, and larynx. Extensive destruction can occur, and secondary bacterial infection is common. Similar syndromes have been reported with some other species in other areas.

4. Infections in patients with AIDS—Leishmaniasis is an opportunistic infection in persons with AIDS seen in southern Europe and other areas. Visceral leishmaniasis can present late in the course of HIV infection, with fever, hepatosplenomegaly, and pancytopenia. The gastrointestinal tract, respiratory tract, and skin may also be involved.

B. Laboratory Findings

Identifying parasites in tissue samples or culture material provides a definitive diagnosis. In **visceral leishmaniasis,** fine-needle aspiration of the spleen for culture and tissue evaluation is generally safe, and yields a diagnosis in over 95% of cases. Bone marrow aspiration is less sensitive but safer and diagnostic in most cases. Giemsa-stained buffy coat of peripheral blood may occasionally show organisms. For all tissue biopsies and touch preparations, Giemsa staining will show amastigotes within macrophages. Cultures with media available from the CDC will grow promastigotes within a few days to weeks. PCR can also identify the infection. Inoculation of laboratory animals can also be used but is time consuming. Species are identified by molecular, isoenzyme, and monoclonal antibody methods. Serologic tests may facilitate diagnosis, but none are sufficiently sensitive or specific to be used alone. Antibody levels are typically high with visceral leishmaniasis but not cutaneous disease. For **cutaneous lesions,** biopsies should be taken from the raised border of a skin lesion, with samples for histopathology, touch preparation, and culture. The histopathology shows inflammation with mononuclear cells. Macrophages filled with amastigotes may be present, especially early in infection. An intradermal leishmanin (Montenegro) skin test is positive in most individuals with cutaneous disease but negative in those with progressive visceral or diffuse cutaneous disease; this test is not approved in the United States. In **mucocutaneous leishmaniasis,** diagnosis is established by detecting amastigotes in scrapings, biopsy preparations, or aspirated tissue fluid, but organisms may be rare. Cultures from these samples may grow organisms. Serologic studies are often negative, but the leishmanin skin test is usually positive.

▶ Treatment

Treatment is not adequate because most drugs are quite toxic, require long courses, and are mostly administered parenterally. The drugs of choice have been pentavalent antimonials, but they are quite toxic, and failures are increasing due to drug resistance. Important newer therapies are amphotericin B, miltefosine, and paromomycin.

A. Visceral Leishmaniasis

The treatment of choice for visceral leishmaniasis is liposomal amphotericin B, which is generally effective and well tolerated but very expensive. Liposomal amphotericin B is approved for this use in the United States; other lipid formulations have been less studied. Standard dosing is 3 mg/kg/d intravenously on days 1–5, 14, and 21, but simpler regimens may be equally effective. Infusion-related side effects include gastrointestinal symptoms, fever, chills, dyspnea, hypotension, and hepatic and renal toxicity. Conventional amphotericin B deoxycholate, which is much less expensive, is also highly effective but with more toxicity. It is administered as a slow infusion of 1 mg/kg/d for 20 days or 0.5–1 mg/kg every second day for up to 8 weeks.

Pentavalent antimonials remain the most commonly used drugs to treat leishmaniasis in most areas. Response rates are good outside India, but in India, resistance is a major problem. Two preparations are available, sodium stibogluconate in the United States and many other areas and meglumine antimonate in Latin America and francophone countries; the compounds appear to have comparable activities. In the United States, sodium stibogluconate can be obtained from the CDC Drug Service, Centers for Disease Control and Prevention, Atlanta, GA 30333; telephone: 404-639-3670.

Treatment is given once daily at a dose of 20 mg/kg/d intravenously (preferred) or intramuscularly for 20 days for cutaneous leishmaniasis and 28 days for visceral or mucocutaneous disease. Toxicity increases over time, with development of gastrointestinal symptoms, fever, headache, myalgias, arthralgias, pancreatitis, and rash. Intramuscular injections can cause sterile abscesses. Monitoring should include serial ECGs, and changes are indications for discontinuation to avoid progression to serious arrhythmias.

Miltefosine is the first oral drug for the treatment of leishmaniasis, and it provides excellent results in India, where resistance to antimonials is increasing. It can be administered at a daily oral dose of 2.5 mg/kg in two divided doses for 28 days and was also effective in regimens including a single dose of liposomal amphotericin followed by 7–14 days of miltefosine. A 28-day course of miltefosine (2.5 mg/kg/d) was also effective for the treatment of New World cutaneous leishmaniasis. Vomiting, diarrhea, and elevations in transaminases and kidney function studies are common, but generally short-lived, side effects. Miltefosine is registered for the treatment of visceral leishmaniasis in India and may become the standard of care in that country, although additional study is needed.

Pentamidine isethionate is an alternative therapy for visceral leishmaniasis, given daily or on alternate days for 15 doses of 2–4 mg/kg intramuscularly or intravenously. Side effects include immediate hypotension; tachycardia; and gastrointestinal symptoms during administration; sterile abscesses; and pancreatic, liver, and kidney abnormalities.

Paromomycin showed some success when applied topically to treat cutaneous leishmaniasis and has recently been developed as a parenteral therapy for visceral disease. The drug was shown to be similarly efficacious to amphotericin B in India. It is much less expensive than liposomal amphotericin B or miltefosine. Approval of an intramuscular preparation for visceral leishmaniasis was received in India in 2006. The drug is well tolerated; side effects include ototoxicity and reversible elevations in liver enzymes.

B. Cutaneous Leishmaniasis

In the Old World, cutaneous leishmaniasis is generally self-healing over some months and does not metastasize to the mucosa, so it may be justified to withhold treatment in regions without mucocutaneous disease if lesions are small and cosmetically unimportant. Lesions on the face or hands are generally treated. New World leishmaniasis has a greater risk of progression to mucocutaneous disease, so treatment is more often warranted. Standard therapy is with pentavalent antimonials for 20 days, as described above. Other treatments include those discussed above for visceral disease, azole antifungals, and allopurinol. Topical therapy has included intralesional antimony, paromomycin ointment, cryotherapy, local heat, and surgical removal. Diffuse cutaneous leishmaniasis and related chronic skin processes generally respond poorly to therapy.

C. Mucocutaneous Leishmaniasis

Cutaneous infections from regions where parasites include those that cause mucocutaneous disease (eg, *L braziliensis* in parts of Latin America) should all be treated to help prevent disease progression. Treatment of mucocutaneous disease with antimonials is disappointing, with responses in only about 60% in Brazil. Other therapies listed above for visceral leishmaniasis may also be used, although they have not been well studied for this indication.

▶ Prevention & Control

Personal protection measures for avoidance of sand fly bites include use of insect repellants, fine-mesh insect netting, long sleeves and pants, and avoidance of warm shaded areas where flies are common. Disease control measures include destruction of animal reservoir hosts, mass treatment of humans in disease-prevalent areas, residual insecticide spraying in dwellings, limiting contact with dogs and other domesticated animals, and use of permethrin-impregnated collars for dogs.

Chappuis F et al. Visceral leishmaniasis: what are the needs for diagnosis, treatment and control? Nat Rev Microbiol. 2007 Nov;5(11):873–82. [PMID: 17938629]

Murray HW et al. Advances in leishmaniasis. Lancet. 2005 Oct 29–Nov 4;366(9496):1561–77. [PMID: 16257344]

Olliaro PL et al. Treatment options for visceral leishmaniasis: a systematic review of clinical studies done in India, 1980–2004. Lancet Infect Dis. 2005 Dec;5(12):763–74. [PMID: 16310148]

Reithinger R et al. Cutaneous leishmaniasis. Lancet Infect Dis. 2007 Sep;7(9):581–96. [PMID: 17714672]

Sundar S. Injectable paromomycin for visceral leishmaniasis in India. N Engl J Med. 2007 Jun 21;356(25):2571–81. [PMID: 17582067]

Sundar S et al. New treatment approach in Indian visceral leishmaniasis: single-dose liposomal amphotericin B followed by short-course oral miltefosine. Clin Infect Dis. 2008 Oct 15;47(8):1000–6. [PMID: 18781879]

MALARIA

 ESSENTIALS OF DIAGNOSIS

▶ Residence or exposure in a malaria-endemic area.

▶ Intermittent attacks of chills, fever, and sweating.

▶ Headache, malaise, myalgia, nausea, vomiting, splenomegaly; anemia, thrombocytopenia.

▶ Intraerythrocytic parasites identified in thick or thin blood smears.

▶ Severe complications of falciparum malaria: cerebral malaria, severe anemia, hypotension, noncardiogenic pulmonary edema, acute kidney injury, hypoglycemia, acidosis, and hemolysis.

▶ General Considerations

Malaria is the most important parasitic disease of humans, causing hundreds of millions of illnesses and probably over a million deaths each year. The disease is endemic in most of the tropics, including much of South and Central America, Africa, the Middle East, the Indian subcontinent, Southeast Asia, and Oceania. Transmission, morbidity, and mortality are greatest in Africa, where most deaths from malaria are in young children. Malaria is also common in travelers from nonendemic areas to the tropics.

Four species of the genus *Plasmodium* classically cause human malaria. *Plasmodium falciparum* is responsible for nearly all severe disease. It is endemic in most malarious areas and is by far the predominant species in Africa. *Plasmodium vivax* is about as common as *P falciparum*, except in Africa. *P vivax* uncommonly causes severe disease, although this outcome may be more common than previously appreciated. *Plasmodium ovale* and *Plasmodium malariae* are much less common causes of disease, and generally do not cause severe illness. *Plasmodium knowlesi*, a parasite of macaque monkeys, is now recognized to cause occasional illnesses, including some severe disease, in humans in Southeast Asia.

Malaria is transmitted by the bite of infected female anopheline mosquitoes. During feeding, mosquitoes inject sporozoites, which circulate to the liver, and rapidly infect hepatocytes, causing asymptomatic liver infection. Merozoites are subsequently released from the liver, and they rapidly infect erythrocytes to begin the asexual erythrocytic stage of infection that is responsible for human disease. Multiple rounds of erythrocytic development, with production of merozoites that invade additional erythrocytes, lead to large numbers of circulating parasites and clinical illness. Some erythrocytic parasites also develop into sexual gametocytes, which are infectious to mosquitoes, allowing completion of the life cycle and infection of others.

Malaria may uncommonly be transmitted from mother-to-infant (congenital malaria), by blood transfusion, and in nonendemic areas by mosquitoes infected after biting infected immigrants or travelers. In *P vivax* and *P ovale,* parasites also form dormant liver hypnozoites, which are not killed by most drugs, allowing subsequent relapses of illness after initial elimination of erythrocytic infections. For all plasmodial species, parasites may recrudesce following initial clinical improvement after suboptimal therapy.

In highly endemic regions, where people are infected repeatedly, antimalarial immunity prevents severe disease in most older children and adults. However, young children, who are relatively nonimmune, are at high risk for severe disease from *P falciparum* infection, and this population is responsible for most deaths from malaria. Pregnant women are also at increased risk for severe falciparum malaria. In areas with lower endemicity, individuals of all ages commonly present with uncomplicated or severe malaria. Travelers, who are generally nonimmune, are at high risk for severe disease from falciparum malaria at any age.

▶ Clinical Findings

A. Symptoms and Signs

An acute attack of malaria typically begins with a prodrome of headache and fatigue, followed by fever. A classic malarial paroxysm includes chills, high fever, and then sweats. Patients may appear to be remarkably well between febrile episodes. Fevers are usually irregular, especially early in the illness, but without therapy may become regular, with 48-hour cycles (*P vivax* and *P ovale*) or 72-hour cycles (*P malariae*), especially with non-falciparum disease. Headache, malaise, myalgias, arthralgias, cough, chest pain, abdominal pain, anorexia, nausea, vomiting, and diarrhea are common. Seizures may represent simple febrile convulsions or evidence of severe neurologic disease. Physical findings may be absent or include signs of anemia, jaundice, splenomegaly, and mild hepatomegaly. Rash and lymphadenopathy are not typical in malaria, and thus suggestive of another cause of fever. When treated appropriately, uncomplicated malaria generally responds well, with a mortality of about 0.1%.

In the developed world, it is imperative that all persons with suggestive symptoms, in particular fever, who have traveled in an endemic area be evaluated for malaria. The risk for falciparum malaria is greatest within 2 months of return from travel; other species may cause disease many months—and occasionally more than a year—after return from an endemic area.

Severe malaria is principally a result of *P falciparum* infection because this species uniquely infects erythrocytes of all ages and mediates the sequestration of infected erythrocytes in small blood vessels, thereby evading clearance of infected erythrocytes by the spleen. Severe falciparum malaria can include dysfunction of any organ system, including neurologic abnormalities progressing to alterations in consciousness, repeated seizures, and coma (cerebral malaria); severe anemia; hypotension and shock;

noncardiogenic pulmonary edema and the acute respiratory distress syndrome; acute kidney injury due to acute tubular necrosis or, less commonly, severe homolysis); hypoglycemia; acidosis; hemolysis with jaundice; hepatic dysfunction; retinal hemorrhages and other fundoscopic abnormalities; bleeding abnormalities, including disseminated intravascular coagulation; and secondary bacterial infections, including pneumonia and *Salmonella* bacteremia. The most common causes of death in children are cerebral malaria and severe anemia; the former a consequence of a single severe infection and the latter often of multiple malarial infections, intestinal helminths, and nutritional deficiencies. Pregnant women are at particular risk during their first pregnancy, probably due to the selection of *P falciparum* strains that preferentially sequester in the placenta; multiparous women are more likely to have antibodies against these strains and thus avoid severe disease. Malaria in pregnancy also increases the likelihood of poor pregnancy outcomes, with increased prematurity, low birth weight, and mortality.

Uncommon disorders resulting from immunologic responses to chronic infection are massive splenomegaly and, with *P malariae* infection, immune complex glomerulopathy with nephrotic syndrome. Although the presentation of malaria is not as markedly affected by HIV infection as are classic opportunistic infections, HIV-infected individuals are at increased risk for malaria and for severe disease, in particular with advanced immunodeficiency.

B. Laboratory Findings

Giemsa-stained blood smears remain the mainstay of diagnosis (Plates 112, 113, 114, and 115), although other routine stains (eg, Wright stain) will also demonstrate parasites. Thick smears provide efficient evaluation of large volumes of blood, but thin smears are simpler for inexperienced personnel and better for discrimination of parasite species. Single smears are usually positive in infected individuals, although parasitemias may be very low in nonimmune individuals. If illness is suspected, repeating smears in 8- to 24-hour intervals is appropriate. The severity of malaria correlates only loosely with the quantity of infecting parasites, but high parasitemias (especially > 10–20% of erythrocytes infected or > 200,000–500,000 parasites/mcL) or the presence of malarial pigment (a breakdown product of hemoglobin) in > 5% of neutrophils are associated with a particularly poor prognosis.

A second means of diagnosis is rapid diagnostic tests to identify circulating plasmodial antigens with a simple "dipstick" format. These tests are not yet well standardized but are increasingly available around the world, including in the United States. At best, they offer sensitivity and specificity near that of high-quality blood smear analysis and are simpler to perform.

Serologic tests indicate history of disease but are not useful for diagnosis of acute infection. PCR is highly sensitive but not available for routine diagnosis. In immune populations, highly sensitive tests, such as PCR, have limited value because subclinical infections, which are of uncertain significance and not routinely treated, are common.

Table 35–2. Major antimalarial drugs.

Drug	Class	Use
Chloroquine	4-Aminoquinoline	Treatment and chemoprophylaxis of infection with sensitive parasites
Amodiaquine[1]	4-Aminoquinoline	Treatment of *Plasmodium falciparum*, optimally in fixed combination with artesunate
Piperaquine[1]	4-Aminoquinoline	Treatment of *P falciparum* in fixed combination with dihydroartemisinin
Quinine	Quinoline methanol	Oral and intravenous[1] (for severe infections) treatment of *P falciparum*
Quinidine	Quinoline methanol	Intravenous therapy of severe infections with *P falciparum*
Mefloquine	Quinoline methanol	Chemoprophylaxis and treatment of infections with *P falciparum*
Primaquine	8-Aminoquinoline	Radical cure and terminal prophylaxis of infections with *Plasmodium vivax* and *Plasmodium ovale;* alternative for malaria chemoprophylaxis
Sulfadoxine-pyrimethamine (Fansidar)	Folate antagonist combination	Treatment of *P falciparum*, optimally in combination with artesunate
Atovaquone-proguanil (Malarone)	Quinone-folate antagonist combination	Treatment and chemoprophylaxis of *P falciparum* infection
Doxycycline	Tetracycline	Treatment (with quinine) of infections with *P falciparum*; chemoprophylaxis
Halofantrine[1]	Phenanthrene methanol	Treatment of infections with some chloroquine-resistant *P falciparum*
Lumefantrine	Amyl alcohol	Treatment of *P falciparum* malaria in fixed combination with artemether (Coartem)
Artemisinins (Artesunate, artemether, dihydroartemisinin)	Sesquiterpene lactone endoperoxides	Treatment of *P falciparum* in oral combination regimens for uncomplicated disease and parenterally for severe malaria

[1]Not available in the United States.
Modified, with permission, from Katzung BG. *Basic & Clinical Pharmacology*. 11th edition. McGraw-Hill, 2009.

Other diagnostic findings with uncomplicated malaria include thrombocytopenia, anemia, leukocytosis or leukopenia, liver function abnormalities, and hepatosplenomegaly. Severe malaria can present with the laboratory abnormalities expected for the advanced organ dysfunction discussed above.

▶ Treatment

Malaria is the most common cause of fever in much of the tropics and in travelers seeking medical attention after return from endemic areas. Fevers are often treated presumptively in endemic areas, but ideally, treatment should follow definitive diagnosis, especially in nonimmune individuals.

Symptomatic malaria is caused only by the erythrocytic stage of infection. Available antimalarial drugs (Table 35–2) act against this stage, except for primaquine, which acts principally against hepatic parasites.

A. Uncomplicated Falciparum Malaria

Decisions about how to treat malaria are affected by the potential for drug resistance, especially with *P falciparum;* the high cost and limited availability of newer agents for developing world populations; and potential toxicity. The drug sensitivity of individual strains can be determined, but such testing is slow and not useful clinically. Rather, therapeutic decisions are made based on the infecting species and geography. *P falciparum* is now commonly resistant to chloroquine and sulfadoxine-pyrimethamine in most areas, with the principal exceptions of Central America west of the

Panama Canal and Hispaniola. Falciparum malaria from other areas should not be treated with these older drugs, and decisions regarding appropriate chemoprophylaxis should follow the same geographic considerations.

In the developing world, malaria is often treated with suboptimal regimens due to the high cost and limited supplies of newer agents. Chloroquine is still widely used in Africa, and its poor efficacy may be underappreciated due to its antipyretic properties, the ability of some immune individuals to recover from acute malaria without effective therapy, and the fact that recrudescences may not lead to symptoms until weeks after partially effective therapy. Sulfadoxine-pyrimethamine is slower acting than most other agents, and suffers from increasing resistance in most areas. Antimalarial therapy in the developing world has undergone major change in recent years, with increasing advocacy of combination regimens as first-line therapies. Most of these regimens are combinations of highly potent but short-acting artemisinin derivatives with longer-acting partner drugs. The World Health Organization (WHO) currently lists five combination therapies as desirable treatments for falciparum malaria in most areas (Table 35–3), but the efficacy of these regimens varies. Other combination therapies are under development. Another drug that remains generally effective for falciparum malaria is quinine, but it must be taken for an extended period to cure disease and is quite poorly tolerated. Thus, in the developing world, quinine is generally reserved for the treatment of severe malaria and for treatment after another regimen has failed.

Table 35–3. Modified WHO recommendations for the treatment of malaria.

Regimen	Notes
Artemether-lumefantrine (Coartem, Riamet)	Coformulated, first-line therapy in multiple African countries. Approved in the United States.
Artesunate-amodiaquine (ASAQ)	Coformulated, first-line therapy in multiple African countries.
Artesunate-mefloquine	Standard therapy in parts of Southeast Asia.
Artesunate-sulfadoxine-pyrimethamine	Efficacy low compared with other regimens in most areas.
Amodiaquine-sulfadox-ine-pyrimethamine	Less expensive; efficacy varies, but remains good in some areas; recommended as an interim option when efficacy established and other regimens are not available.
Dihydroartemisinin-piperaquine	Newer coformulated combination. Highly effective in most areas, but not yet part of WHO recommendations.

World Health Organization: Guidelines for the Treatment of Malaria. World Health Organization. Geneva 2006. *ISBM* 924 1546948.

In developed countries, malaria is an uncommon but potentially life-threatening infection of travelers and immigrants, many of whom are nonimmune, so they are at risk for rapid progression to severe disease. Nonimmune individuals with falciparum malaria should generally be admitted to the hospital due to risks of rapid progression of disease. Options for the treatment of uncomplicated falciparum malaria in the United States have increased with the approval of artemether-lumefantrine in 2008; this drug will likely become the standard for this indication (Table 35–4).

B. Treatment of Non-Falciparum Malaria

The first-line drug for non-falciparum malaria remains chloroquine. Resistance of *P vivax* to chloroquine has increased, but the drug remains generally effective, and since non-falciparum malaria is uncommonly severe, it is reasonable to accept a small risk of treatment failure. For *P vivax* or *P ovale*, eradication of erythrocytic parasites with chloroquine should be accompanied by treatment with primaquine (after evaluating for glucose-6-phosphate dehydrogenase (G6PD) deficiency; see below) to eradicate dormant liver stages (hypnozoites), which may lead to relapses with recurrent erythrocytic infection and malaria symptoms after weeks to months if left untreated. *P malariae* infections need only be treated with chloroquine.

C. Treatment of Severe Malaria

Severe malaria can be defined as presentation with any signs of severe illness or organ dysfunction (including prostration, impaired consciousness, convulsions, respiratory distress, shock, acidosis, severe anemia, excessive bleeding, hypogly-

cemia, jaundice, hemoglobinuria, or kidney impairment) or a high parasite load (generally peripheral parasitemia > 5% or > 200,000 parasites/mcL). It is a medical emergency. Indications for parenteral treatment include severe malaria, as defined above, and inability to take oral drugs. With appropriate prompt therapy and supportive care, rapid recoveries may be seen in even very ill individuals.

In the developing world, severe malaria and deaths from the disease are mostly in young children, in particular from cerebral malaria, severe anemia, and pulmonary disease. In the developed world, mortality from malaria is mostly in adults, and often follows extended illnesses and secondary complications long after eradication of the malarial infection. Standard therapy for severe malaria has been intravenous quinine in most areas and, in the United States, intravenous quinidine, which is equally effective. However, the standard of care is now changing, since intravenous artesunate has shown superiority over quinine.

Patients receiving intravenous quinine or quinidine should receive continuous cardiac monitoring; if QTc prolongation exceeds 25% of baseline, the infusion rate should be reduced. Blood glucose should be monitored every 4–6 hours, and 5–10% dextrose may be coadministered to decrease the likelihood of hypoglycemia. Appropriate care of severe malaria includes maintenance of fluids and electrolytes; respiratory and hemodynamic support; and consideration of blood transfusions, anticonvulsants, antibiotics for bacterial infections, and dialysis. With high parasitemia (> 5–10%), exchange transfusion has been used, but beneficial effects have not clearly been demonstrated, and its role remains uncertain.

Recent studies indicate that intravenous artesunate has superior efficacy and better tolerability than intravenous quinine for severe malaria. Intravenous artesunate became available in the United States in 2007 on an investigational basis through the CDC (for enrollment call 770-488-7788); if approved, the drug is provided emergently from CDC Quarantine Stations. The drug is administered in four doses of 2.4 mg/kg over 3 days, every 12 hours on day 1, and then daily. If artesunate cannot be obtained promptly, severe malaria should be treated with intravenous quinidine. In endemic regions, if parenteral therapy is not available, intrarectal administration of artemether or artesunate is also effective.

D. Antimalarial Drugs

1. Chloroquine—Chloroquine remains the drug of choice for the treatment of sensitive *P falciparum* and other species of malaria parasites. Chloroquine is active against erythrocytic parasites of all human malaria species. It does not eradicate hepatic stages, so must be used with primaquine to eradicate *P vivax* and *P ovale* infections. Chloroquine-resistant *P falciparum* is widespread in nearly all areas of the world with falciparum malaria, with the exceptions of Central America west of the Panama Canal, Mexico, and Hispaniola. Chloroquine-resistant *P vivax* has been reported from a number of areas, most notably Southeast Asia.

Chloroquine is the drug of choice for the treatment of non-falciparum and sensitive falciparum malaria. It rapidly

Table 35–4. Treatment of malaria.

Clinical Setting	Drug Therapy[1]	Alternative Drugs
Chloroquine-sensitive *Plasmodium falciparum* and *Plasmodium malariae* infections	Chloroquine phosphate, 1 g, followed by 500 mg at 6, 24, and 48 hours -or- Chloroquine phosphate, 1 g at 0 and 24 hours, then 0.5 g at 48 hours	
Plasmodium vivax and *Plasmodium ovale* infections	Chloroquine (as above), then (if G6PD normal) primaquine, 30 mg base daily for 14 days	
Uncomplicated infections with chloroquine-resistant *P falciparum*	Coartem (artemether 20 mg, lumefantrine 120 mg, four tablets twice daily for 3 days Malarone, four tablets (total of 1 g atovaquone, 400 mg proguanil) daily for 3 days Quinine sulfate, 650 mg three times daily for 3-7 days Plus one of the following (when quinine given for < 7 days)- Doxycycline, 100 mg twice daily for 7 days -or- Clindamycin, 600 mg twice daily for 7 days	Mefloquine, 15 mg/kg once or 750 mg, then 500 mg in 6-8 hours -or- ASAQ[2] (artesunate 100 mg, amodiaquine 270 mg), two tablets daily for 3 days
Severe or complicated infections with *P falciparum*[3]	Artesunate 2.4 mg/kg IV every 12 hours for 1 day, then daily[3,6]	Quinidine gluconate,[4-6] 10 mg/kg IV over 1-2 hours, then 0.02 mg/kg IV/min -or- Quinidine gluconate,[4-6] 15 mg/kg IV over 4 hours, then 7.5 mg/kg IV over 4 hours every 8 hours -or- Quinine dihydrochloride,[2,4-6] 20 mg/kg IV over 4 hours, then 10 mg/kg IV every 8 hours -or- Artemether,[2,6] 3.2 mg/kg IM, then 1.6 mg/kg/d IM

[1]All dosages are oral and refer to salts unless otherwise indicated. See text for additional information on all agents, including toxicities and cautions. See Centers for Disease Control and Prevention's guidelines (phone: 877-FYI-TRIP; http://www.cdc.gov) for additional information and pediatric dosing.
[2]Not available in the United States.
[3]Available in the United States only on an investigational basis through the CDC (phone: 770-488-7788).
[4]Cardiac monitoring should be in place during intravenous administration of quinidine or quinine.
[5]Avoid loading doses in persons who have received quinine, quinidine, or mefloquine in the prior 24 hours.
[6]With all parenteral regimens, change to an oral regimen (most commonly doxycycline in adults or clindamycin in children) as soon as the patient can tolerate it.
G6PD, glucose-6-phosphate dehydrogenase.
Modified, with permission, from Katzung BG. *Basic & Clinical Pharmacology.* 11th edition. McGraw-Hill, 2009.

terminates fever (in 24–48 hours) and clears parasitemia (in 48–72 hours) caused by sensitive parasites. Chloroquine is also the preferred chemoprophylactic agent in malarious regions without resistant falciparum malaria. Eradication of *P vivax* and *P ovale* requires a course of primaquine.

Chloroquine is usually well tolerated, even with prolonged use. Pruritus is common, primarily in Africans. Nausea, vomiting, abdominal pain, headache, anorexia, malaise, blurring of vision, and urticaria are uncommon. Dosing after meals may reduce some adverse events.

2. Amodiaquine and piperaquine—Amodiaquine is a 4-aminoquinoline that is closely related to chloroquine. Amodiaquine has been widely used to treat malaria because of its low cost, limited toxicity and, in some areas, effectiveness against chloroquine-resistant strains of *P falciparum*. Use of amodiaquine decreased after recognition of rare but

serious side effects, notably agranulocytosis, aplastic anemia, and hepatotoxicity. However, serious side effects are rare with short-term use, and amodiaquine is increasingly advocated as a replacement for chloroquine, particularly in combination regimens (Table 35–3). Chemoprophylaxis with amodiaquine is best avoided because of its apparent increased toxicity with long-term use.

Piperaquine is another 4-aminoquinoline that was previously heavily used in China and has been coformulated with dihydroartemisinin in a new artemisinin-based therapy. Piperaquine appears to be well tolerated, to have minimal problems with resistance (despite prior reports of resistance in China), and in combination with dihydroartemisinin to offer a highly efficacious therapy for falciparum malaria.

3. Mefloquine—Mefloquine is effective therapy for many chloroquine-resistant strains of *P falciparum* and against other malarial species. Although toxicity is a concern, mefloquine is also a recommended chemoprophylactic drug. Resistance to mefloquine has been reported sporadically from many areas, but it appears to be uncommon except in regions of Southeast Asia with high rates of multidrug resistance (especially border areas of Thailand).

For treatment of uncomplicated malaria, mefloquine is rapidly active and can be administered as a single dose or in two doses over 1 day. It is used in combination with artesunate in Southeast Asia, where resistance to mefloquine has been seen but the combination remains effective in most areas. It should be taken with meals and swallowed with a large amount of water. For chemoprophylaxis, mefloquine is effective against most strains of *P falciparum* and probably all other malarial species. It is recommended by the CDC for chemoprophylaxis in all malarious areas except those with no chloroquine resistance (where chloroquine is preferred) and some rural areas of Southeast Asia with a high prevalence of mefloquine resistance. As with chloroquine, eradication of *P vivax* and *P ovale* requires a course of primaquine.

Adverse effects with weekly dosing of mefloquine for chemoprophylaxis include nausea, vomiting, dizziness, sleep and behavioral disturbances, epigastric pain, diarrhea, abdominal pain, headache, and rash. Despite anecdotal reports of seizures and psychosis, a number of controlled studies have found the frequency of serious adverse effects from mefloquine to be no higher than that with other common chemoprophylactic regimens. Nonetheless, mefloquine should be avoided in persons with histories of psychiatric disease or seizures.

Adverse effects are much more common (up to 50% of treatments) with the higher dosages of mefloquine required for treatment. These effects may be lessened by splitting administration of the drug into two doses separated by 6–8 hours. Serious neuropsychiatric toxicities (depression, confusion, acute psychosis, or seizures) have been reported in less than 1 in 1000 treatments, but some authorities believe that these are more common. Mefloquine can also alter cardiac conduction, and so it should not be coadministered with quinine, quinidine, or halofantrine, and caution is required if quinine or quinidine is used to treat malaria after mefloquine chemoprophylaxis. Mefloquine is generally considered safe in young children and pregnant women.

4. Quinine and quinidine—Quinine dihydrochloride and quinidine gluconate remain first-line therapies for falciparum malaria, especially severe disease, although toxicity concerns complicate therapy. Quinine acts rapidly against the four species of human malaria parasites. Quinidine, the dextrorotatory stereoisomer of quinine, is at least as effective as quinine in the treatment of severe falciparum malaria.

Resistance of *P falciparum* to quinine is common in some areas of Southeast Asia, where the drug may fail if used alone to treat falciparum malaria. However, quinine still provides at least a partial therapeutic effect in most patients.

Quinine and quinidine are effective treatments for severe falciparum malaria, although intravenous artesunate is becoming the standard of care (see Artemisinins section below). Quinine can be administered slowly intravenously

or, in a dilute solution, intramuscularly, but parenteral quinine is not available in the United States, where quinidine is used. The drugs can be administered in divided doses or by continuous intravenous infusion; treatment should begin with a loading dose to rapidly achieve effective plasma concentrations. Intravenous quinine and quinidine should be administered with cardiac monitoring because of their cardiac toxicity and the relative unpredictability of their pharmacokinetics. Therapy should be changed to oral quinine as soon as the patient has improved and can tolerate oral medications.

In areas without newer combination regimens, oral quinine sulfate is appropriate first-line therapy for uncomplicated falciparum malaria, although poor tolerance may limit compliance. Quinine is commonly used with a second drug (most often doxycycline) to shorten the duration of use (usually to 3 days) and to limit toxicity. Therapeutic dosages of quinine and quinidine commonly cause tinnitus, headache, nausea, dizziness, flushing, and visual disturbances, a constellation of symptoms termed "cinchonism." Mild symptoms of cinchonism do not warrant the discontinuation of therapy. Hypersensitivity reactions include rash, urticaria, angioedema, and bronchospasm. Hematologic abnormalities include hemolysis (especially with G6PD deficiency), leukopenia, agranulocytosis, and thrombocytopenia. Therapeutic doses may cause hypoglycemia; this is a particular problem in severe infections and in pregnant patients. Quinine can stimulate uterine contractions, especially in the third trimester, but this effect is mild, and quinine and quinidine are considered safe in pregnancy. Intravenous infusions of the drugs may cause thrombophlebitis. Overly rapid infusions can cause severe hypotension. ECG abnormalities (QT prolongation) are fairly common, especially with quinidine, but dangerous arrhythmias are uncommon when the drugs are administered appropriately in a monitored setting. Blackwater fever is a rare severe illness, probably due to hypersensitivity, that includes marked hemolysis and hemoglobinuria in the setting of quinine therapy for malaria. Quinine should not be given concurrently with mefloquine and should be used with caution in a patient who has previously received mefloquine. Absorption may be blocked by aluminum-containing antacids. Quinine can raise plasma levels of warfarin and digoxin. Dosage must be reduced in renal insufficiency.

5. Primaquine—Primaquine phosphate, a synthetic 8-aminoquinoline, is the drug of choice for the eradication of dormant liver forms of *P vivax* and *P ovale*. Primaquine is active against hepatic stages of all human malaria parasites. This action is optimal soon after therapy with chloroquine or quinine. Primaquine also acts against erythrocytic stage parasites, although this activity is too weak for the treatment of active disease, and against gametocytes.

For *P vivax* and *P ovale* infections, chloroquine is used to eradicate erythrocytic forms, and if the G6PD level is normal, a 14-day course of primaquine is initiated to eradicate liver hypnozoites and prevent a subsequent relapse. Some strains of *P vivax*, particularly in New Guinea and Southeast Asia, are relatively resistant to primaquine. For this reason, the CDC has recently doubled the recommended dosage for primaquine to eradicate liver forms (to 52.6 mg primaquine phosphate, or 30 mg base/day), but it remains possible that liver forms may not be eradicated by a single treatment.

Standard chemoprophylaxis does not prevent a relapse of *P vivax* or *P ovale* infections, since the hypnozoite forms of these parasites are not eradicated by chloroquine or other standard treatments. To diminish the likelihood of relapse, some authorities advocate the use of a treatment course of primaquine after the completion of travel to an endemic area.

Primaquine has also been studied as a daily chemoprophylactic agent. Daily treatment with 0.5 mg/kg of base (to a maximum of 30 mg/day) provides protection against malaria caused by *P falciparum* and *P vivax*, but should only be used in persons with documented normal levels of G6PD. In addition, potential toxicities of long-term use remain a concern, and primaquine is not a first-line choice for this purpose.

Primaquine in recommended doses is generally well tolerated. It infrequently causes nausea, epigastric pain, abdominal cramps, and headache, especially when taken on an empty stomach. Rare adverse effects include leukopenia, agranulocytosis, leukocytosis, and cardiac arrhythmias. Standard doses of primaquine may cause hemolysis or methemoglobinemia (manifested by cyanosis), especially in persons with G6PD deficiency or other hereditary metabolic defects. Patients should be tested for G6PD deficiency before primaquine is prescribed. When a patient is deficient in G6PD, treatment strategies may consist of (1) withholding therapy and treating subsequent relapses, if they occur, with chloroquine; (2) treating patients with standard dosing, paying close attention to their hematologic status; or (3) treating with weekly primaquine (45 mg base) for 8 weeks. G6PD-deficient individuals of Mediterranean and Asian ancestry are most likely to have severe deficiency, while those of African ancestry usually have a milder biochemical defect. This difference can be taken into consideration in choosing a treatment strategy. Primaquine should be discontinued if there is evidence of hemolysis or anemia and should be avoided in pregnancy.

6. Inhibitors of folate synthesis—Inhibitors of two parasite enzymes involved in folate metabolism, dihydrofolate reductase (DHFR) and dihydropteroate synthase (DHPS), are used, generally in combination regimens, for the treatment and prevention of malaria. These include the DHFR inhibitors pyrimethamine, proguanil, and chlorproguanil, and the DHPS inhibitors sulfadoxine and dapsone. All described antifolates act relatively slowly against erythrocytic forms of susceptible strains of all four human malaria species. They are not reliably effective against hepatic stages or gametocytes. Fixed-dosed antifolate combinations to treat malaria are sulfadoxine-pyrimethamine (Fansidar) and chloroproguanil/dapsone (Lapdap). These drugs will be discussed only as combinations, as they are not otherwise used to treat or prevent malaria. Malarone, a combination of proguanil with atovaquone, is discussed below.

Fansidar is a fixed combination of sulfadoxine (500 mg) and pyrimethamine (25 mg). The long half-lives of its components allow weekly dosing for chemoprophylaxis, but due to rare serious side effects with long-term dosing, this drug is no longer recommended for this purpose. Sulfadoxine-pyrimethamine became a common back-up drug after chloroquine in many malaria-endemic areas, and replaced chloroquine as the first-line therapy in a number of countries. Advantages of sulfadoxine-pyrimethamine include ease of administration (a single oral dose) and low cost. However, resistance to sulfadoxine-pyrimethamine is rapidly limiting its efficacy. In addition, it is not reliably effective in *P vivax* infections, and its usefulness against *P ovale* and *P malariae* infections has not been adequately studied, limiting its utility outside of Africa.

Sulfadoxine-pyrimethamine is a component of two combination regimens for uncomplicated malaria recommended by the WHO (Table 35–3). Sulfadoxine-pyrimethamine plus artesunate has shown efficacy in some areas but is best replaced by more effective combination regimens in most areas. Amodiaquine plus sulfadoxine-pyrimethamine has shown surprisingly good efficacy in many parts of Africa, despite increasing resistance to both components, and probably offers the most practical treatment for uncomplicated malaria in many endemic areas without access to artemisinin-based therapies.

Lapdap, a fixed combination of chlorproguanil (80 mg) and dapsone (100 mg), was developed as an inexpensive treatment of falciparum malaria for Africa, and a combination with artesunate was under development. However, the drug was withdrawn in 2008 due to unacceptable rates of hematologic toxicity.

7. Artemisinins—Artemisinin (qinghaosu) is a sesquiterpene lactone endoperoxide, the active component of an herbal medicine that has been used as an antipyretic in China for over 2000 years. Analogs have been synthesized to increase solubility and improve antimalarial efficacy. The most important of these analogs are artesunate, artemether, and dihydroartemisinin. A number of artemisinins are available in many countries, although they are more expensive than older therapies. The WHO is encouraging availability of oral artemisinins only in coformulated combination regimens.

Artemisinins act very rapidly against all erythrocytic-stage human malaria parasites. Artemisinin resistance is not yet an important problem, but *P falciparum* isolates with diminished in vitro susceptibility to artemether have been described from South America, and delayed clearance of parasites has been seen after treatment with artesunate in parts of Cambodia.

Artemisinins are playing an increasing role in the treatment of malaria, including multidrug-resistant *P falciparum* malaria. However, due to their short plasma half-lives, recrudescence rates are unacceptably high after short-course therapy, and they are best used in conjunction with another agent. Also because of their short-half lives, they are not useful in chemoprophylaxis.

Artemisinins should be used for uncomplicated malaria in combination regimens including a longer-acting partner drug, known as artemisinin-based combination therapy. Artesunate plus mefloquine has demonstrated excellent efficacy against multidrug resistant parasites in Thailand, but this regimen is too expensive for widespread use in Africa and other areas. The artemisinin-based combination regimens that are currently most advocated in Africa are artesunate plus amodiaquine (ASAQ) and artemether plus lumefantrine (Coartem), each of which is available as a coformulated product and is the recommended therapy for uncomplicated malaria in a number of countries in Africa. However, implementation of treatment guidelines has been slowed due to the high cost of the new therapies, limited drug availability, and other factors. A third available coformulated regimen that has performed well in clinical trials is dihydroartemisinin plus piperaquine.

In studies of severe malaria, intramuscular artemether was at least as effective as intramuscular quinine, and intravenous artesunate was superior to intravenous quinine in terms of efficacy and tolerability. Thus, the standard of care for severe malaria is intravenous artesunate, when it is available, although parenteral quinine remains an acceptable alternative. Artesunate and artemether have also been effective in the treatment of severe malaria when administered rectally, offering a valuable treatment modality when parenteral therapy is not available.

Artemisinins appear to be very well tolerated. The most commonly reported adverse effects have been nausea, vomiting, and diarrhea, which may often be due to acute malaria, rather than drug toxicity. Irreversible neurotoxicity has been seen in animals after very high doses, but this problem has not been recognized in humans after widespread use. Artemisinins are teratogenic in animals, and they should be avoided in the first trimester of pregnancy for uncomplicated malaria. However, for severe malaria, for which all available treatments entail some risk, the WHO endorses the use of intravenous artesunate or quinine while additional data are gathered on artesunate safety.

8. Atovaquone plus proguanil (Malarone)—Atovaquone, a hydroxynaphthoquinone, is not effective when used alone, due to rapid development of drug resistance. However, Malarone, a fixed combination of atovaquone (250 mg) and proguanil (100 mg), is highly effective for both the treatment and chemoprophylaxis of falciparum malaria, and it is approved for both indications in the United States. It also appears to be active against other species of malaria parasites. Unlike most other antimalarials, Malarone provides activity against both erythrocytic and hepatic stage parasites.

For treatment, Malarone is given at an adult dose of four tablets daily for 3 days. For chemoprophylaxis, Malarone must be taken daily. It has an advantage over mefloquine and doxycycline in requiring shorter periods of treatment before and after the period at risk for malaria transmission, due to activity against liver-stage parasites, but it is more expensive than the other agents. It should be taken with food.

Malarone is generally well tolerated. Adverse effects include abdominal pain, nausea, vomiting, diarrhea, headache, and rash, and these are more common with the higher dose required for treatment. Reversible elevations in liver enzymes have been reported. The safety of atovaquone in pregnancy is unknown.

9. Antibiotics—A number of antibacterials in addition to the folate antagonists and sulfonamides are slow-acting antimalarials. None of the antibiotics should be used as single agents for the treatment of malaria due to their slow rate of action.

Tetracycline and doxycycline are active against asexual erythrocytic forms of all human malaria parasites. Doxycycline is commonly used in the treatment of falciparum malaria in conjunction with quinidine or quinine, allowing a shorter and better-tolerated course of those drugs. Doxycycline is also a standard chemoprophylactic drug, especially for use in areas of Southeast Asia with high rates of resistance to other antimalarials, including mefloquine. Doxycycline side effects include gastrointestinal symptoms, candidal vaginitis, and photosensitivity. The drug should be taken while upright with a large amount of water to avoid esophageal irritation. Its safety in long-term chemoprophylaxis has not been extensively evaluated.

Clindamycin can be used in conjunction with quinine or quinidine in those for whom doxycycline is not recommended, such as children and pregnant women. The most common toxicities with clindamycin are gastrointestinal. Azithromycin also has antimalarial activity and is now under study for treatment and chemoprophylaxis.

10. Halofantrine and lumefantrine—Halofantrine hydrochloride, a phenanthrene-methanol related to quinine, is effective against erythrocytic stages of all four human malaria species. Oral absorption is variable and is enhanced with food. Because of toxicity concerns, it should not be taken with meals. Halofantrine is rapidly effective against most chloroquine-resistant strains of *P falciparum,* but its use is limited by irregular absorption and cardiac toxicity. As treatment for falciparum malaria, halofantrine is given orally in three 500-mg doses at 6-hour intervals, and this course is repeated in 1 week for nonimmune individuals. Halofantrine is generally well tolerated. The most common adverse effects are abdominal pain, diarrhea, vomiting, cough, rash, headache, pruritus, and elevated liver enzymes. Of greater concern, the drug alters cardiac conduction, with dose-related prolongation of QT and PR intervals. This effect is worsened by prior mefloquine therapy. Rare instances of dangerous arrhythmias and some deaths have been reported. The drug is contraindicated in patients with cardiac conduction defects and should not be used in those who have recently taken mefloquine. It is also contraindicated in pregnancy.

Lumefantrine, an aryl alcohol related to halofantrine, is available only as a fixed-dose combination with artemether (Coartem or Riamet). As with halofantrine, oral absorption is highly variable and improved when the drug is taken with food. Use of Coartem with a fatty meal is recommended. Coartem is highly effective for the treatment of falciparum malaria, but it is expensive and requires twice-daily dosing. Despite these limitations, due to its reliable efficacy against falciparum malaria, Coartem has recently been selected as the first-line therapy for malaria in many African countries. Coartem is well tolerated; side effects include headache, dizziness, loss of appetite, gastrointestinal symptoms, and palpitations. Importantly, Coartem does not appear to cause the cardiac toxicity seen with halofantrine.

Prevention

Malaria is transmitted by night-biting anopheline mosquitoes. Measures to prevent malaria include control of mosquitoes using ecologic measures and insecticides, and optimal use of these modalities is now under study. Bed nets, in particular nets treated with permethrin insecticides, are heavily promoted as inexpensive means of antimalarial protection, and improvement in mortality rates has been demonstrated. Extensive efforts are also underway to develop a malaria vaccine, and partial protection of African children has been demonstrated, but a vaccine offering complete protection is not anticipated in the near future.

When travelers from nonendemic to endemic countries are counseled on the prevention of malaria, it is imperative to emphasize measures to prevent mosquito bites (insect repellents, insecticides, and bed nets), since parasites are increasingly resistant to multiple drugs and no chemoprophylactic regimen is fully protective. Chemoprophylaxis is recommended for all travelers from nonendemic regions to endemic areas, although risks vary greatly for different locations, and some tropical areas entail no risk; specific recommendations for travel to different locales are available from the CDC (www.cdc.gov). Current recommendations from the CDC include the use of chloroquine for chemoprophylaxis in the few areas with only chloroquine-sensitive malaria parasites (principally the Caribbean and Central America west of the Panama Canal), mefloquine or Malarone for most other malarious areas, and doxycycline for areas with a high prevalence of multidrug-resistant falciparum malaria (principally parts of Southeast Asia) (Table 35–5). Recommendations should be checked regularly (Phone: 877-FYI-TRIP; Internet: www.cdc.gov/travel/) because they may change in response to changing resistance patterns and increasing experience with new drugs. In some circumstances, it may be appropriate for travelers to not use chemoprophylaxis but to carry supplies of drugs with them in case a febrile illness develops and medical attention is unavailable. Regimens for self-treatment include artemisinin-based combinations, Malarone, and quinine. Most authorities do not recommend routine terminal chemoprophylaxis with primaquine to eradicate dormant hepatic stages of *P vivax* and *P ovale* after travel, but this may be appropriate in some circumstances, especially for travelers with major exposure to these parasites.

Regular chemoprophylaxis is not a standard management practice in developing world populations due to the expense and potential toxicities of long-term therapy. However, there is increasing interest in intermittent preventive therapy, whereby at-risk populations receive antimalarial therapy at certain intervals. This strategy may decrease the incidence of malarial morbidity and mortality while allowing antimalarial immunity to develop. Intermittent preventive therapy has been best studied with sulfadoxine-pyrimethamine, a long-acting drug that is administered in a single dose. The two high-risk populations that have been studied are pregnant women and infants. During pregnancy, sulfadoxine-pyrimethamine provided once during both the second and third trimesters has improved pregnancy outcomes. In infants, intermittent therapy with sulfadoxine-pyrimethamine has offered benefits, but dosing schedules are not standardized. With increasing resistance to sulfadoxine-pyrimethamine, it is not clear if the drug will retain prophylactic efficacy or if other drugs with shorter half-lives will be effective for intermittent preventive therapy.

When to Refer

Referral to an expert on infectious diseases or travel medicine is important with all cases of malaria in the United States, and in particular for falciparum malaria, as management can be complex, but referral should not lead to a

Table 35–5. Drugs for the prevention of malaria in travelers.[1]

Drug	Use[2]	Adult Dosage (all oral)[3]
Chloroquine	Areas without resistant *Plasmodium falciparum*	500 mg weekly
Malarone	Areas with multidrug-resistant *P falciparum*	1 tablet (250 mg atovaquone/100 mg proguanil) daily
Mefloquine	Areas with chloroquine-resistant *P falciparum*	250 mg weekly
Doxycycline	Areas with multidrug-resistant *P falciparum*	100 mg daily
Primaquine[4]	Terminal prophylaxis of *Plasmodium vivax* and *Plasmodium ovale* infections; alternative for *P falciparum* prophylaxis	30 mg base daily for 14 days after travel

[1]Recommendations may change, as resistance to all available drugs is increasing. See text for additional information on toxicities and cautions. For additional details and pediatric dosing, see Centers for Disease Control and Prevention's guidelines (phone: 800-CDC-INFO; http://www.cdc.gov). Travelers to remote areas should consider carrying effective therapy (see text) for use if a febrile illness develops, and they cannot reach medical attention quickly.

[2]Areas without known chloroquine-resistant *P falciparum* are Central America west of the Panama Canal, Haiti, Dominican Republic, Egypt, and most malarious countries of the Middle East. Malarone or mefloquine is currently recommended for other malarious areas except for border areas of Thailand, where doxycycline is recommended.

[3]For drugs other than primaquine, begin 1–2 weeks before departure (except 2 days before for doxycycline and Malarone) and continue for 4 weeks after leaving the endemic area (except 1 week for Malarone). All dosages refer to salts unless otherwise indicated.

[4]Screen for glucose-6-phosphate dehydrogenase deficiency before using primaquine.

Reproduced, with permission, from Katzung BG. *Basic & Clinical Pharmacology*. 11th edition. McGraw-Hill, 2009.

delay in initial diagnosis and therapy, since delays in therapy can lead to severe illness or death.

▶ When to Admit

- Non-falciparum malaria generally does not cause severe disease and responds well to therapy, and so admission is only warranted if a patient presents with specific problems that require hospital management.

- Patients with falciparum malaria are generally admitted because the disease can progress rapidly to severe illness; exceptions may be made with individuals who are from malaria-endemic areas, and thus expected to have a degree of immunity, who are without evidence of severe disease, and who are judged able to return promptly for medical attention if their disease progresses.

Baird JK. Effectiveness of antimalarial drugs. N Engl J Med. 2005 Apr 14;352(15):1565–77. [PMID: 15829537]

Chen LH et al. Prevention of malaria in long-term travelers. JAMA. 2006 Nov 8;296(18):2234–44. [PMID: 17090770]

Freedman DO. Clinical practice. Malaria prevention in short-term travelers. N Engl J Med. 2008 Aug 7;359(6):603–12. [PMID: 18687641]

Greenwood PM et al. Malaria. 2005 Apr 23–29;365(9469):1487–98. [PMID: 15850634]

Griffith KS et al. Treatment of malaria in the United States: a systematic review. JAMA. 2007 May 23;297(20):2264–77. [PMID: 17519416]

Nosten F et al. Artemisinin-based combination treatment of falciparum malaria. Am J Trop Med Hyg. 2007 Dec;77(6 Suppl):181–92. [PMID: 18165491]

Rosenthal PJ. Artesunate for the treatment of severe falciparum malaria. N Engl J Med. 2008 Apr 24;358(17):1829–36. [PMID: 18434652]

Whitty CJ et al. Malaria: an update on treatment of adults in non-endemic countries. BMJ. 2006 Jul 29;333(7561):241–5. [PMID: 16873859]

World Health Organization: Guidelines for the treatment of malaria. Geneva. 2006. www.who.int/malaria/docs/Treatment Guidelines2006.pdf

BABESIOSIS

ESSENTIALS OF DIAGNOSIS

- ▶ History of tick bite or exposure to ticks.
- ▶ Fever, flu-like symptoms, anemia.
- ▶ Intraerythrocytic parasites on Giemsa-stained blood smears.
- ▶ Positive serologic tests.

▶ General Considerations

Babesiosis is an uncommon intraerythrocytic infection caused mainly by two *Babesia* species and transmitted by *Ixodes* ticks. In Europe, where only 31 cases of babesiosis have been reported, infection is caused by *Babesia divergens*, which also infects cattle. In the United States, hundreds of cases of babesiosis have been reported, and infection is caused by *Babesia microti*, which also infects wild mammals. Most babesiosis in the United States occurs in the coastal northeast, with some cases also in the upper midwest, following the geographic range of the vector *Ixodes scapularis*, and Lyme disease and anaplasmosis, which are spread by the same vector. Rare episodes of illnesses caused by *B microti*, *B divergens*, and other Babesia-like organisms have been reported from other areas. Babesiosis can also be transmitted by blood transfusion.

▶ Clinical Findings

A. Symptoms and Signs

With *B microti* infections, symptoms appear 1 week to several weeks after a tick bite; parasitemia is evident after 2–4 weeks. Patients usually do not recall the tick bite. The typical flu-like illness develops gradually and is characterized by fever, fatigue, headache, arthralgia, and myalgia. Other findings may include nausea, vomiting, abdominal pain, sore throat, depression, emotional lability, anemia, thrombocytopenia, and splenomegaly. Parasitemia may continue for months to years, with or without symptoms, and the disease is usually self-limited. Severe complications are most likely to occur in older persons or in those who have had splenectomy. Serious complications include respiratory failure, hemolytic anemia, disseminated intravascular coagulation, congestive heart failure, and acute kidney injury. In a study of hospitalized patients, the mortality rate was 6.5%. Most recognized *B divergens* infections in Europe have been in patients who have had splenectomy. These infections progress rapidly with high fever, severe hemolytic anemia, jaundice, hemoglobinuria, and acute kidney injury, with death rates over 40%.

B. Laboratory Findings

Identification of the intraerythrocytic parasite on Giemsa-stained blood smears establishes the diagnosis (Plate 116). These can be confused with malaria parasites, but the morphology is distinctive. Repeated smears are often necessary because well under 1% of erythrocytes may be infected, especially early in infection, although parasitemias can exceed 10%. An indirect immunofluorescent antibody test for *B microti* is available from the CDC; antibody is detectable within 2–4 weeks after the onset of symptoms and persists for months. Diagnosis can also be made by PCR or by inoculation of hamsters or gerbils.

▶ Treatment

Most patients have a mild illness and recover without therapy. Standard therapy is a 7-day course of quinine (650 mg orally three times daily) plus clindamycin (600 mg orally three times daily). An alternative is a 7-day course of atovaquone (750 mg orally every 12 hours) plus azithromycin (600 mg orally once daily). Exchange transfusion has been used successfully in severely ill asplenic patients and those with parasitemia greater than 10%.

Gubernot DM et al. *Babesia* infection through blood transfusions: reports received by the US Food and Drug Administration, 1997–2007. Clin Infect Dis. 2009 Jan 1;48(1):25–30. [PMID: 19035776]

Krause PJ et al. Persistent and relapsing babesiosis in immuno-compromised patients. Clin Infect Dis. 2008 Feb 1;46(3):370–6. [PMID: 18181735]

Vannier E et al. Human babesiosis. Infect Dis Clin North Am. 2008 Sep;22(3):469–88. [PMID: 18755385]

TOXOPLASMOSIS

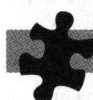

ESSENTIALS OF DIAGNOSIS

▶ Infection confirmed by isolation of *Toxoplasma gondii* or identification of tachyzoites in tissue or body fluids.

Primary infection

▶ Fever, malaise, headache, sore throat.

▶ Lymphadenopathy.

▶ Positive IgG and IgM serologic tests.

Congenital infection

▶ Follows acute infection of seronegative women and leads to CNS abnormalities and retinochoroiditis.

Infection in immunocompromised persons

▶ Reactivation leads to encephalitis, retinochoroiditis, pneumonitis, myocarditis.

▶ Positive IgG but negative IgM serologic tests.

▶ General Considerations

T gondii, an obligate intracellular protozoan, is found world-wide in humans and in many species of animals and birds. The definitive hosts are cats. Humans are infected after ingestion of cysts in raw or undercooked meat, ingestion of oocysts in food or water contaminated by cats, transplacental transmission of trophozoites or, rarely, direct inoculation of trophozoites via blood transfusion or organ transplantation. *Toxoplasma* seroprevalence varies widely. It has decreased in the United States to about 20–30%, but it is much higher in other countries in both the developed and developing worlds, where it may exceed 80%.

▶ Clinical Findings

A. Symptoms and Signs

The clinical manifestations of toxoplasmosis may be grouped into four syndromes.

1. Primary infection in the immunocompetent person—After ingestion, *T gondii* infection progresses from the gastrointestinal tract to lymphatics, and then dissemination. Most acute infections are asymptomatic. About 10–20% are symptomatic after an incubation period of 1–2 weeks. Acute infections in immunocompetent persons typically present as mild, febrile illnesses that resemble infectious mononucleosis. Nontender cervical or diffuse lymphadenopathy may persist for weeks to months. Systemic findings may include fever, malaise, headache, sore throat, rash, myalgias, hepatosplenomegaly, and atypical lymphocytosis. Rare severe manifestations are pneumonitis, meningoencephalitis, hepatitis, myocarditis, polymyositis, and retinochoroiditis. Symptoms may fluctuate, but most patients recover spontaneously within at most a few months.

2. Congenital infection—Congenital transmission occurs as a result of infection, which may be symptomatic or asymptomatic, in a nonimmune woman during pregnancy. Fetal infection follows maternal infection in 30–50% of cases, but this risk varies by trimester: 10–25% during the first, 30–50% during the second, and 60% or higher during the third trimester. In the United States, an estimated 400 to 4000 congenital infections occur yearly. While the risk of fetal infection increases, the risk of severe fetal disease decreases over the course of pregnancy. Early fetal infections commonly lead to spontaneous abortion, stillbirths, or severe neonatal disease, including neurologic manifestations. Neurologic findings can include seizures, psychomotor retardation, deafness, and hydrocephalus. Retinochoroiditis and other sight-threatening eye lesions may develop. Systemic findings include fever or hypothermia, jaundice, vomiting, diarrhea, hepatosplenomegaly, pneumonitis, myocarditis, and rash. Infections later in pregnancy less commonly lead to major fetal problems. Most infants appear normal at birth, but they may have subtle abnormalities and progress to symptoms and signs of congenital toxoplasmosis later in life. Hepatosplenomegaly and lymphadenopathy may develop in the first few months of life; CNS and eye disease often present later. The most common late presentation of congenital toxoplasmosis is retinochoroiditis.

3. Retinochoroiditis—This manifestation of congenital toxoplasmosis presents weeks to years after congenital infection, commonly in teenagers or young adults. Retinochoroiditis also is seen in persons who acquire infection early in life, and these patients more often present with unilateral disease. Uveitis is also seen. Disease presents with pain, photophobia, and visual changes, usually without systemic symptoms. Signs and symptoms eventually improve, but visual defects may persist. Rarely, progression may result in glaucoma and blindness.

4. Reactivated disease in the immunocompromised person—Reactivated toxoplasmosis occurs in patients with AIDS, cancer, or those given immunosuppressive drugs. In patients with advanced AIDS, the most common manifestation is encephalitis, with multiple necrotizing brain lesions. The encephalitis usually presents subacutely, with fever, headache, altered mental status, focal neurologic findings, and other evidence of brain lesions. Less common manifestations of toxoplasmosis in patients with AIDS are chorioretinitis and pneumonitis. Chorioretinitis presents with ocular pain and alterations in vision. Pneumonitis presents with fever, cough, and dyspnea. Toxoplasmosis can develop in seronegative recipients of solid organ or bone marrow transplants due to reactivation or transmission of infection. Reactivation also can occur in those with hematologic malignancies or treated with immunosuppressive drugs. Toxoplasmosis is similar to that in individuals with AIDS, but with immunodeficiency due to malignancy or immunosuppressive drugs, pneumonitis and myocarditis are more common. Less commonly, generalized toxoplasmosis in immunocompromised individuals can involve other organ systems.

B. Diagnostic Testing

1. Identification of parasites—Organisms can be seen in tissue or body fluids, although they may be difficult to identify; special staining techniques can facilitate identification. The demonstration of tachyzoites indicates acute infection; cysts may represent either acute or chronic infection. With lymphadenopathy due to toxoplasmosis, examination of lymph nodes usually does not show organisms. Parasite identification can also be made by inoculation of tissue culture or mice. PCR can be used for sensitive identification of organisms in amniotic fluid, blood, CSF, aqueous humor, and bronchoalveolar lavage fluid.

2. Serologic diagnosis—Multiple serologic methods are used, including the Sabin-Feldman dye test, enzyme-linked immunosorbent assay (ELISA), indirect fluorescent antibody test, and agglutination tests. IgG antibodies are seen within 1–2 weeks of infection, and usually persist for life. IgM antibodies peak earlier than IgG and decline more rapidly, although they may persist for years. In immunocompromised individuals in whom reactivation is suspected, a positive IgG assay indicates distant infection, and thus the potential for reactivated disease; a negative IgG argues strongly against reactivation toxoplasmosis. With reactivation in immunocompromised persons, IgM tests are generally negative.

3. During pregnancy and in newborns—Conversion from a negative to positive serologic test or rising titers are suggestive of acute infection, but tests are not routinely performed during pregnancy. When pregnant women are screened, negative IgG and IgM assays exclude active infection, but indicate the risk of infection during the pregnancy. The pattern of positive IgG with negative IgM is highly suggestive of chronic infection, with no risk of congenital disease unless the mother is severely immunocompromised. A positive IgM test is concerning for new infection because of the risk of congenital disease. Confirmatory testing should be performed before consideration of treatment or possible termination of pregnancy due to the limitations of available tests. Tests of the avidity of anti-IgG antibodies can be helpful, but a battery of tests is needed for confirmation of acute infection during pregnancy. When acute infection during pregnancy is suspected, PCR of amniotic fluid offers a sensitive assessment for congenital disease; this test should optimally be performed at 18 weeks of gestation. In newborns, positive IgM or IgA antibody tests are indicative of congenital infection, although the diagnosis is not ruled out by a negative test. Positive IgG assays may represent transfer of maternal antibodies without infection of the infant. Organisms may be identified by PCR; smears; or culture of blood, CSF, or tissue.

4. In immunocompetent individuals—Individuals with a suggestive clinical syndrome should be tested for IgG and IgM antibodies. Seroconversion, a 16-fold rise in antibody titer, or an IgM titer > 1:64 are suggestive of acute infection, although false-positive results may occur. Acute infection can also be diagnosed by detection of tachyzoites in tissue, culture of organisms, or PCR of blood or body fluids. Histologic evaluation of lymph nodes can show characteristic morphology, with or without organisms.

5. In immunodeficient individuals—A presentation consistent with toxoplasmic encephalitis warrants imaging of the brain. CT and MRI scans typically show multiple ring-enhancing cerebral lesions, most commonly involving the corticomedullary junction and basal ganglia. MRI is the more sensitive imaging modality. In AIDS patients with a positive IgG serologic test and no recent antitoxoplasma or antiviral therapy, the predictive value of a typical imaging study is about 80%. The other common diagnosis in this setting is CNS lymphoma, which more typically causes a single brain lesion. The differential diagnosis also includes tuberculoma, bacterial brain abscess, fungal abscess, and carcinoma. Diagnosis of CNS toxoplasmosis is most typically made after a therapeutic trial, with clinical and radiologic improvement expected within 2–3 weeks. Definitive diagnosis requires brain biopsy and search for organisms and typical histology. In retinochoroiditis, funduscopic examination shows vitreous inflammatory reaction, white retinal lesions, and pigmented scars. Diagnosis of other clinical entities in immunocompromised individuals is generally based on histology.

▶ Treatment

A. Approach to Treatment

Therapy is generally not necessary in immunocompetent persons, since primary illness is self-limited. However, for severe, persistent, or visceral disease, treatment for 2–4 weeks may be considered. Treatment is appropriate for primary infection during pregnancy because the risk of fetal transmission or the severity of congenital disease may be reduced. For retinochoroiditis, most episodes are self-limited, and opinions vary on indications for treatment. Treatment is often advocated for episodes with decreases in visual acuity, multiple or large lesions, macular lesions, significant inflammation, or persistence for over a month. Immunocompromised patients with active infection must be treated. For those with transient immunodeficiency, therapy can be continued for 4–6 weeks after cessation of symptoms. For those with persistent immunodeficiency, such as AIDS patients, full therapy for 4–6 weeks is followed by maintenance therapy with lower doses of drugs. Immunodeficient patients who are asymptomatic but have a positive IgG serologic test should receive long-term chemoprophylaxis.

B. Choice of Drugs

Drugs for toxoplasmosis are active only against tachyzoites, so they do not eradicate infection. Standard therapy is the combination of pyrimethamine (200 mg loading dose, then

50–75 mg (1 mg/kg) orally once daily) plus sulfadiazine (1–1.5 g orally four times daily), with folinic acid (10–20 mg orally once daily) to prevent bone marrow suppression. Patients should be screened for a history of sulfonamide sensitivity (skin rashes, gastrointestinal symptoms, hepatotoxicity). To prevent crystal-induced nephrotoxicity, good urinary output should be maintained; alkalinization with sodium bicarbonate may also be useful. Pyrimethamine side effects include headache and gastrointestinal symptoms. Even with folinic acid therapy, bone marrow suppression may occur; platelet and white blood cell counts should be monitored at least weekly. A first-line alternative to sulfadiazine is clindamycin (600 mg orally four times daily). Other possible alternatives are trimethoprim-sulfamethoxazole or combining pyrimethamine with atovaquone, clarithromycin, azithromycin, or dapsone. Pyrimethamine is not used during the first trimester of pregnancy due to its teratogenicity. Standard therapy for the treatment of acute toxoplasmosis during pregnancy is with spiramycin (1 g orally three times daily until delivery). This therapy is used only to decrease the risk of fetal infection; it reduces the frequency of transmission to the fetus by about 60%. Spiramycin does not cross the placenta, so when fetal infection is documented or for acute infections late in pregnancy (which commonly lead to fetal transmission) treatment with combination regimens as described above is indicated.

▶ Prevention

Prevention of primary infection centers on avoidance of undercooked meat or contact with material contaminated by cat feces, particularly for seronegative pregnant women and immunocompromised persons. For meat, irradiation, cooking to 66 °C kills tissue cysts. Thorough cleaning of hands and surfaces is needed after contact with raw meat or areas contaminated by cats. Oocysts passed in cat feces can remain infective for a year or more, but fresh oocysts are not infective for 48 hours. For best protection, litter boxes should be changed daily and soaked in boiling water for 5 minutes. In addition, gloves should be worn when gardening, fruits and vegetables should be thoroughly washed, and ingestion of dried meat should be avoided.

Universal screening of pregnant women for *T gondii* antibodies is conducted in some countries but not the United States. Pregnant women should ideally have their serum examined for IgG and IgM antibody, and those with negative titers should adhere to the prevention measures described above. Seronegative women who continue to have environmental exposure should undergo repeat serologic screening several times during pregnancy.

For immunocompromised individuals, chemoprophylaxis to prevent primary or reactivated infection is warranted. For transplant recipients, pyrimethamine (25 mg daily for 6 weeks) has been used. For advanced AIDS patients and others, chemoprophylaxis with trimethoprim-sulfamethoxazole (one double-strength tablet daily or two tablets three times weekly), used primarily for protection against *Pneumocystis*, is also effective against *T gondii*. Alternatives are pyrimethamine plus either sulfadoxine or dapsone (various regimens). In AIDS patients,

chemoprophylaxis can be discontinued if antiretroviral therapy leads to immune reconstitution.

Assi MA et al. Donor-transmitted toxoplasmosis in liver transplant recipients: a case report and literature review. Transpl Infect Dis. 2007 Jun;9(2):132–6. [PMID: 17461999]

Miro JM. Discontinuation of primary and secondary *Toxoplasma gondii* prophylaxis is safe in HIV-infected patients after immunological restoration with highly active antiretroviral therapy: results of an open, randomized, multicenter clinical trial. Clin Infect Dis. 2006 Jul 1;43(1):79–89. [PMID: 16758422]

Montoya JG et al. Management of *Toxoplasma gondii* infection during pregnancy. Clin Infect Dis. 2008 Aug 15;47(4):554–66. [PMID: 18624630]

Montoya JG et al. Toxoplasmosis. Lancet. 2004 Jun 12;363(9425):1965–76. [PMID: 15194258]

AMEBIASIS

 ESSENTIALS OF DIAGNOSIS

▶ Organisms or antigen present in stools or abscess aspirate.

▶ Positive serologic tests with colitis or hepatic abscess but may represent prior infections.

Mild to moderate colitis

▶ Recurrent diarrhea.

Severe colitis

▶ Severe bloody diarrhea with fever, abdominal pain, and tenderness.

▶ Prostration.

▶ Progression to hemorrhage or perforation.

Hepatic abscess

▶ Fever, abdominal pain.

▶ Hepatomegaly, hepatic abscess on imaging studies.

▶ General Considerations

The *Entamoeba* complex contains two morphologically identical species: *Entamoeba dispar*, which is avirulent, and *Entamoeba histolytica*, which may be an avirulent intestinal commensal or lead to serious disease. Disease follows penetration of the intestinal wall, resulting in diarrhea, and with severe involvement, dysentery or extraintestinal disease, most commonly liver abscess.

E histolytica infections are present worldwide but are most prevalent in subtropical and tropical areas under conditions of crowding, poor sanitation, and poor nutrition. Of the estimated 500 million persons worldwide infected with *Entamoeba*, most are infected with *E dispar* and an estimated 10% with *E histolytica*. Mortality from invasive *E histolytica* infections is estimated at 100,000 per year.

Humans are the only established *E histolytica* host. Transmission occurs through ingestion of cysts from fecally contaminated food or water, facilitated by person-to-person spread, flies and other arthropods as mechanical vectors, and use of human excrement as fertilizer. Urban outbreaks have occurred because of common-source water contamination.

▶ Clinical Findings

A. Symptoms and Signs

1. Intestinal amebiasis—In most infected persons, the organism lives as a commensal, and the carrier is without symptoms. With symptomatic disease, diarrhea may begin within a week of infection, although an incubation period of 2–4 weeks is more common, with gradual onset of abdominal pain and diarrhea. Fever is uncommon. Periods of remission and recurrence may last days to weeks or longer. Abdominal examination may show distention, tenderness, hyperperistalsis, and hepatomegaly. Microscopic hematochezia is common. More severe presentations include colitis and dysentery, with more extensive diarrhea (10–20 stools per day) and bloody stools. With dysentery, physical findings include high fevers, prostration, vomiting, abdominal pain and tenderness, hepatic enlargement, and hypotension. Severe presentations are more common in young children, pregnant women, those who are malnourished, and those receiving corticosteroids. Thus, in endemic regions, corticosteroids should not be started for presumed inflammatory bowel disease without first ruling out amebiasis. Fulminant amebic colitis can progress to necrotizing colitis, intestinal perforation, mucosal sloughing, and severe hemorrhage, with mortality rates over 40%. More chronic complications of intestinal amebiasis include chronic diarrhea with weight loss, which may last for months to years; bowel ulcerations; and amebic appendicitis. Localized granulomatous lesions (amebomas) can present after either dysentery or chronic intestinal infection. Clinical findings include pain, obstructive symptoms, and hemorrhage and may suggest intestinal carcinoma.

2. Extraintestinal amebiasis—The most common extraintestinal manifestation is amebic liver abscess. This can occur with colitis, but more frequently presents without history of prior intestinal symptoms. Patients present with the acute or gradual onset of abdominal pain, fever, an enlarged and tender liver, anorexia, and weight loss. Diarrhea is present in a small number of patients. Physical examination may show intercostal tenderness. Abscesses are most commonly single and in the right lobe of the liver, and they are much more common in men. Without prompt treatment, amebic abscesses may rupture into the pleural, peritoneal, or pericardial space, which is often fatal. Amebic infections may rarely occur throughout the body, including the lungs, brain, and genitourinary system.

B. Laboratory Findings

Laboratory studies with intestinal amebiasis show leukocytosis and hematochezia, with fecal leukocytes not present in all cases. With extraintestinal amebiasis, leukocytosis and elevated liver function studies are seen.

C. Diagnostic Testing

Diagnosis is by finding *E histolytica* or its antigen or by serologic tests. However, each method has limitations.

1. Intestinal amebiasis—Diagnosis is most commonly made by identifying organisms in the stool. *E histolytica* and *E dispar* cannot be distinguished, but the identification of amebic trophozoites or cysts in a symptomatic patient is highly suggestive of amebiasis. Stool evaluation for organisms is not highly sensitive (~30–50% for amebic colitis), and at least three stool specimens should be evaluated after concentration and staining. Multiple serologic assays are available; these tests are fairly sensitive, although sensitivity is lower (~70% in colitis) early in illness, and they cannot distinguish recent and old disease, as they remain positive for years after infection. A commercially available stool antigen test (TechLab II) offers improved sensitivity (> 90% for colitis); it requires fresh or frozen (not preserved) stool specimens. PCR-based tests are available but not used routinely. Colonoscopy of uncleansed bowel typically shows no specific findings in mild intestinal disease; in severe disease, ulcers may be found with intact intervening friable mucosa, resembling inflammatory bowel disease (Plate 117). Examination of fresh ulcer exudate for motile trophozoites and for *E histolytica* antigen may yield a diagnosis.

2. Hepatic abscess—Serologic tests for anti-amebic antibodies are almost always positive, except very early in the infection. Thus, a negative test in a suspicious case should be repeated in about a week. The stool *E histolytica* antigen test is positive in ~40% of cases. The TechLab II test can also be used to test serum, with good sensitivity if used before the initiation of therapy. Examination of stools for organisms or antigen is frequently negative. As imaging studies cannot distinguish amebic and pyogenic abscesses, when a diagnosis is not available from serologic studies, percutaneous aspiration may be indicated, ideally with an image-guided needle. Aspiration typically yields brown or yellow fluid. Detection of organisms in the aspirate is uncommon, but detection of *E histolytica* antigen is very sensitive and diagnostic. The key risk of aspiration is peritoneal spillage leading to peritonitis from amebas or other (pyogenic or echinococcal) organisms.

D. Imaging

Liver abscesses can be identified by ultrasonography, CT, or MRI, typically with round or oval low-density nonhomogeneous lesions, with abrupt transition from normal liver to the lesion, and hypoechoic centers. Abscesses are most commonly single, but more than one may be present. The right lobe is usually involved.

▶ Treatment

Treatment of amebiasis generally entails the use of metronidazole or tinidazole to eradicate tissue trophozoites and a luminal amebicide to eradicate intestinal cysts (Table 35–6). Asymptomatic infection with *E dispar* does not require therapy. This organism cannot be differentiated morphologically from *E histolytica*, but with negative serology *E dispar* colonization is likely, and treatment is not indicated. Colonization with *E histolytica* is generally treated with a luminal agent. Effective luminal agents are diloxanide furoate (500 mg orally three times daily with meals for 10 days), iodoquinol (diiodohydroxyquin; 650 mg orally three times daily for 21

Table 35–6. Treatment of amebiasis.[1]

Clinical Setting	Drugs of Choice and Adult Dosage	Alternative Drugs and Adult Dosage
Asymptomatic intestinal infection	Luminal agent: Diloxanide furoate,[2] 500 mg orally three times daily for 10 days –or– Iodoquinol, 650 mg orally three times daily for 21 days –or– Paromomycin, 10 mg/kg orally three times daily for 7 days	
Mild to moderate intestinal infection	Metronidazole, 750 mg orally three times daily (or 500 mg IV every 6 hours) for 10 days –or– Tinidazole, 2 g orally daily for 3 days –plus– Luminal agent (see above)	Luminal agent (see above) –plus either– Tetracycline, 250 mg orally three times daily for 10 days –or– Erythromycin, 500 mg orally four times daily for 10 days
Severe intestinal infection	Metronidazole, 750 mg orally three times daily (or 500 mg IV every 6 hours) for 10 days –or– Tinidazole, 2 g orally daily for 3 days –plus– Luminal agent (see above)	Luminal agent (see above) –plus either– Tetracycline, 250 mg orally three times daily for 10 days –or– Dehydroemetine[3] or emetine,[2] 1 mg/kg SC or IM for 3–5 days
Hepatic abscess, ameboma, and other extraintestinal disease	Metronidazole, 750 mg orally three times daily (or 500 mg IV every 6 hours) for 10 days –or– Tinidazole, 2 g orally daily for 3 days –plus– Luminal agent (see above)	Dehydroemetine[3] or emetine,[2] 1 mg/kg SC or IM for 8–10 days, followed by (liver abscess only) chloroquine, 500 mg orally twice daily for 2 days, then 500 mg daily for 21 days –plus– Luminal agent (see above)

[1]See text for additional details and cautions.
[2]Not available in the United States.
[3]Available in the United States only from the CDC Drug Service, Centers for Disease Control and Prevention, Atlanta (404-639-3670).

days), and paromomycin (30 mg/kg base orally, maximum 3 g, in three divided doses after meals daily for 7 days). Side effects associated with luminal agents are flatulence with diloxanide furoate, mild diarrhea with iodoquinol, and gastrointestinal symptoms with paromomycin. Relative contraindications are thyroid disease for iodoquinol and kidney disease for iodoquinol or paromomycin.

Treatment of intestinal amebiasis requires metronidazole (750 mg orally three times daily for 10 days) or tinidazole (2 g orally once daily for 3 days for mild disease and 5 days for serious disease) plus a luminal agent (Table 35–6). Metronidazole has most commonly been used in the United States, but tinidazole, which is now available, offers simpler dosing and less side effects. Metronidazole often induces transient nausea, vomiting, epigastric discomfort, headache, or a metallic taste. A disulfram-like reaction may occur if alcohol is coingested. Metronidazole should be avoided in pregnant or nursing mothers if possible. The same toxicities and concerns probably apply for tinidazole, although it appears to be better tolerated. Fluid and electrolyte replacement is also important for patients with significant diarrhea. Surgical management of acute complications of intestinal amebiasis is

best avoided whenever possible. Successful therapy of severe amebic colitis may be followed by postdysenteric colitis, with continued diarrhea without persistent infection; this syndrome generally resolves in weeks to months.

Alternatives for the treatment of intestinal amebiasis are tetracycline (250–500 mg orally four times daily for 10 days) plus chloroquine (500 mg orally daily for 7 days). Emetine or dehydroemetine can be given subcutaneously (preferred) or intravenously in a dose of 1–1.5 mg/kg/d; the maximum daily dose is 90 mg for dehydroemetine and 65 mg for emetine. These agents are effective but cardiotoxic with a narrow therapeutic range and should be used only until severe disease is controlled. They cause nausea, vomiting, and pain at the injection site. Emetine is not available in the United States and dehydroemetine is only available from the Centers for Disease Control and Prevention Drug Service.

Amebic liver abscess is also treated with metronidazole or tinidazole plus a luminal agent (even if intestinal infection is not documented; Table 35–6). Metronidazole can be used intravenously when necessary. With failure of initial response to metronidazole or tinidazole, chloroquine, emetine or dehydroemetine may be added. Needle aspiration may be helpful for large abscesses (over 5–10 cm), in particular if the diagnosis remains uncertain, if there is an initial lack of response, or if a patient is very ill, suggesting imminent abscess rupture. With successful therapy, abscesses disappear slowly (over months).

▶ Prevention & Control

Prevention requires safe water supplies; sanitary disposal of human feces; adequate cooking of foods; protection of foods from fly contamination; handwashing; and, in endemic areas, avoidance of foods that cannot be cooked or peeled. Water supplies can be boiled, treated with iodine (0.5 mL tincture of iodine per liter for 20 minutes; cysts are resistant to standard concentrations of chlorine), or filtered.

Bercu TE et al. Amebic colitis: new insights into pathogenesis and treatment. Curr Gastroenterol Rep. 2007 Oct;9(5):429–33. [PMID: 17991346]

Fotedar R et al. Laboratory diagnostic techniques for *Entamoeba* species. Clin Microbiol Rev. 2007 Jul;20(3):511–32. [PMID: 17630338]

Haque R et al. Amebiasis. N Engl J Med. 2003 Apr 17;348(16):1565–73. [PMID: 12700377]

Pritt BS et al. Amebiasis. Mayo Clin Proc. 2008 Oct;83(10):1154–9. [PMID: 18828976]

Stanley SL Jr. Amoebiasis. Lancet. 2003 Mar 22;361(9362):1025–34. [PMID: 12660071]

INFECTIONS WITH PATHOGENIC FREE-LIVING AMEBAS

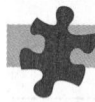 ESSENTIALS OF DIAGNOSIS

- ▶ Acute meningoencephalitis or chronic granulomatous encephalitis after contact with warm fresh water.
- ▶ Keratitis, particularly in contact lens users.

The free-living amebas that cause disease in humans are of the genera *Acanthamoeba*, *Naegleria*, and *Balamuthia*. The organisms are widely distributed in soil and fresh and brackish water. *Acanthamoeba* and *Naegleria* species have been found to harbor *Legionella*, *Vibrio cholerae*, and other endosymbiotic bacteria and may serve as a reservoir for these organisms.

1. Primary Amebic Meningoencephalitis

Primary amebic meningoencephalitis is a fulminating, hemorrhagic, necrotizing meningoencephalitis that occurs in healthy children and young adults and is rapidly fatal. It is caused by free-living amebas, most commonly *Naegleria fowleri*, but also *Balamuthia mandrillaris* and *Acanthamoeba* species. *N fowleri* is a thermophilic organism found in fresh and polluted warm lake water, domestic water supplies, swimming pools, thermal water, and sewers. Most patients give a history of exposure to warm fresh water. The incubation period varies from 2 to 15 days. Early symptoms include headache, fever, stiff neck, and lethargy, often associated with rhinitis and pharyngitis. Vomiting, disorientation, and other signs of meningoencephalitis develop within 1 or 2

days, followed by coma and then death within 7–10 days. No distinctive clinical features distinguish the infection from acute bacterial meningoencephalitis. CSF shows hundred to thousands of leukocytes and erythrocytes per cubic millimeter. Protein is usually elevated, and glucose is normal or moderately reduced. A fresh wet mount of the CSF may show motile trophozoites. Staining with Giemsa or Wright stain will identify the trophozoites. Species identification is based on morphology and immunologic methods. Primary amebic meningoencephalitis is nearly always fatal. Amphotericin B appears to be the drug of choice; one survivor was treated with intravenous and intrathecal amphotericin B, intravenous miconazole, and oral rifampin.

2. Granulomatous Amebic Encephalitis

Acanthamoeba species and *B mandrillaris* can cause an encephalitis that is more chronic in nature than primary amebic meningoencephalitis. Neurologic disease may be preceded by skin lesions, including ulcers and nodules. After an uncertain incubation period neurologic symptoms develop slowly, with headache, meningismus, nausea, vomiting, lethargy, and low-grade fevers progressing over weeks to months to focal neurologic findings, mental status abnormalities, and eventually coma and death. CT and MRI show single or multiple nonspecific lesions. Lumbar puncture is dangerous due to increased intracranial pressure. CSF shows a lymphocytic pleocytosis with elevated protein; amebas are not typically seen. Diagnosis can be made by biopsy of skin or brain lesions. Information on the treatment of granulomatous amebic encephalitis is limited. Some patients have been successfully treated with various combinations of flucytosine, pentamidine, fluconazole or itraconazole, sulfadiazine, trimethoprim-sulfamethoxazole, and azithromycin.

3. Acanthamoeba Keratitis

Acanthamoeba keratitis is a painful, sight-threatening corneal infection. It is associated with corneal trauma, most commonly after use of contact lenses and contaminated saline solution. Symptoms include severe eye pain, photophobia, tearing, and blurred vision. The keratitis progresses slowly, with waxing and waning clinical findings over months, and can progress to blindness. Lack of response to antibacterial, antifungal, and antiviral topical treatments and potential use of contaminated contact lens solution are suggestive of the diagnosis. Ocular examination shows corneal ring infiltrates, but these can also be caused by other pathogens. The diagnosis can be made by examination or culture of corneal scrapings. Available diagnostic techniques include examination of a wet preparation for cysts and motile trophozoites, examination of stained specimens, evaluation with immunofluorescent reagents, culture of organisms, and PCR.

Acanthamoeba keratitis can be cured with local therapy. Topical propamidine isethionate (0.1%), chlorhexidine digluconate (0.02%), polyhexamethylene biguanide, neomycin-polymyxin B-gramicidin, miconazole, and combinations of these agents have been used successfully. Oral itraconazole or ketoconazole can be added for deep keratitis. Drug resistance has been reported. Use of corticosteroid therapy is controversial. In some cases, debridement and penetrating keratoplasty have been performed in addition to medical therapy. Corneal grafting can be done after the amebic infection has been eradicated.

Grate I. Primary amebic meningoencephalitis: a silent killer. CJEM. 2006 Sep;8(5):365–9. [PMID: 17338852]

Hammersmith KM. Diagnosis and management of *Acanthamoeba* keratitis. Curr Opin Ophthalmol. 2006 Aug;17(4):327–31. [PMID: 16900022]

Matin A et al. Increasing importance of *Balamuthia mandrillaris*. Clin Microbiol Rev. 2008 Jul;21(3):435–48. [PMID: 18625680]

Patel A et al. Contact lens-related microbial keratitis: recent outbreaks. Curr Opin Ophthalmol. 2008 Jul;19(4):302–6. [PMID: 18545011]

Visvesvara GS et al. Pathogenic and opportunistic free-living amoebae: *Acanthamoeba* spp., *Balamuthia mandrillaris*, *Naegleria fowleri*, and *Sappinia diploidea*. FEMS Immunol Med Microbiol. 2007 Jun;50(1):1–26. [PMID: 17428307]

COCCIDIOSIS (Cryptosporidiosis, Isosporiasis, Cyclosporiasis, Sarcocystosis) & MICROSPORIDIOSIS

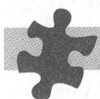 ESSENTIALS OF DIAGNOSIS

- ▶ Acute diarrhea, especially in children in developing countries.
- ▶ Outbreaks of diarrhea secondary to contaminated water or food.
- ▶ Prolonged diarrhea in immunocompromised persons.
- ▶ Diagnosis mostly by identifying organisms in specially stained stool specimens.

General Considerations

The causes of coccidiosis are *Cryptosporidium* species (*C parvum*, *C hominis*, and others); *Isospora belli*; *Cyclospora cayetanensis*; and *Sarcocystis* species. Microsporidiosis is caused by at least 14 species, most commonly *Enterocytozoon bieneusi* and *Encephalitozoon intestinalis*. These infections occur worldwide, particularly in the tropics and in regions where hygiene is poor. They are causes of endemic childhood gastroenteritis (particularly in malnourished children in developing countries); institutional and community outbreaks of diarrhea; traveler's diarrhea; and acute and chronic diarrhea in immunosuppressed patients, in particular those with AIDS. They are all notable for the potential to cause prolonged diarrhea, often lasting for a number of weeks. Clustering occurs in households, day care centers, and among sexual partners.

The infectious agents are oocysts (coccidiosis) or spores (microsporidiosis) transmitted from person to person or by contaminated drinking or swimming water or food. Ingested oocysts release sporozoites that invade and multiply in enterocytes, primarily in the small bowel. Coccidian oocysts and microsporidian cysts can remain viable in the environment for years.

I belli and *C cayetanensis* appear to infect only humans. *C cayetanensis* has caused a number of food-borne outbreaks in the United States in recent years, most commonly associated with imported fresh produce. *Sarcocystis* infects many species; humans are intermediate hosts (infected by ingestion of fecal sporocysts) for some species but definitive hosts for *Sarcocystis bovihominis* and *Sarcocystis suihominis* (infected by ingestion of tissue cysts in undercooked beef and pork, respectively).

Cryptosporidiosis is a zoonosis (*C parvum* principally infects cattle), but most human infections are acquired from humans, in particular with *C hominis*. Cryptosporidia are highly infectious and readily transmitted in day care settings and households. They have caused large community outbreaks due to contaminated water supplies (causing ~400,000 illnesses in Milwaukee in 1993) and are the leading cause of recreational water–associated outbreaks of gastroenteritis. Of note, coccidia and microsporidians will generally be missed on routine evaluations of stool for ova and parasites, as they require special staining techniques for identification.

▶ Clinical Findings

A. Symptoms and Signs

1. Cryptosporidiosis—The incubation period appears to be about 1–14 days. In developing countries, disease is seen primarily in children under 5 years of age, where cryptosporidiosis causes 5–10% of cases of childhood diarrhea. Presenting symptoms in children include acute watery diarrhea, abdominal pain, and cramps, with rapid resolution in most patients; however, symptoms quite commonly persist for 2 weeks or more. In developed countries, most patients are adults. Diarrhea in immunocompetent individuals typically lasts from 5 to 10 days. It is usually watery, with accompanying abdominal pain and cramps, nausea, vomiting, and fever. Relapses may follow initial resolution of symptoms. Mild illness and asymptomatic infection may also be common.

Cryptosporidiosis is a well-characterized cause of diarrhea in those with AIDS. It was common in this population before the advent of highly active antiretroviral therapy, particularly in those with advanced immunosuppression. Clinical manifestations are variable, but patients commonly have chronic diarrhea with frequent foul smelling stools, malabsorption, and weight loss. Severe, life-threatening watery diarrhea may be seen. Cryptosporidiosis also causes extraintestinal disease with AIDS, including pulmonary infiltrates with dyspnea and biliary tract infection with sclerosing cholangitis and AIDS cholangiopathy.

2. Isosporiasis—The incubation period for *I belli* is about 1 week. In immunocompetent persons, it usually causes a self-limited watery diarrhea lasting 2–3 weeks, with abdominal cramps, anorexia, malaise, and weight loss. Fever is unusual. Chronic symptoms may persist for months in some patients. In immunocompromised patients, isosporiasis more commonly causes severe and chronic diarrhea, with complications including marked dehydration, malnutrition, and hemorrhagic colitis. Extraintestinal disease has been reported rarely.

3. Cyclosporiasis—*C cayetanensis* oocysts must undergo a period of sporulation of 7 days or more after shedding before they become infectious. Therefore, person-to-person spread is unlikely, and spread has typically been due to contaminated food (especially fresh produce) and water. The incubation period is 1–11 days. Infections can be asymptomatic. Cyclosporiasis causes an illness similar to that described for the other pathogens described in this section, with watery diarrhea, abdominal cramps, nausea, fatigue, and anorexia. Fever is seen in 25% of cases. Symptoms typically continue for 2 weeks or longer and may persist for months. Relapses of diarrhea are common. Diarrhea may be preceded by a flu-like prodrome and followed by persistent fatigue. In immunocompromised patients, cyclosporiasis is typically more severe and prolonged, with chronic fulminant watery diarrhea and weight loss.

4. Sarcocystosis—*Sarcocystis* infection may be common in some developing countries, but it is usually asymptomatic. Infection appears to most commonly follow the ingestion of undercooked beef or pork, leading to the development of cysts in muscle, with myalgias, fever, bronchospasm, pruritic rash, lymphadenopathy, and subcutaneous nodules. Ingestion of fecal sporocysts may lead to gastrointestinal symptoms.

5. Microsporidiosis—Microsporidia are obligate intracellular protozoans that cause a wide spectrum of diseases. Many infections are of zoonotic origin, but human-to-human transmission has been documented. Infection is mainly by ingestion of spores, but also by direct inoculation of the eyes. In immunocompetent hosts, microsporidian infections most commonly present as self-limited diarrhea. Ocular infections have also been described. Disease from microsporidia is seen mainly in immunocompromised persons, particularly those with AIDS. Infections in AIDS patients are most commonly with *E bieneusi* and *E intestinalis*. They cause chronic diarrhea, with anorexia, bloating, weight loss, and wasting, especially in those with advanced immunodeficiency. Fever is usually not seen. Other illnesses in immunocompromised persons associated with microsporidians (including the genera *Enterocytozoon, Encephalitozoon, Brachiola, Vittaforma, Pleistophora, Trachipleistophora,* and *Microsporidium*) include biliary tract disease (AIDS cholangiopathy), genitourinary infection with cystitis, kidney disease, hepatitis, peritonitis, myositis, respiratory infections including sinusitis, central nervous system infections including granulomatous encephalitis, and disseminated infections. Ocular infections with *Encephalitozoon* species cause conjunctivitis and keratitis, presenting as redness, photophobia, and loss of visual acuity.

B. Laboratory Findings

1. Cryptosporidiosis—Typically, stool is without blood or leukocytes. Diagnosis is traditionally made by detecting the organism in stool using a modified acid-fast stain; this technique is relatively insensitive, and multiple specimens should be evaluated before ruling out the diagnosis. Of note, routine evaluation for ova and parasites typically does not include a modified acid-fast stain, so this must be

specifically requested in many laboratories. Antigen detection offers improved sensitivity and specificity, both of which are well over 90% with a number of available assays, and these methods may now be considered the optimal means of diagnosis.

2. Isosporiasis—Diagnosis of isosporiasis is by examination of stool wet mounts or after modified acid-fast staining, in which the organism is clearly distinguishable from other parasites. Other stains also show the organism. Shedding of oocysts may be intermittent, so the sensitivity of stool evaluation is not high, and multiple samples should be examined. The organism may also be identified in duodenal aspirates or small bowel biopsies.

3. Cyclosporiasis—Diagnosis is made by examination of stool wet mounts or after modified acid-fast staining. Multiple specimens may need to be examined to make a diagnosis. The organism can also be identified in small bowel aspirates or biopsy specimens.

4. Sarcocystosis—Eosinophilia and elevated creatine kinase may be seen. Diagnosis is by identification of the acid-fast organisms in stool or by identification of trophozoites or bradyzoites in tissue biopsies.

5. Microsporidiosis—Diagnosis can be made by identification of organisms in specially stained stool, fluid, or tissue specimens, for example with Weber chromotrope-based stain. Electron microscopy is helpful for confirmation of the diagnosis and speciation. PCR and culture techniques are available but not used routinely.

▶ Treatment

Most acute infections with these pathogens in immunocompetent persons are self-limited and do not require treatment. Supportive treatment for severe or chronic diarrhea includes fluid and electrolyte replacement and, in some cases, parenteral nutrition.

1. Cryptosporidiosis—Treatment of cryptosporidiosis is challenging. No agent is clearly effective. Modest benefits have been seen in some (but not other) studies with paromomycin, a non-absorbed aminoglycoside (25–35 mg/kg orally for 14 days has been used), and nitazoxanide (500 mg–1 g orally twice daily for 3 days in nonimmunocompromised and 2–8 weeks in advanced AIDS patients), which is approved in the United States for this indication. It can cause mild gastrointestinal toxicity. Other agents that have been used with mixed success in AIDS patients with cryptosporidiosis include azithromycin, spiramycin, bovine hyperimmune colostrum, and octreotide. Reversing immunodeficiency with effective antiretroviral therapy is of greatest importance.

2. Isosporiasis—Isosporiasis is effectively treated in immunocompetent and immunosuppressed persons with trimethoprim-sulfamethoxazole (160 mg/800 mg orally 2–4 times daily for 10 days, with higher doses for patients with AIDS). An alternative therapy is pyrimethamine (75 mg orally in four divided doses) with folinic acid (10–25 mg/d orally). Maintenance therapy with low-dose trimethoprim-sulfamethoxazole (daily or three times per week) or Fansidar (weekly) prevents relapse in those with persistent immunosuppression.

3. Cyclosporiasis—Cyclosporiasis is also treated with tri-methoprim-sulfamethoxazole (dosing as for isosporiasis). With AIDS, long-term maintenance therapy (three times weekly) helps prevent relapse. For patients intolerant of trimethoprim-sulfamethoxazole, ciprofloxacin (500 mg orally twice daily for 7 days) showed efficacy, albeit with less ability to clear the organism than trimethoprim-sulfamethoxazole.

4. Sarcocystosis—For sarcocystosis, no specific treatment is established, but sulfadiazine cleared intestinal cysts in one study.

5. Microsporidiosis—Treatment of microsporidiosis is complex. Infections with most species, including those causing gastrointestinal and other manifestations, should be treated with albendazole (400 mg orally twice daily for 2–4 weeks), which has activity against a number of species, but relatively poor efficacy (about 50%) against *E bieneusi*, the most common microsporidial cause of diarrhea in AIDS patients. Fumagillin, which is used to treat honey-bees and fish with microsporidian infections, has shown benefit in clinical trials at a dose of 20 mg three times per day for 14 days; treatment was accompanied by reversible thrombocytopenia. As with cryptosporidiosis, the best means of controlling microsporidiosis in AIDS patients is to restore immune function with effective antiretroviral therapy. Ocular microsporidiosis can be treated with fum-agillin solution (3 mg/mL); this probably should be given with concurrent systemic therapy with albendazole. Adjunctive management may include corticosteroids to decrease inflammation and keratoplasty.

▶ Prevention

Water purification is important for control of these infections. Chlorine disinfection is not effective against cryptosporidial oocysts, so other purification measures are needed. Immunocompromised patients should boil or filter drinking water and should consider avoidance of lakes and swimming pools. Routine precautions (hand-washing, gloves, disinfection) should prevent institutional patient-to-patient spread. Optimal means of preventing microsporidial infections are not well understood, but water purification as discussed above and body substance precautions for immunocompromised and hospitalized individuals are likely effective.

Abubakar I et al. Prevention and treatment of cryptosporidiosis in immunocompromised patients. Cochrane Database Syst Rev. 2007 Jan 24;(1):CD004932. [PMID: 17253532]

Bobak DA. Use of nitazoxanide for gastrointestinal tract infections: treatment of protozoan parasitic infection and beyond. Curr Infect Dis Rep. 2006 Mar;8(2):91–5. [PMID: 16524544]

Didier ES et al. Microsporidiosis: current status. Curr Opin Infect Dis. 2006 Oct;19(5):485–92. [PMID: 16940873]

Lewthwaite P et al. Gastrointestinal parasites in the immuno-compromised. Curr Opin Infect Dis. 2005 Oct;18(5):427–35. [PMID: 16148530]

Wiwanitkit V. Intestinal parasite infestation in HIV infected patients. Curr HIV Res. 2006 Jan;4(1):87–96. [PMID: 16454714]

GIARDIASIS

 ESSENTIALS OF DIAGNOSIS

▶ Acute diarrhea, which may be profuse and watery.
▶ Chronic diarrhea with greasy, malodorous stools.
▶ Abdominal cramps, distention, flatulence, and malaise.
▶ Cysts or trophozoites in stools.

▶ General Considerations

Giardiasis is a protozoal infection of the upper small intestine caused by the flagellate *Giardia lamblia* (also called *Giardia intestinalis* and *Giardia duodenalis*). The parasite occurs worldwide, most abundantly in areas with poor sanitation. In developing countries, young children are very commonly infected. In the United States and Europe, the infection is the most common intestinal pro-tozoal pathogen; the US estimate is of 100,000 to 2.5 million new infections leading to 5000 hospital admissions yearly. Groups at special risk include travelers to *Giardia*-endemic areas, those who swallow contaminated water during recreation or wilderness travel, men who have sex with men, and persons with impaired immunity. Out-breaks are common in households, children's day care centers, and residential facilities, and may occur as a result of contamination of water supplies.

The organism occurs in feces as a flagellated trophozo-ite and as a cyst. Only the cyst form is infectious by the oral route; trophozoites are destroyed by gastric acidity. Humans are a reservoir for the pathogen; dogs, cats, beavers, and other mammals have been implicated but not confirmed as reservoirs. Under suitable moist, cool condi-tions, cysts can survive in the environment for weeks to months. Cysts are transmitted as a result of fecal contam-ination of water or food, by person-to-person contact, or by anal-oral sexual contact. The infectious dose is low, requiring as few as ten cysts. After the cysts are ingested, trophozoites emerge in the duodenum and jejunum. Epi-thelial damage and mucosal invasion are uncommon. Hypogammaglobulinemia, low secretory IgA levels in the gut, achlorhydria, and malnutrition favor the develop-ment of infection.

▶ Clinical Findings
A. Symptoms and Signs

It is estimated that about 50% of infected persons have no discernable infection, about 10% become asymptomatic cyst passers, and 25–50% develop an acute diarrheal syn-drome. Acute diarrhea may clear spontaneously but is commonly followed by chronic diarrhea. The incubation period is usually 1–3 weeks but may be longer. The illness may begin gradually or suddenly. Cysts may not be detected in the stool at the onset of the illness. The acute phase may last days or weeks, and is usually self-limited, although cyst excretion may be prolonged. The initial illness may include profuse watery diarrhea, and hospitalization may be required due to dehydration, particularly in young children. Typical symptoms of chronic disease are abdominal cramps, bloating, flatulence, nausea, malaise, and anorexia. Fever and vomiting are uncommon. Diarrhea is usually not severe in the chronic stage of infection; stools are greasy or frothy and foul smelling, without blood, pus, or mucus. The diarrhea may be daily or recurrent; intervening periods may include constipation. Symptoms can persist for weeks to months. Weight loss is frequent. Chronic disease can include malabsorption, including fat- and protein-losing enteropathy and vitamin deficiencies.

B. Laboratory Findings

Most patients seek medical attention after having been ill for over a week, commonly with weight loss of 5 kg or more. Stool is generally without blood or leukocytes. Diagnosis is traditionally made by the identification of trophozoites or cysts in stool. A wet mount of liquid stool may identify motile trophozoites. Stained fixed specimens may show cysts or trophozoites. Sensitivity of stool analysis is not ideal, estimated at 50–80% for a single specimen and over 90% for three specimens. Sampling of duodenal contents with a string test or biopsy is no longer generally recommended, but biopsies may be helpful in very ill or immunocompromised patients. When giardiasis is highly suspected, antigen assays may be simpler and cheaper than repeated stool examinations, but these tests will not identify other stool pathogens. Multiple tests, which identify antigens of trophozoites or cysts, are available. They are generally quite sensitive (85–98%) and specific (90–100%).

▶ Treatment

The treatments of choice for giardiasis are metronidazole (250 mg orally three times daily for 5–7 days) or tinidazole (2 g orally once). The drugs are not universally effective; cure rates for single courses are typically about 80–95%. Toxicities are as described for treatment of amebiasis, but the lower dosages used for giardiasis limit side effects. Nitazoxanide (500 mg orally twice daily for 3 days) is generally well tolerated but may cause mild gastrointestinal side effects. Other drugs with activity against *Giardia* include furazolidone (100 mg orally four times a day for 7 days), which is about as effective as the other named drugs but causes gastrointestinal side effects; albendazole (400 mg orally daily for 5 days), which appears to have similar efficacy but has been less studied; and paromomycin (500 mg orally three times a day for 7 days), which appears to have somewhat lower efficacy but may be the safest drug (considering potential mutagenicity of metronidazole, tinidazole, and furazolidone) in pregnant women. Symptomatic giardiasis should always be treated. Treatment of asymptomatic patients should be considered, since they can transmit the infection to others. With a presumptive diagnosis but negative diagnostic studies, an empiric

course of treatment is sometimes appropriate. Household or day care contacts with an index case should be tested and treated if infected.

▶ Prevention

Community chlorination (0.4 mg/L) of water is relatively ineffective for inactivating cysts, so filtration is required. For wilderness or international travelers, bringing water to a boil for 1 minute or filtration with a pore size less than 1 mcm are adequate. In day care centers, appropriate disposal of diapers and frequent hand washing are essential.

Huang DB et al. An updated review on *Cryptosporidium* and *Giardia*. Gastroenterol Clin North Am. 2006 Jun;35(2):291–314. [PMID: 16880067]

OTHER INTESTINAL FLAGELLATE INFECTIONS

Balantidium coli is a large ciliated intestinal protozoan found worldwide, but particularly in the tropics. Pigs are the main reservoir. The infection is rare in humans, and results from ingestion of cysts passed in stools of humans or swine. In the new host, the cyst wall dissolves and the trophozoite may invade intestinal mucosa, causing abscesses and ulcerations. Many infections are asymptomatic. Chronic infections may cause recurrent diarrhea or dysentery. Deaths have occurred from intestinal perforation and hemorrhage.

Dientamoeba fragilis is a protozoan that commonly causes infection without symptoms, so its role in human disease remains somewhat controversial. Symptoms attributed to the pathogen include diarrhea, abdominal pain, and anorexia. Other flagellates may infect humans, are generally considered nonpathogens, but may be markers for fecal-oral contamination.

Diagnosis of balantidiasis is established by finding trophozoites or cysts in stool, or in ulcer scrapings of the large bowel. *D fragilis* infection can be hard to diagnose because it only exists in the trophozoite form; the sensitivity of evaluation of three stools is 70–90%. The treatment of choice for balantidiasis is tetracycline, 500 mg orally four times daily for 10 days. The alternative is iodoquinol (diiodohydroxyquin), 650 mg orally three times daily for 21 days, and metronidazole, paromomycin, and nitazoxanide have also been used successfully. *D fragilis* infections have been successfully treated with metronidazole, iodoquinol, and tetracycline; all the regimens are the same as for balantidiasis.

Schuster FL et al. Current world status of *Balantidium coli*. Clin Microbiol Rev. 2008 Oct;21(4):626–38. [PMID: 18854484]
Stark DJ et al. Dientamoebiasis: clinical importance and recent advances. Trends Parasitol. 2006 Feb;22(2):92–6. [PMID: 16380293]

TRICHOMONIASIS

ESSENTIALS OF DIAGNOSIS

▶ Copious vaginal discharge in women.

► Nongonococcal urethritis in men.

► Motile trichomonads on wet mounts.

General Considerations

Trichomoniasis is caused by the protozoan *Trichomonas vaginalis* and is among the most common sexually transmitted diseases, causing vaginitis in women and nongonococcal urethritis in men. It can also occasionally be acquired by other means, since it can survive in moist environments for several hours.

Clinical Findings

A. Symptoms and Signs

T vaginalis is often harbored asymptomatically. For women with symptomatic disease, after an incubation period of 5 days to 4 weeks, a vaginal discharge develops, often with vulvovaginal discomfort, pruritus, dysuria, dyspareunia, or abdominal pain. Examination shows a copious discharge, which is usually not foul smelling but is often frothy and yellow or green in color. Inflammation of the vaginal walls and cervix with punctate hemorrhages are common. Most men infected with *T vaginalis* are asymptomatic, but it can be isolated from about 10% of men with nongonococcal urethritis. In men with trichomonal urethritis, the urethral discharge is generally more scanty than with other causes of urethritis.

B. Diagnostic Testing

Diagnosis is typically made by identifying the organism in vaginal or urethral secretions. Examination of wet mounts will show motile organisms. Tests for bacterial vaginosis (pH > 4.5, fishy odor after addition of potassium hydroxide) are often positive with trichomoniasis. Rapid antigen and nucleic acid amplification tests that are highly specific and much more sensitive than wet mounts are available but are not yet widely used.

Treatment

The treatment of choice is metronidazole (2 g single oral dose). Tinidazole is also approved for this indication at the same dose, and it may be better tolerated and active against some resistant parasites. Toxicities of these drugs are discussed in the section on amebiasis. If the large single dose cannot be tolerated, an alternative metronidazole dosage is 500 mg orally twice daily for 1 week. All infected persons should be treated, even if asymptomatic, to prevent subsequent symptomatic disease and limit spread. Treatment failure suggests reinfection, but metronidazole-resistant organisms have been reported. These may be treated with tinidazole, longer courses of metronidazole, or some experimental therapies.

Nanda N et al. Trichomoniasis and its treatment. Expert Rev Anti Infect Ther. 2006 Feb;4(1):125–35. [PMID: 16441214]

Wendel KA et al. Trichomoniasis: challenges to appropriate management. Clin Infect Dis. 2007 Apr 1;44 Suppl 3:S123–9. [PMID: 17342665]

HELMINTHIC INFECTIONS

TREMATODE (FLUKE) INFECTIONS

SCHISTOSOMIASIS (Bilharziasis)

 ESSENTIALS OF DIAGNOSIS

► History of fresh water exposure in an endemic area.

► Acute schistosomiasis: fever, headache, myalgias, cough, malaise, urticaria, diarrhea, and eosinophilia.

► Intestinal schistosomiasis: abdominal pain, fatigue, diarrhea, and hepatomegaly, progressing to anorexia, weight loss, and features of portal hypertension.

► Urinary schistosomiasis: hematuria and dysuria, progressing to hydroureter, hydronephrosis, urinary infections, and kidney injury.

► Diagnosis based on characteristic eggs in feces or urine; biopsy of rectal or bladder mucosa; positive serology.

General Considerations

Schistosomiasis, which affects more than 200 million persons worldwide, leads to severe consequences in 20 million persons and about 100,000 deaths annually. The disease is caused by five species of trematode blood flukes. Four species cause intestinal schistosomiasis, with infection of mesenteric venules: *Schistosoma mansoni*, which is present in Africa, the Arabian peninsula, South America, and the Caribbean; *Schistosoma japonicum*, which is endemic in China and Southeast Asia; *Schistosoma mekongi*, which is endemic near the Mekong River in Southeast Asia; and *Schistosoma intercalatum*, which occurs in parts of Africa. *Schistosoma haematobium* causes urinary schistosomiasis, with infection of venules of the urinary tract, and is endemic in Africa and the Middle East. Transmission of schistosomiasis is focal, with greatest prevalence in poor rural areas. Control efforts have diminished transmission significantly in many areas, but high level transmission remains common in sub-Saharan Africa and some other areas. Prevalence of infection and illness typically peaks at about 15–20 years of age.

Humans are infected with schistosomes after contact with fresh water containing cercariae released by infected snails. Infection is initiated by penetration of skin or mucous membranes. After penetration, schistosomulae migrate to the portal circulation, where they rapidly mature. After about 6 weeks, adult worms mate, and migrate to terminal mesenteric or bladder venules, where females deposit their eggs. Some eggs reach the lumen of the bowel or bladder and are passed with feces or urine, while others are retained in the bowel or bladder wall or transported in the circulation to other tissues, in particular the liver. Disease in endemic areas is primarily due to a host response to eggs, with granuloma formation and inflammation, eventually leading to fibrosis.

Chronic infection can result in scarring of mesenteric or vesicular blood vessels, leading to portal hypertension and alterations in the urinary tract. In previously uninfected individuals, such as travelers with fresh water contact in endemic regions, acute schistosomiasis may occur, with a febrile illness 2–8 weeks after infection.

► Clinical Findings

A. Symptoms and Signs

1. Cercarial dermatitis—Following cercarial penetration, localized erythema develops in some individuals, which can progress to a pruritic maculopapular rash that persists for some days. Dermatitis can be caused by human schistosomes and, in non-tropical areas, by bird schistosomes that cannot complete their life cycle in humans (swimmer's itch).

2. Acute schistosomiasis (Katayama syndrome)—A febrile illness may develop 2–8 weeks after exposure in persons without prior infection, most commonly after heavy infection with S mansoni or S japonicum. Presenting symptoms and signs include acute onset of fever; headache; myalgias; cough; malaise; urticaria; diarrhea, which may be bloody; hepatosplenomegaly; lymphadenopathy; and pulmonary infiltrates. Localized lesions may occasionally cause severe manifestations, including CNS abnormalities and death. Acute schistosomiasis usually resolves in 2–8 weeks.

3. Chronic schistosomiasis—Many infected persons have light infections and are asymptomatic, but an estimated 50–60% have symptoms and 5–10% have advanced organ damage. Asymptomatic infected children may suffer from anemia and growth retardation. Symptomatic patients with intestinal schistosomiasis typically experience abdominal pain, fatigue, diarrhea, and hepatomegaly. Over years, anorexia, weight loss, weakness, colonic polyps, and features of portal hypertension develop. Late manifestations include hematemesis from esophageal varices, hepatic failure, and pulmonary hypertension. Urinary schistosomiasis may present within months of infection with hematuria and dysuria, most commonly in children and young adults. Fibrotic changes in the urinary tract can lead to hydroureter, hydronephrosis, bacterial urinary infections and, ultimately, kidney disease or bladder cancer.

B. Laboratory Findings

Microscopic examination of stool or urine for eggs, evaluation of tissue, or serologic tests establish the diagnosis. Characteristic eggs can be identified on smears of stool or urine, but filtration or concentration techniques can improve yields. Quantitative tests that yield > 400 eggs per gram of feces or 10 mL of urine are indicative of heavy infections with increased risk of complications. Diagnosis can also be made by biopsy of the rectum, colon, liver, or bladder. Serologic tests include an ELISA available from the CDC that is 99% specific for all species. The test is 99% sensitive for S mansoni, 95% sensitive for S haematobium, but < 50% sensitive for S japonicum. Species-specific immunoblots can increase sensitivity. In acute schistosomiasis, leukocytosis, and marked eosinophilia may occur; serologic tests may become positive before eggs are seen in stool or urine. After therapy, eggs may be shed in stool or urine for months, and so the identification of eggs in fluids or tissue or positive serologic tests cannot distinguish past or active disease. Tests for egg viability are available. With a diagnosis of schistosomiasis, evaluation for the extent of disease is warranted, including liver function studies and imaging of the liver with intestinal disease and ultrasound or other imaging studies of the urinary system in urinary disease.

► Treatment

Treatment is indicated for all schistosome infections. In areas where recurrent infection is common, treatment is valuable in reducing worm burdens and limiting clinical complications. The drug of choice for schistosomiasis is praziquantel. The drug is administered for 1 day at an oral dose of 40 mg/kg (in one or two doses) for S mansoni, S haematobium, and S intercalatum infections and a dose of 60 mg/kg (in two or three doses) for S japonicum and S mekongi. Cure rates are generally > 80% after a single treatment, and those not cured have marked reduction in the intensity of infection. Praziquantel is active against invading cercariae but not developing schistosomulae. Therefore, the drug may not prevent illness when given after exposure and, for recent infections, a repeat course after a few weeks may be appropriate. Praziquantel may be used during pregnancy. Resistance to praziquantel has been reported. Toxicities include abdominal pain, diarrhea, urticaria, headache, nausea, vomiting, and fever, and may be due both to direct effects of the drug and responses to dying worms. Alternative therapies are oxamniquine for S mansoni infection and metrifonate for S haemotobium infection. Both of these drugs currently have limited availability (they are not available in the United States), and resistance may be a problem. No second-line drug is available for S japonicum infections. The antimalarial drug artemether has activity against schistosomulae and adult worms and may be effective in chemoprophylaxis; however, it is expensive, and long-term use in malarious areas might select for resistant malaria parasites. With severe disease, use of corticosteroids in conjunction with praziquantel may decrease complications. Treatment should be followed by repeat examinations for eggs about every 3 months for 1 year after therapy, with re-treatment if eggs are seen.

► Prevention

Travelers to endemic areas should avoid fresh water exposure. Vigorous toweling after exposure may limit cercarial penetration. Chemoprophylaxis with artemether has shown efficacy but is not standard practice. Community control of schistosomiasis includes improved sanitation and water supplies, elimination of snail habitats, and intermittent administration of treatment to limit worm burdens.

Fenwick A et al. Schistosomiasis: challenges for control, treatment and drug resistance. Curr Opin Infect Dis. 2006 Dec;19 (6):577–82. [PMID: 17075334]

Gryseels B et al. Human schistosomiasis. Lancet. 2006 Sep 23;368(9541):1106–18. [PMID: 16997665]

Meltzer E et al. Schistosomiasis among travelers: new aspects of an old disease. Emerg Infect Dis. 2006 Nov;12(11):1696–700. [PMID: 17283619]

Ross AG et al. Katayama syndrome. Lancet Infect Dis. 2007 Mar;7(3):218–24. [PMID: 17317603]

LIVER, LUNG, AND INTESTINAL FLUKES

FASCIOLIASIS

Infection by *Fasciola hepatica*, the sheep liver fluke, results from ingestion of encysted metacercariae on watercress or other aquatic vegetables. Infection is prevalent in sheep-raising areas in many countries, especially parts of South America, the Middle East, and southern Europe. *Fasciola gigantica* has a more restricted distribution in Asia and Africa and causes similar findings. Eggs are passed from host feces into fresh water, leading to infection of snails, and then deposition of metacercariae on vegetation. In humans, metacercariae excyst, penetrate into the peritoneum, migrate through the liver, and mature in the bile ducts, where they cause local necrosis and abscess formation.

Two clinical syndromes are seen, related to acute migration of worms and chronic infection of the biliary tract. Symptoms related to migration of larvae present 6–12 weeks after ingestion. Typical findings are abdominal pain, fever, malaise, weight loss, urticaria, eosinophilia, and leukocytosis. Tender hepatomegaly and elevated liver function tests may be seen. Rarely, migration to other organs may lead to localized disease. The symptoms of worm migration subside after 2–4 months, followed by asymptomatic infection by adult worms or intermittent symptoms of biliary obstruction, with biliary colic and, at times, findings of cholangitis. Early diagnosis is difficult, as eggs are not found in the feces during the acute migratory phase of infection. Clinical suspicion should be based on clinical findings and marked eosinophilia in at risk individuals. CT and other imaging studies show hypodense migratory lesions of the liver. Serologic assays may be positive about 1 month before eggs are seen in stool, but specificities of available tests are not ideal. Definitive diagnosis is made by the identification of characteristic eggs in stool. Repeated examinations may be necessary. In chronic infection, imaging studies show masses obstructing the extrahepatic biliary tract.

Fascioliasis is unusual among fluke infections, in that it does not respond well to treatment with praziquantel. The treatment of choice is triclabendazole, which is also used in veterinary medicine, but is not available in the United States. Standard dosing of 10 mg/kg orally in a single dose or two doses over 12 hours achieves a cure rate of about 80%, but repeat dosing is indicated if abnormal radiologic findings or eosinophilia do not resolve. The second-line drug for fascioliasis is bithionol (30–50 mg/kg/d orally in three divided doses on alternate days for 10–15 days; available in the United States from the CDC Drug Service, Centers for Disease Control and Prevention, Atlanta, GA 30333; telephone: 404-639-3670). Treatment with either drug can be accompanied by abdominal pain and other gastrointestinal symptoms. Prevention of fascioliasis involves avoidance of ingestion of raw aquatic plants.

CLONORCHIASIS & OPISTHORCHIASIS

Infection by *Clonorchis sinensis*, the Chinese liver fluke, is endemic in areas of Japan, Korea, China, Taiwan, Southeast Asia, and the far eastern part of Russia. Millions of people are affected and, in some communities, prevalence can reach over 80%. Opisthorchiasis is principally caused by *Opisthorchis felineus* (regions of the former Soviet Union) or *Opisthorchis viverrini* (Thailand, Laos, Vietnam). Clonorchiasis and opisthorchiasis are clinically indistinguishable. Parasite eggs are shed into water in human or animal feces, where they infect snails, which release cercariae, which infect fish. Human infection follows ingestion of raw, undercooked, or pickled freshwater fish containing metacercariae. These parasites excyst in the duodenum and ascend into the biliary tract, where they mature and remain for many years, shedding eggs in the bile.

Most patients harbor few parasites and are asymptomatic. An acute illness can occur 2–3 weeks after initial infection, with fever, abdominal pain, tender hepatomegaly, urticaria, and eosinophilia. The acute syndrome is difficult to diagnose, since ova may not appear in the feces until 3–4 weeks after onset of symptoms. In chronic heavy infections, findings include abdominal pain, anorexia, weight loss, and tender hepatomegaly. More serious findings can include recurrent bacterial cholangitis and sepsis, cholecystitis, liver abscess, and pancreatitis. An increased risk of cholangiocarcinoma has been documented.

Early diagnosis is presumptive, based on clinical findings and epidemiology. Subsequent diagnosis is made by finding characteristic eggs in stool or duodenal or biliary contents. Repeated concentration tests of stool may be necessary. Imaging studies show characteristic biliary tract dilatations with filling defects due to flukes. Serologic tests can be helpful but are limited by suboptimal specificity.

The drug of choice is praziquantel. A dosage of 25 mg/kg orally three times daily for 2 days provides cure rates over 95%. One day of treatment may be sufficient. Re-treatment may be required, especially in some areas with known decreased praziquantel efficacy. The second-line drug is albendazole (400 mg orally twice daily for 7 days), which appears to be somewhat less effective.

PARAGONIMIASIS

Eight species of *Paragonimus* lung flukes cause human disease. The most important is *Paragonimus westermani*. *Paragonimus* species are endemic in East Asia, Oceania, West Africa, and South America, where millions of persons are infected. Eggs are released into fresh water, where parasites infect snails, and then cercariae infect crabs and crayfish. Human infection follows consumption of raw, undercooked, or pickled freshwater shellfish. Metacercariae then excyst, penetrate into the peritoneum, and pass into the lungs, where they mature into adult worms over about 2 months.

Most persons have moderate worm burdens and are asymptomatic. In symptomatic cases, abdominal pain and diarrhea develop 2 days to 2 weeks after infection, followed by fever, cough, chest pain, urticaria, and eosinophilia. Acute symptoms may last for several weeks. Chronic infection can cause cough productive of brown sputum, hemoptysis, dyspnea, and chest pain, with progression to chronic bronchitis, bronchiectasis, bronchopneumonia, lung abscess, and pleural disease. Ectopic infections can cause disease in other organs, most commonly the CNS, where disease can present with seizures, headaches, and focal neurologic findings due to parasite meningitis, and intracerebral lesions.

The diagnosis of paragonimiasis is made by identifying characteristic eggs in sputum or stool or identifying worms in biopsied tissue. Multiple examinations and concentration techniques may be needed. Serologic tests may be helpful; an ELISA available from the CDC has sensitivity and specificity > 95%. Chest radiographs may show varied abnormalities of the lungs or pleura, including infiltrates, nodules, cavities, and fibrosis, and the findings can be confused with those of tuberculosis. With CNS disease, skull radiographs can show clusters of calcified cysts, and CT or MRI can show clusters of ring-enhancing lesions.

Treatment is with praziquantel (25 mg/kg orally three times daily for 2 days), which provides efficacy of at least 90%. Alternative therapies are bithionol and triclabendazole. As with cysticercosis, for cerebral paragonimiasis, praziquantel should generally be used with corticosteroids. Chronic infection may lead to permanent lung dysfunction and pleural disease requiring drainage procedures.

INTESTINAL FLUKES

The large intestinal fluke, *Fasciolopsis buski*, is a common parasite of pigs and humans in eastern and southern Asia. Eggs shed in stools hatch in fresh water, followed by infection of snails, and release of cercariae that encyst on aquatic plants. Humans are infected by eating uncooked plants, including water chestnuts, bamboo shoots, and watercress. Adult flukes mature in about 3 months and live in the small intestine attached to the mucosa, leading to local inflammation and ulceration. Other intestinal flukes that cause similar syndromes include *Heterophyes* (North Africa and Turkey) and *Metagonimus* (East Asia) species; these species are transmitted by undercooked freshwater fish.

Infections with intestinal flukes are often asymptomatic, although eosinophilia may be marked. In symptomatic cases, after an incubation period of 1–2 months, manifestations include epigastric pain and diarrhea. Other gastrointestinal symptoms, ileus, edema, and ascites may be seen uncommonly. Diagnosis is based on identification of characteristic eggs or adult flukes in the stool. In contrast to other fluke infections, illness more than 6 months after travel in an endemic area is unlikely. The drug of choice is praziquantel, 25 mg/kg orally as a single dose. Alternative therapies are triclabendazole and niclosamide (for most species).

Jeon K et al. Clinical features of recently diagnosed pulmonary paragonimiasis in Korea. Chest. 2005 Sep;128(3):1423–30. [PMID: 16162738]

Marcos LA. Update on hepatobiliary flukes: fascioliasis, opisthorchiasis and clonorchiasis. Curr Opin Infect Dis. 2008 Oct;21(5):523–30. [PMID: 18725803]

Rana SS et al. Parasitic infestations of the biliary tract. Curr Gastroenterol Rep. 2007 Apr;9(2):156–64. [PMID: 17418062]

CESTODE INFECTIONS

The four major tapeworms that cause noninvasive infections in humans are the beef tapeworm *Taenia saginata*, the pork tapeworm *Taenia solium*, the fish tapeworm *Diphyllobothrium latum*, each of which can reach many meters in length, and the dwarf tapeworm *Hymenolepis nana*. *Taenia* and *Hymenolepis* species are broadly distributed, especially in the tropics; *D latum* is most prevalent in temperate regions. Other tapeworms that can cause noninvasive human disease include the rodent tapeworm *Hymenolepis diminuta*, the dog tapeworm *Dipylidium caninum*, and other *Taenia* and *Diphyllobothrium* species. Invasive tapeworm infections, including *T solium* (when infective eggs, rather than cysticerci are ingested) and *Echinococcus* species, will be discussed separately.

NONINVASIVE TAPEWORM INFECTIONS

1. Beef Tapeworm

Infection is most common in cattle breeding areas. Humans are the definitive host. Gravid segments of *T saginata* are passed in human feces to soil, where they are ingested by grazing animals, especially cattle. The eggs then hatch to release embryos that encyst in muscle as cysticerci. Humans are infected by eating raw or undercooked infected beef. Most individuals infected with *T saginata* are asymptomatic, but abdominal pain and other gastrointestinal symptoms may be present. Eosinophilia is common. The most common presenting finding is the passage of proglottids in the stool.

2. Pork Tapeworm

T solium is transmitted to pigs that ingest human feces. Humans can be either the definitive host (after consuming undercooked pork, leading to tapeworm infection) or the intermediate host (after consuming food contaminated with human feces containing *T solium* eggs, leading to cysticercosis, which is discussed under invasive tapeworm infections). As with the beef tapeworm, infection with *T solium* adult worms is generally asymptomatic, but gastrointestinal symptoms may occur. Infection is generally recognized after passage of proglottids. Autoinfection with eggs can progress to cysticercosis.

3. Fish Tapeworm

Infection with *D latum* follows ingestion of undercooked freshwater fish, most commonly in temperate regions. Eggs from human feces are taken up by crustaceans, these are eaten by fish, which are then infectious to humans. Infection with multiple worms over many years can occur. Infections are most commonly asymptomatic, but nonspecific gastrointestinal symptoms, including diarrhea, may occur. Diagnosis usually follows passage of proglottids. Prolonged heavy infection can lead to megaloblastic anemia and neuropathy from vitamin B_{12} deficiency, which is due to infection-induced dissociation of the vitamin from intrinsic factor and to utilization of the vitamin by worms.

4. Dwarf Tapeworm

H nana is the only tapeworm that can be transmitted between humans. Infections are common in warm areas, especially with poor hygiene and institutionalized populations. Infection follows ingestion of food contaminated with human feces. Eggs hatch in the intestines, where oncospheres penetrate the mucosa, encyst as cysticercoid larvae, and then rupture after about 4 days to release adult worms. Autoinfection can lead to amplification of infection. Infection with *H nana,* the related rodent tapeworm *H diminuta,* or the dog tapeworm *D caninum* can also follow accidental ingestion of infected insects. *H nana* are dwarf in size relative to other tapeworms but can reach 5 cm in length. Heavy infection is common, especially in children, and can be accompanied by abdominal discomfort, anorexia, and diarrhea.

▶ Laboratory Findings

Diagnosis is usually made based on the identification of characteristic eggs or proglottids in stool. Egg release may be irregular, so examination of multiple specimens or concentration techniques may be needed.

▶ Treatment

The treatment of choice for noninvasive tapeworm infections is praziquantel. A single dose of praziquantel (5–10 mg/kg orally) is highly effective, except for *H nana,* for which the dosage is 25 mg/kg. Treatment of *H nana* is more difficult, as the drug is not effective against maturing cysts. Therefore, with heavy infections with this parasite a repeat treatment after 1 week, and screening after therapy to document cure are appropriate. Therapy can be accompanied by headache, malaise, dizziness, abdominal pain, and nausea.

The alternative therapy for these infections is niclosamide. A single dose of niclosamide (2 g chewed) is effective against *D latum, Taenia,* and *D caninum* infections. For *H nana,* therapy is continued daily for 1 week. Niclosamide may cause nausea, malaise, and abdominal pain.

Craig P et al. Intestinal cestodes. Curr Opin Infect Dis. 2007 Oct;20(5):524–32. [PMID: 17762788]
Willingham AL et al. Control of *Taenia solium* cysticercosis/taeniosis. Adv Parasitol. 2006;61:509–66. [PMID: 16735172]

INVASIVE CESTODE INFECTIONS

1. Cysticercosis

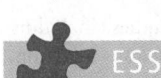

ESSENTIALS OF DIAGNOSIS

▶ Exposure to *T solium* through fecal contamination of food.

▶ Seizures, headache, and other findings of a focal CNS lesion.

▶ Brain imaging shows cysts; positive serologic tests.

▶ General Considerations

Cysticercosis is due to tissue infection with cysts of *T solium* that develop after humans ingest food contaminated with eggs from human feces, thus acting as an intermediate host for the parasite. Prevalence is high where the parasite is endemic, in particular Mexico, Central and South America, the Philippines, and Southeast Asia. An estimated 20 million persons are infected with cysticerci yearly, leading to about 400,000 persons with neurologic symptoms and 50,000 deaths. Antibody prevalence rates up to 10% are recognized in some endemic areas, and the infection is one of the most important causes of seizures in the developing world and in immigrants to the United States from endemic countries.

▶ Clinical Findings

A. Symptoms and Signs

Neurocysticercosis can cause intracerebral, subarachnoid, and spinal cord lesions and intraventricular cysts. Single or multiple lesions may be present. Lesions may persist for years before symptoms develop, generally due to local inflammation or ventricular obstruction. Presenting symptoms include seizures, focal neurologic deficits, altered cognition, and psychiatric disease. Symptoms develop more quickly with intraventricular cysts, with findings of hydrocephalus and meningeal irritation, including severe headache, vomiting, papilledema, and visual loss. A particularly aggressive form of the disease, racemose cysticercosis, involves proliferation of cysts at the base of the brain, leading to alterations of consciousness and death. Spinal cord lesions can present with progressive focal findings.

Cysticercosis of other organ systems is usually clinically benign. Involvement of muscles can uncommonly cause discomfort and is identified by radiographs of muscle showing multiple calcified lesions. Subcutaneous involvement presents with multiple painless palpable skin lesions. Involvement of the eyes can present with ptosis due to extraocular muscle involvement or intraocular abnormalities.

B. Laboratory Findings

CSF examination may show lymphocytic or eosinophilic pleocytosis, decreased glucose, and elevated protein. Serologic tests can indicate prior exposure to *T solium,* but both sensitivity and specificity are limited.

C. Imaging

The diagnosis of neurocysticercosis can be difficult. With neuroimaging by CT or MRI, multiple parenchymal cysts are most typically seen. Parenchymal calcification is also common. Ventricular cysts may be difficult to visualize, with MRI offering better sensitivity than CT.

▶ Treatment

The medical management of neurocysticercosis is controversial, as the benefits of cyst clearance must be weighed against potential harm of an inflammatory response to dying worms. Antihelminthic therapy hastens radiologic improvement in parenchymal cysticercosis. However, some randomized trials have shown that corticosteroids alone are as effective as specific therapy plus corticosteroids for controlling seizures, and some reports have shown exacerbation of disease after antihelminthic therapy. Considering active lesions, disease with a high likelihood of progression, such as intraventricular cysts, may benefit from therapy. At the other end of the spectrum, inactive calcified lesions probably do not benefit from therapy. Overall, it remains difficult to determine when treatment is indicated. When treatment is deemed appropriate, standard therapy consists of albendazole (10–15 mg/kg/d orally for 8 days) or praziquantel (50 mg/kg/d orally for 15–30 days). Albendazole is probably preferred, since it has shown better efficacy in some comparisons and since corticosteroids appear to lower circulating praziquantel levels but increase albendazole levels. Increasing the dosage of albendazole to 30 mg/kg/d orally may improve outcomes. Corticosteroids are usually administered concurrently but dosing is not standardized. Patients should be observed for evidence of localized inflammatory responses. Anticonvulsant therapy is provided if needed, and shunting is performed if required for elevated intracranial pressure. Surgical removal of cysts may be helpful for some difficult cases of neurocysticercosis and for symptomatic non-neurologic disease.

Del Brutto OH et al. Meta-analysis: Cysticidal drugs for neurocysticercosis: albendazole and praziquantel. Ann Intern Med. 2006 Jul 4;145(1):43–51. [PMID: 16818928]

Garcia HH. Antiparasitic drugs in neurocysticercosis: albendazole or praziquantel? Expert Rev Anti Infect Ther. 2008 Jun;6(3):295–8. [PMID: 18588494]

Garcia HH et al; Cysticercosis Working Group in Peru. Neurocysticercosis: updated concepts about an old disease. Lancet Neurol. 2005 Oct;4(10):653–61. [PMID: 16168934]

Matthaiou DK et al. Albendazole versus praziquantel in the treatment of neurocysticercosis: a meta-analysis of comparative trials. PLoS Negl Trop Dis. 2008 Mar 12;2(3):e194. [PMID: 18335068]

Nash TE et al. Treatment of neurocysticercosis: current status and future research needs. Neurology. 2006 Oct 10;67(7):1120–7. [PMID: 17030744]

2. Echinococcosis

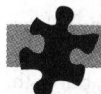

ESSENTIALS OF DIAGNOSIS

▶ History of exposure to dogs or wild canines in an endemic area.

▶ Large cystic lesions, most commonly of the liver or lung.

▶ Positive serologic tests.

▶ General Considerations

Echinococcosis occurs when humans are intermediate hosts for canine tapeworms. Infection is acquired by ingesting food contaminated with canine feces containing parasite eggs. The principal species that infect humans are *Echinococcus granulosus*, which causes cystic hydatid disease, and *Echinococcus multilocularis*, which causes alveolar hydatid disease. *E granulosus* is transmitted by domestic dogs in areas with livestock (sheep, goats, camels, and horses) as intermediate hosts, including Africa, the Middle East, southern Europe, South America, Central Asia, Australia, New Zealand, and the southwestern United States. *E multilocularis*, which much less commonly causes human disease, is transmitted by wild canines, and endemic in northern forest areas of the northern hemisphere, including central Europe, Siberia, northern Japan, northwestern Canada, and western Alaska. An increase in the fox population in Europe has been associated with an increase in human cases. The disease range has also extended southward in Central Asia and China. Other species that cause limited disease in humans are endemic in South America and China.

After humans ingest parasite eggs, the eggs hatch in the intestines to form oncospheres, which penetrate the mucosa, enter the circulation, and encyst in specific organs as hydatid cysts. *E granulosus* forms cysts most commonly in the liver (65%) and lungs (25%), but the cysts may develop in any organ, including the brain, bones, skeletal muscles, kidneys, and spleen. Cysts are most commonly single. The cysts can persist and slowly grow for many years.

▶ Clinical Findings

A. Symptoms and Signs

Infections are commonly asymptomatic and may be noted incidentally on imaging studies or present with symptoms caused by an enlarging or superinfected mass. Findings may include abdominal or chest pain, biliary obstruction, cholangitis, portal hypertension, cirrhosis, bronchial obstruction leading to segmental lung collapse, and abscesses. Cyst leakage or rupture may be accompanied by a severe allergic reaction, including fever and hypotension. Seeding of cysts after rupture may extend the infection to new areas.

E multilocularis generally causes a more aggressive disease than *E granulosus*, with initial infection of the liver, but then local and distant spread commonly suggesting a malignancy. Symptoms based on the areas of involvement gradually worsen over years, with the development of obstructive findings in the liver and elsewhere.

B. Laboratory Findings

Serologic tests, including ELISA and immunoblot, offer sensitivity and specificity over 80% for *E granulosus* liver infections, but lower sensitivity for involvement of other organs. Serologic tests may also distinguish the two major echinococcal infections.

C. Imaging

Diagnosis is usually based on imaging studies, including ultrasonography, CT, and MRI. In *E granulosus* infection, a large cyst containing daughter cysts is highly suggestive of the diagnosis. In *E multilocularis* infection, imaging shows an irregular mass, often with areas of calcification.

▶ Treatment

Treatment of cystic hydatid disease has traditionally involved cautious surgical resection of cysts, with care not to rupture cysts during removal. Injection of a cysticidal agent was used to limit spread in the case of rupture. Recently, new management algorithms include treatment with albendazole, often in conjunction with surgery. When used alone, as in cases where surgery is not possible, albendazole (10–15 mg/kg/d orally) has demonstrated efficacy, with courses of 3 months or longer duration, in some cases with alternating cycles of treatment and rest. Mebendazole (40–50 mg/kg/d orally) is an alternative drug, and praziquantel may also be effective. In some cases, medical therapy is begun, with surgery performed if disease persists after some months of therapy. Another approach, in particular with inoperable cysts, is percutaneous aspiration, injection, and reaspiration (PAIR). In this approach (which should not be used if cysts communicate with the biliary tract), patients receive antihelminthic therapy, and the cyst is partially aspirated. After diagnostic confirmation by examination for parasite protoscolices, a scolicidal agent (such as 95% ethanol or 0.5% cetrimide) is injected. Treatment of alveolar cyst disease is challenging, generally relying on wide surgical resection of lesions. Therapy with albendazole before or during surgery may be beneficial and may also provide improvement or even cure in inoperable cases.

3. Other Invasive Cestode Infections

Ingestion of aquatic copepods infected with larvae of *Spirometra* canine or feline tapeworms can lead to sparganosis, especially in South America and East Asia. Infection can also come from ingestion of undercooked infected meat (including mammals, birds, reptiles, and amphibians) or from use of frog or snake-meat poultices. The worms penetrate the intestinal wall or skin and migrate to various tissues. Inflammatory lesions, most commonly of the skin or eyes, are typically present. In cerebral sparganosis, an intense inflammatory response to worms can lead to severe neurologic disease. Diagnosis is by biopsy or visualization of the parasite. Treatment consists of surgical resection or local injection of ethanol. Antihelminthics do not appear to be helpful. Other non-human tapeworms can also cause localized and CNS inflammatory lesions. These are also managed with surgical resection.

Craig PS et al. Prevention and control of cystic echinococcosis. Lancet Infect Dis. 2007 Jun;7(6):385–94. [PMID: 17521591]

Garcia HH et al. Zoonotic helminth infections of humans: echinococcosis, cysticercosis and fascioliasis. Curr Opin Infect Dis. 2007 Oct;20(5):489–94. [PMID: 17762782]

Junghanss T et al. Clinical management of cystic echinococcosis: state of the art, problems, and perspectives. Am J Trop Med Hyg. 2008 Sep;79(3):301–11. [PMID: 18784219]

Moro P et al. Echinococcosis: a review. Int J Infect Dis. 2008 Oct 18. [Epub ahead of print] [PMID: 18938096]

INTESTINAL NEMATODE (ROUNDWORM) INFECTIONS

ASCARIASIS

ESSENTIALS OF DIAGNOSIS

► Transient cough, urticaria, pulmonary infiltrates, eosinophilia.

► Nonspecific abdominal symptoms.

► Eggs in stool; adult worms occasionally passed.

Ascaris lumbricoides is the most common of the intestinal helminths, infecting about a quarter of the world's population, with estimates of over a billion infections, 12 million acute cases, and 10,000 or more deaths annually. Prevalence is high wherever there is poor hygiene and sanitation or where human feces are used as fertilizer. Heavy infections are most common in children.

Infection follows ingestion of eggs in contaminated food. Larvae hatch in the small intestine, penetrate into the bloodstream, migrate to the lungs, and then travel via airways back to the gastrointestinal tract, where they develop to adult worms, which can be up to 40 cm in length, and live for 1–2 years.

► Clinical Findings

Most persons with *Ascaris* infection are asymptomatic. A small proportion develop symptoms during migration of worms through the lungs, with fever, nonproductive cough, chest pain, dyspnea, and eosinophilia, occasionally with eosinophilic pneumonia. Rarely, larvae lodge ectopically in the brain, kidney, eye, spinal cord, and other sites and may cause local symptoms.

Light intestinal infections usually produce no symptoms. With heavy infection, abdominal discomfort may be seen. Adult worms may also migrate and be coughed up, be vomited, or may emerge through the nose or anus. They may also migrate into the common bile duct, pancreatic duct, appendix, and other sites, which may lead to cholangitis, cholecystitis, pyogenic liver abscess, pancreatitis, obstructive jaundice, or appendicitis. With very heavy infestations, masses of worms may cause intestinal obstruction, volvulus, intussusception, or death. Although severe manifestations of infection are uncommon, the very high prevalence of ascariasis leads to large numbers of individuals, especially children, with important sequelae. Moderate to high worm loads in children are also associated with nutritional abnormalities due to decreased appetite and food intake, and also decreased absorption of nutrients.

The diagnosis of ascariasis is made after adult worms emerge from the mouth, nose, or anus, or by identifying characteristic eggs in the feces. Due to the very high egg burden, concentration techniques are generally not needed. Imaging studies demonstrate worms, with filling defects in contrast studies and at times evidence of intestinal or biliary obstruction. Eosinophilia is marked during worm migration but may be absent during intestinal infection.

► Treatment

All infections should ideally be treated. Treatments of choice are albendazole (single 400 mg oral dose), mebendazole (single 500 mg oral dose or 100 mg twice daily for 3 days), or pyrantel pamoate (single 11 mg/kg oral dose, maximum 1 g). These drugs are all well tolerated but may cause mild gastrointestinal toxicity. They are now considered safe for children above 1 year of age and in pregnancy, although use in the first trimester is best avoided. Intestinal obstruction usually responds to conservative management and antihelminthic therapy. Surgery may be required for appendicitis and other gastrointestinal complications.

TRICHURIASIS

Trichuris trichiura, the whipworm, infects about a billion persons throughout the world, particularly in humid tropical and subtropical environments. Infection is heaviest and most frequent in children. Infections are acquired by ingestion of eggs. The larvae hatch in the small intestine and mature in the large bowel to adult worms of about 4 cm in length. The worms do not migrate through tissues.

Most infected persons are asymptomatic. Heavy infections may be accompanied by abdominal cramps, tenesmus, diarrhea, distention, nausea, and vomiting. The *Trichuris* dysentery syndrome may develop, particularly in malnourished young children, with findings resembling inflammatory bowel disease including bloody diarrhea and rectal prolapse. Chronic infections in children can lead to iron deficiency anemia, growth retardation, and clubbing of the fingers.

Trichuriasis is diagnosed by identification of characteristic eggs and sometimes adult worms in stools. Concentration techniques are not needed. Eosinophilia is common. Treatment is with albendazole (400 mg/d orally) or mebendazole (200 mg/d orally), for 1–3 days for light infections or 3–7 days for heavy infections.

HOOKWORM DISEASE

ESSENTIALS OF DIAGNOSIS

▶ Transient pruritic skin rash and pulmonary symptoms.
▶ Anorexia, diarrhea, abdominal discomfort.
▶ Iron deficiency anemia.
▶ Characteristic eggs and occult blood in the stool.

General Considerations

Infection with the hookworms *Ancylostoma duodenale* and *Necator americanus* is very common, especially in most tropical and subtropical regions. Both worms are broadly distributed. Prevalence is estimated at about 1 billion, causing approximately 65,000 deaths each year. When eggs are deposited on warm moist soil they hatch, releasing larvae that remain infective for up to a week. With contact, the larvae penetrate skin and migrate in the bloodstream to the pulmonary capillaries. In the lungs, the larvae penetrate into alveoli and then are carried by ciliary action upward to the bronchi, trachea, and mouth. After being swallowed, they reach and attach to the mucosa of the upper small bowel, where they mature to adult worms. *Ancylostoma* infection can also be acquired by ingestion of the larvae in food or water. Hookworms attach to the intestinal mucosa and suck blood. Blood loss is proportionate to the worm burden.

Clinical Findings

A. Symptoms and Signs

Most infected persons are asymptomatic. A pruritic maculopapular rash (ground itch) may occur at the site of larval penetration, usually in previously sensitized persons. Pulmonary symptoms may be seen during larval migration through the lungs, with dry cough, wheezing, and low-grade fever, but these symptoms are less common than with ascariasis. Eosinophilia is common, especially during worm migration. About 1 month after infection, as maturing worms attach to the small intestinal mucosa, gastrointestinal symptoms may develop, with epigastric pain, anorexia, and diarrhea, especially in previously unexposed individuals. Persons chronically infected with large worm burdens may have abdominal pain, anorexia, diarrhea, and findings of marked iron-deficiency anemia and protein malnutrition. Anemia can lead to pallor, weakness, dyspnea, and congestive heart failure, and protein loss can lead to hypoalbuminemia, edema, and ascites. These findings may be accompanied by impairment in growth and cognitive development in children. Infection with the dog hookworm *Ancylostoma caninum* can uncommonly lead to abdominal pain, diarrhea, and eosinophilia, with intestinal ulcerations and regional lymphadenitis.

B. Laboratory Findings

Diagnosis is based on the demonstration of characteristic eggs in feces; concentration techniques are usually not needed. Microcytic anemia, occult blood in the stool, hypoalbuminemia, and eosinophilia are common.

Treatment

Treatment is with albendazole (single 400 mg oral dose) or mebendazole (100 mg orally twice daily for 3 days). These drugs are teratogenic, but experience suggests that they are safe in children over 1 year of age and during the second and third trimesters of pregnancy. Occasional adverse effects are diarrhea and abdominal pain. Pyrantel pamoate and levamisole are also effective. Anemia should be managed with iron replacement and, for severe symptomatic anemia, blood transfusion. Mass treatment of children with single doses of albendazole or mebendazole at regular intervals limits worm burdens and the extent of disease and is advocated by the WHO.

STRONGYLOIDIASIS

ESSENTIALS OF DIAGNOSIS

▶ Transient pruritic skin rash and pulmonary symptoms.
▶ Anorexia, diarrhea, abdominal discomfort.
▶ Hyperinfection syndrome with varied severe presentations in the immunocompromised.
▶ Larvae detected in stool.

▸ With hyperinfection, larvae detected in sputum or other fluids.

▸ Eosinophilia.

General Considerations

Strongyloidiasis is caused by infection with *Strongyloides stercoralis*. Although much less prevalent than ascariasis, trichuriasis, or hookworm infections, strongyloidiasis is nonetheless a significant problem, infecting tens of millions of individuals in tropical and subtropical regions. Infection is also endemic in some temperate regions of North America, Europe, Japan, and Australia. Of particular importance is the predilection of the parasite to cause severe infections in immunocompromised individuals due to its ability to replicate in humans. A related parasite, *Strongyloides fuelleborni*, infects humans in parts of Africa and New Guinea.

Among nematodes, *S stercoralis* is uniquely capable of maintaining its full life cycle both within the human host and in soil. Infection occurs when filariform larvae in soil penetrate the skin, enter the bloodstream, and are carried to the lungs, where they escape from capillaries into alveoli, ascend the bronchial tree, and are then swallowed and carried to the duodenum and upper jejunum, where maturation to the adult stage takes place. Females live embedded in the mucosa for up to 5 years, releasing eggs that hatch in the intestines as free rhabditiform larvae that pass to the ground via the feces. In moist soil, these larvae metamorphose into infective filariform larvae. Autoinfection can occur in humans, when some rhabditiform larvae develop into filariform larvae that penetrate the intestinal mucosa or perianal skin, and enter the circulation.

Clinical Findings

A. Symptoms and Signs

As with other intestinal nematodes, most infected persons are asymptomatic. An acute syndrome can be seen at the time of infection, with a pruritic, erythematous, maculopapular rash, usually of the feet. These symptoms may be followed by pulmonary symptoms (including dry cough, dyspnea, and wheezing) and eosinophilia after a number of days, followed by gastrointestinal symptoms after some weeks, as with hookworm infections. Chronic infection may be accompanied by epigastric pain, nausea, diarrhea, and anemia. Maculopapular or urticarial rashes of the buttocks, perineum, and thighs, due to migrating larvae, may be seen. Large worm burdens can lead to malabsorption or intestinal obstruction. Eosinophilia is common but may fluctuate.

The most dangerous manifestation of *S stercoralis* infection is the **hyperinfection syndrome,** with dissemination of large numbers of filariform larvae to the lungs and other tissues in immunocompromised individuals. Mortality with this syndrome approaches 100% without treatment and has been about 25% with treatment. The hyperinfection syndrome is seen in those receiving corticosteroids and other immunosuppressive medications, those with hematologic malignancies, malnutrition, or alcoholism, or

those with AIDS. The risk seems greatest for those receiving corticosteroids, and considering the large number of at risk individuals, the risk in those with AIDS seems relatively low. With hyperinfection large numbers of larvae can migrate to many tissues, including the lungs, CNS, kidneys, and liver. Gastrointestinal symptoms can include abdominal pain, nausea, vomiting, diarrhea, and more severe findings related to intestinal obstruction, perforation, or hemorrhage. Bacterial sepsis, probably secondary to intestinal ulcerations, is a common presenting finding. Pulmonary findings include pneumonitis, cough, hemoptysis, and respiratory failure. Sputum may contain adult worms, larvae, and eggs. CNS disease includes meningitis and brain abscesses; the CSF may contain larvae. Various presentations can progress to shock and death.

B. Laboratory Findings

The diagnosis of strongyloidiasis can be difficult, as eggs are seldom found in feces. Diagnosis is usually based on the identification of rhabditiform larvae in the stool or duodenal contents. These larvae must be distinguished from hookworm larvae, which may hatch after stool collection. Repeated examinations of stool or examination of duodenal fluid may be required for diagnosis because the sensitivity of individual tests is only about 30%. Hyperinfection is diagnosed by the identification of large numbers of larvae in stool, sputum, or other body fluids. An ELISA from the CDC offers about 90% sensitivity and specificity, but cross-reactions with other helminths may occur. Eosinophilia and mild anemia are common, but eosinophilia may be absent with hyperinfection. Hyperinfection may include extensive pulmonary infiltrates, hypoproteinemia, and abnormal liver function studies.

Treatment

Full eradication of *S stercoralis* is more important than with other intestinal helminths due to the ability of the parasite to replicate in humans. The treatment of choice for routine infection is ivermectin (200 mcg orally daily for 1–2 days). This treatment has replaced thiabendazole (25 mg/kg orally twice daily for 3 days), which is relatively poorly tolerated, and albendazole (400 mg orally twice daily for 3 days), which is less effective. For hyperinfection, ivermectin should be administered daily until the clinical syndrome has resolved and larvae have not been identified for at least 2 weeks. Follow-up examinations for larvae in stool or sputum are necessary, with repeat dosing if the infection persists. With continued immunosuppression, eradication may be difficult, and regular repeated doses of antihelminthic therapy (eg, monthly ivermectin) may be required. It is important to be aware of the possibility of strongyloidiasis in those with even a distant history of residence in an endemic area, since the infection can be maintained for decades. Screening of at-risk individuals for infection is appropriate before institution of immunosuppressive therapy. Screening can consist of serologic tests, with stool examinations in those with positive serologic tests, but consideration of presumptive treatment even if the stool evaluations are negative.

ENTEROBIASIS

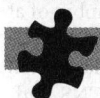

► Nocturnal perianal pruritus.
► Identification of eggs or adult worms on perianal skin or in stool.

General Considerations

Enterobius vermicularis, the pinworm, is a common cause of intestinal infections worldwide, with maximal prevalence in school-age children. Enterobiasis is transmitted person-to-person via ingestion of eggs after contact with the hands or perianal region of an infected individual, food or fomites that have been contaminated by an infected individual, or infected bedding or clothing. Auto-infection also occurs. Eggs hatch in the duodenum and larvae migrate to the cecum. Females mature in about a month, and remain viable for about another month. During this time they migrate through the anus to deposit large numbers of eggs on the perianal skin. Due to the relatively short lifespan of these helminths, continuous reinfection, as in institutional settings, is required, for long-standing infection.

Clinical Findings

A. Symptoms and Signs

Most individuals with pinworm infection are asymptomatic. The most common symptom is perianal pruritus, particularly at night, due to the presence of the female worms or deposited eggs. Insomnia, restlessness, and enuresis are common in children. Perianal scratching may result in excoriation and impetigo. Many mild gastrointestinal symptoms have also been attributed to enterobiasis, but associations are not proven. Serious sequelae are uncommon. Rarely, worm migration results in inflammation or granulomatous reactions of the gastrointestinal or genitourinary tracts. Colonic ulceration and eosinophilic colitis have been reported.

B. Laboratory Findings

Pinworm eggs are usually not found in stool. Diagnosis is made by finding adult worms or eggs on the perianal skin. A common test is to apply clear cellophane tape to the perianal skin, ideally in the early morning, followed by microscopic examination for eggs. The sensitivity of the tape test is reported to be about 50% for a single test and 90% for three tests. Nocturnal examination of the perianal area or gross examination of stools may reveal adult worms, which are about 1 cm in length. Eosinophilia is rare.

Treatment

Treatment is with single oral doses of albendazole (400 mg), mebendazole (100 mg) or pyrantel pamoate (11 mg/kg, to a maximum of 1 g). The dose is repeated in 2 weeks due to frequent reinfection. Other infected family members should be treated concurrently, and treatment of all close contacts may be appropriate when rates of reinfection are high in family, school, or institutional settings. Standard handwashing and hygiene practices are helpful in limiting spread. Perianal scratching should be discouraged. Washing of clothes and bedding should kill pinworm eggs.

Bethony J et al. Soil-transmitted helminth infections: ascariasis, trichuriasis, and hookworm. Lancet. 2006 May 6;367(9521): 1521–32. [PMID: 16679166]

Hotez PJ et al. Hookworm infection. N Engl J Med. 2004 Aug 19;351(8):799–807. [PMID: 15317893]

Keiser J et al. Efficacy of current drugs against soil-transmitted helminth infections: systematic review and meta-analysis. JAMA. 2008 Apr 23;299(16):1937–48. [PMID: 18430913]

Ramanathan R et al. *Strongyloides stercoralis* Infection in the immunocompromised host. Curr Infect Dis Rep. 2008 Mar;10(2):105–10. [PMID: 18462583]

Reddy M et al. Oral drug therapy for multiple neglected tropical diseases: a systematic review. JAMA. 2007 Oct 24;298(16):1911–24. [PMID: 17954542]

INVASIVE NEMATODE (ROUNDWORM) INFECTIONS

DRACUNCULIASIS

► Tender cutaneous ulcer and worm protruding from the skin of an individual who has ingested untreated water in rural Africa.

General Considerations

Dracunculiasis is caused by the nematode *Dracunculus medinensis,* or Guinea worm. It causes chronic cutaneous ulcers with protruding worms in rural Africa. It occurs only in humans and is a major cause of disability, although recent control efforts have been remarkably successful, with decreased annual incidence from about 3.5 million cases in the late 1980s to under 10,000 reported cases in 2007. Dracunculiasis has been eradicated from Asia, but remains endemic in 11 countries in West and Northeast Africa, most notably in southern Sudan. The disease occurs almost exclusively in isolated rural areas; all ages are affected, and prevalence may reach 60%.

Infection occurs after swallowing water containing the infected intermediate host, the crustacean *Cyclops* (known as copepods or water fleas). In the stomach, larvae escape from the copepods, and migrate through the intestinal mucosa to the retroperitoneum, where mating occurs. Females then migrate to subcutaneous tissue, usually of the legs, over about a year. A subcutaneous ulcer then forms. Upon contact with water, the parasite discharges large numbers of larvae, which are ingested by copepods. Adult worms, which can be up to a meter in length, are gradually extruded. Worm death and disintegration in tissue may provoke a severe inflammatory reaction.

Clinical Findings

Patients are usually asymptomatic until the time of worm extrusion. At that time a painful papule develops, with erythema, pruritus, and burning, usually on the lower leg. Multiple lesions may be present. At this time, some patients may also develop a short-lived systemic reaction, which may include fever, urticaria, nausea, vomiting, diarrhea, and dyspnea. The skin lesion vesiculates over a few days, followed by ulceration. The ulcer is tender, often with a visible worm. The worm is then extruded or absorbed over a few weeks, followed by ulcer healing. Secondary infections, including infectious arthritis and tetanus, are common. The disease causes significant disability; lesions commonly prevent walking for a month or more.

Diagnosis follows identification of a typical skin ulcer with a protruding worm. When the worm is not visible, larvae may be identified on smears or seen after immersion in cold water. Eosinophilia is usually present.

Treatment

No drug cures the infection, but metronidazole and mebendazole are sometimes used to limit inflammation and facilitate worm removal. Wet compresses may relieve discomfort. Occlusive dressings improve hygiene and limit shedding of infectious larvae. Worms are typically removed by sequentially rolling them out over a small stick. When available, simple surgical procedures can be used to remove worms. Corticosteroid ointments may hasten healing. Topical antibiotics may limit bacterial superinfection.

Prevention

Dracunculiasis has proven to be easier to control than most parasitic infections. The disease is prevented by avoidance of contaminated drinking water. This can be accomplished by boiling, chlorination, or filtration through finely woven cloth. A WHO dracunculiasis eradication program, initiated in 1986, has been highly successful.

Barry M. The tail end of guinea worm–global eradication without a drug or a vaccine. N Engl J Med. 2007 Jun 21;356(25):2561–4. [PMID: 17582064]

Hopkins DR et al. Dracunculiasis eradication: neglected no longer. Am J Trop Med Hyg. 2008 Oct;79(4):474–9. [PMID: 18840732]

TRICHINOSIS

ESSENTIALS OF DIAGNOSIS

▶ Ingestion of inadequately cooked pork or game.

▶ Transient intestinal symptoms followed by fever, myalgias, and periorbital edema.

▶ Eosinophilia and elevated serum muscle enzymes.

General Considerations

Trichinosis (or trichinellosis) is caused worldwide by *Trichinella spiralis* and related *Trichinella* species. The disease is spread by ingestion of undercooked meat, most commonly pork in areas where pigs feed on garbage. When infected raw meat is ingested, *Trichinella* larvae are freed from cyst walls by gastric acid and pass into the small intestine. The larvae then invade intestinal epithelial cells, develop into adults, and the adults release infective larvae. These parasites travel to skeletal muscle via the bloodstream. They invade muscle cells, enlarge, and form cysts. These larvae may be viable for years. Pigs and other animals become infected by eating infected uncooked food scraps or other animals, such as rats.

The worldwide incidence of trichinosis has decreased, but human infections continue to occur sporadically or in outbreaks. In addition to undercooked pork, infections have been transmitted by ingestion of game and other animals, including bear and walrus in North America and wild boar and horse in Europe. In the United States, about 100 infections are reported annually, about three-fourths from pork and the remainder from game animals.

Clinical Findings

A. Symptoms and Signs

Most infections are asymptomatic. In symptomatic cases, gastrointestinal symptoms, including diarrhea, vomiting, and abdominal pain, develop within the week after ingestion of contaminated meat. These symptoms usually last for less than a week but can occasionally persist for much longer. During the following week, symptoms and signs related to migrating larvae are seen. These findings include, most notably, fever, myalgias, periorbital edema, and eosinophilia. Additional findings may include headache, cough, dyspnea, hoarseness, dysphagia, macular or petechial rash, and sub-conjunctival and retinal hemorrhages. Systemic symptoms usually peak within 2–3 weeks, and commonly persist for about 2 months. In severe cases, generally with large parasite burdens, muscle involvement can be pronounced, with severe muscle pain, edema, and weakness, especially in the head and neck. Muscle pain may persist for months. Uncommon severe findings include myocarditis, pneumonitis, and meningoencephalitis, sometimes leading to death.

B. Laboratory Findings

The clinical diagnosis is supported by findings of elevated serum muscle enzymes (creatine kinase, lactate dehydrogenase, aspartate aminotransferase). Serologic tests become positive 3 or more weeks after infection; a variety of techniques are used, including ELISA, immunofluorescence, indirect hemagglutinin, precipitin, and bentonite flocculation assays. Rising antibody titers are highly suggestive of the diagnosis. Muscle biopsy can usually be avoided, but if the diagnosis is uncertain, biopsy of a tender, swollen muscle may identify *Trichinella* larvae. For maximal yield, biopsy material should be examined histologically, and a portion should be enzymatically digested to release larvae, but evaluation before about 3 weeks after infection may not show muscle larvae.

Treatment

No effective specific therapy for full-blown trichinosis has been identified. However, if infection is suspected early in the course of illness, treatment with mebendazole (2.5 mg/kg orally twice daily) or albendazole (5–7.5 mg/kg orally twice daily) will kill intestinal worms and may limit progression to tissue invasion. Supportive therapy for systemic disease consists of analgesics, antipyretics, bed rest and, in severe illness, corticosteroids. Disease is prevented by adequate cooking or long-term freezing of pork and game. Irradiation of meat is also effective in eliminating *Trichinella* larvae.

McIntyre L et al. Trichinellosis from consumption of wild game meat. CMAJ. 2007 Feb 13;176(4):449–51. [PMID: 17296956]
Puljiz I et al. Electrocardiographic changes and myocarditis in trichinellosis: a retrospective study of 154 patients. Ann Trop Med Parasitol. 2005 Jun;99(4):403–11. [PMID: 15949188]
Watt G et al. Areas of uncertainty in the management of human trichinellosis: a clinical perspective. Expert Rev Anti Infect Ther. 2004 Aug;2(4):649–52. [PMID: 15482227]

ANGIOSTRONGYLIASIS

Nematodes of rats of the genus *Angiostrongylus* cause two distinct syndromes in humans. *Angiostrongylus cantonensis*, the rat lungworm, causes eosinophilic meningoencephalitis, primarily in Southeast Asia and some Pacific islands. *Angiostrongylus costaricensis* causes gastrointestinal inflammation. In both diseases, human infection follows ingestion of larvae within slugs or snails (and also crabs or prawns for *A cantonensis*) or on material contaminated by these organisms. Since the parasites are not in their natural hosts, they cannot complete their life cycles, but they can cause disease after migrating to the brain or gastrointestinal tract.

In *A cantonensis* infection, disease appears to be caused primarily by worm larvae migrating through the CNS and an inflammatory response to dying worms. After an incubation period of 1 day to 2 weeks, presenting symptoms and signs include headache, stiff neck, nausea, vomiting, cranial nerve abnormalities, and paresthesias. Most cases resolve spontaneously after 2–8 weeks, but serious sequelae and death have been reported. The diagnosis is strongly suggested by the finding of eosinophilic CSF pleocytosis (leukocytosis with over 10% eosinophils) in a patient with a history of travel to an endemic area. Peripheral eosinophilia may not be present. A cantonensis larvae have rarely been recovered from the CSF and the eyes. There is no specific treatment. Antihelminthic therapy is probably not indicated, since responses to dying worms may worsen with therapy. Corticosteroids have been used in severe cases.

In *A costaricensis* infection, parasites penetrate ileocecal vasculature and develop into adults, which lay eggs, but do not complete their life cycle. Disease is due to an inflammatory response to dying worms in the intestinal tract, with an eosinophilic granulomatous response, at times including vasculitis and ischemic necrosis. Common findings are abdominal pain, vomiting, and fever. Pain is most commonly localized to the right lower quadrant, and a mass may be appreciated, all mimicking appendicitis. Symptoms may recur over months. Uncommon findings are intestinal perforation or obstruction, or disease due to migration of worms to other sites. Many cases are managed surgically, usually for suspected appendicitis. Biopsy of inflamed intestinal tissue may show worms localized to mesenteric arteries and eosinophilic granulomas. It is not known if antihelminthic therapy is helpful, but diethylcarbamazine, thiabendazole, and mebendazole have been used.

Wang QP et al. Human angiostrongyliasis. Lancet Infect Dis. 2008 Oct;8(10):621–30. [PMID: 18922484]

GNATHOSTOMIASIS

A number of species of *Gnathostoma*, which are parasites of carnivores, can occasionally infect humans. Most cases have been seen in Southeast Asia, but the disease has also been described in many other areas. Eggs shed in the feces of mammals are ingested by marine crustaceans, which are then ingested by fish, frogs, snakes, or mammals. Larvae then encyst in muscles. Human infection follows eating undercooked fish, shellfish, chicken, or pork and can also be transmitted by ingesting copepods in contaminated water. After ingestion, larvae cannot complete development in humans, but rather migrate through tissues.

Acute gastrointestinal symptoms, including nausea, vomiting, abdominal pain, and fever, may develop soon after infection and persist for 2–3 weeks. The disease may then progress to findings consistent with cutaneous or visceral larva migrans. Migratory subcutaneous erythematous swellings may be painful or pruritic. Migrating larvae may also invade other tissues, leading to findings in the eyes, lungs, intestines, and elsewhere. The most serious complications are due to invasion of the CNS, leading to eosinophilic meningoencephalitis and other serious findings. Although a less common cause of eosinophilic meningitis than *A cantonensis* infection, gnathostomiasis tends to be more severe. Severe pain due to migration through spinal roots and focal neurologic findings may be seen. Symptoms are highly variable over time. CSF eosinophilic pleocytosis and peripheral eosinophilia are seen.

The diagnosis of gnathostomiasis is suggested by the history of intermittent subcutaneous swellings and typical CNS findings. Worms can occasionally be identified in skin lesions. Serologic tests may be helpful in establishing a diagnosis. Treatment is with ivermectin (200 mcg/kg orally single dose) or albendazole (400 mg/kg orally daily for 21 days); both treatments have reported cure rates over 90%.

Bhattacharjee H et al. Intravitreal gnathostomiasis and review of literature. Retina. 2007 Jan;27(1):67–73. [PMID: 17218918]
Bussaratid V et al. Efficacy of ivermectin treatment of cutaneous gnathostomiasis evaluated by placebo-controlled trial. Southeast Asian J Trop Med Public Health. 2006 May;37(3):433–40. [PMID: 17120960]
Nontasut P et al. Double-dose ivermectin vs albendazole for the treatment of gnathostomiasis. Southeast Asian J Trop Med Public Health. 2005 May;36(3):650–2. [PMID: 16124432]

TOXOCARIASIS

▶ General Considerations

The dog roundworm *Toxocara canis,* the cat roundworm *Toxocara cati,* and less commonly other helminths may cause visceral larva migrans. *T canis* is highly prevalent in dogs. Humans are infected after ingestion of eggs in material contaminated by dog or other feces. With *T canis,* infection is spread principally by puppies and lactating females, and the eggs must be on the ground for several weeks before they are infectious. After ingestion by humans, larvae migrate to various tissues but cannot complete their life cycle.

▶ Clinical Findings

Visceral larva migrans is seen principally in young children. Most infections are asymptomatic. The most commonly involved organs are the liver and lungs. Presentations include cough, fever, wheezing, hepatomegaly, splenomegaly, lymphadenopathy, pulmonary infiltrates, and eosinophilia. Involvement of the CNS can occur rarely, leading to eosinophilic meningitis and other abnormalities. Ocular larva migrans is a distinct syndrome, usually in children older than is typical for visceral larva migrans. Children present with visual deficits, pain, and a retinal mass, which can be confused with retinoblastoma. *Baylisascaris procyonis,* a roundworm of raccoons, can rarely cause visceral larva migrans in humans, with typically more severe manifestations than those with *T canis,* including eosinophilic meningitis and eye disease.

The diagnosis of visceral larva migrans is suggested by the finding of eosinophilia in a child with hepatomegaly or other signs of the disease, especially with a history of exposure to puppies. The diagnosis is confirmed by the identification of larvae in a biopsy of infected tissue, usually performed when other diseases are suspected. Serologic tests may be helpful; an available ELISA was estimated to have 78% sensitivity and 92% specificity. Most patients recover without specific therapy, although symptoms may persist for months.

▶ Treatment

Treatment with antihelminthics or corticosteroids may be considered in severe cases. No drugs have been proven to be effective, but albendazole (400 mg twice daily for 5 days), mebendazole, thiabendazole, diethylcarbamazine, and ivermectin have been used, and albendazole has been recommended as the treatment of choice.

Despommier D. Toxocariasis: clinical aspects, epidemiology, medical ecology, and molecular aspects. Clin Microbiol Rev. 2003 Apr;16(2):265–72. [PMID: 12692098]

Gavin PJ et al. Baylisascariasis. Clin Microbiol Rev. 2005 Oct; 18(4):703–18. [PMID: 16223954]

Good B et al. Ocular toxocariasis in schoolchildren. Clin Infect Dis. 2004 Jul 15;39(2):173–8. [PMID: 15307025]

CUTANEOUS LARVA MIGRANS (Creeping Eruption)

Cutaneous larva migrans is caused principally by larvae of the dog and cat hookworms, *Ancylostoma braziliense* and *A caninum.* Other animal hookworms, gnathostomiasis, and strongyloidiasis may also cause this syndrome. Infections are common in warm areas, including the southeastern United States. They are most common in children. The disease is caused by the migration of worms through skin;

the non-human parasites cannot complete their life cycles, so only cause cutaneous disease.

▶ Clinical Findings

Intensely pruritic erythematous papules develop, usually on the feet or hands, followed within a few days by serpiginous tracks marking the course of the parasite, which may travel several millimeters per day (Plate 118). Several tracks may be present. The process may continue for weeks, with lesions becoming vesiculated, encrusted, or secondarily infected. Systemic symptoms or eosinophilia are uncommon.

The diagnosis is based on the characteristic appearance of the lesions. Biopsy is usually not indicated.

▶ Treatment

Without treatment, the larvae eventually die and are absorbed. Mild cases do not require treatment. Thiabendazole (10% aqueous suspension) can be applied topically three times daily for 5 or more days. Systemic therapy with albendazole (400 mg orally once or twice daily for 3–5 days) or ivermectin (200 mcg/kg orally single dose) is highly effective.

Heukelbach J et al. Epidemiological and clinical characteristics of hookworm-related cutaneous larva migrans. Lancet Infect Dis. 2008 May;8(5):302–9. [PMID: 18471775]

ANISAKIASIS

Anisakiasis is caused by infection with larvae of saltwater fish and squid. Multiple species of the family *Anisakidae* may occasionally infect humans. Definitive hosts for these parasites are marine mammals. Eggs are passed in the feces and ingested by crustaceans, which are then eaten by fish and squid. When ingested by humans in undercooked seafood, larvae penetrate the stomach or intestinal wall but cannot complete their life cycle. The disease is most common in Japan.

▶ Clinical Findings

Clinical manifestations of anisakiasis follow burrowing of worms into the stomach or intestinal wall, leading to localized ulceration, edema, and eosinophilic granuloma formation. Symptoms usually occur within 2 days of parasite ingestion and include severe epigastric or abdominal pain, nausea, and vomiting. Intestinal involvement can mimic appendicitis. Allergic symptoms, including urticaria, angioedema, and anaphylaxis, have also been attributed to acute infection. Acute symptoms generally resolve within 2 weeks, but chronic symptoms may also be seen, suggesting chronic intestinal diseases such as inflammatory bowel disease, diverticulitis, or carcinoma. Rarely, worms may migrate to other sites or be coughed up. Eosinophilia is usually not seen.

The diagnosis of anisakiasis is suggested in those with acute abdominal symptoms after ingestion of raw fish. Radiographic studies may identify stomach or intestinal lesions, and endoscopy may allow visualization and removal of the worm. When surgery is performed due to consideration of other diagnoses, eosinophilic inflammatory lesions and the invading worms are found.

▶ Treatment

Specific therapy is not indicated, but endoscopic worm removal hastens recovery. The parasites are killed by cooking or deep freezing fish.

Pellegrini M et al. Acute abdomen due to small bowel anisakiasis. Dig Liver Dis. 2005 Jan;37(1):65–7. [PMID: 15702863]
Takei H et al. Intestinal anisakidosis (anisakiosis). Ann Diagn Pathol. 2007 Oct;11(5):350–2. [PMID: 1787002]

FILARIASIS

LYMPHATIC FILARIASIS

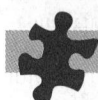

ESSENTIALS OF DIAGNOSIS

▶ Episodic attacks of lymphangitis, lymphadenitis, and fever.

▶ Chronic progressive swelling of extremities and genitals; hydrocele; chyluria; lymphedema.

▶ Microfilariae in blood, chyluria, or hydrocele fluid; positive serologic tests.

Lymphatic filariasis is caused by three filarial nematodes: *Wuchereria bancrofti*, *Brugia malayi*, and *Brugia timori*, and is among the most important parasitic diseases of man. Approximately 120 million people are infected with these organisms in tropical and subtropical countries, about a third of these suffer clinical consequences of the infections, and many are seriously disfigured. *W bancrofti* causes about 90% of episodes of lymphatic filariasis. It is transmitted by *Culex, Aedes,* and *Anopheles* mosquitoes and is widely distributed in the tropics and subtropics, including subsaharan Africa, Southeast Asia, the western Pacific, India, South America, and the Caribbean. *B malayi* is transmitted by *Mansonia* and *Anopheles* mosquitoes and is endemic in parts of China, India, Southeast Asia, and the Pacific. *B timori* is found only in islands of southeastern Indonesia.

Humans are infected by the bites of infected mosquitoes. Larvae then move to the lymphatics and lymph nodes, where they mature over months to thread-like adult worms, and then can persist for many years. The adult worms produce large numbers of microfilariae, which are released into the circulation, and infective to mosquitoes, particularly at night (except for the South Pacific, where microfilaremia peaks during daylight hours).

▶ Clinical Findings

A. Symptoms and Signs

Many infections remain asymptomatic despite circulating microfilariae. Clinical consequences of filarial infection are principally due to inflammatory responses to developing, mature, and dying worms. The initial manifestation of infection is often acute lymphangitis, with fever, painful lymph nodes, edema, and inflammation spreading peripherally from involved lymph nodes (in contrast to bacterial lymphangitis, which spreads centrally). Lymphangitis and lymphadenitis of the upper and lower extremities is common (Plate 119); genital involvement, including epididymitis and orchitis, with scrotal pain and tenderness, occurs principally only with *W bancrofti* infection. Acute attacks of lymphangitis last for a few days to a week and may recur a few times per year. Filarial fevers may also occur without lymphatic inflammation.

The most common chronic manifestation of lymphatic filariasis is swelling of the extremities or genitals due to chronic lymphatic inflammation and obstruction. Extremities become increasingly swollen, with a progression over time from pitting edema, to nonpitting edema, to sclerotic changes of the skin that are referred to as elephantiasis. Genital involvement, particularly with *W bancrofti*, occurs more commonly in men, progressing from painful epididymitis to hydroceles that are usually painless but can become very large, with inguinal lymphadenopathy, thickening of the spermatic cord, scrotal lymphedema, thickening and fissuring of the scrotal skin, and occasionally chyluria. Lymphedema of the female genitalia and breasts may also occur.

Tropical pulmonary eosinophilia is a distinct syndrome principally affecting young adult males with either *W bancrofti* or *B malayi* infection but typically without microfilaremia. This syndrome is characterized by asthma-like symptoms, with cough, wheezing, dyspnea, and low-grade fevers, usually at night. Without treatment, tropical pulmonary eosinophilia can progress to interstitial fibrosis and chronic restrictive lung disease.

B. Laboratory Findings

The diagnosis of lymphatic filariasis is strongly suggested by characteristic findings of lymphangitis or lymphatic obstruction in persons with risk factors for the disease. The diagnosis is confirmed by finding microfilariae, usually in blood, but this may be difficult. In addition, microfilariae may be absent, especially early in the disease progression (first 2–3 years) or with chronic obstructive disease. To increase yields, blood samples are obtained at about midnight in most areas, but not in the South Pacific, where microfilaremia is diurnal. Smears are evaluated by wet mount to identify motile parasites and by Giemsa staining; these examinations can be delayed until the following morning, with storage of samples at room temperature. Of note, the periodicity of microfilaremia is variable, and daytime samples may yield positive results. Microfilariae may also be identified in hydrocele fluid or chylous urine. Eosinophilia is usually absent, except during acute inflammatory syndromes. Available serologic tests, including bentonite flocculation, indirect hemagglutination, ELISA, and indirect fluorescent antibody tests, may be helpful but cannot distinguish between past and active infections. Rapid antigen tests with sensitivity and specificity over 90% are available. Adult worms may also be found in lymph node biopsy specimens (although biopsy is not usually clinically indicated) or by ultrasound of a scrotal hydrocele or lymphedematous breast. When microfilaremia is lacking, especially if sophisticated techniques are not available, diagnoses may need to be made on clinical grounds alone.

Treatment & Control

A. Drug Treatment

Treatment is somewhat controversial, as no drug can fully control or reverse the disease, and treatment may cause serious acute inflammatory symptoms. Diethylcarbamazine is the drug of choice, but it cannot cure infections due to its limited action against adult worms. Asymptomatic infection and acute lymphangitis are treated with this drug (2 mg/kg orally three times daily) for 10–14 days, leading to a marked decrease in microfilaremia. Therapy may be accompanied by allergic symptoms, including fever, headache, malaise, hypotension, and bronchospasm, probably due to release of antigens from dying worms. For this reason, treatment courses may begin with a lower dosage, with escalation over the first 4 days of treatment. Single annual doses of diethylcarbamazine (6 mg/kg orally), alone or with ivermectin (400 mcg/kg orally) or albendazole (400 mg orally) may be as effective as longer courses of diethylcarbamazine. When onchocerciasis or loiasis is suspected, it may be appropriate to withhold diethylcarbamazine to avoid severe reactions to dying microfilariae; rather, ivermectin plus albendazole may be given, although these drugs are less active than diethylcarbamazine against adult worms. Appropriate management of advanced obstructive disease is uncertain. Drainage of hydroceles provides symptomatic relief, although they will recur. Therapy with diethylcarbamazine cannot reverse chronic lymphatic changes but is typically provided to lower worm burdens. An interesting approach under study is to treat with doxycycline (100–200 mg/d orally for 4–6 weeks), which kills obligate intracellular *Wolbachia* bacteria, leading to death of adult filarial worms. Secondary bacterial infections must be treated. Surgical correction may be helpful in some cases.

B. Disease Control

Avoidance of mosquitoes is a key measure; preventive measures include the use of screens, bed nets (ideally treated with insecticide), and insect repellents. Community-based treatment with single annual doses of effective drugs offers a highly effective means of control. The current WHO strategy for control includes mass treatment of at risk communities with single annual doses of diethylcarbamazine plus albendazole or, for areas with onchocerciasis, albendazole plus ivermectin.

Hoerauf A. Filariasis: new drugs and new opportunities for lymphatic filariasis and onchocerciasis. Curr Opin Infect Dis. 2008 Dec;21(6):673–81. [PMID: 18978537]

Johnston KL et al. *Wolbachia* in filarial parasites: targets for filarial infection and disease control. Curr Infect Dis Rep. 2007 Jan;9(1):55–9. [PMID: 17254505]

Ottesen EA et al. The global programme to eliminate lymphatic filariasis: health impact after 8 years. PLoS Negl Trop Dis. 2008 Oct 8;2(10):e317. [PMID: 18841205]

Supali T et al. Doxycycline treatment of *Brugia malayi*-infected persons reduces microfilaremia and adverse reactions after diethylcarbamazine and albendazole treatment. Clin Infect Dis. 2008 May 1;46(9):1385–93. [PMID: 18419441]

Tisch DJ et al. Mass chemotherapy options to control lymphatic filariasis: a systematic review. Lancet Infect Dis. 2005 Aug;5(8):514–23. [PMID: 16048720]

ONCHOCERCIASIS

 ESSENTIALS OF DIAGNOSIS

▶ Severe pruritus, skin excoriations, pigment changes, nodules, and thickening.

▶ Conjunctivitis progressing to severe eye disease and blindness.

▶ Microfilariae in skin snips and on slit-lamp examination; adult worms in subcutaneous nodules.

General Considerations

Onchocerciasis, or river blindness is caused by *Onchocerca volvulus*. An estimated 18 million persons are infected, of whom 3–4 million have skin disease, 500,000 have severe visual impairment, and 300,000 are blinded. Over 99% of infections are in subsaharan Africa, especially the West African savanna, with about half of cases in Nigeria and Congo. In some hyperendemic African villages, close to 100% of individuals are infected, and 10% or more of the population is blind. The disease is also prevalent in the southwestern Arabian peninsula and Latin America, including southern Mexico, Guatemala, Venezuela, Colombia, Ecuador, and northwestern Brazil. Onchocerciasis is transmitted by simulium flies (blackflies). These insects breed in fast-flowing streams and bite during the day.

After the bite of an infected blackfly, larvae are deposited in the skin, where adults develop over 6–12 months. Adult worms live in subcutaneous connective tissue or muscle nodules for a decade or more. Microfilariae are released from the nodules and migrate through subcutaneous and ocular tissues. Disease is due to responses to worms and to intracellular *Wolbachia* bacteria.

Clinical Findings

A. Symptoms and Signs

After an incubation period of up to 1–3 years, the disease typically produces an erythematous, papular, pruritic rash, which may progress to chronic skin thickening and depigmentation. Itching may be severe and unresponsive to medications, such that more disability-adjusted life years are lost to onchocercal skin problems than to blindness. Numerous firm, nontender, movable subcutaneous nodules of about 0.5–3 cm, which contain adult worms, may be present. Due to differences in vector habits, these nodules are more commonly on the lower body in Africa but on the head and upper body in Latin America. Inguinal and femoral lymphadenopathy is common, at times resulting in a "hanging groin," with lymph nodes hanging within a sling of atrophic skin. Patients may also have systemic symptoms, with weight loss and musculoskeletal pain.

The most serious manifestations of onchocerciasis involve the eyes. Microfilariae migrating through the eyes elicit host responses that lead to pathology. Findings include punctate keratitis and corneal opacities, progressing to sclerosing keratitis and blindness. Iridocyclitis, glaucoma, choroiditis, and optic atrophy may also lead to vision loss. The likelihood of blindness after infection varies greatly based on geography, with the risk greatest in savanna regions of West Africa.

B. Diagnostic Testing

The diagnosis is made by identifying microfilariae in skin snips, by visualizing microfilariae in the cornea or anterior chamber by slit-lamp examination, by identification of adult worms in a biopsy or aspirate of a nodule or, uncommonly, by identification of microfilariae in urine. Skin snips from the iliac crest (Africa) or scapula (Americas) are allowed to stand in saline for 2–4 hours or longer, and then examined microscopically for microfilariae. Deep punch biopsies are not needed, and if suspicion persists after a skin snip is negative, the procedure should be repeated. Ultrasound may identify characteristic findings suggestive of adult worms in skin nodules. When the diagnosis remains difficult, the Mazzoti test can be used. In this test, a 50-mg dose of diethylcarbamazine is given. A positive test, with exacerbation of skin rash and pruritus, usually within 3 hours, is highly suggestive of the diagnosis. This test should only be used in suspected lightly infected patients (after other tests are negative), as this treatment can elicit severe skin and eye reactions in heavily infected individuals. A related and safer test using topical diethylcarbamazine is available in some areas. Eosinophilia is a common, but inconsistent finding. Serologic tests are poorly standardized, nonspecific, and generally unhelpful, as in endemic areas positivity is not indicative of acute disease.

▶ Treatment & Control

The treatment of choice is ivermectin, which has replaced diethylcarbamazine due to a much lower risk of severe reactions to therapy. Ivermectin kills microfilariae, but not adult worms, so disease control requires repeat administrations. Treatment is with a single oral dose of 150 mcg/mL, but schedules for re-treatment have not been standardized. One regimen is to treat every 3 months for 1 year, followed by treatment every 6–12 months for the suspected lifespan of adult worms (about 15 years). Treatment results in marked reduction in numbers of microfilariae in the skin and eyes, although its impact on the progression of visual loss remains uncertain. Toxicities of ivermectin are generally mild; fever, pruritus, urticaria, myalgias, edema, hypotension, and tender lymphadenopathy may be seen, presumably due to reactions to dying worms. Ivermectin should be used with caution in patients also at risk for

loiasis, since it can elicit severe reactions including encephalopathy. In patients with severe skin findings not controlled by ivermectin, therapy with suramin may be considered. This is the only drug known to kill adult worms, but it is very toxic. As with other filarial infections, doxycycline acts against *O volvulus* by killing intracellular *Wolbachia* bacteria. A course of 100 mg/day for 6 weeks kills the bacteria and prevents parasite embryogenesis for at least 18 months. Doxycycline is under study for onchocerciasis control but has no clear role in treatment of individual affected patients.

Protection against onchocerciasis includes avoidance of biting flies. Major efforts are underway to control insect vectors in Africa. In addition, mass distribution of ivermectin for intermittent administration at the community level is ongoing, and the prevalence of severe skin and eye disease is decreasing.

Basáñez MG et al. Effect of single-dose ivermectin on *Onchocerca volvulus*: a systematic review and meta-analysis. Lancet Infect Dis. 2008 May;8(5):310–22. [PMID: 18471776]

Boatin BA et al. Control of onchocerciasis. Adv Parasitol. 2006;61:349–94. [PMID: 16735169]

Osei-Atweneboana MY et al. Prevalence and intensity of *Onchocerca volvulus* infection and efficacy of ivermectin in endemic communities in Ghana: a two-phase epidemiological study. Lancet. 2007 Jun 16;369(9578):2021–9. [PMID: 17574093]

Udall DN. Recent updates on onchocerciasis: diagnosis and treatment. Clin Infect Dis. 2007 Jan 1;44(1):53–60. [PMID: 17143815]

LOIASIS

ESSENTIALS OF DIAGNOSIS

▶ Subcutaneous swellings; adult worms migrating across the eye.

▶ Encephalitis, which may be brought on by treatment.

▶ Microfilariae in the blood.

▶ General Considerations

Loiasis is a chronic filarial disease caused by infection with *Loa loa*. The infection occurs in humans and monkeys in rainforest areas of West and central Africa. An estimated 3–13 million persons are infected. The disease is transmitted by chrysops flies, which bite during the day. Over 6–12 months after infection, larvae develop into adult worms, which migrate through subcutaneous tissues, including the subconjunctiva (leading to the term "eye worm"). Adults can live for up to 17 years.

▶ Clinical Findings

A. Symptoms and Signs

Many infected persons are asymptomatic, although they may have high levels of microfilaremia and eosinophilia. Transient subcutaneous swellings (Calabar swellings) develop in symptomatic persons. The swellings are nonerythematous, up to 20 cm in diameter, and may be preceded by local pain or pruritus. They usually resolve after 2–4 days but occasionally persist for several weeks. Calabar swellings are commonly seen around joints and may recur at the same or different sites. Visitors from nonendemic areas are more likely to have allergic-type reactions, including pruritus, urticaria, and angioedema. Adult worms may be seen to migrate across the eye, with either no symptoms or conjunctivitis, with pain and edema. The most serious complication of loiasis is encephalitis, which is most common in those with high level microfilaremia and microfilariae in the CSF. Symptoms may range from headache and insomnia to coma and death. Encephalitis may be brought on by treatment with diethylcarbamazine or ivermectin. Other complications of loiasis include kidney disease, with hematuria and proteinuria; endomyocardial fibrosis; and peripheral neuropathy.

B. Laboratory Findings

The diagnosis is established by identifying microfilariae in blood. Blood is evaluated as for lymphatic filariasis, but for loiasis blood should be obtained during the day. The failure to find microfilariae does not rule out the diagnosis. Identification of a migrating eye worm is also diagnostic. Serologic tests may be helpful in persons from nonendemic areas who may be acutely ill without detectable microfilaremia, but such tests have limited utility for residents of endemic areas because most of them will have positive test results. Diagnostic PCR methods have been described.

▶ Treatment

The treatment of choice is diethylcarbamazine, which eliminates microfilariae and has some activity against adult worms. Treatment with 8–10 mg/kg/d orally for 21 days is curative in about 50% of amicrofilaremic patients, and repeat courses increase efficacy. Mild side effects are common with therapy, including fever, pruritus, arthralgias, nausea, diarrhea, and Calabar swellings. These symptoms may be lessened by administration of antihistamines or corticosteroids. Patients with large worm burdens are at greater risk for serious complications of therapy, including kidney injury, shock, encephalitis, coma, and death. Treatment with ivermectin, which is highly active against microfilariae, but not adult worms, also entails a high risk of severe reactions. To attempt to avoid these sequelae, pretreatment with corticosteroids and antihistamines, and escalating dosage of diethylcarbamazine have been used, but this strategy does not prevent encephalitis. The circulating parasite load that indicates particular risk for severe complications with therapy has been estimated at 2500/mL or greater. Strategies to treat patients with high parasite loads include (1) no treatment; (2) apheresis, if available, to remove microfilariae prior to therapy with diethylcarbamazine; or (3) therapy with albendazole, which appears to be well tolerated due to its slow antiparasitic effects, prior to therapy with diethylcarbamazine or ivermectin.

Boussinesq M. Loiasis. Ann Trop Med Parasitol. 2006 Dec;100(8):715–31. [PMID: 17227650]

Padgett JJ et al. Loiasis: African eye worm. Trans R Soc Trop Med Hyg. 2008 Oct;102(10):983–9. [PMID: 18466939]

Mycotic Infections

Samuel A. Shelburne, MD

Richard J. Hamill, MD

Fungal infections have assumed an increasingly important role as use of broad-spectrum antimicrobial agents has increased and the number of immunodeficient patients has risen. Some pathogens (eg, *Cryptococcus, Candida, Pneumocystis, Fusarium*) rarely cause serious disease in normal hosts. Other endemic fungi (eg, *Histoplasma, Coccidioides, Paracoccidioides*) commonly cause disease in normal hosts but tend to be more aggressive in immunocompromised ones. Superficial mycoses are discussed in Chapter 6.

Successful management of most systemic fungal infections requires knowledge of the natural history of these diseases as well as familiarity with the unique pharmacokinetics, adverse effects, and drug interactions of the various therapeutic agents. Furthermore, most affected individuals usually have significant underlying illnesses. Consequently, clinicians with extensive experience in the management of these disorders should be consulted.

CANDIDIASIS

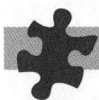 ESSENTIALS OF DIAGNOSIS

▶ Common normal flora but opportunistic pathogen.

▶ Gastrointestinal mucosal disease, particularly esophagitis, most common.

▶ Catheter-associated fungemia occurs in patients who have sustained mucosal injury or received broad-spectrum antibiotics.

▶ General Considerations

Candida albicans can be cultured from the mouth, vagina, and feces of most people. Cutaneous and oral lesions are discussed in Chapters 6 and 8, respectively. The risk factors for invasive candidiasis include prolonged neutropenia, recent abdominal surgery, broad-spectrum antibiotic therapy, advanced chronic kidney disease, the presence of intravascular catheters (especially when providing total parenteral nutrition), and injection drug use. Cellular immunodeficiency predisposes to mucocutaneous disease.

When no other underlying cause is found, persistent oral or vaginal candidiasis should arouse a suspicion of HIV infection.

▶ Clinical Findings & Treatment

A. Mucosal Candidiasis

Esophageal involvement is the most frequent type of significant mucosal disease. Presenting symptoms include substernal odynophagia, gastroesophageal reflux, or nausea without substernal pain. Oral candidiasis, though often associated, is not invariably present. Diagnosis is best confirmed by endoscopy with biopsy and culture. Therapy depends on the severity of disease. If patients are able to swallow and take adequate amounts of fluid orally, fluconazole, 100 mg/d (or itraconazole solution, 10 mg/mL, 200 mg/d), for 10–14 days will usually suffice. In the individual who is more ill or in whom esophagitis has developed while taking fluconazole, options include oral or intravenous voriconazole, 200 mg twice daily; intravenous amphotericin B, 0.3 mg/kg/d; intravenous caspofungin, 50 mg/d; intravenous anidulafungin, 100 mg on day 1, then 50 mg/d; or intravenous micafungin, 150 mg/d. Relapse is common with all agents when there is underlying HIV infection without adequate immune reconstitution.

Vulvovaginal candidiasis occurs in an estimated 75% of women during their lifetime. Risk factors include pregnancy, uncontrolled diabetes mellitus, broad-spectrum antimicrobial treatment, corticosteroid use, and HIV infection. Symptoms include acute vulvar pruritus, burning vaginal discharge, and dyspareunia. Various topical azole preparations (eg, clotrimazole, 100 mg vaginal tablet for 7 days, or miconazole, 200 mg vaginal suppository for 3 days) are effective. One 150 mg oral dose of fluconazole has been shown to have equivalent efficacy with better patient acceptance. Disease recurrence is common but can be decreased with weekly fluconazole therapy (150 mg weekly).

B. Candidal Funguria

Candidal funguria frequently resolves with discontinuance of antibiotics or removal of bladder catheters. Clinical benefit from treatment of asymptomatic candiduria has not been demonstrated, but persistent funguria should raise the suspicion of disseminated infection. When symptomatic funguria persists, oral fluconazole, 200 mg/d for 7–14 days, can be used. Rare complications of candidal urinary tract infections are ureteral obstruction and dissemination.

C. Disseminated Candidiasis

The diagnosis of disseminated *Candida* infection is problematic because *Candida* species are often isolated from mucosal sites in the absence of invasive disease while blood cultures are positive only 50% of the time in disseminated infection. Serologic tests have not proved useful for distinguishing colonization from invasive disease. Thus, the decision to treat for *Candida* when organisms are isolated from urine or sputum (or both) needs to be individualized for each patient. A randomized trial of empiric fluconazole for patients at high risk for, but not proven to have, disseminated candidiasis showed no clinical benefit compared with placebo. Disseminated candidiasis may represent a benign, self-limited process, but until proven otherwise it should be considered a sign of serious, complicated disease.

Organ system involvement in invasive disease may include the eyes, skin, brain, meninges, and myocardium. Antifungal therapy for invasive candidiasis is rapidly evolving with the addition of new agents and the emergence of non-*albicans* species causing significant disease. Options for treatment include fluconazole, 400–800 mg daily; amphotericin B, 0.7 mg/kg/d; liposomal amphotericin B, 3 mg/kg/d; voriconazole, 200 mg twice a day; caspofungin, 50 mg/d; micafungin, 100 mg daily; or anidulafungin, 100 mg/d after 200 mg intravenously once. Therapy for disseminated candidiasis should be continued for 2 weeks after the last positive blood culture and resolution of symptoms and signs of infection. Once patients have become clinically stable, parenteral therapy can be discontinued and oral fluconazole, 200–800 mg orally given as one or two doses daily, is used to complete treatment. Removal or exchange of intravascular catheters is generally recommended and substantially decreases the duration of candidemia and overall mortality, which approaches 30%.

Another form of invasive disease is hepatosplenic candidiasis. This results from aggressive chemotherapy and prolonged neutropenia in patients with underlying hematologic cancers. Typically, fever and variable abdominal pain present weeks after chemotherapy, when neutrophil counts have recovered. Blood cultures are generally negative. Hepatic enzymes reveal an alkaline phosphatase elevation that may be marked. Fluconazole, 400 mg daily, or a lipid formulation of amphotericin B should be given until clinical and radiographic improvement occurs.

D. Candidal Endocarditis

Candidal endocarditis rarely is a complication of transient fungemia. It usually results from direct inoculation at the time of valvular heart surgery or repeated inoculation with injection drug use. Candidal endocarditis occurs with increased frequency on prosthetic valves in the first few months following surgery. Splenomegaly and petechiae are common, and there is a predilection for large-vessel embo-

lization. The diagnosis is established definitively by culturing *Candida* from emboli or from vegetations at the time of valve replacement. Valve destruction (usually aortic or mitral), myocardial ring abscess, and systemic embolization are common. Amphotericin has long been considered the optimal therapy, given in a dosage of 0.5–1 mg/kg/d intravenously, although there are now more and more data regarding the utility of echinocandin and imidazole.

Non-*albicans* species of *Candida* now account for over 50% of clinical bloodstream isolates and are often resistant to imidazole antibiotics such as fluconazole. The widespread use of these agents for prophylaxis in immunocompromised patients can lead to the emergence of pathogens such as *Candida krusei*. Azole-resistant *C albicans* has increased in frequency in immunocompromised patients, particularly in patients with late-stage AIDS receiving long-term suppressive fluconazole.

In all forms of invasive candidiasis, an important element of therapy is reversal of the underlying predisposing factor when possible. In high-risk patients undergoing induction chemotherapy, bone marrow transplantation, or liver transplantation, prophylaxis with antifungal agents has been shown to prevent invasive fungal infections although the effect on mortality and the preferred agent remain debated.

Baddley JW et al; International Collaboration on Endocarditis-Prospective Cohort Study Group (ICE-PCS). Candida infective endocarditis. Eur J Clin Microbiol Infect Dis. 2008 July;27(7):519–29. [PMID: 18283504]

Schuster MG et al. Empirical fluconazole versus placebo for intensive care unit patients: a randomized trial. Ann Intern Med. 2008 Jul 15;149(2):83–90. [PMID: 18626047]

Vazquez JA et al. A phase 2, open-label study of the safety and efficacy of intravenous anidulafungin as a treatment for azole-refractory mucosal candidiasis. J Acquir Immune Defic Syndr. 2008 Jul 1;48(3):304–9. [PMID: 18545153]

HISTOPLASMOSIS

ESSENTIALS OF DIAGNOSIS

▶ Epidemiologically linked to bird droppings and bat exposure; common along river valleys (especially the Ohio River and the Mississippi River valleys).

▶ Most patients asymptomatic; respiratory illness most common clinical problem.

▶ Widespread disease especially common in AIDS or other immunosuppressed states, with poor prognosis.

▶ Biopsy of affected organs with culture or urinary polysaccharide antigen most useful in disseminated disease.

▶ General Considerations

Histoplasmosis is caused by *Histoplasma capsulatum*, a dimorphic fungus that has been isolated from soil contaminated with bird or bat droppings in endemic areas (central and eastern United States, eastern Canada, Mexico, Central America, South America, Africa, and southeast Asia). Infection presumably takes place by inhalation of conidia. These convert into small budding cells that are engulfed by phagocytes in the lungs. The organism proliferates and is carried hematogenously to other organs.

▶ Clinical Findings

A. Symptoms and Signs

Most cases of histoplasmosis are asymptomatic or mild and thus go unrecognized. Past infection is recognized by pulmonary and splenic calcification noted on incidental radiographs. Symptoms and signs of pulmonary involvement are usually absent even in patients who subsequently show areas of calcification on chest radiographs. Symptomatic infection may present with mild influenza-like illness, often lasting 1–4 days. Moderately severe infections are frequently diagnosed as atypical pneumonia. These patients have fever, cough, and mild central chest pain lasting 5–15 days.

Clinically evident infections occur in several forms: (1) **Acute histoplasmosis** frequently occurs in epidemics, often when soil containing infected bird or bat droppings is disturbed. It is a severe disease manifested by marked prostration, fever, and relatively few pulmonary complaints even when radiographs show diffuse pneumonia. The illness may last from 1 week to 6 months but is almost never fatal. (2) **Progressive disseminated histoplasmosis** is usually fatal within 6 weeks or less. Symptoms usually consist of fever, dyspnea, cough, loss of weight, and prostration. Ulcers of the mucous membranes of the oropharynx may be present. The liver and spleen are nearly always enlarged, and all the organs of the body are involved, particularly the adrenal glands, though this infrequently results in adrenal insufficiency. Gastrointestinal involvement may mimic inflammatory bowel disease. (3) **Chronic progressive pulmonary histoplasmosis** is usually seen in older patients with various lesions including apical cavities, infiltrates, and nodules found on radiographs. (4) **Disseminated disease** usually occurs in the profoundly immunocompromised person but can affect immunocompetent persons as well. This form is commonly seen in patients with underlying HIV infection—with CD4 cell counts usually < 100 cells/mcL—and is characterized by fever and multiple organ system involvement. Chest radiographs may show a miliary pattern. Presentation may be fulminant, simulating septic shock, with death ensuing rapidly unless treatment is provided.

B. Laboratory Findings

Most patients with progressive pulmonary disease show anemia of chronic disease. Bone marrow involvement may be prominent in disseminated forms with occurrence of pancytopenia. Alkaline phosphatase and marked lactate dehydrogenase (LDH) and ferritin elevations are also common as are mild elevations of serum aspartate aminotransferase, although alanine aminotransferase is often normal.

In pulmonary disease, sputum culture is rarely positive except in chronic disease; antigen testing of bronchoalveolar lavage fluid may be helpful in acute disease. Blood or bone marrow cultures from immunocompromised patients with acute disseminated disease are positive more than 80% of the time but may take several weeks. A urine antigen assay has a sensitivity of greater than 90% for disseminated disease in AIDS patients and can be used to follow response to therapy. The sensitivity of screening immunodiffusion is 70% in acute pulmonary histoplasmosis, and complement fixation titers are positive in about 80% of cases. Patients with disseminated histoplasmosis may have a false-positive *Aspergillus* galactomannan assay.

▶ Treatment

For progressive localized disease and for mild to moderately severe nonmeningeal disseminated disease in immunocompetent or immunocompromised patients, itraconazole, 200–400 mg/d orally divided into two doses, is the treatment of choice with an overall response rate of approximately 80%. The oral solution is better absorbed than the capsule formulation. Duration of therapy ranges from weeks to several months depending on the severity of illness. Amphotericin B is reserved for individuals who cannot take oral medications; for those who have not responded to itraconazole therapy; for those with meningitis; and for management of severe disseminated disease in an immunocompromised person. Up to 2.5 g total may need to be given in the latter two situations, though this course of treatment can be abbreviated and oral itraconazole instituted once clinical stabilization has occurred. Liposomal amphotericin B in a dosage of 3 mg/kg/d intravenously may be more effective and safer than conventional amphotericin B in seriously ill individuals. Patients with AIDS-related histoplasmosis require lifelong suppressive therapy with itraconazole, 200–400 mg/d orally, although secondary prophylaxis may be discontinued if immune reconstitution occurs in response to antiretroviral therapy.

Huber F et al. AIDS-related *Histoplasma capsulatum* var. *capsulatum* infection: 25 years experience of French Guiana. AIDS. 2008 May 31;22(9):1047–53. [PMID: 18520348]

Wheat LJ et al. Clinical practice guidelines for the management of patients with histoplasmosis: 2007 update by the Infectious Diseases Society of America. Clin Infect Dis. 2007 Oct;45 (7):807–25. [PMID: 17806045]

COCCIDIOIDOMYCOSIS

ESSENTIALS OF DIAGNOSIS

- ▶ Influenza-like illness with malaise, fever, backache, headache, and cough.
- ▶ Erythema nodosum common with acute infection.
- ▶ Dissemination may result in meningitis, bony lesions, or skin and soft tissue abscesses.
- ▶ Chest radiograph findings vary widely from pneumonitis to cavitation.
- ▶ Serologic tests useful; spherules containing endospores demonstrable in sputum or tissues.

General Considerations

Coccidioidomycosis should be considered in the diagnosis of any obscure illness in a patient who has lived in or visited an endemic area.

Infection results from the inhalation of arthroconidia of *Coccidioides immitis* or *Coccidioides posadasii*; both organisms are molds that grow in soil in certain arid regions of the southwestern United States, in Mexico, and in Central and South America.

Less than 1% of immunocompetent persons show dissemination, but among these patients, the mortality rate is high.

In HIV-infected people in endemic areas, coccidioidomycosis is a common opportunistic infection. In these patients, disease manifestations range from focal pulmonary infiltrates to widespread miliary disease with multiple organ involvement and meningitis.

Clinical Findings

A. Symptoms and Signs

Symptoms of primary coccidioidomycosis occur in about 40% of infections. Symptom onset (after an incubation period of 10–30 days) is usually that of a respiratory tract illness with fever and occasionally chills, and coccidioidomycosis is a common etiology of community-acquired pneumonia in endemic areas.

Arthralgia accompanied by periarticular swelling, often of the knees and ankles, is common. Erythema nodosum may appear 2–20 days after onset of symptoms. Persistent pulmonary lesions, varying from cavities and abscesses to parenchymal nodular densities or bronchiectasis, occur in about 5% of diagnosed cases.

Disseminated disease occurs in about 0.1% of white and 1% of nonwhite patients. Filipinos and blacks are especially susceptible, as are pregnant women of all races. Any organ may be involved. Pulmonary findings usually become more pronounced, with mediastinal lymph node enlargement, cough, and increased sputum production. Lung abscesses may rupture into the pleural space, producing an empyema. These may also extend to bones and skin, and pericardial and myocardial involvement has been occasionally observed. Fungemia may occur and is characterized clinically by a diffuse miliary pattern on chest radiograph and by early death. The course may be particularly rapid in immunosuppressed patients. Physicians caring for immunosuppressed patients in endemic areas need to consider that patients may be latently infected.

Bone lesions most often occur at bony prominences. Meningitis occurs in 30–50% of cases of dissemination. Subcutaneous abscesses and verrucous skin lesions are especially common in fulminating cases. Lymphadenitis may occur and may progress to suppuration. HIV-infected persons with disseminated disease have a higher incidence of miliary infiltrates, lymphadenopathy, and meningitis, but skin lesions are uncommon.

B. Laboratory Findings

In primary coccidioidomycosis, there may be moderate leukocytosis and eosinophilia. Serologic testing is useful for both diagnosis and prognosis. The immunodiffusion tube precipitin test detects IgM antibodies and is useful for diagnosis early in the disease process. Historically, a persistent rising IgG complement fixation titer ($\geq$ 1:16) has been considered suggestive of disseminated disease; in addition, complement fixation titers can be used to assess the adequacy of therapy. Serum complement fixation titer may be low when there is meningitis but no other disseminated disease. In patients with HIV-related coccidioidomycosis, the false-negative rate may be as high as 30%.

Demonstrable complement-fixing antibodies in spinal fluid are diagnostic of coccidioidal meningitis. These are found in over 90% of cases. Spinal fluid findings include increased cell count with lymphocytosis and reduced glucose. Spinal fluid culture is positive in approximately 30% of meningitis cases. Spherules filled with endospores may be found in biopsy specimens; though they are not infectious, they convert to the highly contagious arthroconidia when grown in culture media. Blood cultures are rarely positive. A urine antigen test similar to that for histoplasmosis has been developed for coccidioidomycosis; however, there is cross-reactivity of this test for the two diseases.

C. Imaging

Radiographic findings vary, but patchy, nodular pulmonary infiltrates and thin-walled cavities are most common. Hilar lymphadenopathy may be visible and is seen in localized disease; mediastinal lymphadenopathy suggests dissemination. There may be pleural effusions and lytic lesions in bone with accompanying complicated soft-tissue collections.

Treatment

General symptomatic therapy is given as needed for disease limited to the chest with no evidence of progression. For progressive pulmonary or extrapulmonary disease, amphotericin B intravenously is used although oral azoles may be used for mild cases (see Chapter 30). Therapy should be continued, with duration of therapy determined by a declining complement fixation titer and a favorable clinical response. For meningitis, treatment usually is with high-dose oral fluconazole (400–800 mg/d) although lumbar or cisternal intrathecal administration of amphotericin B daily in increasing doses up to 1–1.5 mg/d is used initially by some physicians or in cases refractory to fluconazole. Systemic therapy with amphotericin B, 0.6 mg/kg/d intravenously, is generally given concurrently with intrathecal therapy but is not sufficient alone for the treatment of meningeal disease. Voriconazole or posaconazole may be alternatives to intrathecal amphotericin B in patients who do not respond to fluconazole. Once the patient is clinically stable, oral therapy with an azole, usually lifelong, is the recommended alternative to intrathecal amphotericin B therapy.

Fluconazole, 200–400 mg orally once daily, or itraconazole, 400 mg orally daily divided into two doses, may be given for disease in the chest, bones, and soft tissues; however, therapy must be continued for 6 months or longer after the disease is inactive to prevent relapse. Response to therapy should be monitored by following the progressive decrease in serum complement fixation titers.

Thoracic surgery is occasionally indicated for giant, infected, or ruptured cavities. Surgical drainage is necessary for management of soft tissue abscesses and bone disease. Amphotericin B, 1 mg/kg/d intravenously, is advisable following extensive surgical manipulation of infected tissue until the disease is inactive, whereupon therapy may be continued with an azole.

Prognosis

The prognosis for patients with limited disease is good, but persistent pulmonary cavities may cause complications such as hemoptysis or rupture producing pyopneumothorax. Nodules, cavities, and fibrotic residuals may rarely progress after long periods of stability or regression. Serial complement fixation titers should be performed after therapy for patients with coccidioidomycosis; rising titers warrant reinstitution of therapy because relapse is likely. Late central nervous system complications of adequately treated meningitis include cerebral vasculitis and hydrocephalitis that may require shunting. Disseminated and meningeal forms still have mortality rates exceeding 50% in the absence of therapy.

Blair JE. Approach to the solid organ transplant patient with latent infection and disease caused by *Coccidioides* species. Curr Opin Infect Dis. 2008 Aug;21(4):415–20. [PMID: 18594295]
Durkin M et al. Diagnosis of coccidioidomycosis with use of the *Coccidioides* antigen enzyme immunoassay. Clin Infect Dis. 2008 Oct 15;47(8):e69–73. [PMID: 18781884]

PNEUMOCYSTOSIS
(*Pneumocystis jiroveci* Pneumonia)

ESSENTIALS OF DIAGNOSIS

▶ Fever, dyspnea, nonproductive cough.

▶ Bilateral diffuse interstitial disease without hilar adenopathy by chest radiograph.

▶ Bibasilar crackles on auscultation in many cases; others have no findings.

▶ Reduced partial pressure of oxygen.

▶ *P jiroveci* in sputum, bronchoalveolar lavage fluid, or lung tissue.

General Considerations

Pneumocystis jiroveci, the *Pneumocystis* species that affects humans, is distributed worldwide. Although symptomatic *P jiroveci* disease is rare in the general population, serologic evidence indicates that asymptomatic infections have occurred in most persons by a young age. The overt infection is an acute interstitial plasma cell pneumonia that occurs with high frequency among two groups: (1) as epidemics of primary infections among premature or debilitated or marasmic infants on hospital wards in underdeveloped parts of the world, and (2) as sporadic cases among older children and adults who have an abnormal or altered cellular immune status. Cases occur most commonly in patients with cancer or severe malnutrition and debility, in patients treated with immunosuppressive or cytotoxic drugs or irradiation for the management of organ transplants and cancer and, most frequently, in patients with AIDS (see Chapter 31).

The mode of transmission in primary infection is unknown, but the evidence suggests airborne transmission. Following asymptomatic primary infection, latent and presumably inactive organisms are sparsely distributed in the alveoli. Whether acute infection in older children and adults results from de novo infection or from reactivation of latent infection is not entirely clear, although both mechanisms probably contribute.

Pneumocystis pneumonia occurs in up to 80% of AIDS patients not receiving prophylaxis and is a major cause of death. Its incidence increases in direct proportion to the fall in CD4 cells, with most cases occurring at CD4 cell counts below 200/mcL. Dissemination of the infection to tissues other than the lung is rare. In non-AIDS patients receiving immunosuppressive therapy, symptoms frequently begin after corticosteroids have been tapered or discontinued.

Clinical Findings

A. Symptoms and Signs

Findings are usually limited to the pulmonary parenchyma; extrapulmonary disease is reported rarely. In the sporadic form of the disease associated with deficient cell-mediated immunity, the onset is abrupt, with fever, tachypnea, shortness of breath, and usually nonproductive cough. Pulmonary physical findings may be slight and disproportionate to the degree of illness and the radiologic findings; many patients have bibasilar crackles, but others do not. Without treatment, the course is usually one of rapid deterioration and death. Adult patients may present with spontaneous pneumothorax, usually in patients with previous episodes or those receiving aerosolized pentamidine prophylaxis. Patients with AIDS will usually have other evidence of HIV-associated disease, including fever, fatigue, and weight loss, for weeks or months preceding the illness.

B. Laboratory Findings

Chest radiographs most often show diffuse "interstitial" infiltration, which may be heterogeneous, miliary, or patchy early in infection. There may also be diffuse or focal consolidation, cystic changes, nodules, or cavitation within nodules. Pleural effusions are not seen. About 5–10% of patients with *Pneumocystis* pneumonia have normal chest films. High-resolution chest CT scans may be quite suggestive of *P jiroveci* pneumonia, helping distinguish it from other causes of pneumonia.

Arterial blood gas determinations usually show hypoxemia with hypocapnia but may be normal; however, rapid desaturation occurs if patients are exercised before samples are drawn. Isolated elevation or rising levels of serum LDH are very sensitive but not specific findings for *P jiroveci*.

Lymphopenia with depleted CD4 lymphocytes is common. Serologic tests, including tests to detect antigenemia, are not helpful in diagnosis.

Specific diagnosis depends on morphologic demonstration of the organisms in clinical specimens using specific stains. The organism cannot be cultured. Adequate specimens can sometimes be obtained with induced sputum by having patients inhale an aerosol of hypertonic saline (3%) produced by an ultrasonic nebulizer. Specimens are then stained with Giemsa stain or methenamine silver, either of which allows detection of cysts. The use of monoclonal antibody with immunofluorescence has increased the sensitivity of diagnosis. Alternative techniques for obtaining specimens include bronchoalveolar lavage (sensitivity 86–97%) followed by transbronchial lung biopsy (85–97%), if necessary. Open lung biopsy and needle lung biopsy are infrequently done but may need to be performed to diagnose a granulomatous form of *Pneumocystis* pneumonia. The polymerase chain reaction (PCR) test for the detection of *P jiroveci* appears to be overly sensitive in that many patients without *Pneumocystis* pneumonia will have a positive PCR on respiratory samples.

► Treatment

See Table 31–5. It is appropriate to start empiric therapy for *P jiroveci* pneumonia if the disease is suspected clinically; however, in both AIDS patients and non-AIDS patients with mild to moderately severe disease, continued treatment should be based on a proved diagnosis because of clinical overlap with other infections, the toxicity of therapy, and the possible coexistence of other infectious organisms. Oral trimethoprim-sulfamethoxazole (TMP-SMZ) is the preferred agent because of its low cost and excellent bioavailability in both AIDS patients and non-AIDS patients with mild to moderately severe disease. Patients suffering from nausea and vomiting or intractable diarrhea should be given intravenous TMP-SMZ until they can tolerate the oral formulation. The best-studied second-line option is a combination of clindamycin and primaquine, although dapsone/trimethoprim, pentamidine, and atovaquone have also been used. Therapy should be continued with the selected drug for at least 5–10 days before considering changing agents, as fever, tachypnea, and pulmonary infiltrates persist for 4–6 days after starting treatment. Some patients have a transient worsening of their disease during the first 3–5 days, which may be related to an inflammatory response secondary to the presence of dead or dying organisms. Early addition of corticosteroids may attenuate this response (see Chapter 31). Some clinicians prefer to treat episodes of AIDS-associated *Pneumocystis* pneumonia for 21 days rather than the usual 14 days recommended for non-AIDS cases.

A. Trimethoprim-Sulfamethoxazole

The dosage is TMP 20 mg/kg (12–15 mg/kg may decrease side effects without decreasing efficacy) and SMZ 100 mg/kg given orally or intravenously daily in three or four divided doses for 14–21 days. Adverse reactions are generally those of the sulfonamide component. Patients with AIDS have a high frequency of hypersensitivity reactions (approaching 50%), which may include fever, rashes (sometimes severe), malaise, neutropenia, hepatitis, nephritis, thrombocytopenia, hyperkalemia, and hyperbilirubinemia.

B. Clindamycin/Primaquine

Although there are strong data indicating that trimethoprim-sulfamethoxazole is optimal first-line therapy for *Pneumocystis* pneumonia, the data on alternative agents is less clear. A meta-analysis suggested that clindamycin, 600 mg three times daily, plus primaquine, 15 mg/d, is the best second-line therapy with superior results when compared with pentamidine. Primaquine may cause hemolytic anemia in patients with glucose-6-phosphate dehydrogenase (G6PD)-deficiency.

C. Pentamidine Isethionate

The use of pentamidine has decreased as alternative agents have been studied. This drug is administered intravenously (preferred) or intramuscularly as a single dose of 3 mg (salt)/kg/d for 14–21 days. Pentamidine causes side effects in nearly 50% of patients. Hypoglycemia (often clinically inapparent), hyperglycemia, hyponatremia, and delayed nephrotoxicity with azotemia may occur. Rarely, a variety of other severe adverse reactions may occur, including anemia, thrombocytopenia, ventricular arrhythmias, and fatal pancreatitis. Blood glucose levels should be monitored. Inadvertent rapid intravenous infusion may cause precipitous hypotension.

D. Atovaquone

Atovaquone has been approved by the US Food and Drug Administration (FDA) for patients with mild to moderate disease who cannot tolerate TMP-SMZ or pentamidine, but failure is reported in 15–30% of cases. Mild side effects are common, but no serious reactions have been reported. The dosage is 750 mg three times daily for 21 days.

E. Other Drugs

Dapsone, 100 mg/d, plus trimethoprim 15 mg/kg/d, in three divided doses daily, is an alternative oral regimen for mild to moderate disease or for continuation of therapy after intravenous therapy is no longer needed.

F. Prednisone

Prednisone is given for moderate to severe pneumonia (when Pao_2 on admission is < 70 mm Hg or oxygen saturation is < 90%) in conjunction with antimicrobials; its use during the first 72 hours of therapy for severe *Pneumocystis* pneumonia prevents deterioration in oxygenation and improves survival. The dosage of prednisone is 40 mg twice daily for 5 days, then 40 mg daily for 5 days, and then 20 mg daily until therapy is completed.

G. Supportive Care

Oxygen therapy is indicated to maintain the oxygen saturation over 90% by pulse oximetry.

Prevention

Primary prophylaxis for *Pneumocystis* pneumonia in HIV-infected patients should be given to persons with CD4 counts < 200 cells/mcL, a CD4 percentage below 14%, or weight loss or oral candidiasis (see Table 31–4). Primary prophylaxis is often used in patients with hematologic malignancy and transplant recipients. The occurrence of *P jiroveci* pneumonia while on prophylaxis may be associated with development of resistance to TMP-SMZ. Patients with a history of *Pneumocystis* pneumonia should receive secondary prophylaxis until they have had a durable virologic response to antiretroviral therapy for at least 3–6 months and maintain a CD4 count of > 250 cells/mcL.

Prognosis

In the absence of early and adequate treatment, the fatality rate for the endemic infantile form of *Pneumocystis* pneumonia is 20–50%; for the sporadic form in immunodeficient persons, the fatality rate is nearly 100%. Early treatment reduces the mortality rate to about 3% in the former and 10–20% in AIDS patients. The mortality rate in other immunodeficient patients is still 30–50%, probably because of failure to make a timely diagnosis. In immunodeficient patients who do not receive prophylaxis, recurrences are common (30% in AIDS).

Benfield T et al. Second-line salvage treatment of AIDS-associated *Pneumocystis jirovecii* pneumonia: a case series and systematic review. J Acquir Immune Defic Syndr. 2008 May 1;48(1):63–7. [PMID: 18360286]

Davis JL et al. *Pneumocystis* colonisation is common among hospitalised HIV-infected patients with non-*Pneumocystis* pneumonia. Thorax. 2008 Apr;63(4):329–34. [PMID: 18024536]

CRYPTOCOCCOSIS

ESSENTIALS OF DIAGNOSIS

▶ Most common cause of fungal meningitis.

▶ Predisposing factors: Hodgkin disease, corticosteroid therapy, HIV infection, transplant recipients.

▶ Symptoms of headache, abnormal mental status; meningismus seen occasionally, though rarely in HIV-infected patients.

▶ Demonstration of capsular polysaccharide antigen in cerebrospinal fluid diagnostic; 95% of HIV-infected and solid-organ transplant patients also have a positive serum antigen.

General Considerations

Cryptococcosis is mainly caused by *Cryptococcus neoformans,* an encapsulated budding yeast that has been found worldwide in soil and on dried pigeon dung. *Cryptococcus gattii* is a closely related species that also causes disease in humans although *C gattii* may affect more immunocompetent persons.

Infections are acquired by inhalation. In the lung, the infection may remain localized, heal, or disseminate. Clinically apparent cryptococcal pneumonia rarely develops in immunocompetent persons. Progressive lung disease and dissemination most often occur in the setting of cellular immunodeficiency, including underlying hematologic cancer under treatment, Hodgkin disease, long-term corticosteroid therapy, solid-organ transplant, or HIV infection.

Clinical Findings

A. Symptoms and Signs

Pulmonary disease ranges from simple nodules to widespread infiltrates leading to respiratory failure. Disseminated disease may involve any organ, but central nervous system disease predominates. Headache is usually the first symptom of meningitis. Confusion and other mental status changes as well as cranial nerve abnormalities, nausea, and vomiting may be seen as the disease progresses. Nuchal rigidity and meningeal signs occur about 50% of the time but are uncommon in HIV-infected patients. Communicating hydrocephalus may complicate the course. Primary *C neoformans* infection of the skin may mimic bacterial cellulitis, especially in immunocompromised persons. Clinical worsening associated with improved immunologic status has been reported in HIV-positive and transplant patients with cryptococcosis; this entity has been labeled the immune reconstitution inflammatory syndrome (IRIS).

B. Laboratory Findings

Respiratory tract disease is diagnosed by culture of respiratory secretions or pleural fluid. For suspected meningeal disease, lumbar puncture is the preferred diagnostic procedure. Spinal fluid findings include increased opening pressure, variable pleocytosis, increased protein, and decreased glucose, though as many as 50% of AIDS patients have no pleocytosis. Gram stain of the cerebrospinal fluid usually reveals budding, encapsulated fungal cells. Cryptococcal capsular antigen in cerebrospinal fluid and culture together establish the diagnosis over 90% of the time. Patients with AIDS often have the antigen in both cerebrospinal fluid and serum, and extrameningeal disease (lungs, blood, urinary tract) is common. In patients with AIDS, the serum cryptococcal antigen is also a sensitive screening test for meningitis, being positive in over 95% of cases. MRI is more sensitive than CT in finding central nervous system abnormalities such as cryptococcomas.

Treatment

Because of decreased efficacy and development of resistance, initial therapy with an azole is not recommended for treatment of acute cryptococcal meningitis. Consequently, treatment regimens using amphotericin B should be started. However, there has been a trend away from prolonged amphotericin B therapy regimens, particularly in HIV-infected patients. Thus, amphotericin B, 0.7–1 mg/kg/d intravenously is used for 14 days, followed by an additional 8 weeks of fluconazole, 400 mg/d orally. This regimen has been quite effective, achieving clinical responses and cerebrospinal fluid sterilization in about 70% of patients. The addition of flucytosine has been associated with improved survival, but toxicity is common. Flucytosine is administered orally at a dose of 100 mg/kg/d divided into four equal doses and given every 6 hours. Hematologic parameters should be closely monitored during flucytosine therapy. Repeated lumbar punctures or ventricular shunting should be performed to relieve high cerebrospinal fluid pressures or if hydrocephalus is a complication. Failure to adequately relieve raised intracranial pressure is a major cause of morbidity and mortality. The end points for amphotericin B therapy and for switching to oral fluconazole are a favorable clinical response (decrease in temperature; improvement in headache, nausea, vomiting, and mini-mental status scores), improvement in cerebrospinal fluid biochemical parameters and, most importantly, conversion of cerebrospinal fluid culture to negative.

A similar approach is reasonable for patients with cryptococcal meningitis in the absence of AIDS, though the mortality rate is considerably higher. Lipid amphotericin B preparations appear to have equivalent efficacy with reduced nephrotoxicity. Therapy is generally continued until cerebrospinal fluid cultures become negative and cerebrospinal fluid antigen titers are below 1:8.

Maintenance antifungal therapy is important after treatment of an acute episode in HIV-related cases, since otherwise the rate of relapse is greater than 50%. Fluconazole, 200 mg/d, is the maintenance therapy of choice, decreasing the relapse rate approximately tenfold compared with placebo and threefold compared with weekly amphotericin B in patients whose cerebrospinal fluid has been sterilized by the induction therapy. After successful therapy of cryptococcal meningitis, it is possible to discontinue secondary prophylaxis with fluconazole in individuals with AIDS who have had a satisfactory response to antiretroviral therapy (eg, CD4 cell count > 100–200 cells/mcL for at least 6 months). Among practitioners treating patients without AIDS, there has been a trend in recent years to prescribe a course (eg, 6–12 months) of fluconazole as maintenance therapy following successful treatment of the acute illness; recently published guidelines suggest this as an option.

▶ Prognosis

Factors that indicate a poor prognosis include the activity of the predisposing conditions, older age, organ failure, lack of spinal fluid pleocytosis, high initial antigen titer in either serum or cerebrospinal fluid, decreased mental status, increased intracranial pressure, and the presence of disease outside the nervous system.

Dromer F et al; French Cryptococcosis Study Group. Major role for amphotericin B-flucytosine combination in severe cryptococcosis. PLoS ONE. 2008 Aug 6;3(8):e2870. [PMID: 18682846]
Singh N et al. Pulmonary cryptococcosis in solid organ transplant recipients: clinical relevance of serum cryptococcal antigen. Clin Infect Dis. 2008 Jan 15;46(2):e12–18. [PMID: 18171241]

ASPERGILLOSIS

ESSENTIALS OF DIAGNOSIS

▶ Most common cause of invasive fungal infection in stem cell or organ transplant patients.

▶ Predisposing factors: leukemia, bone marrow or organ transplant, late HIV infection.

▶ Pulmonary, sinus, and CNS are most common disease sites.

▶ Demonstration of galactomannan or β-D-glucan in serum or other body fluid samples contributes to early diagnosis and treatment.

▶ General Considerations

Aspergillus fumigatus is the usual cause of aspergillosis, though many species of *Aspergillus* may cause a wide spectrum of disease. The lungs, sinuses, and brain are the organs most often involved. Clinical illness results either from an aberrant immunologic response or tissue invasion.

▶ Clinical Findings

A. Allergic Bronchopulmonary Aspergillosis

This form of aspergillosis occurs in patients with preexisting asthma who develop worsening bronchospasm and fleeting pulmonary infiltrates accompanied by eosinophilia, high levels of IgE, and IgG *Aspergillus* precipitins in the blood. It also may complicate cystic fibrosis.

B. Invasive Aspergillosis

Invasive manifestations may be seen in immunocompetent or only mildly immunocompromised adults. These include chronic **sinusitis**, colonization of preexisting pulmonary cavities (**aspergilloma**), and chronic necrotizing pulmonary aspergillosis.

1. Sinusitis—Sinus involvement is usually diagnosed histologically after patients with chronic sinus disease undergo surgery.

2. Aspergillomas—Aspergillomas of the lung occur when preexisting lung lesions become secondarily colonized with *Aspergillus* species. These may be found by incidental radiographic studies but may also present with significant hemoptysis.

3. Chronic necrotizing aspergillosis—This invasive manifestation is a relatively rare disease seen in patients with some degree of immunocompromise and presents with a protracted course compared with the more common acute invasive form of the disease. Fibrosis and cavity formation may be prominent.

4. Life-threatening invasive aspergillosis—Severe invasive aspergillosis most commonly occurs in profoundly immunodeficient patients, particularly in patients who have undergone hematopoietic stem cell transplants and in those with prolonged, severe neutropenia. Specific risk factors in patients who have undergone a hematopoietic stem cell transplant include cytopenias, corticosteroid use, iron overload, cytomegalovirus disease, and graft-versus-host disease. Pulmonary disease is most common, with patchy infiltration leading to a severe necrotizing pneumonia. Invasive sinus disease also occurs. There is often tissue infarction as the organism grows into blood vessels; clues to this are the development of pleuritic chest pain and elevation of serum LDH. At any time, there may be hematogenous dissemination to the central nervous system, skin, and other organs. Early diagnosis and reversal of any correctable immunosuppression are essential. Blood cultures have very low yield. Detection of galactomannan by enzyme-linked immunosorbent assay (ELISA) or β-D-glucan, or both, has been used for the early diagnosis of invasive disease, though multiple determinations should be done. Higher galactomannan levels are correlated with increased mortality. False-positive galactomannan tests have been reported in patients receiving β-lactam antibiotics. Isolation of *Aspergillus* from pulmonary secretions does not necessarily imply invasive disease, although its positive predictive value increases with more advanced immunosuppression. Therefore, a definitive diagnosis requires demonstration of *Aspergillus* in tissue or culture from a sterile site. CT scan of the chest may show characteristics quite suggestive of invasive aspergillosis (eg, "halo sign").

▶ Prevention

The high mortality rate and difficulty in diagnosis of invasive aspergillosis often leads clinicians to institute prophylactic therapy for patients with profound immunosuppression. The best-studied agents include fluconazole, itraconazole, voriconazole, and posaconazole, although patient and agent selection criteria remain undefined. Widespread use of broad-spectrum azoles raises concern for development of invasive disease by highly resistant fungi.

▶ Treatment

A. Allergic Bronchopulmonary Aspergillosis

For acute exacerbations, oral prednisone is begun at a dose of 1 mg/kg/d and then tapered slowly over several months. Itraconazole at a dose of 200 mg daily for 16 weeks appears to improve pulmonary function and decrease corticosteroid requirements in these patients, although voriconazole may become the preferred oral agent.

B. Invasive Aspergillosis

1. Sinusitis—These patients may require protracted courses of antifungals (itraconazole, 200 mg twice daily, for weeks to months) in addition to the surgical debridement.

2. Aspergilloma—The most effective therapy for symptomatic aspergilloma remains surgical resection.

3. Chronic necrotizing aspergillosis—Although it would be reasonable to institute therapy targeting *Aspergillus*, response to such therapy is not clear.

4. Life-threatening invasive aspergillosis—When severe invasive aspergillosis is considered clinically likely or is demonstrable by laboratory testing, rapid institution of voriconazole, high doses of amphotericin B, or caspofungin may be life-saving. Voriconazole (6 mg/kg intravenously twice on day 1, then 4 mg/kg/d thereafter) has been shown to be more effective, improve survival, and be associated with fewer severe side effects than conventional amphotericin B when used as initial therapy in invasive aspergillosis. Oral dosing of voriconazole at 4 mg/kg twice daily can be used for less serious infections or as a step-down strategy after intravenous therapy. Some experts believe that intravenous lipid preparations of amphotericin B (3–5 mg/kg/d) should be used preferentially in this setting because they are better tolerated and can be given at higher doses.

Caspofungin (70 mg intravenously on day 1, then 50 mg/d thereafter) is approved for the treatment of invasive aspergillosis in patients who do not respond to or are intolerant of other treatments. Other options include micafungin (100–150 mg/d intravenously) and posaconazole (200 mg orally four times daily). In critically ill patients who are not responding to conventional antifungal treatment, there may be a role for the addition of caspofungin to amphotericin B or voriconazole therapy, although randomized trials are lacking. Based on promising results in neutropenic patients with invasive pulmonary aspergillosis, surgical resection warrants further study. The mortality rate of pulmonary or disseminated disease in the immunocompromised patient remains well above 50%, particularly in patients with refractory neutropenia.

Penack O et al. *Aspergillus galactomannan* testing in patients with long-term neutropenia: implications for clinical management. Ann Oncol. 2008 May;19(5):984–9. [PMID: 18227109]

Raad II et al. Novel antifungal agents as salvage therapy for invasive aspergillosis in patients with hematologic malignancies: posaconazole compared with high-dose lipid formulations of amphotericin B alone or in combination with caspofungin. Leukemia. 2008 Mar;22(3):496–503. [PMID: 18094720]

Walsh TJ et al. Treatment of aspergillosis: clinical practice guidelines of the Infectious Diseases Society of America. Clin Infect Dis. 2008 Feb 1;46(3):327–60. [PMID: 18177225]

MUCORMYCOSIS

The term "mucormycosis" (zygomycosis, phycomycosis) is applied to opportunistic infections caused by members of the genera *Rhizopus, Mucor, Absidia*, and *Cunninghamella*. Predisposing conditions include diabetic ketoacidosis, chronic kidney disease, desferoxamine therapy, and treatment with corticosteroids or cytotoxic drugs. These organisms appear in tissues as broad, branching nonseptate hyphae. Biopsy with histologic examination is almost always required for diagnosis; cultures are frequently negative. Invasive disease of the sinuses, orbits, and the lungs may occur. Widely disseminated disease is seen in patients who have received aggressive chemotherapy and broad-spectrum antifungal prophylaxis. A prolonged course of high-dosage amphotericin B (1–1.5 mg/kg/d intravenously) or a lipid preparation of amphotericin B should be started early. Based on in vitro susceptibility and reports of successful salvage therapy, there may be a role for posaconazole in the treatment of these infections, but other azoles are likely to be ineffective. There are limited data suggesting beneficial synergistic activity when amphotericin and caspofungin are used in combination for mucormycosis. Ongoing studies are assessing whether iron chelation therapy with deferasirox may also be helpful. Control of diabetes and other underlying conditions, along with extensive repeated surgical removal of necrotic, nonperfused tissue, is essential. Even when these measures are introduced in a timely fashion, the prognosis is poor, with a 30–50% mortality rate for localized disease and higher rates in disseminated cases.

Ibrahim AS et al. Iron acquisition: a novel perspective on mucormycosis pathogenesis and treatment. Curr Opin Infect Dis. 2008 Dec;21(6):620–5. [PMID: 18978530]
Reed C et al. Combination polyene-caspofungin treatment of rhino-orbital-cerebral mucormycosis. Clin Infect Dis. 2008 Aug 1;47(3):364–71. [PMID: 18558882]

BLASTOMYCOSIS

Blastomycosis occurs most often in men infected during occupational or recreational activities out of doors and in a geographically limited area of the south central and midwestern United States and Canada. Disease usually occurs in immunocompetent individuals.

Pulmonary infection is most common and may be asymptomatic. When dissemination takes place, lesions are most frequently seen in the skin, bones, and urogenital system.

Cough, moderate fever, dyspnea, and chest pain are common. These may resolve or progress, with bloody and purulent sputum production, pleurisy, fever, chills, loss of weight, and prostration. Radiologic studies, either chest radiographs or CT scans, usually reveal airspace consolidations or masses.

Raised, verrucous cutaneous lesions are commonly present in disseminated blastomycosis. Bones—often the ribs and vertebrae—are frequently involved. Lesions appear to be both destructive and proliferative on radiography. Epididymitis, prostatitis, and other involvement of the male urogenital system may occur. Although they do not appear to be at greater risk for acquisition of disease, infection in HIV-infected persons may progress rapidly, with dissemination common.

Laboratory findings usually include leukocytosis and anemia, though these are not specific. The organism is found in clinical specimens, such as expectorated sputum or tissue, as a thick-walled cell 5–20 mcm in diameter that may have a single broad-based bud. It grows readily on culture. Serologic tests are not well standardized. A urinary antigen test is available, but it has some cross reactivity with *Histoplasma*; consequently, its usefulness in diagnosis and in assessing response to therapy is unclear.

Itraconazole, 200–400 mg/d orally for at least 2–3 months, is the therapy of choice for nonmeningeal disease, with a response rate of over 80%. Amphotericin B, 0.7–1.0 mg/kg/d intravenously (or lipid formulation amphotericin

B), is given for severe disease, treatment failures, or central nervous system involvement.

Clinical follow-up for relapse should be made regularly for several years so that therapy may be resumed or another drug instituted.

Chapman SW et al. Clinical practice guidelines for the management of blastomycosis: 2008 update by the Infectious Diseases Society of America. Clin Infect Dis. 2008 Jun 15;46(12):1801–12. [PMID: 18462107]
Hussein R et al. Blastomycosis in the mountainous region of Northeast Tennessee. Chest. 2008 Nov 18 2009 April;135(4):1019–23. [PMID: 19017881]

PARACOCCIDIOIDOMYCOSIS (South American Blastomycosis)

Paracoccidioides brasiliensis infections have been found only in patients who have resided in South or Central America or Mexico. Long asymptomatic periods enable patients to travel far from the endemic areas before developing clinical problems. Weight loss, pulmonary complaints, or mucosal ulcerations are the most common symptoms. Cutaneous papules may ulcerate and enlarge both peripherally and deeper into the subcutaneous tissue. Differential diagnosis includes mucocutaneous leishmaniasis and syphilis. Extensive coalescent ulcerations may eventually result in destruction of the epiglottis, vocal cords, and uvula. Extension to the lips and face may occur. Eating and drinking are extremely painful. Skin lesions may occur, usually on the face. Variable in appearance, they may have a necrotic central crater with a hard hyperkeratotic border. Lymph node enlargement may follow mucocutaneous lesions, eventually ulcerating and forming draining sinuses; in some patients, it is the presenting symptom. Hepatosplenomegaly may be present as well. The extensive ulceration of the upper gastrointestinal tract may prevent caloric intake and result in cachexia.

Laboratory findings are nonspecific. Serology by immunodiffusion is positive in 98% of cases. Complement fixation titers correlate with progressive disease and fall with effective therapy. The fungus is found in clinical specimens as a spherical cell that may have many buds arising from it. If direct examination does not reveal the organism, biopsy with Gomori staining may be helpful.

Itraconazole, 100 mg twice daily, is the treatment of choice and generally results in a clinical response within 1 month and effective control after 2–6 months. Voriconazole, 200 mg twice daily, appears to be as effective as itraconazole.

de Camargo ZP. Serology of paracoccidioidomycosis. Mycopathologia. 2008 Apr–May;165(4–5):289–302. [PMID: 18777635]

SPOROTRICHOSIS

Sporotrichosis is a chronic fungal infection caused by *Sporothrix schenckii*. It is worldwide in distribution; most patients have had contact with soil, sphagnum moss, or decaying wood. Transmission from animals to humans has also been reported. Infection takes place when the organism is inoculated into the skin—usually on the hand, arm, or foot, especially during gardening.

The most common form of sporotrichosis begins with a hard, nontender subcutaneous nodule. This later becomes adherent to the overlying skin and ulcerates. Within a few days to weeks, similar nodules develop along the lymphatics draining this area, and these may ulcerate as well.

Disseminated sporotrichosis is rare in the immunocompetent person but may present with widespread cutaneous, lung, bone, joint, and central nervous system involvement in immunocompromised patients, especially those with AIDS and alcohol abuse.

Cultures are needed to establish diagnosis. Antibody tests may be useful for diagnosis of disseminated disease, especially meningitis.

Itraconazole, 200–400 mg orally daily for several months, is now the treatment of choice for localized disease and some milder cases of disseminated disease. Terbinafine, 500 mg twice daily, also appears to have good efficacy in lymphocutaneous disease. Amphotericin B intravenously, 1–2 g, is used for severe systemic infection. Surgery is usually contraindicated except for simple aspiration of secondary nodules. Joint involvement may require arthrodesis.

The prognosis is good for lymphocutaneous sporotrichosis; pulmonary, joint, and disseminated disease respond less favorably.

Schubach A. Epidemic sporotrichosis. Curr Opin Infect Dis. 2008 Apr;21(2):129–33. [PMID: 18317034]

PENICILLIUM MARNEFFEI INFECTIONS

Penicillium marneffei is a dimorphic fungus, endemic in southeast Asia, that causes systemic infection in both healthy and immunocompromised hosts. There have been reports of travelers with advanced AIDS returning from southeast Asia with disseminated infection. Clinical manifestations include fever, generalized umbilicated papular rash, lymphadenopathy, cough, and diarrhea. Diagnosis is made by identification of the organism on smears or histopathologic specimens or by culture, where the fungus produces a characteristic red pigment. The best sites for isolation of the fungus include the skin, blood, bone marrow, respiratory tract, and lymph nodes. Antigen and antibody tests have been developed in endemic regions. Patients with mild to moderate infection can be treated with itraconazole, 400 mg divided into two doses daily by mouth for 8 weeks. Amphotericin B, 0.5–0.7 mg/kg/d, is the drug of choice for severe disease and should be continued until patients have had a satisfactory clinical response, at which time they can be switched to itraconazole. Because the relapse rate after successful treatment is 30%, maintenance therapy with itraconazole, 200–400 mg daily, is indicated indefinitely.

Ustianowski AP et al. *Penicillium marneffei* infection in HIV. Curr Opin Infect Dis. 2008 Feb;21(1):31–6. [PMID: 18192783]

CHROMOBLASTOMYCOSIS (Chromomycosis)

Chromoblastomycosis is a chronic, principally tropical cutaneous infection usually affecting young men who are agricultural workers and caused by several species of closely related black molds; *Cladophialophora carrionii* and *Fonsecaea pedrosoi* are the most common etiologic agents.

Lesions usually follow puncture wounds and are slowly progressive, occurring most frequently on a lower extremity. The lesion begins as a papule or ulcer. Over months to years, papules enlarge to become vegetating, papillomatous, verrucous elevated nodules. Satellite lesions may appear along the lymphatics. There may be secondary bacterial infection. Elephantiasis may result.

The fungus is seen as brown, thick-walled, spherical, sometimes septate cells in potassium hydroxide preparations of pus or skin scrapings, which are quite sensitive for diagnosis. The type of reproduction found in culture determines the species.

Itraconazole, 200–400 mg/d orally for 6–18 months, achieves a response rate of 65%. Response rates may be improved by the addition to itraconazole of flucytosine, 100–150 mg/kg/d by mouth divided into four doses. Terbinafine at 500 mg/d may have similar efficacy to itraconazole. Cryosurgery alone for smaller lesions or combined with itraconazole for larger lesions is beneficial.

Queiroz-Telles F et al. Chromoblastomycosis: an overview of clinical manifestations, diagnosis and treatment. Med Mycol. 2009 Feb;47(1):3–15. [PMID: 19085206]

MYCETOMA (Maduromycosis & Actinomycetoma)

Mycetoma is a chronic local, slowly progressive destructive infection, usually involving the foot, that begins in subcutaneous tissues, frequently after localized trauma, and then spreads to contiguous structures. Maduromycosis (also known as eumycetoma) is the term used to describe mycetoma caused by the true fungi and by phylogenetically diverse organisms. Actinomycotic mycetoma is caused by *Nocardia* and *Actinomadura* species. The disease begins as a papule, nodule, or abscess that over months to years progresses slowly to form multiple abscesses and sinus tracts ramifying deep into the tissue. Secondary bacterial infection may result in large open ulcers. Radiographs may show destructive changes in the underlying bone. Tissue Gram stain reveals fine branching hyphae with actinomycotic mycetoma. Larger hyphae are seen with fungal mycetoma; the causative species can often be identified by the color of the characteristic grains within the infected tissues.

The prognosis is good for patients with actinomycetoma, since they usually respond well to sulfonamides and sulfones, especially if treated early. TMP-SMZ, 160/800 mg orally twice a day, or dapsone, 100 mg twice daily after meals, has been reported to be effective. Streptomycin, 14 mg/kg/d intramuscularly, may be useful during the first month of therapy. All oral medications must be taken for months and continued for several months after clinical cure to prevent relapse. Debridement assists healing.

The prognosis for maduromycosis is poor, though surgical debridement along with prolonged itraconazole therapy may result in a response rate of 70%. The various etiologic agents may respond differently to antifungal

Table 36-1. Agents for systemic mycoses.

Drug	Dosing	Renal Clearance?	CSF Penetration?	Toxicities	Spectrum of Activity
Amphotericin B	0.3–1.5 mg/kg/d intravenously	No	Poor	Rigors, fever, azotemia, hypokalemia, hypomagnesemia, renal tubular acidosis, anemia	All major pathogens except *Scedosporium*
Amphotericin B lipid complex	5 mg/kg/d intravenously	No	Poor	Fever, rigors, nausea, hypotension, anemia, azotemia, tachypnea	Same as amphotericin B, above
Liposomal amphotericin B	3–6 mg/kg/d intravenously	No	Poor	Fever, rigors, nausea, hypotension, azotemia, anemia, tachypnea, chest tightness	Same as amphotericin B, above
Anidulafungin	100 mg intravenous loading dose, followed by 50 mg/d intravenously in one dose	< 1%	Poor	Diarrhea, hepatic enzyme elevations, histamine-mediated reactions	Mucosal and invasive candidiasis
Caspofungin acetate	70 mg intravenous loading dose, followed by 50 mg/d intravenously in one dose	< 50%[1]	Poor	Transient neutropenia; hepatic enzyme elevations when used with cyclosporine	Aspergillosis, mucosal and invasive candidiasis, empiric antifungal therapy in febrile neutropenia
Micafungin sodium	150 mg intravenously in one dose (treatment) 50 mg (prophylaxis)	No	Poor	Rash, rigors, headache, phlebitis	Mucosal and invasive candidiasis, prophylaxis in hematopoietic stem cell transplantation
Fluconazole	100–800 mg/d in one or two doses intravenously or orally	Yes	Yes	Nausea, rash, alopecia, headache, hepatic enzyme elevations	Mucosal candidiasis (including urinary tract), cryptococcosis, histoplasmosis, coccidioidomycosis
Flucytosine (5-FC)	100–150 mg/kg/d orally in four divided doses	Yes	Yes	Leukopenia,[2] rash, diarrhea, hepatitis, nausea, vomiting	Cryptococcosis,[3] candidiasis,[3] chromomycosis
Itraconazole	100–400 mg/d orally in one or two doses	No	Variable	Nausea, hypokalemia, edema, hypertension	Histoplasmosis, coccidioidomycosis, blastomycosis, paracoccidioidomycosis, mucosal candidiasis (except urinary), sporotrichosis, aspergillosis, chromomycosis
Ketoconazole	200–800 mg/d orally in one or two doses	No	Poor	Anorexia, nausea, suppression of testosterone and cortisol, rash, headache, hepatic enzyme elevations, hepatic failure	Nonmeningeal histoplasmosis and coccidioidomycosis, blastomycosis, paracoccidioidomycosis, mucosal candidiasis (except urinary)
Posaconazole	400–800 mg/d orally in one or two doses	No	Yes	Nausea, vomiting, abdominal pain, diarrhea, and headache	Broad range of activity including zygomycosis
Terbinafine	250 mg/d orally in one dose	Yes	Poor	Nausea, abdominal pain, taste disturbance, rash, diarrhea, and hepatic enzyme elevations	Dermatophytes, sporotrichosis
Voriconazole	200–400 mg/d orally in two doses or 12 mg/kg intravenously as loading dose for 2 days followed by 6 mg/kg/d intravenously in two doses[5]	Yes	Yes	Transient visual disturbances, rash, hepatic enzyme elevations[4]	All major pathogens except zygomycetes and sporotrichosis

[1]No dosage adjustment required for chronic kidney disease; dosage adjustment necessary with moderate to severe hepatic dysfunction.
[2]Use should be monitored with blood levels to prevent this or the dose adjusted according to creatinine clearance.
[3]In combination with amphotericin B.
[4]Administration with drugs that are metabolized by the cytochrome P450 system is contraindicated or requires careful monitoring.
[5]Because of polymorphisms affecting metabolism, some authorities advocate therapeutic drug monitoring in patients who are not responding to therapy.

agents, so culture results are invaluable. Amputation is necessary in far advanced cases.

Ameen M et al. Developments in the management of mycetomas. Clin Exp Dermatol. 2009 Jan;34(1):1–7. [PMID: 19076788]

OTHER OPPORTUNISTIC MOLD INFECTIONS

Fungi previously considered to be harmless colonizers, including *Pseudallescheria boydii* (*Scedosporium apiospermum*), *Scedosporium prolificans*, *Fusarium*, *Paecilomyces*, *Trichoderma longibrachiatium*, and *Trichosporon*, are emerging as significant pathogens in immunocompromised patients. This occurs most often in patients being treated for hematopoietic malignancies and in those receiving broad-spectrum antifungal prophylaxis. Infection may be localized in the skin, lungs, or sinuses, or widespread disease may appear with lesions in multiple organs. Colonization of old cavitary disease may cause minimal symptoms or may precede dissemination with meningitis or brain abscesses. Endocarditis occurs more commonly in injection drug users. Sinus infection may cause bony erosion. Infection in subcutaneous tissues following traumatic implantation may develop as a well-circumscribed cyst or as an ulcer.

Nonpigmented septate hyphae are seen in tissue and are indistinguishable from those of *Aspergillus* when infections are due to *S apiospermum* or species of *Fusarium*, *Paecilomyces*, *Penicillium*, or other hyaline molds. Spores or mycetoma-like granules are rarely present in tissue.

Infection by any of a number of black molds is designated as phaeohyphomycosis. These black molds (eg, *Exophiala*, *Bipolaris*, *Cladophialophora*, *Curvularia*, *Alternaria*) are common in the environment, especially on decaying vegetation. Human disease due to these agents is rarely encountered but may result in soft tissue abscesses due to traumatic inoculation or may occur as a sequela of chronic sinusitis or profound immunosuppression. In tissues of patients with phaeohyphomycosis, the mold is seen as black or faintly brown hyphae, yeast cells, or both. Culture on appropriate medium is needed to identify the agent. Histologic demonstration of these organisms is definitive evidence of invasive infection; positive cultures must be interpreted cautiously and not assumed to be contaminants in immunocompromised hosts. Some isolates are sensitive to antifungal agents. The differentiation of *S apiospermum* and *Aspergillus* is particularly important, since the former is uniformly resistant to amphotericin B but may be sensitive to azole antifungals (eg, voriconazole).

Stanzani M et al. Update on the treatment of disseminated fusariosis: Focus on voriconazole. Ther Clin Risk Manag. 2007 Dec;3(6):1165–73. [PMID: 18516266]

Troke P et al; Global Scedosporium Study Group. Treatment of scedosporiosis with voriconazole: clinical experience with 107 patients. Antimicrob Agents Chemother. 2008 May;52(5):1743–50. [PMID: 18212110]

ANTIFUNGAL THERAPY

Table 36–1 summarizes the major properties of currently available antifungal agents. Several different lipid-based amphotericin B formulations are used to treat systemic candidiasis, invasive aspergillosis and other disseminated mold infections, disseminated histoplasmosis, and cryptococcal meningitis. Their principal advantage appears to be substantially reduced nephrotoxicity, allowing administration of much higher doses. Because of their expense, use of these agents is often reserved for individuals in whom significant nephrotoxicity develops during amphotericin B therapy. Three agents of the echinocandin class, caspofungin acetate, anidulafungin, and micafungin sodium, are currently approved. The echinocandins have relatively few adverse effects and are useful for the treatment of invasive *Candida* infections. Caspofungin acetate is also approved for use in refractory cases of invasive aspergillosis. Voriconazole has excellent activity against a broad range of fungal pathogens and has been FDA approved for use in invasive *Aspergillus* cases, *Fusarium* and *Scedosporium* infections, *Candida* esophagitis, deep *Candida* infections, and candidemia. Posaconazole has good activity against a broad range of filamentous fungi, including some of the zygomycetes. Cytokine therapy (such as with interferon-γ) and use of growth factors such as granulocyte macrophage-colony-stimulating factor (GM-CSF) (sargramostim or molgramostim) have been shown in animal models to increase clearance of fungi and result in better clinical outcomes and are being evaluated in human disease.

Lipp HP. Antifungal agents—clinical pharmacokinetics and drug interactions. Mycoses. 2008;51(Suppl 1):7–18. [PMID: 18471156]

Sable CA et al. Advances in antifungal therapy. Ann Rev Med. 2008;59:361–79. [PMID: 17967129]

Disorders Due to Physical Agents

Jacqueline A. Nemer, MD, FACEP
Brent R.W. Moelleken, MD, FACS

▼ COLD & HEAT

The human body maintains a steady temperature through the balance of internal heat production and environmental heat loss. In extreme temperatures, the body's thermoregulation may fail. This results in the body's internal temperature moving toward the temperature of the external environment. Heat exchange between the body and environment occurs via four common processes: radiation, evaporation, conduction, and convection. Cold and heat tolerance vary considerably among individuals, depending on physiological and environmental factors.

Cold- and heat-related conditions may arise in any individual, regardless of sex, race, age, or underlying health status. Exposure to cold or heat may cause a wide spectrum of conditions. Factors that increase the likelihood of extreme temperature-related conditions include underlying cardiopulmonary, vascular, neurologic or musculoskeletal diseases; poor physical conditioning; nonacclimatization; advanced age; altered mental status; poor tissue perfusion; inappropriate clothing; concurrent injury; poor peripheral vascular function; inadequate thermoregulation; systemic illness; pharmacologic effects of tobacco, alcohol, and drugs (ie, recreational drugs, sedatives, or drugs that affect sweating).

ACCIDENTAL SYSTEMIC HYPOTHERMIA

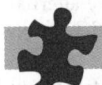 ### ESSENTIALS OF DIAGNOSIS

- ► Hypothermia is a reduction of core body temperature below 35 °C.
- ► An esophageal or rectal probe that measures as low as 25 °C is required; oral, axillary, and otic temperatures are inaccurate.
- ► Resuscitative measures must be continued until the core temperature is over 32 °C.

► General Considerations

Systemic hypothermia is defined as core body temperature less than 35 °C. This may be primary (from exposure to prolonged ambient extremely low temperature) or secondary (due to thermoregulatory dysfunction). Primary and secondary hypothermia may be present at the same time. Hypothermia risk factors include malnutrition, hypothyroidism, adrenal insufficiency, hypopituitarism, diabetes mellitus, uremia, sedentary lifestyle, homelessness, inadequately heated housing, inadequate clothing, occupational or recreational exposure, prior cold weather injury, substance use or overdose, antipsychotic drug use, sepsis, infection, hypoglycemia, as well as the factors listed above. Heat loss occurs more rapidly with high wind velocity ("windchill factor"); water immersion or wet clothing; or direct contact with a cold surface (ie, stone, concrete, soil or the ground).

Accidental hypothermia may occur in the hospital setting due to prolonged postoperative hypothermia or administration of large amounts of refrigerated stored blood products (without rewarming), rapid infusion of intravenous fluids, or prolonged exposure of an undressed patient during resuscitation or procedures.

The human body generates internal heat through muscle activity (ie, shivering or increased physical exertion) and preserves heat loss via peripheral vasoconstriction. In prolonged or repetitive cold exposure, these thermoregulatory responses can become impaired; hypothermia ensues. Hypothermia diagnosis can be easily overlooked and delayed in a critically ill or injured patient. Hypothermia should be considered in any patient with prolonged exposure to ambient or cold environment, trauma, or inadequate clothing.

Systemic hypothermia alters physiologic function. This results in decreased respiratory drive, oxygen consumption, peripheral nerve conduction, gastrointestinal motility, myocardial repolarization, and coagulation cascade.

► Clinical Findings

Symptoms and signs of hypothermia are typically nonspecific and markedly variable based on the patient's underly-

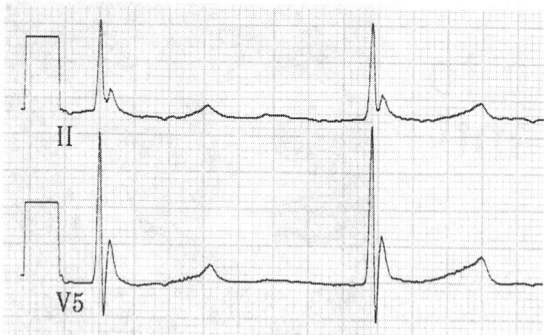

▲ **Figure 37–1.** Electrocardiogram shows leads II and V5 in a patient whose body temperature is 24 °C. Note the bradycardia and Osborn waves. These findings become more prominent as the body temperature lowers, and gradually resolve with rewarming. Osborn waves have an extra deflection at the end of the QRS complex. These are best seen in the inferior and lateral precordial leads.

ing health and circumstances of hypothermia. In mild cases with core temperature between 32 °C and 35 °C, symptoms include tachypnea, tachycardia, hypertension, shivering, impaired coordination, poor judgment, and apathy. With core temperature between 28 °C and 32 °C, the body slows down. Shivering stops; bradycardia, dilated pupils, slowed reflexes, cold diuresis, and confusion and lethargy ensue. Electrocardiogram (ECG) may reveal J wave or Osborn wave (positive deflection in the terminal portion of the QRS complex, most notable in leads II, V_5, and V_6) (Figure 37–1). Below 28 °C, the skin may appear blue or puffy; coma, apnea, loss of reflexes, asystole, or ventricular fibrillation may lead the clinician to assume that patient is dead. Prolonged hypothermia may lead to dysrhythmias and conduction abnormalities, acidemia, hyperkalemia, rhabdomyolysis, pulmonary edema, chronic kidney disease, pneumonia, pancreatitis, hypoglycemia or hyperglycemia, and coagulopathy. Death in systemic hypothermia is usually due to ventricular fibrillation, asystole, or chronic kidney disease.

▶ **Treatment**

Resuscitation begins with assessment and support of airway, breathing and circulation, initiation of rewarming, and prevention of further heat loss. Rewarming is the initial, imperative treatment. The patient should be evaluated for secondary causes of hypothermia, trauma, and peripheral cold injury. Rewarming methods are determined by the degree of hypothermia and the resources available.

During rewarming, continuous monitoring of temperature and other vital signs, cardiac rhythm, and blood sugar must be done. Common complications of rewarming occur as colder peripheral blood returns to central circulation. This may result in core temperature afterdrop, rewarming acidosis from shunting lactate into the circulation, rewarming shock from peripheral vasodilation and

hypovolemia, ventricular fibrillation and other cardiac arrhythmias. Extreme caution must be taken when handling the hypothermic patient to avoid triggering arrhythmias. During the rewarming process, essential testing includes ECG, chest radiograph, arterial blood gases, and bedside glucose. Laboratory evaluation should assess for potential complications of lactic acidosis; rhabdomyolysis; electrolyte abnormalities; infection; and dysfunction of the pancreas, liver, kidneys, and coagulation. False laboratory values will occur if the blood sample is warmed to 37 °C for the testing. Antibiotics are not routinely given. Comatose patients have a high risk of aspiration pneumonia.

A. Passive and Active External Rewarming Methods

Patients with mild hypothermia (rectal temperature > 33 °C) who have been otherwise healthy usually respond well to passive and active external warming. **Passive external rewarming** involves removal of cold wet clothing and covering the patient with blankets to prevent further heat loss. The patient will rewarm due to the body's internal heat production through shivering and increased metabolism. **Active external rewarming** is highly effective and safe for mild hypothermia. This is a noninvasive method of applying external heat to the patient's skin. Examples include warm bedding, heated blankets, heat packs, and immersion into a 40 °C bath. Afterdrop can be lessened by active external rewarming of the trunk but not the extremities and by avoiding any muscle movement by the patient.

B. Active Internal (Core) Rewarming Methods

Active internal core rewarming methods are required for patients with core temperatures of < 33 °C. Patients with milder degrees of hypothermia may also benefit from these methods. Warm humidified oxygen (43–46 °C) is an easy, safe, and highly effective method. Warmed intravenous saline infusions (43 °C) should be used instead of lactated Ringer solution. Volume resuscitation is needed to prevent shock as vasodilation occurs during rewarming. Other methods (including warm solution lavage of the stomach, colon, thoracic cavity, peritoneum, or bladder; extracorporeal blood rewarming by cardiopulmonary, arteriovenous femorofemoral, or venovenous bypass; and hemodialysis) are based on the availability of equipment and skilled personnel. Esophageal rewarming tubes are used abroad and may soon become available in the United States. Endovascular warming devices are a less invasive alternative than extracorporeal methods but are not widely available in hospitals.

For patients with core temperature < 30 °C, treatment includes active rewarming, cardiopulmonary resuscitation (CPR), one shock attempt for dysrhythmia, and withholding of intravenous medications. Once the core temperature reaches 30 °C, cardiac medications can be given but at longer than standard intervals because metabolism is slowed and there is a risk of toxic accumulation as circulation is restored. Defibrillation may be performed as needed. Resuscitative efforts should be continued until the patient's core temperature increases to at least 32 °C.

Prognosis

Prognosis is directly related to the patient's underlying health and comorbidities, the severity of associated conditions, circumstances surrounding the hypothermia, and degree of metabolic acidosis. Prognosis is poor with low pH (≤ 6.6), elevated potassium (≥ 4.0 mEq/L), serious underlying condition, or treatment delay. If treated early, most otherwise healthy patients may survive moderate or severe hypothermia.

HYPOTHERMIA OF THE EXTREMITIES

 ESSENTIALS OF DIAGNOSIS

▶ Cold-induced injuries should not be rubbed or massaged during rewarming.

▶ Rewarming of cold-induced injuries must be performed as soon as possible after there is no risk of refreezing.

Clinical Findings

Cold exposure of the extremities produces immediate localized vasoconstriction followed by generalized vasoconstriction. When the skin temperature falls to 25 °C, tissue demand for oxygen is greater than what is supplied by the slowed circulation: the area becomes cyanotic. At 15 °C, tissue damage occurs due to marked reduction in tissue metabolism and in oxyhemoglobin dissociation. This gives a deceptive pink, well-oxygenated appearance to the skin. Tissue death may result from ischemia and thromboses in the smaller vessels or by actual freezing. Freezing (frostbite) may occur when the skin temperature drops below -4 to -10 °C or at higher temperatures in the presence of wind, immobility, malnutrition, or vascular disease. Cold-induced injuries to the extremities (frostnip, chilbain, trench foot, and frostbite) range from mild to severe.

Prevention

"Keep warm, keep dry, and keep moving." Individuals should wear warm, dry clothing, preferably several layers, with a windproof outer garment. Arms, legs, fingers, and toes should be exercised to maintain circulation. Wet clothing, socks, and shoes should be replaced with dry ones. Extra socks, mittens, and insoles should always be carried in a pack during travel in cold or icy areas. Caution must be taken to avoid cramped positions; constrictive clothing; prolonged dependency of the feet; use of tobacco, alcohol, and sedative medications; and exposure to wet muddy ground and windy conditions.

FROSTNIP & CHILBLAIN (Erythema Pernio)

Frostnip is a mild temporary form of cold-induced injury. The involved area has local paresthesias that completely resolve with passive external rewarming.

Chilblains or **erythema pernio** are inflammatory skin changes caused by exposure to cold without actual freezing of the tissues. These skin lesions may be red or purple, painful or pruritic, with burning or paresthesias; they may be associated with edema or blistering and aggravated by warmth. With continued exposure, ulcerative or hemorrhagic lesions may appear and progress to scarring, fibrosis, and atrophy.

Treatment consists of elevating and passively externally rewarming the affected part. Caution must be taken to avoid rubbing or massaging injured tissues and to avoid applying ice or heat. The area must be protected from trauma and secondary infection.

IMMERSION FOOT OR TRENCH FOOT

Immersion foot (or hand) is caused by prolonged immersion in cool or cold water or mud, usually less than 10 °C. Early symptoms include cold and anesthesia of the affected area (prehyperemic stage). This is followed by hot sensation, intense burning, shooting pains (hyperemic stage). With ongoing cold exposure, the affected part becomes pale or cyanotic with diminished pulsations due to vasospasm (posthyperemic stage). This may result in blistering, swelling, redness, ecchymoses, hemorrhage, necrosis, peripheral nerve injury, or gangrene and secondary complications such as lymphangitis, cellulitis, and thrombophlebitis.

Treatment is best instituted during the hyperemic stage. Treatment consists of air drying, protecting the extremities from trauma and secondary infection, and gradual rewarming by exposure to air at room temperature (not ice or heat). Caution must be taken to avoid massaging or moistening the skin and to avoid water immersion. Bed rest is required until all ulcers have healed. Affected parts are elevated to aid in removal of edema fluid, and pressure sites (eg, heels) are protected with pillows. Prevention involves properly fitting footwear, improved foot hygiene, and sock changes to keep feet clean and dry.

FROSTBITE

Frostbite is injury from tissue freezing and formation of ice crystals in the tissue. In mild cases, only the skin and subcutaneous tissues are involved; the symptoms are numbness, prickling, itching, and pallor. With increasing severity, deep frostbite involves deeper structures. The skin appears white or yellow, loses its elasticity, and becomes immobile. Edema, hemorrhagic blisters, necrosis, and gangrene may appear. This may cause paresthesias and stiffness.

Treatment

A. Immediate Treatment

Evaluate and treat the patient for associated systemic hypothermia and injury. Fluids and electrolytes should be monitored.

1. Rewarming—Rapid rewarming at temperatures slightly above body heat may significantly decrease tissue necrosis. If there is any possibility of refreezing, the frostbitten part should not be thawed. Refreezing results in increased tissue necrosis. Rewarming is best accomplished by warm bath immersion. The frozen extremity is immersed for several minutes in a moving water bath heated to 40–42 °C until the distal tip of the part being thawed flushes. Dry heat (eg, stove or open fire) is more difficult to regulate, increases likelihood of accidental burns and is not recommended. Thawing may cause tenderness and burning pain. Once the frozen part has thawed and returned to normal temperature (usually in about 30 minutes), discontinue external heat. Rewarming by exercise, rubbing, or friction is contraindicated in the early stage. The patient is kept at bed rest with the affected parts elevated and uncovered at room temperature. Casts, occlusive dressings, or bandages are not applied. Blisters should be left intact unless signs of infection supervene.

2. Anti-infective measures and wound care—Frostbite increases susceptibility to tetanus and infection. Tetanus prophylaxis must be considered. Infection risk may be reduced by aseptic wound care and protection of skin blebs from physical contact. Wounds should be kept open and allowed to dry before applying dressings. Nonadherent sterile gauze and fluffy dressing should be loosely applied to wounds and cushions used for all areas of pressure. Antibiotics should not be administered empirically. Systemic antibiotics are reserved for deep infections not responding to local wound care.

B. Medical and Surgical Treatment Options

Debridement and amputation should be considered only after it is established that the tissues are necrotic. Magnetic resonance imaging with angiography and technetium scintigraphy have been used to assess the extent of frostbite and to distinguish viable from nonviable tissue. Eschar formation without evidence of infection may be conservatively treated. The underlying skin may heal spontaneously with the eschar acting as a biologic dressing. Intra-arterial thrombolytic administration within 24 hours of exposure has resulted in improved tissue perfusion and has reduced amputation.

C. Follow-Up Care

Gentle, progressive physical therapy to promote circulation should be instituted as tolerated.

▶ Prognosis

Recovery from frostbite depends on the extent of initial tissue damage, the rewarming reperfusion injury, and the late sequelae (such as chronic kidney disease or postinjury infections) and underlying comorbidities. There may be increased susceptibility to discomfort and injury in the involved extremity upon reexposure to cold. Neuropathic sequelae such as pain, numbness, tingling, hyperhidrosis, and cold sensitivity of the extremities, and nerve conduction abnormalities may persist for many years after the cold injury.

AORN Recommended Practices Committee. Recommended practices for the prevention of unplanned perioperative hypothermia. AORN J. 2007 May;85(5):972–88. [PMID: 17533677]

Aslam AF et al. Hypothermia: evaluation, electrocardiographic manifestations, and management. Am J Med. 2006 Apr; 119(4):297–301. [PMID: 16564768]

Aslan S et al. The Osborn wave in accidental hypothermia. J Emerg Med. 2007 Apr;32(3):271–3. [PMID: 17394990]

Bruen KJ et al. Reduction of the incidence of amputation in frostbite injury with thrombolytic therapy. Arch Surg. 2007 Jun;142(6):546–51. [PMID: 17576891]

Castellani JW et al. American College of Sports Medicine position stand: prevention of cold injuries during exercise. Med Sci Sports Exerc. 2006 Nov;38(11):2012–29. [PMID: 17095937]

Centers for Disease Control and Prevention (CDC). Hypothermia-related mortality–Montana, 1999–2004. MMWR Morb Mortal Wkly Rep. 2007 Apr 20;56(15):367–8. [PMID: 17443122]

Jurkovich GJ. Environmental cold-induced injury. Surg Clin North Am. 2007 Feb;87(1):247–67. [PMID: 17127131]

Laniewicz M et al. Rapid endovascular warming for profound hypothermia. Ann Emerg Med. 2008 Feb;51(2):160–3. [PMID: 17681640]

van Marum RJ et al. Hypothermia following antipsychotic drug use. Eur J Clin Pharmacol. 2007 Jun;63(6):627–31. [PMID: 17401555]

Young AJ et al. Exertional fatigue and cold exposure: mechanisms of hiker's hypothermia. Appl Physiol Nutr Metab. 2007 Aug;32(4):793–8. [PMID: 17622297]

DISORDERS DUE TO HEAT

 ESSENTIALS OF DIAGNOSIS

▶ There is a spectrum of heat-related illnesses: heat cramps, heat exhaustion, heat syncope, and heat stroke.

▶ General Considerations

Hyperthermia results from the body's inability to maintain normal internal temperature through heat loss. The body's heat source is a result of internal metabolic function and environmental conditions. Heat loss occurs through sweating and peripheral vasodilation. The common comorbidities and risk factors leading to heat-related conditions are listed in the chapter's introduction. Additional risk factors include inhibition of sweat production or evaporation, obesity, skin disorders (miliaria), reduced cutaneous blood flow, dehydration, hypotension, reduced cardiac output, and use of drugs that increase metabolism or muscle activity or impair sweating, prolonged seizures, and withdrawal syndromes.

▶ Prevention

Public education is necessary to improve prevention and early recognition of heat-related disorders. Individuals should take steps to reduce personal risk factors (ie, physical inactivity, obesity, tobacco and drug use) and to acclimatize to the hot environment. Proper acclimatization must be achieved before heavy physical exertion (ie, occupational or exercise) is performed in hot environments.

Medical evaluation and monitoring should be used to identify the individuals and the weather conditions that increase risk of heat-related disorders. Athletic events should be organized with attention to thermoregulation: the wet bulb globe temperature (WBGT) index should be monitored. Competition is not recommended when the WBGT exceeds 26–28 °C. Guidance regarding heat hazard is found in the National Weather Service's Heat Index that rates weather conditions based on humidity and temperature measurements (www.weather.gov/om/heat/index.shtml). The US Army provides guidance regarding activity levels according to WBGT levels (www.usariem.army.mil/heatill/appendc.htm).

Those who are physically active in a hot environment should increase fluid consumption. Fluid consumption should include balanced electrolyte fluids and water. Water consumption alone may lead to electrolyte imbalance, particularly hyponatremia. It is not recommended to have salt tablets available for use without medical supervision. Close monitoring of fluid and electrolyte intake and early intervention are recommended in situations necessitating exertion or activity in hot environments. Exertional heat-related disorders are common in unconditioned participants in strenuous activities in hot humid conditions (ie, military drills, marathons, triathlon competitions, or exercise during heat waves).

SPECIFIC SYNDROMES DUE TO HEAT EXPOSURE

1. Heat Syncope or Collapse

Sudden collapse or unconsciousness may result from volume depletion and cutaneous vasodilation with consequent systemic and cerebral hypotension. Exercise-associated postural hypotension is usually the cause of this: it may occur during or immediately following exercise. There is usually a history of prolonged vigorous physical activity. Typically, the skin is cool and moist, the pulse is weak, and the systolic blood pressure is low.

Treatment consists of rest and recumbency in a cool place and fluid and electrolyte rehydration by mouth (or intravenously if necessary).

2. Heat Cramps

Fluid and electrolyte depletion may result in slow, painful skeletal muscle contractions ("cramps") and severe muscle spasms lasting 1–3 minutes, usually of the muscles most heavily used. The skin is moist and cool. The muscles are tender, hard and lumpy, and muscle twitching may be present. The patient is alert, with stable vital signs, and may be agitated and complaining of pain. The body temperature may be normal or slightly increased. There is almost always a history of vigorous activity just preceding the onset of symptoms. Laboratory evaluation may show low serum sodium, hemoconcentration, and elevated urea and creatinine.

The patient should be moved to a cool environment and given oral saline solution (4 tsp of salt per gallon of water) to replace both salt and water. *Oral salt tablets are not recommended.* The patient may have to rest for 1–3 days with continued dietary salt supplementation before returning to work or resuming strenuous activity in the heat.

3. Heat Exhaustion

Heat exhaustion results from prolonged strenuous activity with inadequate water or salt intake in a hot environment. It is characterized by dehydration, sodium depletion, or isotonic fluid loss with accompanying cardiovascular changes.

The diagnosis is based on prolonged symptoms and a rectal temperature over 37.8 °C, increased pulse (> 150% of the patient's normal) and moist skin. Symptoms are similar to those associated with heat syncope and heat cramps. Additional symptoms include nausea, vomiting, malaise, myalgias, hyperventilation, thirst, and weakness. Central nervous system symptoms include headache, dizziness, fatigue, anxiety, paresthesias, impaired judgment, hysteria, and occasionally psychosis. Hyperventilation secondary to heat exhaustion can cause respiratory alkalosis; lactic acidosis may also occur due to poor tissue perfusion. Heat exhaustion may progress to heat stroke if sweating ceases and mental status declines.

Treatment consists of moving patient to a shaded, cool environment, providing adequate hydration (1–2 L over 2–4 hours), oral salt replenishment, and active cooling (ie, fans, cool packs) if necessary. Physiologic saline or isotonic glucose solution should be administered intravenously when oral administration is not appropriate. At least 24 hours of rest and rehydration are recommended.

4. Heat Stroke

Heat stroke is a life-threatening medical emergency. The hallmarks of heat stroke are cerebral dysfunction with core temperature over 40 °C and absence of sweating. It presents in one of two forms: classic and exertional. **Classic heat stroke** occurs in patients with impaired thermoregulatory mechanisms; **exertional heat stroke** occurs in healthy persons undergoing strenuous exertion in a hot or humid environment. Persons at greatest risk are the very young, the elderly, the chronically debilitated, and those taking medications that interfere with heat-dissipating mechanisms (ie, anticholinergics, antihistamines, phenothiazines).

Heat stroke is associated with high morbidity and mortality from cerebral, cardiovascular, liver, or kidney damage. A high Simplified Acute Physiology Score II, high body temperature, prolonged prothrombin time, use of vasoactive drugs within the first day in the intensive care unit (ICU), and an ICU without air conditioning all were associated with increased mortality.

▶ Clinical Findings

A. Symptoms and Signs

Heat stroke may present with dizziness, weakness, emotional lability, nausea and vomiting, diarrhea, confusion, delirium, blurred vision, convulsions, collapse, and unconsciousness. The skin is hot, initially covered with perspiration; later it dries. The pulse is strong initially. Widened pulse pressure is present. Blood pressure may be slightly elevated at first, but hypotension develops later. Tachycardia and hyperventilation (with subsequent respiratory alkalosis) occur. The core temperature is usually over 40 °C.

Exertional heat stroke may present with sudden collapse and loss of consciousness followed by irrational behavior. Anhidrosis may not be present. Multiorgan dysfunction or injury is a common and serious complication.

B. Laboratory Findings

Laboratory evaluation may reveal dehydration; leukocytosis; elevated blood urea nitrogen (BUN); hyperuricemia; hemoconcentration; acid-base abnormalities (eg, lactic acidosis, respiratory alkalosis); decreased serum potassium, sodium, calcium, and phosphorus; thrombocytopenia, fibrinolysis, and coagulopathy; elevated creatine kinase (CK); elevated aminotransferase levels and liver dysfunction; and elevated cardiac markers. Urine is concentrated, with proteinuria, hematuria, tubular casts, and myoglobinuria. ECG findings may include ST–T changes consistent with myocardial ischemia. Pco_2 may be less than 20 mm Hg.

► Treatment

Treatment is aimed at reducing the core temperature rapidly (within 1 hour) while supporting organ system function. Care must be taken to avoid shivering, which will increase internal heat production and inhibit effectiveness of cooling. Benzodiazepines may be used to suppress shivering. Evaporative cooling is a noninvasive, effective, quick and easy way to reduce temperature. The patient is undressed and the entire body sprayed with lukewarm water (20 °C) while large fans circulate the room air. The patient should be in the lateral recumbent position or supported in a hands-and-knees position to expose as maximum skin surface to the air. Alternatively, the use of cold wet sheets accompanied by fanning may be used. Inhalation of cool air or oxygen, and infusion of cool intravenous fluids are also effective.

Immersion in an ice-water bath (1–5 °C) is effective but impractical method due to its physical requirements and limitations to patient access and monitoring. Other cooling alternatives include hand and forearm immersion in cold water, localized ice or ice slush application (groin, axillas, neck), and iced gastric lavage. These are much less effective than evaporative cooling and usually less tolerated in the awake patient. Skin massage is recommended to prevent cutaneous vasoconstriction. Intravascular heat exchange catheter systems as well as hemodialysis using cold dialysate (30–35 °C) have been successful in reducing core temperature. Research suggests that brain cooling may lessen cerebrovascular injury from heat stroke. *Antipyretics (aspirin, acetaminophen) have no effect on environmentally induced hyperthermia and are contraindicated.* Treatment should be continued until the rectal temperature drops to 39 °C.

All patients with suspected heat stroke must be admitted to the hospital for close monitoring, including vital signs, temperature, and cardiac rhythm, and observation for 24 hours. The patient should also be monitored for potential complications of electrolyte abnormalities, acute kidney injury due to rhabdomyolysis, cardiac arrhythmias, coagulopathy, hepatic failure, acute respiratory distress syndrome (ARDS), hypoglycemia, seizures, and infection. Intravascular volume status should be assessed and man-

aged. Hypovolemic and cardiogenic shock must be carefully distinguished, since either or both may occur. Oral or intravenous fluid administration must be provided to ensure a high urinary output (> 50 mL/h). Fluid output should be monitored through the use of an indwelling urinary catheter. Mannitol administration (0.25 mg/kg), and alkalinizing the urine (intravenous administration of 250 mL of 4% bicarbonate administration) may be needed.

Multiorgan dysfunction is the usual cause of heat stroke–related death, and it can be predicted by CK > 1000 units/L, metabolic acidosis, and elevated liver enzymes. Multiorgan dysfunction and inflammation may continue after temperature is normalized. Hypokalemia frequently accompanies heat stroke but may not appear until rehydration. Maintenance of extracellular hydration and electrolyte balance should reduce the risk of chronic kidney disease due to rhabdomyolysis.

Because sensitivity to high environmental temperature may persist for prolonged periods following an episode of heat stroke, immediate reexposure should be avoided.

American College of Sports Medicine; Armstrong LE et al. American College of Sports Medicine position stand. Exertional heat illness during training and competition. Med Sci Sports Exerc. 2007 Mar;39(3):556–72. [PMID: 17473783]

Bouchama A et al. Prognostic factors in heat wave related deaths: a meta-analysis. Arch Intern Med. 2007 Nov 12;167(20):2170–6. [PMID: 17698676]

Howe AS et al. Heat-related illness in athletes. Am J Sports Med. 2007 Aug;35(8):1384–95. [PMID: 17609528]

Hsiao SH et al. Resuscitation from experimental heatstroke by brain cooling therapy. Resuscitation. 2007 Jun;73(3):437–45. [PMID: 17300862]

Kenefick RW et al. Heat exhaustion and dehydration as causes of marathon collapse. Sports Med. 2007;37(4–5):378–81. [PMID: 17465613]

Lewis AM. Emergency: heatstroke in older adults. In this population it's a short step from heat exhaustion. Am J Nurs. 2007 Jun;107(6):52–6. [PMID: 17519606]

LoVecchio F et al. Outcomes after environmental hyperthermia. Am J Emerg Med. 2007 May;25(4):442–4. [PMID: 17499664]

Misset B et al. Mortality of patients with heatstroke admitted to intensive care units during the 2003 heat wave in France: a national multiple-center risk-factor study. Crit Care Med. 2006 Apr;34(4):1087–92. [PMID: 16484920]

Noakes TD. A modern classification of the exercise-related heat illnesses. J Sci Med Sport. 2008 Feb;11(1):33–9. [PMID: 17524793]

▼ BURNS

The incidence and severity of burn injuries has been declining, with both deaths and acute hospitalizations attributable to burns down about 50%. Over three-fourths of burns involve less than 10% of total body surface area. Aggressive, early excision (24–72 hours postburn) of deeply burned tissues and skin grafting, early enteral feeding, and improved infection control have contributed to significantly lower mortality rates and shorter hospitalizations. Nonetheless, an estimated 1.25 million burn injuries and 51,000 acute hospitalizations of burn victims occur each year in the United States. Approximately 12,500 patients per year are admitted to dedicated burn units. Overall, 62% of all patients with burns seen in burn centers had minor burns that affected less than 10% of the total body surface area, and 6.5% of patients admitted had inhalation injury. Among burn patients, 70% were male and had a mean age of 33 years. Flame and scald burns accounted for 78% of injuries.

The first 48 hours of hemodynamic shifts offer the greatest opportunity to impact the survival of the multiply injured patient with burn injuries. Related injuries include smoke inhalation, fractures, and blast injuries. Subsequent problems include bacterial superinfection, sepsis, and multiorgan failure. Finally, scar contractures and disfigurement occur during the later stages of burn injury.

CLASSIFICATION

Burns are classified by extent, depth, patient age, and associated illness or injury. Accurate estimation of burn size and depth is important since this figure will quantify the parameters of resuscitation.

A. Extent

The "rule of nines" (Figure 37–2) is useful for rapidly assessing the extent of a burn. More detailed charts based on age are available when the patient reaches the burn unit. Therefore, it is important to view the entire patient after cleaning soot to make an accurate assessment, both initially and on subsequent examinations. On average, the degree of burn is overestimated by 75% by referring doctors. This becomes important when air transport is instituted to a burn center for minor injuries. One rule of thumb is that the palm of the hand, open, constitutes 1% total body surface area in adults. Only second- and third-degree burns are included in calculating the total burn surface area, since first-degree burns usually do not represent significant injury in terms of prognosis or fluid and electrolyte management. However, first- or second-degree burns may convert to deeper burns, especially if treatment is delayed or bacterial colonization or superinfection occurs.

B. Depth

Judgment of depth of injury is difficult. The **first-degree burn** may be red or gray but will demonstrate excellent capillary refill. First-degree burns are not blistered initially. If the wound is blistered, this represents a partial-thickness injury to the dermis, or a **second-degree burn**. As the degree of burn is progressively deeper, there is a progressive loss of adnexal structures. Hairs can be easily extracted or are absent, sweat glands become less visible, and the skin appears smoother.

Deep second- and third-degree burns are treated in a similar fashion, since neither will heal appropriately without early debridement and grafting; the resultant skin is thin and scarred.

The benefits of hyperbaric oxygen for treatment of acute burns remain unproven and anecdotal.

C. Survival after Burn Injury

The Prognostic Burn Index is the sum of the patient's age and percentage of full thickness or deep partial thickness burn. An additional 20% mortality is added if inhalation injury is present. Recently, patients with a 90–100% predicted mortality rate now have an estimated mortality rate of 50–70%. The Prognostic Burn Index is most useful at the extremes of age. Recent treatment advances have significantly reduced mortality rates, including early burn excision, skin substitute usage, and early enteral feeding. Transfer to a burn unit with its support staff is indicated when burns are large, when there are comorbidities, and when smaller burns occur in high risk areas. According to the 2005 Burn Repository Statistics, mortality rates among all burn victims have decreased from 6.2% in 1995 to 4.7% in 2005.

D. Associated Injuries or Illnesses

An injury commonly associated with burns is smoke inhalation (see Chapter 9). Suspicion of inhalation injury is aroused when the nasal hairs are singed, the mechanism of burn involves closed spaces, the sputum is carbonaceous, or the carboxyhemoglobin level exceeds 5% in nonsmokers. This suspicion should lead the clinician to institute early intubation before airway edema occurs. The products of combustion, not heat, are responsible for lower airway injury. When carbon monoxide poisoning is suspected, pure oxygen is administered for 45 minutes. Early extubation is avoided for the first 48–72 hours since there is a risk of continued airway edema during the dynamic fluid shift period of early resuscitation. Electrical injury that causes burns may also produce cardiac arrhythmias that require immediate attention. Pancreatitis occurs in severe burns. Prior alcohol exposure may exacerbate the pulmonary components of burn injury.

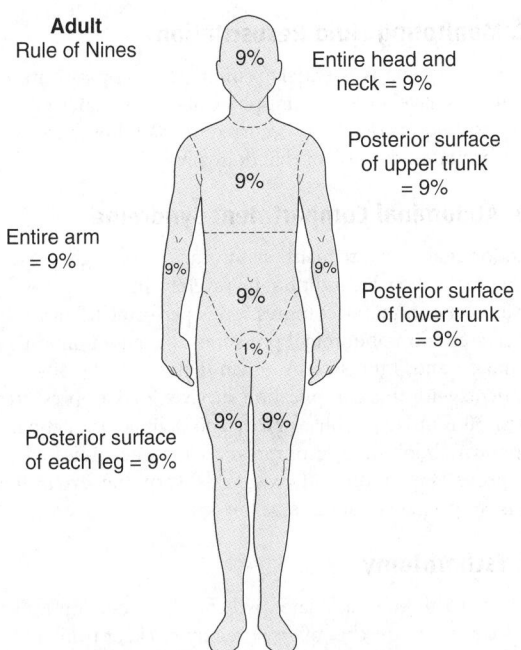

Adult
Rule of Nines

9% — Entire head and neck = 9%

Posterior surface of upper trunk = 9%

9%

Entire arm = 9%

9%   9%

9%

Posterior surface of lower trunk = 9%

1%

9% 9%

Posterior surface of each leg = 9%

▲ **Figure 37–2.** Estimation of body surface area in burns.

Toxic epidermal necrolysis (TEN) occasionally occurs following sulfonamide or phenytoin administration (see Chapter 6). If TEN is severe, patients are best transferred to a burn unit and treated as having severe burn injury. Corticosteroid therapy should be avoided.

SYSTEMIC REACTIONS TO BURN INJURY

The actual burn injury is only the incipient event in a cascade of deleterious local tissue and systemic inflammatory reactions leading to multiorgan system failure in the severely burned patient. When burns greater than approximately 20% of total body surface area are present, systemic metabolic alterations occur and require intensive support. The inflammatory cascade can result in shock.

INITIAL MANAGEMENT

A. Airway

The practitioner or emergency medical technician should proceed as with any other trauma using standard Advanced Trauma Life Support (ATLS) guidelines. The priorities are first to establish an airway, recognizing the frequent necessity to intubate a patient who may appear to be breathing normally but who has sustained an inhalation injury; next, to evaluate the cervical spine and head injuries; and finally, to stabilize fractures. Fluid resuscitation by the Parkland formula (see below) may be instituted simultaneously with initial resuscitation. Endotracheal intubation or tracheotomy should be considered for major burn cases regardless of the area of the body involved, because as fluid resuscitation proceeds generalized edema develops, including edema of the soft tissues of the upper airway and perhaps the lungs as well. Chest radiographs are typically normal initially but may develop an ARDS picture in 24–48 hours with severe inhalation injury. Supplemental oxygen should be administered. Inhalation injuries should be monitored with serial blood gas determination and bronchoscopy. The use of corticosteroids or routine use of antibiotic therapy is not indicated.

B. Vascular Access

A thorough examination is performed to assess the extent of burn and associated injuries. Large bore venous catheter access is established. Subclavian lines are avoided in the emergency setting because of the risk of pneumothorax and subclavian vein laceration when such a line is placed in a volume-depleted patient. Femoral lines provide good temporary access during resuscitation. *Venous access catheters placed in the emergency department should be changed within 24 hours because of the high risk of nonsterile placement.* An arterial line is useful for monitoring mean arterial pressure and for drawing blood in critically ill patients.

FLUID RESUSCITATION

A. Crystalloids

Generalized capillary leak results from burn injury over more than 20% of total body surface area. This often necessitates replacement of a large volume of fluid.

There are many guidelines for fluid resuscitation. The **Parkland formula** relies on the use of lactated Ringer injection. The fluid requirement in the first 24 hours is estimated as 4 mL/kg body weight per percent of body surface area burned. Half the calculated fluid is given in the first 8-hour period. The remaining fluid, divided into two equal parts, is delivered over the next 16 hours. An extremely large volume of fluid may be required. For example, an injury over 40% of the total body surface area in a 70-kg victim may require 11.2 L in the first 24 hours [4 mL × 40(%) × 70 (kg) = 11,200 mL]. The first 8-hour period is measured from the hour of injury. These guidelines may be inadequate, since crystalloid solutions alone may be insufficient to restore cardiac preload during the period of burn shock.

Deep electrical burns and inhalation injury increase the fluid requirement. Adequacy of resuscitation is determined by clinical parameters, including urinary output and specific gravity, blood pressure, pulse, temperature, and central venous pressure. The need for fluid replacement of more than 150% of calculated values indicates possible unrecognized injury, possible comorbidities, and a worse prognosis and may indicate the need for a Swan-Ganz catheter to assist in management.

B. Colloids

Overly aggressive crystalloid administration must be avoided in patients with pulmonary injury, since significant pulmonary edema can develop in patients with normal pulmonary capillary wedge and central venous pressures. In addition, routine colloid administration, previously commonplace, is no longer warranted in routine burn resuscitation in view of its deleterious effect on glomerular filtration and its association with pulmonary edema.

C. Monitoring Fluid Resuscitation

A Foley catheter is essential for monitoring urinary output. Diuretics have no role in this phase of patient management unless fluid overload has occurred or mannitol diuresis is performed in the case of rhabdomyolysis.

D. Abdominal Compartment Syndrome

Abdominal compartment syndrome is emerging as a potentially lethal condition in severely burned patients, even if abdominal decompression is performed. Markedly increased intra-abdominal pressures can cause pulmonary damage and multisystem organ failure. Only 40% of patients with this complication survive. Bladder pressures over 30 mm Hg establish the diagnosis in at-risk patients. Surgical abdominal decompression may be indicated to improve ventilation and oxygen delivery, but even after this, surgery survival remains low.

E. Escharotomy

As edema fluid accumulates, ischemia may develop under any constricting eschar of an extremity, neck, or trunk if the full-thickness burn is circumferential. Escharotomy incisions through the anesthetic eschar can save life and limb and can be performed in the emergency department or operating room.

F. Fasciotomy in Electrical Burns or Crush Injuries

When high-voltage electrical injury occurs, extensive deep tissue necrosis should be suspected. Deep tissue necrosis leads to profound tissue swelling. Because deep tissue compartments in the arms and legs are contained by unyielding fascia, these compartments must be opened by surgical fasciotomy to prevent further soft tissue, vascular, and nerve death.

Electrical burn injuries remain the most devastating and underrecognized burn injuries, causing amputations (often because of unrecognized compartment syndromes) and acute kidney injury, resulting in part from rhabdomyolysis.

THE BURN WOUND

Minor burn wounds should be debrided at bedside to determine the depth of the burn and then thoroughly cleansed. Thereafter, the wound should be debrided daily and dressed with a topical antibiotic such as silver sulfadiazine (Silvadene) or bacitracin ointment. Patient compliance and adequate pain treatment is essential for successful outpatient treatment. The wound should be reevaluated by the treating surgeon if possible within 72 hours to evaluate for signs of infection.

Biobrane and Tegaderm should be reserved for clean scald burns. Acute burns caused by hydrofluoric acid should be treated by water rinsing followed by application of topical calcium. Treatment of the burn wound is based on protecting the wound from desiccation and avoiding further injury of those burned areas that will spontaneously reepithelialize in 7–10 days by application of topical antibiotic such as silver sulfadiazine (Silvadene). It is painless, easy to apply, and effective against most strains of *Pseudomonas*. For severely burned patients, Integra, a temporary skin substitute that can create a thin neodermis, may provide temporary coverage (and may even reduce hospitalization) but it is very expensive. Regular and thorough cleansing of burned areas is a critically important intervention in burn units. Early excision and grafting of burned areas may be performed as soon as 24 hours after burn injury or when the patient can hemodynamically tolerate the excision and grafting procedure. Meticulous prevention of seromas, hypergranulation tissue formation, and malnutrition all decrease time to complete wound healing in skin-grafted patients.

Systemic infection remains a leading cause of morbidity among patients with major burn injuries, with nearly all severely burned patients having one or more septicemic episodes during the hospital course. Antibiotic usage should be targeted to specific organisms obtained by culture. Healthcare-associated infections are increasingly common. Obtaining pharmacologic expertise is useful in choosing appropriate antibiotic therapy, interpreting varying drug levels, and assessing drug-drug interactions. Coagulase-negative staphylococci (63%) and *Staphylococcus*

aureus (20%) are commonly cultured from burn wounds. Methicillin-resistant *S aureus, vancomycin-resistant Enterococcus,* and *Pseudomonas aeruginosa* are also commonly cultured but usually later in the hospital course. *P aeruginosa* infections are associated with the highest mortality rate (33% vs 9% in nonpseudomonal infections), with aminoglycoside-resistant *Pseudomonas* infections particularly morbid. Routine use of blood culture in the severely burned population is indicated to elucidate systemic blood infections that do not manifest these clinical predictors of sepsis.

Wound Closure

The goal of therapy after fluid resuscitation is rapid and stable closure of the wound. Wounds that will not heal spontaneously in 7–10 days (ie, deep second-degree or third-degree burns) are best treated by excision and autograft; otherwise, granulation and infection may develop, and the quality of the skin in regenerated deep partial thickness burns is marginal because of the very thin dermis that emerges.

Cultured allogeneic keratinocyte grafts can provide rapid early coverage for superficial burn injuries. With severe burns, skin substitution with such cultured grafts can be lifesaving. However, although the replaced dermis does have nearly normal histologic dermal elements, there are no adnexal structures present and very few, if any, elastic fibers. Intraoperative use of topical fibrin sealants may reduce blood loss, improve cosmetic results, and improve postoperative graft adherence.

PATIENT SUPPORT

Burn patients require extensive support. An attempt must be made to maintain normal core body temperature (by maintaining environmental temperature at or above 30 °C) in patients with burns over more than 20% of total body surface area, since the hypermetabolic state of burns is exacerbated by subnormal temperatures. Respiratory injury, sepsis, and multiorgan failure are common. Enteral feedings may be started once the ileus of the resuscitation period has resolved, usually the day after the injury. There is often a markedly increased metabolic rate after burn injury, due in large part to whole body synthesis and increased fatty acid substrate cycles. If the patient does not tolerate low-residue tube feedings, total parenteral nutrition should be started without delay through a central venous catheter. Contrary to conventional teachings, data indicate that most patients can be fed adequately with energy equal to 100% to 120% of estimated basal energy expenditure (BEE). A useful guide is to provide 25 kcal/kg body weight plus 40 kcal per percent of burn surface area. Early aggressive enteral nutrition reduces infections, noninfectious complications, length of hospital stay, impaired healing, and mortality. Anticatabolic treatments such as β-blockade, growth hormone, insulin, oxandrolone, and synthetic testosterone have been advocated. Melatonin, which appears to possess multifaceted antioxidant properties, may reduce proinflammatory cytokines and have beneficial chronobiotic effects in severely burned patients.

Careful control of the postinjury blood glucose has been associated with improved hepatic function and better survival after severe burns. Occasionally, ARDS or respiratory failure unresponsive to maximal ventilatory support may develop in burn patients. In addition, the incidence of venous thromboembolism in the lower extremities is high among burn patients. Duplex ultrasonography is the best method for identifying venous thromboembolism.

Prevention of long-term scars remains a formidable problem in seriously burned patients. The V-beam pulsed dye laser and intense pulsed light are emerging as adjunctive treatments to the usual regimen of corticosteroid injections, silicone patches, compression, and scar revision. Permanent sequelae can be avoided by prevention of infection, early aggressive rehabilitation, compressive garments, and early psychological support. Facial transplantation has become a controversial but potential treatment for those patients with devastating unreconstructable facial burns.

Complex microsurgical reconstructions, including prefabricated reconstructive flaps, now benefit severely burned patients with injuries to neck, hand, and arm.

Armour AD et al. The impact of nosocomially-acquired resistant *Pseudomonas aeruginosa* infection in a burn unit. J Trauma. 2007 Jul;63(1):164–71. [PMID: 17622885]

Baker CP et al. Physical and psychologic rehabilitation outcomes for young adults burned as children. Arch Phys Med Rehabil. 2007 Dec;88(12 Suppl 2):S57–64. [PMID: 18036983]

Esselman PC. Burn rehabilitation: an overview. Arch Phys Med Rehabil. 2007 Dec;88(12 Suppl 2):S3–6. [PMID: 18036978]

Foster K. The use of fibrin sealant in burn operations. Surgery. 2007 Oct;142(4 Suppl):S50–4. [PMID: 18019939]

Grunwald TB et al. Acute burns. Plast Reconstr Surg. 2008 May;121(5):311e–319e. [PMID: 18453944]

Houle JM et al. A prefabricated, tissue-engineered Integra free flap. Plast Reconstr Surg. 2007 Oct;120(5):1322–5. [PMID: 17898607]

Jacobs LM et al. Trauma deaths: views of the public and trauma professionals on death and dying from injuries. Arch Surg. 2008 Aug;143(8):730–5. [PMID: 18711031]

Jeschke MG et al. Effect of insulin on the inflammatory and acute phase response after burn injury. Crit Care Med. 2007 Sep;35(9 Suppl):S519–23. [PMID: 17713402]

Jewell L et al. Rate of healing in skin-grafted burn wounds. Plast Reconstr Surg. 2007 Aug;120(2):451–6. [PMID: 17632348]

Maldonado MD et al. Melatonin as pharmacologic support in burn patients: a proposed solution to thermal injury-related lymphocytopenia and oxidative damage. Crit Care Med. 2007 Apr;35(4):1177–85. [PMID: 17312564]

Murray CK et al. Evaluation of white blood cell count, neutrophil percentage, and elevated temperature as predictors of bloodstream infection in burn patients. Arch Surg. 2007 Jul;142(7):639–42. [PMID: 17638801]

Oda J et al. Acute lung injury and multiple organ dysfunction syndrome secondary to intra-abdominal hypertension and abdominal decompression in extensively burned patients. J Trauma. 2007 Jun;62(6):1365–9. [PMID: 17563650]

Pidcoke HF et al. Insulin and the burned patient. Crit Care Med. 2007 Sep;35(9 Suppl):S524–30. [PMID: 17713403]

Plante T et al. Carboxyhemoglobin monitored by bedside continuous CO-oximetry. J Trauma. 2007 Nov;63(5):1187–90. [PMID: 17993970]

Sauerbier M et al. Microvascular reconstruction in burn and electrical burn injuries of the severely traumatized upper extremity. Plast Reconstr Surg. 2007 Feb;119(2):605–15. [PMID: 17230097]

Trottier V et al. Survival after prolonged length of stay in a trauma intensive care unit. J Trauma. 2007 Jan;62(1):147–50. [PMID: 17215746]

White CE et al. Advances in surgical care: management of severe burn injury. Crit Care Med. 2008 Jul;36(7 Suppl):S318–24. [PMID: 18594259]

ELECTRICAL INJURY

 ESSENTIALS OF DIAGNOSIS

▶ Extent of injury is determined by the type, amount, duration, and pathway of electrical current.

▶ Resuscitation must be attempted on an electrical injury victim before assuming the patient is dead; clinical findings are unreliable.

▶ Skin findings may be misleading, and not indicative of the degree of deeper injury.

► General Considerations

Electricity-induced injury occurs by exposure to electrical current of low voltage, high voltage, or lightning. Direct current (DC) is unidirectional electrical flow. It is more likely to cause a single intense muscle contraction and asystole. Alternating current (AC) is bidirectional electrical flow that reverses direction in a sine wave pattern. This may cause muscle tetany, which prolongs the duration and amount of current exposure. If AC current passes through the thoracic area, it may lead to respiratory arrest or ventricular fibrillation. Low voltage is less than 1000 volts, and high voltage is more than 1000 volts. High voltage is most often related to occupational exposure and associated with higher morbidity and mortality. Fatal injury and significant damage may also occur with exposure to low voltage of household AC current. Lightning differs from high-voltage electrical shock in that lightning is massive high voltage (millions of volts) lasting a very brief duration (a small fraction of a second).

Electricity causes damage by various means: direct tissue damage, muscle tetany, direct thermal injury and coagulation necrosis, and trauma from associated falls or violent muscle contractions. The degree of injury depends on the following factors: current type, voltage, and pathway; duration of exposure; tissue resistance; associated trauma; and comorbidities. Tissue resistance varies through the body. Nerve cells are the most vulnerable and bone is the most resistant to electrical current. Skin resistance depends on thickness and condition of skin.

► Clinical Findings

The type and degree of injury is highly dependent on the current pathway. Symptoms and signs may range from tingling, superficial skin burns, and myalgias to paralysis, massive tissue damage, or death. Skin damage does not correlate with the degree of injury. Not all electrical injuries cause skin damage; only very minor skin damage may be present with massive internal injuries. Electrical burns are of three distinct types: flash (arcing) burns, flame (clothing) burns, and the direct heating effect of tissues by the electrical current. The latter lesions are usually sharply demarcated, round or oval, painless yellow-brown areas (Joule burn) with inflammatory reaction. Significant subcutaneous damage can be accompanied by little skin injury, particularly with larger skin surface area electrical contact.

A victim of electrical current injury may appear dead due to dysrhythmia, respiratory arrest, or autonomic dysfunction resulting in pupils that are fixed, dilated, or asymmetric. Resuscitation must be initiated on all victims of electrical injury since clinical findings are deceptive.

Complications

Complications include seizures, paralysis, headache, dysrhythmias, pneumothorax, tissue edema and necrosis, compartment syndrome, fractures from falls or muscle contractions, rhabdomyolysis, acute kidney injury, hypovolemia from third spacing, ruptured ear drums, and acute or delayed cataract formation.

Treatment

A. Emergency Measures

The victim must be separated from the electrical current prior to initiation of CPR or other treatment. The rescuer must be protected. Turn off the power, or separate the victim using nonconductive implements such as dry clothing. Resuscitation must then be initiated since clinical findings of death are unreliable.

B. Hospital Measures

The initial assessment involves airway, breathing, and circulation followed by trauma protocol. Fluid resuscitation is important to maintain adequate urinary output (0.5 mL/kg/h if no myoglobinuria is present, 1.0 mL/kg/h if myoglobinuria is present). Initial evaluation includes cardiac monitoring and ECG, complete blood count, electrolytes, renal function tests, liver biochemical tests, urinalysis, urine myoglobin, serum CK, and CK-MB. Victims must be evaluated for hidden injury (eg, ophthalmic, otologic, muscular, compartment syndromes), organ injury (myocardium, liver, kidney, pancreas), blunt trauma, dehydration, skin burns, hypertension, posttraumatic stress, acid-base disturbances, and neurologic damage.

Prognosis

Prognosis depends on the degree and location of electrical injury, initial damage, and complications. Psychiatric support may be necessary following lightning or severe electroshock exposures.

When to Refer

Fasciotomy may be needed for compartment syndrome. Research suggests some benefit from microvascular reconstruction.

When to Admit

Indications for hospitalization include arrhythmia or ECG changes; high voltage exposure; large burn; neurologic, pulmonary, or cardiac symptoms; suspicion of significant deep tissue or organ damage; transthoracic current pathway; history of cardiac disease; and need for surgery.

Ceber M et al. Pneumothorax due to electrical burn injury. Emerg Med J. 2007 May;24(5):371–2. [PMID: 17452717]

Fordyce TA et al. Thermal burn and electrical injuries among electric utility workers, 1995–2004. Burns. 2007 Mar;33(2):209–20. [PMID: 17116371]

Kidd M et al. The contemporary management of electrical injuries: resuscitation, reconstruction, rehabilitation. Ann Plast Surg. 2007 Mar;58(3):273–8. [PMID: 17471131]

Maghsoudi H et al. Electrical and lightning injuries. J Burn Care Res. 2007 Mar–Apr;28(2):255–61. [PMID: 17351442]

Ofer N et al. Current concepts of microvascular reconstruction for limb salvage in electrical burn injuries. J Plast Reconstr Aesthet Surg. 2007;60(7):724–30. [PMID: 17482533]

Sauerbier M et al. Microvascular reconstruction in burn and electrical burn injuries of the severely traumatized upper extremity. Plast Reconstr Surg. 2007 Feb;119(2);605–15. [PMID: 17230097]

Spies C et al. Narrative review: Electrocution and life-threatening electrical injuries. Ann Intern Med. 2006 Oct 3;145(7):531–7. [PMID: 17015871]

RADIATION EXPOSURE

Radiation exposures occur from both nonionizing and ionizing radiation sources. Nonionizing radiation is low energy, resulting in injuries related to local thermal damage (ie, microwave and radiowave). Ionizing radiation is high energy, causing cellular disruption, DNA damage, and mutations. Ionizing radiation is either electromagnetic (ie, x-rays and gamma rays) or particulate, (ie, alpha or beta particles, neutrons, and protons).

Exposure to radiation may occur from environmental, occupational, medical care, accidental, or intentional (ie, terrorism) exposure. The extent of damage due to radiation exposure depends on the type, quantity, and duration of radiation exposure, the organs exposed, the degree of disruption to DNA, metabolic and cellular function, and the age and underlying condition of the victim.

In 2008, the International Commission on Radiological Protection (ICRP) issued new recommendations for radiologic protection, justification for radiation use, and optimization of protection, and application of dose limits. ICRP uses the term "tissue reaction" to describe the biologic effects of radiation exposure.

In **acute radiation exposure**, medical care includes close monitoring of the gastrointestinal, cutaneous, hematologic, and cerebrovascular symptoms and signs from initial exposure and over time. Radiation dose may be estimated by the timing of symptom onset and severity of symptoms, (particularly nausea and vomiting), decrease in absolute lymphocyte count over hours and days after exposure, and chromosomal abnormalities in circulating lymphocytes.

Radiation exposure results in early and delayed effects. Early effects involve damage of the rapidly dividing cells (ie, the mucosa, skin, and bone marrow). Delayed effects include malignancy, reproduction abnormalities, liver, kidney, and central nervous system and immune system dysfunction. The short-term and long-term outcomes of Chernobyl, Hiroshima, and Nagasaki illustrate these various radiation effects.

IMMEDIATE & DELAYED EFFECTS OF RADIATION EXPOSURE ON NORMAL TISSUES

▶ Clinical Findings

A. Injury to Superficial Structures

Radiation exposure to the skin and mucous membranes may cause erythema, epilation, destruction of fingernails, or epidermolysis, and burns that appear similar to thermal burns usually have a slower onset and course. Chronic damage includes skin scarring, atrophy, telangiectasis, and xerostomia. Radiation effects on the eyes include cataracts, dry eye syndrome, and retinopathy.

B. Injury to Deep Structures

1. Hematopoietic system—Injury to the bone marrow may vary from transient decreases to complete destruction of blood elements. Lymphocytes are most sensitive, followed by polymorphonuclear leukocytes; erythrocytes are the least sensitive. Hematopoietic effects consisting of anemia, thrombocytopenia, and bone marrow suppression can occur 1–3 weeks after radiation exposures exceeding 100 cGy. Bone marrow failure is the main cause of death within the first few months following exposure.

2. Nervous system—The brain and spinal cord are much more sensitive than the peripheral nerves to the acute and delayed effects of radiation. Effects include neuropathy, myelopathy, and cerebral injury. Radiofrequency fields emitted by mobile telephones have been linked to the formation of benign and malignant brain tumors.

3. Cardiovascular system—Ionizing radiation damages the heart and coronary arteries. Smaller vessels (the capillaries and arterioles) are more susceptible to damage than larger blood vessels. Delayed effects from radiation include obliterative endarteritis; coronary artery disease; pericarditis with effusion; or constrictive pericarditis, which may occur months or years later. Myocarditis is less common.

4. Pulmonary system—High or repeated moderate doses of radiation may cause pneumonitis or pulmonary fibrosis, which is often delayed for weeks or months.

5. Gastrointestinal system—Mucositis and mucosal edema may occur within hours or days after exposure. Symptoms include odynophagia, anorexia, nausea, vomiting, dehydration, and weakness. High doses of radiation inhibit gastric secretion and cause inflammation and ulceration of the bowels. Hepatitis, liver dysfunction, and intestinal stenosis may occur as delayed effects.

6. Genitourinary and reproductive systems—Genitourinary radiation effects are dose-dependent, varying from transient decrease in fertility to permanent sterility, chromoso-mal aberrations, fetal damage, or demise. Nephritis and kidney dysfunction may occur as immediate or delayed effects. In men, small single doses of radiation (200–300 cGy) cause temporary aspermatogenesis, and larger doses (600–800 cGy) may cause permanent sterility. In women, single doses of 200 cGy may cause temporary cessation of menses, and 500–800 cGy may cause permanent castration. Moderate to heavy irradiation of the embryo results in injury to the fetus (eg, mental retardation) or in embryonic death and spontaneous abortion. Microcephaly and other congenital abnormalities may occur in children exposed in utero, especially if the fetus was exposed during early pregnancy.

7. Endocrine system—The endocrine system is relatively resistant to low or moderate doses of radiation. Delayed effects of exposure include thyroid dysfunction.

C. Systemic Reaction (Radiation Sickness)

The basic mechanisms of radiation sickness are not known. Symptoms include anorexia, nausea, vomiting, weakness, exhaustion, lassitude and, in some cases prostration; these symptoms may occur singly or in combination. Dehydration, anemia, and infection may follow.

▶ Prevention

Persons handling radiation sources must minimize exposure to radiation by recognizing the importance of time, distance, and shielding. Occupational safety policies and procedures must be followed. This will reduce occupational risk of radiation exposure and improve the emergency response to accidental exposure.

▶ Accidental or Intentional Radiation Exposure

There is an increase in likelihood of accidental or intentional radiation exposure due to the increased use of radiation equipment, radioactive materials, and threat of nuclear terrorism. Prehospital and hospital disaster plans are required for optimal management of radiation exposure. The Radiation Assistance Center (1-865-576-1005) provides 24-hour access to expert information. The Centers for Disease Control and Prevention "Radiation Emergency" website (www.bt.cdc.gov/radiation/index.asp) is also helpful.

▶ Treatment

Treatment is focused on decontamination, symptomatic relief, supportive care, and psychosocial support. Specific treatment options focus on the dose, route, and effects of exposure. Options include administration of fluids and electrolytes, blood product transfusion, antimicrobials, prophylaxis against malignancy, blood stem cell transplantation, and bone marrow transplantation.

▶ Prognosis

Prognosis is determined by the radiation dose, duration, and frequency as well as by the underlying condition of the victim. Approximate dose of exposure correlates with the early onset and severity of symptoms (ie, nausea, vomiting, anorexia, abdominal pain, bloody diarrhea, weight loss) and laboratory findings, particularly the decline in lymphocyte count on the complete blood count. Death is usually due to hematopoietic failure (ie, hemorrhage, anemia, and immunosuppression), gastrointestinal mucosal damage, central nervous system damage, widespread vascular injury, or secondary infection.

The International Agency for Research on Cancer (IARC) reviews the increasing evidence linking radiation exposure to increased cancer risk. Carcinogenesis is related to the total dose, duration, frequency of exposure and to the susceptibility of the victim. There are age-related sensitivities to radiation; prenatal and younger age victims are more susceptible to carcinogenesis.

When to Admit

Most patients with significant ionizing radiation exposure require admission for close monitoring and care.

Brusin JH. Radiation protection. Radiol Technol. 2007 May–Jun;78(5):378–92. [PMID: 17519374]

Cardis E et al. The 15-Country Collaborative Study of Cancer Risk among Radiation Workers in the Nuclear Industry: estimates of radiation-related cancer risks. Radiat Res. 2007 Apr;167(4):396–416. [PMID: 17388693]

Chao NJ. Accidental or intentional exposure to ionizing radiation: biodosimetry and treatment options. Exp Hematol. 2007 Apr;35(4 Suppl 1):24–7. [PMID: 17379083]

Clapp RW et al. Environmental and occupational causes of cancer: new evidence 2005–2007. Rev Environ Health. 2008 Jan–Mar;23(1):1–37. [PMID: 18557596]

Finch SC. Radiation-induced leukemia: lessons from history. Best Pract Res Clin Haematol. 2007 Mar;20(1):109–18. [PMID: 17336261]

Kusunoki Y et al. Long-lasting alterations of the immune system by ionizing radiation exposure: Implications for disease development among atomic bomb survivors. Int J Radiat Biol. 2007 Aug 31;1–14. [PMID: 17852558]

Little MP et al. A systematic review of epidemiological associations between low and moderate doses of ionizing radiation and late cardiovascular effects, and their possible mechanisms. Radiat Res. 2008 Jan;169(1):99–109. [PMID: 18159955]

Mettler FA Jr et al. Health effects in those with acute radiation sickness from the Chernobyl accident. Health Phys. 2007 Nov;93(5):462–9. [PMID: 18049222]

Prysyazhnyuk A et al. Twenty years after the Chernobyl accident: solid cancer incidence in various groups of the Ukrainian population. Radiat Environ Biophys. 2007 Mar;46(1):43–51. [PMID: 17279359]

Rodemann HP. Responses of normal cells to ionizing radiation. Semin Radiat Oncol. 2007 Apr;17(2):81–8. [PMID: 17395038]

Wrixon AD. New recommendations from the International Commission on Radiological Protection—a review. Phys Med Biol. 2008 Apr 21;53(8):R41–60. [PMID: 18364557]

Zenk JL. New therapy for the prevention and prophylactic treatment of acute radiation syndrome. Expert Opin Investig Drugs. 2007 Jun;16(6):767–70. [PMID: 17501689]

NEAR DROWNING

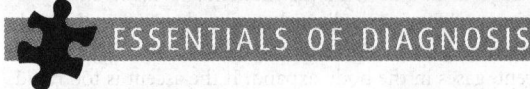

ESSENTIALS OF DIAGNOSIS

▶ The first requirement of rescue is immediate CPR.

▶ Clinical manifestations are hypoxemia, pulmonary edema, and hypoventilation.

General Considerations

Near drowning describes a submersion event leading to injury. Submersion injury may result in aspiration, laryngospasm, hypoxemia, and acidemia. Drowning describes submersion resulting in death. "Wet" drowning is due to aspiration of fluid or foreign material. "Dry" drowning is due to laryngospasm or airway obstruction. The primary effect is hypoxemia due to perfusion of poorly ventilated alveoli, intrapulmonary shunting, and decreased compliance.

Conditions that increase risk of submersion injury include the following: (1) use of alcohol or other drugs, (2) extreme fatigue, (3) poor physical health, (4) hyperventilation, (5) sudden acute illness (eg, hypoglycemia, seizure, dysrhythmia, myocardial infarction), (6) acute brain or spinal cord injury (or both), (7) venomous stings, bites, or injury in the water, and (8) decompression sickness.

A patient may be deceptively asymptomatic during the initial recovery period only to deteriorate or die as a result of acute respiratory failure within the following 12–24 hours.

Clinical Findings

A. Symptoms and Signs

The patient's appearance may vary from asymptomatic, to abnormal vital signs, anxiety, dyspnea, cough, wheezing, trismus, cyanosis, chest pain, dysrhythmia, hypotension, vomiting, diarrhea, headache, altered level of consciousness, neurologic deficit, and apnea. With cold water or prolonged submersion, hypothermia is likely.

B. Laboratory Findings

Arterial blood gas results are helpful in determining the degree of injury since initial clinical findings may appear benign. Pao_2 is usually decreased; $Paco_2$ may be increased or decreased; pH is decreased. Bedside blood sugar must be checked rapidly. Other testing is based on clinical scenario and may include kidney function, electrolytes, urinalysis, blood count, lactate, cardiac markers, coagulation studies, and alcohol and toxicology levels. Metabolic acidosis is common.

Prevention

Prevention is multi-faceted. Physical barriers (ie, fences) should be placed around pools and other accessible bodies of water. Safety flotation devices and rescue supplies must be immediately available. Use of alcohol or sedative drugs must be avoided during swimming, boating, or other water-based activities. There must be close supervision of those who cannot swim, and personal flotation devices must be worn when boating or water skiing. Swimming lessons, water safety, and basic life support education is necessary for anyone involved in water-based activities.

► Treatment

A. First Aid

The first requirement of rescue is immediate basic life support (BLS) treatment and CPR. At the scene, immediate measures to combat hypoxemia are critical to improve outcome. BLS care includes sustained ventilation, oxygenation, and circulatory support. Hypothermia and cervical spine injury should always be suspected.

1. Standard BLS is initiated. CPR is provided if pulse and respirations are absent.
2. Rescuer should not attempt to drain water from the victim's lungs. The Heimlich maneuver (subdiaphragmatic pressure) should be used only if foreign material airway obstruction is suspected. The cervical spine must be immobilized if neck injury is possible.
3. Resuscitation and BLS efforts must be continued until core temperature reaches 32 °C even for seemingly "hopeless" patients. Complete recovery has been reported after prolonged resuscitation of hypothermic patients.

B. Subsequent Management

Careful inpatient monitoring of the patient's condition must occur for 24 hours following near drowning. This includes continuous monitoring of cardiorespiratory and neurologic function; maintenance of oxygenation, serial determination of arterial blood gases, pH, kidney function (serum creatinine), and electrolytes; and measurement of urinary output. Pulmonary edema may not appear for 24 hours.

1. Ensure optimal ventilation and oxygenation—The danger of hypoxemia exists even in the alert, conscious patient who appears to be breathing normally. Oxygen should be administered immediately at the highest available concentration. Oxygen saturation should be maintained at 90% or higher. Endotracheal intubation and mechanical ventilation are necessary for patients unable to maintain an open airway, adequate oxygenation, or ventilation. Nasogastric suctioning can decompress the stomach, aid in removal of swallowed water and reduce the risk of aspiration. Continuous positive airway pressure (CPAP) is an effective noninvasive way of reversing hypoxia and hypercarbia in patients with spontaneous respirations and a patent airway. Positive end-expiratory pressure (PEEP) is also effective for treating respiratory insufficiency. Serial physical examinations and chest radiographs should be carried out to detect possible pneumonitis, atelectasis, and pulmonary edema. Bronchodilators may be used to treat wheezing and bronchospasms due to aspiration. Antibiotics are reserved for clinical evidence of infection and should not be given prophylactically.

2. Cardiovascular support—Intravascular volume status must be monitored to determine whether vascular fluid replacement and pressors or diuretics are needed. Standard therapy for hypotension and pulmonary edema is administered.

3. Correction of blood pH and electrolyte abnormalities—Metabolic acidosis is present in 70% of near-drowning victims, but it is usually corrected through adequate

ventilation and oxygenation. Glycemic control improves outcome.

4. Cerebral injury—Central nervous system damage may progress despite apparently adequate treatment of hypoxia and shock. Standard treatment for brain and spinal cord injury must be followed.

5. Hypothermia—Core temperature should be measured and managed as appropriate (see Systemic Hypothermia, above).

► Course & Prognosis

Victims of near drowning who have had prolonged hypoxemia should remain under close hospital observation for 2–3 days after all supportive measures have been withdrawn and clinical and laboratory findings have been stable. Long-term complications of near drowning may include neurologic impairment, seizure disorder, and pulmonary or cardiac damage.

Papadodima SA et al. Cardiovascular disease and drowning: autopsy and laboratory findings. Hellenic J Cardiol. 2007 Jul–Aug;48(4):198–205. [PMID: 17715610]
Schnitzer PG. Prevention of unintentional childhood injuries. Am Fam Physician. 2006 Dec 1;74(11):1864–9. [PMID: 17168342]

▼ DISORDERS DUE TO ENVIRONMENTAL FACTORS

DYSBARISM & DECOMPRESSION SICKNESS

 ESSENTIALS OF DIAGNOSIS

► Symptoms temporally related to recent diving, altitude or pressure changes.

► Early recognition and prompt treatment of decompression sickness are extremely important.

► Consultation with diving medicine or hyperbaric oxygen specialist is indicated.

► General Considerations

Dysbarism and decompression sickness (DCS) are physiologic problems that result from environmental pressure effects in gases in the body during underwater descent and ascent. These are hazards for fliers and for divers who are involved in recreational diving (eg, scuba diving), deepwater exploration, rescue or salvage operations, or construction. These may also occur in an air traveler when the aircraft cabin in not adequately pressurized during rapid ascent or descent between sea level and high altitudes.

Physics laws describe the mechanisms involved in dysbarism and DCS. As a diver descends, the gases in the body compress; gases dissolve in blood and tissues. During the ascent, gases in the body expand. If the ascent is too rapid, gas bubbles will form and cause damage depending on their location. DCS symptoms depends on the size and number and location of gas bubbles released (notably nitrogen).

Risk of DCS depends on the dive details (depth, duration, number of dives, and interval surface time between dives, water conditions) as well as the diver's age, weight, physical condition, physical exertion, and the rate of ascent. Predisposing factors for DCS include obesity, injury, hypoxia, lung or cardiac disease, right to left cardiac shunt, diver's overall health, dehydration, alcohol and medication effects, and panic attacks. DCS also occurs in those who take hot showers after cold dives, or take air travel too soon.

► Clinical Findings

The range of clinical manifestations varies depending on the location of the gas bubble formation or the compressibility of gases in the body. Symptom onset may be immediate, within minutes or hours (in the majority), or present up to 36 hours later. DCS symptoms include pain in the joints ("the bends"); skin pruritus or burning (skin bends); rashes; spinal cord or cerebral symptoms ("dissociation" symptoms that do not follow typical distribution patterns); labyrinthine DCS ("the staggers," central vertigo); pulmonary DCS ("the chokes," inspiratory pain, cough, and respiratory distress); arterial gas embolism (cerebral, pulmonary); barotrauma of the lungs, ear and sinus; dysbaric osteonecrosis; and coma.

► Treatment

Early recognition and prompt treatment are extremely important. DCS must be considered if symptoms are temporally related to recent diving or altitude or pressure changes. Immediate consultation with diving medicine or hyperbaric oxygen specialist is indicated even if mild symptoms resolved, since relapses with worse outcomes have occurred. Continuous administration of 100% oxygen is indicated and beneficial for all patients. Aspirin may be given for pain. Opioids should be used very cautiously, since these may obscure the response to recompression. Rapid transportation to a hyperbaric treatment facility for recompression is imperative for DCS. If air transportation is chosen, the aircraft must maintain pressurization near sea level to avoid worsening DCS. The clinician should be familiar with the nearest hyperbaric facility. The Divers Alert Network (DAN) is an excellent worldwide resource for emergency advice 24 hours daily for the management of diving-related conditions (www.diversalertnetwork.org, DAN USA 1-919-684-8111, see website for other international phone numbers).

Bennett MH et al. Recompression and adjunctive therapy for decompression illness. Cochrane Database Syst Rev. 2007 Apr 18;(2):CD005277. [PMID: 17443579]

Benton PJ et al. Diving medicine. Travel Med Infect Dis. 2006 May–Jul;4(3-4):238–54. [PMID: 16887745]

MacDonald RD et al. Interfacility transport of patients with decompression illness: literature review and consensus statement. Prehosp Emerg Care. 2006 Oct–Dec;10(4):482–7. [PMID: 16997779]

McMullin AM. Scuba diving: What you and your patients need to know. Cleve Clin J Med. 2006 Aug;73(8):711–16. [PMID: 16913196]

Vann RD et al. Influence of bottom time on preflight surface intervals before flying after diving. Undersea Hyperb Med. 2007 May–Jun;34(3):211–20. [PMID: 17672177]

ALTITUDE-RELATED ILLNESS

► The severity of the altitude illness correlates with the rate and height of ascent, and the individual's susceptibility.

► Prompt recognition and medical attention of early symptoms of altitude illness should prevent progression.

► General Considerations

High altitude medical problems are due to hypobaric hypoxia at high altitudes (greater than 2000 meters or 6560 feet). This usually results from increased physical activity with insufficient acclimatization, inadequate education and preparation, and individual susceptibility (preexisting medical conditions and medication use). Individual susceptibility is a key determinant of the risk of high altitude illness.

The severity of the altitude-related illness correlates with the rapid rate and height of ascent and the individual's susceptibility. High altitude illness comprises a spectrum of conditions based on end-organ effects. Manifestations of altitude illness are: (1) acute mountain sickness (AMS), (2) high-altitude pulmonary edema (HAPE), (3) high-altitude cerebral edema (HACE), (4) subacute mountain sickness, and (5) chronic mountain sickness (Monge disease).

Preventive measures include participant education, medical prescreening, pre-trip planning, and optimal physical conditioning before travel; adequate rest and sleep the day before travel; reduced food intake; and avoidance of alcohol, tobacco, and unnecessary physical activity during travel; slow ascent to allow acclimatization; and a period of rest and inactivity for 1–2 days after arrival at high altitudes. Prophylactic medications may be prescribed if no contraindications exist. Acetazolamide, 250 mg orally every 8–12 hours, may be started on the day before ascent and continued for 48–72 hours at high altitude. Dexamethasone, 4 mg orally every 12 hours beginning on the day of ascent, continuing for 3 days at the higher altitude, and then tapering over 5 days, is an alternative.

1. Acute Mountain Sickness (AMS)

Initial manifestations of AMS include headache (most severe and persistent symptom), lassitude, drowsiness, dizziness, chilliness, nausea and vomiting, facial pallor, dyspnea, and cyanosis. Later symptoms include facial flushing, irritability, difficulty concentrating, vertigo, tinnitus, visual and auditory disturbances, anorexia, insomnia, increased dyspnea and weakness on exertion, increased headaches (due to cerebral edema), palpitations, tachycardia, Cheyne-Stokes breathing, and weight loss. More severe manifestations include pulmonary and cerebral edema (HAPE and HACE; see below).

Initial treatment involves oxygen administration, voluntary periodic hyperventilation, which will often relieve acute symptoms. If immediate descent is not possible, portable hyperbaric chambers can provide symptomatic relief.

Acetazolamide (250 mg orally every 8–12 hours) remains the most effective medication for treatment of AMS and for more severe forms of altitude-related conditions. Dexamethasone (8 mg orally initially followed by 4 mg every 6 hours) is effective for treatment of AMS and acute cerebral edema. Both are recommended therapy for as long as symptoms persist and may be used together in severe cases. In most individuals, symptoms clear within 24–48 hours.

Definitive treatment is immediate descent. Descent is essential if the symptoms are persistent, severe, or worsening or if HAPE or HACE are present.

2. Acute High-Altitude Pulmonary Edema (HAPE)

HAPE is a serious complication and the leading cause of death from altitude illness. The hallmark is markedly elevated pulmonary artery pressure followed by pulmonary edema. It usually occurs at levels above 3000 meters (9840 feet). Early symptoms may appear within 6–36 hours after arrival at a high-altitude area. These include incessant dry cough, shortness of breath disproportionate to exertion, headache, decreased exercise performance, fatigue, dyspnea at rest, and chest tightness. Recognition of the early symptoms may enable the patient to descend before incapacitating pulmonary edema develops. Strenuous exertion should be avoided. An early descent of even 500 or 1000 meters may result in improvement of symptoms. Later, wheezing, orthopnea, and hemoptysis may occur as pulmonary edema worsens. Physical findings include tachycardia, mild fever, tachypnea, cyanosis, prolonged respiration, and rales and rhonchi. The clinical picture may resemble severe pneumonia. The patient may become confused or comatose. Diagnosis is usually clinical; ancillary tests are nonspecific or unavailable on site.

Treatment must often be initiated under field conditions. Prompt recognition and medical attention of early symptoms prevent progression. The patient must rest in the semi-Fowler position (head raised), and 100% oxygen must be administered. *Immediate descent (at least 610 meters [2000 feet]) is essential.* Recompression in a portable hyperbaric bag will temporarily reduce symptoms if rapid or immediate descent is not possible. To conserve oxygen, lower flow rates (2–4 L/min) may be used until the victim recovers or is evacuated to a lower altitude and $SaO_2 \geq 90\%$. Treatment for ARDS (see Chapter 9) may be required for some patients. Calcium channel blockers and selective phosphodiesterase type 5 (PDE5) inhibitors are effective for symptomatic relief. Nifedipine, 10 mg initially followed by 30 mg slow-release tablets every 12 hours is recommended. Dexamethasone, 4 mg every 6 hours, has been recommended if central nervous system symptoms are present. Acetazolamide, 250 mg every 8–12 hours, should be administered if AMS is suspected.

3. Acute High-Altitude Cerebral Edema (HACE)

HACE appears to be an extension of the central nervous system symptoms of AMS and results from cerebral vasogenic edema and hypoxia. It usually occurs at elevations above 2500 meters (8250 feet) and is more common in unacclimatized individuals. Hallmarks are altered consciousness and ataxic gait. Severe headaches, confusion, truncal ataxia, urinary retention or incontinence, focal deficits, papilledema, nausea, vomiting, and seizures may also occur and progress to obtundation and coma.

Treatment is immediate descent for at least 610 meters (2000 feet), continuing until symptoms improve. Oxygen (100% 2–4 L/min) should be administered by mask. Dexamethasone, 4–8 mg orally every 6 hours, is recommended thereafter. If immediate descent is impossible, a portable hyperbaric chamber should be used until symptomatic improvement occurs.

4. Subacute Mountain Sickness

This occurs most frequently in unacclimatized individuals and at altitudes above 4500 meters (14,764 feet). Symptoms of dyspnea and cough are probably due to hypoxic pulmonary hypertension and secondary congestive heart failure. Dehydration, skin dryness, and pruritus also can occur. Treatment consists of rest, oxygen administration, diuretics, and return to lower altitudes.

5. Chronic Mountain Sickness (Monge Disease)

This uncommon condition is seen in residents of high-altitude communities who have lost their acclimatization to such an environment. The disorder is characterized by somnolence, mental depression, cyanosis, clubbing of fingers, chronic hypoxia, hemoglobin > 22 g/dL, polycythemia (hematocrit often > 75%), signs of right ventricular failure, ECG evidence of right axis deviation and right atrial and ventricular hypertrophy, and radiographic evidence of right heart enlargement and central pulmonary vessel prominence, and pulmonary hypertension in some cases. There is no radiographic evidence of structural pulmonary disease. Pulmonary function tests usually disclose alveolar hypoventilation and elevated $PaCO_2$ but fail to reveal defective oxygen transport. There is a diminished respiratory response to CO_2.

Almost complete disappearance of all abnormalities eventually occurs when the patient returns to sea level. Recommended treatments include phlebotomy, oxygen supplementation, respiratory training, medroxyprogesterone (20–60 mg/d orally for 10 weeks), acetazolamide (250 mg/d orally for 3 weeks) and enalapril (5 mg orally daily).

► **When to Admit**

- All patients with HAPE or HACE should be hospitalized for further observation.
- Hospitalization should also be considered for any patient who remains symptomatic after treatment and

descent. Pulmonary symptoms and hypoxia may be worsened by pulmonary embolism, bacterial pneumonia, or bronchitis.

Luks AM et al. Medication and dosage considerations in the prophylaxis and treatment of high-altitude illness. Chest. 2008 Mar;133(3):744–55. [PMID: 18321903]

Maggiorini M. High altitude-induced pulmonary oedema. Cardiovasc Res. 2006 Oct 1;72(1):41–50. [PMID: 16904089]

Plant T et al. Travelling to new heights: practical high altitude medicine. Br J Hosp Med (Lond). 2008 Jun;69(6):348–52. [PMID: 18646420]

Rodway GW et al. Supplemental oxygen and hyperbaric treatment at high altitude: cardiac and respiratory response. Aviat Space Environ Med. 2007 Jun;78(6):613–7. [PMID: 17571664]

Wright A et al. High hopes at high altitudes: pharmacotherapy for acute mountain sickness and high-altitude cerebral and pulmonary oedema. Expert Opin Pharmacother. 2008 Jan;9(1):119–27. [PMID: 18076343]

SAFETY OF AIR TRAVEL & SELECTION OF PATIENTS FOR AIR TRAVEL

The medical safety of air travel depends not only on the nature and severity of the traveler's condition but also on other factors such as the duration and frequency of traveler's air travel, cabin pressurization, availability of medical supplies, presence of health care professionals on board, and traveler's preflight condition. Air travel passengers are susceptible to a wide range of problems: pulmonary (eg, thromboembolism), cardiovascular, gastrointestinal, ocular, immunologic, syncope, neuropsychiatric, metabolic, and substance related. Occupational and frequent flyers are at risk for these as well as radiation, infection, circadian disturbance, and pressurization problems.

Hypobaric hypoxia is the underlying etiology of most serious medical emergencies in flight. Despite commercial aircraft pressurization requirements, there is significant hypoxemia, dyspnea, and stress in travelers with underlying serious cardiopulmonary and other conditions.

Research also demonstrates an association between venous thrombosis and air travel. The risk of severe pulmonary embolism occurring after air travel increases proportionally with the flight duration. Travelers can take preventive measures by wearing support hose and engaging in in-flight leg exercises and walking. Air travel complications may be reduced by the following preventive measures: passenger education, passenger prescreening (especially those who have had recent surgery or an emergency condition, and those with chronic serious medical conditions). Travelers with pulmonary disease must have preflight medical assessment to determine whether supplemental oxygen is required. This is determined by an arterial oxygen tension of less than 70 mm Hg or pulse oximetry less than 92%.

The Air Transport Association of America defines an incapacitated passenger as "one who is suffering from a physical or mental disability and who, because of such disability or the effect of the flight on the disability, is incapable of self-care; would endanger the health or safety of such person or other passengers or airline employees; or would cause discomfort or annoyance of other passengers." Air travel is not advised for anyone with an active pneumothorax, class III and IV pulmonary hypertension, acute worsening of an underlying lung disease, or any unstable conditions. Unstable conditions include poorly controlled hypertension, dysrhythmias, angina, valvular disease, congestive heart failure, or psychiatric condition; severe anemia or sickle cell disease; recent myocardial infarction, cerebrovascular accident, or deep venous thrombosis; postsurgery, especially heart surgery (unless approved by surgeon); and any active communicable disease (tuberculosis, measles, chickenpox, or other communicable virulent infections). Small meals of easily digested food and avoidance of carbonated beverages before and during the flight may reduce the tendency to nausea and vomiting.

Pregnancy and Infancy

Pregnant women may be permitted to fly during the first 8 months of pregnancy unless there is a history of pregnancy complications or premature birth. Infants less than 1 week old should not be flown at high altitudes or for long distances.

Abramowitz HB et al. Venous stasis, deep venous thrombosis and airline flight: can the seat be fixed? Ann Vasc Surg. 2007 May;21(3):267–71. [PMID: 17484958]

Bradford A. The role of hypoxia and platelets in air travel-related venous thromboembolism. Curr Pharm Des. 2007; 13(26):2668–72. [PMID: 17897010]

Cocks R et al. Commercial aviation in-flight emergencies and the physician. Emerg Med Australas. 2007 Feb;19(1):1–8. [PMID: 17305654]

Kim JN et al. Risk factors, health risks, and risk management for aircraft personnel and frequent flyers. J Toxicol Environ Health B Crit Rev. 2007 Apr–May;10(3):223–34. [PMID: 17454553]

Kuipers S et al. The absolute risk of venous thrombosis after air travel: a cohort study of 8,755 employees of international organisations. PLoS Med. 2007 Sep 25;4(9):e290. [PMID: 17896862]

Kuipers S et al. Travel and venous thrombosis: a systematic review. J Intern Med. 2007 Dec;262(6):615–34. [PMID: 18028182]

Mohr LC. Hypoxia during air travel in adults with pulmonary disease. Am J Med Sci. 2008 Jan;335(1):71–9. [PMID: 18195588]

Muhm JM et al. Effect of aircraft-cabin altitude on passenger discomfort. N Engl J Med. 2007 Jul 5;357(1):18–27. [PMID: 17611205]

Philbrick JT et al. Air travel and venous thromboembolism: a systematic review. J Gen Intern Med. 2007 Jan;22(1):107–14. [PMID: 17351849]

Poisoning

Kent R. Olson, MD

▼ INITIAL EVALUATION: POISONING OR OVERDOSE

Patients with drug overdoses or poisoning may initially have no symptoms or they may have varying degrees of overt intoxication. The asymptomatic patient may have been exposed to or may have ingested a lethal dose of a poison but not yet exhibit any manifestations of toxicity. It is important to: (1) quickly assess the potential danger, (2) consider gut decontamination to prevent absorption, and (3) observe the patient for an appropriate interval.

▶ Assess the Danger

If the drug or poison is known, its danger can be assessed by consulting a text or computerized information resource (eg, Poisindex) or by calling a regional poison control center. (In the United States, dialing 800-222-1222 will direct the call to the regional poison control center.) Assessment will usually take into account the dose ingested; the time interval since ingestion; the presence of any symptoms or clinical signs; preexisting cardiac, respiratory, kidney, or liver disease; and, occasionally, specific serum drug or toxin levels. Be aware that the history given by the patient or family may be incomplete or unreliable.

The manufacturer or its local representative may be able to provide information over the phone concerning the toxic ingredients in question and can be contacted directly or via the regional poison control center.

▶ Gut Decontamination

The choice of gut decontamination procedure depends on the toxin and the circumstances. (See below for a more detailed discussion of methods.)

IMMEDIATE 24-HOUR TOXICOLOGY CONSULTATION

Call your regional poison control center
U.S. toll-free 1-800-222-1222

▶ Observation of the Patient

Asymptomatic or mildly symptomatic patients should be observed for at least 4–6 hours. Longer observation is indicated if the ingested substance is a sustained-release preparation or is known to slow gastrointestinal motility or if there may have been exposure to a poison with delayed onset of symptoms (such as acetaminophen, colchicine, or hepatotoxic mushrooms). After that time, the patient may be discharged if no symptoms have developed and adequate gastric decontamination has been provided. Before discharge, psychiatric evaluation should be performed to assess suicidal risk. Intentional ingestions in adolescents should raise the possibility of unwanted pregnancy or sexual abuse.

▼ THE SYMPTOMATIC PATIENT

In symptomatic patients, treatment of life-threatening complications takes precedence over in-depth diagnostic evaluation. Patients with mild symptoms may deteriorate rapidly, which is why all potentially significant exposures should be observed in an acute care facility. The following complications may occur, depending on the type of poisoning.

COMA

▶ Assessment & Complications

Coma is commonly associated with ingestion of large doses of antihistamines, benzodiazepines and other sedative-hypnotic drugs, γ-hydroxybutyrate (GHB), ethanol, opioids, antipsychotic drugs, or antidepressants. The most common cause of death in comatose patients is respiratory failure, which may occur abruptly. Pulmonary aspiration of gastric contents may also occur, especially in victims who are deeply obtunded or convulsing. Hypoxia and hypoventilation may cause or aggravate hypotension, arrhythmias, and seizures. Thus, protection of the airway and assisted ventilation are the most important treatment measures for any poisoned patient.

▶ Treatment

A. Emergency Management

The initial emergency management of coma can be remembered by the mnemonic *ABCD*, for *A*irway, *B*reathing, *C*irculation, and *D*rugs (dextrose, thiamine, and naloxone or flumazenil), respectively.

1. Airway—Establish a patent airway by positioning, suction, or insertion of an artificial nasal or oropharyngeal airway. If the patient is deeply comatose or if there is no gag or cough reflex, perform endotracheal intubation. These airway interventions may not be necessary if the patient is intoxicated by an opioid or a benzodiazepine and responds rapidly to intravenous naloxone or flumazenil (see below).

2. Breathing—Clinically assess the quality and depth of respiration, and provide assistance if necessary with a bag-valve-mask device or mechanical ventilator. Provide supplemental oxygen. The arterial blood CO_2 tension is useful in determining the adequacy of ventilation. The arterial blood PO_2 determination may reveal hypoxemia, which may be caused by respiratory arrest, bronchospasm, pulmonary aspiration, or noncardiogenic pulmonary edema. Pulse oximetry provides an assessment of oxygenation but is not reliable in patients with methemoglobinemia or carbon monoxide poisoning, unless a newer oximetry device capable of detecting these forms of hemoglobin is used (eg, the Masimo Rad-57 pulse CO-oximeter).

3. Circulation—Measure the pulse and blood pressure and estimate tissue perfusion (eg, by measurement of urinary output, skin signs, arterial blood pH). Place the patient on continuous ECG monitoring. Insert an intravenous line, and draw blood for glucose, electrolytes, serum creatinine and liver tests, and possible quantitative toxicologic testing.

4. Drugs

A. Dextrose and thiamine—Unless promptly treated, severe hypoglycemia can cause irreversible brain damage. Therefore, in all comatose or convulsing patients, give 50% dextrose, 50–100 mL by intravenous bolus, unless a rapid bedside blood sugar test is available and rules out hypoglycemia. In alcoholic or very malnourished patients who may have marginal thiamine stores, give thiamine, 100 mg intramuscularly or over 2–3 minutes intravenously.

B. Narcotic antagonists—Naloxone, 0.4–2 mg intravenously, may reverse opioid-induced respiratory depression and coma. It is often given empirically to any comatose patient with depressed respirations. If opioid overdose is strongly suspected, give additional doses of naloxone (up to 5–10 mg may be required to reverse the effects of potent opioids or propoxyphene). **Note:** Naloxone has a much shorter duration of action (2–3 hours) than most common opioids; repeated doses may be required, and continuous observation for at least 3–4 hours after the last dose is mandatory. Nalmefene, a newer opioid antagonist, has a duration of effect longer than that of naloxone but still shorter than that of the opioid methadone.

C. Flumazenil—Flumazenil, 0.2–0.5 mg intravenously, repeated every 30 seconds as needed up to a maximum of 3 mg, may reverse benzodiazepine-induced coma. **Caution:** Flumazenil should **not** be given if the patient has coingested a tricyclic antidepressant, is a user of high-dose benzodiazepines, or has a seizure disorder because its use in these circumstances may precipitate seizures. *In most circumstances, use of flumazenil is not advised as the potential risks outweigh its benefits.* **Note:** Flumazenil has a short duration of effect (2–3 hours), and resedation requiring additional doses is common.

HYPOTHERMIA

▶ Assessment & Complications

Hypothermia commonly accompanies coma due to opioids, ethanol, hypoglycemic agents, phenothiazines, barbiturates, benzodiazepines, and other sedative-hypnotics and central nervous system depressants. Hypothermic patients may have a barely perceptible pulse and blood pressure. Hypothermia may cause or aggravate hypotension, which will not reverse until the temperature is normalized.

▶ Treatment

Treatment of hypothermia is discussed in Chapter 37. Gradual rewarming is preferred unless the patient is in cardiac arrest.

HYPOTENSION

▶ Assessment & Complications

Hypotension may be due to poisoning by many different drugs and poisons, including antihypertensive drugs, β-blockers, calcium channel blockers, disulfiram (ethanol interaction), iron, trazodone, quetiapine, and other antipsychotic agents and antidepressants. Poisons causing hypotension include cyanide, carbon monoxide, hydrogen sulfide, arsenic, and certain mushrooms.

Hypotension in the poisoned or drug-overdosed patient may be caused by venous or arteriolar vasodilation, hypovolemia, depressed cardiac contractility, or a combination of these effects. The only certain way to determine the cause of hypotension in any individual patient is to insert a pulmonary artery catheter and calculate the cardiac output and peripheral vascular resistance. Alternatively, a central venous pressure (CVP) monitor may indicate a need for further fluid therapy.

▶ Treatment

Most patients respond to empiric treatment with repeated 200 mL intravenous boluses of 0.9% saline or other isotonic crystalloid up to a total of 1–2 L; much larger amounts may be needed if the victim is profoundly volume depleted. If fluid therapy is not successful, give dopamine, 5–15 mcg/kg/min by intravenous infusion. Consider pulmonary artery catheterization if hypotension persists.

Hypotension caused by certain toxins may respond to specific treatment. For hypotension caused by overdoses of tricyclic antidepressants or related drugs, administer sodium bicarbonate, 50–100 mEq by intravenous bolus injection. Norepinephrine 4–8 mcg/min by intravenous infusion is more effective than dopamine in some patients with overdoses of tricyclic antidepressants or of drugs with predominantly vasodilating effects. For β-blocker overdose, glucagon (5–10 mg intravenously) may be of value. For calcium channel blocker overdose, administer calcium chloride, 1–2 g intravenously (repeated doses may be necessary; doses of 5–10 g and more have been given in some cases). High-dose insulin euglycemic therapy may also be used (see Calcium Channel Blockers, below). Intralipid 20% lipid emulsion has been reported to improve hemodynamics in human case reports or animal studies of intoxication by highly lipid-soluble drugs such as bupivacaine, bupropion, clomipramine, and verapamil.

Sirianni AJ et al. Use of lipid emulsion in the resuscitation of a patient with prolonged cardiovascular collapse after overdose of bupropion and lamotrigine. Ann Emerg Med. 2008 Apr;51(4):412–5. [PMID: 17766009]

HYPERTENSION

▶ Assessment & Complications

Hypertension may be due to poisoning with amphetamines, anticholinergics, cocaine, yohimbine-containing performance-enhancing products, monoamine oxidase (MAO) inhibitors, and other drugs.

Severe hypertension (eg, diastolic blood pressure > 105–110 mm Hg in a person who does not have chronic hypertension) can result in acute intracranial hemorrhage, myocardial infarction, or aortic dissection.

▶ Treatment

Treat hypertension if the patient is symptomatic or if the diastolic pressure is greater than 105–110 mm Hg—especially if there is no prior history of hypertension.

Hypertensive patients who are agitated or anxious may benefit from a sedative such as lorazepam, 2–3 mg intravenously. For persistent hypertension, administer phentolamine, 2–5 mg intravenously, or nitroprusside sodium, 0.25–8 mcg/kg/min intravenously. If excessive tachycardia is present, add propranolol, 1–5 mg intravenously, or esmolol, 25–100 mcg/kg/min intravenously, or labetalol 0.2–0.3 mg/kg intravenously. **Caution:** Do not give β-blockers alone, since doing so may paradoxically worsen hypertension as a result of unopposed α-adrenergic stimulation.

Wang NE et al. Hypertensive crisis and NSTEMI after accidental overdose of sustained release pseudoephedrine: a case report. Clin Toxicol (Phila). 2008 Nov;46(9):922–3. [PMID: 18608273]

ARRHYTHMIAS

▶ Assessment & Complications

Arrhythmias may occur with a variety of drugs or toxins (Table 38–1). They may also occur as a result of hypoxia, metabolic acidosis, or electrolyte imbalance (eg, hyperkale-

Table 38–1. Common toxins or drugs causing arrhythmias.[1]

Arrhythmia	Common Causes
Sinus bradycardia	β-Blockers, calcium channel blockers, clonidine, digitalis glycosides, organophosphates
Atrioventricular block	β-Blockers, calcium channel blockers, class Ia antiarrhythmics (including quinidine), carbamazepine, clonidine, digitalis glycosides, lithium
Sinus tachycardia	β-Agonists (eg, albuterol), amphetamines, anticholinergics, antihistamines, caffeine, cocaine, pseudoephedrine, tricyclic and other antidepressants
Wide QRS complex	Class Ia and class Ic antiarrhythmics, phenothiazines (eg, thioridazine), potassium (hyperkalemia), propranolol, tricyclic antidepressants, diphenhydramine (severe overdose)
QT interval prolongation and torsades de pointes	Arsenic, class Ia and class III antiarrhythmics, droperidol, lithium, methadone, pentamidine, sotalol, thioridazine, venlafaxine, and many other drugs (see http://www.azcert.org/medical-pros/drug-lists/drug-lists.cfm)
Ventricular premature beats and ventricular tachycardia	Amphetamines, cocaine, ephedrine, caffeine, chlorinated or fluorinated hydrocarbons, digoxin, aconite (found in some Chinese herbal preparations), fluoride, theophylline. QT prolongation can lead to atypical ventricular tachycardia (torsades de pointes)

[1]Arrhythmias may also occur as a result of hypoxia, metabolic acidosis, or electrolyte imbalance (eg, hyperkalemia or hypokalemia, hypocalcemia).

mia, hypokalemia, hypomagnesemia or hypocalcemia), or following exposure to chlorinated solvents or chloral hydrate overdose. Atypical ventricular tachycardia (torsades de pointes) is often associated with drugs that prolong the QT interval.

▶ Treatment

Arrhythmias are often caused by hypoxia or electrolyte imbalance, and these conditions should be sought and treated. If ventricular arrhythmias persist, administer lidocaine or amiodarone at usual antiarrhythmic doses. **Note:** Wide QRS complex tachycardia in the setting of tricyclic antidepressant overdose (or quinidine and other class Ia drugs) should be treated with sodium bicarbonate, 50–100 mEq intravenously by bolus injection. (See discussion of tricyclic antidepressant poisoning.) **Caution:** Avoid class Ia agents (quinidine, procainamide, disopyramide), which may aggravate arrhythmias caused by tricyclic antidepressants. Torsades de pointes associated with prolonged QT interval may respond to intravenous magnesium (2 g intravenously over 2 minutes) or overdrive pacing. Treat digitalis-induced arrhythmias with digoxin-specific antibodies (see discussion of cardiac glycoside poisoning).

For tachyarrhythmias induced by chlorinated solvents, chloral hydrate, Freons, or sympathomimetic agents, use propranolol or esmolol (see doses given above in Hypertension section).

Tarabar AF et al. Citalopram overdose: late presentation of torsades de pointes (TdP) with cardiac arrest. J Med Toxicol. 2008 Jun;4(2):101–5. [PMID: 18570170]

SEIZURES

▶ Assessment & Complications

Seizures may be due to poisoning with many poisons and drugs, including amphetamines, antidepressants (especially tricyclic antidepressants, bupropion, and venlafaxine), antihistamines (especially diphenhydramine), antipsychotics, cocaine, isoniazid (INH), and theophylline.

Seizures may also be caused by hypoxia, hypoglycemia, hypocalcemia, hyponatremia, withdrawal from alcohol or sedative-hypnotics, head trauma, central nervous system infection, or idiopathic epilepsy.

Prolonged or repeated seizures may lead to hypoxia, metabolic acidosis, hyperthermia, and rhabdomyolysis.

▶ Treatment

Administer lorazepam, 2–3 mg, or diazepam, 5–10 mg, intravenously over 1–2 minutes, or—if intravenous access is not immediately available—midazolam, 5–10 mg intramuscularly. If convulsions continue, administer phenobarbital, 15–20 mg/kg slowly intravenously over no less than 30 minutes; or phenytoin, 15 mg/kg intravenously over no less than 30 minutes (maximum infusion rate, 50 mg/min). For drug-induced seizures, phenobarbital is generally preferred over phenytoin. Propofol infusion has also been reported effective for some resistant drug-induced seizures.

Seizures due to a few drugs and toxins may require antidotes or other specific therapies (as listed in Table 38–2).

Thundiyil JG et al. Evolving epidemiology of drug-induced seizures reported to a Poison Control Center System. J Med Toxicol. 2007 Mar;3(1):15–9. [PMID: 18072153]

HYPERTHERMIA

▶ Assessment & Complications

Hyperthermia may be associated with poisoning by amphetamines (especially methylenedioxymethamphetamine [MDMA; "Ecstasy"]), atropine and other anticholinergic drugs, cocaine, salicylates, strychnine, tricyclic antidepressants, and various other medications. Overdoses of serotonin reuptake inhibitors (eg, fluoxetine, paroxetine, sertraline) or their use in a patient taking an MAO inhibitor may cause agitation, hyperactivity, myoclonus, and hyperthermia ("serotonin syndrome"). Antipsychotic agents can cause rigidity and hyperthermia (neuroleptic malignant syndrome [NMS]). (See section on schizophrenia and other psychotic disorders in Chapter 25.) Malignant hyperthermia is a rare disorder associated with general anesthetic agents.

Hyperthermia is a rapidly life-threatening complication. Severe hyperthermia (temperature > 40–41 °C) may

Table 38–2. Seizures related to toxins or drugs requiring special consideration.[1]

Toxin or Drug	Comments
Methylenedioxymethamphetamine (MDMA; "Ecstasy")	Seizures may be due to hyponatremia.
Isoniazid	Administer pyridoxine.
Lithium	May indicate need for hemodialysis.
Organophosphates	Administer pralidoxime (2-PAM) and atropine.
Strychnine	"Seizures" are actually spinally mediated muscle spasms and usually require neuromuscular paralysis.
Theophylline	Seizures indicate need for hemodialysis.
Tricyclic antidepressants	Hyperthermia and cardiotoxicity are common complications of repeated seizures; paralyze early with neuromuscular blockers to reduce muscular hyperactivity.

[1]See text for dosages.

rapidly cause brain damage and multiorgan failure, including rhabdomyolysis, advanced chronic kidney disease, and coagulopathy (see Chapter 37).

▶ Treatment

Treat hyperthermia aggressively by removing all clothing, spraying the patient with tepid water, and fanning the patient. If this is not rapidly effective, as shown by a normal rectal temperature within 30–60 minutes, or if there is significant muscle rigidity or hyperactivity, induce neuromuscular paralysis with a nondepolarizing neuromuscular blocker (eg, rocuronium, vecuronium). Once paralyzed, the patient must be intubated and mechanically ventilated. In patients with seizures, absence of visible muscular convulsive movements may give the false impression that brain seizure activity has ceased; however, this must be confirmed by electroencephalography.

Dantrolene (2–5 mg/kg intravenously) may be effective for hyperthermia associated with muscle rigidity that does not respond to neuromuscular blockade (ie, malignant hyperthermia). Bromocriptine, 2.5–7.5 mg orally daily, has been recommended for neuroleptic malignant syndrome. Cyproheptadine, 4 mg orally every hour for three or four doses, has been used to treat serotonin syndrome.

Dvir Y et al. Serotonin syndrome: a complex but easily avoidable condition. Gen Hosp Psychiatry. 2008 May–Jun;30(3):284–7. [PMID: 18433663]

▼ ANTIDOTES & OTHER TREATMENT

ANTIDOTES

Give an antidote (if available) when there is reasonable certainty of a specific diagnosis (Table 38–3). Antidotes

Table 38–3. Some toxic agents for which there are specific antidotes.[1]

Toxic Agent	Specific Antidote
Acetaminophen	N-Acetylcysteine
Anticholinergics (eg, atropine)	Physostigmine
Anticholinesterases (eg, organophosphate pesticides)	Atropine and pralidoxime (2-PAM)
Benzodiazepines	Flumazenil (rarely used; see warning in text)
Carbon monoxide	Oxygen, hyperbaric oxygen
Cyanide	Sodium nitrite, sodium thiosulfate; hydroxocobalamin
Digitalis glycosides	Digoxin-specific Fab antibodies
Heavy metals (eg, lead, mercury, iron) and arsenic	Specific chelating agents
Isoniazid	Pyridoxine (vitamin B_6)
Methanol, ethylene glycol	Ethanol (ethyl alcohol) or fomepizole (4-methylpyrazole)
Opioids	Naloxone, nalmefene
Snake venom	Specific antivenin

[1]See text for indications and dosages.

themselves may have serious side effects. The indications and dosages for specific antidotes are discussed in the respective sections for specific toxins.

DECONTAMINATION OF THE SKIN

Corrosive agents rapidly injure the skin and eyes and must be removed immediately. In addition, many toxins are readily absorbed through the skin, and systemic absorption can be prevented only by rapid action.

Wash the affected areas with copious quantities of lukewarm water or saline. Wash carefully behind the ears, under the nails, and in skin folds. For oily substances (eg, pesticides), wash the skin at least twice with plain soap and shampoo the hair. Specific decontaminating solutions or solvents (eg, alcohol) are rarely indicated and in some cases may paradoxically enhance absorption. For exposure to chemical warfare poisons such as nerve agents or vesicants, some authorities recommend use of a dilute hypochlorite solution (household bleach diluted 1:10 with water).

DECONTAMINATION OF THE EYES

Act quickly to prevent serious damage. Flush the eyes with copious amounts of saline (preferred) or water. (If available, instill local anesthetic drops in the eye before beginning irrigation.) Remove contact lenses if present. Direct the irrigating stream so that it will flow across the eyes after running off the nasal bridge. Lift the tarsal conjunctiva to look for undissolved particles and to facilitate irrigation. Continue irrigation for 15 minutes or until each eye has been irrigated with at least 1 L of solution. If the toxin is an

acid or a base, check the pH of the tears after irrigation, and continue irrigation until the pH is between 6.5 and 7.5.

After irrigation is complete, perform a careful examination of the eye, using fluorescein and a slit lamp or Wood lamp to identify areas of corneal injury. Patients with serious conjunctival or corneal injury should be immediately referred to an ophthalmologist.

GASTROINTESTINAL DECONTAMINATION

Removal of ingested poisons was a routine part of emergency treatment for decades. However, prospective clinical studies have failed to demonstrate improved outcome after gastric emptying. For small or moderate ingestions of most substances, toxicologists generally recommend oral activated charcoal alone without prior gastric emptying. Exceptions are large ingestions of anticholinergic compounds and salicylates, which often delay gastric emptying, and ingestion of sustained-release or enteric-coated tablets, which may remain intact for several hours.

Gastric emptying is not generally used for ingestion of corrosive agents or petroleum distillates, because further esophageal injury or pulmonary aspiration may result. However, in certain cases, removal of the toxin may be more important than concern over possible complications. Consult a medical toxicologist or regional poison control center (800-222-1222) for advice.

► Emesis

Emesis using syrup of ipecac can partially evacuate gastric contents if given very soon after ingestion (eg, at work or at home). However, it may increase the risk of pulmonary aspiration and delay or prevent the use of oral activated charcoal. Therefore, it is no longer used in the routine management of ingestions.

A. Gastric Lavage

Gastric lavage is more effective for liquid poisons or small pill fragments than for intact tablets or pieces of mushroom. It is most useful when started within 60 minutes after ingestion. However, the lavage procedure may delay administration of activated charcoal and may stimulate vomiting and pulmonary aspiration in an obtunded patient.

1. Indications—Gastric lavage is sometimes used after very large ingestions (eg, massive aspirin overdose), for collection and examination of gastric contents for identification of poison, and for convenient administration of charcoal and antidotes.

2. Contraindications—Do *not* use lavage for stuporous or comatose patients with absent gag reflexes unless they are endotracheally intubated beforehand. Some authorities advise against lavage when caustic material has been ingested; others regard it as essential to remove liquid corrosives from the stomach.

3. Technique—In obtunded or comatose patients, the danger of aspiration pneumonia is reduced by performing endotracheal intubation with a cuffed tube before the procedure. Gently insert a lubricated, soft but noncollapsible stomach tube (at least 37–40 F) through the mouth or nose into the stomach. Aspirate and save the contents, and then lavage repeatedly with 50- to 100-mL aliquots of fluid until the return fluid is clear. Use lukewarm tap water or saline.

B. Activated Charcoal

Activated charcoal effectively adsorbs almost all drugs and poisons. Poorly adsorbed substances include iron, lithium, potassium, sodium, mineral acids, and alcohols.

1. Indications—Activated charcoal should be used for prompt adsorption of drugs or toxins in the stomach and intestine. Studies in volunteers show that activated charcoal given alone may be as effective as or more effective than ipecac-induced emesis or gastric lavage. However, evidence of benefit in clinical studies is lacking. Administration of charcoal, especially if mixed with sorbitol, can provoke vomiting, which could lead to pulmonary aspiration in an obtunded patient.

2. Contraindications—Activated charcoal should not be used for comatose or convulsing patients unless it can be given by gastric tube and the airway is first protected by a cuffed endotracheal tube. It is also contraindicated for patients with ileus or intestinal obstruction or those who have ingested corrosives for whom endoscopy is planned.

3. Technique—Administer activated charcoal, 60–100 g orally or via gastric tube, mixed in aqueous slurry. Repeated doses may be given to ensure gastrointestinal adsorption or to enhance elimination of some drugs (see below).

C. Catharsis

1. Indications—Cathartics are used by some toxicologists for stimulation of peristalsis to hasten the elimination of unabsorbed drugs and poisons and the activated charcoal slurry. There is no clinical evidence to support their use, and some agents (eg, sorbitol) can provoke vomiting, increasing the risk of pulmonary aspiration.

2. Contraindications and cautions—Do not give a cathartic to patients with suspected intestinal obstruction. Avoid sodium-based cathartics in patients with hypertension, advanced chronic kidney disease, and congestive heart failure and magnesium-based cathartics in patients with advanced chronic kidney disease. Sorbitol (an osmotic cathartic found in some prepackaged activated charcoal slurry products) can cause hypotension and dehydration due to third-spacing and also causes intestinal cramping and vomiting.

D. Whole Bowel Irrigation

Whole bowel irrigation uses large volumes of balanced polyethylene glycol-electrolyte solution to mechanically cleanse the entire intestinal tract. Because of the composition of the irrigating solution, there is no significant gain or loss of systemic fluids or electrolytes.

1. Indications—Whole bowel irrigation is particularly effective for massive iron ingestion in which intact tablets are visible on abdominal radiographs. It has also been used

for ingestions of lithium, sustained-release and enteric-coated tablets, and swallowed drug-filled packets.

2. Contraindications—Do not use in patients with suspected intestinal obstruction. Use with caution in patients who are obtunded or have depressed airway protective reflexes.

3. Technique—Administer a balanced polyethylene glycol-electrolyte solution (CoLyte, GoLYTELY) into the stomach via gastric tube at a rate of 1–2 L/h until the rectal effluent is clear. This may take several hours. It is most effective when patients are able to sit on a commode to pass the intestinal contents.

E. Increased Drug Removal

1. Urinary manipulation—Forced diuresis is hazardous; the risk of complications (pulmonary edema, electrolyte imbalance) usually outweighs its benefits. Acidic drugs (eg, salicylates, phenobarbital) are more rapidly excreted with an alkaline urine. Acidification (sometimes promoted for amphetamines, phencyclidine) is *not* very effective and is contraindicated in the presence of rhabdomyolysis or myoglobinuria.

2. Hemodialysis—The indications for dialysis are as follows: (1) Known or suspected potentially lethal amounts of a dialyzable drug (Table 38–4). (2) Poisoning with deep coma, apnea, severe hypotension, fluid and electrolyte or acid-base disturbance, or extreme body temperature changes that cannot be corrected by conventional measures. (3) Poisoning in patients with severe kidney, cardiac, pulmonary, or hepatic disease who will not be able to eliminate toxin by the usual mechanisms.

Continuous renal replacement therapy (also known as continuous venovenous hemodiafiltration) is of uncertain

Table 38–4. Recommended use of hemodialysis in poisoning.

Poison	Indications[1]
Carbamazepine	Seizures, severe cardiotoxicity; serum level > 60 mg/L
Ethylene glycol	Acidosis, serum level > 50 mg/dL
Lithium	Severe symptoms; level > 4 mEq/L more than 12 hours after last dose
Methanol	Acidosis, serum level > 50 mg/dL
Phenobarbital	Intractable hypotension, acidosis despite maximal supportive care
Salicylate	Severe acidosis, CNS symptoms, level > 100 mg/dL (acute overdose) or > 60 mg/dL (chronic intoxication)
Theophylline	Serum level > 90-100 mg/L (acute) or seizures and serum level > 40-60 mg/L (chronic)
Valproic acid	Serum level > 900-1000 mg/L or deep coma, severe acidosis

[1]See text for further discussion of indications.
CNS, central nervous system.

benefit for elimination of most poisons but has been used successfully in the management of lithium intoxication.

3. Repeat-dose charcoal—Repeated doses of activated charcoal, 20–30 g orally or via gastric tube every 3–4 hours, may hasten elimination of some drugs (eg, phenytoin, carbamazepine, dapsone) by absorbing drugs excreted into the gut lumen ("gut dialysis"). However, clinical studies have failed to prove better outcome using multiple-dose charcoal. Sorbitol or other cathartics should *not* be used with each dose, or resulting large stool volumes may lead to dehydration or hypernatremia.

Brahmi N et al. Influence of activated charcoal on the pharma-cokinetics and the clinical features of carbamazepine poisoning. Am J Emerg Med. 2006 Jul;24(4):440–3. [PMID: 16787802]

de Pont AC. Extracorporeal treatment of intoxications. Curr Opin Crit Care. 2007 Dec;13(6):668–73. [PMID: 17975388]

Isbister GK et al. Activated charcoal decreases the risk of QT prolongation after citalopram overdose. Ann Emerg Med. 2007 Nov;50(5):593–600. [PMID: 17719135]

▼ DIAGNOSIS OF POISONING

The identity of the ingested substance or substances is usually known, but occasionally a comatose patient is found with an unlabeled container or the patient is unable or unwilling to give a coherent history. By performing a directed physical examination and ordering common clinical laboratory tests, the clinician can often make a tentative diagnosis that may allow empiric interventions or may suggest specific toxicologic tests.

▶ Physical Examination

Important diagnostic variables in the physical examination include blood pressure, pulse rate, temperature, pupil size, sweating, and the presence or absence of peristaltic activity. Poisonings with many drugs fit into one of four common syndromes.

A. Sympathomimetic Syndrome

The blood pressure and pulse rate are elevated, though with severe hypertension reflex bradycardia may occur. The temperature is often elevated, pupils are dilated, and the skin is sweaty, though mucous membranes are dry. Patients are usually agitated, anxious, or frankly psychotic.

Examples: Amphetamines, cocaine, ephedrine and pseudoephedrine.

B. Sympatholytic Syndrome

The blood pressure and pulse rate are decreased and body temperature is low. The pupils are small or even pinpoint. Peristalsis is usually decreased. Patients are usually obtunded or comatose.

Examples: Barbiturates, benzodiazepines and other sedative hypnotics, GHB, clonidine and related antihypertensives, ethanol, opioids.

C. Cholinergic Syndrome

Stimulation of muscarinic receptors causes bradycardia, miosis, sweating, and hyperperistalsis as well as bronchorrhea, wheezing, excessive salivation, and urinary incontinence. Nicotinic receptor stimulation may produce initial hypertension and tachycardia as well as fasciculations and muscle weakness. Patients are usually agitated and anxious.

Examples: Carbamates, nicotine, organophosphates (including nerve agents), physostigmine.

D. Anticholinergic Syndrome

Tachycardia with mild hypertension is common, and the body temperature is often elevated. Pupils are widely dilated. The skin is flushed, hot, and dry. Peristalsis is decreased, and urinary retention is common. Patients may have myoclonic jerking or choreoathetoid movements. Agitated delirium is frequently seen, and severe hyperthermia may occur.

Examples: Atropine, scopolamine, other naturally occurring and pharmaceutical anticholinergics, antihistamines, tricyclic antidepressants.

▶ Laboratory Tests

The following clinical laboratory tests are recommended for screening of the overdosed patient: measured serum osmolality and osmol gap, electrolytes, glucose, creatinine, blood urea nitrogen (BUN), urinalysis (eg, oxalate crystals with ethylene glycol poisoning, myoglobinuria with rhabdomyolysis), and electrocardiography. Serum acetaminophen and ethanol quantitative levels should be determined in all patients with drug overdoses.

A. Osmol Gap

The osmol gap is defined and calculation of the gap is described in Table 38–5. It is increased in the presence of large quantities of low-molecular-weight substances, most commonly ethanol. Common poisons associated with increased osmol gap are acetone, ethanol, ethylene glycol, isopropyl alcohol, methanol, and propylene glycol. **Note:** Severe alcoholic ketoacidosis and diabetic ketoacidosis can also cause an elevated osmol gap resulting from the production of ketones and other low-molecular-weight substances.

B. Anion Gap

Metabolic acidosis associated with an elevated anion gap is usually due to an accumulation of lactic acid or other acids (see Chapter 21). Common causes of elevated anion gap in poisoning include carbon monoxide, cyanide, ethylene glycol, medicinal iron, INH, methanol, metformin, ibuprofen and salicylates.

The osmol gap should also be checked; combined elevated anion and osmol gaps suggests poisoning by methanol or ethylene glycol, though this may also occur in patients with diabetic ketoacidosis and alcoholic ketoacidosis.

C. Toxicology Laboratory Examination

A comprehensive toxicology screen is of little value in the initial care of the poisoned patient—on the contrary, it is

Table 38–5. Use of the osmol gap in toxicology.

The osmol gap (Δosm) is determined by subtracting the calculated serum osmolality from the measured serum osmolality.

$$\text{Calculated osmolality (osm)} = 2[Na^+(mEq/L)] + \frac{\text{Glucose (mg/dL)}}{18} + \frac{\text{BUN (mg/dL)}}{2.8}$$

Δosm = Measured osmolality − Calculated osmolality

Serum osmolality may be increased by contributions of circulating alcohols and other low-molecular-weight substances. Since these substances are not included in the calculated osmolality, there will be a gap proportionate to their serum concentration and inversely proportionate to their molecular weight:

$$\frac{\text{Serum concentration (mg/dL)}}{} = \Delta\text{osm} \times \frac{\text{Molecular weight}}{10}$$

	Molecular Weight	Toxic Concentration	Approximate Corresponding Δosm (mosm/L)
Ethanol	46	300	65
Methanol	32	50	16
Ethylene glycol	60	100	16
Isopropanol	60	150	25

Note: The normal osmol gap may vary by as much as ± 10 mosm/L; thus, small osmol gaps may be unreliable in the diagnosis of poisoning.
Adapted, with permission, from Stone CK, Humphries RL (editors): *Current Emergency Diagnosis & Treatment,* 5th ed. McGraw-Hill, 2004.

Table 38–6. Specific quantitative levels and potential therapeutic interventions.[1]

Drug or Toxin	Treatment
Acetaminophen	Specific antidote (*N*-acetylcysteine) based on serum level
Carbon monoxide	High carboxyhemoglobin level indicates need for 100% oxygen, consideration of hyperbaric oxygen
Carbamazepine	High level may indicate need for hemodialysis
Digoxin	On basis of serum digoxin level and severity of clinical presentation, treatment with Fab antibody fragments (Digibind) may be indicated
Ethanol	Low serum level may suggest nonalcoholic cause of coma (eg, trauma, other drugs, other alcohols). Serum ethanol may also be useful in monitoring ethanol therapy for methanol or ethylene glycol poisoning.
Iron	Level may indicate need for chelation with deferoxamine
Lithium	Serum levels can guide decision to institute hemodialysis
Methanol, ethylene glycol	Acidosis, high levels indicate need for hemodialysis, therapy with ethanol or fomepizole
Methemoglobin	Methemoglobinemia can be treated with methylene blue intravenously
Salicylates	High level may indicate need for hemodialysis, alkaline diuresis
Theophylline	Immediate hemodialysis or hemoperfusion may be indicated based on serum level
Valproic acid	Elevated levels may indicate need to consider hemodialysis or L-carnitine therapy, or both

[1]Some drugs or toxins may have profound and irreversible toxicity unless rapid and specific management is provided outside of routine supportive care. For these agents, laboratory testing may provide the serum level or other evidence required for administering a specific antidote or arranging for hemodialysis.

time-consuming and expensive. Specific quantitative levels of certain drugs may be extremely helpful (Table 38–6), however, especially if specific antidotes or interventions (eg, dialysis) would be indicated based on the results.

If a toxicology screen is required, urine is the best specimen. Many hospitals can perform a quick but limited screen for "drugs of abuse" (typically these screens include only opiates, amphetamines, and cocaine, and some add benzodiazepines, barbiturates, and tetrahydrocannabinol [marijuana]). There are numerous false-positive and false-negative results. For example, synthetic opioids, such as fentanyl, oxycodone, and methadone are usually not detected by routine opiate screening. Blood samples may be saved for possible quantitative testing, but blood is not generally used for screening purposes since it is relatively insensitive for many common drugs, including psychotropic agents, opioids, and stimulants.

Abdominal Radiographs

A plain film of the abdomen may reveal radiopaque iron tablets, drug-filled condoms, or other toxic material. Studies suggest that few tablets are predictably visible (eg, ferrous sulfate, sodium chloride, calcium carbonate, and potassium chloride). Thus, the radiograph is useful only if abnormal.

▶ When to Refer

Consultation with a regional poison control center (1-800-222-1222) or medical toxicologist is recommended when the diagnosis is uncertain; there are questions about what laboratory tests to order; dialysis is being considered to remove the drug or poison; or advice is needed regarding the indications, dose, and side effects of antidotes.

▶ When to Admit

- The patient has symptoms and signs of intoxication that are not expected to clear within a 6–8 hour observation period.
- Delayed absorption of the drug might be predicted to cause a later onset of serious symptoms (eg, after ingestion of a sustained-release product).

- Continued administration of an antidote is required (eg, *N*-acetylcysteine for acetaminophen overdose).
- Psychiatric or social services evaluation is needed for suicide attempt or suspected drug abuse.

Bronstein AC et al. 2007 Annual Report of the American Association of Poison Control Centers' National Poison Data System (NPDS): 25th Annual Report. Clin Toxicol (Phila). 2008 Dec;46(10):927–1057. [PMID: 19065310]

Goldfrank LR (editor): *Goldfrank's Toxicologic Emergencies*, 9th ed. McGraw-Hill, 2006.

Lynd LD et al. An evaluation of the osmole gap as a screening test for toxic alcohol poisoning. BMC Emerg Med. 2008 Apr 28;8:5. [PMID: 18442409]

Olson KR (editor): *Poisoning & Drug Overdose*, 5th ed. McGraw-Hill, 2007.

SELECTED POISONINGS

ACETAMINOPHEN

Acetaminophen (paracetamol in the United Kingdom, Europe) is a common analgesic found in many nonprescription and prescription products. After absorption, it is metabolized mainly by glucuronidation and sulfation, with a small fraction metabolized via the P450 mixed-function oxidase system (2E1) to a highly toxic reactive intermediate. This toxic intermediate is normally detoxified by cellular glutathione. With acute acetaminophen overdose (> 150–200 mg/kg, or 8–10 g in an average adult), hepatocellular glutathione is depleted and the reactive intermediate attacks other cell proteins, causing necrosis. Patients with enhanced P450 2E1 activity, such as chronic alcoholics and patients taking INH, are at increased risk of developing hepatotoxicity. Hepatic toxicity may also occur after long-term overuse of acetaminophen—eg, as a result of taking two or three acetaminophen-containing products concurrently or exceeding the recommended maximum dose of 4 g/d for several days.

▶ Clinical Findings

Shortly after ingestion, patients may have nausea or vomiting, but there are usually no other signs of toxicity until 24–48 hours after ingestion, when hepatic aminotransferase levels begin to increase. With severe poisoning, fulminant hepatic necrosis may occur, resulting in jaundice, hepatic encephalopathy, advanced chronic kidney disease, and death. Rarely, massive ingestion (eg, serum levels over 500–1000 mg/L) can cause early onset of acute coma, hypotension, and metabolic acidosis unrelated to hepatic injury.

The diagnosis after acute overdose is based on measurement of the serum acetaminophen level. Plot the serum level versus the time since ingestion on the acetaminophen nomogram shown in Figure 38–1. Ingestion of sustained-release products or coingestion of an anticholinergic agent, salicylate, or opioid drug may cause delayed elevation of serum levels and may render the nomogram useless. The nomogram is not useful after chronic overdose.

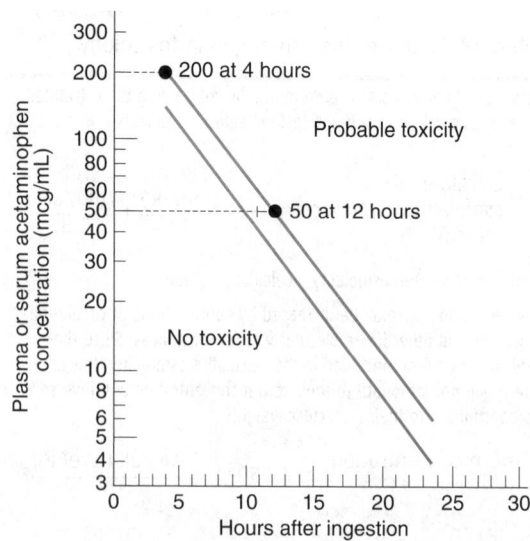

▲ **Figure 38–1.** Nomogram for prediction of acetaminophen hepatotoxicity following acute overdosage. The upper line defines serum acetaminophen concentrations associated with a risk of hepatotoxicity; the lower line defines serum levels 25% below those expected to cause hepatotoxicity. In uncomplicated cases, the upper line can be used as an indication for therapy with *N*-acetylcysteine. However, to provide a margin for error in the estimation of the time of ingestion and for patients at higher risk for hepatotoxicity, the lower line is often used as a guide to treatment. (Adapted, with permission, from Rumack BH et al. Acetaminophen poisoning and toxicity. Pediatrics. 1975 Jun;55(6):871–6.)

▶ Treatment

A. Emergency and Supportive Measures

Administer activated charcoal (see p 1425) if it can be given within 1–2 hours of the ingestion. Although charcoal may interfere with absorption of the oral antidote acetylcysteine, this is not considered clinically significant.

B. Specific Treatment

Although the general recommendation is to treat if the serum acetaminophen level is above the toxic line on the nomogram (Figure 38–1), many clinicians and published guidelines prefer to use the lower line as a guide to treatment, as it provides a 25% safety margin. If the precise time of ingestion is unknown or if the patient is at higher risk for hepatotoxicity (eg, alcoholic, liver disease, long-term use of P450-inducing drugs), then use a lower threshold for initiation of *N*-acetylcysteine (in some case reports, a level of 100 mg/L at 4 hours was suggested in very high-risk patients).

The antidote *N*-acetylcysteine can be given orally or intravenously. Oral treatment begins with a loading dose of *N*-acetylcysteine, 140 mg/kg, followed by 70 mg/kg every 4 hours. Dilute the solution to 5% with water, juice, or soda.

If vomiting interferes with oral *N*-acetylcysteine administration, consider giving the antidote intravenously (see below). The most widely used oral *N*-acetylcysteine protocol in the United States calls for 72 hours of treatment. However, other regimens have demonstrated equivalent success with 20–48 hours of treatment.

A 20-hour intravenous regimen was recently approved by the FDA (Acetadote). It calls for a loading dose of 150 mg/kg given intravenously over 60 minutes, followed by a 4-hour infusion of 50 mg/kg, and a 16-hour infusion of 100 mg/kg. (If Acetadote is not available, the conventional oral formulation may also be given intravenously using a micropore filter and a slow rate of infusion. Call a regional poison control center or medical toxicologist for assistance.)

Treatment with *N*-acetylcysteine is most effective if it is started within 8–10 hours after ingestion.

Betten DP et al. A prospective evaluation of shortened course oral *N*-acetylcysteine for the treatment of acute acetaminophen poisoning. Ann Emerg Med. 2007;50(3):272–9. [PMID: 17210206]

Heard KJ. Acetylcysteine for acetaminophen poisoning. N Engl J Med. 2008 Jul 17;359(3):285–92. [PMID: 18635433]

Kanter MZ. Comparison of oral and i.v. acetylcysteine in the treatment of acetaminophen poisoning. Am J Health Syst Pharm. 2006 Oct 1;63(19):1821–7. [PMID: 16990628]

ACIDS, CORROSIVE

The strong mineral acids exert primarily a local corrosive effect on the skin and mucous membranes. Symptoms include severe pain in the throat and upper gastrointestinal tract; bloody vomitus; difficulty in swallowing, breathing, and speaking; discoloration and destruction of skin and mucous membranes in and around the mouth; and shock. Severe systemic metabolic acidosis may occur both as a result of cellular injury and from systemic absorption of the acid.

Severe deep destructive tissue damage may occur after exposure to hydrofluoric acid because of the penetrating and highly toxic fluoride ion. Systemic hypocalcemia and hyperkalemia may also occur after fluoride absorption, even following skin exposure.

Inhalation of volatile acids, fumes, or gases such as chlorine, fluorine, bromine, or iodine causes severe irritation of the throat and larynx and may cause upper airway obstruction and noncardiogenic pulmonary edema.

▶ Treatment

A. Ingestion

Dilute immediately by giving a glass (4–8 oz) of water to drink. Do *not* give bicarbonate or other neutralizing agents, and do *not* induce vomiting. Some experts recommend immediate placement of a small flexible gastric tube and removal of stomach contents followed by lavage, particularly if the corrosive is a liquid or has important systemic toxicity.

In symptomatic patients, perform flexible endoscopic esophagoscopy to determine the presence and extent of injury. CT scan or plain radiographs of the chest and abdomen may reveal esophageal or gastric perforation.

Perforation, peritonitis, and major bleeding are indications for surgery.

B. Skin Contact

Flood with water for 15 minutes. Use no chemical antidotes; the heat of the reaction may cause additional injury.

For hydrofluoric acid burns, soak the affected area in benzalkonium chloride solution or apply 2.5% calcium gluconate gel (prepared by adding 3.5 g calcium gluconate to 5 oz of water-soluble surgical lubricant, eg, K-Y Jelly); then arrange immediate consultation with a plastic surgeon or other specialist. Binding of the fluoride ion may be achieved by injecting 0.5 mL of 5% calcium gluconate per square centimeter under the burned area. (**Caution:** *Do not use calcium chloride.*) Intra-arterial infusion of calcium is sometimes required for extensive burns or those involving the nail bed; consult with a hand surgeon or poison control center (1-800-222-1222).

C. Eye Contact

Anesthetize the conjunctiva and corneal surfaces with topical local anesthetic drops (eg, proparacaine). Flood with water for 15 minutes, holding the eyelids open. Check pH with pH 6.0–8.0 test paper, and repeat irrigation, using 0.9% saline, until pH is near 7.0. Check for corneal damage with fluorescein and slit lamp examination; consult an ophthalmologist about further treatment.

D. Inhalation

Remove from further exposure to fumes or gas. Check skin and clothing. Treat pulmonary edema.

Flammiger A et al. Sulfuric acid burns (corrosion and acute irritation): evidence-based overview to management. Cutan Ocul Toxicol. 2006;25(1):55–61. [PMID: 16702054]

Vohra R et al. Recurrent life-threatening ventricular dysrhythmias associated with acute hydrofluoric acid ingestion: observations in one case and implications for mechanism of toxicity. Clin Toxicol (Phila). 2008 Jan;46(1):79–84. [PMID: 17906993]

ALKALIES

The strong alkalies are common ingredients of some household cleaning compounds and may be suspected by their "soapy" texture. Those with alkalinity above pH 12.0 are particularly corrosive. Disk (or "button") batteries are also a source. Alkalies cause liquefactive necrosis, which is deeply penetrating. Symptoms include burning pain in the upper gastrointestinal tract, nausea, vomiting, and difficulty in swallowing and breathing. Examination reveals destruction and edema of the affected skin and mucous membranes and bloody vomitus and stools. Radiographs may reveal evidence of perforation or the presence of radiopaque disk batteries in the esophagus or lower gastrointestinal tract.

▶ Treatment

A. Ingestion

Dilute immediately with a glass of water. Do *not* induce emesis. Some gastroenterologists recommend immediate placement of a small flexible gastric tube and removal of stomach contents followed by gastric lavage after ingestion of liquid caustic substances to remove residual material.

Prompt endoscopy is recommended in symptomatic patients to evaluate the extent of damage. If radiograph reveals the location of ingested disk batteries in the esophagus, immediate endoscopic removal is mandatory.

The use of corticosteroids to prevent stricture formation is of no proved benefit and is definitely contraindicated if there is evidence of esophageal perforation.

B. Skin Contact

Wash with running water until the skin no longer feels soapy. Relieve pain and treat shock.

C. Eye Contact

Anesthetize the conjunctival and corneal surfaces with topical anesthetic (eg, proparacaine). Irrigate with water or saline continuously for 20–30 minutes, holding the lids open. Check pH with pH test paper, and repeat irrigation, using 0.9% saline, for additional 30-minute periods until the pH is near 7.0. Check for corneal damage with fluorescein and slit lamp examination; consult an ophthalmologist for further treatment.

Palmer M et al. A,B,Cs of caustic ingestions in suicidal adults. Ann Emerg Med. 2007 Feb;49(2):246–7. [PMID: 17236911]
Schmidt SM et al. Corneal injury due to a calcium hydroxide containing food preparation product ("cal"). Pediatr Emerg Care. 2008 Jul;24(7):468–70. [PMID: 18633308]

AMPHETAMINES & COCAINE

Amphetamines and cocaine are widely abused for their euphorigenic and stimulant properties. Both drugs may be smoked, snorted, ingested, or injected. Amphetamines and cocaine produce central nervous system stimulation and a generalized increase in central and peripheral sympathetic activity. The toxic dose of each drug is highly variable and depends on the route of administration and individual tolerance. The onset of effects is most rapid after intravenous injection or smoking. Amphetamine derivatives and related drugs include methamphetamine ("crystal meth," "crank"), MDMA ("Ecstasy"), ephedrine ("herbal ecstasy"), and methcathinone ("cat"). Nonprescription medications and nutritional supplements may contain stimulant or sympathomimetic drugs such as ephedrine, yohimbine, or caffeine (see Theophylline, below).

▶ Clinical Findings

Presenting symptoms may include anxiety, tremulousness, tachycardia, hypertension, diaphoresis, dilated pupils, agitation, muscular hyperactivity, and psychosis. Muscle hyperactivity may lead to metabolic acidosis and rhabdomyolysis. In severe intoxication, seizures and hyperthermia may occur. Sustained or severe hypertension may result in intracranial hemorrhage, aortic dissection, or myocardial infarction. Hyponatremia has been reported after MDMA use; the mechanism is not known but may involve excessive water intake, syndrome of inappropriate antidiuretic hormone (SIADH), or both.

The diagnosis is supported by finding amphetamines, cocaine, or the cocaine metabolite benzoylecgonine in the urine. Blood screening is generally not sensitive enough to detect these drugs.

▶ Treatment

A. Emergency and Supportive Measures

Maintain a patent airway and assist ventilation, if necessary. Treat coma or seizures as described at the beginning of this chapter. Rapidly lower the body temperature (see hyperthermia, p 1423) in patients who are hyperthermic (temperature > 39–40 °C).

B. Specific Treatment

Treat agitation, psychosis, or seizures with a benzodiazepine such as lorazepam, 2–3 mg intravenously. Add phenobarbital 15 mg/kg intravenously for persistent seizures. Treat hypertension with a vasodilator drug such as phentolamine (1–5 mg intravenously) or a combined α- and β-adrenergic blocker such as labetalol (10–20 mg intravenously). Do *not* administer a pure β-blocker such as propranolol alone, as this may result in paradoxic worsening of the hypertension as a result of unopposed α-adrenergic effects.

Treat tachycardia or tachyarrhythmias with a short-acting β-blocker such as esmolol (25–100 mcg/kg/min by intravenous infusion). Treat hyperthermia as described above. Treat hyponatremia as outlined in Chapter 21.

Mathias S et al. Substance-induced psychosis: a diagnostic conundrum. J Clin Psychiatry. 2008 Mar;69(3):358–67. [PMID: 18278990]
Rusyniak DE et al. Hyperthermic syndromes induced by toxins. Clin Lab Med. 2006 Mar;26(1):165–84. [PMID: 16567230]
Takekawa K et al. Methamphetamine body packer: acute poisoning death due to massive leaking of methamphetamine. J Forensic Sci. 2007 Sep;52(5):1219–22. [PMID: 17680794]

ANTICOAGULANTS

Warfarin and related compounds (including ingredients of many commercial rodenticides) inhibit the clotting mechanism by blocking hepatic synthesis of vitamin K–dependent clotting factors.

Anticoagulants may cause hemoptysis, gross hematuria, bloody stools, hemorrhages into organs, widespread bruising, and bleeding into joint spaces. The prothrombin time is increased within 12–24 hours (peak 36–48 hours) after a single overdose. After ingestion of brodifacoum, difenacoum, and related rodenticides (so-called "super-warfarins"), inhibition of clotting factor synthesis may persist for several weeks or even months after a single dose.

▶ Treatment

A. Emergency and Supportive Measures

Discontinue the drug at the first sign of gross bleeding, and determine the prothrombin time (international normalized ratio, INR). If the patient has ingested an acute overdose, administer activated charcoal (see p 1425).

B. Specific Treatment

Do *not* treat prophylactically with vitamin K—wait for evidence of anticoagulation (elevated prothrombin time). If the INR is elevated, give phytonadione (vitamin K_1), 10–25 mg orally, and additional doses as needed to restore the prothrombin time to normal. Doses as high as 200 mg/d have been required after ingestion of "superwarfarins." Give fresh-frozen plasma or activated Factor VII as needed to rapidly correct the coagulation factor deficit if there is serious bleeding. If the patient is chronically anticoagulated and has strong medical indications for being maintained in that status (eg, prosthetic heart valve), give much smaller doses of vitamin K (1 mg orally) and fresh-frozen plasma (or both) to titrate to the desired prothrombin time.

If the patient has ingested brodifacoum or a related superwarfarin, prolonged observation (over weeks) and repeated administration of large doses of vitamin K may be required.

Olmos V et al. Brodifacoum poisoning with toxicokinetic data. Clin Toxicol (Phila). 2007 Jun–Aug;45(5):487–9. [PMID: 17503253]

Spahr JE et al. Superwarfarin poisoning: a report of two cases and review of the literature. Am J Hematol. 2007 Jul;82(7):656–60. [PMID: 17022046]

Wiedermann CJ et al. Warfarin-induced bleeding complications - clinical presentation and therapeutic options. Thromb Res. 2008;122 Suppl 2:S13–8. [PMID: 18549907]

ANTICONVULSANTS

Anticonvulsants (carbamazepine, phenytoin, valproic acid, and many newer agents) are widely used in the management of seizure disorders. In addition, carbamazepine and valproic acid are increasingly used for treatment of mood disorders.

Phenytoin can be given orally or intravenously. Rapid intravenous injection of phenytoin can cause acute myocardial depression and cardiac arrest owing to the solvent propylene glycol (fosphenytoin does not contain this diluent). Chronic phenytoin intoxication can occur following only slightly increased doses because of zero-order kinetics and a small toxic-therapeutic window. Phenytoin intoxication can also occur following acute intentional or accidental overdose. The overdose syndrome is usually mild even with high serum levels. The most common manifestations are ataxia, nystagmus, and drowsiness. Choreoathetoid movements have been described.

Carbamazepine is used for treatment of trigeminal neuralgia, temporal lobe epilepsy, and other seizure disorders. Intoxication causes drowsiness, stupor and, with high levels, coma and seizures. Dilated pupils and tachycardia are common. Toxicity may be seen with serum levels greater than 20 mg/L, though severe poisoning is usually associated with concentrations greater than 30–40 mg/L. Because of erratic and slow absorption, intoxication may progress over several hours to days.

Valproic acid intoxication produces a unique syndrome consisting of hypernatremia (from the sodium component of the salt), metabolic acidosis, hypocalcemia, elevated serum ammonia, and mild liver aminotransferase elevation. Hypoglycemia may occur as a result of hepatic metabolic dysfunction. Coma with small pupils may be seen and can mimic opioid poisoning. Encephalopathy and cerebral edema can occur.

The newer anticonvulsants **gabapentin**, **levetiracetam**, **vigabatrin,** and **zonisamide** generally cause somnolence, confusion and dizziness; **felbamate** can cause crystalluria and kidney dysfunction after overdose, and may cause idiosyncratic aplastic anemia with therapeutic use; **lamotrigine, topiramate,** and **tiagabine** have been reported to cause seizures after overdose.

▶ Treatment

A. Emergency and Supportive Measures

For recent ingestions, give activated charcoal orally or by gastric tube. For large ingestions of carbamazepine or valproic acid—especially of sustained-release formulations—consider whole bowel irrigation (see p 1425). Multiple-dose activated charcoal and whole-bowel irrigation may be beneficial in ensuring gut decontamination for selected large ingestions.

B. Specific Treatment

There are no specific antidotes. Naloxone was reported to have reversed valproic acid overdose in one anecdotal case. Carnitine may be useful in patients with valproic acid–induced hyperammonemia. Consider hemodialysis for massive intoxication with valproic acid or carbamazepine (eg, carbamazepine levels > 60 mg/L or valproic acid levels > 800 mg/L).

Brahmi N et al. Influence of activated charcoal on the pharmacokinetics and the clinical features of carbamazepine poisoning. Am J Emerg Med. 2006 Jul;24(4):440–3. [PMID: 16787802]

Katiyar A et al. Case files of the Children's Hospital of Michigan Regional Poison Control Center: the use of carnitine for the management of acute valproic acid toxicity. J Med Toxicol. 2007 Sep;3(3):129–38. [PMID: 18072149]

Thundiyil JG et al. Lamotrigine-induced seizures in a child: case report and literature review. Clin Toxicol (Phila). 2007; 45(2):169–72. [PMID: 17364635]

ARSENIC

Arsenic is found in some pesticides and industrial chemicals, and arsenic trioxide has recently been reintroduced as a chemotherapeutic agent. A massive epidemic of chronic arsenic poisoning has occurred in Bangladesh due to naturally occurring arsenic in deep aquifers. Symptoms of acute poisoning usually appear within 1 hour after ingestion but may be delayed as long as 12 hours. They include abdominal pain, vomiting, watery diarrhea, and skeletal muscle cramps. Profound dehydration and shock may occur. In chronic poisoning, symptoms can be vague but often include pancytopenia, painful peripheral sensory neuropathy, and skin changes including melanosis, keratosis, and desquamating rash. Urinary arsenic levels may be falsely elevated after certain meals (eg, seafood) that contain large quantities of a nontoxic form of organic arsenic.

► Treatment

A. Emergency Measures

After recent ingestion (within 1–2 hours), perform gastric lavage and administer 60–100 g of activated charcoal (see p 1425). Administer intravenous fluids to replace losses due to vomiting and diarrhea.

B. Antidote

For patients with severe acute intoxication, give dimercaprol injection (British anti-Lewisite, BAL), 10% solution in oil, 3–5 mg/kg intramuscularly every 4–6 hours for 2 days. The side effects include nausea, vomiting, headache, and hypertension. Follow dimercaprol with oral succimer (dimercaptosuccinic acid, DMSA), 10 mg/kg every 8 hours, for 1 week. Consult a medical toxicologist or regional poison control center (800-222-1222) for advice regarding chelation.

Kapaj S et al. Human health effects from chronic arsenic poisoning—a review. J Environ Sci Health A Tox Hazard Subst Environ Eng. 2006;41(10):2399–428. [PMID: 17018421]
Khandpur S et al. Chronic arsenic toxicity from Ayurvedic medicines. Int J Dermatol. 2008 Jun;47(6):618–21. [PMID: 18477160]

ATROPINE & ANTICHOLINERGICS

Atropine, scopolamine, belladonna, diphenoxylate with atropine, *Datura stramonium*, *Hyoscyamus niger*, some mushrooms, tricyclic antidepressants, and antihistamines are antimuscarinic agents with variable central nervous system effects. The patient complains of dryness of the mouth, thirst, difficulty in swallowing, and blurring of vision. The physical signs include dilated pupils, flushed skin, tachycardia, fever, delirium, myoclonus, ileus, and flushed appearance. Antidepressants and antihistamines may induce convulsions.

Antihistamines are commonly available with or without prescription. Diphenhydramine commonly causes delirium, tachycardia, and seizures. Massive overdose may mimic tricyclic antidepressant poisoning.

► Treatment

A. Emergency and Supportive Measures

Administer activated charcoal (see p 1425). Tepid sponge baths and sedation, or neuromuscular paralysis in rare cases, are indicated to control high temperatures (see p 1423).

B. Specific Treatment

For pure atropine or related anticholinergic syndrome, if symptoms are severe (eg, agitated delirium or excessively

rapid tachycardia), give physostigmine salicylate, 0.5–1 mg slowly intravenously over 5 minutes, with ECG monitoring; repeat as needed to a total dose of 2 mg. Bradyarrhythmias and convulsions are a hazard with physostigmine administration, and it should be avoided in patients with tricyclic antidepressant overdose.

Pragst F et al. Poisonings with diphenhydramine—a survey of 68 clinical and 55 death cases. Forensic Sci Int. 2006 Sep 12;161(2–3):189–97. [PMID: 16857332]
Spina SP et al. Teenagers with Jimson weed (*Datura stramonium*) poisoning. CJEM. 2007 Nov;9(6):467–8. [PMID: 18072995]

β-ADRENERGIC BLOCKERS

There are a wide variety of β-adrenergic blocking drugs, with varying pharmacologic and pharmacokinetic properties (see Table 11–7). The most toxic β-blocker is propranolol. Propranolol competitively blocks β_1 and β_2 adrenoceptors and also has direct membrane-depressant and central nervous system effects.

► Clinical Findings

The most common findings with mild or moderate intoxication are hypotension and bradycardia. Cardiac depression from more severe poisoning is often unresponsive to conventional therapy with β-adrenergic stimulants such as dopamine and norepinephrine. In addition, with propranolol and other lipid-soluble drugs, seizures and coma may occur. Propranolol, oxprenolol, acebutolol, and alprenolol also have membrane-depressant effects and can cause conduction disturbance (wide QRS interval) similar to tricyclic antidepressant overdose.

The diagnosis is based on typical clinical findings. Routine toxicology screening does not usually include β-blockers.

► Treatment

A. Emergency and Supportive Measures

Initially, treat bradycardia or heart block with atropine (0.5–2 mg intravenously), isoproterenol (2–20 mcg/min by intravenous infusion, titrated to the desired heart rate), or an external transcutaneous cardiac pacemaker. However, these measures are often ineffective, and specific antidotal treatment may be necessary (see below).

For ingested drugs, administer activated charcoal (see p 1425).

B. Specific Treatment

If the above measures are not successful in reversing bradycardia and hypotension, give glucagon, 5–10 mg intravenously, followed by an infusion of 1–5 mg/h. Glucagon is an inotropic agent that acts at a different receptor site and is therefore not affected by β-blockade. Membrane-depressant effects (wide QRS interval) may respond to boluses of sodium bicarbonate (50–100 mEq intravenously) as for tricyclic antidepressant poisoning.

Kerns W 2nd. Management of beta-adrenergic blocker and calcium channel antagonist toxicity. Emerg Med Clin North Am. 2007 May;25(2):309–31. [PMID: 17482022]

Shepherd G. Treatment of poisoning caused by beta-adrenergic and calcium-channel blockers. Am J Health Syst Pharm. 2006 Oct 1;63(19):1828–35. [PMID: 16990629]

CALCIUM CHANNEL BLOCKERS

Calcium channel blockers are used to treat angina pectoris, hypertension, supraventricular tachycardia, migraine, and other disorders. In therapeutic doses, nifedipine, nicardipine, amlodipine, felodipine, isradipine, nisoldipine, and nimodipine act mainly on blood vessels, while verapamil and diltiazem act mainly on cardiac contractility and conduction. However, these selective effects are lost after acute overdose. Patients may present with bradycardia, atrioventricular (AV) nodal block, hypotension, or a combination of these effects. Hyperglycemia is common due to blockade of insulin release. With severe poisoning, cardiac arrest may occur.

▶ **Treatment**

A. Emergency and Supportive Measures

For ingested drugs, administer activated charcoal (see p 1425). In addition, whole bowel irrigation should be initiated as soon as possible if the patient has ingested a sustained-release product.

B. Specific Treatment

If bradycardia and hypotension are not reversed with atropine (0.5–2 mg intravenously), isoproterenol (2–20 mcg/min by intravenous infusion), or a transcutaneous cardiac pacemaker, administer calcium chloride intravenously. Start with calcium chloride 10%, 10 mL, or calcium gluconate 10%, 20 mL. Repeat the dose every 3–5 minutes. The optimum (or maximum) dose has not been established, but there are reports of success after as much as 10–12 g of calcium chloride. Calcium is most useful in reversing negative inotropic effects and is less effective for AV nodal blockade and bradycardia. Epinephrine infusion (1–4 mcg/min initially) and glucagon (5–10 mg intravenously) have also been recommended. In addition, high doses of insulin (0.5–1 units/kg intravenous bolus followed by 0.5–1 units/kg/h infusion) along with sufficient dextrose to maintain euglycemia have been reported to be beneficial but there are no controlled studies. Infusion of Intralipid 20% lipid emulsion has been reported to improve hemodynamics in an animal model of verapamil poisoning.

Bania TC et al. Hemodynamic effects of intravenous fat emulsion in an animal model of severe verapamil toxicity resuscitated with atropine, calcium, and saline. Acad Emerg Med. 2007 Feb;14(2):105–11. [PMID: 17267527]

Greene SL et al. Relative safety of hyperinsulinaemia/euglycaemia therapy in the management of calcium channel blocker overdose: a prospective observational study. Intensive Care Med. 2007 Nov;33(11):2019–24. [PMID: 17622512]

Patel NP et al. Hyperinsulinemic euglycemia therapy for verapamil poisoning: a review. Am J Crit Care. 2007 Sep;16(5):498–503. [PMID: 17724247]

CARBON MONOXIDE

Carbon monoxide is a colorless, odorless gas produced by the combustion of carbon-containing materials. Poisoning may occur as a result of suicidal or accidental exposure to automobile exhaust, smoke inhalation in a fire, or accidental exposure to an improperly vented gas heater or other appliance. Carbon monoxide avidly binds to hemoglobin, with an affinity approximately 250 times that of oxygen. This results in reduced oxygen-carrying capacity and altered delivery of oxygen to cells (see also Smoke Inhalation in Chapter 9).

▶ **Clinical Findings**

At low carbon monoxide levels (carboxyhemoglobin saturation 10–20%), victims may have headache, dizziness, abdominal pain, and nausea. With higher levels, confusion, dyspnea, and syncope may occur. Hypotension, coma, and seizures are common with levels greater than 50–60%. Survivors of acute severe poisoning may develop permanent obvious or subtle neurologic and neuropsychiatric deficits. The fetus and newborn may be more susceptible because of high carbon monoxide affinity for fetal hemoglobin.

Carbon monoxide poisoning should be suspected in any person with severe headache or acutely altered mental status, especially during cold weather, when improperly vented heating systems may have been used. Diagnosis depends on specific measurement of the arterial or venous carboxyhemoglobin saturation, although the level may have declined if high-flow oxygen therapy has already been administered, and levels do not always correlate with clinical symptoms. Routine arterial blood gas testing and pulse oximetry are not useful because they give falsely normal PaO_2 and oxyhemoglobin saturation determinations, respectively. (A newer pulse oximetry device, the pulse CO-oximeter [Masimo Rad-57] is capable of distinguishing oxyhemoglobin from carboxyhemoglobin.)

▶ **Treatment**

A. Emergency and Supportive Measures

Maintain a patent airway and assist ventilation, if necessary. Remove the victim from exposure. Treat patients with coma, hypotension, or seizures as described at the beginning of this chapter.

B. Specific Treatment

The half-life of the carboxyhemoglobin (CoHb) complex is about 4–5 hours in room air but is reduced dramatically by high concentrations of oxygen. Administer 100% oxygen by tight-fitting high-flow reservoir face mask or endotracheal tube. Hyperbaric oxygen (HBO) can provide 100% oxygen under higher than atmospheric pressures, further shortening the half-life; it may also reduce the incidence of subtle neuropsychiatric sequelae. Recent studies disagree about the benefit of HBO, but generally recommended indications for HBO in patients with carbon monoxide poisoning include a history of loss of consciousness, CoHb greater than 25%, metabolic acidosis, age over 50 years, and cerebellar findings on neurologic examination.

Hampson NB et al. Carboxyhemoglobin levels in carbon monoxide poisoning: do they correlate with the clinical picture? Am J Emerg Med. 2008 Jul;26(6):665–9. [PMID: 18606318]
Hampson NB et al. Risk factors for short-term mortality from carbon monoxide poisoning treated with hyperbaric oxygen. Crit Care Med. 2008 Sep;36(9):2523–7. [PMID: 18679118]
Prockop LD et al. Carbon monoxide intoxication: an updated review. J Neurol Sci. 2007 Nov 15;262(1–2):122–30. [PMID: 17720201]

CHEMICAL WARFARE: NERVE AGENTS

Nerve agents used in chemical warfare work by cholinesterase inhibition and are most commonly organophosphorus compounds. Agents such as **tabun** (GA), **sarin** (GB), **soman** (GD), and **VX** are similar to insecticides such as malathion but are vastly more potent. They may be inhaled or absorbed through the skin. Systemic effects due to unopposed action of acetylcholine include miosis, salivation, abdominal cramps, diarrhea, and muscle paralysis producing respiratory arrest. Inhalation also produces severe bronchoconstriction and copious nasal and tracheobronchial secretions.

▶ Treatment

A. Emergency and Supportive Measures

Perform thorough decontamination of exposed areas with repeated soap and shampoo washing. Personnel caring for such patients must wear protective clothing and gloves, since cutaneous absorption may occur through normal skin.

B. Specific Treatment

Give atropine in an initial dose of 2 mg intravenously, and repeat as needed to reverse signs of acetylcholine excess. (Some victims have required several hundred milligrams.) Treat also with the cholinesterase-reactivating agent pralidoxime, 1–2 g intravenously initially followed by an infusion at a rate of 200–400 mg/h. United States military personnel in the Iraq invasion were equipped with autoinjectable units containing 2 mg of atropine plus 600 mg of the cholinesterase-reactivating agent pralidoxime.

Barelli A et al. The comprehensive medical preparedness in chemical emergencies: 'the chain of chemical survival'. Eur J Emerg Med. 2008 Apr;15(2):110–8. [PMID: 18446078]
Yoshida T. Preparedness response to hazard and toxic incidents and food terrorism. Yakugaku Zasshi. 2008 Jun;128(6):851–7. [PMID: 18520132]

CHEMICAL WARFARE: RICIN

Ricin is a naturally occurring toxin found in minute quantities in the castor bean (*Ricinus communis*). It can cause toxicity if castor beans are thoroughly chewed or blenderized, although the quantity of ricin is small and it is poorly absorbed from the gastrointestinal tract, so symptoms following castor bean ingestion are usually limited to diarrhea and abdominal pain. Less commonly, severe gastroenteritis can lead to volume depletion and advanced chronic kidney disease. On the other hand, purified ricin is extremely toxic if administered parenterally: the LD_{50} for injected ricin in animals is as low as 0.1 mcg/kg. A fatal case of suspected ricin poisoning by homicidal injection of an estimated 0.28 mg of ricin was associated with diffuse organ damage and death from cardiac failure after 2 days. Inhalation of ricin powder has not been reported in humans, but animal studies suggest it could cause hemorrhagic tracheobronchitis and pneumonia.

▶ Treatment

A. Emergency and Supportive Measures

After suspected ricin inhalation or exposure to powdered ricin, remove clothing and wash skin with water. Personnel caring for such patients should wear protective respiratory gear, clothing, and gloves.

B. Specific Treatment

There is no known antidote or other specific treatment. A vaccine has been developed and is undergoing clinical trials. Provide supportive care for volume loss due to gastroenteritis and cardiac and respiratory support as needed.

Schier JG et al. Public health investigation after the discovery of ricin in a South Carolina postal facility. Am J Public Health. 2007 Apr;97(Suppl 1):S152–7. [PMID: 17413057]

CLONIDINE & OTHER SYMPATHOLYTIC ANTIHYPERTENSIVES

Overdosage with these agents (clonidine, guanabenz, guanfacine, methyldopa) causes bradycardia, hypotension, miosis, respiratory depression, and coma. (Transient hypertension occasionally occurs after acute overdosage, a result of peripheral α-adrenergic effects in high doses.) Symptoms are usually resolved in less than 24 hours, and deaths are rare. Similar symptoms may occur after ingestion of topical nasal decongestants chemically similar to clonidine (oxymetazoline, tetrahydrozoline, naphazoline). Brimonidine is used as an ophthalmic preparation for glaucoma. Tizanidine is a centrally acting muscle relaxant structurally related to clonidine; it produces similar toxicity in overdose.

▶ Treatment

A. Emergency and Supportive Measures

Give activated charcoal (see p 1425). Maintain the airway and support respiration if necessary. Symptomatic treatment is usually sufficient even in massive overdose. Maintain blood pressure with intravenous fluids. Dopamine can also be used. Atropine is usually effective for bradycardia.

B. Specific Treatment

There is no specific antidote. Although tolazoline has been recommended for clonidine overdose, its effects are unpredictable and it should not be used. Naloxone has been reported to be successful in a few anecdotal and poorly substantiated cases.

Rangan C et al. Central alpha-2 adrenergic eye drops: case series of 3 pediatric systemic poisonings. Pediatr Emerg Care. 2008 Mar;24(3):167–9. [PMID: 18347496]
Sklerov JH et al. Tizanidine distribution in a postmortem case. J Anal Toxicol. 2006 Jun;30(5):331–4. [PMID: 16839471]

COCAINE

See Amphetamines & Cocaine.

CYANIDE

Cyanide is a highly toxic chemical used widely in research and commercial laboratories and many industries. Its gaseous form, hydrogen cyanide, is an important component of smoke in fires. Cyanide-generating glycosides are also found in the pits of apricots and other related plants. Cyanide is generated by the breakdown of nitroprusside, and poisoning can result from rapid high-dose infusions. Cyanide is also formed by metabolism of acetonitrile, a solvent found in some over-the-counter fingernail glue removers. Cyanide is rapidly absorbed by inhalation, skin absorption, or ingestion. It disrupts cellular function by inhibiting cytochrome oxidase and preventing cellular oxygen utilization.

▶ Clinical Findings

The onset of toxicity is nearly instantaneous after inhalation of hydrogen cyanide gas but may be delayed for minutes to hours after ingestion of cyanide salts or cyanogenic plants or chemicals. Effects include headache, dizziness, nausea, abdominal pain, and anxiety, followed by confusion, syncope, shock, seizures, coma, and death. The odor of "bitter almonds" may be detected on the victim's breath or in vomitus, though this is not a reliable finding. The venous oxygen saturation may be elevated (> 90%) in severe poisonings because tissues have failed to take up arterial oxygen.

▶ Treatment

A. Emergency and Supportive Measures

Remove the victim from exposure, taking care to avoid exposure to rescuers. For suspected cyanide poisoning due to nitroprusside infusion, stop or slow the rate of infusion. (Metabolic acidosis and other signs of cyanide poisoning usually clear rapidly.)

For cyanide ingestion, administer activated charcoal (see p 1425). Although charcoal has a low affinity for cyanide, the usual doses of 60–100 g are adequate to bind typically ingested lethal doses (100–200 mg).

B. Specific Treatment

In the United States, the conventional cyanide antidote package (Taylor Pharmaceuticals) (Table 38–7) contains nitrites (to induce methemoglobinemia, which binds free cyanide) and thiosulfate (to promote conversion of cyanide to the less toxic thiocyanate). Administer amyl nitrite by crushing an ampule under the victim's nose or at the end of the endotracheal tube, and administer 3% sodium nitrite solution, 10 mL intravenously. **Caution:** Nitrites may induce hypotension and dangerous levels of methemoglobin. Also administer 25% sodium thiosulfate solution, 50 mL intravenously (12.5 g). Hydroxocobalamin, a newer and potentially safer alternative antidote, was approved by the FDA in December 2006. The dose of hydroxocobalamin (Cyanokit, EMD Pharmaceuticals) is 5 g intravenously (children, 70 mg/kg).

Eckstein M. Enhancing public health preparedness for a terrorist attack involving cyanide. J Emerg Med. 2008 Jul;35(1):59–65. [PMID: 17976798]
Hall AH et al. Sodium thiosulfate or hydroxocobalamin for the empiric treatment of cyanide poisoning? Ann Emerg Med. 2007 Jun;49(6):806–13. [PMID: 17098327]
Shepherd G et al. Role of hydroxocobalamin in acute cyanide poisoning. Ann Pharmacother. 2008 May;42(5):661–9. [PMID: 18397973]

DIGITALIS & OTHER CARDIAC GLYCOSIDES

Cardiac glycosides are derived from a variety of plants and are widely used to treat heart failure and supraventricular arrhythmias. These drugs paralyze the Na^+-K^+-ATPase pump and have potent vagotonic effects. Intracellular effects include enhancement of calcium-dependent contractility and shortening of the action potential duration. Digoxin and ouabain are highly tissue-bound, but digitoxin has a volume of distribution of just 0.6 L/kg, making it potentially accessible to enhanced removal procedures such as hemoperfusion or repeated doses of activated charcoal. There are a number of plants (eg, oleander, foxglove, lily-of-the-valley) that contain cardiac glycosides. Bufotenin, a cardiotoxic steroid found in certain toad secretions and used as an herbal medicine and a purported aphrodisiac, has pharmacologic properties similar to cardiac glycosides.

Table 38–7. Currently available cyanide (CN) antidote kits.

Antidote	Contents	Action
Conventional cyanide antidote kit[1]	Amyl nitrite, 0.3 mL aspirol for inhalation; sodium nitrite 300 mg in a 10-mL vial; sodium thiosulfate 12.5 g in a 50-mL vial	Nitrites induce methemoglobinemia, which binds CN; thiosulfate hastens CN conversion to less toxic thiocyanate
Cyanokit[2]	Hydroxocobalamin 5 g in two 2.5-g vials	Converts CN to cyanocobalamin (vitamin B_{12})

[1]In the United States, manufactured by Taylor Pharmaceuticals.
[2]Manufactured by EMD Pharmaceuticals.

Clinical Findings

Intoxication may result from acute single exposure or chronic accidental overmedication. After acute overdosage, nausea and vomiting, bradycardia, hyperkalemia, and AV block frequently occur. Patients in whom toxicity develops gradually during long-term therapy may be hypokalemic and hypomagnesemic owing to concurrent diuretic treatment and more commonly present with ventricular arrhythmias (eg, ectopy, bidirectional ventricular tachycardia, or ventricular fibrillation). Digoxin levels may be only slightly elevated in patients with intoxication from cardiac glycosides other than digoxin because of limited cross-reactivity of immunologic tests.

Treatment

A. Emergency and Supportive Measures

After acute ingestion, administer activated charcoal (see p 1425). Monitor potassium levels and cardiac rhythm closely. Treat bradycardia initially with atropine (0.5–2 mg intravenously) or a transcutaneous external cardiac pacemaker.

B. Specific Treatment

For patients with significant intoxication, administer digoxin-specific antibodies (digoxin immune Fab [ovine]; Digibind or DigiFab). Estimation of the Digibind dose is based on the body burden of digoxin calculated from the ingested dose or the steady-state serum digoxin concentration:

1. From the ingested dose—Number of vials = approximately 1.5–2 × ingested dose (mg).

2. From the serum concentration—Number of vials = serum digoxin (ng/mL) × body weight (kg) × 10^{-2}. **Note:** This is based on the equilibrium digoxin level; after acute overdose, serum levels are falsely high before tissue distribution is complete, and overestimation of the Digibind or DigiFab dose is likely.

3. Empiric dosing—Empiric dosing of Digibind or Digi-Fab may be used if the patient's condition is relatively stable and an underlying condition (eg, atrial fibrillation) suggests a residual level of digitalis activity. Start with one or two vials and reassess the clinical condition after 20–30 minutes. For cardiac glycosides other than digoxin or digitoxin, there is no formula for estimation of vials needed and treatment is empiric.

Note: After administration of digoxin-specific Fab antibody fragment, serum digoxin levels may be falsely elevated depending on the assay technique.

Lapostolle F et al. Assessment of digoxin antibody use in patients with elevated serum digoxin following chronic or acute exposure. Intensive Care Med. 2008 Aug;34(8):1448–53. [PMID: 18389220]

Lapostolle F et al. Digoxin-specific Fab fragments as single first-line therapy in digitalis poisoning. Crit Care Med. 2008 Nov;36(11):3014–8. [PMID: 18824911]

Tsai YC et al. Cardiac glycoside poisoning following suicidal ingestion of *Cerbera manghas*. Clin Toxicol (Phila). 2008 Apr;46(4):340–1. [PMID: 18363136]

ETHANOL, BENZODIAZEPINES, & OTHER SEDATIVE-HYPNOTIC AGENTS

The group of agents known as sedative-hypnotic drugs includes a variety of products used for the treatment of anxiety, depression, insomnia, and epilepsy. Ethanol and other selected agents are also popular recreational drugs. All of these drugs depress the central nervous system reticular activating system, cerebral cortex, and cerebellum.

Clinical Findings

Mild intoxication produces euphoria, slurred speech, and ataxia. Ethanol intoxication may produce hypoglycemia, even at relatively low concentrations. With more severe intoxication, stupor, coma, and respiratory arrest may occur. Carisoprodol (Soma) commonly causes muscle jerking or myoclonus. Death or serious morbidity is usually the result of pulmonary aspiration of gastric contents. Bradycardia, hypotension, and hypothermia are common. Patients with massive intoxication may appear to be dead, with no reflex responses and even absent electroencephalographic activity. Diagnosis and assessment of severity of intoxication are usually based on clinical findings. Ethanol serum levels greater than 300 mg/dL (0.3 g/dL; 65 mmol/L) can produce coma in persons who are not chronically abusing the drug, but regular users may remain awake at much higher levels. Phenobarbital levels greater than 100 mg/L usually cause coma.

Treatment

A. Emergency and Supportive Measures

Administer activated charcoal (see p 1425). Repeat-dose charcoal may enhance elimination of phenobarbital, but it has not been proved to improve clinical outcome. Hemodialysis may be necessary for patients with severe phenobarbital intoxication.

B. Specific Treatment

Flumazenil is a benzodiazepine receptor-specific antagonist; it has no effect on ethanol, barbiturates, or other sedative-hypnotic agents. If used, flumazenil is given slowly intravenously, 0.2 mg over 30–60 seconds, repeated in 0.5 mg increments as needed up to a total dose of 3–5 mg. **Caution:** Flumazenil may induce seizures in patients with preexisting seizure disorder, benzodiazepine addiction, or concomitant tricyclic antidepressant overdose. If seizures occur, diazepam and other benzodiazepine anticonvulsants will not be effective. As with naloxone, the duration of action of flumazenil is short (2–3 hours) and resedation may occur, requiring repeated doses.

Chudnofsky CR. Safety and efficacy of flumazenil in reversing conscious sedation in the emergency department. Emergency Medicine Conscious Sedation Study Group. Acad Emerg Med. 1997 Oct;4(10):944–50. [PMID: 9332625]

Thomson JS et al. Use of flumazenil in benzodiazepine overdose. Emerg Med J. 2006 Feb;23(2):162. [PMID: 16439763]

γ-HYDROXYBUTYRATE (GHB)

GHB has become a popular drug of abuse. It originated as a short-acting general anesthetic and is occasionally used in the treatment of narcolepsy. It gained popularity among bodybuilders for its alleged growth hormone stimulation and found its way into social settings, where it is consumed as a liquid. It has been used to facilitate sexual assault ("date-rape" drug). Symptoms after ingestion include drowsiness and lethargy followed by coma with respiratory depression. Muscle twitching and seizures are sometimes observed. Recovery is usually rapid, with patients awakening within a few hours. Other related chemicals with similar effects include butanediol and γ-butyrolactone (GBL). A prolonged withdrawal syndrome has been described in some heavy users.

▶ Treatment

Monitor the airway and assist breathing if needed. There is no specific treatment. Most patients recover rapidly with supportive care. GHB withdrawal syndrome may require very large doses of benzodiazepines.

Abanades S et al. Relative abuse liability of gamma-hydroxybutyric acid, flunitrazepam, and ethanol in club drug users. J Clin Psychopharmacol. 2007 Dec;27(6):625–38. [PMID: 18004131]
Anderson IB et al. Trends in gamma-hydroxybutyrate (GHB) intoxication: 1999–2003. Ann Emerg Med. 2006 Feb;47(2):177–83. [PMID: 16431231]

IRON

Iron is widely used therapeutically for the treatment of anemia and as a daily supplement in multiple vitamin preparations. Most children's preparations contain about 12–15 mg of elemental iron (as sulfate, gluconate, or fumarate salt) per dose, compared with 60–90 mg in most adult-strength preparations. Iron is corrosive to the gastrointestinal tract and, once absorbed, has depressant effects on the myocardium and on peripheral vascular resistance. Intracellular toxic effects of iron include disruption of Krebs cycle enzymes.

▶ Clinical Findings

Ingestion of less than 30 mg/kg of elemental iron usually produces only mild gastrointestinal upset. Ingestion of more than 40–60 mg/kg may cause vomiting (sometimes with hematemesis), diarrhea, hypotension, and acidosis. Death may occur as a result of profound hypotension due to massive fluid losses and bleeding, metabolic acidosis, peritonitis from intestinal perforation, or sepsis. Fulminant hepatic failure may occur. Survivors of the acute ingestion may suffer permanent gastrointestinal scarring.

Serum iron levels greater than 350–500 mcg/dL are considered potentially toxic, and levels over 1000 mcg/dL are usually associated with severe poisoning. A plain abdominal radiograph may reveal radiopaque tablets.

▶ Treatment

A. Emergency and Supportive Measures

Treat hypotension aggressively with intravenous crystalloid solutions (0.9% saline or lactated Ringer solution). Fluid losses may be massive owing to vomiting and diarrhea as well as third-spacing into injured intestine.

Perform whole bowel irrigation to remove unabsorbed pills from the intestinal tract (see p 1425). Activated charcoal is not effective but may be appropriate if other ingestants are suspected.

B. Specific Treatment

Deferoxamine is a selective iron chelator. It is not useful as an oral binding agent. For patients with established manifestations of toxicity—and particularly those with markedly elevated serum iron levels (eg, greater than 800–1000 mcg/dL)—administer 10–15 mg/kg/h by constant intravenous infusion; higher doses (up to 40–50 mg/kg/h) have been used in massive poisonings. Hypotension may occur. The presence of an iron-deferoxamine complex in the urine may give it a "vin rosé" appearance. Deferoxamine is safe for use in pregnant women with acute iron overdose. **Caution:** Prolonged infusion of deferoxamine (> 36–48 hours) has been associated with development of acute respiratory distress syndrome (ARDS)—the mechanism is not known.

Goldstein LH et al. Ingestion of slow-release iron treated with gastric lavage—never say late. Clin Toxicol (Phila). 2006; 44(3):343. [PMID: 16749558]
Ng HW et al. Endoscopic removal of iron bezoar following acute overdose. Clin Toxicol (Phila). 2008 Nov;46(9):913–5. [PMID: 18608283]

ISONIAZID

INH is an antibacterial drug used mainly in the treatment and prevention of tuberculosis. It may cause hepatitis with long-term use, especially in alcoholic patients and elderly persons. It produces acute toxic effects by competing with pyridoxal 5-phosphate, resulting in lowered brain γ-aminobutyric acid (GABA) levels. Acute ingestion of as little as 1.5–2 g of INH can cause toxicity, and severe poisoning is likely to occur after ingestion of more than 80–100 mg/kg.

▶ Clinical Findings

Confusion, slurred speech, and seizures may occur abruptly after acute overdose. Severe lactic acidosis—out of proportion to the severity of seizures—is probably due to inhibited metabolism of lactate. Peripheral neuropathy and acute hepatitis may occur with long-term use.

Diagnosis is based on a history of ingestion and the presence of severe acidosis associated with seizures. INH is not usually included in routine toxicologic screening, and serum levels are not readily available.

▶ **Treatment**

A. Emergency and Supportive Measures

Seizures may require higher than usual doses of benzodiazepines (eg, lorazepam, 3–5 mg intravenously) or administration of pyridoxine as an antidote (see below).

Administer activated charcoal (see p 1425). Do *not* induce emesis, because of the risk of abrupt onset of seizures.

B. Specific Treatment

Pyridoxine (vitamin B₆) is a specific antagonist of the acute toxic effects of INH and is usually successful in controlling convulsions that do not respond to benzodiazepines. Give 5 g intravenously over 1–2 minutes or, if the amount ingested is known, give a gram-for-gram equivalent amount of pyridoxine. Patients taking INH are usually given 25–50 mg of pyridoxine orally daily to help prevent neuropathy.

Preziosi P. Isoniazid: metabolic aspects and toxicological correlates. Curr Drug Metab. 2007 Dec;8(8):839–51. [PMID: 18220565]

Tai WP et al. Coma caused by isoniazid poisoning in a patient treated with pyridoxine and hemodialysis. Adv Ther. 2008 Oct;25(10):1085–8. [PMID: 18807228]

LEAD

Lead is used in a variety of industrial and commercial products, such as storage batteries, solders, paints, pottery, plumbing, and gasoline and is found in some traditional Hispanic and Ayurvedic ethnic medicines. Lead toxicity usually results from chronic repeated exposure and is rare after a single ingestion. Lead produces a variety of adverse effects on cellular function and primarily affects the nervous system, gastrointestinal tract, and hematopoietic system.

▶ **Clinical Findings**

Lead poisoning often goes undiagnosed initially because presenting symptoms and signs are nonspecific and exposure is not suspected. Common symptoms include colicky abdominal pain, constipation, headache, and irritability. Severe poisoning may cause coma and convulsions. Chronic intoxication can cause learning disorders (in children) and motor neuropathy (eg, wrist drop). Lead-containing bullet fragments in or near joint spaces can result in chronic lead toxicity.

Diagnosis is based on measurement of the blood lead level. Whole blood lead levels less than 10 mcg/dL are usually considered nontoxic. Levels between 10 and 25 mcg/dL have been associated with impaired neurobehavioral development in children. Levels of 25–50 mcg/dL may be associated with headache, irritability, and subclinical neuropathy. Levels of 50–70 mcg/dL are associated with moderate toxicity, and levels greater than 70–100 mcg/dL are often associated with severe poisoning. Other laboratory findings of lead poisoning include microcytic anemia with basophilic stippling and elevated free erythrocyte protoporphyrin.

▶ **Treatment**

A. Emergency and Supportive Measures

For patients with encephalopathy, maintain a patent airway and treat coma and convulsions as described at the beginning of this chapter.

For recent acute ingestion, if a large lead-containing object (eg, fishing weight) is still visible in the stomach on abdominal radiograph, whole bowel irrigation (see p 1425), endoscopy, or even surgical removal may be necessary to prevent subacute lead poisoning. (The acidic gastric contents may corrode the metal surface, enhancing lead absorption. Once the object passes into the small intestine, the risk of toxicity declines.)

Conduct an investigation into the source of the lead exposure.

Workers with a single lead level greater than 60 mcg/dL (or three successive monthly levels greater than 50 mcg/dL) or construction workers with any single blood lead level greater than 50 mcg/dL must by federal law be removed from the site of exposure. Contact the regional office of the United States Occupational Safety and Health Administration (OSHA) for more information. Several states mandate reporting of cases of confirmed lead poisoning.

B. Specific Treatment

The indications for chelation depend on the blood lead level and the patient's clinical state. A medical toxicologist or regional poison control center (800-222-1222) should be consulted for advice about selection and use of these antidotes.

Note: It is impermissible under the law to treat asymptomatic workers with elevated blood lead levels in order to keep their levels under 50 mcg/dL rather than remove them from the exposure.

1. Severe toxicity—Patients with severe intoxication (encephalopathy or levels greater than 70–100 mcg/dL) should receive edetate calcium disodium (ethylenediamine-tetraacetic acid, EDTA), 1500 mg/m²/kg/d (approximately 50 mg/kg/d) in four to six divided doses or as a continuous intravenous infusion. Some clinicians also add dimercaprol (BAL), 4–5 mg/kg intramuscularly every 4 hours for 5 days.

2. Less severe toxicity—Patients with less severe symptoms and asymptomatic patients with blood lead levels between 55 and 69 mcg/dL may be treated with edetate calcium disodium alone in dosages as above. An oral chelator, succimer (DMSA), is available for use in patients with mild to moderate intoxication. The usual dose is 10 mg/kg orally every 8 hours for 5 days, then every 12 hours for 2 weeks.

Karri SK et al. Lead encephalopathy due to traditional medicines. Curr Drug Saf. 2008 Jan;3(1):54–9. [PMID: 18690981]

Sabouraud S et al. Lead poisoning following ingestion of pieces of lead roofing plates: pica-like behavior in an adult. Clin Toxicol (Phila). 2007 Sep 28:1–3. [PMID: 17906991]

Saper RB et al. Lead, mercury, and arsenic in US- and Indian-manufactured Ayurvedic medicines sold via the Internet. JAMA. 2008 Aug 27;300(8):915–23. [PMID: 18728265]

LSD & OTHER HALLUCINOGENS

A variety of substances—ranging from naturally occurring plants and mushrooms to synthetic substances such as phencyclidine (PCP), toluene and other solvents, dextromethorphan, and lysergic acid diethylamide (LSD)—are abused for their hallucinogenic properties. The mechanism of toxicity and the clinical effects vary for each substance.

Many hallucinogenic plants and mushrooms produce anticholinergic delirium, characterized by flushed skin, dry mucous membranes, dilated pupils, tachycardia, and urinary retention. Other plants and mushrooms may contain hallucinogenic indoles such as mescaline and LSD, which typically cause marked visual hallucinations and perceptual distortion, widely dilated pupils, and mild tachycardia. PCP, a dissociative anesthetic agent similar to ketamine, can produce fluctuating delirium and coma, often associated with vertical and horizontal nystagmus. Toluene and other hydrocarbon solvents (butane, trichloroethylene, "chemo," etc) cause euphoria and delirium and may sensitize the myocardium to the effects of catecholamines, leading to fatal dysrhythmias.

▶ Treatment

A. Emergency and Supportive Measures

Maintain a patent airway and assist respirations if necessary. Treat coma, hyperthermia, and seizures as outlined at the beginning of this chapter. For recent large ingestions, consider giving activated charcoal orally or by gastric tube.

B. Specific Treatment

Patients with anticholinergic delirium may benefit from a dose of physostigmine, 0.5–1 mg intravenously, not to exceed 1 mg/min. Dysphoria, agitation, and psychosis associated with LSD or mescaline intoxication may respond to benzodiazepines (eg, lorazepam, 1–2 mg orally or intravenously) or haloperidol (2–5 mg intramuscularly or intravenously). Monitor patients who have sniffed solvents for cardiac dysrhythmias (most commonly premature ventricular contractions, ventricular tachycardia, ventricular fibrillation); treatment with β-blockers such as propranolol (1–5 mg intravenously) or esmolol (250–500 mcg/kg intravenously, then 50 mcg/kg/min by infusion) may be more effective than lidocaine.

Jamison SC et al. A 60-year-old woman with agitation and psychosis following ingestion of dextromethorphan and opioid analgesics. J Psychopharmacol. 2008 Jun 26 [Epub ahead of print]. [PMID: 18583439]

Vural M et al. Dilated cardiomyopathy associated with toluene abuse. Cardiology. 2006;105(3):158–61. [PMID: 16479101]

MERCURY

Acute mercury poisoning usually occurs by ingestion of inorganic mercuric salts or inhalation of metallic mercury vapor. Ingestion of the mercuric salts causes a burning sensation in the throat, discoloration and edema of oral mucous membranes, abdominal pain, vomiting, bloody diarrhea, and shock. Direct nephrotoxicity causes acute kidney injury. Inhalation of high concentrations of metallic mercury vapor may cause acute fulminant chemical pneumonia. Chronic mercury poisoning causes weakness, ataxia, intention tremors, irritability, and depression. Exposure to alkyl (organic) mercury derivatives from contaminated fish or fungicides used on seeds has caused ataxia, tremors, convulsions, and catastrophic birth defects.

▶ Treatment

A. Acute Poisoning

There is no effective specific treatment for mercury vapor pneumonitis. Remove ingested mercuric salts by lavage, and administer activated charcoal (see p 1425). For acute ingestion of mercuric salts, give dimercaprol (BAL) at once, as for arsenic poisoning. Unless the patient has severe gastroenteritis, consider succimer (DMSA), 10 mg/kg orally every 8 hours for 5 days and then every 12 hours for 2 weeks. Unithiol is a chelator that can be given orally or parenterally, but is not commonly available in the United States. Maintain urinary output. Treat oliguria and anuria if they occur.

B. Chronic Poisoning

Remove from exposure. Neurologic toxicity is not considered reversible with chelation, although some authors recommend a trial of succimer or uniothiol (contact a regional poison center or medical toxicologist for advice).

Mozaffarian D et al. Fish intake, contaminants, and human health: evaluating the risks and the benefits. JAMA. 2006 Oct 18;296(15):1885–99. [PMID: 17047219]

Needleman HL. Mercury in dental amalgam—a neurotoxic risk? JAMA. 2006 Apr 19;295(15):1835–6. [PMID: 16622146]

METHANOL & ETHYLENE GLYCOL

Methanol (wood alcohol) is commonly found in a variety of products, including solvents, duplicating fluids, record cleaning solutions, and paint removers. It is sometimes ingested intentionally by alcoholic patients as a substitute for ethanol and may also be found as a contaminant in bootleg whiskey. Ethylene glycol is the major constituent in most antifreeze compounds. The toxicity of both agents is caused by metabolism to highly toxic organic acids—methanol to formic acid; ethylene glycol to glycolic and oxalic acids.

▶ Clinical Findings

Shortly after ingestion of either of these agents, patients usually appear "drunk." The serum osmolality (measured with the freezing point device) is usually increased, but acidosis is often absent early. After several hours, metabolism to toxic organic acids leads to a severe anion gap metabolic acidosis, tachypnea, confusion, convulsions, and coma. Methanol intoxication frequently causes visual disturbances, while ethylene glycol often produces oxalate crystalluria and advanced chronic kidney disease.

Treatment

A. Emergency and Supportive Measures

For patients presenting within 30–60 minutes after ingestion, empty the stomach by gastric lavage (see p 1424). Charcoal is not very effective but should be administered if other poisons or drugs have also been ingested.

B. Specific Treatment

Patients with significant toxicity (manifested by severe metabolic acidosis, altered mental status, and markedly elevated osmol gap) should undergo hemodialysis as soon as possible to remove the parent compound and the toxic metabolites. Treatment with folic acid, thiamine, and pyridoxine may enhance the breakdown of toxic metabolites.

Ethanol blocks metabolism of the parent compounds by competing for the enzyme alcohol dehydrogenase. Fomepizole (4-methylpyrazole; Antizol) blocks alcohol dehydrogenase and is easier to use than ethanol. A regional poison control center (800-222-1222) should be contacted for indications and dosing.

Cook MD et al. Creatinine elevation associated with nitromethane exposure: a marker of potential methanol toxicity. J Emerg Med. 2007 Oct;33(3):249–53. [PMID: 17976551]

Hovda K et al. Expert opinion: fomepizole may ameliorate the need for hemodialysis in methanol poisoning. Hum Exp Toxicol. 2008 Jul;27(7):539–46. [PMID: 18829729]

Kraut JA et al. Toxic alcohol ingestions: clinical features, diagnosis, and management. Clin J Am Soc Nephrol. 2008 Jan;3(1):208–25. [PMID: 18045860]

Lepik KJ et al. Adverse drug events associated with the antidotes for methanol and ethylene glycol poisoning: a comparison of ethanol and fomepizole. Ann Emerg Med. 2008 Jul 17 2009 Apr;53(4):439–450. [PMID: 18639955]

METHEMOGLOBINEMIA-INDUCING AGENTS

A large number of chemical agents are capable of oxidizing ferrous hemoglobin to its ferric state (methemoglobin), a form that cannot carry oxygen. Drugs and chemicals known to cause methemoglobinemia include benzocaine (a local anesthetic found in some topical anesthetic sprays and a variety of nonprescription products), aniline, propanil, nitrites, nitrogen oxide gases, nitrobenzene, dapsone, phenazopyridine (Pyridium), and many others. Dapsone has a long elimination half-life and may produce prolonged or recurrent methemoglobinemia.

► Clinical Findings

Methemoglobinemia reduces oxygen-carrying capacity and may cause dizziness, nausea, headache, dyspnea, confusion, seizures, and coma. The severity of symptoms depends on the percentage of hemoglobin oxidized to methemoglobin; severe poisoning is usually present when methemoglobin fractions are greater than 40–50%. Even at low levels (15–20%), victims appear cyanotic because of the "chocolate brown" color of methemoglobin, but they have normal P_{O_2} results on arterial blood gas determinations. Pulse oximetry gives inaccurate oxygen saturation measurements; the reading is often between 85% and 90%. Severe metabolic acidosis may be present. Hemolysis may occur, especially in patients susceptible to oxidant stress (ie, those with glucose-6-phosphate dehydrogenase deficiency).

► Treatment

A. Emergency and Supportive Measures

Administer high-flow oxygen. If the causative agent was recently ingested, administer activated charcoal (see p 1425). Repeat-dose activated charcoal may enhance dapsone elimination (see p 1425).

B. Specific Treatment

Methylene blue enhances the conversion of methemoglobin to hemoglobin by increasing the activity of the enzyme methemoglobin reductase. For symptomatic patients, administer 1–2 mg/kg (0.1–0.2 mL/kg of 1% solution) intravenously. The dose may be repeated once in 15–20 minutes if necessary. Patients with hereditary methemoglobin reductase deficiency or glucose-6-phosphate dehydrogenase deficiency may not respond to methylene blue treatment.

BheemReddy S et al. Methemoglobinemia following transesophageal echocardiography: a case report and review. Echocardiography. 2006 Apr;23(4):319–21. [PMID: 16640711]

Kwok S et al. Benzocaine and lidocaine induced methemoglobinemia after bronchoscopy: a case report. J Med Case Reports. 2008 Jan 23;2:16. [PMID: 18215265]

Prasad R et al. Dapsone induced methemoglobinemia: intermittent vs continuous intravenous methylene blue therapy. Indian J Pediatr. 2008 Mar;75(3):245–7. [PMID: 18376092]

MONOAMINE OXIDASE INHIBITORS

Overdoses of MAO inhibitors (isocarboxazid, phenelzine, selegiline, moclobemide) cause ataxia, excitement, hypertension, and tachycardia, followed several hours later by hypotension, convulsions, and hyperthermia.

Ingestion of tyramine-containing foods may cause a severe hypertensive reaction in patients taking MAO inhibitors. Foods containing tyramine include aged cheese and red wines. Hypertensive reactions may also occur with any sympathomimetic drug. Severe or fatal hyperthermia (serotonin syndrome) may occur if patients receiving MAO inhibitors are given meperidine, fluoxetine, paroxetine, fluvoxamine, venlafaxine, tryptophan, dextromethorphan, tramadol, or other serotonin-enhancing drugs. This reaction can also occur with the newer selective MAO inhibitor moclobemide, and the antibiotic linezolid, which has MAO-inhibiting properties. The serotonin syndrome has also been reported in patients taking selective serotonin reuptake inhibitors (SSRIs) in large doses or in combination with other SSRIs, even in the absence of an MAO inhibitor or meperidine.

► Treatment

Administer activated charcoal (see p 1425). Treat severe hypertension with nitroprusside, phentolamine, or other rapid-acting vasodilators (see p 1422). Treat hypotension with fluids and positioning, but avoid use of pressor agents if possible. Observe patients for at least 24 hours, since hyperthermic reactions may be delayed. Treat hyperthermia with aggressive cooling; neuromuscular paralysis may be required (see p 1423). Cyproheptadine, 4 mg orally (or by gastric tube) every hour for three or four doses, has been reported to be effective against serotonin syndrome.

Sun-Edelstein C et al. Drug-induced serotonin syndrome. Expert Opin Drug Saf. 2008 Sep;7(5):587–96. [PMID: 18759711]

MUSHROOMS

There are thousands of mushroom species that cause a variety of toxic effects. The most dangerous species of mushrooms are *Amanita phalloides*, *Amanita verna*, *Amanita virosa*, *Gyromitra esculenta*, and the *Galerina* species, all of which contain amatoxin, a potent cytotoxin. Ingestion of even a portion of one mushroom of a dangerous species may be sufficient to cause death.

The characteristic pathologic finding in fatalities from amatoxin-containing mushroom poisoning is acute massive necrosis of the liver.

▶ ## Clinical Findings (Table 38–8)

A. Symptoms and Signs

1. Amatoxin-type cyclopeptides—(*A phalloides*, *A verna*, *A virosa*, and *Galerina* species.) After a latent interval of 8–12 hours, severe abdominal cramps and vomiting begin and progress to profuse diarrhea, followed in 1–2 days by hepatic necrosis, hepatic encephalopathy, and frequently acute kidney injury. The fatality rate is about 20%. Cooking the mushrooms does not prevent poisoning.

2. Gyromitrin type—(*Gyromitra* and *Helvella* species.) Toxicity is more common following ingestion of uncooked mushrooms. Vomiting, diarrhea, hepatic necrosis, convulsions, coma, and hemolysis may occur after a latent period of 8–12 hours. The fatality rate is probably less than 10%.

3. Muscarinic type—(*Inocybe* and *Clitocybe* species.) Vomiting, diarrhea, bradycardia, hypotension, salivation, miosis, bronchospasm, and lacrimation occur shortly after ingestion. Cardiac arrhythmias may occur. Fatalities are rare.

4. Anticholinergic type—(Eg, *Amanita muscaria*, *Amanita pantherina*.) This type causes a variety of symptoms that may be atropine-like, including excitement, delirium, flushed skin, dilated pupils, and muscular jerking tremors, beginning 1–2 hours after ingestion. Fatalities are rare.

5. Gastrointestinal irritant type—(Eg, *Boletus*, *Cantharellus*.) Nausea, vomiting, and diarrhea occur shortly after ingestion. Fatalities are rare.

6. Disulfiram type—(*Coprinus* species.) Disulfiram-like sensitivity to alcohol may persist for several days. Toxicity is characterized by flushing, hypotension, and vomiting after coingestion of alcohol.

7. Hallucinogenic—(*Psilocybe* and *Panaeolus* species.) Mydriasis, nausea and vomiting, and intense visual hallucinations occur 1–2 hours after ingestion. Fatalities are rare.

8. *Cortinarius orellanus*—This mushroom may cause acute kidney injury due to tubulointerstitial nephritis. *Amanita smithiana* has also been reported to cause acute kidney injury.

Table 38–8. Poisonous mushrooms.

Toxin	Genus	Symptoms and Signs	Onset	Treatment
Amanitin	*Amanita (A phalloides, A verna, A virosa)*	Severe gastroenteritis followed by delayed hepatic failure and acute kidney injury after 48–72 hours	6–24 hours	Supportive. Correct dehydration. Give repeated doses of activated charcoal orally. Consider silymarin (silibinin) (see text).
Muscarine	*Inocybe, Clitocybe*	Muscarinic (salivation, miosis, bradycardia, diarrhea)	30–60 minutes	Supportive. Give atropine, 0.5–2 mg intravenously, for severe cholinergic symptoms and signs.
Ibotenic acid, muscimol	*Amanita muscaria* ("fly agaric")	Anticholinergic (mydriasis, tachycardia, hyperpyrexia, delirium)	30–60 minutes	Supportive. Give physostigmine, 0.5–2 mg intravenously, for severe anticholinergic symptoms and signs.
Coprine	*Coprinus*	Disulfiram-like effect occurs with ingestion of ethanol	30–60 minutes	Supportive. Abstain from ethanol for 3–4 days.
Monomethyl-hydrazine	*Gyromitra*	Gastroenteritis; occasionally hemolysis, hepatic failure, and acute kidney injury	6–12 hours	Supportive. Correct dehydration. Pyridoxine, 2.5 mg/kg intravenously, may be helpful.
Orellanine	*Cortinarius*	Nausea, vomiting; acute kidney injury after 1–3 weeks	2–14 days	Supportive.
Psilocybin	*Psilocybe*	Hallucinations	15–30 minutes	Supportive.
Gastrointestinal irritants	Many species	Nausea and vomiting, diarrhea	1/2–2 hours	Supportive. Correct dehydration.

▶ Treatment

A. Emergency Measures

After the onset of symptoms, efforts to remove the toxic agent are probably useless, especially in cases of amatoxin or gyromitrin poisoning, where there is usually a delay of 12 hours or more before symptoms occur and patients seek medical attention. However, induction of vomiting or administration of activated charcoal is recommended for any recent ingestion of an unidentified or potentially toxic mushroom (see p 1425).

B. General Measures

1. Amatoxin-type cyclopeptides—A variety of antidotes (eg, thioctic acid, penicillin, corticosteroids) have been suggested for amatoxin-type mushroom poisoning, but controlled studies are lacking and experimental data in animals are equivocal. Aggressive fluid replacement for diarrhea and intensive supportive care for hepatic failure are the mainstays of treatment. Silymarin (silibinin), a derivative of milk thistle, is commonly used in Europe but is not available in the United States as a pharmaceutical grade intravenous preparation.

Interruption of enterohepatic circulation of the amatoxin by the administration of activated charcoal or by cannulation and drainage of the bile duct may be of value.

Liver transplant may be the only hope for survival in gravely ill patients—contact a liver transplant center early.

2. Gyromitrin type—For gyromitrin poisoning, give pyridoxine, 25 mg/kg intravenously.

3. Muscarinic type—For mushrooms producing predominantly muscarinic-cholinergic symptoms, give atropine, 0.005–0.01 mg/kg intravenously, and repeat as needed.

4. Anticholinergic type—For anticholinergic type, physostigmine, 0.5–1 mg intravenously, may calm extremely agitated patients and reverse peripheral anticholinergic manifestations, but it may also cause bradycardia, asystole, and seizures. Alternately, use a benzodiazepine such as lorazepam, 1–2 mg intravenously.

5. Gastrointestinal irritant type—Treat with antiemetics and intravenous or oral fluids.

6. Disulfiram type—For *Coprinus* ingestion, avoid alcohol. Treat alcohol reaction with fluids and supine position.

7. Hallucinogenic type—Provide a quiet, supportive atmosphere. Diazepam or haloperidol may be used for sedation.

8. *Cortinarius*—Provide supportive care and hemodialysis as needed for acute kidney injury.

Escudié L et al. *Amanita phalloides* poisoning: reassessment of prognostic factors and indications for emergency liver transplantation. J Hepatol. 2007 Mar;46(3):466–73. [PMID: 17188393]

Krenová M et al. Survey of *Amanita phalloides* poisoning: clinical findings and follow-up evaluation. Hum Exp Toxicol. 2007 Dec;26(12):955–61. [PMID: 18375639]

Tong TC et al. Comparative treatment of alpha-amanitin poisoning with *N*-acetylcysteine, benzylpenicillin, cimetidine, thioctic acid, and silybin in a murine model. Ann Emerg Med. 2007 Sep;50(3):282–8. [PMID: 17559970]

Yang WS et al. Acute renal failure caused by mushroom poisoning. J Formos Med Assoc. 2006 Mar;105(3):263–7. [PMID: 16520846]

OPIOIDS

Prescription and illicit opioids (morphine, heroin, codeine, oxycodone, fentanyl, hydromorphone, etc) are popular drugs of abuse and the cause of frequent hospitalizations for overdose. These drugs have widely varying potencies and durations of action; for example, some of the illicit fentanyl derivatives are up to 2000 times more potent than morphine. All of these agents decrease central nervous system activity and sympathetic outflow by acting on opiate receptors in the brain. Tramadol is an analgesic that is unrelated chemically to the opioids but acts on opioid receptors. Buprenorphine is a partial agonist-antagonist opioid used for the outpatient treatment of opioid addiction.

▶ Clinical Findings

Mild intoxication is characterized by euphoria, drowsiness, and constricted pupils. More severe intoxication may cause hypotension, bradycardia, hypothermia, coma, and respiratory arrest. Pulmonary edema may occur. Death is usually due to apnea or pulmonary aspiration of gastric contents. Propoxyphene may cause seizures and prolongation of the QRS interval. Methadone has been associated with QT interval prolongation and torsades de pointes. Tramadol, dextromethorphan, and meperidine also occasionally cause seizures. With meperidine, the metabolite normeperidine is probably the cause of seizures and is most likely to accumulate with repeated dosing in patients with chronic kidney disease. While the duration of effect for heroin is usually 3–5 hours, methadone intoxication may last for 48–72 hours or longer. Many opioids, including fentanyl, tramadol, oxycodone, and methadone, are not detected on routine urine toxicology "opiate" screening. Wound botulism has been associated with skin-popping, especially involving "black tar" heroin. Buprenorphine added to an opioid regimen may produce acute narcotic withdrawal symptoms.

▶ Treatment

A. Emergency and Supportive Measures

Protect the airway and assist ventilation. Administer activated charcoal (see p 1425).

B. Specific Treatment

Naloxone is a specific opioid antagonist that can rapidly reverse signs of narcotic intoxication. Although it is structurally related to the opioids, it has no agonist effects of its own. Administer 0.4–2 mg intravenously, and repeat as needed to awaken the patient and maintain airway protective reflexes and spontaneous breathing. Very large doses (10–20 mg) may be required for patients intoxicated by some opioids (eg, propoxyphene, codeine, fentanyl derivatives). **Caution:** The duration of effect of naloxone is only about 2–3 hours; repeated doses may be necessary for patients intoxicated by long-acting drugs such as methadone. Continuous observation for at least 3 hours after the last naloxone dose is mandatory.

Bailey JE et al; The RADARS System Poison Center Investigators. The underrecognized toll of prescription opioid abuse on young children. Ann Emerg Med. 2008 Sep 5 2009 Apr;53(4):419–24. [PMID: 18774623]

Piper TM et al. Evaluation of a naloxone distribution and administration program in New York City. Subst Use Misuse. 2008;43(7):858–70. [PMID: 18570021]

Schumann H et al. Fentanyl epidemic in Chicago, Illinois and surrounding Cook County. Clin Toxicol (Phila). 2008 Jul;46(6):501–6. [PMID: 18584361]

Shadnia S et al. Tramadol intoxication: a review of 114 cases. Hum Exp Toxicol. 2008 Mar;27(3):201–5. [PMID: 18650251]

PARAQUAT

Paraquat is used as a herbicide. Concentrated solutions of paraquat are highly corrosive to the oropharynx, esophagus, and stomach. The fatal dose after absorption may be as small as 4 mg/kg. If ingestion of paraquat is not rapidly fatal because of its corrosive effects, the herbicide may cause progressive pulmonary fibrosis, with death ensuing after 2–3 weeks. Patients with plasma paraquat levels above 2 mg/L at 6 hours or 0.2 mg/L at 24 hours are likely to die.

► Treatment

Remove ingested paraquat by immediate induced emesis, or by gastric lavage if the patient is already in a health care facility (see p 1424). Clay (bentonite or fuller's earth) and activated charcoal are effective adsorbents. Administer repeated doses of 60 g of activated charcoal by gastric tube every 2 hours for at least three or four doses. Charcoal hemoperfusion, 8 hours per day for 2–3 weeks, has been anecdotally reported to be lifesaving, but clinical and animal studies are equivocal. Supplemental oxygen should be withheld unless the PaO$_2$ is less than 70 mm Hg because oxygen may contribute to the pulmonary damage, which is mediated through lipid peroxidation. Immunosuppressive therapy (cyclophosphamide with dexamethasone) has shown possible benefit in anecdotal reports.

Chomchai C et al. Fetal poisoning after maternal paraquat ingestion during third trimester of pregnancy: case report and literature review. J Med Toxicol. 2007 Dec;3(4):182–6. [PMID: 18072174]

Dinis-Oliveira RJ et al. Paraquat poisonings: mechanisms of lung toxicity, clinical features, and treatment. Crit Rev Toxicol. 2008 Jan;38(1):13–71. [PMID: 18161502]

Lin JL et al. Repeated pulse of methylprednisolone and cyclophosphamide with continuous dexamethasone therapy for patients with severe paraquat poisoning. Crit Care Med. 2006 Feb;34(2):368–73. [PMID: 16424716]

PESTICIDES: CHOLINESTERASE INHIBITORS

Organophosphorus and carbamate insecticides (organophosphates: parathion, malathion, etc; carbamates: carbaryl, aldicarb, etc) are widely used in commercial agriculture and home gardening and have largely replaced older, more environmentally persistent organochlorine compounds such as DDT and chlordane. The organophosphates and carbamates—also called anticholinesterases because they inhibit the enzyme acetylcholinesterase—cause an increase in acetylcholine activity at nicotinic and muscarinic receptors and in the central nervous system. There are a variety of chemical agents in this group, with widely varying potencies. Most of them are poorly water-soluble, are formulated with an aromatic hydrocarbon solvent such as xylene, and are well absorbed through intact skin. Most chemical warfare "nerve agents" (see above) are organophosphates.

► Clinical Findings

Inhibition of cholinesterase results in abdominal cramps, diarrhea, vomiting, excessive salivation, sweating, lacrimation, miosis (constricted pupils), wheezing and bronchorrhea, seizures, and skeletal muscle weakness. Initial tachycardia is usually followed by bradycardia. Profound skeletal muscle weakness, aggravated by excessive bronchial secretions and wheezing, may result in respiratory arrest and death. Symptoms and signs of poisoning may persist or recur over several days, especially with highly lipid-soluble agents such as fenthion or dimethoate.

The diagnosis should be suspected in patients who present with miosis, sweating, and hyperperistalsis. Serum and red blood cell cholinesterase activity is usually depressed at least 50% below baseline in those victims who have severe intoxication.

► Treatment

A. Emergency and Supportive Measures

If the agent was recently ingested, empty the stomach by gastric lavage and administer activated charcoal (see p 1424–5). If the agent is on the victim's skin or hair, wash repeatedly with soap or shampoo and water. Providers must take care to avoid skin exposure by wearing gloves and waterproof aprons. Dilute hypochlorite solution (eg, household bleach diluted 1:10) is reported to help break down organophosphate pesticides and nerve agents on equipment or clothing.

B. Specific Treatment

Atropine reverses excessive muscarinic stimulation and is effective for treatment of salivation, bronchial hypersecretion, wheezing, abdominal cramping, and sweating. However, it does not interact with nicotinic receptors at autonomic ganglia and at the neuromuscular junction and has no effect on muscle weakness. Administer 2 mg intravenously, and if there is no response after 5 minutes, give repeated boluses in rapidly escalating doses as needed to dry bronchial secretions and decrease wheezing; as much as several hundred milligrams of atropine has been given to treat severe poisoning.

Pralidoxime (2-PAM, Protopam) is a specific antidote that reverses organophosphate binding to the cholinesterase enzyme; therefore, it is effective at the neuromuscular junction as well as other nicotinic and muscarinic sites. It is most likely to be effective if started very soon after poisoning, to prevent permanent binding of the organophosphate to cholinesterase. Clinical studies are conflicting regarding the effectiveness of pralidoxime in reducing mortality. It appears to be more effective for chlorpyrifos compared with dimethoate poisoning. Administer 1–2 g intravenously as a loading dose, and begin a continuous infusion (200–500 mg/h, titrated to clinical response). Continue to give pralidoxime as long as there is any evidence of acetylcholine excess. Pralidoxime is of questionable benefit for carbamate poisoning, because carbamates have only a transitory effect on the cholinesterase enzyme. High-dose sodium bicarbonate (5 mEq/kg intravenously over 5 minutes) has been reported effective although the mechanism is unclear and the treatment has not been widely adopted.

Eddleston M et al. Management of acute organophosphorus pesticide poisoning. Lancet. 2008 Feb 16;371(9612):597–607. [PMID: 17706760]

Pawar KS et al. Continuous pralidoxime infusion versus repeated bolus injection to treat organophosphorus pesticide poisoning: a randomised controlled trial. Lancet. 2006 Dec 16;368(9553):2136–41. [PMID: 17174705]

Peter JV et al. Adjuncts and alternatives to oxime therapy in organophosphate poisoning—is there evidence of benefit in human poisoning? Anaesth Intensive Care. 2008 May; 36(3):339–50. [PMID: 18564794]

PETROLEUM DISTILLATES & SOLVENTS

Petroleum distillate toxicity may occur from inhalation of the vapor or as a result of pulmonary aspiration of the liquid during or after ingestion. Acute manifestations of aspiration pneumonitis are vomiting, coughing, and bronchopneumonia. Some hydrocarbons—ie, those with aromatic or halogenated subunits—can also cause severe systemic poisoning after oral ingestion. Hydrocarbons can also cause systemic intoxication by inhalation. Vertigo, muscular incoordination, irregular pulse, myoclonus, and seizures occur with serious poisoning and may be due to hypoxemia or the systemic effects of the agents. Chlorinated and fluorinated hydrocarbons (trichloroethylene, Freons, etc) and many other hydrocarbons can cause ventricular arrhythmias due to increased sensitivity of the myocardium to the effects of endogenous catecholamines.

► Treatment

Remove the patient to fresh air. For simple aliphatic hydrocarbon ingestion, gastric emptying and activated charcoal are not recommended, but these procedures may be indicated if the preparation contains toxic solutes (eg, an insecticide) or is an aromatic or halogenated product. Observe the victim for 6–8 hours for signs of aspiration pneumonitis (cough, localized rales or rhonchi, tachypnea, and infiltrates on chest radiograph). Corticosteroids are not recommended. If fever occurs, give a specific antibiotic only after identification of bacterial pathogens by laboratory studies. Because of the risk of arrhythmias, use bronchodilators with caution in patients with chlorinated or

fluorinated solvent intoxication. If tachyarrhythmias occur, use esmolol intravenously 25–100 mcg/kg/min.

Aziz AA et al. Lung abscess rather than pneumatocele following kerosene ingestion. Br J Hosp Med (Lond). 2007 Nov; 68(11):616–7. [PMID: 18087856]

Domej W et al. Successful outcome after intravenous gasoline injection. J Med Toxicol. 2007 Dec;3(4):173–7. [PMID: 18072172]

Wick R et al. Inhalant deaths in South Australia: a 20-year retrospective autopsy study. Am J Forensic Med Pathol. 2007 Dec;28(4):319–22. [PMID: 18043019]

PHENOTHIAZINES & OTHER ANTIPSYCHOTIC AGENTS

Promethazine, prochlorperazine, chlorpromazine, haloperidol, droperidol, risperidone, olanzapine, ziprasidone, quetiapine, and aripiprazole are used as antiemetics and antipsychotic agents and as potentiators of analgesic and hypnotic drugs.

Phenothiazines (particularly chlorpromazine) induce drowsiness and mild orthostatic hypotension in as many as 50% of patients. Larger doses can cause obtundation, miosis, severe hypotension, tachycardia, convulsions, and coma. Abnormal cardiac conduction may occur, resulting in prolongation of QRS or QT intervals (or both) and ventricular arrhythmias. (Droperidol now has a "black box" warning about prolonged QT interval and the risk of torsades de pointes.) Among the newer agents, quetiapine is more likely to cause coma and hypotension.

With therapeutic or toxic doses, an acute extrapyramidal dystonic reaction may develop in some patients, with spasmodic contractions of the face and neck muscles, extensor rigidity of the back muscles, carpopedal spasm, and motor restlessness. This reaction is more common with haloperidol and the butyrophenones and less common with newer atypical antipsychotics such as ziprasidone, olanzapine, aripiprazole, and quetiapine. Severe rigidity accompanied by hyperthermia and metabolic acidosis ("neuroleptic malignant syndrome") may occasionally occur and is life-threatening (see Chapter 25).

► Treatment

A. Emergency and Supportive Measures

Administer activated charcoal. For severe hypotension, treatment with intravenous fluids and pressor agents may be necessary. Treat hyperthermia as outlined on p 1423. Maintain cardiac monitoring.

B. Specific Treatment

Hypotension and cardiac arrhythmias associated with widened QRS intervals on the ECG in a patient with thioridazine poisoning may respond to intravenous sodium bicarbonate as used for tricyclic antidepressants. Prolongation of the QT interval and torsades de pointes is usually treated with intravenous magnesium or overdrive pacing.

For extrapyramidal signs, give diphenhydramine, 0.5–1 mg/kg intravenously, or benztropine mesylate, 0.01–

0.02 mg/kg intramuscularly. Treatment with oral doses of these agents should be continued for 24–48 hours.

Bromocriptine (2.5–7.5 mg orally daily) may be effective for mild or moderate neuroleptic malignant syndrome. Dantrolene (2–5 mg/kg intravenously) has also been used for muscle contractions but is not a true antidote.

Flanagan RJ. Fatal toxicity of drugs used in psychiatry. Hum Psychopharmacol. 2008 Jan;23(Suppl 1):43–51. [PMID: 18098225]

Klein-Schwartz W et al. Prospective observational multi-poison center study of ziprasidone exposures. Clin Toxicol. 2007 Oct–Nov;45(7):782–6. [PMID: 17926152]

Ngo A et al. Acute quetiapine overdose in adults: a 5-year retrospective case series. Ann Emerg Med 2008;52:541–7. [PMID: 18433934]

QUINIDINE & RELATED ANTIARRHYTHMICS

Quinidine, procainamide, and disopyramide are class Ia antiarrhythmic agents, and flecainide and propafenone are class Ic agents. These drugs have membrane-depressant effects on the sodium-dependent channel responsible for cardiac cell depolarization. Manifestations of cardiotoxicity include arrhythmias, syncope, hypotension, and widening of the QRS complex on the ECG (> 100–120 ms). With type Ia drugs, a lengthened QT interval and atypical or polymorphous ventricular tachycardia (torsades de pointes) may occur. The antimalarials chloroquine and hydroxychloroquine have similar effects in overdose.

▶ Treatment

A. Emergency and Supportive Measures

Administer activated charcoal (see p 1425); consider gastric lavage after large recent overdose. Assist ventilation if needed. Perform continuous cardiac monitoring.

B. Specific Treatment

Treat cardiotoxicity (hypotension, QRS interval widening) with intravenous boluses of sodium bicarbonate, 50–100 mEq. Torsades de pointes may be treated with intravenous magnesium or overdrive pacing.

Hasdemir C et al. Brugada-type ECG pattern and extreme QRS complex widening with propafenone overdose. J Cardiovasc Electrophysiol. 2006 May;17(5):565–6. [PMID: 16684037]

Huston M et al. Are one or two dangerous? Quinine and quinidine exposure in toddlers. J Emerg Med. 2006 Nov;31(4):395–401. [PMID: 17046481]

White NJ. Cardiotoxicity of antimalarial drugs. Lancet Infect Dis. 2007 Aug;7(8):549–58. [PMID: 17646028]

SALICYLATES

Salicylates (aspirin, methyl salicylate, etc) are found in a variety of over-the-counter and prescription medications. Salicylates uncouple cellular oxidative phosphorylation, resulting in anaerobic metabolism and excessive production of lactic acid and heat, and they also interfere with several Krebs cycle enzymes. A single ingestion of more than 200 mg/kg of salicylate is likely to produce significant acute intoxication. Poisoning may also occur as a result of chronic excessive dosing over several days. Although the half-life of salicylate is 2–3 hours after small doses, it may increase to 20 hours or more in patients with intoxication.

▶ Clinical Findings

Acute ingestion often causes nausea and vomiting, occasionally with gastritis. Moderate intoxication is characterized by hyperpnea (deep and rapid breathing), tachycardia, tinnitus, and elevated anion gap metabolic acidosis. Serious intoxication may result in agitation, confusion, coma, seizures, cardiovascular collapse, pulmonary edema, hyperthermia, and death. The prothrombin time is often elevated owing to salicylate-induced hypoprothrombinemia.

Diagnosis is suspected in any patient with metabolic acidosis and is confirmed by measuring the serum salicylate level. Patients with levels greater than 100 mg/dL (1000 mg/L) after an acute overdose are more likely to have severe poisoning. On the other hand, patients with subacute or chronic intoxication may suffer severe symptoms with levels of only 60–70 mg/dL. The arterial blood gas typically reveals a respiratory alkalosis with an underlying metabolic acidosis.

▶ Treatment

A. Emergency and Supportive Measures

Administer activated charcoal (see p 1425). Gastric lavage followed by administration of extra doses of activated charcoal may be needed in patients who ingest more than 10 g of aspirin (see p 1424). The desired ratio of charcoal to aspirin is about 10:1 by weight; while this cannot always be given as a single dose, it may be administered over the first 24 hours in divided doses every 2–4 hours. Treat metabolic acidosis with intravenous sodium bicarbonate. This is critical because acidosis (especially acidemia, pH < 7.40) promotes greater entry of salicylate into cells, worsening toxicity. Brief hypoventilation during rapid sequence intubation may cause sudden and severe deterioration if the pH is allowed to fall.

B. Specific Treatment

Alkalinization of the urine enhances renal salicylate excretion by trapping the salicylate anion in the urine. Add 100 mEq (two ampules) of sodium bicarbonate to 1 L of 5% dextrose in 0.2% saline, and infuse this solution intravenously at a rate of about 150–200 mL/h. Unless the patient is oliguric or hyperkalemic, add 20–30 mEq of potassium chloride to each liter of intravenous fluid. Patients who are volume-depleted often fail to produce an alkaline urine (paradoxical aciduria) unless potassium is given.

Hemodialysis may be lifesaving and is indicated for patients with severe metabolic acidosis, markedly altered mental status, or significantly elevated salicylate levels (eg, > 100–120 mg/dL [1000–1200 mg/L] after acute overdose or > 60–70 mg/dL [600–700 mg/L] with subacute or chronic intoxication).

Kuzak N et al. Reversal of salicylate-induced euglycemic delirium with dextrose. Clin Toxicol (Phila). 2007 Jun–Aug;45(5):526–9. [PMID: 17503260]

Table 38–9. Common seafood poisonings.

Type of Poisoning	Mechanism	Clinical Presentation
Ciguatera	Reef fish ingest toxic dinoflagellates, whose toxins accumulate in fish meat. Commonly implicated fish in the United States are barracuda, jack, snapper, and grouper.	1–6 hours after ingestion, victims develop abdominal pain, vomiting, and diarrhea accompanied by a variety of neurologic symptoms, including paresthesias, reversal of hot and cold sensation, vertigo, headache, and intense itching. Autonomic disturbances, including hypotension and bradycardia, may occur.
Scombroid	Improper preservation of large fish results in bacterial degradation of histidine to histamine. Commonly implicated fish include tuna, mahimahi, bonita, mackerel, and kingfish.	Allergic-like (anaphylactoid) symptoms are due to histamine, usually begin within 15–90 minutes, and include skin flushing, itching, urticaria, angioedema, bronchospasm, and hypotension as well as abdominal pain, vomiting, and diarrhea.
Paralytic shellfish poisoning	Dinoflagellates produce saxitoxin, which is concentrated by filter-feeding mussels and clams. Saxitoxin blocks sodium conductance and neuronal transmission in skeletal muscles.	Onset is usually within 30–60 minutes. Initial symptoms include perioral and intraoral paresthesias. Other symptoms include nausea and vomiting, headache, dizziness, dysphagia, dysarthria, ataxia, and rapidly progressive muscle weakness that may result in respiratory arrest.
Puffer fish poisoning	Tetrodotoxin is concentrated in liver, gonads, intestine, and skin. Toxic effects are similar to those of saxitoxin. Tetrodotoxin is also found in some North American newts and Central American frogs.	Onset is usually within 30–40 minutes but may be as short as 10 minutes. Initial perioral paresthesias are followed by headache, diaphoresis, nausea, vomiting, ataxia, and rapidly progressive muscle weakness that may result in respiratory arrest.

O'Malley GF. Emergency department management of the salicylate-poisoned patient. Emerg Med Clin North Am. 2007 May;25(2):333–46. [PMID: 17482023]

Stolbach AI et al. Mechanical ventilation was associated with acidemia in a case series of salicylate-poisoned patients. Acad Emerg Med. 2008 Sep;15(9):866–9. [PMID: 18821862]

SEAFOOD POISONINGS

A variety of intoxications may occur after eating certain types of fish or other seafood. These include scombroid, ciguatera, paralytic shellfish, and puffer fish poisoning. The mechanisms of toxicity and clinical presentations are described in Table 38–9. In the majority of cases, the seafood has a normal appearance and taste (scombroid may have a peppery taste).

▶ Treatment

A. Emergency and Supportive Measures

Caution: Abrupt respiratory arrest may occur in patients with acute paralytic shellfish and puffer fish poisoning. Observe patients for at least 4–6 hours. Replace fluid and electrolyte losses from gastroenteritis with intravenous saline or other crystalloid solution.

For recent ingestions, it may be possible to adsorb residual toxin in the gut with activated charcoal, 50–60 g orally (see p 1425).

B. Specific Treatment

There is no specific antidote for paralytic shellfish or puffer fish poisoning.

1. Ciguatera—There are anecdotal reports of successful treatment of acute neurologic symptoms with mannitol, 1 g/ kg intravenously, but this approach is not widely accepted.

2. Scombroid—Antihistamines such as diphenhydramine, 25–50 mg intravenously, and the H_2-blocker cimetidine, 300 mg intravenously, are usually effective. For severe reactions, give also epinephrine, 0.3–0.5 mL of a 1:1000 solution subcutaneously.

Noguchi T et al. Tetrodotoxin—distribution and accumulation in aquatic organisms, and cases of human intoxication. Mar Drugs. 2008 May 28;6(2):220–42. [PMID: 18728726]

Schwarz ES et al. Ciguatera poisoning successfully treated with delayed mannitol. Ann Emerg Med. 2008 Oct;52(4):476–7. [PMID: 18809112]

Wang DZ. Neurotoxins from marine dinoflagellates: a brief review. Mar Drugs. 2008 Jun 11;6(2):349–71. [PMID: 18728731]

SNAKE BITES

The venom of poisonous snakes and lizards may be predominantly neurotoxic (coral snake) or predominantly cytolytic (rattlesnakes, other pit vipers). Neurotoxins cause respiratory paralysis; cytolytic venoms cause tissue destruction by digestion and hemorrhage due to hemolysis and destruction of the endothelial lining of the blood vessels. The manifestations of rattlesnake envenomation are mostly local pain, redness, swelling, and extravasation of blood. Perioral tingling, metallic taste, nausea and vomiting, hypotension, and coagulopathy may also occur. Neurotoxic envenomation may cause ptosis, dysphagia, diplopia, and respiratory arrest.

▶ Treatment

A. Emergency Measures

Immobilize the patient and the bitten part in a neutral position. Avoid manipulation of the bitten area. Transport the patient to a medical facility for definitive treatment. Do *not* give alcoholic beverages or stimulants; do *not* apply ice;

do *not* apply a tourniquet. The trauma to underlying structures resulting from incision and suction performed by unskilled people is probably not justified in view of the small amount of venom that can be recovered.

B. Specific Antidote and General Measures

1. Pit viper (eg, rattlesnake) envenomation—For local signs such as swelling, pain, and ecchymosis but no systemic symptoms, give 4–6 vials of crotalid antivenin (CroFab) by slow intravenous drip in 250–500 mL saline. Repeated doses of 2 vials every 6 hours for up to 18 hours has been recommended. For more serious envenomation with marked local effects and systemic toxicity (eg, hypotension, coagulopathy), higher doses and additional vials may be required. Monitor vital signs and the blood coagulation profile. Type and cross-match blood. The adequacy of venom neutralization is indicated by improvement in symptoms and signs, and the rate that swelling slows. Prophylactic antibiotics are not indicated after a rattlesnake bite.

2. Elapid (coral snake) envenomation—Give 1–2 vials of specific antivenom as soon as possible. To locate antisera for exotic snakes, call a regional poison control center (800-222-1222).

Açikalin A et al. The efficacy of low-dose antivenom therapy on morbidity and mortality in snakebite cases. Am J Emerg Med. 2008 May;26(4):402–7. [PMID: 18410806]
McNally J et al. Toxicologic information resources for reptile envenomations. Vet Clin North Am Exot Anim Pract. 2008 May;11(2):389–401. [PMID: 18406394]
Richardson WH et al. Rattlesnake envenomation with neurotoxicity refractory to treatment with crotaline Fab antivenom. Clin Toxicol (Phila). 2007 Jun–Aug;45(5):472–5. [PMID: 17503249]

SPIDER BITES & SCORPION STINGS

The toxin of most species of spiders in the United States causes only local pain, redness, and swelling. That of the more venomous black widow spiders *(Latrodectus mactans)* causes generalized muscular pains, muscle spasms, and rigidity. The brown recluse spider *(Loxosceles reclusa)* causes progressive local necrosis as well as hemolytic reactions (rare). Stings by most scorpions in the United States cause only local pain. Stings by the more toxic *Centruroides* species (found in the southwestern United States) may cause muscle cramps, twitching and jerking, and occasionally hypertension, convulsions, and pulmonary edema. Stings by scorpions from other parts of the world are not discussed here.

▷ Treatment

A. Black Widow Spider Bites

Pain may be relieved with parenteral narcotics or muscle relaxants (eg, methocarbamol, 15 mg/kg). Calcium gluconate 10%, 0.1–0.2 mL/kg intravenously, may relieve muscle rigidity, though its effectiveness is questionable. Antivenin is available, but because of concerns about acute hypersensitivity reactions (horse serum-derived), it is often reserved for very young or elderly patients or those who do not respond to the above measures. Horse serum sensitivity testing is required. (Instruction and testing materials are included in the antivenin kit.)

B. Brown Recluse Spider Bites

Because bites occasionally progress to extensive local necrosis, some authorities recommend early excision of the bite site, whereas others use oral corticosteroids. Anecdotal reports have claimed success with dapsone and colchicine. All of these treatments remain of unproved value.

C. Scorpion Stings

No specific treatment is available for envenomations by scorpions found in the United States. For *Centruroides* stings, some toxicologists use a specific antivenom developed in Arizona, but this is neither FDA-approved nor widely available.

de Almeida DM et al. A new anti-loxoscelic serum produced against recombinant sphingomyelinase D: results of preclinical trials. Am J Trop Med Hyg. 2008 Sep;79(3):463–70. [PMID: 18784245]
Diaz JH et al. Common spider bites. Am Fam Physician. 2007 Mar 15;75(6):869–73. [PMID: 17390599]
Furbee RB et al. Brown recluse spider envenomation. Clin Lab Med. 2006 Mar;26(1):211–26. [PMID: 16567232]
Goddard J et al. Severe reaction from envenomation by the brown widow spider, *Latrodectus geometricus* (Araneae: Theridiidae). South Med J. 2008 Dec;101(12):1269–70. [PMID: 19005454]
Isbister GK et al. A randomised controlled trial of intramuscular vs. intravenous antivenom for latrodectism—the RAVE study. QJM. 2008 Jul;101(7):557–65. [PMID: 18400776]

THEOPHYLLINE & CAFFEINE

Theophylline may cause intoxication after an acute single overdose, or intoxication may occur as a result of chronic accidental repeated overmedication or reduced elimination resulting from hepatic dysfunction or interacting drug (eg, cimetidine, erythromycin). The usual serum half-life of theophylline is 4–6 hours, but this may increase to more than 20 hours after overdose. Caffeine and caffeine-containing herbal products can produce similar toxicity.

▷ Clinical Findings

Mild intoxication causes nausea, vomiting, tachycardia, and tremulousness. Severe intoxication is characterized by ventricular and supraventricular tachyarrhythmias, hypotension, and seizures. Status epilepticus is common and often intractable to the usual anticonvulsants. After acute overdose (but not chronic intoxication), hypokalemia, hyperglycemia, and metabolic acidosis are common. Seizures and other manifestations of toxicity may be delayed for several hours after acute ingestion, especially if a sustained-release preparation such as Theo-Dur was taken.

Diagnosis is based on measurement of the serum theophylline concentration. Seizures and hypotension are likely to develop in acute overdose patients with serum levels greater than 100 mg/L. Serious toxicity may develop at lower levels (ie, 40–60 mg/L) in patients with chronic intoxication.

▶ **Treatment**

A. Emergency and Supportive Measures

After acute ingestion, administer activated charcoal (see p 1425). Repeated doses of activated charcoal may enhance theophylline elimination by "gut dialysis." Addition of whole bowel irrigation should be considered for large ingestions involving sustained-release preparations (see p 1425).

Hemodialysis is effective in removing theophylline and is indicated for patients with status epilepticus or markedly elevated serum theophylline levels (eg, > 100 mg/L after acute overdose or > 60 mg/L with chronic intoxication).

B. Specific Treatment

Treat seizures with benzodiazepines (lorazepam, 2–3 mg intravenously, or diazepam, 5–10 mg intravenously) or phenobarbital (10–15 mg/kg intravenously). Phenytoin is not effective. Hypotension and tachycardia—which are mediated through excessive β-adrenergic stimulation—may respond to β-blocker therapy even in low doses. Administer esmolol, 25–50 mcg/kg/min by intravenous infusion, or propranolol, 0.5–1 mg intravenously.

Korsheed S et al. Treatment of severe theophylline poisoning with the molecular adsorbent recirculating system (MARS). Nephrol Dial Transplant. 2007 Mar;22(3):969–70. [PMID: 17164319]

Liu PH et al. Acute pancreatitis after severe theophylline overdose. Clin Toxicol (Phila). 2008 Dec;46(10):1103. [PMID: 18949588]

McNamara R et al. Caffeine promotes hyperthermia and serotonergic loss following co-administration of the substituted amphetamines, MDMA ("Ecstasy") and MDA ("Love"). Neuropharmacology. 2006 Jan;50(1):69–80. [PMID: 16188283]

TRICYCLIC & OTHER ANTIDEPRESSANTS

Tricyclic and related cyclic antidepressants are among the most dangerous drugs involved in suicidal overdose. These drugs have anticholinergic and cardiac depressant properties ("quinidine-like" sodium channel blockade). Tricyclic antidepressants produce more marked membrane-depressant cardiotoxic effects than the phenothiazines.

Newer antidepressants such as trazodone, fluoxetine, citalopram, paroxetine, sertraline, bupropion, venlafaxine, and fluvoxamine are not chemically related to the tricyclic antidepressant agents and do not generally produce quinidine-like cardiotoxic effects. However, they may cause seizures in overdoses and they may cause serotonin syndrome (see Monoamine Oxidase Inhibitors, above).

▶ **Clinical Findings**

Signs of severe intoxication may occur abruptly and without warning within 30–60 minutes after acute tricyclic overdose. Anticholinergic effects include dilated pupils, tachycardia, dry mouth, flushed skin, muscle twitching, and decreased peristalsis. Quinidine-like cardiotoxic effects include QRS interval widening (> 0.12 s; see Figure 38–2), ventricular arrhythmias, AV block, and hypotension. Rightward-axis deviation of the terminal 40 ms of the QRS has also been described. Prolongation of the QT interval has been reported with citalopram and venlafaxine. Seizures and

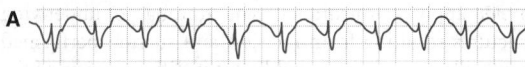
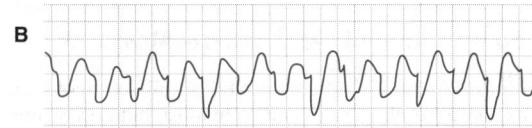
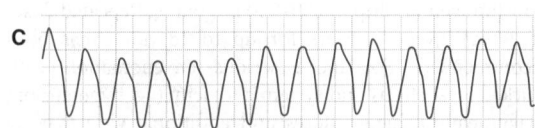

▲ **Figure 38–2.** Cardiac arrhythmias resulting from tricyclic antidepressant overdose. **A:** Delayed intraventricular conduction results in prolonged QRS interval (0.18 s). **B** and **C:** Supraventricular tachycardia with progressive widening of QRS complexes mimics ventricular tachycardia. (Reproduced, with permission, from Benowitz NL, Goldschlager N. Cardiac disturbances in the toxicologic patient. In: Haddad LM, Winchester JF [editors], *Clinical Management of Poisoning and Drug Overdose*, 3rd edition. Saunders/Elsevier, 1998.)

coma are common with severe intoxication. Life-threatening hyperthermia may result from status epilepticus and anticholinergic-induced impairment of sweating. Among newer agents, bupropion and venlafaxine have been associated with a greater risk of seizures.

The diagnosis should be suspected in any overdose patient with anticholinergic side effects, especially if there is widening of the QRS interval or seizures. For intoxication by most tricyclic antidepressants, the QRS interval correlates with the severity of intoxication more reliably than the serum drug level.

Serotonin syndrome should be suspected if agitation, delirium, muscular hyperactivity, and fever develop in a patient taking serotonin reuptake inhibitors.

▶ **Treatment**

A. Emergency and Supportive Measures

Observe patients for at least 6 hours, and admit all patients with evidence of anticholinergic effects (eg, delirium, dilated pupils, tachycardia) or signs of cardiotoxicity (see above).

Administer activated charcoal, and consider gastric lavage after recent large ingestions (see p 1424–5). All of these drugs are highly tissue-bound and are not effectively removed by hemodialysis procedures.

B. Specific Treatment

Cardiotoxic sodium channel-depressant effects of tricyclic antidepressants may respond to boluses of sodium bicarbonate (50–100 mEq intravenously). Sodium bicarbonate provides a large sodium load that alleviates depression of the sodium-dependent channel. Reversal of acidosis may also have beneficial effects at this site. Maintain the pH between 7.45 and 7.50. Alkalinization does not promote excretion of tricyclic antidepressants. Prolongation of the QT interval or torsades de pointes is usually treated with intravenous magnesium or overdrive pacing. Fab antibodies have been developed for some tricyclic antidepressants, but they remain experimental.

Mild serotonin syndrome may be treated with benzodiazepines and withdrawal of the antidepressant. Moderate cases may respond to cyproheptadine (4 mg orally or via gastric tube hourly for three or four doses). Severe hyperthermia should be treated with neuromuscular paralysis and endotracheal intubation in addition to external cooling measures.

Agrawal P et al. Tricyclic antidepressant overdose. J Emerg Med. 2008 Apr;34(3):321–5. [PMID: 18296006]

Barry JD et al. Vasopressin treatment for cyclic antidepressant overdose. J Emerg Med. 2006 Jul;31(1):65–8. [PMID: 16798158]

Heard K et al. A preliminary study of tricyclic antidepressant (TCA) ovine FAB for TCA toxicity. Clin Toxicol (Phila). 2006;44(3):275–81. [PMID: 16749545]

Wood DM et al. Status epilepticus following intentional overdose of fluvoxamine: a case report with serum fluvoxamine concentration. Clin Toxicol (Phila). 2007 Oct–Nov;45(7):791. [PMID: 17952747]

Cancer

Patricia A. Cornett, MD

Tiffany O. Dea, PharmD

The major features of this chapter are the clinical aspects of cancer, including etiology and prevention; staging; diagnosis and treatment of common cancers; and recognition and management of complications from cancer. Additional information may be obtained from the National Cancer Institute (NCI) website at www.cancer.gov/cancerinformation, the American Society of Clinical Oncology website at www.asco.org, and the National Comprehensive Cancer Network (NCCN) website at www.nccn.org. The NCCN website provides detailed, evidence-based recommendations for management of specific cancers as well as guidelines for cancer screening and for supportive care. General reviews in oncology can be obtained from Medscape Hematology/Oncology (www.medscape.com).

▶ Etiology

Cancer is the second most common cause of death in the United States. In 2008, an estimated 1,437,180 cases of cancer were diagnosed, and 565,650 persons died as a result of cancer. Based on cancer rates determined in 2003–2005, more than 40% of people born today will have cancer diagnosed at some point in their lifetime. Table 39–1 lists the 10 leading cancer types in men and women by site.

However, the incidence of cancer in both men and women is decreasing. In 2008, the American Cancer Society, NCI, and the Centers for Disease Control and Prevention reported that the incidence of all cancers for both sexes decreased 0.8% per year from 1999 through 2005. In men, the rate decreased 1.8% per year from 2001 through 2005, largely because the incidence of the three most common cancers (prostate, lung, colorectum) decreased. In women, the rate decreased 0.6% per year from 1998 through 2005 due to the decline in incidence of two of the top three cancers (breast, colorectum); the incidence of the third cancer (lung) was steady.

Over the last two decades, the decreasing incidence of cancer has translated into a decrease in cancer death rates. Ten of the top 15 cancer sites have shown a decrease in mortality events. Only esophageal cancer in men, pancreatic cancer in women, and hepatocellular in both men and women have increased in mortality numbers. This decline in mortality has been seen in all ethnic and racial groups except for American Indians and Alaskan Natives.

Reductions in cancer incidence and mortality reflect a successful implementation of a broad strategy of prevention, detection, and treatment.

▶ Modifiable Risk Factors

Tobacco is the most common preventable cause of cancer death; it is estimated that at least 30% of all cancer deaths in the United States are directly linked to tobacco. A total of 440,000 cancer deaths in the United States and 4.8 million cancer deaths worldwide can be directly attributed to tobacco abuse. Clear evidence links at least 15 cancers to tobacco use. The most dramatic link is with lung cancer, the most common non-dermatologic malignancy; over 90% of lung cancer cases occur in smokers. Any strategy for cancer control must start with the goal of markedly reducing if not eliminating tobacco use.

Strategies for tobacco control should involve a focus on the individual as well as society as a whole. Tobacco cessation directed toward the individual should start with the clinician providing counseling. Simple, concise advice from a clinician can yield cessation rates of 10–20%. Additive strategies include more intensive counseling; nicotine replacement therapy with patches, gum, or lozenges; and prescription medication with bupropion or varenicline. Perhaps a more intriguing phenomenon, with potential for significant impact on cessation rates, is the influence of social contact behavior on an individual smoker's abstinence decision. For instance, analysis of the Framingham Heart Study demonstrated that smoking cessation by a spouse resulted in a 67% decrease in the subject's likelihood of continuing to smoke, and smoking cessation by a friend resulted in a 36% decrease in the subject's likelihood of smoking.

On a societal level, many initiatives have been put into place to actively discourage tobacco use. State or local laws regulating tobacco use in restaurants, the workplace, and other public places have resulted in declines in tobacco use. Countermarketing with aggressive anti-tobacco advertisements has also contributed to tobacco cessation and abstinence. The key recipients of these messages are children; 80%

Table 39–1. Estimated 10 most common cancer cases in the United States in males and females (all races).

Rank	Males (745,180 Total Cases)	Percent	Females (692,000 Total Cases)	Percent
1	Prostate	25	Breast	26
2	Lung and bronchus	15	Lung and bronchus	14
3	Colon and rectum	10	Colon and rectum	10
4	Urinary	7	Uterine corpus	6
5	Lymphoma	5	Lymphoma	4
6	Melanoma	5	Thyroid	4
7	Kidney and renal pelvis	4	Melanoma	4
8	Oral cavity	3	Ovary	3
9	Leukemia	3	Kidney and renal pelvis	3
10	Pancreas	3	Leukemia	3
	Other sites	20	Other sites	23

Data from the American Cancer Society, 2008.

of smokers will start by age 18. Preventing the start of addiction in this vulnerable population should be a top priority.

In fact, there are encouraging signs of success with tobacco control. The prevalence of smoking for United States adults has hit a modern day nadir of 19%, which is a remarkable reduction from the 1955 peak of 57% for males and the 1965 peak of 34% for females. See Chapter 1 for additional material on smoking cessation techniques.

For those Americans who do not abuse tobacco, the most modifiable risk factors would be nutrition and physical activity. Epidemiologic studies suggest that fruit- and vegetable-rich diets lower risks of several gastrointestinal malignancies, including esophageal, stomach, and colon cancers. Excessive consumption of alcohol is linked to increased risks of head and neck cancers as well as cancers of the esophagus and liver. Lastly, being overweight is linked to several malignancies, including breast and uterine cancers in women and colorectal, esophageal, and kidney cancers in both men and women. More importantly, weight reduction can decrease the risks of these cancers.

▶ **Staging**

The most commonly used staging system at the time of diagnosis is the TNM (Tumor, Nodes, Metastasis) system (see www.cancerstaging.org). Rules for staging for individual cancers are established and published by the American Joint Committee on Cancer (AJCC). Elements used for staging include tumor size and level of tumor invasion (T), absence or presence and extent of nodal metastases (N), and presence or absence of systemic metastases (M). Once the TNM designations have been determined, an overall stage is assigned, stage I, II, III, or IV. Clinical staging utilizes physical examination, laboratory and imaging tests as well as results from biopsies; pathologic staging relies on the results from surgery. In some instances, other classifications may be used for certain cancers such as the Ann Arbor staging system for lymphomas or the International Federation of Gynecologists and Obstetricans (FIGO) staging systems for gynecologic malignancies.

Other characteristics of cancers, not reflected in the TNM stage, may be used as another indicator of prognosis. Pathologic features seen on routine histologic examination for some cancers are very important; examples include the Gleason score for prostate cancer and the grade of sarcomas. Special tests done on cancer specimens can also be used to determine prognosis as well as treatment; examples include estrogen and progesterone status and the presence or absence of *HER-2/neu* for breast cancers. Chromosome analysis, now routinely done for patients with hematologic disorders and important in determining prognosis, can occasionally be useful for patients with solid tumors. For example, in patients with carcinoma of unknown primary origin, abnormal findings on chromosome 12 predict a response to chemotherapy and a better prognosis. In the future, as the pathways for oncogenesis and relationships of mutations to treatment and prognosis are better delineated, analysis for detection of chromosomal alterations and oncogene products will be increasingly incorporated into routine practice.

THE PARANEOPLASTIC SYNDROMES

The clinical manifestations of cancer are usually due to pressure effects of local tumor growth, infiltration or metastatic deposition of tumor cells in a variety of organs in the body, or certain systemic symptoms. General problems observed in many patients with advanced or widespread metastatic cancer include anorexia, malaise, weight loss, and sometimes fever. These characteristics must be considered when evaluating a patient with an undiagnosed illness. Except in the case of functioning tumors such as those of the endocrine glands, systemic symptoms of cancer usually are not specific, often consisting of weakness, anorexia, and weight loss. The term paraneoplastic refers to features of disease considered to be due to the remote effects of a cancer that cannot be attributed either to a cancer's direct invasive or metastatic properties and are often considered to be due to aberrant hormonal or metabolic effects not observed in a cancer's normal tissue equivalent. In the paraneoplastic syndromes, clinical findings may resemble those of primary endocrine, metabolic, hematologic, or neuromuscular disorders. At present, the mechanisms for such remote effects can be classified into three groups: (1) effects initiated by a tumor product (eg, carcinoid syndrome, ectopic hormone production), (2) effects of destruction of normal tissues by tumor (eg, hypercalcemia with osteolytic skeletal metastases), and (3) effects due to unknown mechanisms. In paraneoplastic syndromes associated with ectopic hormone production, tumor tissue itself secretes the hormone that produces the syndrome. Ectopic hormones secreted by neoplasms are often pro-hormones of higher molecular weight than those secreted by the more differentiated normal endocrine cell. Such ectopic hormone production by cancer cells is believed to result from activation of genes in the malignant cells that are suppressed in the normal tissue equivalent and in most somatic cells. Autocrine growth factors secreted by neoplastic cells may also result in paraneoplastic syndromes. Small cell lung cancer is the one type of cancer most likely to be associated with paraneoplastic syndromes.

The paraneoplastic syndromes are clinically important for the following reasons:

(1) They sometimes accompany relatively limited neoplastic growth and may provide the clinician with an early clue to the presence of certain types of cancer.

(2) The metabolic or toxic effects of the syndrome may constitute a more urgent hazard to the patient's life than the underlying cancer (eg, hypercalcemia, hyponatremia).

(3) Effective treatment of the tumor should be accompanied by resolution of the paraneoplastic syndrome and, conversely, recurrence of the cancer may be heralded by return of the systemic symptoms. In some instances, rapid response to cytotoxic chemotherapy may briefly increase the severity of the paraneoplastic syndrome in association with tumor lysis (eg, hyponatremia with inappropriate antidiuretic hormone excretion). In some instances the identical symptom complex (eg, hypercalcemia) may be induced by entirely different mechanisms. A single syndrome such as hypercalcemia may be due to any one of a variety of humoral factors, such as secretion of parathyroid hormone precursors or homologs, an osteoclast-activating factor (lymphotoxin), transforming growth factor-α, or prostaglandins. Effective antitumor treatment usually results in return of serum calcium to normal.

Common paraneoplastic syndromes and endocrine secretions associated with functional cancers are summarized in Table 39–2.

▼ TYPES OF CANCER

LUNG CANCER

Sunny Wang, MD; Mark S. Chesnutt, MD;
James A. Murray, DO & Thomas J. Prendergast, MD

BRONCHOGENIC CARCINOMA

 ESSENTIALS OF DIAGNOSIS

▶ New cough, or change in chronic cough.

▶ Dyspnea, hemoptysis, anorexia, weight loss.

▶ Enlarging nodule or mass; persistent opacity, atelectasis, or pleural effusion on chest radiograph or CT scan.

▶ Cytologic or histologic findings of lung cancer in sputum, pleural fluid, or biopsy specimen.

▶ General Considerations

Lung cancer is the leading cause of cancer deaths in both men and women. The American Cancer Society estimated that there were 215,020 new diagnoses and 161,840 deaths from lung cancer in the United States in 2008, accounting for approximately 15% of new cancer diagnoses and 29% of all cancer deaths. More Americans die of lung cancer than of colorectal, breast, and prostate cancers combined. Lung cancer was a previously reportable disease until the widespread use of manufactured cigarettes in the 20th century. The causal connection between cigarettes and lung cancer is now established not only epidemiologically but also through identification of carcinogens in tobacco smoke and analysis of the effect of these carcinogens on specific oncogenes expressed in lung cancer. Even cigarette manufacturers no longer dispute the role of tobacco in this epidemic.

Cigarette smoking causes more than 90% of cases of lung cancer. Since the early 1990s, mortality from lung cancer fell among men while it increased among women and is only now peaking among women, reflecting changing patterns of tobacco use over the past 30 years (see Chapter 1). Other environmental risk factors for the development of lung cancer include exposure to environmental tobacco smoke, radon gas (among uranium miners and in areas where radium in the soil causes significant indoor air contamination), asbestos (60- to 100-fold increased risk in smokers with asbestos exposure), metals (arsenic, chromium, nickel, iron oxide), and industrial carcinogens (bischloromethyl ether). A familial predisposition to lung cancer is recognized. Certain diseases are associated with an increased risk of lung cancer, including pulmonary fibrosis, chronic obstructive pulmonary disease, and sarcoidosis. Second primary lung cancers are more frequent in patients who survive their initial lung cancer.

The median age at diagnosis of lung cancer is 71; it is unusual under the age of 40. After the diagnosis of lung cancer is made, approximately 41% of patients survive 1 year. The combined 5-year survival rate for all stages of lung cancer is now approximately 15%, improved from 12% in 1974–1976.

Five histologic categories of bronchogenic carcinoma account for more than 90% of cases of primary lung cancer. **Squamous cell carcinoma** (20% of cases) arises from the bronchial epithelium, typically as a centrally located, intraluminal sessile or polypoid mass. Squamous cell tumors are more likely to present with hemoptysis and more frequently are diagnosed by sputum cytology. They spread locally and may be associated with hilar adenopathy and mediastinal widening on chest radiography. **Adenocarcinoma** (35–40% of cases) arises from mucus glands or, in the case of **bronchioloalveolar cell carcinoma** (2% of cases), from any epithelial cell within or distal to the terminal bronchioles. Adenocarcinomas usually present as peripheral nodules or masses. Bronchioloalveolar cell carcinoma spreads intraalveolarly and may present as an infiltrate or as single or multiple pulmonary nodules. **Large cell carcinoma** (3–5% of cases) is a heterogeneous group of relatively undifferentiated tumors that share large cells and do not fit into other categories. Large cell carcinomas typically have rapid doubling times and an aggressive clinical course. They present as central or peripheral masses. Tumors that are not better differentiated on pathologic review other than carcinoma unspecified make up about 20–25% of cases. **Small cell**

Table 39–2. Paraneoplastic syndromes associated with cancer.

Hormone Excess or Syndrome	Non-Small Cell Lung Cancer	Small Cell Lung Cancer	Breast Cancer	Renal Cell Carcinoma	Adrenal Cancer	Hepato-cellular Carcinoma	Gastro-intestinal Cancers	Multiple Myeloma	Lymphoma	Thymoma	Prostatic Cancer	Ovarian Cancer	Chorio-carcinoma	Germ Cell Cancers
Endocrine														
Hypercalcemia	++		++	++	++			++	+		++			
Cushing syndrome	+	++		+	++					++	+			
SIADH	++	++												
Hypoglycemia	+			+	+	++	+							
Gonadotropin secretion		++			+	+	+						++	++
Hyperthyroidism													++	+
Hematologic														
Erythrocytosis				++	+	++								
Pure red cell aplasia									+	++				
Coagulopathy			++				++				++	+		
Thrombophlebitis			+				++				++	+		
Neurologic														
Lambert-Eaton myasthenia syndromes	+	++	+				+		+			+		
Subacute cerebellar syndrome		++	+				+		+			+		
Sensory motor peripheral neuropathy		++												
Stiff man syndrome			+											
Dermatologic														
Dermatomyositis	++	++	+				+					+		
Acanthosis nigricans	+		+				++				+			
Fever				++		++			++	+				
Hypertrophic osteoarthropathy	++													

+, reported associated; ++, strong association.
SIADH, syndrome of inappropriate antidiuretic hormone.

carcinoma (10–15% of cases) is a tumor of bronchial origin that typically begins centrally, infiltrating submucosally to cause narrowing or obstruction of the bronchus without a discrete luminal mass. Hilar and mediastinal abnormalities are common on chest radiography.

For purposes of staging and treatment, bronchogenic carcinoma is divided into small cell lung cancer (SCLC) and the other four types, conveniently labeled non–small cell lung cancer (NSCLC). This practical classification reflects different natural histories and different treatment. SCLC is prone to early hematogenous spread. It is rarely amenable to surgical resection and has a very aggressive course with a median survival (untreated) of 6–18 weeks. The four histologic categories comprising NSCLC spread more slowly. They may be cured in the early stages following resection, and they respond similarly to chemotherapy.

▶ **Clinical Findings**

Lung cancer is symptomatic at diagnosis in 75–90% of patients. The clinical presentation depends on the type and location of the primary tumor, the extent of local spread, and the presence of distant metastases and any paraneoplastic syndromes.

A. Symptoms and Signs

Anorexia, weight loss, or asthenia occurs in 55–90% of patients presenting with a new diagnosis of lung cancer. Up to 60% of patients have a new cough or a change in a chronic cough; 6–31% have hemoptysis; and 25–40% complain of pain, sometimes nonspecific chest pain but often referable to bony metastases to the vertebrae, ribs, or pelvis. Local spread may cause endobronchial obstruction with atelectasis and postobstructive pneumonia, pleural effusion (12–33%), change in voice (compromise of the recurrent laryngeal nerve), superior vena cava syndrome (obstruction of the superior vena cava with supraclavicular venous engorgement), and Horner syndrome (ipsilateral ptosis, miosis, and anhidrosis from involvement of the inferior cervical ganglion and the paravertebral sympathetic chain). Distant metastases to the liver are associated with asthenia and weight loss. Brain metastases (10% in NSCLC, more common in adenocarcinoma, and 20–30% in SCLC) may present with headache, nausea, vomiting, seizures, or altered mental status.

Paraneoplastic syndromes are incompletely understood patterns of organ dysfunction related to immune-mediated or secretory effects of neoplasms. These syndromes occur in 10–20% of lung cancer patients. They may precede, accompany, or follow the diagnosis of lung cancer. They do not necessarily indicate metastatic disease. In patients with small cell carcinoma, the syndrome of inappropriate antidiuretic hormone (SIADH) will develop in 10–15%; in those with squamous cell carcinoma, hypercalcemia will develop in 10%. Digital clubbing is seen in up to 20% of patients at diagnosis (Plate 47). Other common paraneoplastic syndromes include increased ACTH production, anemia, hypercoagulability, peripheral neuropathy, and the Eaton-Lambert myasthenia syndrome. Their recognition is important because treatment of the primary tumor may improve or resolve symptoms even when the cancer is not curable.

B. Laboratory Findings

The diagnosis of lung cancer rests on examination of a tissue or cytology specimen. Sputum cytology is highly specific but insensitive; the yield is highest when there are lesions in the central airways. Thoracentesis (sensitivity 50–65%) can be used to establish a diagnosis of lung cancer in patients with malignant pleural effusions. If cytologic examination of an adequate sample (50–100 mL) of pleural fluid is nondiagnostic, the procedure should be repeated once; approximately 30% of the second samples are positive when the first sample is negative. If results remain negative, thoracoscopy is preferred to blind pleural biopsy. Fine-needle aspiration (FNA) of palpable supraclavicular or cervical lymph nodes is frequently diagnostic. Serum tumor markers are neither sensitive nor specific enough to aid in diagnosis.

Fiberoptic bronchoscopy allows visualization of the major airways, cytology brushing of visible lesions or lavage of lung segments with cytologic evaluation of specimens, direct biopsy of endobronchial abnormalities, blind transbronchial biopsy of the pulmonary parenchyma or peripheral nodules, and FNA biopsy of mediastinal lymph nodes. Diagnostic yield varies widely (10–90%) depending on the size of the lesion and its location. Recent advances include fluorescence bronchoscopy, which improves the ability to identify early endobronchial lesions; and endobronchial and transesophageal endoscopic ultrasound, both of which permit more accurate direction of FNA of mediastinal nodes. Transthoracic needle aspiration (TTNA) has a sensitivity between 50% and 97%. Mediastinoscopy, video-assisted thoracoscopic surgery (VATS), and thoracotomy are necessary in cases where less invasive techniques fail to yield a diagnosis.

C. Imaging

Nearly all patients with lung cancer have abnormal findings on chest radiography or CT scan. These findings are rarely specific for a particular diagnosis. Interpretation of characteristic findings in isolated nodules is described in Chapter 9.

D. Special Examinations

1. Staging—Accurate staging is crucial (1) to provide the clinician with information to guide treatment, (2) to provide the patient with accurate information regarding prognosis, and (3) to standardize entry criteria for clinical trials to allow interpretation of results.

There are two essential principles of staging NSCLC. First, the more extensive the disease, the worse the prognosis; second, surgical resection offers the best hope for cure. Staging of NSCLC uses two integrated systems. The **TNM international staging system** attempts a physical description of the neoplasm: T describes the size and location of the primary tumor; N describes the presence and location of nodal metastases; and M refers to the presence or

Table 39–3. Approximate survival rates following treatment for lung cancer.

Non-Small Cell Lung Cancer: Mean 5-Year Survival Following Resection		
Stage	Clinical Staging	Surgical Staging
IA (T1N0M0)	60%	74%
IB (T2N0M0)	38%	61%
IIA (T1N1M0)	34%	55%
IIB (T2N1M0, T3N0M0)	23%	39%
IIIA	9–13%	22%
IIIB[1]	3–12%	
IV[1]	4%	
Small Cell Lung Cancer: Survival Following Chemotherapy		
Stage	Mean 2-Year Survival	Median Survival
Limited	15–20%	14–20 months
Extensive	< 3%	8-13 months

[1]Independent of therapy, generally not surgical patients.
Data from multiple sources. Modified and reproduced, with permission, from Reif MS et al. Evidence-based medicine in the treatment of non-small cell cancer. Clin Chest Med. 2000;21:107.

absence of distant metastases. These TNM stages are grouped into prognostic categories (stages I–IV) using the results of clinical trials. This classification is used to guide therapy. Many patients with stage I and stage II disease are cured through surgery. Patients with stage IIIB and stage IV disease do not benefit from surgery (Table 39–3). Patients with stage IIIA disease have locally invasive disease that may benefit from surgery in certain circumstances.

SCLC is not staged using the TNM system because micrometastases are assumed to be present on diagnosis. SCLC is divided into two categories: **limited disease** (30%), when the tumor is limited to the unilateral hemithorax (including contralateral mediastinal nodes); or **extensive disease** (70%), when the tumor extends beyond the hemithorax (including pleural effusion). This scheme also guides therapy. Patients with limited SCLC benefit from thoracic radiation therapy in addition to chemotherapy as well as prophylactic cranial radiation therapy.

For both SCLC and NSCLC, staging begins with a thorough history and physical examination. A complete examination is essential to exclude obvious metastatic disease to lymph nodes, skin, and bone. A detailed history is essential because the patient's performance status is a powerful predictor of disease course. All patients should have measurement of a complete blood count, electrolytes including calcium, creatinine, liver tests including lactate dehydrogenase (LD) and alkaline phosphatase, and a chest radiograph. Further evaluation will follow the results of these tests. In general, screening asymptomatic lung cancer patients with MRI of the brain, radionuclide bone imaging, and abdominal CT imaging does not change patient outcomes. These tests should be targeted to specific symptoms and signs.

NSCLC patients being considered for surgery require meticulous evaluation to identify those with resectable disease. CT imaging is the most important modality for staging candidates for resection. A chest CT scan precisely defines the size of parenchymal lesions and identifies atelectatic lung or pleural effusions. However, CT imaging is less accurate at determining invasion of the chest wall (sensitivity 62%) or mediastinum (sensitivity 60–75%). The sensitivity and specificity of CT imaging for identifying lung cancer metastatic to the mediastinal lymph nodes are 57% (49–66%) and 82% (77–86%), respectively. Therefore, chest CT imaging does not provide definitive information on staging. CT imaging does help in making the decision about whether to proceed to resection of the primary tumor and sample the mediastinum at thoracotomy (common if there are no lymph nodes > 1 cm) or to use TTNA, mediastinoscopy, esophageal ultrasound with transesophageal needle aspiration, or limited thoracotomy to biopsy suspected metastatic disease (common where there are lymph nodes > 1–2 cm).

Positron emission tomography (PET) using 2-[^{18}F]fluoro-2-deoxyglucose (FDG) is a noninvasive alternative for identifying metastatic foci in the mediastinum or distant sites. The sensitivity and specificity of PET for detecting mediastinal spread of primary lung cancer depend on the size of mediastinal nodes or masses. When only normal-sized (< 1 cm) mediastinal lymph nodes are present, the sensitivity and specificity of PET for tumor involvement of nodes are 74% and 96%, respectively. When CT shows enlarged (> 1 cm) lymph nodes, the sensitivity and specificity are 95% and 76%, respectively.

PET imaging is being incorporated into diagnostic algorithms that take advantage of both its positive and negative predictive values. Many lung cancer specialists find PET most useful to confirm lack of metastatic disease in NSCLC patients who are candidates for surgical resection. There is also evidence that PET imaging reduces futile thoracotomies by identifying mediastinal and distant metastases in patients with NSCLC. Disadvantages of PET imaging include limited resolution below 1 cm; the expense of FDG; limited availability; and false-positive scans due to sarcoidosis, tuberculosis, or fungal infections.

2. Preoperative assessment—See Chapter 3.

3. Pulmonary function testing—Many patients with NSCLC have moderate to severe chronic lung disease that increases the risk of perioperative complications as well as long-term pulmonary insufficiency following lung resection. All patients considered for surgery require spirometry. In the absence of other comorbidities, patients with good lung function (preoperative $FEV_1 \geq 2$ L) are at low risk for complications from lobectomy or pneumonectomy. If the FEV_1 is less than 2 L, then an estimated postoperative FEV_1 should be calculated. The postresection FEV_1 may be estimated from considering preoperative spirometry and the amount of lung to be resected; in severe obstructive disease, a quantitative lung perfusion scan may improve the estimate. A predicted post-lung resection FEV_1 > 800 mL (or > 40% of predicted FEV_1) is associated with a low incidence of perioperative complications. High-risk patients include those with a predicted postoperative FEV_1 < 700 mL (or < 40%

of predicted FEV_1). In these patients and in those with borderline spirometry, cardiopulmonary exercise testing may be helpful. A maximal oxygen uptake ($\dot{V}O_2$) of > 15 mL/kg/min identifies patients with an acceptable incidence of complications and mortality. Patients with a $\dot{V}O_2$ of < 10 mL/kg/min have a very high mortality rate at thoracotomy. Hypoxemia and hypercapnia are not independent predictors of outcome.

4. Screening—The optimal screening of smokers for lung cancer is unclear. Both chest radiographs and analysis of expectorated sputum is ineffective. Recent studies have tried to assess the role of chest CT scans. A study by Bach et al showed that CT screening of populations increases the diagnosis of lung cancer but does not reduce the risk of advanced lung cancer or reduce mortality. The investigators of the International Early Lung Cancer Action Program, however, suggested that there is a role for screening with chest CT. These studies highlight how complex and confusing the analysis of screening for lung cancer can be. At the present time, there are inadequate data to recommend the use of chest CT to screen smokers for lung cancer. The National Lung Screening Trial is an ongoing National Cancer Institute funded multicenter trial to determine whether using low-dose helical CT to screen current or former heavy smokers for lung cancer will improve mortality in this population. Information is available at http://www.cancer.gov/NLST/.

▶ **Treatment**

A. Non–Small Cell Carcinoma

Cure of NSCLC is unlikely without resection. Therefore, the initial approach to the patient is determined by the answers to two questions: (1) Is complete surgical resection technically feasible? (2) If yes, is the patient able to tolerate the surgery with acceptable morbidity and mortality? Clinical features that preclude complete resection include extrathoracic metastases or a malignant pleural effusion; or tumor involving the heart, pericardium, great vessels, esophagus, recurrent laryngeal or phrenic nerves, trachea, main carina, or contralateral mediastinal lymph nodes. Accordingly, stage I and stage II patients are treated with surgical resection where possible. Stage II, and possibly a subset of stage IB, are additionally recommended to receive adjuvant chemotherapy. Stage IIIA patients have poor outcomes when treated with resection alone. They should be referred to multimodality protocols, including chemotherapy and radiotherapy. Stage IIIB patients treated with concurrent chemotherapy and radiation therapy have improved survival. Selected stage IIIB patients who undergo resection after multimodality therapy have shown long-term survival and may be cured. Stage IV patients are treated with chemotherapy or symptom-based palliative therapy, or both (see below).

Surgical approach affects outcome. The North American Lung Cancer Study Group conducted a prospective trial of stage IA patients randomized to lobectomy versus limited resection. They reported a threefold increased rate of local recurrence in the limited resection group ($P = 0.008$) and a

trend toward an increase in overall death rate (increase of 30%, $P = 0.08$) and increase in death rate due to cancer (increase of 50%, $P = 0.09$), compared with patients receiving lobectomy. There are inadequate outcome data on which to base a comparison of VATS with standard thoracotomy. Radiation therapy following surgery improves local control but does not improve survival.

Patients with small early-stage primary lung cancers who are not candidates for surgery because of significant comorbidity or other surgical contraindication may be candidates for stereotactic radiosurgery or radiotherapy. This technology, which is composed of multiple non-parallel radiation beams that converge, allows the delivery of a relatively large dose of radiation to a small, well-defined target. Referral to a radiation oncologist is appropriate in such cases. Patients with locally advanced disease (stages IIIA and IIIB) who are not surgical candidates have improved survival when treated with concurrent chemotherapy and radiation therapy compared with no therapy, radiation alone, or even sequential chemotherapy and radiation.

Neoadjuvant chemotherapy consists of giving antineoplastic drugs in advance of surgery or radiation therapy. There is no consensus on the impact of neoadjuvant therapy on survival in stage I and stage II NSCLC. Such therapy is not recommended outside of ongoing clinical trials. Neoadjuvant therapy is more widely used in selected patients with stage IIIA or stage IIIB disease. Some studies suggest a survival advantage. This remains an area of active research.

Adjuvant chemotherapy consists of administering antineoplastic drugs following surgery or radiation therapy. Cisplatin-containing regimens have been shown to confer an overall survival benefit in at least stage II disease and possibly a subset of stage IB disease. The Lung Adjuvant Cisplatin Evaluation Collaborative Group just published a meta-analysis of the five largest cisplatin-based adjuvant trials. They reported a 5% absolute benefit in 5-year overall survival with a cisplatin-containing doublet regimen following surgery ($P = 0.005$) in patients with at least stage II disease. There is no evidence of a survival benefit, and it may even be detrimental in patients with poor performance status (Eastern Cooperative Oncology Group Score ≤ 2). Novel targeted agents with less toxicity are in clinical trials, and gene expression profiling has shown promise in defining a subset of patients with stage IA disease who may benefit from adjuvant therapy.

Although not curative, chemotherapy has been shown in multiple clinical trials to provide a modest increase in overall survival in patients with stage IIIB and stage IV NSCLC and good performance status compared with supportive care alone, with median survival increased from 5 months to a range of 7–11 months. Palliative chemotherapy also leads to improved quality of life and symptom control. A platinum-based regimen is most often used to treat such cases, with a multitude of active agents from which to choose. A recent randomized trial has now shown a survival benefit of adding bevacizumab (a monoclonal antibody to vascular endothelial growth factor [VEGF]) to a traditional platinum doublet regimen. Another targeted agent, erlotinib (an epidermal growth factor receptor [EGFR] tyrosine kinase inhibitor) has been shown to improve survival as second-line treatment for advanced NSCLC and is especially effective in cases affecting women, nonsmokers, and persons of Asian ethnicity as well as cases involving adenocarcinoma and bronchioalveolar carcinoma histology.

B. Small Cell Carcinoma

Response rates of SCLC to cisplatin and etoposide are excellent: 80–90% response in limited-stage disease (50–60% complete response), and 60–80% response in extensive stage disease (15–20% complete response). However, remissions tend to be short-lived with a median duration of 6–8 months. Once the disease has recurred, median survival is 3–4 months. Overall 2-year survival is 20–40% in limited-stage disease and less than 5% in extensive-stage disease. Thoracic radiation therapy improves survival in patients with limited SCLC but not those with extensive disease. There is a high rate brain metastasis in patients with SCLC, even following a good response to chemotherapy, because chemotherapy does not adequately penetrate the blood-brain barrier. Prophylactic cranial irradiation has been shown to decrease the incidence of central nervous system disease and improve survival in patients with limited stage disease who respond to chemotherapy and possibly in a subset of patients with extensive stage disease who have had an excellent response to chemotherapy.

Occasionally, a patient may have a peripheral nodule resected that turns out to be SCLC. Five-year survival following resection of the equivalent of stage I and stage II SCLC is higher than in patients treated with chemotherapy.

C. Palliative Therapy

Photoresection with the Nd:YAG laser is sometimes performed on central tumors to relieve endobronchial obstruction, improve dyspnea, and control hemoptysis. External beam radiation therapy is also used to control dyspnea and hemoptysis, pain from bony metastases, obstruction from superior vena cava syndrome, and symptomatic brain metastases. Resection of a *solitary* brain metastasis improves quality of life when combined with radiation therapy, and if there is no evidence of other metastatic disease, it may improve survival. Intraluminal radiation (brachytherapy) is an alternative approach to endobronchial disease. Pain syndromes are very common in advanced disease. As patients approach the end of life, meticulous efforts at pain control are essential (see Chapter 5). Consultation with or referral to a palliative care specialist is recommended in advanced disease to aid in symptom management and to facilitate referrals to hospice programs.

▶ Prognosis

The overall 5-year survival rate for lung cancer is 15%. Predictors of survival are the type of tumor (SCLC versus NSCLC), the stage of the tumor, and the patient's performance status, including weight loss in the past 6 months. These are independent predictors in both early and late stage disease. Most data suggest that there is no difference among non–small cell carcinomas when adjusted for stage and performance status.

American College of Chest Physicians; Health and Science Policy Committee. Diagnosis and management of lung cancer. ACCP evidence-based guidelines. Chest. 2003 Jan;123(1 Suppl):D–G, 1S–337S. [PMID: 12527560]

Bach PB et al. Computed tomography screening and lung cancer outcomes. JAMA. 2007 Mar 7;297(9):953–61. [PMID: 17341709]

Bach PB et al. Screening for lung cancer: ACCP evidence-based clinical practice guidelines (2nd edition). Chest. 2007 Sep;132(3 Suppl):69S–77S. [PMID: 17873161]

Black WC et al. CT screening for lung cancer: spiraling into confusion? JAMA. 2007 Mar 7;297(9):995–7. [PMID: 17341714]

Collins BT et al. Radical cyberknife radiosurgery with tumor tracking: an effective treatment for inoperable small peripheral stage I non-small cell lung cancer. J Hematol Oncol. 2009 Jan 17;2(1):1. [PMID: 19149899]

Henschke CI et al; International Early Lung Cancer Action Program Investigators. Survival of patients with stage I lung cancer detected on CT screening. N Engl J Med. 2006 Oct 26;355(17):1763–71. [PMID: 17065637]

Hiraoka M et al. Stereotactic body radiation therapy (SBRT) for early-stage lung cancer. Cancer Radiother. 2007 Jan–Feb;11(1–2):32–5. [PMID: 17158081]

Jemal A et al. Cancer Statistics, 2008. CA Cancer J Clin. 2008 Mar–Apr;58(2):71–96. [PMID: 18287387]

Jett JR et al. Treatment of non-small cell lung cancer, stage IIIB: ACCP evidence-based clinical practice guidelines (2nd edition). Chest. 2007 Sep;132(3 Suppl):266S–276S. [PMID: 17873173]

Pignon JP et al. Lung adjuvant cisplatin evaluation: a pooled analysis by the LACE Collaborative Group. J Clin Oncol. 2008 Jul 20;26(21):3552–9. [PMID: 18506026]

Sandler A et al. Paclitaxel-carboplatin alone or with bevacizumab for non-small-cell lung cancer. N Engl J Med. 2006 Dec 14;355(24):2542–50. [PMID: 17167137]

Shepherd FA et al. Erlotinib in previously treated non-small-cell lung cancer. N Engl J Med. 2005 Jul 14;353(2):123–32. [PMID: 16014882]

Ries LAG et al (eds). SEER Cancer Statistics Review, 1975–2005, National Cancer Institute. Bethesda, MD, http://seer.cancer.gov/csr/1975_2005/, based on November 2007 SEER data submission, posted to the SEER web site, 2008.

Slotman B et al. Prophylactic cranial irradiation in extensive small-cell lung cancer. N Engl J Med. 2007 Aug 16;357(7):664–72. [PMID: 17699816]

PULMONARY METASTASES

Pulmonary metastasis results from the spread of an extrapulmonary malignant tumor through vascular or lymphatic channels or by direct extension. Almost any cancer can metastasize to the lung. Metastases usually occur via the pulmonary artery and typically present as multiple nodules or masses on chest radiography. The radiographic differential diagnosis of multiple pulmonary nodules also includes pulmonary arteriovenous malformation, pulmonary abscesses, granulomatous infection, sarcoidosis, rheumatoid nodules, and Wegener granulomatosis. Metastases to the lungs are found in 20–55% of patients dying of various malignancies. Most are intraparenchymal. Endobronchial metastases occur in less than 5% of patients dying of nonpulmonary cancer; carcinoma of the kidney, breast, colon, and cervix and malignant melanoma are the most likely primary tumors.

Lymphangitic carcinomatosis denotes diffuse involvement of the pulmonary lymphatic network by primary or metastatic lung cancer, probably a result of extension of tumor from lung capillaries to the lymphatics. **Tumor embolization** from extrapulmonary cancer (renal cell carcinoma, hepatocellular carcinoma, choriocarcinoma) is an uncommon route for tumor spread to the lungs. Metastatic cancer may also present as a malignant pleural effusion.

▶ Clinical Findings

A. Symptoms and Signs

Symptoms are uncommon but include cough, hemoptysis and, in advanced cases, dyspnea and hypoxemia. Symptoms are more often referable to the site of the primary tumor.

B. Laboratory Findings

The diagnosis of metastatic cancer involving the lungs is usually established by identifying a primary tumor. Appropriate studies should be ordered if there is a suspicion of any primary cancer, such as breast, thyroid, testis, colorectal, or prostate, for which specific treatment is available. For example, an elevated prostate-specific antigen (PSA) may indicate prostate cancer, carcinoembryonic antigen (CEA) tests for colorectal or pancreatic cancer, and β-human chorionic gonadotropin (βHCG) and α-fetoprotein (AFP) test for testicular cancer. Based on the clinical setting, certain imaging studies should be ordered (see below). If the history, physical examination, and initial studies fail to reveal the site of the primary tumor, attention is better focused on the lung, where tissue samples obtained by bronchoscopy, percutaneous needle biopsy, or thoracotomy may establish the histologic diagnosis and suggest the most likely primary cancer. Occasionally, cytologic studies of pleural fluid or pleural biopsy reveal the diagnosis. Sputum cytology is rarely helpful.

If the initial histologic review does not reveal a primary diagnosis, immunohistochemical staining should be done on the biopsy specimen. For example, PSA and thyroglobulin staining are highly specific for prostate and thyroid cancer, respectively. Thyroid transcription factor-1 (TTF-1) is relatively specific for primary lung adenocarcinoma, while also positive for small cell carcinoma and thyroid carcinoma. An adenocarcinoma that demonstrates negative TTF-1 staining strongly suggests a nonpulmonary primary cancer. Positive estrogen receptor (ER) and progesterone receptor (PR) stains suggest primary breast cancer. Finally, the pattern of cytokeratin 7 and 20 staining can also help point toward a primary diagnosis.

C. Imaging

Chest radiographs usually show multiple spherical densities with sharp margins. The size of metastatic lesions varies from a few millimeters (miliary densities) to large masses. Nearly all are less than 5 cm in diameter. The lesions are usually bilateral, pleural or subpleural in location, and more common in lower lung zones. Cavitation suggests primary squamous cell tumor; calcification suggests osteosarcoma. Lymphangitic spread and solitary pulmonary nodule are less common radiographic presentations of pulmonary metastasis. Conventional chest radiography is less sensitive than CT scan in detecting pulmonary metastases. Mammography should be considered in women unless one has been performed recently to search for possible primary breast cancer. CT imaging of the chest, abdomen, and pelvis may reveal the

site of a primary tumor and will help determine feasibility of surgical resection of the metastatic lung tumors. PET scan may also help in identifying the site of a primary cancer or identifying other areas of extrathoracic metastasis.

▶ Treatment

Once the diagnosis has been established, management consists of treatment of the primary neoplasm and any pulmonary complications. Surgical resection of a *solitary* pulmonary nodule is often prudent in the patient with known current or previous extrapulmonary cancer. Local resection of one or more pulmonary metastases is feasible in a few carefully selected patients with various sarcomas and carcinomas (breast, testis, colon, kidney, and head and neck). Surgical resection should be considered only if the primary tumor is under control, if the patient is a good surgical risk, if all of the metastatic tumor can be resected, if nonsurgical approaches are not available, and if there are no metastases elsewhere in the body. Relative contraindications to resection of pulmonary metastases include (1) malignant melanoma primary, (2) requirement for pneumonectomy, and (3) pleural involvement. Data from the International Registry of Lung Metastases report an overall 5-year survival rate of 36% and 10-year survival rate of 26% after complete resection of pulmonary metastases. For patients with progressive disease, diligent attention to palliative care is essential (see Chapter 5).

Avdalovic M et al. Thoracic manifestations of common nonpulmonary malignancies of women. Clin Chest Med. 2004 Jun; 25(2):379–90. [PMID: 15099897]

Kondo H et al. Surgical treatment for metastatic malignancies. Pulmonary metastasis: indications and outcomes. Int J Clin Oncol. 2005 Apr;10(2):81–5. [PMID: 15864692]

Long-term results of lung metastasectomy: prognostic analyses based on 5206 cases. The International Registry of Lung Metastases. J Thorac Cardiovasc Surg. 1997 Jan;113(1):37–49. [PMID: 9011700]

MESOTHELIOMA

 ESSENTIALS OF DIAGNOSIS

- ▶ Unilateral, nonpleuritic chest pain and dyspnea.
- ▶ Distant (> 20 years earlier) history of exposure to asbestos.
- ▶ Pleural effusion or pleural thickening or both on chest radiographs.
- ▶ Malignant cells in pleural fluid or tissue biopsy.

▶ General Considerations

Mesotheliomas are primary tumors arising from the surface lining of the pleura (80% of cases) or peritoneum (20% of cases). About three-fourths of pleural mesotheliomas are diffuse (usually malignant) tumors, and the remaining one-fourth are localized (usually benign). Men outnumber women by a 3:1 ratio. Numerous studies have confirmed the association of **malignant pleural mesothelioma** with exposure to asbestos (particularly the crocidolite form). The lifetime risk to asbestos workers of developing malignant pleural mesothelioma is as high as 10%. Sixty to 80 percent of patients with malignant mesothelioma report a history of asbestos exposure. The latent period between exposure and onset of symptoms ranges from 20 to 40 years. The clinician should inquire about asbestos exposure through mining, milling, manufacturing, shipyard work, insulation, brake linings, building construction and demolition, roofing materials, and a variety of asbestos products (pipe, textiles, paint, tile, gaskets, panels). Although cigarette smoking significantly increases the risk of bronchogenic carcinoma in asbestos workers and aggravates asbestosis, there is no association between smoking and mesothelioma.

Clinical Findings

A. Symptoms and Signs

The mean age at onset of symptoms of malignant pleural mesothelioma is about 60 years. Symptoms include the insidious onset of shortness of breath, nonpleuritic chest pain, and weight loss. Physical findings include dullness to percussion, diminished breath sounds and, in some cases, digital clubbing.

B. Laboratory Findings

Pleural fluid is exudative and often hemorrhagic. Cytologic tests of pleural fluid are often negative. VATS biopsy is usually necessary to obtain an adequate specimen for histologic diagnosis; even then, distinction from benign inflammatory conditions and from metastatic adenocarcinoma may be difficult. The histologic variants of malignant pleural mesothelioma are epithelial and fibrous (sarcomatous). Special stains and electron microscopy may be needed to confirm the diagnosis.

C. Imaging

Radiographic abnormalities consist of nodular, irregular, unilateral pleural thickening and varying degrees of unilateral pleural effusion. Sixty percent of patients have right-sided disease, while only 5% have bilateral involvement. There may be scoliosis toward the side of the lesion. CT scan helps demonstrate the extent of pleural involvement.

Complications

Malignant pleural mesothelioma progresses rapidly as the tumor spreads along the pleural surface to involve the pericardium, mediastinum, and contralateral pleura. The tumor may eventually extend beyond the thorax to involve abdominal lymph nodes and organs. Progressive pain and dyspnea are characteristic. Local invasion of thoracic structures may cause superior vena cava syndrome, hoarseness, Horner syndrome, and dysphagia. Paraneoplastic syndromes associated with mesothelioma include thrombocytosis, hemolytic anemia, disseminated intravascular coagulopathy, hypercalcemia, and migratory thrombophlebitis.

Treatment

Surgery, radiotherapy, chemotherapy, and a combination of methods are attempted, but treatments are generally unsuc-

cessful. Pleurectomy and decortication (surgical stripping of the pleura and pericardium from apex of the lung to diaphragm) is one surgical approach but does not improve survival outcome even with adjuvant therapy. Some surgeons favor a trimodality approach with extrapleural pneumonectomy, adjuvant radiation, and chemotherapy, arguing that it prolongs survival in highly selected patients. Extrapleural pneumonectomy is a radical surgical procedure involving removal of the ipsilateral lung, parietal and visceral pleura, pericardium, and most of the hemi-diaphragm. However, the limited data for extrapleural pneumonectomy comes from retrospective studies and case series, where the patients are younger, have early-stage disease, have epithelial histology, and lack extrapleural nodal disease. In advanced unresectable cases, palliative chemotherapy with cisplatin and pemetrexed can extend survival as well as improve quality of life. Drainage of pleural effusions, pleurodesis, radiation therapy, and even surgical resection may offer palliative benefit in some patients.

Prognosis

Most patients die of respiratory failure and complications of local extension. Median survival time from onset of symptoms ranges from 4 months in extensive disease to 16 months in localized disease. Five-year survival is less than 5%.

Cameron RB. Extrapleural pneumonectomy is the preferred surgical management in the multimodality therapy of pleural mesothelioma: con Argument. Ann Surg Oncol. 2007 Apr;14(4):1249–53. [PMID: 17066226]

Maziak DE et al; Cancer Care Ontario Program in Evidence-based Care Lung Cancer Disease Site Group. Surgical management of malignant pleural mesothelioma: a systematic review and evidence summary. Lung Cancer. 2005 May;48(2):157–69. [PMID: 15829316]

O'Reilly KM et al. Asbestos-related lung disease. Am Fam Physician. 2007 Mar 1;75(5):683–8. [PMID: 17375514]

Tsiouris A et al. Malignant pleural mesothelioma: current concepts in treatment. Nat Clin Pract Oncol. 2007 Jun;4(6):344–52. [PMID: 17534390]

Volgezang NJ et al. Phase III study of pemetrexed in combination with cisplatin versus cisplatin alone in patients with malignant pleural mesothelioma. J Clin Oncol. 2003 July;21(14):2636–44. [PMID: 12860938]

West SD et al. Management of malignant pleural mesothelioma. Clin Chest Med. 2006 Jun;27(2):335–54. [PMID: 16716822]

HEPATOBILIARY CANCERS

Lawrence S. Friedman, MD

HEPATOCELLULAR CARCINOMA

 ESSENTIALS OF DIAGNOSIS

▶ In Western countries, usually a complication of cirrhosis.

▶ Characteristic CT and MRI features and elevated serum α-fetoprotein may obviate the need for a confirmatory biopsy.

General Considerations

Malignant neoplasms of the liver that arise from parenchymal cells are called hepatocellular carcinomas; those that originate in the ductular cells are called cholangiocarcinomas.

Hepatocellular carcinomas are associated with cirrhosis in 80% of cases. Incidence rates are rising rapidly (twofold since 1978) in the United States and other Western countries, presumably because of the increasing prevalence of cirrhosis caused by chronic hepatitis C infection and nonalcoholic fatty liver disease. In Western countries, risk factors for hepatocellular carcinoma in patients known to have cirrhosis are male gender, age > 55 years (although there has been an increase in the number of younger cases), Asian or Hispanic ethnicity, family history in a first-degree relative, overweight, obesity, diabetes mellitus, hypothyroidism, HCV infection, HBsAg and anti-HBc positivity, prothrombin time < 75% of control, low platelet count, and an elevated serum transferrin saturation. In Africa and most of Asia, hepatitis B is of major etiologic significance, whereas in Western countries and Japan, hepatitis C (particularly genotype 1b and sometimes in combination with "occult" HBV infection) and alcoholic cirrhosis are the most common risk factors. Other associations include hemochromatosis (and possibly the *C282Y* carrier state), aflatoxin exposure (associated with mutation of the *TP53* gene), α_1-antiprotease (α_1-antitrypsin) deficiency, and tyrosinemia. Evidence for an association with long-term use of oral contraceptives is inconclusive. Coffee consumption appears to be protective. The fibrolamellar variant of hepatocellular carcinoma occurs in young women and is characterized by a distinctive histologic picture, absence of risk factors, and indolent course. Vinyl chloride exposure is associated with angiosarcoma of the liver.

Clinical Findings

A. Symptoms and Signs

The presence of a hepatocellular carcinoma may be unsuspected until there is deterioration in the condition of a cirrhotic patient who was formerly stable. Cachexia, weakness, and weight loss are associated symptoms. The sudden appearance of ascites, which may be bloody, suggests portal or hepatic vein thrombosis by tumor or bleeding from the necrotic tumor.

Physical examination may show tender enlargement of the liver, occasionally with a palpable mass. In Africa, the typical presentation in young patients is a rapidly expanding abdominal mass. Auscultation may reveal a bruit over the tumor or a friction rub when the process has extended to the surface of the liver.

B. Laboratory Findings

Laboratory tests may reveal leukocytosis, as opposed to the leukopenia that is frequently encountered in cirrhotic patients. Anemia is common, but a normal or elevated hematocrit may be found in up to one-third of patients owing to elaboration of erythropoietin by the tumor. Sudden and sustained elevation of the serum alkaline phosphatase in a patient who was formerly stable is a common finding. HBsAg is present in a majority of cases in endemic areas, whereas in the United States anti-HCV is found in up to 40% of cases. α-Fetoprotein levels are elevated in up to 70% of patients with hepatocellular carcinoma in Western countries (although the sensitivity is lower in blacks); however, mild elevations are also often seen in patients with chronic hepatitis. Serum levels of desgamma-carboxy prothrombin are elevated in up to 90% of patients with hepatocellular carcinoma, but they may also be elevated in patients with vitamin K deficiency, chronic hepatitis, and metastatic cancer. The L3 glycoform of α-fetoprotein (AFP-L3) is under study. Cytologic study of ascitic fluid rarely reveals malignant cells.

C. Imaging

Multiphasic helical CT scanning and MRI with contrast enhancement are the preferred imaging studies for determining the location and vascularity of the tumor. Lesions smaller than 2 cm may be difficult to characterize. Arterial phase enhancement of the lesion followed by delayed hypointensity ("washout") is most specific for hepatocellular carcinoma. Ultrasound is less sensitive and operator dependent but is used to screen for hepatic nodules in high-risk patients. Contrast-enhanced ultrasound has a sensitivity and specificity approaching those of arterial phase helical CT but, unlike CT and MRI, cannot image the entire liver during the short duration of the arterial phase. In selected cases, endoscopic ultrasonography may be useful. PET is under study.

D. Liver Biopsy and Staging

Liver biopsy is diagnostic, although seeding of the needle tract by tumor is a potential risk (1–3%). Biopsy can be deferred if imaging studies and α-fetoprotein levels are diagnostic (eg, serum α-fetoprotein > 200 ng/mL and a hypervascular mass lesion > 2 cm on imaging of a cirrhotic liver) or if surgical resection is planned. Staging in the TNM classification includes the following definitions: T0: no evidence of primary tumor; T1: solitary tumor without vascular invasion; T2: solitary tumor with vascular invasion or multiple tumors none more than 5 cm; T3: multiple tumors more than 5 cm or tumor involving a major branch of the portal or hepatic vein; and T4: tumors with direct invasion of adjacent organs other than the gallbladder or with perforation of the visceral peritoneum. Alternative staging systems also incorporate liver function, tumor aggressiveness and growth rate, general health of the patient, and treatment. The BCLC (Barcelona Clinic Liver Cancer) staging system is now preferred and includes the Child-Turcotte-Pugh stage, tumor stage, and liver function and has the advantage of linking overall stage with preferred treatment modalities and with an estimation of life expectancy.

Screening & Prevention

In the patient with chronic hepatitis B or cirrhosis caused by HCV or alcohol, surveillance for the development of hepatocellular carcinoma is recommended. Although the standard approach is α-fetoprotein testing and ultrasonography every 6 months, the value of α-fetoprotein screening has been questioned because of its low sensitivity. The risk of hepatocellular carcinoma in a patient with cirrhosis is 3–5% a year. The diagnosis of hepatocellular carcinoma is established (without the need for biopsy) for lesions > 2 cm when characteristic arterial hypervascularity is demonstrated on both helical CT and MRI (or on either CT or MRI if the serum α-fetoprotein level is higher than 200 mg/L). In a population of patients with cirrhosis, over 60% of nodules < 2 cm in diameter detected on a screening ultrasound prove to be hepatocellular carcinoma. Mass vaccination programs against HBV in developing countries are leading to reduced rates of hepatocellular carcinoma. Successful treatment of hepatitis C in patients with cirrhosis reduces the subsequent risk of hepatocellular carcinoma.

▶ Treatment

Surgical resection of solitary hepatocellular carcinomas may result in cure if liver function is preserved (Child-Turcotte-Pugh class A or possibly B) and portal vein thrombosis is not present. Laparoscopic liver resection has been performed in selected cases. Treatment of underlying chronic viral hepatitis, adjuvant chemotherapy, and adaptive immunotherapy may lower postsurgical recurrence rates. Liver transplantation may be appropriate for small unresectable tumors in a patient with advanced cirrhosis, with reported 5-year survival rates of up to 75%. The recurrence-free survival may be better for liver transplantation than for resection in patients with well-compensated cirrhosis and small tumors (one tumor < 5 cm or three or fewer tumors each < 3 cm in diameter [Milan criteria]). Patients with stage 2 hepatocellular carcinoma receive an additional 22 points on their Model for End-Stage Liver Disease (MELD) score (see Chapter 16), markedly increasing their chances of a transplant. However, liver transplantation is often impractical because of the donor organ shortage and living donor liver transplantation may be considered in these cases. Patients with larger tumors (3–5 cm), a serum α-fetoprotein level ≥ 455 ng/mL, or a MELD score ≥ 20 have poor posttransplantation survival. Chemotherapy, hormonal therapy with tamoxifen, and long-acting octreotide have not been shown to prolong life, but transarterial chemoembolization (TACE), transarterial chemoinfusion (TACI), and transarterial radioembolization (TARE) via the hepatic artery are palliative and may prolong survival in patients with a large or multifocal tumor in the absence of extrahepatic spread. TACI and TARE are suitable for patients with portal vein thrombosis. Injection of absolute ethanol into, radiofrequency ablation of, cryotherapy of, or microwave ablation of small tumors (< 2 cm) may prolong survival in patients who are not candidates for resection; these interventions may provide a "bridge" to liver transplantation. Radiofrequency ablation is superior to ethanol injection for tumors > 2 cm in diameter and can be performed after TACE in select cases. Sorafenib (an oral multikinase inhibitor of Raf kinase, the VEGF, and the platelet-derived growth factor receptor [and others]), prolongs median survival as well as the time to radiologic progression by 3 months in patients with advanced hepatocellular carcinoma; sorafenib is the standard of care in these patients. New chemotherapy and radiation therapy techniques ("radioembolization") and novel biologic approaches (eg, bortezomib, a proteasome inhibitor; antiangiogenesis agents; other inhibitors of growth-factor signaling; and gene therapy) are under study. For patients whose disease progresses despite treatment or who present with advanced tumors, vascular invasion, or extrahepatic spread, meticulous efforts at palliative care are essential (see Chapter 5). Severe pain may develop in such patients due to expansion of the liver capsule by the tumor and requires concerted efforts at pain management, including the use of opioids (see Chapter 5).

▶ Prognosis

In the United States, overall 1- and 5-year survival rates for patients with hepatocellular carcinoma are 23% and 5%, respectively. Five-year survival rates rise to 56% for patients with localized resectable disease (T1, T2, selected T3 and T4; N0; M0) but are virtually nil for those with localized unresectable or advanced disease. The fibrolamellar variant has a better prognosis than conventional hepatocellular carcinoma, with a 5-year survival rate of up to 75% following resection.

▶ When to Refer

All patients with hepatocellular carcinoma should be referred to a specialist.

▶ When to Admit

- Complications of cirrhosis.
- Severe pain.
- For surgery and other interventions.

Callstrom MR et al. Technologies for ablation of hepatocellular carcinoma. Gastroenterology. 2008 Jun;134(7):1831–5. [PMID: 18486619]

Cheng BQ et al. Chemoembolization combined with radiofrequency ablation for patients with hepatocellular carcinoma larger than 3 cm: a randomized controlled trial. JAMA. 2008 Apr 9;299(14):1669–77. [PMID: 18398079]

Guglielmi A et al. Comparison of seven staging systems in cirrhotic patients with hepatocellular carcinoma in a cohort of patients who underwent radiofrequency ablation with complete response. Am J Gastroenterol. 2008 Mar;103(3):597–604. [PMID: 17970836]

Llovet JM et al; SHARP Investigators Study Group. Sorafenib in advanced hepatocellular carcinoma. N Engl J Med. 2008 Jul 24;359(4):378–90. [PMID: 18650514]

Veldt BJ et al. Increased risk of hepatocellular carcinoma among patients with hepatitis C cirrhosis and diabetes mellitus. Hepatology. 2008 Jun;47(6):1856–62. [PMID: 18506898]

CARCINOMA OF THE BILIARY TRACT

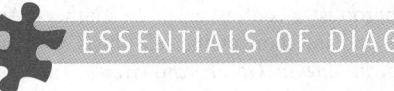
ESSENTIALS OF DIAGNOSIS

▶ Presents with obstructive jaundice, usually painless, often with dilated biliary tree.

- Pain is more common in gallbladder carcinoma than cholangiocarcinoma.
- A Courvoisier (dilated) gallbladder may be detected.
- Diagnosis by cholangiography with biopsy and brushings for cytology.

General Considerations

Carcinoma of the gallbladder occurs in approximately 2% of all people operated on for biliary tract disease. It is notoriously insidious, and the diagnosis is often made unexpectedly at surgery. Cholelithiasis (often large, symptomatic stones) is usually present. Other risk factors are chronic infection of the gallbladder with *Salmonella typhi*, gallbladder polyps over 1 cm in diameter, mucosal calcification of the gallbladder (porcelain gallbladder), and anomalous pancreaticobiliary ductal junction. Genetic factors include *K-ras* and *TP53* mutations. Spread of the cancer—by direct extension into the liver or to the peritoneal surface—may be the initial manifestation. The TNM classification includes the following stages: Tis, carcinoma in situ; T1a, tumor invades lamina propria, and T1b, tumor invades muscle layer; T2, tumor invades perimuscular connective tissue, no extension beyond serosa (visceral peritoneum) or into liver; T3, tumor perforates the serosa or directly invades the liver or adjacent organ or structure; T4, tumor invades the main portal vein or hepatic artery or invades multiple extrahepatic organs or structures; N1, regional lymph node metastasis; and M1, distant metastasis.

Carcinoma of the bile ducts (cholangiocarcinoma) accounts for 3% of all cancer deaths in the United States. It is more prevalent in persons aged 50–70, with a slight male predominance. Two-thirds arise at the confluence of the hepatic ducts (Klatskin tumors), and one-fourth arise in the distal extrahepatic bile duct; the remainder are intrahepatic (peripheral), the incidence of which has risen dramatically since the 1970s. Staging is as follows: T1, solitary tumor without vascular invasion; T2, solitary tumor with vascular invasion or multiple tumors ≤ 5 cm; T3, multiple tumors > 5 cm or involving major branch of portal or hepatic veins; T4, tumor invading adjacent organ (except gallbladder) or perforation of visceral peritoneum; N1, regional lymph node metastasis; and M1, distant metastasis. Other staging systems consider tumor extent, vascular encasement, and hepatic lobe atrophy. The frequency of carcinoma in persons with choledochal cysts has been reported to be over 14% at 20 years, and surgical excision is recommended. There is an increased incidence in patients with bile duct adenoma; biliary papillomatosis; Caroli disease; a biliary-enteric anastomosis; ulcerative colitis, especially those with primary sclerosing cholangitis; biliary cirrhosis; diabetes mellitus; hyperthyroidism; chronic pancreatitis; heavy alcohol consumption; and past exposure to thorotrast, a contrast agent. In southeast Asia, hepatolithiasis and infection of the bile ducts with helminths (*Clonorchis sinensis, Opisthorchis viverrini*) are associated with chronic cholangitis and an increased risk of cholangiocarcinoma. Hepatitis C virus infection, cirrhosis, HIV infection, nonalcoholic fatty liver disease, diabetes mellitus, obesity, and tobacco smoking are additional risk factors for intrahepatic cholangiocarcinoma.

► Clinical Findings

A. Symptoms and Signs

Progressive jaundice is the most common and usually the first sign of obstruction of the extrahepatic biliary system. Pain in the right upper abdomen with radiation into the back is usually present early in the course of gallbladder carcinoma but occurs later in the course of bile duct carcinoma. Anorexia and weight loss are common and may be associated with fever and chills due to cholangitis. Rarely, hematemesis or melena results from erosion of tumor into a blood vessel (hemobilia). Fistula formation between the biliary system and adjacent organs may also occur. The course is usually one of rapid deterioration, with death occurring within a few months.

Physical examination reveals profound jaundice. A palpable gallbladder with obstructive jaundice usually is said to signify malignant disease (Courvoisier law); however, this clinical generalization has been proved to be accurate only about 50% of the time. Hepatomegaly due to hypertrophy of the unobstructed liver lobe is usually present and is associated with liver tenderness. Ascites may occur with peritoneal implants. Pruritus and skin excoriations are common.

B. Laboratory Findings

With biliary obstruction, laboratory examination reveals predominantly conjugated hyperbilirubinemia, with total serum bilirubin values ranging from 5 to 30 mg/dL. There is usually concomitant elevation of the alkaline phosphatase and serum cholesterol. AST is normal or minimally elevated. An elevated CA 19-9 level may help distinguish cholangiocarcinoma from a benign biliary stricture (in the absence of cholangitis).

C. Imaging

Ultrasonography and contrast-enhanced, triple-phase, helical CT may show a gallbladder mass in gallbladder carcinoma and intrahepatic mass or biliary dilation in carcinoma of the bile ducts. CT may also show involved regional lymph nodes and atrophy of a hepatic lobe because of vascular encasement with compensatory hypertrophy of the unaffected lobe. MRI with magnetic resonance cholangiopancreatography (MRCP) and gadolinium enhancement permits visualization of the entire biliary tree and detection of vascular invasion and obviates the need for angiography and, in some cases, direct cholangiography; it has become the imaging procedure of choice but may understage malignant hilar strictures. The sensitivity and image quality can be increased with use of ferumoxide enhancement. In indeterminate cases, PET can detect cholangiocarcinomas as small as 1 cm and lymph node and distant metastases, but false-positive results occur. The most helpful diagnostic studies before surgery are either percutaneous transhepatic or endoscopic retrograde cholangiography with biopsy and cytologic specimens, although false-negative biopsy and cytology results are common. Digital image analysis and fluorescent in situ hybridization of cytologic specimens improve sensitivity. Endoscopic ultrasound (EUS) with FNA of tumors, choledochoscopy, and intraductal ultrasonography may confirm a diagnosis of cholangiocarcinoma in a patient with bile duct stricture and an otherwise indeterminate evaluation.

Treatment

In young and fit patients, curative surgery may be attempted if the tumor is well localized. The 5-year survival rate for carcinoma of the gallbladder invading the lamina propria or muscularis (stage 1, T1a or 1b, N0, M0) is as high as 85% with laparoscopic cholecystectomy but drops to 60%, even with a more extended open resection, if there is perimuscular invasion (T2). The role of radical surgery for T3 and T4 tumors is debatable. If the tumor is unresectable at laparotomy, biliary-enteric bypass (eg, Roux-en-Y hepaticojejunostomy) can be performed. Carcinoma of the bile ducts is curable by surgery in less than 10% of cases. If resection margins are negative, the 5-year survival rate may be as high as 47% for intrahepatic cholangiocarcinomas, 41% for hilar cholangiocarcinoma, and 37% for distal cholangiocarcinomas, but the perioperative mortality rate may be as high as 10%. Palliation can be achieved by placement of a self-expandable metal stent via an endoscopic or percutaneous transhepatic route. Covered metal stents may be more cost-effective than uncovered metal stents because of a lower risk of stent occlusion, but they are not associated with longer survival. For hilar tumors, there is controversy as to whether unilateral or bilateral stents should be inserted. Plastic stents are less expensive but more prone to occlude than metal ones; they are suitable for patients expected to survive only a few months. Photodynamic therapy in combination with stent placement has been demonstrated to prolong survival when compared with stent placement alone in patients with nonresectable cholangiocarcinoma. Radiotherapy may relieve pain and contribute to biliary decompression. There is limited response to chemotherapy such as with gemcitabine. In general, the prognosis is poor, with few patients surviving for more than 12 months after surgery. Although cholangiocarcinoma is generally considered to be a contraindication to liver transplantation because of rapid tumor recurrence, a 75% 5-year survival rate has been reported in patients with stage I and II cholangiocarcinoma undergoing chemoradiation and exploratory laparotomy followed by liver transplantation.

For those patients whose disease progresses despite treatment, meticulous efforts at palliative care are essential (see Chapter 5).

When to Refer

All patients with carcinoma of the biliary tract should be referred to a specialist.

When to Admit

- Biliary obstruction.
- Cholangitis.

Blechacz B et al. Cholangiocarcinoma: advances in pathogenesis, diagnosis, and treatment. Hepatology. 2008 Jul;48(1):308–21. [PMID: 18536057]

Kahaleh M et al. Unresectable cholangiocarcinoma: comparison of survival in biliary stenting alone versus stenting with photodynamic therapy. Clin Gastroenterol Hepatol. 2008 Mar;6(3):290–7. [PMID: 18255347]

Yachimski P et al. Cholangiocarcinoma: natural history, treatment, and strategies for surveillance in high-risk patients. J Clin Gastroenterol. 2008 Feb;42(2):178–90. [PMID: 18209589]

CARCINOMA OF THE PANCREAS & THE PERIAMPULLARY AREA

 ESSENTIALS OF DIAGNOSIS

- ▶ Obstructive jaundice (may be painless).
- ▶ Enlarged gallbladder (may be painful).
- ▶ Upper abdominal pain with radiation to back, weight loss, and thrombophlebitis are usually late manifestations.

General Considerations

Carcinomas involving the head of the pancreas, the ampulla of Vater, the distal common bile duct, and the duodenum are considered together, because they are usually indistinguishable clinically; of these, carcinomas of the pancreas constitute over 90%. Carcinoma is the most common neoplasm of the pancreas. About 75% are in the head and 25% in the body and tail of the organ. They comprise 2% of all cancers and 5% of cancer deaths. Risk factors include age, obesity, tobacco use, heavy alcohol use, chronic pancreatitis, prior abdominal radiation, and family history. New-onset diabetes mellitus after age 45 years occasionally heralds the onset of early pancreatic cancer. About 7–8% of patients with pancreatic cancer have a family history of pancreatic cancer in a first-degree relative, compared with 0.6% of control subjects. Point mutations in codon 12 of the K-ras oncogene are found in 70–100%, inactivation of the tumor suppressor genes INK4A on chromosome 9, TP53 on chromosome 17, and MADH4 on chromosome 18 is found in 95%, 75%, and 55% of pancreatic cancers, respectively, and mutation of the palladin gene is reported to be common. Pancreatic cancer can also occur as part of several hereditary syndromes, including familial breast cancer (carriers of BRCA-2 have a 7% lifetime risk of pancreatic cancer), hereditary pancreatitis (PSS1 mutation), familial cutaneous malignant melanoma (CDKN2A mutation), Peutz–Jeghers syndrome, ataxia-telangiectasia, and hereditary nonpolyposis colorectal cancer. Polymorphisms of the genes for methylene tetrahydrofolate reductase and thymidylate synthase have been reported to be associated with pancreatic cancer. Neuroendocrine tumors account for 1–2% of pancreatic neoplasms and may be functional (producing gastrin, insulin, glucagon, vasoactive intestinal peptide, somatostatin, growth hormone–releasing hormone, adrenocorticotropic hormone, and others) or nonfunctional. Plasma chronogranin A levels are elevated in 88–100% of affected patients.

Cystic neoplasms account for only 1% of pancreatic cancers, but they are important because they are often mistaken for pseudocysts. A cystic neoplasm should be suspected when a cystic lesion in the pancreas is found in the absence of a history of pancreatitis. At least 15% of all pancreatic cysts are neoplasms. Whereas serous cystadenomas (which account for 32–39% of cystic pancreatic neoplasms and also occur in patients with von Hippel–Lindau disease) are benign, mucinous cystic neoplasms (defined by the presence of ovarian stroma) (10–45%), intraductal papillary mucinous neoplasms (21–33%), solid pseudopapillary neoplasms (< 5%), and cystic islet cell tumors (3–5%) may be malignant, although their prognoses are better than the prognosis of adenocarcinoma of the pancreas, unless the neoplasm is locally advanced.

► Clinical Findings

A. Symptoms and Signs

Pain is present in over 70% of cases and is often vague, diffuse, and located in the epigastrium or left upper quadrant when the lesion is in the tail. Radiation of pain into the back is common and sometimes predominates. Sitting up and leaning forward may afford some relief, and this usually indicates that the lesion has spread beyond the pancreas and is inoperable. Diarrhea, perhaps due to maldigestion, is an occasional early symptom. Migratory thrombophlebitis is a rare sign. Weight loss is a common but late finding and may be associated with depression. Occasionally a patient presents with acute pancreatitis in the absence of an alternative cause. Jaundice is usually due to biliary obstruction by a cancer in the pancreatic head. A palpable gallbladder is also indicative of obstruction by neoplasm (Courvoisier law), but there are frequent exceptions. A hard, fixed, occasionally tender mass may be present. In advanced cases, a hard periumbilical (Sister Joseph's) nodule may be palpable.

B. Laboratory Findings

There may be mild anemia. Glycosuria, hyperglycemia, and impaired glucose tolerance or true diabetes mellitus are found in 10–20% of cases. The serum amylase or lipase level is occasionally elevated. Liver biochemical tests may suggest obstructive jaundice. Steatorrhea in the absence of jaundice is uncommon. Occult blood in the stool is suggestive of carcinoma of the ampulla of Vater (the combination of biliary obstruction and bleeding may give the stools a distinctive silver appearance). CA 19-9, with a sensitivity of 70% and a specificity of 87%, has not proved sensitive enough for early detection of pancreatic cancer; increased values are also found in acute and chronic pancreatitis and cholangitis.

C. Imaging

With carcinoma of the head of the pancreas, an upper gastrointestinal series may show a widening of the duodenal loop, mucosal abnormalities in the duodenum ranging from edema to invasion or ulceration, spasm, or compression. Ultrasound is not reliable because of interference by intesti-

nal gas. Multiphase thin-cut helical CT scanning is generally the initial diagnostic procedure and detects a mass in over 80% of cases. CT scanning identifies metastases, delineates the extent of the tumor, and allows for percutaneous FNA for cytologic studies and tumor markers. MRI is an alternative to CT scanning. Preliminary experience suggests that PET is a sensitive technique for detecting pancreatic cancer and metastases. Selective celiac and superior mesenteric arteriography may demonstrate vessel invasion by tumor, a finding that would interdict attempts at surgical resection, but it is less widely used since the advent of multiphase helical CT. Endoscopic ultrasonography is more sensitive than CT scanning for detecting pancreatic cancer and equivalent to CT scanning for determining nodal involvement and resectability. A normal EUS excludes pancreatic cancer. Endoscopic ultrasonography may also be used to guide FNA for tissue diagnosis and tumor markers. Endoscopic retrograde cholangiopancreatography (ERCP) may clarify an ambiguous CT scan or MRI study by delineating the pancreatic duct system or confirming an ampullary or biliary neoplasm. MRCP appears to be at least as sensitive as ERCP in diagnosing pancreatic cancer. In some centers, pancreatoscopy or intraductal ultrasonography can be used to evaluate filling defects in the pancreatic duct and assess resectability of intraductal papillary mucinous tumors. With obstruction of the splenic vein, splenomegaly or gastric varices are present, the latter delineated by endoscopy, endoscopic ultrasonography, or angiography.

Cystic neoplasms can be distinguished by their appearance on CT, endoscopic ultrasonography, and ERCP and features of the cyst fluid on gross and cytologic analysis. For example, serous cystadenomas may have a central scar or honeycomb appearance; mucinous cystadenomas are unilocular or multilocular and contain mucin-rich fluid with high carcinoembryonic antigen levels (> 200 ng/mL); and intraductal papillary mucinous neoplasms are associated with a dilated pancreatic duct and extrusion of gelatinous material from the ampulla.

Staging of pancreatic cancer by the TNM classification includes the following definitions: Tis: carcinoma in situ; T1: tumor limited to the pancreas, 2 cm or less in greatest dimension; T2: tumor limited to the pancreas, more than 2 cm in greatest dimension; T3: tumor extends beyond the pancreas but without involvement of the celiac axis or the superior mesenteric artery; T4, tumor involves the celiac axis or the superior mesenteric artery (unresectable primary tumor).

► Treatment

Abdominal exploration is usually necessary when cytologic diagnosis cannot be made or if resection is to be attempted, which includes about 30% of patients. In a patient with a localized mass in the head of the pancreas and without jaundice, laparoscopy may detect tiny peritoneal or liver metastases and thereby avoid resection in 4–13% of patients. Radical pancreaticoduodenal (Whipple) resection is indicated for lesions strictly limited to the head of the pancreas, periampullary area, and duodenum (T1, N0, M0). Five-year survival rates are 20–25% in this group and as high as 40% in those with negative resection margins and without lymph node involvement. Preoperative endoscopic decompression of an obstructed bile duct is often achieved with a plastic stent or short metal stent but does not reduce operative mortality or morbidity. The best surgical results are achieved at centers that specialize in the multidisciplinary treatment of pancreatic cancer. Adjuvant or neoadjuvant chemotherapy with gemcitabine and fluorouracil, possibly combined with irradiation, appears to be of benefit (Table 39–4). When resection is not feasible, endoscopic stenting of the bile duct is performed to relieve jaundice. A plastic stent is generally placed if the patient's anticipated survival is less than 6 months (or surgery is planned). A metal stent is preferred when anticipated survival is 6 months or greater. Surgical biliary bypass may be considered in patients expected to survive at least 6 months. Surgical duodenal bypass may be considered in patients in whom duodenal obstruction is expected to develop later; alternatively, endoscopic placement of a self-expandable duodenal stent may be feasible. Chemoradiation may be used for palliation of unresectable cancer confined to the pancreas. Chemotherapy has been disappointing in metastatic pancreatic cancer, although improved response rates have been reported with gemcitabine. Novel small molecules (eg, erlotinib), capecitabine (an oral fluoropyrimidine), nucleoside cytidine analogues, and topoisomerase inhibitors are under study. Celiac plexus nerve block or thoracoscopic splanchnicectomy may improve pain control. Photodynamic therapy is under study.

Surgical resection is the treatment of choice for neuroendocrine tumors, when feasible. Metastatic disease may be controlled with long-acting somatostatin analogs, interferon, peptide-receptor radionuclide therapy, and chemoembolization. There is a growing consensus that asymptomatic incidental pancreatic cysts of 2 cm or less are at low risk of invasive carcinoma and may be followed by imaging tests at 6-month intervals, with surgery performed if a cyst enlarges or exceeds 2.5 cm.

Surgical resection is indicated for mucinous cystic neoplasms, symptomatic serous cystadenomas, and cystic tumors larger than 2 cm in diameter that remain undefined after helical CT, EUS, and diagnostic aspiration. All intraductal papillary mucinous neoplasms of the main pancreatic duct should be resected, but those of branch ducts may be followed with serial imaging if they are asymptomatic and exhibit benign features (eg, diameter < 3 cm, absence of nodules or thick walls); most of the latter remain stable on follow-up, but the risk of pancreatic ductal carcinoma and of nonpancreatic cancers may also be increased in this group of patients. In the absence of locally advanced disease, survival is higher for malignant cystic neoplasms than for adenocarcinoma. Endoscopic resection or ablation, with temporary placement of a pancreatic duct stent, may be feasible for ampullary adenomas, but patients must be followed for recurrence.

Prognosis

Carcinoma of the pancreas, especially in the body or tail, has a poor prognosis. Reported 5-year survival rates range

from 2% to 5%. Lesions of the ampulla have a better prognosis, with reported 5-year survival rates of 20–40% after resection; jaundice and lymph node involvement are adverse prognostic factors. In carefully selected patients, resection of cancer of the pancreatic head is feasible and results in reasonable survival. In persons with a strong family history of pancreatic cancer, screening with helical CT and endoscopic ultrasonography should be considered beginning 10 years before the age at which pancreatic cancer was diagnosed in a family member.

For those patients whose disease progresses despite treatment, meticulous efforts at palliative care are essential (see Chapter 5).

▶ When to Refer

All patients with carcinoma involving the pancreas and the periampullary area should be referred to a specialist.

▶ When to Admit

Patients who require surgery and other interventions should be hospitalized.

Belyaev O et al. Intraductal papillary mucinous neoplasms of the pancreas. J Clin Gastroenterol. 2008 Mar;42(3):284–94. [PMID: 18223495]

Brugge WR. The incidental pancreatic cyst on abdominal computerized tomography imaging: diagnosis and management. Clin Gastroenterol Hepatol. 2008 Feb;6(2):140–4. [PMID: 18237864]

Pannala R et al. Prevalence and clinical profile of pancreatic cancer-associated diabetes mellitus. Gastroenterology. 2008 Apr;134(4):981–7. [PMID: 18395079]

Tang RS et al. Evaluation of the guidelines for management of pancreatic branch-duct intraductal papillary mucinous neoplasm. Clin Gastroenterol Hepatol. 2008 Jul;6(7):815–9. [PMID: 18602036]

Zuckerman DS et al. Adjuvant therapy for pancreatic cancer: a review. Cancer. 2008 Jan 15;112(2):243–9. [PMID: 18050292]

ALIMENTARY TRACT CANCERS

Kenneth R. McQuaid, MD

ESOPHAGEAL CANCER

 ESSENTIALS OF DIAGNOSIS

▶ Progressive solid food dysphagia.

▶ Weight loss common.

▶ Endoscopy with biopsy establishes diagnosis.

▶ General Considerations

Esophageal cancer usually develops in persons between 50 and 70 years of age. The overall ratio of men to women is 3:1. There are two histologic types: squamous cell carcinoma and adenocarcinoma. In the United States, **squamous cell cancer** is much more common in blacks than in whites.

Table 39–4. Treatment choices for cancers responsive to systemic agents.

Diagnosis	Current Treatment of Choice	Other Treatments
Acute lymphocytic leukemia (ALL)	Induction combination chemotherapy: Vincristine, prednisone, daunorubicin, asparaginase, intrathecal methotrexate Consolidation combination chemotherapy: Cyclophosphamide, vincristine, doxorubicin, dexamethasone (hyper-CVAD) alternated with cytarabine, methotrexate Maintenance: Methotrexate, 6-mercaptopurine	Imatinib mesylate (Ph positive ALL), autologous or allogeneic transplantation for high risk or at relapse
Acute myelogenous leukemia (AML)	Combination chemotherapy: Cytarabine plus daunorubin or idarubicin	Gemtuzumab ozogamicin, prednisone, doxorubicin
Chronic myelocytic leukemia (CML)	Imatinib mesylate	Dasatinib, nilotinib, allogeneic bone marrow transplantation, hydroxyurea, interferon-α, cytarabine, busulfan
Chronic lymphocytic leukemia (CLL)	Combination chemotherapy: Fludarabine, cyclophosphamide, rituximab (FCR); Fludarabine; or Chlorambucil	Alemtuzumab, bendamustine, pentostatin, cladribine, cyclophosphamide, vincristine, doxorubicin, prednisone
Hairy cell leukemia	Cladribine (2-chlorodeoxyadenosine)	Pentostatin, interferon-α
Hodgkin disease (stages III and IV)	Combination chemotherapy: Doxorubicin, bleomycin, vinblastine, dacarbazine (ABVD); Doxorubicin, vinblastine, mechlorethamine, etoposide, vincristine, bleomycin, prednisone (Stanford V)	Gemcitabine, vinorelbine, ifosfamide, cyclophosphamide, procarbazine, transplantation for relapse
Non-Hodgkin lymphoma (intermediate and high grade)	Combination chemotherapy: Cyclophosphamide, doxorubicin, vincristine, prednisone, rituximab (CHOP-R)	Combination chemotherapy second line: Dexamethasone, cisplatin, cytarabine (DHAP) Etoposide, methylprednisolone, cytarabine, cisplatin (ESHAP) Ifosfamide, carboplatin, etoposide (ICE) Mesna, ifosfamide, mitoxantrone, etoposide (MINE); transplantation for high risk or first relapse
Non-Hodgkin lymphoma (low grade)	Combination chemotherapy: Fludarabine, cyclophosphamide, rituximab (FCR) Cyclophosphamide, vincristine, doxorubicin, prednisone, rituximab (CHOP-R), or Cyclophosphamide, vincristine, prednisone, rituximab (CVP-R) or Chlorambucil	^{131}I tositumomab, ^{90}Y ibritumomab tiuxetan, bendamustine, autologous or allogeneic transplantation
Multiple myeloma	Combination chemotherapy (transplant candidates): Bortezomib, dexamethasone, thalidomide or lenalidomide Dexamethasone, thalidomide or lenalidomide Dexamethasone followed by autologous or miniallogeneic stem cell transplantation Combination chemotherapy (non-transplant candidates): Melphalan, prednisone, bortezomib Melphalan, prednisone	Bortezomib, lenalidomide, thalidomide, dexamethasone, cyclophosphamide
Waldenstrom macroglobulinemia	Combination therapy: Fludarabine, cyclophosphamide, rituximab (FCR), with or without plasmapheresis	Cladribine, thalidomide, bortezomib, chlorambucil, autologous bone marrow transplantation, prednisone
Polycythemia vera	Phlebotomy, hydroxyurea	Anagrelide, radiophosphorus ^{32}P, interferon-α, busulfan, chlorambucil, cyclophosphamide
Non-small cell lung cancer	Combination chemotherapy: Cisplatin, vinorelbine Cisplatin, gemcitabine Cisplatin, etoposide Paclitaxel, carboplatin; all regimens with or without bevacizumab	Docetaxel, vinorelbine, pemetrexed, erlotinib, cetuximab
Small cell lung cancer	Combination chemotherapy: Cisplatin, etoposide	Irinotecan, cyclophosphamide, doxorubicin, vincristine, topotecan
Mesothelioma	Combination chemotherapy: Cisplatin, pemetrexed	Doxorubicin

(continued)

Table 39–4. Treatment choices for cancers responsive to systemic agents. (continued)

Diagnosis	Current Treatment of Choice	Other Treatments
Head and neck cancer	**Combination chemotherapy:** Cisplatin, fluorouracil Paclitaxel, carboplatin Docetaxel, cisplatin, fluorouracil Cisplatin or cetuximab with radiation therapy	Hydroxyurea, bleomycin, methotrexate, cetuximab
Esophageal cancer	**Combination chemotherapy:** Cisplatin, fluorouracil	Paclitaxel, irinotecan, oxaliplatin, capecitabine, docetaxel, epirubicin
Uterine cancer	Progestins, tamoxifen, aromatase inhibitors **Combination chemotherapy:** Cisplatin, doxorubicin, paclitaxel Cisplatin, doxorubicin Carboplatin, paclitaxel	Fluorouracil
Ovarian cancer	**Combination chemotherapy:** Paclitaxel, carboplatin Intraperitoneal cisplatin, paclitaxel Docetaxel, carboplatin Paclitaxel, cisplatin	Gemcitabine, liposomal doxorubicin, topotecan, cyclophosphamide, etoposide, docetaxel
Cervical cancer	**With radiation:** Cisplatin **Combination chemotherapy:** Cisplatin, paclitaxel Cisplatin, topotecan Carboplatin, paclitaxel Cisplatin, gemcitabine	Docetaxel, ifosfamide, vinorelbine, irinotecan, epirubicin, mitomycin, fluorouracil
Breast cancer	**Adjuvant endocrine therapy:** Premenopausal: Tamoxifen Postmenopausal: Aromatase inhibitors (anastrozole, letrozol, exemestane) **Adjuvant chemotherapy (without trastuzumab):** Doxorubicin, cyclophosphamide, docetaxel Doxorubicin, cyclophosphamide, paclitaxel Docetaxel, cyclophosphamide Doxorubicin, cyclophosphamide **Adjuvant chemotherapy (with trastuzumab):** Doxorubicin, cyclophosphamide, paclitaxel, trastuzumab Docetaxel, carboplatin, trastuzumab	Megestrol, aminoglutethimide, capecitabine, mitoxantrone, cisplatin, etoposide, vinblastine, fluorouracil, ixabepilone, gemcitabine
Choriocarcinoma (trophoblastic neoplasms)	*Single agents:* Methotrexate or dactinomycin for low risk disease **Combination chemotherapy:** Etoposide/methotrexate, dactinomycin, cyclophosphamide, vincristine (EMA-CO) for high-risk disease	Vinblastine, cisplatin, mercaptopurine, chlorambucil, doxorubicin
Testicular cancer	**Combination chemotherapy:** Bleomycin, etoposide, cisplatin (BEP) Cisplatin, etoposide (EP)	Vinblastine, ifosfamide, paclitaxel, mesna
Kidney cancer	Sunitinib, temsirolimus, bevacizumab, sorafenib, interleukin-2	Interferon-α, vinblastine, capecitabine, fluorouracil
Bladder cancer	**Combination chemotherapy:** Gemcitabine, cisplatin	Carboplatin, paclitaxel, docetaxel, fluorouracil, pemetrexed, methotrexate
Prostate cancer	Luteinizing hormone-releasing agonist (leuprolide, goserelin, triptorelin) plus an antiandrogen (flutamide, bicalutamide, nilutamide)	Ketoconazole, docetaxel, mitoxantrone, estramustine, prednisone
Brain cancer (anaplastic astrocytoma and glioblastoma multiforme	Temozolomide	Bevacizumab, irinotecan, procarbazine, carmustine, lomustine
Neuroblastoma	**Combination chemotherapy:** Cyclophosphamide, doxorubicin, cisplatin, etoposide	Vincristine, topotecan, irinotecan, ifosfamide, carboplatin, 13-cis-retinoic acid, ^{131}I-MIBG, autologous or allogeneic transplantation
Thyroid cancer	Radioiodine (^{131}I), sorafenib	Doxorubicin, dacarbazine
Adrenal cancer	Mitotane	Doxorubicin, etoposide, cisplatin
Stomach cancer	**Combination chemotherapy:** Epirubicin, cisplatin, fluorouracil Docetaxel, cisplatin, fluorouracil Fluorouracil, leucovorin, oxaliplatin	Capecitabine, sorafenib

(continued)

Table 39–4. Treatment choices for cancers responsive to systemic agents. (continued)

Diagnosis	Current Treatment of Choice	Other Treatments
Pancreatic cancer	Combination chemotherapy: Gemcitabine, cisplatin; Gemcitabine, erlotinib; Gemcitabine	Capecitabine, fluorouracil, oxaliplatin
Colon cancer	Combination chemotherapy: Fluorouracil, leucovorin, oxaliplatin (FOLFOX6) Capecitabine, oxaliplatin (CapeOx) Fluorouracil, leucovorin, irinotecan (FOLFIRI); each regimen with or without bevacizumab	Cetuximab, irinotecan, panitumumab
Rectal cancer	Chemotherapy with radiation: Fluorouracil; for advanced disease same regimens used with colon cancer	Cetuximab, irinotecan, panitumumab
Anal cancer	Combination chemotherapy with radiation: Fluorouracil, mitomycin	Cisplatin
Carcinoid	Combination chemotherapy: Streptozocin, fluorouracil; Cisplatin, etoposide	Doxorubicin, dacarbazine, octreotide, interferon-α
Insulinoma	Interferon, streptozocin	Doxorubicin, fluorouracil, mitomycin
Osteogenic sarcoma	Combination chemotherapy with two of these agents: Doxorubicin, cisplatin, ifosfamide, high-dose methotrexate	Cyclophosphamide, dacarbazine
Soft tissue sarcomas	Combination chemotherapy: Doxorubicin, dacarbazine (AD) Doxorubicin, ifosfamide, mesna (AIM) Mesna, doxorubicin, ifosfamide, dacarbazine (MAID)	Liposomal doxorubicin, methotrexate, gemcitabine, docetaxel
Melanoma	Dacarbazine, temozolomide, high-dose interleukin-2	Paclitaxel, cisplatin, carboplatin, interferon-α, vinblastine
Hepatocellular cancer	Sorafenib	Doxorubicin
Kaposi sarcoma	Liposomal doxorubicin, liposomal daunorubicin	Paclitaxel, vinblastine, vincristine, etoposide, doxorubicin

Chronic alcohol and tobacco use are strongly associated with an increased risk of squamous cell carcinoma. The risk of squamous cell cancer is also increased in patients with tylosis, achalasia, caustic-induced esophageal stricture, and other head and neck cancers. Squamous cell cancer has a high incidence in certain regions of China and Southeast Asia. Half of all cases occur in the distal third of the esophagus. **Adenocarcinoma** is more common in whites. It is increasing dramatically in incidence and now is as common as squamous carcinoma. The majority of adenocarcinomas develop as a complication of Barrett metaplasia due to chronic gastroesophageal reflux. Thus, most adenocarcinomas arise in the distal third of the esophagus. Obesity also is strongly associated with adenocarcinoma, even after controlling for gastroesophageal reflux; however, no causal relationship has been convincingly shown.

Clinical Findings

A. Symptoms and Signs

Most patients with esophageal cancer present with advanced, incurable disease. Over 90% have solid food dysphagia, which progresses over weeks to months. Odynophagia is sometimes present. Significant weight loss is common. Local tumor extension into the tracheobronchial tree may result in a tracheoesophageal fistula, characterized by coughing on swallowing or pneumonia. Chest or back pain suggests mediastinal extension. Recurrent laryngeal involvement may produce hoarseness. Physical examination is often unrevealing. The presence of supraclavicular or cervical lymphadenopathy or of hepatomegaly implies metastatic disease.

B. Laboratory Findings

Laboratory findings are nonspecific. Anemia related to chronic disease or occult blood loss is common. Elevated aminotransferase or alkaline phosphatase concentrations suggest hepatic or bony metastases. Hypoalbuminemia may result from malnutrition.

C. Imaging

Chest radiographs may show adenopathy, a widened mediastinum, pulmonary or bony metastases, or signs of tracheoesophageal fistula such as pneumonia. A barium esophagogram may be the first study obtained to evaluate dysphagia. The appearance of a polypoid, infiltrative, or ulcerative lesion is suggestive of carcinoma and requires endoscopic evaluation. However, even lesions believed to be benign by radiography warrant endoscopic evaluation.

D. Upper Endoscopy

Endoscopy with biopsy establishes the diagnosis of esophageal carcinoma with a high degree of reliability. In some cases, significant submucosal spread of the tumor may yield nondiagnostic mucosal biopsies. Repeated biopsy may be necessary.

Staging

After confirmation of the diagnosis of esophageal carcinoma, the stage of the disease should be determined since doing so influences the choice of therapy. Patients should undergo evaluation with CT of the chest and abdomen to look for evidence of pulmonary or hepatic metastases, lymphadenopathy, and local tumor extension. If there is no evidence of distant metastases or extensive local spread on CT, endoscopic ultrasonography with guided FNA biopsy of lymph nodes should be performed, which is superior to CT in demonstrating the level of local mediastinal extension and local lymph node involvement. PET with fluorodeoxyglucose or integrated PET-CT imaging is more sensitive (and expensive) than CT for detection of distant metastasis. It is increasingly used to look for regional or distant spread in patients thought to have localized disease after other diagnostic studies. Bronchoscopy is sometimes required in proximal esophageal cancer to exclude tracheobronchial extension. Apart from distant metastasis (M1b), the two most important predictors of poor survival are adjacent mediastinal spread (T4) and lymph node involvement. Whereas cure may be achieved in patients with regional lymph node involvement (stages IIB and III), involvement of nodes outside the chest (M1a) is indicative of metastatic disease (stage IV) that is incurable.

Differential Diagnosis

Esophageal carcinoma must be distinguished from other causes of progressive dysphagia, including peptic stricture, achalasia, and adenocarcinoma of the gastric cardia with esophageal involvement. Benign-appearing peptic strictures should be biopsied at presentation to exclude occult malignancy.

Treatment

The approach to esophageal cancer depends on the tumor stage, patient preference and functional status, and the expertise of the attending surgeons, oncologists, gastroenterologists, and radiotherapists. There is no consensus about the optimal treatment approach. It is helpful, however, to classify patients into two general categories.

A. Therapy for "Curable" Disease

Superficial esophageal cancers confined to the epithelium (high-grade dysplasia or carcinoma in situ [Tis]), lamina propria (T1a), or submucosal (T1b) are increasingly recognized in endoscopic screening and surveillance programs. Esophagectomy achieves high cure rates but is associated with mortality (2%) and morbidity. If performed by experienced physicians, endoscopic mucosal resection of superficial cancers (especially Tis and T1a) achieves equivalent long-term survival with less morbidity. For a full discussion of management options in superficial adenocarcinoma, see the section on Barrett Esophagus in Chapter 15. The management of other invasive but potentially "curable" esophageal cancers (stage I, II, or IIIA) is controversial and depends on institutional experience.

1. Surgery with or without neoadjuvant chemoradiation therapy—There is debate over the optimal surgical approach. The procedure with the lowest morbidity is transhiatal esophagectomy with anastomosis of the stomach to the cervical esophagus; however, this approach does not involve sampling or removal of mediastinal lymph nodes. Alternatively, surgeons may perform en bloc transthoracic excision of the esophagus with extended dissection of lymph nodes in the mediastinum and upper abdomen. In a randomized controlled trial comparing these two approaches, en bloc resection was associated with higher perioperative morbidity but a nonsignificant trend toward improved 5-year survival (39% vs 27%). Transhiatal resection may be more appropriate for patients who are elderly or have comorbid illness, and en bloc resection more appropriate in younger or healthier patients with a better prognosis.

Patients without regional lymph node spread (stage I and stage IIA) have high cure rates with surgery alone and require no other radiation or chemotherapy. If regional lymph node metastases have occurred (stage IIB and stage IIIA), the rate of cure with surgery alone is reduced to less than 20%. Meta-analysis of trials comparing neoadjuvant therapy followed by surgery with surgery alone suggests a 13% absolute improvement in 2-year survival with combined therapy. Therefore, in many centers, preoperative (neoadjuvant) chemoradiation therapy is recommended. The most commonly used chemotherapeutic agents are cisplatin and 5-fluorouracil (5-FU), although the optimal regimen is unclear. Furthermore, the superiority of this combined approach compared with surgery alone, or surgery with postoperative adjuvant chemotherapy is unproven.

2. Chemotherapy plus radiation therapy without surgery—Combined treatment with chemotherapy and radiation therapy is superior to radiation therapy alone and has achieved long-term survival rates in up to 25% of patients. In two randomized trials, there was no difference in long-term survival between patients treated with chemoradiation therapy alone versus chemoradiation therapy followed by surgery, although combination therapy achieves superior control of mediastinal disease with a reduced need for subsequent palliative therapies. Chemoradiation therapy alone should be considered in patients with localized disease (stage II or IIIA) who are poor surgical candidates due to serious medical illness or poor functional status (Eastern Cooperative Oncology Group score > 2).

B. Therapy for Incurable Disease

More than half of patients have either locally extensive tumor spread (T4) that is unresectable or distant metastases (M1) ie, stage IIIB and stage IV tumors. Surgery is not warranted in these patients. Since prolonged survival can be achieved in few patients, the primary goal is to provide relief from dysphagia and pain, optimize quality of life, and minimize treatment side effects. The optimal palliative approach depends on the presence or absence of metastatic disease, patient's expected survival, patient preference, and local institutional experience. Many patients with advanced disease may prefer concerted efforts at pain relief and care directed at symptom management (see Chapter 5).

1. Radiation therapy, chemotherapy, and combined therapy—Combined radiation therapy and chemotherapy (5-FU and cisplatin) may achieve palliation in two-thirds of patients but is associated with significant side effects. It should be considered for patients with locally advanced tumors without distant metastases (stage IIIB) who have good functional status, no significant medical problems, in whom prolonged survival may be achieved. Improvement in dysphagia occurs within 2–4 weeks in almost 90% of patients.

Combination chemotherapy may be considered in patients with metastatic disease who still have good functional status and expected survival of several months. Although there is no consensus on optimal therapy, three drug combinations are commonly used: (1) epirubicin or a taxane (docetaxel or paclitaxel), (2) cisplatin or oxaliplatin, and (3) a fluoropyrimidine (5-FU or capecitabine). For patients with poor functional status, single-agent therapy with a fluoropyrimidine, a taxane, or irinotecan may be used. The role of biologic agents (anti-EGFR, anti-VEGF, kinase inhibitors) requires further study.

Radiation therapy alone may afford short-term relief of pain and dysphagia and may be suitable for patients with poor functional status or underlying medical problems. Because it takes up to 6 weeks to administer and may be complicated by temporary worsening of dysphagia and odynophagia, local antitumor therapies may be preferred.

2. Local antitumor therapy—Patients with advanced esophageal cancer often have a poor functional and nutritional status with an average survival of less than 12 weeks from diagnosis. Radiation or chemoradiation is poorly tolerated. Rapid palliation of dysphagia may be achieved by peroral placement of permanent expandable wire stents, application of endoscopic laser therapy, or photodynamic therapy. Although dysphagia and quality of life are improved significantly, patients can seldom eat normally. The choice of treatment depends on available expertise and equipment. Stents are most commonly used because of their relative ease of placement.

▶ Prognosis

The overall 5-year survival rate of esophageal carcinoma is less than 20%. For those patients whose disease progresses despite chemotherapy, meticulous efforts at palliative care are essential (see Chapter 5).

▶ When to Refer

- Patients should be referred to gastroenterologist for evaluation and staging (endoscopy with biopsy, EUS) and palliative endoscopic antitumor therapy (stent).
- Patients with curable and resectable disease (stage IIB or IIIA) and those with locally advanced or metastatic disease should be referred to an oncologist for consideration of neoadjuvant chemotherapy or consideration of chemoradiotherapy or palliative chemotherapy, respectively.

▶ When to Admit

Patients with high-grade esophageal obstruction with inability to manage oral secretions should be admitted.

Cunningham D et al; Upper Gastrointestinal Clinical Studies Group of the National Cancer Research Institute of the United Kingdom. Capecitabine and oxaliplatin for advanced esophagogastric cancer. N Engl J Med. 2008 Jan 3;358(1):36–46. [PMID: 18172173]

Gebski V et al. Survival benefits from neoadjuvant chemoradiotherapy or chemotherapy in oesophageal carcinoma: a meta-analysis. Lancet Oncol. 2007 Mar;8(3):226–34. [PMID: 17329193]

Kelsen DP et al. Long-term results of RTOG trial 8911 (USA Intergroup 113): a random assignment trial comparison of chemotherapy followed by surgery compared with surgery alone for esophageal cancer. J Clin Oncol. 2007 Aug 20; 25(24):3719–25. [PMID: 17704421]

Mariette C et al. Therapeutic strategies in oesophageal carcinoma: role of surgery and other modalities. Lancet Oncol. 2007 Jun;8(6):545–53. [PMID: 17540306]

Umar SB et al. Esophageal cancer: epidemiology, pathogenesis and prevention. Nat Clin Pract Gastroenterol Hepatol. 2008 Sep;5(9):517–26. [PMID: 18679388]

GASTRIC ADENOCARCINOMA

 ESSENTIALS OF DIAGNOSIS

- ▶ Dyspeptic symptoms with weight loss in patients over age 40 years.
- ▶ Iron deficiency anemia: occult blood in stools.
- ▶ Abnormality detected on upper gastrointestinal series or endoscopy.

▶ General Considerations

Gastric adenocarcinoma remains the second most common cause of cancer death worldwide. Its incidence however has declined rapidly over the last 70 years, especially in western countries, which may be attributable to changes in diet (more fruits and vegetables), food refrigeration (allowing more fresh foods and reduced salted, smoked, and preserved foods), reduced toxic environmental exposures, and a decline in *Helicobacter pylori*. The incidence of gastric cancer remains high (70/100,000) in Japan and many developing regions, including eastern Asia, Eastern Europe, Chile, Colombia, and Central America. In the United States, there were an estimated 21,500 new cases and 10,800 deaths in 2008. The incidence is higher in Latinos, African Americans, and Asian Americans.

There are two main histologic variants of gastric cancer: "intestinal-type" (which resembles intestinal cancers in forming glandular structures) and "diffuse" (which is poorly differentiated, has signet-ring cells, and lacks glandular formation). Although both types are declining in incidence, intestinal-type has had the most dramatic reduction. Intestinal-type is still more common (70–80%), occurs twice as often in men as women, primarily affects older people (mean age 63 years), and is more strongly associated with environmental factors. It is believed to arise through a gradual, multi-step progression from inflammation (most commonly due to *H pylori*), to atrophic gastritis, to intestinal metaplasia, and finally dysplasia or cancer. Chronic *H pylori* gastritis is the strong risk factor for gastric carcinoma, increasing the relative risk 3.5- to 20-fold. It is estimated that 60–90% of cases of gastric carcinomas may be attributable to *H pylori*. Because of its unproven efficacy and cost-effectiveness, screening for *H pylori* infection and treating it to prevent gastric cancer is not recommended for asymptomatic adults in the general population but may be considered in patients who have immigrated from regions with a high incidence of gastric cancer or who have a family history of gastric cancer. Other risk factors for intestinal-type gastric cancer include pernicious anemia, a history of partial gastric resection more than 15 years previously, smoking, and diets that are high in nitrates or salt and low in vitamin C.

Diffuse gastric cancer accounts for 20–30% of gastric cancer. In contrast to intestinal-type cancer, it affects men and women equally, occurs more commonly in young people, is not as strongly related to *H pylori* infection, has a worse prognosis, and has not declined in incidence. Most diffuse gastric cancers are attributable to acquired or hereditary mutations in the genes regulating the E-cadherin cell adhesion protein. Familial diffuse gastric cancer accounts for 1–3% of gastric cancers. The cancer may arise at a young age, is often multifocal and infiltrating, and carries a poor prognosis. Many of these families have a germline mutation of E-cadherin *CDH1,* which is inherited in an autosomal dominant pattern and carries a greater than 60% lifetime risk of gastric cancer.

Most gastric cancers arise in the body and antrum. These may occur in a variety of morphologic types: (1) polypoid or fungating intraluminal masses; (2) ulcerating masses; (3) diffusely spreading (linitis plastica), in which the tumor spreads through the submucosa, resulting in a rigid, atonic stomach with thickened folds (prognosis dismal); and (4) superficially spreading or "early" gastric cancer—confined to the mucosa or submucosa (with or without lymph node metastases) and associated with an excellent prognosis.

In contrast to the dramatic decline in cancers of the distal stomach, a rise in incidence of tumors of the gastric cardia has been noted. These tumors have demographic and pathologic features that resemble Barrett-associated esophageal adenocarcinomas (see Esophageal Cancer).

▶ Clinical Findings

A. Symptoms and Signs

Gastric carcinoma is generally asymptomatic until the disease is quite advanced. Symptoms are nonspecific and are determined in part by the location of the tumor. Dyspepsia, vague epigastric pain, anorexia, early satiety, and weight loss are the presenting symptoms in most patients. Patients may derive initial symptomatic relief from over-the-counter remedies, further delaying diagnosis. Ulcerating lesions can lead to acute gastrointestinal bleeding with hematemesis or melena. Pyloric obstruction results in postprandial vomiting. Lower esophageal obstruction causes

progressive dysphagia. Physical examination is rarely helpful. A gastric mass is palpated in less than 20% of patients. Signs of metastatic spread include a left supraclavicular lymph node (Virchow node), an umbilical nodule (Sister Mary Joseph nodule), a rigid rectal shelf (Blumer shelf), and ovarian metastases (Krukenberg tumor). Guaiac-positive stools may be detectable.

B. Laboratory Findings

Iron deficiency anemia due to chronic blood loss or anemia of chronic disease is common. Liver function test abnormalities may be present if there is metastatic liver spread. Other tumor markers are of no value.

C. Endoscopy

Upper endoscopy should be obtained in all patients over age 55 years with new onset of epigastric symptoms (dyspepsia) and in anyone with dyspepsia that is persistent or fails to respond to a short trial of antisecretory therapy. Endoscopy with biopsies of suspicious lesions is highly sensitive for detecting gastric carcinoma. It can be difficult to obtain adequate biopsy specimens in linitis plastica lesions. Because of the high incidence of gastric carcinoma in Japan, screening upper endoscopy is performed to detect early gastric carcinoma. Approximately 40% of tumors detected by screening are early, with a 5-year survival rate of almost 90%. Screening programs are not recommended in the United States.

D. Imaging

A barium upper gastrointestinal series is an acceptable alternative when endoscopy is not readily available but may not detect small or superficial lesions and cannot reliably distinguish benign from malignant ulcerations. Any abnormalities detected with this procedure require endoscopic confirmation.

Once a gastric cancer is diagnosed, preoperative evaluation with abdominal and chest CT and EUS is indicated to delineate the local extent of the primary tumor as well as nodal or distant metastases. PET or combined PET-CT imaging may be more sensitive than CT for detection of distant metastasis. EUS imaging is superior to CT in determining the depth of tumor penetration and is useful for evaluation of early gastric cancers that may be removed by endoscopic mucosal resection.

▶ Staging

Staging is defined according to the TNM system, in which T1 tumors invade the lamina propria (T1a) or submucosa (T1b), T2 invade the muscularis propria, T3 penetrate the serosa, and T4 invade adjacent structures. Lymph nodes are graded as N0 if there is no involvement, and N1, N2, or N3 if there are is involvement of 1–6, 7–15, or more than 15 regional nodes. M1 signifies the presence of metastatic disease.

▶ Differential Diagnosis

Ulcerating gastric adenocarcinomas are distinguished from benign gastric ulcers by biopsies. Approximately 3% of gastric ulcers initially believed to be benign later prove to be malignant. To exclude malignancy, all gastric ulcers identified at endoscopy should be biopsied. Ulcers that are suspicious for malignancy to the endoscopist or that have atypia or dysplasia on histologic examination warrant repeat endoscopy in 2–3 months to verify healing and exclude malignancy. Nonhealing ulcers should be considered for resection. Infiltrative carcinoma with thickened gastric folds must be distinguished from lymphoma and other hypertrophic gastropathies.

Treatment

A. Curative Surgical Resection

After preoperative staging, about two-thirds of patients will be found to have localized disease (ie, stages I–III). In Japan and in specialized centers in the United States, endoscopic mucosal resection is performed in selected patients with small (< 1–2 cm), early (intramucosal or T1aN0) gastric cancers after careful staging with EUS. For all other patients, surgical resection is the only therapy with curative potential. At surgery, approximately 25% of these patients will be found to have locally unresectable tumors or peritoneal, hepatic, or distant lymph node metastases for which "curative" surgical resection is not warranted (see below). The remaining patients with confirmed localized disease should undergo radical surgical resection with curative intent. For adenocarcinoma localized to the distal two-thirds of the stomach, a subtotal distal gastrectomy should be performed. For proximal gastric cancer or diffusely infiltrating disease, total gastrectomy is necessary. Although lymph node dissection should be performed for curative resections, there has been ongoing debate about whether an extended (perigastric; D1), regional (D2), or distant (porta hepatic and periaortic; D3) lymph node dissection is needed. A 2008 large Japanese trial found no difference in survival between patients treated with D2 and D3 (para-aortic) lymphadenectomy. Current NCCN treatment guidelines recommend regional (D2) node resection. The role of preoperative (neoadjuvant) or postoperative (adjuvant) chemotherapy or radiochemotherapy after curative resection is controversial. In the United States, adjuvant chemoradiotherapy (commonly 5-FU and leucovorin) is recommended, especially for patients with lymph node involvement. Outside of the United States, adjuvant chemotherapy alone (commonly, epirubicin, cisplatin, and 5-FU) is used. Tumors arising in the cardia are treated similar to esophageal cancer.

B. Palliative Modalities

Many patients will be found either preoperatively or at the time of surgical exploration to have advanced disease that is not amenable to "curative" surgery due to peritoneal or distant metastases or local invasion of other organs. In some of these cases, palliative resection of the tumor nonetheless may be indicated to alleviate pain, bleeding, or obstruction. For patients with unresectable disease, gastrojejunostomy may be indicated to prevent obstruction. Alternatively, unresected tumors may be treated with endoscopic laser or stent therapy, radiation therapy, or angiographic embolization to relieve bleeding or obstruction. Chemotherapy may

be considered in patients with metastatic disease who still have good functional status and expected survival of several months. Although there is no consensus on optimal therapy, a combination of epirubicin, cisplatin, and 5-FU commonly is used. A large 2008 trial assigned patients with advanced esophageal and gastric cancer to one of four triplet therapies: epirubicin and cisplatin plus either fluorouracil (ECF) or capecitabine (ECX) or epirubicin and oxaliplatin plus either fluorouracil (EOF) or capecitabine (EOX). No difference in median survival was found among the four regimens (9-11 months); however, toxicity in patients treated with oxaliplatin.

Prognosis

The long-term survival of gastric carcinoma is less than 15%. However, 5-year survival in patients who undergo successful curative resection is over 45%. Survival is related to tumor stage, location, and histologic features. Stage I and stage II tumors resected for cure have a greater than 50% long-term survival. Patients with stage III tumors have a poor prognosis (< 20% long-term survival) and should be considered for enrollment in clinical trials. Tumors of the diffuse type have a worse prognosis than the intestinal type. Tumors of the proximal stomach (fundus and cardia) carry a far worse prognosis than distal lesions. Even with apparently localized disease, proximal tumors have a 5-year survival of less than 15%. For those whose disease progresses despite therapy, meticulous efforts at palliative care are essential (see Chapter 5).

When to Refer

- Patients with dysphagia, weight loss, protracted vomiting, iron-deficiency anemia, or new-onset of dyspepsia (especially if age 55 years or older or associated with other alarm symptoms) in whom gastric cancer is suspected should be referred to a gastroenterologist for endoscopic screening.

- Patients should be referred to a surgeon for attempt at curative resection in stage I, II, or III cancer.

- Patients with unresectable or metastatic disease should be referred to an oncologist for consideration of adjuvant chemotherapy or chemoradiotherapy after curative resection or palliative therapy.

When to Admit

Patients with advanced gastric cancer causing protracted vomiting, inability to maintain oral intake, or acute bleeding should be admitted.

Correa P et al. Carcinogenesis of *Helicobacter pylori*. Gastroenterology. 2007 Aug;133(2):659–72. [PMID: 17681184]

Cunningham D et al; Upper Gastrointestinal Clinical Studies Group of the National Cancer Research Institute of the United Kingdom. Capecitabine and oxaliplatin for advanced esophagogastric cancer. N Engl J Med. 2008 Jan 3;358(1):36–46. [PMID: 18172173]

Kim JH et al. Metallic stent placement in the palliative treatment of malignant gastroduodenal obstructions: prospective evaluation of results and factors influencing outcome in 213 patients. Gastrointest Endosc. 2007 Aug;66(2):256–64. [PMID: 17643698]

McColl KE et al. Sporadic gastric cancer; a complex interaction of genetic and environmental risk factors. Am J Gastroenterol. 2007 Sep;102(9):1893–5. [PMID: 17727430]

Rivera F et al. Chemotherapy of advanced gastric cancer. Cancer Treat Rev. 2007 Jun;33(4):315–24. [PMID: 17376598]

Rogers WM et al. Risk-reducing total gastrectomy for germline mutations in E-cadherin (CDH1): pathologic findings with clinical implications. Am J Surg Pathol. 2008 Jun;32(6):799–809. [PMID: 18391748]

Sasako M et al; Japan Clinical Oncology Group. D2 lymphadenectomy alone or with para-aortic nodal dissection for gastric cancer. N Engl J Med. 2008 Jul 31;359(5):453–62. [PMID: 18669424]

GASTRIC LYMPHOMA

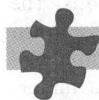 ESSENTIALS OF DIAGNOSIS

▶ Symptoms of dyspepsia, weight loss, or anemia.

▶ Variable abnormalities on upper gastrointestinal series or endoscopy including thickened folds, ulcer, mass or infiltrating lesions; diagnosis established by endoscopic biopsy.

▶ Abdominal CT and EUS required for staging.

General Considerations

Gastric lymphomas may be primary (arising from the gastric mucosa) or may represent a site of secondary involvement in patients with nodal lymphomas. Distinguishing advanced primary gastric lymphoma with adjacent nodal spread from advanced nodal lymphoma with secondary gastric spread can be problematic. Because the prognosis and treatment of primary and secondary gastric lymphomas are entirely different, the distinction is important. Primary lymphoma is the second most common gastric malignancy, accounting for 3% of cancers. More than 95% of these are non-Hodgkin B cell lymphomas. Most primary gastric lymphomas are believed to arise from mucosa-associated lymphoid tissue (MALT). Primary gastric lymphomas comprise two main types: 60% are diffuse large B-cell lymphomas (previously called "high-grade" MALT lymphomas) and 40% are marginal zone B-cell lymphomas of the MALT-type (previously call "low-grade" MALT lymphoma). B cells of nodal origin may be distinguished from those derived from MALT (CD19 and CD20 positive).

Infection with *H pylori* is an important risk factor for the development of primary gastric lymphoma. Chronic infection with *H pylori* causes an intense lymphocytic inflammatory response that may lead to the development of lymphoid follicles. Over 85% of low-grade primary gastric MALT-type lymphomas are associated with *H pylori* infection. It is hypothesized that chronic antigenic stimulation may result in a monoclonal lymphoproliferation that may culminate in low-grade or high-grade lymphoma.

Clinical Findings

The clinical presentation and endoscopic appearance of gastric lymphoma are similar to those of adenocarcinoma.

Most patients have abdominal pain, weight loss, or bleeding. Patients with diffuse large B-cell lymphoma are more likely to have systemic symptoms and advanced tumor stage. At endoscopy, lymphoma may appear as an ulcer, mass, or diffusely infiltrating lesion. The diagnosis is established with endoscopic biopsy. All patients should undergo staging with abdominal and chest CT. EUS is the most sensitive test for determining the level of invasion and presence of perigastric lymphadenopathy.

Treatment

Nodal lymphomas with secondary gastrointestinal involvement usually present at an advanced stage with widely disseminated disease and are seldom curable. Their treatment is addressed in Chapter 13. Treatment of primary gastric lymphomas depends on the tumor histology, grade, and stage. Marginal B-cell lymphomas of the MALT type may be low-grade and localized to the stomach wall (stage IE) and have an excellent prognosis. Where available, EUS should be performed to accurately determine tumor stage. Patients with primary gastric MALT-lymphoma should be tested for *H pylori* infection and treated if positive. Complete lymphoma regression after successful *H pylori* eradication occurs in 75% of cases of stage IE low-grade lymphoma. Remission may take as long as a year. Patients with localized (stage IE) marginal zone MALT-type lymphomas who either are not infected with *H pylori* or do not respond to eradication therapy may be treated with radiation therapy. Patients with diffuse large cell (high-grade) lymphomas and patients with MALT-type lymphomas that extend beyond the gastric wall should be treated with combination chemotherapy (eg, CHOP with rituximab). Because of a low risk of perforation with either radiation therapy or chemotherapy, surgical resection is no longer recommended. The long-term survival of primary gastric lymphoma for stage I is over 85% and for stage II is 35–65%.

Ferrucci PF et al. Primary gastric lymphoma pathogenesis and treatment: what has changed over the past 10 years? Br J Haematol. 2007 Feb;136(4):521–38. [PMID: 17156403]

Fischbach W et al; EGILS (European Gastro-Intestinal Lymphoma Study) Group. Most patients with minimal histological residuals of gastric MALT lymphoma after successful eradication *Helicobacter pylori* can be safely managed by a watch-and-wait strategy: experience from a large international series. Gut. 2007 Dec;56(12):1685–7. [PMID: 17639089]

Morgner A et al. Therapy of gastric mucosa associated lymphoid tissue lymphoma. World J Gastroenterol. 2007 Jul 14;13(26):3554–66. [PMID: 17659705]

GASTRIC CARCINOID TUMORS

Gastric carcinoids are rare neuroendocrine tumors that make up less than 1% of gastric neoplasms. They may occur sporadically or secondary to chronic hypergastrinemia that results in hyperplasia and transformation of enterochromaffin cells in the gastric fundus. Sporadic carcinoids account for 20% of gastric carcinoids. Most are solitary, over 2 cm in size, and have a strong propensity for metastatic spread. Most sporadic carcinoids already have carcinoid syndrome and hepatic or pulmonary metastatic involvement at initial presentation. Localized sporadic carcinoids should be treated with radical gastrectomy.

The majority of carcinoids caused by hypergastrinemia occur in association with either pernicious anemia (75%) or Zollinger-Ellison syndrome (5%). Carcinoids associated with Zollinger-Ellison syndrome occur almost exclusively in patients with MEN 1, in which loss of 11q13 has been reported. Carcinoids caused by hypergastrinemia tend to be multicentric, less than 1 cm in size, and have a low potential for metastatic spread or development of carcinoid syndrome. Small lesions may be successfully treated with endoscopic resection followed by periodic endoscopic surveillance. Antrectomy reduces serum gastrin levels and may lead to regression of small tumors. Patients with large or multiple carcinoids should undergo surgical tumor resection (see Carcinoid Tumors, below).

Landry CS et al. A proposed staging system for gastric carcinoid tumors based on an analysis of 1,543 patients. Ann Surg Oncol. 2009 Jan;16(1):51–60. [PMID: 18953609]

GASTROINTESTINAL MESENCHYMAL TUMORS

Gastrointestinal mesenchymal tumors occur throughout the gastrointestinal tract, but approximately two-thirds occur in the stomach. These tumors (which include stromal tumors, leiomyomas, and schwannomas) derive from mesenchymal stem cells and have an epithelioid or spindle cell histologic pattern, resembling smooth muscle. The most common stromal tumors are gastrointestinal stromal tumors ("GISTs"), which appear to originate from interstitial cells of Cajal. GISTs occur throughout the gastrointestinal tract but most commonly in the stomach (50%) and small intestine (30%). About 85–90% of GISTs have mutations in KIT, a receptor tyrosine kinase that binds stem cell factor, or a homologous tyrosine kinase, platelet-derived growth factor alpha that lead to constitutive activation. Approximately 90% of stromal tumors stain positively for CD117 (part of the KIT protein). Other mesenchymal tumors such as leiomyomas, which derive from smooth muscle cells, stain negative for CD117. Mesenchymal tumors may be discovered incidentally on imaging studies or endoscopy or may cause symptoms, mainly obstruction by large tumors or acute or chronic bleeding due to central ulceration within the tumor. At endoscopy, they appear as a submucosal mass that may have central umbilication or ulceration. EUS (possibly with guided FNA biopsy) is the optimal study for diagnosing mesenchymal tumors and distinguishing them from other submucosal lesions. While almost all GISTs have malignant potential, the risk of developing metastasis is related to the tumor size and mitotic index (> 5 mitoses per high-powered field); however, mitotic index can only be assessed after resection. It is difficult to distinguish with certainty benign from malignant (sarcoma) tumors before resection by EUS appearance or FNA. In general, lesions that are smaller than 2 cm, have a smooth border, and have a homogeneous echo pattern on EUS are more likely benign.

Surgery is recommended for all patients with tumors that are symptomatic, ≥ 2 cm, are increasing in size, or have an EUS appearance suspicious for malignancy. PET-CT scan should be obtained prior to surgery to look for metastatic disease. The management of asymptomatic benign-appearing lesions ≤ 2 cm in size is problematic. Because of a low risk of malignancy, surgical resection should be considered in younger, otherwise healthy patients; however, other patients may be followed up with serial EUS examinations or, in selected cases, endoscopic resections. There is a high risk of metastasis or recurrence when tumors are larger than 5 cm, have an irregular border or cystic spaces, and have increased mitotic activity (more than five mitoses per high-power field). These high-risk tumors have a 50% 5-year survival rate after complete surgical resection. Metastatic tumors are aggressive and carry a poor prognosis. The tyrosine kinase inhibitor imatinib induces disease control in up to 85% of patients with metastatic disease with a progression free-survival of 20–24 months. Resistant tumors may respond to another tyrosine kinase inhibitor, sunitinib.

Badalamenti G et al. Gastrointestinal stromal tumors (GISTs): focus on histopathological diagnosis and biomolecular features. Ann Oncol. 2007 Jun;18 (Suppl 6):vi136–40. [PMID: 17591808]

Heinrich MC et al. Primary and secondary kinase genotypes correlate with the biological and clinical activity of sunitinib in imatinib-resistant gastrointestinal stromal tumor. J Clin Oncol. 2008 Nov 20;26(33):5352–9. [PMID: 18955458]

Rubin BP et al. Gastrointestinal stromal tumour. Lancet. 2007 May 19;369(9574):1731–41. [PMID: 17512858]

MALIGNANCIES OF THE SMALL INTESTINE

1. Adenocarcinoma

These are aggressive tumors that occur most commonly in the duodenum or proximal jejunum. The ampulla of Vater is the most common site of small bowel carcinoma, and the incidence of ampullary carcinoma is increased more than 200-fold in patients with FAP. Ampullary carcinoma may present with jaundice due to bile duct obstruction or bleeding. Surgical resection of early lesions is curative in up to 40% of patients. Periodic endoscopic surveillance to detect early ampullary neoplasms therefore is recommended in patients with this disorder. Nonampullary adenocarcinoma of the small intestine accounts for < 3% of all gastrointestinal cancers but one-third of small bowel cancers. Peak incidence is in the sixth decade. Most cases present with symptoms of obstruction, acute or chronic bleeding, or weight loss. The majority of small bowel cancers have already metastasized at the time of diagnosis. Resection is recommended for control of symptoms. The role of adjuvant therapy is unclear. The prognosis is poor with a 5-year overall survival of 20–30%. Patients with Crohn disease have an increased risk of small intestine adenocarcinoma, most commonly in the ileum, which may be difficult to distinguish from disease-related fibrous strictures.

2. Lymphoma

Gastrointestinal lymphomas may arise in the gastrointestinal tract or involve it secondarily with disseminated disease. In Western countries, primary gastrointestinal lymphomas account for 5% of lymphomas and 20% of small bowel malignancies. They occur most commonly in the distal small intestine. The majority are non-Hodgkin high-grade marginal zone B cell lymphomas. There is an increased incidence of small intestinal lymphomas in patients with AIDS, immunosuppressive therapy, and Crohn disease. T cell lymphomas may arise in patients with celiac sprue. In the Middle East, lymphomas may arise in the setting of immunoproliferative small intestinal disease. In this condition, there is diffuse lymphoplasmacytic infiltration with IgA-secreting B lymphocytes of the mucosa and submucosa that results in weight loss, diarrhea, and malabsorption, which may lead to lymphomatous transformation. A characteristic feature of the disease is the presence of α heavy chains in the serum in 70% produced by clones of IgA plasma cells. Other types of intestinal lymphomas include mantle cell and Burkitt.

Presenting symptoms or signs of primary lymphoma include abdominal pain, weight loss, nausea and vomiting, distention, anemia, and occult blood in the stool. Fevers are unusual. Protein-losing enteropathy may result in hypoalbuminemia, but other signs of malabsorption are unusual. Barium radiography or CT enterography helps localize the site of the lesion. The diagnosis requires endoscopic, percutaneous, or laparoscopic biopsy. To determine tumor stage, patients must undergo chest and abdominal CT, and bone marrow biopsy.

Treatment depends on the tumor histologic grade and stage of disease. Resection of primary intestinal lymphoma, if feasible, is usually recommended. Even in cases of stage III or stage IV disease, surgical debulking may improve survival. In patients with limited disease (stage IE) in whom resection is performed, the role of adjuvant chemotherapy is unclear. Most patients with more extensive disease are treated with combination chemotherapy (eg, CHOP with rituximab) with or without radiation therapy.

3. Carcinoid Tumors

ESSENTIALS OF DIAGNOSIS

▶ Majority are asymptomatic and discovered incidentally at endoscopy or surgery

▶ Carcinoid syndrome occurs in less than 10%; hepatic metastases are generally present.

▶ Risk of metastasis related to tumor size and location.

▶ General Considerations

Gastrointestinal carcinoids are slow growing neuroendocrine tumors that may arise anywhere in the gastrointestinal tract but most commonly occur in the small intestine (30%), rectum (12%), colon (8%), appendix (8%), and stomach (10–30%; see above). Carcinoids may contain a variety of hormones, including serotonin, somatostatin, gastrin, and substance P that may or may not be secreted, and usually display immunoreactivity to chromogranin A.

Although many carcinoids behave in an indolent fashion, the overall 5-year survival rate for patients with carcinoids is 50%, suggesting that most are malignant. The risk of metastatic spread is closely related to tumor size and tumor location. Many small carcinoids are detected incidentally at endoscopy or autopsy. It is not possible by histologic examination to distinguish benign from malignant disease. The best indicator of prognosis is evidence of invasive growth and the presence of regional or distant metastasis.

Carcinoids account for up to one-third of small intestinal tumors. Small intestinal carcinoids most commonly arise in the ileum. Up to one-third are multicentric. Although 60% are less than 2 cm in size, even these small carcinoids may metastasize. Almost all small intestinal carcinoids over 2 cm are associated with metastasis.

Appendiceal carcinoids are identified in 0.3% of appendectomies, usually as an incidental finding. Almost 80% of these tumors are less than 1 cm in size, and 90% are less than 2 cm. Rectal carcinoids are usually detected incidentally as submucosal nodules during proctoscopic examination. Rectal carcinoids less than 1 cm and appendiceal carcinoids less than 2 cm virtually never metastasize and are treated effectively with local excision or simple appendectomy. Tumors larger than 2 cm are associated with the development of metastasis in over 20% of appendiceal carcinoids and 10% of rectal carcinoids. Hence, in younger patients who are good candidates for surgery, a more extensive cancer resection operation is warranted.

▶ Clinical Findings

A. Symptoms and Signs

Most smaller lesions (less than 1-2 cm) are asymptomatic and difficult to detect by endoscopy or imaging studies. When carcinoids present with symptoms, most are at an advanced and incurable stage. Through local extension or metastasis to mesenteric lymph nodes, carcinoids engender a fibroblastic reaction with contraction and kinking of the bowel or encasement of mesenteric vessels. Small intestinal carcinoids may present with abdominal pain, bowel obstruction, or bowel infarction. Abdominal CT or enterography may reveal kinking, but because the lesion is extraluminal the diagnosis may be overlooked for several years. Appendiceal and rectal carcinoids usually are small and asymptomatic but large lesions can cause bleeding, obstruction, or altered bowel habits. Carcinoid involvement of the heart (resulting in right-sided valvular lesions) is a late manifestation of metastatic disease. **Carcinoid syndrome** occurs in less than 10% of patients. More than 90% of patients with carcinoid syndrome have hepatic mestastases, usually from carcinoids of small bowel origin. About 10% of patients with carcinoid syndrome have primary bronchial or ovarian tumors without hepatic metastases. Carcinoid syndrome is caused by tumor secretion of hormonal mediators. The manifestations include facial flushing, edema of the head and neck (especially with bronchial carcinoid), abdominal cramps and diarrhea, bronchospasm, cardiac lesions (pulmonary or tricuspid stenosis or regurgitation), and telangiectases.

B. Laboratory Findings

Plasma chromogranin A (CgA) is the most sensitive screening test for small intestine carcinoids, although its sensitivity for small, localized tumors is unknown. CgA is elevated in almost 90% of patients with advanced small bowel carcinoid. Urinary 5-hydroxyindoleacetic acid (5-HIAA) or platelet serotonin levels are also elevated in patients with metastatic carcinoid; however, these tests are less sensitive than CgA. There is increased urinary 5-HIAA in carcinoid syndrome; symptomatic patients usually excrete more than 25 mg of 5-HIAA per day in the urine. Ideally, all drugs should be withheld for several days prior to the urine collection.

C. Imaging

Abdominal CT may demonstrate a mesenteric mass with tethering of the bowel, lymphadenopathy, and hepatic metastasis. Somatostatin receptor scintigraphy, which is positive in up to 90% of patients with metastatic carcinoid, is superior to all other imaging modalities for the diagnosis of primary and metastatic lesions. Almost all patients with carcinoid syndrome have obvious signs of cancer with liver metastasis on abdominal imaging.

► Treatment

Small intestinal carcinoids are extremely indolent tumors with slow spread. Patients with disease confined to the small intestine should have local excision, for which the cure rate exceeds 85%. In patients with resectable disease who have lymph node involvement, the 5-year disease-free survival is 80%; however, by 25 years, less than 25% remain disease free. Even patients with hepatic metastases may have an indolent course with a median survival of 3 years. In patients with advanced disease, therapy should be deferred until the patient is symptomatic. Surgery should be directed toward palliation of obstructive symptoms.

In patients with carcinoid syndrome, resection of hepatic metastases may provide dramatic improvement. The somatostatin analog octreotide (150–500 mcg subcutaneously three times daily) inhibits hormone secretion from the carcinoid tumor, resulting in dramatic relief of symptoms of carcinoid syndrome, including diarrhea or flushing, in 90% of patients for a median period of 1 year. Thereafter, many patients stop responding to octreotide. Hepatic artery occlusion and chemotherapy may provide symptomatic improvement in some patients with hepatic metastases. Emergency therapy for patients with symptomatic bronchial carcinoids consists of giving prednisone, 15-30 mg orally daily.

4. Small Intestine Sarcoma

Most small intestine sarcomas arise from stromal tumors that stain positive for CD117; a minority arise from smooth muscle tumors (leiomyosarcomas) (see Gastrointestinal Mesenchymal Tumors above).

Kaposi sarcoma was at one time a common complication in AIDS, but the incidence is declining with highly active antiretroviral therapy (HAART). It is strongly associated with infection with human herpesvirus 8. Lesions may be present anywhere in the intestinal tract. Visceral involvement usually is associated with cutaneous disease. Most lesions are clinically silent; however, large lesions may be symptomatic. Interferon-α induces regression in up to one-third of patients who have a CD4 cell count of > 200/mcL. Widespread involvement may be best treated by systemic chemotherapy using combinations of vincristine, bleomycin, or doxorubicin, to which the tumor is very responsive.

Bilimoria KY et al. Small bowel cancer in the United States: changes in epidemiology, treatment, and survival over the last 20 years. Ann Surg. 2009 Jan;249(1):63–71. [PMID: 19106677]

Chambers AJ et al. The palliative benefit of aggressive surgical intervention for both hepatic and mesenteric metastases from neuroendocrine tumors. Surgery. 2008 Oct;144(4):645–51. [PMID: 18847650]

Modlin IM et al. Therapeutic options for gastrointestinal carcinoids. Clin Gastroenterol Hepatol. 2006 May;4(5):526–47. [PMID: 16630755]

Singhal N et al. Adjuvant chemotherapy for small intestine adenocarcinoma. Cochrane Database Syst Rev. 2007 Jul 18;(3):CD005202. [PMID: 17636789]

Yamagami H et al. Usefulness of double-balloon endoscopy in the diagnosis of malignant small-bowel tumors. Clin Gastroenterol Hepatol. 2008 Nov;6(11):1202–5. [PMID: 18799359]

COLORECTAL CANCER

ESSENTIALS OF DIAGNOSIS

► Personal or family history of adenomatous polyps or colorectal cancer are important risk factors.

► Symptoms or signs depend on tumor location.

► Proximal colon: fecal occult blood, anemia.

► Distal colon: change in bowel habits, hematochezia.

► Diagnosis established with colonoscopy.

► General Considerations

Colorectal cancer is the second leading cause of death due to malignancy in the United States. Approximately 6% of Americans will develop colorectal cancer and 40% of those will die of the disease. In 2008, there were an estimated 149,000 new cases and 50,000 deaths. Colorectal cancers are almost all adenocarcinomas, which tend to form bulky exophytic masses or annular constricting lesions. Slightly less than 50% of cancers are located distal to the splenic flexure (within the descending colon or rectosigmoid region). It is currently believed that the majority of colorectal cancers arise from malignant transformation of an adenomatous polyp. Adenomatous polyps that are "advanced" (ie, adenomas at least 1 cm in size, adenomas with villous features, or adenomas with high-grade dysplasia) are associated with a greater risk of cancer.

Approximately 85% of sporadic colorectal cancers have loss of function of one or more tumor suppressor genes (eg, *p53, APC,* or *DCC*) due to a combination of spontaneous mutation of one allele combined with chromosomal instability and aneuploidy (abnormal DNA content) that leads to deletion and loss of heterozygosity of the other allele (eg, 5q, 17q, or 18p deletion). Approximately 15% of colorectal cancers have microsatellite instability due to inactivation of DNA mismatch repair genes. This is most commonly an acquired defect caused by hypermethylation of the promoter region of the MLH1 gene, but may be an indicator of unrecognized HNPCC (see Chapter 15). Colon cancer with high microsatellite instability have distinct clinical and pathologic characteristics, including diploid DNA content, predominance in the proximal colon, poor differentiation, and more favorable prognosis.

▶ Risk Factors

A number of factors increase the risk of developing colorectal cancer. Recognition of these has impact on screening strategies. However, 75% of all cases occur in people with no known predisposing factors.

A. Age

The incidence of colorectal cancer rises sharply after age 45 years, and 90% of cases occur in persons over the age of 50 years.

B. Family History of Neoplasia

A family history of colorectal cancer is present in 20% of patients with colon cancer. Hereditary factors are believed to contribute to 20–30% of colorectal cancers; however, the genes responsible for most of these cases have not yet been identified. Up to 5% of colorectal cancers are caused by inherited germline mutations resulting in polyposis syndromes or hereditary nonpolyposis colorectal cancer (HNPCC) (see Chapter 15). Approximately 6% of the Ashkenazic Jewish population has a missense mutation in the *APC* gene *(APC I1307K)* that confers a modestly increased lifetime risk of developing colorectal cancer (OR 1.4–1.9) but phenotypically resembles sporadic colorectal cancer rather than FAP. Genetic screening is available, and patients harboring the mutation merit intensive screening.

A family history of colorectal cancer or adenomatous polyps is one of the most important risk factors for colorectal cancer. The risk of colon cancer is proportionate to the number and age of affected first-degree family members with colon neoplasia. People with one first-degree family member with colorectal cancer have an increased risk approximately two times that of the general population; however, the risk is almost four times if the family member's cancer was diagnosed at < 45 years of age. Patients with two first-degree relatives have a fourfold, or 25–30% lifetime, risk of developing colon cancer. First-degree relatives of patients with adenomatous polyps also have a twofold increased risk for colorectal neoplasia, especially if the polyp was large (≥ 10 mm) or detected before age 60 years.

C. Inflammatory Bowel Disease

The risk of adenocarcinoma of the colon begins to rise 7–10 years after disease onset in patients with ulcerative colitis and Crohn colitis. The cumulative risk approaches 5–10% after 20 years and 20% after 30 years. Chronic treatment with 5-ASA agents and folate is associated with a lower risk of cancer in patients with ulcerative colitis.

D. Dietary Factors and Chemoprevention

In epidemiologic studies, diets rich in fats and red meat are associated with an increased risk of colorectal adenomas and cancer, whereas diets high in fruits, vegetables, and fiber are associated with a decreased risk. However, prospective, randomized controlled trials failed to demonstrate a risk reduction in the recurrence of adenomatous polyps after treatment with a diet low in fat and high in fiber, fruits, and vegetables, or with fiber supplementation. Calcium carbonate (3 g/d) has been shown in large cohort studies as well as small prospective trials to yield a modest reduction in the relative risk of developing colorectal neoplasia; however, a 2006 prospective study of 36,000 women did not show a protective benefit of calcium (500 mg) and vitamin D (200 international units twice daily) in preventing colon cancer. Similarly, the risk of colon cancer appears to be decreased in persons taking folic acid supplements, but a 2007 prospective trial conducted in patients with a history of adenomas found that folate supplementation did not reduce the incidence of adenoma recurrence compared with placebo. The antioxidant vitamins A, C, E, and beta carotene also have not been shown to be of benefit in prospective controlled studies.

A US Preventive Services Task Force meta-analysis of cohort and case-control studies suggest that prolonged (> 6 years) regular use of aspirin (at least 325 mg twice weekly) and NSAIDs is associated with a 22–33% relative risk reduction in the incidence of colorectal cancer. Two prospective, blinded clinical trials have shown that daily low-dose aspirin (80–325 mg) reduces the number of recurrent adenomas at 1–3 years in patients with a history of colorectal adenomas or cancer; however, two large randomized controlled trials in the United States did not demonstrate a reduction in colorectal cancer incidence in patients taking low-dose aspirin over a 5–10 years. Because long-term aspirin use is associated with a low incidence of serious complications (gastrointestinal hemorrhage, stroke), the US Preventive Services Task Force concluded that it should not be prescribed as a chemopreventive agent in people without polyps or with small adenomas unless there are other medical indications. Long-term administration of low-dose aspirin may be considered in patients with a personal or family history of colorectal cancer or advanced adenomas; however, they do not obviate the need for colonoscopy screening and surveillance.

E. Other Factors

The incidence of colon adenocarcinoma is higher in blacks than in whites. It is unclear whether this is due to genetic or socioeconomic factors (eg, diet or reduced access to screening). Diabetes, metabolic syndrome, obesity, and cigarette smoking are associated with a modest increase in cancer risk.

▶ Clinical Findings

A. Symptoms and Signs

Adenocarcinomas grow slowly and may be present for several years before symptoms appear. However, some asymptomatic tumors may be detected by the presence of fecal occult blood (see Colorectal Cancer Screening, below). Symptoms depend on the location of the carcinoma. Chronic blood loss from right-sided colonic cancers may cause iron deficiency anemia, manifested by fatigue and weakness. Obstruction, however, is uncommon because of the large diameter of the right colon and the liquid consistency of the fecal material. Lesions of the left colon often involve the bowel circumferentially. Because the left colon has a smaller diameter and the fecal matter is solid, obstructive symptoms may develop with colicky abdominal pain and a change in bowel habits. Constipation may alternate with periods of increased frequency and loose stools. The stool may be streaked with blood, though marked bleeding is unusual. With rectal cancers, patients note tenesmus, urgency, and recurrent hematochezia. Weight loss is uncommon. Physical examination is usually normal except in advanced disease. A mass may be palpable in the abdomen. The liver should be examined for hepatomegaly, suggesting metastatic spread. For cancers of the distal rectum, digital examination is necessary to determine whether there is extension into the anal sphincter or fixation, suggesting extension to the pelvic floor.

B. Laboratory Findings

A complete blood count is obtained to look for evidence of anemia. Elevated liver function tests are suspicious for metastatic disease. Carcinoembryonic antigen (CEA) should be measured in all patients with proved colorectal cancer. A preoperative CEA level > 5 ng/mL is a poor prognostic indicator. After complete surgical resection, CEA levels should normalize; persistently elevated levels suggest the presence of persistent disease and warrant further evaluation.

C. Colonoscopy

Colonoscopy is the diagnostic procedure of choice in patients with a clinical history suggestive of colon cancer or in patients with an abnormality suspicious for cancer detected on radiographic imaging. Colonoscopy permits biopsy for pathologic confirmation of malignancy (Plate 20). In patients in whom colonoscopy is unable to reach the cecum (< 5% of cases) or when a nearly obstructing tumor precludes passage of the colonoscope, barium enema or CT colonography examination should be performed.

D. Imaging

Clinicians obtain an abdominal and pelvic CT scan to assist in preoperative staging. CT scans may demonstrate distal metastases but are less accurate in the determination of the level of local tumor extension (T stage) or lymphatic spread (N stage). Intraoperative assessment of the liver by direct palpation and ultrasonography is more accurate than CT scanning for the detection of hepatic metastases. For rectal cancer, pelvic MRI or endorectal ultrasonography provides important accurate information about the depth of penetration of the cancer through the rectal wall and pararectal lymph nodes that may guide preoperative (neoadjuvant) chemoradiotherapy and operative management. A chest CT scan should also be obtained because the systemic blood supply of the distal rectum may promote distal tumor metastasis outside the abdomen. PET is useful to determine recurrent colorectal cancer but currently is not used for staging of primary tumors.

▶ Staging

The TNM system is the commonly used classification to stage colorectal cancer. Staging is important not only because it correlates with the patient's long-term survival but also because it is used to determine which patients should receive adjuvant therapy.

▶ Differential Diagnosis

The nonspecific symptoms of colon cancer may be confused with those of irritable bowel syndrome, diverticular disease, ischemic colitis, inflammatory bowel disease, infectious colitis, and hemorrhoids. Neoplasm must be excluded in any patient over age 40 years who reports a change in bowel habits or hematochezia or who has an unexplained iron deficiency anemia or occult blood in the stools.

▶ Treatment

Resection of the primary colonic or rectal cancer is the treatment of choice for almost all patients who have resectable lesions and can tolerate general anesthesia. Multiple studies demonstrate that minimally invasive, laparoscopically assisted colectomy results in similar outcomes and rates of recurrence to open colectomy. Regional dissection of at least 12 lymph nodes should be performed to determine staging, which guides decisions about adjuvant therapy. Even patients with extensive metastatic disease may benefit from resection of the colonic tumor to reduce the likelihood of intestinal obstruction or serious bleeding.

For rectal carcinoma, the operative approach depends on the level of the tumor above the anal verge, the size and depth of penetration, and the patient's overall condition. Clinical staging by endorectal ultrasound or MRI with endorectal coil is important in guiding the clinical approach. In carefully selected patients with small, mobile (< 4 cm), well-differentiated T1 or T2 rectal tumors that are less than 8 cm from the anal verge and that appear on endosonography to be localized to the rectal wall, transanal excision may be performed. This approach avoids laparotomy and spares the rectum and anal sphincter, preserving normal bowel continence. All other patients will require either a low anterior resection with a colorectal anastomosis or an abdominoperineal resection with a colostomy, depending on how far above the anal verge the tumor is located and the extent of local tumor spread. Careful dissection of the entire mesorectum at the time of surgery has been shown to reduce local recurrence to 8%. With improvements in surgical stapling techniques, it is possible to perform low anterior resection provided there is a margin of at least 2 cm of normal tissue below the tumor. Although low resections obviate a colostomy, they are associated with increased immediate postsurgical complications (leak, dehiscence, stricture) and defecatory complaints (increased stool frequency, defecatory problems, and incontinence). With unresectable rectal cancer, the patient may be palliated with a diverting colostomy, laser fulguration, or placement of an expandable wire stent.

A. Adjuvant Therapy for Colon Cancer

Adjuvant chemotherapy and radiotherapy have been demonstrated to improve overall and tumor-free survival in selected patients with colon cancer.

1. Stage I—Because of the excellent 5-year survival rate (90–100%), no adjuvant therapy is recommended.

2. Stage II (node-negative disease)—The expected 5-year survival rate is 80%. A benefit from adjuvant chemotherapy has not been demonstrated in most controlled trials for stage II colon cancer (see discussion for stage III disease). However, otherwise healthy patients with stage II disease that is at higher risk for recurrence (perforation, T4, poor differentiation on histology) may benefit from adjuvant chemotherapy.

3. Stage III (node-positive disease)—With surgical resection alone, the expected 5-year survival rate is 30–50%. Postoperative adjuvant chemotherapy significantly increases disease-free survival as well as overall survival by up to 30% and is recommended for all patients. In stage III colorectal cancer, patients treated for 6 months with intravenous 5-FU and leucovorin (folinic acid) who have one to three involved nodes have a 5-year survival of 65%, and those with more than three involved nodes have a 5-year survival of up to 40%. Capecitabine is an oral 5-FU analog that obviates the need for intravenous infusions. Monotherapy with capecitabine yields a similar rate of disease-free survival with a lower rate of serious side effects (except for hand-foot syndrome) compared with intravenous 5-FU and leucovorin. Oxaliplatin is an important addition to combination adjuvant therapy. Large, well-designed studies of adjuvant therapy for stage III colon cancer reported a higher rate of disease-free survival at 5 years for patients treated with a combination of oxaliplatin, fluorouracil, and leucovorin (FOLFOX) (66%) than with fluorouracil and leucovorin (FL) alone (59%). The addition of oxaliplatin is associated with an increased incidence of diarrhea and sensory neuropathy, which generally is reversible. Based on these studies, FOLFOX currently is the preferred adjuvant therapy for most patients with Stage III disease. Current studies are evaluating oral capecitabine in combination with oxaliplatin. The role of combination adjuvant therapy of FOLFOX plus a biologic agent (bevacizumab, cetuximab, or panituxumab) also is under investigation.

4. Stage IV (metastatic disease)—Approximately 20% of patients have metastatic disease at the time of initial diagnosis, and another 30% eventually develop metastasis. A subset of these patients have limited disease that is potentially curable with surgical resection. Resection of isolated (one to three) liver or lung metastases may result in long-term (over 5 years) survival in 35–55% of cases. For those with unresectable hepatic metastases, local ablative techniques (cryosurgery, radiofrequency or microwave coagulation, embolization, hepatic intra-arterial chemotherapy) may provide long-term tumor control. The majority of patients with metastatic disease do not have resectable (curable) disease. In the absence of other treatment, the median survival is only 6 months. The goals of therapy are to slow tumor progression while maintaining a reasonable quality of life for as long as possible. Currently, either FOLFOX (the addition of oxaliplatin to 5-FU and folinic acid) or FOLFIRI (the addition of irinotecan to 5-FU and folinic acid) is the preferred first-line treatment regimens for most patients with metastatic colorectal cancer, increasing median survival to 15–20 months. For convenience, oral capecitabine (instead of intravenous 5-FU and leucovorin) can be used in combination with oxaliplatin; however, combination with irinotecan should not be used due to increased toxicity (diarrhea). The role of combination therapy with both oxaliplatin and irinotecan is under investigation. The role of biologic agents (cetuximab, panitumumab, and bevacizumab) is rapidly evolving. Cetuximab and panitumumab are monoclonal antibodies to EGFR; bevacizumab is a monoclonal antibody to VEGF. Combination therapy with bevacizumab and FOLFOX or FOLFIRI prolong mean survival 2–5 months compared with either regimen alone. Therefore, many oncologists are now using one of these combinations for initial therapy of metastatic disease. Bevacizumab may cause serious side effects, including arterial thromboembolic events, bowel perforation, or serious bleeding, in up to 5% of patients.

When disease progresses with FOLFOX or FOLFIRI (often in conjunction with bevacizumab), it is reasonable to switch to the alternative regimen. Patients progressing with one regimen may respond to the alternative regimen, prolonging mean survival to > 20 months. The anti-EGFR agents cetuximab and panitumumab may be used in patients whose disease has progressed despite first-line or second-line therapy. Both agents have modest efficacy when used as single agents for second-line therapy; however, a 2008 study reported that patients whose tumors had *K-ras* mutations did not benefit from anti-EGFR therapy, whereas patients with wild-type *K-ras* had 5 months median improved survival. Patients being considered for anti-EGFR therapy should therefore undergo *K-ras* testing. Cetuximab in combination with FOLFOX or FOLFIRI appears to provide a modest increase in median survival; however, the efficacy of these regimens versus bevacizumab-containing regimens is under investigation. The role of combination therapy of bevacizumab plus cetuximab or panitumumab with or without other agents requires further study.

B. Adjuvant Therapy for Rectal Cancer

Compared with colon cancer, rectal cancer has lower long-term survival rates and significantly higher rates of local tumor recurrence (25%) due to the difficulty of achieving adequate surgical resection margins. When initial imaging studies suggest stage I disease, surgery may be performed first. Combination therapy with fluorouracil (a radiation sensitizing agent) and radiation has been shown to improve the disease-free survival rate and to decrease pelvic recurrence and is recommended for all patients with stage II and stage III rectal cancers. It has long been controversial whether chemoradiation should be administered preoperatively ("neoadjuvant") or postoperatively ("adjuvant"). In 2004, a large, randomized controlled trial reported that preoperative therapy led to better patient treatment compliance, reduced local recurrence and toxicity, and a higher number of sphincter-preserving resections. Therefore, preoperative chemoradiation is recommended for patients with distal rectal cancers that are determined to be stage II or III by endorectal ultrasound or MRI. Following surgical resection with total mesorectal excision, fluorouracil-based therapy may be administered for an additional 4 months.

Follow-Up after Surgery

Patients who have undergone resections for cure are followed closely to look for evidence of symptomatic or asymptomatic tumor recurrence that may be amenable to curative resection in a small number of patients. The optimal cost-effective strategy is not clear. Two randomized trials reported that intense follow-up with yearly colonoscopy, abdominal CT, and chest radiography did not improve overall outcome compared with most standard follow-up protocols. Patients should be evaluated every 3–6 months for 3–5 years with history, physical examination, and CEA determinations. Patients who had a complete preoperative colonoscopy should undergo another colonoscopy 1 year after surgical resection. Patients who did not undergo full colonoscopy preoperatively should undergo colonoscopy within 3–6 months postoperatively to exclude other synchronous colorectal neoplasms and 1 year thereafter. Thereafter, surveillance colonoscopy should be performed every 3–5 years to look for metachronous polyps or cancer. Because of the high incidence of local tumor recurrence in patients with rectal cancer, sigmoidoscopy should be performed every 3–6 months for 3 years. New onset of symptoms or a rising CEA warrants investigation with chest and abdominal CT to look for recurrent or metastatic disease that may be amenable to therapy. For patients with a rising CEA with unrevealing CT imaging, a PET scan is more sensitive for the detection of occult metastatic disease.

Prognosis

The stage of disease at presentation is the most important determinant of long-term survival: stage I, > 90%; stage II, 70–85%; stage III with fewer than four positive lymph nodes, 67%; stage III with more than four positive lymph nodes, 33%; and stage IV, 5–7%. For each stage, rectal cancers have a worse prognosis. For those patients whose disease progresses despite therapy, meticulous efforts at palliative care are essential (see Chapter 5).

▶ Screening for Colorectal Neoplasms

Colorectal cancer is ideal for screening because it is a common disease that is fatal in almost 50% of cases yet is curable if detected at an earlier stage. Furthermore, most cases arise from benign adenomatous polyps that progress over many years to cancer, and removal of these polyps has been shown to prevent the majority of cancers. Colorectal cancer screening is endorsed by the US Preventive Services Task Force, the Agency for Health Care Policy and Research, the American Cancer Society, and every professional gastroenterology and colorectal surgery society. Although there is continued debate about the optimal cost-effective means of providing population screening, there is unanimous consent that screening *of some kind* should be offered to every patient over the age of 50 years. Several analyses suggest that screening is cost effective.

It is important for primary care providers to understand the relative merits of various options and to discuss them with their patients. Despite growing awareness of the importance of screening on the part of medical professionals and the public, less than 50% of patients have undergone screening of any kind. Discussion and encouragement by the primary care provider are the most important factors in achieving patient compliance with screening programs. The potential for harm from screening must be weighed against the likelihood of benefit, especially in elderly patients with comorbid illnesses and shorter life expectancy.

Recommendations for screening from the US Multisociety Task Force are listed in Table 39–5. Patients with first-degree relatives with colorectal neoplasms (cancer or

---

Table 39–5. Recommendations for colorectal cancer screening.[1]

Average-risk individuals ≥ 50 years old[2]
Annual fecal occult blood testing
Flexible sigmoidoscopy every 5 years
Annual fecal occult blood testing and flexible sigmoidoscopy every 5 years
Colonoscopy every 10 years
Barium enema every 5 years
Individuals with a family history of a first-degree member with colorectal neoplasia[3]
Single first-degree relative with colorectal cancer diagnosed at age ≥ 60 years: Begin screening at age 40. Screening guidelines same as average-risk individual; however, preferred method is colonoscopy every 10 years.
Single first-degree relative with colorectal cancer diagnosed at age < 60 years, or multiple first-degree relatives: Begin screening at age 40 or at age 10 years younger than age at diagnosis of the youngest affected relative, whichever is first in time. Recommended screening: colonoscopy every 5 years.

[1]For recommendations for families with inherited polyposis syndromes or hereditary nonpolyposis colon cancer, see Chapter 15.
[2]Colorectal cancer screening and surveillance: clinical guidelines and rationale. Gastroenterology. 2003 Feb;124(2):544–60.
[3]Screening Recommendations of American College of Gastroenterology. Am J Gastroenterol. 2000 Apr;95(4):868–77.

adenomatous polyps) are at increased risk; earlier and more frequent screening is recommended (preferably with colonoscopy) for these individuals. Recommendations for screening in families with inherited cancer syndromes or inflammatory bowel disease are provided in Chapter 15. For patients at average risk for colorectal cancer, the recommendations of the Task Force are discussed below. Screening tests may be classified into two broad categories: stool-based tests and exams that visualize the structure of the colon by direct endoscopic inspection or radiographic imaging.

A. Stool-based Tests

1. Fecal occult blood test—Most colorectal cancers and some large adenomas result in increased chronic blood loss. A variety of tests for fecal occult blood are commercially available that have varying sensitivities and specificities for colorectal neoplasia. These include guaiac-based tests (Hemoccult I and II and Hemeoccult SENSA) that detect the pseudoperoxidase activity of heme or hemoglobin and fecal immunochemical tests (FITs) that detect human globin.

Guaiac-based tests have undergone the most extensive testing and currently have the greatest clinical use. For optimal detection, one specimen card must be prepared from three consecutive bowel movements. To reduce the likelihood of false-positive tests, patients should abstain from aspirin (in doses greater than 325 mg/d), NSAIDs, red meat, poultry, fish, and vegetables with peroxide activity (turnips, horseradish) for 72 hours. Vitamin C may cause a false-negative test. Slides should be developed within 7 days after preparation. The reported sensitivities of a single guaiac-based test for detection of colorectal cancer vary widely, but are lower for Hemeoccult II (35%) than Hemeoccult SENSA (65%). When fecal occult blood test is administered to the general population as part of a screening program, 2–6% of tests are positive. Of those with positive tests, 5–18% have colorectal cancer that is more likely to be at an earlier stage (stage I or II).

Several FITs are commercially available. These tests are highly specific for detecting human globin and therefore eliminate the need for pretest dietary restrictions. As with guaiac-based tests, sampling of three consecutive bowel movements is recommended. In clinical trials that compare FIT with guaiac-based tests, FIT had at least comparable sensitivity to Hemeoccult SENSA for detection of cancers (60–85%) with higher specificity. Because FITs are not affected by diet or medications and have superior accuracy, they are increasingly being substituted for guaiac-based tests despite a higher cost per test ($10-20).

The US Multi-Society Task Force emphasizes that colon cancer prevention should be the primary goal of screening. For that reason, the lower sensitivity of fecal occult blood tests for advanced neoplasia (cancer and advanced adenomatous polyps) makes them a less attractive choice for population-based screening than endoscopic or radiographic tests. Currently, fecal occult blood tests are most suitable in settings where health care resources are limited or in patients who desire a noninvasive method of screen-ing. The Task Force recommends that tests with higher sensitivity for colorectal cancer (Hemeoccult SENSA or FIT) be used rather than less sensitive tests (Hemeoccult II). Regardless of which stool-based test is used, patients should understand that annual testing is required to achieve the maximum screening benefit and that a positive test will require evaluation by colonoscopy accompanied by removal of any polyps identified. If colonoscopy reveals no colorectal neoplasm, further screening for colorectal cancer can be deferred for 10 years. In a meta-analysis of four large, prospective, longitudinal studies, annual or biennial screening with Hemeoccult or Hemeoccult II reduced mortality from colorectal cancer by 25% among those who were compliant with regular testing. Long-term studies with more sensitive stool tests (Heme SENSA or FIT) have not been performed.

2. Multitarget DNA assay—A fecal DNA assay (Pre-Gen Plus) is available for screening for colorectal neoplasia. The test analyzes fecal DNA for 22 gene mutations and DNA integrity. The commercially available first-generation fecal DNA panel detected only one-half of cancers; however, a second-generation assay detected almost 90%. Although the Multisociety Task Force concluded that fecal DNA is an acceptable option for colorectal cancer screening, this test is not yet practical for population-based screening due to its high cost and cumbersome requirements for stool collection and mailing.

B. Endoscopic Examinations of the Colon

1. Flexible sigmoidoscopy—Use of a 60-cm flexible sigmoidoscope permits visualization of the rectosigmoid and descending colon. It requires no sedation and in many centers is performed by a nurse specialist or physician's assistant. Adenomatous polyps are identified in 10–20% and colorectal cancers in 1% of patients. (For management of adenomatous polyps identified at sigmoidoscopy, see Chapter 15.) Case-control studies suggest that screening sigmoidoscopy programs lead to a 60% reduction in colorectal cancer mortality. The risk of serious complications (perforation) associated with flexible sigmoidoscopy is less than 1:10,000 patients.

The chief disadvantage of screening with flexible sigmoidoscopy is that is does not examine the proximal colon. The prevalence of proximal versus distal neoplasia is higher in people over age 65 years of age, African Americans, and women. In men, approximately 50% of advanced neoplasms (cancer, adenomas ≥ 1 cm in size, polyps with villous histology, or high-grade dysplasia) are located in the proximal colon, compared with 60–70% in women. The finding at sigmoidoscopy of an adenomatous polyp in the distal colon increases the likelihood at least twofold that an advanced neoplasm is present in the proximal colon. Therefore, patients found on screening sigmoidoscopy to have an adenomatous polyp of any size should subsequently undergo colonoscopy to evaluate the proximal colon. Using this strategy in men, it is estimated that screening sigmoidoscopy programs will detect approximately 65% of advanced colonic neoplasms. In women, however, sigmoidoscopy screening programs may fail to detect up to 65% of advanced neoplasia.

2. Colonoscopy— Colonoscopy permits examination of the entire colon. In addition to detecting early cancers, colonoscopy allows removal of adenomatous polyps by biopsy or polypectomy, which is believed to reduce the risk of subsequent cancer. Over the past decade, there has been a dramatic increase in screening colonoscopy and a similar decrease in screening sigmoidoscopy due to poor reimbursement and the perceived inferiority of sigmoidoscopy compared with colonoscopy. Colonoscopy requires aggressive bowel cleansing prior to the examination. To alleviate discomfort, intravenous sedation is used for most patients. The incidence of serious complications after colonoscopy (perforation, bleeding, cardiopulmonary events) is 0.1%. In asymptomatic individuals between 50 and 75 years of age undergoing screening colonoscopy, the prevalence of advanced neoplasia is 4–11% and of cancer is 0.1–1%.

Although colonoscopy is believed to be the most sensitive test for detecting adenomas and cancer, it is not infallible. In several studies, the rate of colorectal cancer within 3 years of a screening colonoscopy was 0.7–0.9%, ie, approximately 1 in 110 patients. This may be attributable to adenomatous polyps and early cancers that were overlooked during colonoscopy. Studies of back-to-back colonoscopies confirm that endoscopists overlook 6–12% of polyps > 1 cm and up to 25% of smaller adenomas. Polyps that are small, flat, or located behind folds are easily missed, especially if the bowel preparation is poor. Population-based case-control and cohort studies suggest that colonoscopy is associated with greater reduction in colorectal cancer incidence and mortality in the distal colon than the proximal colon. This may be attributable to incomplete examination of the proximal colon, and differences between the proximal and distal colon that include worse bowel preparation, more aggressive polyp biology, or a higher prevalence of flat polyps. The latter are more common that previously recognized, are more likely to contain advanced pathology, and are more difficult to identify than raised (sessile or pedunculated) polyps. To optimize diagnostic accuracy as well as patient safety and comfort, colonoscopy should be performed after optimal bowel preparation by a well-trained endoscopist who spends sufficient time (at least 7 minutes) carefully examining the colon (especially the proximal colon) while withdrawing the endoscope.

C. Radiographic Examinations of the Colon

1. CT colonography—Using helical CT with computer-assisted image reconstruction, two- and three-dimensional views can be generated of the colon lumen that simulate the view of colonoscopy. CT colonography requires a similar bowel cleansing regimen as colonoscopy as well as insufflation of air into the colon through a rectal tube, which may be associated with discomfort. Nonetheless, this examination is performed rapidly and requires no sedation or intravenous contrast. It has minimal acute risk although there is controversy about potential long-term risks related to radiation exposure from CT examinations. Several large studies have compared the accuracy of virtual colonoscopy with

colonoscopy for colorectal screening. Using current imaging software with multidetector helical scanners, the sensitivity is > 95% for the detection of cancer and > 84–92% for the detection of polyps ≥ 10 mm in size. The sensitivity for polyps 6–9 mm in size ranges from 57% to 84%; for polyps 5 mm or less, the sensitivity is extremely poor.

Patients undergoing screening with CT colonography should be managed appropriately. If no polyps are found, the interval for repeat screening examination is uncertain; however, 5 years may be reasonable. All patients with polyps ≥ 10 mm in size should be referred for colonoscopy with polypectomy because of the high prevalence (30%) of advanced pathology (cancer, high-grade dysplasia, or villous features) within these polyps. The optimal management of patients with polyps < 10 mm in size is controversial. The likelihood of advanced pathology in polyps 6–9 mm in size is 4–7% and in polyps 1–5 mm is < 2%. Studies are ongoing to determine the natural history of polyps within this size range. Pending this information, the US Multisociety Task Force currently recommends that colonoscopy with polypectomy be offered to patients with one or more 6–9 mm polyps. Patients who refuse or who have increased risk of carcinoma should undergo surveillance CT colonography in 3–5 years. At the present time, there is no consensus on the management of patients with polyps < 6 mm; however, some radiologists choose not even to report these findings.

2. Barium enema—Double-contrast barium enema was previously an attractive screening technique because it was widely available, relatively inexpensive, and safe. However, compared to CT colonography, it is more time consuming and difficult to perform, less comfortable, and less accurate. Although it continues to be included among recommended screening options, it has been supplanted CT colonography, where available. A multicenter trial demonstrated that the sensitivity of barium enema is only 50% for polyps ≥ 1 cm and 55–85% for early-stage cancers when compared with colonoscopy. At present, barium enema may be recommended when screening of the entire colon is desired but expertise in CT colonography is unavailable and the patient is unable or unwilling to undergo colonoscopy.

▶ When to Refer

- Patients with symptoms (change in bowel habits, hematochezia), signs (mass on abdominal examination or digital rectal examination [DRE]), or laboratory tests (iron deficiency anemia) suggestive of colorectal neoplasia should be referred for colonoscopy.

- Patients with suspected cancer or adenomatous polyps of any size should be referred for colonoscopy.

- Virtually all patients with proven colorectal cancer should be referred to a surgeon for resection. Patients with stage III or IV disease should be referred to an oncologist.

▶ When to Admit

- Patients with complications of colorectal cancer (obstruction, acute bleeding) requiring urgent evaluation and intervention.

- Patients with severe complications of chemotherapy.
- Patients with advanced metastatic disease requiring palliative care.

Baxter NN et al. Association of colonoscopy and death from colorectal cancer. Ann Intern Med. 2009 Jan 6;150(1):1–8. [PMID: 19075198]

Botteri E et al. Cigarette smoking and adenomatous polyps: a meta-analysis. Gastroenterology. 2008 Feb;134(2):388–95. [PMID: 18242207]

Chan AT et al. Aspirin dose and duration of use and risk of colorectal cancer in men. Gastroenterology. 2008 Jan;134(1):21–8. [PMID: 18005960]

Cole BF et al. Folic acid for the prevention of colorectal adenomas: a randomized clinical trial. JAMA. 2007 June 6;297(21):2351–9. [PMID: 17551129]

Colon Cancer—National Cancer Institute—Cancer Net: http://cancernet.nci.nih.gov.

Dubé C et al. The use of aspirin for primary prevention of colorectal cancer: a systematic review prepared for the U.S. Preventive Services Task Force. Ann Intern Med. 2007 Mar 6;146(5):365–75. [PMID: 17339622]

Grady WM et al. Genomic and epigenetic instability in colorectal cancer pathogenesis. Gastroenterology. 2008 Oct;135(4):1079–99. [PMID: 18773902]

Hewitson P et al. Cochrane systematic review of colorectal cancer screening using the fecal occult blood test (hemeoccult): an update. Am J Gastroenterol. 2008 Jun;103(6):1541–9. [PMID: 18479499]

Imperiale T et al. Five-year risk of colorectal neoplasia after negative screening colonoscopy. N Engl J Med. 2008 Sep 18;359(12):1218–24. [PMID: 18799558]

Johnson CD et al. Accuracy of CT colonography for detection of large adenomas and cancers. N Engl J Med. 2008 Sept 18;359(12):1207–17. [PMID: 18799557]

Kahi CJ et al. Screening, surveillance, and primary prevention for colorectal cancer: a review of the recent literature. Gastroenterology. 2008 Aug;135(2):380–99. [PMID: 18582467]

Karpetis CS et al. K-ras mutations and benefit from cetuximab in advanced colorectal cancer. N Engl J Med. 2008 Oct 23;359(17):1757–65. [PMID: 18946061]

Koopman L et al. Sequential versus combination chemotherapy with capecitabine, irinotecan, and oxaliplatin in advanced colorectal cancer (CAIRO): a phase III randomised controlled trial. Lancet. 2007 Jul 14;370(9582):135–42. [PMID: 17630036]

Lakoff J et al. Risk of developing a proximal versus distal colorectal cancer after a negative colonoscopy: a population-based study. Clin Gastroenterol Hepatol. 2008 Oct;6(10):1117–21. [PMID: 18691942]

Levi Z et al. A quantitative immunochemical fecal occult blood test for colorectal neoplasia. Ann Intern Med. 2007 Feb 20;146(4):244–55. [PMID: 17310048]

Levin B et al. Screening and surveillance for the early detection of colorectal cancer and adenomatous polyps, 2008: a joint guideline from the American Cancer Society, the US Multi-society Task Force on Colorectal Cancer, and the American College of Radiology. Gastroenterology. 2008 May;134(5):1570–95. [PMID: 18384785]

Lieberman D et al. Polyp size and advanced histology in patients undergoing colonoscopy screening: implications for CT colonography. Gastroenterology. 2008 Oct;135(4):1100–5. [PMID: 18691580]

Lieberman DA et al. Prevalence of colon polyps detected by colonoscopy screening in asymptomatic black and white patients. JAMA. 2008 Sep 24;300(12):1417–22. [PMID: 18812532]

Rex D et al. Guidelines for colonoscopy surveillance after cancer resection: a consensus update by the American Cancer Society and the US Multi-Society Task Force on Colorectal Cancer. Gastroenterology. 2006 May;130(6):1865–71. [PMID: 16697749]

Seymour MT et al. Different strategies of sequential and combination chemotherapy for patients with poor prognosis advanced colorectal cancer (MRC FOCUS): a randomised controlled trial. Lancet. 2007 Jul 14;370(9582):143–52. [PMID: 17630037]

Soetikno RM et al. Prevalence of nonpolypoid (flat and depressed) colorectal neoplasms in asymptomatic and symptomatic adults. JAMA. 2008 Mar 5;299(9):1027–35. [PMID: 18319413]

Van Rossum LG et al. Random comparison of guaiac and immunochemical fecal occult blood tests for colorectal cancer in a screening population. Gastroenterology. 2008 Jul;135(1):82–90. [PMID: 18482589]

Wolpin BM et al. Systemic treatment of colorectal cancer. Gastroenterology. 2008 May;134:1296–310. [PMID: 18471507]

CARCINOMA OF THE ANUS

The anal canal is lined from its proximal to distal extent by columnar, transitional and non-keratinized squamous epithelium, which merges at the anal verge with the keratinized perianal skin. Tumors arising from the mucosa of the anal canal are relatively rare, comprising only 1–2% of all cancers of the anus and large intestine. Squamous cancers make up the majority of anal cancers. Anal cancer is increased among people practicing receptive anal intercourse and those with a history of anorectal warts. In over 80% of cases, HPV may be detected, suggesting that this virus is a major causal factor. Anal cancer is increased in HIV-infected individuals, possibly due to interaction with HPV. Bleeding, pain, and local tumor are the most common symptoms. The lesion is often confused with hemorrhoids or other common anal disorders. These tumors tend to become annular, invade the sphincter, and spread upward via the lymphatics into the perirectal mesenteric lymphatic nodes. MR scan and endoluminal ultrasound assist in determining the depth of penetration and local spread.

Treatment depends on the tumor location and histologic stage. Small (< 3 cm) superficial lesions of the perianal skin may be treated with wide local excision. Adenocarcinoma of the anal canal is treated in similar fashion to rectal cancer (see above), commonly by abdominoperineal resection with adjuvant or neoadjuvant chemoradiotherapy. Squamous cancer of the anal canal and large perianal tumors invading the sphincter or rectum are treated with combined-modality therapy that includes external radiation with simultaneous chemotherapy (fluorouracil and either mitomycin or cisplatin). Local control is achieved in 80% of patients. Radical surgery (abdominoperineal resection) is reserved for patients who fail chemotherapy and radiation therapy. The 5-year survival rate is 60–70% for localized tumors and over 25% for metastatic (stage IV) disease.

Anal Cancer (PDQ) Treatment—National Cancer Institute—Cancer Net: http://cancernet.nci.nih.gov.

Das P et al. Current treatment for localized anal carcinoma. Curr Opin Oncol. 2007 Jul;19(4):396–400. [PMID: 17545807]

Peiffert D et al. Cancer of the anal canal. Gastroenterol Clin Biol. 2006 Sep;30 Spec No 2:2S52–2S56. [PMID: 17151563]

CANCERS OF THE GENITOURINARY TRACT

Maxwell V. Meng, MD, FACS

PROSTATE CANCER

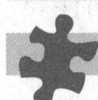 ESSENTIALS OF DIAGNOSIS

▶ Prostatic induration on DRE or elevation of PSA.

▶ Most often asymptomatic.

▶ Rarely: systemic symptoms (weight loss, bone pain).

▶ General Considerations

Prostatic cancer is the most common noncutaneous cancer detected in American men and the second leading cause of cancer-related death. In the United States, over 218,000 new cases of prostate cancer are diagnosed annually, and about 27,000 deaths result. However, the clinical incidence of the disease does not match the prevalence noted at autopsy, where more than 40% of men over 50 years of age are found to have prostatic carcinoma. Most such occult cancers are small and contained within the prostate gland. Few are associated with regional or distant disease. The incidence of prostatic cancer increases with age. Whereas 30% of men aged 60–69 years will have the disease, autopsy incidence increases to 67% in men aged 80–89 years. Although the global prevalence of prostatic cancer at autopsy is relatively consistent, the clinical incidence varies considerably (high in North America and European countries, intermediate in South America, and low in the Far East), suggesting that environmental or dietary differences among populations may be important for prostatic cancer growth. A 50-year-old American man has a lifetime risk of 40% for latent cancer, 16% for developing clinically apparent cancer, and a 2.9% risk of death due to prostatic cancer. Blacks, men with a family history of prostatic cancer, and those with a history of high dietary fat intake are at increased risk for developing prostate cancer.

▶ Clinical Findings

A. Symptoms and Signs

Prostate cancer may manifest as focal nodules or areas of induration within the prostate at the time of DRE. However, currently most prostate cancers are associated with palpably normal prostates and are detected on the basis of elevations in serum PSA.

Patients rarely present with signs of urinary retention or neurologic symptoms as a result of epidural metastases and cord compression. Obstructive voiding symptoms are most often due to benign prostatic hyperplasia, which occurs in the same age group. Nevertheless, large or locally extensive prostatic cancers can cause obstructive voiding symptoms while lymph node metastases can lead to lower extremity lymphedema. As the axial skeleton is the most common site of metastases, patients may present with back pain or pathologic fractures.

B. Laboratory Findings

1. Serum tumor markers—PSA is a glycoprotein produced only by cells, either benign or malignant, of the prostate gland. The serum level is typically low and correlates with the volume of both benign and malignant prostate tissue. Measurement of serum PSA is useful in detecting and staging prostate cancer, monitoring response to treatment, and detecting recurrence before it becomes clinically evident. As a screening test, PSA will be elevated in 10–15% of men. Approximately 18–30% of men with intermediate degrees of elevation (4.1–10 ng/mL) will be found to have prostate cancer. Between 50% and 70% of those with elevations greater than 10 ng/mL will have prostate cancer. (See age-specific PSA reference ranges under Screening for Prostate Cancer, below.) Patients with intermediate levels of PSA usually have localized and therefore potentially curable cancers. It should be remembered that approximately 20% of patients who undergo radical prostatectomy for localized prostate cancer have normal levels of PSA.

In untreated patients with prostate cancer, the level of PSA correlates with the volume and stage of the disease. Whereas most organ-confined cancers are associated with PSA levels less than 10 ng/mL, advanced disease (seminal vesicle invasion, lymph node involvement, or occult distant metastases) is more common in patients with PSA levels in excess of 40 ng/mL. Approximately 98% of patients with metastatic prostate cancer will have elevated PSA. However, there are rare cancers that are localized despite substantial elevations in PSA. Therefore, initial treatment decisions cannot be made on the basis of PSA testing alone. A rising PSA after therapy is usually consistent with progressive disease, either locally recurrent or metastatic.

2. Miscellaneous laboratory testing—Patients in urinary retention or those with ureteral obstruction due to loco-regionally advanced prostate cancers may present with elevations in blood urea nitrogen or creatinine. Patients with bony metastases may have elevations in alkaline phosphatase or hypercalcemia. Laboratory and clinical evidence of disseminated intravascular coagulation can occur in patients with advanced prostate cancers.

3. Prostate biopsy—Transrectal ultrasound-guided biopsy is the standard method for detection of prostate cancer. The use of a spring-loaded, 18-gauge biopsy needle has allowed transrectal biopsy to be performed with little patient discomfort and minimal morbidity. Local anesthesia is routinely used and increases the tolerability of the procedure. The specimen preserves glandular architecture and permits accurate grading. Prostate biopsy specimens are taken from the apex, mid-portion, and base in men who have an abnormal DRE or an elevated serum PSA, or both. Extended-pattern biopsies, including a total of at least ten biopsies, are associated with improved cancer detection and risk stratification of patients with newly diagnosed disease. Patients with abnormalities of the seminal vesicles can have these structures specifically biopsied to identify local tumor invasion.

C. Imaging

Transrectal ultrasonography has been used largely for the staging of prostate carcinomas, where they typically appear as hypoechoic areas. In addition, transrectal ultrasound-guided, rather than digitally guided, biopsy of the prostate is a more accurate way to evaluate suspicious lesions. Use of imaging should be tailored to the likelihood of advanced disease in newly diagnosed cases. Asymptomatic patients with well-differentiated to moderately differentiated cancers, thought to be localized to the prostate on DRE and transurethral ultrasound and associated with modest elevations of PSA (ie, < 10 ng/mL), need no further imaging.

MRI of the prostate allows for evaluation of the prostate lesion as well as regional lymph nodes. The positive predictive value for detection of both capsular penetration and seminal vesicle invasion is similar for transrectal ultrasound and MRI. CT plays little role because of its inability to accurately identify or stage prostate cancers, but it can be used to detect regional lymphatic metastases and intra-abdominal metastases.

Radionuclide bone scan is superior to conventional plain skeletal radiographs in detecting bony metastases. Most prostate cancer metastases are multiple and most commonly localized to the axial skeleton. Those men with more advanced local lesions, symptoms of metastases (eg, bone pain), high-grade disease, or elevations in PSA greater than 20 ng/mL should undergo radionuclide bone scan. Because of the high frequency of abnormal scans in patients in this age group resulting from degenerative joint disease, plain films are often necessary in evaluating patients with indeterminate findings on bone scan. Cross-sectional imaging either by CT or MRI is usually indicated only in those patients in the latter group who have negative bone scans in an attempt to detect lymph node metastases. Patients found to have enlarged pelvic lymph nodes are candidates for FNA.

Intravenous urography and cystoscopy are not routinely needed to evaluate patients with prostate cancer.

Despite application of modern, sophisticated techniques, understaging of prostate cancer occurs in at least 20% of patients.

▶ Screening for Prostate Cancer

Whether screening for prostate cancer results in a decrease in yearly mortality rates due to the disease is the subject of much debate. The screening tests currently available include DRE, PSA testing, and transrectal ultrasound. Depending on the patient population being evaluated, detection rates using DRE alone vary from 1.5% to 7%. Unfortunately, most cancers detected in this manner are advanced (stage T3 or greater). Transrectal ultrasound should not be used as a first-line screening tool because of its expense, low specificity (and therefore high biopsy rate), and minimal improvement in detection rate when compared with the combined use of DRE and PSA testing.

PSA testing increases the detection rate of prostate cancers compared with DRE. Approximately 2–2.5% of men older than 50 years of age will be found to have prostate cancer using PSA testing compared with a rate of approximately 1.5% using DRE alone. PSA is not specific

Table 39–6. Screening for prostatic cancer: Test performance.

Test	Sensitivity	Specificity	Positive Predictive Value
Abnormal PSA (> 4 ng/mL)	0.67	0.97	0.43
Abnormal DRE	0.50	0.94	0.24
Abnormal PSA or DRE	0.84	0.92	0.28
Abnormal PSA *and* DRE	0.34	0.995	0.49

DRE, digital rectal examination; PSA, prostate-specific antigen. Modified, with permission, from Kramer BS et al. Prostate cancer screening: what we know and what we need to know. Ann Intern Med. 1993 Nov 1;119(9):914–23.

for cancer, and there is considerable overlap of values between men with benign prostate hyperplasia and those with prostate cancers. The sensitivity, specificity, and positive predictive value of PSA and DRE are listed in Table 39–6. PSA-detected cancers are more likely to be localized compared with those detected by DRE alone.

To improve the performance of PSA as a screening test, several investigators have developed alternative methods for its use. The serial measurement of PSA over time (PSA velocity) may increase specificity for cancer detection with little loss in sensitivity. A rate of change in PSA greater than 0.75 ng/mL per year is associated with an increased likelihood of cancer detection. In a patient with a normal DRE, an elevated PSA, and a normal transrectal ultrasound, the indications for prostate biopsy may be refined by calculating PSA density (serum PSA/volume of the prostate as measured by ultrasound). Patients with high PSA density are more likely to have disease despite a normal DRE and normal transrectal ultrasound. Some have found measurement of PSA transition zone density (portion of the prostate that enlarges with development of benign prostate hyperplasia) to be more predictive of the presence or absence of cancer than PSA density calculated using the entire prostate volume. As PSA concentration is directly related to patient age, establishment of age-specific reference ranges increases specificity (fewer older men with benign prostate hyperplasia would undergo evaluation) and increases sensitivity (more younger men with cancer would undergo evaluation). Age-specific reference ranges have been established: men 40–49, < 2.5 ng/mL; men 50–59, < 3.5 ng/mL; men 60–69, < 4.5 ng/mL; and men 70–79, < 6.5 ng/mL (based on a previously normal serum PSA of < 4 ng/mL). Black men have lower age-specific reference ranges (age 40–49, < 2 ng/mL; age 50–59, < 4 ng/mL; age 60–69, < 4.5 ng/mL; age 70–79, < 5.5 ng/mL). A more recent attempt at refining PSA has been the measurement of free serum and protein-bound levels (cancer patients have a lower percentage of free serum PSA). Generally, men with free fractions exceeding 25% are unlikely to have prostate cancer, whereas those with free fractions less than 10% have an approximately 50% chance of having prostate cancer. Early reports using cutoffs of 18–20% of free PSA resulted in 5–10% lost sensitivity for 15–40% gains in specificity. The frequency of PSA testing remains a matter of some debate. In men with a normal DRE and a PSA > 2.5 ng/mL, PSA testing should be performed yearly because approximately 50% of these patients convert to having a PSA > 4 ng/mL. Screening can be performed biennially in those with a normal DRE and serum PSA < 2.5 ng/mL; progression in this group is less likely.

▶ **Staging**

The majority of prostate cancers are adenocarcinomas. Most arise in the periphery of the prostate (peripheral zone), though a small percentage arise in the central (5–10%) and transition zones (20%) of the gland. Pathologists utilize the Gleason grading system whereby a "primary" grade is applied to the architectural pattern of malignant glands occupying the largest area of the specimen and a "secondary" pattern is assigned to the next largest area of cancer. Grading is based on architectural rather than histologic criteria, and five "grades" are possible. Adding the score of the primary and secondary patterns gives a Gleason score. Grade correlates with tumor volume, pathologic stage, and prognosis.

▶ **Treatment**

A. Localized Disease

The optimal treatment for patients with clinically localized prostate cancers remains controversial. Patients need to be advised of all treatment options, including active surveillance, with the specific benefits, risks, and limitations. Currently, treatment decisions are made based on tumor grade and stage as well as the age and health of the patient. Although selected patients may be candidates for surveillance based on age or health and evidence of small-volume or well-differentiated cancers, most men with an anticipated life expectancy in excess of 10 years should be considered for treatment. Both radiation therapy and radical prostatectomy result in acceptable levels of local control. A large, prospective, randomized trial compared surveillance with radical prostatectomy in 695 men with clinically localized and well- differentiated to moderately differentiated tumors for a median of 8.2 years. Radical prostatectomy reduced disease-specific mortality, overall mortality, and risks of metastasis and local progression. The absolute reduction in the risk of death after 10 years was small yet statistically significant, but the reductions in the risk of metastasis and local tumor progression were substantial. This trial accrued patients in Sweden between 1989 and 1999, thus likely including patients with greater cancer burden compared with that in patients currently diagnosed using PSA screening.

B. Radical Prostatectomy

During radical prostatectomy, the seminal vesicles, prostate, and ampullae of the vas deferens are removed. Refinements in technique have allowed preservation of urinary

continence in most patients and erectile function in selected patients. Radical prostatectomy can be performed via open retropubic, transperineal, or laparoscopic (with or without robotic assistance) surgery. Local recurrence is uncommon after radical prostatectomy, and the incidence is related to pathologic stage. Organ-confined cancers rarely recur; however, cancers with adverse pathologic features (capsular penetration, seminal vesicle invasion) are associated with higher local (10–25%) and distant (20–50%) relapse rates.

Ideal candidates for prostatectomy include healthy patients with stages T1 and T2 prostate cancers. Patients with advanced local tumors (T4) or lymph node metastases are rarely candidates for prostatectomy alone, although surgery is sometimes used in combination with hormonal therapy and postoperative radiation therapy for select high-risk patients.

Patients with advanced pathologic stage or positive surgical margins are at an increased risk for local and distant tumor relapse. Such patients are candidates for adjuvant therapy (radiation for positive margins or androgen deprivation for lymph node metastases). Although adjuvant radiation appears to reduce local recurrences (0–5% with radiation versus 15–30% without), it has little or no impact on distant failure rates (30–35% with radiation versus 30–45% without). Recent evidence suggests that salvage radiotherapy after radical prostatectomy, within 2 years of PSA relapse, increases prostate cancer-specific survival in men with shorter PSA doubling time (< 6 months).

C. Radiation Therapy

Radiation can be delivered by a variety of techniques including use of external beam radiotherapy and transperineal implantation of radioisotopes. Morbidity is limited, and the survival of patients with localized cancers (T1, T2, and selected T3) approaches 65% at 10 years. As with surgery, the likelihood of local failure correlates with technique and tumor characteristics. The likelihood of a positive prostate biopsy more than 18 months after radiation varies between 20% and 60%. Patients with local recurrence are at an increased risk of cancer progression and cancer death compared with those who have negative biopsies. Ambiguous target definitions, inadequate radiation doses, and understaging of the tumor may be responsible for the failure noted in some series. Newer techniques of radiation (implantation, conformal therapy using three-dimensional reconstruction of CT-based tumor volumes, heavy particle, charged particle, and heavy charged particle) may improve local control rates. Three-dimensional conformal radiation delivers a higher dose because of improved targeting and appears to be associated with greater efficacy as well as lower likelihood of adverse side effects compared with previous techniques. As a result of improvements in imaging, most notably transrectal ultrasound, there has been a resurgence of interest in brachytherapy—the implantation of permanent or temporary radioactive sources (palladium, iodine, or iridium) into the prostate. Brachytherapy can be combined with external beam radiation in patients with higher-grade or higher-volume disease or as monotherapy in those with low-grade or low-volume malignancies. The PSA may rise after brachytherapy because of prostate inflammation and necrosis. This transient elevation (PSA bounce) should not be mistaken for recurrence and may occur up to 20 months after treatment.

D. Surveillance

A beneficial impact of treating localized prostate cancer with respect to survival has not been conclusively demonstrated. Therefore, surveillance alone may be an appropriate form of management for selected patients with prostate cancer. Patients included in observational series are typically older with small volume, well-differentiated cancers. Currently, many men diagnosed with prostate cancer may be candidates for surveillance due to the significant migration to lower stage, as well lower grade, resulting from screening for prostate cancer using PSA testing. Depending on the age and health of the patient, some of these very low-volume, low-grade cancers may never become clinically relevant and can be monitored with serial PSA levels, rectal examinations, and periodic prostate biopsies to assess grade and extent of tumor. The goal of surveillance is to avoid treatment in men who never experience disease progression while recognizing and effectively treating men with early evidence of progression. End points for intervention in patients on surveillance have not been clearly defined and surveillance regimens remain investigational.

E. Cryosurgery

Cryosurgery is a technique whereby liquid nitrogen is circulated through small hollow-core needles inserted into the prostate under ultrasound guidance. The freezing process results in tissue destruction. There has been a resurgence of interest in less invasive forms of therapy for localized prostate cancer as well as several recent technical innovations, including improved percutaneous techniques, expertise in transrectal ultrasound, improved cryotechnology, and better understanding of cryobiology. The positive biopsy rate after cryoablation ranges between 7% and 23%.

F. Locally and Regionally Advanced Disease

Prostate cancers associated with minimal degrees of capsular penetration are candidates for standard irradiation or surgery. Those with locally extensive cancers, including those with seminal vesicle and bladder neck invasion, are at increased risk for both local and distant relapse despite conventional therapy. Currently, a variety of investigational regimens are being tested in an effort to improve cancer outcomes in such patients. Combination therapy (androgen deprivation combined with surgery or irradiation), newer forms of irradiation, and hormonal therapy alone are being tested, as is neoadjuvant and adjuvant chemotherapy. Neoadjuvant and adjuvant androgen deprivation therapy combined with external beam radiation therapy have demonstrated improved survival compared with external beam radiation therapy alone.

G. Metastatic Disease

Since death due to prostate carcinoma is almost invariably the result of failure to control metastatic disease, research has emphasized efforts to improve control of distant disease. It is well known that most prostate carcinomas are hormone dependent and approximately 70–80% of men with metastatic prostate carcinoma will respond to various forms of androgen deprivation. Androgen deprivation may be affected at several levels along the pituitary–gonadal axis using a variety of methods or agents (Table 39–7). Use of luteinizing hormone-releasing hormone (LHRH) agonists (leuprolide, goserelin) achieves androgen deprivation without orchiectomy or administration of diethylstilbestrol and is currently the most common method of reducing testosterone levels. Because of its rapid onset of action, ketoconazole should be considered in patients with advanced prostate cancer who present with spinal cord compression, bilateral ureteral obstruction, or disseminated intravascular coagulation. Although testosterone is the major circulating androgen, the adrenal gland secretes the androgens dehydroepiandrosterone, dehydroepiandrosterone sulfate, and androstenedione. Some

Table 39–7. Androgen deprivation for prostatic cancer.

Level	Agent	Dose	Sequelae
Pituitary, hypothalamus	Diethylstibestrol	1–3 mg orally daily	Gynecomastia, hot flushes, thromboembolic disease, erectile dysfunction
	LHRH agonists	Monthly or 3-monthly depot injection	Erectile dysfunction, hot flushes, gynecomastia, rarely anemia
Adrenal	Ketoconazole	400 mg three times orally daily	Adrenal insufficiency, nausea, rash, ataxia
	Aminoglutethimide	250 mg four times orally daily	Adrenal insufficiency, nausea, rash, ataxia
	Corticosteroids	Prednisone: 20–40 mg orally daily	Gastrointestinal bleeding, fluid retention
Testis	Orchiectomy		Gynecomastia, hot flushes, erectile dysfunction
Prostate cell	Antiandrogens	Flutamide: 250 mg three times orally daily Bicalutamide: 50 mg orally daily	No erectile dysfunction when used alone; nausea, diarrhea

LHRH, luteinizing-hormone-releasing hormone.

investigators believe that suppressing both testicular and adrenal androgens allows for a better initial and longer response than methods that only inhibit production of testicular androgens. Complete androgen blockade can be achieved by combining an antiandrogen with use of an LHRH agonist or orchiectomy. Nonsteroidal antiandrogen agents appear to act by competitively binding the receptor for DHT, the intracellular androgen responsible for prostate cell growth and development. A meta-analysis of trials comparing the use of either an LHRH agonist or orchiectomy alone with the use of either in combination with an antiandrogen agent shows little benefit of combination therapy. However, patients at risk for disease-related symptoms (bone pain, obstructive voiding symptoms) due to the initial elevation of serum testosterone that accompanies the use of an LHRH agonist should receive antiandrogens initially. Bisphosphonates are increasingly being used to prevent osteoporosis associated with androgen deprivation, to decrease bone pain from metastases, and to reduce skeletal related events.

Docetaxel is the first cytotoxic chemotherapy agent to improve survival in patients with hormone-refractory prostate cancer. Current research is underway combining docetaxel with androgen deprivation therapy, radiation therapy, and surgery to determine whether combinations are effective in patients with high-risk prostate cancer. Immune therapies are also under investigation and have shown promise for patients with advanced prostate cancer.

Prognosis

The likelihood of success of surveillance or treatment can be predicted using risk assessment tools that usually combine stage, grade, PSA level, and number and extent of positive prostate biopsies. Several tools are available on the Internet (eg, http://mskcc.org/mskcc/html/5794.cfm). One of the most widely used is the Kattan nomogram; it incorporates tumor stage, grade, and PSA level to predict the likelihood that a patient will be disease-free after radical prostatectomy or radiation therapy.

The CAPRA nomogram uses serum PSA, Gleason grade, clinical stage, percent positive biopsies, and patient age in a point system to risk stratify and predict the likelihood of PSA recurrence 3 and 5 years after radical prostatectomy (Tables 39–8 and 39–9). The CAPRA has been validated on large multicenter and international radical prostatectomy cohorts.

The patterns of prostate cancer progression have been well defined. Small and well-differentiated cancers (grades 1 and 2) are usually confined within the prostate, whereas large-volume (> 4 mL) or poorly differentiated (grades 4 and 5) cancers are more often locally extensive or metastatic to regional lymph nodes or bone. Penetration of the prostate capsule by cancer is common and occurs along perineural spaces. Seminal vesicle invasion is associated with a high likelihood of regional or distant disease, and disease recurrence. Lymphatic metastases can be identified in the obturator and internal iliac lymph node chains. The axial skeleton, as mentioned previously, is the most common site of distant metastases.

Table 39–8. The UCSF Cancer of the Prostate Risk Assessment (CAPRA).

Variable	Level	Points
PSA (ng/mL)	0–6	0
	6.1–10	1
	10.1–20	2
	20.1–30	3
	> 30	4
Gleason grade	1–3/1–3	0
	1–3/4–5	1
	4–5/1–5	3
T-stage	T1 or T2	0
	T3a	1
% positive biopsies (biopsy cores positive divided by the number of biopsies obtained)	< 34%	0
	> 34%	1
Age	< 50 years	0
	> 50 years	1

▶ When to Refer

- All patients should be referred to an urologist. PSA remains integral in prostate cancer diagnosis. Low-risk disease may be managed by active surveillance, surgery, or radiation therapy.

- High-risk disease often requires multimodal treatment strategies.

Albertsen PC et al. 20-year outcomes following conservative management of clinically localized prostate cancer. JAMA. 2005 May 4;293(17):2095–101. [PMID: 15870412]

Bill-Axelson A et al; Scandinavian Prostate Cancer Study Group No. 4. Radical prostatectomy versus watchful waiting in early prostate cancer. N Engl J Med. 2005 May 12;352(19):1977–84. [PMID: 15888698]

Table 39–9. CAPRA: Probability of freedom from PSA recurrence after radical prostatectomy by CAPRA point total.

CAPRA Score	3-Year Recurrence Free Survival (%) (95% CI)	5-Year Recurrence Free Survival (%) (95% CI)
0–1	91 (85–95)	85 (73–92)
2	89 (83–94)	81 (69–89)
3	81 (73–87)	66 (54–76)
4	81 (69–89)	59 (40–74)
5	69 (51–82)	60 (37–77)
6	54 (27–75)	34 (12–57)
7+	24 (9–43)	8 (0–28)

PSA, prostate-specific antigen.

Dall'Era MA et al. Active surveillance for the management of prostate cancer in a contemporary cohort. Cancer. 2008 Jun 15;112(12):2664–70. [PMID: 18433013]

Freedland SJ et al. Risk of prostate cancer-specific mortality following biochemical recurrence after radical prostatectomy. JAMA. 2005 Jul 27;294(4):433–9. [PMID: 16046649]

Meng MV et al. Treatment of patients with high risk localized prostate cancer: results from cancer of the prostate strategic urological research endeavor (CaPSURE). J Urol. 2005 May; 173(5):1557–61. [PMID: 15821485]

Thompson IM et al. Prediction of prostate cancer for patients receiving finasteride: results from the Prostate Cancer Prevention Trial. J Clin Oncol. 2007 Jul 20;25(21):3076–81. [PMID: 17634486]

Trock BJ et al. Prostate cancer-specific survival following salvage radiotherapy vs observation in men with biochemical recurrence after radical prostatectomy. JAMA. 2008 Jun 18;299(23):2760–9. [PMID: 18560003]

Walsh PC et al. Clinical practice. Localized prostate cancer. N Engl J Med. 2007 Dec 27;357(26):2696–705. [PMID: 18160689]

BLADDER CANCER

 ESSENTIALS OF DIAGNOSIS

► Irritative voiding symptoms.
► Gross or microscopic hematuria.
► Positive urinary cytology in most patients.
► Filling defect within bladder noted on imaging.

► General Considerations

Bladder cancer is the second most common urologic cancer; it occurs more commonly in men than women (2.7:1), and the mean age of patients at diagnosis is 65 years. Cigarette smoking and exposure to industrial dyes or solvents are risk factors for the disease and account for approximately 60% and 15% of new cases, respectively. Ninety-eight percent of primary bladder cancers are epithelial malignancies, with the majority being urothelial cell carcinomas (90%). Adenocarcinomas and squamous cell cancers account for approximately 2% and 7%, respectively, of all bladder cancers detected in the United States. The latter is often associated with schistosomiasis, vesical calculi, or prolonged catheter use.

► Clinical Findings

A. Symptoms and Signs

Hematuria—gross or microscopic, chronic or intermittent—is the presenting symptom in 85–90% of patients with bladder cancer. Irritative voiding symptoms (urinary frequency and urgency) occur in a small percentage of patients as a result of the location or size of the cancer. Most patients with bladder cancer do not have signs of the disease because of its superficial nature. Abdominal masses detected on bimanual examination may be present in patients with large-volume or deeply infiltrating cancers. Hepatomegaly or palpable lymphadenopathy may be present in patients with metastatic disease, and lymphe-dema of the lower extremities may be present as a result of locally advanced cancers or metastases to pelvic lymph nodes.

B. Laboratory Findings

Urinalysis reveals microscopic or gross hematuria in the majority of cases. On occasion, hematuria may be accompanied by pyuria. Azotemia may be present in a small number of cases associated with ureteral obstruction. Anemia may occasionally be due to chronic blood loss or to bone marrow metastases. Exfoliated cells from normal and abnormal urothelium can be readily detected in voided urine specimens. Cytology can be useful in detecting the disease at the time of initial presentation or to detect recurrence. Cytology is sensitive in detecting cancers of higher grade and stage (80–90%) but less so in detecting superficial or well-differentiated lesions (50%). There are numerous urinary tumor markers under investigation for screening, assessing recurrence, progression, prognosis or response to therapy; the NMP22 point-of-care assay for a specific urinary protein has shown utility in detecting recurrent tumors.

C. Imaging

Bladder cancers may be identified using ultrasound, CT, or MRI where filling defects within the bladder are noted. However, the presence of cancer is confirmed by cystoscopy and biopsy, with imaging primarily used to evaluate the upper urinary tract and stage more advanced lesions.

D. Cystourethroscopy and Biopsy

The diagnosis and staging of bladder cancers are made by cystoscopy and transurethral resection. If cystoscopy—performed usually under local anesthesia—confirms the presence of bladder cancer, the patient is scheduled for transurethral resection under general or regional anesthesia. Random bladder and, on occasion, prostate urethral biopsies are performed to detect occult disease elsewhere in the bladder and potentially identify patients at greater risk for tumor recurrence and progression.

► Pathology & Staging

Grading is based on cellular features: size, pleomorphism, mitotic rate, and hyperchromatism. Bladder cancer staging is based on the extent of bladder wall penetration and the presence of regional or distant metastases.

The natural history of bladder cancer is based on two separate but related processes: tumor recurrence within the bladder and progression to higher-stage disease. Both are correlated with tumor grade and stage.

► Treatment

Patients with superficial cancers (Ta, T1) are treated with complete transurethral resection and selective use of intravesical chemotherapy. In the subset of patients with large, high-grade, recurrent Ta lesions or T1 cancers and those with carcinoma in situ are good candidates for adjuvant intravesical therapy.

Patients with invasive (T2, T3) but still localized cancers are at risk for both nodal metastases and progression and require radical cystectomy, irradiation, or the combination of chemotherapy and selective surgery or irradiation due to the much higher risk of progression compared with patients with lower-stage lesions.

For patients with muscle invasive (T2 or greater) transitional cell carcinoma, neoadjuvant systemic chemotherapy prior to radical cystectomy is superior to radical cystectomy alone. This is particularly important for higher stage or bulky tumors in order to improve their surgical resectability.

A. Intravesical Chemotherapy

Immunotherapeutic or chemotherapeutic agents delivered directly into the bladder via a urethral catheter can reduce the likelihood of recurrence in those who have undergone complete transurethral resection. Most agents are administered weekly for 6–12 weeks. Efficacy may be increased by prolonging contact time to 2 hours. The use of maintenance therapy after the initial induction regimen is beneficial. Common agents include thiotepa, mitomycin, doxorubicin, and BCG, the last being the most effective agent when compared with the others with respect to reducing disease progression. Side effects of intravesical chemotherapy include irritative voiding symptoms and hemorrhagic cystitis. Patients in whom symptoms or infection develop from BCG may require antituberculous therapy.

B. Surgical Treatment

Although transurethral resection is the initial form of treatment for all bladder tumors since it is diagnostic, allows for proper staging, and controls superficial cancers, muscle-infiltrating cancers require more aggressive treatment. Partial cystectomy is indicated in selected patients with solitary lesions or those with cancers in a bladder diverticulum. Radical cystectomy entails removal of the bladder, prostate, seminal vesicles, and surrounding fat and peritoneal attachments in men and the uterus, cervix, urethra, anterior vaginal vault, and usually the ovaries in women. Bilateral pelvic lymph node dissection is performed in all patients.

Urinary diversion can be performed using a conduit of small or large bowel. However, continent forms of diversion have been developed that avoid the necessity of an external appliance and can be considered in a significant number of patients.

C. Radiotherapy

External beam radiotherapy delivered in fractions over a 6- to 8-week period is generally well tolerated, but approximately 10–15% of patients will develop bladder, bowel, or rectal complications. Local recurrence is common after radiotherapy alone (30–70%) and is therefore combined with systemic chemotherapy in an effort to reduce the need for radical cystectomy or to treat patients who are poor candidates for radical cystectomy.

D. Chemotherapy

Metastatic disease is present in 15% of patients with newly diagnosed bladder cancer, and metastases develop within 2 years in up to 40% of patients who were believed to have localized disease at the time of cystectomy or definitive radiotherapy. Cisplatin-based combination chemotherapy results in partial or complete responses in 15–45% of patients (see Table 39–4).

Combination chemotherapy has been integrated into trials of surgery and radiotherapy. It has been used to decrease recurrence rates with both modalities and to attempt bladder preservation in those treated with radiation. Chemotherapy should be considered before surgery in those with bulky lesions or those suspected of having regional disease, and recent evidence suggests that neoadjuvant chemotherapy may benefit all patients prior to planned cystectomy. Chemoradiation is best suited for those with T2 or limited T3 disease without ureteral obstruction. Alternatively, chemotherapy has been used after cystectomy in patients at high risk for recurrence.

▶ Prognosis

The frequency of recurrence and progression are correlated with grade. Whereas progression may be noted in few grade I cancers (19–37%), it is common with poorly differentiated lesions (33–67%). Carcinoma in situ is most often found in association with papillary bladder cancers. Its presence identifies patients at increased risk for recurrence and progression.

At initial presentation, approximately 50–80% of bladder cancers are superficial: stage Ta, Tis, or T1. When properly treated, lymph node metastases and progression are uncommon in this population and survival is excellent at 81%. Five-year survival of patients with T2 and T3 disease ranges from 50% to 75% after radical cystectomy. Long-term survival for patients with metastatic disease at presentation is rare.

▶ When to Refer

- All patients should be referred to an urologist. Hematuria often deserves evaluation with upper urinary tract imaging and cystoscopy.
- Histologic diagnosis and staging require endoscopic resection of tumor.

Droller MJ. Primary care update on kidney and bladder cancer: a urologic perspective. Med Clin North Am. 2004 Mar;88(2):309–28. [PMID: 15049580]

Grossman HB et al. Surveillance for recurrent bladder cancer using a point-of-care proteomic assay. JAMA. 2006 Jan 18;295(3):299–305. [PMID: 16418465]

Habuchi T et al. Prognostic markers for bladder cancer: International consensus panel on bladder tumor markers. Urology. 2005 Dec;66(6 Suppl 1):64–74. [PMID: 16399416]

Parekh DJ et al. Superficial and muscle-invasive bladder cancer: principles of management for outcomes assessments. J Clin Oncol. 2006 Dec 10;24(35):5519–27. [PMID: 17158537]

Stenzl A et al. The updated EAU guidelines on muscle-invasive and metastatic bladder cancer. Eur Urol. 2009 Jan 13 [Epub ahead of print]. [PMID: 19157687]

Sternberg CN et al. Chemotherapy for bladder cancer: treatment guidelines for neoadjuvant chemotherapy, bladder preservation, adjuvant chemotherapy, and metastatic cancer. Urology. 2007 Jan;69(1 Suppl):62–79. [PMID: 17280909]

CANCERS OF THE URETER & RENAL PELVIS

Cancers of the renal pelvis and ureter are rare and occur more commonly in patients with bladder cancer, smokers, those with Balkan nephropathy, those exposed to Thorotrast (a contrast agent with radioactive thorium in use until the 1960s), or those with a long history of analgesic abuse. The majority are urothelial cell carcinomas. Gross or microscopic hematuria is present in most patients, and flank pain secondary to bleeding and obstruction occurs less commonly. Like primary bladder tumors, urinary cytology is often positive. The most common signs identified at the time of IVU or CT include an intraluminal filling defect, unilateral nonvisualization of the collecting system, and hydronephrosis. Ureteral and renal pelvic tumors must be differentiated from calculi, blood clots, papillary necrosis, or inflammatory and infectious lesions. On occasion, upper urinary tract lesions are accessible for biopsy, fulguration, or resection using a ureteroscope. Treatment is based on the site, size, grade, depth of penetration, and number of tumors present. Most are excised with laparoscopic or open nephroureterectomy (renal pelvic and upper ureteral lesions) or segmental excision of the ureter (distal ureteral lesions). Endoscopic resection may be indicated in patients with limited renal function or focal, low-grade, cancers.

RENAL CELL CARCINOMA

ESSENTIALS OF DIAGNOSIS

▶ Gross or microscopic hematuria.

▶ Flank pain or mass in some patients.

▶ Systemic symptoms such as fever, weight loss may be prominent.

▶ Solid renal mass on imaging.

▶ General Considerations

Renal cell carcinoma accounts for 2.6% of all adult cancers. In the United States, approximately 52,190 cases of renal cell carcinoma are diagnosed and 12,890 deaths result annually. Renal cell carcinoma has a peak incidence in the sixth decade of life and a male-to-female ratio of 2:1. It may be associated with a number of paraneoplastic syndromes (see below and Table 39–2).

The cause is unknown. Cigarette smoking is the only significant environmental risk factor that has been identified. Familial settings for renal cell carcinoma have been identified (von Hippel–Lindau syndrome) as well as an association with dialysis-related acquired cystic disease and specific genetic aberrations (eg, Xp11.2 translocation), but sporadic tumors are far more common.

Renal cell carcinoma originates from the proximal tubule cells. Various histologic cell types are recognized (clear cell, papillary, chromophobe, collecting duct and sarcomatoid).

▶ Clinical Findings

A. Symptoms and Signs

Historically, 60% of patients presented with gross or microscopic hematuria. Flank pain or an abdominal mass was detected in approximately 30% of cases. The triad of flank pain, hematuria, and mass was found in only 10–15% of patients and is often a sign of advanced disease. Fever may be present as a paraneoplastic symptom (see Table 39–2). Symptoms of metastatic disease (cough, bone pain) occur in 20–30% of patients at presentation. Because of the widespread use of ultrasound and CT scanning, renal tumors are frequently detected incidentally in individuals with no urologic symptoms. There has been profound stage migration toward lower stages of disease over the past 10 years, likely due to the increased use of abdominal imaging. However, population mortality rates remain stable.

B. Laboratory Findings

Hematuria is present in 60% of patients. Erythrocytosis from increased erythropoietin production occurs in 5%, though anemia is more common; hypercalcemia may be present in up to 10% of patients. Stauffer syndrome is a reversible syndrome of hepatic dysfunction in the absence of metastatic disease.

C. Imaging

Renal masses are often first identified by abdominal ultrasonography or CT. CT scanning is the most valuable imaging test for renal cell carcinoma. It confirms the character of the mass and further stages the lesion with respect to regional lymph nodes, renal vein, or hepatic involvement. CT also provides valuable information regarding the contralateral kidney (function, bilaterality of neoplasm). Chest radiographs exclude pulmonary metastases, and bone scans should be performed for large tumors and in patients with bone pain or elevated alkaline phosphatase levels. MRI and duplex Doppler ultrasonography are excellent methods of assessing for the presence and extent of tumor thrombus within the renal vein or vena cava.

▶ Differential Diagnosis

Solid lesions of the kidney are renal cell carcinoma until proved otherwise. Other solid masses include angiomyolipomas (fat density usually visible by CT), urothelial cell cancers of the renal pelvis (more centrally located, involvement of the collecting system, positive urinary cytologic tests), adrenal tumors (superoanterior to the kidney) and oncocytomas (indistinguishable from renal cell carcinoma preoperatively), and renal abscesses.

▶ Treatment

Radical nephrectomy is the primary treatment for localized renal cell carcinoma. Patients with a single kidney, bilateral lesions, or significant medical renal disease should be considered for partial nephrectomy. Patients with a normal contralateral kidney and good renal function but a small cancer are also candidates for partial nephrectomy. The use of radiofrequency or cryosurgical ablation is being studied.

No effective chemotherapy is available for metastatic renal cell carcinoma. Vinblastine is the single most effective agent, with short-term partial response rates of 15%. Bevacizumab can prolong time to progression in those with metastatic disease (see Table 39–4). Biologic response modifiers have received much attention, including interferon-α and interleukin-2. Partial response rates of 15–20% and 15–35%, respectively, have been reported. Responders tend to have lower tumor burdens, metastatic disease confined to the lung, and a high performance status. Patients with metastatic kidney cancer and good performance status who have resectable primary tumors should undergo cytoreductive nephrectomy. Two randomized trials have shown a survival benefit of surgery followed by the use of systemic therapy—specifically, biologic response modifiers—compared with the use of systemic therapy alone.

Several targeted drugs, specifically VEGF and Raf-kinase inhibitors, are effective (40% response rates) in patients with advanced kidney cancer. The drugs are oral agents, well tolerated, and particularly active for clear cell carcinoma. The appropriate timing and combination of these agents, with and without surgery and cytokine therapy, remains to be determined.

▶ Prognosis

After radical nephrectomy, tumors confined to the renal capsule (T1–T2) demonstrate 5-year disease-free survivals of 90–100%. Tumors extending beyond the renal capsule (T3 or T4) and node-positive tumors have 50–60% and 0–15% 5-year disease-free survival, respectively. One subgroup of patients with nonlocalized disease has reasonable long-term survival, namely, those with solitary resectable metastases. In this setting, radical nephrectomy with resection of the metastasis results in 5-year disease-free survival rates of 15–30%.

▶ When to Refer

- Patients with solid renal masses require further evaluation and should be referred to an urologist.
- Surgical excision of renal cell carcinoma remains the gold standard.
- Patients with metastatic disease should be referred to an oncologist.

Choueiri TK et al. Clinical factors associated with outcome in patients with metastatic clear-cell renal cell carcinoma treated with vascular endothelial growth factor-targeted therapy. Cancer. 2007 Aug 1;110(3):543–50. [PMID: 17577222]

Escudier B et al. Sorafenib in advanced clear-cell renal-cell carcinoma. N Engl J Med. 2007 Jan 11;356(2):125–34. [PMID: 17215530]

Flanigan RC et al. Nephrectomy followed by interferon alfa-2b compared with interferon alfa-2b alone for metastatic renal-cell cancer. N Engl J Med. 2001 Dec 6;345(23):1655–9. [PMID: 11759643]

Hudes G et al. Temsirolimus, interferon alfa, or both for advanced renal-cell carcinoma. N Engl J Med. 2007 May 31;356(22):2271–81. [PMID: 17538086]

Motzer RJ et al. Sunitinib in patients with metastatic renal cell carcinoma. JAMA. 2006 Jun 7;295(21):2516–24. [PMID: 15479931]

Motzer RJ et al. Sunitinib versus interferon alfa in metastatic renal-cell carcinoma. N Engl J Med. 2007 Jan 11;356(2):115–24. [PMID: 17215529]

OTHER PRIMARY TUMORS OF THE KIDNEY

Oncocytomas account for 3–5% of renal tumors, are usually benign, and are indistinguishable from renal cell carcinoma on preoperative imaging. These tumors are seen in other organs, including the adrenals, salivary glands, and thyroid and parathyroid glands.

Angiomyolipomas are rare benign tumors composed of fat, smooth muscle, and blood vessels. They are most commonly seen in patients with tuberous sclerosis (often multiple and bilateral) or in young to middle-aged women. CT scanning may identify the fat component, which is diagnostic for angiomyolipoma. Asymptomatic lesions less than 5 cm in diameter usually do not require intervention; large lesions can spontaneously bleed. Acute bleeding can be treated by angiographic embolization or, in rare cases, nephrectomy. Lesions over 5 cm are often prophylactically treated with angioembolization to reduce the risk of bleeding.

SECONDARY TUMORS OF THE KIDNEY

The kidney is not an infrequent site for metastatic disease. Of the solid tumors, lung cancer is the most common (20%), followed by breast (10%), stomach (10%), and the contralateral kidney (10%). Lymphoma, both Hodgkin and non-Hodgkin, may also involve the kidney, although it tends to be appear as a diffusely infiltrative process resulting in renal enlargement rather than a discrete mass.

PRIMARY TUMORS OF THE TESTIS

 ESSENTIALS OF DIAGNOSIS

- ▶ Commonest neoplasm in men aged 20–35 years.
- ▶ Typical presentation as a patient-identified painless nodule.
- ▶ Orchiectomy necessary for diagnosis.

▶ General Considerations

Malignant tumors of the testis are rare, with approximately two to three new cases per 100,000 males reported in the United States each year. Ninety to 95 percent of all primary testicular tumors are germ cell tumors and can be divided into two major categories: **nonseminomas**, including embryonal cell carcinoma (20%), teratoma (5%), chorio-carcinoma (< 1%), and mixed cell types (40%); and **semi-nomas** (35%). The remainder of primary testicular tumors are nongerminal neoplasms (Leydig cell, Sertoli cell, gonadoblastoma). The lifetime probability of developing testicular cancer is 0.2% for an American white male. For the purposes of this review, only germ cell tumors will be considered.

Approximately 5% of testicular tumors develop in a patient with a history of cryptorchism, with seminoma being the most common. However, 5–10% of these tumors occur in the contralateral, normally descended testis. The relative risk of development of malignancy is highest for the intra-abdominal testis (1:20) and lower for the inguinal testis (1:80). Placement of the cryptorchid testis into the scrotum (orchidopexy) does not alter the malignant potential of the cryptorchid testis but does facilitate routine examination and tumor detection.

Testicular cancer is slightly more common on the right than the left, paralleling the increased incidence of cryptorchidism on the right side. One to 2 percent of primary testicular tumors are bilateral and up to 50% of these men have a history of unilateral or bilateral cryptorchidism. Primary bilateral testicular tumors may occur synchronously or asynchronously but tend to be of the same histology. Seminoma is the most common histologic finding in bilateral *primary* testicular tumors, while malignant lymphoma is the most common bilateral testicular tumor overall.

In animal models, exogenous estrogen administration during pregnancy has been associated with an increased development of testicular tumors with relative risk ranging from 2.8 to 5.3. Other acquired factors such as trauma and infection-related testicular atrophy have been associated with testicular tumors; however, a causal relationship has not been established.

► Clinical Findings

A. Symptoms and Signs

The most common symptom of testicular cancer is painless enlargement of the testis. Sensations of heaviness are not unusual. Patients are usually the first to recognize an abnormality, yet the typical delay in seeking medical attention ranges from 3 to 6 months. Acute testicular pain resulting from intratesticular hemorrhage occurs in approximately 10% of cases. Ten percent of patients are asymptomatic at presentation, and 10% manifest symptoms relating to metastatic disease such as back pain (retroperitoneal metastases), cough (pulmonary metastases), or lower extremity edema (vena cava obstruction).

A discrete mass or diffuse testicular enlargement is noted in most cases. Secondary hydroceles may be present in 5–10% of cases. In advanced disease, supraclavicular adenopathy may be present, and abdominal examination may reveal a mass. Gynecomastia is seen in 5% of germ cell tumors.

B. Laboratory Findings

Several serum markers are important in the diagnosis and monitoring of testicular carcinoma, including human chorionic gonadotropin (hCG), α-fetoprotein, and LD. α-Fetoprotein is never elevated with pure seminomas, and while hCG is occasionally elevated in seminomas, levels tend to be lower than those seen with nonseminomas. LD may be elevated with either type of tumor. Liver function tests may be elevated in the presence of hepatic metastases, and anemia may be present in advanced disease.

C. Imaging

Scrotal ultrasound can readily determine whether a mass is intratesticular or extratesticular. Once the diagnosis of testicular cancer has been established by inguinal orchiectomy, clinical staging of the disease is accomplished by chest, abdominal, and pelvic CT scanning.

► Staging

In a commonly used staging system for nonseminoma germ cell tumors, a stage A lesion is confined to the testis; stage B demonstrates regional lymph node involvement in the retroperitoneum; and stage C indicates distant metastasis. For seminoma, the M.D. Anderson system is commonly used. In this system, a stage I lesion is confined to the testis, a stage II lesion has spread to the retroperitoneal lymph nodes, and a stage III lesion has supradiaphragmatic nodal or visceral involvement.

► Differential Diagnosis

An incorrect diagnosis is made at the initial examination in up to 25% of patients with testicular tumors. Scrotal ultrasonography should be performed if any uncertainty exists with respect to the diagnosis. Although most intratesticular masses are malignant, a benign lesion—epidermoid cyst—may rarely be seen. Epidermoid cysts are usually very small benign nodules located just underneath the tunica albuginea; occasionally, however, they can be large.

► Treatment

Inguinal exploration with early vascular control of the spermatic cord structures is the initial intervention. If cancer cannot be excluded by examination of the testis, radical orchiectomy is warranted. Scrotal approaches and open testicular biopsies should be avoided. Further therapy depends on the histology of the tumor as well as the clinical stage.

Stage I and IIa **seminomas** (retroperitoneal disease < 10 cm in diameter) are treated by radical orchiectomy and retroperitoneal irradiation. Patients with clinical stage I disease may be candidates for surveillance or single-agent carboplatin. Seminomas of stage IIb (> 10 cm retroperitoneal involvement) and stage III receive primary chemotherapy (etoposide and cisplatin or cisplatin, etoposide, and bleomycin). Surgical resection of residual retroperitoneal masses is warranted if the mass is larger than 3 cm in diameter, under which circumstances 40% will harbor residual carcinoma.

Up to 75% of clinical stage I **nonseminomas** are cured by orchiectomy alone. Selected patients who meet specific criteria may be offered surveillance after orchiectomy. These criteria are as follows: (1) tumor is confined within the tunica albuginea; (2) tumor does not demonstrate vascular invasion; (3) tumor markers normalize after orchiectomy;

(4) radiographic imaging of the chest and abdomen shows no evidence of disease; and (5) the patient is reliable. Patients most likely to experience relapse on a surveillance regimen include those with predominantly embryonal cancer and those with vascular or lymphatic invasion identified in the orchiectomy specimen. Surveillance needs to be considered an active process both by the clinician and by the patient. Patients are followed monthly for the first 2 years and bimonthly in the third year. Tumor markers are obtained at each visit, and chest radiographs and CT scans are obtained every 3 months. Follow-up continues beyond the initial 3 years; however, the 80% of relapses will occur within the first 2 years. With rare exceptions, patients who relapse can be cured by chemotherapy or surgery. Alternatives to surveillance include adjuvant chemotherapy (bleomycin, etoposide, cisplatin) and retroperitoneal lymph nodes dissection.

Patients with bulky retroperitoneal disease (> 3 cm nodes) or metastatic nonseminomas are treated with primary cisplatin-based combination chemotherapy following orchiectomy (etoposide and cisplatin or cisplatin, etoposide, and bleomycin) (see Table 39–4). If tumor markers normalize and a residual mass greater than 1 cm persists on imaging studies, the mass is resected because 20% of the time it will harbor viable cancer and 40% of the time it will harbor teratoma. Even if patients have a complete response to chemotherapy, some clinicians advocate retroperitoneal lymphadenectomy since 10% of patients may harbor residual carcinoma and 10% may have teratoma in the retroperitoneum. If tumor markers fail to normalize following primary chemotherapy, salvage chemotherapy is required (cisplatin, etoposide, ifosfamide).

▶ **Prognosis**

The 5-year disease-free survival rates for stage I and IIa **seminomas** (retroperitoneal disease < 10 cm in diameter) treated by radical orchiectomy and retroperitoneal irradiation are 98% and 92–94%, respectively. Ninety-five percent of patients with stage III disease attain a complete response following orchiectomy and chemotherapy. Patients with bulky retroperitoneal or disseminated disease treated with primary chemotherapy followed by surgery have a 5-year disease-free survival rate of 55–80%. The 5-year disease-free survival rate for patients with stage A **nonseminomas** (includes all treatments, orchiectomy and subsequently) ranges from 96% to 100%. For low-volume stage B disease, 90% 5-year disease-free survival is expected.

▶ **When to Refer**

Patients with solid masses of the testis should be referred to a urologist.

Albers P et al. Randomized phase III trial comparing retroperitoneal lymph node dissection with one course of bleomycin and etoposide plus cisplatin chemotherapy in the adjuvant treatment of clinical stage I noneminomatous testicular germ cell tumors: AUO trial AH 01/94 by the German Testicular Cancer Study Group. J Clin Oncol. 2008 Jun 20;26(18):2966–72. [PMID: 18458040]

Aparicio J et al. Risk-adapted management for patients with clinical stage I seminoma: the Second Spanish Germ Cell Cancer Cooperative Group study. J Clin Oncol. 2005 Dec 1;23(34):8717–23. [PMID: 16260698]
de Wit R et al. Controversies in the management of clinical stage I testis cancer. J Clin Oncol. 2006 Dec 10;24(35):5482–92. [PMID: 17158533]
Einhorn LH et al. High-dose chemotherapy and stem-cell rescue for metastatic germ-cell tumors. N Engl J Med. 2007 Jul 26;357(4):340–8. [PMID: 17652649]
Pettersson A et al. Age at surgery for undescended testis and risk of testicular cancer. N Engl J Med. 2007 May 3;356(18):1835–41. [PMID: 17476009]

SECONDARY TUMORS OF THE TESTIS

Secondary tumors of the testis are rare. In men over the age of 50 years, lymphoma is the most common testis tumor, and overall it is the most common secondary neoplasm of the testis, accounting for 5% of all testicular tumors. It may be seen in three clinical settings: (1) late manifestation of widespread lymphoma, (2) the initial presentation of clinically occult disease, and (3) primary extranodal disease. Radical orchiectomy is indicated to make the diagnosis. Prognosis is related to the stage of disease.

Metastasis to the testis is rare. The most common primary site of origin is the prostate, followed by the lung, gastrointestinal tract, melanoma, and kidney.

▼ CANCER COMPLICATIONS & EMERGENCIES

Cancer is a chronic disease, but acute emergency complications (eg, spinal cord compression, superior vena cava syndrome, malignant effusions) or generalized systemic effects (eg, hypercalcemia, opportunistic infections, disseminated intravascular coagulation, hyperuricemia) may occur as a consequence of local invasion of the cancer. Superior vena cava syndrome is discussed in Chapter 12 and disseminated intravascular coagulation is discussed in Chapter 13.

SPINAL CORD COMPRESSION

 ESSENTIALS OF DIAGNOSIS

▶ Occurs as a complication of metastatic solid tumor lymphoma or multiple myeloma.

▶ Back pain is presenting symptom in most patients.

▶ Prompt diagnosis is essential because once a severe neurologic deficit develops, it is generally irreversible.

▶ Emergent treatment may prevent or potentially reverse paresis and urinary and bowel incontinence.

▶ **General Considerations**

Cancers that cause spinal cord compression most commonly metastasize to the vertebral bodies, resulting in physical damage to the spinal cord from edema, hemorrhage, and ischemia. Persistent compression can result in irreversible changes to the myelin sheaths resulting in permanent neurologic impairment.

Prompt diagnosis and therapeutic intervention are essential, since the probability of reversing neurologic symptoms largely depends on the duration of symptoms. Patients who are treated promptly after symptoms appear may have partial or complete return of function and, depending on tumor sensitivity to specific treatment, may respond favorably to subsequent anticancer therapy.

▶ Clinical Findings

A. Symptoms and Signs

Back pain at the level of the tumor mass occurs in over 80% of cases and may be aggravated by lying down, weight bearing, sneezing, or coughing; it usually precedes the development of neurologic symptoms or signs. Since involvement is usually epidural, a mixture of nerve root and spinal cord symptoms often develops. Progressive weakness and sensory changes commonly occur. Bowel and bladder symptoms progressing to incontinence are late findings.

The initial findings of impending cord compression may be quite subtle, and there should be a high index of suspicion when back pain or weakness of the lower extremities develops in cancer patients.

B. Imaging

MRI is usually the initial imaging procedure of choice in a cancer patient with new-onset back pain. When there are neurologic findings suggesting spinal cord compression, an emergent MRI should be obtained. It is important to obtain a survey of the entire spine to define all areas of tumor involvement for treatment planning purposes.

Bone radiographs, if done, may show evidence of vertebral body or pedicle destruction by the cancer. However, bone radiographs are neither sensitive nor specific and therefore are not helpful in diagnosis or treatment planning. If the back pain symptoms are nonspecific, bone scan imaging may be useful as a screening procedure.

▶ Treatment

Patients found to have epidural impingement of the spinal cord should be given corticosteroids immediately. The initial dose is 10–100 mg intravenously followed by 4–6 mg every 6 hours intravenously or orally. Patients without a known diagnosis of cancer should have emergent surgery to relieve the impingement and obtain a pathologic specimen. Patients with a single area of compression due to solid tumors are best treated with surgical decompression followed by radiation therapy. A randomized trial comparing surgery followed by radiation therapy with radiation therapy alone showed better outcomes (ie, improved ability to ambulate and improved bladder and bowel functions) in persons who had surgery followed by radiation therapy. If multiple vertebral body levels are involved with cancer, radiation therapy is the preferred treatment option. Corticosteroids are generally tapered toward the end of radiation therapy.

George R et al. Interventions for the treatment of metastatic extradural spinal cord compression in adults. Cochrane Database Syst Rev. 2008 Oct 8;(4):CD006716. [PMID: 18843728]

Walji N et al. Common acute oncological emergencies: diagnosis, investigation and management. Postgrad Med J. 2008 Aug;84(994):418–27. [PMID: 18832403]

White BD et al. Diagnosis and management of patients at risk of or with metastatic spinal cord compression: summary of NICE guidance. BMJ. 2008 Nov 27;337:a2538. [PMID: 19039017]

MALIGNANT EFFUSIONS

 ESSENTIALS OF DIAGNOSIS

- ▶ Occur in pleural, pericardial, and peritoneal spaces.
- ▶ Caused by direct neoplastic involvement of serous surface or obstruction of lymphatic drainage.
- ▶ Half of undiagnosed effusions in patients not known to have cancer are malignant.

▶ General Considerations

The development of an effusion in the pleural, pericardial, or peritoneal space may be the initial finding in a patient with cancer, or an effusion may appear during the course of disease progression. Direct involvement of the serous surface with tumor is the most frequent initiating cause of the accumulation of fluid. The most common malignancies causing pleural and pericardial effusions are lung and breast cancers; the most common malignancies associated with malignant ascites are ovarian, colorectal, stomach, and pancreatic cancers.

▶ Clinical Findings

A. Symptoms and Signs

Patients with pleural and pericardial effusions complain of shortness of breath and orthopnea. Patients with ascites complain of abdominal distention and discomfort. Cardiac tamponade causing pressure equalization in the chambers impairing both filling and cardiac output can be a life-threatening event. Signs of tamponade include tachycardia, pulsus paradoxus, and hypotension. Signs of pleural effusions include decreased breath sounds, egophony, and percussion dullness.

B. Laboratory Findings

Malignancy is confirmed as the cause of an effusion when analysis of the fluid specimen shows malignant cells in either the cytology or cell block specimen.

C. Imaging

The presence of effusions can be confirmed with radiographic studies or ultrasonography.

▶ Differential Diagnosis

The differential diagnosis of a malignant pleural or pericardial effusion includes benign processes, such as congestive heart failure, pulmonary embolism, trauma, and infection.

The differential diagnosis of malignant ascites includes similar benign processes, such as congestive heart failure and infections; cirrhosis and pancreatic disease also cause ascites.

Bloody effusions are usually due to cancer, but a bloody pleural effusion can also be due to pulmonary embolism or trauma. Chylous pleural or ascitic fluid is generally associated with obstruction of lymphatic drainage as might occur in lymphomas.

► Treatment

In some cases, treatment of the underlying cancer with chemotherapy can cause regression of the effusions; however, not uncommonly, the presence of an effusion is an end-stage manifestation of the disease. In this situation, decisions regarding management are in large part dictated by the patient's symptoms and goals of care.

A. Pleural Effusion

A pleural effusion that is symptomatic may be managed initially with a **large volume thoracentesis**. With some patients, the effusion slowly reaccumulates, which allows for periodic thoracentesis when the patient becomes symptomatic. However, in most patients, the effusion reaccumulates quickly, causing rapid return of symptoms of shortness of breath. For those patients, several options exist for management. **Chest tube drainage followed by pleurodesis** is the preferred option for patients with a reasonable life expectancy. Patients are generally hospitalized for 3–7 days. The procedure involves placement of a chest tube that is connected to closed water seal drainage. Fluid is allowed to drain over several days. After lung expansion is confirmed on a chest radiograph, a sclerosing agent (such as talc slurry) is injected into the catheter. Other agents that can be used include doxycycline or bleomycin. Patients should be premedicated with analgesics and placed in a variety of positions in order to distribute the drug through the pleural spaces. Pleurodesis will not be successful if the lung cannot be reexpanded; these patients may be treated with the placement of a shunt or continued use of catheter drainage. Until recently, standard management had been to hold sclerosis until the chest tube drainage had decreased to less than 100 mL/d; a recent randomized trial comparing immediate pleurodesis after initial drainage with waiting until drainage had decreased to 100 mL/d showed no difference in pleurodesis efficacy between the two groups.

B. Pericardial Effusion

Fluid may be removed by a needle aspiration or by placement of a catheter for more thorough drainage. As with pleural effusions, most pericardial effusions will reaccumulate. Management options for recurrent, symptomatic effusions include catheter drainage followed by sclerosis with such agents as doxycycline or bleomycin or by pericardiectomy.

C. Malignant Ascites

Patients with malignant ascites not responsive to chemotherapy are generally treated with repeated large volume

paracenteses. As the frequency of drainage to maintain comfort can compromise the patient's quality of life, other alternatives include placement of a catheter or port so that the patient, family member, or visiting nurse can drain fluid as needed at home. Another option is placement of a peritoneovenous shunt; this can be considered for a select group of patients with life expectancy greater than 3 months and fluid that is nonviscous, nonbloody, and nonloculated.

Antunes G et al; Pleural Diseases Group, Standards of Care Committee, British Thoracic Society. BTS guidelines for the management of malignant pleural effusions. Thorax. 2003 May;58(Suppl 2):ii29–38. [PMID: 12728148]

Becker G et al. Malignant ascites: systematic review and guideline for treatment. Eur J Cancer. 2006 Mar;42(5):589–97. [PMID: 16434188]

Maisch B et al. Guidelines on the diagnosis and management of pericardial diseases executive summary; The Task Force on the Diagnosis and Management of Pericardial Diseases of the European Society of Cardiology. Eur Heart J. 2004 Apr;25(7):587–610. [PMID: 15120056]

HYPERCALCEMIA

ESSENTIALS OF DIAGNOSIS

► Usually symptomatic and severe (≥ 15 mg/dL).

► Most common paraneoplastic endocrine syndrome, accounting for most cases of hypercalcemia among inpatients.

► The neoplasm is clinically apparent in nearly all cases when hypercalcemia is detected.

► General Considerations

Hypercalcemia affects 20–30% of cancer patients at some point during their illness. The most common cancers causing hypercalcemia are myeloma, breast carcinoma, and non–small cell lung cancer. The presence of bone metastasis is not an essential feature of the syndrome, since hypercalcemia can be caused by systemic effects of tumor-released proteins (see The Paraneoplastic Syndromes above).

► Clinical Findings

A. Symptoms and Signs

Symptoms and signs of hypercalcemia can be subtle; the severity of symptoms not only depends on the degree of hypercalcemia but also the rate at which the calcium level rises. Early symptoms typically include anorexia, nausea, fatigue, constipation, and polyuria; later findings may include muscular weakness and hyporeflexia, confusion, psychosis, tremor, and lethargy.

B. Laboratory Findings

Symptoms and signs are caused by free calcium; as calcium is bound by protein in the serum, the measured serum calcium will underestimate the free or ionized calcium in

patients with low albumin levels. In the setting of hypoalbuminemia, the corrected serum calcium should be calculated by one of several available formulas (eg, corrected
calcium = measured calcium − measured albumin + 4).
Alternatively, the free calcium can be measured. When the
corrected serum calcium rises above 12 mg/dL, sudden
death due to cardiac arrhythmia or asystole may occur.
The presence of hypercalcemia does not invariably indicate
a dismal prognosis, especially in patients with breast cancer, myeloma, or lymphoma.

In the absence of signs or symptoms of hypercalcemia,
a laboratory finding of elevated serum calcium should be
retested immediately to exclude the possibility of error.

C. ECG

Electrocardiography often shows a shortening of the QT
interval.

▶ Treatment

Emergency management should begin with the initiation
of intravenous fluids with 0.9% saline at 100–200 mL/h to
ensure rehydration with brisk urinary output of the often
volume-depleted patient. If kidney function is normal or
only marginally impaired, a bisphosphonate should be
given. Choices include pamidronate, 60–90 mg intravenously over 2–4 hours, or zoledronic acid, 4 mg intravenously over several minutes. Zoledronic acid is more
potent than pamidronate and has the advantage of a
shorter administration time as well as a longer duration of
effect but is more associated with the uncommon but
serious side effect of osteonecrosis of the jaw. Once hypercalcemia is controlled, treatment directed at the cancer
should be initiated if possible. Commonly, though, hypercalcemia occurs in patients with cancers that are unresponsive to treatment. In the event that the hypercalcemia
becomes refractory to repeated doses of bisphosphonates,
other agents that can help control hypercalcemia (at least
temporarily) include gallium nitrate, calcitonin, and mithramycin; corticosteroids can be useful in patients with
myeloma and lymphoma. Salmon calcitonin, 4–8 international units/kg given subcutaneously or intramuscularly
every 12 hours, can be useful in patients with kidney
disease; its onset of action is within hours but its hypocalcemic effect will wane in 2–3 days.

Body JJ et al. International Society of Geriatric Oncology (SIOG)
   clinical practice recommendations for the use of bisphospho-
   nates in elderly patients. Eur J Cancer. 2007 Mar;43(5):852–8.
   [PMID: 17258449]
Drake MT et al. Bisphosphonates: mechanism of action and role
   in clinical practice. Mayo Clin Proc. 2008 Sep;83(9):1032–45.
   [PMID: 18775204]
Mundy GR et al. PTH-related peptide (PTHrP) in hypercalce-
   mia. J Am Soc Nephrol. 2008 Apr;19(4):672–5. [PMID:
   18256357]
Smith GF et al. Primary care of the patient with cancer. Am Fam
   Physician. 2007 Apr 15;75(8):1207–14. [PMID: 17477104]
Walji N et al. Common acute oncological emergencies: diagno-
   sis, investigation and management. Postgrad Med J. 2008
   Aug;84(994):418–27. [PMID: 18832403]

HYPERURICEMIA & TUMOR LYSIS SYNDROME

 ESSENTIALS OF DIAGNOSIS

▶ Complication of treatment-associated tumor lysis of
   hematologic malignancies as well as rapidly proliferating malignancies.

▶ May be worsened by thiazide diuretic use.

▶ Rapid increase in serum uric acid can result in acute
   urate nephropathy caused by uric acid crystallization.

▶ Reducing pre-chemotherapy serum uric acid is fundamental to preventing urate nephropathy.

▶ General Considerations

Tumor lysis syndrome (TLS) is seen most commonly
following treatment of hematologic malignancies, such as
acute lymphoblastic leukemia and Burkitt lymphoma.
However, TLS can develop from any tumor highly sensitive to chemotherapy. TLS is caused by the massive release
of cellular material including nucleic acids, proteins, phosphorus, and potassium. If both the metabolism and excretion of these breakdown products are overwhelmed, hyperuremia, hyperphosphatemia, and hyperkalemia will
develop abruptly. Acute kidney injury may develop from
the hyperuremia, further exacerbating the hyperphosphatemia and hyperkalemia.

▶ Clinical Findings

Symptoms of hyperphosphatemia include nausea and
vomiting as well as seizures. Also, with high levels of
phosphorus, co-precipitation with calcium can cause renal
tubule blockage further exacerbating the kidney injury.
Hyperkalemia, due to release of intracellular potassium
and with excretion impaired by the kidney disease, can
cause arrhythmias and sudden death.

▶ Treatment

Prevention is the most important factor in the management
of TLS. Guidelines for management of TLS have been
developed by the American Society of Clinical Oncology and
include aggressive hydration prior to initiation of chemotherapy as well as during and after completion of the
chemotherapy. Administration of fluid helps keep urine
flowing and facilitate excretion of uric acid and phosphorus.
For the patients with moderate risk of developing TLS,
allopurinol (which blocks the enzyme xanthine oxidase and
therefore the formation of uric acid from purine breakdown) should be given before starting chemotherapy at an
oral dose of 100 mg/m^2 every 8 hours (maximum 800 mg/d)
with dose adjustments for kidney disease. For patients at
high risk for developing TLS or in whom hyperuricemia
develops despite treatment with allopurinol, rasburicase
0.1–0.2 mg/kg/d is given intravenously for 1–7 days. Rasburicase is a recombinant urate oxidase that converts uric acid
into the more soluble form resulting in rapid decline in uric

acid levels. Rasburicase cannot be given to patients with known glucose 6-phosphate dehydrogenase (G6PD) deficiency nor can it be given to pregnant or lactating women. One of the mainstays of TLS management, systemic bicarbonate infusions to alkalinize the urine, is no longer recommended. Laboratory values should be monitored following initiation of chemotherapy; elevated potassium or phosphorus levels need to be promptly managed.

▶ When to Refer

Should urinary output drop or creatinine level rise, a nephrologist should be consulted to evaluate the need for dialysis.

Coiffier B et al. Guidelines for the management of pediatric and adult tumor lysis syndrome: an evidence-based review. J Clin Oncol. 2008 Jun 1;26(16):2767–78. [PMID: 18509186]
Higdon ML et al. Treatment of oncologic emergencies. Am Fam Physician. 2006 Dec 1;74(11):1873–80. [PMID: 17168344]

INFECTIONS

Chapter 30 provides a more detailed discussion of infections in the immunocompromised patient.

ESSENTIALS OF DIAGNOSIS

▶ In patients with neutropenia, infection is a medical emergency.

▶ The presence of fever, although sometimes attributable to other causes, must be assumed to be due to an infection.

▶ General Considerations

Many patients with disseminated neoplasms have increased susceptibility to infection. In some patients, this results from impaired defense mechanisms (eg, acute leukemia, Hodgkin disease, multiple myeloma, chronic lymphocytic leukemia); in others, it results from the myelosuppressive and immunosuppressive effects of cancer chemotherapy or a combination of these factors. Complicating impaired defense mechanisms are the frequent presence of indwelling catheters, impaired mucosal surfaces, and colonization with more virulent hospital-acquired pathogens.

The source of a neutropenic febrile episode is determined in about 30% of cases through blood, urine, or sputum cultures. The bacterial organisms accounting for the majority of infections in cancer patients include gram-negative bacteria (*Escherichia coli, Klebsiella, Pseudomonas, Enterobacter*) and gram-positive bacteria (coagulase-negative *Staphylococcus, Staphylococcus aureus, Streptococcus pneumoniae, Corynebacterium,* and streptococci). There has been a trend over the last decade of an increasing percentage of gram-positive organisms. The risk of bacterial infections rises when the granulocyte count is below 1000/mcL; the risk dramatically increases when the count falls below 100/mcL.

▶ Clinical Findings

Appropriate cultures (eg, blood, sputum, urine, cerebrospinal fluid) should always be obtained before starting therapy. Two sets of blood cultures should be drawn; if the patient has an indwelling catheter, one of the cultures should be drawn from the line. A chest radiograph should also be obtained.

▶ Treatment

Empiric antibiotic therapy needs to be initiated immediately in the febrile, neutropenic patient. The choice of antibiotics depends on a number of different factors including the patient's clinical status and any localizing source of infection. If the patient is clinically well, monotherapy with an intravenous β-lactam with anti-*Pseudomonas* activity (cefepime, ceftazidime, imipenem/cilastatin, piperacillin/tazabactam) should be started. If the patient is clinically ill with hypotension or hypoxia, an aminoglycoside or fluoroquinolone should be added for "double" gram-negative bacteria coverage. If there is a strong suspicion of a gram-positive organism, such as from *S aureus* catheter infection, vancomycin can be given empirically. In some instances, patients may be treated with oral antibiotics and potentially in the outpatient setting. The Infectious Disease Society of America (IDSA) has published recommendations for antibiotic use in these low-risk patients. These patients must have an expected neutropenic timeframe of 7 days or less and not have comorbidities or signs of hemodynamic instability, gastrointestinal symptoms, altered mental status, pulmonary issues (an infiltrate, hypoxia, or underlying chronic obstructive pulmonary disease) and their liver and kidney function must not be impaired. If a patient is to be treated as an outpatient, he or she must also have good support at home and easy access to returning to the hospital if the clinical status worsens.

Antibiotics should be continued until the neutrophil count is rising and greater than 500/mcL for at least 1 day and the patient has been afebrile for 2 days. If an organism is identified through the cultures, the antibiotics should be adjusted to the antibiotic sensitivities of the isolate; treatment should be continued for the appropriate period of time and at least until the neutrophil count recovers.

For the neutropenic patient who is persistently febrile despite broad-spectrum antibiotics, an empiric antifungal drug should be added (amphotericin B, caspofungin, itraconazole, voriconazole, or liposomal amphotericin B).

Segal BH et al. Prevention and treatment of cancer-related infections. J Natl Compr Canc Netw. 2008 Feb;6(2):122–74. [PMID: 18319048]

▼ PRIMARY CANCER TREATMENT

SYSTEMIC CANCER THERAPY

Detailed guidelines from the NCCN for cancer treatment can be found at www.nccn.org.

Use of cytotoxic drugs, hormones, antihormones, and biologic agents has become a highly specialized and increasingly effective means of treating cancer, with therapy usually administered by a medical oncologist. Selection of specific drugs or protocols for various types of cancer has traditionally been based on results of prior clinical trials; however, many patients have drug-resistant tumors. Molecular mechanisms of drug resistance continue to be the subject of intense study. Described mechanisms of drug resistance include impaired membrane transport of drugs, enhanced drug metabolism, mutated target proteins, and blockage of apoptosis due to mutations in cell cycle proteins. Cancer cells may initially be resistant to chemotherapy or acquire resistance when exposed to drugs.

TOXICITY & DOSE MODIFICATION OF CHEMOTHERAPEUTIC AGENTS

Use of chemotherapy to treat cancer is generally guided by results from clinical trials in individual tumor types. The complexity of treating cancer has increased over the last decade as more drugs, including those with novel mechanisms of action, have been approved by the Food and Drug Administration and introduced into general practice. Drug side effects and toxicities must be anticipated and carefully monitored. The short- and long-term toxicities of individual drugs are listed in Tables 39–10 and 39–11. Decisions on dose modifications for toxicities should be guided by the intent of therapy. In the palliative setting where the aim of therapy is to improve symptoms and quality of life, lowering doses to minimize toxicity is commonly done. However, when the goal of treatment is cure, dosing frequency and intensity should be maintained whenever possible. Cancer chemotherapy should be given and monitored by a medical oncologist or hematologist.

A complete blood count consisting of a differential count with particular attention to the absolute neutrophil count and platelet count as well as tests of liver and kidney function should be obtained before the initiation of chemotherapy. In patients with normal blood counts as well as normal liver and kidney function, drugs are started at their full dose. When the intent of chemotherapy is cure, including treatment in the adjuvant setting, every attempt should be made to schedule chemotherapy on time and at full dose. A complete blood count with differential should be checked at mid cycle to determine the nadir of the absolute neutrophil and platelet counts as well as immediately before the next cycle of chemotherapy is due.

Dose reductions may be necessary for patients with impaired kidney or liver function depending on the clearance mechanism of the drug. For patients receiving chemotherapy for palliation, bone marrow toxicity can be managed with dose reductions or delaying the next treatment cycle. A schema for dose modification is shown in Table 39–12.

1. Bone Marrow Toxicity

Depression of the bone marrow and the ability to produce adequate numbers of white cells, red cells, and platelets is usually the most significant limiting toxicity with cancer chemotherapy. Drugs to ameliorate bone marrow suppression have become standard tools in the armamentarium of medical oncologists.

A. Neutropenia

Granulocyte colony-stimulating factor (G-CSF), given as either daily subcutaneous injections (filgrastim, 300 mcg or 480 mcg) or as a one-time dose (pegfilgrastim, 6 mg) beginning 24–72 hours after cytotoxic chemotherapy is completed, has been shown to markedly reduce the duration and severity of granulocytopenia following cytotoxic chemotherapy (Table 39–11). The American Society of Clinical Oncology and NCCN guidelines recommend primary prophylaxis with a G-CSF when there is 20% risk of febrile neutropenia or when the patient's age, medical history, and disease characteristics makes the patient at high risk for complications related to myelosuppression.

B. Anemia

Erythropoiesis-stimulating agents (ESAs) have been shown to ameliorate the anemia and associated symptoms caused by cancer chemotherapy. However, the evidence suggests that these drugs have untoward effects, including an increased risk of thromboembolism, and even more concerning, decreased survival due to cancer-related deaths. These findings have prompted the US Food and Drug Administration and other organizations (American Society of Hematology, American Society of Clinical Oncology, and NCCN) to issue advisories and guidelines limiting their use. The recommendation that these drugs should not be used when the intent of chemotherapy is curative is controversial, although the evidence is mounting that survival is indeed adversely affected by the administration of ESAs. Studies done in patients with potentially curable head and neck, breast, and cervical cancers have shown inferior outcomes when ESAs were used, though the target hemoglobin for patients in these studies was higher than what is currently recommended. The alternative to managing symptomatic anemia in these patients receiving curative chemotherapy is administration of red blood cell transfusions.

Although the details of these recommendations vary, all agree that oncologists should use ESAs in anemic patients receiving chemotherapy and generally should not be given until the hemoglobin is less than 10 g/dL with the medication held when the hemoglobin is greater than 12 g/dL. Epoetin alfa can be given subcutaneously as a weekly dose of 30,000–40,000 units with a target hemoglobin of 11–12 g/dL (see Table 39–11). Darbepoetin alfa is given subcutaneously every 2–3 weeks at a dose of 200–300 mcg with the same target hemoglobin. Patients need to be iron replete to have maximum therapeutic effect. Uncontrolled hypertension is a contraindication to the use of ESAs; blood pressure must be controlled prior to initiation of this therapy.

C. Thrombocytopenia

Drug management of chemotherapy-induced thrombocytopenia is more limited. The only available drug, oprelvekin or

Table 39–10. Chemotherapeutic agents: Dosage and toxicity.

Chemotherapeutic Agent	Usual Adult Dosage	Acute Toxicity	Delayed Toxicity
Alkylating Agents—Nitrogen Mustards			
Bendamustine (Treanda)	100–120 mg/m² intravenously every 3–4 weeks	Hypersensitivity reaction, nausea, vomiting, skin reaction	Myelosuppression, pyrexia, fatigue
Cyclophosphamide (Cytoxan)	500–1000 mg/m² intravenously every 3 weeks; 100 mg/m²/d orally for 14 days every 4 weeks	Nausea and vomiting	Myelosuppression, hemorrhagic cystitis, alopecia, cardiotoxicity with high-dose therapy, SIADH
Estramustine (Emcyt)	14 mg/kg/d orally in three or four divided doses	Nausea, vomiting, diarrhea	Gynecomastia, thromboembolism, edema
Ifosfamide (Ifex)	1200 mg/m² daily for 5 days intravenously every 3 weeks	Nausea and vomiting	Myelosuppression, hemorrhagic cystitis, neurotoxicity, alopecia, SIADH
Mechlorethamine (nitrogen mustard, Mustargen)	0.4 mg/kg intravenously every 3–6 weeks; or 6 mg/m² intravenously on days 1 and 8 every 4 weeks	Severe nausea and vomiting, severe vesicant	Myelosuppression, increased risk of secondary malignancies
Melphalan (Alkeran)	0.25 mg/kg/d or 8–10 mg/m²/d orally for 4 days every 4–6 weeks; 16 mg/m² intravenously every 2–4 weeks; 200 mg/m² intravenously for bone marrow transplant	Nausea, vomiting, diarrhea, hypersensitivity (IV), mucositis (IV)	Myelosuppression, increased risk of secondary malignancies
Alkylating Agents—Platinum Analogs			
Carboplatin (Paraplatin)	Area under the curve (AUC)-based dosing use Calvert equation [Dose (mg) = AUC × (GFR + 25)] AUC = 2–7 mg/mL/min every 2–4 weeks; or 200–400 mg/m² intravenously every 4 weeks	Nausea, vomiting, hypersensitivity reaction	Myelosuppression, electrolyte disturbances, peripheral neuropathy, nephrotoxicity (less common than with cisplatin)
Cisplatin (Platinol)	50–100 mg/m² intravenously every 3–4 weeks; 20 mg/m²/d intravenously for 5 days every 3 weeks	Severe nausea and vomiting	Nephrotoxicity, ototoxicity, peripheral neuropathy, myelosuppression, electrolyte disturbances
Oxaliplatin (Eloxatin)	85–130 mg/m² intravenously every 2–3 weeks	Peripheral neuropathy triggered or exacerbated by cold, nausea, vomiting, diarrhea, rare anaphylactic reactions	Peripheral neuropathy, myelosuppression
Alkylating Agents—Triazenes			
Dacarbazine (DTIC-Dome)	375 mg/m² intravenously on day 1 and 15 every 4 weeks, 250 mg/m² intravenously for 5 days	Severe nausea and vomiting, anorexia	Myelosuppression, photosensitivity, hepatotoxicity, flu-like syndrome
Procarbazine (Matulane)	60–100 mg/m² orally for 14 days every 4 weeks	Nausea and vomiting	Myelosuppression; disulfiram-like reaction with alcohol; caution with tyramine-containing foods, tricyclic antidepressants, and sympathomimetic agents – MAO inhibition; increased risk of secondary malignancies
Temozolomide (Temodar)	75 mg/m² orally daily during radiation for 42 days 150–200 mg/m² orally for 5 days every 4 weeks	Nausea, vomiting, headache, constipation	Myelosuppression
Alkylating Agents—Miscellaneous			
Busulfan (Myleran)	1–8 mg daily orally	Nausea and vomiting	Myelosuppression, mucositis, hyperpigmentation of skin, rare pulmonary fibrosis, hepatic veno-occlusive disease with high doses (> 16 mg/d in transplant patients)

(continued)

Table 39–10. Chemotherapeutic agents: Dosage and toxicity. (continued)

Chemotherapeutic Agent	Usual Adult Dosage	Acute Toxicity	Delayed Toxicity
Chlorambucil (Leukeran)	0.1–0.2 mg/kg/d orally for 3–6 weeks; or 0.4 mg/kg pulse every 4 weeks	None	Myelosuppression, rare pulmonary toxicity, skin reaction, increased risk of secondary malignancies with prolonged use
Lomustine (CCNU)	100–130 mg/m^2 orally every 6 weeks	Nausea and vomiting	Myelosuppression, pulmonary toxicity
Antimetabolites—Folate Antagonists			
Methotrexate (MTX; Trexall)	Intrathecal: 12 mg High dose: 1000–12,000 mg/m^2 intravenously every 2–3 weeks	Nausea, vomiting, mucositis	Myelosuppression, nephrotoxicity, hepatotoxicity, neurotoxicity (with intrathecal administration and high-dose therapy), photosensitivity, pulmonary toxicity, caution multiple drug interactions which may enhance toxicities (avoid aspirin, penicillins, NSAIDs, omeprazole, TMP-SMZ)
Pemetrexed (Alimta)	500 mg/m^2 intravenously every 3 weeks	Fatigue, nausea, vomiting, diarrhea, rash	Myelosuppression, mucositis Avoid NSAIDs which may decrease pemetrexed clearance and enhance toxicities
Antimetabolites—Purine Analogs			
Cladribine (Leustatin)	0.14 mg/kg/d intravenously or subcutaneously daily for 5 days or 0.09 mg/kg/d intravenously via continuous infusion for 7 days	Mild nausea, fatigue, injection site reaction, rash	Myelosuppression, immunosuppression, fever
Clofarabine (Clolar)	52 mg/m^2 intravenously daily for 5 days every 2–6 weeks (for patients < 21 years of age)	Nausea, vomiting, diarrhea, dermatitis, pruritus, headache, rigor	Myelosuppression, hepatotoxicity, nephrotoxicity, capillary leak syndrome, immunosuppression
Fludarabine (Fludara)	25 mg/m^2 intravenously for 5 days every 4 weeks	Asthenia, fever, myalgias, rare hypersensitivity reaction	Myelosuppression, immunosuppression, neurotoxicity, visual disturbances
Mercaptopurine (6-MP; Purinethol)	Induction: 2.5–5 mg/kg/d orally Maintenance: 1.5–2.5 mg/kg/d orally	Diarrhea, hyperpigmentation of skin, rash	Myelosuppression, immunosuppression, hepatotoxicity, mucositis
Pentostatin (Nipent)	4 mg/m^2 intravenously every other week	Nausea, vomiting, rash	Myelosuppression, immunosuppression, hepatotoxicity
Antimetabolites—Pyrimidine Analogs			
Azacitidine (Vidaza)	75 mg/m^2 subcutaneously or intravenously for 7 days every 4 weeks, may increase to 100 mg/m^2 after two cycles if no response	Injection site reaction, nausea, constipation, fever	Myelosuppression, hepatotoxicity, and nephrotoxicity (rare)
Capecitabine (Xeloda)	625–1250 mg/m^2 orally twice a day for 14 days every 3 weeks	Nausea, vomiting, diarrhea	Hand-foot syndrome, mucositis, hyperbilirubinemia, myelosuppression
Cytarabine (Ara-C, Cytosar U)	Standard dose: 100 mg/m^2/d intravenously via continuous infusion for 7 days High dose: 1000–3000 mg/m^2 intravenously every 12 hours on days 1, 3, 5	Nausea, vomiting, rash, flu-like syndrome	Myelosuppression High-dose therapy: neurotoxicity (cerebellar ataxia, lethargy, confusion), ocular toxicities (conjunctivitis and keratitis), hepatotoxicity, pancreatitis, pulmonary toxicity
Cytarabine Liposome (DepoCyt)	50 mg intrathecally every 14 or 28 days		Chemical arachnoiditis
Decitabine (Dacogen)	15 mg/m^2 intravenously every 8 hours for 3 days, repeat every 8 weeks	Nausea, fatigue, hyperglycemia	Myelosuppression

(continued)

Table 39–10. Chemotherapeutic agents: Dosage and toxicity. (continued)

Chemotherapeutic Agent	Usual Adult Dosage	Acute Toxicity	Delayed Toxicity
Fluorouracil (5-FU; Adrucil)	500–600 mg/m^2 intravenous bolus weekly for 6 weeks, repeat every 8 weeks; in combination with oxaliplatin: 400 mg/m^2 intravenous bolus followed immediately by 600 mg/m^2 intravenously over 22 hours on days 1 and 2 or 400 mg/m^2 intravenous bolus followed immediately by 2400 mg/m^2 intravenously over 46 hours; 1000 mg/m^2 intravenously via continuous infusion for 4–5 days every 3–4 weeks	Nausea, diarrhea	Myelosuppression (intravenous bolus), hand-foot syndrome, mucositis, neurotoxicity, ocular toxicity, photosensitivity, cardiotoxicity (rare)
Gemcitabine (Gemzar)	1000–1250 mg/m^2 intravenously on days 1, 8, 15 every 4 weeks	Nausea, rash, flu-like symptoms, fever, diarrhea	Myelosuppression, edema, hepatotoxicity (rare), hemolytic uremic syndrome (rare), pulmonary toxicity (rare)
Antimicrotubules—Vinca Alkaloids			
Vinblastine (Velban)	6 mg/m^2 intravenously on days 1 and 15 every 4 weeks; 0.11 mg/kg on days 1 and 2	Vesicant, bronchospasm and dyspnea (rare)	Myelosuppression, peripheral neuropathy, constipation, mucositis, alopecia, SIADH (rare)
Vincristine (Oncovin)	0.5–1.4 mg/m^2 intravenously every 3 weeks; 0.4 mg/m^2 intravenously via continuous infusion for 4 days; maximum single dose usually limited to 2 mg	Vesicant	Peripheral neuropathy, constipation, alopecia, SIADH (rare)
Vinorelbine (Navelbine)	30 mg/m^2 intravenously on days 1 and 8 every 3 weeks	Vesicant, nausea, vomiting, bronchospasm and dyspnea (rare)	Myelosuppression, peripheral neuropathy, constipation, alopecia, SIADH (rare)
Antimicrotubules—Taxanes			
Docetaxel (Taxotere)	60–100 mg/m^2 intravenously every 3 weeks; 35–40 mg/m^2 intravenously weekly for 3 weeks with 1 week rest	Hypersensitivity reaction, nausea, vomiting	Myelosuppression, peripheral neuropathy, alopecia, edema, fatigue, mucositis, diarrhea
Paclitaxel (Taxol)	135–175 mg/m^2 intravenously every 3 weeks; 50–80 mg/m^2 intravenously weekly	Hypersensitivity reaction, nausea, vomiting, bradycardia and hypotension during infusion	Myelosuppression, peripheral neuropathy, alopecia, mucositis, diarrhea, arthralgias/myalgias
Paclitaxel protein-bound (Abraxane)	260 mg/m^2 intravenously every 3 weeks	Nausea, vomiting, diarrhea, hypersensitivity reaction (less than paclitaxel)	Myelosuppression, peripheral neuropathy, alopecia, mucositis, arthralgias/myalgias
Antimicrotubules—Epothilone			
Ixabepilone (Ixempra)	40 mg/m^2 intravenously every 3 weeks	Hypersensitivity reaction, nausea, vomiting	Peripheral neuropathy, myelosuppression, alopecia, fatigue, mucositis, diarrhea, arthralgias/ myalgias
Enzyme Inhibitors—Anthracyclines			
Daunorubicin (Cerubidine)	30–60 mg/m^2 intravenously for 3 days	Nausea, vomiting, mucositis, diarrhea, red/orange discoloration of urine, cardiotoxicity (ECG changes). - All anthracyclines except for liposomal doxorubicin are potent vesicants. - Liposomal daunorubicin and liposomal doxorubicin may cause infusion-related reactions	Myelosuppression, cardiotoxicity (cardiomyopathy with congestive heart failure–dose related), alopecia. - Liposomal Doxorubicin can also cause hand-foot syndrome
Liposomal Daunorubicin (Daunoxome)	40 mg/m^2 intravenously every 2 weeks		
Doxorubicin (Adriamycin)	15–20 mg/m^2 intravenously weekly; 45–60 mg/m^2 intravenously every 3 weeks		
Liposomal Doxorubicin (Doxil)	20–50 mg/m^2 intravenously every 3–4 weeks		
Epirubicin (Ellence)	35 mg/m^2 intravenously every 2 weeks; 60–120 mg/m^2 intravenously every 3–4 weeks		
Idarubicin (Idamycin)	12 mg/m^2 intravenously for 3 days		

(continued)

Table 39–10. Chemotherapeutic agents: Dosage and toxicity. (continued)

Chemotherapeutic Agent	Usual Adult Dosage	Acute Toxicity	Delayed Toxicity
Enzyme Inhibitors—Topoisomerase Inhibitors			
Etoposide (Vepesid)	50–100 mg/m^2 intravenously for 3–5 days every 3 weeks, oral dose is twice the intravenous dose	Nausea, vomiting, hypersensitivity reaction, fever, hypotension	Myelosuppression, alopecia, fatigue
Etoposide Phosphate (Etopophos)	100 mg/m^2 intravenously for 3–5 days every 3 weeks		
Irinotecan (Camptosar)	60 mg/m^2 intravenously on days 1, 8, and 15 every 4 weeks; 125 mg/m^2 intravenously weekly for 4 weeks every 6 weeks; 180 mg/m^2 intravenously every other week; 350 mg/m^2 intravenously every 3 weeks	Diarrhea and cholinergic syndrome, nausea, vomiting	Myelosuppression, alopecia
Topotecan (Hycamtin)	1.5 mg/m^2 intravenously for 5 days every 3 weeks; 2.3 mg/m^2 orally for 5 days every 3 weeks	Nausea, vomiting, diarrhea	Myelosuppression, alopecia, asthenia
Targeted Therapy—Monoclonal Antibodies			
Alemtuzumab (Campath)	30 mg/m^2 intravenously three times weekly	Infusion-related reaction, nausea, vomiting, hypotension	Myelosuppression, immunosuppression
Bevacizumab (Avastin)	5–15 mg/kg intravenously every 2–3 weeks	Infusion-related reaction	Arterial thromboembolism, wound healing complications, gastrointestinal perforation or fistula, hemorrhage, hypertension, proteinuria
Cetuximab (Erbitux)	Loading dose 400 mg/m^2 intravenously followed by maintenance dose 250 mg/m^2 intravenously weekly	Infusion-related reaction	Acneiform skin rash, hypomagnesemia, asthenia, paronychial inflammation, pulmonary toxicity (rare)
Gemtuzumab ozogamicin (Mylotarg)	9 mg/m^2 intravenously	Infusion-related reaction, nausea, vomiting	Myelosuppression, hepatotoxicity, veno-occlusive disease (rare)
Ibritumomab tiuxetan (Zevalin)	0.4 mCi/kg intravenously on day 8	Infusion-related reaction	Myelosuppression, asthenia, infections, increased risk of secondary malignancies
^{131}I Tositumomab (Bexxar)	450 mg intravenously	Infusion-related reaction	Myelosuppression, asthenia, infections, hypothyroidism, increased risk of secondary malignancies
Panitumumab (Vectibix)	6 mg/kg intravenously every 2 weeks	Infusion-related reaction	Acneiform skin rash, hypomagnesemia, asthenia, paronychial inflammation, pulmonary toxicity (rare)
Rituximab (Rituxan)	375 mg/m^2 intravenously weekly for 4 weeks, or every 3 weeks	Infusion-related reaction	Rare reactions: Hepatitis B reactivation, pulmonary toxicity, tumor lysis syndrome, Stevens-Johnson syndrome, progressive multifocal leukoencephalopathy, cardiac arrhythmias, bowel obstruction
Trastuzumab (Herceptin)	Loading dose 4 mg/kg intravenously followed by 2 mg/kg intravenously weekly; or loading dose 8 mg/kg followed by 6 mg/kg intravenously every 3 weekly	Infusion-related reaction, headache, diarrhea	Cardiotoxicity, pulmonary toxicity, myelosuppression in combination with chemotherapy
Targeted Therapy—Tyrosine Kinase Inhibitors			
Dasatinib (Sprycel)	70 mg orally twice daily; 100–140 mg orally once daily	Diarrhea, nausea, vomiting	Myelosuppression, fluid retention, fatigue, musculoskeletal pain, rash, cardiac dysfunction/congestive heart failure (rare), hemorrhage (rare)

(continued)

Table 39–10. Chemotherapeutic agents: Dosage and toxicity. (continued)

Chemotherapeutic Agent	Usual Adult Dosage	Acute Toxicity	Delayed Toxicity
Erlotinib (Tarceva)	100–150 mg orally once daily	Diarrhea	Acneiform skin rash, fatigue, anorexia, conjunctivitis, gastrointestinal hemorrhage (rare), pulmonary toxicity (rare)
Gefitinib (Iressa)	250 mg orally once daily	Diarrhea	Acneiform skin rash, asthenia, ocular toxicity, myelosuppression, hepatotoxicity (rare), pulmonary toxicity (rare)
Imatinib (Gleevec)	100–800 mg orally once daily	Nausea, vomiting, diarrhea	Myelosuppression, edema, myalgias, rash, congestive heart failure, left ventricular dysfunction (rare), hemorrhage (rare), hepatotoxicity (rare)
Lapatinib (Tykerb)	1250 mg orally once daily in combination with capecitabine	Diarrhea, nausea, vomiting	Hand-foot syndrome, fatigue, hepatotoxicity (rare), left ventricular dysfunction (rare), prolonged QT interval (rare), interstitial lung disease (rare)
Nilotinib (Tasigna)	400 mg orally twice daily	Nausea, vomiting, headache, diarrhea	Edema, rash, arthralgia, fatigue, myelosuppression, electrolyte abnormalities, elevated serum lipase (rare), hepatotoxicity (rare), prolonged QT interval (rare)
Sorafenib (Nexavar)	400 mg orally twice daily	Diarrhea and nausea	Hypertension, hand-foot syndrome, rash, fatigue, gastrointestinal perforation (rare), hemorrhage (rare), cardiac ischemia/infarction (rare)
Sunitinib (Sutent)	50 mg orally once daily for 4 weeks followed by 2 weeks rest.	Diarrhea and nausea	Hypertension, hand-foot syndrome, rash, yellow discoloration of skin, fatigue, hypothyroidism, mucositis, myelosuppression, left ventricular dysfunction (rare), prolonged QT interval (rare), hemorrhage (rare)
Miscellaneous Agents			
Altretamine (Hexalen)	260 mg/m² orally in 4 divided doses for 14–21 days every 4 weeks	Nausea, vomiting, diarrhea	Neurotoxicity, myelosuppression, flu-like syndrome
Arsenic Trioxide (Trisenox)	0.15 mg/kg intravenously daily	Nausea, dizziness	Edema, acute promyelocytic leukemia differentiation syndrome (fever, dyspnea, skin rash, fluid retention, pleural effusions), prolonged QT interval and complete atrioventricular block
Asparaginase (Elspar)	6000–10,000 units/m² intravenously daily on days 17–28; 6000–10,000 units/m² intramuscularly every 3 days for a total of 9 doses	Hypersensitivity reaction (requires test dose), nausea, vomiting	Coagulation abnormalities (hemorrhagic and/or thrombotic events), hepatotoxicity, pancreatitis, neurotoxicity
Bleomycin (Blenoxane)	10 units/m² intravenously on days 1 and 15 every 4 weeks; 30 units on day 2, 9, and 16 every 3 weeks	Hypersensitivity reaction	Skin reaction (rash, hyperpigmentation of skin, striae), pulmonary fibrosis
Bortezomib (Velcade)	1.3 mg/m² intravenous bolus on days 1, 4, 8, 11 followed by a 10 day rest every 3 weeks	Orthostatic hypotension, fever	Peripheral neuropathy, fatigue, myelosuppression, hemorrhage (rare), left ventricular dysfunction (rare), pulmonary toxicity (rare), reversible posterior leukoencephalopathy syndrome (rare), hepatotoxicity (rare)

(continued)

Table 39–10. Chemotherapeutic agents: Dosage and toxicity. (continued)

Chemotherapeutic Agent	Usual Adult Dosage	Acute Toxicity	Delayed Toxicity
Dactinomycin (Cosmegen)	15 mcg/kg intravenously daily for 5 days; 12 mcg/kg intravenously daily for 5 days; 1000 mcg/m² intravenously	Vesicant, nausea, vomiting	Myelosuppression, mucositis, diarrhea, alopecia, hyperpigmentation of skin, hepatotoxicity, hepato-veno-occlusive disease (rare)
Denileukin diftitox (Ontak)	9 or 18 mcg/kg intravenously daily for 5 days every 3 weeks	Flu-like syndrome, hypersensitivity reaction, nausea, vomiting	Diarrhea, decreased visual acuity, fever, increased risk for infection, hypoalbuminemia, capillary leak syndrome (rare)
Hydroxyurea (Hydrea)	20–30 mg/kg orally once daily	Nausea	Myelosuppression, dermopathy
Lenalidomide (Revlimid)	5–25 mg orally once daily for 21 days every 4 weeks	Diarrhea, itching, rash	Myelosuppression, potential for birth defects, thromboembolic events, fatigue
Mitomycin (Mutamycin)	20 mg/m² intravenously every 6–8 weeks; 20–40 mg intravesically weekly	Vesicant, local irritation (cystitis when given intravesically)	Myelosuppression, mucositis, hemolytic uremic syndrome (rare), pulmonary toxicity (rare)
Mitoxantrone (Novantrone)	12–14 mg/m² intravenously every 3 weeks; induction chemotherapy for leukemia 12 mg/m² intravenously for 2–3 days	Blue-green discoloration of urine, nausea, vomiting, diarrhea, intravenous irritant	Myelosuppression, cardiotoxicity, alopecia, mucositis, increased risk of secondary malignancies (rare)
Temsirolimus (Torisel)	25 mg intravenously weekly	Hypersensitivity reaction, rash	Myelosuppression, edema, fatigue, mucositis, hyperglycemia, hyperlipemia, immunosuppression, nephrotoxicity, interstitial lung disease (rare), bowel perforation (rare), abnormal wound healing
Thalidomide (Thalomid)	50–800 mg orally once daily	Sedation, constipation, fatigue	Potential for birth defects, thromboembolic events, peripheral neuropathy, edema
Tretinoin (All-Trans-Retinoic Acid, ATRA, Vesanoid)	45 mg/m² orally divided twice daily for 45–90 days or 30 days past complete remission		Headache, vitamin A toxicity, retinoic acid-acute promyelocytic leukemia syndrome, ototoxicity
Antiandrogens			
Bicalutamide (Casodex)	50 mg orally once daily	None	Hot flashes, decreased libido, impotence, gynecomastia, breast tenderness, fatigue
Flutamide (Eulexin)	250 mg orally every 8 hours	Diarrhea, yellow-green discoloration of urine	Hot flashes, decreased libido, impotence, gynecomastia, breast tenderness, hepatotoxicity (rare)
Nilutamide (Nilandron)	300 mg orally for 30 days then 150 mg orally once daily	Nausea	Visual disturbances (impaired adaptation to dark), hot flashes, decreased libido, impotence, gynecomastia, breast tenderness, disulfiram reaction with alcohol, interstitial pneumonitis (rare), hepatotoxicity (rare)
Selective Estrogen Receptor Modulators			
Tamoxifen (Nolvadex)	20–40 mg orally once daily	None	Hot flashes, vaginal discharge or bleeding, menstrual irregularities, thromboembolic events (rare), endometrial hyperplasia, cataracts, hepatotoxicity, tumor flare
Toremifene (Fareston)	60 mg orally once daily	Nausea	Hot flashes, vaginal discharge, thromboembolic events (rare), tumor flare, endometrial hyperplasia, cataracts, hepatotoxicity

(continued)

Table 39–10. Chemotherapeutic agents: Dosage and toxicity. (continued)

Chemotherapeutic Agent	Usual Adult Dosage	Acute Toxicity	Delayed Toxicity
Aromatase Inhibitors			
Anastrozole (Arimidex)	1 mg orally once daily	Nausea	Hot flashes, peripheral edema, hypercholesterolemia, arthralgia/myalgia, headache, osteoporosis
Exemestane (Aromasin)	25 mg orally once daily		
Letrozole (Femara)	2.5 mg orally once daily		
Pure Estrogen Receptor Antagonist			
Fulvestrant (Faslodex)	250 mg intramuscularly once a month	Injection site reactions, nausea, diarrhea, constipation	Hot flashes, backache, headache
Progestins			
Megestrol acetate (Megace)	40–320 mg orally once daily or in divided doses (four times a day)	Nausea	Hot flashes, tumor flare, weight gain, hyperglycemia, thrombotic events (rare), adrenal insufficiency (rare)
LHRH Analogs			
Goserelin acetate (Zoladex)	3.6 mg subcutaneously once every month; 10.8 mg subcutaneously once every 3 months	Injection site discomfort	Hot flashes, tumor flare, decreased libido, impotence, vaginal bleeding, thromboembolic events (rare), osteoporosis (rare)
Leuprolide (Lupron)	7.5 mg intramuscularly once every month; 22.5 mg intramuscularly once every 3 months; 30 mg intramuscularly once every 4 months	Injection site reaction	Hot flashes, tumor flare, edema, impotence, thromboembolic events (rare), osteoporosis
Triptorelin pamoate (Trelstar)	3.75 mg intramuscularly once every month; 11.25 mg intramuscularly once every 3 months	None	Hot flashes, tumor flare, skeletal pain, impotence
Adrenocorticosteroids			
Dexamethasone	40 mg orally once weekly or 40 mg orally on days 1–4, 9–12, 17–20	None	Hyperglycemia, weight gain, fluid retention, psychiatric symptoms
Ketoconazole	400 mg orally three times daily	Nausea and vomiting	Hepatotoxicity (rare)
Prednisone	5 mg orally twice a day; 100 mg orally daily for 5 days	None	Hyperglycemia, weight gain, gastritis, fluid retention, psychiatric symptoms
Biologic Response Modifiers			
Interferon-α-2b (Intron A)	5 million international units subcutaneously 3 times a week; 2 million international units/m^2 intramuscularly/subcutaneously three times a week; 20 million international units/m^2 5 days a week for 4 weeks then 10 million international units/m^2 three times a week	Hypersensitivity reaction, injection site reaction, flu-like syndrome, nausea, vomiting, diarrhea	Myelosuppression, fatigue, anorexia, alopecia, depression, hyperthyroidism or hypothyroidism (rare), hepatotoxicity (rare), visual disturbances
Aldesleukin (IL-2, Proleukin)	600,000 international units/kg intravenously every 8 hours for 14 doses, repeat after 9 days rest	Hypotension, nausea, vomiting, diarrhea	Capillary leak syndrome (rare), impaired neutrophil function and increased risk of infection, lethargy or somnolence that may result in coma if therapy is not held

GFR, glomerular filtration rate; LHRH, luteinizing hormone–releasing hormone; MAO, monoamine oxidase; NSAIDs, nonsteroidal anti-inflammatory drugs; SIADH, syndrome of inappropriate antidiuretic hormone; TMP-SMZ, trimethoprim-sulfamethoxazole.

recombinant interleukin-11, has modest activity in improving thrombocytopenia associated with chemotherapy; however, the side effects of fluid retention, congestive heart failure, and arrhythmias have limited its use. Thrombopoietin, the protein that stimulates megakaryopoieis in vivo,

was isolated in 1994. Despite much work attempting to produce a clinically effective thrombopoietin drug for therapeutic use, no such drug is commercially available for this indication. Two drugs approved for use in idiopathic thrombocytopenia romiplostim and eltrombopag have not

Table 39–11. Supportive care agents: Dosage and toxicity.

Agent	Indication	Usual Dose	Acute Toxicity	Delayed Toxicity
Allopurinol (Xyloprim)	Prevent hyperuricemia from tumor lysis syndrome	300 mg orally once daily	None	Rash, Stevens-Johnson syndrome (rare), myelosuppression (rare)
Rasburicase (Elitek)	Prevent hyperuricemia from tumor lysis syndrome	0.17–0.17 mg/kg intravenously for pediatric patients; 3–6 mg intravenously once	Hypersensitivity reaction in patients with G6PD deficiency, nausea, vomiting, diarrhea, fever, headache	Rash
Mesna (Mesnex)	Prevent ifosfamide-induced hemorrhagic cystitis	20% of ifosfamide dose intravenously immediately before ifosfamide and at 4 hours and 8 hours after (total dose is 60% of ifosfamide dose); 100% of ifosfamide dose mixed with ifosfamide in same intravenous bag	Nausea and vomiting	Fatigue, hypotension
Leucovorin	Rescue after high-dose methotrexate; in combination with fluorouracil for colon cancer	10 mg/m² intravenously or orally every 6 hours until serum methotrexate level is below 0.01 micromolar; 20 mg/m² or 200–500 mg/m² intravenously before fluorouracil	Nausea	None
Amifostine (Ethyol)	Prevent cisplatin nephropathy; prevent radiation-induced xerostomia	910 mg/m² intravenously before cisplatin; 200 mg/m² intravenously before radiation	Nausea, vomiting, hypotension, infusion-related reaction	Hypocalcemia
Dexrazoxane (ZInecard)	Prevent cardiomyopathy secondary to doxorubicin; anthracycline-induced injection site extravasation	10 times the doxorubicin dose intravenously before doxorubicin	Nausea	Myelosuppression
Palifermin (Kepivance)	Prevent mucositis following chemotherapy	60 mcg/kg/d intravenously for 3 days before and 3 days after chemotherapy	None	Edema, rash, pruritus, erythema, fever, enlargement or discoloration of tongue, altered taste sensation
Pilocarpine (Salagen)	Radiation-induced xerostomia	5 mg orally 1 hour before chemotherapy, then 5 mg once daily for 7 days; 5–10 mg orally three times a day	Flushing, sweating, nausea, dizziness, increased urinary frequency, rhinitis	None
Samarium (Quadramet)	Pain from bone metastasis	1 milliCurie/kg intravenously	Pain flare, diarrhea, hematuria	Myelosuppression, spinal cord compression
Strontium (Metastron)	Pain from bone metastasis	148 megabecquerels (4 milliCuries) intravenously; or 1.5–2.2 megabecquerels/kg (40–60 microcuries/kg)	Flushing, pain flare	Myelosuppression
Pamidronate (Aredia)	Osteolytic bone metastasis, hypercalcemia of malignancy	90 mg intravenously every 3–4 weeks; 60–90 mg intravenously, may repeat after 7 days	Injection site reaction	Electrolyte disturbances (hypocalcemia), anemia, arthralgia, bone pain, osteonecrosis of the jaw, nephrotoxicity
Zoledronic acid (Zometa)	Osteolytic bone metastasis, hypercalcemia of malignancy	4 mg intravenously every 3–4 weeks	Injection site reaction	Electrolyte disturbances (hypocalcemia), anemia, arthralgia, bone pain, osteonecrosis of the jaw, nephrotoxicity

(continued)

Table 39–11. Supportive care agents: Dosage and toxicity. (continued)

Agent	Indication	Usual Dose	Acute Toxicity	Delayed Toxicity
Growth Factors				
Epoetin alfa (Epogen, Procrit)	Chemotherapy-induced anemia	40,000 units subcutaneously once weekly; 150 units/kg subcutaneously 3 times a week	Injection site reaction	Hypertension, thrombotic events, increased risk of tumor progression or recurrence, seizures, rash
Darbepoetin alfa (Aranesp)	Chemotherapy-induced anemia	2.25 mcg/kg subcutaneously weekly; 500 mcg subcutaneously every 3 weeks Alternative dosing: 200 mcg subcutaneously every 2 weeks or 300 mcg subcutaneously every 3 weeks	Injection site reaction	Hypertension, thrombotic events, increased risk of tumor progression or recurrence, seizures, rash
Filgrastim (Neupogen)	Febrile neutropenia prophylaxis	5–10 mcg/kg/d subcutaneously or intravenously once daily, treat past nadir	Injection site reaction	Bone pain, enlarged spleen, leukocytosis
Pegfilgrastim (Neulasta)	Febrile neutropenia prophylaxis	6 mg subcutaneously once per chemotherapy cycle	Injection site reaction	Bone pain, enlarged spleen, leukocytosis
Sargramostim (Leukine)	Myeloid reconstitution following bone marrow transplant, febrile neutropenia prophylaxis	250 mcg/m² intravenously daily until the absolute neutrophil count is greater than 1500 cells/mcL for 3 consecutive days	Rash, pruritus, injection site reaction, dyspnea, fever	Bone pain, myalgia, fluid retention, supraventricular tachycardia, capillary leak syndrome (rare)
Oprelvekin (Neumega)	Chemotherapy-induced thrombocytopenia	50 mcg/kg subcutaneously every day for 14–21 days or until post-nadir platelet count is greater than 50,000/mcL	Nausea, vomiting, headache, dizziness, blurred vision, dyspnea, injection site reaction	Candidiasis, rash, fluid retention, arrhythmias, febrile neutropenia

G6PD, glucose 6-phosphate dehydrogenase.

been shown to benefit patients with chemotherapy-associated thrombocytopenia.

2. Chemotherapy-Induced Nausea & Vomiting

A number of cytotoxic anticancer drugs can induce nausea and vomiting, which can be the most anticipated and stressful side effects for patients. Chemotherapy-induced nausea and vomiting is mediated in part by the stimulation of at least two central nervous system receptors, 5-hydroxytryptamine subtype 3 (5HT$_3$) and neurokinin subtype 1 (NK$_1$). Chemotherapy-induced nausea and vomiting can be acute, occurring within minutes to hours of chemotherapy administration, or delayed until the second day and lasting up to 7 days. Anticipatory nausea and vomiting may even occur before the administration of chemotherapy. Chemotherapy drugs or drug regimens are classified into high, moderate, low, and minimal likelihoods of causing emesis (90%, 30–90%, 10–30%, < 10%, respectively). Highly emetogenic chemotherapy drugs include cisplatin, carmustine, cyclophosphamide at doses over 1.5 g/m², dacarbazine, mechlorethamine, and streptozocin. Chemotherapy drugs that are moderately emetogenic include doxorubicin, daunomycin, idarubicin, epirubicin, cyclophosphamide, irinotecan, oxaliplatin, ifosfamide, cytarabine, and carboplatin. Drugs with low emetic potential include bortezomib, docetaxel, etoposide, fluorouracil, gemcitabine, methotrexate, mitomycin, mitoxantrone, paclitaxel, pemetrexed, temsirolimus, and topotecan. Drugs with minimal risk of emesis include bevacizumab, bleomycin, cladribine, fludarabine, vinblastine, vincristine, and vinorelbine.

By understanding the physiology of chemotherapy-induced nausea and vomiting, major advances have occurred with the development of new, highly effective antiemetic drugs. Antagonists to the 5HT$_3$-receptor include ondansetron, granisetron, dolasetron, tropisetron, and palonosetron. Each of these drugs have similar efficacy. Ondansetron can be

Table 39–12. A common scheme for dose modification of cancer chemotherapeutic agents.

Granulocyte Count (cells/mcL)	Platelet Count (/mcL)	Suggested Drug Dosage (% of Full Dose)
> 2000	> 100,000	100%
1000–2000	75,000–100,000	50%
< 2000	< 50,000	0%

given either intravenously (8 or 0.15 mg/kg) or orally (24 mg for highly emetogenic chemotherapy, 8 mg twice daily for moderately emetogenic chemotherapy). Doses of 8 mg can be repeated parenterally or orally every 8 hours. Dosing of granisetron is 1 mg or 0.01 mg/kg intravenously or 1–2 mg orally. Dolasetron is given 1.8 mg/kg or a fixed dose of 100 mg intravenously or 100 mg can be given orally. Tropisetron is given at a dose of 5 mg either orally or intravenously. Palonosetron, a long-acting $5HT_3$ with high affinity for the $5HT_3$-receptor given at a dose of 0.25 mg intravenously, is effective for not only acute but also delayed emesis. The efficacy of the $5HT_3$-blockers is improved by adding 6–10 mg of either oral or intravenous dexamethasone.

Aprepitant is an antagonist to the NK_1 receptor. When given as a 125-mg oral dose followed by 80 mg on the second and third day with a $5HT_3$-receptor antagonist (such as ondansetron or granisetron), the immediate and delayed protective effect for highly emetogenic chemotherapy is increased.

Standard therapy for highly emetogenic chemotherapy includes a $5HT_3$-antagonist given on the first day and both dexamethasone and aprepitant given on the first day as well as the second and third days. Moderately emetogenic chemotherapy regimens are best managed with a two-drug regimen of a $5HT_3$-antagonist and dexamethasone. Doses of the $5HT_3$ may be given on days 2 and 3 to prevent delayed emesis.

Other adjunctive medications that may be helpful include lorazepam, 0.5–1.0 mg given orally every 6–8 hours, and prochlorperazine, 5–10 mg orally or intravenously every 8 hours. Lorazepam, in addition to antianxiety effects, has an antinausea effect. Prochlorperazine is generally sufficient to treat patients receiving low emetogenic chemotherapy. A suppository form of prochlorperazine, 25 mg, may be used for patients who are unable to swallow oral medications.

The importance of treating chemotherapy-induced nausea and vomiting expectantly and aggressively beginning with the first course of chemotherapy cannot be understated. Patients being treated in the clinic setting should always be given antiemetics for home use with written instructions as well as contact numbers to call for advice.

3. Gastrointestinal Toxicity

Untoward effects of cancer chemotherapy include damage to the more rapidly growing cells of the body such as the mucosal lining from the mouth through the gastrointestinal tract. Oral symptoms range from mild mouth soreness to frank ulcerations in the mouth. Not uncommonly, mouth ulcerations will have superimposed candida or herpes simplex infections. In addition to receiving cytotoxic chemotherapy, a significant risk factor for development of oral mucositis is poor oral hygiene and existing caries or periodontal disease. Toxicity in the gastrointestinal tract usually manifests as diarrhea. Gastrointestinal symptoms can range from mild symptoms of loose stools to life-threatening diarrhea due to dehydration and electrolyte imbalances. Drugs most commonly associated with causing mucositis in the mouth and the gastrointestinal tract are cytarabine, 5-fluorouracil, and methotrexate.

Patients undergoing treatment for head and neck cancer with concurrent chemotherapy and radiation therapy have a very high risk of developing severe mucositis.

Preventive strategies for managing oral mucositis includes a pretreatment dental examination, particularly for all head and neck cancer patients and any cancer patient with poor dental hygiene who will be receiving chemotherapy. For patients receiving fluorouracil, simple measures such as ice chips in the mouth for 30 minutes during infusion can reduce the incidence and severity of mucositis. Once mucositis is encountered, superimposed fungal infections should be treated with topical antifungal medications (oral nystatin mouth suspensions, or clotrimazole troches) or systemic therapy (fluconazole 100–400 mg orally daily). Suspected herpetic infections can be treated with acyclovir (up to 800 mg orally five times daily) or valacyclovir (1 g orally twice daily). Mucositis may also be managed with mouthwashes; it is also important to provide adequate pain medication.

Newer strategies for prevention of oral mucositis includes the recombinant keratinocyte growth factor inhibitor palifermin. Practice guidelines recommend its use in patients undergoing high-dose chemotherapy because when intravenous palifermin (60 mcg/kg/d) is given prophylactically to patients undergoing high-dose chemotherapy for hematologic diseases, both the incidence and length of mucositis is decreased.

Diarrhea is most associated with fluorouracil, capecitabine, and irinotecan as well as the tyrosine kinase inhibitors (sorafenib, sunitinib, imatinib, dasatinib) and epithelial growth factor inhibitors (cetuximab, panitumumab, and erlotinib). Mild to moderate diarrhea can be managed with oral antidiarrheal medication (loperamide, 4 mg initially followed by 2 mg every 2–4 hours until bowel movements are formed). Occasionally, the diarrhea will be overwhelming causing dehydration, electrolyte imbalances, and acute kidney injury. These patients require inpatient management with aggressive intravenous hydration and replacement of electrolytes.

4. Skin Toxicity

Dermatologic complications from cancer chemotherapy can include hyperpigmenation (liposomal doxorubicin, busulfan, hydroxyurea) alopecia, photosensitivity, nail changes, acral erythema, and generalized rashes. Acral erythema, otherwise known as hand-foot syndrome and most commonly associated with administration of fluorouracil, capecitabine, and liposmal doxorubicin, manifests as painful palms or soles accompanied by erythema, progressing to blistering desquamation and ulceration in its worst forms. Management can include attempts at prevention with oral pyridoxine, 200 mg daily, and applying cold packs to the extremities while the chemotherapy is being administered. The newer agents targeting the epidermal growth factor pathway can cause an acne like rash; interestingly, the development of the rash may identify those who will respond to the drug. Inhibitors of the tyrosine kinase pathway are also associated with a high incidence of dermatologic complications, such as rash and acral erythema.

5. Miscellaneous Drug-Specific Toxicities

The toxicities of individual drugs have been summarized in Tables 39–10 and 39–11; however, several of these warrant additional mention, since they occur with frequently administered agents, and special measures are often indicated.

A. Hemorrhagic Cystitis Induced by Cyclophosphamide or Ifosfamide

Metabolic products of cyclophosphamide that retain cytotoxic activity are excreted into the urine. Some patients appear to metabolize more of the drug to these active excretory products; if their urine is concentrated, severe bladder damage may result. Patients receiving cyclophosphamide must maintain a high fluid intake prior to and following the administration of the drug and be counseled to empty their bladders frequently. Early symptoms suggesting bladder toxicity include dysuria and increased frequency or urination. Should microscopic hematuria develop, it is advisable to stop the drug temporarily or switch to a different alkylating agent, to increase fluid intake, and to administer a urinary analgesic such as phenazopyridine. With severe cystitis, large segments of bladder mucosa may be shed, resulting in prolonged gross hematuria. Such patients should be observed for signs of urinary obstruction and may require cystoscopy for removal of obstructing blood clots. The cyclophosphamide analog ifosfamide can cause severe hemorrhagic cystitis when used alone. However, when its use is followed by a series of doses of the neutralizing agent mesna, bladder toxicity can be prevented. Mesna can also be used for patients taking cyclophosphamide in whom cystitis develops.

B. Neuropathy Due to Vinca Alkaloids and Other Chemotherapy Drugs

Neuropathy is caused by a number of different chemotherapy drugs, the most common being vincristine. The peripheral neuropathy can be sensory, motor, autonomic, or a combination of these effects. In its mildest form, it consists of paresthesias of the fingers and toes. Occasionally, acute jaw or throat pain can develop after vincristine therapy. This may be a form of trigeminal neuralgia. With continued vincristine therapy, the paresthesias extend to the proximal interphalangeal joints, hyporeflexia appears in the lower extremities, and significant weakness can develop. Other drugs in the vinca alkaloid class as well as the taxane drugs (paclitaxel and docetaxel) and the newer agents to treat myeloma (thalidomide and bortezomib) cause similar toxicity. The presence of neurologic symptoms is not in itself a reason to stop therapy; the severity of the symptoms must be balanced against the goals of therapy. Usually though, the presence of moderate to severe paresthesias or the detection of motor impairment would result in the decision to discontinue the drug.

Constipation is the most common symptom of autonomic neuropathy associated with the vinca alkaloids. Patients receiving these drugs should be started on stool softeners and mild cathartics when therapy is begun; otherwise, severe impaction may result from an atonic bowel.

More serious autonomic involvement can lead to acute intestinal obstruction with signs indistinguishable from those of an acute abdomen. Bladder neuropathies are uncommon but may be severe. These two complications are absolute contraindications to continued vincristine therapy.

C. Methotrexate Toxicity

Methotrexate, a folate antagonist, is a commonly used drug and a key component of regimens to treat patients with leptomeningeal disease, acute lymphoblastic leukemia, and sarcomas. The dose used in intrathecal therapy is 12 mg. Methotrexate is almost entirely eliminated by the kidney. The methotrexate toxicity affects cells with rapid turnover, including the bone marrow and mucosa resulting in myelosuppression and mucositis. Methotrexate can also damage the liver and kidney manifesting as elevated liver enzymes and creatinine. High-dose methotrexate, usually defined as a dose of 500 mg/m^2 or more given over 4–36 hours, would be lethal without "rescue" of the normal tissues. Leucovorin, a form of folate, will reverse the toxic effects of methotrexate and is given until serum methotrexate levels are in the safe range (less than 0.05 mmol/L). It is crucial that high-dose methotrexate and leucovorin are given precisely according to protocol as deviations of the timing of methotrexate delivery or delay in rescue can result in patient death. Lower doses of methotrexate can be problematic in patients with kidney disease who cannot clear the drug normally or with patients who have effusions. In the latter instance, methotrexate distributes itself in effusions and will leak out continuously, exposing normal tissue to small but cumulatively toxic amounts of the drug. If methotrexate is given to a patient who either has or develops kidney disease or to a patient with an effusion, prolonged rescue with leucovorin will be necessary.

Vigorous hydration and bicarbonate loading also appear to be important in preventing crystallization of high-dose methotrexate in the renal tubular epithelium and minimizing the possibility of nephrotoxicity. Daily monitoring of the serum creatinine is mandatory. Drugs impairing methotrexate excretion include aspirin, nonsteroidal anti-inflammatory drugs, amiodarone, omeprazole, penicillin, phenytoin, and sulfa compounds; these drugs should be stopped if possible before methotrexate administration.

D. Bleomycin Toxicity

Bleomycin is used for the treatment of testicular cancer, Hodgkin disease, and non-Hodgkin lymphoma. Bleomycin produces edema of the interphalangeal joints and hardening of the palmar and plantar skin. The more serious toxicities include an anaphylactic or serum sickness-like reaction and a serious or fatal pulmonary fibrotic reaction (seen especially in elderly patients receiving a total dose of over 300 units). If nonproductive cough, dyspnea, and pulmonary infiltrates develop, the drug is discontinued, and high-dose corticosteroids are instituted as well as empiric antibiotics pending cultures. Fever alone or with chills is an occasional complication of bleomycin treatment and is not an absolute contraindication to continued treatment. The fever may be avoided by intravenous premedication with hydrocortisone administration. Moreover, fever alone is not predictive of pulmonary toxicity. About 1% of patients (especially those with lymphoma) may have a severe or even fatal hypotensive reaction after the initial dose of bleomycin. In order to identify such patients, a test dose of 5 units of bleomycin is administered first with adequate monitoring and emergency facilities available should they be needed. Patients exhibiting a hypotensive reaction should not receive further bleomycin therapy.

E. Anthracycline Cardiotoxicity

A number of cancer chemotherapy drugs can cause cardiotoxicty. The most common class of drugs associated with cardiotoxicity is the anthracycline antibiotics, including doxorubicin, daunomycin, idarubicin, and epirubicin. They can produce acute (during administration), subacute (days to months following administration), and delayed (years following administration) cardiac toxicity. The most feared complication is the delayed development of congestive heart failure. Risk factors for this debilitating toxicity include the anthracycline cumulative dose, age over 70, previous or concurrent irradiation of the chest, preexisting cardiac disease, and concurrent administration of chemotherapy drugs such as trastuzumab. The problem is greatest with doxorubicin because this drug is the most commonly administered anthracycline due to its major role in the treatment of lymphomas, sarcomas, breast cancer, and certain other solid tumors. Patients receiving anthracyclines should have a baseline multiple-gated radionuclide cardiac scan (MUGA) to calculate the left ventricular ejection fraction (LVEF). If the LVEF is greater than 50%, anthracyclines can be administered; if the LVEF is less than 30%, these drugs should not be given. For patients with intermediate cardiac function, anthracycline dosing, if necessary, should be cautiously done with LVEF monitoring between doses. Studies of left ventricular function and endomyocardial biopsies indicate that some changes in cardiac dynamics occur in most patients by the time they have received 300 mg/m^2 of doxorubicin. In general, patients should not receive a total dose of doxorubicin in excess of 450 mg/m^2; the dose should be lower if prior chest radiotherapy has been given. The appearance of a high resting pulse may herald the appearance of overt cardiac toxicity. Unfortunately, toxicity may be irreversible and frequently fatal at dosage levels above 550 mg/m^2. At lower doses (eg, 350 mg/m^2 of doxorubicin), the symptoms and signs of cardiac failure generally respond well to medical therapy as well as the discontinuation of anthracycline. Laboratory studies suggest that cardiac toxicity may be due to a mechanism involving the formation of intracellular free radicals in cardiac muscle. The iron chelator dexrazoxane has been approved for use as a cardioprotectant for patients receiving anthracyclines; however, some evidence suggests that the anthracycline anticancer effect may be compromised by the coadministration of dexrazoxane. In general, dexrazoxane should not be used when the goal of chemotherapy is for curative intent either in the settings of adjuvant or definitive treatment. Doxorubicin and daunomycin have been formulated as liposomal products; these drugs, approved for use in patients with Kaposi sarcoma and sometimes used in certain cancers as a substitute for conventional anthracyclines, appear to have minimal potential for cardiac toxicity.

F. Cisplatin Nephrotoxicity and Neurotoxicity

Cisplatin is effective in treating a wide range of malignancies, including testicular, bladder, lung, and ovarian cancers. Although nausea and vomiting are the side effects most commonly associated with cisplatin, the more serious side effects of nephrotoxicity and neurotoxicity must also be anticipated and aggressively managed. Patients must be vigorously hydrated prior, during, and after cisplatin administration. Both kidney function and electrolytes must be monitored. Low magnesium and potassium levels as well as hyponatremia can develop. The neurotoxicity is usually manifested as a peripheral neuropathy of mixed sensorimotor type and may be associated with painful paresthesias. Development of neuropathy typically occurs after cumulative doses of 300 mg/m^2. Ototoxicity is a potentially serious manifestation of neurotoxicity and can progress to deafness. Amifostine, developed initially as a radioprotective agent and given intravenously at a dose of 910 mg/m^2 over 15 minutes prior to cisplatin, is used to protect against nephrotoxicity and neuropathy. Use of amifostine does not appear to compromise the antineoplastic effect of cisplatin. The second-generation platinum analog carboplatin is non-nephrotoxic, although it is myelosuppressive. In the setting of preexisting kidney disease or neuropathy, carboplatin is occasionally substituted for cisplatin.

PROGNOSIS

A valuable sign of clinical improvement is the general well-being of the patient. Although this finding is a combination of subjective and objective factors and may be partly a placebo effect, it nonetheless serves as a sign of clinical improvement in assessing some of the objective observations listed above. Factors included in the assessment of general well-being are improved appetite and weight gain and increased "performance status" (eg, ambulatory versus bedridden). Evaluation of factors such as activity status enables the clinician to judge whether the net effect of chemotherapy is worthwhile palliation (see Chapter 5).

Clinical Genetic Disorders

Reed E. Pyeritz, MD, PhD

ACUTE INTERMITTENT PORPHYRIA

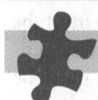 **ESSENTIALS OF DIAGNOSIS**

▶ Unexplained abdominal crisis, generally in young women.

▶ Acute peripheral or central nervous system dysfunction.

▶ Recurrent psychiatric illnesses.

▶ Hyponatremia.

▶ Porphobilinogen in the urine during an attack.

▶ General Considerations

Though there are several different types of porphyrias, the one with the most serious consequences and the one that usually presents in adulthood is acute intermittent porphyria (AIP), which is inherited as an autosomal dominant, though it remains clinically silent in most patients who carry the trait. Clinical illness usually develops in women. Symptoms begin in the teens or 20s, but onset can begin after menopause in rare cases. The disorder is caused by partial deficiency of porphobilinogen deaminase activity, leading to increased excretion of aminolevulinic acid and porphobilinogen in the urine. The diagnosis may be elusive if not specifically considered. The characteristic abdominal pain may be due to abnormalities in autonomic innervation in the gut. In contrast to other forms of porphyria, cutaneous photosensitivity is absent in AIP. Attacks are precipitated by numerous factors, including drugs and intercurrent infections. Harmful and relatively safe drugs for use in treatment are listed in Table 40–1. Hyponatremia may be seen, due in part to inappropriate release of antidiuretic hormone, although gastrointestinal loss of sodium in some patients may be a contributing factor.

▶ Clinical Findings

A. Symptoms and Signs

Patients show intermittent abdominal pain of varying severity, and in some instances it may so simulate acute abdomen

as to lead to exploratory laparotomy. Because the origin of the abdominal pain is neurologic, there is an absence of fever and leukocytosis. Complete recovery between attacks is usual. Any part of the nervous system may be involved, with evidence for autonomic and peripheral neuropathy. Peripheral neuropathy may be symmetric or asymmetric and mild or profound; in the latter instance, it can even lead to quadriplegia with respiratory paralysis. Other central nervous system manifestations include seizures, psychosis, and abnormalities of the basal ganglia. Hyponatremia may further cause or exacerbate central nervous system manifestations.

B. Laboratory Findings

Often there is profound hyponatremia. The diagnosis can be confirmed by demonstrating an increased amount of porphobilinogen in the urine during an acute attack. Freshly voided urine is of normal color but may turn dark upon standing in light and air.

Most families have a different mutation in the porphobilinogen deaminase gene causing AIP. Mutations can be detected and used for presymptomatic and prenatal diagnosis.

▶ Prevention

Avoidance of factors known to precipitate attacks of AIP—especially drugs—can reduce morbidity. Sulfonamides and barbiturates are the most common culprits; others are listed in Table 40–1 and on the Internet (www.drugs-porphyria.org). Starvation diets or prolonged fasting also cause attacks and so must be avoided. Hormonal changes during pregnancy can precipitate crises.

▶ Treatment

Treatment with a high-carbohydrate diet diminishes the number of attacks in some patients and is a reasonable empiric gesture considering its benignity. Acute attacks may be life-threatening and require prompt diagnosis, withdrawal of the inciting agent (if possible), and treatment with analgesics and intravenous glucose and hematin. A minimum of 300 g of carbohydrate per day should be provided orally or intravenously. Electrolyte balance requires close attention. Hematin therapy is still evolving and should be undertaken with full

Table 40–1. Some of the "unsafe" and "probably safe" drugs used in the treatment of acute porphyrias.

Unsafe	Probably Safe
Alcohol	Acetaminophen
Alkylating agents	β-Adrenergic blockers
Barbiturates	Amitriptyline
Carbamazepine	Aspirin
Chloroquine	Atropine
Chlorpropamide	Chloral hydrate
Clonidine	Chlordiazepoxide
Dapsone	Corticosteroids
Ergots	Diazepam
Erythromycin	Digoxin
Estrogens, synthetic	Diphenhydramine
Food additives	Guanethidine
Glutethimide	Hyoscine
Griseofulvin	Ibuprofen
Hydralazine	Imipramine
Ketamine	Insulin
Meprobamate	Lithium
Methyldopa	Naproxen
Metoclopramide	Nitrofurantoin
Nortriptyline	Opioid analgesics
Pentazocine	Penicillamine
Phenytoin	Penicillin and derivatives
Progestins	Phenothiazines
Pyrazinamide	Procaine
Rifampin	Streptomycin
Spironolactone	Succinylcholine
Succinimides	Tetracycline
Sulfonamides	Thiouracil
Theophylline	
Tolazamide	
Tolbutamide	
Valproic acid	

recognition of adverse consequences, especially phlebitis and coagulopathy. The intravenous dosage is up to 4 mg/kg once or twice daily. Liver transplantation may provide an option for patients with disease poorly controlled by medical therapy.

▶ When to Refer

- For management of severe abdominal pain, seizures, or psychosis.
- For preventive management when a patient with porphyria contemplates pregnancy.
- For genetic counseling and molecular diagnosis.

▶ When to Admit

The patient should be hospitalized when he or she has an acute attack accompanied by mental status changes, seizure, or hyponatremia.

Anderson KE et al. Recommendations for the diagnosis and treatment of the acute porphyrias. Ann Intern Med. 2005 Mar 15;142(6):439–50. [PMID: 15767622]

Desnick RJ et al. Inherited porphyrias. In: *Emery and Rimoin's Principles and Practice of Medical Genetics*, 5th ed. Rimoin DL et al (editors). Churchill Livingstone, 2007.

Kauppinen R. Porphyrias. Lancet. 2005 Jan 15–21;365(9455):241–52. [PMID: 15652607]

Norman RA. Past and future: porphyria and porphyrins. Skinmed. 2005 Sep–Oct;4(5):287–92. [PMID: 16282750]

Seth AK et al. Liver transplantation for porphyria: who, when and how? Liver Transpl. 2007 Sep;13(9):1219–27. [PMID: 17763398]

Thunell S et al. Guide to drug porphyrogenicity and drug prescription in the acute porphyrias. Br J Clin Pharmacol. 2007 Nov;64(5):668–79. [PMID: 17578481]

ALKAPTONURIA

ESSENTIALS OF DIAGNOSIS

- ▶ Ochronosis (gray-black discoloration of connective tissue, including the sclerae, ears, and cartilage).
- ▶ Characteristic radiologic changes in the spine, with radiodense intervertebral discs.
- ▶ Arthropathy.
- ▶ Urine darkens on standing.

▶ Clinical Findings

A. Symptoms and Signs

Alkaptonuria is caused by a recessively inherited deficiency of the enzyme homogentisic acid oxidase. This acid derives from metabolism of both phenylalanine and tyrosine and is present in large amounts in the urine throughout the patient's life. An oxidation product accumulates slowly in cartilage throughout the body, leading to degenerative joint disease of the spine and peripheral joints. Indeed, examination of patients in the third and fourth decades shows a slight darkish blue color below the skin in areas overlying cartilage, such as in the ears, a phenomenon called **ochronosis**. In some patients, a more severe hyperpigmentation can be seen in the sclera, conjunctiva, and cornea. Accumulation of metabolites in heart valves can lead to aortic or mitral stenosis. A predisposition to coronary artery disease may also be present. Although the syndrome causes considerable morbidity, life expectancy is reduced only modestly. Symptoms are more often attributable to spondylitis with back pain, leading to a clinical picture difficult to distinguish from that of ankylosing spondylitis, though on radiographic assessment the sacroiliac joints are not fused in alkaptonuria.

B. Laboratory Findings

The diagnosis is established by demonstrating homogentisic acid in the urine, which turns black spontaneously on exposure to the air; this reaction is particularly noteworthy if the urine is alkaline or when alkali is added to a specimen. Molecular analysis of the homogentisic acid oxidase gene, recently mapped to chromosome 3, is available but not necessary for diagnosis.

► **Prevention**

Carrier screening and prenatal diagnosis are possible by testing for genetic mutations.

► **Treatment**

Treatment of the arthritis is similar to that for other arthropathies. Though, in theory, rigid dietary restriction might reduce accumulation of the pigment, this has not proved to be of practical benefit.

Keller JM et al. New developments in ochronosis: review of the literature. Rheumatol Int. 2005 Mar;25(2):81–5. [PMID: 15322814]
Perry MB et al. Musculoskeletal findings and disability in alkaptonuria. J Rheumatol. 2006 Nov;33(11):2280–5. [PMID: 16981292]

DOWN SYNDROME

ESSENTIALS OF DIAGNOSIS

► Typical craniofacial features (flat occiput, epicanthal folds, large tongue).

► Mental retardation.

► Congenital heart disease (eg, atrioventricular canal defects) in 50% of patients.

► Three copies of chromosome 21 (trisomy 21) or a chromosome rearrangement that results in three copies of a region of the long arm of chromosome 21.

► **Clinical Findings**

A. Symptoms and Signs

Down syndrome is usually diagnosed at birth on the basis of the typical craniofacial features, hypotonia, and single palmar crease. Several serious problems that may be evident at birth or may develop early in childhood include duodenal atresia, congenital heart disease (especially atrioventricular canal defects), and hematologic malignancy. The intestinal and cardiac anomalies usually respond to surgery. A transient neonatal leukemia generally responds to conservative management. The incidences of both acute lymphoblastic and myeloid leukemias are increased in childhood. Intelligence varies across a wide spectrum. Many people with Down syndrome do well in sheltered workshops and group homes, but few achieve full independence in adulthood. Other frequent complications include atlanto-axial instability, celiac disease, and hypothyroidism. An Alzheimer-like dementia usually becomes evident in the fourth or fifth decade and, for those who survive childhood, accounts for a reduced life expectancy.

B. Laboratory Findings

Cytogenetic analysis should always be performed—even though most patients will have simple trisomy for chromosome 21—to detect unbalanced translocations; such

patients may have a parent with a balanced translocation, and there will be a substantial recurrence risk of Down syndrome in future offspring of that parent and potentially that parent's relatives.

► **Prevention**

The presence of a fetus with Down syndrome can be detected in many pregnancies in the first or early second trimester through screening maternal serum for α-fetoprotein and other biomarkers ("multiple marker screening") and by detecting increased nuchal thickness and underdevelopment of the nasal bone on fetal ultrasound. The risk of bearing a child with Down syndrome increases exponentially with the age of the mother at conception and begins a marked rise after age 35. By age 45 years, a mother has one chance in 40 of having an affected child. The risk of other conditions associated with trisomy also increases, because of the predisposition of older oocytes to nondisjunction during meiosis. There is little risk of trisomy associated with increased paternal age. However, older men do have an increased risk of fathering a child with a new autosomal dominant condition. But because there are so many distinct conditions, the chance of fathering an offspring with any given one is extremely small.

► **Treatment**

Duodenal atresia should be treated surgically. Congenital heart disease should be treated as in any other patient. No medical treatment has been proven to affect the intellectual capacity.

► **When to Refer**

• For comprehensive evaluation of infants to investigate congenital heart disease, hematologic malignancy, and duodenal atresia.

• For genetic counseling of the parents.

• For signs of dementia in an adult patient.

► **When to Admit**

An affected young patient should be hospitalized when he or she has failure to thrive, regurgitation, breathlessness, or easy bruising.

Andriolo RB et al. Aerobic exercise training programmes for improving physical and psychosocial health in adults with Down syndrome. Cochrane Database Syst Rev. 2005 Jul 20;(3):CD005176. [PMID: 16034968]
Cohen WI. Current dilemmas in Down syndrome clinical care: celiac disease, thyroid disorders, and atlanto-axial instability. Am J Med Genet C Semin Med Genet. 2006 Aug 15;142(3):141–8. [PMID: 16838307]
Dierssen M et al. Pitfalls and hopes in Down syndrome therapeutic approaches: in the search for evidence-based treatments. Behav Genet. 2006 May;36(3):454–68. [PMID: 16520905]
Dixon N et al. Clinical manifestations of hematologic and oncologic disorders in patients with Down syndrome. Am J Med Genet C Semin Med Genet. 2006 Aug 15;142(3):149–57. [PMID: 17048354]
Driscoll DA et al; Professional Practice and Guidelines Committee. First trimester diagnosis and screening for fetal aneuploidy. Genet Med. 2008 Jan;10(1):73–4. [PMID: 18197059]

Galley R. Medical management of the adult patient with Down syndrome. JAAPA. 2005 Apr;18(4):45–6, 48, 51–2. [PMID: 15859488]

Tolmie JL et al. Down syndrome and other autosomal trisomies. In: *Emery and Rimoin's Principles and Practice of Medical Genetics*, 5th ed. Rimoin DL et al (editors). Churchill Livingstone, 2007.

FRAGILE X MENTAL RETARDATION

 ESSENTIALS OF DIAGNOSIS

▶ Expanded trinucleotide repeat in the *FMR1* gene.

▶ Mental retardation and autism in males.

▶ Large testes after puberty.

▶ Learning disabilities or mental retardation in females.

▶ Premature ovarian failure.

▶ Late-onset tremor and ataxia in males and females with moderate trinucleotide repeat expansion (premutation carriers).

▶ Clinical Findings

A. Symptoms and Signs

This X-linked condition accounts for more cases of mental retardation in males than any condition except Down syndrome; about 1 in 4000 to 1 in 6000 males is affected; the condition also affects intellectual function in females, although less severely and about 50% less frequently than in males.

B. Laboratory Findings

The first marker for this condition was a small gap, or fragile site, evident near the tip of the long arm of the X chromosome. Subsequently, the condition was found to be due to expansion of a trinucleotide repeat (CGG) near a gene called *FMR1*. All individuals have some CGG repeats in this location, but as the number increases beyond 52, the chances of further expansion during spermatogenesis or oogenesis increase.

Being born with one *FMR1* allele with 200 or more repeats results in mental retardation in most men, and in about 60% of women. The more repeats, the greater the likelihood that further expansion will occur during gametogenesis; this results in anticipation, in which the disorder can worsen from one generation to the next. Affected (heterozygous) young women show no physical signs other than early menopause, but they may have learning difficulties or frank retardation. Affected males show macroorchidism (enlarged testes) after puberty, large ears and a prominent jaw, a high-pitched voice, autistic characteristics, and mental retardation. Some males show evidence of a mild connective tissue defect, with joint hypermobility and mitral valve prolapse.

Women who are premutation carriers (55–200 CGG repeats) are at increased risk for premature ovarian failure and mild cognitive or behavioral abnormalities. Male and female premutation carriers are at risk for the development of tremor and ataxia beyond middle age (fragile-X tremor-ataxia syndrome, FXTAS). Changes in the cerebellar white matter on MRI may be evident before symptoms appear. Because of the relatively high prevalence of premutation carriers in the general population, older people in whom any of these behavioral or neurologic problems develop should undergo testing of the *FMR1* locus.

▶ Prevention

DNA diagnosis for the number of repeats has supplanted cytogenetic analysis for both clinical and prenatal diagnosis. This should be done on any male or female who has unexplained mental retardation.

▶ Treatment

No specific treatments have been developed. Attention-deficit and hyperactivity symptoms can respond to standard therapy, and a recent trial of L-acetylcarnitine showed promise.

▶ When to Refer

• For otherwise unexplained mental retardation or learning difficulties in boys and girls.

• For otherwise unexplained tremor or ataxia in middle-aged individuals.

• For premature ovarian failure.

• For genetic counseling.

Berry-Kravis E et al. Fragile X-associated tremor/ataxia syndrome: clinical features, genetics, and testing guidelines. Mov Disord. 2007 Oct 31;22(14):2018–30. [PMID: 17618523]

Gatchel JR et al. Diseases of unstable repeat expansion: mechanisms and common principles. Nat Rev Genet. 2005 Oct;6 (10):743–55. [PMID: 16205714]

Hagerman RJ. Lessons from fragile X regarding neurobiology, autism, and neurodegeneration. J Dev Behav Pediatr. 2006 Feb; 27(1):63–74. [PMID: 16511373]

Martin JR et al. Fragile X and reproduction. Curr Opin Obstet Gynecol. 2008 Jun;20(3):216–20. [PMID: 18460934]

Raymond FL. X linked mental retardation: a clinical guide. J Med Genet. 2006 Mar;43(3):193–200. [PMID: 16118346]

Sutherland GR et al. Fragile X syndrome and other causes of X-linked mental handicap. In: *Emery and Rimoin's Principles and Practice of Medical Genetics*, 5th ed. Rimoin DL et al (editors). Churchill Livingstone, 2007.

GAUCHER DISEASE

 ESSENTIALS OF DIAGNOSIS

▶ Deficiency of β-glucocerebrosidase.

▶ Anemia and thrombocytopenia.

▶ Hypersplenism.

▶ Pathologic fractures.

Clinical Findings

A. Symptoms and Signs

Gaucher disease has an autosomal recessive pattern of inheritance. A deficiency of β-glucocerebrosidase causes an accumulation of sphingolipid within phagocytic cells throughout the body. Anemia and thrombocytopenia are common and may be symptomatic; both are due primarily to hypersplenism, but marrow infiltration with Gaucher cells may be a contributing factor. Cortical erosions of bones, especially the vertebrae and femur, are due to local infarctions, but the mechanism is unclear. Episodes of bone pain (termed "crises") are reminiscent of those in sickle cell disease. A hip fracture in a patient with a palpable spleen—especially in a Jewish person of Eastern European origin—suggests the possibility of Gaucher disease.

Two uncommon forms of Gaucher disease, called type II and type III, involve neurologic accumulation of sphingolipid and a variety of neurologic problems. Type II is of infantile onset and has a poor prognosis. Heterozygotes for Gaucher disease may be at increased risk for developing Parkinson disease.

B. Laboratory Findings

Bone marrow aspirates reveal typical Gaucher cells, which have an eccentric nucleus and periodic acid–Schiff (PAS)-positive inclusions, along with wrinkled cytoplasm and inclusion bodies of a fibrillar type. In addition, the serum acid phosphatase is elevated. Definitive diagnosis requires the demonstration of deficient glucocerebrosidase activity in leukocytes. Over 200 mutations have been found to cause Gaucher disease and some are highly predictive of the neuronopathic forms. Thus, mutation detection, especially in a young person, is of potential value. Only four mutations in glucocerebrosidase account for more than 90% of the disease among Ashkenazi Jews, in whom the carrier frequency is 1:15.

Prevention

Most clinical complications can be prevented by early institution of enzyme replacement therapy. Carrier screening, especially among Ashkenazi Jews, detects those couples at 25% risk of having an affected child. Prenatal diagnosis through mutation analysis is feasible.

Treatment

For many years, treatment was supportive and included splenectomy for thrombocytopenia secondary to platelet sequestration. A recombinant form of the enzyme glucocerebrosidase (imiglucerase) for intravenous administration on a regular basis now permits a reduction in total body stores of glycolipid and improvement in orthopedic and hematologic manifestations. Unfortunately, the neurologic manifestations of types II and III have not improved with enzyme replacement therapy. The major drawback is the exceptional cost of imiglucerase, which can exceed $350,000 per year for a severely affected patient. Administration of less enzyme (30 units/kg per month) is effective for most adults and reduces the cost to about $100,000–150,000 annually. Alternative or complementary therapies, including methods to reduce substrate and to provide a chaperone for a defective enzyme, are being developed.

Beck M. New therapeutic options for lysosomal storage disorders: enzyme replacement, small molecules and gene therapy. Hum Genet. 2007 Mar;121(1):1–22. [PMID: 17089160]

Beutler E. Lysosomal storage diseases: natural history and ethical and economic aspects. Mol Genet Metab. 2006 Jul;88(3):208–15. [PMID: 16515872]

Cox TM et al. Management of non-neuronopathic Gaucher disease with special reference to pregnancy, splenectomy, bisphosphonate therapy, use of biomarkers and bone disease monitoring. J Inherit Metab Dis. 2008 Jun;31(3):319–36. [PMID: 18509745]

Vom Dahl S et al. Evidence-based recommendations for monitoring bone disease and the response to enzyme replacement therapy in Gaucher patients. Curr Med Res Opin. 2006 Jun; 22(6):1045–64. [PMID: 16846538]

Weinreb N et al. Imiglucerase (Cerezyme) improves quality of life in patients with skeletal manifestations of Gaucher disease. Clin Genet. 2007 Jun;71(6):576–88. [PMID: 17539908]

DISORDERS OF HOMOCYSTEINE METABOLISM

 ESSENTIALS OF DIAGNOSIS

► For homocystinuria, dislocated ocular lenses.
► Elevated homocysteine in the urine or plasma.

General Considerations

Considerable evidence has accumulated to support the 20-year-old observation that patients with clinical and angiographic evidence of coronary artery disease tend to have higher levels of plasma homocysteine than persons without coronary artery disease. The relationship has been extended to cerebrovascular and peripheral vascular diseases. Although this effect was initially thought to be due at least in part to heterozygotes for cystathionine β-synthase deficiency (see below), there is little supporting evidence. Rather, the major factor leading to hyperhomocysteinemia is folate deficiency. Pyridoxine (vitamin B_6) and vitamin B_{12} are also important in the metabolism of methionine, and deficiency of any of these vitamins can lead to accumulation of homocysteine. A number of genes influence utilization of these vitamins and can predispose to deficiency. For example, having one—and especially two—copies of an allele that causes thermolability of methylene tetrahydrofolate reductase predisposes people to elevated fasting homocysteine levels. However, both nutritional and most genetic deficiencies of these vitamins can be corrected by dietary supplementation of folic acid and, if serum levels are low, vitamins B_6 and B_{12}. In the United States, cereal grains are now fortified with folic acid. Studies are ongoing to determine the long-term utility of routine vitamin supplementation in people at risk for arterial occlusive disease, but many workers in this field recommend, at a minimum, taking 1 mg of folic acid per day. Recent studies showed that therapy with B vitamins lowered homocysteine levels significantly, but did not reduce the risk of either venous thromboembolism or complications of coronary artery disease. The role of lowering homocysteine as primary prevention for sequelae of atherosclerosis is still undetermined. Hyperhomocysteinemia occurs with end-stage chronic kidney disease.

Clinical Findings

A. Symptoms and Signs

Homocystinuria in its classic form is caused by cystathionine β-synthase deficiency and exhibits an autosomal recessive pattern of inheritance. This results in extreme elevations of plasma and urinary homocystine levels, a basis for diagnosis of this disorder. Homocystinuria is similar in certain superficial aspects to Marfan syndrome, since patients may have a similar body habitus and ectopia lentis is almost always present. However, mental retardation is often present in homocystinuria, and the cardiovascular events are those of repeated venous and arterial thromboses whose precise cause remains obscure. Life expectancy is reduced, especially in untreated and pyridoxine-unresponsive patients; myocardial infarction, stroke, and pulmonary embolism are the most common causes of death. This condition is diagnosed by newborn screening for hypermethioninemia; however, pyridoxine-responsive infants may not be detected. The diagnosis should be suspected in patients in the second and third decades of life who show evidence of arterial or venous thromboses and have no other risk factors.

B. Laboratory Findings

Although many mutations have been identified in the cystathionine β-synthase gene, amino acid analysis of plasma remains the most appropriate diagnostic test. Patients should be studied after they have been off folate or pyridoxine supplementation for at least 1 week. Relatively few laboratories currently provide highly reliable assays for homocysteine. Processing of the specimen is crucial to obtain accurate results. The plasma must be separated within 30 minutes; otherwise, blood cells release the amino acid and the measurement will then be artificially elevated.

Prevention

About 50% of patients have a form of cystathionine β-synthase deficiency that improves biochemically and clinically through pharmacologic doses of pyridoxine and folate. For these patients, treatment from infancy can prevent retardation and the other clinical problems. Patients who are pyridoxine nonresponders must be treated with a dietary reduction in methionine and supplementation of cysteine, also from infancy. The vitamin betaine is also useful in reducing plasma methionine levels by facilitating a metabolic pathway that bypasses the defective enzyme.

Treatment

Patients with classic homocystinuria who have suffered venous thrombosis receive anticoagulation therapy, but there are no studies to support prophylactic use of warfarin or antiplatelet agents.

Bazzano LA et al. Effect of folic acid supplementation on risk of cardiovascular diseases: a meta-analysis of randomized controlled trials. JAMA. 2006 Dec 13;296(22):2720–6. [PMID: 17164458]

Cattaneo M. Hyperhomocysteinemia and venous thromboembolism. Semin Thromb Hemost. 2006 Oct;32(7):716–23. [PMID: 17024599]

Ebbing M et al. Mortality and cardiovascular events in patients treated with homocysteine-lowering B vitamins after coronary angiography: a randomized controlled trial. JAMA. 2008 Aug 20;300(7):795–804. [PMID: 18714059]

Lawson-Yuen A et al. The use of betaine in the treatment of elevated homocysteine. Mol Genet Metab. 2006 Jul;88(3):201–7. [PMID: 16545978]

McCully KS. Homocysteine, vitamins, and vascular disease prevention. Am J Clin Nutr. 2007 Nov;86(5):1563S–8S. [PMID: 17991676]

Ray JG et al. Homocysteine-lowering therapy and risk for venous thromboembolism: a randomized trial. Ann Intern Med. 2007 Jun 5;146(11):761–7. [PMID: 17470822]

KLINEFELTER SYNDROME

 ESSENTIALS OF DIAGNOSIS

► Males with hypogonadism and small testes.
► 47,XXY karyotype.

Clinical Findings

A. Symptoms and Signs

Boys with an extra X chromosome are normal in appearance before puberty; thereafter, they have disproportionately long legs and arms, a female escutcheon, gynecomastia, and small testes. Infertility is due to azoospermia; the seminiferous tubules are hyalinized. The diagnosis is often not made until a couple is evaluated for inability to conceive. Mental retardation is somewhat more common than in the general population. Many men with Klinefelter syndrome have learning problems. However, their intelligence usually tests within the broad range of normal. As adults, detailed psychometric testing may reveal a deficiency in executive skills. The risk of breast cancer and diabetes mellitus is much higher in men with Klinefelter syndrome than in 46,XY men.

B. Laboratory Findings

Low serum testosterone is common. The karyotype is typically 47,XXY.

Prevention

Screening for cancer, especially of the breast, and for glucose intolerance are indicated.

Treatment

Treatment with testosterone after puberty is advisable but will not restore fertility. However, men with Klinefelter syndrome have had mature sperm aspirated from their testes and injected into oocytes, resulting in fertilization. After the blastocysts have been implanted into the uterus of a partner, conception has resulted. However, men with Klinefelter syndrome do have an increased risk for aneuploidy in sperm, and therefore chromosome analysis of a blastocyst should be considered before implantation.

Bojesen A et al. The metabolic syndrome is frequent in Klinefelter's syndrome and is associated with abdominal obesity and hypogonadism. Diabetes Care. 2006 Jul;29(7):1591–8. [PMID: 16801584]

Ferlin A et al. Chromosome abnormalities in sperm of individuals with constitutional sex chromosomal abnormalities. Cytogenet Genome Res. 2005;111(3–4):310–6. [PMID: 16192710]

Graham GE et al. Sex chromosome abnormalities. In: *Emery and Rimoin's Principles and Practice of Medical Genetics*, 5th ed. Rimoin DL et al (editors). Churchill Livingstone, 2007.

Ross JL et al. Cognitive and motor development during childhood in boys with Klinefelter syndrome. Am J Med Genet A. 2008 Mar 15;146A(6):708–19. [PMID: 18266239]

Simm PJ et al. The psychosocial impact of Klinefelter syndrome—a 10 year review. J Pediatr Endocrinol Metab. 2006 Apr;19(4):499–505. [PMID: 16759035]

Swerdlow AJ et al. Cancer incidence and mortality in men with Klinefelter syndrome: a cohort study. J Natl Cancer Inst. 2005 Aug 17;97(16):1204–10. [PMID: 16106025]

MARFAN SYNDROME

 ESSENTIALS OF DIAGNOSIS

▶ Disproportionately tall stature, thoracic deformity, and joint laxity or contractures.

▶ Ectopia lentis and myopia.

▶ Aortic dilation and dissection.

▶ Mitral valve prolapse.

▶ General Considerations

Marfan syndrome, a systemic connective tissue disease, has an autosomal dominant pattern of inheritance. It is characterized by abnormalities of the skeletal, ocular, and cardiovascular systems; spontaneous pneumothorax; dural ectasia; and striae atrophicae. Of most concern is disease of the ascending aorta, which begins as a dilated aortic root. Histology of the aorta shows diffuse medial degeneration. Mitral valve leaflets are also abnormal and mitral prolapse and regurgitation may be present, often with elongated chordae tendineae, which on occasion may rupture.

▶ Clinical Findings
A. Symptoms and Signs

Affected patients are typically tall, with particularly long arms, legs, and digits (arachnodactyly). However, there can be wide variability in the clinical presentation. Commonly, scoliosis and anterior chest deformity, such as pectus excavatum, are found. Ectopia lentis may lead to severe myopia and retinal detachment. Mitral valve prolapse is seen in about 85% of patients. Aortic root dilation is common and leads to aortic regurgitation or dissection with rupture. To diagnose Marfan syndrome, people with an affected relative need features in at least two systems. People with no family history need features in the skeletal system, two other systems, and one of the major criteria of ectopia lentis, dilation of the aortic root, or aortic dissection. Patients with homocystinuria due to cystathionine synthase deficiency also have dislocated lenses; tall, disproportionate stature; and thoracic deformity. They tend to have below normal intelligence, stiff joints, and a predisposition to arterial and venous occlusive disease. Males with Klinefelter syndrome do not show the typical ocular or cardiovascular features of Marfan syndrome and are generally sporadic occurrences in the family.

B. Laboratory Findings

Mutations in the fibrillin gene (*FBN1*) on chromosome 15 cause Marfan syndrome. Nonetheless, no simple laboratory test is available to support the diagnosis in questionable cases because related conditions may also be due to defects in fibrillin. The nature of the *FBN1* mutation has little predictive value in terms of prognosis. The pathogenesis of Marfan syndrome involves aberrant regulation of transforming growth factor (TGF)β activity. Mutations in either of two receptors for TGFβ (TGFBR1 and TGFBR2) can cause conditions that resemble Marfan syndrome in terms of aortic aneurysm and dissection and autosomal dominant inheritance.

▶ Prevention

There is prenatal and presymptomatic diagnosis for patients in whom the molecular defect in fibrillin has been found and for large enough families in whom linkage analysis using polymorphic markers around *FBN1* can be performed.

▶ Treatment

Children with Marfan syndrome require regular ophthalmologic surveillance to correct visual acuity and thus prevent amblyopia, and annual orthopedic consultation for diagnosis of scoliosis at an early enough stage so that bracing might delay progression. Patients of all ages require echocardiography at least annually to monitor aortic diameter and mitral valve function. All patients should use standard endocarditis prophylaxis. Long-term β-adrenergic blockade, titrated to individual tolerance but enough to produce a negative inotropic effect (atenolol, 1–2 mg/kg), retards the rate of aortic dilation. A clinical trial comparing the effectiveness of atenolol and losartan, a drug that reduces activity of TGF-β, is underway. Restriction from vigorous physical exertion protects from aortic dissection. Prophylactic replacement of the aortic root with a composite graft when the diameter reaches 45–50 mm in an adult (normal: < 40 mm) prolongs life. A procedure to reimplant the patient's native aortic valve and replace just the aneurysmal sinuses of Valsalva shows promise and also avoids the need for lifelong anticoagulation.

Prognosis

People with Marfan syndrome who are untreated commonly die in the fourth or fifth decade from aortic dissection or congestive heart failure secondary to aortic regurgitation. However, because of earlier diagnosis, lifestyle modifications, β-adrenergic blockade, and prophylactic aortic surgery, life expectancy has increased by several decades in the past 25 years.

When to Refer

- For detailed ophthalmologic examination.
- For at least annual cardiologic evaluation.
- For moderate scoliosis.
- For pregnancy in a woman with Marfan syndrome.
- For genetic counseling.

When to Admit

Any patient with Marfan syndrome in whom severe or unusual chest pain develops should be hospitalized to exclude pneumothorax and aortic dissection.

Brooke BS et al. Angiotensin II blockade and aortic-root dilation in Marfan's syndrome. N Engl J Med. 2008 Jun 26;358(26):2787–95. [PMID: 18579813]

Faivre L et al. Effect of mutation type and location on clinical outcome in 1,013 probands with Marfan syndrome or related phenotypes and *FBN1* mutations: an international study. Am J Hum Genet. 2007 Sep;81(3):454–66. [PMID: 17701892]

Ladouceur M et al. Effect of beta-blockade on ascending aortic dilatation in children with the Marfan syndrome. Am J Cardiol. 2007 Feb 1;99(3):406–9. [PMID: 17261408]

Pyeritz RE. Marfan syndrome and related disorders. In: *Emery and Rimoin's Principles and Practice of Medical Genetics*, 5th ed. Rimoin DL et al (editors). Churchill Livingstone, 2007.

HEREDITARY HEMORRHAGIC TELANGIECTASIA

ESSENTIALS OF DIAGNOSIS

- ► Recurrent epistaxis.
- ► Mucocutaneous telangiectases.
- ► Visceral arteriovenous malformations (especially lung, liver, brain, bowel).

Clinical Findings

A. Symptoms and Signs

Hereditary hemorrhagic telangiectasia (HHT), formerly termed "Osler-Weber-Rendu syndrome," is an autosomal dominant disorder of development of the vasculature. Epistaxis may begin in childhood or later in adolescence. Punctate telangiectases of the lips, tongue, fingers, and skin generally appear in later childhood and adolescence. Arter-iovenous malformations (AVMs) can occur at any age in the brain, lungs, and liver. Bleeding from the gastrointestinal tract is due to mucosal vascular malformations and usually is not a problem until mid-adult years or later. Pulmonary AVMs can cause hypoxemia (with peripheral cyanosis, dyspnea, and clubbing) and right-to-left shunting (with embolic stroke or brain abscess). The criteria for diagnosis require presence of three of the following four features: (1) recurrent epistaxis, (2) visceral AVMs, (3) mucocutaneous telangiectases, and (4) being the near relative of a clearly affected individual. Mutation analysis can be used for presymptomatic diagnosis or exclusion of the worry of HHT.

B. Laboratory Findings

MR or CT arteriography detects AVMs. Mutations in at least five genes can cause HHT. Three have been identified and molecular analysis to identify them is available; these mutations in *ENG*, *ALK1*, and *SMAD4* account for about 70% of families with HHT.

Prevention

Embolization of pulmonary AVMs reduces the risk of stroke and brain abscess. Treatment of brain AVMs reduces the risk of hemorrhagic stroke. All patients with HHT should practice routine endocarditis prophylaxis. All intravenous lines should have an air-filter to prevent embolization of an air bubble. Prenatal diagnosis through mutation detection is possible.

Treatment

All patients in whom the diagnosis of HHT is considered should have an MRI of the brain with contrast. A contrast echocardiogram will detect most pulmonary AVMs when "bubbles" appear on the left side of the heart after 3–6 cardiac cycles. A positive contrast echocardiogram should be followed by a high-resolution CT angiogram for localization of pulmonary AVMs. Patients who have AVMs with a feeding artery of 1 mm diameter or greater should undergo embolization. After successful embolization of all treatable pulmonary AVMs, the CT angiogram should be repeated in 3 years. A person with a negative contrast echocardiogram should have the test repeated every 5 years.

Cohen JH et al. Cost comparison of genetic and clinical screening in families with hereditary hemorrhagic telangiectasia. Am J Med Genet A. 2005 Aug 30;137(2):153–60. [PMID: 16059938]

Gallione CJ et al. *SMAD4* mutations found in unselected HHT patients. J Med Genet. 2006 Oct;43(10):793–7. [PMID: 16613914]

Guttmacher AE et al. Hereditary hemorrhagic telangiectasia. In: *Emery and Rimoin's Principles and Practice of Medical Genetics*, 5th ed. Rimoin DL et al (editors). Churchill Livingstone, 2007.

Nawaz A et al. Digital subtraction pulmonary arteriography versus multidetector CT in the detection of pulmonary arteriovenous malformations. J Vasc Interv Radiol. 2008 Nov;19(11):1582–8. [PMID: 18774307]

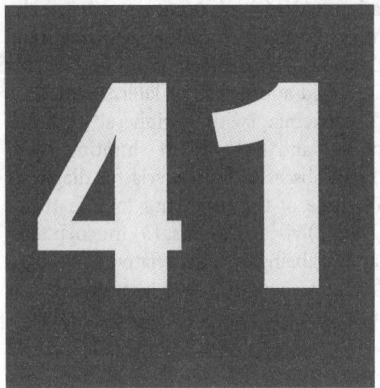

Complementary & Alternative Medicine

Ellen F. Hughes, MD, PhD

Kevin Barrows, MD

The use of complementary and alternative medicine (CAM) has become common in the United States. To maintain effective clinician-patient communication and ensure responsible clinical practice, it is important that clinicians learn the theory, practice, and scientific evidence associated with these therapies. This chapter provides an overview of four alternative medicine therapies: herbal medicine, nonherbal dietary supplements, acupuncture, and mind-body medicine.

► General Considerations

CAM is defined by the National Institutes of Health (NIH) as a group of diverse health care systems, practices, and products that are not presently considered to be part of conventional medicine. CAM therapies may be used alone as an alternative to conventional therapies or in addition to conventional, mainstream medicine to treat conditions and promote well being.

CAM modalities have been classified by NIH into five major categories:

1. **Biologically based practices** use substances found in nature, such as herbs, special diets, or vitamins (in doses outside those used in conventional medicine).
2. **Energy medicine** involves the use of energy fields, such as magnetic fields or biofields (energy fields that some believe surround and penetrate the human body). Examples include Reiki, external qigong, and therapeutic touch.
3. **Manipulative and body-based practices** use manipulation or movement of one or more body parts (massage, chiropractic, Feldenkrais method and other "body work" systems).
4. **Mind-body medicine** uses a variety of techniques designed to enhance the mind's ability to affect bodily function and symptoms, such as biofeedback, meditation, prayer, art and music therapy, hypnosis, and guided imagery.
5. **Whole medical systems** are built on complete systems of theory and practice that have evolved apart from— and often earlier than—the conventional medical approach used in the United States. Systems such as

traditional Oriental medicine, acupuncture, homeopathy, naturopathy, Ayurveda, and Tibetan medicine often use one or more of the methods listed above.

The Centers for Disease Control and Prevention conducted National Health Interview Surveys (NHIS) in 2002 and 2007. Overall, 23,300 American adults from diverse populations were asked about their use of CAM in the 2007 survey. Thirty-eight percent reported using some form of CAM in the previous 12 months, essentially unchanged from 36% in 2002. The most commonly used CAM therapies were nonvitamin, nonmineral natural products (17.7%), with fish oil, glucosamine, echinacea, flaxseed and ginseng being the most common; deep breathing exercises (12.7%); meditation (9.4%); chiropractic or osteopathic manipulation (8.6%); massage (8.3%); and yoga (6.1%). CAM use was higher among women, adults aged 30–69 years, those with higher levels of education, who were not poor, who live in the West and who have quit cigarette smoking. The most common conditions for which adults used CAM were similar to those seen in most primary care offices: musculoskeletal complaints, such as back, neck, and joint pain. Similar to 2002, CAM usage in 2007 was positively associated with the number of health conditions and number of doctor visits in the past 12 months. Most people who use CAM combine it with conventional medicine because they perceive the combination to be superior to either alone. Dissatisfaction with conventional medicine has not previously been found to predict greater CAM use, but more than 25% of US adults in the 2002 survey said they used CAM because they believed conventional medicine could not help them. No questions on health care spending were asked during NHIS interviews, but a smaller national phone survey conducted in 1997 estimated that the US public paid $36 billion on CAM therapies, much of it out-of-pocket.

In January 2005, the Institute of Medicine of the National Academies released a report on the use of CAM in the United States. They recommended "health profession schools incorporate sufficient information about complementary and alternative medicine (CAM) into the standard curriculum at all levels to enable licensed professionals to competently advise their patients about CAM." Indeed, despite the growing numbers of patients seeking CAM, less than 40% of alternative therapies used are disclosed to physicians. In one survey of 1559 patients age 50 or older, 70% who used CAM did not tell their physician. A lack of communication may be dangerous because some CAM therapies can interact adversely with conventional treatments.

Funding for biomedical research in this field increased when the NIH established the Office of Alternative Medicine in 1992 with an annual budget of $2 million. In 1998, its role was expanded as the National Center for Complementary and Alternative Medicine (NCCAM). NCCAM's budget for fiscal year 2008 was $122 million. Although some CAM modalities are not easily evaluated using randomized control trial methodology, the 2005 Institute of Medicine report recommends that conventional and CAM treatments both be held to similar standards of safety and efficacy.

Barnes PM et al. Complementary and alternative medicine use among adults and children: United States, 2007. CDC National Health Statistics Report Number 12, Dec 2008. Available at: http://www.cdc.gov/nchs/data/nhsr/nhsr012.pdf

Gardiner P et al. Factors associated with dietary supplement use among prescription drug users. Arch Intern Med. 2006 Oct 9;166(18):1968–74. [PMID: 17030829]

Institute of Medicine. Complementary and Alternative Medicine in the United States 2005. http://www.nap.edu/books/0309092701/html/

▼ HERBAL MEDICINES

▷ Epidemiology

For thousands of years, plants have been used worldwide for medicinal purposes, dispensed by traditional herbalists who have been involved with their cultivation and preparation as well as assessment of their potency. At present, most herbal products are commercially cultivated, processed in unregulated environments, and purchased over-the-counter without the counseling of a qualified health practitioner.

The use of herbs in the United States has increased dramatically over the past decade, although sales have leveled off over the past several years. Herbal products are used by one of five Americans at an annual total cost of more than $4 billion, but fewer than half of those individuals discuss the matter with a conventional health care provider. Consumers hold strong views about the efficacy of the supplements they take. Seventy percent state that they would continue to take their favorite supplement even if a government study claimed it was not effective.

▷ Regulatory Issues

In 1994, the United States Congress unanimously passed the Dietary Supplement and Health Education Act. This legislative act classifies vitamins, minerals, herbs, and amino acids as nutritional or dietary supplements. Under this law, supplements can be marketed without proof of safety or efficacy as long as no claim is made for their use in the diagnosis, treatment or cure, or prevention of disease. Manufacturers can, however, make "structure and func-

tion" claims that a product enhances a normal body function or state such as thinking, mood, or immune function. For example, saw palmetto can be marketed to support urinary tract health but not to treat benign prostatic hyperplasia. In contrast to prescription drugs, the US Food and Drug Administration (FDA) must first prove that an herbal preparation is *unsafe* before it can order that a product be taken off the market.

▷ Quality Assurance

In the past, consumers had no guarantee of the quality of the products they purchased. They could not be certain that the plant was accurately identified; that the product was free of microbial, pesticide, and heavy metal contamination; or that all batches contained the same ingredients in the same strengths.

Such lack of consistency prompted the Institute of Medicine to call on the government to implement improved quality-control manufacturing standards for supplements, more accurate labeling requirements, and greater consumer protections. In June 2007, the FDA announced that dietary supplement manufacturers must now evaluate the identity, purity, strength, and composition of their products and report all serious adverse events. These new good manufacturing practices must be phased in by June 2010.

Patients should be advised to follow certain guidelines when considering whether to use herbal medicines (Table 41–1).

▷ Product Formulations & Standardization

Herbal formulations include liquids (extracts, tinctures, infusions, and decoctions) and fresh, dried, and powdered preparations. The potency of herbs varies widely depending on which part of the plant is used, where it is cultivated, and what variations there may be in growing conditions and methods of preparation.

To ensure a consistent percentage of the primary active ingredients across batches and brand names, standardized extracts have been developed. Since multiple constituents may have pharmacologic activity, determining the active ingredients for standardization purposes can be a difficult task. In addition, ensuring stability of these active ingredients can be challenging. In a recent study of St John's wort for attention deficit/hyperactivity disorder in children, the product used in the trial was retested at the end of the trial and found to deliver only 50% of the intended dose. The European scientific community has played a significant role in producing and investigating high-quality standardized extracts that contain consistent quantities of marker compounds (ideally, the active ingredients). This work has laid the foundation for conducting phase 2 and phase 3 clinical trials. The quality of research in the field is improving, but most herbal remedies have not been evaluated in controlled clinical trials.

▷ Safety of Herbal Medicines

Although many medicinal herbs are relatively safe, some have significant toxicity. Herbs themselves can have unan-

Table 41-1. Advice to patients using herbal medicines.

Communication
Discuss use of all therapies with your health care provider.

Product Quality
Manufacturers are not required to submit evidence to the FDA or any regulatory body to demonstrate product safety, effectiveness, or product quality but must begin to do so (at least for adverse events) by 2010.
Ask your primary care provider, a pharmacist, or a trained herbalist regarding the specific herbs you are using.
Use herbs that are standardized to contain a specific quantity of the active ingredients.
Select formulations that have been studied in clinical trials.
Select formulations that have been independently tested for quality.

Labeling
Look for a seal of approval from an independent testing agency such as National Products Association (formerly National Nutritional Food Association), NSF International (formerly National Sanitation Foundation), or ConsumerLab.
It should state the common and scientific names of herb(s).
It should state the concentration or dose of the herb(s) and provide instructions on dose and frequency.
It should state that the product is "standardized" to contain a certain amount of the active ingredient(s).
It should state the methods used to ensure product quality.
It should state the name and address of the manufacturer.
It should state the batch or lot number and the expiration date.
It should list potential side effects and interactions.

Pregnancy
Few herbs have been studied for safety during pregnancy.
Seek advice from your primary care provider before using herbs during pregnancy.

Interactions
Discuss with your health care provider the safety profile and interactions that may occur when combining herbs and when taking herbs plus drugs.

Reporting
Report any adverse reactions to your state poison control program or the FDA.

FDA, Food and Drug Administration.

ticipated effects such as hepatotoxicity as seen with chaparral and germander. Ten of twenty patients with fulminant hepatic failure referred to a liver transplant service over a 21-month period were recent or active users of potentially hepatotoxic supplements. Ma-huang contains ephedrine and was sold as a component of many weight loss products and in a banned euphoriant called "herbal ecstasy." Over 800 adverse events associated with ma-huang have been reported, including the widely publicized death of a US major league baseball player in 2003, causing the FDA to ban ephedra-containing products from the market. Herbal products may also be intentionally adulterated with prescription drugs or contaminated with harmful substances such as pesticides or heavy metals. Prescription drugs such as prednisone, nonsteroidal anti-inflammatory drugs (NSAIDs), antibiotics, and testosterone have been detected in imported Chinese patent medicines. In December 2008, the FDA issued a warning that 25 weight loss products available over the counter and on the Internet contained

undeclared, active pharmaceutical ingredients, such as sibutramine, that could put consumers' health at risk.

Twenty-five percent of patients who take prescription medications also take at least one nonvitamin dietary supplement, creating a potential risk for adverse drug-herb or drug-supplement interactions. This figure increases to 50% in older US adults who take prescription medications, putting 1/25 of them at risk for developing a major drug-supplement interaction. Proving that a side effect experienced by a patient taking a dietary supplement is caused by that supplement is often difficult. Practitioners should take a detailed history from the patient and, if possible, obtain a sample of the product to facilitate further analysis, if needed. All suspected adverse events should be reported to the FDA's Medwatch Program (http://www.fda.gov/medwatch), although it is estimated that less than 1% are actually reported.

Ashar BH et al. Advising patients who use dietary supplements. Am J Med. 2008 Feb;121(2):91–7. [PMID: 18261493]

Qato DM et al. Use of prescription and over-the-counter medications and dietary supplements among older adults in the United States. JAMA. 2008 Dec 24;300(24):2867–78. [PMID: 19109115]

Ulbricht C et al. Clinical evidence of herb-drug interactions: a systematic review by the Natural Standard Research Collaborative. Curr Drug Metab. 2008 Dec;9(10):1062–119. [PMID: 19075623]

▶ Review of the Evidence for Selected Herbal Medicines

Table 41–2 provides an overview of selected herbal medicines.

A. St. John's Wort (*Hypericum perforatum*)

Over the past two decades, St. John's wort has been studied in thousands of patients for the treatment of mild to moderate depression. Most preparations are standardized to hypericin or hyperforin. The precise mechanisms of action are not known but are postulated to include selective inhibition of serotonin, γ-aminobutyrate, norepinephrine, and dopamine reuptake in the central nervous system.

Most of the 60-plus randomized controlled clinical trials, systematic reviews, and meta-analyses, including a 2008 Cochrane review, have shown that St. John's wort is more effective than placebo and as effective as prescription antidepressants for the treatment of mild to moderate depression. In addition, a standardized European hypericum extract helped prevent relapse of depression in patients who responded initially to the extract. Pooled analyses of six recent, large trials restricted to patients with major depression, however, showed only minimal effects of St. John's wort compared with placebo. A 4-year NIH study of 300 patients with mild symptoms of depression began in 2003. Patients are being randomized to St. John's wort, placebo, or citalopram for 12 weeks.

St. John's wort is generally well tolerated. Side effects are not common but include mild headache, photosensitivity, gastrointestinal upset, and restlessness. Data from 35 double-blind randomized trials show that drop out and adverse event rates in patients receiving *Hypericum* extracts

Table 41–2. Overview of selected herbal medicines.

	Leading Indications	Dosage	Level of Evidence[1]	Safety[2]	Interaction; Side Effects	Comments
Echinacea (purple coneflower)	1. Treatment of URIs 2. Prevention of URIs	300 mg, or 3 mL q3-4h	1. B 2. C	I	None known: rash, pruritus, nausea	Avoid in immunocompromised patients; avoid use > 4 weeks
Black cohosh	Menopausal symptoms (hot flashes)	Depends on formulation (Remifemin = 20 mg twice daily)	B	I		Case reports of hepatitis, so avoid in liver disease
Garlic (Allium sativum)	1. Cholesterol 2. Hypertension 3. Coronary artery disease	600–900 mg once daily	1. B 2. C 3. C	I	1. Odor, flatulence 2. May have antiplatelet activity	
Ginkgo biloba (EGb 761, GBE)	1. Dementia 2. Claudication	60 mg three times daily	1. A 2. A	II	May have anticoagulant effect	Do not use in patients taking anticoagulants and use caution if allergic to urushiols (mango rind, sumac-poison ivy, cashew nuts)
Asian ginseng (Panax ginseng)	Stamina, aphrodisiac, fertility, "tonic," "energy-booster," "adaptogen"	200–600 mg once daily extract; 1–2 g crude drug	C: multiple studies but few for any given indication	I	Previous reports of toxicity have been attributed to adulterants	
St. John's wort (Hypericum perforatum)	1. Depression: mild to moderate 2. Depression: major	300 mg three times daily	1. A 2. B	I (but significant drug-herb interaction)	Induces cytochrome P450, leading to lower serum levels of certain drugs	Cyclosporine, protease inhibitors, oral contraceptives, warfarin, digoxin levels reduced
Saw palmetto (Serenoa repens)	Benign prostatic hyperplasia	160 mg twice daily	B: small or none	I	Mild GI upset and headaches (rare)	Does not effect PSA levels or prostate size

[1]Level of evidence: A, high quality: consistent evidence from randomized trials or overwhelming evidence from other sources; B, moderate quality: evidence from randomized trials with important limitations or very strong evidence of some other form; C, low quality: evidence from observational studies or randomized trials with serious methodologic flaws.
[2]Safety: I, generally safe; II, relatively safe; III, insufficient evidence; IV, may be harmful; V, clear evidence of harm.
GI, gastrointestinal; PSA, prostate-specific antigen; URI, upper respiratory infection.

were similar to placebo, lower than with older antidepressants, and slightly lower than with selective serotonin reuptake inhibitors (SSRIs). Patients are advised to avoid taking St. John's wort in combination with prescription antidepressants, as there have been case reports of the serotonin syndrome. St. John's wort also induces the cytochrome P450 system (isozyme CYP3A4), which may lower the blood levels of nearly 50% of prescription medications that are metabolized by this system (eg, ethinyl estradiol, warfarin, cyclosporine, statins, and indinavir). St John's wort can also lower the serum level of other medications by affecting the p-glycoprotein transporter system. Several cases of cardiac and renal organ rejection have been reported in patients whose previously stable level of cyclosporine was lowered after initiation of St. John's wort. Of further concern is that this herb-drug interaction may persist even after St. John's wort is discontinued. A 40%

decrease in serum levels of the chemotherapeutic agent irinotecan noted in five patients taking concurrent St. John's wort persisted for 3 weeks after St. John's wort was discontinued.

Jurcic J et al. St John's wort versus paroxetine for depression. Can Fam Physician. 2007 Sep;53(9):1511–3. [PMID: 17872882]

Kasper S et al. Continuation and long-term maintenance treatment with Hypericum extract WS 5570 after recovery from an acute episode of moderate depression: a double-blind, randomized, placebo-controlled long-term trial. Eur Neuropsychopharmacol. 2008 Nov;18(11):803–813. [PMID: 18694635]

Kasper S et al. Efficacy of St John's wort extract WS® 5570 in acute treatment of mild depression. A reanalysis of data from controlled clinical trials. Eur Arch Psychiatry Clin Neurosci. 2008 Feb;258(1):59–63. [PMID: 18084790]

Linde K et al. St John's wort for major depression. Cochrane Database Syst Rev. 2008 Oct;(4):CD000448. [PMID: 18843608]

Zhou SF et al. An update on clinical drug interactions with the herbal antidepressant St John's wort. Curr Drug Metab. 2008 Jun;9(5):394–409. [PMID: 18537576]

B. Garlic

Garlic is one of the top-selling herbs in Europe and the United States. It has been used since antiquity for the treatment of cardiovascular and infectious diseases. The German Federal Health Agency Commission E and the European Scientific Cooperative on Phytotherapy have approved its use for the treatment of hyperlipidemia and atherosclerosis. Garlic is available in multiple over-the-counter formulations (dried, powdered, oils). Many products are standardized to yield 0.6% allicin, the ingredient believed responsible for its odor and therapeutic benefit. Allicin is formed by the action of allinase enzymes when garlic is crushed. Both heat and acid destroy these enzymes, so some experts recommend that garlic is best ingested raw. The best-studied form is an enteric-coated capsule of dehydrated garlic. Freeze-drying helps retain most of the active ingredients found in raw garlic. Enteric coating permits allicin to be released in the small intestine, thereby enhancing absorption and reducing the breath odor. Allicin yield among powdered preparations varies as much as 230-fold in brands used in trials. This lack of standardization may contribute to inconsistent results in dozens of clinical trials.

Several mechanisms for garlic's beneficial effects on cardiovascular disease have been proposed: decreased low-density lipoprotein cholesterol (LDL-C) synthesis and oxidation, decreased platelet aggregation, decreased inflammation, lowered blood pressure, and antibacterial activity.

Doses of 600–900 mg of freeze-dried garlic (equivalent to one-half to one clove) taken for 4–6 weeks lower total cholesterol and LDL-C levels by 4–12%, have minimal effect on blood pressure (< 10 mm Hg, with greater decreases in subjects with hypertension), and no effect on glucose levels. In a well-designed 2007 trial, 192 adults with moderate hypercholesterolemia were randomized to one of four treatment arms for 6 months: raw garlic, two popular garlic supplements, or placebo. None of the three forms of garlic given at approximate doses of a 4-g clove garlic/d, 6 days/week for 6 months had statistically or clinically significant effects on plasma lipids in adults with initial LDL-C levels of 130–160 mg/dL. In addition, a double-blind randomized study in which 90 overweight smokers were randomized to 2.1 g/d garlic powder, 40 mg/d atorvastatin, or placebo for 3 months, showed no significant effect of garlic on inflammatory biomarkers, endothelial function, or lipid profile compared with placebo. Numerous observational studies have suggested that regular consumption of garlic might reduce the risk of developing certain malignancies, but no prospective controlled trials have been performed.

Garlic is well tolerated and apparently safe for long-term use. In addition to the well-known breath and body odor, common side effects include gastrointestinal upset, nausea, and flatulence.

A more than 50% reduction in blood levels of saquinavir after garlic supplementation has been reported. Although the induction of the cytochrome P450 system was hypothe-sized as the mechanism of action of this significant herb-drug interaction, a recent study of healthy volunteers did not reveal an effect of garlic on isozymes CYPP2D6 or CYP3A4. Garlic has been shown to have some antiplatelet activation activity, so there is a theoretical risk of increased bleeding, especially if taken with aspirin, anticoagulants, or NSAIDs. However, a 2006 study of 48 patients taking warfarin randomized to aged garlic extract or placebo for 12 weeks did not report any increased bleeding in those taking garlic. In addition, a 2008 study showed no effect of garlic on warfarin pharmacokinetics in healthy volunteers. No changes in platelet function were noted in healthy volunteers after ingesting raw garlic and garlic oil, but some clinicians recommend stopping garlic 1–2 weeks prior to undergoing elective surgery.

Gardner CD et al. Effect of raw garlic vs. commercial garlic supplements on plasma lipid concentrations in adults with moderate hypercholesterolemia. A randomized, clinical trial. Arch Intern Med. 2007 Feb 26;167(4):346–53. [PMID: 17325296]
Kim JY et al. Garlic intake and cancer risk: an analysis using the Food and Drug Administration's evidence-based review system for the scientific evaluation of health claims. Am J Clin Nutr. 2009 Jan;89(1):257–64. [PMID: 19056580]
Pittler MH et al. Clinical effectiveness of garlic (Allium sativum). Mol Nutr Food Res. 2007 Nov;51(11):1382–85. [PMID: 17918163]
Reid K et al. Effect of garlic on blood pressure: a systematic review and meta-analysis. BMC Cardiovasc Disord. 2008 Jun 16;8:13. [PMID: 18554422]
Reinhardt KM et al. Effects of garlic on blood pressure in patients with and without systolic hypertension: a meta-analysis. Ann Pharmacother. 2008 Dec;42(12):1766–1771. [PMID: 19017826]
Scharbert G et al. Garlic at dietary doses does not impair platelet function. Anesth Analg. 2007 Nov;105(5):1214–8. [PMID: 17959943]

C. Ginkgo

The dried leaf of the ginkgo tree has been used medicinally for thousands of years. More than 400 studies over the past 30 years have investigated ginkgo's ability to improve blood flow in a variety of conditions, including memory impairment, dementia, peripheral vascular disease, vertigo, tinnitus, asthma, SSRI-induced sexual dysfunction, anxiety and acute mountain sickness. It is the sixth best selling herb in the United States with greater than $250 million in sales per year. The German Commission E has approved a standardized form of ginkgo leaf extract (EGb 761) for the treatment of cognitive impairment and intermittent claudication. Multiple pharmacologically active compounds have been isolated from ginkgo. Flavonoids have antioxidant and free radical scavenging ability and terpene lactones have platelet-activating factor antagonist activity. In addition, ginkgo extracts increase the production of nitric oxide and activate certain central neurotransmitters, including the cholinergic system, which may contribute to their beneficial effects on memory and cognition. EGb 761—the formulation that has been studied most extensively—is standardized to contain 24% flavonoid glycosides and 6% terpene lactones.

Early studies that assessed ginkgo's efficacy on cognitive function in the elderly showed a modest improvement when compared with placebo. The longest of these studies (1 year) showed stabilization of cognitive and functional abilities in 309 demented patients treated with EGb 761 compared with placebo, with no differences in adverse outcomes. A 2007 systematic review, however, concluded that ginkgo did not have predictable and clinically significant benefits in patients with dementia. A well-designed NIH-funded study also showed that ginkgo (120 mg EGb721 twice a day) did not prevent dementia in more than 3000 elderly subjects with normal or mildly impaired cognitive function who were monitored for a mean of 6 years. A smaller study also failed to show any reduction in progression to dementia in 118 subjects 85 years of age or older who were randomized to 80 mg of a different formulation of ginkgo three times a day or placebo for 42 months. When researchers took into account participant's adherence, however, the group that actually took their ginkgo had a smaller decline in memory compared with those taking a placebo. There is conflicting evidence about ginkgo's ability to enhance memory in healthy individuals. In general, ginkgo is well tolerated in healthy adults at recommended doses for up to 6 months. Allergic skin reactions, gastrointestinal disturbances, and headache occur in less than 2% of patients. There are theoretical concerns about a risk of increased bleeding because antiplatelet activating factor activity has been demonstrated in vitro. Nearly 20 cases of increased bleeding in patients taking ginkgo have been reported, but establishing a causal relationship is challenging because many of these patients had other risk factors including age and use of medications, such as warfarin, aspirin, or NSAIDs. Of note, no excess bleeding complications have been reported in clinical trials and no differences in coagulation, platelet function, or pharmacokinetics of warfarin have been reported in healthy volunteers. Caution should still be exercised in patients with bleeding disorders or who are taking anticoagulants, aspirin, or other herbs that may increase the risk of bleeding. In one study, ginkgo (90 mg/d) did not show any adverse effects on the pharmacokinetics of donepezil (5 mg/d) when administered together, but potential interactions with other medications used to treat dementia are not known.

Ginkgo has also been evaluated for its effect on intermittent claudication. A meta-analysis of nine randomized, placebo-controlled, double-blinded trials of patients treated with EGb761 showed a modest treatment effect in the increase of pain-free walking distance in favor of ginkgo over placebo. There is insufficient evidence to support ginkgo's efficacy in treating tinnitus, acute mountain sickness, vertigo, or SSRI-associated sexual dysfunction.

Beckert BW et al. The effect of herbal medicines on platelet function: an in vivo experiment and review of the literature. Plas Reconstr Surg. 2007 Dec;120(7):2044–50. [PMID: 18090773]

Birks J et al. Ginkgo biloba for cognitive impairment and dementia. Cochrane Database Syst Rev. 2007 Apr 18;(2):CD003120. [PMID: 17443523]

DeKosky ST et al. Ginkgo biloba for prevention of dementia: a randomized controlled trial. JAMA. 2008 Nov;300(19):2253–2262. [PMID: 19017911]

Dodge HH et al. A randomized, placebo-controlled trial of Ginkgo biloba for the prevention of cognitive decline. Neurology. 2008 May 6;70(19 Pt2):1809–17. [PMID: 18305231]

Gardner CD et al. Effect of Ginkgo biloba (EGb 761) on treadmill walking time among adults with peripheral artery disease: a randomized clinical trial. J Cardiopulm Rehabil Prev. 2008 Jul–Aug;28(4):258–65. [PMID: 18628657]

Gardner CD et al. Effects of Ginkgo biloba (EGb 761) and aspirin on platelet aggregation and platelet function analysis among older adults at risk of cardiovascular disease: a randomized clinical trial. Blood Coagul Fibrinolysis. 2007 Dec;18(8):787–93. [PMID: 17982321]

Kennedy DO et al. Modulation of cognitive performance following doses of 120 mg Ginkgo biloba extract administration to healthy young volunteers. Hum Psychopharmacol. 2007 Dec;22(8):559–66. [PMID: 17902186]

D. Echinacea

Echinacea ranks third among the top-selling herbs in the United States, accounting for more than $300 million in sales annually. Three of nine Echinacea species are currently used for the treatment and prevention of upper respiratory infections. Preparations are made from roots (Echinacea pallida and Echinacea angustifolia), above-ground parts (stems, leaves, and flowers of Echinacea purpurea), or a combination of both. Multiple forms are available over-the-counter, including capsules, fresh pressed juice, tinctures, and teas. Differences in species, growing conditions, plant parts used, and extraction procedures can result in differences in chemical composition and biologic activity. Several active ingredients have been identified, including polysaccharides, glycoproteins, alkaloids, and flavonoids. In vitro, animal, and human studies suggest that these ingredients cause stimulation of the immune system and that they possess anti-inflammatory, free radical-scavenging, and antiviral activity.

The quality of most clinical trials has been limited by use of multiple products and doses (including formulations containing multiple herbs) and the lack of rigorous methodology.

The majority of early trials reported that echinacea is effective in reducing the duration and severity of colds if started within several days of the onset of symptoms but no more effective than placebo when taken to prevent infection. A well-designed, 2005 trial studied three different E angustifolia root preparations for the prevention and treatment of laboratory-induced rhinovirus infections. Four hundred thirty-seven volunteers were randomized to receive either prophylaxis (beginning 7 days before a challenge with rhinovirus) or treatment (beginning at the time of viral challenge), with one of the three different echinacea preparations. No statistically significant effects were seen on rates of infection or severity of symptoms in patients taking the herb. The echinacea used in this trial was well characterized and of high quality, but some clinicians feel that the dose used was lower than that used in routine practice. In contrast, an updated meta-analysis of echinacea monopreparations found that 10 of 16 trials showed the herb to be more effective than placebo for the treatment of colds, particularly preparations made from above-the-ground parts of E purpurea. Authors of a 2007 meta-analysis of 14 clinical trials also conclude that echinacea is beneficial in decreasing both the incidence and duration of the common cold. The herb decreased the odds of developing a upper respiratory tract infection by 58% and the duration of a cold by 1.4 days. In contrast, E pallida was no more effective than placebo in decreasing the risk of ear infections in children prone to otitis media. In general, echinacea is well tolerated, with few reported adverse events. Rare allergic reactions including rash have been reported (especially in patients with ragweed allergies), and there was a single case of recurrent erythema nodosum. The German Commission E recommends that patients who are pregnant, have autoimmune disease, or who are immunocompromised not take echinacea because of its immune-stimulating effects. The Commission also recommends that its use be limited in others to less than 4 weeks. The data supporting these recommendations are not clear.

Linde K et al. Echinacea for preventing and treating the common cold. Cochrane Database Syst Rev. 2006 Jan 25;(1):CD000530. [PMID: 16437427]

Schoop R et al. Echinacea in the prevention of induced rhinovirus colds: a meta-analysis. Clin Ther. 2006 Feb;28(2):174–83. [PMID: 16678640]

Shah SA et al. Evaluation of Echinacea for the prevention and treatment of the common cold: a meta-analysis. Lancet Infect Dis. 2007 Jul;7(7):473–80. [PMID: 17597571]

Wahl RA et al. Echinacea purpurea and manipulative treatment in children with recurrent otitis media: a randomized controlled trial. BMC Complement Altern Med. 2008 Oct 2;8:56. [PMID: 18831749]

Woelkart K et al. Echinacea for preventing and treating the common cold. Planta Med. 2008 Jan;74(6):633–37. [PMID: 18186015]

E. Ginseng

Ginseng root has been used for medicinal purposes in Asia for over 2000 years and is consumed by up to 5% of the population in Western countries. Two major forms of ginseng are in use today: Asian ginseng (*Panax ginseng*) and American ginseng (*Panax quinquefolius*). *Eleutherococcus senticosus* (previously known as Siberian ginseng), is not a member of the *Panax* genus and does not contain ginsenosides that are thought to be the active ingredients in true ginseng. The German Commission E monograph on ginseng root approves its use as "a tonic to counteract weakness and fatigue, as a restorative for declining stamina and impaired concentration, and as an aid to convalescence." Extracts are made from dried roots and contain more than 25 ginsenosides, each with unique and sometimes oppositional effects on the cardiovascular, central nervous, and immune systems. The mechanisms of action have not been clearly delineated.

Multiple indications have been studied using different ginseng species, often with poor methodologic rigor. One European study identified 57 randomized controlled trials of ginseng in the world's literature, but only 16 studies were of good enough quality to be included in their systematic review. Insufficient evidence was available to support or refute the use of ginseng for any of the purported indications, including improvement of physical performance, cognitive functioning, and quality of life. In contrast, a small open label 2008 trial suggests that Korean red ginseng (unskinned Panax ginseng before it is steamed and dried) may improve cognitive function in patients with Alzheimer disease. Some early studies suggest that ginseng causes small reductions in blood pressure, but there was no effect on 24-hour blood pressure or kidney function in 52 hypertensive

patients who took North American ginseng for 12 weeks. A 2006 systematic review of 34 studies also did not support the use of ginseng to treat cardiovascular risk factors, although at least 7 human studies since 2000 report that American and Asian ginseng may lower blood glucose in both healthy and diabetic patients. Ginseng is believed by many to enhance sexual function. A systematic review of 7 randomized clinical trials of Korean red ginseng concluded there was suggestive evidence for effectiveness in treating erectile dysfunction, although the quality of these studies was low.

Ginseng is well tolerated at recommended doses, with few adverse effects. A recent systematic review of adverse reactions reports that the incidence is similar in ginseng monopreparations and placebo. Possible drug interactions have been reported between *P ginseng* and warfarin, phenelzine, calcium channel blockers, digoxin, and alcohol. A potential risk of hypoglycemia exists in diabetic patients taking medications. Earlier reports of "ginseng abuse syndrome" and other toxicities are now attributed to adulterants found in earlier unregulated over-the-counter ginseng products. Indeed, 13 of 21 ginseng products recently evaluated for quality and purity failed because they contained unacceptable levels of pesticides or heavy metals or inadequate concentrations of ginsenosides.

Buettner C et al. Systematic review of the effects of ginseng on cardiovascular risk factors. Ann Pharmacother. 2006 Jan; 40(1):83–95. [PMID: 16332943]

DeAndrade E et al. Study of the efficacy of Korean Red Ginseng in the treatment of erectile dysfunction. Asian J Androl. 2007 Mar;9(2):241–4. [PMID: 16855773]

Heo JH et al. An open label trial of Korean red ginseng as adjuvant treatment for cognitive improvement in patients with Alzheimer's disease. Eur J Neurol. 2008 Aug;15(8):865–68. [PMID: 18684311]

Jang DJ et al. Red ginseng for treating erectile dysfunction: a systematic review. Br J Clin Pharmacol. 2008 Oct;66(4):444–50. [PMID: 18754850]

Ma SW et al. Effect of *Panax ginseng* supplementation on biomarkers of glucose tolerance, antioxidant status and oxidative stress in type 2 diabetic subjects: results of a placebo-controlled human intervention trial. Diabetes Obes Metab. 2008 Nov;10(11):1125–27. [PMID: 18355331]

Stravo PM et al. Long-term intake of North American ginseng has no effect on 24-hour blood pressure and renal function. Hypertension. 2006 Apr;47(4):791–6. [PMID: 16520410]

Vuksan V et al. Korean red ginseng (*Panax ginseng*) improves glucose and insulin regulation in well-controlled, type 2 diabetes: results of a randomized, double-blind, placebo-controlled study of efficacy and safety. Nutr Metab Cardiovasc Dis. 2008 Jan;18(1):46–56. [PMID: 16860976]

F. Saw Palmetto

Saw palmetto is used by over 2 million men in the United States to treat benign prostatic hyperplasia (BPH), and in Europe, it is often the first-line therapy for lower urinary tract symptoms. Lipophilic extracts are prepared from the berries of the dwarf palm tree (*Serenoa repens*) and are standardized to sterols and free fatty acids. Several mechanisms of action have been proposed, including inhibition of 5α-reductase activity, as well as antiandrogenic, anti-inflammatory, and antiproliferative activity. More than 350 saw palmetto products are marketed in the United

States; however, the most studied brand of saw palmetto (Permixon) is not available.

Early studies showed that saw palmetto was more effective than placebo and only slightly less effective than α-blockers for the treatment of BPH. In a 2008 trial of 92 Chinese men with lower urinary tract symptoms associated with BPH, those treated with saw palmetto for 3 months had significantly greater urine flow rates and improved symptoms relative to those taking the placebo. In contrast, a well-designed 2006 trial showed no difference in symptom scores, flow rates, prostate size, postvoid residual volume, quality of life, or prostate-specific antigen in 225 men with moderate to severe BPH treated with saw palmetto (160 mg twice daily) or placebo for 1 year. An even larger (3000 patient), 4–6 year long, multicenter, three-arm randomized, controlled trial of saw palmetto, the herb *Pygeum africanum*, and placebo is being sponsored by the NIH.

Saw palmetto is very well tolerated by most patients, with only mild and rare gastrointestinal symptoms being reported. It has not been shown to reduce prostate size or lower the serum level of prostate-specific antigen. No herb-drug interactions have been reported.

Avins AL et al. A detailed safety assessment of a saw palmetto extract. Complement Ther Med. 2008 Jun;16(3):147–54. [PMID: 18534327]

Avins A et al. Saw palmetto and lower urinary tract symptoms: what is the latest evidence? Curr Urol Rep. 2006 Jul;7(4):260–5. [PMID: 16930496]

Bent S et al. Saw palmetto for benign prostate hyperplasia. N Engl J Med. 2006 Feb 9;354(6):557–66. [PMID: 16467543]

Dedhia RC et al. Phytotherapy for lower urinary tract symptoms secondary to benign prostatic hyperplasia. J Urol. 2008 Jun;179(6):2119–25. [PMID: 18423748]

Shi R et al. Effect of saw palmetto soft gel capsules on lower urinary tract symptoms associated with benign prostatic hyperplasia: a randomized trial in Shanghai, China. J Urol. 2008 Feb;179(2):610–5. [PMID: 18082217]

G. Black Cohosh

Black cohosh, a member of the buttercup family, is a plant native to North America that has gained popularity as a nonhormonal treatment for menopause-related symptoms. Preparations made from its roots and rhizomes were used by Native Americans to treat malaise, genitourinary complaints, colds, and rheumatism. Its mechanism of action remains unclear, but it does not appear to have significant estrogenic effects in vitro or in vivo. A recent report suggests that it acts on the human opioid mu receptor, which may play a role in regulating body temperature.

Black cohosh has been studied in more than 3000 women. The most widely used formulations are two German-manufactured preparations. Fifteen clinical trials have shown efficacy for Remifemin, an isopropanoic extract available since the mid-1950s, and six trials have studied a different product, marketed as Klimadynon. Many clinical trials published since 2003 demonstrate efficacy of black cohosh for reducing menopausal symptoms such as hot flashes, including a 2007 study in which it was as effective as tibolone (a synthetic steroid only available in Europe). In contrast, a year-long trial published in late 2006 did not show that black cohosh alone or in combination with other herbs was any more effective than placebo in reducing hot flashes or night sweats. In this five-arm trial, 351 women, age 45–55 with at least two hot flashes per day, were randomized to receive black cohosh, a combination of black cohosh and nine other herbs, the combination product along with counseling to increase soy consumption, placebo, and conventional hormone replacement therapy (HRT). (The HRT arm was terminated when the Women's Health Initiative trials were prematurely halted in 2002.) A smaller 2008 trial of a preparation containing black cohosh and Chinese herbs also showed no reduction in hot flashes compared with placebo.

Black cohosh is generally well tolerated at recommended doses. Rare case reports of hepatitis have been reported (some severe enough to require liver transplantation), causing the Medicines and Healthcare Registry Agency in Britain to join Australia in requiring that products be labeled with a safety warning. The NIH held a workshop on the safety of black cohosh in 2004 and concluded that there was inadequate evidence of a causal relationship between black cohosh and hepatotoxicity, although they did recommend that liver enzymes be monitored in all participants in NIH-sponsored trials of black cohosh. No significant drug-herb interactions have been reported.

A 2006 analysis of 11 black cohosh products available in the United States revealed that 4 contained a cheaper Asian species, which has different chemical properties, either as the sole ingredient or in combination with North American black cohosh.

Bai W et al. Efficacy and tolerability of a medicinal product containing an isopropanolic black cohosh extract in Chinese women with menopausal symptoms: a randomized, double-blind, parallel-controlled study versus tibolone. Maturitas. 2007 Sep 20;58(1):31–41. [PMID: 17587516]

Borelli F et al. Black cohosh (Cimicifuga racemosa): a systematic review of adverse events. Am J Obstet Gynecol. 2008 Nov;199(5):455–66. [PMID: 18984078]

Nedrow A et al. Complementary and alternative therapies for the management of menopause-related symptoms. A systematic evidence review. Arch Intern Med. 2006 Jul 24;166(14):1453–65. [PMID: 16864755]

Newton KM et al. Treatment of vasomotor symptoms of menopause with black cohosh, multibotanicals, soy, hormone therapy or placebo. Ann Intern Med. 2006 Dec 19;145(12):869–79. [PMID: 17179056]

Raus K et al. First-time proof of endometrial safety of the special black cohosh extract (Actacea or Cimicifuga racemosa extract) CRBNO1055. Menopause. 2006 Jul–Aug;13(4):678–91. [PMID: 16837890]

Ruhlen RL et al. Black cohosh does not exert an estrogenic effect on the breast. Nutr Cancer. 2007;59(2):269–77. [PMID: 18001221]

Van der Sluijs CP et al. A randomized placebo-controlled trial on the effectiveness of an herbal formula to alleviate menopausal vasomotor symptoms. Menopause. 2009 Mar–Apr; 16(2):336–44. [PMID: 19057416]

▼ DIETARY SUPPLEMENTS

Sales of dietary supplements have increased dramatically over the past decade. The Dietary Supplement Health

Education Act of 1994 has made it possible for manufacturers to sell dietary supplements directly to the public without FDA approval or oversight. Reports of adulteration and contamination are available, but the magnitude of this problem remains unknown. Furthermore, there have been several reports of the dose printed on the label being different from the actual dose provided. (See section on herbal medicines, above, for further details on regulatory and quality assurance issues and advice for patients to follow when purchasing these products.) Table 41-3 provides an overview of selected dietary supplements commonly used in the United States today.

▶ Dehydroepiandrosterone

Dehydroepiandrosterone (DHEA) and its metabolite, DHEAS, are secreted by the adrenal cortex and serve as precursors for the synthesis of more than 40 different hormones, including male and female sex hormones. In healthy individuals, DHEA levels fall 10–15% per decade from age 20 until age 70, when they are at 30% of lifetime peak levels. Normal circulating levels vary widely by age, sex, and ethnicity and are affected by body mass index, medications (insulin, corticosteroids, opioids), and thy-

roid function. Reduced levels of DHEA have been reported in people who suffer from a wide variety of chronic illness, including depression, cancer, type 2 diabetes, HIV infection, Alzheimer disease, lupus erythematosus, chronic kidney disease, anorexia, and atherosclerosis. Low levels of DHEA associated with aging and medical illness have been cited in the popular press as evidence that DHEA supplementation might be beneficial.

The mechanism of action of DHEA remains unknown. Animal studies suggest that DHEA and DHEAS have excitatory effects on the central nervous system, which may account for their influence on mood and sense of well-being. A 6-week clinical trial randomized 52 persons with major or minor depression to monotherapy with DHEA or placebo and found DHEA to be superior as measured by multiple well-validated depression scales.

Low DHEA levels in men and women with systemic lupus erythematosus (SLE) and reduction in interleukin-10 levels after supplementation compared with placebo suggest that DHEA may play a causative role. A 2007 systematic review of seven clinical trials of DHEA in SLE patients concluded that it had modest but clinically significant impact on health-related quality of life measures in the short term. Several studies suggest that DHEA supplementation

Table 41-3. Overview of selected dietary supplements.

	Leading Indications	Dosage	Level of Evidence[1]	Safety[2]	Interactions; Side Effects	Comments
Melatonin	1. Insomnia 2. Jet lag	0.1-5 mg	1. B 2. B	I	None	
Dehydroepi-androsterone (DHEA, DHEAS)	1. Depression, dysthymia 2. Lupus 3. Adrenal insufficiency	50 mg once daily	1. C 2. B 3. C	IV (with long-term use)	None reported; androgenic effects	Theoretical concerns that long-term use may result in hormone-dependent malignancies
Omega-3 fatty acids (fish oil)	1. High triglycerides 2. Coronary heart disease 3. Inflammatory conditions	Fish twice weekly for general health (300-500 EPA plus DHA) 1 g/d for heart disease	1. A 2. B 3. C	I I I	Theoretical risk of bleeding at high doses	
Glucosamine sulfate and chondroitin	Osteoarthritis (knee)	Glucosamine 500 mg three times daily; chondroitin 400 mg three times daily	B	I	None reported; rare reports of constipation, diarrhea, drowsiness	Insulin resistance not seen in clinical trials
Coenzyme Q10 (ubiquinone, ubidecarenone, Co-Q10)	Congestive heart failure, cardiac arrest, angina, acute myocardial infarction, migraine prophylaxis	50 mg once daily–150 mg three times daily; goal is to achieve serum level of 2.1 mcg/mL	C	I	Patients taking statins noted to have lower serum levels of Co-Q10	Fat-soluble, so absorption improved when taken with meals

[1]Level of evidence: A, high quality: consistent evidence from randomized trials or overwhelming evidence from other sources; B, moderate quality: evidence from randomized trials with important limitations or very strong evidence of some other form; C, low quality: evidence from observational studies or randomized trials with serious methodologic flaws.
[2]Safety: I, generally safe; II, relatively safe; III, insufficient evidence; IV, may be harmful; V, clear evidence of harm.
DHA, docosahexaenoic acid; EPA, eicosapentaenoic acid.

improves physical and psychological well being in healthy persons, but several well-designed trials have shown that DHEA supplementation has no effect on cognitive performance, body composition, physical performance, or well-being in healthy older adults.

DHEA modestly increases testosterone levels in women, but not in men, unless they have hypogonadism. Side effects include acne, deepening of the voice, and facial hair growth. No serious adverse events have been reported. The long-term effects of DHEA supplementation remain unknown. The safety issue of most concern is that DHEA—as a potent precursor of sex steroids—may increase the risk of estrogen- or androgen-dependent malignancies. Therefore, if supplementation is used, patients should be screened carefully and monitored closely. Furthermore, patients at high risk for prostate, ovarian, breast, or uterine cancer should be counseled against DHEA supplementation.

Bhagra S et al. Dehydroepiandrosterone in adrenal insufficiency and aging. Curr Opin Endocrin Diabetes Obes. 2008 Jun;15(3):239–43. [PMID: 18438171]

Crosbie D et al. Dehydroepiandrosterone for systemic lupus erythematosus. Cochrane Database Syst Rev. 2007 Oct 17;(4):CD005114. [PMID: 17943841]

Kritz-Silverstein D et al. Effects of dehydroepiandrosterone supplementation on cognitive function and quality of life: the DHEA and well-ness (DAWN) trial. J Am Geriatr Soc. 2008 Jul;56(7):1292–8. [PMID: 18482290]

Von Muhlen D et al. Effect of dehydroepiandrosterone supplementation on bone mineral density, bone markers, and body composition in older adults: the DAWN trial. Osteoporos Int. 2008 May;19(5):699–707. [PMID: 18084691]

▶ Glucosamine & Chondroitin

Glucosamine and chondroitin have been used in Europe alone and in combination to treat osteoarthritis since the 1980s. Glucosamine is an amino sugar synthesized by chondrocytes that serves as a substrate for the synthesis of cartilage. In addition to providing structural support, it may also have anti-inflammatory activity. Chondroitin is a glycosaminoglycan normally present in the cartilage matrix that helps maintain articular fluid viscosity, inhibit enzymes that break down cartilage, and stimulate cartilage repair. Glucosamine is prepared commercially from crustacean shells. Chondroitin is extracted from bovine tissues such as cow trachea.

A 2007 meta-analysis concluded that use of chondroitin by itself to treat knee or hip osteoarthritis was not warranted in routine clinical practice.

Two meta-analyses and a 2005 Cochrane Review of 20 randomized, double-blind, placebo-controlled trials involving more than 2570 patients with osteoarthritis support the use of glucosamine (or glucosamine and chondroitin) in the treatment of osteoarthritis of the knee. The Cochrane Review identified efficacy only for trials using a once daily proprietary formulation manufactured by Rotta Pharmaceuticals. In the longest trial using the Rotta formulation, glucosamine not only reduced the symptoms of osteoarthritis of the knee but also slowed the progression of the disease. Reginster and coworkers randomized 212 patients to receive 1500 mg/d of glucosamine or placebo. After 3 years, patients taking glucosamine reported a 24% reduction in symptoms versus a 10% increase in the placebo group. Radiographs revealed that the treatment patients experienced a loss of only 0.06 mm joint space versus 0.31 mm in the placebo group after 3 years. A 2006 randomized controlled trial that examined the efficacy of a non-Rotta glucosamine preparation, however, came to a different conclusion. The Glucosamine/chondroitin Arthritis Intervention Trial (GAIT) was a multicenter randomized double-blind placebo-controlled clinical trial in which 1583 persons were randomized to glucosamine hydrochloride, chondroitin sulfate, glucosamine hydrochloride plus chondroitin sulfate, celecoxib, or placebo. Investigators found no difference overall between the supplements alone or in combination and the placebo at 24 weeks. In a predefined subgroup of patients with moderate to severe pain, however, combined therapy with glucosamine and chondroitin did provide greater pain relief than placebo. When joint-space narrowing was evaluated in a subset of patients who continued in the study for a total of 2 years, glucosamine and chondroitin, alone or in combination, were no better than placebo in slowing the loss of knee cartilage. The generalizability of these results may be limited by the fact that glucosamine hydrochloride was used and patients in the placebo group had less cartilage loss than predicted. In contrast, the 2007 European GUIDE Trial (Glucosamine Unum in Die Efficacy Trial) studied the once daily proprietary formulation of crystalline glucosamine sulfate and found that after 6 months it was more effective than placebo in relieving the symptoms of knee osteoarthritis.

Fewer clinical data are available for patients with osteoarthritis of other joints. In a well-designed 2008 study, 222 patients with mild to moderate osteoarthritis of the hip were randomized to 1500 mg/d of glucosamine sulfate or placebo. Glucosamine had no clinically significant effect on pain, function, or joint space narrowing after 2 years.

Oral glucosamine is generally well tolerated and does not elevate serum glucose levels in humans. No significant drug-herb interactions have been reported, except a possible increase in INR in patients taking glucosamine and warfarin together. In contrast to NSAIDs, glucosamine may take weeks to months before improvement in symptoms is noticed. In summary, clinical trial literature suggests that glucosamine with or without chondroitin is well tolerated and safe with fewer side effects than NSAIDs. However, the efficacy of formulations other than a proprietary European product in the treatment of osteoarthritis remains in question.

Albert SG et al. The effect of glucosamine on serum HDL cholesterol and apolipoprotein A1 levels in people with diabetes. Diabetes Care. 2007 Nov;30(11):2800–3. [PMID: 17682119]

Clegg DO et al. Glucosamine, chondroitin sulfate, and the two in combination for painful knee osteoarthritis. N Engl J Med. 2006 Feb 23;354(8):795–808. [PMID: 16495392]

Herrero-Beaumont G et al. Glucosamine sulfate in the treatment of knee osteoarthritis symptoms: A randomized, double-blind, placebo-controlled study using acetaminophen as a side comparator. Arthritis Rheum. 2007 Feb;56(2):555–67. [PMID: 17265490]

Monfort J et al. Chondroitin sulfate for symptomatic osteoarthritis: critical appraisal of meta-analyses. Curr Med Res Opin. 2008 May;24(5):1303–8. [PMID: 18416884]

Reichenbach S et al. Meta-analysis: chondroitin for osteoarthritis of the knee or hip. Ann Intern Med. 2007 Apr 17;146(8):580–90. [PMID: 17438317]

Rozendaal RM et al. Effect of glucosamine sulfate on hip osteoarthritis. A randomized trial. Ann Intern Med. 2008 Feb 19;148(4):268–277. [PMID: 18283204]

Sawitzke AD et al. The effect of glucosamine and/or chondroitin sulfate on the progression of knee osteoarthritis: a report from the glucosamine/chondroitin arthritis intervention trial. Arthritis Rheum. 2008 Sep;58(10):3183–91. [PMID: 18821708]

Coenzyme Q_{10}

Coenzyme Q_{10} (also known as ubiquinone-10) is a fat-soluble provitamin that resides in the lipid layer of the mitochondria. It plays a crucial role in electron and proton transfer during oxidative phosphorylation and production of adenosine triphosphate (ATP), so it is necessary for the basic functioning of all cells. It also has antioxidant, free radical scavenging, and membrane stabilizing activities. Coenzyme Q_{10} levels decrease with age. Deficiencies have been observed among patients with certain chronic medical conditions, including cardiovascular disease (hypertension, acute coronary syndromes, congestive heart failure), renal failure, male infertility, periodontal disease, cancer, HIV/AIDS, muscular dystrophies, Parkinson disease, and Alzheimer disease. Certain prescription medications may also lower coenzyme Q_{10} levels, including HMG-CoA reductase inhibitors, diabetes medications, β-blockers, diuretics, and antidepressants. Serum levels of coenzyme Q_{10} are increased by taking supplements, but there are conflicting data about whether this results in clinical benefit.

In parts of Russia, Europe, and Japan, coenzyme Q_{10} is part of standard therapy for congestive heart failure, although it is not recommended for treatment of congestive heart failure by the American College of Cardiology or the American Heart Association. Other studies have evaluated coenzyme Q_{10} for acute myocardial infarction, angina, diabetes mellitus, hypertension, migraine prophylaxis, muscular dystrophy, Parkinson disease and periodontal disease with mixed results. A 2006 Cochrane systematic review of treatments for mitochondrial disorders describe two trials of coenzyme Q_{10}, one reporting subjective improvement and significant increase in a scale of muscle strength but the other showing no benefit. Although other medical conditions are also associated with low levels of coenzyme Q_{10}, additional randomized controlled clinical trials are needed before supplementation with coenzyme Q_{10} can be routinely recommended to improve outcomes for any particular condition.

Because coenzyme Q_{10} is lipophilic, it is often formulated with vegetable oil or vitamin E to enhance its absorption. Its bioavailability is also enhanced when it is taken with meals, especially fat-rich foods. No serious adverse events have been noted with coenzyme Q_{10} use, and it is generally well tolerated. Insomnia, elevated liver enzymes, rash, and abdominal complaints are among the mild adverse reactions reported in clinical trials. No significant drug-herb interactions have been reported, but coenzyme Q_{10} is chemically similar to vitamin K and so theoretically may reduce the effectiveness of warfarin.

Chinnery P et al. Treatment for mitochondrial disorders. Cochrane Database Syst Rev. 2006 Jan 25;(1):CD004426. [PMID: 16437486]

Galpern WR et al. Coenzyme Q treatment of neurodegenerative diseases of aging. Mitochondrion. 2007 Jun;7 Suppl:S146–53. [PMID: 17485247]

Pepe S et al. Coenzyme Q10 in cardiovascular disease. Mitochondrion. 2007 Jun;7(Suppl):S154–67. [PMID: 17485243]

Rosenfeldt FL et al. Coenzyme Q10 in the treatment of hypertension: a meta-analysis of the clinical trials. J Hum Hypertens. 2007 Apr;21(4):297–306. [PMID: 17287847]

Schaars CF et al. Effects of ubiquinone (coenzyme Q10) on myopathy in statin users. Curr Opin Lipidol. 2008 Dec;19(6):553–7. [PMID: 18957876]

Omega-3 Fatty Acids

Interest in omega-3 fatty acids began 30 years ago, when it was discovered that the Inuit population of Greenland had low rates of cardiovascular disease, despite consuming a high protein and high fat diet (mostly in form of fish). Evidence from multiple large-scale observational studies and randomized controlled trials indicates that intake of fish or fish oil supplements (or both) containing the omega-3 fatty acids eicosapentaenoic acid (EPA) and docosahexaenoic acid (DHA) is associated with many health benefits. A recent review concluded that modest consumption of fish (1–2 servings per week), especially species higher in the omega-3 fatty acids EPA and DHA, reduces the risk of coronary death by 36% and total mortality by 17%. Multiple mechanisms have been proposed for the beneficial effects of omega-3 fatty acids for both primary and secondary prevention of cardiac disease. These include reductions in triglyceride levels, inflammation, blood pressure (2–5 mm Hg), blood clotting, arrhythmias, atherosclerotic plaque formation, and improvements in arterial and endothelial function. The reduction in triglyceride levels appear to be dose-dependent, with effects at doses as low as 2 g/d. Higher doses have greater effects, and 4 g/d can lower triglyceride levels by 25–40%.

Several well-conducted, randomized controlled trials report that in individuals with a history of heart attack, regular consumption of oily or fish oil/omega-3 supplements reduces the risk of nonfatal heart attack, fatal heart attack, sudden death, and all-cause mortality. Benefits have been reported beginning after 3 months of use, and for as long as 3.5 years of follow-up. Recent data suggest that omega-3 fatty acids may be more effective than statins in treating congestive heart failure. Although fish oils have been studied primarily in patients at risk for cardiovascular disease as well as those with established cardiovascular disease, they are also being investigated in treatment of other conditions such as diabetes, dementia, depression, obesity, inflammatory bowel disease, and attention deficit/hyperactivity disorder.

Animal sources of omega-3 fatty acids (EPA and DHA) include fish, especially cold-water fatty fish such as salmon, mackerel, halibut, anchovies, and sardines. A proprietary plant-based source of DHA is manufactured from algae. Vegetable sources of the omega-3 fatty acid alpha-linolenic acid (ALA) include English walnuts; flaxseeds; tofu/soy and some vegetable oils, such as canola, soy, flaxseed, and olive oil. Dietary intake of omega-3 fatty acids has declined by 80% over the past century, while intake of omega-6 fatty acids has greatly increased. Omega-6 fatty acids come from the common use of other vegetable oils (corn, safflower, and sunflower oils) containing linoleic acid; these compete with omega-3 fatty acids to be converted to active pro-inflammatory metabolites in the body.

In 2003, the American Heart Association recommended that healthy people eat fish at least twice a week as well as consume plant-derived sources of omega-3 fatty acids, such as tofu/soybeans, walnuts, flaxseed oil, and canola oil. People with known coronary heart disease should take in approximately 1 g/d of EPA and DHA (combined). The FDA regards intake of up to 3 g/d of omega-3 fatty acids from fish as safe. Fish oil supplements are widely available over the counter and should be dosed based on their content of EPA and DHA. Omega-3 fatty acid 1 g prescription capsules, containing 465 mg of EFA and 375 mg of DHA, are also FDA-approved for the treatment of hypertriglyceridemia. In a 2007 trial, addition of 4 g/d of prescription omega-3 acids to 40 mg/d simvastatin improved lipid parameters to a greater extent than simvastatin alone.

The most common side effects of fish oil supplementation are gastrointestinal upset, burping, fishy taste, loose stools, and nausea. High doses may also have harmful effects, such as an increased risk of bleeding, so the FDA recommends no more than 3 g of EPA plus DHA per day and no more than 2 g from the diet. The potential for harm from mercury, dioxins, and polychlorinated biphenyls (PCBs) present in some fish was addressed in a recent review which concluded that, in general, the benefits of fish intake exceed the potential risks.

Davidson MH et al. Efficacy and tolerability of adding prescription omega-3 fatty acids 4 g/day to simvistatin 40 mg/day in hypertriglyceridemic patients: an 8-week, randomized, double-blind, placebo-controlled study. Clin Ther. 2007 Jul;29(7):1354–67. [PMID: 17825687]

GISSI-HF Investigators. Effect of n-3-polyunsaturated fatty acids in patients with chronic heart failure (the GISSI-HF trial): a randomized, double-blind, placebo-controlled trial. Lancet. 2008 Oct;372(9645):1223–30. [PMID: 18757090]

Lee JH et al. Omega-3 fatty acids for cardioprotection. Mayo Clin Proc. 2008 Mar;83(3):324–32. [PMID: 18316000]

León H et al. Effect of fish oil on arrhythmias and mortality: systematic review. BMJ. 2008 Dec;337:a2931. [PMID: 19106137]

Mozaffarian D et al. Fish intake, contaminants, and human health. Evaluating the risks and benefits. JAMA. 2006 Oct 18;296(15):1885–99. [PMID: 17047219]

Saremi A et al. The utility of omega-3 fatty acids in cardiovascular disease. Am J Ther. 2009 May 19 [Epub ahead of print]. [PMID: 19092647]

▶ Melatonin

Melatonin (N-acetyl-5-methoxytryptamine) is a hormone synthesized by the pineal gland from the amino acid tryptophan that is released into the circulation in response to environmental light-and-dark signals. Serum levels in humans vary 10- to 20-fold over 24 hours from a low of 2–10 pg/mL during daylight hours to a high of 100–200 pg/mL at night.

Melatonin is used to treat a variety of medical conditions, particularly insomnia and jet lag, given its role in regulating the body's circadian rhythm. Although available as an over-the-counter sleep aid in this country, it is available only by prescription in much of the rest of the world (European Union, Australia, and New Zealand).

A 2005 meta-analysis of 17 clinical trials involving 284 subjects concluded that melatonin was effective in reducing the time it took them to fall asleep and increasing the amount of time they remained asleep. The authors concluded that exogenous melatonin was helpful in treating insomnia, particularly in older individuals and those with low nocturnal levels of melatonin. An NIH State-of-the-Science Panel Report that same year also concluded that melatonin was effective in the management of chronic insomnia in subsets of the adult population.

In contrast, a 2006 meta-analysis, which included patients of all age-groups, failed to document clinically meaningful effects of exogenous melatonin on sleep quality, time to fall asleep, and hours slept per night. Nightly melatonin (2.5 mg) combined with daytime bright light was shown to modestly improve cognitive and noncognitive function in 189 elderly Dutch residents of 12 group care facilities. Melatonin was noted to have adverse effects on mood when used alone in these elderly subjects, but these effects were not observed when melatonin was used in combination with bright light.

Melatonin is believed to have antioxidant, antineoplastic, and immunomodulatory activity, but there are insufficient clinical trial data to support its use for conditions other than insomnia and jet lag. Of interest, melatonin receptors have recently been demonstrated on pancreatic islet cells, which may help explain a link between disturbed sleep and glucose intolerance.

Three melatonin receptors have been identified in mammals: MT1, MT2, and MT3. MT1 and MT2 appear to regulate the circadian sleep-wake cycle. Ramelteon, a selective MT1 and MT2 receptor agonist, was approved by the FDA in 2005 to treat insomnia.

Considerable person-to-person variability in serum levels after taking the same dose of melatonin has been reported. Physiologic doses (0.1–0.3 mg) have been shown to decrease time until sleep, increase duration of sleep, and decrease daytime fatigue. Commonly available over-the-counter doses (1–10 mg) have been reported to raise plasma concentrations to levels 3–60 times greater than normal peak levels.

Melatonin is generally considered safe at recommended oral doses of 5 mg or less for up to 2 years. No hangover effect has been noted, even after 1 month of taking high doses.

Side effects of fatigue, sleepiness, headache, dizziness, and irritability are no more commonly reported than with placebo. Caution is advised in patients taking immunosuppressants or those with vascular disorders or infertility problems.

Lack LC et al. Chronobiology of sleep in humans. Cell Mol Life Sci. 2007 May;64(10):1205–15. [PMID: 17364140]

Lemoine P et al. Prolonged-release melatonin improves sleep quality and morning alertness in insomnia patients aged 55 years and older and has no withdrawal effects. J Sleep Res. 2007 Dec;16(4):372–80. [PMID: 18036082]

Riemersa-van der Lek RF et al. Effect of bright light and melatonin on cognitive and non-cognitive function in elderly residents of group care facilities: a randomized controlled trial. JAMA. 2008 Jun 11;299(22):2642–55. [PMID: 18544724]

Sateia MJ et al. Efficacy and clinical safety of ramelteon: an evidence-based review. Sleep Med Rev. 2008 Aug;12(4):319–32. [PMID: 18603221]

▼ ACUPUNCTURE

In acupuncture, anatomic points on the surface of the body are stimulated by a variety of techniques, often with needles, to treat illness and promote health. Many styles exist and are practiced as part of the thousands of years old medical traditions of China, Japan, Korea and other countries. Practitioners trained in Oriental medicine believe that a vital energy called chi (pronounced "chee") circulates in the body through 12 virtual pathways called meridians. Disease occurs when the flow of chi in the body is not in balance. Each meridian is named after a particular organ or "official." In addition to describing the structure and function of the organ itself, the naming of each meridian also reflects a broader energetic function in Traditional Chinese Medicine.

▶ Mechanism of Action

The mechanism of action of acupuncture is not well understood, but physiologic effects can be measured when acupuncture points are stimulated, such as the release of endorphins and enkephalins. Functional MRI studies reveal that different areas of the brain are activated and deactivated during needling.

Stux G, Berman B, Pomeranz B (editors). *Basics of Acupuncture.* 5th ed. Springer, 2003.

▶ Training, Licensure, & Regulation

Typical acupuncture training for nonphysicians in the United States involves completion of a 4-year (2500 hours) master's degree training program accredited by the Accreditation Commission for Acupuncture and Oriental Medicine (ACAOM). In order to become a licensed acupuncturist (LAc), a national and, frequently, state board examination must be passed. Although many states do not require physicians to obtain additional training, many encourage a minimum of 200 hours of training in an accredited program. There are currently approximately 18,000 licensed acupuncture practitioners and more than 3000 physician acupuncturists in the United States. In 22 of the 43 states that license, register, or certify acupuncturists, these practitioners are permitted to work independently.

▶ Clinical Practice

In the United States and Europe, Oriental medicine-trained practitioners conduct a comprehensive multisystem history, observation, and physical examination during the initial consultation. Examination consists of palpation of the abdomen and selected acupuncture points; examination of the tongue to assess color, shape, and coating; and palpation of the pulse along the wrist at three locations on both arms to assess its quality, rhythm, and strength. In classic acupuncture, each patient is viewed as having a unique constellation of symptoms and signs. What this means is that ten patients presenting with migraine headaches might receive ten unique Chinese medical diagnoses and ten different treatments. Because acupuncture is just one part of a comprehensive system, patients are also often prescribed Chinese herbal therapy, diet, and exercise. Western-style practitioners will conduct a conventional examination and include variable components of the Oriental medicine approach depending on the individual's depth of training. Treatment typically utilizes a fixed combination of acupuncture points for a given medical diagnosis, such that a cohort of migraine sufferers will be treated in a similar way.

Treatment typically involves inserting four to fifteen needles at selected acupuncture points for 10–30 minutes—though certain schools leave the needles in place for only a few seconds to minutes. Virtually all acupuncture is performed with thin, solid, stainless steel, sterile disposable needles that are stimulated manually or with electricity or heat. Follow-up consultations last from 20 minutes to 45 minutes. A course of treatment usually consists of weekly or biweekly visits for 4–10 weeks, followed by less frequent visits as the condition improves.

▶ Adverse Events

The current practice of acupuncture in the United States and Europe is associated with a very low incidence of adverse events (as low as 1 in 10,000 to 1 in 100,000 needle insertions). Reactions such as presyncope, syncope, and drowsiness can be easily prevented by having the patient lie flat on the table, monitoring them during their initial visit, and permitting them to remain in the office until a normal state of awareness is achieved. Serious complications in the literature over the past 30 years are very rare but include spread of infection and pneumothorax from needling patients with emphysema.

▶ Clinical Uses of Acupuncture

More than 1000 English-language reviews of the clinical use of acupuncture in humans have been published in the last 20 years, many pointing out the challenge of designing high-quality trials with effective placebo controls. Several types of placebos have been tried: needling at nonacupuncture points, using a retractable sham needle that does not penetrate the skin, and needling at true acupuncture points that are inappropriate for the condition being treated. Data analysis is complicated by the fact that sham treatments can have physiologic effects in and of themselves. Acupuncture has been shown to be most effective in treating pain and nausea. A 2009 systematic review, however, concluded that "whether needling at acupuncture points or at any site reduces pain independent of the psychological impact of the ritual is unclear." Recent reviews have also concluded that acupuncture is not effective (or that data were inconclusive for) treating hypertension, hot flashes, epilepsy, insomnia, allergic rhinitis, Parkinson disease, restless leg syndrome, and dyspnea. What follows is a selection of some conditions for which patients commonly seek acupuncture care.

Ernst E. Acupuncture: what does the most reliable evidence tell us? J Pain Symptom Manage. 2009 Apr;37(4):709–14. [PMID: 18789644]

Madsen MV et al. Acupuncture treatment for pain: systematic review of randomized clinical trials with acupuncture, placebo acupuncture and no acupuncture groups. BMJ. 2009 Jan 27;338:a3115. [PMID: 19174438]

Park J et al. The status and future of acupuncture clinical research. J Altern Complement Med. 2008 Sep;14(7):871–81. [PMID: 18803496]

A. Low Back Pain

More than 50 clinical trials of acupuncture for the treatment of low back pain were reviewed by the American Pain Society and American College of Physicians as part of clinical practice guidelines that were published in 2007. They concluded that there was a fair level of evidence supporting a moderate benefit of acupuncture in treating subacute (4–8 weeks) or chronic low back pain. In most studies, acupuncture has not been shown to be more effective when compared with other active treatments, but provides additional benefit when added to conventional therapies. A 2008 systematic review of 23 randomized controlled trials involving more than 6000 patients concluded that acupuncture versus no treatment and as an adjunct to conventional care should be advocated in the European Guidelines for the treatment of chronic low back pain.

Ammendolia C et al. Evidence-informed management of chronic low back pain with needle acupuncture. Spine J. 2008 Jan–Feb;8(1):160–72. [PMID: 18164464]

Chou R et al. Nonpharmacologic therapies for acute and chronic low back pain: a review of the evidence for an American Pain Society/American College of Physicians clinical practice guideline. Ann Intern Med. 2007 Oct 2;147(7):492–504. [PMID: 17909210]

Furlan AD et al. Acupuncture and dry-needling for low back pain: an updated systematic review within the framework of the Cochrane Collaboration. Spine. 2005 Apr 15;30(8):944–63. [PMID: 15834340]

Yuan J et al. Effectiveness of acupuncture for low back pain: a systematic review. Spine. 2008 Nov 1;33(23):E887–900. [PMID: 18978583]

B. Osteoarthritis

A 2006 systematic review and meta-analysis of 18 randomized controlled trials concluded that "sham-controlled trials suggest specific efficacy of acupuncture for pain control in patients with osteoarthritis of peripheral joints. The favorable safety profile makes acupuncture a worthy option of consideration, particularly for knee osteoarthritis." Acupuncture plus routine care was associated with marked clinical improvement in a German trial in which 632 patients with osteoarthritis of the hip or knee were randomized to up to 15 sessions of physician-delivered acupuncture or wait-list control for 3 months. The treatment protocol was individualized for each patient at the discretion of the physician, more closely reflecting how acupuncture is practiced clinically. One-third (34.5%) of the acupuncture-treated group had a good response after 3 months, compared with 6.5% of the wait-list control group. The improvement in pain and quality of life was maintained at 6-month follow-up.

A 2007 meta-analysis of nine clinical trials revealed clinically relevant short-term (but not long-term) improvements in pain and function compared with those in wait-list control groups. Authors concluded that some of acupuncture's clinically relevant benefits might be due to placebo and expectation effects.

A 2007 cost effectiveness trial involving almost 500 German patients who were randomized to routine care or routine care plus acupuncture concluded that acupuncture was a cost-effective treatment for osteoarthritis.

Kwon YD et al. Acupuncture for peripheral joint osteoarthritis: a systematic review and meta-analysis. Rheumatology (Oxford). 2006 Nov;45(11):1331–7. [PMID: 16936326]

Manheimer E et al. Meta-analysis: acupuncture for osteoarthritis of the knee. Ann Intern Med. 2007 Jun 19;146(12):868–77. [PMID: 17577006]

Reinhold T et al. Quality of life and cost-effectiveness of acupuncture treatment in patients with osteoarthritis pain. Eur J Health Econ. 2008 Aug;9(3):209–19. [PMID: 17638034]

Scharf HP et al. Acupuncture and knee osteoarthritis: a three-armed randomized trial. Ann Intern Med. 2006 Jul 4;145(1):12–20. [PMID: 16818924]

Witt CM et al. Acupuncture in patients with osteoarthritis of the knee or hip. A randomized controlled trial with an additional nonrandomized arm. Arthritis Rheum. 2006 Nov;54(11):3485–93. [PMID: 17075849]

C. Postoperative Pain

Acupuncture was helpful in reducing pain intensity, opioid consumption, and opioid-associated side effects in a 2008 systematic review of 15 randomized clinical trials comparing acupuncture with sham control for acute postoperative pain. In contrast, a systematic review of 9 trials of auricular acupuncture concluded that the evidence was "promising but not compelling" in its reducing postoperative pain.

Sun Y et al. Acupuncture and related techniques for postoperative pain: a systematic review of randomized controlled trials. Br J Anesth. 2008 Aug;101(2):151–60. [PMID: 18522936]

Usichenko TI et al. Auricular acupuncture for postoperative pain control: a systematic review of randomized clinical trials. Anaesthesia. 2008 Dec;63(12):1343–8. [PMID: 19032304]

D. Headache

Mixed results were reported early on about acupuncture's efficacy in the treatment of headaches, but more recent reviews conclude that it is a safe and effective option for treating both tension and migraine headaches. A 2008 study also concluded that acupuncture was cost effective when compared with routine care in patients with primary headache.

Davis MA et al. Acupuncture for tension-type headache: a meta-analysis of randomized controlled trials. J Pain. 2008 Aug;9(8):667–77. [PMID: 18499526]

Linde K et al. Acupuncture for migraine prophylaxis. Cochrane Database Syst Rev. 2009 Jan 21;(1):CD001218. [PMID: 19160193]

Linde K et al. Acupuncture for tension-type headache. Cochrane Database Syst Rev. 2009 Jan 21;(1):CD007587. [PMID: 19160338]

Sun Y et al. Acupuncture for the management of chronic headache: a systematic review. Anesth Analg. 2008 Dec;107(6):2038–47. [PMID: 19020156]

Witt CM et al. Cost-effectiveness of acupuncture treatment in patients with headache. Cephalalgia. 2008 Apr;28(4):334–45. [PMID: 18315686]

E. Nausea & Vomiting

Based on multiple randomized controlled trials involving more than 6000 patients, there is strong evidence that acupuncture is effective in the treatment of pregnancy-induced, chemotherapy-induced, and postoperative nausea and vomiting. A 2006 systematic review identified 43 trials using a particular acupuncture point (P6) for treatment of nausea and vomiting. P6 is located on the anterior surface of the forearm, several inches proximal to the wrist between the tendons of palmaris longus and flexor carpi radialis. Results across trials were the most consistent for postoperative nausea and vomiting. Compared with sham procedures, P6 stimulation was more effective than comparison in preventing nausea (RR 0.72, 95% CI 0.59–0.89) and vomiting (RR 0.71, 95% CI 0.56–0.91). For example, in the 9 trials that compared P6 stimulation to antiemetic medication, P6 was superior in preventing nausea and equivalent in preventing vomiting. Electroacupuncture was reported to be effective for first-day vomiting after chemotherapy. Trials using noninvasive electrostimulation (primarily with wristwatch type devices) showed no benefit above and beyond control treatment with antiemetic medications.

Arnberger M et al. Monitoring of neuromuscular blockade at the P6 acupuncture point reduces the incidence of postoperative nausea and vomiting. Anesthesiology. 2007 Dec;107(6):903–8. [PMID: 18043058]

Ezzo JM et al. Acupuncture point stimulation for chemotherapy-induced nausea and vomiting. Cochrane Database Syst Rev. 2006 Apr 19;(2):CD002285. [PMID: 16625560]

Streitberger K et al. Acupuncture for nausea and vomiting: an update of clinical and experimental studies. Auton Neurosci. 2006 Oct 30;129(1–2):107–17. [PMID: 16950659]

F. Nicotine, Heroin, Cocaine, & Alcohol Addiction

There is good evidence suggesting that acupuncture is not effective in maintaining abstinence from nicotine addiction. A 2006 Cochrane systematic review of 24 trials concluded "there is no consistent evidence that acupuncture or acupressure, laser therapy or electrostimulation are effective for smoking cessation."

Despite insufficient evidence to support its use, auricular acupuncture is in widespread use throughout American drug treatment facilities. Although heroin, alcohol, and cocaine addiction studies have frequently reported positive outcomes, serious methodologic flaws have been found in these studies. A 2006 Cochrane systematic review of seven studies in which 1433 patients were treated with ear acupuncture for cocaine dependence concluded that there is currently no evidence to support its use.

Bearn J et al. Auricular acupuncture as an adjunct to opiate detoxification treatment: effects on withdrawal symptoms. J Subst Abuse Treat. 2009 Apr;36(3):345–9. [PMID: 19004596]

Gates S et al. Auricular acupuncture for cocaine dependence. Cochrane Database Syst Rev. 2006 Jan 25;(1):CD005192. [PMID: 16437523]

Jordon JB. Acupuncture treatment for opiate addiction: a systematic review. J Subst Abuse Treat. 2006 Jun;30(4):309–14. [PMID: 16716845]

White AR et al. Acupuncture and related interventions for smoking cessation. Cochrane Database Syst Rev. 2006 Jan 25;(1):CD000009. [PMID: 16437420]

G. Infertility

Conflicting results have been reported about the efficacy of acupuncture in improving the outcomes of women undergoing in vitro fertilization. A systematic review of seven clinical studies of acupuncture given with embryo transfer suggested that it may improve rates of pregnancy and live births. In contrast, a review of eight trials published later in 2008 concluded there were insufficient data that adjunctive acupuncture improved in vitro fertilization–related pregnancy rates.

El-Toukhy T et al. A systematic review and meta-analysis of acupuncture in in vitro fertilization. BJOG. 2008 Sep;115(10):1203–13. [PMID: 18652588]

Manheimer E et al. Effects of acupuncture on rates of pregnancy and live birth among women undergoing in vitro fertilization: systematic review and meta-analysis. BMJ. 2008 Mar 8;336(7643):545–9. [PMID: 18258932]

▼ MIND-BODY MEDICINE

▶ Definition

Mind-body medicine is commonly described as the field of medicine that uses processes of the mind to influence the health of the body. While this is a useful initial concept, it still can perpetuate the notion that mind and body are separate, and it fails to acknowledge the bidirectional relationship of mind and body (eg, exercise improves mood). It may be more accurate to think of *mind/body* as a single entity, with the health of one part necessarily influencing the health of the other. The NIH has defined mind-body medicine as "behavioral, psychological, social, and spiritual approaches to medicine not commonly used." This definition distinguishes mind-body medicine therapies from therapies that are more established or mainstream but that may have similar mechanisms of action (eg, psychotherapies, behavioral training, support groups, education). Traditionally defined mind-body therapies include biofeedback, hypnosis, meditation, guided imagery, relaxation techniques, yoga, tai chi, and chi gung.

▶ History

The relationship between mind and body and its importance to health has been recognized for thousands of years by all major healing traditions, including the ancient Greek system that gave rise to modern Western medicine. With the ascendancy in the West of the scientific method and the biomedical model of illness, however, the relationship between mind and body has often been neglected. In the 19th century, interest in hypnosis began and later Freud championed the theory of the unconscious mind, which helped establish the paradigm that processes of the mind profoundly affect health. In the early 20th century, the American physiologist Walter Cannon began exploring the physiologic effects of emotional stimuli. In the 1930s, Dr. Clark Hull began studies of hypnosis, and research into hypnosis greatly expanded in the 1950s. The first biofeedback experiments also occurred in the 1950s. Since then, there has been considerable research evaluating mind-body phenomena and therapies. It has been established, for example, that certain emotions such as anger, anxiety, and depression affect clinical outcomes (including mortality) for conditions such as cardiovascular disease, cancer, and HIV infection. The new field of psychoneuroimmunology has documented, at the physiologic level, the powerful effect of the mind on the nervous, endocrine, and immune systems, and vice versa. Studies have demonstrated that certain forms of mental training, in addition to affecting health, can affect brain function and even structure, leading to a reevaluation of previously held beliefs about neuroplasticity.

▶ Clinical Applications of Mind-Body Medicine

Mind-body medicine is popular. Over 20% of the US adult population has used one or more mind-body therapies in the past year. Data from the 2007 National Health Interview Survey show that use of most mind-body therapies has increased since 2002. The more conventional mind-body therapies already are established, supported by evidence, and widely available. For example, multimodal mind-body interventions that use some combination of cognitive behavioral therapies, support groups, education, relaxation and skills training have been proven effective for coronary artery disease, cancer, and chronic pain conditions. Mind-body therapies also work well as adjunctive treatments, for example with surgery, cancer treatment, and stress-exacerbated conditions (Table 41–4). They also offer the psychological benefit of increasing sense of control for the patient. Finally, mind-body therapies can be recommended because they have a very favorable safety profile.

Fried RG et al. Nonpharmacologic management of common skin and psychocutaneous disorders. Dermatol Ther. 2008 Jan–Feb;21(1):60–8. [PMID: 18318887]

Monti DA et al. Potential role of mind-body therapies in cancer survivorship. Cancer. 2008 Jun 1;112(11 Suppl):2607–16. [PMID: 18428193]

Sierpina V et al. Mind-body therapies for headache. Am Fam Physician. 2007 Nov 15;76(10):1518–22. [PMID: 18052018]

BIOFEEDBACK

▶ Definition

Biofeedback is a behavioral therapy method that teaches a patient to gain greater awareness and control over physiologic functions, including some not normally under conscious control. This is achieved by using technology that presents to the patient in visual or auditory form the level of activity of a physiologic parameter, such as muscle tension,

skin temperature, sweat gland activity, respiratory muscle activity, P_{CO_2}, heart rate variability, or brain wave pattern.

▶ History

Biofeedback began in the 1950s with the work of the experimental psychologist Dr. Neil Miller. He demonstrated that rats could learn to regulate autonomic functions when motivated by painful or pleasurable stimuli. The idea that autonomic function could be volitionally controlled was contrary to the scientific dogma of the time. In the 1960s, other researchers began to examine the human ability to consciously alter physiologic function.

▶ Training & Certification

Certification is obtained through the Biofeedback Certification Institute of America (BCIA) and is open to professionals from clinical health care areas including, but not limited to, psychology, nursing, and counseling. Requirements for certification are: (1) 48 hours of didactic education, (2) 20 hours of contact spent with a BCIA approved mentor, 50 patient/client sessions, and case conference presentations, and (3) successful completion of a written certification examination. There is also a continuing education requirement.

When treating a medical or psychological disorder, biofeedback practitioners are required to hold a current state license in a BCIA-approved health care field or, if without this license, work under the supervision of an appropriately credentialed health care professional. Separate, additional certificates are required for electroencephalographic (EEG) biofeedback (neurofeedback) and pelvic muscle dysfunction work.

▶ Clinical Practice

Since biofeedback is a taught, self-regulatory skill, the patient should be motivated; prepared to take an active role in their treatment; respond well to visible, quantifiable information; or have aptitude or familiarity with technology. Typical biofeedback sessions last 50 minutes, with half or more of that time in active monitoring. To begin a biofeedback session, the therapist applies sensors to the patient that monitor the physiologic parameters of interest. For example, in a case of chronic tension headache, an electromyographic (EMG) sensor may be applied to the skin of the forehead. Information from the sensor feeds back to the patient as sound or as an image on a computer screen in real time, so he or she can begin to learn to reduce tension in the forehead muscle. Multiple sessions are usually required and the patient is asked to practice the learned skills between sessions. The goal of biofeedback is to help the patient train himself to produce the desired response at other times. Some biofeedback software programs and sensors are available for use on a home computer or with portable electronic devices.

▶ Adverse Events & Contraindications

There are no reported adverse effects of biofeedback therapy. Benzodiazepines, opioids, other sedating medicines,

Table 41–4. Overview of mind-body therapies for various clinical conditions.

Condition	Mind-Body Therapy	Level of Evidence[1]	Comment
Surgery/Procedure: Pain	Hypnosis	A	Guided imagery may reduce length of hospital stay
	Guided imagery	B	
Surgery/Procedure: Anxiety	Hypnosis	B	
	Guided imagery	B	
Cancer: Pain	Hypnosis	A	Guided imagery "B" when combined with other therapies
	Guided imagery	B	
Cancer: nausea and vomiting (chemotherapy)	Guided imagery	A	Guided imagery "A" when combined with other therapies
	Hypnosis	B	
Cancer: Psychological symptoms (eg, mood, anxiety, stress)	Guided imagery	A	
	Mindfulness meditation	A	
Chronic pain (various etiologies)	Guided imagery	B	
	Mindfulness meditation	B	
	Hypnosis	B	
Fibromyalgia	Mindfulness meditation	B	
	Guided imagery	C	
Migraine headache	Biofeedback	A	EMG biofeedback or thermal biofeedback plus relaxation
	Guided imagery	C	
Tension headache (recurrent)	Biofeedback	B	
	Guided imagery	C	
Irritable bowel syndrome	Hypnosis	A	
	Guided imagery	C	
Hypertension	Biofeedback	B	Thermal or electrodermal biofeedback best, add relaxation or cognitive therapy to biofeedback
Raynaud phenomenon (primary)	Biofeedback	B	
Anxiety disorders	Mindfulness meditation	B	
Depression	Mindfulness meditation	A	MBCT or MBSR
Insomnia	Mindfulness meditation	B	Progressive muscle relaxation and combination of mind-body therapies also shown effective
	Biofeedback	C	
	Hypnosis	C	
Urinary incontinence	Biofeedback	B	Stress, urge, mixed or post-prostatectomy
Fecal incontinence	Biofeedback	B	First-line therapy
Chronic constipation (pelvic floor dyssynergia)	Biofeedback	A	First-line therapy
Asthma	Biofeedback	C	
	Hypnosis	C	
Smoking cessation	Hypnosis	C	
	Mindfulness meditation	C	

[1]Level of evidence: A, high quality: consistent evidence from randomized trials or overwhelming evidence from other sources; B, moderate quality: evidence from randomized trials with important limitations or very strong evidence of some other form; C, low quality: evidence from observational studies or randomized trials with serious methodologic flaws.
EMG, electromyographic; MBCT, mindfulness-based cognitive therapy; MBSR, mindfulness-based stress reduction.

and even caffeine can sometimes impair the efficacy of biofeedback training.

▶ Clinical Uses of Biofeedback

A. Hypertension

Studies on the blood pressure lowering effect of biofeedback have been published for over 40 years. Meta-analyses consistently show that compared with wait-list or other inactive control groups, biofeedback can significantly lower patients' systolic and diastolic blood pressures (approximately 5–8 mm Hg systolic and 3–5 mm Hg diastolic pressure). However, when biofeedback is compared with active control group (eg, sham biofeedback or nonspecific behavioral control), it is usually not statistically superior in its effect on blood pressure except when coupled with relaxation training or cognitive therapy. One exception is a randomized controlled trial that compared active biofeedback to sham biofeedback and found significant reductions in systolic and mean blood pressure at 12-week follow-up. This study used direct blood pressure biofeedback, although the literature taken as a whole favors thermal and electrodermal (galvanic skin response) biofeedback methods over EMG or direct blood pressure biofeedback methods. In general, the degree of blood pressure reduction with biofeedback strongly correlates with pretest blood pressure. Persons with higher baseline blood pressures show larger beneficial effects from biofeedback.

Because most patients in studies of nonpharmacologic treatment of hypertension have only mild hypertension, the effect of treatments like biofeedback may be more difficult to detect. Also, it is worth noting that, as is the case for all antihypertensive therapies, small reductions in blood pressure yield important clinical benefits.

Also noteworthy in recent years is research on respiratory biofeedback training, in contrast to traditional thermal or electrodermal biofeedback methods for blood pressure reduction. A particular pattern of device-assisted respiration practiced for 15 minutes daily has been shown in seven of eight small studies to lower ambulatory blood pressure. In 2002, the FDA approved a simple device (RESPeRATE) to enable respiratory training for home use.

B. Coronary Artery Disease

There have been clinical studies of the effect of biofeedback on heart rate variability. Heart rate variability is considered to be an indicator of autonomic tone and has been postulated to be the mediator of the effects of cognitive and mind-body therapies on cardiovascular conditions. Cardiac electrophysiology studies have shown that poor heart rate variability is predictive of both short-term and long-term mortality after myocardial infarction. One randomized controlled trial of 63 patients with established coronary artery disease showed that biofeedback significantly increases heart rate variability. Another randomized controlled trial showed an 86% reduction in post-myocardial infarction mortality at 2 years from a psychosocial intervention that included biofeedback training of heart rate variability. However, this study did not show a significant change in heart rate variability with the intervention unless individuals with high heart rate variability at baseline were excluded. Thus, it remains unanswered whether improved heart rate variability from biofeedback training indeed affects important cardiovascular outcomes.

C. Raynaud Phenomenon

There have been seven randomized controlled trials of the efficacy of biofeedback on Raynaud phenomenon. Two show biofeedback to be superior to active control (eg, autogenic training), and four show benefit from biofeedback but equal to active control. One large study showed thermal biofeedback to be equivalent to EMG biofeedback treatment and to treatment with sustained-release nifedipine. However, there was a nonsignificant trend showing superiority of nifedipine over thermal biofeedback.

D. Headache

Biofeedback and other behavioral techniques have been extensively studied in prevention of recurrent migraine and tension headaches, with more than 50 studies including many randomized controlled trials. Several meta-analyses concur there is a significant reduction (30–55%) in headache frequency with biofeedback and other behavioral interventions. Other outcomes with significant improvement in several studies are anxiety, depression, self-efficacy and medication usage. The American Academy of Neurology practice guidelines state that there is grade "A" evidence for the use of thermal biofeedback with relaxation or EMG biofeedback for prevention of migraine. Biofeedback compares favorably with pharmaceutical treatments in several studies. There are also studies showing enhanced efficacy from adding medications to biofeedback therapy. The American Academy of Neurology practice guidelines state that there is grade "B" evidence for behavioral therapy (eg, biofeedback and relaxation techniques) when combined with prophylactic drug therapy (eg, propranolol and amitriptyline) to achieve additional clinical improvement for migraine relief.

E. Urinary Incontinence

There are at least 20 randomized controlled trials of biofeedback for stress, urge, and mixed types of incontinence in mostly postmenopausal women. In all of these trials, biofeedback produced improvement in symptoms; however, when compared with other treatment methods (eg, assisted or unassisted pelvic floor muscle training, use of vaginal cones), biofeedback was superior in less than half of these trials. It could be argued, however, that methods such as assisted pelvic floor muscle training or the use of vaginal cones are themselves forms of biofeedback. Therefore, while it is clear that training of the pelvic muscles is beneficial for reducing incontinence, it is less clear whether biofeedback-enhanced pelvic floor muscle training offers a significant advantage. The same conclusion can be drawn from the 11 randomized controlled trials of urinary incontinence in post-prostatectomy men, which show a benefit for pelvic floor muscle training whether assisted by biofeedback or not. Also noteworthy is a recent secondary analysis of an ongoing study of biofeedback for urinary incontinence, which importantly showed not only improvement in continence but also significant reduction of depression.

F. Fecal Incontinence

There are more than 40 experimental trials of biofeedback for fecal incontinence in adults and all but 2 of these report moderate to large benefit. However, the methodologic quality of many of these publications is low. A 2006 Cochrane review of biofeedback and sphincter exercises for fecal incontinence included 11 randomized controlled trials and concluded that the efficacy of biofeedback for fecal incontinence remained in question. Nonetheless, many authors and clinicians in this field consider it a first-line therapy. A report of 513 consecutive patients seen at a tertiary colorectal referral clinic showed that more than

70% of patients received benefit. American College of Gastroenterology Practice Guidelines consider biofeedback safe and effective and recommend it for treatment of fecal incontinence.

G. Chronic Constipation

About 30–50% of cases of chronic constipation are due to pelvic floor dyssynergia, a failure of the pelvic floor and anal muscles to relax during straining. Pelvic floor dyssynergia may be less amenable to laxative and fiber treatment but appears to be successfully treated with biofeedback. This indication has been studied in adults in at least nine randomized controlled trials. In three trials, biofeedback was superior to sham biofeedback, polyethylene glycol, diazepam, and placebo. Because of its success rate (70–80%) and safety, biofeedback is widely recommended as first-line therapy alone or in combination with other measures.

H. Stroke Rehabilitation

Biofeedback for stroke rehabilitation has been difficult to evaluate for several reasons, including nonstandardized outcome measures and variability in the time post-stroke at which biofeedback is offered. There are over 20 randomized controlled trials, all with small sample sizes. Some individual studies show benefit in motor strength, gait quality, and functional recovery with EMG biofeedback. A Cochrane review concludes EMG biofeedback cannot be recommended as a routine treatment but due to its safety and possible efficacy its use can be reasonably considered.

I. Psychiatric Disorders

EEG biofeedback, also known as neurofeedback, was first used to reduce seizure frequency in epilepsy in the 1970s. Since then, it has been applied to attention-deficit hyperactivity disorders, anxiety disorders, affective disorders, substance use disorders, other psychiatric conditions, and traumatic brain injury. However, there are still few methodologically rigorous trials investigating this form of biofeedback. A recent pilot study suggests that a portable heart-rate variability biofeedback device produces additive benefit when combined with cognitive behavioral therapy (CBT) for patients with anxiety disorders.

J. Asthma

Evidence for the efficacy of biofeedback in asthma is tentatively favorable. Of the 11 small, randomized controlled trials, 5 show clear and significant benefit for clinical (eg, frequency of attacks, medication use) and physiologic (eg, peak expiratory flow, respiratory resistance) parameters, 3 fail to show benefit, and 3 have mixed results. EMG, PCO_2, heart rate variability, and trachea noise methods have all been used.

Chatoor DR et al. Faecal incontinence. Br J Surg. 2007 Feb;94(2):134–44. [PMID: 17221850]

Koh CE et al. Systematic review of randomized controlled trials of the effectiveness of biofeedback for pelvic floor dysfunction. Br J Surg. 2008 Sep;95(9):1079–87. [PMID: 18655219]

Nestoriuc Y et al. Efficacy of biofeedback for migraine: A meta-analysis. Pain. 2007 Mar;128(1–2):111–27. [PMID: 17084028]

Tadic SD et al. Effect of biofeedback on psychological burden and symptoms in older women with urge urinary incontinence. J Am Geriatr Soc. 2007 Dec;55(12):2010–5. [PMID: 18028340]

Tsai PS et al. Blood pressure biofeedback exerts intermediate-term effects on blood pressure and pressure reactivity in individuals with mild hypertension: a randomized controlled study. J Altern Complement Med. 2007 Jun;13(5):547–54. [PMID: 17604559]

Woodford H et al. EMG biofeedback for the recovery of motor function after stroke. Cochrane Database Syst Rev. 2007 Apr;18(2):CD004585. [PMID: 17443550]

HYPNOSIS

▶ Definition

Hypnosis is a procedure that induces an altered state of consciousness in which the patient's mind is more accepting of suggestion. It is believed that during hypnosis the usual evaluative, critical function of the conscious mind is bypassed and more direct communication with the subconscious mind occurs.

▶ History

Hypnotic phenomena, including trancelike states for medical purposes, have been practiced around the world throughout human history. It was the Scottish surgeon, James Braid, in 1843, however, who coined the term "hypnosis" and laid the foundation for the use of hypnosis in modern medicine. Braid believed the effects of hypnosis were mediated by the mind of the patient. Important early research was conducted in the 1930s by Dr. Clark Hull and his student, Dr. Milton Erickson. In the mid-1950s, the British and American Medical Associations suggested that hypnosis be incorporated into the medical curriculum. In 1960, the American Psychological Association endorsed hypnosis as a branch of psychology. In 1996, an NIH Technology Assessment Panel judged hypnosis to be an effective intervention for alleviating pain.

▶ Mechanism of Action

The mechanism of action of hypnosis has not been fully elucidated, but its effects are seen at multiple levels, including somatosensory cortex, anterior cingulate cortex (modulation of pain affect via limbic system), spinal cord and autonomic nervous system (eg, hypnosis can reduce colonic motility in irritable bowel syndrome). Additional recent evidence of mechanism includes upregulation of immune-related gene expression (eg, effects on tumor necrosis factor [TNF]-α) and reduction of mucosal inflammatory response in ulcerative colitis. Hypnotic trance is a state distinct from sleep or relaxation, and hypnotic analgesia is distinct from placebo analgesia.

▶ Training & Certification

Certification for hypnosis, granted through the American Society of Clinical Hypnosis, has the following requirements: (1) health professional degree, (2) 40 hours of workshop training, (3) 20 hours of supervised clinical training, and (4) 2 years of independent practice using clinical hypnosis.

Other certification programs exist. Patients and clinicians should inquire about the training and certification of any practitioner of hypnosis because there are no restrictions limiting its use to licensed health care practitioners.

► Clinical Practice

The procedure of hypnosis can be divided into three phases: induction (or pre-suggestion), suggestion, and post-suggestion. The induction of a trance is accomplished in a variety of ways with the intention of developing relaxation and focused attention. Once the trance is induced, therapeutic suggestions are offered. In the post-suggestion phase, the patient returns to their usual state of consciousness and the suggestions may be discussed and reinforced. Self-hypnosis may be taught to further reinforce the therapeutic suggestions between sessions.

Although most people can respond to hypnosis, there is great variability in hypnotic susceptibility ("suggestibility") in the population. This can be measured with standard instruments such as the Harvard Group Scale of Hypnotic Susceptibility and the Stanford Hypnotic Susceptibility Scale. Studies have shown a positive correlation between hypnotic susceptibility and its efficacy.

The ideal candidate for hypnosis is a patient with high suggestibility and motivation, with a condition for which hypnosis has proven benefit. Course of treatment can vary from a single session to several. Sessions are usually 45–60 minutes, with the first session typically lasting 90–120 minutes. It is helpful when referring patients to dispel common myths about hypnosis. For example, it is not true that one loses consciousness in trance nor that one cedes control to the hypnotist. Trance state may best be described as a voluntary state of mind not unlike the one experienced when absorbed in reading a book or when daydreaming. It may be useful to explain to patients that the purpose of referral to hypnosis is to learn skills to use the mind-body connection.

► Adverse Events

Adverse events from hypnosis have not been well studied. As with any psychological therapy, distressing emotions or thoughts may occur. These can manifest as somatic symptoms, such as dizziness, headache, or nausea. Occasionally, uncovering repressed psychic content can evoke strong emotional response, known as abreaction. A minority of hypnosis practitioners believe abreaction is therapeutic. Also, as with other mind-body medicine modalities that include deliberate relaxation, paradoxical anxiety reactions can rarely occur.

► Contraindications

There is no consensus on contraindications to hypnosis; however, the use of hypnosis in patients with severe psychiatric disease is controversial. Also, patients who have very low scores on hypnotic susceptibility scales are less likely to derive therapeutic benefit.

► Clinical Uses of Hypnosis

A. Pain

There are at least 40 controlled studies of variable methodologic quality on the use of hypnosis for treating acute pain in adult and pediatric populations. All but 3 studies show superiority of hypnosis over a control condition (usual care, no treatment, or attentional control). Hypnosis has been shown effective for peri-procedural and perioperative pain in patients undergoing breast lumpectomy, excisional and core breast biopsy, bone marrow aspiration, pectus excavatum repair (Nuss procedure), percutaneous transluminal coronary angioplasty and other percutaneous vascular and renal procedures, burn wound care, and plastic surgery. Many studies also report less procedure-related anxiety and lower analgesic medication requirement.

For chronic pain, individual studies have shown efficacy for headache, orofacial pain, dyspepsia, vulvodynia, pain from sickle cell disease, fibromyalgia, and low back pain.

B. Cancer-related Symptoms

There are at least four randomized controlled trials specifically evaluating the efficacy of hypnosis for cancer-related pain and anxiety in adults. All four trials show benefit compared with no treatment or usual care. In addition, two of three randomized controlled trials show significant benefit of hypnosis for reducing anticipatory nausea and vomiting from chemotherapy. Other recent randomized controlled trials concluded (1) hypnosis decreased hot flash scores by 68% in breast cancer survivors; (2) self-hypnosis plus empathic attention was superior to empathic attention alone (for reducing pain, anxiety and medication usage) in 201 patients undergoing percutaneous tumor treatment; and (3) hypnosis preoperatively reduced institutional costs for breast cancer patients.

C. Irritable Bowel Syndrome

There are 14 studies of hypnosis for irritable bowel syndrome, 6 of which are controlled (placebo pill, CBT, or wait-list control). All 6 controlled studies show reduction in pain and bowel symptoms and some show improved quality of life and reduced anxiety. There are also 3 follow-up studies showing maintenance of benefits for 1 to 5 years in duration. The American College of Gastroenterology recommends behavioral therapies including hypnosis for the treatment of irritable bowel syndrome.

D. Smoking Cessation

A Cochrane review of 9 trials, distilled from a literature of over 50 studies, concluded that hypnosis is ineffective for smoking cessation. However, a more recent randomized controlled trial comparing hypnosis plus nicotine patch with behavioral counseling plus nicotine patch showed superiority of hypnosis, especially in those with a history of depression.

De Jong AE et al. Non-pharmacological nursing interventions for procedural pain relief in adults with burns: a systematic literature review. Burns. 2007 Nov;33(7):811–27. [PMID: 17606326]

Flory N et al. Practical hypnotic interventions during invasive cancer diagnosis and treatment. Hematol Oncol Clin North Am. 2008 Aug;22(4):709–25. [PMID: 18638697]

Montgomery GH et al. A randomized clinical trial of a brief hypnosis intervention to control side effects in breast surgery patients. J Natl Cancer Inst. 2007 Sep 5;99(17):1304–12. [PMID: 17728216]

Whorwell PJ. Hypnotherapy for irritable bowel syndrome: the response of colonic and noncolonic symptoms. J Psychosom Res. 2008 Jun;64(6):621–3. [PMID: 18501263]

MINDFULNESS MEDITATION

Definition

Meditation is broadly defined as the self-regulation of attention. There are two general types of meditation: mindfulness meditation and concentration meditation. In health care settings, the most widely available form of meditation is the mindfulness-based stress reduction (MBSR) program. This program was specifically designed for medical populations.

The essential exercise of meditation is focusing one's full attention on a designated object of meditation, such as one's breath. When it is noticed that the mind has wandered from this object, attention is returned to the object. Training the mind, beginning with this basic exercise, has many effects including relaxation, metacognition, and revelation of previously subconscious content. In mindfulness meditation, after initial training with the breath, the objects of meditation can include other aspects of human experience, such as physical sensations (eg, pain) or mental and emotional states (eg, anxiety).

History

Mindfulness meditation originated 2500 years ago in northern India from the tradition of Buddhism. It is a deliberate, sustained, nonjudgmental way of paying attention to one's experience that is said to enhance self-awareness, change maladaptive thinking, increase the capacity for skillful response to challenges, and reduce suffering. In 1979, mindfulness meditation practice was first introduced into American medical settings with the development of the MBSR program by Dr. Jon Kabat-Zinn. MBSR is an intensive 8-week program that introduces mindfulness practice in a secular, practical form to participants in the context of their life circumstances. There are now over 250 MBSR programs throughout the United States and many in other countries throughout the world. More recently, a close derivative of MBSR, mindfulness-based cognitive therapy (MBCT), has been developed exclusively for people with recurrent major depression. Mindfulness has also been adapted for use in programs for borderline personality disorder (Dialectical Behavior Therapy), eating disorders, substance abuse, and childbirth preparation.

Mechanism of Action

There have been extensive cardiac, respiratory, metabolic, endocrine, and functional central nervous system studies of individuals during meditation. Though much remains unknown, it is clear that meditation works in part through modulation of the autonomic nervous system, and that its effects are different from and more complex than simple relaxation. From a psychological perspective, it is thought that meditation enables the mind to establish a stable platform from which all events in the field of awareness can be viewed (eg, emotions, thoughts, physical sensations) without reactivity. At the psychological level, proposed mechanisms of mindfulness meditation include metacognition, exposure, uncoupling of maladaptive thoughts from physical stimuli (eg, pain), enhancing cognitive flexibility, relaxation, self-regulation, and reperceiving. At the physiologic level, studies of mindfulness meditation have found effects on the immune system (increased antibody response to vaccination, reduction in proinflammatory cytokines, possible slowed decline of CD4+ lymphocytes in HIV disease), nervous system (enhanced cortical thickness in specific brain regions, enhanced left prefrontal activation on EEG, characteristic functional MRI findings), and endocrine system (reduced cortisol, increased melatonin levels). There is evidence of a dose-response relationship with mindfulness meditation.

Training & Certification

Certification is not required to teach MBSR, but in 2005 the Center for Mindfulness at the University of Massachusetts Medical School, where MBSR began, established a professional certification program. Ideally, an MBSR teacher should have a long-standing daily mindfulness meditation practice, a history of silent meditation retreats, experience leading groups, and a health professional degree.

Clinical Practice

The best candidate for an MBSR program is someone who is motivated and has a medical, surgical, or psychiatric condition with a significant component of psychological distress. Motivation is essential for two reasons. First, participation in an MBSR program requires as much as 28 hours of classroom time over 8 weeks (including an all-day silent retreat) and 30–45 minutes of formal guided mindfulness practice each day. Second, an important part of mindfulness practice is to directly explore any unpleasant physical or mental experiences as they arise. Often, MBSR programs offer free informational sessions that precede the 8-week series so patients can evaluate the program before they decide to enroll.

Adverse Events

There are no adverse effects of mindfulness meditation specifically reported in experimental trials, but meditation can allow previously subconscious, distressing psychic content to come into consciousness. Patients with psychiatric disorders should consult with a mental health care professional before starting a program of meditation.

Contraindications

Untreated psychosis, mania and intoxication from active substance abuse are relative contraindications because these conditions may impair the fundamental exercise required for mindfulness training (ie, repeatedly returning one's attention to a desired object of awareness).

▶ Clinical Uses of Mindfulness Meditation

There are over 60 experimental trials assessing mindfulness-based interventions, approximately half of which are controlled trials. Most of the research examines the efficacy of MBSR programs, but there are also studies of MBCT, shorter mindfulness interventions and vipassana residential retreats. Two meta-analyses of MBSR show average effect sizes of 0.5–0.6.

A. Cancer-related Symptoms

There are 15 studies of mindfulness meditation in patients with cancer, including 4 randomized controlled trials. All 11 studies that measured psychological variables showed significant improvement (mood disturbance, anxiety, symptoms of stress, quality of life). Two studies assessed sleep problems and both found improvement. In a nonrandomized comparison of MBSR and a healing-through-creative-arts program, the mindfulness intervention was superior in reducing symptoms of stress, anxiety, mood disturbance, and increasing sense of spirituality. The two groups were equal in increasing a measure of posttraumatic growth. Two other cancer studies showed that psychological benefits from MBSR were sustained at 6-month and 12-month follow-up, respectively. Interestingly, the first inpatient study of a mindfulness intervention, an uncontrolled pilot study of 20 adults undergoing hematopoietic stem cell transplantation, showed reduced pain, anxiety, and physiological arousal from pre- to post-intervention.

B. Depression

Four studies, two of which are randomized controlled trials, specifically examined the effect of MBCT on patients with major depression and demonstrated relapse reduction of almost 50% in patients who have a history of more than two relapses. One uncontrolled study of MBCT showed that the measured level of mindfulness attained after the intervention successfully predicted depression relapse. An additional randomized controlled trial of MBCT showed improvement in depression and anxiety for bipolar patients with suicidal ideation or behavior. A pilot study using MBCT for 51 patients with treatment-resistant depression (defined as two or more adequate trials of antidepressants) found significantly decreased depression and anxiety levels. A randomized controlled trial of MBSR for women with fibromyalgia showed improvement in depression maintained at 2-month follow-up. Multiple other MBSR studies show improvement in mood in various populations; however, two studies found mindfulness interventions to be equal to comparison groups (CBT and relaxation therapy) and a 2007 review of 15 of these studies concludes overall evidence of benefit is equivocal.

C. Anxiety Disorders

Two early uncontrolled studies specifically examined the effect of MBSR on patients with anxiety disorders and found significant benefits that were maintained at 3 year follow-up. Two uncontrolled studies examined MBCT for generalized anxiety disorder and found pre-to-post changes in anxiety but in one study the effect size was less than that commonly found in CBT studies. A randomized controlled trial of MBSR versus cognitive behavioral group therapy for social anxiety disorder showed cognitive behavioral group therapy was more effective at reducing symptoms of social anxiety; however, the CBT intervention was 50% longer in duration and results for functionality, quality of life, and mood were equal in the two groups. A randomized controlled trial of 31 pregnant women showed reduction of anxiety, perceived stress, and an improvement in mood. A small controlled study showed a significant reduction of symptoms in patients with obsessive-compulsive disorder. An uncontrolled study of adults and adolescents with attention deficit hyperactivity disorder showed significant benefit with MBSR; however, an intensive 10-day mindfulness (vipassana) retreat did not improve symptoms of posttraumatic stress disorder in an incarcerated population.

D. Fibromyalgia

There are four studies of mindfulness interventions for fibromyalgia, including two randomized controlled trials. All four studies show improvement in psychological measures; three showed improvement in pain, although one of the randomized controlled trials did not find MBSR to be superior to an education and support comparison group. One study showed maintenance of most benefits (pain, quality of life, anxiety, depression) at 3-year follow-up.

E. Other Chronic Pain

Seven studies, including almost 700 patients, have been conducted using MBSR in chronic pain populations. All studies showed significant improvement in mental health parameters, such as quality of life, acceptance, pain tolerance, and mood. Six of these studies (three controlled, three uncontrolled) showed pain reduction. One follow-up study showed that improvements were maintained up to 4 years later. A randomized controlled trial of MBSR for patients with rheumatoid arthritis showed improvement in psychological distress and well-being at 6-month follow-up, but no improvement in disease activity. A second randomized controlled study of patients with rheumatoid arthritis compared a mindfulness-based intervention (that was much less intensive than standard MBSR) with a CBT intervention and an education control group. Both experimental groups were significantly superior to the control group, although overall the CBT group showed the greatest reduction in pain and IL-6 levels. In the subset of patients with a history of recurrent depression, however, the mindfulness-based intervention yielded greatest reduction in pain and improvement in mood. Interestingly, a comparison of distant (via videoconferencing) versus on-site mindfulness-based programs for chronic pain showed significant gains for both groups, but the on-site group rated superior in physical quality of life and pain reduction.

F. Other Conditions

Other studies have been conducted on organ transplant recipients, patients suffering from psoriasis, tinnitus, type 2 diabetes, eating disorders, women with sexual arousal disorder, inner city residents, nursing home residents, incarcerated individuals, smokers, nurses and nursing students, college students, and medical students. Nearly all of these studies showed mental health benefit from mindfulness meditation and most showed index symptom reduction. Interestingly, a randomized controlled trial of psychotherapists in training showed improvement in the patients of those therapists who were taught mindfulness.

Grossman P et al. Mindfulness training as an intervention for fibromyalgia: evidence of postintervention and 3-year follow-up benefits in well-being. Psychother Psychosom. 2007;76(4):226–33. [PMID: 17570961]

Williams JM et al. Mindfulness-based Cognitive Therapy (MBCT) in bipolar disorder: preliminary evaluation of immediate effects on between-episode functioning. J Affect Disord. 2008 Apr;107(1–3):275–9. [PMID: 17884176]

Witek-Janusek L et al. Effect of mindfulness based stress reduction on immune function, quality of life and coping in women newly diagnosed with early stage breast cancer. Brain Behav Immun. 2008 Aug;22(6):969–81. [PMID: 18359186]

Zautra AJ et al. Comparison of cognitive behavioral and mindfulness meditation interventions on adaptation to rheumatoid arthritis for patients with and without history of recurrent depression. J Consult Clin Psychol. 2008 Jun;76(3):408–21. [PMID: 18540734]

GUIDED IMAGERY

► Definition

Guided imagery uses the imaginative capacity of the mind to affect one's physical, emotional, or spiritual state. As is the case with psychotherapeutic techniques, guided imagery can be applied in a variety of ways. It may be directive, with the therapist providing specific images, or it may be more receptive, inviting the patient to find their own images. It may be supportive, with the intention to create a relaxed, pleasant or specifically positive feeling (eg, trust or patience) or it may intend to directly work with an area of active challenge (eg, anxiety or pain). Classically, in guided imagery, the therapist is less directive and the patient has a more active role than in hypnosis; however, this distinction is not always true in clinical practice and guided imagery can closely resemble hypnosis, especially when suggestion is used. Guided imagery can be conducted live with a therapist one-on-one, in a group setting (less common), or via audio recording.

► History

Imagery has been used throughout history and can be found in the origins of all ancient healing systems still extant today. In contemporary Western medicine, the psychiatrist Dr. Carl Jung recognized the importance of imagery as an expression of the subconscious and in 1915 developed a psychotherapeutic technique called "active imagination." With the similar intention to aid psychoanalytic exploration, the French psychotherapist Dr. Robert Desoille in the late 1930s created a method he called "directed daydreaming,"

and in the 1950s Dr. Hanscarl Leuner introduced "guided affective imagery." Medical research on guided imagery began in the 1970s and increased greatly in the 1980s. In 1989, the physician Dr. Martin Rossman and the psychologist Dr. David Bresler founded the Academy for Guided Imagery which began certifying health professionals. In recent years, some health insurance companies and surgical programs have been providing free guided imagery recordings for patients undergoing surgery.

► Mechanism of Action

The mechanism of action of guided imagery is not well known, but some physiologic effects have been demonstrated. Three of five studies examining cortisol levels in relation to guided imagery have found that serum levels decreased after the intervention. Studies of the effect of guided imagery on immune function have shown mixed results. However, a recent randomized controlled trial of women with breast cancer showed increased NK cell cytotoxicity and increased IL-2-activated NK cell activity. One study documented reduced physiologic arousal around chemotherapy sessions, as measured by heart rate and systolic blood pressure. Some proposed psychological mechanisms postulated to explain the effects of guided imagery include cognitive restructuring, increased sense of control, increased adaptive coping, distraction, and relaxation.

► Training & Certification

The leading certifying organization, the Academy for Guided Imagery, generally limits certification to licensed health care professionals or health professional students, but exceptions are allowed. To obtain the certification known as "interactive guided imagery," 150 total hours of training is required, including 52 hours of small group supervision. Applicants are also required to adhere to the American Psychological Association code of ethics. Another certifying organization is Beyond Ordinary Nursing, which requires 110 total hours of training, including ten documented imagery sessions.

► Clinical Practice

The length of a typical guided imagery session with a therapist is 50 minutes, with 20–30 minutes spent in active imagery. The imagery portion of the appointment often begins with imagining a place of comfort and safety, then proceeding to the desired area of specific clinical attention. Polysensory recruitment is often used (ie, the patient is asked to imagine visual, auditory, tactile, olfactory cues in imagining the safe place and then in focusing attention). Examples of specific clinical techniques used by the therapist might include dialoging with the symptom ("If your back pain had a voice, what would it say?"), consulting a wisdom figure or inner advisor ("What does your wisdom figure say about how to approach this cancer treatment?"), and visualizing a desired outcome ("Imagine yourself waking up after surgery feeling calm and comfortable."). Interactive Guided Imagery is a type of imagery that more deliberately aims to enhance awareness of subconscious content.

Predictors of favorable outcome from guided imagery, based on three studies, are previous experience with guided imagery, imaging ability of the patient, perceived credibility of the therapist, and rapport of the patient with the therapist. Age, gender, and education level have not shown significant correlation with outcomes, suggesting that this technique can be applied widely.

▶ Adverse Events

Adverse events have not been reported with guided imagery. However, as is the case with any psychotherapeutic technique, distressing psychological content can arise.

▶ Contraindications

There are no contraindications based on outcomes studies. However, due to the potential risk of reexperiencing original trauma, caution is advised in using guided imagery in patients with posttraumatic stress disorder or history of severe trauma or abuse.

▶ Clinical Uses of Guided Imagery

A. Surgery

There are many studies examining the use of guided imagery on outcomes related to such surgeries and procedures as heart surgery, colorectal surgery, abdominal surgery, laparoscopic gynecologic surgery in adults, bone marrow aspiration, lumbar puncture, burn wound debridement, and administration of immunizations in children. Although many of the studies have methodologic limitations, reviews and meta-analyses have found overall benefit of small to moderate effect sizes for reducing psychological distress and reducing postoperative pain. However, a randomized controlled trial of guided imagery for peri-procedural pain and anxiety conducted with 170 women undergoing colposcopy did not show a significant effect. Two of the three randomized controlled trials assessing its effect on average length of hospital stay found a significant decrease with guided imagery intervention. Other studies have shown significant decreases in total opioid use and average pharmacy costs.

B. Cancer-related Symptoms

Most of the studies in patients with cancer use guided imagery in combination with another modality, such as progressive muscle relaxation, meditation, hypnosis, biofeedback, or music therapy. These studies vary in methodologic quality. There are at least 18 randomized controlled

trials in this category and all show benefit for psychological outcomes, such as quality of life, anxiety, and depression. Studies that assessed the effect of guided imagery in combination with other modalities on nausea and vomiting also showed uniform benefit for this symptom. With respect to nonprocedural, cancer-related pain, there are at least 6 randomized controlled trials using guided imagery as part of a combination intervention. Three studies showed significant pain reduction with guided imagery intervention, 2 showed no pain reduction, and 1 showed significant benefit in patients' self-reported ability to decrease pain but not in measured pain intensity.

There are also several randomized controlled trials of guided imagery as a sole adjunctive treatment for patients with cancer. All of these studies again showed that guided imagery led to improvement in psychological outcomes, and in approximately half of the studies, the improvement was superior to other comparison interventions, such as progressive muscle relaxation or hypnosis. The evidence for guided imagery alone in preventing chemotherapy-related nausea and vomiting is mixed.

A single study has examined the effect of guided imagery directly on cancer disease regression using clinical (UICC criteria) and pathologic (biopsy) measures and found no effect.

C. Chronic Pain

There are several studies of guided imagery for various chronic pain conditions, such as osteoarthritis, headache, low back pain, fibromyalgia, and interstitial cystitis. Some of the studies are controlled and all show benefit in either pain, psychological distress, or both.

D. Stroke Rehabilitation

Four randomized controlled trials report efficacy of motor imagery for rehabilitation post-stroke.

Carrico DJ et al. Guided imagery for women with interstitial cystitis: results of a prospective, randomized controlled pilot study. J Altern Complement Med. 2008 Jan–Feb;14(1):53–60. [PMID: 18199015]

León-Pizarro C et al. A randomized trial of the effect of training in relaxation and guided imagery techniques in improving psychological and quality-of-life indices for gynecologic and breast brachytherapy patients. Psychooncology. 2007 Nov;16(11):971–9. [PMID: 17311247]

Zimmermann-Schlatter A et al. Efficacy of motor imagery in post-stroke rehabilitation: a systematic review. J Neuroeng Rehabil. 2008 Mar 14;5:8. [PMID: 18341687]

Appendix: Therapeutic Drug Monitoring & Laboratory Reference Intervals

C. Diana Nicoll, MD, PhD, MPA

Chuanyi Mark Lu, MD

Table 1. Therapeutic drug monitoring.[1]

Drug	Effective Concentrations	Half-Life (hours)	Dosage Adjustments	Comments
Amikacin	Peak: 20–30 mg/L; trough: < 10 mg/L	2–3; ↑ in uremia	↓ in renal dysfunction	Concomitant kanamycin or tobramycin therapy may give falsely elevated amikacin results by immunoassay.
Amitriptyline	95–250 ng/mL	9–46		Drug is highly protein-bound. Patient-specific decrease in protein binding may invalidate quoted therapeutic reference interval for effective concentration.
Carbamazepine	4–12 mg/L	10–15		Induces its own metabolism. Metabolite 10,11-epoxide exhibits 13% cross-reactivity by immunoassay. Toxicity: diplopia, drowsiness, nausea, vomiting, and ataxia.
Cyclosporine	100–300 mcg/L (ng/mL) whole blood	6–12	Need to know specimen and methodology used	Cyclosporine is lipid-soluble (20% bound to leukocytes; 40% to erythrocytes; 40% in plasma, highly bound to lipoproteins); the binding is temperature-dependent in vitro and concentration-dependent in vivo. Obtain whole blood sample in a lavender (EDTA) tube for monitoring. HPLC and LC-tandem mass spectrometry methods are highly specific for parent drug and considered as the gold standard assays. Monoclonal fluorescence polarization immunoassay (FPIA) also measures cyclosporine reliably; polyclonal FPIAs are less specific due to cross-reaction with drug metabolites. Anticonvulsants and rifampin increase metabolism. Erythromycin, ketoconazole, and calcium channel blockers decrease metabolism. The main adverse reaction is dose-related nephrotoxicity.
Desipramine	100–250 ng/mL	13–23		Drug is highly protein-bound. Patient-specific decrease in protein binding may invalidate quoted therapeutic reference interval for effective concentration.
Digoxin	0.8–2 ng/mL	42; ↑ in uremia, CHF	↓ in renal dysfunction, CHF, hypothyroidism ↑ in hyperthyroidism	Bioavailability of digoxin tablets is 50–90%. Specimen must not be drawn within 6 hours of dose. Dialysis does not remove a significant amount. Hypokalemia potentiates toxicity. Digitalis toxicity is a clinical and not a laboratory diagnosis. Digibind (digoxin-specific antibody) therapy of digoxin overdose can interfere with measurement of digoxin levels depending on the digoxin assay. Elimination reduced by quinidine, verapamil, and amiodarone.
Ethosuximide	40–100 mg/L	Child: 30 Adult: 50		Levels used primarily to assess compliance. Toxicity is rare and does not correlate well with plasma concentrations.

(continued)

Table 1. Therapeutic drug monitoring.[1] (continued)

Drug	Effective Concentrations	Half-Life (hours)	Dosage Adjustments	Comments
Gentamicin	Peak: 4–8 mg/L; trough: < 2 mg/L	2–5; ↑ in uremia (7.3 on dialysis)	↓ in renal dysfunction	Draw peak specimen 30 minutes after end of infusion. Draw trough just before next dose. In uremic patients, carbenicillin may decrease gentamicin half-life from 46 hours to 22 hours.
Imipramine	180–350 ng/mL	10–16		Drug is highly protein-bound. Patient-specific decrease in protein binding may invalidate quoted therapeutic reference interval for effective concentration.
Lidocaine	1–5 mg/L	1.8; ↔ in uremia, CHF; ↑ in cirrhosis	↓ in CHF, liver disease	Levels increased with cimetidine therapy. CNS toxicity common in the elderly.
Lithium	0.7–1.5 mmol/L	22; ↑ in uremia	↓ in renal dysfunction	Thiazides and loop diuretics may increase serum lithium levels.
Methotrexate		8.4; ↑ in uremia	↓ in renal dysfunction	Therapeutic concentrations depend on the treatment protocol (low versus high dose) and time of specimen collection. 7-Hydroxymethotrexate cross-reacts 1.5% in immunoassay. To minimize toxicity, leucovorin should be continued if methotrexate level is > 0.1 mcmol/L at 48 hours after start of therapy. Methotrexate > 1 mcmol/L at > 48 hours requires an increase in leucovorin rescue therapy.
Nortriptyline	50–140 ng/mL	18–44		Drug is highly protein-bound. Patient-specific decrease in protein binding may invalidate quoted therapeutic reference interval for effective concentration.
Phenobarbital	10–40 mg/L	86; ↑ in cirrhosis	↓ in liver disease	Metabolized primarily by the hepatic microsomal enzyme system. Many drug-drug interactions.
Phenytoin	10–20 mg/L; 5–10 mg/L in uremia, hypoalbuminemia	Dose/concentration-dependent		Drug metabolite cross-reacts in immunoassays; the cross-reactivity may be of significance only in the presence of advanced chronic kidney disease. Metabolism is capacity-limited. Increase dose cautiously when level approaches therapeutic reference interval, since new steady-state level may be disproportionately higher. Drug is very highly protein-bound; protein binding is decreased in uremia and hypoalbuminemia. Free drug level may be indicated in certain circumstances.
Primidone	5–10 mg/L	8		Phenobarbital cross-reacts 0.5%. Metabolized to phenobarbital. Primidone/phenobarbital ratio > 1:2 suggests poor compliance.
Procainamide	4–8 mg/L	3; ↑ in uremia	↓ in renal dysfunction	30% of patients with plasma levels of 12–16 mcg/mL have ECG changes; 40% of patients with plasma levels of > 16 mcg/mL have severe toxicity. Metabolite N-acetylprocainamide is active.
Quinidine	1–4 mg/L	7; × in CHF; ↑ in liver disease	↓ in liver disease, CHF	Effective concentration is lower in chronic liver disease and nephrosis, where binding is decreased.
Salicylate	150–300 mg/L	Dose-dependent		
Sirolimus	Trough: 4–12 ng/mL when used in combination with cyclosporine A; 12–20 ng/mL if used alone	62	↓ in liver dysfunction and with drugs affecting CYP3A4 activity	Sirolimus is an immunosuppressant used in combination with cyclosporine and corticosteroids for prophylaxis of organ rejection after kidney transplantation. It has also been used in liver and heart transplantation. When used in combination with cyclosporine, careful monitoring of kidney function is required. Once the initial dose titration is complete, monitoring sirolimus trough concentrations weekly for the first month and every 2 weeks for the second month appears to be appropriate.

(continued)

Table 1. Therapeutic drug monitoring.[1] (continued)

Drug	Effective Concentrations	Half-Life (hours)	Dosage Adjustments	Comments
Tacrolimus	Trough: 5–20 ng/mL	8.7–11.3	↓ in liver dysfunction and with drugs affecting CYP3A4 activity	Tacrolimus is used for prophylaxis of organ rejection in adult patients undergoing liver or kidney transplantation and in pediatric patients undergoing liver transplantation. It has also been used to prevent rejection in heart, small bowel, and allogeneic bone marrow transplant patients and to treat autoimmune diseases. Antacid or sucralfate administration should be separated from tacrolimus by at least 2 hr.
Theophylline	5–20 mg/L	9	↓ in CHF, cirrhosis, and with cimetidine	Caffeine cross-reacts 10%. Elimination is increased 1.5–2 times in smokers. 1,3-Dimethyl uric acid metabolite increased in uremia and, because of cross-reactivity, may cause an apparent slight increase in serum theophylline.
Tobramycin	Peak: 5–10 mg/L; trough: < 2 mg/L	2–3; ↑ in uremia	↓ in renal dysfunction	Tobramycin, kanamycin, and amikacin may cross-react in immunoassay.
Valproic acid	55–100 mg/L	13–19		95% protein-bound. Decreased binding in uremia and cirrhosis.
Vancomycin	Trough: 5–15 mg/L	6; ↑ in uremia	↓ in renal dysfunction	Toxicity in uremic patients leads to irreversible deafness. Keep peak level < 30–40 mg/L to avoid toxicity.

[1]Use red-topped tube (not marbled) for therapeutic drug monitoring. In general, the specimen should be drawn just before the next dose (trough).

×, unchanged; ↑, increase(d); ↓, decrease(d); HPLC, high performance liquid chromatography; CHF, congestive heart failure; CNS, central nervous system; ECG, electrocardiogram.

Modified, with permission, from Nicoll D et al. *Pocket Guide to Diagnostic Tests*, 5th ed. McGraw-Hill, 2008.

Table 2. Reference intervals for commonly used tests.[1,2]

		Current metric units × Conversion factor = SI units SI units ÷ Conversion factor = Current metric units			
Test	Specimen	Conventional Units	Conversion Factor	SI Units[2]	Collection
Acetaminophen	Serum	10–20 mg/L Panic: > 50 mg/L	66.16	66–132 mcmol/L	Serum separator tube (SST)
Acetoacetate	Serum or urine	Negative		Negative	SST or urine container
Activated clotting time (ACT)	Whole blood	70–180 seconds (method-specific)			Collect in a plastic syringe without anticoagulant
Adrenocorticotropic hormone (ACTH)	Plasma	9–52 pg/mL (laboratory-specific)	0.22	2–11 pmol/L	Siliconized glass or plastic lavender
Alanine aminotransferase (ALT, SGPT, GPT)	Serum	7–56 units/L (laboratory-specific)	0.02	0.14–1.12 mckat/L (laboratory-specific)	SST
Albumin	Serum	3.4–4.7 mg/dL	10.00	34–47 g/L	SST
Aldosterone	Serum	Salt-loaded (120 mEq Na$^+$/d for 3–4 days): Supine: 3–10 ng/dL Upright: 5–30 ng/dL Salt-depleted (20 mEq Na$^+$/d for 3–4 days): Supine: 12–36 ng/dL Upright: 17–137 ng/dL	27.74	83–277 pmol/L 139–831 pmol/L 332–997 pmol/L 471–3795 pmol/L	SST
	Urine	Salt-loaded (120 mEq Na$^+$/d for 3–4 days): 1.5–12.5 mcg/24 h Salt-depleted (20 mEq Na$^+$/d for 3–4 days): 18–85 mcg/24 h	2.77	4.2–34.6 nmol/d 49.9–235.5 nmol/d	Urine bottle containing boric acid
Alkaline phosphatase	Serum	41–133 units/L (method- and age-dependent)	0.02	0.7–2.2 mckat/L (method- and age-dependent)	SST
Ammonia (NH$_3$)	Plasma	18–60 mcg/dL	0.59	11–35 mcmol/L	Green (iced)
Amylase	Serum	20–110 units/L (laboratory-specific)	0.02	0.33–1.83 mckat/L (laboratory-specific)	SST
Angiotensin-converting enzyme (ACE)	Serum	12–35 units/L (method-dependent)	16.67	200–583 nkat/L (method-dependent)	SST
Antithrombin III (AT III)	Plasma	84–123% (qualitative/activity) 80–130% (quantitative/antigen)			Blue
α_1-Antitrypsin	Serum	110–270 mg/dL	0.01	1.1–2.7 g/L	SST
Aspartate aminotransferase (AST, SGOT, GOT)	Serum	0–35 units/L (laboratory-specific)	0.02	0–0.58 mckat/L (laboratory-specific)	SST
Basophil count	Whole blood	0.01–0.12 × 10^3/mcL	1.00	0.01–0.12 × 10^9/L	Lavender
bcr/abl, t(9;22) translocation by reverse-transcriptase polymerase chain reaction (RT-PCR), qualitative	Whole blood	Negative (Positive: chronic myeloid leukemia, some acute B-lymphoblastic leukemia)			Lavender
β_2 microglobulin	Serum	< 0.2 mg/dL	10	< 2 mg/L	SST
Bilirubin	Serum	Total: 0.1–1.2 mg/dL Direct (conjugated to glucuronide): 0.1–0.5 mg/dL Indirect (unconjugated): 0.1–0.7 mg/dL	17.10	2–21 mcmol/L < 8 mcmol/L < 12 mcmol/L	SST

(continued)

Table 2. Reference intervals for commonly used tests.[1,2] (continued)

		Current metric units × Conversion factor = SI units SI units ÷ Conversion factor = Current metric units			
Test	**Specimen**	**Conventional Units**	**Conversion Factor**	**SI Units[2]**	**Collection**
Blood urea nitrogen (BUN)	Serum	8–20 mg/dL	0.36	2.9–7.1 mmol/L	SST
B-type natriuretic peptide (BNP)	Plasma	< 100 pg/mL	1.0	<100 ng/L	Lavender
C-peptide	Serum	0.8–4.0 ng/mL	0.33	0.27–1.33 nmol/L	SST/iced (fasting) Gold SST
C-reactive protein, high sensitivity (hs-CRP)	Serum	< 1.0 mg/dL	10.00	< 10 mg/L	SST
Calcitonin	Plasma	Male: 0–11.5 pg/mL Female: 0–4.6 pg/mL	1.00	Male: 0–11.5 ng/L Female: 0–4.6 ng/L	Green SST
Calcium (Ca^{2+})	Serum	8.5–10.5 mg/dL **Panic: < 6.5 or > 13.5 mg/dL**	0.25	2.1–2.6 mmol/L	SST
Calcium (ionized)	Serum	4.6–5.3 mg/dL	0.25	1.15–1.32 mmol/L	Green (anaerobic)
Calcium (U_{Ca})	Urine	100–300 mg/24 h	0.025	2.5–7.5 mmol/24 h	Urine bottle containing hydrochloric acid
Carbon dioxide, partial pressure (P_{CO_2})	Whole blood	32–48 mm Hg	0.13	4.26–6.38 kPa	Heparinized syringe (iced)
Carbon dioxide (CO_2), total (bicarbonate)	Serum	22–32 mEq/L **Panic: < 15 or > 40 mEq/L**	1.00	22–32 mmol/L **Panic: < 15 or > 40 mmol/L**	SST
Carboxyhemoglobin (HbCO)	Whole blood	< 9% of total hemoglobin (Hb)	0.01	< 0.09 fraction of total hemoglobin	Heparinized syringe or Green
Carcinoembryonic antigen (CEA)	Serum	0–5 ng/mL	1.00	0–5 mcg/L	SST
Catecholamines	Urine	Norepinephrine: 15–80 mcg/24 h Epinephrine: 0–20 mcg/24 h Dopamine: 65–400 mcg/24 h	5.91 5.46 6.53	89–473 nmol/24 h 0–109 nmol/24 h 425–2610 nmol/24 h	Urine container with hydrochloride acid
CD4 T cell count	Whole blood	$0.36–1.73 \times 10^3$/mcL	1.00	$0.36–1.73 \times 10^6$/L	Lavender (order T-cell subsets and a CBC with differential)
Ceruloplasmin	Serum	20–60 mg/dL (laboratory-specific)	10.00	200–600 mg/L	SST
Chloride (Cl^-)	Serum	101–112 mEq/L	1.00	101–112 mmol/L	SST
Cholesterol	Serum	Desirable: < 200 mg/dL Borderline: 200–240 mg/dL High risk: > 240 mg/dL	0.03	Desirable: < 6.0 mmol/L Borderline: 6.0–7.2 mmol/L High risk: > 7.2 mmol/L	SST
Chorionic gonadotropin, β-subunit (β-hCG), quantitative	Serum	Males and nonpregnant females: undetectable or < 5 mU/mL	1.00	Males and nonpregnant females: undetectable or < 5 units/L	SST
Complement C3	Serum	64–166 mg/dL	10.00	640–1660 mg/L	SST
Complement C4	Serum	15–45 mg/dL	10.00	150–450 mg/L	SST
Complement CH50	Serum	(Laboratory-specific)			Red
Cortisol	Serum	8:00 AM: 5–20 mcg/dL	27.59	140–550 nmol/L	SST

(continued)

Table 2. Reference intervals for commonly used tests.[1,2] (continued)

Test	Specimen	Conventional Units	Conversion Factor	SI Units[2]	Collection
		Current metric units × Conversion factor = SI units			
		SI units ÷ Conversion factor = Current metric units			
Cortisol (urinary free)	Urine	10–110 mcg/24 h	2.76	27.6–303.6 nmol/24 h	Urine bottle containing boric acid
Creatine kinase (CK)	Serum	32–267 units/L (method-dependent)	0.02	0.53–4.45 mckat/L (method-dependent)	SST
Creatine kinase MB (CKMB)	Serum	< 16 units/L or < 4% of total CK (laboratory-specific) Mass units: 0–7 mcg/L	0.04	< 0.27 mckat/L	SST
Creatinine (Cr)	Serum	0.6–1.2 mg/dL	83.3	50–100 mcmol/L	SST
Creatinine clearance (Cl_{cr})	See Collection column	Adults: 90–140 mL/min/1.73 m^2 body surface area (BSA)	0.017	1.5–2.3 mL/s/1.73 m^2 BSA	Carefully timed 24-hour urine and simultaneous serum or plasma creatinine sample
Cryoglobulins	Serum	Negative			Red (transported at 37 °C)
D-dimer, quantitative	Plasma	< 500 ng/mL	1.00	< 500 mcg/L	Blue
Eosinophil count	Whole blood	$0.04–0.5 \times 10^3$/mcL	1.00	$0.04–0.5 \times 10^9$/L	Lavender
Erythrocyte count (RBC count)	Whole blood	$4.7–6.1 \times 10^6$/mcL	1.00	$4.7–6.1 \times 10^{12}$/L	Lavender
Erythrocyte sedimentation rate	Whole blood	Male: < 10 mm/h Female: < 15 mm/h (laboratory-specific)		Same	Lavender (test must be run within 2 h)
Erythropoietin (EPO)	Serum	5–30 mU/mL	1.00	5–30 units/L	SST
Estradiol	Serum	Early follicular: 30–100 pg/mL Late follicular: 100–400 pg/mL Luteal: 50–150 pg/mL Postmenopausal: 2–21 pg/mL	3.67	110–367 pmol/L 367–1468 pmol/L 183–550 pmol/L 7–77 pmol/L	SST
Ethanol	Serum	0 mg/dL Legal "driving under the influence" in many states is defined as > 80 mg/dL (> 17 mmol/L) blood alcohol level; serum alcohol levels are 10–35% higher than whole blood alcohol levels	0.217	0 mmol/L	SST
Factor VIII assay	Plasma	50–150% of normal (varies with age)			Blue (iced)
Fecal fat	Stool	Random: < 60 droplets of fat per high-power field 72-hour: < 7 g/24 h			Qualitative: Random stool sample Quantitative: 72-hour collection following 2-day dietary fat regimen
Ferritin	Serum	Male: 16–300 ng/mL Female: 4–161 ng/mL	1.00	Male: 16–300 mcg/L Female: 4–161 mcg/L	SST
α-Fetoprotein (AFP)	Serum	0–15 ng/mL	1.00	0–15 mcg/L	SST
Fibrinogen (functional)	Plasma	175–433 mg/dL **Panic:** < 75 mg/dL	0.01	1.75–4.3 g/L	Blue

(continued)

Table 2. Reference intervals for commonly used tests.[1,2] (continued)

| | | Current metric units × Conversion factor = SI units | | | |
| | | SI units ÷ Conversion factor = Current metric units | | | |
Test	Specimen	Conventional Units	Conversion Factor	SI Units[2]	Collection
Folic acid (red cells)	Whole blood	165–760 ng/mL	2.27	370–1720 nmol/L	Lavender
Follicle-stimulating hormone (FSH)	Serum	Female: Follicular phase 4–13 mU/mL Luteal phase 2–13 mU/mL Midcycle 5–22 mU/mL Postmenopausal 30–138 mU/mL Male: 1–10 mU/mL (laboratory-specific)	1.00	Female: 4–13 units/L 2–13 units/L 5–22 units/L 30–138 units/L Male: 1–10 units/L (laboratory-specific)	SST
Free erythrocyte proto-porphyrin (FEP)	Whole blood	< 35 mcg/dL (method-dependent)			Lavender
Fructosamine	Serum	190–270 mcmol/L	1.0	190–270 mcmol/L	SST
γ-Glutamyl transpepti-dase (GGT)	Serum	9–85 units/L (laboratory-specific)	0.02	0.15–1.42 mckat/L (laboratory-specific)	SST
Gastrin	Serum	< 100 pg/mL (laboratory-specific)	1.00	< 100 ng/L	SST
Glomerular filtration rate, estimated (eGFR)	Serum	> 60 mL/min/1.73 m^2 (calculated based on serum creatinine)			SST
Glucose	Serum	60–110 mg/dL Panic: < 40 or > 500 mg/dL	0.055	3.3–6.1 mmol/L	(Fasting) SST
Glucose-6-phosphate dehydrogenase (G6PD) screen	Whole blood	5–14 units/g Hb	0.02	0.1–0.28 mckat/L	Lavender
Glutamine	Cerebrospinal fluid (CSF)	6–15 mg/dL Panic: > 40 mg/dL	68.5	411–1028 mcmol/L	Collect CSF in a plastic tube
Glycated (glycosylated) hemoglobin (HbA$_{1c}$)	Serum	3.9–6.9% (method-dependent)			Lavender
Growth hormone (GH)	Serum	0–5 ng/mL	1.00	0–5 mcg/L	SST
Haptoglobin	Serum	46–316 mg/dL	0.01	0.5–3.2 g/L	SST
HDL cholesterol	Serum	Male: 27–67 mg/dL Female: 34–88 mg/dL (HDL cholesterol > 60 mg/dL is thought to lower risk of coronary heart disease)	0.026	0.7–1.73 mmol/L 0.88–2.28 mmol/L	SST
Helicobacter pylori antibody	Serum	Negative			SST
Hematocrit (Hct)	Whole blood	Male: 39–49% Female: 35–45% (age-dependent)	0.01	Male: 0.39–0.49 Female: 0.35–0.45	Lavender
Hemoglobin A$_{1c}$ (See Glycated Hemoglobin)	Serum				
Hemoglobin A$_2$ (HbA$_2$)	Whole blood	1.5–3.5% of total hemoglobin	0.01	0.015–0.035	Lavender
Hemoglobin electro-phoresis	Whole blood	HbA: > 95% HbA$_2$: 1.5–3.5% HbF: < 2% (age dependent)			Lavender

(*continued*)

Table 2. Reference intervals for commonly used tests.[1,2] (continued)

Test	Specimen	Conventional Units	Conversion Factor	SI Units[2]	Collection
		Current metric units × Conversion factor = SI units			
		SI units ÷ Conversion factor = Current metric units			
Hemoglobin, total (Hb)	Whole blood	Male: 13.6–17.5 g/dL Female: 12.0–15.5 g/dL (age dependent) Panic: ≤ 7 g/dL	10.00	Male: 136–175 g/L Female: 120–155 g/L	Lavender
Heparin-associated antibody (heparin-induced thrombocytopenia)	Serum	Negative			SST
HIV antibody	Serum	EIA: Negative Western blot: Nonreactive			SST
HIV RNA, quantitative (viral load)	Plasma	Negative (or < 75 copies/mL, assay-specific)			Lavender
Homocysteine	Plasma	4–12 mcmol/L (method- and age-dependent)	1.00	4–12 mcmol/L	Lavender
5-Hydroxyindoleacetic acid (5-HIAA)	Urine	2–8 mg/24 h	5.23	10–40 mcmol/d	Urine bottle containing hydrochloric acid
IgG index	Serum and CSF	0.29–0.59 ratio (CSF serum ratio)			SST (for serum) and plastic tube (for CSF)
Immunoglobulins (Ig)	Serum	IgA: 78–367 mg/dL IgG: 583–1761 mg/dL IgM: 52–335 mg/dL	0.01	IgA: 0.78–3.67 g/L IgG: 5.83–17.6 g/L IgM: 0.52–3.35 g/L	SST
Insulin, immunoreactive	Serum	6–35 mcU/mL	7.18	42–243 pmol/L	SST
Insulin-like growth factor-1	Plasma	123–463 ng/mL (age- and sex-dependent)	1.0	123–463 mcg/L	SST
Iron (Fe)	Serum	50–175 mcg/dL	0.18	9–31 mcmol/L	SST
Iron-binding capacity, total (TIBC)	Serum	250–460 mcg/dL	0.18	45–82 mcmol/L	SST
Kappa and lambda free light chains, quantitative	Serum	Free kappa: 0.57–2.63 mg/dL Free lambda: 0.33–1.94 mg/dL Free kappa/lambda ratio: 0.26–1.65	0.01	$5.7–26.3 \times 10^{-3}$ g/L $3.3–19.4 \times 10^{-3}$ g/L	SST
Lactate dehydrogenase (LDH)	Serum	88–230 units/L (laboratory-specific)	0.02	1.46–3.82 mckat/L (laboratory-specific)	SST
Lactic acid (lactate)	Venous blood	0.5–2.0 mEq/L	1.00	0.5–2.0 mmol/L	Gray (iced)
LDL cholesterol (calculated or direct)	Serum	Desirable: < 130 mg/dL (< 99 mg/dL for patients with CHD); Borderline: 130–159 mg/dL; High risk: ≥ 160 mg/dL	0.026	< 3.37 mmol/L (< 2.57 mmol/L); 3.38–4.13 mmol/L; > 4.16 mmol/L	SST
Lead (Pb)	Whole blood	Child: < 25 mcg/dL Adult: < 40 mcg/dL	0.05	Child: < 1.21 mcmol/L Adult: < 1.93 mcmol/L	Navy blue (trace metal free)
Leukocyte (white blood cell) count, total (WBC count)	Whole blood	$4.8–10.8 \times 10^3$/mcL Panic: $< 1.5 \times 10^3$/mcL	1.00	$4.8–10.8 \times 10^9$/L	Lavender
Lipase	Serum	0–160 units/L (laboratory-specific)	0.02	0–2.66 mckat/L (laboratory-specific)	SST

(continued)

Table 2. Reference intervals for commonly used tests.[1,2] (continued)

		Current metric units × Conversion factor = SI units SI units ÷ Conversion factor = Current metric units			
Test	**Specimen**	**Conventional Units**	**Conversion Factor**	**SI Units[2]**	**Collection**
Luteinizing hormone (LH)	Serum	Female: Follicular phase 1–18 mU/mL Luteal phase 0.4–20 mU/mL Midcycle 24–105 mU/mL Postmenopausal 15–62 mU/mL Male: 1–10 mU/mL (laboratory-specific)	1.00	Female: 1–18 units/L 0.4–20 units/L 24–105 units/L 15–62 units/L Male: 1–10 units/L (laboratory-specific)	SST
Lymphocyte count	Whole blood	0.8–3.5 × 10³/mcL	1.00	0.8–3.5 × 10⁹/L	Lavender
Magnesium (Mg²⁺)	Serum	1.8–3.0 mg/dL Panic: < 0.5 or > 4.5 mg/dL	0.41	0.75–1.25 mmol/L	SST
Mean corpuscular hemoglobin (MCH)	Whole blood	26–34 pg			Lavender
Mean corpuscular hemoglobin concentration (MCHC)	Whole blood	31–36 g/dL	10.00	310–360 g/L	Lavender
Mean corpuscular volume (MCV)	Whole blood	80–100 fL			Lavender
Metanephrines, free	Plasma	Normetanephrine: < 0.9 nmol/L Metanephrine: < 0.5 nmol/L			Lavender
Metanephrines	Urine	0.3–0.9 mg/24 h	5.46	1.6–4.9 mcmol/24 h	Urine bottle containing hydrochloric acid
Methemoglobin (MetHb)	Whole blood	< 1% of total hemoglobin	0.01	< 0.01 fraction of total hemoglobin	Blood gas syringe, lavender, or green
Methylmalonic acid	Serum	0–0.05 mg/L	8.475	0–0.4 mcmol/L	SST
Monocyte count	Whole blood	0.2–0.8 × 10³/mcL	1.00	0.2–0.8 × 10⁹/L	Lavender
Neutrophil count	Whole blood	2.2–8.6 × 10³/mcL	1.00	2.2–8.6 × 10⁹/L	Lavender
Osmolality	Serum	275–293 mosm/kg H₂O Panic: < 240 or > 320 mosm/kg H₂O	1.00	275–293 mmol/kg H₂O	SST
	Urine	Random: 100–900 mosm/kg H₂O	1.00	Random: 100–900 mmol/kg H₂O	Urine container
Oxygen, partial pressure (Po₂)	Whole blood	83–108 mm Hg	0.13	11.04–14.36 kPa	Heparinized syringe (iced)
Parathyroid hormone (PTH), intact	Serum	Intact PTH: 11–54 pg/mL (laboratory-specific)	0.11	Intact PTH: 1.2–5.7 pmol/L (laboratory-specific)	Red, SST
Partial thromboplastin time, activated (PTT)	Plasma	25–35 seconds (reference interval varies) Panic: ≥ 60 seconds			Blue
pH	Whole blood	Arterial: 7.35–7.45 Venous: 7.31–7.41			Heparinized syringe (iced)
Phosphorus	Serum	2.5–4.5 mg/dL Panic: < 1.0 mg/dL	0.32	0.8–1.45 mmol/L	SST
Plasminogen	Plasma	70–113% (activity)	1.00	70–113%	Blue
Platelet count (Plt)	Whole blood	150–450 × 10³/mcL Panic: < 25 × 10³/mcL	1.0	150–450 × 10⁹/L Panic: < 25 × 10⁹/L	Lavender

(continued)

Table 2. Reference intervals for commonly used tests.[1,2] (continued)

Test	Specimen	Conventional Units	Conversion Factor	SI Units[2]	Collection
		Current metric units × Conversion factor = SI units SI units ÷ Conversion factor = Current metric units			
Platelet-associated IgG	Whole blood	Negative			Lavender
Platelet function test (PFA-100 closure time) (CEPI: collagen/epinephrine cartridge; CADP: collagen/ADP cartridge)	Whole blood	CEPI: 70–170 seconds (laboratory-specific) CADP: 50–110 seconds (laboratory-specific)	1.0	CEPI: 70–170 seconds CADP: 50–110 seconds	Blue
Porphobilinogen (PBG)	Urine	Negative			Protect from light
Potassium (K$^+$)	Serum	3.5–5.0 mEq/L **Panic: < 3.0 or > 6.0 mEq/L**	1.00	3.5–5.0 mmol/L	SST
Prolactin (PRL)	Serum	< 20 ng/mL	1.00	< 20 mcg/L	SST
Prostate-specific antigen (PSA)	Serum	0–4 ng/mL	1.00	0–4 mcg/L	SST
Protein C	Plasma	71–176% (functional) 60–150% (antigenic)			Blue
Protein electrophoresis	Serum	Adults: Albumin: 3.3–4.7 g/dL α_1: 0.1–0.4 g/dL α_2: 0.3–0.9 g/dL β_2: 0.7–1.5 g/dL γ: 0.5–1.4 g/dL (polyclonal)	10.00	33–47 g/L 1–4 g/L 3–9 g/L 7–15 g/L 5–14 g/L (polyclonal)	SST
Protein S (antigen)	Plasma	76–178%			Blue
Protein, total	Serum	6.0–8.0 g/dL	10.00	60–80 g/L	SST
Prothrombin time (PT)	Whole blood	11–15 seconds **Panic: ≥ 30 seconds (laboratory-specific)**			Blue
Red blood cell count	Whole blood	$4.7–6.1 \times 10^6$/mcL (male) $3.5–5.5 \times 10^6$/mcL (female)	1.00	$4.7–6.1 \times 10^{12}$/L $3.5–5.5 \times 10^{12}$/L	Lavender
Renin activity	Plasma	High-sodium diet (75–150 mEq Na$^+$/d): Supine: 0.2–2.3 ng/mL/h Standing: 1.3–4.0 ng/mL/h Low-sodium diet (30–75 mEq Na$^+$/d): Standing: 4.0–7.7 ng/mL/h			Lavender
Reptilase clotting time	Plasma	13–19 seconds			Blue
Reticulocyte count	Whole blood	$33–137 \times 10^3$/mcL	1.00	$33–137 \times 10^9$/L	Lavender
Russell viper venom clotting time (dilute) (RVVT)	Plasma	24–37 seconds			Blue
Salicylate (aspirin)	Serum	20–30 mg/dL **Panic: > 35 mg/dL**	10.00	200–300 mg/L	SST
Sodium (Na$^+$)	Serum	135–145 mEq/L **Panic: < 125 or > 155 mEq/L**	1.00	135–145 mmol/L	SST
Testosterone	Serum	Male: 175–781 ng/dL Female: 10–75 ng/dL	0.0347	Male: 6–27 nmol/L Female: 0.3–2.6 nmol/L	SST

(continued)

Table 2. Reference intervals for commonly used tests.[1,2] (continued)

		Current metric units × Conversion factor = SI units SI units ÷ Conversion factor = Current metric units			
Test	Specimen	Conventional Units	Conversion Factor	SI Units[2]	Collection
Thrombin time	Plasma	8–12 seconds (laboratory-specific)			Blue
Thyroglobulin	Serum	3–42 ng/mL	1.00	3–42 mcg/L	SST
Thyroid-stimulating hormone (TSH)	Serum	0.4–6 mcU/mL	1.00	0.4–6 mU/L	SST
Thyroid-stimulating hormone receptor antibody (TSH-R Ab [stim])	Serum	< 130% of basal activity; based on cAMP generation in thyroid cell tissue culture			
Thyroxine, free (FT₄)	Serum	9–24 pmol/L (varies with method)			SST
Thyroxine (T₄), total	Serum	5–11 mcg/dL	12.80	64–142 nmol/L	SST
Transferrin	Serum	190–375 mg/dL	0.01	1.9–3.75 g/L	SST
Transferrin receptor, soluble (sTfR)	Serum	2.2–5 mg/L (male) 1.9–4.4 mg/L (female) (laboratory-specific)			SST
Triglycerides	Serum	< 165 mg/dL	0.01	< 1.8 mmol/L	SST (fasting)
Triiodothyronine (T₃), total	Serum	95–190 ng/dL	0.015	1.5–2.9 nmol/L	SST
Troponin-I (cTnI)	Serum	< 1.50 ng/mL (method-dependent)			SST
Uric acid	Serum	Male: 2.4–7.4 mg/dL Female: 1.4–5.8 mg/dL	59.48	Male: 140–440 mcmol/L Female: 80–350 mcmol/L	SST
Vanillylmandelic acid (VMA)	Urine	2–7 mg/24 h	5.05	10–35 mcmol/d	Urine bottle containing hydrochloric acid
Vitamin B₁₂	Serum	140–820 pg/mL	0.74	100–600 pmol/L	SST
Vitamin D, 25-hydroxy (25[OH]D)	Serum	20–50 ng/mL	2.5	50–125 nmol/L	SST
Vitamin D, 1,25-dihydroxy (1,25[OH]₂D)	Serum	20–76 pg/mL	2.4	48–182 pmol/L	SST
von Willebrand factor (vWF)	Plasma	50–180% (activity and antigen)			Blue
White blood cell count	Whole blood	4.8–10.8 × 10³/mcL	1.00	4.8–10.8 × 10⁹/L	Lavender

[1]The reference intervals given here in conventional units and in SI units are from several large medical centers. Always use the reference intervals provided by your clinical laboratory, since intervals may be method-dependent.
[2]References: Stein K. Journal adopts use of conventional and SI units. J Am Diet Assoc. 2005 Aug;105(8):1186–7. [PMID: 16182628] Young DS. Implementation of SI units for clinical laboratory data. Ann Intern Med. 1987 Jan;106(1):114–29. [PMID: 3789557]

Table 3. Commonly used specimen collection tubes.

Tube	Tube Contents	Typical Use
Lavender	EDTA	Complete blood count; molecular testing
SST	Serum separator	Serum chemistry tests
Red	None	Blood banking (serum); therapeutic drug monitoring
Blue	Citrate	Coagulation studies
Gray	Inhibitor of glycolysis (sodium fluoride)	Lactic acid
Green	Heparin	Plasma chemistry tests; chromosome analysis
Yellow	Acid citrate	HLA typing; flow cytometry immunophenotyping
Navy	Trace metal free	Trace metals (eg, lead, mercury, arsenic)

EDTA, ethylenediamine tetraacetic acid; SST, serum separator tube.

Index

A antigen, in compatibility testing, 477

A-C ventilation. *See* Assist-control (A-C) ventilation

A cells, pancreatic, 1062

a wave
in AV junctional rhythm, 350
palpitations and, 31
in pulmonary stenosis, 295
in tetralogy of Fallot, 300
in tricuspid stenosis, 313

A3243G mutation, in diabetes mellitus, 1082

AA (Alcoholics Anonymous), 970, 979

AA amyloidosis, 842. *See also* Amyloidosis

A–a Do$_2$ (alveolar-arterial oxygen difference)
in asthma, 219
in COPD, 234
in pulmonary embolism, 267

Abacavir, 1226t, 1228, 1232f. *See also* Antiretroviral therapy
with lamivudine, 1227, 1228, 1231, 1232f
with zidovudine and lamivudine, 1228, 1232f

Abatacept, for rheumatoid arthritis, 751

ABCB4 gene, in idiopathic adulthood ductopenia, 641

ABCD rule, 101

Abciximab. *See also* Glycoprotein IIb/IIIa receptors, drugs blocking
for acute coronary syndromes/myocardial infarction, 327t, 328, 332
platelet function affected by, 490t

Abdominal abscess/infection, 1181t
actinomycosis, 1324
anaerobic, **1322–1323**, 1322t
in Crohn disease, 579
in diverticulitis, 588, 589

Abdominal aortic aneurysms, **423–425**
screening for, **6**, 423

Abdominal compartment syndrome, in burn patient, 1410

Abdominal distention
in acute colonic pseudo-obstruction (Ogilvie syndrome), 565
in acute paralytic ileus, 564
in chronic intestinal pseudo-obstruction/gastroparesis, 566

Abdominal fistulas, in Crohn disease, 578, 579

Abdominal pain/tenderness. *See also* Dyspepsia
in actinomycosis, 1324
in acute angle-closure glaucoma, 157
in acute colonic pseudo-obstruction (Ogilvie syndrome), 565
in acute mesenteric vein occlusion, 422

in aortic aneurysm, 423
in appendicitis, 567
in ascites, 524
in biliary tract carcinoma, 1462
in cholecystitis, 636
in choledocholithiasis/cholangitis, 638
in cholelithiasis/gallstones, 634
in cirrhosis, 619
in Crohn disease, 578, 579
in diverticulitis, 588
in ectopic pregnancy, 713
in erosive/hemorrhagic gastritis (gastropathy), 544
in familial Mediterranean fever, 528
in hepatitis, 605
in irritable bowel syndrome, 569–570, 570
in pancreatic/periampullary carcinoma, 1464
in pancreatitis, 642, 644, 646, 647
in peptic ulcer disease, 502, 549
penetration and, 555
perforation and, 555
in PID, 688
in polyarteritis nodosa, 765
in polycystic kidney disease, 847
in porphyria, 1512
in preeclampsia-eclampsia, 716
in spontaneous bacterial peritonitis, 526, 621
in ulcerative colitis, 583, 585
in visceral artery insufficiency/intestinal angina, 421

Abdominal paracentesis. *See* Paracentesis

Abdominal radiographs, in poisoning/drug overdose, 1427

Abelcet. *See* Amphotericin B lipid complex

Abetalipoproteinemia, vitamin E deficiency and, 1144

ABI/ABPI. *See* Ankle–brachial index

ABIC score, in alcoholic liver disease, 615

Abilify. *See* Aripiprazole

abl gene, in chronic myeloid leukemia, 461

ABLC. *See* Amphotericin B lipid complex

Abnormal illness behaviors, **944–946**

Abnormal movements. *See* Movement disorders

ABO system
compatibility testing for transfusion and, 477
hemolytic transfusion reactions and, 477

Abortion
elective/induced, **700–701**
breast cancer during pregnancy and, 672, 728
C sordellii infection after, 701, 1298

gestational trophoblastic disease and, 715
heart disease during pregnancy and, 724
hypertension during pregnancy and, 724
rubella infection and, 1254
toxoplasmosis testing and, 1364
infection after, 701
anaerobic, 1323
IUD insertion after, 698
recurrent (habitual), **712–713**
spontaneous. *See* Spontaneous abortion

Abortive poliomyelitis, 1252

ABPA. *See* Allergic bronchopulmonary mycosis/aspergillosis

ABPI. *See* Ankle–brachial index

Abraxane. *See* Paclitaxel, protein-bound

Abruptio placentae, third-trimester bleeding caused by, 720

Abscesses, 140–141. *See also specific type and organ or structure affected*
in actinomycetoma, 1400
in actinomycosis, 1323
anaerobic, 1321
of lung, **250**, 1322
in bacterial rhinosinusitis, 170, 194
brain, **901–902**, 1163, 1164, 1181t
deep neck, **206**
in drug users, 1168
in HIV infection/AIDS, 1215
intravascular (septic superficial thrombophlebitis), 429, 429–430
mycobacteria causing, 1324
perianal, 596
peritonsillar, **205**, 1289
ruptured appendicitis and, 568
staphylococcal, 141, 1294–1295

Absence (petit mal) seizures, 879t, 880, 882t. *See also* Seizures

Absence (petit mal) status epilepticus, 884

Absidia infection, 195, 1398–1399

Absorption (digestion)
disorders of. *See* Malabsorption
normal/phases of, 557–558

Absorptive hypercalciuria, 858–859, 858t

Absorptive phase, of digestion/absorption, 558

Abuse
aggression/violence/impulse control disorders and, 976
child. *See* Child abuse
drug/alcohol. *See* Alcohol use/dependency/abuse; Substance use disorders
elder, 19, **75**, 75t

Abuse (*cont.*)
  partner/spousal (domestic violence),
      976, 977
    prevention of, 18–19
    PTSD and, 938
ABVD regimen, for Hodgkin disease, 471
AC regimen, for breast cancer, 665
AC-P regimen, for breast cancer, 666
AC-T regimen, for breast cancer, 666
AC-TH regimen, for breast cancer, 666
Acamprosate, for alcohol use/abuse, 20, 980
Acanthamoeba (acanthamoeba infec-
      tions), 1368
    encephalitis/meningoencephalitis,
      1163, 1164, **1368**
    keratitis, **157**, **1368–1369**
Acanthosis nigricans
    cancer-related, 1453*t*
    insulin resistance and, 1082, 1086
Acarbose, 1091*t*, 1094
Accelerated idioventricular rhythm, **353**
    in myocardial infarction, 337, 353
Acceptance and commitment therapy, for
      schizophrenic/psychotic
      disorders, 960
Accessory atrioventricular pathways,
      supraventricular tachycar-
      dia caused by, 342,
      345–346
Accessory muscles of respiration, in
      asthma exacerbation, 219,
      220*t*
Accidental injury. *See* Trauma
Accommodation, aging affecting (presby-
      opia), 151
ACCORD study, 1089
Accupril. *See* Quinapril
Accutane. *See* Isotretinoin
ACE. *See* Angiotensin converting enzyme
ACE inhibitors. *See* Angiotensin convert-
      ing enzyme (ACE) inhibi-
      tors
Acebutolol, 400*t*
    overdose/toxicity of, 1432
Acellular pertussis vaccine, with tetanus-
      diphtheria toxoid (DTaP/
      Tdap vaccines), 3–4,
      1188–1189*t*, 1190–1191*t*,
      1192–1193*t*, 1194–1197*t*,
      1200, 1298, 1299*t*, 1302,
      1308
    adverse effects/contraindications and,
      1202*t*
    pregnancy and, 1195*t*, 1200
Aceon. *See* Perindopril
Acesulfame potassium, for diabetics, 1090
Acetadote. *See* Acetylcysteine
Acetaldehyde, in alcoholic liver disease,
      614
Acetaminophen, **78**, 79*t*
    in analgesic nephropathy, 845
    with codeine, 78, 83*t*
    for fever, 39
    for osteoarthritis, 731
    overdose/toxicity of, 1424*t*, 1427*t*,
      1428–1429
      hepatotoxicity/hepatic failure and,
      78, 607, 616, 1428, 1428*f*

    for pain management, 78, 79*t*
    reference values for, 1547*t*
Acetazolamide
    adverse ophthalmic effects of, 177*t*
    for altitude-related illness, 1417, 1418
    for glaucoma/ocular hypertension,
      158, 159
    in head injury, 918
    for lithium overdose/toxicity, 972
    renal tubular acidosis caused by, 810
Acetoacetate
    in alcoholic ketoacidosis, 809
    in diabetic ketoacidosis, 808,
      1112–1113
    reference values for, 1547*t*
Acetohexamide, 1090, 1091*t*
Acetone, in diabetic coma/ketoacidosis,
      1112–1113, 1112*t*
Acetone breath odor, in diabetic ketoaci-
      dosis, 1083, 1112
Acetonitrile, cyanide formed by metabo-
      lism of, 1435
Acetylcholine
    aminoglycosides affecting, 934
    in botulism, 933, 1299
    in Huntington disease, 909
    in myasthenic (Lambert-Eaton) syn-
      drome, 933
Acetylcholine receptor antibodies
    in cancer-related neuropathy, 925
    in myasthenia gravis, 932
Acetylcholinesterase inhibitors. *See* Anti-
      cholinesterases
Acetylcysteine
    for acetaminophen overdose/toxicity,
      1424*t*, 1428–1429
      hepatic failure and, 607–608
    contrast media nephrotoxicity medi-
      ated by, 822
Achalasia, 529*t*, **541–542**
Achlorhydria, in pernicious anemia gas-
      tritis, 547
Achromycin. *See* Tetracycline
Acid, caustic/corrosive, **1429**
    esophageal injury caused by, 536,
      1429
    eye injury caused by, 172, 1429, 1430
Acid-antisecretory agents. *See also* Antac-
      ids; H$_2$ receptor blocking
      drugs; Proton pump inhib-
      itors
    for dyspepsia, 503, 504
    for GI bleeding, 519, 554
    for peptic ulcer disease, 550
      bleeding control and, 554
Acid-base disorders, **806–815**. *See also*
      Acidosis; Alkalosis
    in chronic kidney disease, 809,
      827–828
    genetic, 796*t*
    in heat exhaustion, 1407
    in heat stroke, 1407, 1408
    in hypothermia, 1404, 1405
    mixed, **806–807**, 807*t*
    in near drowning, 1416
Acid-fast rods, treatment of infections
      caused by, 1177*t*
Acid refluxate. *See* Gastric acid refluxate

Acidosis, 806. *See also* Ketoacidosis
    anion gap. *See* Anion gap/anion gap
      acidosis
    in chronic kidney disease/renal failure,
      809, 827–828
    dilutional, 810
    dyspnea and, 26
    hyperchloremic normal anion gap,
      808*t*, **809–812**, 809*t*, 811.
      See also Hyperchloremic
      normal anion gap acidosis
    diabetic ketoacidosis and, 808–809,
      1114–1115
    hyperkalemia and, 798, 809*t*
    in hypocitraturic calcium nephrolithi-
      asis, 859
    hypokalemia and, 795, 809*t*
    hyporeninemic hypoaldosteronemic,
      809*t*, 810, 1049
    in hypothermia, 1404, 1405
    lactic, 808, 1112*t*, **1116–1117**. *See also*
      Lactic acidosis
    metabolic, 806, **807–812**, 807*t*, 808*t*.
      See also Metabolic acidosis
    in near drowning, 1416
    parenteral nutritional support and,
      808, 810, 1151*t*
    in poisoning/drug overdose, 809, 1426
      with methanol or ethylene glycol,
      809, 1426, 1439, 1440
      with salicylates, 809, 1426, 1445
    posthypocapnic, 810
    renal tubular, 796*t*, 809*t*, 810, 811. *See
      also* Renal tubular acidosis
    respiratory, 806, 807*t*, **813–814**, 814*t*.
      See also Respiratory acido-
      sis
    rewarming, 1404
    uremic, 809
Aciduria, paradoxic
    in metabolic alkalosis, 812
    in salicylate overdose/toxicity, 1445
Acinetobacter infections, 1176*t*
Acitretin
    adverse ophthalmic effects of, 178*t*
    for psoriasis, 105
    teratogenicity of, 105
Aclovate. *See* Alclometasone
Acne, **120–122**
    antibiotics for, 97*t*, 121
    folliculitis and, 120, 123, 124
    hyperandrogenism and, 120, 1054
    oral contraceptive use and, 121, 694
    rosacea, 120
    steroid (steroid acne/folliculitis), 120
    testosterone replacement therapy and,
      1066
    vulgaris, **120–122**
Acoustic neuroma/neurinoma (vestibular
      schwannoma/eighth nerve
      tumors), **191**, 191*t*, 898*t*,
      904
    hearing loss and, 179, 186, 191, 191*t*
    in neurofibromatosis, 191, 904
Acoustic trauma. *See* Noise trauma
Acquired immunodeficiency syndrome
      (AIDS). *See* HIV infection/
      AIDS

Acral erythema (hand-foot syndrome), chemotherapy-induced, 1480, 1509
Acral lentiginous melanoma, 100, 101
Acrocyanosis, 757
Acrodermatitis chronicum atrophicans, 1344, 1346t
Acromegaly, **997–1000**
Acromioclavicular joint, in rotator cuff disorders, 744
Acropachy, thyroid, 1009
ACS. *See* Acute coronary syndromes
ACT. *See* Activated clotting time
ACTH. *See* Adrenocorticotropic hormone
Actin, in hereditary spherocytosis, 448
Actinic (ultraviolet) keratitis, **172**
Actinic keratoses, **113**
squamous cell carcinoma arising from, 113, 134
Actinobacillus actinomycetemcomitans. See HACEK organisms
Actinomadura species, actinomycotic mycetoma caused by, 1400
Actinomyces/Actinomyces israelii (actino-mycosis), 1177t, **1323–1324**
Actinomycetoma, **1400–1401**
Actinomycotic mycetoma, **1400–1401**
Actiq. *See* Fentanyl
Activated charcoal, for poisoning/drug overdose, 1424, 1425
repeat-dose, 1426
Activated clotting time (ACT), reference values for, 1547t
Activated partial thromboplastin time. *See* Partial thromboplastin time
Activated protein C. *See* Protein C, acti-vated
Activella. *See* Estrogens, with progestins
Activities of daily living–instrumental activities of daily living (ADL–IADL), assessment of ability to perform in elderly, 62, 63
Activity. *See* Exercise/activity
ACTOplus Met. *See* Pioglitazone, with metformin
Actos. *See* Pioglitazone
Acuity, visual. *See* Visual acuity
Acular. *See* Ketorolac
Acupuncture, **1532–1534**
adverse events associated with, 1532
mechanism of action of, 1532
for migraine headache prophylaxis, 874, 1533
Acute angle-closure glaucoma. *See* Angle-closure glaucoma
Acute coronary syndromes, 326. *See also* Myocardial infarction
chest pain in, 28–29, 326
preoperative risk assessment/manage-ment, 50–51, 51t
without ST segment elevation, **325–330**, 327t, 329t
angiography/revascularization in, 328–329, 329t. *See also* Revascularization proce-dures

medical management of, 326–328, 327t
Acute flaccid paralysis (AFP)
coxsackievirus causing, 1279
enterovirus 71 causing, 1280
poliomyelitis and, 1252
Acute idiopathic polyneuropathy. *See* Guillain-Barré syndrome
Acute intermittent porphyria, 923, **1512–1513**, 1513t
Acute interstitial pneumonitis (AIP), 264t
Acute kidney injury (acute renal failure), 816, **819–825**, 820t. *See also* Kidney disease
ACE inhibitor use and, 405
acute tubular necrosis causing, 820t, **821–823**
cirrhosis and (hepatorenal syndrome), 622
glomerulonephritis causing, 820t, **824–825**, 833–834
interstitial nephritis causing, 820t, **823–824**
intrinsic disorders causing, 820t, 821
postoperative, 58–59, 59t
postrenal azotemia causing, 820t, 821
prerenal azotemia causing, 820–821, 820t
Acute leukemia, **464–466**. *See also specific type*
Acute lymphoblastic/lymphocytic leuke-mia (ALL), 464, 465, 466, 1466t
Acute monoblastic leukemia, 465
Acute motor axonal neuropathy (AMAN), 925
Acute motor and sensory axonal neuropa-thy (AMSAN), 925
Acute mountain sickness, **1417–1418**
Acute myeloblastic leukemia, 465
Acute myeloid leukemia (AML), 464, 465, 466, 1466t
bone marrow/stem cell transplanta-tion for, 475, 476
Acute myelomonocytic leukemia, 465
Acute paralytic ileus. *See* Paralytic (ady-namic) ileus
Acute promyelocytic leukemia (APL), 464, 465, 466
DIC associated with, 488
Acute renal failure. *See* Acute kidney injury
Acute respiratory distress syndrome (ARDS), **291–293**, 292t. *See also* Respiratory failure
acute gastric aspiration and, 278
in burn injury, 1412
deferoxamine infusion causing, 1437
in pancreatitis, 644
in SARS, 1275
smoke inhalation and, 277
Acute respiratory failure, **289–291**, 289t. *See also* Acute respiratory distress syndrome; Respi-ratory failure
Acute tubular necrosis. *See* Tubular necro-sis

Acute undifferentiated leukemia, 465
Acute vaccinia syndrome, 1277
Acyclovir, 1238t
for herpes simplex infections, 114, 727, 1157, 1215, 1224t, 1237, 1238t, 1239
esophageal infection and, 535, 1237–1239
keratitis, 173t, 1237
for herpes zoster, 115, 157, 1215, 1225t, 1238t, 1242
during pregnancy, 727, 1237, 1242
prophylactic/suppressive, 1215, 1237, 1242
renal/hepatic failure and, 1184t
for varicella, 1238t, 1242
ADA diet recommendations for diabetes, 1089
ADACEL. *See* Tdap vaccine
Adalat. *See* Nifedipine
Adalimumab. *See also* Anti-TNF agents
for inflammatory bowel disease, 577
Crohn disease, 581
for psoriasis, 105
for rheumatoid arthritis, 751
ADAMTS-13 (von Willebrand factor cleaving protease), in thrombotic microangiopa-thies, 485, 485t
Adapalene gel, for acne, 121
Addiction (drug), 977. *See also* Poisoning/drug overdose; Substance use disorders
pain management in terminally ill/dying patient and, 78
Addison disease, **1047–1050**
acute adrenal crisis in, 1049
hypercalcemia and, 1033, 1050
hyperkalemia and, 797, 1047, 1049
hyponatremia and, 789–790, 790f, 1047
insulin-induced hypoglycemia and, 1103
Adefovir, for hepatitis B, 610, 1238t
Adenitis. *See* Lymphadenitis
Adenocarcinoma. *See specific type and* Cancer
Adenoma sebaceum, 903
Adenomas. *See specific type or structure or organ affected*
Adenomatous polyposis coli gene. *See* APC gene
Adenomatous polyps, 589
colonoscopy in identification/treat-ment of, 589, 590, 1482
colorectal cancer and, 589, 590, 591, 1476, 1477
familial, **591**. *See also* Familial adeno-matous polyposis
FOBT in patients with, 589–590
gastric, 557, 591
malignant, 590
nonfamilial, **589–591**
of small intestine, 567, 589, 591
Adenomyomatosis, biliary tract/gallblad-der, 635t, 636
Adenomyosis, uterine, 683
Adenopathy. *See* Lymphadenopathy

Adenosine, 344t
  for paroxysmal supraventricular
      tachycardia, 342, 344t
Adenosine deaminase, ascitic fluid, in
      tuberculous peritonitis,
      525, 527
Adenosine triphosphatase, copper-trans-
      porting (ATP78), in Wil-
      son disease, 628, 629
Adenosylcobalamin, 445. See also Vitamin
      B$_{12}$
Adenovirus infections, **1275–1276**
  conjunctivitis/keratoconjunctivitis,
      154, 1275
  diarrhea/gastroenteritis, 1172, 1275
ADH. See Antidiuretic hormone
Adherence/nonadherence, patient, **1–2**
  antipsychotic drug administration
      and, 954, 957–958
  antiretroviral therapy and, 1, 1225,
      1231, 1232
  in elderly
      hearing amplification and, 75
      medication regimen and, 74
  lithium therapy and, 972
  tuberculosis therapy and, 254
Adhesion molecules, autoantibodies to, in
      pemphigus, 130
ADHH. See Autosomal dominant hypo-
      calcemia with hypercalci-
      uria
Adipokines
  insulin action in obesity and, 1081
  thiazolidinediones affecting release of,
      1093
Adiponectin
  insulin action in obesity and, 1081
  thiazolidinediones affecting release of,
      1093
Adipose tissue. See Body fat
Adjustment (situational) disorders,
      937–938
  with depressed mood, 961, 963
  posthospital, 989
  suicide risk and, 963
Adjuvant chemotherapy. See also Chemo-
      therapy
  for bladder cancer, 1490
  for breast cancer, 665–666, 665t
  for colorectal cancer, 1479–1480
  for esophageal cancer, 1469
  for gastric adenocarcinoma, 1472
  for lung cancer, 1456–1457
Adjuvant pain medications/treatments,
      85–86
ADL–IADL. See Activities of daily liv-
      ing–instrumental activi-
      ties of daily living
Adnexal masses. See Ovarian cancer/
      tumors
Adnexectomy, for PID, 689
ADPKD1/ADPKD2 genes, 847
Adrenal cortex
  diseases of, **1046–1058.** See also spe-
      cific disorder
  in HIV infection/AIDS, 1214
  hyperplasia of
      aldosteronism caused by, 392, 1056

amenorrhea and, 1068
  congenital, 1048, 1049, 1055
  Cushing syndrome caused by, 1051
  hirsutism/virilization and, 1054,
      1055
  in multiple endocrine neoplasia,
      1076
hypoplasia of
  congenital, 991, 992, 1048
  hypogonadotropic hypogonadism
      and, 991, 992, 1065
tumors of. See Adrenal tumors
Adrenal crisis, **1046–1047**
Adrenal hemorrhage, 1048
Adrenal insufficiency. See Adrenocortical
      insufficiency
Adrenal tumors
  amenorrhea caused by, 1068
  cancer, 1052, 1057, 1467t
  cortical
      aldosterone-secreting, 392, 1056,
          1057
      cortisol-secreting, 1051, 1052,
          1053
  medullary. See Paraganglioma; Pheo-
      chromocytoma
  in multiple endocrine neoplasia, 1076,
      1076t
  paraneoplastic syndromes associated
      with, 1453t
Adrenal vein sampling, in aldosteronism,
      1056, 1057
Adrenalectomy/medical adrenalectomy
  adrenal crisis and, 1046
  for aldosteronism, 1057
  for breast cancer, 668–669
      in male, 673
  for congenital adrenal hyperplasia,
      1054
  for Conn syndrome, 1057
  for Cushing syndrome, 1052, 1053
Adrenergic drugs. See Alpha-adrenergic
      agonists; Alpha-adrener-
      gic blocking drugs; Beta-
      adrenergic agonists; Beta-
      adrenergic blocking drugs
Adrenocortical insufficiency, 992,
      992–993, 994
  acute, **1046–1047**
  chronic, **1047–1050.** See also Addison
      disease
  DHEA for, 1050
  in HIV infection/AIDS, 1214
  hypercalcemia and, 1036
  hyperkalemia and, 797
  hyponatremia and, 789–790, 790f
  perioperative corticosteroid replace-
      ment and, 58
Adrenocorticosteroids. See Corticoste-
      roids
Adrenocorticotropic hormone (ACTH)
  deficiency of, 992, 992–993, 994. See
      also Adrenocortical insuffi-
      ciency
  ectopic/hypersecretion of, 1050–1051,
      1052, 1062
  petrosal sinus levels of, in Cushing
      syndrome, 1052

plasma levels of
  in acute adrenal insufficiency, 1047
  in Addison disease, 1049
  in Cushing syndrome, 1051
  reference values for, 1547t
Adrenoleukodystrophy, 1048, 1049
Adriamycin. See Doxorubicin
Adrucil. See Fluorouracil
Adson test, 932
Adult respiratory distress syndrome. See
      Acute respiratory distress
      syndrome
Adult T cell lymphoma/leukemia (ATL),
      1261. See also Human T
      cell lymphotropic/leuke-
      mia virus
Advance care planning, **90**
Advance directives, **90**
ADVANCE study, 1089
Advil. See Ibuprofen
Adynamic bone disease, 829
Adynamic ileus. See Paralytic (adynamic)
      ileus
Aedes mosquitoes. See Mosquitoes
Aeroallergens, 784
  in allergic rhinitis, 196, 197
  asthma caused by, 216, 221, 223
  avoidance therapy and, 197
  desensitization therapy/immunother-
      apy and, 228
AeroBid. See Flunisolide
Aerodigestive tract. See also specific struc-
      ture
  foreign bodies in, **212, 278**
Aeromonas, diarrhea caused by, 515, 1174
Aerophagia, 510–511
Aerophobia, in rabies, 1255
Affect, in schizophrenic/psychotic disor-
      ders, 953
AFP. See Acute flaccid paralysis; Alpha-
      fetoprotein
AFP-L3, in hepatocellular carcinoma,
      1460
African tick bite fever, 1281t, 1285
African trypanosomiasis, **1348–1349,**
      1349t
Age/aging. See also Older adults
  accommodative loss and (presbyopia),
      151
  benign prostatic hyperplasia and, 866
  breast cancer risk and, 652, 653t
  burn injury survival and, 1409
  colorectal cancer risk and, 1477
  fever/FUO and, 39, 1153
  hearing loss and (presbyacusis), 75,
      179, 186
  maternal, Down syndrome and, 1514
  paternal, mutations and, 1514
  postoperative delirium and, 56, 56t
  postoperative pulmonary complica-
      tions and, 53
  prostate cancer and, 1484
  PSA reference ranges and, 1485
  sleep changes and, 973
  theophyllines affected by, 225t
  weight loss and, 40–41, 72
Age-related macular degeneration,
      162–163

Age-related maculopathy, 162
Agenerase. *See* Amprenavir
Agglutinins
    cold, 453–454
    "febrile," 1154
Aggression, **976–977.** *See also* Violence
    alcohol use/abuse and, 976, 978
    anabolic steroid use and, 976, 984
    phencyclidine use/abuse and, 954,
        976, 982
Aggrestat. *See* Tirofiban
Aging. *See* Age/aging
Agitation, palliation of in terminally ill/
        dying patient, **87**
Agnogenic myeloid metaplasia (myelofi-
        brosis), 457t, **460–461**
Agnosia
    in dementia, 63
    intracranial tumors causing, 899
Agoraphobia, 940, 943
Agranulocytosis. *See also* Neutropenia
    drug-induced, 456
        clozapine causing, 955, 958
        mirtazapine causing, 966
        thiourea therapy causing, 1011
AI. *See* Aromatase inhibitors
AIDS. *See* HIV infection/AIDS
AIDS cholangiopathy, 1245, 1369, 1370
AIDS dementia complex (HIV-associated
        cognitive/motor com-
        plex), 986, 1212
AIDS enteropathy, 1214
AIDS wasting syndrome, 1209–1210
AIP. *See* Acute intermittent porphyria; Acute
        interstitial pneumonitis
Air bronchogram, in ARDS, 292
Air travel
    contraindications to, 1419
    dysbarism/decompression sickness
        and, 1416–1417
    eustachian tube dysfunction/
        barotrauma and, 182, 183
    lower extremity edema and, 37
    medical safety/patient selection and,
        1419
    during pregnancy, 710, 1419
    retinal detachment and, 162
    SARS transmission and, 1274, 1275
Airway disorders, **215–243.** *See also* spe-
        cific type
    allergic bronchopulmonary mycosis,
        241
    asthma, **216–234**
        occupational, 216, 280
    bronchiectasis, **240**
    bronchiolitis, **242–243**
    chronic obstructive pulmonary dis-
        ease (COPD), **234–240,**
        235t
    cystic fibrosis, **241–242**
    lower airway, **215–216**
    obstruction
        in diphtheria, 1302
        dyspnea and, 25, 25t
        by food (café coronary), **277**
        foreign body causing, 212, 278
        in hypoparathyroidism, 1031
        of lower airways, 215–216

    in mononucleosis, 1243
    near drowning and, 1416
    occupational disorders and, **280**
    during sleep (obstructive sleep
        apnea), **288–289**
    tracheostomy and cricothyrotomy
        for, 211–212
    of upper airways, 215
    respiratory failure caused by, 289t
    thermal injury, smoke inhalation and,
        277, 1409
    upper airway, **215**
Airway management. *See also* Intubation
    burn injury and, 1410
    for coma, 915, 1420, 1421
    in hypoparathyroidism, 1032
    tracheostomy and cricothyrotomy in,
        211–212
AIs. *See* Aromatase inhibitors
Akathisia
    antipsychotic drugs causing, 959
    SSRIs causing, 964
Akinesia, in Huntington disease, 908
Akinetic mutism (persistent vegetative
        state), **917**
Akineton. *See* Biperiden
AL amyloidosis, 841. *See also* Amyloidosis
Alanine aminotransferase (ALT),
        599–600, 600t
    in alcoholic liver disease, 614
    in liver disease/jaundice, 599–600, 600t
    in nonalcoholic fatty liver disease, 618
    olanzapine affecting, 956
    in preeclampsia-eclampsia, 717t
    reference/normal values for, 600t,
        1547t
    in viral hepatitis, 602f, 604f, 605
Alarm response, 940
Albendazole
    for ascariasis, 1379
    for clonorchiasis/opisthorchiasis, 1375
    for cysticercosis, 1378
    for enterobiasis/pinworms, 1382
    for filariasis, 1387
    for giardiasis, 1372
    for gnathostomiasis, 1384
    for hookworm disease, 1380
    for hydatid disease, 1379
    for microsporidiosis, 1371
    for trichinosis, 1384
    for trichuriasis/whipworm, 1380
Albinism, 144
Albumin
    ascitic fluid, 525. *See also* Serum-asci-
        tes albumin gradient
    in cirrhosis, 620
    serum levels of
        calcium levels and, 799, 1031,
            1496–1497
        in liver disease/jaundice, 600t
        in myeloma, 472
        in nephrotic syndrome, 838
        postoperative pulmonary compli-
            cations and, 54
        in protein-losing enteropathy, 569
        reference/normal values for, 600t,
            1547t
    urinary. *See* Albuminuria

Albuminuria. *See also* Proteinuria
    in diabetes/diabetic nephropathy, 842,
        1105
Albuterol
    for asthma, 228, 229t
        with ipratropium, 229t
    for cystic fibrosis, 242
    for hyperkalemia, 799t
Alclometasone, 96t
Alcohol addiction, 978. *See also* Alcohol
        use/dependency/abuse
Alcohol use/dependency/abuse (alcohol-
        ism), 19–20, 20t, 21t,
        978–981
    acupuncture for, 1534
    acute intoxication/poisoning, 978,
        985t, 1427t, **1436**
        metabolic acidosis/osmolar gap
            and, 795, 979, 1426
    aggressive/violent behavior and, 976,
        978
    amnestic syndrome and, 986
    anxiety self-treatment and, 942
    atrial fibrillation and, 346
    breast cancer and, 653
    in cardiomyopathy, 370, 371
    cirrhosis and, 614–616, 619, 620
        hepatocellular carcinoma and, 615,
            620, 624, 1460
    coma in diabetic patient and, 1112t
    complications associated with, 979
    Cushing syndrome/hypercortisolism
        and, 1052
    delirium caused by, 978, 985t
    depression and, 962, 970, 978
    differential diagnosis of, 979
    drug therapy for, 19–20, 980–981
    Dupuytren contracture and, 743
    esophageal cancer and, 1468
    fatty liver and, 614–616, 618
    folic acid deficiency and, 446, 447
    gastritis and, 544, 545
    gout/hyperuricemia and, 732, 733,
        734
    hepatitis and, 614–616
    hyperosmolality caused by, 795
    hypertension and, 390, 394, 395t
    hypoglycemia associated with, 981,
        1103, 1117t, 1118, **1121**
    hypophosphatemia and, 802–803
    immunization recommendations and,
        1195t
    incidence of, 19
    ketoacidosis and, 809, 811
    laryngeal squamous cell carcinoma
        and, 210
    lipid abnormalities and, 1125, 1126t
    liver cancer and, 615, 620, 624, 1460,
        1461
    liver disease associated with, **614–616**
        postoperative complications and,
            54
    Mallory-Weiss syndrome/tears and,
        518, 536
    management of, 19–20, 21t, 979–981
    myopathy associated with, 936
    neuropathy associated with, 923
    oral cancer and, 201

Alcohol use/dependency/abuse (alcoholism) (*cont.*)
  in pancreatitis, 642, 646
  in panic disorder, 940
  platelet function affected by, 490t
  porphyria cutanea tarda and, 117
  pregnancy and, 707, 979
  preventable deaths caused by, 2t
  prevention of injury related to, 18
  prevention of/screening tests for, **19–21**, 20t, 21t
  psychotic behavior associated with (alcoholic hallucinosis), 978–979, 979, 980, 986
  sleep disorders and, 974
  thiamin deficiency in, 809, 811, 915, 979, 1140–1141
  trauma outcome/incidence affected by, 18
  Wernicke encephalopathy/Wernicke-Korsakoff syndrome and, 915, 979, 981, 1141
  withdrawal and, 978
    delirium caused by, 978, 985t
    differential diagnosis of, 979
    drug therapy for, 980–981
    seizures caused by, 883, 978, 981
Alcohol Use Disorder Identification Test (AUDIT), 19, 20t
Alcoholic brain syndromes, chronic, 979
Alcoholic cardiomyopathy, 370, 371
Alcoholic (organic) hallucinosis, 978–979, 979, 980, 986
Alcoholic hepatitis, 614–616
  postoperative complications associated with, 54
Alcoholic hyaline (Mallory bodies), 614, 617
Alcoholic ketoacidosis, 809, 811
Alcoholics Anonymous, 970, 979
Aldactazide. *See* Spironolactone, for hypertension, with hydrochlorothiazide
Aldactone. *See* Spironolactone
Aldehyde dehydrogenase deficiency, alcohol use/abuse and, 978
Aldesleukin. *See also* Interleukin-2
  for cancer chemotherapy, 1506t
Aldicarb poisoning, 1443–1444
Aldolase, in polymyositis/dermatomyositis, 760
Aldomet. *See* Methyldopa
Aldosterone. *See also* Aldosteronism; Hypoaldosteronism
  drugs blocking receptors for. *See also* Spironolactone
    for hypertension, 391, 392, 396t, 399t, 405, 411
    for myocardial infarction, 335
  in hypertension, 390, 390–391, 391–392, 405, 411, 1056
  potassium balance/hypokalemia and, 795, 796
  in renal tubular acidosis, 809t, 810
  serum/urine levels of
    in primary aldosteronism, 391, 1056
    reference values for, 1547t

Aldosterone:renin ratio, 391, 394, 1056
Aldosteronism (hyperaldosteronism), **1055–1058**
  glucocorticoid-remediable, 390–391, 796t
  hypertension and, 390–391, 391–392, 393, 1055–1057
  hypokalemia and, 795, 796, 1056, 1057
  renal tubular acidosis and, 809t, 810
  saline-unresponsive metabolic alkalosis and, 813
Aldosteronoma, 392, 1056, 1057
Alefacept. *See also* Anti-TNF agents
  for psoriasis/psoriatic arthritis, 105, 775
Alemtuzumab, 1503t
  for chronic lymphocytic leukemia, 468
Alendronate, 1040, 1046. *See also* Bisphosphonates
  adverse ophthalmic effects of, 178t
  for osteoporosis prevention/management, 1040
  for Paget disease of bone, 1046
Aleukemic leukemia, 465
Aleve. *See* Naproxen
Alfieri procedure, 309
Alfuzosin, for benign prostatic hyperplasia, 869, 869t
Alimentary hypoglycemia, 1117
  functional, 1117, 1117t, **1121**
  postgastrectomy, 1117, 1117t, **1121**
Alimentary tract cancers, **1465–1483**
Alimta. *See* Pemetrexed
Aliskiren/aliskiren with hydrochlorothiazide, 402, 403t
ALK1 gene mutation, in hereditary hemorrhagic telangiectasia, 1519
Alkali administration. *See* Bicarbonate
Alkalies, caustic/corrosive, **1429–1430**
  esophageal injury caused by, 536, 1429–1430
  eye injury caused by, 172, 1430
Alkaline phosphatase
  in alcoholic liver disease, 614
  in cholecystitis, 636
  in choledocholithiasis/cholangitis, 638
  in cirrhosis, 619–620
  in hemochromatosis, 627
  in hepatocellular carcinoma, 1460
  in hypophosphatasia, 1043
  in liver disease/jaundice, 600, 600t
  in osteomalacia, 1043
  in Paget disease of bone, 1045
  reference/normal values for, 600t, 1547t
Alkalinization, urine. *See* Urine, alkalinization of
Alkalosis, 806
  contraction, 813
  in heat exhaustion, 1407
  in heat stroke, 1407, 1408
  metabolic, 806, 807t, **812–813**, 812t. *See also* Metabolic alkalosis
  posthypercapnia, 813, 814
  respiratory, 806, 807t, **814–815**. *See also* Respiratory alkalosis

  salicylate overdose/toxicity causing, 1445
  saline-responsive, 812, 812–813, 812t, 813
  saline-unresponsive, 812, 812t, 813
Alkaptonuria, **1513–1514**
Alkeran. *See* Melphalan
Alkylating agents, 1500–1501t
ALL. *See* Acute lymphoblastic/lymphocytic leukemia
All-Trans-Retinoic Acid. *See* Tretinoin
Allergens, 784. *See also* Allergies/allergic reactions
  anaphylaxis/urticaria/angioedema caused by, 126, 784
  asthma caused by, 216, 221, 223
    desensitization therapy/immunotherapy for, 228
  avoidance of
    for allergic contact dermatitis, 119
    for allergic rhinitis, 197
Allergic alveolitis, extrinsic (hypersensitivity pneumonitis), **279–280**, 280t
Allergic angiitis and granulomatosis (Churg-Strauss syndrome), 276
  leukotriene modifiers for asthma and, 228
  pulmonary involvement in, 276
  renal involvement in, 835f
Allergic bronchopulmonary mycosis/aspergillosis, **241**, 1397, 1398
Allergic conjunctivitis, 155
Allergic contact dermatitis, **118–120**, 784
  impetigo differentiated from, 118, 119
  topical medications causing, 95, 119
  urticarial lesions in, 126
Allergic eye disease, **155**
Allergic rhinitis (hay fever), **196–197**
  conjunctivitis and, 155
  nasal polyps and, 196, 199
Allergic vasculitis, drugs causing, 148t
Allergies/allergic reactions, **784**
  anaphylactic, 784
  angioedema and, 126
  antibody-mediated (cytotoxic), 784
  asthma and, 216, 221, 223
    desensitization therapy/immunotherapy for, 228
  atopic, 784, **784–785**
  to drugs. *See* Drug allergy
  eosinophilic esophagitis and, 537
  in HIV infection/AIDS, 1208
  IgE-mediated (immediate), 784
  immune complex-mediated, 784
  to insulin, 1104
  pseudoallergic (anaphylactoid), **785–786**
  radiocontrast media causing, 786
  T-cell mediated (delayed/cell-mediated), 784
  urticaria caused by, 126
Allergy testing, 784
Allgrove (triple A) syndrome, 1048, 1049
Allicin, 1524. *See also* Garlic
Allium sativum (garlic), 1523t, 1524

Allogeneic stem cell transplantation, **475–476**. *See also* Bone marrow/stem cell transplantation

Alloimmunization, platelet transfusion and, 478

Allopurinol
  drug interactions of, 735
    azathioprine/mercaptopurine dosage adjustments and, 735
  for hyperuricemia/gout, 734, 735
    in cancer patients, 1497, 1507*t*
    in polycythemia, 458
    stone formation and, 859
    in transplant patients, 735
  for tumor lysis syndrome, 1497, 1507*t*

Almonds (bitter), odor of in cyanide poisoning, 1435

Alocril. *See* Nedocromil

Alomide. *See* Lodoxamide

Alopecia, **145–146**
  androgenetic/androgenic (pattern), 145–146
    in women, 146, 1053, 1055
  areata, 146
  chemotherapy-induced, 1509
  nonscarring, **145–146**
  scarring (cicatricial), **145**
  in syphilis, 1334
  totalis, 146
  universalis, 146

Alora. *See* Estradiol transdermal systems

Alosetron, for irritable bowel syndrome, 572

Alpha-adrenergic agonists, for glaucoma/ocular hypertension, 159

Alpha-adrenergic blocking drugs
  for benign prostatic hyperplasia, 869, 869*t*
  for hypertension, 407, 408*t*
  pheochromocytoma surgery and, 1060
  for ureteral stones, 860
  for urinary incontinence, 72

Alpha$_1$-antiprotease/antitrypsin
  in COPD/emphysema, 235
  replacement therapy and, 238
  in protein-losing enteropathy, 569
  reference values for, 1547*t*

Alpha-delta storage pool disease, 489

Alpha-fetoprotein
  in Down syndrome, 1514
  in hepatocellular carcinoma, 1460, 1460–1461
  prenatal testing for, 706
  reference values for, 1549*t*
  testicular tumors producing, 1066, 1493

Alpha-globin gene, 442
  in alpha thalassemia syndromes, 442, 443, 443*t*

Alpha-glucosidase inhibitors, for diabetes mellitus, 1091*t*, 1094–1095, 1101

Alpha interferon. *See* Interferon-α

Alpha-linolenic acid, health benefits of, 1530–1531

5-Alpha-reductase, deficiency of, 1054

5-Alpha-reductase inhibitors. *See also* Finasteride
  for benign prostatic hyperplasia, 870

Alpha-synuclein gene, in parkinsonism, 905

Alpha thalassemia syndromes, 442, 442–443, 443–444, 443*t*
  sickle cell disease and, 451*t*, 452

Alpha thalassemia trait, 443, 443–444, 443*t*

Alphagan. *See* Brimonidine

ALPL gene, in hypophosphatasia, 1043

Alprazolam, 941*t*
  for panic attacks, 942, 943

Alprenolol, overdose/toxicity of, 1432

Alprostadil, for erectile dysfunction, 863, 1108

ALT. *See* Alanine aminotransferase

Altace. *See* Ramipril

Alteplase (tissue plasminogen activator/t-PA). *See also* Thrombolytic therapy
  for acute arterial occlusion of limb, 419
  for myocardial infarction, 333*t*, 334
  for pulmonary embolism, 273, 501*t*
  for stroke, 891

Altered mental status. *See* Mental status, altered

Alternaria, phaeohyphomycosis caused by, 1402

Alternative medicine. *See* Complementary/alternative medicine

Altitude-related illness, **1417–1419**

Altretamine, 1504*t*

Aluminum preparations
  for hyperphosphatemia, 804
    mineral bone disorders of chronic kidney disease and, 830
  osteomalacia caused by, 829, 830, 1043

Alveolar-arterial oxygen difference (A–a Do$_2$)
  in asthma, 219
  in COPD, 234
  in pulmonary embolism, 267

Alveolar hemorrhage syndromes, **276**

Alveolar hydatid disease, 1378–1379

Alveolar hyperventilation, 287–288

Alveolar hypoventilation
  central, 287
  obesity and (Pickwickian syndrome), 287
  primary (Ondine curse), **287**

Alveolar proteinosis, **266**

Alveolitis
  cryptogenic fibrosing (idiopathic fibrosing interstitial pneumonia), **263–265**, 264*t*
  extrinsic allergic (hypersensitivity pneumonitis), **279–280**, 280*t*

Alvimopan, for acute paralytic ileus, 564

Alzheimer disease, 63, 986. *See also* Dementia
  clinical features of, 64, 986
  estrogen replacement therapy and, 1072

ginseng for, 1526
hypertension and, 393
seizures in, 879
treatment of, 65–66, 987–988
  ginkgo in, 1523*t*, 1524–1525

Alzheimer's Association/Alzheimer's Disease and Related Disorders Association, 65, 987–988

AMAN. *See* Acute motor axonal neuropathy

Amanita mushroom poisoning, 1441, 1441*t*, 1442

Amanitin toxin (amatoxin), poisoning with mushrooms containing, 1441, 1441*t*, 1442

Amantadine, 959. *See also* Antiparkinsonism drugs
  influenza/influenza resistance and, 1270, 1271, 1272, 1273
  for neuroleptic malignant syndrome, 959
  for parkinsonism, 906

Amaryl. *See* Glimepiride

Amatoxin (amanitin toxin), poisoning with mushrooms containing, 1441, 1441*t*, 1442

Amaurosis fugax, 165, 420, 889

Ambien. *See* Zolpidem

AmBisome. *See* Liposomal amphotericin B

Amblyomma ticks. *See* Ticks

Ambulatory blood pressure monitoring, 387, 388*t*

Ambulatory electrocardiographic monitoring
  in angina, 320
  in arrhythmia evaluation, seizures and, 881
  in palpitation evaluation, 31–32
  in syncope evaluation, 357

Ambulatory esophageal pH monitoring. *See* Esophageal pH monitoring

Ambulatory peritoneal dialysis, continuous, 831

Amcinonide, 96*t*

Amebas, pathogenic free-living, **1368–1369**
  meningoencephalitis caused by, 1163–1164, **1368**

Amebiasis (entamoeba infection), **1365–1368**, 1367*t*
  extraintestinal, 1366, 1367–1368, 1367*t*
  hepatic (amebic liver abscess), 1366, 1367–1368, 1367*t*
  intestinal, 512, 514, 515, 1172, 1174, 1182*t*, 1366, 1367, 1367*t*

Amebic encephalitis/meningoencephalitis, 1163–1164, **1368**
  granulomatous, 1164, **1368**

Amebic liver abscess (hepatic amebiasis), 1366, 1367–1368, 1367*t*

Amebic ulcers, 1366

Amebicides, 1366–1367, 1367*t*
  adverse ophthalmic effects of, 178*t*

Ameboma, 1366, 1367*t*

Amegakaryocytic thrombocytopenia, 480, 481
Amen. *See* Progesterone
Amenorrhea, **1067–1073**
  in anorexia nervosa, 1139
  in hyperprolactinemia, 1000, 1068, 1069, 1070
  hypogonadism and, 1067–1068, 1068, 1069, 1070
  in polycystic ovary syndrome, 690, 1053, 1069
  pregnancy/lactation causing, 709, 1068, 1068–1069, 1070
  primary, **1067–1068**
  secondary, **1068–1073**. *See also* Menopause; Pregnancy
  in Turner syndrome, 1068, 1074, 1075
American Diabetes Association diet recommendations, 1089
American ginseng, 1526
American trypanosomiasis (Chagas disease), **1349–1351**
  achalasia in, 542
  heart disease/myocarditis in, 368, 1350
Amevive. *See* Alefacept
AMG 531, for myelodysplasia, 463
Amicar. *See* ε-Aminocaproic acid
Amifostine, for chemotherapy/radiation-induced toxicity, 1507*t*
  cisplatin therapy and, 1507*t*, 1511
Amikacin, 1179*t*, 1544*t*
  in renal failure, 1179*t*
Amikin. *See* Amikacin
Amiloride
  for heart failure, 361
  hyperkalemia caused by, 798
  for hypertension, 399*t*
    with hydrochlorothiazide, 399*t*
  lithium interactions and, 972, 972*t*
ε-Aminocaproic acid (EACA), for intracranial aneurysm, 894
Aminoglutethimide, for prostate cancer, 1487*t*
Aminoglycosides, 1179*t*
  contraindications to in myasthenia gravis, 933, 934
  for endocarditis, 1306
  nephrotoxicity/acute kidney injury and, 821
  neuromuscular transmission affected by, **934**
  ototoxicity of, 186
  in renal failure, 1179*t*
Aminolevulinic acid, urinary, in porphyria, 1512
Aminophylline
  for asthma, 228
  lithium interactions and, 972*t*
  for lithium overdose/toxicity, 972
5-Aminosalicylic acid, for inflammatory bowel disease, 575
  colorectal cancer risk and, 586, 1477
  Crohn disease, 580
  ulcerative colitis, 584, 586
Aminotransferase levels. *See also* Alanine aminotransferase; Aspartate aminotransferase

  in acetaminophen toxicity, 607, 1428
  in alcoholic liver disease, 614
  in autoimmune hepatitis, 612
  in cholecystitis, 636
  in choledocholithiasis/cholangitis, 638
  in hepatic failure, 607
  in liver disease/jaundice, 599–600, 600*t*
  in nonalcoholic fatty liver disease, 618
  postoperative complications and, 54, 55
  in viral hepatitis, 602, 602*f*, 604*f*, 605, 609
  zileuton affecting, 228
Amiodarone
  adverse ophthalmic effects of, 177*t*
  for arrhythmias, 343*t*
    atrial fibrillation, 347, 348, 349
    infarct-related, 340
    ventricular tachycardia, 352
  epididymitis and, 856
  hyperthyroidism caused by, 1009, 1010, 1013–1014
  hyponatremia caused by, 790
  hypothyroidism caused by, 1003–1004
  levothyroxine therapy affected by, 1006
Amitriptyline, 966, 968*t*, 1544*t*. *See also* Antidepressants
  for interstitial cystitis, 861
  for migraine prophylaxis, 874*t*
  for neuropathic pain/painful diabetic neuropathy, 85*t*, 1107
  for postherpetic neuralgia, 115, 878
AML. *See* Acute myeloid leukemia
Amlodipine. *See also* Calcium channel blocking drugs
  for angina, 322
  for heart failure, 365, 407
  for hypertension, 406*t*
  lower extremity edema caused by, 37
  overdose/toxicity of, 406*t*, 1432
Ammonia
  in hepatic encephalopathy, 622
  in hepatic failure, 607
  reference values for, 1547*t*
  urine, in hyperchloremic metabolic acidosis/renal tubular acidosis, 809*t*, 810
Amnesia
  in delirium, 986
  dissociative, 940
  in head injury, 918
Amnestic syndrome, 986
Amniocentesis, 707
Amodiaquine, for malaria, 1355*t*, 1357
  with artesunate (ASAQ), 1355*t*, 1356*t*, 1357*t*, 1360
  with sulfadoxine-pyrimethamine, 1356*t*
Amoxapine, 966, 968*t*
Amoxicillin/amoxicillin-clavulanate
  for anthrax, 1301, 1301*t*
  for bacterial rhinosinusitis, 194, 194*t*
  for endocarditis, 1306*t*
  in *H pylori* eradication therapy, 551*t*
  prophylactic, 1158

Amphetamines
  abuse/overdose of, **983–984**, **1430**
  adverse ophthalmic effects of, 177*t*
  during pregnancy, 707
Amphotericin B, 1401*t*
  for aspergillosis, 1158, 1398
  for blastomycosis, 1399
  for candidiasis, 1390, 1391
  for coccidioidomycosis, 1393, 1394
  for cryptococcal meningitis, 1224*t*, 1396–1397
  for histoplasmosis, 1392
  for leishmaniasis, 1352
  lipid-based preparations of, 1401*t*, 1402. *See also* Lipid-based amphotericin B
  for mucormycosis, 195, 1398–1399
  nephrotoxicity/acute kidney injury and, 821–822
  for *P marneffei* infection, 1400
  prophylactic, 1158
  in renal/hepatic failure, 1184*t*
  for sporotrichosis, 1400
Amphotericin B lipid complex, 1401*t*. *See also* Lipid-based amphotericin B
Ampicillin
  allopurinol interactions and, 735
  for endocarditis, 1306, 1306*t*
  rash caused by, 1180
    in mononucleosis, 204, 1243
  renal/hepatic failure and, 1184*t*
  for urinary tract infection, 852*t*
Ampicillin-sulbactam, renal/hepatic failure and, 1184*t*
Amprenavir, 1229, 1232*f*. *See also* Antiretroviral therapy
Ampulla of Vater, carcinoma of (ampullary/periampullary carcinoma), **1463–1465**
Ampullary adenomas, 567
Ampullary carcinoma, 1474
Amputation
  in acute arterial occlusion of limb, 419
  in electrical burns, 1411
  for frostbite, 1406
  in lower leg/foot occlusive disease, 418
AMS. *See* Acute mountain sickness
AMSAN. *See* Acute motor and sensory axonal neuropathy
Amyl nitrite
  abuse of, 984
  for cyanide poisoning, 1435, 1435*t*
Amylase
  ascitic fluid, 525, 528
  in pancreatitis, 644
  in pancreatic enzyme supplements, 647*t*
  pleural fluid, 283
  serum levels of
    in mumps, 1250
    in pancreatitis, 642–643, 644, 646
    reference values for, 1547*t*
Amyloidosis, 841–842
  cardiomyopathy and, 374
  familial Mediterranean fever and, 528
  myeloma and, 472, 848

neuropathy and, 924
renal, **841–842**
Amyotrophic lateral sclerosis, 920, 921
dementia and, 64
Amyotrophy
diabetic, 923, 1106
neuralgic (idiopathic brachial plexus
neuropathy), 930–931
ANA. *See* Antinuclear antibody
Anabolic steroids
abuse of, 984
aggression/violence and, 976, 984
gynecomastia and, 1067
for AIDS wasting, 1210
Anaerobic infections, **1321–1323**
pleuropulmonary (pneumonia/lung
abscess), 244t, **250**, 1322
Anafranil. *See* Clomipramine
Anagrelide
for essential thrombocytosis, 459
for polycythemia, 458
Anakinra, for Still disease, 752
Anal dysplasia/cancer, 1468t, **1483**
in HIV infection/AIDS, 1216, 1483
Anal fissures, 596
in Crohn disease, 578, 579
GI bleeding and, 521
Anal gonorrhea, 594, 1319, 1320
Anal sphincter, disorders of, fecal incontinence and, 595, 595–596
Anal syphilis, 594
Analgesia/analgesics, **78–86**, 79–83t. *See
also specific type or disorder
and* Pain management
acupuncture and, **1532–1534**
breast feeding and, 710t
caffeine-containing, 984
for chronic pain/chronic pain disorders, 78–84, 81–83t, 947
in end-of-life care, 77–78
thrombocytopenia caused by, 483t
tubulointerstitial disease caused by,
845, 846
Analgesic nephropathy, 845, 846
ureteral/renal pelvis cancer and,
1491
Analgesic rebound headache, **876**
Anaphylactic transfusion reactions, 478
Anaphylactoid (pseudoallergic) reactions, **785–786**
Anaphylaxis, 784
insect stings causing, 784
insulin allergy causing, 1104
penicillin allergy causing, 1180
Anaplasma (anaplasmosis), 1281t,
1285–1286
babesiosis coinfection and, 1286
equi, 1281t
Lyme disease coinfection and, 1286,
1346
phagocytophilum, 1281t, 1285
Anaprox. *See* Naproxen
Anasarca, 524–525
Anastrozole, 668t, 1506t
ANCA. *See* Antineutrophil cytoplasmic
antibody
Ancef. *See* Cefazolin
Ancobon. *See* Flucytosine

Ancylostoma
braziliense, 1385
caninum, 1380, 1385
duodenale, 1380
Androderm. *See* Testosterone replacement
therapy
AndroGel. *See* Testosterone replacement
therapy
Androgen deprivation, for prostate cancer, 1487–1488, 1487t
Androgen insensitivity/resistance
male hypogonadism caused by, 865f,
1064
pseudohermaphroditism/amenor-
rhea in, 1068
Androgenetic (androgenic/pattern) baldness, 145–146
in women, 146, 1053, 1055
Androgens. *See also* Antiandrogens; Testosterone
deficiency of, in women, replacement
and, 1070, 1073
excess of. *See* Hyperandrogenism
Androstenedione, in hirsutism/viriliza-
tion, 1054
Anejaculation, 862, 949
Anemias, **439–456**, 440t. *See also specific
cause or type*
in cancer chemotherapy, 1499
in celiac disease, 559
of chronic disease, **441–442**
in cirrhosis, 619, 623
classification of, 439, 440t
in colorectal cancer, 1478
fish tapeworm infection and, 445, 1376
in hairy cell leukemia, 468
in heart failure, 360
hemolytic. *See* Hemolytic anemias/
hemolysis
in hookworm disease, 1380
in hypophosphatemia, 803
in kidney disease, 816, 819, 828–829
macrocytic, 439, 440t
malabsorption and, 558t
in malaria, 1354
microcytic, 439, 440t
in myelodysplasia, 463
in myelofibrosis, 460
in myeloma, 472
during pregnancy, 439, 708, **721**
preoperative evaluation/management
and, 55
refractory, 463
retinal disease associated with, 167
in SLE, 754t
thiazolidinediones causing, 1094
in Waldenström macroglobulinemia,
474
Anergy, skin test. *See* Skin test anergy
Anesthesia/anesthetics
liver function affected by, **54**
local, for eye disorders, precautions
for use of, **172**
Aneuploidy screening, in prenatal testing,
706, 707
Aneurysms, **423–427**. *See also specific type
and artery involved*
mycotic, drug use and, 1168

Angiitis
allergic, granulomatosis and. *See*
Allergic angiitis and granulomatosis
primary, of central nervous system,
772–773
Angina
intestinal (visceral artery insufficiency), **421–422**
Ludwig, 206
pectoris, **317–325**. *See also* Coronary
heart disease
alteration in before myocardial
infarction, 330
in aortic regurgitation, 312, 318
aortic stenosis and, 310, 318
in apathetic hyperthyroidism,
1014–1015
chest pain in, 28–29, 318
change in before STEMI, 330
chronic stable, **317–325**
coronary vasospasm and, 317,
325
differential diagnosis of, 320–321
jaw pain and, 318, 878
postinfarction, 336, 339
preoperative risk assessment/man-
agement and, 49–50, 51f
prevention of further attacks and,
321–324
trial results in, 324
Prinzmetal (variant), 325
prognosis for, 324
in pulmonary embolism, 268t
risk reduction and, 322
treatment of, 321
unstable. *See* Acute coronary syndromes; Unstable angina
Angiodysplasias (vascular ectasias), GI
bleeding and, 518,
520–521
Angioedema, **125–127**
ACE inhibitor/angiotensin II receptor
antagonist therapy and,
126, 405
Angiofibroma
juvenile, 200
in multiple endocrine neoplasia, 1076,
1076t
Angiography/arteriography. *See also specific disorder*
in aortoiliac occlusive disease, 415
cardiac/coronary. *See also* Cardiac
catheterization
in acute coronary syndromes,
328–329, 329t
in angina, 320, 325
cerebral. *See* Cerebral angiography/
arteriography; Neuroim-
aging
CT. *See* Computed tomography; Helical (spiral) CT
in GI bleeding, 520, 521–522, 523
interventional. *See* Embolization
left ventricular, 320
magnetic resonance. *See* Magnetic resonance angiography
in polyarteritis nodosa, 765

Angiography/arteriography (*cont.*)
pulmonary, in pulmonary embolism, 270
helical CT, 30, 269, 270, 271*f*
radionuclide
in angina, 319
in heart failure, 360
in myocardial infarction, 331
in renal artery stenosis/renal vascular hypertension, 391, 833
Angiomas/angiomatosis
bacillary, 1215, 1321
spider, in cirrhosis, 619
in Sturge-Weber syndrome, 904
Angiomyolipomas, of kidney, 1491, 1492
Angioplasty. *See also* Endovascular surgery/prostheses
carotid, 420–421
coronary, for myocardial infarction, 335–336
for hepatic vein obstruction (Budd-Chiari syndrome), 631
percutaneous transluminal coronary. *See* Percutaneous transluminal coronary angioplasty
for renal artery stenosis, 391, 833
for superior vena caval obstruction, 432
for visceral artery insufficiency/intestinal angina, 422
Angiostrongylus cantonensis/costaricensis (angiostrongyliasis), **1384**
Angiotensin II, in hypertension, 390, 402
Angiotensin II receptor blocking agents
angioedema/urticaria and, 126
for heart failure, 362
infarct-related, 340
hyperkalemia caused by, 797, 798
for hypertension, 396*t*, 403–404*t*, 405, 407, 409, 409*f*
in chronic kidney disease/renal failure, 410, 828, 842
in combination regimen, 409, 409*f*
in diabetics, 396*t*, 409–410, 842
for myocardial infarction, 335
for nephrotic syndrome, 839
preoperative cessation of, 52
Angiotensin-converting enzyme (ACE)
in hypertension, 390
reference values for, 1547*t*
in sarcoidosis, 265
Angiotensin-converting enzyme (ACE) inhibitors
for acute coronary syndromes, 327*t*
angioedema/urticaria and, 126, 405
for aortic regurgitation, 312
cough and, 405
for heart failure, 361, 361–362
chronic kidney disease and, 828
infarct-associated, 340
hyperkalemia caused by, 405, 797, 798
for hypertension, 396*t*, 402–405, 403*t*, 407, 409, 409*f*
in combination regimen, 402, 409, 409*f*
contraindications to in pregnancy, 405, 723

in diabetics, 396*t*, 402–405, 407, 409–410, 842, 1088, 1105, 1106, 1108
renal disease and, 405, 410, 820, 828, 842
hyponatremia caused by, 790, 790*f*
lithium interactions and, 972, 972*t*
for myocardial infarction, 327*t*, 335
for nephrotic syndrome, 839
preoperative cessation of, 52
prerenal azotemia caused by, 820
Angle closure, pupillary dilation and, 157, 172
Angle-closure glaucoma
acute, 153*t*, **157–158**
pupillary dilation precipitating, 157, 172
chronic, 157, 159
Angular cheilitis
candidiasis and, 202
in HIV infection/AIDS, 1213
Anhedonia, 961. *See also* Depression
Anhidrosis and asthenia (tropical), 124
Anicteric leptospirosis, 1341
Anidulafungin, 1390, 1391, 1401*t*, 1402
Aniline, methemoglobinemia caused by, 1440
Animal bites, **1165–1166**. *See also* Insect bites/stings
poisonous snake, 1424*t*, **1446–1447**
rabies and, 1165, 1255, 1256
Anion gap/anion gap acidosis, 807, 807–808, 808*t*, 809*t*
alcoholic ketoacidosis and, 809
decreased, 808, 808*t*
diabetic ketoacidosis and, 808–809, 1115
increased, 807, **808–809**, 808*t*, 811
lactic acidosis and, 808, 1117
normal, 807, 808*t*, **809–812**, 809*t*, 811. *See also* Hyperchloremic normal anion gap acidosis
with osmolar gap, 795, 1426
in poisoning/drug overdose, 809, 1426
with methanol or ethylene glycol, 809, 1426, 1439, 1440
with salicylates, 809, 1426, 1445
in renal failure (uremic), 809, 819
in renal tubular acidosis, 809*t*, 810
Anisakiasis (*Anisakis marina*), **1385–1386**
gastritis caused by, 547, 1385
Anismus (pelvic floor dyssynergia), 507–508, 508
biofeedback in management of, 1536*t*, 1538
Ankle–brachial index (ABI/ABPI)
in femoral/popliteal occlusive disease, 416
in lower leg/foot occlusive disease, 418
in venous insufficiency, 37, 143, 144
Ankle sprains, **746–747**
Ankylosing spondylitis, **773–775**
back pain caused by, 738, 739, 773, 774
inflammatory bowel disease and, 777
in reactive arthritis, 776
ANNA-1. *See* Antineuronal nuclear antibodies

Annuloplasty, for tricuspid regurgitation, 314
Anocutaneous reflex, fecal continence and, 595
Anogenital/perianal pruritus, **136–137**, 596–597
in enterobiasis/pinworms, 1382
Anogenital warts. *See* Venereal (genital) warts
Anopheles mosquitoes. *See* Mosquitoes
Anorectal disorders, **593–597**. *See also* Genital ulcers
anal cancer, 1468*t*, **1483**
bleeding in, 521. *See also* Rectal bleeding
chlamydial, 594, 1328
constipation and, 508
in Crohn disease, 578, 579
fecal incontinence and, 595
fissures/abscesses/fistula, 596
gonococcal, 594, 1319, 1320
in granuloma inguinale, 1320–1321
hemorrhoids, **593–594**
in herpes simplex infection, 594–595, 1236
infections, **594–595**
in lymphogranuloma venereum, 1328
in syphilis, 594, 1330
venereal warts, 595
Anorexia
in cirrhosis, 619
nervosa, **1138–1140**
bulimia and (bulimarexia), 1140
Cushing syndrome and, 1052
Anorgasmia. *See* Orgasm, loss of
Anoscopy
in GI bleeding, 521
in hemorrhoids/fecal incontinence, 593, 595–596
Anosmia, 197–198, 899
Anosognosia, intracranial tumors causing, 899
Anovulation
differential diagnosis of, 690
dysfunctional uterine bleeding and, 674
infertility and, 693
ovulation induction and, 693
in polycystic ovary syndrome, 690, 1053
Ansaid. *See* Flurbiprofen
Anserine bursitis, 745
Antacids. *See also* Acid-antisecretory agents
antidepressant drug interactions and, 969*t*
benzodiazepine interactions and, 942*t*
diarrhea caused by, 515
for GERD, 533
hypermagnesemia and, 806
for peptic ulcer disease, 550
Anterior blepharitis, 152
Anterior chest wall syndrome, 321
Anterior communicating artery occlusion, in stroke, 889
Anterior cruciate ligament, of knee, assessment of, 34–35

Anterior drawer sign/test
     in ankle sprain, 746
     in knee pain, 34
Anterior hypopituitarism, **991–995**
Anterior interosseous syndrome, **927**
Anterior ischemic optic neuropathy, 168
     in giant cell arteritis, 168, 766
Anterior talofibular ligament, ankle
          sprains involving, 746
Anterior uveitis, 153t, 160. See also Uveitis
Anthracyclines, 1502t
     for breast cancer, 665
     cardiac toxicity of, 1511
          dexrazoxane for, 1507t, 1511
Anthrax, 1177t, **1300–1302**, 1301t
Anthrax vaccine, 1302
Antiandrogens
     for cancer chemotherapy, 1505t
     for hirsutism/virilization, 1055
     pregnancy and, 1055
     for prostate cancer, 1487–1488, 1487t
Antianginal drugs, 321–322
     preoperative, 50, 51t
Antianxiety drugs, 941–943, 941t, 942t.
          See also specific type
     breast feeding and, 710t
Antiarrhythmic drugs, 343–344t. See also
          specific agent and specific
          arrhythmia
     for arrhythmias in poisoning/drug
          overdose, 1422
     in heart failure, 365
     for infarct-associated arrhythmias,
          335, 340
     overdose/toxicity of, 343–344t, 1422t,
          1445
Antibacterial agents. See also Antibiotics;
          Antimicrobial therapy
     adverse ophthalmic effects of,
          177–178t
     ophthalmic, 173t
Antibiotic-associated colitis/diarrhea,
          511, **573–575**, 1172
     C difficile causing, 511, 573, 574,
          1170t, 1172
Antibiotics, 1176–1178t. See also specific
          type or disorder and Anti-
          microbial therapy
     for acne, 97t, 121
     adverse reactions/toxicity and, 1178
          dermatitis medicamentosa, 148
          ophthalmic, 176, 177–178t
     allergy to, 95
     for asthma, 230
     for bacterial rhinosinusitis, 193–194,
          194t, 1182t
     for bite wounds, 1166
     for brain abscess, 902, 1164
     C difficile colitis/diarrhea and, 511,
          573, 574, 1170t
     for COPD, 238
     cost of, 1180
     for Crohn disease, 580
     for cystic fibrosis, 242
     for diarrhea, 514, 574–575, 1172
     in fever management, 40, 1155
     for gram-negative bacteremia/sepsis,
          1176t, 1311–1312

in H pylori eradication therapy, 550,
          551t, 1176t
in immunocompromised host,
          1158–1159, 1498
for impetigo, 97t, 118, 1182t
infection in cancer patient and, 1498
intravenous administration of,
          1178–1180
for irritable bowel syndrome, 572
for malaria, 1360
for meningitis, 1163t, 1181t
in neutropenic patient, 40, 1158,
          1181t, 1498
ophthalmic, 173t
oral contraceptive failure and, 121
perioperative
     pulmonary complications and, 54
     for surgical site infections, **59–60**,
          60t
for pharyngitis, 204–205, 1182t,
          1289–1290
for PID, 688, 1182t
platelet function affected by, 490t
for pneumonia, 244–245t, 246–247,
          249
prophylactic. See Antimicrobial
          chemoprophylaxis
renal/hepatic failure and, 1184–1185t
resistance to. See Drug resistance
routes of administration for,
          1178–1180
for shock, 437
for spontaneous bacterial peritonitis,
          526, 527, 622
thrombocytopenia caused by, 483t
topical
     for acne, 97t, 121
     for impetigo, 97t, 118
Antibodies. See also Immunoglobulins
     infections associated with defects in,
          1156
     in common variable immunodefi-
          ciency, 786–787
Antibody-mediated (cytotoxic/type II)
          hypersensitivity, 784
Anticancer drugs. See Chemotherapy
Anticardiolipin antibodies, 722, 753, 756.
          See also Lupus anticoagu-
          lant-anticardiolipin-
          antiphospholipid anti-
          body syndrome
     in antiphospholipid antibody syn-
          drome, 753, 756
     pregnancy loss and, 722
     in SLE, 753, 754t
Anti-CCP antibodies, in rheumatoid
          arthritis, 748
Anti-CD3 antibodies, in diabetes delay/
          prevention, 1087
Anticentromere antibody, 754t
     in CREST syndrome/scleroderma,
          754t, 758
Anticholinergic agents
     for allergic disorders/rhinitis, 197
     antidepressant drug interactions and,
          969t
     for asthma, 228, 229t
     for COPD, 237

for irritable bowel syndrome, 572
for nausea and vomiting, 87, 507
overdose/toxicity of, 1424t, **1432**
     ophthalmic effects and, 177t
for parkinsonism, 906, 906t
Anticholinergic syndrome/effects, 1426,
          1432
     of antidepressants, 966–967, 968t,
          1448
     of antipsychotic drugs, 954, 956t, 958
     hallucinogens causing, 1439
Anticholinergic-type mushroom poison-
          ing, 1441, 1441t, 1442
Anticholinesterases/acetylcholinesterase
          inhibitors
     for Alzheimer disease/dementia, 65,
          987
     for myasthenia gravis diagnosis/treat-
          ment, 932, 933
     overdose/toxicity/poisoning with,
          1424t, **1443–1444**
     nerve agents and, 1434
Anticipatory anxiety, in panic disorders,
          940
Anticoagulants, lupus. See Lupus antico-
          agulant
Anticoagulation therapy
     for acute arterial occlusion of limb,
          419
     for acute coronary syndromes,
          326–328, 327t
     antidepressant drug interactions and,
          969t
     for antiphospholipid antibody syn-
          drome, 756
     in SLE, 755
     for atrial fibrillation, 348
          in hyperthyroidism, 1014
          in mitral stenosis, 307
     for atrial flutter, 350
     breast feeding and, 710t
     bridging, 55, 56t, 316
          after cardiac valve replacement, 316
          endocarditis and, 1307
          pregnancy and, 316
     for deep venous thrombosis/pulmo-
          nary embolism (venous
          thromboembolic disease)
          prevention and, 495–496, 496t
          treatment and, 272–273, 496–500,
          497t, 498t, 499t, 500t
     duration of, 499–500, 500t
     in endocarditis, 1307
     ginkgo interactions and, 1525
     for heart failure, 365
     for heparin-induced thrombocytope-
          nia, 487
     for hepatic vein obstruction (Budd-
          Chiari syndrome), 630
     in hypocystinuria, 1517
     investigational oral agents in, 498–499
     for lupus anticoagulant-anticardio-
          lipin-antiphospholipid
          antibody syndrome, 722
     for myocardial infarction, 335, 336,
          340
          after thrombolytic therapy, 334
     for nephrotic syndrome, 840

Anticoagulation therapy (*cont.*)
  overdose/toxicity of, **1430–1431**
  perioperative management of, 55, 56*t*
  for pulmonary hypertension, 275, 381
  for stroke, 891–892
  thrombocytopenia caused by, 483*t*
  for transient ischemic attacks, 888
Anticonstipation agents. *See* Fiber,
    dietary; Laxatives
Anticonvulsant therapy, 881–884, 882*t*
  breast feeding and, 710*t*
  corticosteroid interactions and, 1077
  discontinuing, 883
  drug selection and, 881–883, 882*t*
  for glossopharyngeal neuralgia, 877
  monitoring serum levels during, 883
  for myoclonus, 911
  overdose/toxicity and, 882*t*, 883, **1431**
  for phobic disorder, 943
  for posttraumatic stress disorder, 939
  during pregnancy, 724, 881–883
  for status epilepticus, 884
  for trigeminal neuralgia, 877
Anti-D, for immune thrombocytopenic
    thrombocytopenia, 483,
    484, 484*f*
Antidepressants, 963–970, 965*f*, 968*t*,
    969*t*. *See also specific type*
    and agent
  with antipsychotic agents, 957, 967
  for anxiety, 941, 942
  aripiprazole with, 957
  atypical, 964–966
  breast feeding and, 710*t*
  buspirone as augmenting agent for,
    964
  combination therapy and, 967
  in dementia, 987
  dispensing, 963, 964
  dose tapering and, 967
  drug interactions of, 969*t*
  for dyspepsia, 504
  in elderly, 66–67, 74
  for irritable bowel syndrome, 572
  lithium as augmenting agent for, 964
  lithium interaction and, 969*t*
  maintenance therapy with, 967
  MAOIs, 967, 967*t*, 968*t*, 969*t*. *See also*
    Monoamine oxidase
    inhibitors
  for neuropathic pain/painful diabetic
    neuropathy, 84–85, 85*t*,
    1107
  for OCD, 943, 964
  overdose/toxicity of, 968*t*, **1448–1449**,
    1448*f*
    arrhythmias and, 967, 1448, 1448*f*
    hypotension caused by, 1421–1422
    seizures and, 967, 1423*t*, 1448
    suicidal, 963, 1448
  for panic attacks, 943
  for personality disorder, 951
  for phobic disorder, 943
  for posttraumatic stress disorder, 939
  during pregnancy, 966
  for psychotic depression, 964, 966
  selection of, 964
  sexual dysfunction caused by, 965, 967

  SSRIs, 964–966, 968*t*. *See also* Seroto-
    nin-selective reuptake
    inhibitors
  switching agents and, 967
  thyroid medication/liothyronine as
    augmenting agent for,
    964
  tricyclic, 966–967, 968*t*. *See also* Tri-
    cyclic antidepressants
Antidiabetic agents, 1090–1096, 1091*t*. *See*
    also specific type and agent
    and Insulin therapy
  adverse ophthalmic effects of, 178*t*
  combination regimens and, 1096,
    1101
  with insulin therapy, 1101
  intensive therapy with, 1087–1088
  intraoperative requirements/adminis-
    tration of, 57–58, 57*t*, 58*t*
  for obese type 2 diabetic, 1101
  during pregnancy, 722, 1110
  in prevention/delay of diabetes,
    1086–1087
Antidiarrheal agents, 514, 517, 1172
  for Crohn disease, 580
  for fecal incontinence, 596
  for irritable bowel syndrome, 572
  for traveler's diarrhea, 1174
  for ulcerative colitis, 584
Antidiuretic hormone (ADH). *See also*
    Vasopressin
  in hyponatremia, 789–793
  inappropriate secretion of (SIADH).
    See Syndrome of inappro-
    priate ADH secretion
  volume overload and, 794
Anti-DNase B, in rheumatic fever/heart
    disease, 375
Antidotes, **1423–1424**, 1424*t*. *See also spe-*
    cific agent
Anti-double-stranded (anti-ds)-DNA
  in hyperthyroidism, 1010
  in lupus, 110, 753, 754*t*
Antidromic tachycardia, 341, 345
Antiemetics, 506–507, 506*t*
  for chemotherapy-induced nausea
    and vomiting, 1508–1509
  in HIV infection/AIDS, 1210
  for hyperemesis gravidarum, 711
  phenothiazines as, overdose/toxicity
    of, 1444–1445
Antiendomysial antibodies, in celiac dis-
    ease/dermatitis herpetifor-
    mis, 559, 560
Antiepilepsy drugs. *See* Anticonvulsant
    therapy
Antifolates, for malaria, 1359
Antifreeze. *See* Ethylene glycol poisoning
Antifungal agents, 1401*t*, **1402**. *See also*
    specific agent or disorder
  for dermatologic disorders, 98*t*
  in neutropenia, 1158
  for ophthalmic disorders, 173*t*
  prophylactic, 1158
  for systemic disorders, 1401*t*, **1402**
Anti-GBM antibodies. *See* Anti-glomeru-
    lar basement membrane
    antibodies

Antigen-antibody complexes, 784, 785.
    See also Immune complex-
    mediated hypersensitivity
  in glomerulonephritis, 824, 835*f*
  membranous nephropathy and, 841
  in SLE, 752
Antigenic drift/shift, influenza epidemics/
    pandemics and, 1269
Antiglaucoma agents, 159, 175–176*t*
Antigliadin antibody, in celiac disease,
    559–560
Anti-glomerular basement membrane
    antibodies, in glomerulo-
    nephritis/Goodpasture
    syndrome, 276, 824, 835*f*,
    837–838
Anti-HAV, 602, 602*f*
Anti-HBc, 602*f*, 603, 603*t*
  in hepatocellular carcinoma, 1460
  screening blood for, 478
Anti-HBe, 602*f*, 603, 603*t*, 609
Anti-HBs, 602*f*, 603, 603*t*, 609
  after vaccination, 606
Anti-HCV, 604, 604*f*, 609
  in hepatocellular carcinoma, 1460
  screening blood for, 478, 491
Anti-HDV, 603, 609
Antihistamines, 94–95
  for allergic eye disease, 155, 173*t*
  for allergic rhinitis, 196
  for desensitization reactions, 1183,
    1186
  for insomnia, 974, 984
  MAOI interactions and, 969*t*
  for nausea and vomiting, 87, 507
  for ophthalmic disorders, 155, 173*t*
  in OTC medications, 984
  overdose/toxicity of, 984, 1432
  for pruritus, 94–95, 136
  for urticaria, 126
Anti-Hu antibody
  achalasia and, 542
  in cancer-related neuropathy, 885, 925
Antihypertensive drug therapy, 388*t*,
    395–398, 396*t*, **398–411**.
    See also specific class or
    agent
  aldosterone receptor antagonists in,
    391, 392, 396*t*, 399*t*, 405
  α-adrenoceptor antagonists in, 407,
    408*t*
  angiotensin II receptor blocking
    agents in, 396*t*, 403–404*t*,
    405, 407, 409, 409*f*
  angiotensin-converting enzyme
    (ACE) inhibitors in, 396*t*,
    402–405, 403*t*, 407, 409,
    409*f*
    in diabetics, 396*t*, 402–405,
    409–410, 1088, 1105, 1106,
    1108
  in aortic dissection, 427
  arteriolar dilators in, 407, 408*t*
  β-adrenergic blocking agents in, 396*t*,
    398–402, 400–401*t*,
    407–409, 409*f*
  in blacks, 410, 410*t*
  breast feeding and, 710*t*

calcium channel blocking drugs in, 396*t*, 405–407, 406*t*, 407, 409, 409*f*
combination regimens and, 409, 409*f*
depression caused by, 962
developing regimen for, 407–409, 409*f*, 410*t*
in diabetes mellitus, 396*t*, 409, 409–410, 1088, 1108
complication rate/diabetic nephropathy affected by, 393, 409–410, 842, 1088, 1105, 1106, 1108
diuretics in, 396*t*, 398, 399*t*, 407, 409, 409*f*
in combination products, 398, 399*t*, 409, 409*f*
for urgencies/emergencies, 412
follow-up and, 410–411
goals of, 395–397
heart disease prevention and, 9–12
parenteral, 411–412, 412–414, 413*t*
patient selection for, 387, 388*t*, 389*f*, 390*t*, 395, 396*t*, 397*f*
perioperative, 52
peripheral sympathetic inhibitors in, 407, 408*t*
pheochromocytoma surgery and, 1060–1061, 1061
for preeclampsia/eclampsia, 718, 723
during pregnancy, 723
for prehypertension, 388*t*, 395
in renal disease/failure, 396*t*, 410, 828
renin inhibitors in, 402, 403*t*
stroke/stroke prevention and, 9–12, 396*t*, 407, 891, 894
urgencies/emergencies, 412
sympatholytics in, 407, 408*t*
overdose/toxicity of, 407, 408*t*, **1434–1435**
for urgencies/emergencies, 412–414, 413*t*
vasodilators in, 407, 408*t*
Anti-IgA antibodies, 786
Anti-inflammatory drugs. *See also* Corticosteroids; Nonsteroidal anti-inflammatory drugs
for asthma, 223
ophthalmic, 173–175*t*
for osteoarthritis, 731
Anti-insulin antibodies
in factitious hypoglycemia, 1122
in immune insulin resistance, 1104
in immunopathologic hypoglycemia, 1117*t*, 1118, 1122
insulin therapy causing, 1104
in type 1 diabetes, 1080, 1080*t*
Anti-insulin receptor antibodies, in immunopathologic hypoglycemia, 1117*t*, 1118, 1122
Anti-integrins, in inflammatory bowel disease, 577
Anti-Itch lotion. *See* Pramoxine
Anti-Jo-1 antibody, in polymyositis/dermatomyositis, 754*t*, 760
Antileukotriene agents
for allergic rhinitis, 197

for asthma, 224–225*t*, 228
Anti-liver cytosol type 1, in autoimmune hepatitis, 613
Anti-LKM1, in autoimmune hepatitis, 613
Anti-MAG antibodies, in cancer-related neuropathy, 925
Antimalarial agents, 1355–1360, 1355*t*, 1356*t*, 1357*t*
for lupus, 111, 754
for malaria
chemoprophylaxis, 1361, 1361*t*
combination therapies, 1355, 1356*t*
non-falciparum, 1356, 1357*t*
nonimmune populations and, 1356, 1360
self-treatment, 1361
severe disease, 1356, 1357*t*, 1360
treatment, 1355–1360, 1355*t*, 1356*t*, 1357*t*
uncomplicated falciparum, 1355–1356, 1356*t*, 1357*t*
ophthalmic side effects of, 178*t*
for porphyria cutanea tarda, 117
rabies vaccination and, 1201, 1257
resistance to, 1355, 1356, 1358, 1359
for rheumatoid arthritis, 750
Antimania therapy, 970–973, 972*t*
Antimetabolites, 1501–1502*t*
Anti-Mi-2 antibody, in polymyositis/dermatomyositis, 760
Antimicrobial chemoprophylaxis. *See also* *specific agent and* Antimicrobial therapy
for abortion, 701
for anthrax, 1301, 1301*t*, 1302
for aspergillosis, 1158, 1398
for bite wounds, 1165–1166
for bronchiectasis, 240
candidiasis, 1223
for CMV infection, 1222
in COPD, 238
for cryptococcosis, 1223–1224
for cystitis, 851
for endocarditis, 1305, 1305*t*, 1306*t*
in Marfan syndrome, 1518
during pregnancy, 385
for esophageal varices, 539
for group B streptococcal infection, in pregnancy, 708, 1291
for herpes simplex infection, 114, 1157, 1237–1239
in HIV infection/AIDS, 1219–1220, 1219*t*, 1222–1223, 1222*t*
in immunocompromised host, 1157–1158
for influenza, 1270
for Lyme disease, 1345
for MAC infections, 1222, 1325
for malaria, 1361, 1361*t*. *See also* Antimalarial agents
for meningococcal meningitis, 1309
for opportunistic infections, 1219–1220, 1219*t*, 1222–1223, 1222*t*
for *P jiroveci* infection, 286, 1157, 1210, 1222, 1222*t*, 1396
for peritonitis, 526–527

for plague, 1201, 1318
in rape/sexual assault, 702, 1167
for relapsing fever, 1340
of rheumatic fever, 376
for surgical site infections, **59–60**, 60*t*
for toxoplasmosis, 1222, 1365
for traveler's diarrhea, 1174
for tuberculosis, 4, 257–258, 1158, 1219–1220, 1222
in HIV infection/AIDS, 4, 257, 1219–1220, 1222
Antimicrobial therapy, **1175–1186**, 1176–1178*t*. *See also specific type or disorder and* Antimicrobial chemoprophylaxis
adverse reactions/toxicity and, 1178
allergic reactions/desensitization and, **1180–1186**
for asthma, 230
breast feeding and, 710*t*
clinical response to, 1175
promptness of, 1175–1178
cost of agents and, 1180
duration of, 1178
empiric, 1175, 1181*t*, 1182–1183*t*
in febrile drug user, 1169
in immunocompromised host, 1158, 1498
in fever management, 40, 1155
in immunocompromised host, 1158–1159, 1498
in neutropenic patient, 40, 1158, 1181*t*, 1498
parenteral, 1178
for pneumonia, 244–245*t*, 246–247, 249, 251
renal/hepatic failure and, 1184–1185*t*
resistance to. *See* Drug resistance
routes of administration for, 1178–1180
for shock, 437
susceptibility testing and, 1175
thrombocytopenia caused by, 483*t*
Antimicrotubule agents, in cancer chemotherapy, 1502*t*
Antimigrainous agents, 873–874
Antimitochondrial antibodies, in biliary cirrhosis, 625
Antimitochondrial antibody-negative primary biliary cirrhosis, 626
Antimony. *See* Stibogluconate
Antimotility drugs. *See* Antidiarrheal agents
Anti-nAChR, in cancer-related neuropathy, 925
Anti-native DNA antibody, 754*t*
Antineoplastic agents. *See* Chemotherapy
Antineuronal nuclear antibodies, neurologic paraneoplastic syndromes caused by, achalasia and, 542
Antineutrophil cytoplasmic antibody (ANCA), 754*t*, 835*f*
in autoimmune hepatitis, 613
in Churg-Strauss syndrome, 835*f*
in glomerulonephritis (pauciimmune), 824, 835*f*, **837**

Antineutrophil cytoplasmic antibody (ANCA) (*cont.*)
in inflammatory bowel disease, 579
in interstitial (diffuse parenchymal) lung disease, 262
in microscopic polyangiitis, 770, 824, 835f
in primary sclerosing cholangitis, 641
in Wegener granulomatosis, 754t, 768, 769, 835f
Antinuclear antibody (ANA), 754t
in autoimmune hepatitis, 613
in biliary cirrhosis, 625
in CREST syndrome, 754t, 758
in Graves disease/hyperthyroidism, 1008, 1010
in interstitial (diffuse parenchymal) lung disease, 262
in lupus, 110, 752, 753, 754t, 835f
in mixed connective tissue disease/overlap syndrome, 762
in polymyositis/dermatomyositis, 754t, 760
in rheumatoid arthritis, 748, 754t
in scleroderma, 754t, 758
in Sjögren syndrome, 754t, 762
in Wegener granulomatosis, 754t
Antioxidants. *See also* Vitamin C; Vitamin E
in atherosclerosis/heart disease prevention, 12, 1130
Antiparkinsonism drugs, 906–908, 906t
for antipsychotic-induced side effects/parkinsonism, 959
for neuroleptic malignant syndrome, 959
Antiphlebitic stockings. *See* Compression stockings
Antiphospholipid antibody syndrome/antiphospholipid antibodies, 722, 755–756
factor II antibodies and, 494
false-positive syphilis tests and, 753, 756
livedo reticularis in, 755, 773
pregnancy loss and, 722, 755
SLE and, 753, 754t, 755
Antiplatelet antibody
heparin-associated, 486, 487
reference values for, 1551t
in immune thrombocytopenic purpura, 482
in posttransfusion purpura, 488
Antiplatelet therapy. *See also* Aspirin
for acute coronary syndromes, 326–328, 327t
for angina, 322
bleeding associated with, 78, 548–549
for myocardial infarction, 332, 340
peptic ulcer disease and, 552, 553
for stroke, 892
thrombocytopenia caused by, 483t
for transient ischemic attacks, 888
α_1-Antiprotease/antitrypsin
in COPD/emphysema, 235
replacement therapy and, 238
in protein-losing enteropathy, 569
reference values for, 1547t

Antipruritic agents
systemic, 94–95
topical, 94, 98t
Antipsychotic drugs (neuroleptics), 954–960, 955t, 956t, 958t.
See also specific type and agent
abnormal movements caused by, 911
adherence/nonadherence and, 954, 957–958
for aggressive/violent behavior, 976
for alcoholic hallucinosis, 980
with antidepressants, 957, 967
atypical. *See* Atypical antipsychotics
for bipolar disease/mania, 970
breast cancer and, 958
clinical indications for, 957
for delirium, 67, 87, 987
for dementia, 66, 987
dosage forms and patterns of, 957–958
in elderly, 957
for Huntington disease, 909
for mania, 970
neuroleptic malignant syndrome caused by, 39, 959, 1423, 1444
overdose/toxicity/side effects of, 956t, 958–960, 958t, **1444–1445**
for parkinsonism, 907–908
parkinsonism (reversible) caused by, 905, 959
for personality disorders, 951
in pregnancy, 959
for psychedelic abuse/overdose, 982
relative potency of, 956t
seizure threshold affected by, 959
for Tourette syndrome, 912, 957
Antipyretic drugs, 39
Antireflux surgery. *See* Fundoplication
Antiretroviral therapy, 1223–1234, 1226–1227t, 1232f. *See also specific agent*
adherence with regimen for, 1, 1225, 1231, 1232
antituberculous drug interactions and, 255–256, 1211
CMV retinitis and, 167–168, 1223
combinations/regimens for, 1225, 1227, 1231–1233, 1232f
drug holidays and, 1227, 1233
drug resistance and, 1223, 1225–1227, 1232, 1233
highly active. *See* Highly active antiretroviral therapy
immune reconstitution disease and, 1216–1217
lipid abnormalities caused by, 1216, 1229
myopathy caused by, 1213
opportunistic infection/malignancies and, 1205, 1223, 1225
postexposure
after needle stick, 1221
after sexual assault/rape, 1167
after sexual/drug use exposure, 1221
pregnancy/newborn and, 726, 1207

Anti-Rh$_o$ (D) antibody, in hemolytic disease of newborn, 709
Anti-ribonucleoprotein (anti-RNP) antibody, 762
Anti-SCL-70 antibody, 754t, 758
Antisecretory agents. *See* Acid-antisecretory agents
Antiseizure therapy. *See* Anticonvulsant therapy
Anti-signal recognition particle (anti-SRP) antibody, in polymyositis/dermatomyositis, 760
Anti-SLA/LP, in autoimmune hepatitis, 613
Anti-Smith (anti-Sm) antibody, in SLE, 753, 754t
Anti-smooth muscle antibodies, in autoimmune hepatitis, 613
Antisocial personality disorder, 950, 951, 951t
Antispasmodic agents, for irritable bowel syndrome, 572
Anti-SRP antibody, in polymyositis/dermatomyositis, 760
Anti-SS-A/Ro antibody, 754t
in lupus, 110, 754t
in Sjögren syndrome, 754t, 762
Anti-SS-B/La antibody, 754t
in Sjögren syndrome, 754t, 762
Antistreptolysin O (ASO) titers
in postinfectious glomerulonephritis, 834
in rheumatic fever, 375
Antisynthetase syndrome, 760
Antithrombin III, reference values for, 1547t
Antithrombotic therapy, **495–501**, 496t, 497t, 498t, 499t, 500t, 501t.
See also Anticoagulation therapy; Antiplatelet therapy; Thrombolytic therapy
for myocardial infarction, 335
Antithymocyte globulin
for aplastic anemia, 455
for myelodysplasia, 464
Antithyroid (antithyroglobulin/antithyroperoxidase) antibodies, 1003t
in goiter, 1029
in Graves disease/hyperthyroidism, 1003t, 1008, 1010
amiodarone-induced, 1009, 1010
in hypothyroidism, 1003t, 1005
in pregnancy, 722
in thyroid cancer diagnosis/surveillance, 1024, 1026
in thyroid nodules, 1003t, 1019t, 1020
in thyroiditis, 1017
Hashimoto, 1016, 1017
postpartum, 1016, 1017
Anti-TNF agents. *See also specific agent*
adverse effects of, 577
for ankylosing spondylitis, 774
for gram-negative bacteremia/sepsis, 1312
for inflammatory bowel disease, 576–577

Crohn disease, 581
ulcerative colitis, 585
for psoriasis, 105
for rheumatoid arthritis, 750–751
in combination regimen, 751
for septic shock, 1312
Antitoxin
botulinus, 934, 1300
diphtheria, 1302
α₁-Antitrypsin/antiprotease
in COPD/emphysema, 235
replacement therapy and, 238
in protein-losing enteropathy, 569
reference values for, 1547t
Anti-tTG (transglutaminase/tissue transglutaminase) antibody, in
celiac disease/dermatitis
herpetiformis, 118, 516,
559, 560
Antituberculous drugs, 254–258, 255t,
256t, 1177t
antiretroviral drug interactions and,
255–256, 1211
directly observed therapy (DOT) and,
254
for drug-resistant disease, 252, 256
for extrapulmonary disease, 256
hepatotoxicity and, 4
in HIV-negative persons, 254–255
in HIV-positive persons, 255–256,
1211
prophylactic, 4, 257, 1219–1220,
1222
in latent disease/chemoprophylactic,
4, 257–258, 1158,
1219–1220, 1222
for meningitis, 1326
monitoring therapy with, 256–257
during pregnancy/lactation, 256, 726
resistance to, 252, 256
for tuberculous pericarditis, 378
Anti-VEGF therapy
for age-related macular degeneration,
163
for renal cell carcinoma, 1492
Antivenin
for black widow spider bites, 1447
for scorpion stings, 1447
for snake bites, 1424t, 1447
Antiviral agents, 1238–1239t. See also specific agent or infection
for ophthalmic disorders, 173t
Antizol. See Fomepizole
Anton syndrome, 899
Anus. See also under Anal
carcinoma of, 1468t, 1483
in HIV infection/AIDS, 1216, 1483
rectum protruding through (rectal
prolapse), 593
Anxiety/anxiety disorders, 939–944
anticipatory, 940
chronic pain and, 946
drugs for management of, 941–943,
941t, 942t
generalized, 940
hospitalization/illness and, 988, 989
mind-body therapies for, 1536t
mind-body therapies for, 1536t

biofeedback, 1538
meditation, 1536t, 1541
palpitations in, 31, 32
personality disorder and, 950
in pheochromocytoma, 1058
pre- and postsurgical, 988, 989
mind-body therapies for, 1536t
guided imagery, 1536t, 1543
in schizophrenic/psychotic disorders,
953
Anxiolytic drugs, 941–943, 941t, 942t. See
also specific type
breast feeding and, 710t
Aorta
atherosclerotic/occlusive disease of,
415–416
coarctation of. See Coarctation of
aorta
in Marfan syndrome, 383, 1518
Aortic aneurysms
abdominal, 423–425
screening for, 6, 423
atherosclerosis and, 425
back pain caused by, 423, 425, 738
inflammatory, 423, 424
in Marfan syndrome, 383, 1518
ruptured, 423, 424, 425
in syphilis, 425
thoracic, 425–426
giant cell arteritis and, 766, 767
in Turner syndrome, 1074, 1075
Aortic arch
abnormalities of in tetralogy of Fallot,
300
aneurysm of, 425
Aortic dissection, 426–427
aortic regurgitation and, 312
chest pain in, 29, 321, 426
hypertension and, 393, 426, 427
in Marfan syndrome, 1518
in pregnancy, 385
Aortic regurgitation, 303–305t, 311–313
in Marfan syndrome, 311–312,
312–313, 1518
preoperative evaluation/management
and, 52
rheumatic fever/heart disease and, 311
Aortic root dilation, in Marfan syndrome,
1518
Aortic sclerosis, 302, 310
Aortic stenosis, 302, 303–305t, 309–311
interventions affecting murmur in,
306t
preoperative evaluation/management
and, 52
Aortic valve rupture, 384
Aortitis, in rheumatoid arthritis, 748
Aortoenteric fistula, GI bleeding and,
518
Aorto-femoral bypass, for aortoiliac
occlusive disease, 416
Aortoiliac occlusive disease, 415–416
APACHE system
in pancreatitis, 642
prognosis at end of life and, 88
septic shock and, 437, 1312
Apallic state (persistent vegetative state),
917

Apathetic hyperthyroidism, 1010,
1014–1015
APC gene, 591, 1476–1477, 1477
screening for, 1477
APCED/APECED. See Autoimmune poly-
endocrinopathy-candidia-
sis-ectodermal dystrophy
Aphasia
intracranial tumors casing, 899
stroke causing, 889
Aphthous ulcer, 203
in Behçet syndrome, 772
in Crohn disease, 578
in HIV infection/AIDS, 1213
Apical ballooning syndrome. See Tako-
Tsubo (stress/catechol-
amine-induced) cardiomy-
opathy
Apical impulse
in aortic regurgitation, 312
in cardiomyopathy, 373
Apicitis, petrous, 185
Apidra. See Insulin glulisine
APL. See Acute promyelocytic leukemia
Aplastic anemia, 454–456, 454t, 455t
thrombocytopenia in, 480, 481–482
Aplastic crises
in hereditary spherocytosis, 448
in sickle cell disease, 450, 451
Apley "grind" test, 35
Apnea, sleep. See Sleep apnea
Apnea test, 917
Apneustic breathing, in coma or stupor,
916
Apparent mineralocorticoid excess
genetic mutation in, 796t
hypertension and, 391
Appearance, in schizophrenic/psychotic
disorders, 953
Appendectomy, 568
antibiotic prophylaxis for, 60t
for carcinoids, 1475
during pregnancy, 728
ulcerative colitis risk and, 583
Appendiceal carcinoids, 1475
Appendicitis, 567–568
amebic, 1366
in pregnancy, 568, 728
Appetite, genes affecting control of, 1136
Apraclonidine, for glaucoma/ocular
hypertension, 159, 175t
Apraxia
in dementia, 63
intracranial tumors causing, 899
Aprepitant, 506, 1509
Apresoline. See Hydralazine
APS. See Antiphospholipid antibody syn-
drome
Aptivus/Norvir. See Tipranavir/ritonavir
aPTT. See Partial thromboplastin time
Aqua glycolic, 98t
Aquaphor, 94, 99t
Aquaporin-4, in neuromyelitis optica, 914
Aquinil. See Hydrocortisone
Ara-C. See Cytarabine
Arachnodactyly, in Marfan syndrome,
1518
Aranesp. See Darbepoetin alfa

Arbovirus encephalitides, **1257–1259**
ARBs. *See* Angiotensin II receptor blocking agents
Arch aneurysms, 425
Arcing (flash) burns, 1413
ARDS. *See* Acute respiratory distress syndrome
Aredia. *See* Pamidronate
Arfonad. *See* Trimethaphan
Arg133Trp (PAX-4) mutation, in idiopathic type 1 diabetes mellitus, 1081
Argatroban, for heparin-induced thrombocytopenia, 486t, 487
Arginine vasopressin, in diabetes insipidus, 995, 996
Argyll Robertson pupils, in tabes dorsalis, 1336
Arimidex. *See* Anastrozole
Aripiprazole, 954, 955t, 956t, 957, 967
    for bipolar disease/mania, 970
    overdose/toxicity of, 956t, 957, 1444–1445
Arm edema, in breast cancer/postmastectomy, 671–672
Arnold-Chiari malformation
    cough headache and, 875
    syringomyelia and, 920
Aromasin. *See* Exemestane
Aromatase inhibitors/inactivators, 1506t
    for breast cancer treatment/prevention, 654, 666, 668, 669
    in male, 673
    for endometriosis, 686
Arousal (excitement) stage of sexual activity, 948
    disorders related to, 948, 949–950. *See also* Sexual dysfunction
    in female, 691, 692
Arrhythmias, **340–354**, 343–345t. *See also specific type and* Electrocardiogram
    antidepressants causing, 967, 1448, 1448f
    in cardiomyopathy, 370, 371, 373
    in COPD, 235, 238
    in electrical injury, 1409
    in heart failure, 365
    in hypothermia, 1404
    myocardial infarction and, 336–337
        antiarrhythmic prophylaxis and, 335, 340
    palpitations and, 31, 32
    in pheochromocytoma, 1058, 1059
    in poisoning/drug overdose,
        1422–1423, 1422t. *See also specific agent*
        with antiarrhythmic drugs, 1422t, 1445
        with antidepressants, 967, 1448, 1448f
        with antipsychotic drugs, 958, 1444
        with digitalis glycosides, 1436
        with phenothiazines, 1444
    preoperative evaluation/management of, 52
    seizures differentiated from, 881
    sinus, **340–341**

in SLE, 753
in sleep apnea, 288, 289
syncope caused by, 356, 357
in tetralogy of Fallot, 300, 301
treatment of. *See* Antiarrhythmic drugs
Arsenic poisoning, 1424t, **1431–1432**
Arsenic trioxide
    in cancer chemotherapy, 1504t
    toxicity of, 1431, 1504t
Arsenical melanosis, 144
ART. *See* Antiretroviral therapy; Assisted reproductive technologies
Art therapy, 1520
Artane. *See* Trihexyphenidyl
Artemether
    for malaria, 1355t, 1357t, 1359–1360
        with lumefantrine (Coartem/Riamet), 1355t, 1356, 1356t, 1357t, 1360
    for schistosomiasis, 1374
Artemisinins (qinghaosu)/artemisinin derivatives, for malaria, 1355t, 1359–1360
    in combination regimens, 1355t, 1359–1360
    self-treatment and, 1361
Arterial aneurysms. *See specific type and* Aneurysms
Arterial blood gases
    in acid-base disorders, 806
    in asthma, 219
    in COPD, 234
    in cystic fibrosis, 241
    in dyspnea, 26
    home oxygen therapy and, 236, 236t
    in near drowning, 1415
    in *Pneumocystis* pneumonia, 1210, 1394
    in pneumonia, 246, 248–249
    preoperative, 54
    in pulmonary embolism, 267
    in respiratory failure, 289
Arterial embolism. *See also* Thromboembolism; Thrombosis
    acute occlusion of limb caused by, 419
    atrial fibrillation/cardiac sources and, 346, 347t
    carotid sources of, 420
    in myocardial infarction, 339
    in transient monocular blindness, 165, 420
Arterial graft/prosthesis. *See* Bypass grafting
Arterial lines
    in burn care, 1410
    hospital-associated infection and, 1161
    in shock management, 435
Arterial occlusion
    acute, **418–419**. *See also* Arterial embolism; Arterial thrombosis
    atherosclerotic, **415–422**. *See also* Atherosclerosis
Arterial thrombosis. *See also* Thrombosis
    acute occlusion of limb caused by, 419
    in antiphospholipid antibody syndrome, 755

in homocystinuria, 1517
Arteriography. *See specific type and* Angiography
Arteriolar dilators. *See also* Vasodilator therapy
    for hypertension, 407, 408t
Arteriopathy, plexogenic pulmonary (idiopathic/primary pulmonary hypertension), 274, **380–381**, 381t
Arteriovenous fistulae, spinal dural, 897
Arteriovenous malformations
    gastrointestinal (vascular ectasias), bleeding from, 518, 520–521
    in hereditary hemorrhagic telangiectasia, 1519
    intracranial, 890t, **895–896**. *See also* Stroke
    pulmonary, 1519
    spinal cord, 897
Arteriovenous sheathotomy, for retinal vein occlusion, 164
Arteritis. *See also* Polyarteritis
    coronary artery, in Kawasaki disease, 383, 1288
    giant cell. *See* Giant cell (temporal/cranial) arteritis
    in thromboangiitis obliterans (Buerger disease), 422
Artesunate, for malaria, 1355t, 1356, 1357t, 1359–1360
    with amodiaquine (ASAQ), 1355t, 1356t, 1357t, 1360
    with mefloquine, 1356t, 1358, 1359–1360
    with sulfadoxine-pyrimethamine, 1355t, 1356t
Arthritis/arthralgia
    acupuncture for, 1533
    in alkaptonuria, 1513, 1514
    in ankylosing spondylitis, 774, 775
    arthroplasty/joint replacement for, 731
        osteomyelitis and, 780
    back pain caused by, 738
    in Behçet syndrome, 772
    bursitis differentiated from, 743
    cancer-associated, 783
    chondroitin/glucosamine for, 731, 1528t, 1529–1530
    in coccidioidomycosis, 781, 1393
    in Crohn disease, 578, 776–777
    crystal deposition, **732–736**
    degenerative, **729–732**. *See also* Osteoarthritis
    diagnosis and evaluation of, 729, 730t, 731t
    exercise/activity in management of, 13
    glucosamine/chondroitin for, 731, 1528t, 1529–1530
    gonococcal, **778–779**, 1319
    gouty. *See* Gout/gouty arthritis
    in hemophilia, 491
    in hepatitis, 779
        rheumatoid arthritis differentiated from, 748

in HIV infection/AIDS, 779,
1212–1213
infectious, **777–780**
in drug users, 777, 1168–1169
inflammatory intestinal diseases and,
776–777
leukemic, 783
Lyme, 1343, 1346, 1346*t*
rheumatoid arthritis differentiated
from, 748
mutilans, 775
neck pain caused by, 737
nongonococcal bacterial. *See* Arthritis/arthralgia, septic
in parvovirus B19 infection, 779, 1276
rheumatoid arthritis differentiated
from, 748
pattern of joint involvement and, 729,
730*t*
pneumococcal, 1292
pseudoseptic, 777
psoriatic, 104, **775–776**
reactive. *See* Reactive arthritis
in rheumatic fever, 375
rheumatoid arthritis differentiated
from, 748
rheumatoid. *See* Rheumatoid arthritis
rubella/rubella vaccination and, 779,
1254, 1255
in sarcoidosis, **782**
septic (nongonococcal acute bacterial), **777–778**, 1181*t*
in drug users, 777, 1168–1169
rheumatoid arthritis and, 748, 777,
778
in SLE, 753
rheumatoid arthritis differentiated
from, 748
in Still disease, 751
streptococcal, 1290–1291
surgery for, 731
tophaceous, 732, 733, 735
rheumatoid arthritis differentiated
from, 733
tuberculous, **782**
in ulcerative colitis, 776–777
viral, **779–780**
in Wegener granulomatosis, 768, 769
in Whipple disease, 561, 777
Arthrocentesis, 729, 730*t*, 731*t*. *See also*
Synovial fluid examination
of knee, 35–36
Arthropathy, neurogenic. *See* Neurogenic
arthropathy
Arthroplasty, osteomyelitis and, 780
Arthropods
in encephalitis, 1257–1259
skin lesions caused by, **138–140**. *See
also specific cause*
Artificial insemination, in azoospermia,
694
Artificial nutrition. *See* Nutritional support
Artificial sweeteners, for diabetics, 1090
Artificial tears, for dry eye, 154–155, 763
Arytenoid cartilage, contact ulcers/granulomas of, 209
5-ASA. *See* 5-Aminosalicylic acid

Asacol. *See* Mesalamine
ASAQ (artesunate-amodiaquine), 1355*t*,
1356*t*, 1357*t*, 1360
Asbestosis (asbestos exposure), 279, 279*t*,
280
lung cancer and, 279, 280, 1452
mesothelioma and, 280, 528, 1459
pleural effusion and, 281
smoking and, 279, 280
ASC-US. *See* Atypical squamous cells of
unknown significance
ASCA. *See* Saccharomyces cerevisiae antibodies
Ascaris lumbricoides (ascariasis),
1379–1380
eosinophilic pulmonary syndromes
and, 266, 1379
Ascites, **524–525**, 524*t*. *See also specific
causative disorder*
bile, 528–529
chylous, 528, 621, 1496
in cirrhosis, 620–621
malignant, 524, **527–528**, 1495–1496
neutrocytic, 526
pancreatic, 525, 528, 644, 648
spontaneous bacterial peritonitis and,
526–527, 621
tuberculous, 527
Ascites albumin gradient, serum (SAAG).
See Serum-ascites albumin
gradient
Ascitic fluid analysis/examination, 525.
See also Paracentesis
in ascites, 525
in bacterial peritonitis, 526, 621
in bile ascites, 528–529
in chylous ascites, 528
in cirrhosis, 620–621
culture/Gram stain, 525
in malignant ascites, 528
in pancreatic ascites, 525, 528
in peritoneal carcinomatosis, 528
in tuberculous peritonitis, 525, 527
Ascorbic acid. *See* Vitamin C
ASD. *See* Atrial septal defect
Asendin. *See* Amoxapine
Aseptic meningitis, 1162*t*, 1163. *See also*
Meningitis
coxsackieviruses causing, 1279
echoviruses causing, 1279
leptospiral, 1163, 1341
in Lyme disease, 1163, 1343, 1345
mumps vaccine and, 1251
in syphilis, 1163, 1334
in tick-borne encephalitis, 1266
Ash leaf spots (hypopigmentation), in
tuberous sclerosis, 903
Asherman syndrome, 1069
Asian ginseng, 1523*t*, 1526
ASO titers. *See* Antistreptolysin O (ASO)
titers
Asparaginase, 1504*t*
Aspartame, for diabetics, 1090
Aspartate aminotransferase (AST),
599–600, 600*t*
in alcoholic liver disease, 614
in cirrhosis, 619–620
in hemochromatosis, 627

in liver disease/jaundice, 599–600,
600*t*
in nonalcoholic fatty liver disease, 618
in preeclampsia-eclampsia, 717*t*
reference/normal values for, 600*t*,
1547*t*
in viral hepatitis, 605
Aspergilloma, 1397, 1398
Aspergillus/Aspergillus fumigatus
(aspergillosis), **1397–1398**
allergic bronchopulmonary, **241**,
1397, 1398
chronic necrotizing, 1397, 1398
in HIV infection/AIDS, 192
invasive, 1397–1398, 1398
opportunistic mold infection differentiated from, 1402
prevention of, 1158, 1398
sinusitis and, 195, 1397, 1398
Asphyxia
aspiration of inert material causing,
277
in severe asthma exacerbation, 233
Aspiration, **277–278**
caustic esophageal injury and, 536
in drowning/near drowning, 1415
enteral nutritional support and,
1150
of food (café coronary), **277**
foreign body, 212
retention of, **278**
of gastric contents
acute (Mendelson syndrome), **278**,
1160
chronic, **278**
in comatose patient, 1420
in pneumonia. *See* Pneumonia,
aspiration
of inert material, **277**
of toxic material, **277**
Aspirin, 78. *See also* Antiplatelet therapy;
Salicylates
for acute coronary syndromes, 326,
327*t*
in analgesic nephropathy, 845
for angina, 322
for atrial fibrillation, 348
bleeding caused by, 78, 548–549
after cardiac valve replacement surgery, 316
for chemoprevention, 3*t*, 12
atherosclerosis/heart disease prevention and, 12, 1130
in diabetics, 12, 1089, 1108
in colorectal cancer, 1477
with codeine, 78, 83*t*
for essential thrombocytosis, 459
for fever, 39
GI bleeding associated with, 78,
548–549, 749
iron deficiency and, 439
for myocardial infarction, 327*t*, 332,
335, 336, 340
after thrombolytic therapy, 334
nasal polyps and asthma as contraindication to, 199
overdose/toxicity of, 1445–1446
for pain management, 78

Aspirin (*cont.*)
in peptic ulcer disease, 548–549, 552,
553. *See also* Peptic ulcer
disease, NSAID-induced
platelet function affected by, 490,
490*t*, 548, 749
for polycythemia, 458
reference values for, 1553*t*
Reye syndrome and, 78, 1198, 1270
for rheumatic fever, 376
for stroke, 892
for transient ischemic attacks, 888
Asplenia, immunization recommendations in, 1195*t*
pneumococcal vaccine and, 1195*t*,
1199
Assist-control (A-C) ventilation, for respiratory failure, 290
Assisted reproductive technologies, 694,
866
Assistive devices, fall prevention and,
69–70
AST. *See* Aspartate aminotransferase
Astemizole, antidepressant drug interactions and, 966, 969*t*
Astereognosis, intracranial tumors causing, 899
Asterixis, 524, 622
Asthma, **216–234**
allergic, 216, 221, 223
desensitization therapy/immuno-
therapy for, 228
allergic bronchopulmonary mycosis/
aspergillosis and, 241, 1397
aspirin triggering (triad asthma), 199
β-adrenergic agents for
long-acting, 224*t*, 227, 228
short-acting, 228
bronchial provocation testing in, 219
cardiac, 217
catamenial, 216
classification/diagnosis of, 217–221,
217*f*, 218*t*, 219*t*, 220*t*
complications of, 221
controller medications for, 223,
223–228, 224–225*t*,
226–227*t*
COPD differentiated from, 235
cough and, 22, 23*t*
differential diagnosis of, 221
drugs causing, 216, 281*t*
estrogen replacement therapy and,
1072
exacerbations of
classification of severity of,
217–221, 217*f*, 218*t*, 219*t*,
220*t*, 221, 222*f*
treatment of, 217*f*, 218*t*, 230–233,
231*f*, 232*f*
exercise-induced, 216–217. *See also*
Exercise-induced asthma
hypophosphatemia and, 803
mediator inhibitors for, 223
NAEPP 3 diagnosis/management
guidelines for, 217*f*, 218*t*,
221–223, 222*f*, 230–233,
231*f*, 232*f*
occupational, 216, 280

postoperative pulmonary complications and, 53, 54
during pregnancy, **724**
pulmonary function testing in,
219–221
reliever medications for, 223,
228–230, 229–230*t*
severity/control of, assessing/monitor-
ing, 217–221, 217*f*, 218*t*,
219*t*, 220*t*, 221, 222*f*
treatment of, 223–233
desensitization/immunotherapy in,
228
for exacerbations, 217*f*, 218*t*,
230–233, 231*f*, 232*f*
long-term control medications for,
223, 223–228, 224–225*t*,
226–227*t*
mind-body therapies in, 1536*t*
biofeedback, 1536*t*, 1538
NAEPP 3 guidelines for, 217*f*, 218*t*,
221–223, 222*f*, 230–233,
231*f*, 232*f*
pharmacologic, 223, 223–233
quick relief medications for, 223,
228–230, 229–230*t*
stepwise approach to, 222*f*
triad, 199
vaccinations for patients with, 228
Asthma action plan, 223, 230
Astigmatism, 151
Astrocytoma, 898*t*, 1467*t*
Astroviruses, diarrhea/gastroenteritis
caused by, 1172
Asymptomatic renal disease, 833, 843
Atabrine. *See* Quinacrine
Atacand. *See* Candesartan
Atactic breathing, in coma or stupor, 916
Ataxia
in acute high-altitude cerebral edema,
1418
fragile X tremor-ataxia syndrome and,
1515
Friedreich, 923
intracranial tumors causing, 899
in varicella, 1241
Ataxia-telangiectasia mutation
breast cancer risk and, 653
pancreatic/periampullary carcinoma
and, 1463
Atazanavir, 1226*t*, 1229, 1230, 1232*f*. *See
also* Antiretroviral therapy
Atelectasis
in airway obstruction, 216
pleural effusion and, 283
postoperative, prevention of, 54
in right middle lobe syndrome, 216
Atenolol
for alcohol withdrawal, 980–981
for hypertension, 400*t*
in diabetics, 1088
for Marfan syndrome, 1518
ATG. *See* Antithymocyte globulin
Atherosclerosis, **415–422**. *See also specific
artery affected and* Cardio-
vascular disorders; Vascular disorders
acute limb occlusion and, 419

aneurysms and, 425
aortoiliac disease caused by, **415–416**
cerebrovascular occlusive disease
caused by, 420. *See also*
Stroke
cholesterol/lipoproteins in,
1123–1124, 1124
screening tests for levels of,
1126–1129, 1127–1128*t*,
1129*t*
coronary artery disease caused by. *See*
Coronary heart disease
in diabetes mellitus, 1108, 1108–1109
femoral/popliteal disease caused by,
416–417
garlic for, 1523*t*, 1524
homocysteine/hyperhomocysteine-
mia and, 1516, 1517
hypertension and, 391, 393
lipid-lowering therapy affecting
course of, 1124–1125
lower leg/foot disease caused by,
417–418
renal artery stenosis caused by, 391,
832
transient ischemic attacks and, 886,
888
visceral artery insufficiency and, 421
Atherosclerotic (multi-infarct) dementia,
63, 986
hypertension and, 393
Atherosclerotic plaques. *See* Atherosclerosis
Athletes
cardiovascular screening of, **385–386**
exertional heat stroke in, 1407
sports medicine injuries and, **744–747**
sudden death of, 385–386
cardiomyopathy causing, 373, 386
Athlete's foot, **108–109**
cellulitis and, 109, 129
Ativan. *See* Lorazepam
ATL. *See* Adult T cell lymphoma/leukemia
Atlantoaxial subluxation, neck pain
caused by, 737
Atonic seizures (epileptic drop attacks),
880. *See also* Seizures
Atopic dermatitis (eczema), **101–103**, 784
in food allergy, 101
herpes simplex infection (eczema herpeticum) and, 103, 1236,
1240*t*
smallpox vaccination (eczema vaccinatum) and, 103, 116,
1277
vesiculobullous hand (pompholyx),
116–117
Atopic disease (atopy), 784, **784–785**. *See
also specific disorder and*
Allergies/allergic reactions
asthma and, 216, 221
COPD and, 234
eosinophilic esophagitis and, 537
Atopic keratoconjunctivitis, 155
Atopic-like dermatitis, 102
Atorvastatin, 1131, 1132*t*. *See also* Statin
drugs
in HIV infection/AIDS, 1229

Atovaquone
  for malaria, with proguanil
    (Malarone), 1355t, 1357t,
    1360
  chemoprophylaxis and, 1355t,
    1360, 1361, 1361t
  self-treatment and, 1361
  for *P jiroveci* infection, 1222t, 1224t,
    1395
ATP1A2 gene, in familial hemiplegic
  migraine, 873
ATP78 in Wilson disease, 628, 629
ATRA. *See* Tretinoin
Atrial fibrillation, **346–349**, 347t
  arterial emboli and, 346, 347t
    anticoagulation in prevention/
      management of, 348
    limb occlusion and, 419
    transient ischemic attacks and, 886,
      888
    transient monocular blindness and,
      165
  in atrial septal defect, 297
  in cardiomyopathy, 373
  in hyperthyroidism/thyrotoxicosis,
    346, 1009, 1014
  in mitral regurgitation, 307
  in mitral stenosis, 306, 307
  in myocardial infarction, 336–337
  in preexcitation syndromes, 345
  recurrent paroxysmal, 349
  refractory, 349
Atrial flutter, **349–350**
  in COPD, 238, 349
  in reentry/preexcitation and, 345,
    349–350
Atrial gallop. *See* Heart sounds
Atrial myxoma, 382–383
  herpes simplex virus and, 1236
Atrial (supraventricular) premature beats
    (atrial extrasystoles), **341**
  in myocardial infarction, 336
Atrial septal aneurysm, 297
Atrial septal defect, **297–298**
Atrial septal lipoma, 383
Atrial tachycardia, multifocal (chaotic),
    350
Atrioventricular (heart) block, **355**
  in atrial septal defect, 298
  lithium use and, 971
  in Lyme disease, 1343, 1346, 1346t
  in myocardial infarction, 337
  in poisoning/drug overdose, 1422t
  sudden death and, 353
Atrioventricular canal defect, 297
Atrioventricular dissociation, **355–356**
Atrioventricular junctional rhythm,
    350–351
Atrioventricular nodal reentry tachycardia
    (AVNRT), 342
Atrioventricular pathways, accessory,
    supraventricular tachycar-
    dia caused by, 342,
    345–346
Atrioventricular reentrant tachycardia
    (AVRT), 342, 345
Atripla. *See* Efavirenz, with tenofovir and
  emtricitabine

Atrophic age-related macular degenera-
    tion, 162, 163
Atrophic gastritis
  H pylori infection and, 547
  in pernicious anemia, 547
Atrophic urethritis, urinary incontinence
    and, 70
Atrophic vaginitis
  in menopause, 703, 704, 1071
  urinary incontinence and, 70
Atrophie blanche, 37
Atropine
  for cholinesterase inhibitor (anticho-
    linesterase) poisoning,
    1424t, 1443
    nerve agents and, 1434
  with diphenoxylate. *See* Diphenoxy-
    late with atropine
  for muscarinic-type mushroom poi-
    soning, 1442
  overdose/toxicity of, 1424t, **1432**
  in terminally ill/dying patient, 92
Atypical absences, 879t, 880
Atypical antidepressants, 964–966. *See*
    also Antidepressants
Atypical antipsychotics, 954, 955–957,
    957, 958t. *See also* Antipsy-
    chotic drugs
  for dementia-associated behavior
    problems, 66
  in elderly, 957
  for mania, 970
  for parkinsonism, 907–908
Atypical facial pain, **877**
Atypical measles, 1240t, 1248
Atypical mycobacteria. *See* Nontuberculous
    (atypical) mycobacteria
Atypical nevi/mole, **100**
Atypical psychoses, 953
Atypical squamous cells of unknown sig-
    nificance (ASC-US), 680,
    680t, 681
Audiology, **179–180**
Audiovestibular disorders, 191, 191t. *See*
    also Vestibular disorders
  autoimmune pattern of, 187
AUDIT (Alcohol Use Disorder Identifica-
    tion Test), 19, 20t
Auditory canal. *See* Ear canal
Auditory hallucinations. *See also* Halluci-
    nations
  intracranial tumors causing, 899
  in schizophrenic/psychotic disorders,
    953
Auer rods, in acute leukemia, 465
Augmentation mammoplasty. *See* Breast
    implants
Augmentin. *See* Amoxicillin/amoxicillin-
    clavulanate
Auricle, **180**
Austin Flint murmur, 312
Austrian triad, 1292
Autoimmune cholangitis, 626
Autoimmune disorders/autoimmunity,
    747–764. *See also specific*
    disease
  cognitive disorders/delirium caused
    by, 985t

common variable immunodeficiency
    and, 787
  in diabetes, 1079, 1079–1081, 1080t
  fever/FUO and, 1153, 1154
  hearing loss in, 187
  in HIV infection/AIDS, 1208
  silicone gel breast implants and, 652
Autoimmune hemolytic anemia,
    452–453
  with thrombocytopenia (Evans syn-
    drome), 453
Autoimmune hepatitis, **612–614**
Autoimmune pancreatitis, 646
Autoimmune polyendocrinopathy-candi-
    diasis-ectodermal dystro-
    phy, 1048
Autoimmune thyroiditis. *See* Hashimoto
    (chronic lymphocytic/
    autoimmune) thyroiditis
Autoinflation, for eustachian tube dys-
    function/barotrauma, 182,
    183
Autologous packed red cells, transfusion
    of, 477
Autologous stem cell transplantation, **475.**
    See also Bone marrow/
    stem cell transplantation
Autologous tissue flaps, for breast recon-
    struction, 672
Automatism, postepileptic, 880
Automobile accidents
  cardiac trauma and, 384
  preventable deaths caused by, 2t
  prevention of injury caused by, 18
Automobile driving, by patients with syn-
    cope/ventricular tachycar-
    dia/aborted sudden death,
    357–358
Autonomic dysfunction (dysautonomia),
    884–885
  in Guillain-Barré syndrome, 885, 925
  in polyneuropathies, 922
Autonomic failure, pure, 885
Autonomic neuropathy
  cancer-related, 885
  chemotherapy-induced, 1510
  in diabetes, 923, 1107–1108
    hypoglycemia and, 1103–1104,
      1107
  dysautonomia and, 885
  in porphyria, 923, 1512
Autonomic testing
  in dysautonomia, 885
  in syncope, 357
Autophony, patulous eustachian tube and,
    182
Autosomal dominant hypocalcemia with
    hypercalciuria (ADHH),
    1030, 1031
Autosomal dominant polycystic kidney
    disease, **847–848**, 847t
  intracranial aneurysms and, 848, 894
AV block. *See* Atrioventricular (heart)
    block
AV dissociation, **355–356**
AV junctional rhythm, **350–351**
AV nodal reentry tachycardia (AVNRT),
    342

AV reentrant tachycardia (AVRT), 342, 345
Avalide. *See* Irbesartan
Avandamet. *See* Rosiglitazone, with metformin
Avandaryl. *See* Rosiglitazone, with glimepiride
Avandia. *See* Rosiglitazone
Avapro. *See* Irbesartan
Avascular necrosis of bone, **783–784**
  corticosteroid use and, 1078
Avastin. *See* Bevacizumab
Aveeno, 98t
Aveeno Anti-Itch lotion. *See* Pramoxine
Avelox. *See* Moxifloxacin
Aventis. *See* Insulin glargine
Aventyl. *See* Nortriptyline
Aversive conditioning. *See* Behavior modification
Avian influenza (H5N1), 5, 1269, 1271, **1271–1272**. *See also* Influenza
Avinza. *See* Morphine
Avita. *See* Tretinoin
AVNRT (AV nodal reentry tachycardia), 342
Avoidance therapy
  for allergic contact dermatitis, 119
  for allergic rhinitis, 197
Avoidant personality disorder, 951t
AVRT (AV reentrant tachycardia), 342, 345
Axilla, radial nerve lesions in, 927
Axillary lymph nodes, in breast cancer, 657
  dissection of, 664, 665
    arm edema and, 671–672
    in breast-conserving therapy, 664
  palpation for evaluation of, 656, 656f
  prognosis and, 670
  recurrence and, 671
  sentinel node biopsy and, 664
Axillary vessels, compression of in thoracic outlet/cervical rib syndromes, 737
Axillo-femoral bypass, for aortoiliac occlusive disease, 416
Axonal neuropathies, 921, 925. *See also specific type and* Neuropathies
Aygestin. *See* Norethindrone
Azacitidine, 1501t
  for myelodysplasia, 464
Azactam. *See* Aztreonam
Azathioprine
  with allopurinol, dose adjustments and, 735
  for autoimmune hepatitis, 613
  for inflammatory bowel disease, 576
    Crohn disease, 581
    ulcerative colitis, 584, 585
  for Wegener granulomatosis, 769
Azelastine, for allergic eye disease, 155, 173t
Azidothymidine. *See* Zidovudine
Azithromycin. *See also* Macrolides
  for endocarditis, 1306t

for MAC prophylaxis/treatment, 1222, 1325
for pharyngitis, 205, 1290
renal/hepatic failure and, 1184t
for syphilis, 1333
Azo compounds, for inflammatory bowel disease, 575
Azoospermia, 864
  artificial insemination for infertility caused by, 694
  in cystic fibrosis, 241
  genetic causes of, 865
  in Klinefelter syndrome, 1064, 1517
Azopt. *See* Brinzolamide
Azotemia, 816, 819. *See also* Kidney disease/injury
  in diabetic ketoacidosis, 1112
  heart failure and, 360
  in hepatorenal syndrome, 622
  in hyperglycemic hyperosmolar state, 1015
  pancreatitis and, 644
  parenteral nutritional support and, 1151t
  postrenal, 820t, 821
  prerenal, 820–821, 820t
  in tubulointerstitial disease, 845
AZT. *See* Zidovudine
Aztreonam, renal/hepatic failure and, 1184t

B19 parvovirus infection. *See* Parvovirus B19 infection
B antigen, in compatibility testing, 477
B cell lymphoma. *See also* Non-Hodgkin lymphoma
  gastric, 1473
  small intestine, 1475
B cells, pancreatic, 1062
  in diabetes mellitus, 1079, 1080t, 1081
    latent autoimmune diabetes of adulthood, 1080–1081
  hypoglycemia caused by tumors of, 1062, 1063, **1118–1120**, 1119t. *See also* Insulinomas; Islet cell tumors
B lymphocytes
  clonal malignancy of (chronic lymphocytic leukemia), **467–468**
  in common variable immunodeficiency, 787
  in HIV infection/AIDS, 1208
B-type natriuretic peptide (BNP/beta)
  in deep venous thrombosis/pulmonary embolism, 267–268
  in dyspnea, 26
  in heart failure, 360
  recombinant. *See* Nesiritide
  reference values for, 1548t
Babesia divergens/microti (babesiosis), **1362–1363**
  Lyme disease coinfection and, 1346
Bacillary angiomatosis, 1215, 1321
Bacillary dysentery (shigella dysentery/gastroenteritis), 512, 1171t, 1172, 1174, 1182t, 1314

Bacillus, 1177t
  anthracis, 1177t, 1300. *See also* Anthrax
  cereus, food poisoning/gastroenteritis caused by, 512, 1170t, 1172
Bacillus Calmette-Guérin (BCG)
  for bladder cancer, 1490
  for interstitial cystitis, 861
Bacillus Calmette-Guérin (BCG) vaccine, 257–258
  tuberculin skin test affected by, 253, 257–258
  tuberculosis blood tests and, 4
Bacitracin, for ophthalmic disorders, 173t
Back pain, **738–740**, 739t
  acupuncture for, 1533
  in ankylosing spondylitis, 738, 739, 773, 774
  in aortic aneurysm, 423, 425, 738
  in aortic dissection, 426
  in cancer-related spinal cord compression, 1495
  disk-related, 738, 739
  epidural/subdural hemorrhage causing, 897
  in osteoporosis, 1039
  radiographic evaluation in, 739
  spinal cord lesions/tumors causing, 738, 739, 901
  spinal stenosis causing, 740
  spinal tuberculosis causing, 782
  tumor mass causing, 738, 739
Background retinopathy, 166
Bacteremia. *See also* Sepsis/septic shock
  anaerobic, **1323**
  campylobacter causing, 1316
  catheter-associated, 1160, 1161
  endocarditis and, 1304
  gonococcal, 1319
  gram-negative, 1177t, **1311–1312**
  hospital-associated, 1160, 1161
  in listeriosis, 1303
  in Lyme disease, 1343
  in neutropenic patient, 1158
  osteomyelitis from, 780
  salmonella, 1177t, 1312, **1314**
  staphylococcal, **1296**
  in streptococcal toxic shock syndrome, 1291
  in typhoid fever, 1313
  vibrios causing, 1316
Bacterial infections, **1289–1327**. *See also specific type*
  actinomycosis, **1323–1324**
  anaerobic, **1321–1323**
  diarrhea in, 512t. *See also* Diarrhea, infectious
  drugs for. *See* Antibiotics; Antimicrobial therapy
  endocarditis, **1303–1307**, 1305t, 1306t
  gram-negative, 1176t, 1176–1177t, **1307–1323**
  gram-positive, 1176t, 1177t, **1289–1303**
  mycobacterial, **1324–1327**
  myocarditis in, 368, 369t
  nocardiosis, **1324**
  rhinosinusitis (sinusitis), **192–195**, 194t

shock and. *See* Sepsis/septic shock
vaginosis, 678, 679, 1167
   rape/sexual assault in transmission of, 1167
Bacterial overgrowth, 516, **561–562**
   irritable bowel syndrome and, 570
   vitamin B_{12} deficiency and, 445, 562
Bacterial synergistic gangrene, 1323
Bacteriuria
   asymptomatic, screening for, 5
   catheter-associated, 1161
   in cystitis, 851
   during pregnancy, 725
Bacteroides
   fragilis, 1322
   gastrointestinal strains of, 1176t, 1321
   melaninogenicus. See Prevotella, melaninogenica
   resistant strains of, 1322
Bactrim. *See* Trimethoprim-sulfamethoxazole
Bactroban. *See* Mupirocin
Baden-Walker system, 687
Bagassosis, 280t
Baker (popliteal) cyst, 33, 744
BAL. *See* Dimercaprol
Balamuthia mandrillaris, 1163, 1368
Balance. *See* Disequilibrium; Falls; Vestibular disorders
Balanitis
   candidal, 125
   in chancroid, 1320
Balantidium coli (balantidiasis), 1372
Baldness, **145–146**. *See also* Alopecia
Balint syndrome, 899
Balkan nephropathy, ureteral/renal pelvis cancer and, 1491
Balloon tube tamponade, for esophageal varices, 540
Balloon valvuloplasty. *See* Valvuloplasty
Balsalazide, for inflammatory bowel disease, 575
   ulcerative colitis, 584, 584t
Bamboo spine, 774
Band keratopathy, in hypercalcemia/hyperparathyroidism, 1034
Banding, gastric, for obesity, 15, 1138
Banding (band/variceal ligation)
   for esophageal varices, 539, 540
      prevention of first bleeding episode and, 541
      prevention of rebleeding and, 540
   for hemorrhoids, 594
Barakat syndrome, 1030–1031
Barbiturates. *See* Opioids/opioid analgesics; Sedative-hypnotics
Bariatric surgery, for obesity, 15, 1138
   hypoglycemia after, 1117, 1121
Baritosis, 279t
Barium enema
   in adenomatous polyp identification, 590
   in cancer screening/evaluation, 17t, 1482
   in diverticular disease, 587, 588
Barium esophagography, 530
   in achalasia, 542

   in esophageal cancer, 1468
   in esophageal webs and rings, 538
   in GERD, 531
   in motility disorders, 543
Barium upper gastrointestinal series. *See* Upper gastrointestinal series
Baroreceptors, in volume overload, 794
Barotrauma, **183**
   decompression sickness and, 183, 1417
   mechanical ventilation and, 290–291
Barrett esophagus, 532
   esophageal carcinoma and, 532, 1468
Bartholin duct cyst/abscess, **679**
Bartonella henselae/quintana (bartonellosis), **1321**
   bacillary angiomatosis caused by, 1215, 1321
Bartter syndrome, 796t
Basal body temperature charting, in contraception, 700
   symptothermal natural family planning and, 699
Basal cell carcinoma
   of skin, **133–134**
   of vulva, 685
Basal energy expenditure (BEE)
   exercise and, 1137
   nutritional support and, 1148
Basedow disease, 1008. *See also* Graves disease; Hyperthyroidism
Basilar artery migraine, 873
Basilar artery occlusion, stroke caused by, 891
Basilar meningitis, in syphilis, 1334
Basilar skull fracture, 918
   vertigo caused by, 190
Basophil count, 1547t
Bathing, in dermatologic therapy, 94
Battered elderly, 19, **75**, 75t
Battered woman, 976, 977
   prevention of abuse and, 18–19
Batteries (disk), ingested, alkali injuries caused by, 1429, 1430
Battle sign, 918
Baylisascaris procyonis, visceral larva migrans caused by, 1385
BCG, for bladder cancer, 1490
BCG vaccine, 257–258
   tuberculin skin test affected by, 253, 257–258
   tuberculosis blood tests and, 4
bcl-2 expression, in non-Hodgkin lymphoma, 469
bcr/abl fusion gene
   in chronic myeloid leukemia, 461, 462
   reference values for, 1547t
Beano, for gastrointestinal gas, 511
Beau lines, 146
Becaplermin, for leg/foot ulcers, 144, 1106
Becker muscular dystrophy, 934, 934t, 935
Beclomethasone, for asthma, 226t
Bed rest. *See also* Immobility
   back pain and, 740
   hazards of, 68
      deep venous thrombosis/pulmonary embolism and, 267, 270t

   for preeclampsia-eclampsia, 717
   for third-trimester bleeding, 720
Bedbugs, skin lesions caused by, 139
Bedside tracheostomy, 212
Bedsores (decubitus ulcers), **72–74**, 73t
   bed rest/immobility and, 68, 73
BEE. *See* Basal energy expenditure
Beef. *See* Meat
Beef tapeworm *(T saginata)*, 1376, **1376**
Beer consumption, gout/hyperuricemia and, 733, 734
Beer potomania, 791
Behavior
   abnormal
      illness, **944–946**
      during sleep (parasomnias), **975–976**
   in demented patients, 64, 65–66
   insulin-induced hypoglycemia and, 1103
   in schizophrenic/psychotic disorders, 953
Behavior modification. *See also* Cognitive behavior therapy
   for alcohol use/abuse, 20, 980
   in Alzheimer disease, 988
   for chronic fatigue syndrome, 43
   for obesity management, 15, 1137
   for personality disorders, 951
   for psychiatric problems associated with hospitalization/illness and, 990
   for schizophrenic/psychotic disorders, 960
   for substance use disorders, 21
   for urinary incontinence management, 71
Behçet syndrome, **771–772**
   uveitis in, 160, 772
Bejel (endemic syphilis), 1339
Belching (eructation), 510–511
Bell palsy, **928–929**
   herpes simplex infection and, 928, 1236, 1237
   Lyme disease and, 1343, 1345, 1346t
   varicella-zoster virus infection and, 1241
Belladonna
   MAOI interactions and, 969t
   overdose/toxicity of, 1432
Benazepril, 403t
Bence Jones proteinuria (light chain in urine), 817
   in myeloma, 472, 817, 848
   renal toxicity and, 822
Bendamustine, 1500t
Bends, 1417
Benicar. *See* Olmesartan
Benign essential (familial) tremor, **904–905**
   parkinsonism differentiated from, 905–906
Benign mole, 99
Benign paroxysmal positioning vertigo (BPPV), 189, 191t
Benign prostatic hyperplasia, **866–871**, 867t, 868f, 869t
   phytotherapy/saw palmetto for, 870, 1523t, 1526–1527

Benign prostatic hyperplasia (*cont.*)
  postrenal azotemia caused by, 821
  testosterone replacement therapy and, 1065
  tubulointerstitial disease caused by, 845
  urinary incontinence and, 71, 72
Bentall procedure
  for aortic regurgitation, 313
  for aortic stenosis, 311
BenzaClin. *See* Clindamycin, with benzoyl peroxide
Benzamycin. *See* Erythromycin, with benzoyl peroxide
Benzisothiazolyl piperazine, 955t, 956t. *See also* Antipsychotic drugs
Benzisoxazoles, 954, 955t, 956t. *See also* Antipsychotic drugs
Benznidazole, for Chagas disease, 1350
Benzocaine, methemoglobinemia caused by, 1440
Benzodiazepines, 941–943, 941t, 942t. *See also specific agent*
  for aggressive/violent patient, 976
  for alcohol withdrawal, 19, 883, 980
  with antipsychotic agents, 957
  for anxiety, 941–942, 941t
  for delirium, 987
  drug interactions of, 942t
  for hallucinogen overdose/toxicity, 1439
  for insomnia, 941t, 942
  for nausea and vomiting, 87, 507
  in older adult, 941, 942
  overdose/toxicity of, 942, 1421, 1424t, **1436**. *See also* Flumazenil
  for panic attacks, 942, 943
  for posttraumatic stress disorder, 939
  for sleep disorders, 942, 975–976
  withdrawal from, 942
Benzoyl peroxide
  for acne, 121
    with clindamycin, 97t, 121
    with erythromycin, 97t, 121
  for rosacea, 123
Benztropine, 906t. *See also* Antiparkinsonism drugs
Beraprost, for pulmonary hypertension, 275, 381
Berger disease (IgA nephropathy), **834–835**, 835f, 836t
Beriberi, 1141. *See also* Thiamine (vitamin B₁), deficiency of
  neuropathy associated with, 923, 1141
Bernard-Soulier syndrome, 489, 489–490
Berry aneurysms, 894. *See also* Intracranial aneurysm
Berylliosis, 281
Beta-adrenergic agonists
  for asthma
    exacerbation management and, 230, 231f, 232f, 233
    long-acting, 224t, 227, 228
    short-acting, 228, 229t, 230, 231f, 232f, 233
  for COPD, 237
  for hyperkalemia, 798
  for preterm labor prevention, 719

Beta-adrenergic blocking drugs
  for acute coronary syndromes, 327t, 328
  for aggressive/violent behavior, 976, 987
  for angina, 321
  for anxiety/stress disorders, 943
  for aortic dissection, 427
  for aortic regurgitation, 312–313
  for arrhythmias, 343t
    atrial fibrillation, 347
      in hyperthyroidism, 1014
      infarct-related, 336
    in heart failure, 365
    in hyperthyroidism, 1014
    paroxysmal supraventricular tachycardia, 342, 345
    ventricular tachycardia, 352
  for cardiomyopathy, 373
  depression caused by, 962
  for esophageal varices
    prevention of first bleeding episode and, 541
    prevention of rebleeding and, 540
  for glaucoma/ocular hypertension, 159, 175t
  for Graves disease/hyperthyroidism, 1010–1011, 1014
  in heart failure, 362–363, 365, 402
  for hypertension, 396t, 398–402, 400–401t, 407–409, 409f
    in aortic dissection, 427
    in combination regimen, 409, 409f
    in diabetics, 396t, 402, 1088
    pregnancy and, 723
  hypoglycemic symptoms affected by, 1103
  lipid abnormalities associated with use of, 1126t
  for Marfan syndrome, 1518
  for myocardial infarction, 327t, 335, 336, 340
  overdose/toxicity of, 402, 1422, **1432–1433**
  for panic attacks, 943
  perioperative, 50, 51t
  pheochromocytoma and, 402, 1061
  for phobic disorder, 943
Beta-carotene
  in atherosclerosis/heart disease prevention, 12
  in cancer prevention, 12
  excess intake of, 1144
Beta-catenin, hepatic adenoma and, 633
Beta-globin gene, 442
  in beta thalassemia syndromes, 442, 443t
  in sickle cell syndromes, 450
Beta-glucocerebrosidase, in Gaucher disease, 1516
Beta-hemolytic streptococci. *See specific type under* Group
Beta-hydroxybutyrate/hydroxybutyric acid
  in alcoholic ketoacidosis, 809
  in diabetes mellitus, 1083
  in diabetic ketoacidosis, 808, 809, 1113

Beta interferon. *See* Interferon-β
Beta-lactam antibiotics, for pneumonia, 247, 249
Beta₂-microglobulin, in myeloma, 472, 1547t
Beta-natriuretic peptide. *See* B-type natriuretic peptide
Beta thalassemia syndromes, 442, 443, 443t, 444
  sickle cell disease and, 451t, 452
Betagan. *See* Levobunolol
Betaine, for homocystinuria, 1517
Betamethasone, 97t, 1077t
  for fetal lung maturity, 719
Betaxolol
  for glaucoma/ocular hypertension, 159, 175t
  for systemic hypertension, 400t
Bethesda assay, 491, 494
Bethesda criteria, for HNPCC, 592
Bethesda System, for Pap smear classification, 680–681, 680t
Betimol. *See* Timolol
Betoptic S. *See* Betaxolol
Bevacizumab, 668, 1503t
  for breast cancer, 668
  for colorectal cancer, 1479
  for diabetic eye disease, 1105
  for lung cancer, 1456
  for renal cell carcinoma, 1492
  for retinal vein occlusion, 164
Bexarotene, TSH affected by, 993
Bexxar. *See* Tositumomab
Bezafibrate, 1131–1132
Bezold-Jarisch reflex, in angina, 318
Biaxin. *See* Clarithromycin
Bicalutamide, 1505t
  for prostate cancer, 1487t
Bicarbonate
  for acidosis
    alkalosis caused by, 813
    in chronic kidney disease, 828
    diabetic ketoacidosis, 808, 1114
    increased anion gap acidosis, 811
    lactic acidosis, 1117
    normal anion gap/renal tubular acidosis, 811
  arterial, 806
  contrast media nephrotoxicity mediated by, 822
  in fluid management, 815t
  gastrointestinal loss of, acidosis caused by, 809–810, 809t
  for hyperkalemia, 797, 798, 799t
  lithium interactions and, 972t
  for lithium overdose/toxicity, 972
  plasma/serum levels of
    in acid-base disorders, 806
    in alcoholic ketoacidosis, 809
    in diabetic ketoacidosis, 1112, 1112t
    in hyperchloremic normal anion gap acidosis/renal tubular acidosis, 809–810, 809t, 810
    in lactic acidosis, 1016
    in metabolic acidosis, 806, 807t
    in metabolic alkalosis, 806, 807, 807t, 812, 812t, 813

in respiratory acidosis, 806, 807*t*, 813, 814
in respiratory alkalosis, 806, 807*t*, 814
reference values for, 1548*t*
for salicylate poisoning, 811, 1445
for shock, 437
for tricyclic antidepressant overdose, 1422, 1448–1449
venous, 806
Bicycle riding, injury prevention and, 18
Bifascicular block, 356
Bifidobacterium infantis probiotic, for irritable bowel syndrome, 572–573
Bigeminy, 351
Biguanides, for diabetes mellitus, 1091*t*
Bile acid-binding resins, for lipid modification/heart disease prevention, 1131, 1132
Bile ascites, 528–529
Bile ducts
carcinoma of. *See* Cholangiocarcinoma
common, stones in. *See* Choledocholithiasis
Bile salts, decreased concentration of, malabsorption and, 558
in short bowel syndrome, 562
Bilharziasis, **1373–1375**. *See also Schistosoma*
Biliary cirrhosis, 620, **625–627**
Biliary colic
in choledocholithiasis/cholangitis, 638
in cholelithiasis/gallstones, 634
Biliary obstruction, 598, 599*t*
biliary tract carcinoma causing, 598, 1462
in choledocholithiasis/cholangitis, 638
Biliary pain, 634, 635*t*, 638
Biliary pancreatitis, 643, 644
Biliary sludge (microlithiasis), 634
pancreatitis and, 642, 645
Biliary stricture, **639–640**
cholangitis and, 639–640; 640, 641
Biliary tract
diseases of, **634–641**, 635*t*. *See also specific disease*
carcinoma, 598, **1461–1463**
cholecystitis, **635–637**, 635*t*
choledocholithiasis/cholangitis, 635*t*, **638–639**
cholelithiasis (gallstones), **634–635**, 635*t*
in clonorchiasis/opisthorchiasis, 1375
cytomegalovirus infection and, 1245
dyspepsia and, 502
in fascioliasis, 1375
in HIV infection/AIDS, 1214
inflammation. *See* Cholangitis
pre- and postcholecystectomy syndromes, **637**
primary sclerosing cholangitis, **640–641**
strictures, **639–640**

surgery on, antibiotic prophylaxis for, 60*t*
Bilirubin levels. *See also* Hyperbilirubinemia
in alcoholic liver disease, 614
ascitic fluid, 525
in autoimmune hepatitis, 612
in biliary tract carcinoma, 1462
in cholecystitis, 636
in choledocholithiasis/cholangitis, 638
in cirrhosis, 620
in glucose-6-phosphate dehydrogenase deficiency, 450
in hemolytic anemia, 448
in liver disease/jaundice, 598, 600*t*
reference/normal values for, 598, 600*t*, 1547*t*
urine, 600*t*
in vitamin B$_{12}$ deficiency, 446
Bilirubinate, calcium, in gallstones, 634
Bilivist. *See* Ipodate sodium
Billowing mitral valve. *See* Mitral valve prolapse
Biloma, 639
Bimatoprost, for glaucoma/ocular hypertension, 159, 175*t*
Bimatoprost/timolol, for glaucoma/ocular hypertension, 159, 176*t*
Binge eating, in bulimia nervosa, 1140
Biobrane, for burn wounds, 1411
Biofeedback, 1520, **1535–1538**, 1536*t*
for fecal incontinence, 596, 1536*t*, 1537–1538
for somatoform disorders, 945
for urinary incontinence, 1536*t*, 1537
Biofields, in energy medicine, 1520
Biologic response modifiers, 1506*t*. *See also specific agent*
for renal cell carcinoma, 1492
Biologic therapies
in CAM, 1520. *See also* Dietary supplements; Herbal medicines
for inflammatory bowel disease, 576–577
Biomarkers
in breast cancer, 657, **663–664**. *See also* Hormone receptor sites
prognosis and, 665*t*, 670
cardiac, 326, 331. *See also* Cardiac biomarkers/enzymes
Bioprostheses, for cardiac valve replacement, 315–316. *See also* Valve replacement
Bioterrorism
anthrax and, 1300, 1301, 1302
botulinum toxin and, 1299
chemical warfare agents and nerve agents, **1434**
ricin, **1434**
skin decontamination for, 1424
plague and, 1318
Rickettsia prowazekii and, 1281
smallpox/smallpox vaccination and, 116, 1277
tularemia (*Francisella tularensis*) and, 1317

Biperiden, 906*t*. *See also* Antiparkinsonism drugs
Bipolar disorders, 962. *See also* Depression; Mania
lithium for, 970–972, 972*t*
Bipolaris, phaeohyphomycosis caused by, 1402
Bird-fancier's lung (pigeon-breeder's disease), 280*t*
Bird mites. *See* Mites
Birds
avian influenza and, 1271, 1272
psittacosis (ornithosis) and, 1329
West Nile virus in, 1257
Birth classes, 707
Birth control pills. *See* Oral contraceptives
Bisacodyl, 509*t*, 510
Bisferiens pulse, in cardiomyopathy, 373
Bismuth compounds
for diarrhea, 514
in *H pylori* eradication therapy, 550
for peptic ulcer disease, 550
Bisoprolol
for heart failure, 363
with hydrochlorothiazide, for hypertension, 400*t*
perioperative, 50
Bisphosphonates, 1040. *See also specific agent*
adverse ophthalmic effects of, 178*t*, 1040
in breast cancer management, 667–668
hypercalcemia associated with use of, 1036, 1040
for hypercalcemia/hyperparathyroidism, 801, 1037, 1497
for myeloma-related bone disease, 473
osteonecrosis of jaw and, 783, 1040, 1045
for osteoporosis, 12, 704, 1040, 1070
androgen deprivation therapy and, 1488
chronic corticosteroid treatment and, 1040, 1078
for Paget disease of bone, 1045–1046
Bite cells, in glucose-6-phosphate dehydrogenase deficiency, 450
Bites. *See* Animal bites; Human bite wounds; Insect bites
Bithionol, for fascioliasis, 1375
Bitolterol, for asthma, 228
Bitot spots, in vitamin A deficiency, 1143
Bitter almonds, odor of in cyanide poisoning, 1435
Bivalirudin
for acute coronary syndromes, 327–328, 327*t*
for heparin-induced thrombocytopenia, 486*t*, 487
Biventricular pacing (resynchronization), for heart failure, 365–366
Black cohosh, 1523*t*, 1527
Black eye, 171
in nasal trauma, 199
Black fever. *See* Visceral leishmaniasis
Black molds
chromoblastomycosis caused by, 1400
phaeohyphomycosis caused by, 1402

Black patients. *See also* Racial/ethnic background
cardiomyopathy in, 370
colorectal cancer risk in, 1477
diuretics in, 398
glaucoma in, 158
glucose-6-phosphate dehydrogenase deficiency in, 449
hypertension in, 387, 388, 390
management of, 410, 410*t*
PSA reference values in, 1485
sarcoidosis in, 265
sickle cell anemia/syndromes in, 450
Black plague, 1177*t*, 1318
Black widow spider bite, 139, 1447
Blackwater fever, in malaria, 1358
Bladder
biopsy of, in bladder cancer, 1489
cancer of, 1467*t*, **1489–1491**
hematuria in, 1489
disorders/dysfunction of. *See also specific type and* Urinary incontinence
chronic kidney disease and, 827*t*
postrenal azotemia caused by, 821
spinal trauma causing, 919
infection of. *See* Cystitis
neuropathic, chemotherapy-induced, 1510
Bladder catheterization, intermittent, for incontinence management, 72
Bladder toxicity
cyclophosphamide/ifosfamide causing, 1510
mesna for, 1507*t*, 1510
neuropathies, chemotherapy-induced, 1510
Bladder training, for urinary incontinence, 71
Blalock/Blalock-Taussig shunt, for tetralogy of Fallot, 300
Blast cells
in acute leukemia, 465
refractory anemia with (RAEB), 463
Blastomycosis, **1399**
pneumonia and, 246, 1399
South American (paracoccidioidomycosis), **1399**
Bleach. *See* Hypochlorite
Bleeding/blood loss. *See also specific cause or structure affected and* Thrombocytopenia
acquired disorders causing, **494–495**
in acute leukemia, 464–465
anticoagulant overdose/toxicity and, 272–273, 1430
in Bernard-Soulier syndrome, 489, 490
in chronic kidney disease, 829
in cirrhosis, 620, 623
coagulation factor deficiencies causing. *See also specific factor*
congenital disorders causing, 393*t*, **490–494**, 492*t*
in DIC, 487, 488, **495**
evaluation of, 480, 481*t*
factor II antibodies and, 494
factor V antibodies and, 494

factor VIII/IX antibodies/inhibitors causing, 491, 494
in factor XI deficiency, 493–494
gastrointestinal. *See* Gastrointestinal bleeding
in Glanzmann thrombasthenia, 489
in hemophilia, 491
heparin use/contamination and, 272, 483*t*, **486–487**, 486*t*, **495**
iron deficiency and, 439, 522, 523
in liver disease, **494–495**, 623
lupus anticoagulant and, **495**
malabsorption and, 558*t*
normal hemostasis and, **495**
ovulation, 674
perioperative risk evaluation/management and, 49, 50*t*, 55
in platelet disorders, **480–490**, 481*t*
in polycythemia, 457, 458
during pregnancy
ectopic pregnancy and, 713
in gestational trophoblastic disease, 714–715
third-trimester, **720**
premenopausal/postmenopausal. *See* Vaginal bleeding
rectal. *See* Rectal bleeding
in storage pool disease, 489, 490
thrombolytic therapy for myocardial infarction and, 333
vaginal. *See* Menstruation; Vaginal bleeding
in vitamin K deficiency, 494
in von Willebrand disease, 493
Bleeding history, directed, preoperative, 49, 50*t*, 55
Blenoxane. *See* Bleomycin
Bleomycin, 1504*t*
for malignant pleural effusions, 1496
Raynaud phenomenon caused by, 757
toxicity of, 1504*t*, 1510–1511
for wart removal, 132
Blepharitis, **152**
marginal, 106
Blepharospasm, 910
Blind loop syndrome, vitamin B_{12} deficiency in, 445
Blind spot, enlargement of in optic disk swelling, 169
Blindness. *See also disorders causing and* Visual impairment/loss
age-related macular degeneration causing, 163
in basilar artery migraine, 873
cataract causing, 161
cortical, occipital lobe lesions causing, 899
diabetic eye disease and, 166, 1105
fleeting (amaurosis fugax), 165, 420, 889
in giant cell arteritis, 766, 767
glaucoma causing, 158, 159
onchocerciasis causing, 1387, 1388
river, **1387–1388**
snow, 172
trachoma causing, 154
transient monocular, **165–166**, 420
vitamin A deficiency and, 1143

Blister, burn, 1409
Blistering (bullous) skin disorders, 95*t*, **130–131**. *See also specific type*
Blocadren. *See* Timolol
Blood
contaminated, transfusion of, 478
disorders of, **439–479**. *See also* Hematologic disorders
screening, 478
for arboviruses, 1258
for drugs, 1427
for hepatitis, 478, 491
for HIV, 4–5, 478, 1207, 1219
for HTLV, 1262
in stool. *See* Diarrhea, bloody; Dysentery; Fecal occult blood testing
for toxicology testing, 1427
transfusion of. *See* Transfusions
in urine. *See* Hematuria; Hemoglobinuria
Blood alcohol level
in acute intoxication/poisoning, 978, 1436
reference values for, 1549*t*
Blood culture
central venous catheter sepsis and, 1160
in disseminated candidiasis, 1391
in endocarditis, 1304
in fever/FUO, 1154
in gonococcal arthritis, 778
in gram-negative bacteremia/sepsis, 1311
in hospital-associated infection, 1160
in Lyme disease, 1345
in nongonococcal acute bacterial (septic) arthritis, 777
in pneumonia, 246, 248–249
in staphylococcal osteomyelitis, 1295
in travel-related infectious disease, 1173
in typhoid fever, 1313
Blood dyscrasias. *See also* Bleeding
retinal disorders associated with, **167**
Blood flukes, schistosomiasis caused by, 1373–1375
Blood gases. *See* Arterial blood gases; Venous blood gases
Blood glucose levels. *See* Glucose, blood levels of
Blood glucose meters, 1085
Blood loss. *See* Bleeding
Blood pressure. *See also* Hypertension; Hypotension
biofeedback affecting, 1536–1537, 1536*t*
classification/management and, **387**, 388*t*, 389*f*
exercise/activity affecting, 13
in GI bleeding, 518
health maintenance recommendations/guidelines for, 3*t*, 387, 388*t*, 389*f*
in hypertension, 387, 388*t*, 389*f*, 394
treatment goals and, 395–396

in hypertensive urgencies/emergencies, 387, 411
measurement of, **387**, 394
orthostatic changes in. *See* Orthostatic (postural) hypotension
in preeclampsia-eclampsia, 716, 717t, 718
in shock, 435, 436
Blood specimen, tubes for collection of, 1555t
Blood transfusions. *See* Transfusions
Blood (compatibility) typing, for transfusions, 477
Blood urea nitrogen (BUN), 818, 818t
in acute kidney injury, 819, 820t
in chronic kidney disease, 826–827
reference values for, 1548t
in SIADH, 792
Blood urea nitrogen:creatinine ratio, 818, 820, 820t
Blood vessels. *See specific type and under Vascular*
Blowout fracture, of orbital floor, 171
Blue bloaters, 234, 235t
Blue nevi, **100**
melanoma and, 100
Blue sclera, in osteogenesis imperfecta, 1039
Blue top tubes, 1555t
Blumer shelf, 1471
Blunt trauma, cardiac, 384
Blurred vision. *See* Visual impairment/loss
BMI. *See* Body mass index
BMPR1A gene, in familial juvenile polyposis, 592
BNP. *See* B-type natriuretic peptide
Bocavirus, 1276
BODE index, 239
Body cavity (primary effusion) lymphoma, 1247
Body fat. *See also* Obesity
distribution of in obesity, 1136
in diabetics, 1081, 1083
Body fluid precautions (universal). *See* Body substance isolation
Body image disturbances
in anorexia nervosa, 1139
postsurgical anxiety states and, 988
Body lice, 138
Body mass index, 14, 1136
cancer risk and, 14
in overweight/obese patient, 14, 1136
Body ringworm, **107–108**
Body substance isolation (universal precautions), 1161
in hemorrhagic fevers, 1262–1263
in herpes simplex prevention, 1237
HIV infection/AIDS prevention and, 1219
in SARS, 1275
in swine-origin influenza, 1273–1274
Body temperature
basal. *See* Basal body temperature
in burn injury, maintaining, 1411
elevated, 38–40, 39t. *See also* Fever; Hyperthermia
cholinergic urticaria caused by, 126

in heat exhaustion, 1407
in heat stroke, 1407, 1408
in hyperthermia, 1423
in hypothermia, 1403
normal, 38
in pulmonary embolism, 268t
Body water, 788, 789t
water deficit calculation and, 794
Body weight. *See* Weight
"Body work" systems, 1520
Boerhaave syndrome, 506
Boils (furunculosis), **140–141**, 1182t, 1294
in HIV infection/AIDS, 1215
Boletus (gastrointestinal-irritant type) mushroom poisoning, 1441, 1441t, 1442
Bone
adynamic disease of, 829
avascular necrosis of, **783–784**
corticosteroid use and, 1078
blastomycosis involving, 1399
coccidioidomycosis involving, **781**, 1393
defective mineralization of, in osteomalacia, 1042, 1043
in histoplasmosis, **781**
in hypercalcemia/hyperparathyroidism, 827, 829, 1033, 1035, 1038
infections of, **780–782**. *See also* Osteomyelitis
metabolic disease of, **1038–1046**. *See also specific disorder*
in chronic kidney disease (renal osteodystrophy), 827, 829–830, 1033, 1035, 1038
mycotic infection of, **781**
myeloma involving, 472, 473
Paget disease of, **1044–1046**
in syphilis, 1335
tuberculosis of, 256, **781–782**
Bone density measurements/bone densitometry
cellulose phosphate administration and, 858
in male hypogonadism, 1065
in osteomalacia, 1039, 1043
in osteoporosis, 12, 1039
Bone marrow
depression/failure of
in aplastic anemia, 454
in cancer chemotherapy, **1499–1508**, 1508t
infections and, 1498
with methotrexate, 750, 1510
in myelofibrosis, 460
in myeloma, 472, 473
in neutropenia, 456
radiation exposure and, 1414
thrombocytopenia caused by, **480–482**
examination/morphology of
in acute leukemia, 465
in chronic lymphocytic leukemia, 467
in chronic myeloid leukemia, 461
in essential thrombocytosis, 459

in hairy cell leukemia, 468
in leishmaniasis, 1352
in myelodysplasia, 463
in myelofibrosis, 460
in myeloma, 472
in non-Hodgkin lymphoma, 470
in polycythemia, 458
in sideroblastic anemia, 444–445
in vitamin B$_{12}$ deficiency, 445–446
in Waldenström macroglobulinemia, 474
infiltration of, thrombocytopenia caused by, **482**
stem cells in, for transplantation, 475
Bone marrow/stem cell transplantation, **474–476**
for acute leukemia, 466, 475, 476
adenovirus infection and, 1275, 1276
allogeneic, **475–476**
for aplastic anemia, 455, 476, 481–482
aspergillosis after, 1158, 1397–1398
autologous, **475**
for breast cancer, 669
for cancer, **474–476**
chemotherapy and, 475, 476
for chronic lymphocytic leukemia, 468
for chronic myeloid leukemia, 462, 476
cytomegalovirus infection and, 1157–1158
for Hodgkin disease, 471, 475
immunizations and, 5
infection and, 1156
for lymphoma, 470, 475
for myelodysplasia, 464
for myelofibrosis, 460
for myeloma, 473, 475
for thalassemia, 443, 444
for Waldenström macroglobulinemia, 474
Bone pain
adjuvant modalities for, 85–86
in Gaucher disease, 1516
in hyperparathyroidism, 1033
malabsorption and, 558t
in mineral bone disorders of chronic kidney disease, 829
in myeloma, 472, 473
in osteomalacia, 1043
in Paget disease, 1045
Bone scanning
for breast cancer metastases, 657
for prostate cancer metastases, 1485
BOOP (bronchiolitis obliterans with organizing pneumonia). *See* Cryptogenic organizing pneumonitis
Boosting, tuberculin skin testing and, 254
BOOSTRIX. *See* Tdap vaccine
Borderline personality disorder, 950, 951, 951t
Bordetella infection
bronchiseptica, 1308
pertussis (whooping cough), **1307–1308**
cough in, 22, 23, 24, 1308

Bordetella infection (*cont.*)
  prevention/immunization and,
    3–4, 1200, 1308. *See also*
      Pertussis vaccine
Boredom, in schizophrenic/psychotic dis-
    orders, 953
Bornholm disease, 1279
Borrelia (borreliosis)
  afzelii, 1342, 1343, 1344
  burgdorferi, 1177*t*, 1342, 1343, 1344.
    See also Lyme disease
    myopericarditis caused by, 377,
      1343, 1346, 1346*t*
  garinii, 1342, 1344
  lonestari, 128
  recurrentis, 1177*t*
  relapsing fever caused by, 1177*t*, 1339
Bortezomib, 1504*t*
  for myeloma, 473
  neuropathy caused by, 1510
Bosentan, for pulmonary hypertension,
    275, 381
Botulinum toxin, 933, 1299
Botulinum toxin therapy
  for achalasia, 542
  for focal torsion dystonias, 910
  for migraine headache, 874
Botulinus antitoxin, 934, 1300
Botulism, **933–934, 1299–1300**
Bouchard nodes, 730
Bougie dilators. *See* Esophageal dilation
Boutonneuse fever, 1281*t*, 1285
Boutonnière deformity, 751
Bouveret syndrome, 634
Bovine spongiform encephalopathy (mad
    cow disease), 1260
Bowen disease, **113**
BPH. *See* Benign prostatic hyperplasia
BPPV. *See* Benign paroxysmal positioning
      vertigo
Brachial plexus
  lesions of, **929–932**
  in thoracic outlet/cervical rib syn-
      dromes, 737, **931–932**
Brachial plexus neuropathy, **929–931**
Brachytherapy. *See also* Radiation therapy
  for lung cancer, 1457
  for prostate cancer, 1486–1487
Braden scale, for pressure ulcers, 73
Bradycardia/bradyarrhythmias, 341,
      354–358
  in myocardial infarction, 330, 336
  persistent (sick sinus syndrome), **354**
  in poisoning/drug overdose, 1422*t*
  sinus. *See* Sinus bradycardia
  in sleep apnea, 288, 289
Bradykinesia
  in Lewy body dementia, 64
  in parkinsonism, 905, 906
BRAF gene mutation, in papillary thyroid
      carcinoma, 1022
Brain abscess, **901–902**, 1163, 1164, 1181*t*
  anaerobes causing, 1322
  bacterial rhinosinusitis and, 195
  cancer-related, 902
  in nocardiosis, 1324
  otitis media and, 185
  seizures and, 879

Brain biopsy
  in cerebral lymphoma, 1212
  in primary angiitis of central nervous
      system, 773
Brain cancer, **897–902**, 898*t*, 1467*t*. *See
      also* Intracranial masses/
      tumors
Brain death, **917**
Brain edema. *See* Cerebral edema
Brain natriuretic peptide. *See* B-type
      natriuretic peptide
Brain stimulation
  for idiopathic torsion dystonia, 910
  for parkinsonism, 908
Brain tumors, **897–902**, 898*t*, 1467*t*. *See
      also* Intracranial masses/
      tumors
Brainstem
  arteriovenous malformations in, 895
  ischemia of, seizures differentiated
      from, 881
  lesions/tumors/infarction of, 899
    coma or stupor caused by, 916, 917
    gliomas, 898*t*, 899
    vertigo caused by, 190
Bran, dietary (bran powder), 509*t*. *See
      also* Fiber, dietary
Branch retinal artery occlusion, **164–165**
Branch retinal vein occlusion, **163–164**
Branchial cleft cysts, 213
  deep neck abscesses and, 206
Brandt-Daroff exercises, 189
BRCA1/BRCA2 genes
  breast cancer and, 653, 653*t*
    in male, 673
  ovarian cancer and, 689
  pancreatic/periampullary carcinoma
      and, 1463
Breast, **649–673**
  abscess of, **651–652**
    nipple discharge caused by, 651
    puerperal mastitis and, 651, 720
  augmented. *See also* Breast implants
    disorders of, **652**
  benign disorders of, **649–652**
  biopsy of
    in breast mass evaluation, 655,
      657–658, 658*f*, 659*f*
    in fat necrosis, 651
    in fibroadenoma, 650
    in fibrocystic condition, 649, 650
    mammographic localization, 659
    stereotactic, 659
  cancer of. *See* Breast cancer
  examination of, in cancer screening/
      early detection, 17*t*,
      654–655
  fat necrosis of, **651**
  fibroadenoma of, **650–651**
  fibrocystic condition and, **649–650**
    breast cancer risk and, 649, 653
    nipple discharge in, 649, 651
  male, disorders of. *See* Breast cancer,
      in male; Gynecomastia
  mass/lump in. *See* Breast cancer;
      Lump (breast)
  nipple discharge and, **651**
  phyllodes tumor of, 650

pregnancy affecting, 705
reconstruction of after mastectomy,
    652, 672
  local recurrence and, 652
self-examination of, in cancer screen-
    ing, 16, 17*t*, 655
Breast cancer, **652–672**, 1467*t*
  anatomic locations of, 656, 656*f*
  antipsychotic drug use and, 958
  arm edema and, 671–672
  bilateral, 660–662
  biomarkers/hormone receptor sites
      and, 657, **663–664**
    prognosis and, 665*t*
    treatment and, 663–664
  biopsy in diagnosis of, 655, 657–658,
      658*f*, 659*f*
  breast reconstruction/implants and,
      652
    local recurrence and, 652
  clinical examination in detection/eval-
      uation of, 17*t*, 654–655,
      656–657, 656*f*, 657*f*
  clinical findings in early detection of,
      656–660, 656*f*, 657*f*, 658*f*,
      659*f*
  cytology in evaluation of, 658, 660
  diet and, 653
  differential diagnosis of, 660
  ductal
    invasive/infiltrating, 663*t*
    in situ, 652, 662–663, 663*t*
  early detection/screening for, 16, 17*t*,
      654–656
    genetic testing and, 653
    pregnancy and, 728
  endometrial cancer and, 653
  estrogen replacement therapy and,
      653, 704, 1071, 1072
  exercise affecting risk of, 654
  fibrocystic condition and, 649, 653
  genetic mutations associated with,
      653, 653*t*. *See also BRCA1/
      BRCA2* genes
    prevention and, 653
    screening for, 653
  HER-2/*neu* oncogene overexpression
      in, 663, 664
    prognosis and, 665*t*
    therapy and, 664, 665, 666, 668
  incidence/risk/mortality of, 652–653,
      653*t*
    in male, 673
  inflammatory, **660**
  in situ, 652, 662–663, 663*t*
  lactation and, 660
  lobular
    invasive, 662, 663*t*
    in situ, 662–663, 663*t*
  in male, **673**
    in Klinefelter syndrome, 1064, 1517
  mammography in detection/evalua-
      tion of, 16, 17*t*, 654–655,
      655, 658*f*, 659*f*
    biopsy and, 655, 659
    breast implants and, 652
  metastatic
    imaging for, 657

lymph node assessment and, 657
    treatment of, 667–669, 668t
nipple discharge in, 651, 657
noninvasive, 662–663, 663t
oral contraceptive use and, 653, 696
Paget, 657, **660**
    nipple involvement and, 113, 657,
        660
pancreatic/periampullary carcinoma
    and, 1463
paraneoplastic syndromes associated
    with, 1453t
pathologic types of, 660, 663t
    prognosis and, 660, 665t, 670
pleural effusion in, 285
pregnancy affecting risk of, 653, 653t
pregnancy and, 660, 672, **728**
prevention of, 653–654
    chemoprevention and, 663
    genetic risk factors and, 653
prognosis for, 665t, 670–671, 670t
    in male, 673
    recurrence and, 665t, 671
recurrence of, 665t, 671
    biomarkers and, 665t
    breast reconstruction/implants
        and, 652
    Oncotype Dx assay in assessment
        of, 664, 670
self-examination in prevention/
    screening of, 16, 17t, 655
staging of, 660, 661–662t
    prognosis and, 670, 670t, 671
    therapy choices and, 664
treatment of, 664–670, 1467t
    adjuvant systemic, 665–667, 665t
    biomarkers/hormone receptor sta-
        tus and, 663–664
    breast-conserving, 664
    chemotherapy in, 665–666, 665t,
        669
        pregnancy and, 660, 672
    choice of primary therapy and, 664
    curative, 664–667, 665t
    follow-up, 671–672
    hormone therapy in, 666–667, 667,
        668–669
    in male, 673
    neoadjuvant, 667
    palliative, 664, 667–669, 668t
    during pregnancy/lactation, 660,
        672, 728
    radiation therapy in, 664, 665, 667
    surgical resection, 664–665
    targeted therapy in, 666–667,
        667–669, 668t
    ultrasonography in evaluation of, 659
Breast-conserving therapy, for breast can-
    cer, 664
    local recurrence and, 652
    during pregnancy/lactation, 660
Breast feeding. See Lactation
Breast implants
    breast cancer in patient with, 652
    for breast reconstruction, 652, 672
    local cancer recurrence and, 652
    disorders associated with, **652**
    rupture of, 652

Breast milk. See Lactation
Breast pain, in fibrocystic condition, 649,
    650
Breast surgery, 664–665. See also Lumpec-
    tomy; Mastectomy
    antibiotic prophylaxis for, 60t
Breath odor
    in cyanide poisoning, 1435
    in diabetic ketoacidosis, 1083, 1112
    in uremia, 826
Breath sounds
    in asthma exacerbation, 219
    in heart failure, 360
Breathing. See also under Respiratory
    abnormalities of in coma or stupor,
        916, 1421
    muscles/accessory muscles of, in
        asthma exacerbation, 219,
        220t
    sleep-related disorders of. See Sleep
        apnea
Breathing exercises
    for COPD, 238
    prevention of postoperative pulmo-
        nary complications and, 54
Brevibloc. See Esmolol
Brief psychotic disorders, 953
Brill-Zinsser disease, 1281, 1282
Brimonidine
    for glaucoma/ocular hypertension,
        159, 175t
    overdose/toxicity of, 1434
Brimonidine/timolol, for glaucoma/ocu-
        lar hypertension, 159,
        176t
Brinzolamide, for glaucoma/ocular
        hypertension, 159, 175t
Briquet syndrome, 944
British anti-Lewisite (BAL). See Dimer-
        caprol
Brodifacoum poisoning, 1430–1431
Bromfenac, for ophthalmic disorders,
        174t
Bromocriptine. See also Dopamine ago-
        nists
    for cocaine withdrawal, 983
    for neuroleptic malignant syndrome,
        959, 1423, 1445
    for ovulation induction, 693
    for parkinsonism, 907
Bronchi, foreign body in, **212**
Bronchial carcinoid tumors (bronchial
        adenomas), 261
Bronchial gland carcinoma, 261
Bronchial obstruction, 215–216
Bronchial provocation testing, in asthma,
        219
Bronchiectasis, **240**
    COPD differentiated from, 235
    cough in, 22, 240
    cystic fibrosis and, 240, 241, 242
    in measles, 1249
    nontuberculous mycobacterial infec-
        tion and, 258
Bronchiolitis, **242–243**
    adenoviruses causing, 1275
    constrictive (obliterative/bronchioli-
        tis obliterans), 243

with organizing pneumonia
        (BOOP/cryptogenic orga-
        nizing pneumonitis/COP),
        243, 264t
    silo-filler's disease and, 280
    measles causing, 1248
    proliferative, 243
    respiratory, 243
        interstitial lung disease associated
            with (RB-ILD), 243, 263,
            264t
    RSV, 1268, 1269
Bronchioloalveolar cell carcinoma, 1452.
    See also Lung cancer
Bronchitis
    chlamydial, 1329
    chronic, 234, 235t. See also Chronic
        obstructive pulmonary
        disease
    complications of, 236
    imaging findings in, 235
    industrial, 280
    management of, 238
Bronchoalveolar lavage, for respiratory
        secretion analysis
    in eosinophilic pneumonia, 266
    in immunocompromised host, 251
    in interstitial (diffuse parenchymal)
        lung disease, 263
    in Pneumocystis pneumonia, 251,
        1210, 1395
    in pneumonia, 249
    in pulmonary alveolar proteinosis,
        266
    in sarcoidosis, 265
Bronchoconstriction. See Asthma; Bron-
        chospasm
Bronchodilators
    adverse ophthalmic effects of, 177t
    for asthma
        exacerbation management and,
            230–233, 231f, 232f
        long-acting, 223, 228–230,
            229–230t
        short-acting, 223, 228–230,
            229–230t
    for COPD, 237
    for cystic fibrosis, 242
Bronchogenic carcinoma, **1452–1457**,
        1455t. See also Lung can-
        cer
    cough in, 22
Bronchopneumonia, in measles, 1248
Bronchoprovocation testing. See Bron-
        chial provocation testing
Bronchopulmonary mycosis/aspergillo-
        sis, allergic, **241**, 1397,
        1398
Bronchoscopy. See also Bronchoalveolar
        lavage
    in bronchial carcinoid tumors, 261
    in hemoptysis, 27, 28
    in interstitial (diffuse parenchymal)
        lung disease, 263
    in lung cancer, 1454
    in pneumonia, 249
    in solitary pulmonary nodule, 260
    in tuberculosis, 252

Bronchospasm/bronchoconstriction. *See also* Asthma
　adenosine causing, 342
　in COPD, 234
　in desensitization therapy, 1186
　exercise-induced. *See* Asthma, exercise-induced
　in pulmonary edema, 368
Brown recluse spider bites, 139, 1447
Brown-Séquard syndrome, 919
Brown tumors of bone, in hyperparathyroidism, 1033
Bruce protocol, for exercise testing, 319, 324
Brucella abortus/melitensis/suis (brucellosis), 1176*t*, **1316–1317**
Brudzinski sign, 1309
Brugia
　malayi, 1385
　　eosinophilic pulmonary syndromes and, 266, 1386
　timori, 1385
Bruits
　in aortoiliac occlusive disease, 415
　carotid, 420
　in cerebral arteriovenous malformation, 895
　in occlusive cerebrovascular disease, 420
Brush border enzyme deficiency, 558. *See also* Lactase deficiency
Bruxism, earache and, 186
BSE. *See* Bovine spongiform encephalopathy; Breast, self-examination of
Buboes
　in lymphogranuloma venereum, 594, 1328
　in plague, 1318
Budd-Chiari syndrome (hepatic vein obstruction), 525, **630–631**
Budesonide
　for asthma, 226*t*
　　with formoterol, 224*t*
　for inflammatory bowel disease, 576
　　Crohn disease, 580–581
　　microscopic colitis, 587
Buerger disease (thromboangiitis obliterans), **422–423**
　Raynaud phenomenon and, 757
Bufotenin, toxicity of, 1435
Bulbar palsy, progressive, 920, 921
Bulbar poliomyelitis, 1252
Bulbospinal neuronopathy, X-linked, 921
Bulimia nervosa, **1140**
　with anorexia nervosa (bulimarexia), 1140
Bullectomy, for emphysema, 239
Bullous impetigo, in HIV infection/AIDS, 1215
Bullous pemphigoid, **131**
Bullous (blistering) skin disorders, 95*t*, **130–131**. *See also specific type*
Bumetanide, 399*t*
　for heart failure, 361

for hypertensive urgencies/emergencies, 412
　for pulmonary edema, 367–368
Bumex. *See* Bumetanide
BUN. *See* Blood urea nitrogen
Bundle branch block, 356
　in atrial septal defect, 298
　in myocardial infarction, 337
Buprenorphine, 84
　for opioid addiction, 21, 982, 1442
　overdose/toxicity of, 1442–1443
Bupropion, 964, 968*t*
　for drug-induced erectile dysfunction, 965
　overdose/toxicity of, 968*t*
　for smoking cessation, 7, 11*t*, 1450
Burin variant of MEN 1, 1076
Burkholderia
　mallei (glanders), 1177*t*
　pseudomallei (melioidosis), 1177*t*
　　infection in drug users and, 1169
Burkitt lymphoma, 469, 470, 1475
　Epstein-Barr virus in, 1244
Burkitt type ALL, 465
Burn blister, 1409
Burn surface area, estimating, 1409, 1409*f*
Burning mouth syndrome, **202–203**
Burns, **1408–1412**
　abdominal compartment syndrome and, 1410
　chemical. *See* Chemical injury
　classification of, **1409–1410**, 1409*f*
　depth of, 1409
　electric, 1409, 1410, 1412–1413
　　fasciotomy in, 1411, 1413
　extent of, 1409, 1409*f*
　flash (arcing), 1413
　injuries/illnesses associated with, 1409–1410
　Joule, 1413
　management of
　　fluid resuscitation in, 1410, **1410–1411**
　　initial, **1410**
　　patient support and, **1411–1412**
　　Stevens Johnson syndrome/toxic epidermal necrolysis treatment and, 127, 1410
　　wound care, **1411**
　psychiatric/psychologic problems associated with hospitalization and, 989
　radiation, 1414
　smoke inhalation and, 277, 1409
　survival after, 1409
　systemic reactions to, **1410**
Bursitis, **743–744**. *See also specific type or location affected*
Buruli ulcer, 1325
Buspar. *See* Buspirone
Buspirone, 941*t*
　for aggressive/violent behavior, 976
　antidepressant drug augmentation and, 964
　for anxiety, 941*t*, 942
　for OCD, 943
Busulfan, 1500*t*
Butane, toxicity of, 1439

Butanediol, overdose/toxicity of, 1437
Butenafine, 98*t*
Butoconazole, for vulvovaginal candidiasis, 678
Butorphanol, 84
Butterfly rash, in SLE, 753, 753*t*
Butyrophenones, 954, 955*t*, 956*t*. *See also* Antipsychotic drugs; Haloperidol
　for nausea and vomiting, 506
　overdose/toxicity of, 956*t*, 1444
Byetta. *See* Exenatide
Bypass grafting
　for aortic dissection, 427
　for aortoiliac occlusive disease, 416
　coronary artery. *See* Coronary artery bypass grafting
　for erectile dysfunction, 863
　for femoral/popliteal occlusive disease, 417
　for lower leg/foot occlusive disease, 418
　for superior vena caval syndrome, 432
　for visceral artery insufficiency/intestinal angina, 422
Bypass surgery, for obesity, 15, 1138
　hypoglycemia after, 1117, 1121
Byssinosis, 280

C3
　in bullous pemphigoid, 131
　in IgA nephropathy, 836
　in postinfectious glomerulonephritis, 834
　reference values for, 1548*t*
C3 nephritic factor, in membranoproliferative glomerulonephropathy, 835*f*, 844
C3b
　in autoimmune hemolytic anemia, 452
　in cold agglutinin disease, 453–454
C4, reference values for, 1548*t*
C5A, in familial Mediterranean fever, 528
C282Y mutation, in hemochromatosis, 627, 628. *See also HFE* gene
　hepatocellular carcinoma and, 615, 1460
C$_{cr}$. *See* Creatinine clearance
c-*erb*B-2. *See* HER-2/*neu* overexpression
c-*myc* gene, in Burkitt lymphoma, 469
13C-octanoic acid breath test, in nausea and vomiting, 505
C-peptide
　in factitious hypoglycemia, 1118, 1122
　insulinoma secreting, 1062, 1118
　reference values for, 1548*t*
C-reactive protein, 1548*t*
　coronary heart disease and, 317, 1126
　in Crohn disease, 578
C-urea breath testing. *See* Urea breath testing
c-*v* wave
　in pulmonary stenosis, 295
　in tetralogy of Fallot, 300
14C-xylose test, in bacterial overgrowth, 516
Ca. *See* Calcium

CA 15-3, in breast cancer, 657
CA 19-9
   in cholangiocarcinoma, 641, 1462
   in pancreatic/periampullary carci-
      noma, 1464
CA 27-29, in breast cancer, 657
CA 125, in ovarian tumors, 689, 690
CA-MRSA. *See* Community-associated
      methicillin-resistant *S*
      aureus
Cabergoline
   for GH secreting tumors, 998–999
   for hyperprolactinemia, 1001–1002
CABG. *See* Coronary artery bypass graft-
      ing
Cachectin. *See* Tumor necrosis factor
Cachexia
   diabetic neuropathic, 1107
   in protein-energy malnutrition, 1135
CACN1A gene, in familial hemiplegic
      migraine, 873
CACNA1S gene, in periodic paralysis, 936
CACNL1A3 gene, in periodic paralysis,
      936
CAD (coronary artery disease). *See* Coro-
      nary heart disease
Cadherin cell adhesion protein, gastric
      cancer and, 1471
Cadmium, tubulointerstitial disease
      caused by, 846
CADP test, 1553*t*
Café au lait spots, 904
Café coronary, **277**
Cafergot, for migraine headache, 874
Caffeine, **984**
   fibrocystic breast condition and, 650
   overdose/toxicity of, **984, 1447–1448**
Caffeinism, 984
cagA gene, in *H pylori* gastritis, 546
CAGE screening test, 19, 20*t*
Cajal, interstitial cells of, gastrointestinal
      stromal tumors and, 1474
Calabar swellings, in loiasis, 1388–1389
Calan. *See* Verapamil
Calcaneofibular ligament, ankle sprains
      involving, 746
Calcifediol (25-hydroxyvitamin D₃)
   for hypoparathyroidism/tetany, 1032
   for osteomalacia, 1044
   reference values for, 1554*t*
   serum levels of in osteoporosis, 1039
   for vitamin D deficiency, 1044
Calciferol. *See* Ergocalciferol
Calcific (degenerative) aortic stenosis, 310
Calcimar. *See* Calcitonin
Calcimimetic agents. *See* Cinacalcet
Calcinosis
   cardiac, 383
   tumoral, in mineral bone disorders of
      chronic kidney disease,
      829
Calciphylaxis, 1034, 1035, 1037
Calcipotriene, for psoriasis, 104
Calcitonin
   reference values for, 1548*t*
   in thyroid cancer, 1024
Calcitonin/nasal calcitonin-salmon
   for hypercalcemia, 801, 1497

for osteoporosis, 1041
for Paget disease of bone, 1046
Calcitriol (1,25-dihydroxycholecalciferol)
   for hypocalcemia/hypoparathyroid-
      ism/tetany, 1032, 1032*t*
   for mineral bone disorders of chronic
      kidney disease, 830
   for parathyroid hyperplasia, 1037
   after parathyroidectomy, 1037
   reference values for, 1554*t*
   for vitamin D-dependent rickets, 1043
Calcium
   deficiency of in osteomalacia/rickets,
      829, 1043
   dietary/supplementary, 1146–1147
     for calcium channel blocker over-
       dose, 1423, 1433
     in colorectal cancer prevention,
       1477
     high-calcium diet and, 1146–1147
     hypercalcemia caused by, 801, 1036
     hypercalciuria and, 859
     for hyperkalemia, 798, 799*t*
     for hypermagnesemia, 806
     for hyperoxaluric calcium neph-
       rolithiasis, 859
     for hyperphosphatemia, 804
     for hypertension, 394
     for hypocalcemia/hypoparathy-
       roidism/tetany, 800, 1032
     milk-alkali syndrome and, 800
     for mineral bone disorders of
       chronic kidney disease,
       829
     for osteomalacia, 1044
     for osteoporosis prevention/man-
       agement, 12, 704, 1040
     after parathyroidectomy, 1037
     during pregnancy/lactation, 708
     requirements for in nutritional
       support, 1149
     urinary stone formation and, 857,
       858
   disorders of concentration/metabo-
      lism of, **798–802**. *See also*
      Hypercalcemia; Hypocal-
      cemia
   in chronic kidney disease (renal
      osteodystrophy), 829–830,
      1033
   genetic disorders associated with,
      796*t*, 798
   intracellular, in hypertension, 390
   reference/normal values for, 798,
      1548*t*
   serum levels of
     albumin levels and, 799, 1031,
       1496–1497
     in hypercalcemia/hyperparathy-
       roidism, 801, 1034, 1034*f*
     in hypercalciuria, 858*t*
     in hypocalcemia/hypoparathyroid-
       ism, 799, 800, 1031,
       1034*f*
     magnesium serum levels and, 800,
       805
     parathyroid hormone affecting,
       799, 1030, 1034, 1034*f*

     phosphorus/phosphate affecting,
       802, 803
     reference values for, 1548*t*
   urinary excretion of, 857, 858–859,
      858*t*. *See also* Hypercalci-
      uria
     reference value for, 1548*t*
   in urinary stones, 857, 858–859. *See*
      also Calcium nephrolithia-
      sis; Hypercalciuria
Calcium acetate. *See* Calcium, dietary/
      supplementary
Calcium bilirubinate, in gallstones, 634
Calcium carbonate. *See* Calcium, dietary/
      supplementary
Calcium channel blocking drugs
   for acute coronary syndromes, 328
   for angina, 321–322
   for arrhythmias, 344*t*
     atrial fibrillation, 347
     paroxysmal supraventricular tachy-
       cardia, 342, 345
   for bipolar disease/mania, 973
   for cardiomyopathy, 373
   in heart failure, 365
   for hypertension, 396*t*, 405–407, 406*t*,
      407, 409, 409*f*
     in combination regimen, 409, 409*f*
     in diabetes, 396*t*
     during pregnancy, 723
   for intracranial aneurysm, 894–895
   lower extremity edema caused by, 37
   for migraine prophylaxis, 875
   for myocardial infarction, 335, 340
   overdose/toxicity of, 405, 406*t*, 1422,
      1433
   pheochromocytoma surgery and,
      1060–1061
   for pulmonary hypertension, 381
   for Raynaud phenomenon, 757
Calcium chloride. *See* Calcium, dietary/
      supplementary
Calcium citrate. *See* Calcium, dietary/sup-
      plementary
Calcium disodium edetate (EDTA), for
      lead poisoning, 846, 1438
Calcium gluconate. *See also* Calcium,
      dietary/supplementary
   for calcium channel blocker overdose,
      1433
   for hydrofluoric acid burns, 1411, 1429
   for hypocalcemia/hypoparathyroid-
      ism/tetany, 800, 1032
Calcium load test, in urinary stone dis-
      ease, 857
Calcium nephrolithiasis, 857, 858–859
   hypercalcemia/hyperparathyroidism
      and, 858*t*, 859, 1033
   hypoparathyroidism treatment and,
      1032
Calcium polycarbophil, 509*t*. *See also*
      Fiber, dietary
Calcium pyrophosphate dihydrate deposi-
      tion disease (pseudogout),
      733, **735–736**
Calcium-sensing receptor, 798
   mutations in gene for, 796*t*, 798
   in hypercalcemia, 796*t*, 798

Calcium-sensing receptor (*cont.*)
in hypocalcemia, 796*t*, 798, 799, 1030, 1031
in hypoparathyroidism, 1030
Calculus formation. *See specific type or structure or organ affected*
Calderol. *See* Calcifediol
Calendar method of contraception, 699–700
Caliciviruses, gastroenteritis caused by, 1171*t*
California encephalitis, 1257–1259
California flea rickettsiosis, 1281*t*
Callosities of feet or toes, **133**
in diabetes/vascular disorders, 133, 1106
Caloric testing
in coma or stupor, 916
in Ménière syndrome, 189
Calorie requirements, in nutritional support, 1148–1149
Calorie restriction, in obesity management, 15, 1137
Calorimetry, for energy expenditure measurement, 1148, 1149
Calprotectin, in Crohn disease, 578
Calymmatobacterium (Donovania) granulomatis, 1320
CAM. *See* Complementary/alternative medicine
Cameron erosions, 523
Campath-1H. *See* Alemtuzumab
Camphor/menthol preparations, 94, 98*t*
Camptosar. *See* Irinotecan
Campylobacter, 1176*t*, **1316**
diarrhea/gastroenteritis caused by, 512, 1171*t*, 1172, 1174, 1182*t*, 1316
Guillain-Barré syndrome and, 925
fetus subsp *fetus*, 1316
jejuni, 1171*t*, 1174, 1176*t*, 1316
Campylobacter-like organisms, 1316
Canasa. *See* Mesalamine
Canavan disease, prenatal testing for, 706
Cancer, **1450–1511**. *See also specific type and under Malignant*
cognitive disorders/delirium caused by, 985*t*
complications of, **1494–1498**
DIC in, 487
early detection/screening tests for, 16–18, 17*t*
effusions associated with, **1495–1496**
emergencies associated with, **1494–1498**
etiology of, 1450–1451, 1451*t*
fever/FUO and, 1153, 1154, 1453*t*
guided imagery in patients with, 1536*t*, 1543
HIV infection/AIDS and, 1208, 1215–1216, 1224–1225*t*
hypercalcemia associated with, 801, 1035, 1453*t*, 1454, **1496–1497**
hyperuricemia associated with, **1497–1498**
allopurinol for, 1497, 1507*t*
rasburicase for, 1497–1498, 1507*t*

incidence/risk/mortality of, 1450, 1450–1451, 1451*t*
obesity and, 14, 1451
infectious complications of, **1498**
lipid abnormalities associated with, 1126*t*
meditation in patients with, 1541
neuropathies associated with, 885, 902, **925**
nonmetastatic neurologic complications of, **902–903**
oral contraceptive use and, 694, 696
paraneoplastic syndromes and, **1451–1452**, 1453*t*
pericarditis associated with, 377, 378
pleural effusions in (malignant pleural effusions), 284*t*, 285, 1495–1496
in polymyositis/dermatomyositis, 760, 761, 783, 902
prevention of, **16–18**, 17*t*, 1450–1451. *See also* Cancer, early detection/screening tests for
chemoprevention and, 16
lifestyle modifications and, 1450–1451
prognosis for, 1511
radiation exposure and, 1415
rheumatic manifestations of, **783**
SIADH and, 791, 791*t*, 1453*t*
smoking/smoking cessation and, 7, 1450–1451
spinal cord compression and, **1494–1495**
staging of, 1451
stem cell transplants for, **474–476**
treatment of, **1498–1511**. *See also* Chemotherapy
systemic, **1498–1499**. *See also* Chemotherapy
tumor lysis syndrome and, **1497–1498**
venous thrombosis/pulmonary embolism and, 270*t*
Cancer pain, mind-body therapies for, 1536*t*
guided imagery, 1536*t*, 1543
hypnosis, 1536*t*, 1539
Cancer-related checkup, 17*t*
Cancidas. *See* Caspofungin
Cancuas. *See* Caspofungin
Candesartan/candesartan with hydrochlorothiazide, 403*t*
for heart failure, 362
Candida (candidiasis), **124–125**, **1390–1391**
albicans, 1390
disseminated, 125, 1391
endocarditis in, 1391
esophageal, 535, 1390
in HIV infection/AIDS, 1210, 1213, 1215, 1224*t*, 1390
hepatic, 632, 633
hepatosplenic, 1391
in HIV infection/AIDS, 125, 202, 1215, 1223, 1224*t*, 1390
krusei, 1391

mucocutaneous/mucosal, **124–125**, 1390
nail infection and, 125
non-albicans, 125, 1391
oral (thrush), 125, **202**, 1390
in HIV infection/AIDS, 125, 202, 1213, 1390
osteomyelitis caused by, **781**
prevention of, 1158, 1223
resistant strains of, 1391
tinea cruris differentiated from, 108
in urine, 1390–1391
vulvovaginal, 125, 678, 1390
in diabetes mellitus, 1082*t*, 1083, 1109
in HIV infection/AIDS, 1216, 1224*t*
rape/sexual assault and, 1167
Candida antigen, for wart removal, 132
Candidal funguria (candiduria), 1390–1391
Canker sore (aphthous ulcer), **203**
in Behçet syndrome, 772
in Crohn disease, 578
in HIV infection/AIDS, 1213
Cannabinoids
for nausea and vomiting, 87, 507. *See also* Dronabinol
in pain management, 86
Cannabis sativa, 982. *See also* Marijuana
"Cannon" A waves
in AV junctional rhythm, 350
palpitations and, 31
Cantharellus (gastrointestinal-irritant type) mushroom poisoning, 1441, 1441*t*, 1442
CAPD. *See* Continuous ambulatory peritoneal dialysis
Capecitabine, 1501*t*
for breast cancer, 668, 669
for colorectal cancer, 1479
for gastric adenocarcinoma, 1472
Capillary angiomas, in Sturge-Weber syndrome, 904
Caplan syndrome, 278
Capoten. *See* Captopril
CAPRA nomogram, for prostate cancer assessment, 1488, 1488*t*
Capsaicin
for osteoarthritis, 731
for painful diabetic neuropathy, 1107
for postherpetic neuralgia, 115, 878
Capsule imaging/endoscopy
in Crohn disease, 578–579
in GI bleeding, 522, 523
Captopril, 403*t*
in diabetics, 1105, 1106
for heart failure, 362
for hypertensive urgencies/emergencies, 413*t*, 414
for myocardial infarction, 335
Car accidents. *See* Automobile accidents
Car driving, by patients with syncope/ventricular tachycardia/aborted sudden death, **357–358**
Carac. *See* Fluorouracil
Carbamate poisoning, 1443–1444

Carbamazepine, 881, 882t, 972, 1544t. See
        also Anticonvulsant ther-
        apy
    for alcohol withdrawal, 980
    for bipolar disease/mania, 972
    overdose/toxicity of, 882t, 972, 1427t,
        1431
        hemodialysis for, 1425t, 1431
    for personality disorder, 951
    for seizures, 881, 882t
    during pregnancy, 883
    theophylline affected by, 225t
Carbaryl poisoning, 1443–1444
Carbidopa, for parkinsonism, 906
Carbidopa/levodopa, for parkinsonism,
        906–907
    with entacapone, 907
Carbimazole, for Graves disease/hyper-
        thyroidism, 1011
Carbohydrate deficient transferrin, alco-
        hol use/abuse and, 979
Carbohydrates
    dietary. See also High-carbohydrate
        diet; Low carbohydrate
        diets
        absorption/digestion of, 557–558
        in diabetic diet, 1089
        for islet cell tumors, 1120
        malabsorption of, diarrhea and,
            515, 516, 558t
        in porphyria, 923, 1512
        non-digestible, for constipation, 509
Carbon dioxide
    partial pressure of. See PaCO₂; PCO₂
    reference values for, 1548t
    respiratory failure and, 289t
    venous, 806. See also Bicarbonate
Carbon dioxide laser therapy
    for CIN, 681
    for condylomata acuminata, 679
    for wart removal, 132
Carbon monoxide, diffusing capacity for
        (DL_CO). See Diffusing
        capacity for carbon mon-
        oxide
Carbon monoxide poisoning, 1424t,
        1427t, 1433–1434
    dyspnea in, 26, 1433
    headache in, 44, 1433
    smoke inhalation and, 277, 1409
Carbonic anhydrase inhibitors
    adverse ophthalmic effects of, 177t
    for glaucoma/ocular hypertension,
        159, 175t
    renal tubular acidosis caused by, 810
Carboplatin, 1500t, 1511
    for breast cancer, 666
Carboxyhemoglobin levels
    in carbon monoxide poisoning, 277,
        1433
    reference values for, 1548t
    in smoke inhalation, 277, 1409
Carbuncles, 140–141, 1294
Carcinoembryonic antigen (CEA)
    in breast cancer, 657
    in colorectal cancer, 1478, 1480
    reference values for, 1548t
    in thyroid cancer, 1024

Carcinoid heart disease, 313, 315, 383,
        1475
    pulmonic regurgitation and, 315
    tricuspid stenosis and, 313
Carcinoid syndrome, 261, 1062, 1473,
        1474, 1475, 1476
Carcinoid tumors, 1468t
    bronchial, **261**
    gastric, **1473–1474**, 1475
    intestinal, **1475–1476**
    in multiple endocrine neoplasia, 1075,
        1076, 1076t, 1474
    pancreatic, 1062
    pernicious anemia gastritis and, 547,
        1474
Carcinoma in situ
    of breast, 652, 662–663, 663t
    of cervix, 680t, 682, 682–683
    of vulva, 685
Carcinomatosis
    lymphangitic, 1457
    peritoneal, 527–528
Carcinomatous meningitis (leptomenin-
        geal metastases), 900–901,
        1163
Card agglutination test (CATT), in Afri-
        can trypanosomiasis,
        1349
Cardene. See Nicardipine
Cardiac arrhythmias. See Arrhythmias
Cardiac asthma, 217
Cardiac biomarkers/enzymes
    in acute MI (STEMI), 331
    in cardiac trauma, 384
    in infectious myocarditis, 369
    in non-ST elevation acute coronary
        syndromes, 326
Cardiac calcinosis, 383
Cardiac catheterization
    in acute coronary syndromes,
        328–329, 329t
    in cardiomyopathy, 370t, 371, 373
    in constrictive pericarditis, 379–380
    in coronary artery disease, 320
    in heart failure, 360–361
    in myocardial infarction, 332,
        335–336
Cardiac cirrhosis, 620
Cardiac dysrhythmias. See Arrhythmias
Cardiac failure. See Congestive heart (car-
        diac) failure
Cardiac glycosides. See Digitalis/digitalis
        glycosides
Cardiac index
    in myocardial infarction, 331t
    in shock, 435–436
Cardiac magnetic resonance imaging. See
        Magnetic resonance imag-
        ing (MRI), cardiac
Cardiac murmurs. See Heart murmurs
Cardiac output
    PEEP affecting, in ARDS, 292
    prerenal azotemia and, 820
    in shock liver, 631
Cardiac risk assessment, preoperative,
        49–53, 50t, 51f, 51t, 384
Cardiac risk index, revised, 49, 50t
Cardiac rupture, 384

Cardiac-specific markers (cardiac
        enzymes). See Cardiac bio-
        markers
Cardiac tamponade. See Tamponade
Cardiac transplantation, for heart failure,
        366
Cardiac trauma, **384**
Cardiac tumors, **382–383**
Cardiac valves. See also Prosthetic heart
        valves; Valve replacement;
        Valvular heart disease
    endocarditis affecting, 1303. See also
        Endocarditis
Cardiobacterium hominis. See HACEK
        organisms
Cardiogenic pulmonary edema, 359,
        367–368
    perioperative, 52
Cardiogenic shock, 338, 434, 434t, 435,
        436
    in heat stroke, 1408
    in infectious myocarditis, 369
Cardiogenic syncope, 356–357
Cardiomegaly
    in heart failure, 360
    in hypothyroidism (myxedema heart),
        1005
Cardiomyopathy, **370–374**, 370t
    adenovirus infection and, 1276
    catecholamine-induced. See Cardio-
        myopathy, Tako-Tsubo
    cirrhotic, 620
    coxsackieviruses causing, 1279
    dilated, **370–372**, 370t
    heart failure and, 358, 370, 371
    in hyperthyroidism, 1009, 1014
    hypertrophic/hypertrophic obstruc-
        tive, 370t, **372–374**
        heart murmurs in, 306t
        sudden death and, 373
        of athlete, 373, 386
    infiltrative, 383
    mitral regurgitation and, 308
    palpitations and, 31
    of pregnancy (peripartum cardiomy-
        opathy/heart failure), **385**,
        724, 1000
    restrictive, 370t, **374**
        constrictive pericarditis differenti-
            ated from, 374
    Tako-Tsubo (stress/catecholamine-
        induced), 370, **372**
        myocardial infarction mimicked by,
            330
    trastuzumab causing, 666
Cardiomyoplasty, for heart failure, 366
Cardiomyotomy, Heller, for achalasia, 542
Cardiopulmonary resuscitation
    in electrical injury, 1413
    for hypothermia, 1404
    in near drowning, 1416
    orders regarding in end-of-life care,
        90
Cardiovascular disorders. See also under
        Cardiac; Coronary; Myo-
        cardial and Heart disease;
        Stroke
    in athletes, screening for, **385–386**

Cardiovascular disorders (*cont.*)
bupropion for smoking cessation and, 11*t*
in Chagas disease, 368, 1350
chemoprevention in, **12**
in chronic kidney disease/uremia, 826*t*, 827*t*, 828
cocaine abuse and, 325, 330, 370
coenzyme Q$_{10}$ for, 1528*t*, 1530
cognitive disorders/delirium caused by, 985*t*
COX-2 inhibitors and, 78, 548, 552–553
in diabetes mellitus, 1108–1109
aspirin chemoprevention and, 12, 1089, 1108
glycemic control and, 1087, 1088–1089
hypertension control and, 1088, 1108
homocysteine/hyperhomocysteinemia/homocystinuria in, 1516, 1517
in hypercalcemia, 1034
hypertension affecting morbidity/mortality in, 387, 407
hypertension caused by, 389
hypertensive, 393
in hyperthyroidism, 360, 1009, 1014–1015
in hypothyroidism, 360, 1005
immobility/bed rest and, 68
in Lyme disease, 377, 1343, 1346, 1346*t*
nicotine replacement therapy and, 10*t*, 11*t*
NSAIDs and, 78, 548, 552–553
pregnancy and, **384–385, 724**
preoperative evaluation/management and, **49–53**, 50*t*, 51*f*, 51*t*
prevention of, **6–12**
abdominal aortic aneurysm screening in, **6**, 423
cholesterol screening and, 1126–1129, 1127–1128*t*, 1129*t*
exercise/activity and, 13
hypertension prevention/management and, **9–12**
lipid disorder prevention/management and, **9**, 1124–1125, 1126, 1128, 1129. *See also* Lipid-lowering therapy
omega-3 fatty acids in, 1528*t*, 1530–1531
smoking cessation and, **6–9**, 8*t*, 9*t*, 10*t*, 11*t*
radiation causing, 1414
syphilis and, 1183*t*, 1335–1336
Cardiovascular system
abnormal development of, hypertension and, 389
thiamin deficiency affecting, 1141
Cardioversion
electrical
for atrial fibrillation, 347, 347–348
in hyperthyroidism, 1014
infarct-related, 337
rate control compared with, 348–349

for atrial flutter, 350
in hypothermia, 1404
in myocardial infarction, 337
for paroxysmal supraventricular tachycardia, 344
for ventricular arrhythmias/tachycardia, 352
pharmacologic
for atrial fibrillation, 348–349
for atrial flutter, 350
transesophageal echocardiography-guided, 347–348
Cardioverter defibrillator, implantable. *See* Implantable cardioverter defibrillator
Carditis, rheumatic, 375
Cardizem. *See* Diltiazem
Cardura. *See* Doxazosin
Caregiver issues, in care of elderly, **62–63**
dementia and, 65
Carey-Coombs murmur, in rheumatic carditis, 375
Carisoprodol, overdose/toxicity of, 1436
Carmol, 99*t*
Carney complex/syndrome, 382, 997, 1077
Cushing syndrome and, 1051
Caroli disease, 1462
β-Carotene/carotenoids
in atherosclerosis/heart disease prevention, 12
in cancer prevention, 12
excess intake of, 1144
Carotid angioplasty, 420–421
Carotid artery occlusive disease (carotid stenosis/insufficiency), 420–421
headache associated with, 45, 876
postoperative complications associated with, 57
recurrent, 421
stroke/transient ischemic attacks caused by, 420, 887, 888, 889, 890*t*
transient monocular blindness caused by, 165, 420
Carotid bruits, 420
postoperative stroke and, 57
Carotid endarterectomy/thromboendarterectomy, 420
prophylactic, 57
preoperative, 57
transient monocular blindness and, 165
for transient ischemic attacks and stroke, 420, 888
Carotid insufficiency. *See* Carotid artery occlusive disease
Carotid pulse
in cardiomyopathy, 373
in heart failure, 360
Carotid sinus hypersensitivity, syncope in, 356
Carotid sinus massage/pressure
for paroxysmal supraventricular tachycardia, 342
in syncope evaluation, 357

Carotid stenosis. *See* Carotid artery occlusive disease
Carotid stenting, 420–421
Carpal compression test, 742
Carpal spasm. *See* Trousseau sign
Carpal tunnel syndrome, **742**
in acromegaly/gigantism, 997
Raynaud phenomenon and, 757
Carrier (genetic)
for acute intermittent porphyria, 1512
for cystic fibrosis, 241
for fragile X mental retardation, 1515
for Gaucher disease, 1516
for glucose-6-phosphate dehydrogenase deficiency, 449–450
for hemophilia, 491
for sickle cell disease, **451–452**, 451*t*
for thalassemia, 442, 443, 443*t*
Carrier state (infection)
for amebiasis, 1366
in giardiasis, 1371, 1372
in group B streptococcal infection, 725
in hepatitis B, 602, **726–727**
in hepatitis C, **726–727**
in meningococcal meningitis, 1309
staphylococcal, 1294
nasal vestibulitis and, 195
surgical site infection associated with, 59
in trench fever, 1321
in trichomoniasis, 1373
in typhoid fever, 1313
Carteolol, for glaucoma/ocular hypertension, 159, 175*t*
Cartia. *See* Diltiazem
Carvedilol, 400*t*
for heart failure, 362–363
for myocardial infarction, 335, 340
Cascara, 509*t*, 510
Casodex. *See* Bicalutamide
Caspofungin, 1401*t*, 1402
for aspergillosis, 1398
for candidiasis, 535, 1390, 1391
prophylactic, 1158
renal/hepatic failure and, 1184*t*
CaSR. *See* Calcium-sensing receptor
Castleman disease, 1154, 1247
Castor bean (*Ricinus communis*), ricin toxicity and, 1434
Casts, urinary. *See* Urinary casts
Cat bites, 1165–1166
cat-scratch disease and, 1321
Cat feces, toxoplasmosis and, 1363, 1365
Cat fleas. *See* Fleas
Cat hookworm, cutaneous larva migrans caused by, 1385
Cat roundworm (*T cati*), 1384–1385
Cat-scratch disease, 1321
lymphadenitis/lymphadenopathy in, 433, 1321
Cataflam. *See* Diclofenac
Catamenial asthma, 216
Catamenial pneumothorax, 286
Cataplexy, in narcolepsy, 975
Catapres. *See* Clonidine
Cataract, **161–162**
diabetic, 1104

hypoparathyroidism and, 1031
quetiapine use and, 956
Catastrophic antiphospholipid syndrome, 755, 756
Catatonic schizophrenia, 952, 954, 957
Catatonic syndrome (catatonia), 954, 957
neuroleptic-induced, 959
Catcher's mitt hand, 743
Catecholamine-O-methyltransferase (COMT) inhibitors, for parkinsonism, 907
Catecholamine myocarditis, pheochromocytoma and, 1060, 1061
Catecholamines
in pheochromocytoma, 1058, 1059
reference values for, 1548t
Tako-Tsubo cardiomyopathy and, 370
β-Catenin, hepatic adenoma and, 633
Caterpillars, skin lesions caused by, 139
Cathartics
abuse of in bulimia nervosa, 1140
for poisoning/drug overdose, 1425
Catheter ablation techniques. See Radiofrequency ablation techniques
Catheterization
bladder/urinary. See Bladder catheterization
cardiac. See Cardiac catheterization
Catheters
infections associated with, 1151, 1159, 1160, 1161, 1180
for parenteral nutritional support, 1148
complications associated with, 1151
septic phlebitis and, 429, 1181t
CATT (card agglutination test), in African trypanosomiasis, 1349
Cauda equina injury, 919
Cauda equina tumor, back pain caused by, 738, 739
Cauliflower ear (auricular hematoma), 180
Caustic/corrosive agents
acids, **1429**
alkalies, **1429–1430**
esophageal injury caused by, **536**, 1429
eye injury caused by, 172, 1429, 1430
Cauterization, for CIN, 681
Cavernous hemangioma, of liver, 633
Cavernous sinus thrombosis, bacterial rhinosinusitis and, 195
Cbir 1 antibodies, in inflammatory bowel disease, 579
CC-5013. See Lenalidomide
cCJD. See Classic Creutzfeldt-Jakob disease
CCLE. See Chronic cutaneous lupus erythematosus
CCNU. See Lomustine
CCP antibodies, in rheumatoid arthritis, 748
CCPD. See Continuous cyclic peritoneal dialysis
C$_{cr}$. See Creatinine clearance
CCR5
in HIV infection/AIDS, 1208

in tick-borne encephalitis, 1266
in West Nile virus, 1258
CCR5 co-receptor antagonist, for HIV infection/AIDS, 1231
in combinations, 1227
CD markers. See also specific marker
in hematologic neoplasia
acute leukemia, 465
chronic lymphocytic leukemia, 467
hairy cell leukemia, 468
CD2, in acute lymphoblastic leukemia, 465
CD4/CD8 cell ratio, in sarcoidosis, 265
CD4 T cells
in HIV infection/AIDS, 1205, 1208, 1208–1209, 1209f, 1217–1218
absolute count, 1217–1218, 1217t
antiretroviral therapy initiation/monitoring and, 1223, 1225
CMV retinitis and, 167, 168, 1223
immune reconstitution and, 1217
MAC infections and, 1324, 1325
neurosyphilis and, 1337, 1338
opportunistic infection/course of disease and, 1205, 1209, 1209f, 1217, 1225
percentage of, 1217t, 1218
Pneumocystis pneumonia and, 1210, 1394, 1395, 1396
reference values for, 1548t
CD5
in acute lymphoblastic leukemia, 465
in chronic lymphocytic leukemia, 467
CD7, in acute lymphoblastic leukemia, 465
CD8 T cells, in common variable immunodeficiency, 787
CD10, in acute lymphoblastic leukemia, 465
CD11c, in hairy cell leukemia, 468
CD13, in acute myeloid leukemia, 465
CD19
in acute lymphoblastic leukemia, 465
in chronic lymphocytic leukemia, 467
CD20
in acute lymphoblastic leukemia, 465
in mantle cell lymphoma, 467
CD22, in hairy cell leukemia, 468
CD23, in mantle cell lymphoma, 467
CD33, in acute myeloid leukemia, 465
CD34, in nephrogenic systemic fibrosis, 849
CD38, in chronic lymphocytic leukemia, 467
CD55 deficiency, in paroxysmal nocturnal hemoglobinuria, 449
CD56, in nasal/paranasal tumors, 201
CD59 deficiency, in paroxysmal nocturnal hemoglobinuria, 449
CD117, in gastrointestinal stromal tumors, 1474
CdA. See Cladribine
CDH-1 mutation, gastric cancer and, 1471
CDKAL1/CDKN2A/B gene, in type 2 diabetes, 1082

CDKAL1 gene, in type 2 diabetes, 1082
CDKN2A gene
pancreatic/periampullary carcinoma and, 1463
in type 2 diabetes, 1082
CDKN2B gene, in type 2 diabetes, 1082
CEA. See Carcinoembryonic antigen
Ceclor. See Cefaclor
Cecum, dilation of, in colonic pseudo-obstruction (Ogilvie syndrome), 565
CEE. See Conjugated equine estrogens
Cefaclor, 1179t
Cefadroxil, 1179t
Cefamandole, 1179t
Cefazolin, 1179t
for endocarditis, 1306, 1306t
for surgical site infection prophylaxis, 60t
Cefdinir, for pharyngitis, 1290
Cefditoren, 1179t
Cefepime, 1179t
Cefizox. See Ceftizoxime
Cefonicid, 1179t
Cefoperazone, 1179t
Ceforanide, 1179t
Cefotaxime, 1179t
Cefotetan, for surgical site infection prophylaxis, 60t
Cefoxitin, 1179t
for surgical site infection prophylaxis, 60t
Cefpodoxime, 1179t
for pharyngitis, 1290
Cefprozil, 1179t
Ceftazidime, 1179t
Ceftibuten, 1179t
Ceftin. See Cefuroxime
Ceftizoxime, 1179t
Ceftriaxone, 1179t
for abdominal infections, 1322t
for endocarditis, 1306, 1307
for syphilis, 1333, 1333t
for urinary tract infection, 852t
Cefuroxime, 1179t
Cefzil. See Cefprozil
Celebrex. See Celecoxib
Celecoxib, 78, 79t
cardiovascular complications and, 78, 548
for familial adenomatous polyposis, 591
for hemophilic arthritis, 491
for pain management, 78, 79t
peptic ulcers/peptic ulcer prevention and, 548
for rheumatoid arthritis, 749
Celexa. See Citalopram
Celiac disease/sprue (gluten-sensitive enteropathy), 516, **559–560**
dermatitis herpetiformis and, 118, 559
microscopic colitis and, 587
osteoporosis and, 559, 560
pancreatitis and, 642
Cell-mediated (delayed/type IV) hypersensitivity, 784

Cell-mediated (cellular) immunity, infections associated with defects in, 1156
Cell surface antigens, immune cell. *See under* CD
Cellophane tape test, in enterobiasis/pinworms, 1382
Cellulitis, **129–130**, 1182*t*
  anaerobic, 1323
  of auricle, 180
  deep venous thrombosis differentiated from, 129
  in drug users, 1168
  lymphangitis/lymphadenitis and, 432, 433
  lymphedema and, 433
  necrotizing fasciitis differentiated from, 129
  nonclostridial crepitant, 1323
  orbital, 170
    in bacterial rhinosinusitis, 170, 194
  peritonsillar, **205**
  sublingual/submaxillary space (Ludwig angina), 206
  superficial (erysipelas), **128–129**, 1182*t*, 1290
  synergistic necrotizing, 1323
  tinea pedis and, 109, 129
  vibrios causing, 1316
Cellulose phosphate, for absorptive hypercalciuria, 858
Cenesthetic hallucinations. *See also* Hallucinations
  in schizophrenic/psychotic disorders, 953
Centor criteria, for streptococcal pharyngitis, 204, 1289, 1290
Central alveolar hypoventilation, 287
Central cord syndrome, 919
Central nervous system disorders. *See also* Neurologic disorders
  infections, **1162–1165**, 1162*t*, 1163*t*. *See also* Encephalitis; Meningitis
    anaerobic, 1322
    otitis media and, 185
    primary angiitis, **772–773**
Central nervous system lupus, 753, 754
Central neurogenic hyperventilation, in coma or stupor, 288, 916
Central pontine myelinolysis, hyponatremia treatment and, 792
Central retinal artery occlusion, **164–165**
Central retinal vein occlusion, **163–164**
Central sleep apnea, 288
Central vein nutritional support (total parenteral nutrition/hyperalimentation), 1148, 1148*f*
  acidosis caused by, 808, 810, 1151*t*
  in burn injury, 1411
  catheter-associated infection and, 1151
  complications of, 1151, 1151*t*
  in Crohn disease, 580
  hepatic steatosis caused by, 618
  in HIV infection/AIDS, 1210

patient monitoring during, 1151–1152
  in short bowel syndrome, 563
  solutions for, 1150, 1150*t*
  for ulcerative colitis, 585
Central venous catheters, infection/infection prevention and, 1151, 1160, 1161
Central venous pressure, in shock, 435–436
Centruroides (scorpion) stings, 1447
Cephalexin, 1179*t*
  for endocarditis, 1306*t*
  for urinary tract infection, 852*t*
Cephalosporins, 1178*t*, 1179*t*
  allergy to, penicillin allergy cross-reactivity and, 1181
  for pharyngitis, 205, 1290
  for pneumonia, 247
  for surgical site infection prophylaxis, 59, 60*t*
Cephalothin, platelet function affected by, 490*t*
Cephapirin, 1179*t*
Cephradine, 1179*t*
CEPI test, 1553*t*
Ceratopic, 99*t*
Cercariae/metacercariae
  in clonorchiasis/opisthorchiasis, 1375
  in fascioliasis, 1375
  in fasciolopsiasis, 1376
  in paragonimiasis, 1375
  in schistosomiasis, 1373
Cercarial dermatitis, in schistosomiasis, 1374
Cerclage, for incompetent cervix, 712
Cerebellar arteriovenous malformations, 895
Cerebellar artery obstruction, in stroke, 891
Cerebellar degeneration, paraneoplastic, 902, 1453*t*
Cerebellar hemorrhage, in stroke, 892
Cerebellar tonsils, herniation of, intracranial tumors causing, 898
Cerebellar tumors, 899
  hemangioblastoma, 898*t*
Cerebral aneurysm. *See* Intracranial aneurysm
Cerebral angiography/arteriography. *See also* Neuroimaging
  in brain death determination, 917
  in carotid occlusive disease, 420
  in primary angiitis of central nervous system, 772
Cerebral arteriovenous malformations, 895
Cerebral artery occlusion, in stroke, 889
Cerebral contusions/lacerations, 918*t*
Cerebral edema
  acute high-altitude, **1418**
  in CNS infections, 1164
  in hepatic failure, 608
  hypernatremia treatment and, 794
  in stroke, 891
Cerebral hemorrhage. *See* Intracerebral hemorrhage

Cerebral infarction/ischemia, **889–892**. *See also* Stroke
Cerebral injury, **918**, 918*t*
  in near drowning, 1416
Cerebral ischemia. *See* Cerebral infarction; Transient ischemic attacks
Cerebral lymphoma, primary, in HIV infection/AIDS, 898*t*, 901, 1212, 1216
Cerebral malaria, 1354, 1356
Cerebral metastases, 900
Cerebral salt wasting, 789, 790*f*, 792
Cerebral sparganosis, 1379
Cerebral toxoplasmosis, in HIV infection/AIDS, 901, 1211–1212, 1363, 1364. *See also* Toxoplasma
Cerebrospinal fluid analysis
  in African trypanosomiasis, 1348–1349
  in amebic encephalitis/meningoencephalitis, 1162*t*, 1368
  in anthrax, 1301
  in cancer-related neurologic disorders, 902
  in CNS infections, 1162, 1162*t*, 1164
  in cryptococcosis, 1396
  in cysticercosis, 1377
  in eosinophilic meningoencephalitis (angiostrongyliasis), 1384
  in Guillain-Barré syndrome, 925
  in headache evaluation, 45
  in herpes simplex encephalitis/meningitis, 1236
  in, arbovirus encephalitides, 1258
  in intracranial aneurysm, 894
  in leptomeningeal metastases (carcinomatous meningitis), 900, 1163
  in listeriosis, 1303
  in Lyme disease, 1344, 1345
  in lymphocytic choriomeningitis, 1259
  in meningitis, 1162*t*, 1164
  in meningococcal meningitis, 1309
  in multiple sclerosis, 913
  in pneumococcal meningitis, 1293
  in poliomyelitis, 1252
  in purulent/bacterial meningitis, 1162*t*
  in rabies, 1256
  in spinal tumors, 901
  in syphilis, 1336, 1337
    in HIV infection/AIDS, 1220, 1337, 1338
    indications for, 1336–1337
    treatment failure and, 1334
  in tick-borne encephalitis, 1266
  in tuberculous meningitis, 1162*t*, 1326
Cerebrospinal fluid leakage, in head injury, 918
Cerebrovascular accident. *See* Stroke
Cerebrovascular disorders
  headache in, 44, 45, 876
  hypertensive, 393
  occlusive, **420–421**. *See also* Stroke; Transient ischemic attacks
    homocysteine in, 1516
    oral contraceptive use and, 696

Certolizumab, for inflammatory bowel disease, 577
  Crohn disease, 581
Cerubidine. *See* Daunorubicin
Ceruloplasmin
  reference values for, 1548*t*
  in Wilson disease, 629
Cerumen impaction, 179, **180–181**
Ceruminous gland adenoma, 182
Cervical cap, **699**
Cervical carcinoma. *See* Cervix (uterine), cancer of
Cervical intraepithelial neoplasia (CIN/ dysplasia of cervix), **680–682**, 680*t*
  cytologic (Pap smear) testing for, 680–681, 680*t*
  DES exposure and, 680
  in HIV infection/AIDS, 681, 1216
  HPV tests in screening for, 681
  HPV vaccination in prevention of, 4, 681, 682, 1187–1198, 1190–1191*t*, 1192–1193*t*, 1194–1197*t*
  oral contraceptive use and, 696
Cervical lymph nodes, normal, 213
Cervical lymphadenopathy, reactive, **213**
Cervical mucus/secretions, evaluation of
  in symptothermal natural family planning, 699
  in TwoDay method of contraception, 700
Cervical rib syndrome, 737–738, **931–932**
Cervical spine/disk disease, **929**, 930–931*f*. *See also* Spine
  arthritic/degenerative, 737, 929
  chest pain in, 321
  herniation/protrusion, 737, **929**, 930–931*f*
  neck pain in, 737, **929**, 930–931*f*
  vertigo and, 190, 191*t*
Cervical spondylosis, 737, **929**
Cervical strain, 736
Cervical vertigo, 190, 191*t*
Cervical warts, 678. *See also* Venereal (genital) warts
Cervicitis
  chlamydial, **1328**
  gonococcal, 1319, 1320
  postgonococcal, 1320
Cervicocolpopexy, for pelvic organ prolapse, 687
Cervicofacial actinomycosis, 1323
Cervix (uterine)
  anaerobic infection of, 1323
  biopsy of
    in abnormal premenopausal bleeding, 674
    in CIN/cervical cancer, 681, 682
  cancer of, **682–683**, 1467*t*
    HIV infection/AIDS and, 1216
    HPV infection and, 682, 1216
    screening tests for, 681
    vaccine in prevention of, 4, 682, 1187–1198, 1190–1191*t*, 1192–1193*t*, 1194–1197*t*
    invasive, 680*t*, 683
    oral contraceptive use and, 696

Pap smears in screening for, 16, 17*t*, 680–681, 680*t*
  preinvasive (carcinoma in situ), 680*t*, 682, 682–683
  cauterization of, for CIN, 681
  conization of, for CIN/cervical cancer, 681, 682, 683
  dysplasia (CIN) of, **680–682**, 680*t*. *See also* Cervical intraepithelial neoplasia
  incompetent, 711
    cerclage/activity restriction for, 712
  polyps of, **679**
Cesarean section
  antibiotic prophylaxis for, 60*t*
  for cardiac patient, 385
  for prevention of disease transmission to fetus/newborn
    herpes genitalis, 727, 1237
    HIV, 726, 1207
Cestode infections, **1376–1379**. *See also* *specific type*
  invasive, **1377–1379**
  noninvasive, **1376–1377**
Cetuximab, 1503*t*
  for colorectal cancer, 1479
CFTR. *See* Cystic fibrosis transmembrane conductance regulator (CFTR) protein
CH50 (complement)
  in gonococcal arthritis, 778
  reference values for, 1548*t*
Chagas disease (American trypanosomiasis), **1349–1351**
  achalasia and, 542
  heart disease/myocarditis in, 368, 1350
Chagoma, 1350
Chalazion, **152**
Chancre
  differential diagnosis of, 1332
  syphilitic, 1330, 1332
    anal/anorectal, 594, 1330
  trypanosomal, 1348
Chancroid, **1320**
Channelopathies, periodic paralysis, 936
Chaotic (multifocal) atrial tachycardia, **350**
Charcoal, activated, for poisoning/drug overdose, 1424, 1425
  repeat-dose, 1426
Charcot joint (neurogenic arthropathy), **783**
  in diabetes mellitus, 783, 1106
  in tabes dorsalis, 783, 1336
Charcot-Marie-Tooth disease, 922–923
Charcot triad, 638
CHD. *See* Coronary heart disease
Cheilitis, angular
  candidiasis and, 202
  in HIV infection/AIDS, 1213
Cheiropathy, diabetic, 759
Chelation therapy. *See also specific type*
  adverse ophthalmic effects of, 178*t*
  for arsenic poisoning, 1432
  for heavy metal poisoning, 1424*t*
  for hemochromatosis/iron poisoning/ overload, 444, 628

for iron overdose/toxicity, 1437
  for lead poisoning, 846, 1438
  for mercury poisoning, 1439
  for Wilson disease, 629
Chemical injury
  acids causing, **1429**
  alkalies causing, **1429–1430**
  of esophagus, 536, 1429
  of eye (conjunctivitis/keratitis), **172**, 1429, 1430
  of lung, **280**
    aspiration and, 278
    smoke inhalation and, 277, 1409
Chemical warfare agents. *See also* Bioterrorism
  nerve agents, **1434**
  ricin, **1434**
  skin decontamination and, 1424
Chemoembolization, transcatheter arterial, for hepatocellular carcinoma, 1461
Chemoinfusion, transcatheter arterial, for hepatocellular carcinoma, 1461
Chemokine co-receptors, in HIV infection/AIDS, 1208
Chemoprevention/chemoprophylaxis, 3*t*. *See also specific agent*
  antibiotic/antimicrobial. *See* Antimicrobial chemoprophylaxis
  for cancer, 16
    breast cancer and, 663
    colorectal cancer and, 1477
  for cardiovascular disease, **12**
  for stress gastritis, 545
  for venous thromboembolic disease, **495–496**, 496*t*
Chemoprotection, ototoxic, 187
Chemoradiation therapy
  for bladder cancer, 1490
  for esophageal cancer, 1469, 1470
  for laryngeal squamous cell carcinoma, 210
  for rectal cancer, 1480
Chemoreceptor trigger zone, 504
Chemosclerosis, for malignant effusions, 1496
Chemosis
  in allergic eye disease, 155
  in dysthyroid eye disease, 170, 1009
Chemotherapy (cancer), 1499–1511, 1500–1506*t*, 1507–1508*t*, 1508*t*. *See also specific agent and cancer type*
  adverse ophthalmic effects of, 178*t*
  bone marrow/stem cell transplantation after, 475, 476
  breast feeding and, 710*t*
  cancers responsive to, 1466–1468*t*
  dosages of agents used in, 1500–1506*t*, 1507–1508*t*
  modification of, **1499–1511**, 1508*t*
  high dose. *See* High dose chemotherapy
  hypercalcemia and, **1496–1497**
  hyperuricemia associated with, **1497–1498**

Chemotherapy (cancer) (*cont.*)
infections in neutropenic patients
and, 1181t, 1498
leukemia caused by, 464
nausea and vomiting caused by, 505t,
1508–1509
acupuncture for, 1534
mind-body therapies for, 1536t
guided imagery, 1536t, 1543
ototoxicity and, 186–187
with radiation therapy. *See* Chemoradiation therapy
supportive agents/care and, 1507–1508t
thrombocytopenia and, **482**, 483t,
1499–1508
toxicity of agents used in, **1499–1511**,
1500–1506t
ophthalmic effects and, 178t
Chen sign, 295
Chenodeoxycholic acid, for cholelithiasis/
gallstones, 635
Chest pain, 28–30, 29t, 320–321, 326
in achalasia, 542
in acute coronary syndromes, 28–29,
326
in angina, 28–29, 318
alteration in before myocardial
infarction, 330
coronary vasospasm causing, 317,
325
Prinzmetal (variant), 325
in aortic dissection, 29, 321, 426
in aortic regurgitation, 312
in cardiomyopathy, 373
in cervical/thoracic spine disease, 321,
543
dyspnea and, 25
in esophageal disorders, 29, 321, 543
GERD, 531, 543
infectious esophagitis, 535
motility disorders, 543
pill-induced esophagitis, 536
ischemic, 28–29. *See also* Acute coronary syndromes; Angina
in myocardial infarction, 28–29, 29t,
330
management of, 334–335
in myocarditis, 368
noncardiac, 321, 543, **543–544**. *See
also* Chest pain, in esoph-
ageal disorders
palpitations and, 31
in panic disorders, 29, 30, 544, 944
in pericarditis, 29, 377, 1279
pleuritic (pleuritis), 29, **282**
in epidemic pleurodynia (Bornholm disease), 1279
in pericarditis, 377
in thoracic actinomycosis, 1323
in pneumothorax, 286, 321
psychologic causes of, 544
in pulmonary embolism, 28, 29, 30,
267, 268t, 321
in thoracic outlet syndrome, 321
visceral sensitivity causing, 543–544
Chest pain observation units, 326
Chest percussion
in bronchiectasis, 240

in chronic bronchitis, 238
in cystic fibrosis, 242
Chest tube drainage (tube thoracostomy)
for empyema, 285
for hemothorax, 285
for malignant effusions, 1496
for parapneumonic effusion, 285, 1293
for pneumothorax, 286, 287
Chest wall
breast cancer recurrence in, 671
disorders of, chest pain in, 543
anterior chest wall/Tietze syndrome, 321
respiratory failure caused by disorders of, 289t
Cheyne-Stokes respiration, in coma or
stupor, 916
CHF. *See* Congestive heart (cardiac) failure
Chi, in acupuncture, 1532
Chibroxin. *See* Norfloxacin
Chickenpox. *See* Varicella
Chiggers, skin lesions caused by, 139
Chikungunya fever, **1267–1268**
Chilblain (erythema pernio), **1405**
Child abuse
Munchausen by proxy and, 945
PTSD and, 938
sexual, 976
intrafamilial (incest), 948
Child-Turcotte-Pugh classification for cirrhosis, 624, 624t
hepatocellular carcinoma and, 1460,
1461
surgery and, 55
variceal hemorrhage and, 541
Childbirth preparation classes, 707
Chinese liver fluke infection, 1375
Chiropractic, 1520
Chlamydia (chlamydial infections),
1177–1178t, **1327–1329**.
See also Chlamydophila
dysuria in, 46
gonococcal coinfection and, 1319,
1320, 1328
inclusion conjunctivitis, 154
keratoconjunctivitis, 154
screening/prevention and, 1167
trachoma, 154
trachomatis, 1177t, 1327, **1327–1329**,
1328
anorectal involvement and, 594
epididymitis, 856, 1182t
lymphogranuloma venereum,
1327–1328
pelvic infection/PID, 688, 1177t,
1182t, 1328
during pregnancy, **727**
rape/sexual assault in transmission
of, 702, 1167
urethritis and cervicitis, 1177t,
1182t, **1328–1329**
Chlamydophila, 1327. *See also Chlamydia*
pneumoniae, 1178t, 1327, **1329**
pneumonia caused by, 244t, 1182t,
1329
psittaci, 1177t, 1327, **1329**
Chloasma (melasma), 144
oral contraceptive use and, 144, 697

Chloral hydrate, 941t
Chlorambucil, 1501t
adverse ophthalmic effects of, 178t
for chronic lymphocytic leukemia,
467–468
Chloramphenicol
adverse ophthalmic effects of, 177t
for ophthalmic disorders, 173t
renal/hepatic failure and, 1184t
Chlordane, poisoning caused by,
1443–1444
Chlordiazepoxide, 941t
Chlorguanide. *See* Proguanil
Chloride
in fluid management of, 815, 815t
reference values for, 1548t
requirements for in nutritional support, 1149
serum levels of, in hypercalcemia/
hyperparathyroidism, 801,
1034
urinary, in metabolic alkalosis, 812,
813
2-Chlorodeoxyadenosine. *See* Cladribine
Chlorophenothane (DDT), poisoning
caused by, 1443–1444
Chloroquine, 1356–1357, 1357t
adverse ophthalmic effects of, 178t
for amebiasis, 1367, 1367t
arrhythmias caused by, 1445
for lupus, 111
for malaria, 1355, 1355t, 1356–1357
chemoprophylaxis, 1355t, 1357,
1361, 1361t
for non-falciparum malaria, 1356,
1356–1357, 1357t
in pregnancy, 710
resistance to, 1355, 1356
for uncomplicated falciparum
malaria, 1355, 1356–1357,
1357t
rabies vaccination affected by, 1201,
1257
Chlorproguanil, with dapsone (Lapdap),
1359
Chlorpromazine, 954, 955t, 956t. *See also*
Antipsychotic drugs
overdose/toxicity of, 956t, 959,
1444–1445
Chlorpropamide, 1090, 1091t
adverse ophthalmic effects of, 178t
intensive therapy with, 1088
Chlorthalidone, 398, 399t
Chokes, 1417
Cholangiocarcinoma, 1460, 1462, 1463
in clonorchiasis/opisthorchiasis, 1375,
1462
in primary sclerosing cholangitis, 641,
1462
Cholangiography. *See* Endoscopic retrograde
cholangiopancreatography;
Percutaneous transhepatic
cholangiography
Cholangiopancreatography. *See* Endoscopic retrograde cholangiopancreatography;
Magnetic resonance cho-
langiopancreatography

Cholangiopathy, AIDS, 1245, 1369, 1370
Cholangitis
  autoimmune, 626
  biliary stricture and, 639–640, 640,
    641
  choledocholithiasis and, **638–639**
  in clonorchiasis/opisthorchiasis, 1375
  drugs/toxins causing, 616
  in fascioliasis, 1375
  liver abscess and, 632
  during pregnancy, 727
  primary sclerosing, **640–641**
    cholangiocarcinoma and, 641, 1462
    in HIV infection/AIDS, 1214
Cholecalciferol (vitamin D₃), for hypo-
    parathyroidism, 1032,
    1032t
Cholecystectomy
  for cholecystitis, 637
  for choledocholithiasis/cholangitis,
    638
  for cholelithiasis/gallstones, 634–635
  for gallbladder cancer, 1463
  pancreatitis and, 644, 645
  for precholecystectomy syndrome, 637
  pregnancy and, 728
  symptom persistence after (postchole-
    cystectomy syndrome), **637**
Cholecystitis, **635–637**, 635t, 1181t
  acalculous, 636
    in HIV infection/AIDS, 1214
    parenteral nutritional support and,
      1151t
  acute, **635–637**, 635t
  cholelithiasis/gallstones and, 635–636,
    636
  chronic, 635t, 636
  in HIV infection/AIDS, 1214
  during pregnancy, **727–728**
  xanthogranulomatous, 636
Cholecystostomy, 637
  pancreatitis and, 645
Choledocholithiasis, 635t, **638–639**
  pancreatitis and, 638, 639, 645
  during pregnancy, **727–728**
Cholelithiasis (gallstones), **634–635**, 635t
  cholecystitis and, 635–636, 636
  in Crohn disease, 578, 634
  gallbladder cancer and, 1462
  in hereditary spherocytosis, 448
  pancreatitis and, 642, 643, 645
  during pregnancy, 634, 727
  in short bowel syndrome, 562–563
Cholera, 1171t, 1177t, **1315–1316**
  prevention/immunization and, 1200,
    1315
Cholestasis, 598
  in biliary cirrhosis, 625
  drugs/toxins causing, 616
  hereditary/intrahepatic, 598, 599t
  of pregnancy, 599t, **727–728**
Cholestatic jaundice, 598
  androgens causing, 1065
Cholesteatoma, **184**
Cholesterol, 1123, 1124. See also specific lipo-
    protein and Lipoproteins
  in atherogenesis/coronary heart dis-
    ease, 316, 1123, 1124

  in diabetes mellitus, 1089, 1108
  dietary, 1130, 1146
  elevated levels of, 1123. See also
    Hypercholesterolemia
    screening tests for, 1126–1129,
      1127–1128t, 1129t
  in gallstones, 634
  garlic affecting, 1523t, 1524
  lowering levels of. See Lipid-lowering
    therapy
  protease inhibitors affecting, 1229
  reference/normal values for, 1124,
    1548t, 1550t
  rosiglitazone therapy and, 1093
Cholesterol-lowering diet, 1130, 1146
  in diabetes, 1089, 1146
Cholesterolosis of gallbladder, 635t, 636
Cholestyramine
  for diarrhea, 517
    in Crohn disease, 580
  for idiopathic cholestasis of preg-
    nancy, 728
  for lipid modification/heart disease
    prevention, 1131, 1132t
Choline magnesium salicylate, 79t
Cholinergic rebound, 967
Cholinergic syndrome, 1426
Cholinergic urticaria, 126
Cholinesterase inhibitors. See Anticho-
    linesterases
Chondritis. See Polychondritis
Chondrocalcinosis, **735–736**
Chondroitin/chondroitin plus glu-
    cosamine sulfate, 1528t,
    1529–1530
  in osteoarthritis, 731, 1528t,
    1529–1530
Chordae tendineae
  in mitral regurgitation, 308
  in mitral stenosis, 306
  rupture of, 309
Chorea
  drug-induced, 911
  in Huntington disease, 908
  Sydenham, 375, 909
Chorioamnionitis, **720–721**
Choriocarcinoma, **714–715**, 1467t. See
    also Gestational tropho-
    blastic disease
  hyperthyroidism and, 1009
  paraneoplastic syndrome associated
    with, 1453t
  testicular, 1492
Choriomeningitis, lymphocytic,
    1259–1260
Chorionic gonadotropin. See Human
    chorionic gonadotropin
Chorioretinitis
  in lymphocytic choriomeningitis,
    1259
  toxoplasmic, in HIV infection/AIDS,
    1363, 1364
Choroidal circulation, hypertension
    affecting (hypertensive ret-
    inochoroidopathy), 167
Choroidal neovascularization, in age-
    related macular degenera-
    tion, 162–163

Chromatographically purified rabies vac-
    cine, 1256
Chromoblastomycosis (chromomycosis),
    1400
Chromoendoscopy, in ulcerative colitis,
    586
Chromogranin A (CgA)
  in carcinoid tumors, 1475, 1476
  in pancreatic/periampullary carci-
    noma, 1463
  in pheochromocytomas, 1059
Chronic cutaneous lupus erythematosus,
    110–111
Chronic disease
  anemia of, **441–442**
  mood disorders and, 962
Chronic fatigue syndrome, **41–43**, 42f
  enterovirus infection in development
    of, 1279
  fibromyalgia and, 741
  Q fever, 1287
Chronic inflammatory polyneuropathy,
    926
Chronic kidney disease (CKD), 816,
    825–833, 825t, 826t, 827f,
    827t. See also Renal failure
  acid-base disorders and, 809, 827–828
  anemia in, 441, 816, 828–829
  cardiovascular complications and,
    826t, 827t, 828
  coagulopathy of, 829
  congestive heart failure and, 360, 827t,
    828
  diabetes and, 830, 842, 1104. See also
    Diabetic nephropathy
  dietary management in, 830
  endocrine disorders and, 830
  gout and, 732, 849
  hematologic complications and,
    828–829
  hepatitis C infection and, 844
  hypercalcemia/hyperparathyroidism
    and, 827, 829, 1033, 1034,
    1035, 1038
  hyperglycemia and, 830
  hyperhomocysteinemia in, 1517
  hyperkalemia and, 797, 827
  hypermagnesemia and, 806
  hyperphosphatemia in, 804, 829
  hypertension/hypertension manage-
    ment and, 393, 396t, 410,
    826, 827t, 828
  hypocalcemia and, 799, 800
  hypoglycemia and, 830, 1104
  hyponatremia in, 790f, 792
  immunization recommendations in,
    1195t
  lipid abnormalities and, 1126t
  mineral bone disorders of (renal
    osteodystrophy), 827,
    829–830, 1033, 1035, 1038
  in nephrogenic systemic fibrosis, **849**
  neurologic complications of, 829
  neuropathy associated with, 829, 923
  pericarditis and (uremic pericarditis),
    377, 378, 828
  postoperative complications in
    patients with, 58–59, 59t

Chronic kidney disease (*cont.*)
protein-restricted diet for, 830, 1146
reversible causes of, 826, 827*t*
stages of, 825*t*
surgery in patients with, 59
Chronic lymphocytic leukemia (CLL), **467–468**, 1466*t*
Chronic lymphocytic thyroiditis. *See* Hashimoto (chronic lymphocytic/autoimmune) thyroiditis
Chronic mountain sickness (Monge disease), **1418**
Chronic myeloid leukemia (CML), 457*t*, **461–462**, 1466*t*
bone marrow/stem cell transplantation for, 462, 476
Chronic myelomonocytic leukemia (CMML), 463
Chronic obstructive pulmonary disease (COPD), **234–240**, 235*t*
acidosis in, 234, 814
atrial flutter in, 238, 349
cough in, 22, 23, 234
dyspnea in, 24–25, 26, 234
hypophosphatemia and, 803
immunization recommendations in, 1195*t*
postoperative pulmonary complications and, 53, 54
pulmonary function tests in, 234, 235*t*
pulmonary heart disease (cor pulmonale) and, 238, 382
respiratory failure in, 234, 238
smoking and, 6, 7, 236
surgery for, 238–239
Chronic pain disorders, **946–948**, 947*f*. *See also* Pain
mind-body therapies for, 946–947, 1536*t*
opioids in management of, 78–84, 81–83*t*, 947
Chronic pelvic pain syndrome, **855**, 855*t*
Chronic prolymphocytic leukemia, 467
Chronic renal failure. *See also* Chronic kidney disease
Chronic venous insufficiency. *See* Venous insufficiency/stasis
Chrysotherapy. *See* Gold therapy
Churg-Strauss syndrome (allergic angiitis and granulomatosis), 276
leukotriene modifiers for asthma and, 228
pulmonary involvement in, 276
renal involvement in, 835*f*
Chvostek sign
in hypocalcemia/hypoparathyroidism, 800, 1031
malabsorption and, 558*t*
Chylomicronemia. *See* Hyperchylomicronemia
Chylous ascites, 528, 621, 1496
Chylous pleural effusion, 283, 1496
Cialis. *See* Tadalafil
Cicatricial alopecia, **145**
Ciclopirox, 98*t*
Cidofovir, 1238*t*
for cytomegalovirus infection, 167, 1238*t*

for herpes simplex infection, 1237
for recurrent respiratory papillomatosis, 208
Cigarette/cigar smoking. *See* Smoking
Ciguatera poisoning, 1446, 1446*t*
Ciloxan. *See* Ciprofloxacin
Cimetidine, 550. *See also* H_2 receptor blocking drugs
antidepressant drug interactions and, 969*t*
benzodiazepine interactions and, 942*t*
theophyllines affected by, 225*t*
Cimex lectularius bites, 139
CIN. *See* Cervical intraepithelial neoplasia
Cinacalcet
for hypercalcemia/hyperparathyroidism, 801–802, 1037
for mineral bone disorders of chronic kidney disease, 830, 1037
Cinchonism (quinine toxicity), 1358
Cingulotomy, for OCD, 943
Cipro. *See* Ciprofloxacin
Ciprofibrate, 1131–1132
Ciprofloxacin, 1180*t*
for abdominal infections, 1322*t*
for anthrax, 1301, 1301*t*
for cyclosporiasis, 1371
for ophthalmic disorders, 173*t*
prophylactic, 1158
theophyllines affected by, 225*t*
for urinary tract infection, 852*t*
Circadian rhythm, melatonin affecting, 1531
Circadian rhythm dysfunction, in seasonal affective disorder, 962
Circumcision, HIV infection risk and, 1219
Cirrhosis, **619–625**, 624*t*
alcoholic liver disease/hepatitis and, 614–616, 619, 620
biliary, 620, **625–627**
cardiac, 620
drugs/toxins causing, 617
Dupuytren contracture and, 619, 743
esophageal varices in, 538, 539, 541, 620
prevention of first bleeding episode and, 541
GI bleeding in, 517–518, 538, 539, 620
hemochromatosis and, 620, 627, 628
hepatic coagulopathy and, 494–495
hyponatremia in, 790*f*, 791
Laennec, 619
lipid abnormalities and, 1126*t*
liver cancer and, 615, 620, 624, 1460, 1461
nonalcoholic fatty liver disease and, 617, 618, 620
hepatocellular carcinoma and, 618, 1460
postoperative complications and, 55
spontaneous bacterial peritonitis and, 526, 621–622
theophyllines affected by, 225*t*
viral hepatitis and, 602, 603, 604, 609, 611–612, 620
Cirrhotic cardiomyopathy, 620

Cisapride, antidepressant drug interactions and, 966, 969*t*
Cisplatin, 1500*t*
for bladder cancer, 1490
for gastric adenocarcinoma, 1472
for laryngeal squamous cell carcinoma, 210
for lung cancer, 1456, 1457
for testicular cancer, 1493, 1494
toxicity of, 1500*t*, 1511
amifostine for, 1507*t*
neuropathy, 1511
ototoxicity, 187, 1511
Citalopram, 964, 966, 968*t*
overdose toxicity of, 966, 968*t*, 1448
Citracal (calcium citrate). *See* Calcium, dietary/supplementary
Citrate, in hypocitraturic calcium nephrolithiasis, 859
CJD. *See* Creutzfeldt-Jakob disease
CK. *See* Conductive keratoplasty; Creatine kinase
CK-MB. *See* Creatine kinase-MB
CKD. *See* Chronic kidney disease
Cl⁻. *See* Chloride
Cladophialophora/Cladophialophora carrionii
chromoblastomycosis caused by, 1400
phaeohyphomycosis caused by, 1402
Cladribine (2-chlorodeoxyadenosine), 1501*t*
for hairy cell leukemia, 468
Clarithromycin. *See also* Macrolides
for anthrax, 1301*t*
for endocarditis, 1306*t*
in *H pylori* eradication therapy, 551*t*
for MAC treatment/prophylaxis, 1222, 1224*t*, 1324–1325
renal/hepatic failure and, 1184*t*
theophyllines affected by, 225*t*
Classic Creutzfeldt-Jakob disease, 1260–1261. *See also* Creutzfeldt-Jakob disease
Claudication
in aortoiliac occlusive disease, 415
in femoral/popliteal occlusive disease, 416
ginkgo for, 1523*t*, 1525
jaw (masticatory), in giant cell arteritis, 164, 766
Cl$_{cr}$. *See* Creatinine clearance
Clean-catch urine specimen, for dysuria evaluation, 47
Cleaning agents, poisoning caused by. *See* Caustic/corrosive agents
Clear cell carcinoma of vagina, DES exposure and, 680
Clear liquid diet, 1145
Cleocin. *See* Clindamycin
Clicks. *See also* Heart murmurs
in mitral valve prolapse, 309
in pulmonic regurgitation, 315
in pulmonic stenosis, 295
Climacteric, 1069. *See also* Menopause
Climara. *See* Estradiol transdermal systems
Clindamycin
for acne, 97*t*, 121

for anthrax, 1301t
for bacterial vaginosis, 679
with benzoyl peroxide, 97t
for endocarditis, 1306t
for malaria, 1357t, 1360
for *Pneumocystis* pneumonia, 1395
renal/hepatic failure and, 1184t
for rosacea, 123
for toxoplasmosis, 1224t, 1365
Clinician–patient relationship. *See* Doctor–patient relationship
Clinoril. *See* Sulindac
Clitocybe (muscarinic) mushroom poisoning, 1441, 1441t, 1442
CLL. *See* Chronic lymphocytic leukemia
Clobetasol, 97t
Clock draw, in dementia screening, 64
Clocortolone, 96t
Cloderm. *See* Clocortolone
Clofarabine, 1501t
Clofazamine, for leprosy, 1327
Clolar. *See* Clofarabine
Clomiphene
for male infertility, 994
for ovulation induction, 693, 994, 1055
Clomipramine, 966, 968t. *See also* Antidepressants
for OCD, 943, 966
Clonazepam, 941t. *See also* Benzodiazepines
for bipolar disease/mania, 970
for panic attacks, 942, 943
for seizures, 882t
Clonic seizures, 880. *See also* Seizures
Clonidine
for alcohol withdrawal, 980
antidepressant drug interactions and, 969t
for diarrhea, 517
for hypertension, 407, 408t
urgencies/emergencies, 413t, 414
for menopausal symptoms, 704
for migraine prophylaxis, 874t
for opioid withdrawal, 21, 982
overdose/toxicity of, 408t, 413t, **1434–1435**
Clonorchis sinensis (clonorchiasis), **1375**
cholangiocarcinoma and, 1462
Clopidogrel
for acute coronary syndromes, 327t, 328
for angina, 322
for myocardial infarction, 327t, 332, 335, 340
peptic ulcer disease and, 552, 553
platelet function affected by, 490t
Clorazepate, 941, 941t
Clostridium (clostridial infections), 1177t, **1297–1300**, 1321, 1322
bifermentans, 1297
botulinum (botulism), **933–934**, 1170t, **1299–1300**
difficile, colitis/diarrhea caused by, 511, 512, 573, 574, 1170t, 1172
histolyticum, 1297
myonecrosis/gas gangrene, 1177t, **1297**

novyi, 1297
perfringens, 1297
diarrhea/food poisoning/gastroenteritis caused by, 512, 1170t, 1172
ramosum, 1297
sordellii (endometritis/toxic shock), 701, **1297–1298**
tetani, 1177t, 1298. *See also* Tetanus
Clotrimazole, 98t
for esophageal candidiasis, 535
for oral candidiasis, 202
for vulvovaginal candidiasis, 678, 1390
Clotting factors. *See* Coagulation factors
Clotting time, activated (ACT), reference values for, 1547t
Clozapine, 954, 955, 955t, 956t. *See also* Antipsychotic drugs
agranulocytosis caused by, 955, 958
neuroleptic malignant syndrome and, 959
overdose/toxicity of, 955, 956t, 958–959
in parkinsonism, 908
type 2 diabetes and, 956
Clozaril. *See* Clozapine
Clubbed fingers (digital clubbing), 146
in bronchiectasis, 240
in interstitial (diffuse parenchymal) lung disease, 262
in lung cancer, 1454
Clue cells, in bacterial vaginosis, 678
Cluster headache, 872, **875**
Clusters of differentiation (CD). *See* CD markers
CMF regimen, for breast cancer, 665
CML. *See* Chronic myeloid leukemia
CMML. *See* Chronic myelomonocytic leukemia
CMV. *See* Controlled mechanical ventilation
CMV immune globulin, 1246, 1246–1247
CMV inclusion disease, 1245
CMV infections. *See* Cytomegalovirus infections
Co-Q10 (coenzyme Q10), 1528t, 1530
CO2 laser therapy. *See* Carbon dioxide laser therapy
Coagulase-negative staphylococci, **1296–1297**
burn-associated infection caused by, 1411
endocarditis caused by, 1296–1297, 1306
Coagulation disorders. *See* Bleeding; Coagulopathy; Disseminated intravascular coagulation
Coagulation factors. *See also specific type under Factor*
for anticoagulant overdose, 1431
in liver disease, 494–495
Coagulation necrosis techniques, for benign prostatic hyperplasia, 871
Coagulopathy. *See also specific type and* Bleeding
acquired disorders causing, **494–495**

cancer-related, 1453t
of chronic kidney disease, 829
congenital disorders causing, 393t, **490–494**, 492t
consumptive (DIC), **487–488**, 488t, **495**. *See also* Disseminated intravascular coagulation
in gram-negative bacteremia/sepsis, 1311
of liver disease, **494–495**, 623
hepatic failure and, 607
variceal hemorrhage and. *See* Esophageal varices
preoperative screening for, 49, 50t
Coal worker's pneumoconiosis, 278, 279t
Coarctation of aorta, **296–297**
hypertension and, 296
in Turner syndrome, 1074
Coartem (artemether-lumefantrine/ Riamet), for malaria, 1355t, 1356, 1356t, 1357t, 1360
Cobalamin. *See* Vitamin B12
Cocaine. *See also* Cocaine abuse
toxicity of, 983–984, **1430**
cardiac, 325, 330, 370
Cocaine abuse, 20, 966, **983–984**, **1430**
acupuncture for, 1534
epistaxis and, 198, 983
myocardial ischemia/infarction/myocarditis and, 325, 330, 370
during pregnancy, 707
pulmonary disorders caused by, 281
Coccidioides immitis/posadasii (coccidioidomycosis), **1392–1394**
bone and joint infection in, **781**, 1393
Coccidiosis, **1369–1371**
Cochlea
hearing loss caused by disorders of, 179, 180, 186
noise trauma affecting, 186
recruitment/hyperacusis caused by disorders of, 188
tinnitus caused by disorders of, 187–188
Cochlear implants, 180
pneumococcal vaccination and, 1199
Cochlear otosclerosis, 185
Cockcroft-Gault formula, 818
Codeine, 78, 83t
with aspirin or acetaminophen, 83t
for diarrhea, 517
overdose/toxicity of, 1442–1443
in pain management, 78, 83t
Coenzyme Q10, 1528t, 1530
Coffee grounds emesis/aspirate
in erosive/hemorrhagic gastritis (gastropathy), 544
in GI bleeding, 517, 518, 521, 554
in peptic ulcer disease, 554
Cogan syndrome, 187
Cogentin. *See* Benztropine
Cognitive ability
estrogen replacement therapy and, 704, 1072
ginkgo affecting, 1523t, 1524–1525
ginseng affecting, 1526
impairment in. *See* Cognitive disorders

Cognitive behavior therapy. *See also*
   Behavior modification
   for anxiety disorders, 943
   for chronic fatigue syndrome, 43
   for depression, 970
   for insomnia, 974
   for irritable bowel syndrome, 573
   for schizophrenic/psychotic disor-
      ders, 960
Cognitive disorders, **985–988**. *See also*
   specific type and Delirium;
   Dementia
   decision-making capacity and, 64
   in elderly, 63–66
   mild impairment, 65
   postoperative, 56, 56t
   screening for, 64
   treatment of, 65
Cognitive remediation therapy, for
   schizophrenic/psychotic
   disorders, 960
Cohosh, black, 1523t, 1527
Coin lesion. *See* Solitary pulmonary nodule
Coitus. *See* Sexual intercourse
Colchicine
   for familial Mediterranean fever, 528
   for gout, 733, 734
   neuropathy/myopathy caused by, 761
Cold (common cold/viral rhinitis), **192**,
   1275
   bacterial rhinosinusitis and, 192, 193
   cough in, 22
   echinacea for, 1523t, 1525–1526
Cold agglutinin disease, **453–454**
   Waldenström macroglobulinemia
      and, 454, 474
Cold exposure, 1403, **1403–1406**
   hypothermia caused by
      of extremities, **1405–1406**
      rhabdomyolysis and, 763
      systemic, **1403–1405**, 1404f
   Raynaud phenomenon and, 756
Cold/fever sore (herpes simplex),
   113–114, 1235–1236. *See*
   also Herpes simplex infection
Cold urticaria, 126
Colectomy
   for colorectal cancer, 1478–1479
   in familial adenomatous polyposis,
      591
   for GI bleeding, 522
   for HNPCC, 592–593
   prophylactic, 591
   in ulcerative colitis, 586
Colesevelam, 1131, 1132t
   for diarrhea in Crohn disease, 580
Colestid. *See* Colestipol
Colestipol, 1131, 1132t
   for diarrhea in Crohn disease, 580
Colic. *See* Biliary colic; Renal colic
Colitis. *See also* Diarrhea
   amebic (intestinal amebiasis), 512,
      514, 515, 1172, 1174, 1366
   postdysenteric, 1367
   severe (dysentery), 1366, 1367t. *See*
      also Dysentery

antibiotic-associated, 511, **573–575**,
   1172
   C difficile causing, 511, 573, 574,
      1170t, 1172
collagenous, 587
Crohn, 578
ischemic, 421–422
   GI bleeding and, 521
lymphocytic, 587
microscopic, **587**
postdysenteric, 1367
pseudomembranous, 574. *See also*
   Colitis, antibiotic-associated
ulcerative. *See* Ulcerative colitis
Collagen
   in nephrogenic systemic fibrosis, 849
   type I, mutations in gene for in osteo-
      genesis imperfecta, 1039
Collagenomas, in multiple endocrine
   neoplasia, 1076, 1076t
Collagenous colitis, 587
Collateral ligaments, of knee, assessment
   of, 34–35
Colloids, for fluid management/volume
   replacement
   in burn injuries, 1410
   in shock, 436
Colography, CT (virtual colonoscopy).
   See Colonoscopy, virtual
Colon
   anaerobic flora of, 1322
   biopsy of, in diarrhea, 516
   cancer of, 1468t, 1476–1483. *See also*
      Colorectal cancer
      adjuvant therapy for, 1479
      GI bleeding and, 521, 1478
   carcinoid tumors of, 1475
   dilation of. *See also* Megacolon
      in acute colonic pseudo-obstruc-
         tion (Ogilvie syndrome),
         565
   disorders of, **569–593**. *See also specific*
      disorder
      amebic ulcers, 1366. *See also* Coli-
         tis, amebic
      constipation and. *See* Constipation
   diverticular, **587–589**. *See also*
      Diverticulosis
   fecal impaction and, 510
   GI bleeding and, 520–521
   polyps of, **589–593**
Colon cutoff sign, in pancreatitis, 643
Colon transit time, 507, 508
Colonic inertia (slow colonic transit),
   constipation and, 507, 508,
   508t
Colonic pseudo-obstruction
   acute (Ogilvie syndrome), **565–566**
   chronic, 566
Colonography, CT (virtual colonoscopy).
   See Colonoscopy, virtual
Colonoscopy
   in amebiasis, 1366
   for colon decompression in acute
      colonic pseudo-obstruc-
      tion (Ogilvie syndrome),
      565–566

in colorectal cancer screening/evalua-
   tion, 16, 17t, 59, 1478,
   1480, 1482
in Crohn disease, 578
in diarrhea, 516
in diverticular disease, 587, 588
in GI bleeding
   diagnostic, 521
   obscure bleeding and, 523
   occult bleeding and, 523
   therapeutic, 522
in HNPCC, 592
hyponatremia after, 790
in irritable bowel syndrome, 571
in ischemic colitis, 421
in polyp identification/removal, 589,
   590, 1482
surveillance, 1480
in ulcerative colitis, 583, 586
virtual
   in colorectal cancer screening/eval-
      uation, 16, 1478, 1482
   in polyp identification, 590
Color flow Doppler ultrasound. *See* Echocardiography; Ultrasonog-
   raphy
Color perception, loss of, in optic neuritis,
   168
Colorado tick fever, 1257–1259, **1267**
Colorectal cancer, **1476–1483**, 1480t
   adjuvant therapy for, 1479–1480
   aspirin/NSAIDs in prevention of,
      1477
   calcium supplements in prevention of,
      1477
   chemoprevention and, 1477
   chemotherapy for, 1479–1480
   Crohn disease and, 579, 1477
   diet and, 1477
   familial adenomatous polyposis and,
      591, 1477
   family history affecting risk of, 591,
      1477
   genetic mutations associated with,
      591, 1476–1477, 1477
   fecal DNA assay in identification
      of, 589–590, 1481
   GI bleeding and, 521, 1478
   hamartomatous polyposis syndromes
      and, **591–592**
   hereditary, **591–593**, 1477
   hereditary nonpolyposis (HNPCC),
      592–593, 1477
      endometrial carcinoma and, 592,
         593, 684
      pancreatic/periampullary carci-
         noma and, 1463
   incidence/risk/mortality of, 1450,
      1476, 1477, 1480
   inflammatory bowel disease and, 1477
   nonfamilial adenomatous polyps and,
      589
   pancreatic/periampullary carcinoma
      and, 1463
   polyps/polyposis and, 589, 590, 591,
      1476, 1477
   primary sclerosing cholangitis and,
      641

screening for, 16, 17*t*, 1480–1482, 1480*t*
staging of, 1478
ulcerative colitis and, 586, 641, 1477
Colorectal surgery, 1478–1479
adjuvant therapy and, 1479–1480
antibiotic prophylaxis for, 59, 60*t*
follow-up after, 1480
Colostomy
after colorectal surgery, 1478
diverting, for colorectal cancer, 1479
Colostrum, 709
Colpocleisis, for pelvic organ prolapse, 687
Colposcopy, 675*t*
in CIN, 681
CoLYTE. *See* Polyethylene glycol
Coma, **915–918**
assessment/emergency management of, 915–916, 1421
diabetic/hyperglycemic, 1083, 1111, **1111–1117**, 1112*t*. *See also specific cause*
diabetic ketoacidosis and, 1112, 1112*t*, 1113
hyperglycemic hyperosmolar state and, 1112*t*, 1115–1116
lactic acidosis and, 1111, 1112*t*
hypoglycemic, 1111, 1112*t*
in poisoning/drug overdose, 1112*t*, 1421
hypothermia and, 915, 917, 1421
metabolic disturbances causing, **917.** *See also* Metabolic encephalopathy
myxedema, 1005, 1006
in poisoning/drug overdose, 1112*t*, **1420–1421**
reversible, brain death differentiated from, 917
in stroke, 891
diabetes and, 1112*t*
structural lesions causing, **916–917**
in subarachnoid hemorrhage, 893
Coma vigil (persistent vegetative state), **917**
Combigan. *See* Brimonidine/timolol
Combination antiretroviral therapy, 1225, 1227, 1231–1233, 1232*f*
Combined pituitary hormone deficiency (CPHD), 992
CombiPatch. *See* Estradiol transdermal systems
Combivir. *See* Zidovudine (AZT), with lamivudine
Comedo extraction, for acne, 121
Comedones, in acne, 120, 121
Commissurotomy
mitral, 306, 307
for pulmonary stenosis, 296
Common ALL antigen, 465
Common cold. *See* Cold (common cold/viral rhinitis)
Common duct stones. *See* Choledocholithiasis
Common peroneal nerve palsy, **928**
Common variable immunodeficiency, **786–787**

Commotio cordis, 386
Communicating artery, anterior, occlusion of in stroke, 889
Community-acquired pneumonia, **243–248**, 1181*t*. *See also* Pneumonia
in HIV infection/AIDS, 1210
Community-associated methicillin-resistant *S aureus* (CA-MRSA), 118, 130, 1294
Compartment syndrome, abdominal, in burn patient, 1410
Compatibility testing, for transfusion, 477
Complement. *See also specific component*
in autoimmune hemolytic anemia, 452
in cold agglutinin disease, 453–454
in familial Mediterranean fever, 528
in gonococcal arthritis, 778
in paroxysmal nocturnal hemoglobinuria, 449
in postinfectious glomerulonephritis, 834
reference values for, 1548*t*
in SLE, 110, 753, 754*t*
in urticaria, 126
Complement fixation tests, in coccidioidomycosis, 1393
Complementary/alternative medicine, **1520–1543**. *See also specific type of therapy*
acupuncture, **1532–1534**
dietary supplements, **1527–1532**, 1528*t*
herbal medicines, **1521–1527**, 1522*t*, 1523*t*
mind-body medicine, **1534–1543**, 1536*f*
Complete abortion, 712
Complete (third-degree) heart block, 355
in atrial septal defect, 298
in myocardial infarction, 337
Complex 15, 99*t*
Complex partial seizures, 879, 879*t*. *See also* Seizures
schizophrenia differentiated from, 954
Complex partial status epilepticus, 884
Complex regional pain syndrome (reflex sympathetic dystrophy), **743**
Compliance. *See* Adherence/nonadherence
Compound nevi, 99
Compression chambers/centers. *See* Hyperbaric oxygen therapy; Recompression
Compression fractures. *See* Vertebral/compression fracture
Compression neuropathy. *See* Entrapment/compression neuropathy; Neuropathies
Compression sclerotherapy, for varicose veins, 428–429
Compression stockings
for lymphedema, 433
for varicose veins, 428
for venous insufficiency/leg ulcers, 38, 143, 430, 431

for venous thromboembolic disease, 501
Compromised host. *See* Immunocompromised host
Compulsions, 940. *See also* Obsessivecompulsive disorder
Compulsive water drinking. *See* Psychogenic polydipsia
Computed tomography (CT scans). *See also specific disorder and* Neuroimaging
in angina, 320
in aortic dissection, 426
in aortoiliac occlusive disease, 415
in appendicitis, 567, 568
in carotid occlusive disease, 420
in colorectal cancer evaluation/screening, 1478, 1482
in headache, 45
in hemoptysis, 27–28
in liver disease/jaundice, 600–601
in lung cancer screening, 18, 259, 1456
in lung cancer staging, 1455
in pancreatic/periampullary carcinoma, 1464
in pancreatitis, 643, 643*t*
in pheochromocytoma/paraganglioma, 1059–1060
in pulmonary embolism, 30, 269, 270, 271*f*
in renal artery stenosis, 833
in renal cell carcinoma, 1491
in solitary pulmonary nodule, 260
in thyroid cancer, 1024, 1028
in visceral artery insufficiency, 421
Computed tomography colography/colonography (virtual colonoscopy)
in colorectal cancer screening/evaluation, 16, 1478, 1482
in polyp identification, 590
Computerized stereotactic guided core needle breast biopsy, 659
COMT (catecholamine-*O*-methyltransferase) inhibitors, for parkinsonism, 907
Concentration meditation, 1540
Concussion, 918*t*
labyrinthine, vertigo caused by, 190, 191*t*
Condoms, **699**
for contraception, **699**
for genital wart prevention, 679
for gonorrhea prevention, 1319
for HIV infection/AIDS prevention, 4, 699, 1218–1219, 1220
for syphilis prevention, 1332
Conduction disturbances, **354–358**. *See also specific type*
in hyperkalemia, 798
intraventricular, **356**
in myocardial infarction, 337
in restrictive cardiomyopathy, 374
Conduction velocity studies
in motor neuron diseases, 921
in neuropathies, 922
Conductive hearing loss, 179, 180. *See also* Hearing loss
ossicular disruption causing, 179, 185

Conductive keratoplasty, 152
Condylomas (condylomata)
   acuminata (venereal/genital warts),
         131, 132, 678, 679
      anorectal involvement and, 595
      cervical/vaginal/vulvar, 678, 679
      HPV vaccination in prevention of,
            4, 132, 595, 1187–1198,
            1190–1191t, 1192–1193t,
            1194–1197t
      imiquimod for removal of, 132
      podophyllum resin for removal of,
            132, 679
   lata, 1334
      anorectal involvement and, 594
Conformal radiation therapy, three-
      dimensional, for prostate
      cancer, 1486
Confusion, 986. See also Cognitive disor-
            ders; Delirium
   ECT causing, 969
Congenital adrenal hyperplasia, 1048,
      1049, 1055
Congenital adrenal hypoplasia, 991, 992,
      1048, 1065
Congenital rubella syndrome, 1254, 1255
Congestive heart (cardiac) failure (CHF),
      358–367, 359f
   acute, 367–368
   angiotensin-converting enzyme
         (ACE) inhibitors for, 361
   angiotensin II receptor blockers for,
         362
   antiarrhythmic therapy in, 365
   anticoagulation therapy for, 365
   antihypertensive therapy and, 396t,
         405, 407
   in aortic regurgitation, 312
   in aortic stenosis, 310, 311
   asthma/wheezing caused by (cardiac
         asthma), 217
   in atrial septal defect, 297
   β-blocker therapy in, 362–363, 365,
         402
   biventricular pacing (resynchroniza-
         tion) for, 365–366
   calcium channel blockers for, 365
   cardiac transplantation for, 366
   cardiomyopathy and, 358, 370, 371
   in Chagas disease, 1350
   chemotherapy-induced, 1511
   chronic kidney disease, 360, 827t, 828
   cirrhosis and, 620
   classification of, 358, 359, 359f
   in coarctation of aorta, 296
   coenzyme Q₁₀ for, 1528t, 1530
   combination therapies in manage-
         ment of, 364
   coronary revascularization for, 366
   cough in, 23, 359
   in coxsackievirus myocarditis, 1279
   diet in management of, 366
   digitalis glycosides for, 363–364
   diuretic therapy for, 361
      chronic kidney disease and, 828
   drug management in, 361–365
   dyspnea in, 25, 25t, 26, 358–359
   edema in, 359, 360

exercise/activity in management of,
      366
   hypertension and, 358, 393, 396t, 405,
         407
   in hyperthyroidism, 360, 1009, 1014
   hyponatremia in, 790f, 791
   in hypothyroidism/myxedema, 360,
         1005
   implantable cardioverter defibrilla-
         tors for, 365
   in infectious myocarditis, 368, 369
   liver in, 359, 360, 631
   management of, 359f, 361–366
   myocardial infarction and, 330
   nonpharmacologic management of,
         365–366
   palliative care in, 366
   in patent ductus arteriosus, 301
   in pneumococcal pneumonia, 1292,
         1293
   positive inotropic agents for, 364–365
   in pregnancy/postpartum period
         (peripartum cardiomyopa-
         thy), 385, 724, 1000
   preoperative evaluation/management
         and, 51
   prognosis for, 366
   pulmonary edema in, 359, 367–368
   pulmonary hypertension and, 274,
         275, 360
   refeeding for protein-energy malnu-
         trition and, 1135
   reversible causes of, correction of, 361
   rheumatic fever and, 375
   in SLE, 753
   spironolactone for, 361, 362
   statin therapy in, 365
   surgical interventions in, 366
   theophyllines affected by, 225t
   thiamin deficiency and, 1141
   thiazolidinediones use and, 1094, 1101
   in tricuspid regurgitation, 314
   in tricuspid stenosis, 313
   vasodilator therapy for, 364
   in ventricular septal defect, 299
Congo-Crimean hemorrhagic fever,
      1262–1263
Conivaptan, for hyponatremia/SIADH,
      793
Conization of cervix, for CIN/cervical
      cancer, 681, 682, 683
Conjugated equine estrogens, 1070
Conjunctiva
   foreign body of, 71
   lacerations of, 172
Conjunctivitis, 153–155, 153t. See also
            Keratoconjunctivitis
   adenovirus, 154, 1275
   allergic, 155
   bacterial, 154
   chemical, 172
   chlamydial, 154
   coxsackievirus infection and, 1279
   dry eyes and, 154–155
   enterovirus 70 causing, 1280
   gonococcal, 154, 1319
   inclusion, 154
   viral, 154

Conn syndrome, 1056, 1057
Connective tissue disorders
   cardiac/pericardial involvement in,
         383
   cognitive disorders/delirium caused
         by, 985t
   interstitial (diffuse parenchymal) lung
         disease and, 262
   mixed/overlap syndrome, 762
Connexin-26 mutation, hearing loss and,
         187
Consciousness, inconsistent evidence of,
            in minimally conscious
            state, 917
Constipation, 87, 507–510, 508t, 509t
   alarm symptoms in, 508
   anogenital pruritus and, 136–137
   biofeedback in management of, 1536t,
         1538
   in chemotherapy-induced neuropa-
         thy, 1510
   in diabetic autonomic neuropathy,
         1107
   fecal impaction and, 510, 595
   in hypercalcemia, 801
   in irritable bowel syndrome, 570
   opioids causing, 84, 87
   overflow incontinence and, 510, 595
   palliation of, 87
   in terminally ill/dying patient, 87
   in typhoid fever, 1313
Constitutional epilepsy, 878
Constrictive bronchiolitis, 243. See also
            Bronchiolitis
Constrictive pericarditis, 379–380
   cirrhosis and, 620
   restrictive cardiomyopathy differenti-
         ated from, 374
Contact dermatitis
   allergic, 118–120, 784
      impetigo differentiated from, 118,
            119
      topical medications causing, 95,
            119
      urticarial lesions in, 126
   irritant, 119
Contact lenses, 151
   cleaning solutions for, toxic and
            hypersensitivity reactions
            to, 151
   corneal infections/ulcers/acan-
            thamoeba keratitis and,
            151, 156, 157, 1368
Contact photosensitivity, 142
Contact ulcers, of arytenoid cartilage, 209
Contagious pustular dermatitis (orf), 1277
Continuous ambulatory peritoneal dialy-
         sis, 831
Continuous cyclic peritoneal dialysis, 831
Continuous positive airway pressure
            (CPAP)
   nasal, for sleep apnea, 289
   for near drowning, 1416
   prevention of postoperative pulmo-
            nary complications and, 54
Continuous renal replacement therapy,
            for poisoning/drug over-
            dose, 1425–1426

Continuous subcutaneous insulin infusion (CSII), 1099, 1102. *See also* Insulin infusion pumps
Contraception, 694–701. *See also specific method*
  antibiotic use affecting efficacy of, 121
  emergency/postcoital, **700**
  IUD for, 698, 700
  fertility awareness and, **699–700**
  after gestational trophoblastic disease, 715
  sterilization for, **701**
Contraceptive foam/cream/film/sponge/jelly/suppository, **699**
Contraceptive injections/implants, **697**
Contraceptive-related hypertension, 392, 696–697
Contraceptive transdermal patch, 697–698
Contraceptive vaginal ring, 698
Contraction alkalosis, 813
Contrast media
  iodinated, for Graves disease/hyperthyroidism, 1011–1012
  reactions to, 786
    nephrotoxicity/acute kidney injury and, 822
Contrast nephropathy, 822
Contrast venography, in deep venous thrombosis/pulmonary embolism, 269–270
Controlled mechanical ventilation (CMV), for respiratory failure, 290
Contusions
  cerebral, 918t
  of eye, **171**
  myocardial, 384
Conversion disorder (hysterical conversion), 944
  pseudoseizures and, 881, 944
Convulsions. *See* Seizures
Cooling
  for heat exposure syndromes, 1407, 1408
  for hyperthermia in poisoning/drug overdose, 1423
Coombs test/micro-Coombs test
  in autoimmune hemolytic anemia, 453
  in cold agglutinin disease, 454
COP. *See* Cryptogenic organizing pneumonitis
COPD. *See* Chronic obstructive pulmonary disease
Copepods
  in dracunculiasis, 1382
  in gnathostomiasis, 1384
  in sparganosis, 1379
Copper
  accumulation of in Wilson disease, 628–629
  parenteral nutritional support and, 1149, 1151t
Copper TCu380A intrauterine device, 698
  for emergency/postcoital contraception, 698, 700

Copper-zinc superoxide dismutase gene mutation, in amyotrophic lateral sclerosis, 921
Coprine (*Coprinus*) mushroom poisoning, 1441, 1441t, 1442
Coprolalia, in Tourette syndrome, 911
Coproporphyrins, in porphyria cutanea tarda, 117
Cor pulmonale, **381–382**
  in COPD, 238, 382
  in pulmonary hypertension, 275, 382
  theophyllines affected by, 225t
Coral snake envenomation, 1446–1447
Cord blood, stem cells in, for transplantation, 475
Cord cavitation (syringomyelia), **920**
Corditis, polypoid, 209
Cordran. *See* Flurandrenolide
Core-binding factor leukemias, 465
Core needle (large-needle) biopsy, for breast lump evaluation, 658. *See also* Breast, biopsy of
  stereotactic guided, 659
Core rewarming, for systemic hypothermia, 1404
Core temperature
  in burn injury, maintaining, 1411
  in heat exhaustion, 1407
  in heat stroke, 1407, 1408
  in hypothermia, 1403, 1416
  in near drowning, 1416
Coreg. *See* Carvedilol
Corgard. *See* Nadolol
Corlopam. *See* Fenoldopam
Cornea
  exposure of, in dysthyroid eye disease, 170, 1009
  foreign body of, **171**
  infection of. *See* Keratitis; Keratoconjunctivitis
  trauma to, 153t
    abrasions, **171**
    lacerations, 172
  ulcers of, **156–157**. *See also* Keratitis
    contact lens wear and, 151
  ultraviolet burns of (ultraviolet keratitis), **172**
Corneal transplantation, rabies transmission and, 1255
Corns, of feet or toes, **133**
Coronary angioplasty. *See* Percutaneous transluminal coronary angioplasty
Coronary arteries
  disorders of. *See also* Coronary heart disease
    in Kawasaki syndrome, 383, 1288
    in pregnancy, **385**
    sudden death of athlete and, 386
    in tetralogy of Fallot, 300
    traumatic injury to, 384
Coronary artery aneurysm, in Kawasaki syndrome, 383, 1288
Coronary artery bypass grafting (CABG), 322–323, 323
  platelet function affected by, 490t
  prophylactic/preoperative, 51

Coronary artery disease (CAD). *See* Coronary heart disease
Coronary artery revascularization procedures. *See* Revascularization procedures
Coronary heart disease, **316–340**. *See also* Acute coronary syndromes; Angina; Myocardial infarction
  acute coronary syndromes without ST segment elevation and, **325–330**, 327t, 329t
  acute myocardial infarction with ST segment elevation and, **330–340**, 331t, 333t. *See also* Myocardial infarction
  angina pectoris (chronic stable) and, **317–325**
  antihypertensive drug therapy and, 396t, 407
  aortic stenosis and, 310
  biofeedback in management of, 1537
  cholesterol/lipoproteins in, 316, 1123–1124, **1124**
    screening tests for levels of, 1126–1129, 1127–1128t, 1129t
  in diabetes mellitus, 1108
  heart failure and, 360–361, 366
  in HIV infection/AIDS, 1216
  homocysteine/hyperhomocysteinemia in, 1516, 1517
  hypertriglyceridemia and, 9, 1124, 1133
  metabolic syndrome (syndrome X) and, 14, 317, 318, 325
  myocardial hibernation/stunning and, 317
  in pregnancy, **385**
  preoperative evaluation/management and, 50–51, 51t
  prevention of, 6–12
    aspirin in, 12, 1130
    exercise/activity in, 13
    hypertension control and, 9–12
    lipid disorder prevention/management and, 9, 1124–1125, 1126, 1128, 1129. *See also* Lipid-lowering therapy
    omega-3 fatty acids in, 1528t, 1530–1531
    smoking/smoking cessation and, 6–9, 8t, 9t, 10t, 11t, 316
  revascularization procedures for, 322–323. *See also* Revascularization procedures
  risk factors for, 316–317
    lipoproteins/lipid fractions and, 1123, 1124
    modification/risk reduction and, 1124–1125, 1126, 1128, 1129
  sudden death and, 330, 353
    in athletes, 386
  vasospasm and, 317, **325**
Coronary reperfusion. *See* Reperfusion therapy
Coronary sinus atrial septal defect, 297

Coronary stents, 322, 323. *See also* Percu-
taneous coronary inter-
vention
Coronary vasospasm, 317, **325**
Coronaviruses
diarrhea caused by, 1172
SARS caused by, 1274
Corpus luteum cyst, 728
Corrigan pulse, 312
Corrosive agents. *See* Caustic/corrosive
agents
Corti, organ of, hearing loss caused by
disorders of, 179
Cortical-basal ganglionic degeneration,
parkinsonism and, 906
Cortical blindness, occipital lobe lesions
causing, 899
Corticospinal lesions, coma or stupor
caused by, 916
Corticosteroids. *See also specific agent and
disease*
acne/folliculitis caused by, 120
for ACTH deficiency, 994
adverse effects of, 576, 1078
ophthalmic, 94, **172**, 177*t*
for allergic conjunctivitis/keratocon-
junctivitis, 155
for allergic rhinitis, 196–197
for alopecia, 146
amebiasis in patients taking, 1366
for asthma, 222*f*, 223, 224*t*, 226–227*t*,
228–230, 229–230*t*
exacerbation management and,
230, 231*f*, 232*f*, 233
inhaled, 222*f*, 223, 226–227*t*
systemic, 222*f*, 223, 224*t*, 228–230,
229–230*t*, 231*f*, 232*f*, 233
for atopic dermatitis, 102, 102–103
for back pain, 740
for Bell palsy, 929
for bronchiolitis, 243
in cancer chemotherapy, 1506*t*
for cancer-related hypercalcemia,
1497
for chronic inflammatory polyneuropathy, 926
clinical use of, **1077–1078**, 1077*t*,
1078*t*
for contact dermatitis, 119
for COPD, 237
Cushing syndrome caused by, 1050
for cysticercosis, 1378
for eosinophilic pneumonia, 266
in erythema multiforme, 128
for exfoliative dermatitis/erythro-
derma, 112
for fetal lung maturity, 717, 719
for giant cell arteritis, 165, 168, 767
for gout, 733, 735
for gram-negative bacteremia/sepsis,
1312
in HIV infection/AIDS, 1223
for hypopituitarism, 994
for immune thrombocytopenic
thrombocytopenia, 483,
484*f*
for inflammatory bowel disease,
575–576

Crohn disease, 580–581
ulcerative colitis, 584, 585
intra-articular, for osteoarthritis, 731
for lichen planus, 135
lipid abnormalities associated with
use of, 1126*t*
for lupus, 111, 754
management of patient receiving, 1078*t*
for multiple sclerosis, 913
for myasthenia gravis, 933
for nausea and vomiting, 87, 506, 506*t*
for ophthalmic disorders, 155,
174–175*t*
precautions for use of, **172**
osteoporosis/osteoporosis prevention
and, 576, 1040, 1041, 1078
in pain management, 86
for pemphigus, 131
perioperative, **58**
for polyarteritis nodosa, 765
for polymyositis/dermatomyositis,
761
for prostate cancer, 1487*t*
for psoriasis/psoriatic arthritis, 104,
775
relative potencies of, 1077, 1077*t*
for rheumatic fever/heart disease, 376
for rheumatoid arthritis, 749–750
rosacea exacerbated by, 99, 122
for shock, 437
for skin disorders, 94, 96–97*t*
for spinal cord compression, 1495
for spinal trauma, 919
strongyloidiasis in patients taking, 1381
surgery in patients taking, perioperative replacement and, **58**
topical, 94, 96–97*t*
ophthalmic, 174–175*t*
CORTICUS trial, in shock management,
437
Cortinarius orellanus mushroom poisoning, 1441, 1441*t*, 1442
Cortisol, 1077. *See also* Corticosteroids
excess of, **1050–1053**. *See also* Cushing
syndrome
familial resistance to, 1052
insufficiency of, 992, 994. *See also*
Adrenocortical insuffi-
ciency
acute, 1046–1047
chronic, 1047–1050. *See also* Addison disease
salivary, in Cushing syndrome, 1051
serum levels of
in ACTH deficiency, 992, 994
in acute adrenal insufficiency, 1047
in Addison disease, 1049
in Cushing syndrome, 1051
reference values for, 1548*t*
urine free
in Cushing syndrome, 1051
reference values for, 1549*t*
Cortisol withdrawal syndrome, 1053
Cortisone, 1077
Corynebacterium
diphtheriae, 1177*t*, 1302. *See also*
Diphtheria
jeikeium, 1177*t*

Cosmegen. *See* Dactinomycin
Cosopt. *See* Dorzolamide/timolol
Cosyntropin test
in adrenal insufficiency/Addison disease, 992, 1047, 1049
adrenal vein sampling in, in aldosteronism, 1057
in hirsutism/virilization, 1054
Cotton dust, byssinosis caused by inhalation of, 280
Cotton wool spots
in HIV infection/AIDS, 167
in retinal artery occlusion, 164
in retinal vein occlusion, 163
in SLE, 753
Cough, **22–24**, 23*f*, 23*t*
in anaerobic pneumonia/lung abscess,
250
angiotensin-converting enzyme
(ACE) inhibitors causing,
405
in asthma, 22, 23*t*
in *Bordetella pertussis* infection
(whooping cough), 22, 23,
24, 1308
in bronchiectasis, 22, 240
in COPD, 22, 23, 234
drugs causing, 281*t*
dyspnea and, 22, 23, 25
in GERD, 22, 23, 23*t*, 531
headache associated with, 872, **875**
in heart failure, 23, 359
in lung cancer, 22, 1454
postnasal drip causing, 22, 23*t*
in pulmonary embolism, 268*t*
in tuberculosis, 252
Counseling, health maintenance recom-
mendations/guidelines for,
3*t*
Counterpulsation, extracorporeal, for
angina, 324
Courvoisier law/sign, 598, 1462, 1464
Covera. *See* Verapamil
Cowden syndrome/disease, 592, 1023,
1077
COX-1/COX-2, aspirin/NSAIDs affecting,
78, 548
peptic ulcer disease and, 548, 552
COX-2 inhibitors (coxibs), 78, 749
cardiovascular complications associated with, 78, 548,
552–553
for familial adenomatous polyposis,
591
for gout, 733
lithium interactions and, 972*t*
in pain management, 78
peptic ulcers/peptic ulcer prevention
and, 548, 552, 552–553
recommendations for use of, 552–553
for rheumatoid arthritis, 749
"Coxibs." *See* COX-2 inhibitors
Coxiella burnetii, 1281*t*, 1286, 1287
Coxsackievirus infections, **1278–1279**
herpetic stomatitis differentiated
from, 203
myocarditis, 368, 1279
pericarditis, 376, 1279

Cozaar. *See* Losartan
CPAP. *See* Continuous positive airway
    pressure
CPHD. *See* Combined pituitary hormone
    deficiency
CPPD. *See* Calcium pyrophosphate dihy-
    drate deposition disease
CPR. *See* Cardiopulmonary resuscitation
CPRV. *See* Chromatographically purified
    rabies vaccine
Cr. *See* Creatinine
"Crab yaws," 1339
Crabs (pubic lice), 138
Crack cocaine. *See* Cocaine abuse
Crackles (rales)
    in heart failure, 360
    in interstitial (diffuse parenchymal)
        lung disease, 262
    in pulmonary embolism, 268t
CRAG (cryptococcal antigen) test, 1212,
    1396
Cramps. *See* Dysmenorrhea; Muscle
    cramps
Cranial arteritis. *See* Giant cell (temporal/
    cranial) arteritis
Cranial nerve VIII (acoustic nerve)
    lesions. *See* Schwannoma,
    vestibular
Cranial nerve palsies. *See also specific type*
    brainstem lesions causing, 899
    in diabetes, 1106
    in head injury, 918
    in malignant external otitis, 181
    in Paget disease of bone, 1045
    in sarcoidosis, 924
    stroke causing, 891
Craniopharyngioma, 898t, 993
Creatine kinase
    in acute coronary syndromes, 326
    in electrical burns, 1413
    in polymyositis/dermatomyositis, 760
    reference values for, 1549t
    in rhabdomyolysis, 763, 822
        hypophosphatemia and, 803
        after seizure, 881
Creatine kinase-MB (CK-MB)
    in infectious myocarditis, 369
    in myocardial infarction, 331
    in non-ST elevation acute coronary
        syndromes, 326
    reference values for, 1549t
Creatinine, 817
    ascitic fluid, 525
    serum levels of
        in acute kidney injury, 819
        in chronic kidney disease, 826–827,
            827f
        conditions affecting, 818, 818t
        in hepatorenal syndrome, 622
        reference values for, 1549t
    urinary
        in pheochromocytoma, 1059
        ratio of to urinary protein, 817. *See
            also* Proteinuria
Creatinine:blood urea nitrogen ratio, 818,
    820, 820t
Creatinine clearance, 817–818
    aminoglycoside dosing and, 1179t

GFR measurement and, 817–818, 818t
in hepatorenal syndrome, 622
reference values for, 1549t
Creeping eruption, **1385**
CREST syndrome, 758. *See also* Sclero-
    derma
    autoantibodies in, 754t, 758
Crestor. *See* Rosuvastatin
Cretinism, 1029. *See also* Hypothyroidism
Creutzfeldt-Jakob disease, 986, 1260–1261
    myoclonus in, 910
    parkinsonism and, 906
Cricothyrotomy, **211–212**
Crigler-Najjar syndrome, 598
Crimean-Congo hemorrhagic fever,
    1262–1263
Critical illness
    fever/hospital-associated infection
        and, 1159, 1160, 1161
    hypercalcemia and, 1036
    neuropathy associated with, **924–925**
    psychosis associated with, 988
    stress gastritis associated with,
        544–545
    thyroid tests affected in, 1002
Crixivan. *See* Indinavir
CroFab, for snake bites, 1447
Crohn disease, 575, **577–582**. *See also*
    Inflammatory bowel dis-
    ease
    arthritis in, 578, 776–777
    cholelithiasis/gallstones and, 578, 634
    colorectal cancer and, 579, 1477
    drug therapy for, 580–582
    primary sclerosing cholangitis and,
        640
    small intestinal carcinoma and, 579,
        1474
    social support and, 577
Crolom. *See* Cromolyn
Cromolyn
    for asthma, 223, 224t
    for ophthalmic disorders, 155, 174t
Cross-dressing, 948
Cross-reactivity, in drug allergies, 1181
Cross-resistance, in antiretroviral therapy,
    1230, 1232
Crossed straight leg sign, 738
Crotalid antivenin (CroFab), 1447
CRP. *See* C-reactive protein
CRT. *See* Conformal radiation therapy
Cruciate ligaments, of knee, assessment
    of, 34–35
Crush injuries
    fasciotomy in, 1411
    rhabdomyolysis/renal failure and, 763
Crusted/weeping skin lesions, 95t,
    118–120. *See also specific
    type*
    drying agents for, 94
Cryoglobulins/cryoglobulinemia,
    770–771
    glomerulonephritis and, 771, 835f,
        838
    in hepatitis C, 604, 611, 770, 771, 844
    neuropathies and, 771, 924
    Raynaud phenomenon and, 757
    reference values for, 1549t

Cryoplasty, for femoral/popliteal occlu-
    sive disease, 417
Cryoprecipitate, 479
    for DIC, 488, 488t
Cryotherapy/cryosurgery. *See also* Liquid
    nitrogen
    for CIN/cervical cancer, 681, 683
    for condylomata acuminata, 679
    for fibroadenoma of breast, 650
    for prostate cancer, 1487
    for retinal detachment, 162
    for wart removal, 132
Cryptococcal antigen (CRAG) test, 1212,
    1396
Cryptococcomas, 1396
Cryptococcus gattii/neoformans (crypto-
    coccosis), **1396–1397**
    in HIV infection/AIDS, 901, 1212,
        1224t, 1396, 1397
    prophylaxis of, 1222–1223, 1397
    meningitis caused by, 901, 1212,
        1224t, 1396, 1397
Cryptogenic fibrosing alveolitis (idio-
    pathic fibrosing interstitial
    pneumonia), **263–265**,
    264t
Cryptogenic organizing pneumonitis
    (COP/idiopathic bronchi-
    olitis obliterans with orga-
    nizing pneumonia/
    BOOP), 243, 264t
Cryptogenic stroke. *See* Stroke
Cryptorchism, **1066**
    pseudohermaphroditism and, 1068
    testicular cancer and, 1066, 1493
Cryptosporidium hominis/parvum
    (cryptosporidiosis), 511,
    1172, 1214, **1369–1371**
Crystal deposition arthritis, **732–736**
Crystalloids, for fluid management/vol-
    ume replacement
    in burn injuries, 1410
    hypotension in poisoning/drug over-
        dose and, 1421
    in shock, 436
CSF-VDRL test, 1337
    in HIV infection/AIDS, 1220
CSII. *See* Continuous subcutaneous insu-
    lin infusion
CT angiography. *See* Computed tomogra-
    phy; Helical (spiral) CT
CT scans. *See* Computed tomography
CTCL. *See* Cutaneous T cell lymphoma
Cubicin. *See* Daptomycin
Cubital tunnel, ulnar nerve lesions and,
    927
Cuirass (negative-pressure) ventilation,
    intermittent, for COPD,
    238
Culdocentesis
    in ectopic pregnancy, 714
    in PID, 688
Culex mosquitoes. *See* Mosquitoes
Cultural issues, in end-of-life care, **91**
Cultured grafts, for burn wound closure,
    1411
Cunninghamella infection, 1398–1399
Cup-disk ratio, in chronic glaucoma, 158

Cupping, optic disk, in chronic glaucoma, 158

Cupulolithiasis, vertigo associated with, 190

Curative efforts, withdrawal of, in terminally ill/dying patient, **91–92**, 92t

Curettage. See D&C; Endocervical curettage; Endometrial biopsy

Curettage and electrodesiccation
for basal cell carcinoma, 134
for squamous cell carcinoma, 134

Curvularia, phaeohyphomycosis caused by, 1402

Cushing disease, 1050. See also Cushing syndrome

Cushing syndrome (hypercortisolism), **1050–1053**
amenorrhea in, 1068, 1069
cancer-related, 1453t
corticosteroid-induced, 1050
hypertension and, 392, 1052, 1054
lipid abnormalities associated with, 1126t
obesity in, 1051, 1052, 1136

Cutaneous anthrax, 1300, 1301, 1301–1302, 1302

Cutaneous candidiasis, 125

Cutaneous drug reactions, **147–150**, 148–149t

Cutaneous larva migrans, **1385**

Cutaneous leishmaniasis, 1351–1352, 1352, 1353
post-kala azar, 1351

Cutaneous lupus erythematosus, chronic, **110–111**

Cutaneous T cell lymphoma (mycosis fungoides), **111–112**
exfoliative dermatitis/erythroderma and, 112

Cutaneous tests. See specific type and Skin tests

c-v wave
in pulmonary stenosis, 295
in tetralogy of Fallot, 300

CVP. See Central venous pressure

CXCR4, in HIV infection/AIDS, 1208

Cyanide antidotes, 1424t, 1435, 1435t

Cyanide poisoning, 1424t, **1435**
dyspnea in, 26
smoke inhalation and, 277

Cyanocobalamin. See Vitamin B₁₂

Cyanokit, 1435, 1435t

Cyanosis
digital, in Raynaud phenomenon, 756
in hypothermia, 1405
in pulmonary embolism, 268t

Cyberknife radiosurgery, for pituitary adenoma, 994, 999, 1002, 1052

Cyclic citrullinated peptide (CCP) antibody, in rheumatoid arthritis, 748

Cyclic thrombocytopenia, **482**

Cyclin D1, in mantle cell lymphoma, 467

Cycling, in bipolar disease, 962
lithium use and, 970

Cyclocort. See Amcinonide

Cyclooxygenase-1 and 2 (COX-1/COX-2), aspirin/NSAIDs affecting, 78, 548
peptic ulcer disease and, 548, 552

Cyclooxygenase-2 (COX-2) inhibitors. See COX-2 inhibitors

Cyclophosphamide, 1500t. See also CMF regimen; Immunosuppressive therapy
for aplastic anemia, 455
for breast cancer, 665, 666
for chronic lymphocytic leukemia, 467
hemorrhagic cystitis caused by, 1510
mesna for amelioration of, 1507t, 1510
for microscopic polyangiitis, 770
for Wegener granulomatosis, 769

Cycloserine (DCS), for phobic disorder, 943

Cyclospora cayetanensis (cyclosporiasis), 511, 515, 1172, **1369–1371**

Cyclosporine, 1544t
adverse ophthalmic effects of, 177t
for aplastic anemia, 455
hyperkalemia caused by, 798
nefazodone interaction and, 966
nephrotoxicity/acute kidney injury/graft rejection caused by, 822
for ophthalmic disorders, 155, 175t
for psoriasis, 105
St. John's wort interaction and, 1523
for ulcerative colitis, 585

Cyclothymic disorders, 962

Cycrin. See Progesterone

Cymbalta. See Duloxetine

CYP17 deficiency, 1049

Cyproheptadine
for drug-induced anorgasmia, 965
for migraine prophylaxis, 874t
for serotonin syndrome, 1423, 1440, 1449
for urticaria, 126

Cyproterone, for hirsutism/virilization, 1055

Cystadenocarcinoma, of liver, 633

Cystadenoma
of liver, 633
pancreatic, 1464, 1465

Cystathionine β-synthase deficiency, in homocystinuria, 1516, 1517

Cystectomy, for bladder cancer, 1490

Cysteine, supplementary, for homocystinuria, 1517

Cystic fibrosis, **241–242**
bronchiectasis and, 240, 241, 242
COPD differentiated from, 235
genetic/prenatal testing for, 242, 706

Cystic fibrosis transmembrane conductance regulator (CFTR) protein, 241
genetic/prenatal testing for mutations of, 242
in pancreatitis, 642, 646

Cystic hydatid disease, 1378–1379

Cysticercosis, 1376, **1377–1378**

Cystine urinary stones, 857, 860

Cystinuria, 857

Cystitis, 46, 47f, **851–852**, 852t, 1182t
in epididymitis, 856
in female, 46, 47f, 851
hemorrhagic. See Hemorrhagic cystitis
interstitial, **861–862**

Cystocele, 687

Cystoscopy, 850
in benign prostatic hyperplasia, 867
in bladder cancer, 1489
in interstitial cystitis, 861

Cystourethroscopy, in bladder cancer, 1489

Cytadren. See Aminoglutethimide

Cytarabine, 1501t

Cytarabine liposome, 1501t

Cytochrome P450. See P450 system

Cytokeratin 8 gene, cirrhosis and, 620

Cytokines
in ARDS, 291
in fever, 38
for fungal infection, 1402

Cytolytic snake venom, 1446

Cytomegalovirus immune globulin, 1246, 1246–1247

Cytomegalovirus inclusion disease, 1245

Cytomegalovirus infections, **1245–1247**
esophageal, 535, 1245
gastritis/diarrhea, 513, 547, 1245
in immunocompetent host, 1245, 1246
in immunocompromised host/HIV infection/AIDS, 1224t, 1245, 1245–1246, 1246
prophylaxis of, 1222, 1246
mononucleosis, 1245, 1246
perinatal/congenital, 1245
posttransplant, 1157–1158, 1245, 1246
prevention of, 1157–1158, 1222, 1246
retinitis, 167–168, 1213, 1223, 1245, 1246

Cytomel. See also Triiodothyronine
RAI therapy for thyroid cancer and, 1026
TSH/T₄ levels affected by, 993

Cytopenia
methotrexate causing, 750
in myelodysplasia, 463

Cytosar-U. See Cytarabine

Cytotoxic drugs. See specific agent and Chemotherapy

Cytotoxic (antibody-mediated/type II) hypersensitivity, 784

Cytotoxicity assay, in antibiotic-associated diarrhea, 574

Cytovene. See Ganciclovir

Cytoxan. See Cyclophosphamide

d4T. See Stavudine

D antigen, in compatibility testing, 477

D&C, 675t
for abnormal premenopausal bleeding, 675
for postmenopausal bleeding, 676

D cells, pancreatic, 1062

D-cycloserine (DCS), for phobic disorder, 943
D-dimer fibrin
in deep venous thrombosis/pulmonary embolism, 30, 267, 270, 271f
in DIC, 487
reference values for, 1549t
D state sleep, 973
D-xylose absorption, in bacterial overgrowth, 516, 562
Dacarbazine, 1500t
Dacogen. See Decitabine
Dacryocystitis, 153
Dacryocystorhinostomy, 153
Dactinomycin, 1505t
for gestational trophoblastic disease, 715
Dairy intolerance. See Lactose (milk) intolerance
Dalfopristin/quinupristin. See Quinupristin/dalfopristin
"Dallas" criteria, in infectious myocarditis, 369
Dalmane. See Flurazepam
Dalrymple sign, 1009
Dalteparin, 496t, 497t
Danazol
for abnormal premenopausal bleeding, 675
for endometriosis, 686
Dandruff, 106
Dantrolene
for neuroleptic malignant syndrome/malignant hyperthermia, 959, 1160, 1423, 1445
for spasticity, 914
Dapsone
for actinomycetoma, 1400
for leprosy, 1327
for malaria, with chlorproguanil (Lapdap), 1359
methemoglobinemia caused by, 1440
for P jiroveci infection, 1157, 1222t, 1224t, 1395
prophylactic, 1157, 1222t, 1224t
for toxoplasma prophylaxis, 1222, 1365
Daptomycin, renal/hepatic failure and, 1184t
Darbepoetin alfa
for anemia of chronic kidney disease, 828
for chemotherapy-induced anemia, 1499, 1508t
Darier disease, vaccinia and, 116
Darifenacin, for urinary incontinence, 71
Darkfield microscopic examination
in leptospirosis, 1341
in syphilis, 1331
Darunavir, 1230, 1232f
with ritonavir, 1227t, 1230
Dasatinib, 1503t
for chronic myeloid leukemia, 462
DASH diet, in hypertension/hypertension prevention, 394, 395t
"Date-rape" drug (gamma-hydroxybutyrate/GHB), 1437
Cushing syndrome and, 1052

Datril. See Acetaminophen
Datura stramonium, overdose/toxicity of, 1432
Daunorubicin/daunomycin, 1502t
liposomal, 1502t, 1511
toxicity of, 1502t, 1511
Daunoxome. See Liposomal daunorubicin
Dawn phenomenon, 1102, 1103, 1103t
DAX-1 gene mutation, in congenital adrenal hypoplasia/hypogonadism/azoospermia, 991, 992, 1065
Daypro. See Oxaprozin
Daytime somnolence. See Somnolence
DBE. See Deep breathing exercises
DC cardioversion. See Cardioversion, electrical
DCC gene, in colorectal cancer, 1476–1477
DCCT (Diabetes Control and Complications Trial), 1087, 1110
DCIS. See Ductal carcinoma in situ
DCS. See D-cycloserine; Decompression sickness
DDAVP. See Desmopressin
ddC. See Zalcitabine
ddI. See Didanosine
DDT (chlorophenothane), poisoning caused by, 1443–1444
de Morsier syndrome (septo-optic dysplasia), 991
De Quervain (subacute) thyroiditis, 1008, 1010, 1016, 1017, 1018
hypothyroid phase in, 1003, 1017, 1018
"Deadly quartet." See Metabolic syndrome
Deafness. See Hearing loss
Death. See also End of life
Kübler-Ross' stages of, 92
patient expectations about, 88
preventable causes of, 2, 2t. See also Preventive care
sudden. See Sudden death
tasks after, 93
Decerebrate posturing, 916
Decision making, medical
advance directives and, 90
determination of older patient's capacity for, 64
Decitabine, 1501t
for myelodysplasia, 464
Decompression sickness, 1416–1417
barotrauma and, 183, 1417
Decompressive laminectomy
for cancer-related cord compression, 1495
for spinal trauma, 919
Decongestants
for bacterial rhinosinusitis, 193
overdose/toxicity of, 1434
ophthalmic effects and, 177t
for viral rhinitis (common cold), 192
Decontamination
eye, 1424
gastrointestinal, 1420, 1424–1426, 1425t
caustic/corrosive agent ingestion and, 1429, 1429–1430

skin, 1424
for caustic/corrosive burns, 1424, 1429, 1430
nerve agents in chemical warfare and, 1424
Decorticate posturing, 916
Decubitus ulcers (bed/pressure sores), 72–74, 73t
bed rest/immobility and, 68, 73
De-efferented state (locked-in syndrome), 917–918
Deep brain stimulation
for idiopathic torsion dystonia, 910
for parkinsonism, 908
Deep breathing exercises, prevention of postoperative pulmonary complications and, 54
Deep neck infections, 206
Deep sulcus sign, in pneumothorax, 286
Deep venous thrombosis, 36–37, 37t. See also Venous thromboembolic disease
in antiphospholipid antibody syndrome, 755
Baker cyst differentiated from, 744
cellulitis differentiated from, 129
detection of, 269–270
estrogen replacement therapy and, 1072
hypercoagulability and, 267
lower extremity edema and, 36–37, 37t
prevention of, 495–496, 496t
pulmonary embolism and, 267, 269, 270, 270t. See also Pulmonary venous thromboembolism
superior vena caval obstruction and, 431
treatment of, 496–501, 497t, 498t, 499t, 500t, 501t
venous insufficiency/stasis and, 36–37, 430
in Wegener granulomatosis, 768
Deer ticks. See Ticks
Defecation, dyssynergic (pelvic floor dyssynergia), 507–508, 508
biofeedback in management of, 1536t, 1538
Deferasirox, for transfusional hemosiderosis, 628
Deferoxamine
for hemochromatosis/iron toxicity, 628, 1437
for transfusional hemosiderosis, 444
Defibrillator cardioverter, implantable. See Implantable cardioverter defibrillator
Defibrotide, for sinusoidal obstruction syndrome, 630
Deflazacort, 1077, 1077t. See also Corticosteroids
Degenerative (calcific) aortic stenosis, 310
Degenerative joint disease/arthritis, 729–732. See also Osteoarthritis
Dehydration
blood urea nitrogen (BUN) affected in, 818

Dehydration (*cont.*)
calculating water deficit in, 794
in cholera, 1315
chronic kidney disease and, 827*t*
in diabetes insipidus, 996
in diabetic ketoacidosis, 1112, 1113
diarrhea and, 514, 1172
in heat exposure syndromes, 1047
hypernatremia and, 793
enteral nutritional support and, 1150
hyperosmolality and, in hyperglycemic hyperosmolar state, 1115
hyperosmolar nonketotic, parenteral nutritional support and, 1151*t*
management of. *See* Fluid management/hydration
saline-responsive metabolic alkalosis and, 812
vomiting and, 506
Dehydroemetine, for amebiasis, 1367, 1367*t*
Dehydroepiandrosterone/dehydroepiandrosterone sulfate (DHEA/DHEAS), 1528–1529, 1528*t*
for Addison disease, 1050
hirsutism/virilization and, 1054, 1529
for hypopituitarism and hypogonadism, 994, 1529
serum levels of, in Addison disease, 1049
for SLE, 754, 1528, 1528*t*
Dejerine-Sottas disease, 923
Delavirdine, 1227*t*, 1230–1231, 1232*f. See also* Antiretroviral therapy
Delayed (T-cell mediated/type IV) hypersensitivity, 784
Delayed puberty. *See* Puberty
Delirium, **67–68, 87,** 985–988
alcohol use/abuse and, 978, 985*t*
anticholinergic, 1439. *See also* Anticholinergic syndrome/effects
clinical findings in, 67, 986
dementia and, 63, 65, 67, 985*t*
in elderly, **67–68**
dementia and, 63, 65, 67
postoperative, 56, 56*t*
urinary incontinence and, 70
hospitalization/illness and, 988
lithium-induced, 971
palliation of, **87**
postoperative, 56, 56*t*
in terminally ill/dying patient, 87
treatment of, 67, 87, 987–988
Delirium tremens, 978
Delivery. *See* Labor and delivery
Delta agent (hepatitis D virus/HDV), 601, 603. *See also* Hepatitis D
ΔF508 mutation, in cystic fibrosis, 241
Delta sleep, 973
Delta wave, in preexcitation syndromes, 345
Delusional disorders/delusions, 952, 953
Demadex. *See* Torsemide
Demeclocycline, for hyponatremia, 793

Dementia, **63–66, 912,** 985–988. *See also* Alzheimer disease
assessment of/screening for, 64
behavioral problems and, 64, 65–66
caregiver issues and, 65
clinical findings in, 64, 986
cognitive impairment assessment/treatment and, 64, 65
cortical, 986
in Creutzfeldt-Jakob disease, 986, 1260
decision-making capacity and, 64
delirium and, 63, 65, 67, 985*t*
depression and (pseudodementia), 63, 986
in Down syndrome, 1514
in elderly, **63–66**
estrogen replacement therapy and, 704, 1072
frontotemporal, 64
ginkgo for, 1523*t*, 1524–1525
in HIV infection/AIDS, 986, 1212
in Huntington disease, 908, 986
hypertension and, 393
with Lewy bodies, 63, 64
motor findings and, 64
multi-infarct (vascular), 63, 986
in niacin deficiency, 1142
postoperative delirium and, 56
subcortical, 64
treatment of, 65–66, 987–988
Demerol. *See* Meperidine
Demyelinating neuropathies/polyneuropathies, 921–922. *See also* specific type and Neuropathies
chronic inflammatory, **926**
in HIV infection/AIDS, 924, 1212
optic neuritis and, 168, 169
paraproteinemias and, 923–924
Demyelination. *See also* Demyelinating neuropathies/polyneuropathies
in Guillain-Barré syndrome, 925
hypernatremia and, 793
hyponatremia complications/treatment and, 792
in multiple sclerosis, 912
in progressive multifocal leukoencephalopathy, 1261
Dengue, 1257–1259, **1263–1264**
Dengue shock syndrome, 1263, 1264
Denileukin diftitox, 1505*t*
Denosumab, for osteoporosis, 1041
Dental disorders
actinomycosis and, 1323
anaerobic pleuropulmonary infections and, 250, 1322
bacterial rhinosinusitis and, 193
bisphosphonate use and, 783, 1040
deep neck infections and, 206
earache and, 186
facial pain caused by, 878
in Sjögren syndrome, 762, 763
Dental procedures, endocarditis prophylaxis and, 1305, 1305*t*, 1306*t*
Dentatorubral-pallidoluysian atrophy, 909

Dentition, poor. *See* Dental disorders
Dentures, foreign body aspiration and, 212
Deoxyribonuclease, human (rhDNase), for cystic fibrosis, 242
Dependence (drug), 977. *See also* specific drug and Substance use disorders
in opioid therapy, 78
physiologic, 78, 84, 977
psychologic, 977
Dependent personality disorder, 951*t*
Depersonalization, 940
in schizophrenic/psychotic disorders, 953
Depigmentation disorders, 144. *See also* Hypopigmentation
DepoCyt. *See* Cytarabine liposome
Depression, **961–973**
adjustment disorder with, 961
alcohol dependency and, 962, 970, 978
with atypical features, 962, 964
bipolar disorder and, 962
chronic pain and, 946
complications of, 963
in cyclothymic disorders, 962
dementia and (pseudodementia), 63, 986
DHEA for, 1528, 1528*t*
differential diagnosis of, 962–963
dispensing medications and, 963, 964
drug-induced, 962
drug therapy for, 963–970, 965*f*, 968*t*, 969*t. See also* Antidepressants
dysthymia, 962
ECT for, 963–964, 967–969
in elderly, **66–67**
caregiver issues and, 62–63
screening for, 66
stimulants for, 964
urinary incontinence and, 70
experimental treatments for, 969
headache associated with, **873**
hospitalization/illness and, 962, 988, 989, 990
hypercortisolism in, 1052
illness causing, 962
lithium for, 970
major depressive disorder, 961–962, 964
OCD and, 940
oral contraceptive use and, 607
panic disorder and, 940
parkinsonism differentiated from, 905
perimenopausal, estrogen replacement therapy and, 1071–1072
personality disorder and, 950
phototherapy for, 969
with postpartum onset, 962
in premenstrual dysphoric disorder, 676–677, 962
reserpine causing, 407, 408*t*, 962
schizophrenic/psychotic disorders/ideation and, 953, 964, 966
screening for, 3*t*
in elderly, 66

with seasonal onset, 962, 964, 969
sleep disorders and, 974
somatization disorder and, 944
St. John's wort (Hypericum perforatum) for, 1522, 1523t
suicide and, 963
in terminally ill/dying patient, 92
treatment of, 963–970, 965f, 968t,
969t. See also Antidepressants
meditation in, 1536t, 1541
Dermabrasion, for acne scars, 122
Dermacentor ticks. See Ticks
Dermatitis
atopic. See Atopic dermatitis
cercarial, in schistosomiasis, 1374
contact
allergic, **118–120**, 784
impetigo differentiated from,
118, 119
topical medications causing, 95,
119
urticarial lesions in, 126
irritant, 119
contagious pustular (orf), 1277
drugs causing, **147–150**, 148–149t
exfoliative (exfoliative erythroderma), **112–113**
drugs causing, 112, 148t
psoriatic, 104, 105, 112. See also
Psoriasis
hand, vesiculobullous (pompholyx),
116–117
herpetiformis, **118**
celiac disease and, 118, 559
in HIV infection/AIDS, 1215
medicamentosa (drug eruption),
147–150, 148–149t
in niacin deficiency, 1142
seborrheic. See Seborrheic dermatitis
stasis, 37, 428. See also Venous insuffi-
ciency/stasis
leg ulcers and, 143
Dermatologic therapy, **94–99**, 96–99t
adverse ophthalmic effects of, 178t
Dermatomal herpes zoster, 114–115, 1241
Dermatomyositis, **759–762**
autoantibodies in, 754t, 760
cancer-related, 760, 761, 783, 902,
1453t
sine myositis, 760
Dermatop. See Prednicarbate
Dermatopathic lymphadenopathy, 111
Dermatophytosis, **108–109**. See also Tinea
furunculosis differentiated from, 141
in HIV infection/AIDS, 1215
nail changes in, 147
Dermopathy
in Graves disease (pretibial myxedema), 1008, 1009, 1015
nephrogenic fibrosing, 759
Dermoscopy, in melanoma evaluation,
101
DES. See Diethylstilbestrol
Des-gamma-carboxy prothrombin, in hepatocellular carcinoma, 1460
Desensitization techniques
for phobic disorder, 943

for psychiatric problems associated
with hospitalization/ill-
ness, 990
Desensitization therapy. See also Immunotherapy
for asthma, 228
for drug allergies, 1183–1186
to penicillin, 1180, 1183–1186
Desferrioxamine, adverse ophthalmic
effects of, 178t
Designer drugs, 984
Desipramine, 964, 966, 968t, 1544t. See
also Antidepressants
for neuropathic pain/painful diabetic
neuropathy, 85, 85t, 1107
Desmoid tumors, in familial adenomatous polyposis, 591
Desmopressin (DDAVP)
for bleeding in chronic kidney disease/
uremia, 519, 829
in diabetes insipidus diagnosis, 996
in diabetes insipidus treatment,
996–997
for enuresis, 976
for hemophilia, 491, 492t
for von Willebrand disease, 492t, 493
Desogestrel, in combination oral contraceptives, 695t
thromboembolism and, 696
Desonide, 96t
Desquamative interstitial pneumonia
(DIP), 243, 263, 264t
Desvenlafaxine, 966, 968t
Desynchronization sleep disorder, 973
Desyrel. See Trazodone
Detergent worker's lung, 280t
Detrusor muscle disorders, urinary
incontinence and, 70–71,
71, 72. See also Overflow
incontinence; Urge incon-
tinence
DeVega annuloplasty, 314
Devic syndrome (neuromyelitis optica),
914
optic neuritis in, 168, 914
Dexamethasone, 1077, 1077t. See also
Corticosteroids
for altitude-related illness, 1417, 1418
in cancer chemotherapy, 1506t
for fetal lung maturity, 719
for nausea and vomiting, 87, 506,
506t, 1509
for ophthalmic disorders, 174t
in pain management, 86
for pneumococcal meningitis, 1164,
1294
for spinal tumors/cord compression,
901
Dexamethasone suppression test, in
Cushing syndrome diag-
nosis, 1051
Dexrazoxane, for chemotherapy-induced
cardiac toxicity, 1507t,
1511
Dextroamphetamine
for depression, 964
for narcolepsy, 975
for opioid-induced sedation, 84

Dextromethorphan
MAOI interactions and, 969t, 1440
overdose/toxicity of, 1439
Dextrose
for coma, 1421
in fluid management, 815, 815t
for hypernatremia, 794
for shock, 435
DHA. See Docosahexaenoic acid
DHEA/DHEAS. See Dehydroepiandros-
terone/dehydroepiandros-
terone sulfate
DiaBeta. See Glyburide
Diabetes Control and Complications Trial
(DCCT), 1087, 1110
Diabetes insipidus, **995–997**
craniopharyngioma and, 993
hypernatremia in, 793–794, 996
nephrogenic, 796t, 996, 997
hypercalcemia/hyperparathyroid-
ism and, 801, 1034
lithium causing, 971
in Wolfram syndrome, 995, 1082
Diabetes mellitus, **1079–1117**. See also
under Diabetic
antipsychotic drug use and, 956, 958,
958t
aspirin in chemoprevention and, 12,
1089, 1108
β-blocker use in, 402
blood glucose levels in diagnosis of,
1083–1085, 1084t
blood glucose self-monitoring in,
1085, 1100–1101,
1102–1103
blood-testing procedures in,
1083–1085, 1084t
cardiovascular complications of,
1108–1109
glycemic control and, 1087,
1088–1089
hypertension control and, 1088,
1108
cholelithiasis/gallstones in, 634
chronic kidney disease and, 830, 842,
1104. See also Diabetic
nephropathy
dialysis for, 830, 1106
cirrhosis and, 620, 624
classification and pathogenesis of,
1079–1082, 1080t
clinical findings in, 1082–1086, 1082t,
1084t
clinical trials in, 1086–1089
complications of, 1104–1110
clinical studies of glycemic control
and, 1086–1089
hypoglycemia and, 1104
insulin therapy causing, 1103–1104
continuous glucose monitoring systems in, 1085
diagnostic examination in, 1100
differential diagnosis of, 1086, 1086t
emphysematous pyelonephritis in,
853
enterovirus infection in development
of, 1279
epidemiologic considerations in, 1079

Diabetes mellitus (cont.)
  erectile dysfunction in, 1107–1108
  estrogen replacement affecting risk of, 1071
  exercise and, 13, 1087, 1100, 1101, 1102
  foot disorders/foot care in, 133, 1106
  gastroparesis in, 1107
    hypoglycemia and, 1104
  gestational, 707, 722–723, 723t
  glaucoma in, 158, 159, 1105
  glucose tolerance test in, 1083–1084, 1084t
  glucosuria/glycosuria in, 1083, 1106
  glycated hemoglobin (hemoglobin A₁) measurements in, 1084–1085, 1084t, 1087, 1089, 1103
  glycemic control in
    acceptable levels of, 1103
    blood glucose self-monitoring in, 1085, 1100–1101, 1102–1103
    clinical studies in evaluation of, 1086–1089
    glycated hemoglobin (hemoglobin A₁) measurements in evaluation of, 1084–1085, 1084t, 1087, 1089, 1103
    intensive insulin therapy for. See Insulin therapy, intensive
    pregnancy and, 722–723, 1110
    surgery and, 57–58, 57t, 58t, 1109
  heart disease in, 1108
  HLA in, 1080, 1080t
  hypernatremia and, 793
  hypertension in, 396t, 842, 1083, 1106
    angiotensin-converting enzyme (ACE) inhibitors for, 396t, 402–405, 407, 409–410, 1088, 1105, 1106, 1108
    antihypertensive therapy regimens for, 396t, 409, 409–410
    benefits of control of, 409–410, 1088, 1108
    calcium channel blocking agents and, 396t
  immunization recommendations in, 1195t
  insulin resistance and, 1081, 1082. See also Insulin resistance/insulin insensitivity; Insulin resistance syndrome
  ketonuria in, 1083
  laboratory findings in, 1083–1086, 1084t, 1100
  latent autoimmune of adulthood (LADA), 1080–1081, 1102
  lipid/lipoprotein abnormalities in, 1085–1086, 1108, 1125, 1126t
  maturity-onset of young (MODY), 1080t, 1081–1082
  mitochondrial DNA mutations and, 1080t, 1082
  mucormycosis in, 195, 1398, 1399
  mutant insulin receptors causing, 1082
  mutant insulins causing, 1082

nephrotic syndrome and, 839, 842. See also Diabetic nephropathy
neurogenic arthropathy (Charcot joint) in, 783, 1106
neuropathy and, 923, 1082t. See also Diabetic neuropathy
nonalcoholic fatty liver disease and, 617, 618
occult (late hypoglycemia), 1121
ocular complications of, 166, 1104–1105. See also Diabetic retinopathy
ocular examinations in, 166
osteomyelitis in, 780
pancreatic/periampullary carcinoma and, 1463
patient education (self-management training) in, 1100–1101
polycystic ovary syndrome and, 690, 1053
prebreakfast hyperglycemia in, 1102–1103, 1103t
during pregnancy, 722–723, 723t, 1110
  continuous glucose monitoring and, 1085
prevention of
  exercise and, 13, 1087
  immune intervention therapy and, 1086–1087, 1087
prognosis for, 1110
Schmidt syndrome and, 1048, 1086
self-monitoring of blood glucose and, 1085, 1100–1101, 1102–1103
serum fructosamine levels in, 1085
skin/mucous membrane disorders and, 1083, 1109
surgery in patients with, 57–58, 57t, 58t
treatment of, 1089–1104
  clinical studies in evaluation of, 1086–1089
  combination regimens and, 1096, 1101
  diet in, 1089–1090, 1100, 1146. See also Diet
  drugs in, 1090–1096, 1091t. See also Antidiabetic agents
  general considerations in, 1100
  insulin in, 1096–1099, 1096t, 1097f, 1102–1103, 1102t, 1103t. See also Insulin therapy
  steps in, 1100–1103
  transplantation in, 1099–1100
type 1, 1079, 1079–1081, 1080t, 1102–1103, 1102t, 1103t
  clinical findings in, 1082t, 1083
  clinical trials in, 1086–1087
  HLA in, 1080, 1080t
  idiopathic (type 1B), 1080t, 1081
  immune-mediated (type 1A), 1079, 1079–1081, 1080t
  insulin therapy for, 1096–1099, 1096t, 1097f, 1102–1103, 1102t, 1103t
  prognosis for, 1110
type 2, 1079, 1080t, 1081, 1101–1102
  clinical findings in, 1082t, 1083
  clinical trials in, 1087–1089

drugs for management of, 1090–1096, 1091t. See also Antidiabetic agents
  hepatitis C and, 604
  insulin therapy for, 1087, 1101
  in nonobese patients, 1080t, 1081, 1082, 1101–1102
  in obese patients, 14, 1080t, 1081, 1083, 1101
  prognosis for, 1110
  urinalysis findings in, 1083
  vascular disorders in, 1108–1109
    glycemic control and, 1087, 1088–1089
    hypertension control and, 1088, 1108
  weight loss (unintended) in, 1082t, 1083
    diabetic neuropathic cachexia and, 1107
  in Wolfram syndrome, 1082
Diabetes Prevention Program (DPP), 1087
Diabetes Prevention Trial-1 (DPT-1), 1086–1087
Diabetic amyotrophy, 923, 1106
Diabetic cataracts, 1104
Diabetic cheiropathy, 759
Diabetic coma, 1083, 1111–1117, 1112t. See also specific cause
  diabetic ketoacidosis and, 1112, 1112t, 1113
  hyperglycemic hyperosmolar state and, 1112t, 1115–1116
  lactic acidosis and, 1111, 1116–1117
Diabetic diarrhea, 1107
Diabetic dyslipidemia, 1085–1086, 1108, 1126t
Diabetic ketoacidosis, 808–809, 1083, 1111–1115, 1112t
  coma caused by, 1112, 1112t, 1113
  hyperchloremic normal anion gap acidosis and, 808–809, 1114–1115
  hypophosphatemia in, 803, 1114
  insulin infusion pump use and, 1099, 1112, 1113
Diabetic maculopathy/macular edema, 166, 1105
Diabetic nephropathy, 842, 1104, 1105–1106
  glycemic control and, 842, 1087, 1088, 1105
  hypertension/hypertension control and, 393, 409–410, 842, 1088, 1105, 1106
Diabetic neuropathic cachexia, 1107
Diabetic neuropathy, 923, 1082t, 1106–1108
  foot disorders/ulcers/gangrene and, 1106, 1108–1109
  glycemic control and, 1087
  neurogenic arthropathy (Charcot joint) and, 783, 1106
Diabetic retinopathy, 166–167, 1104, 1105
  glycemic control and, 1087, 1088
  hypertension/hypertension control and, 1088

Diabetic shin spots, 1109
Diabinese. *See* Chlorpropamide
Diagnostic/laboratory tests. *See also specific disorder*
in poisoning/drug overdose, 1426–1427, 1427t
in prenatal care, 706, 707–708. *See also* Prenatal testing
reference values for, 1547–1554t
for screening. *See* Screening tests
specimen collection for, tubes for, 1555t
Dialectical behavioral therapy, for personality disorders, 951
Dialysis, 830–831
for acute tubular necrosis/kidney injury, 823
for bleeding in chronic kidney disease, 829
"gut" (repeat-dose charcoal), 1426
for heat stroke, 1408
for hypercalcemia, 801
hypercalcemia/hyperphosphatemia associated with, 802
for hyperkalemia, 798, 799t
for hypermagnesemia, 806
for hypernatremia, 794
for hyperphosphatemia, 804
for hyponatremia, 792
iron supplementation and, 829
for kidney disease/injury, 823
coagulopathy and, 823
in diabetic, 830, 1106
postoperative, 58–59
for poisoning/drug overdose, 1425–1426, 1425t
with carbamazepine, 1425t
with lithium, 972, 1425t
with methanol or ethylene glycol, 1425t, 1440
with salicylates, 1425t, 1445
with theophylline, 1425t, 1448
with valproic acid, 1425t
preoperative, 59
prognosis for patient undergoing, 832
pruritus associated with, 136
skin lesions and (porphyria cutanea tarda-like), 117
for uremic pericarditis, 378
Diaphragm, respiratory failure caused by disorders of, 289t
Diaphragm (contraceptive), **699**
DIAPPERS mnemonic, 70
Diarrhea, **511–517**, 512t, 513f, 516f, **1169–1172**, 1170–1171t.
See also specific cause and Colitis; Gastroenteritis
acidosis associated with, 810
acute, **511–514**, 512t, 513f, **1169–1172**, 1170–1171t
antibiotic-associated, 511, **573–575**, 1172
antibiotics for, 514, 574–575
in bacterial overgrowth, 516, 562
bloody, 512–513, 513. *See also* Dysentery
campylobacter causing, 512, 1171t, 1172, 1174, 1182t, 1316
Guillain-Barré syndrome and, 925

in carcinoid syndrome, 1475, 1476
in celiac disease, 516, 559
chemotherapy/radiation-induced, 1509
in cholera, 1171t, 1315
chronic, 512t, **514–517**, 516f
clostridial, 511, 512, 1170t, 1172
coccidial and microsporidial, 1369–1371
in Crohn disease, 515, 516, 517, 578, 579, 580
in cryptosporidiosis, 511, 1172, 1214, 1369
in cyclosporiasis, 511, 515, 1172, 1370
in diabetic autonomic neuropathy, 1107
diet in management of, 514
drugs in management of, 514, 517. *See also* Antidiarrheal agents
E coli causing, 512, 513, 1170t, 1172, 1315
endoscopy/mucosal biopsy in, 516
enteral nutritional support and, 1150
factitious, 512t, 515
fecal impaction and, 510, 595
fluid management in, 514, 815t, 1172
in giardiasis, 511, 512t, 515, 1172, 1174, 1371, 1372
in hyperoxaluric calcium nephrolithiasis, 859
in hypocitraturic calcium nephrolithiasis, 859
hypokalemia caused by, 795
in immunocompromised host/HIV infection/AIDS, 511, 515, 516, 1214, 1369–1371
infectious
acute, 511, 512t, **1169–1172**, 1170–1171t
chronic, 512t, 515
inflammatory. *See also* Dysentery
acute, 512–513, 512t, 1169–1172
chronic, 512t, 515
in intestinal amebiasis, 512, 514, 515, 1172, 1366
in irritable bowel syndrome, 515, 570
in isosporiasis, 1172, 1369
in lactase deficiency, 515, 563
in malabsorption, 512t, 515, 516, 558t
in measles, 1249
in microscopic colitis, 516, 587
motility disorders and, 512t, 515
in niacin deficiency, 1142
noninflammatory, 512, 512t, 1172
Norwalk virus causing, 1172, 1278
osmotic, 512t, 514–515
rotaviruses causing, 1171t, 1172, 1278
salmonella causing, 512, 1171t, 1172, 1174, 1182t, 1312, 1314
secretory, 512t, 515, 516
shigella causing, 512, 1171t, 1172, 1174, 1182t, 1314
in short bowel syndrome, 563
stool analysis in, 513–514, 515–516
traveler's, 511, **1173–1175**. *See also* Traveler's diarrhea
in typhoid fever, 1313
in ulcerative colitis, 583, 583t

in vibrio infection, 1170t, 1172, 1315, 1316
VIP/VIPoma causing, 1062
viral, 511, 512t, 1172. *See also specific virus*
in Zollinger-Ellison syndrome (gastrinoma), 556, 1062
Diastolic blood pressure. *See also* Blood pressure
in hypertension, 387, 388t, 389f
treatment goals and, 395–396
in hypertensive urgencies/emergencies, 387, 411
in preeclampsia-eclampsia, 716, 718
Diastolic dysfunction/heart failure, 358, 360. *See also* Congestive heart (cardiac) failure
hypertension and, 358, 393
Diastolic murmurs. *See* Heart murmurs
Diazepam, 941, 941t, 942. *See also* Benzodiazepines
adverse ophthalmic effects of, 177t
for aggressive/violent patient, 976
for alcohol withdrawal, 883, 980
for anxiety, 941, 941t, 942
for nausea and vomiting, 506t
for status epilepticus, 884
Diazoxide
for hypertensive urgencies/emergencies, 412, 413t
for islet cell tumors, 1120
Dibenzodiazepines, 955t, 956t. *See also* Antipsychotic drugs
Dibenzothiazepine, 955t, 956t. *See also* Antipsychotic drugs
Dibenzoxazepines, 954, 955t, 956t. *See also* Antipsychotic drugs
DIC. *See* Disseminated intravascular coagulation
Dichuchwa (endemic syphilis), 1339
Diclofenac, 79t
for ophthalmic disorders, 174t
Didanosine (ddI), 1226t, 1228, 1232, 1232f. *See also* Antiretroviral therapy
neuropathy caused by, 1212, 1228
DIDMOAD (Wolfram syndrome), 995, 1082
Dientamoeba fragilis, 1372
Diet. *See also* Nutrition
acne and, 120
breast cancer risk and, 653, 654
in cancer prevention, 1451
cholelithiasis/gallstones and, 634
cholesterol/lipid-lowering, 1130, 1146
in chronic kidney disease, 830
in cirrhosis, 620
colorectal cancer and, 1477
consistency alterations and, **1145**
constipation and, 508
in Crohn disease, 580
in diabetes mellitus, 1089–1090, 1100, 1146
for obese type 2 diabetic, 1101
pregnancy and, 722
prevention and, 1087
in diarrhea control, 514
in GERD management, 533

Diet (*cont.*)
gluten-free, for celiac disease/dermatitis herpetiformis, 118, 560
in gout, 734, 734*t*
health maintenance recommendations/guidelines for, 3*t*
in heart failure management, 366
in hemochromatosis, 628
in hypertension/hypertension prevention, 394, 395*t*
in hypertriglyceridemia, 1133
in irritable bowel syndrome, 571
for islet cell tumors, 1120
MAOI interactions and, 967*t*, 1440
Mediterranean, 1130
nutrient-restricting, **1145–1146**. *See also specific type*
nutrient-supplementing, **1146–1147**
obesity management/prevention and, 15, 1137
in pancreatitis, 644, 647
in porphyria, 923, 1512
during pregnancy, 706–707
diabetes mellitus and, 722
preventable disease/deaths and, 2*t*
theophyllines affected by, 225*t*
therapeutic, **1145–1147**
urinary stone formation and, 857
in Wilson disease, 629
Diet therapy, **1145–1147**. *See also* Diet; Nutrition
Dietary Supplement and Health Education Act, 1521, 1527–1528
Dietary supplements, **1527–1532**, 1528*t*
oral nutritional supplements, 1147
regulation/quality assurance/safety and, 1521, 1527–1528
Diethylcarbamazine
for filariasis, 1387
for loiasis, 1389
Diethylpropion, for obesity, 1137
Diethylstilbestrol (DES)
for breast cancer, 668*t*
in male, 673
for prostate cancer, 1487*t*
in utero exposure to, effects of, **679–680**
Dieulafoy lesion, 518
Difenacoum poisoning, 1430–1431
Diffuse cutaneous leishmaniasis, 1351–1352, 1353
Diffuse esophageal spasm, 529*t*, 543
Diffuse idiopathic skeletal hyperostosis (DISH), 774
Diffuse panbronchiolitis, 243
Diffuse parenchymal lung disease, **262–266**, 262*t*. *See also specific disorder and* Interstitial lung disease
Diffusing capacity for carbon monoxide ($D_{L_{CO}}$)
in interstitial (diffuse parenchymal) lung disease, 262
in *Pneumocystis* pneumonia, 1210
Diflorasone, 96*t*
Diflucan. *See* Fluconazole
Diflunisal, 79*t*
DiGeorge syndrome, hypoparathyroidism in, 1031

Digestion
disorders of. *See* Malabsorption
normal/phases of, 557–558
Digibind. *See* Digoxin-specific Fab antibody
DigiFab. *See* Digoxin-specific Fab antibody
Digital clubbing, 146
in bronchiectasis, 240
in interstitial (diffuse parenchymal) lung disease, 262
in lung cancer, 1454
Digital cyanosis, in Raynaud phenomenon, 756
Digital ischemia
in Raynaud phenomenon, 756, 757
in scleroderma, 758, 759
Digital mammography, 16, 655
Digital rectal examination. *See* Rectal examination
Digitalis/digitalis glycosides. *See also* Digoxin
antidepressant drug interactions and, 969*t*
for heart failure, 363–364
overdose/toxicity of, 363–364, 1424*t*, **1435–1436**, 1435*t*
hypokalemia and, 796
ophthalmic effects and, 177*t*
Digitoxin, overdose/toxicity of, 1435–1436
Digoxin, 344*t*, 1544*t*. *See also* Digitalis/digitalis glycosides
for arrhythmias, 344*t*
atrial fibrillation, 347
in hyperthyroidism, 1014
in myocardial infarction, 336
benzodiazepine interactions and, 942*t*
for heart failure, 363–364
overdose/toxicity of, 344*t*, 363–364, 1427*t*, 1435–1436
perioperative, 52
Digoxin-specific Fab antibody (digoxin immune Fab), for digitalis toxicity, 364, 1424*t*, 1436
Dihydroartemisinin, for malaria, 1355*t*, 1359–1360
with piperaquine, 1355*t*, 1356*t*, 1357, 1360
Dihydroergotamine
for cluster headache, 875
for migraine headache, 874
Dihydrofolate reductase, antimalarial drugs affecting, 1359
Dihydroindolones, 954, 955*t*, 956*t*. *See also* Antipsychotic drugs
Dihydropteroate synthase, antimalarial drugs affecting, 1359
1,25-Dihydroxycholecalciferol. *See* Calcitriol
Diiodohydroxyquin. *See* Iodoquinol
Dilacor. *See* Diltiazem
Dilated cardiomyopathy. *See* Cardiomyopathy
Dilation and curettage. *See* D&C
Dilaudid. *See* Hydromorphone
Diloxanide, for amebiasis, 1366, 1367, 1367*t*

Diltiazem. *See also* Calcium channel blocking drugs
for angina, 322
for arrhythmias, 344*t*
atrial fibrillation, 347
infarct-related, 336
for hypertension, 405, 406*t*
overdose/toxicity of, 344*t*, 406*t*, 1432
Dilutional acidosis, 810
Dimebon, for dementia, 987
Dimercaprol (BAL)
for arsenic poisoning, 1432
for lead poisoning, 1438
for mercury poisoning, 1439
Dimercaptosuccinic acid (DMSA). *See* Succimer
1,1-Dimethylbiguanide hydrochloride. *See* Metformin
Dimethyltryptamine, 982
Diovan. *See* Valsartan
DIP. *See* Desquamative interstitial pneumonia
Dipeptidyl peptidase 4 (DPP 4) inhibitors, 1095
Diphenhydramine. *See also* Antihistamines
for insomnia, 974
for nausea and vomiting, 87
overdose/toxicity of, 1432
Diphenoxylate with atropine, 517. *See also* Antidiarrheal agents
overdose/toxicity of, 1432
Diphtheria, **1302–1303**
myocarditis in, 368, 1302
neuropathy in, 925, 1302
pharyngitis in, 204, 1289, 1302
prevention/immunization and, 3, 1200, 1302. *See also* Diphtheria and tetanus toxoids and pertussis vaccine
Diphtheria antitoxin, 1302
Diphtheria-tetanus toxoid. *See* Tetanus-diphtheria toxoid
Diphtheria and tetanus toxoids and pertussis vaccine (DTaP/Tdap vaccines), 3–4, 1188–1189*t*, 1190–1191*t*, 1192–1193*t*, 1194–1197*t*, 1200, 1298, 1299*t*, 1302, 1308
adverse effects/contraindications and, 1202*t*
pregnancy and, 1195*t*, 1200
Diphyllobothrium latum (fish tapeworm), 1376, **1376**
vitamin B_{12} deficiency and, 445, 1376
Dipiperazines, 955*t*, 956*t*. *See also* Antipsychotic drugs
Dipivefrin, for glaucoma/ocular hypertension, 159, 175*t*
Diplopia
in dysthyroid eye/Graves disease, 170, 1009
vertigo and, 189
Diprolene. *See* Betamethasone
Dipstick urinalysis, 816. *See also specific disorder*
in dysuria evaluation, 46
in proteinuria evaluation, 817

Dipylidium caninum (dog tapeworm), 1376
  echinococcosis and, 1378
Dipyridamole, platelet function affected by, 490t
Dipyridamole-thallium scintigraphy. *See* Myocardial perfusion scintigraphy
Directed bleeding history, preoperative, 49, 50t, 55
Directly observed therapy (DOT), for tuberculosis, 254
  in drug-resistant tuberculosis, 256
  in HIV-positive persons, 256
Discoid lupus erythematosus, **110–111**
Disease-modifying antirheumatic drugs (DMARDs), 749
  biologic, 750–751
  combination regimens for, 751
  synthetic, 750
Disease prevention. *See* Health maintenance/disease prevention
Disequilibrium (imbalance). *See also* Vertigo
  falls/immobility in elderly and, 68
  in multiple sclerosis, 191, 191t
  in vestibular schwannoma (acoustic neuroma), 191, 191t
DISH. *See* Diffuse idiopathic skeletal hyperostosis
Disipal. *See* Orphenadrine
Disk batteries, ingested, alkali injuries caused by, 1429, 1430
Disk diffusion tests, drug susceptibility, 1175
Disk disease
  cervical. *See* Cervical spine/disk disease
  lumbar/sacral, herniation, 738, 739
  thoracic, chest pain in, 321, 543
Disopyramide, 343t
  for cardiomyopathy, 373
  overdose/toxicity of, 343t, 1445
Disorganized (hebephrenic) schizophrenia, 952
Dissection. *See* Aortic dissection
Disseminated cutaneous leishmaniasis, 1352
Disseminated intravascular coagulation (DIC), **487–488**, 488t, **495**
  in acute leukemia, 465
  in cancer, 487, 902
  in gram-negative bacteremia/sepsis, 487, 1311
  in meningococcal meningitis, 1309
Dissociated sensory loss, 886
  in spinal cord infarction, 897
Dissociative disorder, 940
Dissociative identity disorder (multiple personality disorder), 940
Distal muscular dystrophy, 934t
Distal renal tubular acidosis, 809t, 810. *See also* Renal tubular acidosis
  genetic defects associated with, 796t
  in hypocitraturic calcium nephrolithiasis, 859
  urinary stone formation and, 810, 857

Distal symmetric polyneuropathy, diabetic, 1106
Distributive shock, 434–435, 434t, 435, 436
Disulfiram
  for alcohol use/abuse, 18–20, 980
  antidepressant drug interactions and, 969t
  benzodiazepine interactions and, 942t
Disulfiram-like reactions, *Coprinus* mushroom poisoning causing, 1441, 1441t, 1442
Diulo. *See* Metolazone
Diuresis, forced, in poisoning/drug overdose, 1425
Diuretics. *See also specific agent*
  abuse of in bulimia nervosa, 1140
  for acute tubular necrosis, 823
  adverse effects of, 398
    ophthalmic, 177t
    ototoxic, 186
  for cardiomyopathy, 373, 374
  for cirrhotic ascites, 621
  for constrictive pericarditis, 380
  contraction alkalosis and, 813
  for heart failure, 361
    chronic kidney disease and, 828
    left ventricular (infarct-related), 337
  hypercalcemia and, 801, 1036
  for hypercalciuria, 858–859
  for hyperkalemia, 797, 799t
  for hypernatremia, 794
  for hypertension, 396t, 398, 399t, 407, 409, 409f
    in blacks, 398, 410t
    in combination products, 398, 399t, 409, 409f
    during pregnancy, 723
    urgencies/emergencies, 412
  hypokalemia and, 398, 796
  for hyponatremia, 792
  hyponatremia caused by, 790, 790f
  lipid abnormalities associated with use of, 1126t
  lithium interactions and, 972, 972t
  for lithium overdose/toxicity, 972
  for nephrotic syndrome, 840
  perioperative, 52
  for pulmonary edema, 367–368
Divalproex. *See* Valproic acid/valproate
Diverticula
  colonic, **587–589**
  esophageal/Zenker, **538**
Diverticular bleeding, 520, **589**
Diverticulectomy, for Zenker diverticulum, 538
Diverticulitis, **588–589**
Diverticulosis, **587–588**
  GI bleeding in, 520, **589**
  infection and (diverticulitis), **588–589**
Diving (underwater). *See* Scuba/deep sea diving
Dix-Hallpike testing, 188
Dizziness. *See also* Disequilibrium (imbalance); Vertigo; Vestibular disorders
  falls/immobility in elderly and, 68
DJ1 gene, in parkinsonism, 905

DL$_{CO}$ (diffusing capacity for carbon monoxide)
  in interstitial (diffuse parenchymal) lung disease, 262
  in *Pneumocystis* pneumonia, 1210
DLE. *See* Discoid lupus erythematosus
DMARDs. *See* Disease-modifying antirheumatic drugs
DML, 99t
DMPA. *See* Medroxyprogesterone
DMSA. *See* Succimer
DNA
  double-stranded, antibodies to. *See* Anti-double-stranded (anti-ds)-DNA
  hepatitis B virus, 602, 602f, 603, 609
  native, antibodies to, 754t
DNA amplification tests, in tuberculosis, 252
DNA analysis/diagnosis/probes (molecular genetics). *See also* Genetic testing
  in colorectal cancer screening, 589–590, 1481
  in muscular dystrophy, 935
  in tuberculosis, 252
"Do not attempt resuscitation" (DNAR) orders, **90**
Dobrava virus, 1264
Dobutamine
  for heart failure, 365
    left ventricular (infarct-related), 338
  for shock, 436
Dobutamine stress echocardiography. *See* Echocardiography
Docetaxel, 1502t
  for breast cancer, 666, 669
  neuropathy caused by, 1510
  for prostate cancer, 1488
Docosahexaenoic acid
  health benefits of, 1530
  platelet function affected by, 490t
Docosanol cream, for herpes simplex infection, 1237
Doctor–patient relationship
  adherence and, 1–2
  CAM information and, 1520–1521, 1522t
  chronic pain disorders and, 947
  psychiatric problems associated with hospitalization/illness and, 989
  smoking cessation and, 7, 8t, 9t, 1450
  somatoform disorders and, 945
Docusate sodium, 509t
Dofetilide, 344t
  for atrial fibrillation, 348, 349
Dog bites, 1165–1166
  rabies and, 1165, 1255, 1256
Dog feces
  echinococcosis and, 1378
  toxocariasis/visceral larva migrans and, 1385
Dog fleas. *See* Fleas
Dog hookworm, 1380
  cutaneous larva migrans caused by, 1385

Dog roundworm (*T canis*), 1384–1385
Dog tapeworm (*D caninum*), 1376
　echinococcosis and, 1378
Dog ticks. *See* Ticks
Dolasetron, 506, 506*t*, 1509. *See also* Antiemetics
Doll's-head eye response, in coma or stupor, 916
Dolobid. *See* Diflunisal
Dolophine. *See* Methadone
Domestic violence, 976, 977
　elder abuse and, 19, **75**, 75*t*
　prevention of, 18–19
Donepezil, for dementia, 65, 987
Donovan bodies, 1320
Dopamine
　depletion of in parkinsonism, 905, 907
　in Huntington disease, 909
　for hypotension/shock, 436
　　in poisoning/drug overdose, 1421
　for left ventricular (infarct-related) failure, 338
　positive and negative schizophrenic symptoms and, 952
Dopamine agonists
　for acromegaly/gigantism, 998–999
　for cocaine withdrawal, 983
　for hyperprolactinemia, 1000, 1001–1002
　for neuroleptic malignant syndrome, 959
　for parkinsonism, 907
Dopamine antagonists. *See also* Antipsychotic drugs
　for nausea and vomiting, 506, 506*t*
Doppler ultrasound. *See* Echocardiography; Ultrasonography
Dor procedure, 308
Doral. *See* Quazepam
Doripenem, for abdominal infections, 1322*t*
Dornase alpha (rhDNase), for cystic fibrosis, 242
Dorzolamide, for glaucoma/ocular hypertension, 159, 175*t*
Dorzolamide/timolol, for glaucoma/ocular hypertension, 159, 176*t*
Dose-dense/dose-intense chemotherapy. *See* Chemotherapy
DOT. *See* Directly observed therapy
Double-stranded DNA antibodies
　in hyperthyroidism, 1010
　in lupus, 110, 753, 754*t*
Double vision. *See* Diplopia
Down syndrome (trisomy 21), **1514–1515**
　prenatal screening for, 706, 1514
Doxazosin
　for benign prostatic hyperplasia, 869, 869*t*
　for hypertension, 407, 408*t*
Doxepin, 98*t*, 968*t*. *See also* Antidepressants
　topical, 94, 98*t*
Doxercalciferol, for hyperparathyroidism, 1037
Doxil. *See* Liposomal doxorubicin
Doxorubicin, 1502*t*
　for bladder cancer, 1490

　for breast cancer, 665, 666
　liposomal, 1502*t*, 1511
　　for Kaposi sarcoma, 135, 1216, 1225*t*
　　toxicity of, 1502*t*, 1511
Doxycycline
　for acne, 121
　adverse ophthalmic effects of, 177*t*
　for anthrax, 1301, 1301*t*
　for bacterial rhinosinusitis, 194*t*
　for Lyme disease, 1345, 1346*t*
　for malaria, 1355*t*, 1357*t*, 1360
　　for chemoprophylaxis, 1355*t*, 1360, 1361, 1361*t*
　for malignant pleural effusion, 1496
　for pleurodesis, 285
　for pneumonia, 247
　renal/hepatic failure and, 1184*t*
　for rosacea, 123
　for syphilis, 1333, 1333*t*
　for urinary tract infection, 852*t*
　for *Wolbachia* eradication
　　in filariasis, 1387
　　in onchocerciasis, 1388
DPI. *See* Dry powder inhalers
DPOA-HC. *See* Durable Power of Attorney for Health Care
DPP 4 inhibitors, 1095
DPP (Diabetes Prevention Program), 1087
DPT-1 (Diabetes Prevention Trial-1), 1086–1087
Dracunculus medinensis (dracunculiasis), **1382–1383**
DRE (digital rectal examination). *See* Rectal examination
Dream sleep, 973
DRESS mnemonic, 148
Dressler syndrome (postmyocardial infarction/postcardiotomy pericarditis), 339, 377, 378
Drinking. *See* Alcohol use/dependency/abuse
Driving (automobile), by patients with syncope/ventricular tachycardia/aborted sudden death, **357–358**
Dronabinol (Δ9-tetrahydrocannabinol), for nausea and vomiting, 87, 507
　for AIDS wasting, 1210
Drooling, in esophageal foreign body, 212
"Drop arm" signs, 744
Drop attacks
　epileptic (atonic seizures), 880. *See also* Seizures
　vertebrobasilar ischemic attacks and, 887
Droperidol
　for migraine headache, 874
　for nausea and vomiting, 506
　overdose/toxicity of, 1444–1445
　torsades de pointes caused by, 506, 1444
Drospirenone, in combination oral contraceptives, 695*t*
Drotrecogin alfa (activated protein C), for bacteremia/sepsis/shock, 437, 1312

Drowning, 1415
Drug addiction. *See* Addiction
Drug allergy, 784, **1180–1186**. *See also* specific agent
　cross-reactivity and, 1181
　desensitization therapy for, 1183–1186
　testing for, 1180, 1183
　in topical dermatologic therapy, 95, 147
Drug dependency, 977. *See also* specific drug and Substance use disorders
　in opioid therapy, 78
　physiologic, 78, 84, 977
　psychologic, 977
Drug eruptions, **147–150**, 148–149*t*
　fixed, 149*t*
Drug-induced disorders/side effects
　abnormal movements, **911**
　agranulocytosis, 456, 955, 958, 966
　allergic reactions. *See* Drug allergy
　angioedema, 126
　anion gap acidosis, 809
　asthma, 216, 281*t*
　cognitive disorders/delirium, 67, 985*t*
　constipation, 508, 508*t*
　depression, 962
　dermatitis (dermatitis medicamentosa), **147–150**, 148–149*t*
　diarrhea, 514
　dyspepsia, 502
　in elderly, **74**
　　depression, 66
　　falls and, 68, 69*t*
　eosinophilic pulmonary syndromes, 266
　erectile/sexual dysfunction, 862, 958, 965
　erythema multiforme, 127, 148*t*
　erythema nodosum, 140, 148*t*
　exfoliative dermatitis/erythroderma, 112, 148*t*
　fatty liver disease (hepatic steatosis), 617
　fetotoxicity, 706*t*
　gastritis/gastropathy, 544, 545
　glucose-6-phosphate dehydrogenase deficiency, 450
　gout/hyperuricemia, 732, 733, 734
　gynecomastia, 1064*t*, 1067
　hallucinations/hallucinosis, 986
　Hashimoto thyroiditis, 1016
　headache (analgesic rebound/medication overuse headache), **876**
　hepatic failure, 607
　hepatitis, **616–617**
　hyperglycemia, 1086
　hyperkalemia, 797, 798
　hyperpigmentation, 145, 149*t*
　　nail, 146, 149*t*
　hyperprolactinemia, 1001
　hypoglycemia, 1117*t*, **1122**
　hyponatremia, 790, 790*f*
　hypothyroidism, 1003–1004
　interstitial lung disease, 262*t*, 281*t*
　interstitial nephritis, 824

lichenoid/lichen planus-like, 134, 148*t*
liver disease, **616–617**
long QT syndrome, 354
lung disease, 262*t*, 281*t*
lupus, 111, 148*t*, 281*t*, 752, 752*t*
male infertility, 864
meningeal irritation, 1163
microscopic colitis, 587
microscopic polyangiitis, 770
myocarditis, **369–370**
nail hyperpigmentation, 146, 149*t*
nausea and vomiting, 505*t*
neutropenia, 456
nonalcoholic fatty liver disease, 617
ototoxicity, 186–187
overdoses. *See* Poisoning/drug overdose
pancreatitis, 642
parkinsonism, 905, 911, 959
pemphigus, 130
photosensitivity/photodermatitis, 142, 143, 148*t*
pigmentary changes, 145, 149*t*
platelet dysfunction, 490, 490*t*
porphyria, 1512, 1513*t*
cutanea tarda, 117
psychotic behavior, 954
pulmonary disorders, **281**, 281*t*
pure red cell aplasia, 447
rhabdomyolysis/myopathy/myositis, 761, 763–764, 936
SIADH, 791*t*
sick sinus syndrome, 354
Stevens-Johnson syndrome, 127
teratogenicity, 706*t*
thrombocytopenia, 482, 482–483, 483, 483*t*
tubulointerstitial nephritis, 845, 845*t*
urticaria, 126, 149*t*
Drug monitoring (therapeutic), 1544–1546*t*. *See also* specific agent
Drug overdose. *See* Poisoning/drug overdose
Drug resistance. *See also* specific agent
in anaerobic infections, 1322
in antiretroviral therapy, 1223, 1225–1227, 1232, 1233
in enterococcal infections, 1291
in gonococcal infection, 559, 1320
in HIV infection/AIDS, 1223, 1225–1227, 1232, 1233
hospital-associated infections and, 1159
in influenza, 1270, 1271, 1272, 1273
in leishmaniasis, 1352
in leprosy, 1327
in malaria, 1355, 1356, 1358, 1359
in meningococcal infection, 1309
pharyngitis treatment and, 204, 205
in pneumococcal infections, 246–247, 1293, 1294
in staphylococcal infections, 1294, 1295, 1306–1307
susceptibility testing and, 1175
in HIV infection/AIDS, 1225–1227, 1233
in tuberculosis, 252, 256
in tuberculosis, 252, 255, 256

Drug susceptibility testing, 1175. *See also* Drug resistance
in HIV infection/AIDS, 1225–1227, 1233
in tuberculosis, 252
Drug tolerance, 977. *See also* Substance use disorders
in opioid therapy, 78, 84
Drusen
in age-related macular degeneration/maculopathy, 162
optic disk, 169
Dry drowning, 1415
Dry eye (keratoconjunctivitis sicca), **154–155**
in Sjögren syndrome, 762, 763
Dry mouth. *See* Xerostomia
Dry powder inhalers, for asthma therapy, 223
Dry skin
atopic dermatitis and, 101, 102
emollients for, 94, 98–99*t*
Drying agents, for weepy dermatoses, 94
DTaP vaccines, 1188–1189*t*, 1192–1193*t*, 1308
DTIC-Dome. *See* Dacarbazine
Dual-chamber pacing, 355
for cardiomyopathy, 373
for heart block, 355
for sick sinus syndrome, 354
Dual energy x-ray absorptiometry, in osteoporosis, 1039
Dubin-Johnson syndrome, 599*t*
Duchenne muscular dystrophy, 934–935, 934*t*
cardiomyopathy in, 383
Ductal carcinoma in situ, 652, 662–663, 663
Paget carcinoma and, 113, 660
Ductal lavage, in breast mass evaluation, 660
Ductography, in nipple discharge/breast cancer, 651, 659, 660
Ductopenia, idiopathic adulthood, 641
Ductoscopy, in nipple discharge/breast cancer, 651, 659
Ductus arteriosus, patent, **301–302**, 302*t*
Duetact. *See* Pioglitazone, with glimepiride
Duke criteria (modified), for endocarditis, 1304
Duke Treadmill Score, 324, 324*t*
Duloxetine, 964, 966, 968*t*
for anxiety, 942
for neuropathic pain/diabetic neuropathy, 85, 85*t*, 1107
for urinary incontinence, 71–72
Duncan disease, 1244
Duodenal neuroendocrine tumors, **1062–1063**
in multiple endocrine neoplasia, 1062
Duodenal ulcers, 547–553. *See also* Peptic ulcer disease
Duodenotomy, for Zollinger-Ellison syndrome (gastrinoma), 557
Duodenum. *See also* Small intestine
disorders of, **544–557**
DuoTrav. *See* Travoprost/timolol

Duplex ultrasonography. *See* Ultrasonography
Dupuytren contracture, **742–743**
in cirrhosis, 619, 743
Durable Power of Attorney for Health Care (DPOA-HC), 90
Duroziez sign, 312
Dust mites, atopic dermatitis (eczema) caused by, 102
Dutasteride, for benign prostatic hyperplasia, 870
DVT. *See* Deep venous thrombosis
Dwarf tapeworm (*H nana*), 1376, **1377**
Dwarfism, in GH deficiency, 992
DXA. *See* Dual energy x-ray absorptiometry
Dyazide. *See* Triamterene, with hydrochlorothiazide
Dying patient, care of. *See* End of life, provision of care at
Dymelor. *See* Acetohexamide
DynaCirc. *See* Isradipine
Dysarthria, in motor neuron disease, 921
Dysautonomia (autonomic dysfunction), **884–885**
in Guillain-Barré syndrome, 885, 925
in polyneuropathies, 922
Dysbarism, **1416–1417**
Dysentery, 512–513
amebic, 1366, 1367*t*
colitis after (postdysenteric colitis), 1367
bacillary (*Shigella*). *See* Bacillary dysentery
enteroinvasive *E coli* causing, 1315
reactive arthritis and, 776
Trichuris, 1380
Dysesthesias, 886
Dysfunctional uterine bleeding, 674, 675
estrogen replacement therapy and, 675, 1071
Dysgeusia, **202–203**
Dyshidrosis/dyshidrotic eczema. *See* Vesiculobullous hand eczema
Dyskinesia
in Huntington disease, 908, 909
levodopa-induced, 906, 907
tardive, 959–960
Dyslipidemia. *See also* Hyperlipidemia
antiretroviral therapy and, 1216, 1229
in diabetes mellitus, 1085–1086, 1108, 1126*t*
exercise affecting, 1130
Dysmenorrhea, **677**
endometriosis and, 677, 686
IUD use and, 677, 698
oral contraceptive use and, 677, 694
Dysmotility. *See* Motility disorders
Dysnomia, intracranial tumors causing, 899
Dysorgasmia. *See* Orgasm, loss of
Dyspareunia (painful intercourse), 691–692, 692
Dyspepsia, **502–504**. *See also* Abdominal pain/tenderness
functional (nonulcer), 503
in gastric cancer, 502, 1471

Dyspepsia (*cont.*)
GERD and, 502, 531
in NSAID gastritis, 545
in peptic ulcer disease, 502, 549
Dysphagia, 529, 529*t*, 543
in achalasia, 529*t*, 542
in eosinophilic esophagitis, 529*t*, 537
in esophageal cancer, 529*t*, 1468
in esophageal stricture, 529*t*, 533
in esophageal webs and rings, 537
in GERD, 531, 543
in infectious esophagitis, 535
in motility disorders, 529, 529*t*, 543
in motor neuron disease, 921
in pill-induced esophagitis, 536
in polymyositis/dermatomyositis, 760
in scleroderma, 529*t*, 758
in Zenker diverticulum, 538
Dysphasia, in stroke, 889, 892
Dysphonia, **207**
in laryngopharyngeal reflux, 208
in vocal fold paralysis, 211
Dysphoric disorder, premenstrual, 676–677, 962
Dysplastic nevi. *See* Atypical nevi/mole
Dyspnea, **24–27**, 25*t*, **86**
in acute respiratory failure, 290
in ARDS, 291
in cardiomyopathy, 370, 373
in cirrhosis, 623–624
in COPD, 24–25, 26, 234
cough and, 22, 23, 25
in heart failure, 25, 25*t*, 26, 358–359
in hepatopulmonary syndrome, 623
in interstitial (diffuse parenchymal) lung disease, 262
in malignant pleural effusion, 285, 1495
palliation of, **86**
in pneumothorax, 26, 286
in pulmonary alveolar proteinosis, 266
in pulmonary embolism, 26, 267, 268*t*
in terminally ill/dying patient, 26, 86
Dysrhythmias. *See* Arrhythmias
Dyssomnias, **973–975**. *See also* Insomnia
Dyssynergia, pelvic floor (dyssynergic defecation), 507–508, 508
biofeedback in management of, 1536*t*, 1538
Dysthymia, 962, 964. *See also* Depression
Dysthyroid eye disease, **170**, 1008, 1009
Dystonia
drug-induced, 911
antipsychotics, 911, 959, 1444
oromandibular, 910
torsion
focal, **910**
idiopathic, **909–910**
Dystrophin, in muscular dystrophy, 935
Dysuria (painful voiding), **46–48**, 47*f*. *See also* Irritative voiding symptoms
DYT1 gene, in idiopathic torsion dystonia, 909
DYT6/DYT7 genes, in focal torsion dystonia, 910

E-cadherin cell adhesion protein, gastric cancer and, 1471

E coli. See Escherichia coli
E-tests, drug susceptibility, 1175
EACA. *See* ε-Aminocaproic acid
Ear, **179–192**. *See also* Hearing; Hearing loss
barotrauma affecting, **183**
cauliflower, 180
in HIV infection/AIDS, **191–192**
inner, **186–190**
middle, **183–186**
infection of. *See* Otitis, media
neoplasia of, **185–186**
trauma to, **185**
painful. *See* Earache
Ear canal, **180–182**
bony overgrowths (exostoses/osteomas) of, **182**
foreign body in, **181**
neoplasia of, **182**
pruritus of, **181**
Ear drops
for cerumen removal, 180
for external otitis, 181
ototoxic, avoidance of with perforated tympanic membrane, 187
Earache (otalgia), **186**
in acute otitis media, 183, 184, 186
in external otitis, 181, 186
in malignant external otitis, 181
East African trypanosomiasis, 1348, 1349, 1349*t*
Eastern (equine) encephalitis, 1257–1259
Eating disorders, **1138–1140**
OCD and, 940
Eaton-Lambert syndrome. *See* Lambert-Eaton (myasthenic) syndrome
EBCT. *See* Electron beam CT
Ebola hemorrhagic fever, 1262–1263
Ebstein anomaly, 314
lithium use during pregnancy and, 971
EBV. *See* Epstein-Barr virus
EC regimen, for breast cancer, 665
Ecchymosis, of eye (black eye), 171
in nasal trauma, 199
ECG. *See* Electrocardiogram
Echinacea angustifolia/pallida/purpurea, 870, 1523*t*, 1525–1526
Echinocandins, 1402. *See also specific agent*
Echinococcus granulosus/multilocularis (echinococcosis), **1378–1379**
Echocardiography. *See also* Ultrasonography/Doppler ultrasonography/duplex ultrasonography
in angina, 319
in aortic regurgitation, 305*t*, 312
in aortic stenosis, 305*t*, 310
in cardiac tumors, 383
in cardiomyopathy, 370*t*, 371, 372, 373, 374
cardioversion for atrial fibrillation and, 347–348
in coarctation of aorta, 296
in constrictive pericarditis, 379

in cor pulmonale, 382
in endocarditis, 1304
in heart failure, 360
in hypertension, 394
in infectious myocarditis, 369
in mitral regurgitation, 305*t*, 307–308
in mitral stenosis, 305*t*, 306
in myocardial infarction, 331
in patent ductus arteriosus, 301–302
in pericardial effusion, 378, 379
preoperative, 50
in pulmonary hypertension, 275, 381
in pulmonary stenosis, 295
stress/dobutamine stress
in angina, 319
in heart failure, 360
preoperative, 50
in tetralogy of Fallot, 300–301
in tricuspid regurgitation, 305*t*, 314
in tricuspid stenosis, 305*t*
in valvular heart disease, 305*t*
in ventricular septal defect, 299
Echolalia
in schizophrenic/psychotic disorders, 953
in Tourette syndrome, 911
Echopraxia, in Tourette syndrome, 911
Echovirus infections, **1279–1280**
Eclampsia, 71, 392, 716, 717*t*, 718. *See also* Preeclampsia-eclampsia
hypermagnesemia associated with treatment of, 806
Econazole, 98*t*
ECP. *See* Extracorporeal counterpulsation
"Ecstasy," 984, 1430
"herbal" (ephedrine), 1430
safety/toxicity of, 1522
hyponatremia caused by, 790
seizures caused by, 1423*t*
ECT. *See* Electroconvulsive therapy
Ectasias, vascular. *See* Vascular ectasias
Ecthyma, 118
contagiosa (orf), 1277
Ectopia lentis
in homocystinuria, 1517
in Marfan syndrome, 1518
Ectopic pregnancy, **713–714**
hCG levels in, 705, 713
IUDs and, 698
ruptured, appendicitis differentiated from, 568
Ectropion, **152–153**
Eculizumab, for paroxysmal nocturnal hemoglobinuria, 449
Eczema, **101–103**. *See also* Atopic dermatitis
dyshidrotic. *See* Eczema, vesiculobullous hand
in food allergy, 101
herpeticum, 103, 1236, 1240*t*
vaccinatum, 103, 116
vesiculobullous hand (pompholyx), **116–117**
Edecrin. *See* Ethacrynic acid
Edema
arm, in breast cancer/postmastectomy, 671–672
in burn injury, 1410

in cirrhosis, 620–621
in filariasis, 1386
in glomerulonephritis, 833
in heart failure, 359, 360
hyponatremia and, 790f, 791–792
lower extremity, **36–38**, 37t. *See also*
    Lower extremity edema
malabsorption and, 558t
in nephrotic syndrome, 37, 838, 840
optic disk. *See* Optic disk, swelling of
in preeclampsia-eclampsia, 716
refeeding, 1135
in superior vena caval obstruction,
    431
thiazolidinediones causing, 1094,
    1101
in venous insufficiency, 36–38, 430
    leg ulcers and, 36, 37, 143, 144, 430,
        431
    volume overload and, 794
Edetate calcium disodium (EDTA), for
    lead poisoning, 846, 1438
EDIC (Epidemiology of Diabetes Inter-
    ventions and Complica-
    tions) study, 1087
Edrophonium, for myasthenia diagnosis,
    932
EDTA. *See* Edetate calcium disodium
EEG biofeedback, 1535, 1539
Efalizumab, for psoriasis, 105
Efavirenz, 1227t, 1230, 1232f. *See also*
    Antiretroviral therapy
    fetal anomalies caused by, 726, 1230
    with tenofovir and emtricitabine,
        1228, 1230, 1231, 1232f
Effexor. *See* Venlafaxine
Effusions. *See* Malignant effusions; Peri-
    cardial effusions; Pleural
    effusions
Eflornithine
    for African trypanosomiasis, 1349,
        1349t
    for hirsutism/virilization, 1055
Egatin. *See* Triclabendazole
Egb761 (ginkgo extract), 1523t,
    1524–1525
EHEC. *See Escherichia coli*, enterohemor-
    rhagic
Ehlers–Danlos syndrome
    aortic disorders/aneurysm in, 383, 425
    mitral valve prolapse in, 309, 383
Ehrlichia canis/chaffeensis/ewingii (ehr-
    lichiosis), 1240t, 1281t,
    1285–1286
    babesiosis coinfection and, 1286
    Lyme disease coinfection and, 1286,
        1346
EIC. *See* Epidermal inclusion cysts
Eicosapentaenoic acid, health benefits of,
    1530
EIEC. *See Escherichia coli*, enteroinvasive
Eighth nerve lesions. *See* Schwannoma,
    vestibular
Eikenella corrodens. See HACEK organ-
    isms
Eisenmenger physiology, 297
    in atrial septal defect, 297
    in patent ductus arteriosus, 301

pregnancy and, 724
in ventricular septal defect, 299
Ejaculate, for semen analysis. *See* Semen
    analysis
Ejaculation disturbances, 862, 949. *See
    also* Erectile dysfunction/
    impotence
    in infertility, 865, 865f, 866
Ejaculatory ducts, obstruction of, in infer-
    tility, 866
Ejection clicks. *See* Clicks
Ektacytometry, in hereditary spherocyto-
    sis, 448
Elapid (coral snake) envenomation,
    1446–1447
Elastic compression stockings. *See* Com-
    pression stockings
Elastography, in liver disease/cirrhosis,
    600, 620
Elavil. *See* Amitriptyline
Elbow
    tennis or golf, **745**
    ulnar nerve lesions at, 927
Elder abuse, 19, **75**, 75t
Elderly patients. *See* Geriatric medicine;
    Older adults
Electric burns, 1409, 1410, 1412–1413
    fasciotomy in, 1411, 1413
Electrical alternans, in pericardial effu-
    sion, 378
Electrical cardioversion. *See* Cardiover-
    sion, electrical
Electrical injury, **1412–1413**
Electrocardiogram (ECG). *See also specific
    disorder*
    in acute coronary syndromes, 29–30,
        326
    in acute kidney injury, 819
    ambulatory monitoring of
        in angina, 320
        in arrhythmia evaluation, seizures
            and, 881
    in angina, 318–319
    antidepressants affecting, 967, 1448,
        1448f
    antipsychotic drugs affecting, 957, 958
    in aortic dissection, 426
    in atrial fibrillation, 347
    in atrial flutter, 350
    in atrial septal defect/patent foramen
        ovale, 298
    in cardiomyopathy, 370t, 371, 372, 373
    in chest pain evaluation, 29–30, 29t
    in coarctation of aorta, 296
    in COPD, 235
    in cor pulmonale, 382
    exercise/stress
        in angina, 318–319
        before exercise program initiation,
            13
    in heart failure, 360
    in hyperkalemia, 798
    in hypertension, 393, 394
    in hypokalemia, 796
    in hypothermia, 1404, 1404f
    in infectious myocarditis, 369
    lithium affecting, 971
    in myocardial infarction, 331

in non-ST elevation acute coronary
    syndromes, 326
in palpitations, 31
in paroxysmal supraventricular tachy-
    cardia, 342
in patent ductus arteriosus, 301
in pericardial effusion, 378
in pericarditis, 377
preoperative, 49
in pulmonary embolism, 267
in pulmonary hypertension, 275, 381
in pulmonary stenosis, 295
in syncope, 357
in tetralogy of Fallot, 300
in valvular heart disease, 304t
in ventricular septal defect, 299
Electroconvulsive therapy (ECT),
    963–964, 967–969
    for catatonia, 957
    for neuroleptic malignant syndrome,
        959
Electrodermal biofeedback, 1536t, 1537
Electrodesiccation and curettage
    for basal cell carcinoma, 134
    for squamous cell carcinoma, 134
Electroencephalogram (EEG)
    in epilepsy, 880–881
        absence (petit mal) seizures and,
            880
        nonconvulsive status epilepticus
            and, 884
        solitary seizure and, 883
    in intracranial tumors, 899
    isoelectric, in brain death determina-
        tion, 917
    in pseudoseizure identification, 881, 944
Electroencephalographic (EEG) biofeed-
    back, 1535, 1539
Electrolytes. *See also specific type*
    disorders of concentration of, 766. *See
        also* Fluid and electrolyte
        disorders
    genetic disorders and, 796t
    replacement guidelines for, 815, 815t
    requirements for in nutritional sup-
        port, 815, 1149
Electromyographic biofeedback, 1535,
    1536t, 1537, 1538
Electromyography
    in motor neuron disease, 921
    in muscular dystrophy, 934–935
    in myasthenia gravis, 932
    in myotonic dystrophy, 935
    in polymyositis/dermatomyositis, 760
Electron beam CT (EBCT), in angina, 320
Electronystagmography (ENG), in ver-
    tigo, 189, 190
Electrophoresis. *See* Hemoglobin electro-
    phoresis; Immunofixation
    electrophoresis; Serum
    protein electrophoresis
Electrophysiologic testing
    in multiple sclerosis, 913
    in myasthenia gravis, 932
    in syncope evaluation, 357
Electrovaporization of prostate, trans-
    urethral, for benign pros-
    tatic hyperplasia, 871

Elemental nutritional support solutions, 1150

Elephantiasis
in chromoblastomycosis, 1400
in filariasis, 1386

Elestat. *See* Epinastine

Eletriptan, for migraine headache, 874

Eleutherococcus senticosus, 1526

Elidel. *See* Pimecrolimus

ELISA. *See* Enzyme-linked immunosorbent assay

Elitek. *See* Rasburicase

Ellence. *See* Epirubicin

Elmiron. *See* Pentosan

Elocon. *See* Mometasone

Elongation factor, diphtheria and, 1302

Eloxatin. *See* Oxaliplatin

Elspar. *See* Asparaginase

Eltrombopag
for cirrhosis-related bleeding, 623
for immune thrombocytopenic purpura, 483, 484

Elvitegravir, 1231. *See also* Antiretroviral therapy

Emadine. *See* Emedastine

Embolectomy
in acute arterial occlusion of limb, 419
pulmonary, 273

Embolism. *See also* Thromboembolism
acute occlusion of limb caused by, 419
arterial. *See* Arterial embolism
atrial fibrillation and, 346, 347t
in atrial septal defect/patent foramen ovale, 297
cerebrovascular occlusion and, 420, 889. *See also* Stroke
in endocarditis, 1304, 1305
in mitral regurgitation, 307
in mitral stenosis, 307
in myocardial infarction, 339
paradoxic. *See* Paradoxic embolism
pulmonary. *See* Pulmonary venous thromboembolism
in transient ischemic attacks, 886, 888

Embolization
for GI bleeding, 520, 522, 523
for hemoptysis, 28
for intracranial arteriovenous malformations, 896

Embryo. *See* Fetus

Embryonal cell carcinoma, of testis, 1492

Emcyt. *See* Estramustine

Emedastine, for allergic eye disease, 155, 173t

Emergencies, hypertensive. *See* Hypertensive emergencies

Emergency/postcoital contraception, **700**
IUD for, 698, 700

Emery-Dreifuss muscular dystrophy, 934t

Emesis. *See also* Nausea and vomiting
for poisoning/drug overdose, 1424

Emetine, for amebiasis, 1367, 1367t

EMG biofeedback, 1535, 1536t, 1537, 1538

Emission, loss of, 862. *See also* Erectile dysfunction/impotence

Emmetropia, 151

Emollients, 94, 98–99t

Emotional challenges, for terminally ill/dying patient, 92

Emotive imagery. *See* Guided/emotive imagery

Emphysema, 234, 235t. *See also* Chronic obstructive pulmonary disease
α_1-antiprotease deficiency in, 235
replacement therapy and, 238
bullectomy for, 239
complications of, 236
imaging findings in, 235
panacinar bibasilar, 235

Emphysematous pyelonephritis, 853

Empyema
anaerobes causing, 250, 1322
group A streptococci causing, 1291
middle ear, 183–184. *See also* Otitis, media
pleural, 250, 283, 284t, 285
in pneumococcal pneumonia, 1292

Emsam. *See* Selegiline, transdermal

Emtricitabine, 1226t, 1228, 1232f. *See also* Antiretroviral therapy
for hepatitis B, 1228
resistance to, 1233
with tenofovir, 1227, 1228, 1232f
with tenofovir and efavirenz, 1228, 1230, 1231, 1232f

Emtriva. *See* Emtricitabine

Enalapril, 403t
for heart failure, 362

Enalaprilat, for hypertensive urgencies/emergencies, 412, 413t

Enbrel. *See* Etanercept

Encephalitis, 1163. *See also* Meningoencephalitis
acanthamoeba, 1163, 1164
amebic, 1163–1164, **1368**
granulomatous, 1164, **1368**
arbovirus, **1257–1259**
in coxsackievirus infection, 1279
cytomegalovirus, 1246
enterovirus 71 causing, 1280
herpes simplex, 1236, 1237
inclusion body, 1248
in loiasis, 1389
measles, 1248
mumps, 1251
parkinsonism after, 905
rabies, 1255–1256
tick-borne, 1257–1259, **1266–1267**
toxoplasma, in HIV infection/AIDS, 1363, 1364
West Nile, 1257–1259
yellow fever vaccine-associated, 1203, 1265–1266

Encephalitozoon/Encephalitozoon intestinalis, 1369, 1370

Encephalomyelitis
in Lyme disease, 1344
measles and, 1248
optic neuritis and, 168
yellow fever vaccine-associated, 1203

Encephalopathy
alcohol use/abuse and (chronic alcoholic brain syndromes), 979

bovine spongiform (mad cow disease), 1260
in cancer, 902
hepatic. *See* Hepatic encephalopathy
HIV, 1212
hypertensive, 393, 411
hyponatremic, 792
in hypophosphatemia, 803
in influenza, 1270
lead, 1438
gasoline sniffing and, 984
lithium causing, 971
in Lyme disease, 1343–1344
melarsoprol causing, 1349
metabolic. *See* Metabolic encephalopathy
in Reye syndrome. *See* Reye syndrome
in rubella, 1254
spongiform
bovine (mad cow disease), 1260
transmissible, 1260–1261
uremic, 829
Wernicke, **915**, 979, 981, 1141

End of life
Kübler-Ross' stages of, 92
patient expectations about, **88**
prognosis at, **87–88**, 88f
provision of care at, 76, **87–93**. *See also* Palliative care
advance care planning/advance directives and, **90**
care of family and, **89**, 89t
clinician self-care and, **89**
communicating with patient and, **88–89**, 89t
cultural issues in, **91**
decision-making and, **90**
DNAR orders and, **90**
in hospice/palliative care program, **90–91**
nutrition/hydration needs and, **91**
pain management, **77–78**
patient's wishes regarding, 90
psychologic/social/spiritual issues and, **92–93**, 92t
withdrawal/withholding curative efforts and, **91–92**, 92t

End-stage renal disease (ESRD). *See also* Chronic kidney disease; Renal failure
GFR calculation in, 818
hepatitis C infection and, 844
kidney transplantation for. *See* Kidney transplantation

Endarterectomy, carotid. *See* Carotid endarterectomy/thromboendarterectomy

Endemic flea-borne (murine) typhus, 1281t, **1282–1283**

Endemic goiter, **1029–1030**

Endemic syphilis, **1339**

Endocarditis
infective, 1181t, **1303–1307**, 1305t, 1306t
anaerobic, **1323**
anticoagulation and, 1307
antimicrobial chemoprophylaxis and, 1305, 1305t, 1306t

in Marfan syndrome, 1518
   during pregnancy, 385
aortic regurgitation and, 312
back pain in, 738
C psittaci causing, 1329
candidal, 1391
in drug user, 1168, 1181*t*, 1304
fever/FUO in, 1154
gonococcal, 1319, 1320
HACEK organisms causing, 1304,
   1307
in mitral regurgitation, 307, 308
native valve, 1303–1304, 1307
pneumococcal, 1292, 1293
prosthetic valve, 1296–1297, 1304,
   1307
   anticoagulation and, 1307
in Q fever, 1286, 1287
staphylococcal, 1303, 1304, 1305,
   1306–1307
   coagulase-negative organisms
      causing, 1296–1297, 1306
streptococcal, 1291, 1304,
   1305–1306
   viridans streptococci causing,
      1304, 1305
surgical management of, 1307
tricuspid regurgitation and, 314
valve replacement for, 1307
in ventricular septal defect, 299
Libman-Sacks, in SLE, 753
Endocervical curettage, 675*t*
in abnormal premenopausal bleeding, 674
in CIN/cervical cancer, 681, 682
in endometrial carcinoma, 684
Endoclips, for GI bleeding, 519, 522, 554
for Mallory-Weiss syndrome/tears,
   537
in peptic ulcer disease, 554
Endocrine disorders, **991–1078**. *See also*
         *specific gland and specific
         disorder*
cancer-related, 1453*t*
in chronic kidney disease, 830
cognitive disorders/delirium caused
   by, 985*t*
in HIV infection/AIDS, 1214
in multiple endocrine neoplasia,
   1075–1077, 1076*t*. *See also*
      Multiple endocrine neo-
      plasia
preoperative evaluation/management
   and, **57–58**, 57*t*, 58*t*
radiation and, 1414
Endocrine therapy. *See* Hormone therapy
Endogenous unipolar disorder, 961. *See
         also* Depression
Endoleaks, after abdominal aneurysm
   repair, 424
Endolymphatic hydrops (Ménière syn-
         drome), 189, 191*t*
hearing loss and, 187, 189, 191*t*
Endometrial ablation, for abnormal pre-
         menopausal bleeding, 675
Endometrial biopsy, 675*t*
in abnormal premenopausal bleeding, 674

in endometrial carcinoma, 684
in infertility workup, 693
in postmenopausal vaginal bleeding,
   676
Endometrial carcinoma/cancer of uterus,
         684–685, 1467*t*
breast cancer risk and, 653
estrogen replacement therapy and,
   684, 703, 1072
HNPCC and, 592, 593, 684
incidence/risk/mortality of, 684
oral contraceptive use and, 684, 694,
   696
polycystic ovary syndrome and, 690,
   1053
postmenopausal bleeding and, 676,
   684
tamoxifen and, 669, 684
Endometrial curettage. *See* Endometrial
         biopsy
Endometrial hyperplasia
estrogen replacement therapy and,
   703, 1071
postmenopausal vaginal bleeding
   caused by, 676
Endometriosis, **686–687**
dysmenorrhea and, 677, 686
infertility and, 686
Endometritis, **687–689, 720–721**. *See also*
         Pelvic inflammatory dis-
         ease
amenorrhea and, 1069
C sordellii causing, 701, 1298
postpartum, **720–721**
   streptococcal, 725
Endomyocardial biopsy, in infectious
         myocarditis, 369
Endomyocardial fibrosis, 374
Endomyometritis, 720. *See also*
         Endometritis
Endomysial antibodies, in celiac disease/
         dermatitis herpetiformis,
         559, 560
Endoscopic retrograde cholangiopancre-
         atography (ERCP)
in biliary stricture, 640
in choledocholithiasis/cholangitis,
   638, 639
in liver disease/jaundice, 601
in pancreatic/periampullary carcinoma, 1464
in pancreatitis, 645, 646
during pregnancy, 727
in primary sclerosing cholangitis, 640
Endoscopic ultrasonography
in gastric adenocarcinoma, 1471
in gastric lymphoma, 1473
in gastrointestinal mesenchymal
   tumors, 1474
in liver disease/jaundice, 601
in pancreatic/periampullary carcinoma, 1464
in pancreatitis, 648
in Zollinger-Ellison syndrome/gastri-
   noma, 557
Endoscopy
in achalasia, 542
in celiac disease, 560

in colorectal cancer screening,
   1481–1482. *See also*
      Colonoscopy; Sigmoidos-
      copy
in Crohn disease, 578
in diarrhea, 516
in dyspepsia, 503
in erosive/hemorrhagic gastritis (gastropathy), 544
in esophageal disorders, 530
   Barrett esophagus, 532
   benign neoplasms, 538
   bleeding varices, 539, 539–540
      prevention of first bleeding epi-
         sode and, 541
   cancer, 1468
   caustic injury, 536, 1429, 1430
   eosinophilic esophagitis, 537
   GERD, 531, 533
      treatment and, 533, 534
   infectious esophagitis, 535
   motility disorders, 543
   stricture, 533
in gastric adenocarcinoma, 1471
in gastric lymphoma, 1473
in gastric outlet obstruction, 555
in GI bleeding, 519, 522, 554
   obscure bleeding and, 523
   occult bleeding and, 523
   in peptic ulcer disease, 554
in *H pylori* detection/assessment, 546
in Mallory-Weiss syndrome/tears, 537
in pancreatitis, 647–648
in peptic ulcer disease, 549
   bleeding management and, 554
in pernicious anemia gastritis, 547
in polyp identification, 590, 591
in small intestinal tumors, 567
in ulcerative colitis, 583
in Whipple disease, 561
Endothelial growth factor, vascular. *See*
         Vascular endothelial
         growth factor
Endotracheal aspiration cultures, in
         pneumonia, 249
Endotracheal intubation. *See* Intubation
Endovaginal ultrasound. *See* Ultrasonog-
         raphy
Endovascular surgery/prostheses. *See also*
         Angioplasty; Stents/stent
         grafts
for abdominal aortic aneurysm, 424
for acute arterial occlusion of limb,
   419
for aortoiliac occlusive disease,
   415–416
for carotid occlusive disease, 420–421
for femoral/popliteal occlusive disease, 417
for intracranial aneurysm, 894
for lower leg/foot occlusive disease,
   418
for renal artery stenosis, 391, 833
for thoracic aortic aneurysm, 425
for visceral artery insufficiency/intes-
   tinal angina, 422
Endovascular warming, for hypothermia,
   1404

Endovenous ablation, for varicose veins, 428
Endurance exercise
    heat-related disorders and, 1407
    hyponatremia after, 790f, 791
Enemas
    barium. *See* Barium enema
    for constipation, 509t
Energy deficiency (protein-energy malnutrition), **1134–1135**
Energy medicine, 1520
Energy requirements, in nutritional support, 1148–1149
Enfuvirtide, 1227t, 1231, 1232f. *See also* Antiretroviral therapy
ENG. *See* Electronystagmography
ENG gene mutation, in hereditary hemorrhagic telangiectasia, 1519
Engerix B. *See* Hepatitis B vaccine
Enolase, neuron-specific, in pheochromocytoma, 1059
Enoxacin, theophyllines affected by, 225t
Enoxaparin, 496t, 497t
    for acute coronary syndromes, 326–327
    after thrombolytic therapy for myocardial infarction, 334
Entacapone, with levodopa and carbidopa, for parkinsonism, 907
Entamoeba. See also Amebiasis
    dispar, 1365, 1366
    histolytica, 515, 1172, 1174, 1182t, 1365, 1366
        stool antigen tests for, 514, 515, 1366
Entecavir, for hepatitis B, 610, 1238t
Enteral nutritional support (tube feedings), 1147–1148, 1148f.
        See also Nutritional support
    in burn injury, 1411
    complications of, **1150**
    for Crohn disease, 580
    for elderly, 72
    in pancreatitis, 644
    patient monitoring during, 1151–1152
    for protein–energy malnutrition, 1135, 1147
    solutions for, **1149–1150,** 1149t
    for terminally ill/dying patient, 91
Enteric (typhoid) fever, 1312, **1312–1314**
    prevention/immunization and, 1201, 1313
Enteric infection, irritable bowel syndrome after, 570
Enteritis. *See* Gastroenteritis
Enterobacter infections, 1176t
Enterobius vermicularis (enterobiasis/pinworms), **1382**
Enterocele, 687
Enterococcus faecalis/faecium (enterococcal infection), 1176t, **1291–1292**
    burn-associated infection, 1411
    endocarditis, 1304, 1306
Enterocolitis. *See also* Diarrhea; Gastroenteritis
    in HIV infection/AIDS, 511, 515, 516, 1214

Enterocytozoon/Enterocytozoon bieneusi, 1369, 1370
Enteropancreatic tumors, in multiple endocrine neoplasia, 1076
Enteropathy
    AIDS, 1214
    gluten-sensitive. *See* Celiac disease
    protein-losing. *See* Protein-losing enteropathy
Enteroscopy, in GI bleeding, 522, 523
Enterostomies, tube, 1148, 1148f. *See also* Enteral nutritional support
Enterovirus 72. *See* Hepatitis A virus
Enterovirus infections, 1240t, **1278–1280**
Enterovirus 70/enterovirus 71, **1280**
Enthesopathy/enthesitis
    in ankylosing spondylitis, 774
    in psoriatic arthritis, 775
    in reactive arthritis, 776
Entocort. *See* Budesonide
Entrapment/compression neuropathy, 926. *See also* Neuropathies
    in amyloidosis, 924
    common peroneal nerve, **928**
    femoral nerve, **927**
    lateral femoral cutaneous nerve (meralgia paresthetica), **927–928**
    median nerve (carpal tunnel syndrome), **742**
    pronator teres or anterior interosseous nerve, **927**
    radial nerve (Saturday night palsy), 926, **927**
    in rheumatoid arthritis, 747, 924
    sciatic nerve, **928**
    tibial nerve (tarsal tunnel syndrome), **928**
    ulnar nerve, **927**
Entropion, **152–153**
    in trachoma, 154
Entry inhibitors, for HIV infection/AIDS, 1227t, 1231, 1232f. *See also* Antiretroviral therapy
    in combinations, 1227, 1232f
Enuresis, 975, 976
    in diabetes insipidus, 996
    in diabetes mellitus, 1082t
    imipramine for, 966, 976
Environmental factors
    in asthma, control of, 223
    in diabetes mellitus, 1080, 1081
Environmental lung disorders, **277–282.** *See also specific disorder*
Environmental tobacco smoke. *See* Passive smoking
Enzyme inhibitors, in cancer chemotherapy, 1502–1503t
Enzyme-linked immunosorbent assay (ELISA). *See also specific disorder*
    in HIV infection/AIDS, 1217, 1217t
        blood screening and, 1207
    in Lyme disease, 1344, 1345
Eosinophil count, 1549t

Eosinophilia
    in allergic angiitis and granulomatosis (Churg-Strauss syndrome), 276
    in ascariasis, 1379
    in fascioliasis, 1375
    in hookworm disease, 1380
    in pulmonary disorders. *See* Eosinophilic pulmonary syndromes
    sputum, in asthma, 221
    in toxocariasis/visceral larva migrans, 1385
    in trichuriasis/whipworm, 1380
Eosinophilic esophagitis, 529t, **537**
Eosinophilic fasciitis, 758–759
Eosinophilic folliculitis, 123, 124, 1208
Eosinophilic gastritis, 547
Eosinophilic meningitis/meningoencephalitis
    in angiostrongyliasis, 1384
    in gnathostomiasis, 1384
Eosinophilic pulmonary syndromes, **266**
    ascariasis causing, 266, 1379
    drugs causing, 266
    filariasis causing, 266, 1386
EPA. *See* Eicosapentaenoic acid
Ependymoma, 898t, 901
Ephedra (Ma-huang), 1522
Ephedrine ("herbal ecstasy"), 1430
    safety/toxicity of, 1522
Ephelides (freckles), **100**
Epicondylitis, lateral and medial, **745**
Epidemic encephalitis, enterovirus 71 causing, 1280
Epidemic keratoconjunctivitis
    adenovirus, 154, 1275
    coxsackievirus, 1279
Epidemic louse-borne typhus, **1280–1282,** 1281t
Epidemic pleurodynia, 1279
Epidemiology of Diabetes Interventions and Complications (EDIC) study, 1087
Epidermal inclusion cysts (EIC), **141–142**
    furuncles differentiated from, 141
Epidermoid cyst, testicular, 1493
Epididymitis, 852t, **856–857,** 1182t
    chlamydial, 856, 1182t
    in filariasis, 1386
    gonococcal, 856, 1182t
Epidural abscess
    back pain and, 738, 1295
    bacterial rhinosinusitis and, 195
    otitis media and, 185
    vertebral osteomyelitis and, 781, 1295
Epidural hemorrhage
    cerebral, 918t
    spinal, 897
Epifrin. *See* Epinephrine
Epigastric pain. *See* Abdominal pain/tenderness; Dyspepsia
Epiglottitis (supraglottitis), **208,** 1289
    H influenzae causing, 1310
Epi-LASIK, 151
Epilepsia partialis continua, 911

Epilepsy, **878–884**, 879*t*, 882*t*. *See also* Seizures
  biofeedback in management of, 1538
  drug therapy for, 881–884, 882*t*. *See*
    also Anticonvulsant therapy
  idiopathic/constitutional, 878
  myoclonus/myoclonic jerks and, 910
  photosensitive, 880
  posttraumatic, 878
  pregnancy and, **724**
  surgical management of, 883
  vagal nerve stimulation in manage-
    ment of, 883
Epileptic drop attacks (atonic seizures),
  880. *See also* Seizures
Epinastine, for allergic eye disease, 155,
  173*t*
Epinephrine
  deficiency of, 993
  for desensitization reactions, 1183,
    1186
  endoscopic injection of
    for GI bleeding/peptic ulcer, 519,
      522
    for Mallory-Weiss syndrome, 537
  for glaucoma/ocular hypertension, 159
  in pheochromocytoma, 1058, 1059
  for shock, 436
Epi-pen. *See* Epinephrine
Epirubicin, 1502*t*
  for breast cancer, 665
  for gastric adenocarcinoma, 1472
  toxicity of, 1502*t*, 1511
Epistaxis, **198–199**
  cocaine abuse and, 198, 983
  in hereditary hemorrhagic telangiec-
    tasia, 198, 1519
  juvenile angiofibroma and, 200
  nasal trauma and, 198, 199
Epithelial cells/casts, in urine, 816, 817*t*
Epithelial LASIK (epi-LASIK), 151
Epivir. *See* Lamivudine
Eplerenone, 399*t*, 405, 1057
  for adrenal hyperplasia/Conn syn-
    drome, 1057
  for myocardial infarction, 335
Epley maneuver, 189
EPO. *See* Erythropoietin
Epoetin alfa. *See* Erythropoietin
Epogen (epoetin alfa). *See* Erythropoietin
Epoprostenol, for pulmonary hyperten-
  sion, 275, 381
Epothilones, in cancer chemotherapy,
  1502*t*
Eprosartan/eprosartan with hydrochloro-
  thiazide, 403*t*
Epsom salts. *See* Magnesium sulfate
Epstein-Barr virus, **1243–1245**
  Burkitt lymphoma and, 1244
  mononucleosis caused by, 1240*t*,
    1243–1244
  nasopharyngeal carcinoma and, 200,
    1244
Eptifibatide
  for acute coronary syndromes, 327*t*,
    328
  platelet function affected by, 490*t*
Epzicom. *See* Abacavir, with lamivudine

Equianalgesic dosing, 81–83*t*, 84
Equine encephalitis, 1257–1259
Equine rabies antiserum, 1256
Erb (limb-girdle) muscular dystrophy,
  934, 934*t*
Erbitux. *See* Cetuximab
ERCP. *See* Endoscopic retrograde cholangiopancreatography
Erec-Aid System. *See* Vacuum constriction
  device
Erectile dysfunction/impotence, **862–864**,
  949, 950. *See also* Sexual
    dysfunction
  in chronic kidney disease, 830
  in diabetes mellitus, 1107–1108
  drugs causing, 862
    antidepressants, 965, 967
    antipsychotics, 958
  endocrine causes of, 863
  ginseng for, 1526
  phosphodiesterase inhibitors/sildena-
    fil for, 863, 950, 1107–1108
  psychologic, 862, 863, 949
  vascular disease and, 862, 863
Erections
  loss of, 862. *See also* Erectile dysfunc-
    tion/impotence
  prolonged painful. *See* Priapism
Ergocalciferol (vitamin D₂). *See also* Vitamin D
  for hypoparathyroidism/tetany, 1032,
    1032*t*
  for osteomalacia, 1044
Ergosterol. *See* Ergocalciferol
Ergotamine
  for cluster headache, 875
  for migraine headache, 874
Ergotoxine alkaloids, for dementia, 987
Erlotinib, 1504*t*
  for lung cancer, 1456–1457
Erosive esophagitis. *See* Esophagitis
Erosive gastritis. *See* Gastritis
Erosive skin disorders, 95*t*
Ertaczo. *See* Sertaconazole
Ertapenem
  for abdominal infections, 1322*t*
  renal/hepatic failure and, 1184*t*
  for surgical site infection, 60*t*
Eructation (belching), 510–511
Eruptive psoriasis, 104. *See also* Psoriasis
Eruptive xanthoma, 1125
  in diabetes mellitus, 1083, 1109
Erysipelas, **128–129**, 1182*t*, 1290
Erysipeloid, 129
Erythemas, 95*t*, **125–130**. *See also specific*
  type
  acral (hand-foot syndrome), chemo-
    therapy-induced, 1480,
      1509
  in dermatomyositis, 760
  figurate (shaped), 95*t*
  induratum, 140
  infectiosum (parvovirus B19), 1240*t*,
    1276
  infectious, **128–130**
  marginatum, in rheumatic fever, 375
  migrans, **128**, 1343, 1345, 1346*t*. *See*
    also Lyme disease

multiforme, **127–128**
  drugs causing, 127, 148*t*
  herpes-associated, 127, 128, 1236,
    1239
  major. *See* Stevens-Johnson syn-
    drome; Toxic epidermal
      necrolysis
nodosum, **140**
  in coccidioidomycosis, 1393
  drugs causing, 140, 148*t*
  leprosum, 1327
  in sarcoidosis, 265–266
palmar
  in cirrhosis, 619
  in rheumatoid arthritis, 748
pernio (chilblain), **1405**
reactive, **125–128**
toxic, drugs causing, 148*t*
Erythrasma, 108, 136
Erythroblastosis fetalis, prevention of, **709**
Erythrocyte count
  in pleural fluid, 283, 284*t*
  reference values for, 1549*t*
Erythrocyte sedimentation rate, 1549*t*
Erythrocytes. *See also under Red cell*
  in myeloproliferative disorders, 457*t*
  in pleural fluid, 283, 284*t*
  in sickle cell syndromes, 450, 451
  in urine. *See* Hematuria; Red cell casts
Erythrocytosis, 457
  cancer-related, 1453*t*
  testosterone replacement therapy and,
    1066
Erythroderma, exfoliative, **112–113**
  drugs causing, 112, 148*t*
  psoriatic, 104, 105, 112. *See also* Psori-
    asis
Erythrodermic psoriasis, 104, 105
Erythrogenic toxin (pyrogenic erythrotoxin)
  scarlet fever caused by, 1291
  toxic shock syndrome caused by, 1291
Erythroleukemia, 465
Erythromelalgia, 783
  in essential thrombocytosis, 459
Erythromycin. *See also* Macrolides
  for acne, 97*t*, 121
  for amebiasis, 1367*t*
  for anthrax, 1301*t*
  with benzoyl peroxide, 97*t*
  for ophthalmic disorders, 173*t*
  for pharyngitis, 204–205, 1290
  renal/hepatic failure and, 1184*t*
  for surgical site infection prophylaxis,
    60*t*
  theophyllines affected by, 225*t*
Erythroplakia, **201–202**
Erythropoiesis-stimulating agents, for
  chemotherapy-associated
    anemia, 1499
Erythropoiesis-stimulating protein
  (NESP). *See* Darbepoetin
    alfa
Erythropoietin (EPO)
  in polycythemia, 457, 458
  reference values for, 1549*t*
Erythropoietin (epoetin alfa)
  for anemia of chronic disease, 442

Erythropoietin (epoetin alfa) (*cont.*)
  for anemia of chronic kidney disease, 828–829
  for chemotherapy-induced anemia, 1499, 1508*t*
  for HIV infection/AIDS, 1223
  for myelodysplasia, 463
Erythrotoxin, pyrogenic. *See* Erythrogenic toxin
ESAs. *See* Erythropoiesis-stimulating agents
Eschar formation
  in burn injury, 1410–1411
  in frostbite, 1406
Escharotomy, in burn care, 1410–1411
Escherichia coli, 1176*t*
  antibodies to, in inflammatory bowel disease, 579
  enterohemorrhagic (EHEC), 1170*t*, 1315
  enteroinvasive (EIEC), 1315
  enterotoxigenic (ETEC), 512, 1170*t*, 1172, 1315
  gastroenteritis/food poisoning caused by, 1170*t*, 1172, 1174, **1315**
  pneumonia caused by, 244*t*
Escherichia coli O157:H7, 512, 513, 1170*t*, 1172, 1315
  diarrhea caused by, 512, 513, 1170*t*, 1172, 1315
    antibiotics contraindicated in, 514, 1172, 1315
  hemolytic-uremic syndrome caused by, 485, 1315
Escitalopram, 964, 968*t*
Esclim. *See* Estradiol transdermal systems
Esidrix. *See* Hydrochlorothiazide
Esmolol
  for arrhythmias, 343*t*
    atrial fibrillation, 347
    infarct-related, 336
    paroxysmal supraventricular tachycardia, 342
  for hypertension
    in aortic dissection, 427
    urgencies/emergencies, 412, 413*t*
Esomeprazole, 550, 554. *See also* Proton pump inhibitors
Esophageal clearance, abnormal, in GERD, 531
Esophageal dilation
  for achalasia, 542
  for esophageal webs and rings, 538
  for stricture, 533
Esophageal diverticula, **538**
Esophageal dysphagia, 529, 529*t*. *See also* Dysphagia
Esophageal manometry. *See* Manometry
Esophageal motility disorders, **541–543**
  chest pain in, 543
  dysphagia in, 529, 529*t*, 543
Esophageal pH monitoring, 530
  in chronic aspiration of gastric contents, 278
  in gastroesophageal/laryngopharyngeal reflux, 209, 503, 531, 534
Esophageal (Schatzki) rings, 529*t*, **537–538**

Esophageal spasm, diffuse, 529*t*, 543
Esophageal sphincter, lower
  in achalasia, 541, 542
  chronic aspiration of gastric contents and, 278
  in GERD, 530
  hypertensive, 543
  hypotensive, 530
Esophageal varices, **538–541**
  cirrhosis and, 538, 539, 541, 620
  GI bleeding from, 517–518, 538–541
  prevention of first bleeding episode and, 541
  prevention of rebleeding from, 540–541
Esophageal webs, **537–538**
  iron deficiency anemia and (Plummer-Vinson syndrome), 440, 537
Esophagectomy
  for Barrett esophagus, 532
  for esophageal cancer, 1469
Esophagitis
  bisphosphonates and, 1040, 1045, 1046
  candidal, 535, 1390
    in HIV infection/AIDS, 1210, 1213, 1224*t*, 1390
  chest pain in, 321, 535, 536
  cytomegalovirus, 535, 1245
  eosinophilic, 529*t*, **537**
  erosive/reflux. *See also* Gastroesophageal reflux disease
    chest pain in, 321
    GERD and, 530, 531, 534
    GI bleeding and, 518
    strictures and, 533
  herpetic, 535, 1236, 1237–1239
  in HIV infection/AIDS, 1210, 1213, 1224*t*
  infectious, **535–536**
  pill-induced, **536**
Esophagogastroduodenoscopy, in cirrhosis, 620
Esophagography, barium. *See* Barium esophagography
Esophagus
  Barrett, 532
    esophageal carcinoma and, 532, 1468
  benign tumors of, **538**
  cancer of, **1465–1470**, 1467*t*
    adenocarcinoma, 1468
    Barrett esophagus and, 532, 1468
    dysphagia in, 529*t*, 1468
    incidence/mortality of, 1450, 1470
    squamous cell, 1465–1468
  disorders of, **529–544**. *See also under* *Esophageal and* Esophagitis
    benign, **536–541**
    caustic injury, **536**, 1429, 1429–1430
    chest pain in, 29, 321, 543
    GERD, **530–535**
    motility and, **541–543**
    in scleroderma, 529*t*, 758, 759
    foreign body in, **212**
  nutcracker, 543

resection of, for cancer, 1469
rupture of
  pleural effusion in, 284*t*
  vomiting and (Boerhaave syndrome), 506
sigmoid, 542
strictures of
  caustic injury causing, 536
  dysphagia in, 529*t*, 533
  peptic, 529*t*, 532–533
Espundia (mucocutaneous leishmaniasis), 1352, 1353
ESRD. *See* End-stage renal disease
Essential fatty acids, in nutritional support, 1149
Essential hypertension, 388–390. *See also* Hypertension
  in pregnancy, 391, 392, 723–724
Essential thrombocytosis, 457*t*, **459–460**
Essure, for tubal interruption, 701
Estazolam, 941*t*
Estrace. *See* Estrogen vaginal creams
Estraderm. *See* Estradiol transdermal systems
Estradiol. *See also* Ethinyl estradiol
  in estrogen replacement therapy, 703, 1070
    transdermal, 1070–1071
  reference values for, 1549*t*
  serum levels of, in menopause, 1069
Estradiol transdermal systems (skin patches), 1070–1071
Estradiol vaginal ring
  contraceptive, 698
  in estrogen replacement therapy, 704, 1071
Estradiol vaginal tablets, 1071
Estramustine, 1500*t*
Estratab. *See* Estrogens, oral
Estratest. *See* Estrogens, with methyltestosterone
Estring. *See* Estradiol vaginal ring
EstroGel. *See* Estradiol transdermal systems
Estrogen-progesterone therapy. *See* Estrogen (hormone) replacement therapy
Estrogen receptor modulators, selective (SERMs). *See* Selective estrogen receptor modulators
Estrogen (hormone) replacement therapy, 703–704, 1070–1073. *See also* Estrogens; Selective estrogen receptor modulators
  for atrophic urethritis/vaginitis, 703–704, 1071
  benefits of, 703–704, 704, 1071–1072
  breast cancer risk and, 653, 704, 1071, 1072
  endometrial hyperplasia/carcinoma and, 684, 703, 1071, 1072
  hypercalcemia/hyperparathyroidism affected by, 1038
  lipid modification/heart disease and, 704, 1072
  oral, 703–704, 1070

for osteoporosis prevention/management, 704, 1040–1041
ovarian cancer risk and, 1072
without progestins, 1071, 1072
with progestins, 703, 704, 1070, 1071, 1072–1073
risks of, 704, 1072–1073
after surgical menopause, 704
transdermal, 1070–1071
in Turner syndrome, 1074
vaginal, 704, 1071
for vasomotor symptoms of menopause, 703–704, 1071
Estrogen vaginal creams, 704, 1071
Estrogens. *See also* Estrogen (hormone) replacement therapy
for abnormal premenopausal bleeding, 675
adverse ophthalmic effects of, 177t
for bleeding in chronic kidney disease, 829
in fibrocystic breast condition, 649, 650
hypertension and, 392
in menopause, 703, 1069, 1070
with methyltestosterone, 1073
oral, 703, 703–704, 1070
in oral contraceptives, 695t
plant-derived, 1070
with progestins, 703, 704, 1070, 1071, 1072–1073
receptors for
antagonist of, in cancer chemotherapy, 1506t
in breast cancer, 663
in male, 673
prognosis and, 665t, 670
therapy and, 663, 666, 667
testicular tumors producing, 1065, 1066
transdermal, 1070–1071
in utero exposure to, testicular cancer and, 1493
vaginal, 704, 1071
Estrone, serum levels of
in menopause, 1069
in polycystic ovary syndrome, 690
Estropipate, 1070
Eszopiclone, 941t, 974
Etanercept. *See also* Anti-TNF agents
for asthma, 228
for psoriasis, 105
for rheumatoid arthritis, 751
ETEC. *See Escherichia coli*, enterotoxigenic
Ethacrynic acid, 399t
Ethambutol, 255t, 256t
adverse ophthalmic effects of, 178t
for MAC infections, 1224t, 1325
for tuberculosis, 254, 255, 255t, 256t
in pregnancy, 255, 256, 726
Ethanol (ethyl alcohol). *See also* Alcohol use/dependency/abuse
blood levels of
in acute intoxication/poisoning, 978, 1436
reference values for, 1549t
for methanol or ethylene glycol poisoning, 1424t, 1440
for thyroid nodules, 1021

Ethanol intoxication/poisoning, 978, 985t, 1427t, **1436**. *See also* Alcohol use/dependency/abuse
metabolic acidosis/osmolar gap and, 795, 979, 1426
Ethics, principles of care and, 2
Ethinyl estradiol. *See also* Estradiol; Estrogens
for emergency/postcoital contraception, 700
in estrogen replacement therapy, 1070
in oral contraceptives, 695t
in transdermal contraceptive patch, 697
in vaginal contraceptive ring, 698
Ethmoiditis/ethmoid sinusitis, 193
Ethnicity. *See* Racial/ethnic background
Ethosuximide, 882t, 1544t
Ethyl alcohol. *See* Alcohol use/dependency/abuse; Ethanol
Ethylene glycol poisoning, 1424t, 1427t, **1439–1440**
anion gap/osmolar gap in, 795, 809, 1426, 1439, 1440
hemodialysis for, 1425t, 1440
Ethylenediaminetetraacetic acid (EDTA), for lead poisoning, 846, 1438
Ethynodiol diacetate, in combination oral contraceptives, 695t
Ethyol. *See* Amifostine
Etodolac, 79t
Etonogestrel
in contraceptive implant, 697
in contraceptive vaginal ring, 698
Etopophos. *See* Etoposide
Etoposide/etoposide phosphate, 1503t
for lung cancer, 1457
Etravirine, 1227t, 1230, 1231, 1232f. *See also* Antiretroviral therapy
Etretinate, adverse ophthalmic effects of, 178t
Eucerin, 94, 99t
Eulexin. *See* Flutamide
Eumycetoma (maduromycosis), **1400–1401**
Euphoria
marijuana-induced, 983
opioid-induced, 84
EUS. *See* Endoscopic ultrasonography
Eustachian tube, **182–183**
dysfunction of, **182**
barotrauma and, 183
cholesteatoma and, 184
hearing loss and, 179, 182
in HIV infection/AIDS, 192
patulous, 182
Euthyroid sick, 1002
Euvolemic hypernatremia, 794
Euvolemic hypotonic hyponatremia, 789–791, 790f
Evans syndrome, 453
Evaporative cooling, for heat stroke, 1408
Event recording
in atrial fibrillation, 349
in seizure evaluation, 881
in syncope evaluation, 357

Evista. *See* Raloxifene
Exanthema subitum (roseola infantum), 1240t, **1247**
Exanthems, 1240t
rickettsial, 1240t
viral, 1240t, **1276–1278**
Exchange lists, diabetic diet, 1089
Exchange transfusion
for malaria, 1356
for sickle cell crises, 451
for thrombotic microangiopathies, 485
Excitement (arousal) stage of sexual activity, 948
disorders related to, 948, 949–950. *See also* Sexual dysfunction
in female, 691, 692
Exclamation hairs, in alopecia areata, 146
Executive function, impaired, dementia causing, 63
Exelderm. *See* Sulconazole
Exemestane, 668t, 1506t
Exenatide, 1091t, 1095, 1101
Exendin-4, 1095
Exercise/activity
angina precipitated by, 318
asthma/bronchoconstriction precipitated by, 216–217. *See also* Asthma
back pain and, 740
in cancer prevention, 13, 1451
in constipation management, 508
for COPD, 238
in diabetes prevention/management, 13, 1087, 1100, 1101, 1102, 1103
for fatigue/chronic fatigue syndrome, 43
in health maintenance, 3t, **12–14**
heart disease prevention and, 13
in heart failure management, 366
heart murmurs affected by, 306t
heat exposure syndromes and, 1407
hypertension/hypertension management and, 13, 390, 394, 395t
hyponatremia and, 790f, 791
migraine headache exacerbated by, 45t
in obesity management/prevention, 13, 14, 1137
for osteoarthritis, 13, 731
for osteoporosis prevention/management, 12, 13, 704, 1041
during pregnancy, 707
reduced. *See* Bed rest; Immobility
ventricular premature beats and, 351
Exercise challenge (bronchial provocation) testing, in asthma, 219
Exercise-induced asthma, 216–217. *See also* Asthma
Exercise-induced hypoglycemia, 1100, 1103
Exercise testing. *See also* Stress testing
in asthma, 219
in chest pain/angina, 318–319
echocardiography, 319
electrocardiography, 318–319

Exercise testing (*cont.*)
  before exercise program initiation, 13
  in heart failure, 360
  postinfarction, 339–340
  preoperative, 49–50, 51*f*
  radionuclide angiography, 319
  in syncope evaluation, 357
Exertional heat stroke, 1407, 1408
Exfoliative dermatitis/erythroderma, 112–113
  drugs causing, 112, 148*t*
  psoriatic, 104, 105, 112. *See also* Psoriasis
Exhibitionism, 948
Existential challenges, for terminally ill/dying patient, 92–93, 93*t*
Exophiala, phaeohyphomycosis caused by, 1402
Exophthalmos (proptosis), in dysthyroid eye/Graves disease, 170, 1008, 1009, 1012, 1014
Exostoses, ear canal, 182
Exposure (cold). *See* Cold exposure
Exposure keratitis, 156
External hordeolum (sty), 152
External otitis, 181
  earache in, 181, 186
  malignant, 181–182
External qigong, 1520
Extinction (behavior), personality disorders and, 951
Extracorporeal counterpulsation, for angina, 324
Extracorporeal shock wave lithotripsy
  for renal stones, 860
  for ureteral stones, 860
Extramammary Paget disease, 113
Extraocular movements. *See* Eye (extraocular) movements
Extrapyramidal disorders/effects
  antipsychotic drugs and, 954, 956*t*, 959, 1444–1445
  lithium and, 971
Extrasystoles. *See* Atrial (supraventricular) premature beats; Ventricular premature beats
Extrauterine pregnancy. *See* Ectopic pregnancy
Extremities
  hypothermia of, 1405–1406
  lower. *See under* Lower extremity
  swelling of, in filariasis, 1386
  traumatic injury to, complex regional pain syndrome and, 743
Extrinsic allergic alveolitis (hypersensitivity pneumonitis), 279–280, 280*t*
Exubera, 1099
Exudates, pleural fluid, 283, 283*t*, 284*t*
Eye, 151–156, 177–178*t*. *See also under* Ocular; Optic; Visual
  chemical burns involving, 172, 1429, 1430
  decontamination of, 1424
  disorders of, 151–156, 177–178*t*. *See also specific type and* Visual impairment/loss
    allergic, 155

in Behçet syndrome, 160, 772
  bisphosphonates causing, 178*t*, 1040
  in blood dyscrasias, 167
  diabetes and, 166–167, 1104–1105
  drugs (systemic) causing, 176, 177–178*t*
  dysthyroid, 170, 1008, 1009
  gonococcal, 154, 1319
  headache and, 45
  herpetic, 156, 1236
  in HIV infection/AIDS, 167–168
  hypertension and, 167
  inflammation, 153*t*. *See also* Conjunctivitis; Uveitis
  in loiasis, 1388, 1389
  management of
    ophthalmic agents in, 173–176*t*
    precautions in, 172–176
  in microsporidiosis, 1370, 1371
  in onchocerciasis, 1387, 1388
  refractive errors, 151–152
  in rheumatoid arthritis, 748
  in SLE, 753
  in syphilis, 1335
  systemic disease associations and, 166–168
  in toxocariasis/visceral larva migrans, 1385
  traumatic, 171–172
  in vitamin A deficiency, 1143
  in Wegener granulomatosis, 768
  dry (keratoconjunctivitis sicca), 154–155
    in Sjögren syndrome, 762, 763
  examination of
    after decontamination, 1424
    in diabetes patients, 166, 1105
    in glaucoma prevention, 159
    in Marfan syndrome, 1518
  foreign body in
    conjunctival/corneal, 171
    intraocular, 171
  painful. *See* Ocular/orbital pain
  systemic drugs affecting, 176, 177–178*t*
  in uremia, 826*t*
Eye (extraocular) movements
  in coma or stupor, 916
  disorders of
    in myasthenia gravis, 932
    in ocular motor palsies, 169–170
"Eye worm" (*Loa loa*), 1388–1389
Eyedrops. *See also* Ophthalmic medications
  allergic/toxic reaction to, 155, 176
  contaminated, 172–176
Eyelids
  disorders of, 152–153
  lacerations of, 171
  retraction of, in dysthyroid eye disease, 170, 1009
  seborrheic dermatitis affecting margins of, 106
  tumors of, 153
Ezetimibe, 1132, 1132*t*

ΔF508 mutation, in cystic fibrosis, 241
F cells, pancreatic, 1062

FAC regimen, for breast cancer, 666
Face. *See also under* Facial
  herpes zoster affecting. *See* Ramsay Hunt syndrome
  seborrheic dermatitis affecting, 106
Facial neuropathy, 928–929. *See also* Bell palsy
Facial pain, 876–878
  atypical, 877
  in bacterial rhinosinusitis, 193
  in rhinocerebral mucormycosis, 195
Facial paralysis/palsy, 928–929. *See also* Bell palsy
  in herpes zoster infection (Ramsay Hunt syndrome), 192, 1241
  otitis media and, 185
Facial transplantation, after burn injury, 1412
Facioscapulohumeral muscular dystrophy, 934*t*
Factitious disorders, 944–945, 945
  diarrhea, 512*t*, 515
  fever, 1154
  hypoglycemia, 1118, 1122
  thyrotoxicosis, 1008
Factiv. *See* Gemifloxacin
Factor II antibodies, 494
Factor II deficiency, 494
Factor V antibodies, 494
Factor V deficiency, 494
Factor V Leiden, deep venous thrombosis/pulmonary embolism and, 267
Factor VII deficiency, 494
Factor VIII
  acquired antibodies/inhibitors to, 491, 491–492, 494
  deficiency of
    in hemophilia, 491
    in von Willebrand disease, 493
  reference values for, 1549*t*
Factor VIII concentrate
  for hemophilia, 491, 492*t*
  for von Willebrand disease, 493
Factor IX
  deficiency of in hemophilia, 491
  inhibitor formation and, 491, 491–492
Factor IX concentrate, for hemophilia, 491, 492*t*
Factor X deficiency, 494
Factor XI deficiency, 492*t*, 493–494
Factor XII deficiency, 494
Factor XIII deficiency, 494
Factor concentrates, for hemophilia, 491, 492*t*
  disease transmission and, 491
Faget sign, 1265
Failure to thrive (unintended weight loss), in elderly, 40–41, 72
Fainting, 356, 357. *See also* Syncope
Fallot, tetralogy of, 300–301
Falls, in elderly, 68–70, 69*t*
  fear of, 69
    immobility and, 68
  prevention/injury prevention and, 18, 69–70, 69*t*
  screening for, 68, 69*t*

Famciclovir, 1238*t*
    for herpes simplex infections, 114,
            1215, 1224*t*, 1237, 1238*t*
        esophageal, 535
    for herpes zoster, 115, 157, 1215,
            1225*t*, 1238*t*
    prophylactic/suppressive, 1215, 1237
    renal/hepatic failure and, 1184*t*
Familial adenomatous polyposis, **591**
    colorectal cancer and, **591**, 1477
    genetic mutations associated with, 591
    hepatic tumors and, 591
    small intestinal adenocarcinoma and,
            1474
    small intestinal polyps and, 589, 591
Familial (benign essential) tremor,
            904–905
    parkinsonism differentiated from,
            905–906
Familial combined hyperlipidemia, 1123
Familial hemiplegic migraine, 873
Familial hypercholesterolemia, 1123
Familial hyperchylomicronemia, 1123
Familial hypocalcemia, 796*t*, 798, 1031
Familial hypocalciuric hypercalcemia,
            796*t*, 798, 801, 1034, 1036
Familial juvenile polyposis, 592
Familial Mediterranean fever, **528**
Familial melanoma, 100
Familial paraganglioma, 1058
Family/significant others, of patient at
            end of life, caring for, **89**,
            89*t*
Family counseling
    for anxiety disorders, 943
    chronic pain disorders and, 947–948
    for depression, 970
    for schizophrenic/psychotic disor-
            ders, 960
    for somatoform disorders, 945
Family planning. *See also* Contraception
    symptothermal natural, 699
Famotidine, 550. *See also* H₂ receptor
            blocking drugs
Famvir. *See* Famciclovir
Fanconi syndrome, 802, 803
Fansidar (pyrimethamine-sulfadoxine),
            1355, 1355*t*, 1359
    with amodiaquine, 1356*t*, 1359
    with artesunate, 1355*t*, 1356*t*, 1359
    for isosporiasis, 1371
    for prophylaxis in pregnancy/infants,
            1361
    resistance to, 1355, 1359
FAP. *See* Familial adenomatous polyposis
Fareston. *See* Toremifene
Farmer's lung, 280*t*
Fasciitis
    eosinophilic, 758–759
    necrotizing, 1160, 1291, 1294, 1323
        cellulitis differentiated from, 129
    palmar
        cancer and, 783
        in Dupuytren contracture, 742, 743
    plantar, **747**
Fasciola hepatica/gigantica (fascioliasis),
            1375
Fasciolopsis buski (fasciolopsiasis), 1376

Fasciotomy, in electric burns/crush inju-
            ries, 1411, 1413
Faslodex. *See* Fulvestrant
Fasting, in insulinoma diagnosis,
            1118–1119, 1119*t*
Fasting hyperglycemia, 1084
Fasting hypoglycemia, 1117, 1117*t*. *See
            also* Hypoglycemia
    postethanol, 1121
Fasting plasma glucose, 1083–1084, 1084*t*,
            1100
Fat. *See also* Lipid disorders/lipids
    body. *See* Body fat; Obesity
    dietary, 1146. *See also* Lipid disorders/
            lipids
        absorption/digestion of, 557–558
        colorectal cancer and, 1477
        lowering. *See* Lipid-lowering ther-
            apy
    fecal. *See* Fecal fat
    intravenous, in nutritional support,
            1149, 1151
Fat necrosis of breast, **651**
Fat-restricted diet, 1146. *See also* Low-fat
            diet
    for pancreatitis, 644, 647
Fatal familial insomnia (FFI), 1260
Fatigue, **41–43**, 42*f*
    in Addison disease, 1050
    in diabetes mellitus, 1082*t*
    Q fever causing, 1287
Fatty acids
    in nutritional support, 1149
    omega-3, 1528*t*, 1530–1531
Fatty liver (hepatic steatosis)
    alcoholic, 614–616
    drugs/toxins causing, 617
    hepatic failure and, 607
    hepatitis C and, 604
    nonalcoholic, **617–619**
    of pregnancy, 617, **718–719**
    in Reye syndrome. *See* Reye syndrome
FBN1 gene mutation, in Marfan syn-
            drome, 1518
5-FC. *See* Flucytosine
FE. *See* Fractional excretion
Febrile agglutinins, 1154
Fecal antigen assay, in *H pylori* infection,
            546, 549
Fecal DNA tests, in colorectal cancer
            screening, 589–590, 1481
Fecal examination. *See* Stool analysis
Fecal fat
    in diarrhea, 515
    reference values for, 1549*t*
Fecal immunochemical test (FIT)
    in colorectal cancer screening, 17*t*,
            589–590, 1481
    constipation and, 508
    in GI bleeding, 522, 523
Fecal impaction, 510
    "overflow" fecal incontinence/diar-
            rhea and, 510, 595
    urinary incontinence and, 70
Fecal incontinence, **595–596**
    biofeedback in management of, 596,
            1536*t*, 1537–1538
    fecal impaction and, 510, 595

Fecal leukocytes, in diarrhea, 513, 515, 1172
Fecal occult blood testing, 16, 17*t*, 522,
            523, 1471
    in cancer screening, 16, 17*t*, 589–590,
            1478, 1481
    in constipation, 507
    in GI bleeding, 522, 523
    in pancreatic/periampullary carci-
            noma, 1464
    in polyp identification, 589–590
Fecal osmolality, in diarrhea, 514–515, 515
Feces. *See* Stool analysis
Feeding tubes, 1147. *See also* Enteral
            nutritional support
Feet
    atherosclerotic/occlusive disease and,
            417–418
    callosities and corns of, **133**
        in diabetes/vascular disorders, 133
    in diabetes mellitus, 133, 1100,
            1108–1109
    immersion/trench, **1405**
    mycetoma affecting, 1400
    plantar fasciitis causing pain in, 747
    tinea of, **108–109**
        cellulitis and, 109, 129
    vesiculobullous dermatitis of (pom-
            pholyx), 116–117
Felbamate
    overdose/toxicity of, 882*t*, 1431
    for seizures, 881, 882*t*
Feldene. *See* Piroxicam
Feldenkrais method, 1520
Felodipine, 406*t*
    lower extremity edema caused by, 37
    overdose/toxicity of, 406*t*, 1432
Felty syndrome, 456, 748
Fem-fem bypass, for aortoiliac occlusive
            disease, 416
Female condom, 699
Female infertility. *See* Infertility
Female sex hormones. *See* Estrogens
Femara. *See* Letrozole
Femhrt. *See* Estrogens, with progestins
Femoral arteries, atherosclerotic/occlusive
            disease of, **416–417**
Femoral cutaneous nerve, lateral, lesions
            of (meralgia paresthetica),
            927–928
Femoral neuropathy/femoral nerve palsy,
            927
Femoral-popliteal bypass, 417
Femoral pulses, in aortoiliac occlusive dis-
            ease, 416
FemPatch. *See* Estradiol transdermal sys-
            tems
Femring. *See* Estradiol vaginal ring
Femtosecond laser assisted LASIK
            (IntraLASIK), 151
Fenofibrate, 1131–1132, 1132*t*
Fenofibric acid, 1132*t*
Fenoldopam, for hypertensive urgencies/
            emergencies, 412, 413*t*
Fenoprofen, 79*t*
Fentanyl/fentanyl oral transmucosal and
            buccal/fentanyl transder-
            mal, 78, 81*t*, 84
    overdose/toxicity of, 1442–1443

Fentora. *See* Fentanyl
FEP. *See* Free erythrocyte protoporphyrin
Ferric gluconate. *See* Iron, supplementary
Ferriman-Gallwey scale, 1053
Ferritin, 439
   in anemia of chronic disease, 442
   in hemochromatosis, 627, 628
   in iron deficiency anemia, 440
   reference values for, 1549*t*
   in Still disease, 751
Ferroprotein, in hemochromatosis, 627
Ferrous sulfate. *See* Iron, supplementary
Fertility awareness, contraception based
   on, **699–700**
Fertility disorders. *See* Infertility
Fertilization, in vitro, 694, 866
Fetal alcohol syndrome, 707, 979
Fetal fibronectin, in false versus true labor,
   719
Fetal hemoglobin. *See* Hemoglobin F
Fetal lung maturity
   delivery in preeclampsia/eclampsia
      and, 717
   delivery in third-trimester bleeding
      and, 720
   preterm labor and, 719
Fetal monitoring
   in diabetes, 723
   in preeclampsia-eclampsia, 717, 718
   in third-trimester bleeding, 720
Fetal-placental unit, in preeclampsia-
      eclampsia, 717*t*
Fetal testing. *See* Prenatal testing/diagno-
      sis
α-Fetoprotein. *See* Alpha-fetoprotein
Fetotoxic drugs, 706*t*
Fetus. *See also* Pregnancy
   hepatitis transmission to, 602, 606,
      726–727
   HIV transmission to, 726, 1207, 1221
   radiation affecting, 1414
   rubella affecting, 1254, 1255
   toxoplasmosis transmission to, 1363,
      1365
   VZV transmission to, 725
FEV$_1$ (forced expiratory volume in first
      second)
   in asthma, 217*f*, 218*t*, 219, 219*t*
      bronchial provocation testing and,
      219
      exacerbation classification/man-
      agement and, 218*t*, 219*t*,
      230, 232*f*
   in COPD, 234
   lung cancer surgery and, 1455–1456
   preoperative, 53
FEV$_1$/FVC ratio
   in asthma, 217*f*, 219
   in COPD, 234
Fever, **38–40**, 39*t*
   acute, 1160
   in acute bacterial diarrhea/food poi-
      soning, 1170–1171*t*
   in autoimmune disorders, 1153
   bleomycin causing, 1510–1511
   cancer-related, 1153, 1154, 1453*t*
   in critically ill patient, 1160, 1161
   drug user presenting with, 1169

factitious (self-induced), 1154
giant cell arteritis and, 766–767
in HIV infection/AIDS, 1153, 1154,
   1209
hospital-associated, 1153
infection causing, 38, 39, 1154
   in malaria, 1354, 1355
   in neutropenic patient, 456, 1153,
      1154, 1498
      antimicrobial therapy and, 40,
      1158, 1181*t*, 1498
   postoperative, 1160
   in pulmonary embolism, 268*t*
   in serum sickness, 785
   in Still disease, 751
   subacute, 1160
   theophyllines affected by, 225*t*
   thromboembolic disease causing,
      1160
   in thrombotic microangiopathies,
      485, 485*t*
   travel and, 1173
   of unknown/undetermined origin
      (FUO), 39, 39*t*, **1153–1155**
      in giant cell arteritis, 766–767
Fever/cold sore (herpes simplex),
      113–114, 1235–1236. *See*
      also Herpes simplex infec-
      tion
FFI. *See* Fatal familial insomnia
FGF-23, 802. *See also* Phosphatonin
FHM. *See* Familial hemiplegic migraine
Fiber, dietary, 508, 509*t*, 1146
   for anal fissures, 596
   in colorectal cancer prevention, 1477
   constipation and, 508, 509*t*
   in diabetes mellitus, 1089–1090
   diverticulosis and, 587, 588
   for hemorrhoids, 593–594
   for irritable bowel syndrome, 571
   lipid-modifying effects of, 1130
   for urinary stone disease, 857
Fiber laxatives, 508, 509*t*
Fibric acid derivatives (fibrates), for lipid
      modification/heart disease
      prevention, 1131–1132
Fibrillation. *See* Atrial fibrillation; Ven-
      tricular fibrillation
Fibrillin gene mutation, in Marfan syn-
      drome, 1518
Fibrin D-dimer
   in deep venous thrombosis/pulmo-
      nary embolism, 30, 267,
      270, 271*f*
   in DIC, 487
   reference values for, 1549*t*
Fibrinogen
   in DIC, 487
   reference values for, 1549*t*
   replacement. *See* Cryoprecipitate
Fibroadenoma of breast, **650–651**
Fibroblast growth factor 23, 802. *See also*
      Phosphatonin
Fibrocystic breast condition, **649–650**
   breast cancer risk and, 649, 653
   nipple discharge in, 649, 651
Fibroelastoma, valvular papillary, 383
Fibrogenesis imperfecta ossium, 1043

Fibroid tumor of uterus, **683–684**
Fibromuscular dysplasia/hyperplasia
   renal artery stenosis and, 391, 832, 833
   transient ischemic attacks and, 886
Fibromyalgia, **741–742**
   mind-body therapies for, 1536*t*
      meditation, 1536*t*, 1541
Fibronectin, fetal, in false versus true
      labor, 719
Fibrosing cholestatic hepatitis, 610
FibroSure score, in cirrhosis, 620
Field defects/loss. *See* Visual field defects/
      loss; Visual impairment/
      loss
Fifth disease (erythema infectiosum),
      1240*t*, 1276
Figurate ("shaped") erythema, 95*t*. *See*
      also specific type and
      Erythemas
Filariasis, **1386–1389**
   eosinophilic pulmonary syndromes
      and, 266, 1386
   loiasis, **1388–1389**
   lymphatic, **1386–1387**
   onchocerciasis, **1387–1388**
Filgrastim (G-CSF)
   for chemotherapy-induced toxicity,
      666, 1499, 1508*t*
   for HIV infection/AIDS, 1223
   for neutropenia, 456, 1499
Finasteride (5-alpha-reductase inhibitor)
   for androgenetic (pattern) baldness,
      145
   for benign prostatic hyperplasia, 869*t*,
      870
   for hirsutism/virilization, 1055
   for urinary incontinence, 72
Fine-needle aspiration biopsy, thyroid,
      1003*t*, 1012, 1019*t*, 1020
   in thyroiditis, 1017
Fine-needle aspiration cytology
   for breast lump evaluation, 649, 658.
      See also Breast, biopsy of
   in lung cancer, 1454
Fingernails, disorders of. *See* Nail disor-
      ders
Fingers
   in pompholyx (vesiculobullous hand
      eczema), 117
   in Raynaud phenomenon, 756
   thromboangiitis obliterans (Buerger
      disease) involving, 422
Firearms
   preventable deaths caused by, 2*t*
   prevention of injury caused by, 18
First-degree burn, 1409
First-degree heart block, 355
   in myocardial infarction, 337
First heart sound (S$_1$). *See* Heart sounds
Fish. *See also* Shellfish
   anisakiasis and, 1385
   clonorchiasis/opisthorchiasis and,
      1375
   gnathostomiasis and, 1384
   health benefits of, 1530–1531
   intestinal flukes and, 1376
   poisoning caused by, **1446**, 1446*t*
FISH. *See* Fluorescent in situ hybridization

Fish oil. *See* Omega-3 fatty acids
Fish tapeworm *(D latum)*, 1376, **1376**
  vitamin B$_{12}$ deficiency and, 445, 1376
Fistula in ano, 596
Fistulas
  in Crohn disease, 578, 579
  in diverticulitis, 588
  perianal, 596
  perilymphatic, 183, 190, 191*t*
FIT. *See* Fecal immunochemical test
Fitz-Hugh and Curtis syndrome, 688
5q– syndrome, 463
Fixed drug eruptions, 149*t*
Flagellates, intestinal, **1372**. *See also spe-
    cific type*
Flagyl. *See* Metronidazole
Flail leaflet, 309
Flame (clothing) burns, electrical, 1413
Flank pain
  in polycystic kidney disease, 847
  in renal cell carcinoma, 1491
  in urinary stone disease, 857
Flash (arcing) burns, 1413
Flashbacks, psychedelic drug use and, 982
Flashing lights (photopsia), in migraine
    headache, 873
Flatus, 511
  in lactase deficiency, 511, 563
Flavopiridol, for chronic lymphocytic leu-
    kemia, 468
Fleas
  in bacillary angiomatosis, 1215, 1321
  in California rickettsiosis, 1281*t*
  in endemic typhus, 1281*t*, **1282–1283**
  in plague, 1318
  skin lesions caused by, 139
Flecainide, 343*t*
  for atrial fibrillation, 348, 349
  overdose/toxicity of, 343*t*, 1445
FleetsPhospho-soda. *See* Sodium phos-
    phate
Flexible sigmoidoscopy. *See* Sigmoidos-
    copy
Fliers. *See* Air travel
Flies
  in African trypanosomiasis, 1348
  in amebiasis, 1365
  in leishmaniasis, 1351, 1353
  in loiasis, 1388
  in onchocerciasis, 1387, 1388
Floaters, in vitreous hemorrhage, 162
Flolan. *See* Epoprostenol
Floppy mitral valve. *See* Mitral valve pro-
    lapse
Flower cells, in adult T cell lymphoma/
    leukemia, 1261
Floxin. *See* Ofloxacin
FLT3 gene, in acute leukemia, 465
Flu. *See* Influenza
Flu shots. *See* Influenza virus vaccine
Fluconazole, 107, 1401*t*
  for candidiasis
    disseminated disease, 1391
    esophageal, 535, 1224*t*, 1390
    funguria, 1391
    oral, 202, 1223, 1390
    vulvovaginal, 125, 1223, 1224*t*,
      1390

for coccidioidomycosis, 1393,
    1393–1394
for cryptococcal meningitis,
    1222–1223, 1224*t*,
    1396–1397
prophylactic, 1158, 1223
renal/hepatic failure and, 1184*t*
Flucytosine, 1401*t*
  for chromoblastomycosis, 1400
  for cryptococcal meningitis, 1224*t*,
    1397
  renal/hepatic failure and, 1184*t*
Fludara. *See* Fludarabine
Fludarabine, 1501*t*
  for chronic lymphocytic leukemia,
    467
Fludrocortisone
  for adrenal insufficiency/Addison dis-
    ease, 1050
  for renal tubular acidosis, 811
Fluid and electrolyte disorders, **788–815**.
    See also specific type
  assessment of, **788**, 789*t*
  in diabetic ketoacidosis, 1113
Fluid management/hydration, **815**, 815*t*.
    See also Water/fluid intake
  in ARDS, 292
  in burns, 1410, **1410–1411**
  in cholera, 1315
  for diabetic ketoacidosis, 1114
  for diarrhea/gastroenteritis, 514, 815*t*,
    1172
  for electrical injury, 1413
  in GI bleeding/variceal hemorrhage,
    518, 539
  gout and, 734
  for heat exposure syndromes, 1407
  for hypercalcemia, 1037, 1497
  for hyperglycemic hyperosmolar state,
    1015–1016
  for hypernatremia, 794
  hyponatremia and, 789, 792
  hypotension in poisoning/drug over-
    dose and, 1421
  in hypothermia, 1404
  in malaria (severe infection), 1356
  for methotrexate toxicity, 1510
  in nausea and vomiting, 506
  nutritional support and, 1148
  for pancreatitis, 644
  in protein-energy malnutrition, 1135
  for rhabdomyolysis, 764
  for saline-responsive metabolic alka-
    losis, 813
  in shock, 436
  for terminally ill/dying patient, **91**
  for tumor lysis syndrome/hyperurice-
    mia, 1497
  water deficit calculation and, 794
Fluid volume alterations. *See also* Dehy-
    dration
  hyperosmolality with and without,
    795
  overload, **794–795**
  saline-responsive metabolic alkalosis
    and, 812
Flukes, infections caused by, **1373–1376**.
    See also specific type

blood flukes (schistosomiasis),
    1373–1375
liver/lung/intestinal flukes, **1375–1376**
Flumazenil
  for benzodiazepine overdose/coma,
    942, 1421, 1424*t*, 1436
  for hepatic encephalopathy, 623
Flunisolide, for asthma, 226*t*
Fluocinolone, 96*t*, 1077*t*
Fluocinonide, 96*t*
Fluorescent in situ hybridization (FISH),
    for HER-2/*neu* assessment
    in breast cancer, 663
Fluorescent treponemal antibody absorp-
    tion (FTA-ABS) test. *See*
    FTA-ABS test
Fluorometholone, 1077*t*
  for ophthalmic disorders, 174*t*
Fluoroquinolones
  for anthrax, 1301, 1302
  for diarrhea, 514
  for pneumonia, 247
Fluorouracil, 1502*t*. *See also* CMF regimen
  for actinic keratoses, 113
  adverse ophthalmic effects of, 178*t*
  for colorectal cancer, 1479, 1480
  for gastric adenocarcinoma, 1472
Fluoxetine, 964, 966, 968*t*. *See also* Seroto-
    nin-selective reuptake
    inhibitors
  contraindications to in elderly, 66
  lithium interactions and, 972*t*
  for migraine prophylaxis, 874*t*
  for OCD, 943
  overdose/toxicity of, 966, 968*t*
  for psychosexual disorders, 950
Fluoxymesterone, 1065
Fluphenazine, 954, 955*t*, 956*t*. *See also*
    Antipsychotic drugs
  enanthate or decanoate forms of,
    957–958
Fluprednisolone, 1077*t*
Flurandrenolide, 97*t*, 103
Flurandrenolone, 1077*t*
Flurazepam, 941–942, 941*t*, 974
Flurbiprofen, 79*t*
  for ophthalmic disorders, 174*t*
Flutamide, 1505*t*
  for hirsutism/virilization, 1055
  for prostate cancer, 1487*t*
Fluticasone, for asthma, 226*t*
  with salmeterol, 224*t*
Flutter valve breathing devices
  for bronchiectasis, 240
  for chronic bronchitis, 238
  for cystic fibrosis, 242
Fluvastatin, 1131, 1132*t*. *See also* Statin
    drugs
Fluvoxamine, 964, 966, 968*t*. *See also*
    Serotonin-selective reup-
    take inhibitors
  overdose/toxicity of, 966, 968*t*
"Fly agaric" (anticholinergic-type) mush-
    room poisoning, 1441,
    1441*t*, 1442
Flying. *See* Air travel
FML/FML Forte/FML S.O.P. *See* Fluo-
    rometholone

FMR1 gene, in fragile X mental retardation, 1515

FNA cytology, for breast lump evaluation, 649, 658. *See also* Breast, biopsy of

Foam sclerotherapy, for varicose veins, 428–429

FOBT. *See* Fecal occult blood testing

Focal nodular hyperplasia of liver, 633

Focal segmental glomerular sclerosis, 839*t*, **841**

Focal seizures. *See* Partial (focal) seizures; Seizures

Focal torsion dystonia, **910**

Folate. *See* Folic acid

Foley catheter
  fluid resuscitation in burn care and, 1410
  hospital-associated urinary tract infection and, 1159, 1161
  in shock management, 435

FOLFIRI regimen, 1479

FOLFOX regimen, 1479

Folic acid (folate), 446
  antagonists of in cancer chemotherapy, 1501*t*. *See also* Methotrexate
  deficiency of, **446–447**, 446*t*
    hereditary spherocytosis and, 448
    in homocystinuria/hyperhomocysteinemia, 1516
    in pregnancy, 721
    thrombocytopenia and, 482
  inhibition of synthesis of, for malaria, 1359
  reference values for, 1550*t*
  supplementary, 446, 447
    in colorectal cancer prevention, 586, 1477
    hearing loss and, 75
    for hemoglobin H disease, 444
    for hereditary spherocytosis, 448
    for homocystinuria/hyperhomocysteinemia, 1516, 1517
    in pregnancy, 708–709

Folinic acid (leucovorin) rescue
  with 5-fluorouracil, 1479, 1507*t*
  with methotrexate, 750, 1507*t*, 1510
  with pyrimethamine, 1224*t*, 1365

Follicle-stimulating hormone (FSH)
  in amenorrhea, 1067–1068, 1068, 1069
  deficiency of, 991–992, 1063. *See also* Hypogonadism
  in hirsutism/virilization, 1054
  in hypogonadism, 991–992, 1063, 1065
  in infertility workup, 693, 864, 865*f*
  for male infertility, 994
  in menopause, 703, 1069
  in polycystic ovary syndrome, 690, 1053, 1054
  reference values for, 1550*t*

Follicular lymphoma, 469

Folliculitis, **123–124**, 1294
  acne and, 120, 123, 124
  eosinophilic, 123, 124, 1208
  in HIV infection/AIDS, 123, 1215
  nasal vestibulitis and, 195
  steroid (steroid acne), 120, 123

Follitropins, for male infertility, 994

Fomepizole, for methanol or ethylene glycol poisoning, 1424*t*, 1440

Fomivirsen, 1238*t*

Fondaparinux, 496*t*, 497*t*
  for acute coronary syndromes, 327
  after thrombolytic therapy for myocardial infarction, 334

Fonsecaea pedrosoi, chromoblastomycosis caused by, 1400

Food
  allergy/intolerance to
    anaphylaxis caused by, 784
    atopy and, 784
      food allergy and, 101
    dyspepsia caused by, 502
  aspiration of (café coronary), **277**
  contaminated. *See specific disease and* Food poisoning
  esophageal foreign body, 212
  inadequate, in protein-energy malnutrition, 1134
  MAOI interactions and, 967*t*, 1440
  supplementing oral intake and, 1147. *See also* Nutritional support
  theophyllines affected by, 225*t*
  withholding, in terminally ill/dying patient, 91

Food poisoning, 1170–1171*t*, 1172. *See also* Gastroenteritis
  botulism, **933–934**, 1170*t*, 1299, 1300
  seafood contamination/toxicity and, **1446**, 1446*t*
  vibrios causing, 1170*t*, 1172, 1316

Foot. *See* Feet

Foramen ovale, patent, **297–298**

Forced diuresis, in poisoning/drug overdose, 1425

Forced expiratory volume in one second. *See* FEV$_1$

Forced expiratory volume in one second/forced vital capacity ratio. *See* FEV$_1$/FVC ratio

Forced vital capacity. *See* FVC

Forced vital capacity/forced expiratory volume in one second ratio. *See* FEV$_1$/FVC ratio

Foreign body
  aspiration of, 212. *See also* Aspiration
  retention and, **278**
  conjunctival/corneal, **171**
  in ear canal, 181
  esophageal, 212
  intraocular, 171
  in trachea and bronchi, **212**
  in upper aerodigestive tract, **212**

Formaldehyde, marijuana soaked in ("AMP"), 983

Formoterol, for asthma, 224*t*, 227
  with budesonide, 224*t*

Fortaz. *See* Ceftazidime

Forteo. *See* Teriparatide

Fortovase. *See* Saquinavir

Fosamprenavir, 1226*t*, 1229, 1229–1230, 1232*f*. *See also* Antiretroviral therapy
  with ritonavir, 1229

Fosaprepitant, 506

Foscarnet, 1238*t*
  for cytomegalovirus infection, 167, 1224*t*, 1238*t*, 1246
  for herpes simplex infections, 1224*t*, 1238*t*
    esophageal, 535
  for herpes zoster, 115, 1225*t*, 1238*t*, 1242
  renal/hepatic failure and, 1184*t*

Foscavir. *See* Foscarnet

Fosfomycin, renal/hepatic failure and, 1184*t*

Fosinopril, 403*t*

Fosphenytoin, 884

Fourth heart sound (S$_4$/atrial gallop). *See* Heart sounds

Fourth nerve paralysis, 169

Fractional excretion, 788
  of magnesium, in hypomagnesemia, 805
  of sodium, in acute kidney injury, 820, 820*t*

Fracture-dislocation, spinal, 919

Fractures. *See also under* Bone
  in elderly, falls and, 18, 68, 69
  in hypercalcemia/hyperparathyroidism, 1033, 1035
  in osteomalacia, 1043
  in osteoporosis, 12, 1038, 1039
    prevention of, 12, 704
  in Paget disease of bone, 1045
  pathologic. *See* Pathologic fractures
  skull, **918**

Fragile X mental retardation, **1515**

Fragile X tremor-ataxia syndrome, 1515

Fragility fractures. *See* Pathologic fractures

Fragmin. *See* Dalteparin

Frailty, in elderly, **72**

Frambesia (yaws), 1177*t*, **1339**

Framingham projections, 1126, 1127–1128*t*

Francisella tularensis (tularemia), 1177*t*, **1317–1318**

Freckles (ephelides), **100**

Free erythrocyte protoporphyrin, 1550*t*

Free-living amebas. *See* Amebas

Free thyroxine assay (FT$_4$), 1003*t*
  factors affecting, 1002
  in hyperthyroidism, 1010
    amiodarone-induced, 1010
    during pregnancy, 722, 1010
    thyroiditis and, 1017
    after treatment, 1011, 1012
  in hypothyroidism, 1005
  reference values for, 1554*t*
  in thyroid cancer surveillance, 1026
  in thyroid nodules, 1020

Free thyroxine index (FT$_4$I), factors affecting, 1002

Free triiodothyronine, 1003*t*

Frequency, urinary. *See* Irritative voiding symptoms

Fresh-frozen plasma, transfusion of, **478–479**
  for cirrhosis-related bleeding, 495, 623
  for DIC, 488, 488*t*

for GI bleeding/variceal hemorrhage, 519, 539
for platelet disorders, 492t
for thrombotic microangiopathies, 485
Fresh whole blood, transfusion of, 476
Friction rubs. *See* Pericardial friction rub; Pleural friction rub
Fried rice, *Bacillus cereus* contamination of, 1172
Friedreich ataxia, 923
Frigidity, 949
Frontal lobe lesions, 898–899
Frontal sinusitis, 193
Frontotemporal dementias, 64
Frostbite, 1405, **1405–1406**
Raynaud phenomenon and, 757
Frostnip, **1405**
Frovatriptan, for migraine headache, 874
Frozen red cells, transfusion of, 477
Frozen shoulder, 744
Fructosamine, serum levels of
in diabetes mellitus, 1085
normal/reference values for, 1085, 1550t
Fructose
for diabetics, 1090
in ejaculate, in infertility workup, 865f
intolerance to, flatus caused by, 511
FSH. *See* Follicle-stimulating hormone
FT₃. *See* Free triiodothyronine
FT₄. *See* Free thyroxine assay
FT₄I. *See* Free thyroxine index
FTA-ABS test, 1331t, 1332
in HIV infection/AIDS, 1220
for neurosyphilis, 1337
FTO gene, in type 2 diabetes, 1081
FU. *See* Fluorouracil
Fucithalmic. *See* Fusidic acid
Fugue, 940
Fukuda test, 188
Full liquid diet, 1145
Full-thickness burn, survival and, 1409
Fulminant ulcerative colitis, 583, 585
Fulvestrant, 668t, 669, 1506t
Fumagillin, for microsporidiosis, 1371
Functional alimentary hypoglycemia, 1117, 1117t, **1121**
Functional capacity/status, assessment of
in elderly, 61–62, 63
Functional (nonulcer) dyspepsia, 503
Functional hyperventilation. *See* Hyperventilation
Functional proteinuria, 816
Fundoplication
for erosive esophagitis/GERD, 534
with myotomy, for achalasia, 542
Fungal infections, **1390–1402**. *See also* specific type
of bones and joints, **781**
drugs for, 1401t, **1402**. *See also* Antifungal agents
in HIV infection/AIDS
otologic, 191–192
rashes, 1215
invasive, sinusitis, **195–196**
keratitis, **157**
myocarditis in, 369t

opportunistic, 1390, 1398–1399, **1402**
prevention of, 1222–1223
superficial, **107–110**. *See also* Tinea
Fungemia
in candidiasis, 125, 1391
in coccidioidomycosis, 1393
Funguria, candidal (candiduria), 1390–1391
FUO. *See* Fever, of unknown/undetermined origin
Furazolidone, for giardiasis, 1372
Furosemide. *See also* Diuretics; Loop diuretics
in acute tubular necrosis, 823
for cirrhotic ascites, 621
for heart failure, 361
for hypercalcemia, 801
for hypertension, 399t
urgencies/emergencies, 412, 413t
hypokalemia and, 796
for pulmonary edema, 367–368
Furuncles/furunculosis, **140–141**, 1182t, 1294
in HIV infection/AIDS, 1215
Fusarium, in opportunistic infection, 1402
Fusidic acid, for ophthalmic disorders, 173t
Fusion inhibitors. *See* Entry inhibitors
Fusobacteria/*Fusobacterium necrophorum*, 1321, 1322
Fuzeon. *See* Enfuvirtide
FVC (forced vital capacity)
in asthma, 219
in COPD, 234
in cystic fibrosis, 241
ratio of to forced expiratory volume in one second. *See* FEV₁/FVC ratio
FXTAS (fragile X tremor-ataxia syndrome), 1515

G6PD deficiency. *See* Glucose-6-phosphate dehydrogenase deficiency
G20210A prothrombin mutation
in hepatic vein obstruction (Budd-Chiari syndrome), 630
in noncirrhotic portal hypertension, 631
GA. *See* Tabun poisoning
GABA. *See* Gamma-aminobutyric acid
Gabapentin, 881, 882t. *See also* Anticonvulsant therapy
for menopausal symptoms, 704, 1070
for neuropathic pain/painful diabetic neuropathy, 85, 85t, 1107
overdose/toxicity of, 882t, 1431
for phobic disorder, 943
for postherpetic neuralgia, 115–116, 878, 1242
for seizures, 881, 882t
GABHS. *See* Group A β-hemolytic streptococcal infection
GAD 65 antibodies, in type 1 diabetes, 1080, 1080t
Gadolinium, nephrogenic systemic fibrosis caused by, 849

Gait/gait disorders. *See also* Falls
in elderly, **68–70**, 69t
screening for, 68, 69t
in parkinsonism, 905
in spinal stenosis, 740
in tabes dorsalis, 1336
Galactomannan, in invasive aspergillosis, 1398
Galactorrhea, 1000, 1001
α-D-Galactosidase enzyme (Beano), for gastrointestinal gas, 511
Galantamine, for dementia, 65, 987
Galerina (amatoxin/aminitin toxin) mushroom poisoning, 1441, 1441t, 1442
Gallaverdin phenomenon, 310
Gallbladder
carcinoma of, 1462, 1463
cholesterolosis of, 635t, 636
disorders of
in clonorchiasis/opisthorchiasis, 1375
during pregnancy, **727–728**
gangrene of, 636
hydrops of, 636
porcelain, 635t, 636, 1462
removal of. *See* Cholecystectomy
stones in. *See* Cholelithiasis
strawberry, 636
Gallium nitrate, for cancer-related hypercalcemia/toxicity/bone pain, 1497
Gallium scanning, in infectious myocarditis, 369
Gallstone ileus, 634
Gallstones. *See* Cholelithiasis
GalNac-Gd1a antibodies, in Guillain-Barré syndrome, 925
Gamete intrafallopian transfer (GIFT), 694
Gamma-aminobutyric acid (GABA), in Huntington disease, 909
Gamma-globin, in sickle cell syndromes, 450
Gamma globulin
intravenous. *See* Intravenous immune globulin
serum
in autoimmune hepatitis, 613
in cirrhosis, 620
Gamma-glutamyl transpeptidase (GGTP) levels
alcohol use/abuse and, 979
in liver disease/jaundice, 600
reference values for, 1550t
Gamma-hydroxybutyrate, overdose/toxicity of, **1437**
Cushing syndrome and, 1052
Gamma-hydroxybutyrolactone, overdose/toxicity of, 1437
Gamma interferon. *See* Interferon-γ
Gamma knife radiation/gamma radiosurgery
for acromegaly, 999
for intracranial arteriovenous malformations, 896
for pituitary adenoma, 994, 999, 1002, 1052

Gamma knife radiation/gamma radiosurgery (*cont.*)
for thyroid cancer brain metastases, 1026
for trigeminal neuralgia, 877
Gammopathy, monoclonal. *See* Monoclonal gammopathy
Ganciclovir, 1238*t*
for cytomegalovirus infection, 167, 1157, 1222, 1224*t*, 1238*t*, 1246
renal/hepatic failure and, 1184*t*
Ganfort. *See* Bimatoprost/timolol
Ganglioneuromas, in multiple endocrine neoplasia, 1076*t*, 1077
Gangrene
bacterial synergistic, 1323
of feet, in diabetes mellitus, 1108–1109
of gallbladder, 636
gas, 1177*t*, **1297**
Gardasil. *See* Human papillomavirus (HPV) vaccine
Gardner syndrome, epidermal inclusion cysts in, 142
Gardnerella infection (bacterial vaginosis), 678, 679, 1167
rape/sexual assault in transmission of, 1167
Garlic, 1523*t*, 1524
Gas, gastrointestinal, **510–511**
Gas gangrene, 1177*t*, **1297**
Gasoline, sniffing, 984
Gastrectomy
for carcinoids, 1474
for gastric cancer, 1472
hypoglycemia after, 1117, 1117*t*, **1121**
vitamin B_{12} deficiency and, 445
Gastric acid/gastric contents
aspiration of. *See also* Aspiration
acute (Mendelson syndrome), **278**, 1160
chronic, **278**
in comatose patient, 1420
health care-associated pneumonia and, 248
hypersecretion of, in Zollinger-Ellison syndrome/gastrinoma, 556
inhibition of secretion of. *See* Acid-antisecretory agents; Antacids; H_2 receptor blocking drugs; Proton pump inhibitors
radiation affecting secretion of, 1414
reflux of. *See* Gastric acid refluxate; Gastroesophageal reflux disease
Gastric acid refluxate. *See also* Gastroesophageal reflux disease
abnormal clearance of, 531
irritant effects of, 531
Gastric banding surgery, for obesity, 15, 1138
Gastric bypass, for obesity, 15, 1138
hypoglycemia after, 1117, 1121
Gastric cancer, 1467*t*, **1470–1474**
adenocarcinoma, **1470–1473**
H pylori infection and, 546

pernicious anemia gastritis and, 547, 1471
carcinoid tumors, **1473–1474**, 1475
dyspepsia in, 502
GI bleeding in, 518, 1471
H pylori gastritis and, 546, 1471
lymphoma, **1473**
H pylori infection and, 546, 1473
mesenchymal tumors, **1474**
peptic ulcer disease and, 553, 1471–1472
pernicious anemia gastritis and, 547, 1471
Gastric emptying
delayed, in GERD, 531
in poisoning/drug overdose, 1424
Gastric lavage, for poisoning/drug overdose, 1424–1425
Gastric mucosal biopsy, in gastric adenocarcinoma, 1471
Gastric neoplasms
benign, **557**
malignant. *See* Gastric cancer
Gastric outlet obstruction
in peptic ulcer disease, **555**
vomiting and, 504, 505*t*, 555
Gastric pH
health care-associated pneumonia and, 248
in Zollinger Ellison syndrome/gastrinoma, 556
Gastric polyps, 557, 591
Gastric ulcers, 547–553. *See also* Peptic ulcer disease
gastric cancer and, 553, 1471–1472
refractory, 553, 1472
Gastric varices, GI bleeding from, in portal hypertension, 517–518
Gastrin
D cells secreting, 1062
hypersecretion of
carcinoid tumors and, 1473, 1474
in pernicious anemia gastritis, 547
in Zollinger-Ellison syndrome/gastrinoma, 556, 1062
proton pump inhibitors affecting, 550, 556
reference values for, 1550*t*
Gastrinoma (Zollinger-Ellison syndrome), **556–557**, 1062
carcinoid tumors and, 1474
in multiple endocrine neoplasia, 556, 1062, 1076
peptic ulcer disease and, 552, 553, 556
refractory GERD and, 534, 556
Gastritis, **544–547**. *See also* Gastropathy
alcoholic, 544, 545
in anisakiasis, 547, 1385
atrophic
H pylori infection and, 547
in pernicious anemia, 547
cytomegalovirus, 547, 1245
eosinophilic, 547
erosive/hemorrhagic, **544–545**
GI bleeding and, 518, 544
H pylori, 546
gastric cancer and, 546, 1471
nonerosive/nonspecific, **546–547**

NSAID, 544, 545
in pernicious anemia, 547
phlegmonous/necrotizing, 547
stress, 544, 544–545
Gastroduodenal surgery, antibiotic prophylaxis for, 60*t*
Gastroenteritis, 1182*t*. *See also* Diarrhea
adenovirus causing, 1172, 1275
amebic (intestinal amebiasis), 512, 514, 515, 1172, 1174, 1366, 1367, 1367*t*
appendicitis differentiated from, 568
Bacillus cereus causing, 512, 1170*t*, 1172
campylobacter, 512, 1171*t*, 1172, 1174, 1182*t*, 1316
Guillain-Barré syndrome and, 925
clostridial, 511, 512, 1170*t*, 1172
coccidial and microsporidial, 1369–1371
E coli causing, 512, 513, 1170*t*, 1172, 1315
food-borne. *See* Food poisoning
hypokalemia and, 795
in immunocompromised host/HIV infection/AIDS, 511, 515, 516, 1214, 1369–1371
irritable bowel syndrome and, 570
in measles, 1249
nausea/vomiting in, 504, 505*t*
Norwalk virus causing, 1172, 1278
reactive arthritis and, 776
rotaviruses causing, 1171*t*, 1172, 1278
salmonella causing, 512, 1171*t*, 1172, 1174, 1182*t*, 1312, **1314**
shigella causing (shigellosis), 512, 1171*t*, 1172, 1174, 1182*t*, 1314
staphylococcal, 512, 1170*t*, 1172
viral, 1172, **1278**. *See also specific virus*
Yersinia enterocolitica causing, 512, 1171*t*, 1172
Gastroesophageal junction
mucosal laceration of. *See* Mallory-Weiss syndrome/tears
stricture at. *See* Esophagus, strictures of
Gastroesophageal reflux disease (GERD), **530–535**
alarm features/troublesome symptoms and, 531, 533
Barrett esophagus and, 532
chest pain in, 531, 543
chronic gastric aspiration and, 278
cough and, 22, 23, 23*t*, 531
dyspepsia in, 502, 531
erosive (reflux) esophagitis/GI bleeding and, 518, 530, 531, 534
esophageal webs and rings and, 537
extraesophageal manifestations of, 531, 533–534
heartburn in, 529, 531
laryngopharyngeal reflux and, **208–209**
peptic stricture and, 532–533
Gastrointestinal adenocarcinoma, **1474**

Gastrointestinal bleeding, **517–524,**
   553–555. *See also specific*
   cause
   abdominal aortic aneurysm repair
      and, 424
   acute
      lower, **520–522**
      upper, **517–520**
   anorectal disease causing, 521
   aspirin and, 78, 548–549
   in cirrhosis, 517–518, 538–539, 620
   colorectal cancer and, 521, 1478
   diverticular, 520, **589**
   in erosive/hemorrhagic gastritis (gas-
      tropathy), 518, 544
   in gastric cancer, 518, 1471
   from gastrointestinal/esophageal
      varices, 517–518, 538–541
   hemorrhoids causing, 521, 593
   hepatic encephalopathy and, 539, 622
   in hereditary hemorrhagic telangiec-
      tasia, 1519
   iron deficiency and, 439, 522, 523
   Mallory-Weiss syndrome/tears and,
      518, 536–537
   noncirrhotic portal hypertension and,
      631
   NSAIDs and, 78, 545, 548, 749
   obscure, **523–524**
   occult, **522–523.** *See also* Fecal occult
      blood testing
   in peptic ulcer disease, 517, 548,
      553–555
   in portal hypertension/portal hyper-
      tensive gastropathy,
      517–518, 545
   small intestinal tumors causing,
      566–567
   source location and, 519, 521
   in stress gastritis, 544, 545
   in typhoid fever, 1313
   from vascular ectasias, 518, 520–521
Gastrointestinal carcinoids, **1475–1476**
Gastrointestinal fluid losses, replacement
      guidelines for, 815*t*
Gastrointestinal gas, **510–511**
Gastrointestinal irritant-type mushroom
      poisoning, 1441, 1441*t*,
      1442
Gastrointestinal lymphoma, **1474–1475**
Gastrointestinal mesenchymal tumors,
      1474
Gastrointestinal stromal tumor (GIST),
      557, 567, 1474
Gastrointestinal system, **502–597.** *See also*
      specific structure or organ
      and under Intestinal
   anaerobic flora of, 1322
   decontamination of, in poisoning/
      drug overdose, 1420,
      1424–1426, 1425*t*
      caustic/corrosive agent ingestion
         and, 1429, 1429–1430
   disorders of, **502–597**
      Angiostrongylus causing, 1384
      in anisakiasis, 1385
      in anthrax, 1301, 1302
      in ascariasis, 1379

bleeding. *See* Gastrointestinal
      bleeding
cancer, **1465–1483**
   paraneoplastic syndromes asso-
      ciated with, 1453*t*
   chemotherapy-induced, **1509**
   in common variable immunodefi-
      ciency, 787
   constipation and, **507–510,** 508*t*,
      509*t*
   cytomegalovirus infection and,
      1245, 1246
   diarrhea and, **511–517,** 512*t*, 513*f*,
      516*f*
   dyspepsia in, **502–504**
   flukes causing, 1376
   functional
      dyspepsia (nonulcer dyspepsia),
         503
      irritable bowel syndrome,
         569–573
   gastrointestinal gas and, **510–511**
   in gnathostomiasis, 1384
   hiccups and, **507**
   in HIV infection/AIDS, 1213–1214
   in hookworm disease, 1380
   in hypercalcemia/hyperparathy-
      roidism, 1034
   in hyperoxaluric calcium nephroli-
      thiasis, 859
   motility. *See* Motility disorders
   mushroom poisoning causing,
      1441, 1441*t*, 1442
   nausea and vomiting in, **504–507,**
      505*t*, 506*t*
   noncardiac chest pain and, 321,
      543–544
   radiation causing, 1414
   in schistosomiasis, 1373, 1374
   in scleroderma, 758, 759
   in strongyloidiasis, 1381
   in syphilis, 1335
   in trichinosis, 1383
   in trichuriasis/whipworm, 1380
   in uremia, 826*t*
   mesenchymal tumors of, **1474**
Gastroparesis, 505–506, **566**
   in diabetics, 1107
   hypoglycemia and, 1104
   vomiting and, 505–506, 566
Gastropathy, **544–547.** *See also* Gastritis
   erosive/hemorrhagic, **544–545**
      GI bleeding and, 518, 544
   in HIV infection/AIDS, 1214
   hypertrophic (Ménétrier disease), 547
   portal hypertensive, 544, 545. *See also*
      Portal hypertension
Gastroplasty, for obesity, 15
Gastrostomies, 1148
GATA3 gene mutations, HDR/Barakat
      syndrome caused by,
      1030
Gatifloxacin
   blood glucose in diabetics and, 1122
   ophthalmic, 173*t*
Gaucher cells, 1516
Gaucher disease, **1515–1516**
GB. *See* Sarin poisoning

GB surgery. *See* Gastric banding surgery
GBE. *See* Ginkgo biloba
GBL (gamma-hydroxybutyrolactone),
      overdose/toxicity of, 1437
GBM antibodies. *See* Anti-glomerular
      basement membrane anti-
      bodies
GBP. *See* Gastric bypass
G-CSF (granulocyte colony-stimulating
      factor). *See* Filgrastim
GD. *See* Soman poisoning
GD1a antibodies, in Guillain-Barré syn-
      drome, 925
Gefitinib, 1504*t*
Gemcitabine, 1502*t*
   for breast cancer, 669
Gemfibrozil, 1131–1132, 1132*t*, 1133
   in HIV infection/AIDS, 1229
Gemifloxacin, 1180*t*
   renal/hepatic failure and, 1180*t*, 1184*t*
Gemtuzumab ozogamicin, 1503*t*
Gemzar. *See* Gemcitabine
Gender identity disorder/gender dyspho-
      ria, 948–949, 949–950
Gene therapy, for hemophilia, 491
Generalized anxiety disorder, 940,
      941–942, 941*t*, 942*t*
Generalized seizures, 879*t*, 880, 882*t*. *See*
      also Seizures
   differential diagnosis of, 881
Genetic disorders, **1512–1519.** *See also*
      specific type
Genetic instability
   in colorectal cancer, 1477
   in HNPCC, 592
Genetic testing/counseling. *See also spe-*
      cific disorder and Prenatal
      testing
   for cancer susceptibility genes/cancer
      screening
      APC gene mutation, 591
      breast cancer and, 653
      colorectal cancer and, 591, 592,
         1481
      MYH gene mutation, 591
      ret mutation, 1076
   for Duchenne muscular dystrophy,
      935
   for familial Mediterranean fever, 528
   for hemochromatosis, 628
   for Huntington disease, 909
   in male infertility, 865
   for MEN 1, 1075
   for pancreatitis, 646
   for pheochromocytoma/paragan-
      glioma, 1059
   prenatal, 706, 707
Genital herpes, **113–114,** 1235, 1236. *See*
      also Herpes simplex infec-
      tion
   during pregnancy/neonatal infection,
      727, 1236, 1237
Genital reconstruction surgery, for trans-
      sexuals, 950
Genital ulcers, 1167
   adenovirus causing, 1275
   in Behçet syndrome, 772
   in chancroid, 1320

Genital ulcers (*cont.*)
  in granuloma inguinale, 1321
  herpetic. *See* Genital herpes
  in lymphogranuloma venereum, 1328
  STDs causing, 1167
Genital warts. *See* Venereal (genital) warts
Genitourinary system. *See also specific
    organ or structure*
  anaerobic flora of, 1323
  disorders of, **850–871**. *See also specific
    type*
    anaerobic infection in women, **1323**
    benign prostatic hyperplasia,
      866–871, 867*t*, 868*f*, 869*t*
    in blastomycosis, 1399
    cancer, **1484–1494**
    hematuria in, **850–851**
    infections, **850–857**, 852*t*
    interstitial cystitis, **861–862**
    male erectile and sexual dysfunc-
      tion, **862–864**
    male infertility, **864–866**, 865*f*
    radiation exposure causing, 1414
    in schistosomiasis, 1373, 1374
    ulcers. *See* Genital ulcers
    in uremia, 826*t*
    urinary incontinence, **70–72**
    urinary stone disease, **857–860**, 858*t*
Genotypic resistance testing, in antiretro-
      viral therapy, 1233
Gentamicin, 1179*t*, 1545*t*. *See also* Ami-
      noglycosides
  for endocarditis, 1306, 1307
  for ophthalmic disorders, 173*t*
  in renal failure, 1179*t*
  for urinary tract infections, 852*t*
Geodon. *See* Ziprasidone
GERD. *See* Gastroesophageal reflux dis-
      ease
Geriatric medicine, **61–75**. *See also* Age/
      aging; Older adults
  assessment of older adult and, **61–63**,
      62*f*, 62*t*, 63*t*
  management of common problems
      and, **63–75**
  principles of care and, **61**
Germ cell tumors
  paraneoplastic syndrome associated
      with, 1453*t*
  testicular, 1066, 1492
    bone marrow/stem cell transplan-
      tation for, 475
    gynecomastia and, 1066, 1067,
      1493
Germline testing, in HNPCC, 592
Gerstmann syndrome, 899
Gerstmann-Sträussler-Scheinker syn-
      drome (GSS), 1260
Gestational diabetes, 707, 722–723, 723*t*
Gestational hyperthyroidism. *See* Hyper-
      thyroidism (thyrotoxico-
      sis), during pregnancy
Gestational thrombocytopenia, **489**
Gestational trophoblastic disease,
      714–715, 1467*t*
  hyperthyroidism in, 715, 1009
Gestodene, in oral contraceptives, throm-
      boembolism and, 696

GFR. *See* Glomerular filtration rate
GGTP levels. *See* Gamma-glutamyl
      transpeptidase (GGTP)
      levels
GH. *See* Growth hormone
GHB (gamma hydroxybutyrate), over-
      dose/toxicity of, **1437**
  Cushing syndrome and, 1052
Ghon complex, in tuberculosis, 252–253
Giant cell (temporal/cranial) arteritis,
      164, **766–767**
  headache in, 45, 766, **875–876**
  ischemic optic neuropathy in, 168,
      766
  retinal artery occlusion and, 164
Giant cell myocarditis, 368
Giant cell thyroiditis. *See* Subacute (de
      Quervain) thyroiditis
Giardia antigen assay, stool, 514, 515,
      1372
Giardia lamblia/intestinalis/duodenalis
      (giardiasis), 511, 512*t*, 515,
      1172, 1174, **1371–1372**
GIFT. *See* Gamete intrafallopian transfer
Gigantism, **997–1000**
Gilbert syndrome, 598, 599*t*
Gilles de la Tourette syndrome, **911–912**,
      940
Gingivitis
  in HIV infection/AIDS, 1213
  necrotizing ulcerative, **203**, 1289
Gingivostomatitis. *See also* Gingivitis; Sto-
      matitis
  herpetic, **203**, 1235
Ginkgo biloba, 1523*t*, 1524–1525
Ginseng, 1523*t*, 1526
"Ginseng abuse syndrome," 1526
GIP1. *See* Glucose-dependent insulino-
      tropic polypeptide
GIST. *See* Gastrointestinal stromal
      tumor
Gitelman syndrome, 796*t*
Glanders, 1177*t*
Glanzmann thrombasthenia, 489, 490
Glasgow alcoholic hepatitis score, 615
Glatiramer, for multiple sclerosis, 913
Glaucoma
  acute angle-closure, 153*t*, **157–158**
    pupillary dilation precipitating,
      157, 172
  chronic, **158–159**
    angle-closure, 157, 158, 159
  in diabetes mellitus, 158, 159, 1105
  facial pain caused by, 878
  neovascular (rubeotic), retinal vein
      occlusion and, 164
  normal-tension, 158, 159
  treatment of, 158, 159, 175–176*t*
Gleason grading system, for prostate can-
      cer, 1486
  in CAPRA assessment tool, 1488,
      1488*t*
Gleevec. *See* Imatinib
Gliclazide, 1091*t*, 1092
Glimepiride, 1091*t*, 1092
  with pioglitazone, 1096
  with rosiglitazone, 1096
Glioblastoma multiforme, 898*t*, 1467*t*

Gliomas, 897
  brainstem, 898*t*, 899
  spinal, 901
Gliosis, in multiple sclerosis, 912
Glipizide, 1091*t*, 1092
  with metformin, 1096
Globin chain synthesis, in thalassemias,
      442
γ-Globin, in sickle cell syndromes, 450
α-Globin gene, in alpha thalassemia syn-
      dromes, 442, 443, 443*t*
β-Globin gene
  in beta thalassemia syndromes, 442,
      443*t*
  in sickle cell syndromes, 450
Glomerular filtration rate, 817–818, 818*t*,
      1550*t*
  alkalosis in alkali administration and,
      813
  in chronic kidney disease, 825*t*, 826
  dialysis indications and, 830
  estimated, 1550*t*
  hypertension and, 410
  in prerenal azotemia, 820
  uremic acidosis and, 809
Glomerular proteinuria, 817
Glomerular sclerosis/glomerulosclerosis
  in diabetic nephropathy, 842
  focal segmental, 839*t*, **841**
Glomerulonephritis, 820*t*, **824–825**,
      833–834, 835*f*, 836*t*
  acute kidney injury caused by, 820*t*,
      824–825, 833–834
  anti-glomerular basement membrane
      (anti-GBM), 276, 824,
      835*f*, **837–838**
  autoantibodies in, 276, 824
  cryoglobulin-associated, 771, 835*f*,
      838
  in Goodpasture syndrome, 276, 824,
      835*f*, **837–838**
  IgA nephropathy, **834–835**, 835*f*, 836*t*
  immune-complex, 824
  lupus, 753, 754, 835*f*
  membranoproliferative, 835*f*, 839*t*,
      844
    hepatitis C infection and, 604, 844
    idiopathic, **844**
  in microscopic polyangiitis, 770, 835*f*
  nephritic presentation of, 833–834,
      835*f*, 836*t*
  nephrotic presentation of, 833,
      838–840, 839*t*
  pauci-immune (ANCA-associated),
      824, 835*f*, **837**
  peri-infectious, 835*f*
  postinfectious, **834**, 835*f*, 836*t*, 1289
  rapidly progressive, 833, 836*t*
  in SLE, 753, 754, 843
  in Wegener granulomatosis, 769, 835*f*
Glomerulonephropathies, 826*t*, **833–840**.
      See also Glomerulonephri-
      tis; Nephropathy
  membranoproliferative, 835*f*, 839*t*, **844**
    hepatitis C infection and, 604, 844
  sickle cell, 849
Glomerulosclerosis. *See* Glomerular scle-
      rosis/glomerulosclerosis

Glomus tumors (tympanicum/jugulare), 185–186
  tinnitus and, 186, 188
Glossitis, **202–203**
Glossodynia, **202–203**
Glossopharyngeal neuralgia, **877**
  earache in, 186
  headache in, 872
Glottic (true vocal fold) cancer, 210
GLP-1. *See* Glucagon-like peptide 1
Glucagon
  A cells secreting, 1062
  for β-blocker overdose/toxicity, 1422, 1432
  contraindications to use of in pheochromocytoma, 1059
  for hypoglycemia, 1104
  in insulinoma diagnosis/treatment, 1119
  lack of response to, hypoglycemia and, 1103
Glucagon emergency kit, 1104
Glucagon-like peptide 1 (GLP-1), 1095
Glucagonomas, 1062
β-Glucocerebrosidase, in Gaucher disease, 1516
Glucocorticoid deficiency. *See also* Adrenocortical insufficiency
  familial, 1048
Glucocorticoid-remediable hyperaldosteronism, 390–391, 796*t*.
  See also Aldosteronism
  hypertension and, 390–391
Glucokinase gene defect, in MODY, 1081
Glucophage. *See* Metformin
Glucosamine/glucosamine sulfate plus chondroitin, 1528*t*, 1529–1530
  in osteoarthritis, 731, 1528*t*, 1529–1530
Glucose. *See also* Glucose tolerance/intolerance
  ascitic fluid, 525
    bacterial peritonitis and, 526
  blood levels of. *See also* Hyperglycemia; Hypoglycemia
    acceptable, 1103
    in alcoholic ketoacidosis, 809
    in diabetes mellitus, 1083–1085, 1084*t*
      continuous monitoring of, 1085
      control of. *See* Glycemic control in diabetes
      pregnancy and, 707, 722–723, 723*t*, 1110
      self-monitoring of, 1085, 1100–1101, 1102–1103
      surgery and, 57–58, 57*t*, 58*t*, 1109
    in diabetic ketoacidosis, 1112, 1112*t*
    ginseng affecting, 1526
    hemoglobin A$_{1c}$ levels and, 1084, 1084*t*
    in hyperglycemic hyperosmolar state, 1112*t*, 1115
    hyponatremia and, 789, 790*f*, 792

in insulinoma, 1119
monitoring/management of during surgery, 57–58, 57*t*, 58*t*
prebreakfast hyperglycemia and, 1102–1103, 1103*t*
reference values for, 1550*t*
testing, 1083–1085, 1084*t*
  in pregnancy, 707, 722, 723, 723*t*
cerebrospinal fluid, in CNS infection, 1162*t*
in diabetic ketoacidosis management, 1114
drugs affecting absorption of, for diabetes mellitus, 1091*t*, 1094–1095
hyperosmolality caused by, 795
for hypoglycemia, 1104
hypophosphatemia caused by administration of, 803
intraoperative administration of, 58*t*
pleural fluid, 283, 284*t*
  in parapneumonic effusion, 284*t*, 285
in urine. *See* Glycosuria
Glucose-dependent insulinotropic polypeptide (GIP1), 1095
Glucose-6-phosphate dehydrogenase deficiency, **449–450**
  dapsone therapy and, 1157, 1222
  primaquine therapy and, 1359
  sulfasalazine therapy and, 750
Glucose-6-phosphate dehydrogenase screen, 1550*t*
Glucose tolerance/intolerance, 1083–1084, 1084*t*. *See also* Diabetes mellitus
  in chronic kidney disease, 830
  in Cushing syndrome, 1051
  in diabetes mellitus, 1083–1084, 1084*t*
  functional hypoglycemia and, 1121
  lithium affecting, 971
  prediabetes and, 1087
  in pregnancy, 722, 723*t*
  reference values for, 1550*t*
  testing, 1083–1084, 1084*t*
    in pregnancy, 707, 722, 723, 723*t*
Glucose transporters, thiazolidinediones affecting expression of, 1093
α-Glucosidase inhibitors, for diabetes mellitus, 1091*t*, 1094–1095, 1101
Glucosuria. *See* Glycosuria
Glucotrol. *See* Glipizide
Glucovance. *See* Glyburide, with metformin
GLUT 1/GLUT 4. *See* Glucose transporters
Glutamic acid decarboxylase antibodies, in type 1 diabetes, 1080, 1080*t*
Glutamine, 1550*t*
γ-Glutamyl transpeptidase (GGTP) levels
  alcohol use/abuse and, 979
  in liver disease/jaundice, 600
  reference values for, 1550*t*
Glutathione reductase, in riboflavin deficiency, 1141

Gluten, in celiac disease/sprue, 559, 560
Gluten-free diet, for celiac disease/dermatitis herpetiformis, 118, 560
Gluten-sensitive enteropathy. *See* Celiac disease
Glyburide, 1090–1092, 1091*t*
  with metformin, 1096
  during pregnancy, 722, 1110
Glycated (glycosylated) hemoglobin. *See* Hemoglobin A$_1$/A$_{1a}$/A$_{1b}$/A$_{1c}$
Glycemic control in diabetes
  acceptable levels of, 1103
  complications rate and, clinical studies of, 1086–1089
  exercise/activity and, 13, 1100
  glycated hemoglobin (hemoglobin A$_1$) measurements in evaluation of, 1084–1085, 1084*t*, 1087, 1089, 1103
  nephropathy development/progression and, 842, 1087, 1088, 1105
  pregnancy and, 722–723, 1110
  retinopathy development/progression and, 1087, 1088
  self-monitoring of blood glucose and, 1085, 1100–1101, 1102–1103
  surgery and, 57–58, 57*t*, 58*t*, 1109
Glycohemoglobins. *See* Hemoglobin A$_1$/A$_{1a}$/A$_{1b}$/A$_{1c}$
Glycoprotein-D vaccine, for HSV-2, 1237
Glycoprotein Ib/IX, in Bernard-Soulier syndrome, 489
Glycoprotein IIb/IIIa receptors
  drugs blocking
    for acute coronary syndromes, 327*t*, 328
    for myocardial infarction, 327*t*, 332
    platelet function affected by, 490*t*
  Glanzmann thrombasthenia and, 489
Glycopyrrolate, in terminally ill/dying patient, 92
Glycosuria/glucosuria
  in diabetes mellitus, 1083, 1106
    ketoacidosis and, 1112, 1112*t*
  in hyperglycemic hyperosmolar state, 1016, 1112*t*
  hypernatremia and, 793
  nondiabetic (renal), 1086
  in pregnancy, 1086
Glycosylated (glycated) hemoglobin (hemoglobin A$_1$). *See* Hemoglobin A$_1$/A$_{1a}$/A$_{1b}$/A$_{1c}$
Glycosylphosphatidylinositol (GPI) anchor deficiency, in paroxysmal nocturnal hemoglobinuria, 449
Glycyrrhetinic/glycyrrhizinic acid, hypertension/hypokalemia and, 391, 1057
Glynase. *See* Glyburide
Glyset. *See* Miglitol
GM1/GM1b antibodies, in Guillain-Barré syndrome, 925

GM-CSF (granulocyte macrophage colony-stimulating factor). *See* Sargramostim
Gnathostoma (gnathostomiasis), **1384**
GnRH analogs. *See* Gonadotropin-releasing hormone (GnRH) analogs
Goeckerman regimen, for psoriasis, 105
Goiter, 1019
  endemic, **1029–1030**
  fetal, 1013
  hyperthyroidism and, 1008, 1009
  hypothyroidism/cretinism and, 1003, 1004, 1029
  lithium causing, 971
  multinodular (nodular), **1019–1021**
    toxic, 1008, 1010, 1012, 1013
  substernal, 1029
  thyroid surgery for, 1012, 1021, 1030
Gold therapy, adverse ophthalmic effects of, 178t
Golf elbow, **745**
GoLYTELY. *See* Polyethylene glycol
Gonadal dysgenesis. *See* Turner syndrome
Gonadoblastoma, testicular, 1492–1493
Gonadotropin-releasing hormone (GnRH), deficiency/low pulse frequency of, in amenorrhea, 1067–1068, 1069
Gonadotropin-releasing hormone (GnRH) analogs. *See also* Luteinizing hormone-releasing hormone (LHRH) analogs
  for abnormal premenopausal bleeding, 675
  for endometriosis, 686
  hypogonadism caused by, 993, 1063
Gonadotropins
  cancer-related production of, 1453t
  deficiency of, 991, 991–992. *See also* Hypogonadism
    in amenorrhea, 1067–1068, 1069
  human chorionic (hCG). *See* Human chorionic gonadotropin
  human menopausal (hMG), for ovulation induction, 693
Gonococcal infections/gonorrhea, 1176t, **1319–1320**
  anorectal involvement and, 594, 1319, 1320
  arthritis and, **778–779**, 1319
  chlamydial coinfection and, 1319, 1320, 1328
  conjunctivitis, 154, 1319
  drug resistant, 779, 1320
  epididymitis in, 856, 1182t
  pelvic infection/PID, 688, 1182t, 1319, 1320
  during pregnancy, **727**
  rape/sexual assault in transmission of, 702, 1167
  screening/prevention and, 1167, 1319–1320
Goodpasture syndrome, 276, 824, **837–838**
  alveolar hemorrhage in, 276
  glomerulonephritis in, 276, 824, 835f, **837–838**

Gordon syndrome, 796t
Goserelin, 1506t. *See also* Luteinizing hormone-releasing hormone (LHRH) analogs
  for breast cancer, 668t
  for prostate cancer, 1487
GOT. *See* Aspartate aminotransferase
Gottron sign, 760
Gout/gouty arthritis, **732–735**, 732t, 734t
  kidney disease and, 732, **849**
  rheumatoid arthritis differentiated from, 733, 748
  saturnine, in lead poisoning, 733
  in transplant patient, 735
gp120/160, HIV vaccine development and, 1219
GPI (glycosylphosphatidylinositol) anchor deficiency, in paroxysmal nocturnal hemoglobinuria, 449
GPT. *See* Alanine aminotransferase
GRACE risk score, 339
Gradenigo syndrome, 185
Graft-versus-host reaction, 476
Graft-versus-malignancy effect, 475, 476
Graham patch, for ulcer perforation, 555
Graham–Steel murmur, 315
Gram-negative infections, 1176t, 1176–1177t, **1307–1323**. *See also specific causative agent*
  bacteremia and sepsis, **1311–1312**
  in cancer patient, 1498
  folliculitis, acne and, 120, 123, 124
Gram-positive infections, 1176t, 1177t, **1289–1303**. *See also specific causative agent*
  in cancer patient, 1498
Gram stain
  ascitic fluid, 525
  in pneumonia diagnosis, 246, 249
  synovial fluid
    in gonococcal arthritis, 778
    in nongonococcal acute bacterial (septic) arthritis, 777
Grand mal (tonic-clonic) seizures, 879t, 880, 882t. *See also* Seizures
Grand mal (tonic-clonic) status epilepticus, 880, 883–884
Granisetron, 506, 506t, 1509. *See also* Antiemetics
Granular urinary casts, 816, 817t
Granulocyte colony-stimulating factor (G-CSF). *See* Filgrastim
Granulocyte count
  cancer-related infections and, 1498
  chemotherapy dosage modification and, 1508t
Granulocyte macrophage colony-stimulating factor (GM-CSF). *See* Sargramostim
Granulocyte transfusion, **478**
Granulocytic ehrlichiosis/anaplasmosis, 1281t, 1285, 1286
Granulocytopenia. *See also* Neutropenia
  in cancer chemotherapy, 1499, 1508t
  infections and, 1156

Granuloma. *See also* Granulomatosis; Granulomatous disorders
  arytenoid cartilage, 209
  in Crohn disease, 578
  hepatic, drugs/toxins causing, 617
  inguinale, **1320–1321**
  lethal midline, 201
  pulmonary, in sarcoidosis, 265
  swimming pool, 1325
Granulomatosis
  allergic angiitis and. *See* Allergic angiitis and granulomatosis
  infantisepticum, 1303
  Wegener. *See* Wegener granulomatosis
Granulomatous disorders. *See also specific type and* Granuloma; Granulomatosis
  amebic encephalitis, 1164, **1368**
  hypercalcemia in, 801, 1036
  meningitis, 1162t
  neck masses, 213
  of nose and paranasal sinuses, **199–201**
Granulomatous thyroiditis. *See* Subacute (de Quervain) thyroiditis
Graves dermopathy (pretibial myxedema), 1008, 1009, 1015
Graves disease, 170, 1008, 1009, 1010–1012, 1014, 1015. *See also* Hyperthyroidism
  thyroid antibodies/TSH receptor antibody in, 1008, 1010
Graves ophthalmopathy/exophthalmos, 170, 1008, 1009, 1012, 1014
Gray top tubes, 1555t
Great toe, in gout, 733
Green top tubes, 1555t
Grief reaction/grieving, 961
Grind tests
  Apley, 35
  patellar, 35
Grip (handgrip), heart murmurs affected by, 306t
Grippe, summer, 1278
Griseofulvin, 107, 147
Ground itch, 1380
Group A β-hemolytic streptococcal infection, 1176t
  cellulitis, 129, 1182t
  endocarditis, 1291, 1305–1306
  erysipelas, **128–129**, 1182t, 1290
  glomerulonephritis and, 834, 1289
  pharyngitis, 204, 1182t, 1289–1290
  rapid antigen tests for, 204, 1289, 1290
  rheumatic fever and, 375, 1289
  scarlet fever, 1289
  skin infections, **1290**
Group B streptococcal infection, 1176t, 1291
  endocarditis, 1305–1306
  in pregnancy/neonate, 708, **725**, 1291
Group C streptococcal infection, 1176t, 1291
  endocarditis, 1305–1306
Group D streptococcal infection, 1291
  endocarditis, 1304

Group G streptococcal infection, 1176t, 1291
  endocarditis, 1305–1306
Group therapy. See also Support groups
  for anxiety disorders, 943
  for chronic pain disorders, 948
  for personality disorders, 951
  for somatoform disorders, 945
Growth factors. See also Filgrastim; Sargramostim
  for chemotherapy-induced toxicity, 1508t
  for neutropenia, 456
  platelet-derived, in myelofibrosis, 460
Growth hormone (GH)
  deficiency of, 992, 993, 994–995
  excess of, acromegaly and gigantism caused by, 997–1000
  phosphate metabolism affected by, 802
  replacement therapy with, 994–995
    for AIDS wasting, 1210
    during pregnancy, 995
    for Turner syndrome, 1074
  serum levels of
    in acromegaly/gigantism, 998
    reference values for, 1550t
  tumors secreting, 994, 997, 998
GSS. See Gerstmann-Sträussler-Scheinker syndrome
Guaiac testing. See Fecal occult blood testing
Guanabenz, 407, 408t
  overdose/toxicity of, 408t, 1434
Guanadrel, for hypertension, 407
Guanethidine
  antidepressant drug interactions and, 969t
  for hypertension, 407
  MAOI interactions and, 969t
Guanfacine, 407, 408t
  overdose/toxicity of, 408t, 1434
Guargum, 509t. See also Fiber, dietary
Guided/emotive imagery, 1520, 1536t, 1542–1543
  for anxiety disorders, 943, 1536t
Guillain-Barré syndrome (acute idiopathic polyneuropathy), 925–926
  dysautonomia in, 885, 925
  influenza/influenza vaccination and, 1270
  poliomyelitis differentiated from, 1252
  yellow fever vaccination and, 1203
Guinea worm infection (dracunculiasis), 1382–1383
Gum disease. See Gingivitis
Gummas, in syphilis, 1330, 1335
Guns. See Firearms
Gut. See Gastrointestinal system
Gut dialysis, (repeat-dose charcoal), 1426
Guttate psoriasis, 104. See also Psoriasis
GVM. See Graft-versus-malignancy effect
Gynecologic disorders, 674–704. See also specific disorder
  appendicitis differentiated from, 568
  diagnostic procedures used in, 675t
  in HIV infection/AIDS, 1216

Gynecomastia, 1064t, 1066–1067
  carcinoma of male breast and, 673
  in hyperprolactinemia, 1000, 1067
  in hypogonadism, 1065, 1067
  in Klinefelter syndrome, 1064, 1067, 1517
  testicular tumors causing, 1066, 1067, 1493
  testosterone replacement therapy and, 1066
Gypsy moths, skin lesions caused by, 139
Gyromitra (monomethylhydrazine) mushroom poisoning, 1441, 1441t, 1442

H₁ receptor blocking drugs. See Antihistamines
H₂ receptor blocking drugs
  for GERD, 533
  for peptic ulcer disease, 550
  for stress gastritis, 545
H1N1 influenza (swine-origin), 1198, 1269, 1270, 1271, 1273–1274. See also Influenza
H3N2 influenza, 1269, 1270, 1271
H5N1 avian influenza, 5, 1269, 1271, 1271–1272. See also Influenza
H63D mutation, in hemochromatosis, 627, 628. See also HFE gene
H1069Q mutation, in Wilson disease, 629
H pylori infection. See Helicobacter pylori infection
HAART regimens. See Highly active antiretroviral therapy
Habitrol. See Nicotine, for replacement therapy
Habitual (recurrent) abortion, 712–713
Habituation techniques
  for benign paroxysmal positioning vertigo, 189
  for tinnitus, 188
HACE. See High-altitude cerebral edema
HACEK organisms, endocarditis caused by, 1304, 1307
HAEM. See Herpes-associated erythema multiforme
Haemophilus, 1176t, 1310
  aphrophilus. See HACEK organisms
  ducreyi, 1320
  influenzae, 1310
    immunization against, 1188–1189t, 1192–1193t
    pneumonia caused by, 244t, 1310
  parainfluenzae. See HACEK organisms
Hair
  excess of. See Hirsutism
  exclamation, in alopecia areata, 146
  loss of, 145–146. See also Alopecia
    chemotherapy-induced, 1509
Hair analysis, for drug detection, 977
Hair cells, hearing loss caused by loss of, 179
Hairy cell leukemia, 468–469, 1466t
  aplastic anemia differentiated from, 455
  rheumatic manifestations of, 783

Hairy leukoplakia, 202, 1213
Halcion. See Triazolam
Haldol. See Haloperidol
Hallucinations/hallucinosis
  alcoholic (organic), 978–979, 979, 980, 986
  in delirium tremens, 978
  in dementia, 64, 986
  intracranial tumors causing, 899
  luminous, in migraine headache, 873
  in narcolepsy, 975
  psychedelic drug use and, 982, 1439
  in schizophrenic/psychotic disorders, 952, 953
  substance-induced, 986, 1439
Hallucinogenic mushroom poisoning, 1439, 1441, 1441t, 1442
Hallucinogens, 982, 986, 1439
Hallucinosis. See Hallucinations/hallucinosis
HALO (radiofrequency wave electrocautery) probe, for Barrett esophagus, 532
Halo sign, in invasive aspergillosis, 1398
Halobetasol, 97t
Halofantrine, for malaria, 1355t, 1360
Haloperidol, 954, 955t, 956t, 957. See also Antipsychotic drugs
  for aggressive/violent behavior, 976
  for alcoholic hallucinosis, 980
  antidepressant drug interactions and, 969t
  for bipolar disease/mania, 970
  decanoate form of, 957–958
  for delirium, 56, 67, 87, 987
  for dementia-associated behavior problems, 66, 987
  for hallucinogen overdose/toxicity, 1439
  for Huntington disease, 909
  intravenous, 958
  for opioid-induced nausea and vomiting, 86
  overdose/toxicity of, 956t, 958, 1444–1445
    ophthalmic effects and, 177t
  for personality disorder, 951
  for Tourette syndrome, 912
HAM. See Human T cell lymphotropic/leukemia virus (HTLV), myelopathy caused by
Hamartomatous polyposis syndromes, 591–592
Hamburger. See Meat
Hamman-Rich syndrome (acute interstitial pneumonitis/AIP), 264t
HAMP gene, in juvenile-onset hemochromatosis, 627
Hampton hump, in pulmonary embolism, 268
Hand
  in complex regional pain syndrome, 743
  in immersion syndrome, 1405
  in porphyria cutanea tarda, 117
  in Raynaud phenomenon, 756
Hand dermatitis, vesiculobullous (pompholyx), 116–117

Hand disinfection/washing, in infection control, 1161

Hand-foot-mouth disease
coxsackieviruses causing, 1279
enterovirus 71 causing, 1280
herpetic stomatitis differentiated from, 203

Hand-foot syndrome (acral erythema), chemotherapy-induced, 1480, 1509

Handgrip, heart murmurs affected by, 306t

Hansen disease (leprosy), 1177t, **1326–1327**
neuropathy associated with, 924, 1327

Hantavirus pulmonary syndrome, 1264–1265

Hantaviruses/Hantaan virus, 1262, **1264–1265**

HAPE. See High-altitude pulmonary edema

Haptoglobin
in hemolytic anemia, 447
reference values for, 1550t

Harris-Benedict equation, 1148

Hartley-Dunhill operation, 1012

Hashimoto (chronic lymphocytic/autoimmune) thyroiditis, 1008, 1013, 1016, 1017, 1018
hyperthyroidism caused by, 1008, 1013, 1016, 1017, 1017–1018
hypothyroidism caused by, 1003, 1007, 1016, 1018
thyroid antibodies in, 1016, 1017

Hashitoxicosis, 1013, 1017. See also Hashimoto (chronic lymphocytic/autoimmune) thyroiditis

HAV. See Hepatitis A virus

Havrix. See Hepatitis A vaccine

Hay fever. See Allergic rhinitis

Hb. See Hemoglobin

HbA$_1$. See Hemoglobin A$_1$/A$_{1a}$/A$_{1b}$/A$_{1c}$

HbA$_2$. See Hemoglobin A$_2$

HBcAg, 602
antibody to (anti-HBc), 602f, 603
screening blood for, 478

HbCO. See Carboxyhemoglobin levels

HBeAg, 602f, 603, 603t, 609
antibody to (anti-HBe), 602f, 603, 603t, 609

HbF. See Hemoglobin F

HBIG. See Hepatitis B immune globulin

HBsAg, 602, 602–603, 602f, 603t, 609
antibody to (anti-HBs), 602f, 603, 603t, 609
after vaccination, 606
in hepatocellular carcinoma, 1460
inactive carrier state, 609
maternal carrier state/transmission to newborn and, 602, 726–727
vaccination recommendations and, 606, 706, 726
screening blood for, 478

HBV. See Hepatitis B virus

hCG. See Human chorionic gonadotropin

HCO$_3^-$. See Bicarbonate

Hct. See Hematocrit

HCTZ. See Hydrochlorothiazide

HCV. See Hepatitis C virus

HDAg, 603, 609
antibody to (anti-HDV), 603, 609

HDCV (human diploid cell) rabies vaccine, 1201, 1256

HDL. See High-density lipoproteins/cholesterol

HDL disorders. See Huntington disease-like (HDL) disorders

HDL1/HDL2/HDL3 genes, in Huntington disease-like disorders, 909

HDR syndrome, 1030–1031

HDV. See Hepatitis D virus

Head injury, **918–919**, 918t
coma in diabetic patient and, 1112t
headache associated with, **875**
hearing loss associated with, 186
hypopituitarism associated with, 991
seizures associated with, 878
vertigo associated with, 190

Head lice, 138

Head and neck cancer, 1467t
lymphoma, **214**
metastatic, **214**
squamous cell carcinoma of larynx, **209–211**

Head and neck infections, anaerobic, **1321–1322**

Head and neck surgery, antibiotic prophylaxis for, 60t

Head-up tilt table testing, in syncope, 357

Headache, **44–46**, 44t, 45t, **872–876**. See also Migraine headache
acupuncture for, 1533
acute, **44–46**, 44t, 45t
in altitude-related illness, 1417, 1418
bacterial rhinosinusitis and, 193, 872
in carbon monoxide poisoning, 44, 1433
cerebral arteriovenous malformations causing, 895
chronic, **872–876**
ECT causing, 969
in giant cell arteritis, 45, 766, **875–876**
hypertension and, 44, 45, 393
in intracerebral/subarachnoid hemorrhage, 44, 45, 876, 892, 893
from intracranial aneurysm leak, 894
mind-body therapies for, 1536t
biofeedback, 1536t, 1537
ocular disorders and, 45
oral contraceptive use and, 697
in patent foramen ovale, 298
in pheochromocytoma, 44, 1058
in preeclampsia-eclampsia, 716
in pseudotumor cerebri, 876, 903

Health care-associated infections. See Hospital (health care)-associated infections

Health care providers
HIV transmission risk and, 1220–1221
HSV transmission prevention and, 1236–1237

immunization recommendations for, 1187, 1195t, 1198, 1199
radiation safety and, 1414
relationship of with patient. See Doctor–patient relationship
SARS transmission prevention and, 1275
swine-origin influenza transmission prevention and, 1273–1274

Health care proxy. See Advance directives

Health literacy, adherence and, 1

Health maintenance/disease prevention, **1–21**. See also specific disease
adherence and, **1–2**
principles of care and, 2
recommendations for, 2, 3t

Hearing, evaluation of, **179–180**
in elderly, 75

Hearing aids/hearing amplification, 180
adherence and, 75
in recruitment, 188

Hearing loss, **179–180**. See also specific type
aminoglycosides causing, 186
autoimmune, 187
barotrauma and, 183
cisplatin causing, 187, 1511
conductive, 179, 180
diabetes mellitus and, 1082
in elderly (presbyacusis), **75**, 179, 186
in endolymphatic hydrops (Ménière syndrome), 187, 189, 191t
eustachian tube dysfunction causing, 179, 182
glomus tumors causing, 186
head trauma causing, 186
hereditary, 187
in HIV infection/AIDS, 192
in labyrinthitis, 189, 191t
long QT syndrome and, 353
in multiple sclerosis, 191
mumps causing, 1251
neural, 179
noise trauma causing, 186
ossicular chain disruption causing, 179, 185
in otitis media, 183, 184
in otosclerosis, 179, **185**
ototoxicity and, 186–187. See also Ototoxicity
physical trauma causing, 186
sensorineural, 179, 180
sensory, 179, **186–187**
sudden, 179, 180, 187
tinnitus and, 187–188
vertigo and, 188, 191t
vestibular schwannoma (acoustic neuroma) causing, 179, 186, 191, 191t

Hearing rehabilitation, **180**

Heart, **294–386**. See also under Cardiac; Coronary; Myocardial and Cardiovascular disorders; Heart disease
examination of
in cardiomyopathy, 370t, 371

in cardiovascular screening of athletes, 386
in heart failure, 360
in hypertension, 394
in myocardial infarction, 330
holiday, 346
in hypertension, 393, 394
myxedema, 1005
sarcoidosis involving, 266
systemic diseases affecting, 383–384
traumatic injury of, 384
tumors of, 382–383
Heart block. *See* Atrioventricular (heart) block
Heart disease, 294–386. *See also specific disorder*
acute heart failure/pulmonary edema, 359, 367–368
anthracycline-induced, 1511
dexrazoxane for, 1507t, 1511
in athletes, screening for, 385–386
biofeedback in management of, 1537
bradycardias, 354–358
carcinoid, 313, 315, 383, 1475
cardiomyopathies, 370–374, 370t
in hyperthyroidism, 1009, 1014
peripartum, 385, 724, 1000
in Chagas disease, 368, 1350
chest pain in, 28–29, 326, 330
cholesterol/lipoproteins in, 316, 1123–1124, 1124
screening tests for levels of, 1126–1129, 1127–1128t, 1129t
coenzyme Q₁₀ for, 1528t, 1530
conduction disturbances, 354–358
congenital, 294–302
pregnancy and, 385, 724
congestive heart failure, 358–367, 359f. *See also* Congestive heart (cardiac) failure
coronary (atherosclerotic CAD/ischemic), 316–340. *See also* Coronary heart disease
in diabetes mellitus, 1108
dyspnea in, 25, 25t, 26
endocarditis prophylaxis and, 1305, 1305t
functional classification of, 294
pregnancy and, 724, 724t
in HIV infection/AIDS, 1216
homocysteine/hyperhomocysteinemia in, 1516, 1517
hypertension and, 358, 393
in hyperthyroidism, 360, 1009, 1014–1015
hypertriglyceridemia and, 9, 1124, 1133
in hypothyroidism, 360, 1005
immunization recommendations in, 1195t
in Lyme disease, 377, 1343, 1346, 1346t
in Marfan syndrome, 311–312, 312–313, 383, 1518, 1519
metabolic syndrome (syndrome X) and, 14, 317, 318, 325

myocarditis, 368–370, 369t
neoplastic, 382–383
pericardial disorders and, 376–380
in polyarteritis nodosa, 765
pregnancy and, 384–385, 724, 724t, 1000
preoperative evaluation/management and, 49–53, 50t, 51f, 51t
prevention of
aspirin in, 12, 1130
exercise/activity and, 13
hypertension control and, 9–12
lipid disorder prevention/management and, 9, 1124–1125, 1126, 1128, 1129. *See also* Lipid-lowering therapy
omega-3 fatty acids in, 1528t, 1530–1531
smoking/smoking cessation and, 6–9, 8t, 9t, 10t, 11t, 316
pulmonary (cor pulmonale), 381–382. *See also* Pulmonary heart disease
pulmonary hypertension and, 275, 382
rate and rhythm disturbances, 340–354, 343–345t. *See also* Arrhythmias
rheumatic/rheumatic fever and, 374–376
risk factors for, 316–317
lipoproteins/lipid fractions and, 1123, 1124
modification/risk reduction and, 1124–1125, 1126, 1128, 1129
in scleroderma, 758, 759
in SLE, 753
spondylitic, 774
surgery in patient with, 384
preoperative evaluation/management and, 49–53, 50t, 51f, 51t
systemic disorders and, 383–384
thiazolidinediones contraindicated in, 1094, 1101
traumatic, 384
in Turner syndrome, 1074
valvular, 302–316, 303–305t, 306t. *See also* Valvular heart disease
Heart failure
acute, 367–368
congestive, 358–367, 359f. *See also* Congestive heart (cardiac) failure
Heart-lung transplant, for cystic fibrosis, 242
Heart murmurs, 303–304t
in aortic regurgitation, 303–304t, 312
in aortic stenosis, 303–304t, 306t, 310
atrial myxoma causing, 383
in atrial septal defect/patent foramen ovale, 297
bedside maneuvers/interventions affecting, 306t
in cardiomyopathy, 306t
in coarctation of aorta, 296

in endocarditis, 1304
in heart failure, 360
in mitral regurgitation, 303–304t, 306t, 307
in mitral stenosis, 303–304t, 306
in mitral valve prolapse, 306t, 309
in myocardial infarction, 330
in patent ductus arteriosus, 301
in pulmonary stenosis, 295
in pulmonic regurgitation, 315
in rheumatic carditis, 375
in tetralogy of Fallot, 300
in tricuspid regurgitation, 303–304t, 314
in tricuspid stenosis, 303–304t, 313
in ventricular septal defect, 299
Heart rate
in asthma exacerbation, 220t
disturbances of, 340–354, 343–345t. *See also* Arrhythmias
in GI bleeding, 518
in pulmonary embolism, 268t
Heart rate variability, biofeedback affecting, 1537
Heart rhythm, disturbances of, 340–354, 343–345t. *See also* Arrhythmias
Heart sounds
in aortic regurgitation, 303t
in aortic stenosis, 303t
in atrial septal defect, 297
in heart failure, 360
in hypertension, 394
in mitral regurgitation, 303t, 307
in mitral stenosis, 303t, 306
in myocardial infarction, 330
in patent ductus arteriosus, 301
in pulmonary embolism, 268t
in pulmonary stenosis, 295
in pulmonic regurgitation, 315
in tetralogy of Fallot, 300
in tricuspid regurgitation, 303t, 314
in tricuspid stenosis, 303t
in valvular heart disease, 303t
Heart transplantation, for heart failure, 366
Heart valves. *See also* Prosthetic heart valves; Valve replacement; Valvular heart disease
in alkaptonuria, 1513
endocarditis affecting, 1303. *See also* Endocarditis
Heartburn (pyrosis), 502, 529, 531
Heat
disorders caused by exposure to, 1403, 1406–1408. *See also* Burns; Hyperthermia
cholinergic urticaria, 126
miliaria (heat rash), 124
prevention of, 1406–1407
reduction/removal of, 39, 1403
for heat exposure syndromes, 1407, 1408
Heat cramps, 1407
Heat exhaustion, 1407
Heat rash, 124
Heat stroke, 1407–1408
Heat syncope/collapse, 1407

Heavy metals. *See also specific type*
overdose/poisoning and, 1424*t*
ophthalmic effects and, 178*t*
tubulointerstitial disease caused by, 845–846
Hebephrenic (disorganized) schizophrenia, 952
Heberden nodes, 730
Hectorol. *See* Doxercalciferol
Heel, plantar hyperkeratosis of, 133
Hegar dilators, for vaginismus, 950
Heimlich maneuver, for foreign body removal, 212, 277
Heinz bodies
in glucose-6-phosphate dehydrogenase deficiency, 449, 450
unstable hemoglobins and, 452
Helical (spiral) CT. *See also* Computed tomography
in colorectal cancer screening. *See* Virtual colonoscopy
in lung cancer screening, 18, 259, 1456
in pulmonary embolism, 30, 269, 270, 271*f*
in renal artery stenosis, 833
Helicobacter pylori infection, 1176*t*
dyspepsia and, 502
eradication therapy for, 550, 550–552, 551*t*, 1176*t*
dyspepsia management and, 503, 504
gastric cancer/MALT lymphoma and, 470, 1473
gastritis management and, 546
peptic ulcer management and, 550, 550–552, 551*t*
NSAID-induced ulcers and, 551*t*, 552
perforation prevention and, 555
rebleeding prevention and, 554
gastric cancer/MALT lymphoma and, 546, 1473
gastritis, 546
gastric cancer and, 546, 1471
peptic ulcer disease and, 548, 549, 550–552, 551*t*
HSV infection and, 1236
perforation and, 555
refractory, 553
testing for, 546, 549, 552, 1471
in dyspepsia, 503
reference values for, 1550*t*
Heliotrope rash, in dermatomyositis, 760
Helium-oxygen mixture (Heliox), for smoke inhalation, 277
Heller cardiomyotomy, for achalasia, 542
HELLP syndrome, 487, 488, 716
Helmet cells, in microangiopathic hemolytic anemia, 454
Helminthic infections, 1373–1389. *See also specific type*
cestodes causing, 1376–1379
eosinophilic pulmonary syndromes caused by, 266, 1379, 1386
myocarditis in, 369*t*
nematodes causing, 1379–1389
trematodes (flukes) causing, 1373–1376

Helper-inducer T cells. *See* CD4 T cells
Helvella (gyromitrin) mushroom poisoning, 1441, 1441*t*, 1442
Hemangioblastoma, cerebellar, 898*t*
Hemangioma, cavernous, of liver, 633
Hemarthroses, in hemophilia, 491
Hematemesis
in erosive/hemorrhagic gastritis (gastropathy), 544
in GI bleeding, 517, 554
in Mallory-Weiss syndrome/tears, 536
in peptic ulcer disease, 554
Hematin, for porphyria, 923, 1512–1513
Hematochezia, 517
in constipation, 508
in lower GI bleeding, 520, 521
in peptic ulcer disease, 554
in upper GI bleeding, 517, 554
Hematocrit. *See also specific disorder*
in anemia, 439
in myeloproliferative disorders, 457*t*
in polycythemia, 457, 457*t*, 458
reference values for, 1550*t*
Hematogenous osteomyelitis, 780
Hematologic disorders, 439–479. *See also specific type and* Hemostasis disorders
anemias, 439–456, 440*t*
cancer-related, 1453*t*
in chronic kidney disease, 828–829
leukemias/myeloproliferative disorders, 457–469, 457*t*
lymphomas, 469–474, 469*t*
neutropenia, 456–457, 456*t*
in preeclampsia-eclampsia, 717*t*
preoperative evaluation/management and, 55–56, 56*t*
radiation exposure and, 1414
Hematoma
auricular (cauliflower ear), 180
myocardial, 384
perianal, thrombosed hemorrhoid causing, 594
septal, in nasal trauma, 199
subdural. *See* Subdural hemorrhage/hematoma
Hematometra, in endometrial carcinoma, 684
Hematopoiesis, extramedullary, in myelofibrosis, 460
Hematopoietic progenitor cell transplantation. *See* Bone marrow/stem cell transplantation
Hematopoietic stimulating factors. *See* Filgrastim; Growth factors; Sargramostim
Hematuria, 817, 850–851
in bladder cancer, 1489
in cystitis, 46, 851
dysuria and, 46
in focal segmental glomerular sclerosis, 841
hemorrhagic cystitis and, 1510
in IgA nephropathy, 836
in polycystic kidney disease, 847
in renal cell carcinoma, 1491
in sickle cell disease, 849

in SLE, 754*t*, 843
synpharyngitic, 836
in ureteral/renal pelvis cancer, 1491
in urinary stone disease, 858
Hemoccult testing. *See* Fecal occult blood testing
Hemianopia. *See* Visual field defects
Hemiplegia, in stroke, 889, 891, 892
Hemiplegic migraine, familial/sporadic, 873
Hemobilia, 518
Hemoccult. *See* Fecal occult blood testing
Hemochromatosis, 627–628
cirrhosis and, 620, 627, 628
hepatocellular carcinoma and, 615, 627, 628, 1460
hypopituitarism caused by, 993
Hemodiafiltration, continuous venovenous, for poisoning/drug overdose, 1425
Hemodialysis, 831. *See also* Dialysis
for chronic kidney disease, 831
postoperative, 58–59
for heat stroke, 1408
for hyperkalemia, 798, 799*t*
emergent postoperative, 59
for hypermagnesemia, 806
for hypernatremia, 794
iron supplementation and, 829
for poisoning/drug overdose, 1425–1426, 1425*t*
with carbamazepine, 1425*t*, 1431
with lithium, 972, 1425*t*
with methanol or ethylene glycol, 1425*t*, 1440
with salicylates, 1425*t*, 1445
with theophylline, 1425*t*, 1448
with valproic acid, 1425*t*, 1431
preoperative, 59
pruritus associated with, 136
for uremic pericarditis, 378
Hemodynamic status
in atrial fibrillation, management and, 347–348
in COPD, 235*t*
GI bleeding and, 518
in myocardial infarction, 331, 331*t*
Hemoglobin
in anemia, 439
glycated/glycosylated. *See* Hemoglobin $A_1/A_{1a}/A_{1b}/A_{1c}$
nephrotoxicity/acute tubular necrosis and, 822
reference values for, 1550*t*, 1551*t*
in sickle cell syndromes, 450, 451, 451*t*. *See also* Sickle cell anemia/syndromes
unstable, 452
Hemoglobin A, 442
in beta thalassemia syndromes, 442, 443*t*, 444
in sickle cell syndromes, 451, 451*t*
Hemoglobin $A_1/A_{1a}/A_{1b}/A_{1c}$ (glycated/glycosylated hemoglobin)
in diabetes mellitus, 1084–1085, 1084*t*, 1087, 1089, 1103
acceptable levels of, 1103
capillary glucose and, 1084, 1084*t*

postoperative complications and, 57

pregnancy and, 722, 723, 1110

reference values for, 1550t

Hemoglobin A$_2$, 442

in beta thalassemia syndromes, 442, 443t, 444

reference values for, 1550t

in sickle cell syndromes, 451t

Hemoglobin AS genotype (sickle cell trait), **451–452**, 451t

Hemoglobin C disorders, **452**

in pregnancy, 721

Hemoglobin electrophoresis

in hemoglobin H disease, 444

in prenatal care, 706

reference values for, 1550t

in sickle cell syndromes, 451, 451t

in thalassemias, 443, 444

Hemoglobin F (fetal hemoglobin), 442

in beta thalassemia syndromes, 442, 443t, 444

glycated hemoglobin values affected by, 1084–1085, 1084t

reference values for, 1550t

in sickle cell syndromes, 450, 451, 451t

Hemoglobin H/hemoglobin H disease, 442, 443, 443t, 444

Hemoglobin S, 450, 451, 451t

Hemoglobin saturation. See SaO$_2$

Hemoglobin SC disease, 452

retinopathy in, 167, 452

Hemoglobinemia, in hemolytic anemia, 447–448

Hemoglobinuria, 817

in hemolytic anemia, 447

iron deficiency and, 440

paroxysmal nocturnal, **448–449**

Hemojuvelin, in juvenile-onset hemochromatosis, 627

Hemolytic anemias/hemolysis, **447–448**, 448t. See also specific type or cause

autoimmune, **452–453**

in cold agglutinin disease, 453

in glucose-6-phosphate dehydrogenase deficiency, 450

in hemoglobin C disease, 452

in hereditary spherocytosis, 448

in hypophosphatemia, 803

microangiopathic, **454**

thrombotic microangiopathies and, 485, 485t

in sickle cell syndromes, 450, 451

unstable hemoglobins and, 452

Hemolytic crises, in sickle cell disease, 450, 451

Hemolytic disease of newborn, prevention of, **709**

Hemolytic streptococcus. See specific type under Group

Hemolytic transfusion reactions, 477

Hemolytic-uremic syndrome, 485–486, 485t, 1315

E coli O157:H7 causing, 485, 1315

Hemopericardium, 384

Hemophagocytosis, 489

Hemophilia A and B, **490–492**, 492t

Hemophilia C (factor XI deficiency), 492t, **493–494**

Hemoptysis, **27–28**

in bronchiectasis, 240

in cystic fibrosis, 241

in lung cancer, 27, 1454

in pulmonary embolism, 268t

in tuberculosis, 252

Hemorrhage. See specific type or structure affected and Bleeding

Hemorrhagic conjunctivitis

acute, enterovirus 70 causing, 1280

coxsackievirus infection and, 1279

Hemorrhagic cystitis

adenovirus causing, 1275, 1276

chemotherapy-induced, 1510

mesna for, 1507t, 1510

Hemorrhagic effusion, pleural, 283, 1496. See also Hemothorax

Hemorrhagic fevers, 1257–1259, **1262–1263**

dengue, 1257–1259, **1263–1264**

hantavirus, 1262, 1264, 1265

Hemorrhagic (erosive) gastritis. See Gastritis

Hemorrhagic shock, 434, 436. See also Hypovolemic shock

Hemorrhoidectomy, 594

Hemorrhoids, **593–594**

bleeding and, 521, 593

fecal soiling/incontinence and, 593, 594, 595

pruritus ani caused by, 136

thrombosed, **594**

Hemosiderin, 439

accumulation of, 627. See also Hemochromatosis

urine

in hemolytic anemia, 447

in paroxysmal nocturnal hemoglobinuria, 449

Hemosiderosis

idiopathic pulmonary, 276

transfusional, in thalassemia, 443

Hemostasis disorders, **480–501**, 481t. See also specific type and Bleeding

antithrombotic therapy and, **495–501**, 496t, 497t, 498t, 499t, 500t, 501t

coagulation disorders, **490–495**

platelet disorders, **480–490**, 481t, 490t

preoperative evaluation of, 49, 50t, 55

Hemosuccus pancreaticus, 518

Hemothorax, 283, 285

Hemotympanum, 183, 185

Henderson-Hasselbalch equation, 806

Henoch-Schönlein purpura, **771**, 836t, **837**

HepA. See Hepatitis A vaccine

HepB. See Hepatitis B vaccine

Hepacare. See Hepatitis B vaccine

Hepar lobatum, 1335

Heparin/low-molecular weight heparin, 272, 273, 496t, 497, 497t

for acute arterial occlusion of limb, 419

for acute coronary syndromes, 326–327, 327t

for antiphospholipid antibody syndrome, pregnancy and, 755, 756

after cardiac valve replacement surgery, 316

coagulopathy caused by, **495**

for deep venous thrombosis/pulmonary embolism (venous thromboembolic disease)

prevention and, 495, 496t

treatment and, 272–273, 497, 497t

for DIC, 488

hyperkalemia and, 798

for lupus anticoagulant-anticardiolipin-antiphospholipid antibody syndrome, 722

for myocardial infarction, 327t, 336

after thrombolytic therapy, 334

perioperative management of, 55, 56t

for stroke, 891–892

thrombocytopenia caused by, 272, 483t, **486–487**, 486t

reference values in, 1551t

for transient ischemic attacks, 888

Heparin-associated/PF-4 antibody, 486, 487

reference values for, 1551t

Heparin-induced thrombocytopenia, 272, 483t, **486–487**, 486t

reference values in, 1551t

Hepatic abscess

amebic, 1366, 1367–1368, 1367t

pyogenic, **632–633**

Hepatic adenoma, 633

oral contraceptive use and, 633, 696

Hepatic biopsy. See Liver, biopsy of

Hepatic candidiasis, 632, 633

Hepatic coagulopathy, **494–495**

in cirrhosis, 494–495

hepatic failure and, 607

Hepatic cysts, hydatid, 1378

Hepatic disease. See Liver, disorders of

Hepatic encephalopathy, 608, **622–623**

in cirrhosis, 620, 622–623

GI bleeding/esophageal varices and, 539, 622

in hepatic failure, 608

protein-restricted diet for, 620, 622, 1146

Hepatic (liver) failure, **607–608**

acetaminophen causing, 607

acute, **607–608**

fatty liver of pregnancy and, 617, **718–719**

antimicrobial dosage adjustment and, 1184–1185t

herbal supplement use and, 1522

in HIV infection/AIDS, 1214

in mushroom poisoning, 608, 1441

nefazodone causing, 966

Hepatic fibrosis

in cirrhosis, 619, 620

drugs/toxins causing, 617

Hepatic iminodiacetic acid (HIDA) scan, in cholecystitis, 636

Hepatic steatosis. See Fatty liver

Hepatic vein obstruction (Budd-Chiari syndrome), 525, **630–631**

Hepatitis
  alcoholic, 614–616
    postoperative complications associated with, 54
  autoimmune, **612–614**
  black cohosh causing, 1527
  drugs/toxins causing, **616–617**
  fibrosing cholestatic, 610
  postoperative complications associated with, 54–55
  radiation exposure and, 1414
  in syphilis, 1334
  viral. See also Hepatitis A; Hepatitis B; Hepatitis C; Hepatitis D; Hepatitis E; Hepatitis G
    acute, **601–607**, 602f, 603t, 604f
      arthritis in, 779
        rheumatoid arthritis differentiated from, 748
    chronic, 606, **608–612**
      postoperative complications associated with, 54–55
    cirrhosis and, 602, 603, 604, 609, 611–612, 620
    in drug users, 601, 602, 603, 604, 1168
    hepatic failure and, 607
    in HIV infection/AIDS, 602, 604, 609, 1214
    HSV causing, 1236
    liver cancer and, 602, 603, 609, 611–612, 1460, 1461
    in liver transplant patients, adenoviruses causing, 1276
    postoperative complications associated with, 54–55
    prevention of, 605–606
    transfusion-associated, 478, 491, 601, 602, 603–604
Hepatitis A, 601–602, 602f
  prevention/immunization and, 4, 601, 605–606, 1186, 1201. See also Hepatitis A vaccine
  screening for, in STD patients, 1167
Hepatitis A and B vaccine, 606, 1197t
Hepatitis A immune globulin, 4, 605, 1186, 1201
  during pregnancy/for newborn, 710
Hepatitis A vaccine, 4, 601, 605–606, 1186, 1188–1189t, 1190–1191t, 1192–1193t, 1194–1197t, 1201
  adverse effects/contraindications and, 1202t
  in immunocompromised host/HIV infection/AIDS, 606, 1195t, 1201
  during pregnancy, 710, 1195t
  for travelers, 605, 1186, 1201
Hepatitis A virus (HAV), 601
Hepatitis B, 602–603, 602f, 603t
  antiretroviral agents for, 1228
  arthritis in, 779
  cancer associated with, 602, 609, 611, 1460
  chronic, 602, 603, 603t, 608–609, 609–610
  cirrhosis and, 602, 603, 609, 611–612, 620

delta agent (hepatitis D) and, 603, 609
HIV infection/AIDS and, 602, 609, 1214
maternal carrier state/transmission to newborn and, 602, **726–727**
vaccination recommendations and, 606, 706, 726, 1187, 1195t
polyarteritis nodosa and, 765
prevention/immunization and, 3, 4, 606, 1186–1187, 1200–1201. See also Hepatitis B vaccine
sexual assault/rape in transmission of, 1167
transfusion in transmission of/screening blood for, 478
Hepatitis B core antigen (HBcAg), 602
  antibody to (anti-HBc), 602f, 603, 603t
  screening blood for, 478
Hepatitis B e antigen (HBeAg), 602f, 603, 603t, 609
  antibody to (anti-HBe), 602f, 603, 603t, 609
Hepatitis B immune globulin, 606, 1187
  during pregnancy/for newborn, 606, 726, 1187
Hepatitis B surface antigen (HBsAg), 602, 602–603, 602f, 603t, 609
  antibody to (anti-HBs), 602f, 603, 603t, 609
    after vaccination, 606
  in hepatocellular carcinoma, 1460
  inactive carrier state, 609
  maternal carrier state/transmission to newborn and, 602, 726–727
  vaccination recommendations and, 606, 706, 726, 1187
  screening blood for, 478
Hepatitis B vaccine, 3, 4, 606, 1186–1187, 1188–1189t, 1190–1191t, 1192–1193t, 1194–1197t, 1200–1201
  adverse effects/contraindications and, 1202t
  in cancer prevention, 16, 1461
  in HIV infection/AIDS/immunocompromised host, 606, 1187, 1195t, 1220
  for newborn/pregnant patient, 4, 606, 726, 1187, 1195t
  after rape/sexual assault, 702, 1167
  for travelers, 1187, 1200–1201
Hepatitis B virus (HBV), 601, 602
Hepatitis B virus DNA, 602, 602f, 603, 609
Hepatitis C, 603–604, 604f
  arthritis in, 779
    rheumatoid arthritis differentiated from, 748
  cancer associated with, 612, 1460, 1461
  chronic, 604, 604f, 609, 610–611, 612
  cirrhosis and, 604, 609, 612, 620, 1460
  cryoglobulinemia in, 604, 611, 770, 771, 844
  hemophilia and, 491

HIV infection/AIDS and, 604, 1214
  immune thrombocytopenic purpura in, 482, 484
  in pregnancy, 604, **726–727**
  renal disease and, 844
  thyroiditis and, 1004
  transfusion in transmission of/screening blood for, 478, 491, 603–604
Hepatitis C virus (HCV), 601, 603
  antibodies to (anti-HCV), 604, 604f, 609
  screening blood for, 478, 491
Hepatitis C virus RNA, 604, 604f, 609
Hepatitis D, 603
  chronic, 609, 611
  hepatitis B and, 603, 609
Hepatitis D antigen (HDAg), 603
  antibody to (anti-HDV), 603, 609
Hepatitis D virus (HDV/delta agent), 601, 603
Hepatitis D virus RNA, 603
Hepatitis E, 604
  prevention/immunization and, 4
Hepatitis E vaccine, 4
Hepatitis E virus (HEV), 601, 604
Hepatitis G, 604
Hepatitis G virus (HGV), 601, 604
Hepatobiliary cancers, **1459–1465**. See also specific type
Hepatobiliary CMV, 1245
Hepatoblastomas, in familial adenomatous polyposis, 591
Hepatocellular carcinoma, **1459–1461**, 1468t. See also Liver, cancer of
  cirrhosis and, 615, 620, 624, 1460, 1461
  hemochromatosis and, 615, 627, 628, 1460
  hepatitis and, 602, 603, 609, 611–612, 1460, 1461
  incidence/mortality of, 1450, 1460, 1461
  paraneoplastic syndromes associated with, 1453t
Hepatocellular disease. See also Cirrhosis; Liver, disorders of
  jaundice in, 598, 599t
Hepatocyte nuclear factor 1α (HNF1α), hepatic adenomas and, 633
Hepatojugular reflux, 360
Hepatolenticular degeneration. See Wilson disease
Hepatomegaly
  in chronic lymphocytic leukemia, 467
  in cirrhosis, 619
  in fatty liver, 617–618
  in hairy cell leukemia, 468
  in hepatitis, 605
Hepatopathy, ischemic, 631
Hepatopulmonary syndrome, 623–624
Hepatorenal syndrome, 622
Hepatosplenic candidiasis, 1391
Hepatotoxicity, **616–617**
  of acetaminophen, 78, 607, 616, 1428, 1428f
  antimicrobial dosage adjustment and, 1184–1185t

of antituberculous agents, 4
of black cohosh, 1527
direct, **616**
of herbal supplements, 1522
of methotrexate, 750, 1510
of thiazolidinediones, 1094, 1101
Hepcidin
in anemia of chronic disease, 441
in hemochromatosis, 627
HER-2/*neu* overexpression, in breast cancer, 663, 664
prognosis and, 665t, 670
therapy and, 664, 665, 666, 668
Herald patch, in pityriasis rosea, 105–106
"Herbal ecstasy" (ephedrine), 1430
safety/toxicity of, 1522
Herbal medicines, **1521–1527**, 1522t, 1523t.
See also specific preparation
during pregnancy, 1522t
product formulations/standardization and, 1521
quality assurance and, 1521, 1522t
regulatory issues regarding, 1521
safety of, 1521–1522
Herbicide poisoning. *See* Pesticide poisoning
Herceptin. *See* Trastuzumab
Hereditary angioedema, 126
Hereditary hearing loss, 187
Hereditary hemorrhagic telangiectasia, **1519**
epistaxis in, 198, 1519
Hereditary motor and sensory neuropathy (HMSN), types I to IV, 922–923
Hereditary nonpolyposis colorectal cancer (HNPCC), **592–593**, 1477
endometrial carcinoma and, 592, 593, 684
pancreatic/periampullary carcinoma and, 1463
Hereditary spherocytosis, **448**
Hernias
hiatal
esophageal webs and rings and, 537
GERD and, 531
surgery for, antibiotic prophylaxis for, 60t
vaginal (pelvic organ prolapse), **687**
Herniated nucleus pulposus. *See* Nucleus pulposus, herniation of
Herniation syndromes
intracranial tumors causing, 897–898, 900
lumbar puncture and, 893, 1163, 1164
Heroin use/abuse, 981–982, 1442–1443
acupuncture for, 1534
Herpangina, 1278–1279
Herpes-associated erythema multiforme, 127, 128, 1236, 1239
Herpes genitalis. *See* Genital herpes
Herpes labialis, 1235–1236
esophagitis and, 535
Herpes simplex infection, **113–114**, **1235–1239**
acyclovir prophylaxis/treatment and, 114, 1157, 1215, 1237, 1238t

anorectal involvement and, 594–595, 1236
Bell palsy and, 928, 1236, 1237
chemoprophylaxis for, 114, 1157, 1237–1239
disseminated/generalized, 1215, 1236, 1237
dermatitis in (eczema herpeticum), 103, 1236, 1240t
encephalitis, 1236, 1237
erythema multiforme associated with, 127, 128, 1236, 1239
esophagitis in, 535, 1236, 1237–1239
gladiatorum, 1235
in HIV infection/AIDS, 114, 1157, 1215, 1224t, 1237
esophageal, 535, 1236
keratitis, **156**, 1236, 1237
during pregnancy/neonatal infection, **727**, 1236, 1237
stomatitis/gingivostomatitis in, **203**, 1235
treatment/prevention of, 1157, 1236–1239, 1238–1239t
type 1, 113, **1235–1239**
type 2, 113, **1235–1239**
Herpes zoster (shingles), **114–116**, **1239–1243**
earache in, 186
eye involvement and, 115, **156–157**, 1241
facial paralysis in (Ramsay Hunt syndrome), 192, 1241
in HIV infection/AIDS/immunocompromised host, 115, 1215, 1225t, 1236, 1241
neuralgia after, 115, 115–116, **877–878**, 1241, 1242
prevention and, 1241, 1242. *See also* Herpes zoster vaccine
Herpes zoster ophthalmicus, 115, **156–157**, 1241
Herpes zoster oticus, 186
Herpes zoster vaccine, 5, 115, 877–878, 878, 1187, 1194–1197t, 1242
adverse effects/contraindications and, 1203t
HIV infection/AIDS and, 1195t, 1220
Herpesviruses, **1235–1247**. *See also specific type*
Herpesviruses 1 and 2. *See* Herpes simplex infection
Herpetic stomatitis/gingivostomatitis, **203**, 1235
Herpetic whitlow, 1235, 1237
Herplex. *See* Idoxuridine
Heterophil antibody tests, in mononucleosis, 1243
Heterophyes species, 1376
Heterotopic pregnancy, 713. *See also* Ectopic pregnancy
HEV. *See* Hepatitis E virus
Hexalen. *See* Altretamine
Hexosaminidase deficiency, in juvenile spinal muscular atrophy, 921
HFE gene, in hemochromatosis, 627

hGH. *See* Human growth hormone
HGV. *See* Hepatitis G virus
HHEX-IDE gene, in type 2 diabetes, 1082
HHT. *See* Hereditary hemorrhagic telangiectasia
HHV. *See* Human herpesviruses
5-HIAA. *See* 5-Hydroxyindoleacetic acid
Hiatal hernia
esophageal webs and rings and, 537
GERD and, 531
Hib vaccine, 1188–1189t, 1192–1193t
Hibernation, myocardial, 317
Hiccups, **507**
HIDA scan, in cholecystitis, 636
Hidradenitis suppurativa, 141
High-altitude cerebral edema, **1418**
High-altitude pulmonary edema, **1418**
High blood pressure. *See* Hypertension
High-calcium diet, 1146–1147
High-carbohydrate diet
cholesterol lowering and, 1130
in porphyria, 923, 1512
High-density lipoproteins/cholesterol, 1124
atherogenesis/coronary heart disease and, 316, 1123, 1124
cholesterol-lowering diets and, 1130
in diabetes mellitus, 1085–1086
estrogen replacement affecting, 1071
pioglitazone affecting levels of, 1093
raising levels of
fibric acid derivatives for, 1132
niacin for, 1131, 1133, 1142
reference values for, 1550t
rosiglitazone affecting levels of, 1093
screening tests for levels of, 1126, 1128
testosterone replacement affecting, 1065
High dose chemotherapy, with bone marrow/stem cell transplantation, 475, 476. *See also* Bone marrow/stem cell transplantation
High-fiber diet. *See* Fiber, dietary
High molecular-weight kininogen deficiency, 494
High-potassium diet, 1146
Highly active antiretroviral therapy (HAART), 4, 1205. *See also* Antiretroviral therapy
in cytomegalovirus disease control, 168, 1223, 1246
drug resistance and, 1223, 1225–1227, 1232, 1233
immune reconstitution disease and, 1216–1217
nephropathy progression and, 843
opportunistic infection/malignancies and, 1205, 1223, 1225
during pregnancy, 726
after rape/sexual assault, 1167
Hill sign, 312
Hip
arthritis of
nongonococcal acute bacterial (septic), 777
obesity and, 730
osteonecrosis of, 783

Hip fracture
  falls in elderly and, 18, 68, 69
  osteoporosis and, 1038
  postoperative delirium and, 56
Hip protectors, fracture prevention and, 18
Hirschsprung disease, in multiple endocrine neoplasia, 1077
Hirsutism, **1053–1055**
  in polycystic ovary syndrome, 690, 691, 1053
His-ventricular interval, long, 356
Histamine
  in bronchial provocation testing for asthma, 219
  drugs blocking receptors for. *See* Antihistamines; H$_2$ receptor blocking drugs
Histiocytosis, Langerhans cell, 991, 995
Histoplasma capsulatum (histoplasmosis), **1391–1392**
  bone and joint involvement in, **781**
Histrionic (hysterical) personality disorder, 951*t*
HIT. *See* Heparin-induced thrombocytopenia
HIV/HIV-1, 1208. *See also* HIV infection/AIDS
  drug resistance and, 1223, 1225–1227, 1232, 1233
  drugs blocking entry of into cells (entry inhibitors), 1227*t*, 1231, 1232*f*
    in combinations, 1227, 1232*f*
  screening blood for antibody to, 4–5, 478, 1207, 1219
  serologic tests in identification of. *See* HIV testing
HIV-2, 1208. *See also* HIV infection/AIDS
HIV-associated cognitive/motor complex (AIDS dementia complex), 986, 1212
HIV-associated nephropathy, **843**
HIV infection/AIDS, 4–5, **1205–1234**. *See also* Immunocompromised host
  adenovirus infection and, 1275
  adrenal insufficiency in, 1214
  anal cancer and, 1216, 1483
  arthritis in, 779, 1212–1213
  autoimmunity in, 1208
  bacillary angiomatosis/bartonellosis in, 1215, 1321
  biliary disease in, 1214
  breast feeding in transmission of, 726, 1207, 1221
  campylobacter/campylobacter-like organisms causing disease in, 1214, 1316
  cancer associated with, 1208, 1215–1216, 1224–1225*t*
  candidiasis in, 125, 202, 1215, 1223, 1224*t*, 1390
    esophageal, 1210, 1213, 1224*t*, 1390
    oral (thrush), 125, 202, 1213
    vulvovaginal, 1216, 1224*t*
  CD4 T cells in. *See* CD4 T cells
  CDC definitions and, 1205, 1206*t*

cerebral lymphoma in, 898*t*, 901, 1212, 1216
  EBV DNA and, 901
Chagas disease and, 1350
cholecystitis in, 1214
CIN/cervical cancer in, 681, 1216
clinical findings in, 1208–1217, 1209*f*
coccidial and microsporidial infection in, 1369, 1370, 1371
coccidioidomycosis in, 1393
coronary heart disease in, 1216
counseling and, 1220
  postexposure prophylaxis and, 1221
cryptococcosis/cryptococcal meningitis in, 901, 1212, 1224*t*, 1396, 1397
  prevention of, 1222–1223, 1397
cryptosporidiosis in, 1214, 1369, 1370
cytomegalovirus infections in, 1224*t*, 1245, 1245–1246
  esophagitis, 535, 1245
  prophylaxis of, 1222, 1246
  retinitis, 167–168, 1213, 1223, 1245, 1246
dementia associated with, 986, 1212
diarrhea/enterocolitis in, 511, 515, 516, 1214, 1369–1371
differential diagnosis of, 1218
drug use and, 1168, 1207, 1219, 1220
  postexposure prophylaxis and, 1221
endocrinologic manifestations of, 1214
eosinophilic folliculitis in, 123, 1208
esophagitis in, 535, 1210, 1213, 1224*t*
etiology of, 1208
extrapyramidal effects in patients with, 959
fever/FUO and, 1153, 1154, 1209
folliculitis and, 123, 1208, 1215
gastrointestinal manifestations of, 1213–1214
gastropathy in, 1214
gynecologic manifestations of, 1216
hairy leukoplakia in, 202, 1213
health care maintenance for patients with, 1219–1220, 1219*t*
hemophilia and, 491
hepatic disease/hepatitis in, 602, 604, 609, 1213–1214
hepatitis A vaccine in, 606, 1195*t*
hepatitis B vaccine in, 606, 1187, 1195*t*, 1220
herpes simplex infection in, 114, 1224*t*
  acyclovir treatment/prophylaxis and, 1157, 1215, 1237
  esophagitis, 535, 1236
herpes zoster and, 115, 1215, 1225*t*, 1241
histoplasmosis in, 1392
Hodgkin disease in, 1216
hyperkalemia in, 798, 1214
hyponatremia in, 790
immune thrombocytopenic purpura in, 482, 484
immunization recommendations in, 5, 1195*t*, 1220

incidence/prevalence of, 4, 1207
infections in, 1205, 1206*t*, 1208. *See also specific type and* Opportunistic infections
  CD4 T cell levels and, 1205, 1208–1209, 1209*f*, 1217–1218
  prevention of, 1219–1220, 1219*t*, 1222–1223, 1222*t*
  treatment of, 1223, 1224–1225*t*
inflammatory reactions in, 1216–1217
influenza vaccination and, 5, 1195*t*, 1198, 1220, 1270
intracranial tumors in, **901**
Kaposi sarcoma in, 135, 1208, 1211, 1215–1216, 1225*t*, 1476
laboratory findings in, 1217–1218, 1217*t*
lactic acidosis and, 808
leishmaniasis and, 1352
lymphadenopathy in, eustachian tube dysfunction/serous otitis media and, 192
lymphoma in, 214, 1211, 1212, 1216, 1224*t*
MAC infections in, 258, 1224*t*, 1324–1325
  prevention of, 1222, 1325
malabsorption in, 1214
malaria in, 1354
measles in, 1248
  vaccination against, 1195*t*, 1220, 1249
meningococcal vaccine in, 1195*t*, 1199
mental status changes in. *See* HIV-associated cognitive/motor complex
MMR vaccination and, 1195*t*, 1220, 1249
molluscum contagiosum in, 133, 1215, 1277
myelopathies in, 1212
myocarditis in, 368
myopathy in, 779, 1213
nephropathy in, **843**
neurologic manifestations of, 1211–1212
neuropathy, 924, 1212
nontuberculous mycobacterial infection in, 258, 259, 1211, 1324–1325
ocular manifestations of, **167–168**
oral lesions in, 1213
otitis media and, 192
otologic manifestations of, **191–192**
P marneffei infection in, 1400
parvovirus infection in, 1276, 1277
pathogenesis of, 1208
pathophysiology of, 1208
perinatal transmission of, 726, 1207, 1221
  breast feeding and, 726, 1207, 1221
pneumonia in, 251, 1210. *See also Pneumocystis jiroveci* pneumonia
  CD4 T cell count and, 1210
  immunization against. *See* Pneumococcal vaccine

pneumonitis in, nonspecific interstitial, 1211
postexposure prophylaxis and, 1221
in pregnancy, **726**, 1207, 1221
prevention of. *See* HIV infection/
AIDS, transmission of,
prevention of
prognosis of, 1205, 1233
progressive multifocal leukoencephalopathy in, 1212, 1261
psoriasis/psoriatic arthritis in, 104,
779, 1213, 1215
pulmonary manifestations of, **251**,
1210–1211. *See also* HIV
infection/AIDS, pneumo-
nia in
reactive arthritis and, 776, 779, 1213
retinitis in, 167–168, 1213, 1223
rheumatic manifestations of, **779**,
1212–1213
scabies in, 137, 138
sclerosing cholangitis in, 1214
screening for. *See* HIV testing
seizures in, 879
sinusitis in, 195, 1211
skin disorders in, 1215
sporotrichosis in, 1400
strongyloidiasis in, 1381
syphilis and, 1220, 1333, **1337–1338**
syphilis tests affected by, 1332, 1337
systemic complaints associated with,
1209–1210
T cells in. *See* CD4 T cells
toxoplasmosis in, 901, 1211–1212,
1224*t*, 1363–1364, 1364,
1365
prophylaxis of, 1222, 1365
transient ischemic attacks and, 886
transmission of, 1205–1208
bites in, 1166
to fetus/newborn, 726, 1207, 1221
health care providers and,
1220–1221
prevention of, 4–5, 1218–1221,
1219*t*
blood screening/blood treatment and, 4–5, 478, 1207,
1219
condoms for, 4, 699, 1218–1219,
1220
postexposure prophylaxis and,
1221
rape/sexual assault and, 702, 1167
sexual behavior and, 1205–1207
transfusions and, 1207, 1219
treatment of, 1221–1233
adjunctive, 1223
antiretroviral therapy, 1223–1234,
1226–1227*t*, 1232*f. See also*
Antiretroviral therapy
opportunistic infections/malignan-
cies and, 1223, 1224–1225*t*
prophylaxis and, 1222–1223,
1222*t*
during pregnancy, 726, 1207, 1221
tuberculosis and, 255–256, 1211
tuberculin skin test in, 253*t*, 254,
1211, 1219

tuberculosis in, 4, 253, 1210–1211
chemoprophylaxis/prevention and,
4, 257, 1219–1220, 1222
intestinal involvement in, 568
peritoneal involvement and, 527
treatment of, 255–256, 1211
vaccine development and, 1219
varicella zoster virus infection and,
115, 1215, 1225*t*, 1241
VDRL test in, 1220, 1337
weight loss in, 1209–1210
Wernicke encephalopathy in, 915
in women, 726, 1207, 1221. *See also*
HIV infection/AIDS, peri-
natal transmission of
HIV integrase inhibitors, 1227*t*, 1231,
1232*f*
in combinations, 1227, 1232*f*
HIV painful articular syndrome, 779
HIV rapid antibody tests, 1217, 1217*t*
HIV RNA tests, reference values for, 1551*t*
HIV testing, 4–5, 1217–1218, 1217*t*
in blood screening, 4–5, 478, 1207,
1219
influenza vaccine affecting results in,
1217
after needle-stick, 1220
in pregnancy, 706, 708, 726, 1221
after rape/sexual assault, 702, 1167
reference values for, 1551*t*
in STD patients, 1167
in syphilis patients, 1220, 1333
transmission prevention and, 4–5,
1218
HIV viral load tests, 1217*t*, 1218
antiretroviral therapy initiation/mon-
itoring and, 1223, 1225,
1232
blood screening and, 1207
reference values for, 1551*t*
Hives. *See* Urticaria
Hivid. *See* Zalcitabine
HJV gene, in juvenile-onset hemochromatosis, 627
HLA typing. *See* Human leukocyte antigen (HLA) typing
hMG. *See* Human menopausal gonadotropins
HMG-CoA reductase inhibitors. *See*
Statin drugs
HMSN. *See* Hereditary motor and sensory
neuropathy
HNF1α (hepatocyte nuclear factor 1α),
hepatic adenomas and, 633
HNPCC. *See* Hereditary nonpolyposis
colorectal cancer
Hoarseness, **207**
contact ulcers causing, 209
gastroesophageal reflux and, 209
laryngeal leukoplakia causing, 209
laryngitis causing, 208
laryngopharyngeal reflux causing, 208
in recurrent respiratory papillomatosis, 208
vocal fold nodules and, 209
HOCM (hypertrophic obstructive cardiomyopathy). *See* Cardiomyopathy

Hodgkin disease, **471**, 1466*t*
bone marrow/stem cell transplantation for, 471, 475
fever/FUO and, 1154
in HIV infection/AIDS, 1216
Holiday heart, 346
Holosystolic murmurs. *See* Heart murmurs
Holter monitoring. *See* Ambulatory electrocardiographic monitor-
ing
Homans sign, in deep venous thrombosis/
pulmonary embolism,
268*t*
Home environment, of elderly patients,
falls and, 68, 69*t*
Home hemodialysis, 831
Home oxygen therapy, 236, 236*t*
Homeostenosis. *See* Age/aging
Homocysteine
disorders of metabolism of,
1516–1517
reference values for, 1551*t*
Homocystinuria, 1517
Homogentisic acid oxidase deficiency, in
alkaptonuria, 1513
Homonymous field defects. *See* Visual
field defects
Homosexuality
hepatitis B transmission and, 602
HIV infection/AIDS transmission risk
and, 1207
STDs and, 1166, 1167
Honey, infant botulism and, 1299
"Honeycomb" lung, in interstitial (diffuse parenchymal) lung
disease, 263
Hookworm disease, **1380**
cutaneous larva migrans caused by,
1385
eosinophilic pulmonary syndromes
and, 266, 1380
Hordeolum, **152**
Hormone receptor sites, in breast cancer,
663–664
in male, 673
prognosis and, 665*t*
treatment and, 663–664, 666
Hormone replacement therapy (HRT).
See Estrogen (hormone)
replacement therapy
Hormone therapy. *See also* Estrogen (hormone) replacement ther-
apy; Testosterone
replacement therapy
adverse ophthalmic effects of, 177*t*
for breast cancer, 666–667, 667,
668–669, 668*t*
hormone receptor sites and,
663–664, 666
in male, 673
breast feeding and, 710*t*
in contraception, **697–698**
injections/implants, **697**
oral contraceptives, **694–697**,
695–696*t*, 696*t*
for dysfunctional uterine bleeding,
675

Hormone therapy (*cont.*)
for erectile dysfunction, 863
for lactation suppression, **709–710**
for male infertility, 866
for osteoporosis prevention/management, 704, 1040–1041
for prostate cancer, 1487–1488, 1487*t*
Hormones, ectopic production of
by islet cell tumors, 1062
in paraneoplastic syndromes, 1451–1452
Horner syndrome (oculosympathetic paralysis)
in headache, 45, 875
in lung cancer, 1454
Hospice care, **90–91**. *See also* End of life, provision of care at
Hospital (health care)-associated infections, **1159–1162**
bacterial rhinosinusitis, 193, 194
burn injury and, 1411
coagulase-negative staphylococci causing, 1296–1297
fever/FUO and, 1153
hemorrhagic fevers, 1262
hepatitis C, 604
parvovirus B19, 1277
pneumonia, **248–249**, 1181*t*. *See also* Pneumonia
Hospitalization
for alcohol use/abuse/withdrawal, 980
for asthma/asthma exacerbation, 233
for community-acquired pneumonia, 246, 247
for COPD, 238
for depression, 964
infections acquired during. *See* Hospital (health care)-associated infections
for personality disorders, 951
for preeclampsia/eclampsia, 717*t*
prolonged, 989
psychiatric problems associated with, **988–990**
for schizophrenic/psychotic disorders, 954
for suicidal patient, 963, 964
for third-trimester bleeding, 720
for tuberculosis, 254
Host defenses, impairment of. *See* Immunocompromised host
Hot environments, disorders caused by exposure to, 1403, **1406–1408**. *See also under* Heat
Hot flushes
black cohosh for, 1523*t*, 1527
in carcinoid syndrome, 1475, 1476
estrogen replacement therapy for, 703–704, 1071
in menopause, 703, 1070
Hot soaks, for wart removal, 132
Hot tub (*Pseudomonas*) folliculitis, 123, 124
Household cleaning agents, poisoning caused by. *See* Caustic/corrosive agents
Howell-Jolly bodies, in sickle cell anemia, 451

HPC (hematopoietic progenitor cell transplantation). *See* Bone marrow/stem cell transplantation
HPMPC. *See* Cidofovir
HPS. *See* Hantavirus pulmonary syndrome
HPV. *See* Human papillomavirus
HPV (16/18) and HPV (6/11/16/18) L1 virus-like particle vaccine, 4, 132, 595, 681, 682, 1187–1198, 1190–1191*t*, 1192–1193*t*, 1194–1197*t*
adverse effects/contraindications and, 1202*t*
HRIG. *See* Human rabies immune globulin
HRT (hormone replacement therapy). *See* Estrogen (hormone) replacement therapy
HRV. *See* Rotavirus vaccine
HSDD. *See* Hypoactive sexual desire disorder
HSV-1. *See* Herpes simplex infection, type 1
HSV-2. *See* Herpes simplex infection, type 2
5-HT₃ receptor antagonists. *See* Serotonin 5-HT₃-receptor-blocking agents
HTLV. *See* Human T cell lymphotropic/leukemia virus
Humalog. *See* Insulin lispro
Human bite wounds, **1165–1166**
Human chorionic gonadotropin (hCG)
in amenorrhea, pregnancy and, 1068, 1068–1069, 1070
for cryptorchism, 1066
in ectopic pregnancy, 705, 713
in gestational trophoblastic disease, 715
hyperthyroidism and, 715, 1009
gynecomastia and, 1067
hyperthyroidism during pregnancy and, 715, 1008, 1010
for male infertility, 866, 994
pregnancy tests and, 705
reference values for, 1548*t*
spontaneous abortion and, 712
testicular tumors producing, 1066, 1493
Human deoxyribonuclease (rhDNase), for cystic fibrosis, 242
Human diploid cell (HDCV) rabies vaccine, 1201, 1256
Human granulocytic ehrlichiosis/anaplasmosis, 1281*t*, 1285, 1286
Lyme disease coinfection and, 1346
Human growth hormone, 994–995. *See also* Growth hormone
Human herpesvirus 3. *See* Varicella-zoster virus
Human herpesvirus 4. *See* Epstein-Barr virus
Human herpesvirus 1 and 2. *See* Herpes simplex infection
Human herpesvirus 6, 1240*t*, **1247**
aphthous ulcers and, 203

Human herpesvirus 7, 1240*t*, **1247**
Human herpesvirus 8 (Kaposi sarcoma-associated herpes virus), 135, 1208, **1247**
Human herpesviruses, **1235–1247**. *See also specific type*
Human immunodeficiency virus. *See* HIV/HIV-1; HIV-2
Human insulin, 1096, 1096*t*. *See also* Insulin therapy
Human interferons. *See specific type under* Interferon
Human leukocyte antigen (HLA) typing
for granulocyte transfusions, 478
for platelet transfusions, 478
for stem cell transplant, 475
Human menopausal gonadotropins (hMG), for ovulation induction, 693
Human metapneumovirus, 1268
Human monocytic ehrlichiosis, 1281*t*, 1285, 1286
Human-origin influenza, **1269–1271**. *See also* Influenza
Human papillomavirus (HPV)
in anal cancer, 1216, 1483
in CIN/cervical cancer, 681, 682, 1216
screening for, 681
nasal tumors (inverted papillomas) caused by, 200
recurrent respiratory (laryngeal) papillomas caused by, 208
vaccine for. *See* Human papillomavirus (HPV) vaccine
in vulvar carcinoma, 678, 685
warts caused by, 131, 132
anorectal involvement and, 595
vaginal/vulvar involvement and, 678
Human papillomavirus (HPV) vaccine, 4, 132, 595, 681, 682, 1187–1198, 1190–1191*t*, 1192–1193*t*, 1194–1197*t*
adverse effects/contraindications and, 1202*t*
in recurrent respiratory papillomatosis, 208
Human papillomavirus (HPV) virus-like particle (VLP) vaccine, 4, 681, 682, 1187–1198. *See also* Human papillomavirus (HPV) vaccine
Human parechovirus infection, **1280**
Human parvovirus B19 infection. *See* Parvovirus B19 infection
Human rabies immune globulin, 1256
Human T cell lymphotropic/leukemia virus (HTLV), 1207, **1261–1262**
myelopathy caused by, **915**, 1261–1262
transfusion in transmission of/screening blood for, 1261, 1262
Humidifier lung, 280*t*
Humira. *See* Adalimumab
Humoral immunity. *See also* B lymphocytes; Immunoglobulins
infections associated with defects in, 1156

Humulin, 1096. *See also* Insulin therapy
Hungry bone syndrome, 1037
Huntingtin gene, 908
Huntington disease, **908–909**, 986
    parkinsonism differentiated from, 906
Huntington disease-like (HDL) disor-
        ders, 909
Hürthle cell thyroid carcinoma, 1023,
        1025, 1028
HUS. *See* Hemolytic-uremic syndrome
Hutchinson sign, 1241
Hyaline, alcoholic (Mallory bodies), 614,
        617
Hyaline casts, 817*t*
Hybridization, in situ, for HER-2/*neu*
        assessment in breast can-
        cer, 663
Hycamtin. *See* Topotecan
Hydatid disease/cysts, 1378–1379
Hydatidiform mole, **714–715**. *See also*
        Gestational trophoblastic
        disease
    hyperthyroidism in, 715, 1009
Hydralazine
    for heart failure, 364
    for hypertension, 407, 408*t*
        during pregnancy, 718
        urgencies/emergencies, 412, 413*t*
Hydration. *See* Fluid management/hydra-
        tion
Hydrea. *See* Hydroxyurea
Hydrocarbon toxicity/abuse, 1444
    pneumonitis and, 277, 1444
Hydrocele
    in filariasis, 1386
    in testicular cancer, 1493
Hydrocephalus
    arteriovenous malformations caus-
        ing, 895
    intracranial aneurysm causing, 894
    intracranial tumor causing, 900
    normal-pressure, 919
Hydrochlorothiazide, 398, 399*t*. *See also*
        Diuretics; Thiazide diuret-
        ics
    in combination products, 399*t*, 400*t*,
        403*t*, 404*t*
Hydrocodone, 78, 83*t*
Hydrocortisone, 1077. *See also* Corticoste-
        roids
    for ACTH deficiency, 994
        acute adrenal insufficiency, 1047
        Addison disease, 1049–1050, 1050
    for hypopituitarism, 994
    for inflammatory bowel disease/ulcer-
        ative colitis, 575–576, 584,
        584*t*, 585
    perioperative, 58
    topical, 94, 96*t*
Hydro-Diuril. *See* Hydrochlorothiazide
Hydrofluoric acid burns, 1411, 1429
Hydrogen breath test
    in bacterial overgrowth, 562
    in lactase deficiency, 515, 563
Hydrogen cyanide gas, poisoning caused
        by, 1435
Hydromorphone, 78, 81*t*
    overdose/toxicity of, 1442–1443

Hydronephrosis, in tubulointerstitial dis-
        ease, 845, 846
Hydrophobia, in rabies, 1256
Hydrops
    endolymphatic. *See* Endolymphatic
        hydrops
    fetalis, 443*t*
    of gallbladder, 636
Hydroquinone, for hyperpigmentation,
        145
Hydroxocobalamin, for cyanide poison-
        ing, 1424*t*, 1435, 1435*t*
β-Hydroxybutyrate/hydroxybutyric acid
    in alcoholic ketoacidosis, 809
    in diabetes mellitus, 1083
    in diabetic ketoacidosis, 808, 809, 1113
γ-Hydroxybutyrate, overdose/toxicity of,
        1437
    Cushing syndrome and, 1052
Hydroxychloroquine
    adverse ophthalmic effects of, 178*t*,
        750
    arrhythmias caused by, 1445
    for lupus, 111, 754
    for porphyria cutanea tarda, 117
    for rheumatoid arthritis, 750
18-Hydroxycorticosterone, in aldoster-
        onism, 1056
5-Hydroxyindoleacetic acid (5-HIAA)
    carcinoids secreting, 1476
    reference values for, 1551*t*
11-Hydroxylase/P450c11 deficiency, 1054,
        1057, 1068
17-Hydroxylase/P450c17 deficiency, 1057,
        1068
21-Hydroxylase/P450c21 deficiency,
        1053–1054, 1054, 1055,
        1068
Hydroxymethylglutaryl-coenzyme A
        (HMG-CoA) reductase
        inhibitors. *See* Statin drugs
17-Hydroxyprogesterone
    in amenorrhea, 1068
    in hirsutism/virilization, 1054
    in preterm (premature) labor preven-
        tion, 719
11β-Hydroxysteroid dehydrogenase
    in hypertension, 391
    in licorice-induced hypokalemia, 1057
3β-Hydroxysteroid dehydrogenase defi-
        ciency, amenorrhea in,
        1068
17β-Hydroxysteroid dehydrogenase-3
        deficiency, 1054
5-Hydroxytryptamine-3 receptor antago-
        nists. *See* Serotonin 5-HT$_3$-
        receptor-blocking agents
Hydroxyurea
    in cancer chemotherapy, 1505*t*
    for essential thrombocytosis, 459
    for polycythemia, 458
    for sickle cell disease, 451
25-Hydroxyvitamin D$_3$. *See* Calcifediol
Hydroxyzine, 941*t*. *See also* Antihista-
        mines
    for insomnia, 941*t*, 974
    for pruritus, 94–95
    for urticaria, 126

Hygiene hypothesis, for diabetes mellitus,
        1081
Hygroton. *See* Chlorthalidone
Hymen, imperforate, absent menses and,
        1068
Hymenolepis
    diminuta (rodent tapeworm), 1376
    nana (dwarf tapeworm), 1376, **1377**
Hyoscyamus niger, overdose/toxicity of,
        1432
Hyper-IgE syndrome, atopic-like dermati-
        tis in, 102
Hyperacusis, **188**
Hyperadrenergic syndrome, mitral valve
        prolapse and, 309
Hyperaldosteronism. *See* Aldosteronism
Hyperalimentation. *See* Central vein
        nutritional support
Hyperandrogenism, 1053–1055
    acne and, 120, 1054
    amenorrhea caused by, 1068, 1069
    in hirsutism/virilization, 1053–1055
Hyperbaric oxygen therapy
    for altitude-related illness, 1418
    for carbon monoxide poisoning,
        1424*t*, 1433–1434
    for clostridial myonecrosis, 1297
    for dysbarism/decompression sick-
        ness, 1417
Hyperbilirubinemia, 598, 599*t*. *See also*
        Bilirubin levels; Jaundice
    in biliary tract carcinoma, 1462
    in choledocholithiasis/cholangitis, 638
Hypercalcemia, **800–802**, 801*t*, 1034*f*,
        1035–1036. *See also*
        Hyperparathyroidism
    in Addison disease, 1033, 1050
    adrenocortical insufficiency and, 1036
    artifact causing, 1035
    bisphosphonate use causing, 1036, 1040
    bisphosphonates for, 801, 1037, 1497
    cancer-related, 801, 1035, 1453*t*, 1454,
        1496–1497
        pamidronate/zoledronic acid for,
        1037, 1497, 1507*t*
    chemotherapy-induced, **1496–1497**
    familial hypocalciuric, 796*t*, 798, 801,
        1034, 1036
    hypercalciuria and, 801
    hyperparathyroidism and, 800–802,
        801*t*, 1033–1038, 1034*f*
    hypertension and, 392
    in hyperthyroidism, 1036
    hypocalciuria and, 796*t*, 798, 801,
        1034, 1036
    hypoparathyroidism treatment and,
        1032, 1033
    in kidney injury/renal failure/dialysis
        patients, 802, 827*t*, 1034
    lithium use and, 971, 1036
    in multiple endocrine neoplasia, 556
    in myeloma, 472, 848, 1035
    parathyroid carcinoma and, 1033,
        1037
    in sarcoidosis, 265
Hypercalciuria, 857, 858–859, 858*t*. *See also*
        Calcium nephrolithiasis
    hypercalcemia and, 801

Hypercalciuria (*cont.*)
hyperparathyroidism and, 859, 1033
hypocalcemia/hypoparathyroidism
and, 800, 1030, 1031, 1032
with hypomagnesemia, 796*t*
in sarcoidosis, 265
Hypercapnia. *See* Permissive hypercapnia; Respiratory acidosis
Hypercarotenosis, 1144
Hyperchloremic normal anion gap acidosis, 808*t*, **809–812**, 809*t*,
811
alcoholic ketoacidosis and, 809
diabetic ketoacidosis and, 808–809,
1114–1115
dilutional, 810
gastrointestinal bicarbonate loss and,
809–810, 809*t*
parenteral nutritional support and,
810, 1151*t*
posthypocapnia, 810
renal disease/renal tubular acidosis
and, 809*t*, 810, 811
urinary anion gap in assessment of,
809*t*, 810–811
Hypercholesterolemia. *See also* Cholesterol
familial, 1123
heart disease risk and, 316, 1123
management of. *See* Lipid-lowering
therapy
in nephrotic syndrome, 838, 840
screening for, 1126–1129, 1127–1128*t*,
1129*t*
Hyperchylomicronemia, 1123
in diabetes mellitus, 1083
familial, 1123
Hypercoagulability
in acute mesenteric vein occlusion,
422
in Behçet syndrome, 772
deep venous thrombosis/pulmonary
embolism and, 267
in hepatic vein obstruction (Budd-
Chiari syndrome), 630
in nephrotic syndrome, 840
in noncirrhotic portal hypertension,
631
in paroxysmal nocturnal hemoglobinuria, 449
Hypercortisolism, **1050–1053**. *See also*
Cushing syndrome
Hyperemesis gravidarum, **710–711**
thyroid disorders and, 711, 1008
Hypereosinophilic syndromes, cardiac
involvement in, 383
Hypergammaglobulinemia
bronchiectasis and, 240
chronic pancreatitis and, 646
in HIV infection/AIDS, 1208
Hypergastrinemia
carcinoid tumors and, 1473, 1474
in pernicious anemia gastritis, 547
Zollinger-Ellison syndrome (gastrinoma) and, 556, 557
Hyperglycemia. *See also* Diabetes mellitus
in alcoholic ketoacidosis, 809
antipsychotic drug use and, 958
chronic kidney disease and, 830

coma caused by. *See* Diabetic coma
control of. *See* Glycemic control in
diabetes
in diabetic ketoacidosis, 808, 1112
differential diagnosis of, 1086, 1086*t*
drugs causing, 1086
drugs for treatment of, 1090–1096,
1091*t*. *See also* Antidiabetic
agents; Insulin therapy
in hyperglycemic hyperosmolar state,
1115
hyponatremia and, 789, 790*f*
hypophosphatemia associated with
treatment of, 804
insulin resistance and, 1081, 1086,
1086*t*
pancreatitis/pancreatectomy and,
1086
parenteral nutritional support and,
1151, 1151*t*
in pheochromocytoma, 1059
prebreakfast, 1102–1103, 1103*t*
in pregnancy, congenital anomalies
caused by, 722–723
surgery and, prevention of, 57–58,
57*t*, 58*t*, 1109
Hyperglycemic coma. *See* Diabetic coma
Hyperglycemic hyperosmolar state, 1112*t*,
1115–1116
Hyperhomocysteinemia, in coronary
heart disease/occlusive
arterial disease, 1516, 1517
Hypericin/hyperforin/*Hypericum perforatum* (St. John's wort),
1522–1524, 1523*t*
drug interactions and, 1523
Hyperinfection syndrome, in strongyloidiasis, 1381
Hyperinsulinemia
acne and, 120
factitious, 1118
hypoglycemic
insulinoma causing, 1118
islet hyperplasia causing, 1120
in insulin resistance syndrome (syndrome X), 14, 1082
in polycystic ovary syndrome, 690,
1053
Hyperkalemia, **797–798**, 797*t*, 799*t*
in acidosis, 798, 809*t*, 810
adrenocortical insufficiency/Addison
disease and, 797, 1047,
1049
angiotensin-converting enzyme
(ACE) inhibitors causing,
405, 797, 798
in diabetic ketoacidosis, 1112, 1114
genetic disorders and, 796*t*
in HIV infection/AIDS, 798, 1214
in hyporeninemic hypoaldosteronism,
809*t*, 810, 1049
postoperative, 59
renal disorders/failure and, 796, 798,
819, 823, 827
in tumor lysis syndrome, 1497
Hyperkalemic periodic paralysis, 796*t*,
936
Hyperkeratosis, plantar, of heels, 133

Hyperketonemia
in diabetic ketoacidosis, 809, 1112
at end of life, 91
Hyperleukocytosis
in acute leukemia, 465
in chronic myeloid leukemia, 461, 462
Hyperlipidemia
antipsychotic drugs and, 958, 958*t*
antiretroviral therapy causing, 1216,
1229
in diabetes mellitus, 1085–1086, 1108,
1126*t*
familial combined, 1123
garlic for, 1523*t*, 1524
hyponatremia and, 789, 790*f*, 792
in nephrotic syndrome, 838, 840,
1126*t*
treatment of. *See* Lipid-lowering therapy
Hypermagnesemia, **806**
in acute tubular necrosis/kidney
injury, 823
hypomagnesemia treatment and, 805
Hypermetabolism
in burn injury, 1411
in HIV infection/AIDS, 1209
Hypermethioninemia, newborn screening
for, 1517
Hypernatremia, **793–794**
in diabetes insipidus, 793–794, 996
in diabetes mellitus/glucosuria, 793
enteral nutritional support and, 1150
Hyperopia, 151
Hyperosmolality (hyperosmolar disorders), **795**
hyperglycemia and (hyperglycemic
hyperosmolar state),
1112*t*, **1115–1116**
hypernatremia and, 793
Hyperosmolar nonketotic dehydration,
parenteral nutritional support and, 1151*t*
Hyperostosis, diffuse idiopathic skeletal
(DISH), 774
Hyperoxaluric calcium nephrolithiasis,
859
Hyperparathyroidism, **1033–1038**, 1034*f*.
See also Hypercalcemia
chronic kidney disease and, 827, 1035
bone changes and, 827, 829, 1033,
1035, 1038
hypercalcemia and, 800–802, 801*t*,
1033–1038, 1034*f*
hypercalciuria and, 859, 1033
lithium use and, 971
in multiple endocrine neoplasia, 1033,
1075–1076, 1076*t*
after parathyroidectomy, 1037
parathyroidectomy for, 1036–1037
during pregnancy, 1034
Hyperparathyroidism-jaw tumor syndrome, 1033
Hyperpathia
intracranial mass lesions causing, 899
neuropathy causing, 922
stroke causing, 889
Hyperphosphatemia, **804**, 804*t*
in kidney disease, 819, 829

acute tubular necrosis, 823
  hyperparathyroidism and, 829
  hypocalcemia/hypoparathyroid-
      ism and, 799, 800, 1031
  in lactic acidosis, 1117
  parenteral nutritional support and,
      1151t
  in tumor lysis syndrome, 1497
Hyperpigmentation, 144–145. See also
      Pigmented skin lesions
  in Addison disease, 1048, 1049
  in alkaptonuria, 1513
  chemotherapy-induced, 1509
  drugs causing, 145, 149t
  in hemochromatosis, 627
  nail, drugs causing, 146, 149t
  in porphyria cutanea tarda, 117
  postinflammatory, 144
  in venous insufficiency, 37, 143, 430
  in visceral leishmaniasis, 1351
Hyperprolactinemia, **1000–1002**, 1000t
  amenorrhea and, 1000, 1068, 1069,
      1070
  gynecomastia and, 1000, 1067
  hypogonadotropic hypogonadism
      and, 993–994, 994, 1000,
      1063, 1065
  nipple discharge in, 651
  risperidone-induced, 955
Hyperproteinemia, hyponatremia and,
      789, 790f, 792
Hyperreactio luteinalis, 1054
Hyperreninemic hypoaldosteronism, 1049
Hypersensitivity, visceral
  chest pain and, 543–544
  irritable bowel syndrome and, 570
Hypersensitivity pneumonitis, **279–280**,
      280t
Hypersensitivity reactions, **784**. See also
      Allergies/allergic reactions
  in HIV infection/AIDS, 1208
Hypersomnias, **975**
Hyperstat. See Diazoxide
Hypertension, **387–414**
  aldosteronism and, 390–391, 391–392,
      393, 1055–1057
  aortic dissection and, 393, 426, 427
  assessment/diagnosis of, **387**, 388t,
      389f
  atherosclerosis and, 391, 393
  biofeedback in management of,
      1536–1537, 1536t
  cardiovascular disease/risk factors
      and, 387, 389, 393, 395,
      398t, 407
  cerebrovascular disease and, 393
  chronic kidney disease/renal failure
      and, 410, 826, 827t, 828
  classification of, 387, 388–392, 388t,
      390t
  in coarctation of aorta, 296
  complications of untreated disease
      and, 392–393
  in Cushing syndrome, 392, 1052, 1054
  dementia and, 393
  in diabetes mellitus/diabetic nephrop-
      athy, 396t, 842, 1083, 1105,
      1106, 1108

angiotensin-converting enzyme
      (ACE) inhibitors for, 396t,
      402–405, 407, 409–410,
      842, 1088, 1105, 1106, 1108
  antihypertensive therapy regimens
      for, 396t, 409, 409–410,
      842
  benefits of control of, 409–410,
      1088, 1105, 1108
  calcium channel blocking agents
      and, 396t
  estrogen use and, 392
  fibromuscular dysplasia/renal artery
      stenosis and, 391, 832, 833
  genetic factors in, 390–391
  headache and, 44, 45, 393
  in heart disease/failure, 358, 393, 396t,
      405, 407
  hypercalcemia and, 392
  intracerebral hemorrhage and, 387,
      393, 412, 892
  intracranial. See Intracranial hyper-
      tension
  malignant, 411
      headache in, 44
  management of
      in blacks, 410, 410t
      in chronic kidney disease/renal fail-
          ure, 396t, 410, 828
      in diabetic patients, 396t, 409,
          409–410, 1088, 1108
      exercise/activity and, 13, 390, 394,
          395t
      heart disease prevention and, 9–12
      lifestyle modifications/nonphar-
          macologic therapy and, 13,
          388t, 394, 395t
      mind-body therapies in, 1536t
      pharmacologic, 388t, 395–398,
          396t, **398–411**. See also
          Antihypertensive drug
          therapy
      preoperative, 52
      for urgencies/emergencies,
          412–414, 413t
  metabolic syndrome (syndrome X)
      and, 14, 390, 1082
  ocular. See Ocular hypertension
  oral contraceptive use and, 392,
      696–697
  in pheochromocytoma, 392, 393,
      1058, 1059, 1061
  in poisoning/drug overdose, **1422**
  in polyarteritis nodosa, 765
  in polycystic kidney disease, 847, 848
  portal. See Portal hypertension
  portopulmonary, 623–624
  during pregnancy, 391, 392, **715–718**,
      717t, **723–724**. See also
      Preeclampsia-eclampsia
  preoperative evaluation/management
      and, 52
  prevention of, **9–12**
      exercise/activity in, 13, 390
  primary (essential), 388–390
  pulmonary. See Pulmonary hyperten-
      sion
  renal disease caused by, 393, 827t

renal disease causing, 389, 391, 826,
      828
  renal vascular, 391
  resistant, **411**, 411t
  retinochoroidopathy in, **167**
  secondary, 390–392, 390t
  sodium restriction and, 390, 394,
      395t, 1145
  stroke/stroke prevention and, 9–12,
      387, 393, 396t, 407
  emergencies/urgencies, 412
Hypertension exacerbated in pregnancy,
      391
Hypertensive emergencies, **411–414**, 413t
  MAOIs causing, 967, 1440
  in pheochromocytoma, 1059, 1061
      diagnostic imaging and, 1059–1060
  in scleroderma, 759
Hypertensive encephalopathy, 393, 411
Hypertensive nephropathy, 393, 411
Hypertensive urgencies, **411–414**, 413t.
      See also Hypertensive
      emergencies
Hyperthecosis. See Polycystic ovary syn-
      drome
Hyperthermia, **39**, 39t. See also Fever;
      Heat; Serotonin syndrome
  antipsychotic drugs causing. See Neu-
      roleptic malignant syn-
      drome
  for benign prostatic hyperplasia, 871
  heat exposure syndromes and,
      1406–1408
  malignant, 39, 1160, 1423
  in poisoning/drug overdose, **1423**. See
      also Serotonin syndrome
  prevention of, 1406–1407
Hyperthyroidism (thyrotoxicosis),
      1007–1015
  amiodarone-induced, 1009, 1010,
      1013–1014
  apathetic, 1010, 1014–1015
  atrial fibrillation in, 346, 1009, 1014
  cancer-related, 1009, 1453t
  cardiac disorders/failure and, 360,
      1009, 1014–1015
  eye disease associated with, 170, 1008,
      1009, 1012, 1014
  factitious, 1008
  in gestational trophoblastic disease,
      715, 1009
  goiter/thyroid nodules and, 1008,
      1010, 1012, 1013, 1019,
      1020
  in Graves disease, 1008, 1009,
      1010–1012, 1014, 1015
  Hashimoto thyroiditis and, 1008,
      1013, 1016, 1017,
      1017–1018
  hypercalcemia and, 1036
  iodine-induced (jodbasedow disease/
      phenomenon), 1008
  lactation and, 1013
  lipid abnormalities and, 1126t
  lithium causing, 1008
  muscle weakness and, 761
  osteoporosis and, 1009, 1039
  after parathyroidectomy, 1037

Hyperthyroidism (thyrotoxicosis) (*cont.*)
periodic paralysis and, 936, 1010, 1015
pituitary tumor/hyperplasia causing, 1008, 1013
postpartum, 1008, 1015
during pregnancy, 722, 1008–1009, 1009, 1010, 1013
preoperative evaluation/management and, 58
struma ovarii causing, 1008, 1010
subacute thyroiditis and, 1008, 1010, 1013, 1017, 1018
subclinical, 1015
thyroid carcinoma and, 1009
thyroid testing in, 1003*t*, 1004*t*, 1010
toxic adenoma/solitary nodule causing, 1008, 1012–1013
TSH levels in, 1003*t*
Hypertonic hyponatremia, 789, 790*f*
Hypertonic saline
for cystic fibrosis, 242
for hyponatremia, 792–793
Hypertrichosis
lanuginosa, 1054
minoxidil therapy and, 1055
in porphyria cutanea tarda, 117
Hypertriglyceridemia, 1124, **1133**
alcohol use/abuse and, 1125, 1126*t*
antiretroviral therapy and, 1229
in diabetes mellitus, 1085, 1125
hyponatremia and, 792
management of, 1133
in coronary heart disease prevention, 9, 1133
omega-3 fatty acids in, 1528*t*, 1530
in nephrotic syndrome, 838, 840
nonalcoholic fatty liver disease and, 617
pancreatitis and, 643, 1133
Hypertrophic/hypertrophic obstructive cardiomyopathy. *See* Cardiomyopathy
Hypertrophic gastropathy (Ménétrier disease), 547
Hypertrophic osteoarthropathy/hypertrophic pulmonary osteoarthropathy, 783, 1453*t*
Hypertrophic pulmonary osteoarthropathy, rheumatoid arthritis differentiated from, 748–749
Hyperuricemia, 732, 732*t*, 733
acute tubular necrosis/kidney injury and, 822
cancer-related/chemotherapy-induced, **1497–1498**
allopurinol for, 1497, 1507*t*
rasburicase for, 1497–1498, 1507*t*
chronic kidney disease and, 827*t*
in diabetes insipidus, 996
drugs causing, 732, 733
in gout, 732, 732*t*, 733
in polycythemia, 458
in transplant patient, 735
urinary stone formation and, 732, 859. *See also* Uric acid urinary stones

Hyperuricosuric calcium nephrolithiasis, 859
Hyperventilation, **287–288**
for acute mountain sickness, 1418
lactic acidosis and, 1016
in metabolic acidosis, 811
neurogenic, in coma or stupor, 288, 916
respiratory alkalosis (hypocapnia) and, 287, 814
Hyperviscosity syndrome
in myeloma, 472, 848
in Waldenström macroglobulinemia, 474
Hypervitaminosis A, 1144
Hypervolemic hypernatremia, 793, 794
Hypervolemic hypotonic hyponatremia, 790*f*, 791–792, 792
Hyphema, 171
Hypnagogic hallucinations. *See also* Hallucinations
in narcolepsy, 975
Hypnosis/hypnotherapy, 1520, 1536*t*, **1538–1540**
for chronic pain, 946–947, 1536*t*, 1539
for conversion disorders, 945
for irritable bowel syndrome, 573, 1536*t*, 1539
Hypnotic drugs. *See* Sedative-hypnotics
Hypoactive sexual desire disorder (HSDD), 1070, 1073
Hypoadrenalism. *See* Adrenocortical insufficiency
Hypoalbuminemia
ascites and, 524*t*
calcium levels and, 799, 800, 1497
in protein-losing enteropathy, 569
Hypoaldosteronism, 1049
Addison disease and, 1049
in renal tubular acidosis, 809*t*, 810, 1049
Hypobaric hypoxia, 1417. *See also under* High-altitude
air travel emergencies and, 1419
Hypocalcemia, **798–800**, 800*t*, 1031
familial, 796*t*, 798, 1031
with hypercalciuria, 800, 1030, 1031, 1032
hyperphosphatemia and, 799
hypomagnesemia and, 799, 800, 805, 1031
hypoparathyroidism and, 799, 800, 1030, 1031, 1034*f*. *See also* Hypoparathyroidism
kidney disease/acute tubular necrosis and, 799, 800, 822
muscle cramps caused by, 800, 1031
after parathyroidectomy, 1037
in pseudohypoparathyroidism, 1031, 1034*f*
tetany and, 800, 1031
Hypocalciuria, 801
hypercalcemia and (hypocalciuric hypercalcemia), 796*t*, 798, 801, 1034, 1036
Hypocapnia. *See* Respiratory alkalosis
Hypochloremia, in respiratory acidosis, 814

Hypochlorite, for skin/clothing decontamination, 1424, 1443
Hypocholesterolemic drugs. *See* Lipid-lowering therapy
Hypochondriasis, 940, 944
Hypocitraturic calcium nephrolithiasis, 859
Hypocomplementemia
in hepatitis C-related renal disease, 844
in SLE, 110, 753, 754*t*
Hypogammaglobulinemia
in bronchiectasis, 240
in chronic lymphocytic leukemia, 467
common variable immunodeficiency causing, 786–787
infection and, 1156
Hypoglycemia, 1112*t*, **1117–1122**, 1117*t*
adrenocortical insufficiency/Addison disease and, 1047
alcohol-related, 981, 1103, 1117*t*, 1118, **1121**
in alcoholic ketoacidosis, 809
alimentary, 1117
altered awareness of, 1103, 1118
cancer-related, 1453*t*
chronic kidney disease and, 830, 1104
coma caused by, 1111, 1112*t*
in poisoning/drug overdose, 1112*t*, 1421
drug-induced, 1117*t*, **1122**
exercise-induced, 1100, 1103
extrapancreatic tumors causing, **1120–1121**
factitious, 1118, **1122**
fasting, 1117, 1117*t*
functional, 1117, 1117*t*, **1121**
glucagon response to, lack of, 1103
immunopathologic, 1117*t*, 1118, **1122**
insulin-induced/intensive glycemic control and, 1087, 1103–1104
late (occult diabetes), **1121**
pancreatic B cell tumors/insulinoma causing, 1062, 1063, **1118–1120**, 1119*t*
pentamidine-induced, 1122, 1395
persistent islet hyperplasia causing, 1120
postgastrectomy, 1117, 1117*t*, **1121**
postprandial (reactive), 1117, 1117*t*, **1121–1122**
postethanol, 1121
status epilepticus caused by, 884
surgery and, prevention of, 57–58, 57*t*, 58*t*
Hypoglycemic agents. *See* Antidiabetic agents; Insulin therapy
Hypoglycemic unawareness, 1103, 1118
Hypogonadism
in Addison disease, 1048
female
amenorrhea in, 1067–1068, 1068, 1069, 1070
hormone replacement therapy for, 1068, 1070–1073
premature (premature ovarian failure), 1069
in Turner syndrome, 1074

GH-secreting pituitary tumor causing, 997
in HIV infection/AIDS, 1214
hypergonadotropic, 1063, 1063–1064, 1063t, 1065
hyperprolactinemia and, 993–994, 1000
hypogonadotropic, 865f, 866, 991–992, 993, 994, 1063, 1063t, 1065
in hypopituitarism, 991–992
male, 1063–1066, 1063t
gynecomastia and, 1065, 1067
hormone replacement therapy for, 863, 866, 1065–1066
infertility and, 864, 865f, 866
sexual dysfunction and, 863
osteoporosis and, 1039, 1041
Hypokalemia, 795–797, 795t
aldosteronism and, 795, 796, 1056, 1057
in diabetic ketoacidosis, 1112, 1114
diuretic use and, 398, 796
genetic disorders and, 796t
in heat stroke, 1408
in hyperchloremic metabolic acidosis/renal tubular acidosis, 809t, 810
in hyperglycemic hyperosmolar state, 1016
hypomagnesemia and, 796, 805
in metabolic alkalosis, 812, 813
parenteral nutritional support and, 1151t
renal disorders and, 796, 827t
vitamin B$_{12}$ replacement therapy and, 446
Hypokalemic hyperchloremic metabolic acidosis, 810
Hypokalemic periodic paralysis, 796t, 936
in hyperthyroidism, 936, 1010, 1015
Hypomagnesemia, 805–806, 805t
hypocalcemia/hypoparathyroidism and, 799, 800, 805, 1031
hypokalemia and, 796, 805
parenteral nutritional support and, 1151t
Hypomagnesemia-hypercalciuria syndrome, 796t
Hypomania, 962, 970. See also Mania
in cyclothymic disorders, 962
drug therapy for, 970–973, 972t
Hyponatremia, 789–793, 790f, 791t
adrenocortical insufficiency/Addison disease and, 789–790, 790f, 1047
drugs causing, 790, 790f
endurance exercise causing, 790f, 791
in HIV infection/AIDS, 790
hormone abnormalities causing, 789–790
in hyperglycemic hyperosmolar state, 1015
in hypopituitarism, 992, 993
in hypothyroidism/myxedema, 790f, 1003
nausea/pain/surgery/procedures causing, 790, 790f

after pituitary surgery, 993, 998, 1002
in porphyria, 1512
psychogenic polydipsia/beer potomania causing, 790f, 791, 953
reset osmostat causing, 791, 792
in schizophrenic/psychotic disorders, 953
in SIADH, 790f, 791, 792
Hypoparathyroidism, 1030–1033, 1032t
fetal, maternal hyperparathyroidism and, 1034
hypercalciuria and, 1031, 1032
hypocalcemia and, 799, 800, 1030, 1031, 1034f
hypomagnesemia and, 805, 1031
after parathyroid surgery, 1012, 1025
Riedel thyroiditis causing, 1017
tetany and, 1031, 1032
after thyroidectomy, 1012, 1025, 1030
Hypophosphatasia, osteomalacia in, 1043, 1044
Hypophosphatemia, 802–804, 803t
in diabetic ketoacidosis, 803, 1114
in hyperglycemic hyperosmolar state, 1016
hyperparathyroidism and, 1034
osteomalacia/rickets and, 796t, 1043, 1044
Hypophysectomy, for breast cancer, 668–669
Hypopigmentation, 144–145
in atopic dermatitis, 101
in tinea (pityriasis) versicolor, 110
in tuberous sclerosis, 903
Hypopituitarism, 991–995
amenorrhea and, 1069, 1070
after pituitary surgery, 998, 999
Hypopnea, 288. See also Apnea
Hypoprothrombinemia
in cirrhosis, 623
factor II antibodies and, 494
salicylate-induced, 1445
Hypopyon
in anterior uveitis, 160
in bacterial keratitis, 156
in Behçet syndrome, 772
Hyporeninemic hypoaldosteronism, 1049
in renal tubular acidosis, 809t, 810, 1049
Hyposmia, 197–198
Hypotension, 435
in Addison disease, 1049
bleomycin-induced, 1511
in desensitization therapy, 1186
in diabetes mellitus, 1083
dysautonomia (autonomic dysfunction) and, 884–885, 885
myocardial infarction and, 338
orthostatic (postural). See Orthostatic (postural) hypotension
palpitations and, 31
pheochromocytoma/pheochromocytoma removal and, 1058, 1060, 1061
in poisoning/drug overdose, 1421–1422
right ventricular infarction and, 338

in shock, 435
syncope and, 356
transient ischemic attacks and, 886–887
Hypotensive agents. See Antihypertensive drug therapy
Hypothalamic disorders, 991–1002
amenorrhea caused by, 1067–1068, 1069
Hypothermia
coma and, 915, 917, 1421
of extremities, 1405–1406
near drowning and, 1415, 1416
in poisoning/drug overdose, 1421
prevention of, 1405
rhabdomyolysis and, 763
systemic (accidental), 1403–1405, 1404f
Hypothyroidism, 994, 1003–1007, 1004t
amiodarone-induced, 1003–1004
cardiac disorders/failure and, 360, 1005
congenital/fetal, 1003, 1006, 1029
maternal hyperthyroidism and, 1013
cretinism and, 1029
goiter/thyroid nodules and, 1003, 1004, 1019, 1019–1020
Hashimoto thyroiditis and, 1003, 1007, 1016, 1018
after hyperthyroidism treatment, 1011, 1012, 1013
hyponatremia in, 789, 790f
lipid abnormalities in, 1126t
lithium causing, 971
muscle weakness and, 761
myxedema pericardial effusions and, 377, 1005
obesity and, 1136
during pregnancy, 722, 1003, 1005, 1006–1007
preoperative evaluation/management and, 58
after radioiodine therapy, 1012
Riedel thyroiditis causing, 1017
in subacute (de Quervain) thyroiditis, 1003, 1017, 1018
thyroid testing in, 1003t, 1004t
after thyroidectomy, 1015, 1025
TSH deficiency/levels in, 992, 993, 994, 1003t
Hypotonic hyponatremia, 789–792, 790f
Hypouricemia, in SIADH, 792
Hypoventilation
alveolar
central, 287
primary (Ondine curse), 287
obesity and (Pickwickian syndrome), 287
respiratory acidosis and, 813
Hypovolemic hypernatremia, 793, 794
Hypovolemic hypotonic hyponatremia, 789, 790f, 792
Hypovolemic shock, 434, 434t, 435, 436
in heat stroke, 1408
in myocardial infarction, 338
Hypoxemia
in ARDS, 292

Hypoxemia (*cont.*)
  in asthma, 219
  in COPD, 234
    oxygen therapy and, 236, 236*t*
  in cystic fibrosis, 241
  in interstitial (diffuse parenchymal)
    lung disease, 262
  in malignant pleural effusion, 285
  near drowning and, 1415, 1416
  in respiratory failure, 290
Hypoxia
  hypobaric, 1417. *See also under High-altitude*
  air travel emergencies and, 1419
  lactic acidosis and, 808
  near drowning and, 1416
  in pulmonary embolism, 267
  theophyllines affected by, 225*t*
Hypoxis rooperi, for benign prostatic
    hyperplasia, 870
Hypoglycemia, fasting, postethanol, 1121
Hysterectomy. *See also* Menopause, surgical
  for abnormal premenopausal bleeding, 675
  antibiotic prophylaxis for, 60*t*
  for cervical cancer, 682–683, 683
  for endometrial carcinoma, 684–685
  for endometriosis, 687
  for ovarian cancer, 690
  for pelvic organ prolapse, 687
  for PID, 689
  premature ovarian failure and, 1069
  prophylactic, in HNPCC, 593
  for uterine leiomyoma, 684
Hysteria (somatization disorder), 944
Hysterical conversion. *See* Conversion disorder
Hysterical (histrionic) personality disorder, 951*t*
Hysterosalpingography, 675*t*
  in infertility workup, 692, 693
Hysteroscopy, 675*t*
  in abnormal premenopausal bleeding, 674–675, 675
Hytrin. *See* Terazosin
Hyzaar. *See* Losartan

^{123}I
  for thyroid scanning, 1003*t*, 1019*t*. *See
    also* Radioiodine thyroid
    scans and uptake
  for whole body scanning, in thyroid
    cancer surveillance,
    1027–1028
[^{123}I]mIBG, in pheochromocytoma, 1060,
    1061
^{131}I
  for goiter, 1012, 1013, 1030
  for Graves disease/hyperthyroidism,
    1012
    ophthalmopathy flares and, 1012,
    1014
  for thyroid cancer treatment,
    1025–1026
  for thyroid nodules, 1013, 1021
  for thyroid scanning. *See* Radioiodine
    thyroid scans and uptake

  for whole body scanning, in thyroid
    cancer surveillance,
    1027–1028
^{131}I Tositumomab, 1503*t*
IA-2/IA2-β antibodies, in type 1 diabetes,
    1080, 1080*t*
IAA. *See* Insulin, antibodies to
IADL. *See* Instrumental activities of daily
    living
Iatrogenic pneumothorax, 286
Ibandronate, for osteoporosis prevention/
    management, 1040
Ibotenic acid (anticholinergic-type)
    mushroom poisoning,
    1441, 1441*t*, 1442
Ibritumomab tiuxetan, 1503*t*
  for non-Hodgkin lymphoma, 470
Ibuprofen, 79*t*
  lithium interactions and, 972*t*
  platelet function affected by, 490*t*
Ibutilide, 344*t*
  for atrial fibrillation, 348
  for atrial flutter, 350
ICA. *See* Islet cell antibodies
ICD. *See* Implantable cardioverter
    defibrillator
Ice water bath, for heat stroke, 1408
ICSI. *See* Intracytoplasmic sperm injection
Icteric leptospirosis (Weil syndrome),
    1341
Icterus. *See* Jaundice
Idamycin. *See* Idarubicin
Idarubicin, 1502*t*
  toxicity of, 1502*t*, 1511
Idiogenic osmoles, hypernatremia treatment and, 794
Idiopathic adulthood ductopenia, 641
Idiopathic brachial plexus neuropathy
    (neuralgic amyotrophy),
    930–931
Idiopathic bronchiolitis obliterans with
    organizing pneumonia. *See*
    Cryptogenic organizing
    pneumonitis
Idiopathic cholestasis of pregnancy, 599*t*,
    727–728
Idiopathic epilepsy, 878
Idiopathic fibrosing interstitial pneumonia (idiopathic pulmonary
    fibrosis), **263–265**, 264*t*
Idiopathic membranoproliferative glomerulonephritis, **844**. *See
    also* Membranoproliferative glomerulonephritis
Idiopathic midline destructive disease,
    201
Idiopathic polyneuropathy, acute. *See*
    Guillain-Barré syndrome
Idiopathic pulmonary fibrosis. *See* Idiopathic fibrosing interstitial
    pneumonia
Idiopathic pulmonary hemosiderosis, 276
Idiopathic (primary) pulmonary hypertension, 274, **380–381**,
    381*t*
Idiopathic skeletal hyperostosis, diffuse
    (DISH), 774
Idiopathic torsion dystonia, **909–910**

Idiosyncratic drug reactions, liver disease
    caused by, **616**
Idioventricular rhythm, accelerated, **353**
  in myocardial infarction, 337, 353
Idoxuridine, 1238*t*
IFA. *See* Immunofluorescence assay
Ifex. *See* Ifosfamide
Ifosfamide, 1500*t*
  hemorrhagic cystitis caused by, 1510
  mesna for amelioration of, 1507*t*,
    1510
IgA
  in celiac disease/dermatitis herpetiformis, 118, 559, 560
  in common variable immunodeficiency, 786–787
  in mononucleosis, 1243
  in myeloma, 472, 473
  reference values for, 1551*t*
  selective deficiency of, **786**
  serum levels of, in IgA nephropathy,
    836
IgA nephropathy (Berger disease),
    834–835, 835*f*, 836*t*
IgE, 784. *See also* Allergies/allergic reactions
  in anaphylaxis/urticaria/angioedema,
    126, 784
  atopy/atopic disease and, 784
  tests for, 785
IgE-mediated (immediate/type I) hypersensitivity, 784. *See also*
    Allergies/allergic reactions
IGF-1. *See* Insulin-like growth factor-1
IGF-2. *See* Insulin-like growth factor-2
IGF2BP2 gene, in type 2 diabetes, 1082
IgG
  in antibody-mediated/cytotoxic
    hypersensitivity, 784
  in autoimmune hemolytic anemia,
    452, 453
  in bullous pemphigoid, 131
  in common variable immunodeficiency, 786–787
  deficiency of, with IgA deficiency, 786
  in hepatitis A, 602, 602*f*
  in hepatitis B, 602*f*, 603
  in IgA nephropathy, 836
  in immune complex hypersensitivity,
    784
  intravenous. *See* Intravenous immune
    globulin
  in Lyme disease, 1344
  in mononucleosis, 1243
  in multiple sclerosis, 913
  in myeloma, 472, 473
  in pancreatitis, 646
  platelet-associated, 1553*t*
  in postinfectious glomerulonephritis,
    834
  reference values for, 1551*t*
  in toxoplasmosis, 1364
IgG index, 1551*t*
IgG$_4$-associated cholangitis, 641
IGIV. *See* Intravenous immune globulin
IgM
  in antibody-mediated/cytotoxic
    hypersensitivity, 784

in cold agglutinin disease, 453
in common variable immunodeficiency, 787
in hepatitis A, 602, 602f
in hepatitis B, 602f, 603
in immune complex hypersensitivity, 784
in Lyme disease, 1344
in mononucleosis, 1243
reference values for, 1551t
in toxoplasmosis, 1364
in Waldenström macroglobulinemia, 474
IL. See under Interleukin
IL2RA/IL7RA genes, in multiple sclerosis, 912
Ileitis/ileocolitis, in Crohn disease, 578
Ileum. See also Small intestine
resection of
short bowel syndrome and, 562–563
vitamin B₁₂ deficiency and, 445
Ileus
gallstone, 634
in pancreatitis, 642, 646
paralytic (acute/adynamic), 564
Iliac arteries, atherosclerotic/occlusive disease of, 415–416
Iliotibial band syndrome, 745–746
Illicit drug use. See Substance use disorders
Illness behaviors, abnormal, 944–946
Illusions
psychedelic drug use and, 982
in schizophrenic/psychotic disorders, 953
Iloprost, for pulmonary hypertension, 275, 381
Imagery. See Guided/emotive imagery
Imatinib, 1504t
for chronic myeloid leukemia, 462
for gastrointestinal mesenchymal tumors, 1474
Imbalance. See Disequilibrium; Falls; Vertigo; Vestibular disorders
Imidazoles, topical, 98t
Imiglucerase, for Gaucher disease, 1516
Imipenem
for abdominal infections, 1322t
for anthrax, 1301t
renal/hepatic failure and, 1184t
Imipramine, 966, 968t, 1545t. See also Antidepressants
for enuresis, 966, 976
for migraine prophylaxis, 874t
Imiquimod
for actinic keratoses, 113
for genital warts, 132
Immediate (IgE-mediated/type I) hypersensitivity, 784. See also Allergies/allergic reactions
Immersion (trench) foot/hand, 1405
Immobility
decubitus ulcers (pressure sores) and, 68, 73
deep venous thrombosis/pulmonary embolism and, 267
in elderly, 68

hypercalcemia and, 1036
rhabdomyolysis and, 763
urinary incontinence and, 70
Immune alveolar hemorrhage, 276
Immune clearance hepatitis B, 609
Immune complex-mediated hypersensitivity (type III), 784
glomerulonephritis and, 824
Immune globulin. See specific type and Intravenous immune globulin
Immune insulin resistance, 1104
Immune intervention trials, for diabetes prevention/delay, 1086–1087, 1087
Immune reconstitution syndromes (IRIS), 1216–1217
"Immune recovery" uveitis, 168
Immune thrombocytopenic purpura, 482–484, 483t, 484f. See also Thrombocytopenia
Immune tolerant hepatitis B, 609
Immunity/immune response, disorders of. See Autoimmune disorders; Immunocompromised host; Immunodeficiency
Immunizations (vaccines), 3, 1186–1204, 1202–1203t. See also specific type
recommended types/schedules for
for adults, 3–4, 3t, 1186–1200, 1194–1197t
catch-up schedule and, 1192–1193t
in HIV infection/AIDS/immunocompromised patients, 5, 1195t, 1220
for infants/children/adolescents, 4, 1186, 1188–1193t
during pregnancy, 4, 710, 1195t
for travelers, 4, 1200–1204
safety (adverse effects/contraindications) and, 1202–1203t, 1204
Immunocompromised host. See also HIV infection/AIDS; Immunodeficiency
adenovirus infection in, 1275, 1276
aspergillosis in, 1397–1398
bronchiectasis in, 240
cancer-related infection and, 1498
coccidial and microsporidial infection in, 1369, 1370, 1371
cognitive disorders/delirium and, 985t
cytomegalovirus infection in, 1157–1158, 1245, 1245–1246, 1246
diarrhea in, 511, 515, 516, 1214, 1369–1371
fever/FUO and, 1153, 1154
antimicrobial therapy and, 40, 1158
fungal sinusitis in, 195, 1402
gram-negative bacteremia/sepsis in, 1311
herpes simplex in, 1157, 1236
herpes zoster in, 115, 1241
herpetic stomatitis in, 203
histoplasmosis in, 1392

immunizations in, 5, 1195t
influenza virus vaccine, 5, 1195t, 1198, 1270
MMR vaccine, 1195t, 1249
pneumococcal vaccine, 1195t, 1199
infections in, 1155–1159. See also Opportunistic infections
infectious esophagitis in, 535
mold infections in, 1402
nocardiosis in, 1324
parvovirus infection in, 1276, 1277
Pneumocystis infections in, 1157, 1210, 1394
pulmonary infiltrates/pneumonia in, 251, 1210
scabies in, 137, 138
squamous cell carcinoma in, 134
strongyloidiasis in, 1381
toxoplasmosis in, 1363–1364, 1364, 1365
varicella in, 1242
Immunodeficiency. See also Immunocompromised host
acquired, in HIV infection/AIDS, 1208. See also HIV infection/AIDS
common variable, 786–787
infections associated with, 1155–1159. See also Opportunistic infections
primary, 786–787
selective IgA, 786
Immunofixation electrophoresis, in myeloma, 472
Immunofluorescence assay, in Lyme disease, 1344
Immunoglobulins. See also specific type under Ig and Antibodies
in colostrum/breast milk, 709
reference values for, 1551t
Immunomodulating therapy. See also Immunotherapy
adverse ophthalmic effects of, 177t
for asthma, 225t
for inflammatory bowel disease, 576
Crohn disease, 581
ulcerative colitis, 584–585
for myeloma, 473
for ophthalmic disorders, 175t
thrombocytopenia caused by, 483t
Immunopathologic hypoglycemia, 1117t, 1118, 1122
Immunosuppressive therapy. See also Immunocompromised host; Immunomodulating therapy
for aplastic anemia, 455, 482
for autoimmune hemolytic anemia, 453
breast feeding and, 710t
fever/FUO and, 1154
hyperkalemia caused by, 798
infections and, 1156
Kaposi sarcoma complicating, 135
for multiple sclerosis, 913
for myelodysplasia, 464
for polyarteritis nodosa, 765
for pure red cell aplasia, 447

Immunosuppressive therapy (*cont.*)
for SLE, 754
thrombocytopenia caused by, 483*t*
after transplant
infections and, 1156
kidney transplant and, 831
squamous cell carcinoma and, 134
Immunotherapy. *See also* Immunomodulating therapy
for allergic rhinitis, 197
for asthma, 228
intravesical, for bladder cancer, 1490
in wart removal, 132
Impedance plethysmography, in venous thrombosis/pulmonary embolism, 269
Impedance testing, in esophageal disorders, 530
Imperforate hymen, absent menses and, 1068
Impetiginization, in allergic contact dermatitis, 119
Impetigo, **118**, 1182*t*, **1290**
allergic contact dermatitis differentiated from, 118, 119
antibiotics for, 97*t*, 118, 1182*t*
glomerulonephritis and, 834
in HIV infection/AIDS, 1215
Implanon, 697
Implantable cardioverter defibrillator
for cardiomyopathy, 373
for heart failure, 365
for long QT syndrome, 353–354
postinfarction, 340
for ventricular fibrillation/sudden death, 353
for ventricular tachycardia, 352
Impotence. *See* Erectile dysfunction/impotence
Impulse conduction, disturbances of. *See* Conduction disturbances
Impulse control disorders
aggressive/violent behavior and, 976
in dementia, 986
in personality changes due to general medical condition, 986
In vitro fertilization, 694, 866
acupuncture affecting outcome of, 1534
Inactivated enhanced-potency poliovaccine (IPV/Salk vaccine), 1188*t*, 1190–1191*t*, 1192–1193*t*, 1201, 1252–1253
pregnancy and, 710
for travelers, 1201, 1253
Inactive HBsAg carrier state, 609
Inactivity, physical
lipid abnormalities and, 1126*t*
preventable disease/deaths caused by, 2*t*
prevention of, **12–14**
Incentive spirometry, prevention of postoperative pulmonary complications and, 54
Incest, 948
Inclusion body encephalitis, measles and, 1248
Inclusion body myositis, 761, **935**

Inclusion conjunctivitis, 154
in newborn, 727
Inclusion cysts, epidermal (EIC), **141–142**
furuncles differentiated from, 141
Inclusion disease, cytomegalovirus, in newborn, 1245
Incompetent cervix, 711
cerclage/activity restriction for, 712
Incomplete abortion, 712
Incontinence. *See* Fecal incontinence; Urinary incontinence
Increased intracranial pressure. *See* Intracranial hypertension
Incretins, for diabetes mellitus, 1091*t*, 1095
Indanedione rodenticides (superwarfarins), poisoning caused by, 1430–1431
Indapamide, 399*t*
Inderal. *See* Propranolol
Indian tick typhus, 1281*t*
Indigestion. *See* Dyspepsia
Indinavir, 1226*t*, 1229, 1232*f*. *See also* Antiretroviral therapy
Indocin. *See* Indomethacin
Indometh. *See* Indomethacin
Indomethacin, 79*t*
adverse ophthalmic effects of, 178*t*
for gout, 733
lithium interactions and, 972*t*
in pain management, 79*t*
for patent ductus arteriosus, 301
Industrial bronchitis, 280
Inevitable abortion, 711–712, 712
Infant. *See* Newborn
Infant botulism, 1299
Infarcts. *See specific type*
Infection/infectious diseases, **1153–1175**. *See also specific type or organ system affected*
in acute leukemia, 465
arthritis and, **777–780**
bacterial, **1289–1327**
bite wounds and, **1165–1166**
burn injury and, 1411
in cancer patients, **1498**. *See also* Immunocompromised host; Opportunistic infections
catheter-associated, 1151, 1160, 1161, 1180
chlamydial, 1177–1178*t*, **1327–1329**
cognitive disorders/delirium caused by, 985*t*
in diabetic patient, insulin requirements and, 1100
in drug users, **1168–1169**
HIV infection/AIDS, 1168, 1207, 1219, 1220
postexposure prophylaxis and, 1221
fever/FUO and, 38, 39, 1154
after frostbite, prevention of, 1406
gastritis caused by, 547
headache and, 44, 45
helminthic, **1373–1389**
hospital-associated, **1159–1162**
immunization against, 3, **1186–1204**, 1202–1203*t*. *See also* Immunizations

in immunocompromised host, **1155–1159**. *See also* HIV infection/AIDS; Opportunistic infections
mycotic, **1390–1402**
of bones and joints, **781**
superficial, **107–110**
in myeloma, 472
myocarditis and, **368–369**, 369*t*
neuropathies associated with, **924**
neutropenia and, 456, 1156, 1158, 1498
opportunistic. *See* Opportunistic infections
osteomyelitis and, 780
during pregnancy, **724–727**
prevention of, **3–6**, 1157–1158. *See also* Immunizations
in cancer patient/immunocompromised host, 1157–1158. *See also* HIV infection/AIDS
protozoal, **1348–1373**
reactive arthritis and, 776
rickettsial, 1178*t*, **1280–1287**, 1281*t*
seizures and, 879
sexually transmitted, **1166–1168**
shock associated with. *See* Sepsis/septic shock
spirochetal, 1177*t*
surgical site, 1160
antibiotic prophylaxis for, **59–60**, 60*t*
thrombocytopenia and, **489**
travel and, **1172–1173**
vaccine-preventable, 3–4, **1247–1255**
viral, **1235–1280**
Infection control
handwashing and, 1161
hospital-associated infection prevention and, 1161
Infectious mononucleosis. *See* Mononucleosis
Infective endocarditis. *See* Endocarditis, infective
Inferior vena cava filters/interruption, for pulmonary embolism, 273, 501
Infertility, 692–693, 864
acupuncture for, 1534
female, **692–694**
in chronic kidney disease, 830
endometriosis and, 686
in polycystic ovary syndrome, 690
hyperprolactinemia and, 1000
in hypopituitarism, 991–992
male, **864–866**, 865*f*
cryptorchism and, 1066
in cystic fibrosis, 241
in Klinefelter syndrome, 865, 1064, 1517, 1517–1518
marijuana use and, 983
radiation causing, 1414
Inflammation. *See also specific type and structure/systems affected*
coronary heart disease and, 317
in HIV infection/AIDS, 1216–1217
Inflammatory adenoma of liver, 633
Inflammatory aneurysm, 423, 424

Inflammatory bowel disease, **575–587**. *See also* Crohn disease; Ulcerative colitis
  arthritis and, **776–777**
  colorectal cancer and, 1477
  diarrhea in, 515, 516
  drug therapy for, 575–577
  GI bleeding and, 521
  hyperoxaluric calcium nephrolithiasis and, 859
  primary sclerosing cholangitis and, 640
  social support for patient with, 577
Inflammatory breast carcinoma, **660**, 728. *See also* Breast cancer
Inflammatory eye disease, 153*t*. *See also* Conjunctivitis; Uveitis
Inflammatory myopathy, 936
Inflammatory pericarditis, acute, **376–378**. *See also specific cause and* Pericarditis
Inflammatory polyneuropathy, chronic, **926**
Inflammatory skin nodules, **140–141**. *See also specific type*
Infliximab. *See also* Anti-TNF agents
  for inflammatory bowel disease, 576–577
    Crohn disease, 581
    ulcerative colitis, 584–585, 585
  for psoriasis, 105
  for rheumatoid arthritis, 751
Influenza, **1269–1271**
  avian (H5N1), 5, 1269, 1271, **1271–1272**
  drug resistance and, 1270, 1271, 1272, 1273
  human-origin, **1269–1271**
  neuraminidase inhibitors (oseltamivir/zanamivir) in, 1198, 1238*t*, 1239*t*, 1270, 1271, 1272, 1273
  prevention of, 1270, 1272, 1273–1274. *See also* Influenza virus vaccine
  swine-origin (H1N1/A/California/04/ 2009), 1198, 1269, 1271, **1273–1274**
Influenza A/California/04/2009 (swine-origin influenza), 1198, 1269, 1271, **1273–1274**. *See also* Influenza
Influenza virus vaccine, 3, 3*t*, 5, 1188–1189*t*, 1190–1191*t*, 1194–1197*t*, 1198, 1270
  adverse effects/contraindications and, 1202*t*, 1270
  in asthma patients, 228
  avian (H5N1) influenza and, 5, 1272
  in HIV infection/AIDS/immunocompromised host, 5, 1195*t*, 1198, 1220, 1270
  HIV screening tests affected by, 1217
  pneumonia prevention and, 247
  pregnancy and, 706, 710, 1195*t*
  swine-origin (H1N1) influenza and, 1273
Infratentorial arteriovenous malformations, 895

Infusion pumps
  for enteral nutritional support, 1150
  insulin. *See* Insulin infusion pumps
Ingrown hairs, pseudofolliculitis caused by, 123
Ingrown nails, 146
INH. *See* Isoniazid
Inhalation injury/smoke inhalation, **277**, 1409
Inhalational anthrax, 1301, 1302
Inhaled insulin, 1099
Inhalers
  for asthma therapy, 223, 228, 229*t*
  for COPD therapy, 237
Inhibin A, prenatal screening for, 706
Injection drug use. *See also* Substance use disorders
  febrile patient and, 1169
  infections and, **1168–1169**
    endocarditis, 1168, 1181*t*, 1304
    hematogenous osteomyelitis, 780
    hepatitis, 601, 602, 603, 604, 1168
    HIV infection/AIDS, 1168, 1207, 1219, 1220
      postexposure prophylaxis and, 1221
    wound botulism, 1168, 1299–1300, 1442
Injury. *See* Trauma
INK4A gene, pancreatic/periampullary carcinoma and, 1463
Inner ear, **186–190**
Innocent murmurs. *See* Heart murmurs
Innohep. *See* Tinzaparin
Inocybe (muscarinic) mushroom poisoning, 1441, 1441*t*, 1442
Inotropic agents. *See also* Digitalis/digitalis glycosides
  for heart failure, 364–365
    left ventricular (infarct-related), 338
  for shock, 436
Insect bites/stings, **138–140**. *See also specific type of insect*
  anaphylaxis caused by, 784
  scorpion stings, **1447**
  spider bites, 139, **1447**
  urticaria caused by, 126, 139
Insecticide poisoning
  cholinesterase inhibitors, **1443–1444**
  paraquat, **1443**
Insemination, artificial, in azoospermia, 694
Insomnia, **973–975**
  drug therapy for, 941*t*, 942, 974–975
  fatal familial (FFI), 1260
  melatonin for, 1528*t*, 1531
  mind-body therapies for, 1536*t*
Inspra. *See* Eplerenone
Instability. *See* Falls; Gait/gait disorders; Genetic instability
Instrumental activities of daily living (IADL), assessment of ability to perform in elderly, 62, 63
Insulin. *See also* Insulin therapy
  antibodies to
    in factitious hypoglycemia, 1122

    in immune insulin resistance, 1104
    in immunopathologic hypoglycemia, 1117*t*, 1118, 1122
    insulin therapy causing, 1104
    in type 1 diabetes, 1080, 1080*t*
  B cell tumors/insulinomas secreting, 1062, 1118
  B cells secreting, 1062
  blood levels of
    chronic kidney disease and, 830
    in insulinoma diagnosis, 1118, 1119
    prebreakfast hyperglycemia and, 1102–1103, 1103*t*
  drugs affecting action of, 1091*t*, 1092–1094
  drugs affecting secretion of, 1090–1092, 1091*t*
  factitious hypoglycemia caused by administration of, 1118, 1122
  immunoreactive, reference values for, 1551*t*
  insensitivity to. *See* Insulin resistance/insulin insensitivity
  mutant, in diabetes mellitus, 1082
  receptors for. *See* Insulin receptors
  resistance to. *See* Insulin resistance/insulin insensitivity
Insulin aspart, 1096, 1096*t*, 1097*f*. *See also* Insulin therapy
  in mixtures/combination therapy, 1096*t*, 1099
  in pregnancy, 1110
Insulin detemir, 1096, 1096*t*, 1097*f*, 1098, 1101, 1102, 1102*t*, 1103. *See also* Insulin therapy
Insulin gene, in diabetes mellitus, 1080
Insulin glargine, 1096, 1096*t*, 1097*f*, 1098, 1101, 1102, 1102*t*, 1103. *See also* Insulin therapy
  in pregnancy, 1110
Insulin glulisine, 1096, 1096*t*, 1097–1098. *See also* Insulin therapy
Insulin hypoglycemia test, in GH deficiency, 993
Insulin infusion pumps, 1099, 1102
  continuous glucose monitoring and, 1085
  ketoacidosis and, 1099, 1112, 1113
  during pregnancy, 722, 1110
  rapidly acting analogs used in, 1098, 1102
Insulin-like growth factor-1 (IGF-1)
  in GH deficiency/rhGH therapy, 993, 994, 995
  in GH excess, 997, 998
  reference values for, 1551*t*
Insulin-like growth factor-2 (IGF-2), hypoglycemia due to extrapancreatic tumors and, 1120
Insulin lispro, 1096, 1096*t*, 1097–1098, 1102. *See also* Insulin therapy
  in mixtures/combination therapy, 1096*t*, 1099, 1102
  in pregnancy, 1110

Insulin pens, 1099
Insulin receptors
    antibodies to, in immunopathologic
            hypoglycemia, 1117t, 1118,
            1122
    mutant, diabetes caused by, 1082
Insulin resistance/insulin insensitivity,
            1082. See also Insulin resis-
            tance syndrome
    acanthosis nigricans and, 1082, 1086
    acne and, 120
    cholelithiasis/gallstones and, 634
    in Cushing syndrome, 1051
    in diabetes, 1080t, 1081, 1082
    hyperglycemia and, 1081, 1086, 1086t
    immune, 1104
    in polycystic ovary syndrome, 690,
            1053
    during pregnancy, 722
    thiazolidinediones for, 1091t,
            1093–1094, 1101
Insulin resistance syndrome (metabolic
            syndrome/syndrome X),
            14, 1082
    coronary heart disease/angina and, 14,
            317, 318, 325
    diabetes and, 14, 1082
    fatty liver and, 617
    hypertension and, 14, 390, 1082
    hypophosphatemia and, 803
    obesity and, 14, 1136
    triglycerides in, 1082, 1133
Insulin syringes and needles, 1099
Insulin therapy, 1096–1099, 1096t, 1097f,
            1102–1103, 1102t, 1103t
    administration methods/regimens for,
            1099
    allergy to, 1104
    antidepressant drug interactions and,
            969t
    bioavailability of preparations and,
            1096t
    complications of, 1103–1104
    concentrations of insulin and, 1096
    continuous subcutaneous infusion
            (CSII), 1099, 1102. See also
            Insulin infusion pumps
    for diabetic ketoacidosis, 1113–1114
    exercise affecting, 1100
    factitious hypoglycemia and, 1118,
            1122
    for hyperglycemic hyperosmolar state,
            1016
    for hyperkalemia, 798, 799t
    hypoglycemia and, 1087, 1103–1104
    immunopathology of, 1104
    inhalation for administration of, 1099
    injection sites for, 1099
    intensive, 1102–1103, 1102t, 1103t
        acceptable levels of glycemic con-
            trol and, 1103
        clinical studies of long-term com-
            plications and, 1087, 1088
        diabetic nephropathy develop-
            ment/progression and,
            842, 1087, 1088
        diabetic retinopathy development/
            progression and, 1087, 1088

during pregnancy, 722, 1110
    self-monitoring of blood glucose
            and, 1085, 1100–1101,
            1102–1103
    surgery and, 1109
    in type 2 diabetics, 1087, 1101
    intraoperative requirements/adminis-
            tration of, 57–58, 58t
    lipodystrophy/lipohypertrophy and,
            1104
    MAOI interactions and, 969t
    mixtures for, 1096t, 1098–1099, 1101,
            1102
    during pregnancy, 722, 723, 1110
    preparation types available,
            1096–1099, 1096t, 1097f
    in prevention/delay of diabetes,
            1086–1087
    purified insulin and, 1096
    self-monitoring of blood glucose and,
            1085, 1100–1101,
            1102–1103
    species of insulin and, 1096
    surgery and, 57–58, 57t, 58t, 1109
    for type 1 diabetics, 1096–1099, 1096t,
            1097f, 1102–1103, 1102t,
            1103t
    for type 2 diabetics, 1101
        intensive control and, 1087, 1101
Insulinomas, 1062, 1076, 1118–1120,
            1119t, 1468t. See also Islet
            cell tumors
    localization of, 1062, 1119
INTACS. See Intrastromal corneal ring
            segments
Intal. See Cromolyn
Integra, for burn wound closure, 1411
Integrase inhibitors, for HIV infection/
            AIDS, 1227t, 1231, 1232f
    in combinations, 1227, 1232f
Integrilin. See Eptifibatide
Intelence. See Etravirine
Intensive care unit, patient in. See Critical
            illness
Intensive care unit psychosis, 988
Intercostal neuritis, 321
Intercourse, sexual. See Sexual intercourse
Interdigital (toe web) tinea pedis, cellulitis
            and, 109, 129
Interferon-α/interferon alfa, 1238t
    for cancer chemotherapy, 1506t
    for hepatitis B, 609, 610, 1238t
    for hepatitis C, 606, 610–611, 1238t
    for hepatitis D, 611
    for Kaposi sarcoma, 1225t, 1476
    pegylated. See Peginterferon
    for renal cell carcinoma, 1492
    thyroid dysfunction caused by, 1003,
            1007, 1008
    toxicity of, 1506t
Interferon-β/interferon beta
    for multiple sclerosis, 913
    thyroid dysfunction caused by, 1003,
            1008
Interleukin-2 (IL-2)
    in cancer chemotherapy, 1506t
    for renal cell carcinoma, 1492
    thyroid dysfunction caused by, 1008

Interleukin-2 receptor α gene, in multiple
            sclerosis, 912
Interleukin-6 (IL-6)
    in Addison disease, 1048
    in amiodarone-induced hyperthyroid-
            ism, 1010
Interleukin-7 receptor α gene, in multiple
            sclerosis, 912
Interleukin-8 (IL-8), in familial Mediter-
            ranean fever, 528
Interleukin-11 (neumega/IL-11), recom-
            binant (oprelvekin), for
            chemotherapy-induced
            thrombocytopenia,
            1499–1506, 1508t
Intermediate-acting insulin, 1096t, 1097f.
            See also Insulin therapy
Intermediate uveitis (pars planitis), 160.
            See also Uveitis
Intermittent claudication. See Claudication
Intermittent mandatory ventilation, syn-
            chronized (SIMV), for res-
            piratory failure, 290
Intermittent negative-pressure (cuirass)
            ventilation, for COPD, 238
Intermittent positive-pressure breathing
            (IPPB), prevention of
            postoperative pulmonary
            complications and, 54
Internal hordeolum, 152
Interosseous nerve, anterior, lesion of, 927
Interpersonal relationships, social issues
            for terminally ill/dying
            patient and, 92, 92t
Interstitial cystitis, 861–862
Interstitial lung disease, 262–266, 262t.
            See also specific disorder
    acute pneumonitis (AIP), 264t
    cryptogenic organizing pneumonitis
            (COP/bronchiolitis oblit-
            erans organizing pneumo-
            nia/BOOP), 243, 264t
    desquamative pneumonia (DIP), 243,
            263, 264t
    drug-related, 262t, 281t
    eosinophilic, 266
    idiopathic fibrosing pneumonia,
            263–265, 264t
    nonspecific pneumonia/pneumonitis
            (NSIP), 263, 264t
        in HIV infection/AIDS, 1211
    pulmonary alveolar proteinosis, 266
    respiratory bronchiolitis-associated
            (RB-ILD), 243, 263, 264t
    sarcoidosis, 265–266
    usual pneumonia/pneumonitis (UIP),
            263–265, 264t
Interstitial nephritis, 820t, 823–824
    in SLE, 753, 843
Intertriginous area
    miliaria affecting, 124
    seborrhea of, 106
Intertrigo, 113
    tinea differentiated from, 108
Interventricular septum
    hypertrophy of, in cardiomyopathy, 372
    rupture of, in myocardial infarction,
            338–339

Intervertebral disk disorders. *See* Cervical spine/disk disease; Lumbar spine/disk disease
Interview (medical), 1–2
Intestinal adenocarcinoma, **1474**
Intestinal amebiasis, 512, 514, 515, 1172, 1174, 1366, 1367, 1367t
Intestinal angina (visceral artery insufficiency), **421–422**
Intestinal bacterial overgrowth. *See* Bacterial overgrowth
Intestinal carcinoids, **1475–1476**
Intestinal disorders. *See* Gastrointestinal system, disorders of
Intestinal flagellate infections, **1372.** *See also specific type*
Intestinal flukes, **1376**
Intestinal ischemia, 421–422
GI bleeding and, 521
Intestinal lymphoma, **1474–1475**
Intestinal motility disorders. *See* Motility disorders
Intestinal obstruction. *See also* Motility disorders
in acute colonic pseudo-obstruction (Ogilvie syndrome), **565–566**
in chronic intestinal pseudo-obstruction, **566**
in Crohn disease, 578, 579
in gastroparesis, **566**
tumors causing, 1478
vomiting and, 505t
Intestinal polyps, 567
Intestinal sarcoma, **1476**
Intestinal transplantation, for short bowel syndrome, 563
Intestinal tuberculosis, **568–569**
Intoxication. *See also specific substance causing*
acute alcohol, 978, 985t, 1427t, **1436**
metabolic acidosis/osmolar gap and, 795, 979, 1426
cognitive disorders/delirium caused by, 985t
Intra-arterial embolization. *See* Embolization
Intracerebral hemorrhage, 890t, **892–893**, 918t. *See also* Stroke
arteriovenous malformations causing, 895, 895–896
in coarctation of aorta, 296
headache in, 44, 45, 892
hypertension and, 387, 393, 412, 892
thrombolytic therapy for myocardial infarction and, 333
trauma and, 918t
Intracoronary stents, 322, 323. *See also* Percutaneous coronary intervention
Intracranial aneurysm, 890t, **894–895.** *See also* Stroke
in polycystic kidney disease, 848, 894
Intracranial bleeding. *See* Intracerebral hemorrhage; Subarachnoid hemorrhage
Intracranial hypertension
benign (pseudotumor cerebri), 903

headache and, 876, 903
lithium use and, 971
brain abscess/infection causing, 902
cerebral injury and, 918
ECT contraindicated in, 969
headache and, 44, 45
optic disk swelling and (papilledema), 169
headache and, 45
tumors causing, 897, 899. *See also* Intracranial masses/tumors
vomiting caused by, 505t
Intracranial masses/tumors, **897–902**, 898t, 1467t
abscess causing. *See* Brain abscess
coma or stupor caused by, 916–917
false localizing signs and, 899
headache caused by, 44, 872, **876**
cough headache and, 875
in HIV infection/AIDS, **901**
metastatic, **900–901**
nonmetastatic neurologic complications and, **902–903**
ocular motor palsies and, 170
primary, 897–900, 898t
seizures caused by, 878–879
vocal fold paralysis caused by, 211
Intracranial venous thrombosis, **896.** *See also* Stroke
Intracytoplasmic sperm injection (ICSI), 694, 866
Intraepidermal squamous cell carcinoma (Bowen disease), **113**
Intrahepatic cholestasis, 598, 599t
Intrahepatic portosystemic shunts. *See* Transvenous (transjugular) intrahepatic portosystemic shunts
IntraLASIK (femtosecond laser assisted LASIK), 151
Intralipid. *See* Intravenous fat
Intraluminal phase, of digestion/absorption, 557–558
Intraocular foreign body, **171**
Intraocular hypertension. *See* Ocular hypertension
Intraocular inflammation, 153t. *See also* Uveitis
Intraocular lenses, multifocal/accommodative, 152
after cataract removal, 161
Intraocular pressure, elevated. *See* Ocular hypertension
Intrastromal corneal ring segments (INTACS), 152
Intrathecal pumps, for pain medications, 86
Intrauterine devices (IUDs), **698–699**, 698t
dysmenorrhea and, 677, 698
for emergency/postcoital contraception, 698
levonorgestrel-releasing, 698
for abnormal premenopausal bleeding, 675
pelvic infection/PID and, 688, 698, 1324
progesterone-releasing, 1071

Intrauterine insemination, 866
Intravascular abscesses (septic superficial thrombophlebitis), 429, 429–430
Intravascular ultrasound, in angina, 320
Intravenous catheters. *See* Intravenous lines
Intravenous drug use. *See* Injection drug use
Intravenous fat, in nutritional support, 1149, 1151
Intravenous gamma globulin. *See* Intravenous immune globulin
Intravenous immune globulin
for autoimmune hemolytic anemia, 453
for common variable immunodeficiency, 787
for immune thrombocytopenic purpura, 483, 484, 484f
for pure red cell aplasia, 447
for toxic epidermal necrolysis, 128
Intravenous lines. *See also* Catheters
in burn care, 1410
in GI bleeding, 518
hospital-associated infection and, 1159, 1160, 1161, 1180
for parenteral nutritional support, 1148, 1148f
Intraventricular conduction defects, **356**
Intraventricular cysts, in cysticercosis (neurocysticercosis), 1377
Intravesical chemotherapy, for bladder cancer, 1490
Intrinsic renal failure, 820t, 821. *See also specific cause*
Intron A. *See* Interferon-α/interferon alfa
Intubation. *See also* Airway management; Mechanical ventilation
in asthma, 233
for burn injuries, 1410
in comatose patient, 1421
conversion to tracheostomy and, 212
for near drowning, 1416
pneumonia associated with, 248
for respiratory failure, 290
for smoke inhalation, 277, 1409
Invalidism. *See* Sick role
Invasive fibrous (Riedel) thyroiditis, 1016, 1017, 1018
Invasive fungal sinusitis, **195–196**
Invasive mole, 714. *See also* Gestational trophoblastic disease
Inverse pityriasis rosea, 105
Inverted papilloma, 200
Invirase. *See* Saquinavir
Iodinated contrast agents, for Graves disease/hyperthyroidism, 1011–1012
Iodine
in amiodarone-induced thyroid disease
hyperthyroidism, 1009
hypothyroidism, 1004
deficiency of, **1029–1030**
goiter and, 1029–1030
thyroid nodules caused by, 1019

Iodine (*cont.*)
dietary restriction for thyroid cancer and, 1025
jodbasedow disease/phenomenon and, 1008, 1009
radioactive. *See* Radioactive iodine; Radioiodine thyroid scans and uptake
supplementary, in goiter prevention/treatment, 1029–1030
Iodized salt, goiter prevention/treatment and, 1029–1030
Iodobenzylguanidine ([^{123}I]mIBG) scanning, in pheochromocytoma/paraganglioma, 1060, 1061
Iodochlorhydroxyquin, adverse ophthalmic effects of, 178*t*
Iodoquinol, for amebiasis, 1366–1367, 1367, 1367*t*
Ionizing radiation, 1413. *See also under* Radiation
Iontophoresis sweat test, in cystic fibrosis, 242
Iopanoic acid, for Graves disease/hyperthyroidism, 1011–1012
Iopidine. *See* Apraclonidine
Ipecac, for poisoning/drug overdose, 1424
iPledge, 121
Ipodate sodium, for Graves disease/hyperthyroidism, 1011
IPPB. *See* Intermittent positive-pressure breathing
Ipratropium
for asthma, 228, 229*t*
with albuterol, 229*t*
for COPD, 237
IPV (inactivated poliovaccine/Salk vaccine), 1188*t*, 1190–1191*t*, 1192–1193*t*, 1201, 1252–1253
pregnancy and, 710
for travelers, 1201, 1253
Iquix. *See* Levofloxacin
Irbesartan/irbesartan with hydrochlorothiazide, 403*t*
Iressa. *See* Gefitinib
Iridodialysis, 171
Iridoplasty/iridotomy/iridectomy, for angle-closure glaucoma, 158, 159
Irinotecan, 1503*t*
for colorectal cancer, 1479
St. John's wort interactions and, 1523
IRIS (immune reconstitution syndromes), 1216–1217
Iritis, 153*t*
Iron
accumulation of
in hemochromatosis, 627
in sideroblastic anemia, 444
deficiency of/iron deficiency anemia, **439–441**, 440*t*
celiac disease and, 559
in chronic kidney disease, 828, 829
in cirrhosis, 623
esophageal webs and (Plummer-Vinson syndrome), 440, 537

GI bleeding and, 439, 522, 523
in idiopathic pulmonary hemosiderosis, 276
in paroxysmal nocturnal hemoglobinuria, 440, 449
in polycythemia, 458
during pregnancy, 439, 721
thrombocytopenia and, 482
dietary, 439
nutritional support requirements and, 1149
overdose/toxicity of, 1424*t*, 1427*t*, **1437**. *See also* Hemosiderosis
serum levels of
in anemia of chronic disease, 442
in iron deficiency anemia, 440
in overdose, 1437
reference values for, 1551*t*
supplementary
in dialysis patients, 829
for iron deficiency anemia, 441
for paroxysmal nocturnal hemoglobinuria, 449
in pregnancy, 439, 708–709, 721
total body, 441
Iron-binding capacity, total (TIBC), 1551*t*
Iron deficiency anemia. *See* Iron, deficiency of
Iron overload. *See* Hemochromatosis; Hemosiderosis
Irritable bowel syndrome, **569–573**
alarm symptoms in, 570
mind-body therapies for, 573, 1536*t*
hypnosis, 573, 1536*t*, 1539
Irritant contact dermatitis, 119
Irritative voiding symptoms
in benign prostatic hyperplasia, 867
in bladder cancer, 1489
in cystitis, 46, 47*f*, 851
in epididymitis, 856
in interstitial cystitis, 861
in prostatitis, 853, 854
in pyelonephritis, 852
IS. *See* Incentive spirometry
Ischemia
acute tubular necrosis caused by, 821
brainstem, seizures differentiated from, 881
intestinal, 421–422
GI bleeding and, 521
mesenteric, 421–422
myocardial. *See* Coronary heart disease; Myocardial ischemia
visceral, 421–422
Ischemia testing, noninvasive, preoperative, 49–50, 51*f*
Ischemic chest pain, 28–29. *See also* Angina
Ischemic colitis, 421–422
GI bleeding and, 521
Ischemic heart disease. *See* Angina, pectoris; Coronary heart disease
Ischemic hepatopathy, 631
Ischemic optic neuropathy, **168**
in giant cell arteritis, 168, 766
Ischemic rest pain. *See* Rest pain
Isentress. *See* Raltegravir

Islet cell antibodies, in diabetes mellitus, 1080, 1080*t*
Islet cell tumors, **1062–1063**
hypoglycemia caused by, 1062, 1063, **1118–1120**, 1119*t*
in multiple endocrine neoplasia, 1062, 1076, 1118, 1119, 1120
Islet cells, pancreatic. *See also* B cells
hyperplasia of, persistent, **1120**
transplantation of, for diabetes, 1100
Ismelin. *See* Guanethidine
Isocarboxazid, overdose/toxicity of, 1440–1441
Isoniazid, 255*t*, 256*t*
benzodiazepine interactions and, 942*t*
overdose/toxicity of, 1424*t*, **1437–1438**
neuropathy and, 925, 1438
ophthalmic effects and, 178*t*
pyridoxine (vitamin B$_6$) for, 256, 1142–1143, 1211, 1219, 1424*t*, 1438
seizures and, 1423*t*, 1437, 1438
renal/hepatic failure and, 1184*t*
for tuberculosis, 254, 255, 255*t*, 256*t*
in latent disease/prophylactic, 257, 1219, 1219–1220, 1222
in pregnancy, 254–255, 256, 726
resistance and, 254, 256
Isoniazid/rifampin, for tuberculosis, 255
Isoniazid/rifampin/pyrazinamide, for tuberculosis, 255
Isophane (NPH) insulin. *See* Insulin therapy; NPH insulin
Isopropanol, overdose/toxicity of, osmolar gap in, 809, 1426
Isoptin. *See* Verapamil
Isosorbide. *See also* Nitrates
for angina, 321
for heart failure, 364
left ventricular (infarct-related), 337
for pulmonary edema, 368
Isospora belli (isosporiasis), 1172, **1369–1371**
Isosthenuria, in sickle cell disease, 849
Isotonic hyponatremia, 789, 790*f*
Isotretinoin
for acne, 121–122
adverse ophthalmic effects of, 178*t*
for lupus, 111
for rosacea, 123
teratogenicity of, 111, 121–122
Isradipine, 406*t*
overdose/toxicity of, 406*t*, 1432
Itch-scratch cycle. *See also* Pruritus
in lichen simplex chronicus, 103
Itch-X-Gel. *See* Pramoxine
Itching. *See* Pruritus
Itchy red bump syndrome, 1208
Itopride, for functional dyspepsia, 504
ITP. *See* Immune thrombocytopenic purpura
Itraconazole, 1401*t*
for blastomycosis, 1399
for candidiasis, 535, 1390
for chromoblastomycosis, 1400
for histoplasmosis, 1392

for *P marneffei* infection, 1400
renal/hepatic failure and, 1184*t*
for sporotrichosis, 1400
IUDs. *See* Intrauterine devices
IVC filters. *See* Inferior vena cava filters/
    interruption
Ivermectin
    for filariasis, 1387
    for gnathostomiasis, 1384
    for loiasis, 1389
    for onchocerciasis, 1388
    for scabies, 138
    for strongyloidiasis, 1381
IVF. *See* In vitro fertilization
IVIG. *See* Intravenous immune globulin
IVUS. *See* Intravascular ultrasound
Ixabepilone, 669, 1502*t*
Ixempra. *See* Ixabepilone
Ixodes ticks. *See* Ticks

J stents, ureteral, after shock wave litho-
    tripsy, 860
J wave, in hypothermia, 1404, 1404*f*
JAK2 mutation
    in essential thrombocytosis, 459
    in hepatic vein obstruction (Budd-
        Chiari syndrome), 630
    in myelofibrosis, 460
    in noncirrhotic portal hypertension,
        631
    in polycythemia, 457, 458
Janeway lesions, in endocarditis, 1304
Janumet. *See* Sitagliptin, with metformin
Januvia. *See* Sitagliptin
Japanese B encephalitis, 1257–1259
    immunization against, 1203–1204, 1258
Jarisch-Herxheimer reaction
    in leptospirosis, 1341–1342
    in relapsing fever, 1340
    in syphilis, 1333
Jaundice (icterus), **598–601**, 599*t*, 600*t*
    biliary stricture causing, 639
    in biliary tract cancer, 1462
    in cholecystitis, 636
    in choledocholithiasis/cholangitis, 638
    cholestatic, 598
    in cirrhosis, 619
    hepatic failure and, 607
    in hepatitis, 602*f*, 604*f*, 605
    in idiopathic cholestasis of pregnancy,
        728
    in leptospirosis, 1341
    obstructive, 638, 639
    in sclerosing cholangitis, 640
    travel and, 1173
Jaw
    osteonecrosis of, bisphosphonate use
        and, 783, 1040, 1045
    tumors of, hyperparathyroidism and,
        1033
Jaw claudication, in giant cell arteritis,
    164, 766
Jaw pain
    in acute coronary syndromes, 326
    in angina, 318, 878
JC virus, progressive multifocal leukoen-
    cephalopathy caused by,
    1261

Jejunostomies, 1148
Jervell-Lange-Nielsen syndrome, 353
Jet lag, melatonin for, 1528*t*, 1531
Jo-1 antibody, in polymyositis/dermato-
    myositis, 754*t*, 760
Jock itch, **108**
Jodbasedow disease/phenomenon, 1008,
    1009. *See also* Graves dis-
    ease; Hyperthyroidism
Joint fluid examination. *See* Synovial fluid
    examination
Joints
    bleeding into, in hemophilia, 491
    Charcot. *See* Charcot joint
    coccidioidomycosis involving, **781**,
        1393
    in decompression sickness, 1417
    disorders/inflammation of
        in Chikungunya fever, 1268
        degenerative, **729–732.** *See also*
            Arthritis; Osteoarthritis
        diagnosis and evaluation of, 729,
            730*t*, 731*t*
        in HIV infection/AIDS, 1212–1213
        palindromic, **783**
        pattern of, 729, 730*t*
    histoplasmosis involving, **781**
    mycotic infections of, **781**
    replacement of, 731
        coagulase-negative staphylococcal
            infection and, 1296
        osteomyelitis and, 780
    in sarcoidosis, **782**
    tuberculosis of, **782**
Jones criteria, for rheumatic fever, 375
Joule burn, 1413
Jugular venous pulsations
    in constrictive pericarditis, 379
    in heart failure, 360
    in myocardial infarction, 330
    in tetralogy of Fallot, 300
    in tricuspid regurgitation, 314
    in tricuspid stenosis, 313
Junctional nevi, 99
Junctional rhythm, atrioventricular,
    350–351
Junin hemorrhagic fever, 1262–1263
Juvenile angiofibroma, 200
Juvenile polyposis, familial, 592
Juvenile spinal muscular atrophy, 921
JVP. *See* Jugular venous pulsations

K⁺. *See* Potassium
K103 mutation, NNRTI resistance and,
    1230
K-*ras* oncogene
    colorectal cancer treatment and, 1479
    gallbladder cancer and, 1462
    pancreatic/periampullary carcinoma
        and, 1463
Kadian. *See* Morphine
Kal 1/Kal 2/Kal 3 genes, in Kallmann syn-
    drome, 991
Kala azar. *See* Visceral leishmaniasis
Kaletra. *See* Lopinavir/r
Kallmann syndrome, 991, 991–992, 1067,
    1068
Kaolin pneumoconiosis, 279*t*

Kaposi sarcoma, **135–136**, 1208,
    1215–1216, 1225*t*
    chemotherapy for, 135, 1216, 1225*t*,
        1468*t*, 1476
    cutaneous, 135, 1225*t*
    ear involvement in, 191
    in HIV infection/AIDS, 135, 1208,
        1211, 1215–1216, 1225*t*,
        1476
    intestinal/visceral, 135, 1216, 1225*t*,
        1476
    oral, 1213, 1215
    pulmonary, 135, 1211, 1225*t*
    virus causing, 135
Kaposi sarcoma-associated herpes virus
    (human herpesvirus 8),
    135, 1208, **1247**
Kappa free light chains, reference values
    for, 1551*t*
Karyotyping, in male infertility, 865
Kasabach-Merritt syndrome, 633
Katayama syndrome, 1374
Kattan nomogram, for prostate cancer
    assessment, 1488
Kawasaki disease, 383, 1240*t*, **1287–1288**
Kayexalate. *See* Sodium polystyrene sul-
    fonate
Kayser-Fleischer ring, in Wilson disease,
    629
KCNE3 gene, in periodic paralysis, 936
KCNJ2 gene, in periodic paralysis, 936
KCNJ11 gene, in type 2 diabetes, 1082
Keflex. *See* Cephalexin
Kegel (pelvic muscle) exercises
    for fecal incontinence, 595, 596
    for urinary incontinence, 71
Kemadrin. *See* Procyclidine
Kent bundles, in preexcitation syndromes,
    345
Kenya tick typhus, 1281*t*
Kepivance. *See* Palifermin
Keratectomy, photorefractive (PRK), 151
Keratic precipitates, 160
Keratinocytes, cultured, for burn wound
    closure, 1411
Keratitis, 153*t*, 156–157
    acanthamoeba, **157**, **1368–1369**
    adenovirus, 1275
    bacterial, **156**
    chemical, **172**
    contact lens wear and, 151, 156
    fungal, **157**
    herpes simplex, **156**, 1236, 1237
    in herpes zoster ophthalmicus,
        156–157
    ultraviolet (actinic), **172**
Keratoconjunctivitis. *See also* Conjunc-
    tivitis
    adenovirus, 154, 1275
    atopic, 155
    chlamydial, 154
    epidemic
        adenovirus, 154, 1275
        coxsackievirus, 1279
    herpes simplex, **156**, 1236
    sicca (dry eye), **154–155**
        in Sjögren syndrome, 762, 763
    vernal, 155

Keratolytic agents, for wart removal, 132
Keratomalacia, in vitamin A deficiency, 1143
Keratomileusis
    laser assisted in situ (LASIK), 151–152
    laser epithelial (LASEK), 151
Keratopathy, band, in hypercalcemia/hyperparathyroidism, 1034
Keratoplasty, conductive, 152
Keratoses
    actinic, **113**
        squamous cell carcinoma arising from, 113, 134
    seborrheic, **100**
Kerlone. *See* Betaxolol
Kernig sign, 1309
Ketamine, in pain management, 86
Ketek. *See* Telithromycin
Ketoacidemia, in diabetic ketoacidosis, 1112–1113
Ketoacidosis
    alcoholic, 809, 811
    diabetic, 808–809, 1083, **1111–1115**, 1112*t. See also* Diabetic ketoacidosis
Ketoconazole, 107, 1401*t*
    for ACTH-secreting adrenal tumor, 1052
    in cancer chemotherapy, 1506*t*
    for prostate cancer, 1487, 1487*t*
    renal/hepatic failure and, 1184*t*
    for tinea versicolor, 110
    topical, 98*t*
Ketonemia
    in diabetic ketoacidosis, 809, 1112
    at end of life, 91
Ketones, in urine. *See* Ketonuria
Ketonuria
    in diabetes mellitus, 1083
    in diabetic ketoacidosis, 809, 1112, 1113
Ketoprofen, 79*t*
Ketorolac, 79*t*, 80*t*
    for ophthalmic disorders, 155, 174*t*
Ketosis, in diabetes mellitus, 1080, 1080*t*, 1113. *See also* Diabetic ketoacidosis
17-Ketosteroid reductase deficiency, in hypogonadotropic hypogonadism, 1065
Ketotifen, for allergic eye disease, 155, 174*t*
Kidney. *See also under Renal and* Kidney disease/injury
    abnormal development of, hypertension and, 389
    acute injury of (acute renal failure), 816, **819–825**, 820*t. See also* Renal failure
    biopsy of. *See* Renal biopsy
    calculus formation in. *See* Nephrolithiasis; Urinary stone disease
    cancer of, 1467*t*, **1491–1492**
        paraneoplastic syndromes associated with, 1453*t*
    chronic disease of, 816, **825–833**, 825*t*, 826*t*, 827*f*, 827*t. See also* Chronic kidney disease

cystic diseases of. *See* Renal cysts
disorders of, **816–849**. *See also* Kidney disease/injury
    dysuria caused by disorders of, 46, 47
    in gout, 732, 849
    medullary cystic, 847*t*
    medullary sponge, 847*t*, **848**
    metastatic disease of, **1492**
    methotrexate eliminated by, 1510
    in myeloma, 472, 848–849
    NSAIDs affecting, 78, 749
    in phosphate regulation, 802
    polycystic, **847–848**, 847*t*
        intracranial aneurysms and, 848, 894
    in preeclampsia-eclampsia, 717*t*
    in SLE, 753, 754, **843**
    toxic drug effects on. *See* Nephrotoxicity
    transplantation of. *See* Kidney transplantation
    tumors of, 1467*t*, **1491–1492**
Kidney disease/injury, **816–849**. *See also under Renal and* Nephritis; Nephropathy; Nephrotoxicity
    ACE inhibitor use and, 405, 410, 820, 828
    acid-base disorders in, 809, 809*t*, 810, 811, 819, 827–828. *See also* Renal tubular acidosis
    acute, 816, **819–825**, 820*t*
        postoperative, 58–59, 59*t*
    amyloidosis, **841–842**
    anion gap acidosis and, 809, 819
    assessment of, **816–819**, 817*t*, 818*t*
    asymptomatic, 833, 843
    chronic, 816, **825–833**, 825*t*, 826*t*, 827*f*, 827*t. See also* Chronic kidney disease
    cystic. *See* Renal cysts
    in diabetes. *See* Diabetic nephropathy
    dysuria and, 46, 47
    GFR in, 817–818, 818*t*
    glomerular, 826*t*, **833–840**
    in gout, 732, **849**
    heart failure and, 360, 827*t*, 828
    hematuria in, 817
    in Henoch-Schönlein purpura, 771, 836*t*, **837**
    hepatitis C infection and, 844
    hypercalcemia/hyperparathyroidism and, 827, 829, 1033, 1034, 1035, 1038
    hyperkalemia and, 797, 798, 819, 823, 827
    hypermagnesemia and, 806
    hyperphosphatemia in, 804, 829
    hypertension and, 389, 391, 393, 827*t*
        treatment of, 396*t*, 410
    hypokalemia and, 796
    hypomagnesemia and, 805
    hyponatremia in, 790*f*, 792
    intrinsic, 820*t*, 821
    lithium associated with, 971
    lower extremity edema and, 37
    mercury causing, 1439
    methotrexate and, 1510

in microscopic polyangiitis, 770, 824, 835*f*
in myeloma, 472, **848–849**
myoglobinuria/rhabdomyolysis and, 763, 822
nephritic, 833, **833–834**, 836*t. See also* Nephritic syndrome
nephrotic, 833, 838–840, **838–840**, 839*t. See also* Nephrotic syndrome
neuropathy associated with, 829, 923
NSAIDs causing, 78, 749
in polyarteritis nodosa, 765
in preeclampsia-eclampsia, 717*t*
preoperative evaluation/management and, **58–59**, 59*t*
proteinuria in, 816–817
pruritus associated with, 136
renal biopsy in, **818–819**
in scleroderma, 758, 759
sickle cell syndromes and, **849**
in SLE, 753, 754, **843**
surgery in patients with, 59
in thrombotic microangiopathies, 485, 485*t*
toxic drug effects and. *See* Nephrotoxicity
in tuberculosis, **849**
tubulointerstitial, 826*t*, **844–846**, 845*t*
in tumor lysis syndrome, 1497
urinalysis in, 816, 817*t*
in Wegener granulomatosis, 768, 769, 835*f*
Kidney stones. *See* Nephrolithiasis; Urinary stone disease
Kidney transplantation, 831–832
    adenovirus infection and, 1276
    for IgA nephropathy, 836
Kikuchi disease, 213
Killip classification, 330
Kimmelstiel-Wilson nodules, 842
Kindling, in substance abuse disorders, 977, 983
Kingella kingae. See HACEK organisms
Kininogen, high molecular-weight, deficiency of, 494
Kiesselbach plexus, epistaxis and, 198
KIT protein, in gastrointestinal stromal tumors, 1474
Klatskin tumors, 1462
Klebsiella/Klebsiella pneumoniae, 1176*t*
    pneumonia caused by, 244*t*
Kleine-Levin syndrome, 975
Klimadynon. *See* Black cohosh
Klinefelter syndrome, 1063–1064, 1065, **1517–1518**
    gynecomastia in, 1064, 1067, 1517
    infertility and, 865, 1064, 1517, 1517–1518
Klonopin. *See* Clonazepam
Knee
    arthritis of
        nongonococcal acute bacterial (septic), 777
        obesity and, 730
        radiographic assessment of, 35
    complex regional pain syndrome and, 743

medial meniscus injuries of, **746**
overuse syndromes of, **745–746**
painful, **33–36**, 33*t*, 34*t*, 35*t*, 745–746
in patella-femoral (patellofemoral)
    syndrome, 35, 36, **745**
Knee fracture, radiologic assessment of,
    35
Kocher sign, 1009
Koebner phenomenon
    in lichen planus, 135
    in psoriasis, 104
KOH preparation, 107
Koplik spots, 1248
Korsakoff psychosis/syndrome, 979, 986
KPs. *See* Keratic precipitates
Krukenberg tumor, 1471
KSHV. *See* Kaposi sarcoma-associated
    herpes virus
Kübler-Ross, stages of dying described by,
    92
Kumamoto study, 1087
Kupffer cells
    in autoimmune hemolytic anemia,
        452
    in cirrhosis, 620
    in cold agglutinin disease, 454
Kuru, 1260
Kussmaul respirations, in metabolic aci-
    dosis, 811
Kussmaul sign
    in constrictive pericarditis, 379
    in myocardial infarction, 330
Kwashiorkor/kwashiorkor-like secondary
        protein-energy malnutri-
        tion, 1134, 1135
Kyphoscoliosis, in syringomyelia, 920

L-AmB. *See* Liposomal amphotericin B
La belle indifférence, 944
La/SSB antibody, 754*t*
    in Sjögren syndrome, 754*t*, 762
Labetalol, for hypertension, 400*t*
    in aortic dissection, 427
    pheochromocytoma and, 402, 1061
    in pregnancy, 718
    urgencies/emergencies, 412, 413*t*
Labor and delivery
    for cardiac patient, 385
        endocarditis prophylaxis and, 385
    for diabetic patient, 723
    herpes simplex transmission during,
        1236, 1237
    induction of, after 41 weeks, 708
    preeclampsia/eclampsia and, 717, 718
    preterm (premature), prevention of,
        719–720
    varicella transmission and, 1241
Laboratory tests. *See* Diagnostic/labora-
        tory tests
Labyrinthine concussion, vertigo caused
        by, 190, 191*t*
Labyrinthitis, 189, 191*t*
Lacerations
    cerebral, 918*t*
    ocular, **171–173**
    scalp, 918
Lachman test, in knee pain, 34
Lac-Hydrin-Five, 99*t*

Lacrimal apparatus, disorders of, **152–153**
Lacrimal sac, infection of (dacryocystitis),
    153
Lacrosse agent, California encephalitis
        caused by, 1257–1259
β-Lactam antibiotics. *See* Beta-lactam
        antibiotics
Lactase deficiency, 515, **563–564**. *See also*
        Lactose (milk) intolerance
Lactase enzyme replacement, 564
Lactate. *See* Lactic acid
Lactate dehydrogenase (LD/LDH)
    ascitic fluid, 525
        bacterial peritonitis and, 526
        tuberculous peritonitis and, 527
    in hemolytic anemia, 448
    in non-Hodgkin lymphoma, 470
    in paroxysmal nocturnal hemoglobin-
        uria, 449
    pleural fluid, 283
        in parapneumonic effusion, 285
    in *Pneumocystis* pneumonia, 1210,
        1394
    in preeclampsia-eclampsia, 717*t*
    reference values for, 1551*t*
    in testicular cancer, 1493
    in vitamin B₁₂ deficiency, 446
Lactated Ringer solution. *See* Fluid man-
        agement/hydration
Lactation/breast feeding, **709–710**, 710*t*
    breast abscess and, 651
    breast cancer/breast cancer risk and,
        660, 672, 728
    drug/medication use/avoidance dur-
        ing, **709**, 710*t*. *See also* spe-
        cific agent
    HIV infection/AIDS transmission
        and, 726, 1207, 1221
    iron requirements/supplementation
        during, 439
    IUD insertion and, 698
    mastitis and, **720**
    oral contraceptive use and, 697
    progestin minipill and, 697
    suppression of, **709–710**
Lactic acid (lactate), 808
    in alcoholic ketoacidosis, 809
    in lactic acidosis, 808, 1117
    reference values for, 1551*t*
Lactic acidosis, 808, **1016–1017**, 1112*t*
    alcoholic ketoacidosis and, 809
    metformin causing, 1093
Lactoferrin, fecal
    in Crohn disease, 578
    in diarrhea, 513
Lactose (milk) intolerance, 558*t*,
        563–564
    diarrhea caused by, 515, 563
    flatus caused by, 511, 563
Lactulose
    for constipation, 509, 509*t*
    for hepatic encephalopathy, 539, 608,
        623
Lacunar infarction, **889**, 890*t*. *See also*
        Stroke
LADA. *See* Latent autoimmune diabetes
        mellitus of adulthood
Laennec cirrhosis, 619

Lambda free light chains, reference values
        for, 1551*t*
Lambert-Eaton (myasthenic) syndrome,
        933
    in cancer, 902–903, 933, 1453*t*
Laminectomy, decompressive
    for cancer-related cord compression,
        1495
    for spinal trauma, 919
Lamisil. *See* Terbinafine
Lamivudine (3TC), 1226*t*, 1228, 1232*f*,
        1238*t*. *See also* Antiretrovi-
        ral therapy
    with abacavir, 1227, 1228, 1231, 1232*f*
    for hepatitis B, 610, 1228, 1238*t*
        during pregnancy, 610, 726
    resistance to, 610, 1233
    with zidovudine, 1227, 1228, 1231,
        1232*f*
        postexposure, 1220
    with zidovudine and abacavir, 1228,
        1232*f*
Lamotrigine, 881, 882*t*, 973
    for bipolar disease/mania, 973
    overdose/toxicity of, 882*t*, 973, 1431
    for seizures, 881, 882*t*
    pregnancy and, 883
Langerhans cell histiocytosis, 991, 995
Language. *See* Speech/language
Lanreotide, for acromegaly/gigantism,
        999
Lansoprazole, 550. *See also* Proton pump
        inhibitors
Lanthanum, for hyperphosphatemia, 804
    mineral bone disorders of chronic
        kidney disease and, 830
Lantus. *See* Insulin glargine
Laparoscopy
    in ascites, 525
    in ectopic pregnancy, 714
    in gynecologic disorders, 675*t*
    in PID, 688
    for tubal ligation, 701
    for ulcer perforation closure, 555
Lapatinib, 668, 1504*t*
Lapdap (chlorproguanil plus dapsone),
        for malaria, 1359
Large cell carcinoma of lung, 1452. *See
        also* Lung cancer
Large-needle (core needle) biopsy, for
        breast lump evaluation,
        658. *See also* Breast, biopsy
        of
    stereotactic guided, 659
Large-volume paracentesis. *See* Paracente-
        sis
Laron syndrome/dwarfism, 992, 995
Larva migrans
    cutaneous, **1385**
    visceral, 1384–1385
Laryngeal carcinoma, **209–211**
Laryngeal leukoplakia, **209**
Laryngeal nerve, recurrent
    damage to during thyroid surgery,
        1012, 1025
    vocal fold paralysis caused by damage/
        lesions of, 211, 1012
Laryngeal papillomas, 208

Laryngectomy, for squamous cell carcinoma of larynx, 210, 211
Laryngitis, **208**
Laryngopharyngeal reflux, **208–209**. *See also* Gastroesophageal reflux disease
Laryngospasm
in drowning, 1415
in hypocalcemia, 800
Larynx, **207–211**
tumors of, **209–211**
LASEK (laser epithelial keratomileusis), 151
Laser assisted in situ keratomileusis (LASIK), 151–152
Laser epithelial keratomileusis (LASEK), 151
Laser-induced prostatectomy, transurethral (TULIP), for benign prostatic hyperplasia, 871
Laser therapy
for acne scars, 122
for age-related macular degeneration, 163
for benign prostatic hyperplasia, 871
for burn reconstruction, 1412
for CIN/cervical cancer, 681, 683
for condylomata acuminata, 679
for diabetic retinopathy, 166, 1105
for esophageal cancer palliation, 1470
for glaucoma, 158, 159
for hair removal, 1055
in pseudofolliculitis, 123
for lung cancer palliation, 1457
for pigmentary disorders, 145
for refractive errors, 151–152
for retinal detachment, 162
for retinal vein occlusion, 164
for sickle cell retinopathy, 167
for wart removal, 132
LASIK (laser assisted in situ keratomileusis), 151–152
Lasix. *See* Furosemide
Lassa fever, 1262–1263
Latanoprost, for glaucoma/ocular hypertension, 159, 176t
Latanoprost/timolol, for glaucoma/ocular hypertension, 159, 176t
Late hypoglycemia (occult diabetes), **1121**
Late life psychosis, 953
Latent autoimmune diabetes mellitus of adulthood (LADA), 1080–1081, 1102
Lateral collateral ligament, of knee, assessment of, 34
Lateral epicondylitis, **745**
Lateral femoral cutaneous nerve lesions (meralgia paresthetica), **927–928**
Lateral ligament complex, of ankle, ankle sprains involving, 746
Lateral sclerosis
amyotrophic, 920, 921
dementia and, 64
primary, 920
Latex allergy, anaphylaxis and, 784

Latissimus dorsi flap, for breast reconstruction, 672
Latrodectus mactans (black widow spider), 139, 1447
Lavage
bronchoalveolar. *See* Bronchoalveolar lavage
gastric, for poisoning/drug overdose, 1424–1425
Lavender top tubes, 1555t
Laxative abuse, 515, 984
diarrhea caused by, 515
Laxatives, 509–510, 509t
hypermagnesemia and, 806
for irritable bowel syndrome, 572
LCHAD deficiency. *See* Long-chain 3-hydroxyacylcoenzyme A dehydrogenase deficiency
LCIS. *See* Lobular carcinoma in situ
LCM. *See* Lymphocytic choriomeningitis
LD. *See* Lactate dehydrogenase
LDCT. *See* Low-dose helical computed tomography
LDH. *See* Lactate dehydrogenase
LDL. *See* Low-density lipoproteins/cholesterol
Lead, reference values for, 1438, 1551t
Lead encephalopathy, 1438
gasoline sniffing and, 984
Lead nephropathy, 845–846, 846
Lead poisoning, 1424t, **1438**
gout and, 733
ophthalmic effects of, 178t
tubulointerstitial disease caused by, 845–846, 846
Leflunomide, for rheumatoid arthritis, 750
Left-to-right shunts. *See* Shunts
Left ventricular aneurysm
coronary artery trauma and, 384
myocardial infarction and, 339
Left ventricular angiography, in angina, 320
Left ventricular end-diastolic pressure, in dyspnea, 25, 25t, 26
Left ventricular failure/dysfunction, 358, 358–359. *See also* Congestive heart (cardiac) failure
hypertension and, 358, 393
in myocardial infarction, 337–338, 340
preoperative evaluation/management and, 51
Left ventricular hypertrophy
in coarctation of aorta, 296
hypertensive, 393, 394
sudden death of athlete and, 386
Leg. *See also under* Lower extremity
acute arterial occlusion of, 419
appearance of
in femoral/popliteal occlusive disease, 416
in varicose veins, 428
in venous insufficiency, 36, 37, 143, 430
Leg elevation
for lymphedema, 433
for venous insufficiency, 38, 430–431

Leg pain. *See also* Claudication
in acute arterial occlusion, 419
in pulmonary embolism, 268t
in spinal stenosis, 740
Leg ulcers, in venous insufficiency/varicose veins/lower extremity occlusive disease, 36, 37, **143–144**, 418, 430, 431
osteomyelitis and, 780
Legal blindness. *See also* Blindness
age-related macular degeneration causing, 163
Legionella/Legionella pneumophila, 1176t, 1310, 1311
Legionnaires disease (legionella pneumonia/legionellosis), 244t, 249, 1176t, 1182t, **1310–1311**
Leiden mutation, deep venous thrombosis/pulmonary embolism and, 267
Leiomyomas
esophageal, 538
gastrointestinal, 567, 1474
of uterus (fibroid tumor), **683–684**
Leiomyosarcoma
gastrointestinal (stromal tumors), 557, 567, 1474
of uterus, 683
Leishmania (leishmaniasis), **1351–1353**
cutaneous, 1351–1352, 1352, 1353
post-kala azar, 1351
mucocutaneous (espundia), 1352, 1353
post-kala azar dermal, 1351
recidivans, 1351
visceral (kala azar), 1351, 1352, 1352–1353
Leishmanin skin test, 1352
Lemierre syndrome, 1322
Lenalidomide, 1505t
for chronic lymphocytic leukemia, 468
for myelodysplasia, 463
for myelofibrosis, 460
for myeloma, 473
Lens opacity. *See* Cataract
Lente insulin (not available), 1097
Lentigines, **100**, 144
solar (liver spots), 100, 145
Lentigo maligna melanoma, 100
Lepirudin, for heparin-induced thrombocytopenia, 486t, 487
Leprechaunism, 1080t, 1082
Lepromatous leprosy, 924, 1327. *See also* Leprosy
Lepromin skin test, 1327
Leprosy, 1177t, **1326–1327**
neuropathy associated with, 924, 1327
Leptin/leptin receptor, in obesity, 1136
insulin action and, 1081
Leptomeningeal metastases (carcinomatous meningitis), 900–901, 1163
Leptospira (leptospirosis), 1177t, **1341–1342**
Lescol. *See* Fluvastatin
Lethal midline granuloma, 201

Letrozole, 668t, 1506t
  for endometriosis, 686
Leucovorin (folinic acid) rescue
  with 5-fluorouracil, 1479, 1507t
  with methotrexate, 750, 1507t, 1510
  with pyrimethamine, 1224t, 1365
Leukapheresis
  for acute leukemia, 465
  for chronic myeloid dysplasia, 462
Leukemias, **457–469**, 457t
  acute, **464–466**. See also specific type
    infection and, 1156
    lymphoblastic/lymphocytic (ALL),
      464, 465, 466, 1466t
    megakaryoblastic, 465
    monoblastic, 465
    myeloblastic, 465
    myeloid (AML), 464, 465, 466,
      1466t
    myelomonocytic, 465
    promyelocytic, 464, 465, 466
      DIC associated with, 488
    undifferentiated, 465
  adult T cell (ATL), 1261. See also
      Human T cell lymphotro-
      pic/leukemia virus
  aleukemic, 465
  chronic
    lymphocytic (CLL), **467–468**, 1466t
    myeloid (CML), 457t, **461–462**, 1466t
    myelomonocytic (CMML), 463
    prolymphocytic, 467
  exfoliative dermatitis/erythroderma
      and, 112
  fever/FUO and, 1154
  hairy cell, **468–469**, 1466t
  meningeal, 465
  plasma cell, 472
  rheumatic manifestations of, 783
  secondary to chemotherapy or radia-
      tion therapy, 464
  stem cell transplants for, 462, 466,
      468, 475, 476
Leukemic arthritis, 783
Leukeran. See Chlorambucil
Leukine. See Sargramostim
Leukoagglutinin transfusion reactions,
      477–478
  leukocyte-poor blood in prevention
      of, 476–477
Leukocyte casts, 816, 817t
Leukocyte count. See White blood cell
      count
Leukocyte-poor blood, transfusion of,
      476–477
Leukocytes
  fecal, in diarrhea, 513, 515, 1172
  pleural fluid, 283, 284t
Leukocytosis
  in antibiotic-associated (C difficile)
      colitis, 574
  in cellulitis, 129
  in lymphangitis/lymphadenitis, 432
  in Still disease, 751
Leukoderma, 145
Leukoencephalopathy, progressive multi-
      focal (PML), 1212, **1261**
  natalizumab causing, 913, 1261

Leukopenia, in SLE, 754t
Leukoplakia
  hairy, 202, 1213
  laryngeal, **209**
  oral, **201–202**
Leukotriene modifiers
  for allergic rhinitis, 197
  for asthma, 224–225t, 227–228
Leuprolide, 1506t. See also Luteinizing
      hormone-releasing hor-
      mone (LHRH) analogs
  for abnormal premenopausal bleed-
      ing, 675
  for endometriosis, 686
  for male infertility, 994
  for prostate cancer, 1487
Leustatin. See Cladribine
Levalbuterol, for asthma, 228, 229t
Levaquin. See Levofloxacin
Levatol. See Penbutolol
Levemir. See Insulin detemir
Levetiracetam
  overdose/toxicity of, 882t, 1431
  for seizures, 881, 882t
  pregnancy and, 724
Levitra. See Vardenafil
Levo-Dromoran. See Levorphanol
Levobunolol, for glaucoma/ocular hyper-
      tension, 159, 175t
Levocabastine, for allergic eye disease,
      155, 173t
Levodopa
  benzodiazepine interactions and, 942t
  MAOI interactions and, 907, 969t
  for parkinsonism, 906–907
    with carbidopa and entacapone,
      907
Levofloxacin, 1180t
  for anthrax, 1301
  for bacterial rhinosinusitis, 194t
  for ophthalmic disorders, 173t
Levonorgestrel
  in combination oral contraceptives,
      695t
  for emergency/postcoital contracep-
      tion, 700
  with estradiol, 703
  in Mirena intrauterine device, 698
Levonorgestrel-releasing IUD
  for abnormal premenopausal bleed-
      ing, 675
  for dysmenorrhea, 677
Levorphanol, 82t
Levothyroxine (thyroxine)
  for goiter, 1020–1021
  for hypothyroidism/myxedema, 994,
      1005–1007
    in Hashimoto thyroiditis, 1018
    during pregnancy, 722, 1006
  RAI therapy/surveillance for thyroid
      cancer and, 1026
  thyroid nodules and, 1019t
  after thyroidectomy, 1025, 1025t
Lewy bodies, dementia with, 63, 64
Lexapro. See Escitalopram
Lexiva. See Fosamprenavir
Leydig cell tumors/hyperplasia, 1054,
      1066, 1492

Lhermitte sign, 737
LHRH analogs. See Luteinizing hormone-
      releasing hormone
      (LHRH) analogs
Lialda. See Mesalamine
Libido, loss of, 862, 949. See also Sexual
      dysfunction
  in chronic kidney disease, 830
Libman-Sacks endocarditis, in SLE, 753
Librium. See Chlordiazepoxide
Lice, 138
  in epidemic typhus, **1280–1282**, 1281t
  in relapsing fever, 1339, 1340
  in trench fever, 1321
Lichen planus, **134–135**
  drugs causing eruptions similar to,
      134, 148t
  oral, **201–202**
Lichen planus-like drug eruptions, 134, 148t
Lichen sclerosus, vulvar, 685
Lichen simplex chronicus (circumscribed
      neurodermatitis), **103**
Lichenoid eruptions, drugs causing, 148t
Licorice, hypertension/hypokalemia and,
      391, 1057
Lid. See Eyelids
Lid lag, in dysthyroid eye disease, 170
Liddle syndrome, 391, 796t
Lidex. See Fluocinonide
Lidocaine, 1545t. See also Lidocaine patch
  for arrhythmias, 343t, 1545t
    infarct-related, 337
    ventricular tachycardia, 337, 352
Lidocaine patch, for postherpetic neural-
      gia/neuropathic pain, 85,
      85t, 115, 878
Lidoderm. See Lidocaine patch
Life expectancy
  assessment/prognosis of older adult
      and, **61**, 62f, 62t, 63t
  obesity affecting, 15, 1136
Life support, withdrawal/withholding, in
      end-of-life care, **91–92**, 92t
Lifestyle
  modifications of
    adherence and, 1
    cancer prevention and, 1450–1451
    in constipation management, 508
    in dyspepsia management, 503–504
    in GERD management, 533
    in heart failure management, 366
    in hypertension management/pre-
      vention, 13, 388t, 394, 395t
    in obesity management, 15, 1137
    in urinary incontinence manage-
      ment, 71
  sedentary
    lipid abnormalities and, 1126t
    preventable disease/deaths caused
      by, 2t
    prevention of, **12–14**
Ligamentous laxity, testing, in knee pain,
      34–35
Light, pupillary reaction to. See Pupillary
      reactions
Light chains
  in myeloma, 472
  in urine. See Bence Jones proteinuria

Light eruption, polymorphous (PMLE), 142, 143
Light therapy. *See* Phototherapy
Light visors, for depression with seasonal onset, 969
Lightning injuries, 1412–1413
Ligneous (Riedel) thyroiditis, 1016, 1017, 1018
Limb-girdle (Erb) muscular dystrophy, 934, 934t
Limb loss. *See* Amputation
Linear scleroderma, 759
Linezolid
    for enterococcal infection, 1292
    serotonin syndrome caused by, 1440
    for staphylococcal skin infection, 1295
Linitis plastica, 1471
Linoleic acid, in nutritional support, 1149
Lioresal, for spasticity, 914
Liothyronine. *See also* Thyroid hormone
    antidepressant drug augmentation and, 964
    for myxedema coma, 1006
Lipase
    in absorption/digestion, 558
    lipoprotein, abnormality of, 1123
    in pancreatic enzyme supplements, 647t
    serum levels of
        in pancreatitis, 642–643, 646
        reference values for, 1551t
Lipemia retinalis, 1083, 1125–1126
Lipid-based amphotericin B, 1401t, 1402
    for aspergillosis, 1158, 1398
    for cryptococcal meningitis, 1397
    for mucormycosis, 195, 1398–1399
Lipid disorders/lipids, 1123–1133. *See also* Fat; Lipoproteins
    antiretroviral therapy and, 1216, 1229
    atherogenesis/coronary heart disease and, 1123–1124, 1124
    cholesterol lowering and, 1124–1125, 1129t, 1130–1133, 1132t
    cholesterol screening and, 1126–1129, 1127–1128t, 1129t
    clinical presentations in, 1125–1126
    in diabetes mellitus, 1085–1086, 1108, 1126t
    health maintenance recommendations/guidelines for, 3t
    pharmacologic therapy affecting. *See* Lipid-lowering therapy
    secondary conditions and, 1125, 1126t
    thiazolidinediones affecting, 1093
Lipid fractions, coronary heart disease risk and, 1124. *See also* Lipoproteins
Lipid-lowering therapy, 9, 1124–1125, 1126, 1128, 1129, 1129t, 1130–1133, 1132t
    for acute coronary syndromes, 327t, 328
    in cardiovascular disease prevention, 9, 1124–1125, 1126, 1128, 1129
    cholesterol screening and, 9, 1126–1129, 1127–1128t, 1129t
    in older patients, 1128–1129
    in women, 1128

in diabetes, 1108
    diet and, 1130, 1146
    exercise/activity and, 1130
    goals of, 1126, 1129t, 1130–1131
    for high LDL cholesterol, 1124–1125, 1129t, 1130–1133, 1132t
    for high triglycerides, 1133
    in HIV infection/AIDS, 1229
    in hypertension, 396–397
    pharmacologic, 1130–1133, 1132t. *See also specific type of therapy* and Statin drugs
        rhabdomyolysis/myopathy/myositis caused by, 761, 763–764
    selection of agents for, 1132–1133
    therapeutic effects of, 1124–1125
Lipid-modifying diet, 1130, 1146
    in diabetes, 1089, 1146
Lipiduria, 816
Lipitor. *See* Atorvastatin
Lipoatrophic diabetes, 1080t
Lipoatrophy, antiretroviral therapy and, 1228, 1229
Lipodermatosclerosis, 37
Lipodystrophy
    antiretroviral therapy causing, 936, 1228, 1229
    Cushing syndrome differentiated from, 1052
    at insulin injection sites, 1104
Lipohypertrophy, at insulin injection sites, 1099, 1104
Lipoid nephrosis (minimal change disease), 839t, 840
Lipoid pneumonia, 277
Lipomas
    atrial septal, 383
    epidermal inclusion cysts differentiated from, 142
    intestinal, 567, 592
    in multiple endocrine neoplasia, 1076, 1076t
Liponyssoides sanguineus mites. *See* Mites
Lipoprotein lipase, abnormality of, 1123
Lipoproteins. *See also specific type and* Cholesterol
    atherogenesis/coronary heart disease and, 1123–1124, 1124
    in diabetes mellitus, 1085–1086
    estrogen replacement affecting, 1071
    lowering. *See* Lipid-lowering therapy
    remnant, 1133
    screening tests for levels of, 1126–1129, 1127–1128t, 1129t
    testosterone replacement affecting, 1065
    thiazolidinediones affecting, 1093
Liposomal amphotericin B, 1401t. *See also* Lipid-based amphotericin B
    for candidiasis, 1391
    for histoplasmosis, 1392
    for leishmaniasis, 1352
Liposomal daunorubicin, 1502t, 1511
Liposomal doxorubicin, 1502t, 1511
    for Kaposi sarcoma, 135, 1216, 1225t
5-Lipoxygenase inhibitor, for asthma, 225t, 227–228

Liquid diets, 1145
Liquid nitrogen. *See also* Cryotherapy
    for actinic keratoses, 113
    for condylomata acuminata, 679
    for wart removal, 132
Liquid oxygen systems, for home oxygen therapy, 236
Lisinopril, 403t
    for heart failure, 362
Lispro insulin. *See* Insulin lispro
Listeria monocytogenes (listeriosis), 1177t, **1303**
Literacy (health), adherence and, 1
LITH gene, in cholelithiasis/gallstones, 634
Lithium, 970–972, 972t, 1545t
    antidepressant drug augmentation and, 964
    antidepressant drug interactions and, 969t
    breast feeding and, 710t
    drug interactions of, 972, 972t
    hypercalcemia and, 971, 1036
    hyperthyroidism/thyrotoxicosis/thyroiditis and, 1008
    hypothyroidism and, 971
    monitoring levels of, 1545t
    overdose/toxicity of, 971–972, 1427t
        hemodialysis for, 972, 1425t
        ophthalmic effects and, 177t
        seizures and, 1423t
    in pregnancy, 971
    for unipolar depression, 970
Lithotripsy
    for choledocholithiasis/cholangitis, 639
    for cholelithiasis/gallstones, 635
    for pancreatic duct stones, 648
    for renal stones, 860
    for sialolithiasis, 207
    for ureteral stones, 860
Livedo reticularis, 755, 765, **773**
Liver
    abscesses of
        amebic, 1366, 1367–1368, 1367t
        pyogenic, **632–633**
    anesthesia/surgery affecting function of, **54**
    biopsy of, 600
        in alcoholic liver disease, 614
        in cirrhosis, 620
        in hemochromatosis, 627–628
        in hepatic vein obstruction (Budd-Chiari syndrome), 630
        in hepatocellular carcinoma, 1460
        in nonalcoholic fatty liver disease, 618
    cancer of, **1459–1461**, 1468t. *See also* Hepatocellular carcinoma
        cirrhosis and, 615, 620, 624, 1460, 1461
        hemochromatosis and, 615, 627, 628, 1460
        hepatitis and, 602, 603, 609, 611–612, 1460, 1461
        incidence/mortality of, 1450, 1460, 1461
        paraneoplastic syndromes associated with, 1453t

cavernous hemangioma of, 633
disorders of, **601–634**. *See also specific
disorder and under Hepatic*
acute hepatic failure, **607–608**
alcoholic, **614–616**
ascites in, 524, 524*t*
spontaneous bacterial peritonitis and, 526, 621–622
biliary cirrhosis, **625–627**
black cohosh causing, 1527
bleeding associated with, 494–495,
623
cirrhosis, **619–625**, 624*t*
in clonorchiasis/opisthorchiasis,
1375
coagulopathy, **494–495**
diagnosis of, 599–601, 600*t*
drug- and toxin-induced, **616–617**.
See also Hepatotoxicity
esophageal varices in, 538, 539, 541
in fascioliasis, 1375
hemochromatosis, **627–628**
hepatic vein obstruction (Budd-
Chiari syndrome),
630–631
hepatitis
autoimmune, **612–614**
viral
acute, **601–607**, 602*f*, 603*t*,
604*f*
chronic, 606, **608–612**
in HIV infection/AIDS, 1213–1214
hyponatremia in, 790*f*, 791
immunization recommendations
and, 1195*t*
jaundice in, 598, 599*t*
lipid abnormalities and, 1126*t*
neoplastic. *See also* Liver, cancer of
benign tumors, **633–634**
drugs/toxins causing, 617
oral contraceptive use and, 633,
696
nonalcoholic fatty liver disease,
617–619. *See also* Fatty
liver
noncirrhotic portal hypertension,
631–632
NSAIDs causing, 749
parenteral nutritional support and,
1151*t*
in preeclampsia-eclampsia, 717*t*
preoperative evaluation/manage-
ment and, **54–55**
pruritus associated with, 136
in syphilis, 1335
Wilson disease, **628–630**
enlarged. *See* Hepatomegaly
fatty. *See* Fatty liver
fibrosis of. *See* Hepatic fibrosis
focal nodular hyperplasia of, 633
in heart failure, 359, 360, **631**
in HIV infection/AIDS, 1213–1214
hydatid cyst of, 1378
passive congestion of, 631
resection of, for hepatocellular carcinoma, 1461
shock, 631
transplantation of, 624

adenovirus infection and, 1276
for autoimmune hepatitis, 613
for biliary cirrhosis, 626
biliary stricture and, 639, 640
for cholangiocarcinoma, 1463
for cirrhosis, 620, 624
cytomegalovirus infection and,
1245
esophageal varices and, 541
for hepatic failure, 608
for hepatic vein obstruction (Budd-
Chiari syndrome), 631
for hepatocellular carcinoma, 1461
for hepatopulmonary syndrome/
portopulmonary hyper-
tension, 623–624
for hepatorenal syndrome, 622
for mushroom poisoning, 1442
for Wilson disease, 629
Liver cell adenoma. *See* Hepatic adenoma
Liver failure. *See* Hepatic (liver) failure
Liver flukes, **1375**
Chinese, 1375
sheep, 1375
Liver function tests, 599–600, 600*t*
Liver-kidney microsomes, antibody to, in
autoimmune hepatitis, 613
Liver spots (solar lentigines), 100, 145
Livial. *See* Tibolone
Living will (advance directives), **90**
Livostin. *See* Levocabastine
Lixivaptan, for hyponatremia/SIADH,
793
LMWH (low-molecular-weight heparin).
See Heparin
Loa loa (loiasis), **1388–1389**
Lobectomy, pulmonary, for lung cancer,
1456. *See also* Lung resec-
tion
Lobular carcinoma in situ, 662–663, 663*t*
Local anesthetics, for eye disorders, pre-
cautions for use of, **172**
Locked-in syndrome (de-efferented state),
917–918
Lodine. *See* Etodolac
Lodoxamide, for allergic eye disease, 155,
174*t*
Löffler syndrome, 266, 374
Logiparin. *See* Tinzaparin
Loiasis, **1388–1389**
Lomustine (CCNU), 1501*t*
"Lone atrial fibrillation," 348
Lone Star tick. *See* Ticks
Long-acting insulin, 1096*t*, 1097*f*, 1098,
1101, 1102. *See also* Insulin
therapy
in pregnancy, 1110
Long-chain 3-hydroxyacylcoenzyme A
dehydrogenase deficiency,
acute fatty liver of preg-
nancy and, 718, 719
Long His-ventricular interval, 356
Long QT syndrome, **353–354**. *See also* QT
interval, long
palpitations and, 31
Long-term care facility, caregiver issues
related to placement in,
62–63

Loniten. *See* Minoxidil
Loop diuretics. *See also* Diuretics; Furosemide
for acute tubular necrosis, 823
for heart failure, 361
chronic kidney disease and, 828
for hyperkalemia, 797, 799*t*
for hypernatremia, 794
for hypertension, 398, 399*t*
urgencies/emergencies, 412
hypokalemia and, 796
hyponatremia caused by, 790
ototoxicity of, 186
Loop excision, for CIN, 681
Loperamide, 514, 517, 1174. *See also*
Antidiarrheal agents
for fecal incontinence, 595, 596
for irritable bowel syndrome, 572
Lopid. *See* Gemfibrozil
Lopinavir/r (lopinavir/ritonavir), 1226*t*,
1230, 1232*f*. *See also* Antiretroviral therapy
Lopressor. *See* Metoprolol
Loprox. *See* Ciclopirox
Lorabid. *See* Loracarbef
Loracarbef, 1179*t*
Lorazepam, 941, 941*t*. *See also* Benzodiazepines
for alcohol withdrawal, 883
with antipsychotics, 957
for anxiety/stress disorders, 941, 941*t*
for delirium, 987
for hallucinogen overdose/toxicity,
1439
for insomnia, 942, 974
for nausea and vomiting, 506*t*, 1509
for panic attacks, 942
for personality disorder, 951
for status epilepticus, 884
Lorazepam interview, in conversion disorder, 945
Lorcet. *See* Hydrocodone
Lortab. *See* Hydrocodone
Losartan/losartan with hydrochlorothiazide, 404*t*, 405
for Marfan syndrome, 1518
Lotemax. *See* Loteprednol
Lotensin. *See* Benazepril
Loteprednol, for ophthalmic disorders,
174*t*
Lotrimin Ultra. *See* Butenafine
Louse. *See* Lice
Lovastatin, 1124, 1131, 1132*t*. *See also*
Statin drugs
protease inhibitor interactions and,
1229
for thyroid cancer, 1026
Lovenox. *See* Enoxaparin
Low back pain, **738–740**, 739*t*. *See also*
Back pain
Low carbohydrate diets, in obesity man-
agement, 15, 1137
Low-cholesterol diet, 1130, 1146
in diabetes, 1089, 1146
Low-density lipoproteins/cholesterol,
1124
atherogenesis/coronary heart disease
and, 316, 1123, 1124

*-density lipoproteins/cholesterol
(*cont.*)
in diabetes mellitus, 1085–1086, 1108
diet affecting, 1130
in familial hypercholesterolemia, 1123
garlic affecting, 1130, 1524
lowering levels of, 9, 1124–1125, 1129*t*,
1130–1133, 1132*t*. *See also*
Lipid-lowering therapy
reference values for, 1551*t*
rosiglitazone affecting levels of, 1093
screening tests for levels of, 1126,
1128, 1129*t*
Low-dose helical computed tomography
(LDCT), in lung cancer
screening, 18, 259, 1456
Low-fat diet, 1130, 1146
in diabetes, 1089, 1146
in obesity management, 15, 1137
for pancreatitis, 644, 647
Low-molecular-weight heparin. *See* Heparin
Low-salt diet. *See* Sodium-restricted diet
Low-saturated-fat diet, 1130, 1146
Low-sodium diet. *See* Sodium-restricted
diet
Low vision. *See* Visual impairment/loss
Lower airway/respiratory tract disorders,
215–216. *See also* Pneumonia
Lower esophageal sphincter. *See* Esophageal sphincter, lower
Lower extremity edema, **36–38**, 37*t*
in chronic venous insufficiency,
36–38, 430
leg ulcers and, 36, 37, 143, 144, 430,
431
Lower gastrointestinal bleeding,
520–522. *See also* Gastrointestinal bleeding
Lower leg/foot arteries, atherosclerotic/
occlusive disease of,
417–418
leg ulcers and, 418
osteomyelitis and, 780
Lower motor neuron lesions, weakness in,
886, 921
Lown-Ganong-Levine syndrome, 345
LOX. *See* Liquid oxygen systems
Loxapine, 954, 955*t*, 956*t*
Loxitane. *See* Loxapine
Loxosceles laeta/reclusa (brown recluse
spider), 139, 1447
Lozol. *See* Indapamide
LRRK2 gene, in parkinsonism, 905
LSD, 982, **1439**
Lubiprostone, 509*t*, 510
for irritable bowel syndrome, 572
Lubriderm, 99*t*
Ludiomil. *See* Maprotiline
Ludwig angina, 206
Lues maligna, 1335
Lumbar motion, Schober test of, 739
Lumbar puncture. *See also* Cerebrospinal
fluid analysis
in CNS infections, 1162*t*, 1164
headache after, 876
in headache evaluation, 45

herniation syndromes and, 893, 1163,
1164
Lumbar spine/disk disease, 738. *See also*
Spine
back pain and, 738, 739
herniated disk, 738, 739
stenosis, **740–741**
tuberculosis (Pott disease), 782
Lumbosacral plexus lesions, **932**
Lumefantrine-artemether (Coartem/
Riamet), 1355*t*, 1356,
1356*t*, 1357*t*, 1360
Lumigan. *See* Bimatoprost
Luminous hallucinations. *See also* Hallucinations
in migraine headache, 873
Lump (breast), 656. *See also* Breast cancer
detection/evaluation of, 16, 17*t*,
654–656, 658*f*, 659*f*
biopsy in, 655, 657–658, 658*f*, 659*f*
clinical examination in, 17*t*, 654–655,
656–657, 656*f*, 657*f*
cytology in, 649, 658, 660
mammography in, 16, 17*t*,
654–655, 655, 658*f*, 659*f*
biopsy and, 655, 659
self-examination in, 16, 17*t*, 655
ultrasonography in, 659
differential diagnosis of, 660
fat necrosis causing, 651
fibroadenoma, 650
in fibrocystic condition, 649
in male, 673
removal of. *See* Lumpectomy
Lumpectomy, 664
for ductal carcinoma, 662
local recurrence and, 652
Lunesta. *See* Eszopiclone
Lung, **215–293**. *See also under* Pulmonary
and Respiratory
abscess of, **250**
aspergilloma of, 1397, 1398
cancer of. *See* Lung cancer
collapse of. *See* Atelectasis
fibrosis of. *See* Pulmonary fibrosis
hydatid cyst of, 1378
radiation injury of, **281–282**
toxic/chemical injury of, **280**
aspiration and, 278
smoke inhalation and, 277, 1409
Lung biopsy
in interstitial (diffuse parenchymal)
lung disease, 263
in lung cancer, 1454
in nontuberculous mycobacterial
infection, 259
in *Pneumocystis* pneumonia, 1395
in pulmonary alveolar proteinosis,
266
in sarcoidosis, 265
in solitary pulmonary nodule, 260
in tuberculosis, 252
in Wegener granulomatosis, 768–769
Lung cancer, **1452–1459**, 1455*t*, 1466*t*
adenocarcinoma, 1452, 1454, 1458
asbestosis and, 279, 280, 1452
bronchogenic carcinoma, **1452–1457**,
1455*t*

chemical carcinogens and, **280**, 1452
cough in, 22, 1454
hemoptysis in, 27, 1454
incidence/risk/mortality of, 1450,
1452
mesothelioma, **1458–1459**
metastatic, **1457–1458**
myasthenic syndrome in, 933
palliative therapy for, 1457
paraneoplastic syndromes associated
with, 1453*t*, 1454
pleural effusion in, 285, 1454
screening for, 18, **259–260**, 1456
smoking/smoking cessation and, 6, 7,
1450, 1452
as co-carcinogen, 280
screening and, 18, 259, 1456
solitary pulmonary nodule, **260–261**
squamous cell carcinoma, 1452, 1454
staging of, 1454–1455, 1455*t*
superior vena caval obstruction in,
431
survival rates for, 1452, 1454, 1457
treatment of, 1456–1457, 1466*t*
Lung capacity, total (TLC). *See also* Pulmonary function tests
in COPD, 234
in cystic fibrosis, 241
Lung flukes (*Paragonimus*), **1375–1376**
Lung resection, for lung cancer, 1456
metastatic disease and, 1458
pulmonary function testing and,
1455–1456
Lung scanning
in pulmonary embolism, 268–269
in pulmonary hypertension, 275
Lung sounds. *See* Breath sounds
Lung transplantation
for COPD, 238–239
for cystic fibrosis, 242
for pulmonary hypertension, 275, 381
Lung volume reduction surgery (LVRS),
for COPD, 239
Lung volumes. *See also* Pulmonary function tests
in COPD, 234
Lungworm, rat (*A cantonensis*), 1384
Lupron. *See* Leuprolide
Lupus anticoagulant, **495**, 753, 754*t*, 756
in antiphospholipid antibody syndrome, 756. *See also* Lupus
anticoagulant-anticardiolipin-antiphospholipid
antibody syndrome
pregnancy loss and, 721, 722
in SLE, 753, 754*t*
Lupus anticoagulant-anticardiolipin-antiphospholipid antibody syndrome, **721–722**.
See also Antiphospholipid
antibody syndrome
pregnancy loss and, 711, 713, 721, 722
SLE and, 721–722, 753, 754*t*, 755
Lupus cerebritis, 754
Lupus erythematosus
autoantibodies in, 110, 752, 753, 754*t*
chronic cutaneous (discoid/subacute),
110–111

drug-related, 111, 148t, 281t, 752, 752t
systemic, **752–755**, 753t, 754t. *See also* Systemic lupus erythematosus
Lupus nephritis, 753, 754, 835f
Lupus panniculitis, 140
Luteinizing hormone (LH)
  in amenorrhea, 1068, 1069
  deficiency of, 991–992, 1063. *See also* Hypogonadism
  gynecomastia and, 1067
  in hirsutism/virilization, 1054
  in hypogonadism, 991, 1063, 1065
  in infertility workup, 693, 864, 865f
  in menopause, 703
  in polycystic ovary syndrome, 690, 1053, 1054
  reference values for, 1552t
Luteinizing hormone-releasing hormone (LHRH) analogs
  in cancer chemotherapy, 1506t
  for prostate cancer, 1487, 1487t, 1488
Luteoma of pregnancy, 1054
Luvox. *See* Fluvoxamine
LVEDP. *See* Left ventricular end-diastolic pressure
LVRS. *See* Lung volume reduction surgery
Lyme disease (Lyme borreliosis), 1177t, **1342–1347**, 1346t
  anaplasmosis/ehrlichiosis and, 1286, 1346
  arthritis in, 1343, 1346, 1346t
    rheumatoid arthritis differentiated from, 748
  babesiosis and, 1346
  chronic (post-Lyme disease syndrome), 1346t, 1347
  coinfections and, 1286, 1346
  congenital, 1343
  diagnosis/overdiagnosis of, 1342
  erythema migrans in, 128, 1343, 1345, 1346t
  head and neck symptoms in, **214**
  myopericarditis in, 377, 1343, 1346, 1346t
  neuropathy associated with, 924, 1343
  during pregnancy, 1343, 1346
  prevention of, 1345
  prognosis of, 1346–1347
  serologic testing in, 1342, 1344–1345
  treatment of, 1345–1346, 1346t
  treponemal tests for syphilis and, 1332
Lymph nodes. *See also specific nodes and* Lymphadenitis; Lymphadenopathy
  in filariasis, 1386
  in Hodgkin disease, 471
Lymphadenectomy
  selective (sentinel lymph node biopsy)
    in breast cancer, 663, 664
      arm edema avoidance and, 671
    in melanoma, 101
    in testicular cancer, 1494
Lymphadenitis, **432–433**
  in cat-scratch disease, 433, 1321
  in chancroid, 1320
  in filariasis, 1386

histiocytic necrotizing (Kikuchi disease), 213
mycobacterial (tuberculous and nontuberculous), **213–214**, **1325**
  in plague, 1318
Lymphadenopathy
  in African trypanosomiasis, 1348
  in American trypanosomiasis/Chagas disease, 1350
  in cat-scratch disease, 1321
  cervical, reactive, **213**
  in chronic lymphocytic leukemia, 467
  in cutaneous T cell lymphoma (mycosis fungoides), 111
  dermatopathic, 111
  in exfoliative dermatitis/erythroderma, 112
  HIV, eustachian tube dysfunction/serous otitis media and, 192
  in leishmaniasis, 1351
  in lymphogranuloma venereum (buboes), 1328
  in mononucleosis, 1243
  in non-Hodgkin lymphoma, 469
  in onchocerciasis, 1388
  in pharyngitis, 204, 1289
  in plague, 1318
  in sarcoidosis, 265
  in toxoplasmosis, 1363, 1364
Lymphangitic carcinomatosis, 1457
Lymphangitis, **432–433**, 1182t
  in filariasis, 1386, 1387
Lymphatic channel diseases, **432–434**
  in filariasis, 1386
  in sporotrichosis, 1400
Lymphatic filariasis, **1386–1387**
Lymphedema, **433–434**
  chronic venous insufficiency differentiated from, 431
  in filariasis, 1386
Lymphoblastic lymphoma, 470
Lymphocyte count, 1552t
Lymphocyte-white blood cell count ratio, differentiation of tonsillitis from mononucleosis and, 204
Lymphocytic choriomeningitis, **1259–1260**
Lymphocytic colitis, 587
Lymphocytic meningitis, benign recurrent (Mollaret meningitis), 1236
Lymphocytosis, in chronic lymphocytic leukemia, 467
Lymphogranuloma venereum, 594, **1327–1328**
Lymphoma, **469–474**, 469t, 1466t. *See also* Burkitt lymphoma; Hodgkin disease; Non-Hodgkin lymphoma
  in celiac disease/dermatitis herpetiformis, 118
  cerebral, primary, in HIV infection/AIDS, 898t, 901, 1212, 1216
  classification of, 469, 469t

cutaneous T cell (mycosis fungoides), **111–112**
exfoliative dermatitis/erythroderma and, 112
fever/FUO and, 1154
follicular, 469
gastric, **1473**
  H pylori infection and, 546, 1473
head and neck, **214**
in HIV infection/AIDS, 214, 1211, 1212, 1216, 1224t
of kidney, 1492
large cell (Richter syndrome), 467
lymphoblastic, 470
mantle cell, 467, 470, 475
mucosa-associated lymphoid tissue (MALToma)
  Crohn disease and, 579
  gastric, 470, 1473
  of thyroid, 1023, 1026, 1029
nose and paranasal sinus involvement and, 201
paraneoplastic syndromes associated with, 1453t
primary effusion (body cavity), 1247
in Sjögren syndrome, 763
small intestine, **1474–1475**
stem cell transplantation for, 470, 475
T cell. *See* Human T cell lymphotropic/leukemia virus; T cell lymphoma
testicular, 1493, 1494
of thyroid, 1023, 1026, 1029
thyroiditis and, 1018
Lymphoproliferative disorder, posttransplant, 1243, 1244
Lynch syndrome (hereditary nonpolyposis colorectal cancer/HNPCC), **592–593**, 1477
  pancreatic/periampullary carcinoma and, 1463
Lysergic acid diethylamide (LSD), 982, **1439**

M2 inhibitors (amantadine/rimantadine), influenza/influenza resistance and, 1270, 1271, 1272, 1273
M184V mutation, antiretroviral drug resistance and, 1233
Ma-huang (ephedra), 1522
MAC (*Mycobacterium avium* complex) infections. *See Mycobacterium* (mycobacterial infections), *avium* complex
Machupo virus, 1263
Macroglobulinemia
  neuropathy associated with, 924
  Waldenström. *See* Waldenström macroglobulinemia
Macrolides. *See also specific agent and* Erythromycin
  for pharyngitis, 205, 1290
  for pneumonia, 247
  theophyllines affected by, 225t
Macrophages, in HIV infection/AIDS, 1208

roprolactin/macroprolactinemia,
1001,1002
Macular degeneration, age-related, **162–163**
Maculopathy/macular edema
   age-related, 162
   diabetic, 166, 1105
   rosiglitazone use and, 1094
Mad cow disease (bovine spongiform
      encephalopathy), 1260
MADH4 gene
   in familial juvenile polyposis, 592
   pancreatic/periampullary carcinoma
      and, 1463
Maduromycosis, **1400–1401**
Magnesium
   dietary/supplementary
      for hypocalcemia, 800
      for hypomagnesemia, 805
      for hypoparathyroidism/tetany, 1032
      requirements for in nutritional
         support, 1149
      restriction of for chronic kidney
         disease, 830
   disorders of concentration of,
         805–806. *See also* Hyper-
         magnesemia; Hypo-
         magnesemia
   genetic disorders and, 796t
   in hypocalcemia, 799, 800, 805, 1031
   potassium balance/hypokalemia and,
      796, 805
   reference values for, 805, 1552t
   serum levels of
      calcium serum levels and, 800, 805
      in hypermagnesemia, 806
   urinary excretion of, in hypo-
      magnesemia, 805
Magnesium-ammonium-phosphate
      (struvite) urinary stones,
      857, 859–860
Magnesium chloride. *See* Magnesium,
      dietary/supplementary
Magnesium citrate, for constipation/
      bowel cleansing, 509t, 510
Magnesium hydroxide, 509, 509t
Magnesium oxide. *See* Magnesium,
      dietary/supplementary
Magnesium salicylate, 80t
   choline, 79t
Magnesium sulfate
   for asthma, 233
   for eclampsia, 716, 718
      hypermagnesemia and, 806
   for hypomagnesemia, 805
   for hypoparathyroidism/tetany, 1032
   for preterm labor prevention, 719
Magnetic fields, in energy medicine, 1520
Magnetic resonance angiography (MRA)
   in aortoiliac occlusive disease, 415
   in carotid occlusive disease, 420
   in renal artery stenosis, 391, 833
   in visceral artery insufficiency, 421
Magnetic resonance cholangiopancre-
      atography (MRCP)
   in biliary stricture, 640
   in liver disease/jaundice, 601
   in pancreatic/periampullary carci-
      noma, 1464

in pancreatitis, 645
in primary sclerosing cholangitis, 640
Magnetic resonance elastography, in liver
      disease/cirrhosis, 600, 620
Magnetic resonance imaging (MRI). *See
      also specific disorder and*
      Neuroimaging
   for breast cancer evaluation/screen-
      ing, 655, 657, 659
   cardiac
      in angina, 320
      in cardiomyopathy, 370t, 371, 373,
         374
      in myocardial infarction, 331
   in deep venous thrombosis/pulmo-
      nary embolism, 270
   in liver disease/jaundice, 600–601
   in pancreatic/periampullary carci-
      noma, 1464
   in pheochromocytoma/paragan-
      glioma, 1060
   in prostate cancer, 1485
   in seizure evaluation, 880
   in thyroid cancer, 1024, 1028
Mahaim fibers, in preexcitation syn-
      dromes, 345
Major depressive disorder, 961–962, 964.
      See also Depression
Major outer surface protein A (OspA), in
      Lyme disease, 1343, 1345
Major outer surface protein B (OspB), in
      Lyme disease, 1343
Malabsorption, **557–564**, 558t. *See also
      specific disorder or cause*
   bacterial overgrowth causing,
      561–562
   in celiac disease, **559–560**
   in Crohn disease, 579
   diarrhea caused by, 512t, 515, 516,
      558t
   HIV infection/AIDS, 1214
   hyperoxaluric calcium nephrolithiasis
      and, 859
   in lactase deficiency, 515
   in protein-losing enteropathy, 569
   in scleroderma, 759
   in short bowel syndrome, **562–563**
   in Whipple disease, **560–561**
Malar rash
   in dermatomyositis, 760
   in SLE, 753, 753t
Malaria, **1353–1362**
   cerebral, 1354, 1356
   congenital, 1354
   drug resistance in, 1355, 1356, 1358,
      1359
   in drug users, 1169
   during pregnancy, 1354
      treatment/chemoprophylaxis and,
         1358, 1359, 1360, 1361
   prevention of, 1361, 1361t. *See also*
      Antimalarial agents
   self-treatment and, 1361
   treatment of, 1355–1360, 1355t,
      1356t, 1357t. *See also* Anti-
      malarial agents
   nonimmune populations and,
      1356, 1360

Malarone (atovaquone plus proguanil),
      1355t, 1357t, 1360
   for malaria chemoprophylaxis, 1355t,
      1360, 1361, 1361t
   self treatment and, 1361
Malassezia furfur
   seborrheic dermatitis in HIV caused
      by, 1215
   tinea versicolor caused by, 109
Malathion lotion, for pediculosis, 138
Malathion poisoning, 1443–1444
Male breast
   carcinoma of, **673**
   enlargement of. *See* Gynecomastia
Male erectile dysfunction. *See* Erectile
      dysfunction/impotence
Male infertility. *See* Infertility
Malignant ascites, 524, **527–528**,
      1495–1496
Malignant effusions, **1495–1496**. *See also
      specific type*
Malignant external otitis, **181–182**
Malignant hypertension, 411
   headache in, 44
Malignant hypertensive retinopathy, 167
Malignant hyperthermia, 39, 1160, 1423
Malignant melanoma. *See* Melanoma
Malignant neoplastic disease. *See* Cancer
Malingering, pseudoseizures and, 881
Mallory bodies (alcoholic hyaline), 614,
      617
Mallory-Weiss syndrome/tears, 506, 518,
      536–537
Malnutrition. *See also* Nutritional disorders
   alcoholic liver disease/cirrhosis and,
      614, 615
   in anorexia nervosa, 1139
   in elderly, 40–41, **72**
   neuropathy associated with, 923
   protein–energy, **1134–1135**
Malocclusion (dental)
   earache and, 186
   facial pain and, 878
MALT lymphoma (MALToma)
   Crohn disease and, 579
   gastric, 470, 1473
   thyroid, 1023, 1026, 1029
Maltese crosses, 838
Mammographic localization biopsy, 659
Mammography, 16, 17t, 654–655, 655,
      658f, 659f
   breast implants and, 652
   computerized stereotactic guided core
      needle biopsy and, 659
   estrogen replacement therapy and,
      1072
   localization biopsy and, 659
Mammoplasty, augmentation. *See* Breast
      implants
Mania/manic episodes, 961, 962
   drug therapy for, 970–973, 972t
   ECT for, 969
   schizophrenia differentiated from, 954
   sleep disorders and, 974
Mannitol
   for hepatic failure, 608
   hyponatremia caused by, 789, 790f, 792
   lithium interactions and, 972t

Manometry
  anal, 596
  esophageal, 530
    in achalasia, 530, 542
    in GERD, 531, 534
    in motility disorders, 530, 543
Mansonia mosquitoes. *See* Mosquitoes
Mantle cell lymphoma, 467, 470, 1475
  bone marrow/stem cell transplantation for, 470, 475
Mantoux test, 253, 253*t*. *See also* Tuberculin skin test
MAO inhibitors (MAOIs). *See* Monoamine oxidase inhibitors
Maple bark stripper's disease, 280*t*
Maprotiline, 968*t*
Marasmus/marasmus-like secondary protein-energy malnutrition, 1134, 1135
Maraviroc, 1227*t*, 1231, 1232*f*. *See also* Antiretroviral therapy
Marburg hemorrhagic fever, 1262–1263
Marfan syndrome, **1518–1519**
  aortic disorders (dissection/aneurysm/regurgitation) in, 311–312, 312–313, 383, 425, 1518, 1519
  pregnancy and, 385
  mitral valve prolapse and, 309, 383, 1518
Marginal blepharitis, 106
Marijuana, **982–983**
  for nausea and vomiting, 87, 507. *See also* Dronabinol
  in AIDS wasting, 1210
MARS. *See* Molecular adsorbent recirculating system
Mask of pregnancy. *See* Melasma
Masochism, sexual, 948
Massage therapy, 1520
Mast cell stabilizers/mediator inhibitors
  for asthma, 223
  for ophthalmic disorders, 155, 174*t*
Mastectomy, 664–665
  antibiotic prophylaxis for, 60*t*
  arm edema after, 671–672
  breast conserving therapy and, 664
  breast reconstruction/implants after, 652, 672
    local recurrence and, 652, 671
  for ductal carcinoma, 662
  for inflammatory carcinoma, 660
  local recurrence after, 652, 671
  in male, 673
  for phyllodes tumor of breast, 650
  prophylactic, 653
Masticatory (jaw) claudication, in giant cell arteritis, 164, 766
Mastitis, puerperal, **720**
  candidal, 125
Mastoidectomy, 184
Mastoiditis, 184
Maternal age, Down syndrome and, 1514
Maternally inherited diabetes and deafness (MIDD), 1082
Matulane. *See* Procarbazine
Maturity-onset diabetes of young (MODY), 1080*t*, 1081–1082

Mavik. *See* Trandolapril
Maxillary sinusitis, 193
Maximal oxygen uptake, lung cancer surgery and, 1456
Maxipime. *See* Cefepime
Maxzide. *See* Triamterene, with hydrochlorothiazide
Maze procedure, 307
Mazindol, for obesity, 1137
Mazzotti test, for onchocerciasis, 1388
MBC (minimal bactericidal concentration), 1175
MC4R gene, in type 2 diabetes, 1081
McCune-Albright syndrome, 997, 998, 1077
MCH. *See* Mean corpuscular hemoglobin
MCHC. *See* Mean corpuscular hemoglobin concentration
MCKD1/MCKD2 genes, in medullary sponge kidney, 848
McMurray test, 35, 746
MCTD. *See* Mixed connective tissue disease
MCV. *See* Mean cell/corpuscular volume
MCV/MCV4 vaccine. *See* Meningococcal vaccine
MDIs. *See* Metered-dose inhalers
MDMA (methylenedioxymethamphetamine), 984, 1430
  hyponatremia caused by, 790
  seizures caused by, 1423*t*
MDR. *See* Multidrug resistance
MDRTB. *See* Multidrug resistance, in tuberculosis
Meal replacement diets, 1137
"Meals on Wheels" mnemonic, 41
Mean cell/corpuscular volume (MCV), 1552*t*
  alcohol use/abuse and, 979
  in anemia classification, 439. *See also specific disorder*
Mean corpuscular hemoglobin concentration (MCHC), 1552*t*
Mean corpuscular hemoglobin (MCH), 1552*t*
Measles (rubeola), 1240*t*, **1247–1250**
  atypical, 1240*t*, 1248
  prevention/immunization and, 1198, 1249. *See also* MMR (measles-mumps-rubella) vaccine
Measles encephalitis, 1248
Measles-mumps-rubella vaccine. *See* MMR (measles-mumps-rubella) vaccine
Measles-mumps-rubella-varicella vaccine (MMRV), 1241, 1249, 1251
Measles vaccine, 1198, 1248, 1249. *See also* MMR (measles-mumps-rubella) vaccine
Meat
  bovine spongiform encephalopathy/variant Creutzfeldt-Jakob disease and, 1260
  brucellosis and, 1316
  contaminated, in sarcocystosis, 1370
  E coli gastroenteritis and, 1315

  gnathostomiasis and, 1384
  sparganosis and, 1379
  tapeworm infection and, 1376
  toxoplasmosis and, 1363, 1365
  trichinosis and, 1383
Mebendazole
  for ascariasis, 1379
  for enterobiasis/pinworms, 1382
  for hookworm disease, 1380
  for hydatid disease, 1379
  for trichinosis, 1384
  for trichuriasis/whipworm, 1380
Mecasermin, for Laron syndrome, 995
Mechanical ventilation
  for ARDS, 292
  for asthma, 233
  for comatose patient, 1420, 1421
  complications of, 290–291
  for COPD, 238
  for near drowning, 1416
  pneumonia and, 248, 249
  for respiratory failure, 290–291
  for shock, 435
  tracheostomy for, 211–212
  withdrawal of, in end-of-life care, 92, 92*t*
Mechlorethamine, 1500*t*
Meclofenamate, 80*t*
Meclomen. *See* Meclofenamate
Medial collateral ligament, of knee, assessment of, 34
Medial epicondylitis, **745**
Medial meniscus injuries, **746**
Median nerve compression, in carpal tunnel syndrome, 742
Mediastinal masses, **261–262**
  superior vena caval obstruction and, 431
Mediastinal widening, drug-induced, 281*t*
Mediastinitis, superior vena caval obstruction and, 431
Mediator inhibitors, for asthma, 223
Medical (advance) directives, **90**
Medical interview, 1–2
Medicare prescription drug benefit, 74
Medication overuse headache, **876**
Medications. *See also under Drug*
  adherence to regimen for, 1–2
  Medicare payment for, 74
Medicinal herbs. *See* Herbal medicine
Meditation, 1520, 1536*t*, **1540–1542**
Mediterranean diet, 15, 1130
Mediterranean fever, familial, **528**
Mediterranean spotted fever, 1281*t*, 1285
Medroxyprogesterone
  for abnormal premenopausal bleeding, 675
  for contraceptive injection, 697
  for endometriosis, 686
  in hormone replacement therapy, 703, 704, 1070, 1072
  for postmenopausal vaginal bleeding, 676
  for psychosexual disorders, 950
Medullary cystic kidney, 847*t*
Medullary sponge kidney, 847*t*, **848**
Medulloblastoma, 898*t*
Mefenamic acid, 80*t*

quine, 1355t, 1357–1358, 1357t
  with artesunate, 1356t, 1358, 1359–1360
  for malaria chemoprophylaxis, 1355t,
    1358, 1361, 1361t
  rabies vaccination and, 1201
Mefoxin. See Cefoxitin
MEFV gene, 528
Megace. See Megestrol
Megacolon
  in Chagas disease, 1350
  toxic
    acute colonic pseudo-obstruction
      (Ogilvie syndrome) differ-
      entiated from, 565
    in ulcerative colitis, 585
Megaesophagus, in Chagas disease, 1350
Megakaryoblastic leukemia, 465
Megakaryocytes
  in essential thrombocytosis, 459
  in myelodysplasia, 460
Megaloblastic anemia
  in celiac disease, 559
  folic acid deficiency causing, 447
  subacute combined degeneration of
    spinal cord and, 915
  vitamin B$_{12}$ deficiency causing, 445
    fish tapeworm infection and, 445,
    1376
Megestrol
  for AIDS wasting, 1210
  for breast cancer, 668, 668t
  in cancer chemotherapy, 1506t
  corticosteroid activity of, 1077
  for elderly, 72
Meglitinide analogs, for diabetes mellitus,
    1091t, 1092
Meglumine antimonate, for leishmaniasis,
    1352
Meibomian gland
  abscess of (internal hordeolum), 152
  inflammation of
    blepharitis and, 152
    chalazion and, 152
Melancholia, 961. See also Depression
Melanocytic nevi (normal moles), 99
Melanoma, 100–101, 1468t
  atypical nevi and, 100
  blue nevi and, 100
  familial, 100
  incidence/mortality of, 100
  pancreatic/periampullary carcinoma
    and, 1463
Melanosis
  arsenical, 144
  coli, 516
Melarsoprol, for African trypanosomia-
    sis, 1349, 1349t
MELAS syndrome, 935
Melasma (chloasma), 144
  oral contraceptive use and, 697
Melatonin, 1528t, 1531–1532
MELD (Model for End-Stage Liver Dis-
    ease) score, 624
  hepatocellular carcinoma and, 1461
  postoperative complications and, 55
Melena
  in erosive/hemorrhagic gastritis (gas-
    tropathy), 544

in GI bleeding, 517, 521, 554
  in peptic ulcer disease, 554
Melioidosis, 1177t
  in drug users, 1169
Mellaril. See Thioridazine
Melphalan, 1500t
Memantine, for dementia, 65, 987
Membranoproliferative glomerulonephri-
    tis/glomerulonephropa-
    thy, 835f, 839t, 844
  hepatitis C infection and, 604, 844
  idiopathic, 844
Membranous nephropathy, 839t, 840–841
  hepatitis C infection and, 844
Memory impairment
  in dementia/delirium, 63, 64, 986
  ECT causing, 969
  ginkgo affecting, 1523t, 1524–1525
  in mild cognitive impairment, 65
MEN. See Multiple endocrine neoplasia
MEN1 gene mutation, thyroid tumors
    and, 1023
Menarche, 1067
  age at, breast cancer risk and, 653,
    653t
  failure of. See Amenorrhea
Mendelson syndrome, 278, 1160
Menest. See Estrogens, oral
Ménétrier disease (hypertrophic gastropa-
    thy), 547
Ménière syndrome (endolymphatic
    hydrops), 189, 191t
  hearing loss and, 187, 189, 191t
menin gene, in multiple endocrine neo-
    plasia, 1075
Meningeal irritation, noninfectious, 1163
Meningeal leukemia, 465
Meningiomas, 898t, 901
Meningismus, 1163. See also specific infection
Meningitis, 1162, 1162t, 1163, 1163t,
    1181t. See also Meningoen-
    cephalitis
  in anthrax, 1301
  aseptic/viral, 1162t, 1163. See also spe-
    cific causative agent and
    Aseptic meningitis
  bacterial rhinosinusitis and, 195
  carcinomatous (leptomeningeal
    metastases), 900–901, 1163
  chronic, 1162
  in coccidioidomycosis, 1393, 1394
  coxsackieviruses causing, 1279
  cryptococcal, 901, 1212, 1224t, 1396,
    1397
    prophylaxis of, 1222–1223, 1397
  CSF analysis in, 1162t, 1164
  echoviruses causing, 1279
  in gnathostomiasis, 1384
  gonococcal, 1319
  H influenzae causing, 1176t, 1310
  headache in, 45, 876
  herpes simplex, 1163, 1236
  in HIV infection/AIDS (cryptococcal),
    901, 1212, 1224t, 1396, 1397
    prophylaxis of, 1222–1223, 1397
  in listeriosis, 1303
  in Lyme disease, 1163, 1343, 1345
  meningococcal, 1201, 1308–1309

prevention/immunization and,
    1309. See also Meningo-
    coccal vaccine
  in mumps, 1250, 1251
  otogenic, 185
  in paragonimiasis, 1376
  in plague, 1318
  pneumococcal, 1164, 1293–1294
    prevention of. See Pneumococcal
    vaccine
  purulent/bacterial, 1162, 1162t, 1163t,
    1164, 1181t
    partially treated, 1163
  in syphilis, 1163, 1334, 1336
  in tick-borne encephalitis, 1266
  tuberculous, 1326
  viral. See Meningitis, aseptic
Meningococcal (Neisseria meningitidis)
    infections, 1176t
  drug resistance and, 1309
  meningitis, 1201, 1308–1309
  prevention/immunization and. See
    Meningococcal vaccine
Meningococcal vaccine, 1188–1189t,
    1190–1191t, 1194–1197t,
    1199, 1201, 1309
  adverse effects/contraindications and,
    1202t
  HIV infection/AIDS and, 1195t, 1199
  pregnancy and, 1195t, 1199
  for travelers, 1199, 1201
Meningococcemia, 1240t, 1309
Meningoencephalitis, 1162t. See also
    Encephalitis; Meningitis
  acanthamoeba, 1163, 1164
  in African trypanosomiasis,
    1348–1349
  amebic, 1163–1164, 1368
  in American trypanosomiasis/Chagas
    disease, 1350
  in angiostrongyliasis, 1384
  in gnathostomiasis, 1384
  travel and, 1173
Meningovascular syphilis, 1334, 1336. See
    also Neurosyphilis
Meniscal cartilage, of knee, 33
  tears of, 746
    assessment of, 35
Menopause, 703–704, 1068–1073
  age at
    average, 703, 1069
    breast cancer risk and, 653, 653t
  amenorrhea in, 1069
  black cohosh for symptoms of, 1523t,
    1527
  depression and, estrogen replacement
    therapy and, 1071–1072
  estrogen replacement therapy for. See
    Estrogen (hormone)
    replacement therapy
  libido and, 949
  osteoporosis and, 703, 704, 1038
  premature, 703. See also Ovarian failure
  surgical, 704
    estrogen replacement therapy after,
    704
  vaginal bleeding after. See Postmeno-
    pausal vaginal bleeding

Menorrhagia, 674
   iron deficiency anemia and, 439
   IUD use and, 698
Menostar. *See* Estradiol transdermal systems
Menstruation/menstrual cycle, 674. *See also* Vaginal bleeding
   abnormalities of, in polycystic ovary syndrome, 690, 1053
   age of onset of, breast cancer risk and, 653*t*
   asthma associated with (catamenial asthma), 216
   cessation of, 703. *See also* Amenorrhea; Menopause
   depression associated with, 676–677, 962
   failure to appear. *See* Amenorrhea
   iron deficiency anemia and, 439
   pain associated with. *See* Dysmenorrhea
   pneumothorax associated with (catamenial pneumothorax), 286
Mental retardation
   in Down syndrome, 1514
   fragile X, **1515**
   in homocystinuria, 1517
   in Klinefelter syndrome, 1064, 1517
   in tuberous sclerosis, 903
Mental status, altered
   in chronic kidney disease/uremia, 826
   after head injury, 919
Mentax. *See* Butenafine
Mepacrine. *See* Quinacrine
Meperidine, 82*t*, 84
   MAOI interactions and, 969*t*, 1440
Meralgia paresthetica, **927–928**
Mercaptopurine, 1501*t*
   for inflammatory bowel disease, 576
      Crohn disease, 581
      ulcerative colitis, 584, 585
Mercury poisoning, 1424*t*, **1439**
   marijuana use and, 983
Meridians, in acupuncture, 1532
Meropenem
   for abdominal infections, 1322*t*
   renal/hepatic failure and, 1184*t*
Merrem. *See* Meropenem
MERRF syndrome, 935
Mesalamine, for inflammatory bowel disease, 575
   Crohn disease, 580
   ulcerative colitis, 584, 584*t*, 585
Mescaline, 982, 1439
Mesenchymal tumors, gastrointestinal, **1474**
Mesenteric ischemia/mesenteric artery occlusive disease, 421–422
Mesenteric vasculitis, 765
Mesenteric vein occlusion, **422**
Mesna, for hemorrhagic cystitis, 1507*t*, 1510
Mesnex. *See* Mesna
Mesoridazine, 955*t*, 956*t*
Mesothelioma, **528**, **1458–1459**, 1466*t*
   asbestos exposure and, 280, 528, 1459

Metabolic acidosis, 806, **807–812**, 807*t*, 808*t*. *See also specific type*
   anion gap. *See* Anion gap/anion gap acidosis
   in chronic kidney disease/renal failure, 809, 827–828
   dyspnea and, 26
   in hypocitraturic calcium nephrolithiasis, 859
   in hypothermia, 1404, 1405
   in near drowning, 1416
   parenteral nutritional support and, 810, 1151*t*
   in poisoning/drug overdose, 809, 1426
      with methanol or ethylene glycol, 809, 1426, 1439, 1440
      with salicylates, 809, 1426, 1445
   posthypocapnic, 810
Metabolic alkalosis, 806, 807*t*, **812–813**, 812*t*
   alcoholic ketoacidosis and, 809
   posthypercapnia, 813, 814
Metabolic bone disease, **1038–1046**. *See also specific disorder*
   in chronic kidney disease (renal osteodystrophy), 827, 829–830, 1033, 1035, 1038
Metabolic disturbances
   cognitive disorders/delirium caused by, 985*t*
   coma or stupor caused by, **917**
   neuropathies associated with, **923–924**
   nutritional support and, 1151, 1151*t*
   seizures caused by, 878
Metabolic encephalopathy
   cancer-related, 902
   coma or stupor caused by, 917
Metabolic syndrome (syndrome X/insulin resistance syndrome), 14, 1082
   coronary heart disease/angina and, 14, 317, 318, 325
   diabetes and, 14, 1082
   fatty liver and, 617
   hypertension and, 14, 390, 1082
   hypophosphatemia and, 803
   obesity and, 14, 1136
   triglycerides in, 1082, 1133
Metacercariae. *See* Cercariae/metacercariae
Metaglip. *See* Glipizide, with metformin
Metagonimus species, 1376
Metanephrines
   in pheochromocytoma/paraganglioma, 1059, 1061
   reference values for, 1552*t*
Metapneumovirus, human, 1268
Metastron. *See* Strontium
Metered-dose inhalers
   for asthma therapy, 223, 228, 229*t*
   for COPD therapy, 237
Metformin
   for diabetes mellitus, 1088, 1091*t*, 1092–1093, 1101
      in combination preparations, 1096
      insulin therapy and, 1101

   intensive therapy with, 1088
   prevention and, 1087
   for hirsutism/virilization, 1055
   lactic acidosis caused by, 1093
Methacholine bronchial provocation testing, in asthma, 219
Methadone, 82*t*, 981–982
   hypogonadism caused by, 993
   for opioid withdrawal/maintenance, 21, 981–982, 982, 1442–1443
   overdose/toxicity of, 1442–1443
   for pain management, 82*t*
Methamphetamine, 1430
Methanol poisoning, 1424*t*, 1427*t*, **1439–1440**
   anion gap/osmolar gap in, 795, 809, 1426, 1439, 1440
   ethanol for, 1426, 1440
   hemodialysis for, 1425*t*, 1440
Methcathinone, 1430
Methedrine, 983
Methemalbuminemia, in hemolytic anemia, 448
Methemoglobinemia, 1427*t*, **1440**
   reference values in, 1552*t*
Methicillin, staphylococcal infections resistant to, 1176*t*, 1294
   in burn injury, 1411
   endocarditis and, 1306–1307
   in HIV infection/AIDS, 1215
   impetigo and, 118
Methimazole
   for Graves disease/hyperthyroidism, 1011
      during pregnancy/lactation, 1011, 1013
      RAI therapy and, 1012
      toxic solitary thyroid nodule and, 1012
   immunopathologic hypoglycemia and, 1122
   for toxic multinodular goiter, 1013
Methionine, in homocystinuria/hyperhomocysteinemia, 1516
Methotrexate, 1501*t*, 1545*t*. *See also* CMF regimen
   for ectopic pregnancy, 714
   for elective abortion, 701
   with folinic acid/leucovorin rescue, 750, 1507*t*, 1510
   for gestational trophoblastic disease, 715
   for inflammatory bowel disease, 576
      Crohn disease, 581
   monitoring levels of, 1510, 1545*t*
   for psoriasis/psoriatic arthritis, 105, 775
   for rheumatoid arthritis, 750
   toxicity of, 750, 1501*t*, 1510
   for Wegener granulomatosis, 769
Methyl alcohol. *See* Methanol
Methyl salicylate. *See also* Salicylates
   overdose/toxicity of, 1445–1446
Methylcellulose, 509*t*. *See also* Fiber, dietary
Methylcobalamin, 445. *See also* Vitamin B$_{12}$

/dopa
antidepressant drug interactions and, 969t
for hypertension, 407, 408t
during pregnancy, 407, 723
lithium interactions and, 972t
MAOI interactions and, 969t
overdose/toxicity of, 407, 408t, 1434
Methylene blue
for methemoglobinemia, 1440
for shock, 437
Methylene tetrahydrofolate reductase
homocysteine levels and, 1516
pancreatic/periampullary carcinoma and, 1463
Methylenedioxymethamphetamine. *See* MDMA
Methylmalonic acid
reference values for, 1552t
in vitamin B$_{12}$ deficiency, 446
Methylnaltrexone, for opioid-induced constipation, 87, 510
Methylphenidate
abuse/overdose of, 983
for depression, 964
for opioid-induced sedation, 84
1-Methyl-4-phenyl-1,2,5,6-tetrahydopyridine, parkinsonism caused by, 905
Methylprednisolone, 1077t. *See also* Corticosteroids
for alcoholic liver disease, 615
for allergic contact dermatitis, inappropriateness of, 119
for asthma, 224t, 229t, 230t
for inflammatory bowel disease, 575–576
Crohn disease, 581
ulcerative colitis, 584, 584t, 585
for nausea and vomiting, 506t
4-Methylpyrazole. *See* Fomepizole
Methyltestosterone, 1065, 1073
Methylxanthines, for asthma, 225t, 228
Metipranolol, for glaucoma/ocular hypertension, 159, 175t
Metoclopramide
for diabetic autonomic neuropathy, 1107
for dyspepsia, 504
for migraine headache, 874
for nausea and vomiting, 86, 506t
Metolazone, 399t
for heart failure, 361
Metoprolol
for aggressive/violent behavior, 987
for arrhythmias, 343t
atrial fibrillation, 347
infarct-related, 336
for heart failure, 363
for hypertension, 400t
for myocardial infarction, 335
perioperative, 50
for pheochromocytoma, 1061
Metritis, 720. *See also* Endometritis
Metronidazole
for abdominal infections, 1322t
alcohol interaction and, 1367
for amebiasis, 1366, 1367, 1367t

for antibiotic-associated colitis, 574, 575
for bacterial vaginosis, 679
for giardiasis, 1372
in *H pylori* eradication therapy, 551t
for leg ulcers, 144
renal/hepatic failure and, 1184t
for rosacea, 123
for trichomoniasis, 678, 1373
Metyrapone, for ACTH-secreting adrenal tumor, 1052
Metyrosine, for pheochromocytoma, 1061
Mevacor. *See* Lovastatin
Mexiletine, 343t
Mg. *See* Magnesium
MGUS. *See* Monoclonal gammopathy, of uncertain significance
MI. *See* Myocardial infarction
Mi-2 antibody, in polymyositis/dermatomyositis, 760
Miacalcin. *See* Calcitonin
MIC (minimal inhibitory concentration), 1175
Micafungin, 1390, 1391, 1398, 1401t, 1402
renal/hepatic failure and, 1185t
Micardis. *See* Telmisartan
Mice
lymphocytic choriomeningitis transmission and, 1259
rickettsialpox transmission and, 1281t, 1284–1285
Miconazole, 98t
for vulvovaginal candidiasis, 678, 1390
Micro-Coombs test. *See* Coombs test
Microalbuminuria, in diabetes/diabetic nephropathy, 842, 1105
Microaneurysms, retinal, in HIV infection/AIDS, 167
Microangiopathic hemolytic anemias, 454
thrombotic microangiopathies and, 485, 485t
Microangiopathy
in diabetes mellitus, 1108
thrombotic, 484–486, 485t
Microbes. *See* Infection/infectious diseases
β$_2$-Microglobulin, in myeloma, 472, 1547t
Microlithiasis (biliary sludge), 634
pancreatitis and, 642
Micronase. *See* Glyburide
Micronor. *See* Norethindrone
Microsatellite instability
in colorectal cancer, 1477
in HNPCC, 592
Microscopic colitis, 587
Microscopic polyangiitis, 769–770, 824, 835f
autoantibodies in, 770, 824, 835f
glomerulonephritis and, 770, 824, 835f
Microsporidiosis, 1369–1371
Microsporum infection, tinea corporis/circinata caused by, 107
Microwave hyperthermia, for benign prostatic hyperplasia, 871
Micturition. *See* Voiding
Midamor. *See* Amiloride

Midazolam, 941t, 942
for delirium, 87
for status epilepticus, 884
MIDD. *See* Maternally inherited diabetes and deafness
Middle cerebral artery occlusion, in stroke, 889
Middle ear, 183–186
infection of. *See* Otitis, media
neoplasia of, 185–186
trauma to, 185
Midline malignant reticulosis, 201
Mifepristone (RU 486)
for elective abortion, 700, 701
C sordellii infection after, 701, 1298
for emergency/postcoital contraception, 700
for psychotic depression, 964
Miglitol, 1091t, 1094, 1094–1095
Migraine equivalent, 873
Migraine headache, 44, 45, 45t, 872, 873–875, 874t
acupuncture for, 1533
mind-body therapies for, 1536t
biofeedback, 1536t, 1537
nausea and vomiting in, 505t
oral contraceptive use and, 697
in patent foramen ovale, 298
transient ischemic attacks differentiated from, 887
vertigo/dizziness and, 188, 190, 191t
Migrainous vertigo, 188, 190, 191t
Mild cognitive impairment, 65
Miliaria, 124
crystallina/pustulosa/rubra, 124
Milk, raw
brucellosis and, 1316
campylobacter infection and, 1316
tick-borne encephalitis and, 1266
Milk-alkali syndrome, 801, 813
Milk intolerance. *See* Lactose (milk) intolerance
Milk thistle (silymarin), for mushroom poisoning, 608, 1442
Milker's nodules (paravaccinia), 1277
Milrinone, for heart failure, 365
Miltefosine, for leishmaniasis, 1352
Mind-body medicine, 1520, 1534–1543, 1536t
biofeedback in, 1535–1538, 1536t
guided imagery in, 1520, 1536t, 1542–1543
hypnosis in, 1536t, 1538–1540
meditation in, 1520, 1536t, 1540–1542
Mindfulness meditation, 1520, 1536t, 1540–1542
Mineral bone disorders of chronic kidney disease (renal osteodystrophy), 827, 829–830, 1033, 1035, 1038
Mineral oil, for constipation, 509t
Mineral oil enema, 509t
Mineralocorticoids. *See also* Aldosterone
apparent excess of
genetic mutation in, 796t
hypertension and, 391

deficiency of, 1048. *See also* Adrenocortical insufficiency
  hyperkalemia and, 797
  in saline-unresponsive alkalosis, 813
Minerals
  chronic kidney disease/renal osteodystrophy and, 827, 829–830
  requirements for in nutritional support, 1149
"Mini-cog," in dementia screening, 64
Minilaparotomy, for tubal ligation, 701
Minimal bactericidal concentration (MBC), 1175
Minimal change disease, 839t, **840**
Minimal inhibitory concentration (MIC), 1175
Minimally conscious state, **917**
Minimally invasive prostate surgery, for benign prostatic hyperplasia, 871
Minipill (progestin), 696t, 697
Minipress. *See* Prazosin
Minnesota tube, for esophageal varices, 540
Minocycline
  for acne, 121
  adverse ophthalmic effects of, 177t
  for rheumatoid arthritis, 750
  for rosacea, 123
Minoxidil
  for androgenetic (pattern) baldness, 145, 146
  for hypertension, 407, 408t
  lower extremity edema caused by, 37
Miotics, for glaucoma/ocular hypertension, 175t
Miralax. *See* Polyethylene glycol
Mirena intrauterine device, 698
Mirizzi syndrome, 636
Mirtazapine, 964, 966, 968t
Miscarriage. *See* Abortion
Mismatch repair gene defects
  in colorectal cancer, 592, 1477
  in HNPCC, 592
Misoprostol
  for elective abortion, 700, 701
  for NSAID toxicity mitigation, 550, 552, 749
Missed abortion, 712
Mites
  atopic dermatitis (eczema) and, 102
  bird and rodent, 139
  rickettsialpox and, 1281t, 1284–1285
  scrub typhus and, 1283
  skin lesions and, 139
  in stored products, 139
  trombiculid, 139
Mithramycin, for cancer-related hypercalcemia, 1497
Mitochondrial DNA mutations
  in diabetes mellitus, 1080t, 1082
  myopathies associated with, **935–936**
Mitomycin, 1505t
  for bladder cancer, 1490
Mitoxantrone, 1505t
  toxicity of, 1505t

Mitral regurgitation/insufficiency, 303–305t, **307–308**
  interventions affecting murmur in, 306t
  in Kawasaki syndrome, 1288
  in myocardial infarction, 308
  preoperative evaluation/management and, 52
Mitral stenosis, **302–307**, 303–305t
  pregnancy and, 306–307
  preoperative evaluation/management and, 52
Mitral valve
  parachute, 306
  in rheumatic fever/heart disease, 306, 375
Mitral valve prolapse ("floppy"/myxomatous mitral valve), **309**
  interventions affecting murmur in, 306t
  in Marfan syndrome, 309, 383, 1518
  panic disorder and, 940
  in polycystic kidney disease, 848
Mitral valve rupture, 384
Mittelschmerz, 568
  in symptothermal natural family planning, 699
Mixed acid-base disorders, **806–807**, 807t
  alcoholic ketoacidosis and, 809
Mixed connective tissue disease, **762**
Mixed sleep apnea, 288
MLH1 gene, in colorectal cancer, 1477
  in HNPCC, 592, 1477
MLL gene, 465
MMR (measles-mumps-rubella) vaccine, 1188–1189t, 1190–1191t, 1192–1193t, 1194–1197t, 1198–1199, 1249, 1251, 1254–1255
  adverse effects/contraindications and, 1202t
  arthritis and, 779, 1255
  in HIV infection/AIDS/immunocompromised host, 1195t, 1220, 1249, 1251
  inclusion body encephalitis and, 1248
  pregnancy and, 1195t, 1199, 1249, 1254–1255
MMRV (measles-mumps-rubella-varicella) vaccine, 1241, 1249, 1251
Moban. *See* Molindone
Mobitz type I (Wenckebach) atrioventricular block, 355
  in myocardial infarction, 337
Mobitz type II atrioventricular block, 355
  in myocardial infarction, 337
Moclobemide, overdose/toxicity of, 1440–1441
Modafinil, for narcolepsy, 975
Model for End-Stage Liver Disease (MELD) score, 624
  hepatocellular carcinoma and, 1461
  postoperative complications and, 55
Modified Duke criteria, for endocarditis, 1304
Moduretic. *See* Amiloride, for hypertension, with hydrochlorothiazide

MODY. *See* Maturity-onset diabetes of young
Moexipril, 403t
Mohs surgery
  for basal cell carcinoma, 134
  for eyelid tumors, 153
  for squamous cell carcinoma, 134
Moisturizers (skin)/emollients, 94, 98–99t
Molar pregnancy. *See* Hydatidiform mole
Molds, opportunistic infections caused by, **1402**
  prevention of, 1158
Mole (skin). *See also* Nevi
  atypical (atypical nevus), **100**
  benign, 99
  normal, **99**
Molecular adsorbent recirculating system (MARS)
  for hepatic failure, 608
  for hepatorenal syndrome, 622
Molindone, 954, 955t, 956t
Mollaret meningitis, 1236
Molluscum contagiosum, **133**, 1277
  in HIV infection/AIDS, 133, 1215, 1277
Mometasone, 96t
  for asthma, 226t
Monge disease, **1418**
Monkeypox, 1277–1278
Monoamine oxidase inhibitors (MAOIs), 967, 968t
  drug/food interactions of, 967t, 969t, 1440
  serotonin syndrome and, 955–956, 1440
  overdose/toxicity of, 967, 968t, **1440–1441**
  ophthalmic effects and, 177t
  for parkinsonism, 907
  for phobic disorder, 943
Monoclonal antibodies, in cancer chemotherapy, 1503t
Monoclonal gammopathy
  motor syndromes in, 921
  neuropathy and, 924
  proteinuria in, 817
  of uncertain significance (MGUS), 472–473
Monoclonal protein. *See also* Paraproteins
  in myeloma, 472
  in Waldenström macroglobulinemia, 474
Monocular blindness, transient, **165–166**, 420
Monocyte count, 1552t
Monocytic ehrlichiosis, 1281t, 1285, 1286
Monomethylhydrazine (*Gyromitra*) mushroom poisoning, 1441, 1441t, 1442
Mononeuritis multiplex, **922–926**. *See also* Neuropathies
  in diabetes mellitus, 1106
  in HIV infection/AIDS, 924
  in Lyme disease, 924, 1343
  microscopic polyangiitis and, 770
  polyarteritis nodosa and, 765

...neuropathies, 922, **926–928**. See also Mononeuritis multiplex; Neuropathies
  in diabetes, 1106
  in HIV infection/AIDS, 924, 1212
  in sarcoidosis, 924
Mononucleosis
  cytomegalovirus, 1245, 1246
  Epstein-Barr virus, 1240t, **1243–1244**
  pharyngitis in, 204, 1243, 1244, 1289
Mononucleosis spot (Monospot) test, 1243
Monopril. See Fosinopril
Montelukast, for asthma, 224t, 228
Montenegro (leishmanin) skin test, 1352
Mood disorders, **961–973**. See also Depression; Mania
Moraxella/Moraxella catarrhalis infections, 1176t, **1310**
  keratitis, 156
  pneumonia, 245t, 1310
Morbilliform skin disorders, 95t
Morganella, 1177t
Morning sickness. See Vomiting, of pregnancy
Morphea, 759
Morphine, 78, 82t
  for dyspnea in terminally ill/dying patient, 82
  for myocardial infarction, 334
  overdose/toxicity of, 1442–1443
    ophthalmic effects and, 177t
  for pulmonary edema, 367
de Morsier syndrome (septo-optic dysplasia), 991
Mosaicism
  Klinefelter syndrome and, 1063, 1065
  premature ovarian failure and, 1069
  in Turner syndrome, 1068, 1075
Mosquitoes/mosquito control
  chikungunya fever and, 1267–1268
  dengue and, 1263
  encephalitis and, 1257
  filariasis and, 1386, 1387
  hemorrhagic fevers and, 1262
  malaria and, 1353–1354, 1361
  yellow fever and, 1265
Moths, skin lesions caused by, 139
Motility disorders. See also specific disorder
  colonic, constipation and, 507, 508, 508t
  esophageal, **541–543**
    chest pain in, 543
    dysphagia in, 529, 529t, 543
  intestinal, **564–566**. See also Intestinal obstruction
    diarrhea and, 512t, 515
    in irritable bowel syndrome, 570
    in scleroderma, 758, 759
    vomiting and, 505t
Motion sickness, air travel and, 1419
Motor activity, in schizophrenic/psychotic disorders, 953
Motor conduction velocity studies. See Conduction velocity studies
Motor neuron diseases, **920–921**
  spasticity caused by, 914
  weakness/paralysis caused by, 886, 920, 921

Motor palsies, ocular, **169–170**
  in myasthenia gravis, 932
Motor tics, in Tourette syndrome, 911
Motor vehicle accidents. See Automobile accidents
Motrin. See Ibuprofen
Mountain sickness
  acute, **1417–1418**
  chronic (Monge disease), **1418**
  subacute, **1418**
Mouth. See Oral cavity
Movement disorders, **904–912**. See also specific type
  drug-induced, **911**
MoviPrep. See Polyethylene glycol
Moxalactam, platelet function affected by, 490t
Moxifloxacin, 1180t
  for abdominal infections, 1322t
  for anthrax, 1301
  for bacterial rhinosinusitis, 194t
  for ophthalmic disorders, 173t
6-MP. See Mercaptopurine
MPGN. See Membranoproliferative glomerulonephritis
MPO-ANCA. See Antineutrophil cytoplasmic antibody; Myeloperoxidase ANCA
MPSV4 vaccine. See Meningococcal vaccine
MPTP, parkinsonism caused by, 905
MRA. See Magnetic resonance angiography
MRCP. See Magnetic resonance cholangiopancreatography
MRI. See Magnetic resonance imaging
MRSA infection. See Methicillin, staphylococcal infections resistant to
MS Contin. See Morphine
MSH2/MSH6 genes, in HNPCC, 592
MSI. See Microsatellite instability
MT1/MT2/MT3 (melatonin receptors), 1531
MTX. See Methotrexate
Mucocutaneous (mucosal) candidiasis, **124–125**, 1390
Mucocutaneous herpes simplex, 1235–1236, 1236
Mucocutaneous leishmaniasis (espundia), 1352, 1353
Mucocutaneous lymph node syndrome (Kawasaki disease), 383, 1240t, **1287–1288**
Mucor infection, 195, 1398–1399
Mucormycosis, **1398–1399**
  rhinocerebral, 195
Mucosa-associated lymphoid tissue lymphoma. See MALT lymphoma
Mucosal associated lymphoid tumors. See MALT lymphoma
Mucosal biopsy
  in celiac disease, 560
  in diarrhea, 516
  in gastric adenocarcinoma, 1471
  in Whipple disease, 561
Mucosal phase, of digestion/absorption, 558

Mucosal protective agents, for peptic ulcer disease, 550
Mucositis, oral, chemotherapy/radiation causing, 1414, 1509
Mucous patches, in syphilis, 1334
Multibacillary (lepromatous) leprosy, 924, 1327. See also Leprosy
Multidetector CT (MCDT), in angina, 308
Multidrug resistance. See also Drug resistance
  hospital-associated infections and, 1159
  in tuberculosis, 252, 256
Multifocal (chaotic) atrial tachycardia, **350**
Multi-infarct (vascular) dementia, 63, 986
  hypertension and, 393
Multinodular (nodular) goiter, **1019–1021**. See also Goiter
  toxic, 1008, 1010, 1012, 1013
Multiple endocrine neoplasia, **1075–1077**, 1076t
  type 1 (Wermer syndrome), **1075–1076**, 1076t
    follicular thyroid carcinoma and, 1023
    gastric carcinoids in, 1075, 1076, 1076t, 1474
    gastrinomas in, 556, 1062, 1076
    insulinoma in, 1062, 1076, 1118, 1119
    islet cell tumors in, 1062, 1076, 1118, 1119, 1120
    neuroendocrine tumors in, 1062, 1076
    parathyroid adenoma/hyperplasia in, 1033, 1075–1076, 1076t
    pituitary adenomas in, 991, 1076, 1076t
    prolactinomas in, 1000
  type 2a (Sipple syndrome), **1076–1077**, 1076t
    medullary thyroid carcinoma in, 1023, 1026, 1028, 1076, 1076t, 1077
    parathyroid adenoma/hyperplasia in, 1033, 1076t
    pheochromocytoma in, 1058, 1076t, 1077
  type 2b, 1076t, **1077**
    medullary thyroid carcinoma in, 1023, 1026, 1028, 1076t, 1077
    parathyroid adenoma/hyperplasia in, 1033, 1076t
    pheochromocytoma in, 1058, 1076t, 1077
Multiple marker screening, in Down syndrome, 1514
Multiple myeloma. See Myeloma
Multiple personality disorder (dissociative identity disorder), 940
Multiple sclerosis, **912–914**
  optic neuritis and, 168, 169
  trigeminal neuralgia in, 877
  vertigo/hearing loss in, **191**, 191t

Multisystem atrophy (Shy-Drager syndrome)
dysautonomia and, 885
parkinsonism and, 906
Multitarget DNA tests, in polyp detection/colorectal cancer screening, 589–590, 1481
Mumps, **1250–1251**
prevention/immunization and, 1198, 1251. *See also* MMR (measles-mumps-rubella) vaccine
Mumps vaccine, 1198, 1251. *See also* MMR (measles-mumps-rubella) vaccine
Munchausen by proxy, 945
Munchausen syndrome, 945
Mupirocin, for impetigo, 97*t*, 118
Mural thrombus, myocardial infarction and, 339
Murine (flea-borne) typhus, 1281*t*, **1282–1283**
Murmurs. *See* Heart murmurs
Murphy sign, in cholecystitis, 636
Murray Valley encephalitis, 1257–1259
Muscarinic mushroom poisoning, 1441, 1441*t*, 1442
Muscimol (anticholinergic-type) mushroom poisoning, 1441, 1441*t*, 1442
Muscle biopsy
in motor neuron diseases, 921
in muscular dystrophy, 935
in polyarteritis nodosa, 765
in polymyositis/dermatomyositis, 761
in trichinosis, 1383
Muscle cramps. *See also* Tetany
heat exposure causing, **1407**
in hypocalcemia/hypoparathyroidism, 800, 1031
Muscle cysticercosis, 1377
Muscle necrosis, in rhabdomyolysis, 763
Muscle-specific tyrosine kinase (MuSK) antibodies, in myasthenia gravis, 933
Muscle wasting, 886. *See also* Weakness
in HIV infection/AIDS, 1209–1210
in malabsorption, 558*t*
in motor neuron disease, 920, 921
in muscular dystrophy, 934
Muscle weakness. *See* Myopathies; Weakness
Muscular dystrophies, **934–935**, 934*t*
cardiomyopathy in, 383
Musculoskeletal disorders, **729–784**. *See also specific type and* Arthritis
arthritis (degenerative and crystal-induced), **729–736**
autoimmune, **747–764**
bone infections, **780–782**
diagnosis and evaluation of, 729, 730*t*, 731*t*
in Lyme disease, 1343
pain syndromes, **736–747**
seronegative spondyloarthropathies, **773–777**
sports injuries and, **744–747**

in syphilis, 1335
in trichinosis, 1383
in tuberculosis, **781–782**
vasculitis syndromes and, **764–773**, 764*t*
Musculotendinous strain, cervical, 736
Mushroom picker's disease, 280*t*
Mushroom poisoning, **1441–1442**, 1441*t*
hepatic failure and, 608, 1441
Music therapy, 1520
MuSK antibodies, in myasthenia gravis, 933
Musset sign, 312
Mustargen. *See* Mechlorethamine
Mutamycin. *See* Mitomycin
Mutations. *See also specific type and specific disorder*
Mutism
akinetic (persistent vegetative state), **917**
in dementia, 64
in schizophrenic/psychotic disorders, 952, 953
Myasthenia gravis, **932–933**
aminoglycosides contraindicated in, 933, 934
Graves disease and, 1009
Myasthenic (Lambert-Eaton) syndrome, **933**
in cancer, 902–903, 933, 1453*t*
Mycamine. *See* Micafungin
Mycetoma, **1400–1402**
Mycobacterium (mycobacterial infections), **1324–1327**
abscessus, 258, 259, 1325
avium complex (MAC), 258, 1177*t*, 1224*t*, **1324–1325**
disseminated disease caused by, 258, 1324–1325
in HIV infection/AIDS, 258, 1224*t*, 1324–1325
prophylaxis of, 1222, 1325
lymphadenitis caused by, 1325
pulmonary disease caused by, 258, 1325
bovis
BCG vaccine made from, 257
intestinal disease caused by, 568
lymphadenitis caused by, 1325
chelonae/chelonei, 259, 1177*t*, 1325
fortuitum, 259, 1177*t*, 1325
gordonae, 1325
haemophilum, 1325
kansasii, 258, 259, 1177*t*, 1325
leprae, 1177*t*, 1326
lymphadenitis, **213–214**, **1325**
malmoense, 258, 1325
marinum, 1325
nontuberculous (atypical), **258–259**, **1324–1325**. *See also* Nontuberculous (atypical) mycobacteria
lymphadenitis caused by, **213–214**, **1325**
scrofulaceum, 1325
szulgai, 1325
tuberculosis, 1177*t*, 1325–1326. *See also* Tuberculosis

bone and joint disease caused by, 256, **781–782**
intestinal disease caused by, 568
lymphadenitis caused by, **213–214**, 1325
meningitis caused by, **1326**
pulmonary disease caused by, **251–258**
resistant strains of, 252, 256
ulcerans, 1325
xenopi, 258, 1325
Mycophenolate mofetil, for autoimmune hepatitis, 613
Mycoplasma, 1177*t*
genitalium, 1328
pneumoniae
pneumonia caused by, 244*t*, 1182*t*
Stevens-Johnson syndrome caused by, 127
Mycosis fungoides (cutaneous T cell lymphoma), **111–112**
exfoliative dermatitis/erythroderma and, 112
Mycotic aneurysms, drug use and, 1168
Mycotic infections (mycoses), **1390–1402**. *See also* Fungal infections
allergic bronchopulmonary, **241**
of bones and joints, **781**
drugs for management of, 1401*t*, **1402**. *See also* Antifungal agents
superficial, **107–110**. *See also* Tinea
Myelinolysis, central pontine, hyponatremia treatment and, 792
Myelitis
in coxsackievirus infection, 1279
in cytomegalovirus infection, 1246
in neuromyelitis optica, 914
in tick-borne encephalitis, 1266
Myelodysplastic syndromes, **462–464**
aplastic anemia differentiated from, 455
rheumatic manifestations of, 783
sideroblasts/sideroblastic anemia and, 444, 463
thrombocytopenia and, 480–481
Myelofibrosis, 457*t*, **460–461**
Myelography
in spinal dural arteriovenous fistulae, 897
in spinal tumors, 901
Myeloid growth factors. *See* Filgrastim; Growth factors; Sargramostim
Myeloid leukemia. *See* Acute myeloid leukemia; Chronic myeloid leukemia
Myeloma, **471–473**, 1466*t*
amyloidosis and, 472, 848
hypercalcemia in, 472, 848, 1035
kidney involvement in, 472, **848–849**
neuropathy associated with, 472, 923–924
nonsecretory, 472
paraneoplastic syndromes associated with, 1453*t*
proteinuria in, 472, 817, 848
stem cell transplantation for, 473, 475

eloma kidney, 472, 848
Myelopathy. *See also specific cause*
  epidural/subdural hemorrhage causing, 897
  in HIV infection/AIDS, 1212
  HTLV (tropical spastic paraparesis), **915**, 1261–1262
  neck pain caused by, 737
Myeloperoxidase ANCA (MPO-ANCA). *See also* Antineutrophil cytoplasmic antibody
  in microscopic polyangiitis, 770
  in Wegener granulomatosis, 768, 769
Myeloproliferative disorders, **457–469**, 457t. *See also* Leukemias
  in hepatic vein obstruction (Budd-Chiari syndrome), 630
  platelet function affected in, 490t
  rheumatic manifestations of, 783
Myeloradiculpathy, in spinal dural arteriovenous fistulae, 897
Myelosuppressive therapy
  infection and, 1156, 1498
  for leukemia, 462, 466
  for polycythemia, 458
Myerson sign, 905
MYH gene mutations
  in familial adenomatous polyposis, 591
  in HIV-associated nephropathy, 843
Mykrox. *See* Metolazone
Myleran. *See* Busulfan
Mylotarg. *See* Gemtuzumab ozogamicin
Myocardial contusions/hematomas, 384
Myocardial dysfunction. *See also* Congestive heart (cardiac) failure
  after myocardial infarction, 337–338
Myocardial failure. *See* Congestive heart (cardiac) failure
Myocardial hibernation, 317
Myocardial hypertrophy. *See* Cardiomyopathy
Myocardial infarction/ST-segment elevation myocardial infarction (STEMI), 326, **330–340**, 331t, 333t. *See also* Coronary heart disease
  abdominal aortic aneurysm repair and, 424
  accelerated idioventricular rhythm in, 337, 353
  antihypertensive therapy and, 396t
  arrhythmias associated with, 336–337
    antiarrhythmic prophylaxis and, 335, 340
  aspirin for, 327t, 332, 335, 340
  atrial fibrillation in, 336–337
  biomarkers in, 331
  chest pain in, 28–29, 29t, 330
    management of, 334–335
  cocaine abuse and, 325, 330, 370, 983
  complications of, 336–339
  conduction disturbances associated with, 337
  coronary artery trauma, 384
  coronary vasospasm causing, 325, 330
  COX-2 inhibitors associated with, 78, 548

  in diabetes mellitus, 1088, 1108
  Dressler syndrome after, 339, 377, 378
  estrogen replacement therapy and, 1072
  general care measures in, 334
  heart failure and, 330
  hemodynamic status and, 331, 331t
  hypotension and, 338
  ischemia after, 336
  left ventricular aneurysm and, 339
  left ventricular failure and, 337–338, 340
  mechanical defects associated with, 338–339
  mitral regurgitation and, 308
  mural thrombus and, 339
  myocardial rupture after, 339
  oral contraceptive use and, 696
  painless, 330
  papillary muscle dysfunction/rupture and, 338–339
  pericarditis after, 329, 377, 378
  perioperative, preoperative risk assessment/management and, 50–51, 51t
  postinfarction risk stratification/modification and, 339–340
  during pregnancy, 385
  prevention and, 340
  Q waves and, 331. *See also* Non-Q wave (non-ST elevation) infarction
  reperfusion therapy for, 332–334, 333t
  revascularization procedures and, 332
    postinfarction, 340
    prophylactic/preoperative, 51
  right ventricular infarction and, 338
  shock and, 338, 434
  sinus bradycardia in, 336
  with ST segment elevation, 326, **330–340**, 331t, 333t
  sudden death and, 330, 353
  supraventricular tachyarrhythmias in, 336–337
  surgery and, 50–51, 51t
  thrombolytic therapy for, 332–334, 333t
  treatment of, 332–336, 333t
    postinfarction management and, 339–340
  ventricular arrhythmias in, 337
  ventricular tachycardia/fibrillation in, 337, 351
    antiarrhythmic prophylaxis and, 335
Myocardial ischemia. *See also* Angina; Coronary heart disease; Myocardial infarction
  in acute coronary syndromes, 326
  chest pain in, 28–29. *See also* Angina; Myocardial infarction
  cocaine abuse and, 325, 370, 983
  coronary vasospasm causing, 325
  dyspnea in, 25, 26
  mitral regurgitation and, 308
  postinfarction, 336, 339
  preoperative evaluation of, 49–50, 51f
  silent, 320
  surgery in patients with, 50–51, 51t

Myocardial perfusion scintigraphy
  in angina, 319
  in myocardial infarction, 331
Myocardial rupture, 339
Myocardial sarcoidosis, 266
Myocardial stress imaging, in angina, 319
Myocardial stunning, 317, 320
Myocarditis, **368–370**
  adenovirus infection and, 1276
  in African trypanosomiasis, 1348
  in American trypanosomiasis/Chagas disease, 368, 1350
  clozapine causing, 955, 958–959
  coxsackievirus infection and, 368, 1279
  in diphtheria, 368, 1302
  drug-induced/toxic, **369–370**
  giant cell, 368
  infectious, **368–369**, 369t
  in Kawasaki syndrome, 1288
  pheochromocytoma and, 1060, 1061
  toxoplasmic, 368
Myoclonic epilepsy, ragged red fiber (MERRF) syndrome, 935
Myoclonic seizures, 879t, 880, 882t. *See also* Seizures
Myoclonus, **910–911**
  nocturnal, 975
  opioid-induced, 84
Myoglobinuria, 817, 822
  acute tubular necrosis/rhabdomyolysis and, 763, 822
  electrical injury and, 1413
Myomas (leiomyomas/fibroid tumors), of uterus, **683–684**
Myomectomy, 683
Myonecrosis, clostridial, **1297**
Myopathies (myopathic disorders), **934–936**, 934t
  HIV, 779, 1213
  idiopathic inflammatory, **759–762**
  lipid-lowering therapy/statin drugs causing, 761
  miscellaneous causes of, **936**
  mitochondrial, **935–936**
  zidovudine causing, 1213
Myopericarditis. *See also* Pericarditis
  Borrelia burgdorferi/Lyme disease causing, 377, 1343, 1346, 1346t
Myopia, 151
  surgical correction of, 151–152
Myositis. *See also* Dermatomyositis; Polymyositis
  HMG-CoA reductase inhibitors (statin drugs) causing, 761, 1131
  inclusion body, 761, **935**
Myotomy
  for achalasia, 542
  for Zenker diverticulum, 538
Myotomy–myomectomy, for cardiomyopathy, 373
Myotonia/myotonic dystrophy, 934t, **935**, 936
  cardiomyopathy in, 383
  congenita, **935**

Myringotomy
  for acute otitis media, 184
  for barotrauma, 183
Myxedema, **1003–1007**. *See also* Hypothy-
      roidism
  pretibial (Graves dermopathy), 1008,
      1009, 1015
Myxedema coma, 1005, 1006
Myxedema crisis, 1005, 1006
Myxedema heart, 1005
Myxedema madness, 1005
Myxedema pericardial effusion, 377, 1005
Myxoma, atrial, 382–383
  herpes simplex virus and, 1236
Myxomatous mitral valve. *See* Mitral valve
      prolapse

Na⁺. *See* Sodium
Nabumetone, 80*t*
Nadolol, 401*t*
Naegleria fowleri, 1163, 1368
NAEPP. *See* National Asthma Education
      and Prevention Program
Nafarelin
  for abnormal premenopausal bleed-
      ing, 675
  for endometriosis, 686
Nafcillin
  for endocarditis, 1306, 1307
  platelet function affected by, 490*t*
  renal/hepatic failure and, 1185*t*
NAFLD. *See* Nonalcoholic fatty liver dis-
      ease
Naftifine, 98*t*
Naftin. *See* Naftifine
Nail atrophy, 146
Nail disorders, **146–147**. *See also* Digital
      clubbing
  candidal infection, 125
  chemotherapy-induced, 1509
  hyperpigmentation, drugs causing,
      146, 149*t*
  local, 146
  pitting/stippling, 146
    in psoriasis, 104
  in Raynaud phenomenon, 756–757
  systemic/generalized skin diseases
      and, 146
  tinea unguium (onychomycosis), 146,
      147
Nalfon. *See* Fenoprofen
Nalmefene, for coma/opioid overdose,
      1421, 1424*t*
Naloxone, 981
  for opioid overdose/withdrawal, 21,
      981, 1421, 1424*t*,
      1442–1443
  for shock, 435
Naltrexone
  for alcohol use/abuse, 20, 980
  for opioid withdrawal, 21, 982
Naphazoline, overdose/toxicity of,
      1434
Naprosyn. *See* Naproxen
Naproxen, 80*t*
  cardiovascular risk and, 552–553
Narcissistic personality disorder, 951*t*
Narcolepsy, 975

Narcotic (opioid) antagonists. *See also*
      Naloxone
  for constipation, 510
  for opioid overdose/withdrawal, 21,
      982, 1421, 1442–1443
Narcotics. *See* Opioids/opioid analgesics
Nardil. *See* Phenelzine
Narrowband UVB (NB-UVB) therapy. *See*
      also Phototherapy
  for lichen planus, 135
  for psoriasis, 105
Nasal biopsy, in Wegener granulomatosis,
      769
Nasal bleeding. *See* Epistaxis
Nasal CPAP, for sleep apnea, 289
Nasal polyps, 199–200
  allergic rhinitis and, 196, 199
Nasal pyramid, fracture of, 199
Nasal septoplasty, for sleep apnea, 289
Nasal sinuses. *See* Paranasal sinuses
Nasal trauma, **199**
  epistaxis and, 198, 199
Nasal tumors, **199–201**
Nasal vestibulitis, **195**
NASH. *See* Nonalcoholic steatohepatitis
Nasoduodenal feeding tube, 1147, 1148*f*
Nasogastric intubation
  for feeding tube, 1147, 1148*f*, 1150
  for GI bleeding, 518, 521
  hospital-acquired bacterial rhinosi-
      nusitis and, 193, 194
  for vomiting, 86, 505, 506
Nasolacrimal duct, obstruction of, dacry-
      ocystitis and, 153
Nasopharynx
  juvenile angiofibroma arising in, 200
  malignant tumors of, **200**
    Epstein-Barr virus and, 200, 1244
    serous otitis media and, 183, 200
Natacyn. *See* Natamycin
Natalizumab
  for inflammatory bowel disease, 577
  for multiple sclerosis, 913
  progressive multifocal leukoencepha-
      lopathy caused by, 913,
      1261
Natamycin, for ophthalmic disorders,
      173*t*
Nateglinide, 1091*t*, 1092
National Asthma Education and Preven-
      tion Program (NAEPP),
      asthma diagnosis/manage-
      ment guidelines of, 217*f*,
      218*t*, 221–223, 222*f*,
      230–233, 231*f*, 232*f*
Native DNA, antibodies to, 754*t*
Natriuresis defects, in hypertension, 390
Natriuretic peptide, B-type (BNP/beta)
  in deep venous thrombosis/pulmo-
      nary embolism, 267–268
  in dyspnea, 26
  in heart failure, 360
  recombinant. *See* Nesiritide
  reference values for, 1548*t*
Nausea and vomiting, **86–87, 504–507**,
      505*t*, 506*t*
  acupuncture for, 1534
  air travel and, 1419

in appendicitis, 567
  chemotherapy-induced, 504, 505*t*,
      506, **1508–1509**
    acupuncture for, 1534
    mind-body therapies for, 1536*t*
      guided imagery, 1536*t*, 1543
  with diarrhea/food poisoning/gastro-
      enteritis, 504, 505*t*,
      1170–1171*t*, 1172
  drugs for management of, 86–87,
      506–507, 506*t*. *See also*
      Antiemetics
  in HIV infection/AIDS, 1210
  hyponatremia caused by, 790, 790*f*
  in intestinal obstruction, 505*t*
  in intracerebral hemorrhage, 892
  in migraine headache, 45*t*, 873
  opioids causing, 84, 86
  palliation of, **86–87**
  in pancreatitis, 505*t*, 506, 642, 646
  in polyarteritis nodosa, 765
  postoperative, acupuncture for, 1534
  in pregnancy, 504, **710–711**
    acupuncture for, 1534
    in gestational trophoblastic disease,
        714
  in subarachnoid hemorrhage, 893
  in terminally ill/dying patient, 86–87
Navane. *See* Thiothixene
Navy top tubes, 1555*t*
NB-UVB therapy. *See* Narrowband UVB
      (NB-UVB) therapy
Nd:YAG laser photoresection. *See also*
      Laser therapy
  for lung cancer palliation, 1457
Near drowning, **1415–1416**
Nebivolol, for heart failure, 363
Nebulizer therapy
  for asthma, 223, 228, 229*t*
  for COPD, 237
Necator americanus, 1380
Neck
  infections of
    anaerobic, **1321–1322**
    deep, **206**
    masses caused by, **213–214**
  masses in, **212–214**
    congenital lesions in adults, **213**
    in Hodgkin disease, 471
    infectious and inflammatory,
        213–214
    lymphoma, **214**
    metastatic, **214**
    thyroid cancer. *See* Thyroid cancer
Neck dissection
  for laryngeal squamous cell carci-
      noma, 210
  for thyroid cancer, 1025
Neck injury, cervical vertigo and, 190
Neck pain, **736–737, 929**
  disk-related, 737, **929**, 930–931*f*
Necrobiosis lipoidica diabeticorum, 1109
Necrolysis, toxic epidermal, 127, 1410
  drugs causing, 127, 149*t*, 1410
Necrotizing cellulitis, synergistic, 1323
Necrotizing fasciitis, 1160, 1291, 1294,
      1323
  cellulitis differentiated from, 129

Necrotizing (phlegmonous) gastritis, 547
Necrotizing pancreatitis, 643, 643*t*, 644, 645
Necrotizing pneumonia, 250
Necrotizing ulcerative gingivitis, **203**, 1289
Nedocromil
    for asthma, 223, 224*t*
    for ophthalmic disorders, 155, 174*t*
Needle ablation of prostate, transurethral (TUNA), for benign prostatic hyperplasia, 871
Needle-stick injury
    hepatitis B vaccine after, 1187
    HIV infection/AIDS transmission risk and, 1207, 1220–1221
Nefazodone, 964, 966, 968*t*
Negative-pressure (cuirass) ventilation, intermittent, for COPD, 238
Neglect/abuse, of elderly, 19, **75**, 75*t*
Negri bodies, in rabies, 1256
Neighborhood reaction, 1162*t*, 1163
Neisseria
    gonorrhoeae, 1176*t*, 1318. *See also* Gonococcal infections
        resistant strains of, 779, 1320
    meningitidis, 1176*t*, 1309. *See also* Meningococcal (*Neisseria meningitidis*) infections
        resistant strains of, 1309
Nelfinavir, 1226*t*, 1229, 1232*f*. *See also* Antiretroviral therapy
Nelson syndrome, 1052
Nematode infections, **1379–1389**. *See also specific type*
    filariasis, **1386–1389**
    intestinal roundworm, **1379–1382**
    invasive roundworm, **1382–1386**
Neoadjuvant chemotherapy. *See also* Chemotherapy
    for bladder cancer, 1490
    for breast cancer, 667
    for colorectal cancer, 1478, 1480
    for esophageal cancer, 1469
    for gastric adenocarcinoma, 1472
    for lung cancer, 1456
Neodymium:yttrium-aluminum-garnet laser photoresection. *See* Nd:YAG laser photoresection
Neologisms, in schizophrenic/psychotic disorders, 953
Neomycin, for surgical site infection prophylaxis, 60*t*
Neonate. *See* Newborn
Neoplasia. *See* Cancer
Neoplastic pericarditis, 377, 378
Neorickettsia sennetsu, 1285
Neostigmine
    adverse ophthalmic effects of, 177*t*
    for myasthenia diagnosis/treatment, 932, 933
Neovascular age-related macular degeneration, 162–163
Neovascular (rubeotic) glaucoma, retinal vein occlusion and, 164

Neovascularization
    in age-related macular degeneration, 162–163
    in diabetic retinopathy, 166
    in retinal vein occlusion, 164
Nepafenac, for ophthalmic disorders, 174*t*
Nephrectomy, for renal cell carcinoma, 1491–1492
Nephritic syndrome, 833, **833–834**, 836*t*. *See also* Glomerulonephritis
    diseases with nephrotic components and, **843**
    in membranoproliferative glomerulonephritis, 835*f*, 844
Nephritis
    interstitial, 820*t*, **823–824**
    lupus, 753, 754, 835*f*
    radiation exposure and, 1414
    tubulointerstitial, 826*t*
Nephrocalcinosis
    in hypercalcemia/hyperparathyroidism, 1033, 1034
    in renal tubular acidosis, 810
Nephrogenic diabetes insipidus. *See* Diabetes insipidus, nephrogenic
Nephrogenic fibrosing dermopathy, 759
Nephrogenic systemic fibrosis (NSF), **849**
Nephrolithiasis (kidney stones), **857–860**, 858*t*. *See also* Urinary stone disease
    calcium, 857
        hypercalcemia/hyperparathyroidism and, 858*t*, 859, 1033, 1034
        hypoparathyroidism treatment and, 1032
    in Crohn disease, 578
    cystine, 857, 860
    in polycystic kidney disease, 848
    in renal tubular acidosis, 810, 857, 859
    in short bowel syndrome, 562
    struvite, 857, 859–860
    uric acid, 732, 849, 857
Nephrolithotomy, 860
Nephropathia epidemica, 1264
Nephropathy
    analgesic, 845, 846
    Balkan, ureteral/renal pelvis cancer and, 1491
    contrast, 822
    diabetic. *See* Diabetic nephropathy
    HIV-associated, **843**
    hypercalcemic, 801
    hypertensive, 393, 411
    IgA (Berger disease), **834–835**, 835*f*, 836*t*
    lead, 845–846, 846
    membranous. *See* Membranous nephropathy
    obstructive, 826*t*
    reflux, 845, 846
    urate/uric acid, 732, 849
Nephrosclerosis, hypertension causing, 393
Nephrosis, lipoid (minimal change disease), 839*t*, **840**

Nephrotic syndrome, 833, **838–840**, 839*t*. *See also specific disease*
    in amyloidosis, **841–842**
    in diabetes mellitus, 839, 842. *See also* Diabetic nephropathy
    diseases with nephritic components and, **843**
    focal segmental glomerular sclerosis and, 839*t*, **841**
    in HIV infection/AIDS, 843
    hyponatremia in, 790*f*, 791–792
    lipid abnormalities and, 838, 840, 1126*t*
    lithium causing, 971
    lower extremity edema and, 37, 838, 840
    in membranoproliferative glomerulonephritis, 839*t*, 844
    membranous nephropathy and, 839*t*, **840–841**
    minimal change disease and, 839*t*, **840**
    primary renal disorders and, **840–841**
    proteinuria in, 838
    systemic disorders causing, **841–843**
Nephrotoxicity. *See also specific agent*
    acute tubular necrosis and, 821–822
    of aminoglycosides, 821
    antimicrobial dosage adjustment and, 1184–1185*t*
    chronic kidney disease and, 827*t*
    of cisplatin, 1511
    of cyclosporine, 822
    endogenous substances causing, 822
    exogenous agents causing, 821–822
    of mercury, 1439
    of methotrexate, 1510
    of NSAIDs, 78
    of radiographic contrast media, 822
Nephroureterectomy, 1491
Nerve agents, for chemical warfare, **1434**
    skin decontamination and, 1424
Nerve biopsy
    in polyarteritis nodosa, 765
    in polyneuropathies, 922
Nerve block
    for pain control, 86
        in complex regional pain syndrome, 743
        in herpes zoster/postherpetic neuralgia, 115
    for spasticity, 914
Nerve conduction velocity studies. *See* Conduction velocity studies
Nervous system. *See under* Neurologic
Nesiritide
    for heart failure, 364
    for pulmonary edema, 368
NESP (erythropoiesis-stimulating protein). *See* Darbepoetin alfa
Netilmicin, 1179*t*
Neulasta. *See* Pegfilgrastim
Neumega. *See* Oprelvekin
Neupogen. *See* Filgrastim
Neural hearing loss, 179. *See also* Hearing loss
Neural tube defects, folic acid in prevention of, 709

Neuralgia
  glossopharyngeal. *See* Glossopharyngeal neuralgia
  postherpetic, 115, 115–116, **877–878**, 1241, 1242
    varicella vaccine in prevention of, 5, 115, 877, 878, 1194–1197t
  trigeminal. *See* Trigeminal neuralgia
Neuralgic amyotrophy (idiopathic brachial plexus neuropathy), 930–931
Neuraminidase inhibitors, for influenza, 1198, 1270, 1271, 1272, 1273
Neuritis
  headache and, 872
  intercostal, 321
  optic, **168–169**
    in neuromyelitis optica, 914
Neuroblastoma, 1467t
Neuroborreliosis, 1344, 1345. *See also* Lyme disease
Neuroclaudication, in spinal stenosis, 740, 741
Neurocutaneous diseases, **903–904**
Neurocysticercosis, 1377, 1377–1378
Neurodermatitis, circumscribed (lichen simplex chronicus), **103**
Neuroendocrine tumors, **1062–1063**, 1463, 1465. *See also* Carcinoid tumors; Islet cell tumors
  diarrhea and, 516, 517
  gastrinoma differential diagnosis and, 557
  in multiple endocrine neoplasia, 1062, 1076
Neurofeedback, 1535, 1539
Neurofibromas, 901, 904
Neurofibromatosis, **904**
  neuroendocrine tumors in, 1062
  pheochromocytoma/paraganglioma in, 1058
  vestibular schwannoma (eight nerve tumors/acoustic neuroma) and, 191, 904
Neurogenic arthropathy (Charcot joint), **783**
  in diabetes mellitus, 783, 1106
  in tabes dorsalis, 783, 1336
Neurogenic hyperventilation, in coma or stupor, 288, 916
Neurogenic shock, 434–435, 434t
Neuroimaging
  in bacterial rhinosinusitis, 193
  in brain abscess, 902
  in cerebral infarction, 891
  in CNS infections, 1164
  in cysticercosis, 1377
  in dementia, 64–65
  in headache, 44, 44t, 45
  in Huntington disease, 908–909
  in intracerebral hemorrhage, 893
  in intracranial aneurysm, 894
  in intracranial arteriovenous malformations, 895–896
  in intracranial tumors, 899

in multiple sclerosis, 913
in pituitary tumors, 993, 998
in schizophrenic/psychotic disorders, 954
in seizure evaluation, 880
in stroke, 891
in subarachnoid hemorrhage, 893
in transient ischemic attacks, 887
in vestibular disorders/vertigo, 189
Neurokinin receptor antagonists, for nausea and vomiting, 506, 1509
Neuroleptic malignant syndrome, 39, 959, 1423, 1444
Neuroleptics. *See* Antipsychotic drugs
Neurologic deficits
  arteriovenous malformations causing, 895
  back pain and, 738, 739
  in brain abscess, 902
  in cerebral infarction, 889–891
  in head injury, 919
  in intracerebral hemorrhage, 892
  in intracranial aneurysms, 894
  intracranial tumors causing, 898–899, 898t
    false localizing signs and, 899
  in lacunar infarct, 889
  in leprosy, 924, 1327
  migraine headache and, 873
  neck pain and, 736, 737
  spinal cord tumors/compression causing, 901, 1495
  spinal trauma causing, 919
  in subarachnoid hemorrhage, 893
  in thrombotic microangiopathy, 485, 485t
  in transient ischemic attacks, 886
Neurologic disorders, **872–936**. *See also specific type and* Neurologic deficits; Neuropathies
  in African trypanosomiasis, 1348–1349, 1349t
  in American trypanosomiasis/Chagas disease, 1350
  Angiostrongylus causing, 1384
  in Behçet syndrome, 772
  in chronic kidney disease/uremia, 826t, 829
  coxsackieviruses causing, 1279
  in cryptococcosis, 901, 1212, 1396, 1397
  in cysticercosis, 1377
  cytomegalovirus causing, 1246
  in Gaucher disease, 1516
  in gnathostomiasis, 1384
  herpes simplex, 1236
  in HIV infection/AIDS, 1211–1212
  in hypercalcemia, 1034
  hypernatremia treatment and, 794
  in hyperosmolality, 795
  hyponatremia treatment and, 792
  infection, **1162–1165**, 1162t, 1163t. *See also* Encephalitis; Meningitis
    anaerobic, **1322**
  in leprosy, 924, 1327
  in loiasis, 1389

in Lyme disease, 924, 1343, 1346t
in malaria, 1354, 1356
measles virus causing, 1248
in near drowning, 1416
nonmetastatic complications of cancer, **902–903**, 1453t
in paragonimiasis, 1376
in porphyria, 923, 1512
postoperative, **56–57**, 56t
in preeclampsia-eclampsia, 717t
primary angiitis and, **772–773**
radiation exposure and, 1414
respiratory failure caused by, 289t
SIADH caused by, 791t
in SLE, 753, 754
in strongyloidiasis, 1381
in syphilis. *See* Neurosyphilis
thiamin deficiency causing, 1141
vertigo and, 190
vitamin E deficiency causing, **914**
in Whipple disease, 561
in Wilson disease, 629
Neurologic evaluation
  in back pain, 738–739, 739t
  in dementia, 64
  in headache, 44, 44t, 45
  preoperative, **56–57**, 56t
Neurologic surgery. *See* Neurosurgery
Neuroma/neurinoma. *See also* Neurofibromatosis
  acoustic. *See* Acoustic neuroma/neurinoma
  mucosal, in multiple endocrine neoplasia, 1077
Neuromodulation, for angina, 324
Neuromuscular/neuromuscular transmission disorders, **932–934**
  in hypercalcemia, 1034
  respiratory failure caused by, 289t
  in uremia, 826t
  weakness in, 886
Neuromyelitis optica (Devic syndrome), **914**
  optic neuritis in, 168, 914
Neuron-specific enolase, in pheochromocytoma, 1059
Neuronal neuropathies, 921. *See also specific type and* Neuropathies
Neuronitis, vestibular, 190, 191t
Neuronopathy, bulbospinal X-linked, 921
Neuropathic bladder, chemotherapy-induced, 1510
Neuropathic pain, **84–85**, 85t, 922. *See also* Neuropathies
Neuropathies, **921–929**
  acute motor axonal/acute motor and sensory axonal (AMAN/AMSAN), 925. *See also* Guillain-Barré syndrome
  alcoholism and nutritional deficiency and, 923
  in amyloidosis, 924
  antiretroviral agents causing, 1212, 1228
  autonomic. *See* Autonomic neuropathy
  brachial plexus, **929–931**
  cancer-related, 885, 902, **925**, 1453t

Neuropathies (*cont.*)
chemotherapy-induced, 1510
in chronic kidney disease/uremia, 829, 923
cisplatin-induced, 1511
compression. *See* Entrapment/compression neuropathy
in critically ill patient, **924–925**
in cryoglobulinemia, 771, 924
diabetic, 923, 1082t, 1106–1108
foot disorders/ulcers/gangrene and, 1106, 1109
glycemic control and, 1087
didanosine therapy and, 1212, 1228
diphtheritic, 925, 1302
dysautonomia and, 885
entrapment. *See* Entrapment/compression neuropathy
facial, **928–929**. *See also* Bell palsy
hereditary motor and sensory (HMSN), types I to IV, 922–923
in HIV infection/AIDS, 924, 1212
infectious/inflammatory disease and, **924**
inherited, **922–923**
in leprosy, 924, 1327
in Lyme disease, 924, 1343
metabolic/systemic disease and, **923–924**
in microscopic polyangiitis, 770
in myeloma, 472, 923–924
nutritional, 923. *See also specific nutrient*
optic
inflammatory (optic neuritis), **168–169**
ischemic, **168**
giant cell arteritis and, 168, 766
in paraproteinemias, 923–924
peripheral, **921–929**. *See also specific type*
in polyarteritis nodosa, 765, 924
in porphyria, 923, 1512
in rheumatoid arthritis, 747, 924
in sarcoidosis, 924
stavudine therapy and, 1212, 1228
in thiamin deficiency, 923, 1141
toxic, **925**
in vitamin B$_{12}$ deficiency, 445, 923
Neuropeptide Y, in pheochromocytoma, 1058
Neuroses, Sunday, 939
Neurosurgery, antibiotic prophylaxis for, 60t
Neurosyphilis, 1183t, **1336–1337**
cerebrospinal fluid examination in, 1336, 1337
indications for, 1336–1337
in HIV infection/AIDS, 1220, 1337–1338
treatment failures and, 1334
Neurotomy, radial optic, for retinal vein occlusion, 164
Neurotoxicity. *See also* Neurologic disorders
of cisplatin, 1511
of snake venom, 1446
Neurotransmitters. *See specific type*

Neurotrophic keratitis, 156
Neurotropic disease
viral, **1255–1262**. *See also specific disorder*
yellow fever vaccine-associated, 1203, 1265–1266
Neutral protamine Hagedorn (NPH) insulin. *See* Insulin therapy; NPH insulin
Neutral protamine lispro (NPL) insulin, 1099
Neutrocytic ascites, 526
Neutrogena, 99t
Neutropenia, **456–457**, 456t
in acute leukemia, 465
aspergillosis and, 1398
cancer chemotherapy causing, 1499
fever/FUO and, 456, 1153, 1154, 1498
antimicrobial therapy and, 40, 1158, 1181t, 1498
gram-negative bacteremia/sepsis and, 456, 1311
granulocyte transfusion for, 478
in hairy cell leukemia, 468
infections and, 456, 1156, 1158
in cancer patients, 1181t, 1498
prevention/treatment and, 1157–1158, 1498
pulmonary, 251
Neutrophil count. *See also* Neutropenia; Neutrophilia
ascitic, 525
in bacterial peritonitis, 526, 621
reference values for, 1552t
Neutrophilia
in cellulitis, 129
in gram-negative bacteremia/sepsis, 1311
Nevanac. *See* Nepafenac
Nevi. *See also* Mole (skin)
atypical (dysplastic), **100**
blue, **100**
compound, 99
junctional, 99
melanocytic, **99**
pigmented, 95t, **99–101**
Nevirapine, 1227t, 1230, 1232f. *See also* Antiretroviral therapy
Nevus. *See* Nevi
New World cutaneous leishmaniasis, 1351, 1352, 1353
Newborn/infant
air travel and, 1419
antiretroviral/zidovudine therapy for, 726
chlamydial infection in, 727
CMV infection/inclusion disease in, 1245
coxsackievirus myocarditis in, 1279
gonococcal infection in, 727
group B streptococcal infection in, 708, **725**, 1291
hemolytic disease of, prevention of, **709**
hepatitis B transmission/vaccine and, 602, 606, 726, 1187
hepatitis C transmission and, 726

herpes simplex infection and, 727, 1236, 1237
HIV transmission to, 726, 1207, 1221
listeriosis in (granulomatosis infantisepticum), 1303
maternal thyroid disease and, 722, 1003, 1008, 1013
rubella infection and, 1254, 1255
syphilis in (congenital syphilis), 727, **1338**
toxoplasmosis during pregnancy and, 1363, 1364
varicella in, 725, 1241
Nexavar. *See* Sorafenib
NH$_3$. *See* Ammonia
Niacin (vitamin B$_3$)
deficiency of, **1142**
for lipid modification/heart disease prevention, 1131, 1132–1133, 1132t, 1142
toxicity of, 1131, **1142**
Niacinamide, 1142. *See also* Niacin
Niaspan. *See* Niacin
Nicardipine, 406t
for hypertensive urgencies/emergencies, 412, 413t
overdose/toxicity of, 406t, 413t, 1432
Niclosamide, for tapeworm infection, 1377
Nicoderm. *See* Nicotine, for replacement therapy
Nicotinamide. *See also* Niacin
for niacin deficiency, 1142
Nicotine, 6. *See also* Smoking
acupuncture for withdrawal from, 1534
for replacement therapy, 7, 9t, 10t, 11t, 1450
Nicotinic acid. *See* Niacin
Nicotrol. *See* Nicotine, for replacement therapy
Nifedipine
for angina, 322
for hypertension, 406t
in urgencies/emergencies, 412, 413t, 414
MOAI-induced, 967
overdose/toxicity of, 406t, 413t, 1432
for preterm labor prevention, 719
Nifurtimox
for African trypanosomiasis, 1349, 1349t
for American trypanosomiasis/Chagas disease, 1350
Night blindness, in vitamin A deficiency, 1143
Nightmares, 975
Nikolsky sign, 130
Nil disease (minimal change disease), 839t, **840**
Nilandron. *See* Nilutamide
Nilotinib, 1504t
for chronic myeloid leukemia, 462
Nilutamide, 1505t
Nimodipine, 894. *See also* Calcium channel blocking drugs
overdose/toxicity of, 1432
Nipent. *See* Pentostatin

NIPHS. *See* Noninsulinoma pancreatogenous hypoglycemia syndrome
Nipple, Paget disease of, 113, 660
Nipple discharge, **651**
  in breast cancer, 651, 657
  cytologic evaluation of, 651, 660
  in fibrocystic breast condition, 649, 651
  in hyperprolactinemia, 651
  in male, 673
Nipride. *See* Nitroprusside
Nisoldipine, 406*t*
  overdose/toxicity of, 406*t*, 1432
Nitazoxanide
  for cryptosporidiosis, 1370
  for giardiasis, 1372
Nitrates. *See also* Nitroglycerin
  for acute coronary syndromes, 328
  for angina
    for acute attack, 321
    prophylactic administration of, 321
  for heart failure, 364
    left ventricular (infarct-related), 337
  for myocardial infarction, 335, 336
  phosphodiesterase inhibitor/sildenafil contraindications and, 863, 950, 1108
  for pulmonary edema, 368
Nitric oxide
  in exhaled breath, in asthma, 221
  ginkgo affecting, 1524
  in shock, 437
Nitric oxide synthetase, in shock, 437
Nitrites
  for cyanide poisoning, 1424*t*, 1435, 1435*t*
  methemoglobinemia caused by, 1440
Nitrobenzene, methemoglobinemia caused by, 1440
Nitrofurantoin, for urinary tract infection, 852*t*
Nitrogen, liquid. *See* Liquid nitrogen
Nitrogen balance, nutritional support and, 1149, 1152
Nitrogen mustards, in cancer chemotherapy, 1500*t*
Nitrogen oxide gases, methemoglobinemia caused by, 1440
Nitroglycerin. *See also* Nitrates
  for acute coronary syndromes, 328
  for angina
    for acute attack, 321
    in diagnosis, 318
    prophylactic administration of, 318
  for heart failure, 364
    left ventricular (infarct-related), 337, 338
  for hypertensive urgencies/emergencies, 412, 413*t*
  for myocardial infarction, 334, 335
  phosphodiesterase inhibitor/sildenafil contraindications and, 863, 950, 1108
  for pulmonary edema, 368
Nitroprusside
  cyanide poisoning caused by, 1435

for heart failure, 364
  infarct-related, 337–338
for hypertension
  in aortic dissection, 427
  urgencies/emergencies, 412, 413*t*
Nix. *See* Permethrin
Nizatidine, 550. *See also* H$_2$ receptor blocking drugs
Nizoral. *See* Ketoconazole
Njovera (endemic syphilis), 1339
NK cell lymphoma, nose and paranasal sinus involvement and, 201
NK$_1$ receptor antagonists, for nausea and vomiting, 506, 1509
NMO-IgG, in neuromyelitis optica, 914
NMS. *See* Neuroleptic malignant syndrome
NNRTIs. *See* Nonnucleoside reverse transcriptase inhibitors
Nocardia asteroides/brasiliensis (nocardiosis), 1177*t*, **1324**
  actinomycotic mycetoma and, 1400
Noctec. *See* Chloral hydrate
Nocturia, 70, 71, 867
  in heart failure, 359
Nocturnal myoclonus, 975
Nocturnal penile tumescence testing, 863, 949
Nodular glomerulosclerosis, in diabetic nephropathy, 842
Nodular goiter. *See* Multinodular (nodular) goiter
Nodular malignant melanoma, 100
Nodules
  milker's (paravaccinia), 1277
  pulmonary, solitary. *See* Solitary pulmonary nodule
  rheumatoid, 747–748
    in coal workers (Caplan syndrome), 278
    gouty tophi differentiated from, 733, 748
  skin, 95*t*. *See also specific type*
    inflammatory, **140–141**
    violaceous to purple, **134–136**
  subcutaneous. *See* Subcutaneous nodules
  thyroid, **1019–1021**, 1019*t*. *See also* Goiter; Thyroid cancer; Thyroid nodules
  vocal fold, 209
    laryngitis and, 208
Noise trauma
  hearing loss caused by, 186
  tympanic membrane perforation caused by, 185
Nolvadex. *See* Tamoxifen
Non-ABCDE hepatitis, transfusion-associated, 601
Nonadherence. *See* Adherence/nonadherence
Nonalcoholic fatty liver disease (NAFLD), **617–619**. *See also* Fatty liver
  cirrhosis and, 617, 618, 620
    hepatocellular carcinoma and, 618, 1460

Nonalcoholic steatohepatitis (NASH), 617, 618
Nonbacterial prostatitis, **855**, 855*t*
Noncirrhotic portal hypertension, **631–632**
Nonclostridial crepitant cellulitis, 1323
Noncompliance. *See* Adherence/nonadherence
Nonconvulsive status epilepticus, 884
Nondiabetic (renal) glycosuria, 1086
Nonerosive/nonspecific gastritis, **546–547**
Nonfamilial adenomatous polyps, **589–591**
Nongonococcal acute bacterial arthritis. *See* Septic (nongonococcal acute bacterial) arthritis
Non-group A streptococcal infections, **1291**
Non-Hodgkin lymphoma, **469–471**, 469*t*, 1466*t*. *See also* Lymphoma
  fever/FUO and, 1154
  gastric, 1473
  hepatitis C and, 604
  in HIV infection/AIDS, 214, 1211, 1212, 1216, 1224*t*
  small intestine, 1475
  thyroid, 1023, 1026, 1029
Noninsulinoma pancreatogenous hypoglycemia syndrome, 1119, **1120**
Noninsulinomas, localization of, 1062
Noninvasive ischemia testing, preoperative, 49–50, 51*f*
Noninvasive positive-pressure ventilation (NPPV)
  for COPD, 238
  for respiratory failure, 290
Nonionizing radiation, 1413
Nonketotic hyperglycemic hyperosmolar coma. *See* Hyperglycemic hyperosmolar state
Nonmyeloablative allogeneic transplant. *See* Bone marrow/stem cell transplantation; Reduced-intensity allogeneic stem cell transplantation
Nonnucleoside reverse transcriptase inhibitors (NNRTIs), 1227*t*, 1230–1231, 1232*f*. *See also* Antiretroviral therapy
  antituberculous drug interactions and, 255–256
  in combinations, 1227, 1230, 1232, 1232*f*
  resistance and, 1230
Nonoliguric acute tubular necrosis, 823
Nonoxynol 9, 699, 1168
  HIV infection/AIDS and, 1218
Nonparalytic poliomyelitis, 1252
Nonparoxysmal junctional tachycardia, 350–351
Nonproliferative retinopathy, 166
Non-Q wave (non-ST elevation) infarction, 331, 332. *See also* Myocardial infarction
Non-rapid eye movement (non-REM) sleep, 973

Nonscarring alopecia, **145–146**
Nonsecretory myeloma, 472
Nonseminomas, 1066, 1492, 1493, 1493–1494, 1494
Non-sexually transmitted treponematoses, **1338–1339**
Non–small cell lung cancer, 1454, 1466t. *See also* Lung cancer
  paraneoplastic syndromes associated with, 1453t
  staging of, 1454–1455, 1455t
  survival rates for, 1454
  treatment of, 1456–1457, 1466t
Nonspecific interstitial pneumonia/pneumonitis (NSIP), 263, 264t
  in HIV infection/AIDS, 1211
Non-ST elevation acute coronary syndromes, **325–330**, 327t, 329t. *See also* Myocardial infarction
Nonsteroidal anti-inflammatory drugs (NSAIDs), **78**, 79–80t. *See also specific agent*
  for abnormal premenopausal bleeding, 675
  for acute coronary syndromes, 327t
  in analgesic nephropathy, 845
  for ankylosing spondylitis, 774
  in cancer prevention, 12
    colorectal cancer and, 1477
  cardiovascular complications and, 78, 548, 552–553
  gastritis/gastropathy caused by, 544, 545
  gastrointestinal side effects/bleeding and, 78, 545, 548, 749
  for gout, 733
  hypertension and, 390
  hyponatremia caused by, 790
  for myocardial infarction, 327t, 334–335
  for ophthalmic disorders, 174t
  for osteoarthritis, 731
  for pain management, 78
    with opioid analgesics, 83t
  in peptic ulcer disease, 548–549, 551t, 552–553, 749
    H pylori eradication therapy and, 551t, 552
    misoprostol coadministration and, 550, 552
    prevention and, 552
  platelet function affected by, 490, 490t, 548, 749
  prerenal azotemia caused by, 820
  recommendations for use of, 552–553
  renal toxicity of, 78, 749, 820
  for rheumatoid arthritis, 749
  topical, 97t
Nonsustained ventricular tachycardia, 352
Nontreponemal antigen tests, for syphilis, 1331, 1331–1332, 1331t
Nontuberculous (atypical) mycobacteria (NTM), **258–259**, **1324–1325**
  adenitis/lymphadenitis caused by, **213–214**, 1325

MAC infections. *See Mycobacterium* (mycobacterial infections), *avium* complex
  pulmonary disease caused by, **258–259**, **1325**
    in HIV infection/AIDS, 258, 1211, 1324, 1325
  skin and soft tissue infections caused by, **1325**
Nonulcer (functional) dyspepsia, 503
Noonan syndrome, 295
Nor-QD. *See* Norethindrone
Norelgestromin, in transdermal contraceptive patch, 697
Norepinephrine
  for hypotension/shock, 436
    in tricyclic antidepressant overdose, 1422
  in pheochromocytoma, 1058, 1059
Norethindrone
  for abnormal premenopausal bleeding, 675
  in combination oral contraceptives, 695t
  in hormone replacement therapy, 1070, 1071
  for postmenopausal vaginal bleeding, 676
  in progestin minipill, 696t, 697
Norflex. *See* Orphenadrine
Norfloxacin
  for ophthalmic disorders, 173t
  for urinary tract infection, 852t
Norgestimate
  in combination oral contraceptives, 695t
  in estrogen replacement therapy, 1070
Norgestrel
  in combination oral contraceptives, 695t
  for emergency/postcoital contraception, 700
  in progestin minipill, 696t, 697
Normal anion gap acidosis, 808t, **809–812**, 809t, 811. *See also* Hyperchloremic normal anion gap acidosis
Normal flora, anaerobic infections caused by, 1321–1323
Normal-pressure hydrocephalus, 919
Normal ranges, for diagnostic/laboratory tests, 1547–1554t. *See also specific test*
Normal-tension glaucoma, 158, 159
Normetanephrine, in pheochromocytoma, 1058, 1059
Normochloremic metabolic (increased anion gap) acidosis, 807, **808–809**, 808t, 811
Normodyne. *See* Labetalol
Normokalemic periodic paralysis, 936
Noroviruses, acute diarrhea/food poisoning caused by, 1172, 1278
Norplant system, 697
Norpramin. *See* Desipramine
Norprolac. *See* Quinagolide
North Asian tick typhus, 1281t, 1285
Norton score, for pressure ulcers, 73

Nortriptyline, 966, 968t, 1545t. *See also* Antidepressants
  for neuropathic pain/diabetic neuropathy, 85, 85t
Norvasc. *See* Amlodipine
Norvir. *See* Ritonavir
Norwalk virus, 1172, 1278
Nose, **192–201**. *See also under* Nasal
  infections of, **192–196**. *See also* Rhinitis; Rhinosinusitis; Sinusitis
  inflammatory disease of, **201**
  traumatic injury of, **199**
  tumors/granulomatous disease of, **199–201**
  in Wegener granulomatosis, 201, 768
Nosebleed. *See* Epistaxis
Nosocomial infections. *See* Hospital (health care)-associated infections
Novantrone. *See* Mitoxantrone
Novel erythropoiesis-stimulating protein (NESP). *See* Darbepoetin alfa
Novolin, 1096. *See also* Insulin therapy
Novolog. *See* Insulin aspart
NPH insulin, 1096, 1096t, 1097f, 1098, 1101, 1102. *See also* Insulin therapy
  in mixtures/combination therapy, 1096t, 1098–1099, 1101, 1102
  in pregnancy, 1110
NPL insulin, 1099
NPM1. *See* Nucleophosmin 1
NPPV. *See* Noninvasive positive-pressure ventilation
NREM sleep, 973
NRTIs. *See* Nucleoside reverse transcriptase inhibitors
NSAIDs. *See* Nonsteroidal anti-inflammatory drugs
NSCLC. *See* Non-small cell lung cancer
NSF. *See* Nephrogenic systemic fibrosis
NSIP. *See* Nonspecific interstitial pneumonia/pneumonitis
NSVT. *See* Nonsustained ventricular tachycardia
NTM. *See* Nontuberculous (atypical) mycobacteria
NTZ. *See* Nitazoxanide
Nuclear bleeding scans, in GI bleeding, 521–522
Nuclear terrorism, 1414
Nuclear transcription factor mutations, in MODY, 1081
Nucleic acid amplification tests
  in chlamydial infection, 1328
  in tuberculosis, 252
Nucleophosmin 1, 465
Nucleoside/nucleotide backbone, for antiretroviral regimens, 1231, 1232
Nucleoside reverse transcriptase inhibitors (NRTIs), 1226t, 1227–1228, 1232f. *See also* Antiretroviral therapy
  in combinations, 1227, 1232, 1232f
  for hepatitis B, 610, 1228

Nucleotide reverse transcriptase inhibitor, 1226t, 1228, 1232f. *See also* Antiretroviral therapy
in combinations, 1227, 1232f
for hepatitis B, 610, 1228
Nucleus pulposus, herniation of
cervical, 737, **929**, 930–931f
lumbar/sacral, 738, 739
NuLYTE. *See* Polyethylene glycol
Numorphan. *See* Oxymorphone
Nursing (breast feeding). *See* Lactation
Nursing homes, caregiver issues related to placement in, 62–63
Nutcracker esophagus, 543
NutraSweet. *See* Aspartame
Nutrients. *See also* Diet; Nutritional disorders; Nutritional support
absorption/digestion of, 557–558
diets restricting, **1145–1146**
diets supplementing, **1146–1147**
requirements for in nutritional support, **1148–1149**
Nutrition. *See also* Diet; Nutrients; Nutritional disorders; Nutritional support
in Crohn disease, 580
in pregnancy, **708–709**
preventable disease/deaths and, 2t
for terminally ill/dying patient, **91**
Nutritional disorders, **1134–1152**. *See also* Eating disorders; Malnutrition; Nutritional support; Obesity
cognitive disorders/delirium caused by, 985t
diet therapy for, **1145–1147**
lactic acidosis and, 808
neuropathy associated with, 923. *See also specific type*
thrombocytopenia associated with, **482**
Nutritional support, **1147–1152**, 1148f, 1149t, 1150t, 1151t. *See also* Central vein nutritional support; Enteral nutritional support; Parenteral nutritional support
in alcoholic liver disease/cirrhosis, 615
in burn injury, 1411
in caustic esophageal injury, 536
in Crohn disease, 580
in elderly, 72
in HIV infection/AIDS, 1210
for involuntary weight loss, 41
in pancreatitis, 644
for protein–energy malnutrition, 1135, 1147
in respiratory failure, 291
in short bowel syndrome, 563
for terminally ill/dying patient, 91
Nystagmus
in coma or stupor, 916
in vertigo, 188–189, 190
in vestibular neuronitis, 190
Nystatin, for candidiasis
esophageal, 535
oral, 202
vulvovaginal, 678

Obesity, **1135–1138**
arthritis and, 730
asthma risk and, 216
cancer risk and, 14, 1451
cholelithiasis/gallstones and, 634
cirrhosis and, 624
coronary heart disease and, 317
in Cushing syndrome, 1051, 1052, 1136
definition of/measurements in, 14, 1136
in diabetes mellitus, 14, 1080t, 1081, 1083, 1101
diet and, 1101
metformin for, 1093, 1101
diet/eating behavior changes and, 15, 1137
esophageal cancer and, 1468
exercise/activity and, 13, 14, 1137
genetic factors in, 1136
health consequences of, 1136
in hypertension, 390
hypnosis in management of, 1536t
hypoventilation and (Pickwickian syndrome), **287**
incidence/prevalence of, 14, 1136
leptin gene and, 1136
lipid abnormalities in, 1126t
medical conditions/evaluation and, 1136–1137
medications in management of, 15, 1137–1138
nonalcoholic fatty liver disease and, 617, 618
in polycystic ovary syndrome, 690, 691, 1053
postoperative pulmonary complications and, 53
prevention of, **14–16**
risks of/risk assessment in, 15
surgery in management of, 15, 1138
treatment of, 15, 1137–1138
weight gain in pregnancy and, 708
Obesity-hypoventilation syndrome (Pickwickian syndrome), **287**
Obliterative bronchiolitis, 243. *See also* Bronchiolitis
OBS. *See* Organic brain syndrome
Obscure gastrointestinal bleeding, **523–524**
Obscure-occult bleeding, 523
Obscure-overt bleeding, 523
Obsessions, 940. *See also* Obsessive-compulsive disorder
Obsessive-compulsive disorder, 940, 943, 964, 966
Tourette syndrome and, 911, 940
Obsessive-compulsive personality disorder, 951t
Obstetrics/obstetric disorders, **705–728**. *See also* Pregnancy
adverse ophthalmic effects of drugs used in, 177t
Obstructive lung disease. *See* Airway disorders, obstruction; Chronic obstructive pulmonary disease
Obstructive shock, 434, 434t, 435

Obstructive sleep apnea, 288, **288–289**
obesity-hypoventilation syndrome and, 287
postoperative pulmonary complications and, 53
Obstructive uropathy, tubulointerstitial disease caused by, 845, 846
Obstructive voiding symptoms
in benign prostatic hyperplasia, 866, 866–867, 867t
in prostate cancer, 1484
in prostatitis, 853
Obturator sign, in appendicitis, 567
Occipital lobe lesions, 899
Occlusive dressings
hydrocolloid, for psoriasis, 104
for topical corticosteroids, 94
Occult diabetes (late hypoglycemia), **1121**
Occult gastrointestinal bleeding, **522–523**. *See also* Gastrointestinal bleeding
stool test for. *See* Fecal occult blood testing
Occupational asthma, 216, 280
Occupational pulmonary diseases, **278–281**. *See also specific disorder*
Occupational therapy, for stroke patient, 892
OCD. *See* Obsessive-compulsive disorder
OCD spectrum, 940
Ochronosis, 1513
^{13}C-Octanoic acid breath test, in nausea and vomiting, 505
Octreotide
for acromegaly/gigantism, 999
for ACTH-secreting tumor identification/treatment, 1052
for carcinoid syndrome, 1476
for diarrhea, 517, 1214
for GH-secreting tumor, 994
for GI bleeding/esophageal varices, 519–520, 539
for islet cell tumors, 1063, 1120
for pheochromocytoma identification, 1060
Ocu-Pred. *See* Prednisolone
Ocu-chlor. *See* Chloramphenicol
Ocuflox. *See* Ofloxacin
Ocular contusions, **171**
Ocular disease. *See* Eye, disorders of
Ocular examination. *See* Eye, examination of
Ocular hemorrhages, vitreous, **162**
Ocular hypertension, 158. *See also* Glaucoma
in acute angle closure glaucoma, 158
in chronic glaucoma, 158
treatment of, 158, 159, 175–176t
Ocular lacerations, **171–172**
Ocular larva migrans, 1385
Ocular medications. *See* Ophthalmic medications
Ocular motor palsies, **169–170**
in myasthenia gravis, 932
Ocular movements. *See* Eye (extraocular) movements
Ocular muscular dystrophy, 934t

Ocular/orbital pain
in acute angle-closure glaucoma, 157
in corneal abrasion, 171
headache and, 45, 873
in ultraviolet (actinic) keratitis, 172
in uveitis, 160
Ocular trauma, **171–172**
Oculocephalic reflex, in coma or stupor, 916
Oculomotor response, in coma or stupor, 916
Oculopharyngeal muscular dystrophy, 934t
Oculosympathetic paralysis. *See* Horner syndrome
Oculovestibular reflex, in coma or stupor, 916
Ocusert. *See* Pilocarpine
Oddi, sphincter of. *See* Sphincter of Oddi
Odontogenic infections. *See also* Dental disorders
deep neck infections and, 206
Odor, breath
in cyanide poisoning, 1435
in diabetic ketoacidosis, 1083, 1112
in uremia, 826
Odor identification/discrimination/threshold, disorders of, **197–198**
Odynophagia, 529
in epiglottitis (supraglottitis), 208, 1289
in esophageal cancer, 1468
in infectious esophagitis, 529, 535
in pharyngitis, 204, 205, 1289
in pill-induced esophagitis, 529, 536
Ofloxacin, 1180t
for ophthalmic disorders, 173t
for urinary tract infection, 852t
Ogen. *See* Estrogen vaginal creams
Ogilvie syndrome, **565–566**
Oka/Merck VZV vaccine. *See* Herpes zoster vaccine
Olanzapine, 954, 955t, 956, 956t, 957. *See also* Antipsychotic drugs
for bipolar disease/mania, 970
overdose/toxicity of, 956, 956t, 1444–1445
for personality disorder, 951
Old World cutaneous leishmaniasis, 1351, 1353
Older adults, **61–75**. *See also specific disorder affecting*
abused, 19, **75**, 75t
advance directives and, **90**
antipsychotic therapy in, 957
appendicitis in, 568
assessment of, **61–63**, 62f, 62t, 63t
benzodiazepine use in, 941, 942
caregiver issues and, **62–63**
cholesterol screening in, 1128–1129
delirium in, **67–68**
postoperative, 56, 56t
dementia in, **63–66**
assessment of/screening for, 64
decision-making capacity and, 64
depressed, **66–67**. *See also* Depression

drug use (pharmacotherapy/polypharmacy) and, **74**
falls and, 68, 69t
urinary incontinence and, 70
exercise/"functional fitness" and, 14
falls and, **68–70**, 69t
fecal incontinence and, 595
fever/FUO in, 39, 1153
frailty and, **72**
functional assessment of, 61–62, 63
gait disorders in, **68–70**, 69t
hearing impairment in, **75**
immobility and, **68**
insomnia/insomnia management in, 973, 974
malnourished, 40–41, **72**
management of common problems in, **63–75**
pneumococcal vaccine in, 1199
pressure ulcers in, **72–74**, 73t
principles of care of, **61**
prognosis/life expectancy and, **61**, 62f, 62t, 63t
psychosis in (late life psychosis), 953
suicide in, 66
undernutrition and, 40–41, **72**
urinary incontinence and, **70–72**
values/preferences and, **61**
vision impairment in, **74**
weight loss in, 40–41, **72**
Olecranon bursitis, 743, 744
Olestra, diarrhea caused by, 515
Olfactory dysfunction, **197–198**
Oligoclonal bands, in multiple sclerosis, 913
Oligodendroglioma, 898t
Oligospermia, 864
genetic causes of, 865
Oliguria, 816, 820
in acute tubular necrosis, 823
in obstructive uropathy, 845
in tubulointerstitial disease, 845
Olmesartan/olmesartan with hydrochlorothiazide, 404t
Olopatadine, for ophthalmic disorders, 155, 174t
Olsalazine, for inflammatory bowel disease, 575
Omalizumab, for asthma, 225t, 228
Omega-3 fatty acids, 1528t, 1530–1531
platelet function affected by, 490t
Omental patch, for ulcer perforation, 555
Omeprazole, 550, 554. *See also* Proton pump inhibitors
intravenous, withdrawal of from market, 554
On-off phenomenon, 906
Onchocerca volvulus (onchocerciasis), **1387–1388**
Oncocytoma, of kidney, 1492
Oncogenic osteomalacia, 1043
Oncotype Dx assay, 664
Ondansetron, 506, 506t, 1508–1509. *See also* Antiemetics
Ondine curse (primary alveolar hypoventilation), **287**
Ontak. *See* Denileukin diftitox
Onycholysis, 146

Onychomycosis (tinea unguium), 146, **147**
Onychophagia, 940
Oophorectomy (salpingo-oophorectomy). *See also* Menopause, surgical
in breast cancer prevention/treatment, 668, 669
for endometrial carcinoma, 684–685
estrogen replacement therapy after, 704
for hirsutism/virilization, 1054
in ovarian cancer prevention/treatment, 689, 690
HNPCC and, 593
for PID, 689
premature ovarian failure and, 1069
Oophoritis, in mumps, 1250, 1251
Opana/Opana ER. *See* Oxymorphone
Open-angle glaucoma, chronic, 158–159
Open biopsy, for breast lump evaluation, 658–659. *See also* Breast, biopsy of
Opening snap, in mitral stenosis, 306
Operant conditioning. *See* Behavior modification
Ophthalmia neonatorum, 727
Ophthalmic medications, 173–176t
contaminated, **172–176**
systemic effects of, **176**
toxic and hypersensitivity reactions to, **176**
Ophthalmopathy, Graves, 170, 1008, 1009, 1012, 1014
Ophthalmoplegia
episodic vertigo in, 189
headache and, 45, 873
Ophthalmoplegic migraine, 873
Opioids/opioid analgesics, **78–84**, 81–83t. *See also specific agent*
addiction and, 78
allergic reaction to, 84
for chronic pain, 78–84, 81–83t, 947
constipation caused by, 84, 87, 510
for COPD, 238
dependence and, 78
for diarrhea, 514
for dyspnea, 26, 82
in end-of-life care, 78
for migraine headache, 874
for myocardial infarction, 334
nausea and vomiting caused by, 84, 86
for neuropathic pain, 84, 85
overdose/abuse of, 20–21, **981–982**, 1424t, **1442–1443**
management of, 21, 1442–1443
narcotic antagonists/naloxone for, 21, 982, 1421, 1442–1443
respiratory acidosis caused by, 814
pseudo-addiction and, 78
tolerance and, 78, 84
withdrawal and, 981–982
Opisthorchis felineus/viverrini (opisthorchiasis), **1375**
cholangiocarcinoma and, 1375, 1462
Opium, tincture of. *See* Tincture of opium
Opportunistic infections, **1155–1159**. *See also specific type*
in cancer patients, **1498**

fungi/molds causing, 1390,
1398–1399, **1402**
prevention of, 1158
in HIV infection/AIDS, 1205, 1206t,
1208
CD4 T cell counts and, 1205, 1209,
1209f, 1217–1218
prevention of, 1219–1220, 1219t,
1222–1223, 1222t
treatment of, 1223, 1224–1225t
prevention of, 1157–1158, 1219–1220,
1219t, 1222–1223, 1222t
in transplant patients, 1156,
1157–1158, 1158–1159
treatment of, 1158–1159
Oprelvekin, for chemotherapy-induced
thrombocytopenia,
1499–1506, 1508t
Optic atrophy
in optic neuritis, 168
in pseudotumor cerebri, 903
Optic disk
cupping of, in chronic glaucoma, 158
drusen of, 169
swelling of, **169**
in ischemic optic neuropathy, 168
in optic neuritis, 168
Optic nerve
compression of, in dysthyroid eye disease, 170, 1009
damage to in glaucoma, 158
Optic neuritis, **168–169**
in neuromyelitis optica, 914
Optic neuropathy
inflammatory (optic neuritis),
168–169
ischemic, **168**
in giant cell arteritis, 168, 766
Optic neurotomy, radial, for retinal vein
occlusion, 164
OptiPranolol. See Metipranolol
Optivar. See Azelastine
OPV (oral/Sabin polio vaccine),
1252–1253
IPV booster and, 1201
Oragrafin. See Ipodate sodium
Oral cavity, **201–206**
anaerobic flora of, 1321, 1322, 1323
pneumonia/lung abscess and, 250,
1322
bullous pemphigoid involving, 131
cancer of, **201–202**
candidiasis involving (thrush), 125,
202, 1390
in HIV infection/AIDS, 125, 202,
1213, 1390
erythema multiforme involving, 127
in HIV infection/AIDS, 1213
lichen planus involving, **201–202**
mucositis of, chemotherapy/radiation
causing, 1414, 1509
pemphigus involving, 130
ulcerative lesions of, **203**
in Behçet syndrome, 772
chemotherapy-induced, 1509
herpes simplex esophagitis and,
535
in HIV infection/AIDS, 1213

Oral contraceptives, **694–697**, 695–696t,
696t
for abnormal premenopausal bleeding, 675
antibiotics affecting efficacy of, 121
benzodiazepine interactions and, 942t
breast cancer risk and, 653, 696
cervical dysplasia/cancer and, 696
contraindications/adverse effects of,
696–697, 696t
depression associated with use of, 697
drug interactions and, 694–696
for emergency/postcoital contraception, 700
endometrial cancer and, 684, 694, 696
endometrial hyperplasia/carcinoma
and, 684
for endometriosis, 686
after gestational trophoblastic disease,
715
hepatic adenoma/liver tumors associated with, 633, 696, 1460
for hirsutism/virilization, 694, 1055
for hormone replacement therapy,
1070
hypertension and, 392, 696–697
lactation/breast feeding and, 697
lipid abnormalities associated with
use of, 1126t
melasma (chloasma) caused by, 144,
697
ovarian cancer prevention and, 694,
696
thromboembolic disease and, 696
Oral hypoglycemic agents. See Antidiabetic agents
Oral nutritional supplements, 1147
in HIV infection/AIDS, 1210
Oral polio vaccine (OPV/Sabin vaccine),
1252–1253
IPV booster and, 1201
Oramorph. See Morphine
Orbital abscess, 170
bacterial rhinosinusitis and, 170, 194
Orbital cellulitis, **170**
bacterial rhinosinusitis and, 170, 194
Orbital floor, blowout fracture of, 171
Orbital tumors, ocular motor palsies and,
170
Orchiectomy
for intra-abdominal testes, 1066
for prostate cancer, 1487t, 1488
for testicular cancer, 1066, 1493,
1494
Orchiopexy/orchidopexy, infertility/tes-
ticular cancer risk and,
1066, 1493
Orchitis
in filariasis, 1386
mumps, 1250, 1251
Orellanine, Cortinarius mushroom poisoning and, 1441, 1441t,
1442
Orf, 1277
Organ of Corti, hearing loss caused by
disorders of, 179
Organ transplantation. See specific type
and Transplantation

Organic brain syndrome, **985–988**. See
also Cognitive disorders
alcoholic, 979
Organic (alcoholic) hallucinosis, 978–979,
979, 980, 986
Organic personality syndrome, **986**
Organophosphate poisoning, 1424t,
1443–1444
nerve agents in chemical warfare and,
1434
seizures caused by, 1423t
Orgasm, 948
loss of/orgasmic dysfunction. See also
Sexual dysfunction
antidepressants causing, 965, 967
in female, 691, 692, 949
in male, 862
Oriental spotted fever, 1285
Orientia tsutsugamushi, 1281t, 1283
Orinase. See Tolbutamide
Orlistat, for obesity, 1137–1138
Ornithosis (psittacosis), 1177t, 1327, **1329**
Oromandibular dystonia, 910
Oropharyngeal anthrax, 1301
Oropharyngeal dysphagia, 529, 529t. See
also Dysphagia
Orphenadrine, 906t. See also Antiparkin-
sonism drugs
Ortho Dienestrol. See Estrogen vaginal
creams
Ortho-Prefest. See Estrogens, with progestins
Orthodeoxia
in hepatopulmonary syndrome, 623
in patent foramen ovale, 298
Orthodromic tachycardia, 345
Orthokeratology, 152
Orthopedic surgery, antibiotic prophy-
laxis for, 60t
Orthopedics. See Musculoskeletal disorders
Orthophosphates, for hypercalciuria, 859
Orthostatic (postural) hypotension
in diabetes mellitus, 1083
dysautonomia (autonomic dysfunction) and, 884–885, 885,
922
falls in elderly and, 68, 69t
MAOIs causing, 967
pheochromocytoma/paraganglioma
and, 1058–1059
syncope and, 356, 357
tricyclic antidepressants causing, 966
Orthostatic proteinuria, 816–817
Orudis. See Ketoprofen
Oruvail. See Ketoprofen
Osborn wave, in hypothermia, 1404,
1404f
OsCal (calcium carbonate). See Calcium,
dietary/supplementary
Oseltamivir, for influenza, 1198, 1238t,
1270, 1271, 1272, 1273
Osler nodes, in endocarditis, 1304
Osler sign, 394
Osler triad, 1292
Osler-Weber-Rendu syndrome. See
Hereditary hemorrhagic
telangiectasia

Osmolality
  fecal/stool, in diarrhea, 514–515, 515
  serum, 788
    in diabetic ketoacidosis, 1113
    in hyperglycemic hyperosmolar
      state, 1015
    in hypernatremia, 793
    in hyponatremia, 789, 790f
    in methanol/ethylene glycol poi-
      soning, 1439
    reference values for, 1552t
  urine
    in acute kidney injury, 820t
    in hypernatremia, 793–794
    in hyponatremia, 791
    reference values for, 1552t
Osmolar/osmol gap, **795**
  calculation of, 1427t
  in metabolic acidosis, 795, 1426
  in poisoning/drug overdose, 1426,
    1427t
    alcohol toxicity and, 795, 979, 1426
    isopropanol toxicity and, 809, 1426
    methanol or ethylene glycol toxic-
      ity and, 795, 1426, 1440
Osmolarity, 788
Osmophobia, in migraine headache, 873
OsmoPrep. See Sodium phosphate
Osmostat, reset, hyponatremia caused by,
    791, 792
Osmotic diarrhea, 512t, 514–515. See also
    Diarrhea
Osmotic diuretics
  for angle-closure glaucoma, 159
  lithium interactions and, 972t
  for lithium overdose/toxicity, 972
Osmotic fragility test, in hereditary
    spherocytosis, 448
Osmotic gap, stool, 515
Osmotic laxatives, 509–510, 509t
OspA antigen, in Lyme disease, 1343,
    1345
OspB antigen, in Lyme disease, 1343
Ossicular disruption, hearing loss and,
    179, 185
Osteitis condensans ilii, 774
Osteitis deformans (Paget disease of
    bone), **1044–1046**
Osteitis fibrosa cystica, 829, 1033
Osteoarthritis, **729–732**. See also Arthritis
  acupuncture for, 1533
  arthroplasty/joint replacement for,
    731
    osteomyelitis and, 780
  of cervical spine, 737
  exercise/activity in prevention/man-
    agement of, 13, 731
  glucosamine/chondroitin for, 731,
    1528t, 1529–1530
  of knee
    obesity and, 730
    radiographic assessment of, 35
  prevention of, 731
  rheumatoid arthritis differentiated
    from, 731, 748
Osteoarthropathy, hypertrophic pulmo-
    nary. See Hypertrophic pul-
    monary osteoarthropathy

Osteodystrophy, renal, 827, 829–830,
    1033, 1035
Osteogenesis imperfecta, 1039
Osteogenic sarcoma. See Osteosarcoma
Osteoma, ear canal, **182**
Osteomalacia, 829, **1042–1044**, 1042t
  in celiac disease, 559, 560
  oncogenic, 1043
  osteoporosis with, 1039, 1040,
    1043–1044
Osteomyelitis, 1181t
  acute pyogenic, **780–781**
  bacterial rhinosinusitis and, 194
  candidal, **781**
  in coccidioidomycosis, **781**
  in drug users, 1168–1169
  hematogenous, 780
  in sickle cell syndromes, 780
  of skull base (malignant external oti-
    tis), **181–182**
  staphylococcal, **1195**
  vertebral, 781, 1295
    back pain and, 738, 739
    epidural abscess and, 781, 1295
Osteonecrosis, **783–784**
  corticosteroid use and, 1078
  of jaw, bisphosphonate use and, 783,
    1040, 1045
Osteopenia, 1040
  in complex regional pain syndrome,
    743
Osteophytes
  in diffuse idiopathic skeletal hyperos-
    tosis, 774
  in neck pain, 737, 929
  in spinal stenosis, 740
Osteoporosis, 703, 704, **1038–1042**, 1039t
  in celiac disease, 559, 560
  circumscripta, 1045
  in cirrhosis, 620
  corticosteroid therapy and, 576, 1040,
    1041, 1078
  fractures/bone pain and, 12, 1038,
    1039
  hyperprolactinemia and, 1000
  in hyperthyroidism, 1009, 1039
  hypogonadism and, 1039, 1041
  in men, 1041, 1065
  in myeloma, 472
  osteomalacia with, 1039, 1040,
    1043–1044
  postmenopausal, 703, 704, 1038
  prevention/treatment of, **12**, 704,
    1040–1041
    bisphosphonates in, 12, 704, 1040
    calcium in, 12, 704
      milk-alkali syndrome and, 800
    chronic corticosteroid treatment
      and, 1040, 1041
    estrogen replacement therapy in,
      1040–1041
    exercise/activity and, 12, 13, 704,
      1041
    selective estrogen receptor modula-
      tors in, 1041
    vitamin D in, 12, 69, 704
Osteoprotegerin, in multiple myeloma,
    472

Osteosarcoma (osteogenic sarcoma),
    1468t
  Paget disease of bone and, 1045
Osteosclerosis, in renal osteodystrophy,
    1035
Ostium primum atrial septal defect, 297,
    298
Ostium secundum atrial septal defect,
    297, 298
Otalgia. See Earache
Otic barotrauma. See Barotrauma
Otic drops
  for external otitis, 181
  ototoxic, avoidance of with perforated
    tympanic membrane, 187
Otitis
  external, **181**
    earache in, 181, 186
    malignant, **181–182**
    facial pain and, 878
  media, 1182t
    acute, **183–184**
    chronic, **184**
    complications of, 184–185
    earache in, 183, 184, 186
    in HIV infection/AIDS, 192
    RSV causing, 1268
    serous, **182–183**
      nasopharyngeal carcinoma and,
        183, 200
Otoconia, vertigo associated with, 189,
    190
Otogenic meningitis, 185
Otorrhea, in acute otitis media, 184
Otosclerosis, 179, **185**
Ototoxic chemoprotection, 187
Ototoxicity
  of aminoglycosides, 186
  of cisplatin, 187, 1511
  hearing loss and, 186–187
"Ottawa Knee Rules," 35, 35t
Ouabain, overdose/toxicity of, 1435
Outer surface protein A (OspA), in Lyme
    disease, 1343, 1345
Outer surface protein B (OspB), in Lyme
    disease, 1343
Ovarian ablation, for breast cancer, 666,
    668
Ovarian cancer/tumors, **689–690**, 1467t
  dermatomyositis and, 760–761
  estrogen replacement therapy and,
    1072
  genetic mutations associated with,
    689. See also BRCA1/
    BRCA2 genes
  HNPCC and, 593
  prevention and, 690
  hirsutism/virilization caused by,
    1054
  incidence/mortality/risk of, 689
  palmar fasciitis and, 783
  paraneoplastic syndromes associated
    with, 1453t
  during pregnancy, **728**
  prevention of
    genetic risk factors and, 689
    oral contraceptive use and, 694, 696
  thyroid hormone secreted by, 1008

Ovarian cyst
    appendicitis differentiated from, 568
    in gestational trophoblastic disease,
        715
Ovarian failure, 703, 1068, 1069
    in Turner syndrome, 1074
Ovarian tumor antigen. *See* CA 125
Ovaries, polycystic. *See* Polycystic ovary
        syndrome
Over-the-counter drugs, use/abuse of,
        984–985
    stimulants and, 1430
Overflow incontinence
    fecal, 510, 595
    urinary, 71
Overlap syndrome, **762**
Overload proteinuria, 817
Overuse syndromes
    of knee, **745–746**
    lateral and medial epicondylitis, **745**
Overweight. *See also* Obesity
    definition of, 14, 1136
    prevention of, **14–16**
Ovide. *See* Malathion
Ovulation
    awareness of
        contraception based on, **699–700**
        in infertility counseling, 693
    induction of, for infertility, 693, 994
    in polycystic ovary syndrome, 691
Ovulation bleeding, 674
Owl's eye inclusions, in CMV infection,
        1246
Oxacillin, for endocarditis, 1306, 1307
Oxalate, in urinary stones, 857, 859. *See
        also* Calcium nephrolithia-
        sis
Oxaliplatin, 1500*t*
    for colorectal cancer, 1479
    for gastric adenocarcinoma, 1472
Oxandrolone, for AIDS wasting, 1210
Oxaprozin, 80*t*
Oxazepam, 941*t*
Oxcarbazepine, 881, 882*t*, 972–973. *See
        also* Anticonvulsant ther-
        apy
    for bipolar disease/mania, 972–973
    for seizures, 881, 882*t*
    pregnancy and, 883
Oxiconazole, 98*t*
Oximetry. *See* Pulse oximetry
Oxistat. *See* Oxiconazole
Oxitriptan, for myoclonus, 911
Oxprenolol, overdose/toxicity of, 1432
Oxybutynin, for urinary incontinence, 71
Oxycodone, 78, 82*t*, 83*t*
    in combination preparation, 83*t*
    overdose/toxicity of, 1442–1443
Oxycontin. *See* Oxycodone
Oxygen, partial pressure of. *See* Pao$_2$; Po$_2$
Oxygen saturation. *See* Sao$_2$
Oxygen tension. *See* Po$_2$
Oxygen therapy
    adverse ophthalmic effects of, 177*t*
    for altitude-related illness, 1418
    for ARDS, 292
    for asthma exacerbation, 230, 233
    for burn injury, 1410

for carbon monoxide poisoning,
        1424*t*, 1433–1434
    for cluster headache, 875
    for comatose patient, 1421
    for COPD, 236–237, 236*t*, 238
    for dysbarism/decompression sick-
        ness, 1417
    for dyspnea, 26, 82
    home, 236, 236*t*
    hyperbaric. *See* Hyperbaric oxygen
        therapy
    for hypothermia, 1404
    for methemoglobinemia, 1440
    for near drowning, 1416
    perioperative, surgical site infection
        and, 59
    for *Pneumocystis* pneumonia, 1395
    for pulmonary edema, 367
    for pulmonary hypertension, 275, 381
    for respiratory failure, 290
    for sleep apnea, 289
    for smoke inhalation, 277, 1409
    transtracheal, 236
Oxygen uptake, maximal, lung cancer
        surgery and, 1456
Oxyhemoglobin saturation. *See* Sao$_2$
OxyIR. *See* Oxycodone
Oxymetazoline, overdose/toxicity of, 1434
Oxymorphone, 83*t*
Oxyuriasis (pinworms), **1382**
Oysters, contaminated, vibrio infection
        caused by, 1316

3P tumor suppressor gene, in thyroid can-
        cer, 1023
p24 antigen assay, in blood screening, 478
P53 gene mutations. *See also* TP53 gene
        mutations
    in breast cancer, 653
    in colorectal cancer, 1476–1477
    smoking and, 7
    in thyroid cancer, 1023
P450 aromatase (P450arom) deficiency,
        amenorrhea in, 1068
P450 system/cytochrome P450
    in acetaminophen hepatotoxicity, 1428
    alcoholic liver disease and, 614
    nefazodone affecting, 966
    protease inhibitors affecting, 1229
    St. John's wort affecting, 1523
P450c11 deficiency, 1054, 1057, 1068
P450c17 deficiency, 1057, 1068
P450c21 deficiency, 1053–1054, 1054,
        1055, 1068
P wave
    in cor pulmonale, 382
    in differentiation of aberrantly con-
        ducted supraventricular
        beats from ventricular
        beats, 341, 352
    in multifocal (chaotic) atrial tachycar-
        dia, 350
    in paroxysmal supraventricular tachy-
        cardia, 342
    in pulmonary stenosis, 295
Pacemaker
    overdrive, for ventricular tachycardia,
        352

permanent
    for atrioventricular block, 355
    biventricular (resynchronization),
        for heart failure, 365–366
    for cardiomyopathy, 373
    preoperative placement of, 52
    for refractory atrial fibrillation, 349
    for sick sinus syndrome, 354
    temporary, for infarct-associated con-
        duction disturbances, 336,
        337
Pacemaker syndrome, 354
Packed red cells, transfusion of, 476
    autologous, 477
Paclitaxel, 666, 669, 1502*t*
    neuropathy caused by, 1510
    protein-bound, 1502*t*
Paco$_2$. *See also* Pco$_2$
    in asthma, exacerbation severity/man-
        agement and, 219, 220*t*
    in near drowning, 1415
Paecilomyces, in opportunistic infection,
        1402
Paget carcinoma of breast, 657, **660**
    nipple involvement and, 113, 657, 660
Paget disease
    of bone, **1044–1046**
    extramammary, **113**
    mammary. *See* Paget carcinoma of
        breast
Pain. *See also specific type and* Pain disor-
        ders; Pain management;
        Pain syndromes
    assessment scales for, 76, 77*t*
    cancer. *See* Cancer pain
    chronic, **946–948**, 947*f*
        mind-body therapies for, 946–947,
            1536*t*, 1541
        opioids in management of, 78–84,
            81–83*t*, 947
    in complex regional pain syndrome,
        742–743
    drug therapy for. *See* Pain manage-
        ment, pharmacologic
    at end of life, **77–78**
    hypersensitivity to, in diabetes,
        1106–1107
    hyponatremia caused by, 790
    ischemic. *See* Rest pain
    neuropathic, **84–85**, 85*t*, 922. *See also*
        Neuropathies
    nonpharmacologic interventions in.
        See Pain management,
        nonpharmacologic
    ocular. *See* Ocular/orbital pain
    otic. *See* Earache
    postoperative
        acupuncture for, 1533
        mind-body therapies for, 1536*t*
    psychologic factors and (somatoform
        pain disorder), 944
    response to, in coma or stupor, 916
    rest. *See* Rest pain
    in sickle cell anemia, 450, 451
Pain disorders. *See also* Pain
    chronic, **946–948**, 947*f*
    with psychologic factors (somato-
        form pain disorder), 944

Pain management, **76–86**. *See also specific disorder and* Analgesia/analgesics
assessment scales and, 76, 77t
barriers to good care and, 77–78
in cancer patients, mind-body therapies for, 1536t
guided imagery, 1536t, 1543
hypnosis, 946–947, 1536t, 1539
for chronic pain/chronic pain disorders, 78–84, 81–83t, 946–948
at end of life, **77–78**
nonpharmacologic, **86**, 946–947, 947–948
acupuncture, **1532–1534**
guided imagery, 1536t, 1543
hypnosis, 946–947, 1536t, 1539
meditation, 1536t, 1541
mind-body therapies, 1536t
pharmacologic, **78–86**, 79–83t
acetaminophen/NSAIDs/COX-2 inhibitors, 78, 79–80t
adjuvant, **85–86**
for neuropathic pain, **84–85**, 85t, 922
opioids, **78–84**, 81–83t
principles of, **76–77**, 77t
in terminally ill/dying patient, 77–78
Pain syndromes, **736–747**. *See also specific type and* Pain
Painful bladder syndrome. *See* Interstitial cystitis
Painful diabetic neuropathy, 1106–1107
Painful intercourse. *See* Dyspareunia
Painful subacute thyroiditis, 1017. *See also* Subacute (de Quervain) thyroiditis
Painless myocardial infarction, 330
Painless postpartum thyroiditis, 1016, 1018. *See also* Postpartum thyroiditis
Painless sporadic thyroiditis, 1016, 1018
PAIR (percutaneous aspiration/injection/reaspiration), for hydatid cysts, 1379
Palifermin, for chemotherapy-induced mucositis, 1507t, 1509
Palilalia, in Tourette syndrome, 911
Palindromic rheumatism, **783**
Palivizumab, 1238t
Palladin gene, pancreatic/periampullary carcinoma and, 1463
Palladone. *See* Hydromorphone
Palliative care, **76–93**
definition and scope of, **76**
at end of life, 76, **87–93**. *See also* End of life, provision of care at
for heart failure, 366
symptom management and, 76
constipation, **87**
delirium and agitation, **87**
dyspnea, **86**
nausea and vomiting, **86–87**
pain, **76–86**
Palliative care institutions, **90–91**. *See also* End of life, provision of care at

Pallidotomy, for parkinsonism, 908
Pallor, in Raynaud phenomenon, 756
Palmar erythema
in cirrhosis, 619
in rheumatoid arthritis, 748
Palmar fasciitis
cancer and, 783
rheumatoid arthritis differentiated from, 749
in Dupuytren contracture, 742, 743
Palms
tinea of, **108–109**
ulnar lesions at, 927
vesiculobullous dermatitis of (pompholyx), 116–117
Palonosetron, 506, 506t, 1509. *See also* Antiemetics
Palpitations, **30–32**, 32t
in pheochromocytoma, 1058
in pulmonary embolism, 268t
Palsies. *See specific type and* Paralysis/palsies
Paludrine. *See* Proguanil
2-PAM. *See* Pralidoxime
Pamelor. *See* Nortriptyline
Pamidronate. *See also* Bisphosphonates
adverse ophthalmic effects of, 178t
for chemotherapy-induced toxicity/bone pain, 1507t
for hypercalcemia/hyperparathyroidism, 1037, 1497, 1507t
for osteoporosis prevention/management, 1040
for Paget disease of bone, 1046
Panacinar bibasilar emphysema, 235. *See also* Emphysema
Panaeolus (hallucinogenic) mushroom poisoning, 1441, 1441t, 1442
Panax
ginseng, 1523t, 1526
quinquefolius, 1526
Panbronchiolitis, diffuse, 243
Pancreas
cancer of, **1463–1465**, 1465, 1468t
incidence/mortality of, 1450, 1463, 1465
pancreatitis and, 646, 1463, 1464
diseases of, **641–648**. *See also specific type and* Diabetes mellitus; Pancreatitis
dyspepsia and, 502
vomiting and, 505t, 506
divisum, 642, 644
functioning/neuroendocrine tumors of, **1062–1063**, 1463, 1465
hypoglycemia caused by, **1118–1120**, 1119t
in multiple endocrine neoplasia, 1076, 1076t
pseudocysts of, 642, 644, 645, 648
cystic carcinoma differentiated from, 1464
transplantation of, for diabetes mellitus, 1099–1100
Pancreatectomy, 648
hyperglycemia and, 1086
for persistent islet hyperplasia, 1120

Pancreatic abscess, 644, 645
Pancreatic ascites, 525, 528, 644, 648
Pancreatic duct, calculus formation in (pancreaticolithiasis), 646
Pancreatic enzyme supplements, 647, 647t
Pancreatic insufficiency, 558
Pancreatic islets, 1062. *See also* B cells, pancreatic
hyperplasia of, persistent, **1120**
transplantation of, for diabetes, 1100
tumors of. *See* Islet cell tumors
Pancreatic polypeptide, F cells secreting, 1062
Pancreatic pseudocysts, 642, 644, 645, 648
cystic carcinoma differentiated from, 1464
Pancreatic secretory trypsin inhibitory (PSTI) gene, in pancreatitis, 646
Pancreaticocholangitis, sclerosing, 641
Pancreaticoduodenal resection, for pancreatic/periampullary carcinoma, 1464–1465
Pancreaticojejunostomy, for pancreatitis, 648
Pancreaticolithiasis, 646
Pancreatitis
acute, **641–645**, 642t, 643t
ascites in, 525, 528, 644, 648
autoimmune, 646
biliary, 643, 644
biliary stricture and, 640
in burn injury, 1409
choledocholithiasis and, 638, 639, 645
chronic, **645–648**, 647t
tumefactive, 646
diarrhea in, 517
didanosine therapy and, 1228
hereditary, 642, 646
hyperglycemia in, 1086
hypertriglyceridemia and, 643, 1133
in hypocalcemia, 799
in mumps, 1250, 1251
necrotizing, 643, 643t, 644, 645
pancreatic/periampullary carcinoma and, 646, 1463, 1464
pleural effusion in, 284t
tropical, 646
Pancytopenia, 455t
in acute leukemia, 465
in aplastic anemia, 455, 455t
in hairy cell leukemia, 468
methotrexate causing, 750
stem cell transplantation and, 475
Panencephalitis, subacute sclerosing, 1248
myoclonus in, 910
Panhypergammaglobulinemia. *See* Hypergammaglobulinemia
Panhypogammaglobulinemia. *See* Hypogammaglobulinemia
Panhypopituitarism, 992
Panic disorders/panic attacks, 940, 942, 942–943
chest pain in, 29, 30, 544, 944
hypochondriasis and, 940, 944
palpitations in, 31, 32
seizures differentiated from, 881, 940
sleep, 940

Panitumumab, 1503*t*
  for colorectal cancer, 1479
Panniculitis
  lupus, 140
  sclerosing, 129
Pannus
  in rheumatoid arthritis, 747
  in trachoma, 154
Pansinusitis, 193
Pantoprazole, 550, 554. *See also* Proton
    pump inhibitors
Panuveitis, 160. *See also* Uveitis
Pao$_2$. *See also* Po$_2$
  in ARDS, 291
  in asthma, exacerbation severity/man-
    agement and, 220*t*, 233
  home oxygen therapy and, 236*t*
  in near drowning, 1415
  in smoke inhalation, 277
Papanicolaou smear (Pap smear), 16–18,
    17*t*, 680–681, 680*t*
  anal, in HIV infection/AIDS, 1216
  in cancer screening, 16, 17*t*, 680–681,
    680*t*
  in CIN, 680–681, 680*t*
  in endometrial carcinoma, 684
  in HIV infection/AIDS, 1216
  for HPV screening, 681
  for rape victim, 702
  in STD patient, 1167
Papillary muscles
  dysfunction/rupture of
    mitral regurgitation and, 308
    in myocardial infarction, 338–339
  in mitral stenosis, 306
Papilledema, 169
  headache and, 45
Papillitis. *See also* Optic disk, swelling of
  in optic neuritis, 168
Papillomas
  intraductal, nipple discharge and, 651
  inverted, 200
  recurrent respiratory (laryngeal), **208**
Papillomaviruses. *See* Human papilloma-
    virus
PAPP-A. *See* Pregnancy-associated plasma
    protein-A
Papular urticaria, 126
  bedbugs causing, 139
Papules, 95*t*, **131–134**
  violaceous to purple, **134–136**
Paracentesis
  in ascites, 525. *See also* Ascitic fluid
    analysis/examination
  in cirrhosis, 620–621
  large-volume
    for cirrhotic ascites, 621
    for malignant ascites, 528, 1496
  ultrasound-guided, 525
Paracetamol, 1428. *See also* Acetamino-
    phen
  in analgesic nephropathy, 845
Parachute mitral valve, 306
Paracoccidioides brasiliensis (paracoccidio-
    idomycosis), **1399**
Paradoxic aciduria
  in metabolic alkalosis, 812
  in salicylate overdose/toxicity, 1445

Paradoxic embolism
  in atrial septal defect/patent foramen
    ovale, 297
  in transient ischemic attacks, 886
Paradoxic pulse. *See* Pulsus paradoxus
Paradoxic sleep, 973
Paraganglioma, **1058–1061**
  familial, 1058
Paragonimus/Paragonimus westermani
    (paragonimiasis),
    1375–1376
Parainfluenza viruses, 1268
Paralysis/palsies, **886**. *See also specific type*
    or structure affected
  acute flaccid
    coxsackievirus causing, 1279
    enterovirus 71 causing, 1280
    poliomyelitis and, 1252
  in botulism, 933, 1300
  in conversion disorder, 944
  facial (Bell palsy), **928–929**
  in motor neuron diseases, 886,
    920–921
  ocular motor, **169–170**
    in myasthenia gravis, 932
  periodic. *See* Periodic paralysis
  in poliomyelitis, 1252
  progressive supranuclear, parkin-
    sonism differentiated
    from, 906
  in rabies, 1256
  sleep, in narcolepsy, 975
  spinal cord infarction causing, 897
  spinal trauma causing, 919
  in tick-borne encephalitis, 1266,
    1266–1267
Paralysis agitans (idiopathic Parkinson
    disease), 905. *See also* Par-
    kinsonism
Paralytic (adynamic) ileus, **564**
Paralytic shellfish poisoning, 1446, 1446*t*
Paramalignant pleural effusion, 285
Paramedian artery occlusion, in stroke,
    889–891
Paramyxovirus respiratory infections,
    1268
Paranasal sinuses, **192–201**
  granulomatous disease of, **199–201**
  infections of, **192–196**. *See also* Rhini-
    tis; Rhinosinusitis; Sinusi-
    tis
  inflammatory disease of, **201**
  malignant tumors of, **200**
  in Wegener granulomatosis, 201, 769
Paraneoplastic cerebellar degeneration,
    902
Paraneoplastic pemphigus, 130
Paraneoplastic syndromes, **1451–1452**,
    1453*t*
  achalasia and, 542
  hypercalcemia and. *See* Hypercalce-
    mia, cancer-related
  in lung cancer, 1453*t*, 1454
  neuropathies and, 925
Paranoid delusion, 952, 953
Paranoid personality disorder, 951*t*
Paranoid schizophrenia, 952
  delusions and, 952, 953

Paraparesis, tropical spastic (HTLV-asso-
    ciated myelopathy), **915**,
    1261–1262
Paraphilias (sexual arousal disorders),
    948, 949–950
  in female, 691, 692
Paraplatin. *See* Carboplatin
Paraplegia. *See also* Paralysis
  spinal cord infarction causing, 897
  spinal trauma causing, 919
  after thoracic aneurysm repair, 425
Parapneumonic pleural effusion, 283,
    284*t*, 285
  in pneumococcal pneumonia, 1292,
    1293
Paraproteins
  in myeloma, 472, 473
  neuropathy associated with, 923–924
  in Waldenström macroglobulinemia,
    474
Paraquat poisoning, **1443**
Parasitic infections
  diarrhea in, 515
    stool analysis for, 513, 514, 515
  myocarditis in, 368
Parasomnias, **975–976**
Parasternal lift
  in heart failure, 360
  in pulmonary stenosis, 295
Parasympathetic nervous system, hypogly-
    cemia and, 1103, 1117
Parathar. *See* Teriparatide
Parathion poisoning, 1443–1444
Parathyroid gland
  disorders of, **1030–1038**. *See also*
    Hyperparathyroidism;
    Hypoparathyroidism
  adenoma/hyperplasia, 1033, 1035,
    1037
  in hypercalciuria, 859
  in multiple endocrine neoplasia,
    1033, 1075–1076, 1076*t*
  carcinoma, 1033, 1037
  resection of (parathyroidectomy),
    1036–1037
  thyroid surgery affecting, 1012
  transplantation of tissue from, for
    hypoparathyroidism/tet-
    any, 1032
Parathyroid hormone (PTH), 1030. *See*
    also Hyperparathyroid-
    ism; Hypoparathyroidism
  bisphosphonates affecting, 1040
  calcium balance/imbalance and, 799,
    1030, 1034, 1034*f*
  in hypercalciuria, 858*t*, 859
  in hypophosphatemia, 803
  magnesium imbalances and, 805, 1031
  phosphate balance/imbalances and,
    802
  reference values for, 1552*t*
  renal resistance to, in pseudohypopar-
    athyroidism, 1031–1032
Parathyroid hormone-related protein
    (PTHrP)
  in cancer-related hypercalcemia, 801,
    1035
  in hypophosphatemia, 803

Parathyroidectomy, 1036–1037

Paravaccinia, 1277

Parechovirus infection, **1280**

Parenchymal lung disease
diffuse, **262–266**, 262t. See also specific disorder and Interstitial lung disease
respiratory failure caused by, 289t

Parenteral fluids. See Fluid management/ hydration

Parenteral nutritional support, 1148, 1148f. See also Nutritional support
acidosis and, 808, 810, 1151t
in burn injury, 1411
complications of, **1151**, 1151t
for Crohn disease, 580
in pancreatitis, 644
patient monitoring during, 1151–1152
for protein–energy malnutrition, 1135, 1147
replacement guidelines and, 815
solutions for, **1150–1151**, 1150t

Paresis (general). See also Weakness
in syphilis, 1336

Paresthesias, 886
chemotherapy-induced, 1510
in diabetes mellitus, 1083
malabsorption and, 558t
in thoracic outlet syndrome, 737

Paricalcitol, for hyperparathyroidism, 1037

Parietal lobe lesions, 899

Parkin gene, in parkinsonism, 905

Parkinson disease, idiopathic (paralysis agitans), 905. See also Parkinsonism

Parkinsonism, **905–908**, 906t
drug-induced, 905, 911, 959
antipsychotic agents, 905, 911, 959

Parkland formula, for fluid resuscitation in burns, 1410

Parnate. See Tranylcypromine

Paromomycin
for amebiasis, 1367, 1367t
for cryptosporidiosis, 1370
for giardiasis, 1372
for leishmaniasis, 1353

Paronychia, 141
candidal, 125

Parotid glands. See also Salivary glands
chronic inflammatory/infiltrative disorders affecting, 207
in mumps, 1250
sialadenitis affecting, 206
tumors of, 207

Parotidectomy, 207

Parotitis, 1250

Paroxetine, 964, 966, 968t. See also Serotonin-selective reuptake inhibitors
overdose/toxicity of, 966, 968t
ophthalmic effects and, 177t
during pregnancy, 966

Paroxysmal atrial fibrillation, recurrent, 349

Paroxysmal nocturnal hemoglobinuria, **448–449**

Paroxysmal supraventricular tachycardia, **341–345**

Pars plana vitrectomy, for retinal detachment, 162

Pars planitis (intermediate uveitis), 160. See also Uveitis

Partial mole, 714. See also Gestational trophoblastic disease

Partial pressure of carbon dioxide. See P_{CO_2}

Partial pressure of oxygen. See Pa_{O_2}; P_{O_2}

Partial (focal) seizures, 879, 879t, 882t. See also Seizures
differential diagnosis of, 881
intracranial tumors causing, 878–879
schizophrenia differentiated from, 954
transient ischemic attack differentiated from, 881, 887

Partial status epilepticus, 884

Partial-thickness burn, 1409

Partial thromboplastin time/activated partial thromboplastin time (PTT/aPTT)
monitoring during heparin therapy, 272
prolonged
acquired factor VIII antibodies causing, 494
in hemophilia, 491
lupus anticoagulant causing, 722, 753, 756
in vitamin K deficiency, 494
reference values for, 1552t

Partner abuse (domestic violence), 976, 977
prevention of, 18–19

Parvovirus B19 infection, **1276–1277**
arthritis in, 779, 1276
rheumatoid arthritis differentiated from, 748
erythema infectiosum and, 1240t, 1276

PAS. See Aminosalicylic acid

Passive smoking (environmental tobacco smoke), health hazards of, 7
asthma, 216
cancer, 7, 1452
COPD, 234
during pregnancy, 707

Pasteurella species, in animal bite infections, 1165

Patanol. See Olopatadine

Patch testing, in allergic contact dermatitis, 119

Patella-femoral (patellofemoral) syndrome, **745**
management of, 36
radiologic evaluation of, 35
testing for, 35

Patellar apprehension test, 35

Patellar compression test, 35

Patellar grind test, 35

Patellar tendinitis, 746

Patellofemoral syndrome. See Patella-femoral (patellofemoral) syndrome

Patent ductus arteriosus, **301–302**, 302t

Patent foramen ovale, **297–298**

Paternal age, mutations and, 1514

Pathergy phenomenon, in Behçet syndrome, 772

Pathologic fractures. See also Fractures
in hypercalcemia/hyperparathyroidism, 1033, 1035
malabsorption and, 558t
in mineral bone disorders of chronic kidney disease, 829
in myeloma, 472, 473
in osteomalacia, 1043
in osteoporosis, 1038, 1039

Patient adherence/nonadherence (compliance/noncompliance). See Adherence/nonadherence

Patient-controlled analgesia, 76

Patient-delivered therapy, for STDs, 1168

Patient–doctor relationship. See Doctor–patient relationship

Patient education
acne and, 120
adherence and, 1–2
antituberculous drug therapy and, 254
asthma management and, 221–223
diabetes and, 1100–1101
fibromyalgia and, 741
in SLE, 753–754

Patient surrogate, Durable Power of Attorney for Health Care designating, 90

Pattern baldness (androgenic alopecia), 145–146
in women, 146, 1053, 1055

Patulous eustachian tube, 182

Paucibacillary (tuberculoid) leprosy, 924, 1327. See also Leprosy

Pauci-immune (ANCA-associated) glomerulonephritis, 824, 835f, **837**

Pavor nocturnus (sleep terror), 975, 975–976

PAX-4 (Arg133Trp) mutation, in idiopathic type 1 diabetes mellitus, 1081

Paxil. See Paroxetine

Pb. See Lead

PBG. See Porphobilinogen

PCA. See Patient-controlled analgesia

PCEC (purified chick embryo cell culture) rabies vaccine, 1201, 1256

PCI. See Percutaneous coronary intervention

P_{CO_2}. See also Pa_{CO_2}
in acid-base disorders, 806, 807t
arterial, 806
in metabolic acidosis, 806, 807t
in metabolic alkalosis, 806, 807t, 813
reference values for, 1548t
in respiratory acidosis, 806, 807t, 813, 814
in respiratory alkalosis, 806, 807t, 814
in respiratory failure, 289
venous, 806

PCOS. See Polycystic ovary syndrome

PCP. See Phencyclidine

PCR. See Polymerase chain reaction

PCV (pneumococcal conjugate vaccine). *See* Pneumococcal vaccine
PCWP. *See* Pulmonary capillary wedge pressure
PDGF. *See* Platelet-derived growth factor
PDT. *See* Photodynamic therapy
PE (pulmonary embolism). *See* Pulmonary venous thromboembolism
Pea soup diarrhea, in enteric (typhoid) fever, 1313
Peak expiratory flow (PEF), in asthma, 219–221
    exacerbation classification/management and, 218t, 219t, 220t, 230, 231f, 232f
Pedal pulses
    absence of in lower leg/foot disease, 418
    in spinal stenosis, 741
Pediculosis, **138**. *See also* Lice
Pediculus humanus
    var *capitis*, 138
    var *corporis*, 138
Pedophilia, 948
    intrafamilial (incest), 948
PEEP. *See* Positive end-expiratory pressure
Peer support groups. *See* Support groups
PEF. *See* Peak expiratory flow
Pefloxacin, theophyllines affected by, 225t
PEG. *See* Polyethylene glycol
Pegasys. *See* Peginterferon
Pegfilgrastim, for chemotherapy-induced toxicity, 666, 1499, 1508t
Peginterferon
    for hepatitis B, 609, 610
    for hepatitis C, 606, 610–611
    for hepatitis D, 611
Pegintron. *See* Peginterferon
Pegvisomant, for acromegaly/gigantism, 999
Pelger-Huet cells, 463
Peliosis hepatis
    in bartonellosis, 1321
    drugs/toxins causing, 617, 1065
Pellagra, 1142
Pelvic abscess, anaerobic, 1323
Pelvic appendicitis, 568
Pelvic examination, in rape victim, 702
Pelvic floor dyssynergia, 507–508, 508
    biofeedback in management of, 1536t, 1538
Pelvic inflammatory disease (PID)/pelvic infection, **687–689**, 1182t. *See also* Endometritis; Salpingitis
    in actinomycosis, 1324
    appendicitis differentiated from, 568, 688
    chlamydial, 688, 1177t, 1182t, 1328
    dysmenorrhea differentiated from, 677
    gonococcal, 688, 1182t, 1319, 1320
    in HIV infection/AIDS, 1216
    IUDs and, 688, 698
Pelvic muscle (Kegel) exercises
    for fecal incontinence, 595, 596
    for urinary incontinence, 71

Pelvic organ prolapse, **687**
Pelvic pain
    chronic (chronic pelvic pain syndrome/nonbacterial prostatitis), **855**, 855t
    in dysmenorrhea, 677
    in ectopic pregnancy, 713
    in endometriosis, 686
    in PID, 688
Pemberton sign, 1019t
Pemetrexed, 1501t
Pemphigoid, bullous, **131**
Pemphigus, **130–131**
    foliaceus/erythematosus, 130
    paraneoplastic, 130
    vulgaris/vegetans, 130
Pen injectors, for insulin administration, 1099
Penbutolol, 401t
Penciclovir, 1237, 1238t. *See also* Famciclovir
Penetration, ulcer, **555**
Penicillamine
    adverse ophthalmic effects of, 178t
    for Wilson disease, 629
Penicillin. *See also specific disorder used in*
    allergy to, 1180
        testing/desensitization treatment for, 1180, 1183, 1183–1186
    for anaerobic pneumonia/lung abscess, 250, 1322
    for anthrax, 1301, 1301t
    for endocarditis, 1306
    for group B streptococcal infection prophylaxis in pregnancy, 708
    for non-sexually transmitted treponematoses, 1339
    for pharyngitis, 204, 1290
    platelet function affected by, 490t
    renal/hepatic failure and, 1185t
    resistance to, in pneumococcal infections, 246–247, 1293, 1294
    for rheumatic fever, 376
    for syphilis. *See* Syphilis
Penicillium marneffei infections, **1400**
Penile discharge. *See* Urethral discharge
Penile prostheses, 863
Penile tumescence testing, nocturnal, 863, 949
Penlac. *See* Ciclopirox
Pentamidine
    for African trypanosomiasis, 1349, 1349t
    hypoglycemia caused by, 1122, 1395
    for leishmaniasis, 1352
    for *P jiroveci* infection, 1222t, 1224t, 1395
    pneumothorax and, 286, 1394
    renal/hepatic failure and, 1185t
Pentasa. *See* Mesalamine
Pentavalent antimonials, for leishmaniasis, 1352, 1353
Pentazocine, 84
Pentosan, for interstitial cystitis, 861
Pentostam. *See* Stibogluconate
Pentostatin, 1501t

Pentoxifylline
    for alcoholic liver disease, 615
    for leg ulcers, 144
PEP. *See* Positive expiratory pressure (PEP) therapy
Peptic stricture of esophagus, 529t, 532–533. *See also* Esophagus, strictures of
Peptic ulcer disease, **547–553**, 551t
    complications of, **553–556**
    dyspepsia in, 502, 549
    gastric cancer and, 553, 1471–1472
    gastric outlet obstruction and, **555**
    GI bleeding in, 517, 548, **553–555**
    H pylori-associated, 548, 549, 550–552, 551t
        HSV infection and, 1236
        perforation and, **555**
    NSAID-induced, 548–549, 551t, 552–553, 749
    pharmacologic/medical management of, 549–553, 551t
    refractory, 553
    silent, 549
    ulcer penetration and, **555**
    ulcer perforation and, **555**
    Zollinger-Ellison syndrome (gastrinoma) and, 552, 553, 556, 1062
Pepto-Bismol. *See* Bismuth compounds
Peptostreptococci, 1322, 1323
Perceptual distortions
    psychedelic drug use and, 982
    in schizophrenic/psychotic disorders, 953
Percocet. *See* Oxycodone
Percodan. *See* Oxycodone
Percussion. *See* Chest percussion
Percutaneous aspiration/injection/reaspiration (PAIR), for hydatid cysts, 1379
Percutaneous coronary intervention (PCI), 323
    for acute coronary syndromes, 327t, 328–329, 329t
    for angina, 323
    for myocardial infarction, 327t, 332, 340
    prophylactic/preoperative, 51
Percutaneous dilational tracheostomy, 212
Percutaneous transhepatic cholangiography (PTC)
    in biliary stricture, 640
    in liver disease/jaundice, 601
Percutaneous transluminal coronary angioplasty (PTCA)/stenting, 323. *See also* Percutaneous coronary intervention
Percutaneous valvuloplasty. *See* Valvuloplasty
Perennial rhinitis, 196
Perforation
    in appendicitis, 568
    of colonic diverticula (diverticulitis), **588–589**
    ulcer, **555**

Performance anxiety, 940, 943
Perfusion scans
  lung. *See* Ventilation-perfusion scans
  myocardial. *See* Myocardial perfusion
    scintigraphy
Pergolide, withdrawal of from market,
  907
Periampullary carcinoma, **1463–1465**
Perianal cellophane tape test, in enterobi-
    asis/pinworms, 1382
Perianal disease. *See also* Anorectal disor-
    ders
  abscesses and fistulas, 596
  anal cancer, 1468*t*, **1483**
  in Crohn disease, 578, 579
  hematoma, thrombosed hemorrhoid
    causing, **594**
  warts, 678. *See also* Venereal (genital)
    warts
Perianal pruritus. *See* Anogenital/perianal
    pruritus
Pericardial disease, **376–380**
  in SLE, 753
Pericardial effusions, **378–379**. *See also*
    Pericarditis
  in Kawasaki syndrome, 1288
  malignant, 379, 1495–1496
  myxedema, 377, 1005
  in pneumococcal pneumonia, 1293
  in postmyocardial infarction/postcar-
    diotomy pericarditis
    (Dressler syndrome), 377
Pericardial friction rub
  in myocardial infarction, 330, 339
  in pericardial effusion, 378
  in pericarditis, 377
Pericardial tamponade. *See* Tamponade
Pericardiectomy/pericardial window
  for constrictive pericarditis, 380
  for malignant effusions/neoplastic
    pericarditis, 378
  in pneumococcal pneumonia, 1293
  for uremic pericarditis, 378
Pericardiocentesis. *See also* Pleural fluid
    analysis
  for pericardial effusion/tamponade,
    378, 379, 1293
Pericarditis
  acute inflammatory, **376–378**
  bacterial, 377
  chest pain in, 29, 377
  constrictive, **379–380**
    cirrhosis and, 620
    restrictive cardiomyopathy differ-
      entiated from, 374
  coxsackieviruses causing, 376, 1279
  myocardial infarction and, 339, 377,
    378
  neoplastic, 377, 378
  pneumococcal, 377, 1292, 1293
  postmyocardial infarction/postcar-
    diotomy (Dressler syn-
    drome), 339, 377, 378
  radiation, 377, 378
  tuberculous, 377, 378, 379
  uremic, 377, 378, 828
  viral, 376–377, 377, 378
Perichondritis, 180

Perihepatitis, Fitz-Hugh and Curtis syn-
    drome and, 688
Peri-infectious glomerulonephritis, 835*f*
Perilymphatic fistula, 183, 190, 191*t*
Perindopril, 403*t*
Periocular pain. *See* Ocular/orbital pain
Periodic paralysis, **936**
  hyperkalemic, 796*t*, 936
  hypokalemic, 796*t*, 936
  in hyperthyroidism, 936, 1010,
    1015
  normokalemic, 936
Periodontal disease, anaerobic, 1322
  pneumonia and, 250, 1322
Perioperative management. *See* Preopera-
    tive evaluation/perioperat-
    tive management
Periorbital pain. *See* Ocular/orbital pain
Peripartum cardiomyopathy, **385**, 724,
    1000
Peripheral intravenous lines, infection/
    infection prevention and,
    1160, 1161, 1180
Peripheral nerve tumors, mononeuropa-
    thy caused by, 927
Peripheral neuropathies, **921–929**. *See
    also specific type and* Neu-
    ropathies
Peripheral pulses. *See* Pulses
Peripheral stem cells, for transplantation,
    475
Peripheral vascular disease. *See* Vascular
    disorders
Peripheral vein nutritional support, 1148,
    1148*f*. *See also* Nutritional
    support
  solutions for, 1150–1151
Peristalsis, disorders of. *See* Motility dis-
    orders
Peritoneal carcinomatosis, 527–528
Peritoneal dialysis, 831. *See also* Dialysis
  for chronic kidney disease, 831
  for hyperkalemia, 799*t*
  for hypermagnesemia, 806
Peritoneal effusions, malignant, 1495–1496
Peritoneovenous shunts, for ascites, 621,
    1496
Peritoneum
  diseases of, **524–529**. *See also specific
    type and* Ascites; Peritoni-
    tis
  nausea and vomiting in, 505*t*
  mesothelioma arising in, **528**, 1458
Peritonitis, 1181*t*
  ascitic fluid analysis in, 526, 527
  dialysis and, 831
  diverticulitis and, 588
  in familial Mediterranean fever, 528
  peptic ulcer perforation and, 555
  perforated appendicitis and, 568
  spontaneous bacterial, **526–527**
    in cirrhosis, 526, 621–622
  tuberculous, **527**
Peritonsillar abscess/cellulitis, **205**, 1289
Periungual warts, 131, 132
Permethrin
  for pediculosis, 138
  for scabies, 137, 138

Permissive hypercapnia, 291
  for asthma, 233
Permitil. *See* Fluphenazine
Permixon. *See* Saw palmetto
Pernicious anemia, 446
  carcinoid tumors and, 547, 1474
  gastritis and, 547
  subacute combined degeneration of
    spinal cord and, 915
Pernicious vomiting of pregnancy,
    710–711
Peroneal nerve, common, injury to, **928**
Peroxisome proliferator-activated recep-
    tor alpha (PPAR-α),
    fibrates affecting, 1132
Peroxisome proliferator-activated recep-
    tor gamma (PPAR-γ)
  thiazolidinediones affecting, 1093
  thyroid cancer and, 1024
Peroxisome proliferator-activated recep-
    tor gamma (PPAR-γ)
    tumor suppressor gene,
    thyroid cancer and, 1023
Perphenazine, 954, 955*t*, 956*t*, 957
Persistent anovulation. *See* Polycystic
    ovary syndrome
Persistent islet hyperplasia, **1120**
Persistent vegetative state, **917**
Personal relationships, social issues for
    terminally ill/dying patient
    and, 92, 92*t*
Personality changes
  in dementia, 64
  due to general medical condition, **986**
  in neurosyphilis, 1336
Personality disorders, **950–952**, 951*t*
Perspiration. *See* Sweating
Pertussis (whooping cough), **1307–1308**
  cough in, 22, 23, 24, 1308
  prevention/immunization and, 3–4,
    1200, 1308. *See also* Pertus-
    sis vaccine
Pertussis vaccine, with diphtheria and tet-
    anus toxoids (DTaP/Tdap
    vaccines), 3–4,
    1188–1189*t*, 1190–1191*t*,
    1192–1193*t*, 1194–1197*t*,
    1200, 1298, 1299*t*, 1302,
    1308
  adverse effects/contraindications and,
    1202*t*
  pregnancy and, 1195*t*, 1200
Pes anserine bursa, knee pain caused by,
    33
Pessary
  for pelvic organ prolapse, 687
  for urinary incontinence, 71
Pesticide poisoning
  cholinesterase inhibitors, **1443–1444**
  paraquat, **1443**
PET. *See* Positron emission tomography
Petit mal (absence) seizures, 879*t*, 880,
    882*t*. *See also* Seizures
Petit mal (absence) status epilepticus, 884
Petroleum products, toxicity/abuse of,
    1444
  aspiration and, 277, 1444
Petrous apicitis, 185

Peutz-Jeghers syndrome, 592
  gynecomastia in, 1067
  pancreatic/periampullary carcinoma
    and, 1463
Peyronie disease, 862
  Dupuytren contracture and, 743
PF-4 heparin antibody. *See* Heparin-asso-
    ciated/PF-4 antibody
PFA-100 closure time, reference values
    for, 1553*t*
PFO. *See* Patent foramen ovale
PFT. *See* Pulmonary function tests
PGA. *See* Polyglandular autoimmune syn-
    drome
PGI₂. *See* Prostacyclin
pH
  in acid-base disorders, 806. *See also*
      specific type
  in acidosis, 806
  in alcoholic ketoacidosis, 809
  in alkalosis, 806
  arterial blood, 806
  in diabetic ketoacidosis, 808
  esophageal, monitoring, 530
    in chronic aspiration of gastric
        contents, 278
    in gastroesophageal/laryngopha-
        ryngeal reflux, 209, 503,
        531, 534
  gastric
    health care-associated pneumonia
        and, 248
    in Zollinger-Ellison syndrome/gas-
        trinoma, 556
  in lactic acidosis, 1117
  in metabolic alkalosis, 812, 813
  in near drowning, 1415, 1416
  pharyngeal, monitoring, in gastro-
      esophageal/laryngopha-
      ryngeal reflux, 209
  pleural fluid, 283
    in parapneumonic effusion, 283, 285
  reference values for, 1552*t*
  in respiratory acidosis, 814
  in respiratory alkalosis, 814
  stool, in diarrhea, 515
  urine
    cystine calculi and, 860
    in hyperchloremic metabolic aci-
        dosis/tubular acidosis,
        809*t*, 810, 811
    hyperuricosuric calcium stones
        and, 859
    stone disease and, 858
    struvite calculi and, 859
    uric acid calculi and, 859
    vaginal, 677, 678
    venous blood, 806
Phacoemulsification, for cataract
    removal, 161
Phaeohyphomycosis, 1402
Phalen sign, in carpal tunnel syndrome, 742
Pharmaceuticals. *See under* Drug
Pharyngeal dysphagia, 529, 529*t*. *See also*
    Dysphagia
Pharyngeal pH monitoring, in gastro-
    esophageal/laryngopha-
    ryngeal reflux, 209

Pharyngitis, **203–205**, 1182*t*, **1289–1290**
  antibiotics for, 204–205, 1182*t*,
      1289–1290
  in diphtheria, 204, 1289, 1302
  gonococcal, 204, 1320
  in mononucleosis, 204, 1243, 1244,
      1289
  nonstreptococcal exudative (adenovi-
      rus), 1275
  in peritonsillar abscess and cellulitis,
      205, 1289
  streptococcal, 204, 1182*t*, **1289–1290**
    glomerulonephritis and, 834, 1289
    rheumatic fever after, 375, 1289
  viral, 1275
Pharyngoconjunctival fever, 154, 1275
Pharynx, **201–206**
Phenacetin, in analgesic nephropathy, 845
Phenazopyridine
  methemoglobinemia caused by, 1440
  for urinary tract infection, 48, 852
Phencyclidine, **982**, 1439
  aggressive/violent/psychotic behavior
      caused by, 954, 976, 982
Phenelzine, 968*t*
  overdose/toxicity of, 968*t*, 1440–1441
Phenmetrazine, abuse/overdose of, 983
Phenobarbital, 881, 882*t*, 941*t*, 1545*t*
  for anxiety, 941*t*, 942
  overdose/toxicity of, 882*t*, 1436
    hemodialysis for, 1425*t*
  for seizures, 881, 882*t*
    during pregnancy, 724, 883
    status epilepticus and, 884
  theophyllines affected by, 225*t*
Phenothiazines, 954, 955*t*, 956*t*. *See also*
    Antipsychotic drugs
  hypocalcemia/hypoparathyroidism
      and, 1032–1033
  for nausea and vomiting, 506
  overdose/toxicity of, 956*t*, **1444–1445**
  ophthalmic effects and, 177*t*
Phenotypic resistance testing, in antiret-
    roviral therapy, 1233
Phenoxybenzamine
  for benign prostatic hyperplasia, 869*t*
  pheochromocytoma surgery and,
      1060
Phentermine, for obesity, 1137
D-Phenylalanine derivative, for diabetes
    mellitus, 1091*t*, 1092
Phenylbutazone
  adverse ophthalmic effects of, 178*t*
  lithium interactions and, 972*t*
Phenylpropanolamine, in OTC medica-
    tions, 984
Phenytoin, 881, 882*t*, 1545*t*
  antidepressant drug interactions and,
      969*t*
  overdose/toxicity of, 882*t*, 1431
    ophthalmic effects and, 177*t*
  for seizures, 881, 882*t*
    pregnancy and, 724, 883
    status epilepticus and, 884
  theophyllines affected by, 225*t*
Pheochromocytoma, 392, **1058–1061**,
      1059*t*
  β-blocker use in, 402, 1061

headache in, 44, 1058
hypertension in, 392, 393, 1058, 1059,
    1061
  in multiple endocrine neoplasia, 1058,
      1076*t*, 1077
PHEX endopeptidase mutation, in osteo-
    malacia/rickets, 1043
Philadelphia chromosome, 461, 462, 465
Phimosis, in chancroid, 1320
Phlebectomy, 428, 429
Phlebitis. *See* Thrombophlebitis
Phlebotomy
  for hemochromatosis, 628
  for polycythemia, 458
  for polycythemia-related pulmonary
      hypertension, 275
  for porphyria cutanea tarda, 117
Phlegmonous (necrotizing) gastritis, 547
Phobic disorder, 940, 943
Phonic tics, in Tourette syndrome, 911
Phonophobia, in migraine headache, 45*t*,
    873
Phosphate. *See* Phosphorus/phosphate
Phosphate enema, 509*t*
Phosphatidylinositol class A (PIG-A) gene
    defect, in paroxysmal noc-
    turnal hemoglobinuria,
    449
Phosphatonin (fibroblast growth factor
    23/FGF-23), 802, 1043
  in oncogenic osteomalacia, 1043
  in X-linked hypophosphatemic rick-
      ets, 1043
Phosphaturia, osteomalacia and, 1043,
    1044
Phosphodiesterase inhibitors
  for asthma, 227, 228
  contraindications to with nitroglyc-
      erin, 863, 950, 1108
  for erectile dysfunction, 863, 950,
      1107–1108
Phosphorus/phosphate
  calcium affected by, 802
  in calcium nephrolithiasis/hypercalci-
      uria, 857, 858*t*, 859
  deficiency of. *See also* Hypophos-
      phatemia
    in osteomalacia/rickets, 1043
  dietary/supplementary
    for diabetic ketoacidosis, 1114
    for hyperglycemic hyperosmolar
        state, 1016
    for hypophosphatemia, 803–804
    for osteomalacia, 1044
    requirements for in nutritional
        support, 815, 1149
    restriction of in mineral bone dis-
        orders of chronic kidney
        disease, 829
  disorders of concentration/metabo-
      lism of, **802–804**. *See also*
      Hyperphosphatemia;
      Hypophosphatemia
    in chronic kidney disease (renal
        osteodystrophy), 829–830
    genetic disorders and, 796*t*
    in hypercalcemia, 801
    in hypocalcemia, 799, 800

Phosphorus/phosphate (*cont.*)
parathyroid hormone affecting, 802
reference values for, 1552*t*
urinary excretion of. *See* Phosphaturia
Photoallergy, 142, 143
Photocoagulation
for age-related macular degeneration, 163
for diabetic retinopathy, 166, 1105
for retinal detachment, 162
for retinal vein occlusion, 164
for sickle cell retinopathy, 167
Photodermatitis/photosensitivity, 95*t*, **142–143**
chemotherapy-induced, 1509
drugs causing, 142, 143, 148*t*
in SLE, 753–754
Photodynamic therapy
for age-related macular degeneration, 163
for Barrett esophagus, 532
for cholangiocarcinoma, 1463
for esophageal cancer palliation, 1470
Photoepilation, 1055
Photophobia
in corneal abrasion, 171
in migraine headache, 45*t*, 873
in ultraviolet (actinic) keratitis, 172
Photopsia (flashing lights), in migraine headache, 873
Photorefractive keratectomy (PRK), 151
Photoresection. *See* Nd:YAG laser photoresection
Photosensitive epilepsy, 880
Photosensitivity. *See* Photodermatitis/photosensitivity
Phototherapy
for atopic dermatitis, 103
for lichen planus, 135
for major depression with seasonal onset, 969
for psoriasis, 104, 105
Phototoxicity, 142, 143
Photovaporization of prostate (PVP), for benign prostatic hyperplasia, 871
Phrenic nerve, hiccups caused by irritation of, 507
Phthirus pubis, 138
Phycomycosis (mucormycosis), **1398–1399**
rhinocerebral, 195
Phyllodes tumor of breast, 650
Physical abuse. *See* Abuse
Physical activity. *See* Exercise/activity
Physical agents, disorders caused by, **1403–1419**
altitude-related, **1417–1419**
burn injury, **1408–1412**
cold causing, 1403, **1403–1406**
dysbarism/decompression sickness, **1416–1417**
electrical injury, **1412–1413**
heat (hot environment) causing, 1403, **1406–1408**
near drowning, **1415–1416**
radiation exposure causing, **1413–1415**

Physical instability. *See* Falls; Gait/gait disorders
Physical therapy
for complex regional pain syndrome, 743
for stroke patient, 892
Physician, relationship of with patient. *See* Doctor–patient relationship
Physiologic drug dependence, 78, 84, 977
Physostigmine
for anticholinergic delirium, 1439
for anticholinergic-type mushroom poisoning, 1442
for atropine/anticholinergic overdose, 1424*t*, 1432
Phytanic acid metabolism, in Refsum disease, 923
Phytoestrogens (plant-derived estrogens), 1070, 1073
Phytonadione
for anticoagulant overdose, 1431
for hypoprothrombinemia, in cirrhosis, 623
for vitamin K deficiency, 494
Phytotherapy, for benign prostatic hyperplasia, 870
PI. *See* Protease inhibitors
Pica, in iron deficiency anemia, 440
Pick disease, 64, 986
Pickwickian syndrome (obesity-hypoventilation syndrome), **287**
PID. *See* Pelvic inflammatory disease
Piebaldism, 144
PIG-A gene defect, in paroxysmal nocturnal hemoglobinuria, 449
Pigeon-breeder's disease (bird-fancier's lung), 280*t*
Pigmentary skin disorders, **144–145**. *See also* Hyperpigmentation; Hypopigmentation; Pigmented skin lesions
drugs causing, 145, 149*t*
in hypercarotenosis, 1144
Pigmented basal cell carcinoma, 133
Pigmented skin lesions, 95*t*, **99–101**. *See also specific type*
Pill-induced esophagitis, **536**
Pilocarpine
for chemotherapy/radiation-induced toxicity, 1507*t*
for glaucoma/ocular hypertension, 158, 159, 175*t*
Pilocarpine iontophoresis sweat test, in cystic fibrosis, 242
Pilopine. *See* Pilocarpine
Pimecrolimus, 97*t*
for atopic dermatitis, 102
T-cell lymphoma and, 102
Pimozide, for Tourette syndrome, 912
Pindolol, 401*t*
for aggressive/violent behavior, 976
Pineal tumor, 898*t*
Pinguecula, **155–156**
Pingueculitis, 155–156
Pink puffers, 234, 235*t*
PINK1 gene, in parkinsonism, 905
Pinta, **1339**

Pinworm infection, **1382**
Pioglitazone, 1091*t*, 1093–1094, 1101
with glimepiride, 1096
insulin therapy and, 1101
with metformin, 1096
Piperacillin, renal/hepatic failure and, 1185*t*
Piperacillin-tazobactam
for abdominal infections, 1322*t*
renal/hepatic failure and, 1185*t*
Piperaquine, for malaria, 1355*t*, 1357
with dihydroartemisinin, 1355*t*, 1356*t*, 1357, 1360
Pipracil. *See* Piperacillin
Pirbuterol, for asthma, 228, 229*t*
Piroxicam, 80*t*
Pit viper envenomation, 1446–1447
Pitting (nail), 146
in psoriasis, 104
Pituitary adenoma, 991
ACTH-secreting, 1050, 1051–1052, 1053
GH-secreting, 994, 997, 998
hypopituitarism caused by, 991
in multiple endocrine neoplasia, 991, 1076, 1076*t*
prolactin-secreting, 1000, 1001, 1002
surgical resection/removal of, 993, 995, 998, 1002, 1052
thyrotrophe (TSH secreting), 1008, 1013
Pituitary apoplexy, 169, 993, 998, 1002
Pituitary gland
destruction/necrosis of, adrenal crisis caused by, 1046
disorders of, **991–1002**
acromegaly/gigantism, 997
amenorrhea caused by, 1067–1068, 1069, 1070
anterior hypopituitarism, **991–995**
diabetes insipidus, **995–997**. *See also* Diabetes insipidus
diabetes mellitus, **1079–1117**. *See also* Diabetes mellitus
hyperprolactinemia, **1000–1002**, 1000*t*
hormones produced by, 992*t*
absence of (panhypopituitarism), 992
hyperplasia of, thyrotrophe, 1005, 1008, 1013
tumors of, 991. *See also* Pituitary adenoma
amenorrhea caused by, 1069
Pityriasis
alba, in atopic dermatitis, 101
rosea, **105–106**
drugs causing eruptions similar to, 149*t*
rubra pilaris, 112
versicolor (tinea versicolor), **109–110**
Pityrosporum ovale. See Malassezia furfur
Pivot shift test, in knee pain, 34
"Pizza-pie" retinopathy, in cytomegalovirus infection, 1245
PKD1/PKD2 gene mutations, 847
Placenta previa, third trimester bleeding caused by, 720

Placental disorders, third-trimester bleeding caused by, 720
Plague, 1177t, **1318–1319**
    chemoprophylaxis for, 1201, 1318
Plan B, for emergency/postcoital contraception, 700
Plantar fasciitis, **747**
Plantar fibromatosis, Dupuytren contracture and, 743
Plantar hyperkeratosis of heels, 133
Plantar warts, 131, 132
Plasma cell leukemia, 472
Plasma cells, in myeloma, 472, 848
Plasma chromogranin A (CgA) screening test. *See* Chromogranin A
Plasma fractions/components. *See also* Fresh frozen plasma
    transfusion of, **478–479**
        for thrombotic microangiopathies, 485
Plasma renin activity
    in Addison disease, 1049
    in aldosteronism, 391, 392, 1056, 1057
    in hypertension, 389–390, 390, 391, 402
    reference values for, 1553t
Plasma renin concentration, in aldosteronism, 1056
Plasmacytomas, 472. *See also* Myeloma
Plasmapheresis
    for multiple sclerosis, 913
    for Waldenström macroglobulinemia, 474
Plasminogen, reference values for, 1552t
Plasmodium, 1353–1362. *See also* Malaria
    falciparum, 1353–1362
        resistant strains of, 1355, 1359
        severe infection caused by, 1353, 1354, 1357t
    malariae, 1353–1362
    ovale, 1353–1362
    vivax, 1353–1362
        resistant strains of, 1356, 1358–1359
Platelet-associated IgG, 1553t
Platelet count
    chemotherapy dosage modification and, 1499, 1508t
    desired/reference values for, 480, 481t, 1552t
    in essential thrombocytosis, 457t, 459
    in myeloproliferative disorders, 457t
    in polycythemia, 457t, 458
    in preeclampsia-eclampsia, 716, 717t
Platelet-derived growth factor
    for diabetic foot ulcers, 1106
    in myelofibrosis, 460
Platelet disorders, **480–490**, 481t, 490t
    qualitative, **489–490**, 490t
    thrombocytopenia, **480–489**, 481t. *See also* Thrombocytopenia
Platelet function test, reference values for, 1553t
Platelet glycoprotein IIb/IIIa receptors. *See* Glycoprotein IIb/IIIa receptors
Platelet-inhibiting agents. *See* Antiplatelet therapy

Platelet transfusion, 478. *See also* Transfusions
    for DIC, 487–488, 488t
    for GI bleeding/variceal hemorrhage, 519, 539
Platelets
    acquired disorders of, **490**, 490t
    aspirin/NSAIDs affecting function of, 490, 490t, 548, 749
    autoantibodies against. *See* Antiplatelet antibody
    in Bernard-Soulier syndrome, 489, 490
    in chronic kidney disease/uremia, 490t, 829
    congenital disorders of, **489–490**
    drugs inhibiting. *See* Antiplatelet therapy
    in Glanzmann thrombasthenia, 489, 490
    in myeloproliferative disorders, 490t
    sequestration of in spleen, 481t, **488–489**
    in storage pool disease, 489, 490
Platinol. *See* Cisplatin
Platinum analogs/platinum-based chemotherapy, 1500t. *See also* Cisplatin
Platypnea
    in hepatopulmonary syndrome, 623
    orthodeoxia, in patent foramen ovale, 298
Plendil. *See* Felodipine
Plerixafor, for stem cell mobilization, 475
Plesiomonas, diarrhea caused by, 515
Plethysmography, impedance, in venous thrombosis/pulmonary embolism, 269
Pleural biopsy
    in lung cancer, 1454
    in tuberculosis, 252, 284
Pleural diseases, **282–287**
    occupational, **280–281**
    respiratory failure caused by, 289t
Pleural effusions, **282–285**, 283t, 284t
    in asbestosis, 281
    drug-induced, 281t
    exudative, 283, 283t, 284t
    in heart disease/failure, 360
    in lung cancer, 285, 1454
    malignant, 284t, 285, 1454, 1495–1496
    paramalignant, 285
    parapneumonic, 283, 284t, 285
        in pneumococcal pneumonia, 1292, 1293
    rheumatoid, 284t
    transudative, 283, 283t, 284
    tuberculous, 252, 283–284, 284t
Pleural fluid analysis, 283–284
    in anthrax, 1301
    in lung cancer, 1454
    in malignant effusion, 284t
    in mesothelioma, 1459
    in pneumonia, 246, 249
    in tuberculosis, 252, 283–284, 284t
Pleural friction rub, in pulmonary embolism, 268t

Pleural mesothelioma (malignant pleural mesothelioma), **1458–1459**
Pleurectomy, for mesothelioma, 1459
Pleuritis/pleuritic chest pain, 29, **282**
    in epidemic pleurodynia (Bornholm disease), 1279
    in pericarditis, 377
    in thoracic actinomycosis, 1323
Pleurodesis, for malignant pleural effusion, 285, 1496
Pleurodynia, epidemic, 1279
Plexiform neuroma, 904
Plexogenic pulmonary arteriopathy (idiopathic/primary pulmonary hypertension), 274, **380–381**, 381t
Plexopathy (diabetic amyotrophy), 923, 1106
Plummer disease (toxic adenoma of thyroid), 1008
Plummer-Vinson syndrome, 440, 537
PML. *See* Progressive multifocal leukoencephalopathy
PML-RARa fusion gene, 464, 465
PMLE. *See* Polymorphous light eruption
PMS. *See* Premenstrual syndrome/tension
PMS2 genes, in HNPCC, 592
Pneumatic compression devices
    for lymphedema, 431
    for venous insufficiency/leg ulcers, 143, 431
    for venous thromboembolic disease, 495–496
Pneumatic dilation. *See also* Esophageal dilation
    for achalasia, 542
Pneumatic retinopexy, for retinal detachment, 162
Pneumococcal (*Streptococcus pneumoniae*) infections, 1176t, **1292–1294**
    drug resistance and, 246–247, 1293, 1294
    endocarditis, 1292, 1293, 1305–1306
    immunization against. *See* Pneumococcal vaccine
    keratitis, 156
    meningitis, 1164, **1293–1294**
    pericarditis, 377, 1292, 1293
    pneumonia, 244t, 1182t, **1292–1293**
Pneumococcal vaccine, 3, 3t, 247, 1188–1189t, 1190–1191t, 1192–1193t, 1194–1197t, 1199–1200
    adverse effects/contraindications and, 1202t
    for asthma patients, 228
    in HIV infection/AIDS/immunocompromised host, 1195t, 1199, 1220
Pneumoconioses, **278–279**, 279t
Pneumocystis carinii. See Pneumocystis jiroveci infection; *Pneumocystis jiroveci* pneumonia
Pneumocystis jiroveci infection, 1224t
    otitis, 192
    pentamidine-induced hypoglycemia and, 1122, 1395

Pneumocystis jiroveci infection (*cont.*)
pneumonia. *See Pneumocystis jiroveci* pneumonia
prevention of, 1157, 1222, 1222*t*
Pneumocystis jiroveci pneumonia (pneumocystosis), 244*t*, 251, 1210, 1223, **1394–1396**
CD4 T cell count and, 1210, 1394, 1395, 1396
pentamidine-induced hypoglycemia and, 1122, 1395
pentamidine treatment/chemoprophylaxis and, 1222*t*, 1224*t*, 1395–1396
pneumothorax and, 286, 1210, 1394
prophylaxis of, 286, 1157, 1210, 1222, 1222*t*, 1396
Pneumocystosis. *See Pneumocystis jiroveci* pneumonia
Pneumomediastinum, 286
Pneumonia, **243–250**, 244–245*t*, 1181*t*, 1182*t*. *See also specific causative agent and* Pneumonitis
adenoviruses causing, 1275, 1276
anaerobic, 244*t*, **250**, 1322
in aspergillosis, 1398
aspiration, 1182*t*. *See also* Aspiration
in anaerobic infections, 250, 1322
in community-acquired disease, 245
drug use and, 1168
in health-care associated disease, 248
hydrocarbon toxicity and, 277, 1444
bronchiolitis obliterans and (BOOP/cryptogenic organizing pneumonitis/COP), 243, 264*t*
chlamydial
C pneumoniae causing, 244*t*, 1329
in newborn, 727
in psittacosis, 1329
community-acquired, **243–248**, 1181*t*
cough and, 22–23, 23*t*
cryptococcal, 1396
cytomegalovirus, 1245, 1246
desquamative interstitial (DIP), 243, 263, 264*t*
eosinophilic, 266. *See also* Löffler syndrome
H influenzae causing, 244*t*, 1310
health-care associated, **248–249**, 1181*t*
in histoplasmosis, 1392
idiopathic fibrosing interstitial, **263–265**, 264*t*
in immunocompromised host/HIV infection/AIDS, 251, 1210. *See also Pneumocystis jiroveci* pneumonia
CD4 T cell count and, 1210
in influenza, 1270
Legionnaires, 244*t*, 249, 1176*t*, 1182*t*, 1310–1311
in leptospirosis, 1341
lipoid, 277
in measles, 1248, 1249
mercury vapor, 1439

mycobacterial (NTM), 258–259
necrotizing, 250
nonspecific interstitial (NSIP), 263, 264*t*
in HIV infection/AIDS, 1211
plague, 1318
pleural effusion in (parapneumonic pleural effusion), 283, 284*t*, 285, 1292, 1293
pneumococcal, 1292, 1293
pneumococcal, 244*t*, **1292–1293**
immunization against. *See* Pneumococcal vaccine
Pneumocystis. See Pneumocystis jiroveci pneumonia
postoperative, 53–54, 53*t*, 1181*t*
risk factors for, 53, 53*t*
prevention of, 247
in Q fever, 1287
RSV, 1268
in SARS, 1274
streptococcal, 244*t*, 1182*t*, 1291
treatment of, 244–245*t*, 246–247, 249, 251
in tularemia, 1317
usual interstitial (UIP), 263–265, 264*t*
varicella zoster virus, 1241
during pregnancy, 725, 726, 1241
ventilator-associated, 248, 249, 291, 1160, 1161
viral, 245
Pneumonitis. *See also* Pneumonia
acute gastric aspiration causing, 278, 1160
acute interstitial (AIP), 264*t*
cryptogenic organizing (COP/idiopathic bronchiolitis obliterans with organizing pneumonia/BOOP), 243, 264*t*
cytomegalovirus, 1245, 1246
hydrocarbon/petroleum distillates/solvents causing, 277, 1444
hypersensitivity, **279–280**, 280*t*
mercury vapor, 1439
nonspecific interstitial (NSIP), 263, 264*t*
in HIV infection/AIDS, 1211
radiation, **282**, 1414
toxoplasmic, in HIV infection/AIDS, 1363
usual interstitial (UIP), 263–265, 264*t*
Pneumoplasty, reduction, for COPD, 239
Pneumothorax, **285–287**
catamenial, 286
in COPD, 236, 286
in cystic fibrosis, 241, 242
iatrogenic, 286
P jiroveci pneumonia/pentamidine prophylaxis and, 286, 1210, 1394
spontaneous, **285–287**
dyspnea in, 26, 286
tension, 286
traumatic, 286
Pneumovax. *See* Pneumococcal vaccine
PNH. *See* Paroxysmal nocturnal hemoglobinuria

PO₂. *See also* PaO₂
in dyspnea evaluation, 26
in pulmonary embolism, 267
reference values for, 1552*t*
in respiratory failure, 289, 290
Podagra, 733
Podophyllum resin (podophyllin/podofilox), for genital warts, 132, 679
Poisindex, 1420
Poison control centers, 1420
Poison ivy/oak, 119, 784. *See also* Allergic contact dermatitis
Poisoning/drug overdose, **1420–1449**. *See also specific drug or agent*
abdominal radiographs in, 1427
anion gap in, 1426. *See also* Anion gap/anion gap acidosis
antidotes for, **1423–1424**, 1424*t*
arrhythmias in, **1422–1423**, 1422*t*
coma caused by, 1112*t*, **1420–1421**
diagnosis of, **1426–1428**, 1427*t*
eye decontamination in, **1424**
gastrointestinal decontamination in, 1420, **1424–1426**, 1425*t*
hypertension in, **1422**
hyperthermia in, **1423**
hypotension in, **1421–1422**
hypothermia in, **1421**
initial evaluation in, **1420**
laboratory tests in, 1426–1427, 1427*t*
osmol gap in, 795, 809, 1426, 1427*t*
patient observation and, 1420
physical examination in, 1426
seizures in, **1423**, 1423*t*
skin decontamination in, **1424**
toxicology screen in, 1426–1427, 1427*t*
Poisonous mushrooms, **1441–1442**, 1441*t*
hepatic failure and, 608, 1441
Poisonous snakes, 1424*t*, **1446–1447**
Poliomyelitis, **1251–1253**
prevention/immunization and, 5, 1201, 1252–1253. *See also* Poliovirus vaccine
Poliovirus vaccine, 5, 1188*t*, 1190–1191*t*, 1192–1193*t*, 1201, 1252–1253
poliomyelitis associated with, 1252, 1253
pregnancy and, 710
for travelers, 1201, 1253
Polyalcohols (polyols), for diabetics, 1090
Polyangiitis, microscopic. *See* Microscopic polyangiitis
Polyarteritis. *See also* Arteritis
neuropathy associated with, 765, 924
nodosa, 140, **764–766**
Polyarthralgia. *See* Arthritis/arthralgia
Polyarthritis. *See* Arthritis/arthralgia
Polycarbophil. *See* Fiber, dietary
Polychondritis, relapsing, 180, **771**
Polycystic kidney disease, **847–848**, 847*t*
intracranial aneurysms and, 848, 894
Polycystic ovary syndrome, **690–691**, 1053, 1054
acne in, 120
amenorrhea in, 690, 1053, 1069

hirsutism in, 690, 691, 1053
infertility and, 690, 1054
obesity in, 690, 691, 1053
Polycythemia, **457–459**, 457t, 458t, 1466t
in cor pulmonale, 382
hypertension and, 390
pulmonary hypertension and, 275
spurious, 458
vera, **457–459**, 457t, 458t, 1466t
hepatic vein obstruction (Budd-Chiari syndrome) and, 630
Polydipsia/thirst
in diabetes insipidus, 996
in diabetes mellitus, 1082t, 1083
in hypercalcemia/hyperparathyroidism, 1034
hyponatremia caused by, 790f, 791
lithium causing, 971
psychogenic, 791, 953, 997
in schizophrenic/psychotic disorders, 953–954, 997
Polyendocrinopathy-candidiasis-ectodermal dystrophy, autoimmune, 1048
Polyethylene glycol/PEG 3350
for constipation/preoperative bowel cleansing, 509, 509, 509–510, 509t, 521
for whole bowel irrigation, 1425
Polyglandular autoimmune syndrome
Addison disease in, 1048
Hashimoto thyroiditis in, 1016
type 1, 1030, 1048
autoimmune hepatitis in, 613
type 2, 1048
Polyglandular failure (Schmidt) syndrome, 1048, 1086
Polymerase chain reaction (PCR) testing
in Lyme disease, 1344, 1345
in syphilis, 1332
Polymerase inhibitors, for hepatitis C, 612
Polymorphic reticulosis, 201
Polymorphonuclear neutrophil count, joint fluid, 730t
Polymorphous light eruption (PMLE), 142, 143
Polymyalgia rheumatica, **766–767**
fibromyalgia differentiated from, 741
rheumatoid arthritis differentiated from, 748
Polymyositis, **759–762**
autoantibodies in, 754t, 760
cancer-related, 760, 761
Polymyxins, for ophthalmic disorders, 173t
Polyneuropathies, 886, 922, **922–926**. See also specific type and Neuropathies
acute idiopathic. See Guillain-Barré syndrome
cancer-related, 902, 925
chronic inflammatory, **926**
in diabetes mellitus, 923, 1106
in HIV infection/AIDS, 924, 1212
in Lyme disease, 924
in polyarteritis nodosa, 765, 924
in sarcoidosis, 924
toxic, 925

Polyneuropathy, in rheumatoid arthritis, 924
Polyols (polyalcohols), for diabetics, 1090
Polypectomy
cervical, 679
colonoscopic, 590
GI bleeding after, 521, 590
Polyphagia with weight loss, in diabetes mellitus, 1082t, 1083
Polypharmacy, in elderly, **74**
falls and, 68
urinary incontinence and, 70
Polypoid corditis, 209
Polyps/polyposis
adenomatous, 589. See also Adenomatous polyps
familial, **591**. See also Familial adenomatous polyposis
nonfamilial, **589–591**
cervical, **679**
of colon, **589–593**
GI bleeding and, 521
colorectal cancer and, 589, 590, 591, 1476, 1477
gastric, 557, 591
hamartomatous, **591–592**
in HNPCC, 592
hyperplastic, 589
juvenile familial, 592
nasal, 199–200
allergic rhinitis and, 196, 199
of small intestine, 567, **589**, 591
vocal fold, 209
Polyradiculoneuropathy
in cytomegalovirus infection, 1246
in Guillain-Barré syndrome, 925
in HIV infection/AIDS, 924
in Lyme disease, 924
Polyradiculopathy, in HIV infection/AIDS, 924
Polysomnography, 288
Polystyrene sulfonate, for hyperkalemia, 799t
Polysurgery (surgery proneness), 988, 989
somatization disorder and, 944
Polyuria
in Cushing syndrome, 1051
in diabetes insipidus, 996
in diabetes mellitus, 1082t, 1083
in hypercalcemia/hyperparathyroidism, 801, 1034
lithium causing, 971
in obstructive uropathy, 845
in tubulointerstitial disease, 845, 846
Pomeroy tubal resection, 701
Pompholyx (vesiculobullous hand eczema), **116–117**
Ponstel. See Mefenamic acid
Popliteal arteries
acute occlusion of, 419
atherosclerotic/occlusive disease of, **416–417**
Popliteal (Baker) cyst, 33, 744
Popliteal tenosynovitis, 746
Porcelain gallbladder, 635t, 636, 1462
Pork. See also Meat
in gnathostomiasis, 1384
in trichinosis, 1383

Pork tapeworm (*T solium*), 1376, **1376**
cysticercosis and, 1376, 1377–1378
Porphobilinogen, urinary
in porphyria, 1512
reference values for, 1553t
Porphobilinogen deaminase, deficiency of in porphyria, 1512
Porphyria
acute intermittent, 923, **1512–1513**, 1513t
cutanea tarda, **117–118**, 142, 143
peripheral nerve involvement in, 923, 1512
variegate, 923
Porphyrins, urine, in porphyria cutanea tarda, 117
Portal decompression, for esophageal varices, 540
Portal hypertension
ascites in, 524, 524t
cirrhosis and, 621
malignant, 527, 528
cirrhosis and, 619, 620, 620–621
esophageal varices and, 517–518, 538–539
GI bleeding in, 517–518, 538–539
in myelofibrosis, 460
noncirrhotic, **631–632**
Portal hypertensive gastropathy, 544, 545. See also Portal hypertension
Portal vein thrombosis, noncirrhotic portal hypertension caused by, 631, 632
Portopulmonary hypertension, 623–624
Portosystemic shunts
emergency/surgical, for esophageal varices, 540
rebleeding prevention and, 541
transvenous (transjugular). See Transvenous (transjugular) intrahepatic portosystemic shunts
Posaconazole, 1401t, 1402
for aspergillosis, 1158, 1398
prophylactic, 1158
renal/hepatic failure and, 1185t
Positioning vertigo, benign paroxysmal (BPPV), 189, 191t
Positive end-expiratory pressure (PEEP)
for ARDS, 290, 292
for near drowning, 1416
Positive expiratory pressure (PEP) therapy, in cystic fibrosis, 242
Positive inotropic agents. See Inotropic agents
Positive-pressure breathing
for COPD, 238
intermittent (IPPB), prevention of postoperative pulmonary complications and, 54
Positive-pressure ventilation
for ARDS, 292
noninvasive (NPPV)
for COPD, 238
for respiratory failure, 290
for respiratory failure, 290

Positron emission tomography (PET)
in angina, 320
for breast cancer screening/evaluation, 655, 657, 659–660
for lung cancer staging, 1455
in myocardial hibernation/stunning, 317, 320
in pancreatic/periampullary carcinoma, 1464
in pheochromocytoma/paraganglioma, 1060
in solitary pulmonary nodule, 260
in thyroid cancer evaluation/surveillance, 1024, 1028
Postcapillary pulmonary hypertension, 274
Postcardiotomy/postmyocardial infarction pericarditis (Dressler syndrome), 339, 377, 378
Postcholecystectomy syndrome, **637**
Postcoital/emergency contraception, **700**
IUD for, 698, 700
Postdysenteric colitis, 1367
Postepileptic automatism, 880
Posterior blepharitis, 152
Posterior cerebral artery occlusion, in stroke, 889
Posterior cruciate ligament, of knee, assessment of, 34–35
Posterior drawer ("sag") test, in knee pain, 34–35
Posterior inferior cerebellar artery obstruction, in stroke, 891
Posterior ischemic optic neuropathy, 168
Posterior nasal cavity, epistaxis originating in, 198–199
Posterior synechiae, in uveitis, 160
Posterior uveitis, 160. See also Uveitis
Postethanol reactive hypoglycemia, 1121
Postgastrectomy alimentary hypoglycemia, 1117, 1117t, **1121**
Postgonococcal urethritis/cervicitis, 1320, 1328
Postherpetic neuralgia, 115, 115–116, **877–878**, 1241, 1242
varicella vaccine in prevention of, 5, 115, 877, 878, 1194–1197t
Posthypercapnia alkalosis, 813, 814
Post-hypnotic suggestion, 1539
Posthypocapnia acidosis, 810
Postictal period, 880
pseudoseizures and, 881, 944
Postinfarction ischemia/angina, 336
Postinfectious glomerulonephritis, **834**, 835f, 836t, 1289
Postinfectious irritable bowel syndrome, 570
Postinflammatory hyperpigmentation, 144
Post-kala azar dermal leishmaniasis, 1351
Post-Lyme disease syndrome, 1346t, 1347
Postmenopausal depression, estrogen replacement therapy and, 1071–1072
Postmenopausal vaginal bleeding, **676**
endometrial carcinoma and, 676
Postmyocardial infarction/postcardiotomy pericarditis (Dressler syndrome), 339, 377, 378

Postnasal drip, cough caused by, 22, 23t
Postoperative cognitive dysfunction, 56, 56t
Postoperative fever, 1160
Postoperative hyponatremia, 790
Postoperative pain
acupuncture for, 1533
mind-body therapies for, 1536t
Postpartum depression, 962
Postpartum infection
anaerobic, 1323
C sordellii causing, 1298
mastitis, **720**
streptococcal, 725
Postpartum psychosis, 962
Postpartum thyroiditis, 1008, 1015, 1016, 1017, 1018
Postphlebitic syndrome, 37
Postpoliomyelitis syndrome, 1253
Postpolypectomy hemorrhage, 521
Postpolypectomy surveillance, 590
Postprandial (reactive) hypoglycemia, 1117, 1117t, **1121–1122**.
See also Hypoglycemia
postethanol, 1121
Postrenal azotemia. See Azotemia
Post-thrombotic syndrome, 430
Posttransfusion purpura (PTP), **488**
Posttransplant lymphoproliferative disorder, 1243, 1244
Posttraumatic epilepsy/seizure disorder, 878
Posttraumatic headache, **875**
Posttraumatic stress disorder, **938–939**
abuse victims and, 938, 976, 977
substance use and, 938, 977
Posttraumatic syringomyelia, 920
Posttraumatic vertigo, 190
Postural drainage
in bronchiectasis, 240
in chronic bronchitis, 238
in cystic fibrosis, 242
Postural hypotension. See Orthostatic (postural) hypotension
Postural instability. See Falls; Gait/gait disorders
Postural tremor, drug-induced, 911
Posture stimulation test, in aldosteronism, 1056
Potassium
dietary/replacement, 1146
for diabetic ketoacidosis, 1114
diuretic use and, 398
in fluid management, 815, 815t
for hyperglycemic hyperosmolar state, 1016
hypertension and, 390, 394
for hypokalemia, 796–798
for metabolic alkalosis, 813
requirements for in nutritional support, 1149
restriction of, in chronic kidney disease, 830
disorders of concentration of, **795–798**. See also Hyperkalemia; Hypokalemia
genetic disorders and, 796t

in hyperchloremic normal anion gap acidosis/renal tubular acidosis, 809t
reference values for, 1553t
Potassium chloride. See Potassium, dietary/replacement
Potassium citrate
for hypocitraturic calcium nephrolithiasis, 859
for uric acid calculi, 859
Potassium concentration gradient, transtubular (TTKG), 796
Potassium iodide, in table salt, goiter prevention/treatment and, 1029–1030
Potassium-sparing diuretics
for heart failure, 361
lithium interactions and, 972, 972t
Potomania, beer, 791
Pott disease (spinal tuberculosis), **781–782**
Pott puffy tumor, 194
Potts shunt, for tetralogy of Fallot, 300
Pouchitis, 586
Poultry, avian influenza and, 5, 1271, 1272
Powassan encephalitis, 1257–1259
Power of attorney, durable, for health care, 90
Poxvirus infections, **1277–1278**. See also specific type
pp65 antigen, in cytomegalovirus infection, 1246
PPAR-α. See Peroxisome proliferator-activated receptor alpha
PPAR-γ. See Peroxisome proliferator-activated receptor gamma
PPARG gene. See also Peroxisome proliferator-activated receptor gamma
in insulin resistance, 1081
PPD (purified protein derivative) test, 253, 253t. See also Tuberculin skin test
PPV (pneumococcal polysaccharide vaccine). See Pneumococcal vaccine
PR3-ANCA. See Antineutrophil cytoplasmic antibody; Proteinase-3 ANCA
PRA. See Plasma renin activity
Pralidoxime, for cholinesterase inhibitor (anticholinesterase) poisoning, 1424t, 1443–1444
nerve agents and, 1434
PrameGel. See Pramoxine
Pramipexole, for parkinsonism, 907
Pramlintide, 1091t, 1095–1096
Pramosone. See Hydrocortisone; Pramoxine
Pramoxine, 94, 98t
Prandin. See Repaglinide
Prasugrel
for acute coronary syndromes, 328
for myocardial infarction, 332, 340
Pravachol. See Pravastatin
Pravastatin, 1124, 1131, 1132t. See also Statin drugs
in HIV infection/AIDS, 1229
in older patients, 1128–1129

Prax. *See* Pramoxine
Prayer, in complementary/alternative medicine, 1520
Praziquantel
    for clonorchiasis/opisthorchiasis, 1375
    for cysticercosis, 1378
    for intestinal flukes, 1376
    for paragonimiasis, 1376
    for schistosomiasis, 1374
    for tapeworm infections, 1377
Prazosin
    for benign prostatic hyperplasia, 869, 869*t*
    for hypertension, 407, 408*t*
    for urinary incontinence, 72
Pre-Gen Plus. *See* Multitarget DNA tests
Prebreakfast hyperglycemia, 1102–1103, 1103*t*
Precholecystectomy syndrome, **637**
Precose. *See* Acarbose
Prediabetes, 1087
PredMild. *See* Prednisolone
Prednicarbate, 96*t*
Prednisolone
    for asthma, 224*t*, 229*t*
    for ophthalmic disorders, 175*t*
Prednisone, 1077, 1077*t*. *See also specific disease and* Corticosteroids
    for allergic contact dermatitis, 119
    for asthma, 224*t*, 229*t*, 230
    for autoimmune hemolytic anemia, 453
    for autoimmune hepatitis, 613
    for Bell palsy, 929
    in cancer chemotherapy, 1506*t*
    for chronic inflammatory polyneuropathy, 926
    for erythema nodosum leprosum, 1327
    for giant cell arteritis, 165, 767
    for inflammatory bowel disease, 575–576
        Crohn disease, 581
        ulcerative colitis, 584, 584*t*
    for microscopic polyangiitis, 770
    for minimal change disease, 840
    in pain management, 86
    perioperative, 58
    for *Pneumocystis* infection, 1395
    for polymyalgia rheumatica, 767
    for prostate cancer, 1487*t*
    for Wegener granulomatosis, 769
Preeclampsia-eclampsia, 392, **715–718**, 717*t*, 723
    antihypertensive therapy in, 718, 723
    in gestational trophoblastic disease, 715
    headache and, 44, 716
    hypermagnesemia associated with treatment of, 806
    late-onset (postpartum), 718
Preexcitation syndromes, **345–346**
    palpitations in, 31
Pregabalin
    for painful diabetic neuropathy/neuropathic pain, 85, 85*t*, 1107
    for seizures, 882*t*

Pregnancy, **705–728**
    acne treatment and, 121–122
    adverse ophthalmic effects of drugs used in, 177*t*
    air travel during, 710, 1419
    alcohol use during, 707, 979
    amenorrhea (primary/secondary) caused by, 709, 1068, 1068–1069, 1070
    anemia during, 439, 708, **721**
    antipsychotic drug use during, 959
    appendicitis during, 568, **728**
    asthma during, **724**
    bleeding during
        ectopic pregnancy and, 713
        in gestational trophoblastic disease, 714–715
        third-trimester, **720**
    breast cancer and, 660, 672, **728**
    breast cancer risk and, 653, 653*t*
    C trachomatis infection and, **727**
    cardiac disease and, **724**
    cardiomyopathy of (peripartum cardiomyopathy), **385**, 724, 1000
    choledocholithiasis during, **727–728**
    cholelithiasis/cholecystitis during, 634, **727–728**
    cholestasis of, 599*t*, **727–728**
    chorioamnionitis and, **720–721**
    in chronic kidney disease, 830
    complications of
        cardiovascular, **384–385**, 724, 1000
        during first and second trimesters, **710–715**
        infectious conditions, **724–727**
        medical conditions, **721–724**
        peripartum, **720–721**
        during second and third trimesters, **715–720**
        surgical complications, **727–728**
    coxsackievirus infection during, neonatal myocarditis and, 1279
    cytomegalovirus infection during, 1246–1247
    diabetes mellitus and, **722–723**, 723*t*, 1110
        continuous glucose monitoring systems and, 1085
    diagnosis/differential diagnosis of, **705**
    drug/medication use/avoidance during, 706, 706*t*, 707. *See also specific agent*
    ectopic, **713–714**
        hCG levels in, 705, 713
        IUDs and, 698
    endocarditis prophylaxis during, 385
    fatty liver of, 617, **718–719**
    fever during, 38–39
    folic acid deficiency during, 721
    gallbladder disease/surgery during, **727–728**
    glycosuria and, 1086
    gonorrhea and, **727**
    group B streptococcal infection and, 708, **725**, 1291

    headache during, preeclampsia and, 44, 716
    heart disease and, **384–385**, 724, 724*t*, 1000
    hepatitis B and, 602, **726–727**
        vaccination recommendations and, 606, 706, 726, 1187, 1195*t*
    hepatitis C and, 604, **726–727**
    hepatitis E and, 604, 606
    herbal medicine use during, 1522*t*
    herpes infection during, **727**, 1236, 1237
    HIV infection/AIDS in, **726**, 1207, 1221
    hyperparathyroidism during, 1034
    hypertension and, 391, 392, **715–718**, 717*t*, 723–724. *See also* Preeclampsia-eclampsia
    hyperthyroidism/Graves disease during, 722, 1008–1009, 1009, 1010, 1013
        thiourea drugs and, 722, 1011
        thyroidectomy for, 1012, 1013
    hypoosmolality of, reset osmostat and, 791
    hypothyroidism during, 722, 1003
    immune thrombocytopenic purpura associated with, 484
    immunizations during, 4, 710, 1195*t*
    influenza vaccination and, 706, 710, 1195*t*
    iron requirements/deficiency anemia during, 439, 721
    IUDs and, 698
    lactation and, **709–710**, 710*t*
    listeriosis during, 1303
    lupus anticoagulant-anticardiolipin-antiphospholipid antibody syndrome and, **721–722**, 755
    Lyme disease and, 1343, 1346
    lymphocytic choriomeningitis and, 1259
    malaria treatment/chemoprophylaxis during, 1358, 1359, 1360, 1361
    manifestations of, 705
    Marfan syndrome and, 385
    mask of. *See* Melasma
    maternal virilization during, 1054
    measles/measles vaccine during, 1248, 1249
    mitral stenosis and, 306–307
    MMR vaccination and, 1195*t*, 1199, 1249
    molar (hydatidiform mole), **714–715**. *See also* Gestational trophoblastic disease
        hyperthyroidism in, 715, 1009
    myomectomy during, 683
    nutrition in, **708–709**
    ovarian tumors during, **728**
    parathyroidectomy during, 1036
    parvovirus B19 infection in, 1276
    preeclampsia-eclampsia in, **715–718**, 717*t*
        hypermagnesemia associated with treatment of, 806

Pregnancy (*cont.*)
  prenatal care and, **705–708**, 706*t*
  preterm (premature) labor and,
    719–720
  prevention of hemolytic disease of
    newborn (erythroblastosis
    fetalis) and, **709**
  prolactinoma in, 1001
  prosthetic heart valves and, 316
  Q fever during, 1286, 1287
  rabies vaccination during, 1256
  radiation exposure during, 707, 1414
  respiratory alkalosis in, 814
  Rh incompatibility and, 706, 708, 709.
    See also Rh$_0$ (D) immune
    globulin
  rubella exposure/rubella vaccination
    and, 1195*t*, 1199, 1254–1255
  scabies during, 137
  screening tests in. *See* Prenatal testing
  seizures/seizure treatment and, **724**,
    881–883
    in eclampsia, 716, 718
  sexually transmitted disorders and,
    727
  sickle cell anemia and, 721
  smoking during, 707
    bupropion therapy for cessation
      and, 11*t*
    nicotine therapy for cessation and,
      10*t*, 11*t*
  streptococcal infection and, 708, **725**
  syphilis during, **727**, **1338**
  termination of
    by delivery
      in acute fatty liver of pregnancy,
        718, 719
      in diabetic patient, 723, 1110
      in preeclampsia-eclampsia, 716,
        717, 718
    by elective abortion. *See* Abortion,
      elective/induced
    by recurrent (habitual) abortion,
      712–713
    by spontaneous abortion, **711–712**
  thrombocytopenia during, **489**
  thrombotic microangiopathies dur-
    ing, 485
  thyroid disease during, **722**
    hyperthyroidism, 722, 1008–1009,
      1009, 1010, 1013
    hypothyroidism, 722, 1003
    thyroid cancer treatment and, 1026
    thyroiditis and, 1008, 1015, 1016,
      1017
  toxoplasmosis during, 1363, 1364,
    1365
  travel and, **710**
  traveler's diarrhea during, 710
  trophoblastic disease and, **714–715**.
    See also Gestational tro-
    phoblastic disease
  tuberculosis/tuberculosis treatment
    during, 256, **726**
  ultrasonography during, ectopic preg-
    nancy and, 713
  urinary tract infection during,
    724–725
    varicella (chickenpox)/varicella vac-
      cine during, **725–726**,
      1195*t*, 1241, 1242
    vomiting of, 504, **710–711**
      acupuncture for, 1534
      gestational trophoblastic disease
        and, 714
    weight gain in, 706, 708
    yellow fever vaccination and, 1203,
      1266
Pregnancy-associated plasma protein-A
    (PAPP-A), testing for, 706
Pregnancy tests, 705. *See also* Human
    chorionic gonadotropin
  in amenorrhea, 1068, 1070
  in ectopic pregnancy, 713
  for rape victim, 702
  in spontaneous abortion, 712
Prehn sign, 856
Prehypertension, **387–388**, 388*t*
  treatment of, 388*t*, 395
Prekallikrein deficiency, 494
Preleukemia, 463. *See also* Myelodysplas-
    tic syndromes
Premarin cream. *See* Estrogen vaginal
    creams
Premature beats. *See* Atrial (supraventric-
    ular) premature beats;
    Ventricular premature
    beats
Premature ejaculation, 862, 949. *See also*
    Erectile dysfunction/impo-
    tence
Premature (preterm) labor, prevention of,
    719–720
Premature ovarian failure, 1069
  in Turner syndrome, 1074
Premenopausal bleeding
  abnormal, **674–676**
    in polycystic ovary syndrome, 690
  normal menstrual, 674. *See also* Men-
    struation; Vaginal bleeding
Premenstrual dysphoric disorder,
    676–677, 962
Premenstrual syndrome/tension, **676–677**
Premphase. *See* Estrogens, with progestins
Prempro. *See* Estrogens, with progestins
Prenatal care, **705–708**, 706*t*
Prenatal testing/diagnosis, 706, 707–708.
    See also Genetic testing
  for Down syndrome, 706, 1514
  for Gaucher disease, 1516
  for muscular dystrophy, 935
  for sickle cell disease, 450
  for syphilis, 706
  for toxoplasmosis, 1364
Prenatal vitamins, 706, 708–709
Preoperative evaluation/perioperative
    management, **49–60**. *See*
    also specific type of disorder
  adverse ophthalmic effects of agents
    used in, 177*t*
  antibiotic prophylaxis and, **59–60**, 60*t*
  asymptomatic patient and, 49, 50*t*
  cardiovascular disorders and, **49–53**,
    50*t*, 51*f*, 51*t*
  endocrine disorders and, **57–58**, 57*t*,
    58*t*
    hematologic disorders and, **55–56**, 56*t*
    kidney disease and, **58–59**, 59*t*
    liver disease and, **54–55**
    neurologic disorders and, **56–57**, 56*t*
    pulmonary disorders and, for non-
      lung resection surgery,
      53–54, 53*t*
Prepatellar bursitis, 33, 743
Prerenal azotemia. *See* Azotemia
Presbyacusis (hearing impairment in
    elderly), **75**, 179, 186
Presbyopia, 151
Preservatives, ocular, toxic/hypersensitiv-
    ity reactions to, 155, 176
Pressure sores (decubitus ulcers), **72–74**,
    73*t*
  bed rest/immobility and, 68, 73
Preterm (premature) labor, prevention of,
    719–720
Pretibial myxedema (Graves dermopa-
    thy), 1008, 1009, 1015
Preven, for emergency/postcoital contra-
    ception, 700
Preventive care, **1–21**. *See also specific dis-*
    ease
  adherence and, **1–2**
  principles of care and, **2**
  recommendations for, 2, 3*t*
Prevotella, 1176*t*, 1321
  melaninogenica, 1321, 1322
  resistant strains of, 1322
Prezista/Norvir. *See* Darunavir, with
    ritonavir
Priapism (prolonged painful erection)
  erectile dysfunction therapy causing,
    863, 1108
  trazodone causing, 967
Primaquine
  for malaria, 1355*t*, 1356, 1357,
    1358–1359
    chemoprophylaxis, 1355*t*, 1359,
      1361, 1361*t*
  for *P jiroveci* infection, 1224*t*, 1395
Primary effusion (body cavity) lym-
    phoma, 1247
Primary lateral sclerosis, 920
Primary sclerosing cholangitis, **640–641**
  cholangiocarcinoma and, 641, 1462
  in HIV infection/AIDS, 1214
Primaxin. *See* Imipenem
Primidone, for seizures, 881, 882*t*, 1545*t*
Prinivil. *See* Lisinopril
Prinzmetal (variant) angina, 325
Prion disease, **1260–1261**
PRK. *See* Photorefractive keratectomy
Probenecid
  allopurinol interactions and, 735
  for gout, 734
Probiotics
  for antibiotic-associated colitis, 575
  for irritable bowel syndrome, 572–578
Problem drinking, 978, 979–980. *See also*
    Alcohol use/dependency/
    abuse
  differential diagnosis of, 979
Procainamide, 343*t*, 1545*t*
  antidepressant drug interactions and,
    969*t*

for arrhythmias, 343t
ventricular tachycardia, 352
overdose/toxicity of, 343t, 1445
Procarbazine, 1500t
antidepressant drug interactions and, 969t
Procardia. See Nifedipine
Prochlorperazine, 506t, 1509. See also Antiemetics
overdose/toxicity of, 1444–1445
Procollagen, in nephrogenic systemic fibrosis, 849
Procrit (epoetin alfa). See Erythropoietin
Proctitis, 594
chlamydial, 594, 1328
diarrhea and, 511–512
herpes simplex, 1236, 1239
radiation, 521
in syphilis, 594
Proctocolectomy
for familial adenomatous polyposis, 591
for ulcerative colitis, 586
Proctocolitis, chlamydial, 594
Proctosigmoiditis, in ulcerative colitis, 582
Proctosigmoidoscopy. See Sigmoidoscopy
Procyclidine, 906t. See also Antiparkinsonism drugs
Prodromal schizophrenia, 952
Profunda femoris artery, atherosclerotic/occlusive disease of, 416
Progesterone. See also Progestins
in estrogen replacement therapy, 1071
receptors for, in breast cancer, 663
prognosis and, 665t, 670
therapy and, 663, 666, 667
serum levels of
in infertility workup, 692–693
for pregnancy testing, 705
ectopic pregnancy and, 713
topical, 1071
Progesterone-releasing IUDs, 1071
Progestin minipill, 696t, 697
Progestin withdrawal test, in amenorrhea evaluation, 1069
Progestins
for abnormal premenopausal bleeding, 675
in cancer chemotherapy, 1506t
in combination oral contraceptives, 695t
in estrogen replacement therapy, 703, 704, 1070, 1071, 1072–1073
long-acting (contraceptive injections/implants), 697
for postmenopausal vaginal bleeding, 676
Prognostic Burn Index, 1409
Progressive bulbar palsy, 920, 921
Progressive massive pulmonary fibrosis, 278
Progressive multifocal leukoencephalopathy, 1212, 1261
natalizumab causing, 913, 1261
Progressive spinal muscular atrophy, 920, 921

Progressive supranuclear palsy, parkinsonism differentiated from, 906
Proguanil
with atovaquone (Malarone), 1355t, 1357t, 1360
for malaria chemoprophylaxis, 1355t, 1360, 1361, 1361t
self-treatment and, 1361
during pregnancy, 710
Proinsulin
in factitious hypoglycemia, 1118
in insulinoma, 1062, 1118
Prolactin (PRL)
GH-secreting tumor cosecretion of, 998, 1001
serum levels of. See also Hyperprolactinemia
in infertility workup, 693, 864
in pseudoseizure identification, 881, 944
reference values for, 1553t
tumors secreting, 1000, 1001, 1002
Prolactinoma, 1000, 1001, 1002
Proleukin. See Aldesleukin
Proliferative bronchiolitis, 243. See also Bronchiolitis
Proliferative indices, in breast cancer, 663
Proliferative retinopathy, 166, 1105
Prolixin. See Fluphenazine
Promethazine, 506t. See also Antiemetics
overdose/toxicity of, 1444–1445
Prometrium. See Progestins
Pronator teres syndrome, 927
PROP1 gene mutation, in hypopituitarism, 991, 992
Propafenone, 343t
for atrial fibrillation, 348, 349
overdose/toxicity of, 343t, 1445
Propanil, methemoglobinemia caused by, 1440
Propecia. See Finasteride
Prophylactic antibiotics. See Antimicrobial chemoprophylaxis
Propine. See Dipivefrin
Propionibacterium acnes, 120. See also Acne
Propoxyphene
benzodiazepine interactions and, 942t
overdose/toxicity of, 1442–1443
Propranolol. See also Beta-adrenergic blocking drugs
for aggressive/violent behavior, 976, 987
antidepressant drug interactions and, 969t
for arrhythmias, 343t
for Graves disease/hyperthyroidism, 1010–1011
for hypertension, 401t
for migraine prophylaxis, 874t
overdose/toxicity of, 343t, 1432
for panic attacks, 943
Proptosis (exophthalmos), in dysthyroid eye/Graves disease, 170, 1008, 1009, 1012, 1014
Propylene glycol, lactic acidosis and, 808

Propylthiouracil, for Graves disease/hyperthyroidism, 1011
during pregnancy/lactation, 722, 1011, 1013
RAI therapy and, 1012
toxic solitary thyroid nodule and, 1012
ProQuad. See MMRV (measles-mumps-rubella-varicella) vaccine
Prosom. See Estazolam
Prosopagnosia, intracranial tumors causing, 899
Prostacyclin, for pulmonary hypertension, 275
Prostaglandin analogs. See also specific agent
for glaucoma/ocular hypertension, 159, 175–176t
Prostaglandins
in erectile dysfunction, 863
vascular evaluation and, 863
hyponatremia caused by, 790
NSAIDs affecting, 548
Prostate cancer, 1467t, 1484–1489, 1485t, 1487t, 1488t
hormone therapy for, 1487–1488, 1487t
incidence/risk/mortality of, 1450, 1484, 1488, 1488t
localized, 1486
locally/regionally advanced, 1487
metastatic, 1487–1488
paraneoplastic syndromes and, 1453t
pathology/staging of, 1486
screening for, 16, 17t, 1484, 1485–1486, 1485t
testosterone replacement therapy and, 1065–1066
Prostate gland
benign hyperplasia of, 866–871, 867t, 868f, 869t. See also Benign prostatic hyperplasia
biopsy of, 1484
cancer of. See Prostate cancer
electrovaporization of, 871
inflammation/infection of. See Prostatitis
minimally invasive surgery on, 871
photovaporization of (PVP), 871
transurethral incision of (TUIP), 869t, 870
transurethral needle ablation of (TUNA), 871
transurethral resection of (TURP), 869t, 870
Prostate-specific antigen (PSA), 1484, 1485–1486, 1485t
in benign prostatic hyperplasia, 867
in prostate cancer, 1484, 1485t
in CAPRA assessment tool, 1488, 1488t
screening and, 16, 17t, 1484, 1485–1486, 1485t
reference values for, 1553t
age-specific, 1485
Prostate-specific antigen (PSA) density, in cancer screening, 1485
Prostate-specific antigen (PSA) velocity, in cancer screening, 1485

Prostatectomy
open, for benign prostatic hyperplasia, 869t, 870–871
radical, for prostate cancer, 1486
transurethral laser-induced (TULIP), for benign prostatic hyperplasia, 871
transurethral (TURP), for benign prostatic hyperplasia, 869t, 870
Prostatic pain, in acute bacterial prostatitis, 853
Prostatitis
acute bacterial, 852t, **853–854**, 855t
chronic bacterial, 852t, **854**, 855t
gonococcal, 1319
nonbacterial, **855**, 855t
Prostatodynia, **855–856**, 855t
Prostep. See Nicotine, for replacement therapy
Prostheses
arterial/endovascular. See Bypass grafting
for joint replacement
coagulase-negative staphylococcal infection and, 1296
osteomyelitis and, 780
penile, 863
Prosthetic heart valves, **315–316**. See also Valve replacement
anticoagulant therapy and, 316
pregnancy and, 316
coagulase-negative staphylococcal infection and, 1296–1297
endocarditis and, 1296–1297, 1304, 1307
anticoagulation and, 1307
Protease
in absorption/digestion, 558
in pancreatic enzyme supplements, 647t
Protease inhibitors, 1226–1227t, 1228–1230, 1232f. See also Antiretroviral therapy
antituberculous drug interactions and, 255–256
in combinations, 1227, 1232f
for hepatitis C, 612
lipid abnormalities caused by, 1216, 1229
ritonavir boosting and, 1229
Protein
ascitic fluid, 525
bacterial peritonitis and, 526, 621
pancreatic ascites and, 528, 644
peritoneal carcinomatosis and, 528
tuberculous peritonitis and, 527
cerebrospinal fluid, in CNS infection, 1162t
dietary, 1146
absorption/digestion of, 557–558
deficiency of (protein–energy malnutrition), **1134–1135**
nephrotic syndrome and, 839
requirements for in nutritional support, 1149
restriction of. See Protein-restricted diet
in urinary stone formation, 857

pleural fluid, 283
total serum
in liver disease/jaundice, 600t
reference/normal values for, 600t, 1553t
urinary. See also Proteinuria
ratio of to urinary creatinine, 817
Protein C
activated
for bacteremia/sepsis/shock, 437, 1312
resistance to, hypercoagulability and, 267
reference values for, 1553t
Protein-calorie undernutrition. See Protein-energy malnutrition
Protein/creatinine urinary concentration, 817. See also Proteinuria
Protein electrophoresis
in myeloma, 472
in protein-losing enteropathy, 569
reference values for, 1553t
urinary, in overload proteinuria, 817
in Waldenström macroglobulinemia, 474
Protein–energy malnutrition, **1134–1135**
Protein-losing enteropathy, **569**
GI lymphoma and, 1475
in measles, 1249
in Whipple disease, 561
Protein malnutrition, in nephrotic syndrome, 839
Protein-restricted diet, 1146
for chronic kidney disease, 830, 1146
for diabetes mellitus, 1089
for hepatic encephalopathy, 620, 622, 1146
for nephrotic syndrome, 839
for urinary stones, 857
Protein S, 1553t
Proteinase-3 ANCA (PR3-ANCA). See also Antineutrophil cytoplasmic antibody
in Wegener granulomatosis, 768
Proteinosis, pulmonary alveolar, **266**
Proteinuria, 816–817
Bence Jones. See Bence Jones proteinuria
in diabetes mellitus/diabetic nephropathy, 842, 1105, 1106
by dipstick, 817
in glomerulonephritis, 825
in IgA nephropathy, 836
membranous nephropathy management and, 841
in nephrotic syndrome, 838
in preeclampsia-eclampsia, 716, 717t
in sickle cell disease/glomerulopathy, 849
in SLE, 754t, 843
in tubulointerstitial disease, 846
Proteus
miribilis, 1176t
vulgaris, 1177t
Prothrombin (factor II)
acquired antibodies to, **494**
deficiency of, 494

des-gamma-carboxy, in hepatocellular carcinoma, 1460
Prothrombin time
in alcoholic liver disease, 614, 615
in anticoagulant overdose/toxicity, 1430, 1431
in liver disease/jaundice, 494, 600t
in monitoring in warfarin therapy, 272
prolonged
in cirrhosis, 494, 619
in vitamin K deficiency, 494
reference/normal values for, 600t, 1553t
Proton pump inhibitors
for Barrett esophagus, 532
for dyspepsia, 503, 504
for dysphagia, 543
gastrin levels affected by, 550, 556
for GERD/esophagitis, 531, 533, 534
in H pylori eradication therapy, 550, 550–551, 551t
H pylori test results affected by, 546, 549
for laryngopharyngeal reflux, 208–209
for NSAID gastritis, 545
for NSAID toxicity mitigation, 78, 552, 749
for peptic stricture, 533
for peptic ulcer disease, 550, 552
bleeding management and, 519, 554
prevention and, 552
refractory ulcers and, 553
for stress gastritis, 545
for Zollinger-Ellison syndrome/gastrinoma, 557
Protopam. See Pralidoxime
Protopic. See Tacrolimus, topical
Protoporphyrin, free erythrocyte, 1550t
Protozoal infections, **1348–1373**. See also specific type and organism
diarrhea in, 512t
myocarditis in, 369t
Protriptyline, 968t
Provera. See Progesterone
Providencia, 1177t
Provocation testing. See also specific test
Proximal renal tubular acidosis, 809t, 810. See also Renal tubular acidosis
genetic defects associated with, 796t
Prozac. See Fluoxetine
Prozone phenomenon, 1332
PrP^C/PrP^{Sc}, in prion disease, 1260
PRSS1 gene, in chronic pancreatitis, 646
Pruritus (itching), 95t, **136–140**. See also specific cause
ani, 136, 596–597
anogenital. See Anogenital/perianal pruritus
in biliary cirrhosis, 625, 626
in cutaneous larva migrans, 1385
in decompression sickness (skin bends), 1417
in diabetes, 136, 1082t, 1083
drugs for
systemic, 94–95
topical, 94, 98t, 137

of ear canal, **181**
in hypercalcemia/hyperparathyroidism, 1034
in lichen simplex chronicus, 103
in onchocerciasis, 1387, 1388
in polycythemia, 457
in renal failure/uremia, 136
vulvae, 136
PRV. *See* Rotavirus vaccine
PSA. *See* Prostate-specific antigen
Pseudallescheria boydii, in opportunistic infection, 1402
Pseudoachalasia, 542
Pseudo-addiction, pain management in terminally ill/dying patient and, 78
Pseudoallergic (anaphylactoid) reactions, **785–786**
Pseudoaneurysm
GI bleeding and, 518
myocardial rupture and, 339
Pseudobacteremia, 1160
Pseudobulbar palsy, 920, 921
Pseudoclaudication, of spinal stenosis, 740, 741
Pseudocysts
pancreatic, 642, 644, 645, 648
vocal fold, 209
Pseudodementia (depression and dementia), 63, 986
Pseudoephedrine, MAOI interactions and, 969t
Pseudoepileptic seizures. *See* Pseudoseizures
Pseudofolliculitis, 123
Pseudogout, 733, **735–736**
Pseudohermaphroditism, 1068
Pseudohypoaldosteronism
type I, 796t
type II, 796t
Pseudohyponatremia, 789, 792
Pseudohypoparathyroidism, 1031–1032, 1034f. *See also* Hypoparathyroidism
Pseudomembrane, in diphtheria, 204, 1302, 1303
Pseudomembranous colitis, 574. *See also* Colitis, antibiotic-associated
Pseudomonas aeruginosa, 1177t
burn-associated infection caused by, 1411
eye medications contaminated by, 172–176
hot tub folliculitis caused by, 123, 124
keratitis caused by, 156
malignant external otitis, 181
pneumonia caused by, 244t
Pseudomonic acid. *See* Mupirocin
Pseudo-obstruction, intestinal
acute (Ogilvie syndrome), **565–566**
chronic, **566**
Pseudopapilledema, 169
Pseudoporphyria, 117
Pseudoprecocious puberty, testicular tumors causing, 1066
Pseudopseudohypoparathyroidism, 1032
Pseudoseizures, 881, 944

Pseudoseptic arthritis, 777. *See also* Septic (nongonococcal acute bacterial) arthritis
Pseudothrombocytopenia, **489**
Pseudotumor
cerebri, **903**
headache and, 876, 903
lithium use and, 971
pleural fluid, 284
Psilocybin, 982
hallucinogenic *(Psilocybe)* mushroom poisoning and, 1441, 1441t, 1442
Psittacosis (ornithosis), 1177t, 1327, **1329**
Psoas sign, in appendicitis, 567
Psoralen plus ultraviolet A (PUVA) therapy
for atopic dermatitis, 103
for lichen planus, 135
for psoriasis, 105
Psoriasiform eruptions, drugs causing, 149t
Psoriasis, **103–105**
arthritis and, 104, **775–776**
drugs causing, 149t
exfoliative dermatitis and (erythrodermic psoriasis), 104, 105, 112
in HIV infection/AIDS, 104, 1215
lithium use and, 971
Psoriatic arthritis, 104, **775–776**
in HIV infection/AIDS, 779, 1213
Psoriatic erythroderma, 104, 105
Psoriatic spondylitis, 775
PSS1 mutation, pancreatic/periampullary carcinoma and, 1463
PSTI gene, in chronic pancreatitis, 646
Psychedelic drug abuse, **982**
Psychiatric/psychologic disorders, **937–990.** *See also specific type*
biofeedback in management of, 1538
chest pain and, 544
in elderly, urinary incontinence and, 70
fatigue/chronic fatigue syndrome and, 43
hospitalization and illness and, **988–990**
irritable bowel syndrome and, 570, 571
in Wilson disease, 629
Psychogenic polydipsia, 791, 953, 997
Psychologic challenges, for terminally ill/dying patient, **92**
Psychologic disorders. *See* Psychiatric/psychologic disorders
Psychologic drug dependence, 977
Psychopathic (antisocial) personality disorder, 950, 951, 951t
Psychosexual disorders, **948–950**
sexual dysfunction and, 949, 950. *See also* Sexual dysfunction
Psychosurgery, for OCD, 943
Psychotic depression, 953, 963, 964, 966
Psychotic disorders (psychoses), **952–961.** *See also* Schizophrenic disorders
alcohol withdrawal and (delirium tremens), 978

alcoholic (organic) hallucinosis, 978–979, 979, 980, 986
atypical, 953
brief, 953
classification of, 952–953
delusions and, 952
depression and, 953, 963, 964, 966
differential diagnosis of, 954
drug-induced/toxic, 954
drug therapy for, 954–960, 955t, 956t, 958t. *See also* Antipsychotic drugs
in hypothyroidism (myxedema madness), 1005
intensive care unit, 988
Korsakoff, 979
late life (in elderly), 953
mania differentiated from, 954
postpartum, 962
suicide risk and, 953, 955, 963
Psychotropic agents. *See also* Antianxiety drugs; Antidepressants; Antipsychotic drugs
for irritable bowel syndrome, 572
thrombocytopenia caused by, 483t
Psyllium fiber, 509t. *See also* Fiber, dietary
PT. *See* Prothrombin time
PTC. *See* Percutaneous transhepatic cholangiography
PTCA. *See* Percutaneous transluminal coronary angioplasty
PTEN multiple hamartoma syndrome (Cowden disease), 592, 1023, 1077
Pteroylmonoglutamic acid. *See* Folic acid
Pterygium, **155–156**
PTH. *See* Parathyroid hormone
PTHrP. *See* Parathyroid hormone-related protein
Ptosis
in myasthenia gravis, 932
in third nerve paralysis, 169
PTP. *See* Posttransfusion purpura
PTSD. *See* Posttraumatic stress disorder
PTT. *See* Partial thromboplastin time
Puberty
delayed, male hypogonadism and, 1064
gynecomastia during, 1067
Pubic lice, 138
Puerperal mastitis, **720**
Puestow procedure, modified, 648
Puffer fish poisoning, 1446, 1446t
Puffy tumor, Pott, 194
Pulmonary alveolar proteinosis, **266**
Pulmonary angiography, in pulmonary embolism, 270
helical CT, 30, 269, 270, 271f
Pulmonary arteriopathy, plexogenic (idiopathic/primary pulmonary hypertension), 274, **380–381**, 381t
Pulmonary arteriovenous malformations, in hereditary hemorrhagic telangiectasia, 1519
Pulmonary artery catheter, in shock management, 435
Pulmonary aspiration syndromes, **277–278.** *See also* Aspiration

Pulmonary capillary wedge pressure (PCWP)
  in myocardial infarction, 331t
  in shock, 435
Pulmonary circulation disorders, **266–276**
  alveolar hemorrhage syndromes, **276**
  pulmonary hypertension, **273–276**, 274t, **380–381**, 381t
  respiratory failure caused by, 289t
  thromboembolism, **266–273**, 268t, 270t, 271f. See also Pulmonary venous thromboembolism
  vasculitis, **276**
Pulmonary cysts, hydatid, 1378
Pulmonary diffusing capacity. See Diffusing capacity
Pulmonary disorders, **215–293**. See also specific disorder and under Respiratory
  acute respiratory distress syndrome (ARDS), **291–293**, 292t
  acute respiratory failure, **289–291**, 289t
  air travel and, 1419
  airway disorders, **215–243**
  in anthrax, 1301, 1302
  in ascariasis, 1379
  in aspergillosis, 241, 1397–1398
  in blastomycosis, 1399
  chronic. See specific disorder and Chronic obstructive pulmonary disease
  circulatory, **266–276**
  in coccidioidomycosis, 1393, 1394
  cognitive disorders/delirium caused by, 985t
  cryptococcal, 1396
  decompression sickness, 1417
  drug-induced, 281, 281t
  environmental, **277–282**
  eosinophilic, **266**
  in filariasis, 266, 1386
  hantaviruses causing, 246, 1264–1265
  in histoplasmosis, 1392
  in HIV infection/AIDS, **251**, 1210–1211. See also Pneumonia; Tuberculosis
  in hookworm disease, 266, 1380
  HSV causing, 1236
  immunization recommendations in, 1195t
  infections, **243–259**. See also Pneumonia
    adenovirus, 1275, 1276
    anaerobic, 1322
    Bordetella bronchiseptica causing, 1308
    cytomegalovirus, 1246
    mycobacterial
      nontuberculous, 258–259, **1325**
      tuberculosis, 251–258. See also Tuberculosis
    viral, **1268–1276**
  interstitial (diffuse parenchymal), **262–266**, 262t
  in measles, 1248–1249
  metastatic, **1457–1458**

  microscopic polyangiitis causing, 770
  neoplastic, **259–262**. See also Lung cancer
  in nocardiosis, 1324
  occupational, **278–281**
  in paragonimiasis, 1376
  pleural diseases and, **282–287**
  postoperative, risk factors for, 53, 53t
  preoperative evaluation/management of, **53–54**, 53t
  radiation causing, 281–282, 1414
  respiratory failure, **289–291**, 289t
  in scleroderma, 758, 759
  SIADH caused by, 791t
  in SLE, 753
  in strongyloidiasis, 1381
  in syphilis, 1335
  toxic, **280**. See also Toxic lung injury
  tropical pulmonary eosinophilia, 266, 1386
  in uremia, 826t
  ventilation control disorders and, **287–289**
  in Wegener granulomatosis, 276, 768, 769
Pulmonary edema, **367–368**
  acute high-altitude, **1418**
  drug-induced, 281t
  in heart failure (cardiogenic), 359, **367–368**
  perioperative, 52
  in near drowning, 1416
  respiratory failure caused by, 289t
Pulmonary embolectomy, 273
Pulmonary embolism. See Pulmonary venous thromboembolism
Pulmonary fibrosis
  in ankylosing spondylitis, 774
  bleomycin-induced, 1510
  idiopathic (idiopathic fibrosing interstitial pneumonia), **263–265**, 264t
  in interstitial (diffuse parenchymal) diseases, 262
  in pneumoconioses, 278–279
  progressive massive, 278
  radiation causing, **282**, 1414
Pulmonary function tests. See also Spirometry
  in asthma, 219–221
  in COPD, 234, 235t
  in cor pulmonale, 382
  in cystic fibrosis, 241–242
  in interstitial (diffuse parenchymal) lung disease, 262
  in lung cancer, 1455–1456
  preoperative, 53–54
Pulmonary heart disease (cor pulmonale), **381–382**
  in COPD, 238, 382
  in pulmonary hypertension, 275, 382
  theophyllines affected by, 225t
Pulmonary hemosiderosis, idiopathic, 276
Pulmonary hypertension, **273–276**, 274t, **380–381**, 381t
  in atrial septal defect, 297
  in cirrhosis, 623–624
  in COPD, 235

  heart failure and, 274, 275, 360
  idiopathic (primary), 274, **380–381**, 381t
  in mitral stenosis, 306, 307
  in patent ductus arteriosus, 301
  pulmonic regurgitation and, 315
  secondary, 274, 274t
  in ventricular septal defect, 299
Pulmonary infarction, pleural effusion in, 284t
Pulmonary infiltrates. See also Pneumonia
  drugs causing, 281t
  in immunocompromised host/HIV infection/AIDS, 251, **1210**
  travel and, 1173
Pulmonary nodule, solitary, **260–261**
  in metastatic disease, 1458
Pulmonary osteoarthropathy, hypertrophic. See Hypertrophic pulmonary osteoarthropathy
Pulmonary radiation fibrosis, 282, 1414
Pulmonary regurgitation. See Pulmonic regurgitation
Pulmonary rehabilitation, for COPD, 238
Pulmonary stenosis, **294–296**
Pulmonary thromboembolism. See Pulmonary venous thromboembolism
Pulmonary vasculitis, **276**
Pulmonary veno-occlusive disease, pulmonary hypertension and, 274
Pulmonary venous thromboembolism, **266–273**
  air travel and, 1419
  assessment/diagnosis of, 267–270, 268t, 270t, 271f, 271t
  chest pain in, 28, 29, 30, 267, 268t, 321
  dyspnea in, 26, 267, 268t
  immobility and, 267
  prevention of, 270–272, 495–496, 496t
  septic, 1322
    in drug users, 1168
  treatment of, 272–273, 496–501, 497t, 498t, 499t, 500t, 501t
    thrombolytic therapy in, 500–501, 501t
  venous thrombosis and, 267, 269. See also Deep venous thrombosis; Venous thromboembolic disease
  in Wegener granulomatosis, 768
Pulmonary ventilation-perfusion scans. See Ventilation-perfusion scans
Pulmonic regurgitation, **315**
Pulmonic stenosis. See Pulmonary stenosis
Pulsatile tinnitus, 186, 188
Pulse deficit, in atrial fibrillation, 347
Pulse oximetry
  in dyspnea evaluation, 26
  in hepatopulmonary syndrome, 623
Pulse rate. See Heart rate
Pulses
  absence of
    in acute arterial occlusion, 419
    in lower leg/foot occlusive disease, 418

in aortic regurgitation, 312
in hypertension, 394
Pulsus paradoxus, 378
asthma exacerbation and, 220t
in pericardial effusion/tamponade,
378
Pulvinar sign, 1260
Pupillary dilation, acute angle-closure
glaucoma and, 157, **172**
Pupillary reactions
in coma or stupor, 916
in third nerve paralysis, 169
Pure autonomic failure, 885
Pure red cell aplasia, **447**
cancer-related, 1453t
Purgatives, for constipation/preoperative
bowel cleansing, 509t, 510
Purified chick embryo cell culture
(PCEC) rabies vaccine,
1201, 1256
Purified insulin, 1096. See also Insulin
therapy
Purified protein derivative (PPD) test,
253, 253t. See also Tuber-
culin skin test
Purine analogs, in cancer chemotherapy,
1501t
Purines, dietary, 734, 734t
in hyperuricemia/gout, 734, 734t
in urinary stone formation, 857
Purinethol. See Mercaptopurine
Purple coneflower. See Echinacea
Purpura
cancer-related, 783
in cryoglobulinemia, 771
fulminans, 487
Henoch-Schönlein, **771**, 836t, **837**
immune thrombocytopenic, **482–484**,
483t, 484f. See also Thrombocytopenia
posttransfusion, **488**
thrombotic thrombocytopenic,
485–486, 485t. See also
Thrombocytopenia
Pursed lip breathing, for COPD, 238
Push enteroscopy, in GI bleeding, 522,
523
Pustular skin disorders, 95t, **120–125**. See
also specific type
Puumala viruses, 1264
PUVA therapy. See also Phototherapy
for atopic dermatitis, 103
for lichen planus, 135
for psoriasis, 105
Pyelonephritis, **852–853**, 852t, 1181t, 1182t
dysuria and, 46
emphysematous, 853
Pygeum africanum, for benign prostatic
hyperplasia, 870
Pylephlebitis, ruptured appendicitis and,
568
Pyoderma
miliaria and, 124
in pediculosis, 138
in scabies, 138
Pyogenic arthritis. See Septic (nongonococcal acute bacterial)
arthritis

Pyogenic hepatic abscess, **632–633**
Pyogenic osteomyelitis, **780–781**
Pyometra, in endometrial carcinoma, 684
Pyrantel pamoate
for ascariasis, 1379
for enterobiasis/pinworms, 1382
Pyrazinamide, for tuberculosis, 254, 255,
255t, 256t
in latent disease/prophylactic, 257,
1219
pregnancy and, 254–255, 256
Pyrazinamide/isoniazid/rifampin, for
tuberculosis, 255
Pyridium. See Phenazopyridine
Pyridostigmine, for myasthenia gravis, 933
Pyridoxine (vitamin B_6)
deficiency of, **1142–1143**
for gyromitrin mushroom poisoning,
1442
homocystinuria/hyperhomocysteine-
mia and, 1516, 1517
for isoniazid overdose/toxicity, 256,
1142–1143, 1219, 1222,
1424t, 1438
toxicity of, **1143**
Pyrimethamine
folinic acid (leucovorin) rescue with,
1224t, 1365
for isosporiasis, 1370
for malaria, with sulfadoxine (Fansidar), 1355, 1355t, 1359
with amodiaquine, 1356t, 1359
with artesunate, 1355t, 1356t,
1359
for prophylaxis in pregnancy/
infants, 1361
resistance to, 1355, 1359
for toxoplasmosis, 1222, 1224t,
1364–1365, 1365
Pyrimidine analogs, in cancer chemotherapy, 1501t
Pyrogenic erythrotoxin. See Erythrogenic
toxin
Pyrosis (heartburn), 502, 529, 531
Pyuria, 816
in cystitis, 851
sterile, in tuberculosis, 849

Q fever, 1281t, **1286–1287**
Q waves, in myocardial infarction, 331.
See also Myocardial infarc-
tion; Non-Q wave (non-ST
elevation) infarction
Qigong (external), 1520
Qinghaosu/qinghaosu derivatives. See
Artemisinins
QRS complex. See also Electrocardiogram
in nonparoxysmal junctional tachycardia, 351
in preexcitation syndromes, 345
wide
differentiation of aberrantly conducted supraventricular
beats from ventricular
beats and, 341, 352
in poisoning/drug overdose, 1422,
1422t
with antiarrhythmics, 1445

with antidepressants, 1448, 1448f
with phenothiazines, 1444
in tetralogy of Fallot, 300
in ventricular premature beats, 351
QT interval. See also Electrocardiogram
long, 353–354
in hypocalcemia, 800
in hypomagnesemia, 805
palpitations and, 31
in poisoning/drug toxicity, 354,
1422, 1422t
antiarrhythmic agents in, 354,
1445
antidepressants in, 354, 1448,
1449
antipsychotics in, 957, 958, 958t,
1444
droperidol in, 1444
opioids in, 1442
phenothiazines in, 1444
quinine/quinidine in, 1356,
1358, 1445
short, in hypercalcemia, 801, 1497
Quad screen, in prenatal testing, 706, 707
Quadramet. See Samarium
Quadrantanopia. See Visual field defects
Quadriplegia. See also Paralysis
spinal trauma causing, 919
in stroke, 891
Quality of life
assessment/prognosis of older adult
and, 61–62, 63
palliative care for improvement of, 76,
87, 88
Quazepam, 941t
Queensland tick typhus, 1281t, 1285
Questran. See Cholestyramine
Quetiapine, 954, 955t, 956, 956t. See also
Antipsychotic drugs
for delirium, 67
overdose/toxicity of, 956, 956t,
1444–1445
Quinacrine, for lupus, 111
Quinagolide, for hyperprolactinemia,
1001
Quinapril, 403t
Quincke pulses, 312
Quinidine, 343t, 1545t
antidepressant drug interactions and,
969t
for arrhythmias, 343t
for malaria, 1355t, 1356, 1357t, 1358
overdose/toxicity of, 343t, 1356,
1445
Quinine, for malaria, 1355, 1355t, 1356,
1357t, 1358
pregnancy and, 1361
self-treatment and, 1361
Quinolones, 1180t. See also Fluoroquinolones
theophyllines affected by, 225t
Quinsy, 205
Quinsy tonsillectomy, 205
Quinupristin/dalfopristin, for E faecium
infection, 1291–1292

R-CHOP regimen, 470
R-CVP regimen, 470

Rabeprazole, 550. *See also* Proton pump inhibitors
Rabies, **1255–1257**
  bite injuries and, 1165, 1255, 1256
  prevention/immunization and, 1201, 1256–1257. *See also* Rabies vaccine
Rabies antiserum, 1256
Rabies immune globulin, 1256
Rabies vaccine, 1201, 1256–1257
  adsorbed, 1201
  antimalarial drugs/chloroquine affecting, 1201, 1257
  postexposure, 1201, 1256
  preexposure, 1201, 1256–1257
Rabson-Mendenhall syndrome, 1080t
Raccoon sign, 918
Racemose cysticercosis, 1377
Racial/ethnic background
  alcoholism and, 978
  antipsychotic drug dosing and, 957
  breast cancer risk and, 653, 653t
  cholelithiasis/gallstones and, 634
  colorectal cancer incidence and, 1477
  diabetes mellitus and, 1079–1080, 1081
  esophageal cancer and, 1465
  gastric adenocarcinoma and, 1470
  gout and, 732
  Hashimoto thyroiditis and, 1016
  hemochromatosis and, 627
  hypertension and, 387, 388, 390
    management and, 410, 410t
  multiple sclerosis and, 912
  obesity and, 1136
  prostate cancer risk and, 1484
  PSA reference values in, 1485
  sickle cell anemia and, 450
  SLE and, 752
Radial nerve lesions, **927**
Radial optic neurotomy, for retinal vein occlusion, 164
Radiation burns, 1414
Radiation exposure/reactions, **1413–1415**. *See also* Radiation therapy
  accidental/intentional, 1414
  acute, 1413
  cancer risk and, 1415
  lung injury caused by, **281–282**, 1414
  during pregnancy, 707, 1414
  thyroid cancer risk and, 1022
Radiation fibrosis, pulmonary, **282**, 1414
Radiation pericarditis, 377, 378
Radiation pneumonitis, **282**, 1414
Radiation proctitis, 521
Radiation sickness, 1414
Radiation therapy. *See also* Radiation exposure/reactions
  for basal cell carcinoma, 134
  for bladder cancer, 1490
  for breast cancer, 664, 665, 667
    arm edema and, 671–672
    breast implants and, 652
    lung injury and, 282
  with chemotherapy. *See* Chemoradiation therapy
  for esophageal cancer, 1470
  for Hodgkin disease, 471

  for intracranial tumors, 900
  for laryngeal squamous cell carcinoma, 210
  for lung cancer, 1457
    pulmonary fibrosis and, 282
  lung injury and, **281–282**
  for myeloma-related bone disease, 473
  pericarditis caused by, 377, 378
  pneumonitis and, **282**
  for prolactinoma, 1002
  for prostate cancer, 1486–1487
  for spinal cord compression, 1495
  thrombocytopenia and, **482**
  for thyroid cancer, 1026
  thyroid cancer risk and, 1022
  toxicity of. *See* Radiation exposure/reactions
Radiculomyelopathy, in HIV infection/AIDS, 924
Radioactive iodine
  contraindications to in pregnancy, 722, 1012
  for goiter, 1012, 1013, 1030
  for Graves disease/hyperthyroidism, 1012
    ophthalmopathy flares and, 1012, 1014
  for thyroid cancer treatment, 1025–1026
  for thyroid nodules, 1013, 1021
  for thyroid scanning. *See* Radioiodine thyroid scans and uptake
  for whole body scanning, in thyroid cancer followup, 1027–1028
Radioactive materials for testing, breast feeding and, 710t
Radiocontrast media
  iodinated, for Graves disease/hyperthyroidism, 1011–1012
  reactions to, 786
    nephrotoxicity/acute kidney injury and, 822
Radioembolization, for hepatocellular carcinoma, 1461
Radiofrequency ablation techniques
  for arrhythmias
    atrial fibrillation, 349
    atrial flutter, 350
    paroxysmal supraventricular tachycardia, 344
    preexcitation syndromes, 345
    ventricular tachycardia, 352
  for benign prostatic hyperplasia (TUNA), 871
  for hepatocellular carcinoma, 1461
  for trigeminal neuralgia, 877
Radiofrequency wave electrocautery (HALO), for Barrett esophagus, 532
Radioiodine. *See* Radioactive iodine
Radioiodine thyroid scans and uptake, 1003t
  in goiter, 1029, 1030
  in Graves disease/hyperthyroidism, 1003t, 1010
  in nodule evaluation, 1003t, 1019t, 1020

  in thyroid cancer, 1024
    false positive/false negative, 1024
    postoperative/surveillance, 1024, 1027–1028
  in thyroiditis, 1017
Radionuclide angiography
  in angina, 319
  in cardiomyopathy, 370t, 371
  in heart failure, 360
  in myocardial infarction, 331
Radionuclide scanning. *See specific type*
Radiosurgery. *See* Cyberknife radiosurgery; Gamma knife radiation/gamma radiosurgery
Radiotherapy. *See* Radiation therapy
Radon, lung cancer associated with exposure to, 1452
RAEB. *See* Refractory anemia with excess blasts
Raf-kinase inhibitors, for renal cell carcinoma, 1492
Rage attacks, seizures differentiated from, 881
Ragged red fibers, in mitochondrial myopathies, 935
RAI scans, thyroid. *See* Radioiodine thyroid scans and uptake
Rai staging system, for chronic lymphocytic leukemia, 467
Rales. *See* Crackles
Raloxifene, 1073
  breast cancer incidence risk and, 653–654, 1041, 1073
  hypercalcemia/hyperparathyroidism affected by, 1038
  for osteoporosis, 704, 1041, 1070, 1073
Raltegravir, 1227t, 1231, 1232f. *See also* Antiretroviral therapy
Ramelteon, 941t, 974, 1531
Ramipril, 403t
  for heart disease prevention, in diabetes, 405, 1108
Ramsay Hunt syndrome, 192, 1241
  myoclonus in, 910
Ranitidine, 550. *See also* H$_2$ receptor blocking drugs
Ranke complex, in tuberculosis, 252–253
Ranolazine, for angina, 322
Ranson criteria, 642, 642t
Rape, **701–703**, 976
  gamma-hydroxybutyrate ("date rape" drug) use and, 1437
  sexually transmitted diseases and, 702, 1167
  statutory, 702
Rape trauma syndrome, 702
Rapid antigen testing
  in filariasis, 1386
  in malaria, 1354
  in pharyngitis, 204, 1289, 1290
  in pneumococcal pneumonia, 1292
Rapid cyclers, in bipolar disorder, 962
  lithium use and, 970
Rapid detoxification, for opioid withdrawal, 21, 982
Rapid eye movement (REM) sleep, 973

Rapid eye movement (REM) sleep behavior disorder, 975
Rapid HIV antibody tests, 1217, 1217t
Rapid plasma reagin (RPR) test. See RPR test
Rapidly acting insulin analogs, 1096t, 1097–1098, 1097f, 1102, 1102t. See also Insulin therapy
    in mixtures/combination therapy, 1096t, 1098–1099, 1102, 1102t
    in pregnancy, 1110
    in pumps, 1098, 1102
Rapidly progressive acute glomerulonephritis, 833, 836t
Raptiva. See Efalizumab
ras oncogene, thyroid tumors and, 1022, 1023
Rasagiline, for parkinsonism, 906, 907
Rasburicase, for tumor lysis syndrome/hyperuricemia, 1497–1498, 1507t
Rashes. See also specific type or cause and Skin disorders
    acute exanthems, 1240t
        rickettsial, 1240t
        viral, 1240t, 1276–1278
    chemotherapy-induced, 1509
    in dermatomyositis, 760
    drugs causing (dermatitis medicamentosa), 147–150, 148–149t
    fungal, in HIV infection/AIDS, 1215
    heat causing (miliaria), 124
    in Lyme disease, 128, 1343, 1345, 1346t
    in mononucleosis, 204, 1243
    in pharyngitis, 1289
    photodistributed (photodermatitis), 95t, 142–143
    in SLE, 753, 753t
    in Still disease, 751
    in strongyloidiasis, 1381
    in syphilis, 1334
    travel and, 1173
Rat-bite fever, 1340–1341
Rat fleas. See Fleas
Rat lungworm (A cantonensis), 1384
Rat poison, anticoagulant toxicity and, 1430, 1431
Rate control
    for atrial fibrillation, 347, 348
        cardioversion compared with, 348–349
    for atrial flutter, 350
Rattlesnake envenomation, 1446–1447
Rauwolfia derivatives, antidepressant drug interactions and, 969t
Raynaud disease, 756
Raynaud phenomenon, 756–758, 757t
    biofeedback in management of, 1536t, 1537
    scleroderma and, 756, 757, 758, 759
    in SLE, 753
RB-ILD. See Respiratory bronchiolitis-associated interstitial lung disease

RBC. See Erythrocyte count
Reactivated chronic hepatitis B, 609
Reactive arthritis/Reiter syndrome, 776
    dysentery and, 776
    HIV infection/AIDS and, 776, 779, 1213
Reactive cervical lymphadenopathy, 213
Reactive erythemas, 125–128
Reactive (postprandial) hypoglycemia, 1117, 1117t, 1121–1122. See also Hypoglycemia
    postethanol, 1121
Rebound headache, analgesic overuse and, 876
Rebound tenderness, in appendicitis, 567
Recall. See Memory
Recklinghausen disease, 904
    pheochromocytoma/paraganglioma in, 1058
Recombinant growth factors. See Growth factors
Recombinant human deoxyribonuclease (rhDNase), for cystic fibrosis, 242
Recombinant human growth hormone (rhGH). See Human growth hormone
Recombinant human TSH/rhTSH. See Thyrotropin-α
Recombinant immunoblot assay (RIBA), in hepatitis C, 604
Recombinant tissue plasminogen activator. See Alteplase
Recombivax-HB. See Hepatitis B vaccine
Recompression. See also Hyperbaric oxygen therapy
    for altitude-related illness, 1418
    for dysbarism/decompression sickness, 1417
Reconstructive surgery
    after burn injury, 1412
    genital, for transsexuals, 950
    after mastectomy, 665
        local recurrence and, 652
    vascular. See Bypass grafting
Recrudescent epidemic typhus (Brill-Zinsser disease), 1281, 1282
Recruitment, in cochlear dysfunction, 188
Rectal bleeding, 521. See also Gastrointestinal bleeding
    hemorrhoids causing, 521, 593
Rectal carcinoids, 1475
Rectal examination
    in acute bacterial prostatitis, 853
    in benign prostatic hyperplasia, 867
    in constipation, 508
    in prostate cancer screening/diagnosis, 17t, 1484, 1485, 1485t
Rectal prolapse, 593
Rectal (Blumer) shelf, 1471
Rectal temperature. See Core temperature
Rectocele, 687
Rectovaginal fistulas, in Crohn disease, 578, 579
Rectum. See also under Rectal
    cancer of, 1468t, 1478. See also Colorectal cancer

adjuvant therapy for, 1479–1480
    surgical excision and, 1478–1479
    disorders of, 569–593. See also Anorectal disorders
    gonococcal infection, 594, 1319, 1320
Recurrent (habitual) abortion, 712–713
Recurrent laryngeal nerve
    damage to during thyroid surgery, 1012, 1025
    vocal fold paralysis caused by damage/lesions of, 211, 1012
Recurrent paroxysmal atrial fibrillation, 349
Recurrent respiratory papillomatosis, 208
Red blood cells. See under Red cell and Erythrocytes
Red bugs, skin lesions caused by, 139
Red cell aplasia, pure, 447
    cancer-related, 1453t
Red cell casts, 816, 817t
    in glomerulonephritis, 825
Red cell count
    in pleural fluid, 283, 284t
    reference values for, 1549t, 1553t
Red cell mass, in polycythemia, 458
Red cell transfusions, 476–478. See also specific type and Transfusions
Red man syndrome, 785–786
Red top tubes, 1555t
Reduced-intensity allogeneic stem cell transplantation, 476
5α-Reductase deficiency, 1054
5α-Reductase inhibitors. See also Finasteride
    for benign prostatic hyperplasia, 870
Reduction pneumoplasty, for COPD, 239
Reduviid bugs, in Chagas disease, 1350
Reed-Sternberg cells, 471
Reentry
    in supraventricular tachycardia, 342, 345
    in ventricular premature beats, 351
    in ventricular tachycardia, 351, 352
Refeeding
    fatal hypophosphatemia and, 803
    for protein-energy malnutrition, 1135
Refeeding edema, 1135
Reference ranges, for diagnostic/laboratory tests, 1547–1554t. See also specific test
Reflex sympathetic dystrophy (complex regional pain syndrome), 743
Reflux
    gastroesophageal. See Gastroesophageal reflux disease
    hepatojugular, 360
    laryngopharyngeal, 208–209
    vesicoureteral, tubulointerstitial disease caused by, 845, 846
Reflux esophagitis. See Esophagitis
Reflux nephropathy, 845, 846
Refractive errors, 151–152
Refractory anemia, 463
Refractory anemia with excess blasts (RAEB), 463

Refractory atrial fibrillation, 349
Refractory ulcers, 553
   gastric cancer and, 553, 1472
   Zollinger-Ellison syndrome (gastrinoma) and, 553, 556
Refsum disease, 923
Regional hyperthermia, for benign prostatic hyperplasia, 871
Regional poison control centers, 1420
Regranex. See Becaplermin; Platelet-derived growth factor
Regular insulin, 1096, 1096t, 1097, 1097f.
   See also Insulin therapy
   for diabetic ketoacidosis, 1097, 1113–1114
   in mixtures, 1096t, 1098–1099, 1101
Regurgitation, 504
   in achalasia, 542
   in GERD, 531
   in Zenker diverticulum, 538
Rehydration. See Fluid management/hydration
Reiki, 1520
Reinke edema, 209
Reiter syndrome. See Reactive arthritis
Rejection (transplant), kidney, 831
Relafen. See Nabumetone
Relapsing fever, 1177t, 1339–1340
Relapsing polychondritis, 180, 771
Relapsing-remitting multiple sclerosis, 912, 913
Relaxation techniques
   for anxiety disorders, 943
   for irritable bowel syndrome, 573
   for psychiatric problems associated with hospitalization/illness, 990
   for tension headache, 872
REM sleep, 973
REM sleep behavior disorder, 975
Remediation therapy, for schizophrenic/psychotic disorders, 960
Remeron. See Mirtazapine
Remicade. See Infliximab
Remifemin. See Black cohosh
Remitting seronegative synovitis with non-pitting edema, cancer and, 783
Remnant lipoproteins, 1133. See also Triglycerides
Renal angiography/arteriography, in renal artery stenosis/renal vascular hypertension, 391, 833
Renal artery stenosis, 391, 832–833
   hypertension caused by, 391, 832
   renal insufficiency/prerenal azotemia and, 820
Renal biopsy, 818–819
   in focal segmental glomerular sclerosis, 839t, 841
   in IgA nephropathy, 836
   in nephritic syndrome, 834
   in nephrotic syndrome, 839, 839t
   in SLE, 843
   in Wegener granulomatosis, 769
Renal cell carcinoma, 1467t, 1491–1492
   paraneoplastic syndromes associated with, 1453t, 1491

Renal colic/pain
   back pain and, 738
   urinary stones causing, 857
Renal cysts, 846–848, 847t
   acquired, 847t
   in autosomal dominant polycystic kidney disease, 847–848, 847t
   complex, 846
   infected, 847–848
   in medullary cystic kidney, 847t
   in medullary sponge kidney, 847t, 848
   simple/solitary, 846, 847t
Renal disorders. See Kidney disease/injury
Renal failure. See also Acute kidney injury; Chronic kidney disease; Kidney disease/injury; Uremia
   acute, 816, 819–825, 820t. See also Acute kidney injury
   antimicrobial dosage adjustments and, 1184–1185t
   chronic, 816. See also Chronic kidney disease
   dialysis for. See Dialysis
   immunization recommendations in, 1195t
   intrinsic, 820t, 821
   lower extremity edema and, 37
   myoglobinuria/rhabdomyolysis and, 763, 822
   transplantation for. See Kidney transplantation
Renal (nondiabetic) glycosuria, 1086
Renal hypercalciuria, 858t, 859
Renal imaging
   in chronic kidney disease, 827
   in dysuria evaluation, 47
Renal osteodystrophy, 827, 829–830, 1033, 1035, 1038
Renal pain. See Renal colic
Renal pelvis
   cancer of, 1491
   obstruction of, postrenal azotemia and, 821
Renal stones, 860. See also Nephrolithiasis; Urinary stone disease
Renal transplantation. See Kidney transplantation
Renal tubular acidosis, 809t, 810, 811
   genetic defects associated with, 796t
   hyperkalemia in, 798, 809t
   in hypocitraturic calcium nephrolithiasis, 859
   hypokalemia in, 809t
   nephrolithiasis/urolithiasis and, 810, 857, 859
   in tubulointerstitial disease, 846
   urinary anion gap in, 809t, 810
Renal tubular cell casts, 816, 817t
Renal tubular necrosis, acute, 820t, 821–823
   in pancreatitis, 644
   rhabdomyolysis and, 763, 764, 822
Renal vascular hypertension, 391. See also Hypertension
Renin activity (plasma). See Plasma renin activity

Renin-angiotensin-aldosterone system. See also Aldosterone
   in hypertension, 389–390, 402
   inhibitors of, 402, 403t. See also Angiotensin II receptor blocking agents; Angiotensin-converting enzyme (ACE) inhibitors
   for heart failure, 361–362
Renin inhibitors, for hypertension, 402, 403t
Renova. See Tretinoin
Repaglinide, 1091t, 1092
Repeat-dose charcoal, 1426
Reperfusion therapy, for myocardial infarction, 332–334, 333t
   assessment of, 334
   percutaneous coronary intervention, 327t, 332
   thrombolytic therapy, 332–334, 333t
Reptilase clotting time, 1553t
Rescriptor. See Delavirdine
Rescula. See Unoprostone
Reserpine
   depression caused by, 407, 408t, 962
   for Huntington disease, 909
   for hypertension, 407, 408t
   MAOI interactions and, 969t
Reset osmostat, hyponatremia caused by, 791, 792
Residential facilities, for schizophrenic/psychotic disorders, 960
Residual schizophrenia, 952
Residual volume (RV), in COPD, 234
Resin T_3/T_4 uptake
   factors affecting, 1002
   in hyperthyroidism, 1010
   pregnancy and, 1010
Resistance, microbial. See Drug resistance
Resistant hypertension, 411, 411t
Resistin
   insulin action in obesity and, 1081
   thiazolidinediones affecting release of, 1093
Resolution stage of sexual activity, 948
Resorptive hypercalciuria, 858t, 859
Respiration. See Breathing; Ventilation
Respiratory acidosis (hypercapnia), 806, 807t, 813–814, 814t
   in asthma, 219
   in COPD, 234, 814
   in cystic fibrosis, 241
   dyspnea and, 26
   metabolic alkalosis and, 813
   permissive, 291
     for asthma, 233
   respiratory failure and, 290, 813
Respiratory alkalosis (hypocapnia), 806, 807t, 814–815
   alcoholic ketoacidosis and, 809
   in asthma, 219
   in heat exhaustion, 1407
   in heat stroke, 1407, 1408
   in hyperventilation syndromes, 287, 814
   mechanical ventilation and, 291
   metabolic acidosis and, 810
   in pulmonary embolism, 267
   salicylate overdose/toxicity causing, 1445

Respiratory biofeedback training, 1537
Respiratory bronchiolitis, 243
Respiratory bronchiolitis-associated
            interstitial lung disease
            (RB-ILD), 243, 263, 264t
Respiratory depression, opioids causing,
            78, 84
Respiratory distress syndrome, acute/
            adult. See Acute respira-
            tory distress syndrome
Respiratory failure, **289–291**, 289t. See
            also Acute respiratory dis-
            tress syndrome
    acidosis in, 290, 813
    in acute aspiration of gastric contents,
            278
    asthma exacerbation and, 219, 220t,
            233
    in botulism, 934, 1300
    in burn injury, 1412
    COPD and, 234, 238
    drug-induced, 281t
    electrical injury causing, 1412
    in near drowning, 1415
    in poliomyelitis, 1252
    in SARS, 1275
    tracheostomy for, 211–212
Respiratory papillomatosis, recurrent, **208**
Respiratory rate
    in asthma exacerbation, 220t
    in pulmonary embolism, 268t
Respiratory syncytial virus, **1268–1269**
Respiratory syncytial virus immune glob-
            ulin, 1269
Respiratory tract infection. See Pulmo-
            nary disorders, infections
Rest. See also Bed rest; Immobility
    requirements for during pregnancy,
            707
Rest pain
    in femoral/popliteal occlusive disease,
            417
    in lower leg/foot occlusive disease, 418
    in thromboangiitis obliterans
            (Buerger disease), 423
Restasis. See Cyclosporine
Restenosis, with PCI, 323
Restless legs syndrome, **911**
Restlessness, terminal, 87
Restoril. See Temazepam
Restraints, for aggressive/violent patient,
            977
Restrictive cardiomyopathy. See Cardio-
            myopathy
Resuscitation. See Cardiopulmonary
            resuscitation
Resynchronization (biventricular pac-
            ing), for heart failure,
            365–366
ret oncogene
    in medullary thyroid carcinoma, 1023
    in multiple endocrine neoplasia, 1076,
            1077
    in papillary thyroid carcinoma, 1022
    in pheochromocytoma/paragan-
            glioma, 1059
    prophylactic thyroidectomy and, 1026
Retardation. See Mental retardation

Retention, urinary. See Urinary retention
Reteplase, for myocardial infarction, 333t,
            334
Reticulocyte count, 1553t
Reticulocytosis
    in glucose-6-phosphate dehydrogen-
            ase deficiency, 450
    in hereditary spherocytosis, 448
    in sickle cell anemia, 451
Reticulosis, polymorphic (midline malig-
            nant), 201
Retin-A/Retin A Micro. See Tretinoin
Retina
    degeneration of, in vitamin E defi-
            ciency, 914
    detachment of, **161–162**
    in hypertension, 167, 394
    systemic diseases affecting, **166–168**
Retinal artery occlusion, central and
            branch, **164–165**
Retinal circulation, hypertension affecting
            (hypertensive retinocho-
            roidopathy), 167
Retinal drusen, in age-related macular
            degeneration, 162
Retinal emboli, transient monocular
            blindness caused by, 165,
            420
Retinal hemorrhage
    in blood dyscrasias, 167
    in HIV infection/AIDS, 167
Retinal tears, detachment and, 161
Retinal vasculitis, 160. See also Uveitis
Retinal vein occlusion, central and
            branch, **163–164**
Retinitis
    in bartonellosis, 1321
    cytomegalovirus, 167–168, 1213,
            1223, 1245, 1246
    in HIV infection/AIDS, 167–168,
            1213, 1223
    hydroxychloroquine causing, 750
Retinochoroiditis, toxoplasmic, 1363, 1364
Retinochoroidopathy, hypertensive, **167**
Retinoic acid. See Tretinoin
Retinoic acid receptor, in promyelocytic
            leukemia, 464
Retinoids. See also specific agent and Vita-
            min A
    for acne, 121
    adverse ophthalmic effects of, 178t
    for psoriasis, 105
Retinopathy
    diabetic, **166–167**, 1104, 1105
        glycemic control and, 1087, 1088
        hypertension/hypertension control
            and, 1088
    in hemoglobin SC disease, 167, 452
    malignant hypertensive, 167
    "pizza-pie," in cytomegalovirus infec-
            tion, 1245
    sickle cell, 167
Retinopexy, for retinal detachment, 162
Retrobulbar optic neuritis, 168
Retrocecal appendicitis, 568
Retrograde ejaculation, 862, 865, 865f,
            866, 949. See also Erectile
            dysfunction/impotence

Retroileal appendicitis, 568
Retrovir. See Zidovudine
Revascularization procedures. See also
            specific type and Bypass
            grafting
    for acute arterial occlusion of limb,
            419
    for aortoiliac occlusive disease, 416
    coronary, 322–323, 323
        for acute coronary syndromes,
            328–329, 329t
        for angina, 322–323
        for heart failure, 366
        for myocardial infarction, 332
            postinfarction, 340
            prophylactic/preoperative, 51
        prophylactic/preoperative, 51
        for traumatic injuries, 384
    for erectile dysfunction, 863
    for femoral/popliteal occlusive dis-
            ease, 417
    for lower leg/foot occlusive disease,
            418
    for renal artery stenosis, 833
Reversal reactions, in leprosy, 1327
Reverse T$_3$, 1002
Reverse transcriptase
    in HIV infection, 1207
    inhibitors of. See Nonnucleoside
            reverse transcriptase
            inhibitors; Nucleoside
            reverse transcriptase
            inhibitors; Nucleotide
            reverse transcriptase
            inhibitor
Revised Cardiac Risk Index (RCRI), 49,
            50t
Revlimid. See Lenalidomide
Rewarming
    for frostbite, 1405–1406
    for immersion syndrome, 1405
    for systemic hypothermia, 1404
Reyataz. See Atazanavir
Reye syndrome, 617, 1241, 1270
    aspirin use and, 78
    influenza vaccination and, 1198
Reynold pentad, 638
Rezulin. See Troglitazone
RF. See Rheumatoid factor
Rh$_o$ (D) immune globulin, 709
    after delivery, 709
    after ectopic pregnancy, 709, 714
    after elective abortion, 701, 709
    prenatal administration of, 708, 709
    after spontaneous abortion, 709, 712
Rh incompatibility
    hemolytic disease of newborn caused
            by, 709
    testing for, 706, 708
Rh typing
    during pregnancy, 706, 708
    for transfusions, 477
Rhabdomyolysis, **763–764**
    acute tubular necrosis and, 763, 764,
            822
    in electric burns/crush injuries, 763
    in hypophosphatemia, 802, 803
    statin drugs causing, 761, 763–764

Rhabdomyoma, cardiac, 383
rhDNase, for cystic fibrosis, 242
Rhegmatogenous retinal detachment, 161, 162
Rheumatic carditis/rheumatic valvulitis, 375
    endocarditis and, 1303
Rheumatic diseases. *See also specific disease*
    cancer and, **783**
    HIV infection/AIDS and, **779**, 1212–1213
Rheumatic fever, **374–376**
    arthritis in, 375
        rheumatoid arthritis differentiated from, 748
    prevention and, 376, 1290
    streptococcal pharyngitis and, 375, 1289, 1290
Rheumatic heart disease, **374–376**
    valvular involvement and, 302, 375
Rheumatism, palindromic, **783**
Rheumatoid arthritis, **747–751**
    autoantibodies in, 748, 754t
    differential diagnosis of, 748–749
        ankylosing spondylitis and, 774
        gouty/tophaceous arthritis and, 733, 748
        osteoarthritis and, 731, 748
    neuropathies associated with, 747, 924
    septic arthritis and, 748, 777, 778
Rheumatoid factor, 748, 754t
    in cryoglobulinemia, 770–771
    in interstitial (diffuse parenchymal) lung disease, 262
    in polymyositis/dermatomyositis, 754t, 760
    in rheumatoid arthritis, 748, 754t
    in Sjögren syndrome, 754t, 762
Rheumatoid nodules, 747–748
    in coal workers (Caplan syndrome), 278
    gouty tophi differentiated from, 733, 748
Rheumatoid pleural effusion, 284t
rhGH. *See* Human growth hormone
Rhinitis
    allergic (hay fever), **196–197**
        conjunctivitis and, 155
        nasal polyps and, 196, 199
    medicamentosa, 192
    nasopharyngeal/paranasal sinus cancer and, 200
    perennial, 196
    vasomotor, 196
    viral (common cold), **192**, 1275
        bacterial rhinosinusitis and, 192, 193
        cough in, 22
        echinacea for, 1523t, 1525–1526
Rhinocerebral mucormycosis, 195
Rhinosinusitis, acute bacterial, **192–195**, 194t, 1182t. *See also* Sinusitis
    facial pain associated with, 193
    headache and, 193, 872
    in HIV infection/AIDS, 195, 1211
    hospital-associated, 193, 194

nasopharyngeal/paranasal sinus cancer and, 200
    orbital cellulitis and, 170, 194
Rhipicephalus sanguineus ticks. *See* Ticks
Rhizopus infection, 195, 1398–1399
Rhizotomy
    for spasticity, 915
    for trigeminal neuralgia, 877
rhTSH/recombinant human TSH. *See* Thyrotropin-α
Rhus (poison ivy/oak) contact dermatitis, 119, 784. *See also* Allergic contact dermatitis
Riamet (artemether-lumefantrine/Coartem), for malaria, 1355t, 1356, 1356t, 1357t, 1360
RIBA. *See* Recombinant immunoblot assay
Ribavirin, 1238t
    for hemorrhagic fevers, 1263
    for hepatitis C, 610–611
    for influenza, 1238t, 1271
    for RSV infection, 1238t, 1269
    teratogenicity of, 611, 1269
Riboflavin (vitamin B$_2$), deficiency of, **1141**
Ribonucleoprotein protein (RNP) antibody, 762
Rice, *Bacillus cereus* contamination of, 1172
Rice water stool, in cholera, 1315
Richter syndrome, 467
Ricin, as chemical warfare agent, **1434**
Ricinus communis (castor bean), ricin toxicity and, 1434
Rickets, 1042
    hypophosphatemic (vitamin D-resistant), 796t, 1043, 1044
    vitamin D-dependent, 1042–1043
Rickettsia (rickettsial diseases), 1178t, **1280–1287**, 1281t
    africae, 1281t, 1285
    akari, 1281t, 1284
    australis, 1281t, 1285
    conorii, 1281t, 1285
    felis, 1281t, 1285
    japonica, 1285
    myocarditis in, 368, 369t
    prowazekii, 1280, 1281, 1281t
    rickettsii, 1281t, 1284
    sibirica, 1281t, 1285
    typhi, 1281t, 1282
Rickettsial fever (tick typhus), 1281t, **1285**
Rickettsialpox, 1281t, **1284–1285**
Rickettsiosis, California flea, 1281t
Riedel thyroiditis/struma, 1016, 1017, 1018
Rifabutin
    antiretroviral agent interactions and, 255–256, 1211
    for MAC prophylaxis/treatment, 1222, 1224t, 1325
Rifamate. *See* Isoniazid/rifampin
Rifampin, 255t, 256t
    for anthrax, 1301t, 1302
    antiretroviral agent interactions and, 255–256, 1211
    benzodiazepine interactions and, 942t

for endocarditis, 1306, 1307
    for leprosy, 1327
    for MAC treatment/prophylaxis, 1325
    renal/hepatic failure and, 1185t
    theophyllines affected by, 225t
    for tuberculosis, 254, 255, 255t, 256t
        in latent disease/prophylactic, 257, 1219
        in pregnancy, 255, 256, 726
Rifampin/isoniazid, for tuberculosis, 255
Rifampin/isoniazid/pyrazinamide, for tuberculosis, 255
Rifater. *See* Isoniazid/rifampin/pyrazinamide
Rifaximin
    for flatus, 511
    for irritable bowel syndrome, 572
    for traveler's diarrhea, 514
Rift Valley fever, 1262–1263
Right heart failure, 358, 359. *See also* Congestive heart (cardiac) failure
    liver in, 359, 360, 631
Right middle lobe syndrome, 216
Right-to-left shunts. *See* Shunts
Right ventricular infarction, 338
Rigidity
    in Huntington disease, 908
    in Lewy body dementia, 64
    lithium use and, 971
    in parkinsonism, 905
Riluzole, for amyotrophic lateral sclerosis, 921
Rimantadine, influenza/influenza resistance and, 1198, 1270, 1271, 1272, 1273
Rimexolone, for ophthalmic disorders, 175t
Rimonabant, for obesity, 15
Ring shadow sign, 845
Ringer lactate. *See* Fluid management/hydration
Ringworm. *See* Tinea
Rinne test, 179
Risedronate
    for osteoporosis prevention/management, 1040
    for Paget disease of bone, 1046
Risperdal. *See* Risperidone
Risperidone, 954, 955, 955t, 956t, 957, 967. *See also* Antipsychotic drugs
    for aggressive/violent behavior, 976
    for bipolar disease/mania, 970
    for delirium, 87
    for dementia-associated behavior problems, 66
    long-acting form of, 958
    overdose/toxicity of, 955, 956t, 1444–1445
    for personality disorder, 951
Ristocetin co-factor, in von Willebrand disease, 493
Ritonavir, 1226t, 1229, 1232f. *See also* Antiretroviral therapy
    for antiprotease inhibitor boosting, 1229
    with darunavir, 1227t, 1230

with fosamprenavir, 1229
with lopinavir (lopinavir/r), 1226t,
1230, 1232f
with saquinavir, 1229
with tipranavir, 1227t, 1230
Rituxan. See Rituximab
Rituximab, 1503t
for autoimmune hemolytic anemia,
453
for chronic lymphocytic leukemia,
467, 468
for cold agglutinin disease, 454
for immune thrombocytopenic purpura, 483, 484f
for non-Hodgkin lymphoma, 470
for rheumatoid arthritis, 751
Rivastigmine
for dementia, 65, 66, 987
for parkinsonism, 908
River blindness, **1387–1388**
RMSF. See Rocky Mountain spotted fever
RNA
hepatitis C virus, 604, 604f, 609
hepatitis D virus, 603
HIV, reference values for, 1551t
RNA amplification tests, in tuberculosis,
252
RNA-dependent DNA-polymerase
(reverse transcriptase). See
Reverse transcriptase
RNP. See Ribonucleoprotein protein
(RNP) antibody
Ro/SSA antibody, 754t
in lupus, 110, 754t
in Sjögren syndrome, 754t, 762
Rocaltrol. See Calcitriol
Rocephin. See Ceftriaxone
Rocky Mountain spotted fever, 1240t,
1281t, **1283–1284**
Rodent excreta
hantavirus transmission and, 1264
hemorrhagic fever transmission and,
1262
lymphocytic choriomeningitis trans-
mission and, 1259
Rodent fleas. See Fleas
Rodent mites. See Mites
Rodent tapeworm (H diminuta), 1376
Rodent ticks. See Ticks
Rodenticide poisoning, anticoagulant tox-
icity and, 1430, 1431
Rogaine. See Minoxidil
Romaña sign, 1350
Romano-Ward syndrome, 353
Romiplostim, for immune thrombocyto-
penic purpura, 483
Ropinirole, for parkinsonism, 907
Rosacea, **122–123**
acne, 120
steroid, 99, 122
Rose spots, in enteric (typhoid) fever,
1313
Roseola infantum (exanthema subitum),
1240t, **1247**
Rosiglitazone, 1091t, 1093–1094, 1101
with glimepiride, 1096
with metformin, 1096
osteoporosis and, 1038

Ross procedure, 316
for aortic regurgitation, 313
for aortic stenosis, 311
postoperative pulmonic stenosis and,
295
Rosuvastatin, 1131, 1132t. See also Statin
drugs
RotaTeq. See Rotavirus vaccine
Rotator cuff disorders/tendinitis, **744**
Rotatrix. See Rotavirus vaccine
Rotavirus vaccine, 1188–1189t,
1192–1193t, 1278
Rotaviruses
diarrhea/gastroenteritis caused by,
1171t, 1172, 1278
immunization against, 1188–1189t,
1192–1193t, 1278
Roth spots, in endocarditis, 1304
Rotor syndrome, 599t
Rouleau formation
in myeloma, 472
in Waldenström macroglobulinemia,
474
Roundworm infections. See also specific
type
intestinal, **1379–1382**
invasive, **1382–1386**
Roux-en-Y gastric bypass, for obesity, 15,
1138
hypoglycemia after, 1117, 1121
Rowasa. See Mesalamine
Roxanol. See Morphine
Roxicodone. See Oxycodone
Rozerem. See Ramelteon
RP. See Raynaud phenomenon
RPR test, 1331–1332
in antiphospholipid antibody syn-
drome, 756
in HIV infection/AIDS, 1220, 1337
RRP. See Recurrent respiratory papillomatosis
RS3PE (remitting seronegative synovitis
with non-pitting edema),
cancer and, 783
RSV. See Respiratory syncytial virus
RSVIG. See Respiratory syncytial virus
immune globulin
rt-PA. See Tissue plasminogen activator
rT₃. See Reverse T₃
RT₃U. See Resin T₃/T₄ uptake
RTA. See Renal tubular acidosis
RU 486. See Mifepristone
Rubber band ligation. See Banding
Rubella, 1240t, **1253–1255**
arthritis associated with, 779, 1254
during pregnancy/congenital, 1254,
1255
prevention/immunization and,
1198–1199, 1254–1255.
See also MMR (measles-
mumps-rubella) vaccine
arthritis and, 779, 1255
pregnancy and, 1195t, 1199,
1254–1255
Rubella virus vaccine, 1198–1199,
1254–1255. See also MMR
(measles-mumps-rubella)
vaccine

Rubeola. See Measles
Rubeotic (neovascular) glaucoma, retinal
vein occlusion and, 164
Rufen. See Ibuprofen
Rugger jersey spine, 1035
Rule of nines, 1409, 1409f
for topical corticosteroid calculation,
94
Rumination, 504
Running, overuse syndromes of knee and,
745–746
Russell viper venom clotting time
for lupus anticoagulant detection,
722, 756
reference values for, 1553t
RV (residual volume), in COPD, 234
RVA (rabies vaccine adsorbed), 1201
RVV/RVVT. See Russell viper venom clot-
ting time
RYGB. See Roux-en-Y gastric bypass

S-OIV. See Swine-origin influenza
S stage sleep, 973
SAAG. See Serum-ascites albumin gradi-
ent
Sabin-Feldman dye test, in toxoplasmosis,
1364
Sabin vaccine (oral/OPV poliovaccine),
1252–1253
IPV booster and, 1201
Saccharin, for diabetics, 1090
Saccharomyces boulardii probiotic, for
antibiotic-associated coli-
tis, 575
Saccharomyces cerevisiae antibodies, in
inflammatory bowel dis-
ease, 579
Saccular (berry) aneurysm, 894. See also
Intracranial aneurysm
Sacral spine/disk disease. See also Spine
herniated disk, 738, 739
Sacroiliac joint/sacroiliitis
in ankylosing spondylitis, 774
reactive arthritis and, 776
SAD. See Seasonal affective disorder
Saddle nose deformity
in nasal trauma, 199
in Wegener granulomatosis, 768
Sadism, sexual, 948
Safer sex
in herpes simplex infection prevention, 1236
in HIV infection/AIDS prevention, 4,
1207, 1218–1219, 1220,
1221
in syphilis prevention, 1332
Sagittal sinus thrombosis, in pseudotumor cerebri, 903
Salagen. See Pilocarpine
Salicylates, 1545t. See also Aspirin
overdose/toxicity of, 1427t,
1445–1446
alkali therapy for, 811, 1445
anion gap/osmolar gap in, 809,
1426, 1445
hemodialysis for, 1425t, 1445
ophthalmic effects and, 178t
platelet function affected by, 490t

Salicylates (*cont.*)
reference values for, 1553*t*
for rheumatic fever/heart disease, 376
Salicylic acid preparations, for wart
removal, 132
Saline, 815, 815*t*. *See also* Fluid manage-
ment/hydration
contrast media nephrotoxicity mediated by, 822
for cystic fibrosis, 242
for diabetic ketoacidosis, 1114
dilutional acidosis and, 810
for eye decontamination, **1424**
for heat exposure syndromes, 1407
for hepatic failure, 608
for hypercalcemia, 801, 1497
for hyperglycemic hyperosmolar state,
1015–1016
for hypernatremia, 794
for hyponatremia, 792–793
for metabolic alkalosis, 813
Saline breast prosthesis. *See* Breast
implants
Saline infusion sonohysterography, 675*t*
for abnormal premenopausal bleeding, 675
Saline purgatives, for constipation/preop-
erative bowel cleansing,
510
Saline-responsive metabolic alkalosis,
812, 812–813, 812*t*, 813
Saline-unresponsive metabolic alkalosis,
812, 812*t*, 813
Salivary glands, **206–207**
infiltrative disorders of, **207**
inflammatory disorders of
acute, **206–207**
chronic, **207**
in mumps, 1250
tumors of, **207**
Salivary stones (sialolithiasis), **206–207**
Salk vaccine (inactivated/IPV poliovaccine), 1188*t*, 1190–1191*t*,
1192–1193*t*, 1201,
1252–1253
pregnancy and, 710
for travelers, 1201, 1253
Salmeterol
for asthma, 224*t*, 227
with fluticasone, 224*t*
for COPD, 237
Salmon calcitonin. *See* Calcitonin
Salmonella enterica subsp *enterica* (salmonellosis), 1182*t*,
1312–1314
bacteremia caused by, 1177*t*, 1312,
1314
choleraesuis, 1312
diarrhea/enterocolitis/gastroenteritis
caused by, 512, 1171*t*, 1172,
1174, 1182*t*, 1312, **1314**
drug resistance and, 1313, 1314
typhi, 1312, 1313
typhimurium, 1312
Salpingectomy, for ectopic pregnancy, 714
Salpingitis, **687–689**. *See also* Pelvic
inflammatory disease
appendicitis differentiated from, 568

chlamydial, 1328
gonococcal, 1319
tuberculous, 688
Salpingo-oophorectomy. *See* Oophorectomy
Salpingostomy, for ectopic pregnancy, 714
Salt restriction. *See* Sodium-restricted diet
Salt tablets, heat exposure syndromes and,
1407
Samarium, for bone pain, 1507*t*
Samter triad, 199
Sand flies. *See* Flies
Sandostatin. *See* Octreotide
SaO₂ (oxygen saturation)
in ARDS, 292
in asthma, exacerbation severity/man-
agement and, 220*t*, 233
in cor pulmonale, 382
in dyspnea evaluation, 26
home oxygen therapy and, 236*t*
in near drowning, 1416
Pneumocystis pneumonia treatment
and, 1395
in respiratory failure, 290
in sleep apnea, 288
in smoke inhalation, 277
SAPE (sentinel acute pancreatitis event),
646
Saphenous vein
superficial thrombophlebitis of, 429
varicose, 427
Saquinavir, 1226*t*, 1229, 1232*f*. *See also*
Antiretroviral therapy
interaction with garlic and, 1524
with ritonavir, 1229
Sarafem. *See* Fluoxetine
Sarcocystis bovihominis/suihominis (sarcocystosis), **1369–1371**
Sarcoidosis, 201, **265–266**
arthritis in, **782**
hypercalcemia/hypercalciuria in, 1036
neuropathy associated with, 924
nose and paranasal sinus involvement
and, **201**
pulmonary involvement and, **265–266**
Sarcoma. *See also* specific type
soft tissue, 1468*t*
Sarcoptes scabiei infection (scabies),
137–138
Sargramostim (GM-CSF)
for chemotherapy-induced toxicity,
1508*t*
for HIV infection/AIDS, 1223
Sarin poisoning, 1434
Sarna. *See* Camphor/menthol preparations
SARS. *See* Severe acute respiratory syndrome
Satavaptan, for hyponatremia/SIADH,
793
Saturday night palsy, 926, 927
Saturnine gout, in lead poisoning, 733
Saw palmetto (*Serenoa repens*), 1523*t*,
1526–1527
for benign prostatic hyperplasia, 870,
1523*t*, 1526–1527
Saxitoxin, paralytic shellfish poisoning
caused by, 1446*t*

Sb. *See* Stibogluconate
Scabies, **137–138**
Scaling skin disorders, 95*t*, **101–113**. *See
also specific type*
Scalp
allergic contact dermatitis involving,
119
injuries of, **918**
in pediculosis, 138
pemphigus involving, 130
psoriasis of, 104
seborrhea of, 106
Scalpicin. *See* Hydrocortisone
Scarlet fever, 1240*t*, 1289, 1291
Scarring, prevention of in burn injury, 1412
Scarring (cicatricial) alopecias, **145**
SCC. *See* Squamous cell carcinoma
SCDs (sequential compression devices).
See Pneumatic compres-
sion devices
Scedosporium apiospermum/prolificans, in
opportunistic infections,
1402
Schatzki rings, 529*t*, **537–538**
Schiller test, in CIN, 681
Schilling test, short bowel syndrome/ileal
resection and, 562
Schirmer test, 154
in Sjögren syndrome diagnosis, 762
Schistocytes
in DIC, 487
in microangiopathic hemolytic anemia, 454
*Schistosoma haematobium/intercalatum/
japonicum/mansoni/
mekongi* (schistosomiasis),
1373–1375
bladder cancer and, 1489
Schizoaffective disorders, 952
Schizoid personality disorder, 951*t*
Schizophrenic disorders, **952–961**. *See
also* Psychotic disorders
classification of, 952
depression and, 953, 964
differential diagnosis of, 954
drug-induced/toxic, 954
drug therapy for, 954–960, 955*t*, 956*t*,
958*t*. *See also* Antipsy-
chotic drugs
mania differentiated from, 954
positive and negative symptoms in,
952, 960
antipsychotic drugs affecting, 957
prodromal, 952
suicide risk and, 953, 955, 963
Schizophreniform disorders, 953
Schizotypal personality disorder, 951*t*
Schmidt syndrome, 1048, 1086
Schneiderian papillomas, 200
Schober test of lumbar motion, 739
Schwannoma
gastrointestinal, 1474
vestibular (acoustic neuroma/neuri-
noma/eighth nerve tumor),
191, 191*t*, 898*t*, 904
hearing loss and, 179, 186, 191,
191*t*
in neurofibromatosis, 191, 904

Sciatic nerve palsy, **928**
Sciatica, 738, 740. *See also* Back pain
Scintigraphy. *See specific type*
SCL-70 (scleroderma) antibody, 754*t*, 758
SCLC. *See* Small cell carcinoma of lung
SCLE. *See* Subacute cutaneous lupus ery-
    thematosus
Sclera
    blue, in osteogenesis imperfecta, 1039
    lacerations of, 172
Sclerectomy, for glaucoma, 159
Scleroderma (systemic sclerosis), **758–759**
    autoantibodies in, 754*t*, 758
    dysphagia in, 529*t*, 758
    limited. *See* CREST syndrome
    linear, 759
    Raynaud phenomenon and, 756, 757,
      758, 759
Scleroderma (anti-SCL-70) antibody,
    754*t*, 758
Scleroderma renal crisis, 758, 759
Scleromyxedema, 759
Sclerotherapy
    for esophageal varices, 539, 540
    for hemorrhoids, 594
    for malignant effusions, 1496
    for varicose veins, 428–429
SCN4A gene, in periodic paralysis, 936
Scoliosis, in syringomyelia, 920
Scombroid poisoning, 1446, 1446*t*
Scopolamine
    for nausea and vomiting, 86, 87
    overdose/toxicity of, 1432
    in terminally ill/dying patient, 92
Scorpion stings, **1447**
Scotch tape test, in enterobiasis/pin-
    worms, 1382
Scotomas. *See also* Visual field defects/loss
    in migraine headache, 873
    in optic neuritis, 168
Scratch-itch cycle. *See also* Pruritus
    in lichen simplex chronicus, 103
Screamer's nodules, 209
Screening tests. *See also specific type and*
    disorder and Diagnostic/
    laboratory tests; Genetic
    testing; Prenatal testing
    in cancer prevention, 16–18, 17*t*
    health maintenance/preventive care
      and, 2, 3*t*
Scrofula, **1325**
Scrotal mass. *See* Testes, masses/tumors of
Scrotal pain. *See also* Testicular pain
    in epididymitis, 856
Scrotal pruritus, 136
Scrotal swelling, in filariasis, 1386
Scrub typhus, 1281*t*, **1283**
Scuba/deep sea diving
    dysbarism/decompression sickness
      and, 1416–1417
    eustachian tube dysfunction/otic
      barotrauma and, 182,
      183
Scurvy, 1143
SDH (succinate dehydrogenase) gene
    mutations, in pheochro-
    mocytoma/paragan-
    glioma, 1058, 1059

Seafood poisonings, 1446, 1446*t*. *See also*
    Fish; Shellfish
Seasonal affective disorder, 962, 964, 969
Seborrheic dermatitis, **106**
    atopic dermatitis differentiated from,
      102
    in HIV infection/AIDS, 1215
    pityriasis rosea differentiated from,
      106
Seborrheic keratoses, **100**
Sebum, in acne, 120
Seclusion rooms, for aggressive/violent
    patient, 977
Second-degree burn, 1409
Second-degree heart block, 355
    in myocardial infarction, 337
Second-hand smoke. *See* Passive smoking
Second heart sound (S_2). *See* Heart
    sounds
Secretin stimulation test, in Zollinger-
    Ellison syndrome/gastri-
    noma, 556
Secretory diarrhea, 512*t*, 515, 516. *See also*
    Diarrhea
Sectral. *See* Acebutolol
Sedation
    antidepressants causing, 964, 966,
      968*t*
    for delirium, 87
    opioids causing, 84
Sedative-hypnotics, 941*t*
    antidepressant drug interactions and,
      969*t*
    for anxiety/stress disorders, 938, 941*t*,
      942
    for insomnia, 941*t*, 974
    for nausea and vomiting, 506*t*, 507
    overdose/toxicity of, **1436**
    sleep affected by, 974
Sedentary lifestyle. *See* Lifestyle, sedentary
Segmental myoclonus, 911
Seizures, **878–884**, 879*t*, 882*t*. *See also spe-*
    cific type and Epilepsy; Sta-
    tus epilepticus
    absence (petit mal), 879*t*, 880, 882*t*
    alcohol withdrawal, 883, 978, 981
    antidepressant use and, 967, 1423*t*,
      1448
    antipsychotic drug use and, 959
    atonic, 880
    biofeedback in management of, 1538
    brain abscess and, 879
    cerebral arteriovenous malformations
      causing, 895, 896
    classification of, 879–880, 879*t*
    clonic, 880
    cognitive disorders/delirium caused
      by, 985*t*
    in cysticercosis, 1377
    degenerative disorders and, 879
    differential diagnosis of, 881
    drug therapy for, 881–884, 882*t*. *See*
      also Anticonvulsant ther-
      apy
    flumazenil causing, 1421, 1436
    generalized, 879*t*, 880, 882*t*
    in hypocalcemia, 800
    hypoparathyroidism and, 1031

    hysterical (pseudoseizures), 881, 944
    infection/infectious diseases and, 879
    intracranial tumors causing, 878–879
    in malaria, 1354
    myoclonic, 879*t*, 880, 882*t*
    panic disorder differentiated from,
      881, 940
    partial/focal, 879, 879*t*, 882*t*
    in poisoning/drug overdose, **1423**,
      1423*t*
    posttraumatic, 878
    during pregnancy, **724**
      eclampsia and, 716, 718
    schizophrenia differentiated from, 954
    serial, 880
    solitary, 883
    in Sturge-Weber syndrome, 904
    surgical management of, 883
    in tetanus, 1298
    theophylline use and, 1423*t*, 1447,
      1448
    tonic, 880
    tonic-clonic (grand mal), 879*t*, 880,
      882*t*
    transient ischemic attacks differenti-
      ated from, 881, 887
    in tuberous sclerosis, 903
    vagal nerve stimulation for, 883
    vascular disorders and, 879
Selective estrogen receptor modulators
    (SERMs), 1073. *See also*
    Tamoxifen
    in breast cancer prevention/treatment,
      653–654, 668
    in cancer chemotherapy, 1505*t*
    for osteoporosis, 1041, 1070, 1073
Selective immunoglobulin A deficiency,
    786
Selective serotonin reuptake inhibitors.
    See Serotonin-selective
    reuptake inhibitors
Selegiline
    overdose/toxicity of, 968*t*, 1440–1441
    for parkinsonism, 907
    transdermal, 968*t*
Selenium, for Hashimoto thyroiditis, 1018
Self-care
    assessment of ability to manage, 62, 63
    asthma management and, 221–223
    clinician, providing end-of-life care
      and, **89**
    diabetes management and, 1100–1101
Self-examination, breast, in cancer
    screening, 16, 17*t*, 655
Self-help groups. *See* Support groups
Self-monitoring of blood glucose, in dia-
    betes mellitus, 1085,
    1100–1101, 1102–1103
    in pregnant patient, 722
Self-mutilation, 963
Self-treatment, for malaria, 1361
Selzentry. *See* Maraviroc
Semen analysis, in infertility workup, 693,
    864, 865*f*
Semicircular canal dehiscence, vertigo
    and, 190
Seminal emission, loss of, 862. *See also* Erec-
    tile dysfunction/impotence

Seminiferous tubule dysgenesis. *See* Klinefelter syndrome

Seminomas, 1066, 1492, 1493, 1494

SEN-V virus, 601

Sengstaken-Blakemore tube, for esophageal varices, 540

Senile cataract, 161

Senile freckles. *See* Lentigines

Senna, 509t, 510

Sennetsu fever, 1285

Sensorimotor peripheral neuropathy. *See* Neuropathies

Sensorineural hearing loss, 179, 180, 186–187. *See also* Hearing loss
  in HIV infection/AIDS, 192
  vestibular schwannoma (acoustic neurinoma) causing, 179, 191, 191t

Sensory conduction velocity studies. *See* Conduction velocity studies

Sensory disturbances/loss, **885–886**. *See also* Neuropathies
  dementia assessment and, 65
  in diabetic neuropathy, 1106
  dissociated, 886, 897
  in intracranial tumors, 899
  in leprosy, 924, 1327
  in spinal cord infarction, 897
  in spinal lesions/tumors, 886, 901
  in spinal trauma, 919
  in syringomyelia, 920

Sensory hearing loss, 179, **186–187**. *See also* Hearing loss
  autoimmune, 187
  in cochlear otosclerosis, 185
  hereditary, 187
  sudden, 179, 180, 187
  tinnitus and, 187

Sentinel acute pancreatitis event (SAPE), 646

Sentinel loop, in pancreatitis, 643

Sentinel lymph node biopsy
  in breast cancer, 663, 664
    arm edema avoidance and, 671
  in melanoma, 101

Sentinel pile, 596

Seoul viruses, 1264

Sepsis/septic shock, 434, 434t, 435, 436. *See also* Bacteremia
  ARDS and, 291
  in burn injury, 1411
  in cancer patients, 1498
  corticosteroids for, 437, 1312
  goal directed therapy of, 436
  gram-negative, 1176t, 1177t, **1311–1312**
  in listeriosis, 1303
  postabortion, anaerobic, 1323
  in pyelonephritis, 853
  in strongyloidiasis, 1381
  thrombocytopenia and, **489**
  vibrios causing, 1177t, 1316

Septal ablation, for cardiomyopathy, 373

Septal hematoma, in nasal trauma, 199

Septal hypertrophy, in cardiomyopathy, 372

Septata species. *See Encephalitozoon*

Septic (nongonococcal acute bacterial) arthritis, **777–778**, 1181t
  in drug users, 777, 1168–1169
  rheumatoid arthritis and, 748, 777, 778

Septic bursitis, 743–744

Septic thrombophlebitis, 429, 1181t
  anaerobic infections and, 1321, 1322
  catheter-associated infection and, 429, 1160, 1181t
  in drug user, 1168
  ruptured appendicitis and, 568
  sigmoid sinus, otitis media and, 185

Septo-optic dysplasia (de Morsier syndrome), 991

Septoplasty, nasal, for sleep apnea, 289

Septra. *See* Trimethoprim-sulfamethoxazole

Sequential compression devices. *See* Pneumatic compression devices

Sequential organ failure assessment (SOFA) score, in pancreatitis, 642

Sequoiosis, 280t

Serax. *See* Oxazepam

Serenoa repens (saw palmetto), 1523t, 1526–1527
  for benign prostatic hyperplasia, 870, 1523t, 1526–1527

Serentil. *See* Mesoridazine

Serial seizures, 880. *See also* Seizures

Serine protease inhibitor (*SPINK1*) gene, 15
  in chronic pancreatitis, 646

Serine threonine kinase gene, in Peutz-Jeghers syndrome, 592

SERMs. *See* Selective estrogen receptor modulators

Seronegative spondyloarthropathies, **773–777**. *See also specific type*
  back pain in, 738

Seronegative synovitis, remitting, with non-pitting edema, cancer and, 783

Seroquel. *See* Quetiapine

Serotonin
  carcinoids secreting, 1476
  islet cell tumors secreting, 1062

Serotonin receptor agonists, for irritable bowel syndrome, 572

Serotonin 5-HT$_3$-receptor-blocking agents. *See also* Serotonin-selective reuptake inhibitors
  for irritable bowel syndrome, 572
  for nausea and vomiting, 506, 506t, 1508–1509

Serotonin-selective reuptake inhibitors (SSRIs), 964–966, 968t
  for anxiety/stress disorders, 942
  for depression, 964–966, 968t
  for irritable bowel syndrome, 572
  MAOI interaction and, 965–966, 1440
  for menopausal vasomotor symptoms, 704
  for neuropathic pain, 85, 85t
  for OCD, 943
  osteoporosis and, 1038
  overdose/toxicity of, 964–965, 968t

for panic attacks, 943
  for personality disorders, 951
  for phobic disorder, 943
  platelet function affected by, 490t
  during pregnancy, 966
  for psychosexual disorders, 950
  serotonin syndrome caused by, 965–966, 1423, 1440, 1448, 1449
  sexual side effects of, 965
  withdrawal from, 966

Serotonin syndrome, 39, 965–966, 1423, 1440, 1448, 1449
  St. John's wort causing, 1523

Serous otitis media, **182–183**
  in HIV infection/AIDS, 192
  nasopharyngeal carcinoma and, 183, 200

Serous retinal detachment, 161

Serpasil. *See* Reserpine

Serrated adenoma, 589

Serratia, 1177t

Sertaconazole, 98t

Sertoli cell tumors, 1066, 1492
  gynecomastia and, 1066, 1067

Sertraline, 964, 966. *See also* Serotonin-selective reuptake inhibitors
  for migraine prophylaxis, 874t
  overdose/toxicity of, 966, 968t
  for panic attacks, 943

Serum-ascites albumin gradient (SAAG), 524t, 525
  in cirrhosis, 620–621
  in mesothelioma, 528
  in pancreatic ascites, 528
  in peritoneal carcinomatosis, 528
  in portal hypertension, 524t, 525

Serum osmolality. *See* Osmolality

Serum protein electrophoresis
  in myeloma, 472
  in protein-losing enteropathy, 569
  reference values for, 1553t
  in Waldenström macroglobulinemia, 474

Serum separator (SST) tube, 1555t

Serum sickness, 784, **785**. *See also* Immune complex-mediated hypersensitivity
  urticarial vasculitis in, 126

Serzone. *See* Nefazodone

Sestamibi scintigraphy, in angina, 319

Sevelamer, for hyperphosphatemia, 804
  in mineral bone disorders of chronic kidney disease, 830

Severe acute respiratory syndrome (SARS), **1274–1275**

Sex. *See* Gender

Sex change surgery, for transsexuals, 950

Sex chromosomes. *See* X chromosome; Y chromosome

Sex steroid replacement therapy. *See also* Estrogen (hormone) replacement therapy; Testosterone replacement therapy
  for hypogonadism, 863, 866, 1065–1066, 1070–1073

Sexual abuse
  child, 976
    intrafamilial (incest), 948
  victims of, 976, 977
Sexual arousal disorders, 948, 949–950.
        See also Sexual dysfunction
  in female, 691, 692
Sexual assault. *See* Rape
Sexual behavior
  hepatitis/hepatitis vaccination and,
        602, 604, 605
  herpes simplex infections and, 1235,
        1236
  HIV infection/AIDS and, 1205–1207
    postexposure prophylaxis and,
        1221
    prevention and, 1207, 1218–1219
  STDs and, 1166, 1167
  syphilis and, 1332
Sexual desire disorders, 949
  in female, 691, 692
Sexual dysfunction
  drugs causing, 862
    antidepressants, 965, 967
    antipsychotics, 958
    lithium, 971
  endocrine causes of, 863
  in female, **691–692**, 949, 950
  in male, **862–864**, 949, 950. *See also*
        Erectile dysfunction/impo-
        tence
    hypogonadism and, 863
  psychosexual, 949, 950
Sexual intercourse
  cystitis associated with, 46, 851
  HIV infection/AIDS transmission
        and, 1207, 1219
    postexposure prophylaxis and, 1221
  painful. *See* Dyspareunia
  unlawful (statutory rape), 702
  unprotected, emergency/postcoital
        contraception and, **700**
  IUD for, 698, 700
Sexual masochism, 948
Sexual sadism, 948
Sexually transmitted diseases, **1166–1168**.
        See also specific disease
  condoms in prevention of, 699
  drug use and, 1168
  epididymitis, 852*t*, 865, 1182*t*
  HIV testing and, 1167
  IUD use and, 688, 698
  during pregnancy, **727**
  rape and, 702, 1167
  reactive arthritis and, 776
  syphilis testing and, 1167, 1332
Sézary cells, in cutaneous T cell lym-
        phoma (mycosis fun-
        goides), 111
Sézary syndrome, exfoliative dermatitis
        and, 112
SFA. *See* Superficial femoral artery
SGOT. *See* Aspartate aminotransferase
SGPT. *See* Alanine aminotransferase
Shagreen patches, in tuberous sclerosis, 903
Shared epitope, in rheumatoid arthritis,
        747
Shaver disease, 279*t*

Shaving, pseudofolliculitis and, 123
Shawl sign, 760
Sheathotomy, arteriovenous, for retinal
        vein occlusion, 164
Sheep cell agglutination tests, in mononu-
        cleosis, 1243
Sheep liver fluke infection, 1375
Shellfish, contaminated
  in angiostrongyliasis, 1384
  in gnathostomiasis, 1384
  in paragonimiasis, 1376
  poisoning by, 1446, 1446*t*
  in vibrio infection, 1316
Shiga-like toxins, *E coli* producing, 513,
        1170*t*, 1315. *See also Esche-
        richia coli* O157:H7
Shigella, dysenteriae/flexneri/sonnei
        (shigellosis/bacillary dys-
        entery), 512, 1171*t*, 1172,
        1174, 1182*t*, **1314**
Shin spots, diabetic, 1109
Shingles. *See* Herpes zoster
Shiny corner sign, 774
Shock, **424–438**, 434*t*
  cardiogenic, 338, 434, 434*t*, 435, 436
  dengue, 1263, 1264
  distributive, 434–435, 434*t*, 435, 436
  in ectopic pregnancy, 713
  in heat stroke, 1408
  hypovolemic, 434, 434*t*, 435, 436
    in myocardial infarction, 338
  in infectious myocarditis, 369
  neurogenic, 434–435, 434*t*
  obstructive, 434, 434*t*, 435
  in pancreatitis, 642, 644
  after pheochromocytoma removal,
        1060, 1061
  septic. *See* Sepsis/septic shock
  vasodilatory (distributive), 434–435,
        434*t*, 435, 436
Shock liver, 631
Shock wave lithotripsy
  for renal stones, 860
  for ureteral stones, 860
Short-acting insulin, 1096–1097, 1096*t*,
        1097–1098, 1097*f*. *See also*
        Insulin therapy
Short bowel syndrome, **562–563**
  lactic acidosis and, 868
Short stature, in Turner syndrome, 1068,
        1074
Shortness of breath. *See* Dyspnea
Shoulder-hand syndrome, 743
Shoulder pain
  in brachial plexus neuropathy, 930
  in polymyalgia rheumatica, 766
  in rotator cuff disorders, 744
SHOX gene, in Turner syndrome, 1075
Shunt procedures, for malignant effu-
        sions, 1496
Shunts
  in atrial septal defect, 297, 298
  in patent ductus arteriosus, 301
  portosystemic. *See* Portosystemic shunts
  in ventricular septal defect, 299
Shy-Drager syndrome (multisystem atrophy)
  dysautonomia and, 885
  parkinsonism and, 906

SIADH. *See* Syndrome of inappropriate
        ADH secretion
Sialadenitis, **206**
Sialolithiasis, **206–207**
Siberian ginseng, 1526
Siberian tick typhus, 1281*t*, 1285
Sibutramine, for obesity, 1137
Sick role (invalidism)
  chronic pain disorders and, 946
  psychiatric problems associated with
        hospitalization/illness and,
        990
Sick sinus syndrome, **354**
Sickle cell anemia/syndromes, **450–451**,
        451*t*
  cholelithiasis/gallstones and, 634
  genetic/prenatal testing for, 450, 721
  osteomyelitis and, 780
  in pregnancy, 721
  renal dysfunction associated with,
        849
  screening test for, 451, 452
Sickle cell glomerulopathy, 849
Sickle cell retinopathy, 167
Sickle cell trait, **451–452**, 451*t*
Sickle thalassemia, 451*t*, **452**
Sideroblasts/sideroblastic anemia,
        444–445
  myelodysplasia and, 444, 463
Siderosis, 279*t*
Sigmoid esophagus, 542
Sigmoid sinus thrombosis, otitis media
        and, 185
Sigmoidoscopy
  in antibiotic-associated colitis, 574
  in cancer screening, 16, 17*t*, 590, 1480,
        1481–1482
  in fecal incontinence, 596
  in GI bleeding, 521
  in polyp identification, 590, 1481
  in ulcerative colitis, 583
Signal recognition particle (SRP) anti-
        body, in polymyositis/der-
        matomyositis, 760
Significant others. *See* Family/significant
        others
SIL. *See* Squamous intraepithelial lesions
Sildenafil
  adverse ophthalmic effects of, 177*t*
  contraindications to with nitroglyc-
        erin, 863, 950
  for erectile dysfunction, 863, 950,
        1107–1108
    antidepressant-induced, 950, 965
    in diabetics, 1107–1108
  for pulmonary hypertension, 275,
        381
Silent myocardial ischemia/angina, 320
  dyspnea in, 25, 26
Silent thyroiditis, 1008, 1017. *See also*
        Subacute (de Quervain)
        thyroiditis
Silent ulcers, 549
Silibinin/silymarin, for mushroom poi-
        soning, 608, 1442
Silicone gel breast implants. *See* Breast
        implants
Silicosis, 279, 279*t*

Silo-filler's disease, 280
Silvadene. *See* Silver sulfadiazine
Silver sulfadiazine, for burn wounds, 1411
Silymarin/silibinin, for mushroom poisoning, 608, 1442
Simple partial seizures, 879, 879t. *See also* Seizures
Simple renal cysts, 846, 847t
Simultagnosia, intracranial tumors causing, 899
SIMV. *See* Synchronized intermittent mandatory ventilation
Simvastatin, 1131, 1132t. *See also* Statin drugs
  for Hashimoto thyroiditis, 1018
  protease inhibitor interactions and, 1229
Sin Nombre virus, 1264
Sinemet. *See* Carbidopa/levodopa
Sinequan. *See* Doxepin
Singer's nodules, 209
Single photon emission computed tomography (SPECT)
  in angina, 319, 320
  in Zollinger-Ellison syndrome/gastrinoma, 556–557
Singultus (hiccups), 507
Sinoatrial exit block (sick sinus syndrome), 354
Sinonasal inflammatory disease, 201
Sinus arrest (sick sinus syndrome), 354
Sinus arrhythmia, 340–341
Sinus bradycardia, 341. *See also* Bradycardia/bradyarrhythmias
  in myocardial infarction, 336
  persistent (sick sinus syndrome), 354
  in poisoning/drug overdose, 1422t
  in sleep apnea, 289
Sinus tachycardia, 341. *See also* Tachycardia/tachyarrhythmia
  in hyperthyroidism, 1009, 1014
  in myocardial infarction, 336
  in poisoning/drug overdose, 1422t
Sinus venosus atrial septal defect, 297
Sinuses. *See* Paranasal sinuses
Sinusitis, 192–195, 194t, 1182t. *See also* Rhinosinusitis, acute bacterial
  in aspergillosis, 195, 1397, 1398
  facial pain in, 878
  headache in, 193, 872
  in HIV infection/AIDS, 195, 1211
  invasive fungal, 195–196
Sinusoidal obstruction syndrome, drugs/toxins causing, 617, 630
Sipple syndrome. *See* Multiple endocrine neoplasia, type 2a
Sirolimus, 613, 1545t
SIRS. *See* Systemic inflammatory response syndrome
Sister Joseph's nodule, 1464
Sister Mary Joseph nodule, 1471
Sitagliptin, 1091t, 1095, 1101
  with metformin, 1096
Siti (endemic syphilis), 1339
Situational (stress and adjustment) disorders, 937–938. *See also* Adjustment (situational) disorders

Sixth disease (exanthema subitum), 1240t, 1247
Sixth nerve paralysis, 169
Sjögren syndrome, 762–763
  autoantibodies in, 754t, 762
Skeletal hyperostosis, diffuse idiopathic (DISH), 774
Skeletal system disorders. *See* Bone; Musculoskeletal disorders
Skin, 94–150
  anaerobic flora of, 1323
  biopsy of
    in cutaneous leishmaniasis, 1352
    in leprosy, 1327
    in Lyme disease, 1344
    in onchocerciasis, 1388
    in polyarteritis nodosa, 765
    in rabies, 1256
    in Rocky Mountain spotted fever, 1284
  caustic/corrosive injuries of, 1429, 1430
  changes in, in chronic venous insufficiency, 36, 37, 143, 430, 431
  decontamination of, 1424
    for caustic/corrosive burns, 1424, 1429, 1430
    nerve agents in chemical warfare and, 1424
  disorders of. *See specific type and* Skin cancer; Skin disorders
  dry
    atopic dermatitis and, 101, 102
    emollients for, 94, 98–99t
  hardening of. *See* Scleroderma
Skin bends, 1417
Skin cancer. *See also specific type*
  basal cell carcinoma, 133–134
  ear involved in, 180
  eyelid involved in, 153
  melanoma, 100–101
  PUVA therapy and, 105
  squamous cell carcinoma, 134
  sun avoidance in prevention of, 16
Skin disorders, 94–150, 95t. *See also specific type and* Dermatitis
  anaerobic infections, 1323
  anthrax, 1300, 1301, 1301–1302, 1302
  arthropod infestations, 138–140
  in blastomycosis, 1399
  blistering (bullous), 95t, 130–131
  cancer. *See* Skin cancer
  cancer-related, 1453t
  candidal infection, 125
  in Chagas disease (chagoma), 1350
  chemotherapy causing, 1509
  chilblain (erythema pernio), 1405
  in chromoblastomycosis, 1400
  cryptococcal, 1396
  in cutaneous larva migrans, 1385
  in cutaneous leishmaniasis, 1351–1352, 1352, 1353
  in decompression sickness, 1417
  in diabetes mellitus, 1083, 1109
  in dracunculiasis, 1382, 1383
  in drug users, 1168

drugs causing (dermatitis medicamentosa/drug eruption), 147–150, 148–149t
epidermal inclusion cysts, 141–142
  erosive, 95t
  erythemas, 95t, 125–130
  frostbite, 1405, 1405–1406
  fungal infections, 107–110. *See also* Tinea
    in HIV infection/AIDS, 1215
  in gnathostomiasis, 1384
  in gonococcal arthritis, 778
  in Graves disease (dermopathy/pretibial myxedema), 1008, 1009, 1015
  in Henoch-Schönlein purpura, 771, 837
  in HIV infection/AIDS, 1215
  in hookworm disease, 1380
  in leprosy, 1327
  in Lyme disease, 128, 1343, 1344
  morbilliform, 95t
  morphologic categorization of, 95t
  in mycetoma, 1400
  mycobacterial infections, 1325
  in nephrogenic systemic fibrosis, 849
  nicotine patch causing, 10t
  nodules, 95t
    inflammatory, 140–141
    violaceous to purple, 134–136
    in onchocerciasis, 1387, 1388
  papules, 95t, 131–134
    violaceous to purple, 134–136
  in paracoccidioidomycosis (South American blastomycosis), 1399
  photodermatitis, 95t, 142–143
  pigmentary, 144–145. *See also* Hyperpigmentation; Hypopigmentation
    drugs causing, 145, 149t
    in hypercarotenosis, 1144
  pigmented lesions, 95t, 99–101
  in polyarteritis nodosa, 765
  pruritus (itching) and, 95t, 136–140.
    See also specific cause
  pustular, 95t, 120–125
  radiation causing, 1414
  scaling, 95t, 101–113
  in schistosomiasis, 1374
  in sporotrichosis, 1399, 1400
  staphylococcal infections, 1294–1295
    in HIV infection/AIDS, 1215
  streptococcal infections, 1290
  in strongyloidiasis, 1381
  in syphilis, 1330, 1334, 1335. *See also* Chancre; Gummas
  treatment of, 94–99, 96–99t
    adverse ophthalmic effects of drugs in, 178t
    complications of, 95–99
  in tularemia, 1317
  ulcers, 95t, 143–144
    decubitus (pressure), 72–74, 73t
      bed rest/immobility and, 68, 73
    in diabetics, 1106
    in dracunculiasis, 1382, 1383
    in mycetoma, 1400

osteomyelitis and, 780
in polyarteritis, 765
venous insufficiency/varicose
        veins/lower extremity
        occlusive disease and, 36,
        37, **143–144**, 418, 430,
        431
in uremia, 826t
venous insufficiency/varicose veins
        and. *See* Skin disorders,
        ulcers; Stasis dermatitis;
        Venous insufficiency/
        stasis
vesicular, 95t, **113–118**
weeping/crusted, 95t, **118–120**
drying agents for, 94
Skin grafts
in burn care, 1411
for leg ulcers, 144
Skin substitutes, in burn care, 1411
Skin test anergy
in HIV infection/AIDS, 1211
measles causing, 1249
in sarcoidosis, 265
tuberculin skin test and, 254, 1211
Skin tests. *See also specific type*
allergy, 784
in asthma, 221
in penicillin allergy, 1180, 1183
Skull fractures, **918**. *See also* Head injury
vertigo caused by, 190
SLC30A8 gene/antibodies
in type 1 diabetes, 1080
in type 2 diabetes, 1082
SLE. *See* Systemic lupus erythematosus
Sleep
abnormal behaviors during (parasom-
        nias), **975–976**
age-related changes in, 973
breathing disorders and, **288–289**. *See
        also* Sleep apnea
disorders of, **973–976**
        chronic fatigue syndrome and, 43
drugs for problems with, 941t, 942,
        974–975
stages of, 973
Sleep apnea, **288–289**, 975
in obesity-hypoventilation syndrome,
        287
postoperative pulmonary complica-
        tions and, 53
testosterone replacement therapy and,
        1066
Sleep attacks, in narcolepsy, 975
Sleep hygiene, 974
Sleep panic attacks, 940
Sleep paralysis, in narcolepsy, 975
Sleep terror (pavor nocturnus), 975,
        975–976
Sleepiness. *See* Somnolence
Sleeping sickness, **1348–1349**, 1349t
Sleepwalking (somnambulism), 940, 975,
        976
SLITRK1 gene, in Tourette syndrome, 911
Sm antibody, in SLE, 753, 754t
SMAD4 gene mutation, in hereditary hem-
        orrhagic telangiectasia,
        1519

Small cell carcinoma of lung, 1452–1454,
        1454, 1466t. *See also* Lung
        cancer
paraneoplastic syndromes associated
        with, 1453t, 1454
staging of, 1455
survival rates for, 1454
treatment of, 1457, 1466t
Small intestine. *See also under Intestinal*
absorption/digestion in, 557–558
adenocarcinomas in, **1474**
        Crohn disease and, 579, 1474
bacterial overgrowth in, **561–562**. *See
        also* Bacterial overgrowth
biopsy of
        in bacterial overgrowth, 562
        in celiac disease, 560
        in Whipple disease, 561
carcinoid tumors in, **1475–1476**
disorders of, **557–569**
        appendicitis and, **567–568**
        benign tumors, **566–567**
        malabsorption and, **557–564**, 558t
        malignant tumors, **1474–1476**
        motility disorders, **564–566**. *See
                also* Intestinal obstruction
        protein-losing enteropathy and, **569**
        tuberculosis, **568–569**
lymphomas in, **1474–1475**
polyps in, 567, **589**, 591
resection of, short bowel syndrome
        and, **562–563**
Small intestine push enteroscopy, in GI
        bleeding, 522, 523
Small intestine transplantation, for short
        bowel syndrome, 563
Smallpox (variola), **116**, 1240t, 1277
Smallpox (variola) vaccination, 116, 1277
atopic dermatitis/eczema and, 103,
        116, 1277
for monkeypox prevention, 1277–1278
Smell, disorders of sensation of, **197–198**
Smith antibody, in SLE, 753, 754t
Smoke inhalation, **277**, 1409
cyanide poisoning and, 277
Smoking
abdominal aortic aneurysms and, 423
asbestosis and, 279, 280
bladder cancer and, 1489
cancer and, 1450–1451
cataract development and, 161
cessation of, 7–9, 8t, 9t, 10t, 11t
        acupuncture for, 1534
        acute coronary syndromes and, 327t
        bupropion for, 7, 11t, 1450
        in cancer prevention, 1450–1451
        in cardiovascular/cerebrovascular
                disease prevention, 7–9, 8t,
                9t, 10t, 11t
        in COPD prevention/manage-
                ment, 6, 7, 236
        for hypertension, 394
        mind-body therapies for, 1536t
        hypnosis, 1536t, 1539
        nicotine replacement therapy for, 7,
                9t, 10t, 11t
        postoperative pulmonary compli-
                cations reduced by, 54

for thromboangiitis obliterans
        (Buerger disease), 423
in COPD, 234
coronary heart disease and, 6–9, 8t, 9t,
        10t, 11t, 316
Crohn disease and, 578
environmental exposure and. *See* Pas-
        sive smoking
esophageal cancer and, 1468
Graves ophthalmopathy and, 170,
        1012, 1014
health hazards of, 6–7
hemoptysis and, 27
hypertension and, 390, 394
laryngeal leukoplakia and, 209
laryngeal squamous cell carcinoma
        and, 210
lung cancer and, 6, 7, 1450, 1452
        as co-carcinogen, 280
        screening for, 18, 259, 1456
oral cancer and, 201
pneumothorax and, 286, 287
postoperative pulmonary complica-
        tions and, 53, 54
during pregnancy, 707
preventable disease/deaths caused by,
        2t
in renal cell carcinoma, 1491
respiratory bronchiolitis and, 243
sleep disorders and, 974
theophyllines affected by, 225t
thromboangiitis obliterans (Buerger
        disease) and, 422
ulcerative colitis and, 583
ureteral/renal pelvis cancer and, 1491
vocal fold changes and, 209
Smooth muscle antibodies, in autoim-
        mune hepatitis, 613
Snails, in disease transmission. *See* Cer-
        cariae/metacercariae
Snake bites, 1424t, **1446–1447**
Sneddon syndrome, 773
Sniffing (solvents/gases), 984, 1444
Snoring, in sleep apnea, 288
Snow blindness, 172
Soapsuds enema, 509t
Social challenges, for terminally ill/dying
        patient, **92**, 92t
Social phobias, 940, 943
Social support. *See* Support groups
Sodium
dietary, 1145
        hypertension and, 390, 394, 395t,
                1145
        during pregnancy, 708
        requirements for in nutritional
                support, 1149
        restriction of. *See* Sodium-
                restricted diet
        in urinary stone formation, 857
disorders of concentration of,
        789–795. *See also* Hyper-
        natremia; Hyponatremia
in fluid management, 815, 815t. *See
        also* Saline
fractional excretion of, in acute kidney
        injury, 820, 820t
hyperosmolality caused by, 795

Sodium (*cont.*)
    intracellular, in hypertension, 390
    reference values for, 1553*t*
    retention of in volume overload, 794
    serum
        in hypernatremia, 793, 794
        in hyponatremia, 789, 792
    urine
        in acute kidney injury, 820, 820*t*
        in hyponatremia, 791, 792
Sodium bicarbonate. *See* Bicarbonate
Sodium channel blocking drugs, for
        arrhythmias, 343*t*
Sodium iodide I 131. *See* ^{131}I
Sodium ipodate. *See* Ipodate sodium
Sodium nitrite, for cyanide poisoning,
        1424*t*, 1435, 1435*t*
Sodium nitroprusside. *See* Nitroprusside
Sodium phosphate, for constipation/
        bowel cleansing, 509*t*, 510
Sodium phosphate enema, 509*t*
Sodium polystyrene sulfonate, for hyper-
        kalemia, 799*t*
Sodium-restricted diet, 1145–1146
    for chronic kidney disease, 828, 830
    in cirrhosis, 620, 621
    for heart failure, 366
    for hypertension, 390, 394, 395*t*, 1145
    for nephrotic syndrome, 840
    for urinary stones, 857
Sodium salicylate, in pain management, 80*t*
Sodium stibogluconate (antimony), for
        leishmaniasis, 1352
Sodium sulfacetamide. *See* Sulfacetamide
Sodium thiosulfate, for cyanide poison-
        ing, 1424*t*, 1435, 1435*t*
SOFA score, in pancreatitis, 642
Soft diet, 1145
Soft tissue infections
    anaerobic, **1323**
    mycobacterial, **1325**
    staphylococcal, **1294–1295**
Soft tissue sarcoma, 1468*t*
Solar lentigines (liver spots), 100, 145
Soles of feet
    tinea of, **108–109**
    vesiculobullous dermatitis of (pom-
        pholyx), 116–117
Solifenacin, for urinary incontinence, 71
Solitary pulmonary nodule, **260–261**
    in metastatic disease, 1458
Solitary (simple) renal cysts, **846**, 847*t*
Solitary seizures, 883
Solitary thyroid nodule, 1019
    toxic (thyroid adenoma), 1008,
        1012–1013, 1076*t*
Soluble liver antigen–liver pancreas anti-
        bodies, in autoimmune
        hepatitis, 613
Soluble transferrin receptor, 1554*t*
Solvents
    bladder cancer caused by exposure to,
        1489
    toxicity/abuse of, 984, 1439, **1444**
Soma. *See* Carisoprodol
Soman poisoning, 1434
Somatization disorder (Briquet syn-
        drome/hysteria), 944

Somatoform disorders, **944–946**
Somatoform pain disorder, 944
Somatostatin/somatostatin analogs. *See
        also* Octreotide
    D cells secreting, 1062
    for esophageal varices, 539
Somatostatin receptor scintigraphy
    for ACTH-secreting tumor identifica-
        tion, 1052
    in carcinoids, 1476
    in islet cell tumors, 1062
    in pheochromocytoma/paragan-
        glioma, 1060
    in Zollinger-Ellison syndrome/gastri-
        noma, 556–557
Somatostatinomas, 1062
Somatuline. *See* Lanreotide
Somnambulism (sleepwalking), 940, 975,
        976
Somnolence, excessive, **975**
    restless legs syndrome causing, 911
    in sleep apnea, 288
Somogyi effect, 1102, 1103, 1103*t*
Sonata. *See* Zaleplon
Sonography. *See* Ultrasonography
Sonohysterography, saline infusion, 675*t*
    for abnormal premenopausal bleed-
        ing, 675
Sorafenib, 1504*t*
Sorbitol
    for constipation, 509, 509*t*
    diarrhea caused by, 515
Sore throat. *See* Pharyngitis
Sotalol, 344*t*
    for atrial fibrillation, 348, 349
South African tick fever, 1281*t*
South American blastomycosis, **1399**
Southern tick-associated rash illness
        (STARI), 128
Sparganosis, 1379
Spasmodic torticollis, 910
Spasticity, **914–915**
    spinal trauma causing, 919
    in tetanus, 1298
Specimen collection, tubes for, 1555*t*
SPECT. *See* Single photon emission com-
        puted tomography
Spectazole. *See* Econazole
Spectracef. *See* Cefditoren
Spectrin, in hereditary spherocytosis, 448
Speech/language
    dementia affecting, 63
    in schizophrenic/psychotic disorders,
        953
Speech discrimination
    in neural hearing loss, 191
    in presbyacusis/sensory hearing loss,
        186
    testing, 180
    vestibular schwannoma affecting, 191
Speech therapy, in stroke patient, 892
SPEP. *See* Serum protein electrophoresis
Sperm, deficiencies of, infertility and, 864,
        865*f*
Sperm analysis, in infertility workup, 693,
        864, 865*f*
Spermatogenesis, hormone therapy for
        improvement of, 994

Spermicides, in contraceptive products,
        699
Sphenoid sinusitis, 193
Spherocytes
    in autoimmune hemolytic anemia,
        452
    in hereditary spherocytosis, 448
Spherocytosis, hereditary, **448**
Sphincter of Oddi dilation, for choledo-
        cholithiasis/cholangitis,
        639
Sphincter of Oddi dysfunction
    pancreatitis and, 642
    in postcholecystectomy syndrome,
        637
Sphincterotomy
    for choledocholithiasis/cholangitis,
        638, 639
        during pregnancy, 727
    in pancreatitis, 645, 648
    for sphincter of Oddi dysfunction, 637
Sphincters. *See specific type*
Sphingolipid, accumulation of in Gaucher
        disease, 1516
Spider angiomas, in cirrhosis, 619
Spider bites, 139, **1447**
Spinal cord
    cavitation of (syringomyelia), **920**
    compression of
        spinal trauma causing, 919
        tumors causing, 901, **1494–1495**
    dural arteriovenous fistulae of, 897
    epidural/subdural hemorrhage and,
        897
    infarction of, 897, 919
    lesions/tumors of, **901**
        back pain caused by, 738, 739, 901
        cord compression by, 901,
            1494–1495
        sensory disturbances and, 886, 901
        syringomyelia and, 920
    subacute combined degeneration of,
        915
    transection of, 919
    traumatic injury of, **919–920**
        syringomyelia and, 920
    vascular diseases of, **896–897**
Spinal cord stimulation, for angina, 324
Spinal dural arteriovenous fistulae, 897
Spinal motion, testing, 739
Spinal muscular atrophy
    juvenile, 921
    progressive, 920, 921
Spinal poliomyelitis, 1252
Spinal shock. *See* Neurogenic shock
Spinal stenosis, lumbar, **740–741**
Spinal tumors. *See* Spinal cord, lesions/
        tumors of
Spine. *See also* Spinal cord
    bamboo, 774
    infection of. *See* Vertebral osteomyeli-
        tis
    tuberculosis of (Pott disease),
        781–782
    tumors of. *See* Spinal cord, lesions/
        tumors of
SPINK1 gene, in chronic pancreatitis,
        646

Spinocerebellar degeneration, in vitamin E deficiency, 914
Spiral (helical) CT. *See* Computed tomography; Helical (spiral) CT
Spiramycin, for toxoplasmosis during pregnancy, 1365
Spirillum minus, 1340
Spiritual challenges, for terminally ill/dying patient, **92–93,** 93*t*
Spirochetal infections, 1177*t,* **1330–1347.** *See also specific type*
    anaerobic, periodontal infection caused by, 1321–1322
    meningitis caused by, 1162*t*
    myocarditis in, 369*t*
    non-sexually transmitted, **1338–1339**
    syphilis, **1330–1338,** 1331*t,* 1333*t*
Spirometra tapeworms, 1379
Spirometry. *See also* Pulmonary function tests
    in asthma, 219
    in COPD, 234
    incentive, prevention of postoperative pulmonary complications and, 54
    in lung cancer, 1455–1456
Spironolactone
    for adrenal hyperplasia/Conn syndrome, 1057
    for cirrhotic ascites, 621
    for heart failure, 361, 362
        infarct-related, 335
    for hirsutism/virilization, 1055
    for hypertension, 399*t,* 405
        with hydrochlorothiazide, 399*t*
    lithium interactions and, 972, 972*t*
Splenda. *See* Sucralose
Splenectomy
    for autoimmune hemolytic anemia, 453
    for Gaucher disease, 1516
    for hereditary spherocytosis, 448
    for immune thrombocytopenic purpura, 483–484, 484*f*
    for myelofibrosis, 460
Splenic rupture, in infectious mononucleosis, 1244
Splenic vein thrombosis, noncirrhotic portal hypertension caused by, 632
Splenomegaly, 488–489, 489*t*
    in chronic lymphocytic leukemia, 467
    in chronic myeloid leukemia, 461
    in cirrhosis, 619
    in essential thrombocytosis, 459
    in hairy cell leukemia, 468
    in hepatitis, 605
    in mononucleosis, 1243
    in myelofibrosis, 460
    in noncirrhotic portal hypertension, 631
    in polycythemia, 457
    thrombocytopenia in, 482
    in visceral leishmaniasis, 1351
Splinter hemorrhages, in endocarditis, 1304
Spondylitic heart disease, 774

Spondylitis
    in alkaptonuria, 1513
    ankylosing. *See* Ankylosing spondylitis
    in inflammatory bowel disease, 777
    psoriatic, 775
Spondyloarthropathies, seronegative, **773–777.** *See also specific type*
    back pain in, 738
Spondylolisthesis, back pain in, 739
Spondylosis, cervical, 737, **929**
Spongiform encephalopathies
    bovine (mad cow disease), 1260
    transmissible, 1260–1261
Spongiosis, in prion diseases, 1260
Spontaneous abortion, **711–712**
    with IUD in place, 698
    in lupus anticoagulant-anticardiolipin-antiphospholipid antibody syndrome, 711, 713
Spontaneous bacterial peritonitis, **526–527**
    in cirrhosis, 526, 621–622
Spontaneous fractures. *See* Pathologic fractures
Spontaneous pneumothorax, **285–287.** *See also* Pneumothorax
Spoon nails, 146
Sporadic hemiplegic migraine, 873
Sporadic thyroiditis, painless, 1016, 1018
Sporanox. *See* Itraconazole
Sporothrix schenckii (sporotrichosis), **1399–1400**
Sports medicine injuries, **744–747**
Spotted fevers, 1240*t,* 1281*t,* **1283–1285**
Spousal abuse (domestic violence), 976, 977
    prevention of, 18–19
Sprains, ankle, **746–747**
Sprue, celiac. *See* Celiac disease
Sprycel. *See* Dasatinib
Sputum eosinophilia, in asthma, 221
Sputum examination
    in asthma, 221
    blood found on (hemoptysis), **27–28**
    in bronchiectasis, 240
    in COPD, 235
    in cough evaluation, 23
    in lung cancer, 1454
    in nontuberculous mycobacterial infection, 258–259
    in paragonimiasis, 1376
    in pneumonia, 246, 249
        anaerobic/lung abscess, 250
        in immunocompromised host, 251
        pneumococcal, 1292
        Pneumocystis, 251, 1210, 1395
    in solitary pulmonary nodule, 261
    in strongyloidiasis, 1381
    in tuberculosis, 252
Sputum induction
    in pneumonia, 246
        in immunocompromised host, 251
    in tuberculosis, 252
Squamous cell carcinoma
    of anus, 1483
        in HIV infection/AIDS, 1216, 1483

of bladder, 1489
cervical, 682
of ear canal, 182
of esophagus, 1465–1468
intraepidermal (Bowen disease), **113**
of larynx, **209–211**
    laryngeal leukoplakia and, 209
of lung, 1452, 1454
nasopharyngeal, 200
    inverted/schneiderian papillomas and, 200
oral, 201, 202
of skin, **134**
    actinic keratoses and, 113, 134
of vulva, 685
Squamous intraepithelial lesions (SIL), 680–681, 680*t*
"Square root" sign, 379
Squaric acid dibutylester, for wart removal, 132
Squatting, heart murmurs affected by, 306*t*
SRP antibody, in polymyositis/dermatomyositis, 760
SRS. *See* Somatostatin receptor scintigraphy
SS-A/Ro antibody, 754*t*
    in lupus, 110, 754*t*
    in Sjögren syndrome, 754*t,* 762
SS-B/La antibody, 754*t*
    in Sjögren syndrome, 754*t,* 762
SSc. *See* Scleroderma
SSI. *See* Surgical site infection
SSPE. *See* Subacute sclerosing panencephalitis
SSRIs. *See* Serotonin-selective reuptake inhibitors
SST (serum separator) tube, 1555*t*
ST elevation acute coronary syndromes. *See* Myocardial infarction; ST-segment elevation myocardial infarction
St. John's wort *(Hypericum perforatum),* 1522–1524, 1523*t*
    drug interactions and, 1523
St. Louis encephalitis, 1257–1259
ST segment changes. *See also* Electrocardiogram
    in acute coronary syndromes, 326. *See also* Acute coronary syndromes; Myocardial infarction
    in angina, 318
        Prinzmetal (variant), 325
    antipsychotic drugs causing, 958
    in hypokalemia, 796
    in myocardial infarction, 331
        reperfusion assessment and, 334
    in pericarditis, 377
    in Tako-Tsubo cardiomyopathy, 372
ST-segment elevation myocardial infarction (STEMI), 326, **330–340,** 331*t,* 333*t. See also* Myocardial infarction
Tako-Tsubo cardiomyopathy mimicking, 330
Stalevo. *See* Entacapone, with levodopa and carbidopa

Standard days method of contraception, 700
Standing, heart murmurs affected by, 306t
Stannosis, 279t
Stapedectomy, 185
Staphylococcus (staphylococcal infections)
    abscesses, 141, 1294–1295
    aureus, 1294–1297
        abscesses, 1294–1295
        atopic dermatitis and, 102
        bacteremia, 1296
        breast abscess, 651
        in burn injury, 1411
        cellulitis, 129, 130, 1182t
        community-associated methicillin-resistant (CA-MRSA), 118, 130, 1294
        diarrhea/food poisoning/gastroenteritis, 512, 1170t, 1172
        endocarditis, 1303, 1304, 1305, 1306–1307
        furuncles, 140–141, 1182t, 1294
        impetigo, 118
        methicillin-resistant (MRSA), 1176t, 1294, 1305–1307
            in burn injury, 1411
            in HIV infection/AIDS, 1215
            impetigo and, 118
            screening for, hospital-associated infections and, 1161
        nasal vestibulitis, 195
        osteomyelitis, 1295
        pneumonia, 244t
        of skin and soft tissues, 1294–1295
            in HIV infection/AIDS, 1215
        toxic shock syndrome, 1296
    carrier state and, 1294
        nasal vestibulitis and, 195
        surgical site infection associated with, 59
    cellulitis, 129, 130, 1182t
    coagulase-negative, 1296–1297
        burn-associated, 1411
        endocarditis, 1296–1297, 1306
    cohnii, 1296
    drug resistance and, 1294, 1295, 1306–1307
    epidermidis, 1296
    folliculitis and, 123, 1294
    furunculosis/carbuncles and, 141, 1294
    haemolyticus, 1296
    hominis, 1296
    keratitis, 156
    methicillin-resistant, 1176t, 1294, 1306–1307
        in burn injury, 1411
        in HIV infection/AIDS, 1215
        impetigo and, 118
    non-penicillinase-producing, 1176t
    osteomyelitis, 1295
    penicillinase-producing, 1176t
    saccharolyticus, 1296
    saprophyticus, 1296
    warnerii, 1296
STARI (Southern tick-associated rash illness), 128

Starlix. See Nateglinide
Starvation. See Protein-energy malnutrition
Stasis dermatitis, 37, 428. See also Venous insufficiency/stasis
    leg ulcers and, 143
Statin drugs (HMG-CoA reductase inhibitors), 1126, 1131, 1132, 1132t. See also Lipid-lowering therapy
    adverse ophthalmic effects of, 177t
    for Hashimoto thyroiditis, 1018
    hepatotoxicity and, 616
    for lipid modification/heart disease prevention, 9, 1126, 1131
        acute coronary syndromes and, 327t, 328
        heart failure and, 365
        in HIV infection/AIDS, 1229
        hypertension and, 396–397
    in older patients, 1128–1129
    perioperative, 50
    rhabdomyolysis/myopathy/myositis caused by, 761, 763–764, 1131
Statoconia, vertigo associated with, 190
Status epilepticus, 879t
    alcohol withdrawal and, 883
    drug noncompliance and, 883
    nonconvulsive, 884
    in theophylline overdose, 1447, 1448
    tonic-clonic, 880, 883–884
Statutory rape, 702
Stauffer syndrome, 1491
Stavudine (d4T), 1226t, 1228, 1232, 1232f. See also Antiretroviral therapy
    lipid abnormalities caused by, 1216
    neuropathy caused by, 1212, 1228
    resistance to, 1233
STDs. See Sexually transmitted diseases
Steatohepatitis, nonalcoholic (NASH), 617, 618
Steatorrhea, 558, 558t. See also Malabsorption
    in hyperoxaluric calcium nephrolithiasis, 859
    in pancreatitis, 646, 647
Steatosis, hepatic. See Fatty liver
Stein-Leventhal syndrome. See Polycystic ovary syndrome
Stelazine. See Trifluoperazine
Stellwag sign, 1009
Stem cell disorders
    aplastic anemia, 454–455, 454t, 455t
    leukemias/myeloproliferative disorders, 457
    myeloplastic disorders, 463
    paroxysmal nocturnal hemoglobinuria, 449
Stem cell transplantation, 474–476. See also Bone marrow/stem cell transplantation
Steno-2 study, 1088–1089
Stensen duct
    calculus formation in, 206–207
    in mumps, 1250

Stents/stent grafts ("covered stents"). See also Endovascular surgery/prostheses
    for abdominal aortic aneurysm, 424
    for angina, 322, 323
    for aortoiliac occlusive disease, 415–416
    for biliary stricture, 640
    for biliary tract carcinoma, 1463
    carotid, 420–421
    for cholangiocarcinoma, 1463
    for coarctation of aorta, 297
    for esophageal cancer, 1470
    for femoral/popliteal occlusive disease, 417
    for hepatic vein obstruction (Budd-Chiari syndrome), 631
    intracoronary, 322, 323. See also Percutaneous coronary intervention
    for myocardial infarction, 332
    for pancreatic duct disease, 644, 645
    for pancreatic/periampullary carcinoma, 1465
    for primary sclerosing cholangitis, 641
    for renal artery stenosis, 391, 833
    for superior vena caval obstruction, 432
    ureteral, after shock wave lithotripsy, 860
    for visceral artery insufficiency/intestinal angina, 422
Stereotactic core needle biopsies, in breast cancer, 659
Sterile pyuria, in tuberculosis, 849
Sterility. See Infertility
Sterilization, for birth control, 701
Steroid acne/folliculitis, 120, 123
Steroid rosacea, 99, 122
Steroidogenic enzyme defects
    amenorrhea and, 1068
    hirsutism/virilization and, 1053–1054
Steroids. See Anabolic steroids; Corticosteroids
Stevens-Johnson syndrome (erythema multiforme major), 127–128
    drugs causing, 127, 148t
    herpes simplex infection causing, 1236
Stevens-Johnson syndrome/toxic epidermal necrolysis overlap, 127–128
sTfR. See Transferrin receptor, soluble
STI571. See Imatinib
Stibogluconate (antimony), for leishmaniasis, 1352
Stiff man syndrome, 1453t
Stiffness
    in ankylosing spondylitis, 773
    in myotonic dystrophy/myotonia congenita, 935
    in osteoarthritis, 730
    in polymyalgia rheumatica, 766
    in rheumatoid arthritis, 747
Still disease, 751–752
Stimulant laxatives, 509t, 510

Stimulants
    abuse of, **983–984**, 1430
        aggressive/violent behavior and, 976
        kindling and, 977, 983
    for depression, 964
    for narcolepsy, 975
Stings. *See* Insect bites/stings
Stippling (nail), 146
    in psoriasis, 104
Stomach disorders, **544–557**. *See also under Gastric and Gastrointestinal*
    tumors
        benign, **557**
        malignant, 1467*t*, **1470–1474**. *See also* Gastric cancer
        mesenchymal, **1474**
Stomatitis
    herpetic, **203**, 1235
    ulcerative (aphthous ulcers), **203**
        in Behçet syndrome, 772
        in Crohn disease, 578
        in HIV infection/AIDS, 1213
Stool. *See also* Stool analysis
    blood in. *See* Diarrhea, bloody; Dysentery; Fecal occult blood testing
    impacted. *See* Fecal impaction
    incontinence of, **595–596**. *See also* Fecal incontinence
    leukocytes in. *See* Fecal leukocytes
    rice water, in cholera, 1315
Stool analysis
    in amebiasis, 514, 1366
    in antibiotic-associated colitis, 574
    in ascariasis, 1379
    in bacterial overgrowth, 562
    in clonorchiasis and opisthorchiasis, 1375
    in coccidiosis and microsporidiosis, 1370
    in cryptosporidiosis, 1214, 1370
    in cyclosporiasis, 1370
    in diarrhea, 513–514, 515–516, 1214
    for DNA, in colorectal cancer screening, 589–590
    in fascioliasis, 1375
    in giardiasis, 1371–1372, 1372
    in hookworm disease, 1380
    in intestinal fluke infection, 1376
    in isosporiasis, 1370
    for ova and parasites, 515–516. *See also specific disorder*
    in paragonimiasis, 1376
    in protein-losing enteropathy, 569
    in sarcocystosis, 1370
    in schistosomiasis, 1374
    in shigellosis, 1314
    in strongyloidiasis, 1381
    in tapeworm infections, 1377
    in trichuriasis/whipworm, 1380
Stool antigen assay
    for *E histolytica*, 514, 515
    for *Giardia*, 514, 515, 1372
Stool impaction. *See* Fecal impaction
Stool laxative screen, 515

Stool osmolality, in diarrhea, 514–515, 515
Stool surfactants, 509*t*
Stool weight, in diarrhea evaluation, 515
Storage pool disease, 489, 490
Straight leg raising test, 738
Strains (musculotendinous), cervical, 736
Strawberry gallbladder, 636
Strawberry tongue
    in Kawasaki disease, 1288
    in scarlet fever, 1289
Strep throat. *See Streptococcus* (streptococcal infections), pharyngitis
Streptobacillary fever, rat-bite fever differentiated from, 1340
Streptobacillus moniliformis, 1340
Streptococcus (streptococcal infections), **1289–1291**
    bovis, endocarditis caused by, 1291, 1306
    cellulitis, 129, 130, 1182*t*
    endocarditis, 1291, 1304, 1305–1306
    erysipelas, **128–129**, 1182*t*, 1290
    glomerulonephritis after, 834, 1289
    group A. *See* Group A β-hemolytic streptococcal infection
    group B. *See* Group B streptococcal infection
    impetigo, 118, 1182*t*, 1290
    non-group A, **1291**
    pharyngitis, 204, 1182*t*, **1289–1290**
    pneumonia, 244*t*, 1182*t*, 1290
    pneumoniae (pneumococcal infections), 1176*t*, **1292–1294**. *See also* Pneumococcal (*Streptococcus pneumoniae*) infections
        drug resistance and, 246–247, 1293, 1294
    in pregnancy, 708, **725**
    pyogenes. *See* Group A β-hemolytic streptococcal infection
    rheumatic fever after, 375, 1289
    of skin, **1290**
    toxic shock syndrome caused by, 1291
    viridans, 1176*t*, 1291
        endocarditis caused by, 1304, 1305
Streptokinase. *See also* Thrombolytic therapy
    for myocardial infarction, 333–334, 333*t*
    for pulmonary embolism, 273
Streptomycin, 255*t*, 256*t*. *See also* Aminoglycosides
    for actinomycetoma, 1400
    adverse effects of, ophthalmic, 177*t*
    for tuberculosis, 255, 255*t*, 256, 256*t*
        contraindications to in pregnancy, 256
Stress cardiomyopathy. *See* Tako-Tsubo (stress/catecholamine-induced) cardiomyopathy
Stress disorders (psychiatric/psychologic), **937–938**
    depression and, 963
    irritable bowel syndrome and, 570, 571

    posttraumatic, **938–939**
        abuse victims and, 938, 976, 977
        substance use and, 938, 977
        suicide and, 963
Stress gastritis/ulcers, 544, 544–545
Stress incontinence, 71, 71–72
    in pelvic organ prolapse, 687
Stress reduction techniques, 937
Stress testing. *See also* Exercise testing
    in angina/chest pain evaluation, 319
    echocardiography, 319
    electrocardiography, 318–319
    before exercise program initiation, 13
    in heart failure, 360
    perfusion scintigraphy, 319
    postinfarction, 339–340
    preoperative, 49–50, 51*f*
    radionuclide angiography, 319
    in syncope evaluation, 357
Striae distensae, 1052
Stridor, **207**
    recurrent respiratory papillomatosis causing, 208
    vocal fold paralysis causing, 211
Stroke, **888–897**, 890*t*
    arteriovenous malformations causing, 890*t*, **895–896**
    atrial fibrillation and, 346, 347*t*
        anticoagulation in prevention of, 348, 891–892
    biofeedback in rehabilitation after, 1538
    carotid occlusion causing, 420, 889, 890*t*
    cerebral infarct causing, **889–892**
    coma caused by, 891
        in diabetic patient, 1112*t*
    COX-2 inhibitors associated with, 749
    in endocarditis, 1304
    estrogen replacement therapy affecting incidence of, 1072
    guided imagery in rehabilitation after, 1543
    hemorrhagic, 890*t*
    hypertension and, 9–12, 387, 393, 396*t*, 407
        emergencies/urgencies, 412
    intracerebral hemorrhage causing, 890*t*, **892–893**
    intracranial aneurysm causing, 890*t*, **894–895**
    intracranial venous thrombosis causing, **896**
    ischemic (infarcts), 890*t*
    lacunar infarct causing, **889**, 890*t*
    occlusive cerebrovascular disease causing, 420
    olanzapine use and, 956
    oral contraceptive use and, 696
    postoperative, 56–57
    prevention of, 6–12
        antihypertensive treatment and, 9–12, 396*t*, 407
        carotid endarterectomy in, 420
        chemoprevention and, 12
        lipid-lowering therapy and, 1125
    spinal cord vascular disease causing, **896–897**

Stroke (*cont.*)
subarachnoid hemorrhage causing,
890*t*, **893–894**
transient ischemic attacks and, 886,
887, 888
vertebrobasilar occlusion causing,
889–891, 890*t*
Stroke (heat), **1407–1408**
Stroke volume, in aortic regurgitation,
312
Stroke work index, in myocardial infarction, 331*t*
Stromal tumors (gastrointestinal stromal
tumor/GIST), 557, 567,
1474
Strongyloides fulleborni/stercoralis
(strongyloidiasis),
1380–1381
eosinophilic pulmonary syndromes
and, 266
Strontium, for bone pain, 1507*t*
Struma ovarii, 1008, 1010
Struvite urinary stones, 857, 859–860
Strychnine poisoning, seizures caused by,
1423*t*
Stunning, myocardial, 317
Stupor, **915–918**. *See also* Coma
Sturge-Weber syndrome, **904**
Sty (external hordeolum), 152
Subacromial bursitis, 744
Subacute cerebellar degeneration. *See*
Cerebellar degeneration
Subacute combined degeneration of spinal cord, **915**
Subacute cutaneous lupus erythematosus
(SCLE), 110–111
Subacute mountain sickness, **1418**
Subacute sclerosing panencephalitis, 1248
myoclonus in, 910
Subacute (de Quervain) thyroiditis, 1008,
1010, 1016, 1017, 1018
hypothyroid phase in, 1003, 1017,
1018
Subarachnoid hemorrhage, 890*t*,
893–894. *See also* Stroke
arteriovenous malformations/fistulae
causing
intracranial, 895, 895–896
spinal, 897
headache in, 44, 45, 876, 893
hypopituitarism associated with, 991
intracranial aneurysms causing, 894
oral contraceptive use and, 696
Subareolar abscess, 651–652
Subclavian steal syndrome, 886
Subclavian vessels, compression of in thoracic outlet/cervical rib
syndromes, 737, 932
Subclinical hyperthyroidism, 1015
Subclinical thyroiditis, 1016
Subcutaneous insulin infusion, continuous, 1099, 1102. *See also*
Insulin infusion pumps
Subcutaneous nodules
in cysticercosis, 1377
in gnathostomiasis, 1384
in loiasis, 1388–1389
in nocardiosis, 1324

in onchocerciasis, 1387–1388
in rheumatic fever, 375
in rheumatoid arthritis, 747–748
gouty tophi differentiated from,
733, 748
in sporotrichosis, 1400
Subdural hemorrhage/hematoma
cerebral
acute, 918*t*
chronic, 918–919
falls in elderly and, 69
spinal, 897
Suberosis, 280*t*
Sublingual glands. *See* Salivary glands
Submandibular glands. *See also* Salivary
glands
sialadenitis affecting, 206
tumors of, 207
Submersion injury, 1415–1416
Substance use disorders, **19–21, 977–985**.
*See also specific substance
used and* Injection drug
use
acupuncture for, 1534
aggressive/violent behavior and, 976
atypical psychoses and, 953
breast feeding and, 710*t*
cognitive disorders/delirium caused
by withdrawal and, 985*t*
concerns about, pain management in
terminally ill/dying patient
and, 78
febrile patient and, 1169
hallucinations/hallucinosis caused by,
986, 1439
HIV infection/AIDS and, 1168, 1207,
1219, 1220
infections and, **1168–1169**
overdoses. *See* Poisoning/drug overdose
pregnancy and, 706, 706*t*, 707
preventable deaths and, 2*t*
prevention of injury related to, 18
prevention of/screening tests for,
19–21, 20*t*, 21*t*
toxicology screen in, 1427
Subtentorial lesions. *See also* Brainstem
coma or stupor caused by, 917
Subungual capillary pulsations (Quincke
pulses), 312
Succimer (DMSA)
for arsenic poisoning, 1432
for lead poisoning, 1438
for mercury poisoning, 1439
Succinate dehydrogenase (SDH) mutations, in pheochromocy-
toma/paraganglioma,
1058, 1059
Succinylcholine
lithium interactions and, 972*t*
MAOI interactions and, 969*t*
Succussion splash, in gastric outlet
obstruction, 504, 555
Sucralfate
reduction of ventilator-associated
pneumonia and, 248
for stress gastritis, 545
Sucralose, for diabetics, 1090

Sudden death, **352–353**
aborted, driving recommendations
and, 357–358
of athlete, 385–386
cardiomyopathy causing, 373, 386
cardiomyopathy and, 373
myocardial infarction and, 330, 353
ventricular fibrillation causing, 330,
352–353
ventricular premature beats and, 351
ventricular tachycardia and, 352, 353
Sudeck atrophy, 743
Sugar alcohols, for diabetics, 1090
Suggestibility, in hypnosis, 1539
Suicide, 963
acetaminophen overdose/liver failure
and, 607
alcohol use/abuse and, 978
antidepressant overdose in, 963, 1448
carbon monoxide poisoning and,
1433
caustic esophageal injury and, 536
depression associated with hospital-
ization/illness and, 990
dispensing medications and, 963,
964
in elderly, 66
hospitalization for patient threatening, 963
panic disorder and, 940
in schizophrenic/psychotic disorders,
953, 955, 963
Sular. *See* Nisoldipine
Sulconazole, 98*t*
Sulfacetamide, for ophthalmic disorders,
173*t*
Sulfadiazine
silver, for burn wounds, 1411
for toxoplasmosis, 1224*t*, 1365
Sulfadoxine, with pyrimethamine (Fansidar), 1355, 1355*t*, 1359
with amodiaquine, 1356*t*, 1359
with artesunate, 1355*t*, 1356*t*, 1359
for isosporiasis, 1371
for prophylaxis in pregnancy/infants,
1361
resistance to, 1355, 1359
Sulfamethoxazole-trimethoprim. *See* Tri-
methoprim-sulfamethoxa-
zole
Sulfasalazine
for inflammatory bowel disease, 575
ulcerative colitis, 584, 584*t*, 585
for rheumatoid arthritis, 750
Sulfinpyrazone, for gout, 734
Sulfonamides, adverse ophthalmic effects
of, 178*t*
Sulfonylureas, 1090–1092, 1091*t*, 1101.
See also specific agent
factitious hypoglycemia caused by,
1118, 1122
insulin therapy and, 1101
intensive therapy with, 1088
MAOI interactions and, 969*t*
Sulindac, 80*t*
for familial adenomatous polyposis,
591
in pain management, 80*t*

Sumatriptan
  for cluster headache, 875
  for migraine headache, 874
Summer grippe, 1278
Sun exposure. *See* Ultraviolet light/sun-
      light, exposure to
Sunday neuroses, 939
"Sundowning," 986
Sunitinib, 1504*t*
  for gastrointestinal mesenchymal
      tumors, 1474
  hypothyroidism caused by, 1003
Sunscreens, **95**. *See also* Ultraviolet light/
      sunlight, exposure to, pro-
      tection from
  in cancer prevention, 95
  in herpes simplex prophylaxis, 114,
      1237
  for hyperpigmentation disorders, 145
  for lupus, 111, 753–754
  for photodermatitis/photosensitivity,
      143
  for rosacea, 122
Superficial femoral artery (SFA), athero-
      sclerotic/occlusive disease
      of, 416–417
Superficial reflux, in chronic venous
      insufficiency, correction
      of, 431
Superficial spreading melanoma, 100,
      101
Superficial venous thrombophlebitis,
      429–430
Superior semicircular canal dehiscence,
      vertigo and, 190
Superior vena caval obstruction/syn-
      drome, **431–432**
  in lung cancer, 1454
Superoxide dismutase gene, copper-zinc,
      in amyotrophic lateral
      sclerosis, 921
Superwarfarins, poisoning caused by,
      1430–1431
Supplements, dietary. *See* Dietary supple-
      ments
Support groups. *See also* Group therapy
  for alcohol use/abuse, 979
  for anxiety disorders, 943
  for chronic pain, 948
  for depression, 970
  for inflammatory bowel disease, 577
  in obesity management, 1137
  for paraphilias and gender identity
      disorders, 949
  for personality disorders, 950–951
  for schizophrenic/psychotic disor-
      ders, 960
  for somatoform disorders, 945
  for victim of violence, 977
Suppressor T cells, in common variable
      immunodeficiency, 787
Suppurative thyroiditis, 1016, 1017, 1018
Supraclavicular lymph nodes, in breast
      cancer, 657
  palpation for evaluation of, 656
Supraglottic carcinoma, 210
Supraglottitis (epiglottitis), **208**, 1289
  H influenzae causing, 1310

Supranuclear palsy, progressive, parkin-
      sonism differentiated
      from, 906
Supraspinatus tendon, in rotator cuff dis-
      orders, 744
Supratentorial arteriovenous malforma-
      tions, 895
Supratentorial mass lesion, coma or stu-
      por caused by, 916
Supraventricular beats
  aberrantly conducted, differentiation
      of from ventricular beats,
      341, 351–352
  premature. *See* Atrial (supraventricu-
      lar) premature beats
Supraventricular tachycardia
  accessory atrioventricular pathways
      causing, 342, **345–346**
  bradyarrhythmias and, 354
  in myocardial infarction, 336–337
  palpitations in, 31
  paroxysmal, **341–345**
Suramin, for African trypanosomiasis,
      1349, 1349*t*
Surfer's ear, 182
Surgery. *See also specific disorder or proce-
      dure*
  antibiotic prophylaxis and, **59–60**,
      60*t*
  anxiety before/after, 988, 989
    mind-body therapies for, 1536*t*
    guided imagery, 1536*t*, 1543
  cardiac complications of, prosthetic
      heart valve patients and,
      316
  corticosteroid replacement require-
      ment and, **58**
  in diabetic patient, 57–58, 57*t*, 58*t*,
      1109
  evaluation of patient before, **49–60**.
      See also Preoperative eval-
      uation/perioperative man-
      agement
  fever after, 1160
  guided imagery affecting outcome of,
      1543
  hyponatremia after, 790
  insulin needs and, 57–58, 57*t*, 58*t*,
      1109
  liver function and, **54**
  nausea and vomiting after, acupunc-
      ture for, 1534
  pain after, acupuncture for, 1533
  patient management and, **49–60**. *See
      also* Preoperative evalua-
      tion/perioperative man-
      agement
  during pregnancy, **727–728**
  for refractive error correction,
      151–152
  for wart removal, 132
Surgery proneness (polysurgery), 988, 989
  somatization disorder and, 944
Surgical menopause. *See* Menopause, sur-
      gical
Surgical site infection, 1160
  antibiotic prophylaxis of, **59–60**, 60*t*
Surmontil. *See* Trimipramine

Surrogate, Durable Power of Attorney for
      Health Care designating,
      90
Surveillance. *See* Watchful waiting/sur-
      veillance
Susceptibility testing. *See* Drug resistance;
      Drug susceptibility testing
Sustained ventricular tachycardia, 352
Sustiva. *See* Efavirenz
Sutent. *See* Sunitinib
Swallowing disorders. *See* Dysarthria;
      Dysphagia; Odynophagia
Swan-neck deformity, 751
Sweat chloride test, in cystic fibrosis, 242
Sweating
  fluid loss in, replacement guidelines
      for, 815*t*
  in myocardial infarction, 330
  in pheochromocytoma, 1058
Sweet 'N Low. *See* Saccharin
Sweet One. *See* Acesulfame potassium
Sweeteners, artificial, for diabetics, 1090
SWI. *See* Stroke work index
Swimmer's itch, 1374
Swimming pool granuloma, 1325
Swine-origin influenza (H1N1/A/Califor-
      nia/04/2009), 1198, 1269,
      1271, **1273–1274**. *See also*
      Influenza
SWL. *See* Shock wave lithotripsy
Sycosis, **123–124**
Sydenham chorea, 375, 909
Symblepharon, 172
Symlin. *See* Pramlintide
Sympathectomy, for Raynaud phenome-
      non, 757
Sympathetic nervous system
  in hypertension, 388–389
    peripheral inhibitors in manage-
      ment of, 407, 408*t*
  hypoglycemia and, 1103, 1103–1104
Sympatholytic agents, 407, 408*t*
  overdose/toxicity of, 407, 408*t*,
      1434–1435
Sympatholytic syndrome, 1426
Sympathomimetic agents
  adverse ophthalmic effects of, 177*t*
  antidepressant drug interactions and,
      969*t*
  for glaucoma/ocular hypertension,
      175*t*
  MAOI interactions and, 969*t*, 1440
Sympathomimetic syndrome, 1426
Symptom evaluation/management,
      22–48. *See also specific
      symptom*
Symptothermal natural family planning,
      699
Synchronized intermittent mandatory
      ventilation (SIMV), for
      respiratory failure, 290
Syncope/near syncope, **356–357**
  in aortic stenosis, 310
  cardiogenic, 356–357
  in cardiomyopathy, 373
  driving recommendations and,
      357–358
  dysautonomia and, 884, 885

Syncope/near syncope (*cont.*)
heat, **1407**
palpitations and, 31
seizures differentiated from, 881
vasodepressor/vasovagal, 356, 357
Syndrome of apparent mineralocorticoid excess
genetic mutation in, 796t
hypertension and, 391
Syndrome of inappropriate ADH secretion (SIADH), 791, 791t, 792
cancer-related, 791, 791t, 1453t, 1454
Syndrome X. *See* Metabolic syndrome
Synechiae, posterior, in uveitis, 160
Synercid. *See* Quinupristin/dalfopristin
Synergistic necrotizing cellulitis, 1323
Syngeneic stem cell transplant, 476
Synovial fluid examination, 729, 730t, 731t
in gonococcal arthritis, 778
in knee pain evaluation, 35–36
in Lyme arthritis, 1343
in nongonococcal acute bacterial (septic) arthritis, 777
in rheumatoid arthritis, 748
in tuberculous arthritis, 782
Synovitis
remitting seronegative, with non-pitting edema, cancer and, 783
in rheumatoid arthritis, 747
in SLE, 753
Synpharyngitic hematuria, 836
Synthroid. *See* Levothyroxine
Syphilis, 1177t, 1183t, **1330–1338**, 1331t, 1333t
anorectal involvement and, 594
cardiovascular involvement and, 1183t, **1335–1336**
cerebrospinal fluid examination in, 1336, 1337
in HIV infection/AIDS, 1220, 1337, 1338
indications for, 1336–1337
treatment failures and, 1334
congenital, 727, **1338**
contact treatment and, 1333
course/prognosis of, **1330**
drug therapy for, 1332–1333, 1333t, 1336. *See also* Syphilis, penicillin for
complications of, 1333
HIV infection/AIDS and, 1220, 1337
serologic tests in evaluation of, 1332, 1337
early, 1183t, 1330
endemic, **1339**
follow-up care in, 1333–1334
gummatous, 1330, 1335
in HIV infection/AIDS, 1220, 1333, **1337–1338**
late (tertiary), 1330, 1331t, **1335–1336**
latent, 1183t, 1330
early, 1183t, 1330, **1334**
late (hidden), **1335**

meningovascular/meningitis, 1163, 1334, 1336. *See also* Neurosyphilis
microscopic examination in, 1331
mucous membrane involvement in, 1330, 1334, 1335
natural history of, **1330**
neurologic involvement in. *See* Neurosyphilis
PCR testing in, 1332
penicillin for, 1183t, 1332–1333, 1333t, 1336
HIV infection/AIDS and, 1220, 1337
neurosyphilis and, 1183t, 1333, 1337
pregnancy and, 1338
pregnancy and, **727, 1338**
prevention of/screening for, 1167, 1332
in HIV infection/AIDS, 1220, 1333
in pregnancy, 708, 727, 1333, 1338
primary, 1183t, **1330–1334**, 1331t, 1333t
public health measures in management of, 1333
rape/sexual assault in transmission of, 702, 1167
relapses and, 1334. *See also* Syphilis, latent, early
screening blood for, 478
secondary, 1183t, 1331t, **1334**
pityriasis rosea differentiated from, 106
serologic tests for, 1331–1332, 1331t. *See also specific test*
false-negative, 1332
false-positive, 1332
antiphospholipid antibody causing, 752, 753, 754t, 756
in SLE, 752, 753, 754t
follow-up, 1334, 1337
in HIV infection/AIDS, 1220, 1332, 1333, 1337
in neurosyphilis, 1336, 1337
in non-sexually transmitted treponematoses, 1332
in pregnant patient, 708, 727, 1333, 1338
in STD patients, 1167, 1332
treatment affecting, 1332, 1337
stages of, **1330–1337**, 1331t
treatment failures and, 1334
uveitis in, 160
Syringobulbia, 920
Syringomyelia, **920**
Systemic fibrosing syndrome, Dupuytren contracture and, 743
Systemic inflammatory response syndrome (SIRS), shock and, 434
Systemic lupus erythematosus (SLE), **752–755**, 753t, 754t
arthritis in, 753
rheumatoid arthritis differentiated from, 748
autoantibodies in, 752, 753, 754t
cardiac/pericardial involvement in, 383, 753

criteria for, 752, 752t
DHEA for, 754, 1528, 1528t
drugs associated with, 281t, 752, 752t
lupus anticoagulant in, 753, 754t
mixed connective tissue disease/overlap syndrome and, 762
renal involvement in, 753, 754, **843**
Systemic sclerosis, **758–759**. *See also* Scleroderma
Systolic blood pressure. *See also* Blood pressure
in eclampsia, 718
in hypertension, 387, 388t, 389f
treatment goals and, 395–396
in hypertensive urgencies/emergencies, 387, 1434
Systolic dysfunction. *See* Congestive heart (cardiac) failure
Systolic murmurs. *See* Heart murmurs

T$_3$. *See* Triiodothyronine
T$_4$. *See* Thyroxine
T cell lymphoma
adult (ATL), 1261. *See also* Human T cell lymphotropic/leukemia virus
in celiac disease, 560
cutaneous (mycosis fungoides), **111–112**
exfoliative dermatitis/erythroderma and, 112
intestinal, 1475
nose and paranasal sinus involvement and, 201
tacrolimus/pimecrolimus associated with, 102
T cell-mediated (delayed/type IV) hypersensitivity, 784
T cell proliferative assay, in Lyme disease, 1344
T helper cells. *See* CD4 T cells
T lymphocytes
in common variable immunodeficiency, 787
in delayed hypersensitivity, 784
in HIV infection/AIDS. *See* CD4 T cells
t-PA. *See* Tissue plasminogen activator
T pallidum hemagglutination (TPHA) test, 1332
T pallidum particle agglutination (TPPA) test, 1332
T score, 1039, 1040
T tube, for common duct stone extraction/choledochostomy, 639
T waves. *See also* Electrocardiogram
in acute coronary syndromes, 326
antipsychotic drugs affecting, 958
lithium affecting, 971
in myocardial infarction, 331
in pericardial effusion, 378
in pericarditis, 377
in Tako-Tsubo cardiomyopathy, 372
Tabes dorsalis, 1336
neurogenic arthropathy (Charcot joint) in, 783, 1336
Tabun poisoning, 1434

TAC regimen, for breast cancer, 666
TACE. *See* Transcatheter arterial chemo-embolization
Tache noire, in tick typhus, 1285
"Tachy-brady syndrome," 354
Tachycardia/tachyarrhythmia
    antidromic, 341, 345
    atrial, multifocal (chaotic), **350**
    AV nodal reentry, 342
    in hyperthyroidism, 1009, 1014
    nonparoxysmal junctional, 350–351
    orthodromic, 345
    in poisoning/drug overdose, 1422, 1422t
    sinus. *See* Sinus tachycardia
    in sleep apnea, 288
    supraventricular
        accessory atrioventricular pathways causing, 342, **345–346**
        in myocardial infarction, 336–337
        paroxysmal, **341–345**
        ventricular, **351–352**. *See also* Ventricular tachycardia
        in myocardial infarction, 337
Tachypnea, in pulmonary embolism, 267
TACI. *See* Transcatheter arterial chemoinfusion
Tacrine, for Alzheimer disease, 987
Tacrolimus, 97t, 1546t
    adverse ophthalmic effects of, 177t
    hyperkalemia caused by, 798
    topical, 97t
        for atopic dermatitis, 102
        for lichen planus, 135
        T-cell lymphoma and, 102
        for vitiligo, 145
Tadalafil, 863, 950, 1107, 1108
Taenia
    saginata (beef tapeworm), 1376, **1376**
    solium (pork tapeworm), 1376, **1376**
        cysticercosis and, 1376, 1377–1378
Tegaderm, for burn wounds, 1411
Takayasu disease, 383–384
Tako-Tsubo (stress/catecholamine-induced) cardiomyopathy, 370, **372**
    myocardial infarction mimicked by, 330
Talc poudrage, for malignant effusions, 285, 1496
Talcosis (talc exposure), 279t, 280–281
Tall stature
    GH excess causing (gigantism), **997–1000**
    in Klinefelter syndrome, 1064
    in Marfan syndrome, 1518
Talofibular ligament, ankle sprains involving, 746
Tamm-Horsfall urinary mucoprotein, 816
Tamoxifen, 666, 668t, 669, 1505t
    adverse ophthalmic effects of, 177t
    for breast cancer, 666, 668, 668t, 669
        hormone receptor status and, 664
        in male, 673
        as preventive agent, 653, 653–654
    endometrial carcinoma and, 669, 684
    for osteoporosis, 1070
    for Riedel thyroiditis/struma, 1017, 1018

Tamponade, 378, 379
    cancer-related, 1495
    in neoplastic pericarditis, 377
    in pericardial effusion, 378, 379
    in pneumococcal pneumonia, 1292, 1293
    postinfarction/Dressler syndrome, 377
    in traumatic cardiac injury, 384
    in uremic pericarditis, 378
    in viral pericarditis, 378
TAMs (thymidine analog mutations), antiretroviral drug resistance and, 1233
Tamsulosin
    for benign prostatic hyperplasia, 869, 869t
    for urinary incontinence, 72
Tap water enema, 509t
Tapeworm infections, **1376–1379**. *See also* Cysticercosis; *Echinococcus*
    invasive, **1377–1379**
    noninvasive, **1376–1377**
    vitamin B_{12} deficiency in, 445
TAR. *See* Thrombocytopenia-absent radius syndrome
Tarceva. *See* Erlotinib
Tardive dyskinesia, 959–960
Targeted therapy, in cancer chemotherapy, 1503–1504t
    for breast cancer, 666–667, 667–669, 668t
Tarsal tunnel syndrome, **928**
Tasigna. *See* Nilotinib
Taxanes, 1502t
    for breast cancer, 665–666
    neuropathy caused by, 1510
Taxol. *See* Paclitaxel
Taxotere. *See* Docetaxel
Tay-Sachs disease, screening for, 706
Tazarotene, for acne, 121
Tazorac. *See* Tazarotene
TBE (tick-borne encephalitis). *See* Ticks, encephalitis transmitted by
TBII. *See* Thyrotropin-binding inhibitory immunoglobulin
TBP. *See* Thyroid-binding proteins
3TC. *See* Lamivudine
TC regimen, for breast cancer, 666
TCAs. *See* Tricyclic antidepressants
TCF7L2 gene, in type 2 diabetes, 1081
TCH regimen, for breast cancer, 666
TCu380A intrauterine device, 698
Td vaccine, 1192–1193t, 1194–1197t, 1200, 1298, 1299t, 1308
    pregnancy and, 1195t, 1200
    Tdap replacing, 4, 1200, 1308
Tdap vaccine, 3–4, 1190–1191t, 1192–1193t, 1194–1197t, 1200, 1298, 1299t, 1308
    adverse effects/contraindications and, 1202t
    pregnancy and, 1195t, 1200
TdT. *See* Terminal deoxynucleotidal transferase
Tears, artificial, for dry eye, 154–155, 763
Technetium-99m pyrophosphate scintigraphy, in myocardial infarction, 331

Technetium-99m sestamibi scintigraphy, in angina, 319
Technetium-99m thyroid scanning, 1003t
TEE (transesophageal echocardiography). *See* Echocardiography
Teeth, disorders of. *See* Dental disorders
Tegaserod, withdrawal of from market, 572, 1107
Tekturna. *See* Aliskiren
Telangiectasia
    hereditary hemorrhagic, **1519**
        epistaxis in, 198, 1519
    in rosacea, 122, 123
Telbivudine, for hepatitis B, 610
Telepaque. *See* Iopanoic acid
Telithromycin
    for bacterial rhinosinusitis, 194t
    renal/hepatic failure and, 1185t
Telmisartan/telmisartan with hydrochlorothiazide, 404t
Telogen effluvium, 146
Temazepam, 941t, 974
Temodar. *See* Temozolomide
Temovate. *See* Clobetasol
Temozolomide, 1500t
Temperature. *See* Body temperature; Fever
Temporal artery biopsy, in giant cell arteritis, 165, 767
Temporal (giant cell/cranial) arteritis. *See* Giant cell (temporal/cranial) arteritis
Temporal lobe herniation, intracranial tumors causing, 897–898
Temporal lobe lesions, 899
Temporomandibular joint dysfunction
    earache and, 186
    facial pain caused by, 878
    headache and, 872
Temsirolimus, 1505t
TEN. *See* Toxic epidermal necrolysis
Tendinitis. *See specific type*
Tendinous xanthoma, 1125
Tenecteplase (TNK-t-PA), for myocardial infarction, 333t, 334
Tenex. *See* Guanfacine
Tennis elbow, **745**
Tenofovir, 1226t, 1228, 1232, 1232f. *See also* Antiretroviral therapy
    with emtricitabine, 1227, 1228, 1231, 1232f
    with emtricitabine and efavirenz, 1228, 1230, 1231, 1232f
    for hepatitis B, 610, 1228
Tenormin. *See* Atenolol
Tenosynovitis
    in gonococcal arthritis, 778, 1319
    popliteal, 746
    in tuberculous arthritis, 782
Tension headache, 872, **872–873**
    acupuncture for, 1533
    mind-body therapies for, 1536t
        biofeedback, 1536t, 1537
Tension pneumothorax, 286
Teoptic. *See* Carteolol
Tequin. *See* Gatifloxacin

Teratogenic drugs, 706t. *See also specific agent*

Teratomas, testicular, 1492

Terazosin
for benign prostatic hyperplasia, 869, 869t, 870
for hypertension, 407, 408t
for urinary incontinence, 72

Terbinafine, 98t, 1401t
for chromoblastomycosis, 1400
for onychomycosis, 147
for sporotrichosis, 1400

Terbutaline
for asthma/bronchospasm, 228
for preterm labor prevention, 719

Terconazole, for vulvovaginal candidiasis, 678

Terfenadine, antidepressant drug interactions and, 966, 969t

Teriparatide
for hypophosphatasia, 1043
for osteoporosis, 1041

Terlipressin, for GI bleeding/esophageal varices, 520, 539

Terminal deoxynucleotidal transferase, in acute leukemia, 465

Terminal ileal resection, short bowel syndrome and, 562–563

Terminal illness. *See* End of life

Terminal restlessness, 87

Terrorism. *See also* Bioterrorism; Chemical warfare agents
nuclear, 1414

Testes
diseases of, **1063–1066**
examination of in hypogonadism/ infertility, 1064
intra-abdominal
cancer in, 1066, 1493
in pseudohermaphroditism, 1068
masses/tumors of, **1066, 1492–1494**. *See also* Testicular cancer
gynecomastia and, 1066, 1067
secondary/metastatic, **1494**
retractile, 1066
undescended (cryptorchism), **1066**
testicular cancer and, 1066, 1493

Testicular cancer, 1467t, **1492–1494**
cryptorchism and, 1066, 1493
gynecomastia and, 1066, 1067, 1493
hyperthyroidism and, 1009
secondary/metastatic, **1494**

Testicular feminization, 1068

Testicular lymphoma, 1494

Testicular masses. *See* Testes, masses/ tumors of

Testicular pain, cancer causing, 1493

Testim. *See* Testosterone replacement therapy

Testis. *See* Testes

Testoderm. *See* Testosterone replacement therapy

Testosterone. *See also* Androgens; Testosterone replacement therapy
deficiency of, 1063–1066. *See also* Hypogonadism

pseudohermaphroditism/amenorrhea and, 1068
in women, 1070, 1073
excess of, amenorrhea caused by, 1068
insensitivity/resistance to, 1064, 1068
prostate cancer and, 1487
reference values for, 1553t
serum levels of
in gynecomastia, 1067
in hirsutism/virilization, 1054
in hypogonadism, 992, 1064–1065
in infertility workup, 864, 865f

Testosterone gels/transdermal systems. *See* Testosterone replacement therapy

Testosterone replacement therapy
for AIDS wasting, 1210
for erectile dysfunction, 863
for hypogonadism, 1065–1066
in Klinefelter syndrome, 1517–1518
in men, 1065–1066
in women, 1070, 1073

Tetanospasmin, 1298

Tetanus, 1177t, **1298–1299**, 1299t
in drug users, 1169
prevention/immunization and, 1298, 1299t. *See also* Tetanus and diphtheria toxoids and pertussis vaccine
frostbite and, 1406

Tetanus-diphtheria 5-component acellular pertussis (Tdap) vaccine, 3–4, 1190–1191t, 1192–1193t, 1194–1197t, 1200, 1298, 1299t, 1308
adverse effects/contraindications and, 1202t
pregnancy and, 1195t, 1200

Tetanus-diphtheria toxoid (Td vaccine), 1192–1193t, 1194–1197t, 1298, 1299t, 1308
Tdap replacing, 4, 1200, 1298, 1308

Tetanus and diphtheria toxoids and pertussis vaccine (DTaP/Tdap vaccines), 3–4, 1188–1189t, 1190–1191t, 1192–1193t, 1194–1197t, 1200, 1298, 1299t, 1302, 1308
adverse effects/contraindications and, 1202t
pregnancy and, 1195t, 1200

Tetanus immune globulin, 1298, 1298–1299, 1299t

Tetany
in electrical injury, 1412
in hypocalcemia/hypoparathyroidism, 800, 1031, 1032
malabsorption and, 558t
after parathyroidectomy, 1037
in respiratory alkalosis, 814

Tetrabenazine, for Huntington disease, 909

Tetracycline
for acne, 121
adverse ophthalmic effects of, 177t
for amebiasis, 1367, 1367t
in *H pylori* eradication therapy, 551t

for malaria, 1360
for rosacea, 123
for syphilis, 1333t

Tetrafosmin scintigraphy, in angina, 319

Tetrahydroaminoacridine. *See* Tacrine

Δ9-Tetrahydrocannabinol, 507, 983. *See also* Dronabinol

Tetrahydrozoline, overdose/toxicity of, 1434

Tetralogy of Fallot, **300–301**

Tetrodotoxin, puffer fish poisoning caused by, 1446t

Teveten. *See* Eprosartan

Tg. *See* Thyroglobulin

Tg (thyroglobulin) antibodies. *See* Antithyroid (antithyroglobulin/antithyroperoxidase) antibodies

TGF-β. *See* Transforming growth factor β

THA. *See* Tacrine

Thalamic hemorrhage, in stroke, 892

Thalamic stimulation
for benign essential (familial) tremor, 904–905
for parkinsonism, 908

Thalamic syndrome
intracranial tumors causing, 899
in vertebrobasilar obstruction, 889

Thalamotomy
for benign essential (familial) tremor, 904
for idiopathic torsion dystonia, 910
for parkinsonism, 908

Thalassemias, **442–444**, 443t
sickle, 451t, **452**

Thalidomide
for cancer chemotherapy, 1505t
for erythema nodosum leprosum, 1327
for lupus, 111
for myelofibrosis, 460
for myeloma, 473
neuropathy caused by, 1510
teratogenicity of, 111, 1505t

Thaliton. *See* Chlorthalidone

Thallium-201 scintigraphy
in angina, 319
in myocardial infarction, 331
in thyroid cancer surveillance, 1028

Thalomid. *See* Thalidomide

THC. *See* Δ9-Tetrahydrocannabinol

Theater sign, 745

Theophylline, 1546t
for asthma, 225t, 227
for COPD, 237–238
factors affecting concentrations of, 225t
lithium interactions and, 972t
monitoring levels of, 1546t
overdose/toxicity of, 227, 1427t, **1447–1448**
hemodialysis for, 1425t, 1448
seizures and, 1423t, 1447, 1448

Therapeutic abortion. *See* Abortion, elective/induced

Therapeutic diets, **1145–1147**. *See also* Diet; Nutrition

Therapeutic drug monitoring, 1544–1546t. *See also specific agent*
Therapeutic touch, 1520
Thermal biofeedback, 1536t, 1537
Thermal injury. *See* Burns
Thermocoagulation, endoscopic, for bleeding peptic ulcer, 554
Thermoregulation
    heat exposure syndromes and, 1406, 1407
    systemic hypothermia and, 1403
Thiamine (vitamin B₁)
    for alcohol withdrawal, 981
    for coma, 1421
    deficiency of, **1140–1141**
        alcohol use/alcoholic ketoacidosis and, 809, 811, 915, 979, 1140–1141
        amnestic syndrome and, 986
        neuropathy associated with, 923, 1141
        Wernicke encephalopathy/Wernicke-Korsakoff syndrome caused by, 915, 979, 981, 1141
Thiazide diuretics. *See also* Diuretics
    for acute tubular necrosis, 823
    adverse effects of, 398, 399t
        ophthalmic, 177t
    for heart failure, 361
        chronic kidney disease and, 828
    hypercalcemia and, 801, 1036
    for hypercalciuria, 858–859
    for hyperkalemia, 797
    for hypertension, 398, 399t, 407, 409, 409f
        in combination products, 399t, 409, 409f
    hyponatremia caused by, 790
    lithium interactions and, 972, 972t
Thiazolidinediones, for diabetes mellitus, 1091t, 1093–1094, 1101
Thick blood film, for malaria diagnosis, 1354
Thienobenzodiazepines, 955t, 956t. *See also* Antipsychotic drugs
Thienopyridines, platelet function affected by, 490t
Thimerosal-free vaccines, 4
Thin blood film, for malaria diagnosis, 1354
Thioglitazones, lower extremity edema caused by, 37
Thioguanine, 576
Thiopurine methyltransferase, monitoring, 576
Thioridazine, 955t, 956t
    overdose/toxicity of, 956t, 958, 959, 1444
Thiosulfate, for cyanide poisoning, 1424t, 1435, 1435t
Thiotepa, for bladder cancer, 1490
Thiothixene, 955t, 956t
Thioureas
    for Graves disease/hyperthyroidism, 1011
        during pregnancy/lactation, 1011, 1013
        RAI therapy and, 1012
    for toxic multinodular goiter, 1013

Thioxanthenes, 954, 955t, 956t. *See also* Antipsychotic drugs
Third-degree burns, 1409
Third-degree (complete) heart block, 355
    in atrial septal defect, 298
    in myocardial infarction, 337
Third heart sound (S₃/ventricular gallop). *See* Heart sounds
Third nerve paralysis/palsy, 169, 170
    in ophthalmoplegic migraine, 873
Third-trimester bleeding, **720**
Thirst. *See* Polydipsia
Thoracentesis
    in lung cancer, 1454
    for malignant effusions, 1496
    in pleural effusion, 283
    in pneumonia, 246, 249
Thoracic actinomycosis, 1323
Thoracic aortic aneurysms, **425–426**
    giant cell arteritis and, 766, 767
Thoracic outlet syndrome, **737–738**
    chest pain in, 321
    Raynaud phenomenon and, 757
Thoracic spine disease
    chest pain in, 321, 543
    tuberculosis (Pott disease), 782
Thoracic surgery, antibiotic prophylaxis for, 60t
Thoracoscopic surgery, video-assisted (VATS)
    in lung cancer diagnosis, 1454
    for solitary pulmonary nodule, 261
Thoracoscopy, for pneumothorax, 287
Thoracostomy, tube. *See* Tube thoracostomy
Thoracotomy
    for hemothorax, 285
    for pneumothorax, 287
Thorazine. *See* Chlorpromazine
Thorotrast exposure, ureteral/renal pelvic cancer and, 1491
Thought content, in schizophrenic/psychotic disorders, 953
Threatened abortion, 711, 712
Three-dimensional conformal radiation therapy, for prostate cancer, 1486
Three-item word recall, in dementia screening, 64
"3" sign, in coarctation of aorta, 296
Throat culture, in pharyngitis, 204, 1289, 1290
Thrombasthenia, Glanzmann, 489, 490
Thrombin inhibitors, for heparin-induced thrombocytopenia, 486t, 487
Thrombin time, 1554t
Thromboangiitis obliterans (Buerger disease), **422–423**
    Raynaud phenomenon and, 757
Thrombocytopenia, **480–489**, 481t
    amegakaryocytic, 480, 481
    with autoimmune hemolytic anemia (Evans syndrome), 453
    in bone marrow failure, **480–482**
    in bone marrow infiltration, **482**
    in cancer chemotherapy/irradiation, **482**, 483t, **1499–1508**

cyclic, **482**
    decreased platelet production causing, **480–482**, 481t
    DIC and, **487–488**, 488t
    drug-induced, 482, 482–483, 483, 483t
    gestational, **489**
    in gram-negative bacteremia/sepsis, 1311
    in hairy cell leukemia, 468
    heparin-induced, 272, 483t, **486–487**, 486t
        reference values in, 1551t
    in immune thrombocytopenic purpura, **482–484**, 483t, 484f
    increased platelet destruction causing, 481t, **482–488**
    infection/sepsis-related, **489**
    nutritional deficiencies and, **482**
    platelet sequestration and, **488–489**
    platelet transfusion for, 478, 483
    in preeclampsia-eclampsia, 716
    qualitative platelet disorders and, **489–490**, 490t
    retinal disease associated with, 167
    in SLE, 754t
    in thrombotic microangiopathy, 485–486, 485t
    after transfusion, **488**
    in von Willebrand disease type 2B, **488**, 493
Thrombocytopenia-absent radius syndrome, 480
Thrombocytosis
    essential, 457t, **459–460**
    reactive, 459
Thromboembolism. *See also* Embolism; Thrombosis
    in antiphospholipid antibody syndrome, 755
    in atrial fibrillation, 346, 347t
        anticoagulation in prevention of, 348
        transient monocular blindness and, 165
    in Behçet syndrome, 772
    estrogen replacement therapy and, 1072
    in myocardial infarction, 339
    oral contraceptive use and, 696
    perioperative anticoagulation management and, 55, 56t
    prosthetic heart valves and, 316
    pulmonary. *See* Pulmonary venous thromboembolism
    in Wegener granulomatosis, 768
Thromboendarterectomy
    carotid. *See* Carotid endarterectomy/thromboendarterectomy
    for femoral/popliteal occlusive disease, 417
Thrombolytic therapy
    for acute arterial occlusion of limb, 419
    for frostbite, 1406
    for hepatic vein obstruction (Budd-Chiari syndrome), 630
    for myocardial infarction, 332–334, 333t

Thrombolytic therapy (*cont.*)
  for pulmonary embolism, 273,
    500–501, 501*t*
  for retinal artery occlusion, 165
  for stroke, 891
  for venous thromboembolic disease,
    500–501, 501*t*
Thrombophlebitis. *See also* Thrombosis
  cancer-related, 1453*t*
  leg ulcers and, 143
  oral contraceptive use and, 696
  septic. *See* Septic thrombophlebitis
  of superficial veins, **429–430**
  varicosities and, 427, 428
Thrombopoietin, for chemotherapy-
    induced thrombocytope-
    nia, 1506
Thrombosis. *See also* Thromboembolism;
    Thrombophlebitis
  acute occlusion of limb caused by, 419
  in antiphospholipid antibody syn-
    drome, 755
  cancer-associated, 270*t*
  cavernous sinus, bacterial rhinosinusi-
    tis and, 195
  cerebrovascular occlusion and, 420,
    889
  of deep veins. *See* Deep venous throm-
    bosis
  in DIC, 487, 488
  in essential thrombocytosis, 459
  hemorrhoidal, 594
  in heparin-induced thrombocytope-
    nia, 486
  in homocystinuria, 1517
  intracranial, **896**. *See also* Stroke
  in paroxysmal nocturnal hemoglobin-
    uria, 449
  in polycythemia, 457
  prosthetic heart valves and, 316
  sigmoid sinus, otitis media and, 185
  venous. *See* Venous thromboembolic
    disease
  venous sinus, 902
  in Wegener granulomatosis, 768
Thrombotic microangiopathy, **484–486**,
    485*t*. *See also* Hemolytic-
    uremic syndrome
Thrombotic thrombocytopenic purpura,
    485–486, 485*t*
Thrush (oral candidiasis), 125, **202**, 1390
  in HIV infection/AIDS, 125, 202,
    1213, 1390
Thumb sign, 208
"Thunderclap headache," 44
Thymectomy, for myasthenia gravis, 933
Thymidine analog mutations (TAMs),
    antiretroviral drug resis-
    tance and, 1233
Thymidylate synthase gene mutations,
    pancreatic/periampullary
    carcinoma and, 1463
Thymoma
  myasthenia gravis associated with, 932
  paraneoplastic syndromes associated
    with, 1453*t*
  pure red cell aplasia caused by, 447
Thyrogen. *See* Thyrotropin-α

Thyroglobulin
  antibodies against. *See* Antithyroid
    (antithyroglobulin/antithy-
    roperoxidase) antibodies
  serum levels of
    in goiter, 1029
    reference values for, 1554*t*
    in thyroid cancer diagnosis/surveil-
      lance, 1024, 1026–1027
Thyroglossal duct cysts, **213**
Thyroid adenoma (toxic solitary thyroid
    nodule), 1008, 1012–1013,
    1076*t*
Thyroid antibodies. *See* Antithyroid (anti-
    thyroglobulin/antithyrop-
    eroxidase) antibodies
Thyroid-binding proteins (TBP), 1002
Thyroid cancer, **1021–1029**, 1022*t*, 1025*t*,
    1467*t*
  anaplastic/undifferentiated, 1022*t*,
    1023, 1026, 1029
  fine-needle aspiration biopsy in, 1020
  follicular, 1022*t*, 1023, 1028
  functioning, 1009
  incidence/risk/mortality of,
    1021–1022
  long-term followup/surveillance for,
    1026–1028
  lymphoma, 1023, 1026, 1029
  medullary, 1022*t*, 1023, 1026,
    1028–1029
    in multiple endocrine neoplasia,
      1023, 1026, 1028, 1076,
      1076*t*, 1077
  metastatic, 1022, 1022*t*, 1023, 1024,
    1025, 1025*t*, 1026, 1027,
    1028
  micropapillary, 1022–1023
  papillary, 1022, 1022*t*, 1028
    follicular variant of, 1022, 1028
  radiation exposure and, 1022
  staging of, 1025*t*, 1028–1029
  thyroid nodules and, 1019
  thyroid testing in, 1024
  thyroiditis and, 1018
Thyroid crisis/storm, 1015
  during pregnancy, 722, 1009
Thyroid gland
  biopsy of, 1003*t*, 1012, 1017, 1019*t*, 1020
  disorders of, **1002–1030**. *See also*
      Hyperthyroidism;
      Hypothyroidism; Thyroid
      cancer
    eye disease associated with, **170**,
      1008, 1009
    lithium causing, 971, 1008
    neoplastic. *See* Thyroid cancer;
      Thyroid nodules
    during pregnancy, **722**, 1003,
      1008–1009, 1009, 1010,
      1013
    hyperemesis gravidarum and,
      711, 1008
    preoperative evaluation/manage-
      ment and, **58**
    thyroid testing in, **1002–1003**,
      1003*t*. *See also* Thyroid
      testing

enlarged. *See* Goiter
  infection of (suppurative thyroiditis),
    1016, 1017, 1018
  nodular. *See* Multinodular (nodular)
    goiter; Thyroid cancer;
    Thyroid nodules
Thyroid hormone. *See also* Thyroxine;
    Triiodothyronine
  antidepressant drug augmentation
    and, 964
  deficiency/excess of. *See* Hyperthy-
    roidism; Hypothyroidism
  exogenous, excess ingestion of (thyro-
    toxicosis factitia), 1008
  perioperative, 58
  replacement therapy with. *See*
    Levothyroxine
Thyroid nodules, **1019–1021**, 1019*t*. *See*
    also Goiter; Thyroid cancer
  solitary, 1019
  toxic (thyroid adenoma), 1008,
    1012–1013, 1076*t*
  thyroid testing in, 1003*t*, 1019*t*,
    1020
Thyroid radioactive iodine uptake and
    scan. *See* Radioiodine thy-
    roid scans and uptake
Thyroid-stimulating hormone (TSH/thy-
    rotropin), 1003*t*
  deficiency of, 992, 993, 994
  factors affecting, 1002, 1004*t*
  in goiter, 1029
  in hyperthyroidism, 1003*t*, 1010
    amiodarone-induced, 1010
    pituitary adenoma/hyperplasia
      and, 1008
    pregnancy and, 1010
  in hypothyroidism, 992, 993, 994,
    1003*t*, 1005
    amiodarone-induced, 1003–1004
    levothyroxine replacement and,
      994, 1006, 1007
    pregnancy and, 722
  pituitary hypersecretion/hyperthy-
    roidism and, 1008
  pregnancy and, 722, 1010
  reference values for, 1554*t*
  in thyroid cancer
    postsurgical, 1025
    RAI therapy and, 1025–1026
    surveillance and, 1026
  in thyroid nodules, 1020
    levothyroxine therapy and, 1021
  after thyroidectomy, 1025
  in thyroiditis, 1017
Thyroid-stimulating hormone receptor
    antibody (TSAb/TSH-R
    Ab[stim]). *See also* Thy-
    rotropin receptor antibody
  in Graves disease/hyperthyroidism,
    1003*t*, 1008
    amiodarone-induced, 1010
  reference values for, 1554*t*
Thyroid-stimulating immunoglobulin,
    1003*t*
Thyroid storm. *See* Thyroid crisis/storm
Thyroid surgery/thyroidectomy
  for goiter, 1012, 1021, 1030

for Graves disease/hyperthyroidism, 1012
during pregnancy, 1012, 1013
toxic multinodular goiter and, 1013
toxic solitary thyroid nodule and, 1012–1013
hypoparathyroidism after, 1012, 1025, 1030
for thyroid cancer, 1024–1025
for thyroid nodules, 1021
vocal fold paralysis/recurrent laryngeal nerve damage and, 211, 1012, 1025
Thyroid testing, **1002–1003**, 1003*t*
factors affecting, 1002, 1004*t*
in heart failure, 360
in HIV infection/AIDS, 1214
in hyperthyroidism, 1003*t*, 1004*t*, 1010
in hypothyroidism, 1003*t*, 1005
in thyroid cancer, 1024
in thyroid nodules, 1003*t*, 1019*t*, 1020
in thyroiditis, 1017
Thyroid transcription factor-1 (TTF-1), in lung cancer, 1458
Thyroid withdrawal-stimulated serum Tg/radioiodine scanning, thyroid cancer surveillance and, 1027–1028
Thyroidectomy. *See* Thyroid surgery/thyroidectomy
Thyroiditis, **1015–1018**
amiodarone-induced, 1009
Hashimoto. *See* Hashimoto (chronic lymphocytic/autoimmune) thyroiditis
hepatitis C and, 1004
painless, 1016
postpartum, 1008, 1015, 1016, 1017, 1018
during pregnancy, 1017
Riedel, 1016, 1017, 1018
silent, 1008, 1017
sporadic, 1016, 1018
subacute. *See* Subacute (de Quervain) thyroiditis
suppurative, 1016, 1017, 1018
Thyroperoxidase, antibodies against. *See* Antithyroid (antithyroglobulin/antithyroperoxidase) antibodies
Thyrotoxic hypokalemic periodic paralysis, 936, 1010, 1015
Thyrotoxicosis, **1007–1015**. *See also* Hyperthyroidism
factitia, 1008
Thyrotrophe pituitary adenoma, 1013
Thyrotrophe pituitary hyperplasia, 1005, 1008, 1013
Thyrotropin. *See* Thyroid-stimulating hormone
Thyrotropin-α (rhTSH), RAI therapy/surveillance for thyroid cancer and, 1025, 1026
Thyrotropin-binding inhibitory immunoglobulin (TBII), in amiodarone-induced hyperthyroidism, 1010

Thyrotropin receptor antibody (TRAb), in Graves disease/hyperthyroidism, 1008, 1010
Thyrotropin-stimulated serum Tg/radioiodine scanning, thyroid cancer surveillance and, 1027
Thyroxine (T₄)
free. *See* Free thyroxine assay
replacement therapy with. *See* Levothyroxine
serum levels of
factors affecting, 1002, 1004*t*
in goiter, 1029
in hyperthyroidism, 1009
amiodarone-induced, 1010
pregnancy and, 722, 1010
thyroiditis and, 1017
in hypopituitarism, 992
in hypothyroidism, 1005
in thyroid cancer surveillance, 1026
total, reference values for, 1554*t*
uptake of (resin). *See* Resin T₃/T₄ uptake
Thyroxine (T₄) index, free (FT₄I). *See* Free thyroxine index
TIA. *See* Transient ischemic attacks
Tiagabine, 881, 882*t*
overdose/toxicity of, 882*t*, 1431
for seizures, 881, 882*t*
Tiazac. *See* Diltiazem
TIBC. *See* Total iron-binding capacity
Tibial artery, atherosclerotic/occlusive disease of, 417–418
Tibial nerve, entrapment of (tarsal tunnel syndrome), **928**
Tibolone, 1073
Tic douloureux. *See* Trigeminal neuralgia
Ticar. *See* Ticarcillin
Ticarcillin, platelet function affected by, 490*t*
Tick typhus, 1281*t*, **1285**
Ticks
babesiosis transmitted by, 1362
Colorado tick fever transmitted by, 1267
ehrlichiosis/anaplasmosis transmitted by, 1281*t*, 1286
encephalitis transmitted by (tick-borne encephalitis), 1257–1259, **1266–1267**
hemorrhagic fevers transmitted by, 1262
Lyme disease transmitted by, 1342–1343, 1345
relapsing fever transmitted by, 1339, 1340
removal of, 1342–1343
Rocky Mountain spotted fever transmitted by, 1281*t*, **1284**
skin lesions caused by, 139
Southern tick-associated rash illness (STARI) transmitted by, 128
spotted fevers transmitted by (tick typhus), 1281*t*, **1285**
tularemia transmitted by, 1317

Ticlopidine. *See also* Antiplatelet therapy
platelet function affected by, 490*t*
theophyllines affected by, 225*t*
Tics
in OCD, 940
in Tourette syndrome, 911
Tietze syndrome, 321
TIG. *See* Tetanus immune globulin
Tigecycline
for abdominal infections, 1322*t*
renal/hepatic failure and, 1185*t*
Tilt table testing
in dysautonomia, 885
in syncope, 357
Tiludronate, for Paget disease of bone, 1046
TIMI Risk Score, 339
Timolol
for glaucoma/ocular hypertension, 159, 175*t*
in combination agents, 159, 176*t*
for systemic hypertension, 401*t*
Timoptic/Timoptic-XE. *See* Timolol
Tincture of opium, 517
Tinea
circinata, **107–108**
corporis, **107–108**
cruris, **108**
manuum, **108–109**
pedis, **108–109**
cellulitis and, 109, 129
pityriasis rosea differentiated from, 106
profunda, furuncles differentiated from, 141
unguium (onychomycosis), 146, **147**
versicolor (pityriasis versicolor), **109–110**
Tinel sign, in carpal tunnel syndrome, 742
Tinidazole
for amebiasis, 1366, 1367, 1367*t*
for giardiasis, 1372
for trichomoniasis, 678, 1373
Tinnitus, **187–188**
glomus tumors causing, 186, 188
in labyrinthitis, 189
in Ménière syndrome, 189
in pseudotumor cerebri, 903
vertigo and, 188
Tinzaparin, 497*t*
Tioconazole, for vulvovaginal candidiasis, 678
Tiotropium, for COPD, 237
Tipranavir, 1230, 1232*f. See also* Antiretroviral therapy
Tipranavir/ritonavir, 1227*t*, 1230. *See also* Antiretroviral therapy
TIPS. *See* Transvenous (transjugular) intrahepatic portosystemic shunts
Tirofiban
for acute coronary syndromes, 327*t*, 328
platelet function affected by, 490*t*
Tissue plasminogen activator (t-PA/alteplase). *See also* Thrombolytic therapy
for acute arterial occlusion of limb, 419

Tissue plasminogen activator (t-PA/ alteplase) (*cont.*)
for myocardial infarction, 333*t*, 334
for pulmonary embolism, 273, 501*t*
for stroke, 891
"Tissue reaction," in radiation exposure, 1413
Tissue transglutaminase. *See* Transglutaminase
Tizanidine
overdose/toxicity of, 1434
for spasticity, 914
TLC (total lung capacity). *See also* Pulmonary function tests
in COPD, 234
in cystic fibrosis, 241
TLS. *See* Tumor lysis syndrome
TMA. *See* Thrombotic microangiopathy
TMP-SMZ. *See* Trimethoprim-sulfamethoxazole
TNF. *See* Tumor necrosis factor
TNK-t-PA. *See* Tenecteplase
TNM staging classification, 1451. *See also* specific type of cancer
Tobacco use. *See also* Smoking
cancer and, 1450–1451, 1452
esophageal cancer, 1468
laryngeal cancer, 210
oral cancer, 201
health hazards of, 6–7
postoperative pulmonary complications and, 53, 54
preventable disease/deaths caused by, 2*t*
in thromboangiitis obliterans (Buerger disease), 422
Tobramycin, 1179*t*, 1546*t*. *See also* Aminoglycosides
for ophthalmic disorders, 173*t*
in renal failure, 1179*t*
Tobrex. *See* Tobramycin
Tocolytics, 719
adverse ophthalmic effects of, 177*t*
Toe amputations, in lower leg/foot occlusive disease, 418
Toe web (interdigital) tinea pedis, cellulitis and, 109, 129
Toenails, disorders of. *See* Nail disorders
Toes
callosities and corns of, **133**
in diabetes/vascular disorders, 133
in gout, 733
thromboangiitis obliterans (Buerger disease) involving, 422
Tofranil. *See* Imipramine
Tolazamide, 1090, 1091*t*
Tolazoline, clonidine overdose and, 1434–1435
Tolbutamide, 1090, 1091*t*
in insulinoma diagnosis, 1119
Tolcapone, for parkinsonism, 907
Tolectin. *See* Tolmetin
Tolerance (drug), 977. *See also* Substance use disorders
in opioid therapy, 78, 84
Tolinase. *See* Tolazamide
Tolmetin, 80*t*
Tolterodine, for urinary incontinence, 71

Toluene toxicity/abuse, 1439
anion gap and, 809
Tolvaptan, for hyponatremia/SIADH, 793
Tonal tinnitus, 188
Tongue disorders (glossitis/glossodynia), **202–203**
Tonic-clonic (grand mal) seizures, 879*t*, 880, 882*t*. *See also* Seizures
Tonic-clonic status epilepticus, 880, 883–884
Tonic seizures, 880. *See also* Seizures
Tonicity, 788
Tonsillectomy, **205**
for peritonsillar abscess and cellulitis, 205
quinsy, 205
Tonsillitis, **203–205**. *See also* Pharyngitis
Tooth disorders. *See* Dental disorders
Tophus (tophi)/tophaceous arthritis, 732, 733
rheumatoid nodule differentiated from, 733
Topical therapy, for skin disorders, 94
complications of, 95–99
Topiramate, 881, 882*t*
for alcohol use/abuse, 20
overdose/toxicity of, 882*t*, 1431
ophthalmic effects and, 177*t*
for seizures, 881, 882*t*
pregnancy and, 883
Topoisomerase inhibitors, 1503*t*
Topotecan, 1503*t*
Toprol XL. *See* Metoprolol
Toradol. *See* Ketorolac
Toremifene, 668*t*, 1505*t*
Torisel. *See* Temsirolimus
Torsades de pointes, 351, 354
in poisoning/drug toxicity, 351, 1422, 1422*t*
antiarrhythmics in, 1445
antipsychotics/phenothiazines in, 958, 1444
droperidol in, 1444
opioids in, 1442
Torsemide, 399*t*
for heart failure, 361
Torsion dystonia
focal, **910**
idiopathic, **909–910**
Torticollis, 910
Tositumomab, 1503*t*
Total body iron, 441
Total body water. *See* Body water
Total iron-binding capacity (TIBC), 1551*t*
Total lung capacity (TLC). *See also* Pulmonary function tests
in COPD, 234
in cystic fibrosis, 241
Total parenteral nutrition. *See* Central vein nutritional support
Total protein. *See* Protein
Total triiodothyronine, 1554*t*. *See also* Triiodothyronine
Tourette syndrome, **911–912**, 940
Toxic adenoma (toxic solitary thyroid nodule), 1008, 1012–1013, 1076*t*
Toxic epidermal necrolysis, 127–128, 1410
drugs causing, 127, 149*t*, 1410

Toxic erythema, drugs causing, 148*t*
Toxic lung injury, **280**
aspiration and, 277
smoke inhalation and, 277, 1409
Toxic megacolon
acute colonic pseudo-obstruction (Ogilvie syndrome) differentiated from, 565
in ulcerative colitis, 585
Toxic multinodular goiter, 1008, 1010, 1012, 1013
Toxic myocarditis, **369–370**
Toxic neuropathies, **925**
Toxic psychosis, 954
Toxic shock syndrome
clostridial, 701, **1297–1298**
diaphragm/cervical cap use and, 699
staphylococcal, **1296**
streptococcal, 1291
Toxic solitary thyroid nodule (toxic adenoma), 1008, 1012–1013, 1076*t*
Toxicology screen, in poisoning/drug overdose, 1426–1427, 1427*t*
Toxins. *See also* Poisoning/drug overdose
anion gap affected by, 809, 1426
in *C difficile* colitis, 512, 574
in food poisoning/gastroenteritis, 1172
liver disease caused by, **616–617**. *See also* Hepatotoxicity
osmolar/osmol gap affected by, 1426
screening for, 1426–1427, 1427*t*
Toxocara canis/cati (toxocariasis), **1384–1385**
Toxoplasma/Toxoplasma gondii (toxoplasmosis), **1363–1365**
in HIV infection/AIDS, 901, 1211–1212, 1224*t*, 1363–1364, 1364, 1365
prophylaxis of, 1222, 1365
myocarditis in, 368
during pregnancy (congenital), 1363, 1364, 1365
TP53 gene mutations. *See also* P53 gene mutations
gallbladder cancer and, 1462
hepatocellular carcinoma and, 1460
pancreatic/periampullary carcinoma and, 1463
TPHA test, 1332
TPMT. *See* Thiopurine methyltransferase
TPN (total parenteral nutrition). *See* Central vein nutritional support
TPPA test, for syphilis, 1332
TRAb. *See* Thyrotropin receptor antibody
Trabeculectomy, for glaucoma, 159
Trabeculoplasty, laser, for glaucoma, 159
Trace elements, in nutritional support, 1149
Trachea
foreign body in, **212**
obstruction of, 215
stenosis of, 215
Tracheal intubation. *See also* Intubation; Mechanical ventilation
for respiratory failure, 290

Tracheobronchitis, respiratory syncytial virus causing, 1268
Tracheostomy/tracheotomy, **211–212**. See also specific disorder
for sleep apnea, 289
Trachoma, 154
Tractional retinal detachment, 161
TRAM flap (trans-rectus abdominis muscle flap), for breast reconstruction, 672
Tramadol
MAOI interactions and, 1440
for neuropathic pain, 85, 85t
overdose/toxicity of, 1442–1443
Trance state, in hypnosis, 1539
Trandate. See Labetalol
Trandolapril, 403t
Tranquilizers. See specific agent and Antipsychotic drugs
Transbronchial lung biopsy. See Lung biopsy
Transcatheter arterial chemoembolization (TACE), for hepatocellular carcinoma, 1461
Transcatheter arterial chemoinfusion (TACI), for hepatocellular carcinoma, 1025
Transcobalamins, in polycythemia, 458
Transcranial magnetic stimulation
for depression, 969
for tinnitus, 188
Transdermal contraceptive patch, 697–698
Transesophageal echocardiography. See Echocardiography
Transesophageal echocardiography-guided cardioversion, for atrial fibrillation, 347–348
Transferrin
in anemia of chronic disease, 442
carbohydrate deficient, alcohol use/abuse and, 979
in hemochromatosis, 627, 628
in iron deficiency anemia, 440
reference values for, 1554t
Transferrin receptor, soluble, 1554t
Transforming growth factor β (TGF-β), mutations in receptor for, Marfan syndrome and, 1518
Transfusion reactions
anaphylactic, 478
compatibility testing in prevention of, 477
contaminated blood causing, 478
hemolytic, 477
leukoagglutinin, 477–478
leukocyte-poor blood in prevention of, 476–477
Transfusions (blood/blood products), **476–479**. See also specific type
for aplastic anemia, 455
for autoimmune hemolytic anemia, 453
for chemotherapy-associated anemia, 1499
contaminated blood and, 478

for DIC, 487–488, 488t
disease transmission and, 478
arbovirus encephalitides, 1257
Chagas disease, 1350, 1351
donor screening programs and, 478
hepatitis, 478, 491, 601, 602, 603–604
HIV, 1207, 1219
HTLV, 1261, 1262
parvovirus B19, 1276
variant Creutzfeldt-Jakob disease, 1260
for fluid management/volume replacement
in GI bleeding/variceal hemorrhage, 518, 518–519, 539
in shock, 436
for myelodysplasia, 463
preoperative, 55
purpura associated with, **488**
for sickle cell anemia, 451
for thalassemia, 443, 444
for thrombotic microangiopathies, 485–486
Transglutaminase/tissue transglutaminase (tTG), in celiac disease/dermatitis herpetiformis, 118, 516, 559, 560
Transient elastography, in liver disease/cirrhosis, 600, 620
Transient ischemic attacks, **886–888**
carotid, 420, 887, 888
cerebrovascular occlusion/embolization and, 420, 886, 888
seizures differentiated from, 881, 887
strokes/stroke risk and, 886, 887, 888
vertebrobasilar, 887, 888
Transient monocular blindness, **165–166**, 420
Transjugular intrahepatic portosystemic shunts. See Transvenous (transjugular) intrahepatic portosystemic shunts
Transketolase activity coefficient, in thiamine deficiency, 1141
Translocational hyponatremia, 789, 792
Transmetatarsal amputation, in lower leg/foot occlusive disease, 418
Transmissible spongiform encephalopathies (TSE), 1260–1261
Transnasal ventilation, for COPD, 238
Transplantation. See also specific type or organ and Immunocompromised host
fever/FUO and, 1153, 1154
hyperuricemia/gout and, 735
infections following, 1156
adenoviruses causing, 1275, 1276
arbovirus encephalitides, 1257
cytomegaloviruses causing, 1157–1158, 1245, 1246
hepatitis, 610, 1276
parvovirus, 1276
pneumonia, 251
prevention of, 1157–1158
toxoplasmosis, 1363
treatment of, 1158–1159

lymphoproliferative disorder after, 1243, 1244
rabies transmitted by, 1255
squamous cell carcinoma after, 134
Transrectal ultrasound, in prostate cancer, 1485
for biopsy guidance, 1484
Trans-rectus abdominis muscle flap (TRAM flap), for breast reconstruction, 672
Transsexualism, 948, 949, 950
Transthoracic needle aspiration/biopsy (TTNA/TTNB)
in lung cancer, 1454
in solitary pulmonary nodule, 260
Transtracheal oxygen, for COPD, 236
Transtubular potassium concentration gradient (TTKG), 796
Transudates, pleural fluid, 283, 283t, 284
Transurethral electrovaporization of prostate, for benign prostatic hyperplasia, 871
Transurethral incision of prostate (TUIP), for benign prostatic hyperplasia, 869t, 870
Transurethral laser-induced prostatectomy (TULIP), for benign prostatic hyperplasia, 871
Transurethral needle ablation of prostate (TUNA), for benign prostatic hyperplasia, 871
Transurethral resection of bladder, for bladder cancer, 1489, 1490
Transurethral resection of prostate (TURP), for benign prostatic hyperplasia, 869t, 870
Transvaginal sonography/ultrasound. See Ultrasonography
Transvenous (transjugular) intrahepatic portosystemic shunts (TIPS), 621
for cirrhotic ascites, 621
for esophageal varices, 520, 540
rebleeding prevention and, 540–541
for GI bleeding, 520
for hepatic vein obstruction (Budd-Chiari syndrome), 630–631
for hepatorenal syndrome, 622
Transvestism, 948
Tranxene. See Clorazepate
Tranylcypromine, 968t
Trastuzumab, 666, 668, 1503t
Trauma
cardiac injury and, **384**
cognitive disorders/delirium caused by, 985t
complex regional pain syndrome and, 743
fat necrosis of breast caused by, 651
head injury and, **918–919**, 918t. See also Head injury
headache associated with, **875**
hearing loss associated with, 186
hypokalemia and, 795
middle ear, **185**

Trauma (*cont.*)
  nasal, **199**
    epistaxis and, 198, 199
  ocular, **171–172**
  pneumothorax and, 286
  prevention of, **18–19**
  psychologic/psychiatric disorders after (posttraumatic stress disorder), **938–939**
    abuse victims and, 938, 976, 977
    substance use and, 938, 977
  rhabdomyolysis/renal failure and, 763
  seizures caused by, 878
  spinal, **919–920**
  syringomyelia associated with, 920
  vertigo caused by, 190
Travatan. *See* Travoprost
Travel. *See also* Air travel
  immunizations recommended for, 4, **1200–1204**
    hepatitis A, 605, 1186
    hepatitis B, 1187
  infectious disease and, **1172–1173**
  during pregnancy, **710**
  retinal detachment and, 162
  SARS transmission and, 1274, 1275
  tick typhus and, 1285
Traveler's diarrhea, 511, **1173–1175**
  coccidial and microsporidial, 1369
  during pregnancy, 710
Travoprost, for glaucoma/ocular hypertension, 159, 176t
Travoprost/timolol, for glaucoma/ocular hypertension, 159, 176t
Trazodone, 967, 968t. *See also* Antidepressants
  for depression, 967, 968t
  for insomnia, 974
    MAOI-induced, 967
  overdose/toxicity of, 967, 968t
  priapism caused by, 967
Treanda. *See* Bendamustine
Treatment refusal/withdrawal, **91–92**, 92t
  advance directives and, **90**
Trelstar. *See* Triptorelin
Trematode (fluke) infections, **1373–1376**. *See also specific type*
Tremor
  benign essential (familial), **904–905**
    parkinsonism differentiated from, 905–906
  drug-induced, 911
  fragile X tremor-ataxia syndrome and, 1515
  in parkinsonism, 905
  in pheochromocytoma, 1058
Trench fever, 1321
Trench (immersion) foot/hand, **1405**
Trench mouth, **203**
Treponema
  carateum, 1339
  non-sexually transmitted diseases caused by, **1338–1339**
  pallidum, 1177t, 1330. *See also* Syphilis
    endemicum, 1339
    pertenue, 1177t, 1339
Treponemal antibody tests, for syphilis, 1331, 1331t, 1332

Treprostinil, for pulmonary hypertension, 275, 381
Tretinoin. *See also* Retinoic acid
  for acne, 121
  adverse ophthalmic effects of, 178t
  for cancer chemotherapy, 1505t
  teratogenicity of, 121
Trexall. *See* Methotrexate
Triad asthma, 199
Triamcinolone, 96t, 1077t. *See also* Corticosteroids
  for acne, 122
  for alopecia, 146
  for asthma, 226t
Triamterene
  for heart failure, 361
  with hydrochlorothiazide, for hypertension, 399t
  hyperkalemia caused by, 798
  lithium interactions and, 972, 972t
Triatomine bugs, Chagas disease transmitted by, 1350
Triazenes, in cancer chemotherapy, 1500t
Triazolam, 941, 941t, 975
Trichiasis, in trachoma, 154
Trichinella/Trichinella spiralis (trichinosis/trichinellosis), **1383–1384**
  myocarditis in, 368, 1383
Trichloroethylene, toxicity of, 1439
Trichoderma longibrachiatum, in opportunistic infection, 1402
Trichomonas vaginalis (trichomoniasis), 678, 678–679, **1372–1373**
  rape/sexual assault in transmission of, 702, 1167
Trichophyton/Trichophyton rubrum
  tinea corporis/circinata caused by, 107
  tinea pedis caused by, 108
  tinea unguium caused by, 147
Trichosporon, in opportunistic infection, 1402
Trichotillomania, 146, 940
Trichuris trichiura (trichuriasis/whipworm), **1380**
Triclabendazole, for fascioliasis, 1375
Tricor. *See* Fenofibrate
Tricuspid regurgitation, 303–305t, **314–315**
Tricuspid stenosis, 303–305t, **313–314**
Tricyclic antidepressants, 966–967, 968t. *See also* Antidepressants
  contraindications to in elderly, 66–67
  drug interactions of, 969t
  for neuropathic pain/painful diabetic neuropathy, 84–85, 85t, 1107
  overdose/toxicity of, 966–967, 968t, **1448–1449**, 1448f
    arrhythmias and, 967, 1448, 1448f
    ophthalmic effects and, 177t
    seizures and, 967, 1423t, 1448
    suicidal, 963, 1448
Trientine, for Wilson disease, 629
Trifascicular block, 356
Trifluoperazine, 954, 955t, 956t
Trifluridine, for ophthalmic disorders, 173t, 1239t

Trigeminal nerve
  herpes zoster ophthalmicus and, 115, 156–157, 1241
  postherpetic neuralgia and, 115, 115–116, 877
Trigeminal neuralgia (tic douloureux), **876–877**
  chemotherapy-induced, 1510
  headache and, 872
Trigeminy, 351
Triglycerides, 1124, 1133
  antiretroviral therapy affecting, 1229
  in diabetes mellitus, 1085, 1125
  elevated levels of. *See* Hypertriglyceridemia
  lowering levels of, **1133**
  pioglitazone affecting levels of, 1093
  reference/normal values for, 1554t
Trihexyphenidyl, 906t. *See also* Antiparkinsonism drugs
Triiodothyronine (T$_3$)
  RAI therapy for thyroid cancer and, 1026
  serum levels of, 1003t
    factors affecting, 1002, 1004t
    in hyperthyroidism, 1003t, 1010
      amiodarone-induced, 1010
    thyroiditis and, 1017
    reference values for, 1554t
    in thyroid cancer surveillance, 1026
    total, 1554t
  TSH/T$_4$ levels affected by, 993
  uptake of (resin). *See* Resin T$_3$/T$_4$ uptake
Trilafon. *See* Perphenazine
Trilasate. *See* Choline magnesium salicylate
Trimethaphan, for hypertensive urgencies/emergencies, 412–414, 413t
Trimethobenzamide, 506t. *See also* Antiemetics
Trimethoprim
  hyperkalemia caused by, 798
  for *P jiroveci* infection, 1224t, 1395
Trimethoprim/polymyxin B, for ophthalmic disorders, 173t
Trimethoprim-sulfamethoxazole
  for actinomycetoma, 1400
  for bacterial rhinosinusitis, 194t
  for cyclosporiasis, 1371
  for isosporiasis, 1370, 1370–1371
  for *Pneumocystis* infection, 1157, 1222t, 1224t, 1395
  renal/hepatic failure and, 1185t
  for toxoplasma prophylaxis, 1222, 1365
  for urinary tract infection, 852t
Trimetrexate, for *P jiroveci* infection, 1224t
Trimipramine, 968t
Trinucleotide repeats
  in fragile X mental retardation, 1515
  in Huntington disease, 908
  in X-linked bulbospinal neuronopathy, 921
Triple A (Allgrove) syndrome, 1048, 1049
Triplix. *See* Fenofibric acid

Triptans, for migraine headache, 874
Triptorelin, 1506t
Trisenox. *See* Arsenic trioxide
Trismus
    in cervicofacial actinomycosis, 1323
    in mumps, 1250
    in tetanus, 1298
Trisomy 21 (Down syndrome),
        1514–1515
    prenatal screening for, 706, 1514
Trizivir. *See* Abacavir, with zidovudine
        and lamivudine
TRK gene mutation, in papillary thyroid
        carcinoma, 1022
Trochanteric bursitis, 739, 743
Troglitazone, withdrawal of from market,
        1093, 1094
Troleandomycin, theophyllines affected
        by, 225t
Trombiculid mite larvae, skin lesions
        caused by, 139
Trondane. *See* Pramoxine
Tronothane. *See* Pramoxine
Tropheryma whipplii, 561, 1323. *See also*
        Whipple disease
Trophoblastic disease. *See* Gestational tro-
        phoblastic disease
Tropical anhidrosis and asthenia, 124
Tropical pancreatitis, 646
Tropical pulmonary eosinophilia, 266,
        1386
Tropical spastic paraparesis (HTLV-asso-
        ciated myelopathy), **915**,
        1261–1262
Tropisetron, 1509. *See also* Antiemetics
Troponins
    in deep venous thrombosis/pulmo-
            nary embolism, 267–268
    in infectious myocarditis, 369
    in myocardial infarction, 331
    in non-ST elevation acute coronary
            syndromes, 326
    reference values for, 1554t
Trospium, for urinary incontinence, 71
Trousseau sign (carpal spasm)
    in hypocalcemia/hypoparathyroid-
            ism, 800, 1031
    malabsorption and, 558t
Trousseau syndrome, 487, 488
True vocal fold (glottic) cancer, 210
Trusopt. *See* Dorzolamide
Truvada. *See* Tenofovir, with emtricitabine
Trypanosoma (trypanosomiasis)
    African, **1348–1349**, 1349t
    American (Chagas disease),
        1349–1351
        achalasia and, 542
        heart disease/myocarditis in, 368,
            1350
    brucei gambiense, 1348
    brucei rhodesiense, 1348
    cruzi, 1350
Trypsinogen, mutant gene for, in chronic
        pancreatitis, 646
Tryptophan, MAOI interactions and,
        1440
TSE. *See* Transmissible spongiform
        encephalopathies

Tsetse flies. *See* Flies
TSH. *See* Thyroid-stimulating hormone
TSH receptor antibody (TSH-R Ab
        [stim]). *See* Thyroid-stim-
        ulating hormone receptor
        antibody
TSI. *See* Thyroid-stimulating immuno-
        globulin
Tsutsugamushi fever (scrub typhus),
        1281t, **1283**
TT virus (TTV), 601
TT677 mutation, in noncirrhotic portal
        hypertension, 631
TTF-1. *See* Thyroid transcription factor-1
tTG. *See* Transglutaminase/tissue trans-
        glutaminase
TTKG. *See* Transtubular potassium con-
        centration gradient
TTNA/TTNB. *See* Transthoracic needle
        aspiration/biopsy
TTP. *See* Thrombotic thrombocytopenic
        purpura
TTV. *See* TT virus
Tubal ligation/sterilization, 701
Tubal pregnancy, 713. *See also* Ectopic
        pregnancy
Tube enterostomies, 1148, 1148f. *See also*
        Enteral nutritional sup-
        port
Tube feedings. *See* Enteral nutritional
        support
Tube thoracostomy (chest tube drainage)
    for empyema, 285
    for hemothorax, 285
    for malignant effusions, 1496
    for parapneumonic effusion, 285,
            1293
    for pneumothorax, 286, 287
Tuberculin skin test, 4, 253–254, 253t
    BCG vaccine affecting, 253, 257–258
    in HIV infection/AIDS, 253t, 254,
            1211, 1219
    in intestinal tuberculosis, 568
    in pregnancy, 706, 726
    prophylactic/latent tuberculosis treat-
            ment and, 253t, 257
    in spinal tuberculosis, 782
    in tuberculous peritonitis, 527
Tuberculin skin test conversion, 253
Tuberculoid leprosy, 924, 1327. *See also*
        Leprosy
Tuberculosis, 251–258, 1177t, 1325–1326
    Addison disease caused by, 1048
    ascites in, 527
    blood test for exposure to, 4, 1220
    bone and joint infection in, 256,
            781–782
    drug-resistant, 252, 256
    in drug users, 1168
    extrapulmonary, 256. *See also specific
            type or site*
    fever/FUO in, 1154
    in HIV infection/AIDS, 4, 253, 1211
        chemoprophylaxis/prevention and,
            4, 257, 1219–1220, 1222
        intestinal involvement and, 568
        treatment of, 255–256, 1211
    intestinal, **568–569**

latent, 251–252, 257–258
    meningitis and, **1326**
    pericarditis and, 377, 378, 379
    peritoneal involvement in, **527**
    pleural effusion in, 252, 283–284, 284t
    during pregnancy/lactation, 256, **726**
    prevention/control of, 4, 1158
        in HIV infection/AIDS, 4, 253,
            1211, 1219–1220, 1222
    primary, 251
    progressive primary, 252
    pulmonary, **251–258**
    reactivation, 251–252, 253, 1158
    renal manifestations of, **849**
    as reportable disease, 254
    salpingitis and, 688
    silicosis and, 279
    skin test for. *See* Tuberculin skin test
    treatment of, 254–258, 255t, 256t,
            1177t. *See also* Antituber-
            culous drugs
Tuberculous lymphadenitis, **213–214**,
        1325
Tuberculous meningitis, **1326**
Tuberculous pericarditis, 377, 378, 379
Tuberculous peritonitis, **527**
Tuberculous salpingitis, 688
Tuberous sclerosis, **903–904**
    angiomyolipoma of kidney in, 1492
Tuberous sclerosis complex, neuroendo-
        crine tumors in, 1062
Tubo-ovarian abscess, 689
    anaerobic, 1323
    appendicitis differentiated from, 568
Tubular acidosis. *See* Renal tubular acido-
        sis
Tubular necrosis, acute, 820t, **821–823**
    in pancreatitis, 644
    rhabdomyolysis and, 763, 764, 822
Tubular proteinuria, 817
Tubulointerstitial diseases, 826t, **844–846**,
        845t
TUIP. *See* Transurethral incision of pros-
        tate
Tularemia, 1177t, **1317–1318**
TULIP. *See* Transurethral laser-induced
        prostatectomy
Tumefactive chronic pancreatitis, 646
Tumor embolization, pulmonary metas-
        tases and, 1457–1458
Tumor lysis syndrome, **1497–1498**
Tumor necrosis factor (TNF/cachectin)
    agents inhibiting. *See* Anti-TNF agents
    in alcoholic liver disease, 614
    insulin action in obesity and, 1081
Tumor plop, 383
Tumor suppressor gene mutations. *See*
        also specific type
    in breast cancer, 653
    in colorectal cancer, 1476–1477
Tumoral calcinosis, in mineral bone dis-
        orders of chronic kidney
        disease, 829
Tums (calcium carbonate). *See* Calcium,
        dietary/supplementary
TUNA. *See* Transurethral needle ablation
        of prostate
Tungiasis (*Tunga penetrans*), 139

Tuning fork tests, of hearing, 179
Turcot syndrome, 591. *See also* Familial
    adenomatous polyposis
Turner syndrome (gonadal dysgenesis),
    1073–1075, 1074*t*
    amenorrhea caused by, 1068, 1074,
        1075
TURP. *See* Transurethral resection of
    prostate
TVS (transvaginal sonography/ultrasound).
    See Ultrasonography
12-lead ECG. *See* Electrocardiogram
Twinrix (hepatitis A and B vaccine), 606,
    1197*t*
TwoDay method of contraception, 700
Ty21a vaccine. *See* Typhoid vaccine
Tygacil. *See* Tigecycline
Tykerb. *See* Lapatinib
Tylenol. *See* Acetaminophen
Tylox. *See* Oxycodone
Tympanic membrane
    in acute otitis media, 183–184
    in chronic otitis media/cholesteatoma,
        184
    in eustachian tube dysfunction, 182
    in external otitis, 181
    perforation of
        in acute otitis media, 184
        cerumen removal and, 180
        in chronic otitis media, 184
        ototoxic ear drops contraindicated
          in, 187
        traumatic, 185
        underwater diving contraindicated
          in, 183
    reconstruction of, 184
    in serous otitis media, 183
Tympanocentesis, in otitis media, 184
Typhoid (enteric) fever, 1312, **1312–1314**
    prevention/immunization and, 1201,
        1313
Typhoid vaccine, 1201, 1313
Typhus, 1240*t*, **1280–1283**, 1281*t*. *See also*
    specific type
Tyramine, MAOI interactions and, 907,
    1440
Tyrosine kinase inhibitors, 462,
    1503–1504*t*
    hypothyroidism caused by, 1003
Tyrosine phosphatases, antibodies to, in
    type 1 diabetes, 1080, 1080*t*

U-Lactin, 99*t*
Ubiquinone-10/ubidecarenone (coen-
    zyme Q$_{10}$), 1528*t*, 1530
"Ugly duckling sign," 101
Uhl disease, 371
UIP. *See* Usual interstitial pneumonia/
    pneumonitis
UKPDS (United Kingdom Prospective
    Diabetes Study),
    1087–1088, 1110
Ulcer penetration, **555**
Ulcer perforation, **555**
Ulcerative colitis, 575, **582–587**, 583*t*,
    584*t*. *See also* Inflamma-
    tory bowel disease
    arthritis in, 776–777

colorectal cancer and, 586, 641, 1477
drug therapy for, 584–585, 584*t*
fulminant, 583, 585
GI bleeding and, 521, 583
primary sclerosing cholangitis and,
    640
social support and, 577
Ulcerative stomatitis. *See* Stomatitis,
    ulcerative
Ulcers. *See also* Peptic ulcer disease
    amebic, 1366
    anal fissures, 596
    aphthous. *See* Aphthous ulcer
    Buruli, 1325
    contact, of arytenoid cartilage, 209
    corneal, **156–157**. *See also* Keratitis
        contact lens wear and, 151
    genital/genitourinary. *See* Genital
        ulcers
    intraoral, **203**
        in Behçet syndrome, 772
        chemotherapy-induced, 1509
        in HIV infection/AIDS, 1213
    skin. *See* Skin disorders, ulcers
Ulnar nerve lesions, **927**
    in leprosy, 1327
Ultralente insulin (not available), 1097
Ultram. *See* Tramadol
Ultrarapid detoxification, for opioid with-
    drawal, 982
Ultrasonography/Doppler ultrasonogra-
    phy/duplex ultrasonogra-
    phy. *See also*
    Echocardiography
    in abdominal aortic aneurysms, 423
    in abnormal premenopausal bleed-
        ing, 674
    in aortoiliac occlusive disease, 415
    in appendicitis, 567, 568
    in ascites, 525
    in breast mass evaluation, 659
    in cardiomyopathy, 370*t*, 371, 372,
        373, 374
    in carotid occlusive disease, 420
    in chronic kidney disease, 827
    in chronic venous insufficiency, 37,
        143, 430
    in cirrhosis, 620
    in coarctation of aorta, 296
    in deep venous thrombosis/pulmo-
        nary embolism, 37, 269
    in ectopic pregnancy, 713
    fetal, 707
    in gastric adenocarcinoma, 1471
    in gastric lymphoma, 1473
    in gastrointestinal mesenchymal
        tumors, 1474
    in gestational trophoblastic disease,
        715
    in heart disease. *See* Echocardiography
    in infertility workup, 692, 865
    intravascular, in angina, 320
    in leiomyoma of uterus, 683
    in liver disease/jaundice, 600–601
    in mitral regurgitation, 307–308
    in myocardial infarction, 331
    for ovarian cancer screening/evalua-
        tion, 689

in pancreatic/periampullary carci-
    noma, 1464
in patent ductus arteriosus, 301–302
in postmenopausal bleeding, 676
in prostate cancer, 1485
    for biopsy guidance, 1484
in pulmonary hypertension, 275, 381
in pulmonary stenosis, 295
in renal artery stenosis, 391, 832–833
in spontaneous abortion, 712
in testicular cancer, 1493
in tetralogy of Fallot, 300–301
in thyroid disorders
    thyroid cancer, 1024, 1026
    thyroid nodules, 1003*t*, 1019*t*,
        1020
    thyroiditis, 1017
in urinary stone disease, 858
in valvular heart disease, 305*t*
in varicose veins, 428
in ventricular septal defect, 299
in Zollinger-Ellison syndrome/gastri-
    noma, 557
Ultravate. *See* Halobetasol
Ultraviolet (actinic) keratitis, **172**
Ultraviolet light/sunlight
    exposure to
        actinic keratoses and, 113
        basal cell carcinoma and, 133
        hyperpigmentation and, 145
        hypersensitivity to (photodermati-
          tis), 95*t*, **142–143**
        in lupus, 110, 753–754
        for osteoporosis/osteomalacia,
          1040, 1044
    protection from
        in cancer prevention, 95
        in lupus, 111, 753–754
        in porphyria cutanea tarda, 117
        in rosacea, 122
        sunscreens for, **95**
    squamous cell carcinoma and,
        134
    with psoralen. *See* PUVA therapy
Umbilical cord blood, stem cells in, for
    transplantation, 475
Unasyn. *See* Ampicillin-sulbactam
Uncinate (temporal lobe) lesions, 899
Undernutrition. *See also* Malnutrition;
    Nutritional disorders
    in elderly, 40–41, **72**
Underwater diving. *See* Scuba/deep sea
    diving
Undescended testes. *See* Cryptorchism
Undifferentiated schizophrenia, 952
Unipolar disorder, endogenous, 961. *See*
    also Depression
United Kingdom Prospective Diabetes
    Study (UKPDS),
    1087–1088, 1110
Unithiol, for mercury poisoning, 1439
Univasc. *See* Moexipril
Universal precautions, 1161. *See also* Body
    substance isolation
Unlawful sexual intercourse (statutory
    rape), 702
Unoprostone, for glaucoma/ocular hyper-
    tension, 159, 176*t*

Unstable angina, 326. *See also* Acute coronary syndromes
  β-blockers for, 328
  calcium channel blockers for, 328
  chest pain in, 28–29
  clopidogrel for, 328
  revascularization procedures for, 322–323
Unstable hemoglobins, **452**
"Up and Go Test," 68
Upper airway cough syndrome (postnasal drip), 22, 23*t*
Upper airway/respiratory tract disorders, **215**
  echinacea for, 1523*t*, 1525–1526
  foreign body, **212**, 278
  obstruction, 215
  obstructive sleep apnea, **288–289**
  thermal injury, smoke inhalation and, 277, 1409
Upper endoscopy. *See* Endoscopy
Upper gastrointestinal bleeding, **517–520**. *See also* Gastrointestinal bleeding
Upper gastrointestinal series
  in gastric adenocarcinoma, 1471
  in peptic ulcer disease, 549
Upper motor neuron lesions
  spasticity and, 914
  weakness caused by, 886, 921
UPPP. *See* Uvulopalatopharyngoplasty
Urates/urate crystals. *See also* Uric acid
  in gout, 732, 733
Urate (uric acid) nephropathy, 732, 849
Urea
  hyperosmolality caused by, 795
  lithium interactions and, 972*t*
Urea breath testing, in *H pylori* infection, 546, 549
Urea clearance, GFR measurement and, 818
Urea nitrogen. *See* Blood urea nitrogen
Ureacin. *See* Urea
Ureaplasma urealyticum, 1328
Uremia, 819, 826, 826*t*. *See also* Hemolytic-uremic syndrome; Kidney disease/injury; Renal failure
  coma in diabetic patient and, 1112*t*
  neuropathy associated with, 829, 923
  platelet function affected in, 490*t*
  pruritus in, 136
Uremic acidosis, 809
Uremic encephalopathy, 829
Uremic fetor, 826
Uremic frost, 826
Uremic pericarditis, 377, 378, 828
Ureter
  cancer of, **1491**
  obstruction of. *See also* Urinary tract obstruction
    postrenal azotemia and, 821
    stones causing, 860
Ureteral stones, 860. *See also* Urinary stone disease
Ureteroscopic stone extraction, 860
Urethra, incompetence/obstruction of, postrenal azotemia and, 821

urinary incontinence and, 71–72
Urethral discharge, 1167
  in chlamydial urethritis, 1182*t*, 1328
  in epididymitis, 856
  in gonorrhea, 1182*t*, 1319
  STDs causing, 1167
Urethritis, 1167, 1182*t*
  adenovirus causing, 1276
  atrophic, urinary incontinence and, 70
  chlamydial, 1177*t*, 1182*t*, **1328**
  dysuria caused by, 46
  in epididymitis, 856
  gonococcal, 1182*t*, 1319, 1320
  postgonococcal, 1320, 1328
  STDs causing, 1167, 1182*t*
  Trichomonas causing, 1373
Urethrocele, 687
Urge incontinence, 70–71
Urgencies, hypertensive, **411–414**, 413*t*. *See also* Hypertensive emergencies
Urgency, urinary. *See* Irritative voiding symptoms; Urge incontinence
Uric acid. *See also* Hyperuricemia
  acute tubular necrosis/kidney injury and, 822
  calcium nephrolithiasis and, 859
  in gout, 732, 733
    reducing levels of, 734–735
  in preeclampsia-eclampsia, 717*t*, 723
  reference values for, 1554*t*
  in tumor lysis syndrome, 1497
  uric acid nephrolithiasis/nephropathy and, 732, 849
Uric acid crystals. *See* Urates/urate crystals
Uric acid nephropathy. *See* Urate (uric acid) nephropathy
Uric acid urinary stones, 732, 849, 857, 858, 859
Uricosuric drugs, 734–735
Urinalysis, 816–817, 817*t*. *See also specific disorder*
  dipstick, 816
  for drug detection, 977
  in dysuria evaluation, 46
  in fluid and electrolyte disorders, 788
  for marijuana detection, 983
  microscopic, 816
Urinary anion gap. *See also* Anion gap/anion gap acidosis
  in hyperchloremic metabolic acidosis/renal tubular acidosis, 809*t*, 810–811
Urinary antigen detection tests, in Lyme disease, 1344
Urinary bladder. *See* Bladder
Urinary calculi, **857–860**, 858*t*. *See also* Urinary stone disease
Urinary casts, 816, 817*t*. *See also specific type*
  in acute renal failure/tubular necrosis, 823
  in glomerulonephritis, 825
Urinary chloride, in metabolic alkalosis, 812

Urinary cytology
  in bladder cancer, 1489
  in ureteral/renal pelvic cancer, 1491
Urinary diversion, after cystectomy, 1490
Urinary frequency. *See* Irritative voiding symptoms
Urinary incontinence, **70–72**
  biofeedback in management of, 1536*t*, 1537
  in elderly, **70–72**
  enuresis, 975, 976
  estrogen replacement therapy and, 1072
  interstitial cystitis and, 861
  in pelvic organ prolapse, 687
  spinal trauma and, 919
  in tabes dorsalis, 1336
Urinary retention
  in acute bacterial prostatitis, 854
  postpartum, 725
Urinary sphincter, dysfunction of, in spinal trauma, 919
Urinary stone disease, **857–860**, 858*t*. *See also* Nephrolithiasis
  calcium nephrolithiasis and, 857, 858–859
  Crohn disease and, 578
  cystine stones and, 857, 860
  metabolic analysis and, 857
  in renal tubular acidosis, 810, 857
  struvite stones and, 857, 859–860
  uric acid stones and, 732, 849, 857, 858, 859
Urinary tract infection, 46, 47*f*, **850–857**, 852*t*, 1176*t*, 1181*t*. *See also* Cystitis; Pyelonephritis
  dysuria and, 46, 47*f*
  hospital-associated, 1159
  incontinence and, 70
  kidney injury and, 827*t*
  during pregnancy, **724–725**
  in schistosomiasis, 1373, 1374
  struvite calculi and, 859
Urinary tract obstruction
  postrenal azotemia and, 821
  tubulointerstitial disease caused by, 845, 846
Urinary urgency. *See* Irritative voiding symptoms; Urge incontinence
Urination. *See* Voiding
Urine
  acidification of, in poisoning/drug overdose, 1425
  alkalinization of
    for cystine calculi, 860
    in hypocitraturic calcium nephrolithiasis, 859
    for lithium overdose/toxicity, 972
    in poisoning/drug overdose, 1425
    for salicylate toxicity, 1445
    for uric acid calculi, 859
  candida in, 1390–1391
  electrolyte concentration in, 788
  ketones in. *See* Ketonuria
  osmolality of. *See* Osmolality, urine
  pH of
    cystine calculi and, 860

Urine (cont.)
in hyperchloremic metabolic acidosis/tubular acidosis, 809t, 810, 811
hyperuricosuric calcium stones and, 859
manipulation of in poisoning/drug overdose, 1425
stone disease and, 858
struvite calculi and, 859
uric acid calculi and, 859
sodium in. See Sodium, urine
for toxicology screening, 1427
Urine culture, in dysuria evaluation, 46–47
Urine output
in diabetes insipidus, 996, 1083
in gout, 734
incontinence in elderly and, 70
monitoring, in burn care, 1410
in preeclampsia-eclampsia, 717t, 718
Urine protein-to-creatinine ratio, 817. See also Proteinuria
Urodynamic studies, in prostatodynia, 856
Urofollitropins, for male infertility, 994
Urokinase. See also Thrombolytic therapy
for pulmonary embolism, 273, 501t
Urolithiasis, 857–860, 858t. See also Nephrolithiasis; Urinary stone disease
Urologic disorders, 850–871. See also Genitourinary system, disorders of
Urologic surgery, antibiotic prophylaxis for, 60t
Uropathy, obstructive, tubulointerstitial disease caused by, 845, 846
Uroporphyrins, in porphyria cutanea tarda, 117
Urosepsis, 46
Urothelial cell carcinoma
of bladder, 1489
of ureter/renal pelvis, 1491
Ursodeoxycholic acid
for biliary cirrhosis, 626
for cholelithiasis/gallstones, 635
for idiopathic cholestasis of pregnancy, 728
for primary sclerosing cholangitis, 641
Urticaria, 125–127
ACE inhibitor/angiotensin II receptor antagonist therapy and, 126
antihistamines for, 126
cholinergic, 126
cold, 126
drugs causing, 126, 149t
insect bites/stings causing, 126, 139
Urticating hairs, skin lesions caused by, 139
Usual interstitial pneumonia/pneumonitis (UIP), 263–265, 264t
Uterine bleeding. See Menstruation; Vaginal bleeding
Uterine suspension, for pelvic organ prolapse, 687
Uterine tubes, ligation of, 701

Uterus
cancer of. See Endometrial carcinoma
disorders of, amenorrhea in, 1068, 1069
gravid. See Pregnancy
leiomyoma (fibroid tumor) of, 683–684
perforation of by IUD, 698, 699
peripartum infection of, 720–721
UVA therapy, with psoralen. See PUVA therapy
UVB therapy. See also Phototherapy
for atopic dermatitis, 103
for lichen planus, 135
for psoriasis, 105
Uveitis, 159–160
in ankylosing spondylitis, 774
anterior (iritis), 153t, 160
in Behçet syndrome, 160, 772
"immune recovery," 168
in leptospirosis, 1341
posterior, 160
in syphilis, 160
in toxoplasmosis, 1363
Uvulopalatopharyngoplasty, for sleep apnea, 289

V617F mutation
in hepatic vein obstruction (Budd-Chiari syndrome), 630
in noncirrhotic portal hypertension, 631
V-beam laser, for burn reconstruction, 1412
V/Q scans. See Ventilation-perfusion scans
V2 vasopressin receptor antagonists, for hyponatremia/SIADH, 793
v wave
in constrictive pericarditis, 379
in heart failure, 360
VA. See Visual acuity
vacA gene, in H pylori gastritis, 546
Vaccine-associated poliomyelitis, 1252, 1253
Vaccine bacillus Calmette-Guérin. See BCG vaccine
Vaccine-preventable infections, 3–4, 1247–1255. See also specific type
Vaccines. See specific type and Immunization
Vaccinia, 116
in atopic dermatitis/eczema patients, 103, 116
monkeypox prevention and, 1277–1278
smallpox vaccination and, 116, 1277
Vaccinia gangrenosum, 116
Vaccinia immune globulin, 116, 1277
Vaccinia syndrome, acute, 1277
Vacuum constriction device, for erectile dysfunction, 863, 1108
Vagal nerve. See Vagus nerve
Vagal nerve stimulation
for depression, 969
for seizures, 883
Vagifem. See Estradiol vaginal tablets

Vagina. See also under Vaginal
anaerobic flora of, 1323
Vaginal atrophy. See Atrophic vaginitis
Vaginal bleeding
abnormal premenopausal, 674–676
in polycystic ovary syndrome, 690
in cervical cancer, 682
in endometrial carcinoma, 684
leiomyomas causing, 683, 684
normal menstrual, 674. See also Menstruation
postmenopausal, 676
during pregnancy
ectopic pregnancy and, 713
gestational trophoblastic disease and, 714–715
third-trimester, 720
in spontaneous abortion, 711, 712
Vaginal cancer
DES exposure and, 680
Pap smear in screening for, 16–18
Vaginal discharge. See also Vaginitis/vulvovaginitis
STDs causing, 1167
Vaginal dryness. See Atrophic vaginitis
Vaginal estrogen, 704, 1071
Vaginal hernias (pelvic organ prolapse), 687
Vaginal intraepithelial neoplasia, DES exposure and, 680
Vaginal pessary. See Pessary
Vaginal ring
contraceptive, 698
for estrogen replacement therapy, 704, 1071
Vaginal ultrasound. See Ultrasonography
Vaginal vault suspension, for pelvic organ prolapse, 687
Vaginal warts, 678, 679. See also Venereal (genital) warts
Vaginismus, 692, 949, 950
Vaginitis/vulvovaginitis, 677–679. See also Vulvovaginal candidiasis
atrophic. See Atrophic vaginitis
dysuria and, 46
gonococcal, 1319
STD causing, 1167
Trichomonas vaginalis causing, 678, 678–679, 1373
Vaginosis, bacterial, 678, 679, 1167
rape/sexual assault in transmission of, 1167
Vagus nerve
hiccups caused by irritation of, 507
lesion/damage of, vocal fold paralysis and, 211
stimulation of. See Vagal nerve stimulation
Valacyclovir, 1239t
for herpes simplex infections, 114, 1215, 1224t, 1237, 1239, 1239t
esophageal, 535
for herpes zoster, 115, 1215, 1225t, 1239t, 1242
prophylactic/suppressive, 1215, 1237
Valcyte. See Valganciclovir

Valganciclovir, 1239*t*
for cytomegalovirus infection, 167, 1157, 1158, 1224*t*, 1239*t*, 1246
Valgus stress test, 34
Valium. *See* Diazepam
Valproic acid/valproate, 881, 882*t*, 972, 1546*t*
for bipolar disease/mania, 972
lithium interactions and, 972*t*
overdose/toxicity of, 882*t*, 972, 1427*t*, 1431
hemodialysis for, 1425*t*, 1431
for panic attacks, 943
for seizures, 881, 882*t*
Valsalva maneuver
heart murmurs affected by, 306*t*
for paroxysmal supraventricular tachycardia, 342
Valsartan/valsartan with hydrochlorothiazide
for heart failure, 362
for hypertension, 404*t*
for myocardial infarction, 335
Valtrex. *See* Valacyclovir
Valve replacement
anticoagulation after, 316
endocarditis and, 1307
pregnancy and, 316
for aortic regurgitation, 313
for aortic stenosis, 311
choice and management of prosthetic valves for, **315–316**
coagulase-negative staphylococcal infection and, 1296
for endocarditis, 1307
for mitral stenosis, 307
for mitral valve prolapse, 309
preoperative, 52
for pulmonary stenosis, 296
for pulmonic regurgitation, 315
for tricuspid regurgitation, 314
for tricuspid stenosis, 313
Valves
cardiac. *See also* Prosthetic heart valves; Valve replacement; Valvular heart disease
endocarditis affecting, 1303. *See also* Endocarditis
venous, incompetence of
chronic venous insufficiency and, 430, 431
varicose veins and, 427–428
Valvular heart disease, **302–316,** 303–305*t*, 306*t*. *See also* specific type
in alkaptonuria, 1513
endocarditis and, 1303. *See also* Endocarditis
in Marfan syndrome, 309, 311–312, 312–313, 383, 1518
pregnancy and, 316, 724
preoperative evaluation/management of and, 52
Q fever endocarditis and, 1286, 1287
rheumatic fever/rheumatic heart disease and, 302, 375
in Turner syndrome, 1074

Valvular papillary fibroelastoma, 383
Valvular rupture, 384
Valvuloplasty, 315
for aortic stenosis, 311
for mitral stenosis, 307, 315
during pregnancy, 307
for pulmonary stenosis, 295–296
Vancocin. *See* Vancomycin
Vancomycin, 1546*t*
for anthrax, 1301*t*
for antibiotic-associated colitis, 574, 575
for endocarditis, 1305, 1306, 1307
for meningitis, 1163*t*
red man syndrome caused by, 785–786
renal/hepatic failure and, 1185*t*
resistance to, 1291
burn-associated infection and, 1411
Vanicream, 94
Vanillylmandelic acid, urinary
in pheochromocytoma, 1059
reference values for, 1554*t*
Vaniqa. *See* Eflornithine
Vantin. *See* Cefpodoxime
Vaqta. *See* Hepatitis A vaccine
Vardenafil, 863, 950, 1107, 1108
Varenicline, for smoking cessation, 7, 1450
Variant Creutzfeldt-Jakob disease, 1260–1261. *See also* Creutzfeldt-Jakob disease
Variant (Prinzmetal) angina, 325
Varicella (chickenpox), **1239–1243,** 1240*t*
during pregnancy/congenital, **725–726,** 1241
prevention/immunization and. *See* Varicella vaccine
reactivation of, 115–116, 1239. *See also* Herpes zoster
Varicella vaccine, 5, 1188–1189*t*, 1190–1191*t*, 1192–1193*t*, 1194–1197*t*, 1200, 1241–1242
adverse effects/contraindications and, 1203*t*
immunocompromised host/HIV infection/AIDS and, 1195*t*, 1242
postexposure, 1200, 1242
pregnancy and, 1195*t*, 1242
Varicella-zoster immune globulin, 1242
for newborn, 726, 1242
during pregnancy, 725–726
Varicella zoster virus, 1239. *See also* Herpes zoster; Varicella
Bell palsy caused by, 1241
immunization against. *See* Herpes zoster vaccine; Varicella vaccine
infection with during pregnancy, **725–726,** 1241
reactivation of, 115–116, 1239. *See also* Herpes zoster
Varicocele, in infertility, 864, 866
Varicose veins (varicosities/varices), **427–429**
esophageal. *See* Esophageal varices

GI bleeding from, 517–518
portal hypertension/portal hypertensive gastropathy causing, 517–518, 538–539
leg ulcers and, 143
venous insufficiency/stasis and, 428, 430
Variegate porphyria, 923
Variola (smallpox), **116,** 1240*t*, 1277
Variola (smallpox) vaccination, 116, 1277
atopic dermatitis/eczema and, 103, 116, 1277
for monkeypox prevention, 1277–1278
VariZIG. *See* Varicella-zoster immune globulin
Varus ankle sprains, 746
Varus stress test, 34
Vas deferens obstruction, in male infertility, 866
Vasa previa, third trimester bleeding caused by, 720
Vascular access. *See also* Arterial lines; Intravenous lines
in burn care, 1410
Vascular (multi-infarct) dementia, 63, 986
hypertension and, 393
Vascular disorders (vascular occlusion/anomalies), **415–432.** *See also* specific type or vessel affected and Vasculitis
arterial aneurysms, **423–427**
atherosclerotic, **415–422**
homocysteine/hyperhomocysteinemia and, 1516, 1517
in diabetes mellitus, 1108–1109
aspirin in prevention of, 12, 1089, 1108
foot ulcers/gangrene and, 418, 1108–1109
glycemic control and, 1087, 1088–1089
hypertension control and, 1088, 1108
erectile dysfunction and, 863
GI bleeding and, 518, 520–521
headache and, 44, 45
hepatic vein
Budd-Chiari syndrome, 525, **630–631**
sinusoidal obstruction syndrome, 617, 630
nonatherosclerotic, **422–423**
osteomyelitis and, 780
in preeclampsia-eclampsia, 717*t*
seizures caused by, 879
shock and, **424–438,** 434*t*
in sickle cell syndromes, 450, 451
spinal, **896–897**
venous, **427–432**
Vascular ectasias (angiodysplasias), GI bleeding in, 518, 520–521
Vascular endothelial growth factor (VEGF)
in breast cancer, 664, 668
inhibitors of

Vascular endothelial growth factor (VEGF) (*cont.*)
  for age-related macular degeneration, 163
  for renal cell carcinoma, 1492
Vascular loops, vertigo caused by, 191
Vascular reconstruction. *See* Bypass grafting
Vascular surgery, antibiotic prophylaxis for, 60*t*
Vasculitis, **764–773**, 764*t*. *See also specific disorder*
  allergic, drugs causing, 148*t*
  brain and spinal cord involvement and (primary angiitis of central nervous system), **772–773**
  coronary artery involvement and, 383–384
  pulmonary, **276**
  retinal, 160. *See also* Uveitis
  in rheumatoid arthritis, 748
  in SLE, 753
  urticarial, 126
Vasectomy, 701
Vasoactive drug therapy
  in erectile dysfunction, 863, 1108
    diagnosis and, 863
  for GI bleeding/variceal hemorrhage, 520, 539
  for shock, 436–437
Vasoactive intestinal polypeptide (VIP), tumors secreting, 1062, 1063
Vasodepressor syncope, 356, 357
Vasodilator therapy
  for heart failure, 364
    left ventricular (infarct-related), 337–338
  for hypertension, 407, 408*t*
  for pulmonary hypertension, 275
Vasodilatory (distributive) shock, 434–435, 434*t*, 435, 436
Vasography, in male infertility, 865
Vasomotor disorders
  in menopause, 703–704
    black cohosh for, 1523*t*, 1527
  rhinitis, 196
  syncope (vasovagal syncope), 356, 357
Vaso-occlusive episodes, in sickle cell syndromes, 450, 451
Vasopressin. *See also* Antidiuretic hormone; Desmopressin
  in diabetes insipidus, 995, 996
  for GI bleeding, 520
  for shock, 436–437
  in volume overload, 794
Vasopressin challenge test, in diabetes insipidus, 996
Vasopressin V2 receptor antagonists, for hyponatremia/SIADH, 793
Vasopressinase, diabetes insipidus caused by, 996
Vasospasm. *See also* Vasomotor disorders
  coronary, 317, **325**
  intracranial aneurysm and, 894
  in Raynaud phenomenon, 756
Vasotec. *See* Enalapril; Enalaprilat
Vasovagal syncope, 356, 357

Vater, ampulla of. *See* Ampulla of Vater
VATS. *See* Video-assisted thoracoscopic surgery
VC (vital capacity), forced. *See* FVC
vCJD. *See* Variant Creutzfeldt-Jakob disease
VDRL test, 1331–1332, 1331*t*
  on cerebrospinal fluid (CSF-VDRL), 1337
  in HIV infection/AIDS, 1220, 1338
  in HIV infection/AIDS, 1220, 1337
  for rape victim, 702
Vectibix. *See* Panitumumab
Vegetarians/vegans
  diet in pregnancy and, 709
  dietary vitamin B$_{12}$ deficiency in, 445
Vegetative state, persistent, **917**
VEGF. *See* Vascular endothelial growth factor
Vein stripping, for varicose veins, 428
Veins
  deep, thrombosis of. *See* Deep venous thrombosis
  disorders of, **427–432**. *See also under Venous and* Veno-occlusive disease
  superficial, thrombophlebitis involving, **429–430**
  varicose. *See* Varicose veins
Velcade. *See* Bortezomib
VEMPs. *See* Vestibular-evoked myogenic potentials
Vena cava, superior, obstruction of, **431–432**
Vena cava filters/interruption, for deep venous thrombosis/pulmonary embolism, 273, 501
Venereal Disease Research Laboratory test. *See* VDRL test
Venereal infections. *See* Sexually transmitted diseases
Venereal (genital) warts, 131, 132, 678, 679
  anorectal involvement and, 595
  cervical/vaginal/vulvar, 678, 679
  HPV vaccination in prevention of, 4, 132, 595, 1187–1198, 1190–1191*t*, 1192–1193*t*, 1194–1197*t*
  imiquimod for removal of, 132
  podophyllum resin for removal of, 132, 679
Venezuelan equine encephalitis, 1257–1259
Venlafaxine, 964, 966, 968*t*
  for anxiety, 942
  for depression, 964, 966
  MAOI interactions and, 1440
  for neuropathic pain, 85, 85*t*
  overdose/toxicity of, 966, 968*t*, 1448
Venography
  in deep venous thrombosis/pulmonary embolism, 269–270
  in superior vena caval obstruction, 432
Venomous insect bites/stings, **1447**
  anaphylaxis caused by, 784
Venomous snake bites, 1424*t*, **1446–1447**

Veno-occlusive disease
  hepatic
    Budd-Chiari syndrome, 525, **630–631**
    sinusoidal obstruction syndrome, 617, 630
  pulmonary hypertension and, 274
Venous access. *See* Intravenous lines
Venous blood gases, in acid-base disorders, 806
Venous catheterization, hospital-associated infection and, 1160, 1161, 1180
Venous disease, **427–432**. *See also specific type and* Veno-occlusive disease; Venous insufficiency/stasis
Venous insufficiency/stasis, **430–431**
  deep venous thrombosis and, 36–37, 267, 430
    pulmonary embolism and, 267
  leg ulcers and, 36, 37, **143–144**, 430, 431
  osteomyelitis and, 780
  lower extremity edema and, 36–38, 143, 144, 430, 431
  varicose veins and, 428, 430
Venous pressure
  central. *See* Central venous pressure
  elevated, in superior vena cava obstruction/syndrome, 431
Venous sinus thrombosis, 902
Venous stasis. *See* Venous insufficiency/stasis
Venous thromboembolic disease, 495
  air travel and, 1419
  in antiphospholipid antibody syndrome, 755
  in burn injury, 1412
  cancer-associated, 270*t*
  chest pain and, 28, 29, 30
  of deep veins. *See* Deep venous thrombosis
  detection of, 269–270
  in essential thrombocytosis, 459
  estrogen replacement therapy and, 1072
  fever and, 1160
  in homocystinuria, 1517
  intracranial, **896**. *See also* Stroke
  oral contraceptive use and, 696
  prevention of, **495–496**, 496*t*
  pulmonary embolism and, 267, 269. *See also* Pulmonary venous thromboembolism
  of superficial veins, **429–430**
  treatment of, **496–501**, 497*t*, 498*t*, 499*t*, 500*t*, 501*t*
  in Wegener granulomatosis, 768
Venous valves, incompetence of
  chronic venous insufficiency and, 430, 431
  varicose veins and, 427–428
Venovenous hemodiafiltration, continuous, for poisoning/drug overdose, 1425

Ventilation
disorders of control of, **287–289**. See
also Hyperventilation;
Hypoventilation
mechanical. See Mechanical ventilation
Ventilation-perfusion scans
in COPD, 235t
in pulmonary embolism, 268–269,
270, 271t
in pulmonary hypertension, 275
Ventilator-associated pneumonia, 248,
249, 291, 1160, 1161
Ventricular aneurysm, myocardial infarction and, 339
Ventricular arrhythmias. See also specific
type
in cardiomyopathy, 370, 373
differentiation of from aberrantly
conducted supraventricu-
lar beats, 341, 351–352
in myocardial infarction, 337
antiarrhythmic prophylaxis and,
335
in poisoning/drug overdose, 1422t
Ventricular assist devices, 338, 366
Ventricular cysts, in cysticercosis, 1377
Ventricular dysfunction/failure. See Congestive heart (cardiac) fail-
ure
Ventricular fibrillation, **352–353**
electrical injury causing, 1412
in myocardial infarction, 337, 351
antiarrhythmic prophylaxis and,
335
sudden death caused by, 330, 352–353
Ventricular gallop. See Heart sounds
Ventricular noncompaction, 370
Ventricular premature beats (ventricular
extrasystoles), **351**
in myocardial infarction, 337
in poisoning/drug overdose, 1422t
Ventricular rate control. See Rate control
Ventricular reduction surgery, for heart
failure, 366
Ventricular septal defect, **299–300**
Ventricular tachycardia, **351–352**
driving recommendations and,
357–358
in heart failure, 365
in myocardial infarction, 337, 351
antiarrhythmic prophylaxis and,
335
in poisoning/drug overdose, 1422,
1422t
Vepesid. See Etoposide
Verapamil. See also Calcium channel
blocking drugs
for angina, 322
for arrhythmias, 344t
atrial fibrillation, 347
paroxysmal supraventricular tachycardia, 342
for bipolar disease/mania, 973
for hypertension, 405, 406t
for migraine prophylaxis, 874t
overdose/toxicity of, 344t, 406t,
1432

Verbal utterances. See also Speech/lan-
guage
in schizophrenic/psychotic disorders,
953
Verbigeration, in schizophrenic/psychotic
disorders, 953
Verelan. See Verapamil
Vernal keratoconjunctivitis, 155
Verner–Morrison syndrome, 1062
Verocell rabies vaccine, 1256
Verrucae. See Warts
Versed. See Midazolam
Vertebral artery occlusion, in stroke,
889–891
Vertebral compression/fracture
back pain caused by, 738
in osteoporosis, 1038, 1039
in Paget disease, 1045
Vertebral osteomyelitis, 781, 1295
back pain and, 738, 739
epidural abscess and, 781, 1295
Vertebrobasilar insufficiency/obstruction
stroke caused by, 889–891, 890t
transient ischemic attacks caused by,
887, 888
vertigo caused by, 191, 191t
Verteporfin, for age-related macular
degeneration, 163
Vertigo, **188–190**
in audiovestibular disorders, 188, 191,
191t
benign paroxysmal positioning
(BPPV), 189, 191t
central lesions causing, 188–189, 189,
190, 191, 191t
cervical, 190, 191t
episodic, 189
in labyrinthitis, 189, 191t
in Ménière syndrome, 189, 191t
migrainous, 188, 190, 191t
in multiple sclerosis, **191**, 191t
in perilymphatic fistula, 190, 191t
peripheral lesions causing, 188, 189,
189–190
in superior semicircular canal dehiscence, 190
traumatic, 190
vascular compromise causing, **191**,
191t
in vestibular neuronitis, 190, 191t
vestibular schwannoma (acoustic neurinoma) causing, **191**, 191t
Very-low-calorie diets, in obesity management, 15, 1137
Very-low-density lipoproteins/cholesterol,
1124
in atherosclerosis/heart disease, 1124
lowering levels of. See Lipid-lowering
therapy
Vesanoid. See Tretinoin
Vesicoureteral reflux, tubulointerstitial
disease caused by, 845, 846
Vesicular dermatoses, 95t, **113–118**. See
also specific type
Vesiculobullous hand eczema/vesiculo-
bullous dermatitis of
palms and soles (pom-
pholyx), **116–117**

Vestibular disorders (vestibulopathy),
191, 191t
central, 188–189, 189, 190, **191**, 191t
nausea and vomiting caused by, 87,
504, 505t
neuronitis, 190, 191t
peripheral, 188, 189, 189–190
schwannoma. See Schwannoma, vestibular
vertigo in, 188, 191, 191t. See also Vertigo
Vestibular-evoked myogenic potentials
(VEMPs), in vertigo, 189
Vestibulitis
nasal, **195**
vulvar, 691–692
Vexol. See Rimexolone
VFend. See Voriconazole
VHL. See von Hippel-Lindau syndrome
VHL gene, testing for, in pheochromocy-
toma/paraganglioma, 1059
Viagra. See Sildenafil
Vibrio, 1177t
alginolyticus, 1316
cholerae, 1171t, 1172, 1177t, 1315. See
also Cholera
immunization against, 1200, 1315
diarrhea/food poisoning caused by,
1170t, 1172, 1315, 1316
parahaemolyticus, 1170t, 1172, 1316
vulnificus, 1316
Vicodin. See Hydrocodone
ViCPS vaccine. See Typhoid vaccine
Vidarabine, 1239t
Vidaza. See Azacitidine
Video-assisted thoracoscopic surgery
(VATS)
in lung cancer diagnosis, 1454
for solitary pulmonary nodule, 261
Videoesophagography, 530
Videx. See Didanosine
Vidian nerve, in vasomotor rhinitis, 196
Vigabatrin, overdose/toxicity of, 1431
ophthalmic, 177t
Vigamox. See Moxifloxacin
Villous adenomas, of small intestine, 567
VIN. See Vulvar intraepithelial neoplasia
Vinblastine
for Kaposi sarcoma, 1225t
for renal cell carcinoma, 1492
Vinca alkaloids, neuropathy caused by,
1510
Vincent infection, **203**, 1289
Vincristine, 1502t
adverse ophthalmic effects of, 178t
neuropathy caused by, 1510
Raynaud phenomenon caused by, 757
Vioform. See Iodoquinol
Violence, **976–977**. See also Aggression;
Rape
alcohol use/abuse and, 976, 978
domestic, 976, 977
elder abuse and, 19, **75**, 75t
prevention of, 18–19
prevention of, **18–19**
VIP. See Vasoactive intestinal polypeptide
VIPomas, 1062, 1063
Vira-A. See Vidarabine

Viracept. *See* Nelfinavir
Viral infections, **1235–1280**. *See also spe-*
cific type
adenovirus, **1275–1276**
arthritis and, **779–780**
blood transfusion in transmission of,
478
diarrhea/gastroenteritis, 511, 512*t*,
1172, **1278**
drug therapy for, 1238–1239*t*
enterovirus, 1240*t*, **1278–1280**
exanthematous, 1240*t*, **1276–1278**
hepatitis. *See* Hepatitis
herpesvirus, **1235–1247**
myocarditis in, 368, 369*t*
neurotropic, **1255–1262**
pericarditis, 376–377, 378
respiratory, **1268–1276**
rhinitis (common cold), 192, 1275
bacterial rhinosinusitis and, 192,
193
cough in, 22
echinacea for, 1523*t*, 1525–1526
systemic, **1262–1268**
vaccine-preventable, **1247–1255**
Viral load tests (HIV). *See* HIV viral load
tests
Viramune. *See* Nevirapine
Virchow node, 1471
Virchow triad, 267
Viread. *See* Tenofovir
Viridans streptococci, 1176*t*, 1291
endocarditis caused by, 1304, 1305
Virilization, **1053–1055**
in polycystic ovary syndrome, 690,
1053
Viroptic. *See* Trifluridine
Virtual colonoscopy
in colorectal cancer screening/evalua-
tion, 16, 1478, 1482
in polyp identification, 590
Viruses. *See* Viral infections
Visceral artery insufficiency, **421–422**
Visceral hypersensitivity (heightened visceral nociception)
chest pain and, 543–544
irritable bowel syndrome and, 570
Visceral ischemia, **421–422**
Visceral larva migrans, 1384–1385
Visceral leishmaniasis (kala azar), 1351,
1352, 1352–1353
dermal leishmaniasis after, 1351
in HIV infection/AIDS, 1352
Viscerotropic disease
leishmaniasis, 1351
yellow fever vaccine-associated, 1203,
1266
Viscocanalostomy, for glaucoma, 159
Visicol. *See* Sodium phosphate
Vision
double. *See* Diplopia
impaired/blurred. *See* Visual impair-
ment/loss
Visken. *See* Pindolol
Vistaril. *See* Hydroxyzine
Visual acuity
assessment of in elderly, 74
in optic neuritis, 168

reduced. *See* Visual impairment/loss
in retinal artery occlusion, 164
in retinal vein occlusion, 163, 164
in vitreous hemorrhage, 162
Visual field defects/loss. *See also* Visual
impairment/loss
in glaucoma, 158, 159
in headache, 45, 873
intracranial tumors causing, 899
in ischemic optic neuropathy, 168
in optic neuritis, 168
in retinal artery occlusion, 164
Visual impairment/loss. *See also* Visual
field defects/loss
in age-related macular degeneration,
162, 163
in botulism, 933, 1300
cataract causing, 161
in diabetes, 1082*t*, 1083
in elderly, **74**
episodic, in transient monocular
blindness, 165, 420
in giant cell arteritis, 164, 165, 766,
767
in glaucoma, 157, 158, 159
in headache, 45, 873
in ischemic optic neuropathy, 168
onchocerciasis causing, 1387, 1388
in optic neuritis, 168
in pseudotumor cerebri, 903
refractive errors causing, **151–152**
in retinal artery occlusion, 164
in retinal detachment, 161
in retinal vein occlusion, 163, 164
in thyroid disease. *See* Dysthyroid eye
disease
in transient monocular blindness,
165, 420
in uveitis, 160
in vitreous hemorrhage, 162
Visuospatial impairment, in dementia,
64
Vital capacity, forced. *See* FVC
Vitamin A. *See also* Beta-carotene
deficiency of, **1143–1144**
toxicity of, **1144**
ophthalmic effects and, 178*t*
Vitamin B₁. *See* Thiamine
Vitamin B₂. *See* Riboflavin
Vitamin B₃. *See* Niacin
Vitamin B₆ (pyridoxine)
deficiency of, **1142–1143**
for gyromitrin mushroom poisoning,
1442
homocystinuria/hyperhomocysteine-
mia and, 1516, 1517
for isoniazid overdose/toxicity, 256,
1142–1143, 1219, 1222,
1424*t*, 1438
toxicity of, **1143**
Vitamin B₁₂ (cobalamin), 445
deficiency of, **445–446**, 445*t*
in bacterial overgrowth, 445, 562
fish tapeworm infection and, 445,
1376
neuropathy associated with, 445,
923
pernicious anemia and, 446

short bowel syndrome/ileal resection and, 445, 562
subacute combined degeneration
of spinal cord caused by,
915
thrombocytopenia associated with,
482
homocystinuria/hyperhomocysteine-
mia and, 1516
serum levels of
in polycythemia, 458
reference values for, 1554*t*
in vitamin B₁₂ deficiency, 446
supplemental, 446
for short bowel syndrome, 562
for subacute combined degeneration of spinal cord, 915
Vitamin B₁₂ absorption test (Schilling
test), short bowel syn-
drome/ileal resection and,
562
Vitamin C (ascorbic acid)
in atherosclerosis/heart disease prevention, 12
deficiency of, **1143**
toxicity of, **1143**
Vitamin D, 1144
adverse ophthalmic effects of, 178*t*
deficiency of/resistance to
in cirrhosis, 620
in hyperparathyroidism, 1034,
1035, 1037
in hypocalcemia, 799
in osteomalacia, 1042, 1043
in osteoporosis, 1039
dietary/supplementary
for fracture prevention, 18, 69
hypercalcemia caused by, 801, 1036
for hyperparathyroidism, 1037
for hypocalcemia/hypoparathy-
roidism/tetany, 800, 1032,
1032*t*
for mineral bone disorders of
chronic kidney disease,
830
for osteomalacia, 1044
for osteoporosis prevention/man-
agement, 12, 69, 704, 1040
in hypercalciuria, 858*t*
hypophosphatemia/hypophos-
phatemic rickets and, 796*t*,
1044
phosphate metabolism and, 802
reference values for, 1554*t*
Vitamin D₂ (ergocalciferol/ergosterol).
See also Vitamin D
for hypoparathyroidism/tetany, 1032,
1032*t*
for osteomalacia, 1044
Vitamin D₃ (cholecalciferol), for hypoparathyroidism, 1032,
1032*t*
Vitamin D-dependent rickets, 1042–1043
Vitamin D-resistant (hypophosphatemic)
rickets, 796*t*, 1043, 1044
Vitamin E
in atherosclerosis/heart disease prevention, 12

deficiency of, **914, 1144**
toxicity of, **1144**
Vitamin K, 1144
for anticoagulant overdose, 1431
in coagulation, 494
deficiency and, **494**
for esophageal varices, 539
for hypoprothrombinemia, in cirrhosis, 623
in pregnancy, for seizure disorders, 724
Vitamins. *See also specific vitamin*
absorption/digestion of, 558
adverse ophthalmic effects of, 178*t*
in CAM, 1520
deficiency of, in alcoholic liver disease/cirrhosis, 614, 615, 619
disorders of metabolism of, **1140–1145**
prenatal, 706, 708–709
requirements for in nutritional support, 1149
Vitiligo, 144, 145
in Addison disease, 1048
tinea versicolor differentiated from, 110
Vitrectomy
for diabetic retinopathy, 166
for retinal detachment, 162
for retinal vein occlusion, 164
Vitreous hemorrhage, **162**
Vivactil. *See* Protriptyline
Vivelle/Vivelle-Dot. *See* Estradiol transdermal systems
VLDL. *See* Very-low-density lipoproteins/cholesterol
VLP vaccine. *See* Human papillomavirus (HPV) virus-like particle (VLP) vaccine
VlsE, *B burgdorferi*, Lyme disease diagnosis and, 1344
VMA. *See* Vanillylmandelic acid
Vo₂ (maximal oxygen uptake), lung cancer surgery and, 1456
Vocal fold dysfunction syndrome, 215
Vocal folds
cancer of, 210
leukoplakia of, 209
paralysis of, **211**
thyroid surgery and, 211, 1012
traumatic lesions (nodules/polyps/cysts) of, **209**
laryngitis and, 208
Vogt-Koyanagi-Harada syndrome, 160
Voice, abnormal
evaluation of, 207
in lung cancer, 1454
in squamous cell carcinoma of larynx, 210
in vocal fold paralysis, 211
Voiding
dysfunctional, in prostatodynia, 856
increased. *See* Polyuria
painful (dysuria), **46–48**, 47*f*
Voltaren/Voltaren-XR. *See* Diclofenac
Volume depletion. *See also* Dehydration
chronic kidney disease and, 827*t*
saline-responsive metabolic alkalosis and, 812

Volume overload, **794–795**
Volume reduction surgery, for COPD, 239
Volume replacement. *See also* Fluid management/hydration
for shock, 436
Volume status
hypernatremia and, 793, 794
hyperosmolality and, **795**
hyponatremia and, 789–792, 790*f*
metabolic alkalosis, 812–813, 812*t*
Volutrauma. *See* Barotrauma
Vomiting, 86–87, **504–507**, 505*t*, 506*t*. *See also* Nausea and vomiting
in cholecystitis, 636
with diarrhea/food poisoning/gastroenteritis, 1170–1171*t*, 1172
in gastric outlet obstruction, 504, 505*t*, 555
in gastroparesis, 505–506, 566
induced
in bulimia nervosa, 1140
for poisoning/drug overdose, 1424
Mallory-Weiss syndrome/tears and, 536
of pregnancy, 504, **710–711**
acupuncture for, 1534
gestational trophoblastic disease and, 714
Vomiting center, 504
von Graefe sign, 1009
von Hippel-Lindau syndrome
neuroendocrine tumors in, 1062
pheochromocytoma/paraganglioma in, 1058
renal cell carcinoma in, 1491
von Recklinghausen disease, 904
pheochromocytoma/paraganglioma in, 1058
von Willebrand disease, **492–493**, 492*t*, 493*t*
type 2b, **488**, 493, 493*t*
von Willebrand factor, 492–493
reference values for, 1554*t*
in thrombotic microangiopathies, 485
von Willebrand factor cleaving protease (ADAMTS-13), in thrombotic microangiopathies, 485, 485*t*
von Willebrand factor receptor, in Bernard-Soulier syndrome, 489
Voriconazole, 1401*t*, 1402
for aspergillosis, 1158, 1398
for candidiasis, 535, 1390, 1391
prophylactic, 1158
renal/hepatic failure and, 1185*t*
Voyeurism, 948, 949
VPBs. *See* Ventricular premature beats
VRVg. *See* Verocell rabies vaccine
VSD. *See* Ventricular septal defect
VTE. *See* Venous thromboembolic disease
Vulvar carcinoma, **685–686**
Vulvar dystrophy, 685
Vulvar intraepithelial neoplasia (VIN), 685
Vulvar vestibulitis, 691–692
Vulvar warts, 678, 679. *See also* Venereal (genital) warts

Vulvectomy, 685
Vulvodynia, 691, 692
Vulvovaginal candidiasis, 125, 678, 1390
in diabetes mellitus, 1082*t*, 1083, 1109
in HIV infection/AIDS, 1216, 1224*t*
rape/sexual assault and, 1167
Vulvovaginitis. *See* Vaginitis
vWD. *See* von Willebrand disease
vWF. *See* von Willebrand factor
vWFCP. *See* von Willebrand factor cleaving protease
VX poisoning, 1434
VZIG. *See* Varicella zoster immune globulin
VZV. *See* Varicella-zoster virus
VZV vaccine. *See* Herpes zoster vaccine

Waldenström macroglobulinemia, **474**, 1466*t*
cold agglutinin disease and, 454, 474
Walking program
for COPD, 238
for osteoarthritis, 731
Warfarin, 496*t*, 498, 498*t*, 499*t*
for antiphospholipid antibody syndrome, 756
in SLE, 755
for atrial fibrillation, 348
in hyperthyroidism, 1014
in mitral stenosis, 307
benzodiazepine interactions and, 942*t*
after cardiac valve replacement surgery, 316
for deep venous thrombosis/pulmonary embolism (venous thromboembolic disease), 272–273, 496*t*, 498, 498*t*, 499*t*
drug interactions and, 498, 498*t*
for heparin-induced thrombocytopenia, 487
overdose/toxicity of, 1430–1431
postinfarction, 335, 340
pregnancy and, 272, 316
for stroke, 891–892
for transient ischemic attacks, 888
Warts (verrucae), **131–133**
venereal. *See* Venereal (genital) warts
Washout time, in antidepressant drug therapy, 967
Wasting
in HIV infection/AIDS, 1209–1210
in protein-energy malnutrition, 1135
Watchful waiting/surveillance
for benign prostatic hyperplasia, 868, 868*f*, 869, 869*t*
for prostate cancer, 1486, 1487
Water
body. *See* Body water
contaminated
amebiasis and, 1365–1366, 1368
cholera and, 1315
coccidial/microsporidial infection and, 1369, 1371
cyclosporiasis and, 511, 1370
diarrhea and, 511
dracunculiasis and, 1382, 1383

Water (*cont.*)
enteric (typhoid) fever and, 1312, 1313
fascioliasis and, 1375
fasciolopsiasis and, 1376
giardiasis and, 511, 1371, 1372
gnathostomiasis and, 1384
Legionnaires disease and, 1310
leptospirosis and, 1341
paragonimiasis and, 1375
schistosomiasis and, 1373, 1374
Water deficit. *See also* Dehydration
calculation of, 794
Water drinking. *See* Psychogenic polydipsia; Water/fluid intake
Water fleas, dracunculiasis transmitted by, 1382
Water/fluid intake. *See also* Fluid management/hydration
in diabetes insipidus, 996
disorders of/inappropriate
genetic disorders and, 796t
hypernatremia caused by, 793
hyponatremia caused by, 789, 790f, 791
in schizophrenic/psychotic disorders, 953–954, 997
endurance exercise recommendations and, 791, 1407
heat exposure prevention and, 1407
for hypernatremia, 793, 794
requirements for in nutritional support, 1148
restriction of
for chronic kidney disease, 830
for hyponatremia, 792
urinary stone formation and, 857, 858
withholding, in terminally ill/dying patient, 91
Water-hammer pulse, 312
Water shifts, hyperosmolality with and without, 795
Waterhouse-Friderichsen syndrome, 1047
Waterston-Cooley shunt, for tetralogy of Fallot, 300
Weakness/muscle weakness, 886. *See also* Myopathies; Myositis; Paralysis
in diabetes, 1082t
differential diagnosis of, 761
drugs causing, 761
in Guillain-Barré syndrome, 925
in inclusion body myositis, 761, 935
in motor neuron diseases, 886, 920, 921
in multiple sclerosis, 912
in muscular dystrophy, 934
in myasthenia gravis, 932
in myasthenic (Lambert-Eaton) syndrome, 933
in polymyositis/dermatomyositis, 760, 761
spinal trauma causing, 919
Web space tinea pedis, cellulitis and, 109, 129
Weber test, 179
Webs, esophageal. *See* Esophageal webs

Weeping/crusted skin lesions, 95t, 118–120. *See also specific type*
drying agents for, 94
Wegener granulomatosis, 201, 276, 768–769, 824, 835f
autoantibodies/ANCA in, 754t, 768, 769, 824, 835f
nose and paranasal sinus involvement in, 201, 768, 769
pulmonary involvement in, 276, 768, 769
renal involvement in, 768, 769, 824, 835f
Weight
changes in. *See also* Weight gain; Weight loss
water balance and, 788, 815
energy requirements/expenditure and, 1137, 1148
exercise/activity in maintenance of, 13, 14
normal, 14
Weight gain. *See also* Obesity
drugs causing
antipsychotic agents, 958, 958t
lithium, 971
in pregnancy, 706, 708
prevention of, exercise/activity and, 13, 14
smoking cessation and, 7
Weight loss (involuntary/unintended), 40–41. *See also specific disorder and* Weight reduction
in anorexia, 1139
in diabetes, 1082t, 1083
diabetic neuropathic cachexia and, 1107
in elderly, 40–41, 72
in HIV infection/AIDS, 1209–1210
malabsorption and, 558t
in protein-energy malnutrition, 1134, 1135
in Whipple disease, 561
Weight reduction, 1137–1138
in arthritis prevention/management, 731
exercise/activity in, 13, 14
for fatty liver disease, 618
in GERD management, 533
herbal products for, 1522
in hypertension management/prevention, 390, 395t
hypnosis and, 1536t
for obese patient, 15, 1137–1138
obesity-hypoventilation (Pickwickian) syndrome and, 287
with type 2 diabetes, 1101
for polycystic ovary syndrome, 691
for sleep apnea, 289
Weil syndrome, 1341
WelChol. *See* Colesevelam
Wellbutrin. *See* Bupropion
"Wells rule," 37
Wenckebach (Mobitz type I) atrioventricular block, 355
in myocardial infarction, 337

Wermer syndrome. *See* Multiple endocrine neoplasia, type 1
Wernicke aphasia, stroke causing, 889
Wernicke encephalopathy, 915, 979, 981, 1141
Wernicke-Korsakoff syndrome, 615, 979, 981, 985t, 1141
West African trypanosomiasis, 1348, 1349, 1349t
West Nile fever/encephalitis, 1257–1259
Westermark sign, in pulmonary embolism, 268
Western blot assay
in HIV infection/AIDS, 1217, 1217t
reference values for, 1551t
in Lyme disease, 1344
Western (equine) encephalitis, 1257–1259
Wet drowning, 1415
WFS1 gene mutation, in Wolfram syndrome, 1082
Wharton duct, calculus formation in, 206–207
Wheals. *See* Urticaria
Wheezes
in asthma, 220t
in heart failure (cardiac asthma), 217
in pulmonary embolism, 268t
Whiplash injuries, neck pain in, 736
Whipple disease, 560–561
arthritis in, 561, 777
Whipple resection, for pancreatic/periampullary carcinoma, 1464–1465
Whipple triad, 1118
Whipworm infections (trichuriasis), 1380
Whispered voice test, 75, 179
White blood cell count (leukocyte count), 1551t, 1554t
ascitic fluid, 525
in bacterial peritonitis, 526, 621
in peritoneal carcinomatosis, 528
in tuberculous peritonitis, 527
bursal fluid, 743
cerebrospinal fluid, 1162t
chemotherapy dosage modification and, 1499, 1508t
in cholecystitis, 636
in chronic lymphocytic leukemia, 467
in chronic myeloid leukemia, 457t, 461
in essential thrombocytosis, 457t, 459
joint fluid, 729, 730t
in gonococcal arthritis, 778
in nongonococcal acute bacterial (septic) arthritis, 777
in myelofibrosis, 457t, 460
pleural fluid, 283, 284t
in polycythemia, 457t, 458
reference values for, 1551t, 1554t
White blood cells. *See* Leukocytes
White cell casts, 816, 817t
Whitlow, herpetic, 1235, 1237
Whole blood. *See* Fresh whole blood
Whole bowel irrigation, for poisoning/drug overdose, 1425
Whooping cough (pertussis). *See* Pertussis
Wickham striae, 134–135

Wide QRS complex. *See* QRS complex, wide
Wilson disease (hepatolenticular degeneration), **628–630**
    movement disorders in, **911**
    parkinsonism differentiated from, 906
Winterbottom sign, 1348
Wiskott-Aldrich syndrome, 480
Withdrawal. *See also specific substance*
    cognitive disorders/delirium caused by, 985*t*
    seizures caused by, 883, 978, 981
Withdrawal response, in coma or stupor, 916
Withdrawal/withholding of curative effort, in terminally ill/dying patient, **91–92**, 92*t*
Wolbachia bacteria
    filariasis and, 1387
    onchocerciasis and, 1387, 1388
Wolff-Parkinson-White syndrome, 345
    palpitations in, 31
Wolfram syndrome, 995, 1082
Wood alcohol. *See* Methanol
Wood light
    in fungal infections, 108, 109
    in pigmentary disorder evaluation, 145
    in rape victim examination, 702
Woody (Riedel) thyroiditis, 1016, 1017, 1018
Word recall, three-item, in dementia screening, 64
Wound botulism, 1299–1300
    in drug users, 1168, 1299–1300, 1442
Wound care
    for bite wounds, 1165, 1256
    in burn injuries, **1411**
    for frostbite, 1406
    for lymphangitis/lymphadenitis, 433
    tetanus prophylaxis/treatment and, 1298, 1298–1299, 1299*t*, 1308
Wound infections
    clostridial
        botulism, 1299–1300
            in drug users, 1168, 1299–1300, 1442
        myonecrosis/gas gangrene, 1177*t*, **1297**
        tetanus, 1298–1299, 1299*t*, 1308. *See also* Tetanus
    coagulase-negative staphylococci causing, 1296
    surgical, 1160
        antimicrobial prophylaxis for, **59–60**, 60*t*
Wrestlers, epidemic herpes in (herpes gladiatorum), 1235
Wrist, ulnar nerve lesions at, 927
Writer's cramp, 910
Wuchereria bancrofti, 1385
    eosinophilic pulmonary syndromes and, 266, 1386
Wytensin. *See* Guanabenz

X chromosome
    in biliary cirrhosis, 625

in Charcot-Marie-Tooth disease, 922
in Duchenne muscular dystrophy, 934*t*, 935
fragile site on, mental retardation and, 1515
in idiopathic torsion dystonia, 909
in Klinefelter syndrome, 1063, 1517
in Turner syndrome, 1074, 1075
X chromosome mosaicism
    premature ovarian failure and, 1069
    in Turner syndrome, 1068, 1075
x descent, in tricuspid regurgitation, 314
X25 gene, in Friedreich ataxia, 923
X-inactive-specific transcriptase (XIST), in Klinefelter syndrome, 1065
X-linked bulbospinal neuronopathy, 921
X-linked hypophosphatemic rickets, 1043, 1044
X-ray studies. *See specific disorder and under* Radiation
Xalacom. *See* Latanoprost/timolol
Xalatan. *See* Latanoprost
Xanax. *See* Alprazolam
Xanthogranulomatous cholecystitis, 636
Xanthomas
    in biliary cirrhosis, 625
    eruptive, 1125
        in diabetes mellitus, 1083, 1109
    tendinous, 1125
Xeloda. *See* Capecitabine
Xerosis
    in HIV infection/AIDS, 1215
    in vitamin A deficiency, 1143
Xerostomia, in Sjögren syndrome, 762, 763
Xibrom. *See* Bromfenac
XIST. *See* X-inactive-specific transcriptase
XO karyotype, in Turner syndrome, 1074
Xp-, in Turner syndrome, 1075
XXY karyotype, 1063, 1517. *See also* Klinefelter syndrome
XY karyotype, hirsutism/virilization and, 1054
Xyloprim. *See* Allopurinol
^{14}C-Xylose test, in bacterial overgrowth, 516
D-Xylose absorption, in bacterial overgrowth, 516, 562

Y chromosome, in Klinefelter syndrome, 865, 1063
Y chromosome microdeletions, in male infertility, 865
Yaws (frambesia), 1177*t*, **1339**
Yellow fever, **1265–1266**
    prevention/immunization and, 1201–1203, 1258, 1265–1266
Yellow fever virus vaccine, 1201–1203, 1258, 1265–1266
Yellow top tubes, 1555*t*
Yersinia
    enterocolitica, diarrhea/gastroenteritis caused by, 512, 1171*t*, 1172
    pestis, 1177*t*, 1318

Yttrium-90 ibritumomab tiuxetan. *See* Ibritumomab tiuxetan

Z score, 1039
Zaditor. *See* Ketotifen
Zafirlukast, for asthma, 225*t*, 228
Zalcitabine (ddC), 1228, 1232*f*. *See also* Antiretroviral therapy
Zaleplon, 941*t*, 974
Zanamivir, for influenza, 1198, 1239*t*, 1270, 1271, 1272, 1273
ZAP-70, in chronic lymphocytic leukemia, 467
Zaroxolyn. *See* Metolazone
Zelnorm. *See* Tegaserod
Zemplar. *See* Paricalcitol
Zenker diverticulum, 538
Zerit. *See* Stavudine
Zestril. *See* Lisinopril
Zeta-associated protein (ZAP-70), in chronic lymphocytic leukemia, 467
Zetia. *See* Ezetimibe
Zevalin. *See* Ibritumomab tiuxetan
Ziac. *See* Bisoprolol, with hydrochlorothiazide
Ziagen. *See* Abacavir
Zidovudine (AZT), 1226*t*, 1228, 1232, 1232*f*. *See also* Antiretroviral therapy
    with lamivudine, 1227, 1228, 1231, 1232*f*
        postexposure, 1221
    with lamivudine and abacavir, 1228, 1232*f*
    myopathy caused by, 1213
    for prevention of HIV transmission to fetus/newborn, 726, 1221
        postexposure/after needle stick, 1221
    resistance to, 1233
ZIFT. *See* Zygote intrafallopian transfer
Zileuton, for asthma, 225*t*, 227–228
Zinacef. *See* Cefuroxime
Zinc, parenteral nutritional support and, 1149, 1151*t*
Zinc transporter antibodies, in type 1 diabetes, 1080
Zinecard. *See* Dexrazoxane
Ziprasidone, 954, 955*t*, 956*t*, 957
    overdose/toxicity of, 956*t*, 957, 958, 1444–1445
Zithromax. *See* Azithromycin
ZnT8 antibodies, in type 1 diabetes, 1080
Zocor. *See* Simvastatin
Zoladex. *See* Goserelin
Zoledronate/zoledronic acid, 1040, 1046. *See also* Bisphosphonates
    for chemotherapy-induced toxicity/bone pain, 1507*t*
    for hypercalcemia/hyperparathyroidism, 1037, 1497, 1507*t*
    for osteoporosis prevention/management, 1040
    for Paget disease of bone, 1046
Zollinger-Ellison syndrome (gastrinoma), **556–557**, 1062
    carcinoid tumors and, 1474

Zollinger-Ellison syndrome (gastrinoma) (cont.)
   in multiple endocrine neoplasia, 556, 1062, 1076
   peptic ulcer disease and, 552, 553, 556
   refractory GERD and, 534, 556
Zolmitriptan
   for cluster headache, 875
   for migraine headache, 874
Zoloft. See Sertraline
Zolpidem, 941t, 974

Zometa. See Zoledronate/zoledronic acid
Zona-free hamster egg penetration tests, in infertility workup, 693
Zonalon. See Doxepin
Zonisamide
   overdose/toxicity of, 882t, 1431
   for seizures, 881, 882t
Zostavax (herpes zoster vaccine), 5, 115, 877–878, 878, 1187, 1194–1197t, 1242
Zoster. See Herpes zoster

Zoster ophthalmicus, 115, 156–157, 1241
Zoster sine herpete, 1241
"Zoster vaccine." See Herpes zoster vaccine
Zostrix. See Capsaicin
Zosyn. See Piperacillin-tazobactam
Zovirax. See Acyclovir
Zygomycosis (mucormycosis), 1398–1399
   rhinocerebral, 195
Zygote intrafallopian transfer (ZIFT), 694
Zymar. See Gatifloxacin
Zyprexa. See Olanzapine